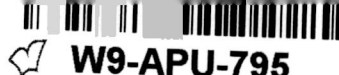

PRINCIPLES AND PRACTICE OF

ADULT
HEALTH
NURSING

PRINCIPLES AND PRACTICE OF

ADULT HEALTH NURSING

SECOND EDITION

Edited by

PATRICIA GAUNTLETT BEARE, RN, PhD
Professor, Louisiana State University, New Orleans, Louisiana

JUDITH L. MYERS, RN, MSN
Assistant Professor, St. Louis University, St. Louis, Missouri

with 955 illustrations

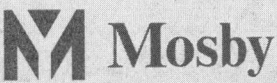 Mosby

St. Louis Baltimore Boston Chicago London Madrid Philadelphia Sydney Toronto

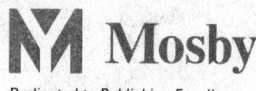 Mosby

Dedicated to Publishing Excellence

Publisher: Alison Miller
Editor-in-Chief: Nancy Coon
Editor: Robin Carter
Developmental Editor: Brian Dennison
Project Manager: Karen Edwards
Production Editor: James W. Russell
Manufacturing Supervisor: Karen Lewis
Designer: Elizabeth Fett
Illustrators: Mark Swindle, Jack Reuter
Cover Designer: Bert Vander Mark

ABOUT THE COVER

This artistic blending of nature and computer imaging reveals the many complex patterns and perspectives of a simple, flawless rose. Adult health nursing strives to reveal the complexities of caring for those who, like this rose in full bloom, are both hardy and fragile.

SECOND EDITION

Printed in the United States of America
Composition by Clarinda Company
Printing/Binding by Rand McNally

Mosby–Year Book, Inc.
11830 Westline Industrial Drive
St. Louis, Missouri 63146

Library of Congress Cataloging-in-Publication Data

Principles and practice of adult health nursing / edited by Patricia
   Gauntlett Beare, Judith L. Myers. — 2nd ed.
       p.   cm.
   Includes bibliographical references and index.
   ISBN 0-8016-6856-5
   1. Nursing. 2. Surgical nursing. I. Beare, Patricia Gauntlett.
II. Myers, Judith L. III. Title: Adult health nursing.
   [DNLM: 1. Nursing Care. 2. Surgical Nursing. WY 150 P957 1994]
RT42.P754 1994
610.73—dc20
DNLM/DLC
for Library of Congress   93-35463
                                                                  CIP

94 95 96 97 98   9 8 7 6 5 4 3 2

Contributors

GRETCHEN AUMANN, RN, MSN
Chapter 10 and Ethical Issues Boxes
Consortium Ethicist and Assistant Professor
Center for Medical Ethics, University of Pittsburgh,
    School of Medicine
Pittsburgh, Pennsylvania

JAN BARRETT, RN, PhD
Chapter 55
Director BSN Program, Deaconess College of Nursing
St. Louis, Missouri

PATRICIA GAUNTLETT BEARE, RN, PhD
Chapter 8
Professor, Louisiana State University,
New Orleans, Louisiana

LASCA BECK, RN, MS
Chapter 53
Instructor, College of Nursing, Arizona State University,
Tempe, Arizona

VIRGINIA TROTTER BETTS, RN, MS, JD
Chapter 9 and Legal Issues Boxes
Vanderbilt Institute for Public Policies Studies,
Nashville, Tennessee

JACQUELINE BIRMINGHAM, RN, MS
Home Care Guides
Director, Discharge Planning, Hartford Hospital,
Hartford, Connecticut

LINDA BOLIN, RN, MSN
Chapter 31
Lecturer/Clinical Instructor, School of Nursing, East
    Carolina University,
Greenville, North Carolina

BARBARA J. BOSS, RN, PhD
Chapter 45
Professor of Nursing, University of Mississippi Medical
    Center,
Jackson, Mississippi

CARROLL CONNER BOUMAN, RN, MS
Chapters 39 and 40
Faculty, School of Nursing, University of Rochester,
Rochester, New York

REBECCA L. BRADLEY, MA, RD
Chapter 16
Associate Professor and Director of Dietetic Internship
    Program, University of Alabama,
Birmingham, Alabama

SHARON A. BRAY, RN, MS
Chapters 35 and 36
Clinical Nurse Educator, Critical Care/Heart, Lung and
    Blood Nursing Service, National Institutes of Health
Bethesda, Maryland

TONI CASCIO, RN, MN, CCRN
Chapter 34
Clinical Educator-Critical Care, Ochsner Foundation
    Hospital,
New Orleans, Louisiana

MARGARET K. COVEY, RN, MS
Chapter 28
Senior Research Specialist, Department of
    Medical-Surgical Nursing, University of Illinois,
Chicago, Illinois

MARILYN NEWCOMER CULP, RN, MN
Chapter 19
School of Nursing, University of Wyoming,
Laramie, Wyoming

CHARMAINE CUMMINGS, RN, MSN
Chapter 51
Director of Nursing Education, National Institutes of
    Health,
Bethesda, Maryland

HETTY L. DEVROOM, RN. BSN, CNRN
Chapter 51
Clinical Research Nurse, National Institute of
    Neurological Disorders and Stroke, National Institutes
    of Health,
Bethesda, Maryland

KATHARINE DONOHOE, RN, MS
Chapters 46 and 48
Nurse Clinician, Department of Neurology, University of
    Rochester,
Rochester, New York

PHYLLIS DUBENDORF, RN, MSN, CCRN, CNRN
Chapter 50
Clinical Nurse Specialist, Thomas Jefferson University
   Hospital,
Philadelphia, Pennsylvania

WANDA DUBUISSON, RN, MN
Chapters 43, 57, and 58
Assistant Professor of Nursing, University of Southern
   Mississippi,
Hattiesburg, Mississippi

FRANCES R. EASON, RNC, EdD
Chapter 57 and 58
Professor, School of Nursing, East Carolina University,
Greenville, North Carolina

LINDA EASTHAM, RN, MSN, FNP
Assessment Content
Family Nurse Practitioner, Department of Internal
   Medicine, University of Virginia,
Charlottesville, Virginia

CAROLE EDELMAN, RN, MS, CS
Chapter 2
Director of Nursing, Osborn Retirement Community
   Associate faculty, School of Nursing, Columbia
   University,
New York, New York

JOYCE ENGEL, RN, MEd
Laboratory and Diagnostic Test Content
Assistant Professor, School of Nursing, University of
   Lethbridge,
Lethbridge, Alberta

ELLEN FLAHERTY, RN, MS, GNP
Chapter 2
Gerontological Nurse Practitioner, Osborn Retirement
   Community,
Rye, New York

KATHLEEN L. FRITSCH, NP, MN
Chapter 60
Nurse Educator, World Health Organization,
Tonga, South Pacific

MARY ANN GILMORE, RN, MSN, CS
Chapter 70
Clinical Nurse Specialist, Oncology, The University of
   Texas M.D. Anderson Cancer Center,
Houston, Texas

MIKEL L. GRAY, RN, CURN, PhD, PNP
Chapter 71
Clinical Urodynamics, Henrietta Egleston Hospital for
   Children, Scottish Rite Children's Hospital, Shepherd
   Spinal Center,
Atlanta, Georgia

DEBRA HAIRE-JOSHU, RN, PhD
Chapter 62
Director, Diabetes Education Center, Diabetes Research
   and Training Center, Washington University School of
   Medicine,
St. Louis, Missouri

MARK C. HAMELINK, CRNA, MSN
Chapter 22, 23, 24
Nurse Anesthetist, Lakeshore Anesthesia,
South Haven, MI

DIANE HAMILTON, RN, PhD
Chapter 18
School of Nursing, University of Rochester,
Rochester, New York

JEANETTE HARTSHORN, RN, PhD, FAAN
Chapter 49
Associate Dean for Academic Administration, University
   of Texas,
Galveston, Texas

LINDA HAYCRAFT, RN, MSN (R)
Chapter 67
Instructor, School of Nursing, St. Louis University

PATRICIA HESS, RN-C, PhD, GNP
Chapter 20
Professor, Department of Nursing, San Francisco State
   University,
San Francisco, California

MARCIA HILL, RN, MSN
Chapter 74
Manager, Dermatology Therapeutics, Methodist
   Hospital, Houston, Texas
Assistant Professor, Department of Dermatology, Baylor
   College of Medicine,
Houston, Texas

JANICE HINKLE, RN, MSN, CNRN
Chapter 47
Instructor, Department of Nursing, Thomas Jefferson
   University,
Philadelphia, Pennsylvania

LINDA C. HODGES, RN, EdD
Chapter 5
Dean and Professor, College of Nursing, The University
   of Arkansas for Medical Sciences,
Little Rock, Arkansas

LISA J. HOPP, RN, PhD
Chapters 27 and 28
Visiting Assistant Professor Purdue University Calumet,
Hammond, Indiana

DEBBIE HUTCHINSON, RN, MSN
Chapter 7
Director of Discharge Planning, The Medical Center of
   Central Georgia, Macon, Georgia

DONNA F.M. JAMIESON, RN, MS
Chapter 28
Faculty, Rush University,
Chicago, Illinois
Nursing Education Coordinator, Elmbrook Memorial
    Hospital,
Brookfield, Wisconsin

KAREN C. JOHNSON-BRENNAN, RN, EdD
Chapter 42
Vice Chair of Baccalaureate Program, Department of
    Nursing, San Francisco State University,
San Francisco, California

MARY KIRKPATRICK, RN, EdD
Chapter 31
Professor, School of Nursing, East Carolina University,
Greenville, North Carolina

JANET L. LARSON, RN, PhD
Chapter 28
Assistant Professor, College of Nursing, University of
    Illinois at Chicago,
Chicago, Illinois

ROBERTA LEE, RN, DrPH
Chapter 4
Professor, School of Nursing, The University of Texas
    Medical Branch,
Galveston, Texas

LORA MCGUIRE, RN, MS
Chapter 14
Nursing Pain Consultant and Instructor, Department of
    Nursing, Joliet Junior College,
Joliet, Illinois

JUDITH L. MYERS, RN, MSN
Chapters 11 and 17
Assistant Professor, St. Louis University,
St. Louis, Missouri

LINDA NAPHOLZ, RN, PhD
Chapter 3
Assistant Professor, Health Restoration Department,
    School of Nursing, University of Wisconsin,
Milwaukee, Wisconsin

VIRGINIA L. NORMAN, RN, MA, MS
Assessment Content
Associate Professor, College of Nursing, University of
    North Dakota,
Grand Forks, North Dakota

JOY M. NORTON, RN, EdD, CS
Chapter 66
Assistant Professor, School of Nursing University of
    Texas Health Science Center,
San Antonio, Texas

CINDY NOWICKI, RN, C, MSN
Chapter 76
Advanced Practice Specialist, Patient-Focused Surgical
    Services, Lakeland Regional Medical Center,
Lakeland, Florida

JANICE NUNNELEE, RNC, MSN
Chapters 30 and 32
Vascular Clinical Nurse Specialist, St. John's Mercy
    Medical Center,
St. Louis, Missouri

BARBARA L. OGDEN, RNC, MSN
Chapter 75
Assistant Professor, College of Nursing, University of
    Florida,
Gainesville, Florida

MELODIE OLSON, RN, PhD
Chapter 1
Associate Professor, College of Nursing, Medical
    University of South Carolina,
Charleston, South Carolina

DEMETRIUS J. PORCHE, RN, MN, CCRN
Chapters 40 and 72
Infection Control (AIDS) Educator/Coordinator, Tulane
    University Medical Center,
New Orleans, Louisiana

CATHERINE RATLIFF, RN, MS, CS, CETN
Chapter 70
Clinical Nurse Specialist, The University of Virginia

PAUL M. READING, BS, RRT
Chapter 26
Affiliate Program Director of Respiratory Care, St John's
    Mercy Medical Center,
St. Louis, Missouri

SUSAN A. REED, RNCS, MSN
Chapter 21
Clinical Nurse Specialist, Fort Howard VA Medical
    Center,
Fort Howard, Maryland

BONITA R. REINERT, RN, MSN, ANP-C
Chapters 69 and 73
Assistant Director of Graduate Program, School of
    Nursing, The University of Southern Mississippi,
Hattiesburg, MS

VEE RICE, RN, PhD
Chapter 13
Critical Care Program Coordinator, The University of
    Tennessee,
Nashville, Tennessee

PATRICIA ROBERTS, PhD
Anatomy and Physiology Content
Associate Professor, School of Nursing, Memorial
    University of Newfoundland,
St. John's Newfoundland

ROBERT E. ST. JOHN, RN, RRT
Chapter 26
Clinical Nurse Specialist, Pulmonary Jewish Hospital at
    Washington University Medical Center
St. Louis, MO.

MARY SAMPEL, RN, MSN
Chapters 64 and 65
Associate Professor, St. Louis University School of
     Nursing,
St. Louis, Missouri

JUDITH K. SANDS, RN, EdD
Chapter 61
Associate Professor, Director of Undergraduate Studies,
     School of Nursing, University of Virginia,
Charlottesville, Virginia

VIRGINIA HUDDLESTON SECOR, RN, MSN, CCRN
Chapter 77
Adjunct Faculty, Vanderbilt University,
Nashville, Tennessee
Critical Care Consultant, Barbara Clark Mims
     Associates,
Lewisville, Texas

KATHLEEN C. SHEPPARD, RN. MSN, CCRN
Chapter 38
Clinical Instructor, The University of Texas M.D.
     Anderson Cancer Center,
Houston, Texas

STARLA TATE, RN MNSc
Chapter 5
Instructor, College of Nursing, University of Arkansas for
     Medical Sciences,
Little Rock, Arkansas

JOAN THIELE, RN, PhD
Chapter 6
Professor, Intercollegiate Center for Nursing Education,
Spokane, Washington

JUDY VENUGOPAL, RN, CNRN
Chapter 71
Coordinator, Continence Center, Emory University
     Hospital Nursing Administration,
Atlanta, Georgia

DEBORAH L. VOLKER, RN, MA, OCN
Chapter 15
Director of Nursing Staff Development, Division of
     Nursing, The University of Texas M.D. Anderson
     Cancer Center,
Houston, Texas

NORMA JEAN WELDY, RN, MS
Chapter 12
Division of Nursing, Goshen College,
Goshen, Indiana

LINDA WILLIAMS, RN, BSN, CPSN
Chapter 76
Administrator Center for Plastic and Reconstructive
     Surgery, P.A.,
Orlando, Florida

Reviewers

IRENE AGUILAR, RN, MEd, MSN
San Antonio College,
San Antonio, Texas

VIRGINIA ARCANGELO, RN, PhD
Thomas Jefferson University,
Philadelphia, Pennsylvania

ELLEN BARKER, MSN, RN, CNRN
Neuroscience Nursing Consultants,
Newark, Delaware

SUSAN J. BENNETT, DNS, RN
Indiana University and Indiana University Medical
    Center,
Indianapolis, Indiana

MARGARET BENZ, RN, MSN
St. Louis University,
St. Louis, Missouri

SHEILA BOLLINGER, EdD, MSN
Houston Community College,
Houston, Texas

JULIA BRONNER, BSN, MS
Northeast Iowa Community College,
Calmar, Iowa

ANN H. CARY, PHD, MPH, RN, A-CCC
Lousiana State University Medical Center,
New Orleans, Louisiana

SUSAN M. CHAPPELL, RN, MSN, CDE
The University of Texas at Arlington, Arlington, Texas
    and Baylor University Medical Center,
Dallas, Texas

SAI CHOON CHOO, RN, BSN, MEd
Douglas College,
New Westminister, British Columbia

ANN S. DELLAIRA, BSN, MSN, PhD
Thomas Jefferson University,
Philadelphia, Pennsylvania

SUSAN DONCKERS, RN, EdD
Radford University,
Radford, Virginia

VIRGINIA M. DOWD, BSN, MEd
San Antonio College,
San Antonio, Texas

DEBORAH OLDENBURG ERICKSON, BSN, MSN
Methodist Medical Center School of Nursing,
Peoria, Illinois

JAMES FAIN, PhD, RN
Yale University School of Nursing,
New Haven, Connecticut

PAULA FELLOWS, RN, MS
Northeastern University,
Boston, Massachusetts

JANET T. GALEENER, BSN, MSN, MA
University of Northern Colorado,
Greeley, Colorado

R. AURORA GARCIA, MSN
San Antonio College,
San Antonio, Texas

DEBORAH EVON GIBSON, DSN, RN
East Arkansas Community College,
Forrest City, Arkansas

DAISY GOULDEN, RN, MS
Southern Nazarene University,
Bethany, Oklahoma

CHERYL GRAFF, RN, MS
Highland Community College
Freeport, Illinois

CAROLYN J. HAISCH, BS, MS
Saint Francis Medical Center,
Peoria, Illinois

JUDITH A. HALSTEAD, RNC, DNS
Indiana University,
Indianapolis, Indiana

WILLIAM O. HOWIE, BSN, MS
Anne Arundel Medical Center,
Maryland

SANDRA IRVIN, BSN, MSN
Purdue University,
West Lafayette, Indiana

User Diary Participants

CAROL F. BAKER, RN, PhD
Ohio State University
Columbus, Ohio

SANDRA CHACKO, PhD, RN
Des Moines Area Community College
Boone, Iowa

SHIRLEY EDEN-KILGOUR, RN, MSN
Memphis State University
Memphis, Tennessee

KATHY HICKEY, RN, MSN
Indiana University
Indianapolis, Indiana

MEG HULL, RN, PhD
Ohio State University
Columbus, Ohio

FRED MAY, RN, MSN
Indiana University
Indianapolis, Indiana

LINDA TENENBAUM, RN, MSN, OCN
Broward Community College
Davie, Florida

JULIA WONG, RN, MScN
Dalhousie University
Halifax, Nova Scotia

Preface

AS WE APPROACH the twenty-first century, nursing practice and nursing education are facing many challenges:

1. The National League for Nursing guidelines for the accreditation of nursing programs have changed to emphasize the evaluation of program outcomes. Nursing faculty are faced with the challenge of writing program evaluation criteria in the areas of critical thinking, communication, and therapeutic interventions.
2. The reform of the health care system is occurring at the municipal, state, and federal levels. Many of these changes in the financing and delivery of health care services indicate a movement toward community-based health care and away from hospital-based care. Health care reform will require increased patient and family participation in care.
3. Population demographics indicate that as we approach the next century the fastest growing segment of the population will be those over age 70. The elderly have needs that are special and require adapting traditional nursing approaches to the care of the adult and creating new approaches to providing nursing care.

This edition of *Principles and Practice of Adult Health Nursing* is designed to help both the student and nursing educator prepare for the changes in nursing practice and nursing education. Content has been updated and extensively rewritten to reflect a contemporary perspective and meet the needs of today's students and tomorrow's practitioners.

CRITICAL THINKING

1. New to this edition are 17 *Critical Thinking Guides.* The algorithms are designed to guide the student through decision-making about patients with specific clinical problems.
2. To help the student utilize research-based knowledge as it applies to patient care, 36 *Research Briefs* have been included throughout the text. Most of these research abstracts come from the latest published research in the nursing literature.

3. *Ethical Issues* boxes (24) present questions that challenge the student to think about his or her own response to ethical issues and decision-making in nursing practice.
4. At the end of each chapter, *Critical Thinking Questions* are included to help the student reflect on what he or she has read. Many of the questions encourage the student to think about how he or she will use the information in providing patient care.
5. *Chapter 6, Clinical Decision Making Using the Nursing Process,* has been completely rewritten to help the student see the relationships between the development of critical thinking skills and clinical decision-making. These essential concepts are applied to the utilization of the nursing process in providing patient care.

COMMUNICATION

1. Ten *Therapeutic Communication Guides* are included in the book. The communication guides provide a model for the student to increase his or her use of therapeutic communication skills with both patients and families.
2. *Documentation* has been retained from the first edition as a subheading under Nursing Management. These sections assist the student in identifying important aspects of nursing care to be recorded in the patient's chart or medical record.

THERAPEUTIC INTERVENTIONS

1. To help the student identify professional accountability guidelines for nursing care, 10 *Standards of Care* boxes are included in this edition. These professional practice standards come from the American Nurses Association and several specialty nursing organizations.
2. *Legal Issues* boxes (11) provide the student with knowledge about the legal aspects of nursing care. This feature helps the student make decisions about his or her legal accountability for patient care.
3. Thirty-six *Nursing Care Plans* are included in this

edition. The care plans use nursing diagnoses and expected outcomes as a format to guide the student in selecting interventions for patients with specific disorders. To help the student apply knowledge to the plan of care, rationales for the interventions are included in the care plans. For this edition the care plans have been revised to a three-column format. This design makes more efficient use of space and more effectively highlights expected outcomes as a key component of practice.

4. New to this edition are the *Preoperative/Postoperative Nursing Intervention* boxes. Each of the 10 boxes provides the student with a summary of the preoperative and postoperative nursing care for patients having specific surgical procedures. Rationales are included to help the student apply knowledge to the care of the surgical patient.

5. To assist the student in developing skill with nursing care procedures *Illustrated Skills* boxes are included in the book. The boxes provide the student with step-by-step guidelines for a procedure with supporting rationales. The illustrations help the student visualize what is being explained.

HEALTH CARE REFORM

1. Chapter 7, *Discharge Planning and Ongoing Care,* has been rewritten to focus the student's attention on preparing the patient to return to the community. Discharge planning is no longer an isolated event in health care delivery; it begins on admission and is incorporated into each aspect of the nursing plan of care.

2. *Ongoing Care* has been retained as a subheading under Nursing Management in each clinical disorder chapter throughout the book. This feature helps the student integrate discharge planning as part of the nursing care for a patient with a specific disorder.

3. An important role the nurse assumes in health care delivery is helping patients prepare to manage their health care at home. *Patient Education Guides* (74) are included in this edition to provide the student with critical information to include in teaching patients as part of discharge planning. In addition, 10 *Home Care Guides* are included. These guides are detailed plans for the more complex, technical skills that patients and families are required to manage in the home.

AGING POPULATION

1. *Geriatric Considerations* boxes (74) are a new feature with this edition. Each box presents information about the older adult's response to changes in health status and his or her special needs for nursing care.

   In the assessment chapters, the geriatric boxes focus the student's attention on the physiologic changes associated with aging. Boxes also present information about modifying assessment skills for the elderly.

2. Chapter 2, *Health Promotion Through the Adult Life Span,* has been rewritten to incorporate more information about health promotion strategies for all adults, including the elderly. The chapter includes current guidelines and goals from *Healthy People 2000.*

CONTENT IN THIS BOOK REPRESENTS A SUBSTANTIAL REVISION

All chapters have been reviewed by medical-surgical generalists and specialists. Additionally, faculty at numerous nursing departments and schools, including associate degree and baccalaureate programs, participated as user diary reviewers. As they prepared lectures and used the book in the classroom, these instructors kept detailed notes on the book over a 2-year period and solicited student input at the end of each semester. These comments were invaluable in improving and refining this book.

Based on this feedback and feedback from other instructors using the book, several *key content areas were targeted for more extensive revision or expansion.* These areas include peripheral and vascular disorders, cardiac disorders, urinary disorders, and, perhaps the most extensive, musculoskeletal disorders. Although the revisions in this edition are substantial throughout, these specific chapters were, in many instances, revised so extensively that they will appear very new to those using the first edition.

Because today's student is an increasingly visual learner, we have significantly expanded our illustration program and adopted a more contemporary, more accessible design. More than *200 illustrations are new* to this edition. Our goal with the expanded illustration program is, foremost, to enable students to visualize key pathophysiologic processes, to "see" the application of therapeutic devices, and to apply physiologic rationales to nursing care. Second, our objective is to achieve consistency and to give the book a more pleasing appearance, thereby engaging student interest. Considered by many to be a real strength of the first edition, the illustration program represents an even greater improvement in this edition.

Finally, the *pedagogy,* again in response to user feedback, has been reconsidered. As in the first edition, each chapter begins with a limited number of measurable learning objectives to focus the student and concludes with review questions to stimulate development of critical thinking skills. The key terms lists, formerly at the ends of chapters, have been moved to the beginnings of chapters. This was done to encourage students to recognize important terminology when first encountered and better prepare them to retain it. Page number references are provided after each key term, and each term is printed in bold face type when defined in the text.

CONTENT IS ORGANIZED LOGICALLY AND PRESENTED UNIFORMLY

Principles and Practice of Adult Health Nursing provides equal emphasis to the disease process and nursing management of the patient to lay a solid foundation for medical-surgical nursing practice. Disorders or conditions are presented in a *consistent format* with separate subheadings, as often as possible, for definition, etiology/epidemiology, pathophysiology, clinical manifestations, and therapeutic management to provide a logical and practical progression of content related to each specific condition. Nursing management is uniformly covered in student-oriented nursing process format of assessment, nursing diagnosis, planning, implementation, and evaluation. Documentation and ongoing care content, for which separate headings are provided, concludes each applicable nursing management section to feature this important role of the nurse. *Color has been used judiciously* to enhance the book's use as a learning tool and a practical reference. Color is used on each disorder heading to facilitate locating content; color is also used on nursing management headings to draw attention to nursing content.

The book is divided into two main sections. Part One, Principles of Adult Health Nursing, establishes a foundation for Part Two, Practice of Adult Health Nursing. We have chosen the term *adult health nursing* over *medical-surgical nursing* for the title of this book for two reasons. First, the term reflects a health-promotion/illness-prevention approach, and second, it corresponds to our inclusion of alternative health care settings in addition to the traditional medical-surgical setting. Because we recognize that each term is commonly used by both faculty and students, *adult health* and *medical-surgical* are used interchangeably throughout the book.

Unit I establishes a foundation for adult health nursing, with chapters on concepts of health and illness, health promotion through the adult life span, stress and adaptation, and epidemiology. Unit II covers dimensions of the nurse's role in adult health nursing. Chapters include nursing roles, clinical decision making and the nursing process, discharge planning and ongoing care, patient and family education, and legal and ethical dimensions. Legal and ethical issues are presented in a manner that encourages nurses to be concerned for the welfare of others and to uphold legal and moral principles.

Unit III presents chapters on physiologic and pathophysiologic factors in nursing, including infection; fluids, electrolytes, and acid-base balance; shock; pain; neoplasia; alterations in nutrition; and sensory overload, deprivation, and sleep disorders. Pathophysiologic alterations or problems that occur as a result of disease processes are discussed as they relate to nursing management presented in the clinical chapters. Immune content formerly in the infection chapter in this unit has been moved to Unit IX and expanded. Unit IV discusses psychosocial dimensions of practice, with separate chapters on caring; altered self-concept; loss, grief, and dying; and substance use disorders. Unit V covers principles of perioperative nursing, in three separate chapters on preoperative, intraoperative, and postoperative patient management.

Part Two comprises the clinical units, Units VI through XVIII, which are organized by biologic system. Each clinical unit begins with a three-part nursing assessment chapter that includes an overview of anatomy and physiology, patient assessment, and nursing implications for related laboratory and diagnostic tests. As mentioned earlier, a consistent format is used to present major medical-surgical disorders.

We have retained numerous features throughout the book that supplement student learning of core content. These content features include patient education guides, legal issues, ethical issues, home care guides, clinical alerts, nursing research briefs, and therapeutic communication guides. All of these aspects were identified by reviewers as assuming increasing importance to the practice of medical-surgical nursing. These content features are listed along with the new features on the endpapers for easy referral.

THE ANCILLARY PACKAGE IS DESIGNED TO SUPPORT INSTRUCTION AND PROMOTE ACTIVE LEARNING

The ancillary package includes an *Instructor's Resource Manual* that relates all three components of the medical-surgical nursing experience: classroom, clinicals, and skills. Included in the resource manual are learning objectives; key terms; three-column chapter outlines with lecture content, active learning activities, and highlighted critical thinking questions; related skills; related clinical activities; student worksheets, including case studies and fill-in-the-blank clinical decision-making guides, and answer section. A 1,000-question *Testbank* is available in NCLEX format in hardcopy or computerized versions. Included for each question are topic, step of the nursing process, cognitive level, NCLEX step, and correct answer with rationale and page number reference to the text. Two-color *Transparency Acetates* are also available in a binder of 200 acetates; several of these transparencies are sequential so that, as the classroom discussion progresses, another layer can be added to communicate progression. A separate *Student Learning Guide* is available either packaged with the text or for separate purchase. This student guide duplicates the worksheets and critical thinking guides found in the Instructor's Resource Manual and is provided for programs in which students use a separate study guide. Finally, a new series of *medical-surgical nursing videos* will be available for course use. Topics will include nursing management and/or patient education for key medical-surgical disorders or conditions.

ACKNOWLEDGMENTS

We have many people to thank for their roles in bringing this book into the classroom, and we can only begin to thank them here. We are especially grateful to our contributors. They have endured tight schedules, demanding editors and reviewers, and endless telephone calls. Without their steadfast efforts, this book would simply not exist. We are also grateful for the freely given advice of our user diary reviewers and their students, who laid the groundwork for the extensive work undertaken by all. We are likewise grateful for the advice of our reviewers, who generously provided constructive comments to further guide this revision. We also thank the contributors who did not participate directly in this edition but whose efforts on the first edition are greatly appreciated:

Julia Wiegand Aucoin, Joyce M. Black, Phyllis A. Bonham, Karen Borchers, Virginia Burggraf, Mary K. Clark, Carolyn Cochrane, Robin Webb Corbett, Patricia Dettenmeier, Susan Dudas, Sally A. Gadow, Gail Gazarian, Mary Jordheim Gokey, Lorraine C. Haertel, Mary Beth Harrington, Judith Hedrick, Linda Heitman, Louis Joffrion, Brenda Johanson, Gertrude Parker Johnson, Jill Kamen, Carol A. Kilmon, Patricia Kreutzer, Patricia L. Lane, Peggy McCall, Bernadette McKay, Mary Meyers-Marquardt, Patricia A. Meehan, Helen Monea, Joyce H. Monk, Mary Courtney Moore, Cynthia Northrop (deceased), Gaye W. Poteet, Alice Poyss, Rosanne Raso, Randi Rutan, Thomas C. Rutan, Nancy Schwab, Kathleen Schwetz, Mary Y. Sieggreen, Phyllis L. Spechko, Mary Ann Spencer-Legler, Marlene Strader, Gail Wiscarz Stuart, Laura Talbot, Poldi Tschirch, Connie Walleck, Cassandra Williamson, Evelyn M. Wills

We are indebted to our editor Robin Carter who worked with us side-by-side and provided sound editorial advice and exceptional problem-solving ability. Our gratitude is also extended to our former editor, Don Ladig, who conceived of this book and saw it through in its successful first edition.

We also thank Brian Dennison, who provided invaluable assistance in the preparation and development of the manuscript, and illustrators Mark Swindle and Jack Reuter, whose original illustrations grace yet even more pages of this book. The production staff at Mosby has also earned our respect for their professionalism and creativity; specifically we wish to thank Karen Edwards, James Russell, Liz Fett, and Karen Lewis. We also appreciate the enthusiasm of the sales and marketing staff of Mosby, specifically Joyce Owen and Bob Boehringer. We appreciate the efforts of Carole Broxson, Carolyn Patiño, Golden Soileau, and Linda and Ken Wendling who prepared the Instructor's Resource Manual and Test Bank, and we thank Bert Vander Mark for his creative cover design.

Last but by no means least, we would like to thank our families, friends, and colleagues for providing continual encouragement and support. This book has been a learning experience and a collaborative effort since its inception. We are indebted to everyone who has contributed his or her expertise in helping students achieve excellence in nursing.

Pat Beare

Judith L. Myers

Contents

Detailed Contents

PART ONE

Principles of Adult Health Nursing

UNIT I

Foundations of Adult Health Nursing

CHAPTER ONE

Health and Illness

LEARNING OBJECTIVES

1 Differentiate the concepts of wellness, illness, and health.
2 Identify factors that influence health and illness.
3 Compare and contrast the ideas of health as a goal, as growth, or as an experience.
4 Describe how the ideas of health as a goal, as growth, or as an experience influence the way one practices nursing.
5 Formulate a personal concept of "health" that will help guide practice and the scholarly pursuit of nursing knowledge.

KEY TERMS

health, p. 10
health belief model, p. 16
health promotion model, p. 17

illness, p. 18
wellness, p. 19

HEALTH IS a concept central to the discipline of nursing as well as to other disciplines involved in giving care. An understanding of health gives direction to nursing practice, assists with formulating a clear understanding of the definition of nursing, and gives structure to the ongoing development of the scholarly base of nursing science.

Health can be considered as a goal, as evidence for growth, or as an experience. The choices that nurses make in assessing, planning, implementing, and evaluating care (the nursing process) depend on which one of these views of health guides their thinking. For example, in the "health as a goal" model, all laboratory test values must be within a standardized set of normal limits for a person to be assessed as healthy. The belief that health is growth suggests that if laboratory values are changing toward normal values, then a person is healthy because growth is in a healthy direction. When health is viewed as experience, laboratory values matter only in relation to a host of other phenomena. In the growth or experience model, mind and body are so integrated that no one piece of information stands

alone. Although all three models consider laboratory values important, the main focus of the model helps the nurse set priorities, determine goals for nursing care, and evaluate outcomes.

Currently, any accepted theory of nursing includes a definition of health, as well as definitions of person (or humanity), environment, and nursing. Table 1-1 compares how some of the more commonly used nursing models define health. Nursing theories provide direction for practice, suggest areas for research, and develop a framework for scholarly inquiry into nursing phenomena.

An early theorist, Virginia Henderson, defines health as "the ability to function independently in relation to 14 identified concepts" (Table 1-1). Nursing care directed by Henderson's concept of health is "a deliberative approach to meet the 14 components of nursing care."

Sr. Callista Roy, Betty Neuman, and Imogene King all cite the fact that health is not static; it is a dynamic state, always changing. Nursing must be carried out in such a way as to influence the direction of that dynamism. For example, the nurse might "de-

5

TABLE 1-1   Comparison Chart of Nursing Models

Nursing models	Definition of nursing	Derivation of nursing activity	Person	Health	Environment
				Conceptualization of	
Nightingale	A profession for women, the goal of which is to discover and use nature's laws governing health in the service of humanity	To put the person in the best condition for nature to restore or preserve health, and to prevent or cure disease and injury	Comprised of physical, intellectual, and metaphysical attributes and potentialities	To be free of disease and to be able to use one's own powers to the fullest	Those elements external to, and which affect, the healthy or sick person
Peplau	A practice discipline designed to facilitate productive energy transformation	A goal-oriented interpersonal process between nurse and patient	A self-system composed of biochemical, physical, and psychological characteristics and needs, with emphasis upon the psychological	Productive level of anxiety such that interpersonal activity and developmental tasks can be accomplished	A microcosm of significant others with whom the patient interacts
Orlando	Interaction with a patient who has a need, involving patient validation with both the need and the help provided, in order to improve the patient's health	Patient's needs determine nursing acts	Behaving human organism; (patients) are persons under medical supervision or treatment	Mental and physical comfort, sense of adequacy and well-being	Time and place, i.e., the context of the nursing situation
Wiedenbach	A deliberate blend of thoughts, feelings, and overt actions . . . practiced in relation to an individual who is in need of help	Patient behavior which indicates a need for help triggers nursing activity	A functioning and competent being, one able to determine if a need for help is being experienced	Specific definition of health is lacking; Wiedenbach implicitly assumes that the nurse's concern for the patient is health related	The environment is not defined; implied that it may contain or produce an obstacle resulting in a need for help
Henderson	The assistance of the individual, sick or well, in activities contributing to health or recovery that she/he would perform had she/he the strength, will, or knowledge	Deliberative approach to meet the 14 components of nursing care	Biological beings with inseparable mind and body	Ability to function independently in relation to 14 components	Not clearly defined; can act on patient in positive or negative way

Levine	Human interaction; incorporates scientific principles in use of the nursing process	Holistic care individualized to each person's needs; nurse supports the person's adaptation	Complex individual in interaction with internal and external environment who responds to change by means of adaptation	A pattern of adaptive change "whole" (Anglo-Saxon term)	Internal environment is the person's physiology whereas external environment has perceptual, operational, and conceptual components
Johnson	Professional discipline with both an art and a science component which functions as an external regulatory force for the behavioral system	Nursing activity derives from a need created by a state of instability or disequilibrium in the behavioral system	Behavioral system identified by actions and behaviors: a totality of 7 interrelated subsystems	Elusive state determined by psychological, social, and physiological factors which is held as a value by all the health professions; a moving state of equilibrium which occurs throughout the health change process	Not explicated in model; implied as all which is external to the behavioral system
Orem	A human service designed to overcome human limitations in self-care action for health-related reasons	Nursing acts are derived from judgments as to why patients require nursing, i.e., by the patient's needs for therapeutic self-care to sustain life and health	Man is an integrated whole, functioning biologically, symbolically, and socially	A state of wholeness or integrity of the individual, his/her parts and modes of functioning	A subcomponent of man, which together comprises an integrated system related to self-care
Roy	A process of analyses and action related to the care of the ill or potentially ill person	Nursing activity derives from the model which prescribes a process of assessment and intervention; nursing intervention is carried out within the context of the nursing process and involves manipulation of stimuli	A biopsychosocial being in constant interaction with a changing environment; the person is an open, adaptive system	The health-illness continuum is a continuous line representing states or degrees of health or illness that a person might experience at a given time; health-illness is an inevitable dimension of the person's life	All conditions, circumstances, and influences surrounding and affecting the development of an organism or group of organisms

Continued.

From Fitzpatrick JJ, Whall AL: *Conceptual models of nursing: analysis and application,* Bowie, Md, 1983, Robert J Brady Co.

TABLE 1-1   Comparison Chart of Nursing Models—cont'd

Nursing models	Definition of nursing	Derivation of nursing activity	Conceptualization of		
			Person	Health	Environment
Paterson and Zderad	Goal-directed response aimed toward nurturing the well-being and more-being of a person with perceived needs related to health/illness	The intersubjective transaction between patient and nurse related to the health/illness quality of living	An incarnate being always becoming in relation with men and things in a world of time and space	Somewhat more than freedom from disease; not defined, nor is the relationship to well-being and more-being delineated	Man's inner world, a biased and shaded reality, and the real world of men and things in time and space
Neuman	Nursing is a unique profession concerned with the total person, i.e., all the variables affecting an individual's response to stressors	The nurse is an intervener who acts in relation to either reduction of encounter with stressors or in relation to mitigating the effect of stressors	A person is a physiologic, psychologic, sociocultural, and developmental being; the person must be viewed as a whole; the wholeness concept is related to the dynamic interrelationship of variables	A person's health is a state of wellness or illness which is determined by the four variables: physiologic, psychologic, sociocultural, and developmental; health is relative and in a dynamic state of flux	There are external and internal environments; the external environment is all that is external to the person; the internal environment is the person's internal state in terms of physiologic, psychologic, sociocultural, and developmental variables
King	A process of human interaction between nurse and client	Nurse and client perceive each other and the situation, communicate information, mutually set goals, and take action to attain goals	An open system exhibiting permeable boundaries permitting an exchange of matter, energy, and information with the environment	Dynamic adjustment to stressors in the internal and external environment through optimum uses of resources to achieve maximum potential for daily living	An open system exhibiting permeable boundaries permitting an exchange of matter, energy, and information with human beings

Rogers	A learned profession whose focus is compassionate concern for maintaining and promoting health and caring for and rehabilitating sick and disabled	Seeks to promote symphonic interaction between environment and man (all people in all settings)	A four-dimensional, negentropic energy field identified by pattern and organization and manifesting characteristics and behaviors that are different from those of the parts which cannot be predicted from knowledge of the parts	Health is a value word broadly defined by cultures and individuals to denote behaviors that are of high value and low value	A four-dimensional, negentropic energy field identified by pattern and organization and encompassing all that (is) outside any given human field
Newman	Nursing science focuses on the health of persons	Nursing practice assists persons to utilize their own resources to attain higher levels of consciousness	Person is an energy field that is part of the life process	Health, as part of the life process, is a fusion of disease and nondisease that is a basic pattern unique to the person, as she/he evolves toward expanded consciousness	Environment is an energy field that is part of the life process; that which is outside of any given human field
Parse	Science and art focusing on man as living unity	Person's qualitative participation with health experiences	Synergistic open being coextensive with universe free to choose in situations	Process of becoming as experienced by person	Co-constitutes becoming in mutual simultaneous energy exchange with person
Fitzpatrick	Science and profession which has as its central concern the meaning attached to life (health)	Focused on enhancing the developmental process toward health	Open system, unified whole, characterized by basic human rhythms	Continuously developing characteristic of humans; full life potential; awareness of meaningfulness of life	Open system in continuous interaction with persons

RESEARCH BRIEF

Kenney J: The consumer's view of health, *J Adv Nurs* 17:829, 1992.

Consumers and health care providers often define and view health differently. Kenney analyzed adults' views of health and compared their views with two current conceptual models of health. She utilized a nonprobability Caucasian sample of 44 female and 21 male adults. Participants completed a questionnaire with 34 definitions of health grouped into 12 nonlabeled categories. Scores were computed for the 12 categories of health, and t-tests were used to analyze gender differences; age and educational differences were analyzed using ANOVA.

Significant gender and educational differences existed in this particular sample of Midwestern, primarily well-educated adults. Women were more likely than men to view social involvement and harmony as definitions of health. The top three categories of definitions of health, ranked by both men and women, included self-concept, fitness, and role performance. Persons with different educational backgrounds also viewed health differently, in terms of body image, fitness, and self-actualization. The researcher's findings suggest that consumers have broad views of health that vary among gender, age, and educational groups.

Quality of care will be enhanced as nurses effectively communicate with patients regarding their views of health and their unique concerns and fears accompanying a chronic alteration in health.

crease the effect of stressors" (Neuman), "manipulate stimuli" (Roy), or "set mutual goals" with the patient (King).

Margaret Newman and Rosemary Rizzo Parse focus on health as "expanded consciousness" or "experience." Nursing focuses on helping the patient understand and use experience to attain higher levels of consciousness, thereby influencing health.

DEFINITIONS

There is not one "correct" definition of **health.** A definition of health is useful if it helps to formulate a clear direction for clinical practice, helps define nursing, gives direction to research, and develops the knowledge of nursing. Smith[25] looked at health from a philosophic perspective and saw four types of definitions of health (Table 1-2). The clinical model of health suggests an absence of disease; the adaptive model suggests an interaction with internal and external environments; the role performance model suggests the ability to perform one's many roles; and the eudaimonistic model suggests a sense of integration with the universe.

Others have written that definitions of health relate to three concepts: actualization, stability, and a combination of actualization and stability.[18,19,34] The actualization category borrows from Maslow's concept of self-actualization,[39] just as Smith's eudaimonistic model does. They both suggest that health is a state of being vigorous, spirited, eager, and excited about life—being the best one can be. Stability relates to adaptation—a purposeful response that takes into account physical, mental, emotional, and social reaction to the environment.[16] The combination of actualization and stability refers to the ability to maintain the actualized state while adjustments to the self are made to maintain stability.[19]

Another way to classify definitions of health is by development. Payne[18] discusses the evolution of the concept of health starting with the idea of humans in harmony with the universe and moving toward holism, a more complex model implying integration

TABLE 1-2   Philosophic Comparison of Health and Illness

Model	Health	Illness
Eudaimonistic	Condition of being the best possible "self" (self-actualized)	Impediment to becoming self-actualized
Adaptive	Ability to interact with social and physical environment	Failure to cope with changes in environment
Role performance	Ability to do one's job or perform role	Inability to carry out one's role
Clinical	Absence of signs or symptoms of disease	Presence of signs or symptoms of disease

Modified from Smith J: The idea of health: a philosophical inquiry, *ANS* 3(3):43, 1981.

with the universe. In using a developmental approach, Payne suggests that later models develop from earlier models and that the concept of health will continue to evolve and be changed as new and more useful definitions are developed (see the box below).

Some definitions of health do not easily fit into a classification system, yet they give a different perspective to the concept of health. Keller[11] found descriptions and definitions of health depend in part on the discipline of the author. An economist, for example, might see health as wealth. Grossman, an economist, as quoted in Pender,[19] suggests that health is "a durable commodity to be purchased." Table 1-3 gives a sample of various definitions of health.

These definitions represent different ideas and have an impact on how health care will be rendered in the future. Where health is defined as a task, response, or goal, the focus of nursing care is on outcomes, such as a temperature of 37° C or ingestion of a diet rich in fiber. If health is perceived as a process, growth, or response, health care focuses more on the process of reaching a defined outcome. Measures to help maintain a normal temperature or a healthy diet pattern are emphasized. If health is seen as integration or unity, the focus may shift even more toward the individual's responsibility to assess body cues (i.e., feeling hot), identify effective measures for decreasing the elevated temperature, and seek out appropriate health care providers. Appropriate health care providers are those who can guide one toward the health promotion techniques necessary to achieve and maintain that sense of well-being.

Current nursing literature reflects the idea that health is most often viewed in a comprehensive manner incorporating a knowledge of disease, but not limited to that knowledge. Disease is an objective fact, a measurable condition verified by laboratory tests, physical examination, and patient history.

When a comprehensive view of health is used, the disease is identified as a cue that the individual can use to gain insight, learn how to avoid the disease in the future, and review life values (a personal concept of mortality and the reasons for being alive). Even acutely ill people are cared for with the idea that they can be helped toward a fuller sense of well-being or connectedness with the universe.

EVOLUTIONARY DEVELOPMENT OF MODELS OF HEALTH

Holistic health
High-level wellness: Dunn
Health based on the normal person
Psychosocial models of health
Adaptation and interaction models
Humanity relates to the environment

Modified from Payne L: Health: a basic concept in nursing theory, *J Adv Nurs* 8:393, 1983.

TABLE 1-3   Selected Definitions of Health

Definitions	Source
Freedom from disease	Traditional usage
"A state of complete physical, mental, and social well-being and not merely the absence of disease"	World Health Organization, 1947
"Adaptation of man to his environment"	Rene Dubos
"Coordinated activity of component parts, each functioning in a normal range"	L. Aubrey
"The effective performance of valued roles and tasks for which an individual has been socialized"	Talcot Parsons[17]
"An integrated method of functioning which is oriented toward maximizing the potential of which the individual is capable; it requires that the individual maintain a continuum of balance and purpose"	Halbert Dunn
"Health is the actualization of inherent and acquired human potential through goal-directed behavior, competent self-care, and satisfying relationships with others while adjustments are made as needed to maintain structural integrity and harmony with the environment"	Nola Pender[19]
"The harmonious balance of body, mind, and spirit in an everchanging environment"	American Holistic Nurses' Association[1]

INFLUENCES

The development of a definition of health is influenced by biologic, psychologic, cultural, economic, political, social, and personal factors. Biologic, psychologic, and personal influences tend to relate to the individual and family, whereas the other factors are related to broader communities, the nation, and the world as they relate to the health of everyone. The adoption of a definition of health relevant to all cultures was achieved in 1947 when the World Health Organization defined health as the "state of complete physical, mental, and social well-being, and not merely the absence of disease and infirmity."[41] By adding an understanding of various "influences" to this most generic of definitions of health, the definition can become more useful. Health as a concept may be used with other terms: health behaviors, health promotion, health care systems, health practices, and health insurance.

Biologic

The biologic influence involves the study of theories of physiology, pathology, and body functioning and disease. It represents the major body of medical science and provides a necessary basis for nursing theory and intervention. This perspective proposes that there are three traditional medical criteria used in identifying a disease:

1. The patient's experience of subjective feelings of sickness
2. The findings that the patient has some disordered function of some body part
3. Symptoms that conform to a recognizable clinical pattern and meet diagnostic criteria[33]

A person is said to be diseased, or ill, from a biologic perspective when the symptoms and indications from physical tests and laboratory tests fit a medical model of disease. A physician makes a medical diagnosis by comparing personal observations of the patient and the reported symptoms with various medical norms based in part on scientific data and in part on clinical experience. If the theory underlying the diagnosis is sound and scientifically confirmed, the cause of disease and the course of treatment can be identified.

Biologic factors must be understood in light of the environments in which they operate. The external environment, such as weather and altitude, makes certain demands on body functioning, and the body adapts to these demands. The way the body adapts can be helpful, or it can cause discomfort and strain, precipitating new problems of health and disease. Illness can be viewed as biologic adaptation, or the body's attempt to accommodate internal stresses and noxious external conditions. It is a poor adaptive response, because it can result in personal pain, discomfort, and decreased activity, and it can threaten to shorten one's life.[4]

Psychologic

The psychologic perspective examines how a person's intrapsychic states and personality traits influence response to health and illness. This emotional component has often been identified in the cause or precipitation of illness and may affect the length and outcome of illness states. This psychologic perspective helps explain why certain people are at risk for illness, suggests reasons why people seek or refuse to seek health care, and proposes ways in which nurses might better educate people and help them comply with nursing and medical treatment plans.

Cognitive appraisal (perception), commitment and beliefs, and individual adaptation are three ways psychology influences health. Stressors and symptoms can be perceived, evaluated, and acted on differently by people. This difference can be related to a person's perception of the significance of the event. Lazarus[37] believes that these cognitive factors play a central role in adaptation, since they affect the impact of stressful events, the choice of coping patterns used, and the variety of emotional, biologic, and behavioral responses the individual displays. His theory suggests that one's cognitive appraisal mediates psychologically between the person and the environment in any stressful encounter. Persons evaluate whether situations are damaging or potentially damaging on the basis of their understanding of how harmful the situations are and what resources are available to neutralize or tolerate the harm.

Lazarus[37] describes three types of primary cognitive appraisals to stress:

1. Harm or loss—referring to actual damage that has already occurred as a result of the event
2. Threat—referring to anticipated damage or the possibility of future harm
3. Challenge—referring to when the focus is placed positively on potential gain, growth, or mastery, rather than on possible risks

Stress seen as a challenge, rather than as a threat or loss, may play a crucial role in psychologic and biologic hardiness, or resistance to disease.[30] One longitudinal study showed that people whose attitude toward life could be rated high on challenge (viewing change as a challenge rather than as a threat), commitment (feeling the opposite of alienation), and control (feeling the opposite of powerlessness) remained healthier than other people.[20]

Other important factors affecting one's response to health and illness are commitments and beliefs.[29] Commitments are an expression of what is important to the individual, and they form the basis of the choices one makes in life. Commitments can thus guide people into or away from situations that threaten or harm, or they can guide people into situations that may potentially be of benefit.

Beliefs also determine how a person evaluates what is happening. Beliefs about personal control are particularly relevant to stress reduction, since they influence both one's emotional response and one's potential coping ability. For example, the psychologic state of helplessness is the belief of an individual that life events are out of one's control. Seligman[24] has shown the similarity between perceived helplessness and states of clinical depression. Many experiments in animals have linked helplessness to ulcer formation, other physical illnesses, and even death. One's beliefs about one's ability to control events do appear to affect overall health and welfare.

Spiritual beliefs and commitments are particularly powerful. Spiritual beliefs relate to a person's sense of the meaning of life and the possibility of the existence of powers greater than oneself. Such beliefs may or may not be tied to a specific religious affiliation, but they affect one's perceptions of health and illness. Beliefs about spirituality include a view of life's goals and convey a sense of purpose to life, which may be hopeful or hopeless. Spiritual beliefs can be divided into three categories of influence: inspiring, ineffectual, and deleterious.[31] Inspiring beliefs are growth producing and provide a sense of peace of mind. Ineffectual beliefs are neutral—they provide neither support nor harm to the individual. Deleterious beliefs are those that can provoke feelings of distress, such as guilt, anger, anxiety, or shame. The nurse's role is to be sensitive to the importance an individual places on spiritual beliefs and to the impact they might have on one's health practices or perceptions of illness.[4]

The phrase *individual adaptation* refers to other psychologic processes that intervene between one's perception and response to stress and illness.[13] The first thing an individual does when facing a stressful event is assess what is happening and try to discover the meaning of it all. This search for meaning is a prerequisite for developing a personal coping strategy. Some life situations are common and familiar and can be quickly evaluated, such as the death of a loved one, the loss of a job, or an automobile accident. Other events, however, are more personal and unique. A sudden, intense dislike of a particular health care worker may be hard to evaluate but may affect compliance with treatment. Individuals experiencing this kind of situation may have more difficulty in arriving at a definition of the experience and the implications of it and in developing a sense of how to respond to it.

The less a particular crisis is shared by others, the more uncertain and problematic is the response. People going through a variety of life crises are often surprised when they join self-help groups and find how typical their experiences are. They come to realize the feelings and behaviors they thought were unique to them are often shared by others in similar situations.

A second psychologic adaptation strategy used by the individual is the attempt to determine the cause of the events being experienced and assign responsibility for their occurrence. The important dimension is whether the person believes the causes are internal or external. Internal causality can be beneficial to the individual. Various studies suggest that individuals with high self-esteem see themselves as more capable of dealing with threatening situations and thus are less vulnerable. People who have a sense of their own power and competence can more readily direct the situation to their own advantage, in contrast to people who see their lives as determined by fate or forces outside their control. Internal attribution can be harmful to the individual if it implies self-blame, guilt, and feelings of worthlessness after failure.

The person who fails in some way but can attribute the failure to outside influences may actually feel better. Blaming external influences for failure must be consistent with reality and supported or validated by others. The person must still work to solve his or her problems.

People come to view their feelings or behavior as a consequence of moral failure or as a punishment for "badness." Victims of acquired immune deficiency syndrome (AIDS), alcoholism, and mental illness are affected by people's perceptions and attributions of illness. Too often, the care the individual receives and the course of the disorder can be negatively affected by these attribution processes (like stereotyping). Most important, nurses and other health care providers need to realize their own assumptions about the causality of illnesses. Negative attributions toward types of patients or illnesses can hamper the ability to provide quality, empathic nursing care.

A final individual adaptation strategy is for the person to compare one's own skills and capacities with those of other people with similar problems. In so doing, the person obtains cues about the meaning of events and ways to respond. By looking to others for comparison, individuals obtain a source of values and a guide for measuring their own progress. How a person feels about self will partly depend on the group selected for comparison.[4]

Cultural

Culture consists of the environment that humans make for themselves.[15] It includes patterns such as language and behavior; interactions with environment and with each other, such as rituals and worship practices; and modifications to the environment, such as with air conditioning or construction.

The culture of a group affects almost every aspect of an individual's growth and development. From conception to death, every major life experience of a person is conditioned to some extent by one's cultural beliefs and orientations. The appropriate marriage partner, the form of birth control one uses, family size and spacing, feeding, and weaning—these and many other decisions depend largely on social customs and taboos. The mother's acquisition of health practices and mothering skills directly influences the health of her baby and may explain in part why mothers in the more advantaged social groups and those who are better educated experience lower infant mortality. Nutrition is a key factor for good health, but food preparation and eating behavior are influenced by cultural norms. Culture determines modes of agriculture, production, food processing, and distribution. Whereas in many areas of the world people are consuming diets deficient in protein, calories, and vitamins, in many developed nations people consume diets rich in fats, sugars, calories, and additives that have been implicated in various diseases, including diabetes, cancer, and heart disease.

The health of a people reflects the way they choose to live. Specifically, patterns of illness and death in a society are influenced by values related to organization of the family, work, and recreation. Humanity's constructed environment may be a major cause of disease. Windowless buildings, for example, may lead to poor ventilation and recirculation of airborne pathogens. Cultural patterns influencing child rearing, the family, social expectations, competition, and sense of social commitment can also be seen as contributing to high rates of psychologic distress, suicide, and violence.

Subcultures within American society have substantially different risks of poor health and death. Although such differences are undoubtedly the result of biologic and genetic factors, they are also influenced by cultural norms.[27] Group norms concerning smoking, drinking, sexual practices, religion, and standards of living can protect or add to one's health-related risks. For example, traditional sex roles in American society discouraged women from smoking and drinking. When fewer women smoked, fewer women had lung cancer. When it became more acceptable for women to smoke, women's rates of lung cancer increased.

An individual must make life-style changes when the subculture called "hospital" is entered. The hospital has a separate language ("void" instead of urinate; "CAT scan" to mean an imaging test instead of a search for a small animal!). Time, values, interactions, and modifications to the environment are all part of the changes an individual submits to on entry into the system, and the individual may in fact experience culture shock because of it.

Blum[2] listed 12 measurable aspects of health, including several culturally determined categories. Disability or incapacity relates to how well a person carries out his or her role. Participation in health care, health-related behaviors, ecologic behavior, social behavior, interpersonal relationships, and the ability to derive pleasure from situations such as work and play are all determinants of a healthy state and are all culturally relevant.

Culture has a major influence on how the individual responds to illness behavior, including when to seek help, what type of practitioner to see, and how illness is viewed by the individual's social group (see research brief). For example, Koos[36] observed that upper-class people were more likely than lower-class people to view themselves as ill when they had particular symptoms. They would also seek a physician's advice sooner than lower-class people. Decisions about health are weighted in relation to family and work needs, finances, and other competing social needs.

Zborowski,[42] in a study of ethnic reactions to pain in a New York City hospital, observed that whereas Jewish and Italian patients responded to pain in an emotional way and tended to exaggerate pain experiences, "old Americans" tended to be more stoic and the Irish more commonly denied pain. He also noted a difference in the attitude underlying Italian and Jewish concerns about pain. Whereas the Italian subjects primarily sought relief from pain, the Jewish subjects were mainly concerned with the meaning and significance of their pain and the consequences of their pain for their future welfare and health.

A nurse is subject to the norms and values of one's own cultural heritage and can evaluate patients based on personal cultural standards. This practice is called ethnocentrism—when one looks at the world from one's own particular cultural viewpoint and believes those norms are best. One should not stereotype individuals based on cultural generalizations. Cultural relativism, in which neither the nurse's cultural values nor the other person's are regarded as superior, helps the nurse to be both sensitive to one's own cultural values and norms and responsive to the cultural values of others.

Economic

The economic environment influences health both on the individual level and on the group level from family to world communities. At the individual level, one's financial status determines health services one can buy, the health-related activities one can afford, and the kinds of food that one can purchase. Extending this concept to the level of communities, the availability of services, activities (and the tools necessary to implement them, such as spas, health clubs, or hiking trails), and food depends on the economics of the community. Crop failures in Third World countries can be devastating, because food storage is nonexistent in some places and no reserves are available.

Economics can also have a devastating effect on the health of nations of affluent people. The growth of the fast-food industry, without a concomitant sufficient understanding of the relationship of fatty foods and disease, is often cited as a major reason for the increase in heart disease and colon cancer in the United States.

The influence and outcome that a conceptual change in health care funding can achieve is evident with the advent of the prospective payment system for government-funded health care. Until the 1980s, health care was funded like most things in a capitalistic economic system, with payment for services rendered. In an attempt to decrease health care costs, the government established a complicated system of payment for services based on patient diagnoses. This system is termed diagnostic related groups (DRGs). Payment to health care providers is made based on the diagnosis or set of diagnoses that the physician identifies for the individual. The reimbursement for treating all individuals in the same DRG (with some other considerations, such as region of the country) is the same, regardless of the actual cost of treating each person. Because it costs less to treat a hospitalized person if the hospital stay is shorter, discharge tends to occur earlier, and a hospital may make money if it can keep costs of treatment below actual reimbursement for the DRG. The hospital loses money if it spends more than it can be reimbursed. This has led to a number of changes in the health care system, including more emphasis on health promotion and maintenance to prevent readmissions, the use of the case management system of delivering nursing care to ensure efficiency and quality of care delivery, the employment of discharge planners to help place people in the community more quickly, the development of support groups in the community, and the movement toward more home health care providers.

Political

Politics influences health. Politicians determine what potential health hazards are allowed in the workplace, what the distribution of resources for health will be, who will be responsible for the health of a nation or for individuals, and which health issues will be studied to improve health care, cure disease, or influence general health. Questions arise as to the right of people to health care and the quality, accessibility, and cost/benefit of health care. Is the country (or state or community) willing to put resources and effort into ensuring all people the means to be all that they can be? Or is sufficient food and the absence of disease enough for the community to provide? The U.S. Public Health Service is coordinating the development of national health objectives for the year 2000. These objectives will focus

---

YEAR 2000 PRIORITY AREAS

Reduce

Tobacco use
Alcohol and other drug use
Environmental health hazards
Violent and abusive behavior
Adolescent pregnancy

Improve

Reproductive health
Nutrition
Mental health
Occupational safety and health
Maternal and infant health
Oral health
Health education and access to preventive health services
Surveillance and data systems

Increase

Physical activity and fitness

Prevent

Mental illness
And control unintentional injuries
And control HIV infection and AIDS
And control sexually transmitted diseases

Detect

And control high blood cholesterol and high blood pressure
And control cancer
And control other chronic diseases and disorders

Immunize

Against and control infectious diseases

Maintain

The health and quality of life of older people

---

on 21 priority areas (see the box labeled "Year 2000 Priority Areas"). The project's goal is to provide direction to planning effective programs at the local, state, and federal levels to promote health and reduce premature death, disease, and disability.

The relationship between politics and economics that influences health is changing. Historically, health care professionals dominated in determining standards of care. Now, special interest groups, financial institutions, third-party insurers of health care, and other groups play an increasing role in defining goals and standards of care. The implementation of the prospective payment system cited earlier is an example. The interrelationship of culture, economics, and politics often determines not only what kind and what level of health is acceptable and affordable, but also the nature of health itself.

Social

Social factors that influence the concept of health include each person's attitudes and actions toward other human beings. It is a widely held assumption that attitudes influence behavior. Negative attitudes of society toward homosexual behavior may have been partly responsible for the low priority of AIDS research in the early 1980s. Societies, family groups, and individuals who thrive in a competitive, aggressive environment tend to develop different health problems (e.g., hypertension) than people from less aggressive settings.

In addition to aggression, other social factors that influence health include attitudes toward change, cooperation and collaboration, societal value of health as contrasted with other social values, the view of "humanity" as basically good or basically evil, and the nature of humans. Many groups behave differently toward people who are not within their own social group.

Attitudes toward health affect health care behaviors. Two people visiting a physician's office may expect different care. The first may want the physician to prescribe medicine to "cure" the problem instantly, believing this is the physician's job. The other may believe the physician does not dispense cures in the form of medicine but assists the individual's own healing processes. This person expects information on self-care, as well as medicine or other procedures. Taking responsibility for self-healing, this person makes appropriate changes in life-style and actively participates in care.

Milio[14] and later Butterfield[3] showed that attitudes and other actions of human beings are limited by policy and other social decisions. They believe that society provides a "range of available health choices," and this range may either limit or enhance how far an individual can go in controlling health. Governmental policies related to availability of abortion illustrate this point, in that where abortion is illegal, it is unavailable as a health choice for some people.

Personal

Personal beliefs are intertwined with culture and social factors, since one acquires beliefs through socialization and culture. However, each competent individual determines when to seek health care intervention, what to do to achieve or maintain health, where to seek care, and whether to follow health care advice. These kinds of decisions are based in

part on norms of society, religious influences, family counseling, and finances.

"Locus of control," a social theory that suggests relationships between outcomes of behaviors that are under the control of an individual and those that are external, is another factor to be considered. Many researchers have attempted to identify other personal factors that influence health behaviors. The most well-known of these is Becker et al.'s Health Belief Model.[32]

HEALTH AS A GOAL
Health Belief Model

All of the influences on the development of a definition and concept of health are incorporated into the **health belief model**, a psychologic and behavioral theory that attempts to explain individual health behaviors.[32] This model assumes that attitudes and beliefs play an important role in health behaviors. The health belief model suggests that health behaviors (such as compliance with treatment protocols) are based on three factors. The first is whether a person perceives a threat ("How susceptible am I to this problem? Is it a serious problem?"). The second factor is whether a person perceives that the recommended behavior is likely to be of value. The third factor is cost or barriers involved in achieving the behavior.

Modifying factors (things that influence the perceptions of threat, value of behavior change, and barriers) include influences mentioned above: cultural, economic, psychologic, and personal belief systems. Social factors include peer group pressure and values, ethnicity, age, and much more demographic data. Modifying factors also include things that might enable the person to change behavior more easily, such as mass media campaigns, friends who have been sick with the same problem, or advice from friends and relatives.

If a person perceives that there is a serious problem that is likely to affect him or her, that actions taken by an individual can limit the extent of that problem, and that the barriers to that problem are not great, the person is likely to take the appropriate action. An example might be the affluent elderly person who fears that a flu virus could cause pneumonia but believes that a vaccine could prevent the flu. That person is likely to go to the physician to get the vaccine injection. A poor person may see the cost of the injection as too high to pay. A person who does not believe that vaccines are effective would not see the injection as useful. These are factors related to belief systems and economics that influence the person's willingness to take health-related action.

If a person believes that a problem is not a threat, that no action can limit the problem anyway, or that the barriers to the action recommended are great, that person is unlikely to take action. Modifying factors, such as information that changes the belief that nothing can help, or helping the person break down barriers (e.g., giving financial assistance if required) can change the outcome.

The health belief model (Figure 1-1) as a guide to nursing practice clearly shows that many modifying factors can be affected within the nursing role. Patient teaching, discharge planning, family counseling, and referrals to other health care professionals (including social service workers) may affect patient information and financial resources, making it possible for patients to comply with treatments and health recommendations.

Nola Pender[19] extended the health belief model into a **health promotion model.** Both models use similar factors as a framework: perception of the individual (including cognition); modifying factors; and variables that suggest how likely one is to take action related to health behaviors. Pender, who has refined her first model, includes seven factors in the cognitive-perception category of the health promotion model. They are the importance of health, per-

ceived control of health, perceived self-efficacy, definition of health, perceived health status, perceived health benefits relating to the health-promoting behavior, and perceived barriers to that behavior.

By considering the importance of health to an individual and the perception of control over health that an individual may have, one can begin to predict how willing the individual may be to develop health promotion behaviors. Pender believes that if it is not important for a person to be healthy, that person will not try to be so. Some people simply are not concerned about health. In addition, some people do not seem to make decisions about health in a manner consistent with their beliefs. Health promotion behaviors include activities such as cessation of cigarette smoking and performing regular exercise—actions taken to improve or maintain good health (Table 1-4). People may believe that smoking may make them sick later but believe they are unable to stop smoking. This is related to self-efficacy, the belief that one can change a specific behavior and maintain that change. Conversely, one may need the support of others in making change related to health promotion behaviors such as cessation of

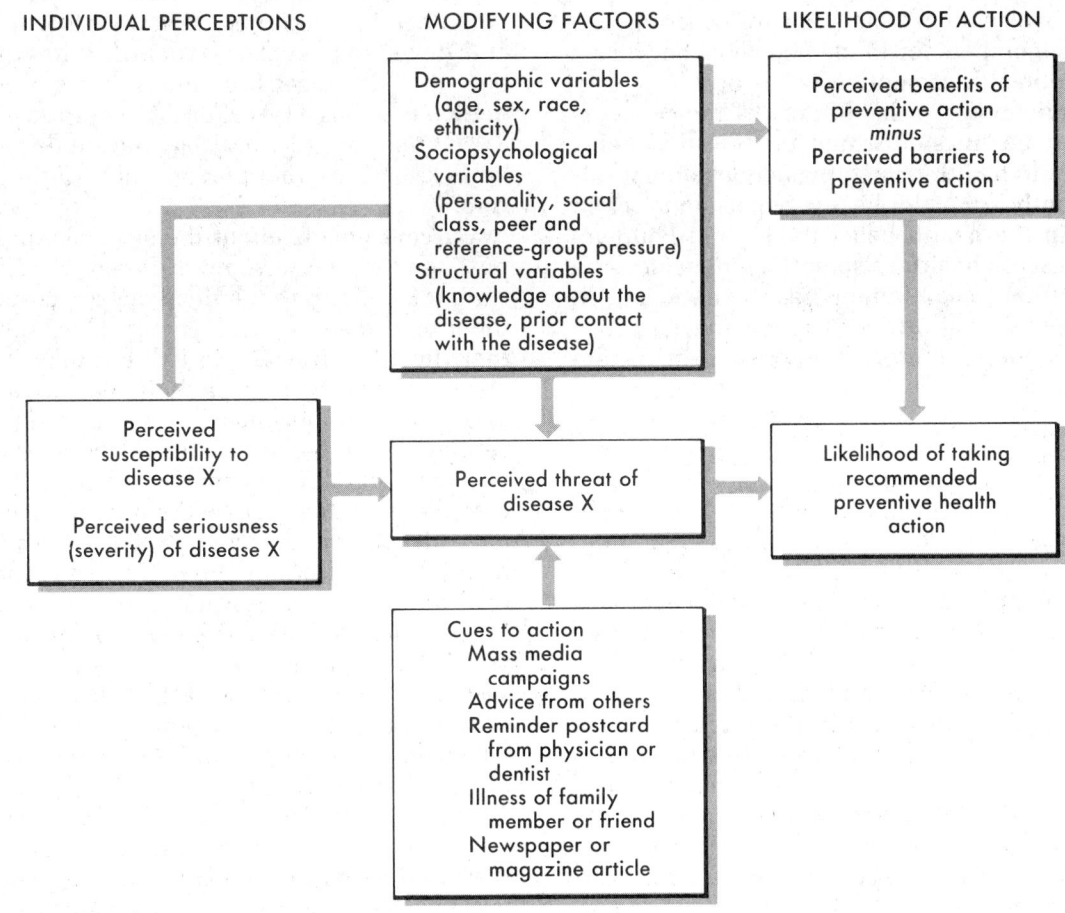

FIGURE 1-1   Health belief model.

TABLE 1-4   Modifying Factors that Influence Health Behaviors

Intrapersonal	Interpersonal	Situational
Age	Significant others	Community resources
Sex	Family patterns of health care	Availability of health-promoting options (e.g., fresh fruit vs. fast foods)
Race	Interactions with health professionals	Access to health-promoting alternatives, such as a safe area to jog in
Ethnicity		
Education		Clean air, environment
Income		Policies promoting health (e.g., nonsmoking areas; regular work breaks to decrease stress)
Weight		
Cognitive skills		
Psychomotor skills		
Past physical fitness		

Modified from Pender N: *Health promotion in nursing practice,* Norwalk, Conn, 1982, Appleton-Century-Crofts.

smoking. This is related to one's perception of control of health behaviors. Some people are self-directed and believe they control their own actions. Others rely on external control, such as support from others. This support can be important to them in changing behaviors related to health. The relationship among decisions about health behaviors, internal and external controls (locus of control), and self-efficacy (competency in the behavior) has direct relevance to health promotion behaviors.

Pender's definition of health, use of the concepts of perceived health status, and perceived benefits and barriers to health-promoting actions do not differ significantly from the health belief model cited earlier. Both the health belief model and Pender's extension discuss health as something to achieve by getting treatment, maintaining healthy habits, or in other ways changing attitudes and behaviors in a specific direction. Therefore health is a goal, a state to be achieved.

Sick Role Model

Talcott Parsons,[17] a sociologist, looked at the problem of **illness** rather than health. For Parsons the "sick role" was defined as the shared expectations of society about how sick people should behave. This set of expectations is central to the understanding of illness and exerted great influence on the understanding of how medicine and health care were to be practiced for many years in the middle part of the twentieth century. Sick people are expected to try to "get well" or achieve the goal of health. They are not required to do things they normally would do (i.e., go to work or complete all of their normal obligations), and they are not responsible for their illness. These beliefs gave health care professionals, especially physicians, great power in society, be-

cause they labeled people as sick, which gave sick persons the "right" not to fulfill obligations or to be responsible for themselves.[35] Physicians identified the sick person who was not trying to get well, sanctioning that person for unproductive behavior.

Some people use the terms illness and disease as synonyms, which they are not. Disease is a defined pathologic condition, such as fever, with measures and deviations from a standard. Illness is the role one who has a disease assumes. In many cultures the person who has a fever (oral temperature more than 38° C) but goes to work may have a disease but not be sick, because that person can carry out his or her role.

Current beliefs about the sick role and about illness tend to refute some of Parsons' basic ideas. A common belief is that individuals are responsible for their own diseases and should be responsible for their health. An example is the smoker who develops cancer of the lung or the noncompliant diabetic individual who becomes blind as a result of diabetic retinopathy. It is important to remember that not all smokers who develop cancer of the lung or all noncompliant diabetic individuals who become blind have developed the condition as a result of poor health habits. Holding the individual responsible for health does not suggest that illness is a punishment for poor health habits. Rather, it suggests a number of nursing actions. Nurses can help individuals assess and modify risk factors, reinforce actions to support the body's own potential healing abilities, and help the patient make decisions that are self-defined as "healthy."

Even though Parsons' theory of the sick role is no longer accepted as it was conceived, its influence on the development of the concept of illness in society is clear. The power of the physician to exempt people from work, for example, made physicians decision makers in industry. Now, consumer groups, nursing organizations, and other health care professionals are establishing standards, policies, and priorities for health care in collaboration with physicians, politicians, and the rest of society. Using beliefs about illness and sick role behavior to examine leadership responsibilities for health care in society is another illustration of the fact that the same things that influence health (culture, economics, politics, demographics, and personal beliefs) influence the concept of illness.

HEALTH AS GROWTH

One idea inherent in the World Health Organization's definition of health, that of complete well-being, leads to a different way of looking at health. If health and illness are considered as two ends of a continuum, one could be healthy and ill at the same time, in varying degrees. One could move from perfect health to health to illness to death in a linear fashion (Figure 1-2). Since both health and illness are multifaceted, this concept is too simplistic. It does not explain, for example, a healthy paraplegic or a psychosomatic illness, in a concise and clear manner.

Some authors equate health with the concept of wellness.[32] But at least one author[10] attempted to differentiate wellness and health. Health is composed of five subgroups: mental health, physical health, social health, spiritual health, and emotional health (Figure 1-3). **Wellness** is the integration of all of these areas of health in a balanced way, so that if a person works on one area of wellness, all other areas must also be improved. This is a useful way of looking at the two concepts, because it explains why one can feel "more well" on some days than on other days. Even in the absence of disease, as Dunn[34] suggested, some days a person feels alive, vivacious, exuberant, and excited. Other days the same person may feel tired, out of sorts, hostile, or melancholy. The difference is not a matter of illness or disease but of levels of wellness.

High-level Wellness

Dunn[34] is credited with developing a model of high-level wellness that has been incorporated into a variety of conceptualizations of health and wellness by nurses. In this model, health develops by stages. Like other kinds of developmental models, progress proceeds in an upward, forward direction toward an ever-increasing potential of function. A constant, open-ended challenge to strive for that higher level of functioning exists, and the result is the total integration of the mind, body, and spirit.

Stages of growth in a health-related direction can be evaluated by measuring what is known of health measurements in each of the five components of wellness (physical, mental, social, spiritual, and emotional health) and then examining the integration of them or relationships among them. For Dunn, these relationships include such things as more energy in each area and a purpose in life that adds a strong "inner life" (e.g., self-esteem) to a strong sense of outer worlds such as family and community.

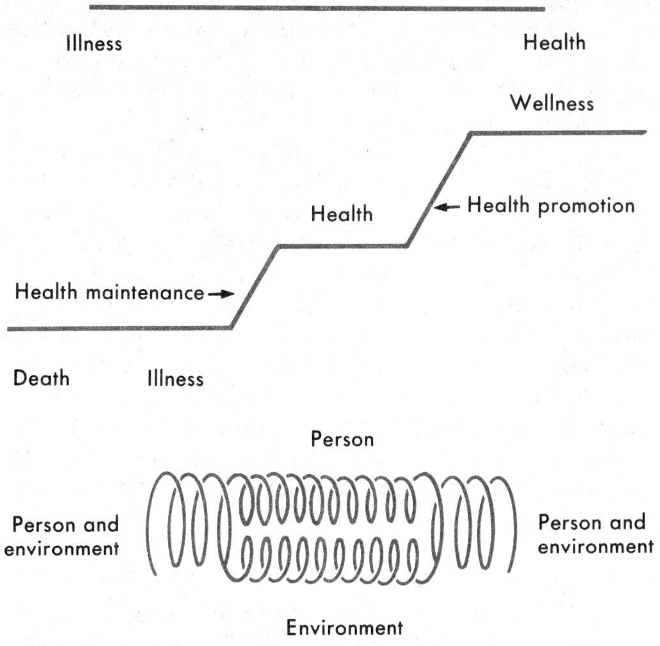

FIGURE 1-2   Comparisons of models of health.

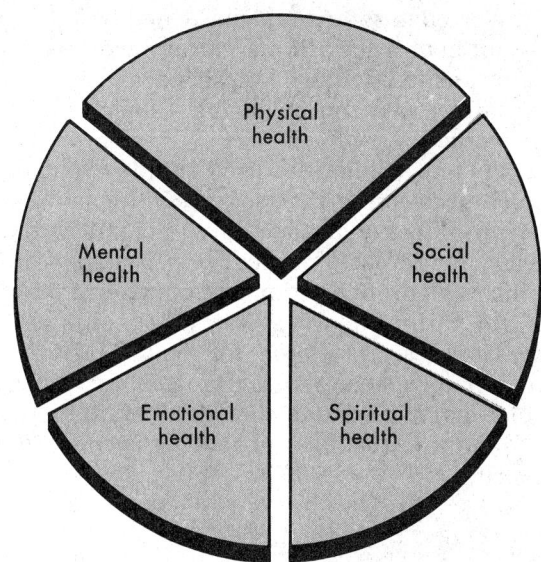

FIGURE 1-3   Wellness: balanced integration of health.

By using this framework, no component of wellness is left out of assessment or treatment plans, and movement toward that final stage of total integration is evaluated (Figure 1-1).

Maslow's Hierarchy of Needs

Dunn's work bears directly on the work of Abraham Maslow.[39] Maslow popularized the term *self-actualization,* using it as the highest level in his conceptualization of the needs of humans. Using a developmental approach, Maslow, like Dunn, saw the growth of humans as a unidirectional progression through several stages to a high level of integration of all the previous stages. However, Maslow organized his model into a pyramid (commonly called a hierarchy) of needs. The lowest level of needs is basic and includes things necessary for survival, such as air, water, and safety. Only when these needs are satisfied can one move to a higher level. Many needs must be continually met—one cannot meet a need for air once and not consider it again! So the model is not meant to be static, but a dynamic interrelationship among steps occurs. One step up from basic physiologic needs and safety needs is a set of needs termed *belongingness and love needs* (including affection and possible sexual expression). The next class of needs is esteem needs, the desire for things such as achievement, competence, independence, and freedom.[12] The highest level of Maslow's hierarchy is self-actualization, which he describes as the need to live up to and within one's potential. "The artist must paint; the poet must write; and the musician must make music." Within this context, he defines health as being self-actualizing; if one is not self-actualized, one must be less than healthy, because all healthy people strive for that highest state of being. A less-than-actualized person must have been thwarted in some of the basic needs and therefore is not healthy. Maslow's hierarchy of needs, as originally posited, followed these stages: physiologic needs, safety, love and belonging, esteem, and self-actualization.

Maslow and Dunn both used the developmental approach to describe (but not really define) health. They view illness as the inability to meet the needs necessary for the achievement of self-actualization, or as incomplete integration or imbalanced integration of the various health systems that comprise humans. The healthy person for both Maslow and Dunn is happy: achieving at the highest potential possible; making positive contributions to the community and the world; and balanced in mind, body, and spirit.

HEALTH AS EXPERIENCE

Health as experience comes from a philosophic basis of total unity with the universe.[5,6] It is not an ob-

jective, it is not attainable, and one does not grow into it in stages. Rather, one acknowledges and focuses one's consciousness on health as a universal element. It is fluid, flowing into, around, and through all of life and beyond life into all structure. Basing definitions and concepts on such philosophic world views is more common to Eastern thought than to Western thought.

HOLISTIC HEALTH AND NURSING PRACTICE

The American Holistic Nurses' Association (AHNA) suggests three ideas in its philosophy that relate to health.[1]

The first idea is the sense that mind, body, and spirit have never been separate, that interconnectedness and balance to greater or lesser degrees are a part of the life process. Rogers[22] has graphically illustrated her concept of humans and environment woven together as a whole by using an illustration of the child's toy known as a Slinky. The spiral along a longitudinal axis shows that human beings evolve in one direction, toward increasing complexity. Each cycle of the Slinky reflects the rhythmic interaction of the individual and the environment. Robin McKarns adapted the illustration to include the concept of health by showing that if the individual and the environment move in different rhythms, the whole is no longer rhythmic, connected, or one (see Figure 1-3). Health reflects interconnectedness. If that interconnectedness is interrupted, the person is no longer healthy, and it is at that place the nurse intervenes to reestablish the rhythmic, flowing, connected whole.

The second idea in the AHNA's philosophy is that of "awareness," or consciousness of the sense of the unity that is implied. The new, interdisciplinary research thrust in psychoneuroimmunology describes ever-increasing evidence that mental attitude affects the immune system, illustrating one of the relationships of consciousness and physiology.[21,26] Nurses use positive mental images in relaxation, guided imagery, and other related nursing actions, thus strengthening "body-mind." In the area of health maintenance, helping people envision good health and what it means for them will help them attain it. Football players, golfers, divers, and people who play sports of all kinds find visualization of success aids them. Conscious thought directs not only attitudes ("I can do it"), but also unconscious action (a smooth golf swing) and choices in behavior related to health maintenance.

The nurse uses the idea of health as expanded consciousness as a part of patient care but also recognizes that his or her own consciousness becomes a part of the environment of the patient. Thus the attitudes, beliefs, self-esteem, and feelings of the nurse become a part of the therapeutic environment, just as those of the patient become a part of the nurse's environment. Introductory courses in nursing commonly include content in self-knowledge to help the nurse understand this relationship. Experienced nurses recognize that part of the reason they have changed through their practice of nursing is because of the mutual environment they have shared with their patients.

The third idea in the AHNA's definition of health is that of personal responsibility for health. Because consciousness, or awareness, is an integral part of the experience of health, the individual is the only one who can give information about the current state of health. The individual "tunes in" intuitively and knows if things feel "right." Certainly laboratory tests, examinations, and the like (quantitative data) are valued as clues to one's diagnosis; but that is a disease-related concept. The ultimate authority on health is the individual.

Using this holistic concept of health and illness to give direction to practice and the study of nursing knowledge suggests that new methods of study of nursing phenomena are needed. Breaking a problem down into its parts is no longer adequate for studying health. Margaret Newman, Martha Rogers, and other nursing theorists have contributed to a new direction by looking at patterns. Patterns describe a wholeness of action that can suggest what to do about a problem. Based on Rogers' theory, nine "human response patterns" have been identified. These patterns are listed in Table 1-5 along with potential areas of nursing intervention for health promotion.[23] These patterns involve mutual exchange between person and environment and serve as one example of the way nursing can be developed based on holistic health definitions.

CRITICAL THINKING QUESTIONS

1 List two reasons why it is important to analyze the term health.
2 What is the difference between the terms health and wellness, and illness and disease?
3 Give one example from your local newspaper of an economic, social, or political issue that influences health today.
4 Analyze the impact social stigma has on the following illnesses: AIDS, alcoholism, and schizophrenia. Identify how social attribution can affect these illnesses.
5 Describe the kind of health meant by the phrases health is a goal, health as growth, and health as experience.
6 Name two models used to describe health as growth.
7 What is holistic health?
8 How has your understanding of the term health changed by reading this chapter?

RESOURCES

1 American Holistic Nurses' Association, 4101 Lake Boone Trail, Suite 201, Raleigh, NC 27607
2 American Public Health Association, 1015 15th St., NW Washington, DC 20005

TABLE 1-5 Patterns of Humanity and Related Areas of Nursing Intervention

Response Patterns	Related Areas of Nursing Intervention
Exchanging	Nutrition
	Elimination
	Tissue perfusion
	Fluid volume
Communicating	Verbal
	Nonverbal
Relating	Role
	Socialization
	Family
	Sexuality
Valuing	Spirituality
Choosing	Coping
Moving	Mobility
	Sleep and rest
	Recreation
	Activities of daily living
Perceiving	Self-concept
	Sensory (visual, auditory)
Knowing	Cognition/learning
Feeling	Pain
	Anxiety
	Violence

Modified from North American Nursing Diagnosis Association (NANDA).

BIBLIOGRAPHY

Current

1. American Holistic Nurses' Association: A new beginning, Raleigh, NC, 1988, The Association (pamphlet).
2. Blum H: *Planning for health: generics for the eighties*, New York, 1981, Human Sciences Press Inc.
3. Butterfield P: Thinking upstream: nurturing a conceptual understanding of the societal context of health behavior, *ANS* 12(2):1, 1990.
4. Cochran C, Stuart G: Psychologic and sociocultural dimensions of health and illness. In Beare PG, Myers J: *Principles and practice of adult health nursing*, St Louis, 1990, Mosby–Year Book.
5. Dossey BM et al: *Holistic nursing: a handbook for practice*, Rockville, Md, 1988, Aspen Publishers Inc.
6. Dossey L: *Beyond illness: discovering the experience of health*, Boston, 1984, Shambhala Publications Inc.
7. Duvall E, Miller B: *Marriage and family development*, New York, 1985, Harper & Row, Publishers, Inc.

8. Edelman C, Mandle CL: *Health promotion throughout the lifespan,* ed 2, St Louis, 1990, Mosby–Year Book.

9. Fawcett J: *Analysis and evaluation of conceptual models of nursing,* ed 2, Philadelphia, 1989, FA Davis Co.

10. Greenberg J: Health and wellness: a conceptual differentiation, *J Sch Health* 55(10):403, 1985.

11. Keller M: Toward a definition of health, *ANS* 3(43):43, 1981.

12. Lowry R: *AH Maslow: an intellectual portrait,* Monterey, Calif, 1973, Brooks/Cole Publishing Co.

13. Mechanic D: Illness behavior, social adaptation, and the management of illness, *J Nerv Ment Dis* 165(2):79, 1977.

14. Milio N: *Promoting health through public policy,* Philadelphia, 1981, FA Davis Co.

15. Moore L et al: *The biocultural basis of health: expanding view of medical anthropology,* Prospect Heights, Ill, 1980, Waveland Press, Inc.

16. Murray R, Zentner J: *Nursing concepts for health promotion,* ed 3, Englewood Cliffs, NJ, 1985, Prentice-Hall, Inc.

17. Parsons T: *The social system,* New York, 1951, Free Press.

18. Payne L: Health: a basic concept in nursing theory, *J Adv Nurs* 8:393, 1983.

19. Pender N: *Health promotion in nursing practice,* Norwalk, Conn, 1982, Appleton-Century-Crofts.

20. Pines M: Psychological hardiness: the role of challenge in health, *Psychology Today* 14:34, 1980.

21. Plotnikoff N: *Stress and immunity,* Boca Raton, Fla, 1991, CRC Press.

22. Rogers ME: *An introduction to the theoretical basis of nursing,* Philadelphia, 1970, FA Davis Co.

23. Roy Sr C: Framework for classification systems development: progress and issues. In *Classification of nursing diagnoses: proceedings of the Fifth National Conference,* St Louis, 1984, Mosby–Year Book.

24. Seligman M: *Helplessness: on depression, development and death,* San Francisco, 1975, WH Freeman & Co, Publishers.

25. Smith J: The idea of health: a philosophical inquiry, *ANS* 3(3):43, 1981.

26. Solomon GF: Psycho-neuroimmunology: interactions between central nervous system and immune system, *J Neurosci Res* 18:1, 1987.

27. Spector R: *Cultural diversity in health and illness,* Norwalk, Conn, 1985, Appleton-Century-Crofts.

28. Starr P: *The social transformation of American medicine,* New York, 1982, Basic Books, Inc, Publishers.

29. Sundeen S et al: *Nurse client interaction: implementing the nursing process,* ed 4, St Louis, 1988, Mosby–Year Book.

30. Wagnild G, Young HM: Another look at hardiness, *Image J Nurs Scholar* 23(4):257, 1991.

Classic

31. Becker MH, Maiman LA: Socio-behavioral determinants of compliance with health and medical care recommendations, *Med Care* 13:10, 1975.

32. Becker MH et al: Selected psychosocial models and correlates of individual health-related behaviors, *Med Care* 15:27-46 1977.

33. Brallier L: *Transition and transformation: successfully managing stress,* San Francisco, 1982, National Nursing Review.

34. Dunn H: *High level wellness,* Thorofare, NJ, 1961, Charles B Slack, Inc.

35. Illich I: *Medical nemesis—the expropriation of health,* New York, 1976, Bantam Books, Inc.

36. Koos E: *The health of Regionville: what people thought and did about it,* New York, 1954, Columbia University Press.

37. Lazarus R: *Psychological stress and the coping process,* New York, 1966, McGraw-Hill, Inc.

38. Lewis A: Health as a social concept, *Br J Sociol* 4:109, 1953.

39. Maslow AH: *Motivation and personality,* New York, 1954, Harper & Row.

40. Twaddle AC, Hessler R: *A sociology of health,* St Louis, 1977, Mosby–Year Book.

41. World Health Organization: *Constitution,* Geneva, 1947, The Organization.

42. Zborowski M: Cultural components in response to pain, *J Soc Issues* 8:16, 1952.

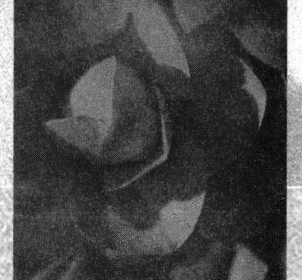

CHAPTER TWO

Health Promotion Through the Adult Life Span

LEARNING OBJECTIVES

1 Discuss three levels of prevention as identified by Leavell and Clark.

2 Describe five age-related physical changes for individuals in young, middle, and older adulthood.

3 Compare health promotion strategies in young, middle, and older adults.

4 Differentiate *Healthy People 2000* national health objectives for young, middle, and older adults.

KEY TERMS

health promotion, p. 23

Healthy People 2000, p. 24

primary prevention, p. 23

specific protection, p. 23

HEALTH PROMOTION has achieved increased recognition as an important component of our health care delivery system. Persons involved in health promotion need to consider the meaning of health promotion since a focused definition clarifies their work and enhances the outcomes of the health care system. Early definitions of health promotion implied negative concepts: preventive health behavior, disease and illness prevention, health promotion, and risk-reducing behavior.[7] More recently health behavior terms are viewed in a more positive way. The definitions linked to positive health outcomes are health behavior, health promotion, health-enhancing behavior, health maintenance, and healthy life-style.[7]

An important historic and lasting influence on the evolution of health promotion is found in the work of Leavell and Clark.[16] In the early 1950s, Leavell and Clark developed a model of prevention that de-

rives from the epidemiology of the natural history of disease. In this model, **primary prevention** includes two distinct categories: health promotion and specific protection. **Health promotion** focused on health education, counseling, and favorable living conditions, whereas **specific protection** emphasized safeguarding individuals and groups from a particular disease by reducing or removing the risk factors of the disease. Table 2-1 shows the Leavell and Clark model of levels of prevention. This chapter uses the primary prevention definition of Leavell and Clark to identify health-promoting and specific protection interventions for the young, middle, and older adult.

HEALTH PROMOTION

Nursing's role in health promotion programs is affecting many organizations and professionals. Well-designed programs focus on a holistic view and re-

TABLE 2-1 Three Levels of Prevention

Primary prevention		Secondary prevention		Tertiary prevention
Health promotion	**Specific protection**	**Early diagnosis and prompt treatment**	**Disability limitations**	**Restoration and rehabilitation**
Health education	Use of specific immunizations	Case-finding measures: individual and mass	Adequate treatment to arrest disease process and prevent further complications and sequelae	Provision of hospital and community facilities for retraining and education to maximize use of remaining capacities
Good standard of nutrition adjusted to developmental phases of life	Attention to personal hygiene	Screening surveys	Provision of facilities to limit disability and to prevent death	Education of public and industry to use rehabilitated persons to fullest possible extent
Attention to personality development	Use of environmental sanitation	Selective examinations to cure and prevent disease process to		
Provision of adequate housing and recreation and agreeable working conditions	Protection against occupational hazards	Prevent spread of communicable disease		Selective placement
Marriage counseling and sex education	Protection from accidents	Prevent complications and sequelae		Work therapy in hospitals
Genetic screening	Use of specific nutrients	Shorten period of disability		Use of sheltered colony
Periodic selective examinations	Protection from carcinogens			
	Avoidance of allergens			

Modified from Leavell H, Clark AE: *Preventive medicine for doctors in the community,* New York, 1965, McGraw-Hill Book Co.

quire teamwork and collaboration. Nurses are uniquely educated to provide holistic care to meet the needs of all age groups, families, and communities. Nurses work with other care providers in implementing health promotion programs. However, nurses must learn the language of health promotion and be able to identify clear goals and objectives. Nurses, as major health providers in the United States, are in an ideal position to coordinate important decision making regarding health promotion. Working with the family and community from a systems perspective, the nurse understands how family members interact and how the family deals with needs and expectations. The nurse's role in health promotion and disease prevention includes the following tasks:

- To become aware of family and community attitudes and behaviors toward health promotion and disease prevention
- To collaborate with the family and community in assessing, improving, enhancing, and evaluating their current health practices
- To assist the family and community in identifying risk-taking behaviors
- To assist the family and community groups in learning healthy life-style habits
- To provide reinforcement for positive health behavior practices
- To serve as a liaison for referral or collaboration between community resources and the family or group

Health promotion programs have a wide array of benefits for individuals, their families, and the larger community. Many recent studies confirm that changes in individual life-style behaviors, such as smoking, diet, and exercise, can reduce the risk of chronic illness.[1] Many life-style practices can be more effective if they go beyond individuals to the larger community. Numerous other studies have shown that multifaceted programs that focus on a range of health risk factors, such as smoking, blood cholesterol levels, and sedentary life-styles, and involve a variety of community agencies and health providers can be effective in reducing the prevalence of disease in specific populations.[2] In this context, health promotion becomes not just information but an active decision-making process at all levels of care.

HEALTHY PEOPLE 2000

In 1979 the U.S. Public Health Service in *Healthy People* identified a trial of national strategies for health: health promotion, specific protection, and preventive health services. However, it was not until the issuance of the 1990 *National Health Objectives: Healthy People 2000* that a subtle but compelling shift was noted in the primary emphasis on health promotion and individual responsibility. **Healthy People 2000** sets broad community health goals for a decade. The principal goals for the 1990s are to (1) increase the span of healthy life of Americans and (2) achieve access to preventive services for all Americans. To meet these goals, 298 specific objectives are identified in 22 separate priority areas. The objectives are also organized by age group in separate chapters. Quantifiable targets have been set for improvements in health status, risk reduction, and service delivery to consolidate the gains made in the 1980s and extend the benefits of improved health to those groups who experience higher morbidity, disability, and mortality than the general population. Organized under three broad approaches of health promotion, health protection, and preventive services, the objectives chart a 10-year course for individual, collective, and environmental change. Implicit throughout the document is the principle that long life, without good health, is insufficient.[12]

YOUNG ADULTHOOD
Physical Development

The young adult years are a period of optimal physical function, the peak years of strength and agility. The 20s are typically unmarred by the presence of acute or chronic illness. Physical growth has halted, but physical condition is maintained. The effects of aging begin to take their toll at about 20 years of age, but it will be another decade before the effects can be noted in the body.[14] Physical changes of young adulthood are summarized in the box below.

Visual acuity and hearing are at their best at 20 years of age and remain keen until 40 years of age, when a gradual decline in function begins. Muscle strength and coordination continue to increase until about age 25 to 30 years old. The teeth achieve dental maturity with the eruption of the adult molars. Hair has its thickest diameter and male hairline usually remains intact through the twenties. The immune system, while still extremely effective, begins to secrete decreased amounts of thymic hormones called thymosins, which control the production and function of lymphocytes. Resistance to infection is virtually undiminished. Height may begin to decrease slightly after 25 years of age as a result of vertebral disintegration. The proportion of body fat increases, even though weight may remain stable.

The young adult years may be the best years to begin a family, since the reproductive systems of both sexes are unlikely to be affected by decreased hormone levels of physical illness. Both sexes respond quickly and repeatedly to sexual stimuli, especially if they are sexually active. Male libido peaks at about 15 to 20 years; women do not reach their peak until the 30s.

There is a slight decrease in cardiac muscle strength after 20 years, but cardiac output remains more than adequate to carry out activities of daily living. Oxygen requirements are slightly diminished because of atrophy of other tissues and decreased physical demand as the young adult ages. The young adult tends to gain weight during the 30s. Most adults exercise less as they age, so they need fewer calories than they did during their teens and 20s. Additionally, an adult's basal metabolic rate decreases during the early 40s so the body requires less food. It is unfortunate that few adults decrease their caloric intake accordingly. Other subtle signs that young adults pass their physical peak as they progress through the 30s are also present. The overall functional capacity of the body decreases slightly

NORMAL PHYSICAL FINDINGS IN THE YOUNG ADULT

Musculoskeletal system—Skeletal growth completed at about 25 years; height increased by 3 to 5 mm by 30 years because of continuing vertebral column growth

Cardiovascular system—Peak strength of musculature at 30 years; larger muscles in men than women; men have greater capacity for carrying oxygen in blood to muscles; young men more likely to have elevated cholesterol levels than young women

Gastrointestinal system—Decrease in digestive juices after 30 years of age; state of physical health influences patterns of digestion and elimination

Mouth—Emergence of "wisdom" teeth, the last four molars; sometimes problematic if wedged between jawbone and other molars

Weight—Weight influenced by life-style, heredity, nutritional habits, gender; desirable weight instead of average weight more appropriate in terms of gender and body build

Reproductive system—Fully mature in the 20s—the best years for reproduction

   Women—Uterus maximum weight 30 years of age; optimal period for reproduction is 20 to 30 years; irregularities not uncommon, such as skipping a menstrual cycle, "spotting," and premenstrual syndrome after significant interruption of cycle

   Men—Leydig cells (male hormones) decrease slowly at about 25 years, as do androgen secretions; no important weight loss in healthy testes; spermatogenesis continues throughout adulthood; ability to father a child not affected

more (.8%) each year. Both sexes start to develop fine wrinkles such as "frown lines" as skin loses elasticity and resilience.

Morbidity and Mortality

The leading causes of death among young adults include injuries, homicide, suicide, cancer, and heart disease[12] (Figure 2-1). The major preventable health concerns of young adults fall into two categories: (1) injuries and violence that kill or disable many young people and (2) developing life-style behaviors. Three quarters of injury deaths among people of this age category are due to automobile accidents, and half of all motor vehicle accidents involve alcohol. The second leading cause of death is homicide. Alcohol and tobacco use, in addition to the use of illicit drugs, has been declining, and awareness among high school seniors has grown. Drinking still is more prevalent among those aged 18 to 24 years than in any other age group. Sexually transmitted diseases, including HIV infection, pose special risks. The highest rate of sexually transmitted diseases is among people 15 to 29 years of age.[6]

Health-promoting Practices

When managing the health care needs of the young adult, the nurse must consider prevention of trauma and untimely deaths, early detection of disease, establishment of lifelong health maintenance, and assistance with reproductive concerns.[20] Young adults are an extremely diverse group of individuals aged 18 to 35 years. Rapid changes, both emotional and physical, accompany a time of learning and experimentation. Health consequences related to tobacco and alcohol use, diet, exercise, sexual practices, and safety habits may be related to attitudes and behaviors that are developed in adolescence.[14]

Health promotion for young adults is an essential component of wellness promotion. Nurses are uniquely qualified to take an active role in providing health monitoring for young adults. A strong focus on prevention at this life stage can have significant positive results later in life. Recommended health promotion guidelines for young adults 18 to 35 years of age are presented in the box on p. 27. See also the box on *Healthy People 2000* objectives for young adults (p. 28).

MIDDLE ADULTHOOD
Physical Development

It is difficult to say when middle age begins. Subtle cues may nudge middle adults into awareness that they are different from young adults but also separate from the older adult. Middle adulthood refers to those individuals between the ages of 36 and 64 years. As adults become middleaged, signs of aging rather than physical development become more apparent. A subtle but gradual decline occurs in most of the body's major systems. The box on p. 28

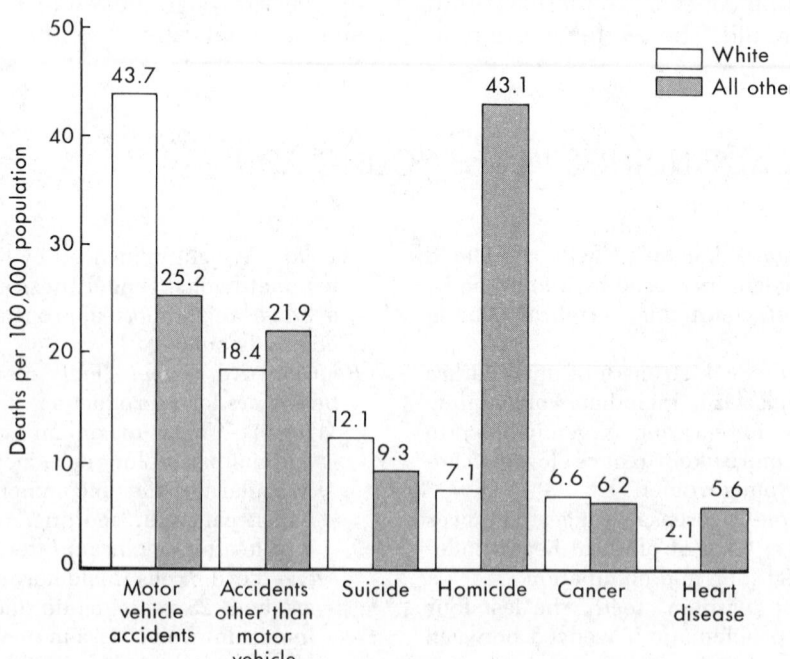

FIGURE 2-1   Major causes of death among young adults. (From Office of Health and Human Services, Washington, DC, 1990.)

HEALTH PROMOTION GUIDELINES FOR THE YOUNG ADULT

Screening

History

Dietary intake
Physical activity
Tobacco/alcohol/drug use
Sexual practices

Physical examination

Height and weight
Blood pressure
High-risk groups
    Complete oral cavity examination
    Palpation for thyroid nodules
    Clinical breast examination
    Clinical testicular examination
    Complete skin examination

Laboratory/diagnostic procedures

Nonfasting total blood cholesterol
Papanicolaou smear
High-risk groups
    Fasting plasma glucose
    Rubella antibodies
    VDRL/RPR
    Urinalysis for bacteriuria
    Chlamydial testing
    Gonorrhea culture
    Counseling and testing for HIV
    Hearing
    Tuberculin skin test
    Electrocardiogram
    Mammogram
    Colonoscopy

Counseling

Diet and exercise

Fat (especially saturated fat), cholesterol, complex carbohydrates, fiber, sodium, iron, calcium
Caloric balance
Selection of exercise program

Substance use

Tobacco: cessation, primary prevention
Alcohol and other drugs
    Limiting alcohol consumption
    Driving/other dangerous activities while under the influence
    Treatment for abuse
High-risk groups
    Sharing/using unsterilized needles and syringes

Sexual practices

Sexually transmitted diseases: partner selection, condoms, anal intercourse
Unintended pregnancy and contraceptive options

Injury prevention

Safety belts
Safety helmets
Violent behavior
Firearms
Smoke detector
Smoking near bedding or upholstery
High-risk groups
    Back-conditioning exercises

Dental health

Regular tooth brushing, flossing, dental visits

Other primary preventive measures

High-risk groups
    Discussion of hemoglobin testing
    Skin protection from ultraviolet light

Immunizations

Tetanus-diphtheria (Td) booster
High-risk groups
    Hepatitis B vaccine
    Pneumococcal vaccine
    Influenza vaccine
    Measles-mumps-rubella vaccine

---

presents normal physical changes in the middle adult.

During the 40s the lens of the eyes gradually becomes less elastic, causing loss of the ability to focus clearly on visual images within close range (presbyopia). Near vision diminishes. Some adults find that they need reading glasses for close work, and others require bifocals. Thickening of the lens also causes a decrease in visual acuity, increased length of time for the adjustment from a light to a dark environment, and diminished peripheral vision.

Fat begins to accumulate in the lower abdomen and the hips, causing a weight gain of about 10 to 20 pounds in most middle-aged adults. If the abdominal muscles also weaken a "pot belly" may result.[3] The skin no longer stretches as tightly across the muscles and bones, and wrinkles are more pronounced. The popularity of the tanned, "healthy" look has accelerated skin changes in many adults, resulting in drier, thinner skin that regenerates less rapidly and is more susceptible to skin cancer.

Hair may begin to grow more slowly and become thin because the diameter of hair follicles decreases. Graying of the hair will be noted as loss of pigmen-

HEALTHY PEOPLE 2000 OBJECTIVES FOR YOUNG ADULTS

Reduce overweight to a prevalence of no more than 20% among people 20 years and older

Reduce deaths among people 15 to 24 years old caused by alcohol-related motor vehicle crashes to no more than 18 per 100,000

Reduce suicides among men 20 to 34 years old to no more than 21.4 per 100,000

Reduce homicides to no more than 7.2 per 100,000 people

Reduce rape of women 12 to 34 years old to no more than 225 per 100,000

Reduce deaths among youths 15 to 24 years old caused by motor vehicles crashes to no more than 33 per 100,000

From US Department of Health and Human Services: *Healthy people 2000: new objectives to promote health and prevent disease,* Washington, DC, 1990, US Government Printing Office.

NORMAL PHYSICAL ASSESSMENT FINDINGS IN THE MIDDLE-AGED ADULT

Skin and hair—Intact: appropriate distribution of pigmentation; slow progressive decrease in skin turgor; graying and loss of hair (baldness patterns in males are established by 55 years of age; hair loss after this time might have other causes)

Head—Symmetry of scalp, skull, face; normal accessory organs of vision

Eyes—Visual acuity by Snellen chart < 20/50; pupillary reaction to light and accommodation; normal visual fields and extraocular movements; normal retinal structures

Ears—Normal auditory structures and acuity

Nose and throat—Patent nares and intact sinuses, mouth, and pharynx; trachea at midline; lateral thyroid lobes nonpalpable

Lungs—Anteroposterior (AP) diameter increased; respiratory rate 16 to 21 breaths per minute and regular; ratio of respiratory rate to heart rate 1:4; normal tactile fremitus, resonance, and breath sounds heard throughout

Heart—Normal heart sounds (systole-S, < S2 at the base; diastole-S, > S2 at the apex), point of maximal impulse at fifth intercostal space in the midclavicular line and 2 cm or less in diameter

Vital signs—Temperature 36.7° to 37.6° C (97° to 99.6° F); pulse 60 to 100 (conditioned athlete = 50); blood pressure: systolic 95 to 140 mm Hg, diastolic 60 to 90 mm Hg; all pulses palpable

Breasts—Decreased size because of decreased muscle mass; normal nipples

Abdomen—No tenderness or organomegaly; decreased strength of abdominal muscles

Reproductive system—Change in menstrual cycle and in duration and quantity of menstrual flow; "hot flashes"; change in cervical mucosa; normal penis and scrotum; prostatic enlargement in some men

Musculoskeletal system—Decreased muscle mass; pathologic fractures resulting from osteoporosis; decreased range of joint motion

Mentation—Appropriate affect, appearance, and behavior; lucidity and appropriate level of cognitive ability; intact cranial nerves; adequate motor response; responsive sensory system

tation occurs. Male pattern hair loss, or balding, is common by middle age. Middle-aged adults have no problem discriminating among sweet, sour, salty, and bitter foods, but they may become less able to detect the more subtle gastronomic differences. The sense of touch begins to decline at about 45 years of age, and sensitivity to pain begins to decline at about 50 years. Tolerance to pain also decreases, so that pain may be perceived more acutely by older adults.[6]

The cardiovascular and pulmonary systems also change with age. The contractility of the heart decreases, resulting in a lower cardiac index. Cardiac function decreases by as much as 15% to 20% from 30 to 49 years.[15] Coronary heart disease is the most common chronic disease condition among men in their 30s and 40s. The usual cause appears to be atherosclerosis. The arteries become less elastic, and hypertension may develop. Respiratory function may also diminish during the 30s and 40s. The lungs and bronchi become less elastic, resulting in decreased maximal lung capacity. It now takes middle-aged adults longer for their heart and respiratory rates to return to normal after exercising. Bowel patterns may change during middle age. Bowel movements may become less frequent because of decreased gastrointestinal motility and physical inactivity.

Sexual needs do not change from earlier years, although sexual function does. Libido varies greatly in both sexes. Male erection takes longer to achieve, and orgasm is slower in coming. Ejaculation is delayed and less forceful. Women may achieve orgasm regularly but less forcefully. A woman's interest in and desire for sex often increase after 35 years of age, whereas a man's desire remains stable or decreases somewhat. During the middle years, sex for procreation is emphasized less. Instead, more emphasis is placed on sexual intimacy and meeting personal desires.

Women experience the climacteric, or menopause, during middle age. Cessation of the menses occurs at about 45 to 50 years. This decrease in ovarian function is often accompanied by symptoms of diminished estrogen production. "Hot flashes" occur in a majority of women. Other symptoms resulting from decreased hormone production include headache, palpitations, and numbness, tingling, or coolness in the extremities. Emotional reactions that may accompany menopause include anxiety, nervousness, and mood swings. When menopause develops, atrophic changes occur in the vagina. The vaginal epithelium becomes thinner and drier from lack of estrogen. The vagina becomes shorter and more narrow. The labia and the clitoris also atrophy, along with the uterus and ovaries. These changes can contribute to vaginal itching and burning, as well as discomfort during intercourse.

Most men are not aware that they too may experience symptoms associated with menopause, including insomnia, fatigue, and the circulatory problems previously mentioned. Most investigators continue to ascribe these problems to various other causes rather than hormonal changes. Since testosterone levels gradually decrease with age, only a small percentage of men are likely to experience hormonal changes similar to those experienced by menopausal women.[2]

Morbidity and Mortality

The health profile of middle-aged adults is substantially determined by behavioral risk factors. Adults have a unique opportunity to take the responsibility for their own personal actions. Positive behavioral changes of the last few decades have reduced rates of related causes of death in cancer, heart disease, stroke, injuries, chronic lung diseases, and liver disease. Table 2-2 presents the seven major causes of death of middle-aged adults in the United States according to frequency of occurrence.

The leading cause of death in middle age is heart disease, followed by malignant neoplasms such as prostatic and colorectal cancer in men and lung and breast cancer in women. Minimizing risk factors for heart disease can be done through exercise, diet, and ceasing cigarette smoking. Recommended risk reduction strategies include exercise such as walking (as opposed to jogging), swimming, biking, or roller skating for 15 to 20 minutes three to four times per week. The possible psychologic benefits include alleviating symptoms of mild or moderate depression and reducing symptoms of anxiety and physiologic response to stress, which lead to improvement of physical well-being.

TABLE 2-2 Major Causes of Death in Middle-Aged Adults

Rank	White	Nonwhite
1	Heart disease	Heart disease
2	Cancer	Cancer
3	Cerebrovascular accident (stroke)	Cerebrovascular accident (stroke)
4	Cirrhosis of liver	Homicide
5	All other accidents	Cirrhosis of liver
6	Motor vehicle accidents	All other accidents
7	Homicide	Motor vehicle accidents

From Edelman C, Mandle C: *Health promotion throughout the lifespan*, St Louis, 1990, Mosby–Year Book.

In 1986 lung cancer surpassed breast cancer as the leading cause of death from cancer in women, and the rate is increasing. Women now have an incidence of lung cancer nearly identical to that of men 30 years ago, which was approximately 20 to 30 years after men began smoking in large numbers. On the contrary, lung cancer in men has begun to level off and is expected to decline as a result of the declining prevalence of smoking among men.

Detecting uterine cancer is important in the 50- to 64-year age group. A careful history in the screening process should include ovulation failure, prolonged estrogen use, obesity, history of infertility, or postmenopausal bleeding. The cure rate for endometrial cancer is high. Although the Pap test is effective in detection of early cervical cancer, it is only 50% effective in detecting endometrial cancer.[9]

Colorectal cancers are the second most common cancer, and the majority occur in persons over 45 years old. At high risk are people with a family history of colorectal polyps, with inflammatory bowel disease, or with a history of a high-fat, low-fiber diet. Despite the fact that the incidence of colorectal cancer increased between 1982 and 1986, the death rate declined an average of 0.9% per year. These changes were accompanied by a shift toward earlier stages of diagnosis for these cancers. The proportion of colorectal cancers diagnosed as advanced disease has been decreasing, whereas the proportion diagnosed in situ and with localized disease has increased from 32% to 43%.[11]

Health-promoting Practices

To promote health and prevent disease during middle age, many adults benefit from a modification of life-style behaviors. Because behavior changes can be difficult to make, supportive social environments are very important. An expanded network of education in health-promoting practices is essential to know the frequencies of these practices. Recommended health promotion guidelines for middle-aged adults are listed in the box below.

A few of the health promotion needs of the middle-aged adult are acceptance of aging, exercise, and weight control. Decreasing or stopping cigarette smoking and alcohol intake also may be identified needs. Preventive health screening is vital. The adult should have input into and control of as many of these behaviors as possible. Health promotion and protection are aimed at the personal habits and lifestyle of adult patients to improve their biologic and psychosocial development. Strategies to help an adult patient achieve a higher level of health include individual or group counseling based on identified risk factors, providing self-help information that is most relevant to the middle-aged adult, and describing available resources. See the box for health promotion guidelines for middle-aged adults.

HEALTH PROMOTION GUIDELINES FOR OLDER ADULTS

Screening
History

Prior symptoms of transient ischemic attack
Dietary intake
Physical activity
Tobacco/alcohol/drug use
Functional status at home

Physical examination

Height and weight
Blood pressure
Visual acuity
Hearing and hearing aids
Clinical breast examination
High-risk groups
    Auscultation for carotid bruits
    Complete skin examination
    Complete oral cavity examination
    Palpation of thyroid nodules

Laboratory/diagnostic procedures

Nonfasting total blood cholesterol
Dipstick urinalysis
Mammogram
Thyroid function tests
High-risk groups
    Fasting plasma glucose
    Tuberculin skin test
    Electrocardiogram
    Papanicolaou smear
    Fecal occult blood/sigmoidoscopy
    Fecal occult blood/colonoscopy

Counseling
Diet and exercise

Fat (especially saturated fat), cholesterol, complex carbohydrates, fiber, sodium, calcium
Caloric balance
Selection of exercise program

Substance use

Tobacco cessation
Alcohol and other drugs
    Limiting alcohol consumption
    Driving/other dangerous activities while under the influence
    Treatment for abuse

Injury prevention

Prevention of falls
Safety belts
Smoke detector
Smoking near bedding or upholstery
Hot water heater temperature
Safety helmets
High-risk groups
    Prevention of childhood injuries

Dental health

Regular dental visits, tooth brushing, flossing

Other primary preventive measures

Glaucoma testing by eye specialist
High-risk groups
    Discussion of estrogen replacement therapy
    Discussion of aspirin therapy
    Skin protection from ultraviolet light

Immunizations

Tetanus-diphtheria (Td) booster
Influenza vaccine
Pneumococcal vaccine
High-risk groups
    Hepatitis B vaccine

HEALTHY PEOPLE 2000 OBJECTIVES FOR MIDDLE-AGED ADULTS

Reduce coronary heart disease deaths to no more than 100 per 100,000 people

Slow the rise in lung cancer deaths to achieve a rate of no more than 42 per 100,000 people

Reduce to no more than 30% the proportion of all pregnancies that are unintended

Reduce the prevalence of mental disorder among adults living in the community to less than 10.7%

Reduce homicides to no more than 7.2 per 100,000 people

Reduce deaths from work-related injuries to no more than 4 per 100,000 full-time workers

Reverse the rise in cancer to achieve a rate of no more than 130 per 100,000 people

Reduce diabetes-related deaths to no more than 34 per 100,000 people

Reduce tuberculosis to an incidence of no more than 3.5 cases per 100,000 people

From US Department of Health and Human Services: *Healthy people 2000: new objectives to promote health and prevent disease,* Washington, DC, 1990, US Government Printing Office.

OLDER ADULTHOOD
Physical Development

Life expectancy has increased dramatically since 1900, and people who reach 65 years of age can expect to live well into their 80s. Maintaining health and functional independence is the most important aspect of health promotion among older adults. Although normal aging is accompanied by inevitable and irreversible changes, many health problems are in fact preventable or can be controlled.

Although the leading causes of death are similar to that of middle age, they also include pneumonia and influenza. The focus, however, for older adults is not only on reducing the risks of life-threatening illness, but also on health problems such as osteoporosis, arthritis, incontinence, dementia, and visual or hearing impairments, all of which have a significant effect on the quality of life.

Normal aging is accompanied by inevitable and irreversible changes over time. Table 2-3 explains these basic changes and the relationship of these to problems typical of the older adult.

Morbidity and Mortality

Intrinsic factors have the greatest influence on normal aging. Some changes are extrinsic, however, and are determined by varying life-styles. Life expectancy has sharply increased as a result of standard of living, nutrition, prevention and treatment of infectious diseases, and progress in medical care. These improvements in living conditions and health care mean that people are living to the "old-old" years (75 years and older). In fact, the population over age 75 has been the fastest growing segment of the total population.

Today the life expectancy is 74.9 years. It is predicted that by the year 2030, 20% of the U.S. population will be over 65 years of age. With this trend continuing the United States will have more old people than ever before.

The leading causes of death in persons over 65 years old are as follows:
- Heart disease
- Malignant neoplasms
- Cerebrovascular disorders
- Chronic obstructive pulmonary disease
- Pneumonia and influenza
- Atherosclerosis
- Diabetes mellitus
- Accidents
- Nephritis, nephrotic syndrome, and nephrosis
- Chronic liver disease[10]

Chronic illness can significantly affect the quality of life for the older adult. An accumulation of the effects of chronic illness increases morbidity in this age group. The 10 most common chronic illnesses in adults over 65 years are as follows:
- Arthritis
- Hypertension
- Hearing impairments
- Heart conditions
- Chronic sinusitis
- Visual impairments
- Orthopedic problems
- Diabetes
- Varicose veins
- Hemorrhoids[10]

Health-promoting Practices

Health promotion for the older adult is directed toward improving and maintaining health at the highest level of function and always toward greater independence. The hallmark of nursing action is health education and promotion of self-care.

The nurse's attitude about aging can hamper care. The nurse must examine personal attitudes about fear of aging and reward from dependency of patients who "need" care, as well as loss of self-esteem of their patients by reinforcing mature adults' strengths, giving them choices and respect. The success of nursing action depends not only on technical skills but also on the abilities to establish rapport and motivate the learner. Communication requires

TABLE 2-3   Physical Changes in the Older Adult

Organ or system	Basic "normal" aging change	Disease(s) or problems
Musculoskeletal system	Decreased synthesis and increased degradation of bone	Osteoporosis and/or fracture
	Diminished muscle size and strength	Fatigue
Eye	Decreased accommodation to light; decreased ability to distinguish between various intensities of light	Accidents
	Increased density of lens	Cataracts
	Loss of elasticity of lens	Presbyopia
	Change in aqueous kinetics	Glaucoma
Mouth and teeth	Resorption of gum and bony tissue surrounding teeth and bone of mandible	Loss of teeth and periodontal disease
	Decreased saliva flow	Malnutrition; disturbing symptom of "burning tongue" (glossopyrosis)
	Decreased number of taste buds	Weight loss
Ears	Anatomic change in inner ear as well as cochlea	Diminished hearing of high-pitched sounds (presbycusis)
Heart	Decreased cardiac muscle and catecholamine level	Diminished cardiac output (50% decrease by 65 yr); increased congestive heart failure
	Increased calcification of valves	Murmurs from aortic and mitral area and/or endocarditis; valve stenosis and/or insufficiency
	Calcification of skeleton of heart	Conduction defects, irritability of the cardiac muscle may result in alterations in rhythm
	Sclerosis of conduction system	Most cases of complete heart block are of unknown origin
Lungs	Decreased elasticity and increased size of alveoli	Changes in lung mechanics, such as decreased vital capacity, maximal voluntary ventilation (MVV), and increased closing volume
	Decreased diffusion and surface area across alveolar-capillary membrane	Diminished Po_2
	Diminished activity of cilia and decreased cough reflex	Impaired bronchoelimination and increased incidence of pneumonia
Immunologic status	Decreased T cell function	Increased negativity in skin tests such as PPD; possible relationship to increased prevalence for malignancies
	Maintenance of secondary immune response (B cell antibody)	
Psychologic status	Role changes	Retirement
	Losses	
	Physical	Correlation with increased death rate within 1 yr of loss of spouse
	Psychologic	Depression
	Social	Loss of significant others, family, and friends
Hormones	Decreased metabolic clearance rate and plasma concentration of aldosterone	Decreased sodium reabsorption
	Decreased estrogen, diminished ovarian function	Postmenopausal decrease of secondary sex characteristics
	Decreased insulin response and peripheral effectiveness	Hyperglycemia
	Increased ADH response to hyperosmolarity	Inappropriate ADH with hyponatremia
	Insensitivity of pituitary gland to TRH in older healthy men	Men less likely to develop hyperthyroidism

TABLE 2-3   Physical Changes in the Older Adult—cont'd

Organ or system	Basic "normal" aging change	Disease(s) or problems
Brain	Probable decrease in brain weight and/or number of cells in specific areas	Memory loss and/or senile dementia
	Alteration in sleep patterns; older persons tend to dream less and have increased periods of wakefulness	Increased complaints of insomnia
	Increased atherosclerosis of cerebral vessels	Multiinfarct dementia
	Increased activity of monoamine oxidase enzyme	Mental depression
	Decreased reaction time	Decrease in IQ scores when speed of response is factor; some aspects of IQ (verbal and vocabulary skills) increase in late life
Arteries	Increased peripheral resistance; diminished aortic elasticity	Abdominal pulsation, bruits, and aneurysms
	Increased systolic and diastolic blood pressure	Positive correlation between blood pressure and morbidity: unclear if this is cause and effect or simply correlation related to third factor; possible protective effect on brain of moderately elevated blood pressure
	Arteriosclerotic and artherosclerotic changes in blood vessels	Occlusion of arteries leading to ischemia
Gastrointestinal tract	Diminished hydrochloric acid secretion (probable)	Association with increased iron deficiency anemia as well as possible association with gastric carcinoma and/or other absorption difficulties
	Diminished large bowel motility	Diminished frequency of bowel movements
	Diminished hepatic synthesis	Diminished serum albumin
	Decreased sensitivity to thirst	Constipation, dehydration
	Decreased absorption of calcium	Malabsorption, osteoporosis
Renal	Decrease in size of urinary bladder	Incontinence and frequency
	Decrease in size of kidneys and number of glomeruli, diminished renal blood flow, glomerular filtration rate, and tubular function	Drug toxicities when kidney is major route of excretion, greater tendency toward at least transient, if not permanent, renal insufficiency in presence of dehydration, diuretics, hypotension, or fever
Genital tract	Enlarged prostate gland	Prostatic obstruction
	Weakening of pelvic floor	Stress incontinence as well as cystocele and urethrocele
	Diminished vaginal and cervical secretions	Pruritus, dyspareunia
	Some, but not total, decrease in sexual function	Fear of impotence; embarrassment at sexual desires
Skin	Decreased response to pain sensation and temperature changes	Accidents
	Decreased response to temperature and vibration; increased pain threshold	Burns
	Decreased subcutaneous fat; loss of fat padding over bony prominences	Decubitus ulcers
	Atrophy of sweat glands	Difficulty in body temperature regulation
	Decreased ability of body to rid itself of heat by evaporation	Heat stroke

Modified from Libow L, Sherman F: *The care of geriatric medicine*, St Louis, 1981, Mosby–Year Book.

consideration of the recipient's ability to understand messages through the sensorium. Because the older adult has diminishing losses of vision and hearing, accommodation to the losses is important. The appropriate use of touch can be a therapeutic communication tool by reducing anxiety, providing reality orientation and sensory stimulation, and reducing physical and psychologic pain. A therapeutic tool to employ in communication is reminiscing. This is an adaptive function in aging that can give the mature adult a sense of security from recalling fond memories.

Exercise is as important in older adults as it is in young and middle-aged adults. Planning appropriate exercise based on past health history and musculoskeletal assessment is crucial to reduce risk of injury. Teaching the importance of self-monitoring (i.e., a warm-up and a cool-down period) will prevent injuries. Modified exercise for the frail older person is part of the daily activities in most day-care centers and nursing homes.

Falling is a common problem. Accidents are the fifth leading cause of death, with falls accounting for two thirds of all accidents. The majority of falls oc-

HEALTH PROMOTION GUIDELINES FOR OLDER ADULTS

Screening
History
Prior symptoms of transient ischemic attack
Dietary intake
Physical activity
Tobacco/alcohol/drug use
Functional status at home

Physical examination
Height and weight
Blood pressure
Visual acuity
Hearing and hearing aids
Clinical breast examination
High-risk groups
    Auscultation for carotid bruits
    Complete skin examination
    Complete oral cavity examination
    Palpation of thyroid nodules

Laboratory/diagnostic procedures
Nonfasting total blood cholesterol
Dipstick urinalysis
Mammogram
Thyroid function tests
High-risk groups
    Fasting plasma glucose
    Tuberculin skin test
    Electrocardiogram
    Papanicolaou smear
    Fecal occult blood/sigmoidoscopy
    Fecal occult blood/colonoscopy

Counseling
Diet and exercise
Fat (especially saturated fat), cholesterol, complex carbohydrates, fiber, sodium, calcium
Caloric balance
Selection of exercise program

Substance use
Tobacco cessation
Alcohol and other drugs
    Limiting alcohol consumption
    Driving/other dangerous activities while under the influence
    Treatment for abuse

Injury prevention
Prevention of falls
Safety belts
Smoke detector
Smoking near bedding or upholstery
Hot water heater temperature
Safety helmets
High-risk groups
    Prevention of childhood injuries

Dental health
Regular dental visits, tooth brushing, flossing

Other primary preventive measures
Glaucoma testing by eye specialist
High-risk groups
    Discussion of estrogen replacement therapy
    Discussion of aspirin therapy
    Skin protection from ultraviolet light

Immunizations
Tetanus-diphtheria (Td) booster
Influenza vaccine
Pneumococcal vaccine
High-risk groups
    Hepatitis B vaccine

cur in or near the home, and they are most commonly caused by a rug or a slippery floor. Other environmental causes associated with falls are snowy or icy surfaces or uneven ground. Age-related conditions that predispose the elderly to falls include dizziness, orthostatic hypotension, musculoskeletal conditions, memory loss, and diminished vision. Statistics show that of elderly patients hospitalized for a fall only one half will be living 1 year later. Prevention via patient education is the key intervention and should include assessment of the home for individual hazards such as waxed floors and rugs. Primary prevention by the nurse should include encouraging the elderly to remove scatter rugs from their homes and stairways. If this is not possible, then the corners of rugs and carpet should be securely taped. Sturdy shoes that offer firm support may also help prevent falls. Hallways should be lighted at night, especially if the elderly person has nocturia.

Adults 65 years or older are the largest users of prescription medication for relief from pain of chronic disorders, constipation, insomnia, and indigestion. Because of fixed incomes, they may use former prescriptions of friends. They are also at high risk for adverse drug reactions or interactions because of the number of prescribed drugs as well as physiologic decline of organ function because of aging. Drug misuse is problematic not only for the older adult who self-medicates or forgets to take medications, but also for the physician who may not recognize the changes in aging and prescribe a standard dosage appropriate for other age groups.[5] Education efforts of the nurse should be aimed at interactions between drugs taken, the relationship of adequate nutrition and fluid intake to how the body distributes and excretes the drug, adverse reactions, and guidelines for remembering to take the medication. Because most older adults have been socialized to "follow doctors' orders," the importance of asking questions must be stressed. A few minutes of role-playing with the older person can be helpful in giving guidelines for communicating with the physician. It is well known that interactions between medications and alcohol have profound reactions, but in the older adult risk is higher because of altered body functions. Although alcohol abuse is less prevalent in the mature years than earlier, it is often underdiagnosed and undertreated. Abuse of alcohol may be unrecognized because symptoms may be identified as a common aging problem: malnutrition, tremors, impaired memory, depression, or fragmented sleep patterns. In assessing a history of alcohol use or abuse, nurses must be nonjudgmental to reduce denial by the family or the older adult. Assessment must include a history of a pattern of alcohol consumption. Appropriate nursing intervention includes a referral of the patient for support through groups such as senior center educational programs and Alcoholics Anonymous.

Although older adults require fewer calories than younger people, older adults need greater amounts of trace elements and vitamins. Changes associated with aging may compound nutritional problems causing malnutrition. Milk and dairy products are an excellent source of protein and calcium for the older adult. However, many people have lactose intolerance. During nutritional counseling, keep in mind that a genetic predisposition toward lactose intolerance occurs in Asians, American Indians, Eskimos, and other ethnic groups in which milk is not a traditional food.

A limited income and a lack of interest in food preparation can promote a diet high in carbohydrates but limited in protein, fresh vegetables, and fruit. Other psychosocial factors that may increase

HEALTHY PEOPLE 2000 OBJECTIVES FOR OLDER ADULTS

Reduce suicides among men aged 65 years and older to no more than 39.2 per 100,000

Reduce deaths among people aged 70 years and older caused by motor vehicle crashes to no more than 20 per 100,000

Reduce deaths among people aged 65 through 84 years from falls and fall-related injuries to no more than 14.4 per 100,000

Reduce deaths among people aged 85 years and older from falls and fall-related injuries to no more than 105 per 100,000

Reduce residential fire deaths among people aged 65 years and older to no more than 3.3 per 100,000

Reduce hip fractures among people aged 65 years and older so that hospitalizations for this condition are no more than 607 per 100,000

Reduce to no more than 90 per 1000 people the proportion of all people 65 years and older who have difficulty in performing two or more personal care activities, thereby preserving independence

Reduce significant hearing impairment among people aged 45 years and older to a prevalence of no more than 180 per 1000 people

Reduce significant visual impairments among people aged 65 years and older to a prevalence of no more than 70 per 1000 people

Reduce epidemic-related pneumonia and influenza deaths among people aged 65 years and older to no more than 7.3 people per 100,000

From US Department of Health and Human Services: *Healthy people 2000: national health promotion and disease prevention objectives,* Washington, DC, 1990, US Government Printing Office.

ETHICAL ISSUES

- Should aging be viewed as a change in situation or a change in self?
- Should certain types of health care be distributed based on the patient's age? For example, should patients over age 55 be denied access to kidney transplants?
- Should geriatric patients be encouraged to execute advance directives that refuse CPR? antibiotics? other therapies? Why or why not?

nutritional risk include living alone, loneliness, forgetfulness, or intentional starvation as a way of suicide. Mechanical high-risk factors are dental changes (loss of teeth, ill-fitting dentures), decreased strength and mobility, diminished vision, or polypharmacy. Diet guidelines to reduce costs can be included in teaching in terms of less expensive foods that still meet requirements for good nutrition such as substituting vegetable proteins for meat.

Mature adults experience both qualitative and quantitative changes in sleep. They take longer to fall asleep, wake more often during the night, and wake more easily. Life-style changes such as retirement may alter rest and sleep patterns. Without the daily pressure of meeting a set schedule, older people have more time to nap. Lack of exercise and boredom may encourage napping. Hypnotics should be avoided on a regular basis because they interfere with REM sleep.

Smoking in the mature adult, who was raised in an era when cigarette smoking was widespread, is a difficult habit to eliminate. The incidence of women smokers 65 years and over has risen during the period of 1965 to 1980.[3] Since smoking can lead to lung cancer, chronic obstructive pulmonary disease, cardiovascular system changes, and a decrease in functioning of the immune system, a strong emphasis on cessation should be part of the self-care teaching. The nurse should provide information on stop smoking programs and reinforce any behavior that decreases smoking.[3] See the box on p. 34 for health promotion guidelines for older adults. See also the box on *Healthy People 2000* objectives for the older adult on p. 35.

CRITICAL THINKING QUESTIONS

1 Define and contrast primary prevention, secondary prevention, and tertiary prevention.
2 What is meant by "healthy people 2000"? What are the nursing implications?
3 Compare the health-promotion objectives for young adulthood, middle adulthood, and mature adulthood.
4 What are the physical changes associated with young adulthood? middle adulthood? mature adulthood?
5 Discuss the leading causes of morbidity and mortality in young adulthood, middle adulthood, and mature adulthood.

BIBLIOGRAPHY

Current

1. American Hospital Association: *Health promotion,* Chicago, 1990, The Association.
2. Bates B: *A guide to physical examination and history taking,* ed 4, Philadelphia, 1987, J.B. Lippincott Company.
3. Burnside I: *Nursing and the aged: a self care approach,* ed 3, New York, 1988, McGraw-Hill, Inc.
4. Ebersole P, Hess P: *Toward healthy aging: human needs and the nursing process,* ed 3, St Louis, 1989, Mosby–Year Book.
5. Flaherty E: Amantadine attack on influenza A, *Geriatr Nurs* 11(5):253, 1990.
6. Katchadourian H: *Fifty: mid-life in perspective,* New York, 1987, WH Freeman & Co, Publishers.
7. Kulbok PA, Baldwin JH: From preventive health behaviors to health promotion: advancing a positive construct of health, *Adv Nurs Sci* 14(4):50-64, 1992.
8. Long NM, et al: *Quality health care for older adults in America: a review of nursing studies,* Kansas City, Mo, 1990, American Nurses' Association.
9. Seligman MEP: Boomer blues, *Psychol Today* 22(10):50, 1988.
10. US Department of Commerce: Statistical abstract of the U.S. ed 110, Washington, DC, 1990, Bureau of the Census.
11. US Department of Health and Human Services: *Healthy People 2000: new objectives to promote health and prevent disease: Public health service,* Washington, DC, 1990, US Government Printing Office.
12. US Department of Health and Human Services: *Prevention report: Public health service,* Washington, DC, Sept 1990, US Government Printing Office.
13. US Preventive Services Task Force: *Guide to clinical prevention services,* Baltimore, 1989, Williams & Wilkins.

Classic

14. Diekelmann N: *Primary health care of the well adult,* New York, 1977, McGraw-Hill, Inc.
15. Frelberg K: *Human development: a life-span approach,* ed 2, Monterey, Calif, 1983, Wadsworth Health Sciences Division.
16. Leavell HR, Clark EG: *Preventive medicine for the doctor in his community,* ed 3, New York, 1965, McGraw-Hill Book Co.
17. Libow L, Sherman F: *The care of geriatric medicine,* St Louis, 1981, Mosby–Year Book.
18. O'Donall MD: Design of workplace health promotion program. *Am J Health Promotion,* 1986.
19. Shamansky SL, Clausen CL: Levels of prevention: examination of the concept, *Nurs Outlook* Feb 1980, p 104.
20. Sundberg MC: *Fundamentals of nursing,* Boston, 1986, Jones & Bartlett Publishers, Inc.
21. World Health Organization Working Group: Health promotion: a discussion document of the concepts and principles, *Pub Health Rev* 14(3-4):245-252, 1986.

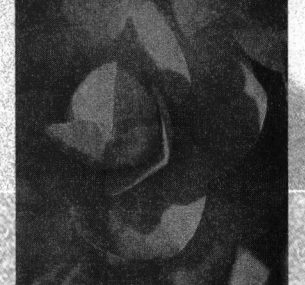

CHAPTER THREE

Promoting Adaptive Responses to Stressors

LEARNING OBJECTIVES

1 Compare and contrast the various theories of stress.
2 Discuss the physiologic response to stress, including the roles of the autonomic nervous system and endocrine system.
3 Discuss the major factors influencing the stress response.
4 Identify the effects of stress.
5 Differentiate adaptive from maladaptive coping mechanisms.
6 Identify the major types of stressors.
7 Apply the nursing process to care of the patient with a stress-related disorder.
8 Describe intervention strategies for managing stress.
9 List common affective, cognitive, and behavioral effects of stress.
10 Discuss common stressors in nursing that affect role performance.

KEY TERMS

adaptation, p. 38
assertiveness, p. 47
autogenic relaxation training, p. 47
biofeedback, p. 47
coping mechanisms, p. 43
defense mechanisms, p. 44
distress, p. 38
eustress, p. 38
fight-or-flight response, p. 40
imagery, p. 48
meditation, p. 48
progressive muscle relaxation (PMR), p. 47
stress, p. 37
stress response, p. 38
stressor, p. 38
therapeutic touch, p. 48

STRESS, a universal phenomenon, has become a household word in the twentieth century. Each individual has unique, highly personalized responses to stress. These responses may be either adaptive or maladaptive and are influenced by the context of the stress, the person's vulnerability, and the stressor. Nurses need to know about the concept of stress and its management to help patients prevent illness, maintain health, and cope with stressors. The topic of stress and its management is a useful starting point for increasing communication about health and nursing interventions.

DEFINITION OF STRESS

Stress is defined as a broad class of experiences in which tension occurs when demanding situations tax the resources, coping, and level of adaptation of the

37

individual. The stimulus for this demand is a **stressor**, which represents a change that often involves a loss of something valued.[4] In fact, the terms stressor and stress stimuli are used interchangeably. Stressors may be categorized as physical, developmental, emotional, environmental, social, cognitive, or spiritual.

Distress may be defined as harmful or unpleasant stress, whereas eustress is stress of a pleasant nature. For example, a person fired from a job experiences distress, whereas a person receiving a promotion feels eustress. Distress includes the physiologic and psychologic results of the demanding situation and can result from understimulation, monotony, boredom, and loneliness. Another factor in distress is overload, or overstimulation, which can result when a demand exceeds the individual's capacity to process or deal with those demands.

Eustress is associated with positive events or situations that are demanding but sought out and are required for personal and professional growth. When the potential outcome is perceived as positive, the individual may perceive the demands as taxing but challenging. Stress perceived as positive may heighten motivation, alertness, and cognitive and behavioral performances.[20]

Adaptation refers to behaviors used by the person to maintain equilibrium when faced with disruptive internal or external stimuli. This process may be unconscious or conscious.[19] Adaptation may be described in terms of responses: behavioral (e.g., fight or flight), physiologic (e.g., increased cardiac output, or secretion of norepinephrine), psychosocial (e.g., anxiety), or sociocultural (e.g., learned helplessness).

Throughout life a person must cope with demands and changes to survive and grow. In addition to the physiologic response to stress, each individual has a personalized stress response. How the individual perceives stress determines his or her ability to tolerate, cope with, and survive stress. This is known as the **stress response** and requires a series of adaptations involving mind and body. A key factor in dealing with the stress response is choice. Whereas one may not be able to control all events or variables in life, one can learn to control one's responses to buffer the effects of stressors on general well-being (see the box above).

THEORIES OF STRESS
Stress as a Stimulus

When defined as a stimulus, stress is conceptualized as a disruptive response. Critical assumptions underlying the stimulus model of stress include (1) life-change events have a similar impact across time and across people; (2) the individual's perception of a stressor as positive or negative is not important; and

---

CHARACTERISTICS OF STRESS RESPONSE

1. The stress response is natural, protective, and adaptive.
2. Physical and emotional stressors trigger specific and nonspecific responses.
3. There are limits in the person's ability to adapt.
4. The magnitude and duration of stressors may be so great that homeostatic mechanisms for adaptation fail, leading to total dysfunction or death.
5. Repeated exposure to stimuli may result in permanent adaptive changes.
6. Individuals differ in response to the same stressor.

---

(3) there is a common threshold beyond which disruption occurs. Stress as a universal phenomenon is important to understanding how it can affect groups and individuals.

Stress is viewed as a stable, additive phenomenon that is measurable by selected life events.[39] Correlations between life events and the onset of diseases have been the model's basic foundation. Prevention of illness is associated with the monitoring and limiting of changes that one is exposed to in a period of time. One use of the stimulus model of stress in nursing practice is to provide an opening for discussion of recent life events.

Stress as a Response

When stress is defined as a response, it represents the disruption caused by a threatening stimulus or stressor. Hans Selye[40] was the first to propose this stress response theory, which he labeled the general adaptation syndrome (GAS). Stress, as defined by Selye, is a nonspecific response of the body to any demands placed on it. Selye's work with laboratory animals showed they exhibited stress responses when subjected to stressors such as learning or performing a difficult task. The responses to prolonged stress included traumatic stomach ulcers and subsequent death.[37]

From this research, Selye proposed the three-stage process of the GAS: the alarm reaction, stage of resistance/adaptation, and stage of exhaustion. In Selye's model, stress is always present, and the response to stress is circular. The system may not move through all stages of the GAS in response to each stressor.

The GAS begins when the person experiences a

physical, emotional, or cognitive stressor. A clear illustration of this syndrome can be found in combat soldiers. Soldiers experience ever-present threats of death or destruction as well as loss of personal freedom and available coping mechanisms. The soldier experiences the alarm stage when first encountering combat. Most soldiers are able to adjust to combat duty. They develop coping abilities to maintain their physical and psychologic well-being. As they do, they enter the next stage of the GAS—resistance—and biologic parameters return to normal. In lengthy combat duty, exhaustion may occur when stress is prolonged. Adaptive energy is depleted, and the body surrenders to stress.

The local adaptation syndrome (LAS) is the result of the stress response occurring in a specific body part. A cut on a hand or a blow to the head is an example of a stressor that initiates the LAS, causing local inflammation. Like the GAS, the body part affected by the stressor may go through the three stages of alarm, resistance, and exhaustion. If the LAS occurs simultaneously in more than one body part or if the LAS is not limited to one body part, the GAS may result. An example of a LAS that results in a GAS response is a local infection that enters the bloodstream and causes sepsis.

The most positive result of the LAS and the GAS is adaptation. With adaptation it is possible to survive, grow, change, and maintain balance in a given situation. However, a common outcome of the stress response is disease. Once a person becomes ill, the illness becomes another stressor, which requires another adaptation. Selye calls many disorders diseases of adaptation, because they result from an incomplete or excessive GAS response induced by pathogens or external agents (see the box above). The GAS may result in two serious consequences. First, it may result in many different forms of disease, both physical and emotional. Second, premature death may occur as a result of depletion of all energy supplies.

Stress as a Transaction

Stress, defined as a transaction, is a concept that encompasses a set of cognitive, affective, and adaptational (coping) variables that arise out of person-environment transactions. The person and environment are seen as constantly intertwined, each affecting and being affected by the other.[36]

The core assumptions of the transactional approach include (1) stress is not measurable as a singular concept, and (2) the person's cognitive appraisal of the situation mediates stress experiences. This model differs from the stimulus and response models, because it allows for individual differences. To quote Lazarus: "The important role of personality factors in producing stress reactions requires that

---

STRESS-RELATED DISORDERS

Hypertension
Ulcers
Skin disorders
Cardiovascular disorders
Elevated cholesterol
Migraine headaches
Eating disorders
Anxiety
Arrhythmias
Raynaud's syndrome
Asthma
Cancer
Alcoholism/drug abuse
Endocrine disorders
Gastrointestinal disorders
Rheumatoid arthritis
Depression
Pancreatitis
Muscular tension
Sleeping difficulties

---

we define stress in terms of transactions between individuals and situations, rather than of either one in isolation."[36] The Lazarus model of stress represents a balance between demands and one's power to deal with them. The transactional orientation to stress is consistent with nursing's view of human experiences by focusing on the individual differences in stress experiences.[13]

According to Lazarus, coping involves both cognitive and behavioral strategies and represents an adjustment to the stressful situation. Coping may be successful when (1) the source of the problem has been dealt with by direct action (i.e., problem solving, assertive communication) or (2) the experience of stress has been directly reduced (i.e., imagery, exercise).

Two important concepts in the Lazarus model are primary appraisal and secondary appraisal. Primary appraisal includes personal judgments about the encounter and whether the situation is likely to cause harm or loss, is threatening, or is challenging. Secondary appraisal involves the individual's assessment of coping abilities and resources to deal adequately with the situation. For example, primary appraisal occurs when an individual acquires all new job responsibilities and determines he or she may risk losing the job if things aren't handled well. Secondary appraisal then would involve an individual reminding himself or herself that he or she has solid knowledge and skills in the new areas of responsibility.

PHYSIOLOGY OF STRESS
Neuroendocrine Physiology of Stress

No simple explanation exists regarding the relationship between stress and the neurophysiologic response of the human body. The body's response to stress occurs not only on a tissue, organ, and systems level, but also on a cellular level.

After the initial perception of a real or imagined stressor, the hypothalamus activates endocrine and neural pathways and functions. The hypothalamus coordinates the homeostatic adjustment and influences three major responses: (1) the sympathetic nervous system discharge as a component of the autonomic nervous system, (2) the release of selected anterior pituitary hormones by way of stimulation from hypothalamic-releasing or release-inhibiting factors, and (3) the release of antidiuretic hormone from the posterior pituitary by the hypothalamic neurons.[12]

Autonomic nervous system

The impulses that arise from the autonomic nervous system are carried through the body by two major subdivisions, the sympathetic and parasympathetic systems. The sympathetic nervous system has become famous for its life-saving functions and is known as the **fight-or-flight response.** Sympathetic arousal results in the body's ability to function beyond its normal everyday function. The sympathetic arousal is summarized in eight effects[32]:

1. Increased blood pressure and heart rate
2. Increased blood flow to the large active muscles coupled with decreased blood flow to internal organs not needed for rapid activity
3. Increased energy consumption throughout the body
4. Increased blood glucose concentration and formation
5. Increased energy release in muscles
6. Increased muscle strength
7. Increased mental activity
8. Increased rate of blood coagulation

Because the fight-or-flight response greatly affects the cardiovascular system, excessive stress over time leads to adverse physiologic effects on this system. Vasoconstriction in small blood vessels, increase in heart rate and arterial pressure, and the addition of lipids can lead to thickening of the walls of blood vessels and eventual hypertension. Hypertension can lead to numerous other disorders of the vascular system, the heart, and the kidneys. Currently researchers are confirming the impact of mental stress specifically on the heart. Such stress may precipitate acute myocardial infarction and sudden death.[11]

When the emergency situation is over, the hypothalamus activates the parasympathetic nervous system. This allows the reparative phase to begin. The parasympathetic system is activated when the body returns to homeostasis. It is impossible for the parasympathetic and sympathetic systems to be working at high levels at the same time. An ebb and a flow exist between the systems. The parasympathetic system seeks relaxation of the smooth muscle fibers; a decrease in heart rate and blood pressure; and increased gastrointestinal functioning, including salivation. Most organs in the body work with both sympathetic and parasympathetic systems acting on them. Some organs, however, are stimulated by only one of these nervous systems. In this case the fluctuation between these two systems determines whether the organ is activated or inhibited.[4]

Endocrine system

The endocrine system, like the nervous system, helps regulate various body activities and systems by the secretion of hormones into the bloodstream. Feedback loops of the central nervous system, autonomic nervous system, and endocrine system make allowances for the ever-changing demands of the internal and external environments (Figure 3-1).

An intimate relationship exists between the hypothalamus and the pituitary gland. The hypothalamus influences both the cortex and the medulla of the adrenal gland. The hypothalamus stimulates the medulla directly through the sympathetic nervous system to release epinephrine into the system. It stimulates the cortex of the adrenals by signaling the pituitary to release adrenocorticotropic hormone (ACTH). The hypothalamus accomplishes this by producing its own hormones. The corticotropin-releasing factor (CRF) signals the anterior pituitary to release ACTH. Release of ACTH moves the adrenal cortex into action with the secretion of cortisol. Almost any kind of stress, whether physical or psychologic, will lead to an instantaneous increase in the level of ACTH. Increased cortisol secretion from the adrenal cortex is the most notable response to increased ACTH. In general, the effect of cortisol is its potentiating effect on glucagon, providing the body with more energy by increasing blood glucose. Cortisol also exerts a permissive effect, resulting in sustained vascular smooth muscle contraction.

The two major hormones secreted by the adrenal medulla are epinephrine and norepinephrine. The general effect of these hormones is the same as that of the sympathetic nervous system. In fact, the action of the adrenals amplifies the action of the sympathetic nervous system. The levels of these hormones vary with the intensity of stimulation of the system. The flooding of epinephrine (adrenergic) and norepinephrine (cholinergic) during high-stress conditions has resulted in research clarifying their

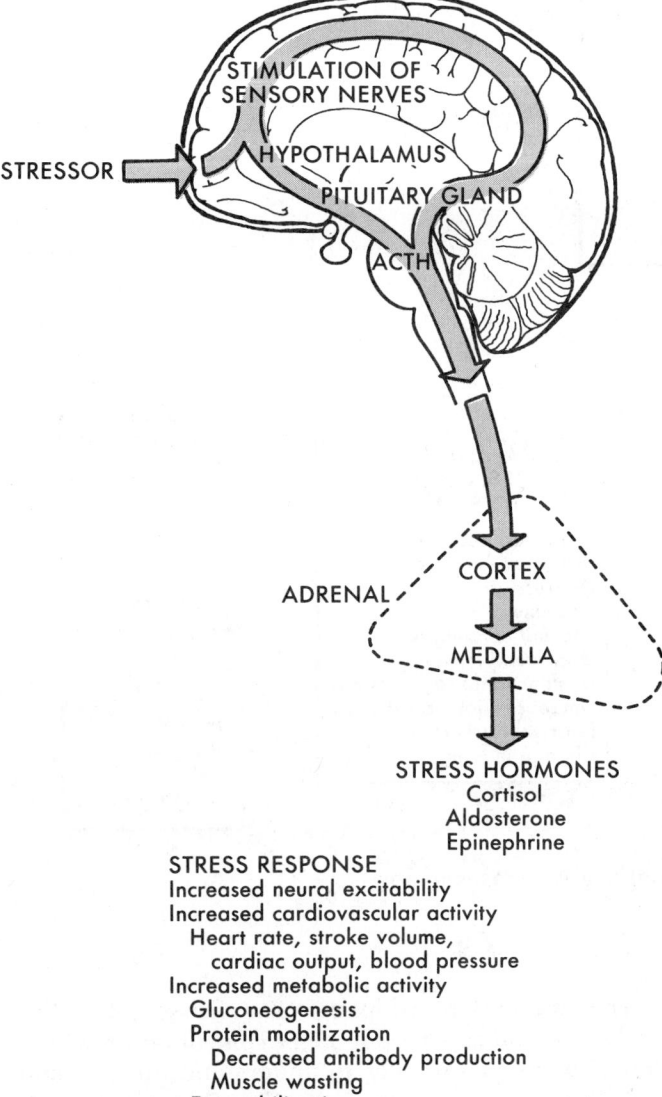

STRESSOR

STIMULATION OF
SENSORY NERVES

HYPOTHALAMUS

PITUITARY GLAND

ACTH

ADRENAL

CORTEX

MEDULLA

STRESS HORMONES
Cortisol
Aldosterone
Epinephrine

STRESS RESPONSE
Increased neural excitability
Increased cardiovascular activity
   Heart rate, stroke volume,
     cardiac output, blood pressure
Increased metabolic activity
   Gluconeogenesis
   Protein mobilization
     Decreased antibody production
     Muscle wasting
   Fat mobilization
Increased sodium retention
Increase in neurological sweating
Change in salivation
Change in GI system tonus and
   motility

FIGURE 3-1   Stress response pathway. (Modified from Girdano E, Jr: *Controlling stress and tension,* ed 2, Englewood Cliffs, NJ, 1986, Prentice-Hall, Inc. With permission.)

respective roles. Research by a team at Stanford University verified that the two hormones behave much differently in speed of reaction and the speed at which they clear out of the bloodstream. Epinephrine is higher when stress is of a mental variety, such as mental arithmetic, continued vigilance, or public speaking. Norepinephrine is associated with physical stressors, such as being immobilized, isometric stress, and physical exercise, and it appears to clear

out of the bloodstream much more slowly than epinephrine.[20]

FACTORS INFLUENCING STRESS RESPONSE

The stress-illness relationship is a complex process that encompasses different factors (Figure 3-2). The same stressor does not have the same effect on all individuals. Further, the same stressor may produce different responses in the same individual at different times. Influencing factors (sometimes called mediating factors) make each individual's response to stressors unique. These factors may be positive and minimize the effects of stress, or they may be negative and actually increase the stress response. Even with positive coping resources, multiple stressors or demands can negatively tip the balance. For example, when Susan was dealing with midterm exams, a paper, and an ill parent, she felt overwhelmed and became ill.

Personal Factors

Personal factors influence the individual's response to stress. These factors include heredity, gender, race, age, personality, and cognitive and prior functioning. An individual's temperament, personal beliefs, attitudes, expectations, and assumptions are other examples of personal factors that affect the stress response. For instance, an individual who has a negative attitude toward life is more likely to have a stronger, more negative response to stress than someone who maintains a positive outlook on life.

Genetic makeup is believed to play a particularly important role in the stress response. Some people are genetically programmed for health and longevity. Others are genetically predisposed to diseases such as high blood pressure, multiple sclerosis, or diabetes.

Another personal factor influencing the stress response is personality type. The type A behavior pattern is a combination of psychologic characteristics, including extreme competitiveness, achievement striving, high job involvement, time urgency, and hostility, whereas type B behavior refers to the absence of this pattern. Research through the 1970s showed a significant link between type A behavior and coronary heart disease. Recent research, however, reveals that type A men are only 58% as likely to die of a second heart attack as are type B men. This suggests that type A behavior alone is not necessarily a killer. Harnessing impatience and hostility and controlling internal stressors are key factors in type A men reducing their potential for a second heart attack, particularly if paired with high cholesterol, high blood pressure, and smoking.

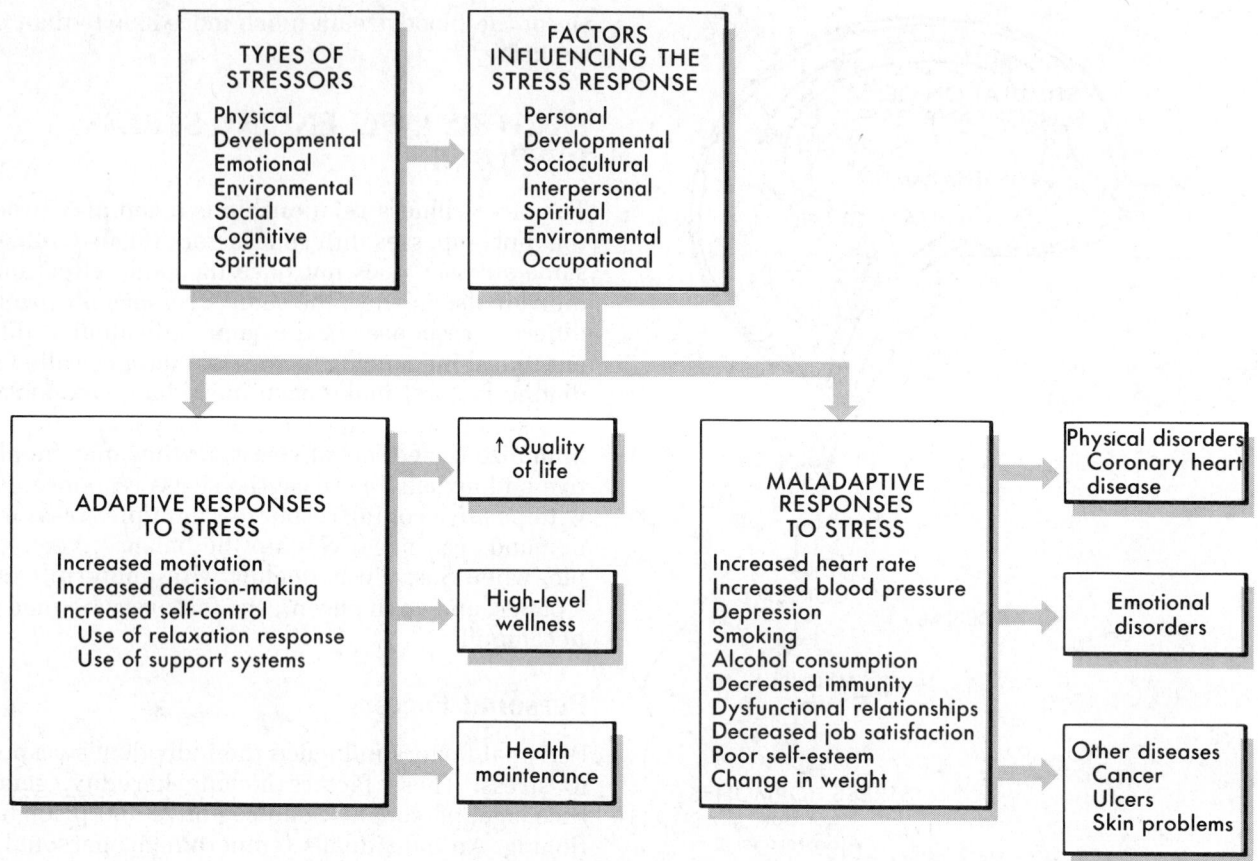

FIGURE 3-2   Adaptive and maladaptive responses to stress.

Sociocultural Factors

Sociocultural factors such as finances, support systems, and social functioning may buffer the effects of stress. The higher incidence of mental disorders or psychologic distress among people of lower socioeconomic status is believed to be caused by their greater exposure to stressful life conditions. Age-related stereotypes and loss of financial and social independence may affect the stress levels of the older adult. Social support resources mediate coping responses and coping effectiveness.[10] It is widely recognized that the perceived degree of control over an individual's environment can affect mental health.

Interpersonal Factors

The quality of interpersonal relationships has the potential to promote or interfere with the person's adaptation to stress. A common line of reasoning is that intimate ties, especially the quality of marital or family resources, are important sources of support. The relationships among an individual's self-esteem, coping response, and later functioning under stress critically depend on his or her partner's corresponding coping level.[10] However, negative in-

terpersonal relationships serve as stressors. One has only to visualize a recent angry confrontation with a loved one or co-worker to understand the stressful effect of a negative encounter. Several stress assessment tools such as the Holmes and Rahe Life Events Scale and the Daily Hassles Scale rank divorce, marriage, and changes in interpersonal relationships as highly stressful.

Spiritual Factors

An individual's spirit is a mediating factor influencing stress. The spiritual part of a person affects perceptions, reactions, and ability to cope with stressors. Brallier[4] defines spirit as "that part of us which can connect with positive forces . . . the universe, God, music, art, environmental surroundings like the mountains or the ocean, other people, animals." Long-established spiritual beliefs as well as the social aspects of religion may provide a positive coping mechanism for the older adult. Spiritual beliefs can help calm emotion and reaction. However, some persons experience emotional and physical distress when they have ambivalent or negative thoughts about their spirituality.

Environmental Factors

The physical environment strongly affects a person's adaptation to stress. Aspects of the environment include air, soil, water, noise, crowding, and climate, esthetic amenities, and quality of the surroundings in which one works and lives. These variables can contribute to a sense of well-being or serve as stressors that may contribute to illness or disease.

Occupational Factors

Some of the conditions that increase stress on the job are fairly common among different groups of workers: fear of job loss, work overload, work underload, lack of control over one's work, unsupportive supervisors or co-workers, limited job opportunities, conflict, boredom, and uncertainty.

Increasing attention has been given to investigating job stress and the staff nurse in the hospital setting. McCranie et al.[16] summarize the common job stressors that staff nurses typically encounter such as death and dying; emotional demands of patients and their families; inadequate staffing and work overload; and conflicts with administrators, physicians, and other nurses. Symptoms of burnout were found to be significantly associated with perceptions of stressful and unrewarding working conditions, as well as a variety of other negative coping mechanisms including tardiness, absenteeism, use of tranquilizing drugs, physical illness, and withdrawal from others. They also investigated whether personality hardiness moderated the impact of job stressors on burnout. The hardiness characteristic is a specific set of attitudes toward challenge, commitment, and control. Their results were consistent with previous research and indicated that burnout was significantly associated with higher levels of perceived job stress and lower levels of personality hardiness. Hardiness as a personality factor alone is not sufficient to prevent burnout. These authors suggest that reducing the frequency and intensity of job stressors experienced by hospital nurses is also required. Adequate staffing, flexible scheduling, implementing conflict management strategies, promoting social support, in-house support groups, and improving the flow of information among nurses, physicians, administrators, and other hospital staff are some of the organizational intervention strategies that should be addressed to prevent staff nurse burnout.

Individual Coping Mechanisms

Coping mechanisms labeled as adaptive are those that promote health while helping the person successfully reduce stress. Maladaptive coping mechanisms may be defined as those that jeopardize a person's health, even though they may temporarily reduce stress. Excessive use of alcohol, addictive drugs, and cigarettes, or avoidance, overeating, and verbally or physically lashing out at others are examples of maladaptive coping.

Coping mechanisms, whether adaptive or maladaptive, focus on one of two possible outcomes. First, coping may be aimed at altering the relationship between the individual and the stressor. Second, coping must assist the person with the psychophysiologic results of stress.

The type of coping strategy that is successful in alleviating the distress depends on the person and the particular situation. The healthy individual is one with a range of adaptive coping strategies (problem focused as well as emotion focused) that are ap-

---

JANIS'S COPING PATTERNS

1. Unconflicted adherence—The person chooses to continue previous behavior and coping mechanisms despite risks or new information. For example, despite learning he is diabetic, John continues to eat an excessive amount of desserts.

2. Unconflicted change—The person indiscriminately follows any new advice or suggestions. George follows his friend's advice to "go out and get drunk" as a way of coping with the stress of his marital conflict.

3. Defensive avoidance—Denial, rationalization, projection, or a number of other cognitive or behavioral coping mechanisms are used to avoid confronting the stressor directly. Susan projects the blame for her high blood pressure onto her stressful job but rationalizes that she's helpless to change the situation.

4. Hypervigilance—In hypervigilance, often known as panic, the person searches frantically for simplistic solutions in coping with the stress. Usually, impulsive decisions are made that are often later regretted. Amy, in a panic over final examinations, quits school after stating that she then will be rid of the source of stress in her life.

5. Vigilance—Vigilance is the most mature coping pattern. The person rationally and systematically assesses the stressors, considers possible alternative sources of stress, decides on appropriate action, and then evaluates the effectiveness. Connie rationally and systematically identifies her conflict with her son as a source of stress. She also decides to sit down and talk assertively but emphatically about her concerns with him. If this does not help she decides to seek counseling for the two of them.

From Janis I: *Stress, attitudes and decisions: selected papers,* New York, 1982, Praeger Publishers.

plied appropriately to the situation. For instance, while awaiting the results of a cancer biopsy, an individual might adaptively use prayer, meditation, relaxation, or distraction. Once the biopsy specimen is known to be cancerous, the individual can use problem solving, seeking support, and counseling.

Defense mechanisms, first defined by Sigmund Freud, are a way of cognitively coping with unpleasant emotions. Everyone uses defense mechanisms, with most people having several in their coping repertoire. These mechanisms remain adaptive until an individual uses them so extensively that rational understanding is impaired. For instance, denial is a normal initial response to coping with a severe loss. However, when extreme denial continues, the individual is prevented from healthy coping. If the individual continues experiencing uninterrupted or overwhelmingly severe stress, these defense mechanisms may not effectively reduce the stress. If this occurs, the person's thought processes may become seriously impaired.

In 1982 Janis[8] described five coping patterns that an individual may use in dealing with stressors. Coping patterns one through four often result in increasing the severity of the stress response, whereas pattern five is effective in reducing the stress response and its negative effects (see the box on p. 43).

CRISIS THEORY AND INTERVENTION

Crisis theory is based on the concept of homeostasis.[6] Emotional balance is maintained by learned coping techniques used to resolve common daily-life stressors. When these stressors become overwhelming, a crisis develops and the people can no longer use previous coping strategies to solve its problems effectively. Periods of disorganization and upset occur during which the system makes unsuccessful attempts to solve the problem. Crises present a danger to the system if it becomes overwhelmed. If the system is overwhelmed and unable to resolve the crises, the system may not recover. However, the crises may provide the opportunity for growth because the individuals are more receptive to therapeutic interventions during times of crisis. Intervention could lead to a higher level of functioning on the part of the individual or family system in crisis. Kus defines crisis intervention as "the systematic application of problem-solving techniques, based on crisis theory designed to help the individual in crisis move through the crisis process as swiftly and painlessly as possible and to achieve the same level of psychologic comfort as experienced before the crisis."[9] The impact of any stressful event largely depends on certain balancing factors, including perception of the event, available situational supports, and coping mechanisms.[2] Any time an individual's problem-solving skills are ineffective in dealing with a stressful situation, crisis intervention may be needed.

When applying the principles of the problem-solving process in the health care setting, the patient must be perceived by the nurse as a basically healthy person able to be actively involved. Problem solving consists of six essential steps that the nurse needs to help the patient through. First, the nurse must help the patient identify and describe the precipitating problem. Second, the nurse must work with the patient to generate possible solutions and list these in writing under the identified problem. Third, the nurse assists the patient in evaluating the possible consequences of the proposed solutions. Fourth, the patient decides which alternative to chose. Fifth, the patient implements the chosen plan. Sixth, the nurse helps the patient evaluate the implementation. Positive changes that have been made by the patient need to be acknowledged and reinforced. It is hoped that the learning that takes place during crisis intervention will allow the patient to cope more effectively with problems in the future. Crisis intervention is a valuable technique in a variety of health care settings. It focuses on the here-and-now, and its time-limited nature make it especially well suited in this era of brief hospitalization and an evolving outpatient health care system.

NURSING MANAGEMENT: THE PATIENT WITH A STRESS-RELATED DISORDER

Nurses are moving away from illness models of care in which patients are "cared for and done to" to wellness models that emphasize personal responsibility and awareness of the interaction among the person's body, mind, spirit, and environment. Brallier[4] states, "In a holistic approach to stress management, great emphasis is placed on the individual's responsibility for his or her own health. That is, locus of control over one's health is within one's self."

In assisting people with stress-related problems, the nurse is concerned with helping these individuals learn to develop increased self-awareness regarding the stressors, learn to modify the number and intensity of existing stressors, and develop effective, healthy, and positive coping skills.

Assessment

It may be unrealistic to expect to obtain a thorough understanding of an individual's stress response immediately on initial contact. Instead, the nurse should expect to increase understanding of the person's stress response and coping patterns through ongoing assessment. During the assessment phase of stress the nurse may use a number of stress identification tools, such as Holmes and Rahe's Life Change Scale,[33] Daily Hassles Inventory, Breeden and Kondo's Anxiety Checklist,[28] or a checklist of physical symptoms, thoughts, and emotions (see the box on p. 45). These tools will help the patient iden-

QUESTIONS FOR ASSESSING STRESSORS AND COPING

- Is the patient able to clarify the source of the stressors?
- Does the patient see the stressor as "uncontrollable"?
- What is the patient's emotional reaction to the stressor?
- What are the possible contributing factors involved (e.g., spiritual distress, disapproval or rejection from others, loss, sudden change in life-style, recent change in health status of self or significant other, or developmental crises)?
- How does the patient perceive the stressor as affecting the future?
- Does the patient see the stressor in a realistic or distorted manner?
- Has the stressor happened before?
- How does the patient usually cope with tension, anxiety, and depression?
- Is the patient prone to labile moods or depressed moods?

- Are feelings communicated directly to others or held inside?
- What methods of coping has the patient tried to deal with the stressor?
- If the method was tried and did not work, why?
- Does the patient feel the previous method or methods would reduce symptoms of stress?
- What support systems are available to help the patient cope?
- Does the patient withdraw from or seek out support systems in times of stress?
- How would the patient describe himself or herself? Or ask "how would a good friend describe you?"
- Ask the patient to rate oneself on a continuum from "being helpless" to "being in control" (1 being helpless, 10 in control of life).

tify specific stressors and more fully examine how demands and changes that affect his or her life. In the older adult the assessment of stressors includes a review of losses such as loss of family or significant others and loss of independence, including physical, financial, social, housing, and self-care.

Self-examination of stressors, which may change events or demands, can increase self-awareness. Developing a clear understanding of the stressors may reduce tension and unrealistic expectations of self. However, focusing on stressors may increase the feeling of apprehension, particularly if the person feels ill equipped to cope with the stress.

The following characteristics of the stressor need to be identified: intensity, duration, probability of the stressor recurring, and pervasiveness of the threat or amount of actual risk to the patient's well-being. The nurse can help the patient focus on ways of handling important stressors. By listening and clarifying coping skills, the nurse can assess adaptation or maladaptation to a stressor. See the box above for examples of questions to help determine how the patient interprets the stressor or stressors.

Each person has a unique coping style and combination of personal strengths and experiences that influence the cognitive appraisal of the stressor and coping resources. According to Brallier,[4] coping styles may include avoidance of stressors, accommodation to stressors, or adjusting mentally and emotionally to stressors. The nurse needs to assess for signs of maladaptive coping. Present or past suicidal and homicidal thoughts indicate poor coping, as does excessive use of alcohol or drugs. In the older adult, maladaptive coping mechanisms can lead to social withdrawal and geropsychiatric manifestations in addition to other signs of maladaptive coping.

Physiologic measures of the stress response may also be included in the stress assessment. Common measures of stress are blood pressure, heart rate, respirations, skin temperature, and muscle tension. Other more complex physiologic measures to assess stress levels include blood glucose levels, urinary excretion of nitrogen, nitrogen balance, indicators of loss of muscle, and ACTH and cortisol levels. These tests may be helpful in determining whether the individual is having an acute stress response, as well as how long the stress response lasts. However, as a result of the expense of a number of these tests, it is unlikely that they would be used to monitor the stress response except in intensive care situations.

Nursing Diagnosis

The stress response is viewed as an individual response and thus may be incorporated into many nursing diagnoses. The nursing diagnoses most likely to reflect the stress response are as follows:

Ineffective individual coping
Anxiety
Sleep pattern disturbance
Powerlessness
Ineffective breathing pattern
Pain

Altered health maintenance
Fear
Ineffective family coping
Altered thought processes
Impaired communication
Knowledge deficit

Planning

Although individuals with a stress-related illness may not be able to control some stressors in their lives, they can exert some control over the stress response. In planning any interventions, it is imperative to reinforce the self-responsibility of the person. One of the first steps in the planning of care for those with stress-related disorders is uncovering the individual, family, or group perception of the stressors and stress response. Then the outcomes or goals they wish to accomplish are reviewed, as well as how they think the nurse and other treatment team members can assist them in that process.[26]

An important step in the planning phase of the nursing process is to develop expected outcomes with the individual. These expected outcomes address the positive change in the individual, family, or group to be achieved through the use of the nursing process. An example of an intervention is a work group that is exhibiting symptoms of severe conflict meeting with the nurse on a weekly basis for 1 month. The expected outcomes of the intervention would be to facilitate positive group cohesion and help decrease the group's stress level.

Implementation

Stress management may be a goal of patients who want to learn self-care. Stress management techniques may be initiated in the clinic, community, or hospital setting. There are many interventions a nurse may offer to help an individual cope with stress, depending on the scope of the problem, the skills of the nurse, and the length of involvement in the nurse-patient relationship.

Individuals hospitalized with serious illnesses are in transition and often face major life-style changes. Interventions aimed at helping to remove stressors within the hospital setting can be implemented by the staff nurse. The staff nurse serves as a stress monitor for the patient in the hospital environment. Volicer[41] has written about stress factors in the experience of hospitalization and has developed an instrument for measuring psychosocial stress factors. Her 49 events, categorized as eight stress factors, include unfamiliarity of surroundings, separation from spouse, financial worries, lack of immediate social support, lack of information, threat of severe illness, separation from family, and loss of control over pain.

Volicer believes the information in this tool can be helpful for the nurse in establishing priorities for nursing interventions.

Some stressors are unalterable. With stressors that cannot be removed, distracting or diversional techniques are encouraged, for instance, relaxation tapes, talking to a supportive person, reading, or watching television. The use of presence or "therapeutic use of self" to listen, show empathy, identify concerns, and provide information is something most nurses can do.

The following interventions can be used by nurses to facilitate self-directed change in individuals, families, or groups to promote healthier living. Several teaching boxes are included in this chapter about various interventions, and the reader is encouraged to see the reference list for excellent books, tapes, and films to further increase understanding of the interventions. An example of another type of self-directed change is use of a self-contract. Self-contracts can be used to identify behaviors the person can change, goals the person wishes to achieve, and the actions necessary to achieve the goals.

Problem solving

Problem solving is a systematic process through which decisions are made. The process of problem solving is similar to the nursing process. For interpersonal problem solving, the six steps of the process are similar to those used for crisis intervention:
1. Gather as much information as possible about the problem.
2. Share the problem with someone else.
3. Brainstorm all possible solutions.
   a. Come up with as many ideas as you can.
   b. Do not critique or throw out any ideas.
   c. Make your list of solutions as long as possible: the longer the list, the more options there are to choose.
4. Select and implement an alternative (possible solution).
5. Evaluate how well the alternative worked.
   a. If it did not work, evaluate why.
   b. Do you need to change "how" you implemented the alternative?
6. If the first alternative does not work, select another alternative from the brainstorming list.

Problem-solving techniques are helpful for the nurse to creatively generate alternatives to health care problems. When the patient is in a transitory state of health or undergoing a stressful situation, the nurse may help the patient mobilize coping abilities by using the problem-solving process. Collaborative problem solving requires the use of listening skills, assertion skills, knowledge of conflict resolution, and evaluation.

Social support

Social support helps the individual cope with stressful events and may help maintain health. Social support is a strong moderator in stress and a person's resilience to illness.[30] The nursing role with this intervention is threefold: assessing the person's social support systems; helping the individual learn to ask for support and feel all right about needing it; and teaching the individual's family or significant others how to be supportive. The nurse needs to work with the individual, family, or group to determine how much social support they will need. The nurse must then compare this with the available amount of social support.

A source of social support and the quality of social support can be measured by a nursing-based instrument, the Norbeck Social Support Questionnaire (NSSQ).[18] The NSSQ provides information about three functional components—affect, affirmation, and aid—and three network properties—number in the network, duration of relationship, and frequency of contact with network members. The NSSQ also includes a component of loss to reflect changes within the individual's network. The NSSQ is an example of a reliable and valid instrument to measure social support. It is currently being tested in a variety of clinical settings and can assist the nurse to assess an individual's social support systems. The strengthening of social supports is a way of buffering the effects of stressors. Factors affecting one's support system are socioeconomic status, the nature of the stressors, the environment, and the acuteness and chronicity of the stressor.

Diaphragmatic breathing

Teaching breath control as a stress management technique can be accomplished by instruction of diaphragmatic breathing. Assessment of whether the individual is "chest" or "belly" breathing is the first step and can be accomplished with the person sitting in a chair or lying in a supine position. If the abdomen expands on inhalation, this indicates partial diaphragmatic breathing. If the abdomen does not move, this is chest breathing. Next, the patient is instructed to exhale completely for the first breath through the mouth to fully evacuate the lungs. Full exhalation pushes all the air out of the lungs, which causes a vacuum and pulls in a deep diaphragmatic breath. Then the patient is encouraged to continue breathing through the nose and imagine the abdomen filling like a balloon on inhalation and letting go of the balloon at exhalation. Encouraging the individual to place his or her hands on the abdomen can aid the individual in learning this technique. Another way of feeling this kind of breath is with a sigh or a yawn. This is the body's way of letting go of tension and stress naturally. Both decreased respiratory rate and increased tidal volume are associated with this type of breathing.

Assertiveness

Assertiveness training is one of the most successful ways of alleviating stress, anxiety, and conflict resulting from interpersonal stressors, although some may view the initial learning and practicing to be assertive as stressful. Changing styles of communicating and behaviors when relating to others is a skill that can be easily learned with positive outcomes. **Assertiveness** is a learned behavior and includes standing up for one's rights without violating the rights of others. The core of assertive behavior is self-responsibility in which the person strives to send clear, direct "I" messages about his or her own thoughts, feelings, and behaviors. According to Jakubowski and Lange[34] assertiveness training is characterized by four distinct features:

1. The person is taught the differences among aggressive, passive, and assertive behavior.
2. The person is assisted in identifying interpersonal rights and responsibilities, as well as those of others.
3. The individual is helped to reduce cognitive and affective barriers to assertive behavior.
4. The person learns specific assertion skills through active practice.

Relaxation training

Relaxation training is particularly useful in treating the stress-related symptoms of insomnia, headaches, pain, general tension, and nervousness. Scandrett and Uecker[23] suggest that relaxation techniques fall into two categories. The first is external, which relies on a more outward focus, and includes **progressive muscle relaxation (PMR),** biofeedback, and hypnosis. The second category includes internally oriented procedures that involve a more inner focus, for example, **autogenic relaxation training,** meditation, and self-hypnosis. The five-step relaxation program that systematically moves patients from externally oriented relaxation techniques to internally oriented ones involves progressive muscle relaxation, shortened muscle relaxation, autogenic heaviness, autogenic warmth, and calming techniques (see patient education guides on pp. 48-49).

Biofeedback

Biofeedback is a type of relaxation training. It is a process for learning voluntary control over automatic, regulated body functions and systems.[29] Biofeedback equipment gives an individual immedi-

PATIENT EDUCATION GUIDE
Progressive Muscle Relaxation

The nurse provides the patient with the following instructions. The patient lies on a flat, firm surface.

Hand—Make a fist, dominant hand first, then nondominant hand.

Lower arm—Press lower arm into the floor, dominant; press lower arm into the floor, nondominant.

Upper arm—"Pull in" upper arm to body, dominant; "pull in" upper arm to body, nondominant.

Forehead—Raise eyebrows toward top of head.

Eyes and nose—Squint your eyes and wrinkle your nose.

Mouth—Purse your lips into a little round O and push out in an accented "kiss."

Neck—Hyperextend your head, grit your teeth, and make a wide smile.

Upper back—Try to touch your shoulder blades, arch your back.*

Abdomen—Suck in your abdomen.

Buttocks—Tighten your buttocks.*

Thigh—Raise your leg about 6 inches off the floor, tighten your upper leg, dominant; raise your leg about 6 inches off the floor, tighten your upper leg, nondominant.

Calf—Pull your foot toward your head, dominant; pull your foot toward your head, nondominant.

Foot—Point your foot away and curl your toes, dominant; point your foot away and curl your toes, nondominant.

*Check for relaxed state. If tense, raise little finger of right or left hand.

ate feedback about body functions such as muscle tension, blood pressure, heart rate, skin surface temperature, and brain wave activity. These selected body systems are monitored via biofeedback instruments that use electrodes to transform the body functions into visual or auditory signals. Any internal body change instantly triggers a signal, such as sound or light. Therefore the person being monitored can see, hear, or see and hear the continual monitoring of body functions, recognize tension areas, and then use this information to modify and control the internal stress response. The goal of the individual is to lower the signal by using any relaxation technique. Home practice is encouraged and may involve using portable biofeedback equipment. A disadvantage of this type of training is possible dependence on equipment. The transfer of learning must be carefully planned and reinforced. Biofeedback is generally used to supplement other relaxation techniques, such as autogenic relaxation and imagery.

Imagery

Imagery is a psychotherapeutic process using an internal state to explore various senses including visual, auditory, kinesthetic, and olfactory. Imagery often begins with a relaxation exercise and then leads the individual into a sensory experience. The content of the imagery exercise is shaped by the person helping with the imagery process. The use of imagery involves an interview, the imagery exercise, and a postimagery discussion.

Meditation

Meditation is a relaxation technique that focuses an individual's attention and alters the individual's level of awareness. Meditation elicits a relaxation response by creating a hypometabolic state of quieting the sympathetic nervous system. When starting to meditate as a stress management technique, beginners describe experiences of relaxation, sleep, and sometimes anxiety (see the patient education guide on p. 49).

Self-hypnosis

Self-hypnosis requires training in hypnotic induction. The trance state of self-induced hypnosis may be achieved in a variety of ways. The basic idea is relaxing into meditation and focusing on suggestions given by a hypnotherapist. Individuals can record hypnotic suggestions and play them back later when they wish to hypnotize themselves. This technique requires disciplined practice. Contrary to popular belief, the person who is hypnotized maintains total self-control. Self-hypnosis is practiced to increase a feeling of inner peace, to reduce performance anxiety in sports or taking examinations, for cessation of cigarette smoking, and for pain control.

Massage

Massage and touch have been used by nurses for decades. These interventions improve circulation, reduce pain and muscular tension, and promote relaxation of the body as well as the mind. Fatigue and chronic muscle tension resulting from effects of stress can be reduced by massage. Therapeutic massage is a technique of systematic rubbing and manipulating tissues of the body. Therapeutic massage increases mobility, flexibility, circulation, and energy. Massage is described as a great way to relax and decrease stress levels.

Therapeutic touch

Therapeutic touch is derived from the ancient art of "laying on of hands." The methodologic process of therapeutic touch has been developed by

PATIENT EDUCATION GUIDE   *Autogenic Relaxation*

The nurse provides the patient with the following instructions:

Sit or lie in a comfortable position with eyes closed.

Say the following:

I am completely at rest, at rest, and my whole body is relaxed.

My thoughts are directed only at this rest. Everything else is immaterial and insignificant; nothing can disturb me.

Rest and relaxation:

Each muscle is relaxed and limp.

Nothing can disturb me.

I am completely at rest.

My right arm is limp and relaxed.

My right arm feels heavy.

My right arm feels relaxed and heavy.

A leaden heaviness spreads through the whole right arm, through the upper arm, through the lower arm, through the hands into the fingertips.

The blood vessels of the right arm are relaxing, the right arm feels beautifully warm.

A pleasant warmth flows through the right arm, through the right upper arm, through the right lower arm, down to the right hand.

The right arm feels beautifully warm and heavy (then to left arm, etc.).

I am completely at rest.

A feeling of rest and well-being is coming over me.

Rest envelops me like an ample cloak—rest protects me.

I surrender completely to the rest and relaxation—I am completely at rest.

This inner rest is of great benefit and helps me relax.

This process deepens with each exercise.

This inner rest will accompany me everywhere.

I will gain confidence and strength from it.

I will feel refreshed as after a deep sleep.

Breathe deeply—pull up your arms—open your eyes.

Sequence: I am very much at rest. My right (left) arm is very heavy. My right (left) arm is very warm. My heart is beating strong and well. My breathing is very relaxed, I breathe peacefully.

From Kleinsorge H, Kliembies G: *Techniques of relaxation*, Bristol, England, 1964, John Wright & Sons, Ltd.

PATIENT EDUCATION GUIDE   *Basic Steps in Meditation*

The nurse provides the patient with the following instructions:

1. Choose a quiet spot where you will not be disturbed by other people or the telephone.
2. Sit in a comfortable position.
3. Close your eyes.
4. Relax all your muscles sequentially from head to feet.
5. Become aware of your breathing, noticing how the breath goes in and out, without trying to control it in any way.
6. Repeat your focus word silently in time with your breathing.
7. Don't worry about how you are doing.
8. Practice at least once every day for 10 to 20 minutes.

Krieger.[35] In this treatment modality, which requires specialized training, a meditative state is used to enter the energy field of the patient and to passively visualize the free flow of energy from the practitioner to the recipient with the intent to support or promote healing. The practitioner focuses on creating a state of harmony and balance and promoting self-healing in the patient. Krieger clearly outlines the healing process as one of centering (a mental state of balance), assessing the energy field, "unruffling" the field, and directing the transfer of energy to the patient. The last point of the process is knowing when to stop the energy flow. The effects of therapeutic touch are similar to the relaxation response. The voice level of the recipient becomes lower, respirations become slower and deeper, the patient may verbalize feeling relaxed, and a peripheral flush may occur in the face.

Psychotherapy

If a person experiences frequent or prolonged psychologic symptoms of stress (i.e., anxiety, difficulty concentrating, blaming others, or worrying) referral to a mental health professional for individual or family psychotherapy may be necessary.

Psychotherapy is a structured relationship between a qualified therapist and an individual, family, or group to accomplish specific interpersonal or emotional goals based on change. In referring an individual or family for psychotherapy, the nurse should know about the education and training of the therapist. In addition, the nurse should encourage the individual or family to choose a therapist with whom they feel comfortable.

Time management

Time management is an effective strategy to reduce the stress of time urgency. It involves allocating appropriate blocks of time for tasks, as well as setting priorities for tasks to be completed. Time management involves matching the best combination of time demands with an individual's supply of available time. High-priority tasks must be dealt with first. If extra time becomes available, then one can do less important tasks. Good time managers consistently plan, prioritize, and delegate. They make maximum use of time but do not take on more tasks than are possible within a given time frame. An individual who takes on more tasks than can be reasonably completed within a limited time frame becomes overloaded and suffers from negative effects of stress. Type A personalities are particularly prone to this "hurry-up" life-style. The stress response is heightened both during the rushing process and later when the frustration of not completing the task is realized.

Nutrition

The food an individual eats has been shown to affect his or her stress response. Some foods deplete the body's ability to cope with stressful situations, either by stimulating the sympathetic nervous system directly or by creating irritability and fatigue. Collectively these diets are known as "stress-prone diets."

Many foods naturally contain sympathomimetic agents—chemical substances that mimic the sympathetic stress response. When eaten, these foods trigger a stress response. The most common of these sympathomimetic stressors in the North American diet is caffeine, which belongs to the xanthine group of drugs. Xanthines are powerful amphetamine-like stimulants that increase metabolism and create a highly alert, awake state. In addition, xanthines trigger release of stress hormones that can increase

heart rate, blood pressure, and oxygen demands. Coffee, teas, colas, and chocolate are the most commonly consumed sources of caffeine. Caffeine consumption in excess of 250 mg per day (approximately two cups of tea or coffee) is considered excessive, with adverse effects on the body.

The second major factor in the stress-prone diet is that of vitamin depletion. Prolonged periods of stress deplete the body's supplies of the B-complex and C vitamins. Both processed flour and refined white sugar have been implicated in the depletion of B-complex vitamins. Particularly during times of severe stress, high levels of vitamin C and the B-complex vitamins are necessary to maintain proper functioning of the endocrine and nervous systems. Deficiencies of vitamins B_1 (thiamin), B_5 (pantothenic acid), and B_6 (pyridoxine hydrochloride) can lead to anxiety, depression, and cardiovascular weakness, whereas vitamin B_2 (riboflavin) and niacin deficiencies can cause muscle weakness and stomach irritability. One way to ensure that a person receives enough essential nutrients is to eat balanced meals that include a high intake of natural rather than processed foods.

Exercise

Along with diet and the use of other positive coping skills, exercise is a healthy way to prevent stress-related disorders, as well as to break chronic stress patterns. Physical activity is a natural and healthy way to release the by-products of the stress response. Pelletier[38] identifies exercise as being beneficial in coping with stress in two ways. First, it produces specific biochemical changes within the body. In fact, if physical activity is vigorous enough, it will cause a parasympathetic nervous system response resulting in feelings of tranquility and relaxation that last long after the activity of exercise is completed. Second, the fact that the individual takes time out to exercise will result in more balance in life and thus enhance the coping of work and demands.

Humor

Humor and laughter are useful coping strategies that can be effective releases for pent-up frustration and anger, as well as for dispelling the anger of others. At times of crisis, humor can be a morale booster. Finding some humor in an overwhelmingly stressful situation can not only help make it seem less stressful, but also help preserve the positive energy needed to cope with the stressor. A bit of levity has often been used to reduce tense situations, put others at ease, and facilitate relaxation in a group situation. Cousins, in his book *Anatomy of an Illness,*[31] writes about healing oneself with humor. Laughter may have an indirect but positive effect on adaptation to illness. Cousins speculates that laughter itself is not the primary healing agent but that intentionally placing oneself in a positive frame of mind can lead to positive health outcomes. Humor may also serve as a necessary "release valve" and has been a vehicle for facilitating cohesion, relaxation, and more productive work relationships for nurses.[5] In addition, humor may be used as a defense mechanism and needs to be explored when used excessively to avoid dealing with a situation. As a nursing intervention, humor can be used based on familiarity with the patient regarding his or her coping style, timing, comfort level, and response to humor.

Evaluation

To evaluate the effectiveness of a stress intervention technique the nurse considers the following:
1. What factors influenced the attainment of the expected outcome?
2. What factors inhibited the attainment of the expected outcome?
3. Has the patient identified the source of stress or threat?
4. Has the patient identified personal strengths and resources to help deal with stress?
5. Does the patient use constructive problem-solving techniques?
6. Is the patient able to attain a level of coping that allows for maximum performance of daily living and social or occupational roles?
7. Does the patient believe he or she has made progress in managing stress? If yes, ask the patient to describe his or her perceptions of the progress made. If no, what does the patient believe has impeded the progress?
8. What interventions did the patient find most helpful in achieving desired outcomes? Least helpful?
9. Does the patient see the need for changes in life-style to maintain health?

CRITICAL THINKING QUESTIONS

1 Write a paragraph describing the similarities and differences in models of stress as a response, stress as a stimulus, and stress as a transaction.
2 Illustrate the differences in a stressor and a stress response by case example. For instance, keep a diary of stress in your life for 1 week, identifying your major stressors, the types of stressors, what factors are influencing your level of stress, and how you respond to each.
3 Describe the nervous system response to a po-

tential car accident. Describe the endocrine system responses to the same accident.
4 List four maladaptive and four adaptive coping mechanisms of an individual in the clinical setting or of a friend, nurse, or patient.
5 List the identified stressors of the individual in question 4.
6 Design a nursing care plan for a patient and list two or more stress management interventions.
7 Choose one intervention strategy and practice it for 1 week. Record effects of this strategy in a stress diary.
8 Interview a staff nurse and ask his or her perception of stressors in the environment.
9 Choose one relaxation technique to practice for 20 minutes each day for 1 week; record effects of this strategy in your stress diary.
10 List three interventions that are appropriate for the registered nurse to utilize in clinical practice.

RESOURCES

The following audiovisual aids are available from these resources:
1 CARE FOR THE CARETAKER Rose Medical Center 4636 East Ninth Ave. Denver, CO 80220 (303) 320-2876
2 CLINICAL CONSEQUENCES OF STRESS: THE IMMUNE CONNECTION Network for Continuing Medical Education One Harmon Place Secaucus, NJ 07094 (800) 223-0272
3 COPING II: GETTING WHAT YOU WANT FilmFair Communications 10900 Ventura Blvd. P.O. Box 1728 Studio City, CA 91604 (213) 877-3191
4 COPING WITH STRESS Journal Video Inc. 930 Pitner Ave. Evanston, IL 60201 (800) 323-5448
5 REST, RELAX AND HEAL University of Cincinnati Medical Center 231 Bethesda Ave. Cincinnati, OH 45267-0574 (513) 872-5627
6 THE TOUCH FILM WITH DR. JESSIE POTTER Sterling Productions 500 N. Dearborn St., Rm. 1119 Chicago, IL 60610 (312) 329-1183

Additional audiovisual aids:
1 Hospital Satellite Network 2020 Avenue of the Stars Los Angeles, CA 90067 (800) 638-3336

BIBLIOGRAPHY
Current
1. Anderson H, Johnson R: Strategies for preventing and coping with burnout. In McFarland GK, Thomas M, editors: *Psychiatric mental health nursing*, Philadelphia, 1991, JB Lippincott Co.

2. Aquilera D, Messick J: *Crisis intervention: theory and methodology,* ed 4, St Louis, 1982, Mosby–Year Book.
3. Barnett R, Beiner L, Baruch G, editors: *Gender and stress,* New York, 1987, Free Press.
4. Brallier L: *Transition and transformation: successfully managing stress,* Los Altos, Calif, 1982, National Nursing Review.
5. Burton-Leiber D: Laughter and humor in critical care, *Dimen Crit Care Nurs* 5(3):162, 1986.
6. Caplan G: *Principles of preventive psychology,* New York, 1964, Basic Books.
7. Courtney C, Escobedo B, A stress management program: inpatient-to-outpatient continuity, *Am J Occup Ther* 44(4):306, 1990.
8. Janis I: *Stress, attitudes and decisions: selected papers,* New York, 1982, Praeger Publishers.
9. Kus R: Crises intervention. In Bulechek J, McCloskey J, editors: *Nursing interventions: treatments for nursing diagnoses,* Philadelphia, 1985, WB Saunders Co.
10. Lazarus R, Folkman S: *Stress, appraisal and coping,* New York, 1984, Springer Publishing Co, Inc.
11. Lewen M, Kennedy H: The role of stress in heart disease, *Hosp Med,* p 125, Aug 1986.
12. Lindsey AM, Carrieri VK: Stress response. In Carrieri V, Lindsey A, West C, editors: *Pathophysiological phenomena in nursing: human responses to illness,* Philadelphia, 1986, WB Saunders Co.
13. Lyon B, Werner J: *Annual review of nursing research,* New York, 1987, Springer Publishing Co.
14. Macinick CG, Macinick JW: Strategies for burnout prevention in the mental health setting, *Int Nurs Rev* 37(2):247, 1990.
15. Manfredi C, Pickett M: Perceived stressful situations and coping strategies utilized by the elderly, *J Commun Health Nurs* 4(2):99, 1987.
16. McCranie E, Lambert V, Lambert C, Jr: Work stress, hardiness, and burnout among hospital staff nurses, *Nurs Res* 36(6):374, 1987.
17. Murray RB, Huelskoetter MW: The person on the health-illness continuum: promoting adaptation to the stress response. In *Psychiatric mental health nursing: giving emotional care,* ed 3, Norwalk, Conn, 1991, Appleton & Lange.
18. Norbeck J, Lindsey A, Carrie V: Further development of the Norbeck social support questionnaire: normative data and validity testing, *Nurs Res* 32(1):4, 1983.
19. Pender N: *Health promotion in nursing practice,* Norwalk, Conn, 1982, Appleton-Century-Crofts.
20. Rice P: *Stress and health: principles and practice for coping and wellness,* Monterey, Calif, 1987, Brooks/Cole Publishing Co.
21. Roberts M: Can what harms also heal? *Psychol Today* 22(5):8, 1988.
22. Robinson JA, Lewis DJ: Coping with ICU work-related stressors: a study, *Crit Care Nurse* 10(5):80, 1990.
23. Scandrett S, Uecker S: Relaxation training. In Bulechek G, McCloskey J, editors: *Nursing interventions: treatments for nursing diagnoses,* Philadelphia, 1985, WB Saunders Co.
24. Sideleau BF: Person-environment interaction. In Haber J, McMahon AL, Price-Hoskins P, Sideleau B, editors: *Comprehensive psychiatric nursing,* ed 4, St Louis, 1992, Mosby–Year Book.
25. Smith E: Fighting cancerous feelings, *Psychol Today* 22(5):22, 1988.
26. Spencer-Legler MA: The nursing process as a framework for psychiatric nursing. In Lancaster J, editor: *Adult psychiatric nursing,* New York, 1987, Medical Examinations Publishing Co, Inc.
27. Weinberger R: Teaching the elderly stress reduction, *J Gerontol Nurs* 17(10):23, 1991.

Classic

28. Breeden S, Kondo C: Using biofeedback to reduce tension, *Am J Nurs* 75(11):2010, 1975.
29. Brown B: *Stress and the art of biofeedback,* New York, 1977, Harper & Row Publishers, Inc.
30. Cobb S: Social support as a moderator of life stress, *Psychosom Med* 38:300, 1976.
31. Cousins N: *Anatomy of an illness,* New York, 1979, WW Norton & Co, Inc.
32. Guyton AC: *Basic human physiology: normal function and mechanisms of disease,* Philadelphia, 1977, WB Saunders Co.
33. Holmes TH, Rahe RH: The Social Readjustment Rating Scale, *J Psychosom Res* 11:213, 1967.
34. Jakubowski P, Lange A: *The assertive option, your rights and responsibilities,* Champaign, Ill, 1978, Research Press.
35. Krieger D: *The therapeutic touch,* Englewood Cliffs, NJ, 1979, Prentice-Hall, Inc.
36. Lazarus R: *Psychological stress and the coping process,* New York, 1966, McGraw-Hill, Inc.
37. MacLean PD: Sensory and perceptive factors in emotional functions of the triune brain. In Grenell RG, Gabay S, editors: *Biological foundations of psychiatry,* vol 1, New York, 1976, Raven Press.
38. Pelletier K: *Holistic medicine: from stress to optimum health,* New York, 1979, Merloyd Lawrence, Inc.
39. Rahe RH: Life change measurement clarification, *Psychosom Med* 40:95, 1977.
40. Selye H: *The stress of life,* New York, 1974, McGraw-Hill.
41. Volicer B: Patient's perceptions of stressful events associated with hospitalization, *Nurs Res* 23:235, 1974.

CHAPTER FOUR

Epidemiology

LEARNING OBJECTIVES

1 Define epidemiology and clinical epidemiology.
2 Calculate common epidemiologic rates.
3 Differentiate among primary, secondary, and tertiary prevention.
4 Describe the major research strategies of epidemiology.
5 List major sources of bias in epidemiologic investigation.
6 Identify major epidemiologic-based intervention strategies in adult health nursing.

KEY TERMS

epidemiology, p. 53
incidence, p. 58
morbidity, p. 57
mortality, p. 57
population, p. 57

prevalence, p. 58
primary prevention, p. 55
rate, p. 57
secondary prevention, p. 55
tertiary prevention, p. 55

ACCORDING to Stallones,[30] **epidemiology** is the study of the "occurrence of disease (and, by inference, health) in groups of people." Clinical epidemiology uses epidemiologic methods to study variation in outcomes of illness and the reasons for variation. It is a way to quantify clinical issues such as nursing diagnosis, intervention, and outcome.[3,17]

The purposes of epidemiology are to (1) identify the etiology of deviations from health, (2) provide the data necessary to prevent or control disease and injuries through community health interventions, and (3) provide data necessary to maximize the timing and effectiveness of clinical interventions and to evaluate interventions. Data derived from epidemiologic investigations are used to identify risk factors for development of disease or occurrence of injuries. Medical-surgical nurses commonly encounter results of epidemiologic investigations. To appropriately use this information in planning care for patients, families, and communities, it is important to understand how these studies are conducted, how they differ from clinical investigations, and how they may be used in nursing practice.

HISTORY

Before World War II, the major causes of mortality in the United States were infectious diseases. Epidemiologists commonly focused their research on identifying the factors associated with disease causation, as well as on specific agents of disease. Study of these epidemics resulted in development of several concepts that continue to be used today. These concepts are agent, host, and environment. In a classic investigation of cholera in London, John Snow[29] reported in 1855 that cholera cases were associated with drinking water, especially from one particular well. Snow recommended closing the well, and the result was a reduction in cholera cases. This demonstrated the concept that one does not need to know the specific pathophysiologic mechanism of disease causation to prevent disease. Knowing environmental factors (risks) associated with diseases provides a basis for prevention.

After World War II, antibiotics became widely available, and the mortality patterns in the United States changed. The population's life expectancy increased, and heart disease, cancer, and stroke were identified as major causes of mortality. Epidemiology shifted its focus to the study of these diseases in populations. Studies such as the Framingham investigation[24] of factors associated with development of coronary heart disease led to identification of risk factors such as hypertension, high serum cholesterol, smoking, and sedentary life-style in the development of heart disease. During this period, epidemiologists debated whether epidemiology of chronic disease (multiple causes) differed from infectious disease (single cause).

Scientists have begun to define epidemiology as a unique science that has a body of research methods and statistical techniques that may be applied to any type of health condition or disease. Thus epidemiologic methods are being applied to a variety of acute health problems, including injuries such as those caused by firearms, as well as chronic health problems such as asthma and infectious diseases such as acquired immune deficiency syndrome (AIDS). Recent textbooks represent a dramatic departure from prior work in terms of clarifying the methods and procedures of epidemiology.[6,13,15]

CONCEPTS OF EPIDEMIOLOGY

The major concepts of epidemiology are agent, host (population), and environment (Figure 4-1). Conceptually, each element in this model affects and is affected by the other elements. When these elements are in balance, the community is "healthy"; that is, it is not experiencing premature mortality or morbidity. This means that "agents" are controlled, the environment is "healthful" or supportive of health, and the "host" is able to function productively. This interaction has important implications for intervention, because implicit within this approach is the idea that prevention of disease may be directed at any component of the model. For example, to prevent AIDS in the United States, you could (potentially) (1) alter the environment by closing businesses where exposure is likely, such as bathhouses in San Francisco, (2) decrease host potential for exposure by health care workers using universal precautions, and (3) quarantine the agent by testing the nation's blood supply and eliminating infected blood. Each of the major concepts (agent, host, and environment) may be described by a number of variables.

Agents may be described as having a high or low ability to cause disease. Bullets (lead) fired from high-velocity handguns result in immediate and of-

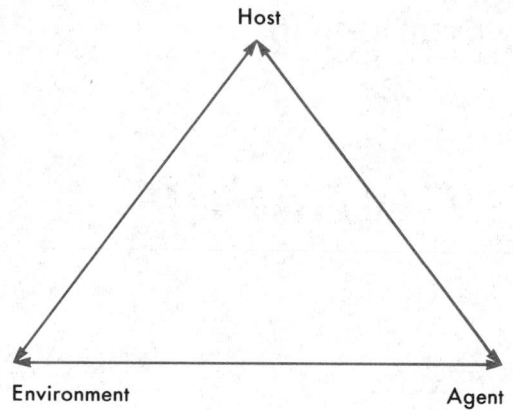

FIGURE 4-1   Concepts in epidemiology.

ten serious injuries (disease), whereas lead that is ingested[28] through food and water supplies requires years of exposure before disease in an individual may be detected. Agents are distributed in the environment, and the patterns of distribution may be detected. For example, one is more likely to find benzene, a known cause of leukemia, in areas of the United States where it is manufactured. Not surprisingly, cases of benzene-induced leukemia are also distributed in this way. This observation led to Aksoy et al.'s research[20] identifying the link between benzene exposure and development of leukemia. Similarly, one is more likely to be exposed to malaria in tropical environments, because the types of mosquitos that carry this disease thrive in tropical environments.

Disease is not distributed in random fashion throughout the United States. Part of epidemiologic study includes identifying areas of concentration of diseases and examining the relationship among concentrations of agents, exposure to them, and disease. Geographic mapping serves multiple purposes in epidemiology, including planning further studies or geographically based intervention strategies.

Some of the many variables associated with hosts include age, gender, race, socioeconomic status, and occupation. Distribution of diseases and health conditions varies according to these characteristics. For example, heart disease, cancer, and stroke are the leading causes of death in the United States. However, this is not the case if the causes of death are described according to the characteristics of age, race, and sex. A landmark publication by the National Research Council and Institute of Medicine[12] noted that injuries, especially motor vehicular, are the leading cause of death among persons 1 to 44 years of age and contribute 40.8% of the potential years of life lost as a result of premature death for persons less than 65 years of age (Figure 4-2). Among African-American males 15 to 24 years of age, homicide is the leading cause of death. Whereas

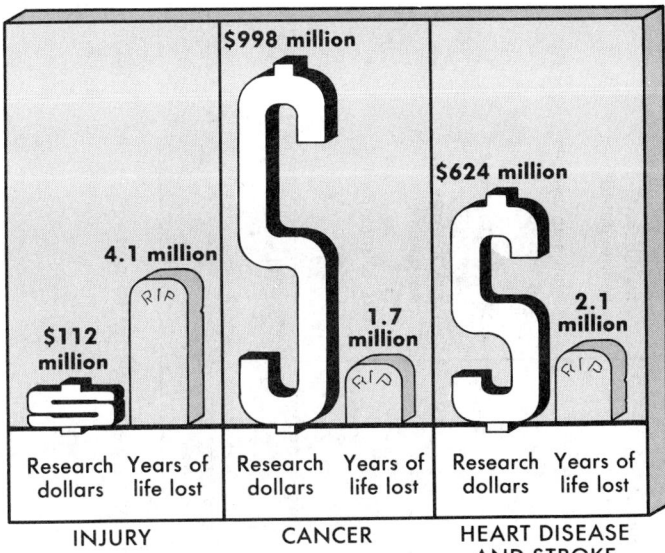

FIGURE 4-2 Years of potential life lost to three causes of death (injury, cancer, and heart disease/stroke) and total federal research funds. (From National Research Council and Institute of Medicine: *Injury in America: a continuing public health problem*, Washington, DC, 1985, National Academy Press.)

investigation of heart disease and other major causes of overall mortality is important, it is also necessary to examine mortality from the perspective of population characteristics to identify the full spectrum of potential prevention strategies.

NURSING AND CLINICAL EPIDEMIOLOGY

This brief presentation of variables used by epidemiologists may sound quite different from those variables customarily considered by nurses. Nurses measure characteristics of individuals, most commonly individuals who are ill. Nurses are concerned with measurement of blood pressure, pulse rate and quality, intake, and so forth. This information is interpreted to provide quality care to the individual measured. Epidemiologists also are interested in obtaining this information, but the intervention focus is the population or some component of it (an aggregate) rather than the individual. The focus of epidemiology is identification of risk factors and agents of disease. The focus of nursing and clinical epidemiology is comparison of interventions and disease outcomes.

Health Promotion and the Nurse

Primary prevention is directed at reducing the probability that a disease will develop before there

is any indication of a pathologic condition. For example, nurses encourage parents to immunize their children, eat a nutritious diet, and avoid drinking and driving. This is one aspect of health promotion, with the specific instructions varying depending on the age and sex of the individuals, families, and groups receiving the information. Another aspect is sanitation of food, air, and water supplied through regulation of industries. Through epidemiologic research, factors associated with an increased chance of developing a particular disease are identified, thus providing the basis for reducing risk of development of disease/injury among persons who do not have indications of disease. This is primary prevention.

Secondary prevention is concerned with early detection of disease (screening) and early treatment to reduce disability and mortality. Nurses encourage Pap tests, blood pressure measurement, and prompt evaluation of symptoms, as well as support compliance with treatment programs that have control or cure of health problems as their intent. Most nursing and medical clinical research is focused on cure or secondary prevention.

Tertiary prevention is concerned with slowing the progress of disease and preventing further disability under the assumption that the individual cannot be completely cured, that is, returned to the previous state of health. Persons who are quadriplegic may never regain use of their arms and legs. However, rehabilitation programs help these individuals and their families develop independent life-styles and reduce the likelihood of developing further health problems, such as bladder infections and skin pressure ulcers.

An idea that underlies these divisions of primary, secondary, and tertiary prevention is natural history of disease (Figure 4-3). Diseases progress through phases of prepathology, pathology, morbidity (disease), and eventually, mortality. The length of time associated with this process varies among diseases. Individual patients receiving nursing care in medical-surgical environments are commonly in a tertiary prevention stage of the disease spectrum. Nursing diagnoses for these persons reflect this. However, part of the nurse's role is to promote health, which, as defined by the World Health Organization,[9] means the attainment by all peoples of the highest possible level of health so that they are capable of working productively and participating in the community. Although it is necessary for the nurse to focus on the specific diagnoses that result in hospitalization, the professional nurse is also expected to evaluate all aspects of the individual's health status and to include prevention in planning nursing care. Information about prevention strategies comes from epidemiology.

Thorough discussion of research methods specific

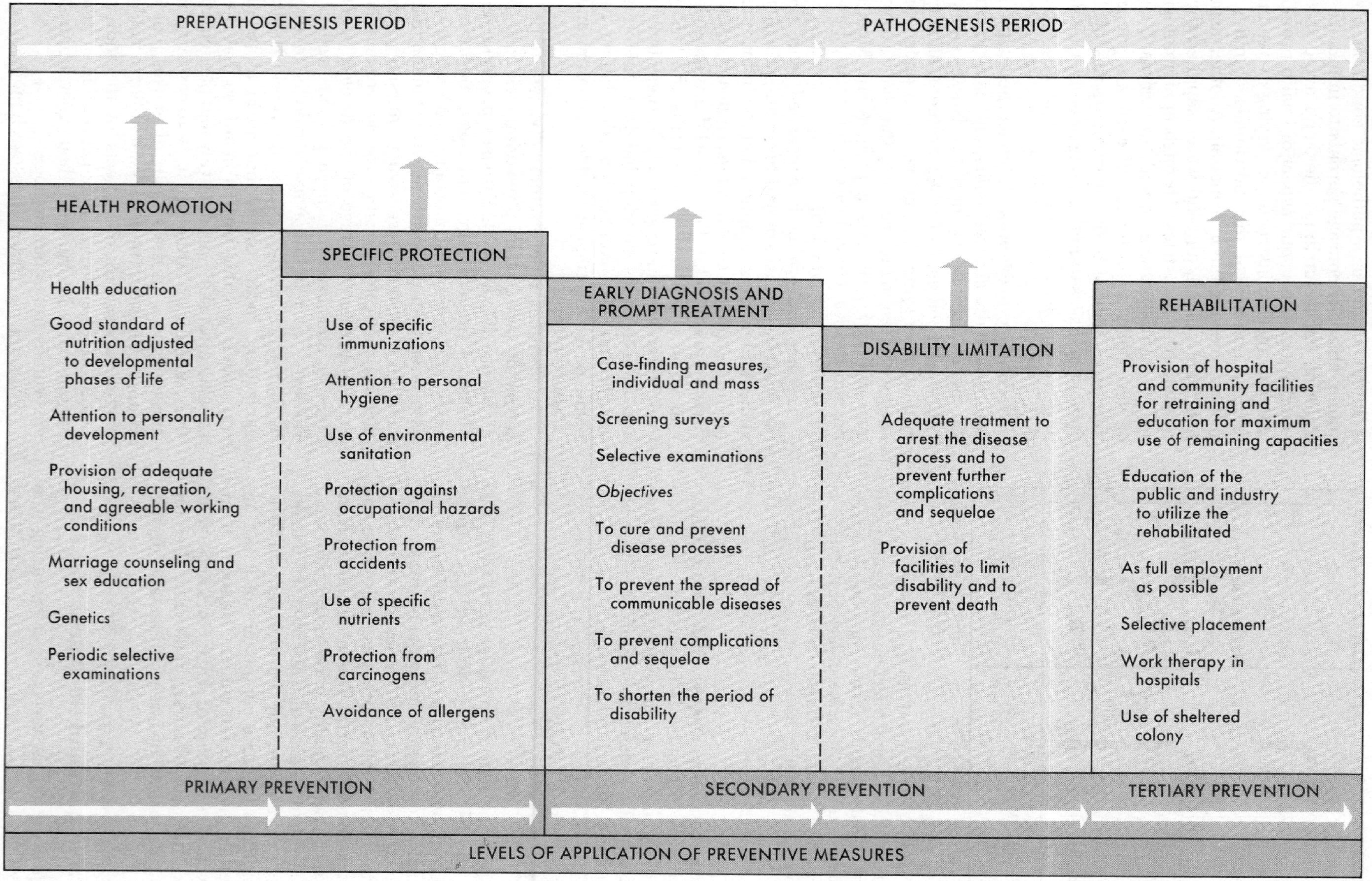

FIGURE 4-3   Levels of prevention and natural history of any disease in humanity. Each level of prevention has a relationship to a stage of the disease process.

to epidemiology is beyond the scope of this chapter. However, nurses commonly encounter this type of research, and it is appropriate to understand whether a study is, in fact, based on principles of epidemiologic research and how nurses can interpret the findings in clinical practice.

Populations in Epidemiologic Research

As noted earlier, epidemiologic research has as its central purpose the determination of factors or exposures associated with states of health. It is therefore population focused. The population selected for study varies depending on how the frequency of the disease varies among people. Sometimes the study population is a community defined by political boundaries such as a city, county, or state. In other situations, the population may be further specified by age, gender, race, or occupation, but a population always forms the base for describing health and disease.

Population measures of health and disease

A **population** may be described as a group of persons who have in common one or more personal or social characteristics and who experience exposure to agents of disease. To summarize this information, rates are constructed using accepted definitions. A **rate** is a measure of disease frequency (case counts) divided by the number of persons in the population for a specific period of time, commonly 1 year. These may be counts of persons with a particular disease **(morbidity)** or persons who have died of a disease **(mortality).** They are commonly expressed as age-specific rates or cause-specific rates. Additional ways to specify rates include gender-specific and occupation-specific rates. Rates are specified to determine whether they change when specific population characteristics are considered. This identifies whether specific groups within a population should be the focus of further research and intervention or whether the entire population is at risk equally. Accurate case counts for the numerator are as important as accurate counts for the denominator. Table 4-1 defines rates commonly encountered in epidemiology.

Observational Epidemiology

Many epidemiologic investigations report observations of health or disease states, summarized as incidence rates. These studies illustrate observational or descriptive epidemiology. The investigator makes no effort to verify etiology (cause and effect) or to experiment. Rather, these studies focus on estimating the relative importance of particular problems and who is affected by them.

TABLE 4-1 Rates for Estimating Health and Disease

Crude mortality	$\dfrac{\text{Number of deaths (100)}}{\text{Total population}}$
Cause-specific mortality	$\dfrac{\text{Number of deaths from specific cause (100,000)}}{\text{Total population}}$
Age-specific mortality	$\dfrac{\text{Number of deaths among persons 35-44 yr (100,000)}}{\text{Number of persons 35-44 yr}}$
Case fatality	$\dfrac{\text{Number of deaths from specific cause (100,000)}}{\text{Number of persons developing the disease}}$
Proportionate mortality	$\dfrac{\text{Number of deaths as result of specific cause (100,000)}}{\text{Total deaths}}$
Incidence	$\dfrac{\text{Number of persons developing a disease (new cases)}}{\text{Population at risk}}$
Prevalence	$\dfrac{\text{Number of persons with a disease}}{\text{Population at risk}}$

Most descriptive epidemiology is based on observation of mortality rather than morbidity. Most rates pertain to mortality because in the United States, a system for counting fatal cases, called the death registration system, exists. Nearly everyone who dies has a death certificate. A dead person cannot be buried in a cemetery or a survivor receive life insurance benefits without one. Death certificates must be signed by a physician or coroner, and they are archived by government agencies. Death certificates include information such as cause of death. These certificates are the major source of information about mortality in the United States and are used for the numerator in mortality. Although the death registration system in the United States is thorough, it is not without error, particularly in coding the cause of death. In many cases, determination of the specific cause of death is done by the physician without autopsy data. In these cases the identified cause may be correct or incorrect. Information routinely collected by the US Census Bureau is commonly used for the denominator.

Measurement of morbidity is often difficult because no system exists that routinely identifies persons with specific disease conditions (except for specific reportable diseases such as rubella, AIDS, and other, usually infectious, diseases). Morbidity is commonly estimated through national surveys such as the National Health Interview Survey, an ongoing survey of a probability sample of residents of the

United States, and through hospital discharge and insurance company data.

Another measure of the effect of a particular disease on a population is the disease's duration. Some diseases are immediately fatal; others are rarely fatal. **Incidence** identifies the number of newly diagnosed cases in a population in a specific period of time, such as a year. **Prevalence** identifies the population proportion that has a particular health condition at a single point in time. The number of persons who are newly diagnosed with heart disease in 1989 in the United States (incidence) will be a much smaller number than the number who have ever been diagnosed by January 1, 1990. When disease duration is short (less than 1 year), incidence and prevalence rates are nearly identical. However, when disease duration is long, the size of the affected population (prevalence) will be much larger than incidence rates would indicate. Case mortality (number of cases who die divided by the number of cases) is a measure of prevalence. Epidemiologists are interested in these measures for two reasons.

First, estimating the number of persons affected provides a measure of the importance of a problem in a community. Generally, when more persons are affected, the problem is of higher importance for the community. It may be argued, however, that case fatality rates are also important, because if everyone who acquires a particular disease dies, that disease is important. Indeed both arguments are common in policy areas where decisions are made about allocation of scarce resources (money) for research and treatment.

The second reason to distinguish between incidence and prevalence is to identify the appropriate baseline measure to monitor to determine the effect of preventive programs. If the purpose of a program is to prevent disease from developing, the appropriate population indicator would be the incidence rate. If the purpose of a prevention program is to provide prompt and adequate care, a more appropriate indicator of program success would be prevalence proportion, or case mortality. Incidence provides a measure of risk of acquiring a health problem. Combining measures of other variables with incidence helps to identify "risk factors" for acquiring and averting specific diseases.

Risk Factors

Many different ways to measure the impact of variables on incidence rates exist. Risk, or the probability of acquiring a particular health problem, varies according to age, race/ethnicity, and gender. When risk is observed, the specific rates may be compared using risk ratios. For example, the risk of developing lung cancer is higher for men than for women. Age, race, and sex, however, are problematic for

prevention efforts, because they are not amenable to change, nor do they describe the complete chain of events leading to disease. They are useful, however, in identifying subgroups for additional research and preventive programs.

Observing a population's experience with specific diseases, estimating rates, and comparing the rates in one community with those of another are done to identify areas for further, more refined studies, to identify "target populations" for intervention, and to establish population baseline information for later use in program evaluation. To compare one community, county, or state with another, it is usually necessary to mathematically adjust the rates obtained in each location for age and possibly race and sex. Fleiss[21] describes the procedures for accomplishing this.

To fully understand the chain of events, it is necessary to first identify and study the relationship between exposure to other variables and the relationship between type and duration of exposures and the disease process. This type of research is called etiologic or analytic epidemiology.

Analytic Epidemiology

In analytic epidemiologic studies, the investigator is interested in determining the relative contribution of factors associated with higher and lower disease rates. These factors are identified through observations about persons who have already been exposed to a suspected agent or who have acquired a particular health problem. Perhaps the observational epidemiology indicates that certain factors such as cigarette smoking describe most of the persons who acquire lung cancer. To determine whether the factor or variable is in fact related to the development of disease, it is necessary to measure or estimate exposure or "dose" over time and whether disease develops. This is generally visualized by a two-by-two table with exposure on one dimension and disease on the other.

Analytic studies based on exposure dimension

In analytic studies based on the exposure dimension the subjects are selected based on whether they can be determined to be exposed or not exposed and whether they can be determined to be free of disease at a point in time. These studies are known as cohort studies. In prospective cohort studies, two or more groups (cohorts) of nondiseased subjects are grouped according to their exposures, observed for a period of time, and monitored for development of disease. The length of the study (commonly 5 years or more), the numbers of subjects required (large), and the problems in maintaining contact with subjects over these long periods make these studies expensive and difficult to complete. Variations on this basic cohort approach are used to reduce research costs and problems. These designs include retrospective cohort and cross-sectional studies.

Analytic studies based on disease dimension

In analytic studies based on the disease dimension the subjects are selected from persons who have been diagnosed with the disease being studied. Generally, they have also been exposed to the potential risk factor. Nondiseased subjects, whose characteristics (usually age, race, and gender) match the "case" subjects, are obtained. The selection of nondiseased subjects for controls is a complex topic and beyond the scope of this chapter. The prior exposures are determined to identify whether exposure seems to be related to development of the disease. This is termed a *case-control study*. This study design is most common for rare diseases and when the disease would likely require medical treatment (facilitating identification of cases).

Experimental Studies

Experimental studies of disease etiology are rare. Conducting such studies requires random assignment to exposed or not exposed groups and subsequent observation to determine whether disease develops. For many diseases the interval between exposure and development of disease is long, and it would be difficult to maintain the experimental conditions over the 10 or 20 years necessary for the experiment. More important, however, ethical issues have an impact on conducting such experiments. If the data from analytical studies indicated that cigarette smoking might cause lung cancer, would it be appropriate to randomly assign subjects to smoking (thus requiring them to begin smoking) and nonsmoking groups? Such a study design would probably not be considered humane.

Community intervention trials are somewhat more common examples of experimental research using epidemiology. A recent example of this is the hypertension detection and follow-up experiment reported by the Hypertension Detection and Follow-up Program Cooperative Group.[23] In this study, hypertensive subjects (n = 10,940) from various communities (n = 14) were randomly assigned to two different treatment programs. One program, called stepped care, followed carefully defined protocols for medical management of hypertension. The other program, called referred care, essentially told the subjects that they were hypertensive and that they should see their physicians for treatment (the accepted instruction after screening at that time). Nearly all of these subjects were observed for 5 years. At the completion of the observation period,

the stepped care group had 17% less overall mortality and 26% less mortality as a result of myocardial infarction than the referred care group. Because of the random assignment of subjects to treatment and control groups, characterizing experimental research, the investigators concluded that rigorous management of hypertension could reduce mortality associated with hypertension, a risk factor for myocardial infarction and cerebrovascular accident.

Sources of Bias in Epidemiologic Research

A hospital or clinic rarely is an appropriate source of subjects for epidemiologic research, because hospitalized subjects do not necessarily reflect the community or population. Using data from multiple sources, White et al.[31] portray health and disease in a hypothetical community of 1000 persons. Over 1 month, only one person would be referred to a university medical center, with nine admitted to other hospitals (five of these referred to other physicians), 250 consulting a physician, and 750 reporting illness or injury. University medical centers tend to admit individuals who have unusual problems requiring sophisticated technology for medical diagnosis and treatment. A 250-bed nonprofit community hospital, in comparison, tends to treat persons who have common, defined health problems and who have financial resources, either personal or through insurance, to pay for services. Nursing students who learn to care for childbearing families at the university medical center are likely to think that childbearing families may be described as single, young, poor, and undereducated, as well as to deliver small-for-gestational-age infants with multiple related medical problems. Nursing students who care for childbearing families in the community hospital (which may be across the street from the first hospital), however, are likely to characterize childbearing families as older, of higher socioeconomic status, married, and educated, as well as having uncomplicated pregnancies and delivering normal infants. Each group is probably correct. However, neither is describing the community. In communities, who is admitted to hospitals or clinics is determined by factors other than residence. This results in a type of selection bias known as Berkson's bias.

A second major source of bias in epidemiologic research is known as the ecologic fallacy, or the tendency to interpret characteristics of a group or population to individuals. For example, if one finds that a particular type of brain cancer is more common in a geographic area that has high levels of air pollution, it may be tempting to conclude that air pollution results in brain cancer. It may also be true that a particular medical center in that same geographic area has a national reputation for treatment of this particular disease and persons with that problem move to that location to receive treatment. These persons may or may not have been exposed to the air pollutants believed to cause the cancer. To establish association between cause and effect, it is essential to determine whether the diseased persons actually experienced exposure to the agent, or air pollution in this case. If not, the ecologic fallacy may bias the findings.

A third source of bias commonly occurring in epidemiologic studies is called statistical bias. In the analysis of two-by-two tables, described earlier, the most common type of statistic is called chi-square. Epidemiologic studies commonly involve large groups of subjects. Statistically, the larger the number of subjects, the more likely it is that you will obtain statistical tests that are considered "significant." In these circumstances, statistically significant findings may be caused by the study design rather than by actual relationships among the data. Studies reported in the popular press suggesting relationships between coffee drinking and breast cancer and studies identifying dietary causes for a variety of health problems are commonly biased as a result of this problem. Too few subjects in a study may result in the obverse conclusion that no relationship exists when, in truth, there is a significant relationship. Determining the proper number of subjects is called statistical power analysis, which requires advanced educational preparation. Generally, studies with less than 40 or more than 250 subjects may present these problems. Evaluating the validity of these reports commonly requires the assistance of statistical experts.

Finally, interpretation bias may result in erroneous conclusions based on the measurement of available but not necessarily interpretable data. For example, Lee et al.[8] conducted a study of firearm mortality and morbidity and found that firearm injuries classified as homicide and attempted homicide were more common among African Americans than among Caucasians or Hispanics in a community. The cases included in this study came from hospital discharge records, emergency medical services records, police records, and death certificates. Is it appropriate therefore to conclude that African Americans are at higher risk of firearms homicide? Or is low socioeconomic status rather than race more likely associated with these high rates? When reading studies, it is essential to think carefully about the procedures used to identify cases to determine whether bias is confounding the findings.

How to Use Epidemiologic Study Findings

As noted previously, epidemiology is concerned with identifying the etiology of disease through research on population level experience with particular health conditions and diseases to identify risk factors, control risk factors, and reduce disease incidence and prevalence. The three major strategies for intervening are education (individual and community), regulation, and services.

Individual education, which focuses on behavioral change to reduce risk, is far more difficult than we would like to think. An underlying assumption in individual education is that persons who engage in risk-taking behavior do so because they do not know or understand the consequences of their behavior. As nurses, we commonly assume that the prudent person, when faced with the epidemiologic facts, would choose to reduce the risk of disease or injury by behavioral change. As nurses, we would be remiss if we did not provide individuals with information that has potential to change behavior and reduce risk of disease. Behavioral change is difficult. Despite the evidence, a significant proportion of the population continues to smoke, lead a sedentary lifestyle, omit wearing seat belts, and so forth. Individual behavioral change is not easy, nor does epidemiology guarantee that individuals who change their behavior will be able to avoid disease and injury. Epidemiology is based on population rather than individual risk factors. The experience of the population may not apply to individuals. Subsequent chapters will discuss risk factors associated with specific types of nursing diagnoses. However, patient education alone is insufficient. From a population perspective, there are additional strategies the nurse can use to promote health.

Community or health education focuses on providing knowledge through programs directed at the community in a general sense. It includes using television, radio, and newspaper as well as providing other written information, such as pamphlets. These materials are developed to meet the learning needs of the average citizen or groups in a community and thus to provide the knowledge basis for behavioral change toward reducing risk within the population.

An additional strategy to reduce risk in a population is regulation. In the case of swimming pool drownings, for example, the nurse could advocate education about cardiopulmonary resuscitation and pool safety. Another approach is to regulate the environment around swimming pools. City or county ordinances that require fences around pools and self-locking gates reduce swimming pool mortality. These solutions require, in part, use of the political process to create change. Any process in the political arena mandates knowledgeable use of power to create coalitions to generate the political strength necessary to create change. Use of this mechanism is important in reducing mortality and morbidity, because regulations potentially affect populations vs. individuals.

The degree to which the political process is effective in reducing mortality and morbidity is partly affected by the political strength of the proponents and antagonists of intervention. A recent book by White[19] describes the political struggle over health promotion through regulation of cigarette production by public health officials vs. the tobacco industry's interest in maintaining production.

The final major approach to intervention is to provide services for populations. Examples range from providing low- or no-cost immunizations to developing national computerized data banks of candidates for organ transplants. Services can be described according to their cost and the number of persons served. Services can be provided to individuals or to entire communities, as in the case of regulating the quality of food and water supplies.

CRITICAL THINKING QUESTIONS

1 What is epidemiology? Discuss its benefits.

2 Define primary, secondary, and tertiary prevention.

3 What are the major research strategies of epidemiology?

4 What are some of the sources of bias in epidemiologic investigation?

5 Describe the major epidemiologic-based nursing intervention strategies.

BIBLIOGRAPHY

Current

1. Anderson B: An overview of drug therapy for chronic adult asthma, *Nurse Pract* 16(12):39-47, 1991.
2. Cherkin DC: Learning to live without practiced denominators, *J Fam Pract* 19(4):437, 1984 (guest editorial).
3. Fletcher RH, Fletcher SW, Wagner EH: *Clinical epidemiology: the essentials,* Baltimore, 1988, Williams & Wilkins.
4. Gage RB: Examining the dynamics of spouse abuse: an alternative view, *Nurse Pract* 16(4):11-16, 1991.
5. Howe RS, Christman C: Outpatient initiation of insulin: a nurse practitioner protocol, *J Am Acad Nurse Pract* 3(1):35-41, 1991.
6. Kelsey JL, Thompson WD, Evans AS: *Methods in observational epidemiology,* New York, 1986, Little, Brown & Co, Inc.
7. Kleinbaum DJ, Kupper LL, Morgenstern: *Epidemiologic research: principles and quantitative methods,* New York, 1982, Van Nostrand Reinhold Co, Inc.
8. Lee RK, Waxweiler RJ, Dobbins JG, Paschetag T: Incidence rates of firearm injuries in Galveston, Texas, 1979-81, *Am J Epidemiol* 134:511-521, 1991.

9. Mahler H: Present status of WHO's initiative "health for all by the year 2000," *Ann Rev Pub Health* 9:71, 1988.
10. Masters R, Sheila FM: The use of restraints, *Rehab Nurs* 15(1):22-25, 1990.
11. Mausner JS, Kramer S: *Epidemiology: an introductory text,* Philadelphia, 1985, WB Saunders Co.
12. National Research Council and Institute of Medicine: *Injury in America: a continuing public health problem,* Washington, DC, 1985, National Academy Press.
13. Rothman KJ: *Modern epidemiology,* Boston, 1986, Little, Brown & Co, Inc.
14. Schaffer SD: Current approaches in adult asthma: assessment, education and emergency management, *Nurse Pract* 16(12):18-34, 1991.
15. Schesselman JJ: Case control studies, New York, 1982, Oxford University Press, Inc.
16. Shamian J: Effect of teaching decision analysis on student nurses' clinical intervention decision making, *Res Nurs Health* 14:59-66, 1991.
17. Weiss NS: *Clinical epidemiology: the study of the outcome of illness,* New York, 1986, Oxford University Press.
18. White JE, Nativio DG, Kobert SN, Engberg SJ: Content and process in clinical decision-making by nurse practitioners, *Image J Nurs Scholar* 24(2):153-158, 1992.
19. White LC: *Merchants of death: American tobacco industry,* New York, 1988, Beech Tree Books.

Classic

20. Aksoy M et al: Acute leukemia due to chronic exposure to benzene, *Am J Med* 52:160, 1972.
21. Fleiss JL: *Statistical methods for rates and proportions,* New York, 1981, John Wiley & Sons, Inc.
22. Haupt A, Kane TT: *Population handbook,* Washington, DC, 1978, Population Reference Bureau, Inc.
23. Hypertension Detection and Follow-up Program Cooperative Group: Five-year findings of the hypertension detection and follow-up program, *JAMA* 242:2562, 1979.
24. Kannel WB et al: Factors of risk in development of coronary heart disease: six year follow-up experience, *Ann Intern Med* 55:33, 1961.
25. Leavell HR, Clark EG: *Preventive medicine for the doctor in his community,* New York, 1958, McGraw-Hill, Inc.
26. Lilienfeld AM: *Foundations of epidemiology,* New York, 1978, Oxford University Press, Inc.
27. MacMahon B, Puggh TF, Ipsen J: *Epidemiologic methods,* Boston, 1980, Little, Brown & Co, Inc.
28. Needleman HL, Landrigan PJ: Health effects of low level exposure to lead, *Annu Rev Pub Health* 2:277, 1981.
29. Snow J: On the mode of communication of cholera. Reprinted in Frost WH, editor: *Snow on cholera,* New York, 1936, Commonwealth Fund.
30. Stallones RA: To advance epidemiology, *Annu Rev Pub Health* 1:69, 1980.
31. White KL, Williams TF, Greenberg BG: The ecology of medical care, *N Engl J Med* 265:885, 1961.

UNIT II

Dimensions of the Nurse's Role in Adult Health Nursing

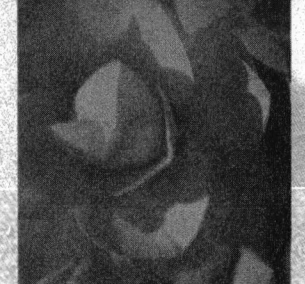

CHAPTER FIVE

Professional Roles of the Nurse

LEARNING OBJECTIVES

1 Discuss the characteristics of a profession as they apply to nursing.
2 Explain the role of the professional organization.
3 Discuss the professional relationship as it applies to nursing.
4 Describe the role of the advocate.
5 Identify the major components of the nursing role.
6 Explain the differences among models of nursing practice.
7 Identify five expanded roles in nursing.
8 Identify four trends that are likely to influence nursing's future.

KEY TERMS

advocate, p. 70
caregiver, p. 69
case management, p. 72
clinical nurse specialist, p. 73
functional model, p. 71
nurse anesthetist, p. 73

nurse clinician, p. 73
nurse midwife, p. 73
nurse practitioner, p. 72
primary nursing, p. 72
profession, p. 65
team nursing, p. 71

THE PROFESSIONALISM of nursing has been a matter of concern and debate within nursing as well as other disciplines for a number of years. Profession is defined in various ways depending on the historic perspective taken, when the definition was developed, society's current view of the profession, and the profession itself. This lack of consensus about the critical elements of a profession makes the exchange of definitions among disciplines difficult without clarification.[19] To enter into and practice a profession one must determine how that specific discipline defines profession and professionalism.

Western society has long valued the notion of a **profession** as a group of individuals who:

Because of the special nature of their activities, "profess" themselves dedicated to moral standards that oblige them to place the good of those they serve above their own self-interest. Traditionally, these groups have been physicians, lawyers, and the clergy, and these pro-

fessionals have been accorded the privileges of self-regulation and discretionary latitude in their actions and decisions.[22]

Perhaps the best-known list of characteristics of a profession is that proposed by Flexner in 1915.[39] He stated that in a profession:

1. The essence of activity is intelligent problem solving resulting in large and personal responsibility for judgment exercised.
2. There is continuous learning from practice to theory.
3. Members are engaged in activities that have practical significance.
4. The profession rests on a specialized body of knowledge, a discipline.
5. Members share a commitment to their work and others in their group.
6. Members are committed to the larger good first and their personal advancement second.

NURSING AS A PROFESSION

At the beginning of the twentieth century, it was generally thought in the United States that the enactment of state registration for nurses would elevate nursing to professional status through the establishment of minimal educational standards for nursing schools. However, as the demand for nurses grew, large numbers of nursing schools of varying quality were established—a circumstance that did little to enhance the professional status of nursing.[10]

With the advent of World War II, nursing increased in importance and stature. In the final days of the war, an article by Bixler and Bixler[36] appeared in the *American Journal of Nursing* appraising nursing's status as a profession. The seven criteria for a profession identified by Bixler and Bixler were applied to nursing as practiced at the time, providing the rationale for considering nursing a profession. Bixler and Bixler[37] reexamined their criteria and nursing's professional status 14 years later and found that both continued to be valid (see box below).

More recently, Hall[14] identified the following five attitudinal components of professionalism:

1. The use of professional organizations as major referents

2. A belief in self-regulation that involves the idea that only professionals in that specific area can set the standards of practice
3. A belief in service to the public that includes the essentiality of the profession
4. A sense of calling to the field or commitment to the profession as a major interest and desire that transcends monetary rewards
5. Autonomy wherein the practitioner should make decisions concerning practice based on the standards of practice and the code of ethics

Adherence to these criteria requires self-discipline by both the profession and the professional. In nursing the profession must set standards of practice and establish procedures to ensure adherence to those standards. The professional nurse must be knowledgeable about standards set by the profession and agree to practice in accordance with them.[11]

Perhaps the best way to view nursing's status as a profession is to think about each of the components of professionalism as a continuum. Within some components of professionalism, nursing can be viewed as highly professional, whereas in others it would fit more closely with the characteristics of an occupation. For example, fewer than 10% of all practicing nurses belong to the American Nurses' Association, yet nursing has one of the highest participation rates in the labor force of any professional group. The last and most important component, autonomy, continues to undergo development in nursing's quest for professionalism.

The Professional Organization

The professional association is that body committed to protect and advance the economic and social welfare of practitioners of a profession.[43] It serves as the official voice of the profession. The primary responsibilities of a professional association are to set standards for the profession and to help enforce those standards (see box on p. 67). In addition, along with statutory agencies, the professional association helps define and expand the scope of practice of the profession and protects the jurisdiction of the profession from encroachment by other disciplines. The American Nurses' Association (ANA) has defined medical-surgical nursing practice as follows:

. . . the nursing care of individuals who have a known or predicted physiological alteration. The nursing process takes into account supportive and potentially disruptive influences on health status, and the related social and behavioral problems resulting from or affecting the patient's response and/or adjustments to the physiological alteration. The practice of medical-surgical nursing is carried out in those settings which deliver primary, acute, and long-term care.

SEVEN CRITERIA FOR A PROFESSION

Criterion One—A profession uses in its practice a well-defined and well-organized body of specialized knowledge that is on the intellectual level of higher learning.

Criterion Two—A profession constantly enlarges the body of knowledge it uses and improves its techniques of education and service by use of the scientific method.

Criterion Three—A profession entrusts the education of its practitioners to institutions of higher education.

Criterion Four—A profession applies its body of knowledge in practical services that are vital to human and social welfare.

Criterion Five—A profession functions autonomously in the formulation of professional policy and in the control of professional activity thereby.

Criterion Six—A profession attracts individuals of intellectual and personal qualities who exalt service above personal gain and who recognize their chosen occupation as a life work.

Criterion Seven—A profession strives to compensate its practitioners by providing freedom of action, opportunity for continuous professional growth, and economic security.

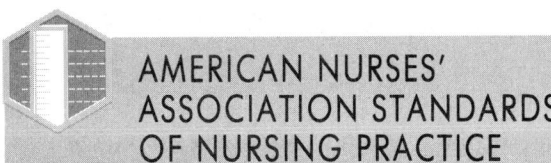

AMERICAN NURSES' ASSOCIATION STANDARDS OF NURSING PRACTICE

Standard I

The collection of data about the health status of the client/patient is systematic and continuous. The data is accessible, communicated, and recorded.

Standard II

Nursing diagnoses are derived from health status data.

Standard III

The plan of nursing care includes goals derived from the nursing diagnoses.

Standard IV

The plan of nursing care includes priorities and the prescribed nursing approaches or measures to achieve the goals derived from the nursing diagnoses.

Standard V

Nursing actions provide for client/patient participation in health promotion, maintenance, and restoration.

Standard VI

Nursing actions assist the client/patient to maximize his health capabilities.

Standard VII

The client/patient's progress or lack of progress toward goal achievement is determined by the client/patient and the nurse.

Standard VIII

The client/patient's progress or lack of progress toward goal achievement directs reassessment, reordering of priorities, new goal setting, and revision of the plan of nursing care.

From American Nurses' Association: Standards of medical-surgical nursing practice, Washington, DC.

In order to implement the nursing process effectively, nurses who are engaged in the practice of medical-surgical nursing should:

1. Base nursing practice on principles and theories of biophysical and behavioral sciences.
2. Continuously update knowledge and skills, applying new knowledges generated by research, changes in health care delivery systems, and changes in social profiles.

3. Determine the range of practice by considering the patient's needs, the nurse's competence, the setting for care, and the resources available.
4. Ensure patient and family participation in health promotion, maintenance, and restoration.

Because of the breadth of the scope of practice reflected in the area designated as medical-surgical nursing, it is the intent of the ANA Executive Committee of the Division on Medical-Surgical Nursing Practice to establish standards of practice in areas of specialized nursing practice; for example, cardiovascular nursing and oncological nursing.*

Professional associations may also engage in activities that enhance the effectiveness of the profession—for example, publication of professional journals, facilitation of research, and accreditation of continuing education. Certification for advanced practice may also be a function of a professional association.

The American Nurses' Association (ANA) in the United States and the Canadian Nurses' Association (CNA) for nurses in Canada are professional organizations. The membership of the ANA or CNA consists of the constituent state or province associations; for the individual nurse, membership comes through joining the state or province association. It is the professional responsibility of the individual nurse to support the professional association through membership and participation in its activities. The association cannot adequately represent all practitioners and therefore the profession as a whole without this support.

Professionhood and Professionalism in Nursing

To fully grasp the meaning of professionhood and professionalism in nursing, it is necessary to examine the differences between these concepts. According to Styles,[25] professionhood focuses on the characteristics of the individual as a member of the profession. The suffix "-hood" connotes a shared specific state or character. Professionhood places the individual nurse at the center of the profession. It emphasizes that the nurse's chief concern must be the individual characteristics he or she brings to the field.

Unlike professionhood, professionalism emphasizes the composite character of the profession. Professionalism moves the focus from ourselves to others. According to Styles, this creates an "I—they" relationship that allows the individual to disown nursing problems and identify nursing problems as belonging to others.

*From American Nurses' Association: *Standards of medical-surgical nursing practice*, Kansas City, Mo, 1974, The Association.

Professional Relationship

A profession may be defined by the methods it uses to acquire and develop knowledge, the standards that it sets for practice and for entry into practice, and the relationship between the discipline and its practitioners. It may be further defined by the nature of its service relationships. Pellegrino[22] asserts that the philosophic grounding of a true profession is described by the nature of the relationship between its practitioners and those who go to them seeking help. He sees five essential characteristics of this relationship.

The most basic characteristic of the professional relationship, according to Pellegrino, is that professionals deal with people who are in a state of vulnerability. These people may seek the restoration of justice, goods, or rights; release from physical illness or pain; or emotional or spiritual comfort or reconciliation. They depend on the professional for the special knowledge and skill that they seek; therefore the initial relationship is a dependent one in which the patient has the need and the professional holds the knowledge.

Second, the patient needs from the professional not only technical knowledge and skill, but also advice, counsel, and assistance with decision making. The professional is expected to enter into the life experience of the patient in such a manner that the assistance rendered will be not only technically correct but also appropriate to that person's values and life-style.

Third, the patient must reveal intimate aspects of his or her life if the professional is to have the information necessary to render assistance. The privacy, dignity, and personal image of the patient may all be compromised. Therefore the nurse must accept the patient as a unique individual who may hold different values, beliefs, and customs and may be of a different race or ethnic orientation.

The fourth characteristic is trust on the part of the patient. The patient must trust that the professional has the level of competence needed to render assistance and that, in a state of vulnerability, he or she will not be exploited. As Pellegrino points out, "Trust is mandatory, and it must be given when one is vulnerable and in the midst of an assault on one's whole person."[22]

The fifth and final characteristic is the promise of help. It is this feature that gives the professional relationship its altruistic, or moral, quality. Implicit in the offer of assistance is the message that the professional has the requisite knowledge and skill to help and that the knowledge and skill will be used to render aid and not to do harm.

NURSE'S ROLE IN ADULT HEALTH NURSING

Nursing's unique role in health care stems from the sustained intimate contact that nurses have with patients. Many other professionals assist patients in the promotion, attainment, and maintenance of health, but no other professional group accepts responsibility as nurses do for the totality of the person's needs across settings and throughout life.

Nursing care is required not only in times of illness but also to promote wellness. At one time the primary focus of nursing was the care of hospitalized patients during the acute or chronic phases of illness and during rehabilitation. Today, however, nursing practice also includes health promotion and maintenance and care of the dying. With this broad scope of practice, nursing care now is delivered in a variety of settings.

Nurses are finding employment in acute care institutions such as hospitals and long-term care facilities such as nursing homes, rehabilitation centers, and hospices. Community settings such as health departments, mental health centers, day-care facilities, outpatient clinics, ambulatory surgery centers, health maintenance organizations (HMOs), and the home also provide practice settings for nurses.

Because of its broad scope, nursing affords an opportunity for all types of personalities to find a practice setting consistent with their personal style, interests, and career goals. Nurses can specialize in a particular type of setting or a particular patient population. Nursing specialties related to particular settings include home health nursing, critical care nursing, community health nursing, and operating room nursing. Specialties based on particular populations include pediatric nursing, gerontology, and maternal-infant nursing. According to Henderson[41]:

> The unique function of the nurse is to assist the individual, sick or well, in the performance of those activities contributing to health, or its recovery (or a peaceful death), that he would perform unaided if he had the necessary strength, will or knowledge. It is likewise the unique contribution of nursing to help the individual to be independent of such assistance as soon as possible.

Because the focus of nursing includes not only the individual, with many unique physical, psychologic, and social needs, but also the family and the community, meeting these multiple needs requires multiple roles: caregiver, coordinator, teacher, advocate, collaborator, discharge planner, researcher, and manager.

In the caregiver role the nurse provides physical care to patients, and in the health care coordinator and manager roles the nurse acquires the resources necessary to ensure that the patient receives quality nursing care in a timely and efficient manner. As a discharge planner the nurse ensures continuity of appropriate care after the patient is discharged from an inpatient setting. As educator and patient counselor, the nurse's duties range from simple instruction in matters of hygiene to organizing and leading patient and family support groups. The nurse also serves in the important role of collaborator, because it is the nurse who provides the vital bridge between the various professional groups and the patient. However, nurses' primary concerns continue to be the promotion and maintenance of the highest level of health and in turn quality of life for each individual served.

Among the health care professions, the nursing profession has the unique distinction of claiming responsibility for the patient at all times during hospitalization. Nurses care for hospitalized patients 24 hours every day with no exceptions. No other professional group comes anywhere close to this sustained level of provider/patient contact. The scope and breadth of nursing's responsibility, combined with nursing's relationship to other health care providers, mandate that nurses encompass the roles of manager and leader. The nurse coordinates the care of the patient while directing the work of other nurses and ancillary workers, including licensed practical nurses.

Nurse as Caregiver

Many of the activities in the caregiver role are concerned with meeting the patient's basic needs of daily life. They include helping the patient meet needs for rest, sleep, food, and water and maintaining basic body functions such as toileting, removing secretions, and maintaining temperature. Another important aspect of this nurturing role is providing comfort and support during illness crises and in the face of death. Thus as a **caregiver**, the nurse not only meets hygiene and life-support needs, but also meets the emotional and psychologic needs that arise with deviation from good health. All the aspects of direct patient care are carried out in such a way that the patient's independence is maintained to the greatest possible extent, within the limitations of illness. In addition, nursing interventions take into consideration the sociocultural background of each patient.

Because of the intimate level of contact required in the caregiver role, a caring aspect is an important component of the nurse's role. The healing aspects of nursing are tied to compassion, understanding, and respect for the patient as a person of worth and dignity.

Nurse as Health Care Coordinator

As the health care provider responsible for patients' care 24 hours each day, the nurse serves as the primary coordinator of all other professional services committed to the care of the patients. In this role the nurse arranges for the necessary diagnostic testing, therapy, counseling, and patient teaching sessions and treatments. The care activities of other professionals are integrated into a nursing plan of care that orchestrates these activities with the cooperation and participation of the patient and the patient's family to allow for the provision of basic nursing and medical care.

Throughout the patient's hospitalization, the nurse must carry out the coordinator role in such a way that the patient's health is not compromised. For example, on the patient's return from a series of gastrointestinal studies, the nurse must notify the dietary department to send the patient's tray to maintain the appropriate nutritional status. During hydrotherapy for the treatment of burns, the proper scheduling of meals and pain medication is crucial to maintain the patient's level of comfort and to prevent nausea and vomiting.

Nurse as Teacher

A major component of the nurse's role is instructing the patient and family in aspects of self-care ranging from health maintenance activities to the care of acute and chronic conditions. The teaching role requires an understanding of learning in a variety of age groups. The nurse must also be aware of the influence of culture when instructing the patient in aspects of care, such as dietary management and the grieving process. For example, cultural norms regarding illness among Jews differ considerably from those of Native Americans.

With the advent of diagnostic related groups (DRGs) as the basis for reimbursement for medical care by both public and private insurers, many patients are being discharged earlier in the recovery stage than in the past. As a result of this trend toward shorter hospital stays, nurses in practice settings must embrace teaching as a primary role. Commonly this teaching not only is directed to the patient but also involves family members or significant others who must provide care during the home rehabilitation phase. For example, a patient may be discharged before having the opportunity to learn crutch walking. In this case a family member must be taught crutch walking to help the patient learn and practice this technique at the appropriate time at home.

The teaching role requires the skill to assess the patient's learning needs and level of learning ability and to design a teaching plan that encompasses cultural, socioeconomic, and personal needs. An important aspect of the teaching role is evaluation. It is not until learning is validated that teaching can be considered successful. Both the aspects taught and the patient's response should be documented in the charts.

Nurse as Discharge Planner

Problems such as inappropriately long inpatient stays, inadequate or inappropriate postdischarge care, and failure to utilize community resources led to the development of the discharge planning role in the health care delivery system.[37] The nurse is an appropriate person to operationalize this role, and today ensuring continuity of patient care during and after hospitalization is a major responsibility of the nurse.

Discharge planning begins on admission to an inpatient facility. On admission the nurse assesses the patient's physical, psychologic, and social needs and develops a plan of care for meeting these needs. This plan draws not only on the resources of the admitting institution but also on the patient's family. As the time for discharge nears the nurse uses information and assessments from throughout the patient's admission to identify postdischarge patient care needs and to develop a plan for meeting those needs. An integral part of that plan is identification of resources, such as family or community agencies, that can assist the patient in recovery or rehabilitation. Thus drawing on the roles of caregiver, coordinator, and teacher, the nurse acting in the discharge planning role helps the patient regain as normal and productive a life as possible. See Chapter 7 for more information.

Nurse as Advocate

As medical knowledge and technology have advanced, the health care system has become more complex. Patients entering the hospital today face a variety of health care providers, electronic devices to monitor body functions, and an environment characterized by many as "high tech/low touch." In this environment of tubes, alarms, and caregivers clad in gowns, goggles, masks, and gloves, the advocacy role of the nurse is more critical than ever.

In the advocacy role the nurse is responsible for defining, defending, and promoting the rights of patients (Table 5-1). For example, the nurse is in a pivotal position to safeguard the patient's right to informed consent before surgery. Also, the nurse is the logical person to interpret the different services offered by other professional health staff and to explain the types of and need for various prescriptions and treatments ordered by the physician. As an **advocate** the nurse is compelled to work on behalf of the patient.

Nurse as Collaborator

Health care today is so complex that care and caring cannot be relegated to any one provider's domain. To carry out the complex treatment plans needed as acuity levels rise and the general population ages, with more and more chronic diseases, collaboration by all involved in care delivery is crucial.

According to Styles,[26] collaboration involves four elements:

1. *Individuals* who share a common interest
2. *Purpose* for the collaborative effort
3. *Principles* or ground rules for the effort
4. *Structure* within which the effort takes place

Using this framework, nurses can effectively work with other members of the health care team to deal with patient care problems. For example, if a patient is unable to swallow medications, the nurse will col-

---

TABLE 5-1   Advocacy Roles in Nursing

	Active	Passive
Patient	Actions by the nurse reflect the nurse's responsibility and obligation to the patient. These actions stem from the nurse's personal and professional beliefs and standards.	Actions by the nurse may or may not reflect personal and professional standards and beliefs. Actions stem from the expectations/obligations imposed by institutional or societal norms and beliefs.
Social	Actions by the nurse reflect a responsibility and obligation to society. These actions stem from the nurse's personal and professional beliefs regarding general human rights and societal needs.	

From Becker PH: Advocacy in nursing: perils and possibilities, *Holistic Nurs Pract* 1(1):54, 1986.

laborate with the physician and the pharmacist to ensure that an appropriate medium for the drug in the right dosage is ordered.

The role of the collaborator can only be expected to grow as the care of patients becomes more complex and life expectancy lengthens while health care resources decline.

Nurse as Researcher

Every profession is built on a body of descriptive knowledge. Like other professions, nursing recognizes the need to identify, verify, and increase the body of scientific knowledge on which practice is based. Although the researcher role is viewed primarily as the responsibility of doctorally prepared nurses, all nurses can participate in the research process. It is appropriate for nurses practicing primarily as caregivers to help identify researchable problems and collect data.

For example, the bedside nurse is in an excellent position to help identify patients prone to falls, respiratory infections, or surgical complications such as phlebitis and urinary tract infections. Identification and validation by nurse researchers of patient profiles prone to complications allow for proactive nursing interventions that reduce the necessity for extended hospitalization and the accompanying costs.

The primary responsibility of the nurse in the caregiving role is to apply research findings in practice. Nursing research provides a theoretic foundation for practice, promoting its advancement and the welfare of those receiving nursing care.

Nurse as Manager

Delivering quality care in today's complex health care system requires managerial knowledge and skill. The nurse manager must know how to assess overall patient care needs, organize patient assignments, delegate work appropriately, and evaluate effectiveness. With the current emphasis on cost effectiveness, when managing patient care assignments, the nurse manager must consider both the efficiency and effectiveness of outcomes and must be knowledgeable about the budget process.

The nurse manager today must make efficient use of scarce resources. He or she must not only do more with fewer material resources, but also in many cases with fewer human resources. Thus nurse managers must know how to assess the strengths and weaknesses of staff and facilitate their ongoing professional development. Acquisition of new skills, as well as refinement of basic skills, can do much to increase staff efficiency and effectiveness.

MODELS FOR NURSING PRACTICE

Current models for the delivery of nursing care include functional nursing, team nursing, primary nursing, and the case management method. In addition, new models of practice are being developed and tested at institutions around the country.

Functional Model

Two factors joined to promote the development of the **functional model** of nursing. The first factor was the time and motion studies conducted in American industry in the 1930s. When models for analyzing industrial tasks were applied to nursing, it was found that nursing care could be described in terms of discrete tasks ranging from simple to very complex. The second factor was economic. As medical care increased in sophistication and therefore costs, it was no longer cost efficient to pay registered nurses to perform the less complex tasks associated with patient care. Thus the functional model of nursing care delivery was developed.

The functional model focuses on nursing jobs or tasks to be completed. Personnel are assigned responsibility for these tasks depending on their preparation and experience, with final responsibility resting with the person making the assignments. A patient receiving care based on this model may have one person to help with the bath and change the bed, another to administer medications, and yet another to perform more complex treatments, such as inserting a nasogastric tube.

The functional model is efficient and economic to administer; however, with the multiplicity of caregivers, care may be fragmented and some aspects of care, such as psychosocial needs, may be overlooked entirely.

Team Nursing

Team nursing grew out of dissatisfaction with the fragmentation that occurs with the functional model. Developed in the early 1950s by Lambertson,[42] team nursing involves the delivery of nursing care by a team of health care providers. The team is led by a professional nurse and usually consists of registered nurses, licensed practical nurses, and nursing assistants. The focus of team nursing is the provision of coordinated, individualized nursing care to a group of patients throughout a shift. The implementation of team nursing requires team conferences, nursing care plans, and the development of leadership skills.

The team method is less fragmented and more humanistic than the functional model. However, the patient may still feel that care is fragmented, and not all registered nurses have the leadership skills necessary to be a team leader.

Primary Nursing

Primary nursing was developed in 1963 by Hall[40] as a further response to the fragmentation of nursing care found in both functional and team nursing. In primary nursing one nurse is responsible for the care of a patient 24 hours each day, 7 days per week.

Ideally, the primary nurse assumes responsibility for a patient on admission and plans, coordinates, and supervises care throughout the admission. Although associates provide care when the primary nurse is off duty, the primary nurse is the frontline manager who communicates with other caregivers and coordinates care. Primary nursing utilizes the nurse in all professional roles—caregiver, coordinator, discharge planner, teacher, and advocate.

Case Management

With increased awareness of health care costs and government spending caps placed on reimbursement for health care, managed care and **case management** have become popular methods of cost containment for health care institutions. According to Brent,[8] managed care is a process that carefully controls health care benefits based on types, levels, and frequency of treatments, access to care, and amount of reimbursement paid for necessary health care services. Included in the managed care system is case management.

Many definitions of case management exist in the current literature. The 1980 Federal Budget Reconciliation Act defined case management as a specific group of services provided for a defined population of people.[15] In a more comprehensive example, Desimone[12] defines case management as "a systematic approach to: identify high-risk/high-cost patients; assessing opportunities to coordinate care; assessing and choosing treatment options; developing treatment plans to improve quality and efficacy; controlling cost; and managing a patient's total care to ensure optimum outcome."

Various case management models were identified by Brault and Kissenger.[7] These include private, social, primary care, insurance, and nursing case management. The registered nurse is identified as the only health care professional qualified to manage within all models. Functions of case management include assessment, planning, linking, monitoring/reassessment, advocacy, case finding, prescreening/gatekeeping, intake, cost containment, capacity building, and termination.[7] Effectiveness of case management within the various models must be addressed to determine feasibility.

A study of 21 case-managed and 21 comparison patients by Bigelow and Young[6] explored questions about implementation and effectiveness of case management services. They found that case-managed clients received more services, had fewer unmet service needs, experienced greater quality of life, and utilized less hospital time.

Developing Models of Practice

Since the early 1980s the Johns Hopkins University Hospital Nursing Department has taken a leading role in the development of innovative models of practice. Anticipating the changes to come in hospital reimbursement, the department sought ways to increase staff satisfaction and retention and thereby reduce the costs of recruitment and orientation of new employees. In addition, they also sought to make more efficient use of nursing personnel.

The first model they developed was the contract model.[34] In this model staff nurses accept responsibility for staffing levels, scheduling and coverage, performance appraisal, and, when necessary, disciplinary action. The nurse manager assumes the role of facilitator. Evaluation of this model revealed lower turnover rates and use of sick time by nurses on the contract unit than in the total institution. In addition, although costs of operation were fairly consistent throughout the institution, the contract model provided more hours of nursing care per patient day.

The second model developed at Johns Hopkins was a group practice model.[34] This model was a response to data indicating that the need for specialty nursing care, such as that provided by nurse practitioners in the emergency department, varies and is not met by rigid, fixed scheduling of nursing specialists. Under this model a group of nurse specialists practicing together shares responsibility with the nurse manager for staffing and scheduling, patient assignment, quality assurance, and peer review. Evaluation of this model showed a 38% increase in productivity per provider, an increase in employee satisfaction, and a decrease in sick days used.

EXPANDED ROLES IN NURSING

An expanded role in nursing is one in which a nurse assumes expanded or increased responsibilities in a practice area and, in most cases, practices with greater autonomy. Qualification for expanded roles comes through additional education and expertise and, in some instances, certification by examination. As the health care delivery system evolves to meet the challenges of rapidly developing scientific and technologic advances in an era of diminishing resources, expanded nursing roles will assume an increasingly important place in the system.

Nurse Practitioner

The **nurse practitioner** role is an expansion of the basic caregiver role. The nurse practitioner has advanced assessment skills and clinical expertise. Most nurse practitioners have masters' degrees in nursing or are graduates of a nurse practitioner program.

Nurse practitioners such as family nurse practitioners are generalists; others specialize in a specific area such as pediatrics or gerontology. They most commonly practice in community health centers, physicians' offices, schools, long-term care facilities, and HMOs. However, an increasing number of nurse practitioners are employed in occupational health settings and in the insurance industry. Their practice, unlike that of other nurses practicing in the advanced role, often includes the prescribing of medication. A nonpublished report from the ANA reported approximately 25,000 to 30,000 nurse practitioners in the United States in 1991.

Clinical Nurse Specialist

The **clinical nurse specialist** (CNS) has advanced clinical skills and knowledge in a particular area of practice, such as adult health or psychiatric/mental health nursing. Preparation for the CNS is usually at the master's level. Six major roles have been identified for the CNS[18]:

1. *Practitioner*—A primary function of the CNS is the provision of direct care to selected patients in any setting, including private practice.
2. *Teacher*—The advanced knowledge and skills inherent in the CNS role make the CNS an excellent teacher for patients, families, and other nursing staff.
3. *Consultant*—Consultant activities of the CNS include promoting collaboration with other professionals and health care agencies, identifying strategies to deliver more cost-effective patient care, establishing standards and definitions of nursing care, and identifying mechanisms of change in various sociopolitical, economic, and legislative arenas and in the system of health care delivery itself.[23]
4. *Researcher*—In this role the CNS conducts original research and replicates studies related to the area of specialization.
5. *Change agent*—The CNS works to bring about changes that improve patient care, promote communication among other health care personnel, and improve nursing practice.[18]
6. *Manager*—Although the management role is a relatively minor one, the CNS functioning in a line or management role contributes indirectly to patient care, usually through the procurement and management of material and human resources necessary for the delivery of care.

The CNS in a hospital setting gives direct patient care, advises other nurses, and coordinates care given by others. In ambulatory settings the CNS functions in a manner similar to the nurse practi-

tioner but limits practice to a specialty area. Recent literature points to the merging of the CNS and nurse practitioner roles.[13]

Nurse Clinician

The **nurse clinician** is a direct-care expert in a particular clinical area who may have advanced educational preparation. Attainment of the role is usually through peer review and may be associated with an institution-specific clinical ladder.

Nurse Midwife

The **nurse midwife** is the oldest of the expanded practice roles; the first school of midwifery opened in 1931.[17] Nurse midwives practice in hospitals or freestanding birthing centers; however, nurse midwives must always function within a medically directed health care system.

Nurse Anesthetist

The **nurse anesthetist** has advanced preparation in an accredited program of anesthesiology and is licensed to administer anesthetic agents under the direct or indirect supervision of an anesthesiologist (physician specializing in the administration of anesthesia). Nurse anesthetists are usually employed by hospitals, ambulatory surgical centers, or private anesthesiology practices.

EMERGING ROLES: LOOKING AT THE FUTURE

A number of social trends will probably play a role in influencing the future of nursing (see box on p. 74). The United States is already experiencing the consequences of decreased financial support for health care. The total cost of health expenditures for 1989 was 666.2 billion dollars. New practice settings such as ambulatory surgical centers and home health agencies have been developed in an effort to find more cost-effective, efficient methods of delivering health care. Likewise, inpatient facilities are developing models of patient care delivery that focus not only on quality nursing care, but also on staff satisfaction, with one goal being the reduction of costs through better staff retention.

Demographic changes in the population are having a major impact on the health care system. Today those over 65 years of age make up close to 13% of the population and generate 31% of national health expenditures.[32] This portion of the population is growing at almost twice the rate of the general population. As this trend progresses, "those making decisions about health-care financing are being forced to consider critically the price tag of on-

SOCIAL TRENDS THAT INFLUENCE NURSING'S FUTURE

Decreased financial support for health care
Demographic changes in the population
Increased cultural diversity in citizens
Proliferation of knowledge and computer information systems

From Poteet GW, Hodges LC: The future of nursing. In Vestal KW, editor: *Management concepts for the new nurse,* Philadelphia, 1987, JB Lippincott.

going and new programs developed to meet the increasing demands of a citizenry that is getting older and poorer."[24]

The United States is also experiencing an increase in cultural diversity among its citizens. It is projected that by 2000 the African-American population (13%) will continue to be the largest minority group in the nation.[30] The percentage of Mexican-American citizens, however, is projected to reach 11.2% of the total population by the year 2000, because of differences in birth rates among Mexican-American (93.2 per 1000), African-American (78.4 per 1000), Caucasian-American (65.2 per 1000), and Asian-American (58.1 per 1000) childbearing women.[27,31] The cultural diversity represented by the various minority groups presents special challenges to the health care system and to nurses striving to meet the health care needs of these populations.

The changing structure of the American family is also exerting an influence on health care. More than 21% of all households are headed by single parents, with 16% of these headed by a single woman,[29] and 56.8% of all women aged 16 years and over are employed outside the home.[27] Almost 24% of all births in 1990 were to unwed mothers; however, almost 57% of all African-American births in 1990 were to single women.[27] These structural changes are shifting family care responsibilities to a group—single women—that often lacks the economic and social supports necessary to carry them out. The health care system, including nursing, must adapt to meet the needs of this growing population.

Finally, the most significant trend influencing the future of nursing is the proliferation of knowledge. If the current increases in both volume and sophistication of new information continue, it is predicted that by the year 2000 we will have instant obsolescence of knowledge.[20] The implications for nursing practice and education are tremendous. Computer networks will be a vital part of health care delivery,

and those professions that embrace this technology will have opportunities to advance that have never before been experienced.

The cumulative effect of these trends is a climate of rapid change. As the health care delivery system adapts to meet the changes and challenges of the future, new roles for nurses will emerge.

The nurse of the future will be a knowledge worker. Job content will be reevaluated and redesigned to meet the demands of increasing knowledge in an environment of decreasing resources, and the gap between professional and technical nurses will widen. The "high tech/low touch" environment spawned by the knowledge explosion will be countered by a renewed emphasis on the humanistic and ethical aspects of health care. Guest relations, a concept borrowed from the hotel industry, will assume a more prominent role in the delivery of health care. Likewise, the advocate role will become increasingly important. Nurses will not only be consumer/patient advocates but also take an increasingly active role in community and political advocacy. If, indeed, nursing pursues the path to independent practice proposed by Orlando,[21] the health care system of the future will be fertile ground for nurse entrepreneurs.

The future offers almost limitless opportunities for nurses and nursing. Nurses of the future will practice in space, in colonies under the world's oceans, and in settings not yet conceived. As new frontiers of practice and health care delivery are opened, nurses will be leaders in the development and application of knowledge.

CRITICAL THINKING QUESTIONS

1 What is a profession?
2 Outline the responsibilities of a practicing medical-surgical nurse.
3 What is the role of the advocate?
4 Explain the differences between models of nursing practice.
5 Discuss what is meant by the expanded role of the nurse.
6 Which four trends are likely to influence nursing's future?

RESOURCES

1 American Nurses Association (ANA) 600 Maryland Ave., SW Suite 100 West Washington, DC 20024-2571 (202) 554-4444
2 American Organization of Nurse Executives (AONE) 840 N. Lake Shore Dr. Chicago, IL 60611 (312) 280-4190
3 Canadian Nurses Association (CNA) 50 The Driveway Ottawa, Ontario K2P 1E2 (613) 237-2133

4 Joint Commission on Accreditation of Health-care Organizations (JCAHO) One Renaissance Blvd. Oakbrook Terrace, IL 60181 (708) 916-5600

5 National League for Nursing (NLN) 350 Hudson St. New York, NY 10014 (212) 989-9393

BIBLIOGRAPHY

Current

1. American Nurses' Association: *Code for nurses with interpretive statements,* Kansas City, Mo, 1985, The Association.
2. American Nurses' Association: *Facts about nursing 86-87,* Kansas City, Mo, 1987, The Association.
3. Baldridge M et al: *National data book and guide to sources: statistical abstract of the United States,* ed 105, Washington, DC, 1985, US Department of Commerce, Bureau of the Census.
4. Bandman EL: The nurse as advocate in everyday ethics, *J NY State Nurses Assoc* 18(1):19, 1987.
5. Becker PH: Advocacy in nursing: perils and possibilities, *Holistic Nurs Pract* 1(1):54, 1986.
6. Bigelow DA, Young DJ: Effectiveness of a case management program, *Community Ment Health J* 27(2):115-123, 1991.
7. Brault GL, Kissenger LD: Case management: ambiguous at best, *J Pediatr Health Care* 5(4):179-182, 1991.
8. Brent NJ: Managed care: legal and ethical implications, *Home Healthcare Nurse* 9(3):8-10, 1991.
9. Brower HT: Advocacy: what it is, *J Gerontol Nurs* 8(3):141, 1982.
10. Crowder ELM: Historical perspectives of nursing's professionalism, *Occup Health Nurs* 33(4):184, 1985.
11. Curtin L: Ethics in nursing practice, *Nurs Management* 19(5):7, 1988.
12. Desimone B: The case for case management, *Contin Care* 3(7):22-23, 1988.
13. Elder RG, Bullough B: Nurse practitioners and clinical nurse specialists: are the roles merging? *Clin Nurse Specialist* 4(2):78-84, 1990.
14. Hall RH: The professions, employed professionals and the professional association. In *Professionalism and the empowerment of nursing,* Kansas City, Mo, 1982, American Nurses' Association.
15. Kane RA: Case management: ethical pitfalls on the road to high quality care, *QRB* 14:161, 1988.
16. Kozier B, Erb G: *Fundamentals of nursing: concepts and procedures,* Menlo Park, Calif, 1987, Addison-Wesley Publishing.
17. Lindberg JB: The nurse person: issues, practice options, and strategies. In Lindberg JB, Hunter ML, Kruszewski AZ, editors: *Introduction to person-centered nursing,* Philadelphia, 1983, JB Lippincott.
18. Menard SW: *The clinical nurse specialist: perspectives on practice,* New York, 1987, John Wiley & Sons.
19. Miller BK: Just what is a professional? *Nurs Success Today* 2(4):21, 1985.
20. Naisbitt J: *Megatrends,* New York, 1984, Warner Communications.
21. Orlando IJ: Nursing in the 21st century: alternate paths, *J Adv Nurs* 12(4):405, 1987.
22. Pellegrino ED: What is a profession? *J Allied Health* 12(3):168, 1983.
23. Poteet GW: Consultation, *Clin Nurse Specialist* 1(2): 1987 (editorial).
24. Poteet GW, Hodges LC: The future of nursing. In Vestal KW, editor: *Management concepts for the new nurse,* Philadelphia, 1987, JB Lippincott.
25. Styles MM: *On nursing: toward a new endowment,* St Louis, 1982, Mosby–Year Book.
26. Styles MM: Reflections on collaboration and unification, *Image* 16(1):21, 1984.
27. US Bureau of Census: *Current population reports,* series P-20, no. 454. *Fertility of American women: June 1990,* Washington, DC, 1991, US Government Printing Office.
28. US Bureau of Labor Statistics: *Employment and earnings and monthly labor review,* Nov, 1983.
29. US Department of Commerce, Bureau of Census: *CD 91-217, 1990 census of population and housing,* Washington, DC, 1991, US Government Printing Office.
30. US Department of Commerce, Bureau of Census: *Current population reports,* series P-25, no. 995. *Projections of Hispanic population: 1983-2080 (from highest series),* Washington, DC, 1986, US Government Printing Office.
31. US Department of Commerce Bureau of Census: *Current population reports,* supplement to P-25, no. 1018 (series 18). *Projections of the population of the United States by age, sex, and race: 1988 to 2080,* Washington, DC, US Government Printing Office (revised 1992).
32. US Department of Health and Human Services, Health Care Financing Administration, Bureau of Data Management and Strategy: *HCFA pub. no. 03325,* Washington, DC, 1991, US Government Printing Office.
33. Webb C: Professionalism revisited, *Nurs Times* 83(35):39, 1987.
34. York D, Fecteau DL: Innovative models for professional nursing practice, *Nurs Economic* 5(4):162, 1987.

Classic

35. American Nurses' Association: *Standards of medical-surgical nursing practice,* Kansas City, Mo, 1974, The Association.
36. Bixler GK, Bixler RW: The professional status of nursing, *Am J Nurs* 45(9):730, 1945.
37. Bixler GK, Bixler RW: The professional status of nursing, *Am J Nurs* 59(8):1142, 1959.
38. Bristow O, Stickney C: *Discharge planning for continuity of care,* Richmond, Va, 1974, Virginia Commonwealth University.
39. Flexner A: Is social work a profession? *School and Society* 1(26):901, 1915.
40. Hall L: A center for nursing, *Nurs Outlook* 11:805, 1963.
41. Henderson V: *The nature of nursing: a definition and its implications for practice, research, and education,* New York, 1966, MacMillan Publishing Co.
42. Lambertson E: *Nursing team organization and functioning,* New York, 1953, Teachers College Press.
43. Merton RK: The functions of the professional association, *Am J Nurs* 58(1):50, 1958.

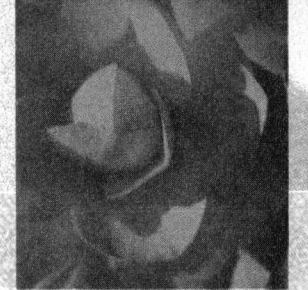

CHAPTER SIX

Clinical Decision Making Using the Nursing Process

LEARNING OBJECTIVES

1 Identify the components involved in clinical decision making.
2 Relate clinical decision making to nursing process.
3 Define the five steps of nursing process.
4 Apply the nursing process to patient situations.
5 Use clinical judgment processes to sort patient cues, formulate tentative hypotheses, and evaluate patient outcomes.
6 Select appropriate NANDA nursing diagnoses based on clinical assessment data.
7 Differentiate between actual and high-risk nursing diagnoses.

KEY TERMS

assessment, p. 80
clinical decision making, p. 77
collaborative problems, p. 87
decision analysis, p. 79
    decision tree, p. 78
North American Nursing Diagnosis Association (NANDA), p. 84

nursing diagnosis, p. 86
nursing process, p. 79
objective data, p. 83
problem-etiology-symptoms (PES), p. 86
subjective data, p. 82
symptom analysis, p. 82

THIS CHAPTER describes clinical decision making in nursing based on nursing process. Nursing process is a five-step cyclic process consisting of assessment of care needs, establishment of nursing diagnoses, planning of patient care, implementation of care, and evaluation of outcomes. Use of computerized systems to manage nursing process data and evaluation of outcomes is also addressed.

CLINICAL DECISION MAKING

Clinical decision making is the heart of nursing practice. Nurses make many crucial decisions regarding patient care. Clinical decision making in

nursing demands application of knowledge, acquisition of data from a myriad of resources, analysis of this information for planning purposes, and evaluation of outcomes. Nursing process provides the framework, or methodology, for clinical decision making in nursing.

Clinical decision making, or clinical problem solving, consists of searching for a solution to a patient problem. The components of clinical decision making are recognition of cues, development of inferences or meaning of the cues, generation of hypotheses or predictions of outcomes, and evaluation of results of interventions.

The first component of clinical decision making

requires identification of the cues, or clinical data, that form patterns identifiable as a patient care problem. Cues are defined as pieces of information; an example of a cue is a patient's statement: "I have pain in my hip when I walk." Other cues are observations made by the nurse, such as noting that a patient's finger joints are red, swollen, and warm to touch and that some of the reported laboratory values are elevated.

The second component of clinical decision making is to develop clinical inferences or to identify patterns that are formed by groups of cues. By synthesizing the cues of joint redness, swelling, and warmth, the pattern of chronic pain related to inflammation resulting from arthritis emerges. At this point the reported pain when walking may be related or may represent a cue to an entirely different patient care problem. A clinical inference is the clinician's speculation as to the pattern or relationship among the various cues, such as speculating that joint redness, swelling, and warmth are related to a single problem while recognizing that hip pain may be a cue representing an entirely different problem.

As a pattern of relationships among cues emerges, the clinician next forms tentative hypotheses as to the diagnostic term that explains the pattern of cues.[20] A nursing diagnosis is "a clinical judgment about individual, family, or community responses to actual or potential health problems/life processes. Nursing diagnoses provide the basis for selection of nursing interventions to achieve outcomes for which the nurse is accountable".[5] A nursing diagnosis is a statement that identifies patient care problems that can be resolved with nursing interventions.

The clinician next continues to seek additional information to confirm or eliminate the various tentative hypotheses being considered. This component of clinical decision making is termed hypothesis testing. At this point the nurse implements nursing interventions appropriate for the identified nursing diagnoses. Additional data are obtained to verify the effectiveness and outcomes of the interventions. The sequence of activities in clinical decision making is illustrated in Figure 6-1.

Developing Clinical Expertise

Both education and experience contribute to development of expertise in clinical decision making. Education provides knowledge of the science of nursing, whereas experience enables the clinician to verify application of nursing knowledge in patient situations. Becoming an expert in nursing practice requires study of the decision-making processes used by others.

Students are often viewed as "novices" in relation to their decision-making skills. Five stages of human performance described by Benner[14] are novice, advanced beginner, competent, proficient, and expert. On completing a basic nursing education program the new graduate is expected to perform as an advanced beginner. At this level the individual has attained sufficient experience to recognize situations that they have seen before. This individual functions at an acceptable level of performance by using learned guidelines to direct decisions. As the advanced beginner achieves a higher level of performance ability, the individual uses guidelines developed through experience as a basis for making clinical decisions.[14] Proficiency and expertise are achieved through experience and are noted by recognition of patterns derived from encountering similar events at some other time.

Clinical practice provides the arena in which the new graduate develops skill, accuracy, and efficiency in making clinical decisions.[8] Analysis of one's own decision and those of more experienced individuals fosters development of clinical expertise. Education and experience of the nurse directly affect clinical decision-making ability.[1,6] Figure 6-2 displays the relationship among education, clinical experience, and development of expertise in clinical decision making.

One method of analyzing decision making is to review clinical situations to identify consequences of alternative actions. Decision analysis using this approach is often represented graphically in an algorithm or **decision tree**. Using a decision tree forces the learner to identify a nursing care problem and its relationship to other situations. For example,

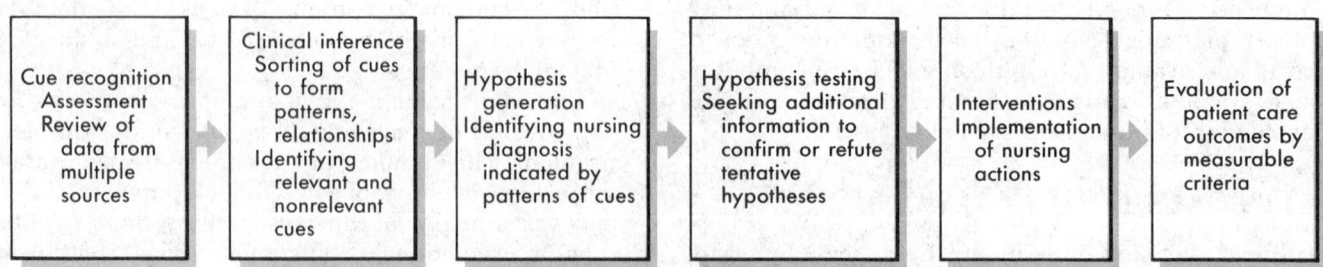

FIGURE 6-1   Steps in clinical decision making.

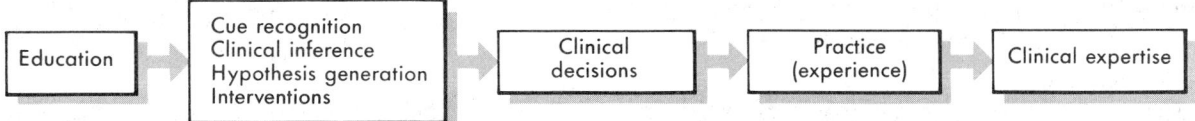

FIGURE 6-2   Application of decision making to clinical situations. Clinical decision making is a learned process. Education provides knowledge needed to identify cues, develop inferences, generate hypotheses, and determine interventions. Clinical decisions improve in efficiency and effectiveness with experience. (Adapted from Thiele JE, Holloway J, Murphy D, et al: Perceived and actual decision making by novice baccalaureate students, *West J Nurs Res* 13:618, 1991. Used with permission.)

suppose that a nurse is working an evening shift in a rehabilitation unit and receives a new patient about 8 PM in the evening. During the initial assessment the patient did not respond correctly to some questions, indicating that the patient was not totally aware of the new surroundings. In addition, a family member comments that "Dad sometimes gets up and wanders around the house at night. Several times he has fallen and bruised himself by running into furniture. We usually leave the lights on so that he won't hurt himself." The decision-making process begins at this point.

Decision analysis

Here is an example of how this hypothetical situation might be viewed using decision analysis. The first step in **decision analysis** is to identify the nature of the problem. From the information obtained in the interview, one appropriate inference is that the individual has altered thought processes with high risk for trauma to himself.

Next, the nurse must identify the alternative interventions available and the consequences of each. In this hypothetical situation, three separate interventions were identified: (1) apply restraints *or* (2) leave subdued lights turned on in the room *or* (3) administer medication for sleep that was prescribed by the admitting physician. Several outcomes may result from each nursing intervention. Figure 6-3 illustrates how this situation might be portrayed on a decision tree.

Each of the three alternative interventions has four potential consequences: (1) prevent injury to the person, (2) result in an injury, (3) prevent an injury but result in another problem, or (4) result in an injury and create an additional problem.

Decision analysis of this hypothetical situation yielded the following three potential nursing care interventions and four different consequences to each intervention. Analyzing clinical problems, alternative interventions, and consequences enables the nurse to recall this information the next time a similar event is encountered.

Review of situations such as this hypothetical event enables one to develop a repertoire of clinical events, including alternatives to care and potential consequences of different treatments. With accumulation of a large number of such events and their outcomes, the probability of certain consequences may be estimated.

NURSING PROCESS

Choosing between alternative actions requires that patient problems be correctly identified, alternatives be considered, and criteria for assessing the value of each outcome be available. These steps form the **nursing process.** The nursing process is a systematic method of delivering individualized nursing care consisting of assessment of patients, identification of nursing care problems, implementation of nursing interventions, and evaluation of the outcomes of care.[10] Nursing process is a thought process, a tool for intellectual decision making based on nursing knowledge. Use of nursing process assists nurses to organize their work and to expand the domain of nursing knowledge and practice. As noted by Henderson,[17] "the nursing process . . . is an analytical process that should be used by all health care providers when their intervention, or the help they offer, is of a problem-solving nature." Identification of actual and high-risk health problems that serve as the focus of care planning, implementation of care, and evaluation of patient care outcomes is the purpose of nursing process.

Nursing process is an interrelated series of steps. These steps are continuous in nature; each step is repeated many times as changes in the patient's health status alter the data base and require additional assessment, nursing diagnoses, planning, implementing, and evaluating of outcomes. The interrelationship of nursing process is shown in Figure 6-4.

Interaction between each step of nursing process is constant; nursing process is dynamic rather than static.[10] Changes in one step of the process affect each of the other steps.

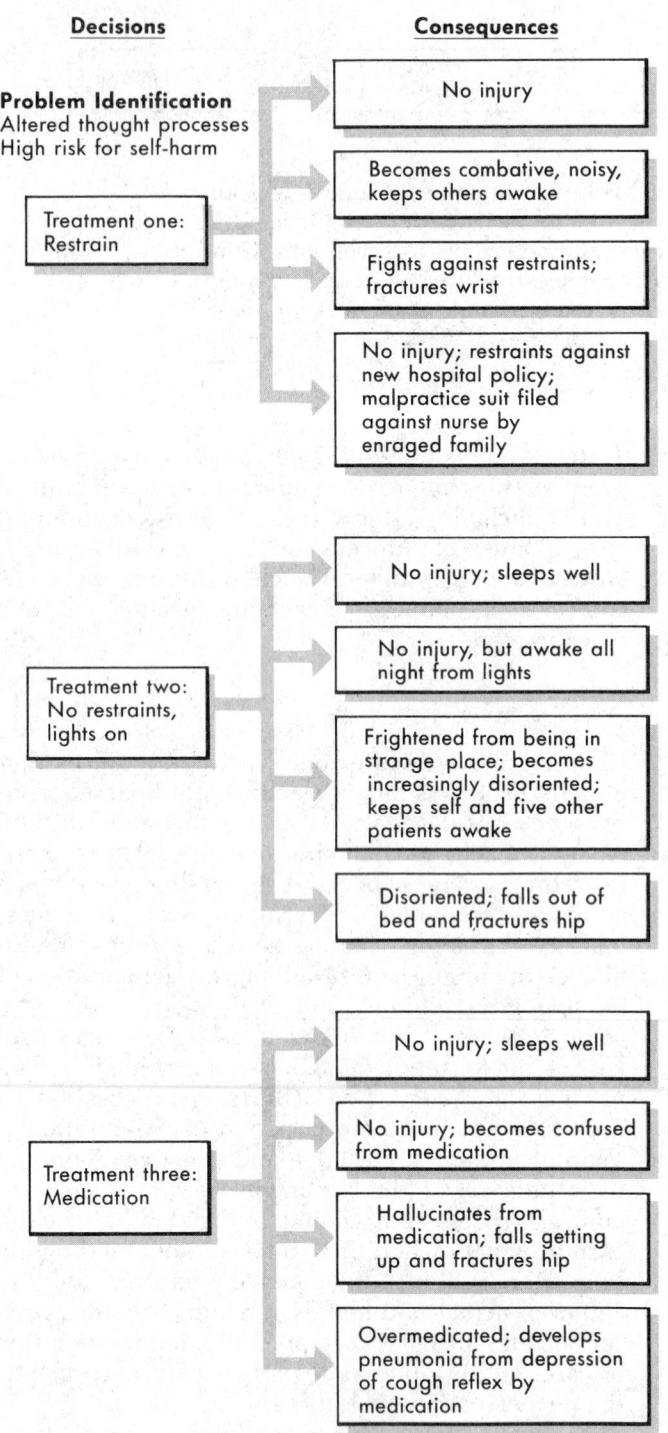

Decisions

Consequences

Problem Identification
Altered thought processes
High risk for self-harm

Treatment one:
Restrain

No injury

Becomes combative, noisy,
keeps others awake

Fights against restraints;
fractures wrist

No injury; restraints against
new hospital policy;
malpractice suit filed
against nurse by
enraged family

Treatment two:
No restraints,
lights on

No injury; sleeps well

No injury, but awake all
night from lights

Frightened from being in
strange place; becomes
increasingly disoriented;
keeps self and five other
patients awake

Disoriented; falls out of
bed and fractures hip

Treatment three:
Medication

No injury; sleeps well

No injury; becomes confused
from medication

Hallucinates from
medication; falls getting
up and fractures hip

Overmedicated; develops
pneumonia from depression
of cough reflex by
medication

FIGURE 6-3   Decision analysis process with possible outcomes.

Assessment

The first step in applying nursing process is assessment, or data collection. **Assessment** is defined as "the systematic observation and reporting of the patient's condition in all five realms of human experience—biological/physiological, environmen-

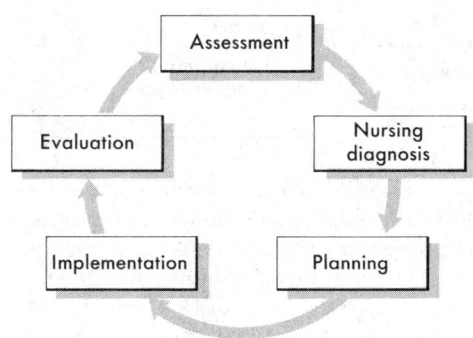

FIGURE 6-4   Steps of nursing process.

tal/safety, sociocultural/interpersonal belonging, psychological/self-esteem, spiritual/self-actualizing realms."[2] Obtaining data from a patient requires that the nurse look beyond obvious cues and clues and systematically seek relevant information pertaining to an individual's health or illness status. As the nurse performs assessments, the clinical cues obtained are categorized as either relevant or nonrelevant in the present situation. Accuracy in deriving clinical inferences is diminished by collecting excessive information and using nonrelevant cues as a basis for nursing decisions.[7] Relevant cues are used to develop nursing diagnoses; nonrelevant cues and those of low relevance are not acted on at the moment. For example, the box on p. 81 contains data obtained from a patient in an outpatient clinic.

In nursing assessment, physiologic, environmental, sociologic, psychologic, and cultural states of the individual are evaluated. Initially, the focus is on carefully observing and accurately documenting health alterations that account for an individual's seeking care. The nurse uses a systematic approach to health assessment to obtain data; most health care facilities provide a health history form for this purpose. The data base outline shown in the box on p. 81 lists the general categories of a thorough health assessment.

In the acute care setting the nurse has limited time for interviewing the patient and performing physical assessments. In many instances a total assessment is completed over several sessions rather than at one lengthy session. The patient may be able to participate in an interview for only a brief period of time. Both the physical assessment and interview questions must focus on identifying the immediate needs of the patient. With the focused interview the nurse begins by clarifying the intent of the interview and the anticipated time frame of the interview. This approach establishes a reason for the interview questions and directs the patient to specific areas of concern.

Once the purpose and time frame of the interview are established, the first few minutes of time are al-

EXAMPLE OF SORTING OF CLINICAL CUES

Clinical cues

Pain in substernal region
Profuse diaphoresis
Blood pressure 130/70
Pulse 122
Wears glasses
Previous cerebrovascular accident (CVA)
Nausea
Burning on urination
Decreased muscle strength in right side caused by CVA
Was watching TV when symptoms started

Sorting of these cues produced the following patterns:

Related cues

Pain in substernal region
Profuse diaphoresis
Blood pressure 130/70
Pulse 122
Was watching TV when symptoms started
Nausea

Clinical inference

Needs to be examined by a physician immediately
Potential acute medical emergency

Low-relevant cues

Burning on urination

Previous CVA
Decreased muscle strength in right side from CVA

Not of immediate concern; other cues potentially life threatening
Document finding; may indicate a potential problem requiring action after acute situation resolved
Same as above; may represent cues with implications for nursing care
Importance decreased, at the moment because of acute threat to life of other findings

Nonrelevant cue:

Wears glasses

Not of concern in present situation

---

lowed for the patient to express the reason for the clinic visit or hospitalization. A nondirective approach allows the patient to use his or her own words and verbal language style in responding to a question such as "What has caused you to seek health care at this time?" In addition to obtaining information, during this initial period the patient and nurse are establishing a nurse-patient relationship based on mutual trust.

Once the patient answers general questions about the present need for health care, focused questions that probe the specific areas of concern are used by the nurse to obtain information. Questions directly related to the symptoms presented and discussed by the patient are the topic of the interview. With the directed approach the nurse is attempting to obtain as much information as possible in a brief period of time. Focusing on the chief complaint, that is, the

DATA BASE OUTLINE

1. Biographic data
2. Reason for visit (chief complaint)
3. Present health status (general summary and symptom analysis; also known as history of present illness [HOPI])
4. Current health data
5. Past health status
6. Family history
7. Review of physiologic systems
8. Psychosocial history
9. Health maintenance efforts
10. Environmental health

From Bowers AC, Thompson JM: *Clinical manual of health assessment,* ed 3, St Louis, 1988, Mosby–Year Book.

specific reason for the present hospitalization, provides an organized approach for the interview.

One method of directing an interview that focuses on the reason or reasons for the present hospitalization or seeking of health care is to conduct a symptom analysis.[3] A **symptom analysis** involves reconstructing from the patient's own words the physical and mental processes underlying the major presenting symptom. For example, the following questions demonstrate the symptoms analysis process undertaken by the nurse during an interview with a 28-year-old male patient admitted to a medical unit with chest pain.

In a nondirective manner the nurse first asked general questions regarding the patient's present hospitalization. For example, the nurse said, "Tell me, what made you come to the hospital today." Nondirective questions provided a focus for the interview and developed mutual trust between the nurse and patient. Next, the nurse asked questions focused on the specific symptoms that resulted in the hospitalization.

"When did the pain begin?" was asked to identify the time of onset of the symptom. Other related questions are "What day did the pain begin?" and "What time did the pain begin?"

"What were you doing before the chest pain began?" This question probed for precipitating factors. Asking "Did the pain begin suddenly or slowly?" continues the refinement of the symptom analysis. As the nurse proceeds with the interview, additional questions such as the following may be asked: "Were you able to continue what you were doing when the pain occurred?"

"What did you do about the pain?"

"Does the pain interfere with other activities? walking? stair climbing? eating? recreation?"

By asking general and then specific questions the nurse identifies the immediate concern and obtains symptom-specific information. The box, left illustrates a general approach to conducting an interview for assessment data.

Use of assessment data requires the examiner to hypothesize or form tentative explanations of alterations in health identified during the course of taking a history and conducting a physical examination. To hypothesize or draw conclusions from the data the examiner must have a knowledge base of physical assessment. Once a full data base is obtained, identifying relevant and nonrelevant data is the next step taken by the nurse.

The nurse must decide which data are relevant and which are nonrelevant or of low relevance at the moment. Only relevant data require interventions at this time. By sorting data the nurse identifies patterns of cues that represent a particular patient problem. Cues that do not fit a pattern may represent a different problem or may be of little relevance to the present situation. For example, assessment of an individual admitted to an acute care facility with a diagnosis of pneumonia resulted in the findings shown in the box below.

When reviewing these findings the nurse realized that the "rash on the left and right elbows and forearms" was not consistent with the pattern of ineffective airway clearance related to tracheobronchial infection. The cues related to the rash require further investigation to determine the importance, if any, of this finding. For instance, the rash could be from working in a garden several days ago and be of no consequence to the present illness. However, the rash could also indicate a drug reaction, although the elbows and forearms are not typical sites for this. In either case, recording the finding prompts the nurse to obtain additional information related to the cause of the impaired skin integrity.

In addition to accurately recording data, the examiner must carefully differentiate between subjective and objective data. **Subjective data** are those pieces of information the patient provides that are the individual's own perceptions of health status. These personal perceptions of the patient cannot be validated by the nurse. Subjective data are state-

ASSESSMENT INTERVIEW PROCESS

Ask general, nondirected questions to:
   Establish mutual trust
   Identify areas for specific focus
Ask directed questions that:
   Focus on symptoms
   Analyze symptoms
   Narrow focus to specific concerns
Probe for precipitating factors that:
   Identify physiologic and mental effects of symptoms
Generate hypotheses that:
   Identify tentative nursing diagnoses

PATIENT CUES/ASSESSMENTS

Oral temperature of 38.3° C (101° F)
Rales, left and right lower lobes
Weakness
Moist cough
Fatigue
Rash on left and right elbows and forearms
Chest pain

ments from the patient such as "I feel tired" or "my throat hurts."

To prevent misinterpretation of information by other health care providers, subjective data are recorded in the patient's own words. For instance, write "The patient stated: 'I feel tired all of the time'" rather than "The patient was tired." Statements of subjective data are recorded as verbatim quotes from the patient.

Objective data are those pieces of information obtained by the examiner through observation, physical assessment techniques, laboratory results, or other physiologic measures. Objective data are verifiable; that is, the data are observable or measurable by other health care providers. Examples of objective data are the patient's weight, blood chemistry studies, and the patient's breath sounds as obtained by auscultation.

Care must be taken to record measurable observations, such as "3 cm bruise that is dark blue in color noted on outer aspect of left thigh." This description is more informative than stating "fairly large bruise seen on thigh." Later observations of the bruised area would result in noting changes in color and size, the basis for determining that healing is occurring. Table 6-1 displays examples of objective and subjective data.

Note that in Table 6-1 not all of the information matches. The statement "I feel I am overweight" is verified by the objective data of the patient's height and weight. The person who said "I'm so tired" has a low hemoglobin and hematocrit that could explain being tired. However, the statement "I feel hot" is not supported by the objective data, the patient's oral temperature. Remember that objective data are based on factual information, whereas subjective data are the individual's perceptions. Both objective and subjective data may be absolutely correct; however, as shown in the examples in Table 6-1 subjective data must be evaluated critically.

Health assessment data recorded by the nurse serve as the basis for planning, providing, and evaluating care. Computerized documentation systems streamline entry of assessment data into a patient's record. Often the physical assessment form used by a facility is entered into the computer. In many integrated computer systems these findings serve as an index to the patient's plan of care and are automatically entered into other appropriate sections of the patient's record. Documentation requirements to meet legal and accreditation standards, hospital policies, and professional standards are often incorporated into automated record-keeping systems.[2] For example, Standard I of the American Nurses' Association's *Standards of Medical-Surgical Nursing Practice*[12] states:

> The collection of data about the health status of the patient is systematic and continuous. These data are communicated to appropriate persons and recorded and stored in a retrievable and accessible system.
>
> Data are obtained by interview, physical examination, review of records and reports, and consultation.
>
> Priority of data collection is determined by the immediate physical condition of the patient.

This standard is augmented by use of computerized information systems that record changes in patient status automatically from physiologic monitoring devices and at specified intervals from manual data entry systems. Automated systems foster nursing process by incorporating the following data entry capabilities[11]:

- Nursing assessment data
- Nursing diagnoses with accompanying descriptors
- Goals and expected outcomes and time frame
- Interventions for each nursing diagnosis
- Progress notes, including evaluation of the plan of care and patient outcomes

The American Nurses' Association's *Standards of Medical-Surgical Nursing Practice*[12] provide criteria for evaluating effective application of nursing process. These standards are listed in the box on p. 84.

A definitive statement of patient care needs is provided by using nursing assessment data as the basis for establishing a nursing diagnosis.

Nursing Diagnosis

History

The concept of a classification scheme of health and illness problems that nurses diagnose and treat entered the nursing literature during the 1950s.[15,18] Diagnosing and treating human responses to illness were formalized by the 1973 *Standards of Nursing Practice* of the American Nurses' Association.[13] As diagnosing and treating health and illness problems became accepted functions of nursing, attention was directed toward development of a taxonomy or classification of human responses that are the purview

TABLE 6-1   Examples of Objective and Subjective Data

Objective data	Subjective data
Weight 65 kg, height 5'2"	"I feel I am overweight."
Hemoglobin 10.5 g, hematocrit 32%	"I'm so tired."
Oral temperature of 36.5° C (97.6° F)	"I feel hot."

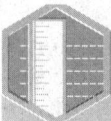

AMERICAN NURSES' ASSOCIATION STANDARDS OF MEDICAL-SURGICAL NURSING PRACTICE

Standard I

The collection of data about the health status of the patient is systematic and continuous. These data are communicated to appropriate persons and recorded and stored in a retrievable and accessible system.

Data are obtained by interview, physical examination, review of records and reports, and consultation.

Priority of data collection is determined by the immediate physical condition of the patient.

Standard II

Nursing diagnosis is derived from health status data.

Nursing diagnosis is a concise statement identifying the patient's problem(s). It is not a summary of all abnormalities.

Standard III

Goals for nursing care are formulated.

A goal is the end state toward which nursing action is directed.

Standard IV

The plan for nursing care prescribes nursing actions to achieve the goals.

The plan for nursing care describes a systematic method to meet the goals.

Standard V

The plan for nursing care is implemented.

The plan must be applied to achieve the goals.

Standard VI

The plan for nursing care is evaluated.

Patient response is compared with observable outcomes, which are specified in the goals.

Standard VII

Reassessment, reordering of priorities, new goal setting, and revision of the plan for nursing care are a continuous process.

The steps of the nursing process are used concurrently and recurrently.

From American Nurses' Association: *Standards of medical-surgical nursing practice,* Kansas City, Mo, 1974, The Association.

CATEGORIES OF HUMAN RESPONSE PATTERNS

- Exchanging: mutual giving and receiving
- Communicating: sending messages
- Relating: establishing bonds
- Valuing: assigning relative worth
- Choosing: selection of alternatives
- Moving: activity
- Perceiving: reception of information
- Knowing: meaning associated with information
- Feeling: subjective awareness of information

From North American Nursing Diagnosis Association (NANDA): *Taxonomy I revised,* St Louis, 1992, The Association.

of nursing. In 1973 the First National Conference for Classification of Nursing Diagnosis coordinated national efforts to develop a standardized classification system. The **North American Nursing Diagnosis Association (NANDA)** emerged from the 1973 meeting. Biennial meetings of NANDA continue the refinement and development of nursing diagnoses. Lists of approved nursing diagnoses are subjected to review and refinement at these conferences as part of national efforts to clarify the nursing diagnosis taxonomy.

In 1987 NANDA adopted Taxonomy 1, which classified each nursing diagnosis under one of nine patterns of human response. The box at left lists the nine patterns of human responses. Additional revisions occurred in 1989, 1990, and 1992. At the present time the complete taxonomy consists of a definition of each diagnostic term accompanied by a list of related factors, identified defining characteristics, desired outcomes, prioritized interventions, and documentation tips. The entire taxonomy of nursing diagnostic terms provides a set of interrelated clinical information that guides the assess-

NANDA-APPROVED NURSING DIAGNOSES

Activity intolerance
Activity intolerance, high risk for
Adjustment, impaired
Airway clearance, ineffective
Anxiety
Aspiration, high risk for
Body image disturbance
Body temperature, high risk for altered
Breastfeeding, effective
Breastfeeding, ineffective
Breastfeeding, interrupted
Breathing pattern, ineffective
Caregiver role strain
Caregiver role strain, high risk for
Communication, impaired verbal
Constipation
Constipation, colonic
Constipation, perceived
Decisional conflict (specify)
Decreased cardiac output
Defensive coping
Denial, ineffective
Diarrhea
Disuse syndrome, high risk for
Diversional activity deficit
Dysreflexia
Family coping, compromised, ineffective
Family coping, disabling, ineffective
Family coping: potential for growth
Family processes, altered
Fatigue
Fear
Fluid volume deficit
Fluid volume deficit, high risk for
Fluid volume excess
Gas exchange, impaired
Grieving, anticipatory
Grieving, dysfunctional
Growth and development, altered
Health maintenance, altered
Health seeking behaviors (specify)
Home maintenance management, impaired

Hopelessness
Hyperthermia
Hypothermia
Incontinence, bowel
Incontinence, functional
Incontinence, reflex
Incontinence, stress
Incontinence, total
Incontinence, urge
Individual coping, ineffective
Infant feeding pattern, ineffective
Infection, high risk for
Injury, high risk for
Knowledge deficit (specify)
Noncompliance (specify)
Nutrition, altered: less than body requirements
Nutrition, altered: more than body requirements
Nutrition, altered: potential for more than body requirements
Oral mucous membrane, altered
Pain
Pain, chronic
Parental role conflict
Parenting, altered
Parenting, high risk for altered
Peripheral neurovascular dysfunction, high risk for
Personal identity disturbance
Physical mobility, impaired
Poisoning, high risk for
Post-trauma response
Powerlessness
Protection, altered
Rape-trauma syndrome
Rape-trauma syndrome: compound reaction
Rape-trauma syndrome: silent reaction
Relocation stress syndrome

Role performance, altered
Self-care deficit, bathing/hygiene
Self-care deficit, feeding
Self-care deficit, dressing/grooming
Self-care deficit, toileting
Self-esteem, chronic low
Self-esteem, situational low
Self-esteem disturbance
Self-mutilation, high risk for
Sensory/perceptual alterations (specify visual, auditory, kinesthetic, gustatory, tactile, olfactory)
Sexual dysfunction
Sexuality patterns, altered
Skin integrity, impaired
Skin integrity, high risk for impaired
Sleep pattern disturbance
Social interaction, impaired
Social isolation
Spiritual distress (distress of the human spirit)
Spontaneous ventilation, inability to sustain
Suffocation, high risk for
Swallowing, impaired
Therapeutic regimen (individual), ineffective management of
Thermoregulation, ineffective
Thought processes, altered
Tissue integrity, impaired
Tissue perfusion, altered (specify type: renal, cerebral, cardiopulmonary, gastrointestinal, peripheral)
Trauma, high risk for
Unilateral neglect
Urinary elimination, altered
Urinary retention
Ventilatory weaning response, dysfunctional
Violence, high risk for: self-directed or directed at others

From North American Nursing Diagnosis Association (NANDA): *Taxonomy I revised*, St Louis, 1992, The Association.

ment, planning, intervention, and evaluation of nursing process applications to patient care situations.

The nursing diagnoses currently approved by NANDA[5] are listed in the box above. Under the leadership provided by NANDA, nursing diagnosis has evolved from a vague concept to standard terminology and classifications subjected to rigorous research for evaluation and validation. Currently more than 60 nursing diagnoses have been identified by NANDA, and more are being tested and evaluated. Continued change in wording, use, and classification of nursing diagnoses may be anticipated.

Definition

A **nursing diagnosis** is a clinical judgment that results from application of nursing process to health problems of patients. The current definition of nursing diagnosis by NANDA is as follows:

> Nursing diagnosis is a clinical judgment about individual, family, or community responses to actual and potential health problems/life processes. Nursing diagnoses provide the basis for selection of nursing interventions to achieve outcomes for which the nurse is accountable.

Writing nursing diagnoses

The purpose of writing nursing diagnoses is to provide consistent, concise statements of the interpretation of nursing assessment data. Nursing diagnosis statements describe the nature, source, and manifestations of health changes that the professional nurse is licensed to identify and to treat by independent and interdependent nursing interventions. A nursing diagnosis identifies by name the conclusions or inferences resulting from the thought processes and clinical judgment of the skilled nurse. Nursing diagnosis is an integral part of nursing process because it provides a common language for identifying patient problems and assists in the selection of nursing interventions.

A nursing diagnosis may be written in relation to

 **RESEARCH BRIEF**

Grant JS, Kinney M: Altered level of consciousness: validity of a nursing diagnosis, *Res Nurs Health* 13:403-410, 1990.

This study describes the processes undertaken to establish the validity of the nursing diagnosis altered level of consciousness (ALC). The methodology included use of four rounds of Delphi technique to obtain data. Magnitude estimation scaling technique was used to ascertain the agreement of neuroscience nursing experts with the defining characteristics of ALC.

Description of the processes used to examine the validity of ALC supports establishment of this nursing diagnosis. Multiple dimensions of the diagnosis of ALC were identified in this study and warrant further investigation. In particular, ALC was found to encompass two dimensions that may be more appropriately applied as separate nursing diagnoses: ALC, content, and ALC, arousal. The authors recommended additional study of the defining characteristics and operational definitions of the nursing diagnoses.

either an actual or a high-risk (formerly potential) nursing problem. The preferred wording of an actual nursing diagnosis is to write a three-part statement beginning with the NANDA diagnostic problem term or terms, the etiologic factor or factors, and the signs and symptoms.

For example, suppose you were caring for an elderly man who had a cerebrovascular accident (CVA) 3 years ago. The man is bedridden and incontinent of urine from lack of muscle tone. As described by Gordon[16]:

> There are three essential components in a nursing diagnosis; they have been referred to as the **PES format.** The three components are the health problem (P), the etiological or related factors (E), and the defining characteristics or cluster of signs and symptoms (S).

The PES format is used to write a diagnostic statement for an actual nursing diagnosis. The words "related to" connect the problem and the etiology, whereas "as manifested by" is used to connect the etiology and the signs and symptoms. The PES format is diagramed as follows:

P: Health problem E: Etiology S: Signs and symptoms
(as related to)   (as manifested by)

Next, the nurse consults a textbook or manual that lists nursing diagnoses. The diagnosis of "altered urinary elimination" matches the health problem, etiology, and signs and symptoms described. The elderly individual described above presents the characteristics of the diagnosis of altered urinary elimination: alteration in patterns of (problem), as related to loss of muscle tone (etiology), as manifested by incontinence, nocturia, and dribbling (signs and symptoms). This nursing diagnosis is an excellent description of health alterations identified by assessment of the individual. If, however, the incontinence is not consistently present or is related to specific activities, this diagnosis would not be appropriate. In such an instance the individual has a health problem, but further assessments are needed to verify the appropriate nursing diagnosis.

An actual nursing diagnosis is written using the PES format when clinical evidence of the descriptive characteristics of the diagnosis is identified through various assessments. High-risk nursing diagnoses describe those events that may occur unless vigorous preventive interventions are initiated by the nurse.

A high-risk nursing diagnosis is written to indicate that a particular nursing diagnosis has a strong likelihood of occurring but is not manifested at present. The elderly gentleman in the previous example is at high risk for developing skin excoriation and irritation from the urine. The nursing diagnosis of high-risk skin integrity impairment related to impaired urinary control is appropriate for this situation. A

EXAMPLE OF HIGH-RISK NURSING DIAGNOSIS

High-risk nursing diagnosis
+
Source or etiology
An example of a high-risk nursing diagnosis is as follows:
High-risk of skin integrity impairment
related to irritation from urinary incontinence

high-risk nursing diagnosis is written as a two-part statement that identifies the potential problem and its cause. Remember that a high-risk nursing diagnosis is likely to occur but has yet to be evidenced by signs and symptoms; therefore the third part of the nursing diagnosis statement, the "as manifested by" is not present. The box above presents an example of a high-risk nursing diagnosis.

Unless vigorous preventive actions are undertaken, tissue impairment or breakdown from urine on the skin is exceedingly likely to occur, thus the designation of a high-risk nursing diagnosis.

Collaborative problems

The term **collaborative problems** is used to describe health problems that require both nursing and medical intervention to diagnose, prevent, and treat. Carpenito[4] defines collaborative problems as "the physiological complications that have resulted or may result from pathophysiological and treatment-related situations. Nurses monitor to detect their onset/status and collaborate with medicine for definitive treatment."

Planning

The third step of nursing process is planning of care. After the nurse has obtained assessment data and interpreted these data into nursing diagnostic statements, the next step is to identify goals or outcomes of care. These statements provide direction to the care given and criteria for the evaluation of that care. Planning is the nursing process step in which the nurse decides how to best provide care that is organized, goal directed, and individualized. Planning of care involves setting priorities for care, de-

RESEARCH BRIEF

Zickuhr MT: American Society of Post Anesthesia Nursing. In Carroll-Johnson RM: *Classification of nursing diagnoses: proceedings of the Ninth Conference,* Philadelphia, 1991, JB Lippincott.

This paper was presented at the Ninth Conference for the Classification of Nursing Diagnoses, held in 1990. The author described a method for using nursing diagnoses as the focus of charting in a rapid care setting. A folding flow sheet was developed to foster nursing process–based charting in a postanesthesia care unit (PACU). Standards of postanesthesia nursing were used as the source of the most common nursing diagnoses for the PACU. The 12 nursing diagnoses most relevant to the PACU were identified and printed on the flow sheet. Charting used the following initials:

P = Problem
E = Etiology
S = Symptoms
EO = Expected outcome
I = Interventions
O = Outcome

Rather than write notes in longhand, identified problems on the printed lists were designated by one of the above initials. Standards of care for each problem served as the basis for designating interventions and outcomes. Use of the flow sheet enabled a combination of initials and check marks to designate the presence of a nursing care problem and the accompanying nursing diagnosis, the intervention, and resolution as shown by the patient's meeting the designated outcome criteria.

Using this PES-EO-IO charting system resulted in nursing process– and nursing diagnosis–based documentation 100% of the time! Documentation of etiology, symptoms, and expected outcomes was accomplished in a timesaving manner. The care plan that resulted was efficient to use, met standards and protocols for the PACU, and avoided duplication of documentation. In this unit the PES-EO-IO charting system integrated nursing diagnosis and nursing process as the structure for development of outcome-based plans of care.

termining expected patient outcomes, identifying nursing actions and interventions, and documenting the care given.

Setting priorities

Planning of care begins with identification of the priority of patient problems. Obviously, life-threatening problems must be dealt with immediately. Prioritize problems that are not life threatening as shown in the box below.

A prioritized list of problems results from careful consideration of non–life-threatening problems. Next, the patient's health status, the nurse's knowledge of actual and high-risk problems, and assignments for the day must be considered. The problems that the nurse and the patient will be able to work on in the time allotted for patient care are selected.

The identified and prioritized nursing care problems are recorded on the care plan. In general, nursing care problems are listed from highest to lowest in priority. Use of a taxonomy of nursing diagnoses assists with determining nursing care priorities in relation to identified assessment data. As changes in the health status of the patient occur, the priorities are reevaluated and the plan of care revised in accord with the new priority listing.

Determining expected patient outcomes

Following identification of patient problems from the assessment data, the expected outcomes or goals of nursing care are written. Goals are always patient centered. Standard II of *Medical-Surgical Nursing Practice* specifies that nursing care goals are formulated. The expected goal or outcome of providing nursing care is manifested as a change, resolution, improvement, or deterioration in the patient's prob-

lem. As a result of nursing interventions, the problem statement portion of the nursing diagnosis is expected to be modified. For example, suppose that the elderly man referred to earlier in this chapter developed dry, cracked mucous membranes of the mouth and lips. The nurse visiting in the home observed that the urine in the urinary collection system was dark in color and small in volume. On talking to family members the nurse was informed that the man had a diagnostic test performed yesterday that required him to go without food or drink for 16 hours. After the test was completed and the individual was home, he was too tired to eat or drink.

Review of NANDA diagnoses and defining characteristics indicated that the nursing diagnosis of altered oral mucous membranes related to NPO (nothing by mouth) status described the grouping of signs and symptoms observed in the individual. One desired outcome for this nursing diagnosis is to identify causes of the disorder. An intervention is to promote fluid intake adequate to prevent dehydration. A textbook of nursing interventions discussed restoring intake, particularly liquids, and monitoring changes in the mouth and mucous membranes and amount and color of urine output as appropriate nursing actions for this nursing diagnosis.

The goals of nursing care indicate a change in the first half of the nursing diagnosis statement. In this situation, effective nursing care would be demonstrated by a change (an improvement) in the altered oral mucous membranes. Outcomes or goals of care should indicate desired changes that are consistent with improvement in health status. Goals are written in clear, concise, measurable terms that serve to monitor progress.

A time frame in which improvement may be observed is included in the goal statement. In this instance the specification of "within 24 hours" is a reasonable time in which to produce an improvement. When feasible, goals should state specific amounts of an intervention. In this situation the goal may state that the individual is to consume 1600 mL of liquids per day (a measurable amount of the intervention).

Stating a realistic time for achieving the goal (such as within 24 hours) and measurable indicators of the changes (urinary output of 1200 to 1500 mL per 24 hours) provides observable, measurable indicators of the effectiveness of the planned interventions for resolution of the health disruption. Expected outcomes or goals are written in clear, concise, measurable, realistic terms that identify changes in the patient's problems that are expected as a result of effective nursing actions. The goals or outcomes of care serve as evaluation criteria, or indicators, of effects of nursing interventions. Many facilities use standards of care as the evaluation criteria for determining effectiveness of nursing care.

PRIORITIZING NON–LIFE-THREATENING PATIENT PROBLEMS

1. Decide which problems are potentially life threatening if not resolved. These problems must be resolved before they become life threatening.
2. Determine which problems are contributing to others. Reduction or resolution of contributory problems may have a positive effect on several other problems.
3. Decide which problems must be resolved *before* others can be addressed. For example, perhaps an individual must understand the nature of diabetes and relationship to insulin use before being willing to learn to administer insulin.

Identifying nursing interventions

Writing nursing interventions becomes easy once the goal is established. Asking the question, "What is needed to achieve the goal?" is useful. In this instance, providing sufficient liquids to increase the moisture to the mucous membranes and to achieve a satisfactory urinary output are all indicated. These activities may be written as separate interventions in this manner:

PLANNED INTERVENTIONS

1. Provide 100 to 200 mL of liquids every 2 hours between 7 AM (awakening time) and 7 PM (2 hours before bedtime).
2. Monitor urinary output for 24 hours. (A written record of the output serves as a portion of the basis for evaluation of effectiveness of nursing interventions.)

Nursing interventions are written to address the etiology or related factors portion of the nursing diagnosis statement. That is, the nursing interventions are directed toward altering the cause of the nursing diagnosis.

The section of the plan of care termed rationale provides a brief explanation of the reason for the nursing diagnoses, goals, and planned interventions. This information is often used for explaining to the patient and others involved in providing care the reason or reasons for performing interventions. For example, the rationale for assessment of specific gravity of urine could be written as follows: specific gravity is elevated (>1.025) when dehydration is present. Textbooks of nursing and biologic sciences are excellent sources for identifying scientific rationales for nursing care.

Writing nursing care plans

In most health care facilities a nursing care plan is written for each patient. Although each facility may use a different format, the typical care plan consists of the following information: assessment data, nursing diagnoses and collaborative problems, nursing actions or interventions, and expected outcomes or goals of nursing care. In addition, some facilities request a list of the rationale for the planned actions. In this text we have chosen to include rationale for action to assist the reader in learning the scientific basis for providing nursing care.

The purpose of written care plans in health facilities is to document patient needs, results of nursing interventions, and outcomes of care. Care plans identify nursing care to be given to each individual patient and direct the focus of documentation of changes in the patient's health status.

Care plans serve as a legal base for verifying that nursing care was provided according to accepted standards of professional practice. Careful attention is given to documentation of nursing interventions; care plans are used to validate costs of care for insurance claims, medicare, and home health care. Documentation on care plans serves as a record of the appropriateness of care and level of practice of individual nurses. Many care settings are beginning to use nursing process as recorded on care plans as a basis for assessing fees for nursing care.

Data obtained in the assessment step of nursing process form the basis for developing nursing care plans. Nursing diagnoses are written after the nursing assessments have been conducted and analyzed. Expected patient outcomes or goals are derived from the problem statement portion of the nursing diagnosis. Reduction or resolution of the identified problem is the expected result of nursing care. Nursing interventions address the etiology portion of the nursing diagnosis and identify nursing actions that are to be implemented to achieve the goals or expected outcomes. Identification of the rationale for nursing care links scientific principles with nursing interventions.

The nursing process step of planning results in a written care plan for a patient. Nursing assessment data and interpretations of assessment data written as nursing diagnoses are the basis for writing a care plan. A care plan consists of the nursing diagnoses, expected outcomes or goals of care, and nursing actions or interventions. In addition, the rationale, evaluation criteria, and nursing assessment data may be placed on the care plan. Clinical judgment processes are activated throughout each aspect of nursing process. Decision making is required to bring order and organization from the multitude of cues present in any patient situation.

Implementation

The fourth phase of nursing process, implementation, is the step in which the care is actually given. Rather than being a totally separate step, implementation requires that the nurse continue all phases of the nursing process. While providing care, the nurse also performs additional assessments; data obtained are used as the basis for identifying other appropriate nursing diagnoses and serve as the source for modifying existing outcomes and interventions.

Nursing interventions include direct patient care given by the nurse, assisting the patient with care, teaching the patient and family, and monitoring the patient. Each of the nursing activities must be accurately documented. Both checklists and narrative documentation are employed for recording nursing interventions; each agency will have forms for documentation purposes and policy guidelines. Many agencies add standards or protocols for interventions to the care plan form. In this way the actual and expected patient outcomes can be quickly compared. Patient progress or alterations in health can be quickly evaluated and acted on by caregivers. Placing standards of care as a concomitant part of the nursing progress record ensures that the standards are met.

In addition to written documentation, verbal reports, such as those reports given at the end of a shift, are based on the results of changes noted in the patient status as interventions are performed. Reports, either written or narrative, are easily organized and presented by following the nursing process steps. The report begins with the nursing diagnoses, including both independent and collaborative (interdependent) problems that have been identified. Next, the nursing interventions that have been delineated are indicated, followed by the expected outcomes and time frame for achieving these goals. Progress noted toward meeting these outcomes is then reported. In this manner, outcomes that have been met or those that are not being achieved can be evaluated and changes in the care plan made according to specific, measurable, observed data.

Evaluation

The last phase of nursing process is evaluation. Evaluation signals the start of nursing process, rather than the end. That is, the evaluation step of nursing process should be considered as recycling, or starting the process anew. The bases for evaluating nursing care are the outcome criteria that are listed on the care plan. Evaluation serves as an indicator of the progress of the patient toward meeting stated goals.

Goal achievement is evaluated by comparing each goal with the patient's actual accomplishments. The results of evaluation indicate whether each goal has been totally met, partially met, or not met. In all three circumstances, comparison of goals and accomplishments provides a basis for modifying goals.

Evaluation of patient outcomes is an essential step in the nursing process. Measures of outcome criteria are used in conjunction with quality assurance programs, nursing audits, standards for nursing practice, and accreditation of hospitals. Objective evaluation requires (1) focusing on the patient to assess the extent to which desired outcomes have been achieved and (2) reviewing the nursing care plan to identify needed changes.

Obtaining assessment data, grouping similar pieces of information, and formulating tentative hypotheses from the grouped information are the most critical aspects of nursing process. Assessment data that the nurse obtains must be sufficient in depth and breadth to enable the nurse to formulate a nursing diagnosis. In like manner, assessment data form the basis for modifying the nursing diagnosis. When evaluating patient care outcomes, the nurse asks:

"What additional patient data are needed? What is the source of these data? Do these data support the tentative nursing diagnosis?" Table 6-2 illustrates the questions to be considered in evaluating nursing process outcomes.

Critical evaluation of nursing care outcomes requires comparison of assessment data obtained from the patient with expected or predicted progress of the patient toward the written outcome criteria. This

TABLE 6-2   Evaluation Considerations for Care Plans

Component	Questions/considerations
Patient assessment	What additional data are needed?
	What is/are the source or sources of data?
	What information has been documented (i.e., recorded)?
Nursing diagnoses	Are these clear? Correctly stated?
	Are the diagnoses supported by the grouping of patient data (i.e., the cues and clues identified as objective and subjective data)?
	Do the identified defining characteristics support the nursing diagnosis?
Outcome criteria	Are these stated in a realistic manner?
	Are these achievable by the patient?
	In the time frame stated?
	Are these stated in such a manner that the nurse can measure achievement toward the goal?
	Do short-term goals and long-term goals reflect progression in health status of the patient?
	How close to being accomplished are the outcome criteria?

review identifies areas in which modification of the recorded plan of care is needed. For instance, if the patient outcome stated "will gain 10 pounds over a 3-month period," weighing the patient provides objective data indicating progress toward this goal. If after 2 months the patient's weight has increased by only 1 pound, reevaluation of the nursing interventions is indicated. Additional data should be obtained to determine why the interventions were not effective. Further assessment may indicate that the patient is being served between-meals snacks of eggnog and milkshakes and does not like either of these beverages. Recording this information on the care plan and modifying the interventions are indicated.

Identification and treatment of patients with actual and high-risk nursing diagnoses occur through systematic application of each step of the nursing process. Evaluation of nursing process is the critical review of actual patient outcomes as compared to expected outcomes and modification based on assessment data. Revision of the care plan occurs as a result of evaluation. Evaluation is often performed concurrently with other phases of nursing process, rather than as a distinctly different step. The results of evaluation are a return to the initial steps of nursing process, obtaining and analyzing data, developing nursing diagnoses, and revising and updating the care plan.

Modifying the care plan

A single nursing diagnosis may have multiple expected outcomes, interventions, and rationales. Once written, a care plan is dynamic rather than static. That is, care plans are reviewed and revised according to changes in the patient's condition. Writing specific, measurable expected outcomes or goals and precise interventions fosters revising care plans. The extent to which outcomes are achieved is determined by matching actual assessments of the patient's response to nursing interventions with the expected outcomes.

If the goals have been totally met, perhaps the goal needs to be increased or is no longer needed. Goals that are partially met or not met at all may need to be discussed with the patient or family; perhaps the goal is unrealistic or misunderstood by the patient. By discussing goals with the patient, the nurse can determine that goals are patient centered and are consistent with the patient's expectation. Review of each goal culminates with a statement indicating progress toward fulfilling it. These statements are written in the patient's record of nursing care. Developing specific outcome criteria is the vital step in evaluating the progress of a patient toward improved health status.

Evaluation is a separate activity when formal evaluations such as chart audits and quality assurance reviews are conducted. The purpose of formal evaluation is to review the quality of nursing care as shown by the written documentation. Such formal evaluation procedures point out the need for consistent, thorough documentation throughout all aspects of nursing process.

Computerization and Nursing Process

With the development of a taxonomy of nursing diagnoses and defining characteristics, computers and nursing process have a lot in common. Use of computers for recording nursing process information is consistent with the American Nurses' Association's *Standards of Nursing Practice,*[13] which stipulates that nursing care is to be based on nursing diagnosis, with specific interventions and evaluation consistent with the nursing diagnosis. Automated patient records systems are available that link nursing assessment data to the care plan and documentation of care.

Computerization of nursing process fosters research and refinement of nursing diagnoses by providing data in legible, consistent, accessible form. Computerization reduces the "manual labor" of recording information by hand and promotes analysis and synthesis of nursing data by professional nurses. Use of nursing process in a diagnostic problem-solving approach is promoted by computerization of nursing records. As nursing process data accumulate, the words of Florence Nightingale[19] may need to be recalled:

> In dwelling upon the vital importance of *sound* observation, it must never be lost sight of what observation is for. It is not for the sake of piling up miscellaneous information or curious facts, but for the sake of saving life and increasing health and comfort.

CRITICAL THINKING QUESTIONS

1 Explain the following steps of clinical nursing decision making:
   a. Recognition of cues
   b. Development of inferences
   c. Generation of hypotheses
   d. Evaluation of results
2 Describe the relationship of clinical decision making to nursing process.
3 Define the five steps of nursing process.
   e. Discuss the relationship between each step.
   f. Discuss the contribution of each nursing process step to patient care outcomes.
4 Describe the differences between subjective and objective data in relation to:
   g. Source or sources
   h. Interpretation

  i. Documentation

  j. Use in planning patient care

5 Describe techniques of a general approach interview for assessment purposes.

6 Discuss nursing diagnoses in relation to:

  k. History of development

  l. Purposes

  m. Uses

  n. Statement (format)

7 Differentiate between the following types of nursing diagnoses:

  o. Actual

  p. High risk

8 Discuss a process for analyzing consequences of clinical decision making.

9 Review the steps to take in determining an appropriate nursing diagnosis for a patient.

BIBLIOGRAPHY

Current

1. Benner P, Tanner CA: Clinical judgment: how expert nurses use intuition. *Am J Nurs* 87:23, 1987.
2. Bircher AC: Nursing diagnosis: an overview. In D'Argenio C, editor: *Implementing nursing diagnosis-based practice: managing the change*, Gaithersburg, Md, 1991, Aspen Publications.
3. Bowers AC, Thompson JM: *Clinical manual of health assessment*, ed 2, St Louis, 1988, Mosby–Year Book.
4. Carpenito LJ: *Nursing diagnosis application to clinical practice*, ed 2, Philadelphia, 1987, JB Lippincott.
5. North American Nursing Diagnosis Association (NANDA): *Taxonomy I revised*, St Louis, 1992, The Association.
6. Pardue SF: Decision making skills and critical thinking ability among associate degree, diploma, baccalaureate and master's prepared nurses, *J Nurs Ed* 26:354, 1987.
7. Radwin LE: Research on diagnostic reasoning in nursing, *Nurs Diagn* 1(2):71, 1990.
8. Tanner C: Teaching clinical judgment. In Holzemer W, editor: *Annual review of nursing research*, New York, 1987, Springer.
9. Thiele JE et al: Perceived and actual decision making by novice baccalaureate students, *West J Nurs Res* 13:618, 1991.
10. Yura H, Walsh MB: *The nursing process*, ed 5, Norwalk, Conn, 1988, Appleton & Lange.
11. Zielstorff RD, McHugh ML, Clinton J: *Computer design criteria*, Kansas City, Mo, 1988, American Nurses' Association.

Classic

12. American Nurses' Association: *Standards of medical-surgical nursing practice*, Kansas City, Mo, 1974, The Association.
13. American Nurses' Association: *Standards of nursing practice*, Kansas City, Mo, 1973, The Association.
14. Benner P: *From novice to expert: excellence and power in clinical nursing practice*, Menlo Park, Calif, 1984, Addison-Wesley.
15. Fry VS: The creative approach to nursing. *Am J Nurs* 53:301, 1953.
16. Gordon M: Nursing diagnosis and the diagnostic process, *Am J Nurs* 76:1298, 1976.
17. Henderson V: The nursing process. *J Adv Nurs* 7:103, 1982.
18. McManus RL: Assumptions of functions of nursing. In *Regional planning for nurses and nursing education*, New York, 1950, Columbia University Teachers College.
19. Nightingale F: *Notes on nursing*, New York, 1969, Dover Publications.
20. Tanner C: Stages of development in diagnostic expertise: characteristics, constraints, strategies. In Carnevali DL et al: *Diagnostic reasoning in nursing*, Philadelphia, 1984, JB Lippincott.

CHAPTER SEVEN

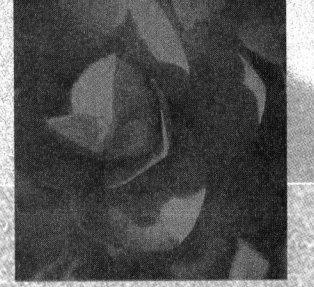

Discharge Planning and Ongoing Care

LEARNING OBJECTIVES

1 Define the process of discharge planning.
2 Explain the nursing role and responsibilities related to facilitating continuity of care.
3 Describe the factors in today's society that are affecting nursing's role in continuity of care.
4 Discuss functional and management activities of daily living and the impact of the nurse's assessment on discharge planning.
5 Define requirements of a discharge planning instruction program for a patient and family.
6 Discuss the roles of the interdisciplinary team.
7 Discuss referral process to community resources in continuity of care.

PREPARING PATIENTS for discharge from an acute care setting requires incorporating the elements of the nursing process. Discharge planning identifies the process by which a health care team facilitates the continuity of care from one health care setting to another. This chapter discusses the process of discharge planning, models of care, factors influencing discharge activities, interdisciplinary team participants and participation, role of the nurse, and referral to community services.

DISCHARGE PLANNING

Discharge planning is a process that incorporates an assessment of the patient's needs with input from the patient, significant other(s), and the health care team, which results in a plan to coordinate available resources to meet the patient's needs.[8] Discharge planning includes:

- An ongoing assessment of anticipated patient care needs (biophysical, psychosocial, environmental, self-care, educational) upon discharge
- Coordination and collaboration with the patient, family, significant other, and caregivers
- Coordination and collaboration with an interdisciplinary health care team
- Knowledge of community resources and services
- Cost-effective use of financial support

Continuing care refers to the mechanism by which a patient transfers from one health care setting to another setting with the end goal of reentry into the community. For example, a patient is discharged with a referral for a home health care nurse to visit and change a dressing or assess self-injection procedures at home. The goal of discharge planning is **continuity of care,** which is the unbroken coordinated provision of health care services. Discharge planning is a process in which nurses and an interdisciplinary team provides coordinated communication of needed services through a referral process to achieve discharge goals.[9,13]

Legislative and Regulatory Influences

One of the greatest factors that has influenced discharge planning is the legislative actions and subsequent interpretations of laws through regulations. Today governmental control of financial reimbursement of health care costs dictates institutional operational practices. Before the prospective reimbursement payment system (1983), patients could remain for unrestricted lengths of time in a hospital. Currently, acute care facilities control lengths of stay by a diagnostic-related payment scale. The primary disadvantage is the "quicker and sicker" discharge of patients from these facilities.

To address this need, postdischarge care services have been developed. Home health agencies have been established to provide a variety of skilled health care interventions. Skilled nursing facility (SNF) units were created to accommodate patients with specific registered nursing care needs. Freestanding rehabilitation facilities and rehabilitation units grew in response to patients' functional deficits at discharge. These services are reimbursed under different governmental programs or guidelines than the prospective payment plan. Part of discharge planning is being aware of the availability of these services and informing the patient and family of these options.

Further legislation directed the development of "guidelines and standards for the discharge planning process in order to ensure a timely and smooth transition to the most appropriate type of setting for posthospital or rehabilitative care."[14] The law mandated that Medicare/Medicaid patients must be assessed upon admission and discharge planning initiated for patients at risk of adverse health consequences. An example is diabetic coma in a patient unable to purchase or prepare meals when discharged to home. In addition, national accrediting commissions reiterate the need for timely discharge planning, ongoing comprehensive assessments, collaboration of interdisciplinary team members, patient, and family, and administrative support of discharge planning activities in their guidelines for quality care. These guidelines also require that a registered nurse ensure that a patient needs assessment and plan of care are completed. An organizational system to support the nurse in achieving this goal is also expected (see box).

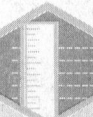

STANDARDS OF CARE

Discharge Planning

The Joint Commission on Accreditation of Health Care Organizations (JCAHO) includes management and administrative as well as nursing care standards for discharge planning. These standards direct hospitals to develop policies and procedures that include mechanisms to identify patients who require discharge planning that promotes continuity of care. The JCAHO standards require hospitals to initiate discharge planning on a timely basis.

Specific nursing care standards from JCAHO include the following:
- Each patient's assessment includes consideration of biophysical, psychosocial, environmental, self-care, educational, and discharge planning factors.
- Nursing staff members collaborate, as appropriate, with physicians and other clinical disciplines in making decisions regarding each patient's need for nursing care.
- The patient's medical record includes documentation of said plan.
- The abilities of the patient and/or, as appropriate, his or her significant other(s) to manage continuing care needs after discharge.

From JCAHO Management and Administrative Service Standards (1993) and Nursing Care Standards (1993).

High-Risk Patients

The "graying of America" is a term used to recognize the increase in the average life expectancy of Americans. Americans 85 years and older today have additional needs because of the aging process (sight and hearing loss) as well as comorbidity of chronic illness (such as bone and joint, cardiovascular, and pulmonary conditions). Combining these factors with changing environmental, financial, and loss of the nuclear American family makes the elderly patient a high-risk patient requiring extensive discharge planning services. Other patients at high risk are listed in the box on p. 95.

Patient and Family Priorities

Hospitalization creates a crisis for the patient and family. In discharge planning, the nurse respects the individual and family needs and incorporates their decisions and priorities into the discharge plan.

HIGH-RISK SCREENING CRITERIA FOR DISCHARGE PLANNING

1. Age 70 or older; any individual who is unable to manage personal, functional, or management activities of daily living (ADLs), is living alone or with a disabled caregiver.
2. Multiple hospitalizations or transfer from another health care facility without established disposition to a health care facility.
3. Social factors include homeless, transient, domestic violence, abuse, neglect, incompetent, mental illness, developmental impairment, no known social support system.

RESEARCH BRIEF

Farren EA: Effects of early discharge planning on length of hospital stay, *Nurs Economics* 9(1):25, 1991.

This article discusses an experimental study design developed by the Baylor Home Care nurses on the impact of proactive intervention for discharge planning assessments. The hypothesis was "discharge planning begun within 24 hours of a patient's hospital admission will facilitate a decrease in LOS of patients hospitalized by 2 or more days" (Farren, p. 26).

During a 3-month investigative period the nurses had 432 patients in their study, 174 in the experimental group and 258 in their control group. Length of stay ranged from 2 to 101 days. The one patient with the exceptionally high length of stay was eliminated from the study. All patients in the experimental group had psychosocial assessment within 24 hours of admission. Using nonparametric procedures for data analysis, the nurses found the experimental group had a median length of stay of 4 days as compared to the control group's 6 days.

The nurses found the study results to be positive for their facility and patients. Significant financial savings for the facility were shown. Additional staff was added and discharge planning assessments upon admission are now protocol for all patients. The author felt one of the most significant results of the study was the possibility to show the financial savings of nursing intervention for the patient's continuity of care.

Nurses also must identify personal barriers to acceptance of the plan, such as finances, time, family needs, and motivation to change. Personal attitudes or knowledge about self-image, prospective community resources, and cultural life-style may influence decisions made for discharge. Recommendations for home modifications may be ignored because of lack of knowledge of resources, lack of transportation or expertise, or lack of financial support. Establishing a rapport with the patient and family facilitates discussion of barriers to accepting the projected plan.[6]

NURSING ROLE IN CONTINUITY OF CARE

The nurse is at the core of patient care within a health care facility. Nursing care provides continuous around-the-clock care. Clinical judgment is required for evaluating and interpreting assessment data. Through an analysis of the interdisciplinary team's progress notes, laboratory and radiology exam results, and the therapeutic regimen, the nurse can anticipate the patient's needs and provide resources to make reentry into a community health care or home setting. Nurses disseminate information about the patient's needs to the interdisciplinary team during the discharge planning process.

Assessment

Upon admission, the nurse assesses the biophysical, psychosocial, educational, self-care, environmental status, and discharge needs of the patient. Psychosocial assessment includes mental health status, social interaction activities (past and present), and family support. The educational evaluation can reveal an expected reading and comprehension level as well as the prospects of returning to an educa-

tional program for vocational training or completion of studies. Self-care deficits can be evaluated through performance of activities of daily living. Living arrangements, including surrounding community and physical attributes of the home, are evaluated during the environmental assessment.

The nurse tries to envision how the patient is going to perform in the post–acute care setting. One way to evaluate a patient's capabilities is to assess the patient's functional abilities and management of activities of daily living (Figure 7-1). Functional abilities describe the patient's performance of an activity. Management skills require higher cognitive processes like problem solving, computation, or judgment. **Activities of daily living (ADL)** can be classified as self-care or instrumental. Traditionally, self-care activities include performing personal hygiene, dressing, eating, and bladder and bowel continence. Depending on which assessment scale is being used, ambulation, communication, and cognitive skills

Patient's Name_____Age_____

Date of Admission_____Anticipated Discharge_____

Available caregiver name and telephone:_____

_____

I.   Patient's Residence for Disposition

    Home:

Bedroom:	_____ upstairs	_____ first floor
Bathroom:	_____ shower	_____ bathtub
Entrance:	_____ steps at entry	_____ garage
	_____ covered entrance	_____ sidewalk to entrance
Kitchen:	_____ gas stove	_____ electric stove
	_____ cupboards above counters	

    Can adaptations be made to the home:_____

    Will a ramp be needed to enter the home:_____

II.   Mental Status

    _____ Oriented   _____ Disoriented

    _____ Unresponsive   _____ Combative

    _____ Other_____

III.   Functional Activities of Daily Living

    EACH OF THE CATEGORIES BELOW IS GRADED ON THE SEVEN-POINT SCALE AS FOLLOWS:

    7-Complete independence
    6-Modified independence—uses adaptive/assistive devices
    5-Needs supervision or setup of activity
    4-Minimal assistance—does 75% of the task by self
    3-Moderate assistance—does 50%-74% of the task by self
    2-Maximal assistance—does 25%-49% of the task by self
    1-Total assistance—does less than 25% of the task by self

	Admission	Update	Discharge
Bathing	_____	_____	_____
Grooming	_____	_____	_____
Dressing - upper body	_____	_____	_____
Dressing - lower body	_____	_____	_____
Toileting	_____	_____	_____
Eating	_____	_____	_____
Modility	_____	_____	_____
Communication - expression	_____	_____	_____
Communication - comprehension	_____	_____	_____

IV.   Instrumental Activities of Living: Independence means performs task without assistance; dependence requires someone else to perform the activity

	Independent	Assistance Needed	Dependent
Medications	_____	_____	_____
Meal Preparation	_____	_____	_____
Shopping for food	_____	_____	_____
Other shopping	_____	_____	_____
Housekeeping	_____	_____	_____
Telephone use	_____	_____	_____
Money Management	_____	_____	_____
Transportation	_____ Independent in own vehicle		
	_____ Independent on public transportation		
	_____ Assistance needed		
	_____ Homebound		

(Continued)

FIGURE 7-1   Assessment of activities of daily living.

Interdisciplinary Team Involved in care:

_____ PT _____ OT _____ ST _____ RT _____ Resp. T _____ Dietitian _____ Social Worker
_____ Spiritual Advisor
_____ Discharge Planning Nurse   _____ Patient / Family Educator
_____ Psychologist   _____ Recreation T   _____ Case Manager
_____ Utilization Review
_____ Resource Team:_____

Discharge Planning Referrals

_____ Rehabilitation facility
_____ Outpatient therapy or clinic
_____ SNF
_____ Nursing home or other residential facility
_____ Home health care
_____ Hospice care
_____ Chronic care facility
_____ Group home
_____ Homemaker services
_____ Other: _____

Community programs:

_____ Public health unit
_____ Visiting nurses service
_____ Meals on wheels
_____ Respite care
_____ Home maintenance

Support programs:

_____ Support group:_____
_____ Day hospital:_____
_____ Adult day care center:_____

Additional needs:

_____ Needs to hire sitter
_____ Needs to hire personal care attendant
_____ Residence needs adaptations
_____ Transportation services:_____
_____ Needs medical supplies:_____
_____ Needs medical equipment:_____
_____ Needs assistive devices:_____

Teaching plans for:	Patient	Family	Caregiver
Diagnosis related	_____	_____	_____
Self-care activities	_____	_____	_____
Instrumental activities	_____	_____	_____
Hiring attendant / sitter	_____	_____	_____
Choosing a rehab center	_____	_____	_____
Choosing a home health agency	_____	_____	_____

Follow up appointments:

_____ Needs transportation
_____ Needs assistance to remember appointment
_____ Needs accessible health care center or office

FIGURE 7-1, cont'd   Assessment of activities of daily living.

may be added. Instrumental activities focus on supportive living activities. These activities can be the ability to use a telephone, manage medication regimen, shop for groceries or clothing, prepare meals, or perform housekeeping chores. Management of instrumental activities of daily living indicate the patient's capability to live alone or degree of dependency on caregivers.

After the nursing assessment, recommendations for interdisciplinary assessment and treatment can be made to the attending physician or discharge planner. Discharge needs of the patient can then be determined following analysis of the total assessment data.

Planning

The nurse and patient jointly identify outcome goals based on patient's needs and therapeutic services needed to achieve those goals. The plan of care is updated periodically. High-priority patients are listed in the box below. Every acute care patient may not need interdisciplinary discharge planning services, however, each patient has a nurse-directed plan of care and discharge plan.

The nurse requires a knowledge base of available community resources, the referral process, and financial support. Building a resource file can also facilitate future discharge planning activities. Most agencies or services are willing to send information packets. Some companies will send professionals to the acute care setting to work with the nurse, patient, and family to explore discharge options. Going home is the goal of most acute care patients; therefore keeping a file of non–health care support services can facilitate achievement of this goal. Services may include, meals-on-wheels services, availability of electric wheelchairs in grocery stores, home delivery of medications, or special appointment accommodations at banks. Maintaining records of current information on available community resources facilitates an appropriate match of the patient's needs with accessible services.

During the planning phase the nurse discusses accessible options with the patient and caregivers. Selection of a particular agency or institution remains the right of the patient and family. Family members are encouraged to tour institutions to gather information and to talk with former and concurrent users of the service. Facilities should be examined and compared to determine if the patient's needs and services match. Introduce possible referrals to alternative sites early so the patient and caregiver have ample time to make their decision.

Implementation

Teaching is an integral part of patient care. Assessment of the teaching needs and educational level of the patient begin the process, but teaching is integrated throughout the therapeutic management. For example, explaining procedures, describing medication side effects, and discussing how to comply or modify risk factors are regular teaching actions by nurses. Formal teaching sessions are not required for every topic. By writing a teaching plan, the nurse can enlist the nursing team to reinforce material or participate in the teaching process. The best evaluation of understanding of presented material is a re-demonstration of the procedure by the patient or caregiver.

Upon agreement to the discharge plan, a referral can be formalized. A transfer to a skilled nursing facility or long-term care facility requires completion of certain forms. Referrals to a home health agency can be completed over the telephone after physician's orders are written. Rehabilitation facilities often send a liaison nurse to assess the patient's potential to benefit from rehabilitative services, explain services to patient and family, and communicate information to the accepting resource. Nurses record these activities and confirm the initiation time and date before discharge.

Confidentiality of medical records prohibits indiscriminate sharing of patient information. Follow the institution's policy and procedure for obtaining the patient's consent to provide information to a refer-

---

HIGH-PRIORITY PATIENTS FOR DISCHARGE PLANNING

- Patients in need of home high-technology therapy (IV therapy, hyperalimentation, chemotherapy, or home ventilator)
- Diagnosis with long-term or terminal implications (HIV positive, cancer, stroke, chronic renal failure, or traumatic brain or spinal cord injury)
- Medication management (complicated medication regimen, new insulin-dependent diabetic, impaired vision, previous failure to follow prescribed medication regimen)
- Patients who will require adaptive equipment at home (hospital beds, oxygen, wheelchairs, assistive devices)
- Patients who require postdischarge skilled nursing care follow-up (home health, special nurse clinic appointments, day care, nursing home)
- Patients who will require rehabilitative therapy
- Elderly patients (65+ years) with additional chronic conditions (arthritis, pulmonary, cardiovascular, DM)
- Patients undergoing major surgical intervention

ral institution. Some agencies will request pertinent information or records to continue a level of care.

A member of the interdisciplinary team may be responsible for the referrals; however, the primary nurse will ensure that the patient has been given discharge instructions and appointments for follow-up care. Discharge instructions (see box) include the nursing actions of teaching, counseling, and appropriate referrals for continuity of care. Clear, concise, accurate documentation of patient's needs on the discharge forms improves the continuity of care. Medication management, which includes dose, frequency, and drug and food interactions and side effects must also be documented. Treatment procedures should be described clearly with type and amount of supplies needed. Any precautions prescribed for the patient are noted; examples are "no weight bearing on left leg (for a patient with a hip replacement)," "cut food into small pieces before serving (if patient has difficulty swallowing)," or "assist patient in transfer from wheelchair to bath chair." In addition, the nurse documents the patient's or family's understanding of and ability to comply with the discharge instruction, as evidenced by verbalization or demonstration.

Follow-up appointments are another necessity, including availability of transportation. Documentation of sources of health care supplies or equipment can be helpful in replacement or return after discharge. A copy of the discharge instructions is given the patient or caregiver.

Evaluation

Finally, the discharge plan is confirmed with the patient or family. Does the patient, family, and/or caregiver still agree to the plan? Have the referral resources accepted transition of services on the agreed upon date? Will needed equipment be available or delivered on discharge day? Has discharge and follow-up transportation been arranged? If the patient is going home alone, have groceries been purchased or will the patient be required to carry out activities on discharge day?

The nurse follows up several days after discharge to answer questions or secure follow-through from a referral agency. At this time an evaluation of the appropriateness of the referral can be completed. Scheduling support groups in the facility or clinic visits are other means of recontacting patients and their families for evaluation of the discharge process.

MODELS OF DISCHARGE PLANNING PROGRAMS

Discharge planning programs and the roles of the various health care professionals are designed by the health care organization. The basic components are institutional and departmental philosophies, goals and objectives, role of the interdisciplinary team members, defined assessment of patient needs, routine of interdisciplinary meetings, mechanism of referral, record of plan, and method for follow-up evaluations.

The discharge planning nurse model uses nurses in an expanded role to assess and coordinate referral to posthospital care. These nurses may assume responsibility for other duties, such as patient/family teaching, quality improvement surveys, and utilization review.[11]

In the discharge planning nurse/social work team model, nurses and social workers are assigned to specific units to collaborate in arranging posthospital care. Divisions of responsibility vary but are usually home care arrangements by nurses and nursing home placement by social workers.

Another model uses a social service or continuing care department to contract with nurses to coordinate postdischarge care for patients dependent on high-technology care. Home health nurses or nurse consultants may function in this role. Responsibilities for discharge planning may be divided between the nurse and the social worker. The final

---

 **PATIENT EDUCATION GUIDE**

Discharge Instruction Topics

Medications: name (generic/trade), dose, frequency, times, purpose, side effects, and food interactions

Treatments: procedure, supplies needed, frequency, location to purchase additional supplies

Diet: type, supplements, eating precautions

Assistive devices: type, usage time, precautions, arrival date, time, location

Durable medical equipment: type, vendor's name and telephone number, arrival date, time, location

Safety precautions: for example, eating or weight bearing

Follow-up appointments: physician, clinics, and outpatient services with date, time, telephone numbers, and transportation arrangements if necessary

Signature of understanding: patient or significant other signs the document to verify understanding of instructions

Signature of the nurse: nurse giving instructions with date

A copy is given to patient/family with original placed in the medical record

A number or person to call in an emergency or to clarify information

model is a social service department that handles all aspects of discharge planning. They complete all referral forms for services recommended by the interdisciplinary team. To ensure accurate communication, the nurse needs to review all nursing care orders that are given to the receiving agency or facility. As the emphasis increases toward care outside the acute care facility, new approaches are continually being taken to the traditional organizational structure for formal discharge planning. The models discussed are examples and are not inclusive of all models of program organization.

INTERDISCIPLINARY RESOURCE TEAM

An interactive interdisciplinary health care team can formulate a comprehensive holistic discharge plan. Members and responsibilities of this team vary with the type and size of each institution. Each discipline contributes an expertise from which the patient benefits. Weekly or biweekly meetings of the team facilitate planning, implementing, reevaluating, and confirming the discharge needs and plans.

As the health care team leader, the physician writes orders that synthesize the interdisciplinary contributions to patient care. Discharge orders for referred services, assistive devices, medications, safety precautions, transportation needs, and diet must be written by the physician. Follow-up appointments are made to evaluate the patient's needs or adjustment after discharge.

The physical therapist plans and administers a treatment plan to restore patients to their previous level of ambulation or mobility and physical performance. The therapist directs training and ordering of assistive ambulatory devices such as canes, walkers, and wheelchairs. Additional interventions may include pain-relief measures, vehicle driving evaluations, and sports and vocational training.

An occupational therapist's responsibilities focus on the patient's occupation. The primary goals are functional improvement in performing activities of daily and instrumental living. They work with the patient on dressing, hygiee feeding, and toileting skills. Assistive devices to accomplish the ADLs are evaluated, and manipulation is taught to the patient or caregiver and ordered by the therapist. To prevent contracture in a paralyzed extremity, the therapist may fabricate a splint to maintain the joints in neutral position. Testing the patient's judgment and problem-solving abilities will conclude the therapeutic interventions. Typical situations are performance of meal preparation, management of financial affairs, and driving evaluations.

A speech pathologist will work with the patient to produce verbal and nonverbal speech. Nonverbal speech may require the use of an assistive device like alphabet lapboards, picture cards, or electronic devices. Speech pathologists also deal with mathematic computations, reading and comprehension, sequencing skills (knowing the order in which activities are done), and ability-to-swallow assessments.

Elimination of secondary pulmonary complications is the primary role of respiratory therapists. They may add their expertise in home care teaching for patients with pulmonary compromise. They can teach pulmonary hygiene techniques, the safe use of oxygen, use of aerosol medications, and the operation and maintenance of ventilator equipment. Since mechanically ventilated patients are leaving acute facilities still ventilator dependent, the respiratory therapist is involved in educating and training the patient, family, or alternative-setting personnel.

Dietitians direct the teaching of restricted, enteral, or special diets. Dietitians may also help people adapt diets to special religious, ethnic, cultural or life-style preferences. In cooperation with the pharmacist, they can advise on food and drug interactions.

Recreational therapists evaluate patients and stimulate them to participate in leisure activities within their physical and cognitive capabilities. Craft projects can provide an alternative intervention for training in maintaining attention span or following directions, as well as building self-esteem. Examples of activities may be management of community resources such as entering a movie theater with a wheelchair, and attainment of physical strength in athletic games.

In some institutions, psychologists or neuropsychologists may supplement counseling provided by the social worker. They can also administer mental testing for determination of mental age, mental status, and cognitive abilities. Family counseling and support groups may be coordinated by these professionals.

Social workers are educated to complete in-depth psychosocial assessments of the patient and family. One aspect of this role is that of a counselor in helping the patient and family adjust and adapt to the illness or injury. Social workers are knowledgeable in financial support systems and regulations, so they can recommend and complete referrals to post-acute care services.[4]

Internal case managers are usually nurses or social workers. Their roles are defined by the activities of those team members. Underlining their activities is management of the patient's financial resources to acquire the services and equipment desired at a cost-efficient price. Case managers employed by insurance companies or alternative settings usually project a lifetime plan, whereas internal case managers focus on the time the patient receives services from that institution. External or internal case managers contribute to discharge plans;

however, case management is considered a separate entry of continuity of care.

The patient may want spiritual comfort during the hospital stay. The spiritual counselor may have a religious affiliation. The health care team should acknowledge this support and seek it.

Numerous other health care professionals may be called into the discharge planning as consultants. They also may be members of the community-service organizations or agencies. They may provide patient/family education, offer interdisciplinary team training or education, or perform unique services. These services may provide medical information (EEG technician or medical specialist [i.e., urologist]) or specialized care (bedside dialysis or behavior management).[10]

Primary nurses remain the patient's primary means of support and coordinator of information and contacts with other professionals. Extended nursing practice roles supplement bedside nursing care.

Some facilities have a designated nurse educator to provide extensive patient/family teaching programs. The most common acute care programs are diabetic, cardiovascular, or dermal/stomal care. Individualized and group teaching classes are held at the bedside or in unit conference rooms. These nurses will document their teaching in the nurses' progress notes.

Utilization review departments have a working knowledge of the reimbursement system, patient criteria for admission, and continuation of inpatient treatment. Nurses performing this job can advise the interdisciplinary team on the cost-efficient status of the patient's inpatient stay.

The discharge planning coordinator may be the patient's primary nurse, designated nurse specialist, or case manager. A social worker or rehabilitation counselor may function in this role, too. This individual is responsible for pulling together the interdisciplinary team communications and designing a discharge plan. Implementation and confirmation of the discharge plan usually is coordinated by this professional. Monitoring of the patient's performance, achievement of goals, and continued needs also will be documented by these professionals. For a summary of services coordinated by the discharge planning team, see the box below.

CONTINUING-CARE FACILITIES

The nurse has specific responsibilities regarding the discharge of a patient to a continuing-care facility. Transfer forms must be completed, and telephoning a verbal report to the receiving facility is mandatory. Faxing copies of the physician's discharge orders and the nursing discharge summary can facilitate a smooth transition. Availability, name, and types of services offered by continuing care facilities vary in different regions of this country. State regulations contribute to the diversity in the availability and variability of continuing care services. Voluntary agency support varies by community and state, usually because of financial funding. Rural vs. urban locations can affect accessibility to some health care facilities.

Rehabilitation Nursing

The primary focus of rehabilitation care is the improvement of performance in activities of daily and instrumental living. An assessment must show the patient's potential to benefit by rehabilitation services, strength to participate in at least 3 hours of therapeutic interventions, and acceptance as a patient by a physician specializing in physical medicine and rehabilitation. Rehabilitation services can be offered on an inpatient or outpatient basis. An interdisciplinary health care team similar to that of an acute care facility implements the care and discharge planning. Coverage of rehabilitation services varies in state medicaid programs and commercial insurance companies.

Rehabilitation nursing is a specialty. As defined by the Association of Rehabilitation Nurses, "Rehabilitation nursing is the diagnosis and treatment of human responses of individuals and groups to actual and potential health problems with the characteris-

SERVICES COORDINATED BY DISCHARGE PLANNING TEAM

Assessments of continuing care needs
Referrals for home health, private-pay nursing services
Medical equipment services
High-tech home care services (TPN, chemotherapy, IV antibiotics)
Referrals for outpatient therapies or clinics
Referrals to residential care facilities (nursing home, group homes, residential schools)
Medical air transport
Rehabilitation facility referrals
Hospice care referrals
Financial assistance
Referrals to volunteer community agencies (Arthritis Foundation, Respite Care)
Referrals to departments of family and children services
Referrals for adoption, foster homes
Referrals for personal care services (meals on wheels, transportation, personal care)

tics of altered functional ability and altered life-style. . . knowledge and skills are appropriate to the magnitude of disruption to the client's physical, social, emotional, economic, and vocational status throughout their lives."[12] The intense nursing and therapeutic needs of the patient often exceed the short course of acute care treatment. Rehabilitation nurses collaborate with an interdisciplinary team led by a physiatrist. The Association of Rehabilitation Nurses delineates the roles of the rehabilitation nurse as (1) teacher, to instruct the patient/caregiver in performing care activities; (2) advocate, to encourage patients to seek new experiences and goals; (3) counselor, to facilitate adjustment and adaptation to a disability; (4) caregiver, to provide assistance until independence in self-care is achieved; and (5) researcher, to enlarge the science of nursing.[3]

Adjusting and adapting to an acquired disability is a lengthy process. Discharge from a rehabilitation facility does occur before the patient has truly accepted the disability. Therefore discharge planning continues to procure needed community services after discharge. The discharge process is similar to that described in an acute care facility. The interdisciplinary rehabilitation team is probably more aware of the physical and attitudinal barriers the patient will confront when returning to the community. By being supportive and encouraging, the team can motivate the patient to implement care activities to prevent readmissions for secondary complications.

To facilitate community reentry, the patient and caregiver(s) will participate in unique learning programs both individually and as a group. Rehabilitation techniques and care activities are demonstrated; redemonstration by the patient and caregiver may be required before some outings. For example, a community visit to a shopping mall or movie theater is a reentry experience. The patient experiences reentry and can discuss feelings and performance with the specialist. Home visits are often arranged to make recommendations for adaptations to ease the patient's return home. Measurement of bathrooms and furniture arrangements can be replicated in the rehabilitation facility so that home activities can be practiced. Patients go to their homes on trial visits to practice care activities and for socialization. Finally, the patient and caregiver may move into a transitional living arrangement to perform total care. These living quarters are usually close to professional nurses for emergency or retraining needs.

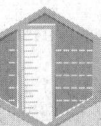

STANDARDS OF CARE

Outcome Criteria in Rehabilitation Nursing

The patient/family/caregiver will demonstrate performance of listed activities after each diagnosis.

Self-care deficit
- Perform self-care activities at a level consistent with capabilities
- Encourage, support, and assist the client as necessary toward achievable self-care

Alteration in neurogenic bladder and/or bowel
- Describe, participate in, and/or direct individual bladder or bowel program
- Monitor and report effects of medication
- Demonstrate capability to adapt a bladder or bowel continence program relative to changes in the environment and health status

Impaired physical mobility
- Demonstrate optimum, safe mobility for the client
- Maintain maximal physical activity for the client

High risk for impaired skin integrity
- Describe etiology and prevention measures
- Explain rationale for preventive measures
- Demonstrate responsibility for prevention program

Impaired verbal communication
- Demonstrate an understanding of the rationale for loss of verbal communication skills
- Use an effective method of communication
- State that there is less frustration with communication

Ineffective individual coping
- Initiate care or ask for help when needed
- Participate in self-care within functional abilities
- Express feelings in a socially acceptable manner
- Verbalize a positive perception of his or her coping abilities
- Ask for information and utilize resources appropriately to cope with problems and assist in decision making

Sexual dysfunction
- Each describes himself or herself as a sexual being
- Demonstrate an understanding of the alterations in sexual function and options available to address those alterations
- Say that sexual activity is satisfying and pleasurable
- Identify resources within the agency/community to support sexuality

From American Nurses Association and Association of Rehabilitation Nurses (1988).

Other Continuing Care Facilities

A patient's need for a minimum of 4.5 hours of skilled nursing care per day is required for admission to a chronic care facility. Close physician monitoring of medical needs is also mandatory. These facilities are not available in all states and financial coverage varies.

Skilled nursing facilities (SNFs) are regulated by state agencies; therefore each state lists acceptable skilled nursing needs for admission. A SNF is usually a unit of a general acute care hospital or nursing home. Social and recreational services are mandatorily provided. Medical testing is customarily covered; however, selected reimbursement may follow in which therapeutic activities will be paid. Length of stay in these units varies depending on if the goal is strengthening or recuperation to participate in rehabilitation programs or disposition to another community residential setting.

The terms *residential care facility, nursing home, personal care home,* and *rest home* are used interchangeably to describe facilities that can provide supervisory care for the patient. These homes provide varying levels of management of ADLs. Management of instrumental activities is usually limited to maintenance of care environment and provision of meals. Due to the comorbidity of elderly patients, placement in a residential care facility may be temporary to regulate medications, increase endurance and performance of ADLs, or await modifications of home environment.

HOME HEALTH NURSING

Home health agencies are capable of providing extensive intermittent nursing care in the home. These services range from dressing changes or insulin injections to intravenous antibiotics or dialysis. The patient needs criteria for coverage follow: (1) must be homebound, (2) require skilled registered professional nurse or physical therapist on an intermittent basis, and (3) services ordered by a physician. Payment for services is outlined in Medicare, Medicaid, or commercial insurance plans (see box at right).

The homebound criteria are defined by the financially responsible party. They generally stipulate that the patient is physically unable to leave the home. Ambulance or selected transportation agencies are required to take the patient to follow-up medical appointments or treatments. There are no exceptions to this rule. The rule is so strict that the patient may not even be allowed to be able to leave for church services.

The American Nurses Association (ANA) stated that "the goal of care (in the home) is to initiate, manage and evaluate the resources needed to promote the client's optimal level of well-being."[7] The

MEDICARE REGULATIONS

Medicare has two parts. Medicare Part A is the hospital insurance, and Part B is the supplementary medical insurance.[7]

Part A Covers:
Some of the costs of hospitalization
Certain related inpatient care
Hospice
Home health care on an intermittent basis
Hospital deductible in 1993 is $676 for the first 60 days; then the patient must pay $169 per day.
After 90 days this increases to $338 per day for up to 60 "lifetime reserve days." The "benefit" period ends 60 days after the patient's discharge from the hospital or skilled nursing facility.
If another hospital admission occurs after that, the patient is responsible for another deductible and cost sharing.
Skilled nursing facility. Coverage for this is for the first 20 days, then the next 80 days the patient is responsible for $84.50 per day. Coverage benefits are exhausted after 100 days in a single benefit period.

Part B Covers:
Doctor's fees
Outpatient hospital services
Certain related services
Therapies such as physical therapy, occupational therapy
Medical equipment services (beds, oxygen, wheelchairs)
Braces, ostomy supplies, artificial limbs (prostheses, orthotics)
Home health services (payment from only A or B, not both)
Medicare is financed in two ways. Part A is paid out of the individual's payroll taxes, whereas Part B is an option billed monthly once the recipient starts to receive Medicare. In 1993 the premiums for Part B are $36.60 per month.

ANA goes on to say that professional nurses have the following responsibilities of care within the home:

- Perform holistic initial and periodic assessment of the client's and family/caregiver's physical and financial resources to develop and support the nursing care plan.
- Identify and coordinate the community resources necessary to support optimal client outcomes.
- Use qualitative and quantitative data to evalu-

ate client responses to care, and monitor the parameters of care according to the nursing care plan.

- Educate and counsel clients, families, and caregivers to promote self-care activities.
- Initiate health-promotion teaching to improve the quality of life, maintain health, and minimize disability.
- Implement the advocacy role through activities that inform, support, and affirm the client and family's self-determination.
- Promote continuity of care through discharge planning, care management, and advocacy.[5]

Home health care promotes active participation of the patient and family in caregiving activities. Teaching and demonstrations of care activities in the acute care setting will be tested in the home. Collaboration with the family and patient on visit time and duration can reduce the disruption of the home routines. The home environment must be respected in a different manner than an institutional environment. An awareness of this issue promotes mutual acceptance of the professional visit.

Home health agencies are responsible for coordinating care from acceptance through discharge. Documentation is important for reimbursement and legal protection. Agencies have a legal responsibility to ensure proper termination of services or may be liable for abandonment if discharge planning conditions are not achieved.

CRITICAL THINKING QUESTIONS

1 Discuss discharge planning, and continuity of care as it relates to the role nursing plays in interactions with the patient.

2 Explain why nursing assessment of activities of daily living is important as it relates to discharge planning. Describe what is different between instrumental and self-care activities of daily living.

3 Describe the roles of the interdisciplinary team members of the discharge planning team to support the patient's needs related to continuing care.

4 Discuss the role of the primary nurse in rehabilitative nursing.

5 Complete the initial assessment tool for a patient who meets high-risk criteria. After completion describe the referrals that could assist the patient to prepare for discharge. What possible community resources could benefit the patient?

BIBLIOGRAPHY

Current

1. *Accreditation manual for hospitals: Management and administrative,* Oakbrook Terrace, IL, 1993, Joint Commission on Accreditation of Healthcare Organizations.
2. American Nurses' Association and Association of Rehabilitation Nurses: *Rehabilitation nursing: Scope of practice; process and outcome criteria for selected diagnoses,* Washington, D.C., 1988, American Nurses' Association.
3. American Nurses Association: *Standards of rehabilitation nursing practice,* Washington, D.C., 1988, American Nurses' Association.
4. Berkman B et al: Screening elder cardiac patients to identify need for social work services, *Health Soc Work* 15(1): 64-72, 1990.
5. Cary AH, ed: *A statement on the scope of home health nursing practice,* Washington, D.C., 1992, American Nurses' Association.
6. Clemen-Stone S et al: *Comprehensive family and community health nursing,* ed 3, St Louis, 1991, Mosby–Year Book.
7. Detlefs DR, Meyers RJ: *1992 Guide to social security and medicare,* Baltimore, Maryland, 1991, Department of Health and Human Services.
8. Hutchinson DR: *Discharge planning for nurses,* 1990, unpublished manuscript.
9. O'Hara PA, Terry MA: *Discharge planning: strategies for assuring continuity of care,* Rockville, Maryland, 1988, Aspen Publishers.
10. Rorden JW, Taft E: *Discharge planning guide for nurses,* Philadelphia, 1990, WB Saunders Co.
11. Volland PJ, ed: *Discharge planning: An interdisciplinary approach to continuity of care,* Owings Mills, Maryland, 1989, National Health Publishing.

Classic

12. American Nurses' Association and Association of Rehabilitation Nurses: *Standards of rehabilitation nursing practice,* Washington, D.C., 1986, American Nurses' Association.
13. McCelland E, Kelly K, Buckwalter KC: *Continuity of care: advancing the concept of discharge planning,* New York, 1985, Grune & Stratton.
14. Public Law, 99-509, October 21, 1986, Federal Register.

CHAPTER EIGHT

Patient and Family Education

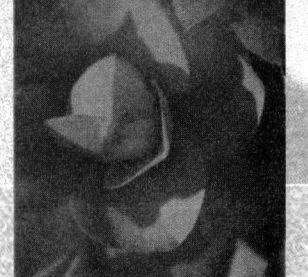

LEARNING OBJECTIVES

1 Describe the components of adult learning theory.
2 Identify the components of the teaching-learning process.
3 Use the nursing process as a format when teaching patients.
4 Identify special learning needs and teaching strategies for the low-literacy patient.
5 Contrast various teaching strategies and their effectiveness for various types of learning.
6 Develop clear and realistic goal statements.
7 Use the teaching-learning process to create an effective learning climate.
8 Compare various media and their effectiveness for various types of learning.
9 Identify appropriate tools to evaluate effectiveness of patient teaching.
10 Identify the legal responsibility of the nurse in patient teaching.

KEY TERMS

abstract conceptualizer, p. 109
active experimenter, p. 109
adult learner, p. 106
auditory accessor, p. 111
concrete experimenter, p. 109
contracting, p. 111
field dependent, p. 111

field independent, p. 111
higher-order questioning, p. 109
kinesthetic accessor, p. 111
reflective observer, p. 109
teaching-learning process, p. 107
visual accessor, p. 111

The teacher . . . if he is indeed wise does not bid you enter the house of his wisdom but rather leads you to the threshold of your own mind.   Kahlil Gibran

AN ESSENTIAL component of nursing care is patient education. Research has demonstrated that effective patient education can promote patient compliance with the therapeutic regimen, as well as reduce hospital admissions, decrease anxiety, and promote and improve patient health. Education can also help the patient assume some responsibility for disease management after hospital discharge. In addition, patient teaching is one of the responsibilities listed in many state nurse practice acts as well as a quality assurance standard listed by the Joint Commission on Accreditation of Hospitals and Organizations (JCAHO). According to Morra,[22] at least five trends will modify our methods and means of educating patients and families:

- Our population will be growing older and living longer. These elders will be more educated because 64% will be high school graduates by the end of the century.

- Minority groups, particularly Hispanics, and disadvantaged people will increase in numbers. One out of four people in the United States will be a member of a racial or ethnic minority in the year 2001.
- The number of people with literacy problems will increase. Fifty-three percent of the US population is currently functionally illiterate or marginally competent in reading, with 50% of young adults unable to understand a newspaper article.
- The health care system will change considerably with less teaching done in the hospitals and an emphasis on teaching patients and families home care skills.

LEARNING THEORY
Adult Learning Theory

Adults differ from children as learners. Knowles[44] describes his adult learning theory model by defining the **adult learner** as a self-directed independent person who becomes ready to learn when the need to know or to perform is experienced. This learner enters the educational activity with an established orientation to learning that is life centered, task centered, or problem centered. The adult learner is internally motivated to learn to increase self-esteem or self-confidence or to seek recognition or a better quality of life. For the adult learner the educator is a facilitator rather than a director of the learning activity. Adult learners wish to be involved in mutual planning of their experiences. They like to participate in diagnosing their needs for learning, formulating their learning objectives, and evaluating their learning. They expect a climate of mutual respect, trust, and collaboration that supports their learning.

The adult learner has a reservoir of experience that serves as a resource for learning. The nurse encourages the use of previous learning whenever possible as the basis for new learning. For example, when teaching pursed-lip breathing, the nurse might compare the technique with blowing bubbles.

Adult education is learner centered. It is dynamic, interactive, and cooperative. It is strengthened through mutual goal setting and is satisfying to both learners and facilitator. The responsibility for success is shared by all participants. The nurse establishes situations that will motivate the patient to learn. Learners also serve as resources for each other and can share experiences and insights. Practical active patient participation using individual, small-group, or large-group learning techniques is an integral part of this teaching-learning process. As the learners progress toward their goals, they feel a sense of reward as they evaluate their learning. The nurse commonly provides positive reinforcement for learning and avoids placing the learners in positions where they may fail. The nurse conveys confidence in the learners' abilities to acquire the necessary skills or knowledge.

Adults learn throughout life to meet emerging needs. The adult's expectation is that learning will be immediately applicable in the life situation. Adults also focus on specific problems to be solved. In other words, adults need information to solve real-life problems and may be uninterested in nonessential content. Other assumptions of adult learning theory include the following:

- The physical learning environment should be conducive to learning, free of distractions, and comfortable.
- Learners should feel the need to learn and share responsibility for planning and implementing the learning process.

Major Theoretic Approaches to Learning

Although an in-depth discussion of learning theories is beyond the scope of this chapter, a brief overview of learning theories is presented in the box below.

LEARNING THEORIES

Trial and error
Law of effect—stresses the importance of the learner's efforts being followed by success.

Classical conditioning
Views learning as a change in behavior occurring as a result of practice. Reinforcement directly satisfies needs or reduces drives. Clear application in learning of skills.

Gestalt psychology
Focuses on learner's thought processes. Learning occurs through organization or interpretation of parts into a whole through the development of new insights or modification of old insights. The learner's past learning and experience serve as the basis for new learning.

Cognitive field theory
Learning is the process of developing new insights and changing old ones through goal-directed, situational, perceptual behaviors. Learning should take place in a realistic environment with situational elements gradually introduced.

Memory

Adults can absorb only a limited amount of new information at once. Short-term memory is limited in its capacity and is lost through new information from sensory memory. For example, if distracting thoughts enter short-term memory from long-term memory, information from short-term memory is lost. This has implications for the learner in that the short-term memory will not be forgotten if the learner is not distracted and if there is opportunity to rehearse or repeat the information. Therefore it is important that the learning environment be free from distractions. Putting material into a story or in practical real-life situations will enhance memory from approximately 20% to 90%.[11]

Long-term memory seems to have unlimited capacity and duration. However, the rate at which new information can be learned is limited to one new item every 4 to 5 seconds. The implication for the adult learner is that the more the learner's experience can be drawn on to organize into familiar patterns, the easier it is to commit the material to memory.

NURSING PROCESS AND TEACHING-LEARNING PROCESS

The nursing process is the means by which nurses deliver systematically planned patient-centered and family-centered care. The nurse uses the problem-solving techniques of the nursing process in patient education to assess patient needs and provide the teaching to promote positive learning outcomes. The **teaching-learning process** is a dynamic entity in which the educator, the learner, and the subject matter are constantly interacting. The nursing process and teaching-learning process are compared in Figure 8-1.

Principles of Patient Education: Teaching-Learning Process

The process of patient teaching includes the following aspects:

- Patient and family assessment, planning, or goal setting
- Determination of teaching methodologies and the teaching intervention itself
- Evaluation of the products of the teaching-learning process to determine if the goals were achieved and learning principles were applied appropriately

Patient education includes both informal and formal teaching. Informal teaching refers to all the unplanned patient-nurse communications. Formal teaching refers to the structured and planned presentations. Traditional patient teaching has focused on the following aspects:

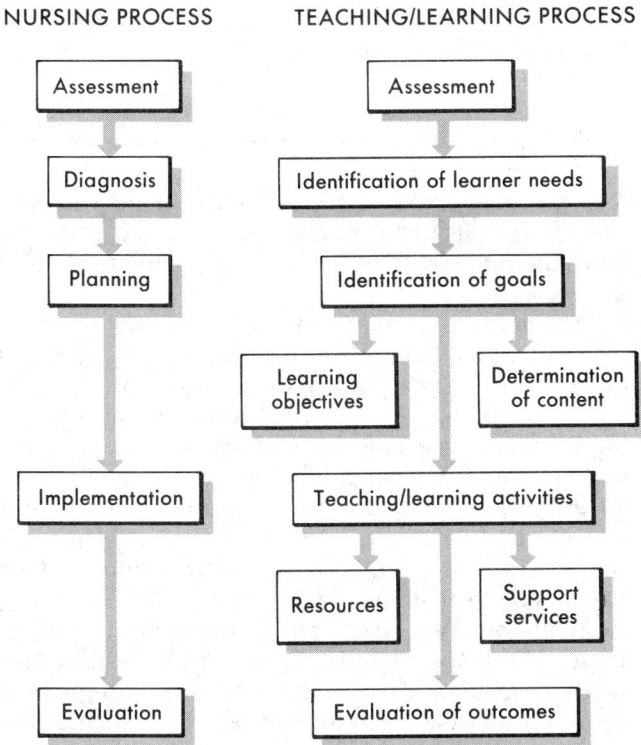

FIGURE 8-1 Comparison of nursing process and teaching-learning process.

- Identifying a particular patient need or problem
- Teaching the patient the knowledge or skills necessary to solve the problem
- Providing encouragement and practice to promote patient accomplishment of the necessary knowledge or skills
- Providing a positive learning experience so the patient values the outcome enough to maintain it

Assessment

Adults enter any new educational experience with previously established ideas, attitudes, and behavior patterns learned over their lifetimes. They also have many responsibilities and problems in life that may have little or nothing to do with what the nurse believes they ought to know. Adults have definite opinions about what is important to them and what they need to change. The first step in the assessment process is to determine what patients and families must know or be able to do to maintain or promote health and prevent further illness. Nurses should not assume patients share their ideas of what they need to learn; they should assess what patients and families feel is necessary to learn. Patient education implies that as a result of learning, patient actions or health behaviors will change. To identify the real educational needs of the patients, the nurse needs to assess *who* needs to change, *what* changes need to occur, *why* they need to occur, and *when* they should occur.

The second step in assessment is to identify what the patient or family already knows about the subject the nurse wishes to teach. By identifying the knowledge base, the nurse can reinforce previous learning and build on what the patient already knows.

Patient learning needs can be assessed with an interview, a questionnaire, tests, or records and reports. The interview allows the patient to express opinions freely, and often the nurse can detect potential teaching problems and negative or positive feelings about learning. The questionnaire has the advantages of being able to reach many people and to yield data that are easily summarized. Unfortunately most questionnaires do not provide for free expression of feelings. Tests may be useful diagnostic tools, but they are often threatening to the patient. Tests are effective when used to diagnose learning needs. Posttests are effective to determine if the content has been learned. Records such as the patient's chart provide the nurse with objective evidence of problems or learning needs of the patient. As part of the data collection, the nurse assesses the functional and psychosocial status of the patient. Functional losses, particularly with the geriatric patient, may impede learning. Hearing, vision, touch, manual dexterity, short-term and long-term memory, and endurance are important considerations. Psychosocial factors such as personal resources, values associated with social roles, anxiety, and support by significant others must be investigated. Consider the life-style factors of the patient. These include family influences, environmental effects, financial resources, and health system factors such as lack of money to buy prescriptions, appointment availability, and poor transportation.

Planning

It is important to remember that all change is voluntary. Nurses are only facilitators of change. Change does not occur by telling people to change or because they should change but by people identifying a need to change or a benefit from the change. Nurses encourage patients to learn to care for their own health needs. They use teaching opportunities to motivate patients to improve their health and longevity.

In the planning phase the nurse identifies goals, objectives, and learning outcomes, selects and sequences subject content, identifies resources, selects instructional methods and materials, and develops an evaluation plan.

Goal setting

Goals provide the framework for measuring the success of teaching. To determine the time, content, methodology, and materials for teaching, realistic goals must be identified. Goals may be cognitive (knowledge), psychomotor (skill learning), and affective, or value and attitudinal. The goal should clearly state the patient outcomes the nurse and patient hope to achieve. The goal should be realistic for the patient to accomplish. The nurse asks the following questions:

- Can the goal be accomplished in this time frame?
- Does the patient have the necessary resources, such as money, transportation, or housing, to accomplish this goal?
- Does the patient have the necessary family or friends as a support system?
- Is the patient mentally able to learn, or must someone else be taught to care for him or her?
- Is the patient physically able to learn, or must someone else be taught the skill?
- Does the patient feel it is valuable and important to learn?
- Is the timing appropriate for learning?

Involving the patient and family in setting goals communicates that the nurse values what they think. For example, the patient may want to lose weight but may not be able to sacrifice potato chips and ice cream. The patient may choose to eliminate other high-caloric foods and substitute a small amount of ice cream and chips. The nurse must be realistic and explain the importance of some goals that must be complied with because of danger to the patient's immediate health. For example, the patient with an infection must recognize the importance of the antibiotic therapy regimen and comply with it. If the overall goal is complex, the nurse breaks it into smaller goals. For example, prioritize the knowledge and skills necessary for a newly diagnosed diabetic patient. Rather than overwhelming the patient with material, consider what the patient needs to know to survive. With the current trend toward shorter stays in the hospital, the nurse may not have time before discharge to teach the patient enough to manage. In that case the nurse provides the patient with resources and makes community resource referrals.

Implementation

Creating a learning climate

Demetrulias and Shaw[38] suggest nurses with creative skills will be more able to meet the challenges of the future and improve the health care of the nation. They define the creative person as one who is "autonomous, self-reliant, internally controlled and self-evaluated. This person is flexible, tolerant of ambiguity, sensitive to problem identification and can make associations among diverse ideas." Creativity, assertiveness, and accountability are valuable assets for nurses, who must be create a nonthreatening atmosphere that encourages the development of the attributes of questioning, active imagination, and support for new ideas. Such an environment results in learners being more spontaneous and open to learning and creativity. One method that develops these attributes is the use of higher-order questioning. **Higher-order questioning** seeks evaluation, inference, and comparison. Examples of this type of questioning are as follows:

1. Quantity questions—"What are all the possible ideas for_____?" These questions encourage fluency and result in the production of a large quantity of ideas.
2. Viewpoint questions—"How could _____ look to a _____ ?" These questions encourage flexibility and develop new perspectives and different categories of ideas.
3. Personal involvement questions—"How would you feel if you were a _____?" These questions aid flexibility by releasing individuals from rigid perceptions.
4. Conscious self-deceit questions—"You have been given the power to _____. How will you use it?" These questions influence flexibility by increasing the ability to create ideal solutions, modify them, and apply them in realistic situations.

5. Reorganization questions—"What would happen if _____ were true?" These questions cause a rethinking of an established pattern and result in altering and reordering of sequences of elements.
6. Forced association—"How is a _____ like a _____?" Associative thinking results in original ideas only when the topics are different from each other.

Learning styles

Rosenbloom[51] describes four basic cognitive styles of learning: *concrete experimentation, reflective observation, abstract conceptualization,* and *active experience.* The **concrete experimenter** is a person who likes to be involved in activities that allow the immediate application or testing of the content to understand it. The **reflective observer** operates in the visual mode and requires visual materials and aids or the opportunity to watch others perform. This person likes to watch others perform and think about the content observed. The **abstract conceptualizer** processes words efficiently so that auditory aids or presentations are sufficient for learning to take place and engage in problem solving. The **active experimenter** wants to apply learning in the real world. Contracts are an effective strategy for this learner. The nurse who recognizes that people learn differently will provide different experiences to satisfy the different cognitive styles of learners. For example, research has indicated that a substan-

TABLE 8-1   Learning Modes, Formats, and Media Examples

Learning mode	Media format	Representative examples of media
Reading	Print materials	Textbooks; reference books; charts; pamphlets; outlines; workbooks and study guides; handouts; crossword puzzles; printed programmed instruction; journals; newspapers; scripts
Seeing	Pictorial materials, visual representations	Filmstrips; film loops; videotapes; television; 8 mm and 16 mm films; displays; exhibits; posters; photographs; slides; overhead transparencies; diagrams; cartoons; simulated activities; demonstrations; flowcharts; graphs; sketches
Listening	Auditory	Lectures; seminars; paired and small-group discussions; skits; audiotapes; videotapes; one-to-one interaction with teacher, peer, or patient; oral presentations; panel discussions; debates; simulations
Manipulating	Tactile, kinesthetic	Practicing with real or simulated items; laboratory activities; manipulating or constructing models; playing games; drawing; filling in work sheets or workbooks; preparing bulletin boards, charts, graphs, or displays

From DeTornay R, Thompson M: *Strategies for teaching nursing,* ed 3, New York, 1987, John Wiley & Sons.

TABLE 8-2 Teaching Strategies

Teaching strategies	Advantages	Disadvantages	Target group	Type of learning
Demonstration/return demo	Presents standards for performance Allows learner to know it can be done	May be difficult to see Limited to small group May make participants nervous	Patients who must learn new skills Patients who need to learn cause/effect FI/FD*—visual, auditory, kinesthetic	Builds skills Changes attitudes Presents standards
Group teaching	Efficient, economical Allows group to support each other Active involvement	Group may digress Difficult to agree on times Transportation may be problem	Participants with common learning needs Patients with chronic disease Preoperative patients School-aged children FD—visual auditory	Explores meaning Increases motivation Creates interest and new attitude Promotes understanding Increases knowledge
Programmed instruction	Active learner involvement Self-paced Provides feedback	Impersonal Lack of one-to-one interaction Learner must be literate and self-motivated	Chronic disease Health promotion FI—visual kinesthetic	Imparts knowledge Develops skills
Lecture	Cost-effective	Limits individuality and personal interaction Boring	Groups of patients Visual, auditory learners	Imparts knowledge
Role-playing	Add or improve skills; opportunity to experience action or anticipate its effects	May be threatening to some learners Time consuming Trust must exist among members	Small groups of patients FD—visual, auditory, kinesthetic	Changes attitudes or feelings Stimulates new ideas
Simulation	Nonthreatening environment creates real-life experience	Time consuming	One-on-one learning FD—visual, auditory, kinesthetic	Builds skills
Case problems	Concrete Real-life situations	Can be boring and too fact oriented	Patients who must apply information FI (FD if used in group)—auditory, kinesthetic	Applies knowledge
Computerized instruction	Interactive review capabilities Free from social restraints	Can be threatening	Individual learns FI—visual, kinesthetic	Applies knowledge

Adapted from Rodriguez L: *Teaching implementation, Ochsner Hospital Patient Teaching Course,* 1988.
*FI = field independent; FD = field dependent.

tial proportion of women with abnormal mammograms have psychologic difficulties even after learning that they do not have cancer. Mailing a psychoeducational booklet on mammography adherence to them had a significant positive impact.[20] Also the learning style inventory is a helpful tool in diagnosing individual learning styles.[44]

Table 8-1 illustrates the use of media in relation to the four main learning modes: reading, seeing, listening, and manipulating. Table 8-2 compares various teaching strategies and their effectiveness for various types of learning.

Teaching strategies and support materials

Media

When used appropriately, media can help the various teaching formats promote effective learning.

Nurses must carefully select media by previewing the material and determining if it is appropriate for the learning experience. Factors to consider are how the media will be used, where they will be used, and whether that particular medium is appropriate for the learner and the learning task. Factors to consider in selecting media or teaching support materials are given in the box below. Table 8-3 summarizes the various forms of media. This table also notes which form of media is effective for the individual's cognitive style and neurolinguistic programming. Cognitive style can be defined as a characteristic manner that structures, organizes, and processes information. **Field independent** is a cognitive style describing the people who are analytic, logical, and concerned with detail. These people tend to be interested in educational and vocational pursuits favoring control and effectiveness, and they like to structure situations on their own. **Field dependent** is the cognitive style describing people who are attentive to social cues, readily reveal their feelings, desire close contact with others, and usually can be found in educational and vocational pursuits requiring working with others.[16]

Neurolinguistic programming is the scientific study of cognitive processing. The different types of cognitive processing can be described as follows:

- **Auditory accessor**—the person who best processes cognitively by hearing
- **Visual accessor**—the person who best processes cognitively by seeing
- **Kinesthetic accessor**—the person who best processes cognitively by touching, feeling, or becoming actively involved in the learning task

FACTORS IN SELECTING MEDIA OR TEACHING SUPPORT MATERIALS

1. Materials are suitable for the purpose of the teaching.
2. Materials are accurate and relevant to the culture and age group.
3. Language is appropriate, understandable, and useful to the audience.
4. Print size is readable.
5. Drawings and diagrams are accurate.
6. Illustrations relate to the audience.
7. Materials are appropriate to the learner's style.
8. Cost is acceptable.
9. Media are suitable to the environment.
10. Ancillary equipment is available.

Contracting

Contracting is a technique in which the patient and nurse agree on mutual goals and specific plans to implement change. The nurse and the patient identify a specific learning goal and the behavior change that will occur as a result of the teaching. The contract specifies the change, when and how it will occur, and how the nurse and patient can evaluate the change. The contract can be verbal or written in clear, sim-

PATIENT EDUCATION GUIDE

1. Make sure your educational objectives are tailored to the needs of the particular patient or family.
2. Let the learners know what kinds of benefits will occur if they change their behaviors or if they participate in teaching. Encourage family support.
3. Show interest and empathy when teaching. Your enthusiasm, listening skills, and knowledge of material will influence the effect of your teaching.
4. Schedule material in short periods that take into consideration the learner's attention span, and break the content into easy-to-understand steps.
5. Organize your teaching so that learning is logical and proceeds at a relaxed pace. Start with the essentials—what the patient needs to know now—then build and reinforce until goals are met.
6. If you demonstrate a skill, accompany it with specific explanations. Allow time for return demonstrations and practice time for the patient.
7. Encourage beginning skills and efforts. Show how your teaching can be incorporated into your learners' daily lives. Help identify obstacles and methods to overcome them.
8. Periodically reassess levels of understanding. Use open-ended questions requiring a response.
9. Use pamphlets or handouts illustrating what you are teaching. Make sure the pamphlet is readable, nonbiased, and up-to-date.
10. Be creative, and use humor appropriately. The learning experience can be enjoyable.
11. If you are using media, such as overheads or slides, use type size large enough to be easily read.
12. Repeat key information at intervals, and summarize at the end.
13. Refer the learner to resources to ask questions or obtain additional information.
14. Keep your language as simple as possible. Explain medical terminology in lay terms.

TABLE 8-3   Media for Teaching

Teaching strategies	Advantages	Disadvantages	Target group	Type of learning
Films, videotapes	Re-create real life Display motion Do not require good reading ability	Too fast for older people Expensive Time to set up and run Teacher attendance	Groups of patients FI*—visual, auditory	Change attitudes Build skills Impart knowledge
Games (e.g., crossword puzzles)	Involve learners No threat Allow for application of knowledge	Not effective if players have difficulty with abstracts or following directions	Adults with acute/chronic disease Health promotion FD*—visual, auditory, kinesthetic	New attitude Application of knowledge Change attitudes or feelings
Handouts, diagrams, models, pamphlets	Consistent Visually reinforce Show relationship Attract attention Direct application Encourage participation	Should be accompanied by verbal explanation Difficult to do correctly Must be accurate depiction Expensive May require artistic skill May require literacy	Well patients Those who must remember detailed information (e.g., titrating medication) Those with limited vocabulary Adults practicing a skill (e.g., breast self-examination) FI/FD—visual, auditory, kinesthetic	Build skills Impart knowledge Teach new skills Apply knowledge and skill Promote understanding
Overhead projectors	Can be used in large and small groups Colorful Focus on thoughts and ideas Prepared ahead of time Transported easily	Accompanied by verbal explanation May be unclear, hard to understand Patient must read	Small or large groups of well or sick patients Reinforcing verbal explanation FI/FD—visual	Promote understanding Impart knowledge
Slides, photographs, filmstrips	Encourage discussion Attract and maintain interest Easily transported Easy to store	Inappropriate for patients with visual problems	Portrayal of real situations Individuals or groups Individuals with poor reading skills FI/FD—visual	Promote understanding of facts
Cassette tapes	Inexpensive Used almost anywhere Require inexpensive recorder Tailored to individual or group	Inappropriate for patients with hearing deficits	Individuals and groups Learning requiring repetition and reinforcement FI/FD—auditory	Reinforce facts

*FI = field independent; FD = field dependent.

ple, measurable terms. An example of a patient goal statement is "I will lose 5 pounds by November 15 using the weight-reduction plan prescribed." Contingency contracts include a specific reinforcer for the behavior. The purpose of contracts between the nurse and patient is to facilitate desired patient behavior by arranging a positive reinforcement or reward. Examples of reinforcers are a back rub in the evening, a game of cards, seeing the doctor in the clinic at the exact scheduled time, or allowing the family extra visiting time. An example of a contingency contract statement where the patients designates the reward would be "I will lose 5 pounds by November 15. My reward will be a movie ticket."

Contracts should always be open to renegotiation. The steps involved in contracting are as follows:

1. Identify the problem.
2. Set goals that will solve the problem. Ask "what can we do together to solve the problem?"
3. Explore what resources are available to meet the mutual goals.
4. Develop a plan. Explore the immediate interventions, time framework, and importance or priority of goals.
5. Determine the activities for which the patient, nurse, or others will be responsible.
6. Set realistic time limits. A time limit can act as a check on progress.
7. Evaluate and modify the contract. If the time limit is up, determine if goals have been met. If the goals have not been met, look to see if new problems developed or if there were other interfering factors. Determine how you can renegotiate the contract.
8. Document progress. State the progress as objective data (i.e., that which was directly observed), for example, "walked from bed to hall three times using a walker."

Special learners

Low-literacy patients

Patients with low-literacy skills are found in every part of the United States and among all population groups. Many people with poor reading skills are highly intelligent and hold important jobs or influential positions in the community. Almost 27 million Americans over 17 years of age can be classified as functional illiterates who cannot read or write well enough to understand a medicine label. Of all adults classified as illiterate, the largest population in the United States is native-born white Americans. Half of all Americans read below the tenth-grade level.

One way to assess patients' comprehension of written material is by using *cloze procedures.* Write a short passage from any instructional material, deleting every fifth word. Replace each word by a blank. Ask the patient to fill in the blanks. When scoring, count all the correct replacement words and divide by the total number of blanks. The patient who scores 60% or better can be considered capable of understanding the material. For assessing reading skill, use a test such as the Wide Range Achievement Test (WRAT), available from Jastak Association, Inc.

Teaching low-literacy patients

Patients with low-literacy levels need simple teaching plans designed to teach the basic information needed to carry out their therapeutic regimen. Patients who cannot read need simply phrased verbal information supplemented with visual aids. Poor readers need simple verbal information supplemented by written information of a low verbal reading level. People with poor reading skills tend to learn best with an anecdotal or story format featuring characters with whom they can identify. Humor is also effective to both hold interest and emphasize the message.[17] Teaching tips for low-literacy patients include the following:

1. Assess the teaching material level with a SMOG or Fry formula.
2. Present the basics of the information.
3. Present no more than three new points at a time.
4. Give the most important information points first and last. This is the how-to knowledge.
5. Sequence information in the way the patient will use it, in a logical, straightforward manner.
6. Give information the patient can use immediately. For example, have the patient do a medication chart.
7. Repeat and summarize the main points of the message at the end of each session.
8. Ask the patient to repeat the information or demonstrate the skill.
9. Use the same words when meanings are the same (e.g., your medicine or drug), not both words.
10. Use the smallest, simplest words when presenting information. Use short sentences.
11. Use technical words sparingly, and never introduce more than five new words in one session.
12. Present written information at a fifth-grade or lower level.
13. Be concrete and time specific (e.g., take one tablet at 6 AM).
14. Keep the information interesting and relevant to the patient's situation or life-style. For example, diabetic exchange lists for a Mexican American should include beans, tacos, tortilla, or other culturally relevant foods.
15. Use written material that gets the reader involved (i.e., how can they use this information in their own situation?).
16. Speak and write in a nonthreatening, conversational style.
17. Avoid long explanations.
18. Do anything you can to decrease anxiety.
19. Reward frequently—even for small accomplishments.

Geriatric patients

The teaching-learning plan for the geriatric patient must be adapted to fit the learning needs and life-styles of the aging person. Special considerations during assessment include the patient's functional

GERIATRIC CONSIDERATIONS

Tips for Teaching the Older Adult

Assess the patient's cognitive potential, considering functional rather than chronologic age, and pace teaching accordingly

Evaluate the patient's self-care abilities

Evaluate the patient's emotional state

Work with the patient to set realistic goals

Assess the patient to ensure what you are trying to teach will fit into his or her life-style (habit structure, finances)

Make sure words you use are clearly understood:

Ask for feedback after each new term used

Use a conversational style

Talk on the patient's level

Use a multisensorial approach (hearing, seeing, touching)

Individualize teaching process to compensate for any impairments:

Aids for impaired hearing:

Use lower-pitched voice

Face patient while speaking

Use nonverbal techniques

Reinforce oral with written

Have patient use hearing aid if patient has one

Supplement hearing by printing new terms on the chalkboard if patient can see

Control outside extraneous noise (e.g., television, radio)

Reemphasize main points

Use appropriate seating

Use clear, concise terminology

Aids for impaired vision:

Prescription glasses

Magnifying glass

Large print

Black on white or black on yellow paper (may be easier to read)

Remember many older people have problems seeing a variety of colors, especially greens and blues

Use large capital letters

Provide adequate lighting

Remove extraneous objects

Avoid glare from objects

Aids to facilitate lower reaction times and limited endurance:

Tailor plans to meet individual patient needs

Keep sessions short (10 to 15 minutes is a good limit)

Schedule sessions for time of day when patient is rested and comfortable

Provide for rest periods as needed

Avoid time pressures

Break down learning process into small steps

Work with only survival-level information in initial session

Aids to facilitate learning for patients with memory loss:

Provide repeated exposure to same message

Provide cues (visual, verbal, written)

Question frequently

Use organizers

Announce topic before discussing it: "I'm going to tell you about how to _____."

Summarize information after the topic has been discussed: "I have told you about how to____."

Encourage the patient to actively participate:

Don't take anything for granted, ask for feedback

Listen carefully to what the older person is saying, both verbally and nonverbally

Get patient's attention

Readiness to learn has a great deal to do with emotional factors—pay attention to them:

Make sure that the patient is comfortable (i.e., basic needs met)

Provide safe environment (e.g., proximity of bathrooms)

Reduce anxiety, depression, grief, and fear as much as possible

Encourage expression of negative feelings

Use *active* listening

Reduce threat to self of learner, such as drawing on past learning strengths (e.g., printed material rather than televised material)

Consider that the patient may lack motivation to learn:

Encourage self-direction (what does the patient want?)

Consider quality vs. quantity of life decision

Focus on problem solving for life satisfaction

Establish mutually realistic goals

Include patient's family or significant others

Teach one step at a time to allow experience of success

Use specific directions that can be followed step by step

Separate "nice to know" from "have to know"

From Fox B: Geriatric patient education: issues and answers, *J Contin Educ Nurs* 19(4):169, 1988.

PATIENT EDUCATION GUIDE   *Basic Medication Rules*

1. Medication instructions must be understood.
   - When, at what time, and how much should be taken?
   - What side effects are possible?
   - How long should the medication be taken?
   - How should the medication be stored (such as refrigerated)?
2. Establish a routine and daily schedule of when to take medication, especially if taking multiple medications.
   - Store medications in one central location, where it is not too hot, too cold, or too wet.
   - Make a schedule of when to take medications and keep in a convenient place.
   - Keep all medications out of the reach of children.
   - Consult a physician about missed doses. Do not assume that taking a double dose the next time is appropriate.
3. Discard medications that have expired or that the physician has terminated.
   - Immediately discard medications that are terminated.

- Check expiration date of all medications every 6 months and discard those that are out-of-date.
4. Take medications only as prescribed by a physician.
   - Never take medicine that is brought in from another country without discussing it with a physician or pharmacist.
   - Never borrow or trade medications. Even medications prescribed for someone else with the same condition may cause harm if not taken under a physician's direct orders.
   - Never discontinue or change medication regimen without consulting a physician or pharmacist.
5. Always carry a list with the names of all current medications.
   - Include all prescribed medicines as well as any topical medications, eye drops, medicines purchased from other countries, herbs, and over-the-counter preparations.

and psychosocial status. Lack of social support may be an important determinant in the decreased compliance that is commonly observed in the elderly. Functional losses in sensory perception, short-term and long-term memory, and dexterity, as well as limitations of mobility will affect the elderly patient's ability to perform skills and may limit learning.

The box on p. 114 lists tips for teaching the older adult. The patient education guide above lists basic medication rules for teaching the low-literacy or elderly patient.

Evaluation

A variety of techniques exist to evaluate learning. Evaluation focuses on the learner and the extent to which the learning goals were accomplished.

Direct observation of the learner can be used to determine whether a skill has been learned. The nurse identifies the essential points of each skill using a checklist and observes whether the patient has partially or totally mastered the skill. The level of mastery may vary. For example, patients must accurately draw up the correct amount of insulin, but it is not essential for them to always correctly calculate calories in their daily diets. The nurse may also observe the patient during a simulation, such as a dressing change, or during a role play to provide im-

mediate feedback or guidance during the activity. The activity may also be recorded using a video or tape recorder.

Written tests are used to measure knowledge and comprehension. Major disadvantages of written tests include test-taking anxiety and the fact that tests can be used only with patients who can read and write adequately. The nurse may choose to ask the question verbally rather than administer a written test if patient anxiety or literacy is a problem. Questions must be clearly phrased and measure what the patient has learned. After giving the test the nurse provides immediate feedback to reinforce learning.

Interviews and questionnaires

Well-constructed questionnaires can be effective. Consider the type of question to be asked, the number of questions and questionnaires, and the literacy level of the patient or group. Construct questions according to the type of information desired. Open-ended questions elicit a different kind of information from objective tests. Whereas the latter can provide information about the knowledge learned or the ability to discriminate inappropriate or incorrect answers, open-ended questions allow the patient to briefly explain answers. Keep questionnaires as brief as possible by asking only relevant questions. Use readable print with a limited number of questions written clearly and at a language level suitable to the patient.

Conduct interviews in an environment where the patient may talk freely. Use open-ended interview questions that allow for communication of information. Interviews are especially appropriate for illiterate patients and family members. Additional questions can be asked during the interview to clarify information or obtain additional information.

Reports

Self-reporting of behaviors can be used as a source of information for such things as measurements of daily weight, medications, pulse and blood pressure, and daily food intake. These reports can be recorded by the patient between clinic visits or patient teaching sessions. The nurse must explain to the patient how to collect and record specific information. The major problem with this type of evaluation is that the data may be inaccurate or not objective.

EVALUATION OF THE TOTAL LEARNING EXPERIENCE

Goals

Were the goals important for the patient to achieve?
Were they realistic for the patient to achieve?
Were they ambiguous?
Were the goals broken into small steps for the learner to accomplish?

Teaching strategy

Was the format appropriate for learning the desired behavior and for the learning ability of the patient?
Did the patient receive the necessary information?
Could the information be augmented with media?
Did the media help the patient learn?
Was the patient given opportunity to practice, ask questions, or clarify information?
Was there opportunity for application of learning?
Was the information clear, concise, and of practical value to the patient?
Did the patient receive feedback and encouragement during the learning experience?
Was there sufficient time for learning to occur?
Was the language or terminology understandable?
Were the data obtained from the evaluation valid and reliable?

Documentation

Document the results of the evaluation, and use them to plan future teaching interventions. If the desired behavior is accomplished, the nurse provides opportunities for reinforcement of the knowledge or skill. If the learning behavior is only partially met or not accomplished, the nurse must reevaluate the total learning experience. Areas to reexamine are given in the box below.

Document individual patient teaching on a form in the patient's chart or medical record. Include the patient's learning needs, what was taught, the patient's learning progress or response to teaching, the materials given to the patient, and the results of the evaluation of the plan. This documentation also serves to plan and implement future teaching. By documenting patient teaching, the nurse can plan for continuity of care from shift to shift or visit to visit. Other nurses or health professionals can reinforce previous teaching, assess the learning already accomplished, or build on previous teaching. An analysis of nursing health care needs to produce specific outcomes rests on accurate, complete, and valid documentation of patient education and information. The patient teaching form promotes professional accountability in that each learner objective is signed by both the nurse and the patient as the objective is met. Each nurse who looks at the form can determine what areas need to be taught. All areas of patient teaching can be covered as the patient masters each area.

LEGAL IMPLICATIONS

In 1972 the American Hospital Association issued a Patient Bill of Rights. According to this bill, patients are entitled to receive information concerning diagnoses, treatment, and prognosis. They are also entitled to receive the information necessary to give informed consent before initiation of treatment or procedures and to refuse treatment. This means patients are free to make decisions based on their needs, value system, and adequate information. The nurse is responsible not only for content taught but also for the materials used for educational purposes. For example, if the materials used are incorrect or cause harm, the nurse is legally responsible. The nurse also has the responsibility to assess the patient's understanding of information.

Courts hold student nurses legally liable for their patient teaching and hold the student to the standards of the competent professional. When the right to know becomes critical to the patient's health, patient teaching becomes a legal duty of the nurse. The courts judge the student in a lawsuit against national and local standards. Local standards include hospital policies, procedure manuals, and testimony from expert witnesses.[49]

It is important to chart patient education—both formal and informal—as well as the patient's questions and the nurse's answers. If patient teaching plans are used, document the teaching plan as part of the nursing care plan. Include documentation of an evaluation of the teaching indicating patient or family understanding of the situation, ability to manage medications, and treatments and response to illness. Substantiation of teaching effectiveness would support standards of care and decrease nurse liability.

CRITICAL THINKING QUESTIONS

1 How do adults learn? What conditions foster adult learning?

2 Compare the teaching-learning process with the nursing process.

3 What factors does the nurse assess in the functional and psychosocial arenas? What other factors are important in data collection?

4 What principles of change must the nurse consider when developing a teaching plan? What are the components of the planning phase?

5 How can the nurse set realistic goals? Write two clear goal statements for knowledge, skill, and value learning.

6 How are teaching strategies selected? Compare media formats for each of the learning modes of reading, seeing, listening, and manipulating.

7 Compare the advantages and disadvantages of five learning strategies. What factors need to be considered in selecting media or teaching support materials?

8 What are the special learning needs of low-literacy and geriatric patients?

9 What techniques can be used to evaluate learning?

10 What are the legal implications for patient teaching? documentation?

RESOURCES

Education

1 GALE RESEARCH COMPANY, Book Tower Dept. 77748, Detroit, MI, 48277-0748 (800) 223-GALE

2 *Medical and Health Information Directory:* $440 for set of three volumes or $175 for each volume

3 Volume 1—organizations; agencies; institutions; voluntary, federal, state, hospital information programs

4 Volume 2—library, audiovisual, data base services

5 Volume 3—health services, treatment centers, hospitals, clinics

Literacy

6 AMERICAN ASSOCIATION OF ADULT AND CONTINUING EDUCATION (AAACE) 1201 16th St., N.W., Suite 230, Washington, DC 20036.

7 US DEPARTMENT OF EDUCATION, DIVISION OF ADULT EDUCATION/ADULT LITERACY INITIATIVE, Reporters Bldg., Room 522, 400 Maryland Ave., S.W. Washington, DC 20202.

8 *Guidelines: Writing for Adults with Limited Reading Skills* (pamphlet, 1988). Available from The Clearinghouse, Division of Adult Education, US Department of Education, 400 Maryland Ave., S.W., Reporters Bldg., Room 522, Washington, DC 20202, (202) 732-2396.

9 *Teaching Patients With Low Literacy Skills* (JB Lippincott Co, 1985, 171 pp.). Available from JB Lippincott Co, Route 3 Box 20-B, Hagerstown, MD 21740, (301) 824-7300 or (800) 638-3030.

BIBLIOGRAPHY

Current

1. Artz K: The patient education workbook: a program development guide for health care practitioners, *Patient Educ Couns* 10(2):191, 1987.
2. Barron S: Documentation of patient education, *Patient Educ Couns* 9:81, Feb 1987.
3. Bartlett EE: The stepped approach to patient education, *Diabetes Educ* 14:130, 1988.
4. Berg BK et al: Patient education needs assessment: constructing a generic guide, *Patient Educ Couns* 9:199, 1987.
5. Boswell E: Training health care professionals to enhance their patient teaching skills, *J Nurs Staff Dev*, pp 233-238, Sept-Oct 1990.
6. Boyd M: A guide to writing effective patient education materials, *Nurs Manage* 18(7):56, 1987.
7. Brockapp D: What is neurolinguistic programming? *Am J Nurse* 83(7):1011, 1983.
8. Cessario L: Utilization of board gaming for conceptual models of nursing, *J Nurs Educ* 26(4):167, 1987.
9. Chan V: Content areas for cardiac teaching: patients' perception of the importance of teaching content after mesocardia infarction, *J Adv Nurs* 15:1139, 1990.
10. Cummings C: Tuning in to learners' style, *Nurs Staff Dev Insider* 1(4):5, July/Aug 1992.
11. Davis A: Developing teaching strategies based on new knowledge, *J Nurs Educ* 27(4):156, April 1988.
12. DeTornay R, Thompson M: *Strategies for teaching nursing,* ed 3, New York, 1987, John Wiley & Sons, Inc.
13. Doak L, Doak C: Lowering the silent barriers to compliance for patients with low literacy skills, *Promoting Health* 8(4):6, 1987.
14. Fournet K: Developing slide/tape presentations for patient education, *DCCN*(7):183, May/June 1988.
15. Fox B: Geriatric patient education: issues and answers, *J Contin Educ Nurs* 19(4):169, 1988.

16. Gilden J, Hendryk M, Clar S, et al: Diabetes support groups improve health care of older diabetic patients, *JAGS* 40:174-150, 1992.

17. Hersch S: Medication education for an elderly black and Hispanic population in the United States, *Hygiene* X:36, 1991.

18. Higgins M: Learning style assessment: a new patient teaching tool, *J Nurs Staff Dev*, p 14, winter 1988.

19. Janz N, Hartman P: Contingency contracting to enhance patient compliance: a review, *Patient Educ Couns* 5(4):165, 1987.

20. Leman C et al: The impact of mailing psychoeducational materials to women with abnormal mammograms, *J Pub Health* 82(5):729-730, May 1992.

21. Mann KV, Sullivan PL: Effect of task-centered instructional programs on hypertensives' ability to achieve and maintain reduced dietary sodium intake, *Patient Educ Couns* 10:53, 1987.

22. Morra M: Future trends in patient education, *Semin Oncol Nurse* 7(2):143-145, 1991.

23. Redman BK: *The process of patient education,* ed 6, St Louis, 1988, Mosby–Year Book.

24. Redman BK, Levine D, Howard D: Organizational resources in support of patient education programs: relationship to reported delivery of instruction, *Patient Educ Couns* 9(2):177, 1987.

25. Sarisley C: Designing a teaching program for outpatient antibiotic therapy, *J Nurs Staff Dev* 3:128, 1987.

26. Smith CE, editor: *Patient education: nurses in partnership with other health professionals,* Orlando, 1987, Grune & Stratton, Inc.

27. Smith CE: Patient teaching: it's the law, *Nurs '87* 17(7):67, 1987.

28. Taylor R: Making the most of your time for patient teaching, *RN,* p 20, Dec 1987.

29. Tilley JD: The nurse's role in patient education: incongruent perceptions among nurses and patients, *J Adv Nurs* 12(3):291, 1987.

Classic

30. Alspach J: The educational process in critical care nursing, St Louis, 1982, Mosby–Year Book.

31. Bartlett EE: Historical glimpses of patient education in the United States, *Patient Educ Couns* 8:135, 1986.

32. Bennett H: Why patients don't follow instructions, *RN* 49:45, March 1986.

33. Brunt B, Scott AL: Factors to consider in the development of self-instructional materials, *J Contin Educ Nurs* 17(3):87, 1986.

34. Clark KM: Recent developments in self-directed learning, *J Contin Educ Nurs* 17(3):76, 1986.

35. Creighton H: Law for the nurse manager: patient teaching, *Nurs Manage* 16(1):12, 1985.

36. Cunningham M, Baker D: How to teach patients better and faster, *RN* 49:50, Sept 1986.

37. Deardorff WW: Computerized health education: a comparison with traditional formats, *Health Educ Q* 13(1):61, 1986.

38. Demetrulias DM, Shaw RJ: Encouraging divergent thinking, *Nurse Educator* 10(6):12, 1985.

39. Duke E: A taxonomy of games and simulations for nursing education, *J Nurs Educ* 25(5):197, 1986.

40. Fox V: Patient teaching: understanding the needs of the adult learner, *AORN J* 44:234, 1986.

41. Garity J: Learning styles—basis for creative teaching and learning, *Nurse Educ,* p 12, March/April 1985.

42. Griesbach EH: Adapting diabetes instruction to patient anxiety levels, *Patient Educ Couns* 8:84, 1986.

43. Jackson B, Gosnell-Moses D: Cognitive style: a guide for selecting teaching strategies for learners in critical care, *Crit Care Q* 7(1):18, 1984.

44. Knowles MS: *Andragogy in action,* San Francisco, 1984, Jossey-Bass, Inc, Publishers.

45. Kolb D: *The learning styles inventory,* Boston, 1985, McBer & Co.

46. Koniak D: Autotutorial and lecture—demonstration instruction: a comparative analysis of the effects upon students' learning of a developmental assessment skill, *West J Nurs Res* 7:80, 1985.

47. Magill K, Williams S, Caspi A: Patient education: progress and problems, *Nurs Manage* 17(2):44, 1986.

48. Managerial Briefs: Patient education: megatrends reinforce its priority, *Nurs Manage* 16(1):23, 1985.

49. Partridge R: Learning styles: a review of selected models, *J Nurs Educ* 22(6):22, 1983.

50. Roberts K, Thurston H: Teaching methodologies: knowledge acquisition and retention, *J Nurs Educ* 23(1):21, 1984.

51. Rosenbloom LL: Learning/teaching styles: cognitive mapping, *J NY State Nurses Assoc* 11(1):32, 1980.

52. Sloan M, Schommer B: Want to get your patient involved in his care? *Nurs '82* 12:49, 1982.

53. Society of Teachers of Family Medicine: *Patient education: a handbook for teachers,* Kansas City, Mo, 1977, Society of Teachers of Family Medicine.

54. Stanton M: Teaching patients: some basic lessons for nurse educators, *Nurs Manage* 16(10):59, 1985.

55. Ward D: Why patient teaching fails, *RN* 49(1):45, 1986.

56. Woldum KM et al, editors: *Patient education: foundations of practice,* Rockville, Md, 1985, Aspen Systems Corp.

CHAPTER NINE

Legal Dimensions

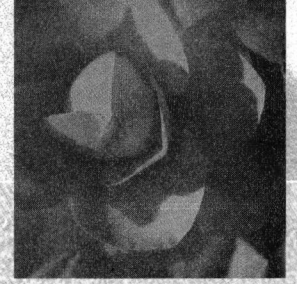

LEARNING OBJECTIVES

1 Outline the legal dimensions of patient care responsibilities.
2 Describe patient rights in the medical-surgical nurse and patient relationship.
3 Define risk management and strategies for avoiding patient injury.
4 Identify the type of employment agreements of the medical-surgical nurse.
5 Describe the state's power to license and regulate the practice of nursing.
6 Name selected aspects of the legal process.

KEY TERMS

administrative laws, p. 130
confidentiality, p. 123
consent, p. 123
contract, p. 128
defendant, p. 120
deposition, p. 131
interrogatories, p. 132
jurisdiction, p. 119

legal standard of care, p. 121
negligence, p. 120
plaintiff, p. 120
state nursing practice act, p. 129
torts, p. 120

THE LEGAL SYSTEM affects medical-surgical nursing in many ways. Four sources of law (constitutions, legislation, regulation, and judicial opinions) are relevant to medical-surgical nursing practice. The relationships among medical-surgical nurses, patients, employers, society, and the profession will determine what laws apply to specific situations. For example, to become a registered nurse, one must successfully complete the required curriculum and pass the licensure examination. The nurse then enters into a special relationship with society, that of a registered nurse. This relationship has obligations, duties, and responsibilities for which the nurse is ac-

countable. State laws in the form of Nurse Practice Acts specify the parameters of legal accountability.

Medical-surgical nurses practice in a variety of settings and are subject to differing federal and state regulations for hospitals, hospices, home health agencies, and long-term care facilities. Regulations may vary according to jurisdiction. A **jurisdiction** is a legally established geographic area, such as a state or country. Laws vary among states and between countries. US Supreme Court decisions and federal regulations are the law across the United States, whereas judicial opinions and laws of an individual state are applicable within that state only. Because

LEGAL TERMS

Administrative law—law pertaining to rules applied to the executive branch of government (e.g., state board of nursing)

Civil law—law concerned with legal rights and obligations between and among citizens

Competency—legal presumption that, when one attains the age of majority, a person is able to make legally enforceable acts

Consent—permission given voluntarily by a person with legal competency

Contract—an agreement between two or more persons that creates, changes, or eliminates a legal right or obligation

Criminal law—substantive field of law defining behaviors prohibited or controlled by society (e.g., murder, robbery)

Deposition—an out-of-court, under-oath statement of a witness

Foreseeability—liability concept that one is responsible for the natural and predictive consequences of one's acts

Legal procedure—rules governing how a lawsuit will proceed

Liability—legal concept that one is responsible and will be held accountable for one's actions (personal liability); that a corporation is responsible and answerable for its own decisions (corporate liability); or that an employer is responsible for an employee's acts done within the scope of employment (vicarious liability known as respondeat superior)

Malpractice—the failure to meet a professional standard of care (to be reasonable and prudent under the circumstances), one involving special knowledge and skill performed by a member of a profession, which leads to harm

Negligence—the failure to meet the ordinary standard of care (to be reasonable and prudent under the circumstances), one not involving special knowledge or skill, which leads to harm

Tort—category of law involving civil wrongs against another's person or property

these variations exist, it is imperative that the medical-surgical nurse seek legal advice on specific questions. This chapter gives general information and should not be relied on to answer a specific legal question. Legal advice and additional reading are essential to resolving specific legal problems. The box above summarizes legal terms related to medical-surgical nursing.

PATIENT CARE DIMENSIONS

Most often the medical-surgical nurse is given responsibility for patient care as an employee of a health care facility or agency, the employer. In such an employment situation the nurse assumes duties to patients through the employment agreement. The nurse enters into an agreement to provide patient care in exchange for salary and benefits from the employer. Part of assuming the job is an agreement to care for a group of patients. This relationship carries with it obligations, responsibilities, and rights of a legal nature. In private duty or independent practice, the nurse assumes duties through a direct nurse/patient relationship. In patient care, legal responsibilities of the medical-surgical nurse include the following duties:

1. Provide safe, competent care.
2. Deliver care according to the legal standard of care.
3. Practice nursing in ways that safeguard patient rights.
4. Prevent violation of patient rights and other laws.

These responsibilities demand that the medical-surgical nurse know the level of care expected, deliver it in a reasonable manner under the circumstances, and understand laws that affect medical-surgical nursing.

Several categories of laws, including torts, contracts, criminal laws, and administrative laws, are enforceable through different legal processes, including civil, criminal, and administrative procedures. This chapter and the legal boxes throughout this text discuss many of these laws and procedures. Figure 9-1 gives a schematic representation of selected legal dimensions of medical-surgical nursing practice.

Several types of law are found in each category. For example, **torts,** which are civil or private wrongs or injuries, are divided into three types: unintentional, intentional, and quasi-intentional. Civil wrongs can be committed against a person or property.

Legal Standard of Care: Negligence/ Malpractice

Negligence involves an unintentional act or a failure to act that leads to injury or harm to a patient. Malpractice is a type of negligence involving an act or a failure to act on the part of a member of a profession (see box on p. 121). The medical-surgical patient who initiates a lawsuit becomes known as the **plaintiff** and must prove all of the following elements: that the nurse (who, if sued, becomes the **defendant**) owed a duty to the patient, that the nurse breached that duty, and that the breach led

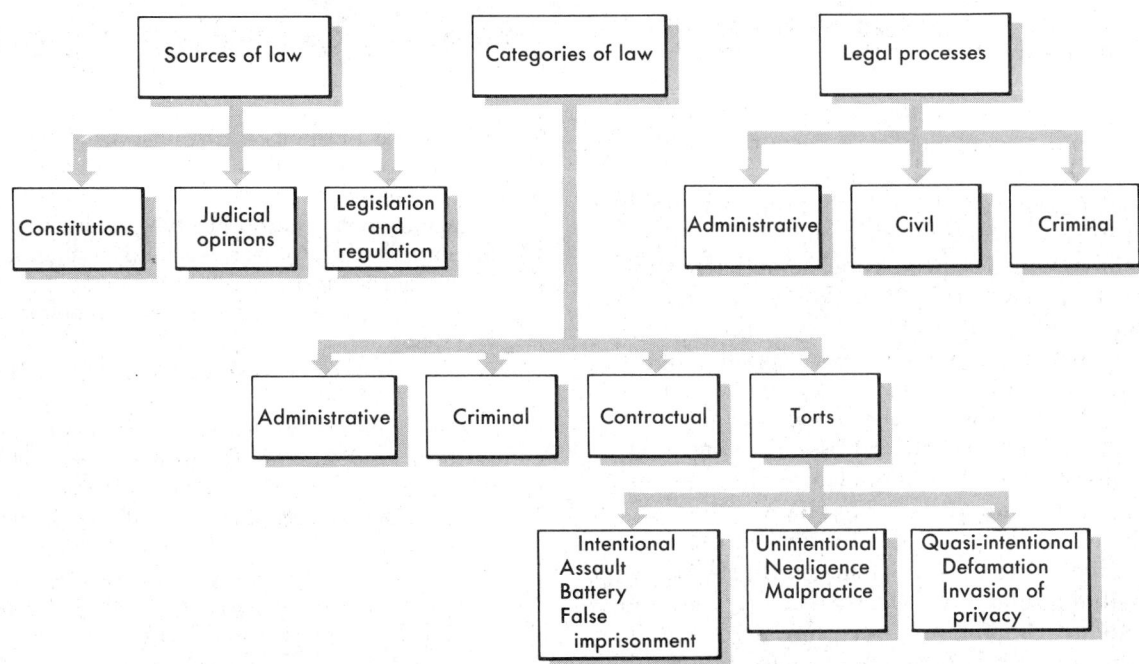

FIGURE 9-1   Selected legal dimensions of medical-surgical nursing practice.

to and was the proximate cause of the patient's specific injuries.

The medical-surgical nurse's duty to a patient with whom there is an established nurse-patient relationship is to provide reasonable, prudent care required by the circumstances. This is known as the nurse's **legal standard of care.** It has several important characteristics.

ELEMENTS TO BE PROVEN IN NEGLIGENCE/MALPRACTICE CASES

1. Duty—defendant owed the plaintiff a reasonable and prudent standard of care under the circumstances; standard of care in a negligence claim is an ordinary standard or in a malpractice claim is a professional standard (one requiring special knowledge and skill possessed by a member of a profession, such as nursing).
2. Breach of duty—either by failure to act (omission) or by committing an act (commission).
3. Proximate cause/causation—required criteria, depending on the jurisdiction: foreseeability plus direct or "but for," or substantial factor.
4. Injury/damages—may be physical or psychologic injuries or both; plaintiff seeks one or more types of money damages: compensable, nominal, punitive.

First, this standard is a reasonable standard, an average, not a standard of excellence or quality. Because this is a professional standard, the plaintiff generally has to produce an expert witness to establish in a malpractice claim that the standard is one requiring the specialized knowledge and skill of a qualified professional.

Second, the exact practice situation or facts of the situation will determine reasonableness. Nursing care is not delivered in a vacuum. Many factors determine what expectations are reasonable. For example, the overall patient care assignment, including the staff/patient ratio and patient acuity level, affects what is reasonable and prudent under the circumstances. The nurse's education, experience, knowledge, and skill are also important factors.

In addition, the standard of care is measured according to what a similarly placed nurse would do in the same situation. Medical-surgical nurses vary their care based on its context, that is, outpatient, inpatient, long-term care, home care, or ambulatory settings. For example, crash carts are an expected part of care in an acute care setting. In home care, however, resources are limited and expected interventions are therefore dissimilar. Thus the reasonable and prudent medical-surgical nurse in an acute care setting would use the crash cart in an emergency; the medical-surgical nurse in a home setting would not use such an intervention but would instead call the rescue squad or ambulance.

Third, the standard of care applied in a malpractice case is the standard that existed at the time of the patient's injury. Current practice standards are not applied to a question of negligence that occurred 3 years ago. The standard of 3 years ago would be applied. Therefore, since the standard evolves with knowledge and experience, it is essential to be familiar with changes in policy and procedure manuals and to stay abreast of current nursing and health care literature.

A case involving acquired immune deficiency syndrome (AIDS) drives this point home. In *Kozup v. Georgetown University*,[1] a hospital was found not liable for transfusing a newborn with blood contaminated with HIV. This result was due to the fact that on January 10, 1983, when the blood was given, the industry standard was such that no screening and no warning of risks or other steps were taken because at the time it was not known that HIV was transmissible in blood. Today's standard is quite different. In 1984 the medical community learned that AIDS was transmissible in blood; in 1985 tests to screen blood were available. Blood banks must now screen all donations properly and store and transfer blood adequately based on the current state of knowledge about AIDS transmission. The standard of care for transfusion has changed dramatically in less than a decade.

A fourth characteristic of the medical-surgical nursing standard is that of variability based on the community, location, or region where care was delivered. Some state laws dictate a national standard to measure reasonable care. Other states require that a regional standard of care be applied.

The plaintiff (the allegedly injured patient) must prove his or her case using evidence, such as the patient records, hospital policy and procedure, and expert testimony, according to legal rules of evidence. To prove what a reasonable and prudent medical-surgical nurse would do under the circumstances, a plaintiff usually presents evidence about the nurse's standard of care, such as that listed in the box above. If the nurse defendant's care does not measure up to the standard and if the nursing care caused or was a factor in the injury, then the patient plaintiff can recover money damages.

Other Torts

Unintentional torts, such as negligence and malpractice, as described on p. 120, are only one type of tort. There are others that are relevant to medical-surgical nursing practice. These include the intentional torts of assault and battery and false imprisonment and the quasi-intentional torts of defamation, invasion of privacy, and breach of confidentiality.

Assault and battery involves behaviors by which one person threatens to touch or harm (assault) or actually touches a person without his or her consent

---

EVIDENCE OF NURSING STANDARDS

1. Practice protocols, contracts, collaborative practice agreements, employment agreements, personnel manuals
2. Agency policy and procedure manuals
3. State Nurse Practice Act and regulations and standards incorporated by reference
4. American Nurses' Association's *Code for Nurses* (1985)
5. American Nurses' Association's *Standards of Practice* (1991)
6. Accreditation criteria of the Joint Commission on Accreditation of Health Care Organizations
7. Other accreditation standards, depending on the practice setting (e.g., National League for Nursing, National Association of Home Care)
8. State and federal licensing laws and regulations governing health care agencies; state, professional, and occupational legislation and regulations
9. Nursing specialty standards of care and certification
10. Nursing literature, textbooks, and journals
11. Education, continuing education, staff development, orientation
12. Experience
13. Expert nurse witnesses; other experts and peers; material witnesses
14. Customary and usual practices of nurses

(battery). Both acts are committed without permission or authorization. Nurses avoid allegations of assault and battery by telling patients about the care to be given and what to expect from the nurse and by asking the patient's permission before carrying out nursing tasks.

Generally, patients have agreed to be hospitalized, and unless the patients object, nurses have an implied permission from which to infer that they want necessary nursing care. However, this implied permission or consent does not mean that patients have consented to everything, that they cannot object, or that they have consented to negligent care. The general consent indicated by voluntary hospital admission does not mean that for medical procedures the patient is not entitled to informed consent (discussed on p. 123) from their physician.

False imprisonment involves acts that have the effect of placing individuals in a confined area against their will. In health care, depending on a patient's individual and therapeutic needs, isolation and restraint may become necessary for the protection of the patient or others. To avoid allegations of false imprisonment, nurses must follow procedures, policies, and state laws governing the use of restraints. The proper use of isolation and restraint is discussed below and is only justified when the patient's safety is in jeopardy or the patient meets assessment criteria defined in law or policy.

The quasi-intentional torts protect an individual's interest in reputation and peace of mind. Defamation literally involves taking from one's reputation by injuring that person's character through false and malicious statements.[5] These statements can be presented in two forms: written (known as libel) and verbal (known as slander). Invasion of privacy and breach of confidentiality involve acts that lead to a violation of a person's peace of mind. Patients are vulnerable to the unauthorized release of private and confidential information about themselves, including, but not limited to, their diagnosis, prognosis, treatment, and care plan. The patient's right to privacy and confidentiality and the precautions nurses should observe are discussed below.

NURSE-PATIENT RELATIONSHIP

Because the nurse's legal duty is to provide competent, reasonable care to patients, some of the most important things the nurse can do to ensure such care is delivered are to know the standard of care, develop consistent patterns of practice that meet the standard, and couple these with accurate documentation, reflecting the standard of care.

Examples of specific nursing actions involved in lawsuits where there was a question of medical-surgical nursing negligence are provided in the box above. This list covers many aspects of medical-surgical nurses' responsibilities in the nurse-patient relationship.

The medical-surgical nurse can employ many steps or strategies to assure that standards are met and documented. These are generally referred to as strategies for risk management. Before employing these, the medical-surgical nurse must consider the duty not to violate patient rights.

Patient Rights

Nursing care should be delivered according to patient and civil rights. Topics pertaining to these rights include the following:
1. Consent
2. Refusing treatment
3. Discharge planning
4. Freedom from restraints
5. Confidentiality

State and federal regulations governing health care facilities mandate that certain rights be afforded patients receiving health care. Hospitals must have established policies for discussing patient

MEDICAL-SURGICAL NURSING ACTIONS INVOLVED IN NEGLIGENCE OR MALPRACTICE LAWSUITS

The following actions constituted a breach of a standard of care that led to injury to a patient. The actions involved failure to:
1. Properly store biopsy needles
2. Use due care as patient's known mental and physical condition required
3. Properly place urinary catheter
4. Assess patient's condition
5. Report patient's worsening condition to physician and supervisor
6. Properly manage emergency resuscitation
7. Take appropriate steps in light of patient's high temperature
8. Properly supervise medicated and incapacitated patients
9. Prevent patient falls
10. Respond promptly to patient's signal for assistance
11. Turn patient every 2 hours per physician's order
12. Properly give an injection
13. Know that medication was contraindicated for asthma patient
14. Recognize signs and symptoms of tight cast
15. Report wound drainage to physician
16. Change dressings properly and frequently
17. Check equipment and use properly
18. Properly assess patient's readiness for discharge

rights and how staff are to adhere to them. A list of rights must be posted in the facility and be available to patients and staff. Hospitals must provide education on and enforcement of patient rights.

Consent

The patient's primary provider is legally obligated to obtain from the adult patient a voluntary and *informed* **consent** before medical treatment. For consent to be valid, the patient must have legal competency to consent. Physicians are obligated to inform patients about the proposed treatment, its risks and benefits, alternatives to it, and the consequences of no treatment. However, if the physician believes that informing a patient will substantially and adversely affect the patient's condition, the physician may withhold information. In an emergency situation, consent is implied, and a health care provider may act to protect patients in life-threatening situations.

Hospitals generally have written policies that reinforce the physician's legal obligation to obtain informed consent to medical treatment. Sometimes, if a hospital fails to ensure that a physician has obtained the patient's informed consent, the hospital can be found liable for breaching a corporate duty to the patients it admits to its facility.

One method of ensuring that physicians obtain the patient's consent is to have another member of the hospital's staff oversee the process. Hospitals often turn to their nursing staff to fulfill this role. Hospitals have established procedures whereby physicians obtain patients' consent, and patients are asked to sign forms documenting that they have received the necessary information from their physician and that they have agreed to the treatment proposed by that physician. According to these policies and procedures, nurses often are put in the position of witnessing the patient's signature.

Assuming the role of witness creates an obligation to later testify if called to do so. A witness is generally one who, being present, personally sees or perceives something. Therefore a witness to a patient signing a consent form could be called to testify in a dispute in which the consent form is relevant. The witness can be asked to relate any information known about the patient's act of signing the form or anything the witness may know about the informed consent.

While obtaining a patient's signature, the medical-surgical nurse may be asked questions by the patient that indicate that the patient has not been adequately or appropriately informed. A nurse who encounters such a situation should immediately discuss the concerns with the treating physician *and* the nursing supervisor. The concerns may center on any aspect of the legal standard for informed consent, including the following:

1. Is the patient voluntarily (without duress) consenting?
2. Does the patient have the ability and lucidity to consent?
3. Has the patient received the appropriate information in a manner that the patient understands?

Since hospitals are held responsible for incompetent medical practice that occurs within their facility and liable for the consequences of incompetent practice, they are obligated to be sure all their patients can give legally defensible informed consent.

Some adult patients are medically, physically, or mentally unable to participate in decisions about their own health needs. However, the patient remains legally competent unless a formal legal procedure declares the patient incompetent.

Opinions provided by physicians and psychiatrists about the patient's mental or physical status are considered by the court when deciding the competency of a patient. If a patient is declared legally incompetent, the court appoints a guardian who makes treatment decisions for the patient.

Since not all situations regarding patient competency go to court, decision making regarding how to proceed with care as the patient would have wanted is left to the physician with involvement of spouses, adult children, or significant others.

There is a legal presumption in all states that an adult, defined as one who has reached the age of majority, is competent to consent to medical treatment, and there is a related presumption of incompetence of those under the age of majority (referred to as minors).[12] State legislatures, however, have defined limited exceptions to the minor's presumed incompetence concerning health care decisions. Hospitals should take these exceptions into consideration and provide policies that govern care of adolescents within the scope of the jurisdiction's laws.

Refusing treatment

Two inherent beliefs basic to the health care professions are respect for each individual and respect for each person's value system. Coinciding with this respect and acceptance is the right of patient autonomy and the freedom to make decisions about one's health care. Implicit in choosing health care options is the right to refuse treatment.

In 1987 the New Jersey Supreme Court expanded the right of individuals to refuse life-sustaining medical treatment and said the patient's interests must come before those of the state. The court's rulings included immunity from civil and criminal liability for those involved in making decisions "in good faith" and provided guidelines for patients, their families, and physicians when approaching such decisions in a care setting.

The court pointed to the Karen Quinlan case and the fact that the patient has a right to refuse invasive medical treatment under a constitutionally protected right of privacy. The court recognized that the state has an interest in preserving life but said those interests weaken—and the individual's right to privacy becomes stronger—as the degree of bodily invasion increases and the prognosis for recovery to a knowledgeable and aware state dims.

Recent court cases around the United States have highlighted the dilemma many health care providers, patients, and family face when trying to balance a belief in the preservation of life with patient wishes. The trend of public opinion and court decisions supporting patient autonomy is exemplified by the passage of the Patient Self-Determination Act of 1990 (see the legal issues box on advance directives on p. 125).

LEGAL ISSUES   *Advance Directives and the Patient Self-Determination Act*

Adults, while legally competent, have the opportunity and the right to make advance decisions concerning the type and extent of health care they wish to receive when they are no longer able to make decisions or express their wishes. The specific tools and options available depend on the laws of the state in which the person resides. However, the two most commonly used tools are the living will and the durable power of attorney for health care.

Of the two, the living will is seen more frequently. It is a written declaration that any competent person may execute at any time, giving specific directions for the withholding or withdrawal of life-prolonging procedures. The person making the declaration must sign and date it and should be as clear as possible about the measures the person wishes used or withheld. If the document is not handwritten, it should be witnessed by at least two persons over 18 years of age, preferably persons who are unrelated to the signer and who do not stand to inherit from the signer's estate.

Specific procedures covered under the living will may be limited by the state. The general definition is any procedure or intervention that serves only to prolong artificially the dying process and where, in the judgment of the attending health care providers applying usual and customary medical standards, death will occur within a short time regardless of whether the procedure or intervention is used. Many living will statutes state that the administration of medication or the performance of any medical procedure to provide comfort or relieve pain are not death-prolonging procedures. A number of states also include artificial nutrition and hydration in this definition; thus persons not wishing tube feedings or total parenteral nutrition should state their desires clearly in the document.

The other tool available is the durable power of attorney for health care, sometimes called a health care proxy. This tool is much broader in scope than the living will. It is a dated, signed, and witnessed statement by a competent adult appointing a person (known as the attorney in fact or health care proxy) to make health care decisions on the signer's behalf if the signer becomes unable to make decisions. The attorney in fact must make decisions within the scope of what the patient would want, not what the person as proxy wants. The durable power of attorney document must be specific for health care. A conventional power of attorney (e.g., for paying bills) is not valid for health care decisions unless it is clearly spelled out in a separate section.

Both instruments can be revoked at any time by the signer and may be rewritten to express new wishes or a new proxy whenever the person feels a change is necessary. Living wills have been available for over 20

years and durable powers of attorney for 10 years. Most adults, when asked, have decided views about what they want done or not done in situations where they might be terminally ill or incapacitated with no hope of recovery, and yet few adults have executed a living will or durable power of attorney. The consequences of inaction are readily apparent in the case of Nancy Cruzan.

On the night of January 11, 1983, Nancy Cruzan lost control of her car, wrecked her car, and was thrown into a ditch. When found, she had no pulse or respiration and was later estimated to have gone 12 to 20 minutes without oxygen to the brain. Heartbeat and respiration were restored by paramedics at the accident site, and Ms. Cruzan was transported to a local hospital. She never regained consciousness but progressed to a persistent vegetative state. A feeding tube was inserted in her stomach, but she did not require help to breathe. She remained in this condition in a nursing facility for 5 years, when her parents petitioned the court to have the feeding tube removed and allow Nancy to die naturally. In 1990 the U.S. Supreme Court upheld a Missouri state Supreme Court ruling that required "clear and convincing evidence" of a patient's wishes before life support measures can be terminated.

Ms. Cruzan had only spoken about her wishes to several people and had not executed an advance directive. Following this decision, her family was able to present enough evidence through testimony of friends to convince the court of Ms. Cruzan's wishes. Nancy Cruzan died in December 1990 following removal of her feeding tube. A direct consequence of this case was the introduction by Senator John Danforth of Missouri of the Patient Self-Determination Act of 1990.

Following the act's enactment on December 1, 1991, all institutions receiving Medicare or Medicaid funds must now ask each newly admitted adult whether or not the individual has an advance directive and must provide information concerning advance directives and the institution's policies governing them. Covered institutions include hospitals, home health agencies, HMOs, hospices, rehabilitation facilities, and nursing homes. Patients do not have to have an advance directive to be admitted to a facility, and the facility may not provide a different or lesser standard of care for patients who have an advance directive.

A copy of the directive must be kept with the patient's medical record. If the patient makes any changes, these must be noted and communicated as quickly as possible to all participating health care providers. Providers are required to honor the patient's wishes to the extent possible and if unable to do so in good conscience, must transfer the patient to a provider who can comply with the patient's directives.

From: The Patient Self-Determination Act of 1990, Sections 4122 and 6157 of the Omnibus Budget Reconciliation Act of 1990, P.L. 101-508. *Cruzan v. Director, Missouri Dept. of Health,* 110 S.Ct. 2841(1990).

Competent adult patients have the right to refuse not only extraordinary treatment but also ordinary treatment. The nurse must remember this and work with the patient to identify reasons for refusal, the options available to the patient, and the consequences of refusal. Careful documentation of these steps demonstrates respect for the patient's values and rights, provides for informed consent, and protects the nurse should legal action arise later.

Death

Regardless of what treatment decisions are made, eventually all people die. Historically, death was synonymous with the cessation of breathing and heartbeat. In 1979 that definition was broadened with passage of the Uniform Determination of Death Act, which utilized the Harvard Medical School's criteria: (1) irreversible cessation of circulatory and respiratory function or (2) irreversible cessation of all functions of the entire brain. The two criteria for the determination of brain death are the absence of all cerebral and brain stem functions, and irreversibility.[6]

No uniform guidelines for the determination of brain death exist. The physician makes the determination based on criteria within a particular locale.[22] Policies and guidelines vary from hospital to hospital. However, the guidelines established by the Harvard Ad Hoc Committee are referred to often.[24] According to the committee the following criteria must be satisfactorily diagnosed in determining that a brain has permanently ceased to function: (1) total unresponsiveness to external applied stimuli, (2) no movement or breathing, (3) no cranial reflexes, and (4) a flat electroencephalogram (EEG).

Institutional policies establish criteria by which death is pronounced and confirmed. The nurse must be aware of the brain death policies of the institution in which she or he is working. Confirming studies such as an EEG, cerebral angiography, and radionuclide brain scans may be ordered to validate brain death. Accurate, clear, concise nursing notes should document the tests, the patient's reactions to these tests, the time of such events, and the time brain death is declared by the physician.

However, prolonged critical observation of a patient may be required in the following circumstances:

- Children younger than 5 years of age should be observed for 24 hours, since they have a greater potential for recovery.
- Hypothermia below 32.2° C can mimic brain death and can protect against neurologic damage as a result of hypoxia.
- Drug intoxication can impair normal response to stimuli.

- Shock, with impaired circulation, can render diagnostic tests invalid.[22]

The duration of clinical observation and testing depends on the cause of the coma and the availability and quality of clinical and laboratory data.[23] Neurologic consultations are extremely important in declaration of brain death.

In all cases in which the death is unexplained or a result of other than natural causes, the death must be reported to the medical examiner or coroner. The date, time, and name of the person from the medical examiner's or coroner's office should be recorded in the patient's medical record. In these cases the coroner must give permission for organ retrieval after the pronouncement of death.[10]

Organ donation

With certified brain death the patient's organs may become available for donation. Only persons with complete and irreversible cessation of brain function may become organ donors.

Laws governing organ donation and transplantation come from both the federal and state levels. The federal statutes have established a network for organ procurement and transplantation, a registry of organ recipients, and have required hospitals to create written protocols for the donation and transplantation process. Federal law also prohibits organ purchases.

State laws affect the procurement and transplantation processes as well. Some states now have an organ donation card or designation with the driver's license. Most states have adopted the Uniform Anatomical Gift Act, which establishes rules about who may make an anatomic gift, how gifts are to be executed, and rights and duties at death. A recent addition to this act by some states is the required request provision. This provision requires the hospital administrator or a designated substitute to request donations of organs from suitable donors. Generally, any competent person over 18 years of age may donate some or all parts of his or her body for transplantation, education, research, advancement of medical science, or therapy. The contribution may be general (to anyone in need) or specific (e.g., to a medical school or hospital).

State statutes also establish a list of persons who can give permission for organ donation at the time of death. This list generally includes the spouse, adult children, parents, siblings, legal guardian, or any other person such as the health care proxy or attorney-in-fact who is authorized to make decisions for the patient or under obligation to make provisions for the body. Organ donation by minors (children under 18 years old) must be by consent of the parent or legal guardian. State statutes also prohibit the physician who pronounces death from participating in the removal or transplantation of organs from that donor, and the surgeon performing the organ removal should not participate in the determination of death.

Medical-surgical nurses may be called on to help ask families for permission to use the organs of the deceased in transplantation or to answer questions concerning the transplant process. Nurses should be well informed about the policies of the institution in which they are working and be supportive of whatever decision the family makes. Careful documentation in the medical record of who was asked and the decision, as well as assuring that the proper releases are signed and in the chart may also be part of the nurse's duties.

Discharge planning

Hospitals are required by regulation to have a mechanism for discharge planning. In fact, utilization review and peer review organizations are mandated to assess the length of stay in the hospital of each patient and to determine its appropriateness. If a longer stay or the hospitalization itself is not medically necessary, the hospital will not be reimbursed for the care costs. Concerned that hospitals might attempt to avoid absorbing these costs, Congress passed laws in 1987 to protect patients from early or inappropriate discharge. These laws create a mechanism for patients to be informed, almost from the day of admission, about their date of discharge. A written plan must be given to the patient, who may object to and appeal the time and medical appropriateness of the discharge.

Freedom from restraints

As mentioned on p. 123, as a general rule, every patient has the right to be free of restraints. However, emergencies and the safety needs of patients may dictate a need to restrain a patient, either physically or chemically. Acceptable practices involving the use of restraints include the following general rules:

1. The least restrictive (to the patient's freedom of movement) means of dealing with the patient's needs should be implemented first, before the more intrusive, more restrictive methods of restraint.
2. Each restraint should be appropriate to the individual needs of a patient; those needs are specifically identified and recorded in the patient record.
3. Restraints are never ordered or used for staff convenience; for discipline; or as substitutes for direct care, activities, or services.[2]

Every state has specific rules about the use of restraints. Generally, unless the situation is an emergency, restraints must be ordered by a physician. Close monitoring of a restrained patient is indicated; for example, regulations may specify that restraints must be released every 2 hours. Frequent monitoring of vital signs may be required by regulations or by hospital policy. The need to apply and continue restraints must be completely documented. Hospital policies and procedures must reflect the applicable laws and regulations within the hospital's jurisdiction.

Confidentiality

It is the duty of every medical-surgical nurse to maintain the patient's right to **confidentiality**. The only information that is made public about patients' hospitalization is their physical presence in the facility and general statements about their condition: stable or critical is all that is said. What part of the facility, such as the AIDS unit; the person's diagnosis, such as cancer; and the expected length of stay are examples of information that *should not* be released to the public.

It is good practice for hospitals to designate a formal spokesperson for the facility. This person can manage press or media requests and be the one to whom nurses can direct public requests for information.

Specific information and the means by which it is released must be with the patient's permission. The patient's instructions about what to release and to whom must be followed to avoid charges of breach of confidentiality. For example, hospitals require patients to sign a release form giving the hospital permission to release the patient's records to insurance companies or Medicare (to receive payment for services) or to release records to other health care providers.

State laws establish rules about patient records. Patients can access their own records and in some situations may amend their records if they disagree with what is written by others. Special rules exist that apply to children's records, psychiatric records, and records maintained by alcohol and drug rehabilitation services. These rules should be part of hospital policy.

State legislatures and court decisions have established that in certain circumstances a health care provider is obligated to breach a patient's right to confidentiality. For example, state statutes, known as reporting statutes, mandate nurses and other health care providers and administrators to report certain health conditions, such as child or elder abuse, patient abuse, gunshot wounds, and communicable diseases. In addition, in many states if the health provider believes that a person will harm another person, the provider may have a duty to breach confidentiality and warn the intended victim. Law on this topic varies tremendously; the medical-surgical nurse should ascertain what laws apply in a specific patient care situation by seeking legal advice.

All states mandate that physicians report cases of AIDS to state health department officials. Those to whom these reports go are under legal obligation to keep the report confidential. The principle of confidentiality is fundamental to successful, voluntary participation in HIV screening programs and the resultant containment of the AIDS epidemic.[8] The American Nurses' Association maintains a forceful position in advocating voluntary, anonymous HIV testing.

Some states have laws passed specifically protecting confidentiality of those who take the AIDS antibody tests.[7] Unauthorized disclosure carries fines, and if disclosure results in economic, bodily, or psychologic harm, the person who disclosed unlawfully shall be liable for actual damages, a misdemeanor punishable by imprisonment, substantial fines, or both.

Documentation

Many types of documents and records are made in the course of normal hospital business. The patient's chart, one of these records, is a legal document. It may be used as evidence in a lawsuit, not only a malpractice or negligence lawsuit, but also other types of lawsuits, such as divorce, proof of immigration, child custody, guardianship, contested wills, and probate.

Hospitals have policies governing documentation of medical-surgical nursing practice. The standards of care of medical-nursing practice also discuss patient records.[4] Documentation should serve the interests of the nurse *and* the patient by recording that the nurse met standards of care and documenting the course of the patient's care, treatment, and response to treatment. The medical-surgical nurse records assessment data, nursing diagnosis plans, interventions, evaluation of care, and the patient's response to interventions.

Rules may exist for recording specific types of care. For example, medications are always recorded *when given.* If restraints are applied, the following should be documented: type of restraint, rationale for using it, the written order for it, the time it was written, how long the order will exist, who placed the restraint, where it was placed, the status of the patient, who monitored the patient and how often, what was done for the patient while restrained, when the restraint was terminated, the patient's condition, and rationale.

Hospitals usually require that an incident, unusual occurrence, or accident report form be completed in certain risk-filled situations, for example, when a patient falls or when a wrong medication is given. These forms usually ask what happened, how the patient was found, and what steps were taken in response to the situation. Complete information should be recorded on the patient's chart such as that an accident occurred, the specific details of what happened, the patient's condition, actions taken by the staff, and all aspects of the incident. Charting that an incident report was filed is not necessary.

Charting should be legible, accurate, in chronologic order, and generally written in black ink. Every entry should be dated, timed, and signed. In busy patient care settings, it is not unusual to forget to chart something. However, it is not good practice to squeeze the information in at a later time when it is remembered. Data added later should be marked with "late entry," dated, and timed at the later time and placed in the record at the next chronologically available place. Generally, during orientation to a nursing position, the specific rules of documentation are covered that apply while practicing within the particular facility.[17]

Liability Insurance

Carrying one's own liability insurance policy is a decision of the practicing medical-surgical nurse. The school of nursing or the clinical facility where the student nurse is assigned patient care responsibilities generally requires students to obtain their own insurance. Employer–health care agencies usually have insurance for their employees' negligent acts done within the scope of their employment. Under the doctrine of *respondeat superior,* employers are liable, along with their employees, for the employee's negligence.

Liability insurance is a mechanism whereby the nurse can shift to an insurance company—the insurer—the financial risk that may result from a nursing action that harms a patient.[15] Insurance is a financial risk management strategy, for without insurance, the nurse's own assets will be considered for compensation for a patient's injuries. When a nurse purchases professional liability insurance, a **contract** is formed. The agreement is that upon the nurse paying the premium, the insurance company agrees to defend the nurse in a negligence or malpractice lawsuit, and if the nurse is found to have committed negligence or malpractice, the insurance company is obligated to compensate the patient to the limits of the insurance policy (the contract). Duties and obligations exist under the insurance contract; the written terms of the insurance policy describe these duties and obligations.

Deciding to purchase insurance involves many factors. The box at right lists several factors to consider. Insurance can be complex; the nurse should ask the insurance company to explain its benefits and coverage *before* the insurance is purchased.

Other Risk Management Strategies

Risk management is a system for identifying, analyzing, and implementing strategies for eliminating, minimizing, and addressing liabilities and malpractice.[14] Many states have laws that mandate that hospitals have risk management programs. These programs usually include a broad range of activities. Many risk management programs emphasize improving communication and making administration and supervision more responsive to staff and patient needs.

State laws often require that hospitals, nursing homes, or other facilities notify the state health department in the event of certain patient situations, such as maternal deaths; deaths caused by factors unrelated to the natural course of illness, disease, or proper treatment; or equipment malfunctions, that did or could have adversely affected a patient or hospital personnel.[18] These reports to the health department are confidential (e.g., they are not accessible to a patient for a malpractice suit in relation to the patient's injury).

NURSE-EMPLOYER RELATIONSHIP

Thus far, this chapter has focused on the important nurse-patient relationship and some of its legal dimensions. In that relationship the nurse or the hospital or both are the usual defendants being sued by the injured person—the plaintiff. In the nurse-employer relationship the nurse may be the plaintiff and the employer the defendant.

Most nurses agree to provide patient services through an employment agreement with a health care facility such as a hospital, nursing home, or home health agency. An essential part of this agreement is the provision of safe, competent nursing services in exchange for payment, benefits, and a safe working environment.

Contracts and Employment Agreements

Most nurses enter a general, flexible employment arrangement with hospital employers. They do not have an employment contract—an express, mutually agreed on arrangement that exists for a specific period of time, such as 1 or 2 years. Nurse employees without an express contract may end their employment arrangement simply by following rules specified in the employer's personnel manual, such as giving 2 weeks' notice. So too can the employer

---

WEIGHING BENEFITS AND RISKS OF PROFESSIONAL LIABILITY INSURANCE

1. Personal assets
2. State laws
3. Immunities
4. Amount of premium
5. Coverage
6. Other insurance policies (employer or business policies)
7. Risks of your practice (including setting, the employer's experience with negligence, and range of nursing interventions employed)
8. Legal rules that may limit a nurse's exposure (such as statute of limitations or other state laws on tort reform measures)
9. Claims made vs. occurrence coverage

From Northrop C: Buy liability insurance?: some factors to consider, *Am Nurse* p 29, Oct 1987.

---

end the employment by following rules about termination of employment in their personnel handbook.

In effect, nurses without express contracts are employed *at will* and may be terminated without cause. Some state and federal labor and employment laws may apply to a nurse's employment situation even in the absence of a contract.

Some nurses do enter into an employment contract, either an express individual contract or an express collective or union contract. The specific terms of the contract govern important employment issues, such as work load and health and safety standards in the workplace. Personnel manuals and state and federal laws also govern this type of employment arrangement.

Collective bargaining is a process involving negotiating a contract and enforcing it.[20] It involves formalizing the relationship between employees and employer and between labor and management. Specific federal laws, primarily the National Labor Relations Act, govern union and management activities.

Nurses have been involved in many types of employment disputes, including sexual harassment, age discrimination, and denial of benefits such as workers' compensation for work-related injuries.[21] For example, a hospital cannot arbitrarily fire a nurse who develops AIDS.[13]

NURSE-SOCIETY RELATIONSHIP
Licensure: Nursing Practice Acts

One aspect of the nurse-society relationship is spelled out in the **state nursing practice act** (NPA).

To practice nursing, one must be licensed. This is one way to protect the public from incompetent, unscrupulous, and illegal behavior.

Every state has laws governing professions or occupations with general provisions for all professionals and specific provisions for each profession, including nursing. The latter is generally known as the state's nursing practice act. This law defines nursing practice, identifies the scope of practice, delineates professional and unprofessional conduct, and creates a board of nursing empowered to make decisions about nursing to protect the public. Board of nursing activities include the following:

1. Approving schools, curriculum, and programs in nursing
2. Defining the scope of nursing and the entry requirements into nursing practice, such as licensure examination
3. Participating in disciplinary actions involving nurses
4. Identifying standards of care

Specific NPA provisions allow graduates of nursing programs who are waiting to take the licensing examination to practice nursing for a limited time between the time of graduation and receiving the results of the licensing examination. During this time (and only for a limited time) the graduate nurse is required by law to practice under the supervision of a registered nurse. Specific provisions describe the scope of student nurse practice while in training.

Administrative Law

Disciplinary decisions or other state board decisions are governed by state **administrative laws** and regulations and by the laws governing professionals and occupations. Administrative laws are those rules and decisions made by administrative bodies and the state administrative procedure act. These government entities are created by the legislature and are in the executive branch of government.

Grounds for Discipline

State legislation and regulations contain the reasons for which a nurse can be disciplined. They generally include negligence, gross negligence, fraud and deceit, criminal acts, unfitness and incompetence, unprofessional conduct, and practicing while impaired.[19]

Legal Actions

In most jurisdictions, hospitals and nurses are required to report incompetent, illegal, or unprofessional conduct of others. Patients may file complaints with the state about a nurse's incompetence or negligence. In addition, being found to have committed negligence or a criminal act or to have committed a violation of the public health laws may be communicated to the state board of nursing.

Regardless of where a complaint may originate, the state agency must investigate it. The state investigator reviews all pertinent documents, including the patient's chart and the nurse's personnel records, and records statements from the nurse being investigated and any other relevant witnesses to the complained-about incident. The investigator recommends, based on the evidence, whether to proceed further against the nurse. Procedurally, several possibilities exist at this point. It is advisable that a nurse who is being investigated obtain legal advice and representation.

Depending on the circumstances, the state board of nursing may decide or recommend that the nurse's license be revoked, suspended, or denied; or the board may recommend that the nurse be placed on probation, specifying that certain conditions be met, such as having the nurse take courses and having the employer submit satisfactory progress reports.

Many states are recognizing the growing problem of drug and alcohol abuse in the nursing profession and are also recognizing that such impairment is a treatable condition from which the nurse can recover and return to competent and safe practice. In a growing number of states, impaired nurses may voluntarily surrender their licenses in exchange for agreeing to enter a treatment and rehabilitation program. Many state nurses' associations provide impaired nurse programs to enhance competent professional practice in their states.[19]

A recent Florida case serves as an example of a board of nursing decision. In this case a nurse's license was revoked for the following acts, which were considered unprofessional conduct:

1. The nurse failed to use proper aseptic techniques in inserting a catheter in a female patient.
2. The nurse failed to respond in a timely fashion to a patient observed to be in distress, and she failed to quickly and expeditiously notify the physician of the patient's situation.
3. The nurse failed to document both the incidents above and her actions.
4. The nurse failed to properly assess and report a broken area on a patient's coccyx and failed to take the steps outlined in the decubitus procedure.[9]

A nurse whose license is revoked or suspended and who wants to practice nursing in the future must initiate a legal action for reinstatement through the state's administrative law procedures. In an action for reinstatement the nurse has the burden of proving that he or she has been rehabilitated and can now practice nursing competently and safely.

Criminal Acts

Nurses have also been involved in criminal acts prohibited by state and federal criminal statutes.[16] These acts include those that are intended to cause bodily harm, including death. The media attention and drama that accompany these care incidents should not override the competent professional performance of most of the nation's 2.1 million professional nurses.

Good Samaritan Laws

All states have Good Samaritan laws. These laws provide immunity from suit for negligence, thereby encouraging those with special knowledge in lifesaving, such as nurses, to render such lifesaving care without fear of liability. For example, The New Jersey Good Samaritan Act reads as follows:

> Any individual, including a person licensed to practice any method of treatment of human ailments, disease, pain, injury, deformity, mental or physical condition, or licensed to render services ancillary thereto, who in good faith renders emergency care at the scene of an accident or emergency to the victim or victims thereof, shall not be liable for any civil damages as a result of any acts or omissions by such person in rendering the emergency care.[11]

Good Samaritan statutes apply only in emergency situations in which the nurse has no legal duty to act. For example, rendering emergency resuscitation while performing one's nursing job would not be a situation to which the Good Samaritan law would apply, whereas the same resuscitation activities at the scene of an accident would.

NURSE-PROFESSION RELATIONSHIP

Medical-surgical nurses also have a special relationship to their profession. The profession defines standards of care, which are published in various documents.[3] The ANA and other nursing organizations develop and promulgate statements and codes that apply to professional nurses. In fact, associations, according to their bylaws and policies, may expel members who practice illegally or unethically.

Importantly, documents of professional associations may be used as evidence in lawsuits. It is a professional responsibility of nurses to maintain standards, improve care, and participate in the development of the profession.

PRINCIPLES OF LEGAL PROCESSES

Basic rules apply to civil dispute resolution: (1) the right to access courts for dispute settlement or legal process and (2) due process rights. Both the defendant and the plaintiff have the right to access the courts as a means of resolving disputes. This is a constitutional right of American citizens. In addition, due process rights mandate that certain procedural principles be followed, such as giving proper notice, providing an opportunity to be heard, presenting evidence, and cross-examining witnesses, all within a fair and just forum.

As mentioned previously, there are two sides to a dispute questioning a nurse's care. The parties to the dispute are the plaintiff and the defendant. The plaintiff is the injured patient who initiated the suit or, in an administrative or criminal action, the plaintiff is the state agency or prosecutor. The defendant is the one accused of violating a standard of care, acting unprofessionally, or committing a criminal act.

Negligence or malpractice disputes take place in a civil law forum; disciplinary disputes are determined within an administrative law forum; and criminal charges are heard in a criminal law forum. Each of these forums has unique rules of procedure and rules of evidence. If the nurse is defendant in any of these forums, it is imperative that legal advice and representation be sought.

The plaintiff begins the process by selecting a lawyer to represent his or her interests. Counsel for the plaintiff (the allegedly injured patient) in a negligence case starts with determining whether there is a basis for the lawsuit or claim. This involves record review, especially the patient's chart, fact gathering, interviews, and review of the case by an expert. The lawyer must also review existing law to determine whether there is a basis for the suit. The lawyer examines the sources and types of law that may be involved in this situation, including constitutions, judicial opinions, legislation, and regulation in all relevant areas of law. The plaintiff has the burden of proving all elements of negligence or malpractice.

Since procedures can vary widely, it is best to review with a lawyer the specifics of what will happen in the lawsuit. The nurse who purchases liability insurance will be provided a lawyer by the company, whereas the nurse who does not will be provided one by the employer or through direct contract. Generally, there are several components to a lawsuit, including filing a complaint, serving the complaint on the defendant, answer by the defendant, discovery, review by an arbitration panel or trial, posttrial decisions, and appeal.

Whether named in a negligence suit or not, a nurse may be called as a witness to the complaint or may be called as an expert witness. As a result, many nurses are involved in two of the tools of discovery: depositions and interrogatories. A **deposition** is an out-of-court, under-oath statement of a witness. It is a formal procedure, and it is advisable for a witness to have an attorney prepare for and be present at the deposition. Generally, the opposing party's lawyer asks questions of the witness. The

GERIATRIC CONSIDERATIONS

Avoiding Chemical Restraints

1. Identify the cause of the behavior such as anxiety, depression, and insomnia.
2. Remove the cause if possible.
   * Establish routines that can help pattern the elder's habits.
   * Decrease lighting and noise at night.
   * Avoid loud noises such as bells, buzzers, or intercoms.
   * Always talk to the elder in a calm, reassuring manner.
   * Provide snacks such as milk and cookies before bedtime.
3. Evaluate use of drug therapy.
   * Do medications interact with each other?
   * Are medications given appropriately (i.e., pain medication for pain, not sleep)?
   * Is the lowest dosage of medication being used?
   * Is the behavior a side effect of medication?
4. Provide exercise activities.

entire exchange is taken down by a court reporter and serves many purposes, such as helping find relevant facts and opinions regarding the dispute. **Interrogatories** are written questions directed to the opposing side.

Other aspects of legal process may also occur in a negligence claim. Most negligence and malpractice suits do not go before a hearing panel or to trial but are settled before trial. The fact that one has settled out of court in a malpractice action can never be introduced in a future case involving another negligence claim. However, insurance companies in many states are required to report settlements to the professional's licensing board. Settlement may not be relevant to other negligence claims, but it is relevant to the board of nursing that regulates one's ability to continue to practice nursing.

SEEKING LEGAL ADVICE

Laws change and differ among states and between state and federal courts. This chapter has provided only an overview and introduction to some of the legal dimensions of medical-surgical nursing practice. It is good practice to obtain legal advice for your specific legal questions. It is also important to keep issues in perspective: nurses and their employers need to seek a partnership in their relationships that enhances legal circumstances. Recognition of the nurse as a valuable and competent professional given adequate resources and a safe environment facilitates positive legal relationships with patients and employers.

CRITICAL THINKING QUESTIONS

1 How can the three categories of torts be differentiated?
2 What are the four elements of negligence/malpractice? What must the patient or plaintiff prove after initiating a lawsuit?
3 What are the legal responsibilities of the nurse after a nurse-patient relationship is established?
4 What are the characteristics of the nurse's legal standard of care?
5 What may be offered as evidence of nursing standards in a malpractice suit to prove what a reasonable and prudent nurse might do in a given circumstance?
6 What is the difference between assault and battery? What are some examples of false imprisonment, defamation, invasion of privacy, and breach of confidentiality?
7 What are the four general areas of patient rights? Who decides the policy on patient rights?
8 What does witnessing to consent mean? Who may sign consent? Are there special exceptions or circumstances?
9 What is the primary concern in a decision regarding a patient's health care?
10 What factors are considered in weighing benefits and burdens of decisions to withdraw or withhold treatment?
11 What information may the nurse legally make public when maintaining patient confidentiality? When must a nurse breach a patient's right to confidentiality?
12 What are the general rules a nurse must follow when using restraints?
13 What factors should the nurse consider in weighing benefits and risks of liability insurance?
14 What constitutes a nurse-employer relationship?
15 Who regulates nursing practice? For what does a nurse practice act provide?
16 What is a Good Samaritan law, and when does it apply?
17 What are the procedural principles of legal process in a lawsuit?

RESOURCES

1 AMERICAN BAR ASSOCIATION 750 North Lake Shore Dr. Chicago, IL 60611, 1-800-621-6159

2 AMERICAN SOCIETY OF LAW & MEDICINE 765 Commonwealth Ave., 16th Floor Boston, MA 02215 (617) 262-4990

3 AMERICAN NURSES ASSOCIATION 600 Maryland Ave., SW Washington, DC 20024 (202) 554-4444

4 THE AMERICAN ASSOCIATION OF NURSE ATTORNEYS 720 Light St. Baltimore, MD 21201 (301) 752-3318

5 THE HASTINGS CENTER 255 Elm Rd. Briarcliff Manor, NY 10510 (914) 762-8500

BIBLIOGRAPHY

1. 663 F. Supp. 1048 (D.D.C. 1987).
2. Adopted from 10 New York Codes, Rules and Regulations §414.20 (October 31, 1984) and New Jersey Administrative Code §8:39-6.2.
3. American Nurses' Association: Code for Nurses with Interpretive Statements, 1985.
4. American Nurses' Association: *Standards of nursing practice,* Kansas City, Mo, 1991, The Association.
5. Black's Law Dictionary 505 (4th ed, 1968).
6. Brent NJ: Uniform determination of death act: implications for nursing practice, *J Neurosurg Nurs* (15):265, 1983.
7. California Health & Safety Code §199.20-.23 (West 1987); Wisconsin Code §146.025 (West 1987).
8. Comment, Protecting Confidentiality in the Efforts to Control AIDS, 24 *Harvard J Legislation* 315, 1986.
9. *Holmes v Department of Professional Regulation, Board of Nursing,* 504 S.2d 1338, 1339 (Florida Appeals, 1987).
10. Mid-American Transplant Association: Organ procurement manual, St Louis, Aug 1986, The Association.
11. New Jersey Statutes Annotated §2A:62A-1 (West 1987).
12. Northrop C: Nursing practice and the legal presumption of competency, *Nurs Outlook* 36:112, March-April 1988.
13. Northrop, Nurses with AIDS—on the firing line? *Nursing 87* 64 August 1987, based on Department of Health and Human Services, Office for Civil Rights Region IV, Complaint No. 04-84-3096, memorandum letter August 5, 1987; See also Pear, U.S. files first AIDS discrimination charge, *The New York Times* August 9, 1987; Rehabilitation Act of 1973, 29 U.S.C. §794 and regulations 45 C.F.R. §84.
14. See Bowyer, Chapter 26, Risk management, *Leg Issues Nurs* 427, 1987.
15. See Feutz, Chapter 27, Professional liability insurance, *Leg Issues Nurs* 441, 1987.
16. See Kelly, Chapter 24, Criminal law overview, *Leg Issues Nurs* 383, 1987.
17. See Mech, Chapter 28, Quality assurance and documentation, *Leg Issues Nurs* 453, 1987.
18. See New York Public Health Law §2805-1 (McKinney 1987).
19. See Northrop, Chapter 25, Licensure revocation, *Leg Issues Nurs* 405, 1987.
20. See Northrop, Chapter 31, Collective bargaining, *Leg Issues Nurs* 501, 1987.
21. See Pohlman, Chapter 30, Employment claims, *Leg Issues Nurs* 487, 1987.
22. Simmons RL, Fulton J, Fulton R: *Manual of vascular access: organ donation and transplantation,* New York, 1984, Springer-Verlag New York.
23. Southeastern Organ Procurement Foundation Report, 1986.
24. Stark JL et al: Attitudes affecting organ donation in the intensive care unit, *Heart Lung* 13(4):400, 1984.

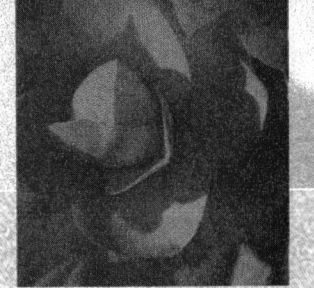

CHAPTER TEN

Ethical Dimensions

LEARNING OBJECTIVES

1 Distinguish among three basic moral positions: utilitarianism, beneficence/paternalism, and advocacy.

2 Identify the different premises underlying the three positions.

3 Critically analyze each position, identifying its difficulties and the way in which one of the other positions handles those difficulties.

4 Define the caring-based theory of ethics and outline its implications for nurses.

5 Explain the role of the nurse in relation to informed consent and truth telling.

6 Distinguish between advocacy and consumerism.

7 List sources of coercion for patients invited to participate in research, and identify the possible contribution of nurses to each form of coercion.

8 Describe application of the advocacy position to the care of patients who cannot participate in decision making.

KEY TERMS

advocacy, p. 140

beneficence, p. 138

caring-based theory, p. 141

consequence-based theory, p. 137

duty-based theory, p. 139

ethics, p. 137

Kantianism, p. 139

paternalism, p. 138

utilitarianism, p. 137

ETHICAL DILEMMAS are familiar to everyone. They are most easily recognized in the form of conflict between different understandings of what is right. An example is the situation in which a family believes it best to withhold a tragic prognosis from the patient when the nurse believes the patient should be told.

Before a concrete ethical problem can be resolved, it is necessary to understand the conflict between different moral views. Such ethical positions or moral views are derived from several ethical theories, including consequence-based theories, duty- or obligation-based theories, and theories of ethics based on caring. It is within these frameworks that nurses struggle to address specific clinical issues such as truth telling, privacy, and confidentiality.

The question of which view a nurse should hold is itself a moral issue that can be resolved in various ways: through the authority of an official document, such as the ANA code of ethics for nurses (see

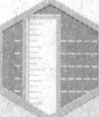

AMERICAN NURSES ASSOCIATION: CODE FOR NURSES

Preamble

A code of ethics makes explicit the primary goals and values of the profession. When individuals become nurses, they make a moral commitment to uphold the values and special obligations expressed in their code. The Code for Nurses is based on a belief about the nature of individuals, nursing, health, and society. Nursing encompasses the protection, promotion, and restoration of health; the prevention of illness; and the alleviation of suffering in the care of clients, including individuals, families, groups, and communities. In the context of these functions, nursing is defined as the diagnosis and treatment of human responses to actual and potential health problems.

Since clients themselves are the primary decision makers in matters concerning their own health, treatment, and well-being, the goal of nursing actions is to support and enhance the client's responsibility and self-determination to the greatest extent possible. In this context, health is not necessarily an end in itself, but rather a means to a life that is meaningful from the client's perspective.

When making clinical judgments, nurses base their decisions on consideration of consequences and of universal moral principles, both of which prescribe and justify nursing actions. The most fundamental of these principles is respect for persons. Other principles stemming from this basic principle are autonomy (self-determination), beneficence (doing good), nonmaleficence (avoiding harm), veracity (truth telling), confidentiality (respecting privileged information), fidelity (keeping promises), and justice (treating people fairly).

In brief, then, the statements of the code and interpretation provide guidance for conduct and relationships in carrying out nursing responsibilities consistent with the ethical obligations of the profession and with high quality in nursing care.

Code for nurses

1. The nurse provides services with respect for human dignity and the uniqueness of the client unrestricted by considerations of social or economic status, personal attributes, or the nature of health problems.
2. The nurse safeguards the client's right to privacy by judiciously protecting information of a confidential nature.
3. The nurse acts to safeguard the client and the public when health care and safety are affected by the incompetent, unethical, or illegal practice of any person.
4. The nurse assumes responsibility and accountability for individual nursing judgments and actions.
5. The nurse maintains competence in nursing.
6. The nurse exercises informed judgment and uses individual competence and qualifications as criteria in seeking consultation, accepting responsibilities, and delegating nursing activities to others.
7. The nurse participates in activities that contribute to the ongoing development of the profession's body of knowledge.
8. The nurse participates in the profession's efforts to implement and improve standards of nursing.
9. The nurse participates in the profession's efforts to establish and maintain conditions of employment conducive to high-quality health care.
10. The nurse participates in the profession's efforts to protect the public from misinformation and misrepresentation and to maintain the integrity of nursing.
11. The nurse collaborates with members of the health professions and other citizens in promoting community and national efforts to meet the health needs of the public.

the box above), through each nurse's individual decision, through a consensus within nursing, or through dialogue between the profession and the public. As each ethical position is described, the reader should reflect at two levels, the personal and the professional: "Is this the moral view from which *I* intend to practice?" and "Is this the ethical position that *nursing as a whole* should endorse?"

ETHICAL THEORIES

Mr. Kramer, an 80-year-old man convalescing from a stroke, has repeatedly resisted therapy and argued that he wants to die, saying that he has lived long enough and cannot endure old age as an invalid. His family is sympathetic to his views and does not insist on treatments that he does not want. They are intensely grieved by his growing unhappiness. Upon entering his room the day he is to be discharged, the nurse finds him without pulse or respiration and an empty barbiturate bottle by his bed.

Reflection on and resolution of ethical problems in health care often progress without formal consideration of ethical theory. Nurses make ethical decisions daily, often without any specific discussion or justification of their basic moral positions or principles. The fact that two people hold different foundations for their views is sometimes irrelevant to resolving the problem. For example, two of Mr. Kramer's nurses may come to the conclusion that his family should not be told of the circumstances surrounding his death. However, one nurse supports the decision by arguing that his duty as a nurse is to respect Mr. Kramer's intrinsic human dignity by respecting his privacy. The other nurse arrived at her conviction by considering that telling the truth to Mr. Kramer's family may damage their view of him, and cause further suffering for them. Thus, they each came to the same resolution of this ethical problem, but from entirely different conceptions of what constitutes right or good. Ethical problems do not always work out this way, however. At times, nurses confront ethical problems that seem unresolvable, perhaps because of the parties holding different ethical principles. In these situations a discussion of the nature and justification of the theories and principles involved can help shed some light on possible resolutions.

Theories of ethics serve several purposes: they provide a general overview of the conception of the good held by the theory; they delineate individual duties and rights held by the framework; and they set the priorities or ordering of the elements within the framework. Whether certain goals, duties, or rights are basic, or they are subordinate, is important in determining the structure of an ethical theory.[3] Theories are, by definition, general in nature. While they provide a general framework and direction for our moral activities and questions, theories are incapable of providing specific direction in particular cases.[1] This type of specific direction is sought through an appeal to the basic principles that grow out of the ethical theories. Although there are many important principles of nursing ethics, those addressed here include beneficence and respect for autonomy. See the box below for a summary of various ethical positions.

Consequence-based Theory

A **consequence-based theory** of ethics locates the rightness or wrongness of actions in the outcome of our actions. An example of this type of ethical reasoning in health care includes making decisions based on a risk-benefit analysis: Do the benefits of particular actions outweigh the risks entailed?

Utilitarianism

A formulation of a consequence-based ethical theory is utilitarianism.[4] Developed by Jeremy Bentham (1748-1832) and John Stuart Mill (1806-1873), the premise of **utilitarianism** is that the combined good of all those involved in a situation has greater importance than the good of a single individual. "The greatest good for the greatest number" is the common formulation of this premise. An action is right or wrong according to its usefulness in promoting the good of all concerned.

In this view, actions such as saving a life or ending a life are neutral, intrinsically neither right nor wrong. Their rightness depends only on their *con-*

SUMMARY OF ETHICAL POSITIONS

Ethics is the systematic investigation of questions about right and wrong. It involves critical analysis of different views of right and wrong, with particular attention paid to the underlying values of each view, its coherence and consistency, and its implications in actual situations.

Morality and morals refer to the common conceptions of what is right and what is wrong. Our morality and morals are reflected in how we live, the decisions we make, and what we hold as valuable.

Utilitarianism is the ethical view that the right action is that which promotes a greater balance of good over harm for everyone concerned in a situation.

Beneficence is the ethical view that the right action is that which promotes the good of the individual patient as that good is understood by the professional.

Paternalism is an extension of beneficence. It is the view that professionals understand patients' best interests better than patients and thus are entitled to act so that a patient's well-being (as professionally defined) is promoted, even when the patient does not agree.

Kantianism is based on Kant's categorical imperative: "Act only on those rules which you can will to be universal law." All specific moral duties are derived from this principle.

Advocacy is the ethical position in which the right action is that which protects and enhances a patient's self-determination regarding health care decisions.

Caring is an ethical framework under study for use as a theoretic basis in clinical nursing practice. It considers relationships as occurring between specific, concrete individuals and emphasizes communication, a desire not to hurt others, and responsiveness as ethical determinants.

sequences, the good or harm that results for everyone involved. Thus utilitarianism is termed a *consequentialist* position, in contrast to positions in which actions are believed intrinsically right or wrong regardless of their results. For the utilitarian, actions are morally inseparable from their results.

What should the nurse do in the case of Mr. Kramer? The moral criterion for her action in the utilitarian framework is that it produce the greatest balance of good over harm for all concerned. The first difficulty or problem for the utilitarian is deciding how large to make the circle of people whose good should be taken into account.

The number of people affected must remain a matter of judgment for the utilitarian. Not only will the number vary with the situation, but it will increase or decrease according to the action the nurse chooses. Mr. Kramer's nurse may decide to pocket (and later destroy) the empty bottle and leave the room, knowing he will not be found until it is too late for resuscitation. Her reasoning would be that his death is a good because it was desired by him, and it releases the family from suffering, provided they think of it as a natural death and not a suicide or a death that cardiopulmonary resuscitation (CPR) could have prevented.

The nurse in this situation has made two decisions. The first is the decision not to attempt resuscitation and thereby ensure the patient's death; the second is a decision to conceal her first decision. Both decisions were made on the same grounds, namely, the greater balance of good over harm that concealment would produce. Although she considers her first decision morally right, she knows that others might not, and thus they could suffer from knowing the actual circumstances of the death. The nurse might suffer by losing her job if the circumstances were known. Through concealment she limits the number of people affected by her action, while still accomplishing what she considers the greatest overall good in the situation.

The second problem for the utilitarian is deciding how to define good in tallying the amount of it that each possible action would achieve. How is the good to be defined? Is it whatever each person in the situation desires? Can death be a good outcome in one case but not in another? Can release from suffering count as a greater good than continued life? Can the pleasure of two persons outweigh the pain of one? How can individual goods be combined to produce a "general" good?

General good is difficult to define. Any situation involving several individuals consists of several discrete individual goods. Averaging those different goods together to calculate the overall good masks the most important thing about them, their individual character. Physical pain for one person will represent a greater harm than for another; continued

life will represent a greater good for some than for others. For a general good to be conceptualized, it would be necessary to regard harms and benefits as comparable for everyone. For example, it would be necessary to decide that a particular good such as preservation of life is the highest good for everyone. There is no way, however, in which such an objective scale could be devised. Definitions of harm and benefit are by nature personal, determined subjectively by each individual.

Beneficence/paternalism

Closely related to utilitarianism, and held as the primary principle in that theoretic framework, is the principle of beneficence. **Beneficence** is the position in which the right action is the one that produces the greatest amount of good for the individual. The patient's well-being is the sole criterion for a good outcome.

Based on that premise, beneficence involves not only acting to promote the patient's best interest, but doing so even when the nurse's view of the patient's good conflicts with the patient's view. Thus beneficence turns into paternalism when a patient disputes the professional's view.

Paternalistic acts and attitudes are those that limit the liberty of individuals for their own good. In nursing, **paternalism** involves the use of some form of coercion to benefit a patient who does not regard the intended outcome as a benefit, or does not regard it as a great enough benefit to outweigh the suffering required to attain it. The coercion need not take overt form. Failing to obtain explicit consent counts as limiting patients' liberty, as does failure to provide patients with adequate information on which to base their consent.

Critics of paternalism claim that only patients themselves can determine what is in their best interest, since that judgment must be based ultimately on subjective, personal values.

Patients cannot know what is best for them without first knowing all of the options available and the objective reasons for and against each one. That information must be provided by the professional. But the professional cannot know which of the options is most consistent with an individual patient's values. That subjective dimension only the patient knows. Objective information itself cannot be the basis for a decision, because it does not take into account a particular patient's fear of anesthesia, fear of blood transfusion, willingness to live with only partial recovery, dedication to following the medical regimen, and so on. These are matters of personal evaluation that only the patient can determine.

A second criticism of paternalism rests on the belief that competent patients have the right to decide what will be done to them. Their freedom of self-determination includes the right to make decisions others consider mistaken or harmful, the right to base decisions on factors others would judge insignificant or irrelevant, and the right even to value an outcome no one else may consider good, namely, death.

The paternalist assumes that illness diminishes the capacity for rational decision making and that the right of self-determination therefore applies only to healthy persons. A person's autonomy definitely is altered by the emergence of physical limitations such as pain or immobility, and the seeking of professional help reflects an awareness of one's own limited understanding. That does not, however, negate the possibility of competent decision making. Patients may be overwhelmed by pain or devastated by a disability, but their limited perspective can be enlarged by access to the different perspective provided by the professional.

In the case of Mr. Kramer, what would the nurse decide if her moral position were beneficence/paternalism? Her concern in this case would be solely with the patient's good. Unlike the utilitarian nurse, she does not take into consideration the consequences for others. But she still faces the problem of defining good. Is death the best outcome for Mr. Kramer? Or are resuscitation and the possibility of continued life in his best interest? The nurse will decide on the basis of *her* evaluation of the various outcomes. Implicit in this evaluation will be her views about death, about aging and disability, about feeling oneself a burden, and about life in a vegetative state. Her view of the patient's best interest will be the basis for her decision, rather than the patient's own self-determination.

Obligation-based Theory

As stated previously, utilitarianism is primarily concerned with raising the quality of life; it holds that persons are morally obligated to increase well-being and to decrease the amount of pain and suffering in the world.[9] These are among the goals of every practicing nurse. Considerations of utility are very important in ethical problems in health care. Who can imagine discussing chemotherapy or surgical procedures, for example, without pondering the risks and benefits involved? Utilitarianism, however, cannot provide a completely adequate moral philosophy. Other ethical viewpoints, based on conceptions of duty or obligation, emerged in response to the inadequacies of utilitarianism. A **duty-based theory** of ethics locates the rightness or wrongness of actions in principles that govern behavior. Such theories take some particular duty or set of duties as fundamental. Examples of duty- or obligation-based theories include those based on a duty to obey God's will, as in the Ten Commandments; the principles set down in the ANA Code of Ethics for Nurses (see box on p. 136); and traditional medical morality rooted in the Hippocratic Oath.

Kantianism

One major ethical viewpoint, known as **Kantianism** (Immanuel Kant, 1724-1804), holds that consequences do not make an action right or wrong. Rather, the moral rightness of a person's actions is dependent upon whether those actions uphold principle, regardless of outcome.[15] For instance, a nurse may administer a drug properly and with the appropriate preparation, and yet, because of some rare and unforeseeable complication, the patient dies. Most individuals would think it unfair to judge the moral worth of the nurse's action solely on the basis of its outcome if the result were unintended and not a result of negligence. Common sense says that the nurse's motive, or the principle behind the action, should determine the judgment of the morality of the action.

Kant believed that nothing is good in itself except a "good will," by which is meant the uniquely human capacity to act according to the concept of law, i.e., principles. In estimating the total worth of one's actions, Kant believed that a good will takes precedence over all else.[19] Contained in a good will is the concept of duty. According to Kantianism, only when persons act from a notion of duty do their actions have moral worth. For instance, nurses have a duty to tell patients the truth. However, merely because a nurse tells a patient the truth does not necessarily mean that the action was morally worthy. Perhaps the nurse told the truth to prevent further difficulties later on, or perhaps the nurse did so to avoid legal problems. Although this nurse may be acting in *accordance with duty*, the nurse is not acting *from duty*. For Kant, actions have true moral worth only when they arise from a recognition of a duty and a choice to perform that duty.

Kant also held that an absolute moral truth had to be consistent and free from internal contradiction. Thus in order for a rule of conduct to be a moral rule, it had to hold universally, in all situations, without exceptions. Further, Kantianism also posits that, in keeping with the idea that humans are rational beings, humans should treat each other as ends in themselves, not as mere means to an end.[5] Thus medical researchers, no matter how lofty their goals, may never use human beings in research without first obtaining their truly informed consent.[8]

A duty-based framework of ethics such as Kant's contains several appealing elements that are applicable to health care. First, Kant's ethics takes much of the "guesswork" out of moral decision making in health care. To act morally is to act on principle. No matter what the consequences or situational nuances, some actions are always wrong. Second, Kant's ethics recognizes humans as intrinsically worthy of respect. Unlike consequentialist ethics, Kant's mandate to treat persons as ends in themselves and not only as means to an end places the individual at the center of moral decisions. In health care, this serves to bring a much needed humanism to care dominated by machines and technology.[6] Third, Kant's concept of duty implies the moral obligation to act from a respect for rights and a recognition of responsibilities. According to Kant, people act morally when they behave according to the concepts of law. Subscribing to this theory necessitates defining and specifying rights and responsibilities clearly and then following the moral imperative in acting with respect to them. Since each individual participating in a nurse-patient relationship has equal claims and duties, Kant's ethics implies a mutuality in relationships between patients and nurses that is not seen in the utilitarian frameworks.

Criticisms of Kant arise from several areas. First, there is no clear method to resolve conflicts of duties. For instance, suppose that by lying to Mr. Kramer's family, the nurse knows he or she can spare them emotional turmoil and pain. The nurse presumably has a duty to tell the truth and a duty to refrain from causing pain to others. Which of these obligations takes precedence when they conflict? Second, how does one resolve the question of who qualifies as a rational autonomous being? Kant is quite clear that duties are owed to beings who are rational and autonomous.[16] Where, though, do children fit in? Or senile adults? How should nurses consider their duties to nonrational, nonautonomous persons? Third, there is no compelling reason that certain actions should hold without exception.[26] In Kant's view, truth telling in nursing practice, therefore, would mean that all patients should be told all the truth all of the time. Clearly, this flies in the face of what nurses experience in their day-to-day practice, as well as it contradicts common sense. The rigidity of Kant's rule, which allows no exceptions, precludes it from being accepted totally as the basis for nursing practice. However, despite its obvious shortcomings, Kantianism holds an appeal for nursing practice precisely because of its recognition of the nature of nursing as more than the scale on which one balances risks and benefits, and of the humanity necessary in health care.

From Kant's view of ethics emerges its primary ethical principle, respect for autonomy. Nurses take respect for autonomy and transform it into advocacy for patients within the practice of nursing.

Advocacy

The term **advocacy** designates the moral position based on the individual right of self-determination.

It is the position in which patient autonomy is the primary value governing the nurse's actions. This means that the nurse, although still concerned with acting in the patient's interest, does not define that interest in any way contrary to the patient's own definition. In advocacy it is not the professional, but the patient, who determines what best interest means.

Advocacy is not a form of consumerism in which the nurse's role is merely to clear a path and stand guard so patients can exercise their autonomy single-handedly. Advocacy recognizes the real limitations imposed by illness and recognizes patients' need for assistance in exercising autonomy in a situation that may be both unfamiliar and frightening. The nurse helps patients with decision making. In consumerism the nurse has no desire to participate in decision making: nurses merely supply patients with the facts, then withdraw, leaving the decision in the patient's hands. The nurse is detached from the decision making, just as in paternalism the patient is removed from decision making. One ethical view—consumerism—dispenses with the nurse, just as the other view—paternalism—dispenses with the patient.

Advocacy, in contrast to consumerism and paternalism, is a partnership. It assumes that patients can be more fully and freely self-determining if they are actively assisted in that endeavor than if they are left to their own devices. The purpose of the partnership is for patients' own values ultimately to be the deciding ones, since only patients can know their personal criteria for health.

Even professionals disagree on the definition of health. The reason for disagreement is the value component of any definition. No concept of health (or disease) is simply a descriptive statement about the presence or absence of a particular condition. Every concept of health includes an evaluation of certain conditions as either desirable or undesirable, worthy of being preserved or calling for a change. In different cultural groups, as in different individuals, the same condition may be evaluated in opposite terms, depending on whether it is consistent with the culture's overall values and goals.

Because health is not a final goal in itself but a means to other ends, a concept of health depends on the specific physical and mental requirements of those ends. Sterility may be a defect in some persons, a treatment for others. A sculptor may not need the same degree of visual acuity as a painter. Loss of a limb may mean insurmountable disability for an athlete, or minimal impairment for a teacher. In each of these cases, a personal or cultural goal provides the framework for a definition of health.

In addition to the goals that health serves for an individual, a concept of health is personal because it involves a determination of the part of the self that will receive care in preference to other parts. In a physiologic concept of health, the physical has priority over the emotional, intellectual, and spiritual aspects of the self. Some patients may assign a higher value to caring for a nonphysical aspect of the self. The health of that part of the person may be attainable only at the expense of the physical self. A paraplegic woman, whose profession as a family therapist requires many hours of sitting, discovers that decubiti develop if she does not lie down every 2 hours, but she may choose to give less priority to physical health to maintain more intense professional involvement. Decisions expressing a personal concept of health reflect the way in which a person values the different aspects of the self. Expression of that individual self-concept is the aim of the nurse-patient partnership of advocacy.

In the case of Mr. Kramer, what would the nurse do in the advocacy framework? Her decision would depend on whether she viewed his near-death condition as an expression of his own freely determined view of death. Her decision will be guided by his decision. Her task is thus to ascertain whether his action truly reflects his autonomy. It is too late to begin this process in an emergency situation. Advocacy is not a position that can suddenly be invoked in crisis. The process of ascertaining the patient's view and providing him with enough information to reach an informed view must begin much earlier. If that has not happened, the nurse cannot be an advocate of Mr. Kramer's personal view, because she does not know it. If the nurse does know it and knows that it has been reached freely and with full information about his options, the obligation as advocate is to respect his decision.

Caring-based Theory

With a theory of universal and abstract principles (e.g., as articulated by Kant or Mill), nurses or patients as moral agents are not particular, concrete individuals with their own life histories, emotions, and desires. Moreover, in such views, moral judgments should not be affected by the particulars in a person's life, including emotions, relationships, and other aspects of persons that distinguish one from any other. Rather, one moral agent is seen as no better or worse than another, and certainly no different from others. This view of morality contradicts all that nurses know about themselves as persons and professionals, and about their patients as persons both within and without the context of health care.

New and exciting work in nursing ethical theory is exploring **caring-based theory** as a foundation of nursing ethics that relies on relationships rather than principles for primary moral reflection. This work is still early in its development, and is presented here as a stimulus for nurses to pursue such research further.

The concept of caring as a framework for ethical reflection in nursing emerged from several authors, each critiquing and building on the other's prior work. Each recognizes the important contributions that nursing, as a primarily female profession, has to offer the further development of such a theory. Starting with the notion that principle-based versions of ethical decision-making do not reflect how many people make ethical decisions,[27] the caring model looks at the moral language of response and caring from a very different perspective: Moral problems are particular, unique situations in which all parties retain their individual identities, values, emotions, feelings, and relationships. Caring and relationship occur between specific, concrete individuals. Moral situations exist within a particular context, both historical and sociologic; they are bound by time and place. This framework for morality places emphasis on concrete situations, people in relationships, caring, communication, a desire not to hurt others, and responsiveness.

When Carol Gilligan published *In A Different Voice* in 1982, she claimed to hear a "distinct moral voice" in the reflections of the women who participated in her research on moral development.[14] Gilligan refers to this as the "voice of care" and contrasts it with the "voice of justice" as represented in principle-based approaches to ethics derived from rationalistic theories such as those of Mill and Kant. Gilligan's research is seen as a corrective to that of Piaget[25] and Kohlberg,[17] whose work in moral development initially excluded women, and later found women to be "less developed" morally than men.

It is most helpful to consider these two moral "voices" as distinct orientations within morality; that is, that the justice and care views are not mutually exclusive. Instead, these perspectives denote different ways of organizing the basic elements of moral judgment: self, others, and the relationships between them. According to Gilligan, the justice orientation construes the moral point of view as impartial, sees particular moral decisions as derived from principles, and emphasizes individual rights in our moral relationships. In contrast, the care orientation rejects impartiality as an essential mark of morality, sees moral decisions occurring in a specific context, and emphasizes responsiveness and responsibility in our relationships with others. In short, the justice views sees us as individuals first, and in relationship with each other only secondarily, while in the care orientation, we are understood as essentially in relationship.

Nel Noddings, in her work on caring,[24] describes a feminine ethical theory that distinguishes between "caring for" and "caring about." Caring about someone distances the nurse from the patient, and involves impersonality and "depersonalization." Caring for focuses on emotion, feelings, and attitudes.

It places reasoning and intellectual processes at the service of emotion and relationship. This shift does not entirely ignore the theoretic contributions of traditional ethics, but assumes that only some aspects of these ethics can inform and enrich the moral lives of those who care for, that is, nurses. Noddings treads a narrow line between the excessive abstractness of traditional ethical views and an overly-particularized view that sees all moral decisions as relative. Others who are pursuing this framework include Sara T. Fry,[10] Jean Watson,[29,30] Sally Gadow,[11,12,13] Mary Carolyn Cooper,[7] and Madeleine Leininger.[18] Research is presently focused on definitions of caring, differentiating nurse caring from physician caring, and postulation of a theory of nursing ethics that is cohesive and coherent.

Development of a framework of caring attempts to reconceptualize some previously accepted notions in a way that accounts for different models of moral thinking. In essence, what is at issue are the goals of morality. Why should a nurse be moral? Ethical frameworks that consist of balancing personal autonomy with the beneficence of others reflect the goal of morality as preventing "collisions" between autonomous individuals. In a framework based on caring in relationship, the goals of morality change to preventing the separation or drawing apart of what Gilligan refers to as women's "spheres of influence"—their networks of relationships with others. This reconceptualization is very important when it comes to working out moral problems, and appeals to nurses because it readily accounts for what nurses experience when they care for patients.

In the case of Mr. Kramer, what would the nurse do in the caring framework? Her decision would depend on the nurse's construction of what it means to care for Mr. Kramer within their patient-nurse relationship. This is shaped by their conversations, their mutual explorations of values and preferences, and so forth. To a large degree, the nurse's decision will depend on how she perceives her relationship with Mr. Kramer. In fact, each of the ethical perspectives discussed here have at their foundation a model of nurse-patient relationship that warrants further explication.

MODELS OF THE NURSE-PATIENT RELATIONSHIP

Nursing care, by definition, takes place within a *relationship* between a patient and a nurse. The nature of that relationship deserves some clarification if one is to develop a fuller view of responsibilities and rights of either participant in decision making.[23]

The diverse ways of viewing such a relationship emerge from the metaphors used to describe it: parent/child, teacher/student, seller/buyer, priest/parishioner, oppressor/victim, friends, contractors, colleagues. Clearly, the choice of an ethical "model" of the nurse-patient relationship will profoundly affect the way in which decisions are made and conflicts are resolved.[31] The relationship model that informs the paternalism perspective, for instance, is clearly that of nurse/parent and patient/child. Within such a construction it is easy to see how a nurse would justify acting only in his/her view of the patient's best interests.[2] The notion of contract is the metaphor for relationships in Kant's duty-based ethics,[28] while covenant is being explored in the context of caring.[20]

The moral basis of nurse-patient relationships is a central issue for nursing ethics. William May[21] examines the concepts of contract and covenant as bases for moral relationships in health care.[22] He describes similarities and differences between the contractual and convenantal bases for communities. Both require mutual respect, agreement between parties, and exchange of some sort. Contractual relationships permit all parties in the relationship to seek information and negotiate agreements that promote mutual benefits. They permit specification of limits, rights, and duties that are legally enforceable. Contracts protect autonomy, and are concerned with the forms of behavior between parties.

Covenants also respect autonomy and regulate behavior. There is a deeper commitment in covenant, however, a concern that goes beyond the specific exchange. This concern arises from a shared history and tradition. Covenant has an element of gift that gives relationships primacy over agreements. The mutuality of covenant, in which the concepts of service and care are deeply rooted, goes beyond the mutual self-interest of contract: that mutuality enriches being for all of the covenanted.

Contract as a basis for relationship, with its high regard for autonomy, holds a strong appeal for nursing: for many nurses, it forms the basis of their patient relationship within the advocacy model. Contract does not, however, take into account the unique and essential feature of nursing, that of caring. Indeed, many nurses feel that contractual nurse-patient relationships tend to strip away the aspects of nursing that actually define the profession. Is it possible to contract to care for someone? When involved in the intimate details of another person's life, is it possible, or, more importantly, moral, to continue on merely because an agreement was made and/or signed? What happens to the relationship if the contract is broken? Is the relationship over also, and if so, did one ever really exist? Caring relationships identify nursing and make it unique among the professions. Contract threatens this identity, and provides a model for nursing practice that is inadequate. Further study of convenantal relationships may be able to provide a richer metaphor for nurse-patient relationships that unites professional autonomy with connectedness.

How a nurse construes the nurse-patient relationship will therefore have a great influence on how and what ethical decisions are made. The types of relationships and their corresponding moral viewpoints can be clarified by comparing their application to truth telling, particularly within the context of informed consent.

INFORMED CONSENT: TRUTH TELLING

From the paternalist perspective, the truth-telling issue is how much information the nurse should disclose to the patient. The question locates responsibility for that decision with the professional rather than with the patient. The answer to the question depends on the nurse's assessment of the patient's best interest. Will disclosure or deception produce the greater good?

Deception traditionally has been the paternalist's treatment of choice, at least for seriously ill patients. Professionals emphasize the dangers of truth telling, the risk that patients may lose hope, relapse, become depressed, refuse treatment or demand excessive treatment, or even attempt suicide on learning their prognosis. In light of these possibilities, truth has been, until recently, administered to patients with great caution.

Deception, however, is not the paternalist's only therapeutic option. A less conservative view now regards candor as clinically indicated in the majority of cases. Truth has become the treatment of choice for several reasons. Professionals have learned that the greater the degree of patient assent in the healing process, the greater the chance of success. Furthermore, deception now is seen as more dangerous than it was formerly, risking harm to the psychologic integrity of patients and endangering their trust and the healing power inherent in that trust.

It must be emphasized that when truth telling is approached by asking how much information will benefit the patient, disclosure is as paternalistic as deception. In the shift from deception to disclosure, all that has changed is the empiric belief regarding the therapeutic value of truth. The underlying moral view is the same, namely, that the decision about information should be made by the professional, according to the criterion of benefit as the professional defines it.

The utilitarian position on truth telling extends the paternalist model beyond the individual patient to everyone who will be affected by the disclosure or deception. Since for both positions an act is right or wrong according to its consequences, deception is intrinsically no worse than disclosure. The amount of good produced is the deciding factor. For utilitarians, good is defined as the group's best interest. As a general practice utilitarians endorse a policy of candor, since the functioning of social groups depends on a presumption of honesty; the simplest communication would be impossible without being able to believe that one is not being lied to.

In nursing, trust is even more crucial than in every-day interaction, since nothing can be done for patients without their willingness to trust professionals. Utilitarian nurses therefore cannot admit holding a moral view in which they do not regard honesty as intrinsically right without making the practice of nursing impossible. This places utilitarians in an interesting paradox. Like paternalists, they regard honesty as neither right nor wrong in itself. For the good of those whose trust they require, however, they must appear to hold the view that honesty is intrinsically right. Behind that appearance, they continue to assess situations according to whether disclosure or deception will produce the greater good.

In contrast to utilitarianism and paternalism, for the advocacy position the truth-telling issue is not a question of whether information will benefit patients, but a question of how much is required for patient decision making.

Advocacy is assistance to patients in determining the selection of information they wish to have, assuming that any information needed will be given freely and with sensitivity. This approach to truth telling also assumes that information other than impersonal data will be discussed if a patient desires. Patients may wish to consider their own feelings and values, as well as those of the people caring for them. In the belief that only scientific data are relevant to clinical judgment, nurses traditionally have considered such intimate information irrelevant or coercive. In the advocacy model, the decision that values and feelings are irrelevant is a determination only the patient can make.

A nurse's refusal to disclose her view to a patient who asks is a form of censorship. The belief behind her refusal is that patient and nurse are such unequal partners that the patient will defer to the nurse. Patients indeed may abstain from decision making if given no assistance in developing their autonomy. The role of the nurse in advocacy is to overcome that initial inequality by helping patients become informed and self-determining rather than to conform out of inexperience or deference.

The practice of obtaining consent from patients before providing treatment depends on full truth telling if the consent is to be a valid expression of patient self-determination. The process of deliberation leading to consent is symbolized (and often legally documented) by the patient's signing an offi-

ETHICAL DECISION-MAKING STEPS

1. Describe all of the relevant factors in the situation: clinical, personal, social, institutional, and so on.
2. Identify the ethical problem in concrete terms, for example, should Mrs. A continue to receive nutritional support, knowing that discontinuing it will result in her death?
3. Identify underlying ethical issues that must be addressed to resolve the concrete problem; for example, is an action that is known to bring about a person's death morally the same as killing?
4. Identify your own ethical position toward patient care in general based on your primary commitment: (a) to achieving the best for everyone involved, (b) to achieving the best in your terms for the patient, or (c) to achieving the best for the patient in the patient's own terms.
5. Identify each of the actions possible in the situation, for example, continue parenteral feeding, reduce quality of feeding, discontinue parenteral feeding and attempt to hand-feed, discontinue all feeding, and so on.
6. Analyze each of the options to determine which is most consistent with the moral position you have identified as your own. This will require having as complete a picture as possible of the situation (step 1) and carefully addressing each of the underlying ethical issues (step 3).

cial form. But such signing, from an ethical perspective, is peripheral. On a moral position that values patient autonomy, the nurse is responsible for helping patients exercise the fullest possible self-determination, regardless of whether a policy exists requiring the signing of consent forms. As nurses well know, the presence in a patient's record of a signed form indicates nothing about the manner in which the signature was obtained. See the box on the left and Figure 10-1 for additional information on ethical decision-making.

RESEARCH AND ETHICS

In clinical experimentation with human subjects, professional responsibilities in regard to consent are more clearly defined than in any other area of health care. Since nurses not only care for patients who are research subjects, but also conduct clinical research themselves, the ethical principle guiding human experimentation is central to nursing ethics. That principle is the same respect for individual autonomy that underlies advocacy. A close look at research ethics will further illuminate the practice of advocacy.

The principle of respect for autonomy of research subjects contrasts with a utilitarian view of research, in which subjects can be used without their consent if the good achieved for society outweighs the harms they suffer. Respect for subjects' autonomy also dif-

FIGURE 10-1 Critical Thinking Guide: ethical decisions.

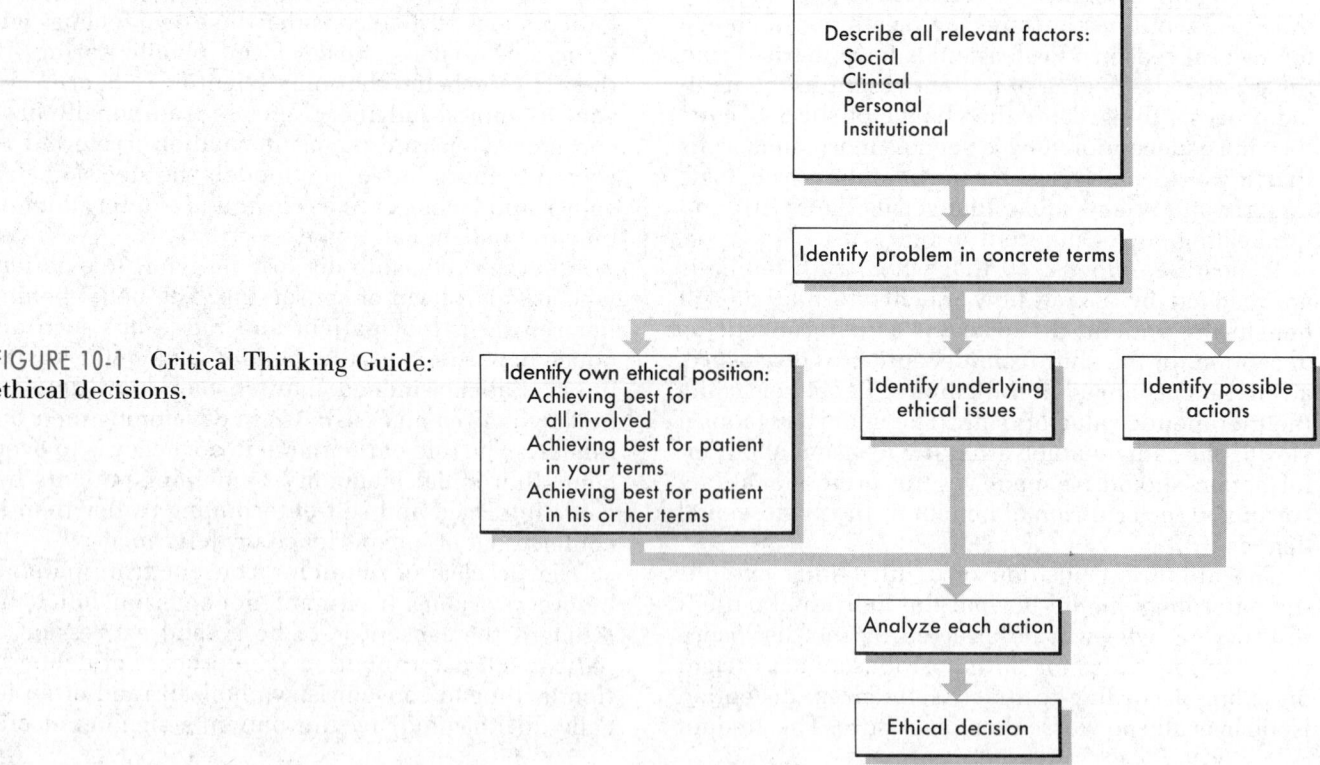

fers from a paternalistic approach, in which professionals rather than subjects decide whether the research in question offers greater possibility of benefit than risk of harm.

In contrast to both utilitarianism and paternalism, contemporary research ethics is based on commitment to individual freedom of self-determination. Participation of research subjects must always be voluntary, never unfree or coerced. Providing subjects with as much information as needed to make a fully informed decision is one means of preventing coercion through ignorance or misunderstanding.

One form of coercion through misinformation can be the patient's inability to distinguish between standard and experimental treatment. Because patients regard the health professional (perhaps the nurse more than any other professional) as someone who has only their best interests at heart, they often assume that a study in which they are invited to participate could be only beneficial. That belief may be false. The experimental therapy may not be expected to benefit the subjects on whom it is tried. Patients whose ignorance in this regard is not corrected have not been adequately informed. A nurse not only must inform prospective subjects about a study, but also must free them of the assumption that because a trusted care-giver is involved, no risk of harm could exist.

Another source of coercion, of which the nurse may be more aware than other professionals, is a patient's fear that good care is contingent on participation in research. This fear may be groundless if all patients receive equally good care. On the other hand, the fear may be grounded in the patient's observation that those who receive experimental treatment receive more meticulous attention and perhaps more sympathetic consideration. In a setting such as a teaching hospital, patients may learn quickly that those who refuse to participate in any study are as suspect as those who refuse treatment; the desire not to seem uncooperative or ungrateful can be a powerful coercion, especially among patients who are unable to pay for their care.

As the modern capability for saving and prolonging life increases, the reluctance to concede to death increases. As a result, patients may experience coercion from yet another source, not a threat of professional abandonment but the pressure of professional interest. As nurses and other professionals become increasingly concerned about particular patients, they may become invested in keeping them alive as long as possible. Formerly professionals may have given up on patients before patients themselves did. Now the professional who can offer further (even if only experimental) treatment may be reluctant to allow a patient to give up. The subtle pressure on such a patient to embark on experimental therapy can be overwhelming.

THE "INCOMPETENT" PATIENT

Even with the broadest definition of competence, there will be patients who fall outside that range and cannot participate in decisions about their care. The typical term for these persons is *incompetent.*

The question of beginning or ending life-sustaining measures for mentally impaired or unconscious persons is perhaps the most common clinical form of ethical nursing problem. For example, how is a decision to be made when such an incompetent patient develops a condition that will prove life-threatening if untreated? Without prior instruction from a formerly competent patient who foresaw that dilemma, what should the health team decide?

The utilitarian approach lends itself especially well to situations in which the wishes of one or more of the participants are unknown. If the patient's view cannot be determined, the decision should be made according to the best outcome that can be achieved for everyone else in the situation. This assumes that the patient is indifferent to any outcome, no longer has (or never has had) the capacity to value one outcome over another. Subtracting the patient from the situation, it follows that the interests of the others involved must be the basis for the decision.

It does not follow necessarily that such a patient will be allowed to die. It may be judged in the best interests of everyone to provide treatment for several reasons: the family is not ready to give up a person they still love, the nurses value caring for the patient, and the hospital does not want to lose the community's trust by allowing patients to die who could have been saved. In other cases, a decision against treatment might serve the overall good: a family may have been bankrupted financially and emotionally by the patient's long care, nurses will be freed by the patient's death to spend more time with patients who are likely to recover, and the institution may be unable to absorb the cost of a nonpaying patient.

Cost containment strikes most people as an unsavory motive for letting patients die. Notice, however, that it is no worse than any other motive concerning the general good, once the premise has been accepted that the patient is indifferent to any good. If no reason whatever can be discerned from the patient's own perspective for believing one outcome preferable to another, then other perspectives must be called on. They will be as varied as financial gain, religious belief, emotional investment, or personnel triage.

Because of the vulnerability of incompetent patients and the ease with which they can be exploited, professionals often avoid allowing anyone's good except that of the patient to enter into their decision. They are then choosing the moral position of beneficence instead of utilitarianism.

The position of beneficence, as pointed out in the

earlier discussion of paternalism, assumes that it is possible for one person to know what is in another's best interest. The advocacy position disputes that possibility. Because a person's best interest can be determined only relative to the individual's own goals and values, only patients themselves can determine their best interest. The role of patients' subjectivity in defining their own good is central to advocacy. In the care of incompetent patients, however, it is just that subjective domain that seems inaccessible. How is anyone able to determine what will benefit or harm these persons?

Beneficence becomes easier rather than harder with incompetent patients. Professionals often believe it is possible to know the patient's best interest because they believe that best interest can be defined objectively. An objective understanding of health and disease is the hallmark of the professional. With these beliefs, nurses practicing beneficence are freed rather than hindered by the lack of knowledge about a patient's subjective views.

The care of incompetent patients provides the most morally clear situation for both utilitarianism and beneficence. On the other hand, it creates the greatest challenge for a position based on patient self-determination. Advocacy must not only be able to promote the self-determination of patients whose autonomy needs little defense, but also be able to illuminate the less accessible self of patients whose subjectivity is all but invisible.

Three avenues are open for attempting this most difficult aspect of advocacy. The first is reference to an unconscious or otherwise incompetent patient's advance directive, such as a preference communicated to family or staff while the patient was lucid. The binding nature of such directives depends in large part on how fully and accurately the patient was able to envision the present situation in reaching an advance decision about it.

In the absence of prior consent, professionals can use a second, less direct approach to patient self-determination, through others' beliefs about what the person would decide if capable of deciding.

The crucial element in this case is the involvement of someone—family member or friend—who can articulate what the patient would have wanted in this situation. This standard for decision making is referred to as "substituted judgment" and aims to implement the subjective preferences of the patient about and for whom decisions must be made. Under this standard, decision making by another on behalf of the patient is guided by that other person's understanding of *what the patient would have wanted,* based on the patient's own values, goals, preferences, and wishes. In the absence of family and friends and any direct or indirect knowledge of what the patient would have wanted, decisions about the care of incompetent patients are based on

a "best interests" standard: what actions, treatments, or other interventions on the patient would advance his or her best interests? Nurses may be able to speak for incompetent patients based on their interactions with and physical care of those patients.

In relation to incompetent patients, advocacy requires that nurses ideally help patients articulate their views before they become incompetent. With patients already incompetent, advocacy requires increased devotion by nurses to the mundane intimacies of physical care as the last—but not least—significant avenue into their personal world.

CRITICAL THINKING QUESTIONS

1 Discuss the desirability of the nursing profession officially adopting one of the three moral positions described in this chapter. Should nursing attempt such a consensus, and if so, which position should it endorse?

2 Criticize each of the positions. Make explicit the different underlying premises to maintain clear distinctions among the three, since in some cases their application may result in the same clinical decision.

3 Using cancer treatment options as an example, describe the nurse's role in facilitating informed consent, contrasting the positions of paternalism, consumerism, and advocacy.

4 Describe the moral differences and similarities between patient consent for standard treatment and for experimental treatment. Discuss the conflict between the utilitarian aspect of clinical research and the position of either beneficence or advocacy that most health professionals hold. What is the best way of resolving the conflict?

5 Discuss the difference between deception and disclosure on the paternalism position.

6 Describe an "incompetent" patient whom you have known, and apply the three basic positions to the question of whether the patient should be placed on a ventilator in the event of respiratory distress.

BIBLIOGRAPHY

1. Arras J, Rhoden N, editors: *Ethical issues in modern medicine,* ed 3, Palo Alto, Calif, 1990, Mayfield Publishing.
2. Ashley J: Hospitals, *paternalism, and the nurse,* New York, 1976, Teachers College Press.
3. Baier A: Doing without moral theory? In: *Postures of the mind,* Minneapolis, 1985, University of Minnesota.
4. Beauchamp TL, Childress JE: *Principles of biomedical ethics,* ed 3, New York, Oxford, 1990, Oxford University Press.

5. Beecher HJ: Ethics and clinical research, *N Engl J Med* 274(24): June 1966.

6. Bursztain HJ, et al: The technological target: involving the patient in clinical choices. In Reiser SJ, Anbar M, editors: *The machine at the bedside: strategies for using technology in patient care,* Cambridge and New York, 1984, Cambridge University Press.

7. Cooper MC: Reconceptualizing nursing ethics, *Scholarly Inquiry for Nursing Practice: An International Journal,* 4(3): 1990.

8. Englehardt HT: Bioethics in pluralist societies, *Perspectives in Biology and Medicine* 26(1):Autumn 1982.

9. Englehardt HT: *The foundations of bioethics,* New York, 1986, Oxford University Press.

10. Fry ST: Toward a theory of nursing ethics, *Advances in nursing science,* Rockville, Md, July 1989.

11. Gadow, S: Toward a new philosophy of nursing, *Nursing Law and Ethics* 1(8): October 1980.

12. Gadow S: Existential advocacy: philosophical foundation in nursing. In Murphy CP, Hunter H, editors: *Ethical problems in the nurse-patient relationship,* Boston, 1983, Allyn & Bacon.

13. Gadow S: The ethics of care and the ethics of cure: synthesis in chronicity, New York, 1988, National League for Nursing.

14. Gilligan C: *In a different voice,* Cambridge, Mass, 1982, Harvard University Press.

15. Hunt R, Arras J: Ethical theory in the medical context. In *Ethical issues in modern medicine,* Palo Alto, Calif, 1977, Stanford University Press.

16. Katz J: Respecting autonomy: the struggle over rights and capacities. In *The silent world of doctor and patient,* New York, 1984, Macmillan.

17. Kohlberg L: *Essays on moral development,* San Francisco, 1981, Harper & Row.

18. Leininger M: *Care: The essence of nursing and health.* Thorofare, NJ, 1984, Charles B Slack.

19. Macklin R: Moral concerns and appeals to rights and duties, *Hastings Cent Rep,* October 1976.

20. Masters R: Is contract an adequate basis for medical ethics, *Hastings Cent Rep,* 5(6): December 1975.

21. May W: Code, covenant, contract, or philanthropy, *Hastings Cent Rep,* 5:29, 1975.

22. May W: *The physician's covenant,* New York, 1986, Oxford University Press.

23. Mitchell C. The nurse-patient relationship: a source of some moral duties. *The Connecticut Scholar: Occasional Papers;* 1986; (no. 8):

24. Noddings N: *Caring: a feminine approach to ethics and moral development,* Berkeley, Calif, 1984, University of California Press.

25. Piaget J: *The moral judgment of the child,* London, 1932, K Paul, Trench, Trubner & Co.

26. Ramsey P: The nature of medical ethics. In: *The teaching of medical ethics,* Veatch R, editor: Hastings-on-Hudson, NY, 1973, Hastings Center.

27. Toulmin S: The tyranny of principles, *Hastings Cent Rep,* 1, December 1981.

28. Veatch R: The principles of contract keeping. In: *A theory of medical ethics,* New York, 1981,

29. Watson J: *Nursing: human science and human care: a theory of nursing.* Norwalk, Conn, 1985, Appleton-Century-Crofts.

30. Watson J, Ray M, editors: *The ethics of care and the ethics of cure: synthesis in chronicity,* New York, 1988, National League for Nursing.

31. Winslow G: From loyalty to advocacy: a new metaphor for nursing, *Hastings Cent Rep,* June 1984.

UNIT III

Physiologic and Pathophysiologic Dimensions of Adult Health Nursing

CHAPTER ELEVEN

Infection

LEARNING OBJECTIVES

1 Characterize the microorganisms that cause infections in the body.

2 Describe the processes involved in host-agent interaction that produce infection.

3 Identify the clinical manifestations associated with the five stages of an acute primary infection.

4 Identify the unique characteristics of nosocomial and opportunistic infections.

5 Compare the clinical manifestations of infection in the older adult with those that occur in the younger adult.

6 Apply the nursing process to the management of the patient with an infection.

7 Identify the immunizations recommended for adults and the elderly.

8 Describe the role of universal precautions and isolation techniques in the prevention and management of infection.

KEY TERMS

carriers, p. 153

incubation, p. 154

isolation, p. 161

methicillin-resistant *Staphylococcus aureus* (MRSA), p. 156

nosocomial infections, p. 155

opportunistic infections, p. 156

pathogenic, p. 152

septicemia, p. 155

shift to the left, p. 158

superimposed infections, p. 156

universal precautions, p. 160

THE RANGE of dysfunction that occurs with an infection is broad, extending from the relatively minor upper respiratory infections to life-threatening myocarditis or hepatitis. The development of an infection depends on exposure to an organism and the degree of susceptibility, which is determined by the effectiveness of the immune system. However, numerous factors influence the interaction between the microorganism (agent) and the host and determine whether infection will occur. Some of these factors involve the characteristics of the pathogen itself, whereas others involve the number of organisms (dose), the mechanisms of their entry and spread through the body, and the resistance produced by the immune system.

INFECTION

Definition/Etiology

Infection refers to those diseases that produce dysfunction because of the presence of a living organism in or on the human body.[31] The microorganisms that cause infectious diseases generally fall into seven categories. Within each group of organisms are those that always produce disease, those that live in the body for mutual benefit, and those that would cause disease if they were not controlled by the immune system. Any organism that has the potential to produce disease is referred to as **pathogenic;** organisms that can exist in the body without causing disease are called *nonpathogenic.*

Viruses

Viruses are probably the most commonly encountered pathogenic organism. Composed of simple nucleic acid surrounded by a protein coat, or "envelope," viruses cannot live on their own; they must invade a cell and use that cell's biochemical machinery to survive. Redirecting the cell's protein synthesis for its own energy and reproduction requirements, the virus eventually kills the cell, either by depleting essential substances or by multiplying so rapidly that the cell membrane breaks open. A few viruses destroy surrounding tissue as well by releasing toxins as the host cell is destroyed. Viruses have also been implicated in the cellular changes that produce certain cancers.

Some viral invasions are rapidly controlled by the immune system; these short acute illnesses result in permanent immunity to the virus. Other viruses, such as herpes simplex or varicella zoster, remain in the body for months or years after the acute infection. Their spread is generally controlled by T and B lymphocytes; however, if the immune system becomes impaired, the disease may reappear.

Bacteria

Bacteria are unicellular organisms with a double cell membrane that protects them against many of the body's defense mechanisms. Although they do not have a nucleus as human cells do, bacteria contain all the mechanisms required for maintaining life and for rapidly replicating themselves. Bacteria are called *aerobic* if they require oxygen and *anaerobic* if they survive only in an oxygen-free environment.

Bacteria damage tissue by directly interfering with essential cell function or by the release of toxins that cause cell damage. During an acute infection, bacteria are attacked by T cells and antibodies produced by B lymphocytes that destroy bacteria. Staphylococcal and streptococcal organisms are the most common sources of bacterial infection in humans.

Mycoplasmas

Mycoplasmas are the smallest organisms that can live outside a host cell. In appearance they are similar to bacteria, except that they lack cell walls and can assume many shapes. Many antibiotics act by destroying the cell membranes of bacteria and are therefore ineffective against mycoplasmas. Only one species, *Mycoplasma pneumoniae,* usually causes disease in humans.

Rickettsiae

Rickettsiae are gram-negative bacilli that cause typhus and Rocky Mountain spotted fever. Being intracellular parasites, they must live off the host cell's nutrients; they cannot live outside the cell. Rickettsiae are transmitted by lice and ticks.

Chlamydiae

Chlamydiae are intracellular parasites that invade a cell and produce offspring released by cell rupture. These offspring, or elementary bodies, are the infectious particles. They are capable of living outside a cell and even resist macrophage destruction. Most researchers believe that Chlamydiae are only partially controlled by the immune system, since *Chlamydia* disease is prolonged and characterized by remissions and exacerbations.

Fungi

Fungi are generally divided into two types: yeasts and molds. They are able to live both inside and outside the human body and are important in the breakdown of plant matter. In a human infection they may assume either form. Superficial fungal invasions are the source of common vaginal infections and athlete's foot. Systemic fungal infections, which occur relatively uncommonly, are caused by *Histoplasma capsulatum,* carried by birds, and *Coccidioides immitis.* If patients do not have adequate T lymphocytes, the organisms can cause major damage and produce extensive fibrotic changes during the healing process.

Protozoa

Protozoa are important parasitic pathogens in worldwide disease; malaria and schistosomiasis are among the significant health problems in developing nations. Other protozoan diseases are *Pneumocystis carinii* (commonly seen in acquired immunodeficiency syndrome [AIDS] patients), toxoplasmosis, and trypanosomiasis (sleeping sickness). These parasites are difficult to control, since they are able to evade the immune response and adapt easily to different host environments. In addition, many parasitic diseases have been shown to depress immune function, limiting the body's defense mechanisms.

Pathophysiology

The process by which organisms produce infectious disease entails exposure, dose, entry, multiplication, dissemination, and damage to host tissues.

Exposure

For people to develop an infection, they must come in contact with an infecting pathogen. Some pathogens are *endogenous*—part of the patient's normal flora. When these normally harmless organisms escape immune system control or are transferred to another site because of surgery or other invasive procedures, they are capable of producing infection. Endogenous organisms from the GI tract, such as the *Escherichia coli* bacteria, are a major source of infection elsewhere in the body.

Exogenous organisms are those that come from the environment. Infection occurs because of direct contact with another person already infected. Individuals with an active infectious disease are easily identified; others, however, serve as **carriers** for pathogens. Their bodies contain pathogens but do not show any symptoms of the disease. Other exogenous sources of infection include contaminated food, water, soil, air, and animals. Hepatitis A, cholera, and gastroenteritis ("travelers' diarrhea") are examples of infections obtained from contaminated food or water.

Dose

The number of organisms required to produce a disease varies widely. Some pathogens such as *Clostridium botulinum* are extremely virulent, and only a small number of organisms is required to cause disease. Other organisms require large numbers to produce disease. The ability of the body's immune system to destroy pathogens plays an important role in determining the disease-producing dose. Generally, however, the larger the dose of organisms, the greater the risk of infection.

Entry

For an invading pathogen to produce an infectious disease within the body, it must be able to overcome or bypass the general protective mechanisms that are part of the immune system: the skin, local chemicals, and the normal bacterial flora prevent pathogenic organisms from establishing themselves within the body. Obviously, any disruption in skin integrity (burns, abrasions, ulcerations, or surgery) provides a convenient entry site. For individuals with intact skin, the mucous membranes are the most common site of entry after inhalation or ingestion of a pathogen.

RESEARCH BRIEF

Conn V: Self-care actions taken by older adults for influenza and colds, *Nurs Res* 40:176, 1991.

This study examined self-care behaviors used by older adults to manage episodes of colds and influenza. Preventive strategies used by the older adult subjects (n = 160) included dressing warmly, obtaining influenza vaccination, and avoiding people with colds or influenza. However, only 38% of the subjects reported regularly obtaining an influenza vaccination.

The subjects reported a variety of self-care actions to manage colds and influenza. Self-administration of over-the-counter medications was the most common self-care activity. Other self-care actions used by the older adults included increasing fluid intake, reducing social interaction, and increasing rest.

Most of the subjects identified no potential health hazards associated with colds and influenza. Only 13% of the older adults identified pneumonia as a potential complication of influenza.

The mechanisms by which organisms penetrate the protective mucous barriers of the respiratory airways, vagina, and GI tracts are not completely clear. It may be that some microorganisms have extremely strong motility that enables them to literally push their way through the mucosal lining; another possibility is that there may be weak spots in the mucous barrier that permit pathogen penetration. It is known that the absence of functioning cilia in the airways (seen in smokers), loss of the normal protective bacteria in the GI tract or vagina (seen in patients receiving oral antibiotics), and mucosal damage (from sexual activity, dental work, or trauma) enhance the ability of organisms to reach the underlying epithelium.

Once the pathogen has passed through the mucosal barrier, its binding sites attach to specific receptors on the epithelium. The binding process may be sufficient for some organisms to begin tissue damage. Other organisms penetrate the epithelial cells, where they replicate and produce signs of the disease. Still others not only penetrate the epithelial cells, but also use these cells as a pathway to the bloodstream. The organisms can then circulate and bind at additional sites.

The body's defenses against pathogen binding on epithelial cells include (1) the normal flora that may cover critical receptor sites, (2) an environmental pH that damages the organisms, and (3) the presence in the mucosal barrier of the antibody IgA, which binds with antigens on the surface of the pathogen and neutralizes its toxins. The antigen-antibody reactions stimulate complement, which in turn heightens the entire inflammatory response and destruction of the organism.

Multiplication

Once inside the body, the organism begins to reproduce. Bacteria, mycoplasmas, and fungi are able to reproduce on their own. Rickettsiae, chlamydiae, and viruses can only live and reproduce inside a host cell. The balance between the rate of pathogen replication and the rate of immune cell destruction determines how quickly tissue dysfunction (and signs of the infection) appears or whether disease occurs at all. The immune system is most effective against organisms that remain outside of the cell, where they can be attacked by antibodies and cytotoxic leukocytes.

Spread

Organisms vary in their methods of dissemination. Some produce chemical substances that not only destroy neighboring tissues but also inhibit immune cell function, enabling the pathogen to escape the immune system's effort to keep the infection localized. Viruses initially spread either along the surface of adjacent cells or through intercellular openings. Interferons, which coat nearby cells with an impenetrable barrier, are the body's primary defense mechanism against viral dissemination. If the organisms cannot be controlled locally and gain access to the bloodstream or lymph channels, the infection may be carried to many different sites in the body; the presence of large numbers of pathogens in the blood or lymph is a dangerous sign.

Tissue damage

Microorganisms produce tissue damage in the body through two primary mechanisms: direct destruction/invasion or the production of chemical toxins. Direct tissue damage may be the result of the pathogen itself or the interaction of the organism with WBCs during the inflammatory response. The lysozymes produced by neutrophils and macrophages during phagocytosis can destroy not only the pathogen, but also nearby cells. In addition, whenever antigen and antibody reactions occur, the inflammatory process is activated. Viruses and other organisms that must invade host cells to live and reproduce inhibit normal cell activities, leading to cell death. The destruction of the host cell releases newly formed viruses, which can then invade and damage nearby cells. The extent of viral virulence (ability to cause disease) is related to the amount of

cell damage created by the virus itself or the immune response that it activates. When viruses bind to other cells in preparation for invasion, they are susceptible to attack from antibodies or complement; the ensuing battle produces inflammation and tissue damage. Also, many virus-infected cells have surface markers that stimulate macrophage activation.

Some viruses are able to rapidly change the shape of their surface antigens. As a result they can continually look "new" to the immune system; formerly successful antibodies or cytotoxic cells no longer work, and new ones must be created. This characteristic of the influenza virus is the reason people can be infected with influenza many times.

The virulence of most bacteria is related to their release of toxins. *Exotoxins,* produced by bacteria directly, damage cell structure and function. *Endotoxins* activate the chemical mediators of the inflammatory response, not only stimulating WBC activity, but also promoting vasodilation and increased vascular permeability. Endotoxins are involved in scarlet fever, cholera, tetanus, and diphtheria. In addition, endotoxins from gram-negative bacteria are often responsible for the circulatory collapse of septic shock (see Chapter 13).

Clinical Manifestations

Because of the varying pathophysiologic processes of each pathogen and the fluctuating strength of people's immunologic defense mechanisms, an infectious disease may take a variety of courses. The most common form of infectious disease is the acute primary infection. However, some infections demonstrate a different progression; these are termed *chronic, latent, secondary,* or *subclinical* infections.

Primary acute infection

A primary acute infection is one that occurs and is resolved within a relatively short period, usually about 14 days. It is characterized by five stages. The first stage is *infection,* characterized by entry of the organism into the body. The second, or **incubation,** stage, encompasses the time between entry of the pathogen and the appearance of clinical symptoms; it can be as short as a few hours or as long as several weeks. During this period the microorganism is actively reproducing. For some infectious diseases, such as chickenpox or gastroenteritis, the incubation period is predictable if the time of exposure is known.

The *prodromal* stage is characterized by the appearance of vague, nonspecific symptoms including a low-grade fever, headache, muscle aches, loss of appetite, and general loss of energy. These symptoms are clinical manifestations of the immune system's battle to control the organism. For example, the fever is the result of interleukin-1 (IL-1) release by macrophages, which changes the temperature "set point" in the hypothalamus.

The fourth stage is referred to as the *acute* stage. It is characterized by the appearance of clinical signs and symptoms associated with the particular tissue or organ system that is damaged by the pathogen and immune response. An infection in the respiratory system may cause a sore throat, cough, or increased sputum production; an infection of the GI tract is characterized by diarrhea and intestinal cramping. During the acute stage the organism is multiplying and spreading.

Convalescence is the fifth stage of an acute primary infection. During this period the organism is first controlled and then destroyed, after which tissue repair begins. Signs and symptoms diminish and the patient's general sense of well-being returns. Some primary infections can be controlled by the immune system alone; others require antimicrobial drugs. Convalescence is followed by *resolution*, the point at which the pathogen has been completely eliminated from the body and tissue repair is complete.

When the primary or secondary site of infection is the bloodstream, the infection is called **septicemia.** Other terms used for the same disorder are *bacteremia, viremia,* and *blood poisoning.* The source of the infection is commonly one of the organisms of the staphylococcal family, normally found on the skin. Another common source is the bacterial flora released from the GI tract after trauma or surgery. Septicemia is a dangerous acute primary infection and may cause death in those patients whose immune systems are compromised.

Unique primary infections

Nosocomial infections

Infections that develop after a patient is admitted to a health care institution are called **nosocomial infections,** and are sometimes referred to as "hospital-acquired infections." For an infection to be defined as nosocomial, there must be no indication that an infection was present or incubating when the patient was admitted. Most nosocomial infections are transmitted by health care workers who fail to wash their hands adequately and change gloves between patients. Signs and symptoms of the nosocomial infections appear either while the patient is in the institution or after the patient has been discharged.

Nosocomial infections develop in the institutionalized patient for a variety of reasons. Any disorder that impairs the body's normal defense mechanisms increases the patient's susceptibility to infection. For example, diagnostic and therapeutic invasive procedures provide an excellent opportunity for microbes

GERIATRIC CONSIDERATIONS

Infections and the Older Adult

Older adults have an increased risk of developing serious infections. The morbidity and mortality associated with infection are higher in the elderly than in younger persons because older adults have poorer outcomes from the treatment of infection. The types of infections that occur frequently in older adults include: pneumonia, tuberculosis (especially in group living situations such as nursing homes), influenza, urinary tract infections, diverticulitis, cholecystitis, and pressure ulcer infections. Nosocomial infections are a special risk for the elderly because they are hospitalized more often and with longer lengths of stay.

Factors that increase the older adult's susceptibility to infection are:

1. A decrease in the function of the immune system and slowed response to antibiotic therapy
2. Physical changes that increase sites for entry and multiplication by infecting microorganisms such as atrophic skin, decreased gastric acid, decreased cough reflex, decreased mucociliary activity, and decreased elasticity of the bronchiolar musculature
3. Decreased protein reserves and decreased serum albumin that slows cellular response to tissue injury caused by invading microorganisms
4. Chronic diseases and drug therapy that can produce immunosuppression
5. Environmental and life-style variables (smoking, air pollution, alcoholism, or delay in seeking health care) that increase anyone's risk for infection but become more important in the older adult because of the interplay of the other risks that increase their susceptibility
6. Changes in mental status and decreased functional ability that can limit the older adult's ability to use preventive health practices to improve resistance to infection

to enter the body. Intravascular lines, tracheal intubation, bladder catheters, and surgical procedures disrupt or bypass the protective barriers of the skin and mucous membranes and provide easy entry for organisms. The most common nosocomial infections are urinary tract infections that develop in patients with indwelling catheters.

In addition, many disease processes and drug treatment regimens can inhibit immune cell function or promote infection in the hospitalized patient. Prostatic hypertrophy, which inhibits the free flow of urine, increases the risk of infection in the urinary tract. Atelectasis (collapse of the alveoli in the lung) is a significant cause of pneumonia. Drugs that slow intestinal peristalsis inhibit the ability of the GI tract to rid itself of the millions of microbes ingested daily, and corticosteroids inhibit macrophage and neutrophil phagocytosis.

Drug-resistant nosocomial infections

Nosocomial infections caused by drug-resistant microorganisms represent a challenge to health care providers in the acute care setting. The increasing prevalence of **methicillin-resistant Staphylococcus aureus (MRSA)** is causing concern that the pathogen may develop resistance to those drugs that are currently effective in treating the infection.[1] The primary mode of transmission of MRSA is by colonized patients and health care workers. Inadequate handwashing by hospital staff has been implicated in the spread of MRSA among patients at risk. Another factor implicated in the transmission of MRSA is transfer of nursing home residents to acute care hospitals. These elderly patients are carriers of MRSA and become reservoirs of the infection when they are hospitalized.

A variety of factors place patients at increased risk for MRSA infection. The older adult is at risk as are those patients with debilitating illnesses. Patients with invasive lines and tubes are also at higher risk for MRSA. Prolonged use of indwelling urinary catheters, endotracheal tubes, mechanical ventilation, and vascular access lines increase the patient's risk for this type of infection.[12]

Opportunistic infections

Opportunistic infections are the result of defective functioning in one or more components of the immune system. Many organisms normally can be controlled easily by the immune system alone. However, when immune function is impaired, these microbes multiply rapidly and produce tissue damage. For example, the bacterial flora of the skin and GI tract are normally harmless to the patient and, indeed, are part of the general protective mechanisms defending the body against more virulent organisms. When the immune system is not functioning adequately, however, these normally present flora are the first to take advantage of decreased host resistance; they become pathogenic and cause infection. Other organisms that commonly cause opportunistic infections are *Candida albicans, Pseudomonas aeruginosa, Pneumocystis carinii, Herpesvirus hominis,* and *Serratia marcescens.*

The number of people who develop opportunistic infections is increasing as a result of immunocompromised states related to diseases or treatment regimens. Patients with disorders of the bone marrow or WBCs (e.g., AIDS and leukemia) and those

with renal disease, liver disease, or diabetes mellitus are particularly susceptible to opportunistic infections caused by immunosuppression. In diabetic patients, for example, neutrophil chemotaxis and phagocytosis are inhibited.

The effects of drugs also contribute to the increased incidence of opportunistic infections. For example, cancer chemotherapy agents and immunosuppressants used in systemic inflammatory disorders affect the production and function of WBCs. Even the antibiotics used to treat many infections destroy normal bacterial flora in the GI tract, thereby promoting increased fungal infections in that area. The opportunistic infection that occurs with antibiotic therapy is called a **superimposed infection.**

The type of opportunistic infection that occurs depends on which body system is most susceptible and the ease with which organisms may gain entry. Thus many of these infections occur in systems open to the environment: the skin, respiratory tract, GI tract, or genitourinary system. Once an organism has established itself, however, it may enter the bloodstream and eventually spread to other parts of the body.

Other types of infection

A *chronic infection* is one in which the appearance of clinical signs and symptoms is prolonged, and there is no definitive resolution. Some chronic infections develop when the organism develops resistance to the treatment or when the treatment is inadequate. For example, when a patient stops taking a prescribed antibiotic before the infection has been completely eliminated, the organism may continue to multiply, producing signs and symptoms of the infection again at a later time.

For other organisms, chronic infection occurs as part of the normal course of events. Clinical signs and symptoms disappear (remission) or reappear (exacerbation), depending on the ability of the immune system to control the infection. Obviously, those factors that influence immune function, such as nutrition, drugs, and stressors, play a significant role in chronic infections.

Latent infections initially follow the same course as does an acute primary infection. However, although the clinical signs disappear, the organism remains in the body in a nonactive state; thus no true resolution occurs. Latent infections may develop into primary infections again if the patient's immune system is compromised in the future. Herpesvirus infections are an example of common latent infections.

A *secondary infection* is one that develops from a second organism after a primary infection has resolved. The primary infection places such a high demand on the immune system that when the second organism appears, the WBCs are unable to control its establishment and multiplication. For example, a patient may develop a secondary bacterial pneumonia after recovering from respiratory viral influenza. Some researchers have determined that certain viruses actually suppress the immune system and inhibit its ability to control other organisms, increasing the risk of secondary infections.

An infection is called subclinical when the organism responsible causes no significant clinical signs or symptoms; instead, the infection is fairly well controlled by the immune system and causes the patient only minimal disturbance. Nevertheless, subclinical infections are a major source for infecting others. Many of the sexually transmitted diseases are spread from person to person because the infected patient is unaware that the infection is present.

NURSING MANAGEMENT OF THE PATIENT WITH AN INFECTION
Assessment

Risk factors

Assessment of the patient for risk factors related to susceptibility to infection begins with determining the status of the patient's external barriers to pathogenic microorganisms. Since the skin is the first line of defense, the nurse needs to inspect all skin surfaces carefully for lesions.

The patient's nutritional status also should be assessed. A decrease in body weight may be an indicator of calorie deficiency. Sources of protein in the patient's diet should be assessed. A serum albumin level provides a measure of the patient's protein adequacy. Protein-calorie malnutrition can lead to an impaired immune response and increase the patient's risk of infection.

The patient is asked about exposure to immunosuppressants such as radiation and medications. Compiling a detailed drug history can reveal medications the patient is taking that suppress immune system function. Chronic diseases such as arthritis, diabetes mellitus, and renal disorders should also be noted in the patient's assessment.

 **CLINICAL ALERT**

The nurse should remember that the patient who is immunocompromised and leukopenic may not exhibit localized signs of infection. Without sufficient WBCs, these patients are unable to initiate a typical response to infection.

Local signs and symptoms

When skin integrity has been disrupted by invasive apparatus, special attention needs to be given to assessing for signs of infection. The nurse inspects insertion sites for redness, edema, increased warmth, and purulent drainage.

Body fluids and secretions are monitored for changes in amount and color. For instance, changes in sputum color and amount are associated with the onset of a respiratory infection. Gastrointestinal infections usually produce a fecal mass that is watery and may contain blood or mucus. For the patient with skin lesions or wounds, the nurse should note changes in the characteristics of wound drainage. The occurrence of localized pain may be the only manifestation of infection in the patient with a fever.

Systemic signs and symptoms

Fever is usually considered the key assessment parameter for the patient with an infection. In the patient with an adequate number of leukocytes, fever is usually an indication of infection. However, patients may develop a fever that is unrelated to the presence of infection. In these patients a fever may be associated with the primary disease process, such as a malignancy, or it may be a side effect of certain treatment modalities. The patient with a head injury may develop a fever unrelated to infection. Any type of brain tissue injury that disrupts the normal temperature regulating function of the hypothalamus can cause a temperature elevation. In either situation, the patient with fever should still be assessed for infection.

The older adult may not have a high fever with an infection. Slight increases in body temperature may occur with a serious infection in the older adult. When the older adult's normal body temperature is at the low end of what is considered normal, an elevation of 0.5° C may represent a fever.[14] Other manifestations associated with infection in the older adult include: weakness, anorexia, changes in mental status, and a decrease in functional ability. For example, the sudden onset of confusion may be the first indication of a respiratory infection in the elderly. Urinary incontinence may be the only manifestation of a urinary tract infection.[2]

During the data collection interview the nurse questions the patient about any history of fever, with special attention given to determining any pattern to the fevers. Documentation of a fever pattern can be useful and may suggest a particular etiologic factor for a fever. For example, a patient with tuberculosis will have characteristic spikes and falls of fever each day, but not return to normal body temperature.[14]

Other systemic manifestations of infection are associated with the presence of a fever. These related signs and symptoms include headache, generalized muscle aches, shivering, and chilling. Assessment of vital signs usually reveals increased pulse, blood pressure, and respiratory rate. The nurse also assesses the patient for changes in fluid balance. Fluid volume deficit can occur with infection because of increased insensible losses and decreased fluid intake.

Laboratory data

Obtaining specimens of body fluids for culture and sensitivity testing is important in planning definitive therapy for the patient with an infection. The patient who spikes a fever greater than 102° F should have specimens of sputum, urine, blood, and wound drainage collected for laboratory examination. The results of these tests will help determine if infection is the cause of the fever.

The white blood cell count (WBC) and differential count can provide the nurse with information about the severity of an infection and the patient's response to therapy (Table 11-1). An elevated WBC count usually indicates an infectious disease. The WBC will begin to rise within 4 to 8 hours after the entry of a pathogenic microorganism. The increase in leukocytes is directly proportional to the severity of the infection. Bacterial infections are associated with an increase in the number of neutrophils and lymphocytes. Patients with an impaired immune response can develop a severe infection with only a mild increase in white blood cells.

The differential count indicates the percentage of each of the five different types of leukocytes. Early in the infectious process, the neutrophil count will be elevated. Neutrophils have a short life span in circulation of 6 to 7 hours. In a severe infection the bone marrow's store of neutrophils is quickly depleted. The bone marrow then releases immature neutrophils called bands or stab cells. The presence of increased numbers of immature forms of white blood cells is called a **shift to the left** in WBC production.[12]

The use of additional diagnostic and laboratory tests depends on the body system affected by the infection. A chest x-ray examination will help in identifying a pulmonary infection. Computerized tomography, magnetic resonance imaging, and ultrasound can be used to document the function of organs affected by infection.

Nursing Diagnosis

Specific nursing diagnoses for the patient with an infection will depend on the tissues, organs, or body systems that are affected by the infection. Nursing diagnoses for the patient with an infection may include:

Altered comfort related to tissue injury and effects of fever

Activity intolerance related to energy demands of infection

Altered health maintenance related to lack of knowledge about measures to prevent infection

Altered nutrition: less than body requirements related to increased caloric needs from fever

Fluid volume deficit related to fever

High risk for infection transmission related to colonization with drug-resistant microorganisms

High risk for injury related to fever

TABLE 11-1   Laboratory Tests

Laboratory test	Normal adult value	Significance in infection
TOTAL WHITE BLOOD CELLS DIFFERENTIAL COUNT	4500-11,000	Elevated
Neutrophils	55%-70%	Elevated within first few hours of infection; decreased in viral infections, in elderly with severe bacterial infection
Bands	3%	Immature neutrophil; levels above 8% represent a shift to the left; seen with acute infections
Lymphocytes	20%-40%	Elevated with viral infections and chronic bacterial infections; decreased in HIV infection
Monocytes	2%-8%	Elevated in viral infections (mononucleosis), tuberculosis, malaria
Eosinophils	1%-4%	Elevated with parasitic infections
Basophils	0.5%-1%	Changes not seen in infections

Planning

Nursing care is planned to support the various protective mechanisms of the patient. Damage to intact defenses should be prevented, and weakened defenses need to be strengthened. Controlling the transmission of pathogens also is an important goal for nursing care of the patient with an infection or at high risk for an infection. Specific outcomes for the patient may include:

Patient will be free of infection

Body temperature will be within normal range

Patient will report increased comfort level

Patient will be able to complete desired activities

Patient will obtain necessary immunizations

Patient and family will demonstrate appropriate measures to control spread of infection

Body weight will be stable

Fluid intake will equal fluid losses

Patient contacts (other patients, health care workers, and family) will be free of infection

Patient will not experience injury or complications of fever

Implementation

Immunizations

Immunizations as a health protective strategy are as important for adults as they are for children. Traditionally there has been less emphasis on immunizations of the adult as part of primary care. Only a small percentage of the adult population are adequately immunized for infectious diseases.[3] The elderly are at particularly high risk for infectious disease and benefit from routine immunization. Many adults did not receive adequate immunizations as children and therefore are at risk for communicable diseases such as measles, mumps, and rubella. The older adult and those people with chronic diseases can benefit from regular immunizations because of their increased infection risk. Health care workers represent a special at-risk population for infectious diseases because of their increased risk of occupational exposure. Nursing personnel, physicians, laboratory technicians, and other health care providers in a variety of health care settings are an important target group for immunizations.[10] Table 11-2 summarizes the immunizations that are recom-

TABLE 11-2 Adult Immunizations

Vaccine	Adults at risk	Comments
Pneumococcal infections	Over age 65 Any adult with chronic health problems, especially respiratory and cardiovascular	Lower respiratory tract infections are fourth leading cause of death in elderly Infections can lead to pneumonia and bacteremia
Hepatitis B	Health care workers Sexually active individuals with multiple partners IV drug users Hemodialysis patients Hemophiliacs Immigrants from countries with high disease rate	Requires separate doses of vaccine given 1 and 6 months after first dose Vaccine recommended for children as part of routine immunization program
Influenza	Health care workers Nursing home residents Over age 65 Any adult with chronic health problems, especially respiratory and cardiovascular	Vaccine given annually in the fall before flu season Used with caution in people with egg allergy Infection can lead to pneumonia
Diphtheria-tetanus	All adults who have not been immunized in prior 10 years	Adults immunized as children require only booster dose
Measles-mumps-rubella (MMR)	Health care workers Adults born after 1956 who were immunized before age 1 Adults who have never had the diseases or been immunized	Used with caution in women of childbearing age Young adults still at risk for the diseases

mended for adults. An adult immunization program should include vaccines for the following infections: pneumococcal infections, influenza, hepatitis B, measles, mumps, rubella, tetanus, and diphtheria.

Nutrition

For the patient with a decreased appetite and decreased activity tolerance, small, frequent feedings may be more acceptable than three large meals. If less energy is expended by eating small meals, the patient may be able to increase the overall intake of food. Nutritional supplements of high nutritional value may be necessary to ensure adequate intake of protein to support the immune system.

Temperature elevations will produce a 7% increase in metabolic needs for each degree of temperature above normal. The patient with a fever will require additional fluids and calories to support the increased metabolic activity.

Sleep and rest

The patient with an infection will benefit from frequent rest periods that allow for conservation of limited energy reserves. Nursing care should be planned to permit several hours of uninterrupted sleep.

Skin integrity

When the protective function of the patient's skin has been diminished by age, invasive procedures, or other types of stressors, special attention should be given to maintaining the remaining integrity of the skin. Daily bathing should be avoided to decrease drying of the skin. Lubricating lotions can be used to prevent further drying. Trauma to oral membranes can be lessened by using a soft toothbrush. Solutions used for mouth care should be evaluated for their potential to cause further drying of the mucous membranes.

The entry sites of invasive lines and catheters should be cared for in such a manner that will decrease the likelihood of these areas becoming a site for bacterial entry into the body. The use of antibiotic ointments and dressings can help decrease microbial contamination. The dressings covering intravascular insertion sites are changed using sterile technique.

Handwashing

Careful handwashing by caregivers is probably the single most effective method of decreasing the transmission of pathogens in the patient's environment. All people having contact with the patient should be reminded to thoroughly wash their hands before entering the patient's room. This group includes not only nursing personnel, but also physicians and other staff, including those from the laboratory, dietary, social service, pastoral care, and housekeeping departments. Handwashing also is done immediately anytime the caregiver's hands come in contact with contaminated material. After contact with the patient, caregivers need to thoroughly wash their hands again. Family members and visitors also are instructed in careful handwashing before and after visiting the patient. The nurse has an important role in promoting effective handwashing procedures by all people who come in contact with the patient.

Universal precautions

Universal precautions are intended to protect health care workers from exposure to bloodborne pathogens. These protective measures are applied to the care of all patients, since it is difficult to know which patients are carriers of bloodborne pathogens. When universal precautions are used in conjunction with effective handwashing by health care providers, the transmission of pathogens from one patient to another can be reduced.

The nurse uses universal precautions anytime there is potential contact with a patient's blood, se-

TABLE 11-3 Universal Precautions

Protective barriers	Examples of situations requiring use
Gloves for all possible contact with blood or body fluid, especially if caregiver's skin is not intact	Parenteral medication administration IV therapy procedures Perineal care Mouth care Wound care Nasopharyngeal suctioning
Gowns for activities when soiling of clothes is possible from splashes of blood or body fluids	Dressing changes and wound care Assisting with invasive procedures involving body fluids (e.g., lumbar puncture, thoracentesis, or chest tube insertion) IV therapy procedures
Masks and protective eyewear for procedures likely to generate droplets of blood or body fluids	Assisting with invasive procedures Airway suctioning

men, vaginal secretions, and other body fluids including cerebrospinal, synovial, pleural, peritoneal, and pericardial. According to Centers for Disease Control guidelines, universal precautions do not apply to feces, nasal secretions, saliva, sputum, sweat, tears, urine, and vomitus unless they contain visible blood. Although universal precautions can protect the nurse from parenteral, mucous membrane, and skin exposure, they cannot prevent exposure to pathogens as a result of penetrating injuries with contaminated needles or other sharp instruments.[8]

Universal precautions involve the use of protective barriers by the nurse and other health care personnel when exposure to the patient's blood or body fluids is likely. These barriers include gloves, gowns, masks, and goggles. Table 11-3 summarizes the universal precaution guidelines. In addition, nosocomial transmission of bloodborne pathogens can be reduced with proper disposal of contaminated materials. Used needles and other single-use sharp instruments should be disposed of immediately after use in a puncture-resistant container. The nurse can ensure that sharps disposal containers are placed in areas where these materials are used. Chemical germicides or solutions of sodium hypochlorite (1:100 or 1:10 dilution of household bleach) can be used to clean and disinfect nondisposable articles and surfaces in the patient care environment that become contaminated with blood or body fluids.

Isolation

The primary goal of **isolation** precautions is to prevent the spread of pathogens from the patient to others. Isolation precautions are part of the infection control procedures for any health care agency. The nurse can initiate isolation precautions whenever a patient's symptoms suggest an infectious disease.[9] The Centers for Disease Control designates seven categories of isolation precautions. Table 11-4 lists the categories of isolation precautions and situations when they are used. Isolation also may be implemented using a disease-specific system of identifying the appropriate precautions.

TABLE 11-4 Isolation Precautions

Isolation type	Precautions indicated	Diseases
Strict	Private room; gown; gloves, mask; discard contaminated articles or bag and label them for disinfecting or sterilizing	Diphtheria (pharyngeal), chickenpox
Contact	Private room; gown and gloves if contact with infective material likely; mask only if close contact with patient; handling of contaminated articles same as strict isolation	Major skin, burn, or wound infection; *S. aureus* or group A *S. pneumonia;* disseminated herpes simplex
Respiratory	Private room; mask only for close contact with the patient; handling of contaminated articles same as strict isolation	Measles; mumps; pertussis; meningitis; meningococcal pneumonia
Acid-fast bacillus (AFB)	Private room with special ventilation; gown if soiling is likely; mask if patient does not cover mouth with coughing; discard or clean and disinfect contaminated articles	Pulmonary tuberculosis
Enteric precautions	Private room is patient hygiene poor; gown and gloves if contact with infective material likely; handling of contaminated articles same as strict	Hepatitis A; gastroenteritis; infectious diarrhea; amebic dysentery
Drainage and secretion precautions	Gown and gloves if contact with infective material likely; handling of contaminated articles same as strict	Limited skin or burn infections
Blood and body fluid precautions	Private room if patient hygiene poor; gown, gloves, and mask if contact with infectious material likely; handling of contaminated articles same as strict; clean blood spills immediately with bleach solution	HIV/AIDS; hepatitis B; hepatitis C; syphilis; malaria

Patients with infectious diseases should be placed in a private room with their own bathroom. Contaminated linen or other materials can be removed from the patient's room in either a single sturdy bag or in double bags, depending on the agency policy. Handwashing before and after contact with the patient is an essential part of isolation.

When a patient is placed on isolation precautions the nurse gives special attention to the psychosocial needs of the patient. Patients with infections requiring isolation may feel dirty or unclean because health care personnel always use some form of barrier protection when providing care. Although the patient is on isolation, nurses may have less frequent contacts and interactions with the patient leading not only to social isolation but also decreased sensory stimulation. Visits from family and friends may be limited during the time isolation precautions are used. This situation adds to the patient's feelings of loneliness. Both the patient and family need to understand the reason for isolation. Family and friends can be encouraged to maintain contact with the patient through phone calls and mail. The nurse also needs to be alert to changes in the patient's condition indicating that isolation is no longer necessary.

Pharmacologic management

Antipyretics

The preservation of the febrile response in the patient with impaired host defenses is important. Minor elevations of body temperature contribute to creating an environment that is unsuitable for pathogen growth. Fever can cause changes in serum iron levels that are detrimental to the activity of some species of microbes. Elevated temperature is also beneficial in preventing viral replication within cells.

The use of antipyretic medications to reduce low-grade fevers may actually further impair the patient's ability to mount a response to infecting microorganisms. Antipyretics are indicated for the patient who experiences significant discomfort with an elevated temperature. Patients with fevers greater than 104° F should also receive antipyretics. When the body temperature exceeds 105° F, central nervous system function can be impaired. Patients with cardiopulmonary disease may not tolerate the increased workload associated with fever. These patients may benefit from the use of antipyretics.

The ultimate selection of an antipyretic agent may be the responsibility of the physician. However, the nurse should recognize that aspirin may not be appropriate because of its antiinflammatory properties. The use of aspirin to lower a fever may further impair the defense mechanisms of the patient. Acetaminophen (Tylenol) may be the antipyretic of choice because it does not possess the antiinflammatory properties of aspirin.

Antimicrobial therapy

Before administering the first dose of an antimicrobial drug, a culture specimen is obtained from the infection site. The results of specimen cultures and drug sensitivity may not be available for several days. The patient who is suspected of having an infection will be started on antimicrobial drug therapy after specimens have been collected. Initially, the patient may be given a broad spectrum antimicrobial agent. In many cases more than one antibiotic will be ordered to give the patient the broadest possible antimicrobial coverage. The physician may select one drug from the group of aminoglycosides and another drug from the group of penicillins and cephalosporins. Adjustments in specific drug selection can be made when culture and sensitivity results are available.

Once the patient has been started on antibiotic therapy, the nurse monitors the patient's response to drug therapy. Nursing actions related to drug therapy include observing for allergic reactions, assessing improvement in the manifestations of infection, obtaining specimens to monitor serum drug levels, and observing for adverse effects of antimicrobials.[23]

Antimicrobials can alter normal microbial flora and contribute to the development of superimposed secondary infections. Superimposed infections are usually caused by fungi. The patient should be assessed frequently for signs of mouth lesions, pulmonary congestion, increased sputum production, changes in sputum color, skin rashes, vaginal discharge, or diarrhea.

Evaluation

The evaluation of nursing care will focus on the patient's response to measures designed to decrease his exposure to pathogens. When the goal of reduced pathogen exposure has been accomplished, the patient should be free of infection.

Documentation

The nurse documents periodic assessments of the patient's status related to the manifestations of infection. Temperature patterns can provide valuable information when they are graphed over time. Administration of antipyretics can be recorded in relationship to the patient's temperature. Other measures used to lower the patient's temperature, such as cooling blankets or ice packs, also need to be documented in the patient's chart.

All nursing measures to protect the patient from infection are documented. The nurse records any patient teaching about immunizations, handwashing, and other protective measures, as well as the patient's response to the teaching. Routine care of invasive lines and catheters can be recorded in the patient's chart.

Ongoing Care

In preparation for discharge the patient and family need to understand the importance of continuing measures to protect the patient from further threats to the immune system. The patient should continue to avoid contact with people who have obvious infections, such as colds or the flu. The patient may need to avoid being around large groups of people in public places. The practice of handwashing should also be continued by the family, especially by those family members responsible for direct care of the patient.

The patient and family should be taught to recognize signs of infection. They need to know what signs and symptoms should be reported to a health care provider. Daily inspection of the skin and oral mucous membranes should become part of the patient's routine. The patient and family should continue measures that support the body's defenses and decrease possible entry of pathogens.

CRITICAL THINKING QUESTIONS

1 Give an example of an infection in each of the seven categories of microorganisms that cause infections.
2 How do the agent and host interact to produce an infection?
3 What factors increase the older adult's susceptibility to infection?
4 Describe the five stages of a primary acute infection in terms of clinical manifestations.
5 Compare the characteristics of nosocomial and opportunistic infections.
6 What is the importance of accurate fever assessment in the patient with an infection?
7 What is the significance of a shift to the left in the patient's differential WBC count?
8 What is the key nursing intervention used to protect the patient from pathogens?
9 Why are immunizations important for adults and the elderly?
10 Discuss the use of pharmacologic agents in the management of the patient with an infection.
11 How are universal precautions and isolation techniques used in the care of a patient with an infection?

BIBLIOGRAPHY

Current

1. American Health Consultants: CDC tracking dramatic upsurge of MRSA in U.S. hospitals, *Hosp Infect Control* 19:29, 1992.
2. Bender P: Deceptive distress in the elderly, *Am J Nurs* 92(10):29, 1992.
3. Bigbee JL, Jansa N: Strategies for promoting health protection, *Nurs Clin North Am* 26:895, 1991.
4. Burke MM, Walsh MB: *Gerontologic nursing: care of the frail elderly,* St Louis, 1992, Mosby–Year Book.
5. Carpenito LJ: *Handbook of nursing diagnosis,* ed 4, Philadelphia, 1991, JB Lippincott.
6. Carpenter DR, Zielinski DA: How do you treat—and control—C. difficile infection? *Am J Nurs* 92(9):22, 1992.
7. Centers for Disease Control: Recommendations for prevention of HIV transmission in health-care settings, *MMWR Suppl* 36(2s):3s, 1987.
8. Centers for Disease Control: Update: universal precautions for prevention of transmission of human immunodeficiency virus, hepatitis B virus, and other bloodborne pathogens in health-care settings, *MMWR* 37:377, 1988.
9. Coleman D: The when and how of isolation, *RN* 50(10):50, 1987.
10. Decker MD, Schaffner W: Immunization of hospital personnel and other health care workers, *Infect Disease Clin North Am* 4:211, 1990.
11. Garner JS et al: CDC definition of nosocomial infections, *Am J Infect Control* 16:128, 1988.
12. Gawlikowski J: White cells at war, *Am J Nurs* 3:44, 1992.
13. Groer MW, Shekleton ME: *Basic pathophysiology: a holistic approach,* ed 3, St Louis, 1989, Mosby–Year Book.
14. Holtzclaw BJ: The febrile response in critical care: state of the science, *Heart Lung* 21:482, 1992.
15. McCloskey JC, Bulechek GM: *Nursing interventions classification (NIC),* St. Louis, 1992, Mosby–Year Book.
16. Mims CA: *The pathogenesis of infectious disease,* ed 3, Orlando, Fla, 1987, Academic Press.
17. Murray RB, Zentner JP: *Nursing assessment and health promotion strategies through the life span,* ed 4, Norwalk, Conn, 1989, Appleton & Lange.
18. Pagana KD, Pagana TJ: *Mosby's diagnostic and laboratory test reference,* St Louis, 1992, Mosby–Year Book.
19. Shovein J, Young MS: MRSA: Pandora's box for hospitals, *Am J Nurs* 92(2):48, 1992.
20. Simmons B et al: The role of handwashing in prevention of endemic intensive care unit infections, *Infect Control Hosp Epidemiol* 11:589, 1990.
21. Van Der Meer JWM: Defects in host-defense mechanisms. In Rubin RH, Young LS, editors: *Clinical approach to infection in the compromised host,* ed 2, New York, 1988, Plenum Publishing.
22. Wade JC, Schimpff SC: Epidemiology and prevention of

infection in the compromised host. In Rubin RH, Young LS, editors: *Clinical approach to infection in the compromised host,* ed 2, New York, 1988, Plenum Publishing.

23. Walsh ML, Johnson CC: Update on antimicrobial agents, *Nurs Clin North Am* 26:341, 1991.

24. Young LS, editor: Fever and septicemia. In Rubin RH, Young LS, editors: *Clinical approach to infection in the compromised host,* ed 2, New York, 1988, Plenum Publishing.

Classic

25. Adams A: External barriers to infection, *Nurs Clin North Am* 20:145, 1985.

26. Baron M, Tafuro P: The extremes of age: the newborn and the elderly, *Nurs Clin North Am* 20:181, 1985.

27. Carrieri VK, Lindsey AM, West CM: *Pathophysiological phenomena in nursing: human responses to illness,* Philadelphia, 1986, WB Saunders.

28. Donovan EW: *Essentials of pathophysiology,* New York, 1985, Macmillan Publishing.

29. Gershwin ME, Beach RS, Hurley LS: *Nutrition and immunity,* Orlando, Fla, 1985, Academic Press.

30. Gurevich I, Tafuro P: Nursing measures for the prevention of infection in the compromised host, *Nurs Clin North Am* 20:257, 1985.

31. Porth CA: *Pathophysiology: concepts of altered health states,* ed 2, Philadelphia, 1986, JB Lippincott.

32. Price SA, Wilson LM: *Pathophysiology: clinical concepts of disease processes,* ed 3, New York, 1986, McGraw-Hill.

33. Roberts R: *Infectious diseases: pathogenesis, diagnosis, and therapy,* St. Louis, 1986, Mosby–Year Book.

34. Roghmann KJ et al: Immune response of elderly adults to pneumococcus: variations by age, sex, and functional impairment, *J Gerontol* 42:265, 1985.

35. Vander AJ, Sherman JH, Luciano DS: *Human physiology,* New York, 1985, McGraw-Hill.

CHAPTER TWELVE

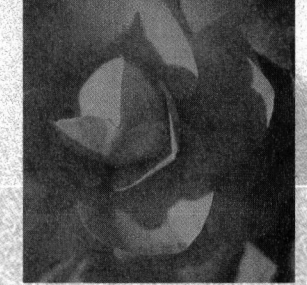

Fluids, Electrolytes, and Acid-Base Balance

LEARNING OBJECTIVES

1 Describe the basic physiologic mechanisms responsible for maintaining fluid, electrolyte, and acid-base balance.

2 Describe the distribution of fluids and electrolytes in the body.

3 Identify the major causes of electrolyte imbalances and their clinical manifestations.

4 List significant nursing assessments for a patient with high risk for or actual fluid-electrolyte imbalance.

5 Describe the nursing management of patients with actual or high risk for fluid imbalances.

6 Describe the nursing management of patients with actual or high risk for electrolyte imbalances.

7 Compare etiology, treatment, and nursing management of acidosis with alkalosis.

8 Discuss the nursing management of the elderly patient with fluid, electrolyte, or acid-base imbalance.

KEY TERMS

BODY FLUIDS are essential to the internal and external environment of healthy cells. Body fluids contain water and dissolved substances, some of which dissociate into two parts or elements and are called electrolytes. Any change in the volume, concentration, or composition of the fluid will affect the function of cells. Acid-base balance is also essential for maintenance of normal functioning cells. Knowledge and understanding of the mechanisms that contribute to fluid, electrolyte, and acid-base balance and imbalance are essential when applying the nursing process to assist the patient to maintain or regain balance. A loss of body fluids can be serious, and a loss of 20% of the fluid content can be fatal. Nearly every illness will be accompanied by some degree of fluid, electrolyte, or acid-base imbalance.

BODY FLUIDS

Water is the largest single constituent of the body. In the average adult the total body water amounts to approximately 60% of the body weight. In the elderly adult, because of changes in body tissues, the total body fluid decreases to 45% to 50% of body weight. Since elderly persons have a much lower percentage of body weight that is fluid, they are highly likely to develop fluid imbalance. There is variation related to the person's age, gender, and amount of body fat. Fat cells contain less fluid than lean tissue.

Body fluids are contained within two major compartments. Most of the body fluid is inside the cells and is called intracellular fluid (ICF). In adults, approximately 40% of the body weight is ICF. In the elderly the ICF is reduced because of tissue loss. Extracellular fluid (ECF) is the fluid outside the cell. The ECF is located in two places. Some of the ECF is within the blood vessels and is called intravascular fluid. Intravascular fluid is about 5% of the body weight. The second place for ECF is the intersititial space, which is outside the cell and between the cells and blood vessels. The interstitial fluid makes up approximately 15% of the body weight in an average adult. The ECF consists of interstitial fluid, intravascular fluid, cerebrospinal fluid, fluids in the gastrointestinal tract, and fluids of the potential spaces. Figure 12-1 shows the distribution of body fluids.

The ECF is in constant movement throughout the body. The ICF in each cell has its own unique composition, but the concentration of the intracellular constituents is similar from one cell to another cell. The fluid compartments are separated by semipermeable membranes. Since the fluids outside the cells (intravascular and interstitial) are constantly moving through capillary walls, the extracellular fluid is contained within a communicating chamber. The ECF supplies the cells with nutrients and other substance needed for cellular function.

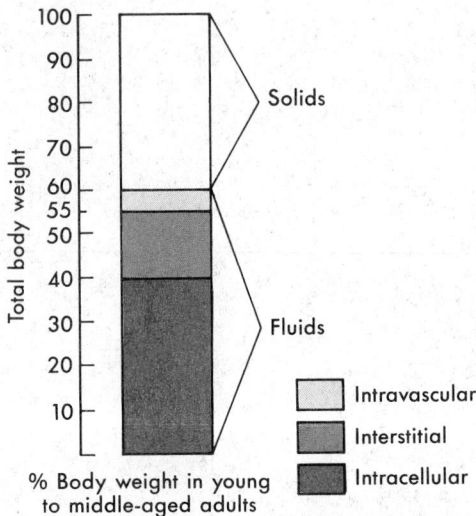

FIGURE 12-1   Distribution of body fluids.

The body fluids consist of water and dissolved substances. Some substances such as glucose, urea, and creatinine do not dissociate in solution. They do not separate from their complex form into simpler substances when they are in solution.

ELECTROLYTES

An atom is the smallest particle of an element that still has the properties of the element. Atoms are composed of particles, namely, the proton, neutron, and electron. The proton carries a positive charge, the electron carries a negative charge, and the neutron is neutral. The proton and the neutron are in the nucleus (center) of the atom. Electrons (which carry negative charges) revolve around the nucleus. Atoms may gain, lose, or share electrons. When an atom carries an electrical charge because it has either gained or lost electrons, it is an ion. When an atom has given away or lost electrons, it will have a positive charge and is called a cation. When an atom has gained (taken on) electrons, it will have a negative charge. An ion that has gained electrons and therefore has a negative charge is called an anion. The combination of two or more atoms to form a substance is called a molecule.

When a substance is dissolved in solution and some of its molecules split (dissociate) into electrically charged atoms called ions, that substance is called an **electrolyte.** For example, when sodium chloride (NaCl) is in a solution, it separates into two parts, sodium (Na^+) and chloride (Cl^-). Sodium is the cation because it carries a positive charge, and chloride carries a negative charge and is called an anion. The volume of fluids is measured in liters (L) or milliliters (mL).

TABLE 12-1 Electrolyte Distribution in Body Fluid

Electrolytes	Extracellular (mEq/L)	Intracellular (mEq/L)
Sodium (Na$^+$)	135 to 154	15 to 20
Potassium (K$^+$)	3.5 to 5	150 to 155
Calcium (Ca^{++})	4.5 to 5.5	1 to 2
Bicarbonate (HCO$_3^-$)	25 to 27	10 to 12
Chloride (Cl$^-$)	98 to 106	1 to 4
Magnesium (Mg^{++})	4.5 to 5.5	27 to 29
Phosphate (HPO$_4^{--}$)	1.7 to 4.6	100 to 104

The unit of measure for an electrolyte is the milliequivalent (mEq), which describes the electrolyte's ability to combine and form other compounds. An equivalent weight is the amount of one electrolyte that will displace or otherwise react with a given amount of hydrogen. One milliequivalent (mEq) of any cation will always react chemically with 1 mEq of an anion. Whenever an electrolyte moves out of a cell, another electrolyte moves in to take its place. The number of cations and anions must be the same for homeostasis to exist in each of the fluid compartments (intracellular, interstitial, and intravascular). The fluid in each of the compartments contains electrolytes. Each compartment has a particular composition of electrolytes that must be in the right compartment in the right amount (Table 12-1).

FLUID AND ELECTROLYTE TRANSPORTATION

Throughout the body the cell membranes and capillary walls are selectively permeable. Selectively permeable membranes allow water and some solutes to pass through them freely. The solute is the substance that is dissolved. One process by which a solute (gas or substance) in solution moves is called diffusion. **Diffusion** is the movement of particles in all directions through a solution. Molecules of a substance dissolved in a solvent spread by diffusion from an area of higher concentration to an area of lower concentration. The solvent is the solution in which the solute is dissolved. Diffusion may also occur across a membrane if the membrane is permeable, or allows free passage. Diffusion occurs within fluid compartments and from one compartment to another if the barrier between the compartments is permeable to the diffusing substances. Oxygen in the air we breathe enters the intravascular compartment and then the cells by diffusion.

Facilitated diffusion involves a carrier system that moves a substance across a membrane faster than it would with simple diffusion. In facilitated diffusion a substance can only move from an area of higher concentration to one of lower concentration. An example of facilitated diffusion is the movement of glucose, which with the assistance of insulin passes through the cell membrane into the cell.

A membrane permeable to water but not to all the solutes present is a selectively permeable membrane. Movement of the solvent or water across this membrane, is called osmosis. **Osmosis** is the movement of solvent molecules across a membrane to an area where there is a higher concentration of solute that cannot pass through the membrane. The reason the solvent moves is that the membrane will not allow the solute through. The result of osmosis is two solutions, separated by a selectively permeable membrane, that are equal in concentration. When a more concentrated solution is on one side of a selectively permeable membrane and a less concentrated solution is on the other side, a pull called osmotic pressure draws the solvent through the membrane to the more concentrated side, or the side with more solute. The amount of osmotic pressure is determined by the relative number of particles of solute on the side of greater concentration (Figure 12-2).

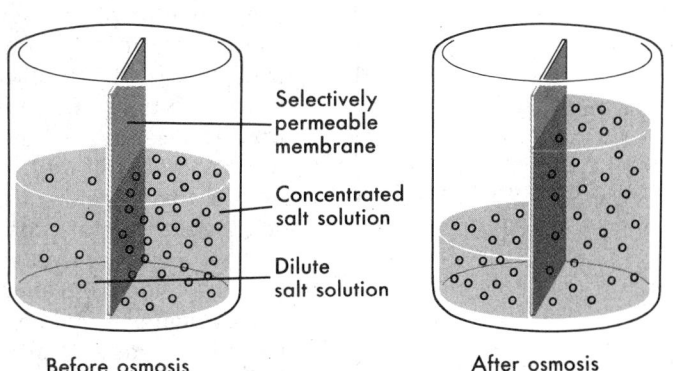

Selectively permeable membrane

Concentrated salt solution

Dilute salt solution

Before osmosis   After osmosis

FIGURE 12-2 Osmosis.

Electrolytes exert ordinary osmotic pressure. However, albumin and other substances with a high molecular weight exert a special kind of osmotic pressure, called colloid osmotic pressure, or *oncotic pressure*. Colloids are of special importance since they cannot pass through the capillary wall, which is the barrier between plasma and the interstitial fluid.

When the solutions on both sides of a selectively permeable membrane have established equilibrium, or are equal in concentration, they are *isotonic*. *Iso*- is a combining form that means alike. The movement of water through the cell membrane normally occurs so rapidly that any lack of osmotic balance is corrected within seconds. When the body is functioning normally, a state of equilibrium is maintained constantly.

The osmotic pressure of a solution is proportional to the number of particles per unit volume of solvent. The unit measure of osmotic pressure is the osmole. The ability of solutes to cause osmosis and osmotic pressure is measured in terms of osmoles. The osmole is too large a unit for satisfactory use in expressing osmotic activity in the body. The term milliosmole (mOsm), which equals 0.001 osmole, is used to measure osmotic pressure in the body. **Osmolality** means the number of osmotically active particles per kilogram of water. The normal osmolality of plasma is 280 to 294 mOsm/kg. Osmolality of ECF is determined by the ECF concentration of sodium (Na). Sodium is the most abundant extracellular cation and therefore provides 90% to 95% of the effective osmotic pressure of the ECF. Because of osmotic equilibrium, the ECF and the ICF normally have nearly the same osmolality.

An example of an isotonic solution is 0.9% sodium chloride, which is referred to as isotonic saline solution, or normal saline solution. This means that it is isotonic to human cells, and thus there will be very little osmosis. Another example of an isotonic solution is 5% glucose.

A solution that contains a lower concentration of salt than another solution is hypotonic, meaning it has less salt or more water than an isotonic solution. If a hypotonic solution is put into the bloodstream, the red blood cells draw water into themselves. This causes the cells to swell and eventually burst, if the situation is not changed, in an attempt to bring about balance.

A solution that has a higher concentration of solutes than another solution is hypertonic. An example of a hypertonic solution is 3% sodium chloride. If a hypertonic solution is infused into the bloodstream, water moves out of the cells into the hypertonic solution. As the cells lose their fluid, they become wrinkled and shriveled like prunes or crenated (see box on intravenous fluids).

Active Transport

Diffusion and osmosis are passive processes since they do not require energy from body cells. The natural tendency of molecules is to move from areas of high concentration to areas of lower concentration. In diffusion the molecules move to areas of lesser solute concentration, and in osmosis the molecules move to areas with less solvent. An active transport system moves molecules or ions "uphill" against concentration and osmotic pressure. Hydrolysis of adenosine triphosphate (ATP) provides the energy needed for active transport. An example of active transport is the **sodium-potassium pump,** which moves sodium to the outside of the cell and then returns potassium to the inside of the cell. However, the concentration of potassium is already much greater inside than outside the cell. In addition to energy, active transport also requires a specific "carrier" molecule as well as a specific enzyme (ATPase) to promote active transport. Sodium, potassium, calcium, magnesium, some sugars, and amino acids use an active transport process (Figure 12-3).

Another factor that influences the movement of fluids and electrolytes is **hydrostatic pressure**, or

---

INTRAVENOUS FLUIDS

Isotonic solutions

5% dextrose in water
Sodium chloride solution (0.9%) (normal saline)

Hypertonic solutions

10% dextrose in normal saline
3% sodium chloride
5% sodium chloride

Hypotonic solutions

One-half hypotonic saline (0.45%)
5% dextrose in 0.45% saline

Isotonic fluids with multiple electrolytes

Plasma-Lyte
Isolyte E
Lactated Ringer's solution (Hartmann's)
Ringer's solution

Hypotonic fluids with multiple electrolytes

Isolyte R
Normosol-M
Plasma-Lyte
Ionosol B

From Weldy NJ: *Body Fluids and electrolytes,* ed 6, St Louis, 1992, Mosby–Year Book.

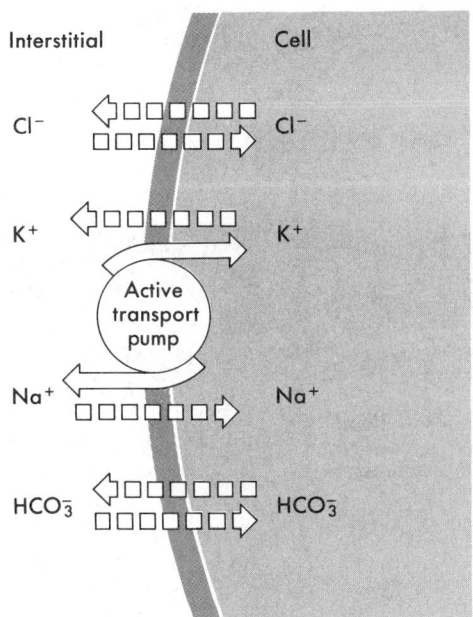

FIGURE 12-3   Sodium-potassium pump.

the force of the fluid pressing outward against the vessel wall. Relating hydrostatic pressure to the blood refers not only to the pressure of the weight of the fluid against the capillary wall, but also to the force with which the blood is propelled by each heartbeat. Because of the force of the blood pressure, the hydrostatic pressure at the arterial end of the capillary is approximately twice as great as at the venous end. When a difference in the hydrostatic pressure exists on two sides of a membrane, water and diffusible solutes move out of the solution with the higher hydrostatic pressure. This is called filtration. **Filtration** is the movement of fluid through a selectively permeable membrane from an area with higher hydrostatic pressure to an area with lower hydrostatic pressure.

In areas where both hydrostatic pressure and osmotic pressure are present, the net result is determined by the pressure differences. At the arterial end of the capillary, the hydrostatic pressure is greater than the osmotic pressure. Therefore fluid and diffusible solutes move out of the capillary. At the venous end of the capillary the osmotic pressure, or pull, is greater than the hydrostatic pressure, and fluids and some solutes move into the capillary. The excess fluid and solutes remaining in the interstitial space are returned to the intravascular compartment by the lymph channels (Figure 12-4).

Fluid Volume Shifts

Fluids may shift from the intravascular compartment into the interstitial space. In some clinical disorders, depletion of the ECF develops because large quantities of fluid are held in an interstitial area, which makes that fluid inaccessible to the body. This is called "third spacing," and the fluid is usually essentially invisible. This shift of fluid into third space may be localized to a single area, or it may spread throughout the body. For example, a person with ascites will have large quantities of fluid in the abdomen.

The reason why fluids may shift into third space includes lowered plasma proteins, increased capillary permeability, or lymphatic blockage. Secondary causes for the intravascular to interstitial fluid shift include trauma, inflammation, or disease. Third spacing is a major factor in the fluid balance of persons who have had abdominal surgery.

The first phase of third spacing is loss. Depending on the cause, it is likely to last for 48 to 72 hours. During this time the symptoms will be those of a fluid volume deficit. The second phase of third spacing is resorption or movement of the fluid from the interstitial space into the intravascular space. Therefore the intravascular volume increases. Usually this shift occurs gradually, and fluid overload does not occur unless extra fluid is given at this time. After the inflammation subsides, the fluid in the tissue spaces begins to be resolved. Nursing actions are aimed at assessment and interventions to prevent severe fluid volume deficit during the first phase and prevent fluid volume overload during the resorption phase. Keep accurate records of intake, output, and daily weights to help identify problems in fluid balance.

REGULATION OF FLUID VOLUME

Normally, fluid enters the body through drinking, water in foods, and water formed by oxidation of foods. Electrolytes are present in both foods and liquids. With a normal diet an excess of essential electrolytes is taken in and the unused electrolytes are excreted. The typical amount of fluid intake over 24 hours for an adult is as follows:

Ingested liquids	1500 mL
Water in foods	700 mL
Water from oxidation	200 mL
	2400 mL

Fluids leave the body by several routes. The average amount of fluid leaving the body in an adult over 24 hours is as follows:

Skin by diffusion	350 mL
Skin by perspiration	100 mL
Lungs through expired air	350 mL
Feces	200 mL
Kidneys	1400 mL
	2400 mL

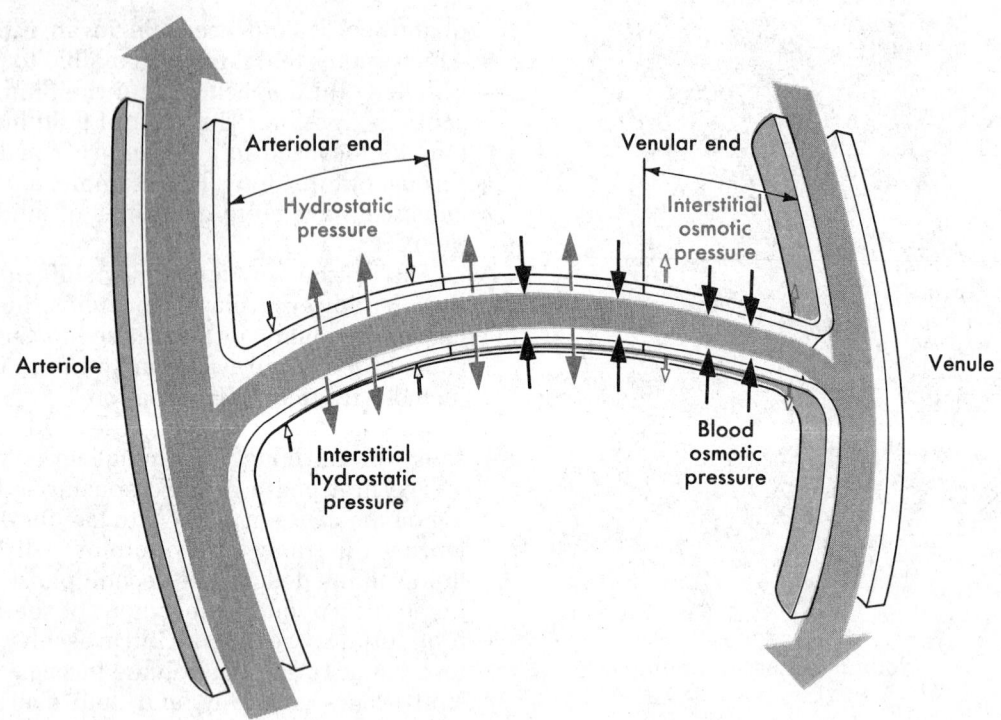

Arterial end of capillary—hydrostatic pressure

Blood hydrostatic pressure	37 mm Hg
Interstitial fluid hydrostatic pressure	– 1 mm Hg
Hydrostatic pressure gradient	36 mm Hg

Arterial end of capillary—osmotic pressure

Blood osmotic (oncotic) pressure	26 mm Hg
Interstitial fluid osmotic pressure	– 1 mm Hg
Osmotic pressure gradient	25 mm Hg

Thus

Filtration force = Hydrostatic pressure gradient	36 mm Hg
Osmotic force = Osmotic pressure gradient	–25 mm Hg
Net filtration force	11 mm Hg

Venous end of capillary—hydrostatic pressure

Blood hydrostatic pressure	17 mm Hg
Interstitial fluid hydrostatic pressure	– 1 mm Hg
Hydrostatic pressure gradient	16 mm Hg

Venous end of capillary—osmotic pressure

Blood osmotic pressure	26 mm Hg
Interstitial fluid osmotic pressure	– 1 mm Hg
Osmotic pressure gradient	25 mm Hg

Thus

Osmotic force	25 mm Hg
Filtration force	–16 mm Hg
Net osmotic pressure	9 mm Hg

FIGURE 12-4   Capillary pressure differences.

As long as all organs are functioning normally, the body is able to balance its fluid content.

REGULATION AND MAINTENANCE OF FLUID AND ELECTROLYTE BALANCE

To maintain health, the volume, concentration, and composition of fluids and electrolytes are maintained within narrow limits. **Homeostasis** indicates the relative stability of the internal environment. The composition of the internal environment may vary from tissue to tissue because of differences in cell activity and metabolism. Because of the move-

ment of substances between the compartments, a relative constancy is maintained. The internal environment is not static but dynamic.

In health the body is able to respond to disturbances in fluids and electrolytes to prevent or repair damage. Thirst, the conscious desire for water, is one of the major factors that determine fluid intake. The osmoreceptors in the hypothalamus are cells that are stimulated by an increase in the osmotic pressure of body fluids to initiate thirst. Eating potato chips makes a person thirsty because the salt on the chips increases the osmotic pressure of body fluids. Thirst is also stimulated by a decrease in the

ECF volume. This is one way the body attempts to regain balance. Another factor that helps to regulate water intake is dryness of the mouth caused by decreased salivary secretion. In a sick person the usual stimuli may be absent.

The volume of water in the body is maintained or restored by adjusting the output to the intake, thus providing homeostasis. The kidneys have the major responsibility to maintain balance of both fluids and electrolytes by controlling output. They remove waste materials or excessive substances from the ECF. The volume of urine is regulated primarily by hormones from the posterior lobe of the pituitary gland (antidiuretic hormone [ADH]) and from the adrenal cortex (aldosterone).

Influenced by these hormones, the kidneys help to regulate the total volume of ECFs, the ratio of water to solutes (concentration), and the specific quantity of different electrolytes (composition). When the ECF volume becomes too high, the blood volume or intravascular volume increases. The venous return to the heart is increased, which then increases cardiac output. This results in an increased arterial pressure. The increased arterial pressure resulting from the increased fluid volume causes the kidneys to excrete the excess fluid. Normally, the interstitial fluid volume is regulated to keep the interstitial fluid spaces filled. However, when this balance is not possible because of disease, the interstitial spaces can become expanded with excess fluid. Excess fluid in the intersitital spaces is called edema. If the ECF volume is decreased because of increased loss or inadequate intake, normally functioning kidneys respond by retaining more fluid so the ECF volume is returned to more nearly normal. However, if the ECF volume deficit is too great or occurs too rapidly, the body may not be able to correct the imbalance, and treatment is necessary.

Aldosterone regulates the ECF volume by affecting the renal control of sodium and potassium. When the production of aldosterone is increased, sodium, chloride, and water are retained. However, potassium is excreted. Aldosterone production is a complex and not entirely understood mechanism. In a healthy person, increased production of aldosterone occurs with a low blood volume, low blood sodium, or high blood potassium.

Antidiuretic hormone (ADH) is the water-conservation hormone. ADH regulates the osmotic pressure of ECF by regulating the amount of water absorbed from the blood by the renal tubules. Increased production of ADH results in increased resorption of water by the kidney through osmosis. The urine volume decreases, but the concentration increases. For example, if a large amount of hypertonic glucose is infused into the body, the osmotic pressure of the ECF increases. This stimulates the production of more ADH so more fluid is retained and the osmotic pressure of the ECF returns to normal.

Role of Organ Systems in Regulating Fluid Volume

Organs involved in homeostatic mechanisms for regulating fluid volume include the kidneys, neuroendocrine system, heart, and blood vessels.

Kidney

The kidneys are essential in regulating fluid and electrolyte balance. They control the quantity of fluids and electrolytes within the body as a whole. The kidneys excrete varying amounts of water and resorb or release sodium, potassium, bicarbonate, and hydrogen ions to regulate intracellular and extracellular concentrations within normal limits.

The kidneys remove excess body fluid by increasing urinary output, or diuresis. On the other hand, if there is a deficit of body fluid, these organs conserve water by decreasing urinary output, or antidiuresis. These organs act not only autonomously, but also in response to other regulatory mechanisms to maintain fluid and electrolyte balance.

Glomerular filtration pressure

The volume and rate of filtration across the glomerular membrane are the result of a balance of various pressures. The filtration pressure is a result of the pressure inside the glomerular capillaries minus the colloid osmotic pressure from plasma proteins, principally albumin, in the blood plus the pressure in Bowman's capsule.

The average glomerular pressure in humans is estimated to be 60 mm Hg. Increases or decreases in this pressure occur under varying conditions. The pressure in Bowman's capsule is estimated to be 18 mm Hg, whereas the average colloid osmotic pressure of blood in the glomerular capillaries is approximately 32 mm Hg. The filtration pressure under these conditions is equal to $60 - (32 + 18) = 10$. At a normal mean filtration pressure of 10 mm Hg, the total filtration rate of both kidneys is 125 mL/min. In general, the higher the glomerular pressure, the greater the filtration rate, whereas the higher the blood colloid osmotic pressure, or Bowman's capsule pressure, the lower the filtration rate.[4]

Colloid osmotic pressure and filtration

When serum colloid osmotic pressure of blood decreases or increases over the normal value, the glomerular filtration rate is affected. For example, drinking only minimal amounts of liquid increases serum osmotic pressure by decreasing intravascular fluid volume. Because the serum osmotic pressure is increased, filtration is decreased, leading to a decrease in urinary output. Based on this information, the net effect of dehydration is oliguria or anuria. The opposite would be evident in the case of over-hydration in that the net effect would be polyuria.

Neuroendocrine system, heart, and blood vessels

Four neuroendocrine mechanisms affect the regulation of ECF volume, which in turn affects the filtration rate of the glomerulus of the kidney nephron. These mechanisms include the central nervous system ischemic response, baroreceptor reflex and volume receptors in the heart and blood vessels, and renin-angiotensin-aldosterone mechanisms.

Central nervous system ischemic response

When afferent arterioles become constricted, the glomerular filtration rate decreases because of a reduction in hydrostatic pressure in the glomerular capillary plexus. For example, massive hemorrhage results in decreased ECF volume, which results in a central nervous system ischemic response. Decreased blood flow interferes with the normal metabolic function of brain tissue with a corresponding increase in the concentration of carbon dioxide in the vasomotor center. Consequently the sympathetic nervous system is stimulated to constrict the afferent arterioles to maintain blood pressure. The decrease in urinary output as a result of such constriction is an effort by the body to conserve ECF volume and thereby correct the hypovolemic state.

Baroreceptor reflex

Baroreceptors are stretch receptors in the large arteries that react to a decrease in ECF by responding to low arterial pressure. As a result the afferent arterioles of the kidneys constrict, decreasing filtration rate and retaining ECF.

Volume receptor mechanism

Volume receptors are stretch receptors in the walls of the right and left atria. Increased pressure in the two atria occurs when intravascular fluid volume becomes excessive. This in turn causes a stretch of the atrial walls, stimulating the receptors to transmit nerve impulses into the brain. The brain responds by inhibiting sympathetic nerve signals to the kidneys, thereby increasing the filtration rate and the urinary output, thus alleviating extracellular excess.

Renin/angiotensin/aldosterone mechanism

Renin is an enzyme that is secreted by the kidneys into the circulatory system in response to decreased pressure in the afferent arteriole or a decrease in ECF volume. Renin then causes splitting of a plasma protein, angiotensinogen, to produce angiotensin I, a vasopressor substance in an inactive form. This in turn is converted to angiotensin II in the lungs. Angiotensin II causes vasoconstriction throughout the body, thereby increasing peripheral resistance. Angiotensin II stimulates aldosterone production and secretion by the adrenal cortex. Aldosterone, a mineralocorticoid hormone, combines with carrier protein enzymes to aid in the transport of sodium from the nephron tubules to the blood, passively followed by water. Potassium is also actively transported in the distal convoluted tubule and collecting ducts. As sodium is reabsorbed into ECF, potassium is excreted into the urine. The net result is an increase in extracellular volume and increased oxygenation of renal cells. When an increase in fluid intake results in increased ECF, renin secretion by the kidney decreases.

The aldosterone negative feedback responds to both extracellular increases and deficits. Three factors are included in this cycle, namely, aldosterone, adrenocorticotropic hormone (ACTH), and sodium. When the sodium level in ECF declines, so does the fluid level. This decrease in sodium stimulates the secretion of ACTH by the pituitary gland, which in turn stimulates the adrenal cortex to release aldosterone. Angiotensin II also stimulates the adrenal cortex to secrete aldosterone. Aldosterone in turn causes the retention of sodium with its corresponding increase in fluid retention. ACTH secretion is thereby reduced, further decreasing the release of aldosterone by the pituitary gland. This cycle is repeated continuously to maintain a balanced ECF level.

NURSING MANAGEMENT OF THE PATIENT WITH FLUID AND ELECTROLYTE PROBLEMS

Assessment
Subjective

In evaluating the history of the patient, the nurse should answer the following questions, which will help ascertain if potential or actual fluid and electrolyte problems exist:

1. Is there any disease process present that might place the patient at risk for potential or actual fluid and electrolyte disturbance? Examples include diabetes mellitus, liver disease, congestive heart failure, intestinal obstruction, and third-space disorders, such as pleural effusion and ascites. What type of imbalance could this condition cause?
2. Is there an abnormal loss of fluids and electrolytes caused by vomiting, diarrhea, or gastric intubation or other types of abnormal fluid loss or excess?
3. Is the patient receiving any medication that could disrupt body fluid balance? Examples in-

clude diuretics, steroids, chemotherapeutic agents, or strong laxatives.

4. Are any of the treatments capable of inducing imbalances? Examples include hyperosmolar tube feedings, gastric suction, or deep radiation treatments.

5. Have any dietary restrictions been imposed? How might fluid balance be altered in this situation?

6. What is the patient's intake of fluids and other nutrients, either orally or by other routes? How do the intake and output compare?

For each question the nurse ascertains the possible types of fluid and electrolyte imbalances that may result, based on an evaluation of the information. It is important to recognize that usually one type of fluid and electrolyte imbalance does not exist alone.

Objective

Review the history and the risk for fluid or electrolyte imbalance. Then assess the signs and symptoms that can be observed (objective) as well as those reported by the patient (subjective). The assessment includes an examination and evaluation of the total fluid intake and output, including urinary output and concentration, characteristics of the skin and mucous membranes, sense of thirst, weight of the patient, signs of edema, vital signs, filling of neck veins and hand veins, neuromuscular irritability, mental status, central venous pressure, and evaluation of laboratory data.

Examination of the total intake and output (I & O) is an important parameter in evaluating the presence of fluid volume excess or deficit. Normally the intake over a 24-hour period is equal to the output. Normal intake includes liquids, water in food, and water produced by metabolism of nutrients. Normal output includes urinary volume, water in feces, sensible loss, and insensible losses of water vapor from the lungs and water evaporation from the skin (see p. 169).

Fluid volume excess is associated with a total intake substantially greater than total output. On the other hand, total intake that is substantially less than that of the output places the patient in danger of fluid deficit.

The accuracy of I & O measurement and recording is vital to ascertain the gains and losses. Accurate intake measurement and recording include all fluids ingested, including water content of foods such as ice cream, gelatin, parenteral fluids (intravenous, intramuscular, and subcutaneous), tube feedings, and irrigating solutions that enter the body.

Accurate measurement and recording of output include the amount of urine output, vomitus, perspiration, diarrhea, and drainage from decubiti, fistu-las, gastric suction, and burned areas; fluid obtained from procedures such as paracentesis and thoracentesis; and an estimation of the amount of water vapor removed via the lungs when hyperpnea is noted. In summary, any loss of fluids via any route should be recorded. If a potential water and electrolyte imbalance is suspected, the nurse initiates an I & O record without waiting for a physician's order.

Urinary output

The average urinary output in adults ranges from 1000 to 2000 mL in 24 hours, which is approximately 40 to 80 mL/hr. Fluid volume deficit is associated with a low urinary output, whereas a high urinary volume indicates fluid volume excess. When urinary output is lower or higher than normal, the nurse considers and assesses the related factors (see the box below).

Examination of the specific gravity (sp gr) of urine is an important consideration in evaluating urinary output. Specific gravity of urine normally ranges from 1.005 to 1.030.

Skin and mucous membranes

Patients with a deficit in ECF volume will exhibit a continued slight elevation of the skin for several seconds after being pinched. However, as one grows

FACTORS RELATED TO ALTERED URINARY OUTPUT

The patient's diagnosis, such as renal disease or diabetes mellitus, which can affect fluid and electrolyte balance

The amount of fluid intake (normal, high, or low)

Fluid losses from other routes

Conditions that lead to higher amount of waste products, such as total parenteral nutrition (TPN) feedings, and increases in body temperature, which require an increase in fluid volume used by the kidney for excretion of these waste products

Urinary volume decrease caused by increase in aldosterone and ADH secretions as a result of stress

Low urinary volume with a high specific gravity indicative of fluid volume deficit

Low urinary volume with a low specific gravity indicative of renal disease

Age of the patient—elderly usually have a decreased renal-concentrating ability

Decreased blood volume (hypovolemia), which causes oliguria because of decreased perfusion of the kidneys; increased blood volume (hypervolemia), which causes an increase in urinary output if there is no kidney damage

older, skin elasticity decreases. Therefore skin turgor of elderly patients should be tested on the skin overlying the sternum or on the inner thighs. Flushed, dry skin may indicate fluid volume deficit.

The mucous membrane in the oral cavity should be examined to determine the amount of moisture present. To determine if a fluid volume deficit exists, the nurse examines the mucous membrane where the gum and inner cheek meet. If this area is dry, fluid volume deficit is suspected. Because of mouth breathing during sleep and age-related changes in the mouth (diminished saliva) the older adult may have a dry mouth without a fluid volume deficit.

Examination of the oral cavity also includes close examination of the tongue. A red and swollen tongue may be caused by an excess of sodium. Fluid volume deficit is suspected when examination of the tongue reveals more than one longitudinal furrow along with a decrease in size.

Thirst

The nurse assesses whether the patient complains of thirst. This phenomenon usually occurs with increased loss of fluid volume, such as in continued bouts of diarrhea. Patients who are unconscious or debilitated cannot respond to thirst. Older persons have a decreased sense of thirst without fluid or electrolyte imbalance. Sodium excess stimulates the sense of thirst.

Weight

Patients with potential or actual fluid and electrolyte problems should be weighed daily, since rapid variations in weight are associated with changes in body fluid volume. Body weight increases when the total fluid intake is greater than the total fluid output. Conversely, body weight rapidly decreases when the total fluid intake is less than the total fluid output. A weight gain of 2.2 pounds is equal to 1 L of retained fluid. Catabolic tissue loss (even in starvation) only accounts for about 0.5 pound of weight loss per day. Therefore any weight loss in excess of this amount is considered fluid loss. The nurse should also be cognizant that when there is a third-space loss of body fluid, as in ascites, the patient's weight may be unchanged even when experiencing severe intravascular fluid volume deficit.

Edema

Edema indicates an expanded volume in the interstitial fluid and is defined as swelling of the interstitial space. It may be localized, as in an area of inflammation, or generalized because of altered capillary hemodynamics with the retention of excess sodium and water. Increased capillary hydrostatic pressure from volume excess or venous obstruction causes edema. Edema is also found in the presence of burns, allergies, or infection because of increased capillary permeability. For example, generalized edema occurs in cirrhosis of the liver and nephrotic syndrome. If periorbital edema is present, the nurse should be alerted to evaluate for significant fluid retention, since the hydrostatic pressure in this region is relatively low. Generalized edema usually is most evident in dependent areas. Therefore lower extremities of ambulatory patients should be checked for the presence of edema, as well as the presacral region of patients on bed rest. Retention of 5 to 10 pounds of excess fluid usually must occur before edema becomes apparent in the adult.

Pitting edema should be assessed over a bony surface, such as the sacrum, or medial malleolus. Use your thumb to press firmly for at least 5 seconds. The depth of depression is estimated in centimeters (1 to 4 cm) to determine severity of the edema.

Vital signs

Changes in body temperature, respiratory rate and depth, heart rate, and blood pressure may signal fluid or electrolyte imbalance. Increased body temperature may cause fluid and electrolyte deficits as a result of increased sweating. For example, body temperature may become elevated with excess serum sodium. Decreased body temperature is seen in sodium deficit and in hypovolemia. The rectal temperature may drop as low as 35° C (95° F) in cases of severe fluid volume deficit.

Increases in respiratory rate and depth may increase insensible fluid loss. Shortness of breath or rales may signify fluid volume excess caused by fluid entrapment in the lungs. Rapid, deep respirations may be part of the compensatory mechanism for metabolic acidosis. Slow, shallow, irregular respirations may occur in metabolic alkalosis and potassium deficit. Stridor is characteristic of calcium deficit. Depressed respirations occur with magnesium deficit.

Increased pulse rate may occur with fluid volume deficit to maintain cardiac output. A bounding pulse may indicate volume excess, since the volume of the pulse depends on the blood volume that is ejected by the left ventricle and its strength of contraction. A weak, irregular, rapid pulse occurs in potassium deficit.

A rapid, weak, thready pulse may indicate fluid volume deficit, the result of intravascular volume deficit or sodium deficit. An irregular pulse may occur with hypokalemia or hypomagnesemia.[5] Pulse volume is increased in fluid volume excess and decreased in fluid volume deficit.

A decrease in blood pressure (BP) is observed in fluid volume deficit, sodium deficit, potassium deficit, and magnesium deficit. An elevated BP may be a result of fluid volume excess or magnesium deficit. Normal BP when lying flat and a drop when the head is elevated occur in fluid volume deficit.

Filling of veins

Normally veins of the posterior aspect of the hand empty within 3 to 5 seconds when elevated. When the hand is placed in a dependent position, the veins fill in 3 to 5 seconds.

When there is a fluid volume deficit, the veins of the lowered hand require more than 3 to 5 seconds to fill. When there is a fluid volume excess, the veins of the elevated hand require more than 3 to 5 seconds to empty.

Assessment of jugular venous distention can provide information about the central venous pressure. Normally when the person is supine, the external jugular veins fill to the anterior border of the sternocleidomastoid muscle. Flat neck veins in the supine position indicate a fluid volume deficit. Position the person with the head of the bed elevated to a 30- to 45-degree angle. Keep the person's neck straight. Provide lighting to visualize the external jugular veins on each side of the neck. Measure the distance between the level of the sternal angle and the point at which the internal and external jugular veins collapse. In a healthy person with the head elevated to a 45-degree angle, the venous distention should not extend higher than 2 to 3 cm above the sternal angle. If the jugular veins are distended more than 3 cm above the sternal angle with the head up 45 degrees, there is likely fluid volume excess or decreased cardiac function.

Behavior

Persons with sodium excess or with fluid deficit may have difficulty forming words without first moistening their tongue and lips. Hoarseness may occur with fluid deficit. Persons with potassium deficit may have difficulty speaking because of muscular weakness. Muscular weakness (especially in legs) occurs in chronic potassium deficit. Soft, flabby muscles may be found in potassium deficit. Flaccid paralysis may occur in either severe potassium deficit or excess. Painful muscle spasms or muscle rigidity may occur in calcium deficit. Hypertonus may occur and is evidenced by tremors that may occur in mild magnesium deficit, whereas convulsions may occur in severe magnesium deficit. Chvostek's sign may be positive in calcium deficit. Trousseau's sign (carpal spasm) may be present in hypocalcemia (see Figure 61-2).

Tingling of fingers and toes may occur in calcium deficit and in potassium deficit. Light-headed feelings and tinnitus may occur with respiratory alkalosis. Abdominal cramping may be present with sodium deficit, calcium deficit, or potassium deficit. Numbness may occur in severe potassium deficit as well as in potassium excess. Deep bone pain may occur with calcium excess. Nausea may occur with potassium excess, sodium deficit, and calcium excess. Abnormal sensitivity to sound may occur with magnesium excess. Dizziness may occur with position change in sodium deficit. Headache may occur in sodium deficit (water intoxication).

The major effect of acidosis is depression of the central nervous system. Acidosis, calcium excess, or sodium excess may cause lethargy and malaise, which may progress to disorientation and on to coma or unconsciousness.

In alkalosis the central nervous system is stimulated, which may result in restlessness or confusion and may progress to convulsions.

Central venous pressure

Central venous pressure (CVP) measures pressure in the right atria or the vena cava and is used to provide information about blood volume, vascular tone, and the heart's pumping action. A normal reading is 2 to 6 mm Hg or 5 to 12 cm H_2O. Pressures below normal indicate a decrease in effective circulating volume caused by volume depletion, such as occurs in bleeding. Pressures below normal occur when fluid shifts out of the vascular space ("third spacing"), in vasodilation, or after administration of specific antihypertensive medications.

A high CVP indicates increased blood volume, poor right ventricular function, or vasoconstriction of the pulmonary vascular bed. Measurements of CVP indicative of fluid imbalance should be evaluated with other clinical data, such as vital signs, heart sounds, and I & O.

Fluid Volume Imbalances

FLUID VOLUME DEFICIT
Definition

Fluid volume deficit is a result of water and electrolyte loss in an isotonic fashion. Serum electrolyte levels basically remain unchanged unless other imbalances are also present.[11] Compensatory mechanisms include increased sympathetic nervous system stimulation, resulting in an increase in heart rate and cardiac contraction, thirst, and release of ADH and aldosterone.

Etiology

Fluid volume deficit (hypovolemia) is often the result of body fluid loss or fluid collection in the third space. This condition is further exacerbated by decreased fluid intake. As a result the extracellular compartment shrinks. This type of deficit is most commonly caused by loss of fluids via the gastrointestinal tract and by conditions that cause polyuria and increase in sensible perspiration, respiratory rate and depth, and body temperature. Depending on the type of fluid lost, fluid volume deficit may be associated with osmolar, acid-base, or electrolyte imbalances. Hypovolemic shock may result from severe loss of ECF volume. Prolonged severe fluid volume deficit may result in renal failure.

Abnormal Gastrointestinal Fluid Loss

Increased losses are caused by abnormal conditions, such as vomiting, diarrhea, presence of fistulas, and drainage of intestinal fluid, bile, or pancreatic fluid. Conditions that interfere with fluid absorption from the gastrointestinal tract, such as obstructions (third-space problem), can be the cause of ECF volume deficit (Table 12-2).

Abnormal Fluid Loss via Skin

Fluid and electrolyte loss increases with an increase in environmental temperature. Sweat losses also occur when body temperature exceeds 101° F.[11] High body temperature and major burns also increase water loss by evaporation.

RESEARCH BRIEF

Fortney SM, Hyatt KH, Davis JF, Vogel JM: Changes in body fluid compartments during a 28-day bedrest, *Aviation Space Environ Med* 62(2):97, Feb 1991.

By the second day of bed rest, plasma volume and extracellular volume decreased significantly by an average of 209 mL and 533 mL, respectively. Total body water decreased more slowly, with an average loss of 1316 mL after 28 days of bed rest.

Early in the bed rest, total body water loss was mostly from the ECV. Later, the total body water deficit was from the intracellular compartment, which decreased an average of 838 mL after 28 days.

These results suggest that losses occur from all fluid compartments during bed rest, with no evidence of restoration of extracellular volume after 1 or 2 weeks.

TABLE 12-2 Causes of Extracellular Fluid Deficit

Cause	Altered function
GASTROINTESTINAL	
Vomiting	Reverse peristalsis causes loss of extracellular secretions, which contain large amounts of sodium and chloride
Diarrhea	Increased forward peristalsis shortens absorption period, preventing ECF absorption
Fistulous drainage	Tubelike passageway between the gastrointestinal tract and an external surface, allowing loss of ECF
Gastrointestinal suction	Evacuation of ECF by mechanical means, such as Levin or Cantor tubes
Excessive tap water enemas	Hypotonic solution draws electrolytes from ECF, causing saline loss when expelled
RENAL	
Overzealous use of diuretics	Excessive loss of Na, Cl, K, and H_2O
Salt-losing nephritis	Tubules, damaged by either chemical or physical means, may allow saline to flow out
DIAPHORESIS	Saline loss caused by hyperthermia or a thermoregulatory response triggered by stress
THIRD SPACE	
Peritonitis	Fluid accumulation in the peritoneal cavity caused by an infectious or inflammatory process
Intestinal obstruction	Fluid accumulation within intestines caused by decreased or absent peristalsis
Postoperative condition	Fluid moves into traumatized operative site because of local inflammatory stress response
Thrombophlebitis	Blood clot(s) with inflammation in vein with resulting venous obstruction
Acute pancreatitis	Inflammatory response with fluid pulled into inflamed site
Ascites	Serous fluid accumulation in the peritoneal cavity related to interference with portal circulation
Fistulous drainage	Tubelike passageway between gastrointestinal tract and internal adjacent cavity allowing loss of ECF
Burns	Fluid accumulation in blisters or interstitial space (Fluid may be lost because of evaporation [white bleeding], which is not a third-space accumulation.)

From Stroot VR et al: *Fluids and electrolytes: a practical approach,* ed 3, Philadelphia, 1984, FA Davis Co.

Increased Water Vapor Loss via Lungs

Water vapor loss increases when conditions exist that are conducive to increasing respiratory rate or depth.[11] An example of increased water vapor loss is hyperpnea caused by body temperature elevation.

Conditions that Increase Renal Excretion of Fluids

Any disorder or treatment that causes increased urine excretion can lead to ECF loss. Examples include diuretic use without careful assessment, conditions such as salt-losing nephritis and hyperglycemia, and hyperosmolar tube feedings (Table 12-3). All these conditions cause polyuria because of the high load of solutes (dissolved substances) causing ECF to be removed from the plasma, tissue spaces, and cells in order for the excess solutes to be excreted in the urine. Elevated body temperature increases the amount of metabolic wastes in the body, which requires extra fluid for its excretion by the kidney.

TABLE 12-3 Pharmacology Summary: Diuretics

Generic name	Trade name	Form	Peak effect (hours)	Potential effect on fluid and electrolyte balance
Aldosterone antagonist (opposes potassium-losing action of aldosterone)				
Spironolactone	Aldactone	PO	72	Hyperkalemia Hyponatremia
Carbonic anhydrase inhibitor				
Acetazolamide	Diamox	PO/IV	2 to 4	Hypokalemia, hyponatremia, increased HCO_3^-
Loop diuretics (act mainly on ascending loop of Henle)				
Furosemide	Lasix	IM or IV	½	Hypokalemia Hyperuricemia Decreased ECF volume
Ethacrynic acid	Edecrin	PO IV	2 to 4 ½	Hyponatremia
Osmotic agent				
Mannitol	Osmitrol	IV		Hyponatremia Hypochloremia Hypokalemia Decreased ECF volume
Potassium-conserving action				
Amiloride hydrochloride	Midamor	PO	3 to 4	Reverses or prevents hyperkalemia
Thiazides				
Chlorothiazide	Diuril	PO	4	Hyponatremia Hypokalemia Decreased ECF volume Hyperglycemia Hyperuricemia
Hydrochlorothiazide	Esidrix HydroDIURIL	PO	3 to 4	Hypochloremia Hyponatremia Hypokalemia

Decrease in Fluid Intake

Any condition that interferes with normal fluid intake, such as deep depression, anxiety, nausea, vomiting, fractured mandible where the jaw is wired, or other oral trauma and surgical procedures, may result in ECF loss.

Third-Space Fluid Loss

Third-space fluid loss occurs when there is a shift of body fluid into a space outside the normal fluid compartments and unavailable to the body, thereby producing a deficit in ECF volume. Examples include peritonitis, ascites, burns, pericarditis, pleural effusion, fluid in joint cavities, acute pancreatitis, traumatic injuries such as fractures, and intestinal obstruction. Third-space fluid loss is usually self-limited to 48 to 72 hours, when the process reverses.

Significant Laboratory Tests

Laboratory tests indicative of fluid deficit include an elevated hematocrit, which results from intravascular fluid loss and elevated blood urea nitrogen (BUN) out of proportion to the serum creatinine. The elevated BUN may be caused by dehydration, decreased perfusion of the renal system, or decreased renal function. The serum electrolyte tests show variable results and depend on the type of fluid lost. Urine sp gr is increased because of compensatory measures of the kidney to conserve water. Serum osmolality will vary. The results depend on the type of fluid that is lost and the compensatory measures to replace fluid volume by sense of thirst and secretion of ADH.

Therapeutic Management

The main goal of treatment is to restore fluid volume and correct any associated electrolyte or acid-base abnormalities. If the deficit is not acute, fluid volume may be restored orally. When fluid losses are severe, fluid volume is replaced via the intravenous route. The type of fluid replacement will depend on the type of fluid lost, severity of the deficit, as well as serum electrolyte values, serum osmolality, and acid-base status.

Isotonic electrolyte solutions, such as lactated Ringer's solution or normal saline, are used to expand plasma volume. These solutions are useful in expanding ECF primarily. Isotonic fluids are usually used as replacement fluids, since fluid losses are generally isotonic.

Dextrose and water solutions are used to provide free water and are used to treat total body water deficits, since they distribute to both ICF and ECF compartments. Mixed saline and hypotonic electrolyte solutions are used to provide additional electrolytes and a buffer once the patient becomes normotensive. This is often used as a maintenance fluid measure and also assists in renal excretion of metabolic wastes. Blood and albumin are used to expand the intravascular fluid compartment primarily.

NURSING MANAGEMENT OF THE PATIENT WITH FLUID VOLUME DEFICIT

Fluid volume deficit can be mild, moderate, or severe depending on the extent of fluid loss. Early recognition and intervention are important, since the problem is potentially life-threatening.

Assessment

ECF volume deficit cannot be determined by serum electrolyte tests. The nurse needs to be aware of signs and symptoms and other laboratory test findings. Signs and symptoms are listed in the box on p. 179.

Nursing Diagnosis

The following nursing diagnosis is suggested:
Fluid volume deficit related to a decrease in circulating volume secondary to ECF loss

Implementation

Assessment of the patient at risk for or actually experiencing fluid volume deficit includes monitoring intake and output (I & O). Depending on the severity of the deficit, I & O may be measured hourly; if less severe, it should be measured at 8-hour intervals. If output is less than 30 mL/hr for 2 consecutive hours, the physician should be contacted immediately. Urine sp gr should be checked at least every 8 hours. With corrective therapy, sp gr should come within the normal range.

Weigh patients daily with a reliable scale. Weight is a critical indicator of fluid status: a weight loss of 2 pounds represents a fluid loss of 1000 mL. The nurse should monitor for hidden fluid losses. Measure and record limb size and abdominal girth and auscultate for egophony. These are indications of fluid in a third space.

Monitor the skin and tongue turgor and the condition of the oral mucous membrane. Monitor laboratory test results for changes and trends, and report significant changes to the physician.

Types of Venous Access Devices and Equipment Necessary for Home Maintenance

Peripheral venous access devices

Peripheral venous access devices are specially designed catheters that can be inserted by a nurse ei-

SIGNS AND SYMPTOMS OF FLUID VOLUME DEFICIT

Dry mucous membranes

Dryness of the mucous membrane where cheek and gum meet is significant in fluid volume deficit. Longitudinal furrows in the tongue indicate fluid volume deficit.

Weight loss

A weight loss of 2% of body weight = a mild deficit; 5% = a moderate deficit; 8% = a severe deficit.

Orthostatic hypotension and increase in pulse rate

A drop in systolic pressure when the patient moves from a lying to a sitting or standing position indicates fluid volume deficit. If the condition becomes more severe, the blood pressure decreases even when the patient is supine. This is a result of loss of compensatory mechanisms.

Increased pulse rate occurs as a result of the action of the heart to compensate for the decrease in intravascular fluid volume.

Body temperature

The body temperature is subnormal in fluid volume deficit unless sodium excess is present. In this latter situation the body temperature is elevated.

Fullness of neck veins

Neck veins are flat with the patient lying supine. Direct measurement of the CVP reveals a decrease in venous pressure. Patients with impaired cardiopulmonary function may have increased venous pressure.

Urinary output

There is decreased urinary output caused by deficit of ECF to perfuse the kidney. In severe cases of fluid volume deficit, oliguria may lead to damage to the renal tubules.

Neurologic symptoms

Patients with prolonged fluid deficit will exhibit altered sensorium caused by a decrease in intravascular fluid volume, which causes a decrease in the perfusion of cerebral cells. The extremities are cold to the touch because of peripheral vasoconstriction.

Other changes

Decreased pulmonary artery pressure, decreased cardiac output, decreased mean arterial pressure, and increased systemic vascular resistance are changes seen in hemodynamic measurements. Moisture in the axilla and groin is absent. Tearing and salivation are decreased. Skin in youth and middle age is inelastic.

---

ther in the hospital or in the home. Some devices are short, and some are relatively long; however, they are not long enough to go into the vena cava, and thus they are considered to be peripheral access devices. These catheters are made of special material that allows them to remain in the vein for prolonged periods of time, are not as irritating as a needle, and require very little care.

The device is usually inserted into the hand or arm and is secured to the skin by tape or a transparent dressing. Site care consists of observing the site, cleansing it with an antiseptic solution, and reapplying a clean dressing. Since there are many different types of peripheral access devices and the material used is different, the plan for site care should be determined for the specific device. The frequency of site care depends on the type of catheter, the condition of the patient's skin, and the patient's general health status.

The same is true for flushing of the catheter. Some catheters do not need flushing because they do not clot and some do. It is advisable to check the manufacturer's guidelines to establish a care plan for flushing the specific device. If flushing is recom-

mended, the nurse should check with the physician or a specially trained intravenous therapy nurse for instructions on flushing.

Peripheral vein intermittent infusion device
Irrigate device with 1 mL of normal saline.
Administer prescribed medication.
Irrigate device with 1 mL of normal saline after medication administration is completed.
Some agencies may recommend a final irrigation with 1 mL of heparin solution (100 units of heparin per milliliter of normal saline).

Central venous catheters

The Hickman and Broviac catheters are two of the many types of central venous catheters. The central venous catheter is a large-bore catheter with one, two, or three ports that can be used for administering intravenous fluids, medications, or parenteral nutrition. The catheter is tunneled under the skin and into the superior vena cava. Medications administered through this catheter are mixed with large quantities of blood, thus decreasing the local reac-

HOME CARE GUIDE   *Intravenous Fluid Hydration*

Intravenous fluid and electrolyte replacement is indicated after hospitalization when a patient cannot take fluids by mouth or through tube feedings. This therapy is sometimes used as a palliative care measure along with other terminal care. Other forms of intravenous therapy, such as total parenteral nutrition or chemotherapy, are discussed elsewhere in this book.

The following information is designed for use for discharge planning for a patient going to a home setting.

Short-term goals

By the time of discharge:
1. All necessary equipment will be available.
2. The caregiver and/or patient will have basic knowledge of the procedures for administering intravenous therapy in the home setting.

Long-term goals

1. The patient will receive adequate hydration to maintain fluid and electrolyte balance.
2. The caregiver will be able to incorporate intravenous therapy into the total care plan with the assistance of a community-based nurse.

Nursing assessment
Health management pattern

A person must be available as a primary caregiver for the duration of the home therapy.

Cognitive pattern

The caregiver and/or patient must demonstrate sufficient skill to be able to learn and manage intravenous therapy equipment and procedures.

Coping/stress tolerance pattern

The total care plan for the patient must be reviewed; since patients needing hydration usually have other care needs, the caregiver may perceive hydration as a "high-tech" procedure and may become overwhelmed and thus unable to manage the basic needs of the patient.

Resources

Financial and insurance resources must be investigated before ordering intravenous therapy for the home; the caregiver and patient need to supply all available insurance information to the home care agencies to determine the source of payment for therapy at home.

Environmental

Evaluation of the home environment may be needed before the patient can be discharged; there is a need for storage space for supplies and bathroom facilities for handwashing; the location of the home and the accessibility for delivery of supplies and provision of 24-hour on-call nursing services by an intravenous therapy nurse must be assessed.

Planning
Therapeutic plan

The therapeutic plan must be decided before discharge; the physician must write orders for the amount and type of fluids and electrolytes and the rate of administration; if the patient is relatively stable, the rate may be such that the 24-hour total volume can be given over an 8-, 10-, or 12-hour period; the schedule can be adapted to the other needs of the patient; for example, the patient can be given fluid for 12 hours during the night to allow flexibility during the day or 12 hours during the day to allow for monitoring of the fluid and allow the caregiver to have uninterrupted sleep during the night.

Caregiver education

Education should begin before discharge and be scheduled to allow the caregiver a minimum of two or three teaching sessions; instruction should be done with the equipment that will be used in the home. Education will be continued in the home by the nurse employed by the home infusion therapy company. The following information should be included in the patient education:

Use of the equipment, including the administration set, needles, syringes, catheter plug, solution bags, and intravenous pump

How to check for sterility of supplies and for particulate matter or cloudiness of the solution

The procedure for site care, either peripheral or central

How to start and discontinue the intravenous therapy

How to calculate and monitor the fluid rate

How to safely discard equipment after use

How and when to reorder supplies

How to monitor for local infection, such as phlebitis or cellulitis

How to monitor intake and output

The necessity for handwashing and the prevention of contamination of the site, the supplies, and the solution

It is advisable to leave instructions in the home.

HOME CARE GUIDE   *Intravenous Fluid Hydration—cont'd*

Agency selection

Options available for each individual hospital are investigated; the referral for intravenous therapy in the home has two parts: one for supplies and equipment and the other for nursing services. The staff nurse should ask for assistance from the discharge planner in agency selection.

Implementation

1. Referral to the appropriate agency should be made at least 1 or 2 working days before planned discharge.
2. All referral forms should be completed, and one copy should be kept for the patient's medical record.
3. Education provided and the caregiver's ability should be included in the referral, as well as areas needing reinforcement.

---

tion to drugs. Because the catheter is placed into a large vein that empties into the heart, the care of this catheter is very important. It is imperative that aseptic technique be used, and at times sterile technique may be used. Vital aspects of care include cleansing the insertion site to prevent infection, flushing with the recommended solution to prevent formation of clots, and keeping the ports capped to prevent introduction of air into the circulatory system.

Equipment needed includes antiseptic solution, such as povidone iodine or alcohol; external dressing, such as a transparent dressing; gloves; and tape (these supplies are available in kits that can be ordered for use by the patient at home); also, heparin flush syringes with needles and saline flush syringes with needles (the quantity needed will depend on the frequency of flushing ordered by the physician and the number of ports).

Central vein intermittent infusion device

Irrigate device with 2 to 5 mL of normal saline (volume depends on type of infusion catheter and agency policy).
Administer prescribed medication.
Irrigate device with 2 to 5 mL of normal saline when medication administration is completed.
Irrigate device with 2 to 5 mL of heparin solution (100 units of heparin per milliliter of normal saline).

Implantable devices

These devices include such brands as Infusaid Implantable Drug Delivery System (Infusaid, Inc., Norwood, Mass.), the Medtronic Drug Administration Device (Medtronic, Inc., Minneapolis, Minn.), Port-A-Cath (Pharmacia Deltec, Inc., St. Paul, Minn.), Infuse-A-Port (Infusaid), or Mediport (Cormed, Mahar, NY). Because these devices are implanted under the skin, the only care needed is a dry, sterile dressing until healed, and then regular observation of the skin over the device.

Equipment needed includes dry, sterile dressings until the wound has healed; special needles may be necessary to fill the device; and alcohol swabs or other antiseptic solution to prepare the skin over the device for the insertion of the needle into the reservoir of the pump.

Administer oral and intravenous fluids as prescribed. (See home care guide on venous access devices.) Signs and symptoms of fluid overload or too rapid administration include rales, shortness of breath, neck vein distention, and edema. Institutional policy regarding fluid challenge should be followed. Document the patient's response to fluid therapy.

Monitor for signs of decrease in cerebral perfusion, checking for signs of confusion, restlessness, anxiety, vertigo, excitability, weakness, and cool, clammy skin.

Take safety precautions, for example, by keeping siderails up, keeping the bed in low position, assisting the patient in ambulation, and changing the patient's position slowly.

Monitor for orthostatic hypotension and increased heart rate. Evaluate capillary refill and check with the physician if refill is delayed more than 5 seconds. Peripheral pulses should be palpated bilaterally in arms and legs, using a Doppler if necessary. The physician should be notified if pulses have recently become very weak or absent.

Teach the patient and family regarding (1) signs and symptoms of fluid volume deficit; (2) maintenance of adequate intake; and (3) use of medications including purpose, dosage, frequency, and potential side effect.

FLUID VOLUME EXCESS
Definition

Fluid volume excess, or hypervolemia, is an expansion of fluid volume in the ECF compartment. It is secondary to an increase in the total body sodium content. The increase in sodium content in turn leads to an increase in total body water. The serum

HOME CARE GUIDE   *Venous Access Devices*

1. *Heparin lock*—This venous access device consists of a short needle or catheter inserted in a peripheral vein, usually in the hand or arm. It is secured to the skin by tape or a transparent dressing. Site care consists of observing the site, cleansing it with an antiseptic solution, and reapplying a clean transparent dressing. The frequency of dressing changes depends on the type of dressing used, the condition of the patient's skin, and the patient's general health status. The frequency of flushing the device depends on the frequency of medications and/or fluids the physician's preference, and the recommendations of the device's manufacturer. The short catheter is flushed after the drug is administered; because it is in a peripheral site there is minimal danger of clotting, therefore frequent flushing with heparin is not necessary. Frequent gentle flushing (at least once every 24 hours at home) may be necessary if the patient has poor vein access and if finding another site would be difficult.

   Equipment needed includes tape; transparent dressings; sterile catheter plug; heparin flush, saline flush in a syringe with needle (if available), or separate disposable syringes; alcohol wipe to clean catheter plug before flushing; and antiseptic solution for cleansing the site. Because this is a peripheral site in a small vein, arrangements must be made before discharge to have the site changed by a skilled IV therapy nurse on a regular basis and as needed. The site should be checked every few days by a home care nurse or on return to a clinic or physician's office.

2. *Central venous catheters*—The Hickman and Broviac catheters are two of the many types of central venous catheters. The central venous catheter is a large-bore catheter with one, two, or three ports that can be used for administering medications and/or fluids. The catheter is tunneled under the skin and into the superior vena cava. Medications admin-istered through this catheter are mixed with large quantities of blood, thus decreasing the local reaction to drugs. Because the catheter is placed into a large vein that empties into the heart, the care of this catheter is very important. It is imperative that aseptic technique be used, and at times sterile technique may be used. Vital aspects of care include cleansing the insertion site to prevent infection, flushing with the recommended solution to prevent formation of clots, and keeping the ports capped to prevent introduction of air into the circulatory system.

   Equipment needed includes antiseptic solution, such as povidone iodine or alcohol; external dressing, such as a transparent dressing; gloves; and tape (these supplies are available in kits that can be ordered for use by the patient at home); also, heparin flush syringes with needles and saline flush syringes with needles (the quantity needed will depend on the frequency of flushing ordered by the physician and the number of ports).

3. *Implantable devices*—These devices include such brands as Infusaid Implantable Drug Delivery System (Infusaid, Inc., Norwood, Mass.), the Medtronic Drug Administration Device (Medtronic, Inc., Minneapolis, Minn.), Port-A-Cath (Pharmacia Deltec, Inc., St. Paul, Minn.), Infuse-A-Port (Infusaid), or Mediport (Cormed, Mahar, NY). Because these devices are implanted under the skin, the only care needed is a dry, sterile dressing until healed, and then regular observation of the skin over the device.

   Equipment needed includes dry, sterile dressings until the wound has healed; special needles may be necessary to fill the device; and alcohol swabs or other antiseptic solution to prepare the skin over the device for the insertion of the needle into the reservoir of the pump.

---

concentration remains the same, since there is isotonic retention of both sodium and water.

Compensatory mechanisms may include the secretion of atrial natriuretic factor, which in turn results in increased excretion of sodium and water via the kidneys and decreased release of aldosterone and ADH.

Etiology

Hypervolemia occurs when the kidney receives a prolonged stimulus to save sodium and water as a result of compromised regulatory mechanisms, as in cirrhosis of the liver, congestive heart failure, renal failure with decreased excretion of sodium and water, and excessive use of intravenous sodium-containing fluid, sodium salts, or drugs with high sodium content. Hypervolemia can lead to heart failure and pulmonary edema.

Significant Laboratory Tests

Laboratory test results vary. The hematocrit may be decreased because of hemodilution. Serum sodium and serum osmolality decrease because of excessive retention of water. The BUN will be increased in the presence of renal failure. Urinary sodium may be elevated and urine sp gr may be decreased if the kidney is functioning adequately, unless there is a prolonged release of aldosterone caused by such conditions as congestive heart failure and cirrhosis of the liver.

Therapeutic Management

The goal of the treatment of fluid volume excess is to treat the primary disorder and return the ECF volume to normal. Treatment includes a restriction of sodium and water intake and the use of diuretics. If hypervolemia is caused by prolonged intravenous administration of sodium-containing fluids, discontinuation of the intravenous line may reduce the fluid volume to its normal state provided that regulatory mechanisms of the body are not compromised. Dialysis may be ordered in life-threatening situations, such as renal failure or severe fluid overload.

NURSING MANAGEMENT OF THE PATIENT WITH FLUID VOLUME EXCESS
Assessment

Early recognition of signs and symptoms of hypervolemia is critical to correct the imbalance before further damage occurs. Signs and symptoms include shortness of breath and orthopnea, presence of edema, weight gain, distended neck veins, tachycardia, distended peripheral veins, increased blood pressure except in the presence of heart failure, crackles, and wheezes. Ascites and pleural effusion in severe hypervolemia as fluid enters third-space areas may occur. CVP may increase.

Nursing Diagnosis

The following general nursing diagnoses are suggested:
  Knowledge deficit related to a lack of understanding of the disease process and/or medical regimen
  Impaired physical mobility related to excessive fluid in tissues of extremities or lungs

Implementation

Assess potential risk and presence of hypervolemia. Monitor I & O hourly, and evaluate for fluid retention. Check the urine sp gr, which should be less than 1.010 if the patient is experiencing diuresis. Check for edema, and measure the depth of pitting. Weigh the patient daily, and document and report any weight gain.

Restrict sodium intake as prescribed. Do not use salt substitutes for patients in renal failure or when potassium-sparing diuretics are used. Limit the patient's intake of fluids. Ice chips may be used to ameliorate thirst, but calculate the amount as part of the fluid intake. Mouth care should be given frequently.

Observe for signs of hypokalemia caused by diuretics, as well as for signs of hyperkalemia if the patient is taking potassium-sparing diuretics. Overcorrection and fluid volume depletion may result from treatment. Signs and symptoms of pulmonary edema may include cough with frothy sputum, anxiety, crackles, tachypnea, tachycardia, gallop rhythm, and increased pulmonary artery pressure. Arterial blood gases are checked for PaO_2 values indicative of hypoxemia and for pH and $PaCO_2$ values indicative of respiratory alkalosis. Placing the patient in a semi-Fowler's position will help decrease dyspnea and increase lung expansion capability.

Electrolyte Imbalances: Sodium

Disturbances in electrolyte balance occur frequently in clinical practice and can result from an excess or deficit in sodium, potassium, chloride, calcium, phosphorus, or magnesium.

The average amount of sodium intake for adults is approximately 6 to 15 g/day. Salt in the form of sodium chloride is by far the most common source of sodium. Sodium is absorbed by the intestines and excreted through the kidneys and the skin.

Sodium is the major cation in ECF. Sodium concentration within the ECF compartment ranges from 135 mEq/L to 148 mEq/L.

Sodium ions are especially important in regulating the voltage of action potentials. Sodium is necessary for the transmission of impulses in nerve and muscle fibers. A deficit in the sodium concentration results in muscle weakness. Since sodium is the most osmotically active solute in the intravascular and interstitial fluid, it is one of the main factors that determine ECF volume. Sodium plays a major role in controlling the size of cells.

The level of sodium in the body is controlled by multiple factors that are not completely understood. These factors include the adrenal gland, the pituitary gland, the skin, the gastrointestinal tract, arterial pressure, and compositional changes in the ECF. The combined effect is that the kidneys are influenced to resorb more or less sodium from the blood and excrete it in the urine. Normally, almost all of the sodium is resorbed and none of it is excreted. However, if the sodium level is high, large amounts can be excreted in the urine. Changes in ECF volume caused by sodium imbalance are illustrated in Figure 12-5.

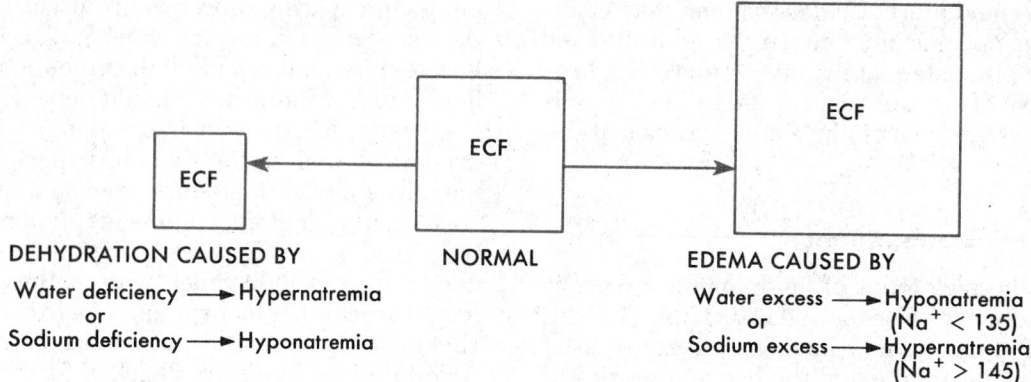

FIGURE 12-5   Changes in extracellular fluid *(ECF)* volume caused by sodium imbalance.

HYPERNATREMIA
Definition

An excess of sodium in ECF is called **hypernatremia.** This is also referred to as a hyperosmolar state in the presence of a fluid deficit. When the amount of water in ECF decreases, the serum sodium value increases even though the amount of sodium remains the same. In other words, when there is a deficit in fluid volume, the concentration of sodium increases.

Etiology

The kidneys regulate sodium excretion in a healthy person according to intake. If the kidneys fail because of hormonal or hemodynamic effects, excess sodium (hypernatremia) may develop. When this occurs, there is also fluid retention, or edema, and therefore an increase in extracellular fluid volume. For the kidneys to perform their regulatory function, blood flow must be adequate and the aldosterone system normal. Therefore the conditions in which hypernatremia may be a problem include renal failure (with sodium retention), inadequate blood circulation to the kidneys (as in congestive heart failure), cirrhosis of the liver, overproduction of aldosterone by the adrenal cortex, and administration of large doses of adrenocorticoids. Elderly persons may have these conditions and are likely to develop sodium excess. Elderly persons may eat more convenience foods, which are often high in sodium. Several studies have demonstrated an age-related decrease in sensitivity for salty tastes, which often leads elderly persons to add more salt to foods.[13]

Even if the kidneys do resorb increased amounts of sodium, the sodium concentration usually will not increase significantly, since the person becomes extremely thirsty and drinks water, which dilutes the sodium that is resorbed. Then the problem becomes fluid volume excess rather than sodium excess, or hypernatremia.

Significant Laboratory Tests

The laboratory data reflective of hypernatremia include a serum sodium value greater than 148 mEq/L, serum osmolality greater than 295 mOsm/kg, and urine sp gr greater than 1.030 when the kidneys are functioning normally. The increase in urine sp gr is a result of the compensatory attempt by the kidneys to conserve water.

Therapeutic Management

Treatment consists of infusion of a hypotonic electrolyte solution, such as 0.3% NaCl or 0.45% NaCl. This method lowers the serum sodium level gradually, thereby decreasing the risk of inducing cerebral edema. If treatment were aimed at a rapid reduction of the serum sodium level, plasma would become temporarily hypo-osmotic. This in turn would allow water to move into brain tissue, causing cerebral edema.

NURSING MANAGEMENT OF THE PATIENT WITH HYPERNATREMIA
Assessment

Initial signs and symptoms of uncompensated hypernatremia are the same as those of dehydration and hyperosmolarity. Signs and symptoms include thirst; a red, dry, swollen tongue; flushed skin; elevated temperature; and neurologic manifestations, such as disorientation, lethargy, irritability, focal or grand mal seizures, and hallucinations. The neurologic manifestations are thought to be caused by cellular dehydration (Figure 12-6).

Nursing Diagnosis

The following general nursing diagnoses are suggested:

High risk for impairment of skin integrity related

Causes

Effects

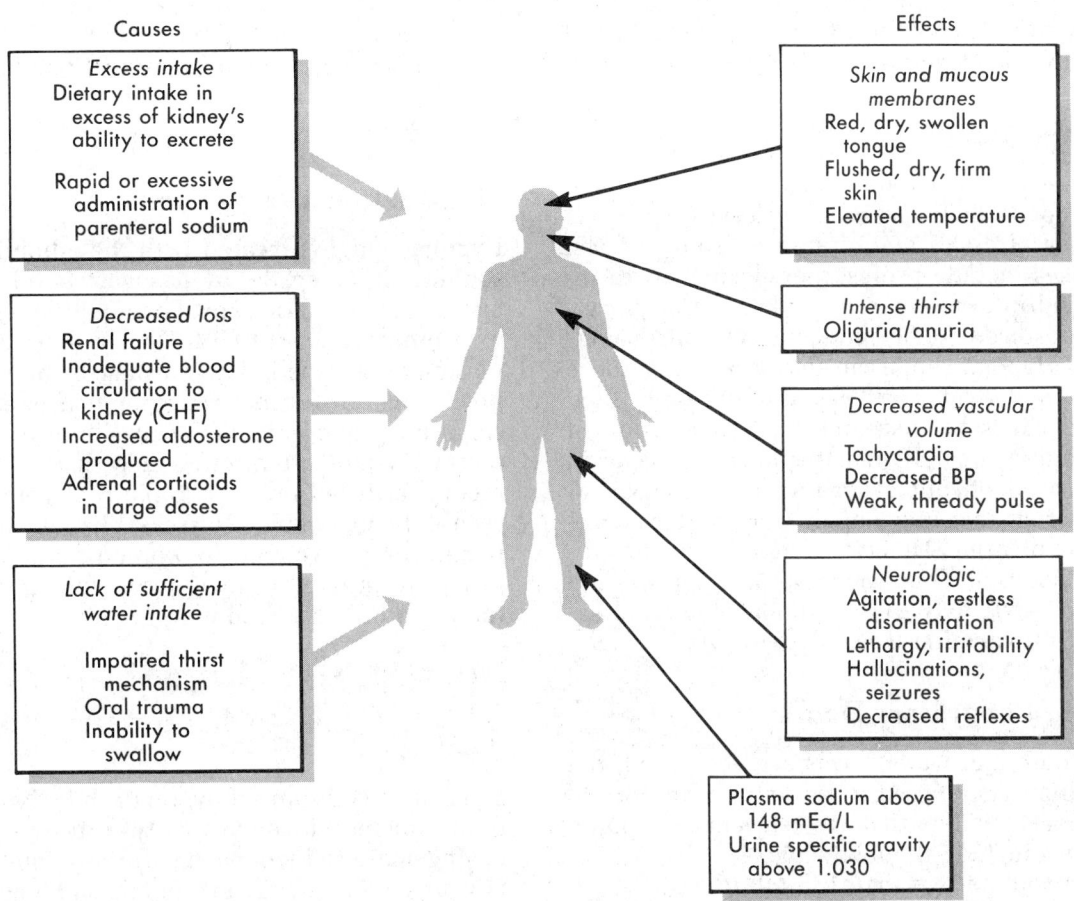

Excess intake
Dietary intake in
excess of kidney's
ability to excrete

Rapid or excessive
administration of
parenteral sodium

Decreased loss
Renal failure
Inadequate blood
circulation to
kidney (CHF)
Increased aldosterone
produced
Adrenal corticoids
in large doses

**Lack of sufficient
water intake**

Impaired thirst
mechanism
Oral trauma
Inability to
swallow

**Skin and mucous
membranes**
Red, dry, swollen
tongue
Flushed, dry, firm
skin
Elevated temperature

Intense thirst
Oliguria/anuria

**Decreased vascular
volume**
Tachycardia
Decreased BP
Weak, thready pulse

Neurologic
Agitation, restless
disorientation
Lethargy, irritability
Hallucinations,
seizures
Decreased reflexes

Plasma sodium above
148 mEq/L
Urine specific gravity
above 1.030

FIGURE 12-6   Causes and effects of hypernatremia.

to peripheral edema secondary to body sodium and water excess

High risk for activity intolerance related to peripheral edema secondary to body sodium and water excess

Implementation

The goal is to prevent hypernatremia by offering fluids at regular intervals or, with physician orders, by using alternate routes, such as tube feedings or parenteral therapy. The nurse should check for excessive thirst and for an increase in body temperature. Elderly persons may not experience thirst sensation with hypernatremia. Accurately monitor fluid losses and gains via I & O recording, daily weights, and specifically watch for low water intake and abnormal losses of water. Check the mouth, tongue, and mucous membranes and give mouth care. Check for ingestion of food and drugs with high sodium content. Also, monitor for changes in sensorium, such as restlessness, increased irritability, disorientation, hallucinations, lethargy, stupor, or coma. Monitor serum sodium levels and urine sp gr values, as well as re-

sponse to parenteral fluid therapy. Laboratory reports of sodium levels and changes in neurologic signs are important indicators of the patient's progress. Sodium levels should be reduced gradually to improve neurologic symptoms.

Provide sufficient water, if tube feedings are used, to keep serum sodium within normal range.

HYPONATREMIA
Definition

Hyponatremia is a condition in which the serum sodium level is below normal. It may be caused by an excessive loss of sodium or by excessive fluid volume. It is generally synonymous with a hypoosmolar state with a relatively greater concentration of water than sodium. It can be thought of as a condition of water excess resulting in a diluted serum. Hyperglycemia leads to a decrease in the serum sodium concentration. Since sodium is primarily an extracellular cation, it becomes diluted as water moves out of cells in response to the osmotic effect of the increased glucose in the blood. Normally, homeostatic mechanisms keep the amount of fluid regulated. However, if renal function is not adequate and the ADH level is elevated, excess water is retained.

Pathophysiology

Sodium losses are related to gastrointestinal, renal, and third-space fluid losses. Skin losses occur via profuse perspiration and drainage from lesions. Other causes include profuse perspiration with increased fluid intake, low salt intake, use of diuretics, and aldosterone deficiency caused by adrenal insufficiency. Hyponatremia can also occur when there is a gain in body water as a result of excessive fluid intake and excessive parenteral administration of dextrose and water. Hyponatremia may occur in heart failure, nephrotic syndrome, and cirrhosis of the liver. Drugs that may impair renal water excretion include nicotine, Diabinese, morphine, barbiturates, and Isuprel. The syndrome of inappropriate secretion of ADH may cause hyponatremia and severe water intoxication (see Chapter 60).

Significant Laboratory Data

If both sodium and water levels are decreased, the serum sodium readings may be within the normal range. Laboratory data that are relevant in hyponatremic states include the following:

- Serum sodium less than 135 mEq/L
- Urinary sodium less than 10 mEq/L and urine sp gr less than 1.010 caused by sodium losses as a result of increased aldosterone secretion stimulated by the low serum sodium level; this process causes renal conservation of sodium

- Urinary sodium greater than 20 mEq/L and urine sp gr higher than 1.012 with increased ADH secretion with no increase in aldosterone secretion

Therapeutic Management

Hyponatremia is treated with the administration of sodium either orally, by nasogastric tube feedings, or via parenteral therapy. Lactated Ringer's solution or isotonic saline (0.9% NaCl) may be given if plasma volume is below normal. If the plasma volume is within normal range or if it is excessive, a small amount of 3% or 5% NaCl may be administered. Careful attention is necessary if this treatment is ordered since too rapid replacement will increase the loss of electrolytes. When the cause of hyponatremia is related to water retention, the preferred treatment is to restrict fluid intake rather than to administer sodium.

NURSING MANAGEMENT OF THE PATIENT WITH HYPONATREMIA
Assessment

Signs and symptoms of hyponatremia depend on the cause, magnitude, and rapidity of the onset. Patients having acute reductions in serum sodium levels usually have more severe symptoms and higher mortality than do those who have a gradual development of hyponatremia. When both sodium and body water are lost, the signs and symptoms are the same as those of ECF deficit.

Early symptoms of chronic hyponatremia caused

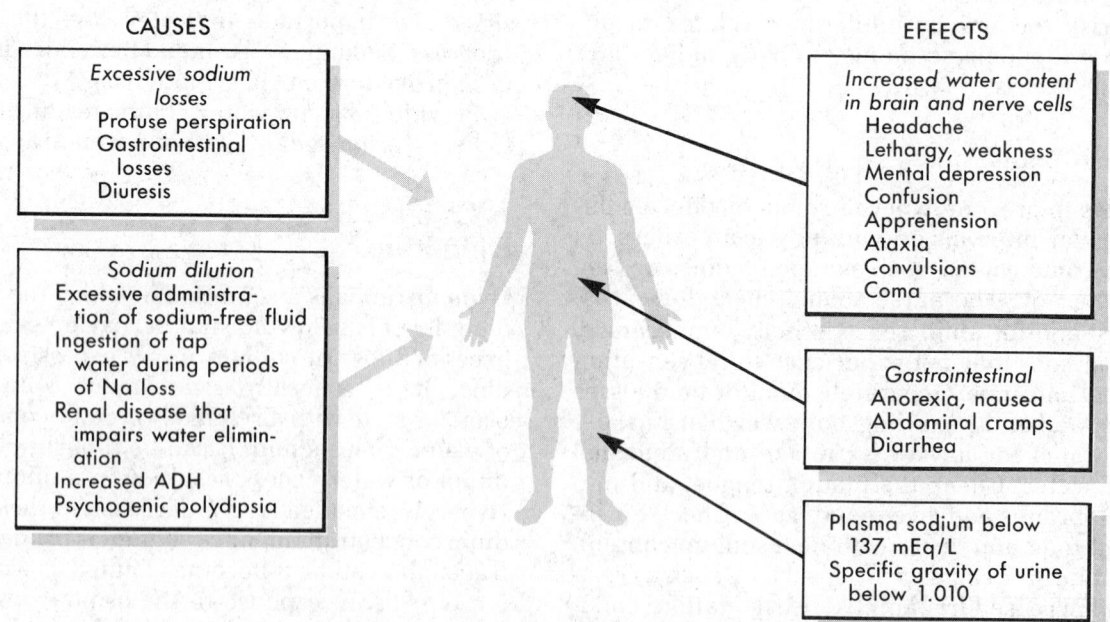

CAUSES

Excessive sodium
losses
Profuse perspiration
Gastrointestinal
losses
Diuresis

Sodium dilution
Excessive administra-
tion of sodium-free fluid
Ingestion of tap
water during periods
of Na loss
Renal disease that
impairs water elimin-
ation
Increased ADH
Psychogenic polydipsia

EFFECTS

Increased water content
in brain and nerve cells
Headache
Lethargy, weakness
Mental depression
Confusion
Apprehension
Ataxia
Convulsions
Coma

Gastrointestinal
Anorexia, nausea
Abdominal cramps
Diarrhea

Plasma sodium below
137 mEq/L
Specific gravity of urine
below 1.010

FIGURE 12-7 Causes and effects of hyponatremia.

by a combination of sodium loss and water gain are those involving the gastrointestinal system (such as anorexia and nausea and vomiting), muscle cramps, fatigue, and dyspnea on exertion. Other signs and symptoms include postural blood pressure changes, poor skin turgor, decreased fullness of neck veins, and flushed skin. Most of the symptoms are related to cellular swelling and cerebral edema, resulting in changes in sensorium with signs of increasing intercranial pressure, headache, lethargy, weakness, depression, confusion, focal weakness, apprehension, ataxia, convulsions, papilledema, and coma. Since the ECF is abnormally dilute, or hypotonic, fluid moves into the cells in an attempt to establish equilibrium. Therefore the volume of the intravascular and interstitial fluid decreases. As the deficit becomes more severe, signs and symptoms such as hypotension as a result of vasomotor collapse, rapid, thready pulse, cold, clammy skin, oliguria, and cyanosis occur.

The symptoms of acute hyponatremia caused by fluid excess are similar to those exhibited by patients with chronic hyponatremia except that the neurologic symptoms are more severe because of the rapid fall in serum sodium levels (Figure 12-7).

Nursing Diagnosis

The following general nursing diagnosis is suggested:
High risk for injury related to ataxia and confusion secondary to severe sodium deficit (<120 to 125 mEq/L)

Implementation

The nurse identifies the patient at risk for potential or actual hyponatremia. Monitor fluid losses and gains by accurate measurement of I & O and daily weights. Check for low sodium intake and loss of sodium-containing fluids, such as gastric fluid, diarrheal fluid, and drainage from fistulas. Monitor gastrointestinal symptoms, and evaluate them relative to total fluid I & O, sodium intake, and laboratory data. Monitor for changes in sensorium and other neurologic disruptions, such as lethargy, confusion, muscle twitching, and convulsions.

Encourage the intake of food and fluid with high sodium content if the patient can eat a regular diet. Monitor patients with conditions such as cardiovascular disease who are receiving fluids with high sodium content either orally or by other routes. Check sodium content of parenteral fluids carefully and check serum sodium levels for increases above normal. Check lungs for crackles, and note other signs of circulatory overload.

Electrolyte Imbalances: Potassium

The mineral potassium is the major electrolyte and principal cation in the ICF compartment. Of the body's potassium, 98% is found in the ICF compartment. Of this, 70% is distributed in skeletal muscle and 28% is in the liver and red blood cells; 2% of the body's potassium is in the ECF. Serum potassium values are based on the portion of potassium in ECF. The amount of potassium in the cells can vary without causing major problems. It is in the ECF compartment where serum potassium values range between 3.5 and 5.0 mEq/L and in which even minor changes become significant in terms of severe potassium imbalance.

The movement of potassium between intracellular and extracellular compartments is controlled mainly by the sodium-potassium pump. Eighty percent of potassium is excreted by the kidneys daily; the remaining 20% is excreted in the feces. Potassium balance is regulated by the kidneys. Potassium and hydrogen ions compete for exchange with sodium ions in the nephron tubules of the kidney. Aldosterone also affects the distal convoluted tubules of the nephrons, thereby regulating sodium and potassium balance. There is a daily potassium loss of approximately 40 mEq/L in urine along with nitrogen waste products. Potassium is not stored in the body. Potassium balance is maintained by a daily intake of 60 to 100 mEq of potassium if there are no abnormal losses occurring and no unusual stress.

Potassium makes up a large part of muscle tissue cells, and the total amount in the human body relates to the size of the individual. Men have approximately 50 mEq of potassium per kilogram of body weight. Women have slightly less.

Potassium is essential for cell metabolism. Since potassium affects the resting potential of nerve and cardiac cells, it is necessary for neuromuscular control and for the precise regulation of skeletal, cardiac, and smooth muscle activity. Potassium contributes to the maintenance of intracellular osmolality and participates in many intracellular enzyme reactions. It plays an important role in the intricate chemical reactions required to transform carbohydrate into energy and to convert proteins into amino acids.

Potassium also plays a part in the body's buffer system. The serum potassium level decreases with alkalosis and increases with acidosis. The potassium level is changed by exchanging hydrogen ions and potassium ions. This in effect compensates for the hydrogen level changes. In acidosis, for example, the body protects itself by moving hydrogen ions from the ECF compartment into the ICF compartment, while potassium ions move out of the cells into the extracellular (serum) compartment to make room for the hydrogen ions. Consequently, the serum level of potassium increases. This level is called false positive, since total body potassium is not elevated; however, a potassium level greater than 5.5 mEq/L may cause toxicity.

Conversely, when alkalosis is present, hydrogen ions in the ECF are low; the cells release hydrogen ions to combat the alkalotic state. Potassium ions from the plasma then enter the cell in exchange for the hydrogen ion release. As a result, serum potassium concentration decreases. Serum potassium levels in this situation are false negative, since total body potassium is unchanged. However, serum levels below 3.0 mEq/L indicate a serious imbalance.

HYPERKALEMIA
Definition

Hyperkalemia is a condition in which there is an increased amount of serum potassium—above 5.0 mEq/L. It is more dangerous than hypokalemia (low serum potassium), since it has a profound effect on the myocardial muscle, which may result in cardiac arrest (Figure 12-8).

Etiology

The major cause of hyperkalemia is renal disease, in which potassium excretion is decreased. Other factors include diarrhea, vomiting, gastric suction, potassium-conserving diuretics, deficiency of adrenal steroids, which causes sodium loss and potassium retention, renal tubular acidosis, extensive tissue trauma including severe infections, lysis of malignant cells caused by the use of chemotherapeutic agents, metabolic or respiratory acidosis, Cushing's syndrome, and osmotic diuresis. The latter occurs in uncontrolled diabetes mellitus. A high intake of potassium in the presence of impaired renal function exacerbates the hyperkalemic state. Intake of oral potassium supplements (when potassium level is normal), excessive use of potassium salt substitutes, rapid transfusion of aged blood in which serum potassium concentration is increased as a result of red blood cell deterioration, rapid parenteral infusion of potassium solutions, and use of potassium penicillin in high doses are other examples of high potassium intake.

Significant Laboratory Tests

The laboratory data reflective of hyperkalemia include a serum potassium level greater than 5.0

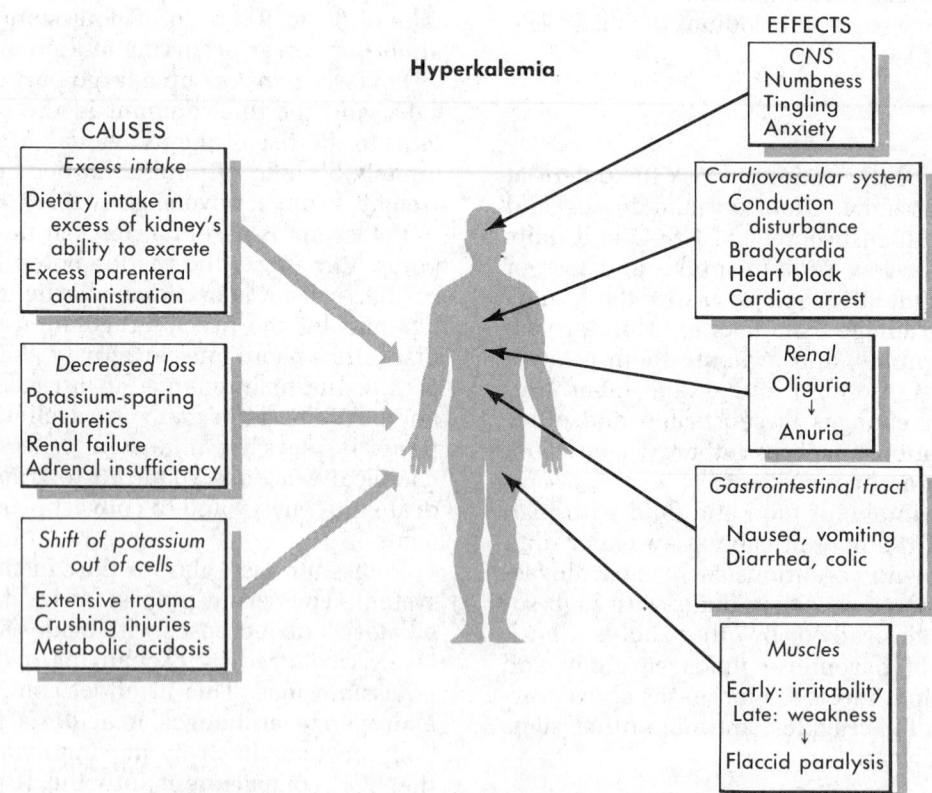

FIGURE 12-8   Causes and effects of hyperkalemia.

mEq/L. Laboratory values may indicate metabolic or respiratory acidosis.

Therapeutic Management

The treatment of hyperkalemia varies according to the severity of the condition. In mild cases, dietary restriction of potassium and/or restricted use of medications containing potassium may be adequate.

Emergency therapy includes rapid IV administration of calcium gluconate to abort serious cardiac symptoms. Calcium acts quickly to protect the myocardium by antagonizing the hyperkalemic action on the heart. The usual dose is 10 mL of a 10% solution administered over 20 minutes (0.5 mL/min). In cardiac resuscitation, 5 to 8 mL may be given and repeated in 10 minutes. Monitoring via ECG is essential so that the infusion can be stopped when the first signs of bradycardia appear. If the patient is receiving digitalis therapy, the nurse needs to be aware that calcium administration sensitizes the heart to digitalis, which may result in digitalis intoxication. The effects of calcium are temporary, lasting 20 to 30 minutes.

Another emergency measure is rapid IV administration of 200 to 300 mL of a 25% hypertonic dextrose solution with 1 unit of insulin per 4 to 5 g of dextrose (1 unit of insulin per 10 g of dextrose if renal failure is present). This treatment causes the potassium to enter the intracellular compartment, thus decreasing serum potassium levels. The dextrose with the accompanying insulin carries the potassium into the cells. As with the administration of calcium gluconate, the effects are temporary. It is important for the nurse to remember that this infusion should not be stopped suddenly because of the stimulation of insulin from the islets of Langerhans. After the infusion of the dextrose/insulin solution, 5% dextrose in water (D_5W) should be administered on a continuous basis.

Sodium bicarbonate (44 mEq) may be added to 500 mL of the D_5W solution to alkalinize the plasma and further result in a temporary shift of potassium into the cells. This medium also furnishes sodium, which acts by antagonizing the effects of potassium on the myocardium. As with the other emergency measures, this treatment is only temporary. If it is deduced that the hyperkalemic condition requires further treatment, measures to remove potassium from the body need to be instituted. These measures include the use of cation-exchange resins, such as hypertonic Kayexalate given orally or rectally, to absorb the potassium into the intestinal tract for removal by feces. Peritoneal dialysis or hemodialysis also may be used.

If necrotic tissue is present as a result of traumatic injuries or large decubitus ulcers, debridement should be considered to remove injured and dead tissue cells, which are releasing potassium into the extracellular compartment. Testosterone propionate injections are sometimes used to assist in the prevention of protein breakdown caused by tissue destruction.

Diet is another important treatment in the management of hyperkalemia. The diet should contain higher amounts of carbohydrate and fats to provide energy and lower amounts of potassium-containing foods.

NURSING MANAGEMENT OF THE PATIENT WITH HYPERKALEMIA
Assessment

The most important symptoms of hyperkalemia relate to its effects on the myocardial muscle. These include changes noted on the ECG, such as tall, peaked T wave, prolonged PR interval, widening of the QRS complex, shortening of the Q-T interval, and disappearance of the P wave. Other cardiac symptoms include ventricular dysrhythmias that may lead to cardiac arrest.

Because potassium plays a major part in neuromuscular activities, elevation in serum potassium initially causes muscle weakness. This can eventually involve facial and respiratory muscles. The muscles innervated by the cranial nerves cause paresthesias of the face and tongue. The patient usually remains alert but apprehensive until cardiac arrest occurs. There is no direct association between serum potassium levels and neuromuscular symptoms. Clinical signs may be absent so that evaluation of the condition is often based on nonspecific signs and symptoms.

Hyperkalemia also affects the gastrointestinal system, causing nausea, intermittent diarrhea, and intestinal colic.

There are times when pseudohyperkalemia should be suspected. This is caused by hemolysis of blood samples before analysis, marked leukocytosis or thrombocytosis, and prolonged use of a tourniquet when obtaining a blood sample. The danger of treating this condition as hyperkalemia is that of dangerously lowering serum potassium levels.

Nursing Diagnosis

The following general nursing diagnosis is suggested:
    Knowledge deficit related to treatment regimen to limit intake of potassium

Implementation

Identify patients at risk for hyperkalemia using knowledge and understanding of the normal and abnormal physiologic processes underlying potassium distribution and potential for increases in serum potassium. Monitor the patient for signs and symptoms of hyperkalemia and prevent hyperkalemia when administering potassium by any route, using standard guidelines.

Causes of pseudohyperkalemia are significant, and prolonged use of a tight tourniquet and exercise of the extremity from which blood samples are obtained should be avoided. Transport blood samples to the laboratory as soon as possible so that hemolysis does not occur before analysis. Do not obtain blood samples from a site above an infusion containing a potassium solution. Check laboratory data for any changes in serum electrolyte values, and monitor ECG tracings for changes in cardiac effects. Monitor kidney function to determine changes in the amount of urine excreted.

If the patient is to receive blood transfusions, check the date that the blood was drawn. Be aware that breakdown of older red blood cells releases potassium and that calcium administration with digitalis can result in digitalis intoxication.

HYPOKALEMIA
Definition

Potassium deficit, or **hypokalemia,** is a condition in which potassium is lost from the body or potassium intake is inadequate, resulting in a serum potassium value below 3.5 mEq/L. Hypokalemia is one of the most common types of electrolyte imbalances. It can occur even when laboratory values fall within the normal range or are borderline.

Etiology

The major cause of potassium loss is increased renal loss. The use of diuretics is the factor most often associated with such loss. Other factors include decreased potassium intake, increased urinary output, gastrointestinal losses, and the presence of alkalosis, either metabolic or respiratory (Figure 12-9). Gastrointestinal losses of potassium are a result of vomiting and gastric suction or draining fistulas

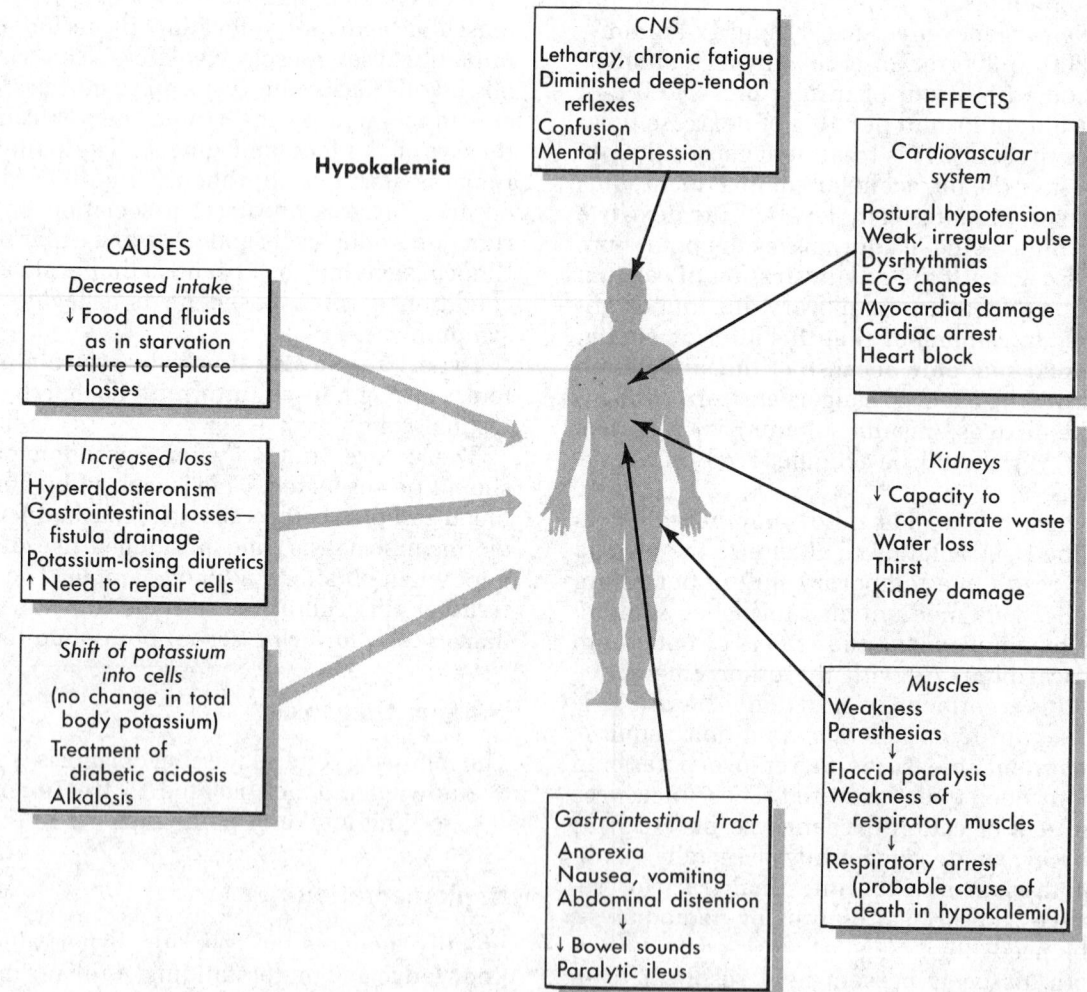

FIGURE 12–9   Causes and effects of hypokalemia.

CLINICAL ALERT

The rate of infusion should not exceed 20 mEq/hr. If the concentration of potassium rises too rapidly, cardiac arrest may occur.

without potassium replacement. Severe potassium loss is often the cause of metabolic alkalosis. Two sodium ions and one hydrogen ion enter the intracellular compartment for every three potassium ions lost from the cell. Because potassium is not conserved by the kidneys, it is not available for the exchange of hydrogen ions in the distal convoluted tubules of the nephron units in the kidneys. To further exacerbate the condition, hydrogen is also excreted, thereby contributing to metabolic alkalosis. Laboratory values show only the amount of extracellular potassium available, so when the laboratory reading of potassium is low, the individual is actually suffering from a serious intracellular potassium deficit.

Significant Laboratory Tests

Significant laboratory tests include serum potassium levels below 3.5 mEq/L and arterial blood gas levels that indicate metabolic alkalosis.

Therapeutic Management

When the imbalance is diagnosed, administration of potassium becomes necessary. In many cases, potassium can be supplemented through the diet in the form of potassium-rich foods. In intravenous and oral potassium replacement, the renal system must be assessed and urine output must be adequate before administration. If potassium is given intravenously, the rate of potassium administration must be limited. Heart muscle is very sensitive to extracellular potassium. For an adult, dilute 40 mEq of potassium in 1000 mL of fluid.

NURSING MANAGEMENT OF THE PATIENT WITH HYPOKALEMIA
Assessment

Hypokalemia can be detected before the imbalance becomes life threatening. Some of the clinical manifestations are anorexia, muscle weakness, weak and irregular pulse, decreased reflexes, decreased bowel sounds, hypotension, dysrhythmias, nausea, vomiting, ileus, paresthesias, and hydrogen ion disturbances. When ECG monitoring is available, the nurse should observe for a flat T wave and ST segment depression.

Nursing Diagnosis

The diagnosis of patients with this imbalance relates to their primary problem identification. As an example, the following general nursing diagnosis is suggested:

Impaired physical mobility related to low potassium level secondary to diuretic therapy

Implementation

The goal of nursing care is to identify the patients at risk and prevent the imbalance. I & O should be monitored hourly. Report urine output of less than 30 mL/hr to the physician. Do not give potassium supplements if the patient has inadequate urine output, since hyperkalemia can result (exception is if the patient is in severe hypokalemia).

Assess digitalized patients for signs of digitalis toxicity. Low potassium levels increase the action of digitalis.

Monitor the ECG tracings for continued signs of hypokalemia, and monitor potassium levels carefully for trends when patients are taking diuretics or on nasogastric suction. Practice caution in the use of salt substitutes if patients are taking potassium-saving diuretics.

Electrolyte Imbalances: Calcium

Calcium and phosphorus are found in the body primarily in the bones and teeth (99%) and dissolved in blood (1%). The amounts of dissolved calcium and phosphate are inversely related. As one increases, the other decreases. This inverse relationship must be maintained, since an increase in both ions would result in an insoluble precipitate.

The dissolved portion of the calcium is carried in the blood in two forms: bound to protein, particularly albumin; and in an ionized form. The serum levels usually reported include total dissolved calcium consisting of both protein-bound and ionized forms. Only the ionized fraction is involved in the promotion of neuromuscular activity. The calcium that is bound to plasma protein cannot pass through the capillary wall and therefore cannot leave the intravascular compartment.

Free, ionized calcium is needed to help maintain the permeability of cell membranes. Calcium is essential for the transmission of nerve impulses and neuromuscular excitability, and it is necessary for normal cardiac function. Calcium is needed for blood coagulation and is important in activating enzyme reactions and hormone secretion. The ionized portion is maintained within fine limits, since a change in ionized calcium can have a profound effect on the body. Within the range that is compatible with life, fluctuations in the concentration of calcium greatly affect the excitability of nerve tissue. Nerve cell membranes are less excitable when sufficient calcium is available.

HYPERCALCEMIA
Definition/Etiology

Hypercalcemia refers to calcium excess in the serum. Two of the primary causes of hypercalcemia are hyperparathyroidism and the presence of a malignancy. Two of the first clinical manifestations reflective of the hypercalcemic condition are anorexia and complaints of "bone pain." Complaints often offered by elderly persons are not always taken seriously, and while the symptoms of anorexia, nausea, and pain continue, the critical problem of hypercalcemia is not treated. Additional symptoms, such as extreme lethargy, confusion, and irritability, and in some cases convulsions, may occur before treatment is instituted (Figure 12-10).

Calcium is an important regulator of the excitation-contraction coupling of the heart and smooth muscles. This is represented by changes in

CLINICAL ALERT

Hypercalcemia exists whenever the serum calcium is over 5.3 mEq/L, or 10.6 mg/dL. An acute increase in serum calcium levels above 8 to 9 mEq/L (17 mg/dL) is an emergency situation.

the individual's ECG tracings, as well as changes in renal function. The ECG tracings show a short Q-T interval and inverted T wave.[9] Such changes are significant in the presence of cardiac disease or when an individual is receiving digitalis preparations. Hypercalcemia precipitates digitalis toxicity. Cardiac standstill can occur when the serum calcium increases to approximately 19 mg/dL.

Significant Laboratory Tests

Significant laboratory tests include total serum calcium levels, ionized calcium values, parathyroid hormone (PTH) levels, and x-ray findings to determine the presence of osteoporosis or urinary calculi. Nor-

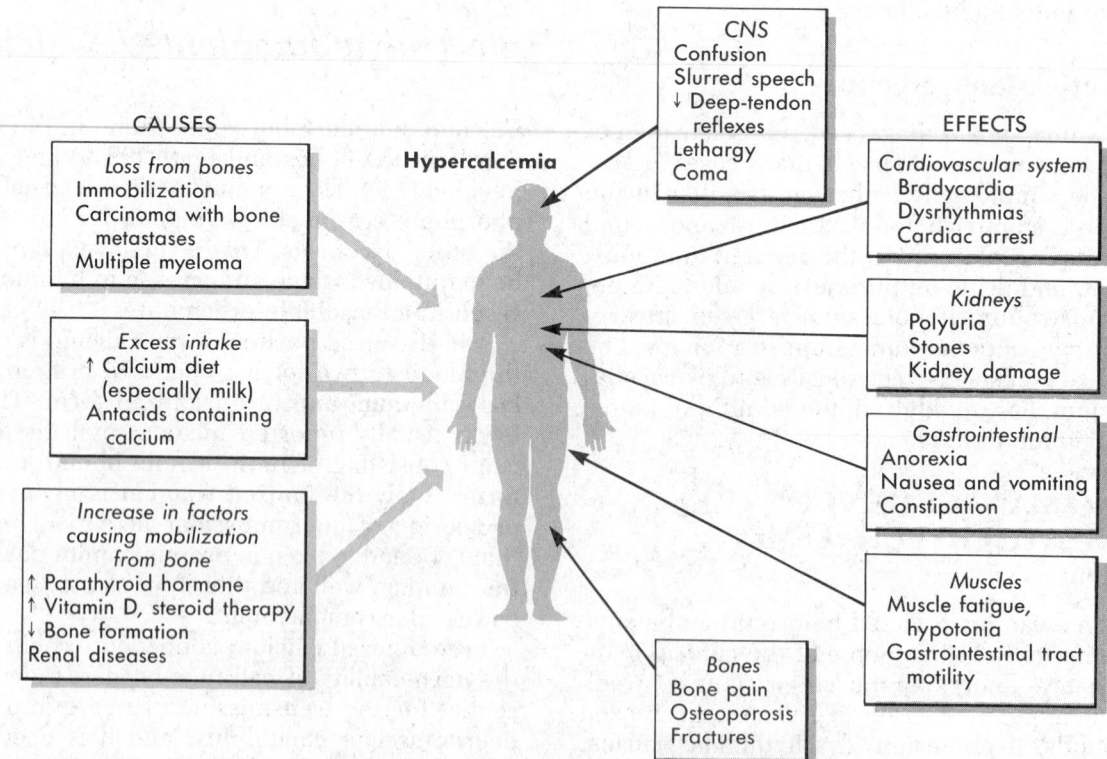

FIGURE 12-10   Causes and effects of hypercalcemia.

mal serum calcium is 4.5 to 5.3 mEq/L (8.5 to 10.5 mg/dL).

Therapeutic Management

Medical treatment is geared toward hydrating the patient. The rationale for this is that volume expansion increases the calcium excretion. The addition of furosemide (Lasix) assists in the inhibition of calcium absorption.[9] One or two liters of isotonic saline (0.9%) may be prescribed every hour along with the intravenous administration of Lasix. It is important to match the rate and amount of saline solution to the patient's output.

Individuals who have associated renal, cardiac, or pulmonary disease are poor candidates for the aforementioned treatment. In such cases, Mithracin and other antineoplastic antibiotics are usually prescribed. These drugs are effective in inhibiting bone resorption and can be repeated for several days. Potential toxic effects of these drugs include bone marrow suppression, nausea, vomiting, and bleeding. Further, these drugs must be used with caution when patients have coexisting renal disease and malignancies.

Patients who have undergone thyroid surgery need to be monitored for symptoms of hypercalcemia, although this is not common today. Patients on bed rest or those who are immobilized over prolonged periods need to be observed for bone mineral loss resulting in hypercalcemia.

NURSING MANAGEMENT OF THE PATIENT WITH HYPERCALCEMIA

Assessment

The symptoms of hypercalcemia are proportional to the degree of elevation of serum calcium. The assessment reveals decreased muscle tone, decreased strength, and depressed reflexes. Clinical findings of muscle weakness, incoordination, anorexia, and constipation are common in hypercalcemic conditions because of the decreased tone in smooth and striated muscle. Polyuria occurs as a result of disturbances in renal tubular function.

Abdominal pain, anorexia, nausea, and vomiting are common complaints of patients with this condition. Symptoms of peptic ulcer are common in individuals with chronically high levels of serum calcium because of increased acid secretions in the stomach.

Nursing Diagnosis

The following general nursing diagnoses are suggested:
    High risk for injury related to muscle weakness and confusion
    Sensory/perceptual alterations related to hyper-

calcemia as evidenced by confusion and lethargy

Implementation

Monitor I & O, and notify the physician for unusual changes in urinary volume. Monitor renal function carefully, since hypercalcemia can impair renal function. Assess for renal stone formation.

Monitor for signs and symptoms of hypercalcemia, and assess orientation to person, place, and time. Monitor for personality changes, and use reality therapy.

Fluids may be given to promote excretion of calcium (administered orally or intravenously). A low-calcium diet should be provided, and medications containing calcium should be avoided. The environment should be safe, since neuromuscular problems may cause poor coordination and abnormal gait.

Monitor for signs of digitalis toxicity, and monitor serum calcium, potassium, and phosphorous values for changes. Check with the physician regarding abnormal values. Mobility should be encouraged to decrease the potential for osteoporosis. Watch for evidence of polyuria caused by increased calcium in urine with potential inhibition of kidney concentration of urine. Watch for signs indicative of impending cardiac arrest.

Excessive intake of milk products should be discouraged. Patients at risk for hypercalcemia (bone diseases, oncology, and osteoporosis) should be educated regarding symptoms of hypercalcemia. A loop diuretic may be prescribed to increase urine production. Inorganic phosphates can be given orally if the patient can tolerate this treatment. Phospho-Soda or Neutra-Phos should be administered as prescribed. Fleet Phospho-Soda may be administered through a nasogastric tube or instilled rectally if the patient cannot tolerate oral preparations.

HYPOCALCEMIA

Definition

Hypocalcemia refers to a lower than normal serum concentration of calcium. Maintainence of normal serum calcium depends on the dietary intake of calcium and vitamin D,[9] adequate levels of phosphorus, and effective functioning of the parathyroid glands (Figure 12-11). An inverse relationship exists between calcium and phosphorus, which normally keeps these two ions in balance. The parathyroid glands are the principal regulators of calcium concentration in the plasma. PTH stimulates the kidney to increase the secretion of phosphorus and reabsorption of calcium into the intravascular compartment. The reabsorbed calcium in the presence of PTH is then absorbed into the bone structure. The

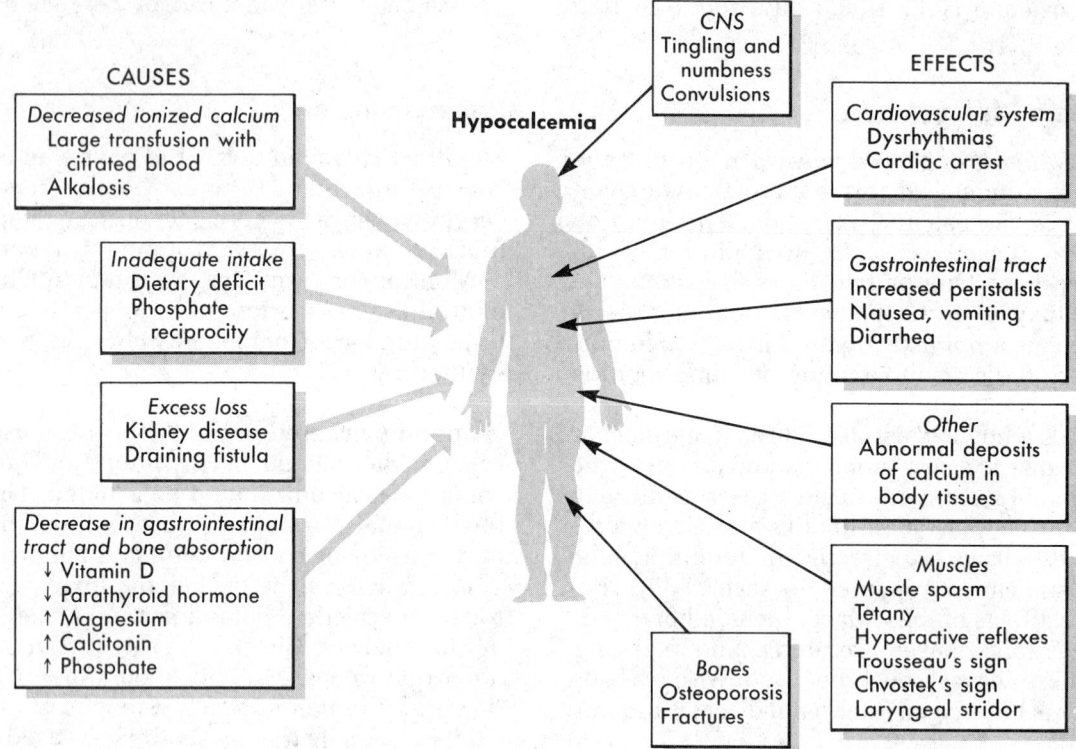

CAUSES

Decreased ionized calcium
Large transfusion with
  citrated blood
Alkalosis

Inadequate intake
Dietary deficit
Phosphate
  reciprocity

Excess loss
Kidney disease
Draining fistula

Decrease in gastrointestinal
tract and bone absorption
  ↓ Vitamin D
  ↓ Parathyroid hormone
  ↑ Magnesium
  ↑ Calcitonin
  ↑ Phosphate

Hypocalcemia

CNS
Tingling and
numbness
Convulsions

EFFECTS

Cardiovascular system
Dysrhythmias
Cardiac arrest

Gastrointestinal tract
Increased peristalsis
Nausea, vomiting
Diarrhea

Other
Abnormal deposits
of calcium in
body tissues

Muscles
Muscle spasm
Tetany
Hyperactive reflexes
Trousseau's sign
Chvostek's sign
Laryngeal stridor

Bones
Osteoporosis
Fractures

FIGURE 12-11   Causes and effects of hypocalcemia.

thyroid gland secretes calcitonin, which metabolizes calcium and lowers the serum calcium level by absorption into bone and excretion via the kidneys. Estrogen stimulates the reabsorption of calcium into the bone. Bone decalcification increases with the onset of menopause, presumably because of the decrease in estrogen secretion. Osteoporosis is a total body calcium deficit, but in some instances patients continue to maintain normal serum calcium levels. Estrogen preparations have been demonstrated to prevent or decrease the initiation of osteoporosis after menopause.[9]

Hypocalcemia is commonly found in patients with renal failure, because these patients frequently have elevated serum phosphate levels. Hyperphosphatemia usually causes a reciprocal drop in the serum calcium level. Other causes of hypocalcemia may be the intake of certain drugs, such as aluminum-containing antacids, aminoglycosides, cisplatin, corticosteroids, Mithracin, phosphates, caffeine, and loop diuretics.

Significant Laboratory Tests

Laboratory tests for hypocalcemic states include total serum calcium levels, ionized serum calcium levels, and PTH, magnesium, and phosphorus levels. In hypocalcemia the serum calcium is below 4.5 mEq/L (8.5 mg/dL).

Therapeutic Management

Calcium is administered safely as an oral supplement. Only in severe hypocalcemia is IV administration of calcium solutions ordered. In this latter case the solution is administered slowly and in small doses in order not to raise the serum calcium levels too quickly.

NURSING MANAGEMENT OF THE PATIENT WITH HYPOCALCEMIA
Assessment

Assess the patient for clinical manifestations of tetany. Tetany is caused by the spontaneous discharge of both sensory and motor fibers in peripherial nerves because of a decrease in serum calcium. Patients with tetany report tingling sensations in the tips of their fingers, around the oral cavity, and less commonly in the feet. A positive Trousseau's sign or Chvostek's sign may be present. Assess the patient for bone fractures.

Assess for prolonged Q-T interval on ECG tracings, as well as mental changes, such as emotional depression, impairment of memory, confusion, delirium, and hallucinations.

Nursing Diagnosis

The following general nursing diagnosis is suggested:
    High risk for injury related to low calcium as evidenced by spasms or tetany

Implementation

Prevention of tetany is the primary goal of nursing care. Monitor the patient for signs and symptoms of hypocalcemia. Administer intravenous calcium slowly and watch for infiltration. Do not infuse intravenous calcium faster than 0.5 mL/min because of hypotension except in cardiac arrest. Never use a central line for calcium infusions. Observe seizure precautions in severe hypocalcemia. Check the airway since laryngeal stridor may occur.

Educate the patient regarding osteoporosis and encourage intake of foods high in calcium. Avoid hyperventilation because metabolic alkalosis may lead to tetany. Monitor ECG tracings for signs and symptoms of digitalis toxicity. Also, observe for signs of heart failure or pulmonary edema, since hypocalcemia can decrease contractility of the myocardium.

Electrolyte Imbalances: Magnesium

Approximately 50% to 60% of the body's magnesium is contained in the bone. Approximately 1% is in the ECF compartment, and the remaining magnesium is located within the cells. It is a major intracellular ion and is closely related to potassium. It acts as a catalyst for many intracellular enzyme functions, especially those relating to carbohydrate and protein metabolism, as well as affecting the sodium-potassium pump. In this latter capacity, magnesium affects intracellular potassium levels. Magnesium also has an effect on neuromuscular activity, on transmission of neural impulses in the central nervous system, and on the functioning of the myocardium.[5]

Even though the exact control of magnesium is unknown, many of the factors that regulate calcium balance also play a role in magnesium balance in the body. The minimum daily requirement of magnesium is 3.6 mg/kg of body weight. It is regulated by several factors, including the presence of vitamin D, for its absorption from the gastrointestinal tract. The kidneys are the major route by which magnesium is excreted from the body. The kidneys can conserve magnesium. The major site of magnesium reabsorption is the ascending limb of Henle's loop. Diuretics

that act on this region of the nephron cause large magnesium losses. The normal serum magnesium level is 1.5 to 2.5 mEq/L. Magnesium is found in two forms—bound to protein and freely ionized. It is the ionized portion that is primarily involved in physiologic processes. Magnesium has an effect on neuromuscular irritability and contractility because of its direct action on the myoneural junction. A magnesium deficit increases neuromuscular irritability, whereas an excess has a sedative effect probably caused by the inhibition of acetylcholine release at the neuromuscular junction.

Magnesium also produces peripheral vasodilation, which can lead to a decrease in blood pressure, resulting in cardiac arrest. Ventricular dysrhythmias may occur because of magnesium imbalances.

Most magnesium imbalances result from a deficit in serum magnesium levels. Such deficits often occur because of excessive ingestion of alcohol secondary to an inadequate dietary intake. Table 12-4 summarizes common manifestations of altered magnesium metabolism.

HYPOMAGNESEMIA
Definition/Etiology

Hypomagnesemia exists when the serum magnesium level falls below 1.5 mEq/L.

Magnesium deficiency is usually caused by decreased absorption from the gastrointestinal tract or by increased urinary excretion (Figure 12-12). Other causes include losses from the gastrointestinal tract via vomiting or diarrhea and with continuous administration of parenteral fluids that do not include magnesium. The majority of patients suffer from alcoholism or are critically ill. Deficits in magnesium level usually are accompanied by deficits in potassium and calcium. Certain medications that affect osmotic diuresis can produce hypomagnesemia. These include mannitol, urea, and glucose. As with calcium, rapid administration of citrated blood causes chelation and may result in a magnesium deficit, especially in the presence of renal or hepatic disease. Other causes include renal disease, pancreatitis, and severe burns. Patients with diabetic ketoacidosis often develop hypomagnesemia because of the osmotic diuresis produced by the glucose overload, which increases the excretion of magnesium by the kidney. Magnesium is also shifted into cells with insulin, which is secreted into the intravascular system because of the glucose overload.

Significant Laboratory Tests

Laboratory tests include serum magnesium levels, serum albumin levels, serum potassium levels, and serum calcium levels (NOTE: Potassium deficiency may be resistant to potassium replacement until

TABLE 12-4   Common Manifestations of Altered Magnesium Metabolism

	Manifestation	Mechanism
MAGNESIUM DEFICIENCY		
Biochemical	Hypocalcemia	Impaired PTH secretion
		PTH resistance of end organs
		Resistance to vitamin D
	Hypokalemia	Renal K^+ wasting
Neuromuscular	Neuromuscular irritability (muscle tremors, weakness, fasciculations, tetany)	Hypocalcemia Hypomagnesemia
	Central nervous system (nystagmus, ataxia, vertigo, psychiatric abnormalities)	
Cardiovascular	Cardiac dysrhythmia (tachycardia, prolonged P-R and Q-T intervals, abnormal T wave)	Hypokalemia Hypomagnesemia
Gastrointestinal	Dysphagia	Neuromuscular irritability
Hematologic	Anemia (reticulocytosis, spherocytosis, microcytosis, erythroid hyperplasia)	Short erythrocyte half-life
MAGNESIUM EXCESS		
Biochemical	Hypocalcemia	Renal calcium wasting
		Impaired PTH secretion
Neuromuscular	Neuromuscular depression (decrease in deep tendon reflexes, paralysis)	Impaired nerve transmission Decrease in postsynaptic response
	Central nervous system (depression, somnolence)	Hypermagnesemia
Cardiovascular	Cardiac dysrhythmias (bradycardia, increased QRS duration)	Hypermagnesemia Hypocalcemia

From Maxwell M et al: *Clinical disorders of fluid and electrolyte metabolism,* ed 4, New York, 1987, McGraw-Hill, Inc.

magnesium has been corrected).[5] ECG evaluations should be assessed and will often reflect magnesium, calcium, and potassium deficiency. In hypomagnesemia the magnesium level is 1.5 mEq/L.

Therapeutic Management

The goal of treatment is to identify and eliminate the cause. Increased dietary intake of magnesium and antacids may be used. If the condition is severe, parenteral infusions of magnesium sulfate may be prescribed. In emergency situations a loading dose of 500 mg of magnesium may be given at an extremely slow rate (15 mg/min) followed by a continuous intravenous infusion of magnesium solution administered slowly over 24 hours. In the latter case it is important to use serial magnesium concentrations to regulate the dose.[11]

NURSING MANAGEMENT OF THE PATIENT WITH HYPOMAGNESEMIA
Assessment

Signs and symptoms of magnesium deficiency are primarily related to the neuromuscular system. Some of the symptoms are a direct result of magnesium deficiency itself, whereas other symptoms are associated with potassium and calcium metabolism. Symptoms include agitation, mood changes, tremors, hallucinations, paresthesias, anorexia, nausea, and vomiting. Other symptoms may include tetany with positive Chvostek's and Trousseau's signs and laryngeal stridor. Tetany is partly a result of the accompanying hypocalcemia. Tachycardia and cardiac dysrhythmias may result, as well as hypotension. Increased sensitivity to digitalis may result in digitalis toxicity.

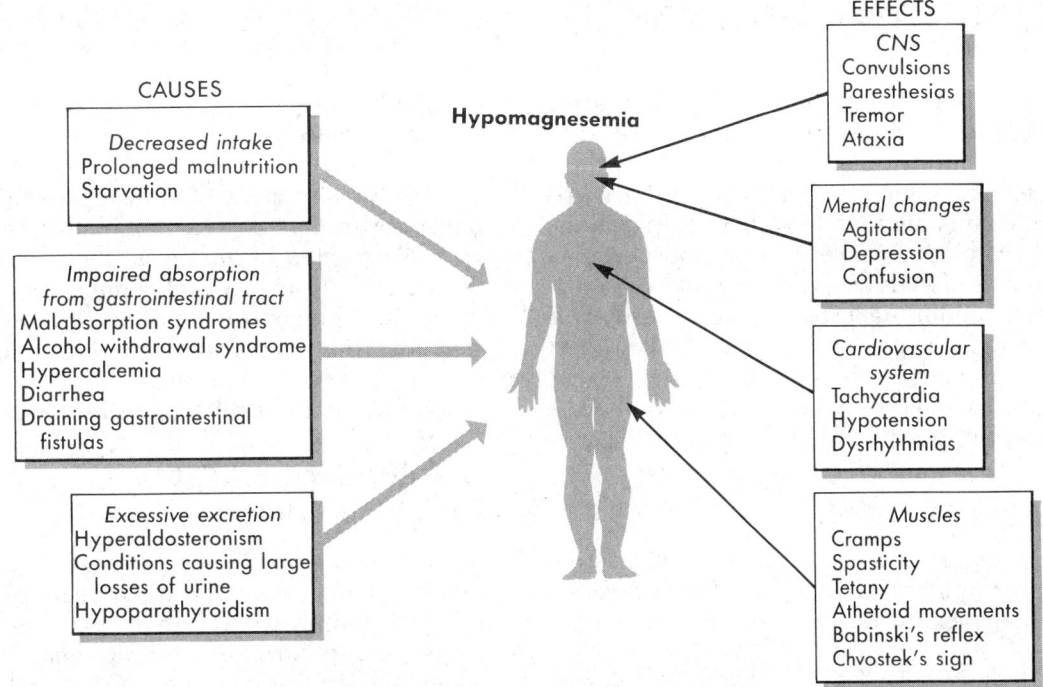

CAUSES

Decreased intake
Prolonged malnutrition
Starvation

*Impaired absorption
from gastrointestinal tract*
Malabsorption syndromes
Alcohol withdrawal syndrome
Hypercalcemia
Diarrhea
Draining gastrointestinal
   fistulas

Excessive excretion
Hyperaldosteronism
Conditions causing large
   losses of urine
Hypoparathyroidism

Hypomagnesemia

EFFECTS

CNS
Convulsions
Paresthesias
Tremor
Ataxia

Mental changes
Agitation
Depression
Confusion

*Cardiovascular
system*
Tachycardia
Hypotension
Dysrhythmias

Muscles
Cramps
Spasticity
Tetany
Athetoid movements
Babinski's reflex
Chvostek's sign

FIGURE 12-12   Causes and effects of hypomagnesemia.

Nursing Diagnosis

The following nursing diagnosis is suggested:
   Potential for injury related to the action of magnesium deficiency on the neuromuscular system

Implementation

Monitor serum magnesium levels of patients at risk, and administer oral magnesium supplements to patients with chronic magnesium deficiency. Provide foods with high magnesium content to patients in nonacute conditions.

Administer intravenous magnesium sulfate ($MgSO_4$) slowly and with caution. Do not leave the patient alone. Monitor for decreased blood pressure, labored respirations, and a decreased patellar reflex. Check every 5 minutes or before each dose for flaccidity and loss of patellar (knee jerk) reflex. Have calcium gluconate available for treatment of tetany or magnesium excess. Be alert for laryngeal stridor. Take safety precautions for patients with neuromuscular symptoms. Assess and document neurologic symptoms and monitor heart rate and check vital signs at regular intervals. Evaluate ECG tracings for dysrhythmias, and check patients receiving digitalis therapy, including monitoring their ECGs.

Educate the patient and family in the use of diuretics, laxatives, and dietary intake of foods high in magnesium.

HYPERMAGNESEMIA
Definition/Etiology

Hypermagnesemia most often occurs in patients with renal failure who are using medications with high magnesium content to control convulsions or who are using antacids with high magnesium content. This condition may also occur in the presence of acute adrenocortical insufficiency. Major symptoms are caused by neurologic depression of peripheral and neuromuscular systems.

Significant Laboratory Tests

Laboratory tests may reveal increased serum magnesium levels over 2.5 mEq/L and ECG changes.

Therapeutic Management

The goal of treatment is prevention if possible. Any magnesium-containing foods or medications are discontinued if the patient is seriously ill. In patients with adequate renal function, diuretics and a 0.45% NaCl solution may be prescribed to excrete excess magnesium via the renal system.

In severe cases with cardiac conduction problems or respiratory difficulties, emergency measures such as intravenous calcium administration with ventilatory support may be required. Hemodialysis with a magnesium-free dialysate may be required.

NURSING MANAGEMENT OF THE PATIENT WITH HYPERMAGNESEMIA
Assessment

Signs and symptoms may be lacking in mild cases. Signs and symptoms of acute magnesium excess include nausea, vomiting, diaphoresis, and alterations in neurologic functioning as evidenced by drowsiness, mental confusion, muscle weakness, paralysis, and coma. Paralysis of the respiratory muscles may occur as a result of sudden overload of serum magnesium. Deep tendon reflexes are depressed. Soft tissue calcification, hypotension, bradycardia, heart block, and cardiac arrest in diastole may occur. Other symptoms include decreased arterial pressure as a result of peripheral vasodilation.

Nursing Diagnosis

The following general nursing diagnosis is suggested:
    High risk for injury related to the effect of excess serum magnesium on the neuromuscular system

Implementation

Assess the patient at risk, monitoring serum magnesium levels. Check vital signs, and be aware of hypotension and apnea potential. Assess neuromuscular symptoms, and document and report abnormal symptoms. Use safety precautions with patients exhibiting neurologic symptoms. Advise the patient and family about medications with high magnesium content.

Electrolyte Imbalances: Phosphorus

Phosphorus is the primary anion in ICF. It is found in the body in the form of inorganic salts. It is mainly distributed in combination with calcium in bones and teeth. The small amount in ECF supports several metabolic functions, including acid-base homeostasis, as the phosphate buffer system. It functions in the formation of energy-storing substances, such as ATP; functions in the formation of red blood cells; and acts as an intermediary in the metabolism of carbohydrates, proteins, and fats. It is critical to normal nerve and muscle function and provides structural support for bones and teeth. Serum phosphate levels vary with gender, age, and diet. Levels decrease with age except for a slight rise in women after menopause. When glucose, insulin, or sugar-containing nutrients are introduced into the plasma, serum phosphate shifts into cells, thereby decreasing its concentration temporarily in ECF.

Acid-base imbalances affect phosphorus levels. For example, respiratory alkalosis causes a shift of serum potassium into cells, potentially resulting in hypophosphatemia.

Approximately 0.8 to 1.5 g of phosphorus is needed daily to maintain a normal balance. The renal system is responsible for approximately 90% of phosphorus that is excreted daily. The remaining 10% is excreted in the feces.

The level of extracellular phosphate is regulated by dietary intake, intestinal absorption, hormonally regulated bone resorption and deposition, and renal excretion. The normal range of serum phosphate in ECF is 1.7 to 2.6 mEq/L (2.5 to 4.5 mg/dL).

HYPERPHOSPHATEMIA
Definition/Etiology

Hyperphosphatemia occurs most often when renal insufficiency exists. There is a decrease in the ability of the kidney to excrete excess phosphorus. Both acute renal failure and chronic renal failure are responsible for the condition of hyperphosphatemia. Other causes include a high phosphate intake. Increased phosphorus intake can occur via intravenous administration. Enemas containing sodium phosphate may increase the absorption of this element via the large intestine. Blood transfusions may increase the phosphorus level in the ECF, since this substance leaks from the blood cells during storage.

Direct injury to muscle tissue causing necrosis and thereby releasing phosphorus into ECF is another cause of hyperphosphatemia. Certain endocrine disorders, such as hypoparathyroidism (in which there is a decrease in the production and release of PTH) result in a serum calcium deficiency and concomitant increase in phosphate concentration.

Hypocalcemia is likely to occur in sudden, severe hyperphosphatemia after intravenous administration of phosphates. A major complication of increased serum phosphate concentration is metastatic calcification (calcium phosphate) into soft tissues, joints, and arteries. Large intake of vitamin D increases phosphorus absorption from the intestinal tract.

Significant Laboratory Tests

Serum phosphate levels will be greater than 2.6 mEq/L (4.5 mg/dL). The parathyroid hormone (PTH) level will be decreased if hypoparathyroidism is present.

X-ray examination may show skeletal changes.

Therapeutic Management

Treatment is directed toward the underlying disorder if possible. Ingestion of high-phosphate sources, such as milk and medications, should be avoided. In severe cases, intravenous administration of calcium and use of dialysis to remove excess phosphorus may be necessary. Administration of phosphate-binding gels, use of dialysis, and restriction of phosphate intake may be prescribed for patients in renal failure. Aluminum hydroxide gels bind with phosphorus in the intestine.

NURSING MANAGEMENT OF THE PATIENT WITH HYPERPHOSPHATEMIA
Assessment

Anorexia, nausea, vomiting, muscle weakness, hyperreflexia, tachycardia, and tetany are some of the signs and symptoms of hyperphosphatemia. Tetany is associated with hypocalcemia, which often occurs with a high increase in serum phosphate. This is the result of the reciprocal relationship between phosphorus and calcium. Usually the majority of symptoms that do occur relate to soft tissue calcifications. Signs of metastatic calcifications include corneal haziness, conjunctivitis, oliguria, irregular heart rate, and papular eruptions. Deposits of calcium phosphate in the heart may cause dysrhythmias.

Nursing Diagnosis

The following general nursing diagnosis is suggested:
   High risk for injury related to risk of calcium phosphate calcifications in soft tissue

Implementation

Monitor serum phosphate and calcium levels in patients at risk for calcium phosphate calcifications. Check with the physician regarding abnormal values. Vitamin D products should be avoided. Observe for symptoms of metastatic calcifications and report them immediately. Monitor for symptoms of tetany, and monitor urine output, BUN, and creatinine, since renal function may be impaired by hyperphosphatemia.

HYPOPHOSPHATEMIA
Definition/Etiology

Hypophosphatemia may occur because of increased urinary losses when there are transient intracellular shifts, decrease in intestinal absorption, or increased use of phosphorus, such as that required in cell functioning and in acid-base regulation. Hyperventilation, use of phosphorus-binding antacids, and increased urinary losses are other causes. Patients in diabetic ketoacidosis lose a significant amount of phosphorus in the urine because of glucose-induced osmotic diuresis.[5] Refeeding after starvation, hyperalimentation, and respiratory alkalosis are other factors that decrease the serum level of phosphorus.

Significant Laboratory Tests

Serum phosphorus will be less than 1.7 mEq/L (2.5 mg/dL). PTH level will be elevated in the presence of hyperparathyroidism. Serum magnesium may be decreased secondary to increased urinary excretion of magnesium because of phosphorus deficiency. X-ray examination may indicate skeletal changes.

Therapeutic Management

Treatment is aimed at the identification and elimination of the underlying cause. If the phosphorus deficiency is mild, the treatment may involve only an increased intake of foods that are high in phosphorus. If the condition is not too severe, oral phosphate supplements might be in order. When the condition is very severe, intravenous administration of sodium phosphate or potassium phosphate may be necessary.

NURSING MANAGEMENT OF THE PATIENT WITH HYPOPHOSPHATEMIA
Assessment

Most of the signs and symptoms are related to a deficiency of ATP or 2,3-diphosphoglycerate (2,3-DPG) or both. An enzyme in red cells, 2,3-DPG interacts with hemoglobin for the promotion of oxygen release. Lack of ATP results in an impairment of cellular energy resources, whereas a deficiency in 2,3-DPG impairs oxygen being delivered to body tissues.[11]

Signs and symptoms of hypophosphatemia include symptoms reflective of sudden deficit in serum phosphorus or symptoms that develop gradually because of chronic deficiency of phosphorus. Acute symptoms include confusion, seizures, and other neurologic signs that are caused by cellular deficiencies of ATP and 2,3-DPG. A deficiency in phosphate causes changes in blood cells, particularly red blood cells, by reducing oxygen-carrying capacity and causing tissue anoxia. Hemolytic anemia can occur because of the fragility of the red blood cells. Symptoms of chest pain may occur as a reflection of myocardial hypoxia, as well as muscle pains and muscle weakness caused by muscle ATP deficiency. Pronounced phosphorus deficiency may be associated with metabolic acidosis. Numbness and tingling of fingers and incoordination are also noted. Chronic signs include memory loss and bone pain.

Nursing Diagnosis

The following general nursing diagnosis is suggested:
   High risk for injury related to confusion, muscle weakness, or seizures

Implementation

Assess the patient at risk for development of hypophosphatemia. Assess for signs of hypoxia, such as restlessness, confusion, chest pain, and cyanosis. Monitor respiratory rate and depth.

Acid-Base Balance

Many disease processes can alter the acid-base balance of the body with the potential for severe alterations, causing alkalosis or acidosis, which in and of themselves may be more devastating than the primary disease itself. To understand the pathophysiologic processes involved in the development of acidotic or alkalotic states and the profound effect on the body system, the nurse needs to have a knowledge of the physiologic processes involved in maintaining an acid-base balance.

Acid-base balance is governed by the regulation of hydrogen ion concentration in the body fluids, and it is the activity of these ions in solution that determines the acidity of fluids within the body. An increased concentration of hydrogen ions (H+) makes a solution more acidic; a decrease makes it more alkaline. Since pH is a negative logarithm (exponent) of the hydrogen ion concentration, the pH falls as the hydrogen ion concentration rises; and as the concentration falls, the pH rises. The balance between acids and bases must be kept within a narrow range of 7.35 to 7.45 pH in the ECF. The pH reflects the hydrogen ion concentration in the body. A pH value less than 7.35 indicates **acidosis,** whereas a pH value greater than 7.45 reflects a state of **alkalosis.** Only slight changes from the normal range of pH are needed to cause marked alterations in the speed of chemical reactions in the cells. Reaction rates may be increased or decreased, and for this reason, the regulation of the acid-base ratio (hydrogen concentration) is one of the most important aspects of homeostasis.[4]

HENDERSON-HASSELBALCH EQUATION

The Henderson-Hasselbalch equation is a mathematical expression of the three parameters reflecting acid-base status. The principle of this equation is that the ratio of base to acid, or HCO_3^- to CO_2 (20:1), determines pH. A simplified form of the equation may be written:

$$pH = pK + \log \frac{Base}{Acid} \text{ or } \frac{Kidney}{Lung}$$

pK is the dissociation constant of a buffer system, which for this system is 6.1:

$$pH = 6.1 + \log \frac{HCO_3^- \text{ mEq/L}}{P_{CO_2} \text{ mm Hg} \times 0.03}$$

To convert partial pressure of carbon dioxide (P_{CO_2}) to the same units as HCO_3^- (either millimoles or milliequivalents), a correction factor of 0.03 is applied. A normal value for HCO_3^- is 24 mEq/L and a P_{CO_2} is normally 40 mm Hg ($40 \times .03 = 1.2$). Therefore:

$$pH = 6.1 + \log \frac{24}{1.2}$$
$$= 6.1 + \log 20$$
$$= 6.1 + 1.30$$
$$= 7.40$$

At the bedside the nurse would not normally be working with logarithmic tables. However, the Henderson-Hasselbalch equation is the foundation on which many acid-base calculations, nomograms, and graphs are constructed, and it is important to understand its application.

Acids are proton donors and give up their hydrogen ions to neutralize or decrease the strength of a base. Bases on the other hand are hydrogen ion acceptors. Bases have fewer hydrogen ions on the pH scale and are responsible for alkalinity of solutions. For example, hydrochloric acid in the body fluids combines with sodium bicarbonate to produce sodium chloride and carbonic acid. This chemical reaction neutralizes the base, sodium bicarbonate, to a salt, namely, sodium chloride, and produces a much weaker acid, carbonic acid. In this process, hydrochloric acid donated its hydrogen proton to the sodium bicarbonate solution. The major method of measuring acid-base balance is the determination of arterial blood gases.

ACID-BASE REGULATORY MECHANISMS
Chemical Buffer Systems

The chemical blood buffers are the first to provide immediate protection against changes in hydrogen ion concentration in ECF. Additionally, these buffers are responsible for transporting excess hydrogen ions to the lungs. The other acid-base regulators do not act as swiftly but do provide a backup system, which results in more thorough protection. Chemical buffers are substances that remove or release hydrogen ions, thereby preventing major changes in the pH. Buffers react only when there is too much acid or base present in the body fluids.

Weakly ionized acids or bases are balanced and paired with a fully ionized salt. Thus when a strong acid or base is present in the body fluid, the buffers act as a sponge that releases or absorbs hydrogen ions as needed to maintain the pH in a range compatible with life. Bicarbonate, phosphate, and the protein buffer are the three primary buffer systems in the ECF. Once these substances react with strong acids or bases, they are in essence "used up" and need to be replaced. This leaves the body vulnerable to continued stress.

Bicarbonate system

Bicarbonate (HCO_3^-) is the metabolic end product of fats and carbohydrates. Sodium, potassium, magnesium, and calcium combine with bicarbonate to form the base bicarbonate.

The major buffer system is the bicarbonate (HCO_3^-)–carbonic acid (H_2CO_3) system. This system maintains the blood pH at 7.35 to 7.45 with a ratio of 20 parts of bicarbonate to 1 part of carbonic acid (Figure 12-13). If this ratio is upset by the addition of a strong acid, some of the bicarbonate will be consumed in the process of neutralizing the strong acid to the weaker carbonic acid. The majority of carbon dioxide diffuses from the cells and combines with plasma proteins. The remaining carbon dioxide dissolved in the blood combines with water to form carbonic acid. Thus when carbonic acid is increased or decreased, producing a different ratio than 20:1, acid-base imbalance results. This system is not especially powerful as a buffer, because 20 times as much bicarbonate buffer is in the form of bicarbonate ion as in the form of dissolved carbon dioxide. Also, the concentration of carbon dioxide and bicarbonate in ECF is not great.[4] However, their role as buffers is very important, since bicarbonate ions are regulated by the kidney and carbon dioxide is regulated by the lungs, which allows the pH concentration of the blood to be increased or decreased via the respiratory and renal systems.

Phosphate system

The phosphate buffer system is composed of $H_2PO_4^-$ and $HPO_4^=$. This system acts in the same manner to regulate acid-base balance as does the bicarbonate system. Strong acids are neutralized to form a weak acid of sodium biphosphate and sodium chloride, resulting in only a very slight change in the pH. When a strong base is added to the system, it is neutralized to form a very weak base and H_2O. This result changes the pH only slightly toward the alkaline side. The total buffering power of this system is less than that of the bicarbonate system, although its role in the kidney tubules does increase the buffering power of the phosphate system.[4]

Protein system

The proteins of the cells and plasma constitute the most plentiful buffer system of the body, mainly because of their high concentration in these locations. Hydrogen ions diffuse in a small amount through cell membranes, bicarbonate diffuses to some extent, whereas carbon dioxide diffuses through the cell membrane readily. The diffusion of the bicarbonate buffer system substance into the cells causes the pH in ICF to change to about the same proportions as the changes in the pH of ECF. The result is that the buffer system inside the cells also assists in buffering the ECF compartment. However, the ability of the intracellular buffer system to assist in regulating acid-base balance in ECF is delayed for several hours because of the slow passage of hydrogen and bicarbonate ions through cell membranes. The protein buffer system acts in a similar fashion as the bicarbonate buffer system. Some amino acids (elements of protein) have free acidic radicals that can dissolve into base and hydrogen ions (Figure 12-14).[4]

Hemoglobin systems

Hemoglobin in red blood cells uses a process called chloride (Cl^-) shift, in which chloride shifts in and out of the red blood cell. This shift is regulated by the level of oxygen in blood plasma. There is an exchange of chloride ions for bicarbonate ions in both

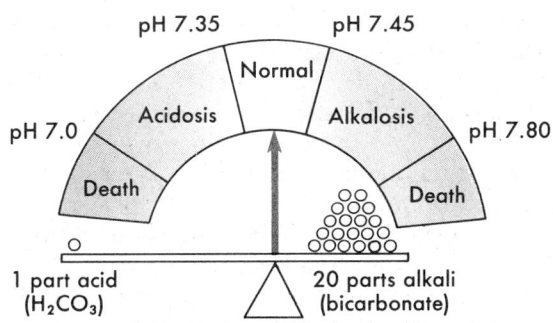

FIGURE 12-13   Relationship of sodium bicarbonate *(BB)* to carbonic acid *(CA)*. Ratio of 20:1 is maintained to achieve a pH of between 7.35 and 7.45.

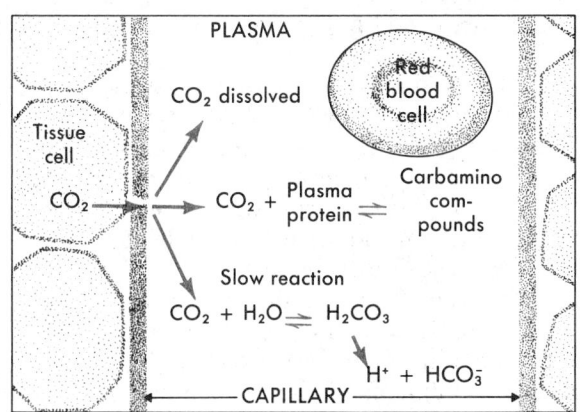

FIGURE 12-14   Carbon dioxide transport in plasma.

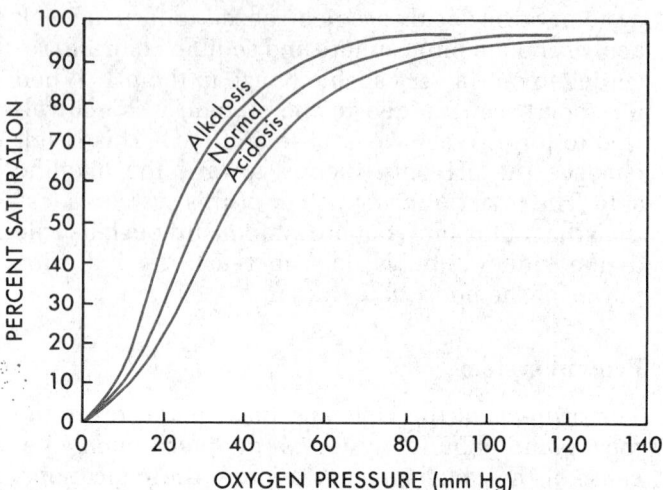

FIGURE 12-15 Oxyhemoglobin dissociation curve showing influence of pH. Acidosis (decrease in pH) shifts curve to right; alkalosis (increase in pH) shifts curve to left.

directions. Figure 12-15 illustrates the oxyhemoglobin dissociation curve.

Lungs

The lungs are the body's next defense in maintaining acid-base balance. This mechanism is one in which the lungs interact with the chemical buffer system to perform their regulatory function. The carbonic acid created by the action of the chemical buffer system in the ECF is transported to the lungs where it is broken down into carbon dioxide and water. These two elements are then exhaled and removed from the body. Hydrogen ions in effect are thereby inactivated. Ventilation is adjusted in response to the amount of carbon dioxide in the blood. A rise in the partial pressure of CO_2 stimulates respiration. A partial pressure of CO_2 greater than 50 mm Hg for a sustained period insensitizes the stimulating effect, and hypoxemia becomes the primary respiratory stimulus.

The lungs also conserve or retain carbon dioxide and thereby assist in compensating for the presence of either metabolic acidosis or alkalosis in the following manner: respirations are increased when metabolic acidosis is present; this results in greater expiration of carbon dioxide, thereby decreasing the acid level; when metabolic alkalosis is present, the lungs retain carbon dioxide by decreasing the respiratory rate, thereby increasing the acid level.

If pulmonary disorders are present, the compensatory mechanisms of the respiratory tract are disrupted. For example, a disorder that obstructs the respiratory tract will cause carbon dioxide retention

and result in respiratory acidosis. In cases of severe pulmonary dysfunction, the lungs cannot compensate for the acid-base imbalance. When conditions cause an increase in respiratory rate and depth, more carbon dioxide is eliminated, resulting in respiratory alkalosis.

Kidneys

The kidneys are the third order of defense in regulating acid-base balance. Compensatory mechanisms of the kidney require hours to several days in which to regulate the acid-base balance. The kidneys regulate acid-base balance by increasing or decreasing bicarbonate concentration in body fluids. Hydrogen ions are excreted and bicarbonate ions retained and reabsorbed because of the action of the renal system. The amount of bicarbonate available for reabsorption can be affected by several different factors. These include the body concentration of acid, stressful situations, use of diuretics, and gastrointestinal losses of bicarbonate and chloride. Another mechanism by which the kidneys compensate for acid-base imbalance is that of acidification of the phosphate buffer by the renal tubule cells. Hydrogen ions in the form of phosphoric acid are excreted in the urine. A third mechanism, the ammonia mechanism, is one in which certain amino acids are chemically changed within the renal tubules into ammonia, which in the presence of hydrogen ions forms ammonium and is excreted in the urine, thereby releasing hydrogen ions from the body. It is noteworthy to mention that the maximum urine acidity is pH 4.0 as compared with pH of blood of 7.4.

In summary, the bicarbonate action is associated with the maintenance of metabolic balance. The carbonic acid action relates to respiratory balance.

ARTERIAL BLOOD GAS ANALYSIS

The analysis of arterial blood gas (ABG) is the primary means by which acid-base imbalances are evaluated.

pH measures the hydrogen ion concentration of the blood and is an indicator of acid-base status. Normal arterial pH is between 7.35 and 7.45. Values less than 7.35 indicate acidosis, whereas values greater than 7.45 indicate a state of alkalosis. (See box on normal blood gas analysis.) Arterial blood gas analysis measures pH, arterial oxygen tension (Pao_2), arterial carbon dioxide tension ($Paco_2$), and either standard plasma bicarbonate (HCO_3^-) or carbon dioxide content (CO_2 content). Table 12-5 summarizes ABG values in disease conditions. $Paco_2$ measures the partial pressure of carbon dioxide in the arterial blood. It is adjusted by means of the rate and depth of respirations. A normal value lies be-

SUMMARY OF NORMAL BLOOD GAS ANALYSIS

pH	7.35 to 7.45
P_{O_2}	80 to 110 mm Hg
P_{CO_2}	35 to 46 mm Hg
CO_2 content	24 to 33 mEq/L
Standard bicarbonate	22 to 26 mEq/L

From Weldy NJ: *Body fluids and electrolytes,* ed 6, St Louis, 1992, Mosby–Year Book.

tween 35 and 45 mm Hg. Values greater than 45 mm Hg indicate alveolar hypoventilation and respiratory acidosis. Values less than 35 mm Hg can result from hyperventilation causing respiratory alkalosis.

Pa_{O_2} is the partial pressure of oxygen in arterial blood. The normal value lies between 80 and 110 mm Hg. A value of less than 60 mm Hg may result in lactic acid production and metabolic acidosis because of anaerobic metabolic processes brought on by hypoxemia. A decrease in the value of Pa_{O_2} occurs with aging.

HCO_3^- is serum bicarbonate, which is the major component of the renal compensatory mechanism. Normal values lie between 22 and 26 mEq/L. It is the main component used by the kidney in regulating acid-base balance. Values less than 22 mEq/L reflect a metabolic acidotic state, whereas values greater than 26 mEq/L indicate the presence of metabolic alkalosis, which may be a primary alkalosis or a response to compensate for respiratory acidosis. The base component may be evaluated by the standard bicarbonate, but some laboratories use the

carbon dioxide content instead. This is a useful test, since it measures both elements of the acid-base proportion and permits an accurate assessment of the clinical problem. The carbon dioxide content represents the sum of all forms of carbon dioxide in the blood, which includes that dissolved in the plasma (measured as P_{CO_2}), that derived from bicarbonate (HCO_3^-), and that derived from plasma carbonic acid (H_2CO_3). Therefore the carbon dioxide content should be thought of as a measure of available base.

Saturation is a measure of the saturation of hemoglobin by oxygen. When the partial pressure of oxygen is decreased below 60 mm Hg, saturation of hemoglobin by oxygen is decreased. The normal saturation values are 95% to 99%.

Acid-Base Imbalance

Acid-base imbalance is reflected in increased acidity or alkalinity of body fluids (Table 12-6). There are two major types of acidosis and alkalosis: respiratory and metabolic. Metabolic acidosis and alkalosis are usually the result of metabolism and utilization of specific types of nutrients. Respiratory acidosis and alkalosis are caused by problems related to pulmonary function or secondary to other disorders that in turn bring about changes in the normal respiratory pattern. Table 12-6 summarizes possible causes of acid-base disturbances.

METABOLIC ACIDOSIS
Definition

Metabolic acidosis is a condition in which there is an increase in hydrogen ion concentration in ECF

TABLE 12-5   ABG Comparisons of Acid-Base Disorders

	Alkalosis			Acidosis		
	Pa_{CO_2}	pH	HCO_3^-	Pa_{CO_2}	pH	HCO_3^-
SIMPLE						
Respiratory	25	7.6	24	50	7.15	25
Metabolic	44	7.54	36	38	7.20	15
COMPENSATED						
Respiratory	25	7.54	21	66	7.37	34
Metabolic	50	7.42	31	23	7.28	9
MIXED DISORDER	40	7.56	38	50	7.20	20

From Horne MM, Swearingen PL: *Pocket guide to fluids and electrolytes,* St Louis, 1989, Mosby–Year Book.

TABLE 12-6   Respiratory and Metabolic Acid-Base Disturbances

Acid-base disturbances	Causes	pH	Pao$_2$	HCO$_3^-$	Mechanisms
Acute respiratory acidosis	Alveolar hypoventilation	Decrease	Increase	Normal range	Increase in CO$_2$, thus H$_2$CO$_3$ and H$^+$; decrease in pH; no time for renal compensation
Chronic respiratory acidosis	Chronic alveolar hypoventilation	Normal range	Increase	Increase	Renal response to increase in CO$_2$: excrete more H$^+$; results in reabsorption of NaHCO$_3$ to restore pH; increased HCO$_3^-$
Acute respiratory alkalosis	Alveolar hyperventilation	Increase	Decrease	Normal range	CO$_2$ "blown off," leaving less end products and excess of base; increased pH
Chronic respiratory alkalosis	Chronic alveolar hyperventilation	Normal range	Decrease	Decrease	Renal response to decreased CO$_2$: excrete more HCO$_3^-$, retain chloride to restore pH; hence less CO$_2$ and less HCO$_3^-$
Metabolic acidosis	Accumulation of (1) lactic acid in circulatory failure, (2) ketoacid in diabetes, or (3) inorganic acids, in renal disease	Decrease	Decrease	Decrease	Addition of large amounts of fixed acids to blood results in loss of base (HCO$_3^-$) and decreased pH; immediate respiratory response results in decreased CO$_2$
Metabolic alkalosis	K$^+$ depletion, vomiting, diarrhea, NaHCO$_3$ excess, or chloride depletion	Increase	Normal range or increase	Increase	Loss of acid or retention of base results in elevated pH and HCO$_3^-$; minimal respiratory response results in normal or elevated CO$_2$

From Wade J: *Respiratory nursing care,* St Louis, 1973, Mosby–Year Book.

that is secondary to an increase in acids produced by the metabolism of nutrients. The ratio of bicarbonate to carbonic acid is decreased from the 20:1 ratio with a decrease in alkaline reserve. The high concentration of hydrogen decreases the pH value to an acidotic level. Metabolic acidosis can be classified as acute and chronic. It is further classified according to the values of the serum anion gap. Serum anion gap refers to unmeasured anions that are negatively charged electrolytes, including sulfates, phosphates, and anions of organic acid, such as lactic acid and ketones. The normal value of these anions is less than 16 mEq/L. When the anion gap value is greater than the normal value, it indicates a greater than normal accumulation of these anions. Figure 12-16 illustrates metabolic acidosis.

Etiology

The primary causes of metabolic acidosis are the result of metabolic and endocrine disorders. Examples include ketoacidosis associated with diabetes melli-

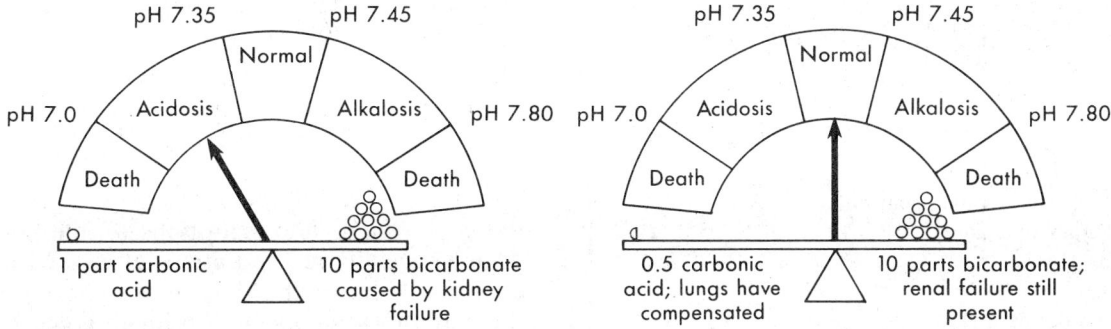

FIGURE 12-16   **A,** Metabolic acidosis. Bicarbonate is decreased because of renal failure. Ratio of carbonic acid to bicarbonate is 10:1; therefore acidosis is present. **B,** Compensation, in which bicarbonate is still decreased but carbonic acid is also decreased. Ratio returns to 20:1, and pH is normal.

tus, use of high fat diets and excessive alcohol intake, lactic acidotic states caused by drug reactions, excessive exercise, respiratory or circulatory failure and renal failure, which causes a decrease in serum bicarbonate below its normal value and a decrease in the pH level. Other causes include normal anion gap acidosis as a direct result of loss of bicarbonate or gain in chlorides, as seen in severe diarrhea, addition of chloride-containing acids (as in parenteral infusions containing isotonic saline or ammonium chloride), and other disorders that result in loss of base. Renal tubular acidosis can cause metabolic acidosis because of the kidney's decreased ability to excrete hydrogen ions. When the nonvolatile acids accumulate at a rate faster than that by which they can be neutralized and regulated by the body's buffer and compensatory systems, metabolic acidosis occurs.

Significant Laboratory Tests

ABG analysis will show a pH value less than 7.35, a serum HCO_3^- level of less than 22 mEq/L (primary acidosis), and a partial pressure CO_2 level less than 38 mm Hg (compensation by lungs). Base excess is always negative. Serum potassium levels may be elevated because of exchange of intracellular potassium for hydrogen ions. Anion gap values are greater than 16 mEq/L (identifies cause). An ECG should be done to detect presence of dysrhythmias caused by increased serum potassium levels.

Therapeutic Management

In most cases, treatment will be aimed at the underlying cause. For example, if the underlying cause is diabetic ketoacidosis, the usual treatment will include insulin and fluids. Insulin increases the passage of glucose out of the intravascular space into the cell. In severe ketoacidosis, IV sodium bicarbonate may be required to increase serum bicarbonate and assist in neutralization of the nonvolatile acid accumulation. An IV solution, such as isotonic saline, 5% dextrose in 0.45% saline, and sodium bicarbonate may be prescribed to increase the serum base levels. Potassium replacement may be required, although hyperkalemia is the usual picture. If hypokalemia should occur, it should be corrected before administration of sodium bicarbonate. If sodium bicarbonate is given in the presence of hypokalemia, the acidosis may be corrected, causing potassium to shift back into the cells and resulting in a severe hypokalemia culminating in cardiac arrest. Mechanical ventilation might be necessary and should be set no lower than the patient's compensatory hyperventilation efforts, which are attempting to compensate for the acidotic state. If the cause is an alcoholic ketoacidosis, IV glucose and saline are usually prescribed. Correction of diarrhea requires addressing other fluid and electrolyte disturbances that may be present.

Hemodialysis or peritoneal dialysis may be prescribed for the patient in acute renal failure to increase the level of serum bicarbonate. If the underlying cause is drug toxicity, the treatment will depend on the compound ingested. Use of dialysis may be prescribed. Lactic acidosis treatment is aimed at the underlying cause. Sodium bicarbonate administration may be prescribed but is only a temporary measure.

NURSING MANAGEMENT OF THE PATIENT WITH METABOLIC ACIDOSIS
Assessment

Signs and symptoms are related to the underlying disorder and the severity of the acid-base imbalance. Table 12-7 compares metabolic acidosis and

POSSIBLE CAUSES OF ACID-BASE DISTURBANCES

Respiratory acidosis

Primary factor: hypoventilation
    Pulmonary disease
    Drugs
    Obesity
    Mechanical asphyxia
    Sleep

Metabolic acidosis

Primary factor: addition of large amounts of fixed acids to body fluids
    Lactic acidosis (circulatory failure)
    Ketoacidosis (diabetes, starvation)
    Phosphates and sulfates (renal disease)
    Acid ingestion (salicylates)
    Secondary to respiratory alkalosis
    Adrenal insufficiency

Respiratory alkalosis

Primary factor: hyperventilation
    Overventilation on a ventilator
    Response to acidosis
    Bacteremia
    Thyrotoxicosis
    Fever
    Hepatic failure
    Response to hypoxia
    Hysteria

Metabolic alkalosis

Primary factor: retention of base or removal of acid from body fluids
    Excessive gastric drainage
    Vomiting
    K^+ depletion (diuretic therapy)
    Burns
    Excessive $NaHCO_3$ administration

From Wade J: *Respiratory nursing care*, St Louis, 1973, Mosby–Year Book.

alkalosis. Examples include headache, drowsiness, vomiting, diarrhea, increased respiratory rate and depth when HCO_3^- value is low, peripheral vasodilation, decreased cardiac output with bradycardia, presence of hyperkalemia, stupor, coma, twitching, and convulsions. Ketone accumulation often produces a fruity-smelling breath. Hyperpnea may be present (Kussmaul's respirations).

Nursing Diagnosis

The following general nursing diagnosis is suggested:
    High risk for injury related to altered sensorium

Implementation

Assess for signs and symptoms of diabetic ketoacidosis especially in the patient at risk with diabetes mellitus. Monitor the degree of hyperglycemia and the patient's response to insulin and bicarbonate administration. Use caution in administration of bicarbonate, and monitor arterial blood gas levels for prevention of metabolic alkalosis.

Blood glucose levels should be monitored to prevent hypoglycemia and cerebral edema. Monitor potassium levels for evidence of hyperkalemia or hypokalemia. Observe for signs of decreased cardiac function and dysrhythmias. Observe rate and depth of respirations (Kussmaul's respirations), and check breath for fruity odor. Observe skin and mucous membrane for redness caused by peripheral vasodilation. The patient may need a retention catheter if in a coma or stuporous. The nurse should monitor neurologic status and should use safety precautions, such as bed rails.

METABOLIC ALKALOSIS
Definition

Metabolic alkalosis is characterized by a decrease in hydrogen ion concentration or an increase in serum bicarbonate. It may result from a metabolic disturbance, causing a rise in serum base, or it may be caused by a decrease in serum acid levels. A compensatory increase in the partial pressure of carbon dioxide will usually be evident. Hypoventilation occurs in an attempt to raise the level of carbonic acid to increase hydrogen ions. Normally functioning kidneys respond by excretion of sodium bicarbonate in the urine. Ammonia formation is restricted by the kidneys, and hydrogen ions in lactic and ketone acids are reabsorbed via the kidneys. Urine pH rises to the alkaline level as a result of the compensatory processes in the kidney.

Etiology

Gastrointestinal loss via emesis or gastric suction is the primary cause of metabolic alkalosis. Such losses include hydrogen and chloride anions. Loss of hydrogen ions occurs from gastric suction. Other causes include overcorrection of metabolic acidosis, potassium deficiency, hyperaldosteronism, and the use of thiazide diuretic therapy, which increases renal excretion of acid.

Parenteral administration of sodium bicarbonate

TABLE 12-7   Summary of Acid-Base Imbalance

Type	Etiology	Compensation
Respiratory acidosis (carbonic acid excess)	Chronic lung disease Surgery	Buffer system Renal system: excrete more H^+
Respiratory alkalosis (carbonic acid deficit)	Increased pulmonary ventilation Encephalitis Hypoxia Fever Salicylate poisoning	Buffer system Renal system: excrete more HCO_3^-
Metabolic acidosis (base deficit)	Diabetic ketoacidosis Uremic acidosis Diarrhea	Buffer system Respiratory system: rapid and deep Renal system: excrete more H^+, retain more HCO_3^-
Metabolic alkalosis (base excess)	Excessive ingestion of base (antacids) Vomiting Gastric suction	Buffer system Respiratory system: slow and shallow Renal system: retain more H^+, excrete more HCO_3^-

From Weldy NJ: *Body fluids and electrolytes,* ed 6, St Louis, 1992, Mosby–Year Book.

in cardiopulmonary resuscitation attempts may result in metabolic alkalosis. Too rapid relief of chronic respiratory acidosis via inappropriate settings on mechanical ventilators also initiates this condition.

Significant Laboratory Tests

ABG values help determine the severity of the alkalotic condition and the patient's response to therapy. The pH value will be greater than 7.45. Serum carbon dioxide content level will increase above 33 mEq/L. Pa_{CO_2} will remain unchanged unless the lungs attempt to compensate for the alkalosis. If compensated, the Pa_{CO_2} will rise in an attempt to increase the carbonic acid level to neutralize the base. Serum bicarbonate will be greater than 21 mEq/L. The serum potassium and chloride levels will be decreased. Base excess will be positive.

Therapeutic Management

Treatment depends on the underlying clinical problem. If the condition is mild, specific therapeutic interventions may not be required. Treatment is directed at improving the patient's ventilation with the procedures geared to the cause of the ventilatory difficulty.

Potassium chloride and normal saline solutions are used to replace gastric losses unless the patient has congestive heart failure. Potassium is indicated

for hypokalemic conditions. Chloride losses can be restored simultaneously by administering potassium chloride.

The administration of sodium and potassium chloride is effective in posthypercapneic alkalosis. This condition occurs when chronic CO_2 retention is corrected too rapidly, as by mechanical ventilation equipment. It is important that potassium and chloride deficits be corrected before definitive treatment for metabolic alkalosis, since if potassium and chloride are not available, the kidneys' ability to excrete excess bicarbonate is compromised. The result would be that the metabolic alkalotic state would continue.

In severe cases, intravenous administration of isotonic hydrochloride or ammonium chloride may be prescribed, especially if potassium and chloride salts are not the appropriate treatment, as in patients with cardiac disorders. This preparation should be administered slowly and be checked frequently for signs of infiltration, since it can damage tissue. This therapy is not appropriate for patients who are in renal or hepatic failure.

NURSING MANAGEMENT OF THE PATIENT WITH METABOLIC ALKALOSIS
Assessment

Signs and symptoms of metabolic alkalosis are usually the result of the body's attempt to compensate acid-base imbalance by decreased alveolar ventilation. The neuromuscular system, lungs, and heart are primarily affected by metabolic alkalosis. Symptoms include numbness and tingling of extremities, nervousness, irritability, disorientation caused by hyperirritability of nerve tissue, and confusion. Seizures may occur. Hypocalcemia may be present, which if severe enough may lead to tetany. This is a result of decreased ionization of calcium compounds.

If hypokalemia is present, signs and symptoms reflective of cardiovascular abnormalities, such as dysrhythmias, postural hypotension, muscle weakness, flaccidity, and paralytic ileus, may occur.

Nursing Diagnosis

Nursing diagnoses and interventions are specific to the underlying clinical problem. An example is as follows:

Knowledge deficit related to precautions needed when taking thiazide diuretics

Implementation

Assess the patient at risk for metabolic alkalosis. Prevent metabolic alkalosis by teaching the patient the use of medications with high bicarbonate content. Use saline solution to irrigate nasogastric tubes.

Monitor for signs and symptoms of metabolic alkalosis, as well as arterial blood gases and report abnormal findings. Monitor the patient with metabolic alkalosis for signs and symptoms of hypokalemia/hypocalcemia. Serum electrolyte values should be monitored to check for changes and trends. Monitor ECG tracings for evidence of dysrhythmias. Monitor the type of diuretic in use and its effects. Measure and document fluid removed by suction and weigh the patient daily to determine fluid volume status.

Hydrogen receptor antagonists should be administered as prescribed to block hydrochloric acid and fluid secretion from the gastric area. Dilute potassium when giving intravenous infusions containing potassium salts, and monitor infusion rates to prevent damage to blood vessels. If ammonium chloride 0.9% is administered, the rate of administration is slow (5 mL of 1% solution/min). Too rapid administration may cause an overcorrection and lead to metabolic acidosis. Seizure/safety precautions should be observed.

RESPIRATORY ACIDOSIS
Definition

Respiratory acidosis is characterized by hypoventilation caused by a reduction in alveolar ventilation manifested by an increase in Pa_{CO_2} greater than 45 mm Hg. In acute respiratory acidosis the hypoventi-

lation results in an elevated Pa_{CO_2}, which occurs because of the inability of the lungs to excrete carbon dioxide satisfactorily. Blood pH is altered by the increase in Pa_{CO_2}; the amount of decrease in the pH value is determined by how quickly the body can compensate acid-base balance via its regulatory mechanisms. The acute type is primarily caused by a sudden failure of ventilation. The prognosis is related to the severity of the underlying disorder, as well as the patient's general condition.

Acute respiratory acidosis is considered a primary type of acidosis, whereas chronic respiratory acidosis is usually a compensated type. Chronic respiratory acidosis is a result of long-standing pulmonary disease, such as bronchitis, or chronic obstructive pulmonary disease (COPD). A near normal pH is often present if renal function is normal, even in the presence of a Pa_{CO_2} greater than 50 mm Hg. Chronic compensatory metabolic alkalosis with serum HCO_3^- greater than 26 mEq/L is present, resulting in compensated respiratory acidosis with a near normal pH. When the patient becomes ill with another clinical disorder, such as pneumonia, the Pa_{CO_2} rises rapidly with a possibility of decompensation and a decrease in pH.

Etiology

Causes of acute respiratory acidosis include acute respiratory failure caused by such conditions as pneumonia, acute pulmonary edema, cardiac arrest, laryngospasms, and oversedation with medications that depress the respiratory center, such as narcotics, sedatives, hypnotics, and anesthetics. Trauma to the medulla or chest wall interferes with the ability of respiratory muscles to ventilate carbon dioxide and take in oxygen. Pharyngeal obstruction leading to asphyxiation and use of mechanical ventilation devices in an inappropriate manner are other causes of acute respiratory acidosis.

Causes of chronic respiratory acidosis include chronic obstructive lung disease, bronchitis, bronchiectasis, advanced multiple sclerosis, and neuromuscular disease, such as myasthenia gravis.

Significant Laboratory Tests

Significant diagnostic tests in acute respiratory acidosis include an evaluation of the findings of ABG measurements. Pa_{CO_2} greater than 45 mm Hg and a pH less than 7.35 are significant. Serum bicarbonate (serum HCO_3^-) initial values are normal unless a mixed disorder is present. Serum electrolyte values are usually normal.

Diagnostic tests that are significant in chronic respiratory acidosis include ABG values with Pa_{CO_2} greater than 45 mm Hg. The pH may be less than 7.35 or within the normal lower range because of renal compensation, except in cases of acute pulmonary infections. If Paco$_2$ shows an abrupt increase, the pH will be lower than normal. Serum HCO$_3^-$ is a primary indicator for the presence of chronic compensated respiratory acidosis. An increased serum HCO$_3^-$ with a pH near normal indicates a fully compensated respiratory acidosis. X-ray examination of the chest should be done to determine extent of pulmonary disease and other changes that may compromise the compensatory mechanisms. ECG is useful in identification of any cardiac involvement. Sputum culture may be ordered to determine if infection is present.

Therapeutic Management

The treatment for respiratory acidosis is geared toward the correction of the underlying source of alveolar hypoventilation. Bronchodilators, oxygen, and antibiotics may be prescribed for pulmonary infections. Removal of foreign bodies that obstruct the airway is another example of correcting the underlying problem. Restoration of normal acid-base balance is the main goal of therapy. If Paco$_2$ is severely elevated and accompanied by signs of cyanosis, supportive mechanisms, such as intubation and mechanical ventilation, may be necessary. Bicarbonate is not used if at all possible, since it may initiate alkalosis when the acidotic state has been corrected.

The treatment for chronic respiratory acidosis includes bronchodilators and antibiotics as indicated. Narcotics and sedatives should be avoided because of their effect on the central nervous system, unless the patient is being mechanically ventilated. Administration of IV fluids for hydration and for facilitating removal of thick pulmonary secretions may be prescribed. Chest physiotherapy measures, such as postural drainage, are useful to aid in the removal of drainage and sputum. Oxygen therapy may be provided. If so, it is absolutely necessary to keep the rate of flow no greater than 3 L/min, because in chronic pulmonary conditions, hypoxia rather than hypercapnia stimulates the respiratory center.

NURSING MANAGEMENT OF THE PATIENT WITH RESPIRATORY ACIDOSIS
Assessment

Acute respiratory acidosis symptoms include central nervous system (CNS) disturbances resulting in restlessness, disorientation, apprehension, somnolence, fine tremors, or coma. Complaints of headache; feelings of fullness in the head; vertigo; warm, flushed skin; dyspnea; and depressed reflexes are other symptoms reflective of acute respiratory acidosis.

Chronic respiratory acidosis symptoms reflect on Paco$_2$ values. If the Paco$_2$ is within a range in which the body can compensate for the imbalance, symptoms may not be specific. When there is a rapid rise

in Paco$_2$, symptoms will include dull headache, weakness, dyspnea, agitation, and insomnia, which may progress to coma. Symptoms of the underlying disease process will be present. Other signs include tachypnea and cyanosis. If severe hypercapnia develops, neurologic symptoms will be caused by cerebral vasodilation. These include increased intracranial pressure, papilledema, dilated conjunctiva, and dilation of facial blood vessels.

Nursing Diagnosis

An example of a nursing diagnosis reflective of respiratory acidosis follows:

Activity intolerance related to insufficient oxygenation secondary to chronic impaired gas exchange

Implementation

Identify the patient at risk for impaired gas exchange with chronic pulmonary dysfunction. Prevent secondary infection, and observe for signs and symptoms of overriding disease processes. Monitor ABG values for changes in values and to assess response to therapy. Observe for critical changes in respiratory, CNS, and cardiovascular status.

Adequate hydration should be maintained. Mechanical ventilation equipment should be used appropriately, checking rate and volume. Provide adequate humidification when giving oxygen. The oxygen rate should be no higher than 3 L/min. In chronic respiratory acidosis, high concentrations of oxygen may precipitate stupor and coma, since hypoxia is the stimulus for the respiratory center in the medulla for patients with chronic CO$_2$ retention.

Compare pretreatment status with posttreatment status. Assess for presence of bowel sounds and gastric distention, which may restrict respiratory function of the diaphragm. Pursed lip breathing should be encouraged.

RESPIRATORY ALKALOSIS
Definition

Respiratory alkalosis is a condition in which there is an increase in the rate of alveolar ventilation. It is marked by a decrease in Paco$_2$ below 35 mm Hg.

Acute respiratory alkalosis is caused by hyperventilation, which is often related to bouts of anxiety. Other conditions that result in acute hypoxia can trigger respiratory alkalosis. There is a rise in pH, which is modified to some degree by intracellular buffering. Hydrogen ions are released from tissue buffers that then lower the plasma HCO$_3^-$ concentration. Usually acute respiratory alkalosis is resolved before kidney compensation can occur because of the slower response of the renal system.

Chronic respiratory alkalosis is a condition

marked by a state of chronic hypocapnea (low $Paco_2$). This low concentration stimulates the renal compensatory mechanism, which results in a decrease in serum bicarbonate. It takes several days for the renal system to respond to this condition.

Etiology

Causes of respiratory alkalosis may be classified into two types: pulmonary and nonpulmonary, which can be either acute or chronic types. Understanding of the mechanisms used by the body to compensate for respiratory alkalosis can be ascertained by using the acute versus chronic classification.

Causes of acute respiratory alkalosis include anxiety; acute episodes of hypoxia caused by pulmonary disorders, such as pneumonia, pulmonary edema, and pulmonary thromboembolism; salicylate toxicity; acute asthma; elevated body temperature; sepsis; excessive mechanical ventilation; and trauma to the respiratory center in the medulla.

Causes of chronic respiratory alkalosis include cerebral disorders, such as tumors or encephalitis; chronic hypoxia caused by heart disease; fibrotic lung disease; chronic hepatic disease; and pregnancy because of the increase in progesterone level, which sensitizes the respiratory center to CO_2.

Significant Laboratory Tests

Significant laboratory tests for the presence of acute respiratory alkalosis include ABG values. The $Paco_2$ value is less than 35 mm Hg. The pH value is greater than 7.45. Serum bicarbonate is within normal range in the acute stage but will decrease within several hours.

Serum phosphate levels may be decreased below 3 mg/dL. ECG tracings may reflect dysrhythmias. Urine pH will be above 7.

Significant laboratory test results for the presence of chronic respiratory alkalosis include ABG values for $Paco_2$ of less than 35 mm Hg with a pH value near normal. The $Paco_2$ value may be decreased in the presence of hypoxia. Serum bicarbonate levels decrease because of renal compensatory measures.

Phosphate levels will be decreased to as low as 0.5 mg/dL in the presence of severe hyperventilation. The alkalotic state causes more phosphate to be transported into cells.

Therapeutic Management

The treatment of acute respiratory alkalosis is aimed at the correction of the underlying clinical problem. If anxiety is the underlying problem, reassurance and making the patient aware that hyperventilation is responsible for the symptoms are the prescribed treatments. If symptoms of anxiety are severe, breathing into a paper bag or rebreathing CO_2

through a special device will increase the $Paco_2$ level.

If hypoxia is the cause, oxygen therapy may be prescribed. Sedatives may be prescribed if the patient is extremely anxious.

The treatment of chronic respiratory alkalosis is geared toward the correction of the underlying cause. Oxygen therapy is administered if hypoxia is present.

NURSING MANAGEMENT OF THE PATIENT WITH RESPIRATORY ALKALOSIS
Assessment

Signs and symptoms of acute respiratory alkalosis include anxiety, apprehension, circumoral numbness, and feeling of lightheadedness caused by a low $Paco_2$, which causes cerebral vasoconstriction and thereby decreases cerebral blood flow. Other symptoms include those of serum calcium deficit, including potential for cardiac dysrhythmias. Symptoms under the rubric of hyperventilation syndrome include palpatations, increased sweating, nausea and vomiting, dry mouth, epigastric pain, blurred vision, feeling of tightness in the chest, and possibly loss of consciousness because of cerebral ischemia.

Nursing Diagnosis

An example of a nursing diagnosis related to acute respiratory alkalosis follows:

Ineffective breathing pattern related to hyperventilation secondary to anxiety

Implementation

Identify the patient at risk, and allay anxiety by reassuring the patient. Encourage the patient to breathe slowly, and monitor the patient's breathing. Administer sedatives or tranquilizers as prescribed. The patient should rebreathe into a paper bag or use a CO_2 rebreathing apparatus. Monitor the patient's cardiac rhythm.

Imbalances in Elderly Persons

It is difficult to separate the effects of age-related changes from those caused by disease processes and life-style. These influences occur over the life span, and because the effects are cumulative, their impact is more evident in older persons. In the older adult who has any condition involving renal function, fluid and electrolyte balance, or plasma volume and osmolality, more serious consequences are likely to occur. Older adults are more likely than younger persons to develop hypovolemia and dehydration secondary to diuretic medications.

A health history can uncover patterns of recent injury or illness that require further investigation. Many elderly people take multiple medications, and a thorough medication history must be made, including over-the-counter medications.

RESPIRATORY

Age-related changes often occur in the upper airway because of calcification of cartilage, altered neuromuscular functioning, and slowing of reflexes. These changes result in mouth breathing, diminished coughing, and a less efficient gag reflex. The increased use of accessory muscles and increased energy necessary for respiratory efficiency are caused by chest wall stiffness and weakened muscular strength. The efficiency of gas exchange is diminished along with decreased Pa_{O_2} because of enlargement of the alveoli, thinning of alveolar walls, and a decreased number of capillaries. A decrease in elastic recoil and early airway closure lead to changes in lung volumes and decreased overall efficiency. Slight amounts of secretions in the alveolar tree can reduce ventilation. The decreased ventilation causes a retention of CO_2, which in turn will elevate bicarbonate levels.

CARDIOVASCULAR

The circulatory system may be difficult to evaluate because of hard, fragile arteries and chronic cardiovascular diseases. Cardiac output diminishes because of the rigid arteries and stasis throughout the vascular system. The pooled blood raises capillary pressure and forces more fluid into the interstitial tissue, producing edema. Systemic blood pressure is elevated. Cerebral blood flow decreases, peripheral resistance increases, and the left ventricular wall hypertrophies. Elderly persons are more susceptible to postural hypotension and to arrhythmias. Overloading the vascular system with fluids can result in congestive heart failure or pulmonary edema. Dependent edema and distended neck veins are found on assessment. Potassium deficiency may occur because of the use of laxatives, furosemide, antibiotics, corticosteroids, licorice, and diarrhea. Hypokalemia results in weakness, cardiac arrhythmias, and digitalis toxicity. Risk factors that may add to the cardiovascular problems in elderly persons include obesity, inactivity, smoking, and dietary habits that lead to hyperlipidemia.

GASTROINTESTINAL

Age-related changes in the gastrointestinal tract include less efficient churning, decreased taste sensation, decreased gastric secretions, loss of elasticity in the intestinal wall, slower motility, and decreased blood flow to the intestine. These changes may lead to malnutrition, dehydration, constipation, and decreased absorption of iron, calcium, vitamin B_{12}, and folic acid.

Elderly persons may be taking medications that may cause adverse reactions such as anorexia, dry mouth, paralytic ileus, diarrhea, or constipation. Investigate medications being taken as well as the type of diet the person usually follows. Use of laxatives and enemas may lead to hypokalemia, hypoalbuminemia, decreased calcium absorption, malabsorption, and acidosis. Assess the nutritional status of older adults, and educate them about basic nutritional needs. Older adults who have an illness or take medications or chemicals that interfere with homeostasis, nutrition, or digestion may need to have their diet modified to compensate for those effects. Tap water enemas until clear can precipitate an electrolyte imbalance and should not be performed.

COGNITIVE-PERCEPTUAL

It is important to assess the cognitive pattern of the elderly patient. Confusion is a common finding that may be the result of a medication or fluid and electrolyte imbalance. A state of confusion can be acute or chronic. The chronic confusion usually described by the patient's family needs to be investigated, because chronic confusion may be a depressive state. Acute confusion may be related to digitalis toxicity, depression, malnutrition, or all in combination.

In beginning an assessment, start with the patient's most recent life changes and current medication regimen. Life changes in elderly persons are stressful and do affect the cognitive state. Focus on the patient's reasoning ability, memory, and orientation. Changes in the patient's mood and affect also need to be investigated.

MUSCULOSKELETAL

Observe the patient's gait. Is the gait steady? Does the individual experience leg cramps, paresthesias? Does the patient report pain, and if so how is it treated? Elderly people often medicate themselves for frequent aches and pains, leading to a potential toxic reaction with their prescribed medications. A common problem is the use of over-the-counter antacids, which can have a high magnesium level. In a patient with an underlying renal pathologic condition, this combination can cause acute confusion, cramping of the legs, and dysrhythmias from hypermagnesemia.

URINARY

Age-related changes in the urinary system may directly affect fluid and electrolyte balance. Some of those changes include a decreased number of nephrons, decreased renal blood flow, decreased glomerular filtration rate, hypertrophy of muscles, relaxation of pelvic floor muscles, contractions during bladder filling, decreased bladder capacity, and degenerative changes in the cerebral cortex. These age-related changes result in a decline in efficiency of homeostatic mechanisms, decreased bladder capacity, nocturia, urinary urgency and frequency, chronic residual urine predisposing to infection, and delayed excretion of water-soluble medications.

Older adults may not experience thirst sensation in response to fluid deprivation. Older adults may not drink enough water to rehydrate their body fluids even when fluids are accessible. When there are conditions that place additional demands on fluid and electrolyte balance, such as elevated body temperature or infection, this reduced thirst sensation may interfere with the normal compensation. Assessing the older person for inadequate hydration is especially important, followed by providing the additional fluids needed in an acceptable way.

CRITICAL THINKING QUESTIONS

1 What are the common causes of fluid volume deficit? overload? clinical signs and symptoms?

2 Name three compartments where fluid is found in the body.

3 What are the means by which fluids move in the body?

4 Describe diffusion, facilitated diffusion, filtration, and osmosis.

5 Describe how aldosterone influences fluid volume.

6 Describe the function of the antidiuretic hormone (ADH).

7 List the important assessment areas to evaluate the fluid status of a patient.

8 When diuretic medications are given, what might be the effect on electrolyte balance?

9 If you are given a report that a 55-year-old patient had 400 mL of urine output for the past 24 hours, what would you want to find out next?

10 If you are caring for Mr. Jones, who weighed 171 pounds yesterday, and today his weight is 180 pounds, what would you find out next? What might this represent?

11 List the function of the following electrolytes: sodium, potassium, calcium, magnesium, and phosphate.

12 Describe the likely causes, signs and symptoms, and expected treatment and nursing care for potassium deficit, sodium excess, magnesium deficit, and calcium excess.

13 Identify factors that might lead to fluid or electrolyte imbalance in elderly persons.

14 Describe the three mechanisms necessary to maintain normal hydrogen ion concentration in the body. Include the following body systems: buffer, respiratory, and renal.

15 Describe the probable causes and effects of metabolic acidosis, metabolic alkalosis, respiratory acidosis, and respiratory alkalosis.

16 Differentiate among simple, compensated, acute, and chronic respiratory or metabolic acidosis and alkalosis.

17 Describe the nursing process for patients with acid-base imbalance.

18 Identify nursing implications for the elderly patient in relationship to fluid, electrolyte, and acid-base imbalance.

BIBLIOGRAPHY

Current

1. Falk B et al: Effects of caffeine ingestion on body fluid balance and thermoregulation during exercise, *Can J Physiol Pharmacol* 68(7):889, July 1990.
2. Fortney SM et al: Changes in body fluid compartments during a 28-day bed rest, *Aviation Space Environ Med* 62(2):97, 1991.
3. Ganong WF: *Review of medical physiology*, ed 13, Los Altos, Calif, 1987, Lange Medical Publications.
4. Guyton RC: *Textbook of medical physiology*, ed 8, Philadelphia, 1991, WB Saunders Co.
5. Horne M, Swearingen PL: *Pocket guide to fluids and electrolytes*, St Louis, 1989, Mosby–Year Book.
6. Howard RL, Schrier RW: A unifying hypothesis of sodium and water regulation in health and disease, *Hormone Res* 34(3-4):118, 1990.
7. Jones DH: Fluid therapy in the PACU, *Crit Care Nurs Clin North Am* 3(1):109, 1991.
8. Lowenstein J: *Acid and bases: a guide to understanding acid-base disorders*, New York, 1992, Oxford University Press, Inc.
9. Maxwell MH, Kleeman CR: *Clinical disorders of fluid and electrolyte metabolism*, ed 4, New York, 1987, McGraw-Hill, Inc.
10. Metheny N: Why worry about IV fluids? *Am J Nurs* 90(6):50, 1990.
11. Metheny N: *Fluid and electrolyte balance: nursing considerations*, Philadelphia, 1992, JB Lippincott Co.
12. Metheny N, Eisenberg P, McSweeney M: Effect of feeding tube properties and three irrigants on clogging rates, *Nurs Res* 37(3):165, 1988.
13. Miller C: *Nursing care of older adults: theory and practice*, Glenview, Ill, 1990, Scott, Foresman/Little, Brown Higher Education.
14. Plumer A, Cosentino F: *Principles and practice of intravenous therapy*, ed 4, Boston, 1987, Little, Brown & Co.
15. Reedy DF: Fluid intake: how can you prevent dehydration? *Geriatr Nurs*, p 224, July/Aug 1988.
16. Sommers M: Rapid fluid resuscitation: how to correct dangerous deficits, *Nurs 90* 20(1):52, 1990.
17. Weldy NJ: *Body fluids and electrolytes: a programmed presentation*, ed 6, St Louis, 1992, Mosby–Year Book.
18. Wyngaarden JB, Smith LH: *Cecil textbook of medicine*, ed 18, Philadelphia, 1988, WB Saunders Co.

Classic

19. Goldberger E: *A primer of water, electrolytes, and acid-base syndromes*, ed 7, Philadelphia, 1986, Lea & Febiger.
20. Wade J: *Respiratory nursing care*, St Louis, 1973, Mosby–Year Book.

CHAPTER THIRTEEN

Shock

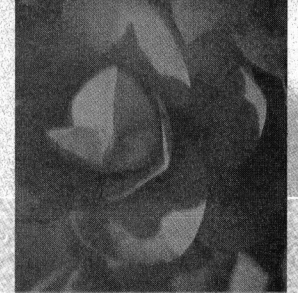

LEARNING OBJECTIVES

1 Differentiate the three types of shock according to definition, etiology, and pathophysiologic alterations.
2 Summarize the cellular changes common to all forms of shock.
3 Compare the characteristics and clinical evidence of the four stages of shock.
4 Explain the neural, hormonal, and chemical changes that occur during the compensatory stage of shock.
5 List the clinical findings and laboratory abnormalities present in the compensatory and progressive stages of shock.
6 Differentiate definitive and supportive therapy for the major types of shock.
7 Review specific nursing actions to prevent the major types of shock.
8 Explain the components of the nursing assessment of the shock patient, including clinical findings and invasive hemodynamic parameters.
9 Identify appropriate nursing diagnoses for the shock patient.
10 Formulate a nursing care plan for the shock patient, including expected patient outcomes and specific nursing interventions.

KEY TERMS

IN TODAY'S world of health care, few clinical problems demand the high level of nursing knowledge and performance of complex technical skills that shock does. A complex disease process, shock affects function of all organs and can deteriorate to multiple organ failure and death. This chapter helps the nurse understand what shock is and what it is not, the major causes of shock, how to recognize shock as it develops and progresses, and what to anticipate in the medical and nursing management of the shock patient.

Nurses must understand shock because almost all hospitalized patients have the potential to develop shock. The causes of shock can be categorized in relation to three major types of shock: hypovolemic, cardiogenic, and distributive. An understanding of the similarities and differences in each classification will help alert the adult health nurse to patients who are at risk to develop specific forms of shock. Study of the progression of the shock state will reveal many of the compensatory mechanisms as sympathetic nervous system stimulation. Progression of the shock state to organ failure incorporates aspects of cardiac failure, respiratory failure, and renal failure. These potential complications of shock underscore the urgency in recognizing and treating this dreaded problem.

DEFINITIONS OF SHOCK

Shock is a life-threatening condition involving almost every organ system. It is not simply a problem of decreased blood pressure; rather, it is a problem of inadequate tissue perfusion. Shock can be defined as a complex syndrome of inadequate blood flow to body tissues resulting in cellular dysfunction and eventual organ failure. Tissue perfusion is inadequate to supply oxygen and nutrients to cells. As the result of an imbalance between oxygen supply and demand, a functional impairment develops in cells, tissues, organs, and eventually body systems.

CLASSIFICATIONS OF SHOCK

Shock can be classified into three major types: hypovolemic, cardiogenic, and distributive. These classifications help the nurse understand the numerous causes of shock and appreciate that all shock is not alike. Differences among the major types influence the clinical picture of shock, the anticipated interventions, and the nursing care.

Hypovolemic Shock

Hypovolemic shock results from decreased intravascular volume. Inadequate fluid volume exists to effectively fill the intravascular compartment. As a result, blood flow and tissue perfusion are decreased.

Hypovolemic shock can develop because of internal fluid shifts or external loss of fluid. Internal fluid shifts occur when fluid moves out of the vascular compartment into another body compartment, such as the interstitial space, but the fluid is not lost from the body. Patients can experience internal fluid shifts because of the following:

1. Internal hemorrhage. Loss of blood from the vascular space can occur with numerous conditions, such as fractures of long bones, ruptured spleen, hemothorax, aortic dissection, ruptured ectopic pregnancy, and hemorrhagic pancreatitis.
2. Pooling of fluid in the interstitial space. This problem develops because of increased capillary permeability. It can develop after thermal injuries, in patients with allergic reactions, and as a result of bacterial toxins.
3. Sequestration of fluid in third spaces. The term *third space* actually refers to the interstitial space; however, its meaning has been expanded to include a closed compartment, such as the peritoneal cavity. Patients with cirrhosis and ascites accumulate fluid in their peritoneal cavities and subsequently can develop inadequate intravascular volume.

External loss of fluid results from the loss of whole blood, the loss of plasma, or the loss of large amounts of any body fluid. The loss of whole blood, or hemorrhage, is the most common cause of hypovolemic shock. External hemorrhage can complicate a patient's postoperative course or can follow a traumatic event, such as a stabbing or amputation.

The loss of plasma (i.e., the fluid part of the blood) occurs when fluid from the blood shifts from the vascular compartment and subsequently is lost from the body. Displaced plasma fluid can be lost from exposed areas, such as thermal injuries or large exudative lesions (e.g., decubiti, extensive dermatitis).

External losses of body fluid from any cause can produce hypovolemic shock if the magnitude of fluid loss is great. Body fluid can be lost via the gastrointestinal tract with vomiting, diarrhea, fistulas, ostomies, and nasogastric suction. Fluid can be lost from the body via excessive sweating, as in heat stroke, and it can be lost through the kidneys because of diuretic administration, diabetes insipidus (a deficiency of antidiuretic hormone), Addison's disease (a deficiency of aldosterone), and hyperglycemic osmotic diuresis (as in diabetic ketoacidosis). If these fluid losses are coupled with inadequate fluid volume replacement, severe dehydration and hypovolemic shock can result.

Pathophysiology

When the intravascular or plasma volume decreases, the body attempts to compensate by mobilizing fluid from the interstitial compartment. Approximately 500 mL of fluid can be mobilized from the interstitial space and moved into the blood vessels. If this fluid shift cannot compensate for the volume deficit, approximately 500 mL of fluid can be mobilized from the intracellular compartment and moved through the interstitial compartment into the vascular space. Because of these fluid shifts a small decrease in the intravascular volume does not produce a decrease in blood pressure. Approximately 15% to 25% of intravascular volume (750 to 1250 mL) must be lost before the deficit in intravascular volume results in a decreased arterial blood pressure.

Figure 13-1 diagrams the sequence of events whereby reduced intravascular volume leads to decreased blood pressure and inadequate tissue perfusion. When the intravascular volume falls, inadequate volume remains to fill the circulatory network. Venous return of blood to the heart falls, and the heart chambers do not fill fully with blood. As a result of decreased filling, stroke volume decreases. Stroke volume is a determinant of cardiac output; therefore when stroke volume decreases, so does cardiac output. As cardiac output falls, the blood pressure decreases. When the blood pressure decreases, capillary blood flow is diminished and oxygen delivery to body cells is inadequate.

Cardiogenic Shock

Cardiogenic shock is a serious form of shock caused by the impaired pumping ability of the heart. Right or left ventricular dysfunction can lead to this form of shock. Left ventricular failure is more commonly involved in the shock process and can reduce blood flow into the systemic circulation.

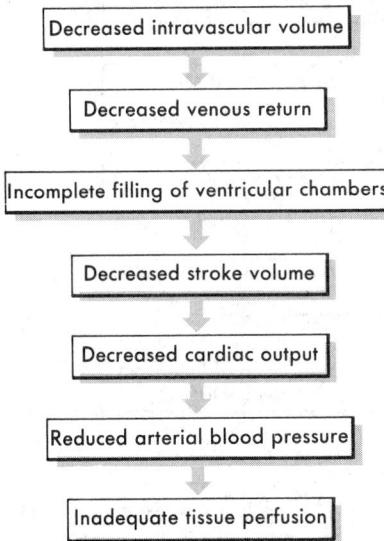

FIGURE 13-1   Pathophysiologic alterations in hypovolemic shock.

Cardiogenic shock is classified according to etiology into two types: coronary and noncoronary. **Coronary cardiogenic shock** is the more common type and is associated with atherosclerotic coronary artery disease. When obstructive coronary artery disease interrupts blood flow and oxygen delivery to heart muscle cells, the cells become ischemic and eventually die. Death of heart muscle, termed myocardial infarction, can place the patient at risk to develop coronary cardiogenic shock. The necrotic heart muscle and the bordering ischemic heart muscle do not contract normally. As a result the heart's ability to pump blood is compromised.

Acute myocardial infarction patients are at greatest risk to develop cardiogenic shock when they have lost 40% or more of the left ventricular muscle mass. This extensive damage occurs with large myocardial infarctions, often involving the anterior wall of the left ventricle. However, the heart muscle damage does not have to occur with a single episode of myocardial damage. The damage can be a cumulative destruction that results from the marginal extension of a recent myocardial infarction or when acute myocardial necrosis occurs in a patient with previous myocardial infarctions.

Myocardial infarctions usually involve the left ventricle. A small percentage of acute myocardial infarctions involve damage to the right ventricle. Right ventricular infarctions can lead to cardiogenic shock, because the damaged right ventricle does not propel sufficient blood forward through the lungs into the left side of the heart. As a result, left ventricular output decreases, and systemic blood flow is inadequate.

The second type of cardiogenic shock is termed noncoronary. **Noncoronary cardiogenic shock** can develop in the absence of coronary artery disease and can be related to a variety of causes, including the following:

1. Cardiomyopathies. Cardiomyopathies are diseases of the heart muscle cell that decrease the ability of the heart muscle to contract. Specific factors associated with the development of cardiomyopathies are hypertension, ischemia, alcohol abuse, vitamin deficiencies, sarcoidosis, viral infection, and familial predisposition.

2. Valvular heart disease. Heart valves can develop one of two major problems. One is stenosis, in which the valve does not open completely and the valve orifice narrows. Stenosis impedes the normal forward flow of blood through the heart chambers. The second problem is regurgitation, in which the valve does not close effectively. Regurgitation allows blood to flow backward rather than being pumped forward. Valvular abnormalities, such as aortic stenosis, mitral stenosis, and aortic regurgitation, can decrease the ability of the

left ventricle to propel blood forward, resulting in cardiogenic shock.

3. Cardiac or pericardial tamponade. Pericardial tamponade is a condition in which blood rapidly fills the pericardial sac. When blood accumulates in the pericardial sac surrounding the heart, the ventricles are compressed and cannot fill adequately with blood. Because the ventricles do not fill adequately, they do not eject a normal stroke volume.

Pathophysiology

The adverse effects of coronary and noncoronary forms of cardiogenic shock are the same (Figure 13-2). When the ventricular chamber cannot propel blood forward, two problems occur. One is decreased stroke volume, with resultant declines in cardiac output, blood pressure, and tissue perfusion. As blood pressure falls, blood flow in the coronary arteries decreases, potentiating myocardial ischemia and predisposing the patient to further cardiac muscle damage. A self-perpetuating cycle of decreased cardiac output and ischemic cardiac muscle damage develops.

The second problem relates to the volume of blood that remains in the left ventricle after systolic ejection. Blood accumulates in the ventricular chamber, increasing ventricular filling pressure and ultimately producing ventricular enlargement. The increased pressure is transmitted passively from the left ventricle to the left atrium into the pulmonary circulation. The pulmonary venous pressure rises, and the high pressure is transmitted to the pulmonary capillaries. Within the pulmonary capillaries, the increased pressure causes fluid to transude from the vascular space into the interstitial and intraalveolar spaces, resulting in pulmonary edema. Subsequently, the high pulmonary pressure is transmitted passively to the right side of the heart and systemic venous circulation. These hemodynamic changes can progress rapidly in minutes or more gradually over several days.

Distributive Shock

Vasogenic or **distributive shock** is characterized by massive vasodilation. The heart can pump blood adequately, and the blood volume is normal; however, the intravascular volume is maldistributed within the circulatory network because of alterations in the blood vessel size. Several types of distributive shock exist, including neurogenic, anaphylactic, and septic.

Neurogenic shock is a form of distributive shock characterized by massive vasodilation as a result of the loss of sympathetic tone. This type of shock is

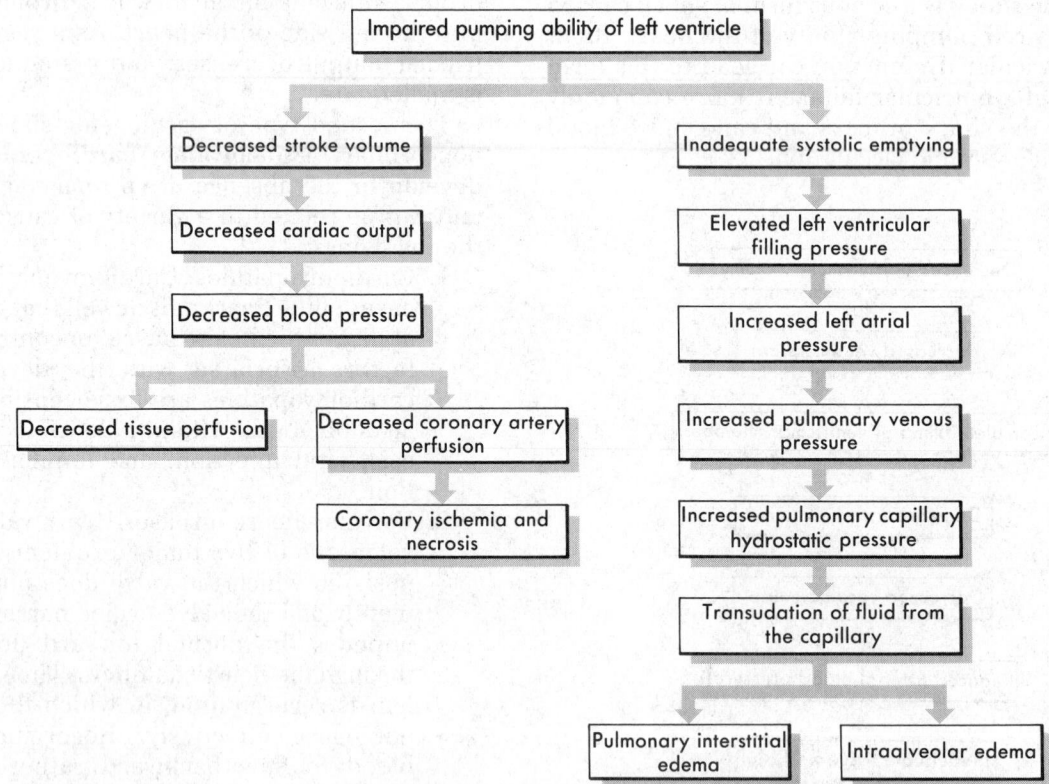

FIGURE 13-2   Pathophysiologic alterations in cardiogenic shock.

rare and usually transitory. Smooth muscle tone within the blood vessel wall normally is mediated by both sympathetic and parasympathetic nerve fibers. The sympathetic nerve fibers carry the message to constrict, whereas the parasympathetic nerve fibers carry the message to dilate. If the sympathetic message is interrupted, the smooth muscle no longer receives the message to constrict. It only receives the message to dilate. Without sympathetic vasoconstrictor tone, massive vasodilation results. Figure 13-3 shows the sympathetic nervous system pathway to vascular smooth muscle.

Loss of sympathetic tone can develop because of injury and disease of the spinal cord above the midthoracic region. High levels of spinal anesthesia, nervous system damage, and ganglionic and adrenergic blocking drugs can impair nerve impulse transmission and decrease sympathetic tone. Sympathetic outflow from the vasomotor center of the medulla of the brain can be blocked intermittently or temporarily decreased by emotional stress, severe pain, and drug overdose.

Pathophysiology

The sympathetic nervous system normally constricts blood vessels to maintain a degree of vascular tone. In neurogenic shock, sympathetic tone is lost. Massive vasodilation of arterioles reduces peripheral vascular resistance and lowers blood pressure. Mas-

sive vasodilation of venules and veins causes blood to pool in the vascular system, decreasing venous return to the right side of the heart. As summarized in Figure 13-4, decreased venous return reduces ventricular filling pressure, stroke volume, cardiac output, and blood pressure. As a result, tissue perfusion is decreased. One unusual aspect of this form of shock is the heart rate. As blood pressure decreases, the sympathetic nervous system usually increases the heart rate. However, in neurogenic shock, the absence of sympathetic outflow prevents an increase in heart rate. The patient manifests a low blood pressure and a normal or slow heart rate. This slow heart rate can further reduce cardiac output and tissue perfusion.

• • •

Anaphylactic shock is characterized by massive vasodilation and increased capillary permeability. It is a severe systemic form of immediate hypersensitivity (allergic reaction) that presents a dramatic, potentially life-threatening clinical picture. Anaphylactic shock follows a severe allergic reaction in which the patient ingests or is injected with an antigen to which he or she has been previously sensitized. Examples of foreign substances that can act as antigens include the following:

1. Drugs (e.g., antibiotics, such as penicillin and its analogs, tetracycline, and sulfonamides; narcotics; and barbiturates)

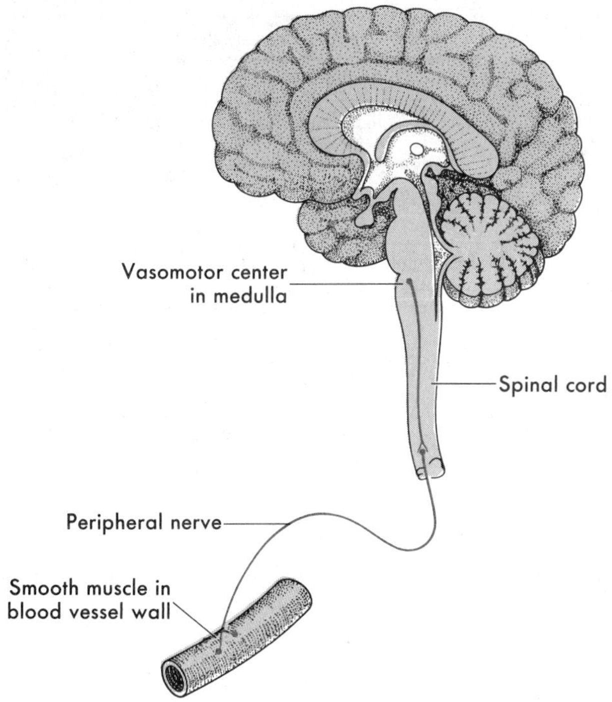

FIGURE 13-3   Pathophysiologic alterations in neurogenic shock.

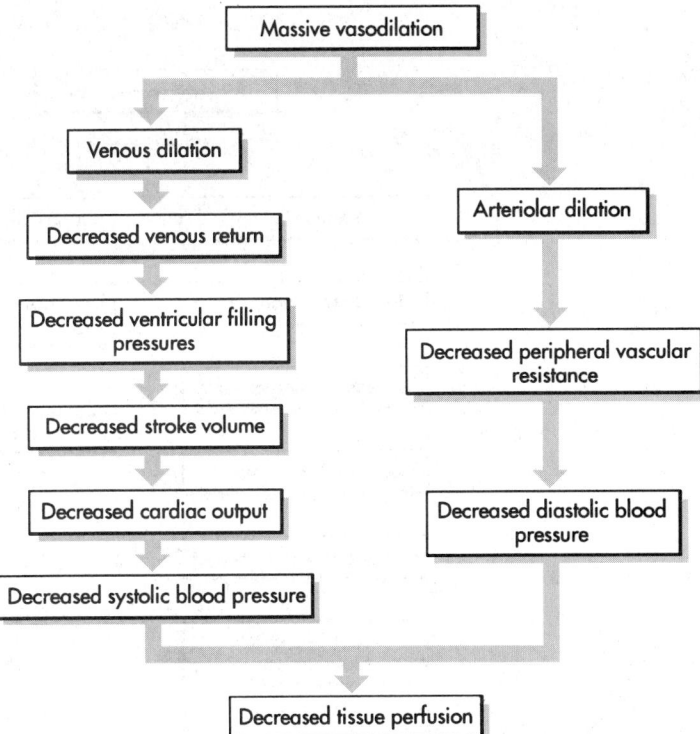

FIGURE 13-4 Sympathetic nervous system pathway to peripheral vascular smooth muscle.

2. Contrast media (as used for diagnostic studies, such as arteriograms, intravenous pyelograms, and computerized tomography scans)
3. Transfused blood and blood products
4. Insect bites or stings (especially from honeybees, bumblebees, hornets, yellow jackets, fire ants, and wasps)

Pathophysiology

The pathophysiologic changes in anaphylactic shock relate to the inflammatory process; antigen-antibody reaction; and release of vasoactive substances, such as histamine, bradykinin, serotonin, and prostaglandins, from activated cells of the immune system. The vasoactive substances produce many effects, including massive vasodilation and increased capillary permeability. (When capillary permeability increases, fluid leaks from the blood capillary into the interstitial compartment.) The net consequences of combined massive vasodilation and increased capillary permeability, summarized in Figure 13-5, decrease peripheral blood flow and tissue perfusion.

• • •

Septic shock, the most common form of distributive shock, is associated with a severe, overwhelming infection. It develops secondary to the invasion of the body by foreign microorganisms and failure of the body's defense system. The incidence of septic shock has increased greatly in the past 20 years, and mortality ranges from 40% to 90%.

The presence of certain conditions and the utilization of specific therapies have been related to an increased incidence of septic shock. These risk factors are summarized in the box on p. 219. See also the box on geriatric considerations.

Causative microorganisms

Any microorganism can produce septic shock if the body's defense systems are impaired and if enough

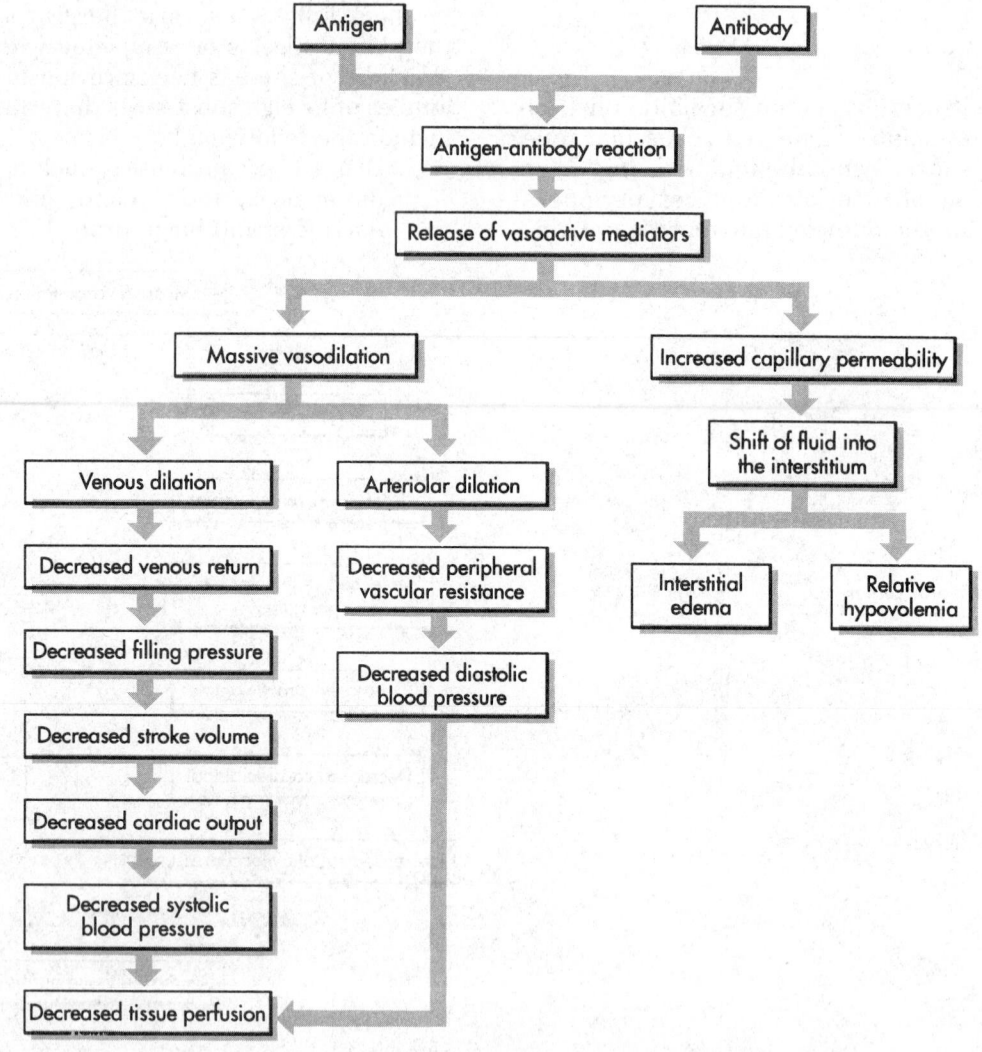

FIGURE 13-5 Pathophysiologic alterations in anaphylactic shock.

RISKS FACTORS FOR SEPTIC SHOCK

Patient-related factors

Extremes of age
Malnutrition
General debilitation
Chronic illnesses
    Congestive heart failure
    Cirrhosis
    Chronic obstructive lung disease
    Cancer
Pregnancy

Treatment-related factors

Insertion of invasive lines and catheters
Surgical procedures, wounds, and drains
Traumatic wounds/thermal injuries
Invasive diagnostic procedures
Drugs
    Antibiotics
    Cytotoxic drugs
    Immunosuppressive drugs

GERIATRIC CONSIDERATIONS

Septic Shock in the Older Adult

Almost half of all septic shock develops in patients over 65 years of age. Elderly patients are at increased risk for septic shock for numerous reasons. With advanced age elderly persons experience impaired organ function and progressive chronic illnesses. For example, the elderly patient may not be able to clear the airways effectively because of decreased mucociliary function, impaired cough reflex, and inadequate hydration. Poor nutrition and general debilitation can weaken respiratory muscles. Thickened retained secretions coupled with respiratory muscle weakness can reduce ventilation and lead to atelectasis and pneumonia. Because of the aging process and chronic illnesses, such as arthritis and heart failure, the elderly patient frequently has impaired physical mobility. Limited activity and sedentary life-styles can lead to skin breakdown and decubitus ulcers in elderly persons. Such skin lesions provide new portals of entry for invading microorganisms to enter the compromised host. Loss of bladder control can necessitate the use of indwelling urinary catheters and predispose the patient to urinary tract infections. Elderly patients in the hospital or long-term care facility also can acquire infections because of exposure to resistant microorganisms, cross contamination, and their own declining immune response.

CAUSATIVE MICROORGANISMS IN SEPTIC SHOCK

Gram-negative bacteria, such as:
    Escherichia coli
    Klebsiella-Enterobacter-Serratia
    Pseudomonas aeruginosa
Gram-positive bacteria, such as:
    Streptococcus pneumoniae
    Staphylococcus aureus
Viruses
Fungi
Rickettsiae

of the microorganism is introduced into the body (see box above). The most common causative microorganisms in septic shock are Gram-negative bacteria. Approximately 50% of all septic shock cases are due to Gram-negative bacteria. The cell walls of these bacteria contain a lipoprotein termed *endotoxin*. Endotoxin is composed of an outer branch chain (which varies with different microorganisms), a middle R core, and an inner lipid A. The lipid A is the toxic portion of the substance that produces adverse effects throughout the body by activating the release of immune mediators.

Pathophysiology

Regardless of the causative microorganism or microorganisms involved, septic shock is a host response that is mediated by complex hormonal and chemical substances produced directly and indirectly through the body's immune system and in response to the adverse effects of endotoxins. The substances are chemically diverse and include peptides, lipids, and aromatic amines. (See box on p. 220.) Three primary pathophysiologic changes characterize septic shock. These changes are (1) massive vasodilation, (2) maldistribution of the intravascular volume, and (3) myocardial depression.

1. Massive vasodilation. Dilation of arterioles decreases peripheral resistance. Dilation of venules and veins reduces venous return and lowers diastolic filling pressures in the heart. The results are decreased cardiac output, peripheral resistance, and blood pressure.

2. Maldistribution of the intravascular volume. The amount of blood or plasma volume initially is normal in septic shock; however, as the shock state progresses, the volume is maldistributed because of increased capillary permeability, selective vasoconstriction, and vascular occlusion.

CHEMICAL MEDIATORS OF SEPTIC SHOCK

Endorphins
Histamine
Interleukins
Kinins (e.g., bradykinin)
Leukotrienes
Myocardial depressant substances
Oxygen radicals
Platelet activating factor
Prostaglandins
Tumor necrosis factor

a. Increased capillary permeability. Increased capillary permeability allows fluid and protein to leave the intravascular compartment and move into the interstitial and intracellular compartments. The results are reduced circulating blood volume, increased blood viscosity, and interstitial and intracellular edema.
b. Selective vasoconstriction. Although vasodilation is a major feature of septic shock, all vascular beds do not dilate. Certain vascular beds, such as those in the pulmonary, renal, and splanchnic circulations, constrict. This constriction occurs in response to sympathetic nervous system activation, selected prostaglandins, and other chemical mediators.
c. Vascular occlusion. Occlusion of small blood vessels is caused by the formation of microemboli and direct endothelial damage. Microemboli result from activation of the clotting system, neutrophil aggregation, and platelet aggregation. Endothelial damage of the blood vessel wall results from the direct toxic effects of certain chemical mediators.

The combined effects of these changes alter hemodynamics, so that some vascular beds receive more blood than they need and other vascular beds do not receive enough blood (Figure 13-6). Tissues that are underperfused do not receive adequate oxygen and nutrients, yet overperfused tissues cannot use all of the nutrients they receive. As a result of maldistribution, nutrients and oxygen remain high in the mixed venous blood.

3. Myocardial depression. Endotoxins and other chemicals released in the septic state depress the force of myocardial contraction. Myocardial depression compounds the vascular changes, decreasing tissue perfusion and oxygen delivery to body cells.

Table 13-1 reviews the three major types of shock.

COMMON CELLULAR CHANGES IN SHOCK

Regardless of the initiating mechanism in shock, all forms of shock share a common denominator, namely, decreased tissue perfusion with altered cellular function. Decreased tissue perfusion reduces oxygen delivery to body cells. Cells cannot produce large amounts of energy without oxygen. To compensate for the energy deficit, cells increase anaerobic metabolism. This form of metabolism produces only small amounts of energy (in the form of aden-

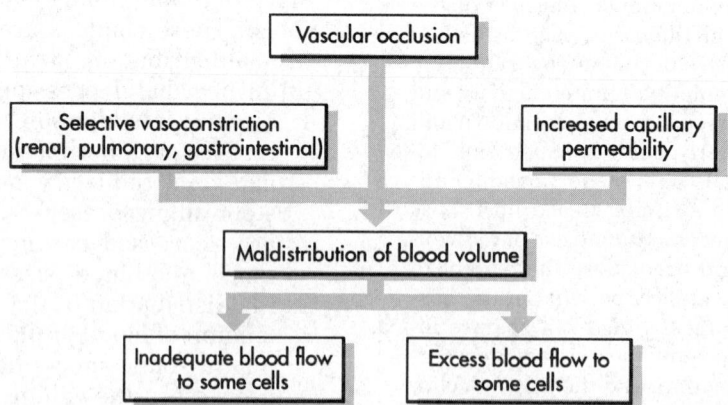

FIGURE 13-6   Maldistribution of blood volume in septic shock.

TABLE 13-1   Shock Classified by Cause

Type of Shock	Cause/Description
Hypovolemic	Decreased intravascular volume as result of internal fluid shifts or external fluid loss
Cardiogenic	Decreased pumping ability of heart, commonly related to death of heart muscle (i.e., myocardial infarction)
Distributive	
Neurogenic	Massive vasodilation as result of loss of sympathetic tone
Anaphylactic	Massive vasodilation and increased capillary permeability as result of severe allergic reaction
Septic	Maldistribution of blood volume and decreased myocardial function caused by overwhelming infection

TABLE 13-2   Stages of Shock

Stage of Shock	Description
Initial	Inadequate oxygen delivery initiates early cellular changes, evidenced by increased blood lactate levels
Compensatory	Decreased cardiac output triggers neural, hormonal, and chemical mechanisms that effectively restore tissue perfusion to vital organs
Progressive	Compensatory mechanisms begin to fail and no longer maintain adequate perfusion to vital organs; organ function begins to deteriorate
Refractory	Shock state is so severe and prolonged that death from multiple organ system failure is imminent

osine 5'-triphosphate, or ATP) and large amounts of pyruvic acid. Pyruvic acid is converted to lactic acid, which accumulates in the cell, causing acidosis. As the cellular pH falls, powerful digestive enzymes are released from the lysosome within the cell. These enzymes destroy the cell membrane and digest the cellular contents. When the integrity of the cell membrane is lost, cellular death is irreversible.

To summarize, the adverse effects of shock on the cell include (1) decreased ATP production, (2) deterioration of cellular function, (3) excess production of lactic acid, (4) eruption of the intracellular lysosomes, and (5) cell death.

PROGRESSION OF SHOCK

The patient in shock manifests specific signs and symptoms as the shock state progresses. To understand the pathophysiologic bases for these clinical changes, it is helpful to follow the progression of shock through four stages. These stages include the initial stage, compensatory stage, progressive stage,

and refractory stage. The nurse should remember that each patient's shock state is unique, and manifestations are highly individualized. The actual timing of the physiologic progression of shock can vary widely. The specific responses described in each stage offer only a guide for correlating the pathophysiology and the clinical manifestations of shock (Table 13-2).

Initial Stage

In the initial stage of shock, cardiac output and tissue perfusion are decreased. Deficiencies in the delivery of oxygen and other nutrients begin to alter cellular function. Aerobic metabolism is decreased, anaerobic metabolism is increased, and excess lactic acid is produced. Although cellular changes are underway, no clinical signs and symptoms are evident in this early stage of shock. In laboratory-induced shock, arterial lactate levels are increased, confirming excess lactic acid production. (Lactate is the resultant anion as lactic acid is neutralized by the body's acid-base buffers.) This stage is a theoretic stage that emphasizes the cellular aspect of shock.

Compensatory Stage

In the compensatory stage of shock, cardiac output is decreased to the degree that compensatory mechanisms are activated. Compensatory mechanisms successfully restore cardiac output and tissue perfusion to vital organs. These homeostatic mechanisms include neural, hormonal, and chemical changes.

Neural compensation

As cardiac output falls, arterial blood pressure decreases, resulting in neural compensation. Within seconds to minutes, pressoreceptors located in the

aorta and carotid arteries sense the decrease in blood pressure. These receptors send a message to the medulla of the brain and activate the sympathetic nervous system.

Activation of the sympathetic nervous system prepares the body for fight or flight. It is the body's response to stress and produces widespread effects in almost all body systems. Sympathetic activation redistributes blood flow to the vital organs, the heart and the brain, and shunts blood away from other organs, such as the kidneys and skin. Specific sympathetic nervous system effects are diagramed in Figure 13-7.

Hormonal compensation

Hormonal compensation stems from activation of the sympathetic nervous system. When renal blood

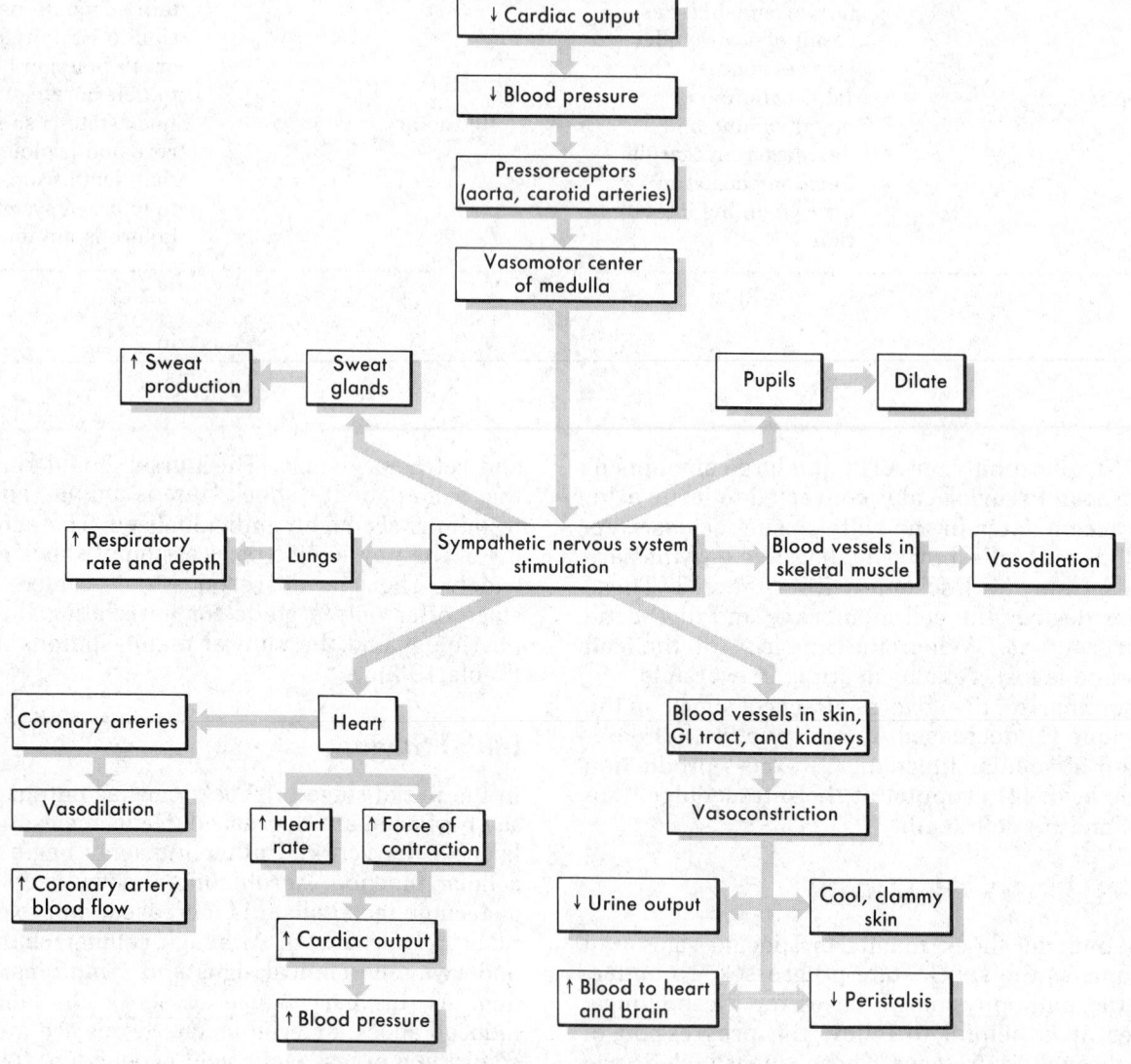

FIGURE 13-7 Neural compensation.

flow is decreased, special sensing cells in the renal nephron (termed juxtaglomerular cells) are stimulated to release renin. Renin activates a substance termed angiotensinogen, or renin substrate, to produce angiotensin 1. Angiotensin 1 circulates via the blood to the lungs, where it is converted to angiotensins 2 and 3. These substances cause direct vasoconstriction and elevate blood pressure. In addition, they stimulate the adrenal cortex to release the hormone aldosterone. Aldosterone, a mineralocorticoid, acts on renal tubules to cause sodium retention. When sodium is retained by the body, the serum sodium increases. As the serum sodium increases, the serum osmolality rises. Increased serum osmolality is sensed by cells in the hypothalamus termed osmoreceptors. These cells stimulate the posterior pituitary gland to release the hormone antidiuretic hormone (ADH), which acts on the renal tubules to cause retention of water. When these mechanisms are activated, the net results are (1) retention of sodium and water, (2) increased blood pressure secondary to increased blood volume and vasoconstriction, and (3) decreased urine volume.

In addition to the renin-aldosterone-ADH mechanism, other hormones are stimulated in the compensatory stage of shock. The sympathetic nervous system stimulation activates the adrenal medulla to secrete the catecholamines epinephrine and norepinephrine. These hormones help sustain the stress response for hours to days.

The anterior pituitary gland is stimulated to secrete adrenocorticotropic hormone (ACTH). ACTH acts on the adrenal cortex to increase the secretion of glucocorticoids, such as cortisol. These hormones stimulate liver cells to increase the breakdown of stored glucose, a process termed glycogenolysis. As glucose is released into the blood, the serum glucose concentration rises. Glucocorticoids also stimulate another hepatic metabolic activity termed gluconeogenesis. In this process liver cells convert fats and proteins into new glucose, which moves into the blood, increasing the serum glucose concentration. Figure 13-8 summarizes the hormonal compensation in shock.

Chemical compensation

Chemical compensation also is related to the sympathetic redistribution of blood to priority organs. When pulmonary blood flow is decreased, some alveoli that contain oxygen are not perfused. The adverse effects are ventilation/perfusion imbalances, impaired gas exchange, and decreased arterial oxygen concentration (i.e., hypoxemia). Hypoxemia, defined as an arterial oxygen tension less than 60 mm Hg, is sensed by peripheral chemoreceptors that increase the rate and depth of ventilation. In the patient with healthy lungs, increased rate and depth of ventilation result in the exhalation of large amounts of carbon dioxide and respiratory alkalosis.

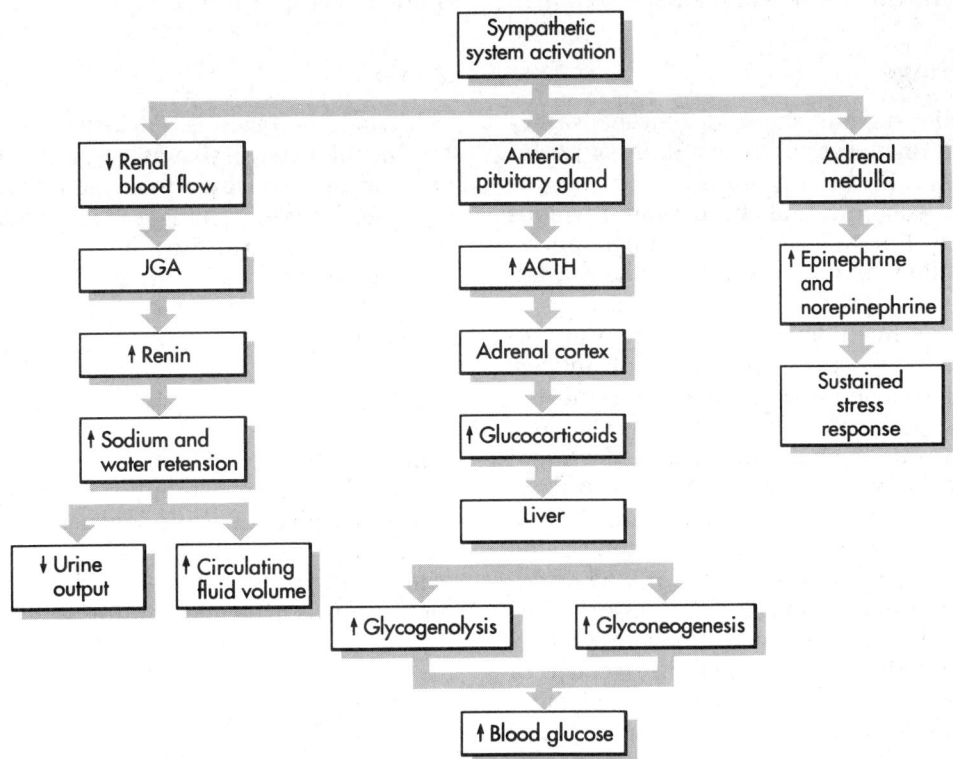

FIGURE 13-8   Hormonal compensation.

Clinical manifestations

The patient in the compensatory stage of shock manifests specific signs and symptoms of the neural, hormonal, and chemical mechanisms just presented. The blood pressure is adequate to perfuse the vital organs. The heart rate is increased to 101 to 150 beats/min. The skin is cool and pale because of peripheral vasoconstriction. The skin feels moist or clammy because of increased secretion of sweat. Peripheral pulses are rapid, weak, and thready as a result of decreased peripheral blood flow. Urine volume is decreased to less than 30 mL/hr as a result of reduced renal blood flow. Because of sympathetic stimulation and decreased gastrointestinal blood flow, bowel sounds are hypoactive. Mild abdominal distention may be noted. The level of consciousness is altered but not severely impaired in this stage of shock. Early hypoxic and hypocapnic changes result in restlessness, confusion, anxiousness, agitation, lethargy, or mental cloudiness. The level of consciousness is decreased, but the patient is able to respond to verbal stimuli and can follow simple commands. The respiratory rate is greater than 20/min, and the depth of ventilation is increased.

Laboratory abnormalities during the compensatory stage of shock include hyperglycemia (an elevated blood glucose concentration), hypoxemia (a decreased arterial oxygen tension), hypocapnia (a decreased arterial carbon dioxide tension), and respiratory alkalosis (the combination of a decreased arterial carbon dioxide tension and an elevated pH).

Progressive Stage

In the progressive stage of shock the compensatory mechanisms are unsuccessful in maintaining perfusion to vital organs. Severe hypoperfusion causes organs to become ischemic, and the patient develops multiple organ system failure. Sustained hypoperfusion reduces cellular oxygen delivery. Ischemic cellular changes lead to production of lactic acid, lysosomal eruption, and cell death. As cells die they release acid metabolic wastes and toxic substances. These ischemic and necrotic changes alter the tissue environment and lead to microvascular changes.

Capillaries lose their ability to regulate flow, and capillary walls become more permeable. Fluid leaves the intravascular compartment and moves into the interstitial compartment. As a result, edema develops in the interstitial compartment, and circulating blood volume is reduced. Fluid also moves from the interstitial compartment into cells, exacerbating cellular edema and dysfunction. Because of fluid displacement from the capillaries, the solid blood components (e.g., red blood cells, white blood cells, and platelets) within the vascular compartment are carried in less fluid. The blood viscosity is increased, and capillary flow is slowed. This combination results in a state of thick or viscous blood (capillary sludging), which predisposes the patient to the development of microemboli and aggregation (clumping) of blood cells, such as neutrophils and platelets. Both problems can further reduce capillary blood flow and impair oxygen delivery to body cells.

Changes in the microcirculation reduce the volume of blood returned to the right side of the heart and consequently decrease cardiac output. As cardiac output decreases, arterial blood pressure falls and coronary artery perfusion suffers. The heart muscle is forced to work harder yet is receiving less oxygen. This imbalance between myocardial oxygen supply and myocardial oxygen demand results in dysrhythmias, ischemia, and even myocardial infarction. Unfortunately, these changes further depress cardiac function and lower cardiac output. A vicious self-perpetuating cycle of decreased cardiac output and cardiac failure develops and leads to deterioration of the circulatory system and inadequate perfusion of all organ systems.

Peripherally, blood flow is reduced, and peripheral pulses are weak, thready, or even absent. Extremities appear cyanotic and feel cold. Sustained hypoperfusion can lead to ischemia of distal areas, such as fingers and toes. Intense ischemia can ultimately result in necrosis and ulceration. Such necrotic lesions can serve as new portals of entry for foreign microorganisms and can increase the shock patient's risk of infection.

Brain

Although the brain is a priority organ, oxygen delivery in the progressive stage of shock is inadequate. The brain is sensitive to oxygen deprivation and undergoes ischemic changes. The patient's level of consciousness deteriorates. The patient no longer responds to verbal stimuli, and his or her response to painful stimuli gradually decreases until he has no response.

Kidneys

The kidneys are damaged because of inadequate blood flow. Renal tubules become ischemic, and acute tubular necrosis ensues. Urine output decreases to less than 20 mL/hr, and the kidneys lose their ability to concentrate urine. Toxic waste products, such as urea and creatinine, cannot be excreted and accumulate in the blood.

Gastrointestinal tract

The gastrointestinal tract suffers adverse consequences from prolonged vasoconstriction. Ischemia

RESEARCH BRIEF

Gutierrez G, Palizas F, Goglio P, et al: Gastric intramucosal pH as a therapeutic index of tissue oxygenation in critically ill patients, *Lancet* 339(8787):195-199, 1992.

Critical illnesses, such as shock, are associated with decreased blood flow to the gastrointestinal tract. When splanchnic tissues are hypoperfused, they generate lactic acid and the gastric mucosal pH (pHi) becomes more acid. The pHi can be measured in the clinical setting with a tonometer, a standard nasogastric tube with a saline-filled silicone balloon attached to the distal end.

This article summarizes the results of a controlled, randomized, multicenter study involving 260 patients admitted to intensive care units. The patients had severe critical illnesses, such as shock, as evidenced by Acute Physiology and Chronic Health Evaluation (APACHE) scores of 15 to 25. The researchers measured gastric mucosal pH (pHi) of the patients on admission to the intensive care unit and randomly assigned patients to a control or protocol group. Patients were stratified by admission pHi to either the low pHi group (when pHi was less than 7.35) or the normal pHi group (when pHi was 7.35 or greater).

Patients in the control groups were treated according to conventional practices for each intensive care unit. Patients in the protocol groups received therapy guided by changes in pHi (measured every 6 hours). When the pHi was below 7.35 or when it fell by 0.10 unit or more from the previous reading, a treatment protocol was initiated. The research design included a treatment protocol with two specific parts: (1) measures to ensure correction of mean arterial blood pressure, arterial oxygen and carbon dioxide tensions, arterial pH, hemoglobin, and temperature; and (2) measures to increase systemic oxygen transport, such as parenteral fluids and dobutamine.

In the patient groups with a normal pHi on admission that then fell to less than 7.35, the therapeutic protocols (guided by pHi) improved survival. In the treatment group, survival was 58%, whereas survival in the control group was 42%.

In the patient groups with a pHi less than 7.35 on admission, survival was similar in both the treatment and control groups. The survival rate in this control group was 36% and in this treatment group was 37%.

The significance of this study centers on the therapeutic end point used to guide therapy. Traditional nonspecific end points, such as blood pressure, pulse, urine output, and cardiac output, may be expanded in the future to include markers of perfusion in specific areas of the body. The pHi (measured with tonometry) may help to guide early therapy in critically ill patients to minimize splanchnic hypoperfusion, prevent its adverse sequelae, and decrease mortality.

---

and ulceration damage the luminal surface of the stomach and intestines. The intestinal walls no longer serve as intact barriers against bacteria and foreign toxins, and bacteria can translocate from the lumen of the gastrointestinal tract into the circulation. Ulceration also increases the incidence of stress ulcers and predisposes the shock patient to gastrointestinal bleeding.

Liver

The liver, as part of the gastrointestinal tract, suffers from prolonged vasoconstriction. Liver cells fail to perform their many functions. Bilirubin, a normal waste product of red blood cell breakdown, cannot be conjugated by the abnormal liver cells. Bilirubin, a yellow pigment, accumulates in the blood and causes jaundice. The hypoperfused liver cannot adequately metabolize drugs or detoxify hormones, such as aldosterone and ADH. Kupffer cells of the liver, which normally filter bacteria from the blood, are depressed. Consequently the patient is more susceptible to bacterial infections. Waste products, such as ammonia and lactic acid, are not metabolized and accumulate in the blood. As hepatic ischemia continues, liver cells die and intracellular enzymes are released and enter the vascular space. Elevations of serum aspartate aminotransferase (AST, formerly SGOT), serum alanine aminotransferase (ALT, formerly SGPT), and lactate dehydrogenase (LDH) confirm liver cell destruction.

Pancreas

The pancreas also suffers from sustained hypoperfusion. Pancreatic cells become ischemic, die, and release enzymes, such as amylase and lipase, into the blood. In addition, pancreatic lysosomal enzymes are released. Some of these pancreatic lysosomal enzymes circulate in the blood and lymphatic system to the heart, where they depress myocardial contractility.

Lungs

In the progressive stage of shock, two pulmonary problems develop: (1) decreased pulmonary capillary blood flow and (2) increased pulmonary capillary permeability. Pulmonary capillary blood flow is decreased, and gas exchange at the alveolar-capillary level is impaired. Arterial oxygen levels decrease, and carbon dioxide levels increase.

With decreased pulmonary capillary blood flow, alveolar cells become ischemic and reduce their production of surfactant. Surfactant is a lipoprotein that normally helps reduce alveolar surface tension and keep alveoli open. Without surfactant, alveoli collapse, producing massive atelectasis. The lungs become stiff, and pulmonary compliance decreases.

The second pulmonary problem is increased pulmonary capillary permeability. Fluid leaves the pulmonary capillaries and produces interstitial and intra-alveolar edema. The presence of edema in the lungs markedly decreases diffusion of oxygen and compounds the severity of the hypoxic state.

The combination of massive atelectasis, widespread interstitial edema, and reduced pulmonary compliance increases the work of breathing. The patient hypoventilates and develops respiratory failure. Specifically, the process is termed shock lung, primary pulmonary edema, or adult respiratory distress syndrome (ARDS). Regardless of the specific name, respiratory failure in the presence of progressive shock is common and is a major clinical problem. (See Chapter 28 for a more complete description of respiratory failure.)

Clinical manifestations

As compensatory mechanisms begin to fail, body system functions deteriorate, as evidenced by the following clinical findings.

The patient's blood pressure is less than his or her normal level and is too low to perfuse the vital organs. The actual blood pressure value in shock varies; however, in the progressive stage of shock, the systolic blood pressure may fall below 80 to 90 mm Hg. The diastolic pressure may remain elevated as a result of sustained vasoconstriction. As a result the pulse pressure (i.e., the difference between the systolic and diastolic pressures) narrows.

The heart rate usually is rapid and often irregular. The skin in the progressive stage of shock is cold, cyanotic, and even mottled. Jaundice can be evident with severe liver ischemia in prolonged shock. Peripheral pulses are weak, thready, and rapid. Often the pulses cannot be palpated and must be assessed with an ultrasound (e.g., Doppler) flowmeter.

Urine volume is less than 20 mL/hr. The level of consciousness is severely depressed in this stage of shock. The patient no longer responds to verbal stimuli. His response to painful stimuli deteriorates from flexion, to extension, to no response.

Respiratory rate continues to be rapid; however, the depth of respirations decreases as the patient hypoventilates. As respiratory failure develops, the patient has shallow breathing patterns because of respiratory muscle fatigue and decreased lung compliance. Auscultation of the lung fields reveals scattered moist crackles caused by widespread interstitial pulmonary edema. Bowel sounds usually are absent as a result of severely decreased intestinal motility.

The laboratory changes in the progressive stage of shock confirm organ damage secondary to hypoperfusion. The abnormalities are summarized in Table 13-3.

Refractory Stage

The refractory stage is the final stage of shock. In this stage the shock state is so profound and cell destruction is so severe that death is inevitable.

TABLE 13-3   Laboratory Changes in Shock

Laboratory Finding	Changes	Etiology
Serum amylase	Increased	Pancreatic ischemia and cell necrosis
Serum lipase	Increased	Pancreatic ischemia and cell necrosis
SGOT	Increased	Liver and/or myocardial cell necrosis
CPK	Increased	Myocardial and/or skeletal muscle cell necrosis
Blood urea nitrogen	Increased	Renal failure, dehydration, and/or gastrointestinal bleeding
Serum creatinine	Increased	Renal failure
Arterial oxygen tension	Decreased	Advanced pulmonary changes
pH	Decreased	Respiratory acidosis as result of hypoventilation; metabolic acidosis as result of increased metabolic wastes

Clinical manifestations

The clinical picture in the refractory stage of shock is a grim picture of multiple organ system failure. The patient demonstrates signs and symptoms of cardiac, respiratory, renal, hepatic, pancreatic, hematologic, gastrointestinal, and neurologic failure. There is profound hypotension that is often unresponsive to potent vasopressor drugs. The patient suffers from severe hypoxemia that does not improve with supplemental oxygen administration. Renal shutdown results in complete anuria and severe metabolic changes caused by accumulation of toxic waste products in the blood. Liver dysfunction alters metabolism of nutrients, the blood glucose concentration, and the degradation of medications. Pancreatic failure indirectly decreases myocardial contractility. Hematologic changes predispose the patient to multiple emboli, diffuse intravascular clotting, and abnormal consumption of clotting factors. Gastrointestinal failure prevents the absorption of nutrients from enteral feedings and predisposes the patient to malnutrition and infectious complications. Neurologic insults reduce responsiveness to environmental stimuli and ultimately diminish the sympathetic stress response. Specifically, the vasomotor center of the medulla fails to continue the sympathetic discharge. As a result the heart rate slows, the blood pressure falls, and the patient suffers cardiac and respiratory arrest. The refractory stage of shock ultimately leads to total body failure and death. Although the progression of events in shock is rather grim, every patient does not progress through all four stages. In many cases the shock state is detected early, appropriate intervention is initiated, and the shock progression is halted. The clinical changes reverse, and the patient recovers. The nurse must understand the possible progression of shock but realize the importance of preventing its development and, when possible, halting its devastating clinical course.

THERAPEUTIC MANAGEMENT

Once shock is recognized, therapy is instituted immediately. Shock therapy can be classified as definitive and supportive.

Definitive Measures

The goal of definitive therapy is to locate and correct the cause or causes of shock. Definitive therapy varies with the causative mechanisms and the specific type of shock.

Hypovolemic shock

Hypovolemic shock is caused by inadequate intravascular volume. It is related to internal fluid shifts or external loss of fluid. Definitive therapy in hypovolemic shock is directed toward maintaining or increasing the intravascular volume. In the immediate postoperative patient who develops hypovolemic shock because of internal hemorrhage, definitive therapy includes returning the patient to the operating suite for surgery to correct the bleeding problem. If external hemorrhage is noted, application of direct pressure to the bleeding site can decrease blood loss. If severe dehydration has resulted from profuse diarrhea and vomiting, antiemetics and antidiarrheal medications can be used to decrease fluid loss.

Parenteral fluids must be administered in hypovolemic shock to replace the volume lost. The choice of parenteral fluid is made by the physician based on the type of fluid lost from the body. (See Chapter 12 for a discussion of parenteral fluid therapy.)

Cardiogenic shock

Cardiogenic shock is caused by the impaired ability of the heart as a pump. Definitive measures include reducing the amount of heart muscle damage and improving the pumping effectiveness of the remaining heart muscle. When cardiogenic shock is caused by myocardial infarction, definitive measures in the early postinfarction period are directed toward improving oxygen supply and decreasing oxygen demand of the heart muscle. The oxygen supply can be increased by administration of supplemental oxygen, usually via a nasal cannula at 3 to 5 L/min. Administration of medications that dilate coronary arteries, such as nitroglycerin, also can improve oxygen delivery. Other definitive measures that can increase oxygen delivery to the heart muscle include administration of thrombolytic agents, such as streptokinase; percutaneous coronary transluminal angioplasty; and emergency coronary artery bypass grafting. (See Chapter 35 for a complete discussion of the management of the patient with acute myocardial infarction.)

Efforts should be instituted to reduce myocardial oxygen demand. Oxygen consumption can be decreased by placing the patient in a position of comfort and restricting activity. Analgesics administered intravenously decrease pain and reduce oxygen consumption. Sedatives, such as diazepam (Valium), can alleviate anxiety and indirectly reduce oxygen demands.

The pumping effectiveness of the heart can be improved by administration of drugs, including positive inotropic agents, vasodilators, and vasopressors.

Positive inotropic agents increase the force of myocardial contraction and improve systolic ejection of blood. Forward stroke volume increases, and consequently cardiac output and blood pressure improve. Specific drugs used to increase the force of contraction in the shock patient are dobutamine (Dobutrex) and dopamine (Intropin). Other drugs with positive inotropic actions include amrinone (Inocor), epinephrine (Adrenalin), and norepinephrine (Levophed). A major disadvantage of positive inotropic drugs is the resultant increase in myocardial oxygen demand. In the severely ill shock patient this increased oxygen demand can potentiate myocardial oxygen supply/demand imbalances.

Vasodilators improve the heart's pumping effectiveness by reducing the workload of the heart. Vasodilation of venules and veins reduces venous return, decreases ventricular filling, and lowers preload. Medications that dilate veins include nitroglycerin (Tridil), nitroprusside (Nipride), morphine, and furosemide (Lasix). Vasodilation of arterioles lowers peripheral vascular resistance and reduces the work of the ventricles in ejecting blood by reducing afterload. Specific afterload reducing agents include nitroprusside, amrinone, and phentolamine (Regitine).

Vasopressor or vasoconstrictor drugs are used to increase peripheral vascular resistance, elevate arterial blood pressure, and maintain coronary artery perfusion. Vasoconstrictor agents are not used in cardiogenic shock unless other measures have failed to maintain adequate coronary perfusion. Potent vasoconstrictor agents include norepinephrine, phenylephrine (Neo-Synephrine), epinephrine, and dopamine (in high doses). Table 13-4 summarizes actions, dosages, and side effects of selected drugs used as positive inotropic agents, vasodilators, and vasoconstrictors.

In some cases of cardiogenic shock, pharmacologic attempts fail to improve the oxygen supply/demand balance. Another method used to improve the heart as a pump is intra-aortic balloon counterpulsation. This invasive technique involves insertion of a dual-chambered polyethylene balloon catheter via the femoral artery into the descending thoracic aorta (see Figure 13-9). The catheter tip is positioned just distal to the left subclavian artery. The catheter is connected to an external counterpulsation unit that senses each cardiac cycle. The balloon is inflated with a gas, such as helium or carbon dioxide, at the beginning of ventricular diastole. When the balloon is inflated, aortic blood pressure rises. Blood is directed into the coronary arteries, and coronary blood flow increases. Balloon inflation also increases perfusion to the brain and other organs.

The balloon is deflated just before ventricular systole, creating a potential intra-aortic space of 30 to 50 mL. Balloon deflation lowers aortic pressure, allowing the aortic valve to open earlier during ventricular contraction. Ventricular emptying is enhanced, so that left ventricular filling pressure decreases, wall tension is minimized, and myocardial oxygen consumption is reduced. With lower pres-

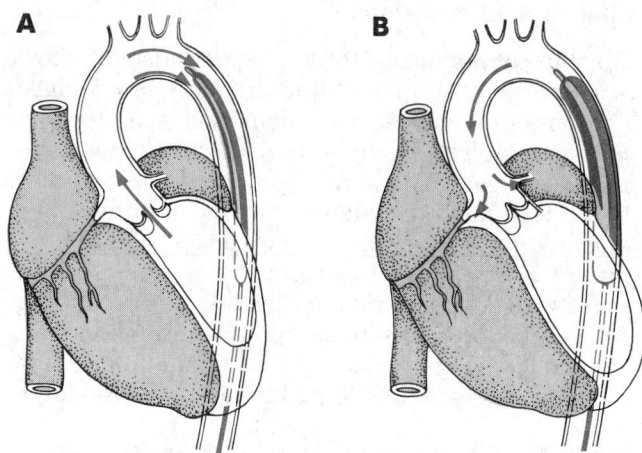

FIGURE 13-9 Position of intra-aortic balloon catheter. **A,** Inflation. **B,** Deflation.

sures in the left side of the heart the pulmonary veins empty more completely, pulmonary blood volume falls, and pulmonary congestion decreases. The beneficial results of intra-aortic balloon counterpulsation are (1) increased myocardial oxygen supply as a result of improved coronary artery perfusion, (2) decreased myocardial oxygen consumption, (3) relief of pulmonary congestion, and (4) improved perfusion to other organs.

Contraindications to the use of the intra-aortic balloon catheter include aortic valve abnormalities and arterial vascular disease. Complications that can result from its use include lower extremity ischemia, femoral and renal artery emboli, trauma to the aortic wall, thrombocytopenia, hemolysis, and deep vein thrombosis. The technique of intra-aortic balloon counterpulsation is confined to intensive care areas. A high degree of technical skill and professional expertise is needed to monitor the operation of the balloon pump, to assess the patient's response, and to detect possible complications.

Other invasive mechanical devices to improve the heart as a pump include left and right ventricular assist devices. Ventricular assist devices consist of either an electrically activated or a pneumatic air-driven pump that supports the function of a single existing ventricular chamber. These devices offer some hope for patients with cardiogenic shock; however, continued research is needed to perfect such devices.

Human heart transplantation is another form of definitive therapy for patients with cardiogenic shock. A transplanted heart recipient requires immunosuppressive drug therapy for life. Immunosuppressive drugs include cyclosporine (Cyclosporin A), azathioprine (Imuran), and antithymocyte globulin. Major complications of heart transplantation are op-

TABLE 13-4   Pharmacology Summary: Vasoactive Drugs

Drug	Actions	Infusion preparation	Dosage	Adverse effects	Nursing considerations
Amrinone (Inocor)	Increases force of myocardial contraction. Dilates arterioles and veins	Add 500 mg to 500 mL of normal saline to achieve 1 mg/mL	Intravenous (IV) bolus: 0.75 to 1.5 mg/kg Follow with continuous IV infusion: 5 to 10 μg/kg/min	Thrombocytopenia, dysrhythmias, hypotension, chest pain, burning at site of infusion	Give IV bolus dose slowly over 2 to 5 minutes to minimize dysrhythmias. Do not mix drug in dextrose solution. Use drug cautiously in patients with profound hypotension. Monitor patient's heart rate and cardiac rhythm during administration, and titrate infusion accordingly
Dobutamine (Dobutrex)	Increases force of myocardial contraction. Mildly dilates arterioles and veins. Increases coronary artery blood flow	Add 500 mg to 250 mL of fluid to achieve 2 mg/mL or 2000 μg/mL	Continuous IV infusion: 2.5 to 20 μg/kg/min	Dysrhythmias, chest pain, nausea, headache, dyspnea, tremors	Monitor patient's blood pressure, heart rate, and cardiac rhythm during administration, and titrate dose accordingly
Dopamine (Intropin)	Small dose: dilates renal, cerebral, and coronary blood vessels. Moderate dose: increases force of myocardial contraction. Large dose: constricts arteries and veins—	Add 200 mg to 250 mL of fluid to achieve 800 μg/mL	Continuous IV infusion: small dose: 2 to 5 μg/kg/min; moderate dose: 5 to 10 μg/kg/min; large dose: greater than 10 μg/kg/min	Dysrhythmias, nausea, vomiting, angina, increased pulmonary congestion	Do not mix drug in alkaline solution. If drug infiltrates, infuse phentolamine (Regitine) into area. Monitor pulmonary capillary wedge pressure during infusion of high dosages. Auscultate breath sounds every hour during continuous infusion. Monitor patient's heart rate, blood pressure, and cardiac rhythm during administration, and titrate dose accordingly

Continued.

TABLE 13-4   Pharmacology Summary: Vasoactive Drugs—cont'd

Drug	Actions	Infusion preparation	Dosage	Adverse effects	Nursing considerations
Epinephrine (Adrenalin)	Increases force of myocardial contraction Constricts arteries and veins (in high doses)	Add 2 mg to 500 mL of fluid to achieve 4 μg/mL	Continuous IV infusion: 20 to 70 μg/min	Dysrhythmias, angina, central nervous system (CNS) excitability (tremors, anxiety, headache, dizziness)	Monitor patient's heart rate and cardiac rhythm during administration, and titrate dose accordingly Do not mix drug in alkaline solution
Nitroglycerin (Tridil)	Dilates veins Dilates arteries (in high doses)	Add 50 mg to 500 mL of 5% dextrose solution to achieve 100 μg/mL	Continuous IV infusion: 5 to 10 μg/min; increase by 5 μg every 3 to 5 minutes (5 to 75 μg/min)	Hypotension, increased heart rate, headache, nausea, vomiting, flushing	Prepare infusion in glass container, because drug readily adsorbs to plastic at unpredictable rate Infuse through special polyethylene tubing to minimize adsorption Use drug cautiously in patients with profound hypotension; administer only in combination with other drugs Monitor patient's heart rate and blood pressure during administration, and titrate dose accordingly

Drug	Action	Preparation	Dosage	Adverse effects	Nursing considerations
Nitroprusside (Nipride)	Dilates arteries and veins	Dilute one 50 mg vial in 2 to 5 mL of 5% dextrose. Add solution to 500 mL of fluid to achieve 0.1 mg/mL	Continuous IV infusion: 3 µg/kg/min	Hypotension, thiocyanate toxicity, cyanide poisoning	Only dilute drug in 5% dextrose; no other fluid should be used. Cover drug-containing IV solution in opaque wrapper, since drug is light-sensitive. Monitor patient's blood pressure, and titrate dose accordingly
Norepinephrine (Levophed)	Increases force of myocardial contraction. Constricts arteries and veins (in high doses)	Add 2 mg to 500 mL of dextrose solution to achieve 4 µg/mL	Continuous IV infusion: 2 to 8 µg/min	Dysrhythmias, oliguria, angina, CNS excitability, tissue necrosis	Avoid mixing drug in saline solutions. If drug infiltrates, infuse phentolamine into area. Do not mix drug in alkaline solution
Phentolamine (Regitine)	Dilates arteries and veins	Add 30 mg to 500 mL of fluid to achieve 60 µg/mL	Continuous IV infusion: 30 µg/min	Hypotension, tachycardia	Use drug cautiously in patients with profound hypotension
Phenylephrine (Neo-Synephrine)	Constricts arteries and veins	Add 60 mg to 500 mL to achieve 120 µg/mL	10 to 30 µg/min	Hypertension, dysrhythmias	Monitor patient's heart rate and cardiac rhythm during administration

portunistic infections, lymphoproliferative malignancies (as a result of long-term immunosuppressive therapy), and occlusive atherosclerosis in the coronary arteries of the transplanted heart (related to an immunologic process that damages the coronary blood vessel wall).

Neurogenic shock

Neurogenic shock, a form of distributive shock, is related to loss of sympathetic innervation to peripheral vessels. It is caused by injury or disease of the spinal cord, interruption of nerve impulse transmission, or vasomotor center depression. Definitive therapy includes minimizing spinal cord trauma by proper stabilization of the trauma victim. If the shock is caused by spinal anesthesia, the nurse ensures proper positioning of the patient in the immediate postoperative period to prevent blockage of sympathetic outflow. (The head of the patient's bed can be elevated to 15 degrees.) Vasomotor center depression cannot be treated with definitive measures unless the cause is ascertained. If it is related to hypoglycemia, elevation of the blood glucose is appropriate. If it is related to extreme pain, the administration of analgesics is definitive. If it is related to anxiety and extreme stress, identification of the stressor and its alleviation are appropriate definitive measures.

Anaphylactic shock

Anaphylactic shock is caused by an extreme hypersensitivity reaction to a specific antigen. Definitive therapy initially includes identification and removal of the causative antigen. In insect bites a tourniquet can be applied to the affected limb in the early prehospital period. If the anaphylactic response occurs during the administration of blood or blood products, the nurse should immediately discontinue the transfusion and keep the intravenous line open with normal saline. In the event of an anaphylactic reaction to the ingestion or injection of a drug or contrast substance, little can be done to remove the antigen. In these cases, measures are used to reverse the effects of the vasoactive immune mediators.

The allergic response can be reversed with the administration of selected drugs. Epinephrine, 0.5 to 1 mg administered intravenously every 5 to 10 minutes, can restore vascular tone and raise the arterial blood pressure. Antihistamines, such as diphenhydramine (Benadryl), 25 to 50 mg intravenously, can reverse the adverse effects of histamine (e.g., vasodilation and bronchoconstriction). In severe cases, methylprednisolone (Solu-Medrol), 60 to 125 mg, is given to reverse the adverse effects of immune mediators and reduce capillary permeability.

Special consideration should be given to patients receiving beta-adrenergic blocking drugs, such as propranolol (Inderal), when they suffer anaphylaxis. These medications decrease the effectiveness of therapeutic interventions, such as epinephrine, and prolong the duration of signs and symptoms of the allergic response. These patients may require a pure beta-adrenergic drug, such as isoproterenol (Isuprel), to enhance the effectiveness of conventional therapy.

The nurse caring for a patient in anaphylactic shock should anticipate the possibility of recurrence of the signs and symptoms as late as 8 hours after exposure to the antigen. These recurrences or delayed reactions require the same therapeutic interventions as the immediate response.

Septic shock

Septic shock is characterized by hemodynamic alterations caused by a severe overwhelming infection. Definitive measures directed toward the cause of the shock include identifying and controlling the source of infection. To locate the origin of the sepsis, specimens of urine, sputum, blood, and wound drainage are obtained according to procedural guidelines and sent to the laboratory for culture and antibiotic sensitivity testing. Radiographic studies of the abdomen and lower chest are taken with the patient in an upright position to rule out the presence of free air beneath the diaphragm. If free air is present below the diaphragm, one must consider the possibility of perforation of the uterine or intestinal viscera. Sinus films are obtained because sinus infections can be the origin of sepsis in patients with nasogastric and nasotracheal tubes. After identification of the septic foci, attempts are made to remove the nidus of infection. Resection and drainage or more invasive surgical techniques are used, when necessary, to drain purulent secretions and remove necrotic tissue.

Another component of definitive therapy in septic shock is administration of appropriate antibiotics. Empiric antibiotic therapy, usually initiated before receiving the culture and sensitivity reports, includes coverage of Gram-negative bacteria and Gram-positive bacteria, including anaerobes. Specific empiric formulas suggest the following:

1. An aminoglycoside, such as gentamicin or tobramycin (Nebcin), for Gram-negative bacteria
2. A third-generation cephalosporin, such as cefotaxime (Claforan) or ceftazidime (Fortaz), for both Gram-negative and Gram-positive bacteria
3. A penicillin agent, such as nafcillin (Nafcil, Unipen) or piperacillin (Pipracil), for Gram-positive bacteria and some Gram-negative bacteria
4. Chloramphenicol (Chloromycetin) or clindamycin (Cleocin) for anaerobic bacteria

Supportive Measures

Definitive therapy specific for each type of shock is directed toward correcting or alleviating the cause of the shock state. Supportive therapy is instituted to establish and maintain adequate tissue perfusion until definitive measures are effective. Aspects of supportive management include the following:

1. Establishment of adequate ventilation and oxygenation
2. Restoration of optimum intravascular volume
3. Maintenance of adequate cardiac output
4. Restoration of normal metabolism

Establishment of ventilation and oxygenation

The first step in establishing adequate ventilation is to open the airway. (See Chapter 34 for specific techniques to establish and maintain a patent airway.) Once an effective airway is established, ventilation must be improved. Simply encouraging the patient to deep breathe and cough can be helpful in increasing the volume of air inspired with each breath. As the shock state progresses and respiratory function deteriorates, respiratory muscles fatigue and the patient hypoventilates. The patient usually requires artificial mechanical ventilatory support to ensure adequate ventilation in the late stages of shock.

Supplemental oxygen is administered to correct the patient's hypoxemia. The route of oxygen administration varies with the form of airway adjunct used and according to the patient's needs. The shock patient usually receives high concentrations of oxygen to correct the hypoxemia evident during the compensatory and progressive stages of shock.

Restoration of intravascular volume

Adequate circulation depends on an optimum intravascular volume. In hypovolemic shock, administration of parenteral fluids is an important part of correcting the cause of shock. However, in other forms of shock, parenteral fluid administration also is important in supporting tissue perfusion. Parenteral fluids used in shock include blood and blood products, pharmaceutical plasma expanders, and crystalloid solutions. Infusion rates of parenteral fluids vary, because cardiac function and vascular capacity are constantly changing in shock. The patient in the intensive care unit frequently has invasive catheters that provide hemodynamic data to guide the rate of fluid therapy.

Maintenance of cardiac output

Providing an adequate intravascular volume is helpful only if the heart can effectively circulate that volume to the tissues. When myocardial contractility is impaired or depressed, cardiac output eventually decreases. Drugs that increase the force of contraction, termed positive inotropic agents, increase stroke volume and improve cardiac output. Positive inotropic drugs, described earlier, include dobutamine and dopamine. To optimize cardiac output the patient's heart rate should be maintained in a normal range (50 to 110 beats/min). If the heart rate is too slow, cardiac output falls because of too few cardiac cycles per minute. If the heart rate is too fast, cardiac output falls because of shortened diastolic filling time and reduced stroke volume. Drugs used to optimize the heart rate include atropine, isoproterenol, lidocaine (Xylocaine), quinidine, procainamide (Pronestyl), and propranolol. In some shock patients, cardiac pacing is used to optimize cardiac output while avoiding potential adverse effects of pharmacologic agents used to correct the heart rate.

No one drug can achieve all of the desired hemodynamic effects in every shock state. The physician must use various combinations of drugs to achieve the precise alterations needed in each patient situation. These numerous combinations of several drugs are referred to as the polypharmacy of shock.

Restoration of normal metabolism

The primary metabolic derangement in shock is acidosis. Acidosis results from both respiratory and metabolic causes. Adequate ventilation to remove carbon dioxide can help correct the acidosis and raise the blood pH. In extreme acidotic states, characterized by a serum bicarbonate less than 10 milliequivalents per liter (mEq/L), sodium bicarbonate is administered intravenously. The dosage is guided by arterial blood gas values and calculation of the patient's base deficit.

The internal environment also is altered because of electrolyte abnormalities. These include hyperkalemia caused by cellular destruction, hypernatremia caused by dehydration and increased aldosterone, and hypophosphatemia caused by malnutrition and administration of phosphate-deficient stored whole blood. Serum electrolytes must be monitored and corrected with appropriate measures during the shock state.

Vitamins, minerals, and other nutritional stores are depleted in shock because of reduced intake, decreased intestinal absorption, and accelerated utilization secondary to stress. The shock patient needs 3000 to 4000 calories per day and supplemental vitamins and minerals to prevent malnutrition and its adverse sequelae.

Supportive measures attempt to improve oxygen delivery to body cells. A patent airway, adequate ventilation, and supplemental oxygen are vital. After oxygen is inspired, it must diffuse into the blood and be carried by adequate numbers of red blood cells. Hemoglobin in red blood cells must bind with

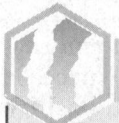

GERIATRIC CONSIDERATIONS

Treating Shock in the Elderly Patient

Avoid administering parenteral fluids rapidly to older patients. The elderly patient may not respond favorably to volume administration because the older heart often is stiff and less compliant. Rapid volume administration can precipitate pulmonary edema in the elderly patient with preexisting heart failure.

Drug metabolism and excretion are impaired in elderly patients who have decreased liver and renal function. For example, some antiarrhythmic drugs, such as lidocaine, are metabolized in the liver. When administering lidocaine to an elderly patient with chronic liver disease, the nurse should consult with the physician about the possible need to reduce the dose. Doses of antibiotics, especially aminoglycosides, are carefully adjusted to avoid adverse effects, such as nephrotoxicity, in elderly patients with diminished renal function.

oxygen to carry it to the tissues and release the oxygen to peripheral cells. When oxygen is delivered to body cells, the cells must be able to use the oxygen to produce energy and restore normal cellular function. Restoration of cellular function is a complex process that cannot be achieved with a single therapeutic intervention. Supportive management of the shock patient requires many drugs and therapies to maintain tissue perfusion and sustain cellular function.

NURSING MANAGEMENT OF THE SHOCK PATIENT
Prevention

One of the most important roles of the nurse is prevention of shock. Because many patients have the potential to develop shock, a constant vigilance must be kept to identify patients at risk to develop any form of shock. For example, multiple trauma victims and postoperative patients are at risk for hypovolemic shock. Patients with acute myocardial infarctions, especially involving the anterior wall of the left ventricle, are at risk to develop cardiogenic shock. Patients with impaired host defenses, such as those with cancer or receiving chemotherapy, can develop septic shock. A thorough nursing history, accurate observations, and continual assessment are key components in identifying patients who are potential shock victims.

Hypovolemic shock

Hypovolemic shock develops when the intravascular volume is decreased. To prevent this form of shock, the nurse constantly assesses the patient's fluid status. Accurate and complete intake and output records are essential in detecting a negative fluid balance. Daily weights provide another gauge of the patient's fluid status. The nurse also considers unmeasured fluid losses, such as insensible loss, profuse perspiration, and copious drainage. Surgical dressings are evaluated in estimating fluid losses. Marking the outline of a stain with a pen or pencil can help in estimating the amount of fluid or blood lost over time from a specific drainage site. Moist dressings may need to be weighed to determine the volume of fluid lost. Measuring and recording the volume of chest tube drainage are other important nursing actions in monitoring the patient's fluid balance.

In a patient with overt bleeding, hypovolemic shock can be prevented by minimizing blood loss. Specific nursing actions include application of direct pressure to the bleeding site and notification of the physician so that more definitive treatment can be initiated. Rapid replacement of intravascular fluid volume can prevent a mild fluid deficit from progressing to a more severe state.

Cardiogenic shock

Cardiogenic shock results from the impaired ability of the ventricles to pump blood. To prevent this form of shock, the nurse caring for the patient with an acute myocardial infarction attempts to decrease or minimize infarction size. A calm, reassuring attitude can do much to alleviate the patient's fears and reduce oxygen needs of the heart. Prompt relief of pain, administration of supplemental oxygen, and restricting physical activity can improve the balance of myocardial oxygen supply and demand.

Neurogenic shock

Neurogenic shock is transient and results from loss of sympathetic tone. The nurse can help prevent neurogenic shock in patients with spinal cord trauma by careful immobilization of spinal cord injuries as early as possible. The nurse attempts to maintain that immobility during transport and diagnostic procedures. After spinal anesthesia, the head of the patient's bed can be kept at a slight elevation of 15 to 20 degrees to prevent spread of the anesthetic agent up the cord to the medulla. Elevations greater than 20 degrees can potentiate spinal headaches.

Anaphylactic shock

Anaphylactic shock occurs as an allergic response to a foreign antigen. The nurse can prevent this type of shock by obtaining a careful, detailed nursing history of the patient's allergies. The nurse should specifically question the patient as to when he or she last experienced a reaction and explore the signs and symptoms the patient develops after he or she receives or is exposed to the substance.

The nurse administers intravenous drugs cautiously. A small amount of the drug should be injected slowly into the vein. If no adverse effects are noted, the remaining amount of the drug can be injected slowly. This deliberate administration is especially important when the patient is receiving a medication for the first time.

When the patient is receiving blood or blood products, the nurse follows hospital procedures in assuring that the patient's blood type and Rh factor have been matched with the transfused blood. The patient is monitored closely during the transfusion for any manifestations of allergic reaction, such as flushing, pruritus, edema, hypotension, and dyspnea.

Septic shock

Septic shock is caused by an overwhelming infection. Considering the impaired defenses of hospitalized patients, the nurse must continuously strive to protect all patients from invading pathogens. Strict aseptic technique during suctioning, dressing changes, and wound care is essential. Careful handwashing between patient contacts can minimize cross contamination. The nurse caring for patients with invasive lines and catheters must use meticulous technique when manipulating the lines, tubings, and portals of entry. The nurse observes all potential portals of entry, noting the presence of local inflammation (e.g., redness, swelling, warmth). Observing for signs and symptoms of systemic infection also is an important nursing role. Monitoring trends in the patient's temperature, white blood cell count, and blood pressure provides important data about the patient's response to invading microorganisms.

Prevention of shock also includes astute assessment of changes in the patient's clinical picture. The nurse must understand the progression of shock to detect early signs and symptoms of shock. For example, early compensation is associated with restlessness, confusion, and elevated blood pressure. Progression of the shock state is associated with hypoventilation and reduced urine output. The nurse must be able to knowledgeably assess the patient's changing clinical condition and interpret assessment findings to prevent progression of shock.

Assessment

The major clinical findings that the nurse assesses in the shock patient are the cardinal parameters of tissue perfusion, namely, level of consciousness, skin, urine output, and vital signs.

The shock patient's level of consciousness decreases because of reduced cerebral blood flow and inadequate oxygen delivery to brain cells. In the early stages of shock the patient displays subtle changes, such as restlessness, agitation, anxiety, and irritability. As cerebral ischemia worsens, the nurse can note confusion, personality changes, paranoia, poor judgment, loss of memory, and altered sleep patterns. The patient's level of consciousness deteriorates during the progression of shock, so that responsiveness to verbal stimuli decreases and eventually is absent. When the patient no longer responds to verbal stimuli, the nurse assesses response to pain. Response to painful stimuli decreases as the patient first flexes to pain, then extends to pain, and finally becomes flaccid, having no response to pain.

Nursing assessment of the skin and mucous membranes should include evaluation of color, temperature, moistness, texture, and turgor. Early in shock, sympathetic nervous system stimulation shunts blood away from nonpriority organs, reducing circulation to the skin. The shock patient's skin becomes cool, pale, and moist. Increased sweat gland activity causes moist clamminess. Capillary refill is reduced. With sustained vasoconstriction, oxygen delivery significantly decreases, and the skin becomes cyanotic, cold, and mottled.

Exceptions to the typical skin changes in shock should be noted. In septic shock the skin often is warm, dry, and pink because of early vasodilation. In the presence of liver ischemia and hepatic failure, the skin and mucous membranes appear jaundiced. In anaphylactic shock the skin may appear flushed with macular or papular rashes. In hypovolemic shock caused by dehydration, the skin is dry with poor skin turgor. The mucous membranes can be pale if hypovolemic shock is related to blood loss.

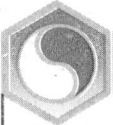 ETHICAL ISSUES

- How should the nurse respond when a man who is hemorrhaging begs her not to administer blood to him because he fears it may be infected with human immunodeficiency virus (HIV) or because he fears everlasting damnation according to religious beliefs that forbid receiving transfusions?

The nurse assesses renal function by measuring and recording the patient's hourly urine output. A minimum hourly urine output is 20 to 30 mL or 0.5 mL/kg. An indwelling urinary catheter is essential in shock states to monitor this parameter.

In addition to measuring urine volume, the nurse notes the composition of urine. Measurements of the urine specific gravity or osmolality reflect concentration of the urine. As early compensatory mechanisms are activated, urine volume falls and urine osmolality rises. The kidneys are able to excrete waste products but are compensating by retaining fluid. (More waste products are dissolved in less water, so the concentration of urine rises.) With progression of the shock state and prolonged renal hypoperfusion, the kidneys excrete fewer waste products. The urine volume remains low, and the urine concentration is either fixed or dilute. The failing kidneys lose their ability to concentrate urine.

The blood pressure in shock initially may be normal or slightly elevated as a result of compensatory mechanisms. The systolic blood pressure can be increased because of increased stroke volume and cardiac output. The diastolic blood pressure can be increased because of peripheral vasoconstriction. As the shock state progresses and compensatory mechanisms fail, the blood pressure decreases and the normal sounds of blood pressure (i.e., the Korotkoff sounds) decrease in intensity. The systolic blood pressure decreases as cardiac output falls. The diastolic blood pressure can remain normal because of sustained vasoconstriction. As a result the pulse pressure (i.e., the difference between the systolic and diastolic blood pressures) narrows.

It is important to remember that shock is a problem of decreased tissue perfusion, not decreased blood pressure. Patients in shock can have a blood pressure that is high, low, or normal, depending on the type of shock, their normal blood pressure range, preexisting health conditions, and compensatory mechanisms. The patient can have a low blood pressure and not be in shock. Examples include patients who are normally hypotensive and patients with aortic stenosis or severe hypothermia.

Blood pressure measurement using a cuff and sphygmomanometer usually is inaccurate in shock. Blood pressure sounds are created as blood flows past the section of artery compressed by the inflated cuff. In shock, decreased stroke volume and sustained vasoconstriction reduce peripheral blood flow, and the cuff blood pressure reading can underestimate the arterial pressure by 15 to 30 mm Hg.

When peripheral blood flow is markedly decreased, flow distal to the inflated cuff can be inadequate to produce audible sounds. When this occurs, the blood pressure is not actually zero. The blood pressure simply is not audible. The nurse may need to palpate the arterial pulse distal to the cuff to estimate the systolic blood pressure. An ultrasound flowmeter (Doppler) can be helpful in obtaining an accurate peripheral blood pressure in shock.

Arterial pulses are palpated in shock to assess peripheral blood flow. The nurse should assess the major arterial pulses, including the carotid, brachial, radial, ulnar, femoral, popliteal, dorsalis pedis, and posterior tibial. Assessment of arterial pulses includes evaluation of rate, rhythm, amplitude, and quality. The rate usually is rapid because of increased heart rate. The rhythm can be irregular because of ischemic dysrhythmias that develop as the shock state progresses. The pulse amplitude is reduced and the quality is thready as a result of decreased peripheral blood flow.

The nurse monitors the patient's respiratory rate and depth. Early in shock, hypoxia stimulates deeper and faster breathing. The respiratory rate commonly exceeds 20/min. Respiratory depth is increased to twice the normal tidal volume. As shock progresses, respiratory muscles fatigue and the patient hypoventilates. Respirations become shallow, though they continue to be rapid. Auscultation of the lung fields reveals moist crackles as progressive pulmonary changes result in interstitial edema. When anaphylactic shock is present, bronchial constriction can produce inspiratory and expiratory wheezes.

As hypoxemia and progressive respiratory changes develop, the nurse must be alert for signs of respiratory distress. The nurse observes for shortness of breath and orthopnea. Flaring nares; downward movement of the trachea; and use of accessory muscles in the neck, shoulders, and abdomen should be recognized and reported.

Temperature in shock usually becomes subnormal because of slowed cellular metabolism and decreased heat production. In septic shock the temperature can be elevated because of the inflammatory response to invading microorganisms. In anaphylactic shock the allergic response can cause an increase in body temperature.

The nurse assesses for associated clinical changes related to shock. Inadequate energy production can lead to complaints of muscle fatigue, weakness, and lassitude. Inadequate blood flow to the heart muscle can precipitate dysrhythmias and episodes of angina. Abnormal heart sounds can include a third heart sound produced by the rapid filling of an untoned failing ventricle or a fourth heart sound caused by atrial filling of a noncompliant injured ventricular chamber. Stasis in the gastrointestinal tract can cause abdominal distention, nausea, anorexia, constipation, and paralytic ileus. Other clinical findings are discussed with each type of shock.

Invasive hemodynamic parameters

The shock patient exhibits many clinical changes that the nurse can detect at the bedside. In addition, invasive catheters are used to gain more information about the patient's cardiopulmonary status. These catheters directly measure pressures within the cardiovascular system and provide data used to calculate additional hemodynamic parameters. The primary hemodynamic parameters include intraarterial blood pressure, central venous (right atrial) pressure, pulmonary artery pressures, cardiac output, and venous oxygen saturation.

Intraarterial blood pressure

The **intraarterial blood pressure** can be measured directly with an indwelling catheter inserted by a physician into an artery. The most common site of insertion is the radial artery. As illustrated in Figure 13-10, the catheter is connected by high-pressure tubing to a transducer and continuous flush system. The transducer transforms the pressure sensed in the catheter to electrical signals visible as a waveform or a digital numeric display or both on the arterial pressure monitor. The arterial pressure monitor provides continuous or intermittent readings of the arterial systolic, diastolic, and mean blood pressures. The continuous flush system delivers small amounts of heparinized normal saline under pressure to maintain patency of the arterial line. Therapeutic advantages of direct arterial pressure monitoring in shock include increased accuracy of blood pressure measurement and access to the arterial circulation. Auscultation or palpation of the blood pressure in shock can be difficult because of the severe reduction in peripheral blood flow. The values obtained with indirect methods are often lower than the true arterial blood pressure. Direct measurement of the arterial blood pressure provides more accurate data on which to base therapy, such as titration of intravenous drug infusions. Access to the arterial circulation also provides a convenient source of arterial blood samples for monitoring arterial blood gases.

Disadvantages of an intraarterial catheter include:
1. Hemorrhage as a result of disconnection of the catheter from the continuous flush system.
2. Ischemia distal to the insertion site. Blood flow can be decreased distal to the site of catheter insertion as a result of occlusion of the artery by vessel spasm or fibrin clots. Ischemia of the fingers can result when the catheter is inserted in the radial artery, whereas femoral artery cannulation can predispose to ischemia of the entire lower limb.
3. Infection related to the presence of an invasive catheter and frequent manipulation of the system to obtain blood samples.
4. Damage to the arterial wall as a result of excessive flushing of the line or manipulation of the arterial catheter.

Technical problems, such as air bubbles in the tubing or a faulty transducer, can produce an inaccurate direct arterial blood pressure reading. It is best to correlate intraarterial pressure measurements

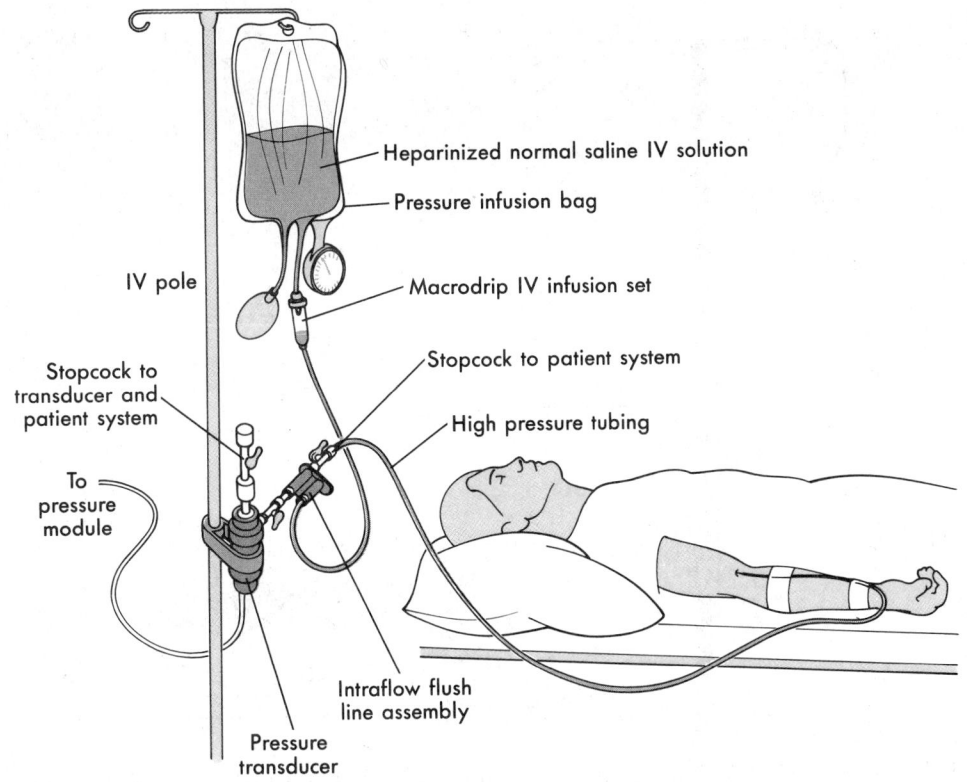

FIGURE 13-10   Equipment setup for intra-arterial pressure monitoring.

with indirect cuff pressures and other assessment data to evaluate perfusion.

Central venous pressure

The **central venous pressure (CVP),** or **right atrial pressure,** is directly monitored using a large-bore indwelling catheter. The catheter is inserted by a physician into a central vein, such as the subclavian or jugular, and advanced until the catheter tip is located in the superior vena cava at the right atrium. The catheter is connected to either (1) a transducer and pressure monitor, which converts the pressure measured in the central circulation to a waveform or a digital numeric display in millimeters of mercury (mm Hg) pressure or both or (2) a plastic or glass water manometer that is used to measure the pressure at the catheter tip in centimeters (cm) of water (Figure 13-11).

Directly measuring the CVP provides an estimate of venous return to the right side of the heart. It reflects right ventricular filling pressure or preload. The CVP is normally 4 to 12 cm of water pressure or −1 to 8 mm Hg. In hypovolemic shock, venous return to the right side of the heart is decreased; therefore the CVP is low. In distributive forms of shock with massive vasodilation, venous return is decreased and right ventricular filling pressure is low. In cardiogenic shock, inadequate systolic emptying elevates filling pressures. Although the primary elevation is in the left ventricle, passive transmission of the high pressure through the pulmonary circula-

tion can eventually increase the right ventricular filling pressure. In addition, right ventricular infarction, although less common than left ventricular infarction, markedly increases right ventricular filling pressure and elevates the CVP.

Potential disadvantages of the CVP catheter include complications related to cannulation of a central vein (e.g., pneumothorax, hemorrhage), infection caused by the indwelling invasive device, and catheter occlusion. The primary limitation of the central venous or right atrial pressure measurement is its inability to reflect left ventricular filling pressure. The data reflect only right heart pressures, which can be normal or low in the presence of left ventricular dysfunction and elevated left ventricular filling pressures.

Pulmonary artery pressures

The pulmonary artery systolic, diastolic, and mean pressures can be measured directly using a balloon-tipped, flow-directed pulmonary artery catheter, such as the Swan-Ganz catheter manufactured by Baxter Health Care Corp. (Figure 13-12). Several types of pulmonary artery catheters have been developed, including double-lumen, triple-lumen, and quadruple-lumen catheters.

The double-lumen pulmonary artery catheter has two lumens. One lumen, termed the *distal lumen,* extends to the catheter tip and is used to measure pressures at the end of the catheter, to infuse fluid, and to obtain blood samples. The second lumen,

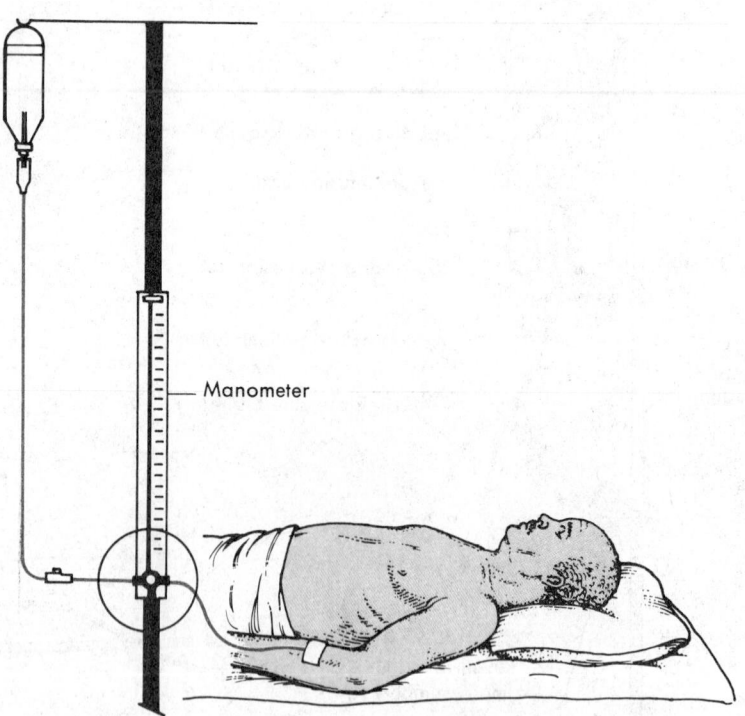

FIGURE 13-11   Measurement of central venous pressure using water manometer.

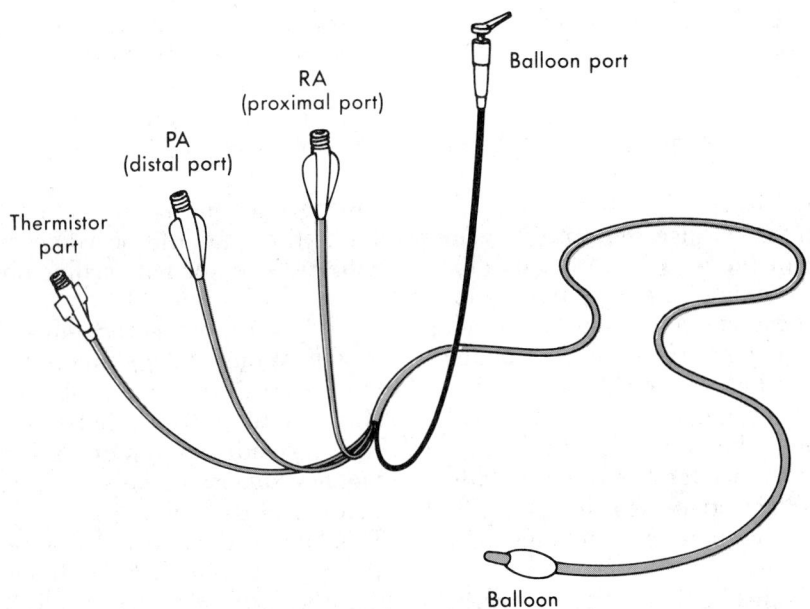

FIGURE 13-12   Pulmonary artery catheter (four-lumen).

termed the *balloon lumen,* extends to a small latex balloon located near the catheter tip. The balloon can be inflated with air introduced into the balloon lumen.

A triple-lumen catheter has the same distal and balloon lumens as a double-lumen catheter. In addition, the catheter contains a third lumen, termed the *proximal lumen,* which extends to approximately 30 cm from the catheter tip. The lumen is used to infuse fluid and monitor pressures.

The quadruple-lumen catheter contains the three lumens just described. In addition, a fourth lumen contains temperature-sensing wires that extend to a small thermistor unit located on the surface of the catheter approximately 4 cm from the tip. This thermistor unit senses temperature and conveys the reading to a bedside computer for calculation of cardiac output. The pulmonary artery catheter is inserted into a vein by a physician and advanced until the catheter tip is located in the superior vena cava or right atrium. The balloon then is inflated, and the catheter is directed with the forward flow of blood from the right atrium, through the right ventricle, and into the pulmonary artery (Figure 13-13.) When the catheter is positioned in the pulmonary artery, the balloon is deflated and is only periodically inflated to obtain specific pressure readings.

The distal lumen of the catheter is connected to a transducer that transforms the pressure sensed at the catheter tip to a waveform or a digital numeric display or both on the pressure monitor. When the catheter is positioned in the pulmonary artery, the distal lumen is used to continuously monitor pulmonary artery pressures. The normal pulmonary artery

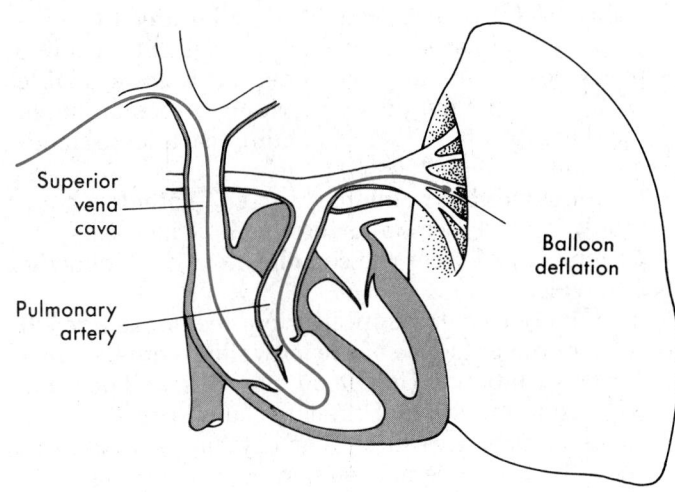

FIGURE 13-13   Pulmonary artery catheter placement.

systolic pressure is 15 to 25 mm Hg, and the normal pulmonary artery diastolic pressure is 8 to 10 mm Hg.

The balloon on the pulmonary artery catheter can be inflated by introducing air into the balloon lumen. Inflation of the balloon facilitates the forward movement of the catheter tip until the balloon comes in contact with the walls of the pulmonary arterial vessel. When this occurs, the balloon becomes wedged, and the catheter can no longer move forward. With the balloon in the wedged position, the distal lumen at the catheter tip can sense only the pressure in the pulmonary capillaries, pulmonary veins, and left atrium. When the mitral valve is open during ventricular diastole, the distal lumen can sense indirectly pressure in the left ventricle (i.e., left ventricular filling pressure or left ventricular end diastolic pressure). The pressure measured in this manner is termed the **pulmonary wedge pressure (PWP),** or pulmonary artery occlusion pressure (PAOP), and normally is 6 to 12 mm Hg.

Although the catheter is inserted into a vein through the right side of the heart into the pulmonary circulation, balloon inflation allows the catheter to provide indirect information about the function of the left heart. In some cases the PWP does not accurately reflect left heart function. Specific examples of conditions that can impair the indirect measurement of left heart function with the pulmonary artery catheter in the wedged position include mitral valve disease, obstructive lung disease, pulmonary venospasm, acute pulmonary embolus, and right ventricular infarction.

When the catheter is positioned so that the catheter tip is in the pulmonary artery, the proximal lumen opens into the right atrium. Connecting the proximal lumen to a transducer or water manometer allows measurement of the central venous or right atrial pressure. This lumen alleviates the need for a second catheter to monitor right heart filling pressures. Pulmonary artery catheters are available with two proximal ports, providing a second lumen for the infusion of fluids and administration of medications.

Although the pulmonary artery catheter commonly is used in monitoring shock, it increases the patient's risk for certain complications, including the following:

1. Increased susceptibility to infection as a result of the presence of the indwelling catheter, manipulation during blood sampling, and possible contamination of the flush solution
2. Disturbances in cardiac rhythm as a result of the presence and motion of the catheter
3. Occlusion of the pulmonary vessel, reduction in pulmonary blood flow, and pulmonary infarction caused by permanent wedging of the balloon
4. Rupture of the pulmonary vessel and subsequent hemorrhage related to overinflation of the balloon
5. Inaccurate pressure readings as a result of displacement of the catheter tip, occlusion of the catheter lumen or lumens, or a faulty transducer/monitor

Cardiac output

The quadruple-lumen pulmonary artery catheter contains a thermistor unit on the catheter tip. The thermistor lumen is connected to a bedside computer and can be used to continuously monitor core temperature. In addition, it can be used to measure cardiac output. In this procedure, iced or room-temperature saline is injected into the proximal lumen of the pulmonary artery catheter so that it enters the right atrium. Based on the temperature changes sensed at the thermistor unit over time following injection of the saline, the computer calculates the patient's cardiac output in liters per minute. The normal cardiac output is 4 to 7 L/min.

Venous oxygen saturation

Modifications of the pulmonary artery catheter have led to the development of a fiberoptic catheter. In addition to the four lumens previously described with a quadruple-lumen catheter, a fiberoptic pulmonary artery catheter contains fiberoptic wires that travel through a fifth lumen to the catheter tip. This lumen is connected to a bedside monitoring device that continuously analyzes light transmitted by the fiberoptic wires as it is reflected by blood cells passing the catheter tip. The light density is affected by the oxygen concentration in the red blood cell. Based on the density and light reflection, the bedside monitor provides a continuous waveform or a numeric digital display or both of the oxygen saturation of hemoglobin in venous blood in the pulmonary artery.

The venous oxygen saturation reflects the amount of oxygen remaining in the venous blood after it has passed through the capillaries. When cells need more oxygen, the body normally increases blood flow by increasing cardiac output. In shock, the body cannot increase cardiac output, and cells are deprived of oxygen. To compensate, cells extract more oxygen than normal from the capillary blood. As a result, the venous oxygen saturation is below the normal value of 60% to 80%.

Septic shock usually increases venous oxygen saturation. One reason is the presence of bacterial toxins that damage cells so that they cannot use oxygen. A second reason relates to maldistribution of blood volume, which results in some areas being hypoperfused and others being hyperperfused. In hyperperfused areas, more oxygen remains in the venous blood. As a result, venous oxygen saturation of mixed venous blood in the pulmonary artery increases.

The pressures and measurements obtained with invasive hemodynamic devices are extremely valuable in monitoring the progression of shock and the patient's response to therapy. Table 13-5 lists some of the measured and derived hemodynamic parameters used in the assessment and management of shock. (Refer to a standard critical care nursing text or a reference text on invasive hemodynamic monitoring for more specific information about equipment setup, operation, and troubleshooting.)

TABLE 13-5   Hemodynamic Parameters

Parameter	How Obtained	Normal Value
Intra-arterial blood pressure	Direct measurement with indwelling arterial catheter	Systolic—greater than 80 to 90 mm Hg Diastolic—greater than 60 to 65 mm Hg
Pulmonary artery pressures	Direct measurement with indwelling pulmo-nary artery catheter	Systolic—15 to 25 mm Hg Diastolic—8 to 10 mm Hg Capillary wedge—6 to 12 mm Hg
Right atrial (central venous) pressure	Direct measurement with indwelling central venous catheter or via proximal lumen of pul-monary artery catheter	−1 to 8 mm Hg or 4 to 12 cm H_2O
Cardiac output (CO)	Determined with quadruple-lumen (thermodi-lution) pulmonary artery catheter and bed-side computer	4 to 7 L/min
Cardiac index (CI)	Calculated according to following formula: $$\frac{\text{Cardiac output}}{\text{Body surface area}}$$	2.5 to 4 L/min/m^2
Stroke volume (SV)	Calculated according to following formula: $$\frac{\text{CO} \times 1000 \text{ mL}}{\text{Heart rate}}$$	60 to 100 mL/beat
Stroke volume index (SVI)	Calculated according to following formula: $$\frac{\text{SV}}{\text{Body surface area}}$$	33 to 47 mL/beat/m^2
Systemic vascular resistance (SVR)	Calculated according to following formula: $$\frac{\text{Mean arterial pressure} - \text{Right atrial pressure}}{\text{Cardiac output}} \times 80$$	800 to 1500 dynes/sec/cm^{-5}
Pulmonary vascular resis-tance (PVR)	Calculated according to following formula: $$\frac{\text{Mean pulmonary artery pressure} - \text{Pulmonary capillary wedge pressure}}{\text{Cardiac output}} \times 80$$	20 to 120 dynes/sec/cm^{-5}
Venous oxygen saturation (SvO$_2$)	Continuous direct measurement with indwell-ing fiberoptic pulmonary artery catheter and bedside computer	60% to 80%

Nursing Diagnoses, Planning, and Interventions

The following section identifies specific nursing di-agnoses appropriate for the shock patient. The ra-tionale for choosing each diagnosis in shock is pre-sented, expected patient outcomes are detailed, and nursing interventions are summarized.

Nursing Diagnosis

Altered tissue perfusion related to decreased car-diac output, inadequate intravascular volume, or maldistribution of blood volume

Rationale

The nursing diagnosis of altered tissue perfusion is appropriate for all shock patients. The specific cause of the alteration varies with the type of shock. In car-diogenic shock the impaired ability of the heart as a pump reduces cardiac output. In hypovolemic shock inadequate intravascular volume reduces cardiac output and tissue perfusion. In distributive forms of shock the intravascular volume is abnormally dis-tributed throughout the body, and tissue perfusion is inadequate. As the shock state progresses, tissue perfusion suffers because of profound hypotension, microvascular changes, and further reductions in cardiac output.

Expected patient outcomes

1. Normal sensorium as evidenced by alert and oriented state, ability to follow simple commands, and response to verbal stimuli
2. Peripheral pulses—full, strong, and regular bilaterally
3. Urine output—greater than 0.5 mL/kg/hr (greater than 30 mL/hr)
4. Skin—warm, dry, and pink
5. Arterial blood pressure—normal for the patient (e.g., systolic—greater than 90 mm Hg and less than 140 mm Hg; diastolic—greater than 65 mm Hg and less than 90 mm Hg)
6. Venous oxygen saturation—60% to 80%
7. Arterial pH—7.35 to 7.45
8. Arterial bicarbonate—24 to 28 mEq/L

Nursing interventions

1. Assess the patient's level of consciousness every hour by questioning orientation, observing responses to verbal stimuli, and observing responses to painful stimuli.
2. Palpate peripheral pulses hourly, including brachial, dorsalis pedis, and posterior tibial. Record presence, equality, rate, rhythm, and quality.
3. Measure and record urine output hourly.
4. Assess skin color and temperature hourly.
5. Continuously monitor patient's arterial blood pressure via the intraarterial catheter. Record reading every 15 minutes or less frequently if stable.
6. Continuously monitor venous oxygen saturation if a fiberoptic pulmonary artery catheter is used. Note changes in the venous oxygen saturation that occur with specific interventions and activities (e.g., suctioning, turning).
7. Assess the adequacy of perfusion by monitoring the arterial blood pH and bicarbonate values as ordered.
8. Administer parenteral fluids and medications as ordered, and assess the patient's response.

Nursing Diagnosis

Decreased cardiac output related to heart muscle damage, toxic metabolic wastes, dysrhythmias, and internal fluid shifts

Rationale

The patient in cardiogenic shock has decreased cardiac output as a result of the loss of functional heart muscle. Patients who have other forms of shock also have decreased cardiac output because of metabolic changes. Renal insufficiency, excess anaerobic metabolism, and respiratory failure create acidosis, which depresses contractility of the heart muscle and decreases cardiac output. As the shock progresses and the heart becomes ischemic, the patient develops dysrhythmias, which also decrease

cardiac output. Changes in the microcirculation result in fluid shifts from the intravascular compartment into the interstitial compartment, decreasing circulating fluid volume and ultimately decreasing cardiac output.

Expected patient outcomes

1. Arterial blood pressure—normal for the patient
2. Heart rate—greater than 50 to 60 beats/min and less than 110 to 120 beats/min
3. Peripheral pulses—full, strong, and regular bilaterally
4. Right atrial pressure—−1 to 8 mm Hg
5. Pulmonary artery pressures: systolic—15 to 25 mm Hg; diastolic—8 to 10 mm Hg; and wedge—6 to 12 mm Hg
6. Cardiac output—4 to 7 L/min
7. Venous oxygen saturation—60% to 80%

Nursing interventions

1. Continuously monitor the patient's arterial blood pressure via the intraarterial catheter. Record the pressure reading every 15 minutes or less frequently if stable.
2. Monitor the patient's cardiac rhythm. Document the rhythm every 8 to 12 hours or more frequently if the rhythm changes.
3. Palpate peripheral pulses hourly, including brachial, dorsalis pedis, and posterior tibial. Record presence, equality, rate, rhythm, and quality.
4. Obtain hemodynamic pressure measurements of right atrial pressure, pulmonary artery pressure, PWP, and cardiac output every hour or as ordered. Continuously monitor venous oxygen saturation.
5. Use invasive hemodynamic measurements to determine systemic vascular resistance, cardiac index, and other derived parameters every 1 to 2 hours or as ordered. Record at least every 2 to 4 hours or after changes in therapy.
6. Maintain the patient on modified bed rest or activity restriction, as ordered, to minimize myocardial oxygen demands.
7. When the patient is receiving vasoactive and inotropic medications, titrate the infusions as ordered to achieve the desired results. Monitor for adverse effects of these potent medications.

Nursing Diagnosis

Impaired gas exchange related to decreased pulmonary blood flow, pulmonary interstitial edema, and hypoventilation

Rationale

The shock patient suffers from impaired gas exchange as progressive changes develop in the lungs. Decreased pulmonary blood flow reduces arterial oxygen tension. As the shock state progresses, fluid transudes from the pulmonary capillaries into the pulmonary interstitium and alveoli, creating pulmonary edema. This problem impairs diffusion of oxygen and further decreases gas exchange. When the patient develops adult respiratory distress syndrome (ARDS), massive atelectasis, decreased lung compliance, and respiratory muscle fatigue reduce effective ventilation. The results are hypoxemia, hypercapnia, and respiratory acidosis.

Expected patient outcomes

1. Respiratory rate—10 to 20 breaths/min
2. Spontaneous ventilations—regular and unlabored
3. Breath sounds—equal bilaterally
4. Absence of crackles
5. Absence of cyanosis
6. Chest x-ray film—free of infiltrates
7. Arterial oxygen tension—greater than 80 mm Hg on 50% oxygen (Fio$_2$ 0.5)
8. Arterial carbon dioxide tension—35 to 45 mm Hg

Nursing interventions

1. Count and record the patient's respiratory rate. Note the depth and regularity of respirations.
2. If the patient is on artificial mechanical ventilation, be aware of the mode and ventilator settings. Record in the nursing record.
3. Observe the symmetry and magnitude of the patient's chest wall movement.
4. Auscultate breath sounds every 1 to 2 hours. Listen anteriorly to evaluate upper and middle lobes and posteriorly to evaluate lower lobes. Auscultate breath sounds more frequently during fluid challenges.
5. Inspect skin and mucous membranes for the presence of cyanosis.
6. Turn the patient at least every 2 hours. Avoid placing the most congested lung areas in the dependent position, since this can potentiate ventilation/perfusion imbalances.
7. Measure endotracheal or tracheostomy tube cuff pressure every 8 to 12 hours. Maintain cuff pressure below 18 to 20 mm Hg.
8. Assist the patient to remove secretions by encouraging the patient to cough and deep breathe if not receiving artificial ventilation. Suction as needed. Maintain adequacy of systemic hydration to decrease viscosity of secretions.
9. Monitor arterial blood gas values as ordered. (See Chapter 26 for detailed information on the nursing care of the patient on artificial mechanical ventilation.)

Nursing Diagnosis

Decreased urinary elimination related to sustained renal vasoconstriction and profound hypotension

Rationale

The shock patient suffers from decreased renal perfusion. Sustained sympathetic vasoconstriction reduces renal blood flow and results in ischemic changes and renal insufficiency.

Expected patient outcomes

1. Urine output—greater than 0.5 mL/kg/hr (greater than 30 mL/hr)
2. Blood urea nitrogen (BUN)—5 to 20 mg/dL
3. Serum creatinine—0.6 to 1.2 mg/dL

Nursing interventions

1. Measure and record urine output hourly.
2. Monitor the patient for progression from the oliguric phase of renal failure to the diuretic (recovery) phase, evidenced by a urine output greater than 400 mL/24 hr and gradual reduction in the BUN.
3. Monitor BUN and serum creatinine values daily or as ordered. Report elevations or trends to the physician.

Psychologic Needs

The patient in shock and the patient's family or significant others have many psychologic and emotional needs. Shock is a life-threatening situation that interrupts the routine daily activities of the patient and family. The patient usually is unfamiliar with the hospital environment and finds the intensive care unit frightening. The patient experiences a sense of powerlessness, fears the possibility of death, and is frustrated about his or her limited power to alter the outcome. The patient in shock has restricted interaction with family and friends because of the seriousness of the condition, intensive care routines, and limited visiting times. The patient whose mental function is decreased due to the hypoperfusion of shock may be confused and unable to distinguish real from unreal. Specific nursing diagnoses related to the patient's psychologic needs include anxiety, fear, impaired verbal communication, impaired social interaction, knowledge deficit, and powerlessness.

Family members of the patient in shock also experience great psychologic stress as they attempt to cope with alterations in their life-styles and family roles created by the critical illness. In addition, they fear the possibility of loss of their loved one, breakdown of their family unit, and great financial burdens from the tremendous cost of intensive care. They too experience a sense of isolation and powerlessness as they wait for news of the patient's condition and fear the final outcome. Because the sequelae of shock can extend the length of hospitalization into weeks and even months, families often suffer physical and emotional exhaustion.

The nurse caring for the shock patient and family

strives to provide emotional support and understand the acute psychologic stress precipitated by the life-threatening illness. Following the steps of the nursing process, the nurse begins with a detailed assessment of the patient's and family's psychologic states, including their perceptions of the events related to the illness, available support systems (e.g., friends, family, church members), usual coping behaviors, spiritual beliefs, and expressed concerns and needs. After adequate information is obtained, the nursing staff should discuss the patient's and family's emotional needs and develop a plan to provide appropriate support. Chaplain or ministerial assistance, social workers, and ethicists may be needed to resolve specific concerns and problems. While the shock patient's physical condition is critical and requires constant monitoring and frequent interventions, the psychologic and emotional needs of the patient and family must not be forgotten.

Additional Nursing Diagnoses

The box below gives nursing diagnoses appropriate for the patient in shock. This listing of nursing diagnoses serves only as a beginning point, since the nurse must individualize each care plan for the specific patient. A total nursing assessment helps the

POSSIBLE NURSING DIAGNOSES FOR SHOCK PATIENT

Activity intolerance
Altered body temperature
Altered nutrition
Altered tissue perfusion
Anxiety
Decreased cardiac output
Fear
Fluid volume deficit
Fluid volume excess
Impaired gas exchange
Impaired physical mobility
Impaired social interaction
Impaired verbal communication
Impaired skin integrity
Ineffective breathing pattern
Ineffective individual and family coping
Infection, high risk for
Injury, high risk for
Knowledge deficit
Pain
Powerlessness
Self-care deficit

nurse incorporate physiologic, pathophysiologic, emotional, psychosocial, and spiritual concerns of the patient and family unit into a holistic plan of care.

Evaluation

Evaluation is an integral component of the nursing process. When caring for the shock patient, the nurse must use assessment data, including clinical findings, hemodynamic parameters, and laboratory abnormalities, to evaluate the patient's response to therapy and progression of the shock state. Measurable expected patient outcomes help the nurse evaluate the impact of nursing interventions. Modifications of specific nursing interventions can be made to more effectively assist the patient achieve the desired outcomes. Evaluation also can help the nurse determine if the original expected outcomes are realistic and achievable. If the goals and outcomes are unrealistic, ongoing evaluation helps the nurse formulate more realistic and appropriate outcome criteria.

For example, the nurse may establish an expected patient outcome of full, strong, and regular pulses for interventions related to decreased cardiac output. However, if potent vasoconstrictor agents are required to maintain a minimum blood pressure, peripheral blood flow will be further diminished and peripheral pulses will not be strong and full. The nurse may need to modify the outcome criteria to include pulses that can be palpated or detected with the Doppler. The pulse characteristics of full and strong may be unrealistic in the severe shock state in the presence of vasoconstrictor medications.

CRITICAL THINKING QUESTIONS

1 Define shock in terms of tissue perfusion.
2 List in separate columns those patients at risk to develop hypovolemic, cardiogenic, neurogenic, anaphylactic, and septic shock.
3 Differentiate the major pathophysiologic changes in hypovolemic, cardiogenic, and septic shock.
4 What causes the massive vasodilation in neurogenic, anaphylactic, and septic shock?
5 Explain the cellular changes in the shock patient.
6 A 65-year-old patient is admitted for an acute myocardial infarction. His blood pressure shortly after admission is 80/50 mm Hg. Is this patient in shock? Explain.
7 A patient's heart rate is 136/min, his peripheral pulses are weak and rapid, his urine output is 25 mL/hr, and his skin is pale and cool. His blood glucose concentration is 200 mg/dL,

and he is lethargic and difficult to arouse. Which stage of shock does he exhibit? Why?

8 Review the effects of compensatory mechanisms by:
   a. Listing five effects of sympathetic nervous system stimulation (refer to Figure 13-7)
   b. Describing the action of three hormones released during compensation
   c. Explaining the effects of decreased pulmonary blood flow on arterial oxygen and carbon dioxide tensions

9 Summarize the effects of shock on the following organs/systems:
   a. Brain
   b. Kidneys
   c. Heart
   d. Liver
   e. Pancreas
   f. Lungs

10 List the laboratory changes that develop in the advanced stage of shock.

11 How can the nurse prevent hypovolemic, cardiogenic, neurogenic, anaphylactic, and septic shock?

12 Differentiate each of the following as either definitive or supportive therapy for shock:
   _____Administering antibiotics
   _____Opening the airway
   _____Initiating mechanical ventilation
   _____Receiving a human heart transplantation
   _____Surgically correcting a bleeding problem
   _____Administering parenteral fluids
   _____Providing adequate nutrition

13 The nurse caring for a patient in shock must monitor many clinical parameters. What findings should the nurse anticipate in advanced shock when checking the:
   a. Blood pressure
   b. Level of consciousness
   c. Urine output
   d. Peripheral pulses
   e. Skin
   f. Bowel sounds

14 Explain why the shock patient may need an intra-arterial catheter to monitor arterial blood pressure. What are potential dangers of this invasive catheter?

15 A pulmonary artery catheter can be used to monitor the cardiovascular status of a shock patient. Explain the purpose of each of the four lumens of the quadruple-lumen pulmonary artery catheter.

16 Compare the advantages and disadvantages of a central venous catheter and a pulmonary artery catheter.

17 List the normal values for the central venous pressure, the pulmonary artery diastolic and systolic pressures, the pulmonary wedge pressure, the cardiac output, and the venous oxygen saturation.

18 A 60-year-old patient with septic shock shows the following changes:
   a. His blood pressure has decreased from 120/90 mm Hg to 70/50 mm Hg.
   b. His skin has changed from pink and warm to cold and pale.
   c. His cardiac output has decreased from 5 L/min to 2.8 L/min.
   Explain the significance of these changes.

19 Review, by listing, possible nursing diagnoses for the shock patient.

20 Summarize specific nursing interventions related to three of the nursing diagnoses listed in question 19.

BIBLIOGRAPHY

Current

1. Ayres SM: The prevention and treatment of shock in acute myocardial infarction, *Chest* 93(suppl 1):17S-21S, 1988.
2. Barone JE, Synder AB: Treatment strategies in shock: use of oxygen transport measurements, *Heart Lung* 20(1):81-86, 1991.
3. Barry SA: Septic shock: special needs of patients with cancer, *Oncol Nurs Forum* 16(1):31-35, 1989.
4. Berron K: Role of the ventricular assist device in acute myocardial infarction, *Crit Care Nurs Q* 12(2):25-37, 1989.
5. Billhardt RA, Rosenbush SW: Cardiogenic and hypovolemic shock, *Med Clin North Am* 70(4):853-876, 1986.
6. Boyd JL, Stanford GG, Chernow B: The pharmacotherapy of septic shock, *Crit Care Clin* 5(1):133-150, 1989.
7. Carlson RW, Weil MH: Managing the patient in shock, *Hosp Med* 21(8):29-66, 1985.
8. Chernow B: *The pharmacologic approach to the critically ill patient,* Baltimore, 1988, Williams & Wilkins.
9. Cunnion RE, Parrillo JE: Myocardial dysfunction in sepsis, *Crit Care Clin* 5(1):99-118, 1989.
10. Dantzker D: Oxygen delivery and utilization in sepsis, *Crit Care Clin* 5(1):81-98, 1989.
11. DePriest JL: Septic shock: what to do until a breakthrough comes along, *Postgrad Med* 86(3):71-77, 1989.
12. Edwards JD: Practical application of oxygen transport principles, *Crit Care Med* 18(1):S45-S48, 1990.
13. Gammage G: Crystalloid versus colloid: is colloid worth the cost? *Int Anesthesiol Clin* 25(1):37-60, 1987.
14. Gawlinski A: Saving the cardiogenic shock patient, *Nurs 89* 19(12):34-42, 1989.
15. Guyton RA, Arcidi JM, Langford DA, et al: Emergency coronary bypass for cardiogenic shock, *Circulation* 76(suppl V):V22-V27, 1987.
16. Hager WD, Katz AM: Management of shock in acute myocardial infarction: changing concepts; past, present, and future, *Cardiology* 74(4):286-296, 1987.
17. Haljamae H: Organ specific metabolic changes in shock, *Prog Clin Biol Res* 264:17-26, 1988.

18. Harnett S: Septic shock in the oncology patient. *Cancer Nurs* 12(4):191-201, 1989.

19. Haustein KO: Review: therapeutic concepts of congestive heart failure, *Int J Clin Pharmacol Therapy Toxicol* 28(7):273-281, 1990.

20. Higgins TL, Chernow B: Pharmacotherapy of circulatory shock, *Disease Month* 33(6):309-361, 1987.

21. Iverson RL: Septic shock: a clinical perspective, *Crit Care Clin* 4(2):215-228, 1988.

22. Jeffries PR, Whelan SK: Cardiogenic shock: current management, *Crit Care Nurs Q* 11(1):48-56, 1988.

23. Kahn RC: Shock as a complication of cancer, *Crit Care Clin* 4(1):129-145, 1988.

24. Katz AM: Changing strategies in the management of heart failure, *J Am Coll Cardiol* 13(3):513-523, 1989.

25. Kelleher RM: Cardiac drugs: new inotropes, *Crit Care Nurs Clin North Am* 1(2):391-397, 1989.

26. Kirby RR: Shock: a systemic or cellular disease? *Int Anesthesiol Clin* 25(1):19-35, 1987.

27. Kuhn MM: Colloids vs. crystalloids, *Crit Care Nurs* 11(5):37-51, 1991.

28. Littleton MT: Pathophysiology and assessment of sepsis and septic shock, *Crit Care Nurs Q* 11(1):30-47, 1988.

29. Luce JM: Pathogenesis and management of septic shock, *Chest* 91(6):883-888, 1987.

30. Matthay MA, Chatterjee K: Bedside catheterization of the pulmonary artery: risks compared with benefits, *Ann Intern Med* 109(10):826-834, 1988.

31. Ormerod AD: Emergency management of anaphylaxis: treatment and clues to diagnosis, *Emergency Decisions* 4(3):31-40, 1988.

32. Parmley WW: Pathophysiology and current therapy of congestive heart failure, *J Am Coll Cardiol* 13(4):771-785, 1989.

33. Parrillo JE, Parker MM, Natanson C, et al: Septic shock in humans: advances in the understanding of pathogenesis, cardiovascular dysfunction, and therapy, *Ann Intern Med* 113(3):227-242, 1990.

34. Perret C: Acute heart failure in myocardial infarction: principles of treatment, *Crit Care Med* 18(1):S26-S29, 1990.

35. Pitt B: Acute myocardial infarction: treatment in the coronary care unit, *Postgrad Med* 85(2):145-154, 1989.

36. Rackow EC, Astiz ME, Weil MH. Cellular oxygen metabolism during sepsis and shock, *JAMA* 259(13):1989-1993, 1988.

37. Rice V: Septic shock: nursing implications of current medical research, *NITA J National Intravenous Therapy Assoc* 10(5):326-333, 1987.

38. Rice V: Cardiogenic shock. In *Advanced critical care nursing*, Rockville, Md, 1989, Aspen Publishers, Inc.

39. Rice V, editor: Shock, *Crit Care Nurs Clin North Am* 2(2):143-342, 1990.

40. Rice V: Shock, a clinical syndrome: an update. I. An overview of shock. II. The stages of shock. III. Therapeutic management. IV. Nursing care of the shock patient, *Crit Care Nurse* 11(4):20-27, 11(5):74-82, 11(6):34-39, 11(7):28-40, 1991.

41. Roberts R: Inotropic therapy for cardiac failure associated with acute myocardial infarction, *Chest* 93(suppl 1):22S-24S, 1988.

42. Roberts SL: Cardiogenic shock: decreased coronary artery tissue perfusion, *Dimen Crit Care Nurs* 7(4):196-209, 1988.

43. Roka L et al: Pathobiochemistry of shock, *J Clin Chem Clin Biochem* 25(4):205-239, 1987.

44. Rosenthal MH: The appropriate use of inotropes in shock, *Can J Anesthesia* 37(4; part II):SIxiv-SIxx, 1990.

45. Schlag G, Redl H, editors: Second Vienna Shock Forum, *Prog Clin Biol Res* 308, 1989.

46. Schreiber TL, Miller DH, Zola B: Management of myocardial infarction shock: current status, *Am Heart J* 117(2):435-443, 1989.

47. Shapiro BA: Blood gas monitoring: yesterday, today, and tomorrow, *Crit Care Med* 17(6):573-581, 1989.

48. Shoemaker WC: Circulatory mechanisms of shock and their mediators, *Crit Care Med* 15(8):787-794, 1987.

49. Shoemaker WC, Kram HB, Appel PL: Therapy of shock based on pathophysiology, monitoring, and outcome prediction, *Crit Care Med* 18(1):S19-S25, 1990.

50. Shoemaker WC, Kram HB, Appel PL, Fleming AW: The efficacy of central venous and pulmonary artery catheters and therapy based upon them in reducing mortality and morbidity, *Arch Surg* 125(10):1332-1338, 1990.

51. Skowronski GA: The pathophysiology of shock, *Med J Australia* 148(11):576-579, 1988.

52. Soto-Aguilar MC, deShazo RD, Waring NP: Anaphylaxis, *Postgrad Med* 82(5):154-170, 1987.

53. Thompson JA, Ayres SM, Hess ML: Cardiogenic shock: causes, diagnosis, and management, *J Crit Illness* 2(10):22-36, 1987.

54. Tuchschmidt J, Oblitas D, Fried JC: Oxygen consumption in sepsis and septic shock, *Crit Care Med* 19(5):664-671, 1991.

55. Vanselow NA: Minutes to counter anaphylaxis, *Emerg Med* 20(15):121-123, 1988.

56. Vincent JL, Leon M, Berre J, et al: Addition of phosphodiesterase inhibitors to adrenergic agents in acutely ill patients, *Int J Cardiol* 28(suppl. 1):S7-S11, 1990.

57. Weg JG: Oxygen transport in adult respiratory distress syndrome and other acute circulatory problems: relationship of oxygen delivery and oxygen consumption, *Crit Care Med* 19(5):650-657, 1991.

58. Weil MH, Rackow EC: A guide to volume repletion, *Emerg Med* 16(8):101-110, 1984.

59. Zimmerman JJ, Dietrich KA: Current perspectives on septic shock, *Pediatr Clin North Am* 34(1):131-163, 1987.

Classic

60. Balakumaran K, Hugenholtz PG: Cardiogenic shock: current concepts in management, *Drugs* 32(4):372-382, 1986.

61. Chernow B, Roth BL: Pharmacologic manipulation of the peripheral vasculature in shock: clinical and experimental approaches, *Circulatory Shock* 18(2):141-155, 1986.

62. Ellrodt AG: Sepsis and septic shock, *Emerg Med Clin North Am* 4(4):809-840, 1986.

63. Gonik B: Septic shock in obstetrics, *Clin Perinatol* 13(4):741-754, 1986.

64. Hagerdal M, Lundberg D, editors: Intravenous fluid therapy: an update, *Acta Anesthesiol Scand* 29(suppl 82):1-100, 1985.

65. Houston MC: Special considerations in the management of septic shock in the elderly, *Geriatr Med Today* 5(1):65-77, 1986.

66. Rice V: Shock management. I. Volume replacement, *Crit Care Nurse* 4(6):69-82, 1984.

67. Rice V: Shock management. II. Pharmacologic intervention, *Crit Care Nurse* 5(1):42-57, 1985.

CHAPTER FOURTEEN

Pain

LEARNING OBJECTIVES

1 Identify three reasons for undertreatment of patients in pain.
2 Describe the nurse's role in pain management.
3 List three factors that influence a patient's pain experience.
4 Differentiate between acute and chronic pain.
5 Explain the transmission of pain.
6 Discuss the two most current theories of pain.
7 Assess a patient in pain using a pain assessment tool.
8 Describe the use of nonopioid analgesics in pain management.
9 Discuss and compare opioid analgesics, using an equianalgesic chart.
10 Discuss four routes of analgesic administration.
11 Describe three major noninvasive pain relief measures and their nursing implications.
12 Describe three invasive pain relief measures and their nursing implications.

KEY TERMS

PAIN is a universal, complex, and subjective experience. Even though it is the most common reason for a patient to seek medical aid, and the number one reason for a person to take medication, the study of pain, or **algology,** is a new field. One of the best definitions of pain is by McCaffery: "Pain is whatever the experiencing person says it is, and exists whenever he says it does."[24] Nurses who approach pain from this perspective can help the patient achieve effective pain management.

Pain is generally related to some type of tissue damage, and serves as a warning signal (e.g., to immediately remove a hand from a hot stove). Although pain is familiar to everyone, it is so complex that it cannot be easily described and there is no single, universal treatment.

SCOPE OF THE PROBLEM

Pain is a major economic problem and a major cause of disability that hampers the lives of many. Bonica states that one third of the American population suffers from chronic pain and estimates that there are 37 million with arthritis, 70 million with back pain, 40 million with headache, and 850,000 with pain related to cancer (two thirds of cancer pain is considered to be moderate to severe). Bonica estimates that 50 million people are partially or totally disabled by pain, and the cost to the American consumer is $70 billion in medical costs, lost work days, and compensation.[1]

According to the World Health Organization, cancer pain can be controlled with proper use of medications in 80% to 90% of the cases, yet 25% of cancer patients in the world die in severe pain.[3]

Reasons for Undertreatment

Nurses and other health care professionals are poorly educated in identifying, assessing, and managing pain, and as a result, a patient's pain often goes unrecognized and untreated. Nurses often cling to outdated beliefs, misconceptions, and biases about patients in pain, including fears of addiction. Ferrell, McCaffery, and Rhiner's recent survey of 14 nursing textbooks found confusing terminology and encouraged fears of addiction when opioids are used for pain relief. This misinformation that nurses receive in their basic education contributes to the exaggerated fear of creating opioid addiction.[7] Factors contributing to these incorrect attitudes are: (1) lack of understanding of the pain process, (2) exaggerated fears of addiction and respiratory depression, (3) denial of pain and its severity, and (4) lack of knowledge of drug pharmacology and the mechanisms of other treatment methods.

Inadequate Education

Historically, nursing education has contained little information on how to adequately assess pain or how to use different treatment methods appropriately (especially medications). Nurses often were given incorrect information, especially that patients in pain have observable signs and symptoms (increased blood pressure, increased pulse, diaphoresis, pallor, dilated pupils), which is generally true only for patients with sudden, severe pain. Some nurses have difficulty believing patients who do not look as if they are in pain.

Not only is education about pain management needed for health care professionals, but the public needs education as well. Nurses can help patients and families maintain successful pain management through education concerning available pain management resources.

Attitudes and Misconceptions

Who is the authority on pain?

Health professionals often assume that they are the authority on pain. Nurses and physicians often discuss how much pain a patient should be having. Statements such as, "You shouldn't hurt that much—it's been 3 days since your surgery," or "You shouldn't be on injections anymore," are far too common. However, each patient's perception of pain is unique because of factors that affect the patient's response, such as past experience, culture, or anxiety.

Because pain is a subjective experience, the patient is the only authority, not the health professional. According to McCaffery's definition of pain, the nurse must believe every patient who says he or she has pain. The nurse needs to keep in mind that some patients may deny pain for a variety of reasons, and that this situation must be explored as well. Some nurses may be afraid to believe every patient, for fear that they may be fooled. In reality, however, it is rare for patients to be malingerers (a person who pretends to have pain).

Because so many practitioners have difficulty with this concept, it must be emphasized repeatedly that there is no test for pain. Even though some nurses with many years of experience think that they can identify patients in pain, it is impossible. Lack of pain expression does not mean lack of pain.[24]

If the nurse's goal is to relieve a patient's pain, holding the attitude that the health professional is the authority will only inhibit accurate assessments, establish adversarial relationships, and impede effective pain management. Because there is no actual proof of pain, the nurse's only recourse is to provide pain relief for every patient.

Addiction, tolerance, and physical dependence

The danger of addiction to pain medication is vastly overrated. Although available data on addiction consistently show it is rarely a result of using opioids for pain relief, health care professionals still have exaggerated fears.

Drug tolerance and physical dependence are involuntary behaviors that involve physiologic changes. Most patients on opioids for a length of time will become physically dependent and possibly drug tolerant. Patients may become physically dependent on several types of medications and may experience physiologic changes if the drug is stopped, but they are never said to be "addicted" to these medications (i.e., digoxin, propranolol, insulin).

Drug abuse and drug addiction are voluntary behaviors that involve active drug seeking. Most people who are addicted to drugs are also physically dependent on them and develop tolerance. However, the reverse is not true.

The data in the literature suggest that the risk of addiction is rare. Porter and Jick's 1980 study[14] of almost 12,000 inpatients receiving opioids for pain discovered only four patients with possible problems with addiction. Likewise, Perry and Heidrich[13] found that none of the 10,000 burn patients had problems with addiction.

Placebos

The word placebo comes from the Latin translation "I will be pleasing." A **placebo** can be defined as any medical treatment (medication or procedure, including surgery) or nursing care that produces an effect in a patient because of its implicit, explicit, or therapeutic intent and not because of its specific nature.[24]

There is no evidence to justify using a placebo to determine whether a patient really has pain. As mentioned earlier, there is no objective test for pain, and placebos are neither the answer nor the test.

It is estimated that one of every three patients will respond positively to a placebo at some time. Studies have shown that many patients with pain such as metastatic bone cancer get some relief after receiving a placebo. Unfortunately, the myth still exists that patients who respond positively to placebos are fakers, and may be viewed negatively by nursing and medical staff.

There are several reasons why placebos may relieve pain; in general, it has to do with the belief system of the patient and the attitude of the nurse administering the placebo. What placebos measure, in fact, is how much trust or confidence the patient has in the nurse or physician.

The patient who responds to a placebo is usually highly motivated to control his or her own pain process. This is important information, because it indicates that other measures besides medications, such as suggestion or relaxation, may help relieve the pain.

Another reason placebos may help control pain is that they reduce a patient's anxiety because the patient trusts that something was done to help. The intent of the placebo is why it may be helpful. It is also postulated that placebos work because they stimulate the production of endorphins.

Many health care professionals believe that using placebos for pain control is unethical because of the deception involved. It destroys the patient/nurse relationship, and it is costly because essentially the patient is charged for an inert substance. The nurse who is uncomfortable administering a placebo for pain control discusses with the patient's physician the rationale for ordering the placebo, and refuses to administer it if deceit or inappropriate rationale is involved.

THE ROLE OF THE NURSE IN PAIN MANAGEMENT

Pain management is a challenge that every nurse faces, regardless of the practice setting. In fact, the nurse's role in pain management is probably more important than that of any other member of the health care team.

Probably no other area of nursing involves patient advocacy as much as pain control. In all nursing fields, the nurse advocates for the patient by clarifying concerns, answering questions, supplying all the information the patient needs to make decisions about his or her care, and supporting the patient's decisions. Effective patient advocacy requires time, patience, and courage. Good listening skills are essential.

At times the nurse may be the only person who believes that the patient has pain. This can be a very frustrating experience for the nurse, requiring patience and energy. But advocacy is critical for effective pain management.

The nurse can provide some pain relief simply by telling the patient, "I believe you are in pain and I will do all I can to help relieve your pain." This statement greatly lowers the patient's anxiety level. A major goal of nursing is to establish trust and rapport with the patient; statements of belief such as the above are of paramount importance in achieving this goal. The patient's statement of pain should be all that is necessary for pain intervention to begin.[24]

The founding principle of effective pain management is Meinhart and McCaffery's statement that "the failure to treat pain is inhumane and constitutes professional negligence."[11] Every person has a right

ETHICAL ISSUES

- How can the nurse's caring relationship with a patient transform the nursing role from pain inflictor to comforter?
- How much voice should the patient have in decisions about pain medication?
- Should all patients be expected to bear a certain amount of pain because it naturally accompanies injury and disease?
- How should the nurse respond to the patient who asks not to be given analgesia?
- Does the nurse have less responsibility for providing pain relief for patients whose injuries are self-inflicted?
- May a patient be given pain medication he or she does not want? May the family consent for the patient in his or her "best interest?"

to freedom from pain; nurses must do everything possible to solve the patient's pain problem.

Many people believe that at least in a hospital a patient's pain will be controlled. Unfortunately, this is not always true. A recent study found that of 353 hospitalized adult medical-surgical patients, 58% said they had excruciating or horrible pain at some time while hospitalized. Fewer than half of the patients had a member of the health care team ask them about their pain or note the pain on the chart.[5]

To control pain, it must be identified. The nurse may be the first person to identify the problem of pain. It is the nurse's role to assess the pain adequately and share this information with the team. The failure to recognize pain is partially the result of an absence of accurate assessments.

The nurse discusses pain management issues with the patient and family and writes a nursing care plan that illustrates the pain problem and includes appropriate and specific interventions. The nurse evaluates the pain-relief measures and documents their effectiveness.

The nurse collaborates with the physician whenever medications or other approaches to pain are not helping. Many patients are afraid or unwilling to tell their physician because they feel uncomfortable about sharing their feelings. Other patients attempt to be "good," and so they do not want to complain or disappoint their physician. The nurse educates the patient about reporting pain and relief from pain control measures.

The nurse coordinating the health care team is also in charge of supervising the activities of nursing assistants and orderlies. It is crucial for these team members to understand the concept of pain management. They must not ignore patients' requests for pain relief, and they should respond quickly. They, too, must be familiar with treatment methods so they can enhance rather than impede the intervention.

FACTORS AFFECTING AN INDIVIDUAL'S RESPONSE TO PAIN

An individual's response to pain is influenced by several factors, which explains why pain is such a complex experience (Figure 14-1).

Anxiety

Anxiety is the most important factor affecting an individual's ability to tolerate and cope with pain. Anxiety can be associated with both acute and chronic pain. According to Sternbach,[28] however, anxiety accompanies acute pain, whereas depression accompanies chronic pain.

Anxiety is also related to what the pain means to the individual. In Henry Beecher's classic work with

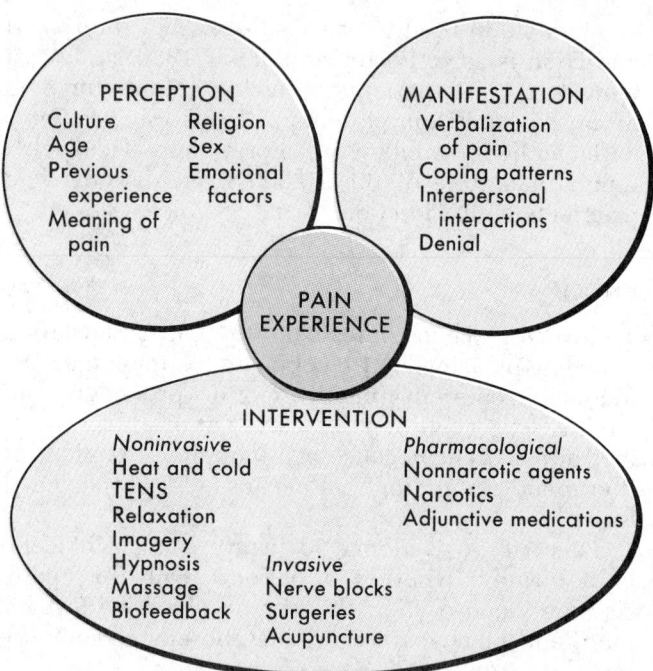

FIGURE 14-1   Conceptual model of pain depicts all three aspects of pain: perception, manifestation, and intervention. *Perception* includes the factors that affect a person's perception of pain, such as culture, religion, age, gender, past experience, and emotional factors such as anxiety. *Manifestation* shows that the most important factor in this aspect of pain is the patient's verbalization, or statement, of pain, or the patient's denial of pain. *Intervention* divides methods of intervention into three types (noninvasive, invasive, and pharmacologic), and itemizes different approaches within these three types. This variety of different approaches is demanded by the complex nature of pain.

soldiers wounded in World War II,[18] he found that their wounds appeared to cause much less pain and distress than one would have thought. The soldiers requested pain medication less frequently than did patients with similar wounds in the general population. According to Beecher, the soldiers' wounds meant that they were ready for discharge. The civilians, on the other hand, did not know what was causing their pain, and so their wounds were a source of anxiety.

Because pain and anxiety work in a circular pattern (decreasing pain tends to lessen anxiety, and decreasing anxiety tends to lessen pain), any strategy the nurse can use to help decrease a patient's anxiety will help control the pain. However, the patient with pain should never be considered "just anxious," and it should never be assumed that decreasing the patient's anxiety will automatically lessen the pain.

Past Experience with Pain

Socially acceptable responses to pain are learned at an early age and are influenced by the way the individual's family copes with pain. In general, the more pain experienced in childhood, the greater the perceptions of pain in adulthood. Studies with patients who have chronic pain have shown that they tend to have had a greater-than-average amount of pain experiences in their families. However, it is not true that the more pain patients experience, the more accustomed they become to it.[11]

The nurse discusses past pain experiences with the patient to find out what measures have helped in the past. Even though some measures may seem unlikely to help, if they are not harmful or contraindicated, they may have a positive effect. The nurse also assesses what measures have not helped a patient's pain in the past. Exploring a person's pain history may remind the patient of how severe pain can be and how difficult it is to obtain relief.

Culture and Religion

As mentioned before, acceptable responses to pain are learned from the individual's environment at an early age. Cultural and religious practices from one's family play an important role in the person's pain experience. Zborowski[29] did a number of studies on the relation of cultural factors to pain experience. In one study, he compared and contrasted four cultural groups—Anglo-Saxons, Italians, Jews, and Irish—and found that the expression of pain was definitely culture-related. For example, some cultures view the expression of pain or suffering as a weakness, so they tend to minimize their pain. Different cultures, on the other hand, believe that pain expression is expected, so they have greater overt manifestations of pain.

Religious beliefs also play a part in the pain experience. Some people may cope with their pain by using their faith and prayer, whereas others may view pain as a punishment for their sins.

It is important for the nurse to realize that not all people manifest pain in the same way and that there is no right or wrong way. The nurse accepts all patients' expressions of pain, regardless of their cultural and religious backgrounds* (see box above).

ACUTE AND CHRONIC PAIN

Pain is generally classified as either acute or chronic (Table 14-1). Pain can also be differentiated by type

*For an in-depth discussion on culture and pain, the reader is referred to Meinhart N, McCaffery M: *Pain: a nursing approach to assessment and analysis*, Norwalk, Conn, 1983, Appleton-Century-Crofts.

SIGNIFICANCE OF THE CULTURAL INFLUENCES ON PAIN FOR NURSING PRACTICE

Avoid stereotyping; do not assume that the characteristics commonly associated with a particular sociocultural group will occur in all patients who are members of that group. Studying the wide variety of cultural expectations with respect to pain helps the nurse appreciate the following:

1. The way one person learned to respond to pain may be not only different from, but quite the opposite from what someone else has learned.
2. Individuals usually consider that the ways they have learned to regard and to respond to pain are both natural and correct. Those behavioral responses are effective methods of communicating about pain with members of their culture.
3. The patient's attitude and behavioral responses to pain may be influenced more by cultural background than by the intensity of pain.
4. Similar responses to pain do not necessarily reflect similar attitudes toward pain.
5. Cultural expectations may be very detailed and varied regarding the following:
   a. Appropriate, acceptable, and effective behavioral responses to pain
   b. When, how, and by whom pain should be treated
   c. The meaning or significance of the pain

Reprinted with permission from Meinhart N, McCaffery M: *Pain: a nursing approach to assessment and analysis*, Norwalk, Conn, 1983, Appleton-Century-Crofts.

(Table 14-2). **Acute pain** is described as temporary, occurring after injury to the body; examples are postoperative pain, labor contractions, and acute renal colic. Acute pain is protective, because it usually causes people to seek treatment. It is addressed by identifying and then treating the cause. Acute pain disappears when the injury is healed.

Chronic pain may be divided into three classes: (1) chronic nonmalignant pain, such as low-back pain and rheumatoid arthritis; (2) chronic intermittent pain, such as migraine headaches; and (3) chronic malignant pain. The ideal treatment for chronic pain is to try to prevent it, but this is not always possible.

PAIN TRANSMISSION

The three types of neurons (nerve cells) involved in pain reception and transmission are afferent or sensory neurons, efferent or motor neurons, and interneurons or connector neurons. All of these nerve cells consist of three parts: cell body, axon, and dendrite. Neurons have receptors on their endings that cause the pain impulse to be conducted to the spinal cord or the brain. These receptors have highly specialized endings that initiate the impulse in response to physical or chemical changes.

Receptors that respond to injury or painful stimuli are called nociceptors. Injury to cells or tissue stimulates the nociceptors to release a variety of chemical substances that initiate pain impulses and mediate pain responses. These substances occur naturally and include histamine, substance P, cho-

linesterase, bradykinin, and prostaglandins. Once released, these substances sensitize nerve endings and transmit pain impulses to higher levels in the brain.

Peripheral nerve fibers conduct the pain impulse to the central nervous system (CNS). These fibers differ in their size and conduction. The A-alpha and A-beta fibers are large myelinated fibers that carry less intense sensations of touch and temperature. A-delta fibers are small, myelinated, and fast; they carry sharp, pricking, painful impulses. The unmyelinated C fibers are small and slow; they are responsible for dull, aching, burning pain, and play a part in chronic pain. The pain response activates the peripheral A-delta fibers. The impulse travels quickly to the substantia gelatinosa in the dorsal horn of the spinal cord where the "gating" mechanism occurs. Later, slower C fibers may carry aching, burning pain impulses of longer duration (Figure 14-2).

The afferent (sensory) impulse enters the dorsal horn of the spinal cord. The impulse exits the spinal cord via the efferent (motor) impulses from the anterior horn. The pain impulse is transmitted over the nerve synapse with the help of neurotransmitters, such as acetylcholine, norepinephrine, epinephrine, serotonin, and dopamine.

Next, the pain impulse crosses over to the opposite side of the spinal cord and ascends to higher centers in the brain via the spinothalamic tract. The spinothalamic tract enters the brain and travels to the thalamus. The thalamus plays a role in memory, recall, and emotional responses. From the thalamus, the impulse goes to the cortex and other areas. All higher levels in the brain play a part in processing the painful stimuli (thalamus, hypothalamus, brainstem, and cortex).

When the pain transmission is relayed to the brain, pain is then perceived subjectively. The de-

TABLE 14-1   Characteristics of Acute and Chronic Pain

Acute	Chronic*
Short duration	Lasts more than several months (usually 5 to 6)
Usually well-defined cause	May or may not be well-defined
Decreases with healing	Begins gradually and persists
Reversible	Exhausting and useless
Mild to severe	Mild to severe
May be accompanied by anxiety	May be accompanied by depression and fatigue

*Chronic malignant, chronic nonmalignant, and chronic intermittent pain.

TABLE 14-2   Source and Description of Types of Pain

Type of pain	Source	Description
Superficial	Arises from localized tissues, usually related to a disturbance of nerve endings	Well-localized, usually described as constant, sharp, tingling, or throbbing
Visceral	Arises from somatic or visceral structures (muscles, periosteum, organs)	Deep pain that is difficult to localize; may be dull or aching
Referred	Felt in another area away from the source of injury; usually originates in the viscera (Figure 14-2)	Common example is when a patient with a myocardial infarction has pain in the shoulder
Central	Caused by destruction or injury to a part of the central nervous system, such as neuralgias, causalgias, or phantom limb pain	Usually very intense, severe, and burning; this pain may not always respond to opioids

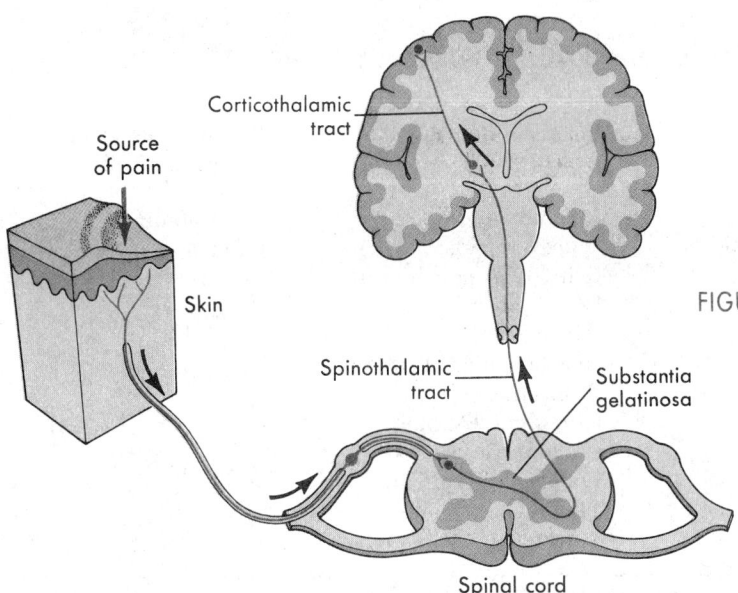

FIGURE 14-2   Neurologic transmission of pain stimulus.

scending paths of the efferent fibers extend from the cortex down to the spinal cord. These descending paths can also influence pain impulses at the level of the spinal cord.

The Gate-Control Theory

The gate-control theory of pain was proposed in 1965 by Melzack and Wall.[26] To put it simply, this theory states that pain impulses from the periphery travel to the gray matter in the dorsal horn of the spinal cord, where a "gating" mechanism exists, called the substantia gelatinosa, which can either open or close the transmission of pain impulses to the brain (Figure 14-3). The gating activity depends on the amount of stimulation large and small nerve

fibers receive. In general, these nerve fibers compete with each other; if more large nerve fibers are stimulated than small, pain transmission is inhibited. In essence, the gate is "closed," and pain impulses are not transmitted to the brain; therefore, no pain is felt. If more small nerve fibers are stimulated than large, pain transmission is facilitated, or the gate is "open."

In addition to the gating mechanism in the spinal cord, there are other places in the CNS where pain impulses can be inhibited. Impulses from the brainstem, caused by sensory input such as distraction or imagery, or those from the cerebral cortex and thalamus, caused by relaxation techniques and anxiety-reduction, may close the gate to painful stimuli.

Melzack and Wall's gate-control theory of pain[26] gives a simple explanation to actions that have been done for years. If a person stubs his toe, he immediately rubs it and it feels better. According to this theory, the rubbing stimulates large nerve fibers to close the gate.

It is postulated that many pain-relief techniques work in just this way, especially the noninvasive techniques. Pain relief occurs because of the stimulation of large nerve fibers that close the gate. The nurse should explain the gate-control theory to the patient to enhance understanding of why a certain technique is being attempted for pain relief.

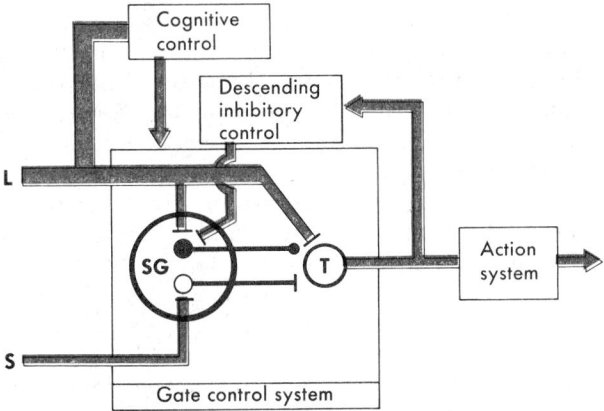

FIGURE 14-3   Gate-control theory. (From Melzack R, Wall PD: *The challenge of pain,* Philadelphia, 1982, Basic Books, Inc. Reprinted with permission.)

The Endorphin/Enkephalin Theory

In 1973 researchers discovered endogenous opioid peptides in the brain. These peptides, called **endorphins,** are naturally occurring compounds that have morphinelike qualities; however, they have no advantages over exogenous opioids, such as morphine.

TABLE 14-3   Simple Representation of Activity at Opiate Receptor Sites

Opiate receptor site	Activity	Primary action site agonist ("on")	Primary action site antagonist ("off")
Mu	Analgesia, decreased respirations, physical dependence, tolerance, constipation, euphoria	Morphine and other "pure" opioids; partially buprenorphine HCl (Buprenex)	Nalbuphine (Nubain) Butorphanol (Stadol) Pentazocine (Talwin)
Kappa	Analgesia, no respiratory depression, no physical dependence	Buprenorphine HCl (Buprenex) Nalbuphine (Nubain) Butorphanol (Stadol) Pentazocine (Talwin)	
Sigma	Psychotomimetic, vasomotor stimulation	Butorphanol (Stadol) Pentazocine (Talwin)	

From McCaffery M, Beebe A: *Pain: clinical manual for nursing practice,* St Louis, 1989, Mosby–Year Book.

Endorphins are the larger, more potent polypeptides found mostly in the pituitary gland and in other areas of the CNS as well. Endorphins modulate pain by preventing the conduction of pain impulses in the CNS. The enkephalins are smaller, specific neurotransmitters that bind with opiate receptors in the dorsal horn of the spinal cord. Enkephalins modulate pain by closing the gate and stopping the pain impulse.

Certain nonpharmacologic interventions help ease pain by stimulating the production of endorphins. These interventions include acupuncture, transcutaneous electrical nerve stimulation (TENS), and placebos.

Some exciting research is currently being done regarding the multiple opioid receptor site theory. An **opioid** is a drug (natural or synthetic) that has properties similar to opium or morphine. Receptors are specialized areas of the cell membrane that are specific binding sites for certain drugs or hormones. There are currently three known classes of opioid receptors: mu, kappa, and sigma (Table 14-3); they are distributed throughout the CNS. The concept of these different receptors helps explain the differences in activity among various opioid analgesics.

There is still controversy regarding the function of the opioid receptors. This field of pain research is rapidly evolving.

PAIN ASSESSMENT

Assessment is the first step toward understanding pain as the patient experiences it, and it provides the framework for a positive patient-nurse alliance. The nurse assesses, documents accurately, and shares this information with the patient's physician as well as other members of the health care team.

In a 1986 study of 207 nurses and nursing students, 96% of the nurses and 91% of the student nurses all recognized the importance of pain assessment. However, only seven of the 207 subjects used a standardized approach (analog scales or flowcharts) to pain assessment in their practice.[16]

Components of Pain Assessment

To accurately gather data and record a pain assessment, it is necessary to use some type of an assessment tool, or at least a visual analog scale (0 to 5) (Figure 14-4).

Location

The nurse has the patient point to or trace the area of pain. The patient may find it helpful to outline the areas of pain on a drawing. The patient may have a localized pain, a radiating pain, or a **referred pain** felt in an area distant from the source (Figure 14-5). The nurse finds out whether the pain is superficial or deep. Also, the nurse determines whether the location of the pain has changed and if the patient has more than one type of pain.

Intensity

A number scale is a helpful and easy way for the patient to give the nurse a clearer understanding of the pain experience. On a scale of 0 to 5, 0 equals no pain and 5 equals the worst pain imaginable. The use of such a scale (some clinicians may use a 0-to-10

PAIN ASSESSMENT TOOL

Name _____

Age _____   Diagnosis _____

Physician _____   Date first seen _____

Medications for pain _____

Location

Have patient point to or trace the area of pain

_____

_____

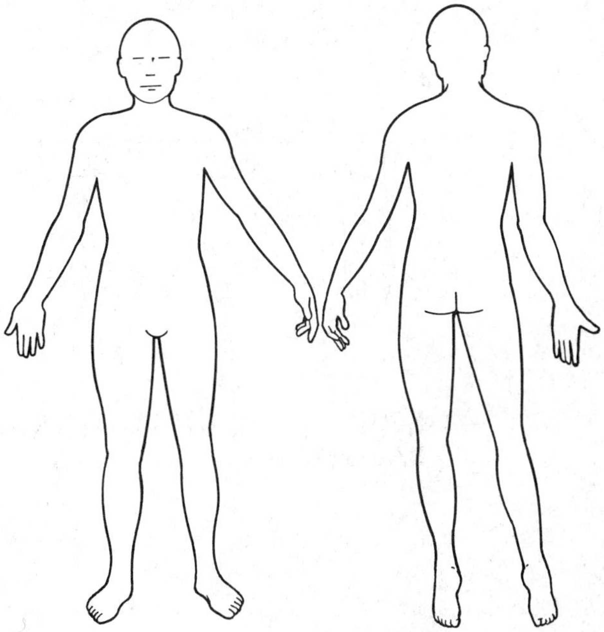

Intensity

Rate pain on a 0 to 5 scale (0 = no pain,
5 = worst pain imaginable):

At present: _____

1 hour after medication: _____

Worst it gets: _____

Best it gets: _____

Comfort

Rate comfort on a 0 to 5 scale (0 = no
relief, 5 = complete relief):

At present: _____

1 hour after medication: _____

Worst it gets: _____

Best it gets: _____

Quality

Have patient describe pain in his words: _____

Chronology

When did the pain start? _____

What time of day does it occur? _____

How often does it appear? _____

How long does it last? _____

Is it constant or intermittent? _____

Has the intensity changed? _____

Patient's view of pain

What makes the pain better? _____

What makes the pain worse? _____

Any associated symptoms? _____

Does pain disturb the patient's sleep? _____

How does the pain affect the patient's mood? _____

What has helped control pain in the past? _____

What is the pain preventing the patient from doing that he would like to do? _____

_____

Signature of person performing assessment _____

FIGURE 14-4   Pain assessment tool.

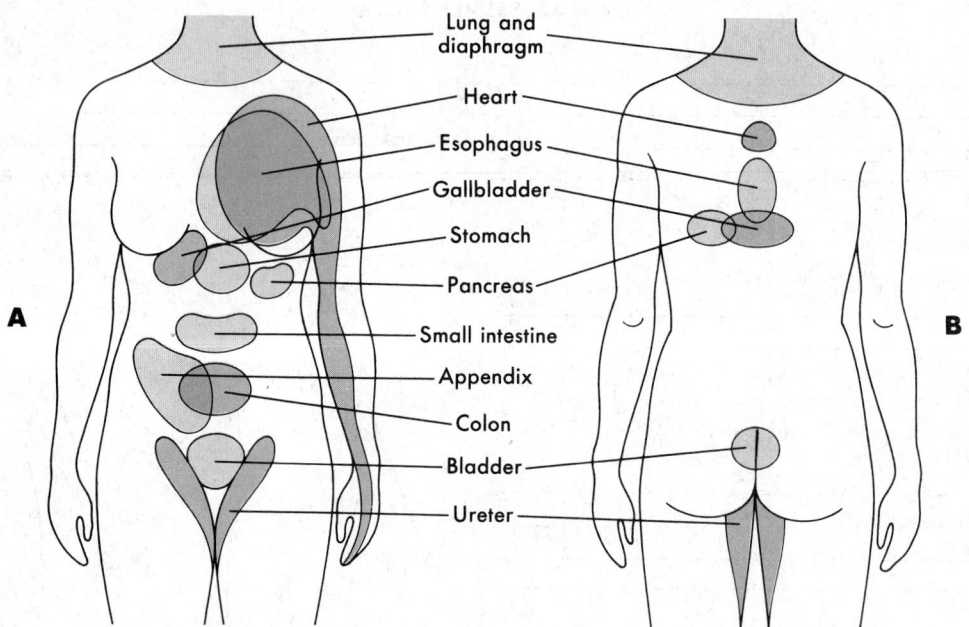

FIGURE 14-5 Surface areas of referred pain from some organs. **A,** Posterior view. **B,** Anterior view.

Patient's name: _____

Room number: _____

Physician: _____

PAIN MEDICATION FLOW SHEET				
Date	Time	Medication	Pain rating (0 to 5)	Respirations

FIGURE 14-6 Pain medication flowsheet.

scale rather than a 0-to-5 scale) affords continuous documentation of the pain rating. The simple number scale also gives nurses a common language for evaluating pain relief. The nurse asks the patient to rate the pain before and after some intervention, such as medication, relaxation techniques, or TENS.

Comfort

Some patients may be better able to describe their pain relief, rather than intensity. For this reason, it is important to assess pain both ways. Again, the nurse uses a number scale as in assessing intensity: 0 equals no relief and 5 equals complete relief.

Quality

The nurse asks the patient to describe the pain in detail. The patient should be encouraged to use his or her own words to fully describe the pain being experienced. Examples may include aching, pricking, soreness, or dullness.

Chronology

The nurse asks the following questions: When did the patient's pain start? What time of day does it occur? How often does it appear? How long does it last? Is it constant or intermittent? Has the intensity changed?

Patient's view of pain

The nurse provides the patient with ample opportunity to discuss what the pain means to him or her. By exploring the following questions about pain, the nurse can complete a thorough pain assessment: What decreases the pain? What aggravates it? What are other associated symptoms? Is sleep disturbed? How does the patient feel? What measures have given relief in the past? What is the patient unable to do because of pain?

Many times the nurse will discover that the associated symptoms are more upsetting than the pain itself. It is important for the nurse to remember that assessment is ongoing. Once an initial pain assessment is completed (using an assessment tool or body chart), the nurse must frequently reevaluate the effectiveness of interventions for pain. A simple way for the nurse to do this is to use a flowsheet (Figure 14-6), which can be filled out hourly, every shift, or at home. Patients and family members may appreciate being asked to perform this themselves.

It may take the nurse only 10 to 15 minutes to complete a pain assessment tool. In the long run, accurate pain assessment saves time. A systematic approach to collecting information about pain enables the nurse to better evaluate and plan interventions for pain relief.

MANAGEMENT OF PAIN
Pharmacologic Approaches to Pain Management

Medications are the most common form of pain control. However, many nurses and other health professionals have inadequate knowledge regarding the pharmacology of drugs used in pain control. This lack of information, together with the misconceptions and attitudes about pain previously discussed, are the two main reasons why patients may have inadequate pain relief.

There are three groups of pain medications (analgesics): (1) nonopioids, (2) opioid agonist-antagonists, and (3) opioids. A fourth group of medications is called adjuvant or coanalgesics. These drugs may be useful in treating other symptoms associated with pain, such as depression, anxiety, or nausea.

Nonopioid analgesics

Nonopioid analgesics work in an entirely different way than opioids. Opioids work at the level of the CNS, whereas nonopioids work at the level of the periphery. It makes sense, then, to deliver both types of analgesics when managing a patient's pain; in that way, the pain can be attacked at two different levels.[24] The nonopioid analgesics are the first step in the analgesic ladder. In other words, they should be tried first for pain that is mild to moderate.

Many nonopioids (except acetaminophen) are potent antiinflammatory agents (Table 14-4). These drugs are very effective with inflammatory type pain, such as rheumatoid arthritis, postoperative pain, dental pain, menstrual pain, episiotomy pain, migraines, low-back pain, sunburn, and particularly bone pain. One cancer pain researcher estimates that approximately 50% of cancer pain can be controlled with nonopioid antiinflammatory agents alone.[9]

The probable reason antiinflammatory agents are so helpful in pain relief is that they inhibit the synthesis of prostaglandins, which are fatty-acid substances found throughout the body. The release of prostaglandins in tissues causes pain, edema, and inflammation. By inhibiting the synthesis of prostaglandins, antiinflammatory drugs decrease inflammation and pain.

The two most common nonopioids are acetylsalicylic acid (aspirin) and acetaminophen. Studies have shown that their analgesic and antipyretic effects are the same in equal doses. The single optimal dose

TABLE 14-4 Pharmacology Summary: Nonopioids

Drug	Recommended dose	Comments
I. Acetaminophen (Tylenol, Panadol, Datril)	650-1000 mg qid	Similar to aspirin in analgesic and antipyretic effects, but slight antiinflammatory effects. No effect on platelet function. Available in liquid. May cause liver toxicity. Can be given with other NSAIDs.*
II. Acetylsalicylic		
a. Acetylsalicylic Acid (aspirin)	650-1000 mg qid	First-choice NSAID if able to tolerate, standard anti-inflammatory, less expensive, increases bleeding time.
b. Choline Magnesium Trisalicylate (Trilisate)	1500 mg bid	Can be given with other NSAIDs. Does not affect platelet aggregation. Available in liquid. Renal sparing.
c. Diflunisal (Dolobid)	500-1000 mg bid	Longer duration of action. Minimal antipyretic effect. Fewer GI effects and no tinnitus.
d. Salsalate (Disalcid)	750 mg qid	No interference with platelet function. No serious GI side effects. Renal sparing.
III. Propionic Acid Derivatives		
a. Ibuprofen (Motrin, Nuprin, Advil)	400-800 mg tid or qid	Fewer side effects than high-dose aspirin. Faster onset of action, short-acting.
b. Fenoprofen (Nalfon)	200-600 mg tid or qid	Short-acting.
c. Naproxen (Naprosyn)	250-500 mg bid	Also available in suspension form. Long duration of action 8-12 hours, so only need to take bid. Better tolerated than Indocin.
d. Naproxen Sodium (Anaprox)	275 mg tid or qid	Available in double-strength 550 mg tablets. Faster onset of action than Naproxen. Long-lasting.
e. Ketoprofen (Orudis)	50-75 mg tid or qid	Rapid onset of action. Long-lasting.
f. Flurbiprofen (Ansaid)	50-200 mg tid or qid	Relatively new NSAID.
IV. Indole Derivatives		
a. Indomethacin (Indocin)	25-50 mg bid or tid	Also available as Indocin SR 75 mg and oral suspension and rectal suppository. High incidence of side effects; headache, edema, GI.
b. Sulindac (Clinoril)	150-200 mg bid	Lower incidence of renal problems than other NSAIDs; although the incidence of side effects is lower than with Indocin, they are still common.
c. Tolmetin (Tolectin)	400-600 mg tid or bid	Weak analgesic effect.
V. Anthranilics		
a. Mefenamic Acid (Ponstel)	250 mg qid	Not recommended for use longer than 7 days. No advantage over other NSAIDs.
b. Meclofenamate (Meclamen)	200-400 mg tid or qid	Diarrhea occurs in one out of six people.
VI. Oxicams		
a. Piroxicam (Feldene)	20 mg once per day	Good for patients who may not comply with multiple daily doses. Not recommended for patients with liver or kidney dysfunction.
VII. Pyrazolones		
a. Phenylbutazone (Butazolidin)	100-200 mg tid	Oldest NSAID with highest incidence of severe side effects such as blood dyscrasias. Not to be given longer than 7-10 days.

NOTE: All NSAIDs must be taken with food or milk to decrease gastric irritation. Cytotec may be given to counteract the GI side effects of the NSAIDs.

*NSAIDs—the NSAIDs decrease the synthesis of prostaglandins, decreasing inflammation and pain.

TABLE 14-4   Pharmacology Summary: Nonopioids—cont'd

Drug	Recommended dose	Comments
VIII. Diclofenac a. (Voltaren)	75-150 mg bid or tid	Thought to produce less GI irritation than does aspirin and comparable in safety to Ibuprofen and Naproxen.
IX. Pyranocarboxylic Acids a. Etodolac (Lodine)	200-400 mg tid or bid	Only NSAID that has no difference in pharmacokinetics in patients more than 65 years of age compared with the general population. Dose should not exceed 1200 mg a day. Patients less than 60 Kg not to exceed 20 mg/Kg/day.
X. Pyrrolo-pyrroles a. Ketorolac tromethamine (Toradol)	30-60 mg IM q6h or 10 mg PO q4-6h	Available parenterally as well as orally. Indicated for acute or postoperative pain, especially bone pain.
XI. Naphthylalkanone a. Nabumetone (Relafen)	1000-2000 mg once per day	Efficacy comparable to aspirin, once-a-day dosing.

of aspirin or acetaminophen is between 650 and 1000 mg.[24]

There is a ceiling to the analgesic effect of the nonopioids. In other words, if the dose of the nonopioid analgesic is greater than 1000 mg, there will be no additional analgesic effect, only more side effects. However, nonopioids do have an additive effect with opioids. Houde's classic study showed that 650 mg of aspirin given orally with 10 mg of morphine sulfate given intramuscularly gave significantly greater pain relief than either drug alone.[22] Combinations of opioids with nonopioid analgesics have the advantage of enhanced pain relief with a decrease in side effects.

In many opioid compounds, for example acetaminophen and codeine (Tylenol #3) or phenacetin with aspirin and caffeine (Empirin compound), the nonopioid dose is insufficient for effective pain relief. Instead of increasing the opioid, it would be wiser to increase the nonopioid to reach the optimal dose of 1000 mg. As mentioned before, because the nonopioids are the first rung in the analgesic ladder, all patients with severe, chronic pain, particularly those with cancer, should receive these drugs. Nonopioids should be continued even when pain is severe enough to warrant the addition of a narcotic.[8]

Acetaminophen

Unlike the rest of the nonopioid analgesics, acetaminophen (Tylenol, Datril, and Panadol) has no antiinflammatory properties. Acetaminophen has some advantages over aspirin in that it is available in a liquid form (which is the best way to take oral analgesics) and it can also be taken on an empty stomach. Acetaminophen causes no adverse gastrointestinal effects, and because of this, it would be preferred for any patient who has a history of ulcer disease. Acetaminophen also has no effect on platelet aggregation as some of the other nonopioids do. This drug would be preferred, then, for patients in whom bleeding is likely, such as preoperative or postoperative patients. Acetaminophen is not without its serious side effects, however; the main one is hepatotoxicity. It should be used cautiously in patients who have a history of liver involvement or liver disease.

Aspirin

Aspirin is probably the most commonly and widely used drug in the world. It is one of the most effective antiinflammatory drugs available. Many studies have shown that 650 mg of aspirin is equal in analgesic effect to some opioids (Table 14-5).

Because aspirin causes gastrointestinal upset, it may be administered with food or on a full stomach. Aspirin is also available in enteric-coated preparations, but this form takes longer to be absorbed and may delay pain relief. In high doses, aspirin also may cause tinnitus. This indicates aspirin toxicity and warrants a reduction of the dosage. The most serious reported side effect of aspirin is gastrointestinal bleeding, but its actual incidence as a result of aspirin consumption is controversial. Although aspirin does prolong bleeding time and impairs platelet ag-

TABLE 14-5 Oral Dosages with Analgesic Effect Equal to 650 mg of Aspirin or Acetaminophen

Meperidine (Demerol)	50 mg
Pentazocine (Talwin)	30 mg
Codeine	32 mg
Dextropropoxyphene (Darvon)	65 mg

gregation, not everyone bleeds when they take aspirin. Bleeding is more of a problem in patients with impaired hemostatic mechanisms.

Nonsteroidal antiinflammatory drugs (NSAIDs)

Antiinflammatory drugs referred to as NSAIDs all inhibit prostaglandin synthesis and are potent antiinflammatory agents. They do differ in their pharmacokinetic effects and duration of action. Drug selection should be made on the basis of many different factors. If the patient has had a prior favorable experience with one of the NSAIDs, then that drug should be tried again.

Dosing is another factor to consider when selecting a particular drug for the patient. Many of these drugs need to be given only once or twice a day, which may be an advantage for certain patients.

Always start at the lowest possible dosage with antiinflammatory drugs (particularly with elderly patients), and give an adequate trial for each drug before switching to another one. The antiinflammatory drug may take 3 to 4 weeks to achieve the optimal analgesic effect in patients with serious inflammatory problems. If the patient does not have effective pain relief after an adequate trial is given, a switch to another class of NSAIDs is recommended because of the similarities in action within each class. According to Foley,[8] the choice of each NSAID must be individualized by using maximal levels of one drug before switching to another.

All NSAIDs can cause gastrointestinal irritation. All of these drugs may be administered on a full stomach or with food. In addition to gastrointestinal irritation, gastrointestinal bleeding can be a serious problem, related to the inhibition of prostaglandin synthesis. Some of the NSAIDs should be used with caution in patients with a history of ulcers.

Opioid agonist/antagonist

The second group of analgesics is the opioid agonist/antagonist. These drugs are opioid (agonists) that antagonize the "pure" agonists (counteract opioid effects). See Table 14-6 for names and dosages of several common opioid agonist/antagonist drugs.

Because of their opioid antagonist properties, administering them after a patient has been receiving opioids may cause withdrawal symptoms. If agonist/antagonist analgesics are given together with an opioid, eventually they will antagonize opioid analgesia; hence, the patient will have poor pain relief.

The major side effects produced by these drugs are drowsiness, occasional nausea, and psychotomimetic effects such as hallucinations and euphoria.

Opioids

The most potent of all analgesics, opioids, act at the CNS level. They reduce pain by binding to specific opiate receptors throughout the CNS. Opioid analgesics are vital in pain management. In general, all opioids are similar, but they do differ in potency and duration of action. The most important point to remember about opioids is that their oral and parenteral dosages vary. In other words, oral and intramuscular dosages are NOT INTERCHANGEABLE.

Equianalgesic chart

The nurse must become familiar with a comparison chart of equivalent opioid dosages (Table 14-7). This chart is useful when switching opioids or routes of administration of opioids, and enables the nurse to learn the dosage of the drugs being administered for pain. After assessing the patient's response to an opioid, the nurse can use the equianalgesic chart to make appropriate recommendations or adjustments. NOTE: When reading about each opioid, the reader is asked to note the equianalgesic doses of the oral and intramuscular routes.

Side effects of opioids
Nausea and vomiting
Nausea and vomiting often are mistaken for allergic reactions, and patients may be denied opioids. The side effect of nausea or vomiting in patients taking opioids varies from patient to patient and with opioid to opioid. If a patient is nauseated after receiving an opioid, the nurse determines the cause and the appropriate treatment.

Nausea and vomiting occur as a side effect in only a minority of patients taking opioids for pain relief. Treating the nausea and vomiting with an appropriate antiemetic usually helps. In addition, if the patient needs to continue the opioid therapy longer than 1 week, the problem usually resolves on its own.

Constipation
Although constipation may seem like a minor side effect, it is not to the patient. Often the discomfort

TABLE 14-6   Pharmacology Summary: Opioid Agonist/Antagonists Equal to 10 mg Morphine IM

Name	Route	Duration of action (hours)	IM dosage (mg)	Comments
Pentazocine (Talwin)	IM, IV, PO	3	50 to 60	Shorter-acting (3 hours) IM than morphine and irritating to tissues Oral route ineffective (30 mg PO = 650 mg aspirin PO) High incidences of psychotomimetic side effects Contraindicated in cardiac patients because it increases cardiac work load and pulmonary arterial pressure
Nalbuphine (Nubain)	IM, IV	3 to 6	10 to 15	Effect may last 3 to 6 hours IM Has fewer reported psychotomimetic effects than pentazocine May be useful analgesic for burn patients, labor and delivery, ER, and pediatric patients
Butorphanol (Stadol)	IM, IV	3 to 4	2 to 3	Effect may last 3 to 4 hours IM Higher incidence of psychotomimetic effects than nalbuphine Contraindicated in cardiac patients, because it also increases cardiac work load
Buprenorphine HCl (Buprenex)	IM, IV	6	0.3 to 0.6	Longer duration of action IM (6 to 8 hours) Fewer psychotomimetic effects Naloxone must be given in unusually high doses if respiratory depression occurs
Dezocine (Dalgan)	IM, IV	3 to 4	10	

TABLE 14-7 Pharmacology Summary: Equianalgesic Chart of Doses Equal to 10 mg Morphine IM

Drug	Subcutaneous/ intramuscular (mg)	Oral (mg)	Peak effect (hours)	Duration of action (hours)	Comments
Codeine Tylenol #2 Tylenol #3 Tylenol #4 (30 mg PO = 650 mg aspirin)	130	200 15 30 60	2	3 to 4	Short-acting, weak opioid Nausea, vomiting, and constipation occur with greater frequency and in more severity as the dosage increases
Demerol (Meperidine) (50 mg PO = 650 mg aspirin)	75	300	1	2 to 3	Short duration of action (2 hours in some patients) Irritating to tissues Oral analgesic effect low (300 mg PO = 75 mg IM) With repetitive administration, renal dysfunction or high frequent dosage a toxic metabolite (normeperidine) is likely to accumulate and cause CNS excitation, such as muscle twitching, irritability, jerking, and seizures
Dilaudid (Hydromorphone) Dilaudid HP 10 mg/1 mL	1.5	7.5	½ to 1	3 to 4	Fast-acting, useful alternative to morphine or meperidine Available orally, parenterally, and by 3 mg rectal suppository High-potency parenteral strength available (10 mg/1 mL) with shorter duration of action than morphine, so may be more useful with the elderly
Duragesic (Transdermal Fentanyl) (25, 50, 75, or 100 g/hr patches)	—	—	12-24	72	Slow onset and very gradual decline in blood levels after removal
Heroin (Diamorphine)	5	NA	1 to 2	4 to 5	Not available in United States, but widely used in England for treatment of cancer pain Similar to morphine, but shorter acting

Drug					Comments
Levo-Dromoran (Levorphanol)	2	4	1 to 2	4 to 8	Long duration of action (4 to 8 hours), because of long half-life (12 to 16 hours) Careful monitoring and dosage adjustments needed to prevent excessive sedation
Methadone (Dolophine)	10	20	1 to 2	4 to 8	Long duration of action because of long half-life (24 to 36 hours). Cumulative effect with repetitive dosing causing sedation, so careful observation of patient is needed. Use with caution in elderly patients or patients with liver or renal dysfunction.
Morphine	10	30 to 60	1 to 2	3 to 4	Standard opioid with which all other analgesics are compared. Drug of choice for severe pain. Very versatile, because it can be given by many routes: oral, subcutaneous, intramuscular, intravenous, rectal, intraspinal. Available as concentrated oral solution 20 mg/mL and sustained-release (long-acting) 30 mg and 60 mg tablets. Cancer pain experts recommend concentrated oral morphine solution or sustained-release tablets regularly around the clock. Although no limit to the dosing of morphine, most patients can be controlled on 30 to 60 mg orally every 4 hours. Occasionally some patients require much higher doses.
Sustained-release morphine	NA	30 to 60	2 to 3	8 to 12	
Numorphan (Oxymorphone) (rectally) (available in 5 mg suppository)	10	NA	2	4 to 6	Available rectally in 5 mg suppository with 4 to 6 hour duration of action; 10 mg rectally equals 10 mg morphine sulfate IM.
Oxycodone	NA	30	1	3 to 4	Fast-acting oral opioid usually given in combination with nonopioids, which may limit the ability to increase doses. Plain oxycodone oral solution available in 5 mg/5 mL.
Percodan (5 mg oxycodone and 325 mg aspirin)					
Percocet (5 mg oxycodone and 325 mg acetaminophen)					
Tylox (5 mg oxycodone and 500 mg acetaminophen)					

of constipation is more distressing to the patient than the pain itself.

Opioids inhibit peristalsis in the gastrointestinal tract. Patients who take regular doses of opioids almost inevitably become constipated. Also, many patients in pain lack proper exercise and have a poor diet, both making the problem of constipation worse.

Whenever a patient is started on regular doses of opioids, it is essential that the preventive approach be used. The nurse follows a care plan to prevent the problem of constipation, such as:

- Assess previous bowel habits
- Record each bowel movement
- Push oral fluids
- Encourage activity and exercise
- Give foods high in bulk and roughage
- Administer stool softeners daily
- If ineffective, give stool softeners plus a stimulant, such as Pericolase
- If ineffective, administer a suppository such as bisacodyl (Dulcolax)
- If ineffective, try Fleet Enema

Sedation

Because opioids have a depressant effect on the CNS, some drowsiness can be anticipated. However, sedation is not always caused by opioids. If the patient is still in pain, other causes of sedation should be ruled out before cutting the opioid dosage or changing medications. For example, other medications, such as a hypnotic (flurazepam [Dalmane], or triazolam [Halcion]) or a tranquilizer (diazepam [Valium], alprazolam [Xanax], promethazine [Phenergan]), could be causing the sedation. Often the elimination of other CNS depressant medications resolves the sedation problem.

Pain, particularly chronic pain, is exhausting. Sleep deprivation can be a serious problem for patients in pain. Many times, after the first 2 to 3 days of effective pain relief, the patient may appear sedated. This can be mistaken for oversedation caused by the opioid, rather than effective pain control in someone who has not had adequate sleep. The nurse instructs the patient and his or her family that this sedation usually subsides in 2 to 5 days. If sedation continues to be a problem, especially for patients with cancer pain, some experts advise administering stimulants early in the morning to counteract the sedation from opioids.

Tolerance

Tolerance is a physiologic characteristic described as requiring increasingly larger doses of opioid to provide the same effect as was produced by the original dosage. The first sign of tolerance is a decreased duration of the analgesic effect. Next comes a decrease in the total analgesic effect. Increasing the

CLINICAL ALERT

For opioid-induced respiratory depression:
1. A baseline of the respiratory rate should always be taken.
2. Respiratory depression is usually slow in onset and is preceded by sedation.
3. Respiratory depression usually occurs:
   - 7 minutes after intravenous administration
   - 30 minutes after intramuscular administration
   - 90 minutes after subcutaneous administration
4. The patient's response to analgesia must be monitored.
5. A flowsheet should be maintained.
6. Naloxone 0.1 mg to 0.4 mg should be given intravenously over 2 to 4 minutes.

frequency between doses or increasing the dosage itself will help overcome tolerance.

The rate of tolerance development depends on the route of administration of the opioid. Tolerance is slower to develop with oral opioids than with intramuscular or intravenous opioids.

The nurse assesses each patient's response to opioids. A common misconception regarding opioids is that tolerance always occurs. This is not true. In general, for patients with advanced cancer, increases in opioid dosages are the result of increased pain rather than tolerance.[12]

Because tolerance develops irregularly, some patients may need increased doses every few weeks, whereas others may never need an increase in dosage. Still others may need their doses decreased periodically.

Respiratory depression

A main reason for inadequate pain control is the exaggerated fear of respiratory depression. However, this problem rarely occurs, especially in patients taking opioids for chronic, long-term pain.[24]

McCaffery also states that patients develop tolerance to respiratory depression at the same time they become tolerant to the analgesic effect of an opioid. Also, "pain appears to be nature's physiologic antidote to the respiratory depressant effects of opioids."[24]

The nurse observes the patient frequently if there is a possibility of respiratory depression. Naloxone (Narcan) is a fast-acting medication given intravenously to reverse the opioid effect. Naloxone should be administered only when absolutely necessary, because it removes all of the pain-relieving effects of the opioid, and it may lead to withdrawal symptoms.

The respiratory depressant effect of the opioid is

usually longer-acting than Naloxone. The nurse continues to monitor the patient after giving Naloxone because respiratory depression can recur.

Timing of analgesics

PRN comes from the Latin pro re nata, "as the need arises." In practice, this need is usually discovered too late. Generally, patients request analgesics after the pain has begun. That is, if ongoing pain can be predicted, medications should be given on an around-the-clock schedule rather than PRN.

Advantages of scheduled around-the-clock analgesics are the following:
- Prevention of pain
- Decreased dosage, since analgesics are most effective if given before the pain occurs or becomes severe
- Decreased anticipatory pain
- Constantly maintained blood levels of the analgesic
- Decreased anxiety about pain medication
- The patient does not have to request analgesics

Disadvantages of PRN analgesics include the following:
- Reinforcement of certain behaviors (patients think they must "act" as if they are in pain)
- Patient put in a dependent position of having to request pain medication after the pain has begun
- Facilitates a cycle of increased anxiety about pain, leading to increased perception of pain, leading to increased pain, leading to increased anxiety

When analgesics are ordered to be given around the clock, the nurse must not hesitate to wake the patient up, just as the nurse would awaken the patient for any other routine, scheduled medication. If the analgesic is not ordered around the clock, the nurse offers and encourages the patient to take it as if it were on a schedule.

Patients are not used to requesting medications; they take them when the nurse administers them. Often it takes a great deal of teaching to convince the patient to request analgesics for pain. In fact, some patients are not even aware that they are supposed to ask for pain medications. A major role for nursing in pain management is to explain and reinforce this concept to patients and families.

Routes of administration

Oral
The oral (PO) route is preferred for analgesic administration. It is a convenient way to provide consistent and prolonged pain relief because steady blood levels of analgesics can be maintained. Drug levels usually peak in 1 to 2 hours.

The oral route is better for the patient because it fosters independence. The patient can maintain some control by not having to depend on someone to administer parenteral medications. The oral route (if given in adequate doses) can be used to manage severe pain effectively.

For patients with long-term pain, the oral route allows greater mobility, especially for home care. Even if the patient is unable to take medications by mouth, the oral route is still a possibility. If the patient has a feeding tube (nasogastric or gastrostomy), oral analgesics can be crushed or given in liquid form and administered through the tube.

Intramuscular
The intramuscular (IM) route is an acceptable way to manage acute, short-term pain. Although there is a rapid peak effect with this route, the duration of action is short. There can also be problems with erratic absorption through the muscle with this route, as well as problems with deposition of medication into fat tissue rather than muscle. One study showed that intramuscular injections did not provide adequate pain relief in postoperative patients. The researchers concluded that this was caused by unpredictable blood concentrations of the analgesic from erratic absorption.[2]

The IM route should be avoided in the management of chronic, long-term pain (especially cancer pain). This route is painful, can cause muscle or nerve damage, wears off fast, has problems with absorption, is costly, and requires the patient to depend on another to administer the medication.

Rectal
The rectal (PR) route for administering analgesics is underutilized, but it has advantages over the parenteral route. If patients are nauseated or unable to take analgesics by mouth, the rectal route should be considered. Because the rectal route is easier to use than IM, SC, or IV routes, it can be helpful for home care and in elderly patients, especially as a backup to PO or IV routes.

There are three opioid suppositories available: hydromorphone (Dilaudid) 3 mg; oxymorphone 5 mg; and morphine sulfate 5 mg, 10 mg, and 20 mg. Rectal dosages are generally the same as with oral medication. The suppositories are easy for patients to self-administer, and have a somewhat long duration of action of 4 to 6 hours.

Intravenous bolus
The intravenous bolus (IV push) route provides the most rapid onset of analgesia, but it has the shortest duration of action. Most opioids have their peak effect in 5 to 15 minutes and last 60 minutes or less.

This route is not recommended for patients in constant pain because it causes peaks and valleys of medication levels in the bloodstream. Another obvious disadvantage of this route is that it requires IV access. However, the IV push route is recommended for acute, painful conditions or procedures, and it may also be helpful for chronic pain patients in acute pain situations, such as when moving from bed to cart.

Intravenous continuous opioid infusion

This route of medication administration provides a constant infusion of IV opioid to maintain constant blood levels. As worldwide pain expert C. Saunders[27] has said, "Constant pain calls for constant control." **Intravenous continuous opioid infusion (ICOI)** is indicated when there is an inability to relieve pain through use of oral or rectal routes with high dosages of opioids, when there is an inability to use the oral or rectal routes, or when the patient's physical condition makes conventional routes of administration ineffective.

ICOI should not be used just for pain in the final stages of cancer. This method of pain control can be very effective for severe burn pain, postoperative pain, and pain in inflammatory bowel disease (colitis and Crohn's disease), to name a few.

Nursing care requires administering the opioid via an infusion pump with an alarm. Vital signs are taken frequently (every 15 minutes during the initial 2 hours) until stable. A flowsheet should be used to document pain relief and respirations. Opioid dosages are titrated to achieve comfort for the patient.

Unless there is a specific contraindication, morphine is the drug of choice for ICOI. It is relatively inexpensive, and is very effective when titrated correctly. Other opioids that may be used are hydromorphone (Dilaudid), levorphanol (Levo-Dromoran), and methadone (Dolophine).

Patient-controlled analgesia

Since the best way to treat pain is to prevent it, an ideal method of pain control is **patient-controlled analgesia (PCA).** PCA is the administration of all forms of pain relief by a method that allows the patient to control as much as possible within the limits of safety.[24] A common use of PCA is through the intravenous route. PCA allows the patient to receive a predetermined IV bolus of an opioid by hitting a syringe pump mechanism. In this way, the patient can control the administration of his own opioid dose (Figure 14-7).

The physician orders a predetermined dose of opioid (usually morphine) and a set lockout interval (5 to 20 minutes). The pump is calibrated to deliver the specified dose whenever the patient "hits the button." The lock-out mechanism is a safeguard to prevent inadvertent overdosage. The pump can record the number of times the patient hits the button, as well as the total cumulative dose delivered.

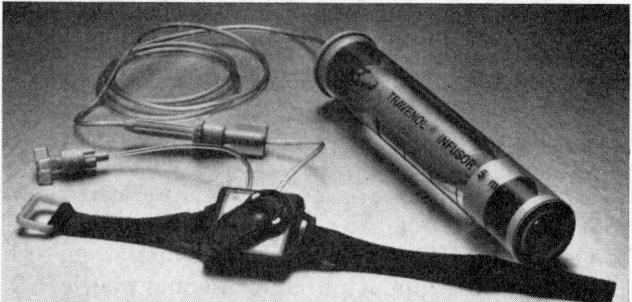
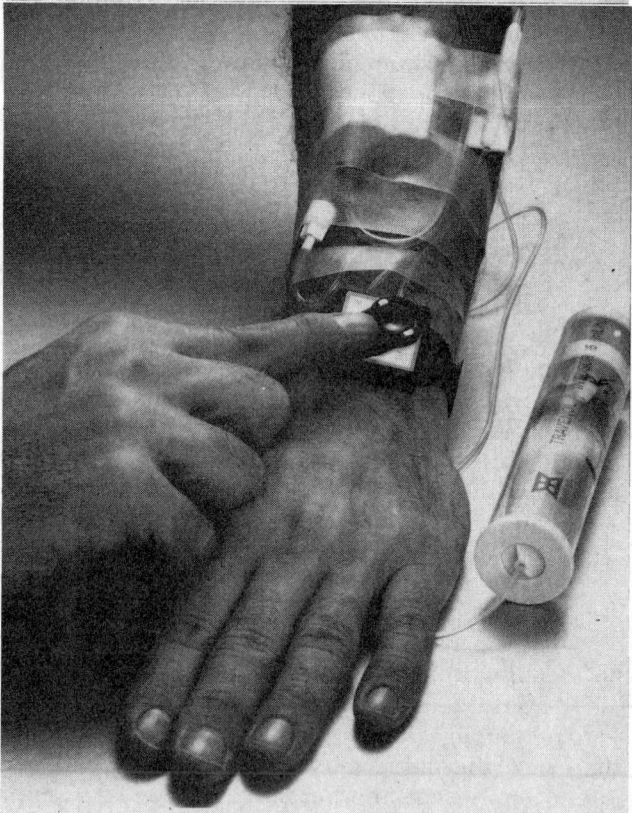

FIGURE 14-7 PCA units. **A,** Portable wrist model. **B,** Patient wearing wrist model. (Courtesy Baxter Healthcare Corporation, Deerfield, Ill.)

Continuous subcutaneous opioid infusion

Continuous subcutaneous opioid infusion (CSI) is a useful alternative for patients who require prolonged administration of parenteral opioids. Most commonly, this route is used for cancer patients who cannot take anything by mouth and in whom intravenous access is not desirable.

Continuous subcutaneous infusion of morphine or hydromorphone (Dilaudid) can provide a constant level of analgesia as well as greater patient mobility. The following are other advantages of CSI:

- Provides prolonged parenteral administration of opioids
- No delay in drug administration
- Avoids repetitive injections

- Avoids peak and trough drug levels
- Avoids need for IV access

The CSI infusion procedure consists of the insertion, using sterile technique, of a small, 27-gauge butterfly needle into the clavicular, abdominal, or thigh area. The needle is connected to an IV pump or portable syringe pump with programmed doses to be titrated to the patient's comfort.

Nursing care consists of inspecting the site every shift for signs of irritation and changing the site as needed (at least every 7 days). The nurse must also instruct the patient and family about the procedure and the pump, because the majority of patients will be discharged with the CSI pump.

Spinal administration

The administration of opioids (such as morphine) via a catheter carefully placed into the epidural or intrathecal (subarachnoid) space is another approach to pain management.

The administration of the opioid is either by intermittent bolus or by a continuous infusion pump. A larger dose of opioid (5 to 10 mg morphine) is required epidurally than intrathecally (1 to 5 mg morphine). Pain relief may last as long as 5 to 16 hours epidurally, and up to 36 hours intrathecally.

Spinal administration of opioids has been successful for postoperative pain, labor contractions, and cancer pain. Careful patient selection is required, especially when considering a catheter for continuous infusion. Usually this is reserved for patients with severe cancer pain who have tried adequate dosages of opioids by other routes without obtaining relief. Until the benefits of this invasive approach to pain management are clearly shown to outweigh the costs and risks, caution should be exercised. The procedure can be very expensive.

Side effects include nausea and vomiting, pruritus, sedation, urinary retention, and respiratory depression.

Nursing care includes monitoring the patient closely immediately after catheter insertion, since respiratory depression may occur up to 24 hours after insertion. Vital signs are taken every 30 minutes, apnea monitors used, and naloxone (Narcan) is made readily available.

Other hazards of epidural analgesia include the possibility of the catheter eroding a blood vessel and causing systemic side effects. There is also a risk of the epidural catheter eroding into the subarachnoid space and causing major respiratory depression.

The nurse inspects the insertion site frequently for signs of redness or swelling. Infection at the site could lead to major complications, such as meningitis.

Nursing care also includes careful pain assessments as well as titration of opioid analgesics (oral as well as spinal), because the physician who inserted the catheter is generally not a pain specialist. It is important for the nurse to monitor these patients carefully and notify the physician as soon as possible if the patient is not comfortable.

Nurses working with spinal administration of opioids must have adequate in-services and hospital or agency policy and procedures to show that they were adequately trained to care for patients with this procedure. Nurses must have clear guidelines so that they are qualified to teach patients and family members (because many of these patients are at home). A nurse should be available by telephone anytime of day or night in case the patient has a question or problem.

Adjuvant analgesics

Adjuvant analgesics can be helpful for the patient in pain. Although not true analgesics, the **adjuvant medications** relieve pain either alone or in combination with analgesics. These drugs can potentiate or enhance the analgesic's effectiveness.

Some nurses and other health professionals confuse potentiators with additives. Additives are drugs that add an effect, either harmful or beneficial.[24] A common example of this is the drug promethazine (Phenergan). Phenergan is a phenothiazine that has been given for years with opioids such as meperidine (Demerol) to enhance the opioid effects. However, it does just the opposite. Phenergan does not have any analgesic or analgesia-potentiating properties. In fact, it is thought to actually have antianalgesic properties.[21,23,25]

The use of adjuvant analgesics not only can provide additional pain relief in some cases but also can help control other discomforts associated with pain (anxiety, depression, nausea, insomnia). These drugs are summarized in Table 14-8.

The home health nurse plays an important role in managing the pain of a patient at home by closely monitoring the patient and the interventions for pain relief through home visits and telephone calls.

Noninvasive Pain-Relief Techniques

Noninvasive pain-relief techniques can be useful alone or as adjuncts in the management of pain. These approaches consist of cutaneous stimulation (heat, cold, massage, and transcutaneous electrical nerve stimulation [TENS]), distraction, relaxation, imagery, hypnosis, biofeedback, and others.

Whether these techniques work because of the gate-control theory or because they decrease a patient's anxiety, they undoubtably have many advantages for pain control; most are inexpensive, easy to perform, have low risks and few side effects, and may not require a physician's order. Probably the best advantage with these techniques is the patient's ability to have some control over the treatment of his or her pain.

TABLE 14-8   Pharmacology Summary: Adjuvant Analgesics

Class	Suggested dosage	Indications	Side effects	Comments
Anticonvulsants				
Phenytoin (Dilantin)	100 mg bid	Chronic neuralgias (trigeminal and postherpetic neuralgias), phantom-limb pain, diabetic neuropathies	Drowsiness, dizziness	Tegretol is the drug of choice for trigeminal and related neuralgia
Carbamazepine (Tegretol)	100 to 400 mg bid or tid			
Valproic Acid (Depakene)	15 mg/kg/day divided into bid			
Corticosteroids				
Prednisone	5-60 mg/day	Bone pain, especially metastasis, nerve root involvement	Weight gain, moon face, hypertension, ulcers	May stimulate mood and appetite
Dexamethasone	1-8 mg/day			
Stimulants				
Caffeine	100 to 200 mg/day	Lethargy, to counteract sedative and respiratory depressant effects of opioids	Excessive stimulation, insomnia, tachycardia, palpitations, anorexia	May produce additive analgesia when given with opioids in high enough doses
Dextroamphetamine (Dexedrine)	5 to 30 mg/day PO in AM	Offsets sedation and respiratory depressant effects of opioids	Restlessness, insomnia, palpitations	May have potentiating effect and analgesic effect of its own
Tricyclic antidepressants				
Amitriptyline (Elavil, Endep)	25 to 300 mg/day PO at hs	Chronic pain, migraine headache, diabetic neuropathy, postherpetic neuralgia, cancer pain, phantom-limb pain	Anticholinergic effects: dry mouth, urinary retention, sedation, hypotension, constipation	Contraindicated in patients receiving MAO inhibitors
Doxepin (Sinequan)	10 to 50 mg/day PO at hs in absence of clinically significant depression; doses must be titrated upward to be effective; dosage will be higher (50 to 300 mg/day) for treatment of depression			Have direct analgesic effects and may potentiate opioids
				Analgesic effects occur sooner and at lower doses than for antidepressant effects
				If given at hs, can benefit patient as a sleeping aid
				Blocks reuptake of neurotransmitter, serotonin, at CNS synapse to help alleviate depression
				Treating the underlying depression in chronic pain helps alleviate some of the pain

McCaffery[24] lists the following general guidelines when using any noninvasive technique:

1. Obtain a physician's order if there is any doubt about the safety of the method or the legality of the nurse's independent action.
2. Inform others (health team members, family, and friends) about how the technique is done, its purpose, and when it might be used.
3. Individualize the technique to suit the needs, preferences, and abilities of the patient.
4. Recognize the importance of the nurse-patient relationship with respect to the patient's confidence in and willingness to try noninvasive technique.
5. Whenever possible, practice the noninvasive pain-relief measure with the patient before the time it is needed.
6. When a noninvasive pain-relief measure is needed, start it either before the pain begins or as soon as possible after the pain begins.

Although not everyone will react successfully to these pain-relief measures, it is worthwhile to attempt any of them before advancing to more invasive techniques. It also enables the nurse to offer options for pain relief to patients.

Cutaneous stimulation

Heat, cold, massage, and transcutaneous electrical nerve stimulation (TENS) are all forms of stimulation to a person's skin to relieve pain.[24] Most of these techniques are used frequently, often without thinking, by the nurse, patient, or family. It is also necessary for the nurse to teach the patient and family the basic rationale behind these techniques to enhance their effectiveness. Simply stated, the technique of **cutaneous stimulation** relieves pain by stimulating the patient's large nerve fibers to "close the gate" to pain-conducting small nerve fibers.

Heat and cold application

Because heat and cold applications are so common, and because they have been used for so long, nurses may underestimate their value in pain control. Both heat and cold decrease pain and muscle spasm. Deciding which therapy to choose should be based on the physiologic effects desired (see box above).

Transcutaneous electrical nerve stimulation

Transcutaneous electrical nerve stimulation (TENS) has been used as a noninvasive pain control measure for almost 20 years. It consists of a pocket-sized, battery-operated device that provides a continuous, mild electrical current to the skin via electrodes. The electrodes are generally placed on or near the painful site.

EFFECTS OF HEAT AND COLD

Heat	Cold
↓ Pain	↓ Pain
↓ Muscle spasm	↓ Muscle spasm
↑ Inflammation	↓ Inflammation
↑ Blood flow	↓ Blood flow
↑ Hemorrhage	↓ Hemorrhage
↑ Edema	↓ Edema

There are many different TENS units available (Figure 14-8); however, they all have the same functioning parts: two to four electrodes to deliver stimulation to the nerves, lead wires to carry the stimulation, and the stimulator itself, small enough for the patient to wear. Patients have described the sensation as being similar to raindrops falling gently on the skin. Other words used to describe the impulse are tapping, buzzing, tingling, and vibrating.

PATIENT EDUCATION GUIDE
TENS

Follow manufacturer's directions carefully, because units vary

Apply electrodes to clean, unbroken skin near area of pain

Observe skin daily for signs of irritation

Make sure the device is turned "OFF" before applying or removing electrodes

Tape electrodes to the skin using hypoallergenic tape

Remember to recharge the batteries or change them as needed

Adjust the controls so that the impulse is a comfortable, pleasant sensation. If muscle contraction occurs, turn down the intensity

Placement of electrodes should never be over the eyes, carotid sinuses, throat, or abdomen during pregnancy

Contraindications for TENS use

People with demand cardiac pacemakers

Patients with a history of cardiac dysrhythmias or myocardial infarction

Pregnancy in the first trimester (may have some benefit for back labor during delivery)

Confused or elderly patients with decreased sensory perception

The units have different dials so that the patient can adjust the intensity, rate, and pulse width (duration) to achieve a soothing, pleasant sensation.

As with all forms of cutaneous stimulation, it is thought that TENS works by stimulating large nerve fibers to "close the gate" in the spinal cord. In addition, TENS may stimulate endorphin production because it has been shown that naloxone (opioid antagonist) reverses the effect. TENS also increases blood flow near the site of electrode placement.

TENS is indicated for various types of acute and chronic pain. Much research has shown TENS to be useful for chronic benign pain such as low-back pain, phantom-limb pain, and neuralgias. More recently, studies have shown TENS to be helpful for acute postoperative pain, especially for abdominal, thoracic, hip, or knee surgeries.

When used for postoperative incisional pain, preoperative teaching is essential for optimal pain control. Since TENS may not completely eliminate the need for analgesics, the patient should be instructed to request pain medications in addition to TENS use.

It is important for the nurse to teach the patient and family the rationale and technique of TENS. Correct electrode placement and optimal adjustment of output are crucial. In addition, it is necessary to have a positive attitude that TENS can be an effective method of pain control.

Massage

Massage is the manipulation of body tissue. Nurses commonly use massage as a form of pain relief or as a muscle relaxant. Although clinical research on massage is scarce, it is well known that a bumped elbow feels better after rubbing it. Although the benefits of massage may seem obvious, some nurses rarely find the time to carry out this simple pain-relieving technique. It is an instinctive, easy, and inexpensive form of cutaneous stimulation that can be a useful pain-relief measure. Also, massage allows the nurse to have time to interact with the patient and to communicate therapeutically.

Distraction

Distraction is anything that diverts the patient's attention from the pain. The use of distraction helps alter the patient's ability to tolerate pain. Structured distraction is probably the easiest and most common way the nurse can help a patient during short periods of pain or painful procedures, such as IV venipunctures, dressing changes for burn patients, bone marrow aspirations, thoracentesis, or paracentesis. Although distraction is simple to use and may benefit many patients, it has a very short duration. Once the technique ends, the pain returns, and sometimes the pain is increased. However, some nurses may mistakenly say, "He can't be having pain. He was just laughing with visitors."

Relaxation

Nurses have been using measures for years to help patients relax (backrubs, quiet environment, and slow, deep breathing). Today, there are many relaxation techniques available to teach patients how to relieve or reduce their anxiety and muscle tension. These techniques also may enhance other pain relief treatments, but relaxation should never be used as a substitute for pain relief measures. Relaxation

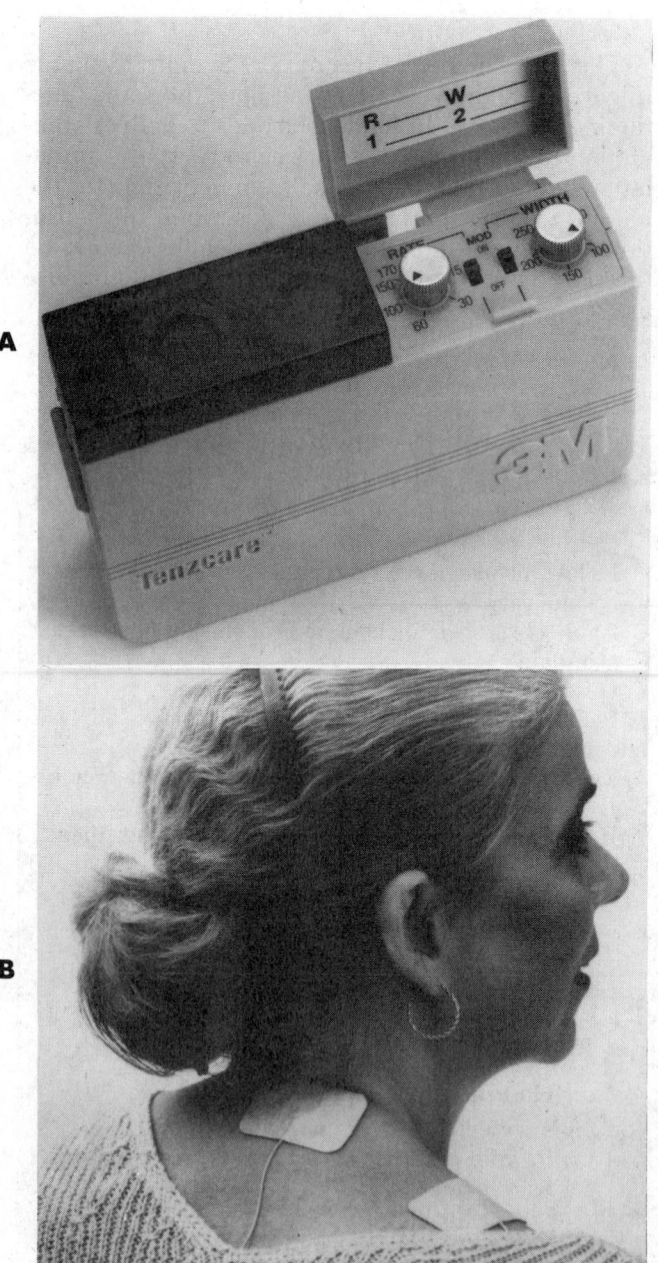

FIGURE 14-8   **A,** TENS unit. **B,** Patient with TENS unit in place. (Courtesy 3M Health Care Group, Home Medical Products Division, Bedford Park, Ill.)

can also act as a form of distraction as well as facilitating sedation or sleep. However, relaxation rarely decreases pain sensation.

Invasive Approaches to Pain Management

Invasive literally means "anything that invades the body." Examples of invasive techniques are nerve blocks, neurosurgical procedures, and acupuncture. Certain invasive techniques can be helpful for the patient with pain. However, careful patient selection and proper technique is essential, because the cost

and risks are high. Invasive techniques generally require a physician's order, and often a surgeon or anesthesiologist's skill.

Nerve blocks

Anyone who has ever received lidocaine (Xylocaine) before a dental procedure is familiar with a nerve block. Nerve blocks consist of injecting an anesthetic agent into or near a nerve to decrease pain pathways (Table 14-9). According to Bonica,[20] nerve blocks may be performed for one of the following reasons:

TABLE 14-9   Types of Nerve Blocks

Nerve block	Definition	Indications	Side effects	Special considerations
Local infiltration	Use of a local anesthetic agent into peripheral nerves	Painful inflammatory conditions, acute musculoskeletal conditions	Minimal	Safest and easiest block; because it is temporary (local), it may need to be repeated several times
Peripheral block	Interruption of peripheral nerve conduction with a local anesthetic or a neurolytic agent	Pain in thoracic area	Because peripheral nerves are mixed, it may cause both sensory and motor losses; if given in intercostal area, most serious complication is pneumothorax	If pain is fairly localized, it is best to use a local anesthetic agent
Celiac plexus block	Interruption of sympathetic and parasympathetic conduction from the abdominal viscera	Visceral pain (especially severe pain caused by pancreatic or upper abdominal cancer)	Hypotension (because of generalized vasodilation), numbness of lower extremities, hematoma, urinary difficulties	Although procedure itself may be painful, it has a high rate of success
Stellate ganglion block	Injection of a local anesthetic agent into a sympathetic nerve group	Pain in upper extremities (shoulder, face, head, or neck), acute herpes zoster, postherpetic neuralgia	Cardiac irregularities, temporary hoarseness, ipsilateral arm weakness, hematoma	May need repeated injections (local)
Lumbar sympathetic block	Injection of a local anesthetic or a neurolytic agent into the spinal cord	Pelvic pain, lower extremity pain, phantom-limb pain	Weakness and paralysis of lower extremities	May need repeated injections if local agent used
Intrathecal (subarachnoid) block	Injection of a neurolytic agent into the spinal cord	Pain in lower chest or upper abdomen	Arachnoiditis, hypotension, bowel and bladder dysfunction	When performed with alcohol or phenol, sometimes called a chemical rhizotomy (see section on neurosurgical pain-relief measures)

1. Prognostic—To predict effects from a permanent block or neurosurgery, including relief of pain as well as possible complications
2. Diagnostic—To determine specific pain pathways and aid in determining the site of pain
3. Therapeutic—To control pain

The nerve block can be performed with either a local temporary anesthetic agent or a permanent neurolytic agent. Local anesthetics are short-acting (procaine), intermediate-acting (lidocaine), or long-acting (bupivacaine). Local anesthetic agents provide pain relief for durations ranging from several hours to several days, and the anesthesia is reversible.

Anesthesiologists generally prefer to perform neurolytic blocks on patients whose life span is shortened because of advanced cancer, rather than for patients with benign pain. Because the procedure is irreversible and associated with serious risks, careful patient selection is required.

Neurosurgical procedures

Neurosurgical procedures for pain relief involve the surgical or chemical (alcohol) interruption of pain pathways. It is essential that patients are carefully selected for these procedures and that they completely understand the potential risks and benefits.

These procedures are most commonly done for cancer patients with severe pain, whose life spans are anticipated to be long enough to warrant such drastic measures. It is necessary for these patients to be given an adequate trial of narcotic analgesics in appropriate dosages and routes before these permanent, risky, and costly procedures are undertaken (Table 14-10).

The nursing care for a patient undergoing neurosurgical procedure for pain control is the same as for any neurosurgical patient. In addition, when performing preoperative teaching, the nurse helps the patient and family understand the procedure and the possible complications. The nurse also informs the patient and family that, unfortunately in some cases, pain relief may diminish over time. Also, just as with nerve blocks, some patients find the numbness or other sensations more uncomfortable than the original pain.

Postoperative care is the same as for any neurosurgical patient: frequent check of vital signs, neurologic assessment, checks for CSF leaks, and checks of the incision and the fluid and electrolyte levels. The nurse also assesses the patient's pain thoroughly (incisional as well as any new sensations) and records all findings.

Acupuncture

Acupuncture, the insertion of needles at various points into the body to relieve pain, comes from the Latin words, *acus* meaning needle, and *pungere* meaning puncture. This invasive technique is based on an ancient Chinese theory of two opposing forces, yin and yang. Each force moves along "meridians" in the body that are associated with particular organs or body parts. The Chinese theory says that pain and illness are caused by an imbalance of yin and yang.

It is believed that there are approximately 1000 known acupuncture points that make up the meridians. These acupuncture points seem to correspond to the same locations as "trigger" points in the body. Trigger points are small, hypersensitive areas in muscle or connective tissue that may cause pain when stimulated and pain relief with sustained pressure.[9]

It is theorized that acupuncture stimulates large nerve fibers to close the gate in the spinal cord to pain impulses. It is also postulated that acupuncture causes the release of endorphins.

Pain Clinics

In 1961 John Bonica, a pioneer in pain research and management, started the first multidisciplinary pain clinic at the University of Washington in Seattle. Because no single treatment for pain exists for all pa-

GERIATRIC CONSIDERATIONS

Pain Management

- Elderly adults have a higher tolerance for cutaneous pain, but a decreased tolerance for deep pain.
- Elderly patients may complain of pain more frequently than younger adults, as the elderly's pain is usually multi-causal.
- Disorders such as musculoskeletal, heart disease, and cancer are more prevalent in the elderly and may produce pain.
- Depression can also masquerade as pain.
- Accurate, in-depth assessment is necessary for effective pain management in the older adult.
- Pain control can be achieved by either pharmacologic or nonpharmacologic means; often a combination of the two can be effective.
- The eldery are at higher risk for drug-related toxicities than younger adults due to multi-drug interactions and the older adult's decline in organ function, especially the kidney.
- Nonpharmacologic pain relief therapies effective in the elderly include application of heat and cold, vibration, biofeedback, and hypnosis.

From Louise Joffrion, RN, C, MSN, DNS Candidate, Baton Rouge General School of Nursing.

TABLE 14-10   Neurosurgical Procedures for Pain Relief

Procedure	Definition	Indications	Possible complications	Special considerations
INTERRUPTION AT THE LEVEL OF THE PERIPHERAL NERVE ROOT (FIRST-ORDER NEURONS)				
Neurectomy	Surgical excision of a peripheral nerve	Pain well-localized in a single peripheral nerve (i.e., trigeminal neuralgia)	Paresthesias; pain may persist	Rarely performed, because it is unusual for pain to involve a single peripheral nerve; also, peripheral nerves regenerate
Rhizotomy	Surgical destruction of posterior nerve roots as they enter the spinal cord	Useful for selective, well-defined nerve root involvement (e.g., pain in upper trunk)	Paresthesias, loss of heat and cold sensations	May be performed through surgical incision (laminectomy) or pericutaneously (more precise and less risky procedure involving local anesthetic and placement of wire electrodes while using x-ray scanning)
Sympathectomy	Interruption of sympathetic afferent nerve fibers either through chemical block or by surgery	Causalgia, phantom-limb pain	Pain may persist	Usually preceded by a local anesthetic block to see if procedure will help
INTERRUPTION AT THE LEVEL OF THE SPINAL CORD (SECOND-ORDER NEURONS)				
Cordotomy	Sectioning of pain pathways in the spinothalamic tract of the spinal cord contralateral (opposite) to the pain	Unilateral cordotomy for pain of extremity or pelvis; bilateral cordotomy for midline pain	Temporary or permanent paralysis, bowel and bladder dysfunction, impotence, loss of pain and temperature sensations; bilateral approach has more complications, including respiratory complications, because of high cervical approach	Most successful neurosurgery for pain (especially cancer pain), may be performed percutaneously or via laminectomy
Tractotomy	Surgical interruption of spinothalamic tract in medulla, contralateral to the pain	Unilateral pain in head, neck, arms	Loss of sensation, complications of craniotomy	Difficult to perform; also rarely done because of high mortality
INTERRUPTION AT THE LEVEL OF THE BRAIN (THIRD-ORDER NEURONS)				
Hypophysectomy	Destruction of the pituitary gland by surgical removal or chemical (alcohol) injection	Metastatic bone pain related to hormone-dependent breast or prostate cancer	Risk of diabetes insipidus and cerebrospinal fluid (CSF) leak	Should be performed only for bone pain related to cancer
Thalamatomy	Surgical interruption of spinothalamic tract at the level of the thalamus	Well-located pain in the head and neck	Complications of craniotomy; pain relief decreases over time	Difficult to find exact location of lesion in the thalamus

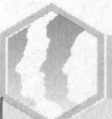

GERIATRIC CONSIDERATIONS

Pain and the Elderly

Pain can be a significant problem for any patient. The lack of education for health professionals on the management of pain in the elderly adds to this problem. [6] The prevalence of pain in the elderly is estimated to be very high. In one study of nursing home patients, 83% reported pain, many in the severe range.[15] Current literature reports that 70% to 80% of the elderly population have at least one chronic condition associated with pain.[4]

The elderly often fail to report pain and even deny it exists. Many deny pain because they believe it is an inevitable part of aging. Other reasons elderly patients may deny pain include fears of cancer, fears of medical treatments, cost issues, and the possibility of being a burden to their families.

Common types of pain in the elderly population include:

1. Headache
2. Low-back pain
3. Neuropathic pain such as diabetic neuropathy, phantom-limb pain, postherpetic neuralgia, trigeminal neuralgia, causalgia
4. Cancer pain—one out of three people in the United States will get cancer, and 50% occurs over the age of 65 years
5. Arthritic pain—degenerative joint disease, rheumatoid arthritis, and other forms of arthritis.

Difficulties with assessing pain in the elderly may be related to sensory or cognitive conditions. The nurse needs to make pain assessment a high priority for the elderly patient, as with any patient.

Difficulties in pain assessment in the elderly may occur with a nonverbal, comatose, or confused patient. It is important for the nurse to keep in mind that these patients often have pain, even though they cannot express it. The nurse can look for any behaviors that may be expressions of pain, such as moaning, restlessness, or withdrawal. Also, any conditions or treatments that a patient may say causes pain will most likely be cues for the nurse when caring for a patient who cannot communicate verbally with similar situations. Whether patients can verbalize pain or not, their reaction to the treatment may be the same. Examples of these conditions are positioning patients with fractures or contractures, dressing changes, and tube feedings.

The pharmacologic management of pain in the elderly is based on the same principles included in this chapter. Several additional points regarding the elderly need to be addressed. Studies show that elderly patients often receive fewer analgesics than do other patients. Although hepatic and renal clearance decreases as a result of aging, analgesics can still be used safely. It is highly recommended to "start low and go slow" when choosing initial nonopioid and opioid doses. Nonopioids recommended are Desalcid, Trilisate, and Dolobid, since they have fewer GI and renal side effects. Opioids recommended are those with short half-lives such as morphine or Dilaudid. Meperidine, Levo-Dromoran, and methadone are avoided because toxic levels may accumulate more easily in the elderly. The duration of action of opioids is usually longer in the elderly, so less frequent dosing is needed. Despite what many people think, pain is not and should not be a normal part of aging. Proper pain management can promote independence, increase function, and greatly improve the quality of life.

---

tients, Bonica believed that a group of specialists as well as a variety of treatment options would provide the best approach to pain management. Bonica's first pain clinic has served as a model for hundreds of others in the United States and abroad.

Most pain clinics accept patients on a referral basis and may be either outpatient or inpatient clinics. The members of the multidisciplinary team usually include a nurse, an anesthesiologist, a neurologist or neurosurgeon, a pharmacist, a social worker, a psychiatrist or psychologist, physical and occupational therapists, and a vocational therapist. Right from the start, the team assures the patient that they believe the pain is real.

Most pain clinic teams have similar goals for their patients:

- Decrease the patient's degree of pain
- Increase the patient's activity and ability to function
- Improve the patient's sleep
- Decrease the patient's dependency on pain medications, if necessary

The pain clinic teams attempt to achieve these goals through a variety of nonpharmacologic approaches (noninvasive and invasive), such as nerve blocks, acupuncture, hypnosis, TENS, biofeedback, psychologic therapies, and group therapies.

The nurse may be asked to help the patient locate a reputable pain clinic. The nurse can refer the patient to the Commission on Accreditation of Rehabilitation Facilities (CARF) to obtain a list of accredited pain clinics in the United States. Generally, pain clinics associated with a major medical center or university are multidisciplinary and have many specialists.

CRITICAL THINKING QUESTIONS

1 Why are some patients in pain undertreated?

2 Discuss some ways the nurse can improve the problems of pain.

3 In caring for two patients with the exact same diagnosis (e.g., first day postoperative cholecystectomy), why may their pain experiences vary? What factors contribute to an individual's perception of pain?

4 A patient in the emergency room has severe, pain in the right side. The physician diagnoses the condition renal colic. Would this be acute or chronic pain? How do these types of pain differ?

5 How are pain impulses carried to the brain? What part of the brain perceives pain?

6 As the nurse is teaching a patient about relaxation techniques, the patient asks, "How will these techniques help my pain?" How might the nurse simply explain the gate-control theory to this patient?

7 Why is assessment of pain an integral component of pain management? What points should be covered when finding out about a patient's pain?

8 What are the similarities between aspirin and acetaminophen? How do they differ? What are NSAIDs? How do they decrease pain?

9 Why are the following opioid doses most likely to be ineffective? Explain the rationale using an equianalgesic chart.

Hydromorphone	1.5 mg PO q4h
Meperidine	50 mg PO q4h
Morphine	15 mg PO q4h

10 What is the nurse's role when administering a continuous opioid infusion? In patient-controlled analgesia?

11 How might TENS, heat and cold, and massage help a patient in pain? What is the nurse's role when using these techniques for pain management?

12 A patient is scheduled for a nerve block for chronic low-back pain. Discuss the different types of nerve blocks and how they might help decrease pain. What types of patients might be considered good candidates for nerve block treatment?

RESOURCES

1 AMERICAN PAIN SOCIETY A multidisciplinary organization composed of clinicians and researchers in the study and treatment of pain. 5700 Old Orchard Road, First Floor Skokie, IL 60077-1057

2 INTERNATIONAL PAIN FOUNDATION Supports public and professional education about pain disorders and their treatment. 909 NE 43rd Street, Room 306 Seattle, WA 98195 206-547-2157

3 INTERNATIONAL ASSOCIATION FOR THE STUDY OF PAIN (IASP) Department of Anesthesiology RN-10 University of Washington School of Medicine Seattle, WA 98195

4 NATIONAL FOUNDATION FOR CHRONIC PAIN A non-profit organization designed to finance research and compile information. 1-800-451-PAIN

5 NATIONAL MIGRAINE FOUNDATION 5252 N. Western Chicago, IL 312-878-7715

6 NATIONAL COMMISSION FOR THE CERTIFICATION OF ACUPUNCTURISTS, INC. To obtain names of practitioners in the reader's area. 1424 16th Street NW Suite 105 Washington, DC 20036 202-232-1404

7 THE AMERICAN SOCIETY OF CLINICAL HYPNOSIS To obtain names of practitioners in the reader's area. 2250 E. Devon Avenue Suite 336 Des Plaines, IL 60018 312-297-3317

8 BIOFEEDBACK SOCIETY OF AMERICA To obtain names of practitioners in the reader's area. 10200 W. 44th Avenue, 304 Wheat Ridge, CO 80033 303-422-8436

BIBLIOGRAPHY

Current

1. Bonica JJ: The importance of education and training in pain diagnosis and therapy: the role of continuing education courses. In Rizzi R, Visentin M, editors: *Pain therapy,* Amsterdam, 1983, Elsevier Biomedical Press.

2. Austin K, et al: Multiple intramuscular injections: a major source of variability in analgesic response to meperidine, *Pain* 8:47, 1980.

3. *Cancer pain relief,* Geneva, 1986, World Health Organization.

4. Butler R, Gastel B: Care of the aged: perspectives on pain and discomfort. In Benich, editor: *Pain, discomfort and humanitarian care,* New York, 1980, Elsevier/North Hall, 297.

5. Donovan MI, Dillon P, McGuire L: Incidence and characteristics of pain in a sample of medical-surgical inpatients, *Pain* 30:69, 1987.

6. Ferrell BA: Pain management in elderly people, *JAGS* 39(1):64, 1991.

7. Ferrell BR, McCaffery M, Rhiner M: Pain and addiction: an urgent need for change in nursing education, *J Pain Symptom Management* 7(2):117, 1992.

8. Foley K: The treatment of cancer pain, *NEJM* 313(2):84, 1985.
9. Kantor TG: Non-steroidal anti-inflammatory analgesics in management of cancer pain. In Management of cancer pain (monograph), *Hosp Pract,* Summer: 30, 1984.
10. McCaffery M, Beebe A: *Pain: clinical manual for nursing practice,* St Louis, 1989, Mosby–Year Book.
11. Meinhart NT, McCaffery M: *Pain: a nursing approach to assessment and analysis,* New York, 1983, Appleton-Century-Crofts.
12. Paice JA: The phenomenon of analgesic tolerance in cancer pain management, *Oncol Nurs Forum* 15(4):455, 1988.
13. Perry S, Heidrich G: Management of pain during debridement: a survey of US burn units, *Pain* 12:267, 1982.
14. Porter J, Jick H: Addiction rare in patients treated with narcotics, *N Engl J Med* 302:133, 1980.
15. Wall RT: Use of analgesics in the elderly, *Clin Geriatr Med* 6(2):345, 1990.
16. Watt-Watson JH: Nurse's knowledge of pain issues: a survey, *J Pain Symptom Management* 2(4):207, 1987.
17. Watt-Watson JH, Donovan MI: *Pain management—nursing perspective,* St Louis, 1992, Mosby–Year Book.

Classic

18. Beecher HK: Relationship of significance of wound to pain experienced, *JAMA* 161:1609, 1956.
19. Benson H: *The relaxation response,* New York, 1976, Avon Books.
20. Bonica JJ: Introduction to nerve blocks. In Bonica JJ, Ventafridda V, editors: *Advances in pain research and therapy,* vol 2, New York, 1979, Raven Press.
21. Dundee JW, Love WJ, Moore J: Alterations in response to somatic pain associated with anesthesia. XV: Further studies with phenothiazine derivatives and similar drugs, *Br J Anesth* 35:597, 1963.
22. Houde RW, Wallensteen SC, Rogers A: Clinical pharmacology of analgesics: a method of assaying analgesic effects, *Clin Pharmacol Ther* 1:163, 1960.
23. Keats AS, Telford J, Kurosu Y: Potentiation of meperidine by promethazine, *Anesthesiology* 22:34, 1961.
24. McCaffery M: *Nursing management of the patient with pain,* ed 2, Philadelphia, 1979, JB Lippincott.
25. McGee JL, Alexander MR: Phenothiazine analgesia: fact or fantasy? *Am J Hosp Pharm* 36:633, 1979.
26. Melzack R, Wall PD: Pain mechanisms: a new theory, *Science* 150:791, 1965.
27. Saunders C: *The management of terminal illness,* London, 1967, London Hospital Medical Publications.
28. Sternbach RA: *Pain: a psychophysiological analysis,* New York, 1963, Academic Press Inc.
29. Zborowski M: *People in pain,* San Francisco, 1969, Jossey-Bass Inc, Publishers.

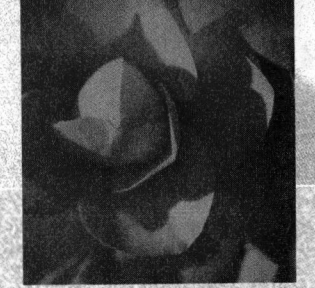

CHAPTER FIFTEEN

Neoplasia

LEARNING OBJECTIVES

1 Compare and contrast cellular characteristics that distinguish cancerous tissue from normal tissue.

2 Relate the process of carcinogenesis to both environmental and host risk factors.

3 Describe the tissue classification system for cancers.

4 List the mechanisms by which cancer cells metastasize.

5 Discuss current incidence of cancers and trends in mortality.

6 Describe screening procedures for early cancer detection.

7 Explain concepts of staging and grading neoplastic disease.

8 Compare and contrast the four major treatment methods, including their indications, limitations, side effects, and safety issues.

9 Explain nursing management for patients with symptoms common to neoplastic disease, treatment, and emergency conditions.

10 Discuss interventions that promote continuity of care, from time of diagnostic workup to the terminal stage of disease.

KEY TERMS

CANCER refers to a large group of potentially lethal disorders characterized by abnormal cell growth and metastasis. Because of its diversity and complexity, cancer has no single treatment, nor can it be attributed to a single etiologic agent. It is the second leading cause of death in the United States; one of every three Americans will probably develop invasive cancer. The economic impact alone is overwhelming; overall costs associated with cancer now exceed $104 billion per year.[1] What is currently known about the disease process, treatment approaches, and methods of prevention changes virtually every day. Fortunately, these advances have changed the entire connotation of the diagnosis of cancer. What was once a uniformly fatal condition is now controllable, if not curable, in many cases.

EPIDEMIOLOGY

The incidence of cancer in the United States, excluding carcinoma in situ and nonmelanoma skin cancers, is estimated to be 1,130,000 in 1992.[4] Figure 15-1 illustrates the estimated cancer incidence in 1992 by site and sex. Cancer occurs more commonly in men than in women and is primarily a disease of advanced age. More than 50% of all cases are diagnosed after the age of 65, with noticeable increases in incidence beginning at age 40.[58] Trends in incidence reveal the following[58]:

- Cancer is increasingly more common among the elderly
- The incidence of cancer has increased overall, but more so in African Americans than in Caucasion Americans.

- The incidence of breast cancer is increasing steadily in women
- The incidence of melanoma has almost doubled in white men and women
- The incidence of lung cancer has increased in all groups, especially women
- The incidence of prostate cancer has increased, especially among black men
- The incidence of colon cancer has increased in all groups
- The incidence of leukemia has decreased
- The incidence of ovarian cancer has decreased slightly
- The incidence of cervical cancer has decreased, although it occurs more commonly in black women

Explanations for general increases in incidence include the increasing overall age of our population and the long-term exposure to environmental risk factors. Decreases in incidence may be the result of earlier detection and better understanding and identification of risk factors.

It is estimated that 520,000 Americans died of cancer in 1992.[4] Lung cancer is now the number-one killer in both sexes. Figure 15-2 illustrates the estimated number of cancer deaths by site and sex. Cancer-related deaths are more common in men than in women and more frequent in older people than in the young. Current trends in mortality are the following[4]:

- Greatest increases in disease-specific mortality rates of all groups are in lung cancer
- Decreases are most notable in stomach and uterine cancer

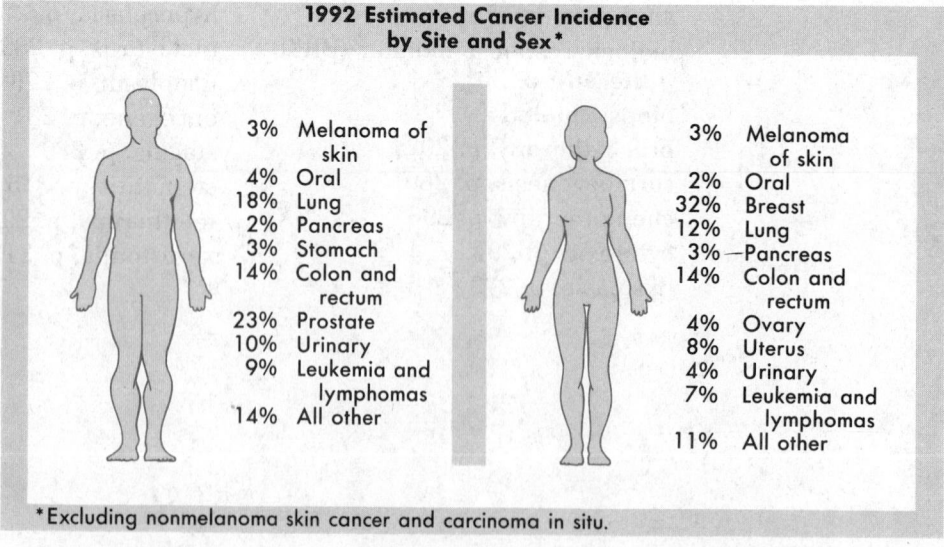

1992 Estimated Cancer Incidence by Site and Sex*

	Men			Women
3%	Melanoma of skin		3%	Melanoma of skin
4%	Oral		2%	Oral
18%	Lung		32%	Breast
2%	Pancreas		12%	Lung
3%	Stomach		3%	Pancreas
14%	Colon and rectum		14%	Colon and rectum
23%	Prostate		4%	Ovary
10%	Urinary		8%	Uterus
9%	Leukemia and lymphomas		4%	Urinary
14%	All other		7%	Leukemia and lymphomas
			11%	All other

*Excluding nonmelanoma skin cancer and carcinoma in situ.

FIGURE 15-1   1992 estimated cancer incidence by site and sex.

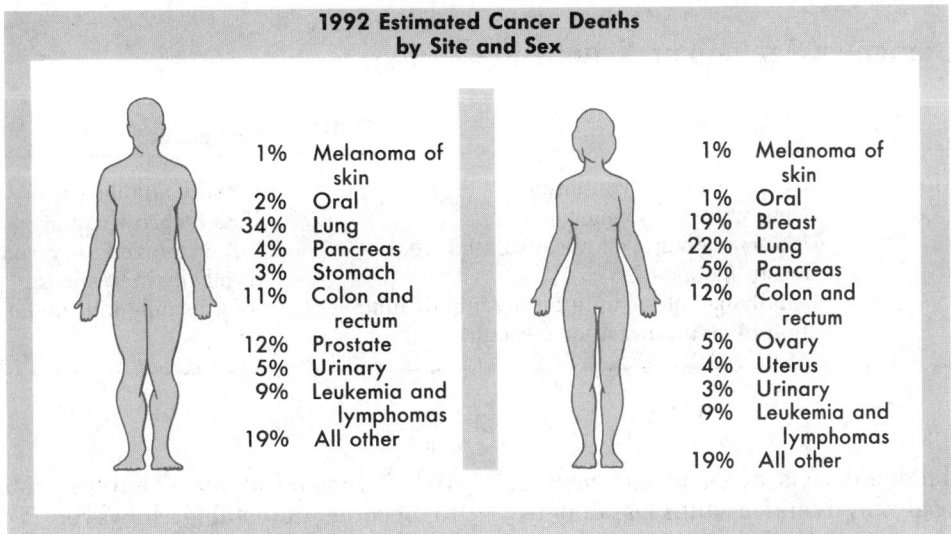

FIGURE 15-2   1992 estimated cancer deaths by site and sex.

- Until 1988, breast cancer was the most common cancer-related cause of death in women: lung cancer has now surpassed it
- Overall survival rates have increased steadily since the turn of the century
- Whites have higher survival rates than do blacks

Survival rates reflect earlier detection measures, improved therapies, and increased availability of care. In terms of cancer epidemiology, the term "survivor" refers to an individual who has survived at least 5 years after being diagnosed with cancer.

CANCER BIOLOGY
Cellular Alterations

Normally, cells grow and divide in a controlled, predictable manner. Their size and number should not exceed that which the body needs to function. One alteration that can occur in this process is that of **hyperplasia,** an increase in the number of normal cells in a tissue or organ. Hyperplasia may be normal or abnormal and can occur in response to a variety of identifiable stimuli. For example, during pregnancy the glandular breast tissue and the uterine musculature both undergo hyperplastic changes that are expected consequences of hormonal stimulation. Abnormal or pathologic hyperplasia, such as chronic irritation of the skin, may also occur. Ultimately, hyperplastic changes cease once the stimuli are removed. Clinically, abnormal hyperplastic changes are significant because they are associated with an increased risk of neoplasia.

Conversion of tissue into an abnormal form is termed metaplasia; in this instance, one fully mature cell type is substituted for another. Metaplasia may occur in response to injury and to chronic irritation or inflammation. In the bronchi of cigarette smok-ers, metaplastic changes are seen when squamous cells replace the ciliated columnar epithelial cells. This response is probably protective, because squamous cells are hardier than ciliated columnar epithelial cells. Usually metaplasia will reverse itself when the cause is removed.

Dysplasia, an alteration in the size, shape, and organization of cells, is another change that occurs. Most often, dysplasia results from chronic irritation or inflammation. Smokers may exhibit dysplastic changes in respiratory tissues and the oral mucosa. As in hyperplasia and metaplasia, dysplasia may also be reversible if the stimulus ceases, but it is much more strongly associated with subsequent neoplastic changes.

Undifferentiated cells (i.e., those that are primitive or poorly developed) that have lost their structural organization are associated with **anaplasia.** Anaplastic changes may vary in degree, but when severe they are considered to indicate cancer.

Neoplasm means "new thing formed" and is used interchangeably with tumor (swelling). A **neoplasm** is an abnormal growth of tissue that serves no function and continues to grow unchecked even if the stimulus is removed. Although often associated with rapid growth, neoplasms may grow slowly for years before detection. Neoplasms may either be benign or malignant, but all are capable of harm because they compete with normal tissue for nutrients and may impinge on adjacent structures. Benign and malignant tumors differ in five key areas (Table 15-1).

Characteristics of Cancer Cells

Metabolism

Normal cells employ aerobic glycolysis for metabolism; that is, oxygen is required for maintenance of

TABLE 15-1   Benign vs. Malignant Neoplasms

Characteristic	Benign	Malignant
Cell differentiation	Usually well differentiated	Usually anaplastic
Growth rate	Usually slow growing	Usually grow rapidly
Invasiveness	Usually remain well encapsulated	Tend to invade adjacent tissue
Metastatic ability	Do not metastasize	Typically metastasize
Prognosis	Usually harmless, unless they impair function of a vital organ or structure	Will usually kill the host if untreated

cell activities. Malignant cells seem to use higher rates of anaerobic glycolysis and are thus less dependent on oxygen. As a result, cells in the core of a tumor can survive, despite poor oxygenation. Differences in intracellular enzyme structure and quantity may account for this difference in metabolism.

Growth and spread

Malignant tumors grow unrestrained. They bypass the normal processes of cell reproduction, thereby exhibiting the property of autonomy. Normally, cell growth is limited by contact inhibition, which occurs when cells stop dividing or moving when they come in contact with each other. Cancer cells also lose the property of adhesion, the normal tendency of cells to stick together. These are key factors in metastatic spread. Loss of contact inhibition and adhesion are a result of increased numbers of degradative surface enzymes that are known to promote invasiveness and metastases. Another change in growth characteristics is the inability of cancer cells to differentiate or mature fully. There is some lack of differentiation in all malignancies, ranging from the fairly well-differentiated cell type to the poorly differentiated. In general, the less differentiated the cells are, the more rapidly the cancer grows, although many exceptions exist.

Ultimately, many factors influence malignant cell replication and the final appearance of a clinically detectable tumor mass. Most tumors weigh at least 1.0 g and are made of 10^9 cells at the time they are clinically detectable. Three key factors govern tumor progression into a detectable mass: (1) the doubling time of the malignant cell (the time for the tumor mass to double its size), (2) the proportion of cells within a tumor mass that continue to remain viable and continue to replicate (also termed "growth fraction"), and (3) the rate at which cells break away and are lost to the original mass. Most cells in tumors are not in the replicating pool. The growth fraction in certain rapidly replicating tumors may approach 20%; normal epithelial tissue is approximately

16%.[10] In general, most cancers probably take years to become detectable; however, a few may arise within months.

Other associated host factors influence tumor growth. Variations in blood supply (and therefore nutrients) are critical. Cells at the tumor surface will thus proliferate faster than those in the core, which tend to die. Hormones may also affect tumor cell proliferation, especially in those tumors that arise in tissues that are normally dependent on hormones for cell function (e.g., prostate, breast, endometrium). Proliferation of some of these tumors may be slowed if the stimulating hormone is reduced. And finally, cancer cells are not as dependent on growth factors as normal cells are; thus cancer cells can proliferate when concentrations of growth factors are much lower than that required by normal cells.[26]

As tumors grow, the individual cells within become increasingly heterogeneous. They develop differences in genetic composition, invasiveness, growth rate, hormonal responsiveness, metastatic potential, and susceptibility to antineoplastic therapy.[34] These changes are caused by random mutations during tumor progression, and can cause the cancer to be highly resistant to any one specific therapy.

Structural changes

In addition to metabolic and growth characteristics, intracellular structural changes are also evident. Abnormalities may occur in cell organelles, such as mitochondria, Golgi apparatus, vacuoles, and centrioles. The nucleus also changes, most notably in chromosomes. The numbers of chromosomes and genes present may change, and translocations of genes between chromosomes may occur.

Carcinogenesis

Carcinogenesis refers to the transformation of normal cells to malignant cells. A carcinogen is a substance that can cause changes in the structure and function of a cell that lead to cancer.[27] The potency and dosage of a carcinogen play a significant role in the development of a malignancy. Although much controversy exists, most authorities agree that carcinogenesis is a complex process involving many interim stages as cells undergo transformation. Environmental and life-style factors may be linked to the majority of malignancies. Additionally, many underlying host factors affect susceptibility to carcinogenic changes.

Various theories of carcinogenesis have been proposed, but most address similar key events: initiation, promotion, and progression (Figure 15-3). Initiation refers to irreversible damage to a cell's DNA following exposure to carcinogenic agents such as chemicals, radiation, or viruses. Much research is now focused on the role that oncogenes play in this process. An **oncogene** is a slightly altered form of a normal gene necessary for cell growth and repair. This oncogene may cause cancer when activated. Although carcinogens may activate oncogenes, other factors yet to be identified may also be triggers. It has even been proposed that a specific oncogene is activated for each tumor type. The oncogene theory provides a common thread or unifying explanation of the nature of all cancers. The initiated or mutated cell then can give rise to daughter cells with the same alteration in DNA. The altered DNA is the critical factor in the ultimate development of a malignant cell. Initiation alone will not result in tumor formation, unless the initiator is a complete carcinogen. That is, the carcinogen is capable of both initiation *and* promotion. Cigarette smoke is an example of a complete carcinogen.

Because of an apparent latency period between initiation and tumor formation, a second stage of carcinogenesis, promotion, has been proposed. Promotion is characterized by the reversible expansion of the initiated cell group and reversible alteration of genetic expression.[31] In other words, promotion enhances the cellular transformation that began during initiation. Promoting factors usually do not alter DNA but exert their effects after initiation; however, certain promoting factors can also act as initiating factors. Unlike initiation, promotion may be reversible, either by removal of the promoting agent or by introduction of reversing factors. Alcohol, asbestos, cigarette smoke, and dietary fat are all potential promoting agents.[31]

Anticarcinogens are substances that may counteract the effects of initiators.[28] Proposed anticarcinogens (also termed "reversing factors") are present in most diets and include vitamin A and betacarotene (retinols), vitamin C, vitamin E, and selenium. Various other drugs, enzymes, and food additives are also under investigation to determine their reversing properties.

After malignant cells are formed by initiation and promotion, a final step, progression, may occur. Progression refers to the evolution of metastatic potential and is technically separate from the first two processes. At this point, the cells undergo further genetic changes that enable them to metastasize.

Risk Factors

Tobacco

Smoking is responsible for 87% of all cases of lung cancer.[1] A link also exists between smoking and cancers of the esophagus, larynx, mouth, bladder, pancreas, and kidneys. Smoking now accounts for at least 30% of all cancer deaths in the United States annually.[1] The popularity of smokeless tobacco is taking an increasing toll as well; the incidence of cancers of the mouth, larynx, throat, and esophagus related to using tobacco in this way is increasing among adolescent males. Tobacco and tobacco smoke contain a variety of known carcinogenic substances that may also act in concert with other carcinogens, such as alcohol and asbestos, to produce an even greater risk. Passive exposure to cigarette

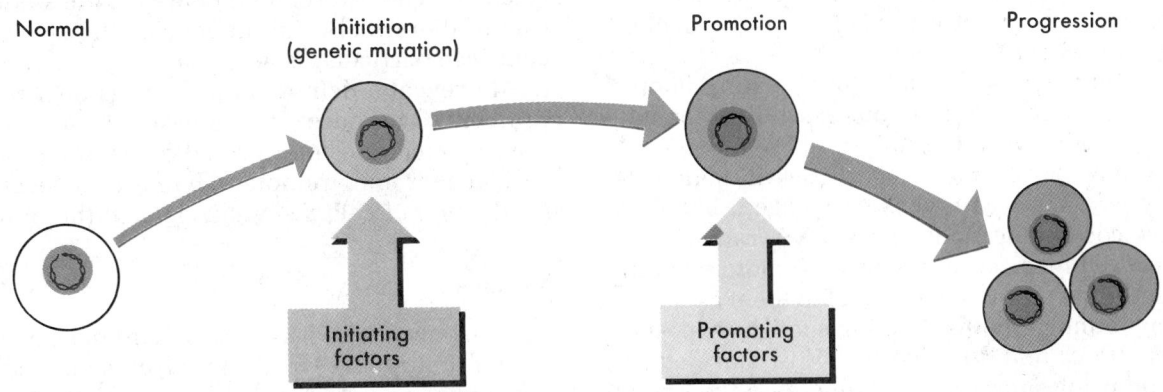

FIGURE 15-3 Carcinogenesis.

smoke is a risk to the nonsmoker. Although study results are mixed, substantial evidence exists to support the increased risk for developing lung cancer.[7]

Alcohol

Alcohol intake may facilitate carcinogenic changes initiated by other carcinogens, especially tobacco. Alcohol enhances the contact between the carcinogen (tobacco) and the cells that line the upper respiratory tract.[27] Use of tobacco and alcohol are well-known risk factors for head and neck cancers.

Occupational exposure

Certain occupations have been linked to an increased risk of cancer. Cigarette smokers who work with asbestos and other industrial carcinogens are at tremendous risk because of the potential for tobacco acting as a "cocarcinogen" or synergist with other compounds. Numerous studies have been conducted that quantify the increased risk. Blot and Fraumeni[39] studied shipyard workers exposed to asbestos and found that the relative risk for lung cancer increased significantly as the number of cigarettes smoked increased. Ultimately, the person who smoked more than two packs a day had a twenty-two fold increased risk for cancer compared to the nonsmoker in the same setting.

Radiation

Ultraviolet (UV) radiation, a component of sunlight has been positively linked with the development of a number of skin cancers, including basal cell carcinoma, squamous cell carcinoma, and malignant melanoma. Persons with fair complexions are at highest risk because they have fewer protective melanocytes in the skin. Although skin cancers only account for approximately 2% of all cancer deaths, melanoma is one of the most rapidly increasing cancers, with an increase by about 4% each year.[16] Approximately 600,000 new cases of nonmelanoma skin cancer occur annually.[1] Those who work outdoors or live in areas with intense sunlight have the highest rate of skin cancers.

The recent popularity of indoor tanning booths may ultimately contribute to increased rates of skin cancers. Tanning units typically emit UV radiation A (UVA) waves, 50% to 55% of which will penetrate the dermis.[63] UVA is a weak carcinogen, but does act as a cocarcinogen. Because UVA radiation is much less likely to cause sunburn, promoters of tanning booths have erroneously labeled them as safe.[63] Avoiding tanning booths, limiting sunlight exposure between 10 AM and 3 PM (when UV rays are strongest), and using sunscreens will decrease the risk of cancers induced by UV radiation exposure.

Ionizing radiation is high-energy radiation associated with cellular damage. It, too, has been linked to the development of malignancies. High doses incurred via occupational exposure or accident (e.g., nuclear plant accidents, atomic weaponry) result in higher incidences of leukemia. Because the hematopoietic system is especially radiosensitive, hematologic malignancies may arise after exposure.

Low-dose radiation exposure incurred during diagnostic radiographic examinations and natural (unavoidable) environmental exposure is less definitely linked to cancer. In the United States, the average exposure to background radiation is approximately 0.7 to 1.5 mGy/year, whereas measurable biologic effects of radiation exposure are not apparent until a dose of 1000 mGy (1 Gy) is incurred.[53] Gray [Gy] refers to the radiation dose absorbed by tissue; it is equivalent to 1 joule/kg.

Earlier use of radiation for non–cancer-related therapies has been linked to an increased incidence of malignancies. In the 1920s through the 1950s, external-beam irradiation was used as a treatment for thymus enlargement and tonsillitis in children. A 7% increase in risk for a thyroid malignancy is now known, as well as a thirteenfold to fortyfold increased risk for a salivary gland neoplasia.[64]

Radon, a gas that forms as a result of radioactive decay of radium and uranium in the earth's crust, is another source of radiation exposure.[27] Exposure to concentrated levels is known to increase the risk of lung cancer in both smokers and nonsmokers. Although the home is the major source of exposure to radon, potential for exposure differs markedly in various parts of the country, depending upon local geologic features.[15]

Diet

Although approximately half of all cancers are believed to be associated with dietary causes (see Table 15-2) studies have yet to reveal details of the process. Certain dietary fats may enhance the production of carcinogens by increasing the amount of bile acids and cholesterol metabolites in the stool.[27] The role of dietary fiber in influencing the risk of colon cancer in particular is not clear; however, most studies do reveal a definite link. Fiber is believed to be protective because it increases fecal bulk and thereby facilitates more rapid excretion of potential carcinogens and promoters. It may also decrease the production of colonic carcinogens in the bowel.[27]

Viruses

Known oncogenic viruses in humans have been identified (Table 15-3). Oncogenic viruses may cause carcinogenic transformation of cells they infect. Although not an oncogenic virus, the human immuno-

TABLE 15-2   Dietary Risk Factors

Risk Factors	Malignancy Site
High fat intake	Breast, colon, prostate, ovary, pancreas, cervix
Nitrates, nitrites (in smoked, pickled, or cured meats)	Stomach, esophagus
Alcohol	Oral cavity, pharynx, larynx, esophagus, liver
Obesity	Breast, prostate, pancreas, ovary
Low fiber intake	Colon, breast

TABLE 15-3   Human Oncogenic Viruses

Virus	Malignancy
Epstein-Barr	Burkitt's lymphoma, nasopharyngeal carcinoma
Herpes simplex II	Cervical carcinoma
Papillomavirus	Cervical carcinoma
Hepatitis B	Hepatocellular carcinoma

deficiency virus (HIV) is associated with the development of opportunistic cancers, such as Kaposi's sarcoma and lymphomas. Although loss of immune surveillance as a result of HIV suppression may contribute to the development of cancers, other contributing factors, such as transmissible agents, have been suggested.[33]

Drugs

Large doses of estrogen and doses given without supplemental progesterone are linked to breast and endocervical cancer; small doses given cyclically in conjunction with progesterone are believed to be safe for the management of estrogen deficiency in postmenopausal women.[41] Diethylstilbestrol (DES), once prescribed for abortion prevention, is now known to be associated with increased risk of vaginal adenocarcinoma in daughters of DES-treated mothers.

In addition to certain hormones, anticancer drugs and immunosuppressive agents are suspect. Alkylating agents used to treat Hodgkin's disease and other malignancies carry an increased risk of causing secondary malignancies many years later. The increased risk of acquiring leukemia after treatment for Hodgkin's disease is especially notable. As survival rates for cancer continue to improve, the incidence of treatment-induced leukemias may also rise alarmingly. Immunosuppressive drugs used to prevent organ rejection after transplantation are linked with increased cancer incidence. The risk of developing lymphoma in particular has been extensively studied. One study estimated that the risk of lymphoma increases twenty-ninefold with cyclosporin, versus thirty-fourfold to fifty-ninefold with conventional immunosuppressive therapy.[43]

Host factors

Host risk factors are endogenous characteristics that appear to predispose the host to cancer. Age, sex, and race influence risk. The incidence of cancer is known to increase with each decade of life, perhaps because of a normal decline in immune defense mechanisms. Indeed, the single greatest risk factor for cancer is age.[14] Females have a lower incidence and a lower death rate associated with cancer than do males.[4] Racial variations do exist, but they are attributed to both environmental and genetic factors. Genetic predisposition to cancer may be a strong factor in certain diseases. Epidemiologic studies of women with breast cancer reveal genetic risks. A woman has a 10% to 50% risk of developing breast cancer if she has two female relatives with the disease.[18]

Tumor Immunology

Tumor immunology is the science that examines the immune system's recognition of and response to cancer cells. The underlying assumption is that cancer cells are formed continuously throughout one's lifetime. An immunomodulated "surveillance network" works to destroy these cells before they can grow into clinically detectable masses. An understanding of this process could lead to advances in both the detection and the treatment of malignancies via manipulation of immune response.

Tumor antigenicity

For an immunologic reaction to occur, cancer cells must have properties that allow the body to distinguish them from normal cells. Because cancer cells and normal cells of the same histologic background have many similar characteristics, the distinction is not always precise. Substances called tumor antigens assist in the recognition process. Two kinds of tumor antigens serve as "red flags" to the immune system. The first are unique antigens that are found

TABLE 15-4   **Classification of Tumors by Tissue Type**

Tissue of origin	Benign	Malignant
EPITHELIUM		
Surface epithelium (nonglandular)	Papilloma	Carcinoma (squamous cell, epidermoid, transitional cell)
Glandular epithelium	Adenoma	Adenocarcinoma
Basal layer of epidermis	—	Basal cell carcinoma
Trophoblasts of placental villi	Hydatidiform mole	Choriocarcinoma
CONNECTIVE TISSUE		
Fibrous tissue	Fibroma	Fibrosarcoma
Cartilage	Chondroma	Chondrosarcoma
Bone	Osteoma	Osteosarcoma
Smooth muscle	Leiomyoma	Leiomyosarcoma
Striated muscle	Rhabdomyoma	Rhabdomyosarcoma
Fat	Lipoma	Liposarcoma
ENDOTHELIAL TISSUE AND ITS DERIVATIVES		
Blood vessels	Hemangioma	Hemangiosarcoma
Lymph vessels	Lymphangioma	Lymphangiosarcoma
Bone marrow		
Granulocytes	—	Myelocytic leukemia
Erythrocytes	Polycythemia vera	Erythrocytic leukemia
Lymphocytes	Infectious mononucleosis	Lymphocytic leukemia
Plasma cells	—	Multiple myeloma
Monocytes	—	Monocytic leukemia
Endothelial lining	—	Ewing's sarcoma
Lymphoid tissue		Hodgkin's disease
		Non-Hodgkin's malignant lymphomas
		Lymphocytic type
		Histiocytic type
		Undifferentiated, pleomorphic type
		Undifferentiated, Burkitt type
Thymus	—	Thymoma
NEURAL TISSUE AND ITS DERIVATIVES		
Glial tissue	"Benign" gliomas (some ependymomas and oligodendrogliomas are considered nonmalignant)	Glioblastoma multiforme, medulloblastoma, astrocytoma, ependymoma, oligodendroglioma
Meninges	Meningioma	Meningeal sarcoma
Neuronal cells	Ganglioneuroma	Neuroblastoma
Nerve sheath	Neurilemmoma	Neurilemmal sarcoma (schwannoma)
Nerve sheath	Neurofibroma	Neurofibrosarcoma
Melanocytes	Pigmented nevus (mole)	Malignant melanoma
Adrenal medulla	Pheochromocytoma	Malignant pheochromocytoma
Retina	—	Retinoblastoma
Specialized nerve endings	Carcinoid tumors	Carcinoid tumors
MIXED TUMORS DERIVED FROM MORE THAN ONE CELL TYPE		
Embryonic kidney	—	Nephroblastoma (Wilms' tumor)
Gonadal tissue	Teratoma	Teratocarcinoma
Gonadal tissue	—	Embryonal carcinoma with choriocarcinoma

From Ruddon RW: *Cancer biology*, New York, 1987, Oxford University Press.

only on cancer cells, not normal cells. Theoretically, a unique antigen may exist for each specific tumor type. Detection of such an antigen could then potentially serve as a diagnostic tool. The other kind of tumor antigen is the oncofetal antigen. These are antigens that are expressed by certain normal cells during fetal development but are subsequently repressed. They are, however, produced by certain cancer cells.

Carcinoembryonic antigen, or CEA, is one example of an oncofetal antigen. It is expressed by fetal gut cells, by colon cancer cells, and, in small amounts, by normal bowel cells. Because CEA may also be produced during inflammatory bowel disease flare-ups and other disorders, it cannot be used solely to diagnose cancer, but CEA can be used to monitor responses to treatment. A rise in serum CEA levels after treatment may indicate recurrence or spread of the cancer.

Failure of the immune response

Clinical experience shows that surveillance activities by the immune system cannot always identify and eradicate malignant cells. Development of disease might result from failure of the immune response. Transplant patients receiving immunosuppressive therapy to avoid rejection of the donated organs develop cancer at a higher rate than the general population (13/2000 vs. 8.2/100,000).[61] A natural decrease in immune function in the aging population has also been correlated with the increased incidence of cancer among the elderly. Several other factors in addition to immunosuppression and age have been cited for inadequate immune control of tumors. Tumor antigens may be either absent or not recognized as being foreign. The immune system may respond inappropriately and actually enhance tumor growth. A malignancy may escape detection by an otherwise healthy immune system by evolving into a nonantigenic form or by residing in a sheltered area where the immune system cannot reach it. Also, the amount of tumor cells may be insufficient to evoke a response; conversely, too many may overwhelm the system.[61]

Classification

Most malignant tumors are classified or named according to their biologic behavior, cellular function, histology, embryonic origin, and anatomic location. The tissue of origin refers to the normal tissue in which the tumor arises. There are four basic tissues in the human body: epithelial tissue, connective tissue, endothelial tissue, and nervous tissue. Each arises from one of the primary germ layers of the embryo, including the ectoderm, mesoderm, and endoderm (Table 15-4).

Metastasis

The spread of a malignancy beyond the primary tumor to distant sites is termed **metastasis.** Metastatic disease remains the primary cause of treatment difficulties and death. If tumors remained localized, surgery alone could increase cure rates drastically. Unfortunately, by the time cancer is diagnosed, metastasis has already occurred in 50% of patients.[13] Critical advances in development of effective cancer therapies may well hinge on a better understanding of metastatic disease.

Mechanisms

Invasion is the spreading of a tumor beyond its boundaries into adjacent tissue. This may be caused by mechanical pressure, migration of individual cells, or release of destructive enzymes. Direct spread is the shedding of cells into body cavities. The cells then travel via that cavity to other organs. Ovarian tumors often metastasize in this manner via the peritoneal cavity. Lymphatic-hematogenic spread refers to dissemination of cancer cells to distant sites via lymphatic vessels or the bloodstream or both (Figure 15-4). Cells adhere to the capillary lining of a distant organ, extravasate through the lining into the tissue, and multiply to form another tumor. The most common target organs for development of metastatic tumors are the lungs, bone, liver, and brain. Table 15-5 outlines metastatic sites common to specific tumor types.

PREVENTION AND EARLY DETECTION

In 1985 a goal of the National Cancer Institute[47] was to reduce the cancer mortality by 50% by the year 2000. Although advances in treatment will help

---

TABLE 15-5   Common Metastatic Sites

Primary tumors	Sites of metastasis
Breast	Bone, lung, liver, lymph nodes, brain
Cervix	Bone, lung, liver, bowel, lymph nodes, kidney
Colon	Lung, liver, lymph nodes
Head/neck	Skin, lung, lymph nodes
Lung	Bone, bone marrow, liver, lymph nodes, kidney, brain
Ovary	Lung, liver, bowel, lymph nodes
Prostate	Bone, lung, liver, lymph nodes

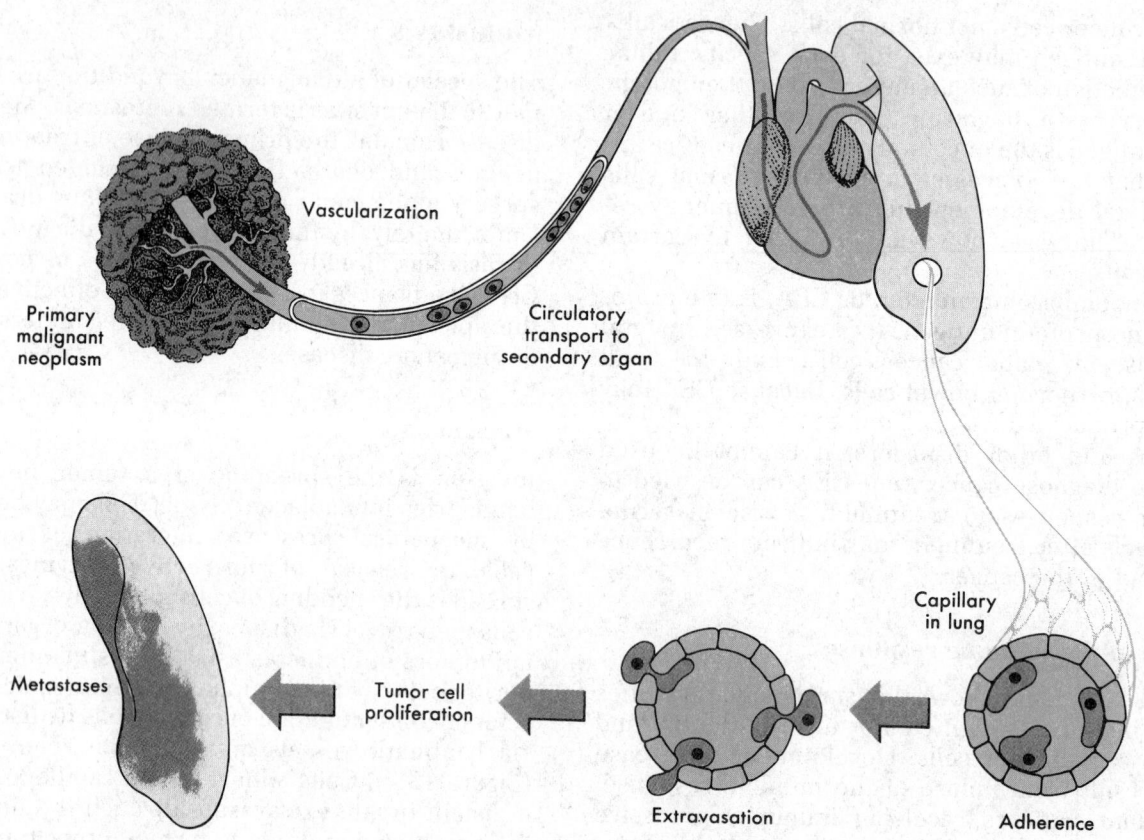

FIGURE 15-4 Lymphatic-hematogenic spread.

achieve this goal, preventive measures are equally important. Increased understanding of the factors associated with cancer has led to many recommendations for reducing individual risk.

Prevention

Because the use of tobacco products currently causes more than 30% of cancer deaths, reduction in use would have a significant impact. Overall, smoking is related to more than 400,000 deaths a year, with an annual economic cost of about $65 billion.[1] Nurses play a key role in reducing tobacco use. Vital activities include the following:

- Educating the public regarding the hazards of tobacco
- Serving as a role model by refraining from tobacco use
- Promoting a smoke-free environment within health care agencies and all work environments
- Promoting smoking cessation programs within the work environment
- Supporting legislation regarding promotion of a smoke-free society; this includes working with professional nursing organizations to achieve this end

- Assisting patients with smoking cessation activities

The American Cancer Society[1] recommends the following nutrition guidelines:

- Maintain desirable weight
- Eat a varied diet
- Include a variety of vegetables and fruits in the daily diet
- Eat more high-fiber foods such as whole-grain cereals, breads, pasta, vegetables, and fruits
- Cut down on total fat intake
- Limit consumption of alcohol
- Limit consumption of salt-cured, smoked, and nitrate-cured foods.

Minimizing exposure to hazardous industrial fibers (asbestos and dust), carcinogenic drugs, chemicals, and ionizing radiation can reduce associated cancer risks. Using sunscreens with a high sun-protection factor (SPF) is highly recommended, along with avoiding the sun during midday, when intensity is greatest.

A healthy life-style that includes a balanced diet, exercise, and adequate rest promotes normal immune function, which plays a role in the destruction of malignant cells.

Both herpes simplex II and papillomaviruses are

TABLE 15-6 Recommendations for Early Detection of Cancer

Examination	Sex	Age	Frequency
Sigmoidoscopy	M and F	50 and older	1 exam every 3 to 5 years
Stool blood test	M and F	50 and older	Every year
Digital rectal examination	M and F	40 and older	Every year
Pap test and pelvic examination	F	18 or older, or sexually active	Every year. After 3 or more satisfactory, consecutive, normal annual examinations, the Pap test may be performed less frequently at the discretion of the physician
Endometrial tissue sample	F	At menopause; women at high risk*	At menopause
Breast self-examination*	F	20 and older	Every month
Clinical breast examination	F	20-39	Every 3 years
		40 and older	Every year
Mammography	F	35-39	Baseline
		40-49	Every 1 to 2 years
		50 and over	Every year
Health counseling†	M and F	20-40	Every 3 years
Cancer checkup‡	M and F	40 and older	Every year

*History of infertility, obesity, failure to ovulate, abnormal uterine bleeding, or estrogen therapy.
†To include counseling about tobacco control, sun exposure, diet and nutrition, risk factors, sexual practices, and environmental and other occupational exposures.
‡To include examination for cancers of the thyroid, testicles, prostate, ovaries, lymph nodes, oral cavity, and skin.
From Fink DJ: Cancer detection: the cancer-related checkup guidelines. In Holleb AI, Fink DJ, Murphy GP, editors: *American cancer society textbook of clinical oncology,* ed 2, Atlanta, 1991, The American Cancer Society

strongly linked to cervical carcinoma. Avoiding exposure to sexually transmitted disease is a critical prevention activity. Barrier contraceptives and careful personal hygiene also are important in cancer prevention.

Early Detection

Cancer-screening activities promote early detection of malignancies and premalignant conditions, and with early detection comes the greater likelihood of successful treatment. Until recently, both private and public health insurance groups were hesitant to cover cancer-screening exams. Medicare coverage is now provided for a Pap smear once every 3 years and a mammogram once every 2 years for women over the age of 65. Cancer detection can and should take place in all settings, including schools, places of employment, physicians' offices, extended care facilities, and day-care centers for the young and old. When interviewing a patient, ask about any previous exposure to known or suspected risk factors. Also ask about the presence of the seven warning signals of cancer, as outlined by the American Cancer Society (see box at right), and watch for any

manifestations of them when examining the patient. Counsel the patient regarding the American Cancer Society's age-specific guidelines for screening activities (Table 15-6).

Ultimately, education is the key to successful screening and detection. The informed consumer who follows preventive life-style and health-care

EARLY WARNING SIGNALS OF CANCER

Change in bowel or bladder habits
A sore that does not heal
Unusual bleeding or discharge
Thickening or lump in breast or elsewhere
Indigestion or difficulty in swallowing
Obvious change in a mole or wart
Nagging cough or hoarseness

From the American Cancer Society: *Cancer facts and figures,* Atlanta, 1992, The Society.

habits will contribute to his or her own well-being. Patient education topics are highlighted in the box at right.

DIAGNOSIS

The diagnosis of cancer is a multiphasic process that includes obtaining a careful history regarding host and environmental risk factors, noting the presence of warning signals, conducting an in-depth physical examination focused on changes indicative of malignancy or a premalignant state, and performing selected diagnostic procedures. A variety of tools can be used to assist with the diagnosis and subsequent monitoring of response to treatment. Categories include cytologic examination, biopsy, imaging, and tumor markers.

Cytologic Examination

Cytologic examination of cells that are sloughed into various body secretions may reveal cancerous changes. Scrapings of organ cavities may also be studied in the same way. George Nicolas Papanicolaou pioneered this field with the study of vaginal and cervical secretions. He developed procedures (e.g., the Pap smear) for obtaining and staining samples and defined guidelines for interpreting the cellular changes observed. In addition to gynecologic cancers, malignancies of the lung, tracheobronchial tree, gastrointestinal tract, and urinary tract may be detected in this manner. Once suspicious cells are found, biopsy may be necessary.

Biopsy

Biopsy refers to the process of obtaining tissue for histologic examination and subsequent diagnosis of disease. Three kinds of biopsy techniques are commonly used: needle, incisional, and excisional. During the needle biopsy cells are aspirated through a needle placed in the tissue. Fine-needle aspiration is especially beneficial for confirming the diagnosis of tumors that are deep-seated or surgically unresectable. Occasionally, fluoroscopy or computed tomography scanning techniques may be used to guide the placement of the needle. Bleeding and infection are potential hazards of any biopsy procedure. An open or incisional biopsy is used for large tumors. This procedure involves removing a small wedge of tissue, usually to include the outer edge of the tumor and a margin of tissue. This allows for comparison of abnormal and normal tissue and cell characteristics. Excisional biopsy is the removal of the entire tumor mass and is best suited for smaller tumors. This approach is optimal in that it allows the pathologist to examine the entire tumor while supposedly lessening the chance of cancer dissemination because the mass is removed intact.

PATIENT EDUCATION TOPICS: CANCER PREVENTION AND DETECTION

- Techniques of breast self-examination
- Techniques of testicular self-examination
- Dietary modifications and weight control
- Decrease of alcohol intake
- Smoking cessation
- Personal hygiene measures
- Techniques of skin self-examination
- Protective measures against sun exposure
- American Cancer Society warning signals of cancer
- Importance and frequency of screening tests
- Importance of early detection

Imaging

Imaging includes conventional radiographic examinations (with or without contrast media), mammography, lymphangiography, tomography, and nuclear imaging. Ultrasound uses high-frequency sound waves instead of x-rays to visualize deep visceral tumors. Advantages include low cost, availability, no use of contrast media, and safety. There is currently no known adverse effect on human tissue related to sound intensities used for diagnostic procedures. A computed tomography scan provides a more complete, three-dimensional view of tumor size, shape, and location than do conventional radiographic examinations. The process involves taking a series of pictures of progressive, cross-sectional slices of the body region. Contrast media may or may not be used. Computed tomography is valuable in the workup for metastatic disease. Magnetic resonance imaging produces images similar to those of computed tomography, but does so by the application of a strong magnetic field. A prime advantage is that it uses no ionizing radiation and hence is better for repeated, frequent follow-up examinations. Although magnetic resonance imaging is primarily used for central nervous system evaluation, tumors of the abdominal and pelvic regions are often well visualized by this means as well.

Tumor Markers

Tumor markers (see Table 15-7) are biochemical substances synthesized and released by tumor cells. These properties can be used as indicators of tumor presence. In many cases, these markers are also manufactured by normal or embryonic cells and may be present in a variety of benign conditions. En-

TABLE 15-7 Tumor Markers

Marker	Associated cancers
Alpha-fetoprotein	Liver, testis
Carcinoembryonic antigen	Colon, lung, breast
Human chorionic gonadotropin	Trophoblastic tumors, germ cell tumors of testis
Calcitonin	Medullary cancer of thyroid
Prostatic acid phosphatase	Prostate
CA-125	Ovary
Immunoglobulins	Multiple myeloma

From Virgi MA, Mercer DW, Heberman RB: Tumor markers in cancer diagnosis and prognosis, *CA* 38(2):104, 1988.

zymes, hormones, antigens, and proteins make up a variety of substances currently known as types of tumor markers. These substances can be used to confirm a diagnosis or a response to therapy, predict or confirm relapse, and assess prognosis.[35]

STAGING AND GRADING OF TUMORS

Staging is the method of describing and classifying the extent of a malignancy at the time of diagnosis. Most solid tumors can be classified according to the TNM system, which refers to tumor, lymph nodes, and metastases. This system describes the presence and extent of local, regional, and distant disease (see box above).

Grading refers to the histopathologic classification of a tumor. It describes the degree of malignancy according to the degree of cellular differentiation present. In some tumor types, the grade is more indicative of prognosis than the stage. Cancers are usually classified as well differentiated, moderately differentiated, or poorly to very poorly differentiated. In general, the more differentiated a tumor is, the better the prognosis. More specific grading systems exist for individual tumor types. Although most solid tumors can be classified according to these staging and grading systems, the hematologic malignancies (leukemias and lymphomas) are notable exceptions (see Chapter 38).

TREATMENT METHODS

The major cancer treatment methods are surgery, radiation therapy, chemotherapy, and biologic response modifier therapy. Because cancers are so varied in their presentation and behavior, selection

TNM SYSTEM OF TUMOR CLASSIFICATION

T—Primary Tumor Classification by Depth of Invasion, Surface Spread, and Size

T0—No evidence of a primary lesion
T1—Superficial lesion confined to organ of origin
T2—Localized lesion with deep invasion into adjacent structure
T3—Advanced lesion confined to an anatomic region of organ of origin
T4—Advanced lesion extending into adjacent organs

N—Lymph Node Involvement

N0—No evidence of disease
N1—Palpable, movable nodes limited to primary site
N2, N3, N4—Progressive increase in size, fixation, and location of palpable nodes

M—Anatomic Extent of Metastasis

M0—No metastasis
M1—Isolated metastasis confined to one organ or site
M2—Multiple metastases confined to one organ or site; no functional impairment
M3—Multiple organs involved; minimal functional impairment
M4—Multiple organ involvement; significant functional impairment

of one or more methods presents a difficult task. Along with consideration of the biologic characteristics of a malignancy must come assessment of the patient's characteristics as well. Personal goals and needs directly affect the decisions to accept or reject suggested treatment plans. Thorough discussion of treatment options, including potential benefits, side effects, risks, and alternatives, is critical for the patient and family to make the best decision.

The major goals of treatment are cure, control, and palliation. The objective of curative therapy is total tumor eradication. Primary therapy describes any treatment that is used as the principal approach for cure. Adjuvant therapy is treatment in addition to the primary approach to control or prevent any micrometastatic disease that may occur. Control refers to the arrest or slowing of tumor growth, without achieving a cure. Survival, as well as quality of life, may be improved.

Palliative treatment can be considered when cures or controls are no longer feasible. The goal of palliation is relief of disease symptoms, such as pain, bleeding, obstruction, or compression of vital structures. Palliation may also be helpful to a patient's psychologic well-being. The purpose of palliative treatment must be clearly understood by the patient and family in terms of comfort as opposed to cure or control.

Surgery

The importance of surgical interventions in the prevention of cancer is often underestimated. One such approach is the excision of premalignant lesions. Such excision is termed prophylactic surgery, which may also be indicated for people with certain congenital or genetic conditions that carry a risk of malignancy. For example, colectomy in the presence of ulcerative colitis, familial colon cancer, or polyposis coli may prevent colorectal cancer later in life.

Diagnosis and staging are greatly facilitated by a variety of surgical approaches. Increasingly, the trend is to separate the biopsy procedure from the surgical removal of a tumor. This allows the patient to assume more control in the decision-making process. The potential danger of tumor spread in the interim is no longer considered to override the patient's rights at this crucial time.

Once a malignancy is accurately diagnosed, staged, and classified, surgery may be the treatment of choice. Considerations governing this decision include biologic characteristics of the tumor, health and age of the patient, feasibility of the procedure, and patient preference. Advanced age is not necessarily a contraindication for cancer surgery. However, older patients have a decreased tolerance of functional changes after major surgery. For example, limb amputation is usually more difficult for an elderly person to adapt to than for a more agile, younger patient.

The "ideal" tumor should be accessible, solid, and have well-defined margins. Excision of the primary tumor may be local or radical in nature. Local excision is used to remove a small tumor and a small margin of surrounding normal tissue. Radical excision refers to a wider dissection of the tumor itself, associated lymphatics and tissue, and surrounding structures; for example, radical cystectomy with urinary diversion. Although radical excisions tend to have a detrimental impact on function, body image, and life-style, such procedures are still warranted when the result can be disease eradication and a chance to live. Increasingly, less radical or modified surgical procedures are undertaken when the radical approach is deemed unnecessary or not the patient's choice.

Palliative surgical approaches can significantly improve the quality of life. Examples of palliative surgery include removal of a tumor that compresses the spinal column and causes pain and neuromuscular dysfunction, colostomy to bypass an intestinal obstruction, removal of isolated metastatic tumors, and tracheostomy to restore an obstructed airway.

Many aspects of nursing care of the surgical oncology patient do not differ from those of any other surgical patient, but a few key considerations warrant discussion. The emotional component of a patient's response to surgical procedures may be tremendous. Diagnostic procedures alone produce extreme anxiety regarding the potential outcome and its implication. Waiting for the biopsy results may seem interminable. The patient and family need the opportunity to discuss questions and fears. Preparatory teaching may need to be constantly reinforced. After surgical interventions, loss of function or body part result in a grieving process. Both the patient and family must be informed that this is a normal event. Support groups can provide invaluable assistance in coping with this need.

Disorders of coagulation accompany certain tumor types and treatments. An abnormal activation of the clotting mechanism as a result of the disease process causes a hypercoagulable state. Postoperative cancer patients are thus at even higher risk than noncancer patients for thromboembolic complications. In particular, venous thrombosis and pulmonary embolism are typical postoperative complications for the geriatric patient undergoing abdominoperineal resection for carcinoma of the colon.[30] Conversely, patients who have received radiation or chemotherapy before a surgical procedure may be platelet deficient (owing to myelosuppression) and at risk for bleeding.

Radiation Therapy

Radiation therapy utilizes ionizing (high-energy) radiation. The purpose is to deliver a precise dose of radiation to a specific area with minimal damage to adjacent, healthy tissue. Radiation is energy that is transmitted in the form of waves or particles. Electromagnetic radiation travels in waves. Examples include radio waves, infrared light, visible light, ultraviolet light, x-rays, and gamma rays. X-rays and gamma rays are types of ionizing radiation. Ionizing radiation refers to high-energy radiation that damages or alters cells. The principal damage is to the DNA in the cell's nucleus.

Energy transmitted in the form of heavy particles is termed particulate radiation. Examples include beta particles, which are emitted from substances such as phosphorus-32 or strontium-90. Beta particles are a form of ionizing radiation as well and are emitted from radioactive substances in solid or liquid form.

Ionizing radiation is the type of radiation delivered in cancer treatment. Exposed cells undergo a variety of responses. At first, the cell's molecular structures become agitated and break. Chemical reactions begin that damage the DNA. The degree of damage will vary greatly. Cells that are more rapidly dividing are more vulnerable or radiosensitive than others. Thus different organ systems in the body will possess differing degrees of radiosensitivity (Table 15-8).

Cells in the mitosis phase are more vulnerable, as are cells that are well oxygenated. Oxygen is a key component for DNA damage. Poorly oxygenated cells at the center of a tumor are not as vulnerable to radiation. Radiation therapy can be effective in these tumor masses, however, because as the peripheral cells are destroyed, revascularization and reoxygenation of the inner cells occur. These cells then become more vulnerable to radiation (Figure 15-5). Additionally, cells that are poorly differentiated are more radiosensitive than well-differentiated cells. In therapeutic doses, radiation tends to kill cells only after a few subsequent cell divisions occur.

Therapeutic ionizing radiation will damage both normal cells and cancer cells. Fortunately, the DNA breakage is more readily repaired in normal cells. Unfortunately, the damage that normal cells incur gives rise to a number of unpleasant side effects.

Therapeutic goals

Radiation therapy is most effective in treating local and regional disease. Treatment can be either curative or palliative and may be used alone or in combination with other methods. For example, radiation may be given preoperatively to shrink a tumor, mak-

TABLE 15-8   Listing of Organs by Radiosensitivity

Radiosensitivity	Organ
High	Lymphoid organs
	Bone marrow
	Testes
	Ovaries
	Intestine
Medium high	Skin
	Cornea
	Oral cavity and esophagus
	Vagina, cervix
	Optic lens
Medium	Fine vasculature
	Growing cartilage
	Growing bone
Medium low	Mature bone
	Mature cartilage
	Kidney
	Liver
	Thyroid
Low	Muscle
	Brain
	Spinal cord

From Leahy IM, St Germain JM, Varricchio CG: *The nurse and radiotherapy: a manual for daily care,* St Louis, 1979, Mosby–Year Book.

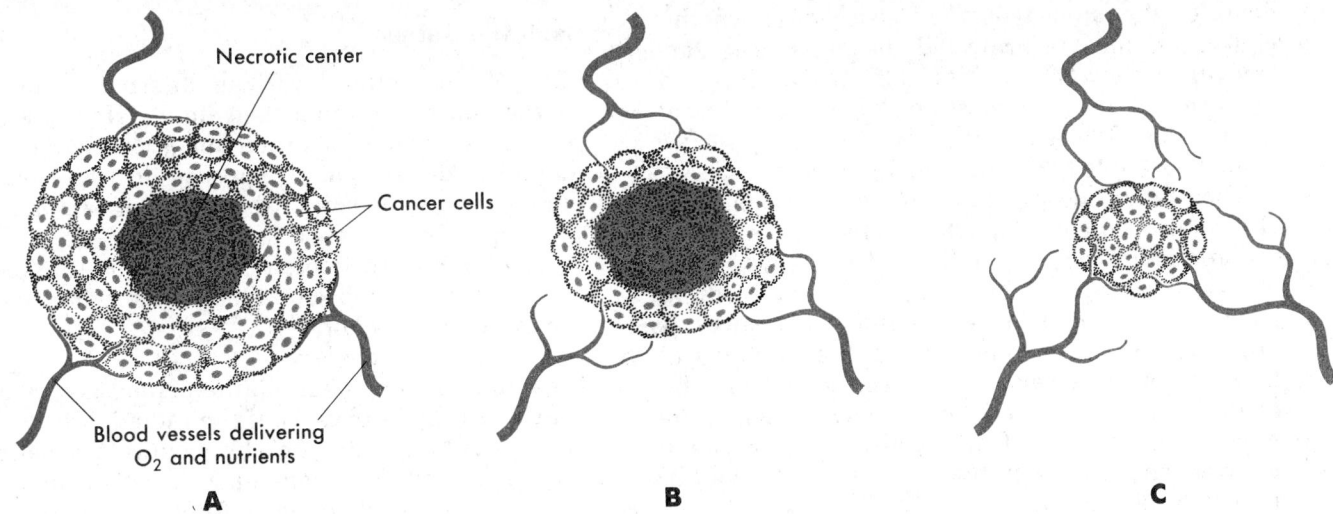

FIGURE 15-5   Reoxygenation of necrotic center of tumor. **A,** Malignant tumor in tumor bed. **B,** During radiation therapy, death of peripheral cell occurs, which allows reoxygenation of necrotic center. **C,** Near completion of therapy, tumor has markedly shrunk because of reoxygenation of center cells.

ing it more surgically resectable. Cancers that can be cured by radiation include Hodgkin's disease, early stage prostate cancer, and early stage head and neck cancers. Many other tumors can be controlled by radiation for extended periods.

Palliative radiation has numerous applications. Pain from bone metastases and tumor pressure can be substantially relieved by radiation. Central nervous system dysfunction secondary to spinal cord compression and brain metastases will abate after radiation, and fungating skin lesions that bleed and ulcerate are also responsive to radiation. Clearly, comfort improves substantially with the use of radiation therapy.

Clinical application

External therapy

External therapy, also termed external beam therapy or **teletherapy,** involves treatment from a source outside the body. Patients eligible for this method first undergo a planning process in which the treatment area is carefully identified and outlined, and specific treatment plans are developed. At this time, the patient may undergo a simulation process, whereby the tumor area is precisely located and marked either by a temporary marker or by permanent tatoos made up of tiny pinpoint dots (Figure 15-6). Anatomic areas that must be shielded or blocked from the radiation beam may also be identified at this time. Lead-lined blocks are then constructed so that the beam will only reach specific body structures.

The actual treatment can be delivered by a linear accelerator or a variety of other machines that may contain various types of isotopes (radioactive sources). The type of machine and isotope used depends on the tumor type, the disease stage, whether vital organs must be protected, the patient's age, and any other concomitant disease.[25] Linear accelerators are now used for most tumors because they almost completely spare the external skin surface while being able to penetrate deeply into the body.[25]

Therapeutic dosage is expressed in units called Grays (also called rads), which refers to the dose of radiation absorbed by the tissue. One Gray is equivalent to absorption of 1 joule/kg. Radiation is administered in fractional doses, meaning that small doses are given over an extended time. Fractionation allows for optimal cancer cell destruction, and because normal cells recover between treatments, side effects are tolerable. Tumor cells, however, cannot recover, and thus each treatment has a cumulative effect on the cancer.

Internal therapy

Internal radiation therapy, or **brachytherapy,** is the use of high-energy radioactive materials placed into

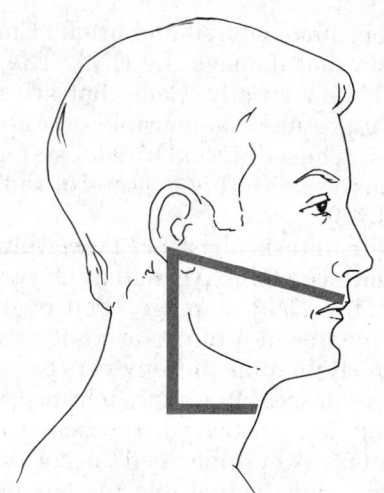

FIGURE 15-6 Portal arrangement for treating buccal mucosa, including salivary glands, alveolar ridge, and mandible.

or directly on the body to treat disease. Three types are used: intracavitary, interstitial, and metabolized. Intracavitary implants involve the insertion of a radioactive source into a body cavity. Many gynecologic cancers are treated in this way. Insertion of a radioactive source directly into tissue via seeds, needles, or capsules is termed interstitial therapy (Figure 15-7). Head and neck lesions and intraabdominal and intrathoracic tumors may all respond to this approach. Metabolized radiotherapy refers to the ingestion, instillation, or injection of radioactive materials that are subsequently metabolized or absorbed.

Radiation safety

Care of the patient with an internal radioactive source can be accomplished quite safely once the principles of radiation protection are understood. To minimize unnecessary exposure to radioactivity, nurses must be aware of the following factors:

- Type of radiation
- Half-life of the isotope, or the time it takes for the source to lose one half of its radioactivity
- Amount of isotope
- Method of delivery

If an implant is being used, the patient is *not* radioactive, but the implant is. If the radiation treatment is given systemically (e.g., by mouth), the patient's secretions and excretions may be radioactive for a specific time based on the half-life of the isotope. Patients receiving brachytherapy are often placed on radiation safety precautions. The necessity of precautions depends on the amount of energy emitted by the isotope in use. A radiation safety officer

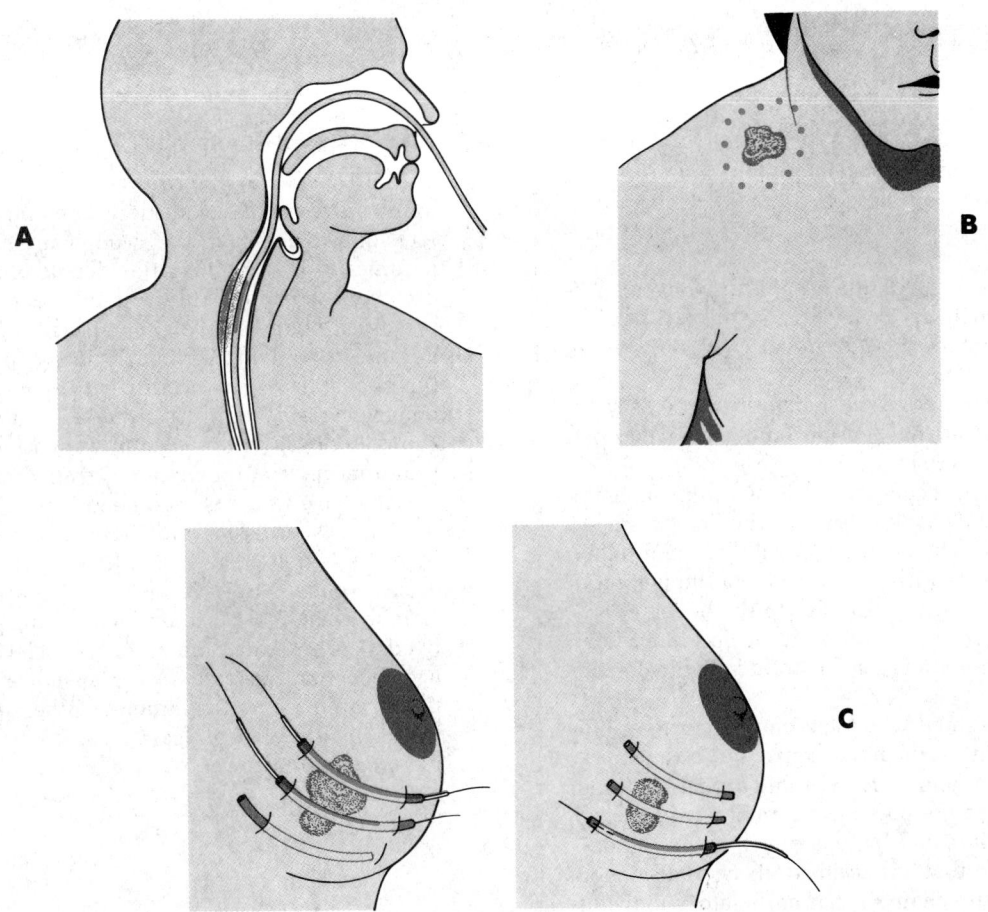

FIGURE 15-7   Examples of internal radiation therapy. **A,** Radium bougie in place for patient with cancer of the esophagus; note that radium is placed next to the tumor. **B,** Iridium seeds implanted for left neck mass. **C,** Iridium seeds implanted for breast cancer.

should always be consulted to determine the necessity of precautions and the time at which they may be discontinued. Visitors and pregnant nurses should be restricted from entering the room until the precautions have been discontinued.

If the patient is receiving radiation therapy via an encapsulated source, his or her room must have a specified, lead-lined container, in which the implant is placed should it become dislodged. In this event, the nurse should use long forceps to handle the source and place it in the container. The nurse must *never* handle the source with bare hands. The safety officer should be notified for removal of the container. The secretions and excretions of patients who received a systemic isotope must be handled carefully. The nurse wears gloves while handling contaminated materials (linens, dressings, etc.). Hands or other affected areas are washed in the event of skin contact.

Care must be efficient and organized because the amount of exposure to the radiation is directly pro-portional to the time spent within a specified distance to the patient. Radiation exposure is governed by the "inverse square law." This states that the radiation dose varies *inversely* with the square of the distance from the radioactive source (Figure 15-8). For example, if a nurse stands twice as far away from the implant in the patient, the exposure will be reduced to one fourth ($2^2 = 4$, the inverse of which is ¼). Therefore maximize the distance from the radioactive source.

Shielding refers to the use of protective barriers. Most implants contain radioactive isotopes that require lead or concrete shielding, so use of barriers is often impossible during direct patient care activities. Lead aprons used in diagnostic radiotherapy settings are not sufficient for protection against gamma rays emitted by radium or cesium.[20] See box on p. 294 for methods to reduce exposure during patient care activities.

The patient who receives external radiation is not radioactive at any time. Be sure the patient, family,

METHODS TO REDUCE RADIATION EXPOSURE

1. Use appropriate radiation precaution signs, wristbands, and tags.
2. Plan care to avoid delays at the person's bedside.
3. Eliminate the bedbath, except for what the person can manage alone.
4. Change linens less frequently or only when soiled.
5. Prepare meal trays outside of the person's room instead of at the bedside (cut up meats, open containers, etc.).
6. Work quickly; concentrate on accomplishing the necessary tasks in as short a time as possible.
7. Position the bedside table, call bell, and television controls within easy reach of the person to avoid frequent return trips to the bedside.
8. Use appropriate monitoring devices, and heed the information regarding total individual exposure.
9. No nurse should care for more than two individuals with radioactive sources at a time.
10. Keep long-handled forceps and a shielded transport cart in the person's room at all times.
11. Use long-handled forceps to retrieve a radioactive source that has accidentally been dislodged.
12. Arrange the chair so that ambulatory individuals can be seated as far from the bed (and thus the caregiver) as possible while linens are being changed.

From Hilderly LJ: Radiotherapy: In Groenwald SL, Frogge MH, Goodman, M, et al, editors: *Cancer nursing: principles and practice,* ed 2, Boston, 1990, Jones and Bartlett.

GERIATRIC CONSIDERATIONS

Radiation Therapy

The elderly patient who receives radiation therapy requires special consideration. Potential side effects and toxicities in this group can be lessened by modifications in fractionation, length of therapy, and area being treated.[3] Skin and mucous membrane integrity and bone marrow function may be more vulnerable to radiation damage owing to the normal functional decline associated with aging. Fatigue secondary to myelosuppression-induced anemia may be compounded by the frequent trips required to the radiotherapy treatment center over prolonged periods. Be sure to assess the need for and availability of supports to assist with both transportation and home activities. Also assess the impact of treatment on the spouse or family. Refer the patient to a social worker if assistance with transportation is needed. The American Cancer Society and other agencies may provide free transportation for patients undergoing treatment. Other referrals to home health agencies can provide invaluable support for home care assistance.

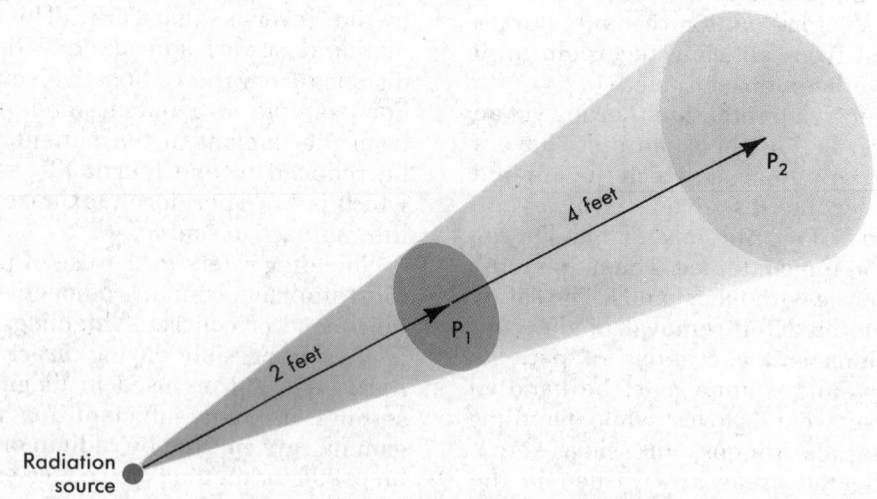

FIGURE 15-8   The inverse square law. As distance from a radiation source increases, exposure decreases by the square of that distance.

TABLE 15-9   Side Effects of Radiation Therapy and Nursing Interventions

Site	Acute effect	Chronic effect	Nursing interventions
Skin	Erythema (30-40 Gy), dry desquamation, moist desquamation (45-60 Gy)	Fibrosis, atrophy, telangiectasis, permanent darkening of skin	Avoid trauma to skin, extremes of temperature, harsh chemicals, soaps
Oral cavity	Change and loss of taste, dryness, mucositis (30-40 Gy)	Permanent xerostomia, permanent taste alterations, dental caries	Monitor weight, and provide artificial saliva, viscous xylocaine, preventive dental care with fluoride, nutritional counseling to maintain dietary status
Esophagus	Pain, esophagitis	Fibrosis	Provide antacids, viscous xylocaine
Stomach	Nausea and vomiting (1.25 Gy)	Obstruction, ulceration, fibrosis	Antiemetics given 1 hour before treatment
Intestines	Diarrhea (20-30 Gy)	Malabsorption, strictures, necrosis (60-70 Gy)	Provide medication for diarrhea, dietary modifications, low-residue diet, good skin care and perineal hygiene
Kidney		Radiation nephritis	
Bladder	Cystitis (30 Gy)	Fibrosis, contracted bladder (65-70 Gy)	Increase fluid intake, may use prophylactic urinary antiseptics
Bone marrow	Decreased white blood cells and platelets	May be chronic anemia especially with combined modality treatment	Initiate bleeding precautions and measures to prevent infection as indicated
Respiratory system	Pneumonitis (25-30 Gy)	Fibrosis	Initiate pulmonary hygiene measures to alleviate cough and dyspnea
Cardiovascular system	Rare reports of pericarditis, myocarditis	Fibrosis	
Central nervous system Brain and spinal cord Peripheral nerves	Edema and inflammation	Infarction, occlusion, necrosis	Monitor sequelae of steroids, assess neurologic status, monitor for headaches
Eyes		Cataracts	
Bone and cartilage Child		Growth disturbances if growth plate of bone is in field (20-30 Gy)	
Gonads Spermatogonia	Decreased sperm count after 90-120 days; temporary sterility (1-3 Gy)		Counsel patient about effect of radiation on fertility
Ovary	Sterility (5-10 Gy) depends on age		

From Strohl RA: The nursing role in radiation oncology: symptom management of acute and chronic reactions, *Oncol Nurs Forum* 15(4):429, 1988.

and staff understand this. No safety precautions are required during the delivery of care.

Quantification of staff exposure to radioactivity can be accomplished by a variety of devices. The film badge is the most common tool used by nurses. This device consists of a small piece of film encased in a badge, which is worn at the body area most likely to be exposed to a radiation source. It is clipped onto the outer clothing and should always be exposed. Increased exposure to radiation results in increased film density. The badges are monitored periodically by the radiation safety officer to determine the amount of exposure. The badge must only be worn while in the patient care area; background environmental radiation (i.e., sunlight) will also change the film, thus altering the accuracy.

Side effects

The site and severity of side effects depend on the body site irradiated, the dose administered, the extent of the treated area, and the method of radiation used. Table 15-9 outlines symptoms and related nursing interventions. Local cutaneous effects are not as pronounced as in the past, owing to use of skin sparing techniques. Skin changes can occur, however, ranging from mild erythema, dry desquamation, or wet desquamation, in which the skin is weeping and may slough. See the box below for patient education guidelines.

Chemotherapy

Both surgery and radiation therapy represent treatment approaches for local or regional disease. Rosenberg[32] notes, however, that when patients with solid tumors are first seen by a physician, about 70% already have micrometastases beyond the primary site. Hence, a more systemic approach is necessary to truly effect a cure in many cases. Additionally, malignancies such as leukemia and lymphoma, which are by nature disseminated cancers, require a systemic treatment as well. **Chemotherapy,** the treatment of cancer with drugs, is an essential weapon for both cure and palliation of many diseases.

 **PATIENT EDUCATION GUIDE**   *Radiation Therapy*

When the patient is receiving radiation therapy, the skin in the area being treated must be given special care. This area will be outlined by purple marks. The skin in this area will be more sensitive and subject to injury, even though it may not look or feel different for several weeks. These guidelines should be followed from the first day of the patient's treatment.

After 2 to 3 weeks, the skin usually becomes reddened and dry. The first set of guidelines applies to skin in that condition. Should some areas open and drain, additional steps must be followed.

Skin Care Guidelines

- During treatment, do not wash the area if possible.
- If the area *must* be washed, use only lukewarm water.
- The patient should not wear constrictive clothing over the area.
- The patient should not expose the treatment area to the sun.
- The patient should not shave the treated area.
- The patient should not use any creams, deodorants, or lotions on the area unless provided by the radiation oncology department.
- If the skin becomes dry and itchy, instruct the patient *not to scratch;* inform the physician, and a topical medication will be prescribed.

- Cornstarch may be used when the skin is dry and itchy.
- Cortisone ointment may be suggested when the skin begins to peel.

If an area of the skin becomes moist and begins to break down, follow the guidelines as developed in the radiation oncology department.

- Mix 1 oz hydrogen peroxide with 3 oz water. Prepare the solution just before you use it. Do not let it stand.
- Using a large syringe, cleanse the area with the solution. The peroxide will bubble. Cleanse the area until clean. Remove any ointment or debris by irrigating the area with the solution.
- Gently pat the area dry.
- If the physician has prescribed an ointment, apply it sparingly to the skin.
- Leave the area uncovered as much as possible. If necessary, cover with a loose dressing of nonadherent material. Do not put tape over the irritated skin.
- Repeat this procedure twice daily unless otherwise instructed by the physician.
- Moisture-permeable dressings also may be suggested.

From Strohl RA: The nursing role in radiation oncology: symptom management of acute and chronic side effects, *Oncol Nurs Forum* 15(4):429, 1988.

Cellular effects

Chemotherapy disrupts the cell life-cycle. The chemotherapeutic agent is **cytotoxic** in nature; that is, it disables a cell, which results in the cell's death. Most agents act either by modifying or interfering with DNA synthesis. Typically, cells that are most vulnerable to chemotherapy are those that are either actively dividing or preparing to divide. As a result, both malignant and normal cells that are most rapidly dividing are the most affected by chemotherapy.

Agents may be classified according to two factors: (1) the specific mechanism by which they disrupt cellular biochemical functions and (2) the point in the cell life cycle where they exert their effects (Figure 15-9). Some drugs are most cytotoxic during a specific phase in the cycle; these are termed cell cycle-specific drugs. These drugs are most effective in malignancies with a large number of actively dividing cells. In general, they are best administered over a prolonged period to allow cells to reach the phase in which the drug acts. Drugs that disable both resting and dividing cells are termed cell cycle-nonspecific agents. These drugs damage the cell at some point in the cycle: death does not occur, however, until the cell attempts to divide. Cell cycle-nonspecific drugs tend to be more dose dependent. This simply means that the number of cells killed is directly proportional to the amount of drug given. Because the exact mechanism of action of many drugs remains unclear, this classification system cannot be considered absolute.

Although the overall goal of chemotherapy administration is to kill all cancer cells present, many obstacles exist. Because most drugs affect rapidly dividing cells, resting cancer cells may remain viable and may reproduce, causing disease recurrence. Theoretically, each time a drug is administered, only a fraction of the malignant cells are killed. Repeated courses must be given to achieve disease remission, because it must be assumed that cancer cells remain behind (Figure 15-10), even when all diagnostic methods show the patient to be free of disease. Obviously, a drug that can kill the highest fraction of cells at one time is the most desirable.

Another potential obstacle relates to tumor growth patterns. In early stages of development, a tumor possesses a large portion of rapidly dividing cells. This results in a short doubling time, the time

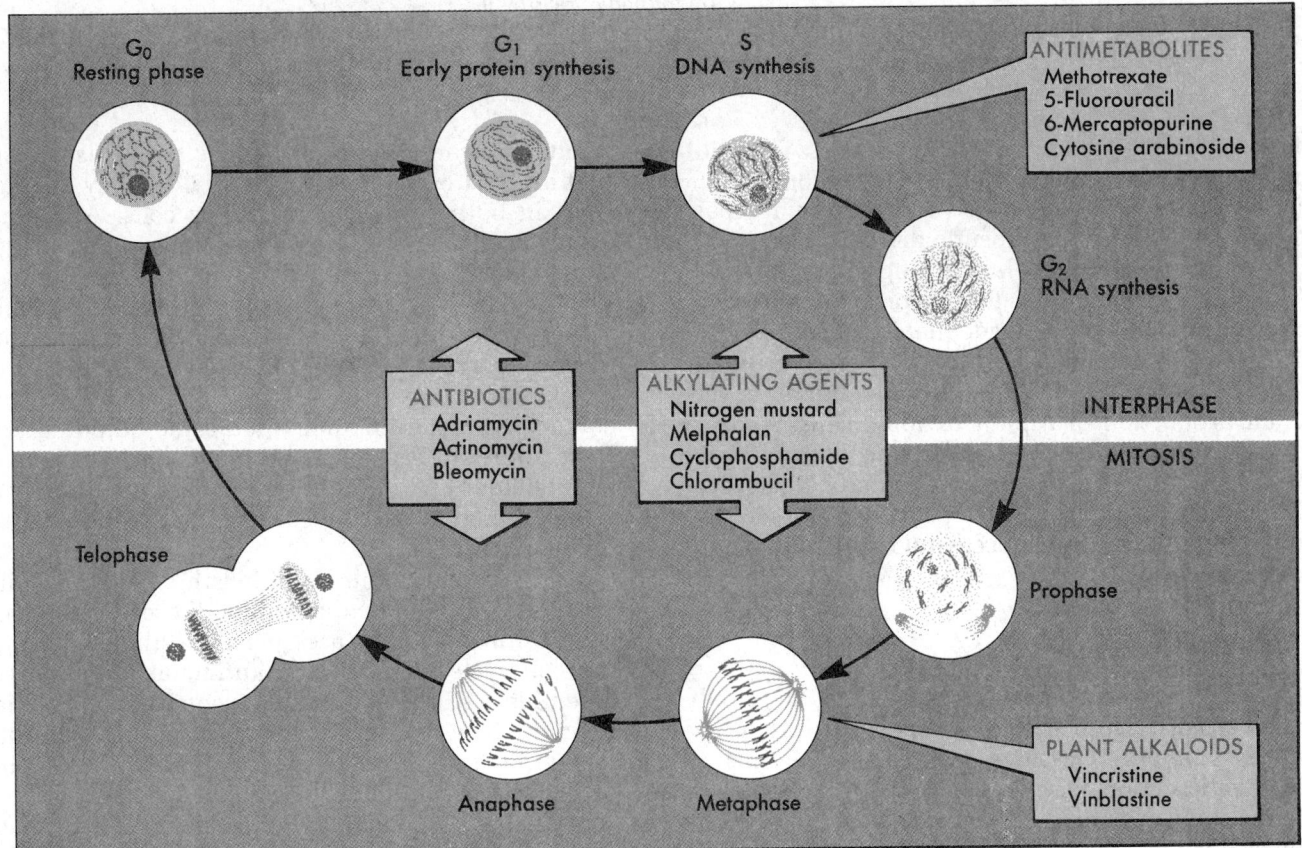

FIGURE 15-9   The cell cycle. Drugs are identified by where they exert their effect.

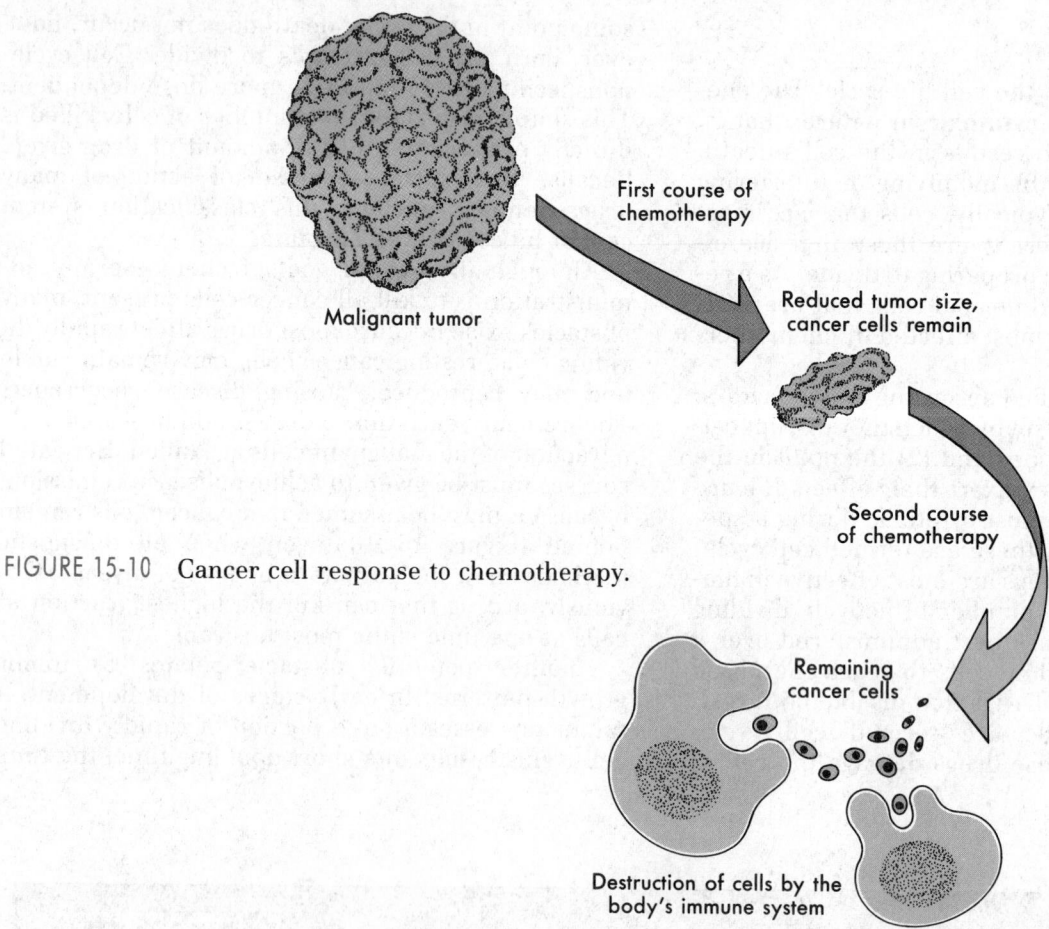

FIGURE 15-10   Cancer cell response to chemotherapy.

it takes for the tumor to double its size. As the tumor grows, its doubling time becomes longer. The cycle of these cells is slower, which may decrease the effect of chemotherapeutic drugs.

Malignant cells may also develop drug resistance. A variety of explanations for this problem have been offered, including: (1) inadequate transport of the drug into the tumor caused by poor vascularity and (2) resistance because the tumor contains a very small proportion of rapidly dividing cells. Another theory proposes that drugs become less effective over time because tumor cells mutate to become drug-resistant. Despite these problems, chemotherapy remains a vital and successful approach to many malignancies.

Classification of agents

Although chemotherapeutic drugs may be subdivided according to cell cycle specificity, they are more commonly classified according to their antineoplastic action (see Table 15-10). Currently five major categories exist, along with a sixth "miscellaneous" category for agents that do not conform to the other five. The first two categories, alkylating

agents and antitumor antibiotics, comprise drugs that are cell cycle-nonspecific; that is, they damage DNA in both resting and dividing cells. Alkylating agents produce breaks and cross-links in the strands of cellular DNA; these breaks and cross-links impair DNA synthesis, thus preventing the cell from replicating. In this regard, alkylating agents are quite similar to radiation therapy, which also produces breaks and cross-links. Alkylating agents have become recognized for their mutagenic potential and their ability to cause second malignancies, particularly leukemia. Antitumor antibiotics bind directly to DNA, changing its configuration and subsequently hindering replication.

In contrast, the third and fourth categories, antimetabolites and vinca alkaloids, are cell cycle specific. Antimetabolites are specific to the S phase of the cell cycle. Structurally, antimetabolites closely resemble natural metabolites required for cellular function. The cell mistakenly incorporates an antimetabolite into the DNA during DNA synthesis. This incorporation ultimately results in disruption of cell replication. Vinca alkaloids, specific to the M phase of the cell cycle, bind to microtubular proteins needed for the formation of the mitotic spindle in

Text continued on p. 305.

TABLE 15-10 Pharmacology Summary: Antineoplastic Agents

Drug	Classification	Major toxicities	Comments
L-Asparaginase	Enzyme (miscellaneous agent)	Hypersensitivity reactions, malaise, anorexia, nausea and vomiting	Nausea and vomiting is usually mild Not toxic to bone marrow, oral mucosa, GI mucosa, or hair follicles Anaphylaxis may occur, especially with IV administration Epinephrine, diphenhydramine, and hydrocortisone must be readily available, as well as physician and resuscitation support Hyperglycemia and coagulation disorders may occur
Bleomycin	Antitumor, antibiotic	Stomatitis, anorexia, fever and chills, pulmonary fibrosis, alopecia	Fever can be controlled by premedication and around-the-clock administration of acetaminophen Skin changes include hyperpigmentation, erythema, nail changes and loss, and inflammation of the palms and hands Oral changes include burning, erythema, and ulceration Pulmonary fibrosis occurs more often with a cumulative dose >300 units; watch for dyspnea, dry cough, and rales Anaphylaxis can occur Increased pain at the tumor site may occur because of local cellular destruction
Busulfan	Alkylating agent	Bone marrow suppression, nausea and vomiting, gonadal changes, pulmonary fibrosis	Reproductive/sexual changes include impotence, azoospermia, amenorrhea, or gynecomastia Pulmonary fibrosis may occur much later (1 to 3 years); watch for dyspnea, dry cough, and rales
Carboplatin	Miscellaneous	Bone marrow suppression, nausea and vomiting, renal toxicity (mild)	Myelosuppression can be a dose-limiting toxicity; both thrombocytopenia and leukopenia may be delayed (14 to 18 days and 18 to 25 days respectively) Nausea and vomiting may have delayed onset; reassure patient that it usually is of short duration
Carmustine	Nitrosourea	Nausea and vomiting, bone marrow suppression, facial flushing, abnormal liver function tests	Bone marrow suppression is usually delayed Nadir typically 3 to 5 weeks Burning and pain may occur along injection site during infusion; application of ice may provide relief Pulmonary fibrosis may occur with cumulative doses over 900 mg/m^2
Chlorambucil	Alkylating agent	Bone marrow suppression, gonadal changes, nausea and vomiting	Myelosuppression is usually moderate, gradual, and rapidly reversible GI effects are usually minimal or absent, unless large doses are given Increased toxicities may occur with prior barbiturate use

Continued.

Data from Becker T: *Cancer chemotherapy: a manual for nurses*, Boston, 1981, Little Brown and Co. Brager BL Yasko JM: *Care of the client receiving chemotherapy*, Reston, Va, 1984, Reston Publishing Co. Carter SK, Bakowski MT, Hellmann K: *Chemotherapy of cancer*, ed 3, New York, 1987, John Wiley & Sons. Fischer DS, Knobf MT: *The cancer chemotherapy handbook*, ed 3, St Louis, 1989, Mosby–Year Book. Perry MC: *The cancer chemotherapy source book*, Baltimore, 1992, Williams & Wilkins.

TABLE 15-10 Pharmacology Summary: Antineoplastic Agents—cont'd

Drug	Classification	Major toxicities	Comments
Cisplatin	Miscellaneous	Nausea and vomiting, renal toxicity, neurotoxicity, anemia	At higher doses, rigorous prehydration and mannitol (for osmotic diuresis) may be given to decrease the risk of renal damage Monitor renal function, including serum electrolytes, BUN and creatinine; 24-hour urine collection for creatinine clearance may be evaluated before therapy Myelosuppression is mild, except at higher doses Ototoxicity (tinnitus or loss of high-frequency hearing) is cumulative and may be permanent Anaphylaxis can occur
Cyclophosphamide	Alkylating agent	Bone marrow suppression, bladder toxicity, nausea, gonadal changes, alopecia	Push fluids (2-3 quarts/day) to maintain urine output; manifestations of bladder toxicity include bladder fibrosis, hemorrhagic cystitis, and bladder carcinoma; check urine for blood at each voiding; administer early in the day (to prevent accumulation of the drug in the bladder and encourage frequent voiding Myelosuppression usually recovers rapidly with sparing of platelets Administer antiemetics for nausea and vomiting Cardiac damage and necrosis can occur with very large single doses May inhibit immune function
Cytarabine	Antimetabolite	Bone marrow suppression, nausea, stomatitis, headaches	Nausea, vomiting, and diarrhea increase in severity with increasing doses Stomatitis and anorexia are common Watch for tumor lysis syndrome (see also Chapter 38) caused by rapid lysis of cells Rash, palmar erythema and desquamation, conjunctivitis, and cerebellar toxicities occur with larger doses
Dacarbazine	Alkylating agent	Nausea and vomiting, bone marrow suppression, alopecia, hepatoxicity, flu syndrome	Flu-like syndrome (headache, malaise, fever, chills, myalgias) may occur 7-10 days after treatment and persist for 1-3 weeks Patient may experience burning sensation at IV site and metallic taste during infusion Vesicant agent; avoid extravasation; burning may or may not be indicative of extravasation in this case Nausea and vomiting (often severe) begins within 1-3 hours and lasts 1-12 hours
Dactinomycin	Antitumor antibiotic	Bone marrow suppression, stomatitis, nausea and vomiting, skin rash, alopecia	Myelosuppression may be severe Vesicant agent; avoid extravasation GI symptoms may be severe Skin changes may include patches of depigmentation with hyperpigmented border (vitiligo), acne, and erythema

Drug	Classification	Toxicities	Comments
Daunorubicin	Antitumor antibiotic	Bone marrow suppression, nausea, stomatitis, cardiac toxicity, alopecia	Skin reactions may develop in previously irradiated areas ("radiation recall"); erythema and desquamation can occur. Reversible skin discoloration may occur along veins used for drug administration. Vesicant agent; avoid extravasation. Cumulative doses >550 mg/m² may cause cardiomyopathy. Patient may experience reversible ECG changes, arrhythmias, and congestive heart failure. Myelosuppression may be severe. Alert patient that urine will turn red until the drug is fully excreted (the drug is red in color; this does not indicate bleeding). Radiation recall can occur
Doxorubicin	Antitumor, antibiotic	Bone marrow suppression, nausea and vomiting, stomatitis, cardiac toxicity, alopecia	Vesicant agent; avoid extravasation. Myelosuppression and nausea/vomiting may be severe. Cardiotoxicity is dose-limiting; cumulative safe dose for adults is 550 mg/m². Flare reaction (facial flushing and local flushing at IV site) may occur especially during rapid drug infusion; slowing infusion rate may resolve symptoms. Alert patient that urine will turn red (see comments under daunorubicin). Radiation recall can occur
Etoposide	Vinca alkaloid	Bone marrow suppression, neurotoxicity, alopecia	Orthostatic hypotension and bradycardia occur if infused too rapidly; most doses can be safely administered over 4 hours. Radiation recall can occur
5-Fluorouracil	Antimetabolite	Diarrhea, bone marrow suppression, stomatitis, nausea, alopecia	Stomatitis and diarrhea are dose-limiting, and can be severe. Skin changes include nail changes and loss, rash, darkening of the veins used for drug administration, and photosensitivity
Hexamethyl melamine	Miscellaneous	Bone marrow suppression, nausea, neurotoxicity	Nausea and vomiting may be severe and dose-limiting. May exacerbate the neurotoxicity of other drugs, especially the vinca alkaloids
Hydroxyurea	Miscellaneous	Bone marrow suppression, nausea, alopecia, diarrhea, stomatitis	Myelosuppression may be dose-limiting, but marrow recovery is rapid after discontinuation of therapy. Renal tubular function can be temporarily impaired. Monitor for hyperuricemia
Ifosfamide	Alkylating agent	Hemorrhagic cystitis, nausea and vomiting, alopecia, CNS (somnolence and confusion), neurotoxicity	Cystitis can be prevented by concomitant administration of Mesna, a uroprotective agent. Maintain rigorous hydration (at least 2 L/day) for 72 hours after treatment. Myelosuppression may be dose-limiting
Lomustine	Alkylating agent	Bone marrow suppression, nausea and vomiting	Myelosuppression is cumulative and may be delayed. Leukopenia may appear about 4-6 weeks after a dose and last 1-2 weeks

Continued.

TABLE 15-10   Pharmacology Summary: Antineoplastic Agents—cont'd

Drug	Classification	Major toxicities	Comments
Mechlorethamine	Alkylating agent	Bone marrow suppression, nausea and vomiting, gonadal changes, stomatitis	To minimize nausea and vomiting, take at bedtime on an empty stomach; premedicate with antiemetic if necessary Crosses blood-brain barrier Short stability; use immediately after reconstitution Potent vesicant; avoid extravasation and any skin or mucous membrane contact Nausea and vomiting are usually severe Chills, fever, and diarrhea may occur immediately after administration Watch for hyperuricemia; maintain adequate hydration of at least 2 L/day for 48 hours after treatment Thrombophlebitis, local irritation, and burning may occur along veins used for administration Patient may experience metallic taste during administration
Melphalan	Alkylating agent	Bone marrow suppression, nausea, gonadal changes, secondary malignancies	Myelosuppression may be delayed up to 30 days after treatment; thrombocytopenia can be persistent Thinning of the hair can occur with repeated doses Nausea and vomiting are uncommon; if they occur, administer the drug with meals and/or antiemetic therapy
6-Mercaptopurine	Antimetabolite	Bone marrow suppression, nausea, hepatic toxicity, stomatitis	Myelosuppression is usually of gradual onset and persistent after the drug is discontinued Allopurinol may be given concomitantly to prevent uric acid nephropathy secondary to hyperuricemia; allopurinol inhibits 6MP degradation; thus 6MP dose must be reduced by $1/3$ in presence of allopurinol administration Cholestatic jaundice may occur after 2-5 months of treatment and is usually reversible after the drug is discontinued
Methotrexate	Antimetabolite	Stomatitis, bone marrow suppression, nausea, renal toxicity	Stomatitis and diarrhea may be severe and warrant interruption of treatment Renal tubular necrosis may occur with high doses During large-dose administration (*100 mg) leucovorin rescue is given concurrently to counteract the immediate hematopoietic toxicity by supplying normal cells with the form of folic acid needed for DNA synthesis Caution patient that urine will turn bright yellow (the color of the drug) and will resolve after the drug is excreted Photosensitivity may occur even without sun exposure; patient may develop erythematous rash and must be cautioned to use sunscreens when outdoors
Mitomycin C	Antitumor, antibiotic	Bone marrow suppression, nausea and vomiting, stomatitis, renal toxicity, alopecia	Vesicant agent; avoid extravasation Myelosuppression is often severe, cumulative, and delayed (up to 8 weeks after therapy) Thrombocytopenia can be especially prolonged Renal toxicity is also cumulative, although rare

Drug	Classification	Common toxicities	Special considerations and comments
Mitoxantrone	Antitumor antibiotic	Nausea and vomiting, myelosuppression, alopecia, stomatitis	Skin reactions include alopecia, dermatitis, pruritus, dark half-circles in nailbeds, and severe phlebitis; nailbed discolorations usually disappear after treatment is discontinued Drug is blue; may cause green discoloration of urine and blue streaking of vein Irritant drug that may cause burning or stinging if infiltration occurs Mild congestive heart failure may occur in patients previously treated with anthracycline antibiotics Transient elevation of hepatic enzymes is seen
Paclitaxel	Miscellaneous	Bone marrow suppression, cardiac toxicity, neurotoxicity, stomatitis	Anaphylaxis: premedicate patient before infusion Watch for bradycardia, hypotension, and arrhythmias; cardiac monitoring may be warranted Myelosuppression is severe in patients who have received prior radiation therapy or chemotherapy Incidence and severity of peripheral neuropathy is usually dose-related
Procarbazine	Miscellaneous	Bone marrow suppression, nausea and vomiting, neurotoxicity	Myelosuppression may be delayed for several weeks after treatment Nausea and vomiting tend to decrease with each subsequent course Adverse reactions are noted with many other substances: Avoid ethyl alcohol, as a disulfiram-like reaction can occur Avoid tyramine (present in foods such as bananas, cheese, yogurt, alcohol, chocolate, and caffeine) as serious hypertensive crisis may result because of monoamine oxidase inhibition activity Avoid CNS depressants and sympathomimetic drugs (i.e., barbiturates, antihistamines, narcotics, phenothiazines, and hypotensive agents) as procarbazine is synergistic with these Neurotoxicity may be manifested by lethargy, fatigue, confusion, stupor, paresthesias, foot drop, headache, dizziness, lack of muscle coordination, and decreased reflexes
Streptozocin	Alkylating agent	Bone marrow suppression, nausea and vomiting, diarrhea, renal toxicity, diabetogenic symptoms	Nausea and vomiting may be severe Dilute and infuse slowly to minimize venous pain during infusion Irritant properties; avoid extravasation Contraindicated in renal disease/dysfunction Renal tubular necrosis, glycosuria, aminoaciduria, and azotemia can result Hepatotoxicity is manifested by abnormalities in liver function studies; this effect is usually mild and reversible Sudden hypoglycemia from a sudden release of insulin can occur (usually within 24 hours of treatment)
Thioguanine	Antimetabolite	Myelosuppression, nausea and vomiting	Other toxicities include hepatic veno-occlusive disease, jaundice, anorexia, diarrhea, stomatitis, and rash

Continued.

TABLE 15-10 Pharmacology Summary: Antineoplastic Agents—cont'd

Drug	Classification	Major toxicities	Comments
Trimetrexate	Antimetabolite	Bone marrow suppression, nausea and vomiting, renal toxicity, hepatic toxicity, stomatitis, skin rash, alopecia	Reduce dose with renal impairment Thrombocytopenia can be severe and prolonged Nausea and vomiting are usually mild Neutropenia may be dose-limiting
Vinblastine	Vinca alkaloid	Bone marrow suppression, neurotoxicity, stomatitis, alopecia, mental depression, nausea	Potent vesicant; avoid extravasation Nausea and vomiting are typically mild and subside within 24 hours Neurotoxicity can be manifested by abdominal pain, diarrhea, constipation, paralytic ileus and obstruction, urinary retention, numbness, paresthesias, loss of deep tendon reflexes, foot drop, headache, convulsions, depression, and Raynaud's phenomenon
Vincristine	Vinca alkaloid	Renal toxicity, hepatic toxicity, skin rash, stomatitis, alopecia	Potent vesicant; avoid extravasation No or minimal bone marrow toxicity Neurotoxicity can be manifested by mild sensor neuropathies that are not dose-limiting Severe paresthesias, jaw pain, loss of deep tendon reflexes, ataxia, foot drop, slapping gait, and muscle wasting would all warrant dose limitation Constipation, paralytic ileus, and abdominal pain can occur, as well as cranial nerve palsies Alopecia can occur Hyponatremia secondary to inappropriate antidiuretic hormone secretion is uncommon, but does occur

dividing cells. The cell is then unable to divide and dies.

The rationale for the fifth category of drugs, hormonal agents, is that tumors arising in hormone-dependent tissue may respond to therapeutic hormones. Unlike other categories of chemotherapeutic agents, hormonal agents are cytostatic rather than cytotoxic; that is, rather than killing the cell they prevent further cell division. Many breast, prostate, endometrial, and adrenocortical tumors respond to hormone therapy. Treatment involves manipulation of the patient's hormonal environment by either adding hormones, using antihormones, or surgically removing the organ that secretes a hormone contributing to tumor growth. For example, estrogen therapy can be used for prostate cancer. Because the prostate gland requires testosterone (an androgen) for normal growth and activity, giving estrogen changes the hormonal environment, affecting tumor activity. Estrogen binds with hypothalamic cell receptor sites, which ultimately results in preventing release of pituitary gonadotropin luteinizing hormone. This decrease in LH level reduces testosterone secretion in the testes, which decreases testosterone available for prostate cancer cell activity.[17]

Corticosteroids, another type of hormonal therapy, may be used in combination with other drugs to treat leukemia, lymphomas, and multiple myeloma. Although the exact mechanism of action is unknown, corticosteroids are synergistic with some antineoplastic drugs.

Therapeutic goals

As with surgery and radiation, chemotherapy may be used for cure, control, or palliation of disease. It is frequently used as an adjunct to both surgery and radiation to eradicate potential micrometastases. Occasionally, tumor size is reduced with chemotherapy, thus rendering it more amenable to surgical resection. Chemotherapy may be indicated to control the disease once the possibility of cure becomes unrealistic. The ability to prolong life for years beyond diagnosis is now a reality. Palliation may also be achieved by chemotherapy-induced tumor reduction.

Combination chemotherapy

In the past, drugs were administered as single agents, resulting in poor responses. Most tumors respond better when treated with a combination of drugs. Typically, combination approaches are developed with the following principles in mind:[12]

- Only drugs that are known to be partially effective when used alone should be selected for combination use
- Drugs with differing toxic effects are selected to

decrease a potentially lethal effect that could result from multiple insults to one organ
- Optimal doses and scheduling are used
- The drug combinations are given as consistently and as frequently as possible while allowing normal tissue to recover between cycles

Side effects and toxic effects

Side effects and toxic effects that accompany chemotherapy result from damage that normal cells incur along with malignant cells. In some cases this presents a major barrier to administration of doses sufficient to effect a cure. Because rapidly dividing cells are the most vulnerable to chemotherapy, bone marrow, gastrointestinal, hair follicle, and gonadal cells suffer the greatest impact. Potential side effects include bone marrow suppression (leading to anemia, bleeding, and infection), stomatitis, mucositis, nausea and vomiting, anorexia, alterations in taste, diarrhea or constipation, alopecia, skin reactions, and reproductive dysfunction. Of course, specific agents affect each body system in varying degrees. Successful assessment and management of side effects is critical.

Elderly patients are at higher risk for toxicities owing to the normal functional deterioration associated with aging. Increased risk for hematopoietic, mucosal, cardiac, and neurologic complications occurs with aggressive chemotherapy.[2] Death due to myelotoxicity and dehydration is a pressing problem in geriatric oncology.[2]

Drug administration

The Oncology Nursing Society[29] states that "only adequately prepared registered professional nurses who are skilled in administering chemotherapy will assume responsibility for its administration in order to ensure quality of patient care and maintain the highest standards of patient and personnel safety." The nurse needs to acquire expertise in both methods and problems of drug administration (Table 15-11). Additional nursing responsibilities include management of drug-delivery devices and patient teaching for self-care management of side effects. The nurse also needs a thorough understanding of specific drug actions, toxic effects, side effects, and dosage ranges. Intravenous administration is the most common route. Drugs can be administered intravenously by both peripheral and central venous access devices.

Handling cytotoxic agents presents a number of potential health hazards. Although much remains unknown, research studies describe instances of increased urine mutagenicity in personnel who handle chemotherapy. Several reports suggest that inhalation or absorption through skin or mucous mem-

TABLE 15-11   Administration of Antineoplastic Agents

Route	Advantages	Disadvantages	Potential complications	Nursing implications
Oral	Ease of administration	Inconsistency of absorption	Drug-specific complications	Evaluate compliance with medication schedule.
Subcutaneous/ intramuscular	Ease of administration Decreased side effects	Adequate muscle mass and tissue required for absorption	Infection Bleeding	Evaluate platelet count (>50,000). Use smallest gauge needle possible. Prepare injection site with an antiseptic solution. Assess injection site for signs and symptoms of infection.
Intravenous	Consistent absorption Required for vesicants	Sclerosing of veins over time	Infection Phlebitis	Check for blood return before and after administration of drugs.
Intraarterial	Increased doses to tumor with decreased systemic toxic effects	Requires surgical procedure for equipment placement	Bleeding Embolism	
Intrathecal/ intraventricular	More consistent drug levels in cerebrospinal fluid	Requires lumbar puncture or surgical placement of reservoir or implanted pump for drug delivery	Headaches Confusion Lethargy Nausea and vomiting Seizures	Observe site for signs of infection. Monitor reservoir or pump functioning.
Intraperitoneal	Direct exposure of intraabdominal metastases to drug	Requires placement of Tenckhoff catheter or intraperitoneal port	Abdominal pain Abdominal distention Bleeding Ileus Intestinal perforation Infection	Warm chemotherapy solution to body temperature. Check patency of catheter or port. Instill solution according to protocol— infuse, dwell, and drain or continuous infusion.
Intravesicular	Direct exposure of bladder surfaces to drug	Requires insertion of Foley catheter	Urinary tract infections Cystitis Bladder contracture Urinary urgency Allergic drug reactions	Maintain sterile technique when inserting Foley catheter. Instill solution, clamp catheter for 1 hour, and unclamp to drain.
Intrapleural	Sclerosing of pleural lining to prevent recurrence of effusions	Requires insertion of a thoracotomy tube	Pain Infection	Monitor for complete drainage from pleural cavity before instillation of drug. Following instillation, clamp tubing and reposition client every 10-15 min × 2 hr. Attach tubing to suction × 18 hr.

From: Bender C: Implications of antineoplastic therapy for nursing. In Clark J, McGee R, editors: *Core curriculum for oncology nursing,* ed 2, Philadelphia, 1992, WB Saunders.

CLINICAL ALERT

Certain chemotherapeutic agents possess vesicant properties. This means that if the drug infiltrates subcutaneous tissue during intravenous administration, severe tissue damage can occur. Manifestations of drug infiltration include pain, tingling, burning, and erythema; tissue ulceration and necrosis can follow. Typically, the degree of damage is directly proportional to the length of exposure. Treatment of extravasation (the resultant tissue damage secondary to infiltration) remains controversial, but may include application of cold or heat or injection of antidotes. Surgical debridement may be required if severe necrosis occurs.

branes of particulate drug matter leads to problems such as skin irritations, headaches, fatigue, and even fetal loss. Even though data are inconclusive, it is recommended that precautions be taken when handling cytotoxic agents and the excreta of patients receiving these drugs. Each clinical agency has a responsibility to adopt procedures based on recommendations of the Occupational Safety and Health Administration (OSHA) and oncology professional organizations.[29,65] Most policies contain the following standards:

- Reconstituting drugs under a class II laminar flow biologic safety cabinet
- Wearing protective clothing during drug reconstitution and administration, including surgical latex gloves and a closed-front, cuffed surgical gown
- Changing protective clothing if it becomes contaminated and after drug administration is completed
- Protecting work surfaces using a plastic-backed absorbent drape
- Washing hands after drug administration and immediately in the event of skin contact
- Careful disposal of drug-contaminated items in designated toxic waste containers

Biologic Response Modifier Therapy

As the mysteries of tumor immunology unravel, increasing interest has developed in the possibility of manipulating the immune system to control or even cure cancer. **Biologic response modifier (BRM)** therapy employs substances capable of stimulating or suppressing the immune system. Recent advances in genetic engineering have resulted in the ability to produce sufficient quantities of BRMs for adequate clinical trials in humans. Ideally, the goal of biologic therapy is to cure cancer with substances that induce little or no toxicity in normal tissue cells. This is an attractive option for patients seeking alternatives to chemotherapy, but most BRMs are still in investigative stages and are not widely available.

Classifications

No clear agreement exists on one ideal classification system for BRMs. Most of the proposed systems base their categories on the modes of action of the various substances. Clark and Longo[42] suggest three functional categories. The first is made of agents that either restore, augment, or modulate immune mechanisms believed to be active in the control of tumor cells; examples include interferons, interleukins, Bacille Calmette-Guerin and *C. parvum*, and tumor antigens. Alpha-interferon is the most extensively investigated BRM to date. It has proved effective in a number of malignancies and is now available for treatment of hairy cell leukemia.

The second category includes cells or cellular products that have direct antitumor effects. Monoclonal antibodies (MoAbs) and tumor necrosis factor fit this classification. MoAbs are proteins designed to attack specific tumor antigens. As a result, MoAbs target tumor cells while ignoring normal cells. Two potential uses of MoAbs are diagnostic and therapeutic. For example, studies are under way to use MoAbs to deliver radioactive isotopes directly to a tumor site, thus allowing better radiographic visualization of the cancer.[22] MoAbs are also being investigated for use as "messengers" that will carry molecules of toxins, such as chemotherapy, directly to a tumor cell, while bypassing healthy cells. Ideally this mechanism could virtually eliminate side effects from exposure of healthy tissue to toxic chemotherapy.

Tumor necrosis factor is a substance produced by activated macrophages. Normally, it plays a role in the inflammatory response. Tumor necrosis factor is also known to be directly toxic to cancer cells and is thus a potential antineoplastic agent.

Other miscellaneous agents that have a variety of other biologic effects make up the third category. This group includes substances that can prevent tumor cells from metastasizing, hormones that stimulate undifferentiated or poorly differentiated cells to mature, and agents that may possibly intervene during carcinogenic changes within a cell. *Cis*-retinoic acid, some anticoagulants, and blood-cell colony stimulating factors all belong in this category (see Chapter 38).

Side Effects and Toxic Effects

Side effects and toxic effects of BRMs are being identified as clinical trials progress. Side effects vary greatly in type and intensity, depending on the specific agent used. For example, side effects of interferon include a flulike syndrome of headache, malaise, chills, and fever; fatigue, leukopenia, and nausea or vomiting may also occur. Interleukin-2, however, can cause severe toxicity, including the flulike syndrome plus capillary leak syndrome, hypotension, confusion, desquamating rash, and renal toxicity. As clinical trials progress, identification of side effects and methods to manage them will continue.

Other Treatment Approaches

Hyperthermia

Hyperthermia is the therapeutic application of heat (greater than 41°C).[55] One underlying assumption for the use of hyperthermia for cancer treatment is that malignant cells are more heat-sensitive than normal cells. As a tumor is heated, the blood flow first increases and then drops, which deprives the tumor of necessary oxygen and nutrients, leading to cell death.[55] Also, heat increases the metabolic rate of tumor cells and thus the need for increased oxygen. As a result, the cells increase anaerobic metabolism, which increases lactic acid production. The now acidic environment causes an increase in cell destruction. A third mechanism of cell kill may be modulated by the immune system. Heat is believed to activate a patient's own lymphocytes against tumor cells.[55]

Hyperthermia can be delivered locally, regionally, or systemically. Agents for local treatment (which may be applied either externally or interstitially) include electromagnetic irradiation (microwaves), electric and magnetic fields, and ultrasound.[59] Regional heating involves the regional perfusion of an organ or limb. Delivery is accomplished by local techniques or by extracorporeal heating of blood that is then recirculated back to the affected limb.[55]

Systemic or "whole body" hyperthermia can be delivered by extracorporeal heating and reinfusion or by conductive methods, such as placing the patient in hot water or a water-heated suit.[55] Hyperthermia may also be used in conjunction with other treatment methods, such as radiation therapy and chemotherapy.

Side effects range from potential skin burning during local therapy to fatigue, hypotension, peripheral neuropathies, nausea, vomiting, and diarrhea with systemic therapy. The clinical results of trials thus far vary greatly. Most focus on control or palliation of disease, with best results in those studies combining hyperthermia with other treatment approaches.

Photodynamic therapy

Photodynamic therapy involves a light-induced destruction of tumor tissue that contains a photosensi-

tizing substance. Typically, hematoporphyrin derivative is used for photosensitization. After intravenous administration, the sensitizer is retained in higher concentrations in the tumor tissue than in normal tissue. Upon application of light (laser beam), the sensitizer interacts with oxygen in the tissue, thus producing a cytotoxic substance.[11] Photodynamic therapy is currently under investigation for palliation and control of a variety of tumors growing on surfaces of the bladder, pleura, head and neck, bronchus, chest wall, and peritoneal cavity.[11] The major side effect of this treatment is that of photosensitivity, which may last from 4 to 6 weeks. To prevent severe sunburn, patients must take precautions to avoid sunlight. Protective clothing that covers *all* skin areas and sunglasses must be worn when outside. Interestingly, many sunscreens are ineffective protection, because they screen out only ultraviolet radiation, not visible sunlight. Opaque sunscreens that block out visible light are a better choice.[11]

Clinical Trials

Only a small number of cancer patients participate in clinical trials; Gross[48] estimates the proportion to be less than 15% of all patients. A patient's decision to enter a clinical trial is influenced by many factors, including fear, anxiety, family pressures, and misconceptions, coupled with the desire to receive the best treatment available. A key nursing action, patient education, helps to clarify and reinforce the patient's comprehension of the nature of the trial and other treatment options (see box p. 309). An excellent teaching tool is also available from the National Cancer Institute, titled *What are Clinical Trials All About?* (Publication no. 85-2706).

Unproven Methods of Treatment

Despite the remarkable advances made in prevention, detection, treatment, and supportive care, cancer patients remain vulnerable targets for the abundant unproven methods of cancer therapy. Unproven methods are those therapies used to treat cancer that are not part of the arsenal currently used by the medical community. Unproven methods are also termed unorthodox or alternative therapies. It is estimated that up to 50% of cancer patients consider or use unorthodox therapies during the course of the disease.[8] Use of these methods can exact a significant medical and economic toll. Exclusive use of an unproven method may allow the disease to progress, which is particularly tragic if the cancer could indeed be responsive to conventional methods. The public spends approximately $4 billion annually on unproven cancer treatments.[8] Understanding the motivations of patients who seek unproven methods and the nature of methods cur-

PATIENT EDUCATION CHECKLIST: CLINICAL TRIAL CONTENT OUTLINE

1. Clinical trials
   a. Definition and phases of research
   b. Purpose
   c. Institution affiliations and sponsor of the study
2. Components of the clinical trial
   a. Study design
   b. Process of randomization
      (1) Treatment possibilities
3. Side effects of the proposed treatment
   a. Known side effects and toxicities
   b. Extent of previous research or use of the treatment proposed
   c. Comparison with prior treatments patient has undergone
   d. Effect on quality of life (duration of side effects, number of follow-up visits and tests, financial costs, limitations)
4. Informed consent process
5. Patient rights
   a. Right to withdraw
   b. Right to information
   c. Confidentiality
6. Costs and reimbursement
7. Expectations of the patient
   a. Compliance with follow-up visits, tests
   b. Reporting of side effects

From Bujorian GA: Clinical trials: patient issues in the decision-making process, *Oncol Nurs Forum* 15(6):779, 1988.

ETHICAL ISSUES

- How should the risk of diminished quality of life with treatment be weighed against the risk of shorter life without treatment? How should such a decision be made?
- Who should have a voice in deciding which risks are worth what benefits?
- Should patients with a life-threatening illness be offered only the most effective treatment available, because time will be lost with less effective therapy? Or should they be offered the widest possible selection of options, including unorthodox ones?
- Do nurses have a responsibility to continue to care for patients who refuse orthodox treatment and resort to alternative remedies?

rently used enables the nurse to formulate some helpful interventions.

Knowing that cancer patients will quite likely explore and engage in alternative methods, the nurse can intervene in several ways:

- Offer factual information about the disease and treatments
- Clarify misconceptions
- Open the door for discussion of alternative methods
- Do not judge or ridicule the person who seeks other choices
- Involve the patient and family in treatment
- Make specific suggestions regarding diet, exercise, and sleep to promote a healthy life-style
- Spend time listening to questions and concerns
- Involve the patient and family in support groups, if desired
- Be aware of alternative therapies the patient may be receiving; watch for any adverse effect

Management of Symptoms and Complications

By instituting measures to prevent and treat symptoms, the nurse directly affects a patient's ability to tolerate and participate in difficult treatment regimens. The ultimate goal of interventions is to improve the patient's and family's quality of life so that they may carry on the business of living.

The American Nurses' Association and the Oncology Nursing Society have generated six professional practice standards that guide the delivery of care to patients and families who experience cancer (see the box on p. 310).[37] The nursing management section of this chapter focuses on those problems most commonly encountered by generalist nurses who provide care to people with cancer. Nursing care for patients with specific malignancies is discussed in each clinical chapter.

ALTERED PROTECTIVE MECHANISMS

Protective mechanisms include immune function, hematopoietic function, integumentary function, and sensorimotor function.[37] Cancer patients experience a variety of altered protective mechanisms within the course of the disease and treatment. The most prevalent and life-threatening outcome of these alterations is that of infection.

Infection is the leading cause of death in cancer patients. Despite advances in treatment and improved overall survival rates, infection remains a significant clinical problem. Drastic compromise of normal defense mechanisms because of treatment and the underlying malignancy increases both the risk and severity of infectious complications. The

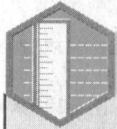

PROFESSIONAL PRACTICE STANDARDS FOR ONCOLOGY NURSING

Standard	Selected Criteria
I. The oncology nurse applies theoretic concepts as a basis for decisions in practice.	Reference materials discussing the conceptual bases for oncology nursing practice are accessible in the practice setting. Nursing actions are consistent with recognized theoretic concepts and established knowledge.
II. The oncology nurse systematically and continually collects data regarding the health status of the patient. The data are recorded, accessible, and communicated to appropriate members of the multidisciplinary team.	The oncology nurse collects data in the following high-incidence areas: prevention and early detection, information, coping, comfort, nutrition, protective mechanisms, mobility, elimination, sexuality, ventilation, circulation.
III. The oncology nurse analyzes assessment data to formulate nursing diagnoses.	The practice setting provides opportunities for documentation of nursing diagnoses by the oncology nurse. The oncology nurse formulates individualized nursing diagnoses that reflect the patient's actual or potential health problems in the eleven high-incidence areas.
IV. The oncology nurse develops an outcome-oriented care plan that is individualized and holistic. This plan is based on nursing diagnoses and incorporates preventive, therapeutic, rehabilitative, palliative, and comforting nursing actions.	Specific measurable goals, described in functional or behavioral terms, are developed for each of the eleven high-incidence problem areas.
V. The oncology nurse implements the nursing care plan to achieve the identified outcomes for the patient.	The oncology nurse coordinates the patient's care using appropriate resources and consultative services to ensure continuity and adequate follow-up. The oncology nurse acts as an advocate to help patients achieve their desired outcomes.
VI. The oncology nurse regularly and systematically evaluates the patient's responses to interventions in order to determine progress toward achievement of outcomes and to revise the data base, nursing diagnoses, and the plan of care.	The oncology nurse reviews the plan of care and revises it based on the evaluation process and critical indicators for the high-incidence problems areas. For example: The patient possesses adequate information about cancer prevention and detection. The patient possesses the knowledge to prevent or manage problems related to alterations in protective mechanisms.

Modified from Standards of Oncology Nursing Practice, 1987, American Nurses' Association and Oncology Nursing Society.

role of colony stimulating factors, used to stimulate repopulation of blood cell progenitors, continues to be investigated. Colony stimulating factors can make a substantial difference in shortening the time that a patient is vulnerable to infection after chemotherapy. (See Chapter 38 for further information.)

Neutropenia, is the single most important factor that predisposes cancer patients to infection. As the neutrophil count falls below 1000/mm³, the risk of infection rises proportionally. The rate of fall of the neutrophil count is also significant; a more rapid decline positively correlates with increased likelihood of infection. Another important factor is the duration of neutropenia. The risk of developing an infection increases the longer neutropenia persists (Figure 15-11).

Neutropenia is most often caused by chemotherapy-induced reduction of white blood cell precursors in the bone marrow. Radiation to flat bones involved in blood cell production (i.e., skull, ribs, sternum, pelvis, vertebrae) may also induce a neutropenic state. Other conditions that lead to neutropenia include underlying malignancies that impair bone marrow function, such as leukemias, lymphomas, and multiple myeloma.

Once the absolute granulocyte count (AGC) drops

below 1000, risk for infection becomes significant. Below 500, risk increases substantially; below 100 risk is severe and will occur in virtually all of these patients. Clinically, the AGC is often used to determine whether a patient is ready for discharge from the hospital or able to withstand further treatment.

Other immune system defects may predispose the patient to infection. Defects in the cellular and humoral components of the immune system can occur because of immunosuppressive drugs, bone marrow transplantation, splenectomy, and impairment secondary to the malignant process (especially in lymphoma and lymphocytic leukemias). Cancer patients frequently receive corticosteroids, which induce defects in the inflammatory response.

Mechanical obstruction caused by tumor mass leads to stasis of secretions and excretions, which in turn leads to infection. Pneumonia secondary to bronchial obstruction (bronchogenic carcinoma) and urinary tract infections secondary to urethral obstruction (prostatic tumors) are typical examples.

Disruption of skin and mucous membranes induced by chemotherapy and radiation toxicities provides a locus for infection. Surgical procedures, cutaneous tumors and metastases, drug extravasation, intravenous therapy devices, invasive diagnostic procedures, and indwelling catheters and drains make up an ever-increasing list of risk factors the cancer patient will encounter in this category.

Because of these risk factors, cancer patients experience an increased incidence of opportunistic infections. Causative microorganisms most often identified are outlined in the box below. The most frequently identified sites include lungs, oral cavity, skin, perianal area, and genitourinary tract.

NURSING MANAGEMENT OF THE PATIENT WITH ALTERED PROTECTIVE MECHANISMS
Assessment

Any patient with suspected infection must be carefully assessed so that any suspicious areas can be identified and secretion or excretion samples cultured. Thus appropriate antibiotic and symptomatic care can be administered. The neutropenic patient may present an extra challenge, because neutropenia diminishes the patient's ability to mount a normal inflammatory reaction. Signs and symptoms of infection may be much more subtle (see Clinical Alert). Fever may be the only sign of a life-threatening septicemia.

COMMON CAUSATIVE ORGANISMS IN THE IMMUNOCOMPROMISED PATIENT WITH CANCER

Classification	Microorganism
Gram-negative bacteria	Pseudomonads
	Escherichia coli
	Klebsiella pneumoniae
	Enterobacter spp.
	Proteus spp.
	Serratia spp.
Gram-positive bacteria	*Staphylococcus aureus*
	Staphylococcus epidermidis
	Streptococcus spp.
	Corynebacteria
	Clostridium difficile
	Enterococcus spp.
Fungi	*Candida* spp.
	Aspergillus spp.
	Cryptococcus neoformans
	Phycomycetes
	Fusarium spp.
Viruses	Herpes simplex
	Herpes zoster
	Cytomegalovirus
Protozoa	*Pneumocystis carinii*
	Toxoplasma gondii

From Volker DL: Infection in the cancer patient with an ostomy, *J ET Nurs* 19:17, 1992.

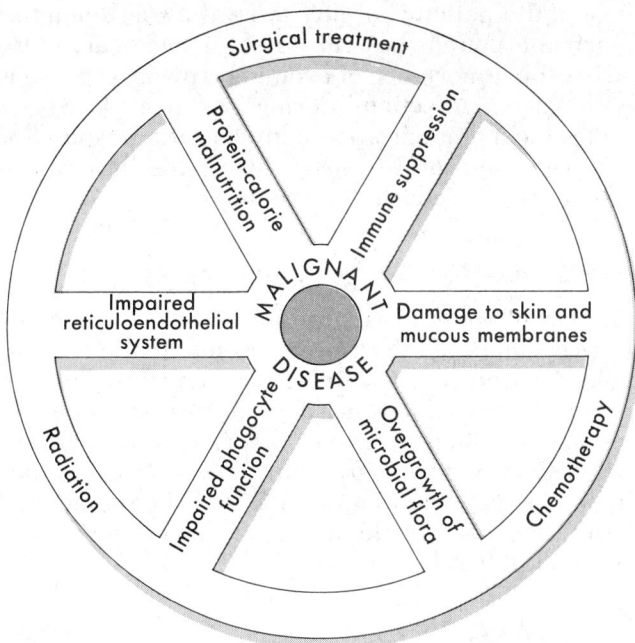

FIGURE 15-11   Risk factors for infection in cancer patients.

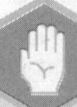

CLINICAL ALERT

Absence of physical signs or symptoms does not rule out infection. In the compromised cancer patient, life-threatening infections can develop and disseminate within hours, leading to septic shock and death.

Assess the patient as follows:

- Skin—examine the entire skin surface and folds for presence of any lesions, cracks, breakdown, rash, or drainage
- Oral—assess for redness, lesions, or tenderness; note presence of any patches, coating, or poor dental hygiene
- Respiratory—watch for cough, pleuritic pain, rhinitis, and tachypnea; also note the presence of adventitious lung sounds and shortness of breath; assess the depth, pattern, and rate of respirations
- Gastrointestinal—inquire about any abdominal tenderness, esophageal pain, nausea, or vomiting; palpate the abdomen and note firmness or tenderness; auscultate bowel sounds; note presence of diarrhea
- Perineal—the rectal area is a frequent locus of infection, so be sure to examine for ulcerations and assess for pain that accompanies bowel movements; vaginal secretions, pain, burning, itching, or odors may indicate infection; also assess for penile or scrotal pain, secretions, edema, and lesions
- Neurologic—changes in sensorium may indicate sepsis

Also note systemic indications such as weakness, chills, and fatigue.

Nursing Diagnosis

The nursing diagnosis is high risk for infection related to the disease or treatment that compromises the host.

Planning

The goal is to prevent infectious complications and promptly detect indications of infection. The expected patient outcome is either that the patient will remain free of infection or that infectious complications will resolve.

Implementation

Institute measures to protect the patient from further infection. If the patient is hospitalized, a private room is desirable; reverse isolation is unnecessary. Meticulous handwashing before any patient contact is usually sufficient. Protect the patient from exposure to visitors and staff with active infections.

Assist with vigorous personal hygiene measures. Institute an oral care regimen (see p. 317) in the presence of potential or actual mucositis. Protect skin barriers by daily bathing and application of emollients. Perineal care includes careful hygiene after defecation. To decrease trauma to the perianal skin, suggest sitz baths or perineal irrigations. Fill a small plastic squeeze bottle with tepid water to cleanse the perineum; then gently pat dry with a towel. Skin abrasions and breakdown secondary to frequent toilet paper use will be minimized. To decrease trauma to the rectal mucosa, avoid the use of rectal temperatures, suppositories, and enemas.

Provide a nutritious, high-calorie, high-protein diet (unless contraindicated) to help restore immune function. Carefully monitor intravenous catheter sites, puncture sites, wounds, and other breaks in skin integrity. Provide care to these sites per institution standards or procedures.

To decrease trauma to the vaginal mucosa, instruct female patients in the use of sanitary napkins instead of tampons; emphasize the importance of changing pads frequently.

Avoid the insertion of indwelling urinary catheters.

Continue to monitor vital signs for impending sepsis.

Teach the patient and family self-care measures. Discharge or home care instructions include information about the signs and symptoms of infection. Assess the patient's ability to read a thermometer; teach the patient how to do so, if necessary. Also stress the importance of avoiding crowds or persons with known infections during risk periods. Other topics include medication administration, wound or skin care, and oral hygiene. Stress the importance of maintaining a clean environment.

Evaluation

Successful patient response to the plan is indicated by prevention of infection or resolution of infectious episodes. Indicators of infection-free status include normal body temperature and the absence of inflammation, purulent drainage, tenderness, or redness. Laboratory and radiographic findings return to normal or remain within normal limits. The patient and family are able to demonstrate or verbalize measures to prevent infection.

BLEEDING

Chemotherapy-induced thrombocytopenia is the most frequent cause of bleeding. As the platelet count decreases, the risk of bleeding increases. A platelet count between 50,000/mm^3 and 100,000/mm^3 indicates minimal risk for bleeding; this level usually requires no treatment but may delay chemotherapy administration until the count exceeds 100,000/mm^3. Between 20,000/mm^3 and 50,000/mm^3, the risk for bleeding is moderate.

Invasive procedures such as central venous catheter placement can be accomplished in the thrombocytopenic patient, but a platelet transfusion may be warranted before the procedure. Once the platelet count drops below 20,000/mm^3, the risk of bleeding is high. Prophylactic platelet transfusions may be given, even in the absence of active bleeding, to decrease the potential for a life-threatening gastrointestinal or central nervous system hemorrhage. Marrow suppression secondary to radiation may also induce thrombocytopenia. As in neutropenia, the risk is greatest when bones involved in active blood cell production are included in the irradiated field. Other sources of myelosuppression include metastatic involvement of the marrow and suppression of platelet production secondary to leukemic cell proliferation.

The spleen normally sequesters one third of the total platelet pool. An enlarged spleen, which may accompany leukemia and lymphoma, may remove the majority of the patient's circulating platelet mass. Disseminated intravascular coagulation is a syndrome of rapid, abnormal consumption of platelets that is often associated with leukemia, adenocarcinoma, sepsis, and hepatic disease. Erosion and subsequent rupture of blood vessels occurs secondary to tumor invasion. Lung cancer and head and neck cancers both induce bleeding in this manner.

NURSING MANAGEMENT OF THE PATIENT WITH BLEEDING

Assessment

Assess the patient's risk for bleeding by identifying underlying risk factors related to disease and treatments. Also note other contributing risks, such as medications (e.g., aspirin, heparin, sodium warfarin, nonsteroidal antiinflammatory drugs, penicillins) known to interfere with hemostasis.

Physical assessment focuses on manifestations of bleeding as follows: note spontaneous petechiae and ecchymoses, prolonged bleeding from sites of invasive procedures, epistaxis, gingival bleeding, and gastrointestinal or genitourinary tract bleeding. Symptoms of organ dysfunction secondary to bleeding are site specific. Particularly note a change in the level of consciousness and the onset of headache, which may indicate central nervous system bleeding. Watch for changes in vital signs indicative of hypovolemia related to blood loss. Erosion of major blood vessels is usually accompanied by frank hemorrhage and subsequent shock. In thrombocytopenic patients, symptoms of spontaneous bleeding typically occur when the platelet count drops below 20,000/mm^3; at counts between 20,000/mm^3 and 50,000/mm^3, prolonged bleeding may occur at invasive procedure sites, as well as following minor trauma.

Monitor diagnostic studies such as platelet count, coagulation profile, and results of guaiac studies of body fluids and excreta for occult blood.

Nursing Diagnosis/Planning

The nursing diagnosis is high risk for injury related to thrombocytopenia or bleeding. Prevention, early detection, and prompt intervention must all be maximized for the patient with bleeding. The patient is encouraged to participate in measures to accomplish these goals.

Implementation

Minimize risk of bleeding by avoiding intramuscular injections, nonessential invasive procedures, straight-edged razors, and other sources of trauma. Prevent rectal bleeding by avoiding rectal suppositories, enemas, or rectal thermometers. Administer stool softeners, lubricants, or laxatives as ordered. Women may receive progestational agents to suppress menstruation.

Apply pressure at venipuncture sites for at least 3 to 5 minutes. Maintain a safe environment to avoid trauma from falls. Frequent oral care and application of lip lubricants will preserve integrity of the oral mucosa. In the event of oral bleeding, instruct the patient to rinse with cool saline or tap water. If the area of bleeding can be localized, apply gentle manual pressure with a dampened gauze. If severe bleeding occurs, application of topical thrombin is most helpful.

Epistaxis is usually halted by application of gentle pressure. If pressure is unsuccessful, nasal packing is suggested. Saline lavage via nasogastric tube halts gastrointestinal bleeding; irrigation via threeway Foley catheter will decrease bladder hemorrhage while facilitating clot removal.

Patients with head and neck cancer who are at risk for erosion of the carotid artery should be placed on carotid precautions. This entails identification of the patient at risk and placing appropriate materials at the bedside. Typical supplies include bedside suction, tracheostomy tray, several packages of gauze dressing, and material for initiation of venous access. Reassure the patient while this equipment remains in the room because the presence of these supplies is a constant reminder of a potential emergency.

Administer platelet transfusions as ordered. Prophylactic transfusions may be given when the platelet count falls below 20,000/mm^3. Teach the patient and family assessment parameters, risk factors, and measures to prevent or control bleeding.

Evaluation

Successful patient response to the plan is indicated by prevention of bleeding or resolution of hemorrhagic episodes. Laboratory values should return to or remain within normal limits. The patient and family can demonstrate or verbalize measures to prevent and control bleeding.

ANEMIA

Anemia is another complication of altered protective mechanisms in the cancer patient. Although anemia can have a substantial impact on the quality of a patient's life, anemia is less often associated with life-threatening problems than neutropenia or thrombocytopenia. The phenomenon of chemotherapy-induced anemia is due to the life span of each cellular element in the peripheral bloodstream, and the drug's impact on the life cycle of bone marrow stem cells. The rate of disappearance of each cell type from the peripheral bloodstream correlates with the half-life of the cell line. The average half-life of a neutrophil is much shorter (6 to 8 hours) than that of a platelet (5 to 7 days); the life span of a red blood cell is 120 days. Because neutrophils disappear very quickly, infection is the first and most profound problem to occur. Anemia may never develop or be only minimal, because circulating cells continue to function despite suppressed bone marrow stem cells.

Anemia represents a significant problem, however, because it can seriously affect self-care ability. Any bone marrow–suppressive disease or therapy, including chemotherapy, radiation therapy, or other drugs (e.g., phenytoin, cephalosporins, sulfa drugs, amphotericin B) may induce anemia. The decreased intake, absorption, or utilization of iron, folic acid, and vitamin B_{12} also contribute to anemia.

NURSING MANAGEMENT OF THE PATIENT WITH ANEMIA

Assessment

Manifestations of anemia are all related to the diminished oxygen-carrying capacity of the blood. Assess the patient for relevant risk factors such as previous and current therapy for cancer, and medications known to cause anemia. Note any history of headache, dyspnea on exertion, dizziness, tachycardia, chest pain, or hypersensitivity to cold. Also note any history of blood loss via stool, emesis, menses, urine, or nasopharynx.

Physical assessment findings may include pallor of the skin, nail beds, conjunctivae, and circumoral tissues. Auscultate the heart for potential murmur or other irregularities. Check for the presence of any active bleeding in the skin (petechiae, purpura), gums, GI tract, vagina, and nasopharynx. Also inspect all wound sites and dressings for active bleeding. Lethargy and a decreased level of responsiveness may occur once the hemoglobin is less than 7.5 g/dL.

Check the patient's vital signs; an increased pulse and respiration rate may accompany anemia as a result of hypoxemia. Blood pressure may be decreased as a result of hypovolemia. In particular, check blood pressure in lying, sitting, and standing positions to detect orthostatic changes. Monitor and report changes in hemoglobin and hematocrit levels.

Nursing Diagnosis/Planning

The nursing diagnosis is fatigue related to anemia. The goal is to conserve the patient's available energy and promote comfort during periods of anemia. The patient and family are taught to identify causes of anemia and participate in measures to reduce fatigue secondary to tissue hypoxia.

Implementation

Comfort measures include provision of adequate rest periods. Identify necessary activities of daily living and ask the patient to prioritize their importance. Provide warm clothing and blankets. Nutritional support is important for the restoration of red blood cells. Assist with oral care before and after meals to promote comfort and enhance appetite. Provide a diet high in protein, vitamins, and iron. Frequent, small meals may be more tolerable for a patient with low energy. Assist with meals if necessary. Administer supplemental iron, vitamin B_{12}, or folic acid as ordered by a physician.

Administer oxygen as ordered. Supplemental oxygen counteracts tissue hypoxia and helps to lessen the workload of the heart. Anticipate the need to transfuse packed red blood cells once the patient's hemoglobin is 8 g/dL or less (see Chapter 38).

Promote safety and emphasize the importance of conserving energy. Advise the patient to ask for assistance if orthostatic changes are present. Assist the family in assessing the home environment for potential hazards and determining the need for devices (e.g., wheelchair, walker) that can minimize the patient's energy expenditure. Arrange for oxygen at home if necessary.

Evaluation

Successful patient response to the plan is indicated by adequate oxygenation of tissues as demonstrated by the absence of symptoms of anemia. The patient and family should be able to verbalize or demonstrate measures that conserve energy during periods of fatigue.

ALOPECIA

Although not critical to a patient's physical well-being, alopecia can have a devastating effect. The term **alopecia** refers to hair loss that occurs as a result of cancer treatments. Scalp hair is most commonly affected, but other body hair may become thin, including eyelashes, eyebrows, pubic hair, and axillary hair. The extent of hair loss is extremely individual and depends, in part, on the type, dosage, and duration of therapy. Potential problems precipitated by alopecia include negative changes in self-image, decreased social activity, and altered interpersonal relationships.

Because most hair follicles are metabolically active at any one time, they are particularly susceptible to the effect of certain chemotherapeutic drugs. The hair bulb atrophies, causing breakage of the hair shaft. Chemotherapy-induced hair loss is temporary; the one exception is androgens used for hormone therapy. The person with a genetic predisposition for baldness who receives androgen therapy may incur permanent alopecia. Otherwise, hair regrowth after chemotherapy typically occurs in 1 to 2 months. Patients may report changes in color or texture of new hair, including increased thickness and curls, along with increased gray hair.

Radiation therapy will induce alopecia in the treatment field. The effect is greatest in the scalp, however. As with that induced by chemotherapy, radiation-induced alopecia is dosage-dependent, but differs from chemotherapy in that it sometimes is permanent in nature. In adults treated with whole brain irradiation greater than 40 Gy (4000 rads), hair loss is usually permanent. At lesser total doses, regrowth should begin about 1 month after treatment.

NURSING MANAGEMENT OF THE PATIENT WITH ALOPECIA
Assessment

Assess the risk for alopecia related to treatment. Determine the meaning of hair loss to the patient. Alopecia may be just as devastating to the 65-year-old man as it is to the 20-year-old woman. Note the patient's usual methods for hair care and practices that can damage hair, such as frequent shampooing and use of heated rollers, blow dryers, curling irons, permanents, and dyes. All of these methods will facilitate hair loss after treatment.

Nursing Diagnosis

The nursing diagnosis is body image disturbance related to treatment-induced alopecia. Other associated nursing diagnoses may include impaired social interactions and altered sexuality patterns.

Planning

The goal is to minimize the effect of alopecia on the patient's well-being. Interventions should enable the patient to describe the potential effect that alopecia may have and to participate in measures to adapt to the condition.

Implementation

Provide information to the patient regarding the potential for hair loss. Emphasize that loss usually occurs over a period of days to weeks, and that regrowth will occur (except as outlined above). Also inform the patient that the color or texture of regrown hair may be different from before treatment. Suggest self-care measures, such as washing with a gentle shampoo every 3 to 4 days, using a wide-toothed comb or soft-bristled brush, and application of a gentle emollient to the scalp (provided it is not receiving radiation) once it is exposed. Discourage use of hair care practices that may damage hair.

Explore strategies that enhance self-image and adaptation. Patients often find that selecting a wig, if desired, is best done before hair loss begins, so that hair color and texture can be matched. Other patients may prefer scarves or hats. Some insurance companies and the American Cancer Society will provide financial assistance with head coverings. Also consider referring the patient to the American Cancer Society's "Look Good, Feel Better" program.

Evaluation

The patient and family should be able to verbalize an understanding that alopecia is a side effect of the treatment being received, and can state whether the effect will be temporary or permanent. Also, they should be able to describe self-care strategies for managing or minimizing the effects of alopecia on body image.

ORAL COMPLICATIONS

Oral complications frequently encountered include **stomatitis,** an inflammation of the oral mucosa surfaces, and **xerostomia,** or drying of the oral cavity. Both directly impact nutritional status, comfort, and potential for additional complications, such as infection and bleeding.

In chemotherapy, epithelial cells in the oral mucosa slough and become denuded owing to cytotoxicity of chemotherapeutic agents. Cell replication and growth are impeded resulting in mucosal atrophy and inflammation. Other indirect effects include the immunosuppressive and myelosuppressive actions of the drugs.

Radiation to the head and neck produces a similar cellular response. Patients experience a change in or even loss of taste, accompanied by xerostomia or stomatitis. Unlike chemotherapy, radiation therapy can induce permanent oral changes. Both xerostomia and taste alterations may persist on a chronic basis.

Other factors include poor oral hygiene, poor nutritional status, dehydration, tumor infiltration of the mucous membranes, oxygen administration, and administration of drugs that induce drying, such as antihistamines or opioids. Direct tumor invasion of the salivary glands also produces xerostomia.

NURSING MANAGEMENT OF THE PATIENT WITH ORAL COMPLICATIONS
Assessment

Assess the patient for risk factors. Particularly note any antecedent oral or dental problems and alcohol or tobacco use. Review the patient's current oral hygiene practices. Assess the impact of any oral changes on comfort, nutritional status, and activities of daily living. Complete an oral examination, noting condition of lips, tongue, mucous membranes, gingiva, and teeth. Note the presence of any redness, tenderness, burning, or pain. Look for lesions, ulcers, and white patches on the mucous membranes. Also assess quality and amount of saliva, ability to swallow, and breathing habits.

Nursing Diagnosis

The nursing diagnosis is altered oral mucous membrane integrity, related to complications of disease or treatment.

Planning

The goal is to promote patient comfort and support nutritional intake. The patient and family should be able to describe risk factors, demonstrate an oral hygiene regimen, and identify complications that need to be reported.

Implementation

If no alterations are present, institute an oral care regimen that includes brushing teeth with a soft-bristled toothbrush after each meal and at bedtime. Ideally, all patients should be examined by a dental oncologist before treatment.

See Table 15-12 for a detailed review of interventions for varying degrees of stomatitis and Table 15-13 for common agents used for oral care. A soft, bland diet will decrease pain and minimize irritation. Other comfort measures for both stomatitis and xerostomia include lip emollients (water-soluble lubricants, lanolin) and artificial saliva.

Teach the patient oral care measures. Emphasize that fresh oral care solutions should be mixed *each time* care is done to eliminate potential for bacterial growth forming in premixed solutions. Decreased salivary production, oral mucosal atrophy, and decreased vascularity are all natural consequences of aging and thus increase the risk of oral problems in the elderly patient. In the presence of oral pathologic conditions, dentures should be worn only for meals. Adequate cleansing can be achieved with diluted hydrogen peroxide.

Evaluation

Successful patient response to the interventions includes prevention or resolution of oral mucositis. Mucous membranes will be intact; the patient will have no complaint of oral pain or discomfort. The patient will also be able to demonstrate oral hygiene measures and verbalize the rationale for meticulous oral care.

NAUSEA AND VOMITING

Nausea and vomiting are the most distressing aspects of treatment for many patients. Even the general public is acquainted with this complication and associate it with treatment, despite the fact that not all drugs cause it and not all patients experience it. Successful control of nausea and vomiting not only promotes patient compliance with treatment regimens, but also vastly improves the quality of life during treatment. Potential complications of protracted, uncontrolled nausea and vomiting include electrolyte imbalances, dehydration, gastritis, and altered nutritional status.

Chemotherapeutic drugs that are emetic in nature (see Table 15-14) are believed to trigger any one of these areas: the chemoreceptor trigger zone (CTZ) in the medulla oblongata, the cerebral cortex, and peripheral receptors in the pharynx and gastrointestinal tract (Figure 15-12). These areas stimulate vomiting when subjected to noxious stimuli. In most instances vomiting ceases within 48 hours after treatment ceases; nausea may last longer, but duration differs among individuals.[60] Chemotherapy-induced nausea and vomiting may be acute, delayed, or anticipatory in nature. Anticipatory nausea and vomiting occur before a given treatment and have often been termed a "Pavlovian" or psychogenic response based on previous negative experience with chemotherapy.

Many patients receiving radiation therapy experience nausea and vomiting in addition to effects specific to the irradiated area. Supposedly, this results from release of toxins into the bloodstream as the tumor is destroyed. Radiation therapy to the abdominal area may also precipitate nausea and vom-

TABLE 15-12	Nursing Interventions: Stomatitis

Assessment	Interventions

GRADE 0:

No stomatitis.

Mucosa is moist, pink, and soft. No ulceration or lesions. No discomfort in mouth.

Instruct the client to stop smoking and reduce the intake of alcoholic beverages.

After each meal and at bedtime, brush teeth with dentifrice and floss (except during periods of thrombocytopenia and neutropenia).

A plaque-disclosing dye can be helpful in identifying plaque to be removed by brushing or flossing. If client is edentulous, frequent oral irrigations should be performed.

GRADE I:

Mild stomatitis.

Whitish gingival area observable, or client mentions slight burning sensation or discomfort in oral cavity.

Every 2 hr, provide normal saline rinses. Brush teeth after meals and at bedtime using dentifrice if not irritating.

Floss at least once a day (except during periods of thrombocytopenia and neutropenia).

Use an ice massage to the web between the thumb and index finger of the hand on the same side as the painful area in the mouth.

Provide a soft, bland diet.

GRADE II:

Moderate stomatitis.

Moderate erythema, shallow ulcerations, or white patches present. Client complains of pain but can continue to eat, drink, and swallow.

Every 1 to 2 hr, provide normal saline rinses. Brush teeth after meals and at bedtime using dentifrice if not irritating. Use Toothettes if toothbrushing is not tolerated. Floss once a day if tolerated (except during periods of thrombocytopenia and neutropenia).

Topical anesthetics may be used if needed.

Provide a soft, bland diet, especially cool foods. A dietitian can help plan meals to meet the nutritional needs of the client.

GRADE III:

Severe stomatitis.

Severe erythema, full thickness ulceration, mucosal necrosis, bleeding, white patches present. Client complains of severe pain and is unable to eat, drink, or swallow.

Every 1 to 2 hr, provide normal saline rinses. Toothbrushing and flossing may not be tolerated, so Toothette or gauze-wrapped finger is used to remove debris and plaque. Oral irrigations gently cleanse the mouth.

An interim dental prosthesis to protect ulcerated mucosa and provide a surface for chewing has been described (DePaola, 1983). It is worn while eating and at night while sleeping.

Topical anesthetics and systemic analgesics may be used as needed.

Topical thrombin may be used.

Tube feeding or parenteral nutrition may be needed.

Note: Following resolution of stomatitis, clients should again brush their teeth after each meal and at bedtime and floss once a day. From Iwamoto R: Alterations in oral status. In Baird SB, McCorkle R, Grant M, editors: *Cancer nursing,* Philadelphia, 1991, WB Saunders.

TABLE 15-13 Agents for Oral Care

Agents	Comments
CLEANSING	
Normal saline	Economical, available, least irritating
Sodium bicarbonate	Decreases odors, buffers acidity, dissolves mucin
Hydrogen peroxide	Germicidal, mechanical cleansing, debriding. Use diluted solution and follow with normal saline or water rinse. Aspiration precautions with foaming action
Commercial mouthwashes	Avoid mouthwashes containing alcohol, oils, astringents, antiseptics, and flavorings
Chlorhexidine gluconate	Antimicrobial: decreases dental plaque and gingival inflammation. Bitter taste, tooth staining
LUBRICATING	
Saliva substitutes	Decreases pain, dryness; protects mucosa
Lemon-glycerin	Mouth irritant, decalcifies teeth
Water-soluble lubricant, lanolin	Lip emollient; if petrolatum used, avoid aspirating
PAIN CONTROL	
Coating	
Kaopectate, milk of magnesia, Orabase	Covers ulcerated mucosa; temporary pain relief; may dry mucosa
Sucralfate	Binds to exposed mucosa for pain relief and protection
Hydroxypropyl cellulose film former (Zilactin)	Binds to oral mucosa forming protective coating; transient stinging with gel application
Vitamin E	Anecdotal reports of pain control; heals stomatitis
Topical Anesthetic	
Lidocaine viscous	Transient pain relief; interferes with gag reflex when swallowed
Dyclonine hydrochloride	Transient pain relief; useful in persons with xerostomia; aspiration precautions if swallowed
Cocaine solution	Transient pain relief; monitor central nervous system effects; tachycardia
Combination mouthwashes	Usually contains nonsteroidal antiinflammatory agent in addition to topical anesthetic
Systemic	
Opioid medications	For severe pain; taken 30-60 min before meals and as needed
Nonsteroidal antiinflammatory agents	
OTHER	
Topical thrombin	To control minor bleeding
Fluoride	To prevent caries; apply to debris-free teeth after thorough mouth care
Allopurinol	To minimize chemotherapy-induced stomatitis
Antibiotic mouthwashes	For prophylaxis and treatment of oral infections such as candidiasis and gram-negative opportunistic organisms

From Iwamoto R: Alterations in oral status. In Baird SB, McCorkle R, Grant M, editors: *Cancer nursing,* Philadelphia, 1991, WB Saunders.

TABLE 15-14   Chemotherapeutic Agents with Emetic Actions

Nausea with low potential for emesis*	Nausea with moderate potential for emesis†	Nausea with high potential for severe emesis‡
L-Asparaginase	Azacytidine	Cisplatin
Bleomycin	Carboplatin	Cyclophosphamide
Chlorambucil	Cytarabine§	Dacarbazine
Hydroxyurea	Daunorubicin	Dactinomycin
L-Phenylalanine	Doxorubicin (Adriamycin)	Ifosfamide
Mercaptopurine	Etoposide (VP-16)	Mitomycin
Methotrexate§	Fluorouracil	Mechlorethamine (nitrogen mustard)
Tamoxifen	Hexamethylmelamine	Nitrosoureas
Thioguanine	Mithramycin	
Thiotepa	Mitoxantrone	
Vinblastine	Procarbazine	
Vincristine	Streptozocin	
Steroids (most)		

*A drug that is associated with a 20% or lower incidence of eliciting nausea or vomiting, or both, has low potential for emesis.
†A drug that is associated with a 25%-70% incidence of eliciting nausea or vomiting, or both, has moderate potential for emesis.
‡A drug that is associated with a 75% or greater incidence of nausea or vomiting, or both, has high potential for severe emesis.
§At low doses. Potential increased at higher doses.
From Ringlein JW: Management of nausea and vomiting and other acute side effects of cancer chemotherapy. In Skeel RT, editor: *Handbook of cancer chemotherapy*, ed 3, Boston, 1991, Little, Brown & Co.

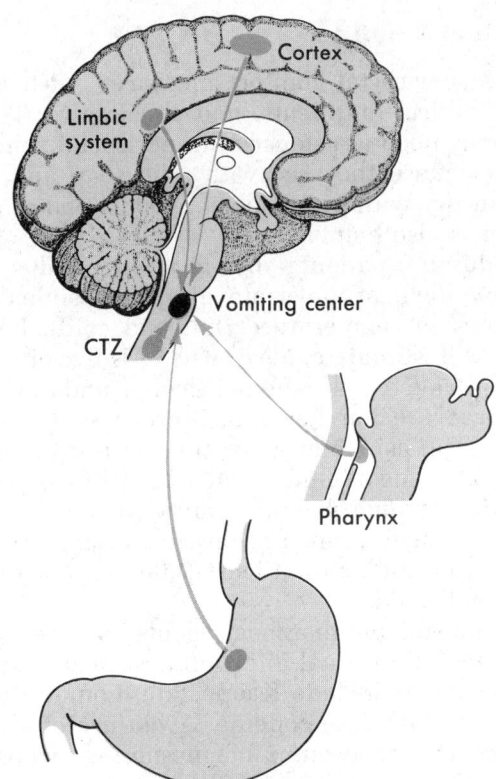

FIGURE 15-12   Vomiting action. Once stimulated, vomiting center acts on cranial nerves, spinal nerves to diaphragm, and abdominal muscles, which results in automatic response of vomiting.

iting owing to the direct effect on the gastric lining. Other causes of nausea and vomiting in cancer patients include hypercalcemia, bowel obstruction, central nervous system tumors, liver metastases, uremia, and infection.

NURSING MANAGEMENT OF THE PATIENT WITH NAUSEA AND VOMITING

Assessment

Assess the patient for potential risk factors associated with nausea and vomiting. Note the patterns of nausea and vomiting, including onset, frequency, and severity. Determine aggravating factors (such as food odors, motion, coughing, drugs, and particular foods) and past measures that have provided relief (both pharmacologic and nonpharmacologic). Also assess the impact of nausea and vomiting on activities of daily living.

Nursing Diagnosis/Planning

The nursing diagnosis is altered nutrition: less than body requirements related to nausea and vomiting. The goal of adequate nutritional intake is promoted along with provision of comfort.

Implementation

If any measures were helpful during previous episodes, institute these measures. Nonpharmacologic approaches are varied. Dietary manipulation, such as eating cold foods, clear liquids, and crackers and avoiding strong or spicy foods. Heated foods may create intolerable odors and precipitate vomiting. Experiment with eating patterns. A few patients may prefer to eat before treatment so that they avoid "dry heaves." Others prefer an empty stomach. Frequent oral care provides comfort and improves intake at mealtime. Distraction, relaxation techniques, and other behavioral approaches may be helpful.

Antiemetic drugs are administered before treatment and liberally thereafter. Use the "around-the-clock" scheduled approach that has proved successful with pain management. A variety of antiemetic drug protocols has been developed that has significantly reduced the incidence and severity of emesis. One combination, intravenous administration of metoclopramide, diphenhydramine, lorazepam, and dexamethasone, provides marked relief. Ondansetron, a newer antiemetic drug, has also proved to provide substantial relief of nausea and vomiting associated with chemotherapy.

Evaluation

Successful response to the care plan is evidenced by the patient's ability to regain or maintain normal weight for body size. The patient should experience either little or no nausea and vomiting. Additionally, evaluate the response to teaching by asking the patient to verbalize measures to maintain nutritional intake.

DIARRHEA

Diarrhea occurs in both chemotherapy patients and radiation therapy patients for reasons similar to those of nausea and vomiting. Both treatments destroy epithelial cells lining the gastrointestinal tract, leading to atrophy of the intestinal mucosa. Vital nutrients and fluids are thus lost. Other treatment methods may precipitate diarrhea. After resection of the bowel, patients may experience a fluid malabsorption syndrome. After a bone marrow transplant, a patient may experience diarrhea as a result of graft-vs.-host disease. In this case, the immunocompetent cells of the donor marrow recognize the GI cells of the patient as foreign and destroy targeted cells that line the bowel. Medications known to cause diarrhea include antibiotics, antacids, and laxatives. Other potential sources of diarrhea in the cancer patient include stress, bowel obstruction secondary to tumor growth, nutritional supplements with high osmolarity, intestinal infection, and stress.

NURSING MANAGEMENT OF THE PATIENT WITH DIARRHEA

Assessment

Assess patient for risk factors and other contributing factors, such as lactose intolerance. Perform an abdominal assessment to include presence of bowel sounds, abdominal distention or rigidity, flatus, cramping, or pain. Determine quantity and frequency of diarrhea, especially noting color, consistency, and odor of stools. Examine the the perianal skin for presence of excoriation or tenderness. Assess hydration status (skin turgor, urine color, intake and output, mucous membranes, electrolytes, presence of thirst). Note any conditions, such as food or fluids, that aggravate the diarrhea. Obtain a nutrition history. Note current weight and assess for recent weight loss.

Nursing Diagnosis/Planning

The nursing diagnosis is diarrhea related to disease or treatment. The patient should be able to return to a normal elimination pattern and avoid the development of complications, such as dehydration and altered nutritional status.

Implementation

Provide perirectal comfort measures, such as sitz baths, topical ointments, and anesthetics. The patient may need assistance with perirectal skin care; gently cleanse the area with mild soap and water and pat dry with a soft towel. Application of a skin barrier is also helpful.

Modify the patient's diet to a low-residue, high-protein, high-carbohydrate diet if possible. Avoid extremes in temperature (hot and cold), because these will stimulate peristalsis. Also avoid spicy, fatty, or fried foods, caffeine, alcohol, and milk products. In severe diarrhea, total bowel rest may be necessary. This is achieved by placing the patient on NPO status and administering all nutrition parenterally. Monitor fluid balance status. Watch for symptoms of dehydration. Encourage the patient to increase fluid intake to at least 3000 mL a day unless contraindicated.

Administer antidiarrheal agents as ordered, unless a gastrointestinal infection is suspected. Examples of agents include Kaopectate, Lomotil, Immodium, and low-dose codeine. Avoid use of antacids that contain magnesium; magnesium works osmotically and draws water into the bowel, which aggravates diarrhea. Antacids that contain aluminum usually are more appropriate. Bulk-forming agents may also be used, such as methylcellulose or other products.

Teach the patient and family appropriate self-

CLINICAL ALERT

Do not administer ordered antidiarrheal agents if gastrointestinal infection is suspected. Interference with elimination of gastrointestinal pathogens could result in overwhelming sepsis.

care measures such as dietary changes, foods that aggravate diarrhea, and medications that may alleviate diarrhea. Review problems to report to the nurse or doctor, such as blood in the stool, signs of dehydration, sudden abdominal distention, fever, and increase in the frequency and quantity of stools. Teach perirectal skin care measures and use of topical anesthetics or skin barriers.

Evaluation

Diarrhea should lessen or resolve after instituting the care plan. Return to normal bowel function will be manifested by a return to the pretreatment pattern of defecation accompanied by normal bowel sounds, stools of normal consistency, and absence of abdominal cramping. The patient should also be able to identify measures to minimize diarrhea.

CONSTIPATION

The major pitfall in management of constipation is failure to recognize it as a potential risk and institute prophylactic management. All too often constipation develops unnecessarily. The vinca alkaloid chemotherapeutic agents can cause a neurotoxic effect, leading to decreased peristalsis. Paralytic ileus is a less frequently seen sequela of vinca alkaloid treatment. Other agents that also decrease peristalsis include opioids, antidepressants, and tranquilizers. Tumors may cause partial obstruction, leading to difficult passage of stool. Ovarian, colorectal, and abdominal lymphomas are most often associated with this problem. Other risk factors include anorexia, decreased activity, lack of privacy, stress, dehydration, and laxative abuse. Metabolic changes that may slow GI motility include hypercalcemia and hyperkalemia.

NURSING MANAGEMENT OF THE PATIENT WITH CONSTIPATION
Assessment

Assess the patient for the presence of risk factors for developing constipation. Assess bowel status, including usual patterns of defecation, discomfort

(such as cramping), distention, and presence of bowel sounds. Watch for signs of fecal impaction (e.g., frequent liquid stools, feeling of pressure in the rectum, abdominal cramping, distended abdomen, hypoactive bowel sounds). Inspect the external rectal area for hemorrhoids. Digital rectal examination may reveal hard stool in the rectum. If neutropenia, thrombocytopenia, or rectal tumor is present, do not check for fecal impaction. Determine current patterns of food and fluid intake; check for presence of dehydration. Evaluate medication regimen and note any drugs that may cause constipation.

Nursing Diagnosis/Planning

The nursing diagnosis is constipation related to disease or treatment. The goal is to help the patient to maintain or regain a normal elimination pattern.

Implementation

Provide adequate hydration by encouraging fluid intake of at least 3000 mL per day, unless contraindicated. Promote mobility and exercise. After consultation with the patient, change the diet to increase the amount of fiber and bulk-forming foods. Administer stool softeners, cathartics, or laxatives as ordered. If a bulk-forming laxative is used, ensure that the patient can drink sufficient water to minimize the risk of causing an intestinal or esophageal obstruction. If the patient is severely constipated, enemas, or digital disimpaction may be necessary. Again, these measures may be contraindicated in the presence of neutropenia, thrombocytopenia, or friable rectal tumor.

Teach the patient and family appropriate self-care measures including factors that contribute to constipation and measures to prevent constipation. Discuss the importance of detecting and reporting early signs of constipation, such as hard, infrequent stools. Teach the patient the rationale for any dietary and medication measures.

Evaluation

Patients should maintain or resume a normal pattern of elimination. They will also be able to verbalize an understanding of the factors related to risk of constipation and to demonstrate measures to promote bowel elimination, such as adequate fluid intake, utilization of stool softeners, and maintenance of physical mobility.

SEXUAL DYSFUNCTION

All the preceding complications, along with a variety of disease processes, may contribute to sexual or reproductive dysfunction. A number of risk factors affect sexuality. Surgical disfigurement, changes in body image secondary to advancing or uncontrolled tumor growth, and functional loss related to chemotherapy, external radiation therapy, or brachytherapy are contributors. Sexual dysfunction can result from any one factor or a combination of factors.

NURSING MANAGEMENT OF THE PATIENT WITH SEXUAL DYSFUNCTION

Assessment

Assess for presence of risk factors for sexual dysfunction. Explore previous sexual history, including preferred sexual role and relationships, perceptions of self as a sexual being, and preferred sexual behaviors (type, frequency, and satisfaction).[9] Also note the patient's reproductive history as appropriate. Assessment parameters include menstrual history (for females), number of children, desire for children in the future, history of difficulty with reproduction, and types of contraceptive use. Also, explore the patient's (and partner's, if appropriate) perceptions of how the disease and treatment will affect sexuality. An assessment of sexual health is incorporated into the overall patient assessment process. The following brief assessment questions are examples that can open a discussion with the patient and lead to a more in-depth assessment if needed:

- Has being ill interfered with your being a (husband, father, wife, mother)?[24]
- Has your illness changed the way you see yourself as a man/woman?[24]
- Has your illness affected your sexual function?[51]

Nursing Diagnosis/Planning

The nursing diagnosis is sexual dysfunction related to disease process or treatment. Other potential associated diagnoses include altered role performance, activity intolerance, anticipatory grieving, and self-esteem disturbance.[9] The goal is to help the patient understand the potential impact of disease or treatment on sexuality. If the patient desires, an additional goal is to assist with attaining a satisfying sexual role.

Implementation

Although the specific concerns of the patient and significant other will guide the nurse's approach, the following general interventions may be helpful[51]:

- Foster open communication regarding sexuality
- Provide anticipatory guidance about probable changes
- Validate normalcy of sexual behavior
- Educate regarding sexuality
- Counsel regarding alternate sexual expressions
- Consult with other professionals equipped to provide more intensive therapy as needed

The ultimate outcome is that the patient is provided with the appropriate milieu and information regarding his sexual health.

Patients undergoing treatment may also require counseling regarding reproductive issues. Ovaries and testes may be damaged by radiation and chemotherapy, so pregnancy is not advised during either treatment. If a fetus is conceived, teratogenic effects may result. Information regarding sperm banking should be provided in the event that permanent sterility or sperm mutation is possible. Prophylactic oophoropexy (surgical displacement of ovaries outside an anticipated radiation field) is another approach that can be suggested.

Evaluation

The patient should be able to verbalize an understanding of the impact of the disease and treatment on sexuality. In the event of a verbalized need, the patient should be able to identify key resource people available for more intensive sexual counseling. Ultimately, the patient should be able to maintain a satisfying sexual role and concept.[21]

ALTERATIONS IN NUTRITION

Alterations in nutritional status can be attributed to nausea and vomiting, bowel elimination problems, pain, psychologic distress, fatigue, treatment-induced anorexia, and a host of other problems. But malnutrition also results from a problem inherent in the cancer process. Indeed, malnutrition occurs in a substantial proportion of hospitalized cancer patients. Although the exact mechanism is unknown, most authorities agree that a malignancy competes with the host for essential nutrients, which results in cachexia. Cachexia is characterized by progres-

RESEARCH BRIEF

Waltman NL et al: Nutritional status, pressure sores, and mortality in elderly patients with cancer, *Oncol Nurs Forum* 18(5):867, 1991.

The impact of nutritional status on the skin integrity of the elderly cancer patient is of particular concern. Waltman et al studied differences in nutritional status, incidence of pressure sores, and incidence of mortality between hospitalized elderly cancer patients and hospitalized elderly patients without cancer. They found that the cancer patients were at greater risk for developing pressure sores, and that the incidence of pressure sores was related to the presence of protein deficiency.

sive loss of body fat, muscle, and weight, and in itself may result in death.

Malnutrition in cancer patients is termed "protein-calorie" in nature because the protein-calorie composition of the diet cannot meet metabolic demands. The metabolism of both carbohydrates and proteins is altered, resulting in depletion of amino acids, glucose intolerance, and protein loss via excretion or leakage. The tumor may also alter lipid metabolism; consequently, fat from host tissues is dislodged and mobilized for use as another energy source. Other contributing factors include altered taste sensation, anorexia, and tumor obstruction of the gastrointestinal tract. Countless psychologic factors affect nutritional status, aside from all the physiologic insults.

Nutritional assessment and interventions are outlined in Chapter 16. When establishing caloric needs and diet, one must consider the metabolic and mechanical impact of the malignancy. Enteral and parenteral approaches are often required, depending on bowel function. Fortunately, increased recognition of the need to treat potential nutrition problems prophylactically (e.g., the initiation of total parenteral nutrition before surgery or chemotherapy) may decrease the morbidity associated with malnutrition.

PAIN

Although not all cancer patients experience chronic pain, it remains a significant but manageable problem for many. No comprehensive national or international epidemiologic studies have been done to determine the incidence and prevalence of cancer pain, but based on local and regional studies, Bonica[40] concluded that 40% to 50% of persons in early or intermediate stages and 70% of those with advanced or terminal cancer have pain. Successful pain management requires an understanding of the causes of pain specific to cancer, the impact on and the meaning to the patient, and proper use of the many therapeutic approaches.

Common pain syndromes occurring in cancer patients can be divided into three categories: (1) pain syndromes associated with direct tumor infiltration, (2) pain syndromes associated with cancer therapy, and (3) pain syndromes not associated with cancer or cancer therapy.[45]

Direct tumor infiltration of bones or infiltration that results in nerve compression or obstruction can cause pain. Metastatic spread of disease to any bone may generate pain, but spinal involvement is of particular concern. Occasionally, bony lytic lesions are not painful and remain undetected until the bone is so weakened that it breaks. The characteristics of bone pain vary, but its presence may be the first indication of either recurrence or spread of disease. Tumor compression of nerve structures can result in

a neuropathy with sharp, localized, or radicular pain. Peripheral nerve involvement manifests as a burning sensation or hypersensitivity in the area. Obstruction of the gastrointestinal and urinary tract is frequently associated with crampy, diffuse pain.[46]

Pain associated with treatment is equally multidimensional. Postradiation fibrosis of targeted tissue may result in lumbosacral and brachial plexopathies, sensorimotor changes, lymphedema, and radiation myelopathy.[46]

Chemotherapy can induce painful syndromes. Administration of vinca alkaloid drugs (e.g., vincristine) can result in a peripheral neuropathy; pain, burning, and tingling sensations occur in addition to muscle weakness. Ulcerated oral and esophageal mucosal surfaces secondary to chemotherapy-induced stomatitis are excruciatingly painful. Chronic, burning pain may develop after acquiring herpetic infections during periods of immunosuppression. This postherpetic neuralgia may persist for the remainder of the patient's life.

Nurses may lose sight of the third syndrome, that of pain unrelated to cancer or its treatment. Cancer patients may have arthritis, back pain, or any of the other pain syndromes that plague the older population. These may become aggravated during treatment or periods of lessened mobility.

The significance of pain to the cancer patient is laden with concerns of relapse, progression, and painful death. Although definitely a unique experience to each individual, the onset of new pain is equated with progression of disease. Certainly, this must be investigated and, if possible, ruled out. Enduring the diagnostic testing process and waiting for results is a fearful process. Thus carefully explain and prepare the patient for procedures and also anticipate any need for extra analgesics so that comfort during this anxiety-laden time can be promoted.

NURSING MANAGEMENT OF THE PATIENT WITH PAIN

Because of the prevalence and seriousness of cancer pain, the Oncology Nursing Society has formulated a position paper that defines the responsibilities of professional nurses in relation to cancer pain (see box on p. 324). Fulfillment of these responsibilities is critical to the successful management of cancer patients' pain.

Nursing care of the cancer patient experiencing pain is not unlike that for other patients who experience pain. Please see Chapter 14 for an in-depth discussion of application of the nursing process for patients who experience pain. Interventions must be implemented with consideration to the underlying pathophysiologic event (or cause). Combination approaches tend to work best, including the use of nonopioid and opioid analgesics, opioid potentiators, antidepressants, tranquilizers, nerve blocks, and

ONCOLOGY NURSING SOCIETY POSITION PAPER ON CANCER PAIN

Nursing responsibilities in cancer pain management
Positions:

- Individuals with cancer pain have a right to obtain optimal pain relief. Nurses caring for them have an ethical obligation to ensure exploration of everything possible within the scope of nursing practice to provide this relief.
- Nurses caring for individuals with cancer pain must exercise leadership in identifying and assessing cancer pain and in planning, implementing, coordinating, and evaluating the interdisciplinary management of cancer pain.
- Nurses are responsible for identifying the problem of inadequate pain management in patients with cancer and for intervening responsibly to achieve optimal pain relief.
- Nurses caring for individuals with cancer pain should perform initial and ongoing pain assessments and communicate assessment data to colleagues.

- After assessing the individual experiencing cancer pain, the nurse develops a plan of care with the individual/significant other that: includes specific measurable goals and effective pain management techniques based on mutual goal setting; specifies a schedule for the timing of interventions, the routes of medication administration, and the ongoing assessment of pain, pain relief, and side effects associated with pain therapy as well as overall effectiveness of the regimen; and addresses nursing responsibilities as well as communication and other collaborative interventions with other health care providers involved in the individual's care.
- Nurses are responsible and accountable for implementation and coordination of the plan for management of cancer pain.
- Nurses are responsible for evaluating patient responses to interventions for cancer pain control and for using evaluation data to revise the care plan. Nurses use all available clinical and administrative resources to ensure progress toward achieving relief or control of cancer pain.

From: Spross JA, McGuire DB, Schmitt RM: Oncology Nursing Society position paper on cancer pain, Pittsburgh, 1991, Oncology Nursing Press.

neurosurgical procedures. Other noninvasive measures, cutaneous stimulation, relaxation, imagery, and hypnosis assist as well.

The patient may also benefit from use of the major cancer treatment methods for palliation of pain. Surgery to repair pathologic fractures (secondary to bone metastases), reduce tumor bulk that obstructs or compresses, or debride fungating lesions contributes to pain relief. Radiation of metastatic bone lesions may produce dramatic, swift results. Other palliative uses of radiation include reduction of tumor bulk, decrease in ulcerative lesions, and reduction of tumor-associated inflammation. Chemotherapy plays a lesser role in palliation of pain, but it can ease patient discomfort related to widely disseminated disease.

Cancer patients no longer need to suffer because of pain. The wide arsenal of therapeutic interventions, coupled with increased understanding of how to use them most effectively, should decrease suffering tremendously.

ONCOLOGIC EMERGENCIES

The use of aggressive treatment methods and sophisticated supportive care has changed the character of the disease course for most cancer patients.

Historically, most patients experienced a short course with a steady decline to death. Now cancer is more akin to a chronic disease, punctuated by acute, often life-threatening complications called "oncologic emergencies." These critical episodes occur because of (1) complications of the underlying disease process and (2) application of the various treatment methods. Anticipation of these potential emergencies, prompt detection, and early intervention are all key factors that promote patient survival. Table 15-15 summarizes approaches to identification and management of common oncologic emergencies.

ONGOING CARE

The diagnosis of cancer has profound consequences on the patient, family, and significant others. The disease course and thus the patient's needs and reactions will vary greatly from person to person. The diagnosis of cancer means different things to each individual. An important nursing role is to explore this meaning, to identify potential needs and stressors, and to determine interventions suited to those needs. Past experiences with other family members or friends who have had cancer will, in part, influence the person's reaction to his or her own diag-

TABLE 15-15 Oncologic Emergencies

Syndrome	Risk factors	Signs/symptoms	Interventions
Hypercalcemia	Bone metastases (especially in breast cancer) Multiple myeloma Dehydration Immobility Lung cancer	Nausea/vomiting Constipation Lethargy, weakness Confusion, stupor Polyuria Electrocardiogram changes, dysrhythmias	Vigorous IV hydration Diuretics Monitor fluid balance status Administer calcium-binding agents Safety precautions Promote mobility
Disseminated intravascular coagulation (DIC)	Acute leukemias Adenocarcinomas (especially prostate) Sepsis Liver failure	Active bleeding Petechiae, ecchymosis Cool, ecchymotic fingertips and toes Shock secondary to blood loss	Blood product replacement Protect from further bleeding or trauma Administer heparin, epsilon amino caproic acid (EACA) Treat shock Frequent vital signs
Superior vena cava syndrome (SVCS)	Lung cancer Other intrathoracic tumors Thrombosed central venous catheter	Dyspnea Headache Venous distention Reddened, swollen face and neck Upper-extremity edema	Radiation therapy to tumor Administer oxygen, diuretics, steroids, tranquilizers Positioning for optimal respiratory effort
Spinal cord compression	Vertebral bone metastases Primary tumor involving spinal cord, vertebrae	Pain Loss of bladder/bowel control Weakness, gait change Sensory loss	Radiation therapy Steroids Pain management Bladder/bowel training Physical therapy Supportive care during immobility
Septic shock	Neutropenia All other risk factors that predispose to infection	Fever, chills Hypotension Tachycardia Tachypnea Decreased urinary output Cool, clammy skin Cloudy sensorium	Fluids, oxygen Antibiotics Ventilatory support Monitor fluid balance status Sodium bicarbonate if acidotic Inotropic drugs
Pericardial effusion/tamponade	Chest radiation Lung, breast cancer Mesothelioma Leukemia/lymphoma	Pain Anxiety Tachycardia, dysrhythmias Dyspnea Hypotension, narrow pulse pressure	Pericardiocentesis Oxygen Hemodynamic monitoring Vasopressors
Syndrome of inappropriate antidiuretic hormone secretion (SIADH)	Lung cancer Vincristine Cyclophosphamide	Irritability Confusion Seizures Fluid retention Weakness	Fluid restriction IV hypertonic saline Seizure precautions Monitor fluid balance status
Tumor lysis syndrome	Leukemia and lymphoma patients receiving chemotherapy	Hypocalcemia Hyperphosphatemia Hyperkalemia Hyperuricemia Weakness, confusion Numbness, tingling Muscle cramps Progressive renal failure	Vigorous IV hydration Allopurinol Sodium bicarbonate Monitor fluid balance status Monitor electrolytes, BUN, creatinine

nosis. Thoughts of death, guilt over past life-style habits, doom, or panic may be conjured. The older patient may have already lost several family members and friends to cancer. People within the patient's primary support system, particularly a spouse, may have already died. Assess what the patient already understands about the disease and treatment; clarify any misconceptions that may be present. The teaching and supportive measures during the diagnostic and treatment phase include:

- Patient and family teaching about the disease process
- Patient and family teaching for diagnostic and treatment methods specific to their plan of care
- Provision of resource materials to supplement above teaching
- Referral to other helpful resources, such as support groups, community agencies, information hotlines, and others as suggested at the end of the chapter
- Provision of positive feedback and reinforcement regarding successful participation in self-care
- Encouragement of activities that foster self-esteem, such as improvement of physical appearance, return to work, return to family roles and activities
- Exploration and encouragement of useful coping strategies (e.g., exercise, relaxation techniques) that the patient used before the illness

The patient in the diagnostic and treatment phase will seek information everywhere. He or she may try unproven methods, change physicians frequently, and seek advice from everyone, including other patients and families. These behaviors are normal and a part of the coping process.

The pattern of disease process will determine some of the stressors and resultant needs encountered. Some patients will undergo treatment and eventually be cured; others may bounce back and forth between remission and recurrence; still others may not respond to treatment and face a steady deterioration of health. For most, however, some degree of disease control is realistic. A common problem encountered is that of fear of relapse. This fear may manifest in different behaviors, ranging from denial to extreme preoccupation with seemingly minor complaints. Again, individuals will respond differently. Reassure the patient that fear of recurrence is normal; clarify the meaning of symptoms and discomforts that arise during treatment so that patients understand the nature of the symptom. The patient who becomes ill because of treatment side effects may believe the problems are caused by disease progression.

Like patients and families, nurses may be vulnerable to misconceptions about the disease and treatments. Some nurses, because of feelings of discom-

THERAPEUTIC COMMUNICATION GUIDE

The Cancer Patient

Assessment

1. Determine the family's knowledge regarding the diagnosis of brain tumor

    Example: Nurse: "Ms. Jones, what do you know about your husband's condition?"

    Patient: "Well, I know that he's been falling a lot and he's been taking a lot of painkillers. Today he says he's seeing double."

    Nurse: "Can you tell me what were his first changes in behavior and how long ago these occurred?"

    Patient: "Well, I guess it started about 2 months ago. He seemed to be angry at the slightest little annoyance."

Intervention

1. Open up feelings

    Example: Nurse: "Have you ever been through anything like this before?"

    Patient: "No, I just can't understand why he's acting like this. He's always been such a gentleman."

2. Assess coping behavior used in the past

    Example: Nurse: What helped you get through these last 2 months?"

    Patient: "Well, we have three sons. They are a great comfort to me. And I have my faith in God. We're a strong family and just don't have much use for outside help."

3. Recognize family's feelings; help family by trying to provide information

    Example: Nurse: "I would like to offer you every support we have. Is there any way that I might meet with you and your sons to explain what we have available to make this a more comfortable time for your husband and the family?"

fort, unintentionally construct barriers to open communication and care. When first working with cancer patients, the nurse may wonder where to begin, what to do or say, how to help. In a classic study, Larson[52] explored what cancer patients believe to be the most important nursing care functions. To a sample of hospitalized cancer patients, Larson provided a list of nursing behaviors that denote caring (e.g., the acts, conduct, and mannerisms enacted by professional nurses that convey to the patient concern, safety, and attention). They were asked to rate the importance of each one in making patients feel cared for. Patients rated behaviors related to "hands-on" clinical competency (giving injections, starting IVs, managing equipment, "gives good physical care") as being most important. Being accessible, following up, and listening were also highly rated. Larson suggests that the need for cancer patients to have skillfully implemented care is critical. Skilled care can form the starting point for development of a trusting relationship, which can lead to exploration of the other, perhaps more difficult needs regarding the psychosocial impact of the illness.

Rehabilitation and Survivorship

Given that over 50% of cancer patients are cured of their disease, rehabilitation becomes an important issue. Those who are cured have multiple needs regarding the resumption of daily living. Although rehabilitation is most often equated with restoration or improvement of physical function, cancer patients face other challenges as well. Coping with attitudes of friends, acquaintances, employers, and coworkers presents a number of challenges. Societal and personal attitudes regarding cancer can significantly affect rehabilitation. Sadly, much of the general public and many health care professionals still view cancer as an inevitably protracted terminal illness. Perhaps this contributes to the fact that aggressive, comprehensive rehabilitation services for cancer patients are still lacking. Because the nurse is frequently the person to whom a patient turns regarding problems or concerns, it is important to be aware of the potential needs, barriers, and resources for assistance.

Physical rehabilitation needs depend on the functional consequences of the disease and treatment. Assistance may be required to restore speech, ambulation, nutritional intake, or bowel/bladder control, with the emphasis placed on achieving some degree of independence in performing activities of daily living. Adaptation to amputation, laryngectomy, mastectomy, colostomy, ileal conduit, peripheral neuropathies, decreased cognitive function, feeding via tubes, and tracheostomy all require significant rehabilitative efforts. The support groups in particular are invaluable for the exchange of practical advice by those who have the most intimate experience.

The psychosocial aspects cannot be underestimated. Individual needs and responses will differ, based on past coping abilities, personal meaning of the diagnosis, available support systems, changes in body image, and overall sense of well-being and state of health. The survivor is keenly aware of reactions and responses of those who are aware of his diagnosis. Social interactions may take on new meaning, particularly if the patient has a permanent, physically obvious disability. The prejudices and misconceptions that other handicapped individuals live with may now be a reality for the cancer patient.

Economic implications for survivors and their families may be a problem. Cancer survivors may face job discrimination owing to misbeliefs regarding ability to work satisfactorily after treatment.

Insurability presents another obstacle. Examples of problems encountered include cancellation of health insurance policies, refusal of new applications, exclusions of cancer-related coverage, and loss of coverage as a result of loss of employment. The person who does retain his job and health insurance may become fearful of ever-changing employers because of the potential of being denied coverage in the new job. Because insurance codes vary from state to state, it is important to be familiar with those that pertain to the person with cancer. Refer patients to local sources of legal aid in the event that questionable insurance practices arise. Cancer is unquestionably an expensive disease. The billions of dollars expended annually undoubtedly contribute to difficulties obtaining and maintaining adequate coverage.

Nurses must be aware of available rehabilitation resources and the need to promote to health professionals and the general public alike the positive aspects of cancer care and improvements in survival. Nurses encourage patients and families to participate in programs such as the American Cancer Society's "I Can Cope" and "Dialogue" groups. Patients are referred to the appropriate team member (e.g., physical therapist, occupational therapist, or social worker) or specialized group depending on the specific rehabilitation need; programs such as "Reach to Recovery" and "CanSurmount" are but a few examples. The patient's employment situation is assessed for potential barriers to returning to work. The patient is helped to prepare for potential responses to diagnosis in social and work situations.

Secondary Malignancy

Development of a second primary malignancy is a relatively new problem in cancer patient care. This presents yet another potential shadow in the patient's life. Exposure to radiation therapy, cytotoxic drugs, or both may predispose the patient to the occurrence of another cancer. In follow-up visits after treatment assess for potential manifestations of another malignancy; teach prevention and detection methods that the patient can practice.

Outpatient and Home Care

Outpatient and home care of the cancer patient are increasingly common. Both treatment (from curative to palliation) and supportive care can be successfully administered in these settings. Thus nurses need to understand the scope, limitations, and benefits of these practices.

The patient who opts for treatment at home needs the services of a nurse who understands the complexity of the disease process, the treatment method and the management of side effects. For example, skilled delivery of chemotherapy is a must, but symptom management becomes equally vital. The home care nurse must be able to provide both services. The advantages of treatment in the home are numerous; many patients feel that their quality of life is improved because there is less disruption of the family routine for trips to treatment centers. In most cases, however, there must also be a competent caregiver or significant other present. The elderly cancer patient may not have this advantage because the spouse, if present, may also be ill or debilitated and unable to participate actively in the patient's care. Reliance on neighbors or friends requires close assessment by the nurse to determine reliability, safety, and feasibility of the situation.

Care in outpatient or ambulatory settings is becoming increasingly popular. Not only do patients receive all of the four major treatment methods in these settings, but follow-up care and monitoring as well. Use of outpatient settings can save the patient the expense and disruption of unnecessary hospitalizations. Ideally, disease- and treatment-related problems are monitored so that they can be alleviated or minimized before requiring inpatient, acute care.

Chemotherapy administration is a mainstay of outpatient care. Patients may come to this setting for short-term (e.g., those less than several hours) infusions, or may even be involved in self-administration of continuous infusion chemotherapy in the home setting. Because of recent advances in portable drug-delivery pumps, chemotherapy treatment in the home can be the most cost efficient and palatable to patients and their life-styles.

THE TERMINALLY ILL PATIENT

Care of the terminally ill patient requires an understanding of the trajectory of terminal illness, symptomatology, therapeutic interventions, and impact on family members. Comfort is the focus and goal of care. Symptoms that the patient experiences may be related to uncontrolled growth of the primary tumor (as in tumor pressure and erosion), complications of metastatic disease (such as pain secondary to bone metastases), side effects of treatments, poor nutritional status, and generalized debilitation. Overall, pain is the most frequently encountered problem in patients with advanced cancer.[19]

Although each patient is unique, nursing research studies[19] do reveal some common trends in characteristics and needs of patients with advanced cancer. Typically, patients are elderly, with two thirds of the group more than 65 years of age. The most frequent cancer diagnoses include lung, breast, rectum and sigmoid, and prostate, with a wide range of illness duration from 2 months to more than 10 years. Bone, liver, lung, and brain are the predominant sites of metastases. The most common patient symptoms include pain, confusion, anorexia, dysphagia, and nausea.

Comfort needs of the terminally ill patient have also been studied. Fleming et al[44] assessed nurses' perceptions of the actions they engage in to comfort the advanced cancer patient. When asked to identify activities that they perform to reduce suffering associated with physical, emotional, or interactive aspects of the patient, nurses' responses included (1) physiologic care, such as activities of daily living; (2) psychologic care, including touching and listening; (3) spiritual aspects, such as facilitating participation in worship services and praying with the patient; (4) symptom management; (5) activities that include families, friends, and other members of the health care team.

The impact of a patient's terminal illness on the caregiver is profound. Stetz[62] explored the demands experienced by spouse caregivers of terminally ill adult cancer patients in the home setting. Management of physical care, treatments, and illness-related changes are especially difficult, even in those situations where patients receive skilled nursing care in the home. In general, male spouses have particular difficulty managing the household, whereas female spouses have more difficulty "standing by" or observing their spouses experiencing physical symptoms. Hays[49] notes that as the number and intensity of uncontrolled symptoms increase, so does the amount of anxiety and fatigue of family members. Uncontrolled pain and nausea and vomiting were described as especially difficult for the caregivers to witness.

NURSING MANAGEMENT OF THE TERMINALLY ILL PATIENT
Assessment

Care of the terminally ill patient begins by assessing the sources and degree of discomforts, the method of pain and symptom management, and the

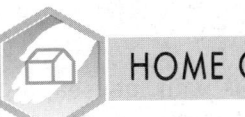

Patients requiring chemotherapy may be discharged with various types of venous access devices. These devices allow patients to receive a series of treatments without needing a new IV site for each treatment, thus preserving the veins for future use.

There are two general types of devices; one is surgically implanted under the skin, and the other is a percutaneous device inserted through the skin into a vein. The former requires very little care after the incision has healed, and is accessed by a needle inserted through the skin into the device. The percutaneous type, such as a heparin lock or a Hickman catheter, requires specific care on a regular basis.

In some cases the venous access device is inserted on an outpatient basis.

Short-Term Goals

1. All necessary supplies and equipment will be available at time of discharge.
2. The patient and caregiver will know basic procedures for caring for the venous access device.

Long-Term Goals

1. The patient will be able to complete the planned chemotherapy without complications from the venous access device.
2. The patient will be able to incorporate care of the venous access device into activities of daily living.

Nursing Assessment Factors

1. The patient's ability to manage care of the venous access site must be assessed. A caregiver may be included for some of the procedures if the patient is acutely ill and unable to manage the procedure alone (if the patient is elderly, caregiver education is essential).
2. Cognitive pattern—Selecting a venous access device for long-term chemotherapy should be done after assessing the patient's ability to care for the device.
3. Coping—stress tolerance pattern—The total patient care plan must be reviewed. The rate of teaching will be affected by the patient's overall ability, the diagnosis, and the total care plan.
4. Resources—Financial and insurance resources must be investigated before ordering the necessary equipment. The reimbursement for equipment varies, depending on the skilled care needs of the patient, the type of insurance, and where the chemotherapy will be administered.
5. Environment—The home environment may need to be evaluated before discharge. There must be handwashing facilities, accessibility for delivery of supplies and equipment, and provisions for emergency assistance.

Planning

1. Start implementing the discharge of a patient with a venous access device as soon as the device is inserted. Some teaching can be started before the device is inserted (see Chapter 12). The length of time needed for teaching and for ordering supplies depends on the type of access device and the teaching needs of the patient.
2. The plan for chemotherapy administration should be made before discharge. The patient may receive chemotherapy as an outpatient in a clinic, in a doctor's office, or at home. In some cases the site care required for a percutaneous device can be done by a nurse at the time of chemotherapy administration. In this case the patient will not need to learn the procedure for site care, but will still need to learn the other aspects of care.
3. Patient and caregiver education should begin before discharge and should allow the patient and caregiver a minimum of one or two teaching sessions. Instruction should be done with the equipment and supplies that the patient will be using at home. The education session should include the following:
   a. How to use the equipment, including needles, syringes, heparin flush syringes, and catheter plugs
   b. How to check for sterility of supplies
   c. The recommended procedure for site care for percutaneous devices
   d. How to safely discard equipment after use
   e. How and when to reorder equipment
   f. How to monitor for local infection, such as phlebitis or cellulitis of either type of device
   g. How to distinguish between reaction to the chemotherapeutic agent and a systemic infection
   h. The necessity for handwashing and for prevention of contamination of the venous access site
   i. The safety precautions regarding capping of the central venous transcutaneous access device
   j. A phone number to call if a problem arises

   If the patient has not learned the procedure or is unable to carry out the procedure safely before discharge, inform the physician. Referral to a home care agency may be necessary to complete the teaching or to provide the skilled care needed.

Implementation

1. Equipment must be ordered 1 to 2 working days before discharge so that the supplies will be delivered in time for the patient to use at home.
2. All necessary forms must be completed before discharge.
3. If the patient is being referred to a home care agency for follow-up nursing visits, include education done and the patient and caregiver's ability.

Documentation

1. The discharge planning process must be documented as it is being developed.
2. The patient and caregiver's ability to manage the care must be documented in the medical record.
3. In the patient's medical record, include the name and phone number of the company contacted for supplies.

effects of the disease and treatment on activity.[38] Explore current coping strategies by both the patient and the family. Ask the patient what concerns him most at this time. Use this answer to plan and prioritize interventions accordingly.

Nursing Diagnosis/Planning

The nursing diagnosis is alteration in comfort related to impact of the terminal disease process. The goal is to alleviate discomfort by assisting the patient to achieve as comfortable a death as possible in accordance with his needs, attitudes, life-style, and desires.

Implementation

After assessing the patient and his or her priorities, work together to establish interventions that will help the patient achieve these goals. Pain management must be explored and facilitated. Austin et al[38] examined variables that could influence home care cancer pain management and found that 50% of patients studied who reported severe pain did not adhere to their prescribed analgesic medication regimens. The patients listed reasons ranging from concern about addiction to the desire to maintain personal control. Thus potential nursing actions could include patient teaching regarding the myths of addiction and helping the patient to maintain control by allowing the patient to determine the desired tolerance level of the pain.

Explore patient and family needs and desires with regard to the setting for provision of terminal care. Both the home and inpatient settings can be appropriate, and care may or may not be administered under the auspices of a hospice approach (see also Chapter 20, Grief, Loss, and Dying, for principles of hospice care). Home care can present a special challenge. The decision to proceed with this plan must be based on careful assessment of the patient's needs and the family's ability to provide for those needs. The physical and emotional strain of home care for the terminal patient may be more than the patient or family can tolerate. Sometimes pressure from family and friends may cause a patient to seek this option without carefully weighing the consequences and alternatives.

Hays[49] examined the relationships among patient symptoms, family anxiety and fatigue, and patterns of hospice service use in the home. Comparisons were made between patients who were and those who were not ultimately hospitalized for inpatient hospice care before death. Study results revealed that patients who required periods of institutionalization experienced more individual symptoms and more combinations of symptoms, and their families exhibited greater anxiety and fatigue in response to uncontrolled symptoms (such as pain, nausea, and vomiting). The implication that certain home care patients may be predisposed to requiring an inpatient admission is of interest. Home care may not be a viable method of care delivery once symptoms pass a certain threshold, particularly in the presence of increases in family fatigue and anxiety.

Nursing interventions to decrease the risk of institutionalization in those who prefer to remain at home include effective symptom control of pain and nausea and vomiting to increase patient comfort and decrease family fatigue and anxiety. Arrange for ancillary services to assist with care in order to reduce family fatigue. In addition, begin anticipatory teaching for the patient and family regarding the disease trajectory and patient deterioration to portray a realistic picture of potential stressors.

Another learning need for families is that of skill acquisition. Although nursing support may be present, family members still voice anxiety and concern over performance of physical care activities.[62] Ultimately, support the patient and family in their choice of care setting. Let them know that it is permissible to change their minds if one setting or another no longer meets their needs.

Other comfort measures for the terminally ill patient are quite basic; care of the dying need not be mysterious, complex, or frightening. Attention to seemingly simple comfort measures, such as a back rub, oral care, or manicure, can do more to comfort than many nurses realize. Patients may have difficult questions or concerns, and nurses thus worry about having the "right" answers. But often the patient wants you to just listen: the expectation is not that you have all the answers. Resist the temptation to label a patient's responses or feelings. This may present a barrier to hearing what he or she wants to tell you. Responses to terminal illness are not nearly as predictable or sequential as many assume.

Spiritual care needs of the cancer patient are often a lesser priority to the nurse than physical care needs.[44,50] Highfield and Cason[50] maintain that each nurse takes one of the following approaches to spiritual care:

1. Defines spirituality as part of the psychosocial dimension and thus subject to psychosocial theoretic principles
2. Denies the existence of the spiritual dimension entirely and does not address patient needs
3. Defines the spiritual dimension as a separate entity that warrants consideration in patient care

The spiritual dimension "encompasses the need for finding satisfactory answers to ultimate questions about the meaning of life, illness, and death."[50] Nursing interventions should thus assess the meaning of these issues to the patient. Some patients may express a belief in God and practice a specific religious doctrine; others may believe this realm exists outside of formal religious activities and does not refer to any specific deity. Give patients permission to discuss this aspect of their being. Access to the opportunity for discussion of spiritual issues with the nurse may be sufficient for some patients; others may desire clerical consultation. Some nurses are comfortable praying with patients as part of spiritual care; others offer to pray for the patient at a later, private time. Opportunities for nursing research abound in the realm of spirituality, especially with the terminally ill patient. Detailed descriptions of patient perceptions of spiritual needs and preferences regarding related spiritual interventions are lacking as yet.

Evaluation

Successful patient and family responses to interventions are evidenced by the achievement of a relatively comfortable death in the setting and manner that they choose. The caregiver and patient (when appropriate) will be able to verbalize or demonstrate comfort measures individualized to identified needs.

CRITICAL THINKING QUESTIONS

1 Discuss trends in cancer incidence.
2 Describe the five differences between benign and malignant tumors.
3 Explain the cellular characteristics of a malignant cell.
4 What are the three events in carcinogenesis?
5 List six environmental risk factors for cancer.
6 Describe dietary modifications suggested to decrease the risk for cancer.
7 Explain how the immune system is believed to be a surveillance network against cancer cells.
8 Describe three potential mechanisms of metastasis.
9 What are some measures that can reduce an individual's risk for cancer?
10 What are the seven warning signals of cancer?
11 What are the three major goals of cancer treatment?
12 Discuss nursing considerations in the care of the patient undergoing brachytherapy.
13 Why is it important to give repeated doses of chemotherapy?
14 Describe the nursing implications of handling chemotherapeutic drugs.
15 What should be included in a patient-teaching plan regarding clinical trials?
16 Explain potential risk factors for infection in the cancer patient.
17 Explain how chemotherapy and radiation therapy can induce diarrhea.
18 List three categories of pain syndromes that occur in cancer patients.
19 What supportive care measures could be used to assist the patient in the diagnostic and treatment phase of disease?
20 What are potential obstacles to successful rehabilitation of the cancer patient?
21 What must be assessed when determining appropriateness of home treatment and care for the patient?
22 What nursing interventions could be used to provide comfort for the terminally ill patient?

RESOURCES

1 American Cancer Society (ACS) ACS sponsors numerous self-help support groups for patients and families, including: CanSurmount, I Can Cope, Reach to Recovery, The International Association of Laryngectomees
2 Cancer Information Clearinghouse, Office of Cancer Communications, National Cancer Institute Building 31, Room 10A18 Bethesda, MD 20205
3 Cancer Information Service 1-800-4-CANCER Alaska: 1-800-638-6070 Hawaii: (808) 524-1234 (in Oahu dial direct; call collect from surrounding islands)
4 The National Coalition for Cancer Survivorship 323 Eighth Street, Southwest Albuquerque, NM 87102
5 Make Today Count P.O. Box 222 Osage, MO 65065

BIBLIOGRAPHY

Current

1. American Cancer Society: *Cancer facts and figures*, Atlanta, 1992.
2. Balducci L et al: Pharmacology of antineoplastic agents in the elderly patient, *Semin Oncol* 16(1):76, 1989.
3. Blesch KS: The normal physiological changes of aging and their impact on the response to cancer treatment, *Semin Oncol Nurs* 4(3):178, 1988.
4. Boring CC, Squires TS, Tong T: Cancer statistics, *CA* 42(1):19, 1992.
5. Brown ML: Special report: the national economic burden of cancer: an update, *JNCI* 82:1811, 1990.
6. Bujorian GA: Clinical trials: patient issues in the decision-making process, *Oncol Nurs Forum* 15(6):779, 1988.
7. Byrd JC, Shapiro RS, Schiedermayer DL: Passive smoking: a review of medical and legal issues. *Am J Public Health* 79:209, 1989.
8. Cassileth BR, Brown H: Unorthodox cancer medicine, *CA* 38(3):176, 1988.

9. Clark JC, McGee RF, Preston R: Nursing management of responses to the cancer experience. In Clark JC, McGee RF, editors: *Core curriculum for oncology nursing,* ed 2, Philadelphia, 1992, WB Saunders.

10. Cotran RS, Kumar V, Robbins SL: *Robbins pathologic basis of disease,* ed 4, Philadelphia, 1989, WB Saunders.

11. Dachowski LJ, DeLaney TF: Photodynamic therapy: the NCI experience and its nursing implications, *Oncol Nurs Forum* 19(1):63, 1992.

12. DeVita VT: Principles of chemotherapy. In DeVita VT, Hellman S, Rosenberg SA, editors: *Cancer: principles and practice of oncology,* ed 3, vol 1, Philadelphia, 1989, JB Lippincott.

13. Dudjak L: Cancer metastasis, *Semin Oncol Nurs* 8(1):40, 1992.

14. Ershler WB, Yarbro JW: Introduction: geriatric oncology comes of age, *Semin Oncol* 16(1):1, 1989.

15. Fry RJM: Principles of carcinogenesis: physical. In DeVita VT, Hellman S, Sosenberg SA, editors: *Cancer: principles and practice of oncology,* ed 3, vol 1, Philadelphia, 1989, JB Lippincott.

16. Garfinkel L: Cancer statistics and trends. In Holleb AI, Fink DJ, Murphy GP: *American Cancer Society textbook of clinical oncology,* Atlanta, 1991, The Society.

17. Goodman MS: Concepts of hormonal manipulation in the treatment of cancer, *Oncol Nurs Forum* 15(5):639, 1988.

18. Goodman MS, Harte N: Breast cancer. In Groenwald SL et al, editors: *Cancer nursing: principles and practice,* ed 2, Boston, 1990, Jones & Bartlett.

19. Gray G et al: A clinical data base for advanced cancer patients: implications for nursing, *Cancer Nurs* 11(2):77, 1988.

20. Hilderly L: Radiotherapy. In Groenwald S et al, editors: *Cancer nursing: principles and practice,* ed 2, Boston, 1990, Jones & Bartlett.

21. Hogan CM: Sexual dysfunction related to disease process and treatment. In *Guidelines for oncology nursing practice,* ed 2, Philadelphia, 1991, WB Saunders.

22. Hood LE, Abernathy E: Biologic response modifiers. In Baird SB, McCorkle R, Grant M, editors: *Cancer nursing: a comprehensive textbook,* Philadelphia, 1991, WB Saunders.

23. Kane N: Implications of unproven methods for nursing. In Clark J, McGee R, editors: *Core curriculum for oncology nursing,* ed 2, Philadelphia, 1992, WB Saunders.

24. Lamb MA: Alterations in sexuality and sexual functioning. In Baird SB, McCorkle R, Grant M, editors: *Cancer nursing: a comprehensive textbook,* Philadelphia, 1991, WB Saunders.

25. Lewis F, Levita M: Understanding radiotherapy, *Cancer Nurs* 11(3):174, 1988.

26. Lind J: Tumor cell growth and cell kinetics, *Semin Oncol Nurs,* 8(1):3, 1992.

27. McMillan S: Carcinogenesis, *Semin Oncol Nurs* 8(1):10, 1992.

28. Mettlin C, Mirand AL: The causes of cancer. In Baird SB, McCorkle R, Grant M, editors: *Cancer nursing: a comprehensive textbook,* Philadelphia, 1991, WB Saunders.

29. Oncology Nursing Society: Cancer chemotherapy guidelines, Module II, Pittsburgh, 1988, The Society.

30. Patterson WB: Surgical issues in geriatric oncology, *Semin Oncol* 16(1):57, 1989.

31. Pitot HC: Principles of carcinogenesis: chemical. In DeVita VT, Hellman S, Rosenberg SA, editors: *Cancer: principles and practice of oncology,* ed 3, vol 1, Philadelphia, 1989, JB Lippincott.

32. Rosenberg SA: Principles of surgical oncology. In DeVita VT, Hellman S, Rosenberg SA, editors: *Cancer: principles and practice of oncology,* ed 3, vol 1, Philadelphia, 1989, JB Lippincott.

33. Safai B, Diaz B, Schwartz J: Malignant neoplasms associated with human immunodeficiency virus infection, *CA* 42(2):74, 1992.

34. Volker DL: Pathophysiology of cancer: In Clark JC, McGee RF, editors: *Core curriculum in oncology nursing,* ed 2, Philadelphia, 1992, WB Saunders.

35. Virji MA, Mercer DW, Heberman RB: Tumor markers in cancer diagnosis and prognosis, *CA* 38(2):104, 1988.

36. Waltman NL et al: Nutritional status, pressure sores, and mortality in elderly patients with cancer, *Oncol Nurs Forum* 18(5):867, 1991.

Classic

37. American Nurses' Association and Oncology Nursing Society: *Standards of oncology nursing practice,* Kansas City, Mo, 1987, The Association.

38. Austin C et al: Hospice home care pain management: four critical variables, *Cancer Nurs* 9(2):58, 1986.

39. Blot WJ, Fraumini JF: Cancer among shipyard workers. In Peto R, Schneiderman M, editors: Banbury report 9: quantification of occupational cancer, Cold Spring Harbor, NY, 1981, Cold Spring Harbor Laboratory.

40. Bonica JJ: Preface: a short course on the management of cancer pain, *J Pain Symptom Management* (suppl) 2(2), 1987.

41. Braunstein GD: Opinion: Pro—The benefits of estrogen therapy to the menopausal woman outweigh the risks of developing endometrial cancer, *CA* 34(4):210, 1984.

42. Clark JW, Longo DL: Biological response modifiers, *Mediguide to Oncol* 6(2):1, 1986.

43. Cockburn I: Assessment of the risks of malignancy and lymphoma developing in patients using Sandimmune, *Transplant Proc* 19(1):1804, 1987.

44. Fleming C, Scanlon C, D'Agostino N: A study of the comfort needs of patients with advanced cancer, *Cancer Nurs* 10(5):237, 1987.

45. Foley KM: Cancer pain syndromes, *J Pain Symptom Management* (suppl) 2(2):513, 1987.

46. Foley KM: Pain syndromes in patients with cancer. In Bonica JJ, Ventafridda V, editors: *Advances in pain research and therapy,* vol 2, New York, 1979, Raven Press.

47. Greenwald P, Sondik EJ, editors: *Cancer control objectives for the nation: 1985-2000,* NCI Monograph No. 2:1, 1986.

48. Gross J: Clinical research in cancer chemotherapy, *Oncol Nurs Forum* 13(1):59, 1986.

49. Hays JC: Patient symptoms and family coping: predictors of hospice utilization patterns, *Cancer Nurs* 9(6):317, 1986.

50. Highfield MF, Cason C: Spiritual needs of patients: are they recognized? *Cancer Nurs* 6(3):187, 1983.

51. Lamb MA, Woods NF: Sexuality and the cancer patient, *Cancer Nurs* 4(2):137, 1981.

52. Larson PJ: Important nurse caring behaviors perceived by patients with cancer, *Oncol Nurs Forum* 11(6):46, 1984.

53. Loken MK: Physicians' obligations in radiation issues, *JAMA* 258(5):673, 1987.

54. Mettler FA, Mosely RD: Medical effects of ionizing radiation, Orlando, Fla, 1985, Grune & Stratton.

55. Moore CL: Hyperthermia: a modern experiment in cancer treatment, *Oncol Nurs Forum* 11(2):31, 1984.

56. Morrow CP: Opinion: Con—The benefits of estrogen to

the menopausal women outweigh the risks of developing endometrial cancer, *CA* 34(4):220, 1984.

57. Norman C, Dickson D: The aftermath of Chernobyl, *Science* 233(4769):1141, 1986.

58. Page HS, Asire AJ: *Cancer rates and risks,* ed 3, Pub No 85-691, Washington, DC, 1985, National Institutes of Health.

59. Perez CA et al: Hyperthermia. In Perez CA, Brady LW, editors: *Principles and practice of radiation oncology,* Philadelphia, 1987, JB Lippincott.

60. Rhodes VA, Watson PA, Johnson MH: Patterns of nausea and vomiting in chemotherapy patients: a preliminary study, *Oncol Nurs Forum* 12(3):42, 1985.

61. Sell S: *Immunology, immunopathology, and immunity,* ed 4, New York, 1987, Elsevier Science Publishing Co.

62. Stetz KM: Caregiving demands during advanced cancer: the spouse's needs, *Cancer Nurs* 10(5):260, 1987.

63. Stewart DS: Indoor tanning: the nurse's role in preventing skin damage, *Cancer Nurs* 10(2):260, 1987.

64. Strome M: Childhood irradiation of pharyngeal lymphoid tissue: management considerations, *Otolaryngol Clin North Am* 20(2):377, 1987.

65. US Department of Labor, Office of Occupational Medicine: Occupational Safety and Health Administration: *Work practice guidelines for personnel dealing with cytotoxic (antineoplastic) drugs,* Pub No 8-1.1, Washington, DC, 1986.

66. Wegman J: Hospice home death, hospital death, and coping abilities of widows, *Cancer Nurs* 10(3):148, 1987.

CHAPTER SIXTEEN

Alterations in Nutrition

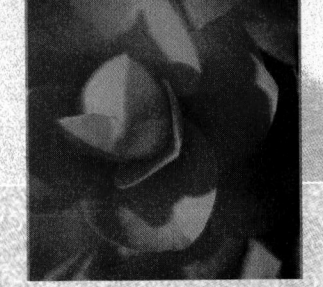

LEARNING OBJECTIVES

1 Identify individuals at risk for undernutrition.

2 Perform a basic nutrition assessment on any patient.

3 Compare and contrast nutrition support methods, including indications, administration, nursing care, and management of complications.

4 Recognize factors contributing to obesity and overweight.

5 State the health risks associated with obesity and overweight.

6 Describe medical, surgical, and behavioral approaches to the management of obesity.

7 Evaluate weight-loss programs according to the criteria provided in the chapter.

8 Describe nutritional assessment techniques that may be used in the elderly.

9 Discuss the food pyramid as it relates to the Dietary Guidelines for Americans.

10 Devise a teaching care plan for a patient with an alteration in nutrition.

KEY TERMS

MALNUTRITION, or alteration in nutritional status, occurs under several circumstances, including **undernutrition,** or inadequate nutrient balance; overweight and obesity, which result from excessive calorie intake; and eating disorders, which may be defined as bizarre behaviors and beliefs related to food and food intake. Primary malnutrition is the result of a poor diet. Secondary malnutrition may occur as the result of gastrointestinal obstruction, malabsorption syndromes, or medications.

UNDERNUTRITION
Definition

Protein-calorie malnutrition (PCM) is a form of undernutrition resulting from lack of protein and calories. There are two forms of PCM—marasmus and kwashiorkor. In **marasmus,** the deficiencies of protein and energy are approximately equal in severity. **Kwashiorkor,** however, is principally a protein deficiency. Individuals with marasmus are thin and obviously underfed, with wasting of the muscles and subcutaneous tissue. The effects of kwashiorkor are somewhat more subtle. Individuals with kwashiorkor have decreased protein synthesis, which is most easily detected by measuring levels of albumin and other serum proteins. Serum oncotic pressure diminishes because of the decrease in serum proteins, and edema is common. Because of this edema, individuals with kwashiorkor may not lose weight and may even appear plump, despite severe undernutrition. Although at first glance individuals with kwashiorkor look healthier than those with marasmus, kwashiorkor is at least as serious as marasmus. Kwashiorkor severely inhibits the body's ability to heal wounds or to make antibodies, lymphocytes, and other factors required for resisting infection.

Deficiencies of vitamins, minerals, trace elements, and essential fatty acids are another form of undernutrition. They rarely occur singly, but instead are found in combination with PCM and other vitamin and mineral deficiencies. The sources and roles of these nutrients are shown in Table 16-1.

Etiology

Although undernutrition, especially PCM, is commonly thought of as a problem of underdeveloped countries, it also occurs in the United States and other industrialized nations. It is most apt to occur under the following four conditions.

Poor diet

Poverty is a classic cause, particularly in the elderly. A variety of other causes—for example, limited income, multiple food allergies, numerous strong food dislikes, poor dentition, loneliness and apathy (e.g., in the elderly person living alone), and ignorance of nutritional needs—can limit diets excessively. Immobility may render an older individual unable to cook, as well as unable to go to the store to obtain food; lack of transportation has been listed as a major cause of poor diet in older adults. The anorexia, nausea, and vomiting often accompanying acute or chronic diseases (such as cancer and its therapies, acquired immune deficiency syndrome, chronic obstructive pulmonary disease, and renal or hepatic failure) may be severe enough to cause undernutrition. Alcohol may displace other, more nutritious

TABLE 16-1   Nutrient Sources and Roles

Nutrient	Best sources	Roles	Effects of deficiency
FAT-SOLUBLE VITAMINS			
Vitamin A (retinol)	Liver, kidney, fortified butter and margarine, dark green leafy vegetables, and yellow fruits and vegetables	Normal growth, development, and maintenance of epithelial tissues; production of rhodopsin (visual purple)	Night blindness; drying of cornea and blindness; rough, dry skin and poor skin healing; respiratory infections
Vitamin D (calciferol)	Skin exposure to sunlight, fortified milk and cereals, fish liver oil	Maintenance of normal calcium and phosphorus metabolism, formation of normal bones and teeth	Rickets (in children), osteomalacia (in adults)
Vitamin E (tocopherol)	Vegetable oils, green leafy vegetables, wheat germ, egg yolk, nuts	Antioxidant, protects unsaturated fatty acids and vitamin A from damage	Hemolytic anemia, neuromuscular disorders

TABLE 16-1 Nutrient Sources and Roles—cont'd

Nutrient	Best sources	Roles	Effects of deficiency
Vitamin K	Green vegetables, beef liver, vegetable oil; also synthesized by gut bacteria	Production of prothrombin, required for blood clotting	Prolonged bleeding

WATER-SOLUBLE VITAMINS

Nutrient	Best sources	Roles	Effects of deficiency
Vitamin B₁* (thiamin)	Pork, liver, legumes, whole grain and enriched breads and cereals	Carbohydrate metabolism	Berberi: fatigue, neuritis, cardiac failure, peripheral edema
Vitamin B₂* (riboflavin)	Milk and dairy products, organ meats, green leafy vegetables, enriched breads and cereals	Energy metabolism	Dermatitis, glossitis (inflamed tongue), cheilosis (cracking at corners of mouth)
Nicotinic acid* (niacin)	Meat, fish, poultry, whole grain and enriched breads and cereals	Energy metabolism	Pellagra: scaly dermatitis, especially in areas exposed to sun; diarrhea; confusion
Vitamin B₆* (pyridoxine)	Pork, wheat germ, milk, egg yolk, legumes, grains	Amino acid metabolism	Hypochromic, microcytic anemia; irritability; convulsions
Folic acid* (Folacin)	Green leafy vegetables, organ meats, legumes	Synthesis of nucleic acids, maturation of red blood cells	Glossitis; macrocytic (megaloblastic) anemia
Vitamin B₁₂* (cobalamin)	Organ meats, meat, milk and dairy products, eggs, brewer's yeast	Synthesis of nucleic acids, maturation of red blood cells, normal function of nervous tissue	Megaloblastic anemia; degeneration of the nervous system with ataxia and neuritis
Pantothenic acid*	All foods, especially eggs, organ meats, yeast	Energy metabolism	Cramps, vomiting, paresthesias
Biotin*	Organ meats, eggs, nuts, meat, fish, poultry, grains, milk, cheese, most vegetables	Energy and amino acid metabolism	Anorexia, dermatitis, hypercholesterolemia
Vitamin C (ascorbic acid)	Citrus fruit, melons, tomatoes, peppers, raw cabbage and pineapple, broccoli, greens, strawberries, potatoes	Production of collagen, promotion of iron absorption, maintenance of intercellular cement substance (promotes firm capillary walls), steroid hormone synthesis, conversion of folic acid to its active form	Scurvy: gingivitis, petechiae, ecchymoses, pains in extremities, poor wound healing, susceptibility to infection; iron deficiency anemia

MINERALS

Nutrient	Best sources	Roles	Effects of deficiency
Calcium	Milk and milk products, sardines, canned salmon, dark green leafy vegetables	Formation of bones and teeth; blood clotting; nerve and muscle function	Acute: tetany (paresthesias and muscle spasms) Chronic: rickets (children), osteoporosis (adults)

*B complex vitamin.

Continued.

TABLE 16-1   Nutrient Sources and Roles—cont'd

Nutrient	Best sources	Roles	Effects of deficiency
Phosphorus	Milk and milk products, meats, whole grains, nuts, legumes	Formation of bones, teeth, nucleic acids; buffer system	Tremor, ataxia, stupor, hemolytic anemia, anorexia, nausea, vomiting, decreased myocardial contractility
Magnesium	Whole grains, nuts, meat, milk, legumes	Formation of bones and teeth; muscle and nerve function	Tremors, convulsions, cardiac dysrhythmia

TRACE ELEMENTS†

Nutrient	Best sources	Roles	Effects of deficiency
Iron	Organ meats, legumes, whole grain or enriched breads and cereals, green leafy vegetables, molasses	Formation of hemoglobin and myoglobin; energy metabolism (cytochrome enzyme system)	Microcytic, hypochromic anemia; fatigue
Zinc	Shellfish, organ meats, meat, milk, legumes, whole grains, eggs	Component of more than 80 enzymes, including carbonic anhydrase, lactic dehydrogenase, and alkaline phosphatase; required for DNA synthesis	Diarrhea, dermatitis, impaired sense of taste, impaired wound healing
Copper	Liver, meat, fish, whole grains, legumes, chocolate, nuts	Component of many enzymes involved in development and maintenance of bone, CNS, hemoglobin synthesis, hair formation and pigmentation	Iron deficiency anemia, neutropenia, hypercholesterolemia
Iodine	Iodized salt, seafood, milk and milk products	Component of thyroxine (thyroid hormone)	Goiter: hypothyroidism, mental sluggishness, decreased metabolic rate
Manganese	Whole grains, legumes, fruits, tea	Protein, carbohydrate, and lipid metabolism	Poorly defined in humans; ataxia, sterility in animals
Molybdenum	Organ meats, pork and lamb, whole grains, legumes	Conversion of purines to uric acid, metabolism of sulfur-containing amino acids	Tachycardia, tachypnea, lethargy, convulsions, central scotomas (blind spots)
Selenium	Organ meat, meat, fish, poultry, molasses, grains	Antioxidant (interacts with vitamin E)	Congestive heart failure, dysrhythmias
Fluorine	Fluoridated water, fish, meat, chicken, tea, eggs	Formation and maintenance of bones and teeth	Dental caries, perhaps accelerated osteoporosis
Chromium	Coffee, nuts, cheese, whole grains	Normal glucose metabolism	Impaired glucose tolerance

LIPIDS

Nutrient	Best sources	Roles	Effects of deficiency
Essential fatty acids (linoleic and linolenic acids)	Fats, vegetable oils (especially safflower, sunflower, corn, soy, cottonseed), and fish oils	Maintenance of integrity of cell membranes; precursors of prostaglandins, prostacyclins, and thromboxanes	Dry, scaly skin; alopecia; thrombocytopenia; delayed wound healing

†Only a few milligrams or micrograms needed per day.

foods in the diet. Also, food fads and exaggerated beliefs about foods (e.g., belief that certain foods will prevent or cure disease, certain foods are harmful, only "natural" foods should be eaten, and specific food combinations will "burn fat") have been known to cause undernutrition.

Inability to assimilate food ingested

Maldigestion and malabsorption accompany many acute and chronic medical and surgical conditions. Inflammatory bowel disease, radiation enteritis, scleroderma affecting the small bowel, and extensive intestinal resection (short bowel syndrome) limit the amount of intestinal surface available for nutrient absorption. In chronic diarrhea, transit time through the bowel may be so short that absorption is incomplete. Insufficient digestive enzymes are released in diseases such as cystic fibrosis and chronic pancreatitis, and cirrhosis of the liver can cause inadequate production of bile salts.

Because fat (triglyceride) digestion and absorption are complex, they are especially likely to be impaired during illness. For fat digestion to proceed normally, bile salts, which are detergent molecules soluble in both water and fat, must surround the fat, forming micelles. Micelles help make fat miscible in the watery environment inside the gastrointestinal (GI) tract and break larger fat globules into smaller ones, thereby increasing the surface area and making it easier for enzymes to attack the triglycerides. Specific enzymes called lipases are required to hydrolyze triglycerides before they can be absorbed. The pancreas is the most important source of lipases in adults. Therefore defects in production of bile salts or pancreatic enzymes tend to reduce fat absorption. Furthermore, most fat absorption occurs in the ileum, so that ileal resection also impedes fat absorption. Malabsorption of fat (steatorrhea) not only causes loss of calories, but also loss of the fat-soluble vitamins A, D, E, and K, which are dissolved in the fat, and loss of minerals and trace elements such as calcium, magnesium, and zinc, which are trapped in the fat as soaps.

Physical stress

Stressors that increase metabolic rate and nutritional requirements include infection, trauma, surgery, and burns. Infection elevates protein requirements as the body accelerates production of immunoglobulins, leukocytes, and complement. Fever has a major impact on the metabolic rate; caloric needs increase by approximately 12% for each elevation in temperature of 1° C (or 7% for each 1° F). Trauma, surgery, and burns increase needs for protein, calories, zinc, and vitamin C for healing. Burn damage to the integument predisposes the patient to infection and increases loss of body heat, further increasing caloric expenditure. Some neoplasms have also been noted to elevate metabolic rate; thus the tumor may grow at the expense of the host, who experiences wasting and protein depletion. Furthermore, some medications, notably corticosteroids, promote catabolism and increase protein needs.

Abnormal nutrient losses

A variety of conditions are associated with nutrient losses. Fistulas and draining wounds, including decubitus ulcers, cause losses of protein, zinc, and fluid. After being burned, the damaged integument allows leakage of serum and the proteins it contains. Losses include not only proteins, but also zinc and other trace minerals that are bound to the proteins. Massive loss of protein may occur in nephrotic syndrome and protein-losing enteropathy.

Epidemiology

Surveys of hospitalized patients have revealed that 12% to 48% have signs of undernutrition at the time of admission.[35,57,66] Furthermore, nutritional status of more than two thirds of medical patients staying in a major teaching hospital for 2 weeks or longer was noted to deteriorate during hospitalization.[66] A reevaluation of hospital malnutrition 12 years later indicates that the identification of patients with malnutrition has improved.[12] Deteriorating nutritional status may have been related to the seriousness of the patients' diseases, because the patients who are most ill are usually referred to teaching hospitals. Other possible contributing factors include lack of communication among the nurses, physicians, and dietitians responsible for the care of these patients; frequent diagnostic testing that caused patients to miss meals or to be too exhausted for meals; medications and other therapies that caused anorexia, nausea, or vomiting and thus interfered with food intake; or inadequate use of tube feedings or total parenteral nutrition (delivery of all nutrients by vein, also known as TPN) to maintain the nutritional status of these patients. With the current emphasis on home care and early discharge of patients from the hospital, it can be anticipated that undernutrition will increase in prevalence among home-care patients.

Pathophysiology

When protein and calorie intake are inadequate for more than a few hours, existing body proteins will be broken down to meet the body's needs. Even when the individual has large fat reserves, catabolism of body proteins will occur. Unlike fat, proteins provide the amino acids that are needed for tissue synthesis and repair, and also serve as a significant source of glucose, which is required for the metabolism of erythrocytes and, over the short term, the central nervous system. The well-nourished individual can tolerate a few days of starvation well when not exposed to stress, but a patient who experiences trauma, surgery, burns, or infection, along with inadequate nutritional intake, will have accelerated catabolism. The previously undernourished patient exposed to stress (for example, a cancer patient with anorexia and weight loss who undergoes surgery) is especially vulnerable.

The skeletal muscles represent a large pool of amino acids, and consequently muscle wasting usually accompanies prolonged undernutrition. Muscle wasting is a serious problem in undernutrition; it may, for example, affect the intercostal muscles and diaphragm, interfering with the ability to breathe deeply and cough effectively after surgery, and thus contribute to pneumonia. However, loss of "visceral" proteins, which include the blood cells and serum proteins, is even more serious than loss of muscle proteins. Erythrocytes are necessary for transporting oxygen to all body tissues, leukocytes are involved in resisting infection, and serum proteins such as albumin and globulins are necessary for both transporting nutrients to the body tissues and resisting infection. Furthermore, serum proteins are essential for maintaining the blood's oncotic pressure. Low levels of serum proteins result in edema and impaired circulation. Undernourished hospitalized patients usually have a combination of kwashiorkor and marasmus, with wasting of muscle and subcutaneous fat, as well as decreases in visceral proteins.

Undernutrition is an ominous finding among critically ill patients. Undernourished patients are three times more likely to experience major surgical complications than well-nourished ones.[57] Wound dehiscence, decubitus ulcers, sepsis, and pulmonary infections are more common among the undernourished.[34,57] Immunosuppression resulting from undernutrition makes the patient especially vulnerable to secondary infections. Hospital stays of medical patients with evidence of undernutrition are approximately two-thirds longer than those of well-nourished patients, and mortality is 3 times greater.[66] Moreover, undernutrition contributes to **inanition,** a state of exhaustion resulting from nutritional depletion. This impairs the patient's ability to participate in self-care, plan for the future, and tolerate or remember patient teaching.

Clinical Manifestations

Common physical findings that are characteristic of undernutrition are listed in Table 16-2. In addition, there are a number of normal changes that occur as a result of aging that have an impact on the nutri-

tional status of the elderly. The greatest impact is demonstrated by changes in the gastrointestinal tract. Changes in the smooth muscle of the esophagus and diminished function in the esophageal sphincter lead to decreased esophageal motility and cause problems in swallowing high-bulk foods. There is decreased intestinal blood flow and diminished liver size, as well as decreased contractile function of intestinal smooth muscle. The resulting impairment of intestinal metabolism and absorption and impairment of liver metabolism often leads to malnutrition, probably subclinical, and at times constipation. Last, the diminished secretion of HCl (hypochlorhydria) can lead to a defective absorption of nutrients, such as calcium, as well as iron. Pernicious anemia, as well as iron deficiency anemias and osteoporosis, can be directly related.[8]

Therapeutic Management

Drug therapy

Individuals with severe anorexia resulting from chronic illness may benefit from using appetite stimulants, such as cyproheptadine, but pharmacologic therapy alone is usually insufficient to correct most cases of undernutrition. Where undernutrition accompanies serious medical or psychologic illness, correction of the underlying illness, if possible, is an important step in alleviating nutritional problems. Unfortunately, in many cases it is not possible to resolve underlying illnesses completely. Moreover, the patient may be so malnourished that it is dangerous to wait for the disease to respond to therapy before seeing improvement in nutritional status. Also, wound healing and recovery from illness is likely to be delayed in the malnourished person.

Enteral nutrition support

A form of nutritional care known as nutrition support is necessary in moderate to severe undernutrition. **Nutrition support** refers to provision of specially formulated or delivered intravenous (IV) or enteral nutrients to prevent or treat malnutrition.[3]

The GI tract is the preferred route for feedings whenever possible, because enteral feedings are more physiologic than IV feedings. Furthermore, enteral feedings are much more economical, and they are less likely to be associated with serious complications. Enteral nutrition support may be delivered either via mouth or enteral tube feedings.

Oral feedings and supplements
The oral route is preferred for feeding all patients. A diet of ordinary foods is the least expensive way of providing oral nutrition, as well as the most acceptable feeding method to most patients.

TABLE 16-2   Clinical Manifestations of Undernutrition

Area of concern	Possible deficiency	Area of concern	Possible deficiency
HEAD AND NECK		SKIN	
Dull, dry, brittle, easily plucked hair	Protein	Dry, scaly	Vitamin A, zinc, essential fatty acids
Hair loss (alopecia)	Protein, zinc, biotin	Follicular hyperkeratosis (resembles gooseflesh)	Vitamin A
Thyroid enlargement	Iodine	Eczematous lesions	Zinc
EYES		Petechiae, ecchymoses	Vitamin C, vitamin K
Scleral and corneal dryness (xerosis)	Vitamin A	Nasolabial seborrhea (greasy, scaly areas between nose and upper lip)	Nicotinic acid, vitamin B_2, vitamin B_6
Pale conjunctiva or blue sclerae	Iron	Poor wound healing	Protein, zinc, vitamin C
Corneal vascularization	Vitamin B_2	CIRCULATORY SYSTEM	
MOUTH		Tachycardia, heart failure	Vitamin B_1
Cheilosis or angular stomatitis (lesions at the corners of the mouth)	Vitamin B_2	Dysrhythmia	Magnesium, potassium, selenium
Glossitis (red, sore tongue)	Nicotinic acid, folic acid, vitamin B_{12}, other B vitamins	ABDOMEN	
		Hepatomegaly	Protein
Gingivitis (inflamed gums)	Vitamin C	NEUROLOGIC SYSTEM	
Hypogeusia, dysgeusia (diminished sense of taste, foul taste)	Zinc	Paresthesias (pain and tingling or altered sensation in the extremities)	Vitamin B_1, vitamin B_6, vitamin B_{12}, biotin
Dental caries	Fluorine	Weakness	Vitamin C, vitamin B_1, vitamin B_6, vitamin B_{12}, calories
Atrophy of papillae of tongue	Iron, B vitamins		
MUSCULOSKELETAL SYSTEM, EXTREMITIES		Ataxia	Vitamin B_1, vitamin B_{12}
Muscle wasting	Calories	Tremor	Magnesium
Edema	Protein, vitamin B_1	Decreased tendon reflexes	Vitamin B_1
Bone tenderness	Vitamin D, calcium, phosphorus	Confabulation, disorientation	Vitamin B_1

The Dietary Guidelines for Americans developed by the U.S. Department of Agriculture and Health and Human Services are guidelines to stay healthy. The dietary guidelines are:

- Eat a variety of foods.
- Maintain a healthy weight.
- Choose a diet low in fat, saturated fat, and cholesterol.
- Choose a diet with plenty of vegetables, fruits, and grain products.
- Use sugars only in moderation.
- If you drink alcoholic beverages, do so in moderation.

The Food Guide Pyramid (see Figure 16-1) may be used to help patients put the Dietary Guidelines into practice. The grain, cereal, and pasta group forms the base of the pyramid. The next level includes the vegetable group and the fruit group. The third level is the meat group and milk group. At the apex of the pyramid are fat, oils, and sweets, which should be used sparingly.

However, some patients who are able to eat have difficulty consuming enough food. A variety of "defined formula diets" are available to supplement or replace meals for patients with inadequate intake from ordinary foods. Patients with mild to moderate anorexia and those with small to moderate increases in calorie and protein needs, such as patients with burns of less than 20% of the body surface area, are examples of those who may benefit from defined formula diets as supplements.

Defined formula diets have a known composition and are usually liquid; some can be used for both oral and tube feeding. Defined formula diets may

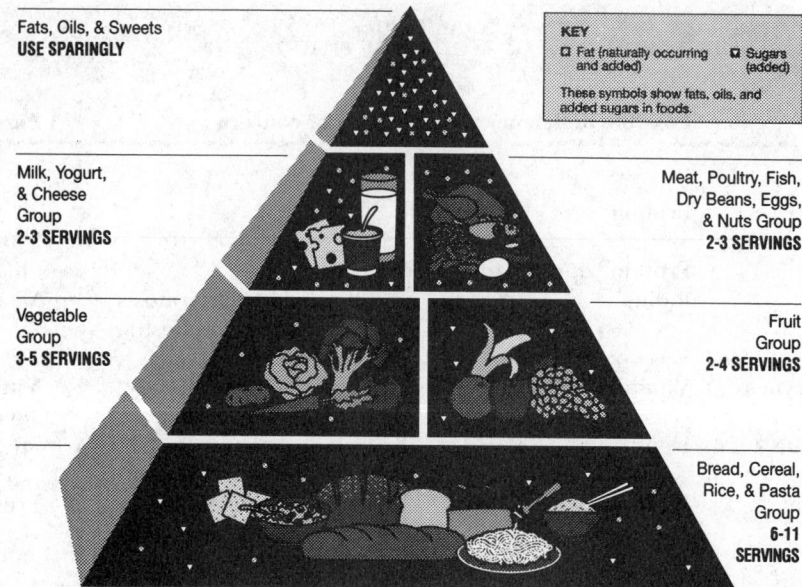

FIGURE 16-1 Food guide pyramid: a guide to daily food choices. (From U.S. Department of Agriculture/U.S. Department of Health and Human Services.)

contain "polymeric" ingredients, which require normal digestive and absorptive ability, or they may be "elemental" (predigested). The major differences between the two types of defined formula diets are their protein and fat composition. The **polymeric formulas** contain unmodified protein, such as soy, milk, or egg white protein. **Elemental formulas** contain amino acids, protein hydrolysates, or peptides (products of protein hydrolysis). The fat source in polymeric products is usually a vegetable oil that contains mostly long-chain triglycerides (LCTs). In contrast, elemental formulas are either low in fat or high in medium-chain triglycerides (MCTs), which are more readily digested and absorbed than LCTs. (The fatty acids in LCTs are longer than 12 carbons, whereas those in MCTs are 8 to 12 carbons in length.) LCTs are suitable for most people with functional GI tracts. MCTs are more easily absorbed than LCTs, and are better suited for people with diminished bile salt or lipase production or those with reduced absorptive area.

Many healthy adults, particularly blacks, native Americans, and Asians, have a deficiency of lactase, the enzyme required to digest lactose. Furthermore, lactase activity is diminished in many disease states, such as radiation enteritis, gastroenteritis, and Crohn's disease. When lactase deficiency is present, lactose ingestion results in abdominal cramping, bloating, and diarrhea. Because of the prevalence of lactase deficiency, almost all defined formula diets are made without lactose. Both polymeric and elemental formulas contain the same carbohydrates usually glucose oligosaccharides (also known as glu-

cose polymers, dextrins, and corn syrup solids, all of which consist of short chains of glucose molecules) and sucrose (table sugar). Table 16-3 lists the types of defined formula diets and their uses.

In addition to the complete defined formula diets, "modular" components or ingredients can be added to foods and beverages and used to prepare liquid supplements and tube feedings. Both carbohydrate and lipid modules are used primarily as calorie supplements. Modular protein and amino acid components are also available to increase the protein content of feedings.

Although oral feedings are the most economical and convenient form of nutrition support and are associated with few complications, they require that the patient be highly motivated and cooperative. Patients with severe anorexia, nausea, or vomiting often fail to consume enough by the oral route, no matter how tasty the food or supplements. Oral supplements can become monotonous, especially if the same product is used continually. Also, elemental formulas are usually unpalatable. Virtually all patients needing these formulas find it impossible to drink enough of them to meet their nutritional needs.

Enteral tube feedings
Enteral tube feedings are used for patients who cannot or will not consume adequate amounts of food by mouth and yet have at least some ability to digest and absorb nutrients. These include patients with severe anorexia, those with malabsorption as a result of pancreatic insufficiency or short bowel

TABLE 16-3   Defined Formula Diets for Enteral Feedings

Formula type	Nutritional problem	Clinical examples	Representative formulas
Complete diet with intact protein and LCT; some contain lactose, some do not	Inability to ingest food Inability to ingest enough food to meet needs	Oral or esophageal cancer Coma Anorexia nervosa Anorexia of chronic illness Trauma and burns	Blended food Compleat; Resource*; Meritene* (Sandoz) Ensure; Enrich; Osmolite (Ross) Isocal; Sustacal (Mead Johnson) Entrition (Biosearch) Travasorb Liquid (Travenol) Instant Breakfast*† (Carnation)
Elemental or "predigested" diet with amino acids and peptides, MCT or minimal fat, no lactose, unpalatable	Impaired digestion and/or absorption	Pancreatitis Cystic fibrosis Inflammatory bowel disease Short bowel syndrome Radiation enteritis	Criticare HN (Mead Johnson) Vital (Ross) Vivonex T.E.N. (Norwich Eaton) Travasorb HN (Travenol) Reabilan (O'Brien)
Specialized diets containing altered proportions of amino acids, no lactose, usually unpalatable	Impaired excretion of nitrogen waste products	Renal failure	Amin-Aid (Kendall McGaw) Travasorb Renal (Travenol) NEPRO (Ross)
	Impaired metabolism of aromatic amino acids	Hepatic failure	Hepatic-Aid II (Kendall McGaw); Travasorb Hepatic (Travenol)
	Increased use of branched-chain amino acids for energy	Trauma	Stresstein (Sandoz) TraumaCal (Mead Johnson) Traum-Aid HBC (Kendall McGaw)
	High fat, low carbohydrate—decreases CO_2 production and respiratory quotient	Pulmonary	Pulmocare (Ross)
Same as any of the above, with more than 1 kcal/mL	Same as any of the above, with need for fluid restriction	Congestive heart failure Inappropriate antidiuretic hormone secretion	Magnacal (Biosearch) Isocal HCN (Mead Johnson) TwoCal HN (Ross) Nutrisource Modular System (Sandoz)

*Ordinarily for oral consumption only.
†Contains lactose.

syndrome (with at least 10% of the small intestine remaining), and those with major stress who simply cannot eat enough to meet their needs. It has become increasingly common to support the nutrition of ailing older persons with oral nutrient-rich supplements or tube feedings.

The tube feeding route may be either intragastric or transpyloric (directly into the small bowel). Intragastric feedings are given by nasogastric (NG) or gastrostomy tube (Figure 16-2). These tubes permit the use of almost the entire GI tract for digestion and absorption, but they are associated with increased potential for pulmonary aspiration, in comparison with transpyloric tubes.[31] NG tubes are easy to insert and are inexpensive, but the proximal end is visible and is not aesthetically pleasing; furthermore, they are easy to dislodge. In contrast, gastrostomy tubes are not easily dislodged, are hidden by cloth-

ing, and are able to bypass esophageal obstruction. They are usually larger in diameter than NG, nasoduodenal (ND), or nasojejunal (NJ) tubes, thus allowing the use of thicker, more viscous formulas, such as those prepared from blended foods. However, they may allow leakage of gastric juices around the tube, thus eroding the skin.

Transpyloric feedings may be given by ND, NJ, or jejunostomy tubes. These tubes tend to reduce the likelihood of gastroesophageal reflux and pulmonary aspiration. However, they bypass the stomach and its acidity, an important antiinfective barrier. Moreover, continuous feedings are almost always necessary when given via the transpyloric route, because the small bowel tolerates rapid infusion of formula poorly. Continuous feedings may be more inconvenient, especially for the home-care patient, and they often necessitate a feeding pump, thus increasing ex-

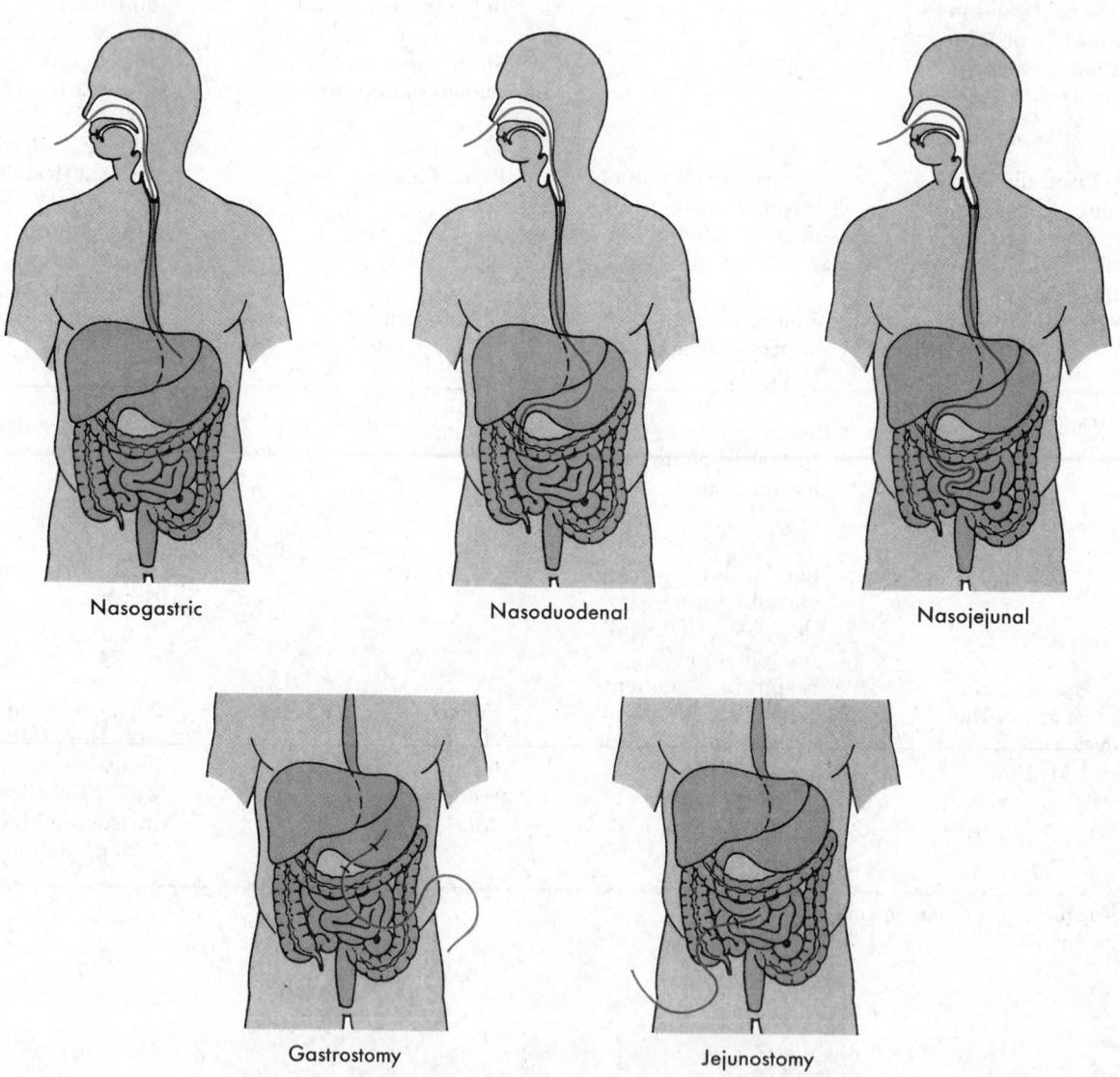

Nasogastric

Nasoduodenal

Nasojejunal

Gastrostomy

Jejunostomy

FIGURE 16-2   Tube feeding routes.

penses. ND and NJ tubes, like NG tubes, are easily dislodged and are readily visible. Their distal ends often become refluxed into the stomach, causing them to become NG tubes. In contrast, jejunostomy tubes are not easily dislodged, are hidden by clothing, and allow bypass of an upper GI obstruction or gastroparesis.

If the duration of feedings is to be only a few weeks, nasoenteral tubes are usually used. If feedings are required for long periods of time, a percutaneous endoscopic gastrostomy (PEG) is preferred over surgical gastrotomies because of lower cost and decreased morbidity. PEG tubes are inserted through the esophagus into the stomach with the aid of an endoscope and there pulled through a stab wound made in the abdominal wall (Figure 16-3). General anesthesia is not required for PEG placement; usually a parenteral sedative is used. PEGs are sometimes performed on an outpatient basis.

A new procedure for long-term feeding into the small bowel is the direct endoscopic jejunostomy

(DEJ). DEJ is not used widely at the present time.[16,40]

The type of formula used is dictated primarily by the patient's need. Individuals with normal digestion, absorption, and metabolism can use polymeric formulas, including blended foodstuffs. Those with impaired digestion, absorption, or metabolism of nutrients require commercial elemental formulas that are tailored to meet their needs (Table 16-3). Many clinicians feel that patients experience less diarrhea if formula **osmolality** (the concentration, which is determined by the number of particles in the solution) is approximately equal to that of blood, or about 300 mOsm/kg. Some formulas, especially the elemental ones, are hypertonic or hyperosmolar, with osmolalities well above 300 mOsm/kg.

The fluid status of patients receiving these formulas should be monitored, especially those who are unable to consume water ad lib or who have increased water requirements. Recent evidence indicates that tube feedings should not be diluted, but

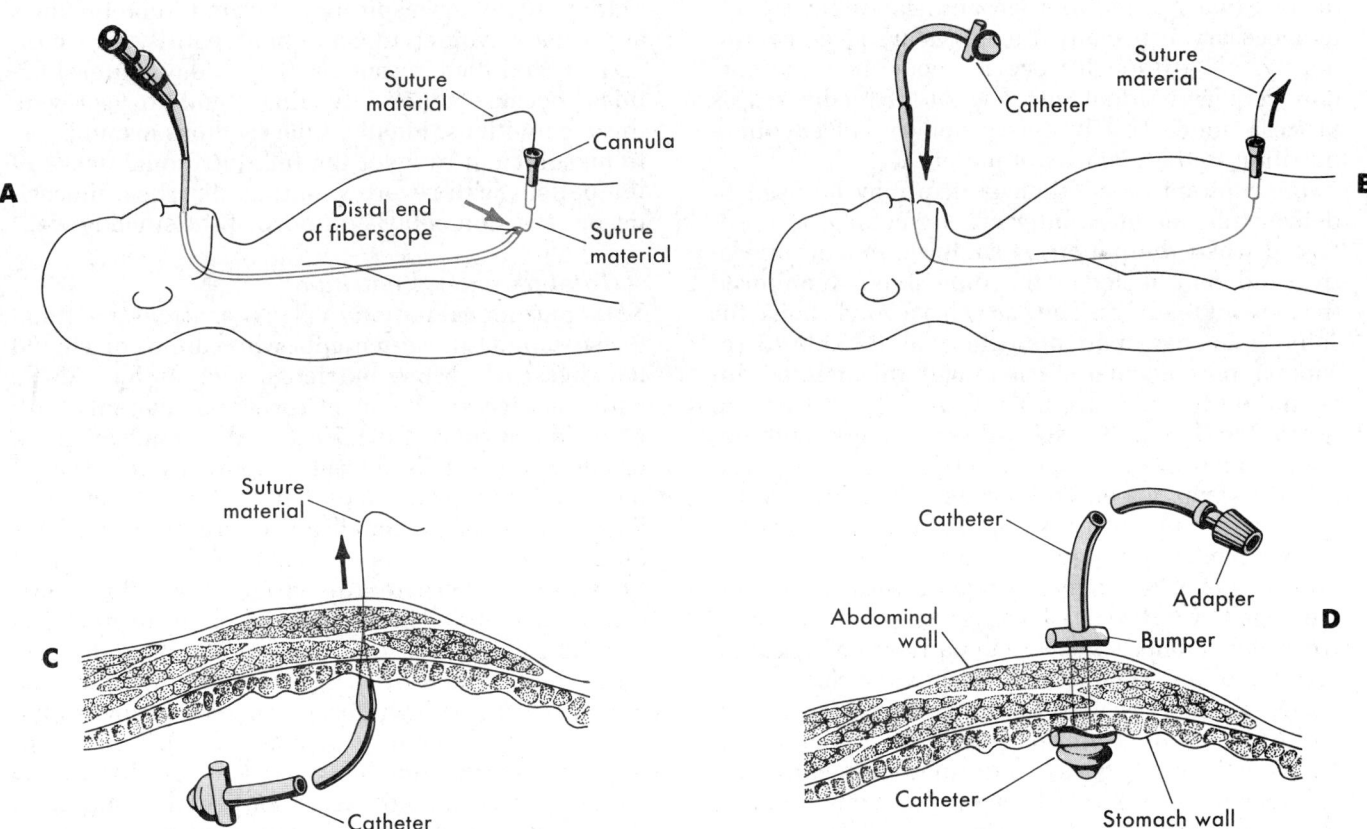

FIGURE 16-3   Ponsky-Gauderer technique for PEG placement. **A,** Anesthetized anterior abdominal wall is penetrated by cannula; suture material is grasped and drawn into the stomach and esophagus via endoscope. **B,** Gastrostomy tube assembly is attached to suture at oral end. **C,** Suture with attached gastrostomy tube is withdrawn through abdominal wall. **D,** External bumper is positioned on skin and capped adapter is attached to tube.

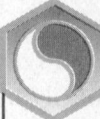

ETHICAL ISSUES

- Because feeding is traditionally part of the cultural meaning of nursing, should nurses have the primary role in making decisions about nutrition support?
- How should a decision be reached, and by whom, regarding removal of a NG tube in an unconscious elderly patient who is not dying, but whose family feels should be allowed the dignity of a natural death, without artificial means of nutrition?
- Is there a morally relevant difference between foregoing artificial nutrition and hydration and foregoing ventilatory support or CPR?

started full strength, gradually increasing the rate. In geriatric patients receiving tube feeding, fluid balance should be monitored since the incidence of dehydration is high.[10,38] However, recent evidence indicates that routine dilution and slow delivery are unnecessary, especially if feedings are given continuously.[29,58] Although very malnourished patients may require gradual introduction of feedings, this process unnecessarily delays delivery of adequate nutrition to the majority of patients.

Intermittent or continuous drip may be used to deliver tube feedings. Intermittent feedings are preferred when the patient is confused or uncooperative and may dislodge the tube if not monitored throughout feedings. They are also a good choice for some home-care patients, who may be able to resume a more normal life-style with this method. Intermittent feedings are usually given by gravity drip over 20 to 30 minutes several times a day. Continuous feedings are used when nutrients are delivered into the small bowel. They are less likely than intermittent feedings to cause discomfort and diarrhea during duodenal or jejunal feedings, thus delivery of nutrients is usually more adequate with continuous feedings.[16] Continuous feedings are also preferred when the patient has severe impairment of digestion or absorption. When the absorptive surface is reduced, as in short bowel syndrome, or its integrity and function are compromised, as in radiation enteritis or Crohn's disease, intermittent feedings are unlikely to be tolerated, and continuous feedings may avert the need for permanent TPN. Even in stressed patients who would be expected to have normal absorptive capacity, such as those with major burns, continuous delivery of nutrients has been shown to decrease diarrhea and permit delivery of larger volumes of formula than intermittent feedings.[29] Continuous feedings may be given through-

out the day or during some portion of the day, such as over 12 to 14 hours at night. Delivery of feedings at night interferes as little as possible with daily activities, an important consideration for the long-term home-care patient. In addition, nocturnal feedings may not depress the appetite as much as feedings given around the clock; this encourages oral intake in patients whose tube feedings are used only as an adjunct to oral feedings. Sometimes continuous feedings can be delivered by gravity drip, but in many instances this results in too irregular a delivery rate. Usually the patient needs a pump to regulate the feedings. Small, lightweight enteral feeding pumps that interfere only slightly with patient mobility have been developed for this purpose. Enteral pumps are less expensive than IV pumps and are easy to operate, making them well suited for both home and hospital use.

Although tube feedings are preferable to TPN whenever possible, they do have limitations. First, tube feedings cannot be used in patients with ileus or severe GI hypomotility, because these patients are unable to absorb the feedings and are likely to have gastroesophageal reflux or vomiting with potential pulmonary aspiration. Second, tube feedings are usually avoided in acute pancreatitis, severe diarrhea, and high-output (>500 mL/day) enteral fistulas, because enteral feedings tend to aggravate these conditions. Finally, tube feedings are unlikely to be sufficient to meet the full nutritional needs of the patient with severe vomiting, diarrhea, mucositis, or resection of 90% or more of the small bowel.[4]

Total parenteral nutrition

Total parenteral nutrition (TPN) provides a method for sustaining those patients who cannot or should not digest or absorb nutrients, such as individuals with massive small bowel resection. Patients with resection of more than 70% of the small intestine usually require TPN at least temporarily until the remaining bowel can adapt. Those with resection of 80% to 90% of the small bowel often require TPN on a permanent basis to sustain life. Other conditions that may create a need for TPN include serious abnormalities of GI motility or absorption (including collagen vascular diseases, Crohn's disease, and radiation enteritis), severe vomiting and diarrhea (such as in high-dosage chemotherapy, radiation, and bone marrow transplantation), severe pancreatitis (enteral feedings worsen the disease by stimulating pancreatic secretion), enterocutaneous fistulae (bowel rest may allow healing of fistulae without surgical intervention), and any condition where it is anticipated that the patient may not be able to tolerate enteral feedings for 7 days or longer.

TPN consists of a solution of amino acids, glucose (dextrose), minerals, trace elements, and vitamins. Patients receiving TPN are subject to a variety of metabolic and nutritional abnormalities. Hyperglycemia and excesses or deficits of sodium, potassium, calcium, phosphorus, magnesium, and trace elements are among the common problems associated with TPN.

TPN can be delivered either through a peripheral or a central vein, such as the subclavian or jugular. As with other peripheral IVs, mechanical complications of peripheral TPN are relatively minor, with the most common being peripheral venous thrombosis. However, use of peripheral TPN requires adequate peripheral venous access; thus it may not be suitable for prolonged use or for those patients who have already had considerable IV therapy. The concentration of glucose in peripheral TPN is limited to 10% to 15%. In contrast, in the central veins with their high blood flow, glucose concentrations of 25% to 35% can be used.

There are significant risks associated with central venous catheters, including catheter-related sepsis (bacterial or fungal); localized infection along the catheter tract through the skin and subcutaneous tissues; pneumothorax or hemothorax resulting from damage to the pleura during placement; air embolus; and subclavian thrombosis. However, the catheter provides reliable venous access, and central venous TPN has been a life-saving therapy for many patients. A central venous catheter is shown in Figure 16-4.

To make IV feedings complete, lipid emulsions are also administered to patients receiving TPN. Lipids, which are isotonic, may be infused via peripheral or central veins. They are usually "piggybacked" with a Y-connector into the TPN line below the level of the in-line filter because the lipid particles are too large to allow for filtration, but lipids are sometimes added directly to the glucose—amino acid TPN solutions, rather than piggybacking the two. Adding lipids to TPN solutions decreases nursing time required for delivery of TPN and makes administration easier for patients receiving treatment at home. Lipids are given daily during peripheral TPN, because the restriction of glucose concentration in the TPN necessitates the patient have additional calories, which the lipid can provide. During central TPN, lipids may be given only once or twice per week to provide essential fatty acids, or they may be given daily to supplement glucose as a calorie source. Excessive carbohydrate intake raises the patient's respiratory quotient, which is the amount of carbon dioxide produced in comparison with the amount of oxygen consumed. The need to rid the body of large amounts of carbon dioxide can produce tachypnea and shortness of breath in the stressed patient, and it can prevent the ventilator-dependent patient from being weaned successfully. Therefore the current trend is to use lipid emulsions to provide approximately one third to one half of the nonprotein calories, even in the patient receiving central venous TPN.

NURSING MANAGEMENT OF THE PATIENT WITH UNDERNUTRITION

A team approach is the most successful means of delivering nutrition support.[30] Patients cared for by a nutrition support team have fewer complications and are more likely to receive the nutrients they require than patients not managed in this way. Most nutrition support teams consist of one or more physicians, nurses, dietitians, and pharmacists. The team may solicit the services of social workers, psychologists, dentists, and others to meet the needs of the individual patient. The team as a whole, or individual members of the team, collect information from the patient, family, and medical record and perform a nutrition assessment. From this information, the team plans the patient's nutrition care, including goals of therapy, calculated nutritional needs, and route of delivery of nutrients. The team evaluates the care continually and updates the plan as needed. The nurse, as the team member with the most patient contact, is an integral part of all phases of nutrition support.

Assessment

Diagnosis of undernutrition, determination of its severity, and evaluation of patient progress toward nutritional goals can be difficult, because there is no

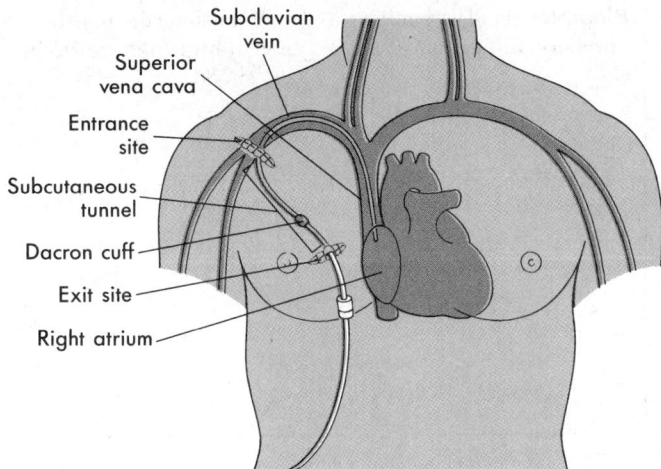

FIGURE 16-4 The Hickman central venous catheter. After distal end of catheter is threaded through subclavian vein and into right atrium, proximal end is tunneled under subcutaneous tissue to increase catheter stability. A Dacron cuff on proximal portion of catheter provides a roughened surface, which encourages subcutaneous tissue to adhere to catheter and further secure it.

TABLE 16-4   Nutrition Assessment Summary

Area of evaluation	Characteristics or causes of undernutrition	Laboratory test	Undesirable finding
PHYSICAL AND ANTHROPOMETRIC DATA		**INDICATORS OF PROTEIN NOURISHMENT**	
Body weight*	Weight <85% of ideal for height	Serum albumin	<3.5 g/dL
Weight loss*	Weight <90% of usual, especially if loss occurred in <6 months	Serum transferrin	<170 mg/dL
		Serum prealbumin	<20 mg/dL
		Nitrogen balance‡	<0
Triceps skinfold	<8 mm in men, <18 mm in women	Urine creatinine excretion	<23 mg/kg ideal body weight in men, <17 mg/kg ideal body weight in women
Clinical manifestations of undernutrition*	Any sign or symptom from Table 16-2 that cannot be explained by other causes	Total lymphocyte count (TLC)§	<1200/mm^3
NUTRITION HISTORY DATA		**INDICATORS OF VITAMIN AND MINERAL NOURISHMENT**	
Inadequate nutrient intake*	Alcoholism, anorexia, dysphagia, limited diet (avoidance of food groups† because of food aversions, inadequate nutrition knowledge), poor dentition, elderly, depression, poverty, coma	Hemoglobin (Hgb)	<14 g/dL in men, <12 g/dL in women (iron deficiency)
		Hematocrit (Hct)	<42% in men, <37% in women (iron deficiency)
		Mean corpuscular volume (MCV)	<80 μm^3 (iron deficiency, "microcytic" anemia); >95 μm^3 (folic acid or vitamin B$_{12}$ deficiency, "macrocytic" anemia)
Excessive nutrient losses or failure to absorb nutrients*	Vomiting, diarrhea, fistula, draining wound, nephrosis (proteinuria), protein-losing enteropathy, intestinal or pancreatic disease causing maldigestion or malabsorption, inflammatory bowel disease, cystic fibrosis, radiation enteritis, pancreatitis, extensive intestinal resection	Mean corpuscular hemoglobin (MCH)	<27 pg (iron deficiency); >31 pg (folic acid or vitamin B$_{12}$ deficiency)
		Mean corpuscular hemoglobin concentration (MCHC)	<32 g/dL (iron deficiency)
		Blood levels of specific vitamins or minerals	Varies according to vitamin/mineral measured
Increased metabolic requirements*	Burns, trauma, surgery, fever, sepsis, abscess, cancer, hyperthyroidism		
Medications causing catabolism; severe nausea, vomiting, or diarrhea; or having "antimetabolic" effects*	Steroids, cancer chemotherapeutic agents		

*Evaluation of parameter is essential for even the most basic nutrition assessment.

†Avoidance of meats, eggs, and legumes: suspect lack of protein, iron, and zinc; avoidance of dairy products: suspect lack of calcium, riboflavin, and possibly protein; avoidance of fruits and vegetables: suspect lack of vitamins A and C; avoidance of breads and cereals: suspect lack of thiamin, riboflavin, iron, and fiber.

‡Nitrogen balance = (protein intake × 0.16) − (24-hour urine urea nitrogen + 4 g). The 4 g is an estimate of fecal, skin, and other nonurinary losses.

§TLC = white blood count × percent lymphocytes.

perfectly reliable diagnostic test or physical sign that correlates with undernutrition. However, a thorough history and physical examination, combined with diagnostic tests, can yield much useful information about nutritional status. Assessment is summarized in Table 16-4, and further information is given below. Every patient should have at least a basic nutrition assessment. Based on the findings from the basic assessment, a more detailed assessment may be warranted.

Nutrition history

The nutrition history can be obtained by any member of the team, depending on the setting. In the hospital it is usually the responsibility of the dietitian, who will communicate pertinent findings to other members of the team. In the home or other outpatient setting, the nurse may be responsible for the nutrition history. The nutrition history requires an in-depth interview of the patient or the patient and family, a review of the patient's record, and possibly a consultation with other members of the health care team. The interviewer explores the patient's eating habits and usual food intake, along with financial, educational, cultural, social, religious, medical, and pharmacologic factors that may have an impact on food intake. A history of recent weight loss should be included. Loss of more than 5% of body weight in a month or 10% in 6 months is significant.

For the older adult, food may have a value far greater than nutritional need. It furnishes a means of marking the passage of time during the day, as well as the sharing of intimate moments with family and friends. The prevalence of loneliness in the elderly population makes it imperative that this history include a social assessment. The person who eats alone probably has only marginal nutrition, and should be observed and inspected for further signs of undernutrition.[8] Also, an important consideration is the elderly person's income level for food, as well as the mobility and strength available for purchasing food and preparing meals (see box).

Anthropometric measurements and physical examination

Height and weight are two anthropometric, or body, measurements that should be measured on every patient if at all possible, because the patient's verbal report of height and weight is likely to be inaccurate. However, body weight measurements may be distorted by edema or dehydration. Furthermore, weight measurement by itself provides only limited information. For instance, a patient may have a decrease in lean body mass (including muscle and all other nonfat tissue, and including the metabolically active tissues of the body that are critical for sur-

GERIATRIC CONSIDERATIONS

Nutrition Assessment

Suggested questions to include when interviewing the older adult about nutritional status:

1. What changes have you noticed in your height or weight?
2. Do you experience any changes in your appetite?
3. Have you had any problems chewing or swallowing food?
4. Do you experience any pain or discomfort during or after eating?
5. What prescription or over-the-counter drugs do you take regularly?
6. Are you able to get groceries when you need them?
7. Do you have someone to help you with grocery shopping and meal preparation?
8. How many times a day do you eat?
9. Do you eat alone?
10. How many times a week do you eat away from home?
11. How much money do you spend a week on groceries or eating away from home?
12. Do you think you have any problems with your nutrition that we should know about?
13. Do you have any leg cramps? Night sweats?
14. How often do you eat fresh fruits and vegetables?
15. How much water do you drink each day?
16. Do you drink alcoholic beverages? If so, how much? What kind?

vival) but a normal body weight for their height if they contain excessive fat.

Height measurement in elderly individuals is often difficult because of inability to stand erect or walk. Recumbent knee height can be used to estimate stature. Knee height is obtained by measuring with a caliper between the apex of the knee and the sole of the foot, with both at a 90° angle. A knee height caliper is available from Ross Laboratories.[11] For a more indepth assessment, skinfold measurements may be obtained with special calipers. These measurements give an indication of subcutaneous fat stores. The triceps skinfold (Figure 16-5) is the most commonly used, because it is accessible and because the most reliable reference ranges are available for the triceps. Also, the triceps measurement, along with the arm circumference measurement at that point, can be used to calculate arm muscle mass, an indicator of protein nourishment. Skin-

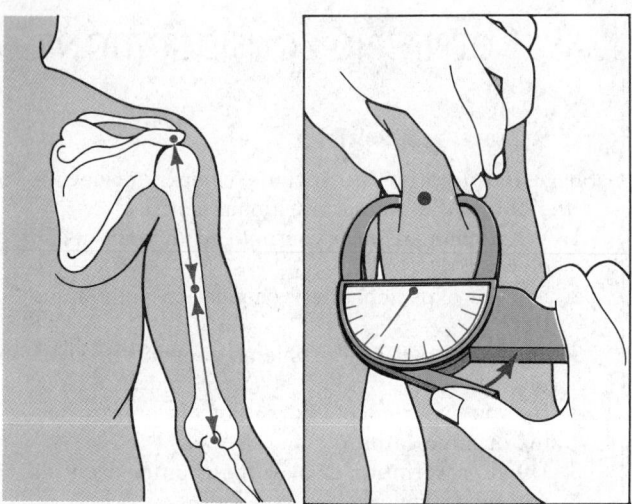

FIGURE 16-5   Triceps skinfold (TSF) is measured at midpoint of upper arm, located by measuring distance from acromion to olecranon process and marking halfway point. TSF is obtained by grasping skin and subcutaneous tissue at back of arm about 1 cm from midpoint. Calipers are then applied to skinfold, and reading is taken to the nearest millimeter.

folds are measured by specially trained dietitians or nurses; measurements obtained by novices tend to be highly variable. New anthropometric standards have recently been derived that are age-adjusted from ages 25 through 74 according to frame size. For frail, elderly persons over age 75, determinations have yet to be made.[63]

A physical examination is a critical part of the nutrition assessment process. Table 16-2 lists signs of undernutrition that the examiner should consider. Needs for protein, vitamin C, and zinc increase during wound healing, and vitamin A is especially important in maintaining epithelial integrity and preventing pulmonary infection in ventilator-dependent, extremely malnourished, or stressed patients. Therefore special care is taken in assessing adequacy of these four nutrients.

Diagnostic tests

Although diagnostic tests provide much valuable information, good judgment should be used in interpreting them. Drugs, anesthesia, stress, aging, and diseases other than undernutrition can alter laboratory values. For example, the liver forms serum proteins, including albumin, transferrin (an iron-transport protein), and prealbumin; thus levels of all these proteins decline in patients with liver failure. Also, serum protein, hemoglobin, and hematocrit levels are falsely elevated in dehydrated patients

and falsely depressed in overhydrated patients. Another problem is that certain tests are difficult to perform accurately. Nitrogen balance and creatinine excretion, for instance, require 24-hour urine collections, which are notoriously difficult to obtain. Moreover, values for diagnostic tests may be altered in the elderly, and in many instances it is not yet clear what the "normal" values are for elderly patients. Certainly laboratory tests should not be substituted for a thorough nutrition and weight loss history, along with a physical examination, because these "subjective" measurements have been shown to be as accurate in predicting nutritional risk as a battery of laboratory tests.[17]

There is a growing trend toward using indirect calorimetry in nutrition assessment. With this technique, the energy expenditure (and thus caloric needs) can be estimated by measuring the amount of oxygen consumed and carbon dioxide produced by the patient. By accurately determining caloric needs, indirect calorimetry helps prevent overfeeding or underfeeding, and so tends to reduce the costs of nutrition support.[23] Unfortunately, indirect calorimetry is not available in many institutions.

Nursing Diagnosis

The primary nursing diagnosis associated with undernutrition is "altered nutrition: less than body requirement." Depending on the patient's underlying disease, physiologic state, environmental circumstances, cognitive and perceptual state, and family and social relationships, a variety of other nursing diagnoses may apply. For example, the diagnoses of "knowledge deficit," "sensory-perceptual alteration: gustatory and/or olfactory," "impaired swallowing," or "fatigue" apply in some, but not all, cases of undernutrition.

Planning

Planning centers around achieving the following goals:
1. Stabilization and improvement of nutrition status as evidenced by
   a. Weight gain or stabilization
   b. Resolution of physical signs of deficiency
   c. Normalization of laboratory parameters
2. Avoidance of complications of nutrition support
3. Independence of the patient and family in performing the necessary tasks, if nutrition support is to be continued at home
4. Smooth transition from tube feedings or TPN to oral feedings, if appropriate
5. Maintenance of psychologic support to patient and caregiver

Implementation

Oral feedings

Whenever possible, the team should rely on oral feedings (foods and supplements) instead of more aggressive forms of nutrition support. For oral feedings to be sufficient in the undernourished patient, the nurse must evaluate patient intake and consult with the dietitian, patient, and family regarding eating problems and possible interventions. In the hospital, the nurse and dietitian work closely together in planning and evaluating these interventions. In the outpatient setting, it is often the nurse's responsibility to instruct the patient and family and to evaluate the patient's response. The nurse may use the Food Guide Pyramid as a guide (Figure 16-1). Suggestions for maximizing the patient's intake of protein and calories from ordinary foods, as well as improving intake of nutritional supplements, are given in Table 16-5.

Enteral tube feedings

When tube feedings are needed, the nurse is often responsible for placing the tube (unless it is a feeding ostomy), depending on institutional policies; she also is responsible for maintaining the tube, administering the formula, and monitoring the patient's response to the feedings.

In selecting a tube, it is well to remember that the smaller the diameter, the more comfortable the tube. Generally, small-bore (8 F) tubes are appropriate for most adults receiving defined formula diets (1 F ≈ 0.34 mm). Mucosal trauma and patient discomfort caused by the tube were common a few years ago when most NG and ND/NJ tubes were 14 F or larger; patient complaints are rare with the current small-bore tubes.[16] If the formula is very viscous or is made of blended foods, it may be necessary to use a 10 F or 12 F tube.

Tubes made of "nonreactive" materials, such as polyurethane and silicone rubber, are soft and do not stiffen with use, so they are the most comfortable tubes. They can be left in place indefinitely. One disadvantage of the small-bore tubes is their tendency to occlude; polyurethane tubes appear to be less likely than silicone rubber to become occluded.[44] Tubes made of polyvinylchloride (PVC) and polyethylene (PE) are sometimes used instead of nonreactive tubes, but these stiffen during use and must be replaced every 3 to 4 days to avoid perforation of the GI tract. They are more likely than nonreactive tubes to irritate the nares and mucosa. Table 16-6 and Figure 16-6 describe nasogastric tube insertion.

Although the gastrostomy tube is normally inserted by the physician, the nurse participates in preoperative teaching and may assist with the insertion. Preoperative teaching for gastrostomy placement includes a description of the procedure, including the postoperative appearance of the site and the tube (drawings or photographs are invaluable in this regard), and an explanation of the type of feeding to be given after surgery. Patients who will be given a general anesthetic need instruction regarding postoperative coughing and deep-breathing, but this is usually not necessary for those with a PEG.

Procedures for administration of intermittent and continuous feedings are given in Table 16-7. In addition to intermittent and continuous drip, there is a third method of delivering nutrients, known as bolus feeding. Bolus feedings are administered in the same way that intermittent ones are except that bolus feedings are infused rapidly, usually in approximately 5 minutes, through the barrel of a syringe attached to the proximal end of the feeding tube. They can cause abdominal discomfort, gastroesophageal reflux with pulmonary aspiration, dumping syndrome, and impaired absorption of nutrients. Bolus feedings are not currently recommended.

The skin around the tube is cleaned every day, and the tape around the tube is replaced whenever it becomes loosened or soiled. Secure taping helps prevent movement of the tube, which may irritate the nares or skin, or result in accidental dislodgment of the tube. Dressings are used around gastrostomy insertion sites initially; they are changed daily and the skin cleansed with half-strength hydrogen peroxide. The external "bumper" holding the PEG in place can be gently pulled up from the skin to allow adequate skin care, and then returned to its former position.[54] If leakage of gastric fluid occurs around a gastrostomy tube, the skin can be protected with karaya powder.

To prevent dryness of the mouth, a common complaint during tube feeding, the patient is encouraged to breathe through the nose as much as possible, drink and eat as much as desired (if compatible with the patient's nutrition orders), suck sugar-free candies or chew sugar-free gum (if allowed), and perform regular mouth care. If the patient is unconscious or otherwise unable to perform mouth care, the nurse should do it or should enlist the family in performing it. Patients commonly report that they can "taste" the tube feedings, and frequent mouth care will clear the palate of unpleasant flavors from the formula, as well as cleaning the teeth, tongue, and oral mucous membranes.

Enteral tube feeding complications

Complications of tube feedings include pulmonary aspiration of formula, diarrhea, fluid volume deficit or excess, and metabolic derangements such as hy-

TABLE 16-5   Increasing Oral Protein and Calorie Intake

Intervention	Rationale
Increasing Intake of Ordinary Foods:	
Arrange for patient to have several small meals and three snacks daily. Use milk or cream. Try putting it in cream sauces, gravies, puddings, custards, hot soups, hot cereals, mashed potatoes.	Large meals may seem overwhelming to the ill or anorexic patient.
Add extra margarine. Add 2 tablespoons skim milk powder to milk or soups, hot cereals, and mashed potatoes.	Fat is a good source of concentrated calories if fat is tolerated. Adds extra protein.
Add peanut butter to crackers, breads, or in milkshakes, or use instant breakfast mix alone or add to milkshake.	Adds protein and calories.
Have snacks containing concentrated calories available at all times; such as meat, cheese, or peanut butter sandwiches, milkshakes, sherbet floats, nuts, fruit-flavored yogurt, ice cream, dried fruits, and puddings.	Make it easy for the patient to snack when hunger occurs.
Use jam or jellies on bread, biscuits.	
Improving Intake of Defined Formula Diets Used as Oral Supplements:	
Serve supplements thoroughly chilled or over ice. Offer small amounts frequently, and encourage patient to sip them slowly.	The flavor is better when cold. Most defined formula diets are rich in easily digested carbohydrates; rapid hydrolysis of the carbohydrates in the duodenum increases the osmotic concentration in the bowel, contributing to "dumping syndrome," a malady characterized by weakness, tachycardia, abdominal cramping, and diarrhea; drinking the supplements quickly makes **dumping syndrome** more likely.
Choose supplements that offer at least 1.5 cal/mL; these include Magnacal (Biosearch), TwoCal HN (Ross), and Sustacal HCW (Mead Johnson)	Most supplements contain only 1 calorie/mL; this is so dilute that the patient has difficulty taking enough.
Allow the patient to taste several supplements before selecting one or more for use.	Personal preferences vary, and supplements are available in a variety of flavors. Some may prefer unflavored.
Using Modular Ingredients to Increase Intake:	
Add carbohydrate modules such as Polycose and Moducal to any beverage except soft drinks (in which they may dissipate the carbonation) and to cooked or ready-to-eat cereals, mashed potatoes, soups, and puddings; usually add 1 tablespoon (15 mL/120 mL of food).	Carbohydrate modules have little sweetness and thus do not distort the flavors of foods to which they are added.
Combine MCT oil with fruit juice or use it in frying, sauteeing, or baking.	MCT oil can be used just as any other oil, which means that the patient's food often needs to be prepared separately from the rest of the family's.
Administer Lipomul, a fat supplement, after or between meals; it is usually given in 15 to 30 mL doses several times a day.	Avoid decreasing appetite; Lipomul is flavored and requires no disguising.
Protein supplements can be added to milk, soups, mashed potatoes, cooked cereals, sandwich fillings, or meat loaf.	Some protein supplements do not dissolve well and may be easier to serve in textured foods such as cereals and potatoes than in beverages.

These suggestions are general guidelines. Needs of individual patient must be considered. For instance, the patient with arteriosclerotic heart disease who needs to increase caloric intake would need to avoid consuming foods containing saturated fats. Instead substitute products containing polyunsaturated fats.

TABLE 16-6 Insertion of an Enteral Feeding Tube

Procedure	Rationale

Describe the procedure, including expected sensations, to the patient; explain what the patient can do to help:
   Swallow when told to do so to help advance the tube; sipping a beverage or chewing ice chips, if allowed, may help the patient do this
   Signal with the hands if a respite is needed or if discomfort becomes extreme
   Some patients may want to advance the tube themselves, and they should be allowed to do so
	Tolerance of the procedure is improved if the patient knows what to expect; tube insertion causes a gagging sensation, but it should not be extremely uncomfortable or cause choking

If metoclopramide is ordered, administer it at least 15 minutes before tube insertion	Metoclopramide stimulates motility in the pyloric region and helps encourage transpyloric passage of the tube; however, it is only effective when given before tube insertion, rather than after the distal tip is already in the stomach[57]
Measure the tube to determine how much to insert; mark the distance on the tube with tape or indelible ink. Length to be inserted for an NG tube is equal to: $$\frac{(NEX - 50\ cm)}{2} + 50\ cm$$ where NEX is the distance in cm from the nose to the earlobe to the xiphoid process[61]	Inserting too short a length can cause formula to be infused into the esophagus, where it can readily enter the respiratory tract; if amount of tube inserted is too long, the tube can coil and knot in the stomach
If a nonreactive tube is used, insert the stylet (do not remove the stylet and reinsert it while the tube is inside the patient); place PE or PVC tubes in ice for a few minutes	Stiffening the tube may make it easier to advance; an alert, cooperative patient may find it more comfortable to forego this step; if the stylet is reinserted while in the patient, there is the potential for passage of the stylet through the feeding holes and damage or even perforation of the GI tract, although major manufacturers have modified their tubes to prevent this
Lubricate the tip of the tube with a water-soluble lubricant; some tubes have a coating that becomes slippery when wet; these only need to be dipped in water	This promotes patient comfort
Place the patient in Fowler's position, if possible	Gravity aids the tube in passing through the esophagus
Gently advance the tube slightly upward and dorsally through the nostril, then downward through the esophagus; if it is difficult to advance the tube through one nostril, try the other; antihistamine nasal sprays may make tube passage more comfortable; encourage the patient to swallow while the tube is passing down the esophagus	Sometimes there is obstruction of one nare, rarely are both affected; antihistamines help dilate the nasal passage by shrinking the mucosa
If the tube is difficult to advance or if the patient experiences choking during or after tube passage, remove it and try again	Choking or difficulty advancing the tube often indicates that the tube is in the bronchial tree

When the tube is inserted to the desired length, check to be sure that it is in proper position by one of the following methods:
   Radiography (the surest method)
   Checking the pH of fluid aspirated from the tube
   Injection of air through the tube with a syringe while auscultating over the left upper quadrant of the abdomen
	Almost all tubes have a radiopaque marker, making tubes readily visible on x-ray examination; aspiration of fluid with pH <3 is usually indicative that the tube is in the stomach; an influx of air has been heard even when the tube tip was in the esophagus or pleural space, which makes auscultation a less desirable method of confirmation

Tape the tube securely to the face, with the tube out of the patient's line of vision	Taping helps prevent dislodgement and also minimizes trauma and irritation to the nares from excessive movement of the tube; taping the tube to the forehead places the tube in the patient's line of vision and is very distracting

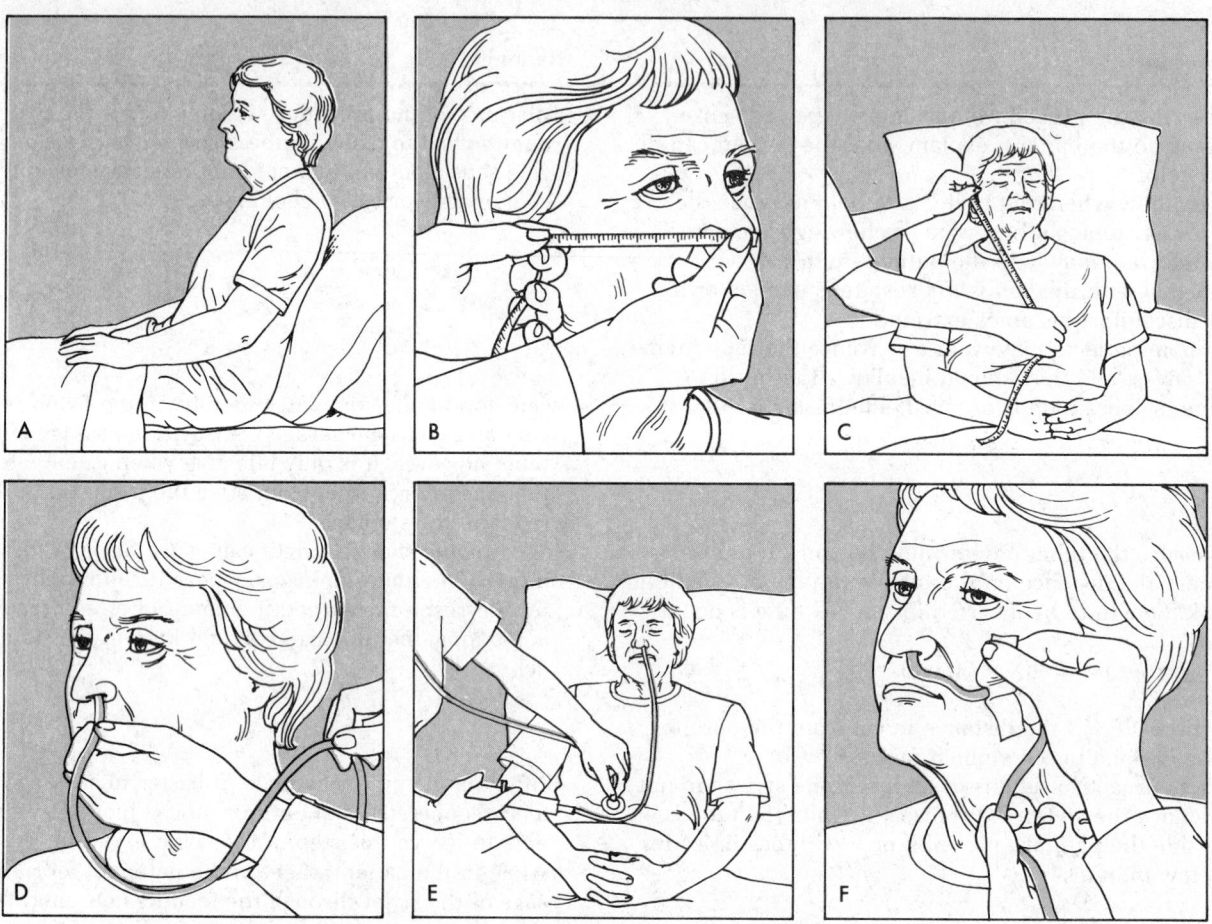

FIGURE 16-6   Insertion of a feeding tube. **A,** Place patient in Fowler's position before tube placement, if possible, so that gravity can facilitate passage of tube. **B** and **C,** Measure the distance from nose to ear and then to xiphoid process and calculate length of tube needed (see Table 16-6). **D,** Encourage patient to sip fluids or chew ice chips during tube insertion. **E,** One method of confirming tube placement is to auscultate patient's abdomen while injecting air through tube. **F,** Tape tube securely to patient's cheek.

perglycemia and electrolyte imbalances. The nurse's role in preventing and managing these complications includes careful attention to tube placement, tube maintenance, and formula delivery to decrease the risk of complications; frequent assessment of the patient's status and response to tube feedings; monitoring of physical and laboratory data; and consultation with the physician and other health care team members to alert them to problems and potential problems. Table 16-8 lists specific measures for managing some of the most common complications.

Total parenteral nutrition

The nurse's role in administering TPN is similar to that in administering tube feedings, including maintaining the infusion catheter, administering the TPN

and lipid solutions safely, and monitoring the patient for adverse effects.

Because the TPN catheter is an indwelling foreign body, it represents an important potential source for infection. The catheter site is kept covered by a dressing composed either of gauze and tape or of a transparent film. Dressing changes are done under aseptic conditions, usually by the nurse. Dressing change protocols vary from institution to institution, but in most instances gauze and tape dressings are changed routinely every 2 to 3 days and transparent ones every 5 to 7 days. Usually the skin is cleansed with a povidone-iodine solution. Cleansing of the skin is always done in a circular manner, beginning at the catheter insertion site and moving outward. It is best to allow the povidone-iodine solution to dry before applying the dressing. A povidone-iodine

TABLE 16-7 Continuous and Intermittent Tube Feedings

Procedure	Rationale
CONTINUOUS TUBE FEEDINGS	
Obtain prescribed formula from refrigerator or storage area	Ready-to-use formulas need no refrigeration; home- or hospital-prepared or reconstituted formulas should be refrigerated until needed; there is no need to warm formulas to room or body temperature before use, because they will slowly warm as they hang and infuse
Wash hands and cleanse any required equipment, such as a can opener, before use	Bacteria proliferate rapidly in enteral formulas and can cause gastroenteritis and even sepsis[12,48]
Pour formula into a feeding pouch or bottle; if possible, use containers and delivery sets designed specifically for enteral feeding	Use of containers and delivery sets designed for parenteral use has resulted in accidental intravenous delivery of enteral formulas
Pour no more formula into the feeding container than will be infused in 4 to 6 hours, unless using sterile formula packaged in ready-to-use feeding pouches; discard disposable containers and tubing every 24 hours	Opened formula held at room temperature is a good medium for bacterial growth, and it is easy to contaminate the formula or delivery system while filling the pouch
Check the feeding tube placement by aspirating GI contents or auscultating the abdomen while injecting air	Ensure that the feeding is delivered into the GI tract
Elevate the patient's head to 30 degrees, if possible.	Elevating the patient's head reduces the risk of reflux and pulmonary aspiration
Prime the delivery tubing and attach it to the enteral feeding pump, or regulate rate with a control clamp; attach the delivery tubing to the proximal end of the feeding tube and begin the feeding	Monitoring the rate carefully prevents overfeeding (with the possibility of causing diarrhea) or failure to deliver sufficient nutrients
Flush the feeding tube every 4 to 6 hours with tap water (or other fluid, if ordered); usually 30 to 60 mL are adequate; fluid-restricted patients may need less.	Flushing the feeding tube prevents clogging
INTERMITTENT FEEDINGS	
Obtain formula from refrigerator or storage area; if formula is in the refrigerator, allow it to warm to room temperature	If delivered rapidly, cold formula may cause abdominal cramping[34]
Wash hands and cleanse any necessary equipment before use	Avoid bacterial contamination of the feeding
Pour the formula into a feeding pouch and prime the delivery tubing, using administration sets designed for enteral use, if possible	Use of administration sets designed for IV fluids has resulted in accidental IV delivery of defined formula diets
Check the feeding tube placement by aspirating GI contents and auscultating during injection of air	Checking the feeding tube's placement ensures that the formula will be delivered into the GI tract
Elevate the patient's head to 30 degrees, if possible	Elevating the patient's head reduces the risk of reflux and pulmonary aspiration
Attach the delivery tubing to the proximal end of the feeding tube and regulate the flow so that the formula infuses at no more than 30 mL/min;[36] if well tolerated, the rate may gradually be increased	Feedings administered more rapidly may cause abdominal cramping; very ill or malnourished patients may not tolerate a feeding given as rapidly as 30 mL/min
When the feeding is completed, flush the feeding tube with tap water (or other fluid, if ordered); usually 30 to 60 mL are adequate; fluid-restricted patients may need less	Flushing the feeding tube prevents clogging
Wash the feeding pouch and tubing thoroughly; disposable administration sets should be discarded every 24 hours[3]	Thorough washing prevents multiplication of microorganisms in an administration set that is to be reused; costs may prohibit discard of administration sets every 24 hours during home-care tube feeding, but special care should be taken to wash administration sets and containers thoroughly if they are to be used longer

TABLE 16-8 Complications of Tube Feeding

Nursing intervention	Rationale
DIARRHEA	
Record frequency and consistency of stools; if stools are frequent and loose, weigh or measure them	Make possible diagnosis of diarrhea, which is defined in terms of both frequency and consistency of stool; >200 g/day of liquid or loose stools is often considered to be diarrhea
Check with the dietitian regarding osmolality of the formula; if it is hypertonic, discuss with the physician the possibility of temporarily diluting the formula, slowing the rate, or giving it continuously (if feedings are currently intermittent)	Hypertonic formula can draw fluid into the bowel to dilute the formula, causing dumping syndrome and diarrhea
Discuss with the physician the possibility of using an elemental diet temporarily, if the patient is very malnourished and hypoalbuminemic[60]	Hypoalbuminemia causes decreased plasma oncotic pressure and may impair absorption; malnutrition also reduces intestinal villi size (reducing the area of absorptive surface) and levels of enzymes located in the brush border (e.g., disaccharidases); thus a predigested diet may improve tolerance of some malnourished patients
Check the patient's medication record for drugs that may cause diarrhea: antibiotics, antacids, laxatives, digitalis, quinidine, lactulose[19,37]; consult the pharmacist if necessary; if appropriate, discuss with the physician the possibility of using a drug with less potential for diarrhea	Diarrhea caused by drugs is sometimes mistakenly attributed to tube feedings
Check with the pharmacist regarding the osmolality of medications the patient receives enterally; dilute them well if they are hypertonic	Hypertonic medications may cause diarrhea in the same way that hypertonic formula does[19]
Evaluate cleanliness of formula administration; be especially careful with transpyloric feedings and those in patients receiving cimetidine or antacids	Ensure that there is no bacterial contamination; gastric acidity provides a barrier to microorganisms in the upper GI tract; bypass of the stomach or decrease in acidity increases the risk of bacterial proliferation[18]
Perform a digital rectal examination if stools are extremely liquid	Rule out the possibility of fecal impaction (with liquid stool seeping around the impaction)
Administer antidiarrheals as ordered	The physician may order antidiarrheals if likely causes of diarrhea have been ruled out or cannot be corrected
PULMONARY ASPIRATION	
Monitor patient for acute respiratory distress, tachypnea, tachycardia, frothy sputum, and new radiographic infiltrates	Identify aspirated material
Tint all formula with blue food coloring	Tinting the formula improves the detection of aspirated material
Keep head elevated at least 30 degrees during feedings if possible; stop feedings for 30 to 60 minutes before any procedure that requires that the head be in a dependent position; keep cuff of endotracheal or tracheostomy tube inflated during feedings, if applicable[46]	Elevating the patient's head prevents formula from entering the airway
Measure gastric residual every 4 to 8 hours or before every intermittent feeding; use a 30 to 60 mL syringe to aspirate residual; follow existing orders regarding	Gastric retention may promote reflux of formula; larger syringes exert less suction than smaller ones and are less likely to cause small-bore nonreactive

TABLE 16-8   Complications of Tube Feeding—cont'd

Nursing intervention	Rationale
residuals; if no orders apply, notify physician of residuals greater than the amount infused in 2 hours of continuous feedings or half the volume of the previous intermittent feeding	tubes to collapse, preventing the measurement of residuals
Discuss with the physician the possibility of using transpyloric feedings in the patient at risk for aspiration (unconscious, with poor gag reflex, or with delayed gastric emptying)	Transpyloric feedings may reduce the risk of aspiration, because they place both the pyloric and cardiac sphincters between the formula and the trachea

CLOGGING OF FEEDING TUBES

Irrigate tube with 30 to 60 mL water (or other fluid as ordered*) every 4 to 8 hours during continuous feedings and after every intermittent feeding	Irrigating the tube maintains patency by flushing potential precipitants in the formula from the tube
Avoid giving medications by tube, if possible; if they must be given by tube, notify the pharmacist so that they can be formulated as suspensions or elixirs, rather than as tablets that must be crushed; irrigate tube well before and after administering any medication; never add medication to the formula unless there is evidence that the two are compatible	Tubes are commonly obstructed by crushed tablets or formula coagulated by medications with which it is incompatible

FLUID VOLUME DEFICIT

Monitor patient for rising BUN and hematocrit levels, poor skin turgor, dry mucous membranes, and thirst	These indicate fluid volume deficit
Irrigate the tube with increased amounts of fluid or encourage the patient to drink fluids (if allowed) if signs of fluid volume deficit occur	Increased intake of free water will help alleviate fluid volume deficit

*Some clinicians recommend use of soft drinks, especially Coca-Cola, or cranberry juice as routine irrigants or for clearing obstructions. However, Coca-Cola has been found to be no more effective than water as an irrigant, and cranberry juice is inferior to both Coca-Cola and water.[47] Acidic products such as soft drinks and cranberry juice could coagulate proteins and thus might actually promote clogging. One laboratory study found that papain, an enzyme from papaya and often used in meat tenderizers, was effective in clearing clogs, but this has not been tested in human subjects.[42,47]

ointment may be applied to the catheter site before applying the new dressing. For patients with allergy to iodine, a noniodine-containing antibacterial scrub solution can be used for skin cleansing, and ointment can be omitted or an antibiotic ointment can be used, if approved by the physician.

Complications of TPN

TPN has many potential complications, including catheter-related sepsis; air embolus; fluid volume excess; pneumothorax; subclavian vein thrombosis; and metabolic derangements such as hypo- and hyperglycemia, hypophosphatemia, and hypo- and hyperkalemia. Nursing care of the patient receiving TPN, including management of the more common or severe complications, is described in the nursing care plan on p. 358.

Patient education

Education of the patient and family regarding nutrition support is summarized in the patient education guide on p. 361.

Transitional feeding

When tube feedings or TPN are discontinued, the patient may have difficulty maintaining an adequate nutritional status. Some patients have a depressed appetite while receiving aggressive nutrition support, and their appetites may not return to normal for a period of time after nutrition support ceases. Patients receiving TPN with no enteral feedings usually have some degree of mucosal atrophy in the bowel; the bowel apparently needs the stimulation of digesting and absorbing nutrients to maintain its normal function.[51] Therefore it is important that

NURSING CARE PLAN   *The Patient Receiving TPN*

Nursing diagnosis/ Expected outcomes	Interventions	Rationale
Altered nutrition: less than body requirements • *Patient will receive adequate nutrients to meet needs*	Administer TPN within 10% of ordered rate Weigh patient daily Monitor laboratory data: serum albumin, transferrin, or prealbumin; vitamins; minerals; trace elements; and electrolytes Monitor patient for physical signs of deficiencies (Table 16-2)	The patient requiring TPN often has preexisting nutritional deficits. It is possible that the patient's nutritional needs have been underestimated, or it may be difficult to deliver all the nutrients needed (e.g., when severe fluid restriction is required); therefore there is a potential for deficiency
Altered nutrition: high risk for more than body requirements • *Patient will not experience ill effects as a result of excess nutrient provision*	Monitor levels of serum glucose, BUN, electrolytes, and triglycerides (if lipids are given) Monitor P_{CO_2} of ventilator-dependent patients Encourage ambulation and other exercise as tolerated; provide passive exercise for patients who cannot exercise	Excess of any nutrient added to TPN can occur; a rising BUN level may indicate excess amino acid intake; serum triglycerides are the best indicator of excess lipid emulsion intake Excess carbohydrate increases P_{CO_2} production, making it difficult to wean patients from ventilators If no exercise is performed, the new tissue formed tends to be fat, rather than muscle
• *Patient is monitored for refeeding syndrome*	Monitor serum phosphorus, O_2 consumption, CO_2 production	If calorie needs (especially with glucose) are exceeded in hypometabolic starved patients, this may cause hypophosphatemia and repletion heart failure. Increase nutrition support gradually with a portion of the fuel as fat
Fluid volume excess, high risk for • *Fluid balance will be maintained*	Administer TPN at the rate ordered Weigh patient daily Monitor respiratory rate, pulse, breath sounds, edema Note electrolyte, BUN, and hematocrit levels Administer medications (diuretics, albumin) as ordered	The malnourished patient is especially prone to pulmonary edema and anasarca as a result of diminished plasma oncotic pressure
Impaired skin integrity • *Infection and sepsis will be avoided* • *If infection or sepsis occurs, it will be detected early and appropriate intervention will be made*	Monitor vital signs Change TPN catheter dressing, tubing, and solutions under aseptic conditions Inspect TPN solutions for cloudiness, cracks, or leaks before hanging Discard TPN solutions after 24 hours and lipid emulsions after 12[51] Use a 0.22 μm filter on TPN lines; do not filter lipids	The TPN catheter breaches the integrity of the skin and increases the likelihood of infection Although glucose–amino acid TPN solutions are not good growth media for most bacteria, lipids are; both fluids are good media for fungi[12,13] Lipids cannot be delivered through an antimicrobial filter because some lipid particles are larger than 0.22 μm

NURSING CARE PLAN   *The Patient Receiving TPN—cont'd*

Nursing diagnosis/ Expected outcomes	Interventions	Rationale
	Change the TPN dressing if it becomes wet, soiled, or nonadherent	Scrupulous asepsis is the only way to avoid infection caused by contamination of the catheter, tubing, or fluids
	Check for redness and drainage at the catheter insertion site during dressing changes	
	Avoid drawing blood or administering other fluids/medications via the TPN catheter	
	Administer antibiotics/antifungals as ordered	
Ineffective breathing pattern, potential for, due to pneumothorax	Before catheter insertion, teach patient what to expect and help him relax and breathe normally	Damage to the pleura during catheter insertion can result in a pneumothorax
• *The patient will have full lung expansion and adequate ventilation*	Observe patient for signs of pneumothorax: diminished or unequal breath sounds, tachypnea, dyspnea, cyanosis, and labored breathing, especially during the first 48 hours after catheter insertion	A frightened patient who moves during insertion or breathes erratically increases the risk of pneumothorax
	Provide chest tube care as required	
Altered tissue perfusion, high risk for	Prevent air embolus:	
	Secure all tubing and catheter connections; use "Luer-Lok" connections whenever possible	An open route into a central vein allows large amounts of air to enter rapidly and may be fatal
• *Patient will have adequate tissue perfusion*	Use air-eliminating filters on TPN lines	
	Teach the patient to perform Valsalva maneuver whenever the tubing is disconnected (e.g., during tubing changes); in the ventilator-dependent patient, disconnect and reconnect the tubing quickly at end expiration	Increased intrathoracic pressure (Valsalva maneuver) prevents air entry
	Clamp or reconnect the tubing quickly if it is disconnected inadvertently	
	Cover the catheter site with an occlusive dressing for 24 hours after catheter removal	The tract created by the catheter can allow air entry even after the catheter is removed
	Observe patient for respiratory distress, hypotension, "mill wheel" heart murmur, neurologic deficits	
	Place the patient in left lateral decubitus and Trendelenburg position, administer O_2 and CPR as needed, and notify physician if air embolus is suspected	If air embolus does occur, positioning may reduce the amount of air that enters the outflow tract from the right ventricle

Continued.

NURSING CARE PLAN   *The Patient Receiving TPN—cont'd*

Nursing diagnosis/ Expected outcomes	Interventions	Rationale
	Avoid subclavian vein thrombosis: Maintain aseptic technique in handling the catheter, tubing, and solutions Assess patient for pain in the insertion site, development of collateral circulation on the chest wall, and edema of the ipsilateral shoulder Remove the catheter and administer anticoagulants and antibiotics as ordered if thrombosis occurs	Subclavian thrombosis is most likely following repeated or traumatic catheterizations, where the intima of the vessel is damaged; prevention of catheter-related sepsis, and thus of the need for recatheterization, is the best way to prevent thrombosis
Sensory-perceptual alterations: gustatory (in patients for whom oral food intake is contraindicated) • *Patient will accept the necessity of not having oral intake* • *Patient will not experience loss of social interaction as a result of food deprivation*	Ensure that the patient and family understand the reason for TPN and exclusion of oral intake	The patient may be helped by being informed of the length of time that food deprivation is likely to last (eventually almost all patients can eat at least small amounts)
	Discuss with the patient the meaning of food and eating for him as an individual Encourage the patient to use sugar-free gum or candies, if allowed by the physician	Eating and the taste of food are basic pleasures, and many patients receiving TPN without oral intake complain of feeling deprived
	Encourage the home-care patient to join other family members at mealtime and to attend social events as he feels able	Much of family and social life revolves around eating; the patient who does not participate in family meals and in social events may experience isolation

tube feedings or TPN not be stopped abruptly but be gradually tapered while oral intake increases. The nurse must record type and amount of all oral intake during this time period to document the patient's ability to meet nutritional needs via the oral route.

Evaluation

Evaluation of progress includes regular measurement of patient weight (daily in TPN patients; every 1 to 3 days in enterally fed patients). Steady gains of no more than 0.22 kg (½ lb) per day, or stabilization of weight at the desired level, are evidence of efficacy of nutrition support. Average gains of more than 0.1 to 0.22 kg (¼ to ½ lb) are more often a re-

sult of fluid retention than of anabolism, or tissue-building. Skinfold measurements and arm muscle circumference should also increase. It may take weeks or even months for anthropometric measurements to reach usual or ideal values.

Laboratory parameters, including serum albumin, transferrin, or prealbumin and total lymphocyte count, should stabilize in the normal range. Serum albumin and total lymphocyte count are slow to change, however, and may take weeks to normalize. Nitrogen balance should become positive within a few days in the undernourished individual who is receiving adequate nutrition support. Blood levels of vitamin C and zinc should be evaluated in the burn or trauma patient, and supplements provided until healing appears complete. The health care team

PATIENT EDUCATION GUIDE *Nutrition Support*

Objective I: To increase the patient's and family's understanding of nutrition support and elicit their cooperation in delivering nutrition support safely

A. Background information (for both home-care and hospital patients receiving tube feedings or TPN)
1. Reasons for tube feeding or TPN (whichever is appropriate) and importance of therapy
2. Need to avoid tension on feeding tube or TPN catheter
3. Importance of accurate intake and output measurements and how the patient/family can help in obtaining these
4. Signs and symptoms to report to the health care team
   a. Fever, chills
   b. Excessive urination or thirst
   c. Shortness of breath
   d. Pain, tenderness, or leakage of fluid around gastrostomy, jejunostomy, or TPN catheter site
   e. Swelling of the shoulder (in TPN patients)

Objective II: To prepare the patient and family to deliver tube feedings safely at home

A. Feeding tube maintenance
1. Insert the feeding tube, if applicable
2. Aspirate GI contents to confirm placement of the feeding tube
3. Cleanse area around insertion site daily
4. Irrigate tube with 30 to 60 mL of water (or other fluid as directed) after each intermittent feeding or every 4 to 8 hours during continuous feedings
B. Formula preparation and administration
1. Prepare formula from pureed foods with the recipe provided or reconstitute concentrated or powdered commercial formula, if appropriate
2. Use prepared or opened formula within 24 hours; store all such formula in the refrigerator until use
3. Hang only enough formula for 4 to 8 hours of infusion (NOTE: formula is sometimes allowed to hang longer than in the hospital setting because many home-care patients receive their feedings during the night, and hanging 8 hours' worth allows them to sleep through the night without having to hang more formula; this is relatively safe, because the patient's home tends to be cooler at night, reducing risk of spoilage)
4. Wash all administration sets thoroughly every 8 hours or discard disposable supplies every 24 hours
5. Deliver intermittent or continuous feedings on the appropriate schedule
6. Operate enteral feeding pump, if applicable
7. Elevate head during feedings (use shock blocks or a wedge under the mattress to elevate head of bed for nocturnal feedings)
8. Avoid administering crushed tablets via tube, flush tube with water before and after administering any medications via tube, and avoid mixing medications with formula
C. Problems to report to the health care team
1. Diarrhea persisting more than 2 to 3 days
2. Fever unexplained by other illness
3. Difficulty breathing, rapid respirations, or frothy sputum (seek emergency assistance)
4. Consistent average weight gain of more than 0.22 kg (½ lb) per day over several days
5. Excessive thirst, frequent urination, weight loss

Objective III: To prepare the patient and family to administer TPN safely at home

A. Catheter care
1. Change the dressing on a regular schedule
2. Cleanse dressing area in a circular motion, starting at the insertion site and working outward
3. Use povidone-iodine or other antimicrobial solution for cleansing skin
4. Irrigate the catheter with heparinized saline and cap the catheter whenever the infusion is stopped, if appropriate (most home-care patients infuse their TPN on a cyclic schedule and stop the infusion for part of the day)

Data from Johndrow PD: Administer hyperalimentation at home? *Home Healthcare Nurse*, p 27, November/December, 1984; Kennedy-Caldwell C and Guenter P: *Nutrition support nursing care curriculum*, ed 2, Silver Springs, Md, 1988, American Society for Parenteral and Enteral Nutrition; Koithan M: Home total parenteral nutrition: complications, *NITA* 8:231, 1985.

Continued.

PATIENT EDUCATION GUIDE   *Nutrition Support—cont'd*

5. Clamp catheter before disconnecting the tubing and applying the cap; use a clamp without teeth; avoid repeatedly clamping in the same place, as this may damage the catheter
6. Do not swim or let catheter site become wet unless allowed by the physician
7. Avoid contact sports where the catheter might be damaged
8. If catheter breaks or is leaking, clamp it or perform temporary repair (as directed by the physician) and notify the health care team

B. TPN solution
1. Prepare the TPN solution from individual ingredients, if applicable (the pharmacist usually instructs the patient in doing this, but the nurse may need to reinforce principles of asepsis and careful measurement of ingredients; some patients obtain premixed solutions from a local pharmacy or from a commercial supplier)
2. Store mixed solutions in a refrigerator until use
3. Inspect all solutions for precipitates, leaking, or cloudiness before hanging them
4. Wash hands before connecting the TPN container to the administration tubing
5. Avoid touch contamination of any connection between the TPN solution and the catheter
6. Use an infusion pump to deliver the solution

C. Lipid emulsions
1. Inspect lipids for separation or "oiling" out before hanging them
2. Deliver lipids on the schedule specified by the health care team
3. Piggyback lipids into the TPN line below the filter (if applicable)
4. Allow lipids to hang for no more than 12 hours

D. Self-monitoring
1. Test blood or urine for sugar every day or as directed
2. Weigh daily, at the same time each day and in approximately the same clothing
3. Check temperature if the patient feels unusually hot, is flushed, has chills, or develops glucose intolerance when the same glucose intake was previously tolerated

E. Awareness of problems/coping with problems
1. Recognize the symptoms of air embolus, subclavian thrombosis, and sepsis
2. Report symptoms of subclavian thrombosis and sepsis to the health care team immediately; clamp the catheter or reconnect the tubing and seek emergency assistance if air embolus is suspected
3. Report to the health care team consistent weight gain of more than 0.22 kg (½ lb) per day; shortness of breath; elevated urine or blood sugar; temperature >101° F for more than 24 hours; redness, swelling, or draining at catheter site; catheter damage
4. Recognize and report to the health care team signs of electrolyte and mineral imbalance (NOTE: Most home-care TPN patients are relatively stable in their electrolyte/mineral needs; imbalances are most likely to occur when an acute illness is superimposed on their chronic problem; For that reason, patients at highest risk will be identified in the following listing to make it clear which patients require the most extensive teaching.)
   a. Sodium
      (1) Hyponatremia
         (a) Symptoms: behavioral changes—inattention, lethargy, confusion, apprehension; abdominal and muscle cramping; muscle twitching
         (b) Causes/patients at most risk: diarrhea (especially increased ileostomy drainage); prolonged vomiting, fistula drainage; diuretic therapy; chronic renal insufficiency; cirrhosis of the liver; Addison's disease; syndrome of inappropriate antidiuretic hormone secretion
      (2) Hypernatremia
         (a) Symptoms: thirst; dry, sticky mucous membranes; decreased urination
         (b) Causes/patients at most risk: prolonged vomiting, profuse diarrhea, inadequate fluid intake to replace losses
   b. Potassium
      (1) Hypokalemia
         (a) Symptoms: muscular weakness, orthostatic hypotension (dizziness/faintness on arising from the sitting or lying position)
         (b) Causes/patients at most risk: severe diarrhea, fistula drainage, prolonged diuretic usage, corticosteroid therapy

PATIENT EDUCATION GUIDE   *Nutrition Support—cont'd*

    (2) Hyperkalemia
        (a) Symptoms: decreased urination, weakness and fatigue, paresthesias
        (b) Causes/patients at most risk: renal failure
  c. Calcium (hypocalcemia)
        (1) Symptoms: paresthesias around mouth and in extremities, muscle spasms and cramps
        (2) Causes/patients at most risk: severe or prolonged diarrhea, especially with steatorrhea
  d. Phosphorus (hypophosphatemia)
        (1) Symptoms: tremor; ataxia; paresthesia; slurred speech; irritability; stupor
        (2) Causes/patients at most risk: carbohydrate providing almost all of TPN calories; alcoholism; diabetic
            ketoacidosis; pregnancy; dialysis; severe malnutrition
  e. Magnesium
        (1) Hypomagnesemia
            (a) Symptoms: tremors, muscle twitching, convulsions, paresthesias
            (b) Causes/patients at most risk: severe and prolonged diarrhea, especially with steatorrhea; fistula
                drainage; alcoholism
        (2) Hypermagnesemia
            (a) Symptoms: lethargy, slurred speech, ataxia
            (b) Causes/patients at most risk: renal failure

must evaluate all nutritional parameters, and especially laboratory analyses, in the light of the patient's overall condition (e.g., state of hydration, level of stress, ongoing illness such as cancer).

Evaluation should also include the presence or absence of any evidence of the complications discussed above, as well as the benefit of nutrition support to the patient. Nutrition support is only worthwhile as long as the benefits outweigh the risks, and consideration of benefits must include patient well-being and quality of life, although these factors may be difficult to measure. In certain individuals, such as terminally ill patients for whom no other treatment is available, nutrition support may only prolong life and suffering. In these cases, nutrition support may not be warranted, or it may be appropriate only if the health care team, the patient (if possible), and the family continually reassess the patient's status and the relative benefit afforded by nutrition support.

Documentation

The nurse documents the following information in the patient's chart to meet standards of care for nutrition support (see box).

Assessment data

The nurse is responsible for obtaining a baseline height and weight measurement for each patient, regardless of whether the physician orders this done. Information required for a basic nutrition assessment (see Table 16-4) should be available on every patient record. In some settings the physician may collect the data; in others, the dietitian may have this responsibility; and in still others, several team members may divide the task. The nurse should be aware of the responsibility and be sure that all information is documented by some member of the team. In the home-care setting, the nurse is apt to be responsible for collecting and updating nutrition assessment data.

Monitoring of nutrition support

This includes regular patient weights, as well as triceps skinfold and arm circumference, if the nurse has been trained to perform these measurements. It also includes any evidence of resolution of clinical manifestations of deficiency. In some settings, the nurse is responsible for routine urine or blood glucose measurements, using testing strips, and these values are recorded. Strict intake and output measurements, with clear records of the intake of tube feeding formula, TPN solutions, and food, are documented daily for the duration of nutrition support. In addition, the nurse documents any signs or symptoms indicating complications of nutrition support or nursing interventions, and note patient response to the interventions.

Patient education

Patient and family teaching regarding the reason for nutrition support, the techniques of nutrition sup-

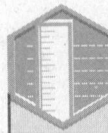

STANDARDS OF CARE

Nutrition Support

Nursing care will include the following:

1. All patients will have documented evidence of at least a basic nutritional assessment.

2. All patients receiving nutrition support will have evidence of daily monitoring of tolerance of feedings, including weight (daily for TPN patients, at least every third day for enterally fed patients); state of hydration; glucose tolerance; presence of bowel sounds and absence of gastric retention of feedings (for enterally fed patients); and indications of infection. Monitoring may be performed by the nurse or, in the home-care setting, by the patient or family members after appropriate teaching by the nurse.

3. All patients receiving nutrition support will have documented evidence of patient teaching regarding the reason for nutrition support and the appropriate method for delivery of nutrition support. Patients to be discharged on TPN or tube feedings will have documentation of teaching regarding maintenance of the catheter or feeding tube, preparation (if necessary) and administration of TPN solution or defined formula diet, and management of problems associated with nutrition support.

port, and symptoms to be alert for should be documented. For patients who are to be discharged, the nurse documents all teaching given, along with the patient and family response. It is important that the patient and family members be able to demonstrate, rather than simply to verbalize an understanding of, all skills that will be required at home and that their demonstration of these skills be described in the patient's record.

OVERWEIGHT AND OBESITY

Definition

Overweight refers to any weight in excess of the desirable body weight, whereas **obesity** is a term applied to an excess of body fat. For simplicity, obesity is often defined as 120% or more of the desirable or ideal body weight (IBW). The severity of obesity may be graded as: (1) mild, 120% to 140% of IBW; (2) moderate, 141% to 200% of IBW; and (3) severe or morbid, >200% of IBW.

The overweight person is not necessarily overly fat, and overweight need not be an undesirable finding. For example, an athlete may have sufficient muscle bulk that he or she exceeds the IBW for height according to standard charts.

Epidemiology/Etiology

Obesity is estimated to affect at least 26% of Americans between the ages of 20 and 75 years, with greatest prevalence among women who are black and poor. Males living in poverty have the lowest incidence of obesity.[66] There is no single cause for obesity. Several factors are known to contribute to the problem, including the following.

Heredity

Children of two obese parents have an 80% chance of being obese, whereas those with one obese parent have a 40% risk, and those without an obese parent have only a 7% chance. Although the correlation between the weight of parents and children can be at least partly a result of the environmental influences within the home, studies of adopted children indicate that there is a strong genetic component involved in obesity. Stunkard and others[66] found that there was no relationship between obesity of adoptees and their adoptive parents. However, there was a very significant correlation between obesity of the adoptees and their biologic parents, particularly the mothers.

Environment

The environment both inside and outside of the home fosters overeating in a variety of ways. In some families, food is used as a reward or as a sign of love and affection. Television watching, a favorite pastime in many homes, is commonly accompanied by snacking; also, its sedentary nature fosters weight gain. Labor-saving devices and sedentary jobs decrease energy expenditure. Furthermore, food—often high in calories and low in nutrient value—is a part of most social gatherings and outings, especially "fast food" in today's fast-paced society.

Physiologic factors

The metabolic rate declines by about 2% per decade after age 30, and unwary adults who do not adjust their food intake or activity levels to compensate may find themselves growing heavier. Other than this known change in metabolic rate, and the relatively few cases of obesity caused by endocrine disorders such as hypothyroidism, the connection between physiologic function and obesity remains unclear. An interesting hypothesis proposes that some obesity may be caused by a defect in the function of brown fat, a body tissue involved in thermogenesis (heat production). Brown fat tends to dissipate calories as heat, rather than to store them.[52] Another hypothesis is the "set-point" or "lipostatic" theory. This theory proposes that the amount of body fat is determined in a manner analogous to thermostatic control of heating or cooling. If the person loses weight so that he is below his set-point, he feels unsatisfied and eats until he regains his usual amount of fat. Similarly, adults who gain weight while being force-fed resume their former eating habits and lose the excess weight without depriving themselves. This theory helps explain why many obese and overweight persons have such difficulty maintaining weight loss.

Psychologic influences

Loneliness, grief, anxiety, depression, and other emotions can lead to overeating. Also, obese people seem to be more responsive than lean individuals to external cues such as food advertisements or the fact that others around them are eating, rather than to their own hunger or satiety.

Pathophysiology

Obesity is a known health risk. Both diabetes mellitus and hypertension, for example, are 2.9 times more likely to occur in obese individuals than in those who are not obese.[56] Other disorders with a clear relationship to obesity are coronary artery disease and certain types of cancer, including cancer of the colon, rectum, and prostate in men and cancer of the gallbladder, biliary passages, breast (postmenopausal), uterus, and ovaries in women. Furthermore, obesity may cause great psychologic distress.[65] Obesity has also been implicated in some pulmonary disorders (dyspnea, alveolar hypoventilation, and sleep apnea), degenerative joint disease, gout, and endocrine disorders such as menstrual irregularities and hirsutism in obese women and infertility in men.

Risks posed by obesity appear to be influenced by three main factors: degree of obesity, age, and fat distribution. The greater the degree of obesity, the greater the risk. Those weighing more than 145% of IBW have a mortality rate more than twice that of normal-weight adults. Moreover, morbidity is greater in obese adults under age 45 than in those over 45. In addition, coronary artery disease is more common in individuals with increased abdominal fat than in those with excessive thigh and gluteal fat.[65]

Clinical Manifestations

Determining whether an individual is obese is not as easy as it may seem. Underwater (hydrostatic) weighing gives a relatively accurate indication of the percentage of body fat. Unfortunately, the stress of the procedure makes it impractical for ill or infirm individuals.

Measurement of height and weight and comparison of these values with standard charts is usually the first step in the process of identifying obesity. However, as mentioned previously, this may produce erroneous results. Body weight is an individual matter, and it must be interpreted as such. For one thing, body weight tends to increase with age, and overweight in the elderly patient may not be as great a problem as in the younger one. Also, weight charts may not be applicable to persons of all socioeconomic levels and ethnic groups. In addition, the individual may have a higher than normal percentage of body fat, along with a low percentage of lean body mass, and be obese although his weight is within the normal range. One way to evaluate the amount of body fat is to measure skinfolds at one or more sites. A triceps skinfold larger than 27 mm in women or 16 mm in men is often taken as an indicator of obesity.[63]

An increasingly popular technique is to calculate the body mass index (BMI) by the following formula:

$$BMI = \frac{Weight\ in\ kg}{(Height\ in\ meters)^2}$$

A BMI greater than 27.8 for men or 27.3 for women is usually considered an indication of excessive fat.[65]

Therapeutic Management

Obesity is a long-term problem, and there are no quick and easy cures. Weight loss requires a great deal of motivation on the part of the patient, as well as support from family, friends, and the health care team. Methods used to treat obesity include diet, behavioral modification, exercise, pharmacologic agents, special devices, and surgical intervention.

Weight-loss diets

Regardless of the cause of obesity, the cure is to consume fewer calories than are needed. Each 0.45 kg, or 1 lb, of body fat represents approximately 3500 stored calories. Therefore to lose just 0.45 kg a week, the dieter must consume 500 calories a day less than needed for energy expenditure. (As a rule of thumb, energy needs are about 20 to 25 calories/kg of desirable body weight if the individual is sedentary, 30 calories/kg if moderately active, and 35 to 45 calories/kg if very active.) Generally, 0.45 to 0.9 kg (1 to 2 lb) per week is the maximum realistic and safe amount of weight loss.

Careful selection of foods with low caloric density from the Food Guide Pyramid allows the person to consume a moderate low-calorie diet (usually 1000 to 1800 calories/day) that will promote gradual weight loss. Foods with low caloric density include most fruits and vegetables; lean meats, poultry, and fish; skim-milk products; and whole-grain breads and cereals, all prepared and served with little or no added sugar or fat. Fats and concentrated sweets are foods of high caloric density. Gradual weight loss may not be as immediately motivating as diets that promise a loss of several pounds a week, but moderate low-calorie diets have the advantages of providing the individual time to make lasting changes in eating habits while eating a satisfying, rather than a deprived, diet.

Very low-calorie diets, or VLCD, are those that provide less than 800 calories/day. It is difficult to make such a diet adequate, and VLCD should not be undertaken without a physician's supervision. Individuals who are moderately or severely obese may become discouraged with the slow results obtainable from moderate low-calorie diets, and thus VLCD may help them remain motivated. The protein-sparing modified fast (PSMF) is one form of VLCD. The PSMF usually includes 400 to 700 calories/day, and most of these calories are in the form of protein. The PSMF can be based on a special liquid formula or on lean meat, poultry, and fish. Much loss of skeletal muscle and other body proteins occurs during total fasting, and the PSMF is designed to preserve body proteins while producing rapid weight loss. Weight loss of 1.5 to 2.3 kg (3.3 to 5.1 lb) per week may be expected during the PSMF. Unfortunately, losses during VLCD are rarely maintained, and patients sometimes have a tendency to indulge in eating binges after discontinuing the diet.[48]

Exercise

Regular and sustained movements of large muscle groups promote the loss of fat while preserving the lean body mass. Exercise also contributes to a feeling of well-being and helps shape and tone the body. It should be a part of every weight-loss regimen.

Behavioral modification

To maintain weight loss, it is important to make permanent changes in eating habits and life-style. Behavioral modification is a way of making these changes and should therefore be an adjunct to every weight and exercise program.

Pharmacologic agents

Amphetamines and other anorexigenic drugs are sometimes prescribed to help patients lose weight. Generally, drugs should only be used as an adjunct to dieting in patients who have been unsuccessful at losing weight without the drugs. If used at all, drugs should be used only for the first 6 to 8 weeks of di-

eting, to help the patient adjust to eating less. Weight loss resulting from the use of appetite suppressants is unlikely to be lasting. Moreover, dependence on amphetamines is a serious possibility. Some of the side effects of amphetamines are hyperactivity, dyskinesia, hypertension, palpitations, and, rarely, psychosis.

The active ingredients in most over-the-counter diet drugs are caffeine or phenylpropanolamine, which have limited benefits when taken at the recommended dosages. Some over-the-counter products provide fiber or bulking agents. A diet of bulky, high-fiber foods is low in concentrated calories and causes the person to become satisfied before consuming as many calories as he would on a diet high in concentrated calories; adding fiber in the form of a medication is not beneficial, however, unless calorie intake is also reduced.

Human chorionic gonadotropin (HCG) has been touted as a mobilizer of fat stores, but a double-blind study of HCG versus a placebo revealed no difference in weight loss between the two treatments. Weight loss in individuals receiving HCG results from the 500-calorie diet prescribed to accompany the drug.[48]

Surgical procedures

Surgical intervention is reserved for patients who are ≥45 kg above ideal body weight and who have failed to lose weight with more conventional methods. Gastric restriction reduces the gastric reservoir to the smallest size and thus limits the amount of food that can be eaten. The most common gastric operation consists of vertical band **gastroplasty,** vertical ring gastroplasty, and gastric banding (see Figure 16-7).

In **gastric bypass** (Figure 16-8), the reservoir is connected to the jejunum, bypassing the distal stomach and the duodenum. Gastric surgery is not a panacea for obesity. Although 90% of gastric bypass patients lose at least 50% of their excess weight, only 30% to 50% of patients will reach a weight of less than 125% of their IBW. Furthermore, almost all of the weight loss occurs within the first year after surgery, and weight gain often begins within 1 to 2 years after surgery.

Suction lipectomy should not be considered a method of weight control, and it is contraindicated in patients with generalized obesity. It should be used only for removing adipose tissue deposits for cosmetic reasons after the patient has achieved the IBW.

Fads and quackery

Fads and quackery abound in the field of weight loss. Claims are made that specific foods, combinations of foods, or diet aids have unique, magical (e.g., "fat

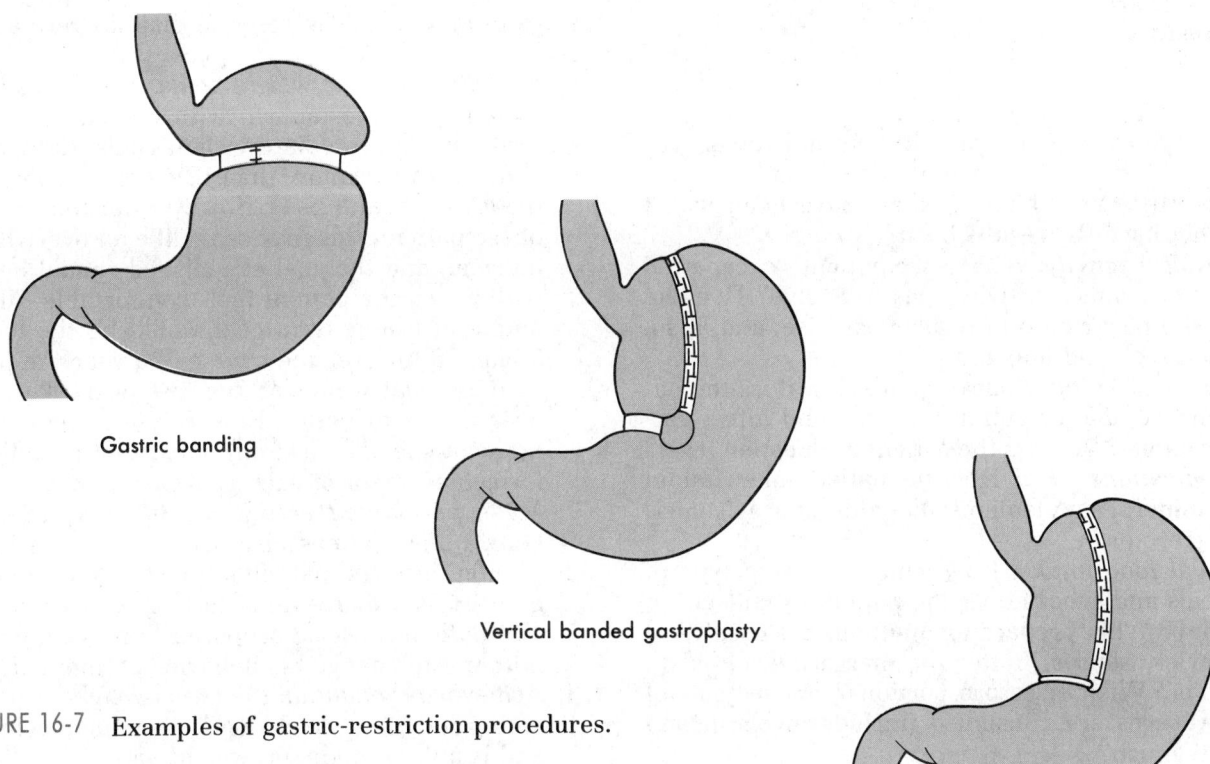

Gastric banding

Vertical banded gastroplasty

Vertical ring gastroplasty

FIGURE 16-7   Examples of gastric-restriction procedures.

burning"), or previously undiscovered qualities.[48] A popular fad is the very low–carbohydrate diet, which includes *The Complete Scarsdale Medical Diet, The Doctor's Quick Weight Loss Diet* (Stillman diet), and *Atkin's Diet Revolution,* among others. These diets induce ketosis, and because diuresis accompanies ketosis, weight loss is rapid. However, the fluid lost is eventually replaced, and because the diets do little to retrain eating habits, all the weight lost is usually regained. Hyperuricemia and increased low density—lipoprotein cholesterol (which may contribute to coronary artery disease) are worrisome consequences of these diets.[67]

Body wraps and clothing designed to "sweat away pounds" are completely ineffective in fat reduction. Massages and passive exercises are also unsuccessful in mobilizing fat. Furthermore, there is no basis to the belief that there is a special type of fat called cellulite, which demands another type of approach than other body fat. Cellulite will only disappear with an effective weight-loss program.

NURSING MANAGEMENT OF THE OBESE PATIENT
Assessment

Assessment of the obese individual is centered around obtaining a detailed diet history and accurate anthropometric measurements.

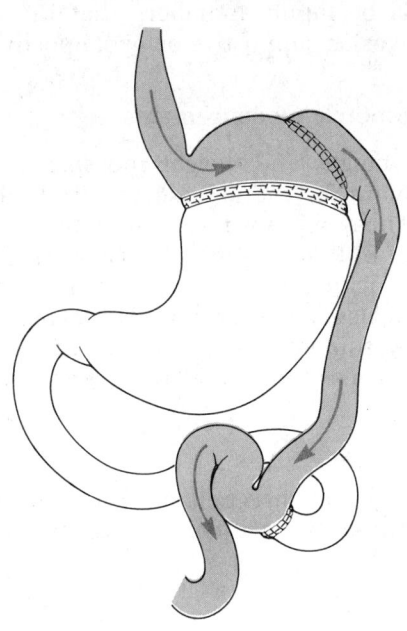

FIGURE 16-8   Roux-en-Y gastric bypass. Stomach reservoir is closed with a line of staples, jejunum is resected from duodenum and anastomosed to stomach reservoir, and duodenal stump is connected to jejunum to allow drainage of duodenal secretions.

Diet history

A diet history interview with an obese individual should cover the following topics:

1. *Diets followed in the past.* Has the individual ever dieted? If so, how many times and how frequently? What kinds of diets have been used? What have the results been?
2. *Physical activity.* What is the patient's occupation and how much activity does it involve? Does he or she participate in regular exercise, and, if so, what type and how much?
3. *Ethnic or cultural background.* How does the patient's ethnic or cultural background affect eating habits? What is the patient's education level?
4. *Medications taken.* Does the patient take vitamin or mineral supplements, diet aids, anorexigenics, or steroids?
5. *Usual food intake.* How many and what type of meals and snacks does the patient usually eat in a day? What preparation methods are used? Are gravies, sauces, butter, or margarine added to foods? What sizes are portions? What types of beverages are consumed (include alcohol), and how much?
6. *Conditions under which eating occurs.* Is the patient happy, sad, lonely, or bored when eating? Does the patient eat alone or with others? When and where does eating take place? What does food mean to the patient—comfort, indulgence, reward, love?
7. *Stresses and support systems.* What types of stress is the individual exposed to? Are there friends or family members that the individual perceives as supportive or unsupportive?

Anthropometric measurements

Accurate height and weight measurements are a starting point for the assessment of all obese individuals. These measurements may be used for calculation of BMI, as described earlier. In some cases, skinfold thicknesses, measured with special calipers, will also be desirable. These are best performed by someone with training and experience, because novices tend to obtain inconsistent results.

Nursing Diagnosis

The nursing diagnosis related to obesity and overweight is: altered nutrition: more than body requirements.

Planning

Because an effective weight-loss regimen requires major changes in deeply ingrained eating habits and life-style, the patient should be involved at every stage of planning. The steps in planning are as follows:

1. *Establish realistic weight goals.* The first step of planning is to establish, with the patient, long-term and intermediate weight goals. Individuals with weights no more than 120% of the IBW have the lowest health risks. However, for the severely obese patient, this may seem like an overwhelming goal, and the goal established should be one with which the patient feels comfortable. An example of a long-term goal would be the loss of 34 kg (75 lb) over the course of a year. An intermediate goal would be the loss of 3.6 kg (8 lb) over the next month. Rewards (e.g., new clothing or a special vacation) should be established for achievement of each goal.
2. *Make permanent eating and life-style changes.* Only a diet and exercise plan that can be incorporated into the patient's life-style on a permanent basis will result in lasting weight control. The patient must be prepared to make the commitment to change his behavior permanently.
3. *Achieve and maintain the target weight.* Through eating and life-style changes, the patient achieves and is able to maintain weight loss.

Implementation

Moderate low-calorie diet

Although the dietitian usually develops a diet plan in conjunction with the patient and instructs the patient in the diet, to reinforce the teachings the nurse should be aware of what the patient has been taught. Most often the dietitian will teach adult patients to use the Exchange Lists for Meal Planning.[20] This has the advantage of allowing patients to individualize their diets without having to count calories. From the diet plan, the patient knows how many servings from each food exchange list (meats, milk, fruits, vegetables, breads, and fats) can be eaten daily.

Control of portion sizes is crucial in achieving and maintaining weight loss, and the patient should be encouraged to weigh or measure all foods initially, until skill in estimating portion sizes is attained. The dieter must be especially careful to limit fat in the diet. Fat is a very concentrated source of calories, and dieters consuming low-fat diets are the most successful in reducing their caloric intake and losing weight.[39] Fried foods, obviously fatty meats, butter, margarine, salad dressings, and mayonnaise are easily recognized sources of fat. Hidden sources of fat include nonskim dairy products, meat with marbled fat (which cannot be trimmed away), bacon, sausage, nuts, seeds, quick breads, and snack crackers and chips. The nurse can review with the patient their usual intake and help him choose alternatives with fewer calories, such as substituting poultry with the skin removed for prime or choice beef, cheeses made from skim milk for higher fat cheese, and fresh vegetables with a low-fat yogurt dip for high-calorie snack foods. Since fat is the purveyor of most of the flavor of foods, dieters may find a low-fat diet tasteless and unsatisfying. Generous use of herbs, spices, and low-calorie seasonings, as well as taking pains to serve foods attractively, helps make low-fat foods more interesting and appealing. A variety of low-fat convenience foods, including complete frozen meals, are now available for those patients who have the inclination and the financial ability to use them. However, commercially prepared foods such as these are often high in sodium; patients should be cautioned to read the labels and avoid serving the high-sodium products frequently, especially if they suffer from hypertension.

Obese and overweight individuals often have poor eating habits. For example, they may skip meals and then be so hungry that they overeat at their next exposure to food. Dieting can be an opportunity to improve eating habits and establish patterns for lasting health. The patient should be taught that there is no one food or group of foods that must be avoided. All foods can be eaten in moderation, but care should be taken not to consume excessive amounts of sweets and fats, which contain few nutrients but many calories. Patients who have dieted many times are often "chronically restrained eaters." They try to avoid specific foods that they find highly desirable, because when they start to eat those foods, they often lose control and binge. They need to practice controlling their intake of these foods so that they do not have to apply this "on-off" attitude toward food.[51]

Aerobic exercise

The obese patient, particularly one with known heart disease or with a family history of heart disease, should be thoroughly evaluated before beginning an exercise program. Exercises such as jogging and rope skipping may worsen degenerative joint disease, so patients with this problem and severely obese patients should be encouraged to choose less stressful activities, such as swimming, bicycling, or walking. To promote fat loss, exercise should involve large muscle groups, be performed at least 3 days/week, and expend at least 300 calories/session (or 4 days/week, with an expenditure of 200 calories/session).[62] The caloric costs of some common exercises are shown in Table 16-9. Obese and overweight patients often find it difficult to commit themselves to exercise regimens on a continuing basis—although they begin exercise programs, they soon allow their participation to lapse. One nursing study, however, has shown that a variety of factors, some of which can be manipulated by the exercise group leader, improve participation and that well-informed nurses may have a major impact on exercise habits. See the research brief below.

In addition to regular aerobic exercise, the patient should be taught to increase his energy expenditure during his usual daily activities. For instance, he can park farther from his office and increase his walking distance, or use the stairs instead of taking the elevator.

TABLE 16-9 Approximate Energy Expenditure During Exercise

Activity	Calories/kg/minute	Calories used during 30 minutes of exercise by a 70 kg (154 lb) person
Bicycling 12 mph	0.17	357
Running 5 mph	0.14	294
Swimming (fast freestyle)	0.13	273
Walking 3 mph	0.06	126

RESEARCH BRIEF

Gillett PA: Self-reported factors influencing exercise adherence in overweight women, *Nurs Res* 37:25-29, 1988.

In a study of factors related to exercise adherence, moderately overweight female volunteers, aged 35 to 58, participated in a 16½-week aerobic dance program. Subjects were randomly assigned to an experimental group (n = 20) that received intensity-controlled, graded exercise and individual and group reinforcement, or to a control group (n = 18) that exercised at a moderate intensity typical of commercial fitness classes and received no special reinforcement. Although attrition rates of 50% to 68% have been reported in similar populations, 94% of both groups adhered to the program. In poststudy interviews, subjects identified factors that had positively influenced adherence: group homogeneity, opportunities for social networking, positive feelings about increased fitness, leader with a nursing background, commitment to a goal, desire to change body image, and desire to improve physical health. Exercise programs appear to offer nurses an interesting opportunity for health promotion.

Behavior modification techniques

The dieter should be taught the following behavioral modification strategies: self-monitoring, controlling stimuli that foster overeating, improving coping skills, and using rewards to reinforce appropriate behaviors. For at least 4 months after beginning the diet and whenever weight rebounds thereafter, the patient should record exercise, food intake, and emotional and environmental conditions related to food intake to provide a basis for planning changes and for evaluating these changes. The dieter will learn to break the associations between environmental cues or external stimuli and eating. In some cases, the dieter is taught to use aversion methods (e.g., visualizing an unappealing scene) to control food intake. The records kept by the patient should help him or her recognize the difference between eating because of hunger and eating because some stimulus reminded them to eat. He or she can then substitute another activity for eating. Improving coping skills will help the patient deal with eating problems. One way of improving coping skills is through assertiveness training. Recruiting friends and family members to provide support and feedback can also improve coping.[67] The patient also should establish positive contingencies or rewards, specified in signed contracts with the nurse or other health care

PATIENT EDUCATION GUIDE   *Weight Control*

Objectives: To promote eating and life-style changes that will result in weight loss and maintenance of weight loss

A. Eating behaviors
   1. Eat regular meals
   2. Weigh or measure foods until skill is established in estimating portion sizes
   3. Limit high-fat foods
   4. Eat bulky, high-fiber foods
   5. Use behavioral modification techniques that slow the rate of eating and reduce uncontrolled eating, for example:
      a. Eat slowly; chew food well and put utensils down between bites; do not pick up utensils until you have swallowed the previous mouthful
      b. Limit temptation during food shopping; never shop for food on an empty stomach; make out a grocery list before shopping and stick to it
      c. Do not put bowls of food on the table; fill plates in the kitchen
      d. Use small dishes (e.g., salad or bread-and-butter plate rather than dinner plate)
      e. Leave a small amount of food on your plate at the end of each meal
      f. Never eat while involved in any other activity, such as reading or watching television; do not eat standing up
      g. Eat only in one or two places, such as the kitchen and dining room tables; never eat or "taste" while cooking
      h. Keep a diary of when and where you eat and under what circumstances (e.g., boredom, loneliness, anxiety); be aware of problem circumstances and substitute another activity for eating
      i. Keep low-calorie snacks available at all times
   6. Practice controlling intake of desired foods, rather than avoiding the foods altogether
   7. Record food intake daily
   8. Enlist family and friends to provide support
B. Exercise
   1. Use large muscle groups in sustained activity
   2. Exercise at least 3 days/week
   3. Utilize at least 300 calories/session
   4. Increase energy expenditure during daily activities
C. Maintenance of weight loss
   1. Know target weight and maximum acceptable weight gain
   2. Weigh at least once weekly
   3. Reduce intake (or increase activity) and record all intake if weight gain occurs
   4. Continue to practice controlled intake of desired foods
   5. Continue to rely on support of family and friends

provider, to be applied in response to desirable eating behaviors (see the patient education guide below).

It is most important that the patient understand that the idea is to structure the environment so that it contributes to success in controlling food intake, rather than to learn these specific strategies. The patient may be able to devise individualized strategies tailored to his or her life-style.

Evaluation of weight-loss programs

Some patients may wish to use one of the many commercial weight-reduction groups available. The nurse can help the patient evaluate these groups, using the following criteria: diets for weight reduction should meet all nutrient needs except calorie requirements, be adaptable to the individual's tastes and habits, be practical in terms of cost and convenience, minimize hunger and fatigue, and be compatible with establishing a lasting change in eating habits. Liquid formula diets and any diet lasting less than 3 to 4 weeks fail to meet at least the last criterion.

Ideally, weight-reduction programs encourage active exercise, which increases energy expenditure, is safe for the participants, and can be incorporated into the patient's life-style on a continuing basis. Successful programs usually include self-monitoring and behavior modification techniques to help participants control eating behaviors, and they provide follow-up for at least 6 months after the end of dieting.[67]

Gastric partitioning

Teaching includes instructions in deep breathing and coughing postoperatively, information about pain control, and a realistic description of the probable results of surgery. The patient should be aware that gastric partitioning is a method of reinforcing changes in eating habits, not a cure for obesity.

Nausea and vomiting are the most common problems after gastric partitioning, and obstruction is a potential problem. Because of this, initial feedings are liquids or strained, blended foods. The nurse gives the patient a 30 mL medication cup once oral fluids are allowed, and encourages intake of 30 mL of fluid/hour. The patient should become accustomed to measuring all intake in the 30 mL cup and avoiding overfilling the gastric reservoir. During the first 6 to 8 weeks after surgery, the diet can be advanced to soft and then to regular foods. Patients are encouraged to develop the habits of eating slowly, chewing all food well, and eating very small meals.

Patients with gastric bypass may experience dumping syndrome. This can be averted by avoiding concentrated sweets, eating slowly, and avoiding liquids during mealtime after the early postoperative period.

During the first 1 to 2 postoperative years, the effects of the surgery will reinforce dieting efforts by decreasing the amount that patients can comfortably eat at one time. After that time, the gastric reservoir has usually stretched to the point that it is of little benefit. During the first 2 years after surgery, patients need to learn to apply behavior modification techniques, limit calorie-dense foods with few nutrients (fats, pastries, candies, sweets, and sweetened beverages), and eat regular, small meals. They should be followed initially at weekly or biweekly intervals; the intervals can gradually be lengthened, but they should be seen at least monthly until they have reached the target weight or stabilized their weight.

Support and positive feedback

Losing weight, whether it is a few pounds or many, is rarely an easy process. The nurse should convey respect and encouragement for the dieter's efforts. Dieters occasionally encounter plateaus, where their weight remains the same despite adherence to the diet. This is most likely caused by a resetting of the metabolic rate, which is the body's response to food restriction and weight loss. Dieters find plateaus very discouraging, and they may go off their diets at this point, never to resume them. Support is especially important during this time. Dieters need to know that if they continue to follow their diets, their weight will eventually begin to decrease again. Decreasing intake by 100 to 200 calories, if this will not reduce the daily allowance below 800 calories, will help the dieter to begin to lose again. As an alternative, increasing the length or intensity of exercise sessions often helps end the plateau.

Evaluation

There are two major outcome criteria for weight reduction: weight loss and maintenance of weight loss. A maximum loss of 0.45 to 0.9 kg (1 to 2 lb) per week is the expected outcome for most diets that are safe and effective in retraining eating habits. Patients are followed weekly or bi-weekly during the dieting process to ensure that loss continues and that they are incorporating new eating and exercise habits into their life-style.

As difficult as it is, losing weight is not usually as difficult as maintaining loss. Patients need to be taught to be aware of "maximal acceptable weight gain,"[67] which varies, but may be 5% to 10% above their target or lowest weight. If they reach maximal acceptable gain, they should return to recording all intake, reducing intake, and evaluating activity patterns. Most formerly obese patients find it necessary to weigh at least weekly for the balance of their lives to regulate their weight adequately.

Where appropriate, it may be possible to use other parameters, such as reduction in blood pressure in the hypertensive patient or of blood glucose in the diabetic patient, to evaluate the success of weight-control measures and reinforce the patient's efforts.

Documentation

Each patient will have documented evidence of the following:

1. A nutrition assessment, consisting of at least height and weight measurements and a diet history
2. A weight-loss goal established jointly by the patient and the health care team
3. An individualized diet and exercise plan
4. Regular monitoring of progress made toward achievement of the goal
5. Periodic follow-up after the patient has achieved the desired weight-loss goal or stabilized his or her weight

CRITICAL THINKING QUESTIONS

1 What patient characteristics would alert you to the possibility of undernutrition? Why would these characteristics lead you to suspect nutritional deficits?

2 Mrs. R., a 79-year-old woman, is hospitalized for a hip fracture. The admission nursing history reveals that she has lived alone since the death of her husband 3 years earlier. She complains that the meals served in the hospital are "so large that they would feed three people." In discussing this with Mrs. R., the dietitian finds that her usual intake consists of toast, jam, and tea for breakfast, with canned soup and crackers for lunch and dinner. What nutritional deficiencies might Mrs. R. be expected to have? What other information would you want to evaluate her nutritional status more fully?

3 A 55-year-old woman is admitted to the hospital for evaluation of an unexplained weight loss of 8 kg (17.6 lb). What information would be necessary to perform a basic nutrition assessment on her? If her serum albumin level is 3.8 g/dL (normal >3.5) and her current weight is 91% of her usual weight, can her nutritional status be described as adequate? Explain.

4 A patient hospitalized for 10 weeks after a motor vehicle accident experienced weight loss, hypoalbuminemia (abnormally low serum albumin), and hair loss. Describe the risks, in terms of morbidity, associated with these nutrition-related deficits.

5 A patient must have radical head and neck surgery because of cancer of the tongue. Oral intake will be impossible for weeks after the surgery. What nutrition support method would you expect to use, and why?

6 A 76-year-old diabetic patient who has suffered a cerebrovascular accident is to receive tube feedings. Design a nursing care plan to promote feeding safety for this patient.

7 A patient with short bowel syndrome and an ileostomy is to be discharged on home TPN. Lipid emulsion will be mixed with his TPN, which will be prepared and delivered by a home-care vendor. What specific areas will be of most concern in teaching him and his wife to deliver home TPN?

8 Define obesity and overweight. What health risks are associated with these disorders?

9 Explain how genetic, family, physical, and psychologic characteristics may interact to cause obesity.

10 Think of an obese or overweight friend or family member, or interview an obese or overweight patient. Devise an individualized teaching plan to help the person use behavioral modification techniques, exercise, and diet changes in a weight control program.

11 Describe surgical procedures that are effective in promoting weight loss. Discuss the preoperative teaching and follow-up care required by patients undergoing these procedures.

12 List the basic criteria for safe and effective weight-loss programs. Choose two popular weight-loss programs and discuss the ways in which they do or do not meet these criteria.

RESOURCES

1 AMERICAN SOCIETY FOR PARENTERAL AND ENTERAL NUTRITION 8605 Cameron St., Suite 500 Silver Spring, MD 20910

2 THE OLEY FOUNDATION 214 Hun Memorial Albany Medical Center Albany, New York 12208
Through the Oley Foundation, patients on long-term (especially home-care) parenteral and enteral nutrition can communicate with and learn more about other patients receiving similar types of nutrition support.

3 WILLIAMS & WILKINS PUBLISHING CO. *Nutrition Today* Teaching Aids 428 E. Preston St. Baltimore, MD 21202

This series of nutrition-related teaching aids (consisting of slides and syllabus) for health professionals includes gastrointestinal absorption, diagnosing nutritional deficiencies, and nutritional care of the cancer patient.

4 HEALTHY LIVING INSTITUTE 402 S. 14th St., Box 612 Hettinger, ND 58639

In its monthly *International Obesity Newsletter* for professionals, the institute reports research in the field of obesity, reviews diet books and programs, and lists upcoming obesity conferences.

5 ODPHP NATIONAL HEALTH INFORMATION CENTER P.O. Box 11-3 Washington, DC 20013

Nutrition and health publications, including the following, are available for a nominal handling fee.

- Nutrition and Your Health: Dietary Guidelines for Americans, ed 3, 1990. Single copy or reproducible available only. To order bulk copies, contact the U.S. Government Printing Office at (202)783-3238 and refer to Stock No. 001-000-5274.
- The Surgeon General's Report on Nutrition and Health, 1988.
- The Surgeon General's Report on Nutrition and Health: Summary and Recommendations, 1988.

BIBLIOGRAPHY

Current

1. Alverdy JC et al: Effect of commercially available chemically defined liquid diets on the intestinal microflora and bacterial translocation from the gut, *J Parent Ent Nutr* 14:1, 1990.
2. Ahmed FE: Effect of nutrition on the health of the elderly, *J Am Diet Assoc* 92:1102, 1992.
3. American Society for Parenteral and Enteral Nutrition: Guidelines for use of total parenteral nutrition in the hospitalized adult patient, *J Parent Ent Nutr* 10:441, 1986.
4. American Society for Parenteral and Enteral Nutrition: Guidelines for the use of enteral nutrition in the adult patient, *J Parent Ent Nutr* 11:435, 1987.
5. American Society for Parenteral and Enteral Nutrition: Standards for nutrition support: hospitalized patients, *Nutr Clin Pract* 3:28, 1988.
6. Bray GA: Pathophysiology of obesity, *Am J Clin Nutr* 55:488S, 1992.
7. Bray GA: Drug treatment of obesity, *Am J Clin Nutr* 55:538S, 1992.
8. Burnside I: *Nursing and the aged: a self-care approach*, ed 3, New York, 1988, McGraw-Hill.
9. Compos A, Mequid MM: A critical appraisal of the usefulness of perioperative nutritional support, *Am J Clin Nutr* 55:117, 1992.
10. Ciocon JO: Indications for tube feedings in elderly patients, *Dysphagsia* 5:1, 1990.
11. Chumlea W et al: Nutritional assessment of the elderly through anthropometry, ed 2, Columbus, 1987, Ross Laboratories.
12. Crocker KS et al: Microbial growth comparison of fine commercial parenteral lipid emulsions, *J Parent Ent Nutr* 8:391, 1984.
13. Crocker KS et al: Microbial growth in clinically used enteral delivery systems, *Am J Inf Control* 14:250, 1986.
14. Coats KG et al: Hospital-associated malnutrition: a reevaluation 12 years later, *J Am Diet Assoc* 93:27, 1992.
15. D'Angio R et al: The growth of microorganisms in total parenteral nutrition admixtures, *J Parent Ent Nutr* 11:394, 1987.
16. DeChicco RS et al: Selection of nutrition support regimens, *Nutr Clin Pract* 7:239, 1992.
17. Desky AS et al: Predicting nutrition-associated complications for patients undergoing gastrointestinal surgery, *J Parent Ent Nutr* 11:440, 1987.
18. Donowitz LG et al: Alterations of normal gastric flora in cimetidine therapy, *Infect Control* 7:23, 1986.
19. Edes T et al: Diarrhea in tube-fed patients: feeding formulas not necessarily the cause, *Am J Med* 88:91, 1990.
20. Exchange Lists for Meal Planning, American Diabetes Association and American Dietetic Association, 1986.
21. Flynn KT, Norton LC, Fisher RL: Enteral tube feeding: indications, practices, and outcomes, *Image* 19(1):14, 1987.
22. Freedland CP et al: Microbial contamination of continuous drip feedings, *J Parent Ent Nutr* 13:18, 1989.
23. Foster G et al: Caloric requirements in total parenteral nutrition, *J Am Coll Nutr* 6:231, 1987.
24. Foster GD et al: A controlled comparison of three very-low-calorie diets: effects on weight, body composition and symptoms, *Am J Clin Nutr* 55:811, 1992.
25. Grace DM: Gastric restriction procedures for treating severe obesity, *Am J Clin Nutr* 55:556S, 1992.
26. Grant JP: *Handbook of total parenteral nutrition*, ed 2, 1992, WB Saunders.
27. Grunow JE et al: Contamination of enteral nutrition systems during prolonged intermittent use, *J Parent Ent Nutr* 13:23, 1989.
28. National Institutes of Health Consensus Development Conference Statement: Gastrointestinal surgery for severe obesity, *Am J Clin Nutr* 15:6155, 1992.
29. Gottschlich MM et al: Diarrhea in tube-fed burn patients: incidence, etiology, nutritional impact, and prevention, *J Parent Ent Nutr* 12:338, 1988.
30. Hamaoui E: Assessing the nutrition support team, *J Parent Ent Nutr* 11:412, 1987.
31. Halverson JD: Metabolic risk of obesity surgery and long-term follow-up, *Am J Clin Nutr* 55:6025, 1992.
32. Heimburger D: Diarrhea with enteral feeding: will the real cause please stand up? *Am J Med* 88:89, 1990.
33. Herfindal ET et al: Survey of home nutritional support patients, *J Parent Ent Nutr* 13:3, 1989.
34. Holmes R et al: Combating pressures sores—nutritionally, *Am J Nurs* 87:1301, 1987.
35. Kamath SK et al: Hospital malnutrition: a 22-hospital screening study, *J Am Diet Assoc* 86:203, 1986.
36. Kennedy-Caldwell C, Guenter P: *Nutrition support nursing core curriculum*, ed 2, Silver Spring, Md, 1988. American Society for Parenteral and Enteral Nutrition.
37. Kohn CL, Keithley JK: Techniques for evaluating and managing diarrhea in the tube-fed patient, *Nutr Clin Pract* 2:250, 1987.
38. Kositzke JA: A question of balance, dehydration in the elderly, *J Gerontol Nurs* 16:4, 1990.
39. Lissner L et al: Dietary fat and the regulation of energy intake in human subjects, *Am J Clin Nutr* 46:886, 1987.
40. Mamel JJ: Percutaneous endoscopic gastrostomy, *Nutr Clin Pract* 2:65, 1987.
41. MacBurney M et al: *Formulas in clinical nutrition: enteral*

and tube feedings, In Rombeau J, Calwell M, eds, Philadelphia, 1990, WB Saunders.

42. Marcuard SP: Dissolution of clotted enteral feedings, *J Parent Ent Nutr* 11:168, 1987.

43. Metheny N: Measures to test placement of nasogastric and nasointestinal feeding tubes: a review, *Nurs Res* 37:324, 1988.

44. Metheny NA, Eisenberg P, McSweeney M: Effect of feeding tube properties and three irrigants on clogging rates, *Nurs Res* 37:165, 1988.

45. Mughal MM, Mequid M: The effect of nutritional status on morbidity after elective surgery for benign gastrointestinal disease, *J Parent Ent Nutr* 11:140, 1987.

46. Mullen H et al: Risk of pulmonary aspiration among patients receiving enteral nutrition support, *J Parent Ent Nutr* 16:160, 1992.

47. Nicholson LJ: Declogging small-bore feeding tubes, *J Parent Ent Nutr* 11:594, 1987.

48. Rock CL, Coulston AM: Weight-control approaches: a review by the California Dietetic Association, *J Am Diet Assoc* 88:44, 1988.

49. Rolls BJ, Phillips PA: Aging and disturbances of thirst and fluid balance, *Nutr Rev* 48:3, 1990.

50. Sahyoun NR et al: Dietary intakes and biochemical indicators of nutritional status in an elderly institutionalized population, *Am J Clin Nutr* 47:524, 1988.

51. Saito H et al: The effect of route of nutrient administered on the nutritional state, catabolic hormone secretion, and gut muscosal integrity after burn injury, *J Parent Ent Nutr* 11:1, 1987.

52. Schulz LO: Brown adipose tissue: regulation of thermogenesis and implications for obesity, *J Am Diet Assoc* 87:761, 1987.

53. Solomon SM, Kriby DF: The refeeding syndrome: a review, *J Parent Ent Nutr* 14:90, 1990.

54. Starkey JF, Jefferson PA, Kirby DF: Taking care of percutaneous endoscopic gastrostomy, *Am J Nurs* 88:42, 1988.

55. Stokes MA et al: Mortality in patients on home parenteral nutrition, *J Parent Ent Nutr* 13:2, 1989.

56. Van Itallie TB: Health implications of overweight and obesity in the United States, *Ann Intern Med* 103:983, 1985.

57. Warnold I, Lundhold K: Clinical significance of preoperative nutritional status in 215 noncancer patients, *Ann Surg* 199:299, 1984.

58. Weinsier, RL et al: *Handbook of clinical nutrition,* ed 2, St. Louis, 1989, Mosby–Year Book.

59. Weiss SR: Obesity: Pathogenesis, consequences, and approaches to treatment, *Psych Clin North Am* 7:307, 1984.

60. Wrobel J, Bodin T: Are serum albumin levels detrimental to enteral formulation tolerance? *J Parent Ent Nutr* 12:215, 1988.

61. Zheng JJ, Rosenberg IH: What is the nutritional status of the elderly, *Geriatrics* 44:57, 1989.

Classic

62. American College of Sports Medicine: The recommended quantity and quality of exercise for developing and maintaining fitness in healthy adults, *Med Sci Sports Exerc* 10:VII, 1978.

63. Frisancho AR: New standards of weight and body composition by frame size and height for assessment of nutritional status of adults and the elderly, *Am J Clin Nutr* 40:808, 1981.

64. Hanson RL: Predictive criteria for length of nasogastric tube insertion for tube feeding, *J Parent Ent Nutr* 3:160, 1979.

65. National Institutes of Health Consensus Development Panel: Health implications of obesity, *Ann Intern Med* 103:1073, 1985.

66. Stunkard AJ et al: An adoption study of human obesity, *N Engl J Med* 314:193, 1986.

67. Weinsier RL et al: Hospital malnutrition: a prospective evaluation of general medical patients during the course of hospitalization, *Am J Clin Nutr* 32:418, 1979.

68. Van Itallie TB: Health implications of overweight and obesity in the United States, *Ann Intern Med* 103:983, 1985.

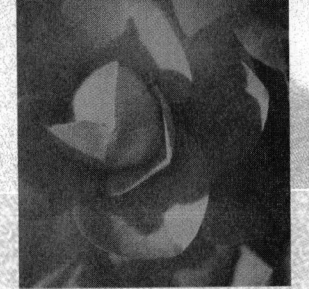

CHAPTER SEVENTEEN

Sensory Deprivation, Sensory Overload, and Sleep Disorders

LEARNING OBJECTIVES

1 Identify risk factors for sensory deprivation in the hospitalized patient.

2 Assess patients for evidence of adverse effects of sensory deprivation.

3 State principles for maintenance of an adequate sensory environment in acute care settings.

4 Describe the behavioral and physiologic responses to sensory overload in the acute care settings.

5 Identify the effects of sensory overload on the older adult.

6 Describe the characteristics of the sleep pattern disturbances of the major sleep disorders.

7 Evaluate the risk factors for sleep pattern disturbance in the hospitalized patient.

8 List the nursing actions appropriate for persons with sleep pattern disturbances.

KEY TERMS

circadian, p. 382
insomnia, p. 383
narcolepsy, p. 384
nonrapid eye movement (NREM), p. 382
rapid eye movement (REM), p. 382

reticular activating system (RAS), p. 382
reticular formation, p. 381
sensory deprivation, p. 376
sensory overload, p. 379

SENSORY-PERCEPTUAL ALTERATIONS are actual or perceived changes in the stimuli received by an individual. These may be visual, auditory, tactile, thermal, or kinesthetic stimuli resulting from alterations in the environment because of an imposed hospital stay or alterations in the individual caused by an illness or physiologic disorder. Nurses play a significant role in monitoring patients' environment to minimize stimuli changes. Nurses assess patients' individual responses and intervene to modulate the effects of unavoidable changes.

Individuals function as integrated systems in constant interaction with the environment. The central nervous system facilitates the amazingly complex task of receiving, processing, and responding to environmental input. Perception, the individual's awareness of the surrounding world, is mediated by physiologic processes that convert environmental stimuli into action potentials in nerve fibers that are then conducted via afferent pathways through the spinal cord or specific portions of the brain to the reticular formation. All sensory input is received by the reticular formation before it is transmitted to the cerebral cortex. The reticular formation is a network of neurons extending from the medulla to the thalamus in the central core of the brainstem, which monitors sensory inputs and outputs and regulates the state of arousal through the reticular activating system, located within the reticular formation. Responses to sensory information are facilitated by the individual's receptivity. The reticular activating system helps maintain the waking state and selectivity of attention.

The alert or waking state is the condition in which the individual is in a state of readiness to receive and process sensory stimuli, thus permitting subjective responses to the environment. The waking state is a necessary prerequisite for the cortical functions of stimulating voluntary movement, learning, intellectual activity, and localizing sensations. Stimulation and maintenance of the wakeful state by the reticular activating system occur in response to any stimulus received by the reticular formation. Whereas the arousal state occurs in response to diffuse or nonspecific signals from the reticular activating system, maintaining arousal and focusing attention during the waking state involves an exchange of signals between the cerebral cortex and the reticular formation in a positive feedback cycle. Quantity and quality of stimuli affect cortical arousal and function.

SENSORY DEPRIVATION

The reticular activating system is believed to serve a homeostatic function in the regulation of sensory input, increasing or decreasing cortical arousal in response to extreme or diminished levels of stimulation. **Sensory deprivation** is a state in which the level of sensory input is insufficient to maintain the degree of cortical arousal necessary for homeostasis. Humans who undergo sensory deprivation may experience a variety of alterations in perception, cognitive function, and behavior. These include disorientation, visual and auditory hallucinations, abnormal tactile or kinesthetic experiences, diminished ability to concentrate or think clearly, decreased cognitive task performance, anxiety, and somatic complaints. Insufficient stimulation can interfere with the positive feedback loop between the cerebral cortex and the reticular activating system, causing problems with maintenance of the arousal state. Disorientation can occur, and hallucinations may result from a compensatory effort to maintain arousal.[29] The cortex may increase its ac-

tivity in the absence of adequate stimulation from the reticular activating system and thus contribute to the behavioral disturbances that may be associated with sensory deprivation.[35]

Risk Factors

Risk factors for sensory-perceptual alterations related to sensory deprivation may include aging, physical debility, social isolation, immobility, and neurologic impairments that alter sensory function (Table 17-1). Immobility places the individual at particularly high risk.[44] Restriction of mobility alone produces many of the classic symptoms of sensory deprivation. Physical and social isolation often associated with hospitalization can increase risk. Wood[42] found that patients cared for in single-occupant hospital rooms were more likely to experience sensory disturbances than those in double-occupant rooms. Conditions that alter sensory input, such as visual or hearing loss, spinal cord injury, and peripheral neuropathies, can contribute to sensory disturbances associated with deprivation.

In general daily activities expose the individual to a variety of stimuli in the external environment. The stimuli may or may not have meaning to the individual. People learn to screen out the stimuli that are meaningless and selectively admit the pertinent stimuli. The healthy person is able to seek a different environment or change the environment as needed. When an individual becomes ill and is hospitalized, he or she is confined in an often unfamiliar, unresponsive environment. The hospital environment has important therapeutic value, but also evokes a variety of emotional and psychologic responses, which can be adaptive or maladaptive. The literature cites a variety of behaviors that occur when the individual's coping system deteriorates. The behaviors include anxiety, panic, confusion, delusions, hallucinations, combativeness, aggressive-

TABLE 17-1   Risk Factors for Sensory Deprivation

Situations that alter sensory input	Stressors in the hospital environment
Aging	Therapeutic isolation
Visual and hearing losses	Disruption of normal diurnal variations
Physical debilitation	Sleep deprivation
Spinal cord injury	Drug effects
Peripheral neuropathies	Electrolyte imbalances
	Prolonged immobility

ness, restlessness, disorientation, and distractibility.*

Many factors in the hospital environment can contribute to sensory deprivation. Patients in private rooms may experience social isolation because of insufficient contact with staff or visitors. Patients who are very ill, confused or disruptive, or immobilized with many appliances are more likely to be assigned to private rooms to reduce the disturbance to other patients and facilitate nursing care delivery. Therapeutic isolation, whether to protect the immunosuppressed patient or to prevent spread of infection, increases social isolation. Intensive care environments create significant risks for sensory disturbances. Patients are often in single-occupant rooms, recumbent much or all of the time, and exposed to visual and auditory cues that are monotonous and provide little meaningful stimulation.[22] The patient's experience of normal diurnal variations or variations over a 24-hour period is disrupted, because care activities progress around the clock, and environmental input remains basically unchanged day and night. The hospitalized patient may experience a variety of stresses that can alter the sensory-perceptual process: sleep deprivation, pain, anxiety, drug effects, or electrolyte imbalances.

Patients having eye surgery are at increased risk because of the presence of an impaired sensory mo-

*References 8, 19, 20, 23, 25.

dality. The elderly patient with impaired vision may have learned to adapt to decreased sensory input in a familiar environment. However, these adaptive behaviors may not be effective when the older adult becomes ill and requires hospitalization.[6] Patients with selected neurologic disorders, spinal cord injury, myasthenia gravis, and other diseases or conditions that cause immobility are also at increased risk because of the loss or impairment of the kinesthetic sense and mobility. Patients with severely restricted mobility because of special beds, such as the Roto-rest, circular electric bed, or Stryker frame, or because of restrictive appliances, such as halo traction or skeletal traction, experience even greater risk of sensory disturbances. Patients transferred to the hospital from other institutional environments, such as nursing homes or institutions for the disabled, may exhibit preexisting sensory deprivation, which can be exacerbated in the hospital environment.

NURSING MANAGEMENT OF THE PATIENT WITH SENSORY DEPRIVATION
Assessment

Development of a plan of care for the patient with sensory-perceptual alterations related to sensory deprivation, actual or potential, requires careful evaluation of the patient's physical status, behavior, and environment. Particular attention must be paid

GERIATRIC CONSIDERATIONS

Sensory Deprivation

Preexisting sensory impairment can increase the risk for the older adult of sensory deprivation in the hospital setting. Nursing interventions can help the elderly adapt to a new environment and limit the incidence of sensory deprivation.

Visual impairment

Controlled lighting can help the older adult see better in the hospital. Increased light intensity can help the person see better. However, glare from bright sunlight can diminish the older adult's visual acuity. Closing curtains or blinds on windows can reduce glare and improve vision for the older adult. Adequate background light can help the older adult adjust to decreased visual accommodation when moving from brightly lit to dimly lit rooms and hallways.

Hearing impairment

Speaking in a controlled, lower pitch can help the older adult respond more appropriately to conversations. Visual cues and contextual cues may help the elderly adapt to auditory stimuli. The visual reinforcement of auditory input can help the older adult remember important information.

Touch

Elderly people who have lost spouses and other family may suffer from touch deprivation. Selective use of touch by the nurse can provide relevant stimuli and help orient the older adult to a strange environment.

Balance

Decreased perception of proprioceptive stimuli from joints and muscles impairs the older adult's balance. Increased mobility can help the older adult respond to kinesthetic sensations and reduce the risk of falls.

to the patient's mental status, including both cognitive and sensory functions. The existence of actual and potential risk factors for sensory deprivation is identified in the initial assessment (see box at right) and incorporated into routine shift assessment activities. Patients may be aware that indeterminate sensory experiences, sensory distortions, and illusions are not real and not related to actual environmental stimuli.[37] They are often reluctant to report unusual sensory experiences to nurses or physicians because of their concerns about being labeled "crazy." The elderly may be particularly reluctant to report these incidents because of their fears of being considered "senile" or incompetent.[36]

Changes in behavior associated with sensory deprivation include boredom, reduced awareness, difficulty concentrating, disorientation to the environment, delusional thoughts, and hallucinations. The patient may become irritable the longer he or she is in a situation of decreased sensory input. Emotional reactions may range from worry and anxiety to fear, depression, and paranoid ideations. The person becomes preoccupied with the passage of time. With sensory deprivation the patient may be increasingly restless or become passive and withdrawn.[11]

Nursing Diagnosis

The diagnosis of high risk for sensory-perceptual alterations related to sensory deprivation can be caused by social isolation, anxiety, impaired mobility, sleep deprivation, or altered thought processes. These etiologies for the diagnosis need to be considered when planning nursing care.

Planning

Prevention is the most effective and desirable strategy for caring for the patient at risk for adverse effects caused by sensory deprivation. Desired patient outcomes for the patient include:

The patient will remain oriented to time, place, and person.

The patient will not report abnormal sensory phenomena such as auditory and visual hallucinations.

The patient will not demonstrate cognitive impairment such as decreased attention span, impaired memory, or reduced task performance.

The patient will not pull at dressings or tubings.

Implementation

Nurses play an important role in the prevention of sensory deprivation. By conducting a careful assessment, managing the patient's sensory and social environment, and being aware of risk factors, the nurse can avert this potential problem for many pa-

---

ASSESSMENT PARAMETERS FOR SENSORY DEPRIVATION

Cognitive function—evaluation of orientation, memory, and thought processes.

Motor function—is mobility impaired? Must the patient remain recumbent?

Sensory function—is there a preexisting sensory alteration, visual, auditory, or tactile? Is the patient experiencing unusual bodily sensations—feeling numb, cold, floating, or "disconnected" sensations?

Has the patient seen or heard things that are unreal or incongruent with environmental stimulation?

Psychologic—what are the patient's coping skills; is he or she anxious or restless?

Behavioral—does the patient demonstrate behavioral disturbances or noncompliance, such as pulling on tubings or dressings?

Environmental—has the patient experienced prehospital deprivation in a home, nursing home, or institutional environment?

Social—what family support is available; what other resources for social support are available?

---

tients. The nurse's presence can do much to minimize the disabling effects of restrictive hospital environments. In addition, the patient will benefit from opportunities for social interaction with visitors, staff, and other patients. Conversations that focus on the patient's interests and experiences provide meaningful stimulation that helps promote cognitive activity. Providing variation in the patient's physical environment supports the brain functions of alertness, concentration, and orientation. A room with a window can help the patient track the normal day/night changes. Calendars, clocks, and pictures of family members can provide meaningful visual stimuli for the patient. Watching television or listening to the radio can be a source of stimulation in the patient's environment. The nurse helps the patient select favorite programs. However if a television or radio is left on all the time, they become monotonous stimuli that contribute to sensory deprivation. The nurse maintains the patient's physical mobility to provide appropriate kinesthetic stimuli. Increasing mobility assists the patient in moving to different locations that promote changing sensory stimulation. For the patient who is immobilized, passive range-of-motion exercises will increase kinesthetic sensations in joints and muscles.

Evaluation

The nurse can determine the effectiveness of the interventions by evaluating the patient's level of consciousness, orientation, attention span, mood, and behavior. The patient will have normal diurnal variations in sleep/wakefulness. The patient will be alert and will respond appropriately to environmental stimuli.

Documentation

Charting for the patient with sensory deprivation includes documentation of preexisting sensory/perceptual deficits such as visual or hearing impairment and cognitive impairment. The nurse records the interventions used to provide meaningful environmental stimuli. The documentation of the patient's response to interventions includes more than "alert and oriented." The nurse charts the appropriateness of the patient's response to changes in the environment.

SENSORY OVERLOAD

Sensory overload, sensory bombardment, sensory stimulation, and environmental overdose are synonymous terms. **Sensory overload** is defined as a situation in which an individual is bombarded by multisensory stimuli at a greater-than-normal intensity level. The response to the stimuli and the type and meaning of stimuli presented affect the individual's adaptive behavior. Sensory overload can disrupt the mechanism of information processing and decrease the meaningfulness of the environment,[18,31] which results in maladaptive responses (see box below).

Risk Factors

Sensory overload is a condition that can arise in the hospital environment, especially in the critical care unit. Sleep loss is a major risk factor for sensory overload. During an acute illness, it is difficult to maintain normal habits, which often help keep one's life organized. Other risk factors in the hospital environment that may cause sensory overload are excessive environmental stimuli and a loss of control for the patient. Patients in the intensive care unit are at particular risk for these problems.

NURSING MANAGEMENT OF THE PATIENT WITH SENSORY OVERLOAD
Assessment

The nurse assesses for sensory overload by collecting subjective and objective data on individual and environmental variables. The individual variables include behavioral and physiologic responses. The amount and intensity of the sensory input from the environment and the alteration in pattern or meaningfulness of the sensory inputs are the two variables to be examined from the environmental perspective.

Individual factors

The physiologic responses to sensory overload resemble the stress response of the general adaptation syndrome described by Selye.[37] The basis of this response is the release of epinephrine and norepinephrine from the adrenal medulla, which results in peripheral vasoconstriction, hypertension, tachycardia, increased cerebral blood flow, sweating, slight increase in skeletal muscle tension, and increase in blood cortisol and cholesterol.[22,26]

The psychologic responses to sensory overload result from a global clouding of consciousness. The internal and external stimuli are processed through the reticular activating system (RAS). Linking the RAS with the cerebral cortex is the corticifugal system, which allows the cortex to be bombarded with stimuli.[32] Perceptual or information processing, learning, judgment, and emotion are affected. The resulting behaviors include experiencing perceptual disorders (hallucinations, sound distortion), time expansion, feelings of unpleasantness and loss of control, the sensation of floating in space, nausea, headache, aggressiveness, anxiety, lability, difficulty with speech, fatigue, paranoia, and somatic effects.[18,33] The patient also may experience decreased problem-solving ability, inability to concentrate, and inappropriate social behavior.[11]

Environmental factors

Two variables are important to consider when assessing environmental factors: (1) the amount and intensity of the environmental stimuli and (2) the patient's perception of the stimuli present in the environment. It is important to determine the significance of these variables to the patient by assessing the adaptive or maladaptive responses of the patient.

SENSORY OVERLOAD BEHAVIORS

Anxiety	Aggressiveness
Panic	Restlessness
Confusion	Disorientation
Delusions	Distractibility
Hallucinations	Sleep loss
Combativeness	

TABLE 17-2	Risk Factors for Sensory Overload		
Cognitive	**Visual**	**Auditory**	**Tactile**
Worrying	Glaring lights	Noise from:	Pain from surgery or invasive
Coping with illness	Unrecognizable faces	Crying	procedures
Anxiety	Rapid movements	Crash of equipment	Increased pressure (e.g., casts)
Nervousness	Numerous visitors	Buzzers	Chest restraints
Sleep loss		Telephones	
Medications (caffeine)		Interrupted schedule	

On entering the hospital, a patient leaves his normal environment. Admission to the hospital represents a significant disruption of the patient's lifestyle. There are foreign sights, sounds, and smells that present new stimuli with which the person must learn to cope. Examples of sensory overload stimuli in the hospital are summarized in Table 17-2.

The hospitalized patient often experiences physical overstimulation and emotional deprivation. The patient is exposed to an enormous amount of sensory input in the form of pain, continuous lighting, machine noises, nurses and doctors talking at the bedside, multiple invasive procedures, and frequent interruptions.[18,24,27,39] Patients are not able to control the inflow of information, nor can they escape from it. Therefore they are unable to use normal adaptive responses to sensory input.

Nursing Diagnosis

The primary nursing diagnosis for the patient experiencing sensory overload is sensory-perceptual alteration related to excessive stimuli. Other nursing diagnoses that can be the focus of planning care for the patient with problems of sensory overload include:

High risk for injury related to disorientation

Altered thought processes related to disorientation and loss of sleep

Impaired communication related to decreased ability to process increased sensory input

Planning

Since sensory overload has a variety of behavioral manifestations, patient outcomes focus on prevention of the physical or psychologic responses previously described. If the suggested nursing actions are implemented, minimal maladaptive responses should occur. Specific outcomes for the plan of care can include:

The patient will remain alert and oriented to the physical environment

The patient will respond appropriately to environmental stimuli

The patient will engage in meaningful conversations

The patient will verbalize decreased anxiety or irritability

Implementation

The responsibility of the nurse in caring for the patient experiencing sensory overload is to control the environment for the well-being of the patient and increase staff awareness of the need to reduce unnecessary sensory stimuli. For any patient experiencing sensory overload and feelings of loss of control in the environment, a calm approach and unconditional acceptance by the nurse can help the patient feel more safe and secure. Interventions can be developed to limit the intensity of various categories of stimuli: noise, lighting, crowding, and touch.

Noise

Woods and Falk[43] found that the noisiest places in the hospital were in two patient care areas: the recovery room and intensive care unit (ICU). Nursing interventions to decrease the sensory input from noise include establishing a private area for patients, families, and health care professionals to talk away from the bedside. Limiting bedside conversation to that directed to the patient also creates less disturbance. Reducing the alarm volumes on infusion pumps and ventilators and reducing the volume on telephones and paging equipment are additional measures that would facilitate a decrease in noise within the patient's environment. Providing soft foam ear plugs for the patient may also tend to blot out the extraneous noise.*

Lighting

Continuous lighting creates sensory confusion, causing patients to lose track of time, interrupt their sleep, and alter their circadian rhythms. This is a problem in both the general hospital unit and the

*References 18, 21, 26, 31, and 36.

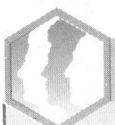

GERIATRIC CONSIDERATIONS

Sensory Overload

Sensory overload can create significant communication problems for the older adult. The ability to manage increased sensory stimuli can be diminished by the presence of cognitive impairments, thus increasing sensory overload. Situations that can contribute to sensory overload during an assessment interview include asking for too much information at one time, too many people trying to talk at one time (such as family members or other health care providers), and environmental noise and distractions. The older adult who uses a hearing aid may be particularly sensitive to environmental noises because the hearing aid magnifies background sounds. Hospital noises (equipment alarms or voice paging systems) that the nurse has become accustomed to may be distracting to the elderly patient and add to the sensory overload.

The nurse can facilitate communication with the older adult by controlling the amount of sensory stimuli. The nurse should limit the number of topics discussed during an assessment interview. Closing the door to the room may screen out some of the potentially distracting environmental noises. If family members are present during the conversation, encourage them to let the older adult speak for himself or herself.

ICU. Dimming or turning out the lights can reduce sensory overload. Providing periods of reduced light can promote more effective periods of sleep for the patient.

A number of actions can be implemented that will maintain adequate lighting while still diminishing sensory input. Machinery that has flashing lights can have tape placed over the lights to decrease their intensity. Grouping patients according to acuity limits sleep disturbances for the less critically ill. Turning off or dimming the overhead lights further reduces visual stimulation and facilitates day and night light fluctuations. Eye patches or a blindfold can also be worn by the patient and may eventually become standard equipment at the bedside. Closing the doors to the patient's room and using adjustable window shades, heavy drapes, or slatted blinds will also diminish light. In some instances night-lights may provide adequate illumination, and when placed below bed level, they will be even less disruptive to the patient's sleep.[21,36]

Crowding

Crowding exists primarily in the ICU. Patients are strangers to each other and to the hospital person-

nel. Being surrounded by unfamiliar faces may precipitate a sense of loss of privacy and control for a patient. Also, it may be difficult for the patient's family to provide meaningful stimuli to the patient because of the barriers posed by the machinery and equipment used in caring for the critically ill. Therefore nursing actions are aimed at fostering family interaction with the patient. The patient's need for family support should be a priority in the plan of care. Teaching the family to use touch and assistive devices, such as paper and pencil and an alphabet board, may enhance communication. Explaining patient care activities to both the patient and family should diminish the patient's feeling of loss of control.

Evaluation

The patient who is effectively coping with environmental stimuli will be alert and oriented. The patient will report feeling rested upon awakening. Responses to environmental stimuli will be appropriate. The patient will report feeling in control with reduced anxiety.

Documentation

The nurse documents the patient's response to interventions that reduce the level of environmental stimulation. Behavioral changes and subjective reports of the patient's feelings are included in the documentation. The nurse also records situations that seem to precipitate sensory overload responses in the patient.

SLEEP DISORDERS
Sleep Physiology

Sleep is an active process in which adults spend about one third of their time. Sleep is not simply the absence of being awake, but rather a complex state necessary for both mental and physical health. Sleep does not provide generalized rest for the whole brain because there is no general inhibition of cerebral neurons during sleep. Blood flow and oxygen consumption (metabolism) do not decrease. There seems to be a reorganization of neuronal activity that provides rest for specific elements of the brain. This process is essential for supporting the long-term structural and chemical changes necessary for learning and memory.

RAS arousal

Sleep is produced by an active process that inhibits neuronal stimulation. Structurally, this takes place in a diffuse group of neurons. They are located in the **reticular formation** that extends as a continuum from the diencephalon through the brainstem and

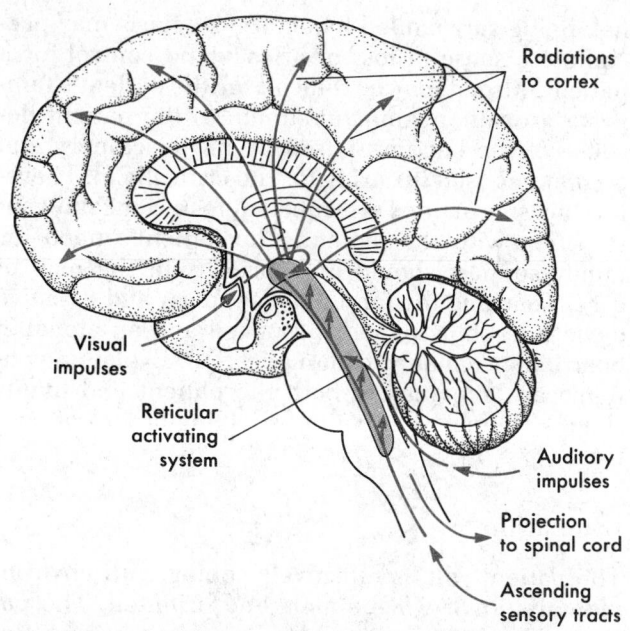

FIGURE 17-1   Reticular activating system. Centers in the brainstem reticular formation relay impulses from the spinal cord and specialized sensory tracts to the cerebral cortex.

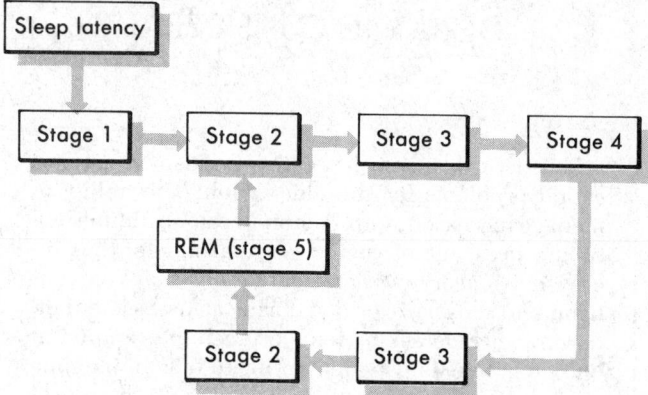

FIGURE 17-2   Adult sleep cycle. Each cycle is approximately 90 minutes long. Normally, four to five cycles are completed per night. (From Barndt-Maglio B: Sleep pattern disturbance, *Dimens Crit Care Nurs* 5(6):347, 1986.)

into the spinal cord. The reticular formation cannot be clearly separated functionally from the basal ganglia, thalamus, cerebellum, and the cerebral cortex. The functional component of the brainstem that exerts influence on consciousness and the wake-sleep cycle is called the **reticular activating system (RAS)** (Figure 17-1). It, along with the thalamus and cerebral cortex, activates the state of consciousness. The reticular activating system may also function as a deactivation mechanism to decrease alertness and produce sleep. Knowledge of the neurochemical influences on sleep is limited, but it is known that alertness is maintained by norepinephrine and the catecholaminergic neurons in the locus ceruleus of the brainstem. Sleep is mediated through serotonin and the raphe nuclei of the brainstem.

Sleep-wake cycles

Sleep is divided into five ultraradian (within a day) stages according to characteristic changes in brain waves, eye movement, and muscle tone (Figure 17-2). Stages I through IV are referred to as **nonrapid eye movement (NREM)** or quiet sleep. In stage I a person experiences a sensation of drifting or floating. The electroencephalogram (EEG) records alpha waves—slow and of low amplitude—in this stage. No dreaming occurs in stage II, and the sleeper can be easily awakened. Sleep spindles appear on the EEG. Sleep deepens in stage III. Breathing slows,

body temperature and blood pressure drop, the heart rate is about 60 beats per minute. Stage IV is characterized by deep, obvious sleep. The brain is still receptive, as evidenced by evoked activity, but there is no waking. Delta waves appear on the EEG during stages III and IV, and growth hormone surges. Stage V, characterized by **rapid eye movement (REM)** and dreaming, is the active stage of sleep. There is a change in respiratory rhythm and rate, reduction in muscle tone, and variation in cardiac rhythm.

There is a cyclic alteration of REM and NREM sleep stages, lasting between 80 and 120 minutes each, throughout the night. The slower NREM sleep stages predominate during the first part of the night, whereas REM sleep dominates the later hours. Daily sleep requirements differ greatly among individuals. However, the proportion of time spent in the various sleep stages remains relatively constant (Figure 17-3).

Circadian (day to day) changes also occur in the sleep-wake cycle. These are probably mediated in the hypothalamus. Altering a regular sleep-wake pattern can disrupt the circadian rhythm. Jobs that require shift rotations and long distance travel through several time zones that results in jet lag both require adjustment of the circadian clock.

Risk Factors

Changes in life-style can be a contributing factor to sleep pattern disturbance. Pleasant changes such as taking a vacation or getting married and unpleasant changes such as taking a test or experiencing the death of a close friend or relative can contribute to a change in a person's sleep. Sleep patterns may also

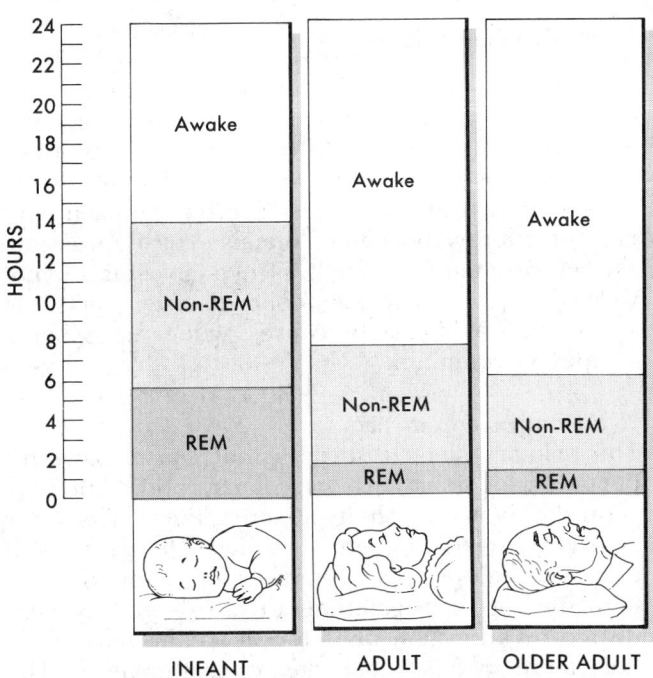

FIGURE 17-3   Sleep-wake cycles across the life span. Infants: approximately 40% of total sleep time is REM. Adults: 20% of total sleep time is REM. Older adults: total sleep time is slightly reduced, REM remains 20% of total.

GERIATRIC CONSIDERATIONS

Sleep Pattern Disturbance

As a person ages, the amount of total sleep time spent in Stage I increases from 5% to 10%. This change in the sleep cycle may account for the older adult's report of more frequent arousals during the night. The elderly person can spend up to 20% of nocturnal time in bed in periods of wakefulness. The total sleep time for older adults remains the same as when they were younger. When the time spent in daytime napping is added to nocturnal sleep time the older adult may have an increased total sleep time. Yet the elderly often complain of decreased sleep efficiency, the time actually asleep. The older adult uses daytime naps to compensate for perceived inadequate nighttime sleep.

In older adults, REM sleep diminishes in length and intensity. REM sleep is distributed throughout the night for the older adult rather than in the second half of the night as seen in younger adults.

The most common factor contributing to sleep pattern disturbance in the elderly is discomfort from illness such as pain or dyspnea. Medications to treat chronic health problems, especially those that affect the central nervous system, also disrupt the normal sleep/wake cycle of the older adult. Anxiety, boredom, fatigue, and depression contribute to the development of sleep pattern disturbance.[11,14]

change with advancing age, hormonal changes in the body, and psychologic disorders (see box above).

A thorough physical examination may reveal risk factors such as an enlarged neck, obesity, diabetes, or thyroid dysfunction. The pain of arthritis, angina, or gastric reflux may interfere with sleep. The respiratory alterations of chronic obstructive lung disease and elimination problems associated with urethritis or enlarged prostate can interfere with sleep. Physical limitations imposed by pregnancy, surgery, or an orthopedic appliance are additional risks that may cause a sleep pattern disturbance.

Insomnia

Insomnia is the most common sleep disorder. It is reported most frequently in women, in the lower socioeconomic classes, and in the elderly. It is not known why these groups are at risk. **Insomnia** is defined as a disorder of initiating and maintaining sleep. Primary insomnia refers to a sleep problem that exists in the absence of any major medical or psychiatric condition. Other types of insomnia are sleep onset (difficulty falling asleep), sleep maintenance (middle-of-the-night awakening), and terminal insomnia (early morning awakening). Knowing the quantity of sleep or the quality of sleep is useful in determining the existence of insomnia. Individual

sleep requirements vary both in the number of hours required and in the depth of sleep, which is determined by how refreshed the individual feels on awakening. Therefore an individual's satisfaction with the length and quality of sleep is the basis for determining the presence of insomnia. For example, if an older adult believes that frequent awakenings during the night are abnormal, they may report problems with insomnia and seek treatment with medications.[14] No specific pathophysiologic cause for insomnia is known. Researchers have suggested that overactivity of the reticular activating system is responsible for some types of insomnia. Others suggest a dysfunction of the neurotransmitter serotonin as a cause of sleep disorders. A number of people who complain of insomnia are not synchronized with their circadian rhythms; thus they try to sleep at inappropriate times. They are unable to sleep at conventional times, but fall asleep easily and sleep well at other times.

Other factors that may lead to insomnia include physical symptoms, environmental disturbances, stress, and drugs. Physical symptoms such as pain, dyspnea, and fever cause discomfort that precludes sleep. Environmental disturbances such as noise, bright light, or general discomfort caused by such things as being too hot or cold may also interfere with sleep. Emotional stress in the form of anxiety or grief may interfere with both the quantity and quality of sleep. Stimulant drugs such as caffeine and nicotine can cause insomnia. Alcohol, a depressant, may help a person fall asleep more quickly but interferes with sleep later in the night. Diuretics taken too close to bedtime may interrupt sleep when their action necessitates a trip to the bathroom. Most hypnotics can cause a rebound insomnia, characterized by sleep of a shorter duration with a high incidence of nightmares, when the medication is suddenly discontinued.

The effects of insomnia or sleep loss have been evaluated mainly by sleep deprivation studies. Sleep deprivation is associated with bizarre behavior and temporary neuroses or psychoses (Table 17-3). Energy mobilization decreases as adenosine triphosphate (ATP) levels in the body decrease. The adrenal cortical or "stress" hormone level increases in the blood. A chemical, similar to having LSD in the blood, may contribute to causing hallucinations. Mental agility decreases, memory fails, the attention span is limited, and reality is distorted. These effects can be relieved by 12 to 14 hours of sleep characterized by increased REM episodes. Ten days of such sleep are required to counteract 4 to 5 days of sleep deprivation.

Extensive physiologic changes occur as a result of sleep deprivation. The degree of change usually correlates with the duration of the sleep loss. Reflexes slow and muscle coordination decreases. Equilibrium and muscle strength may be lost. Nystagmus and ptosis may be observed in the eyes. Respiratory effort may diminish and cardiac dysrhythmias may occur. A general decrease in memory, reasoning, and judgment takes place, and anxiety increases.

TABLE 17-3 Effects of Sleep Deprivation

Physiologic	Psychologic
Slow reflexes	Bizarre behavior
Loss of equilibrium	Temporary neuroses or psychoses
Nystagmus	Sluggishness
Ptosis	Decreased mental agility
Decreased respirations	Memory failure
Cardiac arrhythmias	Limited attention

Excessive somnolence

Persons with excessive daytime somnolence can feel sleepy all the time, have sleep attacks, or both. Sleepiness is a perceived need for sleep. The most common cause of this complaint is inadequate sleep. Excessive daytime sleepiness can be confused with lack of energy, boredom, malaise, or depression. Therefore conditions such as hypoglycemia, hypothyroidism, or other metabolic disorders must be considered as possible causes when assessing a sleepiness complaint.

Primary sleep disorders

The primary sleep disorders that cause excessive daytime sleepiness are narcolepsy and idiopathic central nervous system hypersomnolence. The latter is a rare disorder sometimes called "sleep drunkenness." **Narcolepsy** is a sleep disorder of unknown origin affecting the regulation of REM sleep. It is manifested by an urgent need for sleep and may cause the victim to fall asleep during conversation. The sleep attack may be precipitated by a sudden emotional change such as laughter and may consist of a brief loss of muscle tone, specifically of the face and neck. Both idiopathic central nervous system hypersomnolence and narcolepsy may respond to treatment with central nervous system stimulants.

Secondary sleep disorders

Secondary sleep disorders that cause excessive daytime sleepiness are central and obstructive sleep apnea and nocturnal myoclonus, or periodic movements in sleep. Central sleep apnea occurs when the respiratory rate or tidal volume decreases during sleep. It may be associated with conditions such as obesity, neuromuscular disease, or disorders of the brainstem. Central sleep apnea can be treated with respiratory stimulants.

Nocturnal myoclonus and the related "restless legs syndrome" are characterized by periodic leg movement in sleep and are considered a type of insomnia. Nocturnal myoclonus and the associated leg pain and paresthesias awaken patients from a sound sleep. The patient may report that symptoms are relieved if he or she sleeps sitting up. Some cases of "restless legs syndrome" may be associated with reduced cardiopulmonary compliance and lumbar spinal stenosis.[10] Benzodiazepines and opioids may be used in treatment.

The most serious secondary cause of excessive daytime sleepiness associated with disturbed nocturnal sleep is obstructive sleep apnea. It is an intermittent obstruction of the upper airway at the oropharynx involving the soft palate and tongue. The apneic episodes, which usually last 20 to 40 seconds, may number several hundred per night and cause partial arousal. Obstructive sleep apnea is most common in obese, middle-aged men. Loud snoring and excessive daytime sleepiness are the most common symptoms. The spouse of the patient may also experience sleep pattern disturbance because of the loud snoring, frequent arousals, and anxiety about the periods of apnea. Treatment depends on the severity of symptoms. Weight loss may be effective. In severe cases, a tracheostomy is required. The most commonly used therapy is continuous positive airway pressure (CPAP) administered via a nasal mask worn during sleep. Drugs are not usually effective because of the mechanical nature of the condition. Sedatives and hypnotics must be avoided because they further depress respirations.

NURSING MANAGEMENT OF THE PATIENT WITH SLEEP PATTERN DISTURBANCE
Assessment

A thorough patient assessment is essential for diagnosing any complaint about sleep (see the boxes below). Compiling a sleep history will identify the type of sleep disturbance, its duration, the quality and quantity of sleep, and the person's beliefs about sleep. A patient with a sleep pattern disturbance may report difficulty falling asleep (sleep latency), interrupted sleep, awakening earlier than desired, or not feeling well rested.[2,7] The nurse listens for in-

dications of attitudes toward sleep that are based on misinformation or lack of knowledge about normal variations in sleep/wake cycles. A drug history is relevant because many drugs can disrupt sleep or cause sleepiness. Question the use of over-the-counter medications, caffeine, tobacco, and alcohol. Physical and psychologic symptoms should also be recorded. Bed partners may have answers to questions about sleep problems manifested by the patient. A sleep diary may provide useful information about the amount and pattern of sleep over time (Figure 17-4).

Nursing Diagnosis

The etiologies for the primary diagnosis of sleep pattern disturbance are numerous. A specific etiology can be selected based on the assessment data; for example, sleep pattern disturbance related to chronic joint pain. Other diagnoses that may be ap-

---

ASSESSMENT PARAMETERS FOR SLEEP PATTERN DISTURBANCE

Compiled sleep history, including sleep environment, bedtime routines, and sleep aids from the individual, family, and significant others
Current sleep pattern
Past sleep pattern
Current rest and activity pattern
Past rest and activity pattern
Drug history, including alcohol
History of seizure disorder
Mental status
Pain: assess involved anatomic structures and physiologic systems
Presence of abnormal motor movement
Respiratory status
Cardiovascular status
Blood pressure
Weight
Neck appearance

From American Nurses' Association and American Association of Neuroscience Nurses: *Neuroscience nursing practice*, Kansas City, Mo, 1985, The Association.

ASSESSMENT QUESTIONS FOR THE PATIENT WITH SLEEP PATTERN DISTURBANCE

Do you have trouble falling asleep?
Do you awaken soon after you fall asleep?
  Do you awaken in the middle of the night or the early morning?
How long have you had this difficulty?
  Do you have the same problem every night or in any particular pattern?
Have you found anything that helps?
Does anything make it worse?
Do you feel refreshed when you get up?
Are you sleepy during the day?
Do you nap during the day?
Are your naps planned?
Do you go to bed at the same time each night?
Do you get up at the same time each day?
  How much sleep do you think you need in order to feel rested?
  How long do you think it should take you to fall asleep?
Do you have a regular bedtime ritual?
Do others in your family have difficulty sleeping?
Are you sleeping less than normal?
  Is there something, such as noise, that keeps you awake?
  Has this sleep problem changed your mood or your behavior?
Do you feel anxious at night?
Do you have pain that keeps you awake?

	Day 1	Day 2	Day 3	Day 4	Day 5	Day 6	Day 7
Time went to bed							
Did you feel sleepy?							
Time went to sleep							
Number of awakenings							
Reason for awakenings							
Length of time to return to sleep							
Time of arising							
Did you feel rested?							
Daytime naps: number and length							

FIGURE 17-4   Sleep diary.

propriate for the patient with a sleep pattern disturbance include:

Altered thought processes related to sleep deprivation

Sensory/perceptual impairment related to sleep deprivation

High risk for injury related to excessive daytime sleepiness

Planning

It is the responsibility of the nurse to help the patient determine the nature of the sleep pattern disturbance and develop specific outcomes (see box on p. 387). Specific measures to promote sleep should be employed. Provisions should be made to correct abnormal sleep patterns so the patient awakes feeling rested after undisturbed periods of sleep.

Implementation

For the hospitalized patient the nurse maintains an environment conducive to sleep that includes minimal noise, appropriate room temperature, and a natural cycle of light and darkness. Noise is often reported as the most frequent cause of sleep disturbances by patients.[2] Dimming lights at night can help the patient maintain a more normal sleep/wake cycle. Knowing that the nurse is available during the night increases the patient's sense of security in a strange environment and promotes more restful sleep.

Providing effective pain management achieves a level of comfort that will not disrupt the patient's normal sleep pattern. The patient also may need the nurse's assistance in finding a comfortable position for sleep. The use of additional hygiene and comfort measures at bedtime can promote more effective sleep for the patient. These interventions include back rubs, washing the patient's face, teethbrushing, and voiding.[15] The nurse encourages the patient to use bedtime rituals in the hospital that help the patient prepare for sleep when at home. Minimizing nighttime treatments and using monitoring techniques that will not awaken the patient will allow the patient extended periods of uninterrupted sleep.

Some sleep pattern disturbances are unavoidable. The nurse teaches the patient and family techniques appropriate for dealing with sleep pattern disturbances at home. The patient is instructed to establish a consistent daily schedule, including a set time

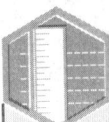

STANDARDS OF CARE: SLEEP PATTERN DISTURBANCE

Defining characteristics

One or more of the following:

   Less sleep than normal
   Continuous environmental stimuli
   Interrupted sleep
   Altered behavior or mood in the presence of any of the above
   Report or observation of difficulty initiating sleep, restlessness during sleep, or daytime somnolence
   Verbal report of not feeling well rested
   Verbal report of altered sleep pattern
   Verbal report of distraction by environmental stimuli
   Verbal report of anxiety or pain at night

Process criteria (interventions)

The nurse institutes measures to promote adequate sleep periods, such as:

   Maintaining a cycle of light and darkness
   Minimizing nighttime noise and treatments
   Using monitoring techniques and equipment that minimize the need to awaken the individual

The nurse identifies the nature of the sleep pattern disturbance

The nurse institutes and teaches measures to promote sleep, such as:

   Managing dietary and chemical substance intake
   Maintaining consistent times to go to bed and arise
   Manipulating the environment
   Positioning
   Managing activity, exercise, and work factors
   Limiting the frequency and length of naps
   Collaborating with the physician regarding the medication regimen

The nurse institutes measures to promote the management of anxiety, such as:

   Encouraging the verbalization of fears and concerns
   Teaching relaxation techniques

The nurse institutes measures to promote the management of pain

The nurse collaborates with the appropriate specialist

The nurse provides information about available resources

Outcome criteria

The individual describes the nature of the sleep pattern disturbance
The individual carries out measures to promote sleep
The individual has undisturbed periods for sleep
The individual reports feeling rested upon awakening

Adapted from American Nurses' Association: *Neuroscience nursing practice*, Kansas City, Mo, 1985, The Association.

to rise and retire. Daytime naps are discouraged if they interfere with sleep at night (see Patient Education Guide on p. 388).

Pharmacologic treatments

Hypnotics are the drugs of choice today in the treatment of sleep disorders. These drugs can shorten sleep onset when the patient has difficulty falling asleep; they can reduce nighttime wakefulness; or they can provide an antianxiety effect when insomnia is accompanied by marked anxiety.[34]

Health care professionals are often the ones who demand that medications be used to quiet patients. However, most of the literature recommends that alternative methods be used to treat insomnia. The reason for this is that hypnotic drugs have a central nervous system depressant effect. Sedation occurs with low doses, and chemical hypnosis results with higher doses. Tolerance may develop with repeated

RESEARCH BRIEF

Edwards GB, Schuring LM: Sleep protocol: a research-based practice change, *Crit Care Nurse* 13(2):84, 1993.

This study identified the number of undisturbed blocks of at least 60 minutes that were allowed for patients to rest or sleep for the first 7 days in a medical ICU. In addition, researchers identified the procedures that disturbed the patients' rest most often. Data analysis indicated that the average number of blocks of at least 60 minutes of undisturbed rest or sleep time per patient per day was 2.2. Only one of these blocks fell during conventional sleep hours. Data indicated that when a patient's rest/sleep time was interrupted, only one procedure was performed by the nursing or respiratory therapy staff.

As a result of the research, nurses in the MICU instituted a sleep protocol to increase the number of uninterrupted blocks of time available to the patient for rest or sleep. The sleep protocol was a coordinated activity that involved nursing staff, medical staff, pharmacy, and respiratory therapy. Patient care activities and treatments were grouped together and scheduled to allow the patient more uninterrupted sleep time, especially during the night.

TABLE 17-4   Drugs Commonly Used in Altering Sleep Patterns

Benzodiazapines	Barbiturates	Nonbarbiturates
Temazepam (Restoril)	Short-acting:	Diphenhydramine (Benadryl)
Triazolam (Halcion)	Secobarbital (Seconal)	Chloral hydrate (Noctec)
Flurazepam (Dalmane)	Pentobarbital (Nembutal)	Ethchlorvynol (Placidyl)
Diazepam (Valium)	Intermediate-acting:	Glutethimide (Doriden)
Oxazepam (Serax)	Amobarbital (Amytal)	
	Phenobarbital (Luminal)	

PATIENT EDUCATION GUIDE   *Sleep Habits*

- Maintain the same daily schedule for waking, resting, activity, and sleeping 7 days a week.
- Avoid staying in bed beyond your usual waking time. Arise at the same time each day, even if you have not slept well.
- Establish a bedtime ritual that works for you. Follow it every night.
- Make sure your bed, mattress, pillow, bed linens, and bedclothes are comfortable.
- Control the ambient temperature, noise, and light in your bedroom if possible.
- Use your bed only for sleep-compatible activities.
- Limit daytime napping to no more than 1-2 hours a day. Avoid naps within 6 hours of your bedtime.
- Avoid all sedatives and stimulants such as caffeine, alcohol, and some over-the-counter medications for pain or colds in the late afternoon or evening.
- If you smoke, do not do so right before bedtime.
- Do not eat a large meal within 3 hours of bedtime. A light snack containing carbohydrates may be beneficial to promote sleep.
- Perform moderate exercise daily, but limit vigorous activity in the evening.
- Perform only quiet activities in the evening to promote relaxation such as praying, meditation, rhythmic breathing, listening to soothing music, reading nonstimulating material, or watching nonstimulating television.
- If you cannot fall asleep within 30 minutes, get out of bed and engage in some form of nonstimulating yet diverting activity. DO NOT WATCH THE CLOCK. DO NOT TRY TOO HARD TO FALL ASLEEP.[1,12,14]

administration. When drug administration is terminated at a high-dose level, a characteristic withdrawal syndrome ensues, with tremor, convulsions, and delirium.[41] There is also the potential for psychologic and physiologic dependence with these drugs. Hypnotics may be prescribed alone or in conjunction with sedatives.

The most commonly used hypnotics are the benzodiazepines (Table 17-4). This group of drugs works in a unique fashion. They potentiate the naturally occurring inhibitory transmitter gamma-aminobutyric acid (GABA) in the limbic system and in other parts of the brain to induce sleep and create an anticonvulsant effect. The duration of action also differentiates these drugs from others. Benzodiazepines potentiate the effect of other central nervous system depressants, including alcohol, narcotics, and barbiturates. The most common side effects of benzodiazepines are drowsiness and ataxia. Gastrointestinal discomfort may also develop. Therefore it is recommended that the drugs be taken with meals. Benzodiazepines can cause REM rebound, characterized by frequent dreams and nightmares that awaken the individual. It is thought that this occurs because of a decrease in REM sleep. However, not all drugs in this group cause this phenomenon. Dalmane, for example, reduces REM sleep but does not cause REM rebound.

Barbiturates have long been used to treat sleep disorders. Their mechanism of action is central nervous system (CNS) depression. However, they currently have limited use in this area because of their disadvantages and dangers, which are threefold. First, barbiturates have an addictive and habituating property with both abuse and regular use. Second, overdose is usually fatal because of the respiratory depressant effect. Third, they tend to interact with other drugs, causing alterations in liver enzymes, which may affect treatment regimens.[38] The various barbiturates differ in their onset and duration of action.

Many other nonbarbiturate drugs exist that can be used to induce sleep. Two of the most popular are diphenhydramine and chloral hydrate. Diphenhydramine is an antihistamine used primarily for the treatment of motion sickness, pruritus, and vestibular-induced vomiting. Its use in sleep disorders is prompted by its side effect of drowsiness. There is weak experimental evidence of a relationship between the proper use of hypnotics and the appearance of withdrawal effects such as worsening of sleep and insomnia, next-day performance impairment, and rebound phenomenon. However, diphenhydramine is often used to treat sleep disorders in the elderly because there appears to be less chance of these effects in this age group.[29] Chloral hydrate is one of the oldest hypnotics and is well tolerated by elderly individuals. A possible reason for the decrease in popularity of this drug may be its

side effects of gastrointestinal irritation, nausea, vomiting, and flatulence. In liquid form it also has an unpleasant taste and is best given with meals. This drug may also produce psychologic and physical dependence.

Evaluation

Subjective evaluation of the interventions for sleep pattern disturbance include the patient's report of feeling rested on awakening. The patient will indicate increased satisfaction with both the quantity and quality of nocturnal sleep. Objectively, the nurse observes infrequent yawning, reduced irritability, decreased fatigue, and improved participation in daily routines. As the patient becomes more successful in establishing sleep routines, there should be less use of pharmacologic agents to promote sleep. The patient will have increased periods of uninterrupted sleep as the hospital environment becomes more conducive to sleep. It may take several days for the patient to achieve uninterrupted sleep periods of several hours.

Documentation

Documentation of the assessment of sleep pattern disturbance and the related plan of care is important to promote continuity of care and produce long-term changes in the patient's sleep/wake cycle. The assessment documents information that will help identify the specific etiology of the sleep pattern disturbance. Specific interventions and bedtime rituals are charted so that all nursing personnel can use a consistent approach in helping the patient at bedtime

CRITICAL THINKING QUESTIONS

1 What are the clinical manifestations of a sensory alteration?
2 Compare the effects of sensory overload and sensory deprivation.
3 How does the hospital environment contribute to sensory alterations and sleep disorders?
4 What measures does a nurse implement to maintain an adequate sensory environment for the hospitalized patient?
5 What are the physiologic and psychologic effects of sleep deprivation?
6 Describe the nursing interventions to promote sleep.

BIBLIOGRAPHY

Current

1. Aronoff MS: *Sleep and its secrets: The river of crystal light,* New York, 1991, Plenum Press.

2. Beyerman K: Etiologies of sleep pattern disturbance in hospitalized patients. In McLane AM: *Classification of nursing diagnoses: proceedings of the seventh conference,* St Louis, 1987, Mosby–Year Book.

3. Burke MM, Walsh MB: *Gerontologic nursing: care of the frail elderly,* St Louis, 1992, Mosby–Year Book.

4. Comptom P: Critical illness and intensive care: what it means to the client, *Crit Care Nurse* 11:50, 1991.

5. Davis-Sharts J: The elder and critical care: sleep and mobility issues, *Nurs Clin North Am* 24:755, 1989.

6. Hahn K: About sensory loss, *Nursing* 19(2):97, 1989.

7. Johnson SE: Sleep pattern disturbance: defining characteristics observable in practice. In Carroll-Johnson RM: *Classification of nursing diagnoses: proceedings of the eighth conference,* Philadelphia, 1989, JB Lippincott.

8. Kales A, Constantin RS, Kales JS: Sleep disorders: Insomnia sleepwalking, night terrors, nightmares, and enuresis, *Ann Intern Med* 106:582, 1987.

9. Kloosterman ND: Cultural care: the missing link in severe sensory alteration, *Nurs Sci Q* 4:119, 1991.

10. LaBan MM, Viola SL: Restless legs syndrome associated with diminished cardiopulmonary compliance and lumbar spinal stenosis—a motor concomitant of "Vesper's curse," *Arch Phys Med Rehab* 71:384, 1990.

11. Maas M, Buckwalter K, Hardy MA: *Nursing diagnoses and interventions for the elderly,* Redwood, CA, 1991, Addison-Wesley.

12. McCloskey JC, Bulechek GM: *Nursing interventions classification,* St Louis, 1992, Mosby–Year Book.

13. Mendelson WB: *Human sleep: research and clinical care,* New York, 1987, Plenum Medical Book Co.

14. Miller CA: *Nursing care of older adults: theory and practice,* Glenview IL, 1990, Scott, Foresman and Co.

15. Reimer M: Sleep pattern disturbance: nursing interventions perceived by patients and their nurses as facilitating nocturnal sleep in hospital. In McLane AM: *Classification of nursing diagnoses: proceedings of the seventh conference,* St Louis, 1987, Mosby–Year Book, Inc.

16. Smith SJ: Sensory deprivation and the ophthalmic patient, *J Ophthal Nurs Tech* 8:148, 1989.

Classic

17. American Nurses Association and American Association of Neuroscience Nurses: *Neuroscience nursing practice,* Kansas City, Mo, 1985, The Association.

18. Baker C: Sensory overload and noise in the ICU: sources of environmental stress, *Crit Care Q* 6:66, 1984.

19. Baker TL: Introduction to sleep and sleep disorders, *Med Clin North Am* 69:1123, 1985.

20. Barry MJ: Sensory alterations, overload and underload: making a nursing diagnosis. In Kennedy M, Pfeifer G: *Current practice in nursing care of the adult,* St Louis, 1979, Mosby–Year Book.

21. Brewer MJ: To sleep or not to sleep: the consequences of sleep deprivation, *Crit Care Nurse* 5:35, 1985.

22. Cantrell R: Physiological effects of noise, *Otolaryngol Clin North Am* 12:537, 1979.

23. Diekstra RFW, Stubbe L, Willemsteyn B: ICU sensory deprivation, *Nurs Success Today* 3:21, 1986.

24. Gowan N: The perceptual world of the intensive care unit: an overview of some environmental considerations in the helping relationship, *Heart Lung* 8:340, 1979.

25. Guilleminault C: Disorders of excessive sleepiness, *Ann Clin Res* 17:209, 1985.

26. Hansell H: The behavioral effects of noise on man: the patient with intensive care unit psychosis, *Heart Lung* 13:59, 1984.

27. Hilton A: Noise in acute patient care areas, *Res Nurs Health* 8:283, 1985.

28. Jahanshahi J: Insomnia, *Nursing* 3:328, 1986.

29. James D: Survey of hypnotic drug use in nursing homes, *J Am Geriatr Soc,* June 1986, p. 436.

30. Kryter K: Non-auditory effects of environmental noise, *Am J Public Health* 62:389, 1972.

31. Lindenmuth J, Breu C, Malooley J: Sensory overload, *Am J Nurs,* August 1980, p. 1456.

32. Lindsley D: Common factors in sensory deprivation, sensory distortion, and sensory overload. In Solomon P, ed: *Sensory deprivation,* Cambridge, Mass, 1961, Harvard University Press.

33. McCorkle R: Effects of touch on seriously ill patients, *Nurs Res* 3:125, 1974.

34. Nicholson A: Hypnotics: their place in therapeutics, *Drugs* 31:164, 1986.

35. Phillips B: Sleep, sleep loss, and breathing, *South Med J* 78:1483, 1985.

36. Rudy EB: *Advanced neurological and neurosurgical nursing,* St Louis, 1984, Mosby–Year Book.

37. Selye H: *Stress without distress,* Philadelphia, 1974, JB Lippincott Co.

38. Smith S: Drugs and sleep, *Nurs Times* 81:36, 1985.

39. Syvalahti E: Drug treatment of insomnia: indications and complications, *Ann Clin Res* 17:265, 1985.

40. Walsh RN, Cumins RA: Neural responses to therapeutic sensory environments, In Walsh RN, Greenough WT, editors: *Environment as therapy for brain dysfunction,* New York, 1976, Plenum Press.

41. Williams RL, Karacan I: Recent developments in the diagnosis and treatment of sleep disorders, *Hosp Community Psychiatry* 36:951, 1985.

42. Wood M: Clinical sensory deprivation: a comparative study of patients in single care and two-bed rooms, *J Nurs Adm* 7:28, 1977.

43. Woods NF, Falk SA: Noise stimuli in the acute care area, *Nurs Res* 23:144, 1974.

44. Zubek JP, Macneill M: Perceptual deprivation phenomena: role of the recumbent position, *J Abnorm Psychol* 72:147, 1967.

UNIT IV

Psychosocial Dimensions of Adult Health Nursing

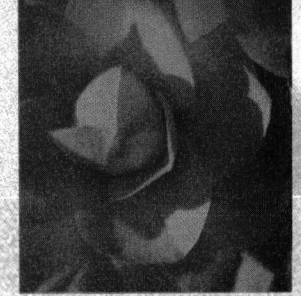

CHAPTER EIGHTEEN

Caring and the Emotional Response to Illness

LEARNING OBJECTIVES

1 Describe the process of caring and how caring may be evidenced by the nurse.
2 Describe common manifestations of loneliness and the appropriate nursing interventions.
3 Differentiate among the different types and levels of anxiety.
4 Describe nursing interventions to help the patient cope with anxiety.
5 Differentiate between anger and hostility.
6 Describe how the nurse may intervene to channel anger constructively.
7 Describe behaviors commonly exhibited by the dependent or manipulative patient and the appropriate caring nursing interventions.

NURSES CARE for and about people. **Caring** may be described as a feeling of liking another person or a feeling of concern for another human being. Yet caring is not just "enjoying another" or having a transient feeling of attraction to a person. Caring for and about a patient is a *process* that involves developing a relationship of mutual respect, knowledge, trust, and courage.

The task of caring for sick "strangers" called "patients" can be difficult. The obligation to care has defined the distinctive art of American nursing since its beginning in 1875.[12] The profession's commitment to receiving through giving, its capacity to view humanity with love, and its sensitivity to suffering have traditionally defined the social function of nursing in American culture.

Caring is demonstrated through an interpersonal process and shared experience between the nurse and the patient. Caring may be demonstrated through three distinctive methods: tangible caring, emotional caring, and informational caring.[13,19] Nurses offer tangible caring when they attend to the physical and environmental needs of the patient. For example, administering a bath or medication involves the nurse giving tangible care to the patient. Tangible care is also evident when the nurse provides a safe and effective environment for the patient. Psychologic interventions such as touch, presence, and verbal or nonverbal communication techniques are examples of a nurse's emotional caring. The assessment, planning, intervention, evaluation, and replanning of the patient's multiple emotional needs are components of emotional caring. When the nurse offers hope, empathy, limit-setting, or humor to the patient, an important aspect of care is provided that helps the patient deal with illness. Health promotion, teaching, resource allocation, and communication are methods of informational caring. As an important part of quality care, nurses teach patients about their diagnostic procedures, medications, and hospital routine. An effective nurse teaches a patient about the physiologic mechanism of the patient's illness, diet, and treatments. When the nurse shares knowledge and expertise with both patients and families and documents the interventions, informational caring is rendered. Whether the nurse serves in the role of teacher, advocate, caregiver, problem solver, or care coordinator, tangible, emotional, and informational caring is given to patients and families.[3]

CARING AND THE EXPERIENCE OF ILLNESS

Although humans have individual and unique responses to illness, generally the experience of illness threatens a person's psychologic, sociologic, and spiritual well-being.

Since the 1970s researchers have explored the notion that social support affects a person's experience of illness. Social supports are resources such as informational, financial, or emotional aid or help provided by other persons.[5] Researchers suggest that social support may enhance health and assist in the recovery from illness. Social support may increase health through promoting self-care practices and mobilizing the immune system. Moreover, social support is associated with recovery and coping with serious illness and injury.[5,7]

The usefulness of tangible support such as money, child care, and emotional backing is readily apparent to nurses. The onset of an illness has an intense impact upon the individual and the family. Whether the illness begins with pain, weakness, or disorientation, the symptoms may frighten patients and families. Thus actual tangible support and the perception of the availability of this support affect the experience of illness.

Nurses must understand that the experience of illness will evoke emotional responses within individuals and families. As patients attempt to regain stability and control over their environment, they will need to manage anxiety, make decisions, and mobilize resources. The nurse's task is to care, understand, and respond to the needs of the persons dealing with health concerns.

When the individual and family enter the health care system, the nurse responds. In an attempt to relieve the discomfort, nurse and patient enter into a dialogue, a relationship, and a shared experience. Knowing that all people are unique and have a right to respond differently to illness, the nurse must remain fully aware that understanding will require acceptance, presence, authenticity, and communication. In this way, the nurse will understand responses to illness from the perspective of the patient and will be able to perform effectively.

PATIENT RESPONSES TO ILLNESS
Loneliness

Individuals experiencing illness often suffer from feelings of **loneliness.** Loneliness is a manifestation of the universal need for intimacy or human contact. Being alone can be acceptable, desirable, or exhilarating; loneliness is usually a painful, even dreaded, experience. Patients are alone in that the actual illness belongs to their life experience. Still, the experience of illness need not produce loneliness. For example, Mr. Lopez, a patient undergoing a spinal tap, knows that a needle will enter his spine and produce discomfort. Although he alone must endure the spinal tap, the touch, presence, and support of the nurse modifies the fear, pain, and anxiety of the procedure. Through touch and sensitivity, the nurse responds to the need for human contact and helps ameliorate the potential for loneliness (see box on p. 395).[15]

Loneliness is a common emotional response to illness; however, the specific causes of loneliness are difficult to determine. A physical illness that results in confinement, immobility, and isolation from significant others may produce loneliness. In the hospital, the patient is given an unfamiliar room, bed, and pillow and is surrounded with strangers called health professionals. The patient has been alienated from familiar people and surroundings and has taken on the sick role. Although convalescing or chronically ill patients remain in their homes, surrounded by familiar people and objects, they may feel loneliness as much as the hospitalized patient does. Isolation and the lack of closeness can occur even in a familiar environment. In aged patients hearing and sight may be impaired, resulting in communication deficits that foster separation and loneliness. Moreover, the loss of a spouse, pet, sibling, or friend through death may deprive the aged patient of meaningful relationships and thus generate loneliness. A homebound patient can lose autonomy, social life, and self-esteem, all of which can ultimately cause loneliness.

THERAPEUTIC COMMUNICATION GUIDE

Loneliness

1. Never assume anything; always validate.
   Example: You observe that Mr. Jones constantly stares out the window. Explore the *meaning* of the behavior, rather than *assuming* that he wishes to be outside the hospital. State: "I notice you staring out the window; does that mean you'd like to be out of the hospital?" The patient now has the opportunity to validate or negate your thought and share his experience with you.
2. Share your observations directly. When Mr. Jones appears sad, tell him what you see. This allows for an exchange of perceptions and information.
   Example: Nurse: Mr. Jones, you look sad.
   Patient: No, I am not, actually. I'm worried that with my broken arm, I can't chop wood and heat my house.
   By validating observations, the nurse can respond to the patient's experience and needs.
3. Do not talk in generalities. If something is implicit, make it explicit. Find the meaning of the patient's experience.
   Example: Patient: My daughter did not visit.
   Nurse: And it feels like she is too busy to spend time with you?
   Patient: In a way, but I think my illness scares her.

4. Use open-ended questions rather than those that can be answered with a "yes" or a "no."
5. When patients talk about people, direct the response to the *relationship* with the person.
6. When patients talk about events, direct the response toward the *meaning* of the experience.
7. Try to direct the communication from the general to the specific. Have the patient describe the experience, *thoughts* about the experience, and then the *feelings* about the experience.
8. Verbal and nonverbal communication should be aimed at helping the patient in the quest for autonomy, self-expression, and self-awareness. The nurse can help the patient expand his or her awareness.
   To diminish the patient's loneliness, the nurse must be present (physically and emotionally), gathering information, giving comfort, and making the patient feel cared about, remembered, and valued.

Behaviors

Patients suffering from loneliness often cannot identify the feeling or articulate it to the nurse. Loneliness is an uncomfortable experience that is frequently hidden, disguised, or expressed in another form. The nurse must be acutely observant, sensitive, and intuitive while assessing the patient. Loneliness may be evidenced by physical complaints such as headaches, backaches, or other vague pain. These complaints are tenacious, and as the nurse attends to one set of complaints, often another is voiced by the patient. The patient may appear withdrawn and depressed and may express guilt feelings over seemingly small mistakes. The nurse must remember that loneliness is an individual human experience, and behaviors that signal loneliness vary widely.

Nursing response

Presence is a nursing intervention that is essential in diminishing loneliness. Presence is simply "being

there."[2,22] Physical and psychologic presence includes availability, attending to needs, physical closeness, and interpersonal rapport. Nurses announce their presence by introducing themselves, by formulating the care plan *with* the patient, and by checking frequently with the patient. The nurse's attitude and approach are aimed at supporting and reinforcing the patient's efforts to explore and resolve the present situation and determine future goals. The nurse does not rescue by attempting to change the patient; rather, the nurse *facilitates*. The motives and abilities to change are within the patient, and the nurse contributes by setting these forces into motion.

The nurse maintains the patient's comfort and diminishes loneliness by attending to basic needs. Disturbed nutrition and appetite, sleep, elimination, and mobility are characteristic of the withdrawal and depression that can accompany loneliness. Listen to the patient's physiologic concerns, alleviate acute symptoms, and help reestablish a normal pattern.

Methods of verbal and nonverbal communication enhance the patient's ability to disclose feelings of loneliness. The nurse actively listens to the patient and must present open, nonverbal communication clues using frequent eye contact, touch, and relaxed posture. Often nurses complete their nursing care tasks by giving "action directions" such as "turn," "cough," "swallow," "eat," and "move." Action directions may reduce the patient to an object and produce isolation and loneliness. Communication *with*, not *to*, patients will provide closeness, not distance. Communication that creates closeness is generally labeled "therapeutic communication." In contrast to "social communication" and giving directions, therapeutic communication techniques such as reflecting, restating, clarifying, focusing, and remaining silent enhance understanding and preserve the self-respect of the patient.[14]

Anxiety and Fear

Individuals experiencing illness usually suffer from fear or anxiety. Many experiences associated with illness threaten the patient's physical, social, financial, emotional, and spiritual patterns, producing tension and apprehension. **Anxiety** is a diffuse, subjective feeling associated with discomfort, helplessness, uncertainty, and isolation. According to Stuart and Sundeen (1991), anxiety is provoked by the unknown and accompanies all new experiences.[14] In contrast, the concept of **fear** suggests that the individual has a specific source or reason for the feeling. Although the literature stresses the difference between fear and anxiety, nurses observe that in most patients fear and anxiety occur together and often potentiate one another. For example, a patient scheduled for cardiac surgery probably will experience anxiety regarding the outcome and will voice fear about the actual procedure.

There are four types of anxiety. The anxiety that nurses observe in patients is often labeled signal anxiety. Very often the source of the anxiety is not consciously realized but is triggered or signaled by the unconscious. Anxiety may be caused by a memory, anticipation of danger, or an unconscious feeling of being threatened. In contrast, Spielberg (1972) compared trait anxiety and state anxiety.[26] Trait anxiety refers to the generalized anxiety that some people feel at all times. These people may be described as "uptight" or "high-strung." State anxiety refers to a specific situation or event and is usually short-lived. Free-floating anxiety is constant anxiety accompanied by a fear or dread. Often free-floating anxiety manifests itself as compulsive ritualistic behaviors such as handwashing or avoidance behaviors such as phobias.

Anxiety can be differentiated by levels as well as by types. Peplau (1963) identified four levels of anxiety.[24] In mild anxiety the person is alert, productive, and motivated. This level of anxiety is considered normal and beneficial to high functioning. Moderate anxiety produces some discomfort, preoccupation, and restlessness. The person experiencing moderate anxiety is less able to learn, focus, or produce work. The third level of anxiety is severe anxiety, in which pacing, insomnia, trembling, tachycardia, and irritability will be observed. Physiologic symptoms of increased blood pressure, pulse, and respirations, diaphoresis, anorexia, dry mouth, and dilated pupils will be evident. In the final level, panic, the individual experiences a loss of control, becomes disorganized, and is resistant to direction. Anxiety can be conceptualized as existing on a continuum from relaxation to panic. The nurse can readily determine the patient's level of anxiety by behaviors observed. To facilitate the patient's well-being, it is necessary for the nurse to determine the cause of the anxiety.

The causes of anxiety may be analyzed from several theoretic perspectives. Many psychoanalytic theorists view anxiety as a conflict between the id (instincts) and the superego (conscience), underscored by the original anxiety of the birth trauma; interpersonal theorists argue that anxiety arises from a fear of disapproval and a lack of emotional bonding. Other approaches regard anxiety as a behavioral response to blocked goals (behaviorist model) or a neurochemical reaction to frustration (biologic model).[1,13,17] Despite the multiple theoretic views, there is a general agreement that anxiety arises when a person encounters a threat.

Behaviors

Patients suffering anxiety exhibit a wide range of symptoms and behaviors. Physiologic symptoms may include rapid heart rate and respirations, elevated blood pressure, slowed digestive processes, dilated pupils, increased blood glucose, skin vasoconstriction, diaphoresis, hives, anorexia, and rigid muscles. The patient may have an inability to concentrate or solve problems, difficulty with abstract thinking, or ineptness at following directions. Emotional signs may include rumination, crying, agitation, withdrawal, negative self-statements, or extreme talkativeness. The spiritual dimension of a patient's discomfort may manifest itself through despair, indifference, reduced creativity, or alienation. Many individuals use a variety of behaviors to express anxiety. The nurse may easily miss the signs and symptoms of mild anxiety because the patient often copes with these feelings by utilizing his or her own resources, but when anxiety approaches the moderate level nursing interventions are often required.

Although mild and moderate anxiety are not necessarily unhealthy situations, severe anxiety interferes markedly with normal functioning and demands intervention.

Nursing response

A responsive nurse will provide comfort, understanding, and tangible interventions to the patient who experiences anxiety. The patient's physiologic needs must be attended to by the nurse. The nurse must also provide a comfortable environment. Excessive noise, poor lighting, undue cold or heat, and clutter are not conducive to preventing anxiety.

Self-awareness and nonverbal and verbal communication are particularly important in dealing with an anxious patient. How and what the nurse says and does may help or hinder the patient in coping with anxiety. Anxiety is contagious. Ideally, the nurse realizes and remembers that the anxiety belongs to the patient. It is important for the nurse neither to lend nor borrow anxiety from the patient. The nurse should exhibit a calm, supportive demeanor and be cognizant of his or her own nonverbal cues. The nurse should move slowly, deliberately, and confidently and should be consistent, congruent, and kind. It is best to speak slowly and clearly and use short, simple sentences. The nurse's presence and behavior gives the patient a message that the situation is manageable and that help is available. Although the nurse's presence and calmness provide an effective start in reducing anxiety,

INTERVENTIONS TO REDUCE ANXIETY

1. Acknowledge the patient's anxiety, and validate its existence within the patient's experience. Often the anxious feelings become more endurable when they are acknowledged. On the other hand, many patients deny, intellectualize, or rationalize their feelings and thus avoid acknowledging anxiety. In this case, continue with supportive confrontation in the patient's language. For example, younger persons may state that they feel "uptight," while denying anxiety. Older persons can often verbalize their "nervousness" or "frustration," but they consider anxiety unacceptable. If an impasse is reached, try to rephrase the observation.
   Example: Nurse: "You appear anxious." (first try)
   "How have you reacted since you learned your diagnosis?" (second try)
   "This must be difficult for you." (third try)
   If the feelings can be approached in a nonthreatening manner, the patient is usually able to verbalize them and most often is relieved. If the patient's denial persists, the patient will handle feelings when the time is right.
2. Discover the cause of the threat and its meaning to the patient. A person with terminal illness may be anxious because of familial responsibilities, not death. Do not assume that patients share the nurse's viewpoint. A nurse may believe that discharge from the hospital is a wonderful experience, but it may be anxiety-provoking for patients who must now cope with illness at home.

3. Discover how the patient has coped with anxiety in the past. Ask directly, "How have you managed nervousness before?" or "What has helped you cope in the past?"
4. Help the patient identify options and strategies for reducing anxiety. What can be done to exert some control over a portion of the situation? What can be "fixed" and what must be "let go?" Teach progressive relaxation, imagery, or meditation. If unskilled in these techniques, the nurse can learn them or locate a consultant. Refocus the patient on positive thinking or on another activity. Occupational activities such as puzzles, music, and art can help the patient refocus.
5. Identify the patient's support system of friends and relatives and use their visits to help the patient feel less alone.
6. Teach the patient. Lack of knowledge regarding routines, diagnostic tests, consequences of illness, and side effects of medications add to the patient's anxiety. Knowledge generally helps the patient feel more control over the treatment and promotes a sense of well-being.
7. Use social communication judiciously. Despite the idea that communication must be therapeutic, not social, most patients *do* respond to talk of motorcycles, boats, movies, or weather. If social communication is effective in giving a 2-year-old an injection, it may also be helpful with an adult experiencing a gallbladder x-ray examination or surgery under a local anesthetic. The rhythm and tone of the nurse's voice can reduce a patient's anxiety no matter what the topic.
8. Medicate. Medication is not necessarily the last resort. Often antianxiety agents are useful in allowing the patient to draw upon coping strategies.

additional responses are often necessary (see box on p. 397).

Anger/Hostility

Anger is a common response of individuals experiencing illness. Although anger is a natural and expected reaction, it is often believed to be inappropriate, frightening, or distasteful. It is important for the nurse to remember that, although anger is a normal response, aggression, hostility, and violence *are* unacceptable.

Anger is a feeling that arises in response to a threat. Individuals often express anger to avoid anxiety. Anger is usually short-lived and compatible with love. For example, a parent may become angry with a child who crosses the street alone. The parent realizes that the love for the child and the fear that the child will be hurt create anger. Similarly, the patient may express anger at the nurse but may appreciate and like the nurse despite the anger. Aggression is any behavior that is aimed at hurting another person psychologically or physically. Aggressive behavior is unacceptable. Hostility is an attitude that usually has a destructive component. **Hostility** may be covert or overt. If a patient states, "You are a bunch of incompetents," he or she is expressing overt hostility. If the same patient smiles and is compliant but tells the physician that the nurses are incompetent, this behavior is an example of covert hostility.

Behaviors

Expressions of anger may be nonverbal, verbal, or physical. Each expression of anger may also be direct or indirect. Direct nonverbal expressions of anger include glaring, "turning the cold shoulder," or clenching the jaw or fists. Indirect nonverbal expressions may manifest as withdrawal, brooding, or passivity or as physical illness, such as ulcer, asthma, or colitis. Although the exact mechanism by which anger causes disease is unclear, it seems to be connected to the stress-related illness mechanism. Direct verbal expression of anger is easily detected. Shouting, cursing, ridiculing, and confronting are readily assessed as angry behaviors. Indirect verbal expression of anger may include rumination, blaming, sarcasm, or gossiping. Direct physical expression of anger includes violent acts upon persons or animals, and indirect physical anger is usually displaced upon objects. Kicking the chair is an example of indirect physical anger. Often nurses are more comfortable with indirect expressions of anger. A patient who gossips is often experienced as amusing, and patients who express anger through somatic complaints are behaving within the illness role that nurses manage daily.

Direct expressions of anger, whether they be verbal, nonverbal, or physical, may produce feelings of helplessness or anxiety in the nurse. Both direct and indirect expressions of anger offer a challenge for creating thoughtful nursing interventions and responding to those experiencing illness.

Moreover, Novaco (1976) observed that the expression of anger has positive functions:

1. Anger energizes behavior.
2. The open expression of anger is characteristic of a healthy relationship.
3. Appropriate expressions of anger project a healthy self-concept.
4. Anger gives individuals a sense of control over situations and alleviates their sense of helplessness.
5. Anger alerts individuals to the need for coping mechanisms to manage and resolve problems.
6. Anger can serve as a defense for feelings of anxiety.[21]

Awareness of the positive functions of anger is necessary for the nurse to respond effectively to ill patients. At times, the nurse will want to encourage the constructive use of anger to enhance a patient's well-being.

Nursing response

Anger is such a common part of a person's reaction to illness that the nurse should carefully consider the patient who does *not* show anger. For example, a patient who suffers from stroke and does not express anger but remains withdrawn may have a poor prognosis. The patient requires some degree of anger as a motivation for recovery.

Initially the nurse directs interventions at preventing anger. Since anger may develop when an individual faces a situation that stimulates anxiety and helplessness, the nurse can direct interventions toward providing a safe and effective environment and attending to the unmet needs of the patient. Caring and environmental nursing actions help prevent anger.

Information-giving and teaching may also prevent an angry response. Human beings generally enjoy control and predictability. If patients and families understand routines, tests, discharge plans, or home care regimens, there is less likelihood of frustration or anger. Clear, concise communication, offering options for care, and a supportive attitude on the part of the nurse can prevent and diffuse anger.

Nurses unable to prevent angry responses must intervene directly. The nurse must keep in mind that anger is normal, that anger may be beneficial to individuals, and that reacting to anger with defensiveness or anger is not helpful. Although nurses encounter a myriad of situations involving anger that call for varied responses, general communication

THERAPEUTIC COMMUNICATION GUIDE

Dealing with Anger

1. Be aware of nonverbal communication. Do not rush, demand, react with hostility, or be overly cheerful. Be calm, move slowly, avoid touch, and maintain eye contact and a firm body posture. A patient who is losing control is frightened. A nurse's appearance of control without rigidity is reassuring.
2. Validate the presence of anger if possible. Say, "I understand why you may be angry." If you use a reflective statement such as "You seem angry," you may receive an angry response. Don't accentuate the obvious, but validate gently.
3. Do not shut the door on anger. Explaining too soon, justifying yourself, or reassuring before the patient can vent anger is not helpful and only serves to escalate anger. Do not condescend ("Tell me about it; I want to help") or interpret ("You are angry because I'm an authority figure"). Do not pass the buck or pretend to be unaccountable ("Wait for the physician" or "It's not my fault"). Anger is a feeling, not logical reasoning.
4. Listen for the cause and meaning of the patient's anger. There may be a reasonable explanation for the anger and the solution may be self-evident. Help the patient locate the source and meaning of the anger. Has the patient lost his or her perceived control? self-esteem? autonomy? role? Most often, an angry patient has lost or believes he or she will lose something of value.
5. Search for a solution to the situation using problem-solving methods.
6. If the patient's anger continues to escalate, the nurse may want to offer a "time-out" or medication, explaining to the patient that anger is permissible but loss of control is not. A quiet environment or medication may promote calmness. A nurse must protect the patient and the staff from harm and minimize destruction of property. Limit setting often provides structure to the patient's experience and lowers the energy that accompanies anger.
7. Refrain from showing fear. When nurses perceive their own anxiety, they require help.
8. If the patient becomes violent (common in psychiatric, delirious, or demented patients) consider using restraints, seclusion rooms, or medication. If the situation has escalated to this point, the nurse needs help. A "show of support" (5 to 8 persons) often calms the patient. Any physical or chemical restraints must have a doctor's order and be used after all other nursing measures fail.
9. Talk about the episode of anger after the patient regains calmness. Teach the patient the interplay between anxiety and anger, look for different ways the situation could be handled, role play, and support the patient. Angry patients must not be rejected.

guidelines can help the nursing care plan (see box above).

Dependence and Manipulation

Dependence and manipulation are behavioral responses common to individuals suffering illness. Patients may believe that they are totally dependent upon the nurse for physical and emotional care. Denying their own abilities and self-direction, patients may use controlling behaviors to gain power over the nurse. The controlling behaviors are called manipulation. If a patient believes he or she is dependent, the patient will act dependently and often manipulate in order to meet perceived needs.

Dependence is a behavior in which one person relies on another for support or nurturance. The individual seeks physical contact, physical and emotional help, attention, and approval. Dependent individuals have a need for security. Although a nurse provides caring and nurturance by virtue of the role, a patient's wellness is achieved by interdependence.

Even very ill patients have the desire to feed or wash themselves. A patient's overdependency is a signal that other nursing intervention or support is needed.

Often, very dependent patients attempt to gain security through manipulation. **Manipulation** is a powerful behavior that either controls other people, protects against anxiety, or uses other people to meet the patient's needs. The manipulator is often charming but insincere. Manipulation may be direct or indirect. An example of direct manipulation is the patient who flatters a nurse and then asks for a back rub. Dependence and manipulation may be conscious or unconscious. Because these behaviors are common emotional responses to illness and often induce negative feelings in the nurse, it is important for the nurse to learn to identify and manage these behaviors in a patient.

Behaviors

Dependency may manifest itself with behaviors such as poor personal hygiene, noncompliance, mistrust

CARE OF MANIPULATIVE AND DEPENDENT PATIENTS

1. Stay nonjudgmental, calm, and objective.
2. Use a kind, but very firm, matter-of-fact attitude. Confront the patient's lies and attempts at being dependent. Encourage the patient to determine what he or she wants and to ask for it directly. Ask kindly and directly "what is it you need?" If the patient wants water every five minutes, negotiate. Tell the patient that he or she may have water every 30 minutes. This helps the patient delay gratification.
3. Make short, frequent visits. Tell the patient why you are there, complete your tasks or contact, and leave. Say what you mean, and mean what you say. Do as you promise, and state what you intend to do.
4. Set limits on touching and attention-seeking behavior.
5. Provide outlets for anger, such as art, music, projects, and reading.
6. Assign the patient simple tasks so he or she can experience success.
7. Facilitate the expression of feelings and explore the meaning of those feelings. Anger and anxiety are often at the base of dependent and manipulative behaviors. If the patient denies a problem with feelings, tell him or her "It appears that you need help with your feelings, but since you disagree, we will continue with your treatment contract." Assure the patient that you are there to help but that he or she must help, too.
8. Reinforce independent behavior and successes.
9. Be sure the daily regimen of the patient is structured, consistent, and continuous. The patient should have a schedule from morning to night. Each shift must abide by the care plan. Tolerate no derogatory remarks regarding other staff members. Refer the patient to the person with whom he or she is unhappy, and continue with the structured care plans.

of staff, inappropriate attention seeking, withdrawal, inappropriate touching, procrastination, indecisiveness, and a low tolerance for frustration. Manipulative, dependent patients generally lack insight regarding their problems and are often demanding, ingratiating, and solicitous. Narcissism and intimidation may also be signs of dependency and manipulation.

Nursing response

The care of dependent and manipulative patients can be frustrating for the nurse. It is important to remember that these patients are in need of caring, understanding, and presence. It is also important to realize that the caring must be tempered with limit setting and firmness. If the nurse is feeling helpless and overwhelmed, it is clear that firmness and limit setting are inadequate. The nurse must be clear, congruent, and consistent. Continuity of care and cohesive teamwork provide the dependent patient with the structure needed to feel secure. The less secure a dependent patient feels, the more the dependency and manipulation will be demonstrated (see box above).

The dependent or manipulative patient is a human being in need and responds to structure, limit setting, and firmness. The goal is to assist the patient in discerning skills and meeting overwhelming security needs through more appropriate channels.

CRITICAL THINKING QUESTIONS

1 What is caring? How can nurses demonstrate caring behavior with their patients? What are the components of the three distinctive methods of caring?

2 What is loneliness? What kinds of behaviors might the patient exhibit? How does the nurse intervene?

3 What is the difference between anxiety and fear? What are the different levels of anxiety? Types? Symptoms? How can the nurse intervene?

4 What is the difference between anger and hostility? What is the basis for anger? How can anger be expressed? What are the positive functions of anger? How can the nurse intervene to channel anger constructively?

5 How can the nurse set limits on manipulative behavior? What other actions might the nurse take to demonstrate caring and help the patient become less dependent?

BIBLIOGRAPHY

Current

1. Beck A, Emery G: *Anxiety disorders and phobias,* New York, 1985, Basic Books.
2. Benner P: *From novice to expert,* London, 1984, Addison Wesley.

3. Benner P, Wrubel J: *The primacy of caring: stress and coping in health and illness,* London, 1988, Addison Wesley.
4. Davis T, Jensen L: Identifying depression in medical patients, *Image* 20(4):191, Winter 1988.
5. Cohen S, Syme SL: *Social support and health,* Orlando, 1985, Academic Press.
6. Drew N: Exclusion and confirmation: a phenomenology of patient's experiences with caregivers, *Image* 18(2):39, Summer 1986.
7. Gottlieb B: *Social networks and social support,* Beverly Hills, 1981, Sage.
8. Hardin S, Halaris A: Nonverbal communication of patients and high and low empathy nurses, *J Psychiatr Mental Health Nurs* 21:14, 1983.
9. Hoffman K: Hunches on childhood, Unpublished manuscript, 1987.
10. Kronberg M: Nursing interventions in the management of assaultive patients. In Lion J, Reid W, editors: *Assaults within psychiatric facilities,* New York, 1983, Grune & Stratton.
11. Leventhal H, Nering D, Steele D: Disease representations and coping with health threats. In Turk D, Kerns R, editors: *Health issues and families,* New York, 1984, John Wiley & Sons.
12. Reverby S: *Ordered to care: the dilemma of American nursing,* Cambridge, 1987, Cambridge University Press.
13. Steeves R, Kahn D: Experience of meaning and suffering, *Image* 19(3):114, Fall 1987.
14. Stuart G, Sundeen S: *Principles and practice of psychiatric nursing,* St. Louis, 1991, Mosby–Year Book.
15. Welt S: The development of roots of loneliness, *Arch Psychiatr Nurs* 1(1):25, February 1987.

Classic

16. Lazarus R: Cognitive and coping process of emotion. In Monat S, Lazarus R, editors: *Stress and coping: an anthology,* New York, 1974, Columbia University Press.
17. Lesse S: *Anxiety: its components, diagnosis and treatment,* New York, 1970, Grune & Stratton.
18. Lorenz K: *On aggression,* New York, 1966, Harcourt, Brace, & World.
19. Mayeroff M: *On caring,* New York, 1971, Harper & Row.
20. Meares R: *The management of anxiety patients,* Philadelphia, 1963, WB Saunders.
21. Novaco R: The functions and regulation of the arousal of anger, *Am J Psychiatry* 133:1124, 1976.
22. Paterson JC, Zerad LT: *Humanistic nursing,* New York, 1976, Wiley & Sons.
23. Peplau H: Loneliness, *Am J Nurs* 55:1576, 1955.
24. Peplau H: A working definition of anxiety. In Bird S, Marshall S, editors: *Clinical approaches to psychiatry,* New York, 1963, Macmillan.
25. Peplau LA, Perlman D: *Loneliness: a source book of current therapy and research,* New York, 1972, Wiley & Sons.
26. Spielberg C: *Anxiety,* New York, 1972, Academic Press.
27. Watson J: *The philosophy of science and caring,* Boston, 1979, 8, Little, Brown & Co.

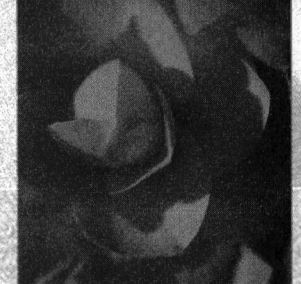

CHAPTER NINETEEN

Altered Self-Concept

LEARNING OBJECTIVES

1 Identify the four components of self-concept.
2 Describe the impact of illness and surgery on self-concept.
3 Recognize verbal or nonverbal cues that might indicate a threat to or alteration in self-concept.
4 Contrast strategies nurses can use to help patients cope with altered body image or threats to their self-concept in the initial adjustment period as well as the rehabilitative phase.
5 Identify types of patients who might be at risk for altered self-concept.
6 Describe the interrelationship of components of self-concept as whole.
7 Discuss the significance of the family in patient adjustment to altered body image.
8 Discuss the role of nursing in facilitating acceptance of altered self-concept or role function.

KEY TERMS

body image, p. 404
personal identity, p. 406
role theory, p. 405

schemata, p. 404
self-concept, p. 404
self-esteem, p. 406

FOR THE WOMAN who experiences a mastectomy or a person with a disfiguring burn scar, alterations in appearance are readily apparent. Yet many other patient situations involve no change in physical appearance and do impact on the self-concept. For example, the middle-aged man who has experienced a stroke and is unable to manipulate his dominant side is at risk for disturbances in self-concept, because he is unable to enact his usual role as provider, husband, and father. Likewise, the young adult college student newly diagnosed with a seizure disorder may withdraw from her usual activities and be unable to interact with peers or participate in the learning environment as a result of low self-esteem.

Each of these individuals presents a uniquely different challenge, although they are each experiencing an alteration to the self-concept. Their potential responses to illness or injury and their needs will vary widely and encompass many diverse nursing diagnoses. Each person continually strives to develop an adequate self-concept to preserve psychic integrity. Perception of self has a tremendous influence in determining behavior. There is seemingly a circular process whereby the self-concept influences behavior, which in turn affects one's self-concept. In clinical practice, nurses are commonly confronted with issues related to self-concept, body image, and self-esteem.

403

SIGNIFICANCE TO NURSING

Coombs identified two major reasons for the helping professions to concern themselves with self-concept. From his perspective the helper's effectiveness in facilitating patient change is seriously impaired if the self-concept is ignored. Second, patients "judge the value of their experience with helpers from the frame of reference of self-concept. What affects the self-concept seems relevant. What appears remote from it seems irrelevant."[50] Examining the self-concept is a multifaceted phenomenon; this chapter focuses on (1) components of self-concept, (2) formation of self-concept, (3) key factors affecting self-concept, (4) application of a nursing model, (5) assessment focus, and (6) nursing diagnosis.

DEFINITION OF SELF-CONCEPT

Our current understanding of self-concept derives from several theoretic perspectives: those of symbolic interactionalists, phenomenologists, and behavioralists. From the viewpoint of symbolic interactionalists, self-concept is continuously evolving from infancy to old age and is influenced by interpersonal interactions as well as the perception of how one appears to others. Cooley, Mead, and Kinch have hypothesized the "looking glass" idea in which self-concept is seen as a reflection of one's perception about how one appears to others.[77] Harry Stack Sullivan expanded this view in 1953.[55] He saw the self-concept as arising out of social interaction with significant others. The key to developing self-concept was in forming a reflected self-appraisal in response to those who provide reward and punishment in a person's life.

This notion of self-concept as not static but continuously redefined was emphasized by Toffler.[79] He proposed a changing nature of self-concept where each person develops "serial selves"—a series of selves developed and discarded in adaptation to a rapidly changing world.

Epstein attempted a more comprehensive definition and proposed that the self-concept is really a "self-theory":

> Self-concept is the theory that the individual has unwittingly constructed about himself as an experiencing, functional individual, and it is part of a broader theory which he holds with respect to his entire range of significant experience. . . . The fundamental purpose of the self-theory is to optimize the pleasure-pain balance of the individual over the course of a lifetime . . . to facilitate the maintenance of self-esteem and to organize the data of experience in a manner that can be effectively coped with.[57]

In applying self-concept theory to nursing practice, Driever[55] has arrived at a definition that incorporates the views of symbolic interactionalists, phenomenologists, and behaviorists: "the self-concept is the composite of beliefs and feelings that one holds about oneself at a given point in time, formed from perceptions, particularly of others' reactions, and directing one's behavior."

The influence of the symbolic interactionalist point of view is evident in the emphasis placed on the role of others in the formation of the self-concept. From this perspective, one becomes, in large measure, what others expect. The contribution of phenomenology's influence can be seen in the reference to the self-concept as an ongoing process. Driever also believes that the function of the self-concept is to direct behavior, thus incorporating a behaviorist principle.

COMPONENTS OF SELF-CONCEPT

Simply stated, **self-concept** is a mental image or picture of the self. It comprises the following components:

1. Body image, or "how I experience my body"
2. Subjective self, or "how I see myself, who I think I am"
3. Ideal self, or "the self I would like to be or who I feel I should be"
4. Social self, or "the way I feel others see me"[1]

In 1978 the Third National Conference on the Classification of Nursing Diagnoses identified four components of self-concept: (1) body image, (2) self-esteem, (3) role, and (4) personal identity.

Body Image

An important aspect of self-concept is that of **body image.** The perception of one's body is recognized as an important determinant of role, self-esteem, feelings of security, self-confidence, and personal identity.[57] However, body image is not simply what we think about our appearance; it also encompasses our perception of our function, sensation, and mobility. One of the first perceptions we have of self is an awareness of the body through sensorimotor experience. Throughout life, physical perceptions are key factors in the developing sense of self. Body image might be defined as a "mental picture" (the conscious information, feelings, and perceptions one uses to identify oneself as being uniquely different from everyone else) and includes one's concept of physical structure and personal space.[65]

Numerous theorists have proposed possible models to explain how body image is acquired. Henry Head explains that each individual builds up a set of references of the body called **schemata,** which are like blueprints.[37] These schemata have a neurologic basis and influence awareness. They contain information about body structure that changes as new information is received through body stimulation to provide integration between permanent and temporary body states. As a result of Head's proposal, body experience began to be recognized as an important determinant in developing behavior, as well as a tool for adjustment and adaptation.

Head's definition of body image includes "the perceptions, attitudes, emotions and personality reactions of the individual in relation to his own body."[62] Body image, then, is perceived as a learned concept formed from our responses to the environment. Kolb divided body image into four components:

1. Body-percept, which establishes the postural model of the body
2. Body concept, which are those beliefs and feelings about the body that arise from interaction with others
3. Body-ego, which is the receiving or viewing aspect of the body
4. Body-ideal, which provides a kind of mental measuring stick against which to judge the actual body[62]

Schoenfield states that body image is a complex of conscious and unconscious elements that represent the following aspects:

1. Actual subjective perceptions of the body, both as it appears and its ability to function
2. The internalized psychologic factors arising out of the individual's personal emotional experience as well as distortions of the body concept expressed as somatic delusions
3. Sociologic factors (parental and societal reaction to the individual) and the interpretation of these reactions
4. Ideal body image formulated by the individual's attitude toward his or her body derived from identification with the body of others[52]

Shontz[78] conceptualized a hierarchy of body image experiences encompassing function as well as fantasy actively integrated by the body ego in relation to the past and present that are intimately interrelated and serve a variety of functions. Shontz's body experience functions include sensory register, instrument for action, source of drives, stimulation to self, stimulation to others, private inner world, and expressive instrument.

Still another significant dimension of body image is the manner in which the individual perceives the body boundary. Some people view their body as a base of support and have strong boundary perceptions, whereas others may perceive the body surface to be fragile and easily permeated.[66]

Other studies exploring body experience and personality have identified three psychologic operations: body experience can dampen or magnify experience; body experience establishes a boundary between self and the environment; and body experience distributes attention to major body sectors—people do not attend equally to all sectors—different body parts may have different significance to each individual.[58]

For example, a surgical patient with extensive dressings has difficulty with a realistic appraisal of body boundaries and might feel threatened by the approach of another individual if body movement and dressing change evoke memories of previously painful events. Utilizing Rorschach picture drawings and other projective psychologic tests, Fisher and Cleveland[58] found the following deviations in body image resulting from illness or surgery: feelings of loss of body boundary; a sense of depersonalization; feelings of alien or extra parts; phantom limb; and confusion between right vs. left.

Murray[70] explains the formation and development of body image as a continuous process that does not end with the approach of adulthood. The infant learns to differentiate the physical self from the environment. When basic needs are met with warmth and acceptance, the infant feels positive. Subsequently the developing child then internalizes (incorporates into the self) the significant other's attitudes toward the self. Ultimately, the individual internalizes the standards of society. Attitudes toward various body parts are developed. Social stimuli impinge on the self and add another dimension to the body image. As middle age approaches, physical changes require adjustment of the body image. The aging process continues with emotional, as well as physical, losses to be experienced. The loss of a previous activity level or functional changes in either eating or elimination patterns are frequently perceived by the elder as negating value or worth. All of these changes must be continually absorbed and integrated into the body image if it is to remain consistent with reality. Thus one's mental picture of body image represents the subjective, as well as objective, experience with the body and is derived from internal, as well as external, experience and perception. This mental picture represents the ideal, as well as the actual; thus there may be some inconsistency with reality.

Role Theory

Our continuous interaction with others provides a source of feedback about our competence and function in the performance of our roles. Thus an understanding of **role theory** contributes to our understanding of the impact of role performance on self-concept. Meleis has developed a conceptual framework derived from the social interactionalist perspective:

> The role that the actor elects to play is a derivative of his voluntary actions that are motivated by the returns expected, and, indeed, received from others. In addition, the role assumed by an interactant in a given sit-

uation is validated when others indicate acceptance of that role allocation.

The roles one chooses to assume reflect the beliefs and feelings an individual has about himself or herself. Thus the interaction with others that creates and modifies one's various roles has a significant impact on the self-concept.[67]

Individuals undergo multiple role transitions in their lifetime. Meleis identifies three conditions that change role relationships, requiring adjustments on the part of both the actor and the significant others. These conditions include developmental, situational, and health-illness transitions. People in the process of health-illness role transition require ongoing nursing assessment and possible intervention to successfully incorporate the new role into the self-concept.[67]

Personal Identity

Personal identity is that part of the self-concept through which we recognize ourselves as unique beings, separate from the rest of the world. It is basically a psychoanalytic concept that relates to the ability to distinguish between self and nonself. In Freudian terms it is the *ego*. It is through the personal identity that we recognize that which belongs to us.[62]

Self-esteem

Self-esteem represents the evaluative component of self-concept. There is an integral relationship between self-esteem and self-concept. Coppersmith[51] elaborated on four bases of self-esteem:

1. Significance: how much an individual is loved, approved of, and appreciated
2. Competence: how well tasks considered important are performed
3. Virtue: the attainment of moral ethical standards
4. Power: how much and how well the individual can control self and influence others

Driever[55] defines **self-esteem** as "the individual's perception of his worth" and posits that a direct relationship exists between self-concept and self-esteem. Rubin[76] has related self-esteem to the ability of individuals to use themselves functionally to achieve a precise goal. Self-esteem is highly equated with control, whereas loss of control results in feelings of shame and failure. Adequacy, competence, and excellence in body function are the essential measures of self-worth and self-esteem. Wholeness depends on synchrony of function. Loss of function or even alteration in functions produces a bereavement for self as a whole integrated person: "To lose or to be threatened with the loss of a complex, coordinated and controlled functional activity that has

been achieved and integrated into the personal system is to lose or be threatened with the loss of self."[76]

Social interaction theorists have encompassed and expanded the concept of self to be a learned process from interaction with self and others.

• • •

Incorporating all of these views, self-concept can thus be defined as one's beliefs about oneself that are derived from others' reactions, as well as self-perception. It includes components of body image, self-esteem, roles and role performance, behavior, and personal identity. As Epstein[57] suggests, it is a theory about oneself; this self-theory continuously changes and evolves as one interacts with others.

CONCEPTUAL FRAMEWORK FOR NURSING
Systems Theory

The Bonham-Cheney model represents a method for organizing the various ideas and concepts from literature and previous research to define a nursing focus for assessment of self-concept.[49] The model uses a systems approach to present self-concept as a two-dimensional process that includes the real self as well as the perceived self. Using a systems approach, self-concept is viewed as an open system composed of two interrelated subsystems of personal identity and self-perspective. The subsystems are divided

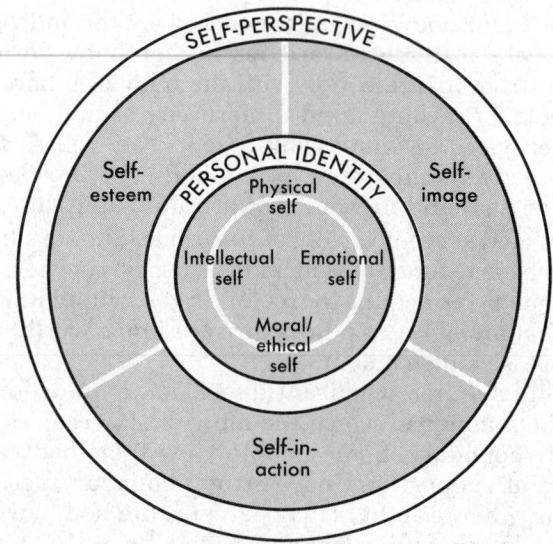

FIGURE 19-1 A model of self-concept. (From Bonham P, Cheney A: Concept of self: a framework for nursing assessment. In Chinn P, editor: *Advances in nursing theory development*, Rockville, Md, 1983, Aspen Systems Corporation. Reprinted with permission of Aspen Publishers, Inc, copyright 1983.)

into component parts. Personal identity is composed of the intellectual self, the physical self, the moral/ethical self, and the emotional self. Self-perspective includes self-image, self-esteem, and self in action. Self-concept is seen as a two-dimensional process that evolves from the interaction between personal identity and self-perspective.[49]

Each subsystem and component part interact to comprise and affect the whole. The system can change and adapt through feedback and transfer of energy to balance negative threats with positive forces. Figure 19-1 illustrates the self-system.

Viewing self-concept from a systems approach helps explain the variations in responses to illness and threats of self-concept. Each person differs in the positive and negative forces within his or her system. Individuals with positive coping skills and strong support systems can compensate for negative threats to their self-concept.

Application of Model

In the Bonham-Cheney model the self-concept depends on the foundation of personal identity comprising the intellectual self, the physical self, the moral/ethical self, and the emotional self.

The intellectual self includes all of the rational and cognitive powers. Creative and artistic skills also fall within this dimension. The physical self is that element of personal identity that encompasses the structure, function, and appearance of the body. The personal belief and values systems is the foundation of the moral/ethical self. It includes the spiritual and ethical dimensions of the self. Such concepts as conscience and personal values are incorporated into this aspect of the self. The final component of personal identity is the emotional self. Included here is the entire spectrum of feeling states. Desires, in terms of dreams and aspirations or ambitions, are part of the emotional self, as are the needs and drives that formulate them. Feelings such as fear, anger, and depression are its contrasting side.

Personal identity is the foundation of self-concept but, taken alone, is not sufficient to explain such a complex phenomenon. A deeper dimension is required. This dimension is supplied by the self as it views each of these components of personal identity from three self-perspectives, namely, self-image, self-esteem, and self in action. The way in which one views one's personal identity defines the perspective of self-image. Self-image is concerned with how one sees oneself and includes the perceived, actual, and ideal selves. The perceived self refers to what one believes is true about personal identity. This may not equate with what is actually true. In addition, this perspective is often influenced by what one wishes were true.

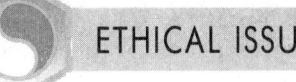

ETHICAL ISSUES

- In what morally relevant ways can illness change a person's self-perception?
- Can a patient who is occasionally disoriented participate in decisions regarding care? If so, under what circumstances?

The perspective of self-esteem identifies a sense of self-worth. Value is placed on each aspect of personal identity. The dichotomies of acceptable/unacceptable and satisfied/dissatisfied are addressed in this perspective.

The interaction with the environment by each element of personal identity is incorporated into the perspective of self in action. This perspective is similar to the traditional concept of roles. It deals with the effect each element of personal identity has on behavior. The various interpersonal and intrapersonal roles one chooses to assume are expressed here. The term *self in action* is used to provide consistency in labeling the model.

In the Bonham-Cheney model, then, self-concept is a two-dimensional phenomenon that evolves from the dynamic interaction between the personal identity with all its elements and the three self-perspectives. The self-concept can be viewed as somewhat fluid, with new information creating changes in beliefs about the self. However, some aspects of this concept may be so valued by the individual as to be difficult or impossible to modify. The ability to identify those areas would have considerable impact on the nursing process.

IMPACT OF ILLNESS ON SELF-CONCEPT

Illness, surgery, or disability can cause major threats to one's overall self-concept, self-esteem, personal identity, and, in particular, one's body image. Perception of wholeness and physical self are important determinants of self-concept. What then happens to a person who is ill, loses a limb, or undergoes surgery (an intense physical assault on the body)? Patients facing surgery have fears related to their body image. In a study of hospitalized patients' perceptions of stressful events, 47 patients were asked to rate stressful events associated with hospitalization. It was found that the possible loss of the function of body senses was listed as third highest, and possible disfigurement was listed as sixth highest out of 45 stressful events.[80]

The loss of a body part, illness, injury, or disfigurement causes a major threat to one's perception of body image. Disturbances occur as the person's uniqueness has been altered, and limits have been imposed on behavior through physical loss or alteration of body structure or function. The person experiences conflict between the way the body is now and the mental perception of the way it was before.[75] Loss of control is likewise a threat to one's self-esteem and overall self-concept. We must be cognizant of how being dependent affects individuals and impedes role performance and individuals' feelings of self-worth.

Changes in physical self can thus cause problems in self-esteem and in role performance. The overall self-concept is threatened. "Confrontation with personal physical mutilation, irrespective of the cause and irrespective of the extent or visibility, will release in the afflicted person feelings of insecurity as identity is threatened and self-esteem lowered."[42] In dealing with threats to self-concept from changes in the body structure, function, or appearance, the impact of loss must be considered. Loss is a situation whereby an individual experiences deprivation of something that was previously present. The manner in which each individual perceives the loss depends on past experience with loss, the value placed on the lost object, and the cultural, psychologic, economic, and family supports available for dealing with the loss.[63] Individual reaction will vary. It is important to note that it is not necessarily the extent or nature of the actual loss, but the individual's perception, that determines the reaction. Refer to Chapter 20 for a discussion on loss.

Patients at Risk

Many patients with varying medical or surgical conditions are at risk of threats to their self-concept, such as those suffering from strokes, amputation, mastectomy, paralysis, blindness, burns, deformity, loss of hair as a result of chemotherapy, and disfigurement as a result of radical surgery, ostomy, or tracheostomy. The changes these patients experience may cause a discrepancy between the actual and ideal body perception, resulting in disturbances in self-image, self-esteem, or role identity.

Studies are limited in areas such as general medical conditions and how they specifically affect self-concept or its component parts. Yet nurses must carefully consider the impact of any illness or disease that causes a change in the body; limits independence or life-style; limits function; or alters appearance, control, or role performance. Some groups have been studied to determine the effects of their disease. For example, patients with rheumatoid arthritis have been noted to experience problems with self-esteem as a result of body changes in structure and function caused by joint deformity, deterioration, and chronic pain.[35]

GERIATRIC CONSIDERATIONS

Self-Concept

The loss of control and independence seems to be the greatest threat to the elderly and their self-concept.

Concentrate on preserving physical function and give choices whenever possible.

Self-esteem may be affected by the loss of role function and independence.

Enhance self-esteem by promoting self-care and social relationships.

Maintain independence by providing support services (i.e., transportation, meals on wheels, home health aides).

Multiple physical changes occur in aging that may affect body image.

Another example of a patient who is especially prone to problems with threats to body image, self-esteem, and overall self-concept is the person having an ostomy. The effect stoma surgery has on anyone is profound. One reason is society's views on elimination. People expect the function of elimination to be carried out in private, and if it occurs in public, harsh sanctions are imposed. The individual who experiences stoma surgery is especially prone to difficulty relating to body image and self-concept, since two assaults on the body image are experienced: the change in structure or loss of an organ, and subsequently a loss of control of bowel or bladder functions.[64]

Other subtle problems that patients perceive as threats, which nurses may not recognize, are reactions to fairly routine procedures, such as having to remove dentures before surgery, having clothing removed, and having to wear hospital gowns.

Also in instances where there is not a specific illness, patients may experience distress from a discrepancy in the actual vs. ideal body image, such as those who see themselves as too tall, too short, too fat, or too thin compared with societal norms.

The patient's perception is the key to understanding the reactions, and that individual with poor self-esteem, altered self-concept, or unsatisfactory body image before being ill will be especially vulnerable to problems with illness. Therefore virtually any illness can affect self-concept if there is any alteration in the appearance, structure, function, or control of the body. Nurses must be keenly aware of changes that may seem insignificant but that may have a major impact on self-esteem or role or body image and consequently on overall self-concept.

Clinical Manifestations of Altered Self-Concept

Formal assessment tools to measure various facets of self-concept are continuously evolving together with our understanding of self-worth; these tools include locus of control scales, Rosenberg's self-esteem scale, and Piers Harris self-concept scale.

Patients may present various verbal and nonverbal cues when faced with threats to their self-concept, and the nurse relies on a general observation of appearance and behavior before employing a formal specific assessment tool. Realize these are only cues and may have causes other than being a specific reaction to the disease, illness, or surgery. It is necessary to validate the meaning of these cues with the patient before a precise interpretation can be inferred.

It is estimated that at least half of our messages are communicated nonverbally and that perhaps two thirds of the spoken and nonverbal communication is not congruent. Cultural and regional differences of expression and meaning must be considered. Verbal language and body language must be evaluated within the context of the entire communication process.[53]

Norris and Kunes-Connell[22] state that the defining characteristics indicating a disturbance in self-esteem are lack of eye contact, head and shoulder flexion, verbal self-negating statements, expressions of guilt, evaluation of self as unable to deal with situations, lack of follow-through, nonparticipation in

SIGNS OF ALTERATION IN SELF-CONCEPT

1. Refuses to look at, touch, or care for affected area
2. Becomes nauseous when looking at or caring for affected area
3. Verbalizes worry over clothing, appearance
4. Verbalizes feeling less feminine or less masculine, less sexually desirable
5. Verbalizes fear of rejection by others
6. Refuses to go out—social isolation
7. Makes derogatory remarks about self
8. Holds misconceptions about body function or structure
9. Rejects others; withdraws
10. Verbalizes feelings of shame or worthlessness
11. Verbalizes feeling mutilated or dirty (unclean) or obsessively cleans
12. Neglects personal hygiene
13. Expresses anger
14. Exhibits depression
15. Verbalizes feeling body is frail or permeable[70,76]

therapy, and self-neglect. Other verbal or nonverbal cues that may indicate alterations in self-concept are included in the box below.

Patient and family reactions

Patients undergoing surgery, illness, or trauma have multiple physical, psychosocial, and sexual needs and threats to their self-concepts. An individual's subjective perception of the experience may vary based on previous self-esteem, self-concept, family and social support, previous coping skills, and the extent or cause of the specific illness. For example, a patient with a long, painful disease might accept a disfiguring operation more readily than a patient who has had very few symptoms before surgery.[45]

In addition, health professionals must recognize the patient's family has problems in adjustment. Family members may also experience a sense of loss in reacting to a major body change or disfiguring disease of the patient. Family members thus have stress and difficulty coping with a loved one's illness. Roles and relationships within the family might also be reversed as a result of an illness, which can cause a patient to experience poor self-esteem. The nurse assesses and observes the hierarchic role relationships and preserves these relationships as much as possible to prevent causing the patient to feel dependent or a loss of control.[74] Family members and spouses therefore need information and support, particularly in the preoperative and postoperative periods, to help them adjust. This is important, since a reciprocal relationship exists whereby the patient affects and is affected by the family.[61]

Nurses need to be cognizant of the factors that influence a patient's ability to adapt, such as the patient's perception of what has happened; the patient's physical status, age, and sex; the symptoms, length, and nature of the disability; the prognosis and other aspects of the treatment that might influence the patient's view; the patient's ability to cope with stress in the past; social, cultural, or family attitudes and values; how life-styles are changed—what roles are changed; how sexual relations will be affected; and perhaps most important of all, how the patient perceives that his or her spouse or family will react. This last point relating to spouse and family acceptance is particularly important. For example, studies have shown that spouse and family acceptance or rejection is a key and critical element in the adaptation and rehabilitation of an ostomate.[56,72]

NURSING MANAGEMENT RELATED TO SELF-CONCEPT
Assessment

In the area of self-concept, it is important to keep in mind that various factors and conditions pose

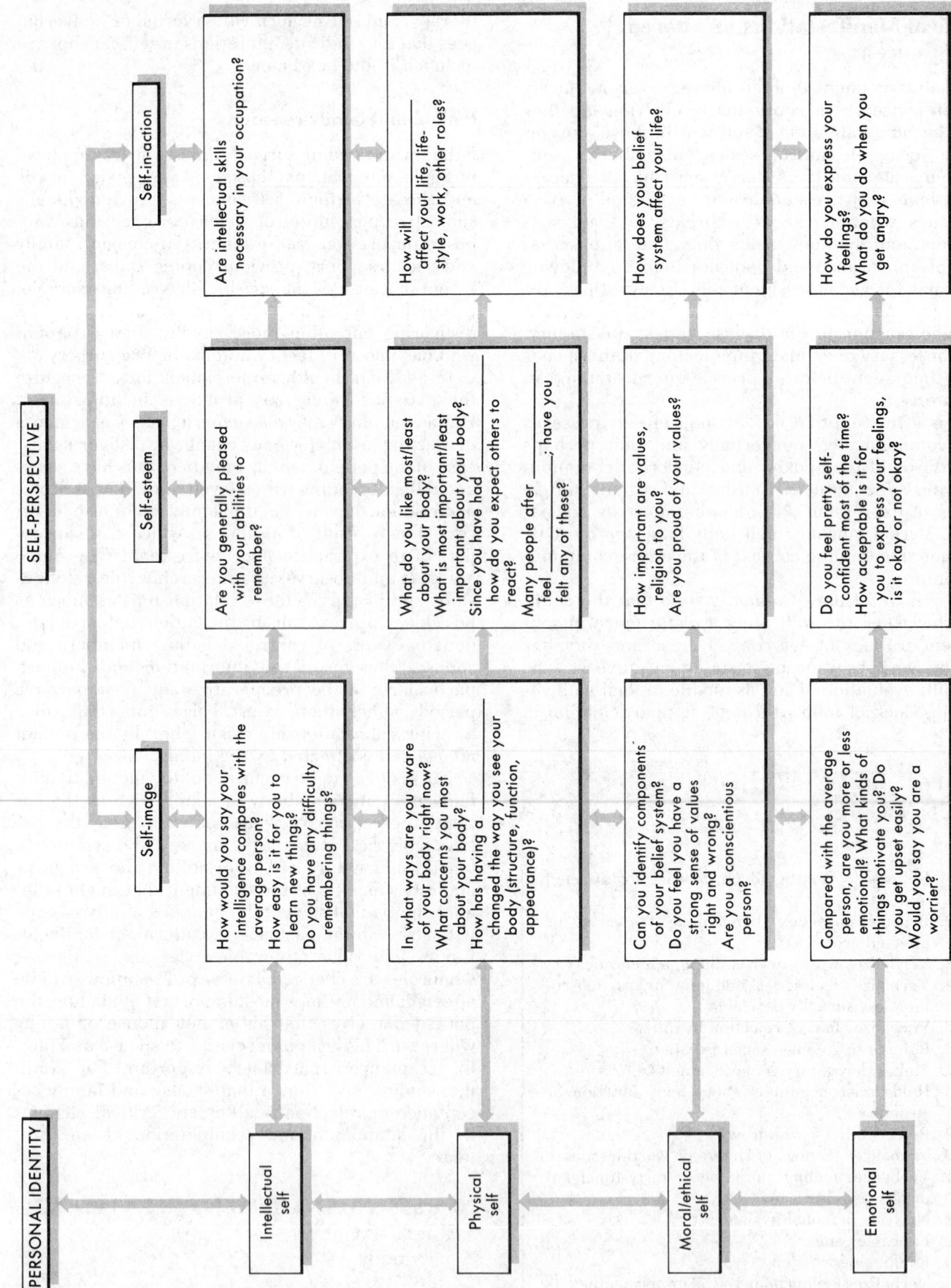

FIGURE 19-2 Sample questions. (From Bonham P, Cheney A: Concept of self: a framework for nursing assessment. In Chinn P, editor: *Advances in nursing theory development*, Rockville, Md, 1983, Aspen Systems Corporation. Reprinted with permission of Aspen Publishers, Inc, copyright 1983.)

threats and put the patient at risk for altered self-concept but that these problems do not automatically cause a negative self-concept. For example, patients may view their physical self-image as unsatisfactory and still have satisfactory self-esteem and overall self-concept.

A study of patients with rheumatoid arthritis found that it is not necessary to view oneself as attractive to have high self-esteem and a satisfactory self-concept.[36] Patients with spinal cord injuries for at least 4 years were found to have a high sense of personal, moral, ethical, and social selves and a lower physical self-image; yet these patients had an overall positive self-concept.[60] Women in treatment for obesity reported more negative body images than normal-weight individuals, yet they had satisfactory overall self-concepts.[83] Likewise, and contrary to ordinary expectations, a study of 30 cancer patients found that cancer patients can cope with threats to their self-concept: over half felt hopeful, worthwhile, calm, in control, useful, accepted, and loved despite their terminal illness.[68] These studies provide evidence that with support and intervention by helping, caring individuals, patients can be aided to maintain or attain satisfactory self-concepts.

Consequently, it is necessary to take note of patients at particular risk to threats to the self-concept, but nurses must not make automatic assumptions as to the final impact of the disease or disability on the individual until a careful assessment is made and validated with feedback from the patient.

In using the Bonham-Cheney model for assessment, the sample questions (Figure 19-2) may serve as a guide to the nurse in conducting an interview of the patient to determine problems and strengths in self-concept. In conducting the assessment interview, the nurse must try to determine the patient's perception of family and significant others' reactions, as well as what support systems or coping mechanisms the patient has available as strengths. Family reaction can be either a problem or a strength depending on a patient's perception.

This information enables the nurse to map out the patient's perceived self-concept and can then be analyzed to determine which areas are problematic and need intervention and which areas are being compensated and do not require intervention.

Nursing Diagnosis

The following diagnoses may apply to the patient with altered self-concept:

Knowledge deficit about body function

Body image disturbance caused by a change in the structure, function, and appearance of the body

Situational low self-esteem because of physical alteration

Fear of dependence resulting from loss of control of body function

Social isolation caused by fear of rejection

Ineffective individual coping resulting from anger and depression about the alteration

Self-care deficit because of difficulty accepting the alteration

Planning

Once the nursing diagnoses are formulated, behavioral goals are developed that encompass the affective, cognitive, and psychomotor domains, such as the following:

Patient accepts the need to look at the altered site

Patient touches and can explain the changed area's appearance and function

Patient accepts the need to learn to care for the area

Patient develops independence and competence in caring for the area

Patient is able to accept altered function and structure and reintegrate these into a positive body image and self-concept and adjust to all alterations in life-styles

In assessing and planning strategies for intervention, the issues of social support and the involvement of family or significant others must be addressed. Social support has been noted to have positive effects on how persons deal with stress, feelings of self-worth, and overall self-concept.

Studies related to social support found that the patient's perception of the support and the perceived value were key factors. The amount or number of supports was not seen as being as important as the degree of the perceived satisfaction with whatever was provided. The history of the relationship between the provider of the help and the recipient is important.[14,43,69]

The help from significant others includes informational help, emotional support, tangible help, and an integrative type of relationship with some sharing and reciprocity of help.[14] The idea of interaction and sharing is an important concept to promote health and wellness. A giving and receiving relationship is seen as the key to health.[73]

Another approach is to encourage patients to participate in self-care and group activities. By providing self-care and involvement with others, the patient exercises control and enhances independence and self-esteem and contributes to a sense of increased competency. "Self-worth develops as we become involved and exercise control through role relationships and group interaction."[31] Interaction with others helps develop a sense of belonging, helps define one's uniqueness, provides an opportunity to make decisions and set goals, and provides examples to see how others have achieved positive actions for coping. A study of spinal cord–injured patients in a rehabilitation program for pain demonstrated significant positive changes in the patients' self-concepts from participating in a group program.[48]

Nurses can positively enhance a patient's self-esteem by valuing the continued abilities of patients, especially elderly patients. People must be given choices in their care and some control over their lives and illnesses to enhance the patient's belief in self-capability and self-adequacy.[44]

On the subject of control and independence, a group of spinal cord–injured patients indicated that perceived independence and provision of one's own transportation, assistance needed, and living arrangements were the key factors in helping them adapt with a positive self-concept. The patients stressed that mobility and transportation had the greatest impact on their self-concepts.[60] To assist patients in positive adaptation to threats to self-concepts, nurses face these main challenges: (1) to effectively involve families and significant others in patient care, (2) to allow patients to make decisions and choices and have control over their care, (3) to have patients provide as much self-care and be as independent as possible, and (4) to allow and provide opportunities for patients to interact and participate with others in a give-and-take relationship.

Implementation

When patients experience alterations in their bodies that can alter their self-concept, the role of nursing becomes very important. An individual with a healthy self-concept before surgery, illness, or disability should regain or maintain that self-concept and achieve a high level of rehabilitation with adequate help.

In implementing a care plan, priorities should be established among the patient's needs. Needs are assessed as to which require immediate intervention and which can be postponed or are more long-term needs.[59] Also, needs may be classified as informational, technical, or emotional.[81] For example, at varying times these needs may vary. Preoperatively a patient may have more informational and emotional needs, whereas postoperatively, technical needs may have a greater priority.

In working with patients, the nurse's reaction is important; patients may test the nurse first. Any withdrawal or sign of repulsion can seriously affect the patient's ability to adjust to threats to the self-concept. The nursing process must be predicated on the nurse's understanding of personal feelings, fears, and values and one's own capacity to put another's needs first and to give freely of self in an open, honest, and supportive way. If a nurse cannot deal with a certain issue, then the patient can be referred to others for assistance.

Patient education

Patients and families must be informed and educated about possible changes they might experience as a result of illness, treatment, or surgery, so they have time to prepare themselves. Nurses must explain the reasons for various physical and other changes to enhance understanding.[47]

Likewise, efforts can be made to minimize the effects of the changes of diseases or treatment by helping obtain various cosmetic or prosthetic devices needed, such as scarves, bonnets, caps, or wigs for

PATIENT EDUCATION GUIDE   *Altered Self-Concept*

Encourage staff, family, and others to provide an environment of acceptance and caring

Encourage patients to express their fears, feelings, concerns, and anger

Be an active listener, and, by reflecting back perceptions, help patients develop insights into their feelings

Provide emotional, informational, and technical support and reassurance

Make patients and families aware that anger, depression, and fear are acceptable and normal reactions to loss

Prepare patients and families in advance of changes, so they know what to expect

Allow patients as much control and independence as possible

Teach patients and families in areas related to their specific needs and questions

Involve patients in as much self-care as possible

Provide direct nursing care in areas where the patient or family is not ready or is unable to assume responsibility

Provide privacy and act as a sounding board

Help patients identify positive aspects of life—help focus on what is left and not just the loss

Help patient and significant others deal with sexual concerns about body changes

Encourage participation with others or group sessions to discuss and share similar needs, problems, and concerns

patients receiving chemotherapy or breast prostheses for patients with mastectomies.

In summary, strategies that can be used to decrease negative factors and enhance positive factors related to altered self-concept are summarized in the box on p. 412.

Preoperative preparation

To begin to deal effectively with the crisis of body image for the surgical patient, proper preparation is needed before the surgery. Learning self-care and acceptance and resolution of an altered body image progress more rapidly in those patients who have been psychologically prepared for surgery.[82] Preoperatively a general learning plan should be outlined to establish goals mutually set by the patient, family, and medical staff to prepare the patient as completely as possible to understand the surgery, terminology, altered anatomy and physiology, equipment needed, and other factors pertinent to the surgery.

Postoperative care

When a care plan is implemented postoperatively to deal with altered self-concept, it is important to recognize that in any loss, a patient may be depressed and unable to cope initially with the changes. During this initial reaction to the loss, much support, listening, and patience are needed. Nurses must allow patients a time for denial and not force prematurely a level of acceptance in patients before they are able to mobilize their coping skills and adapt. As awareness and recognition develop, the patient may express anger. It is vital here that the nurse not react in anger but help the patient realize that anger is normal and acceptable and find appropriate ways to channel or express the anger. Encouragement to talk is helpful, so the patient does not turn the anger inward. As the patient evidences increased readiness, some of the anger passes and the patient begins to progress to the reconciliation stage. The nurse may begin at this point to implement teaching and self-care, since the patient will begin to be interested in learning. The patient begins to address the loss or altered function or structure and can start to deal with assimilating the changes.

Progressive teaching

Recognizing the impact of loss as it affects patient adjustment, Dericks and Donovan suggest four progressive steps that can be implemented to help the patient begin to deal with an altered self-concept:

1. The first step is one of narration, where the nurse demonstrates and explains to the patient what is going on and allows the patient to express feelings and concerns.

2. Next is the look, touch, and talk phase. The patient looks at, touches, and talks more about the care and other concerns. The nurse here is still providing the care as the patient observes.

3. In the third step of participation the patient is ready to begin to assist in the techniques required to perform self-care, while the nurse is there offering support, guidance, and assistance.

4. The last step is exploration, in which the patient has mastered the techniques to competently provide self-care and must go out alone to resume an independent life. Thus the patient is gradually brought to self-care.[54]

Evaluation

Careful consideration is given to the patient's perception of whether care is effective and needs are being met. Evaluation of progress in meeting goals should be done at specific times. Kolb suggests that a healthy adaptation to self-concept changes may be judged by the patient's willingness to verbalize or discuss body changes and feelings and by the patient's ability to care for oneself and accept the help of others.[62] In evaluating the response to care, the nurse observes carefully for subjective and objective expressions of behavior, such as changes in expression of anger, ability to express feelings, family's ability to cope, anxiety of patient or family, inappropriate use of pain medication, expressions of satisfaction or dissatisfaction with body or self-worth, verbal expression of fear, expression of hope or lack of hope, and supportive statements or help from the family.[63]

Documentation

Documentation provides sufficient information to determine the "map" or self theory that the patient is using to guide and direct behavior. The assessment specifically addresses strengths as well as problems. In assessing the self-concept, it is essential to address the patient's subjective perceptions and feelings, as well as objective cues observed by the nurse. Reactions of family and significant others are recorded. Names of resources and significant others are documented, so they may be used as a help system.

Ongoing Care

Discharge planning and follow-up after hospitalization are necessary to continue the support and guidance needed for patients with altered self-concept to adapt to life. Patients and families who have experienced severe threats to their self-concept, such as with major changes in their body and life-style, require special assessment for posthospital needs. Discharge planning is particularly critical for those with cancer, ostomies, mastectomies, amputation, and paralysis, as well as for elderly persons who live alone and other persons with severe debilitating diseases.

Particular clues indicating there may be posthospital problems or care needs are inadequate support systems; inadequate finances for food, medicine, or medical supplies; poor housing or unsafe home environment; inability to carry out treatments or prescribed therapy; inability to perform activities of daily living; and social withdrawal.

Patients should have complete written instructions for special procedures, and if possible the patient's helper should be taught techniques of care before discharge. Teach the patient the signs and symptoms of complications and what to do in case of an emergency. Patients may also need referrals to vocational counseling for job retraining and information about reconstructive surgery available in such instances as burns, mastectomies, and pelvic exenteration. Follow-up exercise therapy may be needed in some instances, such as for patients with neurologic deficits or burns, to minimize disfigurement and enhance mobilization. Also, in cases where patients have experienced severe disfigurement or physical changes, it might be helpful to plan an outing from the hospital before discharge to have the patient get used to facing the public and dealing with the emotional reactions.[65]

CRITICAL THINKING QUESTIONS

1 What are the components of self-concept as defined by the Third National Conference on Nursing Diagnoses?

2 What is the definition of body image, self-esteem, role, and personal identity?

3 How do the components of self-concept interrelate to form the whole?

4 How does illness or surgery affect body image, self-esteem, role, and overall self-concept?

5 What types of patients are at special risk for altered self-concept?

6 What strategies can be used to increase strengths or decrease problems when threats to self-concept occur?

7 What role does the family play in patient adjustment to altered body image or self-concept?

8 What nursing diagnoses may be developed pertaining to altered self-concept?

9 What are indications that a patient needs special discharge planning and follow-up care?

10 What is the role of self-help groups for patients with altered self-concept?

BIBLIOGRAPHY

Current

1. Atwater E: *Psychology of adjustment,* ed 3, Englewood Cliffs, NJ, 1987, Prentice-Hall, Inc.
2. Bednar RL et al: *Self-esteem: paradoxes and innovations in clinical theory and practice,* Washington, DC, 1989, American Psychological Association.
3. Brundage DJ: Self-concept alterations: theory and assessment. In Thelan LT et al: *Nursing diagnosis in critical care,* St Louis, 1990, Mosby–Year Book, Inc.
4. Cohen A: Body image in the person with a stoma, *J Enterostom Ther* 18(2):68, 1991.
5. Cornwell C, Schmitt M: Perceived health status, self-esteem and body image in women with rheumatoid arthritis or systemic lupus erythematosus, *Res Nurs Health* 13(2):99-107, 1990.
6. Diekmann JM: Measuring body image. In Frank-Stromberg M: *Instruments for clinical nursing research,* Norwalk, Conn, 1988, Appleton & Lange.
7. Dropkin MJ: Coping with disfigurement and dysfunction after head and neck cancer surgery: a conceptual framework, *Semin Oncol Nurs* 5(3):213-219, 1989.
8. French JK, Phillips JA: Shattered images: recovery for the SCI client, *Rehabil Nurs* 16(3):134, 1991.
9. Haber J et al: *Comprehensive psychiatric nursing,* ed 4, St Louis, 1992, Mosby–Year Book, Inc.
10. Hopwood P, Maguire GP: Body image problems in cancer patients, *Br J Psychiatry* 153(suppl 2):47-50, 1988.
11. Jureidini J: Psychotherapeutic implications of severe physical disability, *Am J Psychother* 42(2):297-307, 1988.
12. Kilkus SP: Self-assertion and nurses: a different voice, *Nurs Outlook* 38(3):135, 143, 1990.
13. Koehler ML: Relationship between self-concept and successful rehabilitation, *Rehabil Nurs* 14(1):9-12, 1989.
14. Krause N: Satisfaction with social support and self related health in older adults, *Gerontologist* 27(31):301, 1987.
15. LeMone P: Analysis of a human phenomenon: self-concept, *Nurs Diagn* 2(3):126-130, 1991.
16. Lisanti P: Perceived body space and self-esteem in adult males with and without chronic low back pain, *Orthopaedic Nurs* 8(3):49-56, 1989.
17. Markus H: Unresolved issues of self-representation, *Cognitive Ther Res* 14:241-253, 1990.
18. Martocchio B: Authenticity, belonging, emotional closeness, and self-representation, *Oncol Nurs Forum* 14(4):32-37, 1987.
19. Mason KJ: Congenital orthopedic anomalies and their impact on the family, *Nurs Clin North Am* 26(1):1-16, 1991.
20. McFarland GK, McFarlane EA: *Nursing diagnosis and intervention,* ed 2, St Louis, 1993, Mosby–Year Book, Inc.
21. Nelson RB: Social support, self-esteem, and depression in the institutionalized elderly, *Iss Ment Health Nurs* 10:55-68, 1989.
22. Norris J, Kunes-Connell M: Self-esteem disturbance: a clinical validation study. In McLane AM: *Classification of nursing diagnoses: proceedings of the Seventh Conference,* St Louis, 1987, Mosby–Year Book, Inc.
23. Olson B et al: The patient in a halo brace: striving for normalcy in body image and self-concept, *Orthop Nurs* 10(1):44-50, 1991.
24. Pasquali EA et al: *Mental health nursing: a holistic approach,* ed 3, St Louis, 1989, Mosby–Year Book, Inc.
25. Pillow DR et al: Attributional style in relation to self-esteem and depression: mediational and interactive models, *J Res Person* 25:57-69, 1991.

26. Platzner H: Body image—a problem for intensive care patients. I, *Intensive Care Nurs* 3:61-66, 1987.
27. Platzner H: Body image—a problem for intensive care patients. II, *Intensive Care Nurs* 3:125-132, 1987.
28. Price B: *Body image nursing concepts and care,* New York, 1990, Prentice-Hall, Inc.
29. Rawlins RP et al: *Mental health–psychiatric nursing: a holistic life-cycle approach,* ed 3, St Louis, 1993, Mosby–Year Book, Inc.
30. Reed P: An analysis of the concept of self-neglect, *Adv Nurs Sci* 12(1):39, 1989.
31. Rice M, Szoza H: Group intervention for reinforcing self-worth following mastectomy, *Oncol Nurs Forum* 15(1):33, 1988.
32. Rix KJB, Smith RP, editors: The psychopathology of body image, *Br J Psychiatry* 153(suppl 2), 1988.
33. Salter M: *Altered body image—the nurse's role,* New York, 1988, John Wiley & Sons.
34. Samond RJ, Cammermeyer M: Perceptions of body image in subjects with multiple sclerosis: pilot study, *J Neurosci Nurs* 21(3):190-194, 1989.
35. Skevington S et al: Self-esteem and perception of attractiveness: an investigation of early rheumatoid arthritis, *Br J Med Psychol* 60:45, 1987.
36. Slevin A, Roberts A: Discharge planning: a tool for decision making, *Nurs Management* 18(12):47, 1987.
37. Steffenhagen R, Burns J: *The social dynamics of self-esteem,* New York, 1987, Praeger.
38. Stuart GW, Sundeen SJ: *Principles and practice of psychiatric nursing,* ed 4, St Louis, 1991, Mosby–Year Book, Inc.
39. Thompson JM et al: *Mosby's clinical nursing,* ed 3, St Louis, 1993, Mosby–Year Book, Inc.
40. Utz SW et al: Perceptions of body image and health status in persons with mitral valve prolapse, *Image J Nurs Scholar* 22(1):18-22, 1990.
41. Walsh A, Walsh PA: Love, self-esteem, and multiple sclerosis, *Soc Sci Med* 29(7):793-798, 1989.
42. Wassmer A: The impact of mutilating surgery or trauma on body image, *Int Nurs Rev,* p 86, Jan-Feb 1988.
43. Weinert C, Brandt P: Measuring social support with the personal resource questionnaire, *West J Nurs Res* 9(4):589, 1987.
44. Whall A: Self esteem and the mental health of older adults, *J Gerontol Nurs,* p 41, April 1987.
45. Williamson E: Patient perception of the ostomy experience, *J Enterostom Ther* 14(4):146, 1987.
46. Wright J: Self-perception alterations with coronary artery by-pass surgery, *Heart Lung* 16:483, 1987.

Classic

47. Baxley K, Erdman K: Alopecia effect in cancer patient's body image, *Cancer Nurs,* p 499, Dec 1984.
48. Beekman C et al: Self-concept: an outcome of a program for spinal pain, *Pain* 22:59, 1985.
49. Bonham P, Cheney A: Concept of self: a framework for nursing assessment. In Chinn P, editor: *Advances in nursing theory development,* Rockville, Md, 1983, Aspen Systems Corp.
50. Coombs A: Self-concept: product and producer of experience. In Avila D et al: *Helping relationships,* Boston, 1971, Allyn & Bacon, Inc.
51. Coppersmith: *The antecedents of self-esteem,* San Francisco, 1967, WH Freeman.
52. Corbeil M: Nursing process for a patient with a body image disturbance, *Nurs Clin North Am,* March 1971.
53. Davis AJAM: Body talk, *Am J Nurs,* p 931, July 1984.
54. Dericks V, Donovan C: The ostomy patient really needs you, *Nurs '76,* p 30, Sept 1979.

55. Driever M: Theory of self-concept. In Roy C, Sr: *Introduction to nursing: an adaptation model,* Englewood Cliffs, NJ, 1976, Prentice-Hall, Inc.
56. Dyk R, Sutherland A: Adaptation of the spouse and other family members to the colostomy patient, *Cancer,* p 123, Jan-Feb 1956.
57. Epstein S: The self-concept revisited, *Am Psychol* 28(5):404, 1973.
58. Fisher S, Cleveland S: *Body image and personality,* NJ, 1978, Divan and Nustrand Co, Inc.
59. George G: If patient teaching tries your patience, try this plan, *Nurs '82,* p 50, May 1982.
60. Green B et al: Self-concept among persons with long term spinal cord injury, *Arch Phys Med Rehabil,* p 751, Dec 1984.
61. Kobza L: Impact of ostomy on the spouse, *J Enterostom Ther,* p 54, Oct 1983.
62. Kolb L: Disturbances in body image. In Arieti S, Reiser M, editors: *American handbook of psychiatry,* ed 2, New York, 1975, Basic Books Inc, Publishers.
63. Lambert V, Lambert L: *Psychosocial care of the physically ill: what every nurse should know,* ed 2, Englewood Cliffs, NJ, 1985, Prentice-Hall, Inc.
64. Lindensmith S: Body image and the crisis of enterostomy, *Can Nurse,* p 24, Nov 1977.
65. Marvin J: Planning home care of a burn patient, *Nurs '83,* p 65, Aug 1983.
66. McCloskey J: How to make the most of body image theory and nursing practice, *Nurs '76* 6(5):68, 1976.
67. Meleis A: Role insufficiency and role supplementation, *Nurs Res* 24(4):264, 1975.
68. Morris C: Self-concept as altered by the diagnosis of cancer, *Nurs Clin North Am* 20(4):611, 1985.
69. Muhlenkamp A, Sayles J: Self-esteem, social support and positive health practices, *Nurs Res* 35(6):334, 1986.
70. Murray R: Principles of nursing intervention for the adult with body image changes, *Nurs Clin North Am* 7(4):697, 1972.
71. Norris J, Cannell M: Self-esteem disturbance, *Nurs Clin North Am,* p 745, Dec 1985.
72. Prudden J: Psychological problems following ileostomy and colostomy, *Cancer* 28:219, 1971.
73. Riehl J: Application of interaction theory. In Riehl J, Ray C, Sr, editors: *Conceptual models for nursing practices,* ed 2, New York, 1980, Appleton-Century-Crofts.
74. Robbins M, Schacht T: Family hierarchies, *Am J Nurs,* p 284, Feb 1982.
75. Roberts S: *Behavioral concepts and nursing intervention,* Englewood Cliffs, NJ, 1978, Prentice-Hall, Inc.
76. Rubin R: Body image and self-esteem, *Nurs Outlook* 16(6):20, 1968.
77. Schrauger J, Schoeneman T: Symbolic interactionist view of self-concept, *Psychol Bull* 86(3):549, 1979.
78. Shontz F: *The psychological aspects of physical illness and disability,* New York, 1975, MacMillan Publishing Co.
79. Toffler A: *Future shock,* New York, 1970, Bantam Books, Inc.
80. Volicer B: Patients' perceptions of stressful events associated with hospitalization, *Nurs Res,* p 235, May-June 1974.
81. Watson P: Meeting the needs of patients undergoing surgery, *J Enterostom Ther* 12:121, 1985.
82. Watson P et al: Comprehensive care of ileostomy patients, *Nurs Clin North Am,* p 427, Sept 1976.
83. White J, Schroeder M: Femininity, image, feminism and a decision to seek treatment in obese women, *Health Care for Women International,* p 455, 1986.

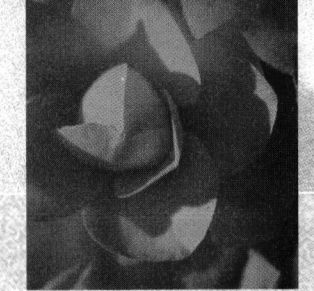

CHAPTER TWENTY

Loss, Grief, and Dying

LEARNING OBJECTIVES

1 Define loss, and describe four types of loss.
2 Discuss factors that affect the loss response.
3 Define three types of grief, and compare the components of various grief theories.
4 Explain the process the nurse uses to cope with the care of dying patients and families.
5 State four strengths the nurse needs to help a grieving individual.
6 Describe the roles of the nurse in assisting the grieving person.
7 Compare the similarities and differences of various dying theories.
8 Describe the effects of impending death on the patient, the family, and the nurse or caregiver.
9 Outline the kind of assessment data needed to develop a plan of care for a dying patient.
10 Outline the kind of assessment data needed to help the family through the dying process.
11 Discuss interventions to maintain the rights of the dying patient and anticipate the needs.
12 Explain the hospice concept.

KEY TERMS

acceptance, p. 426
acute grief, p. 418
anger, p. 426
awareness dying, p. 427
bargaining, p. 426
closed awareness, p. 427
denial, p. 426
depression, p. 426
grief, p. 418

hospice, p. 433
living-dying trajectory, p. 425
loss, p. 418
mutual pretense or awareness, p. 427
open awareness, p. 427
process of mourning, p. 421
suspicion awareness, p. 429

THE UNIVERSALITY of loss, grief, and dying commonly are overpowering experiences that one is unable to stop or control. Everyone responds to these events with their own unique coping mechanisms.

Understanding the dynamics of loss, grief, and dying will not only help nurses better comprehend their own feelings and responses to loss and grief, it will give them an appreciation for the response of their patients to whom they give care, of the patient's family, and of the colleagues with whom they work.

LOSS
Types of Loss

An individual may experience various types of **loss** throughout a lifetime. Depending on the significance of the loss, negligible or intense responses will be generated. Logically, multiple loss experiences will intensify the overall response. Four types of loss exist that individuals will experience singularly or collectively at any time.

Loss of external objects, either physical or material is, perhaps, the most common loss experience. External objects, or material loss, can be tangible, such as the loss of money, house, pets, or possessions, or it can be intangible, as in leaving one's country or homeland or moving from one city to another.

A second type of loss that all individuals experience is maturational loss. Losses of this type occur throughout the life span. This loss begins with weaning the infant from the mother's breast and continues with loss of baby teeth; loss of position in the family as more siblings arrive; loss of relationships, such as first love; going off to college; marriage; and changes in the body with the normal aging process.

Every individual has an overall mental image of his body and persona. When events occur that alter a person physically or psychologically, a third type of loss is evident: loss of body image or some aspect of self (symbolic loss). Loss of body image can be initiated by physical assaults, such as the surgical removal of the breast, ovaries, or uterus; or the loss of an extremity through an accident or surgery. Psychologic losses include loss of ideas one holds dear and feelings about one's attractiveness, lovableness, confidence, and worth. Loss of positive attitudes, such as independence and control, and loss of social role, such as mother, father, or breadwinner, are also examples of this type of loss.

When familiar symptoms of disease are eliminated after medical or surgical intervention, the secondary gains that may have served a particular function for an individual are lost, and that person becomes uncomfortable and may grieve over the loss.

Loss of a loved one or a significant other is perhaps the most difficult loss a person experiences, especially if it is caused by death. This type of loss is the most difficult for nurses and other health care professionals to handle, because they also are confronted with their own mortality and vulnerability.

Each loss carries with it a threat of additional or future losses and secondary losses. The initial loss of health can, for example, precipitate the loss of a job (some aspect of self), money (material objects), family role, self-esteem, or body part. As one begins to assimilate and understand the concept of loss, it becomes increasingly apparent that loss plays a peripheral, as well as a central, role in both the start and outcome of illness and disease. Experiencing a major loss, such as the death of a spouse, may trigger psychosomatic illness or a variety of symptoms in a person, because loss is such a serious body stressor.

Any kind of loss is an integral part of the human experience and can be a stimulus for growth. The discomfort felt when a loss occurs stimulates a need to do something about it or to explore new avenues to lessen the discomfort or make it go away. The response one has or exhibits as a result of loss depends on one's previous loss experiences, the meaning attached to the loss, one's methods of coping, cultural dictates, the means available for handling the loss, environmental factors, and messages from parents and peers.[3] Jackson[20] similarly applied these factors to loss by death. He identified individual personality, social roles, one's personal value structure, and the perceived relative importance of the loss as factors that affect the response to loss and the potential for growth.

GRIEF

The feelings and emotions caused by loss are clinically identified as **grief**. Grief is the hardest work an individual will ever do in his or her lifetime, particularly if the grief involves the loss of a loved one or some aspect of self. Similar to loss, grief is universal; different perhaps in expression, but with common features exhibited by most individuals. Grief, also called bereavement or mourning, is a response to something lost and the process of incorporating the experience of loss into one's ongoing life. Like loss, grief is of several types, including acute, anticipatory, and pathologic, or impaired.

Types of Grief

Acute grief is like a crisis, lasting about 4 to 6 weeks. It occurs after a sudden event, particularly after a death or some major insult to the psyche or soma.

Various theorists have identified the symptoms of acute grief. Symptoms of somatic distress occur in waves lasting varying periods, usually 20 minutes to 1 hour. They occur every time the loss is acknowl-

PHYSIOLOGIC MANIFESTATIONS OF GRIEF

Anorexia and other gastrointestinal distress
Weight loss
Inability to sleep
Crying
Tendency to sigh
Lack of strength
Physical exhaustion
Feeling of emptiness/heaviness
Feeling of a lump in the throat
Heart palpitations (anxiety)
Nervousness/tension
Loss of libido or hyperactive sex drive

edged. Among the many physical symptoms experienced are shortness of breath, a tightening in the throat, sighing, weakness, feelings of exhaustion or detachment, sweating, gastrointestinal upset, and numbness (see the box above). A vivid example of somatic distress is described by C.S. Lewis in his book *A Grief Observed*,[26] the writing of which helped him through the loss of his wife.

> The same flutter in the stomach, the same restlessness, the yawning I keep swallowing . . . it feels like being mildly drunk or confused. There is a sort of invisible blanket between the world and me . . . something inside me tries to assure me . . . then comes a sudden jab of red-hot memories.

Preoccupation with the image (of the deceased or of the lost body part, function, or meaningful object) is a phenomenon similar to daydreaming and is commonly accompanied by a sense of unreality. Feelings of guilt are often present. Self-blame for negligence is common. Depending on the person, these guilt feelings may remain unstated, or they may be verbalized in an attempt to seek validation. Hostility directed toward friendships that the griever normally maintains may result from inner struggles. The person is concerned about the irrational anger he feels. There is a lack or loss of warmth toward others and a struggle to deal with this. The outward behavior might be expressed in stiff or formal social interactions with people who previously had been included in a relaxed and informal relationship. Loss of patterns of conduct are evident in the grieving individual's ability to initiate or maintain activities. People usually have typical ways of accomplishing activities of daily living and job-related responsibilities. The distraction and restlessness of acute grief causes a feeling of being at "loose ends." Motivation and zest disappear; tasks and activities take considerable ef-

fort to accomplish. Things such as dressing that normally take 20 minutes to accomplish may now take hours, and every moment may seem exhausting. The griever may become overwhelmed by the significant number of daily activities he has to perform. The ability to make a decision becomes difficult.

Anticipatory grief is the response to loss before it actually occurs. When a person is dying, families commonly attempt to prepare themselves for the loss. Preparation also occurs in the face of potential loss of belongings, friends moving away, and surgery to remove a body part. A person facing surgery or death grieves for the real or potential losses that these states impose. During anticipatory grief, the individual experiences a sequence of feelings and behaviors similar to those that occur in acute grief. The individual is preoccupied with the particular loss event and anticipates the mode of readjustment that might be necessary.

Anticipatory grief is valuable, since it serves as a form of insulation or protection against the loss. At times, it is a rehearsal for the real event that is destined to occur. Janis[21] notes the "work of worrying" before surgery is a form of anticipatory grief and finds it to be associated with better psychologic and physiologic outcomes. The benefits of anticipatory grief have led caregivers to help patients anticipate future losses, so when they occur, the patients are prepared for them. Futterman, Hoffman, and Sabshin,[14] from their work with parents and dying children, conceptualized anticipatory grief into five functionally related aspects: (1) acknowledgment—convinced the inevitable will occur; (2) grieving—experiencing and expressing the emotional impact of the anticipated loss and the physical, psychologic, and interpersonal turmoil associated with it; (3) reconciliation of the situation; (4) detachment—withdrawal of emotional investment from person or object; (5) memorialization—developing a relatively fixed conscious mental representation of that which will be lost.

Anticipatory grief may have adverse effects. If the event does not occur when expected, those who are awaiting it may become hostile and impatient. In the case of someone who is dying, it may result in premature detachment of the family from the dying patient and prevent the family from reinvesting in the patient. This is known as the Lazarus syndrome. It may deprive friends and families of final close relationships and prevent resolution of unfinished business. Researchers have found that grief after anticipatory grief is no less painful than unanticipated loss, but it does allow for less of an assault on the mourner's adaptive capacity.[31] Anticipatory grief then can be helpful or harmful to the griever, but it must be recognized as a legitimate phenomenon for intervention.[7]

Impaired grief, chronic grief, or pathologic grief

TABLE 20-1   Interrelationship of Grief Theory Models

Theorist	Onset	Grief						Resolution
Bowlby[11]	Protest	Despair			Detachment			Resolution
Engel[13]	Shock		Developing awareness	Restitution		Resolving the loss	Ideation	Outcome
Gorer[17]	Shock	Intensive grief work				Reestablishing physical and mental balance		
Kavnaugh[22]	Shock		Disorganization	Volatile emotions	Guilt	Loss and loneliness	Relief	Reestablishment
Kübler-Ross[25]	Denial		Anger	Bargaining	Depression	Acceptance		
Lindemann[27]	Shock	Acute mourning			Resolution of grief			
Parkes and Weiss[31]	Intellectual recognition and explanation of loss	Emotional acceptance of the loss				Assumption of new identity		
Raphael[33]	Shock Numbness Disbelief	Separation pain			Psychologic mourning process			Reintegration
Weissman and Kamm (1985)	Shock Disbelief Denial		Undoing	Anger	Sadness			Integration
Wooden[35]	Accepting the reality	Experiencing the pain			Adjusting to a changed environment			Withdrawing and reinvesting emotional energy

begins with normal grief responses. However, sometime during the grief work, obstacles occur that interfere with the normal progression of the grieving. These obstacles prolong the grief and delay the reaction to it. Where there should be normal symptoms, there are exaggerated ones and distorted perceptions. Impaired grief may be fostered in situations where there is a lack of social involvement with others. The person who lives alone, socializes little, and has few close friends or an ineffective support network will probably have difficulty grieving. Unresolved guilt is another factor that affects the ability to grieve successfully. When there is ambivalence and guilt involving the loss of a person or related to the loss of a body part or function, impaired grief may ensue. The individual who has difficulty expressing feelings will also have difficulty with normal grief. Feelings and thoughts need to be expressed when there is a major loss. Whatever the reason, when a person does not know how or does not have the capacity to express the loss to others, the ability to grieve successfully will most likely be impaired. If a grief response is delayed for more than 2 weeks, and irrational anger, social outbursts, and insomnia appear, impaired grief should be suspected. A person in impaired grief commonly is not aware that there is a problem. The individual becomes fixated in some phase of the grieving process with real or imagined feelings of intense separation anxiety, self-blame for loss of a body part, or in the case of death, hostility toward the person who has died. A person with this kind of aberrant grief re-quires the professional help of a clinical nurse specialist, hospice nurse, psychologist, or psychiatrist.

Grief Experience

Grief makes the fact of loss real. The **process of mourning** or grieving is essential for personal adaptation to the loss, whether it is the result of death, termination of a relationship, a change in life-style, or a change in situation. Numerous theorists have identified the phases an individual goes through when doing grief work or mourning (Table 20-1). All theories seem to demonstrate that in the normal grief process, there is an onset, active grief work, and a resolution or reorganization of the survivor's life after the loss. Although these theories show a linear progression of the grief experience, the process occurs in individualized ways, including regression and progression through the phases.

John Bowlby's approach[11] provides an illustration of this (Figure 20-1). Imagine his circular diagram as a spiraled bedspring. With each loss experience, the behaviors and feelings repeat themselves. This continues throughout life. The movement around this inclined circle is not easy, and at times the individual slides back and forth between phases. At other times, if there have been previous loss experiences, the individual will readily pass through a phase and linger in another. In essence, what this suggests is that loss is cumulative, and that one can learn, grow, and gain meaning from varied experiences of loss.

The grief process or experience takes time, much

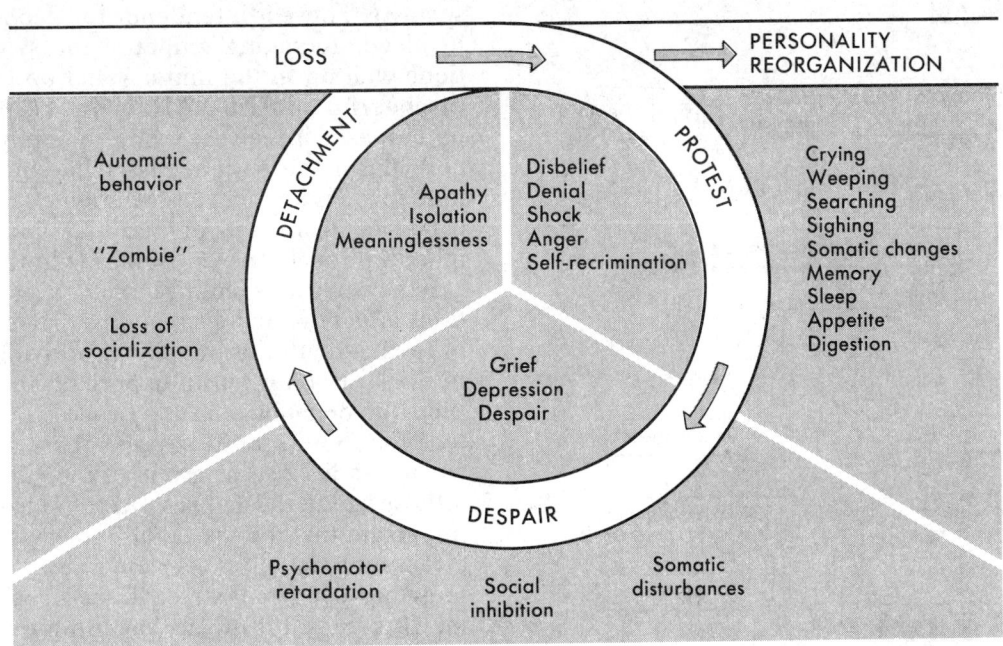

FIGURE 20-1   An illustration of John Bowlby's approach to loss.

longer than a person anticipates and society allows. People return to what appears to a casual observer as normal functioning in a few days or weeks after a major loss, such as death; but the pangs of grief continue for years, although with diminished frequency and intensity. In loss by death, grieving takes at least 1 year; 2 years is not unusual, but in some ways an important loss always remains with us. The pain of grief often is exacerbated on anniversary dates such as birthdays, holidays, and wedding anniversaries. Grieving or mourning is often viewed as a "weakness, a self-indulgence, a reprehensible bad habit instead of a psychologic necessity."[29] However, there are cultural variations. For some cultures outward expression of grief is encouraged. Grieving can be supported in its progress, but anything that forces the natural course of grief work or tests reality too early is likely to impair the process of grief resolution.

Grief work takes an enormous amount of physical and emotional energy. It is the hardest work anyone can do and has been likened to being as exhausting as digging a ditch. Grief may be manifested in many ways: physically, cognitively, affectively, and behaviorally. Often people are not aware that the feelings they experience after a loss are a grief response. All cultures seem to observe a certain set of behaviors after death, but there do not appear to be a set of behaviors when the loss is of another type. A person who loses his home, is seriously ill, or who has lost his job does not know that the feelings he experiences and the behaviors he displays in the weeks afterward are natural and normal reactions to loss. In most instances, the individual is labeled "depressed," rather than grieving. The essential concept of grief is that after any significant loss or change, some degree of grief and grief work will occur (Figure 20-2).

Assessment of Grief

Grief assessment is based on knowledge of the grief and mourning process and on ascertaining that a loss event has occurred or is anticipated (see box, p. 423). Data are obtained through observation of behavior, as well as through questioning the individual about the events (losses and gains) in his life during the past year. In some instances where there may be impaired grief, it is necessary to inquire into events of the past. Knowledge of past losses or present gains that bring with them losses will help the nurse develop a plan of care with the patient that will facilitate the physiologic and psychologic manifestations of the grieving process, regardless of whether they are transient or continuing. Inherent in developing interventions is knowledge about the patient's coping mechanisms (effective and ineffective) and support systems upon which the patient can rely.

Interventions

One of the goals of nursing is to help the person or family in attaining and maintaining a healthy adjustment to the loss experience. Interventions that meet this goal are basic and simple, but because emotions are involved, the simple often becomes difficult.

A nurse who for the first time cares for a dying patient often feels intense discomfort, fear, and insecurity. There is a tendency to become emotionally involved, forsaking empathy for sympathy. Questions well up in the mind: What do I say? Should I be cheerful or serious? How do I respond when the patient asks if they are dying? What if I start to cry? or What if the patient dies while in my care? The nurse who is keeping information about the patient's condition from him or her may find it difficult to maintain touch or eye contact with the patient.

Many negative cultural influences and superstitions affect the nurse's response. Those who are new in caring for the terminally ill or dying patient need to know it is normal to experience a wide range of thoughts or feelings in the process. It is also important for the nurse to express these feelings with a trusted individual or group of individuals.

Loss requires the presence of four strengths. It is important that nurses acquire these strengths before attempting to help those who grieve. First, the nurse must have spiritual strength, or strength from within. This does not mean that the nurse must have a specific religious orientation, but that the nurse must have a positive belief in self. The nurse must also

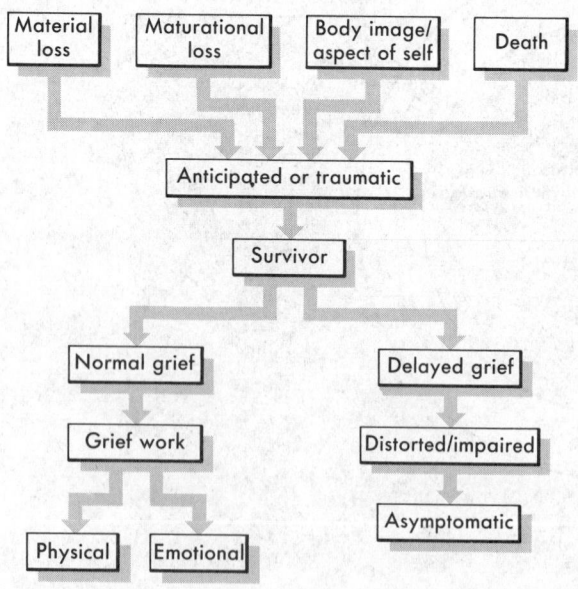

FIGURE 20-2   Grief process.

FACTORS INFLUENCING THE GRIEVING PROCESS

Physical

Illness involves numerous losses

Each loss must be identified

Each loss prompts and requires its own grief response

Importance of the loss varies according to meaning by individual

Sedatives—deprive experience of reality of loss that must be faced

Nutritional state—if inadequate, leads to inability to cope or meet demands of daily living, and numerous symptoms caused by grief

Rest—inadequate leads to mental and physical exhaustion, disease, unresolved grief

Exercise—if inadequate, limits emotional outlet, aggressive feelings, tension, anxiety, and leads to depression

Psychologic

Unique nature and meaning of loss

Individual qualities of the relationship

Role body part/self-image/aspect of self was to the individual and/or family

Individual coping behavior, personality, mental health

Individual level of maturity and intelligence

Past experience with loss or death

Social, cultural, ethnic, religious/philosophic background

Sex-role conditioning

Immediate circumstances surrounding loss

Timeliness of the loss

Perception of preventability (sudden vs. expected)

Number, type, quality of secondary losses

Presence of concurrent stresses/crises

Specific to Dying/Death (in addition to above)

Role deceased occupied in family or social system

Amount of unfinished business

Perception of deceased's fulfillment in life

Immediate circumstances surrounding death

Length of illness before death

Anticipatory grief and involvement with dying patient

Social

Individual support systems and the acceptance of assistance of its members

Individual sociocultural, ethnic, religious/philosophic background

Educational, economic, occupational status

Ritual

---

find meaning in life. A personal philosophy can sustain the self during difficult times. With age, life experiences grow and a person's philosophy may change; but at any particular time, the individual should have a philosophy. The nurse must develop emotional maturity. The person who has always gotten whatever he or she desires will most likely have trouble when confronted with deprivation or loss. Finally, comfort with personal mortality is the fourth strength essential for working with loss and grief.

There are several approaches to working with those who are in grief. In the first approach, the nurse assumes various roles: supporter; facilitator; and advocate in which eye contact, listening, and touch are employed. The second approach employs "talking out," "feeling out," and "acting out."

The nurse assumes the role of supporter, facilitator, or advocate according to the needs of the patient or family. As the supporter, the nurse uses the most potent types of intervention: eye contact, listening, and touch. Eye contact allows and provides an appraisal of the grief situation. It conveys nonverbal encouragement, so that communication can begin. It is also a sign to the patient that the nurse

is ready to listen and to understand his or her feelings.

Listening is an important intervention skill for the nurse, who serves as a support person for the griever. It is far easier to give advice on how to resolve problems than it is to allow the grieving person the time and space to express feelings. Such attempts to resolve problems or situations for the individual who is grieving are presumptuous, even though it is assumed that the nurse "knows what is best."

When listening, the nurse soon discovers that it is not so much the actual loss that concerns the griever as it is the sense of threat to the griever's self. The nurse who listens carefully to both the stated and the implied will hear such phrases as, "How will I get on?" "What do I do now?" "What will become of me?" "I don't know what to do." "How could he (they) do this to me?" or "Help me!" Because the nurse knows that there is resolution, such statements may seem melodramatic, but to the one who is grieving, there seems to be no resolution. The griever cannot yet look ahead and know that the despair and other feelings will indeed resolve. This means that in the process of listening, the nurse will need to clarify what is said to help the person confront fears about the future. When these fears are not dealt with, the griever will tend to exaggerate them beyond the realm of reality and thus intensify the anxiety state. Sometimes the best approach is to give patient and family space and an environment conducive to the work of grieving. The nurse can be available but not intrusive, and can consolidate activities to decrease interruptions.

The nurse can facilitate patient problem solving by exploring how the patient solved problems in the past. Insight into the patient's method of crisis resolution directs the nurse's course of action. In some instances where a patient has difficulty making decisions, it is helpful to ask him "what if" questions or to provide a number of alternatives from which to choose.

It is difficult for the nurse and others to listen to the same thing endlessly repeated, but reminiscing

is important to the griever. It allows for the working through of loss. Reminiscence is a means by which denial can fall by the wayside and allow the reality of the loss to filter slowly into the conscious mind. Reminiscence helps the griever acknowledge that indeed the loss is real, and that life can go on even though it will be difficult.

Early in grief work the nurse will be an advocate for the grieving patient. Energy or motivation may be so low that it is difficult for the patient to function effectively. The nurse may need to actively intervene at these times on behalf of the patient or arrange for a family member to assume responsibility as the patient's advocate.

In talking out, the individual should be encouraged to talk about his or her grief and express any feelings. Most persons do not like to hear the same story over and over and in a relatively short time tune out the individual or withdraw from the situation. When feelings are ventilated or shared with

LEGAL ISSUES   *Advance Directive Laws*

While legally competent, adults have several tools available to them, depending on the state in which they reside, that give advance direction to health care providers about treatment decisions. The medical-surgical nurse may run across them in several contexts: hospitals, nursing homes, or the patient's home.

The most commonly used tool is the "living will." This is a statutorily recognized (meaning there is state legislation defining its use) written declaration that any competent person may execute directing the withholding or withdrawal of death-prolonging procedures. It is signed by the person making the declaration, dated, and if not completely written in the person's handwriting, signed in the presence of two or more witnesses at least 18 years of age.

Death-prolonging procedures are defined by legislation and generally include any medical procedure or intervention that, when applied to a patient, would serve only to prolong artificially the dying process and where, in the judgment of the attending physician pursuant to usual and customary medical standards, death will occur within a short time regardless of whether such procedure or intervention is utilized. Many of the living will statutes state that death-prolonging procedures do not include the administration of medication or the performance of any medical procedure deemed necessary to provide comfort care or to alleviate pain, or the performance of any procedure to provide nutrition or hydration.

Another tool available in many states is the durable

power of attorney, sometimes called health care proxy. This tool is much broader in scope than the living will. It is a written, dated, signed, and witnessed statement of a competent adult appointing a person of his or her choice to make health care decisions on his or her behalf when unable to participate in health care decisions. The appointed person is referred to as the one holding a power of attorney for health care decisions, or the health care proxy, depending on what the state specifies. The appointed person stands in the shoes of the person who made the appointment and is to make decisions as that person would have wanted.

Either of these tools may be revoked by the person making them. State statutes provide immunity for a physician, licensed health care professional, medical care facility, or employee of the facility, who in good faith and pursuant to the usual and customary medical standards, causes or participates in the withholding or withdrawal of death-prolonging procedures that are not otherwise unlawful from a patient pursuant to the declaration made pursuant to legislation. In such a case, that person will not be subject to criminal or civil liability or be found to have committed an act of unprofessional conduct.

Both of these tools should be inserted into the patient's medical record for those authorized to care for the patient to know about and refer to. Each health care agency should have a written policy for staff to follow in conjunction with the living will or durable power of attorney.

Source: Uniform Rights of the Terminally Ill Act, Chapter 459 Declarations, Life Support, Uniform Laws (as of 1988, adopted in Alaska, Iowa, Maine, Missouri, Montana, Oklahoma).

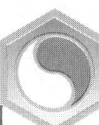

ETHICAL ISSUES

- Is a patient's refusal of life-sustaining treatment a form of suicide? If a nurse cooperates with the patient's refusal, is she assisting in suicide?
- What is the difference between active euthanasia and assisted suicide? Between killing a patient or allowing a patient to die?
- Is there a morally relevant difference between withholding treatment and withdrawing treatment? Is there a legal difference?
- Is there a morally relevant difference between withdrawing a ventilator and withdrawing a NG tube? Is there a legal difference?
- If the amount of pain medication required to relieve a dying patient's pain would also cause the patient to stop breathing, would the nurse who gave the medication have committed active euthanasia? Why or why not?
- What does it mean to say that a patient has a valid DNR order? Should a patient with a "no CPR" order be refused admittance to the ICU?
- What help can an Advance Directive offer in the care of a comatose patient? Should an Advance Directive written 10 years before and never discussed again be considered morally binding?

others, the momentary panics, hysteria, and other sensations accompanying grief are less frightening. Despite the belief that those who are grieving want to be left alone, in actuality, they want to talk about their loss with people who care. Feeling out is a cathartic experience. People today expect stoicism and bravery. Public display of deep feelings is a source of embarrassment for some cultures. The result is that feelings are suppressed and depression may result. In many instances, it is the nurse who encourages the patient or family to express their feelings. The nurse literally has to say "It's okay" to express hurt, anger, or whatever feelings the patient or family has. Acting out is a natural extension of feelings. Intense physical activity gives one some control over emotions. Ancients used to tear their clothes or their hair. Today forms of acting out that are taken include jumping into the car and driving at high speed or throwing things, or for some, feverishly gardening, cleaning house, or engrossing oneself in work. When someone is acting out, it is the role of the caregiver to ascertain that the acting out is safe. If the individual needs to throw things, use of tennis balls or other objects that will not injure the individual, others, or property is suggested. Dr. Elizabeth Kübler-Ross, in her seminars during the late 1960s, would sometimes have angry seminar participants take a piece of rubber hose and beat a pillow or mattress that was provided to dissipate their anger.

DYING
Nature of Dying

The process of dying is the most challenging of life experiences. It is an individual and private experience, and most of all, it is coming to terms with being alone.

How one responds to bad news, extreme stress, change, disappointment, or loss governs coping responses and attitudes toward dying. These coping and defense patterns are established early in life. Thus most people die as they have lived.

The age of the dying person and the dying person's attitude toward life significantly affect coping styles and the way the news of impending death is handled. For example, news of fatal illness in early adulthood is met with outrage and fury, "It isn't fair!" Adults under the age of 40 generally greet the knowledge of dying with severe feelings of disappointment, anger, and frustration, because this is a time in their lives when relationships are still being established, careers are just getting off the ground, and there is still so much to do. After the age of 40, the individual is a little more accepting of fate, although there are still many goals left to accomplish at a time in life when he or she should be enjoying the benefits of years of work. Instead, however, the present now becomes a time in the person's life for introspection, the evaluation of life goals, and the consideration of the quality of life rather than the quantity of life. For many, time perspective changes, because careers have been interrupted and loving relationships will be shortened.[6] Advanced adulthood is a time of goal reevaluation, regardless of whether the person is dying. For the elderly, dying evokes life review and assessment of whether life has been worthwhile. If it has not been worthwhile, an attempt is made to repair former failures in the remaining time; for example, resolving conflict between parent and child or sibling and sibling, or completing a task that has been left undone.

Pattison[32] developed a **living-dying trajectory** that explains patterns of coping with diagnosis of terminal illness that abruptly confronts the individual with crisis. Pattison calls the time between the crisis or knowledge of death and the point of death, the living-dying interval. Medical science may extend the length of terminal illness for a number of years, thus the living-dying interval may be lengthened.

Pattison's living-dying trajectory remains relevant today. Pattison divided the trajectory into three clinical phases that occur along a living-dying interval.[32] The acute phase, associated with recent diagnosis of a terminal illness, is usually the peak time of crisis, when there is great uncertainty. Crisis intervention is most effective here because the individual, family, and caregivers are struggling to come to terms with impending death. Impending death, or the chronic living-dying phase, is a time when work-activity patterns, entertainment, and relationships should be maintained as normally as life-style permits. The terminal phase is ushered in by withdrawal or turning away from the outside world in response to internal body signals that tell the dying person to conserve energy.

Theorists and the Dying Process

In the mid-1960s, researchers began to publish their observations about coping mechanisms during terminal illness (Figure 20-3). Dr. Elizabeth Kübler-Ross' stages have passed into the popular vocabulary of death, in part, because middle-aged persons recognize themselves in her study subjects.[8] Dr. Kübler-Ross[25] describes her five stages of dying as denial, anger, bargaining, depression, and acceptance. **Denial** serves as a buffer after unexpected shock, as in a terminal diagnosis, and provides time to collect and remobilize oneself. Eventually, this temporary defense is replaced by partial acceptance. **Anger** in the form of rage, envy, and resentment is expressed by projecting these feelings at friends, family, and hospital staff. The anger phase of the terminally ill is a difficult phase for caregivers and family to experience because patient anger may be taken personally. **Bargaining** is an attempt by the terminally ill to postpone the inevitable by establishing self-imposed deadlines for accomplishments, attendance at events, or making other promises to themselves. Most of these deadlines and promises are silently made. **Depression** is indicative of dealing with the sense of great loss. It is an essential and beneficial part of preparing for acceptance of inevitable death. Depression is affected by the discrepancy between the patient's wishes, readiness for death, and the expectations of those in the patient's environment. **Acceptance** occurs when one passes through the previous stages. Acceptance is described as the ability to contemplate the coming of death with a certain degree of expectancy. Because of fatigue and weakness with increasing periods of napping or sleep, the dying individual begins to communicate more nonverbally than verbally. Interest in anything diminishes, and the wish to be alone is strong. Retsinas noted that the response of the elderly to dying did not necessarily reflect the stages explained by Kübler-Ross, because time perspective changes and reevaluation of life or life review.[8]

Keleman[23] reconstructed Kübler-Ross's stages of dying into three phases: (1) the resistive stage, which encompasses responses such as anger, denial, bargaining, fight, and avoidance; (2) the review stage, which introduces a new consciousness as one's life flashes by; the struggle or resistance disappears and

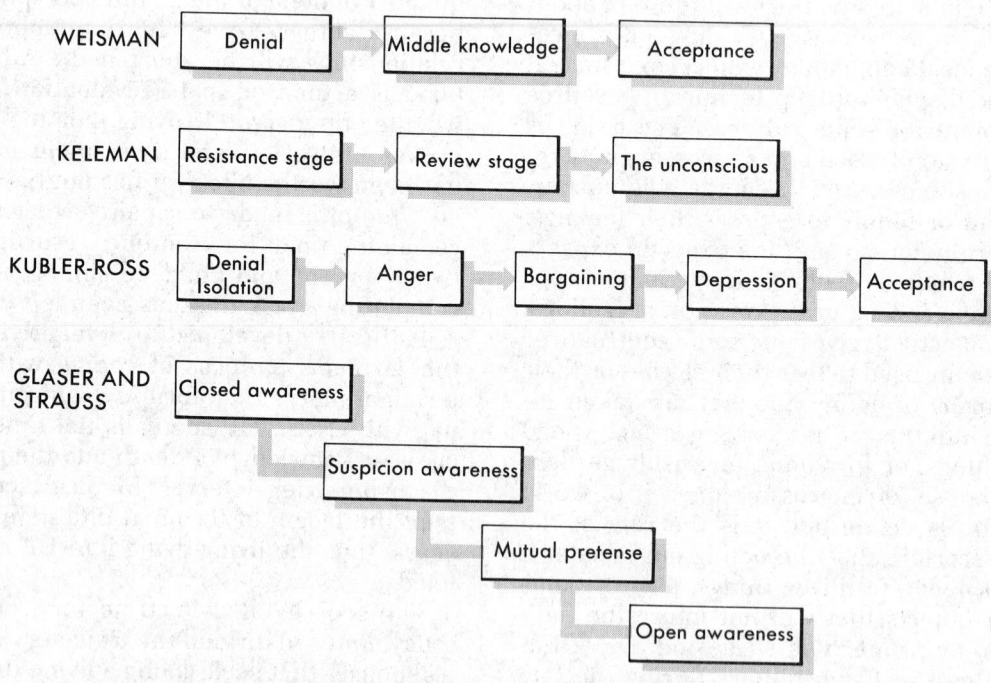

FIGURE 20-3 Theories of stages of dying.

the individual begins to deal with unfinished business and reclaims a part of self, becoming more in tune to self of the present rather than that of the past; and (3) the unconscious stage, which is much like birth or being revived from a cardiac arrest. The individual can talk about dying with calm, and at times, ecstasy.

Nurses and others who deal with the dying process in the home or in institutional settings must be careful not to label the terminally ill as being in one stage or another. Categories can transform the dying person into a nonperson in the eyes of all involved. Nonpersons are talked about and over with the assumption that they are incapable of hearing or making decisions for themselves. It is not intentional; it just happens, and health professionals must be aware of this phenomenon.

Glaser and Strauss[15] considered the dying process from a broader perspective. Their research identified four theoretical models of **awareness dying** that could be applied not only to the patient but to the family, friends, and particularly the health care professionals: closed awareness; suspicion awareness, or suspect awareness; mutual awareness, or mutual pretense; and open awareness. **Closed awareness** is described as "keeping the secret." Medical personnel know that the patient will die prematurely, but the patient does not know it. Generally caregivers invent a fictitious future for the patient to believe in, in hopes that it will boost the patient's morale. In **suspicion awareness,** the patient suspects that he or she is going to die. Hints are bandied back and forth, and a contest ensues for control of the information. In truth, the patient wants his suspicions to be wrong. **Mutual pretense or awareness** is basically called "let's pretend." Everyone knows the patient has a terminal illness and will die, but neither the patient, family, nor medical personnel talk about it—real feelings are kept hidden. **Open awareness** acknowledges the reality of approaching death. The patient, family, and medical staff openly acknowledge the eventual death of the patient. The patient may ask, "Will I die?" and "How and when will I die?" The patient becomes resigned to dying, and the family grieves with the patient rather than for the patient.

Dying Individual

Terminal patients may not see clearly the approach of their death. What is seen with clarity is how far they have come from their former state of well-being. An individual's perception of wholeness is related to his ego integrity, and as more and more losses are sustained, there is a progressively greater constriction of ego strength. At first, physical strength is diminished or is lost. Social isolation occurs because people do not know what to say to someone who has been told he or she is dying. Future plans are threatened as the final stages of illness near. The inability to provide for others and then for one's self leads to total dependence.

In the patient's evaluation of his state of well-being, thoughts turn to what factors are important to the patient based on personal criteria. Often, it is not death itself that is most threatening, but the process of dying. Every individual has a tolerance for physical pain, emotional pain, dependency, physical mutilation, loneliness, and isolation, beyond which death is preferable to living.

Anyone forced to cope with serious illness or injury must make some basic adaptations. Moos and Tsu[28] have established seven such adaptations:

1. To deal with discomfort, incapacity, and other symptoms of the illness or injury
2. To manage stresses of special treatment procedures and the institutional setting
3. To develop and maintain adequate relationships with caregivers
4. To preserve a reasonable emotional balance for managing upsetting feelings aroused by the illness (anxiety, anger, alienation, guilt, and inadequacy)
5. To preserve a satisfying self-image and to maintain a sense of competency and mastery
6. To preserve relationships with family and friends (communication must be kept open)
7. To prepare for an uncertain future which holds the threat of significant losses

In addition, there are a number of tasks that are unique to the terminally ill:

1. Making arrangements or concluding a variety of affairs
2. Coping with the imminent loss of loved ones and self
3. Anticipating future medical care needs
4. Planning the future
5. Anticipating future pain and discomfort and facing possible loss of sensory, motor, and cognitive abilities
6. Coping effectively with loss of self and identifying with the death encounter
7. Making the decision to slow down or speed up the dying process
8. Dealing with numerous psychologic problems, such as guilt, depression, anger, and abandonment

The dying have certain rights and needs that, if respected, can make the final years, months, and days serene or manageable (see boxes on p. 428). Often those who are around the terminal patient think only of themselves and how they will cope with the situation of the dying patient. They forget or are unaware that it is the dying person who must deal with the indignities imposed by others on his or her own personal rights and needs.

DYING PERSON'S BILL OF RIGHTS

I have the right to be treated as a living human being until I die.

I have the right to maintain a sense of hopefulness, however changing its focus may be.

I have the right to be cared for by those who can maintain a sense of hopefulness, however changing this might be.

I have the right to express my emotions and feelings about my approaching death, in my own way.

I have the right to participate in decisions concerning my care.

I have the right to expect continuing medical and nursing attention even though "cure" goals must be changed to "comfort" goals.

I have the right not to die alone.

I have the right to be free of pain.

I have the right to have my questions answered honestly.

I have the right not to be deceived.

I have the right to have help from and for my family in accepting my death.

I have the right to die in peace and dignity.

I have the right to retain my individuality and not be judged for my decisions that may be contrary to the beliefs of others.

I have the right to discuss and enlarge my religious or spiritual experiences, regardless of what they may mean to others.

I have the right to expect that the sanctity of the human body will be respected after death.

I have the right to be cared for by caring, sensitive, knowledgeable people who will attempt to understand my needs and will be able to gain some satisfaction in helping me face my death.

NEEDS OF THE TERMINAL INDIVIDUAL

To feel oneself, a normal person, a part of normal life right to the end

To talk

To be listened to with understanding

To trust those in whose care he or she is

To feel that he or she is being told the truth

To preserve personal identity

To maintain self-respect in the face of increasing weakness

To share and come to terms with the unavoidable future

To be given the opportunity to voice hidden fears

To be loved and to share love

To be secure

To maintain independence

To be free of pain

To conserve energy

To obtain relief from physical symptoms

As the patient enters the final phase of life, two important problems must be faced if death is to occur with dignity and serenity: (1) the patient needs permission to die from the important person or persons who will be left behind, and (2) the dying person must voluntarily let go of all possessions and persons held dear. These two requirements do not come easily. The terminally ill person must deal with feelings of jealousy and resentment toward those who will continue to live on; self-pity must be reduced or eliminated, and the veil of denial must be lifted. Such major tasks cannot be done alone; they require the assistance of endearing and close friends. The permissions sought by the dying are not usually spoken or written, but are seen and felt when family members, friends, and medical personnel have the ability to cope with the dying patient as a person.

Gray[18] and McCracken and Gerdsen[4] describe the physical signs and symptoms that occur during the final days of life and the emotional/spiritual symptoms of approaching death (Tables 20-2 and 20-3). Too often, nurses, families, and patients are unaware and unprepared for these physical responses. Families and friends need to be told about physical changes, such as a detached look in the eyes, cool extremities, dusky color, audible lung congestion, and a change in respirations known as Cheyne-Stokes respiration. The nurse should also be aware that pupils become barely reactive, and that blood pressure may be only audible by a Doppler device. Family and friends should be allowed to participate in the care.

Dying Process and the Family

When a family member becomes seriously or terminally ill and cannot uphold his role and obligations,

TABLE 20-2   Physical Signs and Symptoms Associated with the Final Stages of Dying—Rationale and Interventions

Symptoms	Rationale	Interventions
Coolness, color and temperature change in hands, arms, feet, and legs	Peripheral circulation diminishes to facilitate increased circulation to vital organs	Place socks on feet. Cover with light cotton blanket.
Increased sleeping	Conservation of energy	Spend time with the patient; hold patient's hand; speak normally to the patient even though there may be a lack of verbal response or consciousness.
Disorientation, confusion of time, place, or person	Metabolic changes	Identify self by name before speaking to patient; speak softly, clearly, and truthfully.
Incontinence of urine and feces	Increased muscle relaxation and decreased consciousness	Maintain vigilance and change bedding as appropriate.
Congestion	Poor circulation of body fluids, immobilization, and inability to expectorate secretions causing gurgling, rattles, bubbling	Elevate the head and gently turn the head to the side to drain secretions.
Restlessness	Metabolic changes and a decrease in oxygen to the brain	Calm the patient by speech and action. Reduce light; gently rub back, stroke arms, or read aloud, play soothing music. DO NOT USE RESTRAINTS.
Decreased intake of food and liquids	Body conservation of energy for function	Do not force patient to eat or drink. Give ice chips, soft drinks, juice, and popsicles as appropriate. Apply petroleum jelly to dry lips. If patient is a mouth-breather, apply protective jelly more frequently as needed.
Decreased urine output	Decreased fluid intake and decreased circulation to kidney	None
Altered breathing pattern	Metabolic and oxygen changes to respiratory centers	Elevate the head of bed; hold hand, speak gently.

the homeostatic balance in the family shifts and disequilibrium occurs. The emotional energy of the family becomes focused on regaining equilibrium in the face of change. Krant[24] notes that problems begin to occur in the family at the time of diagnosis. Influencing this is the role of the dying individual in the family and the personal meaning of that individual to the other family members. For example, a dying father may be the breadwinner, the car driver, or the toy repairer; but he also may be the object of love for its own sake—loved for his personal traits or loved and hated simultaneously.

Coping with the realization of a loved one dying and the eventual loss of that person by death also means that it is the death of the family unit as it existed. It is a constant struggle for the family to remain involved with the dying person as they try to withdraw and try to adjust their lives without the dying member. This requires enormous energy from the family members, who are already overburdened with their own anticipatory grief. The conflict is not only grieving for the dying one but for a part of themselves that will be lost with the death of this family member. Anticipatory grief and dealing with imminent change by a family require a number of adaptive tasks to facilitate healthy resolution of the dying.

Family members need to remain involved with the patient. This means sharing and responding to the patient's experience. At times family members have to separate their own identities from that of the patient's and learn to tolerate the reality that this

TABLE 20-3   Emotional/Spiritual Symptoms of Approaching Death—Rationale and Interventions

Symptoms	Rationale	Intervention
Withdrawal	Prepares the patient for release and detachment and letting go of relationships and surroundings	Continue communicating in a normal manner using a normal voice tone. Identify self by name; hold hand, say what you want person to hear from you.
Vision-like experiences (dead friends or family, religious vision)	Preparation for transition	Do not contradict or argue regarding whether this is or is not a real experience. If the patient is frightened, reassure that he or she is not crazy, but that these aberrations do occur.
Restlessness	Tension, fear, unfinished business	Listen to patient express fears, sadness, and anger associated with dying. Give permission to go.
Decreased socialization	As energy diminishes, the patient withdraws and begins to make the transition	Express support; give permission to die.
Unusual communication: out of character statements, gestures, requests	Signals readiness to let go	Say what needs to be said to the dying patient; kiss, hug, or cry with him or her.

Modified from McCracken AL, Gerdsen L: Sharing the legacy: hospice care principles for terminally ill elders, *J Gerontol Nurs* 17 (12), 1991.

family member will die while they live on. The ability of family members to truly support, love, and provide intimacy may lead to exhaustion, impatience, anger, and a sense of futility as the patient's illness drags on and on. Often the family may be at a different grieving stage than the patient. This can hinder communication between patient and family members. As the illness worsens, physical disability increases, and the patient complains more often, intensifying feelings of helplessness and frustration in the family members. Adapting to role changes requires accommodation to the new demands within the family, such as new responsibilities and permanent changes. Bearing the effects of grief requires acknowledgment of the current feelings that surface in anticipatory grief. Coming to terms with the reality of the impending loss means that family members must go through many emotional responses in achieving acceptance of the loved one's approaching death. Family members must begin to plan for their own future without their loved one. Saying good-bye acknowledges leave-taking and may be expressed in verbal, nonverbal, concrete, or symbolic ways. By working through these tasks, the family members are moving toward the completion of unfinished business with the dying patient—business that, if left ignored, will compound the transition through the grieving process.

The family members are extremely pressured during the last days of the patient's life. They are caught between experiencing and remembering the patient as he or she is and was; between pushing for more or letting nature take its course, and at times not wanting to be involved because of distasteful experiences with the patient. These decisions will profoundly affect them for the rest of their lives. Many times, families feel guilt-ridden because they are thinking more about their own needs instead of those of the dying patient. Despite the family's grief and pain, the family must give the patient permission to die, let the patient know that it is all right to let go and leave. It is the last act of love and dignity the family can offer the dying patient. There are times when there is no family to say "it's okay to let go." This task falls to the nurse who has developed a meaningful relationship with the patient throughout care.

Dying Process and the Health Professional

Whenever we lose something or someone in whom we have invested, we have a need to grieve. Similarly, nurses in their daily work environment are confronted with dying patients. By the very nature of the population whom nurses serve, they are forced to confront loss, not only of patients and families, but personal loss as well. Caring for dying patients over time, or watching patients go home and repeatedly return, involves a degree of emotional investment and a feeling of grief that requires resolution.

A social factor that has long affected the nurse's ability to grieve is the assumption that the role of the caregiver is to be emotionally strong. The nurse is told that feelings of ambivalence or guilt toward the patient are inappropriate. The nurse attempts to remain controlled and detached, thwarting the acknowledgment or resolution of feelings. The nurse, too, can experience conflict between wanting to cure the dying patient and yet wanting that patient to be relieved of suffering, if it is a lingering death.

Harper[19] identified a process of adaptation through which health professionals must pass to cope with the stress of caring for the dying. The initial stage, intellectualization, focuses on professional knowledge and facts that at times emphasize philosophic issues. During this period, conversation with the dying is distant, and a flurry of activity ensues as the caregivers busy themselves with physical tasks and reading about the patient's illness in an attempt to allay their own anxieties.

The professional then experiences a sudden jolt that forces him or her out of the intellectual haven into a confrontation with the reality of the patient's impending death and a realization of personal mortality. Grieving is triggered for oneself and at the same time by genuine pity for the patient. The caregiver feels guilty and frustrated for comparing personal health with that of the dying patient. Hostile feelings are not uncommon for caregivers to experience when they attempt to fight their feelings. Harper calls this emotional survival. Depression, pain, mourning, and grief are crucial periods for the health professional. There are times when the caregiver must acknowledge the fact that death does exist and that personal frustration will not make the patient live. The health professional is said to have arrived at self-mastery when he or she is free from identifying with the patient's symptoms and is no longer occupied with personal mortality and feelings of guilt over being healthier than the patient. Self-mastery allows greater sensitivity to the patient without the incapacitating effects to the caregiver. Harper describes this phase as emotional arrival: moderation, mitigation, and accommodation. Finally, the health professional comes to the point of deep compassion: self-realization, self-awareness, and self-actualization. This is a culmination of previous growth and development that enables the caregiver to relate compassionately to the patient and fully accept the impending death. The enhanced dignity and self-respect that the caregiver now feels allows him or her to give respect and dignity to the dying patient. The health professional has learned through this growth process that living can be more painful than dying. Now concern for the dying can be translated into constructive and appropriate care activities for both the patient and the family.

It is important for the caregiver to have outside interests and a support network beyond the work setting to maintain a balanced perspective in life. Without this equilibrium, it will be difficult to grow and accept the death of others and oneself.

Assessment

Dying patient

Few, if any, tools are available to assess dying patients. Caregivers, for the most part, must depend on their understanding of the dying process and the behaviors identified by the various dying theorists. A danger exists among health professionals of superimposing what they think the patient should feel and do in the dying process. This stereotyping, according to phases or stages of dying, should be guarded against. The purpose of knowing about the dying theories is to recognize what emotions and behavior can occur and to plan interventions accordingly as they appear. Rando[7] presents an extensive list of items to assess for the dying patient and the illness (see box on p. 432).

Dying patient's family

The feelings of the family are often neglected when a member of the family is dying. Attention paid to the family revolves around their presence as an obstacle or nuisance to the caregiving staff. More often than not, animosity toward the family develops or prejudgments are made about their behavior during this stressful time.

The ability to do a detailed family assessment depends on the willingness, availability, and degree of stress of the family as well as the time constraints of the nurse who may be caring for a group of patients. Using whatever time is available, the nurse can make an attempt to acquire information early in the dying patient's illness to help the family cope with the dying process as it progresses. Rando[7] outlines data that are important to obtain if effective intervention is to be developed.

Values, norms, beliefs, and priorities of the family must be recognized and accepted. Rarely do major changes in behavior and communication patterns change just because a family member is dying. However, if a health professional plans realistic interventions and outcomes consistent with the existing fam-

ASSESSMENT OF THE DYING PATIENT AND FAMILY

Patient

Age
Gender
Coping styles and abilities
Social, cultural, ethnic background
Previous experience with illness, pain, deterioration, loss, and grief
Mental health
Intelligence
Life-style
Fulfillment of goals
Amount of unfinished business
The nature of the illness (death trajectory, problems particular to this illness, treatment, amount of pain)
Time passed since diagnosis
Response to illness
Knowledge about the illness/disease
Acceptance/rejection of the sick role
Amount of striving for dependence/independence
Feelings of fear about illness
Comfort in expressing thoughts and feelings and amount of expression.
Location of the patient (home, hospital, nursing home)
Relationship with each family member and significant other since diagnosis
Family rules, norms, values, and past experience that might inhibit grief or interfere with a therapeutic relationship

Family

Family makeup (members of family)
Developmental stage of the family
Existing subsystems
Specific roles of each member

Characteristics of Family System

How flexible or rigid
Type of communication style
Rules, norms, and expectations
Values, beliefs
Quality of emotional relationships
Dependence, interdependence, freedom of each member
How close to or disengaged from the dying member
Established extrafamilial interactions
Strengths and vulnerabilities of the family
Style of leadership and decision making
Usual methods of problem solving, crisis resolution
Disciplinary patterns
Family resources (personal, financial, community)
Current problems identified by family
Quality of communication with caregivers
Immediate and long-range anticipated needs

---

ily system, he or she may be able to foster positive growth.

Nursing Diagnosis

The following nursing diagnoses may apply to the dying patient:

Altered body image
Fear
Grieving: Actual or high risk
          Anticipatory
          Dysfunctional
Hopelessness
Impaired adjustment
Impaired denial
Powerlessness
Social isolation
Spiritual distress

Interventions

Care of the dying patient has many facets, and ranges from the simple act of hand-holding to the complexities of dealing with a plethora of emotions. The core of interventions in the care of the dying focus on communication, relief of symptoms and pain, knowledge of available resources, facilitation of problem solving, and fostering involvement in and control of decisions affecting the patient's care.

Communication includes the verbal and nonverbal exchange between the nurse and the patient. Talking with the dying is full of emotional landmines, but it is a vehicle for establishing a trust relationship that can help relieve anxiety. Talking is a way to instruct, explain, divert attention, and amuse a patient. Nonverbal responses are expressed in facial expressions, touch, and behavior. "Touch hunger," or the lack of human contact through tactile stimulation such as holding hands or receiving and giving hugs, is often experienced by the dying. Procedural touch used in bathing and treatments does not fulfill the touch need.

Knowledge of community resources will help the nurse give direction to the patient and family and help them cope with the physical, emotional, socioeconomic, and religious problems that might occur.

A list of resources appears at the end of this chapter.

Loss of health, independence, social contacts, finances, and energy threaten control over oneself and the environment. Nurses can meet a patient's needs by providing choices in care, so that the patient may remain an active participant. Environmental stimulation through social contacts and diversional activity often relieves the sense of isolation and abandonment. It is not feasible for all patients to choose to be cared for at home, but they should be supported if they choose it. Ancillary services must be provided that will cooperate with the patient and family. The patient and family should be aware that if they get into difficulty, they should not consider it defeat to return to the hospital for care.

Hospice

Hospice is a word that has come down from the Middle Ages, when it was used to describe a way station where travelers, pilgrims, and ill people could

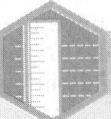

STANDARDS OF HOSPICE NURSING

Standard I. Organization of hospice services

The hospice program identifies and meets the needs of terminally ill patients and their families. The program is centrally administered by an executive officer who may be a nurse.

Standard II. Interdisciplinary collaboration

The nurse collaborates with other members of the hospice interdisciplinary team, including the patient, family, physician, other nurses, social worker, volunteer, and clergy. The team is coordinated by a qualified health care professional from the discipline most appropriate in each case. The team meets regularly to develop and maintain a suitable plan of care for the patient and family.

Standard III. Data collection

The nurse systematically collects data that are comprehensive and accurate.

Standard IV. Nursing diagnosis

The nurse uses assessment data to determine nursing diagnosis.

Standard V. Planning

The nurse participates in the development of the interdisciplinary team's plan of care for each client and family. The nurse's input toward the plan is based on nursing diagnosis. It is congruent with the hospice philosophy, hospice policies, and interdisciplinary concepts. The nurse's input also reflects an appreciation of the importance of the patient's and family's help in developing the plan.

Standard VI. Intervention

The nurse, guided by the interdisciplinary care plan, provides care aimed at maximizing the quality of the patient's life. Pain and symptom control measures are taken, and the nurse acts to facilitate the patient's and family's progress toward the goals they set.*

Standard VII. Evaluation

The nurse continually evaluates the patient's and family's responses to the interdisciplinary team's interventions.

Standard VIII. Continuity of care

The nurse, as a member of the interdisciplinary team, ensures continuity of care for the terminally ill patient and their family.

Standard IX. Research

The nurse participates in research activities that contribute to the profession's continuing development of knowledge about hospice nursing care.

Standard X. Theory

The nurse applies theoretic concepts as a basis for decisions in practice.

Standard XI. Ethics

The nurse uses the American Nurses' Association's Code for Nurses and other appropriate resources as a guide for ethical decision making, such as deciding whether to forego life-sustaining treatment.

Standard XII. Professional development

The nurse participates in peer review and other means of evaluation to ensure the quality of nursing practice. The nurse assumes responsibility for professional development and contributes to the professional growth of the interdisciplinary team members.

*Pain and symptom control measures are taken, and the nurse acts to facilitate the patient's and family's progress toward the goals they set.
With permission of the American Nurses' Association, Kansas City, MO

stop and depend on receiving humane care. It comes from the same root word as hospital and hospitality.

The term *hospice* has come to mean a philosophy of care for the terminally ill. Hospice programs in the United States provide terminally ill patients and their families the choice of humane care in the home rather than institutional care. Each hospice program is unique to the special needs of its own community, but all hospices have the following common features: a focus on supportive care, not cure; an emphasis on controlling pain and other symptoms of terminal diseases; nursing services available 24 hours a day, 7 days a week; a focus on the entire family, rather than just the patient, as the recipient of care; an approach to care that includes trained volunteers and a multidisciplinary team; and follow-up bereavement services for the family after the patient's death.

Hope of remission or cure is never abandoned, but the focus of care is on creating an environment that encourages honesty, compassion, and mutual support. The intimacy of everyone working together establishes an environment where it is safe for patients, family, and hospice personnel to share sad and wonderful moments with one another.

The purposes and goals of hospice are reflected in the following functions of the hospice team of health professionals and volunteers. One function is to reorient the patient and family to the reality that the home is the primary place of care with family members, most often, the caregivers. This is necessary because people generally wish to die at home, but families desire the person to die in the hospital because they fear actually seeing death occur or are afraid they cannot handle the care. A second function is to restore the patient's uniqueness and his place in life. An attempt is made to restore the dying person to the primary decision-maker role regarding his care. Final choices and decisions should be made by the patient and the family. Redefining of relationships is a third function of hospice care. This facilitates the identification of care that will be needed and who will provide that care. It is not always possible for family members or spouses to give care. Thus each individual who is in contact with the dying patient will have a unique role to play. Important too, for the patient and the family, is the knowledge that the hospice team—of health professionals or volunteers—will be available for the patient and family at any time, and that the family will not be alone, even after the death. Reestablishment of control involves one of the prime goals of hospice care, that of relief of pain and other symptoms. The premise is not to wait until complaints arise, but to anticipate and relieve symptoms before they emerge. Last, reeducation of the patient and family is important to enable the dying individual to live as meaningful a life as possible in the remaining time. Hospice personnel find out what the individual and family already know about the illness, care techniques, and support measures, and then augment or teach what is needed.

The American Nurses' Association, in its publication *Standards and Scope of Hospice Nursing Practice,* established criteria for nursing practice (see the box on p. 433). The standards reflect the great strides hospice care has made in the past decade. They have expanded the thinking of the medical and nursing communities, pioneered understanding and methods of pain control, and restored choice to millions of individuals who otherwise would have died in the hospital because there was no choice. Hospice has shown that the dying can live to their fullest until the end.

CRITICAL THINKING QUESTIONS

1 Describe the concept of loss: when does it occur and why? Give examples of the types of loss.

2 Compare acute grief with anticipatory grief.

3 What interventions can you take to help an individual through his grief?

4 Explain the similarities and differences of the grief theories presented in this chapter. Do you think that any one of them is more effective than the others? If so why; if not why?

5 Kübler-Ross and Pattison write about the processes that occur in a person who is aware he or she is dying.
   a. Would you recommend withholding the terminal diagnosis from a dying person? If so, under what circumstances?
   b. If you had a terminal illness, would you want to be told?
   c. If your mother or father had a terminal illness, would you want her (him) to be told?

6 Using Glaser and Strauss, discuss your reasons for your answers above. Consider both the advantages and disadvantages of withholding information from the viewpoint of the patient, the hospital staff, and the family.

7 The patient you are caring for is dying.
   d. What needs would you anticipate the dying patient might have?
   e. What information do you need to help the patient through the dying process?
   f. What kind of assessment information is needed to help the family through its grieving process?
   g. What nursing interventions can be performed to provide comfort from the phys-

ical and emotional signs and symptoms that occur in the terminal days and hours of life?

8 What is hospice and what are its goals?

RESOURCES

Counseling

1 Ackerman Institute for Family Therapy 149 E. 78th Street New York, NY 10021

2 To Life P.O. Box 9354 Charlotte, NC 28299

Hospice

3 National Hospice Organization Suite 402 1901 N. Fort Myer Drive Arlington, VA 22209

The widowed

4 National Association for Widowed People P.O. Box 3564 Springfield, IL 62708

5 Parents without Partners 7910 Woodmont Avenue Washington, DC 20014

6 Society of Military Widows P.O. Box 1714 La Mesa, CA 92041

7 Widowed Persons Service (WPS) NRTA-AARP 1909 K Street Washington, DC 20049

Euthanasia

8 American Euthanasia Foundation 95 N. Birch Road, Suite 301 Ft. Lauderdale, FL 33304

9 Concern for Dying 250 W. 57th Street New York, NY 10107

Education

10 Center for Death Education and Research 1167 Social Science Building University of Minnesota 267 19th Avenue, South Minneapolis, MN 55455

11 Association for Death Education and Counseling 638 Prospect Avenue Hartford, CT 06105

BIBLIOGRAPHY

Current

1. American Nurses' Association: *Standards and scope of hospice nursing practice*, Kansas City, Mo, 1987, The Association.
2. Bledsoe AS: Dying patients: caring makes the difference, *Nursing '87* 17(6):44, June 1987.
3. Despelder LA, Strickland AL: *The last dance*, ed 2, Palo Alto, 1990, Mayfield Publishing Co.
4. McCracken AL, Gerdsen L: Sharing the legacy: hospice care principles for terminally ill elders, *J Gerontol Nurs* 17(12), 1991.
5. Nursing grand rounds, *Nursing '88* 18(6):53, June 1988.
6. O'Conner N: *Letting go with love: the grieving process*, Apache Junction, Ariz, 1984, La Mariposa.
7. Rando TA: *Grief, dying and death*. Champaign, Ill, 1984, Research Press.
8. Retsinas J: A theoretical reassessment of the applicability of Kübler-Ross's stages of dying, *Death Studies* 12:207-216, 1988.
9. Rousseau PC: How fluid deprivation affects the terminally ill, *RN*, 1991.
10. Ufema JK: How to talk to dying patients, *Nursing '87* 17(8):43, August 1987.

Classic

11. Bowlby J: Process of mourning, *Int J Psychoanal* 42:317, 1961.
12. Duda D: *A guide to dying at home*, Sante Fe, NM, 1982, John Muir Publishing.
13. Engel G: Grief and grieving, *Am J Nurs* 64:93, 1964.
14. Futterman EH, Hoffman I, Sabshin M: Parental anticipatory mourning. In Schoenberg B, et al, editors: *Psychosocial aspects of terminal care*, New York, 1972, Columbia University Press.
15. Glaser B, Strauss A: *Awareness of dying*, Chicago, 1965, Aldine.
16. Glaser B, Strauss A: *Time for dying*, Chicago, 1968, Aldine.
17. Gorer G: *Death, grief, mourning*, London, 1965, Cresset Press.
18. Gray VR: Some physical needs. *In dealing with death and dying, nursing 76 books*, Jenkintown, Penn, 1976, Intermed Communications.
19. Harper BC: *Death: the coping mechanisms of the health professional*, Greenville, SC, 1977, Southeastern University Press.
20. Jackson E: *Understanding grief*, Nashville, Tenn, 1957, Abingdon.
21. Janis IL: *Psychological stress*, New York, 1958, John Wiley and Sons.
22. Kavanaugh RE: *Facing death*, Los Angeles, Calif, 1972, Nash Publishing.
23. Keleman S: Stages of dying, *Voices* 10:46, 1974.
24. Krant MJ: *Dying and dignity*, Springfield, Ill, 1974, Charles C Thomas Publishers.
25. Kübler-Ross E: *On death and dying*, New York, 1969, Macmillan.
26. Lewis CS: *A grief observed*, London, 1961, Faber.
27. Lindemann E: Symptomatology and management of acute grief, *Am J Psychiatry* 101: 141, 1944.
28. Moos RH, Tsu VD: Crisis of physical illness: an overview. In Moos RH, ed: *Coping with physical illness*, New York, 1977, Plenum.
29. Parks CM: *Bereavement*, New York, 1972, International Universities Press.
30. Parks CM: *Bereavement: study of grief in adult life*, Middlesex, England, 1975, Penguin Books.
31. Parks CM, Weiss RS: *Recovery from bereavement*, New York, 1983, Basic Books.
32. Pattison EM: The living-dying process. In Garfield CA ed, *Psychosocial care of the dying patient*, New York, McGraw-Hill, 1978.
33. Raphael B: *The anatomy of bereavement*, New York, 1983, Basic Books.
34. Stoddard S: *The hospice movement: a better way of caring for the dying*. Briarcliff Manor, NY, 1978, Stein and Day.
35. Wooden JW: *Grief counseling and grief therapy*, New York, 1982, Springer Publishing.

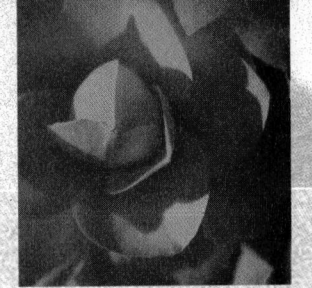

CHAPTER TWENTY-ONE

Substance Use Disorders

LEARNING OBJECTIVES:

1 Discuss the major etiologic factors in the development of substance abuse.
2 Discuss the impact of chemical dependency on the family system and the development of codependency.
3 Identify the key symptoms and interventions in the management of patients experiencing abstinence/withdrawal syndrome or overdose.
4 Apply the nursing process to the acute management of the substance abuse patient.
5 Recognize the physical and psychologic signs and symptoms that may indicate the presence of a substance abuse problem.
6 Discuss the role of the nurse in treating substance abuse patients and their families.
7 Identify community resources available to chemically dependent patients and their families.

KEY TERMS

alcoholism, p. 440
caffeinism, p. 446
codependency, p. 439
cross tolerance, p. 438
delerium tremens (DTs), p. 440
detoxification, p. 450

Johnsonian intervention, p. 451
substance abuse, p. 437
substance dependency, p. 438
tolerance, p. 438
withdrawal, p. 438

SUBSTANCE ABUSE is a major health care problem in the United States today. The National Institute on Alcohol Abuse and Alcoholism (1990) reports that more than 15 million adults have an alcohol abuse problem.[7] At the same time, 14.5 million Americans use illicit drugs on a regular basis.[8] These numbers translate roughly into 18% to 20% of the population; i.e., one of every five Americans will have a serious problem with substance abuse.

Substance abuse occurs in all ages, genders, races, and classes. The ability to assess a substance abuse problem in any patient is paramount to providing appropriate and comprehensive nursing care.

OVERVIEW

Substance abuse disorders fall into two general categories: substance abuse and substance dependency. **Substance abuse** is pathologic use of a chemical substance accompanied by loss of control over when and how much of the substance is used. As a result, social, physical, and occupational functioning are impaired.

Substance dependency or chemical dependency is a more severe form of substance abuse. The chemically dependent person displays a psychologic or physiologic reliance demonstrated by tolerance for the substance and symptoms of withdrawal if it is discontinued. **Tolerance** is a physiologic adaptation to the effect of the chemical substance. Over time, an increased dose or more frequent dose interval is necessary to maintain the intensity of effects. A related phenomenon is that of **cross-tolerance,** in which an increased adaptation to one substance, after prolonged use, leads to tolerance of other substances in the same category. For example, an alcohol-dependent individual will develop a tolerance for other central nervous system (CNS) depressants such as benzodiazepines and surgical anesthetics. Similarly, the narcotic dependent patient will demonstrate a tolerance for "normal" pain medication dosages and need more frequent or higher doses of medication for pain management. **Withdrawal** occurs when there is an abrupt decrease or discontinuation of alcohol or drugs in an individual who is chemically dependent. Substance-specific behavioral and physiologic symptoms develop in response to changes in the CNS as the substance is eliminated from the body. Complete abstinence is not essential for the emergence of withdrawal symptoms.

Early substance dependence is characterized by a psychologic reliance on the chemical for the sense of well-being and pleasure it produces. During later stages, the chemically dependent individual compulsively uses the substance, in spite of adverse consequences, in order to "feel normal" and to avoid the discomfort of withdrawal.

ETIOLOGY

Various theories have been put forth to explain why some people are more prone to abusing substances. These theories focus on biologic, psychologic, behavioral, sociocultural, and family factors.

The biologic model proposes that the cause of chemical dependency is physiologic. Physiologic causes include a genetic propensity, metabolic defect (such as abnormal enzyme levels), or neurobiologic abnormalities.[18,19]

Some psychologic theorists view substance abuse as a response to external or internal stress that cannot be managed in other ways. The substance abuser self-medicates repeatedly in order to escape feelings of inadequacy, depression, or anxiety.

The behavioral model proposes that patterns of behavior are learned and continue because they have been rewarded or reinforced. The use of chem-

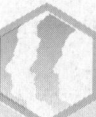

GERIATRIC CONSIDERATIONS

Substance Abuse

1. 70% of all hospitalized older persons and up to 50% of nursing home residents have alcohol-related problems.
2. Most elderly people take prescription drugs including sedatives, which, when combined with alcohol, can be dangerous.
3. Often drinking is at home and hidden. Signs of abuse include more depression or hostility, neglect in personal appearance, unexplained burns or bruises, and often intoxication or slight tipsiness.
4. Symptoms may not be noticed or attributed to other diseases or part of the aging process.
5. Guidelines in talking to the elderly patient:
   a. Avoid confrontation. Be supportive.
   b. Treat the elderly patient as an adult.
   c. Consistently and patiently show respect and caring.
   d. Focus on the effects alcohol and drugs have in combination and effects on personal life.
   e. Try to involve the patient in relationships or activities he or she cares about.
   f. Listen and be supportive.
   g. Since aging slows down processing of information, give information slowly.
6. The response to treatment is highest for this age group, but, because of the toxic effects of alcohol, the recovery process may be slower.

icals to manage stress and deal with problems is modeled by the parents and often reinforced within the peer group.

Sociologic and cultural factors must also be considered. People learn to drink and take drugs within the context of a group, such as the family, community, and society. Their attitudes, beliefs, values, and behaviors are shaped by these groups. For example, subpopulations within American society, such as the Irish, Native Americans, and African Americans, demonstrate a predisposition toward the development of substance abuse problems while others, such as Jewish or Asian cultures, are less likely to do so. Chemical dependency can also be a problem among the elderly and the homeless (see boxes above and on p. 439).

The family systems model views substance abuse as a family, rather than an individual, problem. Members define roles, communication patterns, and interaction processes to achieve an equilibrium that may or may not be healthy. Substance abuse can develop as a maladaptive response to family emotional

SUBSTANCE ABUSE AND THE HOMELESS

For many people, a chronic problem with chemical dependency may eventually lead to homelessness. Preoccupation with drugs and/or alcohol may result in job instability and unemployment, the development of psychiatric problems, and family/support system disintegration. The chemically dependent individual can find himself or herself without resources and "on the streets." In fact, 60% of the homeless have lifetime problems with alcohol and drug use. Homeless substance abusers also experience greater health problems.[2,5,9] The homeless are more likely to experience delerium tremens and to suffer poor physical health from their substance abuse, poor living conditions, and limited access to health care than the general alcoholic population. Traumatic injury as a result of substance abuse and victimization on the streets often serve as reasons for entry to the health care scene. Multiple health problems and placement difficulties make the homeless substance abuser a particularly challenging patient.

---

processes. As the substance abuse progresses, family members become entrenched in rigid and predictable roles to maintain this maladaptive pattern of interaction. Wegscheider-Cruse[30] labeled these family roles as the enabler, scapegoat, mascot, hero, and lonely child.

The "enabler" allows the substance abuser to continue using without experiencing the consequences of substance abuse. For example, the "enabler" may assume all parenting, financial, and household responsibilities; bail the substance abuser out of legal or work difficulties; tolerate the physical or emotional abuse that often accompanies substance abuse; or assume blame for the substance abuser's drinking or use of drugs.[15] The "scapegoat" is the child who seems to draw attention to his or her maladaptive behavior, such as truancy, which serves to defocus from the parental dysfunction. The "mascot" often attempts to divert the family's emotional pain by behaving playfully. The "hero" is the child who gets perfect grades and wins awards to bring a sense of accomplishment to this dysfunctional family. The "lonely" child isolates from the family, assuming that his or her needs will never be met. These roles are as dysfunctional as the substance abuse and are aimed at avoiding rather than confronting the problem of chemical dependency in the family.

Chemical dependency affects all family members.

ETHICAL ISSUES

- What should the nurse's role be in relation to a patient's unhealthy life-style?
- Should access to certain types of health care be denied to patients whose health-abusing habits contributed to their poor health? For example, should liver transplants be denied to a recovering alcoholic? May conditions be placed on a patient's access to such care? For example, if the patient promises to stop smoking, and stays "smoke-free" for 6 months, should the patient then be considered for a heart transplant?

Codependency, the phenomenon that results from living in a dysfunctional family, has predictable stages and begins with denial and rationalization of the problem. The struggle of protecting, controlling, and fighting the addicted person becomes so consuming that the codependent eventually loses interest in self and the outside world. Treatment of the substance abuser must also involve the patient's family.

There is no single cause of substance abuse and no universally accepted model of its development. Just as human beings are multifaceted, so are the substance abuse disorders. More research is needed to further understand the illness and its impact on family members.

COMMONLY ABUSED SUBSTANCES
Central Nervous System Depressants

Alcohol

Alcohol is one of the most widely used and socially accepted drugs in modern society. After ingestion, alcohol is rapidly absorbed from the stomach, small intestine, and colon into the bloodstream. The rapidity of absorption is affected by the alcohol content of the beverage and the presence or absence of food in the stomach. Alcohol is metabolized with the assistance of an enzyme in the liver known as acetaldehyde dehydrogenase (ADH). In the metabolic process, ADH converts alcohol into acetylaldehyde and eventually acetate. The rapidity of metabolism depends on the weight and tolerance of the drinker. When consumption of alcohol exceeds its metabolism, alcohol accumulates and the individual becomes intoxicated.[15]

Alcoholism is the most serious effect of chronic excessive alcohol ingestion. The currently accepted

RESEARCH BRIEF

Abstinence in chemically dependent people, Stefanik-Campasi C: *Ad Nurse* 3(5):16, Sept 1988.

Although chemical dependency is a major health care problem in the United States, it is not understood why some patients recover while others do not. To identify perceived factors that influenced chemically dependent outpatients to maintain abstinence, Stefanik-Campasi conducted a descriptive exploratory research study for the purpose of identifying perceived factors that help people maintain abstinence. The methodology consisted of conducting individual interviews with a sample of 35 court-ordered outpatients from a drug and alcohol program. The mean age of the sample was 27.8 years. Although 57% identified alcohol as their drug of choice, 77% reported polyaddictions. Abstinence ranging from 3 months to 2 years was reported by 68.9% of the respondents. Perceived factors influencing abstinence in priority order were legal implications, health concerns, and AA/NA or religion. Those perceived factors that influenced relapse in priority order consisted of contacting old friends, conflicts with family/significant others, and lack of involvement in AA/NA or religion. In this sample, legal factors as the priority influencing factor suggests the importance of external controls versus internal controls in maintaining abstinence.

definition of **alcoholism** is:

A chronic, progressive, and potentially fatal biogenetic and psychosocial disease characterized by tolerance and physical dependence manifested by a loss of control, as well as diverse personality changes and social consequences.[10]

Because of the strong physical dependence that develops as a result of alcoholism, withdrawal from alcohol is potentially life-threatening. The symptoms of alcohol withdrawal are the result of a hyperexcitability of the CNS, a rebound reaction to the chronically alcohol-induced CNS depressed state. The onset of withdrawal symptoms occurs generally 6 to 12 hours after the last drink, as blood alcohol concentration levels begin to decrease. The amount of alcohol regularly consumed and the length of time the individual has been a chronic drinker will determine the severity of alcohol withdrawal. As a result, each alcoholic's withdrawal response is unique.

The most serious and advanced progression of the alcohol withdrawal syndrome is the potentially fatal **delerium tremens (DTs).** The symptoms and treat-ment of DTs are given in the box on p. 441. Alcohol abuse is more physically damaging than the abuse of any other psychoactive drug. The physical damage is cumulative, in that the alcoholic can drink for years before the effects on the body become grossly apparent. This may permit the alcoholic to deny the physical consequences and the addiction until the damage is permanent. Table 21-1 summarizes selected physical illnesses and possible causes related to excessive alcohol intake.

Benzodiazepines

The class of drugs known as benzodiazepines includes alprazolam (Xanax), lorazepam (Ativan), triazolam (Halcion), chlordiazepoxide (Librium), diazepam (Valium), oxazepam (Serax), and clorazepate (Tranxene). These drugs are widely prescribed as antianxiety medications and are sometimes termed minor tranquilizers. Because of their antianxiety action, the benzodiazepines are the second most common substance abused. Woolf[15] lists three reasons why this class of drugs has achieved particular notoriety: (1) the denial of many physicians of the drugs' addiction potential; (2) the delayed withdrawal syndrome with subtle symptoms; and (3) the fact that the drugs are widely prescribed and therefore available for abuse. The antianxiety effects of benzodiazepines are short-lived. Continued use leads to tolerance and the escalation of anxiety symptoms more intense than had been experienced before use. Because of the many adverse effects (e.g., abdominal cramping, irritability, vomiting, tremors, sleep disturbances and convulsions) that can occur during withdrawal, the abuser should be carefully withdrawn under medical supervision. Rather than discontinuing benzodiazepines altogether, the dose is gradually decreased until the drug is withdrawn totally. Because of the CNS depressant effects of benzodiazepines, they are cross-tolerant to alcohol and are often used in the medical management of alcohol withdrawal. Although few deaths occur from benzodiazepine overdose alone, the synergistic effect that occurs with the combination of benzodiazepines and alcohol can lead to overdose. Table 21-2 lists commonly abused substances and a summary of related nursing interventions.

Barbiturates

Barbiturates include amobarbital (Amytal), pentobarbital (Nembutal), secobarbital (Seconal), and butabarbital. Clinically, these drugs have been widely prescribed as sedatives, hypnotics, anesthetics, and anticonvulsants. Symptom presentation of barbiturate intoxication mimics that of alcohol intoxication. Withdrawal from barbiturates is potentially lethal

ALCOHOL WITHDRAWAL SYMPTOMS AND TREATMENT

Withdrawal symptoms

Tremulousness ("the shakes"); onset 3-36 hours after the last drink
Increased psychomotor hyperactivity with tremors
Insomnia
Acute anxiety and hyperalertness
Tachycardia (120-140 beats/min)
Hypertension
Anorexia
Agitation
Possible nausea, abdominal cramps, vomiting
Weakness
Craving for alcohol or sedative drug
Acute hallucinosis
Auditory or visual hallucinations assume prominence; this may indicate that alcohol withdrawal delirium is impending
Alcohol withdrawal delirium (the horrors, delirium tremens, DTs); onset 24-72 hours after last drink; most serious of withdrawal phases (5%-36% mortality)
Disorientation
Hallucinations
Delusions
Delirium
Severe agitation

Treatment of withdrawal
Impending withdrawal

Monitor vital signs every 3 hours; notify physician of any abnormal readings
Provide a quiet, nonstimulating environment, yet keep a light on in room
Administer sedating medications promptly as ordered (do not undersedate); ensure medications are taken
Frequently orient patient to place, person, time; quietly and simply explain all procedures, routines, expected components of treatment process

Accurately record intake and output (including emesis, diarrhea, estimated loss from diaphoresis)
Do not force fluids until it has been established that patient is dehydrated; however, ensure that patient takes estimated minimum of fluids per 24-hour period
Allow ambulation ad lib if ordered and *if patient is stable,* since this channels excess agitation
Allow patient to express fears regarding withdrawal; provide nonjudgmental, caring concern
Institute seizure precautions (oral airway, upright siderails, remove potentially harmful objects)
Assist patient with activities of daily living (bathing, eating, mouthcare) without overstimulating patient (e.g., no shaving, nail care)
Provide small, frequent, high-carbohydrate feedings that are easily digested; administer antiemetic PRN before meals (offer patient flavored fluids, gelatins); administer vitamins as ordered, such as multivitamin, B-complex including thiamine, vitamin C
Test urine for specific gravity and stools for guaiac to detect GI dysfunction
Be there; spend time with patient and family

Alcohol withdrawal delirium

Monitor vital signs qh
Assess neurologic status qh
Stimulate patient to cough and deep breathe q2h
Carefully evaluate bladder and bowel functions
Inspect skin for signs of breakdown or traumatic injury
IVs, tube feedings, catheter if ordered
Restrain patient to prevent injury if needed
Check patient at least every 15 minutes
Administer anticonvulsant medications as ordered

---

and therefore requires hospitalization. The most serious adverse reaction to barbiturate use is overdose, which may result in accidental death. For chronic barbiturate users, tolerance will develop to the sedating effects, prompting the user to steadily increase the amount or dose of barbiturates. Overdose can occur easily because with increasing dosages, tolerance does not develop to the respiratory depression effects of barbiturates. As a result, the user can experience respiratory arrest.

Narcotics/opiates

This category of CNS depressants includes opium, opiate derivatives (i.e., heroin, codeine, morphine,

hydromorphone), and the synthetic opiates (i.e., meperidine, methadone, propoxyphene [Darvon], and pentazocine [Talwin]). Although chemical dependency can occur with any of the narcotics, heroin is the most common drug of abuse of the opiate group. The stages of effects include the euphoric "rush" and the physically and mentally relaxing "nod." These effects last between 3 and 6 hours.

Withdrawal from heroin is not life-threatening and may be quite mild based on the purity of street-cut heroin. Withdrawal often resembles flulike symptoms, including diaphoresis, vomiting, diarrhea, and musculoskeletal aches, although the subjective experience of withdrawal will be reported as much more severe.

TABLE 21-1   Disorders Related to Excessive Alcohol Intake

Problem	Suspected cause
Hypoglycemia	Limited food intake, depletion of glycogen stores, inhibition of gluconeogenesis
Lactic acidosis	Excessive production of lactic acid by hepatocytes
Hyperuricemia	Reduced renal clearance of uric acid associated with lactic acid accumulation in the body and the need to eliminate it
Esophagitis	Direct toxic effect, vomiting
Gastritis	Direct toxic effect, increased secretin and histamine production
Duodenal ulceration	Increased secretin and histamine production
Malabsorption	Pancreatic insufficiency, mucosal damage associated with reduced transport activity and disaccharidase production, hyperperistalsis
Fatty liver	Triglyceride accumulation in hepatocytes
Hyperlipidemia	Increased lipoprotein production, increased lipoprotein clearance, mobilization of nonhepatic fat stores
Hyperketonemia	Excessive fat metabolism
Alcoholic hepatitis	Hepatocyte inflammation and necrosis related to alcohol and its metabolism
Cirrhosis	Scarification of liver tissue associated with long-term fatty infiltration or hepatitis
Pancreatitis	Alcohol-induced inflammation of the pancreas leading to increased secretin production
Anemias	Direct toxic effect, malabsorption of nutrients, malnutrition, decreased transferrin synthesis
Beriberi heart disease	Thiamine deficiency
Cardiomyopathy	Direct toxic effect, malnutrition
Skeletal myopathies	Direct toxic effect
Reduced bone density with increased fracture risk	Excessive excretion of calcium in the urine, poor diet, malabsorption of vitamin D, reduced liver hydroxylation of vitamin D
Impaired immune response	Malnutrition, direct toxic effect
Hemorrhagic displays	Impaired production of blood-clotting proteins
Wernicke-Korsakoff syndrome	Thiamine deficiency
Tuberculosis/pneumonia	Reduced resistance to infection, atelectasis
Cancer of the gastrointestinal system (neck, throat, stomach, pancreas)	Indirect toxic effects
Impotency	Neuropathy and CNS depressant
Peripheral neuritis	Malnutrition, especially vitamin deficiencies (B complex)
Malnutrition	Alcohol is high in calories and acts as appetite suppressant

Stimulants

Stimulants comprise a category of substances that produces excitation and stimulation of the CNS. The abuse of stimulants has been increasing rapidly in recent years. This is probably the result of a combination of many factors, including their increased availability, the glamorous image of cocaine and other stimulants portrayed in the media, and the demands of today's fast-paced society. CNS stimulants result in psychologic dependence. In addition, all drugs in the category are thought to produce physical dependence and tolerance with the exception of amphetamines. Although not proven, physical dependence is still considered possible with amphetamines.

Cocaine/crack

Cocaine and its derivative, crack, have become more widely abused during the past decade. Cocaine is a

TABLE 21-2   Nursing Interventions Summary for Commonly Abused Substances

Withdrawal symptoms	Nursing interventions	Overdose
Barbiturates		
Withdrawal is potentially fatal	In caring for the patient withdrawing from barbiturates, the nurse should:	*Signs of overdose*
Onset 48-72 hr after last dose	Monitor vital signs and neurologic reflex responses (fluctuations can precede convulsions)	Inebriation Coma Constricted pupils
Increased temperature	Provide a quiet, nonstimulating environment to decrease agitation	Dilated pupils if hypoxic Hypotension/shock
Postural hypotension		Hypothermia
Tachycardia	Frequently reorient the patient to reality and person, place, and time (to decrease anxiety and increase the patient's self-control)	Cyanosis Renal failure
Insomnia		
Agitation		*Treatment of overdose*
Tremors	Administer medication in a careful and timely manner	Maintain adequate airway
Grand mal seizures	Institute seizure precautions (siderails up, potentially harmful objects removed)	Institute CPR if necessary
Psychosis		Induce vomiting only if the patient is alert and taking adequate measures to prevent aspiration
	Carefully observe the patient's response to the withdrawal regimen (i.e., any unusual sedation, increase in hyperactivity, somnolence)	IV fluids as prescribed
	Convey a concerned, caring attitude, and give the patient an opportunity to talk about fears/feelings regarding withdrawal	
	Provide safe recreational/diversional activity (i.e., card games, checkers)	
Benzodiazepines		
Panic attacks	Slow titration of drug(s)	
Depression	Supportive nursing care such as monitoring vital signs and hydration	
Agitation		
Abdominal cramping		
Vomiting		
Insomnia		
Sweating		
Convulsions		
Narcotics/opiates		
Onset 4 to 10 hr after last "fix"	Detoxification using methadone and/or clonidine hydrochloride (Catapres)	*Treatment of overdose*
Drug craving		Do not waste time looking for constricted pupils or needle marks
Restlessness		Establish an open *airway*
Insomnia		*Breathe* for the person by administering mouth-to-mouth resuscitation if necessary
Yawning		
Runny nose		Check pulses (radial, temporal, carotid, and femoral)
		If no pulse is present, begin cardiopulmonary resuscitation
Perspiring		
Muscle cramping		

Continued.

TABLE 21-2   Nursing Interventions Summary for Commonly Abused Substances—cont'd

Withdrawal symptoms	Nursing interventions	Overdose
Narcotics/opiates—cont'd		
Joint pains Tremors Diarrhea Vomiting Hot and cold flashes Increased temperature, blood pressure, and pulse May last 4 to 10 days		If the person is in an emergency medical treatment setting, a narcotic antagonist will be administered (naloxone hydrochloride 0.4-2 mg, levallorphan tartrate 1 mg) Monitor the person closely until he or she is fully responsive
Stimulants/amphetamines		
"Crash"—depression and exhaustion	Teach patient to anticipate symptoms of lethargy, irritability, or hypersomnia	Frequently monitor vital signs and heart (ECG monitoring) If respiratory depression occurs, maintain an open airway, and administer artificial respirations Cardiotoxicity is often treated by intravenous administration of propranolol 1 mg/min up to a maximum of 8 mg Psychosis may be treated by administering up to three 5 mg doses of haloperidol at 1-hr intervals Other nursing interventions for treating cocaine toxic psychosis include those similar to treating cocaine withdrawal symptoms (i.e., creating a quiet, nonstimulating environment, using a calm, reassuring approach with the patient)

ETHICAL ISSUES

- Should patients have the right to decide between the certainty of pain when medication is inadequate and the possibility of dependence if medication is adequate?
- Is there a moral difference between using a narcotic to erase pain and using it to replace pain with euphoria?
- Is there a moral difference between individuals deciding for themselves that their emotional pain warrants "substance abuse" and professionals deciding for patients that their physical pain warrants the prescription of addictive substances?

relatively short-acting drug; its effects last approximately 20 to 30 minutes. Cocaine is a strong CNS stimulant, and the user experiences euphoria, elation, increased energy, and excitation. In high doses, cocaine can lead to agitation, anxiety, and exhaustion. As a result, cocaine abusers often also abuse alcohol, sedatives, or heroin to manage the discomfort of increasing CNS stimulation.

Psychologic dependence can occur quickly with cocaine because the "high" is usually followed by a "crash" in which the user experiences depression and low energy. The crash serves as motivation to use more cocaine, leading to repeated abuse.

"Snorting" or inhaling cocaine through the nose is the most common method of administration, although "freebasing" has gained popularity in recent years. With freebasing, the user smokes the drug after processing it chemically by dissolving it in an alkaline solution to make a solid, smokeable "rock." Cocaine freebase, or "crack," lowers the burning temperature of cocaine so that it can be smoked.

Freebase cocaine reaches the brain in 6 to 7 seconds (intravenous cocaine reaches the brain in 15 to 30 seconds), which increases the intensity of effects that the user experiences. Chronic abuse and/or extremely high doses can provoke intense fear and anxiety, paranoia, hallucinations (visual, tactile, or auditory), and delusions. Cocaine-induced psychosis has caused violent, aggressive behavior.

Sudden cocaine death syndrome results from cardiotoxic effects that may occur when cocaine is used. Shortly after the administration of cocaine, the heart rate increases dramatically, which may result in fatal arrhythmias. Many users report a "pounding" heart and chest pain when under the influence of co-

caine. A second cause of death is depression of the medullary respiratory center after convulsions. The cocaine-induced stroke is becoming an increasing problem. As a result of cocaine's stimulating effect, the body's blood vessels constrict. When this and tachycardia occur, blood pressure increases suddenly and dramatically. If the rise in blood pressure is enough, an aneurysm or cerebrovascular accident, or both, may result.

The myth of cocaine abuse is that it is only psychologically addicting because no gross physiologic abnormalities are evident during withdrawal. However, long-term abuse leads to sustained neurochemical changes in the brain. The changes produce

---

 **NURSING CARE PLAN**   *Patient in Acute Phase of Cocaine Overdose*

Nursing diagnosis/ Expected outcome	Interventions	Rationale
Cardiac output alteration: decreased related to reduced stroke volume • *Heart rate and blood pressure will stabilize*	Monitor and record vital signs q1h until stable, then q3h Administer medications as ordered—IV propranolol 1 mg/min up to 8 mg Provide a quiet, nonstimulating environment	Cocaine intoxication can cause overstimulation of the heart, resulting in an MI or possibly fatal cardiac dysrhythmias
Altered nutrition: less than body requirements related to loss of appetite • *Will regain normal appetite and food and ʃuid intake with no evidence of gastritis following detoxification*	Offer small meals and frequent nutritionally sound snacks Weigh daily Monitor intake	Cocaine is an appetite suppressant; until desire for food returns, nutritional intake needs to be restored and monitored
Sleep pattern disturbance related to CNS stimulant use • *Will sleep at least 4 to 5 hours per night without waking after 1 week*	Relaxation exercises before bedtime Provide comfort measures such as warm bath Do not serve caffeinated beverages or food Administer medications as ordered; give medications with sleep-inducing properties hs Carefully monitor and record sleep patterns	Cocaine is a CNS stimulant; therefore interventions that reduce CNS stimulation are indicated to promote rest
Sensory perception alteration related to drug-induced organicity • *Hallucinations will cease within 72 hours after last dose of cocaine*	Provide nurse's perception of reality Provide quiet nonstimulating environment Provide reassurance often Focus on the "here and now" rather than the hallucinations	Focusing on the "here and now" provides a diversion from the frightening thoughts and decreases anxiety
Thought processes alteration related to cocaine-induced psychosis • *Will show no signs of delusional thinking following detoxification*	Use calm, empathetic approach Point out reality without being judgmental or argumentative	Using an empathetic, quiet approach decreases stimulation and helps build a trusting relationship

a true physiologic cocaine withdrawal, but the clinical expression resembles psychologic symptoms such as craving, irritability, anxiety, fatigue, and depression. Short-term or "recreational" use can cause arrhythmia myopathy and myocardial infarction.

Caffeine

Caffeine is the most widely used and the most socially accepted stimulant. One of the adverse effects of excessive caffeine intake is **caffeinism,** a clinical term for the toxic syndrome caused by acute or chronic overuse. The clinical manifestations of the syndrome include anxiety, nervousness, irritability, tremulousness, and fatigue. Other symptoms include sleep disturbances, diuresis, headache, tachycardia, diarrhea, and lightheadedness.[20]

The nurse should be alert to the symptoms of caffeine withdrawal, which are similar to those of caffeinism. The caffeine withdrawal headache is a particularly common symptom, in which relief tends to occur promptly with renewed caffeine intake, thus perpetuating the dependence.

Nicotine

Nicotine is a mild CNS stimulant, and its abuse is widely recognized. The difficulty in altering the dependence produced by nicotine is equal to that of other highly abused substances today.[22] Although smoking usually begins in response to psychosocial factors, use of tobacco becomes habitual because of the reinforcing effects of nicotine.[12] Of the many drugs that are self-administered, nicotine is one of the most rapidly metabolized in the body, with a half-life of about 40 to 80 minutes. The user must then smoke several times a day to get the desired effect because of this brief period of action.[23]

There are a number of community-based programs to promote smoking cessation. One of the most active nonprofit organizations in the development of smoking cessation programs is the American Cancer Society (ACS). The basic components of the ACS "Quit Smoking Clinic" include participating in group sessions led by a facilitator, viewing and discussing a series of films on smoking and smoking cessation, and practicing abstinence from smoking. Nurses are becoming increasingly active as facilitators by offering programs within hospitals to patients, outpatients, and interested people in the community.

Hallucinogens/Psychedelics

The category of substances known as hallucinogens became popular during the late 1960s and early 1970s when individuals began regarding chemicals as a way to create altered perceptions and con-sciousness. These substances have also been termed psychotomimetic (meaning producer of psychosis), psychedelic, and mind-altering.

Hallucinogens do not cause physical dependence and tolerance. However, psychologic dependence does occur with frequent use. Although marijuana and PCP are still widely used, it is believed that LSD, mescaline, STP, and other hallucinogens have decreased in popularity.

PCP

Sometimes referred to as "angel dust," PCP is an animal tranquilizer that has been diverted to illegal street use. It is often smoked in a mixture with another drug or substance, such as marijuana or even parsley flakes.

PCP acts as a depressant to the CNS, often initially mimicking alcohol intoxication with numbness of extremities, muscular incoordination, dizziness, and flushing. Other physical manifestations of PCP intoxication include hypertension, nausea and vomiting, increased deep-tendon reflexes, hypersalivation, and dysarthria. At higher doses, serious physiologic problems can occur, including seizures, coma, and death.[21]

PCP ingestion should be considered a psychiatric emergency because of the volatile nature of the patient's behavior. The patient is extremely unpredictable, and behavior fluctuates from apathetic, calm immobility to periods of paranoia, hyperactivity, and agitation with the potential for harm to self or others. Careful assessment will help determine the level of supervision and type of care required. Environmental stimulation should be minimal. The nurse should calmly approach the PCP-intoxicated patient and provide frequent reassurance that the patient is safe. Benzodiazepines, especially diazepam (Valium), may be prescribed to reduce the patient's agitation and prevent seizures. The nurse may encourage the intake of fluids, especially cranberry juice, which acidifies the urine and hastens the excretion of PCP.

Inhalants/volatile substances.

The inhalants and volatile substances consist of chemicals, which when inhaled, produce intoxication and an altered state of consciousness. Generally, these chemicals can be divided into three groups: aerosols, commercial solvents, and anesthetics. The most frequently abused inhalants include gasoline, glues, aerosols, paint and paint thinners, sterno, lighter fluid, nitrous oxide, and amyl nitrate. For teenage males, inhalants are often the earliest drugs of abuse. When assessing for inhalant abuse, the nurse looks for clues such as glazed eyes, unusual breath odors, confusion/drunken state without the smell of alcohol, and redness or soreness around the nose or mouth.

Over-the-Counter Drugs

Over-the-counter (OTC) drugs are those available without prescription, intended for the treatment of minor illnesses that are believed to be self-limiting.[27] The use of OTC drugs in the United States is staggering: an estimated 5 billion dollars a year is spent on OTC drugs. Such widespread use is probably because of the belief that OTC medications can actually cure minor illnesses.

Abuse of OTC drugs usually occurs for two reasons: (1) the person taking the OTC drug does not consult a health professional regarding the proper use of the drug, thereby being uninformed regarding the drug or the condition being treated; and (2) the OTC drug user often thinks that if one dose does a little good, two doses will do more good. Occasionally, abuse of OTC drugs will occur when a substance abuser's "primary drug of abuse" is unavailable; for instance, an alcoholic patient will drink alcohol-based cough syrup or mouthwash.

When assessing for potential abuse of OTC drugs, the nurse inquires about the patient's use of any OTC drugs, including frequency, amounts, reason for taking, and effects. Specific information about

GERIATRIC CONSIDERATIONS

Polypharmacy in the Elderly

OTC drugs are thought to be consumed and abused more by the elderly than by younger persons. "Overall, OTC drugs may account for 2 of every 5 drugs taken by the elderly—a consumption pattern 7 times greater than that of younger adults."[25] The reasons for this increased use of OTC drugs in the elderly seem obvious; older persons usually have more medical problems and limited incomes and mobility, increasing the tendency toward self-treatment rather than treatment by a health professional. Unfortunately, the elderly are more susceptible to adverse side effects from all drugs. Oversedation, metabolic imbalances, mental status abnormalities, cardiac dysrhythmias, and worsening of preexisting chronic conditions are a few of the many adverse effects that may be caused by the abuse or misuse of OTC drugs in the elderly. Senior citizens are also the most frequent consumers of prescription medications; therefore the interaction between OTC drugs and prescription medications creates an even greater risk.

the more commonly used OTC drugs and possible adverse effects are briefly covered in Table 21-3.

Multiple Substance Abuse

One of the most startling trends among those with substance use disorders is the rapidly increasing occurrence of multiple substance abuse. This problem usually manifests by the abuse of more than one substance simultaneously or sequential abuse of more than one substance. An example of the former is mixing alcohol and benzodiazepines. Taking cocaine for stimulation and following with alcohol for relaxation is an example of the latter. Needless to say, the assessment and treatment of those who abuse multiple substances becomes increasingly more complicated, particularly when one considers that the abuser will likely experience withdrawal from a number of substances concurrently.

NURSING MANAGEMENT OF THE PATIENT WITH SUBSTANCE ABUSE DISORDER
Assessment

Regardless of the health care setting, nurses will encounter a substantial number of patients with substance abuse disorders. Most of these patients will not have a primary diagnosis of substance abuse, nor will they articulate the problem to their caregivers. Unfortunately, if chemical dependency is not detected, many people will remain undiagnosed and without the benefit of treatment. Because of denial or lack of knowledge, often patients are unaware of the underlying reason for their physical symptoms (e.g., gastritis, insomnia, or impotence) and psychosocial problems such as depression, and family or work difficulties. To facilitate early treatment, the nurse must know the signs and symptoms of substance abuse and be able to accurately assess them. While assessing any patient, signs and symptoms should cue the nurse that a possible problem with substance abuse exists (see box on p. 449).

The nurse cannot expect the patient with a substance abuse disorder to admit this problem readily. Questions such as "How much alcohol do you drink?" and "What drugs do you take or have you tried?" will elicit more revealing responses than "Do you drink or use drugs?" or "Do you have a problem with alcohol or drugs?" which allow for only yes/no responses.

The nurse assesses for current use and pattern of use, amount, date, and time of last use in order to determine the onset of withdrawal and detoxification nursing care and medical needs. The patient is also assessed for physical symptoms of withdrawal and psychosocial problems related to substance

TABLE 21-3 Adverse Effects of Commonly Used Over-the-Counter Drugs

Drug categories	Active ingredient	Adverse effects
Sedatives	Pyrilamine, doxylamine (antihistamine-like substances)	Alteration of normal sleep patterns; paradoxical insomnia; feelings of heaviness and weakness; anticholinergic effects (e.g., dry mouth) Acute toxicity: fixed, dilated pupils; fever; excitement; possible hallucinations
Appetite suppressants	Phenylpropanolamine, caffeine	CNS stimulation: tachycardia, palpitations, insomnia, headache, nervousness, nausea, hypertension
Analgesics	Aspirin, acetaminophen	Disturbances of acid/base balance; hemorrhage; encephalopathy; GI symptoms; fatal hepatic necrosis in acute overdose
Laxatives		Habituation; fluid and electrolyte imbalance; abuse common in elderly
Antihistamines, cold/allergy products	Varied: pyrilamine, doxylamine, alcohol, codeine, dextromethorphan	Dependence, anticholinergic symptoms, sedation, agitation, hypertension, anxiety, palpitations, respiratory depression with overdose

LEGAL ISSUES *Chemically Impaired Nurses*

Nurses' use of alcohol and drugs, both prescription and recreational, mirrors that of society in general. Concern has mounted within the profession over the numbers of chemically impaired nurses coming before boards of nursing for disciplinary action. Drug and alcohol abuse are serious problems in themselves; in impaired professionals, the problems are compounded. There is an added threat to patients when the caregiver's performance and judgment are diminished.

Traditionally, impaired nurses were investigated and faced loss of licensure if allegations of chemical abuse were substantiated. In the past 10 years, with the support of the American Nurses' Association, many states have developed peer-assistance programs to bring impaired nurses into treatment and rehabilitation.

A number of states have also passed legislation under the heading of nursing disciplinary diversion acts. These statutes allow nurses and other professionals to voluntarily or temporarily surrender their licenses in exchange for agreeing to enter a treatment or rehabilitation program. This allows the nurse to be "diverted" from full investigation and disciplinary action. In its place, the nurse receives the treatment and support essential to recovery and a return to practice. During the surrender period, the nurse may not practice, and the nurse's treatment and progress are closely monitored. The nurse typically agrees to supervision by the state usually for a period of 2 years.

With sufficient progress, the license can be reinstated. Reinstatement is generally conditional upon continued monitoring and successful rehabilitation with positive progress reports. The message to all nurses is: if there is reason to suspect a colleague of chemical dependency, document specific incidents and contact either the state nurses' association or the state board of nursing. They can offer advice and assistance in getting the individual into treatment, before tragedy strikes and the nurse loses his or her license permanently.

From: The American Nurses' Association, Suggested State Legislation, 1990; Addictions and Psychological Dysfunctions in Nursing, 1984 and 1992.

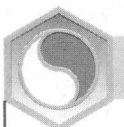

ETHICAL ISSUES

- What is a nurse's responsibility toward a colleague who is chemically dependent but whose professional competence is unimpaired?
- What is the nurse's responsibility toward the patients who are cared for by a nurse who is chemically dependent?
- What is the responsibility of the nurse toward a colleague who refuses help in overcoming addiction? toward a patient?

SIGNS AND SYMPTOMS OF SUBSTANCE ABUSE

Physical signs and symptoms of substance abuse include:

Flushed face
Unsteady or wide gait
Hypertension
Cardiac arrhythmias or complaints of chest pain
Tachycardia
Impotency
Bruises and scars (e.g. fall- or trauma-related, skin tracks)
Weight loss, nausea, vomiting, gastritis
Liver enlargement and elevated liver enzymes
Anemia or evidence of nutritional deficiencies
Insomnia or sleep disturbance
Infections (pneumonia) or abscesses
Poor hygiene and grooming

Psychosocial signs and symptoms of substance abuse:

History of suicide attempts
Complaints of anxiety or depression
Family history of substance abuse
Family complaints of substance use
History of physical or sexual abuse
Poor impulse control
Deterioration of performance at work or school
Alienation of family, friends, co-workers
Defensiveness or reluctance to discuss problems about substance use
Arrests for driving while intoxicated, possession, assault, or other legal problems
Feelings of impending doom
Financial difficulties

abuse in order to assist the patient in admitting the severity of the problem. Substance abuse patients often deny the existence of an alcohol and/or drug problem and can only begin to see the effect this illness has on their lives when confronted with the work, family, financial, and legal problems experienced as a result of substance abuse.

The Short Michigan Alcoholism Screening Test (SMAST) is a tool that has been designed to help identify the chemically dependent person (see box on p. 450). This tool is brief and easy to administer to any patient who presents with physical and psychosocial signs and symptoms of substance abuse or who gives the nurse reason to suspect an underlying substance abuse disorder. Since many drug abusers deny a problem with alcohol, the alcoholism screening test can be adapted by substituting questions about drugs such as heroin, cocaine, or diazepam in addition to questions about alcohol.

Self-assessment

Before working with the substance abuse patient, nurses must assess their own views about alcoholism and drug abuse. If nurses do not carefully examine their feelings, they may unknowingly respond to the patient in a judgmental, rejecting, or even enabling manner, thereby interfering with the patient's treatment. Questions adapted from Estes[17] to assist in the process of self-examination are given in the box on p. 450. Manipulation, denial, dysfunctional anger, impulsiveness, and low frustration tolerance are common patterns of behavior displayed by substance abusers; this behavior often generates feelings of frustration, anger, and helplessness in the nurse caring for them. When the nurse understands the significance of the patient's dysfunctional behaviors as well as the nurses' own reaction to these behaviors, power struggles and feelings of exploitation can be averted.

Nursing Diagnosis

The following diagnoses are common to the patient with a substance abuse disorder:

High risk for altered nutrition related to inadequate intake

High risk for injury related to changes in sensorium or chemical withdrawal or overdose

Sensory-perceptual alteration related to sleep pattern disturbance

High risk for violence directed at self/others, related to chemical alteration

Ineffective coping related to inability to deal with situational or developmental stress

Altered thought processes related to chemical effects and destruction of brain tissue

ALCOHOLISM SCREENING TEST

1. Do you feel you are a normal drinker? (By normal we mean you drink less than or as much as most other people.) (No)*
2. Does your wife, husband, a parent, or other near relative ever worry or complain about your drinking? (Yes)
3. Do you ever feel guilty about your drinking? (Yes)
4. Do friends or relatives think you are a normal drinker? (No)
5. Are you able to stop drinking when you want to? (No)
6. Have you ever attended a meeting of Alcoholics Anonymous? (Yes)
7. Has drinking ever created problems between you and your wife, husband, a parent, or other near relative? (Yes)
8. Have you ever gotten into trouble at work because of drinking? (Yes)
9. Have you ever neglected your obligations, your family, or your work for two or more days in a row because you were drinking? (Yes)
10. Have you ever gone to anyone for help about your drinking? (Yes)
11. Have you ever been in a hospital because of drinking? (Yes)
12. Have you ever been arrested for drunken driving, driving while intoxicated, or driving under the influence of alcoholic beverages? (Yes)
13. Have you ever been arrested, even for a few hours, because of other drunken behavior? (Yes)

*Alcoholism-indicating responses in parentheses.

Scoring: 0-1 points—nonalcoholic

2 points—possible alcoholic

3 points—alcoholic

Short Michigan Alcohol Screening Test (SMAST) reprinted by permission from Selzer AV and van Rooijen L: J *Stud Alcohol* 36:117, 1975. Copyright by Journal of Studies on Alcohol, Inc., Rutgers Center of Alcohol Studies, New Brunswick, NJ 08903.

Planning

In planning care for the substance abuse patient, the nurse is continuously aware that substance abuse can result in life-threatening conditions, such as withdrawal or overdose (see Care Plan on p. 445). The first priority is to medically stabilize the patient. If the patient presents with a physical dependency on a CNS depressant (alcohol, sedative-hypnotics, or opiates), medical management is required to prevent the progression of the signs and symptoms of withdrawal. **Detoxification** is the process in which the substance that is abused is replaced by a longer-

SELF-ASSESSMENT QUESTIONS: SUBSTANCE ABUSE

How do I respond when I believe that another person is angry with me?

How do I respond when unwarranted anger is directed at me?

How do I respond to the patient who keeps returning primarily for drugs?

How do I respond to the drug abuse patient who requests pain medications?

How do I respond when a person is trying to manipulate me?

Do I drink or use drugs? If so, when, where, how often, how much, and for what reasons?

What did I learn about alcohol/drugs when I was growing up?

What are my attitudes about alcohol/drugs?

What is my family history regarding substance abuse?

Do I believe alcoholism or drug dependency is a disease or a sign of moral or emotional weakness?

Do I believe individuals with alcohol or drug abuse problems come from all walks of life?

Do I believe individuals with alcohol or drug abuse problems can change their life-style to exclude chemicals?

acting cross-tolerant substance, in which decreasing doses are given over time to provide for a safe withdrawal with minimal discomfort. After the patient completes detoxification, physical symptoms related to the health problems associated with chronic substance abuse may appear. The nurse must reassess the patient to identify and manage illnesses related to excessive alcoholism or drug abuse.

After the resolution of the patient's physiologic crises, the nurse focuses on helping the patient to accept that a substance abuse problem exists and to plan for rehabilitation. Finally, it should be emphasized that substance abuse is an illness with a high rate of relapse. Many substance abusers try once and sometimes several times to use the substance in a controlled way. For this reason, the nurse and patient must avoid setting unrealistic expectations, while maintaining cautious optimism and encouragement.

Observable outcome goals for the substance abuse patient include[3,13]:

1. Detoxifies without medical complications within 5 days after admission.
2. Verbalizes two medical and psychosocial consequences of substance abuse.

3. Develops aftercare plans addressing his or her problem with substance abuse (inpatient, outpatient, and/or self-help groups).
4. The family will verbalize feelings to the nurse and each other about the impact of substance abuse on individual and group functioning.
5. The family will attend two family self-help group meetings while the patient is hospitalized.

Implementation

Identification, medical and behavior management, health teaching, and referral are major nursing interventions with the substance abuse patient. Nurses who care for these patients need interpersonal, communication, and psychosocial skills as well as a firm knowledge of the medical treatment of substance abuse. Table 21-2 summarizes nursing interventions for patients who are chemically dependent.

The Johnsonian intervention

Substance abusers often deny the severity of their problem even though it may be obvious to the people around them. In the past, it was believed that the substance abuser could not be helped until he or she "hit bottom" and requested assistance. Currently those in the field believe that the dangerous consequences of waiting can be prevented by early detection. The **Johnsonian intervention** consists of a meeting of the patient's significant others to plan a group confrontation regarding the patient's substance abuse problem. The patient's significant others include family, close friends, and perhaps the employer or physician. With the help of a professional in the field of addiction, these people rehearse what they want to say to the patient for the purpose of breaking through the patient's denial that a substance abuse problem exists.

Presenting a united front, they provide concrete examples of the impact of the patient's substance abuse on self and others. The patient is encouraged to accept professional help and treatment plans are made.[11,24] If the patient opts to refuse help, the significant others must identify ways they prevent the substance abuser from experiencing the consequences of chemical dependency, and make plans to minimize their codependent behavior in the future.

Behavior management

The substance abuse patient often presents as manipulative, angry, and with a low tolerance for frustration. Manipulation and an angry affect are means of controlling others and avoiding interpersonal anxiety. The substance abuse patient manages anxiety by making demands for immediate gratification. As a result of the substance abuser's impatience and hostility, the nurse may unconsciously avoid that patient's room or limit the amount of contact with the patient.

While the patient's provocative behavior may anger the nurse, the nurse strives to avoid reacting emotionally. He or she sets firm limits on the patient's behavior. The patient must know what is expected, what behaviors will and will not be tolerated, and the consequences for unacceptable behavior. For example, the nurse should clearly state that drugs and alcohol are not permitted in the hospital and that noncompliance may prompt the treatment team to consider immediate discharge. Another example of limit testing on the part of the substance abuser is the patient who is sexually inappropriate. The nurse needs to address the patient's behavior immediately and firmly, by calmly stating that the behavior is inappropriate and by explaining the role of the nurse relative to the patient. It is essential that the nurse communicates the limits set with the patient to other staff in order to maintain consistency in dealing with the patient.

Health teaching

Health teaching is a critical component of the nursing care of the substance abuse patient. Many of these patients are unaware of the physiologic effects of drugs and alcohol. For example, a patient may not be aware that alcohol elevates liver enzymes, causing destruction of liver tissue. The role of the nurse is to instruct the patient about the medical aspects of substance abuse so that the patient can learn about the deleterious effects of these chemicals. The patient may not know that many substance abusers use drugs and alcohol to self-medicate for anxiety and depression; this practice may provide temporary relief but eventually results in feeling worse. Many substance abusers, especially intravenous drug abusers, are at high risk for transmission of HIV disease. Alcoholics may deny themselves as high risk for HIV exposure. However, the alcoholic may have blackouts or amnesia without a loss of consciousness while drinking, and engage in high risk behaviors such as unprotected sex or using intravenous drugs and sharing needles. Health teaching about HIV transmission and prevention is essential for the substance abuse patient.

The alcoholic who expresses concern about the impulsivity of his or her drinking may use disulfurim (Antabuse) as a deterrent. Antabuse interferes with the metabolism of alcohol. When alcohol is ingested after the patient has taken Antabuse, a reaction including flushing, palpitations, vomiting, and possible shock may occur. The patient needs instruction about the toxic effects of ingesting alcohol or over-the-counter products that may contain alcohol (mouthwash, aftershave, cough syrup) while using Antabuse. To help the patient avoid this pitfall, the nurse reviews with the patient where to find alcohol listed as an ingredient on product labels.

To maintain abstinence and achieve a balanced life-style the patient must learn new behaviors. The nurse can help by addressing these basic patient education needs as identified in the patient teaching guide.

Pain management

The nurse is often in a difficult situation with the patient who has an active addiction and also seeks pain medications for a legitimate medical problem. It is not unusual for the nurse to assume the patient's report of pain lacks credibility and to withhold or delay the patient's pain medications. Pain is a subjective experience and the patient's self-report should be considered the most reliable indicator of pain.

Withholding pain medications does nothing constructive for the patient's addiction and may ultimately have a negative effect on the nurse-patient relationship. It is the nurse's professional responsibility to accept and respond to the patient's report of pain even though it is possible the patient may deceive the nurse. The nurse must conduct a pain assessment and attempt to determine the cause of pain. McCaffery and Vourakis[6] recommend teaching the patient to use a pain scale for reporting and comparing the patient's experience of pain. Using a scale of 1 to 10 or mild, moderate, severe, excruciating, the patient can determine what pain level is manageable without medication and at what level the patient will require analgesia. Establishing a schedule for pain medication administration will reduce the potential for conflict and give the patient a sense of control in his or her care.

For the narcotic dependent patient, the nurse should anticipate that the tolerance for pain medication is truly higher than that of other patients. Larger, more frequent doses will be required to manage the patient's pain. The nurse may be concerned about the potential for overdose in higher doses. However, the patient's tolerance to the respiratory and sedating effects are greater than to the analgesic effects.[6]

Discharge planning

Many alcoholics and drug abusers are admitted to medical and surgical units of general hospitals or emergency rooms, often without a diagnosis of alcohol/drug dependency but suffering from the medical consequences of substance abuse. Nurses in these settings are often the first to detect signs of early withdrawal and to care for patients who are withdrawing or overdosing from various substances. Detoxification alone does nothing for long-term abstinence. After the problem of substance abuse is identified and medically managed, further treatment is encouraged to ensure the likelihood of recovery.

The nurse needs to be aware of the local resources for inpatient and outpatient treatment programs and self-help groups in order to provide comprehensive discharge planning for the patient's substance abuse problem. Alcoholics Anonymous and Narcotics Anonymous are listed in most local telephone directories and may be able to provide inpatient referral suggestions.

 PATIENT EDUCATION GUIDE   *Maintaining Health and Abstinence*

1. Exercise:
   * Maintain regular exercise pattern as leisure time activity.
2. Nutrition:
   * Eat three meals a day selecting foods from the four food groups.
   * Avoid alcohol, which is high in calories and suppresses appetite.
   * Avoid caffeine and high-sugar snacks as craving substitutes.
3. Stress
   * Do relaxation and spiritual exercises daily such as meditation or reading recovery literature.

* Sleep 6 to 8 hours daily.
* Avoid the tendency to overwork in the absence of substance abuse.
* Cultivate new leisure activities and friendships.
* Practice assertiveness techniques to modify anger/manipulation.
4. Medication
   * Take only medication as prescribed.
   * Avoid cross-addiction with other substances of abuse.

Substance abuse rehabilitation programs are generally 3- to 6-week programs located within general hospital, psychiatric hospital, or private addiction hospital settings. Stuckey and Harrison[28] identify that most rehabilitation programs include the following components: (1) a strong Alcoholics/Narcotics Anonymous orientation; (2) an emphasis on education using the disease model; (3) use of group therapy for insight, confrontation, and support; and (4) family involvement.

A critical component of substance abuse treatment is follow-up or aftercare management. Aftercare management is accomplished in a variety of ways: involvement with self-help groups including Alcoholics Anonymous (AA), Narcotics Anonymous (NA) and Chemically Dependents Anonymous (CDA); outpatient counseling that may be combined with methadone maintenance or urine monitoring in which the patient provides urine specimens three times a week for drug testing; day treatment programs that provide education and group counseling daily for 1 to 3 months; and outpatient programs that provide individual, family, and/or group therapy. The nurse begins discharge planning with substance abuse patients as soon as possible because many substance abusers are noncompliant with follow-up, either denying the severity of their problem or the importance of ongoing aftercare.

Self-help groups

Alcoholics Anonymous, Narcotics Anonymous, and Chemically Dependents Anonymous are self-help groups whose intent is to help the substance abuser. The format is the group meeting in which members and leaders, who are nonprofessionals, participate. Anyone who desires help is invited to attend. One of the basic principles of AA is to strive for abstinence one day at a time. All self-help groups have 12 steps and traditions that include an admission that one is powerless over the substance, a reliance on a higher power, and a responsibility to help one another achieve and maintain abstinence through group meetings and sponsorship.

Self-help groups also exist for the family members of the substance abuser. These groups—Al-Anon, Alateen, and Adult Children of Alcoholics—are based on the premise that everyone in the family is affected by the substance abuse of one (or more) members. Family members will often deny the impact of the substance abuse on their lives or view aftercare as the sole responsibility of the substance abuser. The nurse must assist the family in identifying how the substance abuser's behavior interferes with family functioning and that each member has a responsibility to seek help either professionally or through the supportive self-help groups. Without the family's involvement in aftercare activities, members will have difficulty with the patient's abstinence, which will conflict with established and dysfunctional family roles and behaviors.

Evaluation

In evaluating the patient's response to nursing interventions, the nurse refers to those outcome objectives established in the planning phase of the nursing process. If the patient's need was for detoxification, the nurse will want to examine the safety and level of comfort the patient achieved during the withdrawal process through the absence or presence of withdrawal signs and symptoms.

To evaluate the patient's acknowledgment of a substance abuse problem, the nurse considers whether the patient established realistic aftercare plans including attendence at self-help group meetings. The patient who accepts his or her substance abuse problem and need for ongoing treatment will develop specific aftercare plans. If the patient has vague aftercare plans, the nurse may want to assist the patient in refocusing on how substance abuse has been problematic and what the difference will be this time. Sometimes the substance abuse patient enters the treatment setting for medical reasons that may be indirectly related to alcohol or drug abuse. Any attempts the nurse makes to discuss substance abuse as a health concern with the patient meets with resistance. The patient does not want to acknowledge the existence of a substance abuse problem or need for further treatment. The nurse can only provide the patient with education about the effects of substance abuse. Problem patient behaviors, such as manipulation or hostility, and effective nursing interventions should be identified in the nursing care plan and progress notes to enhance consistency of the treatment team. Finally, specific discharge plans should be recorded as the patient and family contract to follow-up with further treatment.

Documentation

The nurse documents the patient's and family member's response to effects of drugs and alcohol on the body; the patient has the responsibility to put this information into action. However, if the patient does not choose recovery, the nurse is careful to avoid responding with anger to the patient's decision.

Finally, the nurse evaluates the family's response to nursing interventions through their involvement in the patient's substance abuse treatment; this includes attending Al-Anon meetings and verbalizing at least three ways substance abuse has affected family functioning.

CRITICAL THINKING QUESTIONS

1 Mr. B. has just been admitted to the medical-surgical unit with the chief complaint of vomiting blood since yesterday. While you interview the patient for the nursing assessment, he tells you that he has been feeling depressed for the past month after his wife announced she was filing for a divorce. His blood pressure is 160/100 and pulse is 100. Plan your care based on the priorities of this patient's needs.

2 While he is undergoing tests, Mr. B.'s wife visits that evening with their three children. When you ask the names of her children, she becomes very tearful and angrily states, "Why do I have to take care of everything? His drinking has destroyed our relationship and he tells me it's my fault for not understanding him!" What factors would you consider in intervening with her?

3 A patient comes into the emergency room claiming that she drinks a pint of whiskey a day, shoots heroin and cocaine three times a day, and uses Valium and Xanax whenever she can purchase them. She claims she wants to stop using drugs and alcohol but is afraid she won't get through withdrawal. How will the nurse plan for the safe management of these simultaneous abstinence/withdrawal syndromes?

RESOURCES

1 Alcoholics Anonymous World Services, Inc. Box 459, Grand Central Station New York, NY 10163

2 Al-Anon Family Group Headquarters P.O. Box 182, Madison Square Station New York, NY 10159

3 Hazelden Educational Materials Pleasant Valley Road Box 176 Center City, MN 55012-0176 (800) 328-9000

4 Narcotics Anonymous World Service Office P.O. Box 622 Sun Valley, CA 91352

5 National Institute on Alcohol Abuse and Alcoholism U.S. Department of Health and Human Services 5600 Fishers Lane Rockville, MD 20857

6 National Institute on Drug Abuse U.S. Department of Health and Human Services 5600 Fishers Lane Rockville, MD 20857

7 National Nurses' Society on Addiction P.O. Box 1014 Skokie, IL 60077

8 National Self-Help Clearing House 33 West 42nd St N.Y., NY 10036

BIBLIOGRAPHY

Current

1. American Nurses' Association and National Nurses' Society on Addictions: PMH-10 standards of addictions nursing practice with selected diagnoses and criteria, Kansas City, Mo, 1988, The Association.
2. Casely R, Morse G: Correlates of problem drinking among homeless men, *Hosp Community Psychiatry* 42(7):721, 1991.
3. Kirk E, Bradford L: Effects of alcohol on the central nervous system: implications for the neuroscience nurse, *J Neurosci Nurs* 19(6):326, 1987.
4. Lanros NE: *Assessment and intervention in emergency nursing,* Norwalk, Conn, 1988, Appleton & Lange.
5. Linn L, Gelberg L, Leake B: Substance abuse and mental health status of homeless and domiciled low-income users of a medical clinic, *Hosp Community Psychiatry* 41(3):306, 1990.
6. McCaffery M, Vourakis C: Assessment and relief of pain in chemically dependent patients, *Orthopaedic Nurs* 11(2):13, 1992.
7. National Institute on Alcohol Abuse and Alcoholism: *Personal communication,* November 12, 1991.
8. National Institute on Drug Abuse: *National household survey on drug abuse: main findings,* 1988, Washington, DC, US Department of Health and Human Services.
9. Padgett D, Struening E: Influence of substance abuse and mental disorders on emergency room use by homeless adults, *Hosp Community Psychiatry* 42(8):834, 1991.
10. Rinaldi RC et al: Clarification and standardization of substance abuse terminology, *JAMA* 259(4):555, 1988.
11. Sullivan E, Bissell L, Williams E: *Chemical dependency in nursing: the deadly diversion,* Menlo Park, Calif, 1988, Addison-Wesley Publishing.
12. Surgeon General: *The health consequences of smoking and nicotine addiction: a report of the surgeon general,* US Department of Health and Human Services, Pub No (CDC) 89-8411, Washington, DC, 1989, US Government Printing Office.
13. Williams E: Strategies for intervention, *Nurs Clin North Am* 24(1):95, 1989.

Classic

14. American Psychiatric Association: *Diagnostic and statistical manual of mental disorders,* ed III-R, Washington, DC, 1985, The Association.
15. Bennett G, Vourakis C, Woolf DS, editors: *Substance abuse: pharmacologic, developmental and clinical perspectives,* New York, 1983, John Wiley & Sons.
16. Blum K: *The handbook of abusable drugs,* New York, 1984, Gardner Press.
17. Estes NJ, Heinemann ME: *Alcoholism: development, consequences, and interventions,* ed 3, St Louis, 1986, Mosby–Year Book.
18. Gold MS, Pottash AC: Neurobiological aspects of opiate addiction and withdrawal. In Gottheil E et al, editors: *Etiologic aspects of alcohol and drug abuse,* Springfield, Ill, 1983, Charles C Thomas Publisher.
19. Goodwin DW: The genetics of alcoholism. In Gottheil E et al, editors: *Etiologic aspects of alcohol and drug abuse,* Springfield, Ill, 1983, Charles C Thomas Publisher.
20. Greden JF: Caffeinism and caffeine withdrawal. In Lowinson JH, Ruiz P, editors: *Substance abuse: clinical problems and perspectives,* Baltimore, 1981, Williams & Wilkins.

21. Grinspoon L, Bakalar JB: Drug dependence: non-narcotic agents. In Kaplan HI, Freeman AM, Saddock BJ, editors: *Comprehensive textbook of psychiatry,* ed 4, Baltimore, 1985, Williams & Wilkins.
22. Holbrook JM: CNS stimulants. In Bennett G, Vourakis C, Woolf DS: *Substance abuse: pharmacologic, developmental and clinical perspectives,* New York, 1983, John C. Wiley & Sons.
23. Jaffe JH, Kanzler M: Nicotine: tobacco use, abuse and dependence. In Lowinson JH, Ruiz P, editors: *Substance abuse: clinical problems and perspectives,* Baltimore, 1981, Williams & Wilkins.
24. Johnson Institute: *Chemical dependency and recovery are a family affair,* Minneapolis, 1979, Johnson Institute.
25. Kofoed LL: OTC drug overuse in the elderly: what to watch for, *Geriatrics* 40(10):55, 1985.
26. Lowinson JH, Ruiz P: *Substance abuse: clinical problems and perspectives,* Baltimore, 1981, Williams & Wilkins.
27. Moore DF: Over-the-counter drugs. In Bennett G, Vourakis C, Woolf DS: *Substance abuse: pharmacologic, developmental and clinical perspectives,* New York, 1983, John C. Wiley & Sons.
28. Stuckey RF, Harrison JS: The alcoholism rehabilitation center. In Pattison M, Kaufman E, editors: *Encyclopedic handbook of alcoholism,* New York, 1982, Gardner Press.
29. Valliant GE: *The natural history of alcoholism: causes, patterns and paths to recovery,* Cambridge, Mass, 1983, Harvard University Press.
30. Wegscheider-Cruse S: *Another chance: hope and health for the alcoholic family,* Palo Alto, Calif; 1983, Science & Behavior Books.

Principles of
Perioperative Nursing

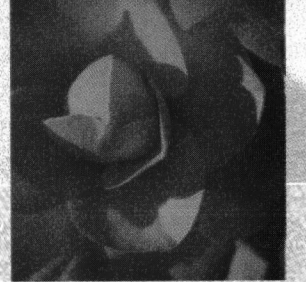

CHAPTER TWENTY-TWO

Preoperative Nursing

LEARNING OBJECTIVES

1 Describe the nursing activities in the preoperative period.
2 Classify surgery according to intent or purpose and degree of urgency.
3 Discuss physiologic disruptions that occur as a result of surgery.
4 Describe common preoperative psychologic concerns and nursing support measures.
5 Identify potential risk factors or abnormalities during a preoperative patient assessment.
6 Formulate an individualized plan of nursing care for the preoperative patient.
7 Prepare an individualized teaching plan for preoperative patients.
8 Evaluate the preoperative patient's readiness for surgery.

KEY TERMS

ambulatory surgery, p. 462
anesthesia, p. 461
outpatient surgery, p. 462

perioperative period, p. 459
preoperative period, p. 459
same-day surgery, p. 462

NURSING CARE of the patient undergoing surgery requires an understanding of the perioperative phase of surgical care. This knowledge is applied within the framework of the nursing process to promote a smooth and safe passage through the **perioperative period,** which is divided into the preoperative, intraoperative, and postoperative periods. This unit discusses general nursing care of patients during the perioperative period, whereas care unique to specific body systems or surgical procedures is discussed in chapters focusing on those areas. Table 22-1 provides examples of activities in perioperative nursing practice identified by the American Association of Operating Room Nurses.

THE PREOPERATIVE ENVIRONMENT

The **preoperative period** begins with the decision to perform surgery and continues until transfer of the patient into the operating room. Primary nursing responsibilities during this time center on collection of data, preparation of the patient for the stress of surgery and anesthesia, and education to reduce anxiety and facilitate postoperative recovery.

Surgery

Surgery has been described as the branch of medicine dealing with operative procedures. In the past, surgery has been divided into minor and major pro-

TABLE 22-1   Examples of Perioperative Nursing Activities

Preoperative phase	Intraoperative phase	Postoperative phase

PREOPERATIVE ASSESSMENT
Home/clinic
  1. Initiates initial preoperative assessment
  2. Plans teaching methods appropriate to patient's needs
  3. Involves family in interview
Surgical unit
  1. Completes preoperative assessment
  2. Coordinates patient teaching with other nursing staff
  3. Explains phases in perioperative period and expectations
  4. Develops a plan of care
Surgical suite
  1. Assesses patient's level of consciousness
  2. Reviews chart
  3. Identifies patient
  4. Verifies surgical site
Planning
  1. Determines a plan of care
Psychologic support
  1. Tells patient what is happening
  2. Determines psychologic status
  3. Gives prior warning of noxious stimuli
  4. Communicates patient's emotional status to other appropriate members of the health care team
	MAINTENANCE OF SAFETY
	  1. Ensures that the sponge, needle, and instrument counts are correct
	  2. Positions the patient
	    a. Functional alignment
	    b. Exposure of surgical site
	    c. Maintenance of position throughout procedure
	  3. Applies grounding device to patient
	  4. Provides physical support
	Physiologic monitoring
	  1. Calculates effects on patient of excessive fluid loss
	  2. Distinguishes normal from abnormal cardiopulmonary data
	  3. Reports changes in patient's pulse, respirations, temperature, and blood pressure
	Psychologic monitoring (before induction and if patient conscious)
	  1. Provides emotional support to patient
	  2. Stands near/touches patient during procedures/induction
	  3. Continues to assess patient's emotional status
	  4. Communicates patient's emotional status to other appropriate members of the health care team
	Nursing management
	  1. Provides physical safety for the patient
	  2. Maintains aseptic, controlled environment
	  3. Effectively manages human resources
		COMMUNICATION OF INTRAOPERATIVE INFORMATION
		  1. Gives patient's name
		  2. States type of surgery performed
		  3. Provides contributing intraoperative factors (i.e., drain, catheters)
		  4. States physical limitations
		  5. States impairments resulting from surgery
		  6. Reports patient's preoperative level of consciousness
		  7. Communicates necessary equipment needs
		Postoperative evaluation
		Postanesthesia care unit
		  1. Determines patient's immediate response to surgical intervention
		Surgical unit
		  1. Evaluates effectiveness of nursing care in the operating room
		  2. Determines patient's level of satisfaction with care given during perioperative period
		  3. Evaluates products used on patient in the operating room
		  4. Determines patient's psychologic status
		  5. Assists with discharge planning
		Home/clinic
		  1. Seeks patient's perception of surgery in terms of the effects of anesthetic agents, impact on body image, distortion, immobilization
		  2. Determines family's perceptions of surgery

Reprinted with permission from *AORN standards and recommended practices for perioperative nursing,* Denver, 1988. Copyright © American Association of Operating Room Nurses, Inc., Denver, Colo.

cedures, but in the eyes of the patient (and ideally the nurse), no surgery is minor. Every surgical procedure results in major physiologic and psychologic disruption of the individual.

Knowledge of the purpose of surgery, as well as the degree of urgency, is a necessary prerequisite for planning nursing care. Surgery may be done for a variety of reasons and is often classified according to the intent or purpose:

Diagnostic or *exploratory* surgery is done to determine the origin of symptoms or the extent of a disease or lesion, such as a biopsy or diagnostic laparoscopy.

Curative surgery attempts to repair, replace, or remove diseased, defective, or infected tissues and to eliminate a disease, such as removal of a diseased appendix, gallbladder, or ulcer.

Restorative surgery returns lost function or corrects deformities, such as stabilizing a fracture, a herniorrhaphy, or mitral valve replacement.

Palliative surgery does not cure but decreases symptoms or slows the disease process, such as a sympathectomy or removing part of a tumor (debulking).

Cosmetic surgery is performed to preserve or improve appearance, such as removal of unsightly scar tissues or recontouring the nose to improve appearance.

Surgery may also be classified by degree of urgency or threatened loss of life, limb, or disability.

Optional surgeries are based on the desires or personal preference of the patient, such as a face-lift, and are arranged at the convenience of the patient.

Elective surgeries are recommended operations with no particular need to proceed quickly with the operation; a delay will not be harmful, and the procedure may be scheduled at the convenience of the patient and surgeon.

Urgent surgeries are operations where a delay could prove detrimental to the patient; they should be performed as expediently as possible.

Emergency surgeries are immediately necessary for preservation of function or life.

Most surgical procedures are given descriptive names based on the organ or body area involved and the type of procedure. For example, tonsillectomy refers to the removal of the tonsils.

Anesthesia

In general terms, the practice of inducing **anesthesia** involves rendering patients insensible to pain during surgical, obstetric, therapeutic, or diagnostic procedures and managing the patients while they are under anesthesia. Anesthesia may be divided into general, regional, or monitored anesthesia care.

Preoperatively the anesthetist will review the patient's medical history, interview the patient, and perform a brief physical examination. The preoperative "workup" is designed to allow the anesthetist to tailor the anesthetic technique to best suit each patient's particular requirements. The decision of which anesthetic technique to use is made by the anesthetist, in conjunction with the patient, only after considering individual patient factors and surgical requirements. In addition to choosing the anesthetic technique, the anesthetist also determines the physical status and risk of anesthesia for the patient. The American Society of Anesthesiologists' Classification of Physical Status is one of the most commonly used systems to estimate patient risk. On the basis of preoperative assessment, the patient is assigned to one of the following categories:

Class I The pathologic process is localized, and the patient has no major physiologic or psycho-

logic systemic disturbances (i.e., the patient is in good general health)

Class II The patient has a mild to moderate systemic disturbance caused either by the condition to be treated surgically or by other processes (e.g., moderate obesity, smoking, or controlled hypertension)

Class III The patient has a severe systemic disturbance that limits physical activity but is not incapacitating (e.g., the patient with coronary artery disease, insulin-dependent diabetes, or uncontrolled hypertension)

Class IV The patient has a severe systemic disorder that is a constant threat to life (e.g., kidney failure, severe vascular disease)

Class V The moribund patient that is not expected to survive 24 hours even with the operation (e.g., a ruptured abdominal aneurysm, multiorgan system failure, or severely injured trauma patient)

Class VI The patient who has been declared brain-dead and whose organs are being removed for donor purposes

Emergency Any patient in one of the above classes who has surgery on an emergency basis. Emergency designation is added to the number classification.

Outpatient Surgery

Historically, most operative procedures took place in the hospital and involved admission to the hospi-

---

OUTPATIENT SELECTION CRITERIA

Patient

Agreeable to concept of outpatient surgery

Adequate home care in the immediate postoperative period

Capable of understanding and following preoperative and postoperative instructions

American Society of Anesthesiologists physical status I or II and medically stable Class III

Procedure

Elective procedure

Produces minimal physiologic derangements

Minimal postoperative nausea and vomiting anticipated

Postoperative pain controllable with oral analgesics

Not expected to involve large blood loss or require transfusion

Does not require continuous postoperative medical or nursing evaluation and patient care

ADVANTAGES OF OUTPATIENT SURGERY

Less psychologic stress associated with hospitalization

Decreased exposure to hospital infections

Patient may return to work earlier

Economic savings

Consumer satisfaction

tal, often for several days. These same procedures are now being performed increasingly on an outpatient basis (also called **same-day surgery** or **ambulatory surgery**) in either a hospital-based operating room or a free-standing surgery center. Some advantages of performing **outpatient surgery** are listed in the box above. Even when the patient must be hospitalized after surgery, admission to the hospital often occurs on the morning of surgery rather than on the day before surgery, as was commonplace in the past. It has been estimated that more than 60% of the operations performed in the United States could be done satisfactorily on an outpatient basis. In determining which patients are candidates for outpatient surgery, the patient goes through a screening process. The box on p. 461 lists several criteria that generally must be met before an outpatient procedure is planned. Exact criteria are established by each institution and staff.

The goal of outpatient surgery is to give high-quality care to the patient requiring surgery and to decrease patient complications with the most efficient use of time and money. This presents a challenge for the nurse to provide highly competent, safe, compassionate nursing care with time for establishing the nurse-patient relationship and applying the nursing process compressed into a few hours. Outpatient nursing care includes all the elements and care involved with inpatient surgery; however, time is often limited in the outpatient setting.

Most outpatient units have a thorough preadmission screening procedure that takes place before the day of surgery. This may take place at the physician's office, hospital, or outpatient center and includes an up-to-date medical history, consultations, laboratory tests, x-ray films, or electrocardiograms. One method of increasing time for nursing interventions is to have the patient visit the nurse at the surgery center before the day of surgery. This allows for a thorough assessment and patient teaching in a less hurried environment and allows a tour of the facility. Preoperative assessment and instructions can also be conducted and given over the telephone. The

use of written instructions is an important part of outpatient nursing care. Research has indicated that in the outpatient setting, and often in the inpatient setting, comprehension and compliance with preoperative and postoperative teaching are greatly enhanced through the use of written materials. Instructions should include when and where to come for surgery, limitations of oral intake, type of clothing to wear, medications to be taken before arrival, and laboratory or radiology reports to be brought with the patient. The patient must be accompanied home by a responsible adult. Documentation for outpatient surgery is facilitated by the use of checklists, which structure the assessment and preparations to include essential information and reduce the time required to complete written documentation.

With the push toward outpatient care a variation of outpatient surgery, often referred to as short-stay surgery, has emerged. Short-stay surgery allows patients having surgery to be observed and treated for additional time, while retaining their outpatient status. Often patients are cared for on an observation or interim unit. These units are designed to comfortably accommodate a patient for a short time following surgery, usually less than 24 hours. As an alternative, patients may be cared for on a general surgical unit for up to 23 hours without being formally admitted as an inpatient. Short-stay surgery is often used for patients who require skilled postoperative care or monitoring during the transition following surgery and their return home. If after sufficient time the patient is not ready for discharge they may be admitted as an inpatient for further care. The short-stay status overcomes some of the risks of premature discharge following surgery, while helping reduce unnecessary admissions and payment denials from third-party payers.

Once the decision is made to perform surgery, preparations begin. The period for preparation may extend over several weeks or, in cases of emergency surgery, last only a few minutes. Included in the preparation may be laboratory studies, diagnostic tests, and x-ray films. Although these tests are generally medical, the role of preparing the patient for the tests and coordinating various studies is often conducted by the nurse. Commonly requested preoperative laboratory tests are listed in Table 22-2.

Preoperative Receiving Area

Most hospitals and surgery centers have a preoperative receiving area (preoperative holding area or presurgical suite) located near the operating rooms. In this area the patient awaits transfer into the operating room. Many facilities allow a family member or friend to stay with the patient while in the preoperative receiving area. Final preparations are conducted here, and a final review of the medical record

TABLE 22-2 Preoperative Laboratory Tests

Test	When indicated
Hemoglobin/hematocrit	All patients
White blood cell (WBC) count	Infection suspected, after radiation, chemotherapy, immunosuppressive or steroid therapy, hypersplenism, aplastic anemia, collagen-vascular diseases
Prothrombin time (PT)/partial thromboplastin time (PTT)	Known or suspected coagulation disorder, anticoagulation therapy or anticipated therapy, hemorrhage or anemia, thrombosis, liver disease, malabsorption or poor nutrition
Platelets	Known platelet abnormality, hemorrhage or purpura, leukemia, hypersplenism, transplant rejection, after radiation or chemotherapy
Electrolytes	Age over 60, diabetes, use of diuretics, dysrhythmias, renal disease, urologic procedures, diarrhea or malnutrition, other fluid or electrolyte disorder
Blood glucose	Diabetes, hypoglycemia
Renal function (blood urea nitrogen [BUN], creatinine)	Proteinurea, urologic procedure, severe hypertension, renal disease
Chemistry panel	Age over 60; diabetes; pancreatic, renal, or liver adrenal disease; radiation or chemotherapy
Pregnancy test	Females of childbearing age unless currently menstruating or surgically sterile
Urinalysis	All patients
Electrocardiogram (ECG)	Men over 40, women over 45, suspected or known cardiac disease
Chest x-ray films	Age over 60, smoker, suspected or known lung disease or infection

is made to ensure documentation is complete. A preoperative checklist, similar to Figure 22-1, is usually used to ensure and document that all preparations are complete. The patient generally wears a clean hospital gown and a special cap covering the hair. The surgeon or anesthetist may visit the patient to make any last minute checks or answer any questions that the patient may have. If preoperative medications have not been previously administered, they may be administered here. An intravenous (IV) infusion may be started here. The patient is monitored closely in the preoperative receiving area for reactions to the preoperative medications and to protect the patient from injury. The preoperative receiving area should be quiet and provide the nurse an opportunity to reassure and support the patient.

PREOPERATIVE PERIOD

Nursing plays an important role in the preoperative period. Nursing care during this time influences the patient's entire perioperative experience. Adequate preparation through assessment, risk management, and education promotes a smooth operative course and recovery. There is no "routine" preoperative experience; it is unique for each patient; and the challenge for nurses is to identify, plan, and provide nursing care to meet the individual needs of each patient.

The experience and perception of surgery differ for each patient. Surgery is an actual or potential threat to body integrity and interferes with normal functioning. The patient is undergoing personal injury or illness and changing personal habits, even if only temporarily. Normal routines of sleeping, eating, exercising, socializing, and performing spiritual activities may be interrupted. Surgery imposes stress on all body systems, which is both physiologic and psychologic. Although discussed separately for clarity, the mind and body are inseparable; stress is best understood and addressed with a holistic approach.

Physiologic Response to Surgery

Homeostasis is maintained in healthy individuals through a complex system of autoregulatory control mechanisms. In an effort to restore health, the stress of surgery initiates the same response pattern that is seen in major trauma. (The stress response is discussed in Chapter 3.) Through the neuroendocrine system, stimuli accompanying injury are sensed, and the neural and hormonal responses, designed to conserve energy and facilitate repair of the injury, are initiated. The metabolic response to surgical stress, as shown in Figure 22-2, is characterized by release of catecholamines, glucocorticoids, growth hormone, and glucagon, with suppression of insulin secretion; all of which lead to a catabolic reaction (Table 22-3). The duration and magnitude of physi-

PREOPERATIVE CHECK LIST

PREOPERATIVE ASSESSMENT		Jones, Robert	SP 403

PREOPERATIVE ASSESSMENT

ALLERGIES _____ WEIGHT _____

Deaf ☐   Mental status: Alert ☐
Blind ☐   Confused ☐

Jones, Robert   SP 403
#123-45-6789   CATH.
Drs. Albert/Watson   11-11-23
NICKNAME:

PRELIMINARY PREOPERATIVE PREPARATION

LAB WORK	N/A	Initiated	Charted	Sent/Called to OR	DIAGNOSTIC WORK-UP	N/A	Initiated	Charted	Sent/Called to OR
CBC		☐	☐	☐	Chest x-ray	☐	☐	☐	☐
SMA$_{12}$		☐	☐	☐	ECG	☐	☐	☐	☐
Urinalysis		☐	☐	☐	History and physical	☐	☐	☐	☐
Electrolytes	☐	☐	☐	☐	Preoperative note		☐	☐	☐
Biocept G	☐	☐	☐	☐	Medical consultation	☐	☐	☐	☐
Type and screen	☐	☐	☐	☐	Consent		☐	☐	☐
Type and cross # Units	☐	☐	☐	☐	Preoperative preparation	☐			

Signature of nurse(s) responsible for completing this segment:

3-11 _____

11-7 _____

7-3 _____

Comments: _____
_____
_____
_____
_____

IMMEDIATE PREOPERATIVE PREPARATION

Check box if present and removed:

Glasses ☐
Nail polish ☐
Contact lenses ☐
Hair pins, beads ☐
Property and valuables ☐
Jewelry ☐
Dentures ☐
Prosthesis ☐

If present check box:

Pace maker ☐
Hearing aid ☐
Caps ☐
Loose teeth ☐
—Location _____
_____

NPO   Yes ☐   No ☐
Voided   Yes ☐   No ☐
Vital signs:
T _____
P _____
R _____
B/P _____

Preoperative medications: Given ☐   Held ☐   Not ordered ☐
Side rails: In place ☐   Addressograph plate ☐   MAR ☐

Special comments _____
_____
_____
_____

Check reviewed by _____

Doctor please call _____ At phone # _____

To OR at _____ Received in OR at _____ Signature: _____

FIGURE 22-1 Example of a preoperative checklist. (From Seneca C: How we streamlined pre-op paperwork, *RN* 49:3, 1986.)

ologic response is modified by the magnitude of surgical injury, preexisting disease, infection, medication, starvation, anesthesia, psychologic state, and a variety of unique individual factors.

Psychologic Response to Surgery

The fear, discomfort, immobilization, dependency, and disruption of life and body that occur with surgery elicit a strong emotional response. Even when considered normal and appropriate to the stress of surgery, the anxiety and fears provoked by surgery can play an important role in influencing the operative course and subsequent recovery. Fears that are commonly associated with surgery and anesthesia include:

1. *Loss of control* associated primarily with anesthesia. Patients may be concerned about their actions or verbalizations while under the effect of drugs and anesthetic. In addition, the patient becomes almost totally dependent on the health care team during the surgical experience, even for the most basic of needs, such as breathing and life support, while under the influence of anesthetic.
2. *Fear of the unknown* is common and may result from uncertainty about the surgical outcome or may stem from a lack of knowledge regarding the surgical experience.
3. *Fear of anesthesia* may include fears of unpleasant induction or emergence from anesthesia. The patient may fear that he or she will wake up during the operation or feel pain while under the effects of anesthetic. This fear is often related to loss of control and fear of the unknown.
4. *Fear of pain* or inadequate postoperative analgesia is common.
5. *Fear of death* is commonly present and constitutes a legitimate fear. Even with the great strides in surgery and anesthesia, no anesthetic or operation is perfectly safe for all patients. However, for many patients, the mere act of driving to the hospital or surgical center exposes them to higher risks of injury than the surgery and anesthesia they are about to undergo.
6. *Fear of separation* from the usual support group is often present. The patient is separated from a spouse, family, or other support group and cared for by strangers during much of this highly stressful period.
7. *Fear of disruption of life patterns* may be present. Surgery and recovery interfere in varying degrees with activities of daily living, social activities, as well as work and professional activities.
8. *Fear of mutilation* or loss of part of the body is also common. Surgery disrupts body integrity and threatens body image.

There is evidence that a relationship exists between preoperative fear and postoperative behavior. The preoperative anxiety level has been shown to influence the amount of anesthesia required, the

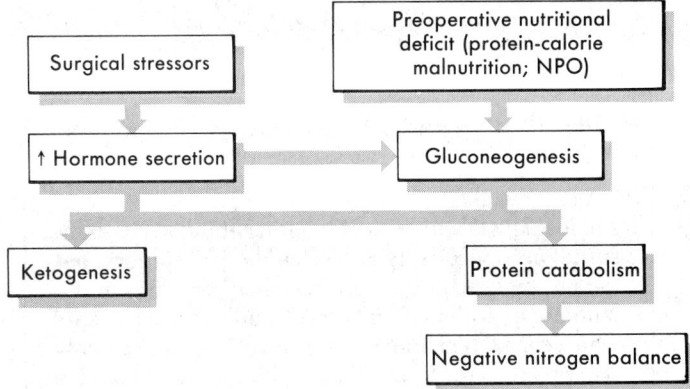

FIGURE 22-2   Metabolic response to surgery.

TABLE 22-3   Responses to Increased Hormone Secretion

Hormone	Physiologic effect	Patient response
Norepinephrine	Peripheral vasoconstriction	Maintained blood pressure
	Decreased gastrointestinal function	Constipation
Glucocorticoids	Gluconeogenesis	Increased energy fuels
	Negative nitrogen balance	Decreased tissue repair
	Decreased immune response	Increased risk of infection
	Increased platelet activity	Increased clot formation
Aldosterone and antidiuretic hormone	Sodium and water reabsorption	Decreased urine output
		Increased circulatory volume

RESEARCH BRIEF

Nyamathi A, Kwashiwabara A: Preoperative anxiety: its effect on cognitive thinking, *AORN J* 47(1):164, 1988.

Anxiety levels and critical thinking ability were measured preoperatively in 60 same-day surgery patients. Analysis of the data revealed that 25% of the patients had high anxiety levels, and of the patients who scored high on anxiety levels, 75% had low scores on critical thinking ability. The data also showed that as anxiety levels rose, cognitive abilities diminished. This result suggests that nurses should consider the effect of anxiety on cognitive thinking ability when they teach patients. Preoperative patients with high anxiety levels may have difficulty making decisions, as well as comprehending instructions and information.

amount of postoperative pain medication needed, and the speed of recovery after surgery. Three distinct coping patterns have been noted in preoperative patients.

1. High anticipatory fear—these patients have a heightened level of anxiety and fear of pain, mutilation, or death, and they may continue to be extremely anxious postoperatively.
2. Moderate anticipatory fear—these patients worry occasionally and are anxious about specific details of the operation; they tend to be cooperative and participate in their postoperative care.
3. Low anticipatory fear—these patients show an absence of anxiety along with an unrealistic, optimistic outlook; they may be preoccupied and difficult to treat and sometimes less compliant with postoperative treatments.

NURSING MANAGEMENT OF THE PREOPERATIVE PATIENT
Assessment

Physical assessment

The physical assessment provides baseline data such as height, weight, and vital signs. The nurse should be alert for signs of dehydration and altered nutrition. Rashes, sores, skin lesions, or signs of infection may be significant findings in the preoperative patient.

Surgical and anesthetic history

Understanding the patient's experiences with previous surgeries helps identify potential problems that may occur. If the patient has experienced surgery before, the date, type of surgery, and reason should be documented, as well as the occurrence of complications, such as infection, hemorrhage, breathing difficulties, or thromboembolism. The presence or absence of complications and family history of anesthesia-related complications, such as prolonged sleep or malignant hyperthermia (a genetically determined hypermetabolic response to certain anesthetic drugs), should be noted. The patient's overall experience with prior surgery and anesthesia is important. Was the experience positive or negative? What in particular did the patient like or dislike? Often this will reveal specific concerns, desires, or expectations of the patient, which the nurse should consider when planning nursing care.

Medications

A careful history will document medications currently used or recently discontinued, drug allergies, and sensitivities. It should obtain information on both prescription and nonprescription drugs and include the name, dose, and route of administration for drugs used during the preceding 6 months. It is important to include drugs used for recreational, as well as therapeutic, purposes and to include alcohol use in the history.

Preexisting disease

As shown in Table 22-4, some preexisting diseases increase the risk of surgery and anesthesia to the patient, contribute to perioperative problems, and may indicate the need for further in-depth assessment of the involved organ systems. Recognition of chronic and acute conditions helps the nurse anticipate potential problems and recognize special needs.

Mental and psychosocial assessment

Patients anticipating surgery may experience a variety of fears and hopes. The nurse must determine each patient's perceptions, emotions, behaviors, and support systems that may help or interfere with the ability to progress through the surgical period. The information that the nurse must gather can be obtained through careful and directed patient interactions. The unhurried and understanding nurse invites confidence and often gains much by listening. Psychosocial assessment of the surgical patient includes:

General perceptions about surgery
Sensorium and thought processes

TABLE 22-4 Preoperative Assessment

Abnormal findings	Relevance to anesthesia
GENERAL	
Obesity	Generally associated with higher surgical morbidity and mortality, greater risk of airway obstruction as a result of abundant soft tissue in upper airway, and a greater risk of aspiration
Anorexia nervosa	Likelihood of metabolic and electrolyte imbalances, and ECG changes
HEENT	
Intracranial disease	Increased incidence of respiratory depression
Otitis media	Risk for perforation of tympanic membrane during masking
Glaucoma, narrow angle	Need to avoid atropine
Lens inserts	Risk of dislodgement
Loose or carious teeth	Risk of dislodgement and aspiration
Mouth or neck mass	May require fiberoptic intubation
Recent upper respiratory infection	Increased risk for airflow obstruction (may persist for 5 weeks after illness)
PULMONARY	
Wheezing	Fourfold increase in perioperative respiratory complications
Smoking	Increased risk of bronchospasm
CARDIAC	
Congestive heart disease	At risk for decompensation as a result of stresses of surgery
Past myocardial infarction (MI)	Risk of reinfarction, especially if MI in past 6 months
Valvular disease	Risk dependent on stage of disease; may require subacute bacterial endocarditis prophylaxis
Bradydysrhythmias	May consider pacemaker management
Hypertension	May cancel if not controlled; may need to evaluate end-organ damage
GASTROINTESTINAL	
Hiatal hernia, esophagitis	May necessitate preoperative medication to control gastric acidity
Esophageal varices	May increase risk to a status IV classification (American Society of Anesthesiologists) because of risk of initiating hemorrhage with intubation
Liver disease	May affect metabolism and excretion of anesthetic agents
RENAL	
Kidney stones	Will need to prevent dehydration
Renal insufficiency	Stress of surgery may initiate failure; drugs may be excreted slowly
ENDOCRINE	
Diabetes	NPO status and/or IV glucose may affect control
Hyperthyroid	At risk for cardiac dysrhythmias, thyroid storm
Hypothyroid	May have decreased anesthetic requirement
Hyperlipidemia	Drug therapy may interact with surgery-related drugs
MUSCULOSKELETAL	
History of back surgery	May deter spinal anesthesia; may increase risks associated with intubation if surgery was in cervical area
Kyphosis	Requires special anesthesia arrangements if lung expansion is compromised
Cervical arthritis	At risk for neck injury during intubation
HEMATOLOGIC	
Anemia	Requires medical workup, may require preoperative treatment
Sickle cell disease	Requires special preoperative hydration
Polycythemia	At risk for perioperative complications
BLEEDING DISORDERS	May require additional preoperative evaluation, or perioperative treatment
NEUROLOGIC	
Seizures	Patients need a check of the therapeutic level of their medications
Myasthenia gravis	May exclude the use of muscle relaxants because of a decreased ability to reverse their effects

From Knight CG, Donnelly MK: Assessing the preoperative adult, *Nurse Pract* 13(1):8, 1988.

Attention and concentration
Attitude and motivation
Anxiety level and specific fears
Self-esteem and self-concept
Support from significant others
Psychologic assets and coping mechanisms

Planning and Implementation

The time for preoperative preparation varies considerably with individual situations and institutional policies. Generally, laboratory studies and medical tests conducted within 30 days of the surgery are acceptable, provided there are no intervening changes in patient status.

Nutrition

Patients who are scheduled for procedures under local or no anesthesia may be allowed a light breakfast or clear liquids only on the day of surgery. Patients scheduled for general or regional anesthesia are not allowed to eat or drink (nothing by mouth) for 6 to 8 hours before surgery. Food and drink are usually withheld from midnight until the time of surgery. This is necessary to minimize the risk of aspiration of gastric contents into the lungs during anesthesia. Patients may be allowed to take oral medications with a small amount (<30 mL) of water. If gastrointestinal obstruction is present, a nasogastric tube may be placed to empty the stomach.

When the surgery involves the abdominal cavity, especially when it involves the stomach, intestine, or rectum, a bowel prep may be ordered. This is done to empty the bowel and reduce the bacterial content, and it may include enemas, laxatives, and antibiotics. The use of bowel preps may deplete body fluids and result in dehydration and electrolyte imbalances, particularly when combined with the restriction of oral intake that occurs before surgery. Fluids may be administered by IV infusion to prevent or correct dehydration. The presence of nutritional deficiencies, dehydration, and electrolyte imbalances may require that additional time be allotted to replace deficits or correct imbalances before surgery.

Obesity greatly increases surgical and anesthetic risk and may make the operation technically more difficult for the surgeon. Fatty tissues heal slowly and are more prone to wound infections and dehiscence (separation). Hypoventilation and postoperative pulmonary complications are more common in the overweight patient, as is thrombophlebitis. If time permits, the severely overweight patient may be placed on a weight-loss program before surgery.

Elimination

Patients should be instructed to empty their bladders immediately before being transferred to the operating room or receiving their preoperative medication. This is done to prevent bladder distention or incontinence during anesthesia and surgery. Enemas and laxatives are not routinely used except as discussed for abdominal surgery. Because of the potential for injury once a patient has received preoperative medications, the patient should not be allowed out of bed without assistance.

Hygiene

The goals of skin preparations are to remove dirt and microbes from the skin and inhibit rebound growth of microbes with the least amount of tissue irritation. A patient may be instructed by the surgeon to shower or scrub the body area involved in the operation with an antibacterial soap or solution. The patient is usually instructed to wash vigorously several times the night before surgery. Removal of hair from the operative site should be done only as necessary. Depilatories and electric clippers may be used for hair removal before arrival in the surgical suite. To decrease the chance of wound infections, shaving of the operative site should be limited to the smallest area reasonable and should be done immediately before surgery, usually in the operating room. Abrasions, nicks, lacerations, or burns from preoperative shaving disrupt the mechanical barrier of the skin. Research has demonstrated an increase in infection rate as the time between the preoperative shave and the operation increases. Depilatories are sometimes used to avoid nicks or cuts, but these may cause skin irritation in sensitive patients, especially in the groin or axilla.

Valuables and prostheses

Jewelry should not be taken into the operating room. Valuables should be left with the patient's family or clearly labeled and stored according to institutional policy. Some patients may strongly object to removing a ring or may wish to take a medal or object of religious significance with them into the operating room. Exceptions may be made, depending on institutional policy, to accommodate the patient's desires. Rings should be taped on the finger or loosely tied to the patient's wrist, other objects should be labeled and care exercised to prevent loss or damage. Many patients are more willing to comply when it is explained to them that the policy is for their own protection and safety. Not only is there risk of loss or damage to jewelry, but it may also endanger the patient (metal objects may cause burns when electrocautery is used, hairpins may cause scalp injury, and rings may compromise circulation to fingers that swell during surgery).

All prostheses should be documented and, if not necessary, removed and stored before surgery. Contact lenses should always be removed; when they are

TABLE 22-5   Drug Management and Preoperative Preparation

Drug	Preoperative preparation	Potential intraoperative problems
Antianginal medications	Sublingual tablets can be continued until induction with IV nitroglycerin or paste administered intraoperatively; methemoglobin levels of heavy nitrate users should be monitored	Potentiate hypotensive effects of some anesthetic agents, particularly in hypovolemic patients
Antidysrhythmics	Continue to day of surgery	Potentiate neuromuscular blockers
Antibiotics	Avoid aminoglycosides (i.e., neomycin)	Aminoglycosides potentiate neuromuscular blockers and anesthetics that provide muscular relaxation
Anticoagulants	Replace oral anticoagulants with subcutaneous heparin to ensure prompt reversal, if necessary, with IV protamine sulfate	Oral anticoagulants are not reversed by protamine sulfate and it takes 24 to 48 hours for IV vitamin K_1 (phytonadione [AquaMEPHYTON]) to return prothrombin time to normal
Antidiabetics	Measure preoperative blood glucose; discontinue chlorpropamide 48 hours before surgery and continue all other oral hypoglycemics until the evening before surgery; begin glucose/insulin infusion before surgery if indicated	Intraoperative fluctuations in blood glucose
Antihypertensives	Continue methyldopa, reserpine, and guanethidine to day of surgery; continue clonidine parenterally to avoid severe rebound hypertension	Unstable blood pressure with wide fluctuations
Antiparkinson medications	Continue levodopa until night before surgery; if antiemetic is needed, antihistamine type (diphenhydramine) preferred over phenothiazine	Phenothiazines nullify antiparkinson effects of levodopa; aminoglycosides may interact to cause neuromuscular blockade
Antiseizure medications	Phenytoin augments nondepolarizing neuromuscular blockade	Continue phenytoin and phenobarbital to day of surgery
Beta-blockers	Continue to day of surgery; may be given IV if oral route contraindicated	Potentiate cardiac depressant effects of some anesthetics
Cardiac glycosides	Continue to day of surgery; assess patient for signs of digitalis toxicity or potassium depletion and correct if present	Potentiate nondepolarizing muscle relaxants
Corticosteroids	Continue to day of surgery; administer 100 mg hydrocortisone 1 hour before surgery	Patients who are on corticosteroid therapy (7.5 mg daily prednisone or equivalent) for at least 2 months preceding surgery require intraoperative and postoperative supplementation
Psychotropes	Monoamine oxidase inhibitors (MAOIs) should be discontinued 2 weeks before surgery	MAOIs interact with narcotic analgesics, (i.e., meperidine [Demerol]), local anesthetic/epinephrine combinations, and other vasopressors
	Continue tricyclic antidepressants, lithium, and phenothiazine antipsychotics to day of surgery	Lithium prolongs the effect of depolarizing muscle relaxants

From Waugaman WR et al: *Principles and practice of nurse anesthesia*, Norwalk, Conn, 1988, Appleton & Lange.

left in the eyes, corneal ulcerations or displacement may result. Chewing gum, partial dentures, or orthodontic appliances should be removed to prevent displacement into the throat where they may be aspirated or may cause obstruction during induction of anesthesia. Removal of dentures, eyeglasses, and hearing aids creates a feeling of helplessness in the patient, increases anxiety, and may make communication with the patient difficult. When possible, they may be permitted in the operating room, but their presence must be made known to the operating team members, who may sometimes remove them and protect them immediately before or after induction of anesthesia.

Medications

As shown in Table 22-5, drug therapy has the potential to create intraoperative problems and must be considered in the preoperative preparation. Administration of most medications should be continued throughout the perioperative period, including the day of surgery. Some of the more notable exceptions that should be discontinued or have dosage adjusted before surgery are anticoagulants and aspirin (may increase operative blood loss), monoamine oxidase inhibitors (dangerous interactions may occur with many anesthetic drugs), and hypoglycemics (may cause severe hypoglycemia when oral intake is stopped). Drug administration may be changed to the intramuscular (IM) or IV route if the oral route is contraindicated.

Special preoperative medications may be ordered by the anesthetist or surgeon. Preoperative medications are given to reduce anxiety and facilitate a smooth and safe induction of anesthesia. For maximum effectiveness, administration should occur about 60 minutes before induction of anesthesia. Traditionally, preoperative medications consisted of a combination of one or more of the following drugs: a narcotic, an antisialagogue/antimuscarinic (drugs that decrease secretions), and a barbiturate/tranquilizer. Preanesthetic medications are still used for specific purposes but with less frequency than in the past. There has been an increase in the use of oral medications rather than IM injections. Table 22-6 lists some of the more commonly used preoperative medications. Pharmacologic preparations are not a substitute for adequate emotional preparation. Often psychologic preparation will decrease or eliminate the need for antianxiety agents or tranquilizers.

When preoperative drugs are administered, the patient should be advised of the drug's effects and protected from injury. Bed rails should be raised, the call button placed near the patient, and the patient instructed to remain in bed. The patient is monitored closely for adverse effects, especially for signs of respiratory depression or excessive sedation after the administration of tranquilizers, barbiturates, or narcotics.

Psychologic preparation of the patient

The short-term effects of psychologic preparation before surgery have been shown to reduce the need for preoperative medications and postoperative pain medication. Preoperative interventions should supply information and reassurance about the events that will occur as well as discuss coping mechanisms the patient can use to handle stress and discomfort. Planning should be based on the patient's desire for information, the patient's attitude toward surgery, and the anticipated effect of the surgery, as perceived by the patient. Some patients may want only the essential information, whereas others may want to know every detail.

Preoperative information allows the patient to mentally "rehearse" and to develop realistic expectations and coping mechanisms. The nurse can provide emotional support by fostering the patient's sense of control over his or her own destiny (e.g., teaching techniques for prevention of postoperative complications and to speed recovery). Reassurance is provided to the patient for many concerns, such as the availability of medications to alleviate postoperative pain. Effective methods for coping with stress may be reviewed while reinforcing methods found particularly effective by the patient in the past.

Preparations should also include family and significant others whenever possible. Before surgery, the anxiety and fears of family influence the patient's own level of anxiety. Patient anxiety also influences the family's anxiety. Many patients find the presence of a supporting and familiar individual comforting. A family member may be permitted to accompany the patient to the preoperative holding area. Waiting can be extremely stressful for the family and friends of a patient in surgery. They should know where to wait while the patient is in surgery, and if possible, how to get periodic updates during a long operation. When the family desires or when they will be involved in the postoperative care of the patient, they should be included in the preoperative instructions.

Teaching

Preoperative instruction should include general information, listed in the box on p. 473, to inform the patient about the perioperative experience and to pave the way for patient participation in the recovery period. Based on needs identified in the nursing assessment, teaching is built on the patient's knowledge, understanding, and expectations.

Patients who are well-informed and aware of

TABLE 22-6   Pharmacology Summary: Preanesthetic Medications

Classification	Trade name	Adult dosage	Route	Purpose
SEDATIVE-HYPNOTICS				
Chloral hydrate		0.25-1 g	PO	Promote sleep the night before surgery
Pentobarbital sodium	Nembutal sodium	50-200 mg	PO, IM	
Secobarbital sodium	Seconal sodium	50-200 mg	PO, IM	
Flurazepam HCl	Dalmane	15-30 mg	PO	
NARCOTICS				
Butorphanol tartrate	Stadol	1-2 mg	IM, IV	Provide preoperative analgesia
Fentanyl citrate	Sublimaze	0.05-0.1 mg	IM	
Meperidine HCl	Demerol	50-100 mg	IM, IV	
Morphine sulfate		5-15 mg	IM, IV	
ANTICHOLINERGICS				
Atropine sulfate		0.4-0.6 mg	IM, IV	Decrease oral secretions and interrupt vagal nerve impulses, which slow the heart
Glycopyrrolate	Robinul	0.2-0.4 mg	IM, IV	
Scopolamine hydrobromide	Hyoscine	0.2-0.6 mg	IM, IV	
TRANQUILIZERS/ANTIANXIETY AGENTS				
Diazepam	Valium	5-15 mg	PO, IM, IV	Decrease anxiety and promote a calm preoperative state
Midazolam HCl	Versed	1-4 mg	IM, IV	
Lorazepam	Ativan	0.5-2 mg	PO, IM	
Hydroxyzine HCl	Atarax	25-100 mg	PO, IM	
H$_2$ RECEPTOR ANTAGONISTS				
Cimetidine	Tagamet	300-600 mg	PO	Decrease the amount of gastric secretions and increase the pH of gastric secretions
		300 mg	IM, IV	
Ranitidine	Zantac	150 mg	PO	
		50 mg	IM, IV	
Famotidine	Pepcid	40 mg	PO	
		20 mg	IV	
Nizatidine	Axid	150-300 mg	PO	
GASTRIC MOTILITY STIMULANT				
Metoclopramide	Reglan	10-20 mg	PO, IM, IV	Decrease volume of gastric contents
ANTACID				
Sodium citrate	Bicitra	15-30 mL	PO	Increase gastric pH
ANTIEMETICS				
Droperidol	Inapsine	0.5-2.5 mg	IM, IV	Prevent postoperative nausea and vomiting; also used as antianxiety agents, will potentiate narcotics
Promethazine HCl	Phenergan	12.5-25 mg	IM, IV	

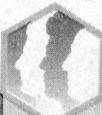

GERIATRIC CONSIDERATIONS

The Older Adult and Surgery

Surgery and anesthesia impose stress with more pronounced effects in the elderly patient, who has a lower ability to adapt or compensate than a younger patient. Studies of surgical risk and outcome often show a higher rate of complications in the older population; however, the results have been generally inconclusive as to the degree of risk, if any, that can be attributed to age alone. Chronologic age is a poor indicator of outcomes, since although a generalized decline in organ function occurs with age, the geriatric patient is more than just a feeble adult. Specific factors that increase surgical risk or the need for nursing interventions are related to disease states, nutritional status, mental health, and functional abilities.

Special preoperative assessment and management of the geriatric patient are essential. The nursing history can reveal age-related changes and coexisting diseases. The elderly often are taking several medications and are particularly at risk for adverse drug interactions or reactions during the perioperative period. All medications, including nonprescription drugs, should be documented. Preoperative medications, when used, are given in reduced dosages. Mental status, general mood, and attitude toward surgery should be documented and considered when planning care. Preoperative teaching is particularly important to allay fears and improve postoperative cooperation. Learning may take longer in the elderly, and sensory impairments and environmental distractions should be considered when teaching. Emphasis should be placed on early postoperative mobility, pulmonary function, safety, and problems with elimination. Because the elderly may not easily adapt to altered routines and schedules, every effort should be made to preserve the normal time schedule and routines of the geriatric patient.

The elderly, commonly compromised by chronic disease, a body that is immunosuppressed, and a foreshortened life, require a nurse advocate. It is the nurse who must intervene on the elderly's behalf with the physician or family. To increase chances for survival, preoperative assessment is imperative:

1. Determine the feasibility of surgical treatment. Which will be longer, the natural prognosis of the disease or life expectancy?
2. If surgery is not performed, what effect will this have on the quality of life?
3. Will aggressive surgical intervention result in death?
4. Can surgery be on an elective basis before an acute exacerbation occurs?
5. Whether the surgery should be extensive (i.e., radical, modified, staged) will depend on the physiologic state of the patient, as well as the disease process.

---

what will be happening during their surgical experience are better able to deal with the stress of surgery. Patients should know what tests will be performed, when and why they should not eat or drink before surgery, what the preoperative preparations entail, and when they will occur (bowel and skin preparations, preoperative medication, transfer to preoperative holding and surgery), as well as an explanation of the postanesthesia care unit (PACU) or recovery room and postoperative care. The patient should be prepared for dressings or other treatments or interventions that are anticipated, such as a nasogastric tube, urinary catheter, chest tube, or wound drains. A tour of the preoperative and postanesthesia areas and introduction of the patient to the personnel who will be involved in patient care promotes continuity of care and helps the patient prepare for the operative experience.

Respiratory care

There is a decline in lung ventilation and gas exchange after surgery. The magnitude of diminished respiratory function varies with the individual patient, the length of anesthesia, and the surgical site. To help eliminate inhaled anesthetics, prevent alveolar collapse, and mobilize secretions after surgery, the patient must be taught deep breathing (or "sustained maximal inspiration") and coughing techniques. Deep breathing or sustained maximal inspiration is done by having the patient take a slow deep breath through the nose, hold the breath for a few seconds, and then slowly exhale through the mouth. Abdominal breathing is most effective for deep breathing and can be taught by instructing the patient to place the hands over the lower ribs and upper abdomen. While deep breathing, the patient should concentrate on feeling the abdominal excursion with each breath. This also serves as an excellent relaxation technique for many patients.

After several deep breaths, the patient should be instructed to cough deeply from the chest, not the throat. Secretions that are in the lungs may be moved up the respiratory tract by deep breathing and stimulate the cough reflex, or the patient may need to voluntarily cough.

PATIENT EDUCATION GUIDE
Preoperative Instruction

General information
Restrictions of oral intake
Bowel or skin preparations
Preoperative testing
Medications
Preoperative holding area
Waiting room for family
General timetable of perioperative events

Outpatients
Where and when to come for surgery
What to wear
Who must accompany patient

Postoperative care
Postanesthesia recovery unit routines
Coughing and deep breathing
Splinting techniques
Turning and body movement
Pain management
Activities and restrictions
Postoperative dressings or drains
Special treatments or checks
Discharge instructions

Patients who undergo abdominal or thoracic operations usually experience the greatest decline in respiratory function after surgery. Splinting is a technique useful for minimizing incisional discomfort while these patients deep breathe and cough. When done by either patient or nurse, splinting is accomplished by pressing the hands, a blanket, a pillow, or a similar soft object on the incision to reduce strain. In addition to splinting a painful incision, analgesics should be administered to control pain before deep breathing and coughing.

Turning and body movement

To prevent venous stasis and to improve muscle tone, circulation, and respiratory function, the patient should be taught and encouraged to move about after surgery. While in bed, the patient should turn from side to side at least every 2 hours. Extremities may be exercised by flexing, extending, and rotating the ankle, knee, hip, wrist, elbow, and shoulder joints, unless contraindicated. The patient should be taught to rhythmically contract and relax the major muscle groups in the body, which helps improve circulation. To be effective, the exercises should be done several times each hour while

awake. The patient should be informed of the anticipated postoperative activity level, encouraged to be out of bed and ambulating as soon as possible after surgery, and informed of any restrictions that may be placed on activities.

Pain management

Most, but not all, patients experience some degree of pain after surgery. Postsurgical pain contributes to patient discomfort, slower recovery, and may compromise patient outcomes. Clinical surveys indicate that routine use of intramuscular injections of narcotics on an "as needed" basis provides inadequate pain relief in about one-half of postoperative patients. A focused and aggressive approach to pain prevention, assessment, and management should be implemented in the perioperative period to effectively treat postoperative pain and improve patient outcomes. Preoperative preparation should include several steps:
- Discuss the patient's previous experience with pain, beliefs about pain, and preferences for pain management.
- Give the patient information about pain management therapies and their rationale for use.
- With the patient, develop a plan for pain assessment and management.
- Select and teach the use of a pain assessment tool and determine preoperatively the level of pain requiring adjustment of analgesia or additional interventions.
- Provide the patient with information and training in nonpharmacologic pain control options.
- Emphasize communication of unrelieved pain; factual reporting of pain rather than stoicism or exaggeration, and that pain prevention and early treatment are easier than relieving established pain.

See Figure 22-3, pain treatment flowchart: Preoperative and intraoperative phases.

Emergencies

Preoperative interventions may be limited by the urgency of the impending surgery or the condition of the patient. Nursing interventions should cover the essentials with a minimal amount of time. During the sometimes hurried preparations, the nurse should take extra care to consider emotional needs and prepare the patient and family for the operation by providing information and reassurance and answering questions.

Evaluation

Evaluation is an ongoing process in preoperative nursing. Goals may be assessed by asking the patient

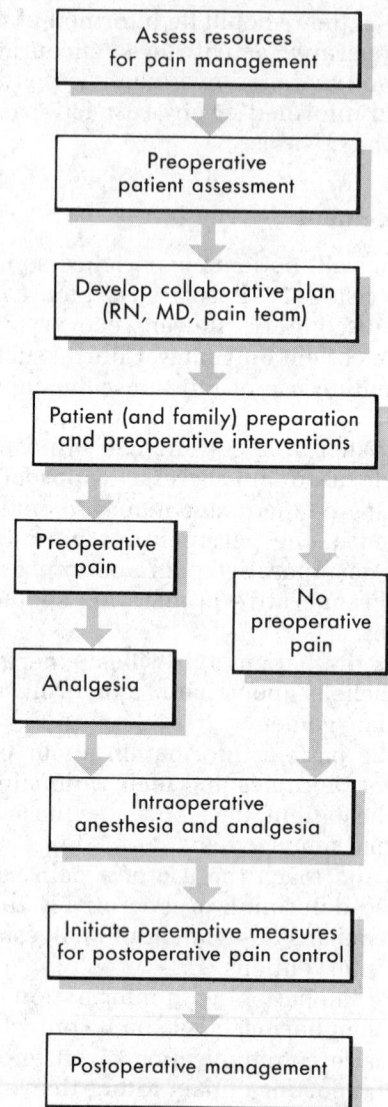

FIGURE 22-3   Critical Thinking Guide: Pain Treatment in the Pre- and Intraoperative Patient. (From US Department of Health and Human Services, Feb 1992.)

to repeat the information back or demonstrate activities, such as splinting an incision or breathing exercises. The preoperative checklist provides a way to check and document that all essential steps of preoperative preparation have been completed before entering the intraoperative period. Evaluation relates to the specific nursing goals established for the preoperative period for each patient and covers the collection of data, preparation for surgery and anesthesia, reduction of anxiety, and preoperative education. All the appropriate data should be clearly documented on the medical record. The patient should be able to demonstrate a general knowledge of the course of perioperative events and postoperative care and an appropriate anxiety level as identified in the nursing care plan. Evaluation relating to the specific nursing goals established for the intra-

operative and postoperative period for each patient is conducted throughout the perioperative period. A final evaluation of goal attainment is not possible until the perioperative period is complete, since the perioperative preparations encompass the entire perioperative period.

Just as preoperative planning takes into account the patient's goals and desires, so must the evaluation assess how well these goals have been attained. The best evaluator of patient goal attainment is the patient. Is he satisfied that his goals have been reached for the preoperative period?

Once the preoperative nursing and patient goals have been met, the patient is ready to enter the next phase of the perioperative period. The preoperative period provides the nurse with the opportunity to establish a firm foundation for the remaining perioperative care. The ultimate success and outcome of the perioperative period depend heavily on the nursing care provided in the preoperative period.

Documentation

Informed consent

Except in unusual situations, informed consent must be obtained before surgery. In order for a surgical consent to be valid, three basic criteria must be met. The patient's decision must be *voluntary,* the patient must be *informed,* and the patient must be *competent* to understand the information and alternatives. Spouses or children are not able to give consent for competent adults.

One of the caveats of preoperative nursing is *no patient should be administered the preoperative medication until the consent has been signed!* A patient is not considered competent to make an informed decision while under the influence of a potentially mind-altering drug. If a narcotic, sedative, or tranquilizing drug has been administered before signing the surgical consent, the drug effects must be allowed to wear off before consent can be given.

A patient may revoke his consent to surgery at any time before the operation. It may become apparent to the nurse that the patient does not understand the procedure or incorrectly believes that there are no risks or adverse consequences involved. When this situation occurs, the nurse should inform the immediate supervisor and the responsible physician of the patient's change of mind or lack of comprehension. Remember that informed consent must be obtained before the patient's preoperative medication to be valid. Informed consent is discussed more thoroughly in Chapter 10.

Patient record

Before transferring the patient to surgery, the patient's record is reviewed for completeness. Re-

quired documentation includes:
>   Vital signs
>   Allergies
>   Prostheses
>   Special patient needs
>   Consent forms—signed, witnessed, and dated
>   Patient teaching
>   Complete health history

If ordered:
>   Radiology studies
>   Laboratory values
>   Electrocardiogram results
>   Administration of preoperative medications
>   Completed consultation reports

Patients will not be able to identify themselves while under general anesthesia. *All patients must be wearing an identification bracelet when they are transferred to the operating room.*

CRITICAL THINKING QUESTIONS

1 Define the perioperative period, and list nursing goals for this time.

2 List two methods of classifying surgery and, using both methods, classify the surgery for a patient scheduled to undergo a laparoscopy to evaluate chronic pelvic pain.

3 What physiologic changes may occur as a result of surgical stress?

4 Identify fears commonly associated with surgery, and explain how you might respond to them.

5 What preoperative laboratory tests would most likely be needed for a 55-year-old male patient who smokes but has no other history suggestive of systemic disease?

6 What criteria must be met for a patient to have surgery as an outpatient?

7 What are some of the advantages of outpatient surgery?

8 Identify nursing care that is commonly performed in the preoperative receiving area.

9 Describe the purpose of the preoperative assessment.

10 What questions would you ask as part of the psychosocial assessment of the preoperative patient?

11 If a patient wanted to wear jewelry into the operating room, what would your response be?

12 List information that you would include in a general teaching plan for the preoperative patient.

13 How would you evaluate a patient's readiness for surgery?

BIBLIOGRAPHY

Current

1. American Association of Operating Room Nurses, Inc: *AORN standards and recommended practices for perioperative nursing,* Denver, 1988, The Association.
2. Applegeet CJ: Nursing aspects of outpatient surgery, *Urol Clin North Am* 14(1):21, 1987.
3. Burden N: Regional anesthesia: what patients—and nurses—need to know, *RN* p 56, May, 1988.
4. Chitwood LB: Unveiling the mysteries of anesthesia, *Nurs '87,* p 53, Feb, 1987.
5. Cruz LD: Ambulatory surgery—the next decade, *AORN J* 53(1):241, 1990.
6. Eddy ME, Coslow BI: Preparation for ambulatory surgery: a patient education program, *J Post Anesthesia Nurs* 6(1):5, 1991.
7. Goulart AE: Preoperative teaching for surgical patients, *Periop Nurs Q* 3(2):8, 1987.
8. Hardy JD: *Hardy's textbook of surgery,* ed 2, Philadelphia, 1988, JB Lippincott.
9. Hill GJ: *Outpatient surgery,* ed 3, Philadelphia, 1988, WB Saunders.
10. Kneedler JA, Dodge GH: *Perioperative patient care,* ed 2, Boston, 1987, Blackwell Scientific Publications.
11. Knight CG, Donnelly MK: Assessing the preoperative adult, *Nurse Pract* 13(1):6, 1988.
12. Llewellyn JG: Short stay surgery, *AORN J* 53(5):1179, 1991.
13. McConnell EA: *Clinical considerations in perioperative nursing: preventive aspects of care,* Philadelphia, 1987, JB Lippincott.
14. Nyamathi A, Kashiwabara A: Preoperative anxiety, its effect on cognitive thinking, *AORN J* 47(1):164, 1988.
15. Omerod BH: Perioperative nursing care of the elderly outpatient, *Periop Nurs Q* 3(2):22, 1987.
16. Squibb CB: Outpatient surgical evaluations, *Nurs Management* 19(1):32L, 1988.
17. Stanfield V: Perioperative education: changing to meet short stay needs, *J Post Anesthesia Nurs* 2(2):74, 1987.
18. Wong CA: Preoperative patient preparation, *J Post Anesthesia Nurs* 5(3):149, 1990.
19. Zambricki CS: Preoperative preparation and evaluation. In Waugaman WR et al: *Principles and practice of nurse anesthesia,* Norwalk, Conn, 1988, Appleton & Lange.

Classic

20. Anand KJS: The stress response to surgical trauma: from physiological basis to therapeutic implications, *Prog Food Nutr Sci V* 10:67, 1986.
21. Devine EC, Cook TD: A meta-analysis of effects of psychoeducational interventions on length of postsurgical stay, *Nurs Res* 32(5):267, 1983.
22. Devine EC, Cook TD: Clinical and cost-saving effects of psychoeducational interventions with surgical patients: a meta-analysis, *Res Nurs Health* 9(2):89, 1986.
23. Johnston M: Pre-operative emotional states and postoperative recovery, *Adv Psychosom Med* 15:1, 1986.
24. McCartney DJ: Implementing wellness philosophy in an ambulatory surgery center, *Periop Nurs Q* 1(1):63, 1985.
25. Mauldin BC: The preoperative assessment carries the patient through the surgical experience, *AORN J* 39(4):770, 1984.
26. Rabinow J: Avoiding legal risks in the short procedure unit (S.P.U.), *Nurs Life* 6(1):24, 1986.

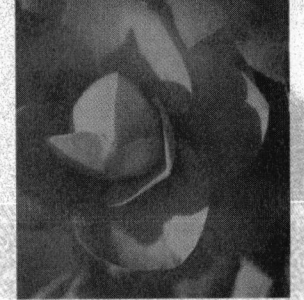

CHAPTER TWENTY-THREE

Intraoperative Nursing

LEARNING OBJECTIVES

1 Describe the roles of the surgical team members and the importance of the team approach.
2 Differentiate among the different forms of anesthesia.
3 Contrast the effects of common surgical positions on the respiratory system, cardiovascular system, peripheral nerves, and skin.
4 Apply the principles of surgical asepsis to intraoperative nursing care.
5 Recognize breaks in surgical aseptic technique.
6 Identify common threats to the safety of the intraoperative patient.
7 List nursing measures to decrease intraoperative heat loss.
8 Demonstrate appropriate emotional support and care of the operative patient.
9 Identify information that should be shared between the operating room and recovery unit when the patient is transferred after surgery.

KEY TERMS

anesthesia, p. 478
caudal anesthesia, p. 481
circulating nurse, p. 478
epidural anesthesia, p. 481
general anesthesia, p. 479
local anesthesia, p. 481

malignant hyperthermia, p. 483
regional anesthesia, p. 479
scrub nurse, p. 478
spinal anesthesia, p. 481
surgical asepsis, p. 487

AFTER PREOPERATIVE preparation and evaluation, the patient enters the intraoperative period. This period begins with the transfer of the patient into the operating room and ends with the admission of the patient to the postanesthesia care unit. Nursing care during this phase may encompass a range of activities directed toward the patient experiencing surgery. The focus of nursing care changes from that of preparing the patient for the operative experience to that of patient protector, advocate, and provider of care because of the patient's increased dependency during the operative period. The general goal of nursing care is to promote an uneventful surgical procedure while protecting the patient from injury.

THE INTRAOPERATIVE ENVIRONMENT

The surgical suite is a unique environment, unlike any other in the hospital or clinic setting. It is an acute care unit designed to provide to the extent possible a controlled and germ-free environment for the conduct of the operative procedures. The physical environment is closely controlled; the flow of personnel, supplies, and equipment is restricted; and the unit is usually close to the postanesthesia care unit, intensive care unit, and other support services, such as laboratory, blood bank, radiology, and surgical pathology.

The Operating Room Environment

Most surgical suites are divided into three areas or zones to regulate traffic. The first area is the semipublic area where people are permitted to wear street clothes and mix with staff in scrub attire. This may include the patient receiving area, some offices, the front desk, and locker rooms. The second area is the semirestricted areas, such as the hallways and work rooms adjacent to the operating room. Required attire includes caps, shoe covers on clean shoes, and scrub clothes. The restricted area includes the operating rooms and areas for preparation of sterile instruments. Proper attire for the restricted area is the same as for the semirestricted area with the addition of face masks.

The Surgical Team

When the patient arrives in the operating room, a team of professionals is present to participate in the care. The surgeon and assistants, the anesthetist, and the intraoperative nurses must function harmoniously to provide a safe, comfortable, and therapeutic environment for the patient, who totally depends on the surgical team for his welfare and safety. The success and ease with which the operation is accomplished greatly depends on group dynamics as professionals work to achieve common goals.

Anesthetist

Anesthesia may be provided either by an anesthesiologist or nurse anesthetist. The anesthesiologist is a physician who administers anesthesia, and the nurse anesthetist is a registered nurse who administers anesthesia. The nurse is a certified registered nurse anesthetist (CRNA). The anesthesiologist or nurse anesthetist may work independently or they may work together as an "anesthesia care team" to provide anesthesia to the patient.

Surgeon

The surgeon is the physician who performs the operative procedure. The surgeon's responsibilities include management of the preoperative medical evaluation, conduct of the operative procedure, and postoperative management of the patient.

Surgical assistants and allied personnel

The surgical assistant, sometimes referred to as "first assistant," aids the surgeon in performing the operation. The **scrub nurse** is assigned duties requiring sterile technique in the operating room. The **circulating nurse** is responsible for the nonsterile nursing functions within the operating room. Examples of nursing activities of the operating room nurse functioning in either the scrub or circulating role are listed in the box below.

Additional members of the operating team or support services may assist with intraoperative care, depending on the needs of the patient. Some of these personnel include blood bank personnel, pharmacists, radiologists, perfusionists, pathologists, and many members of the allied health professions.

Anesthesia

Anesthesia means the absence of pain ("an" meaning without and "esthesia" meaning awareness or feeling). Anesthesia may be divided into three categories: general, regional, and monitored anesthesia care.

OPERATING ROOM NURSING ACTIVITIES

Assurance of information and supportive preoperative teaching specifically related to the surgical intervention and the operating room nursing care

Identification of the individual

Verification of the surgical site

Verification of operative consent and procedure and reports of essential diagnostic procedures

Positioning according to physiologic procedures

Adherence to principles of asepsis

Assurance of appropriate and properly functioning equipment and supplies for the individual

Provision of comfort measures and supportive care to the individual

Environmental monitoring and safety

Psychologic and physiologic monitoring of the individual

Evaluation of outcomes in relation to the identified nursing activities

Communication of intraoperative information to significant others and members of the health care team

From *AORN Standards and Recommended Practices for Perioperative Nursing*, The Association of Operating Room Nurses, Inc., Denver, 1992.

General anesthesia

General anesthesia refers to a drug-induced state in which analgesia, amnesia, muscle relaxation, and unconsciousness occur. General anesthetics may be administered by inhalation or by oral, rectal, or parenteral routes, with the inhalation and intravenous routes most commonly used. Inhalation agents are useful because of their ease of administration and elimination through the respiratory system. They are administered either as gases or as vapors of volatile liquids through an anesthesia delivery system and a face mask or endotracheal tube. With the exception of nitrous oxide, inhalation anesthetics can produce all the required elements of general anesthesia. Currently used inhalation anesthetics are listed in Table 23-1. Anesthesia is also commonly administered by the intravenous route. However, single intravenous drugs generally do not produce all of the elements of general anesthesia. Several intravenous drugs are usually given, each with a specific purpose. The term *balanced anesthesia* has been used to describe the administration of several drugs to produce the desired components of general anesthesia. Neuromuscular blocking drugs may be administered to provide skeletal muscle relaxation or paralysis to facilitate some types of surgery and intubation of the trachea for airway management. Intravenous drugs commonly used in the administration of general anesthesia are presented in Table 23-2.

Anesthetic hazards

Anesthetic hazards to the patient relate to the drugs administered, the equipment used to deliver anesthetic agents, and the process of administering and managing anesthesia. There is inherent toxicity in the drugs used for anesthesia as well as dangers from procedures, equipment, human error, and the operating room environment. The risk of anesthesia is also tied to surgical risk. Complications or untoward reactions may be as small as a sore throat or as significant as death. Current estimates of anesthetic-related mortality are generally less than 1 in 10,000 anesthetics. Although anesthesia-related injuries or death are uncommon, extraordinary measures are used to minimize risk, including careful preoperative evaluation and extensive intraoperative monitoring of patients.

Regional anesthesia

Regional anesthesia refers to techniques that render only a specific region of the body insensitive to pain. Regional anesthesia provides a pain-free state with good operating conditions for certain operative procedures without producing loss of consciousness. Anesthesia results from blocking nerve transmission before the impulses reach the central nervous system; motor block occurs from a block of nerve transmission after the impulses leave the central nervous system. This is accomplished by depositing a local

---

TABLE 23-1   Pharmacology Summary: Inhalation Anesthetic Agents

Agent	Toxicity	Side effects/adverse reactions
VOLATILE LIQUIDS		
Halothane (Fluothane, Somnothane)	May cause liver damage or "halothane hepatitis"	Hypotension, cardiovascular depression, lowered body temperature, respiratory depression, malignant hyperthermia, emergence shivering, trembling, confusion, hallucinations, nervousness, increased excitability
Enflurane (Ethrane)		See halothane
Isoflurane (Forane)	Nephrotoxic (unlikely because of very limited metabolism)	See halothane
COMPRESSED GAS		
Nitrous oxide	May be teratogenic with prolonged exposure	Weak anesthetic, no muscle relaxation, must always be administered with at least 20% oxygen to avoid hypoxia, may cause bowel distention, may contribute to postoperative nausea and vomiting

TABLE 23-2   Injectable Drugs for Anesthesia

Generic name	Trade name	Comments
BARBITURATES		
Methohexital sodium	Brevital	Used for rapid, pleasant induction of anesthesia; has the shortest duration of action (5 to 7 minutes) of the barbiturates
Thiamylal sodium	Surital	Used for rapid, pleasant induction of anesthesia; duration of action about 15 minutes
Thiopental sodium	Pentothal	Used for rapid, pleasant induction of anesthesia, duration of action about 15 minutes
BENZODIAZEPINES		
Diazepam	Valium	Used in low doses for sedation amnesic and anxiolytic properties, high doses may be used for anesthetic induction, do not mix with other liquids, very irritating to tissues when administered IV or IM
Midazolam	Versed	See diazepam; less irritating to tissues with 3 to 4 times the potency of diazepam
NARCOTICS		
Alfentanil hydrochloride	Alfenta	A potent, short-acting narcotic analgesic used with nitrous oxide and a muscle relaxant for general anesthesia or as a supplement to an anesthetic gas
Fentanyl citrate	Sublimaze	See alfentanil; longer acting than alfentanil
Sufentanil citrate	Sufenta	See alfentanil; longer acting than fentanyl
NEUROMUSCULAR BLOCKING DRUGS		
Succinylcholine chloride	Anectine Quelicin Sucostrin	Ultra-short duration of action (2 to 8 minutes); may cause cardiac dysrhythmias, postoperative myalgias; may trigger malignant hyperthermia in susceptible patients
Mivacurium chloride	Mivacron	Short duration; may cause histamine release and transient hypotension
Metocurine iodide	Metubine	Intermediate duration of action
Gallamine triethiodide	Flaxedil	Intermediate duration of action may increase heart rate
Atracurium bresylate	Tracrium	Intermediate duration of action; may cause histamine release
Tubocurarine chloride (curare)	Tubarine	Intermediate duration of action; may cause histamine release and transient hypotension
Vecuronium bromide	Norcuron	Intermediate duration of action
Pancuronium bromide	Pavulon	Long duration of action; may increase heart rate
Pipecuronium bromide	Arduan	Long duration of action
Doxicurium chloride	Nuromax	Long duration of action
MISCELLANEOUS		
Etomidate	Amidate	Nonbarbiturate used for induction (bolus) or maintenance of anesthesia (infusion) during short anesthetics; may transiently suppress adrenal function
Propofol	Diprivan	Nonbarbiturate used for induction (bolus) or maintenance of anesthesia (infusion) during use of short anesthetics
Ketamine	Ketaject	Used for induction and/or maintenance of anesthesia; may be administered IM or IV, produces a cataleptic anesthesia with profound analgesia; during recovery, unpleasant dreams, hallucinations, and delirium may occur

anesthetic solution along the path of a nerve. This form of anesthesia is sometimes called *conduction anesthesia,* because it interrupts nerve impulse conduction. The regional nerve blocks are designated by their site of action.

Spinal anesthesia

Spinal anesthesia, or subarachnoid block, is accomplished by injecting an anesthetic solution into the cerebral spinal fluid that surrounds the lower spinal cord and nerve roots (Figure 23-1). In the adult, the spinal cord terminates at the level of the first or occasionally the second lumbar vertebra. A special needle is placed into the spinal canal below the level of the spinal cord, and the anesthetic is injected into the cerebrospinal fluid. This results in a block of nerve transmission through the spinal nerve roots. Spinal anesthesia is useful for many procedures involving the lower abdomen and extremities.

Epidural and caudal anesthesia

The injection of a local anesthetic into the space adjacent to the dural membrane, also known as the epidural space (see Figure 23-1), of the spinal column is called **epidural anesthesia.** It is useful for many of the same procedures as spinal anesthesia. Epidural anesthesia is commonly used for obstetric procedures as well as surgical procedures. Low con-

centrations of local anesthetics or narcotics can be used for relief of labor discomfort or postoperative pain. When the local anesthetic is injected into the epidural space through the sacral canal, it is referred to as **caudal anesthesia.**

Peripheral nerve blocks

Local anesthetics can be injected around most peripheral nerves. Peripheral nerve blocks provide anesthesia in the area of distribution of the blocked nerve. The decision to use a peripheral nerve block depends on surgical requirements and individual considerations as well as the expertise of the anesthetist who administers the nerve block.

Local anesthesia

Local anesthesia refers to the topical application or infiltration into tissues of an anesthetic agent that

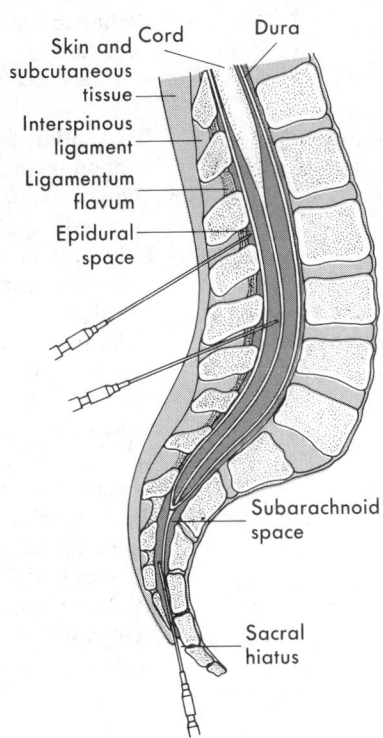

FIGURE 23-1 Sagittal section demonstrating needle placement for spinal (subarachnoid), epidural, and caudal nerve blocks.

TOXIC EFFECTS OF LOCAL ANESTHETICS

Central nervous system

As the blood levels of local anesthetics increase to toxic levels, the initial toxic reactions are excitatory in nature and include the following:
Light-headedness
Dizziness
Tinnitus
Difficulty in mental focusing
Slurred speech
Shivering
Muscular twitching
Tremors
Convulsions
If the blood concentration continues to rise, generalized central nervous system depression will occur, eventually leading to respiratory arrest

Cardiovascular system

At low concentrations, local anesthetics have a stimulatory effect on cardiac and vascular smooth muscle; at high concentrations, myocardial depression and vasodilation occur; if the toxic levels continue to increase, conduction in the heart is slowed and bradycardia develops; if the blood concentration continues to rise, cardiovascular collapse will occur
Some local anesthetics, most notably lidocaine and procaine, have an antidysrhythmic effect that occurs at concentrations well below the toxic range
Cocaine is unique among the local anesthetics in that it consistently causes profound and widespread vasoconstriction

TABLE 23-3   Pharmacology Summary: Selected Injected Local Anesthetics

Generic name	Trade name	Metabolism	Use	Dosage and administration
SHORT-ACTING (½-1 HR)				
Chloroprocaine	Nesacaine Nescaine-CE	Ester compound-metabolized by cholinesterases in plasma and liver to a PABA compound; excretion: kidneys	Nesacaine—infiltration and regional anesthesia. Nescaine-CE for caudal and epidural anesthesia	Usual adult dosage for infiltration nerve blocks: 30-800 mg as 1% or 2% solutions, depending on site and length of surgical procedure. Caudal and epidural: 40-500 mg as 2% or 3% solution (without epinephrine)
Procaine HCl	Novocain	Ester compound—same as above	Infiltration, nerve block, spinal anesthesia, epidural block	Usual adult dosage for infiltration: 0.25%-0.5% solution, 350-600 mg, up to 1 gram. Peripheral nerve block: 500 mg as 0.5%, 1%, or 2% solution. Spinal and epidural dosage vary with individual client, procedure, and degree of anesthesia desired. Pediatric dosage: not available
INTERMEDIATE DURATION (1-3 HR)				
Lidocaine	Xylocaine	Amide compound. Metabolism: liver to active and toxic metabolites. Excretion: kidneys	Infiltration, nerve block, spinal, epidural	Usual adult dosage depends on site and length of surgical procedure. Lidocaine is available with and without epinephrine
Mepivacaine HCl	Carbocaine HCl	Amide compound—see above	Infiltration, nerve blocks, caudal, epidural	Available alone and with levonordefrin (vasoconstrictor); dosage depends on site and length of surgical procedure. Adult maximum dosage: dental, up to 6.6 mg/kg body weight (300 mg maximum per appointment); other usages, up to 7 mg/kg body weight

Modified from McKenry L, Salerno E: *Mosby's pharmacology in nursing*, ed 18, St Louis, 1992, Mosby–Year Book.

TABLE 23-3   Pharmacology Summary: Selected Injected Local Anesthetics—cont'd

Generic name	Trade name	Metabolism	Use	Dosage and administration
Prilocaine HCl	Citanest Citanest Forte	Amide compound—see above	Infiltration, peripheral nerve blocks, caudal, epidural	Available alone or with epinephrine (vasoconstrictor); although dosages vary with site and length of procedure, the adult maximum dosages are as follows: dental, up to 400 mg as a 4% solution in 2-hr period. Other usages, 400 mg maximum in debilitated patients and patients with liver impairment; healthy adults, 600 mg maximum

LONG DURATION (3-10 HR)

Generic name	Trade name	Metabolism	Use	Dosage and administration
Bupivacaine	Marcaine Sensorcaine	Amide type—see above	Infiltration, caudal, epidural, peripheral nerve blocks	Available alone or with dextrose (Marcaine spinal) or with epinephrine; dosages vary with site, additional drugs, and length of procedure
Dibucaine HCl	Nupercaine	Amide type—see above	Caudal, spinal	Available alone and with dextrose (heavy solution Nupercaine); dosage varies with site of injection, additional drugs if ordered, and length of procedure
Etidocaine	Duranest	Amide type—see above	Infiltration, peripheral nerve blocks, caudal and epidural nerve blocks	Available alone and with epinephrine; dosages vary with site and length of procedure
Tetracaine HCl	Prontocaine HCl	Ester compound—see above	Saddle block (low spinal), up to costal margin, spinal anesthesia	Available alone and with dextrose; dosages vary with site and length of procedure

disrupts sensation at the level of the nerve endings. This results in loss of sensation limited to the immediate area of application.

Local anesthetics

Local anesthetics reversibly block nerve conduction. The area where the anesthetic is applied or injected determines the area of anesthesia. An overview of selected local anesthetics is provided in Table 23-3. Local anesthetics are absorbed from the application site; if a sufficient amount is absorbed, systemic toxicity may occur. The box on p. 481 lists some reactions to local anesthetics. Vasoconstrictors are sometimes used with local anesthetics to decrease systemic absorption and prolong the action.

Malignant hyperthermia

The most common cause of anesthetic-induced death in North America is **malignant hyperthermia.**

SIGNS AND SYMPTOMS OF MALIGNANT HYPERTHERMIA

Tachycardia*
Tachypnea*
Muscle rigidity
Cyanosis
Dysrhythmias
Skin mottling
Fever
Profuse sweating
Unstable blood pressure
Not all clinical signs may be seen in an attack of malignant hyperthermia
Symptoms may also be related to causes other than malignant hyperthermia

*Most consistent and pronounced.

The term *malignant* refers to the rapid progressive nature of the condition, which may become fatal if not promptly recognized and aggressively treated. *Hyperthermia* refers to the rapid rise in body temperature that sometimes occurs (as much as 1° C every 5 minutes). Malignant hyperthermia is an inherited disorder of abnormal muscle metabolism characterized by an uncontrollable increase in muscle metabolism and heat production in response to stress or certain anesthetics. The exact pathophysiology of malignant hyperthermia is not completely understood but appears to result from an alteration of the calcium-storing properties of the cellular or intracellular muscle cell membrane. The clinical signs and symptoms of malignant hyperthermia are described in the box above. Patients with known family history of malignant hyperthermia may benefit from referral to the Malignant Hyperthermia Association of the United States (MHAUS), a nonprofit educational organization that provides services for patients and professionals.

The only specific treatment for malignant hyperthermia is administration of dantrolene (Dantrium), a direct-acting skeletal muscle relaxant. Treatment of malignant hyperthermia includes both symptomatic therapy as well as dantroline administration and cessation of anesthesia and surgery. Prompt recognition and aggressive symptomatic therapy are essential to prevent or limit complications and decrease mortality.

Individuals susceptible to malignant hyperthermia have an underlying muscle disorder, which may not manifest itself until a life-threatening crisis occurs. Evaluation for susceptibility to malignant hyperthermia includes a personal and family anesthetic history and a history and physical examination for the existence of clinical muscle abnormalities. The only reliable diagnostic test is the contracture response of muscle, which requires a muscle biopsy with the patient under local anesthesia, performed nationally in only a few centers. All persons identified by their physician as malignant hyperthermia–susceptible should carry identification (i.e., Medic Alert bracelets) indicating their susceptibility. Anesthesia can be safely administered to these patients. However, the anesthetist must be aware of the patient's possible susceptibility to avoid certain anesthetics that could trigger an attack of malignant hyperthermia.

NURSING MANAGEMENT OF THE INTRAOPERATIVE PATIENT

Assessment

When the patient enters the operating room, the nurse identifies the patient (both verbally and by the identification band and medical record) and completes a nursing assessment of the patient's immediate preoperative condition. The planned operative procedure is confirmed, and all documentation is reviewed for completeness.

Nursing Diagnosis

Several nursing diagnoses may be appropriate for each patient related to the perioperative assessment and operative procedure planned. Common diagnoses may include the following:

High risk for impaired skin integrity related to shaving, skin prep, grounding pads, surgical positioning, or surgical incision

Altered thermoregulation related to operative environment and anesthetic medication

Anxiety related to unfamiliar environment and operative procedure

High risk for injury related to loss of protective reflexes and sensation

Impaired verbal communication related to preoperative or intraoperative medications (sedatives and hypnotics)

High risk for infection related to operative wound

Planning

Nursing care is based on goals related to nursing diagnoses established for each patient and may include the following outcome criteria:

Patient will leave operating room with skin integrity maintained except surgical incision and drain sites

Patient will be normothermic on discharge from the operating room

Patient (and/or family) will exhibit decreased

LEGAL ISSUES   *Legal Principles Unique to Operating Room Setting*

On May 27, 1980, a patient underwent surgery to repair a hernia. During the surgery, the physician placed a lap sponge or lap mat measuring 12 inches by 12 inches into the exposed abdominal cavity. The sponge was not removed before the incision was closed.

Two surgical nurses, both employed by the hospital, assisted the surgeon during the procedure. They were responsible for the sponge count and did not tell the physician about the unaccounted sponge before closure of the incision.

The patient was discharged 3 days later. Between June 1 and September 29, the patient experienced a draining wound, diminished appetite, weight loss, edema in his legs, and in September the onset of grayish skin color. He was seen by the surgeon 34 times. X-ray films made on June 20 showed the lap sponge, but the radiologist did not detect it. On October 6, 1980, the patient's wife had him admitted to another hospital, where x-ray films again showed the lap sponge. The patient's condition had deteriorated such that immediate surgery was precluded. The patient was treated to stabilize his condition before surgery; however, his condition deteriorated further, and he died October 24. Autopsy showed the sponge had wadded into a ball,

and the bowel had wrapped around it, resulting in ischemia, perforation of the bowel, and peritonitis. The patient's wife sued for malpractice and wrongful death.

In this case the court ruled that it was obvious the standard of care had been breached. Although the radiologist was negligent for failing to detect the sponge during x-ray examination, the surgeon and the nurses were liable for their own acts. Further, the court stated that the surgeon could not excuse his own liability by pointing to the nurses or the radiologist. The nurses were liable for their own acts and omissions, and thus shared liability. The trial jury's award of $75,000 for wrongful death was affirmed, and the case was remanded for a retrial on the survivor's claim for damages.

This case reflects the trend in recent years for courts to acknowledge nursing as a distinct profession and nurses' own accountability for their acts. Each member of the surgical team shared responsibility for the wrongful death of the patient in this case. Surgical nurses must be vigilant about their performance and must be aware of their legal responsibility and accountability to the patient as well as their duty to care.

Source: Rudeck v Wright, 709 P2d 621, Montana, 1985.

---

level of anxiety during the operative period and after surgery

Patient will remain free of injury while in the operating room

Intraoperative communication will be maintained through the use of both verbal and nonverbal measures: the patient will be able to communicate effectively with the surgery staff, and staff will be able to effectively communicate with the patient

Aseptic technique will be maintained throughout the operative procedure, and operative wound will remain free from signs of infection 48 hours postoperatively

Implementation

Emotional support and care

Nursing care should include warm personal contact to humanize the often cold, aseptic, and highly technical environment of the operating room. During the preparation for anesthesia and surgery, the nurse continues to reassure the patient, reduce anxiety, and provide physical comfort and safety measures. The nurse can describe any sensory stimulation the patient will experience (e.g., placement of the blood

pressure cuff, electrocardiogram, intravenous lines, and protective safety straps) and assure the patient that he or she will be there during the operation. The nurse should use basic communication skills, such as touch, eye contact, and realistic verbal reassurance, to reduce anxiety. This patient-centered nursing care continues throughout the surgical procedure. Even when the patient receives a general anesthetic, it should be remembered that what is said in the operating room may be subconsciously heard by the patient. Intraoperative awareness or postoperative recall has been documented as a contributing factor in postoperative distress and emotional difficulties. The effects of intraoperative recall may not be apparent for several weeks or months.

CLINICAL ALERT

Patients should never be left unattended or unobserved in the operating room.

Patient safety

During surgery, and particularly anesthesia, the patient is unable to protect himself from many sources of possible harm, and the nurse must act for the patient to prevent injury. Normal self-protective mechanisms, such as pain and withdrawal movements, are lost with the induction of anesthesia, while the protective barrier of the skin is disrupted by surgery, increasing risk of infection. Essential elements for monitoring and protecting patient safety are a keen awareness of the potential for harm, recognition of body areas most susceptible to injury, strict adherence to principles of positioning and asepsis, and monitoring sites for breakdown or early signs of injury. Small or potentially dangerous objects, such as needles and syringes, should not be left near the patient. Bedrails and safety straps should be used, even for the fully conscious patient. Restraints may occasionally be necessary to protect the delirious, semicomatose, or disoriented patient from injury.

Positioning the patient

A variety of positions are used for surgery. The more commonly used surgical positions are presented in Figure 23-2. Selection of the position considers the operative site and the patient's condition. Positioning is a responsibility shared among the circulating nurse, anesthetist, and surgeon. The surgical position should provide optimal exposure and access to the operative site without compromising organ function or patient safety. It must also allow access by the anesthetist for induction of anesthesia, airway control, and the administration of intravenous fluids and drugs. Anesthesia is generally begun in the supine position, and the patient is then repositioned for surgery if necessary.

All surgical positions, but some more than others, have been potentially harmful because of their effects on respiration, circulation, peripheral nerves, and the skin (see box, p. 487). Under normal circumstances, the body can compensate for position changes through a variety of reflex mechanisms. However, many of the compensatory reflexes are obtunded by anesthesia. Because protective pain sensations are blocked by anesthesia, muscle strain or areas of increased pressure can occur. Muscle strain from positioning in surgery may contribute to postoperative discomfort.

Safe positioning considers the physiologic derangements brought about by both anesthesia and position. Position changes in the anesthetized patient should be made slowly to allow the circulatory system time to adjust to the changes in blood distribution. Patient limitations, such as reduced joint motion, may be exceeded under the effects of anesthesia, which may result in injury or postoperative pain. Patient limits or restrictions are assessed *before* induction of anesthesia. When moving the head or extremities of an anesthetized patient, the usual direction and range of motion for that particular patient should be followed without forcing movement. Planning and coordination of the operating room team are necessary to prevent disruption of monitoring or dislodgment of vascular cannulas, urinary catheters, or drains while positioning the patient. Body sites especially vulnerable to injury related to surgical positioning are given in Table 23-5.

Asepsis

All persons in the operating room must be alert to contamination of sterile items and must aid in maintaining aseptic conditions. **Surgical asepsis** may be

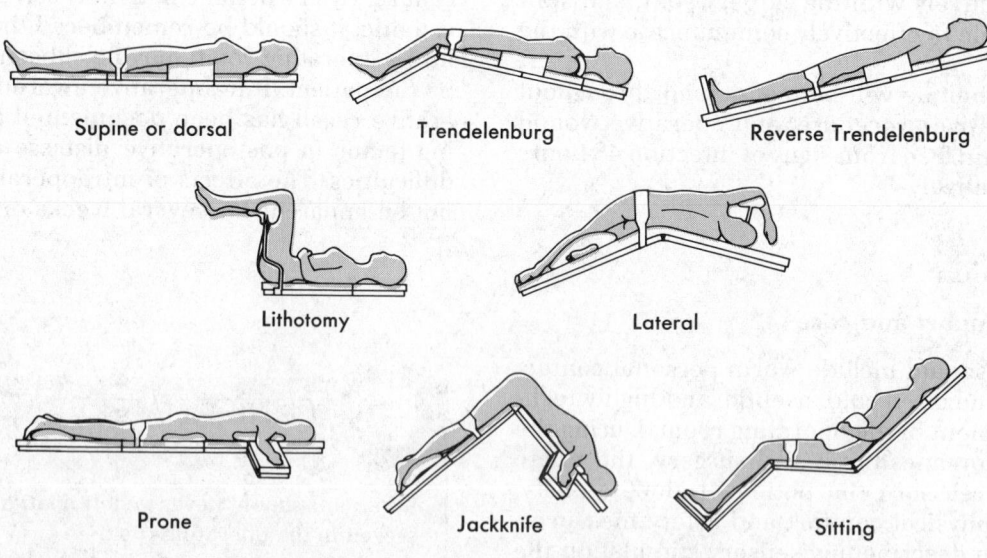

Supine or dorsal   Trendelenburg   Reverse Trendelenburg

Lithotomy   Lateral

Prone   Jackknife   Sitting

FIGURE 23-2   Common surgical positions.

Respiratory system

Movement of the diaphragm or chest wall may be restricted by position or shifting visceral pressure resulting from position. In addition to mechanical interference with respiration, position changes alter distribution of inspired air, change patterns of blood flow throughout the lungs, and affect movement of secretions. (Table 23-4 shows the respiratory effects of specific surgical positions in the normal awake patient. The reduction of vital capacity [vital capacity refers to the amount of air that can be voluntarily exhaled after maximal inhalation and reflects mechanical properties of the lungs] is even greater in the anesthetized patient.)

Circulatory system

Both general and regional anesthesia reduce central nervous system control of vascular constriction. Blood follows the law of gravity in the absence of reflex vasoconstriction, increasing the tendency for blood to pool in the dependent areas of the body. Diminished muscle tone reduces the "milking" action of the muscle and contributes to the pooling of blood.

Peripheral nerves and vessels

Peripheral nerves may be subject to direct mechanical injury. Nerve injuries usually result from stretching or pressure that causes reduced blood flow and ischemia.

Permanent injury may result from only a few minutes of pressure. The most vulnerable time is when muscle relaxation is greatest during anesthesia. Superficial nerves, such as the ulnar and brachial nerves, are at greatest risk for injury. Vessel damage occurs in much the same manner as nerve injury. Circulation is compromised by direct compression, occlusion by hyperextension, or twisting of a limb causing internal compression of a vessel. Potential damages can be avoided or minimized by use of soft pads to prevent compression of peripheral nerves and modifications of extreme positions to prevent stretch of muscles, nerves, and vessels.

Skin pressure

Pressure sores, or decubitus ulcers, may develop if circulation to the skin is inadequate. Blood flow may be compromised by a reduction in capillary pressure, a situation that may result from decreased blood pressure or compression of blood vessels. Most of the body weight is distributed over bony prominences (such as heels, elbows, pelvis, sacrum, and occiput), creating excessive pressure on the skin overlying these areas. Areas of pressure should be thoroughly padded to prevent tissue damage.

TABLE 23-4 Effect of Position on Lung Volumes

Position	Percent decrease in vital capacity (from standing position)
Reverse Trendelenburg	9%
Supine	9.5%
Prone	10%
Lateral	10%
Jackknife	12.5%
Trendelenburg	14.5%
Lithotomy	18%

The effect of position in the normal conscious subject on vital capacity. Changes are greater under the effects of general anesthesia.

Adapted from Little DM: Posture and anesthesia, *Can Anaesth Soc J* 7: 2, 1960.

TABLE 23-5 Body Sites Especially Vulnerable to Injury Related to Surgical Positioning

Site	Type of injury
Eyes	Corneal abrasion; retinal damage by pressure on globe (especially with glaucoma)
Ears	Tympanic membrane perforation by foreign objects; cauliflower ear from folding the pinna
Mouth	Lacerations and bruising of lips and damage to teeth; dislodgment of airway devices
Neck	Neuropathy and impairment of cerebral blood flow by rotation of the neck
Extremities	
Nerves	Neuropathy from stretching, twisting, and compression
Joints	Overextension or dislocation, especially of arthritic joints
Vascular	Distal ischemia and edema from circulatory occlusion

PRINCIPLES OF SURGICAL ASEPSIS

Scrubbed persons should wear sterile gowns and gloves

Gowns are considered sterile only from chest to waist in front and from hands to just above the elbows; all other areas are considered contaminated

Sterile drapes should be used to establish a sterile field

All items used within a sterile field should be sterile

All items introduced into a sterile field should be dispensed by methods that maintain sterility of the item and integrity of the sterile field

Contaminated items should be removed immediately from the sterile field

Tables are considered sterile only at and above table level; items extending below table level are considered unsterile

Unsterile items should not extend over the sterile field

Once opened, the edges of a sterile package are considered contaminated

A margin of safety should be maintained between sterile objects and the unsterile area

The sterile field is created as close as possible to the time of use

A sterile field should be constantly monitored and maintained

If there is any doubt regarding the sterility of an article, it is considered unsterile

Once sterile supplies are opened for use with one patient, they must either be discarded or resterilized before they are used with another patient

Sterile fluids should be poured from a height sufficient to protect from accidental touching of the unsterile container with the sterile receiving container and low enough to prevent splashing

---

described as all efforts to prevent microbial contamination of the operative site. Most surgical infections result from either endogenous or exogenous operating room contamination of the wound. The goal of surgical asepsis is to prevent or minimize postoperative wound infections. Development of wound infection is influenced by the condition of the wound after surgery, patient susceptibility, and microbial contamination. Basic principles of aseptic technique and scrubbing for the operating room are described in the box above, and the box on p. 489. The patient is at risk for introduction of infecting organisms through vascular cannulas, catheters, drains, or the surgical wound. Standards and guidelines for surgical scrubs and skin preparation should be strictly followed.

Skin preparation

To reduce contamination of the surgical wound, the skin around the operative site is prepared to reduce the number of organisms present and inhibit rebound growth. Preoperatively, the skin is prepared and hair removed (Chapter 22).

Electrical hazards

Modern surgery and anesthesia heavily depend on electrical equipment, including monitors, headlamps, microscopes, endoscopic equipment, electrical operating tables, and electrocautery devices, all of which pose a threat to patient safety. Electrical hazards include fire, electric shock, and burns.

Sparks caused by faulty equipment, static electricity, or the use of lasers and electrical cautery devices are possible sources of ignition. Explosive anesthetic gases are no longer used. However, the use of high oxygen concentrations for anesthesia increases fire risk, as does alcohol or other flammable substances occasionally found in the operating room.

The heart and nervous tissues are most susceptible to the effects of electric shock when the protective skin and superficial tissues are violated by surgery. A very small current may affect the normal electrical activity of the heart if applied directly or conducted close to the heart by wires, catheters, or cautery. Nerve damage may result from electrical overstimulation.

Both electrical and thermal burns are possible. They may result from contact with hot electrical wires or passage of electricity through the body when improperly grounded. Electrical burns usually result from the use of electrocautery with inadequate or improper grounding and are the most common electrical hazard in the operating room. Burns result from alternate return pathways for electrosurgical current through body contacts with small surface areas that conduct electricity, such as electrocardiogram electrodes, or contact with the intravenous pole or operating table. Protection from electrical hazards entails proper use and maintenance of all electrical equipment and properly grounding the patient when electrocautery is used.

Laser safety

A variety of lasers are being used with increasing frequency in patient care settings, especially in op-

SCRUBBING FOR AN OPERATION

There are several methods for cleansing and degerming the skin of the hands and forearms before participating in a surgical procedure, referred to as the "surgical scrub." Although there is no practical method of sterilizing the hands, the purpose of a surgical scrub is to:

- Remove soil and transient microbes from the skin
- Reduce resident microbial count as low as possible
- Inhibit rebound growth of microbes

Institutional policies and procedures determine the exact timing and method of surgical scrub for each practice setting or clinical situation. These policies should consider the guidelines outlined below.

Action

1. All jewelry including watches should be removed before the scrub
2. Fingernails should be free of polish and trimmed short, with cuticles in good condition
3. Hands and forearms should be free from lesions and breaks in skin integrity
4. A rapid-acting, broad-spectrum, and long-acting antimicrobial soap or detergent should be used
5. Standardized surgical scrub procedures include:
   a. Hands and arms should be thoroughly moistened, washed, and rinsed before beginning the surgical scrub
   b. Subungual areas should be cleansed with a nail cleaner under running water
   c. An approved antimicrobial agent should be applied to hands and forearms with friction
   d. Hands should be held higher than the elbows and away from surgical attire
   e. Brushes or sponges used in the surgical scrub should be discarded after use
6. An anatomic timed scrub or a counted brush stroke method should be used for all surgical scrubs
   a. The anatomic timed method—a prescribed amount of time is allotted for each anatomic area
   b. The counted brush stroke method—a set number of brush strokes is allotted to each designated surface of the hands and forearms

Rationale

Jewelry is a reservoir for bacteria and prevents effective surgical scrubs

Cracked nails, polish, or artificial nails may harbor bacteria or prevent effective surgical scrubs

Skin infections have the potential to contaminate surgical wounds

Studies have shown that surgical scrub agents reduce indigenous skin microflora and inhibit rebound growth of microbes

   a. Prescrub reduces incidence of skin reactions, loosens surface debris
   b. Dirt and organisms can collect under the nails
   c. The principal action of handwashing is mechanical removal of dirt and microorganisms; antimicrobial agents kill and inhibit rapid rebound growth of microorganisms
   d. This position allows water to run from the cleanest area down and prevents contamination
   e. Disposal of used items prevents cross contamination of the surgical scrub area

The anatomic timed scrub and counted stroke method assure sufficient exposure of all skin surfaces to friction and antimicrobial solution

Modified from *Recommended Practices for Surgical Hand Scrubs*, 1992, The Association of Operating Room Nurses.

erative procedures. Lasers are useful for cutting, coagulating, vaporizing, and welding tissue. Utilization of lasers in surgery continues to increase because of a number of advantages, including reduced tissue damage, less postoperative pain and scarring, and more rapid recovery for patients.

Laser beams deliver energy directly to the tissues, which results in extremely high temperatures. Hazards to both the patient and health care providers include direct damage to the skin and eyes from the laser beam, inhalation of smoke and particulate matter, and fire. Laser warning signs should be placed at all entrances to areas where lasers are in use. When the laser is used in a manner that produces smoke, special high-filtration masks are worn to reduce inhalation of smoke or particulate matter. In addition, smoke and fumes are evacuated through a high-efficiency filter to further reduce exposure. Laser-safe eye protection is used for OR staff and conscious patients. Protective patient eye shields are used for procedures close to the eye. Exposed tissue around the operative field is protected with wet towels or sponges to prevent thermal injury. Nonreflective instruments are used to decrease chances of laser beam reflection, scatter, or disbursement. When possible, backstops or guards are

GUIDE TO FIRE SAFETY DURING LASER SURGERY

- Sterile water or saline should be immediately available to douse a small fire.
- A halon fire extinguisher should be available in the department in case the laser catches on fire.
- Do not place dry combustibles in the vicinity of the laser impact site. Use wet towels or nonflammable drapes near the laser target area. Moisten these items with sterile saline or water to prevent ignition. Constantly monitor the moisture level throughout the procedure.
- Utilize nonreflective instrumentation in or near the laser tissue impact site to decrease accidental direct reflection of the laser beam. Cover larger instruments, such as retractors, with wet sponges or towels to protect against reflection.
- Do not prep with flammable skin preparations, such as alcohol.
- A wet pack may be inserted into the rectum to provide a tamponade to prevent methane gas from escaping into the surgical area.
- Use a specially prepared or a commercially manufactured laser endotracheal tube during laser procedures of the oropharynx. An unprotected PVC endotracheal tube can readily be ignited from an inadvertent laser beam impact. Protect the endotracheal tube cuff with wet gauze sponges.
- Place the laser in the standby mode when not in use.
- Identify the laser footpedal to avoid accidental activation.
- Do not place fluids or solutions on the laser unit. Protect the laser system from spillage or splatter that could cause short-circuiting and fire.

From Meeker MH, Rothrock JC: Alexander's care of the patient in surgery, ed 9, St Louis, 1991, Mosby–Year Book.

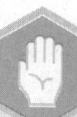

CLINICAL ALERT

Latex Sensitivity

In 1991 the U.S. Food and Drug Administration (FDA) issued an alert on allergic reactions to latex. The FDA reports that allergic reactions to latex (natural rubber) are increasingly being reported. Latex is used in gloves, catheters, intubation tubes, anesthesia masks, dental dams, and many other medical devices. Reactions have ranged from urticaria to systemic anaphylaxis. Several patients have died as the result of anaphylactoid reactions during barium enemas using latex cuffed enema tips. Repeated exposure to latex in medical and other consumer products may be part of the reason that sensitivity reactions appear to be increasing. The FDA reports that 6% to 7% of surgical personnel and 18% to 40% of spina bifida patients are latex sensitive.

The FDA recommends that health care professionals:

- Include questions about latex sensitivity when taking a health history, especially for surgical and radiology and spina bifida patients. Patients should be questioned about itching, rash, or wheezing after blowing up balloons or wearing latex gloves.
- If latex sensitivity is suspected, consider using devices made with alternate materials.
- Be alert to possible allergic reactions whenever latex-containing devices are used, especially when they come in contact with mucous membranes.
- If an allergic reaction occurs and latex sensitivity is suspected, advise the patient. Patients should be advised to inform emergency and health care personnel about the suspected sensitivity before undergoing any treatment. Wearing a Medical ID bracelet should be considered.

---

used to prevent beam reflection toward nontargeted areas. Flammable or combustible material, solutions, or anesthetics are not used near the site of laser use.

Chemical burns

Skin irritation or chemical burns may occur from exposure to antimicrobial prepping solutions, usually as a result of the patient lying in a pool of solution during surgery. These solutions should not pool under the patient. The patient should be kept on a clean, dry surface during surgery.

Temperature

Many patients experience a significant loss of body heat and subsequent decrease in core temperature during surgery and anesthesia. Among the factors contributing to this problem are administration of cold gases, infusion of cool intravenous fluids, altered thermoregulation and decreased metabolism from anesthetic medications, exposure to low operating room temperatures, cold irrigating solutions, and evaporative loss through the operative site. Elderly, thin, and very young patients are at greatest risk for intraoperative hypothermia. Heat loss is usually greater when large sections of the body are exposed, increasing evaporative heat loss, such as abdominal or thoracic operations and during prolonged surgery.

A variety of measures may be used to limit heat loss in the operating room. Passive measures include applying warmed blankets or thermal wrap to the patient on arrival in the operating room, increasing the ambient room temperature while the patient is exposed and skin prepared, and limiting time and skin exposure during positioning, skin preparation, and application of sterile drapes. Active warming measures include warmed irrigating and intravenous fluids, warming mattresses and blankets, and heating and humidifying inhaled gases.

Evaluation

Evaluation of nursing goals developed for the intraoperative period is made before transfer of the patient to the postoperative recovery unit and completes the intraoperative period. Goals, or expected outcomes, that are evaluated may include but are not limited to (1) maintenance of skin integrity; (2) maintenance of fluid and electrolyte balance; (3) absence of adverse effects related to positioning; (4) elimination of extraneous objects and chemical, physical, and electrical hazards; and (5) maintenance of body temperature. Physiologic functions and the condition of the patient (including catheters, drains, intravenous sites, and dressings) are evaluated and documented.

Documentation

The intraoperative record should include the information listed in the box below and reflect nursing assessment and planning, continual evaluation of nursing care and the patient response to nursing care, and care given by other members of the surgical team. Most surgical nurses use a special intraoperative flowsheet for the nursing record.

Transfer from the Operating Room

Movement of the patient from the operating table to the recovery bed or stretcher should be done smoothly with a sufficient number of people to allow proper weight distribution without injuring the patient or staff. The semianesthetized patient should not be roughly dragged or bounced across the table

---

RECOMMENDED DOCUMENTATION OF PERIOPERATIVE NURSING CARE

The method of documenting perioperative nursing care may vary from one practice setting to another. The forms could include, but are not limited to, perioperative checklists, nurses' notes, flowsheets, care plans, and operative count records.[6]

Every practice setting uses a formal system for documenting patient care. Records are different in each setting. The methods selected for documenting perioperative nursing care must fit with the institution's overall philosophy of nursing documentation and its system for record keeping. Perioperative documentation should include:

- identification of persons providing care; name, title, and signature of the person responsible for the entry
- evidence of a patient assessment upon arrival to the perioperative suite including the level of consciousness, psychosocial status, and baseline physical data
- patient's overall skin condition on arrival and discharge from the perioperative suite
- presence and disposition of sensory aids and prosthetic devices accompanying the patient to surgery. Prosthetic devices are defined as artificial substitutes for body parts (e.g., an arm, leg, eye, dentures, hearing aid, wig)
- patient's position, supports, and/or restraints used during the surgical procedure
- placement of the dispersive electrode pad and identification of the electrosurgical unit and settings

- placement of temperature control devices and identification of the unit recording time and temperature
- placement of electrocardiographic or other monitoring electrodes
- medications, irrigations, and solutions administered or dispensed by the registered nurse
- specimens and cultures taken during the procedure
- skin preparation, solutions, area prepared, and any reactions that may have occurred
- placement of drains, catheters, packings, and dressings
- placement of tourniquet cuff and person applying the cuff, pressure, time, and identification of the unit
- urinary output and estimated blood loss, as appropriate
- placement of implants (i.e., tissue, inert, or radioactive material inserted into a body cavity or grafted onto the tissue of the recipient), manufacturer, lot number, type, size, and other identifying information, occurrence and results of surgical item counts
- time of discharge, disposition of patient, method of transfer, and patient status
- intraoperative x-rays and fluroscopy
- wound classification
- other direct patient care issues that are pertinent to patient outcomes

From *AORN Standards and Recommended Practices for Perioperative Nursing*, 1992, Association of Operating Room Nurses, Inc.

edge onto the stretcher, because this may cause injuries to the back, head, neck, or extremities. A coordinated effort by all involved with use of drawsheets or body rollers and attention to extremities, vascular lines, drains, and monitors will promote safe patient transfers. Communication with the receiving unit and nurse before transfer includes essential equipment needed for the patient, such as ventilators, special monitors, and suction equipment.

The transfer between the operating room and recovery area occurs at a time when the patient may be prone to injury, airway difficulties, vomiting and aspiration, or cardiovascular instability because of the effects of residual anesthesia. The transfer should be completed as expediently as possible with the patient accompanied by members of the operating team, including a nurse and anesthetist. On arrival in the postanesthesia unit, the operating nurse reports the procedure, plan of nursing care, and additional information to the nurses who will care for the patient. The nurse in charge of the patient in the postanesthesia care unit should be informed of the following:

1. The operation performed
2. Vital signs
3. Drugs (including anesthetic agents and techniques), fluids, and blood products administered in the operating room
4. Blood loss during surgery, as well as urine output or other drainage
5. Presence of drains or catheters
6. Problems that occurred during surgery or anesthesia
7. Presence of abnormalities or preexisting disease
8. Special observations or interventions recommended
9. Patient concerns or desires for the recovery period
10. Special perioperative nursing care plans

CRITICAL THINKING QUESTIONS

1 What are the roles of the surgical team members? Discuss the importance of the team approach.
2 What are the advantages and disadvantages of the various types of anesthesia?
3 What are the effects of common surgical positions on the following body systems: respiratory, cardiovascular, peripheral nervous, integumentary?
4 What are the common threats to the safety of the intraoperative patient?
5 List nursing measures to decrease intraoperative heat loss.
6 What kind of emotional support should the nurse provide the operative patient?
7 What information should be shared between the operating room and the recovery unit when a patient is transferred after surgery?

RESOURCES

1 AMERICAN ASSOCIATION OF NURSE ANESTHETISTS (AANA) 216 Higgins Road Park Ridge, Il 60069 1-312-692-7050
2 ASSOCIATION OF OPERATING ROOM NURSES (AORN) 10170 E. Mississippi Ave. Denver, CO 80231 1-303-755-6300
3 MALIGNANT HYPERTHERMIA ASSOCIATION OF THE UNITED STATES (MHAUS) Box 3231 Darien, CT 06820 1-203-634-4917 (Phone consultation in malignant hyperthermia emergencies—Medic Alert Foundation International, 1-209-634-4917, ask for INDEX ZERO)

BIBLIOGRAPHY

Current

1. Aitkenhead AR: Awareness during anaesthesia. In Taylor TH, Major E, editors: *Hazards and complications of anaesthesia,* New York, 1987, Churchill Livingstone.
2. Association of Operating Room Nurses: *AORN standards and recommended practices for perioperative nursing,* Denver, 1992, The Association.
3. Association of Operating Room Nurses: RN first assistant 1987 survey update, *AORN* 47(1):238, 1988.
4. CDC Guidelines for prevention of surgical wound infections, Atlanta, 1985, Centers for Disease Control.
5. Chitwood LB: Unveiling the mysteries of anesthesia, *Nurs 87* Feb:53, 1987.
6. Eger II EI: Fetal injury and abortion associated with occupational exposure to inhaled anesthetics, *AANA J* 59(4):309, 1991.
7. Hambrarus A: Aerobiology in the operating room: a review, *J Hosp Infect* 11(Suppl A):68, 1988.
8. Kneedler JA, Dodge GH: *Perioperative patient care,* ed 2, Boston, 1987, Blackwell Scientific Publications.
9. Life-threatening reactions to latex are increasing, FDA warns, *AJN* (7):14, 1991.
10. Meeker MH, Rothrock JC: *Alexander's care of the patient in surgery,* ed 9, St Louis, 1991, Mosby–Year Book.
11. Reed EA, Applegeet CJ: Infection control: AORN recommended practices in ambulatory surgery, *AORN J* 43(5):1002, 1986.
12. Taylor TH, Major E, editors: *Hazards and complications of anaesthesia,* New York, 1987, Churchill Livingstone.
13. Tannenbaum TN, Goldberg RJ: Exposure to anesthetic gases and reproductive outcome, *J Occup Med* 27(9):659, 1985.
14. US Food and Drug Administration reports allergic reactions to latex, *AANA J* 59(4):300, 1991.

Classic

15. Britt BA, Gordon RA: Peripheral nerve injuries associated with anesthesia, *Can Anaesth Soc J* 11:514, 1964.

16. Closs SJ, Macdonald IA, Hawthorn PJ: Factors affecting perioperative body temperature, *J Adv Nurs* 11(6):739, 1986.
17. Ellis FR, Heffron JA: Clinical and biochemical aspects of malignant hyperpyrexia. In Atkinson RS, Adams AP, editors: *Recent advances in anaesthesia and analgesia,* No 15, New York, 1985, Churchill Livingstone.
18. Keenan RL: Anesthesia disasters: incidence, causes, and preventability, *Semin Anesth* 5(3):175, 1986.
19. Little DM: Posture and anesthesia, *Can Anaesth Soc J* 7:2, 1960.
20. Martin JT: *Positioning in anesthesia and surgery,* Philadelphia, 1978, WB Saunders.
21. McConnell EA: *Clinical considerations in perioperative nursing,* Philadelphia, 1987, JB Lippincott.
22. Morley-Forster PK: Unintentional hypothermia in the operating room, *Can Anaesth Soc J* 3(4):515, 1986.
23. Tannenbaum TN, Goldberg RJ: Exposure to anesthetic gases and reproductive outcome, *J Occup Med* 27(9):659, 1985.
24. US Food and Drug Administration reports allergic reactions to latex, *AANA J* 59(4):300, 1991.

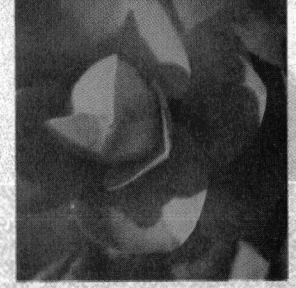

CHAPTER TWENTY-FOUR

Postoperative Nursing

LEARNING OBJECTIVES

1 Describe nursing assessment of the patient in the postanesthesia care unit including postanesthesia recovery score.
2 Discuss the elements and implementation of the postanesthesia "wake-up" regimen.
3 Identify common postanesthesia problems and related nursing care.
4 Describe the process of discharging and transferring a patient out of the postanesthesia care unit.
5 Identify common problems in the later postoperative period.
6 Describe nursing activities to prevent postoperative complications and promote healing.
7 Apply principles of postoperative nursing to develop a plan of nursing care for the postoperative patient.

KEY TERMS

THE POSTOPERATIVE period begins with the end of surgery and admission to a **postanesthesia care unit (PACU),** also called the "recovery room." Some patients receiving a local anesthetic or undergoing operative procedures not requiring anesthesia may be discharged from the operating room to their hospital room or home. The length of the postoperative period varies with the time required to recover from the stress and disruption caused by surgery and anesthesia. This period may only last a few hours, or it may extend for several months.

The postoperative period can be divided into two phases. The first phase is the immediate postoperative period and is characterized by the initial recovery from the stress of anesthesia and surgery during the first postoperative hours. The second phase is the period of resolution and healing. This period may extend for months after major surgery. While there is no distinct dividing line between the initial phase of postoperative recovery and the second phase, nursing care and related considerations will be discussed separately, with the understanding that the two periods overlap.

IMMEDIATE POSTOPERATIVE PERIOD
Recovery from Anesthesia

Cognitive function and motor performance may take up to 48 hours to return to preanesthetic levels after general anesthesia. However, the most pronounced effects of anesthesia have generally dissipated before the patient is discharged from the PACU. Most patients spend from 30 minutes to several hours in the PACU. It is during this time that the patient is stabilized and aroused from the residual anesthetic effects. Primary nursing goals for the immediate postoperative period are to:

1. Maintain a patent airway
2. Recognize and manage complications
3. Ensure patient safety
4. Stabilize vital signs
5. Dissipate residual anesthesia
6. Provide pain relief
7. Provide emotional reassurance and decrease anxiety

During this arousal time the nurse assesses the patient, implements immediate postoperative nursing measures, and evaluates and modifies the perioperative care plan as needed. The American Society of Postanesthesia Nursing (ASPAN) has described the goal of the postanesthesia nurse as being "to assist the patient in returning to a safe physiologic level after an anesthetic by providing safe, knowledgeable, individualized nursing care to patients and their families in the immediate postanesthetic phase." After discharge from the PACU, the nurse's goal is to help the patient in returning to a

RESEARCH BRIEF

O'Connell M: Anxiety reduction in family members of patients in surgery and postanesthesia care: a pilot study, *Postanesth Nurs* 4(1):7, 1989.

This study examines the effects of the postanesthesia nurse's information-giving on family members' anxiety during the patient's intraoperative and postanesthesia experience. In this pilot study, waiting family members of patients undergoing surgery were asked to complete a self-evaluation questionnaire for assessment of anxiety level at the beginning of surgery and again just before the patient was transferred to his own unit. At half-hour intervals during surgery the participants were given information about the patient's status and were given an opportunity to have their questions answered. Data analysis showed a significant reduction in anxiety following the provision of information. While this study is only preliminary, the findings would suggest that by keeping family members informed of the patient's progress throughout the surgical and postanesthesia period, the nurse helps them reduce their anxiety levels.

"safe physiologic level after enabling discharge with an appropriate knowledge base for home care."

Family

The family should be notified when surgery is complete and the patient is admitted to the PACU. Most surgeons will speak with the family immediately after surgery, briefly informing them of what was done and the patient's condition. The nurse should know what the patient and family were told in order to better answer questions and reinforce the information. Family members may be very anxious during this time, and information and reassurance often reduce anxiety. The family should be informed of what to expect when the patient leaves the PACU. Institutional policies generally restrict visitation by families while the patient is in the PACU. Visitation is sometimes allowed after the patient is stabilized and alert and may be particularly helpful for both the patient and family in some instances, particularly with children or very apprehensive patients.

NURSING MANAGEMENT OF THE PATIENT DURING IMMEDIATE POSTOPERATIVE PERIOD
Assessment

The patient is transferred to the recovery room directly from the operating room and is accompanied by a nurse and the anesthetist, as well as by a member of the surgical team. On the patient's admission, the postanesthesia nurse receives a report from both the operating room nurse and the anesthetist. Of particular interest to the postanesthesia nurse are:

1. The patient's preoperative status and relevant preoperative findings
2. The anesthetic technique used
3. Drugs administered in the operating room (including anesthetic drugs)
4. The surgical procedure performed and the length of time required
5. Estimated fluid and blood lost and administered during surgery
6. Complications or unusual occurrences
7. Location of catheters, drains, and dressings
8. The postoperative nursing care plan

When the patient is admitted to the PACU, a nursing assessment is made and documented on the recovery room record. A general postoperative nursing assessment is given in the box on p. 497.

Patients are assessed and monitored frequently in the PACU. Initially, some patients will require constant nursing care until stabilized or awake. Vital signs are recorded on admission and every 5 minutes until stable. After a patient has demonstrated stable vital signs, the vital signs are recorded every 15 to 30 minutes until discharge from the PACU.

GENERAL POSTOPERATIVE ASSESSMENT

Airway and Breathing

Adequacy of airway and airway reflexes (gag, cough, swallow)

Type of airway in place (if artificial airway is used)

Rate and quality of respiration

Breath sounds

Ability to cough and deep breathe (when awake)

Amount and method of oxygen administered, time initiated

Circulation

Pulse rate, peripheral pulses

Cardiac monitor pattern (if applicable)

Pressure readings, including arterial blood pressure and central venous pressure (if monitored)

Skin color and temperature

Metabolic

Skin integrity and turgor

Temperature

Urine output

Type and rate of intravenous fluids administered

General

Location, condition, and output from drains and catheters

Muscle strength and response

Bowel sounds

Surgical incision

   Presence, type, and condition of dressing

   Condition of suture line (if not obscured by dressing)

   Quality and amount of wound drainage (if present)

Position of patient

Pain

   Location, intensity, medication administered, and patient response

Level of consciousness, orientation, condition of sensorium and thought processes, and ability to communicate

Patients Having Spinal Epidural or Other Regional Anesthetic

Location and level of anesthesia in affected area

Ability to move involved extremity

TABLE 24-1   Postanesthesia Scoring System

Postanesthesia recovery score	In	15	30	45	Hrs	Out
ACTIVITY						
4 extremities	2	2	2	2	2	2
2 extremities	1	1	1	1	1	1
0 extremities	0	0	0	0	0	0
RESPIRATION						
Able to deep breathe and cough freely	2	2	2	2	2	2
Dyspnea shallow or limited breathing	1	1	1	1	1	1
Apneic	0	0	0	0	0	0
CIRCULATION						
BP = 20 mm of preanesthesia level	2	2	2	2	2	2
Preoperative BP = 20 to 50 mm of preanesthesia level	1	1	1	1	1	1
BP = 50 mm of preanesthesia level	0	0	0	0	0	0
CONSCIOUSNESS						
Fully awake	2	2	2	2	2	2
Arousable on calling	1	1	1	1	1	1
Not responding	0	0	0	0	0	0
COLOR						
Normal	2	2	2	2	2	2
Pale, dusky, blotchy, jaundiced, other	1	1	1	1	1	1
Cyanotic	0	0	0	0	0	0

DISMISSAL CRITERIA

Total score of 10, plus stable 1 signs.

A physician's order is required for discharge with lower score.   Total

From Wetchler BV: Anesthesia for outpatient surgery *AORN J* 34(2):282, 1981.

Postanesthesia recovery score

Most PACU nurses use a scoring system to document patient status. Table 24-1 shows a widely used scoring system first introduced by Aldrete and Kroulik[16] in 1970. The Aldrete scoring system evaluates the patient regarding activity, respiration, circulation, level of consciousness, and color. Many recent scoring systems evaluate the patient's temperature rather than color since temperature is a more objective assessment.

Nursing Diagnosis

Some of the more commonly encountered nursing diagnoses in the PACU include:

   Fluid volume deficit related to blood loss, output

from drains, postoperative vomiting, or NPO status

Ineffective airway clearance related to anesthesia or surgery

Ineffective breathing pattern related to surgical incision or anesthetic and narcotic drug effects

High risk for aspiration related to altered airway reflexes from surgery, drug effects, or vomiting

Pain

Hypothermia related to cold operative environment or altered thermoregulation

Sensory/perceptual alterations related to regional or general anesthesia or medications administered

Planning

Examples of possible patient outcomes include:

Patient's fluid volume status will be monitored; intake and output will be balanced; electrolytes, urine output, blood pressure and skin turgor will be within normal limits; alterations will be detected and physician notified of significant problems while patient is in PACU

Patient will effectively maintain own airway; cough and clear secretions on discharge from the PACU

Patient will have normal respiratory rate and depth and be able to perform cascade cough and sustained maximal inspiration (SMI) maneuver at discharge from PACU

Patient will have clear breath sounds and be free of signs or symptoms of aspiration

Patient will have no postoperative pain or an acceptable level of postoperative discomfort

Patient will be normothermic at discharge from PACU

Patient will be oriented to person, time, and place; sensory deficits from anesthesia will be receding at time of discharge from PACU

Implementation

"Wake-Up" regimen

An important nursing activity in the PACU is the "wake-up" or "stir-up" regimen. It is designed to mobilize the patient, promote improved gas exchange, and decrease complications. It has been divided into several major activities, including the sustained maximal inspiration maneuver (see Chapter 22), the cascade cough (see Chapter 26), and repositioning every 10 to 15 minutes. Preoperative teaching is an important prerequisite for improved patient acceptance and compliance with the wake-up regimen.

Promoting gas exchange

Because all general anesthetics are potent respiratory depressants, most patients receiving general anesthesia are given supplemental oxygen in the recovery room. A variety of methods are available for administering oxygen (see Chapter 26).

Hypoventilation is common in the PACU after general anesthesia. Diminished ventilation may be the result of residual anesthetics, muscle relaxants, pain, or narcotics. Since inhalation anesthetics are removed from the body through the lungs, encouraging the sleepy postoperative patient to deep breathe promotes more rapid removal of the anesthetic gases and increases wakening. Decreased lung volumes are the major factor contributing to postoperative pulmonary complications. Low lung volumes occur as a result of a shallow, monotonous, sighless breathing pattern that follows anesthesia or that accompanies pain or the administration of narcotic medications. Unless contraindicated, the patient should be stimulated to take several deep breaths every 5 to 10 minutes in the PACU. The sustained maximal inspiration maneuver is most effective in preventing or minimizing postoperative pulmonary complications.

Positioning and mobilization

When patients are first brought to the recovery room, the semiprone and side-lying positions are generally the best. These positions promote maintenance of a patent airway in the partially anesthetized patient, decrease the risk of aspiration, and promote ventilation of the lower lung lobes. Frequent repositioning is needed to reduce or prevent atelectasis and venous stasis. Until patients awake, they are repositioned from side to side. When they are able, they should be encouraged to move and change position frequently. Mobilization and contraction-relaxation of muscles promotes circulation and improves cardiac function. However, care must be exercised to prevent tension on or dislodgment of dressings, drains, or catheters.

Pain relief

Early and effective pain relief reduces reflex muscle splinting and subsequent respiratory compromise. Pain relief actually improves respiratory function and decreases oxygen demand by decreasing myocardial work related to the stress response initiated by pain. Nonpharmacologic methods for reducing pain and pain response (Chapter 14) should be used in conjunction with appropriate medications and often can greatly reduce the need for postoperative pain medication. Pain relief should be prompt and effective to avoid setting up a cycle of pain. Evaluate for cumulative effect of anesthesia and pain medication, especially in the elderly.

Care of patient following anesthesia

Regional or local anesthesia

Nursing care for the patient following regional anesthesia includes assessment and documentation of the extent of nerve block (the area that has been affected). Assessment includes not only determining the location of anesthesia but also the presence of diminished feeling (hypoanesthesia), the adequacy of circulation, and the presence or absence of muscle function and control. Nursing care includes safe physiologic positioning of affected limbs until sensation returns. The affected area is monitored for return of sensation and function. As a regional block wears off, the patient may experience pain and require the administration of analgesics. The patient should be evaluated for signs of local anesthetic toxicity if large amounts of a local anesthetic have been administered.

Spinal or epidural anesthesia

When large regions of the body are involved, such as with spinal or epidural anesthetics, hypotension may result from blockade of autonomic function. If the anesthetic from a spinal or epidural injection spreads excessively, the muscles of respiration may be involved and respiratory function may be compromised. Blood pressure, pulse, and respiration should be monitored closely and the physician notified of any problems. An additional complication of spinal and occasionally epidural anesthesia is the postdural puncture headache, often called the "spinal headache." The postdural puncture headache is generally located in the frontal and occipital regions and is relieved when the patient lies flat. Leakage of cerebrospinal fluid (CSF) from the puncture site and subsequent drop in CSF pressure is believed to be the cause. Because of the risk of headache, some physicians restrict ambulation or have patients lie flat for several hours following spinal anesthesia.

Patient safety

When a patient is experiencing residual effects of anesthetic drugs, the potential for injury is high. Patients may display restless or disoriented behavior on emergence from anesthesia and must be protected from self-inflicted injury or disruption of dressings, IVs, drains, catheters, or monitoring equipment. Attention is given to possible causes of agitation, disorientation, or restlessness, and the causes are treated promptly. While the patient remains on the stretcher, safety straps are secured and the side rails maintained in the upright position. Restraints are used only when necessary to protect the patient. Constant nursing surveillance is essential to detect potential sources of injury. All catheters, IVs, and monitors are secured to prevent being dislodged by movement. As will be discussed in the following sections of the chapter, positioning is maintained to protect the airway from aspiration or obstruction, to maintain circulation, and to promote gas exchange.

Common postanesthesia problems

There are a multitude of possible problems or complications that may be encountered in the PACU. Some of the more commonly encountered problems, or potential problems, are listed in the box below.

Research indicates that no matter what type of anesthetic (regional or general) is administered,

---

COMMON POSTANESTHESIA PROBLEMS

Apnea, Hypoventilation, and Hypoxia

Contributing factors
  Airway obstruction
  Respiratory depressant drugs
  Residual effects of muscle relaxants
  Pain
  Constrictive abdominal or thoracic dressings
Treatment
  Airway maintenance
  Oxygen administration
  Reversal of anesthetic agents by narcotic antagonists and anticholinesterases
  Respiratory stimulants
  Wake-up regimen
  Pain relief

Hypotension

Contributing factors
  Hypovolemia (blood loss; fluid deficit)
  Cutaneous vasodilation with rewarming
  Loss of sympathetic tone
  Myocardial dysfunction
  Drugs
  Technical problems
Treatment
  Determine cause
  Replace volume deficits
  Place patient in Trendelenburg's position
  Administer vasopressors

Hypertension

Contributing factors
  Pain
  Delirium and agitation
  Hypoxia
  Hypercarbia
  Excess fluid administration
  Moderate hypothermia
  Gastric or bladder distention
  Preoperative hypertension
Treatment
  Determine cause
  Drug therapy (analgesics; sedation)

there is some degree of impaired respiratory function in the PACU. Most anesthetic agents are potent respiratory depressants, which lead to respiratory depression in almost all patients receiving general anesthesia. Patients under regional or local anesthesia may have been administered sedative drugs during the procedure, leading to respiratory depression in the postoperative period. Incomplete recovery from muscle relaxants administered with anesthesia or loss of respiratory muscle function as a result of regional anesthesia (spinal or epidural) may contribute to postoperative hypoventilation. The site of the surgical incision also affects the degree of altered respiratory function. Patients who have had upper abdominal or thoracic surgery have a greater decrease in lung volumes postoperatively. Pain also contributes to postoperative hypoventilation. Nursing measures to improve respiratory function in the postoperative period include the stir-up regimen and the administration of supplemental oxygen.

Evaluation

When the patient has recovered from the effects of the anesthesia, vital signs have been stabilized, pain has been effectively managed, and complications have been resolved or stabilized, the patient is ready for discharge from the PACU. Most patients' post-anesthesia scores should be at least a 9 or 10 before transfer (Table 24-1), and they must meet the discharge criteria of the PACU. A final nursing assessment and evaluation of the patient is made and documented on the PACU record.

Ongoing Care

Transfer of patient from PACU

When patients are to be sent home, they may be discharged directly from the PACU or they may be sent first to an intermediate area for discharge. If hospitalization is required, the patient is transferred to the appropriate unit. Before such transfer, the nurse should notify the receiving nurse of the patient transfer and any special equipment that may be required. A nurse accompanies the patient during the transfer, and they are met by the receiving nurse. A nursing report to the receiving nurse includes information about:

1. Operative procedure performed
2. Type of anesthetic and medications administered
3. General patient condition
4. Postoperative course including complications, intake and output, and medications or treatments administered in the PACU
5. Presence and condition of dressings, drains, and catheters
6. Last vital signs recorded in the PACU

Sending patient home

If surgery is performed on an outpatient basis, a nursing assessment and evaluation must demonstrate the readiness of the patient for discharge. Therefore assessment and evaluation before discharge should document:

1. Adequate respiratory function
2. Ability of patient to deep breathe, cough, and exhibit an intact gag reflex
3. Stable vital signs and temperature within normal range
4. Level of consciousness and muscle strength
5. Ability of patient to safely ambulate with assistance, consistent with developmental ability
6. Ability of patient to swallow and retain oral fluids
7. Ability of patient to urinate
8. Skin color and condition
9. Pain (minimal), controllable with oral analgesics
10. Adequate neurovascular status of operative extremity
11. Ability of patient to demonstrate proper care of drains and catheters
12. Ability of patient to describe wound care or changing of dressings
13. Ability of patient to describe or demonstrate the proper administration of prescribed medications (eyedrops, eardrops, topically applied ointments, etc.)
14. Patient and provider understanding of home care instructions
15. Written discharge instructions that have been given to patient/family
16. Availability of safe transportation home

When outpatient surgery is done and complications develop, discharge is delayed or the patient is transferred to an appropriate care facility for inpatient care or short-term observation. Side effects or adverse reactions that commonly delay discharge include excessive bleeding or pain, prolonged emergence from anesthesia, dizziness, and intractable nausea and vomiting.

Specific instructions for each patient being discharged should be discussed with both the patient and the accompanying adult and should be provided in written form. Specific instructions generally include:

1. Warnings about avoiding hazardous activity (such as driving or operating machinery) for at least 24 hours; not making important decisions for at least 24 hours; and not consuming any alcohol for at least 24 hours (it may interact with, or potentiate, residual anesthetic drugs or pain medications)
2. Specific limitations of activity

3. Care of the surgical site
4. Special diet or restrictions
5. Signs and symptoms of infection or other complications to watch for
6. When and how to notify the physician if any questions or complications arise
7. Postoperative medications and treatments
8. Follow-up appointments

Ambulatory surgical patients should be given a written pain management plan as part of the discharge plan. The pain management plan should include specific drugs to be taken, frequency of administration, potential side effects and drug interactions, nondrug strategies for pain control, and an individual to notify about pain control problems.

LATER POSTOPERATIVE PERIOD

During the second postoperative phase, there is resolution of the physiologic and psychologic disruptions and imbalances that followed surgery, anesthesia, and healing. Unless this resolution and healing occurs, the patient will not recover from the stress of the operative experience.

NURSING MANAGEMENT OF THE PATIENT DURING LATER POSTOPERATIVE PERIOD

Assessment

Postoperative assessment continues as the postoperative period progresses. Assessment enables the nurse to follow the postoperative recovery of the patient as well as to detect the development of actual or potential complications. A thorough assessment is essential with attention paid to respiratory, cardiovascular, comfort and safety, and psychosocial needs.

Nursing Diagnosis

Nursing diagnoses in the later postoperative period are related to type of surgery, potential postoperative complications, and unique needs of each patient. Commonly encountered nursing diagnoses in the postoperative period include:

Pain related to incision

Impaired gas exchange related to incisional pain, narcotic administration, immobility, or obesity

Altered nutrition: less than body requirements, related to postoperative NPO status or increased metabolic need

Infection related to surgical wound, drains, or catheters

Fluid volume deficit related to wound or gastric drainage, postoperative vomiting, or NPO status

Planning

Goals during this time are maintenance of physiological functioning, promotion of healing, and return to optimal health. Included in the nursing goals are prevention or treatment of postoperative pain, returning the patient to maximal functional level, and care directed toward actual, potential, or possible complications identified by nursing diagnoses. (Care related to specific operative procedures is discussed in later chapters.) Specific nursing outcomes that may be applicable to the postoperative patient include:

Postoperative pain will be controlled through the use of analgesics and alternate pain control methods

The patient will demonstrate cascade cough, sustained maximal inspiration, and normal respiratory pattern

The patient will consume a well-balanced high protein–high carbohydrate diet and maintain or return to preoperative weight

The patient will not experience signs or symptoms of infection

The patient will maintain adequate fluid volume, urine output, and electrolyte balance

Implementation

Postoperative pain

Postoperative pain is one of the greatest fears of patients undergoing surgery. Pain is an extremely complex phenomenon with a variety of factors influencing its manifestation. Postoperative pain occurs most commonly from tissue damage caused by the incision, manipulation, and injury to tissues during surgery. The restriction of movement and the psychologic and the physiologic alterations that accompany pain can result in serious disturbances in normal functions, particularly in the patient with preexisting pulmonary or cardiovascular disease. The most important factor determining the effect of pain on respiration is the site of the incision, with thoracic and upper abdominal incisions producing the greatest detrimental effects on respiration. Severe postoperative pain has been associated with increased levels of circulating catecholamines, which increase blood pressure and may cause cardiac dysrhythmias. Postoperative pain is known to decrease lung function, increase oxygen consumption, and deplete patient energy. As indicated in Figure 24-1 the management of postoperative pain is an ongoing process. Preoperatively, strategies for pain control should be established and implemented as discussed in Chapter 22. Postoperatively, frequent assessment, intervention, reassessment, and appropriate modifications of the pain control plan ensures adequate pain relief using a balance of drug and nondrug strate-

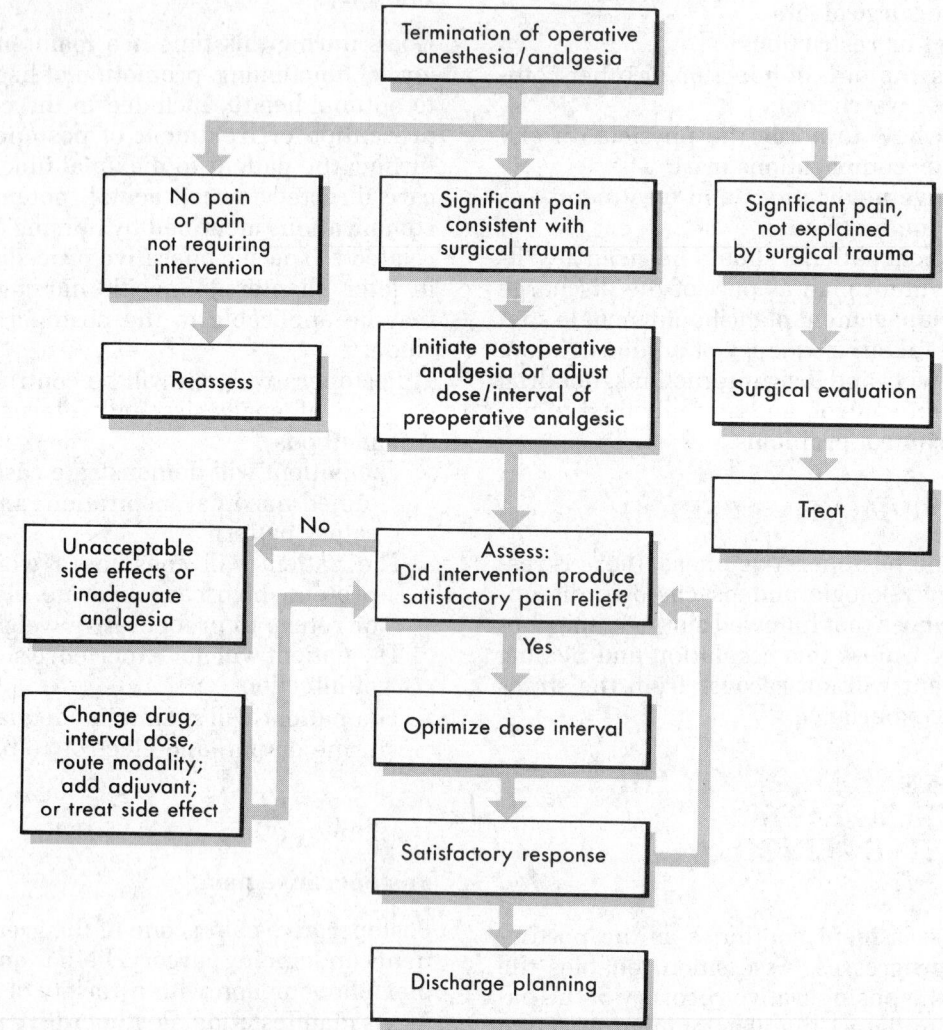

FIGURE 24-1   Critical Thinking Guide: Pain Treatment in the Postoperative Patient. (From US Department of Health and Human Services, Feb 1992.)

gies. Pain and its nursing management are further discussed in Chapter 14.

Alterations in gas exchange

After anesthesia and surgery, patients experience a reduction in pulmonary function. The major factor in decreased pulmonary function is a reduction in lung volumes caused by a shallow, monotonous, sighless breathing pattern in the postoperative period. This breathing pattern results from the effects of pain, analgesic administration, and immobility. Also contributing to reduced pulmonary function is irritation, trauma, or contamination of the tracheobronchial tree during anesthesia and depressed ciliary function and clearance of mucus caused by anesthesia and narcotic administration. Reduction in lung volumes is significant and may persist for many days. As lung volumes decrease, the small airways narrow and become obstructed, and surfactant function is altered. This leads to trapping of air in the alveoli and ultimately to alveolar collapse or **atelectasis.** Atelectasis and retained secretions provide an excellent culture medium for the development of infection or pneumonia. Most patients have adequate reserve to accommodate the altered lung function and recover quickly, although some factors predispose them to the development of impaired gas exchange. Patients at increased risk for postoperative pulmonary complications include chronic cigarette smokers and patients with preexisting pulmonary disease or respiratory infections, obesity, advanced age, an upper abdominal or thoracic incision, or prolonged postoperative immobility.

Nursing measures to prevent or minimize the development of postoperative pulmonary complications include early mobility, SMI, and the cascade cough. Early mobility and frequent position changes facilitate secretion clearance and improve the distribution of ventilation and perfusion in the lungs. Voluntary deep breathing has been used to minimize alveolar collapse and the decrease in lung volumes postoperatively. SMI or maximum inhalation followed by holding the maximal volume for several seconds before exhalation produces high alveolar inflating pressures and is more effective than simple deep breathing in preventing alveolar collapse. Incentive spirometers are devices designed to encourage the patient to perform SMI by providing visual feedback of the inspiratory effort.

Coughing is effective in mobilizing retained secretions that result from anesthesia, surgery, and immobility. The cascade cough (as described in Chapter 26) is most effective in mobilizing secretions. Between cascade coughs, the patient should be encouraged to perform SMI. Practicing SMI dilates the airways during inspiration and compresses the air-

ways when the glottis is closed at maximal inspiration; this "milks" the secretions toward the larger airways where they can be more easily removed by coughing. Chest percussion and postural drainage also facilitate movement of secretions into larger airways.

Wound healing

Healing of surgical wounds takes place in three phases—inflammation, proliferation, and maturation. An hour-by-hour view of the wound healing process is presented in Figure 24-2. The first phase, inflammation, begins at the time of surgery and continues for 4 to 6 days. Initially an exudate containing blood, lymph, and fibrin closely binds the wound edges together. Blood supply and leukocytes (white blood cells) are increased. Strands of fibrin form that hold the tissues together; epithelial cells form a thin layer across the wound and a layer of clotted blood forms a scab. During this phase there is little

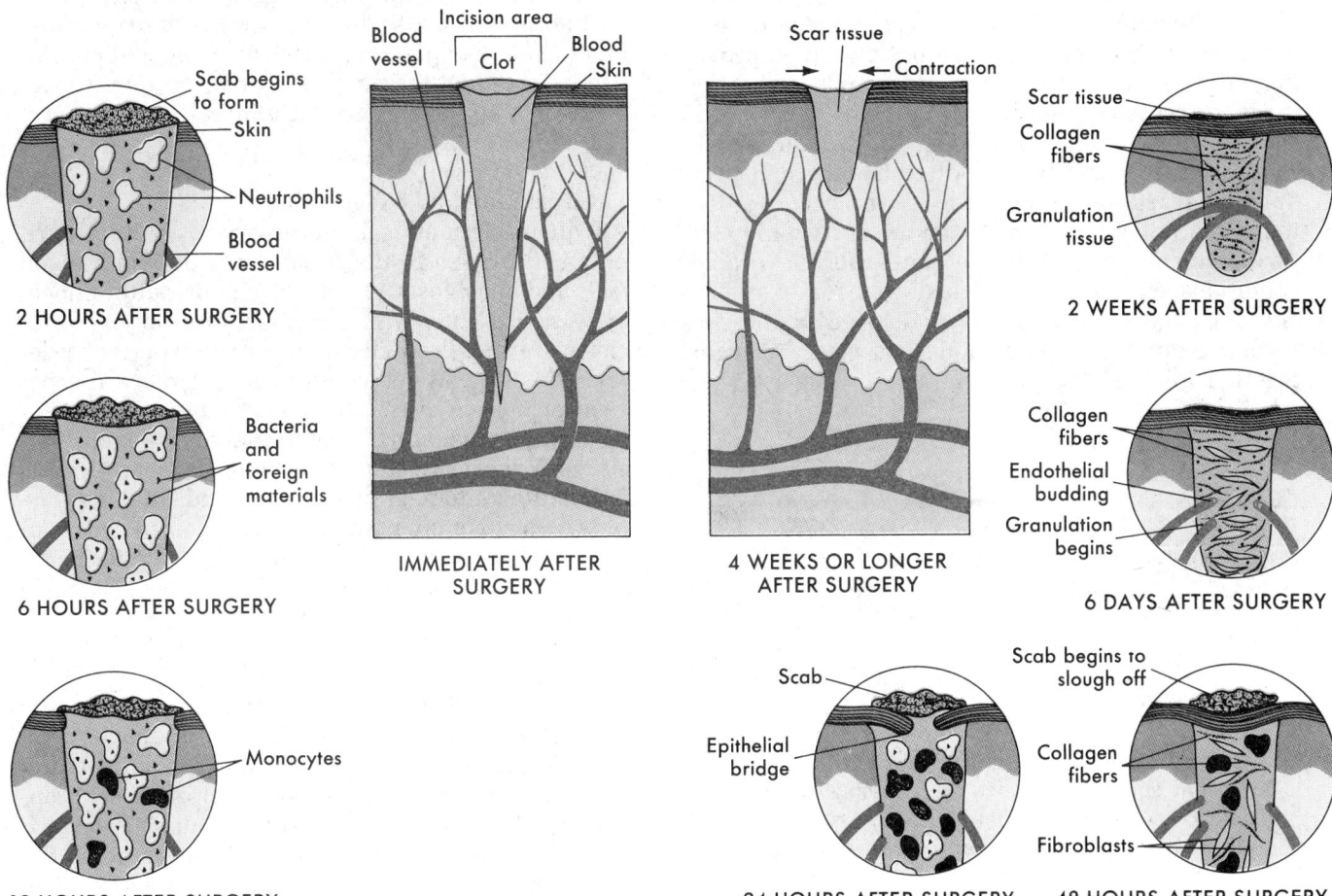

FIGURE 24-2   Hour-by-hour view of the wound healing process—primary intention. (Modified from Johnson & Johnson Products, Inc: *Postoperative wound care*, Part 1, New Brunswick, NJ, 1982.)

increase in wound strength, and sutures hold the wound together.

After the third or fourth day and continuing for about 2 weeks, the proliferative stage of wound healing occurs. During this second phase, there is a rapid proliferation of fibroblasts (connective tissue cells), collagen (a protein fiber), epithelial cells, and blood vessels. This highly vascular connective tissue is called "granulation tissue." The wound becomes progressively stronger during this time, allowing for removal of skin sutures.

Maturation, the third phase of healing, begins in the second or third week following surgery and may continue for up to 2 years. The wound appears healed; however, there continues to be a decrease in fibroblasts, increasing organization of the scar, and increased strength of the wound. Key elements of postoperative wound assessment are listed in the box below.

When the wound edges are closely approximated, with minimal trauma and contamination, the wound heals by **primary intention** or primary healing. Healing by primary intention occurs when there are no complications, such as infection, necrosis, or abnormal scar formation. Healing by **secondary intention** occurs when wound edges are not closely approximated. This is seen in infected wounds or where there is excessive trauma or tissue loss. Healing occurs by granulation tissue filling the wound, which requires more time for complete healing and produces a larger scar. **Tertiary intention** occurs when there is a delay between the injury and wound closure. Suturing may be delayed until more favorable conditions exist for wound healing—for example, clearing of gross infection. With delayed wound closure, two opposing granulation surfaces are brought together for healing.

ASSESSMENT OF THE SURGICAL WOUND

- Examine wound for approximation of suture line
- Observe for edema, bleeding
- Inspect wound for signs of infection: erythema, drainage, odor, pain, induration, suture tension
- Do not generally remove the dressing; drainage and bleeding may be monitored by circling any drainage on the dressing and reevaluating for an increase in size
- Observe wound healing by secondary intention for the presence of granulation tissue; assess tissue integrity and color

Dehiscence and evisceration

Wound healing may be disrupted by **dehiscence** or partial or complete separation of the wound edges. **Evisceration** occurs when the patient's viscera protrude through the disrupted wound. Disruption and evisceration may be caused by problems in suturing the wound or by poor tissue integrity. The patient may report a sensation of "giving" when wound separation occurs. Excessive coughing, straining, malnutrition, obesity, and infection are among the many factors that may predispose a wound to dehiscence. A patient who has experienced dehiscence should be instructed to remain quiet and to avoid coughing or straining. Such a patient should be positioned to remove further stress on the wound. If evisceration occurs, the protruding viscera should be loosely covered with a warm, sterile saline dressing. The surgeon should be notified since treatment consists of reapproximating the wound edges.

Factors altering healing
Nutrition

Nutritional deficiencies are associated with impaired wound healing, and treatment begins with preoperative assessment of adequate nutrition and identification of patients at risk for malnutrition. Nutrients essential for healing include protein, carbohydrates, fats, vitamins, and minerals and are presented in Table 24-2.

Circulation and oxygenation

Adequate circulation is necessary to deliver nutrients and oxygen to the tissue, provide white blood cells and fibroblasts, and remove debris after phagocytosis. Patients with vascular disease or other causes of impaired circulation may experience delayed healing. Major conditions that place the patient at increased risk for inadequate tissue perfusion and oxygenation include diabetes, venous stasis, vascular insufficiency, cardiopulmonary disease, irradiation, edema, hypovolemia, and smoking (one of the most common and least recognized causes of poor wound oxygenation). Since fatty tissue has a relatively poor blood supply, obesity may also delay wound healing.

Drains

When fluid collects within a wound or surgical site, it interferes with wound healing by creating a "dead space" that has no circulation, thus providing a medium for bacterial growth and interfering with approximation of tissues, which may cause tissue irritation. Tissue above this area may break down because of the absence of support and circulation. Fluid collection may result from bleeding, infection, or exudates from the wound. When fluid buildup is anticipated, a drain is often placed within the wound to drain off fluid before it has a chance to accumu-

TABLE 24-2   Function of Key Nutrients Involved in Wound Healing

Specific nutrients	Contribution of wound healing
Amino acids	Needed for neovascularization, lymphocyte formation, fibroblast proliferation, collagen synthesis, and wound remodeling
	Required for certain cell-mediated responses, including phagocytosis and intracellular killing of bacteria
Albumin	Prevents wound edema secondary to low serum oncotic pressure
Glucose	Needed for energy requirement of leukocytes and fibroblasts to function in inhibiting activities of wound infection

Essential unsaturated fatty acids
  Linoleic
  Linolenic
  Arachidonic
	Serve as building blocks for prostaglandins that regulate cellular metabolism, inflammation, and circulation
	Are consituents of triglycerides and fatty acids contained in cellular and subcellular membranes

Ascorbic acid	Needed for hydroxylation of proline and lysine in collagen synthesis
	Enhances capillary formation and decreases capillary fragility
	Is a necessary component of complement that functions in immune reactions and increases defenses to infection
Vitamin B complex	Serve as cofactors of enzyme systems
Pyridoxine, pantothenic and folic acid	Required for antibody formation and white blood cell function
Vitamin A	Enhances epithelialization of cell membranes
	Enhances rate of collagen synthesis and cross-linking of newly formed collagen
	Antagonizes the inhibitory effects of glucocorticoids on cell membranes
Vitamin D	Necessary for absorption, transport, and metabolism of calcium
	Indirectly affects phosphorus metabolism
Vitamin E	No special role known; may be important if there is a fatty acid deficiency
Vitamin K	Needed for synthesis of prothrombin and clotting factors VII, IX, and X
	Required for synthesis of calcium-binding protein
Zinc	Stabilizes cell membranes
	Needed for cell mitosis and cell proliferation in wound repair
Iron	Needed for hydroxylation of proline and lysine in collagen synthesis
	Enhances bactericidal activity of leukocytes
	Secondarily, deficiency may cause decrease in oxygen transport to wound
Copper	Is an integral part of the enzyme lysyl oxidase, which catalyzes formation of stable collagen cross-links

From Schumann D: Preoperative measures to promote wound healing, *Nurs Clin North Am* 14:683, 1979.

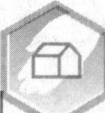

HOME CARE GUIDE   *Postoperative Wound Care*

Each patient who has had a surgical and/or an invasive diagnostic procedure must be evaluated to determine if there is a need for postoperative wound care.

Short-term goals

By the time of discharge:
1. The patient will use, verbalize, and perform basic knowledge of wound care procedures prescribed by the physician.
2. All the supplies and equipment needed to carry out procedures will be available at the time of discharge or will be ordered and delivered to the patient's home in time for the next dressing or procedure.
3. A referral will be made to a home care agency, including specific information about the nursing care procedures that will need to be carried out in the home.

Long-term goals

1. The patient's wound will heal without complications.
2. Wound management will be incorporated into the total care plan of the patient.

Nursing assessment
Health management pattern

The patient's ability to care for his own wound depends on factors such as the location of the wound, which affects the ability to see or reach the wound, the type of wound care involved, such as packing, irrigating, or a simple dry sterile dressing; the patient's energy level; and the total care needs of the patient. Patients with wounds of the lower extremity may have weight-bearing and ambulation restrictions. Wounds of the upper extremity may make it impossible for the patient to do the wound care since most wound care procedures take two hands.

Cognitive pattern

The patient and/or caregiver must be able to learn the procedure, especially if it is a complex wound management plan.

Therapeutic plan

The total medical plan must be assessed so that an overall plan can be established. The physician may want a wound to heal by secondary intention; therefore the packing procedure is very important. The type of antibiotic and the route of administration must be known so that teaching can begin. The physician may plan on an extended course of IV antibiotics and wound care.

Potential for compliance

Wound healing depends on wound management, taking of all prescribed medications, and completion of all procedures. The patient must be aware of the importance of taking medications, especially antibiotics, on a scheduled basis and must be aware of the importance of each of the steps in the irrigation and wound-packing procedure.

Environment

The need for bathroom facilities for handwashing and wound care is very important for patients being discharged.

Planning

For patients needing ongoing wound management:

Planning for discharge

Planning for discharge for a patient needing wound care may need to be done 2 to 3 days before discharge or may be done on the day of discharge, depending on the complexity of the procedure. Some lengths of stay for surgical procedures are relatively short, and some wound management plans are not decided on until discharge. When discharge to a skilled facility or nursing home occurs, a liaison nurse should be provided by the facility to observe the procedure. Continuity of care should also be provided by a well-documented care plan, detailing the wound care procedure.

Patient education

Education of the patient/caregiver for wound management includes understanding:
1. The type of dressings used for all steps in the procedure including the type of dressing for packing a wound, the type for absorbing wound drainage, special dressings that are precut to go around a tube and the type of tape to be used to secure the dressing, and any specific brands of dressings currently used.
2. Wound irrigation procedures, including the type of irrigation solution used, and the equipment needed to flush the wound and catch the solution as it runs out.
3. Instructions in sterile technique using gloves and sterilized equipment (included when there is danger of contamination of an open wound).
4. Discarding of dressings and irrigation solutions especially from an infected wound.

HOME CARE GUIDE *Postoperative Wound Care—cont'd*

5. How to reorder equipment ahead of time. Since the patient will be receiving care other than in the hospital, wound care supplies should not be sent home with the patient; the wound management procedure may change and the supplies may not be needed. In addition, hospital supplies are intended to be used for hospital patients, and the additional cost of sending supplies home is not built into a hospital budget.
6. Instructions in signs and symptoms of infection, dehiscence, or hemorrhage, along with how and when to seek medical care.
7. Instructions in wound healing so that the patient can recognize steps in the wound healing process.

Implementation

For patients needing ongoing wound management:
1. Ordering of supplies can be done through a local pharmacy or home care company. The order can be called into the patient's pharmacy or the nurse can give a list of supplies needed to the patient or caregiver for purchase on the way home. Some irrigation solutions require a prescription.

2. If the patient cannot do the procedure, the patient should be referred to a home care agency for wound management or for additional instructions in the home environment. In some cases the nurse in the hospital can request that dressings be brought to the home by the home care nurse. In this case the patient should still be aware of the need for some dressing supplies in case the dressing becomes disrupted on the way home, or in case the home care nurse is delayed.
3. All necessary referral forms should be completed, including giving patient/caregiver education as well as assessing the patient's and caregiver's understanding of the procedure and the place where supplies are to be ordered.

late and interfere with healing. Drains may also be placed to drain the bladder, stomach, or bowel. When a large amount of drainage is present, the drains may be attached to a collection bottle or bag and are sometimes attached to suction to facilitate drainage.

Some of the drains commonly used include gastrostomy tubes, nasogastric tubes, T-tubes, Foley catheters, and Penrose drains. Nursing interventions include monitoring and recording the type and amount of drainage. To ensure proper function of the drain, kinking or plugging of the drain should be avoided. The patient should generally not lie on the drain, and drains should be secured to prevent dislodging. Indications, use, and nursing care for various drains are discussed throughout the text in relation to specific body systems and operative procedures.

Infection

Bacterial wound contamination is one of the most common causes of altered wound healing. Even though strict aseptic technique is used to minimize bacterial contamination, all wounds are contaminated postoperatively to some extent. Contamination of the wound may occur preoperatively (following trauma, skin infection, or from nicks and abrasions related to preoperative shaving), intraoperatively (by exposure to bowel contents or pus), or

postoperatively. If the amount of bacteria in the wound is sufficient or immune defenses are compromised, clinical infection may result. Infection slows healing by prolonging the inflammatory phase of healing, competing for nutrients in the wound, and producing damaging chemicals and enzymes.

Dressings

Most operative wounds are covered with a dressing in the operating room. Individual physician preferences and differences in the type of wound may affect the type of dressing used. Regardless of the type of dressing, they speed the rate of epithelialization, decrease motion within the wound, decrease postoperative pain, and minimize the potential for infection or bleeding.

Wound dressings may be either occlusive or nonocclusive. The process of epithelial resurfacing is an important part of the healing process and requires a moist environment. When nonocclusive dressings are used or the wound is left exposed, a dry crust-scab forms and slows the process of reepithelialization. Occlusive dressings provide a moist environment, which is more conducive to epithelial regeneration, but have the disadvantage of providing a good environment for growth of microorganisms under the dressing. After the first few days, the wound is covered with epithelium and the dressings serve little purpose except to prevent trauma to the wound, such as chafing from clothes or catching of sutures or skin staples on linens. Other methods of covering surgical wounds include sprays or ointments that leave a thin protective covering to prevent drying or abrasion of the wound.

Maintaining circulation

Thrombosis

Development of clots in the larger veins of the pelvis and lower extremities may occur after surgery. A clot in the vein, also called a "thrombus," may impair circulation, or a section of the clot may break off and move through the bloodstream to the heart or lungs as a pulmonary embolism. Venous thrombosis—associated with an inflammatory response causing pain, swelling, and tenderness—is called thrombophlebitis. When a thrombus within a vessel produces little or no signs or symptoms, the condition is called phlebothrombosis.

Three factors may play a role in the development of venous thrombosis; hypercoagulation, damage to the venous wall, and stasis or slow movement of blood. Postoperatively, venous stasis is probably the most common cause of venous thrombosis. After trauma and tissue damage (i.e., surgery), coagulation products develop in the circulation and may be deposited at sites of venous stasis. Thrombosis most commonly occurs in the calf, thigh, or pelvic veins. A clot may form without any symptoms. If symptoms do occur, they may include increased temperature in the affected limb or, systemically, pain or swelling in the limb. Homans' sign, or calf pain on dorsiflexion of the foot, indicates a probable thrombus, but this sign is not always present. If the thrombus is in a superficial vein, a reddened line along the path of the vessel may be present. Patients may complain of an aching or tender knot or bump in their leg.

Nursing interventions focus initially on prevention of thrombus formation. The box at top, right, lists some of the risk factors associated with the occurrence of deep venous thrombosis. If signs or symptoms suggestive of a venous thrombosis occur, the patient should be confined to bed rest and the physician notified. Elevation, heat, rest, elastic bandages, and anticoagulants are usually prescribed to prevent thrombi from embolizing and to prevent new thrombus formation. The affected extremity should be handled with care to avoid dislodging the clot.

Embolism

Pulmonary embolism is a serious consequence of venous thrombosis and, if large enough, may result in sudden death. Patients with a pulmonary embolism may exhibit dyspnea, wheezing, chest pain, and hemoptysis, or shock. Symptoms of a pulmonary em-

---

RISK FACTORS ASSOCIATED WITH DEVELOPMENT OF POSTOPERATIVE VENOUS THROMBOSIS

Pathologic conditions
Malignancy
Congestive heart failure
History of deep-vein thrombosis
Polycythemia

Type of surgery
Pelvic surgery
Abdominal or thoracic surgery
Fracture of hip or leg

Surgery-related factors
Anesthesia
Shock
Reduced mobility
Sitting for long periods
Pressure on popliteal area
Intestinal distention
Tight dressings or casts on lower extremities

Intrinsic factors
Advanced age
Obesity
Malnutrition
Oral contraceptive use
Hypercoagulation states
Dehydration

---

bolus require immediate notification of the patient's physician. Since pulmonary emboli result from deep-vein thrombosis, prevention is the same as for deep-vein thrombosis. Nursing care and medical management are discussed in Chapter 32.

Maintaining metabolic equilibrium

Nutrition

Malnutrition occurs in many surgical patients and contributes to delayed wound healing, prolonged recovery time, and increased postoperative complications. After surgery, there is a sudden increase in metabolic demand that results in a large mobilization of body proteins, fat, and carbohydrates to supply increased metabolic needs and tissue needs for healing. This is called the **catabolic phase,** when body stores are metabolized in the postoperative patient. Carbohydrate reserves are rapidly exhausted, and then the body must break down protein and fat for energy. Because of the stress response to surgery, the body preferentially uses protein for metabolic needs (protein catabolism) rather than stores of fat. As stress continues, the body adapts and begins to better use fat stores for energy requirements. Later the body turns to an **anabolic phase,** or constructive metabolic state, during which depleted proteins and essential nutrients are restored. This change may occur in a matter of a day or two or take several months in cases of severe tissue injury and trauma.

Adequate nutrition, particularly in the catabolic phase, is important to meet increased needs for metabolism and tissue repair. Insufficient nutritional intake may be classified as either insufficient protein intake (protein malnutrition) or insufficient intake of both proteins and calories (protein-calorie malnutrition). Food and fluid intake records, calorie counts, and daily weights may help the nurse in assessing the patient's nutritional status. A postoperative diet high in protein, calories, vitamins, and minerals is encouraged, unless it is contraindicated for the patient. In the later stages of recovery, when the patient is in the anabolic phase, nutritional intake and needs are assessed again. Patients who experience a prolonged recovery, particularly with reduced activity, may need a reduction of caloric intake to prevent unhealthy weight gain related to decreased energy expenditure. Chapter 16 provides more complete information on nutrition.

Fluid and electrolytes

Maintenance of the body's water and electrolyte balance and distribution are essential to proper functioning of body systems. The response to surgery and anesthesia generally includes conservation of fluid and salt by the kidney resulting from sympathetic stimulation, secretion of antidiuretic hormone (ADH), and activation of the renin-angiotensin system (see Chapter 12). Extracellular fluid volume deficits may result from inadequate fluid replacement during surgery and recovery and increased losses from vomiting, gastric suctioning, diarrhea, wound drainage, diaphoresis, or fever. In addition, loss of fluid into tissues (third spacing) occurs from tissue trauma, manipulation, or shock and is especially pronounced following abdominal or major operative procedures. Fluid overload may occur after surgery, particularly in patients with cardiopulmonary or renal disease, but is much less common then fluid deficits.

Electrolyte alterations may occur postoperatively because of a shift from one body compartment to another or because of excessive intake or losses. The two electrolytes most commonly involved are potassium and sodium. Patients at risk are those with reduced cardiovascular or renal function, fluid volume abnormalities, increased losses from diarrhea, vomiting, fistula, or wound drainage, or those receiving diuretics. Assessment and nursing interventions for patients with electrolyte alterations are discussed in Chapter 12.

Maintaining urinary function

Urinary retention

Postoperative urinary retention sometimes occurs. Causes of postoperative urinary retention include trauma to the bladder or its nerve supply from operations done in close proximity to the bladder, edema around the bladder neck and reflex spasm of sphincters that may accompany pain or anxiety, and drugs, particularly anesthetic-related drugs, which may cause retention. Spinal and epidural anesthesia may cause urinary retention because of delayed recovery of autonomic bladder reflexes.

Nursing interventions to facilitate voiding include ambulation and normal positioning for voiding. Techniques such as running water so the patient can hear the sound, running water over the perineum, having the patient sit in a warm bath, or heat application to the perineum may help the patient void. Another important measure is to reassure the patient and provide a private, stress-free environment to help the patient relax. When these measures fail, catheterization should be performed to relieve distention. Because of a lower infection rate, intermittent catheterization is generally preferred to an indwelling catheter.

Urinary tract infection

The urinary tract is the most common site for nosocomial infections, and these are generally associated with urinary tract catheterization. Single brief catheterizations are associated with lower infection rates. Microorganisms are introduced into the bladder along the outside of the catheter and along the internal lumen of the catheter if the collection system has been contaminated. Prevention of urinary tract infection includes use of strict sterile technique for catheterization, intermittent catheterization rather than indwelling catheters, limiting the use of indwelling catheters to the shortest possible time, maintaining a sterile, closed drainage system, and appropriate catheter and meatal hygiene.

Maintaining gastrointestinal function

Acute parotitis

Acute parotitis, or "surgical mumps," is a staphlylococcal infection that may develop in the parotid glands postoperatively. The signs and symptoms are pain, swelling, and tenderness at the angle of the jaw. An elevated temperature and white blood count may also occur. The infection requires prompt treatment to avoid possible spread to adjacent tissues. The factors that seem to increase risk include poor oral hygiene, dehydration, and the use of anticholinergic drugs. Preventive nursing interventions include adequate hydration, good oral hygiene, and stimulation of salivary flow by having the patient chew gum, hard candy, or lemon slices.

Nausea and vomiting

Nausea and vomiting may develop from a variety of causes including medications, gastric distention, surgical manipulation, pain, shock, electrolyte abnormalities, and psychologic factors. Nursing measures to prevent or treat nausea and vomiting include limiting oral intake until peristalsis has returned, beginning the postoperative diet with liquids and advancing to a normal diet as patient tolerance increases, moving the patient slowly, controlling pain, and reducing patient fear and anxiety. When nonpharmacologic methods are ineffective in controlling nausea and vomiting, antiemetic medications may be prescribed.

Hiccoughs

Factors that may contribute to hiccoughs (singultuses) include surgery near the phrenic nerve, peritonitis, gastric distention, intestinal obstruction, and acid-base and electrolyte disturbances. Hiccoughs may be disturbing to the patient and painful in the presence of an abdominal incision but, if short-lived, are usually not harmful. If hiccoughs persist, they can lead to exhaustion, vomiting, and wound dehiscence.

Paralytic ileus

Paralytic ileus is the condition of diminished or absent peristalsis. Stress response to surgery and anesthesia, manipulation of abdominal organs during surgery, electrolyte imbalances, use of anesthetics and pain medications, wound infections, and postoperative immobility can all contribute to diminished or uncoordinated peristalsis. Paralytic ileus occurs to some degree following all abdominal operations with a gradual return of bowel motility over several days. Signs and symptoms include diminished bowel sounds, abdominal distention, and feelings of fullness. Ileus may be accompanied by vomiting, particularly if there is any oral intake before return of normal peristalsis. Nursing measures include withholding oral intake until bowel sounds return. Ambulation may hasten the return of peristalsis. A nasogastric tube may be placed to prevent distention and vomiting until bowel function returns. In addition to the return of bowel sounds, the passing of flatus or feces per rectum and the return of the patient's appetite signal the return of peristalsis.

Constipation

Constipation is caused by decreased gastrointestinal motility and is often the result of analgesic adminis-

tration or altered dietary intake. The constipated patient may experience abdominal distention, bloating, headaches, or nausea. Nursing measures to prevent or restore normal bowel habits include early ambulation, adequate hydration, increasing bulk and roughage in the diet unless contraindicated, and administering stool softeners and cathartics. Bowel function should be monitored postoperatively and treatment initiated before development of severe constipation or stool impactions.

Evaluation

The patient may achieve either a complete postoperative recovery in a short amount of time without complications, require a prolonged postoperative recovery, or may never return to the preoperative functional level. The goals of periodic postoperative evaluation are to determine the progress the patient has made toward meeting established goals and returning to optimal health. As initial nursing and patient goals are met, new goals may be established to further recovery. Evaluation provides the basis for determining the appropriateness, effectiveness, and need for continuing nursing care with the ultimate goal being to restore the patient to a level of health where nursing interventions are no longer necessary.

CRITICAL THINKING QUESTIONS

1 Discuss nursing assessment of the patient in the postanesthesia care unit (PACU).
2 What is the postanesthesia recovery score? How is it used?
3 What are common postanesthesia problems? Describe the related nursing care.
4 What are the steps in discharging and transferring a patient from the PACU?
5 What are common problems in the later postoperative period?
6 What nursing activities prevent postoperative complications and promote healing?
7 Outline the steps in the wound healing process.

RESOURCES

1 American Society of Postanesthesia Nurses (ASPAN) 11508 Allecingie Parkway, Suite C Richmond, VA 23235 (804) 692-7050

BIBLIOGRAPHY

Current

1. Acute Pain Management Guideline Panel. *Acute pain management: operative or medical procedures and trauma.* AHCPR Pub No 92-0032. Rockville, Md, Feb

1992, Agency for Health Care Policy and Research, Public Health Service, US Department of Health and Human Services.

2. Alsberger DB, Shrewsbury P: Postoperative pain management: the PACU nurse's challenge, *J Postanesth Nurs* 3(6):399, 1988.

3. Drain CB, Christoph SS: *The recovery room, a critical care approach to postanesthesia nursing,* ed 2, Philadelphia, 1987, WB Saunders.

4. Feldman ME: Inadvertent hypothermia: a threat to homeostasis in the postanesthetic patient, *J Postanesth Nurs* 3(2):82, 1988.

5. Hardy EB, Cirello BL, Gutzeit NM: Rewarming patients in the PACU: can we make a difference? *J Postanesth Nurs* 3(5):313, 1988.

6. Isreal SJ, DeKornfeld TJ: *Recovery room care,* ed 2, Chicago, 1987, Mosby–Year Book.

7. Litwack K: Practical points in the management of hypothermia, *J Postanesth Nurs* 3(5):339, 1988.

8. Litwack K, Parnass S: Practical points in the management of postoperative nausea and vomiting, *J Postanesth Nurs* 3(4):275, 1988.

9. McCammon RL: Management of postanesthesia complications in the recovery room, 1987 Review Course Lectures, Cleveland, 1987, p. 90, International Anesthesia Research Society.

10. Mendelson LS: Pain management for ambulatory surgery, *J Postanesth Nurs* 3(2):109, 1988.

11. Nimmo WS: New directions in the management of postoperative pain, 1988 Review Course Lectures, Cleveland, 1988, International Anesthesia Research Society, p. 16.

12. Orgill D, Demling RH: Current concepts and approaches to wound healing, *Crit Care Med* 16(9):899, 1988.

13. Taylor TH, Major E: Hazards and complications of anesthesia, New York, 1987, Churchill Livingstone.

14. Trounson LW: Hypertensive crisis, *J Postanesth Nurs* 3(2):102, 1988.

15. White PF: Management of postoperative pain—use of opioid analgesics, 1987 Review Course Lectures, Cleveland, 1987, International Anesthesia Research Society, p. 84.

Classic

16. Aldrete JA, Kroulik D: A postanesthetic recovery score, *Anesth Analg* 49:924, 1970.

17. Cramer C: The postanesthetic assessment checklist: a clinical nursing assessment tool, *Breathline* 4(3):7, 1984.

18. Drain C: Comparison of two inspiratory maneuvers on increasing lung volumes in postoperative upper abdominal surgical patients, *AANA J* 52(4):379, 1984.

19. Drain C: Postanesthesia lung volumes in surgical patients, *AANA J* 49(3):261, 1981.

20. Luczun ME: *Handbook of postanesthesia nursing,* Rockville, Md, 1981, Aspen Publishers Inc.

21. Standards of Nursing Practice, Richmond, Va, 1986, The American Society of Postanesthesia Nurses.

22. Wetchler BV: Postanesthesia scoring system, discharging ambulatory surgery patients, *AORN J* 41(2):382, 1985.

23. Wetchler BV: Managing pain in the postanesthesia care unit, *J Postanesth Nurs* 1(1):52, 1986.

24. Wysocki AB: Surgical wound healing, a review for perioperative nurses, *AORN J* 49(2):502, 1989.

25. Young ME: Malnutrition and wound healing, *Heart Lung* 17(1):60, 1988.

PART TWO

Practice of Adult Health Nursing

UNIT VI

Respiratory System

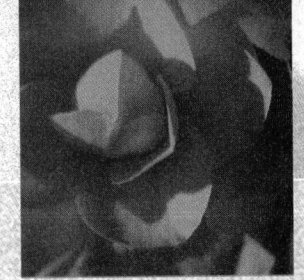

CHAPTER TWENTY-FIVE

Nursing Assessment of the Respiratory System

LEARNING OBJECTIVES

1 Understand the structure and function of the respiratory system.
2 Describe the physical principles of respiratory gas transport.
3 Obtain relevant subjective information from the patient who has a respiratory alteration.
4 Using correct technique, examine the patient to obtain appropriate objective information about the respiratory system.
5 Differentiate abnormal from normal subjective and objective findings related to the respiratory system.
6 Describe procedures and tests used in the detection and diagnosis of disorders of the respiratory system.
7 Describe patient preparation and care related to diagnostic procedures of the respiratory system.

KEY TERMS

THE RESPIRATORY SYSTEM maintains the homeostasis of carbon dioxide and oxygen by adjusting the ventilation of the pulmonary alveoli to maintain a constant concentration of carbon dioxide in arterial blood. This level of ventilation also maintains the homeostasis of oxygen because normally it is greater than is required for hemoglobin to become saturated with oxygen. Respiration can be divided into the processes that (1) result in the ventilation of the alveoli, (2) are responsible for carrying oxygen and carbon dioxide between the alveoli and the tissue cells, and (3) maintain the homeostasis of arterial carbon dioxide and, to a lesser extent, oxygen concentrations.

Assessment of the respiratory system includes examining the nose, sinuses, mouth, throat, tracheobronchial airways, lungs, and thoracic cage. The examination of the thorax and lungs, in particular, is conducted in conjunction with the cardiovascular system assessment.

ANATOMY AND PHYSIOLOGY
Ventilation

Anatomy of respiratory tract

The respiratory tract is often divided into the upper and lower respiratory tracts. The **upper respiratory tract** (Figure 25-1) includes the nose, the paranasal sinuses, and the pharynx. The nasal mucosa is responsible for warming and humidifying the incoming air, and the hairs and mucus are responsible for filtering out any particles suspended in it. This protects the bronchial tree from dehydration, contamination, and irritation. In the upper part of the nose the mucosa contains *olfactory* sensory cells that are able to detect a variety of substances in solution and are responsible for the sense of smell.

The *paranasal sinuses* are blind-ended cavities that connect with the nasal cavity and are lined by nasal mucosa (Figure 25-2). The middle ear connects with the nasopharynx through the *eustachian tubes,* which are also lined with nasal mucosa. The sinuses and the middle ear are susceptible to nasal and throat infections, which spread to them via the mucosa. This can be particularly serious when the infection spreads to the middle ear and mastoid sinuses, because it may cause permanent hearing loss or spread further into the meninges.

The *pharynx* extends from the posterior portion of the nose to the esophagus and larynx. It is divided anatomically according to location: the nasopharynx near the nose, the oropharynx near the mouth, and the laryngeal pharynx near the larynx. The pharynx is very muscular, and its various openings can be closed off to permit passage either of air during inspiration or expiration or food or drink during swallowing or vomiting. These two functions should never occur simultaneously because food could enter the trachea, block it, and cause death by as-

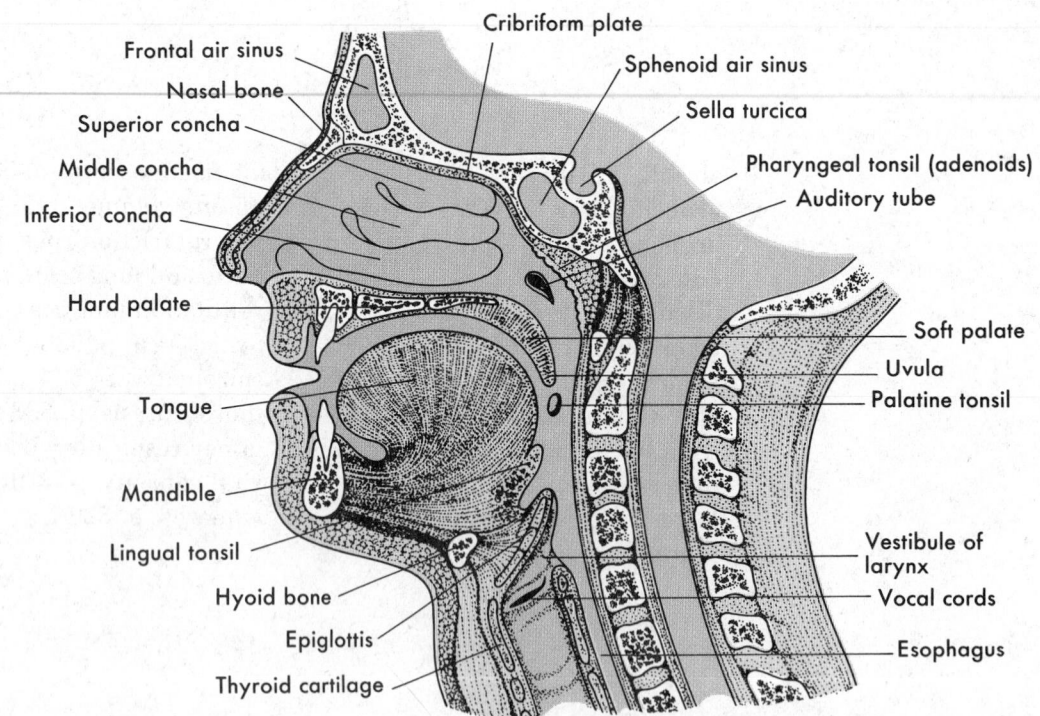

FIGURE 25-1   Upper respiratory tract.

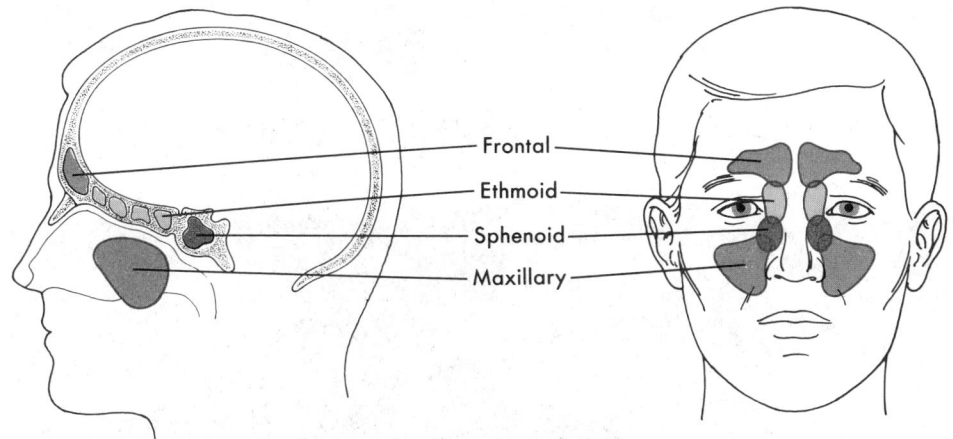

FIGURE 25-2   Location of sinuses.

phyxia. Normally the pharyngeal openings are relaxed for respiration and are closed off by a complex reflex during swallowing or vomiting (see Unit XV). With the exception of the nose and pharynx, the respiratory tract is lined throughout with *ciliated columnar epithelium* and liberally supplied with mucus-secreting goblet cells. The mucus secreted by the respiratory mucosa contains IgA antibodies that protect the lungs against some of the endemic infectious agents, and it also traps particles so they can be carried out of the respiratory tree in the mucus swept toward the pharynx by the cilia of the columnar epithelium.

The **lower respiratory tract** is made up of the larynx, the trachea, the bronchial tree, and the lungs (Figure 25-3).

The *larynx* (voice box) is a strong cartilage tube that forms the upper end of the trachea. Two pairs of folds jut out into its lumen. The lower pair are the true *vocal cords* that can be made to vibrate to produce sounds of different frequencies, as in singing or speaking. The top of the larynx is closed off by a flap of cartilage called the *epiglottis*. This is done by reflex muscle contraction during swallowing or vomiting.

The *trachea* (windpipe) is a tube that is strengthened by C-shaped *hyaline cartilage* rings that keep the airway open. It branches at its inferior end into the right and left *primary bronchi*. (Aspirated foreign objects generally lodge in the right bronchus, because it is larger and more vertical.) Each primary bronchus divides into *secondary* and *tertiary bronchi* and *bronchioles.* All these tubes are also kept patent by cartilaginous rings. The bronchioles divide into smaller and smaller tubes until the smallest, the *alveolar ducts,* lead to the **alveoli,** which form the mass of the lungs.

The right lung is made up of three lobes, the left of two. The lung tissue is very elastic, and the lungs are always stretched to fill the thoracic cavity at both sides of the mediastinum. This creates a negative (subatmospheric) pressure in the *intrapleural* (intrathoracic) space. If air enters this space, the lungs shrink to a considerably smaller size.

The *bronchial tree* distributes air to the alveoli of the various lobes and segments of the lungs. The surface area of the alveoli is approximately 40 times that of the skin and is made up of two layers of squamous epithelium separated by a narrow interstitial space. The bronchial tree provides an extremely large surface area for gas exchange between alveolar air and blood.

Pulmonary ventilation

Pulmonary ventilation mixes the stale air in the alveoli with fresh air from the atmosphere to remove excess carbon dioxide from the blood and replace the oxygen used by metabolism.

Ventilation of the alveoli results from alternately lowering and raising the air pressure within the lungs by alternately increasing and decreasing their volume, so that air is drawn into and forced out of the alveoli. Inasmuch as the lungs are stuck by the negative intrapleural pressure to the walls of the thoracic cavity and the diaphragm, their volume changes with the volume of the thoracic cavity.

For **inspiration,** the volume of the thorax (and the lungs) is increased by contracting the external intercostal skeletal muscles to raise the rib cage and increase the diameter of the thorax, and contracting the diaphragm to lower it and increase the longitudinal dimension of the thorax. This lowers the intrapulmonary pressure, and air is forced into the lungs by the higher exterior air pressure until intrapulmonary pressure rises to equal it.

Expiration is usually a passive process. Relaxing the external intercostal muscles and the diaphragm

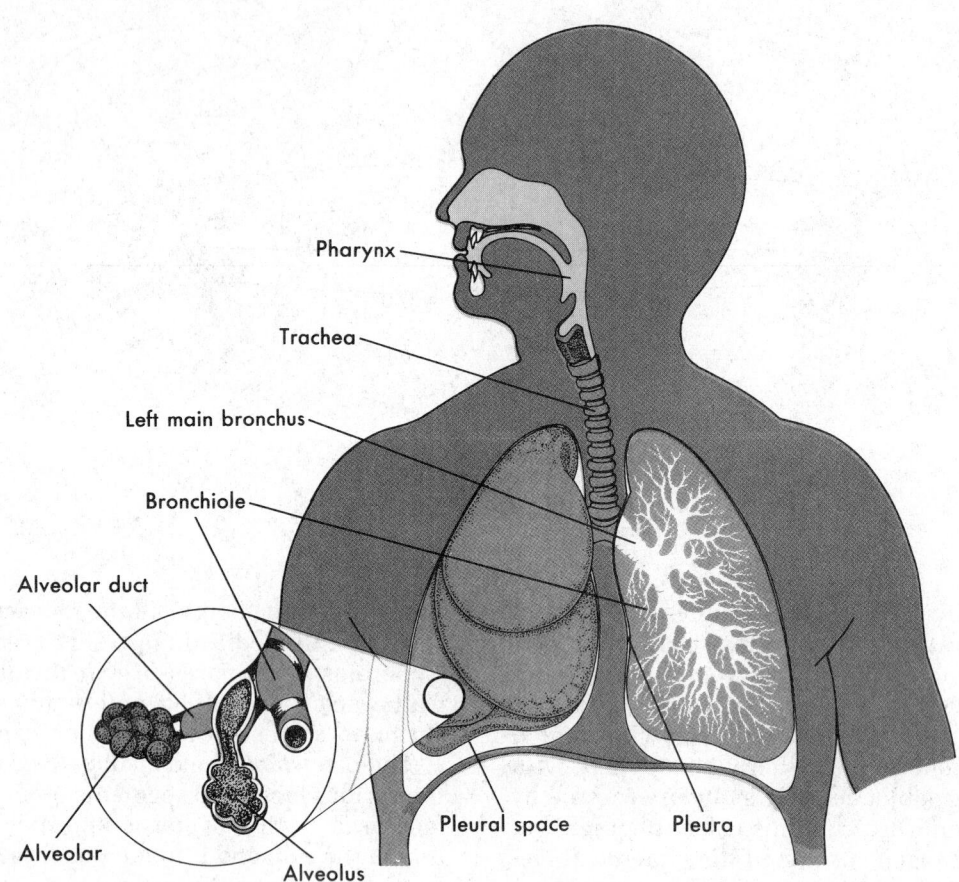

Pharynx

Trachea

Left main bronchus

Bronchiole

Alveolar duct

Alveolar

Alveolus

Pleural space

Pleura

FIGURE 25-3   Lower respiratory tract.

is sufficient because then the elasticity of the lungs and the surface tension of the alveoli compress the lungs and chest wall, increase intrapulmonary pressure, and force air out of the lungs. However, when metabolism is increased and the respiratory system is stressed, expiration may be speeded up by contracting the internal intercostal muscles and, if additional force is required, by contracting the abdominal muscles. For adults the respiratory rate is usually 8 to 16 breaths per minute at rest.

Lung volumes

The maximum amount of air that can be inspired or expired in one breath is called the **vital capacity.** This volume of air can be divided into three components:

1. *Tidal volume* is the amount of air breathed in or out at any particular time. It increases as metabolic activity increases.
2. *Inspiratory reserve volume* is the volume of air that can be forcibly inspired at the end of a normal tidal inspiration.
3. *Expiratory reserve volume* is the volume of air that can be forcibly expired at the end of a normal tidal expiration.

The proportion of the vital capacity taken up by the tidal volume increases with physical activity at the expense of the remaining two volumes. The relationship among these three volumes, vital capacity, and total lung volume is given in Figure 25-4.

After as much air as possible has been expired, air still remains in the lungs trapped in the alveoli. This volume of air is called the *residual volume.* When the thorax is opened, the lungs shrink to a smaller size, and the volume of air that remains is called the *minimal volume.* Only the lungs of a fetus or a stillborn baby do not contain air.

Another important lung volume is the *anatomic dead space,* which is made up of the air in the passageways that do not take part in gas exchange with the blood. The anatomic dead space makes up approximately 30% of the tidal volume and contains stale alveolar air at the end of expiration. This stale air is the first air to enter the alveoli during inspiration, and if the dead space is increased by, for example, breathing through a tube, no fresh air will enter the alveoli until the tidal volume has exceeded the volume of the natural dead space plus the volume of the tube. If the tube volume is large, it is possible that no fresh air will enter the alveoli, and the individual will asphyxiate. For this reason snorkel

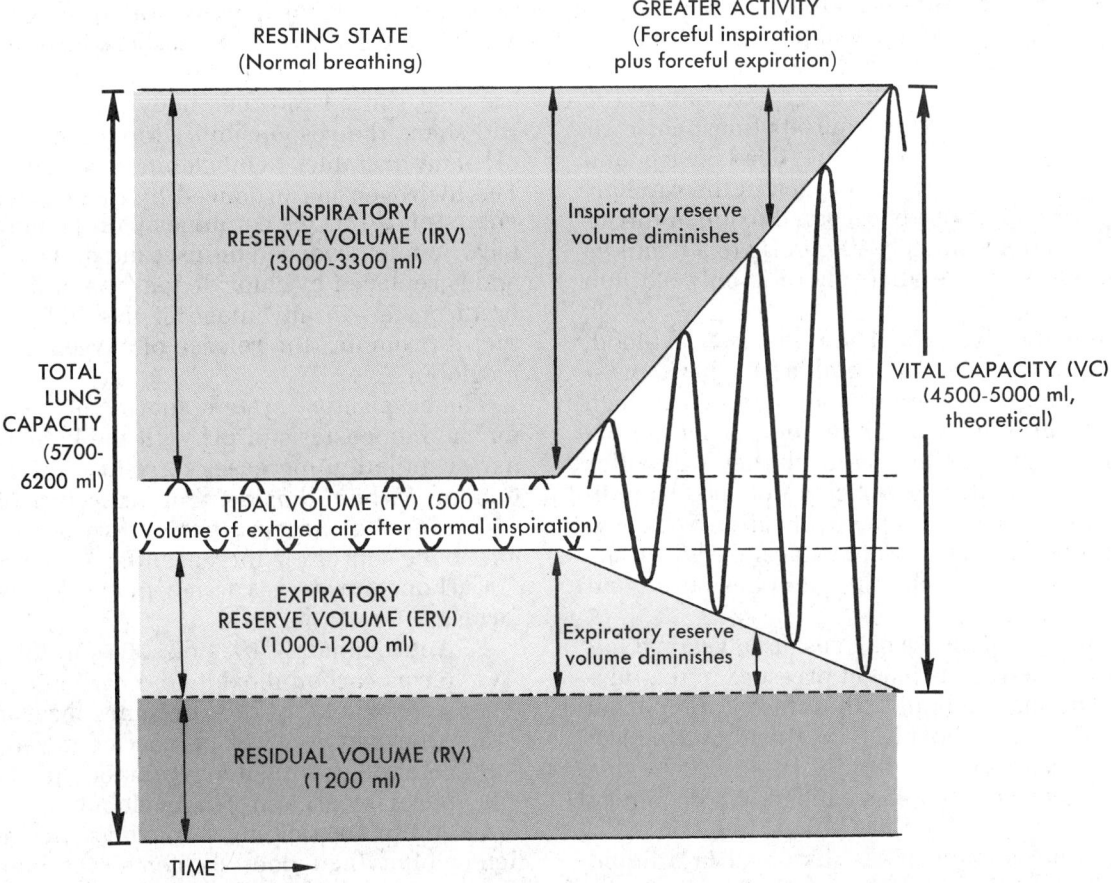

FIGURE 25-4   During normal, quiet respirations, atmosphere and lungs exchange about 500 mL of air *(TV)*. With forcible inspiration, about 3300 mL more air can be inhaled *(IRV)*. After normal inspiration and expiration, approximately 1000 mL more air can be forcibly expired *(ERV)*. Vital capacity is amount of air that can be forcibly expired after maximum inspiration and indicates, therefore, largest amount of air that can enter and leave lungs during respiration. Residual volume is air that remains trapped in alveoli. (From Thibodeau GA: *Anthony's textbook of anatomy and physiology*, ed 13, St Louis, 1990, Mosby–Year Book.)

breathing tubes should not be longer than approximately 10 inches.

Some diseases, such as emphysema, increase the dead space. Affected individuals have abnormally high **minute volumes** (volume inspired per minute) for even minimal levels of activity and may suffer respiratory distress without any additional physical activity if they become excited.

Gas Transport

Physical principles

1. Gas diffuses from an area of high concentration to an area of low concentration. Respiratory gas concentration is usually expressed as mm Hg partial pressure. The partial pressure of oxygen is higher in the alveoli than it is in blood; therefore oxygen diffuses from the alveoli into the blood. Conversely, the partial pressure of oxygen in the tissues is lower than it is in tissue capillaries; therefore oxygen diffuses from the capillaries into the tissues. The reverse is true of the carbon dioxide concentration gradients, so carbon dioxide moves in the reverse direction.

2. The amount of gas diffusing from one area to another depends not only on the concentration gradient, but also on the distance to be traveled. Conditions such as edema and pulmonary congestion increase the distance to be traveled, thereby reducing the amount of oxygen and carbon dioxide that can be moved between the tissues and their capillaries and between the alveoli and their capillaries.

3. The partial pressure of a gas depends on the proportion of the gas found in a mixture of gases and the total pressure of the mixture. For example, when

the atmospheric pressure is 760 mm Hg and oxygen forms 21% of the air, the partial pressure of oxygen (Po_2) is 21% of 760, which is 159.6 mm Hg.

The Po_2 in the alveoli falls to approximately 100 mm Hg (13%) because the inspired atmospheric air mixes with the stale air of the dead space and reaches equilibrium with the oxygen in the capillaries. The partial pressure of carbon dioxide in the alveoli rises to approximately 40 mm Hg (5%), and its partial pressure in the atmosphere is only 0.3 mm Hg (0.003%).

The Po_2 in the alveoli, and hence in arterial blood, is sensitive to the environmental atmospheric pressure. For example, divers may be exposed to high atmospheric pressures, and if the proportions of oxygen and nitrogen are not reduced, they will suffer from oxygen and nitrogen toxicity. Conversely, individuals flying at high altitudes will suffer from oxygen deficiency unless the proportion of oxygen in the air is increased or the aircraft cabin pressure is increased.

4. The partial pressure of a gas dissolved in a liquid is determined by its partial pressure in the mixture surrounding the liquid. Therefore if the partial pressure of carbon dioxide (Pco_2) in the alveoli at the end of inspiration is 40 mm Hg, the Pco_2 dissolved in the alveolar capillary blood will be almost the same.

5. The total amount of gas dissolved in a liquid depends on both its solubility in the liquid and its partial pressure. At high atmospheric pressures, a large amount of oxygen, carbon dioxide, and nitrogen is dissolved in the body fluids. If the high pressure is reduced quickly, as when a diver ascends from great depth too quickly, much of the dissolved gas bubbles out of the body fluids and blocks some of the smaller blood vessels. Anoxia in the tissues supplied by the blocked vessels and swelling resulting from the expansion of air pockets in the various organs cause severe pain. A too rapid fall in pressure can result in death unless the diver is treated in a hyperbaric chamber.

Blood transport of carbon dioxide

Respiratory control mechanisms adjust ventilation so that the partial pressure of carbon dioxide in arterial blood is approximately 40 mm Hg, which produces a pH of 7.45. The partial Pco_2 in venous blood is usually approximately 46 mm Hg, which produces a pH of 7.35. This difference in pH results solely because of the change in the hydrogen ion concentration caused by the change in the concentration of carbon dioxide, because carbon dioxide combines reversibly with water to form carbonic acid:

$$CO_2 + H_2O = H_2CO_3 = H^+ + HCO_3^-$$

Carbonic anhydrase enzyme increases the rate of this vital reaction. An increase in carbon dioxide always results in an increase of hydrogen ions and acidity, and a decrease in carbon dioxide results in a decrease of hydrogen ions. Extra hydrogen ions are also shifted to other body buffer systems that will share the responsibility for the homeostasis of pH. For example, hemoglobin is a protein buffer. The hydrogen ion produced by carbon dioxide that enters erythrocytes combines with hemoglobin; the bicarbonate produced diffuses out of the erythrocyte and is replaced by chloride ions that diffuse into the erythrocyte. An advantage of this buffer system is that it promotes the release of oxygen from the hemoglobin.

The respiratory system shares the responsibility for the homeostasis of pH with the kidneys. Pulmonary ventilation increases to reduce the concentration of carbon dioxide and hence carbonic acid whenever the concentration of hydrogen ions from metabolic sources is increased (see Chapter 12).

Carbon dioxide is carried in the blood in three forms:

1. Approximately 10% dissolves in the body water as carbon dioxide and carbonic acid.
2. Approximately 70% becomes bicarbonate.
3. Approximately 20% is carried in venous blood combined with deoxygenated hemoglobin to become carbaminohemoglobin.

Carbon monoxide has a much greater affinity for hemoglobin than does oxygen or carbon dioxide. The combination of hemoglobin and carbon monoxide, which produces bright red carboxyhemoglobin, is irreversible under normal conditions. Even small amounts of carbon monoxide, when inspired over a long time, render large amounts of hemoglobin useless for oxygen transport and thereby cause death. The red carboxyhemoglobin and the vasodilation caused by tissue hypoxia produce a characteristic pink flush to the skin of the individual with carbon monoxide poisoning. Death or permanent neurologic damage may result without hyperbaric oxygen therapy.

Blood transport of oxygen

Oxygen is carried in the blood in two forms:
1. Dissolved in water (0.3 mL/dL blood)
2. Combined with hemoglobin (20 mL/dL blood)

The **dissolved oxygen** is the only oxygen that can cross the cell membranes and the interstitial fluid for cell respiration. The body's dissolved oxygen would be insufficient to maintain life if it were not constantly and rapidly replaced from the huge reservoir of oxygen carried by hemoglobin.

Hemoglobin has several properties that make it ideal for carrying oxygen for respiration:
1. One gram of hemoglobin can hold 1.34 mL of oxygen, and therefore 100 mL of blood normally carries approximately 20 mL of oxygen.
2. Hemoglobin either combines with or releases

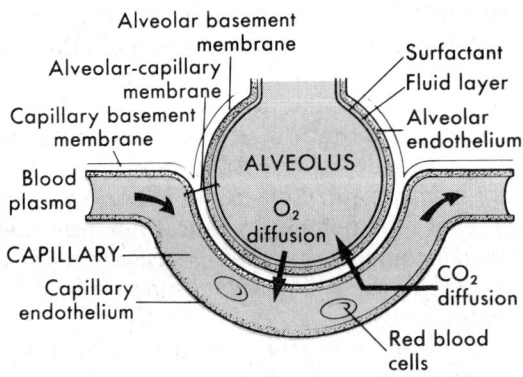

FIGURE 25-5   Blood transport of oxygen.

oxygen quickly, depending on the P_{O_2} surrounding it (Figure 25-5). The affinity of hemoglobin for oxygen is altered by the surrounding pH to release more oxygen where the pH is reduced, as in the tissues, and to combine with more oxygen where the pH is increased, as in the lungs. The affinity of hemoglobin for oxygen is also increased slightly in the lungs by the cooler temperature produced by the incoming air. The affinity is reduced in the tissues by the temperature increase produced by accelerated metabolism, especially with fever or vigorous exercise.

The oxygen saturation curve of hemoglobin (Figure 25-6) shows that when the P_{O_2} is above 90 mm Hg, as in the lungs, hemoglobin is almost completely saturated, and the curve is at a plateau stage. Consequently, hyperventilation will not significantly increase the *maximum* amount of oxygen that can be carried by the blood.

Homeostasis of Carbon Dioxide and Oxygen

The respiratory system has both intrinsic and extrinsic mechanisms to control ventilation and thus the homeostasis of blood, carbon dioxide, and oxygen. Ventilation is also controlled by the cerebral cortex to allow the respiratory system to function appropriately during voluntary activities such as talking, singing, blowing musical instruments, and inflating balloons.

Intrinsic control mechanisms

The lungs have a considerable intrinsic reserve capacity for gas exchange. Normally, the capillary-alveolar exchange of gases is completed quickly before the blood in the alveolar capillaries has passed the alveolar membrane. So more time is still available to complete the exchange when less ideal conditions prevail, for example, when the P_{O_2} in the alveoli is reduced (as at high altitudes or with some

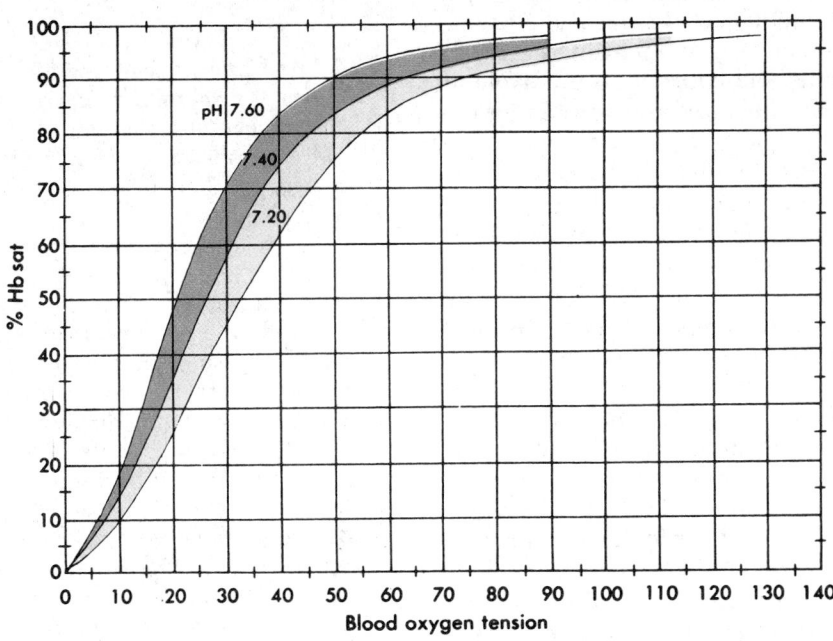

FIGURE 25-6   Oxygen saturation curve of hemoglobin. For given oxygen tension, the higher the blood pH, the more the hemoglobin holds onto its oxygen, maintaining higher saturation. (From Thibodeau GA: *Anthony's textbook of anatomy and physiology,* ed 13, St Louis, 1990, Mosby–Year Book.)

respiratory diseases) or when venous carbon dioxide is increased significantly (as with vigorous exercise or fever).

Blood flow in the lungs is distributed to each segment according to the P_{O_2} in the alveoli. Since the partial pressure in a segment of lung depends on the ventilation of the alveoli, most of the blood is shunted away from poorly ventilated or congested segments to those that are well ventilated. Increasing the volume of inspired air normally increases the number of alveoli that are well ventilated and thus increases the number that are taking part in gas exchange.

Under resting conditions the hydrostatic pressure gradient affects the lungs significantly. The gradient is lower in the capillaries of superior areas of the lungs, and these areas may not exchange gases to their full potential, because less blood is flowing through them. However, whenever pulmonary blood pressure rises, the volume of blood flowing in the upper segments increases, contributing more to the exchange of gases.

Extrinsic control mechanisms

The extrinsic mechanisms involved with the homeostasis of carbon dioxide and oxygen mainly concern the reflex control of the rate and depth (tidal volume) of pulmonary ventilation, and hence the minute volume. When stressed, the respiratory control center also stimulates the cardiovascular control center to increase cardiac output (i.e., blood flow through the lungs).

Pulmonary ventilation is controlled by the respiratory centers in the medulla and pons of the brainstem, which receive sensory input from the brain and peripheral regions and coordinate the skeletal muscles of respiration: the diaphragm and intercostal muscles.

Without any external stimulation, the respiratory center produces an innate breathing rhythm by alternating stimulation and inhibition of two areas in the pons; one promotes inspiration, the other expiration. This innate rhythm is monitored continuously by stretch receptors in the lungs that increase their rate of impulse generation as the degree of inflation of the lungs increases. Inflation is inhibited by a reflex as the lungs approach hyperextension.

An increase in the P_{CO_2} is the most potent respiratory stimulant. It causes an increase in both the rate and depth of respiration and affects the respiratory center directly via neurons in the medulla and indirectly via chemoreceptors in the carotid bodies. An increase in hydrogen ions in the cerebrospinal fluid also stimulates respiration but to a lesser extent.

Under normal conditions arterial oxygen concentration never falls low enough (50 mm Hg) to stimulate respiration. However, when it does, it does so indirectly through the chemoreceptors in the carotid bodies. This reflex stimulation does not increase respiratory minute volume by much, and it only operates after acclimatization at high altitudes or when the carbon dioxide reflex response has been blunted by chronic respiratory diseases. When the arterial oxygen level falls quickly, cerebral function may be depressed so quickly that the respiratory center cannot respond to the reflex stimulation received from the carotid bodies.

The respiratory center can also be affected by other stimuli. Irritants detected by sensory receptors in the epithelium of the airways cause coughing and sneezing. Swallowing or vomiting inhibits respiration. The respiratory center responds to stimulation relayed from the thalamus (pain may temporarily inhibit or stimulate respiration) and from the hypothalamus (strong emotions can stimulate or depress respiration). However, the effect of pain and emotion varies from individual to individual.

Voluntary control of respiration

Respiration can be voluntarily controlled only when the respiratory center is not being stimulated by high arterial concentrations of carbon dioxide.

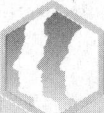

GERIATRIC CONSIDERATIONS

Physiologic Changes in the Respiratory System

At all times during the life cycle the respiratory system is vulnerable to injuries caused by infections, environmental pollutants, and allergic reactions. These are often far more damaging to the system than the decline in function that is a normal component of aging.

Age-related changes include an increased susceptibility to infection because of a decline in the protection normally provided by the intact mucous barrier, a decrease in the effectiveness of the bronchial cilia, and changes in the composition of the connective tissues of the lungs and chest. Elderly persons rely far more on the diaphragm for inspiration, and breathing requires more effort especially when lying down. Vital capacity declines with age, and it takes longer to inspire or expire air because of the decline in the elastic recoil of the lungs and an increase in the stiffness of the chest wall. Although total lung volume does not change significantly, residual volume increases; and although the alveolar partial pressure of oxygen usually does not change, the alveolar-capillary gradient does increase slightly.

Breath holding (voluntary apnea) can be controlled voluntarily only until the P_{CO_2} rises to the critical set point at which resumption of breathing is mandated by the respiratory center. Hyperventilation, which reduces the concentration of carbon dioxide in arterial blood, allows breathing to be stopped for two to three times longer than normal, because it takes longer for the P_{CO_2} to rise to the critical set point. Conversely, strenuous exercise reduces voluntary breath holding to a few seconds, because carbon dioxide production is so rapid that the set point is quickly reached.

The voluntary pattern of respiration for talking and singing involves taking in a larger than normal breath and making expiration last for one or two complete sentences or musical cadenzas. However, after vigorous exercise or during acute respiratory distress, carbon dioxide concentrations may stimulate respiration to such an extent that it is not possible to speak in sentences, and messages must be gasped out one or two words at a time.

ASSESSMENT
Subjective

Patients with respiratory distress may seek health care for a variety of complaints that include cough, shortness of breath, chest pain, and wheezing. Some symptoms may result from a cardiac disorder rather than a respiratory disorder.

An adequate system-specific history for any patient includes a review of related systems and delineation of any positive findings (symptoms of which the patient complains) through exploration of various dimensions. Specific dimensions utilized to delineate positive findings include onset, duration, frequency, alleviating factors, aggravating factors, precipitating events, location, quality, quantity, associated symptoms, and chronology of events. Noting any significant negatives (symptoms the patient denies) is important because it allows other clinicians to know specifically what the interviewer asked. To record "no problems" does not communicate which symptoms the patient denied. The box above lists potential symptoms to review with the patient. In addition to specific symptoms, ask the patient about previous thoracic trauma or surgery; use of oxygen or ventilation-assisting devices; and previous testing such as allergy testing, pulmonary function tests, tuberculin skin tests, or chest x-ray films. Explore any past history of tuberculosis, bronchitis, emphysema, asthma, or cystic fibrosis.

Other appropriate history to explore includes major adult illnesses, hospitalizations, surgeries, injuries or accidents, immunizations, current medications, allergies, and habits. Major adult illnesses relevant to a respiratory disorder include any previous history of illnesses listed above as well as cardiac

---

POTENTIAL SYMPTOMS ASSOCIATED WITH RESPIRATORY DISORDERS

Cough (productive vs. dry)
Chest pain
Cyanosis
Dysphagia (difficulty swallowing may lead to aspiration)
Dyspnea
Hemoptysis
Sputum
Wheezing

---

disease, cancer, or a diagnosis of human immunodeficiency virus (HIV). When recording hospitalizations and surgeries, determine the hospital, attending physician, and dates of the hospital stay. Immunizations for an adult include noting the last tetanus booster (DT), completion of hepatitis vaccine series, and any immunizations for travel abroad. A previous BCG vaccine is also relevant for the patient with a respiratory disorder. Other immunizations particularly relevant to the elderly or immunocompromised population include the pneumonia vaccine and last influenza vaccine. Inquire regarding the tuberculosis (TB) skin test, and record that information with immunizations even though it is not an immunization. When recording current medications include the name of the drug, who prescribed it, for what condition it was prescribed, when the patient began taking it, dosage, and frequency. Habits about which to inquire include alcohol consumption, tobacco use, use of recreational or illicit drugs, caffeine consumption, and exercise.

Family history that is relevant to the respiratory system includes tuberculosis, cystic fibrosis, emphysema, allergy, asthma, atopic dermatitis, and malignancy. A positive finding should include the disease as well as the individual's relationship to the patient (e.g., lung cancer, father; cystic fibrosis, maternal aunt). Family history usually includes grandparents, parents, aunts, uncles, siblings, spouse, and children.

Objective

The nurse determines the appropriate systems to be assessed based on the history obtained and knowledge of pathophysiology. Some patients have more complex symptom involvement than others, and therefore assessment needs may vary from patient to patient. General assessment and evaluation of the integumentary, respiratory, cardiovascular, and gastrointestinal systems are usually included. General assessment is significant in every patient and refers to the examiner's overall impression of the patient's state of health.

General assessment includes height, weight, vital signs, apparent age (relative to chronologic age), nutritional status, general appearance, and stature. Note any obvious abnormalities or assistive devices. Also record whether the patient appears to be comfortable or in distress.

Integumentary

Inspect and palpate the skin noting warmth, color, moisture, turgor, lesions, and vascularity. Inspect the nails noting the presence or absence of clubbing. Also evaluate growth, curvature, adhesion, color, and thickness.

Respiratory

Inspect the neck for position of the trachea, retraction of the sternocleidomastoid or trapezius muscles, and supraclavicular retraction during inspiration. Retraction of the sternocleidomastoid or trapezius muscles and supraclavicular retraction indicate respiratory distress and are referred to as use of accessory muscles.

Inspect the thorax noting configuration and sym-

metry of movement. Observe the patient from the side as well as front and back, carefully evaluating the anteroposterior (AP) to transverse (or lateral) diameter ratio. Normally, the AP diameter is less than the transverse (or lateral) diameter (Figure 25-7, A). However, in the patient with a long history of chronic obstructive pulmonary disease, the AP diameter may increase to equal the transverse diameter (i.e., barrel chest). In the patient with a barrel chest the ribs lose the 45-degree angle and become more horizontal; a slight kyphosis of the thoracic spine develops, and the sternal angle becomes more prominent. Elderly adults may also have an increase of the AP diameter, leading to a more barrel-chested appearance secondary to osteoporosis (Figure 25-7, B). Observe for kyphosis, lordosis, scoliosis, pectus carinatum, and pectus excavatum. Note the presence or absence of intercostal retractions during inspiration. Presence of intercostal retractions indicates respiratory distress and is not seen in normal or eupneic respirations.

Palpate the thorax generally for tenderness, muscle mass, and masses. Assess thoracic expansion (respiratory excursion) by standing behind the patient, placing your thumbs on either side of the spine at approximately the level of the tenth rib, using your hands to encase the lateral thorax (rib cage), and instructing the patient to inhale deeply. Your hands should move with the thorax. Note symmetry of movement as your thumbs diverge (Figure 25-8).

Assess tactile fremitus. **Fremitus** is the palpable vibration transmitted to the chest wall as a result of speech. Stand behind the patient, placing the palmar surfaces of your fingertips on the patient's back. Systematically move your fingertips while the patient

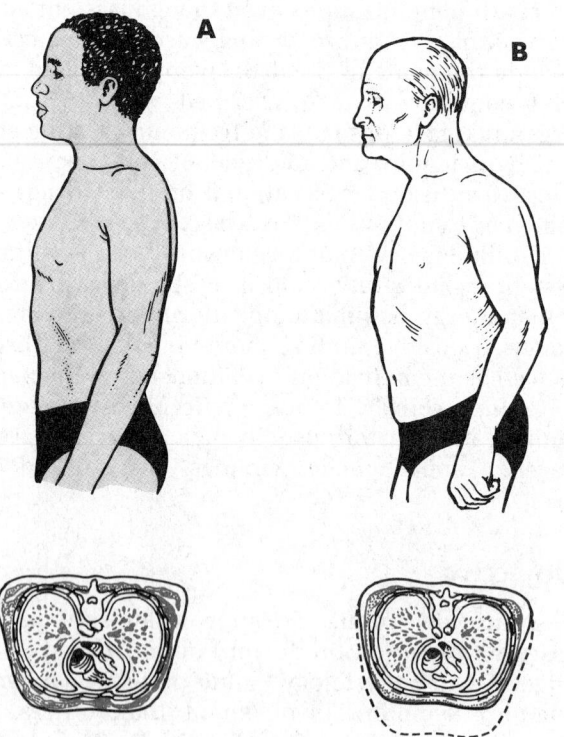

FIGURE 25-7 Anteroposterior (AP) diameter in, **A,** healthy adult male, and, **B,** barrel chest.

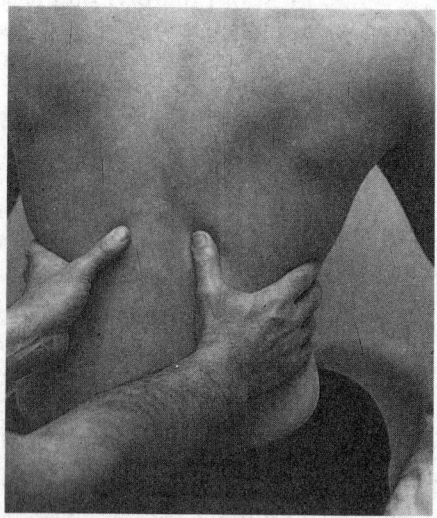

FIGURE 25-8   Thoracic expansion. (From Seidel HM et al: *Mosby's guide to physical examination,* ed 2, St Louis, 1991, Mosby–Year Book.)

repeats a few numbers or words such as "ninety nine" or "Mickey Mouse" each time you touch the back. Move side to side for evaluation of symmetry. The ulnar surface of the hand may be substituted for the palmar surfaces of the fingertips (Figure 25-9). If fremitus is difficult to discern, have the patient speak louder. Fremitus may vary with voice pitch as well as thickness of chest wall.

Do general percussion from side to side and from apices to bases in posterior, lateral, and anterior aspects (Figures 25-10 and 25-11). Resonance is the normal percussion tone in the peripheral lung. If the rib is percussed, it will elicit a flat tone rather than resonance. Hyperresonance is abnormal in an adult but may be noted in the patient with a long history of chronic obstructive pulmonary disease.

Diaphragmatic excursion or expansion may be percussed to determine the level of the diaphragm at inspiration and expiration or movement of the diaphragm. Ask the patient to inhale deeply and hold the breath. Deep inspiration normally moves the di-

aphragm down. Percuss along the scapular line until resonance is replaced with dullness. Mark the point of change. The level of dullness indicates the level of the diaphragm. Allow the patient to breathe normally a few times, and then have the patient exhale as much as possible and hold. Exhalation moves the diaphragm upward. Percuss along the scapular line until resonance is replaced with dullness. The level of dullness indicates the upper level of diaphragmatic movement. Mark this point of change. Measure the distance between the marks. Repeat on the opposite side (Figure 25-12). Diaphragmatic excursion is usually 3 to 5 cm bilaterally.

Auscultate the peripheral lung fields. Instruct the patient to take slow, deep breaths through the mouth. Be careful not to have the patient hyperventilate. Listen systematically, moving from apices to bases posteriorly, laterally, and anteriorly. If the patient is frail or elderly, it may be necessary to begin at the bases to avoid evaluating these areas when the patient is fatigued and unable to breathe deeply. Note pitch, intensity, location, quality, and duration of inspiration and expiration. In the peripheral lung fields the normal breath sounds are low pitched and of low intensity; they are referred to as vesicular, with inspiration being greater (of longer duration) than expiration. Bronchovesicular breath sounds may be normally heard at the first to second intercostal space, at the sternal border, and over the upper right posterior lung field. These breath sounds are of medium pitch, with inspiration equal to expiration. Bronchial breath sounds may be normally heard over the manubrium, are high pitched, and are loud; inspiration is less (of shorter duration) than expiration. Tracheal breath sounds are very loud, high pitched, and audible only over the trachea, and they have a long expiratory phase (Figure

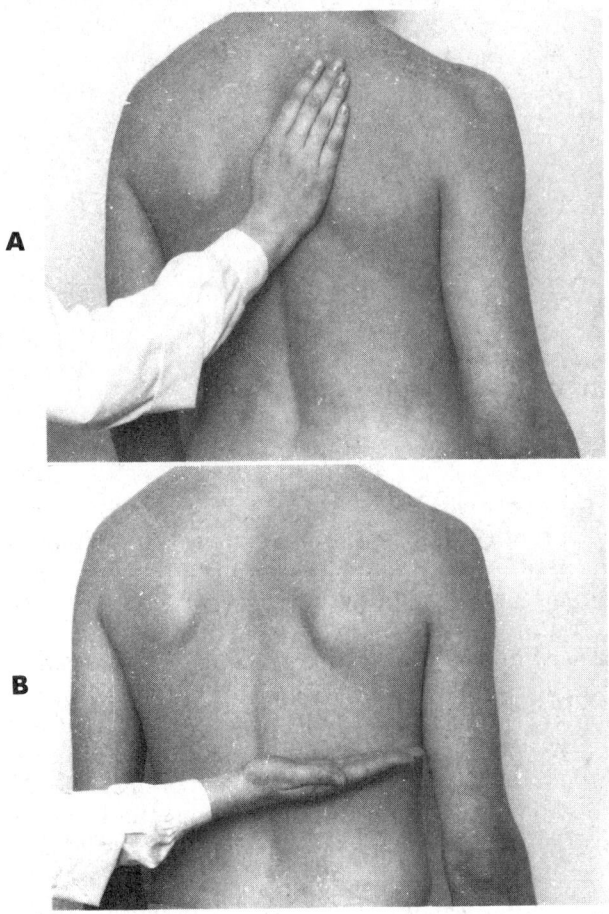

FIGURE 25-9   Palpation for assessment of tactile fremitus using, **A,** palmar surface of fingertips and, **B,** ulnar aspect of hand. (From Malasanos L et al: *Health assessment*, ed 4, St Louis, 1990, Mosby–Year Book.)

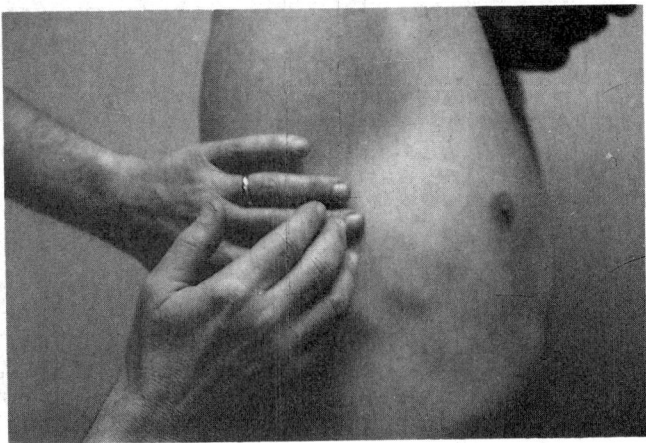

FIGURE 25-10   Indirect percussion. (From Seidel HM et al: *Mosby's guide to physical examination*, ed 2, St Louis, 1991, Mosby–Year Book.)

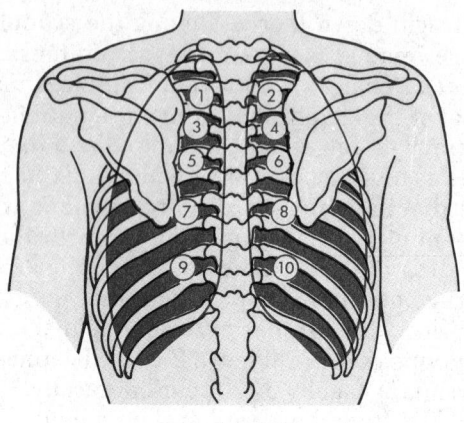
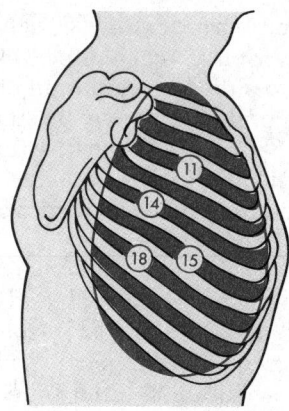

Posterior thorax

Right lateral thorax

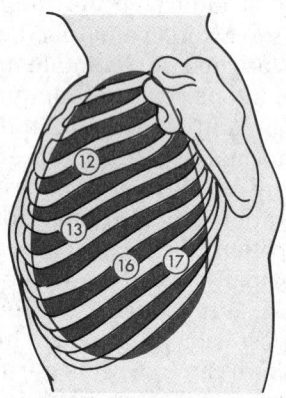
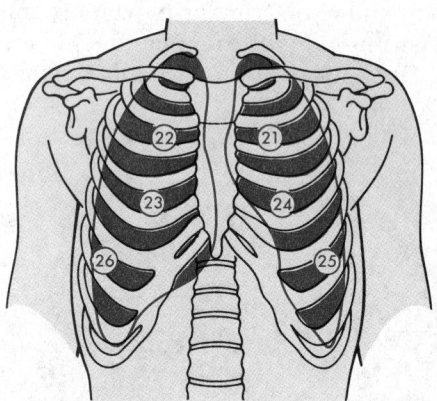

Left lateral thorax

Anterior thorax

FIGURE 25-11   Suggested percussion and auscultation sequence. Stethoscope is moved in systematic numeric sequence.

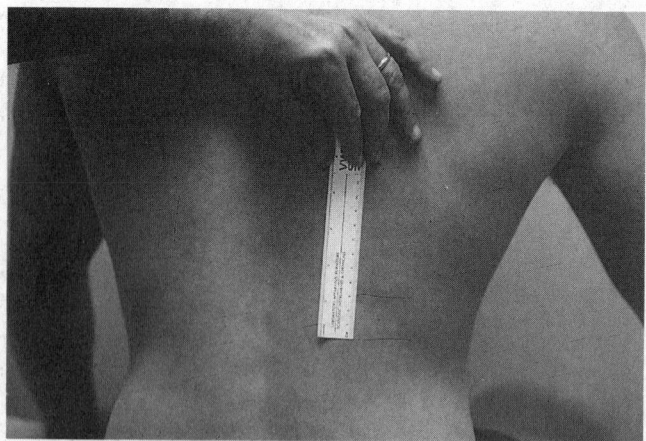

FIGURE 25-12   Diaphragmatic excursion. (From Seidel HM et al: *Mosby's guide to physical examination,* ed 2, St Louis, 1991, Mosby–Year Book.)

25-13). To hear bronchovesicular or tracheobronchial breath sounds in the peripheral lung fields is abnormal. Absent or decreased breath sounds may be due to shallow breathing, obesity, barrel chest, or fluid in the lung tissue.

Auscultate and note the presence or absence of any adventitious breath sounds. Adventitious breath sounds are abnormal and may include crackles (rales), wheezes (rhonchi), and pleural friction rubs (PFRs). When assessing adventitious breath sounds, record the type of adventitious sound, the location, and the timing of the sound. A **crackle** (rale) is a brief, discontinuous sound heard more frequently on inspiration. Crackles have been compared to the sound that is made when opening Velcro or rubbing hair between the fingers. Crackles are caused by the movement of air through fluid in the airways and alveoli. Examples of disorders in which crackles may

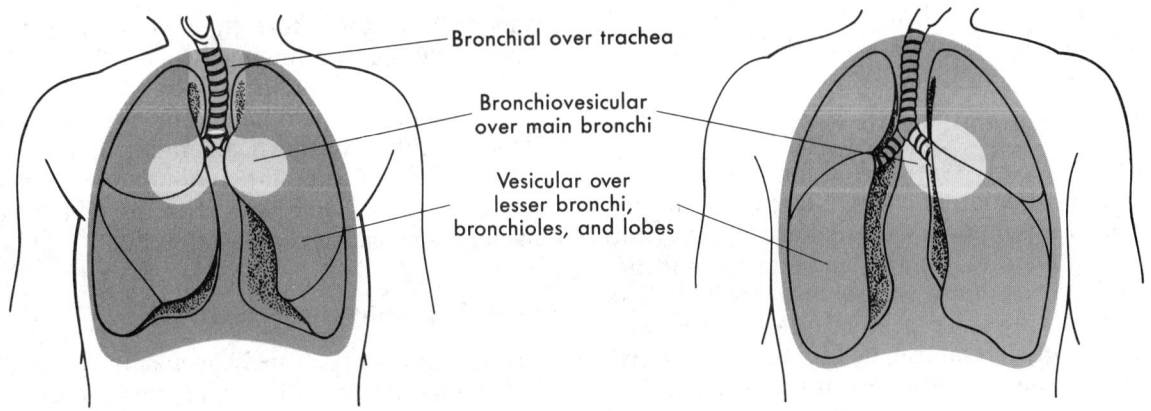

- Bronchial over trachea
- Bronchiovesicular over main bronchi
- Vesicular over lesser bronchi, bronchioles, and lobes

FIGURE 25-13   Normal auscultatory sounds.

be heard include pneumonia, pulmonary edema, and congestive heart failure. **Wheezes** are continuous sounds, occur more frequently in expiration, and have been described as musical or rumbling. Wheezes are caused by the passage of air through constricted bronchi such as in asthma or in the presence of a foreign body. Airways may be constricted because of secretions, spasms, tumor, or swelling. If wheezes are heard, have the patient cough and note if the wheezes cleared with the cough. Wheezes that clear with cough are usually caused by secretions. In asthma, wheezes may be heard on inspiration and expiration. **Pleural friction rubs** are loud grating or creaking sounds produced by the rubbing together of inflamed visceral and parietal pleura and heard in late inspiration and early expiration.

Occasionally, vocal sounds may be abnormally transmitted throughout the lungs. If an increase in tactile fremitus, dullness on percussion, or decreased breath sounds on auscultation is noted, assess transmission of vocal sounds for the presence of bronchophony, egophony, or whispered pectoriloquy. To evaluate the presence of **bronchophony,** auscultate the chest over the suspected area of consolidation while the patient says "ninety nine." Normally the words will be muffled and indistinct. Over an area of consolidation, the intensity of the vocal sounds is increased and the words are distinct ("NINETY NINE"). To evaluate **egophony,** auscultate the chest over the suspected area of consolidation while the patient repeats "e, e, e, e, e." Normally the sounds will be muffled and indistinct. In consolidation the "e, e, e" will sound like "a, a, a." To evaluate the presence of whispered pectoriloquy, auscultate the chest over the suspected area of consolidation while the patient whispers letters or numbers. Normally the sounds will be absent or barely audible. In the presence of consolidation the sounds are distinct and clearly audible.

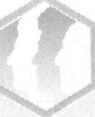

GERIATRIC CONSIDERATIONS

Respiratory Assessment

General approach

Allow more time than for a younger adult.

Articulate clearly; the elderly patient may be hearing impaired.

Remember that impaired sight, comprehension, or mobility may result in less than optimal cooperation.

Provide clear, concise instructions.

History collection

As needed use fewer open-ended questions and provide some choices; for example, "Is your chest pain dull, sharp, aching, or stabbing?"

As needed repeat questions.

Be alert for answers that do not appear appropriate; the patient may not have understood the question correctly because of impaired hearing or impaired comprehension.

Physical assessment

The physical examination itself is not different, but the approach needs to be altered such that the appropriate information is assessed without undue discomfort or embarrassment for the patient.

Provide an environment with minimal noise, distraction, and interruption.

Require as few position changes as possible.

Kyphosis is associated with aging.

Chest expansion may be decreased.

Breathing may be more shallow.

Rales or crackles may be present in the bases in the absence of respiratory or cardiovascular disease secondary to atelectasis or fibrotic lung changes.

LABORATORY AND DIAGNOSTIC TESTS
Radiography

Chest roentgenogram (chest x-ray film)

The basic chest x-ray film is used for screening, diagnosis, and evaluation of change in respiratory disorders. Normal pulmonary tissues are radiolucent, so fluid, foreign bodies, tumors, and other abnormalities will appear as dense contrasts on the film. The most common views are posteroanterior (PA) and lateral (especially left lateral, or LL), but other views such as the oblique, lateral decubitus, or apical lordotic views may be employed for visualization of specific concerns.

Fluoroscopy may also be used to visualize pulmonary structures when evaluation of lung expansion, diaphragmatic movement, or visualization of nodular calcifications is desired. Fluoroscopy permits visualization of the lungs and diaphragm and involves passing a continuous stream of x-rays through the patient's body so shadows of the structure are cast on a fluorescent screen. This procedure is indicated only when visualization of thoracic motion is desired, because it exposes the patient to more radiation than the standard x-ray film.

Patient preparation

Explain the nature of the procedure to the patient. Then instruct the patient to remove all metal objects between the neck and chest and to change into a hospital gown.

Tomography (body-section roentgenography, planigraphy, and laminagraphy)

Tomography is an extension of standard chest radiography that provides clearly focused radiographic images of single layers or planes of lung tissue. Since tomography employs high radiation levels, it is primarily reserved for further evaluation of masses, lesions, and emphysema. Patient preparation is the same as that for the basic chest x-ray film. Tell the patient to remain immobile in a supine position.

Esophagram (barium swallow and esophagraphy)

The esophagram is useful in detecting pharyngeal musculature disorders and displacement of the esophagus, which may indicate mediastinal lymphadenopathy or metastatic disease of the esophagus. After oral administration of barium sulfate or gastrografin, films are taken of the chest.

Patient preparation

Inform the patient that the test allows visualization of the functioning of the pharynx and esophagus. Then tell the patient that fasting is required beginning at midnight before the test and that the procedure includes swallowing two mixtures of barium. Explain that the patient will be secured to a tilt table and that films will be taken with the table in various positions. Remove all metal objects from the x-ray field. Instruct the patient to monitor bowel movements for 2 to 3 days after the test, because the barium may cause constipation.

Bronchography (bronchogram)

Bronchography is a rarely performed procedure, but it remains the definitive test for diagnosing bronchiectasis. A radiopaque iodine contrast medium is introduced into the tracheobronchial tree through a catheter.

Patient preparation

The nurse informs the patient that the test helps to detect bronchial abnormalities. The patient's history is checked for sensitivity to anesthetics, iodine, or contrast media. The patient's mouth is examined for inflammation of the mucosa and the presence of loose or capped teeth. Bridges and dentures are also noted. The nurse instructs the patient to perform good oral hygiene and remove dentures before the test. If the procedure is to be performed with the patient under local anesthetic, the patient is told that a local anesthetic will be sprayed on the throat before the procedure to suppress the gag reflex. The nurse warns the patient that there may be some difficulty breathing during the procedure and coughing may be precipitated. The patient is reassured that there will be no blockage of the airway and enough oxygen will be received. Since relaxation facilitates intubation, the patient is instructed in relaxation techniques and mouth breathing and is told to fast for 12 hours preceding the test.

The nurse obtains an informed consent from the patient and then administers premedication as ordered, ensuring that the patient voids before the test.

Postprocedure care

The patient must avoid oral intake until the gag reflex returns (usually in 2 to 8 hours). If the patient has a sore throat, offer liquid gargles and lozenges when the gag reflex returns. Observe the patient's vital signs, breath sounds, and color for signs of respiratory distress and bleeding, and monitor the patient for signs of pneumonia, bronchospasm, or atelectasis.

Pulmonary angiography

Pulmonary angiography is used to visualize pulmonary vasculature and therefore is particularly useful in locating pathologic conditions or obstruction of the pulmonary vessels. This procedure provides a definitive diagnosis of pulmonary embolism when that diagnosis cannot be established by other means. A catheter is threaded into the pulmonary artery through a peripheral vein, usually in the antecubital fossa. Pressure readings and blood samples are obtained in the right side of the heart and pulmonary artery. Then a radiopaque dye is injected while x-ray films are taken in rapid sequence.

Patient preparation

Tell the patient that the procedure visualizes the blood vessels in the lungs, and instruct the patient to avoid oral ingestion, except for sips of water, for 4 to 6 hours before the test. Review the patient's history for hypersensitivity to contrast media or shellfish. Inform the physician of hypersensitivities, since the physician may decide to cancel the procedure or order administration of prednisone and diphenhydramine (Benadryl) before and after the procedure.

An informed consent is obtained, after which the nurse shaves and prepares the anticipated entry site.

Postprocedure care

Monitor vital signs every 15 minutes, and maintain the patient on bed rest for 2 to 4 hours after the procedure. Observe the pressure dressing over the venous site for bleeding, and observe the urinary output, since a nephrotoxic response to the contrast medium is possible.

Observe the venous puncture site for signs of thrombophlebitis such as warmth, tenderness, swelling, and redness. Sutures are removed from the venous entry site 4 to 5 days after the procedure.

Computed Tomography Scan

Thoracic computed tomography (CT) is useful in differentiating calcified coin lesions from tumors and in detecting small peripheral nodules and effusion. It is particularly valuable in visualizing lesions of the hilus and mediastinum, which are difficult to assess with basic x-ray procedures. CT is performed with or without the injection of a radiopaque contrast medium and provides cross-sectional (layer by layer) views of the thorax by passing narrow x-ray beams from a computerized scanner through it (Figure 25-14). Minimal radiation exposure is necessary.

Patient preparation

Inform the patient that the test provides detailed visualization of the chest. If a contrast medium is used, tell the patient that fasting is required for 4 hours before the test. Check the patient's history for sensitivity to iodine preparations. Inform the patient that a warm, flushed feeling and a salty taste may accompany the injection of the dye and that these effects are temporary. Make the patient aware of the need to lie very still inside a large, noisy, ring-shaped x-ray machine. Instruct the patient to remove all metal objects from the x-ray field. The test takes approximately 20 to 45 minutes.

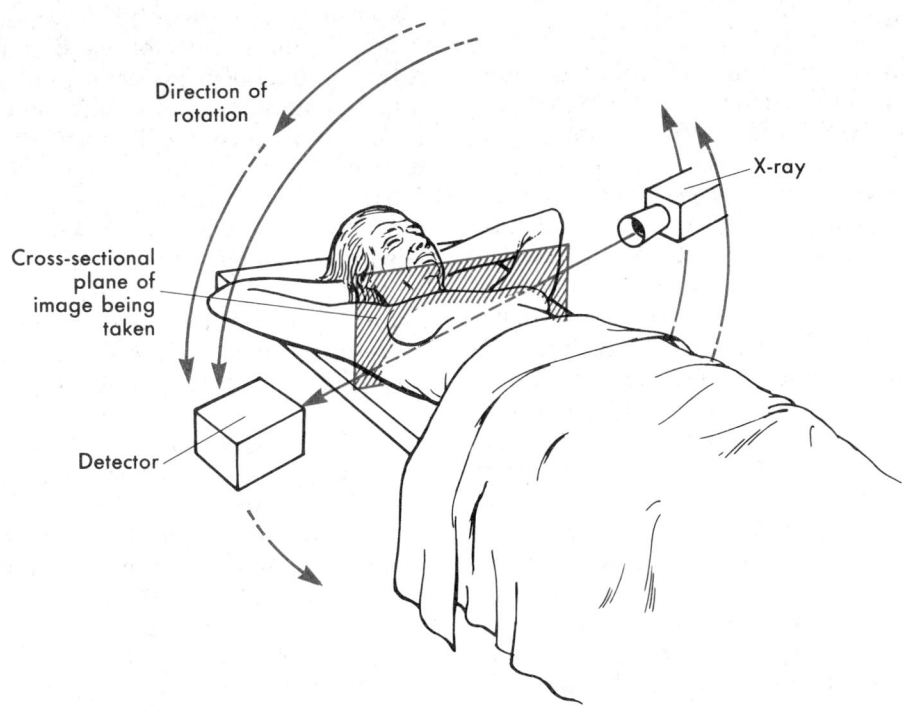

FIGURE 25-14   Positioning for computed tomography (CT) scan of thorax.

Magnetic Resonance Imaging

Magnetic resonance imaging (MRI) is useful in detecting pulmonary emboli, pulmonary edema, hilar masses, and lymph nodes. MRI produces images of soft tissue detail and contrast that are exquisite in quality and that are superior to those of CT in discriminating between vascular structures and mediastinal nodes. MRI is a type of body scan in which an energy field is created with a magnet and radio waves. Changes in the energy field are visualized on a computer screen.

Prepare the patient by explaining that the test provides detailed images of the chest. Tell the patient that he or she will be placed on a moving pallet that is pushed into a cylinder and that there will be a variety of noises during the scan. These noises are loud but not usually unbearable. If the patient wishes, ear plugs can be used. All metal objects such as jewelry or hair clips must be removed before the MRI. MRI is contraindicated for patients with pacemakers. The magnet may also cause movement and damage for patients with surgical clips or heart valves. Patients with dental fillings and bridges may experience an odd sensation in their mouths if these appliances contain ferrous material. If the patient has an intravenous line with a drip regulator, check with the personnel operating the MRI to ensure that the regulator will not be disrupted by the MRI. Since the procedure takes approximately 60 minutes, encourage the patient to void before the MRI.

Radioisotope Procedures

Lung scintiscanning

Lung scintiscanning helps in the screening and detection of thromboembolic disease and obstructive lung diseases and in ventilation-perfusion studies. A scintillation camera takes a radioactivity reading after the patient receives macroaggregated albumin tagged with technetium-99m intravenously **(perfusion lung scan)** or breathes air mixed with xenon through a mask **(ventilation lung scan)**. During perfusion scanning, scans are done as the patient reaches total lung capacity in an initial breath and after the patient resumes breathing (wash-out phase). Information from the scans should be combined with that from blood gas determinations and pulmonary function studies because of the limited specificity of the scans.

Pulmonary ventilation and perfusion scans may be performed in emergencies on pregnant clients using a reduced dose of radioisotope. A chest x-ray film is taken for comparison with results of the scanning and may be performed either before or after the scan. Explain the procedure to the patient. The patient will hear clicking noises as the scan is performed, but the noise is not unbearable and the patient should not experience pain from the procedure. If the patient has pain or dyspnea that may make lying down difficult, reassure that sitting is possible for parts of the procedure and that someone may stay with the patient during the procedure. If the patient is having a ventilation scan, explain that the patient will need to breathe through a ventilation tube or mask. Reassure that the exposure to radiation and the amount of excreted radiation is minimal. If the patient is pregnant, a signed consent may be necessary. The procedure takes 30 to 60 minutes.

Endoscopy Procedures

Bronchoscopy/bronchial biopsy

Bronchoscopy is the direct visualization of the larynx, trachea, and bronchi through the use of a flexible fiberoptic bronchoscope. The bronchoscope is introduced through the nose, mouth, tracheotomy tube, or endotracheal tube (Figure 25-15). A bronchoscopy is performed for the purposes of diagnosis, assessment of changes, specimen collection, and removal of mucous plugs or foreign objects. A brush, biopsy forceps, or a catheter is passed through the bronchoscope if specimens for cytology are required. The procedure is generally contraindicated in patients with asthma, recent myocardial infarction, unstable angina, and uncontrolled dysrhythmia, and it is also contraindicated in pulmonary hypertension, mechanical ventilation or positive end-expiratory pressure (PEEP), and severe anemia. Complications include reaction to the local anesthetic, bronchospasm, aspiration, hypoxemia, bleeding, pneumothorax, and infection.

The patient is placed in a supine position, and the bronchoscope is introduced once the patient's nasopharynx and oropharynx have been anesthetized topically with lidocaine (Xylocaine). This solution is also dropped through the scope onto the epiglottis and vocal cords to depress coughing and diminish pain. The patient is encouraged to remain relaxed and to breathe through the nose. The nurse monitors vital signs throughout the procedure.

Patient preparation

The patient is told the procedure evaluates abnormalities in the respiratory structures, is reassured the airway will not be blocked, and is told medications will be given to decrease coughing. Instruct the patient to fast for 6 to 8 hours before the procedure.

Obtain an informed consent, and administer preprocedure medications as ordered. Usually atropine and a sedative are given to inhibit vagal stimulation (which alleviates symptoms of bradycardia, dysrhythmias, and hypotension), suppress the cough reflex, and relieve anxiety. Make certain that the patient removes glasses, contact lenses, and dentures before the procedure.

Postprocedure care

Keep the patient turned to the side until the patient is able to expectorate secretions. Take vital signs frequently for the first 2 to 4 hours according to institutional protocol. Auscultate for decreased breath sounds, which may signal pneumothorax, and assess the patient for signs and symptoms of bronchospasm, laryngospasm, and dysrhythmias. The sputum may be pink tinged for a few hours if a biopsy has been performed. Immediately report frank bleeding and difficulty in breathing. Withhold oral fluids until the patient's gag reflex returns. Discourage coughing, smoking, talking, and clearing of the throat for the first few hours. Warm, saline gargles and lozenges are effective in relieving throat discomfort.

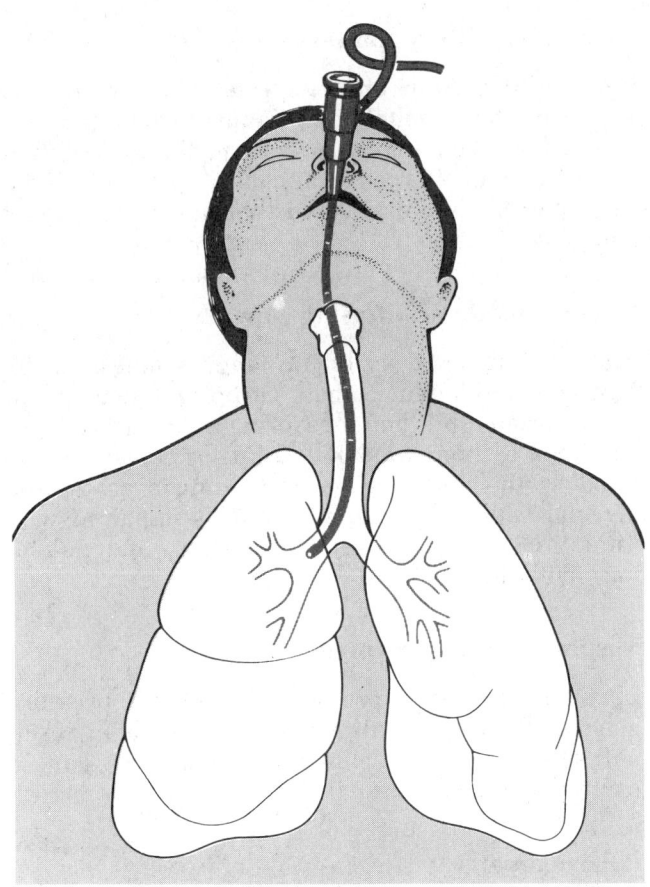

FIGURE 25-15   Bronchoscopy. Bronchoscope is inserted through trachea and into bronchus. (From Pagana KD, Pagana TJ: *Diagnostic and laboratory test reference*, St Louis, 1992, Mosby–Year Book.)

Mediastinoscopy

Mediastinoscopy is an endoscopic examination of the mediastinum for the purposes of exploration and biopsy of the lymph nodes. The procedure is performed through an incision in the suprasternal notch with the patient under general anesthesia. Strict sterile technique is observed. The procedure is useful in the diagnosis of carcinoma, lymphoma, and sarcoidosis and in the staging of lung cancer.

Patient preparation

Explain that the procedure allows visualization of the area between the lungs. Instruct the patient to fast beginning at midnight preceding the test, and obtain an informed consent. Ensure that blood has been typed and cross-matched and is available as ordered in the event of a thoracotomy or hemorrhage. Monitor the patient for pneumothorax, hemorrhage, infection, and damage to the left recurrent laryngeal nerve after the procedure.

Pleural Fluid Examination

Thoracentesis

A **thoracentesis** is performed to obtain pleural fluid for analysis, to remove pleural fluid, or to instill medication. Specimens are examined for gross appearance, consistency, glucose, protein content, cellular composition, and amylase. Specimens are also examined cytologically for malignant cells and cultured for pathogens. During thoracentesis the physician inserts a large-bore needle through the chest wall into the pleural space. The procedure is performed using strict sterile technique. The nurse positions the patient upright with arms and shoulders supported on an overbed table (Figure 25-16). If unable to sit, the patient is placed on the unaffected side. The patient's pulse and response are monitored during the procedure.

Patient preparation

Outline the procedure for the patient, emphasizing the importance of remaining immobile (sudden movement may cause trauma to the visceral pleura). Tell the patient that a feeling of pressure will be experienced during the procedure. Obtain a signed consent and a thoracentesis tray.

Postprocedure care

Place the patient on the unaffected side for 1 hour to allow the puncture site to close. Monitor vital signs frequently, and observe for expectoration of blood. Assess the patient for signs of pneumothorax, shock, subcutaneous emphysema, and pyogenic infection.

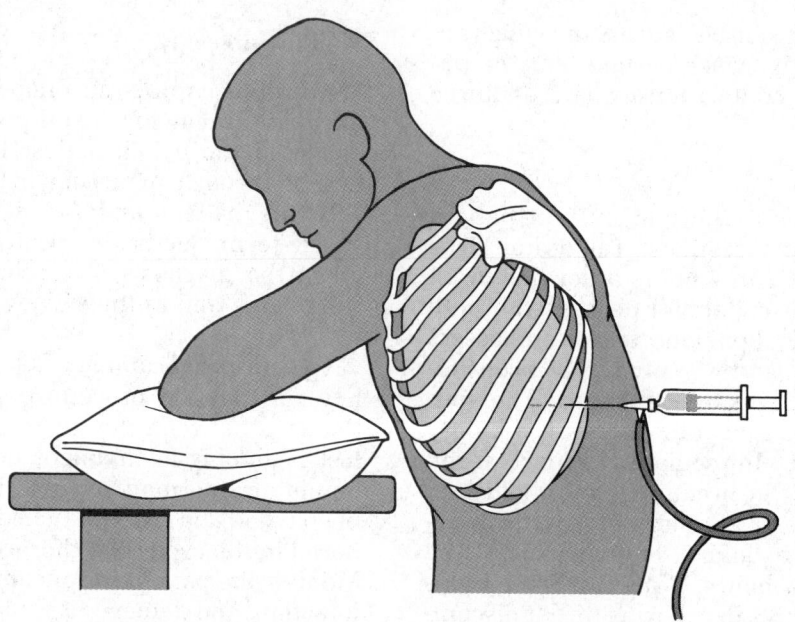

FIGURE 25-16 Thoracentesis.

Lung biopsy (pleural biopsy)

Biopsy specimens of the tracheobronchial structures may be obtained through percutaneous needle biopsy or via a bronchoscope. Needle biopsy specimens may be of lung or pleural tissue. Specimens are commonly obtained to detect malignant growths. Patient preparation is the same as that for bronchoscopy if done via bronchoscope and the same as that for thoracentesis if done percutaneously.

Pulmonary Function Tests

Spirometry

Spirometry measures lung volumes and capacities and flow rates (see the boxes on p. 535). Test results are based on the degree of deviation from normal, taking into consideration the patient's age, height, weight, and sex. Spirometry is used in the diagnosis of lung disease, to evaluate the extent of disability, for preoperative evaluation of respiratory function, to evaluate response to bronchodilator medications, and to detect lung disease in individuals who work in hazardous environments. Values less than 80% of the predicted norm are considered abnormal, and values less than 50% of the predicted norm indicate poor pulmonary function.

During spirometry the patient sits in an upright position and breathes into a mouthpiece attached to a spirometer. A nose clip is used to ensure that no air escapes through the nose. Tight clothing is loosened before the test. The full cooperation of the patient is necessary for accurate results.

Flow-volume loop analysis

Flow-volume loop analysis relates instantaneous expiratory flow to the lung volume at which the particular flow occurs, during rapid maximal inhalation and exhalation (forced vital capacity). Flow-volume loop analysis is more useful than the conventional spirogram.

Determination of diffusing capacity

The diffusing capacity of the lungs is measured by having the individual inhale carbon monoxide in a single breath and then measuring the blood concentration of carbon monoxide. Diffusing capacity is defined as the ability of gases to diffuse across the alveolar-capillary membrane and is impaired with interstitial lung disease, emphysema, and pulmonary embolism.

Maximal inspiratory pressure

Maximal inspiratory pressure (MIP) is the pressure generated on maximal inhalation, starting at residual volume, against a closed system and is useful in evaluating neuromuscular disease.

Pulse oximetry

Pulse oximetry is a quick and convenient method of continuously monitoring a patient's arterial blood saturation (SaO_2). Although it does not replace arterial blood gas (ABG) analysis, it offers a rapid, less expensive method of assessing SaO_2 and is more accurate than visual assessment.

DEFINITIONS OF LUNG CAPACITIES

Total lung capacity (TLC)—Total volume of air that lungs can contain when fully inflated

Vital capacity (VC)—Maximum amount of air that can be exhaled after *maximum* inspiration; sometimes called expiratory vital capacity

Inspiratory capacity (IC)—Maximum amount of air that can be exhaled after *normal* inspiration

Functional residual capacity (FRC)—Volume of air remaining in the lungs after normal expiration

DESCRIPTIONS OF FLOW RATES

Forced expiratory volume in first second of expiration after full inspiration (FEV)—Valuable measurement of airway obstruction; decreases linearly with age and in patients with chronic obstructive disease

Maximal midexpiratory flow (MMEF)—Measures the average rate of flow during the middle half of the forced expiration; useful indicator of early disease of small airways; more sensitive indicator of expired air flow than forced midexpiratory flow (FEV)

Maximal voluntary ventilation (MVV) or maximal breathing capacity (MBC)—Patient breathes as deeply and rapidly as possible for a specified period; the volume of air moved is reported in liters per minute; useful index of airflow, muscle strength, airway resistance, and coordination

The standard pulse oximeter is a photoelectric apparatus that has two diodes that beam light through pigmentation in the skin's outer layer, tissue, nail, venous blood, and arterial blood. A photodetector immediately opposite the diodes receives the red and infrared light emitted by the diodes and measures only the amount of light absorbed by oxygenated and deoxygenated hemoglobin in the pulsating arterial bed. (Deoxygenated hemoglobin absorbs more red light and oxygenated blood more infrared light.) Newer oximeters have flat probes that can be positioned over central sites such as the carotid and measure reflected rather than transmitted light.

Continuous monitoring is also possible through the use of a fiberoptic sensor that is threaded into the artery. This technique, still being refined, involves passing light through the fiber to its tip, which has been treated with indicator chemicals. A camera-like device picks up the light that returns after passing through one of the indicator dyes and gives an indication of the pH and carbon dioxide levels of the blood. These sensors may also be capable of measuring oxygen, electrolytes, and cardiac enzymes.

Patient preparation

The nurse explains that pulse oximetry measures the amount of oxygen in the blood and attaches the oximeter to the patient's toe, finger, nose, earlobe, or forehead. Pediatric and adult adhesive sensors and the finger-clip sensor for adults are placed on the index, middle, or ring fingers. Infant, pediatric, and adult adhesive sensors can be placed on a toe unless the patient has compromised circulation in the lower extremities. The nasal sensor is placed on the cartilaginous area of the nose, immediately below the bridge.

Sputum Examination

Sputum specimens are obtained for culture and sensitivity and cytologic examination. Results of sputum studies help in establishing diagnosis, determining infectiousness, and selecting an appropriate management regimen. A possible source case of tuberculosis is judged potentially infectious if the patient is positive for acid-fast bacilli on direct smear or stained sputum but is considered to have an unlikely chance of infecting others if the patient is positive for tubercle bacilli only on culture and not on smear. Sputum must be raised from the lungs and bronchi. It may be obtained directly through coughing or through a number of indirect methods such as tracheal suctioning, endotracheal aspiration, transtracheal aspiration, bronchoscopic removal, or gastric aspiration. Gastric aspiration is usually performed when tuberculosis is suspected and requires that the patient fast and that the specimen be obtained via a nasogastric tube.

The direct method of obtaining a sputum specimen involves instructing the patient to clear the nose and throat and rinse the mouth with water to decrease contamination of the sputum. Tell the patient to take a few deep breaths and then cough, using the diaphragm. Ask the patient to expectorate into a sterile container. Check to ensure that the specimen of sputum is mucoidlike, not saliva, before taking it to the laboratory. Transport the container to the laboratory immediately, since allowing the specimen to stand in a warm environment promotes overgrowth of the organism. If the patient is unable to cough deeply, an aerosol treatment may be necessary to stimulate coughing. Specimen collection is also facilitated by encouraging the patient to have a liberal intake of fluids and by collecting specimens when the patient first awakens, so that sputum is not swallowed.

Throat Culture

A throat culture is performed primarily to identify group A *betahemolytic streptococci* (GABHS) so that appropriate treatment of pharyngitis may be instituted. It may also be used to screen for carriers of *Neisseria meningitidis* and to detect sore throats associated with *Chlamydia trachomatis, Neisseria gonorrhoeae,* and *Corynebacterium diphtheriae. C. diphtheriae* is plated on Loffler's slant or tellurite agar and *N. gonorrhoeae* on Thayer-Martin media. Routine cultures are plated on sheep-blood agar, which offers preliminary results in 12 to 24 hours. The sensitivity of these cultures ranges from 95% to 99%, and the specificity is 90%. Cultures tend to be less useful if infections are recurrent because the infections are deeply embedded in the lymphoid tissues and may not be accessible to swabbing.

Newer, more rapid tests for detecting GABHS offer results in 10 to 30 minutes. Rapid tests detect GABHS through latex agglutinations, enzyme-linked immunoabsorbent assay (ELISA), or coagglutination. ELISA is also useful for rapid, in-office detection of *Chlamydia.* Since these tests are not as sensitive to GABHS as culture methods, a follow-up throat culture is recommended when rapid test results are negative and clinical symptoms suggest infection.

Patient preparation

Explain to the patient that this test helps to identify the microorganisms that are causing symptoms. Tell the patient to tilt the head back, and swab both tonsillar pillars and the posterior pharynx wall. A tongue depressor is used in the collection of the swab so that the swab is less likely to contact the normal flora of the mouth. If evaluating the presence of *N. gonorrhoeae,* the nurse uses a Dacron swab since cotton will inhibit the growth of the organism. The swab is immediately placed in a labelled culture tube and transported to the laboratory.

Skin Tests

Tuberculin skin testing (Mantoux)

The **Mantoux test** identifies individuals infected with *Mycobacterium tuberculosis.* The test does not differentiate between active and dormant infection.

Using a tuberculin syringe, inject 0.1 mL of intermediate strength purified protein derivative (PPD) into the inner aspect of the forearm. Hold the syringe almost parallel to the skin, with the needle bevel up. A pronounced wheal formation during intradermal injection of PPD indicates that it was properly administered.

Read the test 48 to 72 hours after injection by palpating the area for the presence of induration. Only the induration, and not the erythema, is measured at its widest width. Erythema without induration is not considered significant.

Misleading or false-negative results can result if the injection is not intradermal or if the nurse measures the area of erythema rather than the area of induration. The test may be falsely negative if the vaccine has been denatured by light, heat, or bacteriologic contamination and if the patient is unable to mount a hypersensitivity response. Neoplastic disease, immunosuppressive therapy, sarcoidosis, malnutrition, advanced age, and recent live-virus immunization affect the tuberculin response. For these reasons, a two-step testing procedure, in which the Mantoux is repeated 1 week to 1 month after the initial test, may be recommended for some patients. The second skin test is sufficient to stimulate immunologic recall and produce a positive result (booster phenomenon) in individuals who have been infected with mycobacteria but whose immunity has faded over time.

Patient preparation

Tell the patient that the test helps to determine whether tuberculosis is present and that the test results will be read in 48 to 72 hours.

Interpretation of results

Positive reaction = 10 mm or more of induration.

Doubtful reaction = 5 to 9 mm of induration. Individuals with this reaction who have been in close contact with persons with active tuberculosis are regarded as significant reactors.

Negative reaction = 0 to 4 mm of induration. No further follow-up is necessary.

Schick test

The **Schick test** measures an individual's immunity to diphtheria. Using intradermal injection technique, 0.1 mL of purified diphtheria toxin is injected into the inner aspect of one forearm, and 0.1 mL of inactivated purified diphtheria toxoid is injected into the other arm as a control. The test is read after 24 hours, after 48 hours, and again at 4 to 7 days after injection. Positive reactions begin within 24 hours at the site where the toxin was injected and may develop to greater than 2 cm in size. A positive reaction indicates the patient lacks immunity to diphtheria.

Blood Serum Tests

A number of tests such as the complete blood count and differential, arterial blood gases, and alpha-antitrypsin assay are useful in diagnosing respiratory disorders and determining the extent and cause of respiratory disease. The complete blood count and differential are described in detail in Chapter 37. Table 25-1 includes a general description of collection of arterial blood gases. Chapter 13 includes a more complete description of arterial blood gases.

TABLE 25-1   Blood and Serum Tests for Respiratory Assessment

Determination	Purpose/description	Reference range
Alpha-antitrypsin assay	Alpha-antitrypsin is a plasma protein that is a major inhibitor of trypsin in serum and of enzymatic proteolysis; a deficiency of alpha-antitrypsin leads to major pulmonary disease in adults; test is indicated when emphysema begins at an early age or when there is a family history of emphysema	>250 mg/dL
Arterial blood gases (ABGs)	ABGs are done to determine adequacy of ventilation and metabolic status; arterial blood is collected in a heparinized syringe, from which all air is expelled; specimen is placed on ice and sent immediately to laboratory; direct pressure is applied to the arterial puncture for at least 5 minutes after specimen has been collected	See Chapter 12

CRITICAL THINKING QUESTIONS

1 Describe the homeostatic function of the respiratory system.

2 How is oxygen carried in the blood?

3 Compose at least three questions to ask patients regarding risk factors for respiratory impairment.

4 Discuss possible psychosocial concerns of patients with respiratory alterations.

5 Design a logical plan for assessing the thorax and lungs of a patient in respiratory distress, setting priorities of assessment to allow for immediate intervention if indicated.

6 Discuss the preparation and care of a patient undergoing bronchography.

7 Describe how a throat culture is obtained.

BIBLIOGRAPHY

Current

1. Bowers A, Thompson J: *Clinical manual of health assessment,* ed 3, St Louis, 1988, Mosby–Year Book.
2. Burrell LO: *Adult nursing in hospital and community settings,* Norwalk, Conn, 1992, Appleton & Lange.
3. Gallo JJ et al: *Handbook of geriatric assessment,* Rockville, Md, 1988, Aspen Publishers.
4. Gordon M: *Manual of nursing diagnosis,* New York, 1987, McGraw-Hill.
5. Kane RL et al: *Essentials of clinical geriatrics,* ed 2, New York, 1989, McGraw-Hill.
6. Kenny RA: *Physiology of aging: a synopsis,* St Louis, Mosby–Year Book.
7. LeFever Kee J: *Handbook of laboratory and diagnostic tests with nursing implications,* Norwalk, Conn, 1990, Appleton & Lange.
8. Malasanos L et al: *Health assessment,* ed 4, St Louis, 1990, Mosby–Year Book.
9. Mathews PJ, Mathews LM, Mitchell RR: Airway monitoring and ventilation, *Nurs 92* 22:2, 1992.
10. McDonagh A: Getting your patient ready for a nuclear medicine scan, *Nurs 91* 21:2, 1991.
11. Muhrer JC: Diagnostic considerations in the evaluation and treatment of sore throat, *Nurs Prac* 16:9, 1991.
12. Murray R, Zentner S: *Nursing assessment and health promotion through the life span,* Englewood Cliffs, NJ, 1989, Prentice-Hall.
13. PIOPED investigators: The value of ventilation/perfusion scans in acute pulmonary embolism, *JAMA* 263:20, 1990.
14. Seidel HM et al: *Mosby's guide to physical examination,* ed 2, St Louis, 1991, Mosby–Year Book.
15. Sonnesso G: Are you ready to use pulse oximetry? *Nurs 92* 21:8, 1992.
16. Stiff D: Sensor devised to check blood inside arteries, *Wall Street Journal,* Sept 26, 1991.
17. Swartz MH: *Textbook of physical diagnosis,* Philadelphia, 1989, WB Saunders Co.
18. Thelan LA, Davie JK, Urden LD: *Textbook of critical care nursing: diagnosis and management,* St Louis, 1990, Mosby–Year Book.
19. Wensel M: An alternative to 'two-step' tuberculin skin testing for Southeast Asian refugees, *Nurs Prac* 16:11, 1991.

Classic

20. Bloch B, Hunter M: Teaching physiological assessment of black persons, *Nurs Educ* 6:24, 1981.
21. Block G, Nolan J: *Health assessment for professional nursing: a developmental approach,* New York, 1986, Appleton-Century-Crofts.
22. Carotenuto R, Bullock J: *Physical assessment of the gerontologic client,* Philadelphia, 1981, FA Davis Co.
23. Fields W, McGinn-Campbell K: *Introduction to health assessment,* Reston, Va, 1983, Reston Publishing Co.
24. Price S, Wilson L: *Pathophysiology,* New York, 1986, McGraw-Hill.
25. Prior JA, Silberstein JS, Stang J: *Physical diagnosis: the history and examination of the patient,* ed 6, St Louis, 1981, Mosby–Year Book.

CHAPTER TWENTY-SIX

Nursing Interventions Common to Respiratory Disorders

LEARNING OBJECTIVES

1 Evaluate the effectiveness of deep breathing and coughing techniques in patient care.
2 Discuss the use of chest physical therapy in promoting airway clearance.
3 Identify indications for the use of artificial airways.
4 Compare artificial airways, endotracheal tubes, and tracheostomy tubes.
5 Discuss potential complications of artificial airways.
6 Develop a nursing care plan for the patient with an artificial airway.
7 Describe the key assessment criteria indicating a patient's need for oxygen therapy.
8 Compare and contrast negative and positive pressure ventilators.
9 Describe commonly used negative pressure ventilators.
10 Discuss potential complications of mechanical ventilation.
11 Develop a nursing care plan for the patient using mechanical ventilation.
12 Assess the function of chest tube drainage systems.

KEY TERMS

THIS CHAPTER provides an overview of the procedures and equipment used to treat patients with pulmonary problems. Patients with respiratory disorders may suffer from ineffective airway clearance, ineffective breathing patterns, or impaired gas exchange. Close cooperation between the nurse and respiratory care practitioners will ensure that the patient receives optimal care.

The following is a synopsis of respiratory procedures commonly used to treat patients with specific pulmonary disorders or dysfunctions discussed in Chapters 27 and 28.

Breathing Exercises

Normal inspiration is an active process that uses the diaphragm and external intercostal muscles. The chest wall expands outward and the diaphragm drops, displacing the abdominal contents. Exhalation at rest is a passive or relaxation process. The time required for exhalation is approximately twice the time needed for inspiration; the inspiratory to expiratory (I:E) ratio is normally 1:2. Any change in breathing pattern due to disease, trauma, or surgery may indicate a need for breathing exercises. Ineffective breathing patterns can be manifested by:

- Decreased breath sounds in lung segments
- Hypopnea (decreased lung volume), tachypnea (respiratory rate greater than 20/min), bradypnea (respiratory rate less than 6/min)
- Use of accessory muscles for respiration (neck, intercostals, shoulder, abdomen)
- Paradoxical respiratory movement (abdomen bulges during expiration, retracts during inspiration)
- Dyspnea (patient complaint of shortness of breath) at rest or with activity
- Restlessness, anxiety, diaphoresis (perspiration at rest)
- Tachycardia (heart rate greater than 100 beats per minute)

Breathing exercises promote optimal ventilation and gas exchange.[26] They are usually instituted when the patient's condition is stable such as during the postoperative period or when recovering from an acute exacerbation of a chronic respiratory problem. The nurse helps achieve desired patient outcomes through explanation, demonstration, hands-on assistance, and reinforcement. More than one kind of breathing exercise may be used. It is the nurse's responsibility to assess the patient's ability to perform these techniques, to modify the approach as needed, and to evaluate the patient's clinical response.

For **diaphragmatic breathing** (manually assisted) place the patient in a semi-Fowler or sitting position with the nurse's or patient's hand placed over the epigastric area. Instruct the patient to breathe in deeply through the nose, if possible, and exhale slowly through the mouth. The nurse's hand serves as a visual cue to reinforce effective diaphragmatic movement during inspiration and expiration. Eventually the patient should become independent in monitoring controlled diaphragmatic movement with breathing. This is done about 10 times an hour as needed.

For **resisted breathing** (stimulation of stretch receptors) the patient assumes a semi-Fowler or sitting position with the nurse's hands placed on the lateral thorax. The patient takes a deep breath, trying to push the nurse's hands away. The nurse provides gentle resistance on the chest wall during inspiration.

The patient may be in any position for the inspiratory hold (yawn) maneuver. The patient takes a deep breath and holds it for 3 to 5 seconds. Then the nurse gives a verbal cue to exhale. The exhalation often elicits a cough.

For pursed lip breathing, the patient may also be in any position. The nurse places one hand over the epigastric area. As the patient exhales through pursed lips, contracting the abdominal muscles, the nurse gently pushes up and in to support the diaphragm. This exercise is useful in treating patients with COPD who have air trapping. Pursed lip breathing provides positive pressure in the airways, keeping the airways and alveoli open longer during exhalation.

INCENTIVE SPIROMETRY

The device most commonly used to monitor the ability to take a deep breath is the **incentive spirometer (IS),** a cylinder with volume markings on its outer surface and an indicator or float that rises as the patient inhales air through the spirometer (Figure 26-1). An IS is indicated for patients who are at risk for or have developed **atelectasis** (alveolar collapse). Incentive spirometers are typically ordered following surgery, especially thoracic and upper abdominal procedures. Other factors such as x-ray evidence of atelectasis, history of chronic respiratory disease, neuromuscular disease, obesity, smoking, immobility, or secretion retention are common indicators for an IS to be placed at the patient's bedside. Patients must be alert, cooperative, motivated, understand instructions, have the ability to deep breathe and hold their breath upon command. IS therapy is of no benefit for patients who can meet or exceed their predicted lung volumes.

Ideally, patients are taught to use the IS before surgery. During that session, the preoperative inspiratory volume can be determined and used as a postoperative goal. Postoperatively, the patient

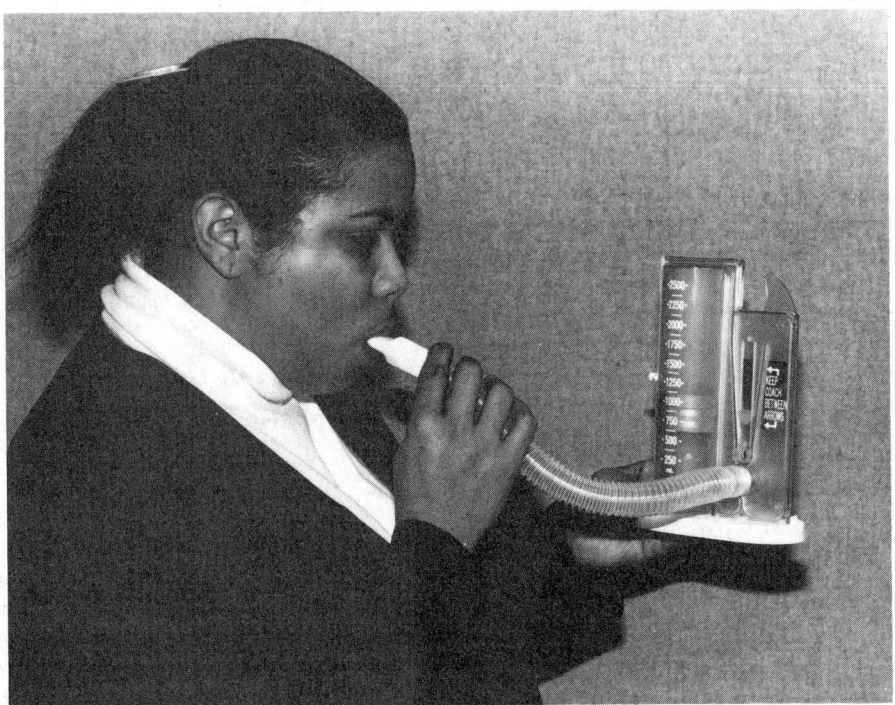

FIGURE 26-1   Patient using a volume-oriented incentive spirometer.

should be able to inhale at least 1 L of air per breath through the device within the first 48 hours after starting treatment.

Patient Care

Early studies of IS therapy showed best results were achieved when patients used the device frequently.[45] In addition, holding the breath at the end of inspiration is important to promote distribution of air throughout the lungs. See patient education guide at right for further information.

Evaluation of Incentive Spirometry

To monitor IS therapy, the nurse records the maximum volume of air the patient was able to inspire, encourages the patient to cough at the end of the session, and auscultates the lung fields before and after the session to assess changes in lung sounds as a result of the deep breaths.

Complications are infrequent and relatively minor. Incisional pain during the IS breath or cough is the most commonly reported complaint. New incisional sites should be splinted with a pillow or blanket during coughing to lessen the pain and chance of dehiscence or evisceration. Patients may complain of dizziness or tingling of the extremities if they take sustained inspirations too rapidly in succession (hyperventilation).

The maximal amount of air a patient can inhale from resting exhalation (inspiratory capacity) should increase daily as the patient's respiratory muscles gradually regain their function or as the lungs reinflate with air. As the patient's condition improves, the frequency of sessions can be reduced. IS is not needed once the patient is ambulating and has clear

PATIENT EDUCATION GUIDE
Using the Incentive Spirometer

1. Sit as upright as can be tolerated.
2. Seal lips around mouthpiece.
3. Inhale as slowly and deeply as possible and watch the spirometer indicator rise.
4. Hold the deep breath for the count of "5" if possible.
5. Remove the mouthpiece from your mouth and breathe out slowly.
6. Aim for a higher number with each successive breath you take.
7. Repeat this process for 10 breaths and cough after the last breath.

breath sounds, a strong cough, and no evidence of pulmonary problems.

Treatment is considered effective when atelectasis or pulmonary complications are reversed or absent. Occasionally, a patient may have difficulty using the IS device and yet be able to breathe deeply. In such a situation, coaching the patient to breathe deeply and cough is a suitable alternative to breathing through the IS.

INTERMITTENT POSITIVE PRESSURE BREATHING

Intermittent positive pressure breathing (IPPB) is a pressurized breath that simulates spontaneous breathing by physically stretching the lung and chest wall. Treatment is indicated with atelectasis that is unresponsive to less intensive techniques, such as IS or deep breathing. Such patients may be unable to breathe deeply and cough effectively because of chronic airway obstruction, neuromuscular limitations, or restriction of lung expansion. On occasion, IPPB has been used for patients with acute respiratory failure as a method of intermittent mechanical ventilatory support to avoid intubation and continuous mechanical ventilation.

COUGHING EXERCISES

An important role of the nurse is to instruct and assist the patient in producing an effective cough. Factors that influence the ability to cough include:

1. *Position*—A sitting position is the most effective and comfortable.

2. *Pain*—The patient may need analgesia before the cough exercise. Pain limits the degree of chest expansion which can both promote atelectasis and limit the volume of air needed to move secretions.

3. *Incisional support*—Splinting a painful area during coughing with gentle hand pressure helps the patient cough. The patient can be taught to "hug" a pillow.

4. *A dry mouth*—Makes coughing more difficult. Oral hydration using ice chips or sips of water can make coughing easier.

Various coughing techniques can be incorporated into the patient's plan of care. For a **cascade cough** the patient is instructed to take a deep breath, then cough several times until he or she feels like there is no air left in the lungs. This cough maneuver moves secretions from smaller to larger airways, since the cough is performed at different lung volumes. The **huff cough** requires the patient to take a deep breath and then, with an open mouth, do a series of expiratory "huffs." After repeating this maneuver several times, the patient should attempt to cough. This maneuver is sometimes performed

when pain limits normal coughing. A **quad-assist** cough is designed to help patients with reduced expiratory muscle ability. The nurse augments the patient's muscle forces by pushing up and in with one hand below the xiphoid process when the patient tries to cough. If possible, the patient should be bent forward at the waist at the same time the cough is augmented. These two movements increase abdominal pressure and diaphragmatic movement upward to facilitate secretion clearance.

Evaluation of the Cough

The nurse records the following information: intensity of the cough (strong or weak); sound (moist or dry); and frequency (intermittent or continuous). If sputum was produced, the nurse also notes the color, amount, consistency (thick or thin), and the presence of blood. Determine if breath sounds improve after the cough as signified by an increase in aeration or clearing of gurgles as assessed by auscultation. Patients who cannot effectively clear their secretions by coughing are suctioned.

CHEST PHYSICAL THERAPY

Chest physical therapy (also called chest physiotherapy or CPT) is indicated for patients who have difficulty clearing their airway secretions by coughing or with suctioning.[47,53,62] Obstruction of the airway by secretions can lead to atelectasis and pneumonia. Although CPT is occasionally performed by nurses, it is usually provided by the respiratory care or physical therapy departments. The CPT treatment usually includes two components: postural drainage (PD), and therapeutic percussion (P) and vibration (VIB).

Postural Drainage

Postural drainage (PD) is accomplished by positioning the patient to promote mucus flow through gravity. The patient is positioned according to the segment or lobe that is affected by mucus accumulation. These positions are illustrated in Figure 26-2. The patient is usually placed in a particular position for at least 5 minutes or as tolerated. Patients are encouraged to breathe deeply while in that position and to cough when turned upright.

PD is indicated for patients who have difficulty clearing secretions due to airway obstruction and/or excessive mucus production.[7,23,53] Signs of airway obstruction include decreased breath sounds with crackles or gurgles, increased respiratory rate, tachycardia, fever, decreasing oxygen saturation, and a weak, nonproductive cough in a patient with a history of bronchial disease or lung abscess. Chest films reveal atelectasis or pneumonia (infiltrates).

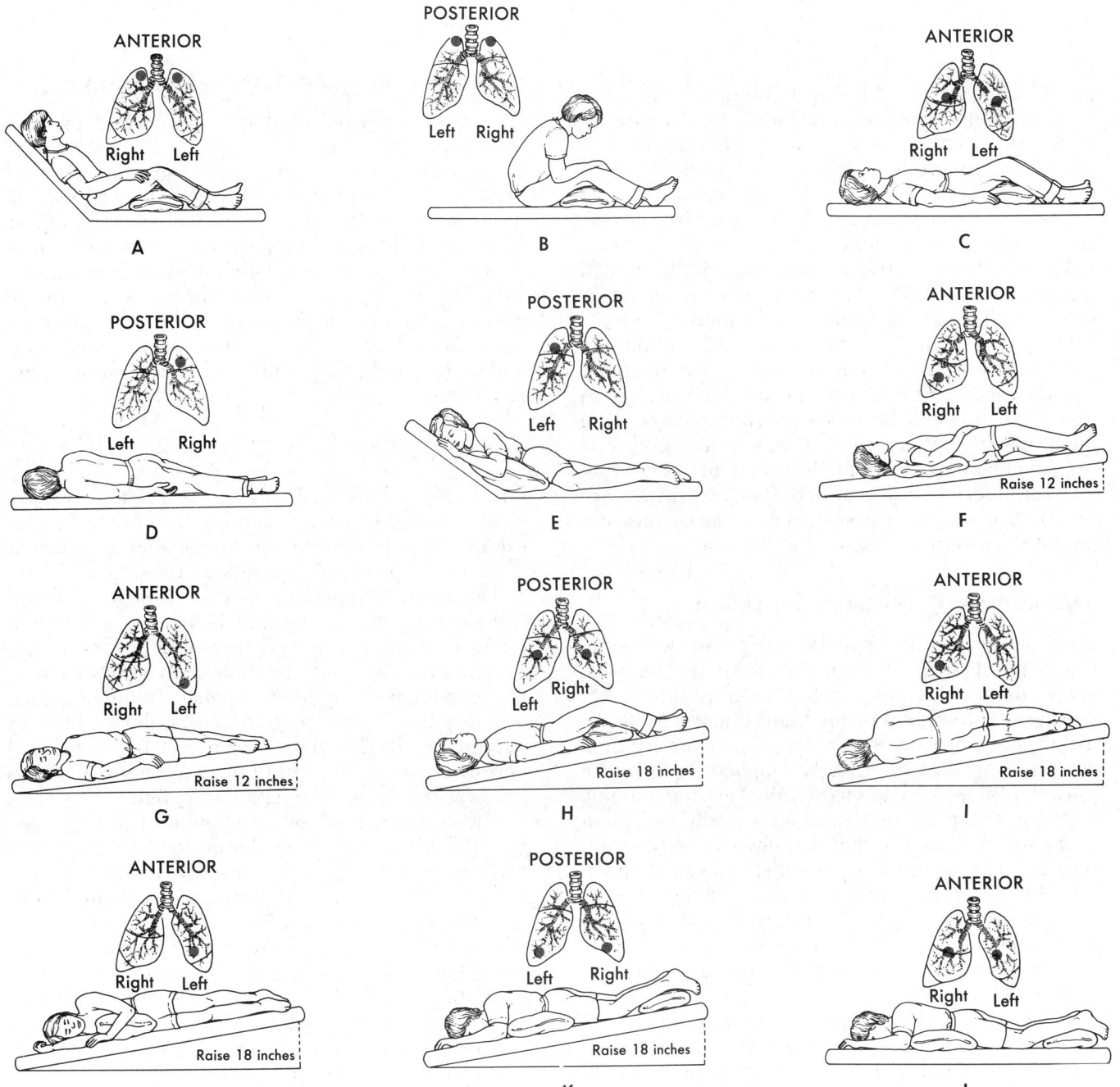

FIGURE 26-2   Positions for postural drainage. **A,** Anterior apical segment. **B,** Posterior apical segment. **C,** Anterior segment. **D,** Right posterior segment. **E,** Left posterior segment. **F,** Right middle lobe. **G,** Left lingula. **H,** Anterior segments. **I,** Right lateral segment. **J,** Left lateral segment. **K,** Posterior segments. **L,** Superior segments. (From Thompson JM et al: *Mosby's manual of clinical nursing,* ed 2, St Louis, 1989, Mosby–Year Book.)

This treatment is most often used for patients with chronic airway diseases such as bronchiectasis or cystic fibrosis (CF). Postural drainage does not slow the progression of CF. However, when it is not done, air flow through the lungs tends to diminish because of retained secretions. Stable patients with CF may substitute an exercise session or program for PD treatment.[5,64] PD is usually administered immediately following an aerosolized bronchodilator treatment or it may be given as a single therapy. The typical treatment lasts at least half an hour and is provided up to four times a day. PD may be administered as often as tolerated for patients with excessive secretion production.

PD is contraindicated for patients with increased intracranial pressure, head, neck, chest, or spinal injuries, cardiovascular instability, pulmonary edema, large pleural effusions and empyema, pulmonary embolism, uncontrolled hypertension, distended abdomen, postesophageal surgery, or blood in sputum related to lung cancer. It is avoided in patients who have recently eaten a meal. If the patient is receiving tube feedings, the pump is turned off at least half an hour before CPT is provided. Patients with severe obstructive airway disease or heart disease may not be able to tolerate some of the PD positions.

Therapeutic Percussion/Vibration

Therapeutic percussion is typically provided while the patient is in the various PD positions. The caregiver's hands are cupped so that an air pocket is created within the palm of the hand (Figure 26-3). To dislodge mucus from the airways the hands are then rhythmically and alternately clapped against the portion of the patient's chest wall overlying the lung segment which is being drained. Usually bed linen or a gown is placed so that the nurse's hands do not directly clap against the patient's exposed skin, especially in the older patient where padding such as a towel may be helpful. Vibration is performed by placing the hands against the chest wall and slightly compressing and "quivering" the hands as the patient exhales.

Percussion and vibration are contraindicated for patients with recent epidural spinal infusion, spinal anesthesia, or pacemaker placements, thoracic skin

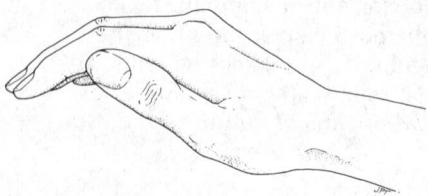

FIGURE 26-3 The nurse uses a cupped hand position for chest percussion.

grafts, burns, infections, or open wounds, subcutaneous emphysema, lung contusion, bronchospasm, osteomyelitis of the ribs, osteoporosis, coagulopathy, suspected pulmonary tuberculosis, or complaints of chest pain.

Evaluation of Chest Physical Therapy

The nurse notes the patient's comments regarding treatment, as well as changes in vital signs, breathing pattern, mental status, skin color, and sputum production. The patient will usually expectorate 30 to 60 minutes after treatment. Patients may suffer from the following complications: hypoxemia (decreased blood oxygen tension), hypotension, pulmonary hemorrhage, pain, vomiting and aspiration of gastric secretions, bronchospasm, or dysrhythmias. The nurse records any such problems and complaints following CPT and immediately notifies the physician.

SUCTIONING

Suctioning is indicated when a patient is unable to clear secretions with coughing. Suctioning is also used to obtain a sputum specimen when the patient is unable to produce a sample by coughing.

The suction catheter is passed through an artificial airway if one is in place. Otherwise, the catheter is inserted through the nose and advanced into the trachea. Although the nurse may receive an order to suction a patient at a specific frequency, such as every hour, frequency should be determined by patient need. The nurse assesses the patient and performs suctioning only when necessary. Guidelines for suctioning are listed on p. 545.

The closed tracheal suctioning catheter system (CTSS) is a new technique for suctioning airway secretions in mechanically ventilated patients.[18,28,42,46] The CTSS consists of a suction catheter enclosed within a plastic sleeve which can be advanced into an endotracheal or tracheostomy tube. The CTSS is attached directly to the ventilator tubing circuit (Figure 26-4) and unlike standard open catheter suctioning, ventilator operation is not interrupted. The catheter system is usually changed every 24 hours.

Complications of Suctioning

Hypoxemia or atelectasis can occur because air (including oxygen) as well as secretions are removed from the lungs by the catheter. Encouraging the patient to take deep breaths of 100% oxygen or providing oxygen with a manual resuscitation bag may minimize the degree of deoxygenation and prevent atelectasis. The airway epithelium may be damaged when the suction catheter makes direct contact with

GUIDELINES FOR NASOTRACHEAL OR OROTRACHEAL SUCTIONING

Procedure

Wash hands

Explain procedure to patient

Adjust suction regulator to 80 to 120 mm Hg and occlude tubing with finger to test suction

Place patient in semi-Fowler position

Apply mask, goggles, and unsterile gloves

Open sterile glove, suction catheter package, and bottled water

Squeeze water-soluble lubricant onto sterile wrapper

Encourage the patient to take five deep breaths (with supplemental oxygen if possible)

Connect the catheter to suction tubing and occlude the suction finger port to test the system

Put the sterile glove on your dominant hand over the examination glove

With the sterile-gloved hand, remove the catheter from its paper wrapping so that it does not touch a potentially contaminated object or surface

Dip catheter tip into lubricant and gently advance catheter through nares during inspiration

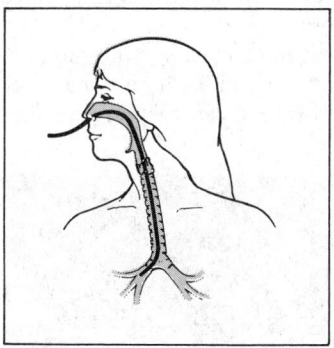

Instruct the patient to cough

Withdraw catheter 2 to 3 cm while applying intermittent suction, and rotate catheter between thumb and index finger

Repeat suction process as tolerated by the patient allowing adequate recovery between attempts

Allow the patient to take several deep breaths

Thoroughly clear catheter and suction tubing by flushing with bottled water

Discard catheter and gloves

Administer mouth care frequently

Auscultate chest; evaluate breath sounds

Wash hands

Document date, time, frequency of suctioning, and patient's responses to suctioning; note nature and amount of secretions, and record pertinent observations or changes in progress notes; secretions should be described with regard to consistency/ease of clearing, amount, color, and odor

Rationale

Excessive vacuum pressures can cause mucosal trauma, tissue grabbing, and bleeding

In accordance with infection control policy

One hand and catheter must remain sterile; two-glove technique is used to avoid contact contamination and to protect second hand from organisms in secretions

Unless contraindicated, catheter should be directed inferiorly and medially along floor of nasal passageway; when resistance is met at posterior nasopharynx, gently rotate catheter downward; if use of oral passage is necessary, inserting oral airway facilitates control of tongue; *do not* force catheter if obstruction is met; insertion of catheter may stimulate gag reflex; be prepared to turn patient to side if vomiting occurs

Continuous suction may cause mucosal damage; 10 seconds is maximum for each aspiration; if catheter "grabs" mucosa, release suction; if any complications occur, discontinue procedure, and instruct patient to breathe deeply

Do not tire patient; observe for signs of cardiac or respiratory distress

Hypoxemia and atelectasis can result from suctioning; both conditions may respond to oxygen administration and deep breathing

Coil catheter around gloved hand; remove glove over coiled catheter

TRACHEAL SUCTIONING OF A PATIENT WITH AN ARTIFICIAL AIRWAY

Procedure

Wash hands

Explain procedure to patient

Adjust suction regulator to 80 to 120 mm Hg (adults)

Set oxygen flowmeter connected to manual resuscitation bag at 15 L or greater/min or connect the bag into the oxygen wall outlet

Apply mask, goggles, and unsterile gloves

Open suction catheter package and sterile gloves

Connect catheter to suction tubing and occlude the suction finger port to test system

Disconnect ventilator or oxygen source and attach manual resuscitator bag

Preoxygenate and hyperinflate at least five deep breaths with manual resuscitator bag

Put sterile gloves onto dominant hand over examination glove

Remove wrapping from catheter, maintaining sterility of one hand

Gently insert catheter through tube as far as it will go

Slowly withdraw catheter while applying intermittent suction: total suctioning time not to exceed 10 to 15 seconds

Hyperinflate the patient with at least five breaths using the manual resuscitator bag

Flush catheter and connective tubing with water

Suction mouth and pharynx

Reconnect the patient to the ventilator or oxygen source

Dispose of suction catheter

Secure suction connection tubing over wall suction so that tip does not contact floor

Administer mouth care, if indicated; this should be performed wearing unsterile gloves

Auscultate chest; evaluate breath sounds

Wash hands

Document date, time, frequency of treatments, and patient's response to treatments; note nature and amount of secretions and record pertinent observations or changes in nursing progress notes; secretions should be described with regard to consistency/ease of clearing, amount, color, and odor

NOTE: Some of these steps will be unnecessary with closed tracheal suction catheter systems

Rationale

Studies show manual resuscitation bags deliver close to 100% oxygen at 15 L/min

In accordance with infection control policy

Catheter should remain protected by package

One hand and catheter must remain sterile; coiling catheter around sterile hand protects catheter; two-glove technique is used to avoid contact contamination and protect second hand from organisms in secretions

Advance without suction to prevent mucosal damage

Remember, patient is not being adequately oxygenated at this time

Application of intermittent suction prevents catheter adherence to mucosal wall; continuous suction may cause mucosal damage; catheter should be withdrawn within 10 seconds; if bradycardia or signs of hypoxia are noted, immediately withdraw catheter and oxygenate manually

Do not reenter trachea after suctioning mouth and pharynx; catheter is contaminated

Coil catheter around gloved hand; remove glove over coiled catheter

Dust and particulate matter contaminate system and may clog vacuum outlets; do not leave tubing on bed; organisms in tubing can further colonize patient environment

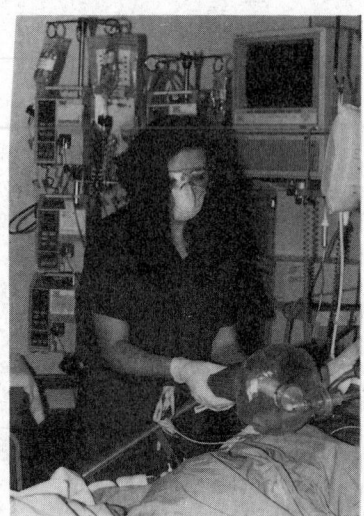

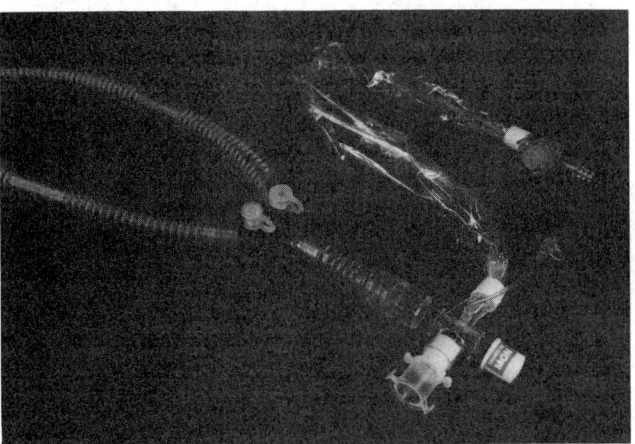

FIGURE 26-4   Closed tracheal suction catheter system.

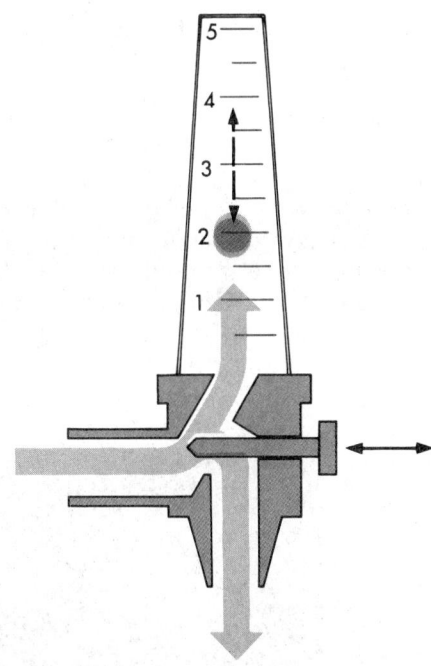

FIGURE 26-5   Oxygen flowmeter.

the tissues. Suctioning may provoke violent coughing, which can cause vomiting and aspiration of gastric contents, as well as induce constriction of pharyngeal, laryngeal, and bronchial muscles.[55] In addition, direct stimulation of vagal nerve fibers in the airway may cause cardiac arrhythmias (premature ventricular contractions or bradycardia). The procedure can also lead to temporary increases in intracranial pressure. Most of these problems can be avoided or minimized by limiting the duration and frequency of suctioning. The nurse pays strict attention to avoiding contamination of suction catheters and equipment to prevent pulmonary infection. The patient's vital signs are closely monitored before and after suctioning.

OXYGEN THERAPY

Oxygen therapy is used for patients who suffer from **hypoxemia** (low arterial oxygen tensions). In acutely ill patients who are breathing room air, an arterial oxygen pressure (PaO_2) less than 60 millimeters of mercury or an oxygen saturation of hemoglobin (SaO_2) less than 90% are common laboratory indications of the need for oxygen therapy. The frail elderly and those with chronic pulmonary diseases may tolerate lower oxygenation levels without impairment of function or clinical signs of respiratory distress. Oxygen may also be administered to patients with pulmonary artery hypertension or to those who suffer hypoxemia during exercise or sleep.

Hypoxemia may be suspected in patients who develop unexplained restlessness, dyspnea, tachycardia, hypertension, diaphoresis, tachypnea, use of accessory muscles for respiration, confusion, impaired judgment and disorientation. Cyanosis (bluish coloring) of the face, lips, or tongue may also indicate a lowered oxygen tension. However, hypoxemia may be present in the absence of cyanosis. Hypoxemia

may develop secondary to changes in air or blood flow through the lung. Diseases that cause alveolar shunting (blood flow through the lung is maintained while air flow is absent) such as pneumonia, airway obstruction, and pulmonary edema, may lead to a reduction in blood oxygen tension. Conditions that promote alveolar deadspace (air flow without blood flow) such as blood loss, cardiac failure, or pulmonary emboli, may also cause hypoxemia. In addition, a lower than expected PaO_2 may result from hypoventilation and hypermetabolism. Many patients have various degrees of these cardiopulmonary problems. It may be inappropriate to simply administer oxygen without conducting a thorough patient assessment to determine the cause of the hypoxemic event. Oxygen therapy is commonly prescribed in the initial treatment of severe trauma, acute myocardial infarction, and immediately following surgery or extubation.

Oxygen Delivery Systems

In the hospital setting, the flow of oxygen to a patient is controlled by a flowmeter that is inserted into a specially designated wall outlet. A flowmeter consists of a dial or knob and a clear tube with markings on its exterior surface, and is usually labelled in increments of liters per minute. A small ball or rod floats inside the clear tube to indicate the rate of gas that is being delivered to the patient. The dial or knob is adjusted until the indicator rises to the center of the prescribed liter flow (Figure 26-5).

One end of the oxygen therapy device is attached to the flowmeter and the opposite end is fitted onto the patient's face. The oxygen therapy device selected depends upon the fractional concentration of inspired oxygen (FIO_2, or oxygen percent expressed as a decimal) that is needed to treat the hypoxemia. Oxygen therapy systems fall into three categories: high-flow, reservoir-type, and low-flow systems. A high-flow system provides all of the gas that the patient inhales. These systems deliver a consistent oxygen concentration that is unaffected by the patient's breathing pattern. High-flow systems are typ-

ically used to deliver oxygen to critically ill patients or those with endotracheal or tracheostomy tubes. Reservoir systems are oxygen masks designed to hold a volume of gas which can be inspired if the patient's inspiratory flow exceeds that of the flowmeter. Low-flow systems provide only a part of the patient's demand for airflow. The patient breathes in room air around the device so that the inspired oxygen concentration lies somewhere between 100% oxygen and room air (21% oxygen).

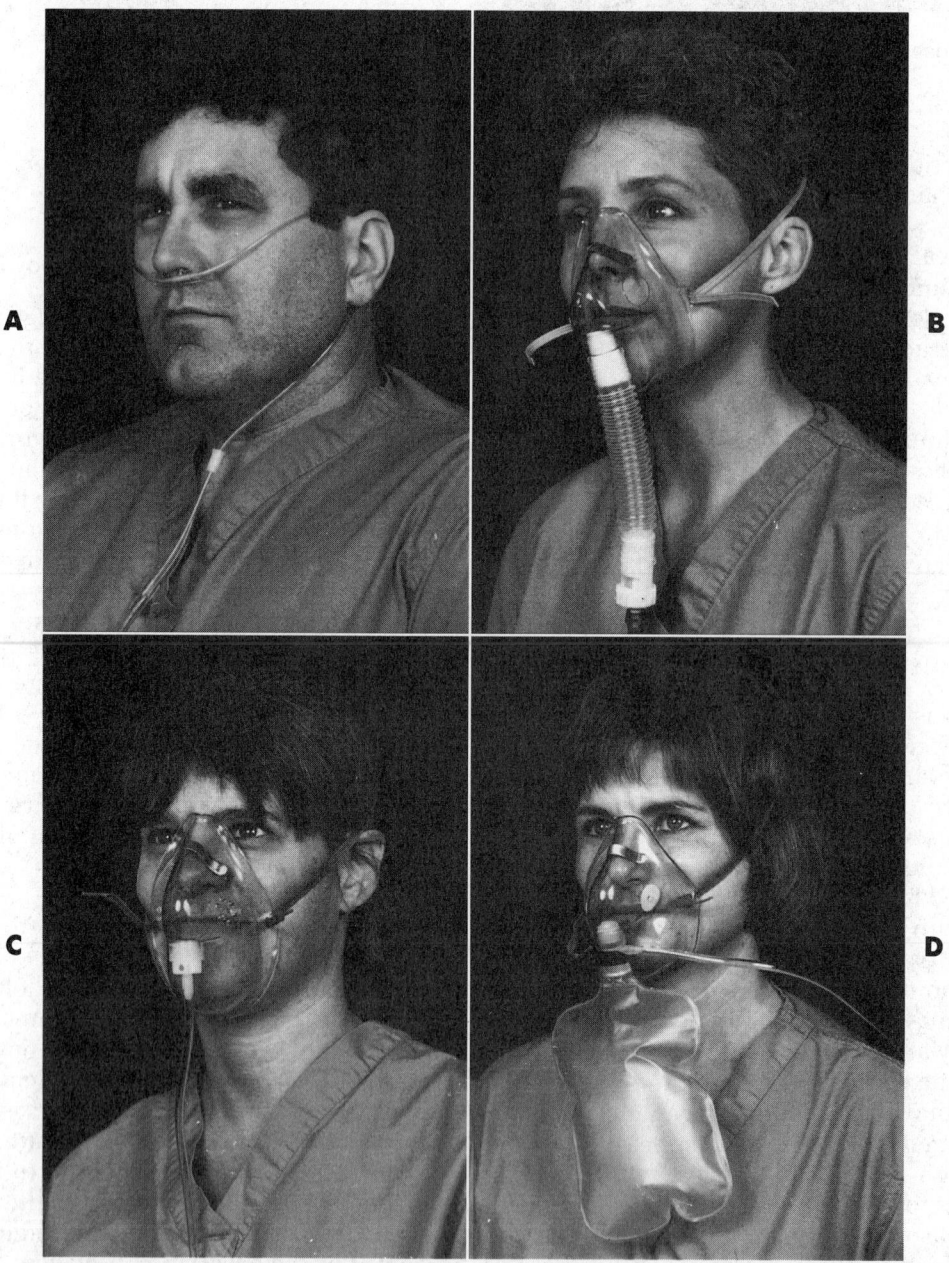

FIGURE 26-6   Oxygen delivery devices for nonintubated patients. **A,** Nasal cannula. **B,** Venturi mask. **C,** Simple oxygen mask. **D,** Nonrebreathing mask.

TABLE 26-1   Oxygen Delivery Devices for Nonintubated Patients

Device	FIo$_2$	Flow rate range (liters/min)	Nursing considerations
Nasal cannula	0.22 to 0.50	0.25 to 5.0	FIo$_2$ varies with breathing pattern, high FIo$_2$s possible with hypoventilation Prongs may irritate the nose and gas flow may dry nasal mucosa Evaluate the nares, face, and ears for signs of pressure sores—padding the tubing and loosening may help Most common and simple oxygen therapy device
Venturi mask	0.24 to 0.50	4 to 12	Delivers a consistent FIo$_2$ regardless of the patient's breathing pattern FIo$_2$ adjusted by changing nozzles which are attached to mask intake tube Flow rate needed for specific FIo$_2$ is stamped on nozzles Interferes with eating and speaking, not well tolerated by alert patients Ensure that air intake tubes are not blocked or covered, FIo$_2$ will increase High flow rates may cause dehydration of airway and thickened secretions
Simple oxygen mask	0.35 to 0.55	5 to 10	To be effective, the mask must fit tightly Should patient vomit, aspiration of gastric secretions likely Inadequate flow may cause CO$_2$ retention Used for short-term or emergency situations Uncomfortable and not well tolerated by alert patients
Partial rebreather mask	0.40 to 0.60	5 to 10	Bag serves as reservoir for oxygen Set flow rate to ensure bag does not collapse when patient inhales If mask is disconnected from gas flow, patient may suffocate Presence of one-way valve between mask and reservoir bag denotes non-rebreathing mask
Non-rebreather mask	0.60 to 1.0	5 to 10	Absence of one-way valve between mask and reservoir bag denotes partial rebreathing mask Patient should be monitored with pulse oximeter Used for critically ill patients Oxygen toxicity is possible Other concerns same as simple mask

Low-flow devices are usually easier to assemble, more comfortable for the patient to use, and less expensive than high-flow ones. The device most commonly used to deliver oxygen to patients is the nasal cannula, which is classified as a low-flow device. Examples and characteristics of the devices commonly used to deliver oxygen to patients are contained in Figure 26-6 and Table 26-1.

Oxygen is delivered through the flowmeter as a dry gas. Those patients receiving oxygen through a nasal cannula may complain of dryness of the nose, sore throat, nasal bleeding, thickened secretions, or other problems related to dehydration of the upper airway. The nurse is alert for signs or symptoms of airway drying when the patient receives oxygen flow greater than 5 liters per minute. A humidifier (a plastic jar filled with water) may be attached to the bottom of the flowmeter, but in most instances is not necessary.[4]

Complications of Oxygen Therapy

The complications of providing supplemental oxygen to patients are those associated with oxygen as a drug and those related to the particular oxygen delivery system. Breathing oxygen concentrations greater than 50% for more than 24 hours can cause injury to lung tissue, or oxygen toxicity. Early signs of oxygen toxicity include cough, restlessness, lethargy, vomiting, dyspnea, and retrosternal chest pain, burning, or tightness. More advanced disease may be present when the patient develops a pneumonia-like presentation, which includes infiltrates on chest x-ray, cyanosis, pulmonary edema, and possibly hemoptysis. In addition, breathing high concentrations of oxygen reduces the quantity of gaseous nitrogen in the alveoli. In the event that the patient's airways become obstructed or the patient hypoventilates, the alveoli are more susceptible to collapse without the stabilizing influence of nitrogen gas. This condition is called absorption atelectasis. Oxygen therapy may induce hypoventilation in patients who have received opioids or sedatives or in certain patients with chronic obstructive airway disease. Oxygen therapy should be titrated so that the patient receives only the amount needed to reverse hypoxemia and discontinued as soon as permitted by the patient's clinical condition.

Evaluation of Oxygen Therapy

The concentration (or flow) of oxygen is titrated to achieve a Pao_2 greater than 60 mm Hg or saturation greater than 90%. The classic method of evaluating the success of oxygen therapy is to obtain an arterial blood gas (ABG). The nurse waits 20 to 30 minutes after changing the FIo_2 before drawing an ABG. In patients who do not have obstructive airway disease, an ABG may be obtained within 10 minutes after changing the FIo_2 or oxygen flow.[34] Recently, portable pulse oximeters have become available so that the oxygen saturation of hemoglobin in a peripheral digit (Spo_2) is now a common method of assessing the degree of oxygenation. The accuracy of these devices may be limited by clinical conditions such as motion artifact, abnormal hemoglobins, room lighting, low blood flow, skin pigmentation, and nail polish.[30] Another limitation is that the Spo_2 is a poor indicator of hyperoxemia, that is, a Pao_2 that is higher than normal (or necessary). In addition, the Spo_2 is not affected to a significant degree by anemia. The patient may have a low blood oxygen content that is not reflected by the Spo_2 reading. In general, an Spo_2 greater than 92% in light-skinned patients, and 94% in dark-skinned patients, will mean that their Pao_2 is greater than 60 mm Hg.[25] In addition to recording the Spo_2, the nurse charts the date and time of the measurement as well as the patient's body position, activity level, oxygen flow or FIo_2, and clinical appearance.

Home Oxygen Therapy

Some patients continue oxygen therapy following discharge (see patient education guide).[31] In addition to treating primary pulmonary conditions such as COPD, home oxygen therapy has been used to treat pulmonary hypertension, recurring congestive heart failure, erythrocytosis (increased numbers of red blood cells due to hypoxia), impaired cognitive processes, and sleep apnea syndrome. Three major types of gas delivery systems are available for home care patients: compressed gas cylinders, liquid oxygen cylinders, and oxygen concentrators. There are advantages and limitations to each of these systems.[29] Normally, when the physician orders home oxygen therapy, the nurse or social worker contacts a home equipment supplier who matches the patient's needs with the appropriate system.

Transtracheal Oxygenation

The transtracheal oxygen (TTo_2) catheter is a thin Teflon-coated tube that is surgically placed into the trachea (Figure 26-7). The TTo_2 catheter is typically used in home care patients who do not wish to use nasal cannulas or as a cost savings measure. There may be other benefits to TTo_2 such as improved taste, smell, appetite, and body image.[1,22,46] Patients with a TTo_2 catheter often maintain adequate oxygenation and are able to decrease their oxygen flow requirements to more than half of the flow used with a nasal cannula. Complications of TTo_2 therapy include inflammation, bleeding, infection of the insertion site and thickened secretions. The catheter has to be routinely cleared of secretions or the flow of oxygen will be inhibited. Therefore the patient who

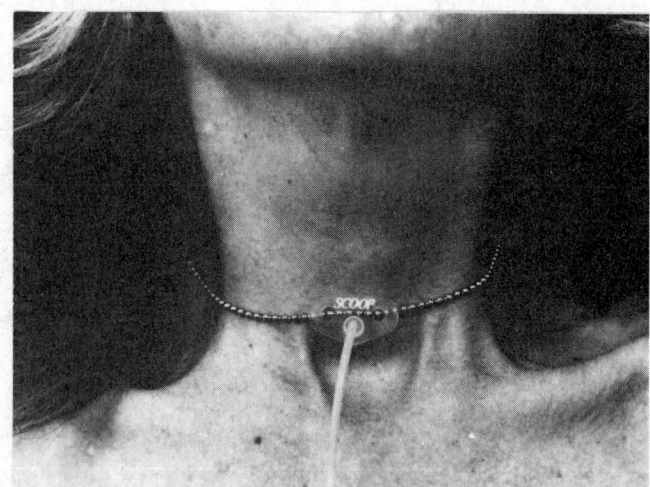

FIGURE 26-7 Transtracheal oxygen catheter.

PATIENT EDUCATION GUIDE   *Home Oxygen Therapy*

Oxygen will be ordered by your doctor only if you need it. It is a medicine and must be used like any other prescription. Follow your doctor's orders exactly. Too much oxygen can be harmful.

The physician order should read as follows:
- Rate of flow (exactly)
- Whether oxygen is to be used all the time, only at night, or while exercising. Make sure you understand your doctor's orders exactly.
- Oxygen flow rates of ½ to 4 L/min are used most frequently. Flow rates greater than 5 L are rarely used.

How can I tell how much oxygen flow I am getting?
- If you are in the hospital receiving oxygen, an oxygen flow meter is used.
- If you are going to use oxygen at home, your home oxygen supply company will talk to you about the equipment.

Safety Tips
Remember, oxygen will not explode but will cause something on fire to burn much faster.
- No smoking in any room where oxygen is being used.
- The oxygen equipment should be at least 10 feet away from any open flame; this includes pilot lights in stoves, furnaces, and water heaters.
- Keep your equipment at least 10 feet away from electrical equipment that may spark.
- Do not use oily lotions, face creams, grease, lip balms, and petroleum jelly around oxygen equipment. These substances are flammable.

Storage and Handling
- Oxygen should be stored in a well-ventilated area away from direct heat or sun. The corner of a room or other out-of-the-way locations are best to avoid accidental breakage.
- Do not try to repair oxygen equipment or let untrained persons try to fix equipment. Always call your service person when a problem arises.
- Oxygen tanks should be secured by a chain, cord, or stand. Handle small tanks carefully when walking.
- Keep oxygen turned off when not in use.

Traveling with Oxygen
By planning ahead of time, you can have a safe, enjoyable trip. When planning a trip:
- First, see your doctor before traveling.
- Ask your doctor to write clearly or type prescriptions of your medicines in case your medicines are lost or stolen.
- Obtain a written summary of your health history from your doctor in case you get sick and have to see another doctor while you are away.
- A medic-alert bracelet or neck chain may be a good idea.
- Depending on how you plan to travel—car, bus, train, plane, or boat—your oxygen supply company can help.

---

is using a TTO_2 catheter must be motivated and able to take care of the device.

HUMIDITY THERAPY

Humidity therapy involves adding moisture, in the form of water vapor and/or aerosols, to a flow of gas that is being administered to the patient. Humidity therapy also helps liquefy secretions. More often, the devices are used to humidify high-flow oxygen that is delivered to patients with artificial airways such as endotracheal or tracheostomy tubes.

Bubble humidifiers have been used to add humidity to low flow oxygen systems (Figure 26-8). Some institutions use these devices with reservoir and Venturi-type oxygen masks as well.

A cascade-type humidifier is a large-volume, heated canister that is used when high flows of gas are administered to patients. Those devices produce a large quantity of water vapor and small aerosol particles that are not visible to the naked eye (Figure 26-9). Usually these types of humidifiers are connected to mechanical ventilators or positive pressure systems to humidify the oxygen for critically ill patients in the ICU.

Another humidification device available for mechanically ventilated patients is the heat and moisture exchanger (HME), also known as a condenser or an artificial nose. The HME is a small canister containing a piece of foam rubber or paper filter that is inserted into the ventilator tubing circuit. The foam or paper traps the moisture and heat as the patient exhales into the device. When the ventilator delivers the next breath to the patient, it blows the

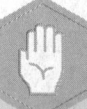

CLINICAL ALERT

There must be no smoking or open flames near a patient receiving oxygen therapy, because oxygen supports combustion. It is important to post caution signs when oxygen is in use.

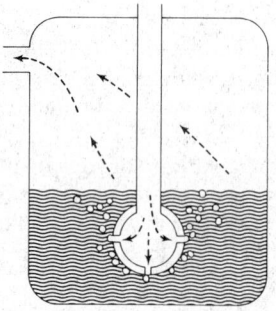

FIGURE 26-8   In a bubble humidifier, gas is directed below the surface of the water and bubbles back to the top. (From McPherson SP: *Respiratory therapy equipment,* ed 3, St Louis, 1985, Mosby–Year Book.)

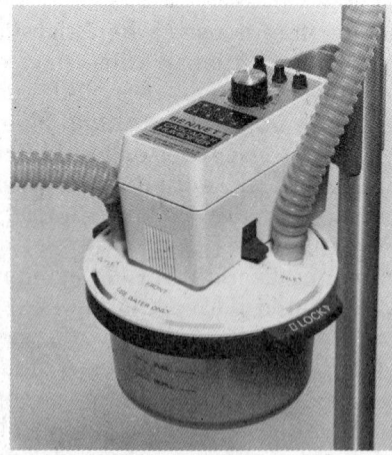

FIGURE 26-9   A cascade humidifier. (From McPherson SP: *Respiratory therapy equipment,* ed 3, St Louis, 1985, Mosby–Year Book.)

moisture and heat back into the patient. These devices eliminate the excess water that often accumulates in the tubing; however, they can become plugged with mucus and can dry secretions in some patients, thus interfering with effective ventilation.

Supplemental humidity can be provided by an aerosol-generating device called a nebulizer. Most nebulizers used in clinical practice are canisters of water that use pressurized oxygen or air to produce the aerosol mist. These nebulizers can be categorized as large- or small-volume types depending upon the size of their liquid reservoirs. Large-volume nebulizers are used to deliver fluids either continuously or for extended periods of time (Figure 26-10). Small-volume nebulizers are used to deliver medications to the airways and lungs (see aerosol therapy). Sterile distilled water is used most of the time as the liquid in large-volume devices. However, half-normal (0.45%) saline may be substituted for water when delivering an aerosol to a patient with reactive airway disease. The devices are usually used when the patient is breathing oxygen or air through a tracheostomy or endotracheal tube without the aid of a positive pressure ventilator. The components of the nebulizers that attach the nebu-

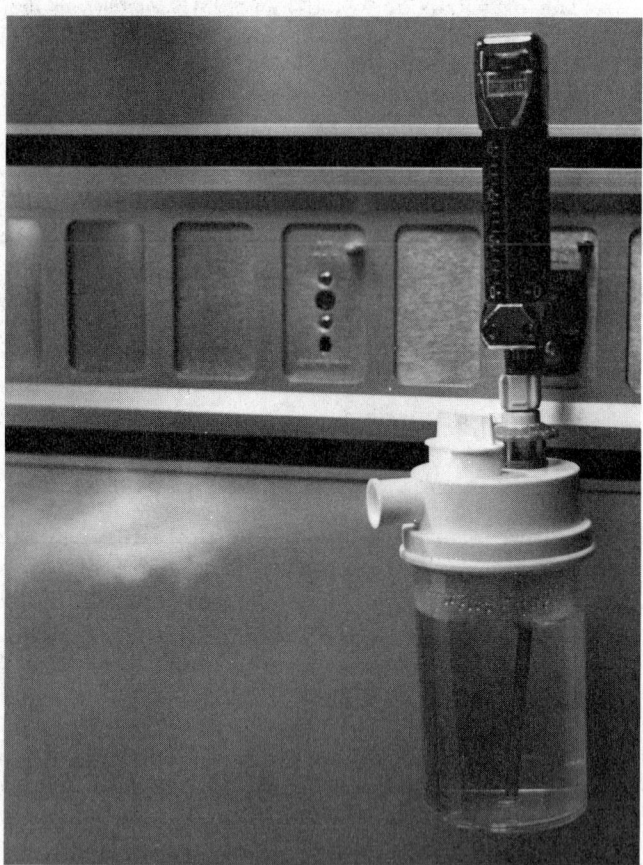

FIGURE 26-10   Large-volume nebulizer.

lizer tubing to the patients are typically referred to as a "Briggs," "t-piece," or "trach-collar" systems. The patient can breathe from a large-volume nebulizer system through an aerosol mask or face tent as well.

All of these systems deliver water to the patient in the form of gas vapor or aerosol. Encouraging the patient to drink water is more economical and may be just as effective as nebulizers or humidifiers in liquifying secretions. The nurse should consult the patient's physician regarding whether there are any fluid restrictions that will limit water intake during the admission and after discharge.

AEROSOL THERAPY
Small-Volume Nebulizers

Drugs can be given as aerosols to be inhaled by the patient into the tracheobronchial tree and possibly into the alveoli (see Table 26-2). There are two types of nebulizers designed for this purpose: small-volume nebulizers (SVNs) and metered-dose inhal-

TABLE 26-2   Pharmacology Summary: Aerosolized Medications

Generic name	Trade name(s)	Solution strength	MDI dose (mg/puff)	Tablet dose (mg/tablet)	Dry powder (mg/capsule)
BETA-AGONISTS:					
Action—relax bronchial smooth muscle. Side effects include tremor, nausea, vomiting, tachycardia, hypotension, decreased serum potassium (hypokalemia), hypoxemia, dysrhythmias, hypoglycemia. Used predominantly to treat patients with mild to severe asthma.					
Terbutaline	Brethine, Bricanyl, Brethaire	1 mg/mL	0.20	2.5 and 5.0	NA
Metaproterenol	Alupent	50 mg/mL	0.65	10.0 and 20.0	NA
Albuterol	Proventil, Ventolin	5 mg/mL	0.09	2.0 and 4.0	0.2
Bitolterol	Tornalate	2 mg/mL	0.37	NA	NA
ANTICHOLINERGICS (VAGAL BLOCKERS):					
Action—prevent bronchospasm and reduce mucus production. Side effects include blurred vision, eye pain, rhinitis, sore throat, cough, wheezing, nausea, gastrointestinal discomfort, reduced urine output, and bradycardia. Used predominantly to treat patients with emphysema, chronic bronchitis, stable asthma.					
Ipratropium Br	Atrovent	NA	0.18		
Glycopyrrolate	Robinul	0.2 mg/mL	N/A		
CORTICOSTEROIDS:					
Action—antiinflammatory, reduces airway swelling. Side effects include adrenal suppression, voice changes, sore throat, oral *Candida* infection (thrush), cough, bone demineralization, cataract formation, increased blood glucose levels, muscle and joint pain. Used to treat patients with stable asthma.					
Dexamethasone	Decadron	NA	0.08	0.25 to 6.0 mg	
Beclomethasone	Beclovent, Vanceril, Beclotide	NA	0.04		
Flunisolide	AeroBid	NA	0.25		
Triamcinolone	Azmacort	NA	0.10	1.0 to 8.0 mg	
MAST CELL STABILIZER:					
Action—reinforce mast cell membrane which diminishes the immune system's response to foreign proteins. Side effects include cough and bronchospasm. Used to treat patients with allergies and asthma.					
Cromolyn Sodium	Intal, Aarane	20 mg	0.80	20.0	
ANTIINFECTIVES:					
Action—treatment of pulmonary infections. Side effects are those associated with the particular antiinfective agents and irritation of the airways as manifested by cough. Ribavirin is used primarily to treat viral infections of the lower respiratory tract and pentamidine is used to treat *Pneumocystis carinii* pneumonia.					
Ribavirin	Virazole	20 g/mL	NA		
Pentamidine	NebuPent	300 mg			

ers (MDIs). Some SVNs are powered by an external gas source such as compressed air or oxygen. Bronchodilators, drugs that increase the diameter of the airways, are the most common type of medication delivered by SVNs. Antibiotics, such as pentamidine (used to treat *Pneumocystis carinii* infections), may also be nebulized by SVNs. Ideally, SVN aerosols are inhaled by the patient through a mouthpiece that is attached to the nebulizer canister. Other devices such as face masks are used with patients who are fatigued, cannot follow instructions, or are unable to use a mouthpiece. Special adaptors are available for patients who have a tracheostomy or endotracheal tube.

An electrically powered "ultrasonic nebulizer" (USN) is another type of aerosol-generating device used in clinical practice. There are large- and small-volume models of USNs. Small-volume USN devices can be used to deliver the same medications as pneumatically powered SVNs. USNs are more expensive and susceptible to breakage than pneumatic nebulizers. They are typically used in the home care setting and to a limited degree in hospital practice.

Patient Care

The purpose of aerosol therapy is discussed with the patient in simple, nontechnical terms before the first treatment session. Patients are encouraged to inhale as slowly as possible through the mouth during treatment. The patient's chest should be auscultated before, during, and after the treatment to assess any changes in breath sounds that occur in response to the treatment. The pulse and respiratory rate before and after the treatment are recorded. The patient is encouraged to cough and produce sputum during and after the therapy. The strength of the cough, quantity, and color of secretions should be recorded also. In addition, when bronchodilators are used, gas flow measurements such as peak expiratory flow rate (PEFR) may be measured before and after the treatment. Most beta-agonist bronchodilators have an onset of action within 5 minutes and reach their peak effect between 30 and 45 minutes after therapy.

If the patient is being monitored by a pulse oximeter, the Spo_2 should be recorded before, during, and after the treatment as well. For those on a cardiac monitor, dysrhythmias that occur during or immediately after the treatment should be promptly reported to a physician. The patient is questioned about any subjective improvements in breathing, clearance of secretions, or adverse side effects such as palpitations, nervousness, and anxiety.

Metered-Dose Inhalers

A **metered-dose inhaler (MDI)** is a pressurized canister which releases an aerosol containing the drug suspended in a fluorocarbon gas stream. It is held between the middle finger and thumb and squeezed by the index finger to eject a single dose of the aerosol. They have been shown to be as effective as SVNs in delivering drugs to patients who properly use the MDI device.[2,3,24,27,40] In addition, MDI therapy is considerably more cost effective, time-saving, and convenient than SVN therapy. Only those patients who are unable to control their breathing pattern, unable to follow instructions, or state a preference for SVN therapy should be given aerosol treatments by that method. In addition, patients with severe respiratory distress are usually treated initially by SVN, or until their respiratory condition stabilizes.

A spacer is a tube, canister, or bag that attaches to the MDI mouthpiece and acts as an artificial extension of the oropharynx. It allows for the evaporation of the propellant gas and removes most of the large aerosol particles that would impact upon the patient's pharynx if the spacer was not in place. However, since many patients have difficulty using the MDI properly, spacers are recommended for all persons treated in the hospital setting. The use of a spacer eliminates some of the problems of coordinating the patient's breathing efforts with hand activation of the MDI. In addition, it helps to promote consistency in the patient teaching and delivery of MDI therapy by a variety of health care practitioners. Spacers are required for inhaled corticosteroid therapy as a means of reducing or eliminating oropharyngeal infections secondary to topical immunosuppression.

Thorough and repeated patient instructions are essential in MDI therapy. Several studies have documented a lack of knowledge about how to use the devices among health care workers[13] as well as inappropriate patient technique associated with MDIs.[13,48,58,59] The nurse has a critical role in either providing or reinforcing instructions given to the patient (see patient education guide). Demonstration and practice with a MDI placebo and leaving written instructions with the patient are optimal teaching methods. In addition, the patient is taught to estimate the amount of remaining medication in the MDI canister by placing it in a pan of water (Figure 26-11). The evaluation of the patient is the same as following a treatment delivered by a SVN.

Evaluation of Aerosol Therapy

The treatment is evaluated against its original purpose. Bronchodilator treatments are usually ordered to alleviate the patient's wheezing or symptoms of respiratory distress. The patient's respiratory distress should be diminished within minutes after the treatment as evidenced by a lower respiratory rate or improved breath sounds. The treatment is considered effective if the patient's condition, symptoms, breath sounds, or flow rates improve. Adverse

PATIENT EDUCATION GUIDE   *Using an MDI*

The nurse provides the patient with the following instructions:
1. Assemble the inhaler.
2. Shake the inhaler to mix the medication and propellant.
3. Remove the cap from the mouthpiece.

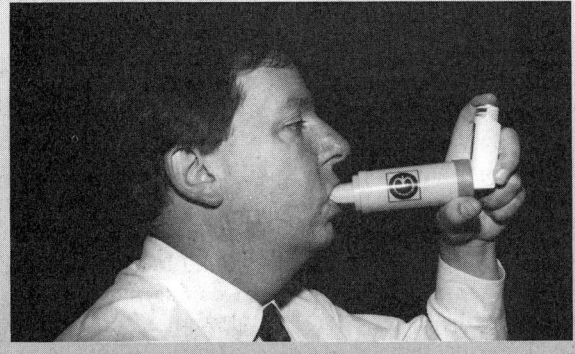

4. Hold both the head and the canister upright with your index finger on top and your thumb on the bottom.
5. Breathe out gently through your mouth.
6. Place the mouthpiece up to your mouth, keeping the mouthpiece about one-half inch away from your face. Keeping your tongue below the opening of the inhaler and your mouth wide open, begin to inhale slowly and deeply and depress the top of the canister with your index finger.
7. Remove the inhaler from your mouth.
8. Hold your breath for a count of 10 or as long as you possibly can.
9. If two puffs are prescribed, wait 3 minutes before taking the second one. This will allow the first puff to dilate the airways so that the second puff will deposit more deeply into the airways.

Have the patient demonstrate the correct procedure for using a MDI placebo.

---

reactions from SVN treatments depend upon the drug being nebulized. The most often reported complaints include tremors, anxiety, insomnia, headache, nausea, cough, and foul taste. Serious side effects are infrequent and minor problems subside usually within 30 to 60 minutes after the treatment. There is no limitation to the frequency of aerosol therapy and beta-agonists have even been nebulized continuously to treat patients with severe asthma.[30]

FIGURE 26-11 Method to determine the amount of medication left in an MDI. An empty canister floats on its side; a full canister sinks to the bottom of a pan of water.

ARTIFICIAL AIRWAYS

Artificial airways are devices designed to maintain patent communication between the tracheobronchial tree and the air supply in the external environment. A variety of devices can be used to maintain airway patency. Some artificial airways only keep the upper airways open. Tracheal patency is maintained by airways placed directly into the trachea (Table 26-3).

Oral Airways

Oral airways are devices that are inserted into the mouth. They are used to prevent occlusion of the airway by the tongue in unconscious patients. The main advantage of the oral airway is ease of insertion; however, it is also easily dislodged. The airway must be the appropriate size for the patient. An airway that is too small will not stay in place. An airway that is too large may depress the glottis, stimulating the "gag" reflex, vomiting, or laryngospasm. An airway that is too long may also force the epiglottis into a position occluding the trachea. An oral airway is the correct size if, when the flange is held parallel to the front teeth with the airway against the patient's cheek, the end of the curve reaches the angle of the jaw. Figure 26-12 illustrates an oral airway in place. Oral airways are not indicated for the conscious patient. They are uncomfortable and are more likely

TABLE 26-3   Artificial Airways

Airway	Indications	Advantages	Disadvantages
Oral airway	Obstruction of the upper airway	Ease of insertion	May stimulate gag reflex Uncomfortable for conscious patients
Nasal airway	Obstruction of nasal passages Protection of nasal mucosa (from trauma caused by multiple insertions of suction catheters)	Ease of insertion Easily tolerated by patients	Does not prevent occlusion of upper airway by the tongue
Endotracheal tube	Temporary measure for airway obstruction Provision of accurate high concentration of oxygen Management of secretions Mechanical ventilation	Direct communication with trachea Relative ease of insertion Oral: larger diameter tube may be used Nasal: easily stabilized; preserves ability to mouth words	Potential for infection Patient inability to speak Potential for laryngeal damage Potential for aspiration Potential for tracheal damage May be uncomfortable for conscious patients Length and inner diameter of tube causes an increase in airway resistance Oral: easily dislodged; may be occluded by biting; difficult to anchor securely Nasal: requires use of narrow diameter; potential for obstruction of sinuses and eustachian tubes
Tracheostomy tube	Long-term measure for airway obstruction Provision of accurate high concentrations of oxygen Management of secretions Mechanical ventilation	Direct communication with trachea Avoidance of trauma to larynx Preservation of protective function of epiglottis Easily tolerated by patients Shorter tube length results in less increased airway resistance than with endotracheal tubes	Surgical procedure with potential for: infection; bleeding Potential tube displacement into subcutaneous tissue Potential for tracheal damage

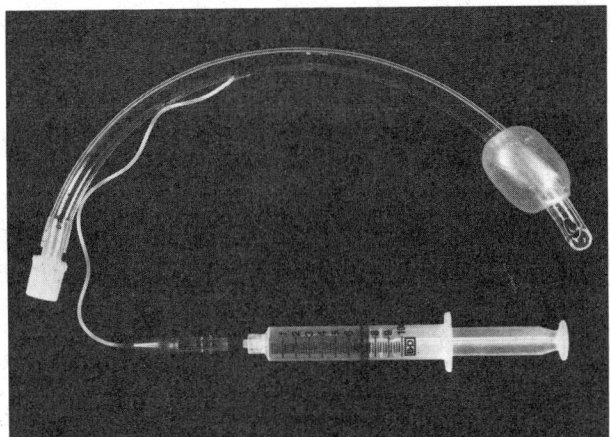

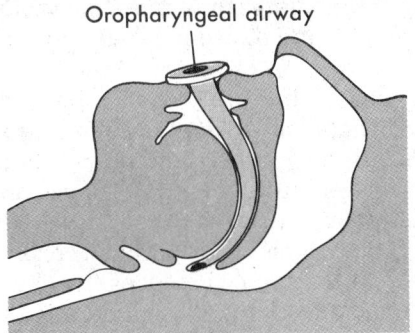

Oropharyngeal airway

FIGURE 26-12   Oral airway in place.

to trigger gagging and vomiting in patients who are awake. Other contraindications to the use of an oral airway include trauma to the lower face and oral surgery.

When the patient has an oral airway in place, mouth care is administered frequently. The goals of mouth care are to increase patient comfort, remove oral debris, maintain sufficient moisture of the oral mucosa, and prevent infection. Although there is much controversy surrounding methods of mouth care, no one method has been proven superior. At present, mouth care using toothpaste and a soft toothbrush is recommended. Any agent that causes drying of the oral mucosa is avoided, because adequate moisture is a major factor in maintaining oral hygiene and comfort and in preventing infection. The patient's tongue, lips, and gums are observed frequently for possible trauma caused by pressure of the airway on these soft tissues. The airway is removed and cleaned every 8 hours. Encrusted secretions are removed by soaking the airway in a solution of equal parts of hydrogen peroxide and normal saline. Despite the ease with which oral airways may be displaced, they should not be taped in place unless absolutely necessary to maintain position. Taping an oral airway in place will decrease the pa-tient's ability to expel vomitus, should vomiting occur.

Nasal Airways

Unlike oral airways, nasal airways are not useful for the prevention of airway occlusion by the tongue. The main indication for the insertion of a nasal airway is to protect the nasal mucosa from the trauma of frequent passage of suction catheters. Nasal airways are useful for airway access in both the conscious and unconscious patient. They are more easily tolerated than oral airways and are not as easily displaced. Nasal airways should always be securely taped to the nose.

Nasal airways should not be used in patients with nasal obstruction or multiple facial fractures. They may also be contraindicated in patients with abnormal coagulation studies. The nasal mucosa has a rich blood supply and bleeds easily and profusely when traumatized. Cannulation of the nares in patients with bleeding disorders should be avoided, if possible. However, if the patient requires frequent nasotracheal suctioning, the one-time insertion of a nasal airway may be indicated to protect the nasal mucosa from multiple passes of suction catheters.

Because the nasal airway may cause some pressure against the nare, the patient must be observed for the development of necrosis in this area. Obstruction of the sinus tracts by a nasal airway may result in sinusitis. Signs and symptoms of this complication, such as temperature elevation and the development of rhinorrhea, should be assessed and reported.

Airway obstructions that occur below the oropharynx or nasopharynx require the use of an airway that terminates in the trachea itself.[7] Airways may be inserted into the trachea by being passed through the epiglottis (endotracheal tubes) or by surgical placement through the neck, directly into the trachea (tracheostomy tubes).

Endotracheal Tubes

Indications for endotracheal intubation are obstruction of the airway at the level of the epiglottis or below, patient inability to clear secretions, delivery of accurate oxygen concentrations, and the institution of mechanical ventilation.[36]

Endotracheal tubes may be inserted orotracheally (via the mouth) or nasotracheally (via the nose). Orotracheal intubation is technically an easier procedure. It allows the use of a larger diameter (i.e., 8 mm ID) endotracheal tube and is therefore the method of choice if measures such as bronchoscopy are anticipated. The larger size of the tube also reduces the work of breathing by decreasing resistance to airflow. However, the presence of the tube in the mouth is uncomfortable for the patient. The tube may also be manipulated by the patient's tongue, resulting in tube movement and possible laryngeal damage. If the patient bites on the tube, airway occlusion may occur.

Nasotracheal intubation is a more difficult procedure than orotracheal intubation, and therefore it is usually not the method of choice in an emergency. When this approach is used, the size of the tube that may be inserted is limited by the diameter of the nares. The required use of a smaller tube increases resistance, thus increasing the work of breathing. The sensation is similar to trying to breathe through a straw. The larger the inner diameter of the tube, the easier it is to move air through it.

Passage of the tube through the nasal passages, with resulting irritation of the nasal mucosa, increases the risk of bleeding. Nasotracheal intubation is therefore discouraged in patients with bleeding disorders. Nasotracheal intubation is more comfortable for the patient, however, and is usually better tolerated than orotracheal intubation. The patient is unable to manipulate the endotracheal tube with the tongue, or to bite down on it, and the nares stabilize the tube at the insertion site. This combination of factors results in less tube movement and possibly less incidence of laryngeal damage.[36,37]

Several types of endotracheal tubes are available. The most commonly used in the acute care setting is the "cuffed" endotracheal tube. Although several cuff designs are available, the most common design has a circular balloon, which forms a symmetric ring around the outside the endotracheal tube, a short distance above the tip.

When the tube is inserted, the cuffed tip is passed through the epiglottis, through the larynx, and into the trachea. Once the tube is in the correct position, the cuff is inflated with air. This causes the cuff to expand and occlude the space between the outside of the endotracheal tube and the tracheal wall (Figure 26-13). With the cuff inflated, a seal is formed and all the air that moves in and out of the patient's lungs must move through the endotracheal tube. The formation of this seal allows complete mechanical control of the patient's ventilation, if necessary. It also allows the delivery of precise concentrations of oxygen to the alveoli by eliminating the possibility of the patient inhaling some room air around the endotracheal tube and diluting the concentration of oxygen delivered.

No matter which route is chosen for endotracheal intubation, the same basic pieces of equipment are needed for the procedure (see box on p. 559).

Before the endotracheal tube is inserted, the cuff should be inflated to verify that there are no leaks in the balloon, which would prevent formation of an adequate seal. In some instances, it may be necessary to briefly anesthetize the patient for the procedure. As soon as the procedure is completed, the cuff is inflated and tube placement is checked by auscultating both sides of the patient's chest while being ventilated with the manual resuscitation bag. Manual ventilation is used to ensure that a sufficient amount of air is moved in and out of the lungs to

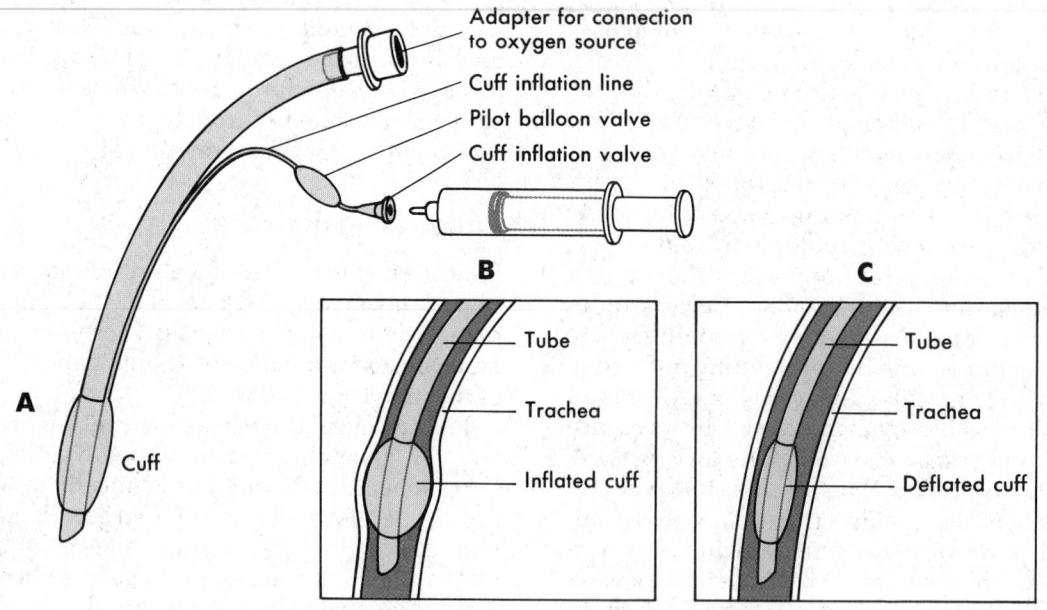

FIGURE 26-13 **A,** Parts of a cuffed endotracheal tube. **B,** Tube in place with the cuff inflated. **C,** Tube in place with the cuff deflated.

ENDOTRACHEAL INTUBATION

Equipment Needed

Sterile endotracheal tube (size specified by physician,
    commonly 7 mm ID, 8 mm ID, or 9 mm ID)
Sterile, water-soluble lubricating gel
10 or 12 mL syringe
Sterile gloves
Oxygen supply with flowmeter and adapter
100% manual resuscitation bag with mask and oxygen
    connecting tubing
Suction bottle with regulator, attached to suction
    source
Sterile suction catheters (usually 14F, although 12F
    may be used)
Tonsil tip suction
Sterile water
Laryngoscope with blade

For nasotracheal intubation

Anesthetic spray/solution (xylocaine spray or gel)
Sterile applicator swabs
Magill forceps

Procedure

Procedure	Rationale
Sedate patient as ordered	Sedation will decrease anxiety and improve patient tolerance of the procedure
Pull bed away from wall and remove headboard	Allows physician easy access to head of bed
Place patient supine or in semi-Fowler's position	
Position head in proper alignment with neck slightly extended	Removes any pillows from behind patient's head
Open endotracheal tube and syringe	
Put on sterile gloves and barriers as required by Infection Control and attach syringe to endotracheal tube cuff valve	Preserve sterility of equipment
Inflate cuff with 10 cc of air	
Leave cuff inflated for several seconds, observing for any leaks or cuff asymmetry	If a leak or asymmetry is observed, discard the tube and use a new one
Aspirate all air from the cuff	
Apply sterile lubricating gel to the tip of the endotracheal tube	
Assist physician with administration of topical anesthetic as needed	Topical anesthetic minimizes pain and gagging
Provide laryngoscope, tube (with syringe), and oral suction to physician as needed	Tonsil tip may be used for oral suctioning; Magill forceps and/or a stylette may also be needed, according to physician's preference
After insertion of tube, assist physician with inflation of cuff and suctioning as needed	
Manually ventilate the patient	
Auscultate for bilateral breath sounds	
Auscultate over abdomen	If the tube is in correct position, breath sounds should be heard bilaterally
Secure endotracheal tube in place noting level of tube at mouth or nose	
Administer oxygen/mechanical ventilation to patient as ordered	
Endotracheal tube placement should be confirmed by chest x-ray films	Endotracheal tube has centimeter markings which should be noted at the gum or lip line; notation should be made in permanent record

Document

Air in cuff (mL)
Level of tube
Breath sounds
Tolerance of procedure

allow easy detection of breath sounds with a stethoscope. If the tube is in the trachea, breath sounds will be heard bilaterally, and the patient will be unable to speak.

Pharmacologic Agents for Intubation

Pharmacologic agents to facilitate intubation are administered only by adequately trained individuals familiar with their actions, hazards, appropriate dosages, and route of administration. These drugs are indicated only if the patient is conscious or semiconscious and are particularly useful when topical anesthesia is ineffective or the patient is agitated or uncooperative or has raised intracranial pressure.[36] Sedative-hypnotic agents reduce patient agitation and anxiety. Benzodiazepine drugs such as diazepam (Valium) and midazolam (Versed) are two agents with excellent amnesic properties. Opioid drugs are useful for their sedative, analgesic, and antitussive effects. Morphine and fentanyl are the most commonly administered. The opiate antagonist (naloxone) should be available whenever an opioid agent is used. Paralytic agents are used if muscle relaxation is required. They are prescribed only if full ventilatory support is immediately available, because they cause paralysis of all striated muscles, including the respiratory muscles, and block protective airway reflexes. Complete sedation is required before these agents are administered.[15] Succinylcholine (Anectine), vecuronium (Norcuron), and pancuronium (Pavulon) are commonly used paralytic agents, but succinylcholine is the most common because of its short duration of action.

Once position is confirmed by physical examination, the endotracheal tube is anchored in place.[36] Placement must be confirmed by chest x-ray films as soon as possible. Correct placement of endotracheal tube tip is 1 to 2 cm above the bifurcation of the trachea (carina).

Tracheostomy Tubes

Tracheostomy tubes are similar in principle and design to endotracheal tubes. The major difference is that tracheostomy tubes are inserted directly into the trachea through an incision in the neck, bypassing the pharynx, epiglottis, and larynx. Use of a tracheostomy tube avoids the risk of damage to these structures. For long-term use, tracheostomy is preferred over endotracheal intubation. Although the structure of the tracheostomy tube most commonly used in the acutely ill patient is similar to the structure of cuffed endotracheal tubes, several other types of tracheostomy tubes are available. If the indication for tracheostomy is airway protection or management of secretions without mechanical ventilation, an uncuffed tracheostomy tube may be used. Tracheostomy tubes may also be of single-lumen or double-lumen design. Although both designs facilitate secretion removal by suctioning, the double-lumen tracheostomy tube allows the removal of the inner cannula for cleaning of encrusted secretions, while the outer cannula preserves the patency of the airway.[51,52] Figure 26-14, A and B, shows two types of tracheostomy tubes.

Complications of Intubation

Complications of intubation can be mechanical and/or physiologic in nature. Mechanical complications include tube displacement, obstruction, and loss of cuff seal. Retained secretions, bacterial colonization, tracheal damage, laryngeal damage, endosinusitis, and aspiration are physiologic complications.[11,21,35,36]

Tube displacement

One of the most common mechanical complications of intubation is tube displacement.[36,60] Although

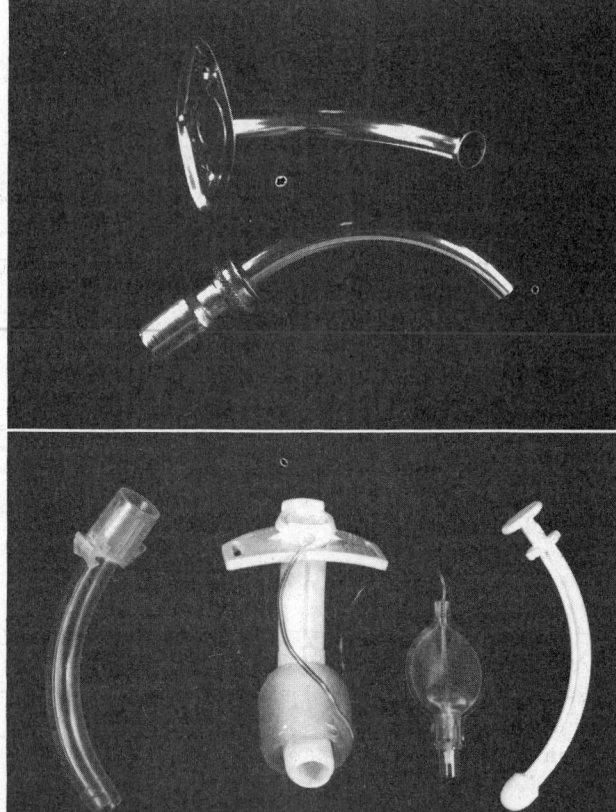

A

B

FIGURE 26-14 **A,** Silver Jackson tracheostomy tube with inner cannula. **B,** Shiley tracheostomy tube, showing the inner cannula and the obturator used for insertion.

proper positioning of the tube is confirmed at the time of intubation, tube placement can change at any time. If the tube is advanced too far, it may terminate in one of the mainstem bronchi. Because the angle of the right mainstem bronchus is less acute than that of the left mainstem bronchus, a tube that has been inserted too far will usually terminate in the right mainstem bronchus. This will result in the movement of air in and out of the right lung, but no air movement in and out of the left lung (Figure 26-15). Breath sounds will be heard over the right side of the patient's chest, but not over the left. In this situation, the physician repositions the tube by pulling it back a few centimeters. Although it can occur at any time, intubation of the right mainstem bronchus usually occurs at the time of tube insertion.

During endotracheal intubation, the tube may inadvertently be advanced into the esophagus, rather than the trachea. This will result in the absence of breath sounds on both sides of the patient's chest. Abdominal distention will occur as air is forced into the stomach, and vomiting may result. An endotracheal tube that has been misplaced into the esophagus must be removed immediately, and intubation of the trachea must be reattempted.[36]

Upward displacement of an endotracheal tube, so that the cuff is at the level of the vocal cords rather than in the trachea, will result in the inability to maintain a cuff seal, despite the addition of large amounts of air. Air will be heard escaping through the patient's nose and mouth. With a large leak, the patient may even be able to speak. Whenever tube displacement is detected, the endotracheal/tracheostomy tube is repositioned or replaced by the physician.

Obstruction

Obstruction of an artificial airway is evidenced by the onset of signs and symptoms of acute respiratory distress: dyspnea, tachypnea, use of accessory muscles of respiration, and cyanosis. Airway obstruction may be caused by kinking of the tube or by the accumulation of secretions, causing a mucous plug. In the case of an oral endotracheal tube, obstruction also may be caused by the patient biting down on the tube. Two less common causes of obstruction are cuff herniation, so that a portion of the inflated cuff occludes the end of the tube, and placement of the bevel of the tube against the tracheal wall. Displacement of a tracheostomy tube out of the trachea and into subcutaneous tissue of the neck is another potential cause of obstruction of tracheostomy tubes.[36]

Regardless of the cause of tube occlusion, the immediate priority is reestablishment of a patent airway. Obstruction of oral endotracheal tubes by biting is usually a transient phenomenon. The nurse explains the purpose of the tube, and if the patient still does not refrain from biting the tube, insertion of a bite block may be required.

For other causes of tube obstruction, the position of the tube and the patient's head and neck are readjusted to bring them into proper alignment and avoid kinking. Ventilation with a manual resuscitation bag is attempted. If the patient cannot be ventilated, the airway is suctioned. If the suction catheter cannot be passed, or if ventilation is still not possible after suctioning, deflate the cuff and reattempt ventilation. Continued inability to ventilate requires immediate removal and replacement of the artificial airway.

Loss of cuff seal

Loss of cuff seal often occurs with the use of endotracheal tubes and, less frequently, with tracheostomy tubes. Loss of seal may be detected by listening for air movement through the nose and mouth, around the tube. If the air leak is large enough, the patient may be able to direct enough air through the vocal cords to speak. Air leaks caused by the loss of cuff seal are often caused by changes in the patient's position or by traction on the tube. Resultant distortion of the cuff makes it asymmetric and unable to completely occlude the space between the outer wall of the tube and the tracheal wall. Displacement of the tube may also result in the inability to achieve an adequate seal. Repositioning of the tube by the physician usually corrects these situations. A hole in the cuff or a crack in the valve on the cuff inflation line will also cause loss of seal. Leaks of this nature

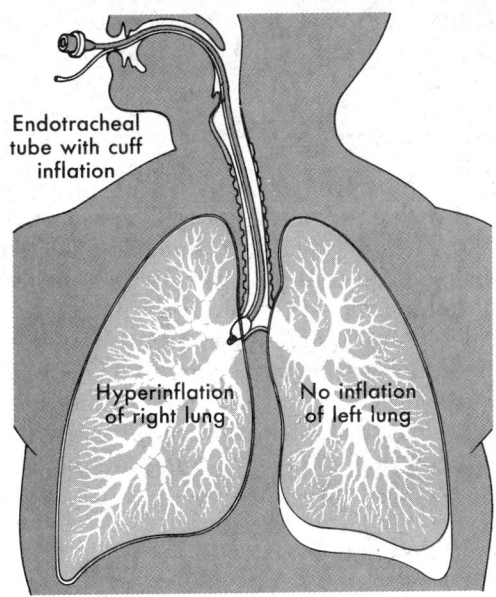

FIGURE 26-15   Migration of an endotracheal tube in the right mainstream bronchus.

Endotracheal tube with cuff inflation

Hyperinflation of right lung

No inflation of left lung

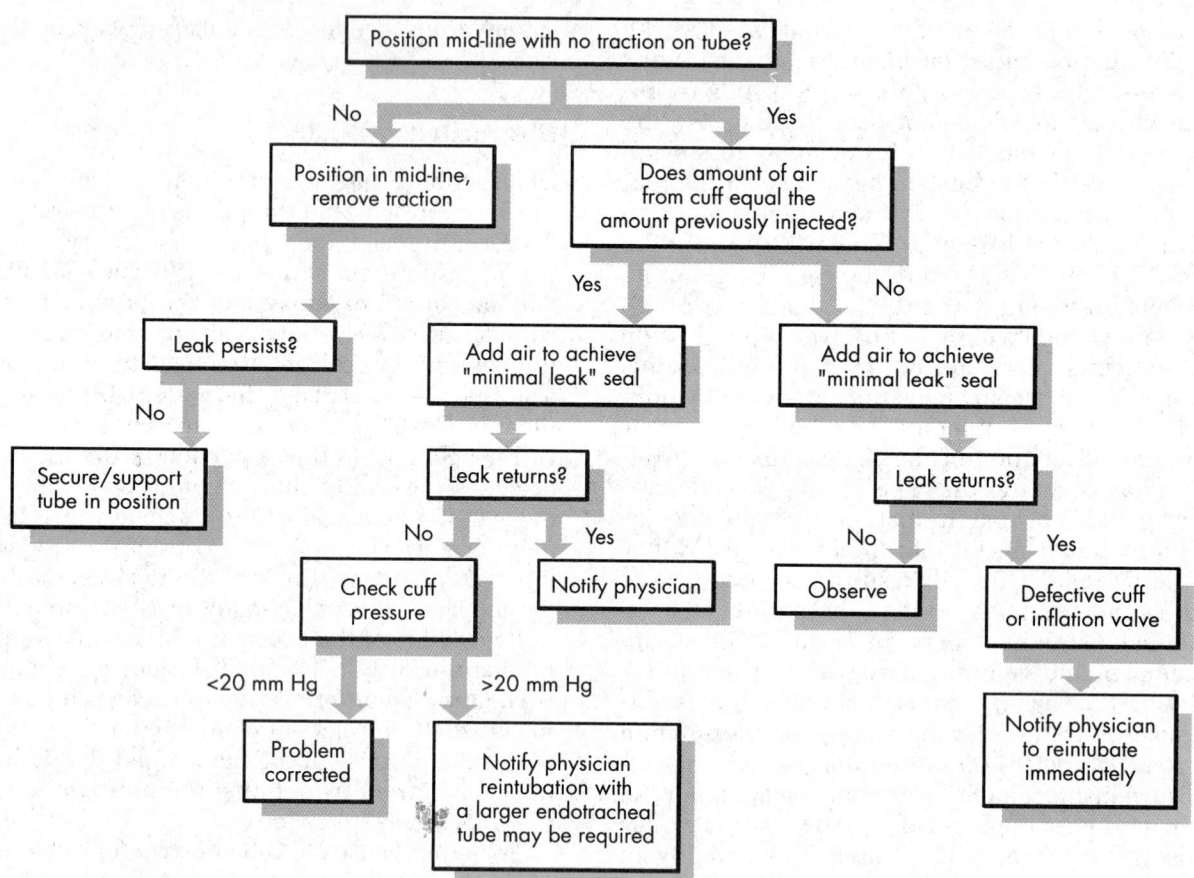

FIGURE 26-16   Critical Thinking Guide: evaluation of cuff leak.

are temporarily corrected by the addition of air to the cuff, but they eventually recur as the cuff continues to lose air. The inability to aspirate an amount of air from the cuff equivalent to the amount injected is a definite indicator of a defect of this type. Whenever cuff leaks are caused by faulty valves, replacement of the tube is advisable. Figure 26-16 shows a critical thinking guide for evaluating loss of cuff seal.

Retained secretions

The presence of an endotracheal or tracheostomy tube within the tracheobronchial tree interferes with the patient's ability to cough and therefore to manage secretions.[35] An effective cough is produced by building up intrathoracic pressure against a closed epiglottis. The epiglottis is suddenly opened, allowing the pressurized air to escape rapidly into the atmosphere, propelling particles and secretions from the trachea. Endotracheal and tracheostomy tubes provide a direct communication between the lungs and the external environment, preventing the accumulation of sufficient intrathoracic pressure to generate an effective cough. For this reason, patients require assistance with secretion removal. The bolus use of normal saline instillations (3 to 5 mL) in the artificial airway as a means of loosening thick secretions during suctioning is of questionable benefit.[43]

Bacterial colonization

Normally, the upper airways warm, filter, and humidify the inspired air. This results in the delivery of sterile, moist air to the tracheobronchial tree, preventing bacterial contamination of the lungs and drying of the mucosa. Air inspired through endotracheal/tracheostomy tubes bypasses the upper airways and these defense mechanisms. Bacterial colonization of the tracheobronchial tree occurs and there is an increased risk of pulmonary infection.[16] Use of sterile technique when suctioning the tube can help minimize risk of infection.

Tracheal damage

Inflation of the tube cuff results in the mechanical displacement of pressure against the tracheal mucosa. Although the mucosa is richly supplied with capillaries, the average pressure in these capillaries is only approximately 25 to 30 mm Hg. If the pressure of the tube cuff is allowed to exceed the pressure in the tracheal capillaries, blood flow will be impeded and tracheal necrosis can occur. Tracheal necrosis may result in scarring and tracheal stenosis after the tube is removed. Occasionally, the resulting stenosis is severe enough to require surgical correction. Erosion of the tracheal wall is also possible, and a tracheoesophageal fistula may result. Patients who have both endotracheal/tracheostomy tubes and nasogastric tubes are at higher risk for this complication, which may require reconstructive surgery of the trachea.

In the past necrosis of the trachea was virtually unavoidable, because the tube cuffs could not achieve a seal at pressures less than tracheal capillary pressure. Modern endotracheal tube cuffs are "high-volume, low-pressure" cuffs. The addition of a relatively large volume of air to the cuff results in only a minor increase in the pressure applied to the trachea. This has resulted in a significant decrease in the incidence of tracheal necrosis. However, if enough air is injected into the cuff, even "high-volume, low-pressure" cuffs can generate cuff pressures higher than tracheal capillary pressure.

Careful monitoring and management of endotracheal/tracheostomy tube cuff pressures minimize the risk of these complications. The smallest amount of air needed to achieve a seal should be used. An adequate seal has been achieved if, during maximal mechanical inspiration (via manual resuscitation bag or ventilator), a slight air leak can be heard with a stethoscope placed over the trachea; this is known as the minimal leak technique. When the minimal leak technique is used, cuff pressures are measured at least daily to ensure that they do not exceed 15 to 20 mm Hg. Cuff pressure of more than 20 mm Hg to achieve minimal leakage may indicate that the tube is too small for the patient. Replacement of the tube with one of larger diameter frequently corrects this problem.

Another technique frequently used for obtaining an adequate tracheal cuff seal is known as the minimal occluding volume technique. This method involves auscultation over the trachea while air is added to the cuff until the leak is obliterated. Cuff pressure is then measured and recorded. Unless a leak is observed or suspected, pressures need not be routinely measured. With either technique, however, the air-filled cuff should be checked when the postoperative patient returns to the critical care unit after general anesthesia, because some inhalation anesthetic gases, including nitrous oxide, diffuse into cuffs, raising cuff pressures to very high levels. In the event of any inadvertent leak, hemostat clamps should *not* be placed on the cuff inflation line.[36]

Endolaryngeal damage

Endotracheal tubes can cause laryngeal damage. Although any patient with an endotracheal tube in place is at risk for this complication, women seem to be predisposed to it. Other factors that increase the risk of laryngeal damage are traumatic intubation, high cuff pressures, tube movement, and prolonged intubation. The precise definition of "prolonged intubation" is controversial; periods as short as 72 hours and as long as 14 days have been proposed. In general, concern regarding potential laryngeal damage usually begins to be raised around 10 days. Prolonged endotracheal intubation is an indication for tracheostomy.[36] Because tracheostomy tubes bypass the larynx, the possibility of laryngeal damage is avoided.

Endosinusitis

Obstruction of the nasal sinuses by the wall of a nasal endotracheal tube may result in the development of sinusitis. Any nasally intubated patient who develops an increase in nasal drainage or a fever of unknown origin should be evaluated for this complication.

Aspiration

Splinting the epiglottis with an endotracheal tube keeps the communication between the oropharynx and the trachea open and makes oral feeding of intubated patients hazardous. Although many particles that pass into the trachea will be trapped above the cuff of the endotracheal tube, a significant amount of food may be aspirated into the lungs. It is critical for the nurse to recognize that even a properly inflated tube cuff does not protect from aspiration of liquids, including enteral formula feedings.[10,11] The placement of the endotracheal tube also interferes with the ability to swallow, especially in the case of oral endotracheal tubes. Therefore, oral feeding of patients with endotracheal tubes is generally not recommended.

Because tracheostomy tubes do not splint the glottis or interfere with swallowing, oral feeding of these patients is possible and encouraged. However, if the patient has been endotracheally intubated before tracheostomy, the function of the glottis and presence of the gag reflex must be evaluated. Prolonged endotracheal intubation may have diminished the gag reflex or resulted in edema of the glottis. Either condition increases the risk of aspiration.

Feeding of these patients always begins with water and the head of the bed is elevated at least 45 degrees. The patient is closely monitored for signs and symptoms of aspiration, such as coughing and gagging. The diet is then advanced as tolerated.

NURSING MANAGEMENT OF THE PATIENT WITH AN ARTIFICIAL AIRWAY
Assessment

Assessment of patients with artificial airways begins with physical assessment of the respiratory system. Special attention is paid to auscultation of the thorax. The presence of bilateral breath sounds indicates that ventilation of both lungs is occurring. Auscultation of crackles (rales) or gurgles (rhonchi) may indicate the presence of secretions in the airways and the need for suctioning. The position and security of the tube are evaluated regularly. For endotracheal tubes, the level of the tube at the nose or mouth is monitored to detect any tube movement as quickly as possible. For tracheostomy tubes, the flange of the tube should be against the patient's neck. The integrity of the ties or tape anchoring the tube is also evaluated.

Frequent assessment of the condition of the skin and mucous membranes around the area of tube insertion will facilitate the detection of any pressure areas caused by the tube and, in the case of tracheostomy tubes, of any signs of infection at the incisional site. Cuff pressure is measured periodically according to hospital or institutional policy and whenever air is added to the cuff. The patient's anxiety and comfort levels are assessed frequently. Anxiety or discomfort will contribute to the work of breathing and to further feelings of dyspnea. Agitated patients, in particular, are at risk for displacement of the tube. The patient may need to be mildly sedated to increase tolerance of the tube.

Nursing Diagnosis

Nursing diagnoses for the intubated patient include the following:

High risk for injury: tube displacement related to patient movement, agitation; tracheal necrosis related to tube cuff pressures, pressure necrosis

High risk for aspiration related to splinting of the glottis, difficulty swallowing, diminished gag reflex and edema of the epiglottis

High risk for infection related to intubation of the tracheobronchial tree incision, retained secretions

Impaired verbal communication related to endotracheal/tracheostomy tube

Altered body image related to endotracheal/tracheostomy tube

Knowledge deficit related to endotracheal/tracheostomy tube

Planning

General goals for the care of patients with endotracheal/tracheostomy tubes are that patients will:

Maintain correct tube placement

Have no tracheal necrosis or pressure necrosis at the tube site

Experience no aspiration

Demonstrate no signs or symptoms of pulmonary infection or local infection at the tracheostomy site

Communicate their needs and desires

Express interest in self-care

Be knowledgeable about the tube, describe appropriate health care measures, and demonstrate tracheostomy care and suctioning

Implementation

Maintenance of proper tube position is one of the primary nursing responsibilities in caring for these patients. The endotracheal/tracheostomy tube must always be anchored securely in place. Tracheostomy tubes may be secured by tying twill tape around the tube and then around the patient's head, or by encircling the endotracheal tube with adhesive tape and applying the end of the tape to the patient's face (see the box on p. 565). If tape is used, the skin beneath the tape should be maintained by some type of protective agent, such as benzoin. There are also numerous anchoring devices commercially available. Regardless of the technique used for securing the endotracheal tube, the level of the tube at the patient's nose or mouth when the tube is appropriately positioned should be noted. All endotracheal tubes have numbered centimeter marks imprinted along the tube. These marks may be used to identify tube position, or a permanent marker may be used to mark the tube at the level of the nose or mouth. Regular monitoring of the mark will allow immediate detection of any tube movement.

For tracheostomy tubes, twill tape is threaded through the holes in the flange of the tube and tied securely around the patient's neck. When the tube is appropriately placed, the flange will lie flat against the patient's neck. The endotracheal/tracheostomy tube should be supported whenever the patient is moved or repositioned. Oxygen or ventilator tubing attached to the tube are positioned in a manner that avoids placing traction on the tube, as well as aspirating water condensate down the tube. The use of swivel adapters may help minimize this problem.

Adequate warming and humidification of inspired air should always be provided for these patients. The respiratory therapy devices discussed elsewhere in this chapter may be adapted easily for use in intubated patients.

Feeding endotracheally intubated patients is best accomplished through the use of a small bore nasointestinal feeding tube.[10] Following feeding tube insertion, correct tube placement should be verified by x-ray examination before any attempt at feeding is started. In addition, the presence of bowel sounds

SECURING AN ENDOTRACHEAL TUBE

Equipment Needed

1- or 1½-inch tape
Scissors
Protective skin barrier (i.e., tincture of benzoin)
Alcohol
4 in. × 4 in. gauze pads
Razor (optional)
Acetone (optional)
Felt-tip marker

Procedure	Rationale
For oral endotracheal tubes, shave patient, if necessary; use benzoin applicator	Promotes adherence of tape
Wet 4 in. × 4 in. gauze pads with one of each of the solutions	
Remove old tape from tube, if necessary	Endotracheal tube must be held in place by an assistant manually until it is secured again
Clean upper lip and cheeks (for oral endotracheal tube) or nose from brow to tip (for nasal endotracheal tube) with alcohol-soaked 4 in. × 4 in. gauze pads	
If necessary, remove old tape with acetone-soaked 4 in. × 4 in. gauze pad	
Using a 4 in. × 4 in. gauze pad, apply protective skin barrier to upper lip and across cheeks, toward angle of jaws	Protective skin barrier should not be sprayed onto patient's face
Allow to air dry	Increases adherence to tape
Cut a strip of 1- to 1½-inch tape long enough to go around the patient's head plus an additional 6 inches	
Cut a second piece of tape long enough to cover the back of the head (approximately 6 inches)	
Lay the long piece of tape with the adhesive side up on a flat surface	
Place the second short piece of tape, sticky side down, on the center of the longer strip	
Position the tape under the patient's head with the double tape portion around the back of the patient's neck	Keeps hair on posterior neck area from sticking to tape and being pulled
Tear or cut a slit, lengthwise, in each end of the tape to the point at which the endotracheal tube meets the mouth or naris	
Turn the tape under ¼-inch on the slit ends	Allows easy access to the ends for tape removal
Secure the tape on one side of the face from ear to corner of mouth (oral) or naris (nasal)	
Pull firmly and hold other side of tape to reduce slack	
Wrap the upper half of the split tape around the tube as close to the mouth or nose as possible	The tape should encircle the tube several times
Secure the lower half piece across the upper lip	Avoid taping directly across the nose since the pulling of tape and tube on this area may lead to skin breakdown
Secure the remaining piece of split tape from the other side of the face in the same fashion	
When the tube position has been verified by x-ray film, mark the point of exit from the mouth or nose with the felt-tipped marker	Facilitates early detection of any endotracheal tube movement

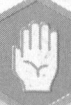

CLINICAL ALERT

In the event of accidental extubation, the patient is immediately assessed for respiratory competence. In the severely compromised patient, inadvertent extubation is a medical emergency. Preservation of the airway and administration of adequate supplemental oxygen are the primary concerns. A manual resuscitation bag and face mask should be kept at the bedside at all times for use if this situation arises. In addition, a tube of the same size or one size smaller than the one currently in place should also be at the bedside to expedite tube replacement. If accidental extubation occurs, the physician is notified immediately to assess the patient and to replace the tube if needed.

and of an adequate cuff seal must be verified before feeding is begun. Elevating the head of the bed to an angle of 45 degrees or more and preventing gastric distention will help minimize the risk of aspiration.[10] Patients with tracheostomy tubes may eat normally, provided they are able to effectively swallow and have an intact gag reflex.

A major factor contributing to anxiety in intubated patients is the inability to speak. Patients and their families require frequent reassurance that the voice loss caused by the tube is only temporary. Effective alternative communication must be provided.[17] Lip reading is an effective alternative for some patients, but some patients are unable to mouth words clearly, and staff inability to understand their requests may increase frustration. Writing with pencil and paper is often an easy, convenient alternative, but it does require a significant energy expenditure that fatigues some patients. Commercially available or homemade word boards that allow the patient to communicate by pointing to letters or words can be employed with great success. Their main disadvantage is that they are slow and tedious to use and require adequate eyesight. Electronic voice simulators and specially designed tubes are also available and may be the method of choice in some cases. A speech pathologist can evaluate for the use of these devices. The patient's abilities and limitations must be considered when selecting communication options, and must be reassessed frequently as the patient's status changes.[17]

Ongoing Care

In addition to the considerations already discussed, patients with a tracheostomy require nursing care specific to the surgical procedure (see box on p.

567). Immediately after a tracheostomy, patients are closely monitored for hemodynamic and respiratory compromise. To minimize bleeding, the tracheostomy tube is not manipulated in any way, including cuff deflation, for the first 24 hours. The tracheostomy site is observed for bleeding and crepitus. Small amounts of each can be expected to occur, but continued bleeding or expansion of the area of crepitus is reported.[51] The dressing at the site is changed as often as necessary, using tracheostomy sponges, which are made with a precut slit for encircling the tracheostomy tube. Regular sponges with a slit cut into them are not recommended, because loose threads of gauze may be aspirated into the tube. The tracheostomy site is cleansed with normal saline whenever the dressing is changed.

Some tracheostomy tubes are constructed with an inner and an outer cannula (a tube inside a tube). The inner cannula can be removed for thorough cleaning while the outer cannula remains in place to protect the patient's airway. When the inner cannula is removed, a special adapter must be used to attach the ventilator to the outer cannula if necessary. The inner cannula may be cleansed by immersion in a solution of equal parts of hydrogen peroxide and sterile normal saline. If necessary, encrusted secretions may be removed from the inner cannula by scrubbing with sterile pipe cleaners or a small brush. The inner cannula is rinsed completely with normal saline before being reinserted into the outer cannula (see the box on p. 569).

Most patients who undergo tracheostomy have already endured prolonged endotracheal intubation. Special attention is given to their ability to communicate and to cope with this long-term intervention. Patients and families require teaching and support if they are expected to care for the tracheostomy themselves. Topics to cover include suctioning technique, care of the stoma, the need for filtering and warming inspired air, and symptoms requiring consultation with health care professionals (see the box on p. 570). The local chapter of the American Lung Association usually has patient teaching materials and support groups available to assist the patient and family in managing care.

MECHANICAL VENTILATION

Patients who lack the ability to sustain spontaneous breathing because of problems with alveolar ventilation, oxygenation, or both, may require some form of mechanical ventilatory support. The decision to use mechanical ventilation is typically made by the physician and based on several factors; i.e., the patient's underlying condition, physical exam findings, and acid-base status including an assessment of oxygenation. It is important to understand, however, that employing artificial or mechanical techniques

NURSING CARE PLAN   *The Patient with a Tracheostomy*

Nursing diagnosis/ *Expected outcome*	Interventions	Rationale
High risk for infection related to contamination of airwaves, and to tracheostomy surgical incision • *Patient will be free from infection as evidenced by:* • *Normal temperature* • *Absence of erythema at incision site, odor, drainage* • *Healing of surgical incision*	Use sterile technique when suctioning Change oxygen tubing/humidifying equipment daily Use sterile water to fill humidifiers Drain any water condensation from oxygen/humidifying tubing, away from the reservoir For double-lumen tracheostomy tubes, inspect inner cannula every shift and clean at least daily and PRN to remove excessive secretions For tracheostomies, cleanse peristomal area gently with normal saline; perform sterile dressing changes when caring for wound; record appearance of wound and drainage; monitor temperature	The skin is a protective environment for many microbes. When there is interruption of skin integrity and moisture is present, the number of bacteria increases. Accumulation of mucus and old blood provides a medium for microorganisms. A clean site and aseptic dressing reduces the possibility of infection.
Altered body image related to presence of tracheostomy tube • *Acceptance of altered body image as evidenced by:* • *Interaction with family and significant others, self-statements indicating beginning acceptance* • *Attention to personal hygiene* • *Expression of feelings about disfigurement*	Help the patient to identify past strengths and coping mechanisms Assess the patient's body image concept and note nonverbal responses to changes that have taken place Provide patient with tissues to absorb oral secretions Provide oral care including mouthwash of half-strength hydrogen peroxide every 8 hours and PRN Allow time for questions, clarification, return demonstration (when applicable), and provide feedback Determine if repetition of information is necessary at a later time	Verbalization of feelings and identification of past coping mechanisms help patient regain self-concept. Attention to personal hygiene may lessen feelings of a poor body image.
Ineffective airway clearance related to decreased effectiveness of cough secretions and edema • *The patient will maintain a patent airway as evidenced by:* • *Absence of gurgles, wheezes, decreased amount of sputum/ secretions* • *Absence of dyspnea or tachypnea* • *Arterial blood gas values within normal range for the patient*	Assess character of respiratory rate and depth Perform oral/pharyngeal suctioning PRN Maintain humidification of inspired air Provide oxygen/mechanical ventilation as ordered Provide chest physical therapy and suctioning as needed	Frequent suctioning is necessary to maintain a patent airway. Edema, resulting from the procedure may compress the trachea. Increased secretions and difficulty swallowing saliva contribute to risk of aspiration. Secretions that accumulate reduce alveolar ventilation and contribute to hypoxemia and increased work of breathing. Chest physical therapy will facilitate mobilization of secretions.

Continued.

NURSING CARE PLAN   *The Patient with a Tracheostomy—cont'd*

Nursing diagnosis/ Expected outcome	Interventions	Rationale
Impaired verbal communication related to presence of artificial airway • *Alternate means of communication* • *Decreased anxiety and frustration*	Explain all alternatives to speech communication Assess patient's ability to perform alternative communication attempts through writing, gesturing, picture books Determine patient's ability to learn esophageal speech Introduce patient to artificial speech aids Consult with family and surgeon about artificial speech aids or surgical prosthetic voice restoration Teach patient, family, or significant other that patience assists in adapting and learning alternative speech communication	

Altered nutrition: less than body requirements related to decreased oral intake, dysphagia, edema
 	
• *Adequate intake of nutrients as evidenced by:*
  • *Maintenance of normal weight*
• *Feeding procedure*
• *Tolerance of tube feedings as evidenced by:*
  • *No gastric distention or nausea*
  • *Absence of diarrhea*
	Administer tube feedings as ordered
	Observe for diarrhea
	Weigh daily
	For patients with tracheostomy tubes:
	  Assess for ability to swallow
	  Auscultate for bowel sounds
	  Keep head of bed at least 30-degree angle or higher
	  If fed in stomach, check for residual and hold feedings according to institutional policy
		Oral feeding with an endotracheal tube in place is not advisable. The endotracheal tube splints the glottis open and increases the risk of aspiration.
		Patients with tracheostomies can be fed orally. However, patients who were endotracheally intubated for a long period before tracheostomy may have a diminished swallowing reflex.

Knowledge deficit related to postoperative care, hospitalization, and routine care of tracheostomy • *The patient will verbalize knowledge of preoperative preparation, intraoperative care, and postoperative care* • *The patient will demonstrate turn, cough, and deep-breathing exercises and state why they are important* • *The patient will verbalize procedure to be performed* • *The patient will demonstrate tracheostomy care*	Explain preoperative preparation: • *Turn, cough, and deep-breathing exercises* • *Preoperative medications* • *Placement of tracheostomy* *Explain/demonstrate tracheostomy care, humidified oxygen to neck, suctioning, inability to speak* *Provide information regarding procedures after surgery (i.e., saline mouth irrigations)*	The need for providing information for the seriously ill patient has been established. Information provides reassurance and decreases anxiety of life-threatening situations. For individuals who have had no experience with previous illness or hospitalizations, lack of knowledge contributes to anxiety, since they have no idea of what to expect from the environment or the persons caring for them.

CLEANING TRACHEOSTOMY TUBE INNER CANNULA

The inner cannula of the tracheostomy tube should be cleaned daily.

Equipment Needed
- Two sterile bowls
- Sterile pipe cleaners
- Sterile gloves
- Sterile 4 in. × 4 in. gauze pads
- Hydrogen peroxide
- Normal saline

For patients on mechanical ventilation:
- Spare inner cannula or special adapter

Procedure

Pour hydrogen peroxide in one sterile bowl, normal saline in the other

Disconnect tracheostomy tube from oxygen source, if present

Hold the tracheostomy tube flange with one hand while unlocking the inner cannula with the other

To remove the inner cannula, pull it out and down simultaneously

Reconnect oxygen source to tracheostomy outer cannula

Rinse the inner cannula with hydrogen peroxide

Brush encrusted secretions off the inner cannula with sterile pipe cleaners

Rinse the inner cannula with normal saline

With a sterile 4 in. × 4 in. gauze pad, wipe all excess moisture from the inner cannula

Disconnect the oxygen source from the outer cannula

Insert the inner cannula back into the tracheostomy tube

Lock the inner cannula in place

Reconnect to oxygen source as indicated

Rationale

The lock must be completely open to allow easy removal of the inner cannula

For patients on mechanical ventilation, a special adapter or a spare inner cannula is required to attach the ventilator to the outer cannula

Hydrogen peroxide will loosen encrusted secretions

Several pipe cleaners may be twisted together to form a scrub brush

All hydrogen peroxide must be rinsed from the inner cannula

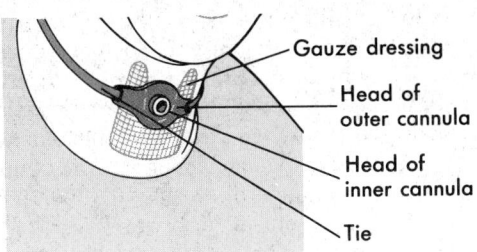

which assist ventilation are only supportive, never curative. Mechanical ventilation is usually provided using either negative pressure or positive pressure devices. Although both methods are described, the vast majority of mechanical ventilators used today deliver positive pressure to the airway.

Negative Pressure Ventilation

Negative pressure ventilation is the type of ventilation that occurs naturally. In the spontaneously breathing patient, contraction of the diaphragm and intercostal muscles increases the volume of the thoracic cage and the lungs. This creates negative pressure within the lungs with respect to atmospheric pressure. The negative pressure pulls air into the lungs. It is the generation of this negative pressure that is the driving force for inspiration. Expiration occurs passively because of the elastic recoil of the lungs and thorax when the inspiratory muscles relax.

Negative pressure ventilators mimic this sequence of events. Although they vary in design, negative pressure ventilators are applied to the pa-

 **PATIENT EDUCATION GUIDE** *Tracheostomy*

The nurse should provide the patient with the following instructions:

1. Bacteria can easily enter the tracheostomy. To avoid infection, always wash your hands before touching your tracheostomy.
2. Observe the stoma daily for any signs of redness, swelling, or drainage.
3. Clean the stoma twice a day using a clean, damp face cloth; do not use soap.
4. A thin coat of petrolatum may be applied to the skin around the stoma; be careful not to let any enter the stoma.
5. Avoid dust, smoke, aerosol sprays, perfumes, car exhaust, powder, and raking leaves. Particles from any of these may enter directly into your tracheostomy. If you must be exposed to any of these agents, cover your tracheostomy with a piece of cotton cloth.
6. Vacuum instead of sweeping. Dust and mop with damp cloths or mops rather than dry ones.
7. Wear a stoma covering to warm and filter the inspired air, especially in cold weather. A variety of clothing and accessories can be worn by men and women over the stoma covering. High-neck sweaters, turtlenecks, and scarves work well. They should fit loosely around the neck, so that there is always easy access to the stoma and so that breathing is not obstructed.
8. Cover your tracheostomy, not your nose and mouth, when coughing or sneezing.
9. Do not use tissues or cotton tip applicators near the stoma, because pieces of these materials may break off and enter the tracheostomy. Use a handkerchief when coughing.
10. Additional humidification of the air, especially during the winter when rooms are heated, will help keep secretions moist enough to be removed by coughing. Commercially available vaporizers or humidifiers may be used. The water (H_2O) in the vaporizer should be changed daily, and the vaporizer cleaned with soapy H_2O at least twice a week. Alternatively, a pan of water can be kept on the stove or radiator. The H_2O should be changed daily. Moist gauze may be used for a stoma cover, rather than the piece of cotton cloth.

11. When taking a bath or shower, stand on a non-slip bath mat, because a fall could cause water to be splashed into your tracheostomy; showers are preferred.
12. When showering, adjust the shower head so that the water is directed to a level on your body below your tracheostomy. A well-wrung towel can be draped around the neck, over the tracheostomy for further protection.
13. Be sure to cover your tracheostomy with your hand or with a commercially available shower guard while rinsing your head.
14. While shaving or having a haircut, wear a protective covering and a towel over the stoma to prevent dust and hair particles from entering.
15. Avoid wearing clothing with small ornaments, such as sequins or small buttons, near the neckline. Women should avoid wearing necklaces with small individual parts (i.e., pearls)
16. Clean mouth and teeth at least three times a day. Use mouthwash often, because the ability to detect mouth odor is lessened.
17. Purchase and wear a medic alert tag indicating that you have a tracheostomy and with instructions should the tracheostomy become obstructed or in the event of a cardiopulmonary arrest.
18. No change in sleep habits is required. You will be able to breathe easily, even with blankets covering your tracheostomy.
19. If your tracheostomy tube has an inner cannula, clean it daily and PRN with a solution of equal parts of hydrogen peroxide and water. Rinse the cannula thoroughly under running water before reinserting it.
20. Change the twill tape holding your tracheostomy in place when needed. Secure the new tape in place before removing the old tape.
21. Suction the tracheostomy using clean technique as needed.

tient's chest wall. The ventilator creates a vacuum, which pulls the chest wall out, expanding its volume and that of the lungs. This creates negative pressure within the lungs, and inspiration of air results. Although negative pressure ventilators fell into disuse with the development of the newer positive pressure ventilators, they are currently regaining popularity in select cases.[9]

Negative pressure ventilators currently in use include the "iron lung," the chest cuirass, the pneumobelt, and the pneumowrap. The "iron lung," one of the earliest negative pressure ventilators, was first used clinically in 1928 at the Children's Hospital in Boston, Massachusetts. The "iron lung" is a metallic cylinder that encases the patient's entire body from the neck down. Negative pressure is provided by the mechanical movement of a diaphragm at the patient's feet. A portable model of the "iron lung" is also available. The cuirass is a negative pressure ventilator that resembles a turtle shell. It is applied to the patient's chest and abdomen. Negative pressure is created by a motor that is attached to the shell by a hose (Figure 26-17). The pneumobelt consists of an inflatable rubber diaphragm that is held in place over the patient's abdomen with straps. When the bladder is inflated with air, it compresses the abdominal contents, pushing the diaphragm up. When the bladder deflates, the abdominal contents return to their normal position and the diaphragm moves down. This downward movement of the diaphragm results in the creation of negative pressure within the thorax, and inspiration. The pneumobelt is less effective than the other ventilators and is unsuitable for obese or very thin individuals. The pneumowrap consists of a poncho that fits over the upper body. This poncho is attached to a motor, which creates a vacuum within the wrap and expands the thoracic cage.

Proper functioning of negative pressure ventilators is evidenced by the patient's inability to speak during the inspiratory portion of the ventilator cycle. Phonation requires exhalation of air through the vocal cords. If the ventilator is truly controlling the patient's respiratory cycle, he or she will be unable to exhale any air during the ventilator's inspiratory phase. Negative pressure ventilation is particularly useful in patients with inadequate ventilation related to neuromuscular weakness or abnormalities of CNS control of respiration. They are well adapted to use by those patients who require ventilator support only while sleeping.

There are two major advantages of negative pressure mechanical ventilation. First, it is the physiologic equivalent of normal respiration and preserves normal intrathoracic pressure changes. Normally, during inspiration the heart and great vessels are also exposed to the negative pressure caused by the contraction of the muscles of respiration. This results in an increase in venous return during inspiration, as the blood flows from areas of higher pressure in the periphery to areas of lower pressure in the heart and great vessels. This increase in venous return contributes to the maintenance of an adequate cardiac output. Negative pressure mechanical ventilation preserves this "bellows" effect on cardiac output. The second major advantage of negative pressure mechanical ventilation is that implementation of the technique does not require intubation of the patient. Therefore, all the potential adverse effects of endotracheal intubation are avoided.

A major limitation of this technique of ventilation is the inability to deliver high concentrations of oxygen to the patient. During negative pressure ventilation, oxygen is delivered by the same methods used for spontaneously breathing patients (i.e., face masks, nasal prongs). For those patients who require high percentages of oxygen to maintain adequate oxygenation, the technique is inadequate.

Use of negative pressure ventilators requires that the patient's thorax be encased in the ventilator

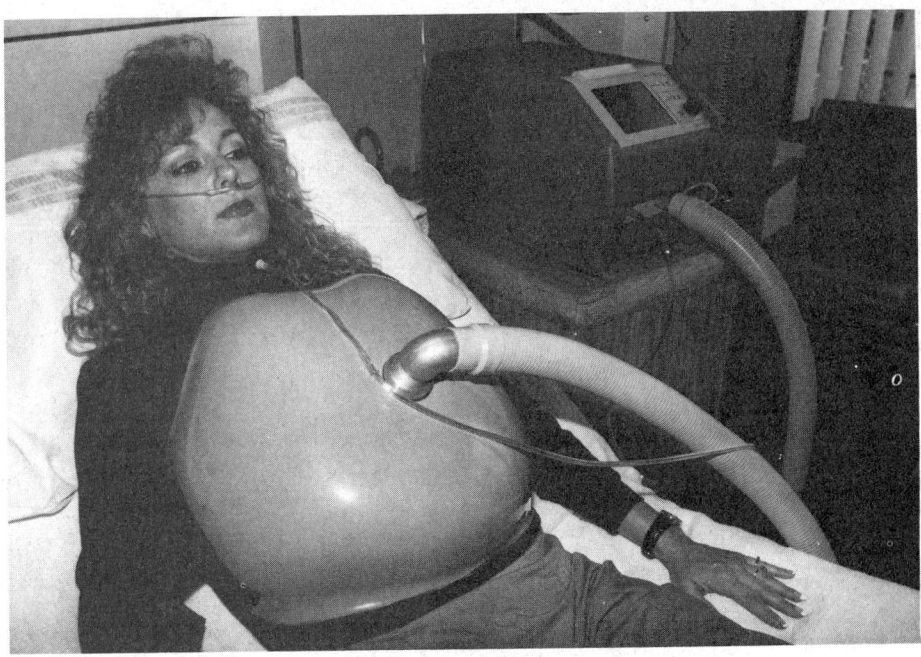

FIGURE 26-17   Chest cuirass.

shell. A tight seal at all points where the patient's body exits the device is necessary to ensure no loss of vacuum. The need to achieve an adequate seal results in some patient discomfort and the potential for decubitus ulcer formation in those areas. The imposed immobility, especially with the use of the "iron lung," places the patient at risk for the complications associated with immobility and may cause some musculoskeletal pain.

Because the ventilator and not the patient regulates the timing of inspiration, the ability to communicate is somewhat compromised. The obvious loss of the ability to phonate may cause some psychologic distress.

Another limitation of negative pressure mechanical ventilators is that precise control of the amount of air moved in and out of the lungs with each breath is not possible. Any changes in the tightness of the seal or in the compliance of the patient's thorax will result in changes in the amount of air delivered. Therefore, this type of ventilatory support is typically used in patients with normal lungs, not those with known chronic obstructive lung disease or obstructive sleep apnea.

Positive Pressure Ventilation

Positive pressure ventilation is the physiologic opposite of negative pressure ventilation. Positive pressure ventilators force air into the lungs. To ensure delivery of air to the lungs, intubation of the patient's airway is usually required. Positive pressure ventilation is typically classified by the method that terminates inspiration. The two most common methods are pressure-limited ventilators and volume-limited ventilation.

Pressure-limited ventilators force air into the lungs until a preset pressure is reached. When that pressure is achieved, the ventilator terminates the inspiratory phase, regardless of how much air has been delivered to the patient. Any increase in airway resistance or decrease in thoracic compliance will decrease the tidal volume delivered by a pressure-cycled ventilator. Changes in airway resistance may be caused by bronchospasm or accumulation of secretions. Decreased compliance may be caused by interstitial edema, atelectasis, or pneumothorax.[49,50]

Volume-limited ventilators (Figure 26-18) force air into the lungs until a preset volume of air has been delivered. The preset tidal volume or minute ventilation is constant in spite of changes in airway resistance or compliance. Increased airway resistance or decreased compliance will, however, increase the pressure required to deliver the tidal volume. To avoid the delivery of extreme pressures to the lungs and problems arising from this, a maximum inspiratory pressure limit is set. The pressure

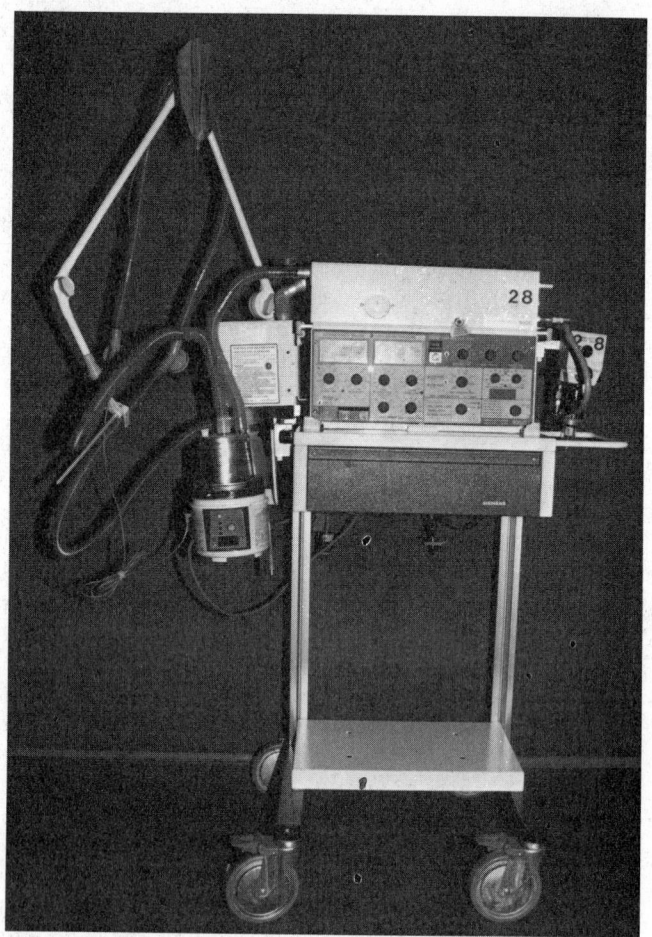

FIGURE 26-18   Volume-limited ventilators.

limit is usually set 10 to 15 cm H_2O above the patient's peak inspiratory pressure. If the pressure limit is reached before the tidal volume has been completely delivered, the ventilator will terminate the inspiratory phase and activate a high-pressure alarm which is usually both visual and audible. Because volume-limited ventilators control the patient's tidal volume more precisely, they are preferred for continuous mechanical ventilation.

Conventional Modes of Ventilation

In the controlled mandatory ventilation (CMV) mode, the ventilator delivers only the number of breaths per minute and the tidal volume for which it has been set. The ventilator will not respond to any spontaneous breathing attempts. Because of the inability for the patient to trigger a machine-generated breath, this mode is rarely used today.

In the assist/control (A/C) mode, the ventilator will respond to the patient's attempts at spontaneous breathing. Although the patient cannot breathe at a rate less than the preset ventilator rate, attempts to breathe faster than the preset rate will result in the ventilator sensing the patient's inspiratory effort and then delivering a preset tidal volume. Thus the patient can increase the number of breaths per minute above the preset rate. However, the volume delivered by either machine- or patient-initiated breaths will be constant.

In the intermittent mandatory ventilation (IMV) mode, the ventilator delivers a preset tidal volume at a predetermined rate. However, in-between the mandatory breaths, the patient is allowed to breathe spontaneously and generate his or her own tidal volume. Therefore the patient's spontaneous tidal volume is determined by the strength and duration of inspiratory effort. The gas source provided to the patient from the ventilator during a spontaneous breath is delivered via either a continuous gas flow through the ventilator circuit or from a demand valve inside the ventilator that responds to spontaneous inspiratory efforts.

The synchronized intermittent mandatory ventilation (SIMV) mode is a further refinement of the IMV mode. All of the previously discussed characteristics of the IMV mode are true of the SIMV mode. In the SIMV mode, however, the ventilator will attempt to sense the patient's inspiratory efforts and synchronize the delivery of the preset breaths during those efforts. The synchronization of the ventilator breaths with the patient's respiratory efforts prevents the ventilator from delivering a breath while the patient is attempting to exhale. Although SIMV would appear to be more beneficial to the patient then IMV, comparisons of the two modes have not indicated its superiority.[39]

It should be noted that there are no studies to date that conclusively demonstrate any one mode of ventilation to be superior over another. Rather, appropriately applied, A/C and IMV are of equal value as ventilatory techniques.

Other Modes of Ventilation

In those circumstances where conventional modes of ventilation fail to achieve adequate alveolar ventilation and oxygenation, alternate techniques may be recommended. The following represent brief operational definitions of less commonly used techniques for assisting ventilation.[32,33]

High-frequency ventilation (HFV) is a form of positive pressure ventilation in which ventilation is provided at very rapid respiratory rates using small tidal volumes. The rate setting in high-frequency ventilation may vary from 60 to 2400 breaths/min. The pressure required to deliver the small tidal volumes of high-frequency ventilation is usually less than the pressure required to deliver traditional tidal volumes. Therefore this technique is usually employed when high positive airway pressures ag-

gravate lung injury. Several methods of HFV are currently in use.

High-frequency positive pressure ventilation (HFPPV) delivers small tidal volumes, using a constant volume positive pressure ventilator. Rate can be varied from 60 to 100 breaths/min.

High-frequency jet ventilation (HFJV) delivers "jets" of air into the patient's airway through a narrow catheter at rates of 100 to 900 breaths/min.

High-frequency oscillation (HFO) delivers air to the patient in waves. The oscillations occur at rates up to 2400/min. This technique differs from other ventilator techniques in that it does not deliver a specified volume of air to the patient at a specified interval. Instead, the oscillations promote the movement of gases in the tracheobronchial tree and thereby enhance diffusion. In addition, oscillators assist the patient to exhale as well as provide inspiratory support.

None of the high-frequency ventilation techniques described are widely used at the present time. To date, no studies have demonstrated high frequency ventilation to be superior to conventional modes of ventilation for most critically ill patients.

Inverse ratio ventilation (IRV) is a ventilatory technique whereby the inspiratory to expiratory ratio (I:E) is reversed from the normal I:E of 1:2 or longer. An I:E ratio of 2:1 is typically used. However, I:E ratios of up to 4:1 have been applied to critically ill patients. Machine breaths are delivered using either a preset pressure, inspiratory time, or tidal volume. IRV is usually recommended as a method of improving oxygenation in select cases when conventional techniques fail. The longer inspiratory time used is thought to be beneficial by recruiting previously closed alveoli while the short expiratory time is thought to prevent alveolar recollapse. This method can be very uncomfortable for patients. Therefore sedation and pharmacologic paralysis are often used while the patient is receiving IRV. The use of IRV remains controversial at the time of this writing and should be utilized only by those clinicians familiar with the ventilator machine settings and potential adverse effects.[32,33]

Adjunctive Measures

In addition to the various modes of ventilation, ventilators are also capable of providing several options to assist with mechanical ventilatory support. These support techniques do not control ventilation, but are used to augment spontaneous breaths and/or improve patient oxygenation.

Positive end-expiratory pressure (PEEP) is positive pressure applied to the tracheobronchial tree at the end of expiration. PEEP increases the resistance to expiration and thereby increases the amount of air remaining in the lungs during the expiratory phase. The increase in functional residual capacity (FRC) prevents the collapse of alveoli that may occur during unopposed expiration, and may help to keep them open for gas exchange. The end result is an elevation of the Pao_2 at the same inspired oxygen level (FIo_2). PEEP is often used in the attempt to decrease the FIo_2 required for adequate oxygenation. It is believed that, in the spontaneously breathing patient, the epiglottis provides 5 cm PEEP normally. Therefore, in many institutions, 5 cm H_2O PEEP (physiologic PEEP) is routinely used.

Continuous positive airway pressure (CPAP) is based on the same physiologic principles as PEEP. Positive pressure is applied to the tracheobronchial tree throughout the respiratory cycle, resulting in increased FRC and improved oxygenation. CPAP is used on the spontaneously breathing patient. CPAP can also be applied on nonintubated patients via either a facemask or a nasal mask. A recently introduced variation of nasal CPAP device is the incorporation of inspiratory pressure support in addition to the end-expiratory pressure feature.[9] This device is referred to as BiPAP (Respironics Inc., Murrysville, Pennsylvania).

Pressure support ventilation (PSV) is defined as a ventilator setting that augments a patient's inspiratory effort as a result of a clinician-selected positive airway pressure.[33] The pressure support level is constant and its duration controlled by the patient's inspiratory effort. Thus tidal volume is not constant and depends predominantly on strength of effort and the level of PSV used. Second, PSV can be clinically used in two ways. First is in conjunction with IMV. The PSV level used is 5 to 10 cm H_2O and is mainly beneficial in overcoming the resistance of the artificial airway and demand valve of the ventilator. Second, PSV can be used as a stand-alone ventilatory mode. PS levels are adjusted to achieve a tidal volume of 10 to 12 mL/kg body weight.

Complications of Ventilation

The requirement for endotracheal intubation exposes the patient to all the risks and potential complications of intubation. Positive pressure ventilation may increase ventilation/perfusion mismatching in the lungs. Gravitational forces can cause uneven distribution of blood flow in the lungs, which results in dependent (lower) lung areas receiving more perfusion than do alveoli in the upper lung fields. Alveoli in dependent lung areas are smaller in the expiratory phase than alveoli located superiorly. Because these alveoli are smaller, they are able to expand more during negative pressure inspiration, and therefore receive more ventilation as well as more blood flow. In the spontaneously breathing patient, these two phenomena result in an optimal matching of ventilation and perfusion. Alveoli located superi-

orly are ventilated less and perfused less than dependent alveoli.

Although the distribution of perfusion is unchanged by positive pressure mechanical ventilation, the distribution of ventilation is altered. Alveoli located superiorly offer less resistance to inflation by positive pressure. Therefore during positive pressure ventilation, alveoli located in the upper lung fields are ventilated more and perfused less, while dependent alveoli are ventilated less and perfused more. The resultant ventilation/perfusion mismatch may exacerbate hypoxemia.

During the inspiratory phase of the mechanical ventilatory cycle, positive pressure is generated in the thorax. The heart and great vessels are exposed to this positive pressure. Blood in the periphery may be unable to enter the heart and great vessels against the high pressure created. This results in a decrease in venous return, during the inspiratory phase. The decrease venous return may cause a decrease in cardiac output. Although many patients are able to compensate adequately for the decrease in cardiac output, some patients will demonstrate signs and symptoms of hemodynamic compromise (i.e., hypotension, tachycardia). The addition of PEEP to the ventilator settings will increase the risk of this complication, especially at PEEP levels of 10 cm H_2O and above.

The decrease in cardiac output caused by positive pressure ventilation causes the baroreceptors in the carotids and the aortic arch to sense low pressure. They trigger reflex responses such as tachycardia, vasoconstriction, and fluid retention. The fluid retention can become a significant problem in any patient who has underlying cardiac disease.

The pulmonary tree is accustomed to low pressures throughout the respiratory cycle. Delivery of high pressures to the lungs may result in rupture of any weakened areas of the lung tissue (i.e., blebs). Even normal lung tissue will rupture if it is exposed to sufficiently high pressures. Rupture of lung tissue results in the escape of air into the pleural space, subcutaneous tissue, or mediastinum. This phenomenon is known as barotrauma and is more likely to occur when ventilator peak inspiratory pressures or PEEP levels are high.[14] With each inspiratory cycle, the ventilator will continue to force more air into the patient's lungs and through the rupture.

Accumulation of air in the pleural space results in the formation of a pneumothorax. Because the ventilator will continue to force air into the pleural space, during each breath, and there is no avenue for its escape, high pressures will be generated in the pleural space. These high pressures will collapse the lung on the affected side (tension pneumothorax). They will also cause compression of the heart and great vessels, severely compromising venous return and reducing cardiac output. Compression of the heart and great vessels and decreased cardiac output may also result from the accumulation of air in the mediastinum (pneumomediastinum). Tension pneumothorax and pneumomediastinum are medical emergencies, requiring immediate insertion of a chest tube or mediastinal tube to evacuate the air from the involved spaces.

Dissection of air into the subcutaneous tissue results in subcutaneous emphysema. Swelling of the soft tissues and palpation of crepitations over the affected areas are indicative of this complication. Although subcutaneous emphysema may cause some patient discomfort and psychologic distress because of the disfigurement, it requires no treatment. The air will eventually be reabsorbed and the tissues will return to normal. However, because subcutaneous emphysema is indicative of an air leak, the patient is closely monitored for the development of signs and symptoms of pneumothorax or pneumomediastinum.

Occasionally, patients have difficulty breathing in synchrony with the ventilator. If the patient is attempting to exhale when the ventilator is attempting to deliver a mechanical inspiration, high inspiratory pressures will result. Continual patient breathing against the ventilator cycle is termed breathing "out of phase" or "bucking" the ventilator, which has serious physiologic consequences. First, the ventilator will be unable to deliver the preset tidal volume. Second, breathing out of phase increases the work of breathing. Finally, the resultant increased intrathoracic pressure predisposes the patient to develop barotrauma and decreases venous return and cardiac output.

One method for eliminating "bucking" or fighting the ventilator is to remove the patient from the ventilator and provide manual ventilation. If this intervention is unsuccessful, sedation may be required. In extreme cases, temporary muscle paralysis achieved by the administration of neuromuscular blocking agents may be necessary.

When a patient is receiving neuromuscular blocking agents to allow effective ventilation, special attention must be given to the psychologic implications of administrating these drugs.[15] Although the patient will be unable to move for the duration of the drug's effect, his or her level of consciousness will not be altered in any way. The ability to hear and process information will remain intact. Therefore the patient should always be included in conversations that take place within earshot. In addition, the experience of being completely paralyzed may be terrifying, despite the reassurances of health care workers that the effects are only temporary. Simultaneous administration of a sedative will help decrease the patient's anxiety. The patient's family may also require frequent reassurance that the paralysis is drug in-

duced and temporary. Special attention to skin integrity and secretion removal must be incorporated into the plan of care.

The ability to administer high oxygen concentrations (>50%) to mechanically ventilated patients is not without inherent risks. The administration of 100% oxygen places the patient at risk for the development of absorption atelectasis. Normally, the alveoli contain oxygen, carbon dioxide, and nitrogen. In the event that all the oxygen and carbon dioxide are absorbed across the alveolar membrane, the remaining nitrogen, which is not absorbable, prevents collapse of the alveolus. When 100% oxygen is administered, no nitrogen is present in the alveoli. Therefore if total absorption of the oxygen and carbon dioxide occurs, the alveoli collapse. If possible, the administration of 100% oxygen for prolonged periods (>24 to 48 hours) should be avoided.

The administration of oxygen concentrations greater than 50% places the patient at risk for the development of oxygen toxicity. Prolonged exposure of the lung tissue to high oxygen levels causes degenerative changes, which in turn decrease the ability of gas (oxygen and carbon dioxide) to diffuse across the alveolar membrane. The goal of oxygen supplementation via mechanical ventilation is to achieve adequate arterial oxygenation at oxygen concentrations less than 50%. PEEP or CPAP is frequently used to decrease the FIO_2 required for adequate oxygenation, and thereby reduce the risk of oxygen toxicity.

Patients who are receiving mechanical ventilation are particularly susceptible to both sensory deprivation and sensory overload. The relative immobility, communication difficulties, and impairment of taste and smell caused by intubation and mechanical ventilation contribute to sensory deprivation. The constant noise from the ventilator and the frequent sounding of ventilator alarms contribute to sensory overload.

The actual physical attachment to the ventilator frequently results in emotional attachment. Patients may demonstrate concern and hypervigilance whenever any ventilator adjustments or manipulations are carried out. The perception that health care workers are more concerned with the machinery than with the patient may lead to feelings of isolation and dehumanization. Fear, anxiety, and sleep deprivation frequently contribute to patients' psychologic reaction to mechanical ventilation. Explanations of all manipulations and procedures, and attention to the patient as an individual will help minimize these problems.[49,50]

Finally the combined physical and psychologic stressors induced by the acute illness and by mechanical ventilation itself may contribute to the development of stress ulcers.

NURSING MANAGEMENT OF THE PATIENT USING MECHANICAL VENTILATION

Assessment

Successful management of the patient on mechanical ventilation requires continuous, careful evaluation of the patient's status.[49,50] Blood pressure, pulse, and respirations are monitored at least every 4 hours, or more frequently as the patient's status changes. Assessment of the respiratory pattern is made whenever the nurse has contact with the patient. Use of the accessory muscles of respiration is an indication of respiratory distress and is reported immediately. Paradoxical respirations (inward movement of the abdomen during inspiration) are inefficient and an indication that the patient is tiring and should also be reported immediately.

All ventilator settings (FIO_2, tidal volume rate, and PEEP) are verified at least every 2 hours and whenever any changes are made (see box below). Peak inspiratory pressures (PIP) generated by the ventilator should also be monitored at least every 2 hours. A sustained increase in PIP is reported.

The patient's temperature is monitored at least every 4 hours, and airway secretions are monitored

---

VENTILATOR SETTINGS

Conventional Modes

FIO_2

The fraction of inspired oxygen concentration may be varied from 0.21 to 1.0. Increasing the FIO_2 should increase the PaO_2.

Tidal volume

The amount of air delivered by each ventilator-controlled breath, usually set at approximately 10 to 15 mL/kg. Increasing the tidal volume should decrease the $PaCO_2$; and possibly increase the PaO_2.

Rate

The number of ventilator-controlled breaths the machine will deliver per minute. Increasing the mechanical rate should decrease the $PaCO_2$.

PEEP

The amount of positive pressure applied at the end of expiration. Typical clinical range is 5 to 10 cm H_2O. Increasing PEEP should increase PaO_2. Higher levels may be used to treat patients with severe hypoxemia.

---

for any signs of infection. Infection or fever increases the metabolic rate, thus increasing the production of carbon dioxide. Increased production of carbon dioxide results in increased ventilatory requirements. Pulmonary infections will increase secretions, increasing the work of breathing, and therefore worsen gas exchange.

Hydration status is assessed by recording intake and output and daily weights. Overhydration may contribute to interstitial pulmonary edema, compromising gas exchange and increasing the work of breathing. Dehydration may render secretions thick and tenacious, decreasing the patient's ability to clear them effectively, even with the assistance of suctioning. Auscultation of all lung fields should be performed at least every 4 hours.

Arterial blood gas values are monitored whenever any changes occur in the patient's status or following major changes in the ventilator settings. Hypoxemia decreases the efficiency of muscle function, including the respiratory muscles. Hypercarbia increases ventilatory demands. The added stress of attempting to compensate for any metabolic acid-base disorders will complicate patient management and decrease the likelihood of successful discontinuation of mechanical ventilation. Use of a pulse oximeter to continuously monitor arterial oxygen saturation is recommended for patients who demonstrate hypoxemia or are at high risk for oxygen desaturation episodes.

Daily evaluations of the patient's nutritional status and caloric intake are made.[10] In starvation states, patients will use their diaphragm as a protein source to meet their metabolic needs. Obviously, any loss of diaphragmatic strength will compromise the patient's respiratory muscle capacity. The usual recommended daily intake for patients on mechanical ventilation is 30 to 35 K calories/kg body weight. Patients who have difficulty with the elimination of carbon dioxide may require some of these calories delivered as fats rather than as carbohydrates. The metabolism of fats yields less carbon dioxide per gram than the metabolism of an equivalent amount of carbohydrate; therefore, calories obtained from fats generate less ventilatory work. When evaluating nutritional status, electrolyte levels should also be monitored. Electrolyte disorders may decrease the strength of the respiratory muscles. In addition to monitoring sodium, potassium, chloride, and carbon dioxide, phosphorus levels should be assessed. Phosphorus is necessary for the formation of adenosine triphosphate (ATP), the energy supply for cellular metabolic processes. Without sufficient stores of ATP, the respiratory muscles will be unable to function at the level needed to support spontaneous respiration.

For patients who have a nasogastric tube in place, gastric pH is monitored at the beginning of each shift or at least every 12 hours. Because of the high risk of stress ulcer formation, a pH less than 5 should be reported. Hemoglobin and hematocrit levels are also monitored as appropriate.

Nursing Diagnosis

Nursing diagnoses for patients on mechanical ventilation include nursing diagnoses common to intubated patients and may include the following:

Inadequate ventilation related to respiratory muscle dysfunction, decreased ventilatory drive, increased ventilatory demand, increased dead space

Inadequate gas exchange related to increased secretions, interstitial edema, shunt

High risk for injury: barotrauma related to positive pressure ventilation, elevated peak inspiratory pressures

High risk for decreased cardiac output related to decreased venous return

High risk for injury: stress ulcer related to mechanical ventilation, stress

Anxiety related to mechanical ventilation, severity of illness

Sensory/perceptual alterations related to monotony of environment, frequency of procedures, equipment noise

High risk for fluid volume excess related to fluid retention

Sleep pattern disturbance related to unfamiliar environment, equipment noise, frequency of procedures

Planning

General goals for the care of patients on mechanical ventilation include goals for the intubated patient and in addition the following:

Patient will maintain adequate ventilation as evidenced by $Paco_2$ <50 mm Hg, and arterial pH in the range of 7.35 to 7.45, respiratory rate 10 to 26 per minute, absence of abnormal respiratory patterns

Patient will maintain Pao_2 >60 mm Hg or within normal limits for the patient

Patient will not experience barotrauma as evidenced by equal breath sounds bilaterally, symmetric chest expansion, absence of subcutaneous emphysema

Patient will maintain acceptable cardiac output as evidenced by blood pressure >90 mm Hg systolic, pulse 60 to 100 BPM, skin warm and dry, urine output >30 mL/hr

Patient will not develop gastrointestinal bleeding related to stress ulcer as evidenced by absence of red or coffee ground gastric aspirate, gastric pH >5, stable hemoglobin and hematocrit levels

Patient will demonstrate decreased anxiety by communication of same and ability to cooperate with treatment

Patient will experience minimal sensory deprivation/overload as evidenced by communication of same and ability to participate in diversional activities

Patient will maintain fluid balance as evidenced by absence of edema, absence or decrease in crackles on auscultation of lung fields, daily intake equal to daily output (plus or minus 500 mL)

Patient will obtain adequate sleep as evidenced by sleeping for periods of at least 2 hours uninterrupted, for a total of at least 6 hours during the night

Implementation

The care of patients on mechanical ventilation includes the interventions described for intubated patients. In addition, special attention is paid to measures to improve ventilation and gas exchange.

Improved ventilation and improved gas exchange may be facilitated by maintaining the head of the bed at a 30-degree angle or higher to facilitate diaphragmatic excursion. Mobilization of the patient with frequent position changes in bed and gradual mobilization to the chair and ultimately to ambulation, as tolerated, will also improve ventilation and mobilization of secretions. In the presence of unilateral lung disease, frequent positioning of the patient with the "good" lung in the dependent position will maximize its blood flow and optimize ventilation/perfusion matching. Chest physical therapy and postural drainage may aid in the mobilization of secretions for suctioning and facilitate optimal gas exchange.

Ventilator alarms should remain on at all times to ensure appropriate functioning of the ventilator (see the box on p. 578). In the presence of signs or symptoms of respiratory distress, accompanied by activation of one or more ventilator alarms, the patient is manually ventilated before and during attempts to adjust the ventilator. The primary concern is adequate ventilation and oxygenation of the patient.

As noted previously, if the patient is observed to be breathing "out of phase" with the ventilator, measures must be taken immediately to correct the situation. The nurse consults the respiratory therapist to ensure that the ventilator is functioning properly and that the settings are appropriate for the patient's condition. In some instances, calm reassurance and coaching of the patient's respiratory efforts may be all that is necessary. For patients who are unable to cooperate with coaching, manual ventilation for a brief period during an acute crisis may be

VENTILATOR ALARMS

High Pressure

The high-pressure alarm sounds when the preset peak inspiratory pressure limit is reached by the ventilator before it has delivered the set tidal volume. When the peak inspiratory pressure limit is reached, the ventilator will terminate the inspiratory phase.

Causes:

Tubing obstructions or kinks
Breathing "out of phase" or "bucking" the ventilator
Accumulation of secretions
Condensation of water in the ventilator tubing
Coughing or Valsalva maneuver
Increased airway resistance, bronchospasm
Decreased pulmonary compliance
Pneumothorax

Low Pressure

The low-pressure alarm sounds when little or no pressure is generated during delivery of a machine breath.

Causes:

Disconnection of the ventilator tubing at any point in the circuit, most frequently occurs at the ventilator/endotracheal tube junction or due to cuff leak

Exaggerated patient inspiratory effort, generating extreme negative pressures

---

used, allowing better synchrony with the patient's respiratory efforts. If none of these methods is successful in returning the patient to breathing "in phase" with the ventilator, sedation may be required.

To minimize anxiety all procedures are explained. Frequent reassurance regarding significance of alarms and that nursing staff are in close proximity at all times will also help to alleviate their fears. The call bell should be kept within easy reach at all times. Patient care should be coordinated to conform to the patient's usual sleep-wake cycle. For most patients, treatment activities are scheduled during the day or "waking" hours. Physical therapy, unless contraindicated, is ordered on all mechanically ventilated patients. However, care should be taken to schedule periods of rest between activities. During the patient's "sleep" cycle, patient care activities should be arranged to allow periods of at least 2 hours for uninterrupted sleep. Periods of at least 2 hours have been shown to be necessary to allow for REM sleep. Lights are dimmed and noise is minimized during this time. The administration of

hypnotics to assist the patient in obtaining adequate sleep may be necessary because of the unfamiliarity of the surroundings and patient anxiety.

WEANING FROM MECHANICAL VENTILATION

The procedure for discontinuing the artificial support of ventilation is commonly described by the term "weaning."[39,41] The weaning process has two distinct phases. During the first phase, the patient is evaluated to determine if he or she might be able to breathe independently of the ventilator. The second phase involves actually separating the patient from the ventilator for a period of time usually referred to as a "weaning trial."

Weaning Parameters

Once the decision to wean a patient from a ventilator has been made, various studies of the ventilator patient's pulmonary function are performed. Typically, these tests assess inspiratory muscle strength, resting ventilation, and may include arterial blood gas analysis to evaluate the efficiency of respiration. Collectively, the data generated from bedside lung function studies are called "parameters."

The bedside parameters usually include the maximum inspiratory pressure (MIP), the vital capacity (VC), resting minute ventilation (VE), and its components, the tidal volume (Vt) and respiratory rate, or frequency (f). Some institutions include the maximum voluntary ventilation (MVV) as part of the parameter assessment.

Maximum inspiratory pressure (MIP) is also called "peak negative pressure" (PNP), "maximum inspiratory force" (MIF), or "negative inspiratory force" (NIF). This is a simple test that evaluates respiratory muscle strength. The patient is disconnected from the ventilator circuit and a pressure manometer is attached to the endotracheal or tracheostomy tube connector. The airway is then occluded and the maximal amount of inspiratory pressure that the patient can "suck" against the manometer is recorded. The patient is supposed to be able to generate at least -20 to -30 cm H_2O to be considered as meeting the minimum criteria for weaning.

The vital capacity (VC) is the maximal amount of air that a patient can inhale and then exhale in a single breath. It is intended to reflect the stiffness (compliance) of lung tissue, the patient's ability to self-sigh, or to inspire enough air for a cough to clear secretions from the airways. In addition, since the test requires a forceful exhalation, it evaluates the efficacy of the abdominal muscles to contract and produce a cough.

The VC is measured by disconnecting the patient from the ventilator circuit and attaching a spirometer to the endotracheal or tracheostomy tube connector. The patient is instructed to fully inhale and then exhale as deeply as possible. The volume of exhaled air is then measured by the spirometer. The VC is supposed to reach a volume of at least 1 L, or from 10 to 15 mL/kg, in order to meet proposed weaning standards for this test.

The minute ventilation (VE) is the volume of air that a patient breathes during a minute's time. It is typically measured by a spirometer that is attached to endotracheal or tracheostomy tube connector. The VE is usually assessed immediately after the patient is disconnected from the ventilator. Therefore it is a resting state measurement. But unlike the VC, the measurement of the VE does not depend upon patient cooperation. The VE is supposed to be less than 10 L/min in order to be compatible with weaning success.

The respiratory rate, or frequency (f), is one of the principal signs of respiratory function that is monitored in the ICU. The f tends to trend inversely with the VE; that is, as the VE drops, the f rises, and vice versa. Although the f may be a simple, objective assessment, the nurse should monitor the patient for other signs or symptoms of respiratory muscle fatigue before deciding to alter the weaning regimen. Even if the f does change during weaning, the influence of f upon arterial blood gas and pH values cannot be predicted. Therefore f alone is not used as the sole limiting criterion for a weaning trial. A sustained respiratory rate greater than 30 to 35 br/min might be used as a standard protocol for drawing an arterial blood gas.

The tidal volume (Vt) is the amount of air that is exhaled after a single resting inhalation. It is either measured by a spirometer or is calculated by dividing the VE by the f. The VE and Vt usually change simultaneously and change inversely with the f. The Vt is supposed to be greater than 5 mL per kg of ideal body weight in order to be compatible with weaning.

The maximum voluntary ventilation (MVV) is the maximum amount of air that can be forcibly inhaled and exhaled per minute. It is supposed to reflect the compliance of the lung and the patient's ability to exercise the respiratory muscles. The patient is usually connected to a spirometer and instructed to breathe as quickly and deeply as possible for a certain time. The MVV is to be equal to twice the resting VE in order to meet the criteria for weaning.

The arterial acid-base and blood gas status (ABGs) may help to predict who will fail a weaning trial. Patients who suffer from clinically serious hypercapnia and hypoxemia, in spite of optimum ventilator settings, will typically deteriorate when artificial support is withdrawn. However, pre-weaning-trial ABGs may not be useful for predicting successful weaning of patients who otherwise seem to be good candidates for the procedure. The patient should have a PaO_2 of 60 mm Hg or greater on an FIO_2 of 0.40 or less before weaning trials. ABG values cannot be predicted given the patient's breathing patterns or physical findings. During a weaning trial, respiratory rates that rise above 30 br/min and/or evidence of paradoxical or asynchronous motion of the abdomen or chest wall may be indicators that an ABG should be drawn and analyzed. If the $PaCO_2$ has risen and caused the pH to fall below 7.30, the patient should be reconnected to the ventilator because the weaning trial has failed. In addition, a low PaO_2 that drops further during a weaning trial probably should be included as a criterion for limiting the duration of a weaning period. It should be noted, however, that changes in body position alone at the time an ABG is drawn can affect oxygenation, depending on the degree of ventilation/perfusion mismatch.[57] Nevertheless, physical findings alone are not always reliable ways to discriminate among patients who are tolerating or failing the weaning attempt.

Noninvasive Monitors of Weaning

Pulse Oximetry

Attaching patients to oximeters during the weaning period to noninvasively monitor the oxygen saturation of hemoglobin (SpO_2%) has become commonplace in intensive care units.[20] Physicians write orders to draw an ABG, titrate the oxygen concentration, or discontinue a weaning trial when the monitor reads a certain SpO_2%. However, there is no agreement about the SpO_2% that should trigger specific activity.

Major changes in a weaning protocol (such as discontinuance of the trial and reconnection to a ventilator) should not be dependent upon oximetry readings alone. Rather, the oximeter may alert the staff that an ABG should be drawn and subsequent action be based upon those results. The applications of an oximeter during weaning should be to match the inspired oxygen concentration with the oxygen needs of the patient, reduce unnecessary ABGs when the patient's clinical status is stable, or to warn the attending staff that the patient's cardiorespiratory status has deteriorated.

Exhaled carbon dioxide

When a patient's alveolar ventilation falls, the arterial carbon dioxide ($PaCO_2$) rises, causing a fall in the arterial pH, a situation described as respiratory acidosis. Theoretically, as the $PaCO_2$ rises, the concentration of CO_2 in the exhaled air measured at the end of a normal tidal breath ($PetCO_2$) rises as well.[31] Carbon dioxide monitors (capnometers) have been used to alert patient attendants about rising CO_2

tensions (hypercapnea) that patients may experience during weaning.

However, the Pet_{CO_2} value is not solely dependent upon ventilation. Rather, pulmonary perfusion has as much influence upon the Pet_{CO_2} as does alveolar ventilation. The concentration of CO_2 in expired air reflects the quality of CO_2 that is delivered to the alveolar air space by pulmonary capillaries. As the blood flow through the capillaries changes, so will the Pet_{CO_2}. If cardiac output falls, or the patient suffers pulmonary emboli, the Pet_{CO_2} will fall. The low Pet_{CO_2} could be misinterpreted as hyperventilation when, in fact, it means that ventilation exceeded perfusion. The Pa_{CO_2} may actually rise under those circumstances and the capnometer would not reflect the Pa_{CO_2} level.[31]

Just as alveolar perfusion may alter the Pet_{CO_2}, metabolism also can influence that indicator. It is not uncommon to see sudden increases in the Pet_{CO_2} following shivering as patients warm themselves. As a patient's core temperature rises, so can the Pet_{CO_2}. These conditions result in an increased CO_2 production causing a concomitant rise in mixed venous P_{CO_2} and Pet_{CO_2}.

NURSING MANAGEMENT OF THE PATIENT BEING WEANED FROM VENTILATION

Nursing Diagnosis

Nursing diagnoses common to patients being weaned from mechanical ventilation are the same as those common to intubated patients and to patients on mechanical ventilation.

Planning

The primary goal for patients being weaned from mechanical ventilation is the following:

Patient will be and will remain extubated with arterial blood gas values within normal limits for the patient.

Implementation

There is no agreement on the best method to wean a patient from mechanical ventilation. However, once the decision has been made to attempt to wean the patient, three methods are available: the "T-piece" technique, the IMV technique, and the PSV technique.

The T-piece technique is the traditional weaning method.[41] In this technique, the patient is removed from the ventilator and placed on a T-piece (Figure 26-19), which passively delivers the specified Fi_{O_2}. Initially, the patient remains on the T-piece for a few minutes after which he or she is reconnected to the

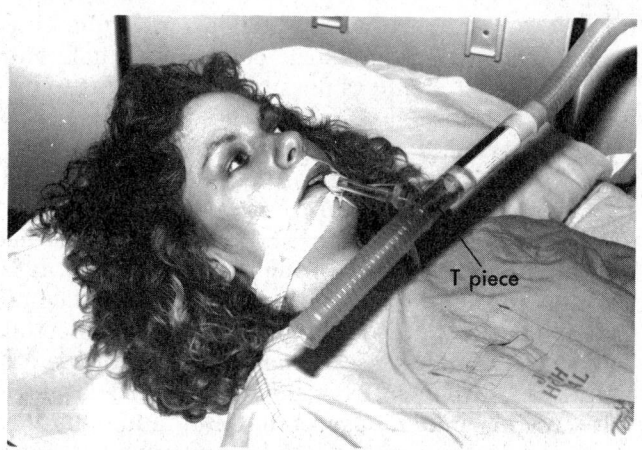

FIGURE 26-19 Patient on a T-piece.

ventilator. Because the patient is totally without mechanical ventilatory support during T-piece weaning, close nursing observation is critical. The period that the patient is on the T-piece is gradually lengthened until the patient is able to breathe spontaneously for a prolonged period (hours). Mechanical ventilation is then discontinued.

The IMV technique for weaning is accomplished by gradual reduction in the number of mechanical breaths the ventilator delivers, until the patient is breathing totally on his or her own.[39] When a patient is weaned by this method, he or she is not required to breathe without some degree of ventilator support until the final stages of weaning.

The pressure support ventilation mode is available on certain modern ventilators.[33,41] When used as a stand-alone mode, the PS is raised to a level which achieves a spontaneous tidal volume of 10 to 12 mL/kg or the lowest respiratory rate. The PS is gradually reduced in 3 to 6 cm H_2O increments as judged by a stable respiratory rate until a level of 5 to 10 cm H_2O is reached. Within that pressure range, extubation of the patient may be possible.

Of prime importance to the weaning effort is the establishment of trust between the patient and the health care team. This may be facilitated by consistency in the health care providers caring for the patient. As the ventilator support is gradually decreased and the patient begins to assume more of the work of breathing, he or she may begin to experience some anxiety. Fear that he or she will once again experience the sensation of being unable to breathe may interfere with the patient's ability to cooperate with the plan. Reassurance that he or she is under constant surveillance and the expression of confidence in the patient's ability will help alleviate this anxiety. It is important that the weaning plan for the day be fully explained and that realistic achievable goals be set. The successful achievement of these goals, no matter how small, will bolster the patient's confidence.

If the patient demonstrates signs or symptoms of tiring, weaning attempts are temporarily halted. When T-piece weaning, the patient is returned to total ventilator support as soon as any indications of weaning failure are observed. If he or she is set on the IMV mode of ventilation, the ventilator rate is increased to its previous setting. If PSV is used, the pressure support level may be raised until the patient's respiratory rate decreases to pre-weaning levels.

Weaning must be terminated before the patient becomes exhausted. A failed weaning attempt can be psychologically devastating. It may shatter the patient's confidence in the health care team's ability to detect and prevent escalating respiratory distress. Persisting in a weaning trial to the point of patient exhaustion will damage any trust the health care providers have established with the patient. In addition, it may take several days for respiratory muscles, which have been exhausted during an unsuccessful attempt, to recover sufficient strength to make another trial feasible.

Home Care

Occasionally, a patient is unable to wean from mechanical ventilation because of the severity of the underlying disease process or general debilitation. Such patients may receive ventilator support at home. Recent studies have demonstrated that home care is a cost-effective and psychologically beneficial alternative to institutionalization for ventilator-dependent individuals.[8,19] This alternative has been particularly beneficial for patients with COPD, chest wall deformity, or neuromuscular disease.

Assessment of the patient and family includes an evaluation of their motivation to undertake the responsibility of home ventilator care. The physical and emotional strength of the patient and family must be considered. Family dynamics are assessed for any areas of conflict, since the stress associated with home care may exacerbate these problems.[38] Home care difficulties may also become the focus of frustrations displaced from other areas of conflict. The availability of professional support services in the patient's community is evaluated. The availability of home health care assistance and professional nursing services is also investigated. Vendors of medical equipment are evaluated with respect to equipment and services provided, 24-hour availability, and acceptance of third-party payment for expenses incurred.

The physical layout of the patient's living area is evaluated for accessibility. In addition, the electrical wiring of the house is assessed for handling the additional load imposed by the ventilator and suction equipment. Finally, the knowledge level of the patient and family regarding all aspects of ventilator care and troubleshooting, tracheostomy care, secretion management, and general health care measures are considered.

Hospital discharge of the ventilator-dependent patient begins with consultation of the physician, nurse, pulmonary clinical nurse specialist, social worker, respiratory therapist, occupational therapist, physical therapist, and dietitian. Together, they constitute the discharge planning team for the patient. It is important that these individuals be consistent throughout the patient's progress toward discharge so that a level of trust and confidence can be established. Patient and family education is initiated as soon as possible. Preliminary discussions should provide a description of the skills and knowledge the patient and family will need to acquire, a tentative time frame for learning, and a tentative discharge date. The patient and family should have input into the most appropriate times for teaching to occur.

A local vendor who is able to supply all of the equipment needed in the home is contacted and arrangements for third-party payment are made. The patient's home should be rewired to provide an independent circuit for the ventilator and other respiratory equipment. An auxiliary power source should also be obtained for use in the event of a power failure. A home health care agency must be contacted for nursing support.

CHEST TUBES
Definition

A chest (or thoracostomy) tube is made from clear, flexible plastic and is approximately 20 inches long (51 cm). Various sizes of chest tubes are available from a few millimeters to a centimeter or wider in diameter. The chest tube is open on both ends; one end is attached to the external drainage system while the other end lies inside the patient. There are several small holes to allow for additional drainage of fluid or air into the section of the tube that lies inside the patient. There is a radiopaque line that runs the length of the chest tube so that it is visible in a chest x-ray.

Chest tubes are usually placed so that they lie between specific tissue sheets that are found inside the thorax. The visceral pleura covers the entire surface of each lung. The parietal pleura separates the lungs from the mediastinum, lines the inside wall of the thorax, and covers the surface of the diaphragm. The pericardium lies on top of the epicardium of the heart. Many of these tissues are pressed flat against each other and are separated only by a thin layer of fluid. The fluid-filled region between the visceral and parietal pleura is called the pleural space.

Air that enters the pleural space is called a pneumothorax. A pneumothorax causes the lung to fall away from the inner chest wall and collapse. A pneumothorax may be considered "open" in which air moves freely into and out of the pleural space, or "closed" in which air has entered and is trapped in the pleural space.

A tension pneumothorax occurs when air pressure in the pleural space becomes greater than atmospheric pressure. This buildup of air pressure causes the lung, heart, and other structures in the mediastinum to be pushed or "shifted" away from the pneumothorax. In addition, the diaphragm may be forced toward the abdominal cavity. Blood flow into the thorax is usually impaired, cardiac output falls, and cardiopulmonary arrest is possible as a result of a tension pneumothorax.

A pneumomediastinum occurs when air enters the area in the thorax which contains the heart, great vessels, esophagus, trachea, and mainstem bronchi. Occasionally, the air will travel up the mediastinum and into the soft tissues of the neck, shoulders, and face. Air that lies under the skin is referred to as subcutaneous emphysema. The crackling sensation that the clinician feels as pressure on the skin is applied is called subcutaneous crepitus. Subcutaneous air does not pose a threat to the patient. However, its presence may indicate that a pneumothorax or pneumomediastinum has occurred and should be reported immediately to the patient's physician. Air may dissect into the pericardial sac and occupy the space between the pericardium and epicardium. This situation is termed a pneumopericardium.

An excess accumulation of fluid in the pleural space is called a pleural effusion. A pleural effusion may result from heart failure, pneumonia, trauma (including surgery), cancer, and/or abdominal organ injury or illness. Pleural effusions may be described in terms of the type of cells found in the fluid, which may include blood (hemothorax), lymph (chylothorax) or infection (empyema). A pericardium effusion consists of fluid that builds up in the space between the pericardium and epicardium. Fluid in the pleural space, mediastinum, or pericardium that interferes with heart function causes a life-threatening situation called a cardiac tamponade. A cardiac tamponade is treated by removing the fluid or prevented by providing for drainage of the effusion from the affected area.

Therapeutic Management

Disorders of the pleural space are usually diagnosed by chest x-ray. Because pneumothoraces and effusions are a result of disease or injury, identification and treatment of a causative disease or injury is undertaken as soon as the disorder is detected. The physician may elect not to treat small pneumotho-

races or pleural effusions unless the problem causes the patient to suffer discomfort, dyspnea, or a decline in either lung or heart function. A needle may be inserted into the affected area in order to relieve the air pressure or remove fluid. A tube can be placed into the area to allow for continuous drainage of air and/or fluid if the pneumothorax or effusion is large or recurring. For instance, a mediastinal tube is routinely used during the postoperative recovery period to drain blood and fluid away from the heart after cardiac surgery.

Placement of the chest tube is important to ensure optimal drainage of fluid or air. Because air rises, a pleural chest tube inserted for a pneumothorax is usually placed in the anterior chest near the apex in the second intercostal space. Conversely, fluid is pulled down by gravity and tends to pool in the base and posterior areas of the lung. Pleural chest tubes inserted to drain fluid are usually placed posteriorly near the base of the lungs, midaxillary in the fourth to sixth intercostal spaces (Figure 26-20). Mediastinal chest tubes are usually placed in the central chest along the anterior and posterior surfaces of the heart.

Following thoracic surgery, a mediastinal chest tube is placed through the chest wall and into position before the chest is closed. The technique used to insert a pleural chest tube depends on the skills and preference of the physician. The procedure generally starts with an injectable analgesic followed by local anesthesia of the insertion site. A small incision, 1 to 3 cm, is made in the chest wall. The intercostal muscles are dissected over the rib to the pleura. A hemostat is used to puncture the pleura. The chest tube is inserted through the opening and into position. At this time the chest drainage system is connected. The physician uses a purse-string suture to help secure the chest tube and applies a pet-

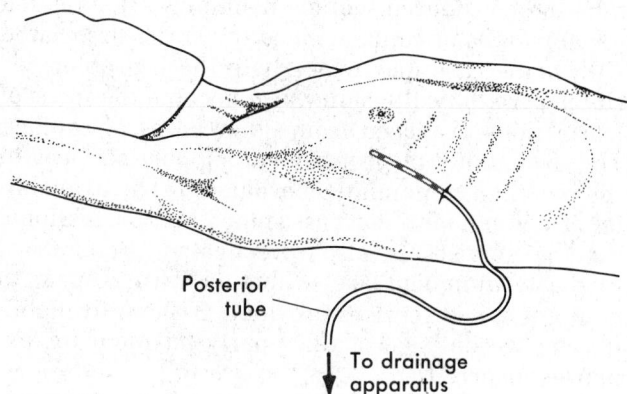

FIGURE 26-20 Placement of an anterior chest tube to drain air, and placement of a posterior tube to drain fluid.

rolatum gauze dressing over the incision. In many cases the chest tube or drainage tubing is also taped to the chest or abdomen. A dry occlusive (airtight) dressing is then applied. When the chest tube is secure a chest x-ray film is taken to determine proper placement of the chest tube.

Chest tube drainage is assessed for the volume of air leak or fluid accumulated over a given period. A pleural chest tube placed for a pneumothorax is not removed until the air leak is gone. Some physicians will leave a pleural chest tube in place in patients receiving mechanical ventilation even though the leak is sealed, because of the risk for recurrent pneumothorax from positive pressure ventilation. A chest tube placed to drain pleural or pericardial fluid is removed when fluid drainage is minimal, usually 50 mL in 24 hours. In most surgical cases, mediastinal and pleural chest tubes are removed by the second or third postoperative day, although this varies with the recovery of the patient.

Several different kinds of commercial drainage systems are commonly used (Figure 26-21). Fortunately, they are all based on the traditional three-bottle system. Understanding the principles of the three-bottle system allows the nurse to apply his or her knowledge to any commercial system.

In the three-bottle system each bottle has a separate function. The first bottle is the collection bottle. This bottle is connected to the chest tube. Fluid drains from the chest into the bottle via a short tube (Figure 26-22). At no time should the short tube be submerged in fluid.

Bottle two is the water-seal bottle. A second short tube in bottle one is connected to the long tube in bottle two. To achieve an effective water seal, the long tube in bottle two must be submerged under at least 2 cm of water throughout inspiration and expiration. The water seal acts as a one-way valve, allowing air out of the chest but not back in. Negative pressure is maintained, promoting lung expansion. Bubbling of air through the water in bottle two indicates that an air leak is present. When the bubbling stops, the air leak is sealed. Fluid in the long tube will fluctuate with the pleural pressure changes of inspiration and expiration (sometimes referred to as tidaling). When no fluctuation is present, the chest tube may be clogged.

Bottle three is the suction-control bottle. A short tube in bottle two is connected to a short tube in bottle three. A second short tube is connected to the suction regulator. A long tube open to the atmosphere is submerged in water to the ordered amount

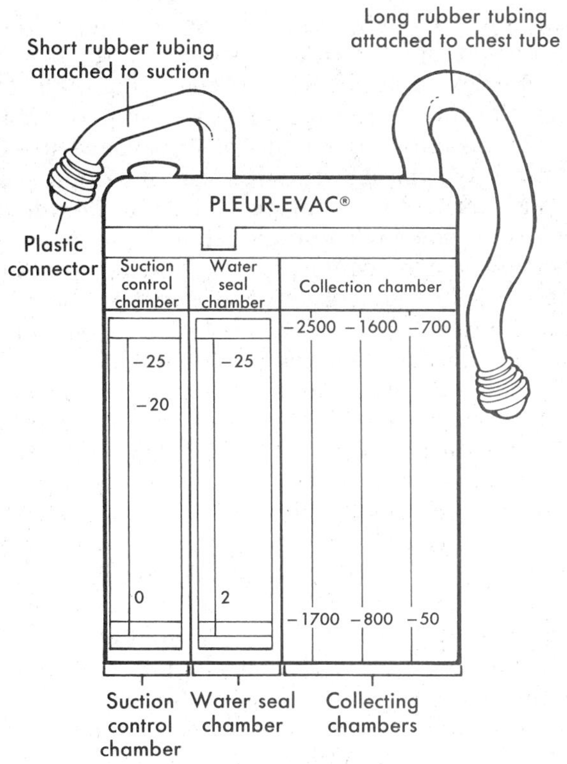

FIGURE 26-21   Pleur-Evac commercial drainage system. (From Thompson JM et al: *Mosby's manual of clinical nursing*, ed 2, St Louis, 1989, Mosby–Year Book.)

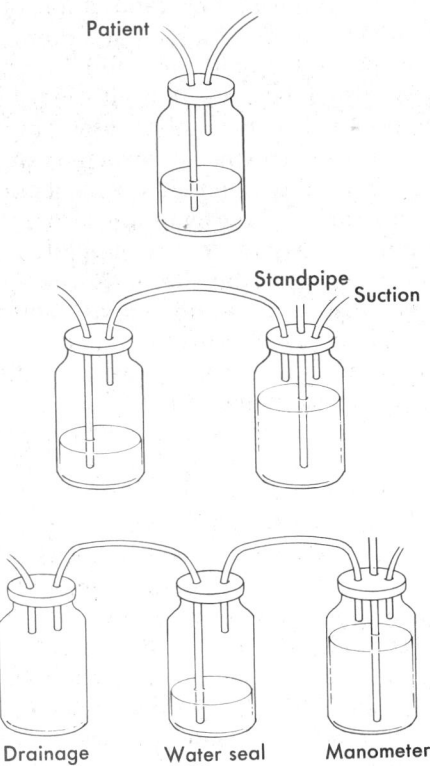

FIGURE 26-22   Three-bottle chest drainage system. (From Thompson JM et al: *Mosby's manual of clinical nursing*, ed 2, St Louis, 1989, Mosby–Year Book.)

of suction (i.e., -20 cm H_2O). The depth the long tube inserted under water is the amount of suction applied to the patient's chest. Bubbling in bottle three indicates that suction is being applied at the level the long tube is submerged. Turning up the suction regulator will result in pulling in atmospheric air and more bubbling, but not more suction pressure or vacuum. Suction is increased or decreased by moving the long tube up or down in the water. The suction-control bottle limits the amount of pressure that can be applied to the chest, regardless of the amount set on the suction regulator.

NURSING MANAGEMENT OF THE PATIENT WITH A CHEST TUBE
Assessment

Nursing assessment of the patient with a chest tube begins before the chest tube is inserted. Establishing a baseline of vital signs, chest examination, and pain symptoms gives the nurse important information for comparison with future assessments. In most cases the chest tube will already be in place when the nurse meets the patient for the first time. When caring for the patient with an existing chest tube, the nurse assesses the patient first and then the chest drainage system.

Patient assessment begins with inquiring how the patient feels, followed by examination of the vital signs. Pain can alter assessment findings. For instance, the patient in pain may splint his or her chest and not take deep breaths, thus altering auscultation and percussion findings. After assessing the vital signs, the nurse performs a thorough respiratory assessment to identify changes via inspection, palpation, percussion, and auscultation.

When patient assessment is completed, the nurse examines the chest tube site and drainage system. The dressing is assessed for drainage and occlusiveness. A wet dressing provides media for bacterial growth and migration. A loose dressing allows air or bacteria to possibly enter the pleural cavity. The chest tube is assessed for a securely taped connection to the drainage tubing. The nurse follows the drainage tubing down to the drainage system, checking for kinks and proper position. The tubing is coiled on the bed and drains directly into the drainage system without dependent looping.

The drainage system is first assessed for secure connections. The volume of fluid that has accumulated in the collection chamber since the last assessment is noted. The color, consistency, and any obvious odor of the fluid drainage is assessed. It should be noted whether the color of the fluid in the tubing is different from that in the collection chamber. A change in color from dark red to bright red may signal fresh bleeding. A change from bloody to serous fluid indicates improvement. It should be noted whether any clots are present in the drainage and

whether the drainage is thick or purulent. Although an odor is normal in the patient with an empyema, it is abnormal in other patients and usually means an infection is present.

The nurse observes the water-seal chamber for tidaling of the fluid column with inspiration and expiration. During spontaneous respirations the fluid column will rise during inspiration and fall during expiration. The opposite is true of a patient receiving positive pressure breaths from a ventilator: the fluid column will fall during inspiration and rise during expiration. Tidaling may be less in the patient receiving positive end-expiratory pressure (PEEP) or absent if the drainage holes are occluded by lung tissue or clots.

The nurse also identifies the presence or absence of air leak in the water-seal chamber. In the patient with a mediastinal chest tube there should not be an air leak in the water-seal chamber because the mediastinum is not in contact with the pleural cavity. An air leak in the water-seal chamber may be from the lung, the insertion site, a loose connection in the drainage system, or a crack in the collection device. When the nurse identifies an air leak, it is important to determine its origin. The nurse uses special chest tube clamps always present at the bedside to perform this assessment.

To assess the origin of the air leak, the nurse begins by momentarily (no more than 10 seconds) clamping the chest tube as close to the patient's chest as possible and working down to the drainage unit. For example, if the air leak or bubbling stops when the tube closest to chest is clamped, air may be coming either from the pleural space itself or from around the chest tube at the insertion site. If an air leak to the drainage system is identified, it must be replaced. The nurse should pay particular attention to connections which can become loose. One common point may be where the chest tube joins the drainage system. If a loose connection exists, tape may be used for reinforcement.

Finally the nurse assesses the suction control chamber for proper fluid volume height, which controls suction pressure. Water that has evaporated from the chamber must be replaced to ensure adequate suction pressure as determined by the physician. Presence of gentle bubbling in the suction control chamber is evidence that suction is being applied to the chest. Absence of bubbling in the suction-control chamber indicates that there may be inadequate suction applied to the patient's chest. If suction is not being used, the suction-control chamber should be open to the atmosphere (i.e., disconnected from the suction regulator).

If the patient also has mediastinal tubes, the nurse performs a complete cardiac assessment in addition to the respiratory assessment. Heart sounds are important to help identify cardiac tamponade. Fluid drainage is assessed more frequently, at least hourly, in the immediate postoperative cardiac patient with mediastinal chest tubes to determine rate of bleeding. The accumulation of more than 100 mL/hr may indicate the need for further medical or surgical intervention. Bubbling or tidaling of mediastinal drainage indicates either a leak in the drainage system or displacement of the chest tube.

Nursing Diagnosis

Many nursing diagnoses are appropriate for the patient with a chest tube, including:

Decreased cardiac output related to cardiac tamponade, tension pneumothorax

Impaired gas exchange related to disease process

Impaired skin integrity related to chest tube incision

Ineffective airway clearance related to pain from compressed lung tissue

Ineffective breathing pattern related to pain

Knowledge deficit related to chest tube insertion and care

Pain related to chest tube insertion

Planning

Specific patient goals related to the age and health of the patient are given priority on the basis of the nursing assessment. Priority is given to goals that promote physical and psychologic integrity of the patient. The nurse is careful to include the patient's assessment of goal importance in developing a plan of care. General patient care goals may include the following:

Patient demonstrates vital signs, color, mentation, level of consciousness that are normal for the patient

Patient verbalizes fears or anxieties and identifies resources for coping

Patient has normal arterial blood gases with or without supplemental oxygen

Patient's incision site is healed without infection present

Patient coughs out secretions with the assistance of a splinting pillow and/or analgesics

Patient breathes at normal rate and depth

Patient is knowledgeable about procedure and care of chest tube

Chest tube does not become dislodged

Patient verbalizes relief of pain with comfort measures or analgesics

Patient has reinflated lung on chest x-ray film

Patient does not develop cardiac tamponade or tension pneumothorax

Implementation

Insertion of a chest tube is a painful, anxiety-producing procedure. The patient must be prepared

for the procedure. The nurse explains to the patient and family what to expect, including positioning (semi-Fowler or side-lying), chest discomfort from the tube, and activity limitations, such as bathing and ambulation constraints. The patient is premedicated according to physician orders. Analgesia is continued after insertion, as ordered. After insertion the nurse instructs the patient in techniques of deep breathing and coughing using a pillow for support.

Care of the chest tube and drainage system is also important. The nurse maintains a dry occlusive dressing at all times. According to institution policy, the nurse reinforces or changes the dressing when it becomes wet or soiled. Tape surrounding the dressing is to be secured to the skin at all times. Adhesive or waterproof tape is ideal; paper tape is not occlusive and not sufficiently secure. If the patient's skin is excoriated from the tape, the nurse may apply a protective barrier, such as benzoin or stomahesive.

Each connection of the chest tube system is checked for secureness on a regular basis at the beginning and end of each shift. The most secure connection is a spiral wrap from each of two directions that allows for visibility of drainage in the tubing (Figure 26-23). The patient is cautioned not to pull on the tubing when moving in the bed or transferring from the bed to the chair.

Fluid drainage from the chest tube is measured and marked directly on the drainage unit according to patient condition and institution policy. Most commercial systems have an opaque area for marking drainage. Tape is applied to the collection chamber area for marking, if necessary. The physician is notified of a significant change in the amount, color, consistency, or odor of fluid drainage, as well as the amount of air leak. When an air leak is present, the nurse determines the origin as discussed in assessment.

In most cases fluid and air easily flow from the chest into the collection chamber as long as there are no dependent loops or kinks. Sometimes the nurse may supplement gravity by milking or strip-

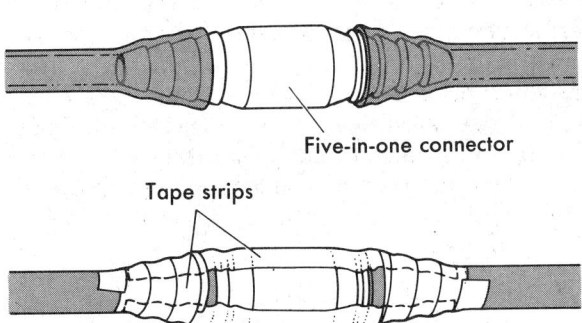

FIGURE 26-23   Method for wrapping chest tube connections.

ping the chest tube. Each institution has its own policy regarding milking and stripping. Milking the chest tube is accomplished by alternately compressing and releasing the drainage tubing between thumb and forefinger. Milking, which applies gentle intermittent suction to the chest, is not to be confused with stripping. Stripping a chest tube can generate negative suction pressures in excess of −200 mm Hg.[54] Fragile blood vessels, lung tissue, and fresh sutures can be "sucked" into the holes of the chest tube. Stripping a chest tube is performed by lubricating the thumb and forefinger. The drainage tubing is grasped and stretched as the thumb and forefinger slide down several inches of the tubing before release.

A key concern of the nurse is what action to take if the chest drainage system becomes accidentally disconnected. In the distant past, nurses were taught to clamp the chest tube immediately. That placed patients with a persistent pneumothorax or copious mediastinal drainage at risk for a tension pneumothorax or cardiac tamponade. Current practice is to not clamp the chest tube. The small amount of air that enters the pleural or mediastinal space can easily be evacuated by syringe or suction. As quickly as possible, the end of the chest tube is placed in a container of sterile water or saline, such as the bottle of water used to fill the suction control chamber, until the drainage system can be replaced.

If the pleural chest tube is accidentally pulled out, the nurse applies an occlusive dressing and notifies the physician immediately. A chest tube can usually be prevented from being accidentally removed by careful attention to secure connections and placement of drainage tubings.

Evaluation

With the implementation of a successful plan of care, the nurse will assess normal indices of oxygenation and ventilation including vital signs, color, level of consciousness, mentation, and blood gases. Drainage or bubbling in the chest tube will be minimal or cease as expected, allowing the chest tube to be discontinued. The patient will not develop complications of the chest tube such as dislodgement, accidental removal, skin infection, pneumonia, recurrent pneumothorax, cardiac tamponade, or tension pneumothorax. The patient will demonstrate knowledge of care of a chest tube or remaining incision. The nurse will also identify that the patient has employed adequate coping mechanisms or located resources to resolve anxieties or fears.

Documentation

Documentation begins with accurate recording of assessment and interventions. The nurse includes assessment of the patient, of the chest tube insertion site, and of the drainage system. The nurse records the patient's comfort level, interventions used to alter comfort level, and the patient's response. A record of the teaching and effectiveness in performing of deep breathing and coughing exercises is made. The nurse documents inspection, palpation, percussion, and auscultation findings from the respiratory assessment as well as heart sounds from the cardiac assessment. Documentation of the chest tube insertion site includes condition of the skin and implemented therapies. The nurse records the appearance of the dressing. It is important to note when loose or soiled dressings were reinforced or changed for infection control.

The nurse records the quality and quantity of drainage from the chest tube. The color, consistency, and odor of fluid in the collection chamber is noted and documents the presence or the absence of an air leak in the water seal chamber. When an air leak is present, the nurse documents the origin of the leak and notes that all connections are securely taped. Tidaling of fluid in the water seal chamber is identified as present or absent in the patient record. The nurse documents the level of fluid or pressure applied by the suction control chamber.

Ongoing Care

The care of a patient being discharged with a chest tube is rare. A patient may, however, be discharged with an empyema tube. An empyema tube is a chest tube that is in the pleural space to drain a pocket of infected secretions. Because the infection has been walled off from the lung, there is no need for a water seal system. The physician usually cuts the chest tube off at the chest wall and very slowly, about 1 cm per week or less, pulls the chest tube out. Some empyema tubes are never discontinued.

CRITICAL THINKING QUESTIONS

1 Describe the signs and symptoms of ineffective breathing.

2 Explain the procedure for using an incentive spirometer.

3 List the interventions that a nurse can perform to improve the patient's ability to cough.

4 Identify the indications for chest physiotherapy.

5 Describe the clinical indications, procedure, and complications of suctioning a patient with and without an artificial airway.

6 Identify the indications, evaluation techniques, and complications associated with oxygen therapy.

7 Match the oxygen delivery system with the patient's clinical condition.

8 Describe the various types of equipment used to provide supplemental humidity to patients.

9 List the instructions that should be given to a patient to properly use a metered-dose-inhaler.

10 Match the types of artificial airways used in clinical practice with their indications and complications.

11 Compare and contrast the various modes of positive pressure ventilation.

12 Describe clinical indications for continuous mechanical ventilation.

13 Differentiate between the pleural disorders for which chest tubes are used.

14 Describe the operation of a modern chest tube collection system.

15 Write nursing care plans for patients receiving incentive spirometry, oxygen therapy, chest physiotherapy, metered-dose-inhalers, artificial airways, continuous mechanical ventilation, weaning trials, and chest tubes.

BIBLIOGRAPHY

Current

1. Adamo JP et al: The Cleveland Clinic's initial experience with transtracheal oxygen therapy, *Respir Care* 35:153, 1990.

2. Berry RB et al: Nebulizer vs. spacer for bronchodilator delivery in patients hospitalized for acute exacerbations of COPD, *Chest* 96:1241, 1990.

3. Bowton DL et al: Substitution of metered-dose-inhalers for hand-held nebulizers; success and cost savings in a large, acute-care hospital, *Chest* 101:305, 1992.

4. Campbell EJ, Baker MD, Crites-Silver P: Subjective effects of humidification of oxygen for delivery by nasal cannula. A prospective study. *Chest* 93:289, 1988.

5. Cerny FJ: Relative effects of bronchial drainage and exercise for in-hospital care of patients with cystic fibrosis, *Phys Ther* 69:633, 1989.

6. Clemmer TP et al: Effectiveness of the kinetic treatment table for preventing and treating pulmonary complications in severely head-injured patients, *Crit Care Med* 18:614, 1990.

7. Dennison RD: Managing the patient with upper airway obstruction, *Nursing* 17:34, 1987.

8. Dettenmeier PA: Planning for successful home mechanical ventilation, *AACN Clin Issues Crit Care Nurs* 1:267, 1990.

9. Dettenmeier PA, Jackson NC: Chronic hypoventilation syndrome: treatment with non-invasive mechanical ventilation, *AACN Clin Issues Crit Care Nurs* 2:415, 1991.

10. Eisenberg PG: Pulmonary complications from enteral nutrition, *Crit Care Nurs Clin North Am* 3:641, 1991.

11. Elpern EH et al: Incidence of aspiration in tracheally intubated adults, *Heart Lung* 16:527, 1987.

12. Gentilello L et al: Effect of a rotating bed on the incidence of pulmonary complications in critically ill patients, *Crit Care Med* 16:783, 1988.

13. Guidry GG et al: Incorrect use of metered-dose-inhalers by medical personnel, *Chest* 101:31, 1992.

14. Haake R et al: Barotrauma: pathophysiology, risk factors and presentation, *Chest* 91:608, 1987.

15. Halloran T: Use of sedation and neuromuscular paralysis during mechanical ventilation, *Crit Care Nurs Clin North Am* 3:651, 1991.

16. Hanley MV, Tyler ML: Ineffective airway clearance related to airway infection, *Nurs Clin North Am* 22:135, 1987.

17. Hargrove S, Mandzak-McCarron K: Respiratory rehabilitation: communication aids for the tracheostomized patient, *Rehabil Nurs* 12:193, 1987.

18. Harshberger S et al: Effect of using a closed airway system catheter when suctioning mechanically ventilated patients, *Heart Lung* 13:216, 1988.

19. Haynes N, Raine SF, Rushing P: Discharging ICU ventilator-dependent patients to home health care, *Crit Care Nurse* 10:39, 1990.

20. Hess D: Noninvasive respiratory monitoring during ventilatory support, *Crit Care Nurs Clin North Am* 3:565, 1991.

21. Hoffman LA, Maszkiewicz RC: Airway management for the critically ill patient. *Am J Nurs* 87:39, 1987.

22. Hoffman LA, Wesmiller SW: Home oxygen. Transtracheal and other options, *Am J Nurs* 88:464, 1988.

23. Hoffman LA: Ineffective airway clearance related to neuromuscular dysfunction, *Nurs Clin North Am* 22:151, 1987.

24. Jasper AC et al: Cost-benefit comparison of aerosol bronchodilator delivery methods in hospitalized patients, *Chest* 91:614, 1987.

25. Jurban A, Tobin MJ: Reliability of pulse oximetry in titrating supplemental oxygen therapy in ventilator-dependent patients, *Chest* 97:1420, 1990.

26. Lareau S, Larson JL: Ineffective breathing pattern related to airflow limitation, *Nurs Clin North Am* 22:179, 1987.

27. Morley TF et al: Comparison of beta-adrenergic agents delivered by nebulizer vs. metered-dose-inhaler with InspirEase in hospitalized asthmatic patients, *Chest* 94:1205, 1988.

28. Noll ML, Hix CD, Scott G: Closed tracheal suction systems: effectiveness and nursing implications, *AACN Clin Issues Crit Care Nurs* 1:318, 1990.

29. Openbrier DR, Hoffman LA: Home oxygen therapy. Evaluation and prescription, *Am J Nurs* 88:192, 1988.

30. Portnoy J et al: Continuous nebulization for status asthmaticus, *Ann Allergy* 69:71, 1992.

31. St. John RE: Exhaled gas analysis: technical and clinical aspects of capnography and oxygen consumption, *Crit Care Nurs Clin North Am* 1:669, 1989.

32. St. John RE, Baker KA: Pressure-controlled inverse ratio ventilation, *Crit Care Nurs Clin North Am* 3:621, 1991.

33. St. John RE, Lefrak SS: Alternate modes of mechanical ventilation, *AACN Clin Issues Crit Care Nurs* 1:248, 1991.

34. Schuch CS, Price JG: Determination of time required for blood gas homeostasis in the intubated post-open heart surgery adult after ventilator changes, *Heart Lung* 16:364, 1987.

35. Shekleton ME et al: Ineffective airway clearance related to artificial airway, *Nurs Clin North Am* 22:167, 1987.

36. Stauffer JL: Medical management of the airway, *Clin Chest Med* 12:449, 1991.

37. Tasota FJ et al: Evaluation of two methods used to stabilize endotracheal tubes, *Heart Lung* 16:140, 1987.

38. Thomas VM et al: Caring for the person receiving venti-

latory support at home: caregivers' needs and involvement, *Heart Lung* 21:180; 1992.

39. Tobin MJ, Dantzker DR: Mechanical ventilation and weaning. In: Dantzker DR, editor: *Cardiopulmonary critical care,* ed 2, Philadelphia, 1991, WB Saunders.

40. Turner JR et al: Equivalence of continuous flow nebulizer and metered-dose-inhaler with reservoir bag for treatment of acute airflow obstruction, *Chest* 93:476, 1988.

41. Weilitz PB: Weaning from mechanical ventilation: old and new strategies, *Crit Care Nurs Clin North Am* 3:585, 1991.

42. Witmer MT, Hess D, Simmons M: An evaluation of the effectiveness of secretion removal with the Ballard closed-circuit suction catheter, *Respir Care* 36:844, 1991.

Classic

43. Ackerman MH: The bolus use of normal saline instillations in artificial airways: is it useful or necessary? *Heart Lung* 14:505, 1985.

44. Anthonisen NR: Long-term oxygen therapy, *Ann Intern Med* 99:519, 1983.

45. Bartlett RH et al: Studies on the pathogenesis and prevention of postoperative pulmonary complications, *Surg Gynecol Obstet* 137:925, 1973.

46. Christopher KL et al: Transtracheal oxygen therapy for refractory hypoxemia, *JAMA* 256:494, 1986.

47. Cosenza JJ, Norton LC: Secretion clearance: state of the art from a nursing perspective, *Crit Care Nurse* 6:23, 1986.

48. Epstein SW et al: Survey of the clinical use of pressurized aerosol inhalers, *Can Med Assoc J* 120:813, 1979.

49. Grossbach I: Trouble-shooting ventilator and patient related problems (part 1), *Crit Care Nurs* 6:58, 1986.

50. Grossbach I: Trouble-shooting ventilator and patient related problems (part 2), *Crit Care Nurse* 6:64, 1986.

51. Heffner JE, Miller KS, Sahn SA: Tracheostomy in the intensive care unit. Part 1: Indications, technique, management, *Chest* 90:269, 1986.

52. Heffner JE, Miller KS, Sahn SA: Tracheostomy in the intensive care unit. Part 2: Complications, *Chest* 90:430, 1986.

53. Kirilloff LH et al: Does chest physical therapy work? *Chest* 88:436, 1985.

54. Knauss PJ: Chest tube stripping: is it necessary? *Focus Crit Care* 12:41, 1985.

55. Knipper JS: Minimizing complications of tracheal suctioning, *Focus Crit Care* 13:23, 1986.

56. Marini JJ: Postoperative atelectasis: physiology, clinical importance and principles of management, *Respir Care* 29:516, 1984.

57. Norton LC Conforti CG: The effects of body position on oxygenation, *Heart Lung* 14:45, 1985.

58. Orehek J et al: Patient error in use of bronchodilator metered aerosols, *Br Med J* 1:76, 1976.

59. Paterson IC, Crompton GK: Use of pressurized aerosols by asthmatic patients, *Br Med J* 1:76, 1976.

60. Rashkin MC et al: Acute complications of endotracheal intubation, *Chest* 89:165, 1986.

61. Sutton PP et al: Assessment of percussion, vibratory-shaking and breathing exercises in chest physiotherapy, *Eur J Respir Dis* 66:147, 1986.

62. Van Der Schans CP, Piers DA, Postma DS: Effect of manual percussion on tracheobronchial clearance in patients with chronic airflow obstruction and excessive tracheobronchial secretion, *Thorax* 41:448, 1986.

63. Wollmer P et al: Inefficiency of chest percussion in the physical therapy of chronic bronchitis, *Eur J Respir Dis* 66:233, 1985.

64. Zach M, Oberwaldner B, Hausler F: Cystic fibrosis: physical exercise versus chest physiotherapy, *Arch Dis Child* 57:587, 1982.

CHAPTER TWENTY-SEVEN

Nursing Management of Adults with Upper Airway Disorders

LEARNING OBJECTIVES

1 Relate principles of nursing management to the care of patients with disorders of the upper airway.

2 Discuss the role of drug therapy in the management of patients with inflammatory disorders of the upper airway.

3 Identify treatment measures for the patient experiencing nasal trauma.

4 List the risk factors that contribute to the development of cancer of the larynx.

5 Identify measures to promote communication for the patient after a laryngectomy.

6 Describe the psychologic impact of laryngeal cancer and its treatment.

KEY TERMS

Caldwell-Luc procedure, p. 591
coryza, p. 592
deviated septum, p. 597
epistaxis, p. 600
esophageal speech, p. 610
hemilaryngectomy, p. 606
laryngitis, p. 593
nasal septoplasty, p. 597

pharyngitis, p. 592
radical neck dissection, p. 607
rhinitis, p. 592
rhinorrhea, p. 592
saddle deformity, p. 597
sinusitis, p. 589
submucosal resection, p. 597
total laryngectomy, p. 606

THE PRIMARY function of the upper airway structures is to provide a direct link between the external environment and the lungs. Besides this role in respiratory function, the upper airways also provide sense organs for taste and smell. Verbal communication is also facilitated by the larynx.

The effects of disorders of the upper airways are not limited to changes in respiratory function. The diseases and injuries of the upper airways also have the potential to affect nutrition, communication, body image, and social interaction. Many of these disease processes are not life-threatening. However, because they can develop into chronic health problems, they can permanently alter a patient's life.

SINUSITIS
Definition

Sinusitis is an inflammation of one or more of the nasal sinuses. The sinuses are air-filled cavities lined

589

with mucous membranes. They decrease the weight of the skull and add resonance to the voice.

Etiology/Epidemiology

Sinusitis may be acute or chronic. Acute sinusitis commonly accompanies or follows an upper respiratory tract infection. Sinusitis, especially of the maxillary sinus, may occur as a sequela of dental abscess or tooth extraction. Commonly all of the anterior sinuses (frontal, ethmoid, and maxillary) are affected. *Haemophilus in; uenzae, Streptococcus pyogenes,* and *Streptococcus pneumoniae,* as well as some anaerobes including bacteroids, are pathogens that commonly cause acute sinusitis. The mucous membranes become thickened from prolonged or repeated inflammation and infection. Anaerobic pathogens are the more common infectious cause of chronic sinusitis. Fungus may also cause chronic infections, particularly in immunosuppressed patients. Noninfectious contributors to chronic sinusitis include smoking, habitual nasal sprays or inhalants, and a history of allergy.

Pathophysiology

The sinuses drain into the middle meatus of the nose. Sinusitis may be caused by blockage of sinus drainage or by spread of infection from the nasal passages. Because the nasal and sinus mucous membranes are continuous, contamination of the sinuses may easily occur via this route.

Any process that impairs sinus drainage may cause accumulation of secretions in the sinuses. Nasal polyps, deviated septum, mucous membrane edema caused by irritation from viral invasion, inhalation of foreign substances, or allergic reactions may impair sinus drainage or cause total sinus obstruction. Bacterial contamination of these pooled secretions produces infection.

Clinical Manifestations

The clinical manifestations of sinusitis are the result of the infectious process and the pressure exerted by the secretions accumulating in the sinus. The patient often complains of a headache and tenderness or pain over the affected sinuses. Acute sinusitis headache or pain is usually constant and severe. Chronic sinusitis pain is described as dull and may be constant or intermittent. Symptoms of sinusitis may worsen for the first 3 to 4 hours after the patient rises and improve later as secretions drain. Coughing may be precipitated by drainage of secretions into the pharynx. Swallowed secretions may induce nausea or vomiting. Fever, elevated white blood cell count, sore throat, and purulent nasal drainage may be present and are worse in acute sinusitis. Foul-smelling, purulent drainage may indicate an anaerobic infection. Periorbital edema and purulent eye drainage are common in small children, although adults may also have these symptoms. Finally, anosmia (absence of sense of smell), hyposmia (decreased sense of smell), and decreased sense of taste may occur.

During physical examination, transillumination of the sinuses should be evaluated. Transillumination is performed by having the patient hold a flashlight bulb inside his or her closed mouth. Normally the sinuses will glow. Purulent secretions accumulating in the sinuses will cause those areas to appear darker than the other sinuses.

Definitive diagnosis of sinusitis is made by x-ray examination. Multiple views of the head are required to allow visualization of all the sinuses. Mucosal thickening of pus in the sinuses results in a cloudy appearance on x-ray film. Only approximately 10% of those patients who think they have sinusitis are actually diagnosed by x-ray examination as having the disorder.

Complications of sinusitis are primarily attributable to the spread of the infection and usually occur after an acute exacerbation of chronic sinusitis. Bacteremia, sepsis, periorbital abscess, or cellulitis may occur. If the maxillary sinus is the site of infection, oroantral fistula (development of a tract connecting the maxillary sinus and the mouth) may occur. Extension of the infection may cause meningitis or subdural, epidural, or brain abscess. Hearing loss may result from edema of the eustachian tube.

Therapeutic Management

The major therapeutic goals in the treatment of sinusitis are to achieve sinus drainage, control the infection, and relieve pain. These goals are achieved with the use of medications or surgery.

Drug therapy

Drug therapy is primarily aimed at resolution of infection and relief of symptoms.

Antibiotics

Broad-spectrum antibiotics to which the infecting organism is sensitive limit the duration and extent of infection. The physician commonly prescribes one of the following drugs: ampicillin, amoxicillin, amoxicillin/potassium clavulanate, erythromycin, cefaclor, cefuroxime, and clindamycin. Antibiotics are used judiciously in chronic sinusitis to prevent organism resistance. A patient with chronic sinusitis with a suspected acute infection will be given a drug, such as clindamycin, that treats anaerobes.

Analgesics

Pain relief may be achieved by using ibuprofen, acetaminophen, or codeine. Aspirin may be associated with polyposis and is usually not recommended. In particularly painful cases of sinusitis, stronger narcotics may be required.

Decongestants

Nasal spray or oral decongestants are used to treat sinusitis to decrease edema in the nasal mucosa. Decreasing edema will decrease the size of the turbinates and minimize obstruction of sinus drainage. Most decongestants (such as pseudoephedrine) exert sympathomimetic effects. In addition to vasoconstriction, they may produce increased heart rate and contractility. These effects are usually of minor importance. However, in patients with preexisting heart disease, such preparations may cause dysrhythmias, hypertension, and increased myocardial oxygen demand. Patients taking other sympathomimetic drugs should be closely monitored for potential drug interactions. Concomitant administration of these drugs and monoamine oxidase inhibitors is contraindicated.

Antihistamines

Antihistamines, such as dexchlorpheniramine or diphenhydramine, may be useful in the management of symptoms of sinusitis. These drugs interfere with the increased capillary permeability and vasodilation caused by histamine. Antihistamines also exert anticholinergic effects that result in decreased nasal congestion and facilitate sinus drainage. Antihistamines may also increase the viscosity of secretions and possibly hinder sinus drainage. Close monitoring is required when administering anticholinergics to patients with endocrine disorders, hypertension, urinary disorders, and glaucoma. Newer antihistamines such as astemizole (Hismanal) and terfenadine (Seldane) have the advantage of longer duration of action, which requires less frequent dosing. In addition, these drugs produce little sedation.

Saline

Some physicians recommend regular use of saline nose drops or sprays to facilitate sinus drainage. Best deposition of the medication occurs when the head is tipped back and to the side on which the drops are to be instilled. Five minutes in each position (right and left side) may be necessary for the drops to reach the posterior nares (Figure 27-1).

Intranasal steroids

Intranasal steroid drops and sprays should not be used during acute sinusitis, since they may impair the local immune response to infection. However, they may reduce tissue edema associated with allergic and inflammatory causes of sinusitis.

Surgical management

If adequate drainage of the sinuses does not occur with medications, surgical intervention may be required. This varies from simple sinus irrigation to removal of the mucous membranes. Drainage may be facilitated by irrigation of the sinuses with normal saline via the natural ostia, or openings, in the nose. Surgical insertion of a trocar into the sinus is an alternative method for performing irrigation and facilitating drainage. Nasal secretions obtained from irrigation of the sinuses may be cultured and tested for sensitivity.

In patients with chronic sinusitis, surgery may be performed to correct any structural abnormalities, such as deviated septum or nasal polyps, that may be obstructing sinus drainage. Surgical removal of the sinus mucous membranes, such as sphenoidectomy, ethmoidectomy, or orosteoplastic flap surgery (frontal), may also improve drainage in chronic sinusitis.

The **Caldwell-Luc procedure** is a surgical procedure used in chronic maxillary sinusitis. The surgical approach is made via an incision in the upper gums into the maxillary sinus. The sinus is cleared of infected secretions and mucous membranes. To promote normal sinus drainage, antrostomy (opening in the midanterior portion of the inferior turbinate) is performed. Temporary numbness of the upper lip and teeth occurs in some patients who receive the Caldwell-Luc procedure, because some nerves supplying these structures are traumatized. Chewing may also be impaired. Because of nasal

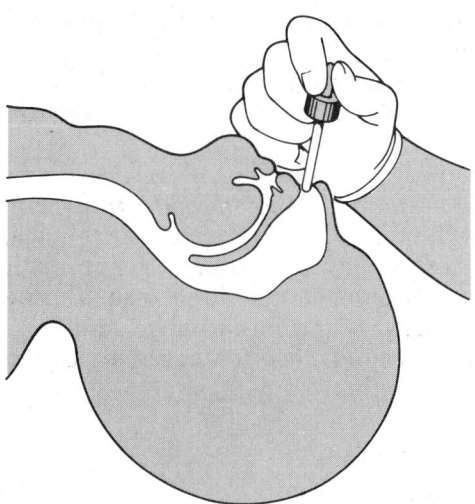

FIGURE 27-1   Instilling nose drops.

packing, the patient must mouth breathe until the packing is removed. Patients are also unable to wear dentures or blow their nose until the incision is healed in about 10 to 14 days.

RHINITIS
Definition/Etiology

Rhinitis is defined as inflammation of the mucous membranes of the nasopharynx. Rhinitis may be acute or chronic. Types of rhinitis include acute viral rhinitis, allergic rhinitis, nonallergic vasomotor rhinitis, and eosinophilic vasomotor rhinitis. Most lay persons refer to rhinitis as a runny nose **(rhinorrhea)** or cold.

Rhinitis is commonly caused by viral infection, as in acute rhinitis or the common cold, **coryza.** Acute viral rhinitis is the most common infectious disease in humanity. Known organisms in acute viral rhinitis include rhinovirus, adenovirus, echovirus, influenza virus, parainfluenza virus, and coxsackievirus. The mode of transmission is by droplet contamination, usually from sneezing. Almost everyone has developed acute viral rhinitis at some time, although children are more susceptible than adults. Crowded conditions, fatigue, and poor nutrition also contribute to the spread of acute viral rhinitis.

Exposure to allergens may cause rhinitis in sensitive individuals. This allergic rhinitis, or "hay fever," may occur in a seasonal or a random pattern, depending on the allergens involved. Sensitivity to allergens such as pollen results in a seasonal pattern. Sensitivity to allergens such as dust or animal dander results in an intermittent pattern.

Psychologic stressors may also trigger rhinitis. This type of rhinitis, nonallergic vasomotor rhinitis, closely resembles allergic rhinitis except for the presence of a precipitating allergen. In nonallergic vasomotor rhinitis, no allergen can be identified.

Finally, eosinophilic nonallergic rhinitis may be precipitated by agents that irritate the nasal mucosa, such as smoke, alcohol, or temperature and humidity changes. Eosinophilic nonallergic rhinitis is similar to nonallergic vasomotor rhinitis, except for the presence of eosinophils in nasal secretions in the former.

Pathophysiology

Irritation of nasal mucosa results in nasal discharge and edema of nasal mucosa. If mucosal edema becomes sufficiently severe, nasal obstruction may occur. Persistent rhinitis may result in fibrous scarring of subepithelial connective tissue and atrophy of mucus-secreting glands. When the causative agent of rhinitis is viral infection, the immune response is triggered. In allergic rhinitis, response to allergens results in histamine release.

Clinical Manifestations

Patients with rhinitis of any type commonly have sneezing and nasal discharge. Although nasal secretions are usually thin and watery, mucoid or purulent drainage may also occur, especially in chronic rhinitis. Frontal or generalized headache may accompany rhinitis. In acute rhinitis, the patient may experience cough, fever, sore throat, and malaise. Sore throat is especially common when the patient mouth breathes or has excessive postnasal drainage. Secondary infection, such as otitis media, bronchitis, or pneumonia, may complicate acute viral rhinitis. Itching and tearing of the eyes and sometimes itching of the nose are observed in early phases of acute viral rhinitis and throughout the course of allergic rhinitis, nonallergic rhinitis, and eosinophilic vasomotor rhinitis.

Mucous membranes in acute forms of rhinitis appear red and swollen. The nasal mucosa of patients with allergic rhinitis is characteristically swollen, pale (gray to dull red), and boggy. Nasal polyps may also be found in patients with allergic rhinitis. When frequent nose blowing is required, skin around the nose and upper lip may become excoriated.

Therapeutic Management

Management of rhinitis is directed at eliminating the precipitating factor and alleviating symptoms. There are no cures for rhinitis.

For acute rhinitis, rest and fluid intake should be encouraged to support the immune system, to mobilize secretions, and to combat viral infection. Antipyretic agents and analgesics are useful in controlling fever and relieving pain, respectively.

Patients commonly use an over-the-counter antihistamine, decongestant, or combination medication to relieve symptoms of itchy, watery eyes, and runny nose. Although many patients believe high doses of vitamin C are useful in treating acute rhinitis, the literature does not support this practice. The physician prescribes antibiotics for treating secondary infections.

For allergic rhinitis, nonallergic vasomotor rhinitis, and eosinophilic nonallergic rhinitis, elimination of the offending agent is the treatment of choice. Antihistamines may give some symptomatic relief; however, prolonged use often results in decreased effectiveness. When nasal polyps are present, surgery (polypectomy) is often necessary to remove the nasal obstruction.

PHARYNGITIS
Definition/Etiology

Pharyngitis is an inflammation of the pharynx or throat. The most common cause of acute pharyngitis is viral invasion. Bacterial infection by streptococci, termed *strep throat,* is a severe form of acute pharyngitis. Staphylococci and the diplococci *Neisseria gonorrhoeae* are other common bacterial causes of pharyngitis. Pharyngitis may accompany mononucleosis.

Pathophysiology

Invasion of a pharyngeal mucosa usually begins by droplet transmission. The incubation period varies from a few hours to several days, depending on the organism. Pharyngitis is communicable. Mucous membranes become inflamed and edematous. The tonsils are often involved.

Clinical Manifestations

A sore throat is the most common complaint. The patient may also complain of a dry or scratchy throat. Severe pain and dysphagia are common with strep throat. A dry, hacking cough may be present. Fever is often present. Examination of the throat reveals redness and edema. White plaques may also be observed. When sinusitis or rhinitis accompanies pharyngitis, secretions may be seen on the posterior wall of the pharynx.

Therapeutic Management

Treatment of viral pharyngitis is symptomatic. The patient is advised to increase fluid intake and get more rest. Analgesics, antipyretics, and anesthetic throat lozenges may be used. An ice collar or warm saline throat gargles may also relieve pain. Humidity via a humidifier or steam vaporizer provides symptomatic relief. A liquid or semisolid diet is preferred, because it may not irritate the throat as does a regular diet.

When the physician suspects a bacterial cause of pharyngitis, a throat culture is performed. Antibiotics, such as penicillin and erythromycin, are used to treat severe infections. The patient with valvular heart disease (rheumatic fever, endocarditis) may take prophylactic antibiotics during viral pharyngitis to prevent infection.

TONSILLITIS
Definition

Acute tonsillitis is an acute inflammation of the tonsils and their crypts.

Etiology

Acute tonsillitis is usually caused by streptococci or less commonly by staphylococci. Tonsillitis is common in children, although adults may also be af-

fected. An episode of tonsillitis occurs more often when the patient's resistance to infection is low, such as after a viral illness or excessive fatigue.

Pathophysiology

Pharyngitis is commonly associated with tonsillitis. Infection in the pharynx drains via the lymphatics to involve the tonsils. An intense inflammatory response occurs, causing edema, hyperemia, and sometimes copious pus. Tonsillar and peritonsillar hypertrophy may progress to occlude the airway. The mucosal epithelium may be destroyed, resulting in superficial or penetrating cryptic abscesses. A peritonsillar abscess is also termed *quinsy sore throat.*

Clinical Manifestations

The first sign of tonsillitis is marked enlargement of the tonsils. The tonsils are reddened and edematous. The patient complains of a sore throat, pain on swallowing that may radiate to the ear, and general muscle aching. A soft, gray-white exudate may be present on the tonsils, signifying abscess. The patient usually has a high-grade fever and leukocytosis.

Therapeutic Management

Treatment of tonsillitis is directed at eliminating infection. A throat culture is usually performed to identify the organism, and therapy with antibiotics is initiated. If tonsillitis progresses to a peritonsillar abscess, incision and drainage are often necessary. Repeated episodes of tonsillitis may require removal of the tonsils (tonsillectomy) 4 to 6 weeks after an acute attack. Complications of untreated tonsillitis are varied. Cardiac and renal damage may occur, as well as pneumonia. Early diagnosis and the use of antibiotics have led to lower incidence of complications.

LARYNGITIS
Definition

Laryngitis is the inflammation of mucous membranes in the lining of the larynx. The common disorder may be either acute or chronic.

Etiology

Acute laryngitis may be a result of a bacterial or viral agent that attacks the larynx, the subglottis area, and the epiglottis. Often, however, laryngitis is not an isolated disorder but a part of a general upper respiratory tract infection, such as the common cold or sore throat. Trauma from irritants, such as inhalation of toxic or irritating fumes (smoking), vocal abuse (public speaking, occupational overuse), endotracheal intubation, and alcohol ingestion can cause acute as well as chronic laryngitis. In addition, chronic laryngitis may be caused by repeated attacks of acute laryngitis, allergies, chronic tonsillitis, and adenoiditis.

Pathophysiology

When acute laryngitis is found in combination with an upper respiratory infection, viruses are the usual infectious agents. Organisms such as *Streptococcus pneumoniae* and beta-hemolytic streptococci will cause acute laryngitis in the form of a sore throat. Laryngitis will also occur in conjunction with pneumonia, influenza, tracheitis, and bronchitis. *Haemophilus influenzae* causes acute epiglottitis in adults. These infectious organisms, along with the noninfectious causes mentioned earlier, result in the acute inflammation of the laryngeal mucosa. The vocal cords become edematous. Chronic laryngitis results in inflammatory changes in the laryngeal mucosa. Over time, serious voice disability occurs.

Clinical Manifestations

The signs and symptoms of acute laryngitis usually begin with hoarseness that progresses to aphonia. Fever, malaise, pain on swallowing, scratchy throat, and dry cough may occur also. In severe cases, stridor and dyspnea can be present. The true vocal cords appear swollen and red rather than white without rounded edges. Secretions can be seen on the vocal cords or in the trachea. The entire laryngeal area is erythematous.

The patient with chronic laryngitis develops progressive hoarseness, which commonly is worse in the morning as dried secretions accumulate in the larynx. Hoarseness improves through the day and worsens again in the evening. Pain is usually not present, nor is there a productive cough. The patient usually clears the throat frequently and has a dry, harsh cough. The laryngeal mucosa appears uniformly red but smooth with no swelling. In some cases polypoid growths will be visualized. This condition, called chronic polypoid laryngitis, is often found in patients who have a long history of smoking.

Laryngitis is usually diagnosed by clinical signs and symptoms, although direct or indirect laryngoscopy can be performed. Indirect, or mirror, laryngoscopy can be quickly and easily performed in the physician's office, clinic, or emergency room, and serves for most diagnostic purposes. Direct laryngoscopy can be performed with the patient under either local or general anesthesia. These examinations will reveal (1) abnormalities in the true cords, (2) reddened, inflamed mucosa, or (3) secretions on the vocal cords.

Therapeutic Management

The treatment of acute laryngitis is usually directed at relief of symptoms. Patient symptoms may be relieved by the use of analgesic/antipyretic agents, such as acetaminophen or aspirin, antitussive medications, throat sprays or lozenges, steam or cool mist inhalations, and rest. The patient should avoid talking and smoking. When infection is present, antibiotics, such as penicillin or ampicillin, are prescribed. Steroids may rarely be used to decrease swelling.

Severe cases of acute laryngitis require hospitalization. Vocal cord edema can become severe enough to close off the airway. An emergency tracheostomy must then be performed.

Chronic laryngitis improves with avoidance or removal of irritants, correction of faulty voice habits, and treatments of chronic tonsillitis and adenoiditis. Stripping vocal cord polyps can be performed with the patient under local or general anesthesia. Measures for symptomatic relief are similar to those for acute laryngitis.

NURSING MANAGEMENT OF THE PATIENT WITH SINUSITIS, RHINITIS, PHARYNGITIS, TONSILLITIS, OR LARYNGITIS

Assessment

The nursing assessment of a patient with suspected sinusitis, rhinitis, pharyngitis, tonsillitis, or laryngitis share many common factors. The nurse questions the patient regarding potential causes of infection or inflammation. The patient is questioned regarding recent upper respiratory tract infections, smoking habits, or history of allergy. Specifically, if the nurse suspects sinusitis, any history of deviated septum or nasal polyps or recent dental work might point to the cause of the disorder. Further, the patient may be able to identify environmental factors that contribute to sinusitis. Some of the patients experience worse sinusitis in chilly, cold, damp environments, whereas others complain that dry, hot air is more irritating.

A complete list of over-the-counter and prescription medications used by the patient is obtained. The nurse carefully questions the patient to determine proper use of antibiotics, analgesics, decongestants, and antihistamines. The nurse identifies improper overuse or underuse of any of these medications.

The nurse assesses the patient for pain, swelling, or tenderness of the facial bones if sinusitis is suspected. A lighted scope or flashlight is used to identify clouding of the sinuses if the cause is infectious sinusitis. Vital signs are taken to identify fever and hemodynamic stability. The throat is examined for erythema, exudate, and swelling of the tonsils. Airway obstruction may exist if any of the upper airway structures become swollen, so the nurse completes a thorough respiratory assessment, paying particular attention to breathing pattern and upper airway auscultation.

The nurse examines the patient for potential complications of any of these disorders. The patient with chronic sinusitis is at risk to develop infections outside the bony structures of the sinuses. Therefore the nurse completes a neurologic assessment if meningitis or brain abscess is suspected.

Nursing Diagnosis

Nursing diagnoses for the patient with sinusitis, rhinitis, pharyngitis, tonsillitis, and laryngitis are similar. The nurse chooses those that are specific to the individual and to the etiology. The etiology and to some degree, the management will depend on the anatomic involvement and whether the underlying cause is infectious or only inflammatory. These diagnoses may include:

Ineffective airway clearance related to increased secretions or nasal packing, or airway obstruction caused by swollen membranes

Pain related to pressure and/or inflammation

Fatigue related to excessive coughing and/or infection

Risk for noncompliance related to knowledge deficit of therapeutic and preventive measures

High risk for hyperthermia related to infection

Sensory alterations (olfactory or gustatory) related to tissue inflammation

Impaired tissue integrity related to frequent nasal drainage or surgical incision

Hemorrhage related to surgical intervention for sinusitis or tonsillitis

Impaired verbal communication related to laryngeal inflammation

Dysphagia related to pharyngeal inflammation or edema

Planning

General goals for the care of the patient with sinusitis, rhinitis, pharyngitis, or laryngitis may include the following:

Sinus drainage and maintenance of a patent airway

Pain relief

Verbalization of knowledge about the disease and its treatment and ability to describe actions and potential side effects of medications

Four to six hours of sleep a day with decreased fatigue

Patient will verbalize and practice health care measures to prevent recurrence of the disorder

Normal temperature before discharge

Improved or normal sense of smell and taste

Normal healing of incision without evidence of infection (for surgical intervention of chronic sinusitis or tonsillitis)

Return of normal voice (laryngitis) and ability to swallow (pharyngitis)

Implementation

The nursing care of a patient begins with teaching the patient about the disease and its treatment, including proper use of antibiotics. The nurse stresses the importance of completing an antibiotic prescription even though symptoms have improved. The intermittent use of decongestants and antihistamines is discussed. The patient is cautioned that antihistamines may cause drowsiness, and decongestants may cause sleeplessness or loss of appetite. Failure of a decongestant, antihistamine, or analgesic to relieve symptoms should be reported to the physician. The patient is instructed in proper use of nasal sprays or drops (see Patient Education Guides on p. 596 and below).

 **PATIENT EDUCATION GUIDE**

Rhinitis

Avoid exposure to viral rhinitis including crowds, people with colds, day care centers

Remove potential allergens from the environment, including animals; woolen products; foods such as eggs, milk, or chocolate; smoke from cigarettes, cigars, or pipes; carpets and throw rugs; and cloth window coverings

Prevent further infection by:

 Disposing of tissues properly

 Avoiding use of cloth handkerchiefs

 Using good hand-washing technique

 Covering mouth and nose when coughing and sneezing

 Blowing nose with both nostrils open to avoid forcing matter into sinuses or ears

 Keeping skin dry under and around nose

Get additional rest

Drink 2 to 4 L of fluids daily

Medications

 Analgesics

 Antihistamines—effective at first sign of cold; use with caution if drowsiness occurs

 Decongestants—use intermittently to prevent rebound congestion

PATIENT EDUCATION GUIDE

Sinusitis

Environmental factors

Stop smoking

Avoid allergens

Avoid exposure to cold, damp conditions (including air conditioning)

Obtain adequate sleep and rest and dietary intake

Drink sufficient amounts of fluids

Notify physician of persistent or increased sinus pain, fever, or change in drainage characteristics

Medications

Continue taking antibiotics as instructed for the duration of the prescription; do not discontinue them when you feel better

Use decongestants and antihistamines for relief of symptoms only when necessary; frequent use may decrease effectiveness

Use nasal irrigation as ordered

Avoid aspirin

The nurse must instruct patients with laryngitis to rest their voices and provide nonverbal alternatives to communication for the duration of voice rest. If the laryngitis is severe and associated with significant airway obstruction, the nurse must be particularly attentive to the patient's breathing pattern, frequently assessing the patient for respiratory distress. An altered breathing pattern or abnormal vital signs usually appear before the development of stridor. If breathing becomes more difficult, the physician is notified immediately. A tracheostomy tray may be kept at the bedside.

Comfort measures may relieve some of the pain associated with sinusitis or the other disorders. These might include application of a moist, warm facecloth over involved sinuses, adequate humidification of the air, or use of cool-mist inhalation therapy to promote drainage of mucus from the sinuses or nose and provide relief of sinus pain or sore throat.

Environmental factors that may aggravate sinusitis or put the patient at risk for infection are discussed with the patient. Exposure to cold and damp conditions should be minimized. Avoiding air-conditioned environments may also be recommended. The patient should not smoke or be around others who smoke. If the patient is susceptible to frequent upper respiratory tract infections, he or she should avoid crowded places. The patient is encouraged also to get adequate rest and hydration.

Evaluation

The patient will be able to demonstrate knowledge of the disease and its treatment(s) by appropriate use of medications, appropriate health-seeking behaviors if symptoms recur or do not improve. The patient's upper airway will drain secretions and remain patent. Vital signs will return to baseline. No signs of infection or hemorrhage will develop if surgery was performed for sinusitis or tonsillitis. Radiologic examination of the sinuses or upper airway will return to normal when indicated. If the larynx was involved in the process, hoarseness should decrease in 2 to 3 days and resolve completely within 2 weeks.

Documentation

Documentation of care for the patient with any of these infectious or inflammatory disorders begins with accurate recording of the patient history, including symptoms and medications used. The nurse records vital signs and pertinent physical assessment readings. The nurse is careful to document color, consistency, and odor of nasal secretions, as well as the presence, location, and quality of pain. The nurse notes patient allergies, especially to antibiotics and pain medications. A record of the patient's response to analgesics is included by the nurse. The nurse notes the patient and family's response to teaching. The nurse records the patient's activity level and assessment of fatigue/rest state. An estimation of fluid intake is placed in the medical record. The nurse reports color and edema of mucous membranes, as well as skin condition and temperatures. If respiratory distress occurs related to airway obstruction, the nurse reports the rate and depth of the breathing pattern and presence of stridor or other upper airway noises.

VOCAL CORD NODULES
Definition

Vocal cord nodules are benign growths that form at the junction of the anterior one third or posterior two thirds of the vocal cords.

Etiology/Epidemiology

Nodules result from chronic vocal abuse and are also referred to as singer's, teacher's, or preacher's nodules. Nodules are more common in females at any age.

Clinical Manifestations

The nodules first appear red and raised over the vocal cord surface, then change into small, white lumps that touch when the cords approximate. Because they are raised, nodules prop the cords apart. A characteristic hoarse, breathy voice is produced.

Therapeutic Management

Conservative treatment is usually effective. Complete voice rest often causes even large nodules to disappear. Speech therapy may be prescribed after voice rest to restore a normal voice and prevent recurrences of nodules. Surgical removal is easily performed by indirect laryngoscopy after the patient receives a local anesthetic. The patient is encouraged to observe complete voice rest or to whisper to cause less trauma.

VOCAL CORD POLYPS
Definition

Polyps are edematous masses of mucous membranes that can appear anywhere on the vocal cords but tend to be unilateral. Most polyps have a broad-base attachment to the cord, which results in permanent interference with voice production. However, some polyps hang under the vocal cord and cause only intermittent symptoms.

Etiology/Epidemiology/Clinical Manifestations

Vocal cord polyps usually develop because of chronic voice abuse, inhalation of toxic irritants such as smoke, allergies, and commonly acute upper respiratory tract infections. They are commonly found in adults who have allergies, live in dry climates, or smoke. Painful hoarseness is the only symptom.

Therapeutic Management

Surgical stripping, which permits firm mucosal regeneration, can be performed with the patient under either local or general anesthesia. During the stripping procedure, care is taken to avoid stripping the cords all the way to the anterior commissure, the point where the vocal cords meet at the midline. A laryngeal web, which is more commonly a congenital disorder, may form where the two raw surfaces meet. Surgical stripping may be performed in two stages to avoid this.

NURSING MANAGEMENT OF THE PATIENT WITH VOCAL CORD NODULES AND POLYPS

Nursing management of the patient with vocal cord nodules and polyps is similar to nursing management of patients with laryngitis.

DEVIATED SEPTUM
Definition

Nasal obstruction is commonly caused by displacement of the nasal septum from the midline position. This condition is termed **deviated septum.**

Etiology/Epidemiology

The nasal septum is usually straight and midline at birth, although a congenital deviated septum may occur. Nasal trauma is the most common cause of deviated septum in both children and adults. Some degree of nasal septal deviation is present in many adults.

Pathophysiology

Septal deviation is not pathologic unless the disorder results in nasal obstruction. Protrusion of the septal cartilage into one nasal passage may cause partial or total obstruction. The severity of nasal obstruction does not correlate well with the observed degree of septal deviation.

Clinical Manifestations

The most common symptom of patients with septal deviation is nasal obstruction. The patient or family member may complain of snoring during sleep. Breathing while awake may also be noisy or difficult. Pressing one nostril against the nose to occlude air flow and asking the patient to inhale through the other nostril is one technique to determine obstruction. Patients may also experience headache, epistaxis, postnasal drip, or sinusitis. Examination of the nose shows protrusion of the septum into one nostril.

Therapeutic Management

Surgical intervention—submucosal resection or nasal septoplasty—is required for the treatment of septal deviation. Patients receive a local anesthetic to undergo these procedures. With **submucosal resection** an incision is made into the nasal mucous membrane, and the bone and cartilage producing the deviation are removed. The nasal mucosa is laid back in place, and both nostrils are packed to prevent bleeding and to maintain the mucosa in the midline position. The packing usually remains in place for 24 to 48 hours. **Nasal septoplasty** involves reconstruction of the septum and may also include rhinoplasty—reconstruction of the external nose (see Chapter 76).

Complications of this procedure include septal tearing and saddle deformity. **Saddle deformity** is the formation of a depression in the bridge of the nose. This depression results from the removal of the support structures (bone and cartilage) or from retraction of the scar tissue over the incisional site.

NURSING MANAGEMENT OF THE PATIENT WITH A DEVIATED SEPTUM
Assessment

Preoperative nursing assessment of the patient with a deviated septum focuses on the patient history, particularly regarding symptoms of nasal obstruction, and patient understanding of the problem and the procedure.

Postoperative nursing assessment focuses on early detection of complications, such as bleeding and airway obstruction. The nurse assesses vital signs, especially pulse, which may indicate blood volume deficit. In addition to bleeding that is visible from the nasal packing drip pad, the patient may also bleed through the posterior nasal pharynx and swallow large, unquantified amounts of blood without the nurse's knowledge.

The nurse also assesses for normal breathing pattern and rate to identify airway obstruction, remembering that the patient will be breathing exclusively from the mouth while the packing is in place. Localized pain, edema, and skin discoloration are usually present for several days after surgery. The nurse identifies increases or decreases in these signs or symptoms.

Finally, the nurse assesses appetite. Postnasal drainage, the presence of old blood in the nose and mouth, dryness of the mouth from mouth breathing, anosmia, and anesthesia contribute to anorexia, nausea, or vomiting.

Nursing Diagnosis

Nursing diagnoses for the patient with septal deviation surgery include but are not limited to the following:
High risk for decreased cardiac output related to bleeding
Ineffective airway clearance related to increased secretions or nasal packing
High risk for infection related to surgical procedure
Noncompliance related to medication usage
Anxiety related to surgical procedure
Body image disturbance related to facial swelling and discoloration
Altered oral mucous membrane related to mouth breathing
Pain related to surgical procedure

Planning

Appropriate goals for the patient with septal deviation surgery include the following:
Normal vital signs
Patent airway
Surgical wounds will remain free of infection without purulent drainage
Patient reports appropriate medication usage including action, side effects, and consequences of overuse or underuse
Patient verbalizes decreased anxiety and demonstrates normalized vital signs
Patient verbalizes body image changes and identifies coping mechanisms
Mucous membranes remain moist and noninfected
Pain relief

Implementation

Preoperative nursing interventions center around patient teaching. The patient is instructed that a nasal pack will be in place postoperatively and that this will require mouth breathing. The patient is encouraged to practice mouth breathing and swallowing with an occluded nose before the procedure. The postoperative routine is fully explained, including the need to expectorate rather than swallow all secretions. Throat-clearing coughs are preferred to deep coughs. The patient learns that a drip pad will be placed under the nose to catch blood and secretions (Figure 27-2). Frequent assessment of drainage and vital signs will be made.

Postoperatively, the patient may be lethargic if sedatives have been administered. Therefore the bed should be in the low position with the siderails up until the patient is fully alert.

The patient may experience some pain, although pain after nasal septal surgery is usually minimal. Administration of mild analgesics generally achieves satisfactory pain control. The application of cold to the area may provide additional pain relief while the resultant vasoconstriction may diminish bleeding. Elevation of the head of the bed may decrease nasal edema and facilitate drainage.

The duration of hospitalization for septal deviation surgery is limited, usually same day or next day discharge. Therefore it is important that the patient be given sufficient self-care home instruction (see box on p. 599).

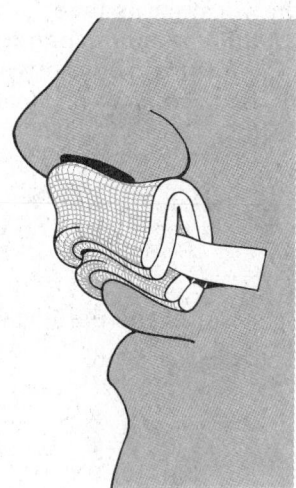

FIGURE 27-2   Nasal drip pad.

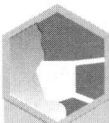

POSTOPERATIVE NURSING INTERVENTIONS

Deviated Septum

Avoid trauma to the nose; do not blow nose or sneeze vigorously

Avoid strenuous activities, such as exercise and vigorous coughing, as well as constipation; in particular, the Valsalva maneuver should be avoided because it increases the blood pressure and may stress the incision

Avoid swimming, at least until the first postoperative visit; this will prevent exposure of the incision to contaminants potentially present in the water

Avoid smoking and the use of nose drops or nasal sprays (unless specifically prescribed)

Change drip pad when soiled

Observe for increased bloody drainage on drip pad, foul-smelling secretions, fever, and bright-red vomitus

Keep ice compresses on nose for 24 hours

Rinse mouth frequently with mouthwash or diluted hydrogen peroxide

Increase fluid intake

Avoid nose blowing and sneezing unless physician gives approval

Evaluation

Several areas should be evaluated. Vital signs indicate normal or insufficient blood volume, as well as presence of anxiety, infection, or compromised airway. Increased swallowing, bright-red blood on the drip pad, or bright-red vomitus indicate possible hemorrhage. The nurse identifies patient response to analgesic administration, as well as other comfort measures, such as elevating the head of the bed and applying cold compresses. The nurse evaluates the patient's ability to chew food and to swallow in order to assess the risk for inadequate nutrition or aspiration.

Documentation

As always, documentation of nursing care begins with recording the patient history, including medication use. The nurse documents vital signs. The amount of drainage from the nose is often estimated by documenting frequency of drip pad changes over a given period. The nurse includes in the progress notes medication administration for sedation or pain relief, as well as comfort or antianxiety measures. Documentation of patient or family teaching preop-

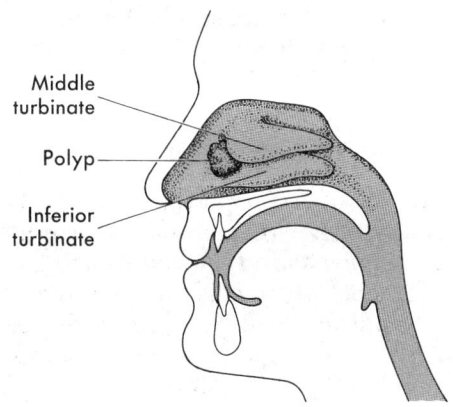

FIGURE 27-3   Nasal polyps.

eratively and postoperatively is an important part of the medical record.

NASAL POLYPS
Definition

Nasal polyps are smooth, round outgrowths from the nasal septum (Figure 27-3). They usually have a stemlike base, which attaches the polyp to the septum and makes them fairly movable.

Etiology/Epidemiology

Nasal polyps originate from mucous membranes of the nose or sinuses as a result of recurrent localized swelling. They commonly occur in patients with chronic allergic rhinitis or asthma. Aspirin sensitivity is suggested in asthma patients with polyps. Although polyps may be unilateral, they are usually bilateral.

Pathophysiology

Polyps are caused by irritation of mucous membranes from an allergy or sinusitis. A polyp is small at first, but with each occurrence of submucosal edema, its size increases. A fully developed polyp protruding into the airway appears as a smooth, pale tumor. In many cases, polyps are multiple and can cause deformity of the nasal bones. Anosmia is a common problem in patients with nasal polyps. The major complications of nasal polyps are nasal obstruction and sinusitis.

Clinical Manifestations

Many patients are unaware of the presence of nasal polyps. Nasal polyps are seen by insertion of a lighted nasal speculum into the nose. The patient may complain of decreased air flow on the side of the polyp; symptoms of sinusitis may also be present.

Therapeutic Management

The treatment of nasal polyps is surgical removal (polypectomy). After the patient receives a local anesthetic, the polyps are removed by using a "snare," or biting forceps, which clips the polyps at the stalk. The nose is packed with gauze for 24 hours. Pain is minimal. Because polyps tend to recur, surgery is often repeated and may include sinus surgery. Corticosteroid nasal sprays are also effective at reducing polyp size. However, once the steroid is discontinued, polyps may grow larger or recur.

NURSING MANAGEMENT OF THE PATIENT WITH NASAL POLYPS

Assessment

The degree of nasal obstruction is assessed in the patient with nasal polyps. The nurse assesses the patient for respiratory distress. An elevated respiratory rate may be present, or the patient may be mouth breathing. Mucous membranes in the mouth may be dry when mouth breathing is predominant.

Nursing Diagnosis

Although many nursing diagnoses may be appropriate, the following are suggested but are not inclusive:

Ineffective airway clearance related to nasal polyps

High risk for infection related to nasal obstruction from polyps

Knowledge deficit related to polypectomy

Pain related to polypectomy

Sensory alterations—olfactory related to nasal polyps

Sleep pattern disturbance related to hospitalization or nasal packing

Planning

Based on the stated nursing diagnoses, goals may include the following:

Patient clears nasal secretions effectively postoperatively

Patient does not develop sinusitis from nasal obstruction, or if sinusitis does develop, the condition will be recognized and treatment initiated

Patient states purpose, technique, complications, and proposed outcome of polypectomy

Pain relief

Improved sense of smell postoperatively

Patient sleeps 4 to 6 hours per day

Implementation

Because same-day discharge is common with nasal polyp surgery, preoperative and postoperative teachings are important. The patient is taught physical signs and symptoms that indicate bleeding or infection. Adequate fluid intake and rest are encouraged for 2 or 3 days.

Evaluation

The nurse evaluates care based on goal achievement. Most important is to evaluate patient knowledge of nasal polyp surgery and follow-up care. Adequate rest and pain relief may be observed by the nurse. Vital signs should indicate absence of hemorrhage (rare) and infections. Nasal secretions are cleared without disturbing the operative site.

Documentation

The nurse records baseline and postoperative vital signs. Preoperative and postoperative teaching are documented in the patient chart. The nurse notes the presence and characteristics of nasal drainage.

EPISTAXIS
Definition

Epistaxis, or nosebleed, is categorized as one of two types: anterior or posterior. Anterior epistaxis originates in the anterior portion of the nasal septum, which receives its blood supply predominantly from the external carotids. Posterior epistaxis originates from the posterior portion of the nasal septum, which receives its predominant blood supply from the anterior ethmoid and internal maxillary arterial systems.

Etiology/Epidemiology

The principal cause of anterior epistaxis is trauma, although chronic infection, violent sneezing or nose blowing, and local irritation of mucous membranes (nose picking) may also cause epistaxis. Mild trauma, such as that caused by nose blowing, may dislodge crusts from the nasal mucosa, resulting in anterior bleeding. Bleeding from this site is usually not severe, since the blood vessels in this area are relatively small.

Although posterior bleeding may also be precipitated by trauma, it less commonly arises from this cause. Posterior epistaxis usually occurs in patients who have some underlying disorder, such as hypertension or atherosclerotic disease. These disorders damage the vessel walls and make them more susceptible to splitting. Posterior epistaxis usually occurs spontaneously and is more severe than anterior epistaxis.

Posterior epistaxis is more common in the elderly. In adults, epistaxis is more common in men than in women. Epistaxis may also be present in patients with thrombocytopenia purpura, leukemia, or rheumatic fever. Epistaxis is rarely an isolated symptom in patients with coagulation disorders.

Therapeutic Management

Complications experienced by patients with nosebleeds are the result of blood loss. In those instances where blood loss is severe, the patient may experience signs and symptoms of volume depletion, hypoxemia, and shock. Death is possible. Therapy of epistaxis is aimed at limiting blood loss. An important part of management is the physician's identification of the precise site of bleeding. Medical measures are attempted before surgery.

Pressure and positioning

Immediate interventions for the patient experiencing a nosebleed include applying pressure to the nose to attempt to stop bleeding. However, in patients who have sustained facial injuries, pressure on the nose should be avoided until the possibility of nasal fracture has been ruled out. Pressure may be required for 5 to 30 minutes. Ice packs applied to the area may help control bleeding by causing reflex vasoconstriction of the capillaries. The patient should be sitting with his head tilted forward. Upright positioning will provide less blood flow to the head than does the supine position, and forward tilt of the head will avoid drainage of blood into the nasopharynx. The patient should be instructed to expectorate any secretions rather than swallowing them so that the extent of bleeding can be evaluated. This also minimizes the possibility that the accumulation of blood in the stomach will precipitate emesis.

Nasal packing

Nasal packing may be employed to apply pressure directly to the involved area. Anterior nasal packing is done using 1/2-inch gauze strips coated with petrolatum. Anterior nasal packs are usually left in place for 24 to 72 hours.

Posterior nasal packing is the treatment of choice for posterior epistaxis. Patients are usually hospitalized because the procedure is painful and additional bleeding may occur. The posterior nasal packing, made of sterile gauze, is held in the desired shape by silk sutures. The suture strings are used to remove the packing. Posterior packing is usually left in place for 2 to 5 days. A gauze pad is placed under the nostril to absorb any blood or other drainage. Patients with nasal packing in place must be carefully monitored for proper pack position, as well as for signs and symptoms of infection. If the pack slips out of position, the airway can become completely occluded and cause hypoxemia and death. Occlusion of the eustachian tube by posterior nasal packs may cause ear discomfort or otitis media.

Balloon tamponade of posterior epistaxis may be employed as an alternative to the more traditional posterior nasal packing. The principles of the nasal packing and balloon tamponade are identical: application of pressure directly to the site of bleeding; however, equipment and technique vary slightly. A balloon-tipped catheter is threaded through the nose into the nasopharynx. The balloon is then inflated in the appropriate position and left in place for 2 to 4 days.

Drug therapy

Although medications are usually not employed for the treatment of epistaxis, topical administration of vasoconstricting agents may be used. Vasoconstrictors decrease blood supply to the area and help control the bleeding. A cotton ball or the nasal pack is saturated with a solution of 1:1000 phenylephrine (Neo-Synephrine) and inserted into the nostril. Pressure is then applied for several minutes. The cotton ball is then removed and the patient is reevaluated for bleeding. Vasoconstricting agents are primarily useful in patients with anterior epistaxis. The posterior vessels are relatively inaccessible via this technique. Broad-spectrum antibiotic solutions may also be applied in this manner.

Surgical management

Cautery of the involved vessels may be attempted if medical measures have been ineffective. Cautery may be achieved by either electrical or chemical means. No matter which technique is chosen, topical anesthesia of the area should be achieved before the procedure is attempted.

Electrocautery is the application of an electric current to the bleeding site. The current produces coagulation of blood in the area and terminates bleeding. Chemical cautery is performed by applying a sclerosing agent, such as silver nitrate or hypertonic saline, to the site. Sclerosis of the involved vessels results. Like the application of vasoconstricting agents, cautery techniques are most useful in patients who have anterior bleeding because the posterior vessels are relatively inaccessible. Refractory posterior epistaxis may require direct surgical arterial ligation. The source of bleeding must be carefully identified.

NURSING MANAGEMENT OF THE PATIENT WITH EPISTAXIS

Assessment

Nursing assessment of the patient with epistaxis begins with an evaluation of the degree of hemodynamic compromise precipitated by bleeding. The nurse also assesses for signs and symptoms of hypoxia. Immediate assessment includes determining vital signs and evaluating the patient's level of consciousness. When posterior packs are in place, the nurse also assesses for ear discomfort caused by blocked eustachian tubes.

Further assessment is directed at obtaining a complete nursing history. The precipitating factors for the nosebleed are investigated. The patient is questioned regarding any trauma or irritation to the nose, as well as history of epistaxis. Pertinent data would also include a patient history of hypertension, atherosclerotic disease of any type, coagulation disorders, leukemia, thrombocytopenic purpura, or active rheumatic fever.

Nursing Diagnosis

Among the nursing diagnoses that may be appropriate for the patient with epistaxis, the most common are:

High risk for decreased cardiac output related to bleeding

Ineffective airway clearance related to increased secretions or blood in the airway and/or nasal packing

Altered nutrition: less than body requirements related to nausea and vomiting from accumulation of blood in the stomach

High risk for infection related to violation of mucosal integrity

Impaired gas exchange related to decreased hemoglobin

Pain related to nasal packing

Anxiety related to epistaxis

Planning

The priority of goals established for the patient with epistaxis will depend on the severity of the problem and the presence or absence of associated complications. Appropriate goals for patients with epistaxis include the following:

Normal vital signs and level of consciousness

Evidence of normal gas exchange and breathing pattern

Adequate caloric intake

Absence of infection or prompt recognition of infection and initiation of appropriate treatment

Hemoglobin greater than 10 g/dL

Pain relief

Patient verbalizes decreased anxiety

Implementation

Commonly the patient with epistaxis is managed in the ambulatory care setting. Nursing interventions in this area are focused on immediate resolution of the problem and patient teaching.

The nurse approaches the patient and family in a calm, reassuring manner. The apparent severity of blood loss in patients with epistaxis can be very alarming. Vital signs are assessed immediately, and if not contraindicated, the patient is positioned with the head of the bed elevated, and pressure is applied to the nose. The patient can be instructed in properly applying pressure. Patients will require coaching in mouth breathing while pressure is applied. Ice compresses may aid in vasoconstriction. An emesis basin is provided for expectorating blood. The patient should not swallow blood so that blood loss can be quantified. A blood transfusion may be required.

Mouth care is performed frequently to moisten mucous membranes, which may dry and crack from mouth breathing. Nutrition is affected not only by nausea from swallowed blood, but also by impaired swallowing and chewing. A liquid or semisolid diet is usually preferred.

The patient may experience a sucking noise when swallowing, caused by occlusion of the nasal airways by the packing. Reassurance that the sound will disappear when the packing is removed should help allay anxiety.

Maintaining an adequate airway and adequate oxygenation are primary nursing concerns, since the nasal pack increases airway resistance even in the proper position. The patient's respiratory rate and pattern must be observed frequently. Color and temperature of the skin, as well as the presence of confusion or diaphoresis, are evaluated to detect respiratory compromises. Tachycardia, hypotension, and confusion develop when cardiac output falls. The nurse can estimate proper placement of the nasal pack by oral examination and proper position of the sutures.

Evaluation

When evaluating care of the patient with epistaxis, the nurse considers assessment parameters first. Maintaining stable vital signs or improving compromised vital signs is imperative. Respiratory accessory muscles should not be used. Cyanosis and diaphoresis should be absent. The patient's level of consciousness should be normal. Bleeding should darken from bright red to reddish brown. Ear discomfort should be absent or minimal. Mucous membranes should remain pink and moist. The patient should appear less anxious, and nasal packs should remain as placed by the physician.

Documentation

Documentation of nursing care begins with recording vital signs and with respiratory assessment. The nurse notes the color and estimates the quantity of bloody drainage. A record of the patient's level of consciousness and signs and symptoms of normal or low cardiac output and oxygen level should be noted. The patient record should indicate condition of mucous membranes. In addition, patient attitude, including anxiety, is documented. The nurse carefully records presence and position of nasal packs and, if present, sutures or balloons.

NASAL FRACTURES
Definition

A nasal fracture is a traumatic injury to the bony structure of the nose.

Etiology/Epidemiology

Nasal fracture can occur independent from other facial injuries and commonly results from athletic or intentional trauma. A nasal fracture may occur also in combination with other facial injuries that result from major trauma, such as a fall, a motor vehicle accident, an explosion, a high-velocity projectile, or a fight. Nasal fracture is not usually a pathologic or stress fracture.

Pathophysiology

A bone is fractured when there is complete or partial interruption of osseous tissue. Nasal fractures may occur on one or both sides of the nose. A unilateral fracture may produce little or no displacement and subsequently no nasal obstruction. A simple crack is evident on x-ray studies.

More common and serious are bilateral fractures producing both external deformity and internal obstruction. The entire nose may be deviated and may have an S or C configuration. A comminuted fracture associated with severe frontal forces applied to the bridge of the nose may flatten the bridge and fracture the nasal septum. These complex fractures are characterized by a marked depression of the nasal and facial bones with accompanying damage to surrounding structures.

Soft-tissue injuries may accompany facial injuries when major trauma is involved. When a patient comes to the hospital with lacerations, contusions, hematomas, abrasions, or accidental tattooing (i.e.,

pavement or debris embedded in facial trauma), a nasal fracture should be suspected.

Clinical Manifestations

The signs and symptoms of a nasal fracture vary with its severity. Displacement of the nasal septum may be present. Edema and bruising of the nose are common.

X-ray studies of the face and nose will reveal fractures and depressions. Nasal films, both lateral and occlusal views, are helpful in diagnosing middle-face fractures. Speculum examination may reveal laceration, septal dislocation or fracture, or a septal hematoma.

Therapeutic Management

For a unilateral nasal fracture, firm pressure on the convex side of the nose will reduce the fracture. External metal splints may be applied to immobilize the displaced fragment in less complex fractures (when the nasal septum and bones are not comminuted). Usually within 10 days sufficient fibrous tissue will form to maintain proper alignment. Splints are padded to prevent skin breakdown. Nasal packing may be used to control brisk bleeding and help stabilize the internal structures. Packing is removed within 72 hours after insertion because of the risk of infection. Splints are removed within 2 weeks.

Surgical open reduction and internal fixation should be scheduled as soon as possible after the injury, because swelling makes identifying landmarks and manipulating tissues for proper reduction difficult. If excessive edema is present, surgery should be delayed for a week to allow swelling to subside. Nasal packing may be inserted postoperatively and should be left in for no more than 72 hours.

Analgesics such as aspirin with codeine or acetaminophen are used to control pain. Intravenous or oral antibiotics, such as ampicillin, may be prescribed, especially when surgery is required.

NURSING MANAGEMENT OF THE PATIENT WITH A NASAL FRACTURE
Assessment

Airway assessment should be the first focus of the nurse. Substantial amounts of blood can drain postoperatively into the nasopharynx with a nasal fracture. Partial or complete airway obstruction can occur, especially if the patient has an altered level of consciousness caused either by possible ingestion of alcohol or head trauma. The patient should be observed for signs of respiratory distress including inspiratory efforts with no corresponding thoracic or abdominal motion, nasal flaring, inspiratory grunting, intercostal retractions, cyanosis, and absence of breath sounds on auscultation. The ability to mouth breathe is also assessed.

If possible, the exact history of the injury should be clarified, as well as a history of previous fractures or nasal deviation. The usual closed reduction techniques may be ineffective in reducing a healed, displaced fracture.

The nurse assesses the nasal area for ecchymosis, tenderness, epistaxis, and soft-tissue injuries. Nasal drainage should be examined for possible cerebrospinal fluid (CSF) leak (clear fluid dripping from the nose and/or ears). Gentle palpation may reveal bony crepitus and abnormal motion of the nasal bones.

Nursing Diagnosis

Nursing diagnoses for nasal fracture are similar to epistaxis, with the following additions:

High risk for infection related to CSF leak or nasal packing

Sensory/perceptual alterations (visual and smell) related to nasal fracture

Body image disturbance related to nasal fracture

Planning

The priority of goals established for the patient with a nasal fracture will depend on the severity of the problem and the presence or absence of associated complications. Appropriate goals for the patient with this problem include the following:

Patent airway and normal blood gas levels

Pain relief

Normal body temperature

Normal vision and ability to smell

Participation in self-care activities postoperatively

Verbalization of acceptance of temporary disfigurement

Implementation

Occasionally the patient with a nasal fracture is managed in the ambulatory care setting. However, more often the patient with a nasal fracture will be admitted to the hospital because of other injuries that require aggressive medical and nursing management. Resuscitation efforts will depend on the nature of these other injuries and their need for priority measures.

The nurse assesses the patient for signs of airway obstruction and respiratory distress, including tachypnea, shortness of breath, decreased level of consciousness, dysphagia, and dyspnea. The patient may need to mouth breathe. Suctioning and frequent oral hygiene may be necessary.

Pain is relieved by administering analgesics as prescribed and applying ice. Elevating the head of the bed reduces edema and decreases bleeding, which may also relieve pain.

The presence of infection is determined by fever, foul drainage, and decreased level of consciousness, in addition to other physical signs and symptoms. Antibiotics and antipyretics may be administered.

Because the patient may develop impaired visual and olfactory sensory perceptions, the nurse assesses pupillary response, periorbital edema, scleral hemorrhage, and sense of smell. Ice packs to the eyes may decrease swelling that impairs vision. The nurse informs the patient that the sense of smell will return gradually. A room deodorizer is provided if nasal packing odor becomes offensive.

The nurse helps the patient cope with temporary disfigurement induced by the nasal fracture by allowing the patient to ventilate feelings. The importance of avoiding further nasal trauma, especially while the splint is in place, is stressed. The nurse also teaches the patient about the injury healing process. The patient learns that swelling will subside in several days. Bruising may persist for several weeks.

Evaluation

The nurse evaluates care based on the attainment of goals. A patent airway, stable vital signs, and normal blood gas levels are indicators that airway clearance is effective. The patient will be relieved of pain. Swelling will begin to subside. Localized infection or meningitis may not develop; however, if they do, the nurse will have contacted the physician for further antibiotic orders. The patient will be afebrile with normal level of consciousness and functions. The patient's vision will be assessed as normal; scleral hemorrhage, if present, will resolve in several weeks. The patient will demonstrate self-care of the nasal packings and splint and will demonstrate acceptance of altered facial features, such as looking in a mirror.

Documentation

Vital signs and the presence, quantity, and quality of nasal drainage are recorded. The nurse documents physical findings, such as periorbital edema, scleral hemorrhage, ecchymosis, and edema. Interventions, such as ice packs and head-of-bed positions, are noted. The nurse documents the assessment of the patient's body image perception, as well as interventions directed at body image acceptance. The administration and effectiveness of pain medications are recorded.

LARYNGEAL CANCER
Definition

Carcinoma of the larynx is customarily grouped with other cancers of the head and neck, since the mucosae of the entire upper aerodigestive and respiratory areas are uniformly exposed to carcinogens. This type of exposure is termed *field cancerization*. When a cancer develops in one area, the likelihood is high that additional lesions will develop in adjacent exposed areas, either simultaneously or sequentially.

Etiology/Epidemiology

The two primary risk factors for laryngeal squamous cell cancer are prolonged use of tobacco and alcohol. Although each substance poses an independent risk, their combined use causes a synergistic effect.[18] Chronic laryngitis, voice abuse, and family predisposition to cancer are also factors. Cancer of the larynx is rare in nonsmokers. Certain dietary factors in various cultures and prior exposure to radiation also have been cited as factors increasing susceptibility to laryngeal cancer. Approximately 12,500 new cases of laryngeal cancer were diagnosed in the United States in 1992, and 80% of them were men. Approximately 3650 people died of laryngeal cancer that year. This accounts for approximately 0.7% of all cancer deaths.[2] The diagnosis usually occurs between 55 and 70 years of age. An increase in smoking by women has led to increased laryngeal cancer in women with the male-to-female ratio decreasing from 11:1 in 1960 to 5:1 more recently.[3]

Pathophysiology

The most common form of laryngeal cancer is squamous cell carcinoma, which develops on the epithelium of the vocal cords. Laryngeal cancer exclusive to the true vocal cords grows slowly because of limited lymphatic distribution. Involvement of the epiglottis, false vocal cords, and pyriform sinuses, which are rich in lymph nodes, commonly results in metastasis to the deep lymph nodes of the neck. Precursors of squamous cell carcinoma are white (leukoplakia) and red (erythroplakia) patches on the epithelium. When these cells grow beyond the epithelium, cancer invades the underlying muscle and other tissues of the larynx and, if undetected, invades the surrounding structures.

Clinical Manifestations

The earliest symptom of laryngeal cancer is hoarseness or voice change. These same symptoms occur in acute or chronic laryngitis. Hoarseness that persists for longer than 2 weeks should be thoroughly investigated to rule out cancer. Tumors on or between the vocal cords deny their mechanical approximation, and therefore they cannot vibrate against each other, producing hoarseness or voice change.

Late symptoms of laryngeal cancer are dysphagia, increasing dyspnea, cough, hemoptysis, weight loss, pain within or around the thyroid or Adam's apple that radiates to the ear on the affected side, and the appearance of enlarged cervical neck nodes. This last symptom may be the reason that a patient finally consults a physician. The presence of such a mass is always evidence of advanced disease. The patient has usually ignored early hoarseness or a persistent tickle in the throat. Blood-stained sputum may also be produced by cough, a result of ulceration of the lesion. If the lesion remains untreated, there may be erosion into major blood vessels with frank hemorrhage.

The diagnosis of laryngeal cancer is achieved by a combination of detailed history and physical examination; x-ray studies of the head, neck, and chest; laryngeal tomography; and laboratory investigations. Indirect laryngoscopy may provide early recognition of mucosal abnormalities (red and white patches). However, a direct laryngoscopy permits a biopsy to be obtained for microscopic examination and diagnostic verification. Needle biopsy of enlarged nodes allows diagnosis of cancer without complicating a subsequent radical neck dissection.

Therapeutic Management

As with all cancers, early diagnosis and treatment of laryngeal cancer can lead to a high cure rate (80% to 90% for small lesions of the cords). Treatment depends primarily on patient condition and tumor size, type, and metastasis. Patient preference is always considered in treatment options.

Staging

Staging is an important step in the decision-making process for the treatment of laryngeal cancer. Staging guidelines developed by the American Joint Commission for Cancer (1977) are widely used by clinicians today. The guidelines are referred to as the TNM system: T is a measure of tumor size and location (e.g., supraglottis, glottis, or subglottis); N is the number of nodes found; and M indicates the presence or absence of distant metastases. A combination of diagnostic tests and physical examination is used to stage the tumor.

Radiation therapy

External beam radiation may be used as solitary or adjuvant treatment to chemotherapy or surgery for laryngeal cancer. The goals of radiation therapy may be curative or palliative. Radiation treatment disrupts the DNA structure and causes the cell to die. It is most effective in cells that rapidly divide. When a tumor is fixed and the vocal cord is freely movable, the cure rate can be as high as 89% to 96% with radiation alone. Radiation therapy[1,6] changes the tone and timbre of speech but does not render the patient voiceless.

As an adjuvant therapy, radiotherapy has several uses. Radiotherapy may follow chemotherapy for a larger tumor that responded well to the latter. Complete eradication of the tumor with voice preservation may occur. However, the incidence and intensity of side effects may be enhanced when radiotherapy and chemotherapy occur concurrently.[23] Intraoperative radioactive implants may be used to eliminate (1) tumor cells that remain despite the excisional margins being free from tumor or (2) a tumor that is not completely resectable. Radiotherapy may be used postoperatively when there is evidence of metastasis to the cervical nodes. Some clinicians have reported no significant difference in cancer recurrence at 2 years between patients who were treated with radiation alone and those who had more radical neck dissection. Postoperative radiotherapy is begun within 6 weeks of surgery.[23]

Chemotherapy

The use of chemotherapeutic agents for treatment of laryngeal cancer continues to be investigated. Methotrexate, bleomycin, vincristine, doxorubicin, and cisplatin, 5-fluorouracil, cyclophosphamide, methylglyoxal bis(guanylhydrazone), mitoxantrone, carboplatin, and fludarabine are among the antineoplastic agents that have been studied either alone or in combination. These agents may be given either before or after surgery for certain types of laryngeal tumors. Recent investigations have used them as the first treatment immediately after diagnosis of advanced tumors, in conjunction, but before, surgery or radiation therapy.[8]

It is theorized that micrometastasis (i.e., clinically undetectable deposits of tumor cells) is present at the time of initial diagnosis. The site of deposit is far enough removed from the primary site to be unaffected by localized radiation or surgical excision. The micrometastasis becomes diagnosable deposits months to years after initial treatment. Animal studies have provided data to support vigorous treatment with chemotherapeutic agents early after diagnosis of a primary site of carcinoma. Some human clinical trials have been conducted after surgical resection, but further investigations are needed before the long-term benefit to patients with laryngeal cancer is revealed.[1,27]

Surgical therapy

The various surgical techniques depend on the location, size, and degree of invasion of the laryngeal tumor. Several of these approaches are discussed here with their possible complications.

Excisional biopsy is confined to small, localized cancers, and the patient can be discharged the same day. The patient is encouraged to practice complete voice rest with whispering for 1 week. No vocal rehabilitation is necessary. Emphasis is placed on educating the patient to the increased probability of recurrence if preoperative unhealthy behaviors are resumed.

Laryngectomy

A **hemilaryngectomy,** also termed a vertical laryngectomy because of the vertical midneck incision, is performed when tumor involvement is confined to one cord. Approximately one half of the larynx is resected along with the false cord, ventricle, and diseased true cord. A supraglottic laryngectomy is performed for carcinoma of the epiglottis and the adjacent structures above the level of the true vocal cords. The upper portion of the larynx is excised via a horizontal incision just above the true vocal cords, which leaves the fold intact. With these partial laryngectomies, a temporary cuffed tracheostomy tube is required to allow for operative swelling to subside and proper tissue healing in the remaining larynx. Nasogastric feedings continue for about 1 week after the procedure, with close monitoring of the patient for aspiration. Swallowing can be difficult at first because of glottic edema. The patient with a supraglottic laryngectomy may have prolonged or permanent dysphagia, resulting in repeated aspiration and the need for a total laryngectomy to protect the lower airway. Removal of the tracheostomy tube usually occurs within the first 5 days. A hemilaryngectomy or supraglottic laryngectomy is desirable because the ability to speak and swallow is preserved, although the voice in the latter is hoarse.

A **total laryngectomy** is performed for advanced laryngeal cancer that involves true vocal cords. The epiglottis, thyroid cartilage, entire larynx, several tracheal rings, and the hyoid bone are removed. Radical neck dissection of muscles, veins, and nerves may accompany a total laryngectomy, or it may be performed independently when the tongue, tonsil, lip, pharynx, or thyroid is cancerous.

After a total laryngectomy, the patient has no voice and has a permanent tracheostomy. The trachea is sewn closed and does not communicate with the pharynx. The sense of smell is severely impaired or absent, because little or no air flows through the nose. The patient may be anorexic. Many patients are poorly nourished before surgery so their nutritional status may deteriorate further postoperatively.

Nutrition needs are met with parenteral hyperalimentation or enteral tube feedings through a nasogastric tube for 7 to 10 days, after which the oral feedings are initiated. Aspiration is not a problem, since the trachea is closed. Broad-spectrum antibi-

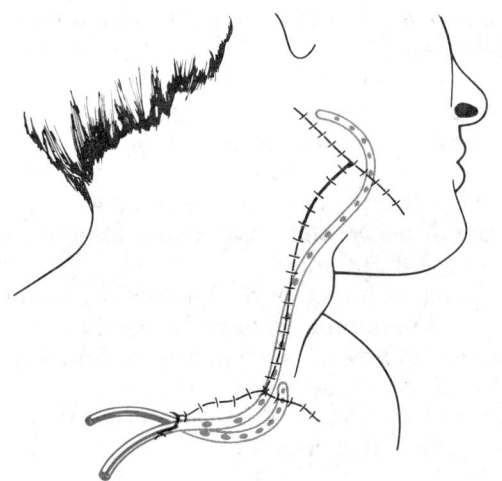

FIGURE 27-4   Neck drains.

otics are used for 10 to 12 days postoperatively. In addition, Jackson-Pratt catheters are used to drain bloody secretions from the operative site (Figure 27-4).

Radical neck dissection

The purpose of **radical neck dissection** is to remove regional metastatic cancer, such as cervical lymph nodes, when there is no evidence of distant metastasis. It is usually performed in conjunction with a supraglottic or total laryngectomy. The primary tumor is often localized preoperatively by irradiation. Neck dissections are also performed on patients without laryngeal cancer, with the primary lesions located on the tongue, tonsil, lip, nasopharynx, or thyroid gland.

The procedure itself involves removal of the cervical lymph nodes, the internal jugular vein, the sternocleidomastoid muscle, and the spinal accessory nerve. The external carotid artery may also be sacrificed. When a radical neck dissection is accompanied by another procedure, it is termed a composite resection and may include removal of all or part of the tongue, mandible, or floor of the mouth.

Complications

Radiation therapy alone may result in persistent laryngeal edema, fibrosis of the neck and larynx, and esophageal stenosis. Nutritional deficits may occur with any of the therapies, but patients report particular difficulty eating after radiotherapy.[25] This difficulty arises from common complications of radiotherapy that include stomatitis, xerostomia (dryness of the mouth), dental caries, osteoradionecrosis, and taste changes.[9] The patient's mouth becomes very painful with these complications so that eating is an unpleasant and difficult experience. Partial and to-

tal laryngectomy can be complicated by infection, carotid artery rupture, cutaneous fistula formation including salivary fistula, dysphagia, and aspiration. Carotid artery rupture may cause massive internal or external hemorrhage. This is a complication in 3.5% of patients who have had radical surgery.[19] When thyroid resection accompanies laryngectomy, hypocalcemia may occur. Chemotherapy is associated with many toxic effects that are independent of the agent, dosage, and duration of therapy. White blood cell function is usually impaired. The patient may also develop gastroenteritis, pulmonary fibrosis, vital organ toxicity (such as cardiomyopathy and hepatotoxicity), as well as hearing loss, confusion, and paralysis.

NURSING MANAGEMENT OF THE PATIENT WITH LARYNGEAL CANCER
Assessment

The assessment of a patient with laryngeal cancer encompasses preoperative, postoperative, and rehabilitative phases. On admission to the hospital, the nurse initiates assessment of the patient's symptoms, health history, habits, living conditions, occupation, and social structure. The nurse may identify problems, such as chronic obstructive pulmonary disease (COPD) from cigarette smoking or alcoholism commonly associated with laryngeal cancer.

The nurse assesses nutritional status. With dysphagia and with the tumor competing for nutrients, the patient may be nutritionally depleted. Surgery, chemotherapy, and radiation will also alter nutritional status. An estimation of caloric requirements and intake can be performed by the nurse or dietitian. Preoperatively, while the medical team makes a diagnosis, the nurse assesses the patient's emotional and knowledge needs related to impending diagnostic procedures or surgery. The nurse assesses the patient's coping mechanisms and support systems. An assessment of postoperative communication needs is also initiated. The nurse identifies the patient's understanding of equipment (nasogastric and tracheostomy tubes) and care (suctioning, tracheostomy care) that will be part of the postoperative care. Models may be used in the preoperative period.

In the immediate postoperative phase the nurse assesses hemodynamic status through vital signs. A complete respiratory assessment is needed and includes the nature of suctioned secretions, as well as the quality of breath sounds. The nurse identifies patency of the tracheostomy and nasogastric tubes. Jackson-Pratt catheters are assessed for amount and quality of drainage (e.g., frank blood, serosanguineous).

When the patient is stable, assessment of swallowing and speech function begins. A speech therapist is often involved in assessments and interventions related to swallowing and speech. The patient's knowledge of the tracheostomy tube and care is assessed with the intent to evaluate self-care for discharge. Using a mirror and the patient's own tracheostomy is more appropriate than using models for assessment of proper tracheostomy care.

In the rehabilitation phase, self-tracheostomy care, communication, and swallowing are assessed. Before discharge the nurse needs to inspect the home environment for adequate care potential, including sleeping, bathing, and toileting facilities. Cleanliness of the home is assessed. In particular, cleanliness of the tracheostomy tube care area and suctioning equipment is examined. Patient technique is assessed. Ideally, the nurse can assess the patient interacting with family members who communicate regularly with the patient, as well as visitors who communicate infrequently, to identify refinements. The effectiveness of the permanent communication device is identified.

Swallowing is again assessed for dysphagia. Esophageal stenosis or esophagitis may be present, especially when radiation therapy is instituted. Weight loss may indicate undernutrition.

Nursing Diagnosis

The patient with a total laryngectomy has multiple nursing care problems. Therefore numerous nursing diagnoses may be appropriate. The following nursing diagnoses are appropriate for the majority of patients undergoing elective laryngectomy for laryngeal cancer. The nurse may also consider nursing diagnoses related to role conflict, ineffective coping mechanisms, and impaired gas exchange.

Ineffective airway clearance related to disease process

Ineffective breathing pattern related to pain

Pain related to operative incision

Impaired verbal communication related to laryngectomy

High risk for infection related to surgical incisions and inadequate nutritional status

High risk for hemorrhage related to carotid artery rupture

Self-esteem disturbance related to mutilating surgery and altered body image

Impaired skin integrity related to tracheostomy and potential salivary fistula

Altered nutrition: less than body requirements related to dysphagia

Knowledge deficit related to tracheostomy care and suctioning

Planning

Goals depend on the needs of the patient in the preoperative, postoperative, and rehabilitative phases

of care. Specific patient outcomes for nursing care are as follows:

Patent airway without mucous plugging and arterial blood gases within normal range

Normal rate and depth of breathing

Patient relates relief of pain

Effective communication without voice

Evidence of decreased anxiety and effective coping by patient and family

No evidence of infection at the operative site

Patient will maintain usual body weight

Acceptance of new appearance as evidenced by self-care and social reintegration

Patient will demonstrate proper care of tracheostomy tube and suctioning

Implementation

The nursing care of a patient with a total laryngectomy spans the preoperative and postoperative phases of illness.

Preoperative care

In the preoperative period, the nurse is concerned with obtaining a complete health and social history, including habits, living conditions, occupation, support system, and symptoms of illness. The patient is introduced via models to tracheostomy care and suctioning. The occupational therapist should be consulted preoperatively to help establish a communication system that can be used immediately after surgery during voice rest and to prepare the patient for postoperative rehabilitation. For example, the patient may try to use electronic voice devices. The patient may visit the intensive care unit to become familiar with the environment and procedures that will occur immediately after surgery. The patient should practice deep breathing and coughing techniques to use postoperatively and may be introduced to chest physical therapy in the event that it is required. The cardiopulmonary medical therapy will be optimized and may include bronchodilators to improve airway clearance.

The nurse clarifies and reinforces physicians' discussions with the patient. After evaluating the patient's physical, mental, and emotional status, the nurse may contact the hospital chaplain, psychiatric nurse, or private clergy to counsel the patient. The nurse may also arrange a visit by a lay laryngectomy volunteer. Many people perceive a diagnosis of cancer to be a sentence to pain, mutilation, or death.

Postoperative care

Postoperatively, the nurse initially helps the patient reach hemodynamic stability by administering intravenous fluids and blood products. Vital signs are assessed frequently. The patient's head is elevated 30 degrees to promote jugular vein drainage and reduce edema, which can compress major blood vessels and nerves. Drainage from catheters and on the dressing is measured. The dressing may need to be reinforced or the physician may need to be notified when drainage is excessive. A complete respiratory assessment is performed. After careful assessment, the nurse aseptically suctions the tracheostomy tube to remove clots and secretions. The patient is turned and helped to deep breathe and cough frequently. Chest physical therapy may be performed if the patient is unable to adequately clear secretions. The stoma is cleansed with peroxide and saline. A dressing is applied to protect skin and sutures from secretions. The inner cannula is aseptically removed, cleaned, and replaced at least every 8 hours. Humidity or humidified oxygen is delivered via a tracheostomy collar to prevent secretions from thickening and mucous membranes from drying. Oral secretions are suctioned with a tonsillar top suction catheter until the patient can swallow. Oral hygiene is performed frequently postoperatively to decrease odor. Nasal secretions may also need suctioning, since the patient cannot blow his or her nose.

When the patient is discharged from the intensive care unit, the nurse initiates self-tracheostomy care and self-suctioning. Whereas the nurse must use aseptic technique, the patient or solitary caregiver learns clean technique in most instances. The patient usually learns removal and cleaning of the inner cannula, followed by stoma care, and finally suctioning. Before discharge the patient learns how to remove, clean, and replace the laryngectomy tube. The nurse teaches the patient signs and symptoms of infection including secretion assessment.

At the same time that tracheostomy care is taught, the nurse instructs the patient in care of feeding tubes if present. Swallowing rehabilitation should be initiated as soon as the patient is able. A speech and swallowing therapist should be consulted if the patient is dysphagic. The therapist will be able to assess what type of swallowing problem exists and can give the appropriate therapy and teaching required. Some patients will have more success swallowing thicker liquids while others will do better with thin liquids. Similarly, depending on the extent of surgery and swallowing dysfunction, a particular head position or exercise may improve swallowing. Tube feedings usually continue until the patient can consume adequate calories orally.

Pain control is usually achieved with narcotics immediately after surgery. As the patient nears discharge, analgesics such as acetaminophen are used.

Care of the operative sutures is necessary to prevent infection. Hydrogen peroxide and normal saline on cotton swabs or gauze are used to gently cleanse the suture line. An antimicrobial ointment is applied as prescribed to reduce infection and decrease scarring. Intravenous antibiotics are also administered

as ordered. Signs of infection are reported promptly to the physician.

Before discharge, the tracheostomy tube is removed and replaced with a laryngectomy tube. A metal or plastic laryngectomy tube, shorter and wider than a tracheostomy tube, may be used to maintain stoma size and enhance pulmonary toilet. Some physicians, however, believe there is less reaction and a better stoma formed if the patient wears no tube unless respiratory insufficiency is a potential problem for the patient. The inner cannula of the tube should be cleaned as frequently as necessary to avoid possible mucus plugs and airway obstruction. One way to keep secretions liquefied is to instill 2 to 3 mL of sterile saline into the stoma before suctioning. Care must be taken when removing the inner cannula so that the outer cannula will not be dislodged. A square knot or double-tied bow should secure the outer cannula to avoid dislodgment.

The patient undergoing laryngectomy and radical neck dissection presents additional nursing care problems. Extensive skin flaps are created in radical neck dissection. The accumulation of drainage and blood beneath the skin provides a medium for bacterial growth, can cause hematoma formation, and interferes with healing. Therefore a Hemovac drainage device will be sutured under the skin to provide a closed, continuous drainage system. The Hemovac must be assessed frequently for proper function (remain compressed) and to empty, measure, and record the amount of drainage. Approximately 70 to 120 mL of serosanguineous drainage will be expected on the first postoperative day; 30 to 50 mL on day 2; and 10 to 30 mL on the third day.

Specific care measures may be prescribed for the skin flap and donor site, and they must be performed meticulously. There should be adequate ventilation to and prevention of pressure or friction on the graft area at all times.

The presence of excessive swelling may indicate hematoma formation, although some edema is normal. The patient is assured that facial and upper body edema will subside as the days progress. Keeping the head of the patient's bed elevated at all times will help decrease the swelling. The nurse should assess the wound hourly the first day after surgery for this condition and possible clogging of the drainage tubing in the Hemovac device(s). This assessment can be combined with other wound care. Other signs of hematoma formation include changes in skin coloration or blanching, changes in type or rate of drainage, or airway compression. In addition, alterations in hemoglobin and hematocrit levels consistent with blood loss should be monitored.

Signs of infection at the suture line must be reported promptly. If infection disrupts the suture line, the patient is at higher risk for development of carotid artery rupture. Therefore, emergency equipment should be at the bedside if this threat exists.[19] If the carotid artery becomes exposed, rupture may not occur for 6 to 10 days longer. Therefore vigilant assessment should be continued for many days after the nurse identifies that the suture line is not intact.

Salivary fistulas are a common problem after laryngeal surgery. Though they are not life threatening, they delay healing of the suture sites. The fistula occurs when there is a break in the pharyngeal suture so that saliva leaks into the surrounding tissue. The saliva erodes the tissue and eventually causes a channel to the skin. They are more likely to occur within the first 3 to 4 postoperative days. They should be treated with sterile or medicated gauze packing.

When the external carotid artery has been sacrificed, there will be a resultant decrease in oxygen to the area, automatically causing variations in the patient's skin color until collateral blood vessels can establish. There may also be a lack of oxygen to the brain. Lightheadedness, gait alterations, and spatial disorientation may occur. The patient should be cautioned to change position slowly and should have assistance with self-care needs and ambulation. An added precaution is to keep siderails up for the first few days after the operation.

During radical neck dissection, the surgeon manipulates the major blood vessels of the neck. This may lead to disruption in the integrity of the vessel and subsequent embolization. Any change in mental status must be reported immediately, since the risk for a cerebrovascular accident exists.

Because strategic muscles and nerves have been removed, the patient will experience difficulty in lifting his or her head. The patient can be taught head support by placing one or both hands behind the head to lift or turn. With resection of the spinal accessory nerve, there is a shoulder droop on one side and an aching pain for several months. The use of head massage and liniments may help reduce the symptoms. Sensory loss may occur in the affected shoulder. The patient should be taught how to prevent accidental trauma caused by numbness. Male patients should be encouraged to use an electric razor when shaving the affected area.

Once the operative wound has fully healed, physical therapy personnel are consulted to instruct the patient in various exercises. These include range-of-motion exercises for the neck and shoulder. Other exercises are used to replace the function of lost muscles with other muscles and include crawling up a wall with the fingers of both hands to stretch the arm on the affected side high above the head.[17,19]

Evaluation

The nurse evaluates care of the laryngectomy patient based on goal achievement. The patient will maintain normal vital signs and arterial blood gas levels. The suture line and tracheostomy site will not become infected. The patient will not develop respiratory distress or a mucus plug.

Preoperative teaching is evaluated postoperatively. The patient will appear less anxious and may communicate less anxiety. Pain relief will be achieved. The patient will adopt one or more alternate means of communication and use them effectively. The patient will also demonstrate proper suctioning and proper care of the tracheostomy tube, suture line, and feeding tube.

Documentation

The nurse documents all assessment data, starting with the patient's health and social history. The nurse records postoperative physical status, especially regarding the neck dressing and drains, integrity of the skin surrounding sutures, pulmonary secretions, and nasogastric or oral feedings.

All preoperative and postoperative teaching is recorded in the chart. The nurse reports on the patient's ability to perform self-care of incision, secretion removal, tracheostomy tube care, and other therapies, including medication administration.

The nurse is careful to report the patient's emotional status and ability to communicate and includes a record of successful *and* unsuccessful communication devices.

Ongoing Care

Before and after discharge, there are two major areas that require extensive patient education: speech rehabilitation and care of the stoma (see box on p. 611).

Speech rehabilitation is begun postoperatively in discussion with the primary nurse, speech therapist, and others. The patient needs to be assured that activities directed toward successful speech rehabilitation will begin as soon as the esophageal suture line is healed. This may be an appropriate time for a representative from the laryngectomy club (through the local chapter of the American Cancer Society) to visit the patient if this has not already occurred. The significant others in the patient's life need to be encouraged to maintain a supportive environment and to maintain communication with the patient.[16]

It should be noted that many people who have had a laryngectomy develop laryngeal, esophageal, or pharyngeal speech without the use of or need for a mechanical or electrical device. For **esophageal speech,** the patient swallows air and then holds it in the upper esophagus. The air is expelled as a belch, which is controlled by the patient. As many as 6 to 10 words may be pronounced before reswallowing air is necessary. The voice is deep but audi-

PATIENT EDUCATION GUIDE   *Laryngectomy and Radical Neck Dissection*

General hygiene

Clean teeth and mouth 3 times daily, since the ability to detect mouth odor is lessened; use mouthwash frequently

Wear a protective cover over the tracheostomy when taking a shower; showers are encouraged for elimination of body odors

Wear a protective cover over the stoma while shaving or having hair cut to prevent hair and dust particles from entering

Stoma care

Observe the stoma daily for signs of redness, secretions, or swelling; observe also for pyrexia

To prevent infection, always wash hands before touching the stoma

Clean the stoma twice daily using a clean, damp washcloth; the use of soaps should be avoided, because they irritate the skin; tissues may obstruct the airway

Apply petrolatum around the exterior of the stoma, if ordered, taking care not to allow any to enter

Cover the stoma with a bib (a piece of cotton cloth) to aid in warming and filtering inspired air; a variety of clothing and accessories can be worn by men and women to cover the bib; high-neck sweaters, turtlenecks, and scarves work well; there should always be easy access to the stoma for inserting a handkerchief or for emergency actions.

Emergency care

Wear a Medic Alert tag, indicating that a laryngectomy has been done and containing instruction regarding first aid should the stoma become obstructed or a cardiopulmonary arrest occur

Swimming may be possible with new commercial covers, but be aware that drowning could easily occur without getting head wet; other people who have been instructed in first aid measures should be present during swimming

Stomal hydration

Additional hydration is needed for airway; use of commercial humidifiers or a pan of water on the stove or radiator will greatly add to comfort

When taking a bath or shower, allow water to accumulate 4 to 6 inches while sitting in the tub or standing in the shower stall on a nonslip mat; a well-wrung towel can be draped around the neck for added moisture and to prevent perspiration from dripping into the stoma

Other healthful behaviors

Moderation is the key rule in all normal activities; move slowly, control emotions, and exercise with moderation to avoid fatigue

When coughing, remember to cover stoma instead of mouth; moisture and secretions can be expelled onto clothing

Report persistent coughing to physician

If there is a history of alcohol intake, moderation or abstinence must be practiced; smokers should stop and should seek assistance to do so

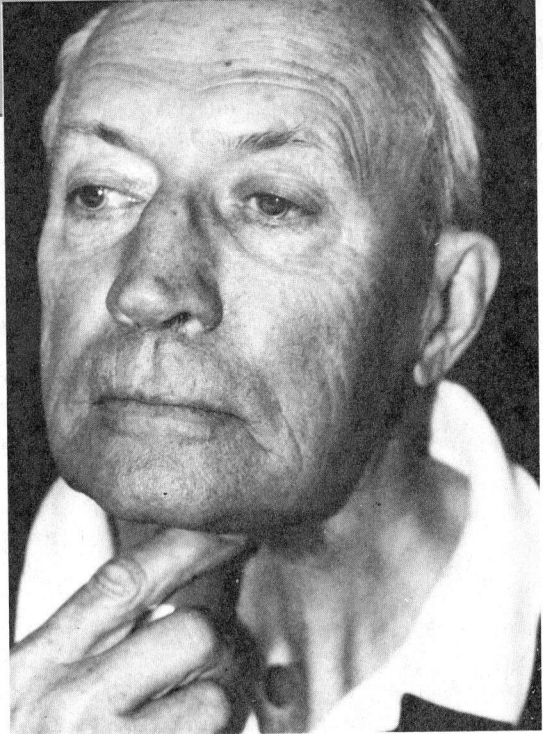

FIGURE 27-5   Electronic larynx. (From Davis JH et al: *Clinical surgery,* vol 2, St Louis, 1987, Mosby–Year Book.)

ble and quite serviceable. Because of air swallowing, the patient may experience some gastric distention and nausea at first, but this problem will subside as the patient masters this speech pattern.

Many factors affect successful speech rehabilitation. The patient's motivation to succeed, emotional status, and age, as well as extent of the surgery, are key factors to be considered. Success also requires continual practice in an environment that is relaxed and in which support is provided by all health care providers, family, and friends.

If esophageal speech is not mastered in 2 to 3 months, an artificial larynx may be prescribed (Figure 27-5). A variety of mechanical devices are available. Newer electronic aids allow for more natural speech by providing for pitch inflection and volume control. Male and female voices can even be approximated.

 **NURSING CARE PLAN** *Postoperative Total Laryngectomy Patient*

Nursing diagnosis/ *Expected outcome*	Interventions	Rationale
Ineffective airway clearance related to glottic resection, secretions, and edema • *Patient will maintain patent airway as evidenced by: absence of rhonchi, wheezes, tachypnea, dyspnea, or accessory muscle use; decreased amount of sputum/secretions; communication that breathing is easier; arterial blood gas levels within normal limits*	Assess respiratory rate and characteristics q1-2h Maintain head of bed at 30 degrees or higher Monitor arterial blood-gas levels, if obtained Turn, cough, and encourage deep breaths q2-4h Provide constant humidity Provide tracheostomy care (see tracheostomy care plan) PRN using aseptic technique	Frequent suctioning is necessary to maintain a patent airway; however, routine suctioning without evidence of secretions or clots may lead to further tracheal trauma; edema from the surgical procedure may compress the trachea; with resection of the glottis and placement of a tracheostomy tube, the patient's inability to increase intrathoracic pressure against a closed glottis decreases cough effectiveness
Ineffective breathing patterns related to newly created airway, anxiety, pain, and immobility • *Patient will maintain effective breathing patterns as evidenced by: normal respiratory rate and skin color; deep breathing exercises, which optimize ventilation; body positions that promote ventilation/perfusion matching; communicating relief of pain*	Assess respiratory rate, pattern, and other characteristics q1-2h Alternate position between side-to-side and supine, with head of bed elevated at least 30 degrees at all times; change position q2-4h Auscultate breath sounds q2-4h Coach patient to take slow deep breaths or use specific techniques if patient has COPD; evaluate effectiveness and repeat q2-4h Suction patient PRN Administer analgesics q4h PRN, and use respiratory depressants, such as codeine and morphine, with caution Advance activity from bed rest to ambulation as soon as possible	Movement in bed facilitates gas exchange and reduces complications, such as atelectasis; work of breathing is decreased in certain positions; coughing clears the airway of excessive secretions; pain control allows the patient to deep breathe and cough and provides needed rest
Pain related to operative incision • *Patient will communicate relief of pain*	Elevate head of bed at all times Teach patient to move his or her head by supporting the back of the neck with one hand each time it is necessary to turn or lift in bed Provide comfort measures, such as back rubs and mouth care Administer analgesics as needed; assess efficacy	Edema is decreased by elevation of head; pain control provides needed rest and promotes mobility; supporting the neck splints the operative tissues

NURSING CARE PLAN *Postoperative Total Laryngectomy Patient—cont'd*

Nursing diagnosis/ Expected outcome	Interventions	Rationale
Impaired verbal communication related to removal of larynx • *Patient will effectively communicate with nursing staff and visitors*	Provide patient with alternate implements for communication, including pencil, paper, Magic Slate, picture books, and electronic voice device Keep call bell by patient's hand at all times Ask patient questions that require a yes or no response, if possible, to avoid fatigue and frustration Keep all intravenous tubing and other equipment free for patient to write/move easily Determine patient's ability to learn esophageal speech; consult with surgeon about prosthetic voice restoration; place IV catheters in the nondominant hand, if possible, to enhance gesture use	Communication difficulties contribute to frustration, anxiety, and depression; an alternative method of communication restores some measure of self-confidence and helps the patient maintain independence
Anxiety or fear related to inability to speak, isolation, mutilating surgery, diagnosis of cancer, drooling • *Patient will experience decreased anxiety as evidenced by: communication of needs and concerns; statements of preference for alternative communication devices*	Keep call bell within easy reach at all times Locate patient close to the nurses' station Answer call light/bell as quickly as possible Check patient frequently Keep oral suction catheter beside patient Allow patient to express feelings of denial or anger Encourage significant others to support patient Provide information about alternative methods of communication Discuss referrals for support group, such as American Cancer Society Introduce patients to ICU before surgery	Increased feelings of anxiety, fear, or anger expend energy needed for the healing process; encouraging expressions of feelings and providing information allows the patient to begin to work through depression and to develop a different perspective in a stressful situation that cannot be changed
Impaired skin integrity related to surgical incision, tracheostomy, and skin contact with wound drainage • *Patient will be free from infection as evidenced by normal temperature; absence of erythema, odor, and drainage at incision site; and healing of surgical incision*	Assess temperature q4h or PRN Administer antibiotics as ordered Maintain aseptic technique when suctioning Observe suture lines and tracheostomy site for signs of infection (redness, pain, swelling, odor, discharge) and record Clean skin around tracheostomy with moist saline gauze Apply sterile Y dressing under tracheostomy tube if present; replace PRN Clean suture lines bid with cotton-tipped applicators dipped in saline and peroxide solution	The skin is a protective environment for many microbes; when there is interruption of skin, the number of bacteria increases; accumulation of mucus and old blood provides a medium for microorganisms; a clean site and aseptic dressing changes reduce the possibility of infection

Continued.

NURSING CARE PLAN   *Postoperative Total Laryngectomy Patient—cont'd*

Nursing diagnosis/ Expected outcome	Interventions	Rationale
Altered nutrition: less than body requirements related to dysphagia, edema, and decreased oral intake • *Patient will have adequate intake of nutrients as evidenced by: tolerating nasogastric/gastrostomy tube feeding; normal bowel function (for the patient); preoperative weight; interest in food and ability to perform tube feeding procedure*	Apply antimicrobial ointment to suture lines after cleansing Maintain patient wound drains, and empty collection bags aseptically Administer tube feedings as ordered Keep head of bed elevated at all times Aspirate gastric residual volume q2-4h Explain to patient that tube feeding is a temporary measure and that when healing occurs in a few weeks, he or she may begin to eat normally again Monitor the patient's intake and output and advance per nursing unit protocol Weigh patient daily Assess hydration status for need for additional fluids: skin turgor; observe for diarrhea Consult occupational therapist to assist with swallowing instruction Provide supplemental feedings if necessary	Learning to swallow and eat after a radical neck dissection with a total laryngectomy requires effort and patience; the patient needs adequate nutrition to effect healing, to participate in rehabilitative activities, and to maintain strength
Self-esteem disturbance related to disfiguring surgery • *Patient will accept altered body image as evidenced by: positive interaction with family and significant others, ability to maintain eye contact, self-statements indicating beginning acceptance; attention to personal hygiene; verbalization of feelings about disfigurement; statement of past accomplishments*	Help the patient identify past strengths and coping mechanisms Assess the patient's body image concept and note nonverbal responses to changes that have taken place Provide patient with tissues to absorb oral secretions Provide oral care including mouthwash of half-strength hydrogen peroxide q2h	Verbalization of feelings and identification of past coping mechanisms help patient regain self-concept; attention to personal hygiene may lessen feelings of poor body image

CRITICAL THINKING QUESTIONS

1 What nursing interventions are appropriate for a patient with inflammation of the sinuses and nasal mucosa?
2 Describe the nursing interventions for a patient experiencing nasal trauma.
3 What is the nurse's role in risk factor management to reduce the incidence of laryngeal cancer?
4 What are the major elements to be included in patient teaching for individuals after a total laryngectomy and radical neck dissection?
5 How can the nurse promote communication for the patient after a laryngectomy?
6 Why do patients with disorders of the upper airways experience problems with nutrition?

RESOURCES

Sources of information and materials for laryngectomized persons:

1 The American Cancer Society International Association of Laryngectomees (IAL) 777 Third Avenue New York, NY 10017

BIBLIOGRAPHY

Current

1. American Cancer Society: *Cancer Manual,* ed 7, Boston, 1986, Massachusetts Division.
2. Boring CC et al: Cancer statistics, 1992, *CA Cancer J Clin* 42:1, 1992.
3. DeRienzo DP et al: Carcinoma of the larynx: changing incidence in women, *Arch Otolaryngol Head Neck Surg* 117, 1991.
4. Dropkin MJ: Coping with disfigurement and dysfunction after head and neck cancer surgery: a conceptual framework, *Sem Oncol Nurs* 5:3, 1989.
5. Grant M et al: Nutritional management in the head and neck cancer patient, *Semin Oncol Nurs* 5:3, 1989.
6. Hargrove S et al: Respiratory rehabilitation: communication aids for the tracheostomized patient, *Rehabil Nurs* July/Aug: 193, 1987.
7. Harmon AR: *Nursing care of the adult trauma patient,* New York, 1985, John Wiley & Sons.
8. Harris LL, Smith S: Chemotherapy in head and neck cancer, *Semin Oncol Nurs* 5:3, 1989.
9. Iwamoto R: Principles of radiation therapy. In Otto SE, editor: *Oncology nursing,* St. Louis, 1991, Mosby–Year Book.
10. Loch EW: Sinusitis, *Prim Care* 17:2, 1990.
11. Logemann JA: Swallowing and communication rehabilitation, *Semin Oncol Nurs* 5:3, 1989.
12. Loos GD: Pharyngitis, croup epiglottis, *Prim Care* 17:2, 1990.
13. Maas A: A model for quality of life after laryngectomy, *Soc Sci Med* 33:12, 1991.
14. Oleson M, King TW: Back to the beginning: nursing case management of the older client with alaryngeal speech needs, *J Gerontol Nurs* 16:12, 1990.
15. Parzuchowski R: Head and neck cancers. In Otto SE, editor: *Oncology nursing,* St. Louis, 1991, Mosby–Year Book.
16. Richardson JL et al: Social environment and adjustment after laryngectomy, *Health Soc Work* Nov, 1991.
17. Sawyer DL, Bruya MA: Care of the patient having radical neck surgery or permanent laryngostomy: a nursing diagnostic approach, *Focus Crit Care* 17:2, 1990.
18. Schleper JR: Prevention, detection, and diagnosis of head and neck cancers, *Semin Oncol Nurs* 5:3, 1989.
19. Schwartz SS, Yuska CM: Common patient care issues following surgery for head and neck cancer, *Semin Oncol Nurs* 5:3, 1989.
20. Sealey L: Nasal obstruction, *Nurs Mirror* 161(5):22, 1985.
21. Serra A: Anterior nasal packs, *Nurs Mirror* July:16, 1985.
22. Singler BA: Nursing care of patients with laryngeal carcinoma, *Semin Oncol Nurs* 5:3, 1989.
23. Strohl RA: Radiation therapy for head and neck cancers, *Semin Oncol Nurs* 5:3, 1989.
24. Thompson JM et al: *Clinical nursing,* ed 3, St. Louis, 1993, Mosby–Year Book.
25. Wilson PR et al: Eating strategies used by persons with head and neck cancer during and after radiotherapy, *Cancer Nurs* 14:2, 1991.

Classic

26. Aiken S: Family structure and utilization of cancer support groups, *Oncol Nurs Forum* 9:22, 1982.
27. Bouchard-Kurtz R, Speese-Owens N: Nursing care of the cancer patient, ed 4, St. Louis, 1981, Mosby–Year Book.
28. *Coping with cancer: a resource for the health professional,* Bethesda, Md, US Department of Health and Human Services, Public Health Service, NIH, 1980.
29. Crissman JD: Laryngeal keratosis preceding laryngeal carcinoma, *Arch Otolaryngol Head Neck Surg* 108:445, 1982.
30. Larsen GL: Rehabilitation for the patient with head and neck cancer, *Am J Nurs* 82:119, 1982.

CHAPTER TWENTY-EIGHT

Nursing Management of Adults with Lower Airway Disorders

LEARNING OBJECTIVES

1 Explain the major alterations in physiologic functioning in specific disorders of the lower respiratory tract.
2 Outline the self-care components for patients with asthma.
3 Differentiate between respiratory failure caused by oxygenation failure and caused by ventilatory failure, including pathophysiologic mechanisms and therapeutic interventions.
4 Discuss symptoms associated with disorders of the lower respiratory system, and describe appropriate nursing interventions.
5 Describe risk factors associated with lung cancer, chronic obstructive pulmonary disease, and lower respiratory tract infections such as pneumonia and tuberculosis.
6 Develop a teaching plan for a patient with stable chronic obstructive pulmonary disease.
7 Develop a care plan for a patient with an acute asthma attack.
8 Describe expected outcomes of therapy for patients with acute respiratory failure.
9 Describe parameters that should be monitored closely for patients with an acute exacerbation of chronic obstructive pulmonary disease, respiratory failure, and an acute asthma attack.
10 Outline nursing care of patients with tuberculosis and pneumonia.
11 Discuss goals of therapy for patients with lung cancer.
12 Describe the nursing care required for the specific types of chest trauma, and explain rationale.

KEY TERMS

airway clearance, p. 627
asthma, p. 628
chronic bronchitis, p. 618
chronic obstructive pulmonary disease (COPD), p. 618
cor pulmonale, p. 620
dyspnea, p. 622
emphysema, p. 618
flail chest, p. 668
hypercapnia, p. 634

hypoxemia, p. 619
pneumonia, p. 648
pulse oximeter, p. 622
respiratory failure, p. 639
shunting, p. 619
status asthmaticus, p. 629
tuberculosis, p. 655
ventilation-perfusion mismatch, p. 619

THE LOWER RESPIRATORY system performs the functions of gas exchange and ventilation, and a wide range of conditions can interfere with these functions. Major disorders of the lower airways can be classified into six categories: chronic obstructive pulmonary disease, asthma, restrictive lung diseases, infectious disease, lung cancer, and traumatic injuries. Respiratory failure can occur with unsuccessful treatment of any one of these disorders. The etiologic factors and pathologic conditions of these disorders vary extensively. They commonly disrupt physiologic functioning of the respiratory system through one or more of the following mechanisms: mismatch of ventilation and perfusion, shunting, impaired diffusion, and impaired ventilation. From the clinical perspective, acutely ill patients often experience severe difficulty with airway clearance, alterations in breathing patterns, and impaired oxygenation, as well as anxiety. Chronically ill patients experience similar problems, although to a lesser degree. Chronically ill patients must learn to cope with their symptoms, however, and live with the condition. Comprehensive nursing care deals with all of these problems.

CHRONIC OBSTRUCTIVE PULMONARY DISEASE
Definition

Chronic obstructive pulmonary disease (COPD) is a broad term used to describe conditions characterized by a chronic obstruction to expiratory airflow.[3] Patients with COPD have difficulty emptying their lungs when asked to rapidly and forcefully exhale. Emphysema and chronic bronchitis are two examples of COPD. Specific pathologic changes are different for emphysema and chronic bronchitis, but most patients initially exhibit a combination of both

conditions. Therapeutic management is the same for both of them. COPD is a chronic, progressive condition characterized by periodic exacerbations. During an exacerbation, symptoms are exaggerated, and patients are acutely ill. Between exacerbations, symptoms are present but to a lesser extent, and the clinical condition is generally stable. In the discussion that follows, the period between exacerbations is referred to as stable COPD.

Emphysema is the enlargement of air spaces distal to the terminal bronchioles and is associated with destruction of the alveolar wall (Figure 28-1). The lung connective tissue is damaged, and this causes an enlargement of air spaces and destruction of gas exchange units. The mechanism of destruction is thought to be an imbalance between proteolytic enzymes, which destroy lung tissue, and protease inhibitors, which inactivate proteolytic enzymes. This concept is known as the protease-antiprotease imbalance hypothesis. Increased levels of proteases, such as elastase, are released from either neutrophils or macrophages in the lung to destroy lung tissue.[31,53]

Chronic bronchitis refers to a clinical condition in which patients produce excessive mucus. Diagnostic criteria include production of excessive tracheobronchial secretions on a daily basis for at least 3 months of the year for 2 consecutive years and no other cause of chronic cough, such as tuberculosis, lung cancer, or congestive heart failure.[3] Under normal conditions the volume of tracheobronchial secretions is small, ranging from 10 to 150 mL/day, and the secretions are removed from the respiratory tract by the mucociliary system. When excessive tracheobronchial secretions are produced, they overwhelm the mucociliary system and must be expectorated as sputum. Normally no sputum is expectorated. Chronic bronchitis is associated with enlarge-

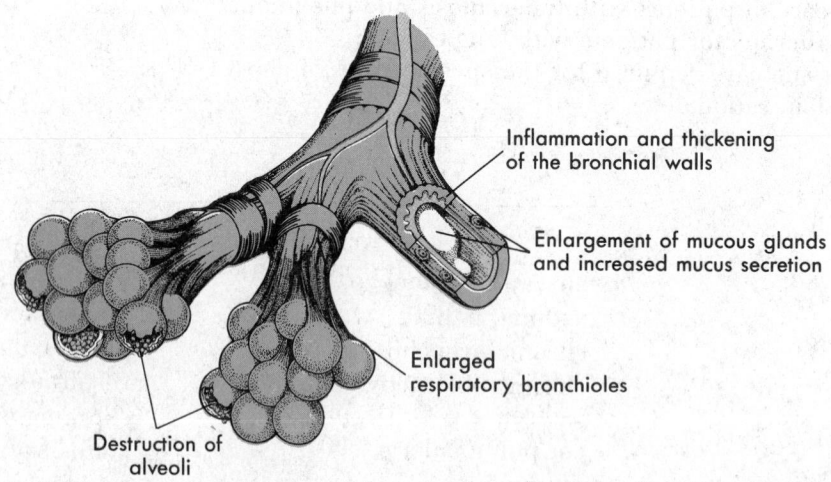

Inflammation and thickening of the bronchial walls

Enlargement of mucous glands and increased mucus secretion

Enlarged respiratory bronchioles

Destruction of alveoli

FIGURE 28-1   Effects of emphysema.

ment, or hyperplasia, of the bronchial mucous glands, and it has been suggested that airflow obstruction may result from encroachment of the bronchial mucous glands on the bronchial lumen.[66]

Etiology/Epidemiology

The risk factors for COPD include cigarette smoking, age, sex, socioeconomic status, and environmental exposure.[67] The most important risk factor is cigarette smoking, which accounts for 80% to 90% of the risk of developing COPD. Male cigarette smokers increase their risk of developing chronic bronchitis by 5.3, and female smokers increase their risk by 4.2 times.[67]

Age is another risk factor for the development of COPD. There is a normal decline in pulmonary function tests in healthy people. The volume of air exhaled in the first second of a forced expiratory maneuver (FEV_1) declines by 25 to 30 mL/yr in healthy adults. In addition to this normal decline in FEV_1, older persons are more likely to develop COPD. This may be an effect of increased exposure to causative agents, or it may be a time-dependent feature of the condition, which progresses slowly and does not manifest itself as COPD for 3 to 4 decades.

Additionally, males and people with lower incomes, less education, and lower occupational status are at increased risk for developing COPD. The specific relationship between individual risk factors and the development of COPD is not well understood. It may be an effect of increased environmental exposure, smoking patterns, and alcohol consumption. Chronic bronchitis and COPD tend to occur with greater frequency in some families. An inherited deficiency in alpha$_1$ protease inhibitor places people at risk for the development of emphysema; but this accounts for less than 1% of the familial COPD. It is believed that the remainder of familial COPD may be related to an interaction between hereditary and environmental factors. Environmental exposure to a wide range of chemicals and dusts can increase the risk of developing COPD. For example, coal miners experience an increased incidence of COPD. People who work around organic dusts, such as grain dust and wood dust, tend to develop hypersensitivities. This is referred to as occupational asthma. Experts suggest many other occupational hazards exist, but they have not been clearly defined.

Pathophysiology

Abnormalities of gas exchange

In patients with COPD, pulmonary abnormalities of gas exchange are related to three mechanisms: mismatch of ventilation and perfusion, shunting of the pulmonary capillary blood, and impaired gas diffusion. For patients with stable COPD the primary problem is ventilation-perfusion inequality. However, shunting may be a problem for COPD patients with an infection-induced exacerbation.

Ventilation-perfusion mismatch

Ventilation-perfusion mismatch is a major cause of **hypoxemia**, which is the subnormal oxygenation of arterial blood. Efficient gas exchange depends on a matching of alveolar ventilation and pulmonary capillary blood flow. The relationship between alveolar ventilation and perfusion is referred to as the V/Q ratio. The normal V/Q ratio is 0.8, and alterations in this ratio among different sections of the lung will cause hypoxemia. In COPD patients, high V/Q ratios can occur in areas of the lung where destruction of alveoli is accompanied by loss of capillary beds. In these regions ventilation remains the same but pulmonary capillary perfusion is reduced. Additionally, evidence suggests low V/Q ratios can occur in areas where the airways are partially occluded by mucus, hypertrophy of smooth muscle, or bronchospasm. The first condition is explained by those changes in the lung attributed to emphysema, whereas the second condition is explained by pathologic changes attributed to chronic bronchitis. However, many patients have both chronic bronchitis and emphysema, and this could explain why they have regions of both high and low V/Q ratios.

In patients with COPD, abnormalities of ventilation are related to an increase in the work of breathing and a decrease in the mechanical efficiency of the respiratory muscles. In patients with COPD, airflow obstruction is associated with an increase in airway resistance, and the respiratory muscles must generate higher pressures to ventilate the lungs. In addition, hyperinflation of the chest wall places the respiratory muscles at a mechanical disadvantage and reduces their effectiveness in generating the forces required to ventilate the lungs.

Shunting of pulmonary capillary blood

In COPD patients, **shunting** occurs when a portion of the cardiac output passes through the pulmonary capillary bed without becoming oxygenated. This has a major effect on gas exchange, because unoxygenated blood is deposited into the arterial circulation. This is not a major occurrence in patients with stable COPD, but it does occur in patients during acute infection-induced exacerbations. This is probably a result of the excessive amounts of pulmonary secretions that totally occlude segments of alveoli.

Impaired gas diffusion

Traditionally it was thought that diffusion was significantly impaired in COPD patients. It was believed that in emphysema the loss of alveolar surface area impaired diffusion by decreasing the surface area available for diffusion, and in chronic bronchitis the accumulation of secretions impaired diffusion by increasing the length of the diffusion path from alveolar gas to capillary blood. Currently, it is thought that impaired diffusion is less important in the pathophysiology of COPD.

Complications

Complications of COPD include acute respiratory failure, cor pulmonale, pneumothorax, and giant bullae. Acute respiratory failure (ARF) is a complication that occurs during an exacerbation of COPD, when both ventilation and oxygenation are inadequate to meet resting requirements of the body. Acute respiratory failure is characterized by a significant decrease in arterial P_{O_2} and/or a combined increase in arterial P_{CO_2} and decrease in pH. Typically, the P_{O_2} is 55 mm Hg or lower and the arterial P_{CO_2} is greater than 50 mm Hg. ARF is presented in greater detail later in this chapter.

Cor pulmonale is an enlargement of the right ventricle caused by pulmonary diseases that overload the right ventricle.[8] Hypoxemia causes vasoconstriction of the pulmonary vascular bed, which increases pulmonary vascular resistance, so the right ventricle has to pump against higher pulmonary artery pressures. Other factors that contribute to increased pulmonary vascular resistance include the loss of pulmonary vascular bed in emphysema and compression of pulmonary capillaries by increased pressure in the alveoli. Continuous low-flow oxygen is administered to treat the underlying cause of cor pulmonale. Diuretics may be administered if there is peripheral edema, but digitalis is used only when cor pulmonale is associated with a concurrent left ventricular failure.

Spontaneous pneumothorax is rare in patients with COPD, but it can create serious clinical problems. The clinical effects of pneumothorax depend on the size of the pneumothorax and the severity of the COPD. The vital capacity will be reduced, and arterial hypoxemia will be worsened.

Giant bullae can occur in patients with chronic bronchitis or emphysema. Giant bullae are air-containing structures within the lung parenchyma that are associated with an increased incidence of spontaneous pneumothorax. When the bullae are large, they compress adjacent lung tissue, rendering it nonfunctional. The extent of pulmonary impairment is related to the size of the bullae and the extent of lung compression.

Clinical Manifestations

History

The severity of symptoms tends to increase as severity of COPD increases, but this does not hold true for all patients. Some patients with severe COPD experience few symptoms, whereas others with mild obstruction may experience severe symptoms. For most patients the onset of symptoms is insidious, and patients with mild COPD generally experience few if any observable clinical symptoms until they have severe COPD (see box below). In the early stages these patients may have a productive cough and some shortness of breath with intensive physical activity; but these symptoms appear so gradually that many patients are unaware of them, and the symptoms are accepted as part of "getting older." Eventually dyspnea becomes so severe that it forces patients to reduce their level of activity.

Patients with COPD gradually become physically disabled. They commonly report limitations in their ability to walk up and down stairs, long distances, or at normal speeds with other people. Because of these difficulties, they tend to limit their travel and stay close to home. Social and recreational patterns are eventually affected, and these patients tend to become isolated. Economic security and family structure may be threatened. They may have to switch jobs, apply for disability, or retire early. They will also experience difficulty performing tasks of home maintenance, such as mowing the lawn and vacuuming. These problems lead to major changes in roles and the division of work among family members. Patients also experience problems with psychosocial adjustment. They report a higher incidence of mood disturbances, such as tension and anxiety, as well as depression.[63]

Many patients with COPD lose weight.[62] Increased levels of morbidity and mortality have been observed among those patients who lose weight. Potential effects of malnutrition on the respiratory system include respiratory muscle weakness and alterations in lung defenses against infection. In addition,

---

PROGRESSION OF SYMPTOMS FOR PATIENTS WITH COPD

Cough and sputum production on arising in the morning
Mild shortness of breath on extreme exertion
Increased cough and sputum production (smoker's cough)
Shortness of breath on exertion
Persistent cough producing large volumes of sputum
Shortness of breath with mild exertion
Inability to perform household maintenance chores
Fatigability

patients with COPD are predisposed to frequent exacerbations, which are often caused by infections of the lower respiratory tract. Many patients experience one or two exacerbations per year characterized by a worsening of dyspnea and cough associated with an increased volume of purulent sputum with no fever.

Physical examination

If the acute exacerbation does not respond to initial therapy, patients will come to the emergency room in respiratory distress. Their breathing is labored, with rapid shallow respirations and recruitment of accessory muscles to breathe. Dyspnea is often so intense and patients are so anxious they cannot breathe in the supine position. Skin color may be pale or dusky.

In contrast, patients with stable COPD come to the physician's office in no acute distress. Those with severe COPD develop a hyperinflated chest, which is visible on inspection as an increase in the diameter of the anteroposterior dimensions of the chest.

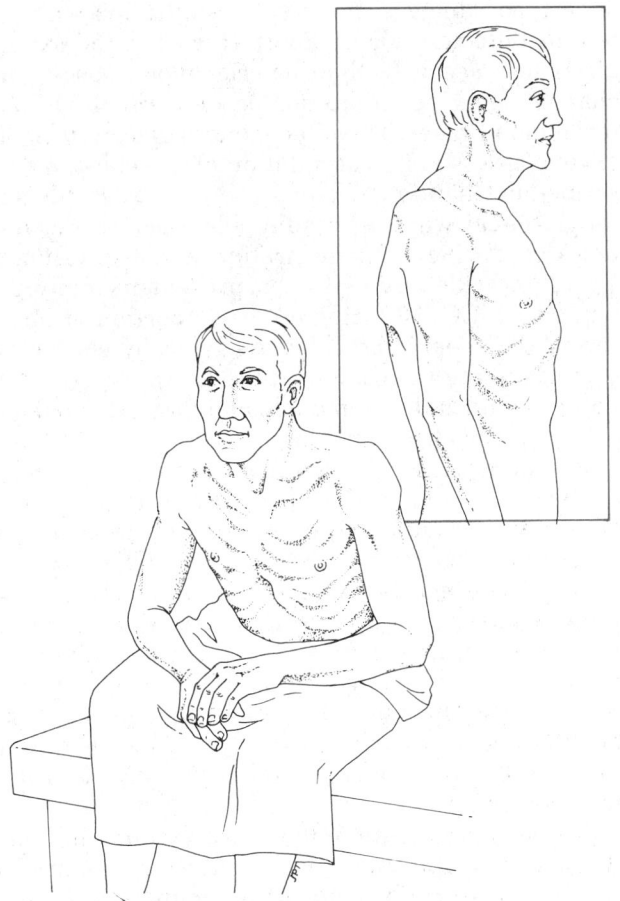

FIGURE 28-2   Patient with severe COPD. Note prominence of accessory muscles of respiration and hyperinflated chest.

This has been referred to as a barrel-shaped chest and is more prominent in some patients than in others (Figure 28-2). Patients may also demonstrate hypertrophy of the accessory muscles of respiration in the upper chest and neck. Cyanosis may be present in some patients, but it is generally not a good indicator of oxygenation. In patients with severe COPD, auscultation of the chest reveals diminished breath sounds and distant heart sounds. Patients with stable COPD have occasional coarse crackles on inspiration and occasional wheezing. They also demonstrate a prolonged expiratory time that exceeds 4 seconds. During an exacerbation the adventitious breath sounds increase, and coarse crackles may be heard bilaterally throughout the lungs.

Laboratory findings

COPD is diagnosed by pulmonary function tests. A reduction in the expiratory airflow is reflected by a decrease in the FEV_1. In patients with increased airway resistance, higher pressures are required in the lungs to produce expiratory airflow. These higher pressures tend to collapse the small conducting airways before the alveoli are emptied, thus causing trapping of air in the lungs. When this occurs, increasing expiratory effort is associated with greater air trapping and reduced expiratory volume.

Hyperinflation of the chest is reflected by an increase in lung volumes. Patients with COPD have an increased total lung capacity and residual volume with a normal or reduced vital capacity. In the earlier stages, patients may have a normal total lung capacity with a slight increase in residual volume and a slight decrease in vital capacity.

In the early stages of COPD arterial blood gases demonstrate mild to moderate hypoxemia with Po_2 in the high 60s to the high 70s (mm Hg) and normal arterial Pco_2. As the condition advances, hypoxemia increases, and hypercapnia may develop. During an acute exacerbation the arterial blood gases deteriorate, with decreasing Po_2 and increasing Pco_2.

Chest x-ray studies are generally normal in the early stages of COPD. Chest x-ray films provide a rough indicator of the extent of emphysema in patients with COPD. Typical chest findings in severe emphysema include increased radiolucency of the lungs, evidence of a low flat diaphragm, and an enlarged retrosternal air space. Vascular markings consistent with attenuation of pulmonary vessels may also be present. Patients with chronic bronchitis do not demonstrate specific changes on the chest x-ray films.

Therapeutic Management

COPD is a progressive condition with no cure. The primary therapeutic goal is to improve quality of life by limiting symptoms and increasing functional ability. Medical interventions are directed toward reducing airflow obstruction and clinical symptoms through the use of medications.

Three major classes of bronchodilators are used for treating COPD patients: anticholinergics, beta-adrenergic agonists, and methylxanthines. Bronchodilation reduces airflow obstruction, making it easier to exhale, but some patients do not respond to bronchodilators. These patients have irreversible airflow obstruction. Both types of bronchodilators can produce cardiovascular side effects, as well as problems with nervousness and tremors; hence they are not indicated on an ongoing basis if they fail to produce bronchodilation and fail to improve subjective symptoms. Intravenous bronchodilators are used routinely to treat acute exacerbations. Other medications commonly used in patients with COPD include anticholinergics, corticosteroids, mucolytics and expectorants, antibiotics, and influenza vaccines. Corticosteroids are used to treat acute exacerbations in combination with intravenous aminophylline. Short courses of antibiotics are often required to treat acute exacerbations of COPD. Annual influenza vaccines are recommended for patients with COPD. Oxygen therapy is routinely prescribed for patients with a resting arterial P_{O_2} below 55 to 60 mm Hg. This applies to stable patients and patients with an acute exacerbation.

NURSING MANAGEMENT OF THE PATIENT WITH COPD

Assessment

When COPD patients are hospitalized for an acute exacerbation, frequent assessments of gas exchange, breathing patterns, and airway clearance will be required until patients begin to respond to medications. Changes in breathing patterns indicate changes in ventilation. For example, an increase in the rate of respirations and a decrease in the depth of respirations suggest a deterioration in ventilation. A lack of coordination in respiratory motion of the chest wall and abdomen suggests heavy inspiratory loads or the presence of respiratory muscle fatigue.

In addition to the direct assessment of breathing patterns, the effectiveness of ventilation can be assessed by the arterial P_{CO_2}. Inadequate ventilation is indicated by an arterial P_{CO_2} that either exceeds 40 mm Hg or exceeds normal baseline levels. It is important to remember that many COPD patients retain CO_2 and in their stable condition live with high levels of CO_2. For these people an increase above baseline suggests acute hypoventilation. Additionally, a noticeable deterioration in mental status may indicate inadequate oxygenation.

In unstable patients a **pulse oximeter** may be used to monitor oxygen saturation. This machine

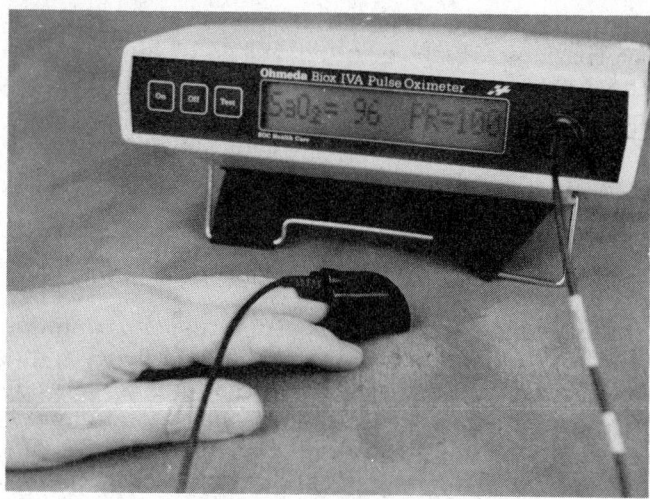

FIGURE 28-3 Portable pulse oximeter displays oxygen saturation and pulse rate. (Courtesy Ohmeda, Boulder, Colorado.)

monitors oxyhemoglobin saturation noninvasively with a probe that gently clips onto either the ear or finger, so changes in oxygen saturation can be readily detected (Figure 28-3). However, the oximeter is less accurate than arterial blood gases, and changes in oxygenations should be verified with arterial blood gases. The effectiveness of airway clearance is assessed by auscultation of the chest, as described in Chapter 25. The presence of secretions in the large airways is readily identified by coarse crackles during both inspiration and expiration.[59] Coarse crackles may also be present in many patients with COPD during the early portion of inspiration. The coarse crackles are typically characterized as discontinuous, interrupted, explosive sounds that are loud and low in pitch, and they often change or disappear after coughing.

An increase in dyspnea may be the first clinical evidence of an exacerbation, and during the course of the exacerbation, dyspnea may be intense and persistent even at rest. **Dyspnea** is a subjective sensation described as unpleasant breathlessness. Patients sometimes describe this sensation as shortness of breath, tightness in the chest, inability to breathe deeply enough, or inability to get the air out.[10,55] The intensity of dyspnea changes throughout the course of the exacerbation, and it is most likely to fluctuate during the early days, when it is most severe.

Nurses monitor the intensity of dyspnea in much the same way they monitor the intensity of pain. The Borg category-ratio scale is commonly used to document the intensity of dyspnea (Figure 28-4). When monitoring dyspnea, it is also important to document the intensity of dyspnea with respect to specific ac-

Breathlessness	
0	Nothing at all
0.5	Very, very slight
1	Very slight
2	Slight
3	Moderate
4	Somewhat severe
5	Severe
6	
7	Very severe
8	
9	
10	Very, very severe (almost maximal)
Maximal	

FIGURE 28-4   Borg category-ratio scale. Using this scale from 0 to 10, how much shortness of breath do you have right now?

tivities. For example, patients may have no dyspnea while sitting quietly in a chair, but they may experience intense levels of dyspnea when walking a short distance across the room.

Activity tolerance is assessed by respiratory rate, heart rate, blood pressure, dyspnea, and oxygen saturation during an activity. Oxygen saturation is easily monitored with a portable oximeter while walking or during routine bedside activities. Desaturation is indicated by a decrease of more than 3% oxygen saturation with any activity or a saturation of less than 85%. Other evidence of activity intolerance includes severe dyspnea, sudden onset of pallor and sweating, marked apprehension, lack of coordination, labored respirations with an increase in respiratory rate, and an excessive increase in heart rate or blood pressure. An increase in heart rate beyond 85% predicted maximal heart rate (predicted maximal heart rate is 220 minus patient age in years) is excessive and suggests the activity should be stopped.[43]

During an acute exacerbation, dyspnea is commonly associated with anxiety. Patients may appear apprehensive, tense, or afraid of being left alone, and some may be panicked. Some patients may not outwardly appear anxious, but they may express anxiety as demanding and hostile behavior.

Nursing Diagnosis

The primary nursing diagnoses associated with an acute exacerbation are as follows:

Ineffective airway clearance related to increased secretions and ineffective cough

Ineffective breathing patterns related to altered pulmonary mechanics and increased work of breathing

Impaired gas exchange related to ventilation-perfusion mismatch

Activity intolerance related to decreased oxygen delivery to tissues

Anxiety related to dyspnea

Altered nutrition: less than body requirements related to anorexia and frequent coughing

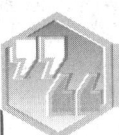

THERAPEUTIC COMMUNICATION GUIDE

The Chain Smoker with Emphysema

1. Confront denial and noncompliance with treatment regimen by describing situation.

   Example   *Nurse:*   "Mr. Jones, you say you want to live to see your grandchildren, yet you still smoke three packs of cigarettes every day. This aggravates your emphysema and your ability to breathe."

   Patient: "I know, but you wouldn't understand. How do you know how hard it is for me to live with emphysema?"

2. Provide support and understanding. Reinforce patient's belief in reality.

   Example   *Nurse:*   "I can understand the frustration you have with trying to quit smoking. You've been smoking almost 20 years. Am I mistaken in my belief that you do want to live longer?"

   Patient: "No, you're right, but I can't seem to quit. You expect too much from me."

3. Use silence and reflection. Provide modification that may be more realistic and elicit patient's cooperation.

   Example   *Nurse:*   (short silence) "I would like to help you quit smoking. What do you think would be more realistic?"

Planning

The priority goals of nursing interventions for patients with an acute exacerbation of COPD are the maintenance of adequate oxygenation, ventilation, and airway clearance. Specific patient outcomes for nursing care include the following:

Breath sounds are clear with no crackles

Effective cough that clears the airways of secretions with ease

Respiratory rate between 12 and 20 breaths/min at rest

Coordinated respiratory motion of abdomen and rib cage

Patient only uses accessory muscles of respiration for increased levels of ventilation

Arterial Po_2 at patient's normal baseline

Patient reports less dyspnea and is breathing comfortably

Patient reports reduced anxiety

Reduced muscle tension in face and upper and lower extremities

Patient reports restful sleep

Patient maintains usual body weight

Implementation

The nurse takes primary responsibility for specific interventions to mobilize secretions, promote efficient breathing patterns, and maintain adequate oxygenation. These interventions include coughing techniques, breathing exercises, and relaxation techniques, as well as other aspects of nursing care that promote comfort and psychosocial adjustment. Also included are teaching activities designed to prepare patients to care for themselves.

GERIATRIC CONSIDERATIONS

Bronchodilator Therapy for COPD

Age-related changes in pharmacokinetics and the presence of other chronic health problems increase the older adult's risk for side effects associated with bronchodilator drugs used to treat COPD. For theophylline preparations the older adult should have drug levels monitored at more frequent intervals than the young adult.

Side effects associated with anticholinergic bronchodilators such as urinary retention and blurred vision may be particularly troublesome for the older adult. Ipratropium bromide administered by inhalation will provide therapeutic benefit with fewer systemic side effects. The older adult should exercise caution in using over-the-counter bronchodilators. These drugs usually contain alpha and beta agonists (epinephrine and ephedrine) that can aggravate preexisting health problems such as hypertension or diabetes.

Although metered dose inhalers may produce fewer side effects, the older adult may have difficulty learning to coordinate drug administration with respiratory activity. Decreased motor function and range of motion in the hands may render the older adult less able to use the device effectively.

TABLE 28-1   Pharmacology Summary: COPD Medications

Medication	Route	Action	Side effects
Anticholinergics	Metered dose inhaler	Bronchodilator	Depend on specific drug
Beta$_2$-adrenergic agents	Metered dose inhaler; oral	Bronchodilator	Rapid heart rate, tremor
Methylxanthines	Intravenous; oral	Bronchodilator	Gastrointestinal toxicity, sleeplessness, cardiac dysrhythmias, convulsions
Corticosteroids	Metered dose inhaler; oral; intravenous	Anti-inflammatory	Major problems are associated with long-term use of steroids: decreased resistance to infection, muscle wasting, and other problems

Drug therapy

To reduce airway resistance the nurse administers antibiotics, bronchodilators (see geriatric box), and steroids as ordered by the physician (Table 28-1). If side effects are severe enough, they may warrant a change of medications; but in the acute phase, patients may have to tolerate some jitters and tremors (although it is important for them to understand and explain the source of the discomfort). In the earliest phase of therapy, medications will be administered intravenously and then converted to oral and inhaled routes as soon as the patient is stabilized. Many patients will require intravenous fluid replacement and nutritional supplements, because they are too dyspneic to consume adequate fluids and nutrients.

Airway clearance

Interventions to improve airway clearance are directed toward mobilizing secretions to make them easier to expectorate. These interventions include deep breathing, chest percussion, and selected cough techniques. Chest percussion and coughing techniques are discussed in Chapter 25. Removal of secretions also promotes comfort, since patients report less dyspnea after removing secretions.

Airway clearance may be enhanced by the administration of bronchodilators before cough routines. This decreases airway resistance and thereby increases the velocity of gas generated during the cough. The higher velocity of airflow enhances airway clearance.

A chronic, productive cough can be annoying, irritating, and fatiguing, but patients must be careful about taking medications such as codeine to suppress the cough. Suppression of a productive cough leads to an undesirable retention of secretions. Similarly, these patients must be careful about taking antihistamines, because these may dry up secretions and make them more difficult to expectorate.

Some patients report relief of dyspnea in the upright leaning forward position, where they lean forward bracing their arms on a stationary object. This is thought to stabilize the rib cage, thereby making it easier to breathe. In the upright position, gravity pulls downward on the abdominal contents, making it easier to take a deep breath. In the supine position, abdominal contents push on the diaphragm. This makes it easier to empty the lungs. The effects of position should be assessed in individual patients, because the overall effect may vary from patient to patient. In the hospital, positioning can be accomplished by either sitting patients at the side of the bed so they can lean over the bedside table or by raising the head of the bed.

Oxygen therapy

For patients with an acute exacerbation, a small increase in the fraction of inspired oxygen (FIO_2) is often required to maintain adequate oxygenation until the underlying condition is treated with antibiotics, bronchodilators, and corticosteroids. The administration of 1 to 2 L of oxygen per minute by nasal cannula should be sufficient to maintain adequate oxyhemoglobin saturation. In most patients an arterial PO_2 of 60 mm Hg will be sufficient to saturate hemoglobin at high levels. See Chapter 26 for further details regarding administration of oxygen.

When administering oxygen to COPD patients, the nurse monitors for retention of CO_2. A small fraction of patients with severe COPD are predisposed to CO_2 retention when breathing high concentrations of oxygen. This may be caused by the loss of the hypoxic stimulus to breathe in patients with a reduced ventilatory response to elevations in CO_2, or it may be related to changes in ventilation and perfusion. Although it is important to recognize this potential hazard, in an emergency situation the nurse should not withhold oxygen because of fear of CO_2 retention.

Rest and activity

During an acute exacerbation, patients should limit physical activity to reduce oxygen consumption and decrease ventilatory requirements. Activities are gradually resumed as tolerated and as respiratory function improves.

Nutrition

Patients often lose their appetite during acute exacerbations. The nurse explores ways to maintain dietary intake. These might include providing small, frequent meals, arranging for favorite foods, or providing supplemental foods, such as high-protein milk shakes. If a consultation with the dietitian is needed, the nurse tries to include the patient's spouse in the consultation, because problems with appetite often persist after discharge from the hospital.

Breathing exercises

Breathing exercises may reduce the intensity of dyspnea. Patients can be instructed to use pursed-lip breathing techniques to increase expiratory time, decrease respiratory rate, and increase tidal volume. This facilitates ventilation by reducing the respiratory rate and increasing tidal volume.

As patients improve, some may benefit from relaxation training to help control alterations in breathing patterns related to anxiety. Progressive relaxation and biofeedback techniques may be used to enhance patients' sense of control over their breathing. The sensation of dyspnea frightens patients and family members, who tend to think dyspnea is caused by low oxygen levels. Such patients can sometimes be reassured death is not imminent when they are informed their oxygen saturation is within normal or acceptable levels. It is also important to keep patients and family members informed of the nature of and rationale for treatment. This gives them confidence they are being appropriately treated. The presence of family members is often reassuring to patients, and the nurse should make the family feel welcome.

Evaluation

During an acute exacerbation the patient's condition must be assessed frequently until the patient stabilizes. Evidence of appropriate progress includes a reduction in the subjective effort required to breathe, along with a return to normal rate and depth of respirations. The patient maintains usual arterial blood gases and reports an absence of dyspnea at rest and minimal dyspnea with activity. The patient is relaxed enough to sleep as needed and feels rested on awakening.

Documentation

Documentation in the nursing notes includes a chronologic record of clinical progress with respect to breathing patterns, breath sounds, characteristics of sputum, and sensations of dyspnea and fatigue. In addition, records document patient teaching with respect to patient understanding of the disease condition and prescribed therapy.

Ongoing Care

Ongoing care of patients with stable COPD is directed toward improving the quality of life by teaching patients to care for themselves, helping them cope with symptoms, encouraging them to exercise and increase their functional ability, and helping them make the necessary adjustments in life-style. When stable, these patients feel much better than during an exacerbation and are capable of functioning at higher levels. Common problems experienced by patients with stable COPD include impaired gas exchange, dyspnea with exertion (causing reduced exercise tolerance), ineffective airway clearance, inadequate nutritional status, and difficulty adjusting to changes in social roles.

Impaired gas exchange

Some patients with stable COPD are hypoxemic. In the most severe cases, patients are hypoxemic at rest; whereas others only desaturate during exercise. If they desaturate at rest, they need to use oxygen 24 hours per day at home. Guidelines for patients who desaturate during exercise are less clear, but these patients will tolerate higher levels of activity if they use oxygen during strenuous activities.

Patients commonly resist the use of home oxygen, stating it is a crutch or an ominous sign of their condition. They may refuse to use oxygen, because they are afraid of becoming dependent on it, thinking that if they hold out until they cannot live without it, they will live longer and maintain better health. However, the opposite is true. Patients with severe hypoxemia have lower death rates and a higher quality of life if they use continuous oxygen.[52] It is important to listen to patients' concerns and provide them with the facts necessary to make their decisions.

Home oxygen is administered by three methods: tanks of compressed gas, liquid oxygen, and oxygen concentrators. Each method has its advantages and disadvantages, and it is best for patients to decide which system is most appropriate for them. The liquid oxygen system offers maximal portability for active patients (Figure 28-5), whereas the oxygen concentrators are convenient for patients who stay at home. Compressed gas is the least expensive method. For further details see Chapter 26.

Dyspnea

Dyspnea is a problem for patients with stable COPD. It is generally experienced with any form of exer-

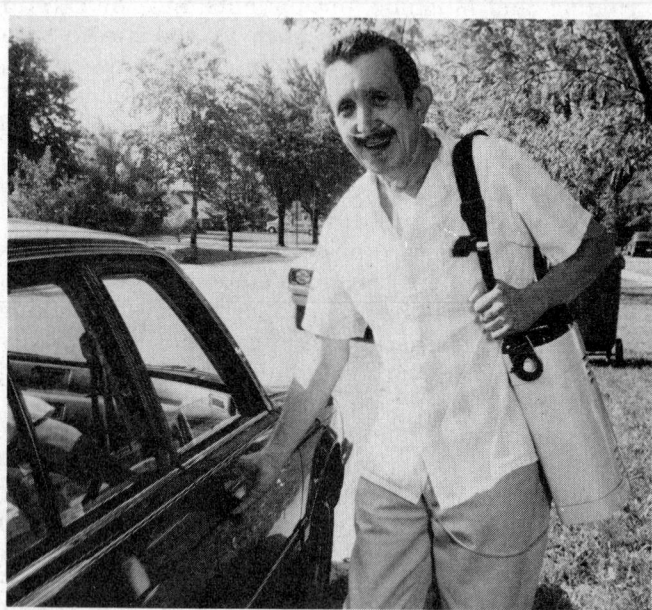

FIGURE 28-5 Patient with severe COPD travels with portable tank of liquid oxygen.

tion, bending over, or lifting heavy objects. There is no intervention that completely relieves dyspnea, but a variety of techniques are used to reduce its intensity. These include diaphragmatic breathing, pursed-lip breathing, and relaxation therapy.

Airway clearance

Airway clearance is a continuing problem for many patients with stable COPD. For most patients, deep breathing and cough techniques are the most appropriate interventions, whereas chest percussion and postural drainage are only useful for patients producing copious amounts of sputum. It is important that patients assess their sputum and understand the importance of expectorating secretions. Patients should be taught to inspect their sputum and report significant changes to their primary caregiver. Changes in color from clear to white to clear can be expected, but yellow or green sputum suggests the presence of a lower respiratory tract infection and should be reported to the primary caregiver. The volume of sputum may fluctuate, but it is important to report either excessive increases or reductions if they are accompanied by an increase in dyspnea or a fever.

Exercise tolerance

Patients will experience rapid deconditioning if they avoid exercise because of dyspnea on exertion. Consequently patients with uncomplicated COPD need to be encouraged to select a form of exercise that appeals to them, to stay active, and to exercise on a regular basis. Both walking and bicycling on a stationary bicycle are appropriate, but walking has the advantage of being less boring. Patients will benefit from exercising regularly at the highest levels they can tolerate.

Inspiratory muscle training is another form of exercise patients can use to improve the strength and endurance of their inspiratory muscles. Patients exercise their inspiratory muscles by breathing against an inspiratory load—either a resistive load or a pressure load (Figure 28-6).

Psychosocial adjustment

As with any chronic illness, it is important to observe COPD patients for problems related to psychosocial adjustment. These problems may include prolonged periods of depressed moods, high levels of anxiety, or increased family tension. As the physical disability increases, COPD patients and their families must redistribute responsibilities for tasks such as home repairs, home maintenance, household income, and housecleaning. This is not easy, because people take pride in performing these tasks and derive self-esteem from them. Patients and family members need emotional support and guidance as they restructure their lives. They need information regarding community services that may increase the patient's independence and decrease the caretaker's burden. Local senior citizens clubs, for example, may provide social contacts for patients who are left at home every day while the spouse works. The local secretary of state's office may provide disabled parking stickers, which make it easier for patients to go shopping. Local organizations may provide "meals on wheels" for patients who cannot cook for themselves. The nurse is in an ideal position to inform patients about available community services and to refer them to a social worker if necessary.

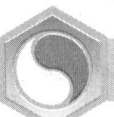

ETHICAL ISSUES

- Should an indigent person with COPD who continues to smoke receive free care and treatment? Should a wealthy person in the same situation continue to receive care and treatment?
- How should the nurse respond when a chronic COPD patient says that at the next hospitalization he or she will refuse to be intubated, even though weaning off the ventilator has been easy during previous admissions?

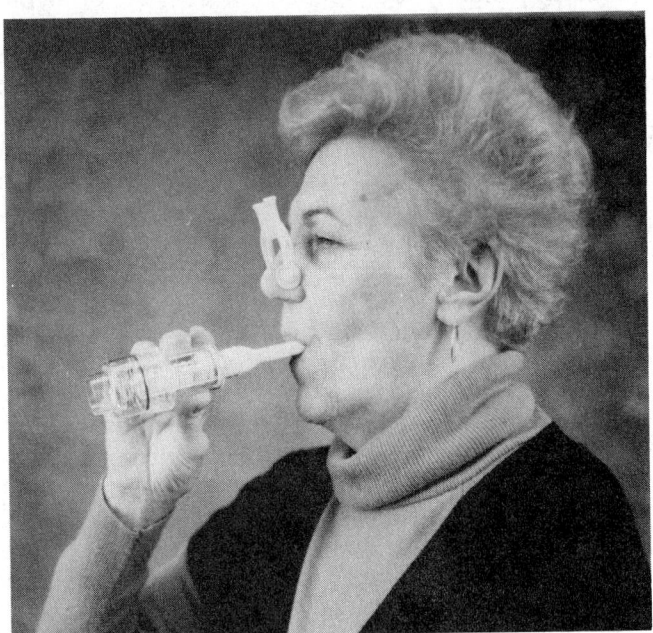

FIGURE 28-6   Patient with COPD exercises her inspiratory muscles using a Threshold Inspiratory Muscles Trainer. (Courtesy Healthscan Inc, Cedar Grove, NJ.)

ASTHMA
Definition

Asthma is characterized by (1) reversible airway obstruction, (2) airway inflammation, and (3) airway hyperresponsiveness.[27]

Etiology/Epidemiology

The etiologic factors of asthma are not completely understood, but it is clear that asthma can develop after exposure to a variety of substances. For some patients asthma results from an allergic reaction to specific allergens. For others it is acquired from exposure to chemicals in the workplace, such as airborne dusts, gases, vapors, or fumes. This is referred to as occupational asthma. Asthma also occurs with no identifiable cause. Patients with allergic asthma are predominantly under 30 years of age, and many have a family history of allergies. Among elderly persons, asthma is commonly of a nonallergic cause; however, evidence exists that past allergies continue to plague individuals, and a mixed form of the disease may be exhibited by older people.[32]

Pathophysiology

The underlying mechanism of asthma is thought to be inflammation of the airways, even in persons with mild asthma. Both airway obstruction and airway hyperresponsiveness are caused by inflammation of the airways.[27]

The acute asthma attack is characterized by increasing airway obstruction caused by bronchospasm, mucosal edema of the airways, and thick, tenacious mucus that has a tendency to plug peripheral airways.[16] For allergy-induced asthma the hyperresponsiveness is a classic IgE-mediated inflammatory response. For asthma triggered by stimuli such as environmental irritants, respiratory tract infection, exercise, and cold air, the response is thought to be related to a more generalized hyperresponsiveness caused by inflammation of the airways.

Pathologic changes in the airways ultimately interfere with gas exchange and ventilation through ventilation-perfusion mismatch, impaired diffusion, hypoventilation, and to some extent shunting. Mismatch of ventilation and perfusion occurs because of varying degrees of airflow obstruction throughout the lungs with portions of the pulmonary circulation being distributed to underventilated sections of the lungs. Diffusion is impaired by excessive secretions in the airways. Shunting occurs in areas of atelectasis. In the early stages of an asthma attack, patients tend to hyperventilate, but hypoventilation eventually occurs if the work of breathing exceeds the ability of the respiratory muscles to ventilate the lungs.

The extent and magnitude of pathophysiologic alterations are related to the severity of the attack and can range from mild increases in airflow obstruction to respiratory failure and death.

Clinical Manifestations

Patients with asthma have a generalized hyperresponsiveness of the airways, and a variety of physical, chemical, and pharmacologic stimuli can precipitate an attack; but these stimuli do not cause breathing problems in other people. Common allergens include dust, pollens, animal dander, and specific foods and additives. Irritants include automobile emissions, industrial pollutants, cigarette smoke, vapors from cleaning solvents, perfume, paint, paint thinner, sprays such as furniture polish, household cleaning products, and cold air. Exercise triggers asthma attacks for some patients, and this is probably related to the effects of cold air on the airways. Respiratory infections also tend to irritate the airways and exacerbate asthma. Beta-adrenergic blockers interfere with the action of beta-agonist bronchodilators and cause bronchoconstriction. Emotional stress can trigger an attack and prolong an existing attack. Despite this extensive list of stimuli, many asthma attacks occur with no apparent precipitating event.

Dyspnea is the major symptom of an asthma attack, and it is commonly accompanied by wheezing. Younger patients tend to report higher levels of dyspnea during an asthma attack, and people with frequent asthma attacks tend to report lower levels of dyspnea than persons with few attacks. Consequently the intensity of dyspnea is not a good indicator of the degree of bronchoconstriction. Nevertheless, it is important, because it reflects the patient's perception of the intensity of the attack and has implications for nursing care.

In addition to dyspnea, patients describe a variety of sensations or symptoms during an asthma attack. Some patients panic and complain of being scared, worried, frightened, and afraid of dying. Many patients feel irritable, cranky, short tempered, and edgy. They also describe a variety of sensations related to hyperventilation, including dizziness, tingling sensations, headaches, numbness, and nausea. Additionally, they describe sensations related to airway obstruction, including chest filling up, chest tightening, rapid shallow breathing, coughing, and choking, as well as shortness of breath. Finally, they complain of having no energy and of feeling weak, worn out, and fatigued. These symptoms are commonly experienced by patients during an asthma attack, but all symptoms are not experienced with each attack.

The severity of the asthma attack is reflected by the degree of airflow obstruction, level of oxygenation, nature of breathing patterns, and changes in level of consciousness. During a severe asthma attack, patients are diaphoretic, anxious, and too dyspneic to talk. Severe attacks are characterized by severe airflow obstruction, hypoxemia, the use of accessory muscles to breathe, a paradoxic pulse, and a decrease in the level of consciousness. Gas exchange is impaired in most patients during an asthma attack, and ventilation increases in all but the most severe asthma attacks and only decreases with the onset of respiratory failure. The paradoxic pulse develops because of large swings in intrathoracic pressure during inspiration and expiration. With severe bronchoconstriction, the respiratory muscles must generate large pressures to ventilate the lungs, and these pressures influence the return of venous blood to the right side of the heart. During inspiration, negative intrathoracic pressures increase venous return, and during expiration, positive intrathoracic pressures decrease venous return. This causes fluctuations in the systolic blood pressure of 10 mm Hg or greater. Finally, it is an ominous sign if patients become lethargic and drowsy and appear to give up from exhaustion, because this commonly accompanies the onset of respiratory failure.

Therapeutic Management

Many asthma attack victims respond to inhaled bronchodilators taken at home and do not require hospitalization, but hospital admission is required when the patient does not respond to inhaled bronchodilators or to drugs administered in the emergency room. This condition is referred to as **status asthmaticus.** Additionally, hospitalization may be required for exacerbations of asthma precipitated by infections such as acute bronchitis, pneumonia, or sinusitis.[3] During the acute phase of an attack, therapeutic interventions are directed toward relieving bronchoconstriction. After recovery from the acute attack, therapeutic interventions are directed toward preventing further attacks by prescribing medication to reduce inflammation of the airways and by teaching patients to care for themselves. Antibiotics are commonly required to treat the infection that precipitated the attack.

Drug therapy is the primary mode of treating asthma. Key drugs are beta agonists, methylxanthines, and corticosteroids. The specific combination of drugs and method of administration depend on the severity of the asthma attack and the response to therapy. In general, the nurse instructs patients to take their inhaled beta agonists at the first evidence of an asthma attack, because this may produce sufficient bronchodilation to stop the attack. However, patients who do not respond to inhaled bronchodilators within a reasonable period should

---

PATIENTS AT INCREASED RISK FOR LIFE-THREATENING ASTHMA ATTACK

Infants less than 1 year old
Prior history of life-threatening asthma attack
Less than 10% improvement in peak expiratory flow rate (PEFR) or FEV_1 in the emergency room
PEFR or FEV_1 below 25% of predicted
P_{CO_2} above 40 mm Hg
Wide daily fluctuation in PEFR or FEV_1

From National Asthma Education Program, Expert Panel Report: *Executive summary: guidelines for the diagnosis and management of asthma,* Pub No 91-3042A, Washington, DC, 1991, USDHHS, National Heart, Lung, and Blood Institutes.

---

seek medical assistance by either calling their physician or going to an emergency room.

When patients arrive at the emergency room, drugs are prescribed in the following order until the patient responds: inhaled beta agonists or subcutaneous beta agonists for three doses followed by systemic corticosteroids. Inhaled medications are administered via nebulizer during the acute phase of the attack. Methylxanthines are not recommended in the emergency room because they have not proven to be any more effective than beta agonists alone, but methylxanthines are commonly administered to patients if they require hospitalization for the exacerbation.

For patients with mild asthma, maintenance therapy may be limited to inhaled beta agonists on an as-needed basis. For patients with moderate to severe asthma a regular regimen of drugs will be prescribed to reduce the frequency of asthma attacks. Inhaled corticosteroids are administered on a routine basis for their anti-inflammatory effects. They seldom produce the systemic side effects seen with oral corticosteroids, but localized side effects can include oropharyngeal candidiasis, dysphonia, and coughing. Inhaled cromolyn sodium is administered for its nonsteroidal anti-inflammatory effects. It produces fewer localized side effects and is beneficial for patients who respond to it. Inhaled beta agonists and theophylline are administered as maintenance therapy for their bronchodilator effects. Inhaled beta agonists may produce side effects from cardiac stimulation in persons with cardiac disease and in elderly persons. Optimal effects of theophylline are derived from serum levels between 10 and 20 µg/mL, but there is a fine line between therapeutic and toxic levels of theophylline. Signs and symptoms of theophylline toxicity include gastrointestinal disturbances, seizures, tachycardia, and arrhythmias. To avoid toxicity some physicians will aim for serum levels between 5 and 15 µg/mL. Individual patients respond differently, and physicians will prescribe medications in the above order until asthma symptoms are controlled. Severe side effects can be experienced from long-term use of oral corticosteroids. They are generally prescribed only when absolutely necessary, although some patients with asthma do require oral corticosteroids on a routine basis to control their symptoms.

NURSING MANAGEMENT OF THE PATIENT WITH ASTHMA
Assessment

During an acute asthma attack the nurse monitors ventilation and the effort required to breathe by assessing breathing patterns. This includes the direct observation of rate and depth of respirations, use of accessory muscles of respiration, auscultation of breath sounds, and pulse rate. During the acute phase of the attack, breathing patterns will be inefficient, and the work of breathing will be high. In addition, gas exchange must be monitored closely. This can be accomplished by using a combination of arterial blood gases and pulse oximetry. If the attack is severe, frequent blood gases can be anticipated, and an indwelling arterial catheter should be inserted to eliminate repeated punctures. During an acute attack, the intensity of dyspnea and the effort required to breathe must be assessed regularly. Assessment of dyspnea is important, because it indicates the patient's perception of the attack.[20] The nurse also monitors fluid balance during a prolonged attack. These patients are often too dyspneic to drink adequate fluids, and they are losing excessive fluids because of high minute ventilation. This places them at risk for an inadequate fluid volume. Once patients have stabilized, the nurse attempts to identify the cause of the attack, because this information is needed to help patients control their attacks. When caring for patients in the community setting, nursing assessment focuses on patterns of symptoms, methods used to prevent attacks, and self-care techniques for management of acute attacks.

Nursing Diagnosis

Nursing diagnoses associated with an acute asthma attack include the following:

Ineffective breathing patterns related to increased airway resistance

Impaired gas exchange related to ventilation-perfusion mismatch, impaired diffusion, or arteriovenous shunting

Fear related to thoughts of impending death

Fatigue related to increased effort to breathe

Fluid volume deficit related to decreased intake and increased insensible loss

Nursing diagnoses associated with chronic asthma include the following:

Activity intolerance related to actual dyspnea or fear of dyspnea

Altered nutrition: less than body requirements related to fatigue and dyspnea

Sexual dysfunction related to dyspnea and fatigue

Planning

Outcome criteria for the patient with asthma include the following:

Patient returns to normal breathing patterns, including rate and depth of respirations

Patient maintains $Paco_2$ at normal baseline (approximately 40 mm Hg for most patients)

Breath sounds are clear on auscultation, with little or no evidence of wheezing

Patient maintains Pao_2 at normal baseline (approximately 100 mm Hg for most patients)

Patient reports no breathlessness at rest and minimal breathlessness with activities

Patient reports feeling rested after scheduled rest periods

Patient expresses realistic expectations regarding current health status

Implementation

For patients having an acute asthma attack, nursing care is similar to nursing care of patients with an acute exacerbation of COPD. To establish adequate ventilation and gas exchange, the nurse administers bronchodilators, corticosteroids, and oxygen as ordered by the physician. The major symptom of asthma is dyspnea, and nursing interventions are directed toward reducing its intensity. Dyspnea will abate with bronchodilation. In addition, the sensation of dyspnea may be partially alleviated by positioning patients in an upright position with the head of the bed elevated so they do not have to hold themselves upright. Additionally, dyspnea may be somewhat attenuated by maintaining an environment that is cool and dry but not too cold. Patients often practice a variety of self-care techniques at home to alleviate dyspnea, and the nurse can help them with any of these techniques if they are not contraindicated under the circumstances.

Fluid balance must be maintained without overloading patients. If fluids cannot be taken orally, they can be administered intravenously, but it is important not to administer excessive amounts of fluid, because this may increase the extravascular lung water and increase mismatch of ventilation and perfusion.[1]

During a prolonged asthma attack, patients become extremely fatigued, and nursing interventions are designed to conserve energy. Most patients demonstrate a natural tendency to limit physical exertion during the attack, and the nurse can help them by arranging their physical environment to conserve energy and by helping them with positioning and other physical tasks. While the patient is in the hospital, the activities of the day should be programmed so that a minimum of fatigue occurs (e.g., morning care and examination followed by a rest period before any major activities). Patients may be easily fatigued for several weeks after an exacerbation of asthma. This must be considered when working with these patients and their families to develop a functional plan for care at home.

Patients can be tense and anxious during the acute asthma attack, but they will feel more secure if the nurse or a family member stays within close proximity until symptoms abate. Coaching **patients** to breathe slower and deeper may also reduce anxiety. The nurse comforts patients by briefly explaining interventions and keeping them informed of their progress.

Evaluation

Evidence of adequate ventilation is established by an arterial Pco_2 less than or equal to 40 mm Hg, and adequacy of gas exchange is established with an arterial oxyhemoglobin saturation greater than 85% and an arterial Po_2 greater than 60 mm Hg. Additionally, improvements in FEV_1 and peak flow provide strong evidence that patients are responding appropriately to therapy. Further clinical evidence of improved ventilation and oxygenation includes normal respiratory rate and tidal volume, clear breath sounds, and quiet breathing without the use of accessory muscles of respiration. As symptoms improve, patients will report a reduction in dyspnea and effort required to breathe, and they will appear alert, relaxed, and less anxious.

Documentation

When documenting the nursing process, it is important to describe the appearance of patients, including the color of skin and use of accessory muscles for breathing, as well as subjective data describing the intensity of dyspnea. In addition, the characteristic of breath sounds and oxyhemoglobin saturation from oximetry will help in documenting clinical progress. Nurses should also document patient teaching, including patient knowledge regarding medication, technique with metered dose inhaler, and avoidance of triggers.

Ongoing Care

To reduce the number of asthma attacks, patients must learn to care for themselves at home. Important aspects of self-care include learning to avoid stimuli that trigger attacks, learning how to take the medication, and learning to monitor peak expiratory airflow. In addition, patients must learn when to seek medical assistance to avoid waiting so long they develop intractable asthma.

Inhaled medication

During hospitalization, patients can be taught how to use a metered dose inhaler for the administration of inhaled bronchodilators, but reinforcement will be required after discharge. Patients must use the metered dose inhalers properly to administer the maximal amount of medication directly into the lungs. They should be taught to hold the mouthpiece approximately 1½ to 2 inches from the mouth; empty the lungs completely and then inhale slowly and deeply through the mouth while pressing down on the metal canister to release a puff of medication; and continue to breathe in slowly and then hold the breath for 10 seconds or as long as possible. This technique is difficult to coordinate, especially for older patients, and these patients should be taught to use a spacer device such as the Optihaler to improve drug delivery deep into the lungs (Figure 28-7).

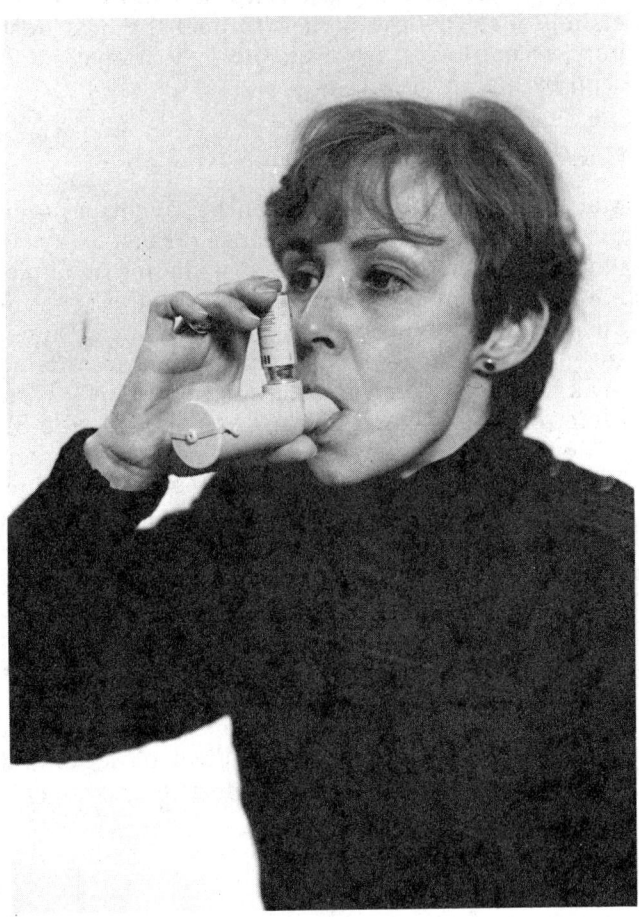

FIGURE 28-7   Patient using spacer device to improve drug delivery. (Courtesy Healthscan Inc, Cedar Grove, NJ.)

Inhaled corticosteroids produce large aerosolized droplets and are therefore best administered with a metered dose inhaler and spacer device to reduce localized side effects that occur with heavy deposition of the aerosol within the mouth. Rinsing the mouth out after each dose will also aid in reducing local side effects.

Theophylline levels

Theophylline clearance from the system is decreased and theophylline levels in the blood are increased by fever, liver disease, congestive heart failure, and commonly used drugs, including cimetidine, quinoline, antibiotics, troleandomycin, and erythromycin. Routine serum theophylline levels are drawn every 6 to 12 months, but therapeutic and toxic levels are so close that the nurse must routinely monitor patients for any of the above factors that may lead to toxicity. Additionally, the nurse routinely observes for clinical evidence of toxicity that would suggest the need for further evaluation. The most common toxic effects are nausea, vomiting, tachycardia, and arrhythmias. In the case of suspected theophylline toxicity the nurse obtains a venous blood sample for analysis of serum theophylline levels and instructs the patient to hold the next dose until serum levels are available and the patient is seen by the physician.

Home monitoring of airway obstruction

Many patients with asthma can be taught to monitor their peak expiratory flow rate (PEFR) on a regular basis at home.[27] The PEFR is the maximal airflow rate during a forced expiration, and it is an indicator of airflow obstruction. PEFR can be measured by patients at home with a small affordable peak flowmeter, such as the Mini-Wright Peak Flow Meter or the Assess Peak Flow Meter (Figure 28-8).

Routine monitoring of PEFR helps patients manage their asthma. Patients can measure peak flow throughout the day to identify diurnal variations. They can monitor response to bronchodilator medications by measuring PEFR, and this can be used to adjust medications. Measures of PEFR can be used to identify early changes in airflow obstruction (which sometimes occur before patients detect any symptoms), thereby allowing early treatment and prevention of severe asthma attacks. It allows them to adjust medications to meet individual needs and thereby provide better protection against asthma attacks.

Avoiding triggers

Avoidance techniques are important for people with asthma triggered by allergies, and the nurse can help

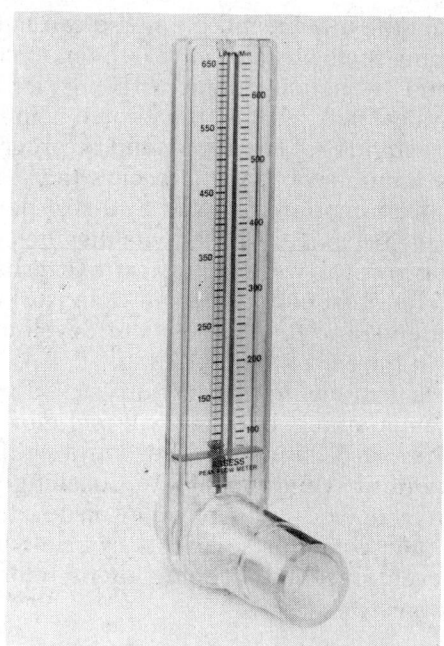

FIGURE 28-8   An Assess Peak Flow Meter. (Courtesy Healthscan Inc, Cedar Grove, NJ.)

patients identify conditions and situations that place them at risk for exposure to allergens. Even if patients cannot completely avoid exposure to allergens, they may improve their symptoms by reducing their exposure. This can be a difficult process, and patients need assistance in planning avoidance techniques. For example, allergies to animal skin, hair, and feathers may require removal of a pet from the local environment. Allergies to pollen may be impossible to avoid, but appropriate furnace air filters and air conditioning may reduce exposure.

Patients with food allergies can learn to cook at home without using the offending food, but it is more difficult to avoid accidental exposure to the allergen in restaurants. These patients will need to learn about typical practices regarding food preparation in restaurants to avoid accidental exposure. Restaurant food preparation techniques vary considerably from home practices, and this requires consultation with a dietitian.

Some patients are allergic to dust mites, which live in household dust found in carpets, furniture, clothing, and bedding. Generalized dust reduction techniques are helpful, and they include vacuuming carpets and furniture once each week, mopping floors instead of dry sweeping them, and damp-dusting furniture.

However, special attention must be given to the bedroom. Effective techniques in the bedroom include the use of plastic mattress and pillow covers, removal of bedroom carpeting and replacement with a surface that can be washed frequently, and removal of wool blankets and replacement with cotton or synthetic materials that can be washed weekly.[41] Dust mites thrive in humid environments; consequently it may be helpful to reduce the relative humidity in the house by closing the bathroom door during showers and baths and avoiding the use of humidifiers.

Air conditioning reduces the relative humidity while reducing indoor pollen and spore counts. It also reduces dust from the outside environment. However, patients should be instructed to clean their air conditioners frequently, because air conditioners can become contaminated with fungi and cause exacerbations of asthma. The same problem can occur with automobile air conditioners.[58]

Exercise

Patients with asthma need to stay physically fit and exercise just like other people. To do this they may be instructed to take an extra dose of their inhaled beta agonist just before exercising. This may limit or prevent severe bronchoconstriction and allow them to enjoy exercise. To avoid overdosing, specific guidelines are worked out with the patient's physician.

Emotional triggers

Intense emotional states such as anger, fear, and anxiety can provoke asthma attacks in some people. For these people, progressive muscle relaxation and biofeedback techniques may be helpful in controlling symptoms.

RESTRICTIVE LUNG DISEASE
Definition

Restrictive lung diseases encompass a vast array of disorders that lead to decreased lung inflation. The hallmark of all restrictive disorders, regardless of the cause, is decreased lung volumes. Lung volumes shrink because of altered mechanics, including changes in pressure-volume relationships, elastic recoil, and work of breathing.

Etiology/Epidemiology

The site of the restriction may be intrapulmonary or extrapulmonary. Intrapulmonary disorders include diseases of the lung tissue or parenchyma, such as interstitial lung disease, atelectasis, and lung resection. Interstitial lung disease has many causes, and representative examples are listed in Table 28-2. Extrapulmonary disorders include abnormalities of the pleura, chest wall, and respiratory muscles. Pleural diseases that affect lung expansion include pleural

TABLE 28-2 Causes of Chronic Interstitial Lung Disease	
Cause	**Example**
Idiopathic	Interstitial pulmonary fibrosis
Occupational exposure	
Asbestos	Asbestosis
Fungi	Farmer's lung
Toxic fumes and coal dust	Pneumoconiosis
Poisons	
Paraquat	Pneumoconiosis
Immunologic diseases	Rheumatoid lung
	Sarcoidosis

effusion, pleural thickening, and pneumothorax. The chest wall may be restricted by increases in chest wall mass, such as in obesity, ascites, and pregnancy. Additionally, spinal deformities may restrict lung expansion, as in scoliosis, kyphosis, and ankylosing spondylitis. Respiratory muscle weakness will limit maximal lung inflation, as in neuromuscular disorders such as Guillain-Barré syndrome, amyotrophic lateral sclerosis, and myasthenia gravis, as well as muscular dystrophies and spinal cord injuries.

Pathophysiology

The reduction in lung volumes can be explained by the pressure-volume relationships of the lungs and chest wall. The lungs and chest wall are elastic tissues, and they behave according to their compliance and elastance properties. Compliance and elastance are reciprocal and therefore cause changes to occur in the opposite direction. Compliance refers to the change in volume for a given unit of change in pressure, and elastance refers to the change in pressure for a given change in volume. A simple analogy is a balloon. A balloon that is flabby and easy to blow up is compliant but not elastic. That is, large changes in the size or volume of the balloon require only a small amount of effort or pressure to inflate the balloon. Similarly, a balloon that is stiff and difficult to inflate is not compliant, but it is highly elastic. It is difficult to blow up because a great deal of effort or pressure results in only small changes in the size or volume of the balloon. The analogy can easily be applied to the lungs and chest wall.

Regardless of whether the source of the restrictive disorder is intrapulmonary or extrapulmonary, the total respiratory system becomes stiffer. The respiratory muscles must work hard to generate large changes in pressure, and this results in only small changes in volume. Because the respiratory muscles must work harder to inflate the stiff respiratory system, work of breathing increases. Consequently increased work of breathing results in an increased oxygen cost of breathing.

Lung volumes may decrease for reasons other than a change in the elastic properties of the respiratory system. Lung inflation decreases because of an actual loss of alveoli, such as in lung resection and atelectasis, or lung inflation decreases because of a loss of inflating force, such as in respiratory muscle weakness.

Hypoxemia often characterizes restrictive disorders. **Hypercapnia,** defined as an arterial CO_2 tension of more than 45 mm Hg, may also be found if the disorder progresses to the point of respiratory failure.

Hypoxemia characterizes intrapulmonary disorders such as interstitial fibrosis and pneumonia. The primary cause of hypoxemia is ventilation-perfusion mismatch. That is, poorly ventilated alveoli receive a disproportionate blood supply. Impaired diffusion of oxygen across the alveolar-capillary membrane may also contribute to the hypoxemia. This occurs because the width of the membrane is increased in interstitial fibrosis by fibrotic changes and in pneumonia by fluid or exudate accumulation. In addition, diffusion may be limited by loss of surface area, which occurs in lung resection or atelectasis. However, mismatch of ventilation and perfusion accounts for most hypoxemia.

Hypercapnia results when the respiratory pump can no longer eliminate adequate CO_2 to maintain normal arterial blood gases. The central nervous system (CNS) may fail to adequately drive the respiratory muscles, as in CNS depression caused by drug effects, or the impulse to stimulate breathing cannot be propagated to the respiratory muscles, as in spinal cord injury. The work of breathing may outstrip the respiratory muscles' ability to maintain adequate ventilation, so that respiratory failure ensues, as in the end stages of interstitial fibrosis or with severe spinal deformation. Finally, respiratory failure occurs when the central drive to breathe becomes depressed and the work of breathing increases to produce hypercapnia, as in obesity hypoventilation syndrome.[65]

The primary complication of a chronic restrictive disorder is cor pulmonale. This occurs particularly in the late stages of interstitial fibrosis and in obesity hypoventilation syndrome. This complication results from pulmonary hypertension probably related to vasoconstriction induced by chronic hypoxemia.

Clinical Manifestations

Dyspnea or shortness of breath is the primary and overwhelming subjective response to the mechanical and gas exchange alterations found in all the restrictive disorders. The progression of dyspnea may be different depending on the cause. For example, in interstitial fibrosis, dyspnea may initially occur only with exertion. As the disease progresses, it begins to plague the individual with only minimal exertion and finally even at rest.[45] In contrast, the onset of dyspnea may be more acute in atelectasis or pneumothorax, because these conditions occur suddenly. Patients with restrictive disorders do not tolerate activity, because of dyspnea. This may have a devastating effect on their ability to work and carry on activities of daily living as they become increasingly disabled by the dyspnea. Subsequently, interpersonal relationships may suffer as the individual is unable to perform usual roles in the family and in other situations. Last, a dry but persistent cough may be present, particularly in interstitial fibrosis. If patients become infected, the cough may produce purulent sputum.

Patients with restrictive disorders tend to breathe faster and more shallowly than normal. This is particularly marked in patients with interstitial fibrosis. The increase in respiratory rate and decrease in tidal volume maintain minute ventilation while decreasing the work of breathing.[45] If patients with stiff lungs shorten the time of inspiration, decrease the depth of inspiration, and increase the respiratory rate to maintain the minute ventilation, the elastic load decreases so the inspiratory muscles do not work as hard with each breath. However, this compensatory breathing pattern is inefficient and incomplete. Respiratory rate must increase to maintain minute ventilation, since tidal volume decreases. However, as tidal volume decreases, the amount of effective alveolar ventilation decreases, and the proportion of ventilation that is wasted as dead space ventilation increases, since tidal volume is equal to the sum of alveolar ventilation and dead space. Dead space refers to the segment of airways with no alveoli (the conducting airways) and no gas exchange. The absolute amount of dead space may not increase, but the proportion of tidal volume that is dead space ventilation increases. Dead space ventilation does not contribute to gas exchange, so the oxygen cost of this change in breathing pattern is still high. Because of the increased work of breathing, patients may need to use accessory muscles to accomplish the task of ventilation.

Therapeutic Management

Interstitial fibrosis cannot be cured, but steroid therapy may slow the progress of diffuse lung inflammation and injury. Steroid therapy is most beneficial if it is administered in the early alveolitis stages of the disease.

Since impaired gas exchange is the primary outcome of the altered mechanics, hypoxemia must be treated. Oxygen therapy may be required only in the acute stages of a pneumonia or atelectasis, but long-term therapy will be required for patients with interstitial fibrosis. Initially, oxygen may be required only with exercise or during sleep, when patients tend to desaturate. The dose will be prescribed based on the outcome of arterial blood gas analysis during exercise, sleep, and rest. If the resting room air arterial Po_2 is less than 55 to 60 mm Hg, patients will require continuous therapy.

If the cause of the restriction is obesity, the main therapy is weight loss. If patients are able to lose a significant amount of weight, lung inflation, as well as the abnormal gas exchange, improves. Even a 5% to 10% decrease in weight may improve the incidence of sleep apnea, which is associated with the pulmonary complications of morbid obesity; and thus the gas exchange problems, including hypercapnia and hypoxemia, improve.

Patients with obesity hypoventilation syndrome, sometimes referred to as pickwickian syndrome, seem to have a decreased central drive to breathe. Therefore physicians prescribe the hormone progesterone. Interestingly, investigators discovered that progesterone is a respiratory stimulant when they noted pregnant women tended to hyperventilate. Subsequently physicians began prescribing progesterone to individuals who are obese, hypoventilate, suffer from sleep apnea, or become hypercapnic. The drug has been shown to significantly improve oxygenation and ventilation. Oxygen may also be prescribed for either continuous or nocturnal use, since these patients are hypoxemic.

Other therapies for patients with obesity hypo-ventilation syndrome include those aimed at improving upper airway obstruction. A tracheotomy can eliminate upper airway obstruction and thus sleep apnea.[38] However, the procedure can prove technically difficult and risky in obese patients with a short neck or mandible. In addition, long-term management, potential complications, and the social and psychologic implications of a tracheotomy may make it an undesirable therapy for some patients.

Because of the problems associated with a tracheotomy, investigators have developed other therapies. Nasal continuous positive airway pressure (nasal CPAP) applied with a mask apparatus (Figure 28-9) has been used in many obstructive sleep-apnea patients. It acts as a "pneumatic splint" by providing positive pressure to the upper airway, so the upper airway tissue cannot collapse and occlude the airway.[38]

Spinal deformities and neuromuscular diseases are the other major causes of extrapulmonary restriction. The major medical treatment for these problems may be mechanical ventilation. Since little can be done to cure these diseases, the care is supportive. Once patients experience ventilatory failure, either external negative pressure ventilators can be used or patients can be intubated and placed on a positive pressure ventilator. The negative pressure device accomplishes ventilation by creating a vacuum pressure against the chest wall. A cuirass or poncho surrounds the chest wall and provides the negative pressure when connected to a vacuum source (Figure 28-10). The rehabilitative and home care implications of artificial ventilation are numerous and will be covered in the nursing management discussion.

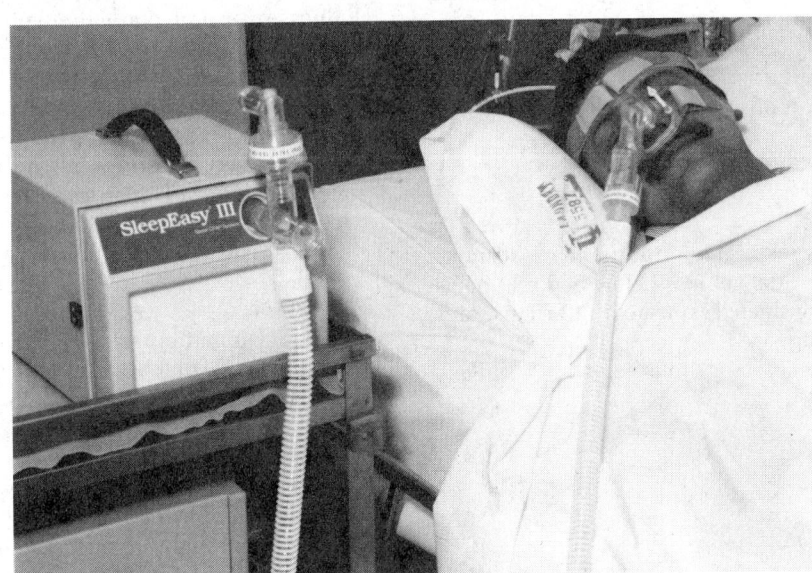

FIGURE 28-9   Patient wearing mask required for administration of nasal CPAP.

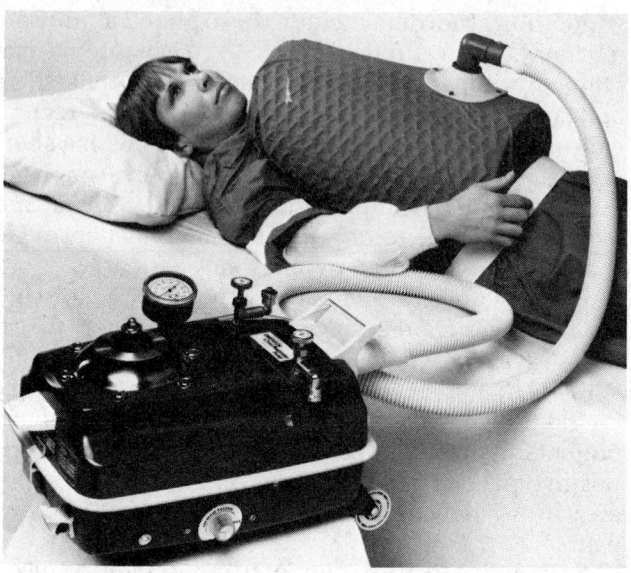

FIGURE 28-10 Patient wearing negative pressure ventilator. (Courtesy JH Emerson Co, Cambridge, Mass.)

NURSING MANAGEMENT OF THE PATIENT WITH RESTRICTIVE LUNG DISEASE

Assessment

Since the goal of the management of restrictive disorders is to ensure adequate gas exchange and improve symptoms, the assessment centers on the factors influencing these goals. Again, the assessment will be based in part on the cause of the disorder. A synopsis of the nursing assessment is listed in the box below, but some parts of the assessment warrant further discussion.

If the respiratory muscles fatigue, the nurse may observe respiratory alternans or paradoxic breathing. Respiratory alternans occurs when patients alternate using the chest wall and abdominal muscles to breathe. Paradoxic breathing occurs when the upper abdomen moves inward during inspiration rather than outward, as normally occurs when the diaphragm descends and pushes abdominal contents outward. These two changes in respiratory pattern require careful observation. The nurse should observe patients from a tangential point of view. The nurse can enhance this assessment by palpating the thorax and upper abdomen to assess which muscles are contracting.

COMMON ASSESSMENT FINDINGS FOR RESTRICTIVE LUNG DISEASE

History

Occupational exposure: toxic chemicals, asbestos, fungus, coal, Paraquat

Systemic diseases: sarcoidosis, rheumatoid arthritis, systemic lupus erythematosus

Subjective findings

Dyspnea with exertion or at rest

Activity intolerance

Objective findings

Observation

Breathing pattern—respiratory rate above 20/min; shallow breaths or tidal volume below 500 mL; periods of apnea during sleep; respiratory alternans; and paradoxic breathing

Work of breathing—accessory muscle use

Palpation

Decreased chest excursion

Percussion

Dullness over atelectatic lung, pleural effusion, or consolidated lung

Auscultation

Diminished breath sounds with decreased tidal volume; absent breath sounds during apnea or over atelectatic lung segment; rales or crackles over fibrotic lung or pneumonia; and absent or diminished breath sounds over pleural effusion

Other data

Pulmonary function tests—lung volumes below 80% of predicted normal airway resistance and FEV_1

Arterial blood gases—Pao_2 below 55 mm Hg; oxyhemoglobin saturation (Sao_2) below 90%

Exercise tolerance—progressive decline in distance walked in 12 minutes or report of decreasing ability to perform activities of daily living

Height and weight—weight above 120% based on height and sex

Apnea, or the absence of respiration, can be classified as a disturbance in breathing pattern. In obesity hypoventilation syndrome, it occurs during sleep. If a sleep-apnea screening is done on the nursing unit using oximetry, the nurse must provide for a private room, a quiet environment, and periods of uninterrupted sleep. In obstruction obesity hypoventilation syndrome, the nurse should also observe for the presence or absence of abdominal and chest excursion with the presence or absence of airflow from the nose and mouth.

Type of sleep apnea	Chest/abdominal movement	Air movement
Central	No	No
Obstruction	Yes	No
Mixed	Yes/no	Yes/no

The nurse can observe sleep apnea and verify absence of respiration by auscultating the patient for breath sounds. Again the nurse must be careful to watch the patient for several minutes to catch a period of apnea. The nurse should document the duration of apnea and the frequency if possible. Diagnosis and evaluation of treatment may require more sophisticated technologic methods to assess the pattern of apnea in the sleep laboratory. Chest wall and abdominal motion can be monitored with a noninvasive instrument called a respiratory inductive plethysmograph. With this device the patient wears two elastic belts, one around the upper rib cage and the other around the abdomen. Alarms can be set for respiratory rate, and breathing patterns can be documented on graphic recordings.

In the hospital setting the nurse observes how patients carry out activities of daily living. The spectrum of independence may vary from fully independent to completely dependent. Generally patients will be limited by dyspnea.

During rehabilitation the nurse might measure patient progress by self-report of the ability to perform activities of daily living or other activities that patients do on a regular basis. Alternatively, patients may complete a submaximal exercise test, such as the 12-minute distance walk. The nurse must carefully monitor patients for signs of oxygen desaturation during this test and may need to use a pulse oximeter, which measures oxygen saturation and heart rate. The distance walked can be used to monitor change in exercise tolerance from one test to the next, rather than as an absolute determination of exercise tolerance.

Since dyspnea is a common and debilitating manifestation of restrictive disorders, the nurse assesses dyspnea to monitor subjective response. The nurse may ask patients to rate their dyspnea on a scale such as the Borg category-ratio scale or on a visual analog scale. Patients can also keep a diary of symptoms to assess the progress of the disease or therapy.

Nursing Diagnosis

Although the etiologic factors are vast, the primary cause of restrictive disorders is based on decreased lung inflation. The nursing diagnoses associated with restrictive disorders include the following:

Ineffective breathing pattern related to decreased lung inflation

Impaired gas exchange related to inadequate surface area for diffusion

Activity intolerance related to impaired gas exchange

Planning

The main goal of nursing intervention in the restrictive disorders is the maintenance of adequate oxygenation and ventilation. An outcome is that patients verbalize improvement of the symptoms of dyspnea and exercise intolerance. Depending on the cause of the restriction, other goals may be realistic, such as significant weight loss in obese patients or adequate airway clearance in patients with pneumonia. Other outcomes include adjustment to altered role performance in patients with chronic debilitation and family and patient exhibiting appropriate coping strategies.

Implementation

Since the primary goal of nursing intervention is the maintenance of adequate gas exchange, the first nursing actions are aimed at this goal. Based on the assessment of oxygenation, the nurse administers oxygen therapy to maintain an arterial oxygen concentration of at least 55 to 60 mm Hg or a saturation of at least 90%. In the acute care setting, oxygen may be delivered invasively via an endotracheal tube or noninvasively via any number of oxygen masks or by nasal cannula. If ventilation fails, as is seen by an increase in arterial P_{CO_2}, patients may require artificial ventilation. Alternatively, patients may receive respiratory stimulants, such as progesterone. The nurse's role in artificial ventilation is complex and is discussed in Chapter 26. The nurse's role in the management of respiratory stimulants includes knowing proper administration of the drug, monitoring its effect on ventilation, observing for side effects, and performing patient teaching.

If atelectasis causes the decreased lung inflation and is related to accumulation of secretions, chest physiotherapy may be indicated and is commonly practiced.

Since oxygenation depends on the supply and demand for oxygen, the nurse intervenes not only to increase the supply of oxygen but also to decrease the demand. In contrast to efforts to keep patients with COPD active to avoid deconditioning, the nurse helps patients with restrictive disease conserve energy to decrease the need for oxygen. These interventions may include helping patients limit the use of the upper extremities during activities of daily living or supporting the arms during these activities, helping plan efficient ways to accomplish tasks, and allowing for adequate rest between activities. The nurse includes family members in this intervention not only to incorporate them in the plan but also to teach them how the disease limits patients so they are unable to perform usual activities.

Since obesity is one extrapulmonary cause of restriction, the nurse may help with a plan for weight loss. This may include dietary management or surgical intervention. If a surgical procedure is performed, the postoperative care in this patient must include attention to the potential pulmonary complications associated with morbid obesity. Obese patients are more prone to atelectasis and pneumonia because of decreased lung expansion. Therefore the nurse must observe closely for these complications and encourage coughing and deep-breathing techniques and ambulation as soon as indicated.

Evaluation/Documentation

The nurse monitors the adequacy of oxygenation in terms of arterial blood gases (PaO_2 above 55 to 60 mm Hg), oxygen saturation (SaO_2 above 90%), and patient color and skin temperature. The long-term outcome may be evaluated in terms of the amount of oxygen required to meet these goals. Patients with interstitial fibrosis unfortunately require increasing oxygen concentrations as the disease progresses.

The nurse must quantify the self-report of a patient's dyspnea to evaluate the outcome of interventions. Since some of the diseases are progressively debilitating, the best the nurse might expect is only mild or subtle improvement in symptoms. The nurse who quantifies and documents the amount of activity patients can tolerate through observation in the acute setting and daily diaries in a long-term setting can evaluate patient progress or decline.

Ongoing Care

Rehabilitation and long-term care

Most of the etiologic factors of restriction cause long-term disability. After an acute setback or exacerbation of the disease, patients may require a phase of rehabilitation to facilitate a return to previous function. However, few data exist to support a particular approach with these patients. They may be en-

rolled in a pulmonary rehabilitation program that combines patient teaching, monitoring of exercise, occupational therapy, and assistance with coping strategies. Oxygen prescriptions are often made by the collaboration of the physician and nurse during rehabilitation or in the outpatient clinic. Patients with interstitial fibrosis may be prescribed steroids, so the outcome of this therapy is monitored in the rehabilitation setting.

Home care

The home care of patients with restrictive disorders primarily involves oxygen use and possibly home ventilation. The nurse helps patients and families find the best oxygen administration system to suit their needs in terms of space, mobility, and cost. When patients return home, the nurse teaches patients and families about the safe use of oxygen. The nurse includes the following in a teaching plan: the oxygen prescription and the reasons for using only the prescribed amount, fire precautions, use of equipment, access to agencies that supply oxygen, and information about agencies that may help pay for the cost of oxygen. Many patients may be embarrassed about wearing oxygen. These feelings may need to be explored, or an alternative oxygen apparatus therapy that is less conspicuous may need to be investigated.

Many of the restrictive disorders cause progressive debilitation. Therefore these individuals may not be able to perform the same roles in the family as before the disease occurred. The home care nurse may need to help the family members adjust to these changes as they shift household and financial responsibilities.

Some patients may require home ventilation. Both positive pressure ventilators, which require a tracheotomy, and negative pressure ventilators, which are noninvasive, may be used at home. The latter intervention is used most commonly in patients with neuromuscular disorders or spinal deformities. Discharge planning is begun far in advance of a patient's expected return home to ensure the equipment and personnel will be available. Most important, the family must be taught many techniques and skills, including tracheostomy care (if positive pressure ventilation is used), care of equipment, and emergency plans. Home ventilation poses many challenges to the nurse and to the patient and family. The impact of this intervention on families has not been investigated. Although potential benefits exist in terms of financial savings and preservation of family integrity, the nurse who cares for these patients must be particularly attuned to the potential deleterious effects of stress on families caring for these patients in the home.

RESPIRATORY FAILURE
Definition

Respiratory failure occurs when the lungs are unable to maintain oxygen and CO_2 homeostasis. Respiratory failure is a significant cause of morbidity and mortality in acute care centers. In the clinical setting, arterial blood gas analysis is used to evaluate and define respiratory failure. Generally, the criteria for respiratory failure include an arterial oxygen tension of less than 50 to 60 mm Hg or an arterial CO_2 tension of greater than 45 to 50 mm Hg.[21] Respiratory failure can be either acute or chronic depending on the underlying cause and rapidity of onset. The pH of the arterial blood gas is used to evaluate whether the respiratory failure is acute or chronic. During acute respiratory failure, patients are in acidosis (pH < 7.30), whereas in chronic respiratory failure the pH is normal or close to normal because of renal compensation. Further, respiratory failure can be categorized by the cause: ventilatory failure, oxygenation failure, and combined ventilatory and oxygenation failure. Table 28-3 differentiates among the three.

Ventilatory failure occurs when the alveolar ventilation is insufficient to maintain arterial P_{CO_2} within normal limits. Pathophysiologic mechanisms include defective ventilatory control mechanisms, altered mechanics of the lungs and chest wall, and impaired respiratory muscle function. Primary ventilatory failure occurs with depression of the central nervous system as in a drug overdose, and it can occur with neuromuscular diseases when the respiratory muscles cease to function adequately as in poliomyelitis, muscular dystrophy, and Guillain-Barré syndrome.

Oxygenation failure occurs when gas exchange is insufficient to maintain arterial P_{O_2} within normal limits given the level of the FIO_2. Pathophysiologic mechanisms include alveolar hypoventilation, impaired diffusion, mismatch of ventilation and perfusion, and right-to-left shunting. In alveolar hypoventilation the decreased P_{O_2} is secondary to the increased P_{CO_2} and can be seen even in the absence of lung tissue abnormalities. In this situation ventilatory failure causes oxygenation failure, resulting in a combination of ventilation and oxygenation failure. Impaired diffusion is a lesser cause of severe hypoxemia, contributing to severe hypoxemia, but it is seldom the primary cause of hypoxemia. Mismatch of ventilation and perfusion is the most common cause of hypoxemia and is found in most forms of oxygenation failure. Right-to-left shunting and severe hypoxemia can be seen in patients with pneumonia when pulmonary capillary perfusion persists to areas of consolidated lung tissue. Oxygenation failure and severe hypoxemia caused by diffuse infiltrates is seen in patients with acute respiratory distress syndrome (ARDS) and in patients with left ventricular failure. Left ventricular failure produces an increase in pulmonary venous pressure and pulmonary capillary pressure, eventually causing an increase in pulmonary blood volume and interstitial pulmonary edema. The increase in pulmonary capillary hydrostatic pressure drives fluid from the capillaries into the interstitial spaces and alveoli. This is referred to as increased pressure pulmonary edema or cardiac pulmonary edema, and it produces diffuse pulmonary infiltrates, decreases compliance of the lung, and increases the work of breathing. Care of the patient with left ventricular failure and increased pressure pulmonary edema is presented in Chapter 34. ARDS is a diffuse noncardiac pulmonary edema characterized by an increased permeability of pulmonary capillaries and is described below in greater detail.

A combined oxygenation and ventilatory failure can occur in COPD and severe asthma, diseases of the lung parenchyma and/or airways. For all patients with oxygenation failure the goal of therapy is to support oxygenation and ventilation while treating the underlying cause of the hypoxemia. Treat-

TABLE 28-3   Oxygenation and Ventilatory Respiratory Failure

Type of respiratory failure	Clinical examples	Blood gas changes		
		Pa_{O_2}	Pa_{CO_2}	$P(A-a)O_2$
Oxygenation	Pneumonia Pulmonary edema	Low	Normal to low	High
Ventilatory	Drug overdose Poliomyelitis	Low	High	Normal
Oxygenation and ventilatory	COPD Severe asthma	Low	High	High

ment of the underlying cause varies with the condition. Methods for supporting oxygenation and ventilation center around supplemental oxygen therapy and if necessary mechanical ventilation. These principles are illustrated in the care of patients with ARDS presented below.

Etiology/Epidemiology

ARDS is a common problem, and 65% of cases are fatal. In many cases the patients are young and otherwise healthy. Patients over 30 years and those with acquired immune deficiency syndrome (AIDS), aspiration pneumonia, multiorgan failure, and concurrent disseminated intravascular coagulation seem to have the poorest prognosis. ARDS is the result of massive injury to the lungs caused by a catastrophic event that triggers the lung injury. ARDS is not caused by abnormalities of the left side of the heart or chronic pulmonary disease.

Pathophysiology

ARDS is usually caused by an acute lung injury and characterized by an increased permeability pulmo-

ETIOLOGY OF ARDS

Major causes
Multiple blood transfusions
Aspiration of gastric contents
Sepsis
Trauma

Other causes
Diffuse pneumonia
Disseminated intravascular coagulation
Venous air embolism
Thrombotic thrombocytopenia purpura
Idiosyncratic drug reaction
Pulmonary contusion
High altitude
Smoke inhalation
Drug overdose
Oxygen toxic reaction
Irritant gas inhalation
Eclampsia
Fat embolism
Near-drowning
Leukemia
Surface burns
Radiation

From Crowley JJ, Raffin TA: Acute lung injury: mechanisms and potential therapy. In Simmons DH, editor: *Current pulmonology*, vol 12, St Louis, 1991, Mosby–Year Book, Inc.

nary edema (Figure 28-11). The acute lung injury involves damage to the endothelial cells of the pulmonary capillaries, increasing the permeability of the pulmonary capillaries and allowing movement of fluid and protein from the capillaries to the interstitial and alveolar spaces. Alveolar spaces become flooded, and surfactant activity is reduced. Proposed mechanisms of endothelial cell damage include direct injury of the cells during the aspiration of toxic chemicals, neutrophil-mediated injury, arachidonic acid metabolite injury, and coagulation product injury.[12] Neutrophils are thought to play an important role in the inflammatory process associated with some forms of acute lung injury.

Clinical Manifestations

Patients all experience marked respiratory distress and hypoxemia (even with supplemental oxygen therapy). Refractory hypoxemia in patients with no previous history of respiratory disease is a hallmark of ARDS. Chest x-ray findings are diffuse. Overall lung compliance is reduced with increased shunt fraction and dead space ventilation. Patients with no prior history of respiratory disease who develop sudden-onset, severe respiratory distress and severe hypoxemia that is refractory to oxygen therapy should be evaluated for ARDS.

Therapeutic Management

The aim of therapy is to support lung function until healing occurs and to prevent the development of complications related to medical therapy and the underlying disease process. The goals of therapeutic management are to optimize gas exchange between the atmosphere and blood, maintain adequate tissue perfusion through fluid balance and stable hemodynamics, and control the underlying problem.

Gas exchange

The first goal of therapeutic management—optimizing gas exchange—is generally approached through the use of mechanical ventilation. Every effort is made to use the lowest fraction of inspired oxygen (FIO_2) possible to avoid the complication of oxygen toxicity. Since patients on an FIO_2 of greater than 0.60 for 2 to 3 days are at a higher risk of developing oxygen toxicity, it is preferable to maintain patients on an FIO_2 of 0.50 or less. Usually treatment is initiated with high concentrations of oxygen to ensure adequate oxygenation, and then the FIO_2 is reduced as rapidly as possible. If greater than 0.50 FIO_2 is needed to correct the hypoxemia, positive end expiratory pressure (PEEP) is instituted in an effort to reduce the FIO_2.

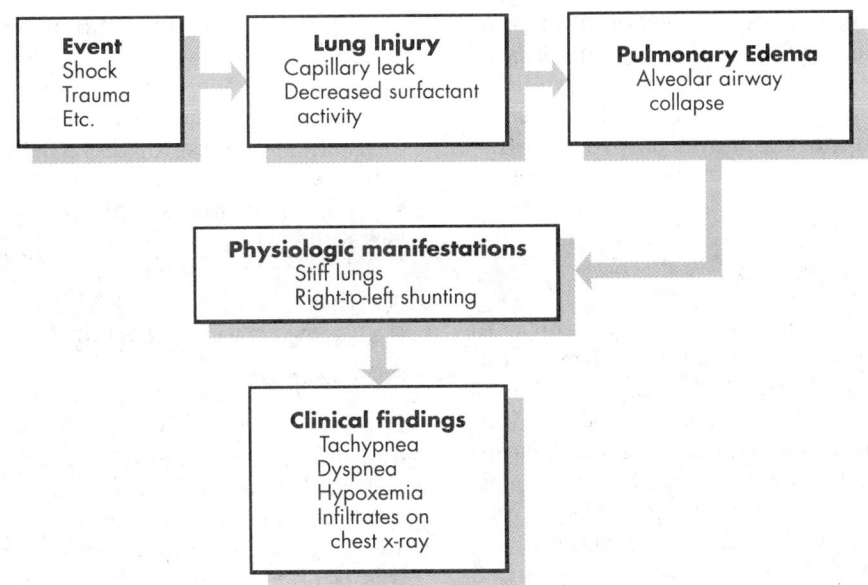

FIGURE 28-11 Pathophysiology of ARDS. (Adapted from Martin L: *Pulmonary physiology in clinical practice,* St Louis, 1987, Mosby–Year Book, Inc.)

PEEP maintains a positive intrathoracic pressure at the end of expiration, which helps to improve gas exchange by increasing ventilation to alveoli with low ventilation/perfusion ratios and expanding atelectatic alveoli. This PEEP is intended to reduce the need for high oxygen concentrations. PEEP is generally instituted if the PaO_2 is 60 mm Hg on 0.50 FiO_2. The level of PEEP should be guided by the ability to reduce inspired oxygen concentration without impairing oxygen delivery to the tissues.

When PEEP is instituted, clinical response is monitored by checking arterial oxygen tension, arterial blood pressure, cardiac output, and percentage of shunt. The level of PEEP is gradually increased by small increments (usually 3 to 5 cm H_2O) while the nurse frequently monitors the clinical response. If cardiac output and blood pressure fall during PEEP, patients may need to be supported by using vasoactive drugs or increased intravenous fluids.

Large tidal volumes are often used, ranging from 10 to 15 mL/kg of body weight. Since ARDS patients have decreased lung compliance (stiff lungs), ventilation with large tidal volumes and high levels of PEEP may result in elevated peak airway pressures. The peak airway pressure refers to the maximal amount of positive airway pressure that develops when the mechanical ventilator delivers a breath. Frequently this can be in excess of 50 to 60 cm H_2O at the end of inspiration in patients with ARDS.

Large tidal volumes, high levels of PEEP, and high peak airway pressures have been implicated as risk factors in barotrauma. High intrapulmonary pressures can rupture alveoli so that air escapes into other structures. Barotrauma is the presence of air outside the alveolus, and it is manifested in a number of ways: pulmonary interstitial emphysema, pneumothorax, pneumomediastinum, subcutaneous emphysema, pneumoperitoneum, tension lung cysts, or subpleural air cysts. It has been reported that inspiratory pressures greater than 70 cm H_2O are associated with a 43% risk of barotrauma, whereas the risk of barotrauma falls to 8% when inspiratory pressure is 50 to 70 cm H_2O.[30]

The choice between intermittent mandatory ventilation and assisted control ventilation is usually based on the personal preference of the physician, since controlled studies comparing the two modes are not available. The control mode of ventilation is usually reserved for patients in whom asynchronous breathing is causing ineffective ventilation and where a reduction in CO_2 production is needed. Conscious patients who require total control of ventilation are typically sedated and sometimes pharmacologically paralyzed.

Newer techniques for mechanical ventilation are employed to improve gas exchange while reducing potential side effects. High-frequency positive pressure ventilation and high-frequency jet ventilation have been used in an attempt to lower peak airway pressures and reduce the risk of barotrauma during mechanical ventilation.[50] These techniques involve rapid respiratory rates (anywhere from 60 to 200 breaths/min) at low tidal volumes. Inverse ratio ventilation is used to improve recruitment of alveoli and optimize alveolar ventilation. This technique increases inspiratory time so that the ratio of inspiratory/expiratory time is greater than one. It remains to be seen whether any of these techniques improve morbidity or mortality in comparison with conventional ventilatory support. Chapter 26 provides further information on the use of mechanical ventilation.

Tissue perfusion

The second goal of therapeutic management is to maintain adequate tissue perfusion and thereby enhance the delivery of oxygen to the tissues. This is achieved via careful fluid volume therapy and maintenance of stable hemodynamics. Increased capillary and alveolar membrane permeability as a result of lung injury promotes fluid extravasation and pulmonary edema. Any mechanism that promotes the formation of pulmonary edema, such as a positive fluid balance, must be avoided. Positive fluid balance (high blood volume) increases hydrostatic pressure, which tends to push fluid into the alveoli through leaky membranes. Conversely, hypovolemia (lower blood volume) must also be avoided. Although hypovolemia reduces pulmonary vascular pressure and pulmonary fluid extravasation, it also decreases cardiac output during PEEP, which impairs tissue perfusion. Therefore normovolemia is the goal of fluid management.

It is controversial whether colloids (e.g., albumin) or crystalloids (e.g., normal saline) are indicated. Since the edema fluid in the lungs is protein rich, it is thought that administration of colloids may worsen edema by leaking into the alveolus, increasing interstitial oncotic pressure, and pulling in more fluid. For this reason, as well as the added cost and lack of documented benefit in comparison with crystalloid therapy, colloids are generally not used.

Regardless of the approach to fluid therapy, patients must be closely monitored for signs of hypervolemia and hypovolemia. Hypervolemia is treated with diuretic therapy. Inotropic drugs, such as dopamine or dobutamine, may also be used to improve systemic oxygen transport by increasing cardiac output.

Management of underlying disease

The third goal of medical management is to control the underlying problem that precipitated the ARDS. For infected patients (i.e., sepsis, pneumonia), the microorganism should be identified and treated with appropriate antibiotic therapy. Controversy exists as to whether corticosteroids should be administered. Corticosteroids have been advocated for their antiinflammatory effects, depression of platelets, and depression of lung fibroblasts. Evidence of improved mortality or morbidity during ARDS with steroid therapy is lacking. In addition, some studies indicate that corticosteroids may worsen lung injury and significantly increase mortality as a result of secondary infection.[6,54] If corticosteroids are used, it is usually early in the course of the ARDS, and they are rapidly tapered off. Careful assessment for signs and symptoms of infection during steroid administration is important.

NURSING MANAGEMENT OF THE PATIENT WITH ARDS
Assessment

Patients at high risk for ARDS, such as those with multiple trauma, sepsis, or aspiration pneumonia, should be monitored for signs and symptoms of acute oxygenation failure. Patients should be assessed for signs and symptoms of hypoxemia, since this is one of the cardinal findings of ARDS. However, clinical signs of hypoxemia are unreliable and should be verified with arterial blood gases. The box below summarizes the signs and symptoms of hypoxemia and indicates how vulnerable the CNS and myocardium are to lowered oxygen tensions. In profound hypoxemia, convulsions, retinal hemorrhages, or brain damage can occur.[46]

Over 96% of ARDS patients require mechanical ventilation.[5] Once mechanical ventilation has been instituted, it is important to assess the adequacy of ventilation. The nurse checks the ventilator settings at frequent intervals including ventilation mode, FIO_2, respiratory rate, tidal volume, peak inspiratory pressure, level of PEEP, and status of alarm settings. The nurse assesses breathing patterns for evidence that the patient is "fighting the ventilator"—asynchronous breathing and triggering the high-pressure alarm by attempting to exhale while the ventilator is delivering a breath.

During the initiation of PEEP, the nurse must carefully evaluate the cardiovascular response as well as the gas exchange. Arterial blood pressure,

---

SIGNS AND SYMPTOMS OF HYPOXEMIA

Respiratory: dyspnea, severe tachypnea
CNS: combativeness, confusion, impaired judgment, restlessness, and diaphoresis
Cardiovascular: dysrhythmias, tachycardia, increased arterial blood pressure and increased pulmonary arterial pressure, eventually hypotension and bradycardia (severe hypoxemia)

heart rate, and cardiac output (if patients have a thermodilution-equipped pulmonary artery catheter) should be assessed after any increase in PEEP level. For patients with fiberoptic pulmonary artery catheters in place, mixed venous oxygen saturation (SVo$_2$) can be monitored to evaluate oxygenation.[70] In nonseptic patients, SVo$_2$ correlates with optimal oxygen delivery to the tissues.[47]

Fluid balance must also be carefully assessed to avoid overhydration or dehydration. Overhydration would increase extravascular lung water, and dehydration would lead to enhanced cardiovascular depression related to PEEP therapy. The balance of intake and output should be assessed on an hourly basis. Decreasing urine output can be a sign of poor renal perfusion related to low cardiac output. Also the humidity in the ventilator circuit is a source of insensible fluid gain (300 to 500 mL/day) and must be calculated into fluid intake. Patients receiving mechanical ventilation have increased levels of antidiuretic hormone (ADH), which also promotes fluid retention. Daily weights can be used to assess trends in fluid status. For patients with a pulmonary artery catheter, the pulmonary capillary wedge pressure (PCWP) and pulmonary artery diastolic (PAD) pressure are used to assess fluid status. These pressures reflect the left ventricular end-diastolic pressure, or filling pressure, of the heart. High pressures correlate with fluid overload, whereas low pressures correlate with low blood volume status. The optimal PCWP is the lowest pressure that can be maintained without adversely affecting the cardiac output. Normal readings of PCWP equal 5 to 12 mm Hg; and normal readings of PAD pressure equal 5 to 10 mm Hg.[26] Usually these two parameters have a high correlation, so the PAD pressure is used for continuous monitoring.

Because patients with ARDS demonstrate decreased lung compliance, they frequently require high peak airway pressures and high levels of PEEP for adequate ventilation. This places them at risk for barotrauma, making it important for the nurse to assess for signs and symptoms of barotrauma. Symptoms of barotrauma are presented in the box below.[21,30] Equipment for chest tube insertion should be readily available.

Mechanically ventilated patients are assessed for signs of gastrointestinal bleeding by testing stools for guaiac. Nutritional status is monitored to detect early evidence of malnutrition secondary to increased metabolism. Since infection increases mortality, the nurse assesses for evidence of infection, including hyperthermia and hypothermia, elevation of white blood cell count, or shift in the differential of the white blood cell count. Chapter 26 addresses nursing interventions related to patients supported by mechanical ventilation.

Nursing Diagnosis

The nursing diagnoses for ARDS patients relate to both the disease process itself and to the need for mechanical ventilation. Nursing diagnoses include the following:

Ineffective breathing pattern related to decreased lung compliance and anxiety

Impaired gas exchange related to increased shunt and ventilation-perfusion mismatch

Ineffective airway clearance related to immobility and artificial airway

Decreased cardiac output related to high PEEP

High risk for injury related to barotrauma

Fluid volume excess related to increased pulmonary membrane permeability and excess ADH secretion

Impaired verbal communication related to artificial airway and pharmacologic paralysis

Altered nutrition: less than body requirements related to altered metabolic demands and disruption of the oral route

Impaired physical mobility related to pharmacologic paralysis and bed rest

Impaired skin integrity related to altered perfusion and immobility

Altered oral mucous membranes related to artificial airway

Sleep pattern disturbance related to critical care environment and need for frequent nursing interventions

Powerlessness related to dependence on high-technology equipment

Ineffective family coping related to increased stress and anxiety of critical illness

---

SYMPTOMS OF BAROTRAUMA

Nonspecific findings

Agitation

Progressive hypoxemia

Hypotension and tachycardia

Cardiovascular collapse

Increased central venous pressure

Chest findings

Crepitation in neck, face, chest, axillae, or abdomen

Absence of breath sounds in conjunction with distended neck veins and distant heart sounds

Mediastinal crunch

Pulmonary interstitial emphysema on chest x-ray studies

Rising peak airway pressure

Planning

Nursing care for the patient with ARDS is planned to maintain respiratory and hemodynamic stability. Preventing complications and minimizing psychologic stressors for the patient and family are important parts of the care plan. Outcome criteria for the patient include the following:

Airway is patent

Breathing is in synchrony with the ventilator at a rate slow enough to maintain a normal level of ventilation ($Paco_2$ 35 to 45 mm Hg)

Pao_2 is above 60 mm Hg on 40% FIo_2 with a shunt fraction of less than 20%

Hemodynamic parameters (cardiac output, blood pressure, and heart rate) are stable

Peak airway pressure stays below 40 to 50 mm Hg

Pulmonary capillary wedge pressure is as low as it will go while maintaining an acceptable cardiac output

Balanced intake and output are maintained

Weight is stable

Needs are communicated through nonverbal means

Skin remains intact

Oral mucous membranes are moist and intact

Implementation

Gas exchange

The nursing interventions are based on the identified nursing diagnoses and goals. For impaired gas exchange it is important to monitor patients for signs of hypoxemia and to obtain arterial blood gases as indicated. When there is a change in ventilator settings, the blood gas should be obtained within 20 to 30 minutes. The use of an indwelling arterial catheter alleviates the need for repeated punctures. Certain nursing interventions, such as suctioning, can impair gas exchange. Suctioning should only be performed when secretions are present (i.e., crackles auscultated over large airways) and *not* on a routine basis, since many ARDS patients do not tolerate this procedure well.[56] Suctioning technique should include preoxygenation, minimal suction time, postsuctioning hyperinflation, and maintenance of PEEP. For patients on 10 cm H_2O PEEP or greater, a "PEEP adaptor" can be attached to the resuscitation bag, so that PEEP can be maintained during suctioning.

Breathing patterns

Asynchronous breathing leads to increased work of breathing, increased oxygen consumption, impaired ventilation, and higher peak airway pressures. It is important to provide emotional support and allay patient anxiety. Helping patients relax and encouraging them to "let the machine do the work" may help reduce tachypnea and oxygen consumption. If patients continue to "fight" the ventilator, sedation may be necessary. In some instances patients are pharmacologically paralyzed with intravenous pancuronium and sedated with either morphine or diazepam. Since patient sensorium is still intact, it is important to allay anxiety by reassuring them the paralysis is temporary and by administering sedatives to promote relaxation. Since paralyzed patients cannot breathe, inadvertent disconnection of the ventilator could result in cardiopulmonary arrest or death. Therefore it is essential the ventilator alarms are *never* turned off and are responded to promptly. The artificial airway should be securely stabilized, and a resuscitation bag with mask should be available at the bedside in the event of ventilator malfunction or accidental extubation. Patients have no cough reflex and must be carefully assessed for retained secretions. The eyes must be kept lubricated to avoid corneal abrasions related to absent corneal reflex.

Cardiac output

Maintaining cardiac output is essential for tissue oxygen delivery. Whenever the level of PEEP is increased, the cardiovascular response must be monitored. If the cardiac output drops and the patient is hypovolemic, fluid may be administered, or inotropic agents such as dopamine or dobutamine may be administered via continuous intravenous infusion. Hemodynamic parameters are monitored every 15 minutes until the patient is stabilized and then every 1 to 2 hours. Continuous monitoring using an electrocardiogram (ECG) monitor, indwelling arterial catheter, and pulmonary artery catheter helps provide early warning of changes in hemodynamic status. The nurse must also monitor perfusion of vital organs: (1) CNS—level of consciousness, movement, and sensation; (2) renal status—urine output, blood urea nitrogen, and serum creatinine; and (3) myocardium—heart rate and rhythm.

Airway clearance

Airway clearance is maintained by use of the artificial airway and suctioning. Chapter 26 discusses this in further detail.

Nutrition

Patients with ARDS are at risk for malnutrition because of increased metabolic needs and disruption of oral intake. Factors such as sepsis, trauma, fever, and increased work of breathing increase nutritional requirements. The presence of the artificial airway prevents intake via the oral route. Unstable hemodynamic status diverts attention from early nutritional support. All of these factors can lead to malnutrition. The amount of calories and protein should be based on the patient's hypermetabolic state. The enteral route is preferred, but poor gastrointestinal perfusion and motility can interfere with absorption of nutrients. Gastric distention should be avoided, since it can contribute to respiratory insufficiency. Regardless of the route of administration used, fluid balance and electrolytes (sodium, potassium, chloride, calcium, phosphate, and magnesium) must be carefully monitored.

Individual and family coping

ARDS is stressful for both patients and their families. Patients may experience feelings of powerlessness as a result of the inability to breathe and dependence on machines. They may feel anxious because of the strange surroundings, the amount of equipment, and the noise level in the critical care unit (Figure 28-12). It is important for the nurse to provide explanations about what is happening, provide opportunities for patients to participate in some decisions, support patients during periods of frustration and anxiety, and promote patient confidence in caregivers.[18] Patients who received pancuronium report that hearing and touch are what they remembered most.[69] Therefore it is important that both speech and touch be used when providing reassurance.

Family members may not be able to cope effectively with the sudden, severe changes in a patient's condition. The shock of seeing a loved one dependent on so many life-support machines is stressful. The nurse must remain calm and reassuring while giving clear explanations of what to expect. It is important to promote a sense of hope without misleading the family. Although the mortality of ARDS is high, the prognosis of ARDS survivors is quite encouraging. Some survivors of ARDS can have residual obstructive or restrictive pulmonary defects, reduced diffusing capacity, oxygen desaturation with exercise, or dyspnea; but the degree is usually mild.[14] Many ARDS survivors resume previous activities and occupations, although some may need to change to easier occupations.[51]

Family awareness of the good prognosis for survivors may help alleviate some of the stress. The nurse should also anticipate the need for family members to express fears and seek clarification of the patient's condition and therapy.

Evaluation

The nurse must evaluate the effectiveness of therapy aimed at improving gas exchange and oxygen transport, efforts to reduce the incidence of compli-

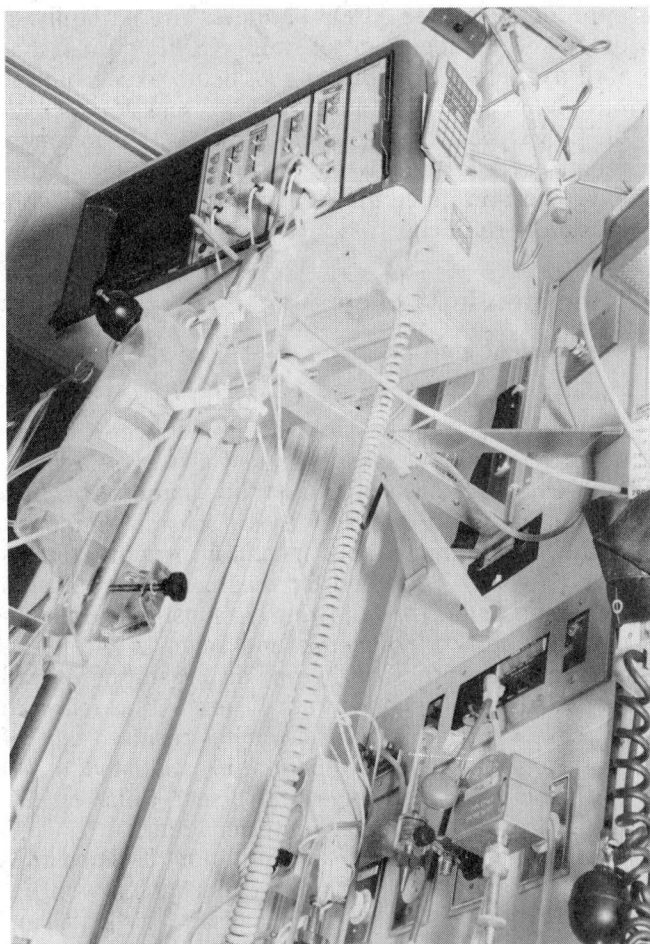

FIGURE 28-12   View from patient's perspective in intensive care unit.

cations (barotrauma, fluid imbalance, nutritional deficit), and interventions aimed at improving the psychosocial adjustment of both patient and family.

Documentation

To chart progress, it is important to document physiologic and psychosocial responses. Physiologic responses include arterial blood gas analysis, hemodynamic parameters, breathing pattern, and nutritional assessment. Changes in the psychosocial adjustment in response to nursing interventions should be documented so the approach of each nurse is consistent.

ACUTE OXYGENATION AND VENTILATION RESPIRATORY FAILURE: EXACERBATION OF COPD

The management of COPD patients with acute ventilatory and oxygenation failure is different from the approach used for ARDS patients. The pathophysiology and management of stable COPD patients, as well as factors precipitating an acute exacerbation, have been presented earlier. This discussion focuses on COPD patients in whom conservative management has failed to correct the acute ventilatory and oxygenation failure and for whom mechanical ventilation is required.

Therapeutic Management

Mechanical ventilation

Generally, mechanical ventilation of COPD patients is avoided if at all possible. The presence of an endotracheal tube causes increased airway resistance and work of breathing and an inability to use pursed-lip breathing. For these reasons, endotracheal intubation without mechanical ventilation is rarely used.[21] The need for mechanical ventilation is defined under the following circumstances: (1) patient has *severe* hypoxemia and acidosis and is unable to cooperate with therapy as a result of altered mental status; (2) conservative therapy has failed to improve hypoxemia/acidosis or has resulted in progressive somnolence; (3) patient is exhausted; or (4) patient is unable to expectorate secretions, resulting in progressive clinical deterioration.[49]

The mode of mechanical ventilation (assisted control ventilation vs. intermittent mechanical ventilation) is determined by the physician. Assisted control ventilation allows patients to select their own minute ventilation. However, rapid triggering of the ventilator can promote lung hyperinflation (because there is insufficient time for complete exhalation) and respiratory alkalosis. Overinflation of bullae can lead to barotrauma, and respiratory alkalosis can lead to cerebral vasoconstriction. The potential advantage of assisted control ventilation is that it may lower the work of breathing. When appropriately applied, intermittent mechanical ventilation reduces the likelihood of alkalosis and hyperinflation and allows patients to support part of the work of breathing.

COPD patients generally respond to oxygen administration; therefore the FIO_2 is adjusted to correct the hypoxemia. PEEP preferentially inflates lung areas with high compliance (such as bullae), which predisposes COPD patients to barotrauma; so it is generally not used. The determination of minute ventilation (tidal volume times rate) is based on the arterial blood gases. The goal is to attain a $PaCO_2$ equivalent to the patient's baseline before the exacerbation rather than a "normal" $PaCO_2$. For the pH, both acidosis and alkalosis should be avoided. Weaning from mechanical ventilation begins when the patient is stabilized (i.e., infection cleared, heart failure corrected, nutritional status improved, and bronchospasm relieved). Successful weaning re-

quires judgment and skill on the part of the clinician (see Chapter 26).

Drug therapy

During acute respiratory failure it is important to optimize bronchodilation. Intravenous aminophylline is commonly used to maintain a therapeutic drug level. Various factors affect the metabolism of aminophylline; therefore the maintenance infusion dosage varies (see discussion of treatment of asthma). Theophylline toxicity can be life threatening; therefore drug levels should be monitored closely. Inhaled beta agonists can be administered via the ventilator circuits. These drugs are administered for bronchodilation, as well as to improve clearance of secretions. Dosage depends on the drug (metaproterenol, albuteral, isoproterenol, isoetharine), and administration is usually every 3 to 4 hours. Unlike in ARDS, the use of corticosteroids in COPD patients with acute respiratory failure seems to speed recovery and decrease the length of mechanical ventilation.[21] Either methylprednisolone or hydrocortisone is given intravenously every 6 hours. Antibiotics are used only to treat specific infections, and the choice of agents relates to the causative organism (e.g., *Haemophilus influenzae, Streptococcus pneumoniae*). Digoxin is used if *left-sided* heart failure is present. Antidysrhythmic agents may be used for dysrhythmias that fail to respond to correction of hypoxemia and acidosis. Low-dose subcutaneous heparin may be used to avoid the complication of pulmonary embolism. Stress ulcer prophylaxis may also be considered (antacids, cimetidine, or ranitidine).

Nutrition

Nutritional support should begin early (as soon as patient is stabilized) to prevent further cachexia and wasting of inspiratory muscles. Since high glucose loads may increase CO_2 production and hypophosphatemia impairs oxygenation, both should be avoided. Generally the nonprotein calories for COPD patients are composed of a higher proportion of lipids than glucose. Extra lipids can be administered intravenously using lipid emulsions or enterally using specially formulated tube feedings or lipid additives.[28]

NURSING MANAGEMENT OF THE PATIENT WITH ACUTE OXYGENATION AND VENTILATORY FAILURE

Assessment

In addition to monitoring for signs and symptoms of hypoxemia, the nurse must assess patients for hypercapnia. Signs of hypercapnia include headache, lethargy, flushed dry skin, increased intracranial pressure, vasodilation, and papilledema. Adequacy of secretion clearance, response to mechanical ventilation, and degree of bronchospasm must be assessed. Since hypoxemia, hypercapnia, and acidosis influence the CNS, the neurologic status of patients should be evaluated. The nurse must also assess patients for signs of drug toxicity. Signs of aminophylline toxicity include CNS stimulation, nausea, diarrhea, insomnia, cardiac dysrhythmias, and seizures. If signs of toxicity occur, the serum drug level should be checked. The patient's cardiac rate and rhythm should be assessed, usually via a continuous cardiac monitor. Increases in cardiac rate may be a result of hypoxemia or beta-agonist administration, whereas rhythm disturbances can be caused by theophylline toxicity or hypoxemia. Fluid balance and nutritional status should also be evaluated.

Nursing Diagnosis

The nursing diagnoses include those previously discussed under the COPD section, as well as the potential for fluid volume excess. COPD patients in acute respiratory failure can have hormonal imbalances that predispose them to hyponatremia and edema.[48]

Planning

The nursing care for COPD patients in acute respiratory failure is planned to achieve the following outcomes:

Airway remains patent
Body weight remains stable
Intake and output remain balanced
Breathing pattern and arterial blood gas levels return to prefailure levels
Lungs clear to auscultation

Implementation

Secretion clearance is an important aspect of patient management. Timing of postural drainage, deep breathing, and suctioning after administration of inhaled beta agonists may improve clearance. The chest should be auscultated to evaluate the effectiveness of therapy. Many intensive care unit patients are kept flat in bed because of hemodynamic instability. However, COPD patients on a ventilator need to have the head of the bed elevated to optimize their pattern of breathing. Ventilated patients can be helped into a chair as soon as they are clinically stable. Length of time in the chair should be increased gradually to avoid fatigue. During weaning trials, patients can be coached to adopt a breathing pattern emphasizing deep inspirations with slow controlled exhalation. Weaning is discussed in more detail in Chapter 26.

Fluid balance in COPD patients with acute respiratory failure can be delicate. Dehydration may promote increased viscosity of secretions and reduce right ventricular filling pressure, and therefore it should be avoided. When filling pressure is low, the right ventricle may be unable to pump effectively against the resistance of pulmonary hypertension, causing decreased cardiac output and hypotension. Hypotensive patients may require judicious fluid therapy despite the presence of peripheral edema. Oxygen therapy can reduce pulmonary hypertension and promote fluid diuresis and improved cardiac output. Since PCWP readings are not reliable in patients with pulmonary hypertension, daily weights and accurate measurement of intake and output are essential. If diuretics are used, the patient's blood pressure should be carefully monitored.[21] Other aspects of care relate to the need for intubation and mechanical ventilation (see Chapter 26). Careful monitoring of the patient's response to therapy (especially during weaning) and early identification of complications by the nurse can positively influence patient outcomes.

Evaluation

The nurse must evaluate the effectiveness of interventions aimed at secretion clearance. The nurse must also evaluate the patient's response to mechanical ventilation and bronchodilator therapy, signs of drug toxicity, ability to tolerate weaning attempts, and fluid balance, as well as the complications, if any, the patient is experiencing.

Documentation

The nurse documents changes in breathing patterns (especially during weaning attempts), evidence of secretion removal (improved breath sounds, character/quantity of secretions), effectiveness of bronchodilation (reduced wheezing and dyspnea), signs related to fluid imbalance (peripheral edema, hypotension, intake/output, daily weights), and tolerance of weaning attempts (respiratory rate/pattern, heart rate, blood pressure, mental status, arterial blood gases).

Ongoing Care

When the underlying cause of the respiratory failure is controlled, most patients are weaned from the mechanical ventilator and discharged home. However, some patients cannot be weaned during the acute hospitalization and require long-term ventilator support. These patients may be transferred to a long-term ventilator unit where further attempts will be made to wean them from the ventilator. To prepare patients for further weaning trials nursing care focuses on improving nutritional status, maintaining skin integrity, and establishing communication and psychologic support, along with efforts to improve lung function. If these efforts are successful the patient is discharged home. If they are not successful in weaning the patient and establishing spontaneous ventilation the patient is evaluated for nursing home placement or home placement with long-term ventilator support.

Home care of the ventilator-dependent patient is attractive, because it is less expensive and it maintains the family unit. The situation is carefully evaluated to be sure that the family caregiver has adequate resources to care for the ventilator-dependent person without unduly straining the family unit. Financial resources and insurance coverage are carefully evaluated to determine if the family can afford to pay for the costs that are not covered by insurance. Utility costs will rise, some medical supplies will not be covered by insurance, and insurance policies may become depleted. Family caregivers report that problems with insurance coverage are very stressful and time consuming; hence a detailed analysis of the insurance coverage is important to avoid potentially serious financial problems for the family caregiver.[15] In addition to mastering the physical care—personal care and pulmonary care—the caregiver must be capable of coordinating services of equipment vendors for wheelchairs, enteral feeding supplies, ventilator equipment, oxygen equipment, and communication devices. The caregiver must also be prepared to coordinate and monitor the quality of home nursing services. To be successful the family caregiver must be prepared for all aspects of the role.

When home placement is requested the nurse initiates and coordinates an assessment of the family situation to determine feasibility of home placement. The nurse teaches the family caregiver how to care for the patient and provides opportunities for the caregiver to participate in the patient's care while in the hospital. The nurse arranges for follow-up support after discharge.

PNEUMONIA
Definition

Pneumonia is an inflammation of the lower respiratory tract that involves the lung parenchyma, including alveoli and supportive structures. It can be caused by a wide variety of etiologic agents including bacteria, viruses, fungi, and mycobacteria.[42] Mode of transmission and clinical manifestations vary depending on the etiologic agent. Pneumonia has been known as the friendly killer of elderly persons. It is often the presenting cause of death in elderly persons, although other chronic conditions are the real reason older adults die of pneumonia.[57]

Pneumonias are classified in a variety of ways. Clinicians classify pneumonias as either community acquired or hospital acquired. They can be further classified by anatomic dissemination of the inflammation or according to the causal agent. Community-acquired pneumonias are pneumonias that occur in the community. They usually begin as common respiratory illnesses and progress to fulminant pulmonary infections. *Streptococcus pneumoniae* is the most common cause of community-acquired pneumonia. Community-acquired pneumonias occur in very young and elderly persons. Hospital-acquired, or nosocomial, pneumonias are most commonly caused by bacteria, such as *Pseudomonas aeruginosa, Klebsiella pneumoniae,* and *Staphylococcus aureus.* Many cases are transmitted by direct contact through the hands of hospital personnel. A recent study reported an incidence of 6.5 cases of hospital-acquired pneumonia per 1000 admissions.[4] Nosocomial pneumonias account for 16% of nosocomial infections, and associated death rates are related to both the etiologic agent and the general clinical status of the patient. The mortality ranges from 30% to 50%, but most of these pneumonias occur in the intensive care units where the critical condition of the patient contributes to the high mortality.

Pneumonias are sometimes classified according to anatomic location. Lobular pneumonias or bronchopneumonias refer to patchy consolidations of the lung, which may be limited to one lobe but generally include both lungs and more than one lobe. Lobar pneumonias refer to infections of an entire lobe or a major portion of the lobe. Pneumonias can also be classified according to the causal agent. For example, they may be referred to as viral, bacterial, or fungal pneumonias. However, once the specific etiologic organism has been identified, it will be used to classify pneumonias such as pneumococcal, staphylococcal, or *Klebsiella* pneumonia.

Etiology/Epidemiology

Pneumonia results from an interaction between pathogen and host. When the respiratory system is exposed to infectious organisms, the outcome depends on the condition of the respiratory defenses, the number of pathogens, and the virulence of the pathogens. Compromised patients are more susceptible to the invasion of pathogens. Virulent pathogens are more likely to succeed in overcoming respiratory defenses. Inoculation with large doses of pathogens is more likely to overwhelm respiratory defenses than small doses. Pathogens can be introduced into the lung by three primary routes: aspiration, inhalation, and circulatory spread.

Mode of transmission

Aspiration transmits microorganisms from the oropharynx and gastrointestinal tract to the lungs by direct contact. The oropharyngeal secretions contain many bacteria, which inoculate the lungs when aspirated. Aspiration is a common cause of bacterial pneumonias, especially nosocomial pneumonias. Patients predisposed to aspiration pneumonia include those with disorders of the esophagus, diminished gag and cough reflexes, and an endotracheal or nasogastric tube.

Inhalation is an important mode of transmission. Microorganisms are suspended in water droplets and sprayed into the air with coughing, sneezing, and talking. If the water droplets are small, they will remain suspended long enough for the water to evaporate, leaving a droplet nucleus that includes the microorganism. The droplet nucleus is a small particle that remains suspended in the air for a long time and can be inhaled deeply into the lungs. If enough microorganisms are inhaled to overcome the lung defenses, the lungs will become infected. The more virulent organisms require smaller doses to infect the lungs. It is difficult to demonstrate airborne transmission of microorganisms, but it is thought that viral infections are transmitted in this manner, whereas most bacterial pneumonias are transmitted in other ways.

Circulatory spread of infections occurs when pathogens are transmitted through the circulatory system to the lungs from preexisting infections in other parts of the body. This occurs in patients with septicemia and endocarditis, but especially in those patients who also have lung disease or are immunosuppressed.

Risk factors

Alterations in respiratory defenses place some people at increased risk for developing pneumonia. Older people have a greater risk of developing pneumonia, and this is attributed in part to an age-related decline in the immunologic system and the prevalence of underlying diseases in this population (see box).[68] Patients with chronic respiratory diseases, such as bronchiectasis, cystic fibrosis, and COPD, experience recurrent bouts of pneumonia, which are attributed to impaired mucociliary clearance. In addition, patients with other chronic debilitating diseases such as chronic congestive heart failure, tricuspid or pulmonary valvular heart disease, diabetes mellitus, hepatic failure, and renal failure are predisposed to pneumonia because of impaired respiratory defenses. Patients with severe nutritional deficits tend to develop recurrent pneumonias that are related to associated deficiencies in the immune system. Alcoholics, drug abusers, and patients with neurologic problems, such as impaired gag reflex or swallowing reflex, are at risk for aspiration pneumonia.

Immunosuppressed patients are at risk for opportunistic infections. Those at risk include patients tak-

GERIATRIC CONSIDERATIONS

Pneumonia

Pneumonia is the fourth leading cause of death among people over 65 years of age. Older adults living in nursing homes are at highest risk. Because the older adult may have other chronic health problems, morbidity and mortality from pneumonia are higher than in younger adults. Several factors contribute to the older adult's increased risk: age-related changes in immune function, decreased cough reflex, decreased functional reserve, and decreased mobility. The bedridden older adult is at increased risk for aspiration pneumonia.

Pneumonia is often overlooked in the older adult because the symptoms do not present a typical clinical picture. Instead of fever and pulmonary symptoms, pneumonia in the older adult may be manifested by lethargy, confusion, tachypnea, and dehydration.

ing chemotherapy for a malignancy, patients taking immunosuppressive drugs for organ transplant, patients taking long-term oral corticosteroids for asthma, and patients with AIDS.

Bacterial pneumonias

Less than one half of all reported pneumonias are caused by bacteria, but most pneumonias found in older people are bacterial in origin. Of those pneumonias requiring hospitalization, at least 80% are caused by bacterial agents.

Gram-positive organisms such as *Streptococcus pneumoniae, Staphylococcus aureus,* and *Streptococcus pyogenes* can cause pneumonias. Most cases occur in winter or early spring and are often preceded by an upper respiratory infection. The exact mode of transmission is unknown. Death rates for all hospitalized patients range from 15% to 20%, but in hospitalized patients over 70 years old, mortality ranges from 50% to 70%.[22]

Mycoplasma pneumoniae, free-living, nonmotile bacteria with no cell walls, produce a relatively mild pneumonia in healthy persons. *Mycoplasma* pneumonia occurs in all age groups and is transmitted from person to person by aerosolized respiratory droplets and can spread rapidly through a family.

Haemophilus influenzae is a Gram-negative bacillus that commonly colonizes the airways of patients with COPD and is thought to spread through aerosolized respiratory droplets. *H. influenzae* pneumonias occur commonly in older persons with COPD, chronic alcoholism, or diabetes mellitus, and they often require hospitalization. Death rates are approximately 30%, especially in older, chronically ill patients.

Anaerobic bacteria are prevalent in the upper respiratory tract and, when aspirated in sufficient quantities, can produce both community- and hospital-acquired pneumonias. The most common anaerobic organisms include *Fusobacterium nucleatum,* pigmented *Bacteroides, Peptostreptococcus,* and microaerophilic *Streptococcus.*[22] Many patients with anaerobic pneumonia have concomitant chronic illnesses, such as malignancy, bronchiectasis, and pulmonary infarction.

Gram-negative pathogens such as *Klebsiella, Pseudomonas, Enterobacter, Escherichia, Proteus,* and *Pseudomonas* species commonly produce pneumonias as secondary infections in immunocompromised patients. *Klebsiella pneumoniae* is the most common cause of Gram-negative pneumonia. It generally results from aspiration of oral secretions, but it can be transmitted by contaminated respiratory therapy equipment.

Pseudomonas aeruginosa, a Gram-negative bacillus, is the most common cause of nosocomial pneumonias. *Pseudomonas* colonizes in the oropharyngeal region and is aspirated into the lungs. It can also be transmitted by contaminated respiratory therapy equipment. *Pseudomonas* pneumonias generally occur in elderly persons with chronic health problems, such as heart disease or COPD.

Viral pneumonia

Influenza virus type A is the most common cause of viral pneumonias in healthy persons and can be community acquired or hospital acquired. Epidemics of influenza virus are associated with an increased incidence of pneumonia. This virus produces a severe pneumonia in previously healthy people and is thought to be transmitted by airborne droplet, which makes it easily spread in a hospital or nursing home environment. As previously mentioned, the influenza virus interferes with pulmonary defenses, making patients more susceptible to a secondary bacterial pneumonia.

Cytomegalovirus is the most common cause of viral pneumonia in immunosuppressed patients. Patients with organ transplants, patients with autoimmune deficiency syndrome, and patients taking antineoplastic drugs are susceptible to cytomegalovirus. Cytomegalovirus affects many organs throughout the body, but its greatest effects are on the lungs. It produces a severe pneumonia with high death rates.

Fungal infections

Histoplasmosis is caused by *Histoplasma capsulatum.* It is transmitted by inhalation of spores. *H.*

capsulatum is a fungus that lives in the soil and requires organic nitrogen for growth.[34] It is endemic in a number of areas in the United States and thrives in soil that is high in nitrogen, such as soil in areas with many bird droppings and compost heaps.

H. capsulatum invades the lungs and spreads throughout the body via the circulatory system. In most cases, histoplasmosis is either asymptomatic or is characterized by a brief infection of the lower respiratory tract that is self-limiting and requires no special treatment. In some cases it produces a severe pneumonia, which is treated with amphotericin B.

Coccidioidomycosis is caused by *Coccidioides immitis. C. immitis* is endemic in the southwest United States and northern Mexico and is transmitted by inhaling spores that live in the soil in these areas. When spores are inhaled into the alveoli, they cause a granulomatous and suppurative response. Most infections are asymptomatic; some produce a mild respiratory illness, and some produce a severe pneumonia. Amphotericin B is the drug of choice when treatment is required.

Other pneumonias

Protozoa and helminths are rare causes of pneumonia, but *Pneumocystis carinii* has recently been noted for its high incidence in patients with AIDS. *P. carinii* is thought to be a unicellular protozoon, but recent evidence suggests it may be a fungus. It is thought to be transmitted by airborne droplets, but there is no research evidence to support this, and it may result from reactivation of a latent infection.[29] Death rates are high.

Pathophysiology

Alterations in pathophysiology vary considerably depending on the causative organism, but pneumonia generally refers to an inflammation of the lung parenchyma associated with the production of exudate. The alveoli, bronchioles, and bronchi are filled with suppurative exudate that consolidates and prevents ventilation of a portion of the lung. This produces arteriovenous shunting and hypoxemia. The severity of hypoxemia is related to the magnitude of the shunt and the extent of compensatory hypoxic vasoconstriction in the affected area.

Clinical Manifestations

Specific clinical manifestations of pneumonia are related to the infectious organism, the patient's prior health status, and the extent of the infection. Some patients experience few symptoms, whereas others become critically ill. Patients are hospitalized if they develop hypoxemia, respiratory or metabolic acidosis, multilobar disease, dehydration, or extrapulmonary complications associated with an underlying condition. Pneumonias can be classified as typical or atypical on the basis of clinical presentation.

Typical pneumonias have an abrupt onset of fever and shaking chills accompanied by a cough that becomes productive with purulent sputum and a pleuritic type of chest pain. However, presenting symptoms in elderly persons may be anorexia, weakness, lethargy or confusion, and a rapid respiratory rate. Temperature is not a reliable sign of infection in older persons. *S. pneumoniae, H. influenzae,* and *K. pneumoniae* are the most common causative organisms for typical pneumonia.

Physical examination of the lungs reveals evidence of consolidations, including dullness to percussion over the affected area of the lungs with increased fremitus, bronchophony, egophony, bronchial breath sounds, and crackles. Typical findings on chest x-ray studies include patchy infiltrates or consolidation over the affected area and a small pleural effusion in some patients. Arterial blood gases show evidence of hypoxemia. The white blood cell count is generally elevated, with an increase in the immature polymorphonuclear leukocytes.

In contrast, atypical pneumonias have a gradual, insidious onset of symptoms, including headache, sore throat, muscle soreness, and fatigue. Patients might experience a dry cough, and some produce mucoid sputum. They generally do not experience fever and chills. Viral infections and *Mycoplasma pneumoniae* are the most common causes of atypical pneumonia, although *Legionella pneumophila* infection also produces an atypical pneumonia.[17] Physical assessment can reveal a few scattered wheezes and crackles with minimal or no evidence of consolidation. Chest x-ray film changes range from minimal infiltrates to substantial bilateral infiltrates. The white blood cell count can be slightly elevated, but it is commonly less than 10,000/mL.

Therapeutic Management

Bacterial pneumonias are treated with antimicrobial drugs and supportive therapy. Treatment for viral pneumonias is limited to supportive therapy with close observation for evidence of respiratory failure and early treatment of secondary bacterial pneumonias. Supportive therapy is directed toward relief of symptoms and generally includes bed rest, maintenance of adequate fluid and nutritional intake, antitussives to relieve coughing, and mild analgesics to relieve muscle soreness.

NURSING MANAGEMENT OF THE PATIENT WITH PNEUMONIA
Assessment

Data required for assessing the adequacy of oxygenation include either arterial blood gases or oxygen saturation as measured by pulse oximetry, respiratory rate, heart rate, blood pressure, and level of consciousness. Evidence of hypoxemia includes a decrease in oxygen saturation accompanied by a change in the level of consciousness and sometimes accompanied by rapid shallow breathing and dyspnea. Persistent severe hypoxemia is associated with an initial increase in heart rate and blood pressure, which, if not treated, is followed by a decline in both. To assess the adequacy of airway clearance, the nurse auscultates the chest for evidence of fluid in the airways, paying special attention to the presence of crackles and wheezes. Other aspects of the nursing assessment that are especially important in planning nursing care for patients with pneumonia include evidence related to fluid balance, nutritional status, activity tolerance, body temperature, anxiety, comfort, sleep, and rest.

Nursing Diagnosis

Specific nursing diagnoses for patients with pneumonia vary depending on the severity of the infection. Appropriate nursing diagnoses might include the following:

Impaired gas exchange related to ventilation-perfusion mismatch or arteriovenous shunting

Ineffective airway clearance related to increased secretions

Activity intolerance related to tissue hypoxia

Altered nutrition: less than body requirements related to inadequate intake

Anxiety related to dyspnea

Sleep pattern disturbance related to frequent coughing

Planning

Priorities for planning nursing care of patients with pneumonia include treatment of the infection, maintenance of adequate oxygenation, and maintenance of patent airways while observing for evidence of complications such as respiratory failure. Appropriate outcome criteria include the following:

Pa_{O_2} greater than 55 mm Hg at rest and with activities

Breath sounds clear with coughing

Sputum expectorated with minimal effort

Patient reports no shortness of breath

Activities produce usual level of fatigue

During activities the rate and depth of respirations remain within usual range for each patient

Appetite returns to normal baseline

Patient consumes regular meals that provide adequate nutrients

Patient sleeps comfortably at night and feels rested in the morning

Implementation

Hypoxemia is an early sign of impaired gas exchange, and it must be identified and treated early to prevent the development of respiratory failure. Administration of supplemental oxygen may be appropriate for patients with hypoxemia. It will increase alveolar oxygen tension and increase the gradient for diffusion, but it will not improve gas exchange in areas of the lung with arteriovenous shunting.

The potential for ineffective airway clearance is greatest for patients with bacterial pneumonia because of the increase in tracheobronchial secretions. The nurse helps the patient with frequent changes in position and deep-breathing exercises to aid in mobilizing secretions. If the patient becomes fatigued with coughing, the effort required for coughing can be reduced by teaching the patient to perform the "huff" cough as described in Chapter 26. The patient may also benefit from chest physiotherapy if he or she can tolerate it.

Dyspnea at rest can make patients uncomfortable in the early stages of pneumonia. Dyspnea may be reduced by positioning patients with the head of the bed elevated, using pursed-lip breathing, limiting physical exertion, and maintaining patent airways. Bronchodilators may also relieve dyspnea for some patients.

As the clinical condition improves, the nurse gradually advances activity levels while monitoring oxygen saturation with a pulse oximeter to make sure the patient tolerates the activity without desaturating more than 4%. It is important for the nurse to accompany the patient during early attempts at ambulation and to explain the function of the pulse oximeter. This reduces anxiety and gives the patient confidence in his or her ability to tolerate exertion. If a pulse oximeter is not available, the nurse must monitor other signs of oxygenation.

During the acute stages of pneumonia, patients lose their appetites and are at risk for developing a nutritional deficit. Consequently assessment and treatment of nutritional status should immediately begin. The nurse closely monitors nutritional intake and changes in weight while consulting with the patient, close family members, and the dietitian to ensure that sufficient nutrients are consumed to meet energy needs and prevent loss of muscle mass. Total parenteral nutrition may be necessary in severe prolonged illnesses.

Older patients may develop an acute confused state and require major intervention to protect their safety. Restraints may have to be applied; however, open dialogue must be maintained not only to assess mentation but also to determine appropriate interventions. The nurse should involve family members at all times.

Patient teaching is an important aspect of patient care, because patients are less anxious and they tend to participate to a greater extent in their own care if they understand their condition and the rationale for therapy. This includes the rationale for an adequate intake of fluids and nutrients, the need to cough and clear secretions from the lungs, and the need to gradually increase activity with planned periods of rest. Patients also need information about their infectiousness and transmission of organisms to avoid unnecessary isolation and to avoid infecting other people at high risk of infection. Moreover,

NURSING CARE PLAN   *Patient with Pneumonia*

Nursing diagnosis/ Expected outcomes	Interventions	Rationale
Ineffective airway clearance related to accumulation of mucus and exudate in response to airway infection; inadequate cough in response to fatigue, pain, or tenacious sputum • *Airway will be free of secretions* • *Breath sounds will be clear throughout lung fields*	Assess sputum production: volume, color, consistency, and clarity; obtain specimens as ordered Assess effectiveness of cough: ability to expectorate sputum; strength of cough Auscultate and percuss lungs for evidence of crackles, rhonchi (low-pitched wheezes), diminished breath sounds, dullness to percussion, presence of pain or guarding that diminishes ability to cough Avoid cough suppressants if patient is producing sputum	Accumulation and stagnation of secretions will delay recovery from pneumonia; deep breathing will help maintain patency of peripheral airways, and it will help mobilize secretions; the huff cough helps mobilize secretions and requires limited energy expenditures; postural drainage is only helpful in patients producing large volumes of secretions. If secretions are thick and tenacious, humidified air may be necessary to loosen mucus

Nursing diagnosis/ *Expected outcomes*	Interventions	Rationale
	Help patient with mobilization of secretions: teach patient huff cough; encourage deep breathing every 1 to 2 hours while awake; maintain normal levels of hydration	Cough suppressants may impair normal mechanisms for airway clearance and contribute to retention of secretions
	Perform chest physiotherapy, including percussion and postural drainage as indicated and tolerated; provide humidity to loosen secretions, including humidified oxygen or ultrasonic nebulizer as prescribed; suction airway if patient unable to mobilize secretions using nasopharyngeal or oropharyngeal airway	
	Have patient support area of pain if it inhibits an effective cough	
	Anticipate need for endotracheal intubation for management of secretions	Intubation may be required if tracheobronchial secretions have to be removed by suctioning
	Teach family member percussion and postural drainage if patient has excessive secretions at time of discharge	
Impaired gas exchange, hypoxemia related to arteriovenous shunting and diffusion • *Arterial Po₂ will remain higher than 55 mm Hg* • *Resume usual breathing pattern* • *Resume or maintain mental status*	Assess adequacy of gas exchange: assess rate, depth, and pattern of respiration on a routine basis	Patient is at risk for developing hypoxemia; increased concentrations of inspired oxygen will increase the rate of oxygen diffusion at the level of the alveolar and capillary membranes
	Monitor arterial blood gases intermittently until patient stabilizes	
	Monitor oxyhemoglobin saturation continuously with oximetry while patient is unstable	
	Assess skin color	
	Monitor for altered mental status: restlessness, lethargy, disorientation	
	Notify physician immediately of deteriorating arterial blood gases or mental status	
	Administer oxygen as ordered	
	Anticipate need for mechanical ventilation to ensure adequate oxygenation	Mechanical ventilation may be needed to ensure oxygenation and ventilation by delivering high concentrations of oxygen at high tidal volumes
	Monitor body temperature on a regular basis	A spike in temperature may be evidence of inadequate antibiotic therapy
Activity intolerance related to dyspnea, fatigue, tissue hypoxia, excessive coughing, disruption of sleep, malnutrition • *Ability to perform activities without excessive fatigue* • *Resume normal sleep patterns*	Provide for ample rest periods: pace and prioritize activities; monitor for excessive fatigue; explain patient's rest needs to family, help them with pacing their visits and encourage them to help patient as indicated	Decreased activity tolerance may be related to decreased delivery of oxygen to the tissues, increased work of breathing, and inadequate nutritional intake

Continued.

NURSING CARE PLAN   *Patient with Pneumonia—cont'd*

Nursing diagnosis/ Expected outcomes	Interventions	Rationale
	Provide for uninterrupted sleep periods: plan nursing activities around hours of sleep; encourage patient to notify nurse when awake to take advantage of wakefulness for necessary assessments/ treatments; use sleep aids cautiously, since they may suppress necessary respiratory drive	
	Use cough suppressants only if patient does not produce sputum	A dry, persistent cough can be fatiguing; under these circumstances a cough suppressant may help conserve energy
	Ensure adequate nutrition: assist with meals if unable to tolerate activity; choose high protein/high carbohydrate foods; patient may prefer small, frequent feedings; use nutritional supplements as required; anticipate need for enteral/parenteral feeding	
Anxiety related to symptoms of fear, dyspnea, and pleuritic chest pain • *Decreased level of anxiety*	Explain common symptoms of pneumonia including pain, dyspnea	Anxiety is often associated with dyspnea and rapid, shallow breathing; relief of dyspnea may reduce anxiety
	Explain procedures	
	Allow significant others time with patient but avoid fatiguing the patient (the presence of family members may provide a sense of security)	
	Reassure and help patient regain control of breathing pattern	
	Assess for evidence of acute impaired gas exchange	Severe hypoxemia can produce anxiety, especially when a mucous plug develops in an intubated patient
	Relieve any mucous plugging	
Knowledge deficit related to new condition and unfamiliarity with the disease process • *Patient and family will demonstrate understanding of treatments and disease process and comply with necessary treatments*	Provide information regarding acute situation to patient and family	Information enables patient to participate to a greater extent in his care
	Provide preventive information: assess risk factors, including age, immunosuppression, and chronic pulmonary disease; teach appropriate avoidance behaviors for patients in high-risk groups; encourage vaccination for influenza and pneumococcus in high-risk groups; provide information and encourage good nutrition in individuals at risk for malnutrition	
	Evaluate effectiveness of patient/ family teaching; reinforce or explore alternative teaching methods	

patients who are susceptible to repeated lower respiratory infections should learn the signs and symptoms of pneumonia. They should know to call their primary caregiver if they experience persistent difficulty in breathing associated with a fever.

Evaluation

The time required for full recovery from pneumonia depends to a great extent on the patient's prior health status. Healthy persons recover much faster than persons with chronic debilitating conditions, such as chronic lung disease or chronic alcoholism, and the nurse must remember this when evaluating the patient's progress. With effective antibiotic therapy, respiratory function gradually improves, but pharmacologic therapy must be changed if there is no improvement or if respiratory function deteriorates. As patients improve, their breathing pattern returns to normal both at rest and during exertion, and they tolerate increasing levels of physical activity. The nurse can also expect to see improvements in the patient's appetite and energy level. Many patients are predisposed to repeated episodes of pneumonia, and it is especially important they demonstrate an understanding of the disease condition and rationale for therapy, as well as the early signs and symptoms of pneumonia so they know when to seek medical attention in the future.

Documentation

An accurate record of assessment data, nursing interventions, and response to therapy is necessary to evaluate patient progress and the effectiveness of nursing interventions. Records of arterial blood gases, breath sounds, and breathing patterns, as well as the color, consistency, and quantity of sputum, are vital in documenting patient progress. Subjective data should also be documented describing intensity of dyspnea, activity tolerance, and psychosocial adjustment. In addition, each nurse must document patient teaching so it can be reinforced by other nurses.

TUBERCULOSIS
Definition

Since antimycobacterial chemotherapy was developed in the 1940s, the incidence of tuberculosis has continued to decrease, until 1986 when it began to rise.[11] In the United States over 20,000 cases of tuberculosis are reported each year. **Tuberculosis** is a disease caused by an infection with *Mycobacterium tuberculosis* bacilli, and it is primarily a disease of the lungs, but it can involve other places such as lymphatic, pleural, genitourinary, disseminated or "miliary," bone and joint, meningeal, and peritoneal sites. Extrapulmonary involvement is common in persons with HIV infection. This discussion will be limited to pulmonary tuberculosis.

Etiology/Pathophysiology

The most common cause of tuberculosis is *M. tuberculosis*, but *M. bovis* and *M. africanum* can also cause tuberculosis. The *M. tuberculosis* is a robust bacillus that is capable of surviving for long periods under adverse circumstances. One study demonstrated that 28% to 32% of bacilli survived for 9 hours in standard room conditions.[60] However, this bacillus can be killed with exposure to ultraviolet light.

Tuberculosis can be highly contagious and is transmitted by airborne mechanisms from infected persons. All persons infected with the tuberculosis bacilli, however, will not necessarily develop tuberculosis, and only 10% of infected people will develop the disease some time in their life.[11] After initial exposure a localized tuberculin infection develops and in most cases automatically heals. A calcified lesion or focus (Ghon's lesion) remains, and the clinical condition of tuberculosis develops many years later.

People at the greatest risk for developing tuberculosis include those who are immunocompromised as in HIV infection; live in overcrowded conditions such as slums, prisons, nursing homes, and shelters for the homeless; and are intravenous drug users, alcoholic, malnourished, or elderly. Moreover, persons living in close contact with an active tuberculosis patient are more likely to become infected and to develop tuberculosis. This in part explains the higher incidence of tuberculosis associated with crowded impoverished living conditions. The high prevalence of active tuberculosis in elderly people is caused by the endogenous reactivation of an old infection that occurred 50 to 70 years ago, before the development of antituberculosis drugs (see geriatric box).[13] In this population, reactivation is associated with many of the risk factors for initial infection. In addition, elderly people can be newly infected while living in the closed environment of a nursing home.

Clinical Manifestations

Symptoms vary from patient to patient depending on the extent of the disease. Patients in the early stages of tuberculosis with small inflammatory lesions will be asymptomatic, whereas patients with advanced bilateral, cavitary, multicentric disease are more likely to experience symptoms. The most common symptom of pulmonary tuberculosis is a cough. Initially the cough is nonproductive, but if the disease progresses without treatment, the cough will become productive with mucoid or mucopurulent sputum. Hemoptysis may eventually develop, but hem-

Tuberculosis

Many factors contribute to the increased incidence of tuberculosis among older adults. Normal age-related changes in immune function and the presence of chronic health problems increase their susceptibility. Many older adults were exposed to tuberculosis when younger because of its former prevalence. The occurrence of tuberculosis in the older adult may represent reactivation of a dormant infection. The decreased immune function limits the usefulness of skin tests in diagnosing the disorder. A chest x-ray film or sputum culture is more accurate.

The classic symptoms may not be present. Instead, the older adult may only have weight loss or anorexia as a clinical manifestation. Drug therapy for tuberculosis is effective in the older adult, but more frequent monitoring for side effects is an important part of nursing management.

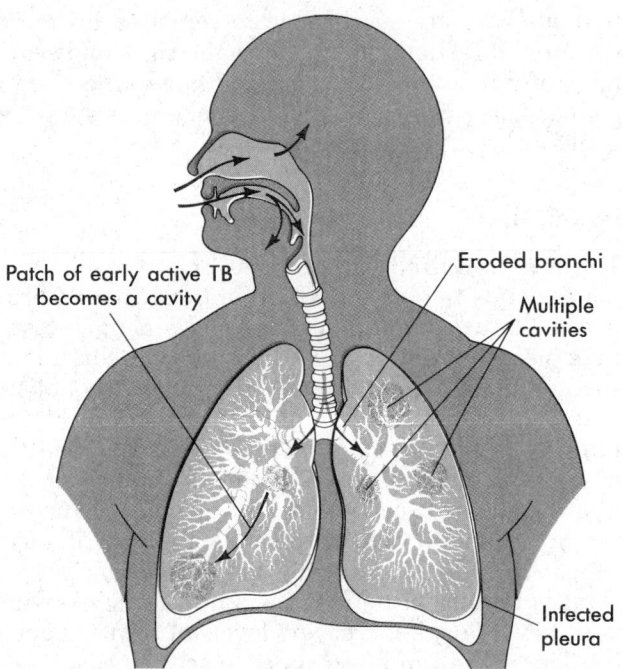

Patch of early active TB becomes a cavity

Eroded bronchi

Multiple cavities

Infected pleura

FIGURE 28-13 Clinical manifestations of active tuberculosis include infection, cavitation, and tissue destruction.

orrhage only occurs in extensive cavitary disease. When the lung tissue adjacent to the pleura is involved, patients will experience a pleuritic type of chest pain. This pain is generally sharp and made worse by a deep breath or a cough. Dyspnea is rare except in advanced cases or in patients with complications, such as pleural effusion or pneumothorax. Systemic effects such as fever, night sweats, malaise, weight loss, anorexia, and fatigue are seen in patients with extensive disease.

As with other infectious diseases, clinical manifestations in elderly persons may be atypical. If the person is mentally confused it may be difficult to get a clear description of symptoms. Moreover, a chronic productive cough may be attributed to a long history of smoking.

In the early stages of tuberculosis, inflammatory lesions are visible on chest x-ray films as small nondescript densities most commonly found in the apical and posterior segments of the right upper lobe or in the apicoposterior segment of the left upper lobe. As the condition progresses, large areas of the lung are infected, and cavitation and tissue destruction occur (Figure 28-13) and are visible on chest radiograph. With treatment the cavity shrinks, leaving a fibrotic scar and calcification that is visible on chest x-ray films, although large cavities may persist. However, chest x-ray studies cannot be used to determine if the tuberculosis is active or inactive, because cavities may be present in patients with inactive tuberculosis, and scars may be present in patients with active tuberculosis. The scar causes a re-

traction of lung tissue, and this creates a restrictive lung disease, which can be seen on pulmonary function tests where patients demonstrate reduced lung volumes. For more information, see the section on restrictive lung disease in this chapter.

In active tuberculosis, organisms can be isolated from sputum by microscopic examination and culture techniques. This is required for a definitive diagnosis. Sputum specimens will become negative after treatment with an effective course of antimycobacterial chemotherapy.

Therapeutic Management

In the 1950s, patients were hospitalized for all or part of their treatment for tuberculosis; it is now recognized that hospitalization is not necessary, and treatment is generally conducted on an outpatient basis. However, tuberculosis patients may be hospitalized for diagnostic evaluation, side effects of antimycobacterial chemotherapy, and complications of tuberculosis, as well as concurrent illness.[37]

Therapy for tuberculosis consists of the use of combinations of drugs. The tuberculosis bacilli are not all susceptible to the same antimycobacterial drugs, and problems can arise with the development of drug-resistant mutants. To avoid these problems it is necessary to treat tuberculosis with multiple drugs at the same time. The Centers for Disease

TABLE 28-4   First-line Drugs Recommended for Treatment of Tuberculosis

Drug	Daily dose	Twice weekly dose	Adverse reactions
Isoniazid	5 mg/kg	15 mg/kg (maximum 900 mg)	Hepatic enzyme elevation, peripheral neuropathy, hepatitis hypersensitivity
Rifampin	10 mg/kg	10 mg/kg (maximum 600 mg)	Orange discoloration of secretions and urine, nausea, vomiting, hepatitis, purpura (rare)
Pyrazinamide	15-30 mg/kg	50-70 mg/kg	Hepatotoxicity, hyperuricemia
Streptomycin	15 mg/kg	25-30 mg/kg	Ototoxicity, nephrotoxicity
Ethambutol	15-25 mg/kg	50 mg/kg	Optic neuritis (decreased red-green color discrimination, decreased visual acuity), skin rash

From *Core curriculum on tuberculosis*, ed 2, Atlanta, 1991, USDHHS, Centers for Disease Control.

Control recommend a minimum of 6 months of therapy with isoniazid, rifampin, and pyrazinamide for the first 2 months, followed by 4 months of isoniazid and rifampin.[3] An alternative regimen is 9 months of therapy with isoniazid and rifampin. The 6-month and 9-month regimens are equally effective if patients are consistent about taking the medication. Other first-line drugs that are less effective include streptomycin and ethambutol (Table 28-4). Ethambutol is used when the bacilli are resistant to isoniazid. Streptomycin can be used in the first 2 months of therapy, but its usefulness is limited, because it is not absorbed through the gastrointestinal tract and must be given parenterally.

Recent outbreaks of multidrug-resistant tuberculosis have been reported in HIV-infected persons.[11] In these patients the *M. tuberculosis* bacilli are not susceptible to two or more commonly used drugs. They must be treated with a combination of drugs to which their *M. tuberculosis* strain is susceptible, but this may be difficult if it requires using second-line drugs that tend to produce toxic side effects.

The effectiveness of therapy is established by examining monthly sputum specimens until they become negative. By the end of 3 months of treatment, 90% of the positive sputums will have become negative for *M. tuberculosis* bacilli. In patients with negative sputum before treatment, follow-up focuses on chest x-ray studies and clinical evaluation of symptoms. The effectiveness of therapy depends greatly on the patient's willingness and ability to take medications on a regular basis as prescribed. Sporadically taking medications is associated with treatment failure and the development of drug-resistant strains of *M. tuberculosis* bacilli. Shorter courses of medication are associated with high relapse rates.[3]

Initial drug resistance is another reason for the failure of treatment. This tends to be a bigger problem in developing countries and is relatively uncommon in the United States and Canada. When drug resistance occurs, it is generally to isoniazid or streptomycin and rarely to rifampin or ethambutol.

PATIENTS AT INCREASED RISK FOR DRUG-RESISTANT TUBERCULOSIS

Foreign-born persons from Asia, Africa, and Latin America

Residents of geographic areas in the United States with a high prevalence of drug resistance

Persons with a history of previous treatment for tuberculosis

Persons with positive bacteriology after 3 months of therapy

Contacts of known or suspected drug-resistant cases

From *Core curriculum on tuberculosis*, ed 2, Atlanta, 1991, USDHHS, Centers for Disease Control.

Isoniazid is also recommended for 6 to 12 months for prevention of tuberculosis in selected high-risk groups of patients.[3] These include persons in close contact with a patient suspected of active tuberculosis, especially if they develop a positive skin test, as well as newly infected persons with a positive skin test within the last 2 years, persons with a history of tuberculosis who have not been adequately treated, and persons with a positive skin test and abnormal chest x-ray films. Finally, these groups include persons under 35 years of age and patients with a positive skin test who have other chronic debilitating diseases such as silicosis, diabetes mellitus, immunosuppressive therapy, hematologic and reticuloendothelial diseases, AIDS, end-stage renal disease, and conditions associated with significant weight loss.

NURSING MANAGEMENT OF THE PATIENT WITH TUBERCULOSIS

Assessment

Nursing assessment of patients suspected of having tuberculosis includes a routine evaluation of the respiratory system as described in Chapter 25. However, no findings are specific to tuberculosis. Clinical findings will depend on the extent of the pulmonary involvement. In the early stages of inflammation there may be evidence of crackles, and as the disease progresses with cavitary lesions there may be dullness to percussion and associated bronchial breath sounds. Similarly, symptoms will depend on the progression of the disease, but the nurse should carefully describe the nature and severity of the cough, the characteristics of sputum, and other pulmonary symptoms. Additionally, for patients with newly diagnosed or suspected tuberculosis, it is important to identify their close personal contacts to determine who is at risk for being infected with the *M. tuberculosis* bacilli. It is also important to evaluate the patient's potential for taking medication on a regular basis and to assess the patient's knowledge of and previous experience with tuberculosis.

Information that is needed to determine the risk of infection to close personal contacts includes the patient's living conditions, such as the number of persons sleeping in a room, the ventilation in the room, and the source of light. The number of close personal contacts, frequency and proximity of the contact, and age and health status of close personal contacts are also helpful in determining the susceptibility to infection.

It is important for the patient to take his or her medication on a regular basis for the entire 6 to 9 months of treatment. The nurse assesses those factors that will indicate the likelihood of the patient's following through with taking prescribed medication. Factors to consider in evaluating the potential for reliably taking medication include past performance, history of alcohol or drug abuse, financial resources or insurance, and stability of living conditions. In elderly persons special attention is given to the potential for memory deficits.

Finally, the nurse assesses the patient's knowledge of and experience with tuberculosis. Tuberculosis is a curable disease, but it kills people in underdeveloped countries if they are not treated with antimycobacterial chemotherapy. If they are not taught otherwise, patients may think of tuberculosis as a deadly disease, and this may influence their willingness to accept the diagnosis and follow through with treatment. Moreover, tuberculosis is associated with poor, crowded living conditions, and patients may perceive a stigma that influences their willingness to accept the diagnosis and follow through with treatment.

Nursing Diagnosis

Patients hospitalized with newly diagnosed or suspected tuberculosis will have potential respiratory problems similar to those of patients with a lower respiratory infection. Nursing diagnoses for the patient with tuberculosis include the following:

Knowledge deficit related to lack of information about measures to prevent transmission of organism

Noncompliance related to length of treatment, cost of treatment, and drug side effects

Planning

Patient teaching is a priority when caring for patients with newly diagnosed or suspected tuberculosis. Nursing care is planned to achieve the following outcomes:

Patient will cover mouth when coughing and wear a mask when close to others

Patient will take antimycobacterial medications as prescribed

Implementation

Nursing care of patients with newly diagnosed or suspected tuberculosis includes preventing the transmission of the *M. tuberculosis* bacilli. The infectious status of patients declines immediately after starting effective chemotherapy, but it is difficult to know precisely when patients are no longer infectious, because the contagious period varies from patient to patient. The degree of infectiousness depends on the extent of the disease and the number of bacilli present in the lungs, as well as on the amount of secretions and frequency of coughing. Effective antimycobacterial chemotherapy reduces the number of bacilli and reduces the tendency to cough, thereby reducing the patient's infectiousness within days. Moreover, it has been demonstrated that patients are not necessarily infectious, even though their sputum cultures are still positive. Consequently most clinicians consider patients not infectious after 1 to 2 weeks of effective chemotherapy; but the nurse must remember this is a rough guideline, and it may vary from patient to patient.

To prevent transmission of tuberculosis, patients need to be taught to cover their mouth and nose with a tissue when coughing or sneezing. Covering the mouth reduces the number of droplets that are sprayed into the air, because they impact on the tissue. Face masks are of limited value.[11]

Ultraviolet light kills the *M. tuberculosis* bacilli, and it can be used to decontaminate the air in areas prone to contamination, such as hospital units with tuberculosis patients and clinic waiting rooms where tuberculosis patients are seen. Special equipment must be installed, and for this reason it is only practical in high-risk areas. Good ventilation with a frequent exchange of the air in the room is another means of reducing the concentration of *M. tuberculosis* bacilli in the environment and thereby reducing the chances of transmitting the organism. The recommended exchange rate is five or six exchanges of room air per hour.[11] However, if a complete system cannot be set up, the use of an exhaust fan at an open window will improve ventilation.

As discussed earlier, it is important that patients take their medication consistently throughout the prescribed 6 or 9 months of therapy. Consequently patient teaching should focus on this, and when possible, family members or close personal friends should be included. Patients and family members need to know about the potentially serious consequences of not treating tuberculosis, and they need to understand that the sporadic use of medications may increase their risk of developing resistant strains of *M. tuberculosis* bacilli. Teaching may be individualized or in group settings, but it is important to spend some time with each patient to develop an individualized plan for remembering to take the medication. Some patients may need to record each dose as it is taken, and some may wish to use special devices that allow them to pour out seven daily doses at a time with one compartment per dose. Other patients, however, may have no difficulty in remembering to take their medication. In a few cases it may be most appropriate to ask a family member to share in the responsibility by administering the medication to the patient. These concepts may be reinforced in the hospital by giving patients responsibility for taking their own medications when appropriate.

In discharge planning it is important to establish the nature of follow-up care. Patients need to be observed on a monthly basis until they have completed the prescribed course of therapy. This is important to identify any adverse reactions to medications and to evaluate their response to therapy. They need to know who to call if they have questions about their progress. Finally, it is also important to verify that patients have adequate financial resources to pay for the medication and follow-up care. If this is a problem, the nurse should refer the patient to a social worker for assistance. The antimycobacterial medications can be expensive, and patients will not follow through if they cannot pay for the medication.

Evaluation

The ultimate test of effective therapy is the absence of *M. tuberculosis* in the sputum, but it may take several months to develop negative sputum. Additionally, the effectiveness of therapy can be determined in part by observing clinical signs and symptoms of pulmonary function with regular assessments of the respiratory system. While the patient is in the hospital, patient teaching can be evaluated by observing patient behavior when coughing and taking medication. The nurse looks for evidence that patients understand the disease process, the prescribed medication schedule, and the effects of treatment, as well as the nature of adverse reactions to treatment and what to do if they occur. Patients are expected to describe their responsibilities in maintaining appointments for routine follow-up appointments. Additionally, it may be beneficial for the nurse to call patients 1 week after discharge to reinforce the importance of taking the medication, to answer any questions they may have, and to evaluate the effectiveness of their individual plans for taking the medication.

Documentation

The nurse documents findings from the respiratory assessment, being careful to describe the volume, color, and consistency of sputum and the frequency of cough. It is also important to document data obtained in the psychosocial assessment, because this may influence patient response to long-term follow-up. The nurse records interventions such as patient teaching and consultations with social work and documents patient response to these interventions. It is important to note if family members were included in patient teaching.

Effective therapy for tuberculosis will take a minimum of 6 to 9 months; consequently it is important to document relevant information for the clinicians in the agency, clinic, or private practice responsible for follow-up care. Most important, this includes a summary of patient teaching and individualized plans made for taking the medication, as well as any other information that will help them in observing the patient.

Ongoing Care

Ongoing care of patients with tuberculosis includes close follow-up to evaluate response to medications and reinforcement of patient teaching as described earlier. The required course of therapy is so long that patients may become careless in taking medications; hence it is important to regularly assess their habits in taking medication and to provide positive reinforcement as necessary. Treatment of the homeless population and short-term jail population is difficult because of transience and noncompliance. Supervised twice weekly therapy is best but is difficult to accomplish in these populations. Major emphasis must be placed on early detection and prevention of tuberculosis in these environments. Providing ventilation with five or six air exchanges per hour and placing ultraviolet lights in large common rooms will reduce the risk of transmission. Ultraviolet lights should be allowed to burn 24 hours per day to disinfect the area. Staff and clientele should be skin tested periodically, and persons with suspicious symptoms should be evaluated medically as soon as possible.

LUNG CANCER
Definition

Lung cancer is a serious health problem in the United States. It is the second most common cause of death, and it is the leading cause of cancer death. The incidence of lung cancer has increased steadily since 1945, and it recently surpassed breast cancer as the leading cause of cancer deaths in women.

Etiology/Epidemiology

It is estimated that 80% of lung cancers are caused by cigarette smoking and are therefore preventable. Smoking is the most important risk factor associated with lung cancer. The relationship between lung cancer and cigarette smoking was first documented in the 1950s. A solid body of evidence gathered since then has established that cigarette smoking increases the risk of lung cancer.

Additionally, the incidence of lung cancer is increased for people with occupational exposure to selected physical and chemical agents, such as asbestos, arsenic fumes, radon, and chromium. In most cases, exposure occurs through inhalation of these toxic chemicals. The combination of cigarette smoking and occupational exposure can produce additive effects, which increase the risk of lung cancer be-

yond the risk for either one alone. For example, smokers exposed to asbestos increase their risk of lung cancer by 64 times.[9] The chances of developing lung cancer are related to the intensity and duration of exposure to the toxic agent. In the case of cigarette smoke the risk of lung cancer is associated with the quantity of tobacco smoked and the duration of smoking. The chances of getting lung cancer are increased 10 times in an average smoker and 15 to 25 times in a heavy smoker.[35] Moreover, the risk of lung cancer is higher in smokers who deeply inhale the cigarette smoke. This is related to the intensity of exposure, because deep inhalation allows smoke to travel further into the airways. Similarly, the intensity and duration of occupational exposure affect the person's chances of developing lung cancer. Since lung cancer occurs after years of exposure, with peak incidence in the fifth and sixth decades, elderly persons are at risk.

The majority of lung cancers are squamous cell carcinomas, adenocarcinomas, large cell carcinomas, and small cell carcinomas.[64] For clinical purposes these cancers are divided into two groups—small cell lung cancers (SCLCs) and non–small cell lung cancers (NSCLCs). The clinical course for each of the NSCLCs is similar, whereas the clinical course for SCLC is quite different.

Approximately 30% to 35% of lung cancers are squamous cell carcinomas. These tumors grow slowly, are least likely to have distant metastasis, and have the best prognosis. Most of these tumors originate centrally at the first bronchus beyond the main-stem bronchus, and they tend to grow both toward the carina and toward the peripheral airways. In late stages they commonly form bulky masses that obstruct the bronchi and invade the bronchial wall, pulmonary parenchyma, bronchiolar and mediastinal lymph nodes, and soft tissues.[61] Approximately 25% to 30% of lung cancers are adenocarcinomas. Most of these tumors originate in the peripheral portions of the lung and have an intermediate growth rate. Most of their growth is in the peripheral portion of the lung. Like the other lung cancers, they are associated with cigarette smoking, but they are the most common lung tumor in nonsmokers.[64] Approximately 15% of lung cancers are large cell carcinomas. These tumors are generally large bulky masses located in the peripheral part of the lung.[61,64] They grow rapidly, invading lymph and vascular channels. Approximately 12% to 25% of lung cancers are SCLCs. These tumors are the fastest growing lung cancers. They originate centrally in the major bronchi and metastasize to the hilar region early in the disease. As the disease progresses, they commonly metastasize to distant sites such as the bone, liver, and brain. Most of these tumors have metastasized at the time of initial diagnosis.

Clinical Manifestations

Local disease

At the time of diagnosis the most commonly reported symptom is a cough. However, most patients with lung cancer are heavy smokers with COPD and long histories of a productive cough. They might experience a change in the nature of their cough, but subtle changes are difficult to detect and may go unnoticed. The cough is commonly productive, especially in heavy smokers, and it may get worse, since these patients are prone to lower respiratory tract infections. The productive cough is likely to continue in the treatment phase as both radiation therapy and chemotherapy interfere with immune responses and predispose patients to lower respiratory tract infections, which are associated with excessive tracheobronchial secretions. Additionally, radiation therapy tends to make tracheobronchial secretions thicker than normal and therefore difficult to expectorate.

Dyspnea is a major problem for many patients with lung cancer, because it can be unrelenting and can persist even at rest. The cause of dyspnea varies from patient to patient, and it varies with the progression of the disease. Dyspnea may be an early symptom of lung cancer, reflecting the effects of tumor invasion into lung tissue or tumor pressure on airways. It may develop as a side effect of medical therapy, as in pneumonitis caused by chemotherapy or fibrosis caused by radiation therapy. Finally, dyspnea may develop or get worse as the tumor enlarges and encroaches on lung tissue or with the development of a pleural effusion. Dyspnea can be associated with intense anxiety, because it often develops over a relatively short period, and patients can interpret it as evidence of an encroaching tumor. It is a major problem for these patients.

Hemoptysis occurs when the tumor erodes the epithelial layer or invades a blood vessel. It occurs more often in squamous cell carcinoma and large cell carcinoma than in SCLC. Chest discomfort can be associated with atelectasis, the collapse of alveoli. Patients with lung cancer develop atelectasis secondary to mechanical obstruction of the airways, compression of lung tissue, and shallow breathing patterns. When the tumor obstructs the airway, it prevents or reduces alveolar ventilation to a region of the lung and produces atelectasis in that region. The size of the atelectatic area depends on the size of the obstructed airway and degree of obstruction. Localized compression of lung tissue occurs with large tumors and with large pleural effusions secondary to metastasis. Patients with lung cancer may adopt a shallow breathing pattern if they experience pain on deep breathing or if they are heavily sedated. With shallow breathing the lungs are never fully expanded, and this leads to atelectasis. Atelectasis causes hypoxemia secondary to ventilation-perfusion mismatch and shunting.

Chest pain occurs as the tumor invades the respiratory structures, especially the chest wall. Patients may experience a sharp pleuritic type of chest pain that is worse with deep breathing and requires narcotics for relief.

Superior vena cava syndrome occurs when a lung tumor presses on the superior vena cava, partially or completely occluding it and impeding venous return from the head, neck, arms, and upper chest. Symptoms are related to venous obstruction, airway obstruction, and increased cerebral venous pressure. The most common symptoms include edema of the face, neck, arms, and upper torso. If severe enough, it may lead to airway obstruction accompanied by dyspnea and respiratory distress. It may also cause increased cerebral vascular pressure with symptoms of headache, visual disturbances, changes in level of consciousness, and seizure.[23]

Metastasis

Some patients initially exhibit evidence of metastasis within the thoracic cavity, to the CNS, and to the spinal cord. Metastasis within the thoracic cavity can cause esophageal compression and dysphagia, recurrent laryngeal nerve palsy, and hoarseness, as well as symptoms of superior vena cava syndrome. Metastasis to the CNS may be accompanied by symptoms of headache; memory problems; focal weakness; and occasionally seizures, ataxia, and aphasia. Metastasis to the spinal cord may be accompanied by pain, motor weakness, sensory changes, autonomic dysfunction, and eventually paralysis.[19]

Fluid may accumulate in the pleural space, causing a pleural effusion. This can be caused by infiltration of the tumor into the pleura or by obstruction of the venous circulation. Pleural effusions will be associated with dyspnea.

Systemic manifestations

Patients may initially exhibit extrapulmonary syndromes associated with lung cancer that are not related to metastasis. They include endocrine, neuromuscular, skeletal, hematologic, and cutaneous disorders (see box, p. 662).[36] The mechanisms of these syndromes are largely unknown, but they can cause serious symptoms that require treatment.

Diagnosis

Early detection is the key to successful resection of the NSCLC tumors, but current screening methods

EXTRAPULMONARY SYNDROMES ASSOCIATED WITH LUNG CANCER

Endocrine

Cushing's syndrome
Hypercalcemia
Syndrome of inappropriate antidiuretic hormone secretion
Gynecomastia
Hypoglycemia

Neuromuscular

Encephalomyelitis
Cerebellar degeneration
Peripheral neuropathy
Eaton-Lambert syndrome
Polymyositis

Skeletal

Hypertrophic pulmonary osteoarthropathy (clubbing of fingers)

Hematologic

Anemia
Disseminated intravascular coagulation
Thrombophlebitis

are inadequate. Mass screening programs with chest x-ray studies and sputum cytology have successfully identified NSCLCs at an earlier stage, but early identification has had no effect on mortality.[33] Most patients are diagnosed after reporting to the physician with one of the previously mentioned physical symptoms.

Definitive diagnosis of lung cancer requires histologic evidence of the type of cancer to differentiate primary lung cancer from a secondary cancer arising from metastasis of some other source. Once a positive diagnosis has been made, it is important to determine the extent of the tumor, the presence of any nodal involvement, and the extent of metastasis. This is referred to as staging the tumor, and it is especially important, because the stage of the tumor influences the nature of the treatment. When metastasis is present, surgical removal of the primary tumor does not improve the prognosis. In this case, accurate staging can prevent unnecessary surgery. To accurately diagnose lung cancer, the physician uses bronchoscopy, mediastinoscopy, transthoracic needle biopsy, or exploratory thoracotomy. These procedures are invasive, but most physicians make every attempt to diagnose the tumor using the least invasive procedure.

The majority of lung cancers produce abnormal chest x-ray studies. For example, when the tumor obstructs a bronchus, it interferes with normal ventilation to that portion of the lung and results in atelectasis. If the tumor is small enough that it does not obstruct the airways, or if it is located in the shadow of the mediastinum or hilum, it may be missed on chest x-ray films. When abnormalities appear on a chest x-ray film, the physician follows up immediately with further diagnostic procedures to establish a definitive diagnosis.

Therapeutic Management

Treatment for lung cancer depends on the type of cancer and the stage of the disease. Surgery, radiation therapy, and chemotherapy are all used. The chances for a cure are much better when the disease is diagnosed in its early stages. Of patients diagnosed with localized disease, 33% have a 5-year survival. However, less than 24% of patients are diagnosed with localized disease, and the remainder have regional or distant metastasis at diagnosis. In general, 13% of all lung cancer patients will survive for 5 years after diagnosis.[2]

Surgical treatment

Surgical removal of lung cancer is appropriate when the cancer is diagnosed in its earliest stages before metastasis. When the disease has progressed, there is little chance that surgery will improve the prognosis. When surgical removal of the tumor fails to cure the disease, it can be because the entire tumor was not removed, or because there was undetected metastasis before surgery.

In addition to considering the stage of the disease, the surgeon evaluates patients for other conditions that might increase the risk of surgery. These patients are generally older, and most of them have been heavy smokers. Consequently they may have COPD or coronary heart disease that would limit their ability to tolerate surgery. Moreover, it may limit their ability to tolerate the loss of lung tissue, and this must be considered when determining the extent of surgery. Surgical treatment ranges from a pneumonectomy to a wedge resection. The surgeon's goal is to remove the entire tumor without seriously compromising lung function. The extent of surgery will be based on the location of the tumor, as well as on the patient's cardiopulmonary status.

Laser surgery

Endoscopic surgery is a new technique in which laser surgery is performed on the lungs, allowing the surgeon to remove peripheral tumors without cutting ribs. Peripheral lung tissue is accessed through an endoscope inserted between the ribs through a small incision in the chest wall. This technique is physically less stressful and can be used on sicker patients who cannot tolerate a thoracotomy. It shortens the postoperative recovery period and reduces the length of hospital stay. It is very useful for small tumors that can be fully accessible through this route.

Thoracotomy for lung resection

Pneumonectomy (removal of a whole lung) and lobectomy (removal of a single lobe) are the most common procedures performed for lung cancer. A pneumonectomy involves the loss of a significant amount of lung tissue along with the accompanying pulmonary vascular bed. The nature of the tumor dictates the procedure, whereas pulmonary function determines if the patient can withstand the procedure. Patients should have an FEV_1 of 1 L after the lung resection; hence patients with severe COPD do not qualify for pneumonectomy. Patients are exercise tested to further determine the adequacy of pulmonary reserve. When a pneumonectomy is planned a ventilation-perfusion scan is performed to more precisely determine the function of the remaining lung.

Segmental resection is the removal of a lung segment, and wedge resection is the removal of a small V-shaped wedge of lung tissue. These techniques are employed to preserve as much lung tissue as possible, and they are used for small tumors located close to the surface of the lung.

Potential complications of a thoracotomy include atelectasis, empyema, bronchopleural fistula, bleeding, atrial fibrillation, and respiratory failure. Atelectasis occurs to some extent in all patients and is treated with vigorous pulmonary physiotherapy, but delayed resolution can require bronchoscopic suctioning. Empyema is caused by an infection of the pleural fluid with an organism that is resistant to the prophylactic antibiotic given postoperatively. Bronchopleural fistula is a serious but rare complication, occurring when the incision forming the bronchial stump does not heal properly. Postoperative bleeding could require surgical exploration of the chest, but this is relatively rare. Atrial fibrillation is commonly seen postoperatively and is treated with digoxin. Respiratory failure is most likely to occur in elderly patients with chronic bronchitis and emphysema, especially if they develop an infection following surgery.

Radiation therapy

Radiation therapy is administered with the hope of cure in select patients with lung cancer. It is used as adjunctive therapy after surgery to improve tumor control, and it is used as palliative therapy to control symptoms in others. Radiation therapy is most effective in rapidly dividing cancer cells and in smaller tumors. However, most lung cancers are diagnosed so late in the course of the disease they require large doses of radiation to eradicate them. In this situation the effective tumoricidal dose may exceed the tolerance of normal lung parenchyma.

Radiation therapy will commonly be offered to patients with inoperable NSCLCs when the cancer has not spread beyond the thorax. The goal is to control the spread of the tumor and improve survival. In this case, asymptomatic patients and patients still functioning at a high level are most likely to benefit. Despite many advances in radiation therapy, its role as a cure for lung cancer has not been well established, although it is still offered to many patients with inoperable tumors to give them every possible chance for a cure.

Additionally, radiation therapy is used to shrink the tumor and control symptoms in inoperable patients and to prevent brain metastasis. Symptoms such as hemoptysis, shoulder and arm pain, chest pain, and dyspnea may be relieved by treating the tumor with radiation therapy. It can be used in superior vena cava obstruction to reduce the tumor size and alleviate obstruction. Low-dose radiation therapy has been applied to the brain to prevent brain metastasis.

Toxic side effects of radiation therapy to the lung include esophagitis, fibrosis, and pneumonitis. Esophagitis with dysphagia commonly occurs during the course of radiation therapy, whereas fibrosis and pneumonitis appear several months after therapy. Esophagitis is generally transient, although it can be associated with esophageal strictures. Fibrosis is a common side effect, and it interferes with diffusion of gases and leaves patients with restrictive lung disease.

Chemotherapy

Chemotherapy provides systemic treatment for lung cancer. It offers the only hope for treatment in advanced disease with distant metastasis, although the best response occurs in patients with localized disease. Chemotherapy is most effective in SCLC, whereas it has a minimal impact on NSCLC, with 5% or fewer of patients responding with a complete remission. In contrast, SCLC is highly responsive to chemotherapy. Most effective combinations of chemotherapy produce complete or partial tumor response in more than 80% of patients. Complete remission occurs in 50% of patients with limited disease and 20% of patients with extensive disease.[19]

Prevention

Smoking is a major health problem, and it is the biggest preventable cause of lung cancer. Smokers have a reduced life expectancy and higher mortality; and both mortality and health status improve for those who quit smoking. Current data suggest 33% of adults in the United States smoke, including 35% of men and 28% of women. The percentage of smokers has declined significantly from a reported 52% in 1964, but it is still a serious national health problem that requires the attention of all health professionals.[35,39] Most smokers report they want to quit but have been unsuccessful or lack confidence in their ability to quit. There are so many strategies available to help smokers quit that it can be confusing to the general public. Hence nurses need to be informed about the available options and the efficacy of each to advise patients.

Therapeutic interventions designed to help people quit smoking can be classified into two groups based on the goal of the intervention. Some interventions are designed to help people with the initial quitting, and some are designed to help people refrain from smoking once they have quit. These are referred to as strategies for cessation and strategies for maintenance.

Strategies can also be classified according to the primary methodology employed. Commonly used methods include self-care, educational approaches, nicotine chewing gum, hypnosis, acupuncture, and behavioral methods. Whereas many different strategies have been tested, there is as yet no proven method that is decidedly superior to other methods.

Self-care methods are those techniques that are used by individuals to quit smoking on their own without the continued support of trained professionals. Self-care methods include personalized strategies designed by the individual, brief instruction provided by health professionals, and aids or self-help guides to quitting smoking. Commonly used aids and self-help resources include instruction booklets, manuals, audiotapes, and correspondence courses. These materials are popular, inexpensive, and convenient. The effectiveness of self-care methods has not been well documented, but most research studies report approximately 16% to 20% of individuals who decide to quit smoking on their own are eventually successful.[39] Consequently nurses must take these methods seriously and use them whenever appropriate. This can be done, for example, by making pamphlets available in clinic waiting rooms, hospital visitors lounges, and local drug stores.

Although most strategies have an educational component, some strategies emphasize education. These programs usually include lectures, informative films, records of smoking, specific instructions on how to quit, and literature that can be read at home. These programs emphasize health education, and they are available in many locations such as hospitals, industrial clinics, high schools, universities, community organizations, and city health departments. Most programs range in length from 1 week to 3 months of classes. Over two thirds of the evaluations report a 33% success rate at 1-year follow-up.[39]

Nicotine chewing gum can be effective for highly motivated people. The nicotine in the gum is absorbed through the oral mucosa so blood levels of nicotine are maintained during smoking cessation. Theoretically this allows people to overcome the psychologic dependence on cigarettes without experiencing the physical symptoms of withdrawal from nicotine; when they have overcome the psychologic dependence, they can gradually reduce the amount of nicotine gum. It is important to note that the manufacturer provides specific instructions for how to chew the gum, and these instructions should be explained to patients. Even though the gum is an effective aid to smoking cessation, there is a strong tendency to start smoking again when the gum is discontinued.

Nicotine can also be administered by transdermal patch to help maintain blood levels during smoking cessation. With the transdermal patch nicotine is gradually absorbed through the skin and blood levels are maintained more evenly than with the nicotine gum. Some patients are sensitive to the transdermal tape, and some have reported problems with insomnia, especially when the patch is worn 24 hours per day. The patch is relatively new and its efficacy is not fully known, but evidence suggests that it is beneficial, especially when accompanied by other strategies for smoking cessation.

Other strategies are classified as either aversive techniques or self-management techniques. Aversive techniques include rapid smoking, satiation, covert sensitization, and shock therapy. Self-management techniques include self-monitoring by keeping records of the number of cigarettes smoked, nicotine fading by cutting down gradually on the number of cigarettes smoked, stimulus control by altering specific situations that tend to make people want a cigarette, contingency management by making contracts with the therapist or peers, and relaxation therapy. Behavioral strategies have a sound theoretical rationale, but reports of their effectiveness are inconsistent. The use of either aversive therapies or self-management techniques by themselves has not been effective. Many programs use a combination of strategies, and this can be helpful if the combined strategies are not so complicated as to confuse patients. Many successful treatment programs combine more than one behavioral strategy or use behavioral techniques combined with other strategies.

Important strategies for maintaining abstinence from smoking include social support, coping skills, and a variety of cognitive approaches. Theoretically, social support reinforces smoke-free behavior and helps people maintain abstinence when confronted with withdrawal symptoms and social pressures to smoke. Social support can come from a variety of sources, such as family and friends, or it can be provided by the treatment program through a therapist or buddy arrangements. Coping strategies are designed to help people deal with high-risk situations that can trigger relapse. Techniques include identifying high-risk situations, rehearsing behaviors to deal with these high-risk situations, and building in rewards for cessation.

NURSING MANAGEMENT OF THE PATIENT WITH LUNG CANCER
Assessment

Assessment of the respiratory system is described in Chapter 25. Typical pulmonary problems experienced by patients with lung cancer include dyspnea, ineffective breathing patterns, ineffective airway clearance, and ineffective gas exchange. Many patients with lung cancer experience dyspnea as a result of multiple disruptions in physiologic function of the respiratory system, and they are predisposed to breathing-pattern disturbances related to chest pain and discomfort. In addition, they may experience difficulties in airway clearance associated with excessive tracheobronchial secretions, thick tenacious secretions, muscle weakness, and chest pain. These problems are significant, because they can lead to the development of atelectasis and pneumonia, which interfere with gas exchange.

Arterial blood gas analysis is required to evaluate effectiveness of gas exchange. The biggest concern in this group of patients is inadequate oxygenation as a result of ventilation-perfusion mismatch and shunting in areas of atelectasis and consolidation. This is reflected in a decrease in arterial Po_2 and oxygen saturation. Arterial punctures are invasive and painful, and the analyses are expensive; hence they will be ordered by the physician when specifically indicated rather than routinely.

When concerned about the level of oxygenation during activities of daily living, the nurse monitors oxygen saturation with a pulse oximeter (see Figure 28-3). This test is noninvasive, it takes little time, and the equipment is readily available in most hospital settings. It is most useful for monitoring acute changes in oxygenation during selected activities.

Dyspnea is assessed from the patient's subjective report. As with other pulmonary conditions, the assessment of dyspnea in lung cancer patients includes a description of the onset, magnitude, and precipitating events. It is especially important to identify any interventions the patient has discovered are helpful in relieving the dyspnea. This includes specific positions, such as elevation of the head of the bed, side-lying positions, or leaning forward. It must

be remembered that the patient's anxiety level does contribute to the degree of perceived and experienced dyspnea. If the tumor does not respond to medical treatment, one can expect dyspnea to gradually become worse.

In addition to sensations of dyspnea, it is important to identify the presence of any other type of discomfort during breathing. Patients may experience chest pain with deep inspiration or coughing. These are significant observations, because they may prevent patients from taking a deep breath or they may interfere with the patient's ability to produce an effective cough.

The intensity of fatigue will vary with the progress of the disease and with treatment regimens. It is important to monitor changes in the level of fatigue. This can be done by asking patients to report intensity of fatigue on a visual analog scale or on a scale from 1 to 10.

Patients with lung cancer commonly experience alterations in their nutritional status that adversely affect their clinical condition and quality of life. Hence it is important for the nurse to assess nutritional status. In the early stages of lung cancer it is especially important to assess appetite, because many of these patients experience anorexia. By assessing appetite the nurse can identify nutritional problems in the early stages, before they become serious clinical problems.

Assessment of clinical evidence of distant metastasis and complications of medical therapy is important because it will help the nurse predict the need for further interventions. For example, early evidence of brain metastasis suggests the need to take protective measures against hazards of memory loss, whereas evidence of bone metastasis may suggest the need to protect against trauma and pathologic bone fractures. Important laboratory data include the calcium levels, which sometimes rise in patients with lung cancer.

Additionally, the nurse assesses the patient's psychosocial adjustment, because these issues may have a major impact on the quality of life. This includes observing for evidence of altered moods, such as anxiety or depression. It also includes observing for evidence of family functioning.

Nursing Diagnosis

Nursing diagnoses vary depending on the progression of the disease and preexisting health status. Common diagnoses include the following:

Chest pain related to invasion of tumor

Ineffective breathing pattern related to chest discomfort

Impaired gas exchange related to ventilation-perfusion mismatch and invasion of tumor

Ineffective airway clearance related to thick tracheobronchial secretions with decreased ability to cough and muscle weakness

Altered nutrition: less than body requirements related to anorexia

Fatigue related to persistent cough and muscle weakness

Anxiety related to inability to function, dependency on others, and poor prognosis

High risk for infection related to diminished immune function

Planning

The priority for nursing care of patients with lung cancer is maintenance of adequate gas exchange and airway clearance while trying to keep patients as comfortable as possible. For patients in the acute phase, outcome criteria might include the following:

Patient reports reduced shortness of breath and increased comfort while breathing

Patient describes increased comfort during coughing and deep breathing

Rate and depth of respirations are within normal limits, and accessory muscles are not used at rest

Pao_2 is greater than 55 mm Hg at rest and with activities

Breath sounds are clear with coughing

Sputum is expectorated with minimal effort

Weight is stable

Patient reports less fatigue

Patient sleeps comfortably at night and feels rested in the morning

Patient maintains realistic level of activity

Patient uses appropriate aids to improve mobility

Patient describes symptoms of a lower respiratory tract infection and identifies appropriate actions to be taken

Implementation

Nursing care of patients with cancer is complex. This section is limited to the nursing management of problems that are unique to lung cancer patients. These include problems related to typical patterns of metastasis, as well as problems of breathing pattern disturbances, ineffective airway clearance, dyspnea, and lung surgery. Nurses must also help patients in dealing with problems related to gastrointestinal symptoms caused by chemotherapy and radiation therapy, as well as nutritional deficits, chronic pain, fatigue, and issues related to psychosocial adjustment.

Airway clearance

Radiation therapy causes tracheobronchial secretions to become thick and difficult to expectorate. In this situation it is important to maintain adequate hydration by providing a variety of fluids. Patients can also be taught techniques such as the huff cough or the cascade cough to improve the efficiency of their cough; if secretions are copious, physical therapy techniques such as postural drainage, percussion, and vibration can be used if patients tolerate them. These procedures can be exhausting, and patients with advanced lung cancer are commonly too weak and frail to tolerate them.

Dyspnea

Interventions for dyspnea related to lung cancer are the same as those described earlier for patients with COPD, and they include positioning, controlling the environment, relaxation techniques, and breathing techniques such as pursed-lip breathing. In addition to these interventions, the nurse can help patients with any other techniques they have found helpful. This might include allowing extra time for performing activities of daily living so patients can move slower.[7] As the disease progresses, dyspnea can become so intense that it can only be relieved by reducing the tumor mass.

The anxiety associated with dyspnea will often be alleviated if and when the dyspnea subsides. However, the nurse may further alleviate anxiety by keeping patients well informed about their condition, explaining procedures, and giving patients as much control as possible over their daily schedule while in the hospital. Family members may also be helpful, and the nurse encourages their participation whenever appropriate. However, family members will need support and guidance to cope with the patient's physical and psychosocial changes, as well as to work through anticipatory loss and grief associated with terminal illness.

Pain

Chest pain interferes with breathing patterns, and it reduces the quality of life. It is treated with medications and other comfort measures such as positioning. When it gets too severe, radiation therapy or chemotherapy may be required to reduce the size of the tumor and alleviate the pain. The goal of therapy is to enhance quality of life while improving breathing patterns. If increasing doses of narcotics are required for pain relief, the narcotics will eventually depress respirations. At this point the health care team, the family, and if possible the patient decide on the appropriate course of action. To withhold medication may improve breathing patterns but produce unreasonable suffering. Many factors must be considered in making this decision, and it is a decision that should be shared among all persons concerned. The nurse can facilitate this process by anticipating it as the time draws near and by calling a conference of those concerned so that adequate time is allowed for the family to participate in making the decision. The management of cancer pain is a major nursing challenge, and the reader is referred to Chapters 14 and 15 for further details.

Preoperative care

Preparation for surgery includes the general preoperative care described in Chapter 22. Emphasis is placed on airway clearance to improve gas exchange before surgery. Coughing and deep breathing are performed at regular intervals to keep the airways cleared of secretions. Postural drainage can be employed if the patient is producing large volumes of secretions. Bronchodilators are administered to assist with airway clearance, and antibiotics are administered if an infection is present. Additionally, patients are taught the rationale for and importance of coughing and deep breathing during the postoperative phase.

Initially the pulmonologist and surgeon explain the medical diagnosis, proposed surgical intervention, and prognosis. Because of the associated stress and anxiety patients may not completely understand and they may forget. This makes it important that the nurse follow up to clarify the patient's level of understanding, to answer additional questions, and to provide general support. To allay fear of the unknown the nurse explains events as they will occur before and after surgery including a description of the environment and the presence of chest tubes postoperatively. The family members are included in these discussions whenever possible, because they will provide ongoing support after the patient leaves the hospital.

Postoperative care

The postoperative physical needs of patients with lung surgery are similar to those of patients with other major types of surgery, with one exception— patients with lung surgery will have chest tubes inserted during the surgery to drain the thoracic cavity and the intrapleural space. Other aspects of the postoperative course are influenced by the patient's health status before surgery. As with other major types of surgery, it is important to prevent atelectasis by helping patients with coughing and deep breathing on a frequent basis. Both procedures are painful; hence it is often helpful to provide adequate pain medication before coughing and deep breathing. The nurse can also reduce the degree of discomfort by splinting the incision while the patient is coughing and deep breathing. Additionally, patient position should be changed frequently by turning the patient from side to side with special attention to the chest tubes to make sure they are not kinked.

The nurse monitors chest tube drainage and ob-

serves for potential complications such as separation of the tubing, occlusion of the tube, or accidental removal of the tube. During the immediate postoperative period, excessive chest tube drainage (generally more than 200 mL/hr for more than 2 to 3 hours) indicates postoperative bleeding, and the surgeon should be notified. The drainage gradually diminishes, and after several days the tube is removed by the physician when it is no longer needed.

It is the nurse's responsibility to gradually increase the patient's activity and begin exercises early in the postoperative period. Early ambulation is important to prevent a number of postoperative complications, and it encourages deep breathing. Patients are first gotten up in a chair at the bedside and helped with walking as soon as possible, making sure to keep the collection system for the chest tube drainage below the level of the chest. Upper extremity exercises are started early to regain strength in the muscles that were incised during the surgery.

Evaluation

Frequent assessments of clinical progress are necessary to determine the response to therapy. The extent of the disease determines realistic goals for the patient. Ideally, the goal is normal arterial blood gases with normal breathing patterns, minimal chest discomfort, and limited dyspnea. When patients become terminally ill, the primary goal is to maintain comfort; this can be judged by the patient's report of comfort and ability to sleep and rest.

Documentation

Patient records include an accurate chronologic record of the patient's symptoms and response to interventions. Documentation of pain includes the nature, location, and intensity, as well as the response to pain medication. Documentation also includes the intensity of dyspnea and the response to interventions such as positioning. Accurate records are kept of the patient's appetite and consumption of food. In addition, nurses need to document physical assessment data and evidence of support for adequate home care.

Ongoing Care

Lung cancer has a major impact on quality of life. Newly diagnosed patients with lung cancer experience an immediate threat to health and well-being, because the course of the disease is generally short. Lung cancer is different from many other cancers in that it tends to progress fairly rapidly. The type of lung cancer influences the rate of disease progression, and this affects the patient's coping response. For patients with SCLC diagnosed with extensive disease, mean survival ranges from 8 to 18 months.

This gives patients and family little time to adjust to the reality of cancer. Time is an important factor because of the number of issues to be dealt with and the nature of the issues.

These patients must cope with major changes in their lives including physical side effects of lung cancer and its treatments; changes in functional status, both physically and socially; changes in psychologic status, such as depression and anxiety; and changes in social interactions at work and at home.[44] For example, as patients become disabled, family roles must be altered, with others assuming responsibility for tasks that patients had fulfilled. Further, patients and families must deal with death, which is a sensitive issue that takes time to work through. It is likely that many of these tasks may be left undone when there is limited time available and much of that time is taken up with the requirements of the medical treatment regimen. The nurse is in a unique position to assess cues, provide for family support, and generally facilitate psychosocial adjustment of patients and their families.

CHEST TRAUMA
Definition

Injuries caused by trauma to the chest can be classified as nonpenetrating and penetrating. Nonpenetrating chest injuries include fractures of the rib cage and sternum, flail chest, pulmonary contusion, pneumothorax, and hemothorax. Penetrating chest wounds cause pneumothorax, hemothorax, and laceration of the parenchyma. These injuries to the chest may be accompanied by injuries to other organs in the thoracic cavity and abdominal cavity, because any force severe enough to damage the chest wall and lungs may also damage adjacent structures.

Etiology/Epidemiology

Traumatic injuries to the chest are caused by direct and indirect effects of the applied force. A blow to the chest can fracture the skeletal structure of the chest wall by the effects of direct force applied to the chest wall. It can injure underlying organs by indirect effects of compression, as in pulmonary contusion, and by shearing forces, as in tears of the tracheobronchial tree. Moreover, the forces of acceleration and deceleration also contribute to these injuries. The most severe injuries from blunt trauma occur in automobile accidents, when the driver impacts with the steering wheel, and in falls from great heights, but chest injuries can also be caused by the impact of shock waves from a massive explosion, by the impact of a gunshot to the chest when wearing protective armor, and by lesser falls. Penetrating chest injuries, such as a gunshot wound and stabbing with a knife, commonly occur in violent crimes.

Pathophysiology/Clinical Manifestations

The effects of a blow to the chest wall depend on the magnitude, velocity, and duration of the force of impact, but effects also depend on the characteristics of the patient. Younger patients are less likely to sustain fractures because of the elasticity of their bones, and patients with preexisting pulmonary disease are more likely to experience impaired pulmonary functioning.

Rib fracture

Simple rib fractures are relatively benign and if uncomplicated will heal within 3 to 6 weeks without medical intervention. Most patients will experience pain related to chest wall motion, and the natural tendency is to splint the chest. This should be avoided, because it interferes with ventilation of the lung and is associated with an increased incidence of atelectasis.

Multiple rib fractures can be caused by severe chest trauma and may therefore be associated with a variety of serious injuries to the organs of the chest, including cardiac contusion, pulmonary contusion, major vascular injury, or injuries to abdominal organs such as the spleen or liver. Because of their close proximity, fractures of the first and second ribs are associated with myocardial contusion and major vascular injury, whereas fractures of the ninth, tenth, or eleventh rib are associated with injury of the spleen and liver.[71]

Flail chest

A **flail chest** can occur when three or more adjacent ribs are fractured in two places (Figure 28-14). This damages the structural integrity of the chest wall, and the affected portion can be sucked inward during inspiration to produce a paradoxic motion, but the paradoxic motion may not be observed initially, because trauma-related muscle spasms splint the chest wall. When the affected portion of the chest wall is pulled inward during inspiration, it interferes with ventilation to the underlying area and can cause the mediastinum to shift to the opposite side, compressing lung parenchyma on the opposite side and interfering with venous return to the right side of the heart.[40] A flail chest can cause considerable pain and splinting, which further interfere with ventilation. A flail chest is generally associated with severe chest trauma and is therefore accompanied by pulmonary contusion.

Pulmonary contusion

Pulmonary contusion is caused by compression of the lung parenchyma during severe trauma to the

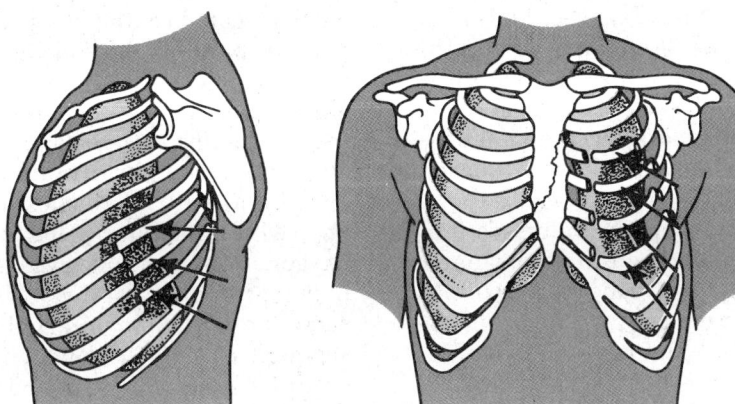

FIGURE 28-14   Two examples of flail chest, one on the lateral and one on the anterior portion of chest wall. Several adjacent ribs are fractured in two places. Arrows indicate direction and force of injury.

chest. Tissue injury causes an increase in permeability of capillary membranes, which is associated with localized pulmonary edema and extravasation of blood into the interstitial and alveolar spaces.[40] It is also associated with an increase in tracheobronchial secretions. Ventilation and gas exchange are impaired, causing hypoxemia and CO_2 retention, and airway clearance mechanisms can be overwhelmed, causing atelectasis. The injury to lung parenchyma is localized, and the extent of pathophysiologic alterations is related to the magnitude of the affected area. Pneumonia is the most common complication, but a massive pulmonary contusion could cause respiratory failure.

The chest wall can be bruised, and patients commonly complain of localized chest pain; some patients experience acute respiratory distress, whereas others do not. The clinical condition can deteriorate over the first 24 to 72 hours. As the clinical condition deteriorates, patients become dyspneic and cyanotic with rapid shallow respirations, rapid pulse, and low blood pressure. Arterial P_{O_2} declines, and P_{CO_2} rises. Chest x-ray findings range from patchy, irregular infiltrates to areas of consolidation.

Pneumothorax

A pneumothorax is the accumulation of air in the pleural space between the visceral and parietal pleura. It can be caused by either blunt trauma or a penetrating chest injury. It can also occur spontaneously in healthy people and in patients with COPD when a subpleural bleb ruptures.[25]

In penetrating chest injuries, air enters the pleural space either through the exterior chest wall or from the lungs, if the injury penetrates into the parenchyma. With blunt trauma, air enters the pleural space when a fractured rib punctures the visceral pleura or when the force of the impact compresses the lung sufficiently to cause rupture of alveoli.

The mechanism of the pneumothorax and the volume of accumulated air determine the clinical manifestations. A simple pneumothorax occurs when air enters the pleural space and does not communicate with the atmosphere. This is associated with a partial or complete collapse of the involved lung. If enough air enters the pleural cavity to increase intrapleural pressure above alveolar pressure, the mediastinum will shift toward the unaffected side and compress the unaffected lung. This is called a tension pneumothorax, and it occurs when air continues to be sucked into the pleural space after the injury.

The pneumothorax increases intrathoracic pressure, reduces the vital capacity, reduces ventilation, and decreases venous return to the heart. It is a serious clinical condition and can lead to hypoxemia, acute respiratory failure, and death if not appropriately treated. Most patients initially exhibit dyspnea and chest pain. They may also initially have other evidence of acute respiratory distress, including cyanosis and rapid shallow respirations. The affected side of the chest can appear hyperinflated, and it will sound hyperresonant to percussion. Breath sounds may be absent over the affected lung and diminished over the opposite lung. Hemodynamic changes include decreased blood pressure, displaced point maximal impulse, and distant heart sounds.

Hemothorax

Hemothorax is the accumulation of blood in the pleural space, and it often occurs with a pneumothorax. Bleeding comes from the pulmonary capillaries of the lung, from the intercostal spaces, and occasionally from the heart or great vessels in the chest.[40] Bleeding may subside on its own if it originates in the low-pressure vessels of the pulmonary circulation, but it can continue until treated if it originates in high-pressure vessels, such as the thoracic aorta or arteries branching from the aorta.

Blood in the intrapleural space compresses lung tissue, reducing ventilation and causing a mismatch in ventilation and perfusion that leads to hypoxemia. If the hemorrhage is large enough, patients can develop hypovolemic shock. Clinical manifestations depend on the volume of the hemorrhage into the intrapleural space, with a small hemothorax causing few clinical changes. A large hemothorax can produce clinical evidence of hypoxemia and shock, including rapid shallow respirations, tachycardia, and low blood pressure. Most patients complain of dyspnea and chest pain. Fluid levels can be seen on an upright chest film, but many of these patients are too sick to sit upright. Arterial P_{O_2} may be reduced and P_{CO_2} elevated.

Early pulmonary complications of rib fracture include pneumothorax and hemothorax caused by penetration of sharp bone fragments into the pleural cavity or into the parenchyma. Later pulmonary complications include atelectasis and pneumonia, which are related to hypoventilation caused by pain on breathing.

Any penetrating chest wound that causes a pneumothorax or hemothorax can introduce bacteria into the pleural space, and if the fluid and air are not drained within 24 to 48 hours, an infection and empyema can ensue. An empyema is an abscess or collection of purulent exudate in the pleural cavity that is generally treated with antibiotics. However, the empyema could become complicated with a bronchopleural fistula, which drains the purulent exudate from the pleural space into the airways of the lungs. The patient would then expectorate the purulent secretions, and thoracostomy drainage would be necessary.

Therapeutic Management

Patients with a simple rib fracture are generally treated at home, but patients with multiple rib fractures are hospitalized for at least 24 to 48 hours to observe for other more serious chest injuries, such as cardiac contusion, pulmonary contusion, and pneumothorax. Goals of treatment for a rib fracture are to reduce pain and maintain adequate ventilation until the fracture heals. These patients were once treated by binding the chest to immobilize the bones, but that practice was discontinued, because it interfered with ventilation, especially in older people and people with pulmonary disease. Current practice is to treat patients with pain medications,

so they can breathe deeply and cough as needed without pain. Pain medications are administered as needed, being careful not to oversedate the patient. When pain is severe, intercostal nerve blocks are used with long-term local anesthetics to relieve pain, so patients can perform deep breathing exercises.

Patients with a flail chest require supportive therapy, which includes relief of pain, maintenance of oxygenation, and airway clearance. These patients may be intubated and ventilated with positive pressure ventilation to internally stabilize the floating segment of the rib cage. This prevents the floating segment from being sucked inward during inspiration. This treatment is somewhat controversial, and some physicians reserve it for patients in respiratory failure.[40]

Patients with pulmonary contusions are treated in the critical care unit with supportive therapy to maintain adequate ventilation, oxygenation, and airway clearance. They may require mechanical ventilation to maintain adequate ventilation and oxygenation. Supplemental oxygen therapy may also be necessary to maintain adequate oxygenation. Chest physiotherapy and coughing with support to the chest wall are used to maintain airway clearance. Endotracheal suctioning can also be used to clear the airway of secretions in intubated patients. Intercostal nerve blocks can be used to relieve pain.

When patients initially exhibit an open sucking chest wound, it must be sealed immediately to prevent the development of a tension pneumothorax. Sterile gauze pretreated with petroleum jelly can be applied to the wound to prevent further air from being sucked into the pleural space. Less air will be trapped in the pleural space if the gauze is applied at the end of a cough or at the end of expiration when intrapleural pressure is higher.

A pneumothorax caused by trauma is generally treated by inserting a chest tube into the pleural space regardless of the size of the pneumothorax. This is referred to as a tube thoracostomy. When patients also have a hemothorax, a second tube may be inserted inferiorly for drainage of fluid. A tension pneumothorax is a medical emergency and may require immediate relief of intrapleural pressure before the tube thoracostomy. This can be accomplished by inserting a large-bore needle into the intrapleural space. When the patient stabilizes, a chest tube is inserted to allow complete evacuation of the pleural space.

Treatment of a hemothorax depends on the volume of fluid collected in the pleural space. A small hemothorax may be allowed to reabsorb over a period of days if it is monitored closely with serial chest x-ray studies, but larger volumes must be drained with a large-bore thoracostomy tube connected to underwater sealed drainage and suction (20 to 30 cm H_2O). When large volumes of blood are lost into the pleural space, volume replacement may be necessary, and if the bleeding persists, the patient may have to be taken to the operating room for a thoracotomy to stop the bleeding.

NURSING MANAGEMENT OF THE PATIENT WITH CHEST TRAUMA
Assessment

Nursing assessment of the patient with chest trauma includes a thorough respiratory assessment, but when the patient is first brought to the hospital, the nurse must conduct a preliminary assessment to establish priorities. This includes inspection for penetrating wounds, rate and depth of respirations, and auscultation of breath sounds. In patients with acute respiratory distress, the need for ventilation and oxygenation must be met before proceeding with a thorough assessment.

Information describing the nature of the traumatic event provides clues to the potential mechanism and severity of the injury. This information directs the nurse in assessing for multiple trauma. In alert patients, it is also important to ascertain the extent of their discomfort, especially the presence of dyspnea and pain with breathing, as well as pain in other parts of the body.

Patients must be completely undressed to the waist for a thorough inspection of the chest. Inspection of the chest focuses on the characteristics of breathing patterns, including rate and depth of respirations, excursion of the chest, and use of accessory muscles to breathe, as well as skin color and evidence of penetration of the chest. Inspection of the chest is especially important when assessing patients with chest trauma. Limitation in chest wall motion may be observed in patients with a fractured rib. Paradoxic chest wall motion may be observed in patients with flail chest, and this is best observed by holding a light tangentially to the chest. Labored breathing with the use of accessory muscles to breathe may indicate serious trauma, including pneumothorax or hemothorax.

When palpating the chest wall, the nurse looks for evidence of chest wall irregularities or deformities, tenderness over ribs or sternum, and the presence of subcutaneous emphysema. The nurse palpates the chest while the patient breathes deeply, and this allows a thorough examination of the chest wall motion including both the anteroposterior dimension and the lateral dimension. This can reveal evidence of paradoxic chest wall motion and uneven or absent motion of the chest during breathing. In patients with a tension pneumothorax a shift of the trachea to the unaffected side of the chest can be identified by palpation of the trachea at the anterior aspect of the neck.

When percussing and auscultating the chest, the nurse looks for evidence of adequate ventilation to all portions of the lung, as well as for evidence of a collapsed lung or fluid in the pleural space. In patients with a pneumothorax, the affected area will be hyperresonant to percussion, with decreased or absent tactile fremitus and decreased or absent breath sounds. If there is fluid in the pleural space, it will sound dull or flat to percussion with decreased breath sounds at the base posteriorly on the affected side. If both pneumothorax and hemothorax are present, the clinical manifestations of pneumothorax will predominate on physical assessment. Later in the course of treatment, the clinical condition may be complicated by atelectasis, and this will be associated with dullness to percussion and decreased or absent breath sounds over the affected area.

Nursing Diagnosis

Common nursing diagnoses for patients with chest trauma include the following:

Ineffective breathing pattern related to pleuritic chest pain

Impaired gas exchange related to retained tracheobronchial secretions and ineffective breathing patterns

Ineffective airway clearance related to increased volume of tracheobronchial secretions

Anxiety related to fear of death related to major accident

Planning

When the patient is admitted to the emergency room, the primary goal of nursing care is to maintain a patent airway, adequate ventilation, and adequate circulation while assessing the extent of injury. Once the patient is stabilized, nursing care is directed toward assessing the clinical condition, maintaining adequate gas exchange, reducing the patient's anxiety, alleviating pain, and helping with medical interventions such as insertion of chest tubes and intubation as necessary. As the clinical condition progresses, nursing care focuses on clearing tracheobronchial secretions from the airway, mobilizing patients to prevent pulmonary complications, maintaining nutritional status, and managing pain and physical discomfort. Outcome criteria include the following:

Patient will demonstrate an ability to take deep breaths

Rate and depth of respirations are within normal limits

Arterial P_{O_2} is maintained above 55 mm Hg

Breath sounds are clear with no adventitious sounds

Patient reports minimal respiratory discomfort

Patient appears relaxed

Patient expresses realistic expectations regarding health status

Patient sleeps appropriate number of hours and reports feeling rested

Implementation

Emergency care

Emergency care is administered to stabilize the patient, assess the extent of injury, and initiate treatment. Once the clinical condition is stabilized, patients are transferred from the emergency room to either a critical care unit or a regular nursing unit. At this stage, care focuses on treating the injury and preventing complications. These different stages of care focus on slightly different goals and therefore are discussed separately.

Patients with severe chest injuries may have other injuries, and the full extent of the damage may not be fully appreciated on admission to the emergency room; some injuries may remain undiagnosed for a while, and the clinical condition may deteriorate rapidly. Consequently the nurse must monitor patients closely until their condition completely stabilizes. This includes cardiovascular and neurologic function, as well as pulmonary function. The adequacy of ventilation, oxygenation, and circulation is of prime concern and will require frequent monitoring of breathing patterns, especially rate and depth of respiration and use of accessory muscles to determine if work of breathing has increased. The cardiovascular status must be monitored closely, including heart rate, blood pressure, and cardiac rhythm. Most patients with severe chest trauma should be connected to a cardiac monitor. Level of consciousness is also monitored closely.

Many patients may require supplemental oxygen, and this is managed and monitored by the nurse as described in Chapter 26. Some patients will need a tube thoracostomy to evacuate air and fluid from the pleural space, and the nurse is responsible for setting up the necessary instruments and equipment and assisting with the procedure. The nurse is also responsible for monitoring the drainage from the chest tube and reporting excessive amounts to the physician, as described in Chapter 26.

Patients may be anxious in the emergency room; consequently the nurse explains all procedures before they are performed. This includes explaining sensory experiences that are associated with a procedure (e.g., the nature and duration of pain associated with the insertion of a chest tube and the discomfort that may be experienced once the tube is in place). This information helps patients cope with the pain of a procedure, it communicates concern for their well-being, and it establishes trust between nurses and patients. It is equally important to explain why procedures are being done (e.g., the need for oxygen therapy or the need for chest tubes). These explanations will help alleviate the patient's anxiety and instill confidence in the caregivers. Additionally, the nurse is responsible for maintaining channels of communication with the family by keeping them informed of the patient's progress. Family members should be allowed to visit as soon as patients are stabilized.

Acute care

Many patients with traumatic pneumothorax or multiple rib fractures will have other injuries that require admission to the critical care unit. These patients must be monitored closely with indwelling arterial lines; they may be intubated and ventilated with a mechanical ventilator, and some will have chest tubes. Nursing care related to ventilators and chest tubes is described in Chapter 26.

Patients with severe chest trauma are admitted to the hospital for observation, even if their injuries appear to be limited. The nurse continues to monitor these patients closely for evidence of respiratory distress, as in the emergency room. Depending on the patient's clinical condition, breathing patterns and vital signs may have to be monitored every 15 minutes until the patient is stable enough to reduce observations to every hour and eventually to every 4 hours.

A penetrating chest injury predisposes patients to infection. Hence the nurse observes for early evidence of an infection and reports positive findings to the physician, because early medical treatment may prevent the development of serious complications. An elevation in temperature accompanied by alterations in breathing patterns and heart rate may indicate the presence of an infection.

Patients with severe chest trauma will produce excessive tracheobronchial secretions, and nursing care is directed toward maintaining adequate airway clearance. A record of fluid intake and output will help in maintaining adequate hydration, which is necessary to prevent the development of excessively thick tracheobronchial secretions. A regular schedule of coughing and deep breathing will help mobilize secretions, but if secretions are retained despite these efforts, intubation may be necessary so the nurse can clear the airways by suctioning the trachea. The use of chest physiotherapy must be evaluated on an individual basis, because it may be contraindicated in some patients depending on the nature of their injuries. In addition to specific techniques for airway clearance, it is important to mobilize patients as soon as possible, because this will force them to take deeper breaths and mobilize secretions. This means turning patients in bed at least every 2 hours if they cannot turn themselves, and it means ambulating them as soon as possible. Patients may be reluctant to move around because of chest pain from the injury or discomfort from the chest tube, but this can be managed by timing pain medications to coincide with the activity schedule. It is also important to teach patients about the benefits of early ambulation to encourage them to participate in their own therapy.

Patients with severe chest trauma may be at risk for developing protein-calorie malnutrition. Consequently it is important for the nurse to monitor the patient for changes in nutritional status by weighing the patient on a regular basis. However, the nurse must remember that body weight may be influenced by factors other than nutritional status, such as the retention of fluid; but if weight is evaluated in conjunction with fluid status, it can be used to identify a reduction in body mass associated with the loss of body mass. Moreover, body weight responds to changes in nutritional status faster than other measures, such as serum albumin and total proteins, which tend to be slow in responding to changes in nutrition. In addition, the nurse should consult with a dietitian and monitor the patient's daily intake of protein and calories. Food supplements may be necessary if the patient cannot maintain an adequate intake.

Patients may experience high levels of generalized pain and discomfort in the first 24 to 48 hours after an injury as a result of massive soft tissue injury. In addition, they will experience sharp localized pain associated with fractured bones. Severe pain of this nature can delay recovery by interfering with sleep and rest, by preventing deep breathing, and by limiting mobility. Consequently pain management is an important aspect of nursing care. Pain medication should be used in conjunction with other techniques to keep patients comfortable enough to maintain adequate rest and to actively participate in therapies such as coughing, deep breathing, and ambulation. Techniques such as relaxation therapy and diversional activities may enhance the patient's level of comfort.

Evaluation

The nurse evaluates patient progress on a regular basis to determine the effectiveness of the treatment plan. Effective breathing patterns are confirmed by the presence of vesicular breath sounds throughout the chest with no adventitious sounds, as well as normal rate and depth of respiration. Evidence of adequate gas exchange includes normal arterial blood gases as measured by arterial puncture or by pulse oximetry. An adequate nutritional status is manifested by the maintenance of a stable weight. Patients should demonstrate an understanding of the need to clear secretions from their lungs by coughing and deep breathing on a regular basis using techniques to minimize discomfort. In addition, the nurse uses subjective data to determine the effectiveness of interventions designed to relieve pain, dyspnea, and anxiety.

Documentation

The nurse documents all phases of the nursing process, but in patients with chest trauma, it is especially important to record a detailed picture of their clinical condition on admission to the emergency room, including the findings of a pulmonary assessment, level of consciousness, and the nature of the accident. The patient's progress is carefully documented in the medical records, including data acquired during frequent observations of breathing patterns, airway clearance, and oxygenation. Records should also reflect subjective data regarding the intensity of pain and dyspnea, as well as evidence of psychosocial adjustment to the injury, because this information is needed to evaluate progress.

Ongoing Care

Patients with a simple rib fracture will be seen in the emergency room and sent home. For these patients, teaching emphasizes the importance of maintaining adequate ventilation to the lungs despite the discomfort associated with breathing. Patients should be instructed to maintain their normal levels of activity and perform routine deep breathing exercises. They will be given a prescription for analgesics, and they need to be encouraged to take the medication before breathing exercises if necessary. The nurse should also arrange a follow-up appointment for the patient either with his or her private physician or in a clinic. Patients with more severe injuries from chest trauma will be discharged from the hospital. These patients must be taught about their medications, including how and when to take them and potential side effects. They need to learn the importance of airway clearance techniques, and they need to learn to perform any therapeutic procedures that will be required at home. Patient teaching includes the importance of maintaining adequate nutrition, rest, and exercise in the early stages of convalescence. Patients also need to understand the importance of follow-up care with their primary caregiver to monitor their progress.

CRITICAL THINKING QUESTIONS

1 What are the three pathophysiologic alterations that impair gas exchange in the patient with COPD?

2 List specific nursing interventions for the pa-

tient with COPD related to drug therapy, airway clearance, rest, nutrition, oxygen therapy, and breathing exercises.

3 What are the major problem areas for the COPD patient that are addressed in planning ongoing care?

4 Describe the progression of an acute asthma attack in terms of triggering stimuli and clinical manifestations.

5 How does the nurse prepare the asthma patient for self-care?

6 What is the effect of lung restriction on pulmonary function and gas exchange?

7 Outline the primary considerations in the therapeutic management of ARDS that influence nursing care for the patient.

8 Discuss the advantages and disadvantages of home ventilator care for the patient with chronic respiratory failure.

9 Develop a care plan for the patient with a nursing diagnosis of ineffective airway clearance related to increased mucous production from a pulmonary infection.

10 What are the primary nursing interventions related to the treatment of tuberculosis and prevention of transmission of the infection?

11 Classify the clinical manifestations of lung cancer according to local disease, metastasis, and systemic effects.

12 Describe strategies useful to prevent lung cancer.

13 Compare the emergency care, acute care, and long-term care for a patient with chest trauma.

BIBLIOGRAPHY

Current

1. Ahmed T: Status asthmaticus. In Dantzker DR, editor: *Cardiopulmonary critical care*, Orlando, Fla, 1986, Grune & Stratton, Inc.
2. American Cancer Society: *Cancer facts and figures—1988*, New York, 1988, The Society.
3. American Thoracic Society: Standards for the diagnosis and care of patients with chronic obstructive pulmonary disease (COPD) and asthma, *Am Rev Respir Dis* 136:225, 1987.
4. Bartlett JG et al: Bacteriology of hospital-acquired pneumonia, *Arch Intern Med* 146:868, 1986.
5. Baumann WR et al: Incidence and mortality of adult respiratory distress syndrome: a prospective analysis from a large metropolitan hospital, *Crit Care Med* 14(1):1, 1986.
6. Bone RC et al: Early methylprednisolone treatment for septic syndrome and the adult respiratory distress syndrome, *Chest* 92(6):1032, 1987.
7. Brown ML et al: Lung cancer and dyspnea: the patient's perception, *Oncol Nurs Forum* 13:19, 1986.
8. Butler J: Cor pulmonale. In Murray JF, Nadel JA, editors: *Textbook of respiratory medicine*, Philadelphia, 1988, WB Saunders Co.
9. Carr DT, Holoye PY: Metastatic malignant tumors. In Murray JF, Nadel JA, editors: *Textbook of respiratory medicine*, Philadelphia, 1988, WB Saunders Co.
10. Carrieri VK, Janson-Bjerklie S: Strategies patients use to manage the sensation of dyspnea, *West J Nurs Res* 8(3):285, 1986.
11. *Core curriculum on tuberculosis*, ed 2, Atlanta, 1991, US-DHHS, Centers for Disease Control.
12. Crowley JJ, Raffin TA: Acute lung injury: mechanisms and potential therapy. In Simmons DH, editor: *Current pulmonology*, vol 12, St Louis, 1991, Mosby–Year Book, Inc.
13. Dutt AK, Stead WW: Tuberculosis. In Simmons DH, editor: *Current pulmonology*, vol 11, St Louis, 1990, Mosby–Year Book, Inc.
14. Elliot CG et al: Prediction of pulmonary function abnormalities after adult respiratory distress syndrome (ARDS), *Am Rev Respir Dis* 135:634, 1987.
15. Findeis A, Larson JL, Gallo A: Caregiver appraisal: family caregivers of home ventilator assisted individuals, *Rehabil Nurs.* (In press.)
16. George RB: Management of the acute asthma attack. In Bone RC, George RB, Hudson LD, editors: *Acute respiratory failure*, New York, 1987, Churchill Livingstone, Inc.
17. Gerberding JL, Sande MA: General principles and diagnostic approach. In Murray JF, Nadel JA, editors: *Textbook of respiratory medicine*, Philadelphia, 1988, WB Saunders Co.
18. Gries ML, Fernster J: Patient perceptions of the mechanical ventilation experience, *Focus Crit Care* 15(2):52, 1988.
19. Iannuzzi MC, Scoggin CH: Small cell lung cancer, *Am Rev Respir Dis* 134(3):593, 1986.
20. Janson-Bjerklie S et al: Predictors of dyspnea intensity in asthma, *Nurs Res* 36:179, 1987.
21. Johanson WG, Peters JI: Pathophysiology and treatment. In Murray JF, Nadel JA, editors: *Textbook of respiratory medicine*, Philadelphia, 1988, WB Saunders Co.
22. Johnson CC, Finegold SM: Pyogenic bacterial pneumonia, lung abscess, and empyema. In Murray JF, Nadel JA, editors: *Textbook of respiratory medicine*, Philadelphia, 1988, WB Saunders Co.
23. Jones LA: Superior vena cava syndrome: an oncologic complication, *Semin Oncol Nurs* 3(3):211, 1987.
24. Larson JL et al: Inspiratory muscle training with a pressure threshold breathing device in patients with chronic obstructive pulmonary disease, *Am Rev Respir Dis* 138:689, 1988.
25. Light RW: Pneumothorax. In Murray JF, Nadel JA, editors: *Textbook of respiratory medicine*, Philadelphia, 1988, WB Saunders Co.
26. Lough ME: Introduction to hemodynamic monitoring, *Nurs Clin North Am* 22(1):89, 1987.
27. National Asthma Education Program, Expert Panel Report: *Executive summary: guidelines for the diagnosis and management of asthma*, Pub No 91-3042A, Washington, DC, 1991, USDHHS, National Heart, Lung, and Blood Institutes.
28. Openbriar DR, Covey MK: Ineffective breathing pattern related to malnutrition, *Nurs Clin North Am* 22(1):225, 1987.
29. Petersen C, Slutkin G, Mills J: Parasitic infections. In Murray JF, Nadel JA, editors: *Textbook of respiratory medicine*, Philadelphia, 1988, WB Saunders Co.
30. Pingleton SK: Complications of acute respiratory failure, *Am Rev Respir Dis* 137:1463, 1988.

31. Pride NB, Macklem PT: Lung mechanics. In Cherniak NS, Widdicombe JG, editors: *Handbook of physiology,* section 3. *The respiratory system,* vol 3, Baltimore, 1986, Williams & Wilkins Co.

32. Rossman I: *Clinical geriatrics,* ed 3, Philadelphia, 1986, JB Lippincott Co.

33. Sanderson DR: Lung cancer screening: the Mayo study, *Chest* 89:324S, 1986.

34. Sarosi GA, Davies SF: Fungal infections. In Murray JF, Nadel JA, editors: *Textbook of respiratory medicine,* Philadelphia, 1988, WB Saunders Co.

35. Schwartz JL: *Review and evaluation of smoking cessation methods: the United States and Canada 1978-1985,* Rockville, Md, 1987, Division of Cancer Prevention and Control, National Cancer Institute.

36. Smith LH: Systemic manifestations of carcinoma of the lung. In Murray JF, Nadel JA, editors: *Textbook of respiratory medicine,* Philadelphia, 1988, WB Saunders Co.

37. Snukst-Torbeck G, Werhane MJ, Schraufnagel DE: Treatment of tuberculosis in a nurse-managed clinic, *Heart Lung* 16:30, 1987.

38. Strohl KP, Cherniack N, Gothe B: Physiologic basis of therapy for sleep apnea, *Am Rev Respir Dis* 134:791, 1986.

39. US Department of Health and Human Services: *Smoking and health: a national status report,* Rockville, Md, 1987, Division of Cancer Prevention and Control, National Cancer Institute.

40. Vukich DJ, Markovchick VJ: Pulmonary and chest wall injuries. In Rosen P et al, editors: *Emergency medicine,* vol 1, ed 2, St Louis, 1988, Mosby–Year Book, Inc.

41. Walshaw MJ, Evans CC: Allergen avoidance in house dust mite sensitive adult asthma, *Q J Med* 58:199, 1986.

42. Washington JA: Microbiologic diagnosis of lower respiratory tract infection. In Murray JF, Nadel JA, editors: *Textbook of respiratory medicine,* Philadelphia, 1988, WB Saunders Co.

43. Wasserman K et al: *Principles of exercise testing and interpretation,* Philadelphia, 1987, Lea & Febiger.

44. Yancik R, Yates JW: Quality of life assessment of cancer patients: Conceptual and methodologic challenges and constraints, *Cancer Bull* 38(5):217, 1986.

Classic

45. Burdon J, Killian K, Jones L: Pattern of breathing during exercise in patients with interstitial lung disease, *Thorax* 38:778, 1983.

46. Chin R, Pesce R: Practical aspects in management of respiratory failure in chronic obstructive pulmonary disease, *Crit Care Q* 6(2):1, 1983.

47. Fahey PJ, Harris K, Vanderwarf C: Clinical experience with continuous monitoring of mixed venous oxygen saturation in respiratory failure, *Chest* 86:748, 1984.

48. Farber MO et al: Hormonal abnormalities affecting sodium and water balance in acute respiratory failure due to chronic obstructive lung disease, *Chest* 85(1):49, 1984.

49. Francis PB: Acute respiratory failure in obstructive lung disease, *Med Clin North Am* 67(3):657, 1983.

50. Griffin JP, Carlon GC: Medical and nursing implications of high-frequency jet ventilation, *Heart Lung* 13:250, 1984.

51. Halevy A et al: Long-term evaluation of patients following the adult respiratory distress syndrome, *Respir Care* 29:132, 1984.

52. Heaton RK et al: Psychologic effects of continuous and nocturnal oxygen therapy in hypoxemic chronic obstructive pulmonary disease, *Arch Intern Med* 143:1941, 1983.

53. Janoff A: Elastases and emphysema, *Am Rev Respir Dis* 132:417, 1985.

54. Kehrer JP et al: Enhanced acute lung damage following corticosteroid treatment, *Am Rev Respir Dis* 130:256, 1984.

55. Kinsman RA et al: Multidimensional analysis of the symptoms of chronic bronchitis and emphysema, *J Behav Med* 6:339, 1983.

56. Knipper J: Evaluation of adventitious sounds as an indicator of the need for tracheal suctioning: IVAC award paper; *Heart Lung* 13:292, 1984.

57. Knudsen F: Respiratory conditions in older adults. In Steffl B, editor: *Handbook of gerontological nursing,* New York, 1984, Van Nostrand Reinhold Co, Inc.

58. Kumar P, Marier R, Leech SH: Respiratory allergies related to automobile air conditioners, *N Engl J Med* 311:1619, 1984.

59. Lehrer S: *Understanding lung sounds,* Philadelphia, 1984, WB Saunders Co.

60. Loudon RG et al: Aerial transmission of mycobacteria, *Am Rev Respir Dis* 100:165, 1969.

61. Matthews MJ, Mackay B, Lukeman J: The pathology of non–small cell carcinoma of the lung, *Semin Oncol* 10:34, 1983.

62. Openbrier DR et al: Nutritional status and lung function in patients with emphysema and chronic bronchitis, *Chest* 83:17, 1983.

63. Prigatano GP, Wright EC, Levin D: Quality of life and its predictors in patients with mild hypoxemia and chronic obstructive pulmonary disease, *Arch Intern Med* 144:1613, 1984.

64. Sarna GP et al: Lung cancer. In Haskell CM, editor: *Cancer treatment,* ed 2, Philadelphia, 1985, WB Saunders Co.

65. Sharp JT: The chest and respiratory muscles in obesity, pregnancy, and ascites. In Roussos C, Macklem PT, editors: *Thorax,* part B, New York, 1985, Marcel Dekker, Inc.

66. Thurlbeck WM: Chronic airflow obstruction correlation of structure and function. In Petty TL, editor: *Lung biology in health and disease: chronic obstructive pulmonary disease,* ed 2, New York, 1985, Marcel Dekker, Inc.

67. Tockman MS, Khoury MJ, Cohen BH: The epidemiology of COPD. In Petty TL, editor: *Lung biology in health and disease: chronic obstructive pulmonary disease,* ed 2, New York, 1985, Marcel Dekker, Inc.

68. Verhese A, Beck SL: Bacterial pneumonia in the elderly, *Medicine* 62:271, 1983.

69. Vitello-Cicciu JM: Recalled perceptions of patients administered pancuronium bromide, *Focus Crit Care* 11(1):28, 1984.

70. White KM: Completing the hemodynamic picture: SVo$_2$, *Heart Lung* 14(3):272, 1985.

71. Wilson RF, Steiger Z: Thoracic injuries. In Tintinalli JE et al, editors: *Emergency medicine,* New York, 1985, McGraw-Hill, Inc.

Peripheral Vascular System

CHAPTER TWENTY-NINE

Nursing Assessment of the Peripheral Vascular System

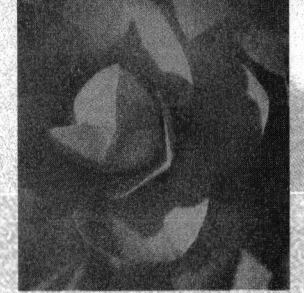

LEARNING OBJECTIVES

1 Know the main structural components of the peripheral vascular system and their functions.
2 Understand the physical and physiologic principles that control blood flow and pressure.
3 Obtain relevant subjective information from the patient who has a peripheral vascular alteration.
4 Using correct technique, examine the patient to obtain appropriate objective information about the peripheral vascular system.
5 Differentiate abnormal from normal subjective and objective findings related to the peripheral vascular system.
6 Describe diagnostic procedures related to the vascular system.
7 Describe the preparation and care of patients undergoing diagnostic procedures for vascular disorders.

THE PERIPHERAL vascular system includes the branching network of vessels that convey blood from the left side of the heart to the tissues and then back to the right side of the heart.

Blood flow to the skin, bones, muscles, viscera, and nervous system is pumped first into the aorta by the heart and then through a series of arteries with decreasing diameters until it passes through the smallest arterioles and enters the tissue capillaries. From the capillaries the blood collects in the venules and flows back to the heart through veins with increasing diameters, until the two venae cavae deliver it back to the right side of the heart to be pumped to the lungs for reoxygenation and removal of the excess carbon dioxide. A portion of the blood plasma filters out of the capillaries into the interstitial space and is returned to the blood through the vessels of the lymph system.

Alterations of the vascular system usually occur in adulthood. Exercise, diet, and other health care practices affect the integrity of the system. Risk factors in relation to peripheral vascular alterations include a sedentary life-style, high lipid dietary intake, smoking, and obesity. Women are particularly prone to obstructed circulation in the lower extremities during pregnancy, and certain disease processes (e.g., diabetes mellitus) are almost invariably associated with the development of peripheral vascular impairment.

Throughout the assessment the nurse notes pertinent positive and negative findings in an attempt to establish if there are any peripheral vascular abnormalities and to identify their causes.

ANATOMY AND PHYSIOLOGY
Blood Vessels

There are three types of blood vessels: arteries, veins, and capillaries. The **capillaries** are the functional units of the system because they are the vessels that allow substances to diffuse to and from the blood into the interstitial space that provides the environment in which the tissue cells live.

Capillary walls are made up of a layer of simple squamous epithelium that also forms the lining (endothelium) of the rest of the cardiovascular system. The endothelial cells not only provide a physical barrier to contain blood, but also react to blood flow–related forces by secreting substances such as prostaglandins and nitric oxide that affect the tone of smooth muscle cells surrounding them, tissue growth factors, and substances that give anticlotting properties to the blood-endothelial surface.

In the arteries and veins the endothelium is surrounded by a layer of elastin and smooth muscle and on the outer surface by a layer of white fibrous connective tissue. The proportions of these components differ significantly in arteries and veins. For example, the amount of elastin is much greater in arter-

ies than veins, allowing them to remain open even when there is no blood in them. Arterial walls are also thicker and stronger, enabling them to withstand the high pressures generated by the heart.

All high-pressure vessels tend to leak fluid out of the lumen. The **arteries** are the high-pressure vessels of the circulatory system, and plasma tends to leak into the subendothelial layers of the arterial wall, especially where the endothelium is damaged. The intrusion of plasma into the wall is one step in the development of atherosclerosis and the formation of calcified plaques in the lumen, which eventually produce a reduction in blood flow. The endothelium is particularly sensitive to damage from the friction of turbulent and fast blood flow. This type of blood flow occurs normally just distal to major arterial bifurcations and, pathologically, just distal to arterial stenoses. As individuals age, these areas have a higher risk of developing atherosclerotic plaques, especially in individuals with high blood pressure. Atherosclerosis carries an increased risk of sudden death where arteries to the heart or brain are involved and an increased risk of peripheral vascular disease where the arteries to the limbs are involved.

The resistance arterioles are the smallest vessels of the arterial tree; their constriction and dilation control the volume of blood flowing into the capillaries. They are called resistance arterioles because they resist the flow of blood.

Figure 29-1 shows the principal arteries. The blood flow to the hands, feet, and brain is protected by arterial anastomoses that ensure that when one of the supplying arteries is damaged, flow is maintained through the anastomoses from the other arteries. This is particularly important for the brain, which is supplied by the right and left internal carotid arteries and the right and left vertebral arteries through an anastomosis called the circle of Willis.

Several arteries supply the liver and the gastrointestinal system. The celiac artery supplies the hepatic and gastric arteries, which supply the liver and stomach with oxygenated blood, and the superior and inferior mesenteric arteries supply the large and small intestines. Deoxygenated blood from all these areas is collected by the hepatic portal vein (Figure 29-2), which supplies the liver capillaries with the concentrated products of digestion and enables the liver to process the nutrients before they enter the general circulation. The portal system also delivers higher concentrations of insulin and glucagon to the liver than to the rest of the body, because in the portal vein these hormones are only diluted by the blood returning from the gastrointestinal tract. In the atria the concentration of the hormones is diluted further by the blood returning from the rest of the body.

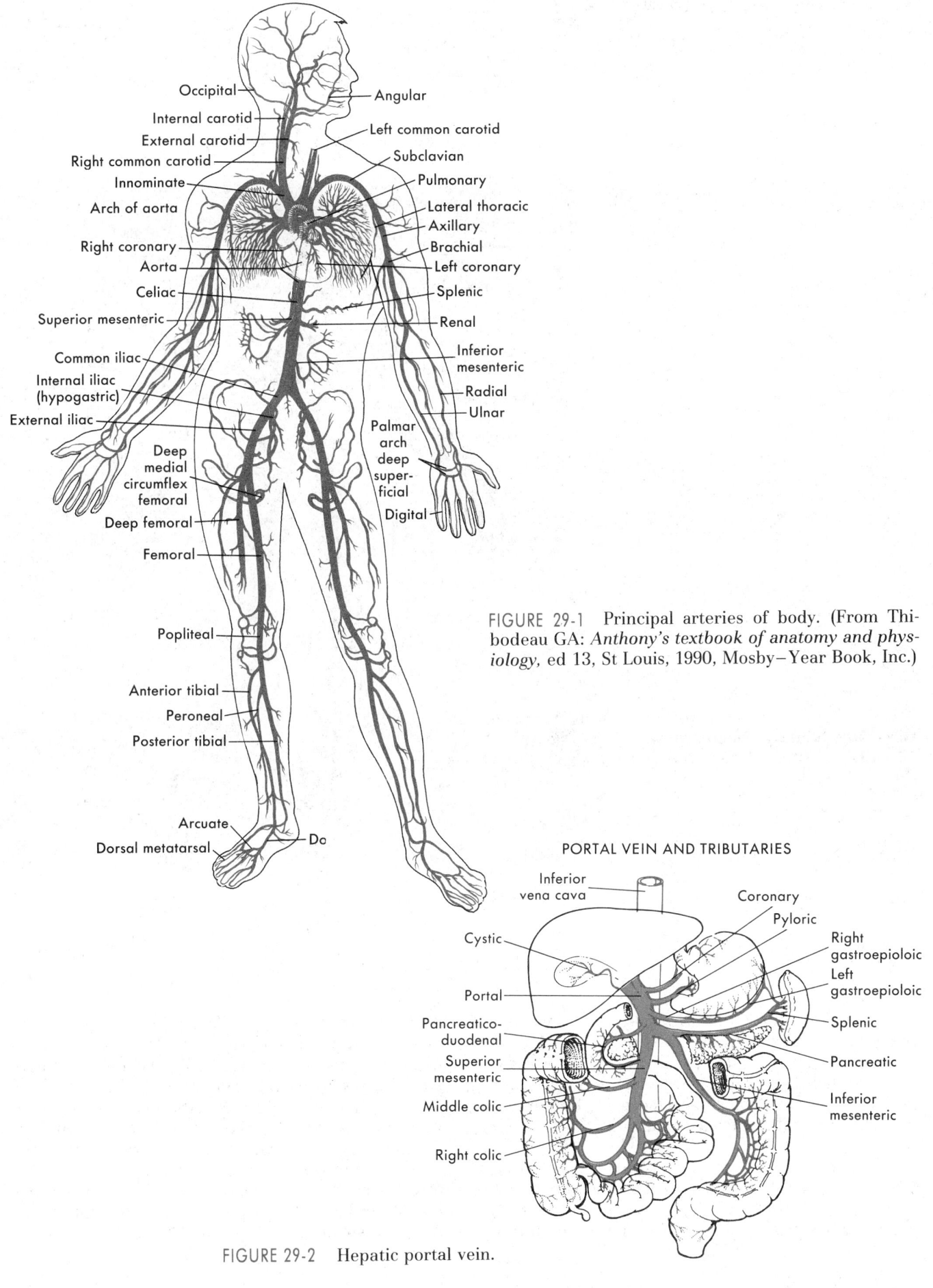

Occipital
Angular
Internal carotid
Left common carotid
External carotid
Subclavian
Right common carotid
Innominate
Pulmonary
Arch of aorta
Lateral thoracic
Axillary
Right coronary
Brachial
Aorta
Left coronary
Celiac
Splenic
Superior mesenteric
Renal
Common iliac
Inferior mesenteric
Internal iliac (hypogastric)
Radial
External iliac
Ulnar
Deep medial circumflex femoral
Palmar arch deep superficial
Deep femoral
Digital
Femoral
Popliteal
Anterior tibial
Peroneal
Posterior tibial
Arcuate
Dorsal metatarsal
Do

FIGURE 29-1 Principal arteries of body. (From Thibodeau GA: *Anthony's textbook of anatomy and physiology,* ed 13, St Louis, 1990, Mosby–Year Book, Inc.)

PORTAL VEIN AND TRIBUTARIES

Inferior vena cava
Coronary
Pyloric
Cystic
Right gastroepioloic
Left gastroepioloic
Portal
Splenic
Pancreatico-duodenal
Pancreatic
Superior mesenteric
Inferior mesenteric
Middle colic
Right colic

FIGURE 29-2 Hepatic portal vein.

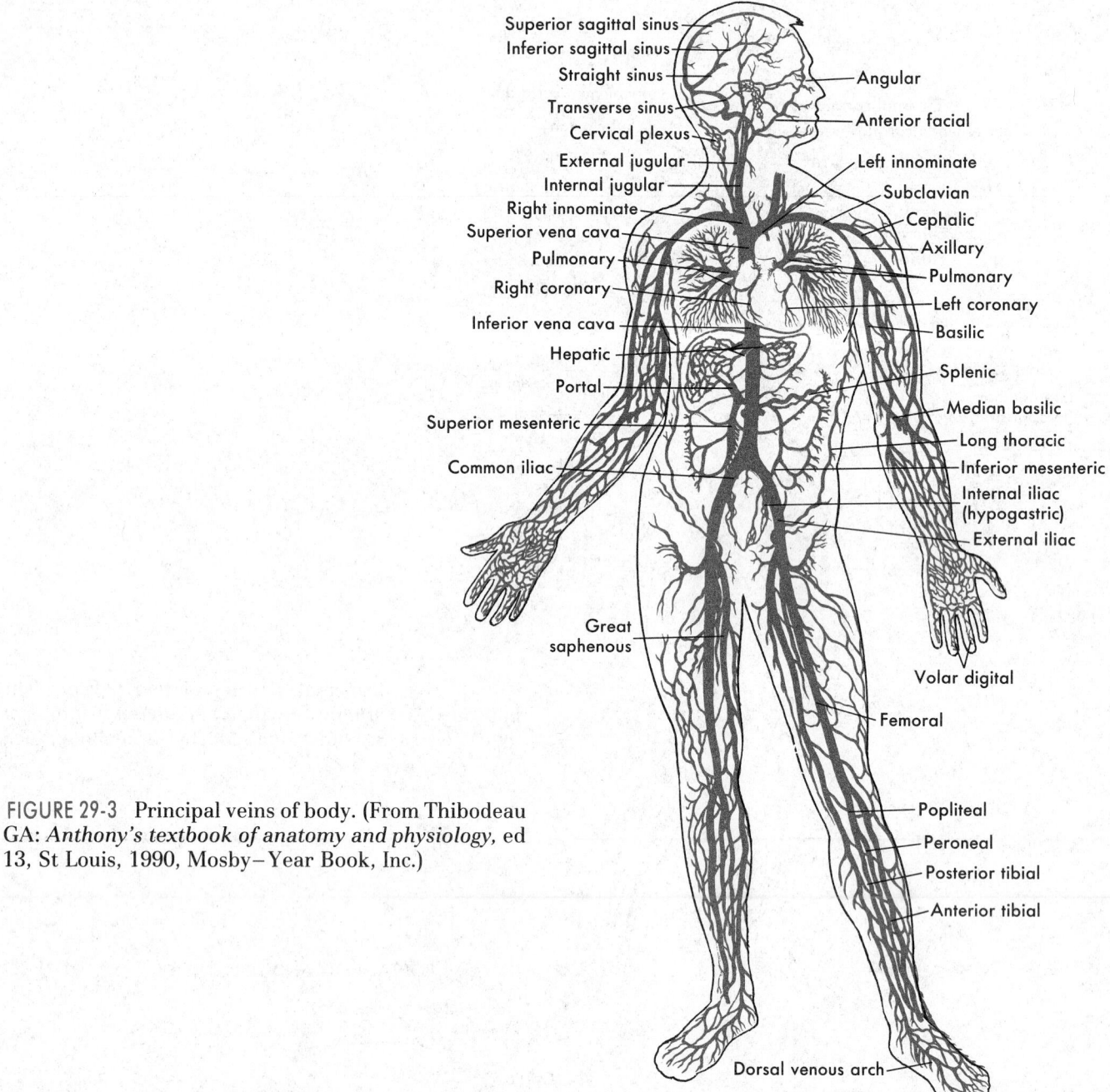

FIGURE 29-3   Principal veins of body. (From Thibodeau GA: *Anthony's textbook of anatomy and physiology,* ed 13, St Louis, 1990, Mosby–Year Book, Inc.)

Figure 29-3 shows the principal veins. There are many more venous anastomoses than there are arterial anastomoses. They connect the deep veins to the superficial veins, the deep veins to each other, and the superficial veins to each other, so that blood can take the route of least resistance back to the heart.

Compared with arteries, **veins** are difficult to see when there is no blood in them because they collapse, have relatively thin walls, and blend with their surroundings. In the upright position the veins in the neck are almost empty because gravity draws blood down toward the right atrium. Prominence of the jugular veins is evidence of a significant rise in **central venous pressure** and usually indicates heart failure. The veins inferior to the heart usually contain approximately 60% of the blood volume. Semilunar valves ensure that the pressure on the walls of the veins of the feet, mainly caused by the force of gravity, is not excessive. They cut the long column of blood that extends from the heart to the feet into small sections. In addition, they help con-

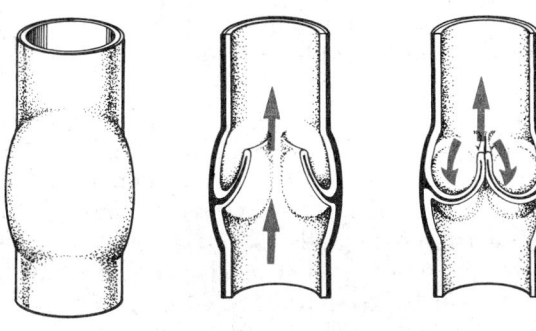

FIGURE 29-4   Action of semilunar valves.

trol the flow of blood by preventing retrograde flow (Figure 29-4).

The blood contained in the veins below the heart must be forced against gravity back to the heart. The most important force opposing gravity is the squeezing action of skeletal muscle contraction. This skeletal muscle pump forces blood out of the veins near the muscles, and the valves ensure that it only moves toward the heart. The skeletal muscle pump is assisted by (1) constriction of the venous smooth muscle, which prevents the capacity of the veins of the limbs from becoming excessive and ensures that the valves are not dilated to the point of incompetence, and (2) the suction created in the veins by the negative thoracic and abdominal pressures associated with respiration. Prominence of the veins of the limbs indicates poor venous tone and insufficient skeletal muscle activity in the limbs.

Physical Principles That Determine Blood Flow

The flow of blood is governed by the physical principles that govern the flow of liquids: the pressure difference along the system and the resistance to flow generated by the blood and the vessels.

The pumping action of the heart creates the pressure difference. Several factors determine the resistance to blood flow **(peripheral resistance).** Peripheral resistance increases as blood viscosity increases, the length of the vessels increases, and the radius of the vessels decreases. In reality, blood viscosity only changes with disease (rises with polycythemia, falls with anemia), and the length of the vessels only changes slowly as the individual grows (peripheral resistance increases as a baby grows) or disease affects the length of the vessels. Therefore neither of these factors is important in short-term changes in peripheral resistance. The body uses small changes in the radius of the blood vessels to produce large changes in peripheral resistance and hence control blood flow to the different regions.

Physiologic Control of Blood Flow and Arterial Pressure

Because peripheral resistance is inversely proportional to the cube root of the radius, doubling the radius of the resistance arterioles by dilation increases flow by a factor of 16. Thus vasoconstriction and vasodilation of the resistance arterioles supplying the various capillary beds control blood flow to the various tissues. The radius of the resistance arterioles is modified by intrinsic and extrinsic mechanisms.

Intrinsic control of blood flow is a property of the tissue itself and does not require stimulation by the nervous system or hormones. The flow of blood through most tissues is directly proportional to the tissue's use of oxygen, because the resistance arterioles are sensitive to the concentration of oxygen in the interstitial fluid around them. (The resistance arterioles of the brain are sensitive to carbon dioxide rather than oxygen.) When the tissue becomes more active, it uses more oxygen and the concentration of oxygen falls; this causes the resistance arterioles to dilate because their smooth muscle relaxes as oxygen concentration falls. The dilation lowers the resistance opposing the flow of blood; thus more blood flows through the active tissue, and more oxygen is delivered until the optimal concentration of oxygen is restored. (When the brain becomes more active, the level of carbon dioxide increases and causes the resistance arterioles to dilate, and the extra blood flow that results washes out the excess carbon dioxide.)

Extrinsic control of blood flow is a property of the sympathetic nervous system and hormones. It overrides the normal intrinsic control exerted by the resistance arterioles and allows the flow of blood to be shunted away from tissues that can survive with less blood to tissues that are essential to maintain life. The brain and heart cannot survive even short periods of deprivation, and the skeletal muscles require extra blood when they are needed to survive a crisis.

The proportion of the cardiac output that flows to the skin, the gastrointestinal tract, and the kidneys can be reduced for periods without any deleterious effects. It is reduced routinely during even moderate exercise, and inasmuch as approximately 20% of the cardiac output normally flows to the kidneys and 25% to the liver and gastrointestinal tract, constriction of the resistance arterioles in these regions of the body makes a significant quantity of blood available for use by other tissues. During exercise, this blood flows rapidly through the skeletal muscles. During crises, such as heart failure or hemorrhage, resistance arterioles of the muscles are also constricted, and blood remains in the arterial system longer. This keeps blood pressure high and provides adequate blood flow to the heart and brain, even when cardiac output is cut to almost half of its normal level. During such crises, if blood flow through the skin is not needed for temperature control, the blood vessels of the skin are also constricted. Poor skin color is one of the signs of sympathetic nervous system activity readily apparent to those providing health care.

Arterial blood pressure increases when cardiac output, peripheral resistance, or blood volume increases. Homeostasis of blood pressure is essential because blood flow to the brain and heart becomes inadequate if it falls too low and there is an increased risk of vessel rupture and damage if it becomes too high. Long-term control of blood volume, and hence pressure, is a function of the kidney (see Unit X). Rapid, short-term control of blood pressure is by cardiac and vascular reflexes.

Reflexes that maintain the homeostasis of arterial blood pressure are initiated by changes that are detected by stretch receptors (baroreceptors) in the walls of the carotid sinuses and the aortic arch. Changes in baroreceptor stimulation are received by the cardiac and vasomotor control centers in the medulla oblongata. If arterial pressure increases above normal, it is lowered by increasing the parasympathetic stimulation to the heart carried by the vagus nerve. This reduces cardiac output by slowing the heart rate. If arterial blood pressure falls markedly, it is raised (1) by increasing cardiac output through increased sympathetic nervous stimulation of heart rate and strength, (2) by vasoconstriction of the venous reservoirs, and (3) by increasing peripheral resistance in the gastrointestinal, renal, and musculocutaneous capillary beds.

Blood pressure is measured to ensure that high blood pressure **(hypertension)** does not exist undiagnosed for a long time and to ensure that blood pressure is not too low **(hypotension)** to provide an adequate perfusion pressure. It is essential for the health care provider to evaluate each individual situation carefully, because blood pressure only gives an indication that blood flow is satisfactory under normal conditions. Under abnormal conditions, blood pressure can be high or within normal limits even when cardiac output is severely impaired, because elevated peripheral resistance diverts blood to the large arteries from the peripheral resistance areas of the kidney, gastrointestinal tract, and skin. To ensure that the risk of such a "normotensive" individual going into shock is not overlooked, the health care provider should check for signs of hyperactivity of the sympathetic nervous system, such as a fast, weak pulse rate and skin that is cold, clammy, and pale or ashen.

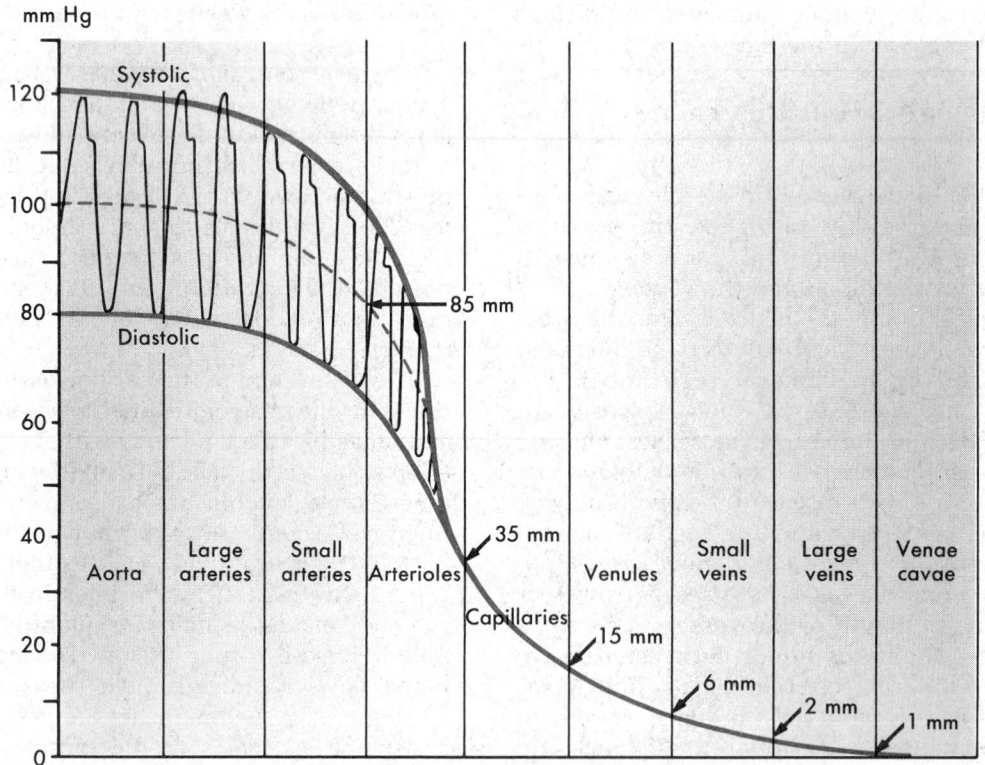

FIGURE 29-5   Blood pressure gradient.

Blood pressure throughout the cardiovascular system (with some exceptions in the major arteries caused by wave reflection) decreases as it moves out along the arterial tree through the arteries and veins. It is lowest in the atria and great veins when the atrioventricular valves first open. The pressure of blood in the systemic vascular system, also referred to as **hydrostatic pressure,** is presented graphically in Figure 29-5.

Capillary dynamics

The capillary walls serve effectively as membranes that allow rapid diffusion of lipid-soluble substances such as oxygen and carbon dioxide and slower diffusion and filtration of water and relatively small molecules (i.e., salts, hormones, amino acids, glucose) to and from the tissue cells. The capillary walls retain the blood proteins and erythrocytes while allowing white blood cells to cross them by diapedesis.

The filtration of water and small molecules into the interstitial fluid is powered by the hydrostatic pressure gradient across the capillary wall and opposed by the colloid osmotic pressure gradient. Capillary hydrostatic pressure is the blood pressure generated by the cardiac contraction that remains after the blood has passed through the resistance arterioles. The pressure is higher in capillaries that are close to arterioles and lower in capillaries close to venules. Therefore filtration of water and small molecules tends to be out of the capillaries that are near the resistance arterioles and into the capillaries near the venules. The colloid osmotic pressure of the blood is the pressure resulting from the concentration of the blood proteins, especially albumen. Excessive interstitial fluid **(edema)** develops when venous hydrostatic pressure is excessive (e.g., during heart failure or venous obstruction), when blood albumen concentration falls (e.g., during kidney disease or acute starvation), and when the lymphatic system is obstructed.

The water that filters out of the capillaries (1) returns any protein that escapes from the capillaries to the cardiovascular system via the lymphatic system; (2) carries debris and infectious material away from the interstitial space to the lymph nodes; and (3) increases the efficiency with which some nutrients are delivered to and waste products are removed from the cells.

Lymph Vessels

The lymphatic system is made up of blind-ended lymph capillaries that collect interstitial fluid (now called lymph), the lymph vessels that transport it to the subclavian veins, and the two lymph organs, the spleen and the thymus gland.

The lymphatic capillaries are more permeable than regular capillaries, and their simple squamous epithelial cells overlap so they act as valves and allow fluid to enter but not leave the capillary. Whenever interstitial fluid pressure rises, the flow from the lymphatic capillaries into the collecting lymphatics increases. The collecting lymphatics and larger lymph vessels contain semilunar valves that prevent retrograde lymph flow. They are also interrupted at frequent intervals by **lymph nodes** that filter out particles and expose the lymph to the action of the many lymphocytes and macrophages within the nodes. The tonsils of the oropharynx and pharynx are large lymph nodes, as are the Peyer patches of the mesentery. Lymph nodes commonly become infected and swollen, especially in younger children.

Lymph is drained from the right side of the head, neck, and thorax and from the right arm into the right subclavian vein close to the jugular vein by way of the right lymphatic duct; lymph is drained from the rest of the body into the left subclavian vein, mostly by way of the thoracic duct. The main lymph vessels and nodes, with the exception of the extensive system draining the gastrointestinal organs, are shown in Figure 29-6. In the intestines the lymph system bypasses the liver and carries absorbed fat from the lymph capillaries (lacteals) directly to the general circulatory system for use by the body tissues. The structure of the main lymph vessels is similar to that of veins, and their transport of lymph is similar (i.e., driven by skeletal muscle pumping and the suction generated by respiratory movements). If

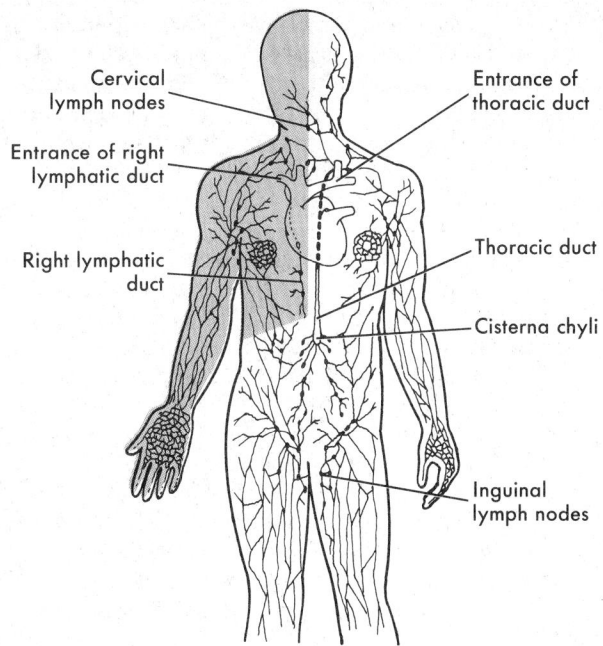

FIGURE 29-6   Lymphatic system.

lymphatic drainage is impaired, the amount of fluid in the interstitial space rises and edema results.

When metastatic cancerous cells enter the lymph system, as with microorganisms, they cause the infected nodes to swell. Some cells may escape into the general circulation or into the tissue surrounding the infected nodes. Once in the general circulation, the cancerous cells are delivered to the lungs by the pulmonary circulation. After lodging and growing in the lung tissue, they enter the pulmonary veins and travel to the heart and to the systemic arteries. Once they reach the left ventricle, the probability that a tissue will receive a metastatic cell depends on the proportion of the cardiac output that flows through that tissue.

The **spleen** and **thymus gland** are organs of the lymphatic system. The spleen is ovoid and is located in the left hypochondrium just above the left kidney. It is made up of a capsule that encloses large venous sinuses and large aggregations of lymphocytes and macrophages. The spleen removes defective red blood cells and platelets from the circulation, stores approximately 150 to 200 mL of blood to be pumped into the general circulation in times of stress, removes microorganisms from the blood, and enlarges significantly as its monocytes and lymphocytes reproduce during infections.

The thymus gland, located in the upper mediastinum and the lower portion of the neck, is made up of two triangular lobes. It is covered by a fibrous capsule, and its cortex and medulla are largely made up of lymphocytes. The thymus gland is relatively large during a person's infancy and begins to atrophy at puberty until it is barely recognizable in old age. It plays a critical role in the immune system. In early infancy the thymus gland is responsible for initiating the proper function of the T-lymphocytes, and it continues to play a role in immunity for older individuals, possibly as an endocrine gland. The function of the immune system is reviewed in Chapter 39.

ASSESSMENT
Subjective

A focused health history for a patient with a suspected or previously diagnosed peripheral vascular problem requires the nurse to use knowledge of pathophysiology to guide questioning in an appropriate and complete manner. Peripheral vascular disease rarely occurs in the absence of other disease processes such as diabetes, coronary artery disease, or hypertension. Patients may seek health care for changes in lower extremities such as swelling, ulceration, or pain.

An adequate system-specific history for any patient includes a review of related systems and delineation of any positive findings (symptoms the patient complains of) through exploring various dimensions. Specific dimensions used to delineate positive findings include onset, duration, frequency, alleviating factors, aggravating factors, precipitating events, location, quality, quantity, associated symptoms, and chronology of events. Noting any significant negatives (symptoms the patient denies) is important because it allows other clinicians to know specifically what the interviewer asked. To record "no problems" does not communicate which symptoms the patient denied. The box on p. 687 lists potential symptoms to review with the patient. In addition to specific symptoms, ask the patient about previous blood clots, strokes, myocardial infarctions, recent surgeries, pregnancy, prolonged inactivity, or trauma.

Other appropriate history to explore includes major adult illnesses, hospitalizations, surgeries, injuries or accidents, immunizations, current medications, allergies, and habits. When recording hospitalizations and surgeries, determine the hospital, attending physician, and dates of the hospital stay. If

GERIATRIC CONSIDERATIONS

Physiologic Changes in the Peripheral Vascular System

A number of changes to the blood vessels develop with advancing age: the distensibility and elasticity of the arterial wall decrease because the proportion of collagen increases and the proportion of elastin decreases. Consequently, the proportion of the stroke volume that can be stored in them during systole is reduced, and the profile of their blood pressure and flow waves changes. Venous elasticity also declines and increases the risk of varicosities in areas where venous pressure is high; and veins become more tortuous with advancing age. An increase in the thickness of the basement membrane of capillaries and a reduction in the density of capillary fenestrations reduce tissue perfusion and increase capillary-tissue diffusion gradients. However, this does not usually result in tissue damage unless oxygen demand is increased or delivery is further impaired by trauma, edema, or disease.

Throughout life, damage to the endothelium reduces its ability to protect the peripheral vascular system and leads to the development of atherosclerotic plaques. The development of some plaques occurs in all individuals as they grow older, and therefore the risk of cerebral and cardiac ischemia from occlusion increases with age. However, accelerated atherosclerosis caused by unhealthy life-style choices or disease should not be considered a normal aging process.

POTENTIAL SYMPTOMS IN PERIPHERAL VASCULAR DISORDERS

Pain in one or both lower extremities with activity (intermittent claudication)

Pain in one or both lower extremities unrelated to activity

Swelling in one or both lower extremities

Change in color of one or both lower extremities

Sore or ulcer on one or both lower extremities that does not heal or heals very slowly

Change in temperature of one or both lower extremities

Feelings of coldness or tingling in the lower extremities

the patient has a history of serious injuries or accidents, determine the injury sustained, how treated, where treated, attending physician, and if there are any sequelae. Immunizations for an adult include noting the last tetanus booster (DT), completion of hepatitis vaccine series, as well as any immunizations for travel abroad. When recording current medications include the name of the drug, who prescribed it, for what condition it was prescribed, when the patient began taking it, dosage, and frequency. Allergies should be recorded with careful attention to the allergic response. Include allergies to contrast material specifically, because some patients may have had previous experience with aller-

gies caused by testing procedures. Habits include alcohol consumption, tobacco use, use of recreational or illicit drugs, caffeine consumption, and exercise.

Family history that is relevant to the peripheral vascular system includes stroke, hypertension, myocardial infarction, hyperlipidemia, and thrombophlebitis. A positive finding should include the disease as well as the individual's relationship to the patient (i.e., cerebrovascular accident [CVA], maternal aunt; myocardial infarction [MI], paternal uncle).

Objective

Based on the history obtained and knowledge of pathophysiology, the nurse determines the appropriate systems to be assessed. Some patients will have more complex symptom involvement than others, and therefore assessment needs may vary from patient to patient. Objective data the nurse may evaluate include general and abdominal assessment and evaluation of the integumentary, cardiovascular, respiratory, neurologic, and peripheral vascular systems. General assessment is significant in every patient and refers to the examiner's overall impression of the patient's state of health. The box below includes potential objective findings that may be noted on examination of a patient with a peripheral vascular disorder.

General assessment

Vital signs are always valuable. Also note height, weight, facial expression, apparent age (relative to chronologic age), nutritional status, general appear-

POTENTIAL OBJECTIVE FINDINGS IN PERIPHERAL VASCULAR DISORDERS

General
Appearance of distress

Cardiovascular
Tachycardia
Irregularly irregular rhythm
Atrial fibrillation on electrocardiogı

Respiratory
Tachypnea
Dyspnea
Area of decreased breath sounds

Abdominal
Renal, iliac, or aortic bruits

Extremities
Pallor
Cyanosis
Erythema
Dependent rubor (dusky redness)
Brownish pigmentation
Decreased hair distribution on lower extremities
Shiny skin
Dry, scaly skin
Scars
Edema
Impaired pulses
Coolness on palpation
Localized area of elevated temperature
Palpable cord
Area of tenderness on palpation
Pallor on elevation of one or both lower extremities

ance, and stature. Any obvious abnormalities or assistive devices are also noted. Note whether the patient appears to be comfortable or in distress.

Cardiovascular

Observe the precordium for any heaves, lifts, or pulsations. Palpate the precordium for thrills and the apical impulse. Note the size and location of the apical impulse. Auscultate the precordium with the bell and the diaphragm noting the rate, rhythm, the first heart sound (S_1), the second heart sound (S_2), any gallops (S_3 or S_4), any murmurs, any pericardial friction rubs, or any other extra sounds. Patients admitted with a deep vein thrombosis (DVT) may have atrial fibrillation that would be noted as an irregularly irregular rhythm on auscultation. Rhythms cannot be diagnosed from auscultation. Rhythms must be diagnosed through electrocardiograms (ECGs) (see Chapter 33).

Respiratory

Inspect the thorax, noting symmetry, configuration, and pattern of respirations, including depth, regularity, and ease of respirations. Palpate the thorax for tenderness and masses. Percuss the thorax generally for quality and symmetry. Auscultate the thorax, noting breath sounds and any adventitious sounds such as crackles (rales), wheezes (rhonchi), or pleural friction rubs. A patient with peripheral vascular disease may also experience a pulmonary embolism. Thus careful attention to respiratory status is important (see Chapter 25).

Abdominal

Inspect the abdomen for lesions, scars, striae, visible peristalsis, symmetry, contour, and umbilicus placement and contour. Auscultate the abdomen for presence of bowel sounds and vascular sounds. Note especially any renal, iliac, or aortic bruits. A renal bruit might reflect renal artery stenosis, whereas an aortic bruit may reflect an aortic aneurysm. Percuss the abdomen generally noting tone and specifically to note liver span in the right midclavicular line. Also percuss the spleen to determine size. Palpate the abdomen lightly and then more deeply, noting muscle tone, tenderness, and the presence or absence of any masses. Palpate deeply to identify liver and spleen borders (see Chapter 63).

Peripheral vascular

Inspect the extremities, noting symmetry, color, pigmentation changes, ulcerations, varicosities, superficial venous patterns, edema, hair presence and distribution, rashes, or scars. If ulcerations are noted,

---

SCALES FOR GRADING PULSES

Example 1

4 = bounding
3 = full, increased
2 = expected
1 = diminished, barely palpable
0 = absent, not palpable

Example 2

3+ = bounding
2+ = normal
1+ = weak, thready
 0 = absent

Example 3

4+ = normal
3+ = mildly impaired
2+ = moderately impaired
1+ = markedly impaired
 0 = absent

---

document location, size, depth, contour, and any drainage. Rashes and scars should also be documented, noting location, size, contour, and color. Observe the nails for growth, curvature, adhesion, color, thickness, and clubbing. (Refer to Chapter 73 for a complete discussion of documentation of integumentary changes.)

Palpate peripheral pulses, noting presence or absence, amplitude, and symmetry. When grading amplitude of pulses, document the scale being used. Various scales have been defined in the literature (see the box above). If a distal pulse is not palpable, note color, warmth, and capillary refill of the extremity and palpate the more proximal pulse or pulses.

If edema is noted on inspection, palpate the extremity, noting the quality of edema as either pitting or nonpitting. Lymphedema is nonpitting and may be unilateral. Pitting edema may be graded as 1+ to 4+ (Figure 29-7). The circumference of the extremities can also be measured bilaterally and over time. Comparisons can be made from side to side to assist in determining and documenting the degree of edema.

Some special examination techniques may be helpful in evaluating the peripheral vascular system. The **retrograde filling (Trendelenburg's) test** is used in evaluating valvular competency in the superficial venous system. With the patient lying supine, elevate the leg 90 degrees for approximately 15 seconds. Then place a tourniquet around the patient's

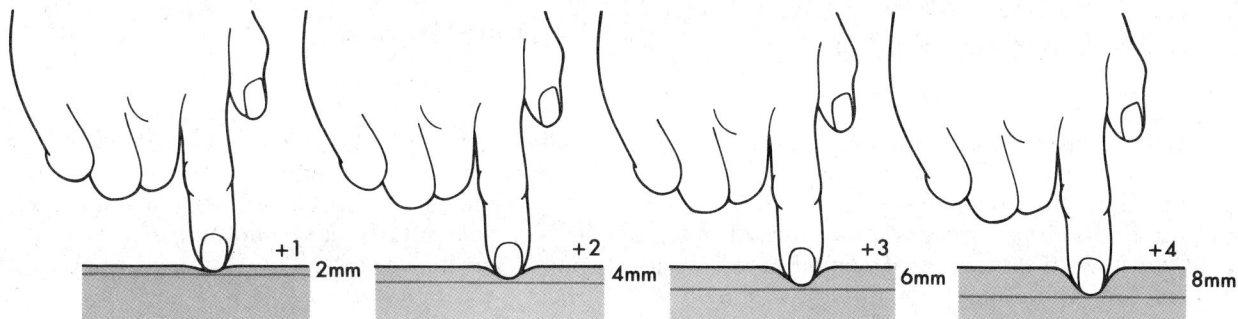

FIGURE 29-7   Grading of edema.

thigh tight enough to occlude superficial veins but not so tight as to occlude the arterial pulse or deeper vessels. Ask the patient to stand. Observe for venous filling in the leg. Venous filling should occur from distal to proximal. After approximately 20 to 30 seconds, release the tourniquet. Note any sudden filling. Sudden filling after release of the tourniquet and filling from proximal to distal indicate venous valvular incompetency or retrograde filling.

Another special technique, **Allen's test,** may be used to evaluate the arterial supply to the hand. Have the patient rest with the hands supinated in the lap. Ask the patient to make a tight fist with one hand. The nurse should compress both radial and ulnar arteries firmly between the thumb and finger. Then ask the patient to open the hand into a relaxed, slightly flexed position. The palm will be pale. Release the pressure over the ulnar artery, and the palm should become pink within 3 to 5 seconds. Persisting paleness indicates occlusion of the ulnar artery or its branches. This procedure can be repeated for both hands and for the radial artery as well.

Throughout the examination, assess for signs of arterial (decreased perfusion to a body part) and venous (sluggish return of blood to the heart from a body part) insufficiency. These conditions may exist alone or simultaneously, making assessment difficult at times.

Neurologic

Neurologic findings in peripheral vascular disease may involve sensory function changes. Sensation of extremities can be evaluated through testing awareness of sharp and dull beginning distally and moving proximally. Light touch is also evaluated. Use a sterile needle for sharp and dull and a cotton ball for light touch. Begin by instructing the patient as to what is sharp and what is dull with the patient's eyes open. With the patient's eyes closed, begin touching the extremities in a systematic manner. Do not alternate sharp and dull in a predictable pattern. Be sure to test sharp in the areas of concern to the in-

dividual patient, because this is the true indicator of function. Checking dull is simply a validation of patient reliability. When testing light touch, begin with the patient's eyes open for directions. Instruct the patient to acknowledge when a light touch is perceived. If desired, testing point localization can be incorporated into testing light touch by having the patient point to the area being touched. (Refer to Chapter 44 for a complete description of neurologic assessment.)

GERIATRIC CONSIDERATIONS

Peripheral Vascular Assessment

General Approach
Allow more time than for a younger adult

Articulate clearly; the geriatric patient may be hearing impaired

Impaired sight, comprehension, or mobility may result in less than optimum cooperation

Provide clear, concise instructions

History Collection
Be alert for answers that do not appear appropriate; the patient may not have understood the question correctly as a result of impaired hearing or impaired comprehension

Some questions may need to be repeated in a different manner

Physical Assessment
The physical examination itself is not different, but the approach needs to be altered such that the appropriate information is assessed without undue discomfort or embarrassment for the patient

Maintain an environment with minimal noise, distractions, and interruption

Arterial walls stiffen with age

DIAGNOSTIC AND LABORATORY TESTS
Noninvasive Diagnostic Studies

Ocular pneumoplethysmography

Ocular pneumoplethysmography (OPPG) is a noninvasive test that provides data about the systolic pressure in the ophthalmic artery. The systolic pressure of the ophthalmic artery is a measure of maximum blood flow to the cerebral hemispheres. This test is useful in evaluating the symptoms of transient ischemic attacks and neurologic defects and in evaluating the efficacy of a carotid endarterectomy. It may be contraindicated in patients who have had eye surgery, eye pathologic conditions, or allergies to topical anesthetics. During the procedure, suction cups are applied to the eyes after they have been anesthetized. Suction is applied to create a vacuum that obliterates the pulses in both eyes. As suction is released, the pulses return and systolic pressure in the ophthalmic artery is estimated. Three readings are taken and averaged. A difference of greater than 5 mm Hg between the right and left eyes can indicate stenosis of the carotid artery.

Patient preparation
The patient is told that drops will be placed in the eyes before the procedure and that the drops may cause temporary stinging. If the patient wears contact lenses, these are removed before the procedure. The patient is told that small cups resembling contact lenses are placed on the eyes and that a pulling sensation and transient loss of vision may be experienced as suction is applied.

Postprocedure care
The patient is instructed to avoid rubbing the eyes for at least 2 hours after the test and to blot tears. Contact lenses should not be inserted for at least 2 hours after the procedure. Bloodshot eyes are a normal response. Artificial tears will help soothe eye irritation. Since corneal abrasions can occur, the nurse monitors the patient for pain and continuing photophobia.

Carotid phonoangiography

Using **carotid phonoangiography** (CPA) helps determine the location and severity of stenosis of the carotid artery. During CPA, a special microphone is placed directly below the mandible (internal carotid artery), on the midneck (carotid bifurcation), and over the clavicle (common carotid artery). The sounds that are picked up are displayed on an oscilloscope. This test is less sensitive than ultrasound arteriography, but it is quick and relatively easy. No special patient preparation is required other than explaining that the test is painless and that it will evaluate the circulation in the neck arteries.

Ultrasound imaging

Ultrasound imaging (Doppler ultrasound; ultrasound angiography) is a noninvasive assessment of individuals with suspected or known carotid artery disease, peripheral artery or venous occlusive disease, venous thrombosis, and valvular insufficiency. It is a particularly easy and safe way of detecting deep vein thrombosis. The Doppler stethoscope directs ultrasonic waves to the artery or vein being evaluated. The waves reflect off red blood cells, producing either a waveform on a recorder or an audible signal. Normal arterial waveforms are pronounced, reflecting the peaks and valleys of systolic and diastolic pressures. A flattened waveform indicates constricted or obstructed blood flow. Venous waveforms are of continuous amplitude and in phase with respirations. No special preparation is required other than explanation of the procedure.

Impedance plethysmography

Impedance plethysmography is used to measure venous outflow in the lower legs when pneumatic cuffs wrapped around the thighs are inflated and deflated. The test is based on the assumption that blood is a good conductor of electricity and that as blood volume is altered electrical resistance is changed. By measuring and recording the resistance through attached electrodes the quality of blood flow is established. Sharp rises in venous volume indicate venous occlusion and aid in diagnosing venous thrombosis. The patient is told that the test helps to detect clots and that the sensation is similar to that of having blood pressure measured. The patient will need to be supine with the leg elevated and the knee flexed. A patient gown is required. The test takes 35 to 45 minutes to complete.

Segmental arterial pressure monitoring

Segmental arterial pressure monitoring (segmental limb systolic pressures; SLPs) measures pressure differences between upper and lower extremities and between like extremities. Conventional sphygmomanometers with appropriately sized cuffs are used. A nondirectional pocket-type Doppler is used, because it is more accurate in detecting systolic pressure. If a slight difference is detected in the upper extremities, the higher reading is recorded. Successive readings, taken with the patient at rest, in both thighs, calves, and ankles should be equal to or slightly higher than those in the upper extremities. A difference of more than 20 mm Hg is considered abnormal. Pressures are equal at similar levels in lower extremities, and pressures of the thigh, calf, and ankle in the same extremity are also equal. A drop in pressure in one calf indicates popliteal or femoral disease; a drop in one thigh indicates unilateral iliac disease. Large collateral circulation may mask pressure differences caused by occlusive disease.

Invasive Diagnostic Studies

Contrast venography

Contrast venography (venogram; plebography; venography) is a fluoroscopic examination of the deep leg veins following intravenous injection of a contrast dye into the extremity being assessed. It is the definitive test in the diagnosis of deep vein thrombosis but is uncomfortable and invasive and should be preceded by noninvasive screening procedures such as Doppler ultrasound. Venography may also be performed on upper extremities. The procedure takes approximately 30 to 60 minutes.

Radionuclide venography may be performed if the patient is allergic to contrast dye or is very ill. Radioactive agents such as technetium 99 and thallium 201 or the radiopharmaceutical I 125 fibrinogen is injected intravenously, and the patient is placed under a gamma camera that counts the radioactive particles in the affected areas. If technetium 99 or thallium 201 is used the scan takes up to 3 hours to complete. If radioactive fibrinogen scanning is used the scanning occurs over 3 days because the radioisotope becomes actively incorporated into a forming thrombus, a process that takes 6 to 72 hours. Venous thrombosis is suspected if radioactivity increases by more than 20% in an area.

Patient preparation
The nurse explains that the test assesses blood flow in the legs and that the patient will be strapped to an x-ray table that may be tilted in various positions. Dye will be injected in the dorsum of the foot, and the patient may feel a slight burning sensation or flushing as the dye is injected. The patient is instructed not to move the leg during injection of the dye or x-ray filming. The patient's history is checked for evidence of past allergic reaction to the contrast medium, and antihistamines or steroids are administered as ordered. If the patient is taking anticoagulants the nurse needs to check with the physician about temporarily discontinuing these medications. Sedatives may be ordered if the patient is extremely apprehensive or has a low pain threshold. Fasting may be required for 4 hours before the test. Baseline vital signs are taken, and the patient is encouraged to void before the test.

Postprocedure care
The nurse monitors vital signs as indicated and checks the dorsalis pedis, popliteal, and femoral pulses. The nurse assesses the patient for an allergic response to the dye (hives, laryngeal stridor, dyspnea, tachycardia [usually within 30 minutes of injection of the contrast medium]); cellulitis (swelling, redness, pain) caused by subcutaneous infiltration of the medium; and bacteremia (fever, chills, cutaneous flush).

Contrast arteriography

Contrast arteriography (contrast arteriogram) is a standard in vascular diagnostic imaging. It is the most invasive test used in evaluating peripheral vascular disease and aids in the diagnosis of arterial emboli or thrombi, arterial trauma, aneurysm, Buerger's disease, and arteriosclerotic vascular occlusive disease and aids in the reevaluation of the patency of arteries following grafting. The procedure involves inserting a radiopaque catheter into the femoral artery and injecting a contrast medium while continuous x-ray films visualize the arterial system from the abdominal aorta to the feet.

Patient preparation
The patient is informed that the test evaluates arterial blood flow in the limb to be assessed. The procedure takes approximately 1½ to 2 hours during which the patient lies flat on his or her back on the examining table. A local anesthetic will be used at the insertion site. The nurse determines if the patient has allergies to iodinated contrast media and warns that the patient may experience a sensation of pressure or burning, nausea, transient flushing, and a metallic taste as the dye is injected. The nurse assesses baseline vital signs and distal pulses (dorsalis pedis in the foot), peripheral artery status, and motor sensory function. It is helpful to place a mark over the distal pulses so that they may be easily located following the procedure. The patient is instructed to eat or drink nothing for 6 to 8 hours before the procedure unless the angiographer directs otherwise. (Some angiographers prefer that the patient maintain a clear fluid intake to prevent dehydration and a resulting hemoconcentration that can precipitate occlusion.) The nurse obtains an informed consent from the patient before administration of sedation as ordered by the physician.

Postprocedure care
The patient is usually kept on bed rest for 4 to 8 hours after the test with the leg straight, and the catheter insertion site is evaluated for hemorrhage, hematoma, and inflammation. If a pressure dressing is in place, the nurse lifts the edge of the dressing and observes the dressing over the site and the skin next to the site. Vital signs are monitored every 15 minutes for the first 2 hours or according to hospital protocol for evidence of bleeding. The involved extremity is assessed for pain, numbness, tingling,

and loss of function, and the color and temperature of the limb are compared with those of the uninvolved extremity. The nurse monitors distal pulses and capillary filling every 15 minutes for the first 2 hours. The patient is asked to describe how the limb feels and to move the toes. Coolness, numbness, tingling, pallor, diminished distal pulses, and loss of function may signal distal embolization or a thrombus and need to be evaluated carefully. The nurse encourages fluids to promote excretion of the contrast medium and to prevent renal damage secondary to the contrast medium.

Digital vascular imaging

Digital vascular imaging (DVI; digital subtraction angiography [DSI]) is a computerized fluoroscopic method that enables good quality visualization of arterial vessels and that is less expensive and quicker than catheter angiography. Contrast medium is injected through a catheter, and x-ray films are taken. An image-intensifying video system displays the vessels on a television monitor, and a computer removes or subtracts images that are not required, so that a final intense image of the desired area remains.

Patient preparation

The patient is told that the procedure enables visualization of blood flow and takes 30 to 60 minutes. The nurse explains that a local anesthetic will be injected at the insertion site and that a contrast medium will be administered. More than one injection may be required, because separate injections are required for each view of the limb. The nurse informs the patient that he or she must remain immobile as directed during the test. The patient's history is checked for evidence of allergic sensitivity to the contrast medium. The patient is instructed to fast for 2 to 6 hours before the test. An informed consent is obtained.

Postprocedure care

A pressure dressing, if applied, is maintained over the catheter insertion site. The nurse assesses the patient for dizziness, nausea, and vomiting that may occur following the procedure. The patient is encouraged to increase fluid intake over the subsequent 24 hours to facilitate excretion of the medium and is instructed in care of the wound.

CRITICAL THINKING QUESTIONS

1 Name the factors that affect peripheral resistance.
2 How does the sympathetic nervous system alter blood flow during a physiologic crisis?
3 Name the pertinent indicators in assessing circulation, motion, and sensation.
4 What manifestations distinguish arterial from venous insufficiency?
5 Formulate at least three questions to assess the psychosocial aspects of a patient's concern about vascular alterations.
6 What observations should be made of a patient following OPPG? Which observation or observations would indicate complications?
7 For what complications would a nurse observe a patient after contrast venography?

BIBLIOGRAPHY

Current

1. Bates B: *A guide to physical examination and history taking*, ed 5, Philadelphia, 1991, JB Lippincott.
2. Blank CA, Irwin JH: Assessment of peripheral vascular disorders, *Nurs Clin North Am* 25:4, 1990.
3. Bowers AC, Thompson JM: *Clinical manual of health assessment*, ed 3, St Louis, 1988, Mosby–Year Book.
4. Burrell LO: *Adult nursing in hospital and community settings*, Norwalk, Conn, 1992, Appleton & Lange.
5. Fellows E, Jocz AM: Getting the upper hand on lower extremity disease, *Nurs 91* 21:8, 1991.
6. Gordon M: *Manual of nursing diagnosis*, New York, 1987, McGraw-Hill Inc.
7. Kenny RA: *Physiology of aging: a synopsis*, St Louis, 1992, Mosby–Year Book.
8. LeFever Kee J: *Handbook of laboratory and diagnostic tests with nursing implications*, Norwalk, Conn, 1990, Appleton & Lange.
9. Malasanos L et al: *Health assessment*, ed 4, St Louis, 1990, Mosby–Year Book.
10. McDonagh A: Getting your patient ready for a nuclear medicine scan, *Nurs 92* 21:2, 1992.
11. Murray R, Zentner S: *Nursing assessment and health promotion through the life span*, Englewood Cliffs, NJ, 1989, Prentice-Hall.
12. Seidel HM et al: *Mosby's guide to physical examination*, ed 2, St Louis, 1991, Mosby–Year Book, Inc.
13. Swartz, MH: *Textbook of physical diagnosis*, Philadelphia, 1989, WB Saunders.
14. Tilkian SM, Conover MB, Tilkian AG: *Clinical implications of laboratory tests*, St Louis, 1987, Mosby–Year Book.

Classic

15. Bloch B, Hunter M: Teaching physiological assessment of black persons, *Nurse Educ* 6(1):24, 1981.
16. Block G, Nolan J: *Health assessment for professional nursing: a developmental approach*, New York, 1986, Appleton & Lange.
17. Carotenuto R, Bullock J: *Physical assessment of the gerontologic client*, Philadelphia, 1981, FA Davis Co.
18. Fields W, McGinn-Campbell K: *Introduction to health assessment*, Reston, Va, 1983, Reston Publishing Company.
19. Massey JA: Diagnostic testing for peripheral vascular disease, *Nurs Clin North Am* 21:2, 1986.
20. Price S, Wilson L: *Pathophysiology*, New York, 1986, McGraw-Hill.
21. Prior JA, Silberstein JS, Stang JM: *Physical diagnosis: the history and examination of the patient*, ed 6, St Louis, 1981, Mosby–Year Book.

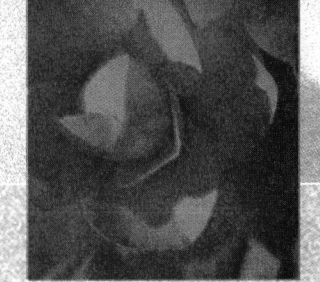

CHAPTER THIRTY

Nursing Management of Adults with Arterial Disorders

LEARNING OBJECTIVES

1 Describe the pathophysiology of arterial occlusive disease.

2 Recognize clinical manifestations of arterial occlusive disease.

3 Describe risk reduction strategies in the management of arterial occlusive disease.

4 Relate nursing management principles to the care of the patient with arterial occlusive disease.

5 Outline nursing management principles for the patient with an abdominal aneurysm.

6 Describe comprehensive nursing care for the patient undergoing arterial surgery.

7 Outline the pathophysiology of the patient with Raynaud's disease and thoracic outlet syndrome.

8 Describe the clinical manifestations of the patient with Raynaud's disease and thoracic outlet syndrome.

9 Relate nursing management principles to the care of the patient with Raynaud's disease and thoracic outlet syndrome.

KEY TERMS

ARTERIAL DISORDERS are most frequently diseases of the elderly. Lifelong habits such as tobacco use, a high-fat diet, obesity, and a sedentary lifestyle contribute to the development of the disorder. Hypertension or arterial endothelial injury may predispose some people to early development of arterial occlusive disease. The effects of arterial disease are seen in the tissues and organs supplied by the diseased arteries. Ischemia may be asymptomatic in the early stages; however, the onset of claudication, rest pain, or gangrene may persuade the patient to seek medical intervention. The severity of the symptoms depends upon the degree of disease, the location of the occlusive lesions, and the adaptive ability of the collateral circulation. Surgical intervention may be necessary to reestablish blood flow to the affected tissues. The least desirable outcome of surgical intervention is amputation. Patient education and nursing intervention in early stages of arterial disease may help to decrease the incidence of amputation.

ATHEROSCLEROSIS
Definition

Atherosclerosis is the major pathologic process by which lipid deposits occur in the intimal and subintimal layers of the artery. Calcium may precipitate out with the lipids, resulting in a calcified plaque. These changes are commonly known as "hardening of the arteries."

Etiology/Epidemiology

The effects of atherosclerosis are most often seen in persons over the age of 50. The development of atherosclerosis begins in infancy. Fatty streaks can be found in the human aorta at age 3 and are found in increasing numbers above age 18. Symptomatic lower-extremity atherosclerosis occurs in approximately 2% of the adult population of the United States with a male-to-female ratio of 2:1.

Risk factors for peripheral arterial occlusive disease may be slightly different from those for coronary artery disease (CAD) (see box above). Smoking, diabetes mellitus, hypertension, and a family history of atherosclerosis may be the primary risk factors. Other contributing factors include hyperlipidemia (especially hypertriglyceridemia), obesity, a sedentary life-style, and stress. Of these risk factors, smoking, diabetes mellitus, hypertension, obesity, exercise, and stress have some elements of patient control. Heredity, as well as age and gender, are uncontrollable elements.

Smoking is the most consistent risk factor in the literature on peripheral vascular occlusive disease. The odds of developing claudication are 15 times higher in men who smoke and seven times higher

---

RISK FACTORS FOR ATHEROSCLEROSIS

Controllable
Hypertension
Smoking
Hyperlipidemia
Stress
Exercise
Diabetes mellitus

Uncontrollable
Family history
Age
Gender

---

in women who smoke than in those who have never smoked. More than 90% of those patients requiring surgery as a result of infrainguinal or aortoiliac occlusive disease are smokers. The severity of the disease and the age of onset are related to the total number of cigarettes smoked.

The mechanisms of injury to the arteries in smoking are many. The two major atherogenic elements are nicotine and carbon monoxide. Nicotine affects the sympathetic nervous system and causes arterial constriction and increased vascular resistance. The combined result is an episode of acute hypertension compounded by an increased need for oxygen. Carbon monoxide lowers the oxygen-carrying capacity of the blood by binding with hemoglobin in place of oxygen. It is presumed that the oxygen supply to the artery itself is compromised, and this results in arterial wall damage.

Hypertensive individuals have an increased risk of developing atherosclerosis. The sustained high intraarterial pressure damages the intima of the artery (see Chapter 31).

Hyperlipidemia has been implicated in the development of arterial occlusive disease. Links between hyperlipidemia, cardiac disease, and lower-extremity occlusive disease seem to exist. Increased levels of low-density lipoproteins (LDLs) seem to increase risk of atherosclerosis, and high-density lipoproteins (HDLs) seem to have a protective function. HDLs may lower the levels of cholesterol in the bloodstream. Smoking decreases the levels of HDLs, which may account for some of the damage caused by smoking.

Pathophysiology

The development of an atherosclerotic plaque begins in infancy. The initial deposits are fatty streaks consisting of lipids, smooth-muscle cells, and lipid-containing macrophages. These lesions have been noted to appear and disappear early in life. Later changes in the intima include fibrous plaques that contain lipids, connective tissue, smooth-muscle cells, cholesterol crystals, and calcium deposits. These plaques do not disappear (though some recent data indicate that they may regress) but may remain stable or progress to an area of intramural hemorrhage and intimal calcification.

There are several theories of plaque development. One theory is that of injury and suggests that endothelial damage causes release of growth factors, platelet adherence, and smooth-muscle migration. This hypothesis implicates hyperlipidemia as a possible source of damage. A second theory of atherosclerosis is that of lipid damage to the arterial wall. This implies that the lipids infiltrate the arterial wall and stimulate smooth-muscle cell proliferation, resulting in a plaque. A final theory is that a single smooth-muscle cell is the beginning of each plaque and that this cell multiplies in tumorlike fashion.

Smoking (see box below) is implicated in the theories of atherosclerosis in many ways. The injury theory is enhanced by evidence that smoking causes vessel-wall hypoxia and injury-induced myointimal thickening. Transient hypertension, which results during smoking, accentuates the process. Hypoxia of the vessel wall increases the permeability of the wall to lipoproteins and increases the plaque deposition. Indirectly, smoking affects arterial occlusive disease by decreasing the synthesis of prostacycline, a natural inhibitor of platelet aggregation. This enhances the tendency to form clots in an already-narrowed arterial lumen.

Once the plaque has begun to form, it may extend into the media with resultant ulceration and hemorrhage. This roughened surface may lead to further deposition of platelets, causing a thrombus (Figure 30-1). In addition, the growth of the plaque creates an increasing obstruction to the flow of blood. The amount of narrowing (stenosis) that causes a decrease in flow is called a critical stenosis. The narrowed arteries are also less elastic, secondary to calcium deposition. The combination of stenosis and loss of elasticity results in the inability of the arterial system to respond to the increased demand for tissue perfusion. The end result is ischemia of the tissues supplied by the involved arteries.

Chronic arterial occlusions (those that develop over time) cause the development of collateral circulation, which is the enlargement of smaller vessels to carry the blood supply to the tissues affected by the stenosis. Collateral circulation may or may not be adequate to maintain tissue viability. In contrast, acute (or sudden) occlusion of an artery does not allow collateral circulation development, and the tissue ischemia is more pronounced and more dangerous to tissue viability.

The most common areas for developing atherosclerotic plaques are at the major arterial bifurcations. It is believed that turbulence and sheer stress at these locations may predispose a patient to this problem (see Figure 30-2 for locations). In addition to the major bifurcations, the aorta and the superficial femoral artery at Hunter's canal are frequently involved.

Clinical Manifestations

Atherosclerosis is asymptomatic until a critical stenosis occurs in an artery. The symptoms that occur at that time are results of decreased blood supply to the tissues. Pain is the most common symptom reported. Intermittent claudication is the name for the pain that develops in any muscle in the body that has inadequate blood supply and is then exercised. Claudication has three important criteria: it must occur after the patient has walked (or exercised) a predictable distance or amount, it must be relieved by rest (not change in position), and it must be replicable

EFFECTS OF SMOKING ON THE VASCULAR SYSTEM

Cardiovascular effects

Increased heart rate
Increased systolic blood pressure
Vasoconstriction
Reduced exercise tolerance
Increased left-ventricular end-diastolic pressure
Lowered threshold for fibrillation

Vessel effects

Decreased oxygenation of vessel walls
Increased permeability of endothelium
Endothelial injury
Increased myointimal proliferation
Less prostacycline production

Blood effects

Shorter platelet survival
Increased platelet stickiness
Hemoconcentration
Anemia
Increased fibrinogen levels
Increased viscosity

Lipid effects

Increased total cholesterol
Lowered HDL cholesterol
Increased permeability of vessel to lipids

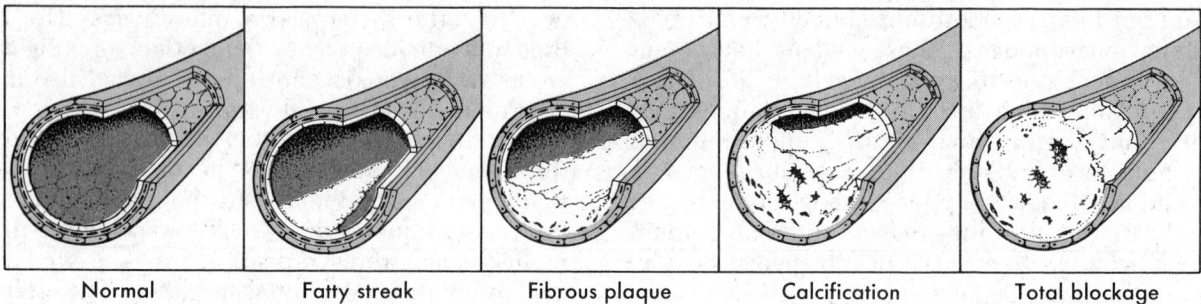

| Normal | Fatty streak | Fibrous plaque | Calcification | Total blockage |

FIGURE 30-1   Progressive development of atherosclerosis.

(occur at the same distance and speed and be relieved by the same measures). This occurs because the oxygen supply is adequate for the resting muscle but not for the exercising muscle.

A more serious manifestation of atherosclerosis is rest pain. This indicates that arterial circulation is inadequate to maintain tissue viability at rest. The pain is severe, occurs most frequently at night, and is relieved by a dependent position. The most common site for rest pain is the toes.

Besides pain and diminished pulses, the patient with atherosclerosis may also have symptoms specific to the tissues that are affected by decreased blood flow (such as abdominal pain after eating secondary to inadequate intestinal blood supply). These symptoms are a result of the dysfunction of the tissue or organ system.

Therapeutic Management

The goal of treatment of atherosclerosis is preventing progression of disease and relieving symptoms. Treatment (including surgery) does not cure the disease, and it is important that patients understand this concept. Risk reduction is another therapeutic goal. This has a secondary benefit of possibly reducing disease progression. Dietary restriction of cholesterol (see box below) and weight control are the first steps in lipid control. Drug therapy, in conjunction with diet, is instituted when diet alone is unsuccessful. Table 30-1 summarizes antihyperlipidemic medications.

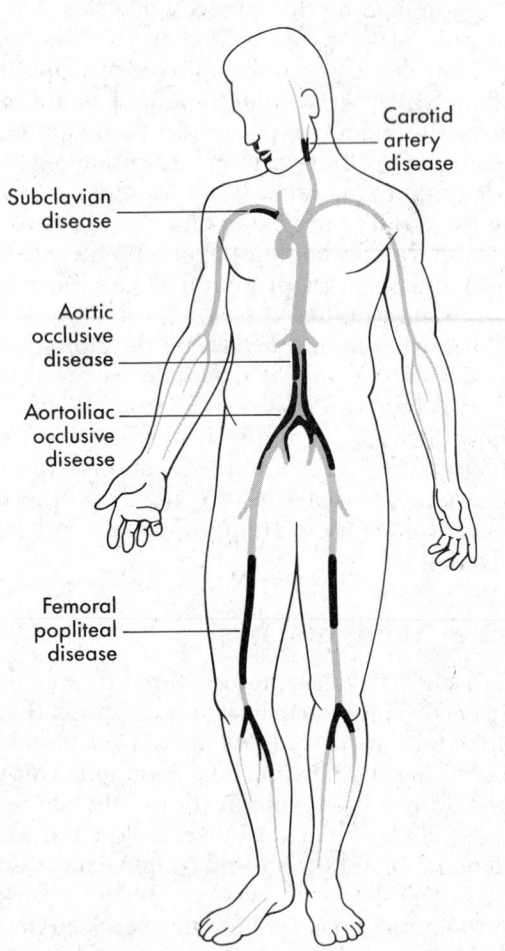

FIGURE 30-2   Common sites of atherosclerotic disease.

Carotid artery disease

Subclavian disease

Aortic occlusive disease

Aortoiliac occlusive disease

Femoral popliteal disease

RECOMMENDATIONS FOR REDUCING CHOLESTEROL

"High-risk" individuals should be treated with intensive diet restriction; drug therapy is added if dietary treatment is inadequate

"Moderate-risk" adults should be treated with intensive diet restriction

Individuals should adopt a diet that reduces dietary fat and limits daily cholesterol intake to 250 to 300 mg or less

Individuals should achieve and maintain ideal body weight

Other risk factors that may contribute to hyperlipidemia should be reduced

From The Consensus Development Panel, National Heart, Lung, and Blood Institute and the Office of Medical Applications of Research (NIH, 1987).

| TABLE 30-1   Pharmacology Summary: Antihyperlipidemic Medications |||||

| Generic/trade name | Effect against | | Precautions |
	Cholesterol	Triglycerides	
Cholestyramine (Questran)	+	+/−	May interfere with normal fat absorption
Colestipol (Colestid)	+	+/−	May increase bleeding caused by vitamin K deficiency
Clofibrate (Atromid-S)	+	+	Contraindicated in patients with liver or renal dysfunction
Probucol (Lorelco)	+	−	Not to be used in combination with other lipid-lowering drugs or in patients with cardiac problems
Dextrothyroxine (Choloxin)	+	−	Avoid in patients with cardiac and liver disease
Gemifibrozil (Lopid)	+	+	Avoid in patients with cardiac, liver, and gallbladder disease
Nicotinic acid (Nicobid)	+	+	Avoid in patients with liver dysfunction and hypotension
Lovastatin (Mevacor)	+	+	Avoid in patients with liver dysfunction

Patients with diabetes mellitus should be treated with the goal of maintaining a blood glucose level in the 120 to 160 range. Vascular disease of the lower extremities occurs in diabetic patients 20 times more often than in nondiabetics. For this reason, optimum control of blood glucose is desirable to prevent occurrence or progression of arterial disease.

Control of underlying medical problems that could contribute to a hyperlipidemic, hypertensive, hyperglycemic, or hypercoagulable state is undertaken. Laboratory studies to monitor these problems include (but are not limited to) serum lipids, fasting blood glucose, hemoglobin, hematocrit, coagulation studies, WBC, SGOT, SGPT, LDH, alkaline phosphatase, BUN, and creatinine. Changes that indicate exacerbation of primary disease processes or medication side effects are reported immediately.

Dietary restriction for weight control can be combined with an exercise program of walking. This has a threefold benefit of burning more calories, increasing cardiac and general conditioning, and developing collateral circulation.

NURSING MANAGEMENT OF THE PATIENT WITH ATHEROSCLEROSIS
Assessment

Assessment of the patient who has atherosclerosis begins with a thorough health history. The association of diseases such as diabetes mellitus, coronary artery disease, hypertension, stroke, and renal insufficiency with atherosclerosis in other sites makes it imperative to obtain a personal and family history of these disorders. A focused interview begins with gathering information on the patient's chief complaint, related symptoms, and how the symptoms cause alterations in daily function. When discussing pain such as claudication, the nurse records the three major criteria related to claudication. In addition, the nurse questions the patient about the effect the problem has upon his or her desired activity level. For example, walking three blocks briskly may not be critical to an 80-year-old retired patient, but it may be essential to the 50-year-old patient who must work an assembly line as a supervisor. Document whether the patient smokes, the number of cigarettes smoked, and for how long the patient has smoked. Record eating habits and alcohol intake as well as the patient's occupation. Family relationships and the patient's support system are important to note and incorporate into interventions.

Specific questions related to arterial disease are critical. Cardiac assessment is covered in Chapter 33. Sexual function in the male patient is important to note and not always a comfortable topic for the patient or the nurse. Sometimes the statement "Hardening of the arteries affects the penis' blood supply which is necessary for sexual functioning" may be a comfortable way to begin questioning. The patient may not be aware that the same disease that makes it difficult to walk any distance also affects sexual performance.

Nursing Diagnosis

Nursing diagnoses for the patient with atherosclerosis include:

Alteration in tissue perfusion related to decreased arterial blood flow

Acute and chronic pain related to decreased tissue perfusion

Impaired health maintenance related to poor risk factor management

Knowledge deficit related to risk factors of atherosclerosis

Alteration in life-style and sexual function

Planning

The nursing management for the patient is planned to achieve the following outcomes:

Patient will adopt protective measures against injury of impaired tissue

Patient will complete desired activities without experiencing pain

Patient will practice behavior to increase collateral circulation

Patient will state the relationship between atherosclerosis and risk factors

Patient will state the relationship between atherosclerosis and decrease in sexual function

Implementation

Nursing interventions for patients with atherosclerosis are primarily for secondary and tertiary prevention. Education is the easiest method for implementing this prevention. However, the patient may be aware of the need for change and choose to do nothing. Behavior modification is more difficult. Risk factor management is the major therapeutic intervention. Determining the patient's understanding of the disease and its effects on people in general and the patient in particular is necessary. Modification of risk factors is difficult because of lifetime habits and cultural definitions of behavior. Multiple behavior changes are also unmanageable. A plan to eliminate one factor at a time may prove more successful. Patient involvement in planning risk-factor reduction is essential, because participation and stratification of factors by the patient may improve cooperation. In addition, the patient's family or support system must be included to ensure long-term assistance with the plan.

The patient should understand that life-style changes are difficult, even with commitment. Smoking cessation is one of the most difficult changes. The patient should know that smoking or use of any tobacco product is harmful and that diet modification is essential for patients with hyperlipidemia. Community support group information and written material is reviewed with the patient at regular intervals. Discharge teaching and risk factor modification are addressed briefly in the initial interview. These are reviewed by all nurses caring for the patient in the hospital, in home health care, and in the outpatient setting.

Evaluation

The plan of treatment and its implementation include a method of evaluation. The patient should be aware of this evaluation tool. Discouragement over the difficulties in treatment should be expected, but positive feedback is essential. Emphasis on minor triumphs, small improvements in health status, and decreased pain will help the patient focus on advancing toward the long-term goal. The patient must also have short-term objectives and goals. Short-term goals are easier to reach and may help achieve long-term goals.

CHRONIC INFRARENAL AND ARTERIAL DISEASE
Definition

Atherosclerosis of the aorta and iliac arteries is one of the most common causes of ischemic symptoms in the lower limbs of elderly Western patients. Atherosclerosis of the extremities (primarily the legs) is responsible for the morbidity most frequently associated with the disease, with the exception of stroke

---

PATIENT EDUCATION GUIDE   *Antihyperlipidemic Agents*

Mix the medication with water or juice; do not take it dry

Take the medication 1 hour before or 6 hours after other medications to avoid interference with absorption of other drugs

Take with meals

Report gastrointestinal symptoms such as nausea and vomiting, abdominal pain, or diarrhea and other symptoms such as dizziness, heart palpitations, sweating, headache, or skin rash to the attending physician (The nurse should be aware that patients taking clofibrate have an increased risk of developing cholelithiasis) (see Chapter 47 for cerebrovascular disease). Loss of limb function, pain, and disability, in addition to amputation, are the complications most often found in arterial occlusive disease of the extremities. These complications occur when the stenosis in an artery supplying an area below the renal arteries is severe enough to limit blood supply to that area. The results are tissue damage and decreased healing.

Etiology/Epidemiology

Atherosclerosis obliterans is the most common arterial disease. At least 95% of arterial occlusive disease is atherosclerotic in origin. It is the leading cause of lower-extremity occlusive disease after age 30. Patients with symptomatic lower-extremity disease have been reported to have a life expectancy of 10 years less than the general population. Several long-term studies have observed patients with arterial-occlusive disease. Notably, the Framingham study documents an increase of symptomatic lower-extremity disease (claudication) with age. It found men to be more symptomatic than were women. Other studies have reinforced this finding. The co-morbidities of diabetes mellitus and heavy cigarette smoking are linked with the highest increase in intermittent claudication. Smoking triples the risk of development of claudication, and hypertension doubles the risk. In addition, smoking increases the potential need for amputation.

Pathophysiology

The pathophysiology of infrarenal and lower-extremity arterial occlusive disease is the same as that discussed earlier. Atherosclerotic lesions generally begin in the aorta and, if unchecked, progress to disease in the distal arteries. In patients with diabetes, the distribution is reversed. Initial occlusions occur distally in the smaller vessels, such as those in the tibial-peroneal region, and only later do lesions occur in the aorta.

Clinical Manifestations

Severity of lower-extremity symptoms are related to the length of time over which an artery is occluded, the level at which the artery is occluded, the presence of more than one stenosis, the degree of stenosis, and the presence of collateral vessels. Pulses may or may not be absent or decreased distal to the stenosis or occlusion, depending upon the degree of collateral circulation. Collateral vessels appear to develop over a period of 6 to 24 months, or faster with appropriate vascular rehabilitation. Some researchers believe that the decrease of symptoms is secondary to metabolic adaptation of the muscle rather than actual increased blood flow.

The reason most patients seek medical attention for arterial disease of a lower extremity is pain. Intermittent claudication is the symptom most frequently reported first. Relatively few of these patients with claudication progress to rest pain, gangrene, or limb loss. Claudication is usually described as a cramping, aching pain that develops in the calf or thigh in a patient with lower-extremity disease. If the lesion is higher than the groin, the patient may report buttock claudication.

If the patient has developed collateral circulation, the body compensates somewhat for the decreased blood supply. However, if the collateral circulation is inadequate, the patient may develop rest pain. This implies that the oxygen supply to the tissues is insufficient even at rest, a sign of serious impairment. Patients with rest pain from lower-extremity arterial disease relate that they have little pain in the daytime but develop severe pain upon going to bed at night. Patients may try to relieve this pain by hanging their feet over the side of the bed or by wal___ pain___ is a ___ of th___

P___ dise___ or i___ skin___ abra___

P___ tual___ pati___ The___ foot___ The___ leg___ over___ tien___ com___ the weight of co___

Pallor is a second manifestation of arterial insufficiency of the lower extremities. With elevation, the veins empty and do not refill, and the limb becomes pale. When the foot is placed in a dependent position the skin becomes red. This is known as dependent rubor. Rubor is a result of dilation of the arterioles, and in chronic disease a permanent reddish-blue discoloration may be present. In addition, hair loss (usually in a sock distribution) occurs, and nails may become deformed or brittle (Figure 30-3). As the tissues become more cadaveric as a result of chronic insufficiency, the color may change from pale or ruddy to a dark blue or purple. The color may change in patchy areas or in one toe and progress to the entire foot or limb.

Coolness of a limb indicates reduced arterial flow. Bilateral assessment of temperature is essential.

TABLE 30-2   Comparison of Symptoms of Claudication and Rest Pain

	Claudication	Rest pain
Location	Distal to stenosis, in muscle	Distal to stenosis, usually in foot (especially toes)
Quality	Crampy, achy	Burning/throbbing
Quantity	Mild to severe	Severe, intolerable
Chronology	Increases/decreases with life-style changes	Increases over time
Aggravating factors	Muscle use	Lying down, elevating feet; pressure; any movement
Alleviating factors	Cessation of activity	Lowering foot, moving about, narcotics later
Setting	Ambulating	Resting, often waking from sleep
Associated activity	Increases with excess body weight or weight carrying; ambulating on an upward incline, walking faster	Any irritation may be constant

FIGURE 30-3   Thick toenails and callus formation on an ischemic foot. Also note toe deformities. A health care professional, not the patient, should perform foot care.

Sometimes a line of temperature differential correlates with the area of arterial occlusion. This temperature differential is more dramatic in acute occlusive disease.

In advanced atherosclerosis, ischemia may lead to necrosis, ulceration, and gangrene (Figure 30-4). Gangrene is a sign of tissue death secondary to inadequate blood supply. Gangrene itself is painless because the nerves are also dead. It is generally an indication for medical or surgical intervention as soon as possible, providing the patient is in a condition to withstand surgery.

Therapeutic Management

Medical management

The primary goal of treatment for arterial occlusive disease is to reduce the imbalance between tissue demands and the present vascular supply. The plan is to increase blood supply and to achieve a balance between rest to reduce oxygen need and activity to promote collateral circulation.

Drug therapy

Pentoxifylline (Trental) is a medication frequently used in lower-extremity arterial occlusive disease. It reduces blood viscosity by altering the membrane flexibility of the red blood cell. This action allows the red blood cells to reshape to fit into smaller vessels. The drug is indicated in patients who experience claudication only or in whom the risks of surgery are extremely high and a conservative method of treatment is desired. The drug requires 4 months to become effective because it affects the red blood cells during their development. This information on time delay in relief of symptoms is essential to relate to patients or they may discontinue the drug, thinking it does not work. Recent studies show that patients with symptoms of claudication for less than 1 year or with an ankle/brachial index of 0.8 (normal is >1.0) or greater seem to have the greatest benefit from the drug. Patients with gangrene or very advanced occlusive disease may receive no benefit from this medication. Various antiplatelet drugs are being studied for use in claudication. Several are under clinical trials at present.

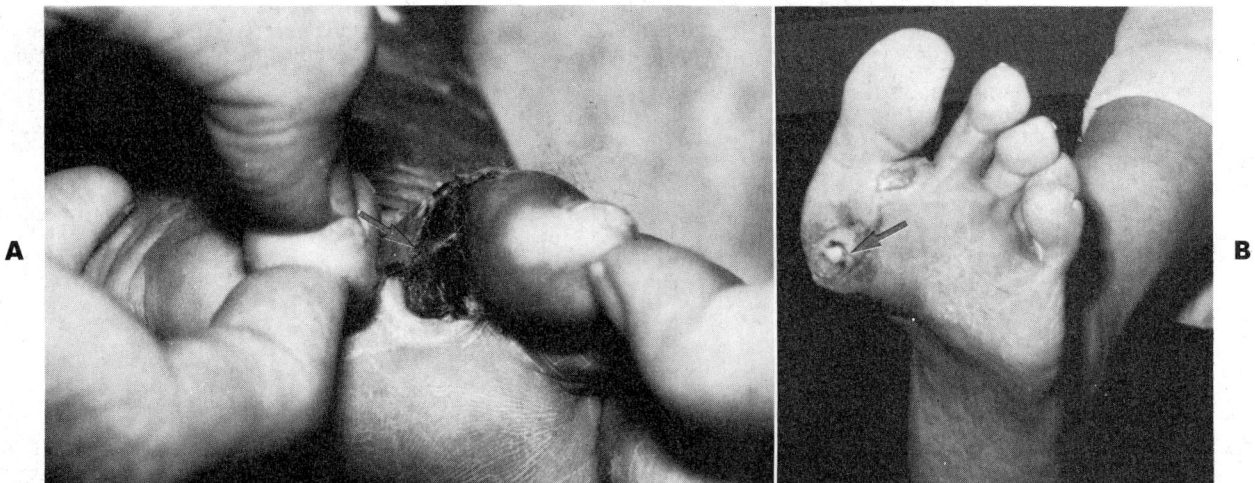

FIGURE 30-4   **A,** Gangrenous ulcer between the fourth and fifth toe of a diabetic patient. The patient had severe neuropathy and did not examine his feet. A common femoral-to-dorsalis pedis bypass was necessary to save the foot. **B,** Malperforans ulcer in a diabetic with insufficient blood supply.

One method of decreasing claudication that has proven temporarily effective is hemodilution with medications such as dextran. Once hemodilution is stopped, the same level of exercise intolerance returns.

Percutaneous transluminal angioplasty
Percutaneous transluminal angioplasty (PTA) is an effective method of treating carefully selected arterial stenoses or very short occlusions. It is most effective in the larger arteries of the lower extremities (iliac and femoral arteries) as well as the renal arteries and the coronary arteries (see Chapter 35 for PTCA for coronary arteries). The goal of the angioplasty is to crush the plaque (shatter it), and then the vessel is dilated. PTA is not always successful, but it may be repeated should the stenosis recur. It is performed in the radiology department under angiographic guidance.

Atherectomy
Atherectomy is a recent method of opening severely stenotic or occluded vessels. It is most often performed in conjunction with an operative procedure but may be the only therapy used and then is performed percutaneously. Ideal sites for atherectomy are isolated lesions in the femoral and tibial vessels and lesions that are difficult to treat with other methods. Atherectomy is done under angiographic and/or angioscopic guidance. During an atherectomy, a high-speed, rotating cutting device is used to cut through the plaque. Some devices have a method of trapping the debris, and others suction debris out of the vessel.

Laser angioplasty
Laser, using light energy, has had some popularity in treatment of vascular lesions. It is frequently used with PTA, and the technique is similar. It is performed percutaneously, under angiographic guidance. A guidewire is threaded to the site of the occlusion and the fiber-optic catheter is inserted. Laser energy is applied to the plaque, which vaporizes it. Long-term results are not as encouraging as early reports, with occlusions occurring frequently at 3-month intervals.

Surgical management

In order to have successful revascularization below the inguinal ligament, there must be adequate blood flow into those vessels. Adequate inflow may negate the necessity to do further surgery. If conservative measures have failed to relieve symptoms and if the patient is committed to life-style changes even after surgery, then workup of the general medical condition of the patient begins. After evaluation and clearance for surgery there are several options available to the vascular surgeon in aortoiliac occlusive disease. The primary choices are aortoiliac endarterectomy, aortoiliac or aortofemoral bypass, and extraanatomic bypass. Choice of the surgical procedure depends on operative indications, the general condition of the patient, and surgeon preference for one procedure over another.

Surgical procedures
An **endarterectomy** is the removal of the atherosclerotic plaque without removing, bypassing, or replac-

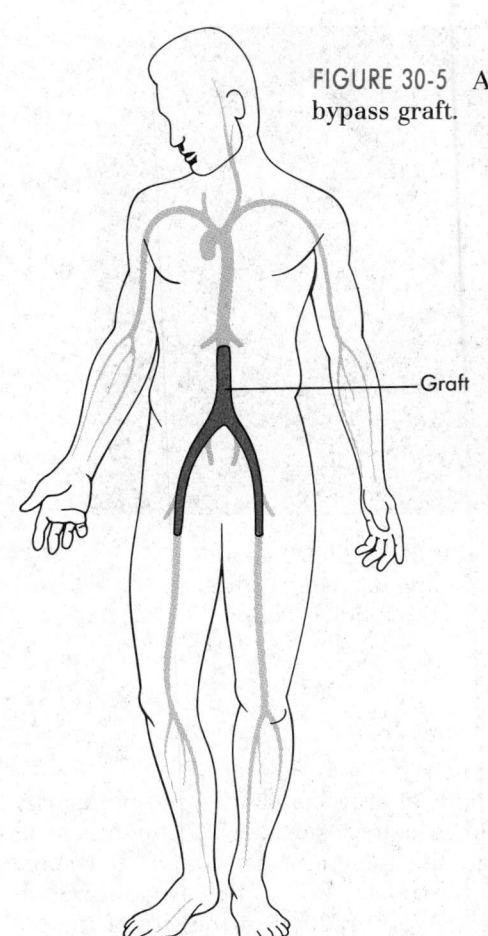

FIGURE 30-5   Aortobifemoral bypass graft.

HIGH-RISK PATIENTS WHO MAY BENEFIT FROM EXTRAANATOMIC BYPASS

- Those with intraabdominal infection or infected graft
- Severe CAD—ejection fraction less than 30%
- Goldman criteria greater than 5
- Life expectancy less than 2 years
- Morbid obesity
- Age over 70 years
- Presence of aortoenteric fistula

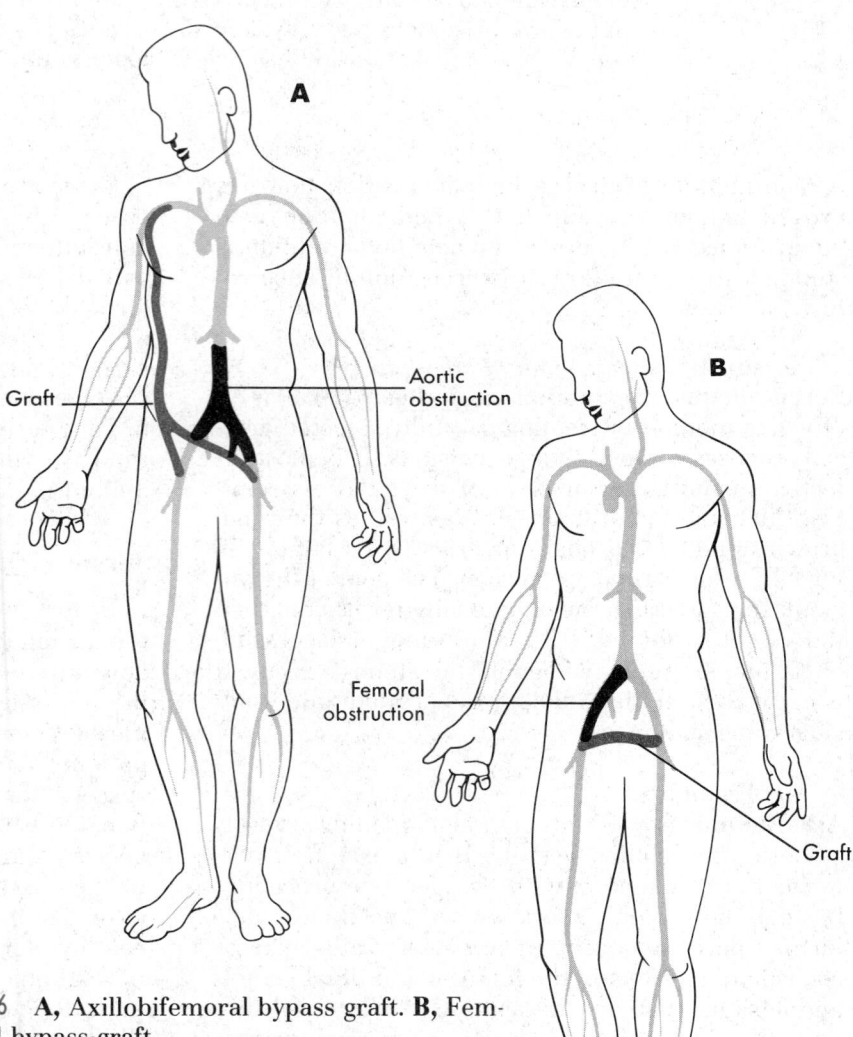

FIGURE 30-6   **A,** Axillobifemoral bypass graft. **B,** Femorofemoral bypass graft.

ing the affected artery. The diseased intima and media are removed, leaving a smooth adventia. Operative mortality is low, and long-term results are favorable. One advantage of the surgery is that there is no prosthetic material introduced into the patient. This reduces the risk of infection, which is minimal even with a bypass graft. This procedure is not performed as commonly as in the past.

The most common operation for aortoiliac disease is the **aortofemoral bypass** graft. This is a prosthetic graft that extends from just below the renal arteries to the femoral arteries in the groin (Figure 30-5).

An **extraanatomic bypass** is a graft in the subcutaneous tissue instead of the abdominal cavity. This procedure is an alternative way to bypass occluded vessels without the risks of an intraabdominal operation. The box on p. 702 lists the indications for extraanatomic bypass. Common types of extraanatomic bypass are the axillobifemoral and the femorofemoral bypass (Figure 30-6).

The most common bypass below the inguinal ligament is the **in situ vein bypass.** This procedure is performed for limb salvage or to treat disabling claudication. More severe indications for surgery generally require a more distal bypass. In the in situ bypass, the venous valve cusps are rendered incompetent (cut), which allows the blood to flow distally through the vein. In contrast, the vein is sometimes removed from the body and reversed top-to-bottom so that the blood can flow through the vein as a conduit. Leaving the vein in situ allows it to keep its own blood supply and permits bypass to smaller-caliber vessels. The in situ bypass seems to have a better rate of patency than does a reversed vein or synthetic bypass for these reasons.

Preoperative preparation for the patient scheduled for an in situ bypass may include duplex ultrasound imaging to map the course of the vein and assess its diameter. The vein is generally marked so that the surgeon can identify it readily during surgery. Postoperatively, the patient will note that the bypass can sometimes be palpated as a result of its superficial course, so the patient may be taught to check the pulse daily.

In situ bypasses may go to any of the infrapopliteal vessels: the popliteal, the anterior or posterior tibial, the dorsalis pedis, and in some cases the plantar (Figure 30-7). Sometimes a surgeon may elect to use prosthetic material to the popliteal vessels or vessels just below the knee. However, the vein offers the only long-term patency for distal vessels in the ankle and foot (see box on p. 704).

Amputation

Amputation is the treatment of last resort for an ischemic limb. Conservative therapy or arterial bypass techniques make amputation in ambulatory pa-

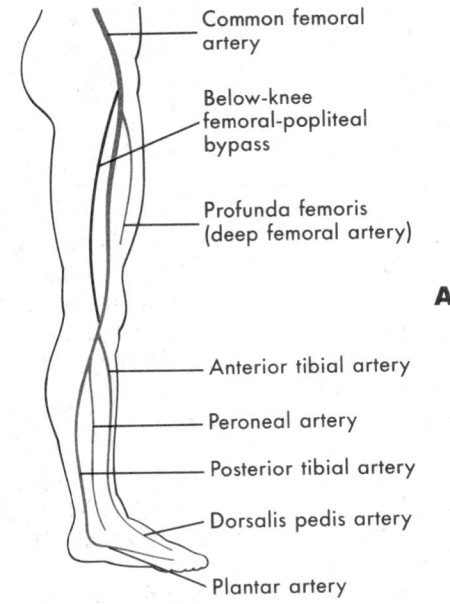

A

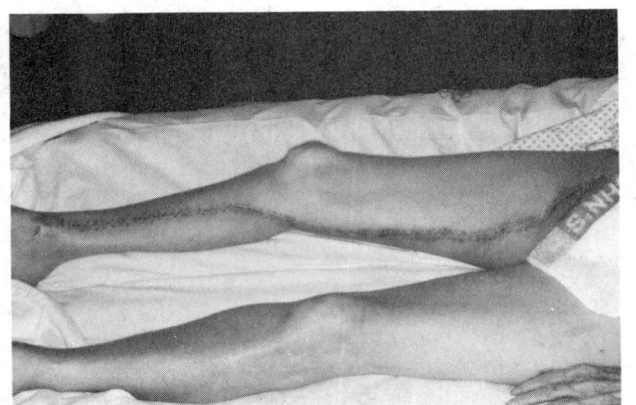

B

FIGURE 30-7   **A,** In situ vein bypass. **B,** Incision for a femoral-to-peroneal artery in situ bypass graft. **C,** Gangrenous toes and subsequent dorsalis pedis bypass graft incision.

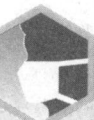

PREOPERATIVE AND POSTOPERATIVE NURSING INTERVENTIONS

THE PATIENT WITH A FEMORAL TO POPLITEAL OR FEMORAL TO DISTAL TIBIAL BYPASS GRAFT

Nursing Intervention	Rationale
Preoperative	
Auscultation and palpation	Establishes patient baseline and basis for postoperative evaluation
Doppler exam of patient	
Record capillary refill time	
Establish walking distance tolerated and compounding factors (e.g., incline, speed)	Establishes preoperative baseline and basis for postoperative or rehabilitation goals
Protect feet with sheepskin or lamb's wool between *all* toes. Use bed cradle	Ischemic skin damages easily, even with weight of bed covers
Elevate head of bed on blocks if ordered	Gravity assists blood flow in the extremities
Maintain adequate fluid intake	Adequate blood pressure, fluid volume, and decreased blood viscosity help prevent occlusion in a stenotic area of the artery
Instruct patient not to smoke	Smoking increases pulmonary risks, causes vasospasm, and increases hypercoagulability
Teach patient activity restrictions or exercises permitted in the postoperative period	May assist with patient compliance
Scrub extremity with bacteriostatic soap if ordered	May decrease skin flora and decrease infections
Postoperative	
Auscultate and palpate or take Doppler pulse in the graft, dorsalis pedis, posterior tibial, and peroneal arteries	Identifies patent graft and outflow vessels
Assess wound for bleeding or swelling from hematoma formation	Patients may experience bleeding from graft anastomoses, venous tributaries of an in situ graft, or oozing from intraoperative anticoagulation
Avoid compression or circumferential dressings	May cause occlusion of graft or decrease blood flow in other areas
Observe suture or staple line for redness, warmth, or infection drainage	May be indicative of incisional or graft infection
Do not allow patient to put powder, lotion, or other material in the groin. Keep groin dry	Groin incisions are warm, moist environments conducive to infection
Do not flex the groin or knees more than 45 degrees for extended periods	May slow wound healing and increase possibility of lymphocele formation
Protect feet with sheepskin or lamb's wool between *all*	Ischemic skin damages easily, even with weight of bed covers
	Long-term protection of feet is essential because, although the symptoms are treated, the disease is not cured

in these patients, neuropathy may prevent perception of a severe infection, which renders the foot unsalvageable. In some cases, a bypass may provide an adequate blood supply for the foot to heal a local amputation such as a toe or transmetatarsal amputation.

NURSING MANAGEMENT OF THE PATIENT WITH CHRONIC ARTERIAL OCCLUSIVE DISEASE OF THE EXTREMITIES

Assessment

Baseline pulses are palpated in all four extremities, even if only one is affected. Pulses of the upper extremity include brachial, radial, and ulnar. Complete vascular assessment includes taking carotid, axillary, and superficial temporal artery pulses bilaterally. Lower-extremity pulses include femoral, popliteal, dorsalis pedis, and posterior tibial pulses. Presence or absence of pulse during palpation and/or Doppler should be recorded. Approximately 5% of the population has a congenitally absent dorsalis pedis pulse, and this alone is not a sign of ischemia. Pulses should be taken with a light pressure of the fingers so that the patient's pulse is not occluded and also so that the nurse's pulse is not mistaken for the patient's.

Color of the extremities should be noted and capillary refill tested. Capillary refill is determined by compressing the tissue between the fingers until the blood is forced out of the tissue being held. The time it takes to cease blanching and to return to normal color should be less than 3 seconds.

A history of exercise tolerance in the affected limb is obtained. The nurse determines how far the patient can walk (measured in blocks or hundreds of feet). It is important to determine the current limits, because patients frequently refer to how far they used to walk. The exact site of discomfort and the relief measures practiced are recorded. In those patients with rest pain, the frequency, precipitating factors, and relief measures are noted. Any recent or sudden change of exercise tolerance or occurrence of pain may indicate an acute event such as a recent arterial occlusion. Treatment may differ for the recent occlusion.

Knowledge assessment is essential to identify risk factors, disease processes, and symptoms. Refer to risk factors and clinical manifestations for question ideas. The support network of the patient is assessed to begin planning for discharge care.

Nursing Diagnosis

Examples of nursing diagnoses common to patients who have peripheral arterial disease caused by atherosclerosis are:

Altered tissue perfusion of the extremity related to decreased arterial flow

Activity intolerance related to imbalance between tissue demand and blood supply

Sleep pattern disturbance related to rest pain

Impaired tissue integrity related to decrease in blood supply

High risk for infection related to decreased tissue oxygenation

Pain related to ischemia

Fear related to possible limb loss

High risk for body image disturbance related to potential loss of body part

Lack of knowledge of self-care activities to reduce risk factors

Planning

The goals will be determined by the nurse and the patient. The order of priority is usually determined by the degree of distress perceived by the patient. The following are examples of goals:

Patient will have maximum tissue perfusion

Patient will manage activity within own limits

Patient will express concerns to significant others

Patient will obtain adequate rest

Patient will have decreased pain

Patient will practice self-care to avoid tissue damage

Implementation

Risk factor management

Risk factor management includes dietary control of lipids, maintaining optimum body weight, weight loss if indicated, and smoking cessation. Dietary consultation and referral to a smoking cessation group may help the patient change habits. Risk factor management is the same for any type of arterial occlusive disease and is discussed in the general overview.

Pain management

The pain associated with arterial insufficiency caused by atherosclerosis ranges from discomfort with claudication to severe rest pain. The nursing care required for this pain is varied. The patient may already be placing the limb in a dependent position. If the patient is not knowlegeable about why this helps, it should be explained. At home, the use of 6- or 8-inch blocks under the head of the bed may help, and in the hospital, the bed may be positioned or placed upon blocks. A bed cradle or bed board may keep covers off of the toes and decrease pain. First the nurse determines if the pain is the cause of sleeplessness. If it is not, the cause is determined and addressed.

In the presence of a severe stenosis, it is essential to maintain an adequate blood pressure and fluid volume to prevent occlusion. The patient should be instructed to maintain this volume by increasing fluid intake unless other medical conditions contraindicate this plan (such as congestive heart failure). This is critical in patients who are not surgical candidates because of poor general health, but who may have an extremely tight stenosis.

For the patient experiencing intermittent claudication, there are several interventions. Encourage the patient to keep a log of exercise tolerance with specific measurements of distance walked. It is important that the patient understand that the pain of claudication does not harm the limb and that exercise is helpful. If there is no use of the limb to induce claudication, no collateral circulation will develop. Once an exercise program is cleared by the medical staff, a consistent walking program is begun. If a vascular rehabilitation program is available, a referral is appropriate.

NURSING CARE PLAN *Patient with Arterial Insufficiency*

Nursing Diagnosis/Expected Outcome	Interventions	Rationale

Altered peripheral tissue perfusion, arterial, related to progressive atherosclerosis
 	
• *Maximum perfusion will be maintained*
	Position affected extremity in a dependent position
	Maintain oral intake to avoid thirst and dehydration
	
	Check color, temperature, sensation, and quality of peripheral pulses initially and at designated intervals; report changes immediately
	Assess causative and contributing factors to arterial insufficiency
	  Activities that cause symptoms
	  Distance individual is able to ambulate before pain occurs
		Gravity enhances arterial flow
		Intravascular fluid volume must be maintained to avoid drop in blood pressure that may occlude an atherosclerotic artery
		Changes in color, temperature, sensation, and quality of peripheral pulses may indicate decrease in arterial flow
		Modification of contributing factors may reduce symptoms

High risk for impaired tissue integrity related to decreased arterial circulation • *Patient will state the activities that promote tissue integrity*	Promote factors that protect the extremity Keep extremity warm (wear warm clothing) Reduce risk for trauma Change positions frequently Avoid crossing legs Avoid circular bands, garters Protect feet	Injury to the extremity will require more blood to heal than to keep the tissue intact; an extremity with compromised circulation may not be able to provide the extra blood that is required Constricting clothing, such as garters and tight elastic bands on stockings, and leg crossing compress the vessels in the legs

Activity intolerance, claudication related to peripheral arterial diseases
 	
• *Patient will increase activity without added discomfort*
• *Patient will be able to manage activity within the limitations of the claudication*
	Assess claudication
	  Monitor distance of claudication
	  Monitor time for claudication to cease
	  Initiate ambulation program
	  Increase ambulation distance over time	

	Reduce or eliminate contributing factors: promote health behavior Increase activity Eliminate smoking Control obesity	Collateral blood flow will improve with increased demand It is not harmful to walk into the pain of claudication; the oxygen requirement of the muscles stimulates the collateral arteries to increase in size Nicotinic receptors on the arterial wall cause arterial constriction when stimulated by nicotine Oxygen requirement increases as weight load is increased

NURSING CARE PLAN   *Patient with Arterial Insufficiency—cont'd*

Nursing Diagnosis/Expected Outcome	Interventions	Rationale

Knowledge deficit of risk factors for arterial insufficiency
 	
•*Patient will describe the relationship of risk factors to arterial insufficiency*
	Teach patient about risk factors
	  Cease smoking (refer to smoking cessation program)
	  Provide warmth
	  Avoid stress
	  Exercise moderately
	  Avoid infection/skin breakdown
	  Modify diet
	  Control blood pressure and blood glucose
		Risk factor modification may reduce the symptoms and prevent the need for an operation

Acute pain related to ischemia
 	
•*Patient will be free of pain or have pain reduced*
	Patient will state the pain is less as a result of:
	  Arterial positioning
	  Decreased oxygen demands
	  Analgesics
	Avoidance of vasoconstriction
	Lamb's wool between all toes
		Arterial blood supply to an extremity can be increased by placing the extremity below the heart
		Analgesic medication may reduce the pain so that the patient is able to tolerate daily activities
		Decreases the skin pressure in the ischemic area and allows more blood flow between the bony prominences

Grieving related to anticipated loss of limb because of arterial insufficiency
 	
•*Patient will express concerns*
	Assess concerns about potential loss
	
	Assess responses of individual
	  Encourage patient to share feelings
	  Support patient's strengths
	Support patient's grief reaction
	If amputation is inevitable:
	  Accept patient's reaction
	  Discuss with patient/family:
	    Surgical procedure
	    Rehabilitation program
	    Postoperative expectations
	    Exercises
	    Phantom sensations
	Provide health teaching and referrals as needed
	  Discuss possible outcomes
	  Discuss coping strategies
	Identify support groups
		Individuals with arterial insufficiency are at risk of loss of limb with or without medical or surgical intervention
		
		Responses to grief are individual
		
		Rehearsal of anticipated events helps promote positive coping strategies
		
		Identification with others who have been in similar situations is supportive

Tissue integrity

Protecting the limb from decreases in blood flow is essential. No constricting garments, such as garters, should be worn. Protection of skin integrity may mean the difference between limb salvage and amputation. Skin and foot care is critical. The family is included in foot care plans. Many times the blood supply may be adequate to maintain intact skin but not to heal a wound. In the hospital and at home, protect the foot with sheepskin at the foot of the bed, lamb's wool between all toes, and a warm sock if necessary. Lamb's wool is woven in and out between the toes. If small pieces are placed between toes, the pieces will fall out. There are also many commercial devices available for foot protection and include the Rooke Boot and the Bunny Boot, among others.

Emotional support

Individuals with arterial insufficiency are told that there is a possibility that amputation may be the final outcome of the disease. This outcome may occur secondary to pain, an unsalvageable foot, or the unavailability of a suitable vessel for bypass. Patients are allowed to express their feelings about any anticipated loss. Even a digit loss is an extreme trauma to some patients. The nurse assesses the concerns and encourages the individual to share feelings. The nurse then supports the strengths of the patient and provides help in the grief reaction. Support group referral is helpful, as is alerting the family and staff to potential feelings (see Nursing Care Plan box on pp. 706 and 707).

Surgical management

Aortic and aortoiliac operations

Preoperative preparation for these types of surgery include all of the standard nursing preparations for abdominal surgery. In addition, preoperative assessment and recording of lower-extremity pulses, BUN, and creatinine are essential. Pulses document the preoperative baseline by which to judge surgical success.

The patient receives standard preoperative teaching about incisional pain, wound splinting, and available pain-control measures. Epidural analgesia may be an option and assists in mobility and pulmonary toilet. Deep breathing exercises should be practiced. The patient is made aware of leg exercises to perform after surgery and the potential for the presence of intermittent compression devices to prevent deep vein thrombosis.

Inform the patient and family that the first few days will be spent in the intensive care unit. The patient will return from surgery with some or all of the following: a nasogastric tube, a urinary catheter, intravenous and intraarterial lines, a pulmonary artery catheter, intermittent compression device on the legs, and an endotracheal tube. Pulses will be taken at regular intervals and loss of pulses reported immediately. If no pulse is expected in one area the surgeon should alert the nursing staff and this should be recorded.

Constantly be alert for complications. These include graft thrombosis, atheromatous emboli, lymphoceles, graft infections, aortoenteric fistulas, and false aneurysms. Atheromatous emboli occur during surgery when debris from the plaque breaks loose and lodges distally. If this occurs in a small-digit artery, the patient may have "blue-toe syndrome" and digit pain. If a larger vessel occludes, the patient may require removal of the embolus in the operating room. This is called an **embolectomy.**

Early graft failure may be caused by graft thrombosis or thrombosis of the vessels past the graft (outflow thrombosis). A graft thrombectomy may be performed and the patient started on anticoagulants.

It is important to distinguish between thrombotic and embolic events. Treatment decisions depend upon an accurate diagnosis. A thrombus occurs at the site of the problem, but an embolus originates from another source. If the source of an embolus is not treated, then other embolic events may occur. Early detection and reporting of changes in circulatory status may save the patient's extremity.

Gastrointestinal complications that may occur after abdominal aortic operations include colon ischemia. This is most often seen after repair of an aortic aneurysm. Symptoms of this ischemia are diarrhea occurring before expected bowel function, white blood cell count greater than 30,000, abdominal distention, abdominal pain (especially left lower quadrant), fever, and acidosis. In the presence of these symptoms, the patient will need to undergo an endoscopic evaluation. When the blood supply to the bowel is blocked, there is mucosal destruction within 30 minutes and gangrene within hours. If ischemia is present to any degree by endoscopy, then immediate surgical intervention is necessary. Minimal areas of ischemia may require no treatment beyond bowel rest.

Lower-extremity bypass
Preoperative preparation

The patient who is undergoing a lower-extremity bypass has an extensive surgery to face and many fears to address. Lower-extremity bypass is performed for severe disability or limb salvage. For these reasons the patient may experience more anxiety than with abdominal bypasses. The patient will be aware that if the bypass is unsuccessful, the most frequent outcome is amputation. However, the nurse should emphasize that, in the hands of a competent vascular surgeon, the results are generally favorable, even long term. It is important to give the patient hope while outlining realistic expectations.

Preoperative pain may cause concerns related to postoperative discomfort. This concern is especially prevalent if the incision will extend from groin to foot. The patient must be assured that medications will be available to alleviate the pain and be instructed to request them for relief.

Cleanliness is essential in the areas of groin incisions. This must be stressed in the preoperative teaching so that the patient will not use powder or other products on the groin wound. Rationale for the teaching is that the primary site of postoperative infection is the groin, more so in the obese patient.

If possible, the surgeon supplies the patient with a drawing of the surgical procedure and anastomotic sites. The nurse reviews this with the patient if he or she has any questions. Activity restrictions or extension exercises (if permitted by the surgeon) are taught preoperatively. A return demonstration of skills by the patient is important. Patients seem to perform these better if they are taught before surgery.

Postoperative management

After surgery the patient may or may not go to a monitored unit, depending upon the patient's condition and the surgeon's preference. In the postoperative period the extremities are assessed for color, temperature, pulses, motor and sensory function, and the status of the incision. All findings must be compared to the preoperative baseline. The patient may be on prophylactic intravenous antibiotics for 3 to 4 days to prevent infection, especially if a prosthetic material is used. Some surgeons prescribe aspirin for antiplatelet action or heparin for a few days. Standard nursing care for patients taking heparin is employed.

Wound care is essential (see box above). Occasionally during vascular reconstructive surgery the lymph channels may be cut. Clear lymphatic drainage may seep through the incision (especially in the groin). Local swelling may occur. Wound disruption may occur in the early or late postoperative period. Early disruption may be related to a technical problem during surgery or severe swelling in the incision. Late disruption may be a result of swelling in the extremity, infection, or from maceration in a moist area such as the groin. Signs of infection should be promptly reported so that therapy can be instituted. Delay may cause infection of the graft.

The graft may occlude at any time. Signs of graft occlusion are the same as for acute arterial occlusion. The six Ps—pain, pulselessness, pallor, paresthesias, paralysis, and polar sensation (cold)—are all signs of graft occlusion and must be reported immediately. Patients should be instructed about these signs before discharge and told specifically to notify

CLINICAL ALERT

Hemorrhage or hematoma formation can occur in the early postoperative period. Oozing blood or rapid swelling around the incision indicates bleeding in the wound. The nurse asks the surgeon how much swelling or bleeding is expected. Rapid swelling may be an indication that the sutures on the artery have come loose. Severe, cramplike pain may occur with occlusion.

the physician. Dehydration, smoking, and compression of a limb may cause occlusion. The patient should maintain adequate fluid intake, stop smoking, and keep a pillow between the legs if the graft goes along the inside of the knee. Graft infection is a rare complication and generally occurs late in the postoperative period, sometimes months or years after surgery. If the graft is of prosthetic material it must be removed. Limb survival will depend on the ability to revascularize the limb or the collateral circulation that has developed.

Activity in the postoperative period depends upon physician orders. The patient's leg should not be elevated unless it is specifically ordered to decrease postoperative limb edema that may threaten the graft. If the patient is allowed to sit, the leg should be propped up to decrease edema. Activity should increasingly progress. Pain management is an important nursing function. Assessment must be done to ascertain if the pain is incisional, ischemic, or a result of edema or some other nonoperative cause. Pain medication and assistance with positioning are provided.

Axillobifemoral bypass

Nursing measures specific to this surgical procedure involve graft protection and assessment for complications. The patient is instructed not to lie on the graft and not to wear constrictive belts. A sign is placed above the bed instructing other personnel not to take brachial blood pressure readings in the affected arm and to take blood samples from the unaffected side. The patient should avoid excessive flexion of the axilla and groin areas to avoid tension on the sutures.

Pulses are obtained in the extremities but may not be present by palpation. Pulsation of the graft is assessed along the thorax, and, in obese patients, a Doppler may be necessary to check the graft pulse. Femoral pulses should be palpable. It is important to reassure the patient that bruising along the side, back, and groin is expected. The genitalia may be ecchymotic and swollen.

Evaluation

Short-term evaluation of interventions to decrease risk factors may only determine the patient's willingness to participate. The long-term evaluation of symptomatology, skin viability, and graft patency will determine the success of the interventions. Unfortunately, nurses often see patients episodically. If possible, communication with the physician's nurse clinician or the outpatient clinic may reassure the nurse that interventions are successful. Vascular rehabilitation nurses or visiting nurses may monitor the success of exercise routines and healing of the patient's wounds. Increased compliance with hospital interventions is seen in the patient followed by nurses in the outpatient setting according to research by Hollier et al. Teaching is an important nursing intervention, and assessment of learning can be performed by nurses who see the patients in their own homes. Reinforcing these teachings is essential.

Ongoing Care

At discharge the patient should understand that the disease has not been cured. The symptoms may be relieved, but ongoing care is necessary. The patient must be seen on a regular basis by the physician, vascular surgeon, or nurse practitioner in order to monitor the status of the surgery and disease progression. Risk management practices should continue, and the patient should be encouraged to seek advice on diet, exercise, and smoking cessation should it be needed.

The individual with atherosclerosis who develops arterial insufficiency must learn the symptoms of disease progression. Self-care is the key to early and prompt treatment. A sudden change in symptoms must be evaluated immediately or the individual may face limb loss. Progression of claudication may indicate the need for further diagnostic evaluation.

Foot care as a lifelong practice cannot be overemphasized. Detailed instructions are given in the hospital and reviewed by nurses in the outpatient setting. Medical attention is obtained immediately for any injury to the affected extremities. The patient must understand that monitoring the circulation of the extremities is a permanent part of life. Assessment of pulses, color, temperature, presence of ulcers or skin lesions, and perception of touch must be performed on a daily basis by the patient or significant other. Any change is reported to the physician. The patient is instructed to check with the vascular surgeon before undergoing any procedure on the feet.

Should the patient have a prosthetic graft placed, additional care is needed. Other medical care that

has a risk of bacterial shower in the blood (such as dental work) requires prophylactic antibiotics. Any evidence of infection in the affected extremity such as redness, warmth, pain, and fever is brought to the physician's attention.

Discharge medications are generally the same as those given preoperatively. The only addition may be aspirin because of its antiplatelet effect.

Aneurysms

An **aneurysm** is the localized, irreversible dilation of an artery secondary to an alteration in the integrity of its wall. The abdominal aorta is the most common site for aneurysm development. There are several classifications of aneurysms (Figure 30-8). True aneurysms are either fusiform or saccular. Fusiform aneurysms are circumferentially dilated, and saccular aneurysms involve outpouching of only one "side" or wall of the artery. The primary discussion of this section is on "true" aneurysms, but a brief mention of other aneurysms is also necessary.

False aneurysms, or *pseudoaneurysms,* involve a division between the layers of the artery itself. It

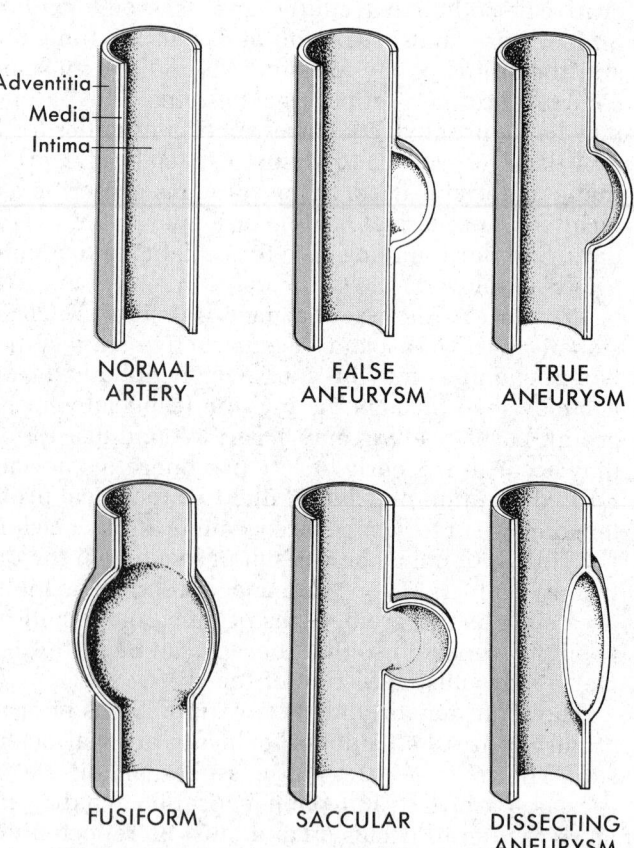

FIGURE 30-8   Types of aneurysms.

would compare to a bubble between the layers. There is a collection of blood between layers or in the connective tissue outside the artery. The pseudoaneurysm pulsates only because of the artery underneath it.

A second type of pseudoaneurysm occurs at the anastomosis of a graft to the native artery. At times the sutures weaken, and the connection between the graft and the artery dilate, forming an aneurysm.

Dissecting aneurysms occur because of an entry tear in the intima and media. This tear can sometimes be traced to trauma, but the cause is generally unknown. Blood enters the tear, forcing a longitudinal separation of the media. The blood pressure forces more blood into the tear, eventually creating a false channel for blood flow. This channel generally involves a part of the arterial wall, not the entire circumference. Approximately 70% of these occur in the ascending aorta, and only 1% occur in the abdominal aorta. Hypertension is a major risk factor. Dissecting aneurysms can be either chronic, with the false channel extending little or clotting completely, or acute, with the false channel extending retrograde or antegrade and eventually rupturing through the outside layer of the artery. Acute dissecting aneurysms require immediate surgical intervention. Chronic dissecting aneurysms may be treated conservatively by control of blood pressure, but the risk of rupture is great.

There are three classes of dissecting aneurysms. Type I begins just above the aortic valve and may extend down the aorta into the abdomen. This type is seen in approximately 60% of dissecting aneurysms. Type II is limited to the ascending aorta and does not extend into the arch. It accounts for 10% of the dissections and occurs most often in Marfan's syndrome and pregnancy. Type III begins distal to the subclavian artery on the arch and extends down into the abdominal aorta and beyond. Older hypertensive patients are more likely to be seen with this type.

ABDOMINAL AORTIC ANEURYSM
Etiology/Epidemiology

An **abdominal aorta aneurysm (AAA)** can be caused by connective tissue disorders, trauma, Marfan's syndrome, infection, cystic medial necrosis, and arteritis. In the majority of cases, the cause is not identified. Recent research seems to indicate a hereditary tendency in aneurysm formation. The risk ratio for persons with a first-degree relative with an AAA compared to a person in the general population is 6:1. The possibility of a specific genetic abnormality or problem with the elastin in the aorta seems high. In the past atherosclerosis was blamed for nonspecific aneurysms; however, recent studies discount this as a primary cause.

The majority of abdominal aortic aneurysms occur in men between the ages of 60 and 70. First-degree relatives of persons with an AAA seem to develop dilation at an earlier age.

The natural course of an untreated AAA is to expand and rupture. Surgery is recommended once the patient's aneurysm measures 5 cm or more. An aneurysm of 6 cm or more has a 20% chance of rupturing in 1 year. Rupture is more common in the obese patient because of difficulties in palpating an AAA through adipose tissue.

Pathophysiology

The cause of nonspecific AAA seems to be a decreased amount of elastin in the arterial wall. The normal amount of elastin found in normal subjects is 12% as opposed to 1% or less in subjects with an aneurysm. The cause of tendency to develop aneurysmal dilation of the infrarenal aorta is uncertain. The normal adult aorta is approximately 2.5 cm in diameter. Once the AAA reaches 5 cm in a nonobese patient, it can be palpated. Some speculated causes are the increased turbulence in the area, lack of nourishment of the artery (less vaso vasorum in this area), slower turnover of smooth muscle cells, and increased tension in an area with fewer elastin units. Inflammatory AAA, which accounts for 5% to 10% of all aortic aneurysms, may be caused by infection or some obscure form of arteritis. Pathologists differ in speculating upon the cause. These aneurysms have a tendency to rupture at smaller sizes than the nonspecific aneurysm.

Clinical Manifestations

In general, the presence of an abdominal aortic aneurysm causes no symptoms. The only complaint may be a prominent pulse felt in the abdomen when reclining. Diagnosis is usually made with a routine examination or by accident while evaluating another problem. An example is the patient with kidney problems who has an intravenous pyelogram and the displacement resulting from aneurysmal dilation is seen, or the calcified outline of the aneurysm is noted. If symptoms are present, the aneurysm is expanding or rupture is imminent. Symptoms include low back pain, abdominal pain (especially with palpation of the aneurysm), or flank pain. Rupture may be heralded by intense back pain, lower abdominal pain, collapse, shock, mottling of the lower extremities, and decreased hemoglobin. Emergency intervention is indicated.

Therapeutic Management

The treatment of choice for an abdominal aneurysm of 6 cm or more is surgical repair. Controversy exists over whether aneurysms of 4 cm or more should be repaired or followed with sequential sonography. The operative mortality rate for elective aneurysm repair is approximately 5% as opposed to 50% to 80% for the ruptured aneurysm. If the patient is in a remote area without rapid access to medical care, the mortality rate is 100%. Obviously, repair before rupture is desirable.

The most common cause of perioperative mortality is cardiac complications. Complete medical evaluation for risk factors is essential. The workup may include evaluation of left ventricular function, stress testing (exercise or dipyridamole thallium), or cardiac catheterization (see Chapter 33 for details on cardiac evaluation). If catheterization indicates the need for coronary bypass surgery, this may be performed before aneurysm resection. Patients who do not require surgery are monitored with pulmonary artery catheters in an intensive care setting. In some cases, preoperative placement of monitoring devices is necessary to optimize cardiac status and obtain baseline parameters.

Pulmonary disease is another cause of perioperative morbidity. Any cessation of smoking that can occur before surgery is of value. Explanation of the rationale and referral to a support group may be helpful. The patient should be aware that a long history of smoking may indicate a prolonged postoperative intubation period.

Renal disease manifested by a creatinine level above 3 or a creatinine clearance of less than 20 mL may require hydration before surgery. This is especially true if the patient has angiography or a contrast CT scan shortly before surgery. Mannitol and a fluid bolus for decreased output may be necessary in the postoperative period.

Some surgeons order an angiography before surgery to determine the vascular supply above and below the aneurysm. Others require only a sonogram or a CT scan. An angiogram may not reveal the true width of the aneurysm because laminated clot frequently lines the dilated area. Occasionally a bowel preparation is ordered before surgery. The type required varies greatly from surgeon to surgeon.

NURSING MANAGEMENT OF THE PATIENT WITH ABDOMINAL AORTIC ANEURYSM
Nursing Diagnosis

Nursing diagnoses in the preoperative phase include the following:

Knowledge deficit of the hereditary nature of the disease and the planned therapy

High risk for pain related to the surgical incision

Fear related to knowledge of risks of surgery and of rupture of the aneurysm

In addition to diagnoses common to any abdominal procedure, the following relate to the patient with aortic surgery:

Increased risk for impaired tissue integrity of the lower extremities secondary to ischemia

Increased risk for fluid volume deficit related to hemorrhage or third spacing of fluid

Increased risk of altered peripheral tissue perfusion related to thrombus or embolus

Knowledge deficit about discharge instructions

Planning

Preoperatively, the patient will:
   Be able to state an understanding of the hereditary nature of the disease and relay the facts to family as well as the plans for therapy
   Describe methods of pain management
   Seek counsel with family or other support groups and relate understanding of the risk/benefit ratio of treatment
Postoperatively, the patient will:
   State signs and symptoms of ischemia of the extremities, if present
   Maintain adequate fluid balance
   Have adequate peripheral tissue perfusion
   Have knowledge of discharge instructions

Implementation

It is the surgeon's responsibility to discuss the risks and potential complications of surgery or alternate therapy. However, the patient will need information about the normal proceedings in the preoperative and postoperative period. Expected events such as length of stay in the intensive care unit, the presence of tubes or monitoring devices, and the possibility of ventilator use are discussed with the patient and the family. Emotional support is essential.

Intraoperatively, the aorta is crossclamped to stop flow so that a graft may be inserted. This increases the risk of stress upon the heart, resulting in a myocardial infarction (MI) or congestive failure. In addition, the hypotension that occasionally occurs following release of the clamp may cause an MI, a stroke, or damage to the kidneys. Fluid volume must be maintained. Postoperatively, fluid volume is most accurately maintained with a pulmonary artery catheter or central line. Urine output is measured hourly. Any output less than 25 to 30 mL/hr is reported immediately.

Heparin is usually given intraoperatively during vascular procedures to prevent clotting during surgery. The effects of heparin are reversed after the operation, but the nurse must be alert for indications that the patient is still bleeding. Indications may include a drop in central venous pressure, decreased urine output, a nondilutional drop in hemoglobin, and a drop in arterial pressure.

In the postoperative period, distal arterial perfusion is closely monitored. Pulses in both lower extremities are assessed and compared with preoperative records. Other signs of changes in color, pain level, motion, sensation, and temperature are noted and reported. Distal arteries may have occluded during surgery secondary to decreased pressure during aortic clamping or to debris broken free during arterial manipulation. Darkened patches in the toes or soles of the feet or pain in these areas may alert the nurse to this possibility (Figure 30-9). Notify the physician if this mottling is noted.

As with aortoiliac reconstruction, the risk of ischemic colitis exists. Diarrhea that occurs before bowel function is expected to return is called to the attention of the physician. Bloody diarrhea may herald this complication. The patient usually complains of left lower-quadrant pain, and sepsis may be present. A colonoscopy is needed to confirm the diagnosis.

In patients who have aneurysm repair that extends above the renal arteries, there is a risk of spinal cord ischemia. Damage to the artery of Adamkiewicz, the main artery to the spinal cord, may result in paralysis of the lower extremities. Assessment for motor and sensory function is essential. Assessment may be complicated in patients who have epidural analgesia.

Pain relief may be difficult because of the length of the incision and the fact that major abdominal muscles are used in moving. Pain medications are given as needed. Some institutions use patient-controlled analgesia or epidural analgesia with success. Patients seem to mobilize and ventilate more easily with decreased pain. Patients are encouraged to ask for medication and not be fearful of habituation.

In general, mobility is encouraged on the first or second postoperative day. Within 2 to 3 days the patient does not require intensive care unless complications ensue. Normal gut function should be expected on the fourth or fifth postoperative day. Most patients who experience no complications are discharged within 7 to 10 days.

Discharge planning includes wound care, which is minimal, and activity instructions. Unless the physician requests otherwise, the patient may shower or bathe, and lotion may be applied to soften the scar. The patient may use stairs. Lifting is restricted to less than 5 pounds. The patient is instructed to avoid driving until cleared by the physician, because braking may increase intraabdominal pressure and disrupt the wound.

Evaluation

Evaluation is based on expected outcomes for the individual. Patient education is evaluated by having the patient redemonstrate or reexplain the material. Activity instructions should be clearly and concisely stated by the patient or significant other.

Documentation

Teaching, patient response, and all patient procedures performed are documented carefully by the nurse. Condition of the wound, medication lists and precautions, life-style changes, and activity are specifically addressed.

ACUTE ARTERIAL OCCLUSION
Definition/Etiology

An **acute arterial occlusion** is the sudden obstruction of an artery, resulting in a decrease in tissue perfusion distal to the obstruction without adequate time for collateral circulation to develop. Acute occlusion usually can be accurately documented by the patient because of the suddenness of symptoms. The causes of acute arterial occlusion are thrombosis and embolization. An arterial thrombus usually develops at the site of an atherosclerotic plaque. A clot may form in an aneurysm and break loose to travel distally. Emboli in the arterial system usually originate from a plaque or from a clot in the left side of the heart. The embolus may be a clot that forms as a result of valvular heart disease (see Chapter 36) or atrial fibrillation (see Chapter 34). Emboli may also originate at any site of trauma (such as a puncture site). This is a complication of arteriography or reconstructive surgery. The most common sites of embolic problems are the extremities and the brain.

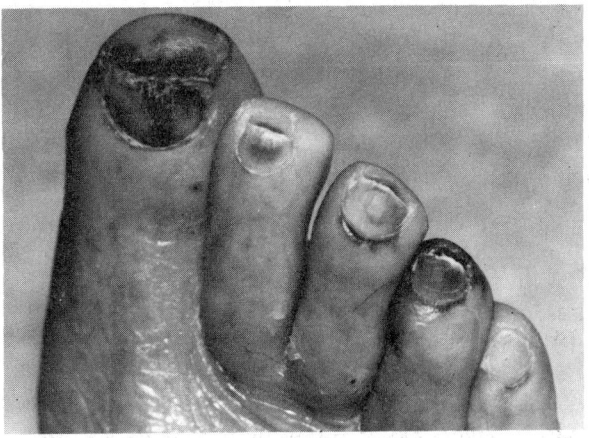

FIGURE 30-9 Blue toes from emboli resulting from emergency resection of an abdominal aortic aneurysm. The areas healed without further therapy.

Pathophysiology/Clinical Manifestations

The primary outcome of acute arterial occlusion is the sudden disruption of arterial blood flow. Decreased tissue perfusion results in acute ischemia distal to the occlusion. With sudden occlusion in an artery, the area fed by the artery will develop symptoms related to ischemia (Figure 30-10). The signs of occlusion noted in the lower extremities are applicable. In the brain, the patient will exhibit symptoms related to the area of loss of brain function (see Chapter 47 on cerebrovascular disease).

Therapeutic Management

The goal of therapy is to reduce symptoms, restore flow to the area, and decrease damage from ischemia. The patient is generally given anticoagulants (heparin or in some cases thrombolytic therapy), and bed rest is prescribed. If an extremity is involved, the extremity is protected from further tissue damage with standard measures, such as sheepskin. If anticoagulants and conservative measures are not immediately successful in increasing blood flow, surgical embolectomy may be necessary to salvage the limb.

NURSING MANAGEMENT OF THE PATIENT WITH ACUTE ARTERIAL OCCLUSION

The nurse is often the first health professional to encounter a person with an acute arterial occlusion. Out of the hospital, the visiting nurse may be the person contacted if the patient is having a problem. The nurse must be able to identify patients at risk for developing thrombi or emboli. Patient reports of

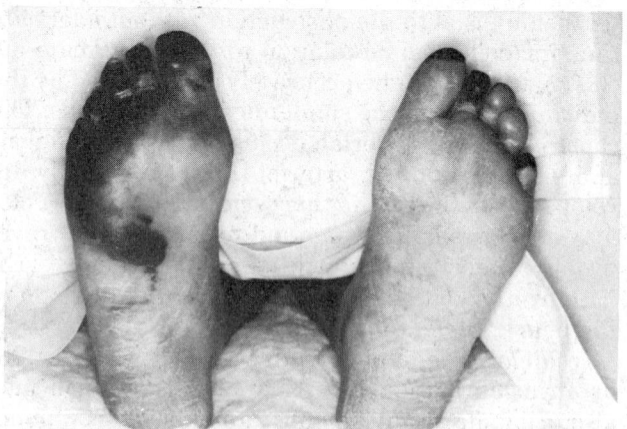

FIGURE 30-10   Severe gangrenous toes and feet secondary to a large arterial embolus.

the sudden onset of pain in an extremity are assessed as soon as possible for associated changes (the six Ps). Peripheral pulses are assessed at regular intervals in the hospital postoperative period (hourly the first day, twice a shift for 2 days, and then every shift until discharge, unless changes in the patient's status warrant more frequent assessment). The patient is also instructed on outpatient monitoring. Visiting nurses regularly check patient compliance in this area.

The patient with an acute arterial occlusion may be restless because of pain. The nurse needs to assist the patient in keeping the limb immobilized to reduce pain and the potential for tissue damage secondary to trauma.

Anticoagulation therapy is appropriate for the patient at risk for arterial clot formation as well as for treatment of that eventuality. Anticoagulants may prevent the occurrence of arterial clots or prevent their extension and embolization to distal sites (see Chapter 32 for patient education related to anticoagulant therapy). Further methods of prevention of arterial clot formation include position changes, mobility, and avoiding tight or restrictive clothing.

Nonatherosclerotic Peripheral Vascular Disease

RAYNAUD'S DISEASE
Definition/Etiology

Raynaud's disease is the condition most often seen in patients with vasospastic disorders. Vasospasm of the upper extremities is seen as a complication of medications, intraarterial manipulation, and angiography; however, the primary cause is Raynaud's disease. By definition, it is intermittent digital vasospasm that occurs as a result of temperature change or emotional stress. Arterial spasm may occur secondary to the use of vibrating tools, but this is more common in males. Raynaud's disease is common in a number of areas in the world. Cool, damp climates are a prime location for the disease. It is estimated that 20% of young adults in the United States have this problem. It can exist as an isolated condition with no underlying disease or can be associated with a connective tissue disorder (Raynaud's phenomenon).

Pathophysiology

Studies suggest that Raynaud's disease results from two different pathologic states. The states may exist separately or may be mixed. In the first state there is abnormal, forceful digital artery contraction in the presence of cold (or even decreased temperatures) or stress. This contraction is strong enough to overcome the normal intraarterial pressure that distends and closes the artery. The second occurs in patients with occlusive disease. These patients have arterial obstructions and decreased pressures. The contractile pressures may not be as great in these individuals, but they may be adequate to overcome an artery with a low-flow state.

Clinical Manifestations

Classic symptoms begin with initial blanching of the digits with or without accompanying numbness (Figure 30-11). This is a result of the arterial spasm and tissue ischemia. Spasm may last only a few minutes or may last until relief measures are taken. Cyanosis follows pallor, and, as the artery relaxes, a reactive hyperemic effect occurs with burning pain and throbbing. The patient may complain that the area feels swollen. In the early stages of the disease it may take dramatic temperature changes to cause symptoms; however, as time passes, minimal drops in temperature may precipitate an episode. If the stimuli are not curtailed, the disease may progress to occlusion of the arteries, accompanied by tissue necrosis and ulceration. These ulcers are often painful and difficult to treat. Digit amputation may result. This occurs in approximately 10% of those with associated occlusive disease.

Therapeutic Management

No single treatment of Raynaud's disease has been uniformly successful. Unfortunately, some physicians regard the disease as a "nuisance," and patients may have delay in therapy. If there is an underlying disease or a medication that is causing symptoms, then this must be treated. Connective tissue disorders must be ruled out. Treatment of the disease must be patient-specific. Avoidance of the causes of symptoms must be encouraged. Education and reassurance are prime treatments. Calcium channel blockers (e.g., nifedipine) may cause vasodilation and provide some relief. Side effects are minimal (chiefly headache). These may be necessary only in the winter months unless stress is a primary precipitating cause. Nitroglycerin in various forms is used by some practitioners, and so is reserpine. Side effects are more severe with these medications (e.g., headaches, dizziness, hypotension). Pentoxifylline does not seem to affect Raynaud's disease, but studies are continuing to judge its effectiveness when arterial occlusive disease accompanies Raynaud's disease.

Cervicothoracic sympathectomy has been used in the past and is occasionally used in the patient with rest pain or gangrene. It is most often used in patients with accompanying connective tissue disorders. It does not seem to affect the long-term course of the disease.

Biofeedback and Pavlovian conditioning are other measures that have been tried as treatment. Plasmapheresis has been tried in some patients with severe symptoms. This is still experimental and is very expensive. Life-style modification is the most effective and simple treatment. Stress management, smoking cessation, and avoidance of cold as well as cessation of work with vibrating tools is necessary.

NURSING MANAGEMENT OF THE PATIENT WITH RAYNAUD'S DISEASE
Assessment

Assessment of contralateral extremities for vascular status is necessary. Color changes, not only in the extremity but in parts of the digits, must be noted. Temperature differential in segments of a digit in an acute episode may be quite dramatic. Patients must be questioned about the digits affected most fre-

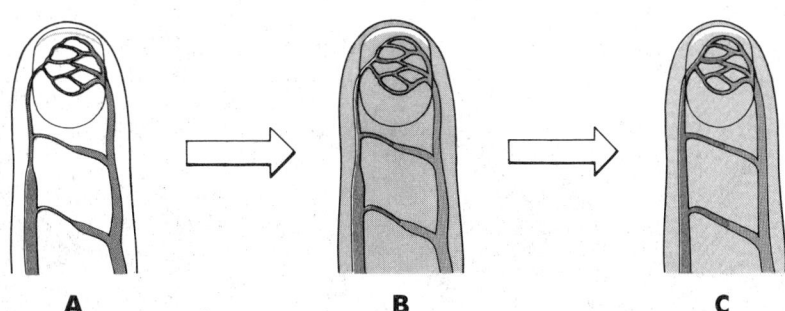

A   **B**   **C**

FIGURE 30-11 Characteristic color changes of Raynaud's disease. **A,** Pallor, or whiteness, occurs with digital artery constriction from cold or stress. **B,** Cyanosis, or blueness, follows as the arteries relax, allowing for limited blood flow. **C,** Rubor, or redness, finally results from reactive hyperemia.

quently. In the nonacute state capillary refill may or may not be delayed. Causative factors must be recorded. Work practices with vibrating tools must be noted.

Nursing Diagnosis

Nursing diagnoses for the patient with Raynaud's disease include:

Acute pain related to tissue ischemia

Impaired tissue perfusion related to decreased arterial flow

Fear of recurring episodes secondary to lack of information about the disease process and treatment options

Planning

The nursing care for the patient will achieve the following outcomes:

Demonstrate knowledge of measures to prevent recurrent episodes

Decrease number of episodes of arterial spasm

Skin temperature, color, and pulses will be within patient's normal limits

Implementation

Patient education and emotional support become important aspects of nursing care of these patients. See the patient education guide below for key points. The patient will need to learn measures to

treat acute episodes. Gradual warming of the affected part is necessary. Warming the digit in lukewarm water or placing it in the mouth or in the axilla are nontraumatic ways to warm. Pain will still be present with warming, but it should be less than if warm water or other methods are used.

Evaluation

The patient should be able to demonstrate methods of treating acute episodes. The patient should stop smoking and should have normal skin temperatures and capillary refill time.

THORACIC OUTLET SYNDROME
Definition

Thoracic outlet syndrome is a set of upper-extremity symptoms resulting from neurovascular compression in the thoracic outlet area. These symptoms result from compression of the brachial nerve plexus and the subclavian artery and vein by the first rib, scalenus anterior muscle, and the clavicle. There are many specific causes of the compression.

Etiology/Pathophysiology

Causes may be related to trauma to the first rib or the scalenus muscle. Congenital causes may be an abnormal first rib or congenital ligaments or bands in the area. Other precipitating factors may include

---

 **PATIENT EDUCATION GUIDE** *Avoiding Raynaud's Disease Symptoms*

Avoiding Cold

Use mittens (wool or cotton) in cold weather

Use gloves to remove articles from the freezer

Avoiding Vibration

If job duties include the use of vibratory tools, request a change in duties

Avoiding Causative Medications

Avoid any medication that seems to precipitate episodes

Managing Stress

Anticipate stressful situations

Examine present coping strategies; determine whether new strategies are indicated

Practice stress-reducing techniques

Identify and attempt to avoid stress-producing activities

Smoking Cessation

The nicotine in cigarette smoke stimulates constriction of the artery—"cutting down" will not improve the situation; complete smoking cessation is necessary

Managing Symptoms

Practice stress-reducing techniques

Warm hands and feet by placing them next to another warm body part or by placing them in warm (not hot) water

Avoid hot water bottles or heating pads

Use prescription medications at the beginning of an attack to reduce the severity

Biofeedback

nonthrombotic subclavian vein occlusion, hyperabduction or the pectoralis minor syndrome, chronic inflammation of the area, and postural defects.

Symptoms are related to what causes the compression and to whether the artery, vein, or the nerve plexus is compressed. If the artery is compressed, then stenosis develops in the area, and a poststenotic dilation may occur. Thrombus formation is more likely in these patients. When venous compression occurs, it is usually secondary to compression by ligaments. The vein narrows, and venous occlusion or thrombosis may occur. Nerve plexus compression is most common. It is believed that many people may have an anatomic predisposition to thoracic outlet syndrome, but that trauma may precipitate its occurrence. Occupations that require abduction and external arm rotation may aggravate the syndrome. Thoracic outlet syndrome occurs in about 1% of the population, mostly in young women.

Clinical Manifestations

The presenting signs and symptoms depend on which structure (nerve, vein, or artery) is affected. Nerve compression is the most common. What results is pressure upon the nerve complex, which produces neck and shoulder pain and occipital headache. Other complaints include pain, numbness, and tingling of the neck, shoulder, upper arm, forearm, and hand. Symptoms associated with subclavian arterial compression are changes in temperature and color of the hand. There may be decreased or absent radial or ulnar pulses. Trauma within the artery may result in atherosclerotic plaque deposition. Emboli to the fingers may result from stenosis, poststenotic dilation, and subsequent clot formation in the vessel. Venous compression is less common. Symptoms include edema of the hand and arm as well as venous distention.

Diagnostic evaluation includes thoracic outlet maneuvers performed in the physician's office. These include the Adson maneuver, the ball-thrower's maneuver, and the military brace position (Figure 30-12). Noninvasive blood-flow testing may be helpful in documenting loss of pulses in certain anatomic positions. Plain x-ray films of the clavicular area may identify a prominent first rib. Angiography is indicated only in severe, disabling cases (see box on p. 718). These are also performed in various anatomic positions to document compression. Nerve conduction studies can document thoracic outlet nerve compression.

Many persons with thoracic outlet syndrome are asymptomatic except for loss of pulses in certain maneuvers or numbness in the hands when working overhead. These patients require careful observation but no intervention.

Therapeutic Management

If the symptoms are caused by nerve compression, only the treatment is conservative. A referral to physical therapy for exercises is the first line of treatment. Exercises are aimed at enlarging the tho-

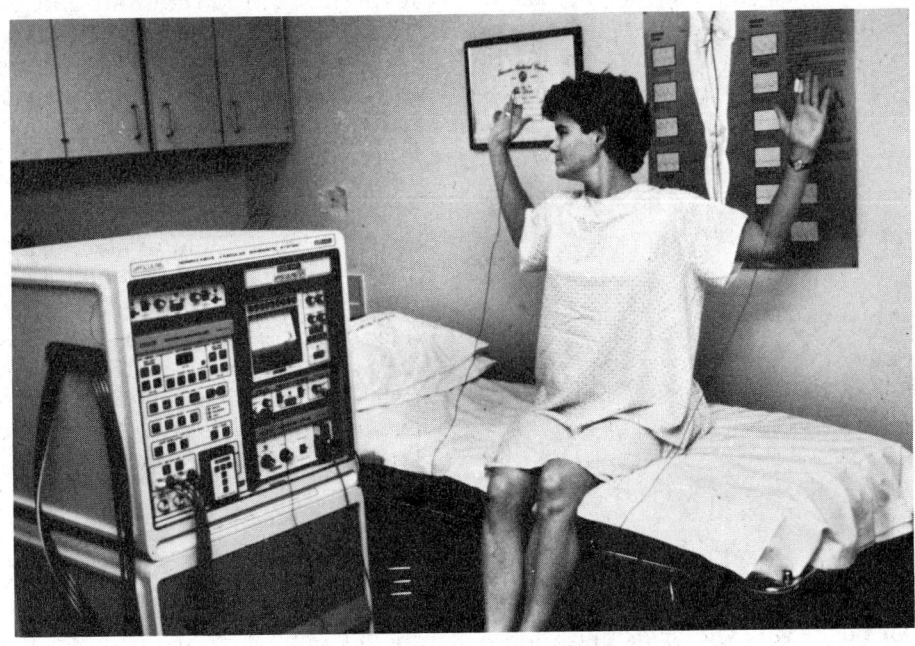

FIGURE 30-12 The military brace position.

ALLEN TEST

This test is done to assess the arterial patency of the palmar arch. It is performed before inserting a needle into the radial artery for obtaining blood or for arterial monitoring. Assurance of an intact palmar arch may protect the hand from ischemia and possible death if the radial artery should thrombose.

Procedure

Both the radial and ulnar pulses are identified

The patient is asked to clench the fist to completely empty the capillaries in the hand

The examiner uses the thumb and forefinger of each hand to occlude the patient's radial and ulnar arteries simultaneously

The patient is asked to open the fist

The examiner then releases the thumb and forefinger over the radial artery while continuing to compress the ulnar artery

If the palmar arch is intact, the capillaries of the hand fill, and the skin will suddenly flush

The maneuver is repeated, compressing the radial artery while the ulnar is released. The resulting skin color change should be the same as during the radial examination

racic outlet by improving posture. If the artery is involved and there is resulting stenosis or emboli, surgery may be indicated. Removal of the cervical or first rib or arterial reconstruction may be necessary. Venous thrombosis may require heparin therapy in the acute phase. Long-term oral anticoagulants may be indicated. Surgical removal of the obstruction may be recommended.

NURSING MANAGEMENT OF THE PATIENT WITH THORACIC OUTLET SYNDROME

Assessment

Because of the complicated anatomy related to thoracic outlet syndrome, patients often have difficulty understanding the problem. Careful explanation is essential. The nurse needs to assess the patient's knowledge of the disorder. The patient is examined for signs of circulatory impairment. The radial and ulnar pulses are palpated. Edema of the arm is recorded. Skin temperature, color, and capillary refill time are assessed. Neurologic symptoms are elicited through changes of position of the arms and shoulder.

Nursing Diagnosis

Based on the assessment data, the following diagnoses may be appropriate:

Knowledge deficit related to lack of information about the disease and its treatment

Pain or numbness related to changes of position of the affected arm

Impaired job performance related to necessity for arm positions that cause symptoms

Planning

Outcomes for the plan of care should include:

Verbalize knowledge of the disease and its treatment

Pain and numbness will be reduced

Will change jobs or explore new methods of job activities

Implementation

The nurse begins teaching the patient about thoracic outlet syndrome. Pictures of anatomy may be helpful. Causes of symptoms must be related to anatomy. Cooperation with treatment may be better if the rationale for treatment is explained. The nurse can reinforce the exercise program and refer the patient to physical therapy if questions in practice occur. The overweight patient may benefit from a weight reduction plan. The patient also may need emotional and financial support as job activities are modified to reduce symptoms.

Postoperative care

If the first rib is removed, the patient may have a transaxillary or supraclavicular incision. The patient will then need a dressing and possibly a small drain in place. Ambulation and activity are important. The patient should receive adequate pain medication to help range-of-motion activities. If arterial reconstruction was performed in addition to rib resection, then assessment for hematoma formation is important. The radial and ulnar pulses must be palpated and documented. This should be done hourly in the first 24 hours. Occasionally injury to the thoracic duct occurs in surgery as a result of the close proximity of the duct to the incision site. If this happens, there will be swelling and a clear (or milky) drainage of lymphatic fluid. This is generally self-limiting but may require pressure dressings or ligation.

Ongoing care

Patients may be discharged on the second to fourth postoperative day. Mobility is encouraged. Patients should take their pain medication, avoid splinting the arm, and perform complete range-of-motion exercises. Lifting heavy objects or strenuous activity is discouraged. Follow-up visits with the physician occur in 2 to 3 weeks, and further activity instructions will be given at that time. The care of visiting nurses is not generally needed.

CRITICAL THINKING QUESTIONS

1 How can people modify their life-styles to reduce risk factors for atherosclerosis?

2 What are the implications for the patient with intermittent claudication and rest pain?

3 Explain the benefit of exercise for the patient with chronic arterial occlusive disease.

4 What is the nursing management for the patient treated medically for chronic arterial occlusive disease?

5 What is the postoperative care for the patient having arterial bypass surgery?

6 What are the different types of abdominal aneurysms?

7 Describe the problems experienced by the patient with thoracic outlet syndrome.

BIBLIOGRAPHY

Current

1. AbuRahma AF, Woodruff BA: Effects and limitations of pentoxifylline therapy in various stages of peripheral vascular disease of the lower extremity, *Am J Surg* 160:266, 1990.
2. Bengtsson H et al: Ultrasonographic screening of the abdominal aorta among siblings of patients with abdominal aortic aneurysms, *Br J Surg* 76:589, 1989.
3. Bensen JL, Karmody AM: In situ artery bypass: Surgery for leg salvage, *AORN J* 45 (1):40, 1987.
4. Bishop A: The use of epidural analgesia in postoperative vascular surgical patients, *J Vasc Nurs* 8(4):2, 1990.
5. Bondy B: Mesenteric ischemia, *J Vasc* 8(3):2, 1990.
6. Brophy CM, Smith GJ, Tilson MD: Pathology of nonspecific abdominal aortic aneurysm. In Ernst CB, Stanley JC, editors: *Current therapy in vascular surgery II*, Philadelphia, 1991, B.C. Decker.
7. Cole CW et al: Abdominal aortic aneurysm: Consequences of a positive family history, *Can J Surg* 32:117, 1989.
8. Criado E et al: Intermittent claudication, *Surg Gynecol Obstet* 173:163.
9. Dixon MB, Nunnelee J: Arterial reconstruction for atherosclerotic occlusive disease, *J Cardiovasc Nurs* 1(2):36, 1987.
10. Edwards JM, Porter JM: Diagnosis of upper extremity vasospastic disease. In Ernst CB, Stanley JC, editors: *Current therapy in vascular surgery II*, Philadelphia, 1991, B.C. Decker.
11. Ernst E, Kollar L, Matrai A: A double blind trial of dextran hemodilution vs. placebo in claudicants, *J Intern Med* 227:19, 1990.
12. Expert panel: Report of the national cholesterol education program expert panel on detection, evaluation and treatment of high blood cholesterol in adults, *Arch Intern Med* 148:36, 1988.
13. Fahey VA: Thoracic outlet syndrome, *J Cardiovasc Nurs* 1:12, 1987.

14. Ford KA: Laser-assisted angioplasty in the patient with peripheral arterial disease, *J Vasc Nurs* 8(3):6, 1990.
15. Helt J: Foot care and footwear to prevent amputation, *J Vasc Nurs* 9(4):2, 1991.
16. Hiatt WR et al: Benefit of exercise conditioning for patients with peripheral arterial disease, *Circulation* 81:602, 1990.
17. Hill S: Discharge planning for the vascular patient: Where does home care fit in? *J Vasc Nurs* 9(3):6, 1991.
18. Hollier L et al: Efficacy of home health care in patients with peripheral vascular disease, *Am J Surg* 160:179, 1990.
19. Hubner C: Exercise therapy and smoking cessation for intermittent claudication, *J Cardiovasc Nurs* 1:2, 1987.
20. Kannel WB, McGee DL: Update on some epidemiologic features of intermittent claudication: the Framingham study, *J Am Geriatr Soc* 33(1):13, 1985.
21. Kontusaari S et al: A mutation in the gene for type II procollagen in a family with aortic aneurysms, *J Clin Invest* 86:1485, 1990.
22. Kowallek D: Symptomatic subclavian artery stenosis: a case study, *J Vasc Nurs* 9(4):9, 1991.
23. Krupski WC, Rapp JH: Smoking and atherosclerosis, *Perspect Vasc Surg*, 103, 1989.
24. LaCroix AZ et al: Smoking and mortality among older men and women in three communities, *N Engl J Med* 324:1619, 1991.
25. Lindgarde F et al: Conservative drug treatment in patients with moderately severe chronic occlusive peripheral arterial disease, *Circulation* 80:1549, 1989.
26. Lovell MB, Harris KA: Abdominal aortic aneurysms, *J Vasc* 9(1):2, 1991.
27. Powell J, Greenhalgh RM: Cellular, enzymatic, and genetic factors in the pathogenesis of abdominal aortic aneurysms, *J Vasc Surg* 9:297, 1989.
28. Pacy PJ, Dodson PM, Taylor MP: The effect of a high-fibre, low-fat, low-sodium diet on diabetics with intermittent claudication, *Br J Clin Prac* 40(8):313, 1986.
29. Reilly JM, Tilson MD: Incidence and etiology of abdominal aortic aneurysms, *Surg Clin North Am* 69:705, 1989.
30. Robinson LC: Chronic arterial occlusive disease of the lower extremity, *J Vasc Nurs* 9(2):2, 1991.
31. Swenson WM, James EC: Left subclavian-common carotid artery anastomosis for correction of the subclavian steal syndrome, *Contemp Surg* 39:21, 1991.
32. Webster MW et al: Ultrasound screening of first-degree relatives of patients with an abdominal aortic aneurysm, *J Vasc Surg* 13:9, 1991.
33. Williams LR et al: Vascular rehabilitation: Benefits of a structured exercise/risk modification program, *J Vasc Surg* 14:320, 1991.
34. Young JR: Treatment of upper extremity vasospastic disorders. In Ernst CB, Stanley JC, editors: *Current therapy in vascular surgery II*, Philadelphia, 1991, B.C. Decker.

Classic

35. Andrews Ekers M, Satiani B: EAB: A new route for vascular revascularization, *Nurs 82* 12:34, 1982.
36. Baum PL: Heed the early warning signs of PVD, peripheral vascular disease, *Nurs 85* 3:50, 1985.
37. Boozer M, Craven RF: Nursing care of the patient with chronic occlusive peripheral artery disease, *Cardiovasc Nurs* 15:13, 1981.
38. Doyle JE: If your patient's legs hurt the reason may be arterial insufficiency, *Nurs 81* 11:74, 1981.
39. Pepper GA: New drug for intermittent claudication, *Nurse Pract* 5:54, 1985.

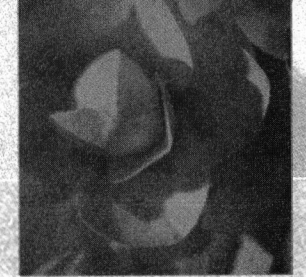

CHAPTER THIRTY-ONE

Nursing Management of Adults with Hypertension

LEARNING OBJECTIVES

1 Describe the types and complications of hypertension and national objectives for hypertension prevention.

2 Explain the multifactorial basis for hypertension.

3 Identify high-risk factors and individuals with increased potential for developing high blood pressure.

4 Assess an individual for the detection, screening, and follow-up of hypertension by listing the essential components.

5 List the benefits and liabilities of therapeutic regimens in treating hypertension.

6 Apply the concept of "self-care" to the preventive/rehabilitative nursing care of a newly diagnosed patient with hypertension.

7 Compare and contrast the pharmacologic and nonpharmacologic approaches to hypertension, noting the controversies of each.

8 Relate the empiric evidence for carrying out pharmacologic vs. nonpharmacologic approaches to hypertension.

9 State the teaching/learning strategies and outcome measures for patient education.

HYPERTENSION IS a major health care issue facing Americans in the 1990s. In the United States alone, over 61 million cases of hypertension have been diagnosed with an estimated 600,000 deaths per year related to hypertension. It is a major factor in the etiology of strokes and costs 600 million dollars per year to the economy. Hypertension, a multifaceted illness, accounts for the largest number of office visits to physicians and the most use of prescription drugs.[33,40] Newly diagnosed cases affected approximately 29,000 women and 32,000 men in 1987 with a predicted rate of one of every four Americans being at risk for this chronic illness. Hypertension is the single most important predictor of cardiovascular risk. It occurs across the life span with both men and women expected to experience hypertension at the same rate after 60 years of age.

"The 1988 Report of the Joint National Committee on Detection, Evaluation, and Treatment of High Blood Pressure" sets forth guidelines emphasizing greater patient involvement, more flexibility in the stepped care approach, increased use of nonpharmacologic approaches, and serious consideration of the effect of a lifetime commitment to antihypertensive agents on quality of life, cost, and compliance.[12] The U.S. Public Health Service has set forth "1990 Objectives for the Nation," of which nine relate to hypertension control (see box).

NATIONAL HEALTH PROMOTION AND DISEASE PREVENTION OBJECTIVES

Increase to at least 50% the proportion of people with high blood pressure whose blood pressure is under control

Increase to at least 90% the proportion of people with high blood pressure who are taking action to help control their blood pressure

Increase to at least 90% the proportion of adults who have had their blood pressure measured within the preceding 2 years and can state whether their blood pressure was normal or high

Reduce overweight to a prevalence of no more than 20% among people aged 20 years and older and no more than 15% among adolescents aged 12 through 19 years

Increase to at least 30% the proportion of people aged 6 years and older who engage regularly, preferably daily, in light to moderate physical activity for at least 30 minutes per day

Reduce cigarette smoking to a prevalence of no more than 15% among people aged 20 years per 100,000 people

Increase to at least 50% the proportion of work sites with 50 or more employees that offer high blood pressure and/or cholesterol education and control activities to their employees

Reduce stroke death to no more than 20 per 100,000 people

Reverse the increase in end-stage renal disease to attain an incidence of no more than 13 per 100,000

From Department of Health and Human Services: *Healthy people 2000*, Washington, DC, 1990, US Government Printing Office.

HYPERTENSION
Definition

Hypertension, or high blood pressure, occurs when the force of blood exerted against the arterial blood vessels exceeds an arterial blood pressure of 140/90 mm Hg. Hypertension is a sustained mean arterial pressure of greater than 100 mm Hg under resting conditions. Hypertension is not diagnosed on a single blood pressure measurement but is reconfirmed on two or more subsequent measurements at about the same time of day. The diastolic pressure is usually crucial and results from the interaction between cardiac output and peripheral vascular resistance. Kaplan suggests that the definition of hypertension be modified to include the conceptual basis of hypertension as "that level of blood pressure at which the benefits (minus the risks and costs) of action exceed the risks and costs (minus the benefits) of inaction."[14]

Hypertension can be classified by stages (see box). In the past, terms such as benign and labile have been used to describe hypertension, but they are no longer appropriate. Terms such as "early primary hypertension" reflect an increased interest in hypertension from a preventive perspective as does the term "isolated systolic hypertension."

Primary hypertension, also called essential or idiopathic hypertension, accounts for over 90% of the cases of hypertension. This chronic elevation in blood pressure occurs without evidence of any other disease process. Primary hypertension has no single known causative etiology but rather is multifactorial in nature.

Secondary hypertension, which accounts for 5% to 10% of hypertension cases, is caused by other pathologic states. Unlike primary hypertension, secondary hypertension has a specific cause in each individual. These causes include renal disease (acute glomerulonephritis, renal tumors); endocrine disor-

---

CLASSIFICATION OF HYPERTENSION

Stage 1: systolic 140 to 159 mm Hg, diastolic 90 to 99 mm Hg

Stage 2: systolic 160 to 179 mm Hg, diastolic 100 to 109 mm Hg

Stage 3: systolic 180 to 209 mm Hg, diastolic 110 to 119 mm Hg

Stage 4: systolic ≥210 mm Hg; diastolic ≥120 mm Hg

From Joint National Committee on Detection, Evaluation, and Treatment of High Blood Pressure (JNC): *Evaluation and treatment of high blood pressure,* Washington, DC, 1992, National Institutes of Health.

ders (primary aldosteronism); vascular disorders (coarctation of the aorta); pregnancy-related disease (preeclampsia, eclampsia); and drug-related disorders (birth control pills, steroids, cyclosporin). The most frequent disease conditions include kidney and vascular disorders, alterations in endocrine function, and acute brain lesions.

Isolated systolic hypertension (ISH) (above 160 mm Hg) is common in elderly persons. Approximately 6% of 60- to 69-year-old people are diagnosed as having ISH. These individuals have a two to three times greater risk of strokes, cardiovascular disease, and death than persons of similar age without ISH.[21] Both systolic and diastolic pressures of 140/90 mm Hg or greater are significant and are associated with increased mortality and morbidity in individuals over 65 years of age. The *National Health and Nutrition Examination Survey* showed the prevalence of these combined types of hypertension to be 64% in individuals 65 years of age and older and 76% in blacks compared with 63% in whites.[45] In contrast to viewing hypertension as part of the aging process, recent studies offer more insight on the special needs of older people with hypertension.

Refractory hypertension refers to hypertension that does not respond to the pharmacologic effects of medication. Refractory hypertension is evidence of the failure of drugs to regulate the patient's blood pressure.

Pregnancy-induced hypertension (above 15 mm Hg above normal pressure during the first trimester) is implicated as a precursor to toxemia, a serious complication of pregnancy. Pregnant patients with a known family history of hypertension need to be aware of their individual risk as weight gain and edema develop.

White coat hypertension is a phenomenon describing those individuals who have normal pressures except at clinic visits. These individuals exhibit an elevated blood pressure especially when examined by a physician, which may contribute to a significant number of misdiagnoses. These individuals are more likely to be younger women, to be recently diagnosed, and to weigh less than patients whose pressure was elevated both in the clinic and during ambulatory monitoring.

Etiology/Epidemiology

Although the etiology of hypertension remains unknown, risk factors have been identified that serve as initiators or accelerators (Figure 31-1). Genetic or nonmodifiable factors relate to family history, gender, age, and ethnic group. Environmental or modifiable factors relate to nutrition, life-style habits, and the individual's stress profile. Determining the patient's risk for this chronic illness is an important role of the nurse. The relative risk for hypertension

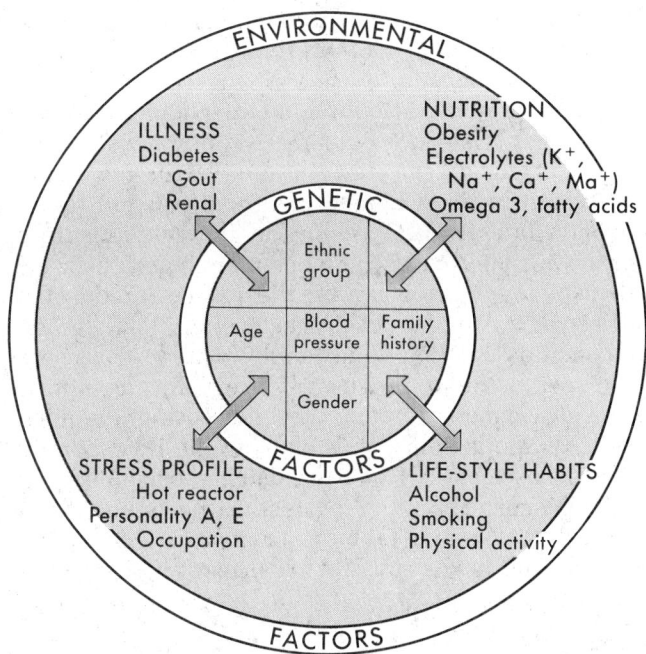

FIGURE 31-1 Factors contributing to hypertension.

depends on the number and severity of modifiable risk factors.

Genetic (nonmodifiable) factors

Family history
Genetic predisposition appears to be associated with elevated intracellular sodium levels and lowered potassium/sodium ratios. This genetic predisposition is particularly prevalent in blacks. Individuals whose parents have hypertension have a greater risk of developing high blood pressure at a younger age. However, even though the familial tendency may be influenced by genetic transmission, it is unclear to what extent genetic elements act in combination with environmental factors.

Gender
Hypertension increases with age in both men and women. However, men experience hypertension at higher rates and at an earlier age than women until after 60 years of age. Men have greater risks than women of both mortality and morbidity caused by cardiovascular disease, and men tend to benefit more from pharmacologic therapy than women.[38] A rapid pulse rate is thought to be a predictor of high blood pressure in men but not in women.[39] Considerable epidemiologic data demonstrate greater prevalence of left ventricular failure and cardiac failure in male patients with hypertension than female patients, but this difference in prevalence disappears following menopause in women.

Those factors significant to high blood pressure in women include use of oral contraceptives, gestational hypertension, postmenopausal estrogen therapy, living alone, attending night school, and experiencing a crisis in the year preceding development of hypertension. Earlier episodic events may cause a woman to be at higher risk for persistent hypertension later in life. Factors in the relationship of oral contraceptive use and postmenopausal estrogen therapy to hypertension are the dosage and duration of estrogen, the use of progesterone, life-style habits such as smoking, and family history. The use of estrogen without the use of progesterone affords cardiovascular protection by increasing the high-density lipoproteins, thus slowing the development of atherosclerosis. However, when estrogen is given with progesterone, this protective mechanism is diminished. Women taking estrogen are encouraged to take the lowest possible therapeutic dosage and not to smoke.

Age

Hypertension occurs across the life span. Age and hypertension are linearly associated in that the arterial blood vessels become less compliant with age, usually because of the buildup of atherosclerotic plaques. Hypertension in childhood and adolescence has great significance to the development of hypertension in later life. Genetics and childhood obesity are two of the best predictors for hypertension in adulthood. Johnson's study showed that body mass was the most consistent predictor of blood pressures in both black and white adolescent females.[11] Risk factors for children who go on to develop adult-onset hypertension include overweight, family history, inadequate physical activity, and increased heart rate and blood pressure with mental stress.

New data suggest that hypertension among American adults is more pervasive than originally thought and the whole population may be at risk. Individuals with "high-normal" blood pressure (systolic 130 to 139 mm Hg or greater or diastolic 80 to 89 mm Hg or greater) are at risk, with 75% to 85% of people experiencing elevations in blood pressure as they move through the middle years.[27]

Black and white males are affected more by hypertension and more severely before 35 years of age; but by 65 years of age the prevalence of hypertension in women exceeds their male counterparts. Not only do women tend to develop hypertension later in life, but also they tend to tolerate it better than men. Women tend to be afflicted more with ISH, with age and weight being the major risk factors. The treatment of hypertension in women has not been shown to be as beneficial as in men.

Sixteen percent of the population will be over 65 years of age by the year 2000. Fifty percent will have a blood pressure reading greater than 160/95 mm Hg, and 20% of hypertensive patients over 55 years of age will have ISH.[25] Systolic hypertension is most prevalent in elderly persons (6% in 60 to 69 year olds; 11% in 70 to 79 year olds; 18% in persons 80 years or older) and is expected to increase to 14.5 million by the year 2025 with the aging population.[22] Factors that contribute to systolic hypertension in elderly persons are included in the box below.

ISH may be more significant as a risk factor for coronary disease, cardiovascular disease, cerebrovascular disease, and cardiac failure.[10] The SHEP (Systolic Hypertension in the Elderly Program) pilot study is the first trial to test the efficacy of antihypertensive drug treatment for persons with ISH in significantly reducing the risk of stroke, lowering the incidence of nonfatal myocardial infarction (MI) and coronary heart disease, and lowering total mortality.[29]

Ethnicity

In the United States the prevalence of hypertension in blacks far exceeds that of whites, and the neglect in treating even mild hypertension in the black population is a more ominous prognosis.[1] One in every three blacks will develop hypertension. Possible explanations for this higher incidence and severity are higher plasma sodium, lower plasma potassium, environmental stressors, and renal lesions—especially nephrosclerosis. In addition, Hispanics are thought to have a high rate of high blood pressure, although studies validating the prevalence is lacking.[19] Death rates for black males and females are higher in the

GERIATRIC CONSIDERATIONS

Hypertension

Aortic distensibility or compliance and the decreased stroke volume and velocity of ejection contribute to hypertension in elderly persons. The diminished compliance from the resistive arterial wall and decreased aortic distensibility found in aged persons contribute to ISH. Other factors associated with aging such as decreased cardiac output and heart rate with increased peripheral resistance, the loss of functioning nephrons, decreased plasma renin concentration, and left ventricular hypertrophy contribute to the development of hypertension.

Aged persons are also at risk because of the number of concomitant diseases (diabetes, renal and heart failure, degenerative diseases) they may have in their later years. Not only are the vessels stiffer, more calcified, and less elastic, but also the complications of hypertension are greater because of the length of exposure to risk factors.

Southeast than in other parts of the United States, in part because of the prevalence of hypertension. Hypertension in black females is significantly higher in the Southeast (44%) than in all other regions.[23] There are also racial differences in terms of response to therapy. For example, weight reduction is very effective in lowering high blood pressure in obese black patients. However, black patients do not obtain the therapeutic response to beta blockers or angiotensin-converting enzyme (ACE) inhibitors found in white patients. Other ethnic groups need further study, since little is known about American Indians, Hispanics, and Asian—Pacific Islanders pertaining to cultural differences and hypertension development.

Environmental (modifiable) factors

Stress profile

Although definitive studies are lacking, it is believed that psychologic factors can chronically alter blood pressure. Stress can increase peripheral vascular resistance and cardiac output and also stimulate sympathetic activity. Stress may be associated with occupational situations, choices, socioeconomic levels, and personality characteristics.

Personality A, the hard-driven, ambitious, time-oriented individual with hidden hostility, has been associated with cardiovascular risks. As early as 1939, Alexander described hypertensive patients as impulsive, hostile, and aggressive.[32] More recently, personality E, the "hot reactor," has been described as characterizing the hypertensive profile. This individual is continually explosive when thwarted in reaching goals. Gentry et al. attributed higher diastolic pressures to both habitually expressed anger and suppressed anger coping styles among both men and women and blacks and whites.[35]

The question of the proposed relationship between blood pressure and personality type remains unanswered. Some individuals diagnosed as having hypertension will have emotional factors, whereas others will not. Although the concept of anger being related to hypertension may not be definitive at this time, studies consistently support the idea that suppressed anger is characteristic of young male patients with borderline hypertension. Other aspects of environment associated with hypertension are urban crowding, combat service, and natural catastrophes, which also suggest the possible role of anger and anxiety in hypertension.[36] Although not a causative agent independent of other considerations, the angry personality may aggravate hypertension.

Occupation

Certain occupations have been characterized as "hypertensive prone" because of the stressful nature of the job. For example, air traffic controllers are often characterized as having severe stress caused by the constant and life-threatening decisions they have to make. Female clerical workers with dissatisfying boss relationships show evidence of more cardiovascular risks. Occupations with high levels of pressure and unsatisfying relationships may be sufficiently stressful to cause muscle tone tension, rapid heart rates, and vasoconstriction.

Socioeconomic status

Another source of stress for specific population groups is their economic level. Groups who are economically deprived often have a high incidence of hypertension. Such factors as poor nutritional habits, low-status jobs, frustration and discontentment, and suppression of hostility contribute to stress-related hypertension.[31] Other factors that may have an impact on one's health include a relatively reduced access to quality health care and poor living conditions.

The economic impact of a therapeutic regimen is an important consideration. Drug therapy can be expensive, ranging from approximately $3.25 to $26 monthly and $100 to $400 yearly depending on the type of medication, such as diuretics or calcium channel blockers. Over 3 decades of a person's life, approximately $9200.00 or more could be spent on antihypertension medication. Being unable to afford drug therapy may result in a decreased level of compliance. Newer drugs tend to cost considerably more. Thus evaluation of newer drugs should include justifying their use in terms of potency, efficacy, and number of side effects in relation to cost.

Nutrition

Nutritional factors have a renewed significance in the control of blood pressure.[26] Caloric and energy expenditure leading to obesity, as well as intake of alcohol, potassium, sodium, calcium, magnesium, and the omega-3 fatty acids, is related to hypertension. A major component in the prevention of hypertension is nutritional, hygienic measures. Hypertension may be a disease of excesses of salt, calories, and alcohol.

The salt controversy is ongoing. The INTERSALT study clearly showed highly significant relations between urinary sodium/potassium excretions and systolic blood pressure.[27] Americans consume between 4 and 6 g of salt daily but need no more than 2 g. Approximately 75% of the daily salt intake comes from food processing, approximately 15% is added at the table, and 10% occurs naturally in foods. The second excess, calories, relates to the body mass index and ratio of waist to hip circumference, which is significantly related to blood pressure elevations. Body mass index is independent of other variables related to blood pressure. Increases in body mass index tend to be associated with age and sedentary life-style. Women have a higher body mass index than men.

Obesity

Obesity independently is a risk factor for cardiovascular disease. Whelton showed weight and salt intake to be the most significant contributors to hypertension.[31] Women who are markedly obese in their fourth decade are seven times more likely to develop hypertension[27]; and the distribution of adipose tissue, particularly when obesity is central or abdominal, confers a higher risk for hypertension.[34] Central obesity is felt to lead to insulin resistance leading to hyperinsulinemia, sodium retention, and an increase in arterial blood pressure. Whereas obesity may not cause hypertension, an association exists between increased weight and an increased incidence of hypertension.[36] This increase may be caused by the increased blood volume associated with weight gain. A loss in weight produces a lower blood pressure. Studies are inconclusive regarding the effectiveness of a limited caloric intake or the sodium restriction that usually accompanies weight reduction.

Nutrients

The HANES studies analyzed the relationship of 17 nutrients to the blood pressure profile of 10,372 American adults, aged 18 to 74 years, providing some of the most significant data on hypertension and cardiovascular disease.[45] Although causality cannot be established, levels of intake of vitamins A and C were implicated as distinguishing hypertensive from normotensive individuals. The Surgeon General's Report on Nutrition of 1988 also noted these same deficiencies in the American diet.[28] From these studies, one can conclude the following:

1. Nutrition deficiencies exist for people with hypertension as compared with those with normal blood pressure.
2. Deficiencies in intake of calcium, potassium, vitamins A and C, and sodium are associated with hypertension (sodium remains controversial).
3. Reduced consumption of dairy products or lower calcium intake is related to hypertension.
4. Controversies remain regarding the role of calcium and sodium in hypertension.

Calcium. Both calcium excess and calcium deficiency have been implicated in several chronic conditions (hypertension, osteoporosis, and cardiovascular dysrhythmias). In hypertension, increased intracellular calcium produces a vasoconstrictive effect, raising the blood pressure. Despite the conflicting evidence, according to Kaplan, "There are good data showing that hypertensives ingest less calcium."[39] Studies indicate that after 10 years of age, most Americans eat well below the recommended dietary calcium allowance.[45] It is reasonable to assume that nurses can help individuals at high risk for hypertension in the maintenance of adequate calcium intake.

Sodium. The role of sodium in hypertension remains controversial. Normotensive subjects do not experience a fall in blood pressure during sodium restriction, and only a proportion of any population on high sodium intake develops hypertension. Therefore the causal relationship is not clear. With a positive history of hypertension, there appears to be a salt-sensitive group, especially among blacks.

Potassium. Various minerals are implicated as being possible causes of hypertension, particularly a deficiency in dietary potassium. By releasing *renin,* potassium activates the angiotensin I to II conversion, retaining sodium and vasoconstricting the arterial network and thus elevating the blood pressure. Repeatedly, hypokalemia is found in untreated hypertensive patients, so it is prudent to encourage individuals to consume more high-potassium foods such as oranges, bananas, and parsley, especially if taking a diuretic, which depletes sodium and potassium.

Life-style habits
Alcohol

As early as 1915 a relationship between alcohol consumption and blood pressure elevations was suspected. Specific guidelines recommend a moderate intake of alcohol and state that more than 2 oz/day can elevate blood pressure. Alcohol on a frequent basis has a positive relationship to blood pressure elevation. Newer studies suggest that drinking frequency may contribute more than the consumption of alcohol to blood pressure elevation.[24] A threshold effect of 1 mm Hg increase appears to exist for those individuals having more than 2 oz of ethanol per day. The exact mechanism of the effect of alcohol on blood pressure is unclear, although increased cardiac output, increased cortisol secretion, increased free intracellular calcium levels, renal vasoconstriction, and cerebrovascular spasms have all been mentioned as possible explanations.

Smoking

The association between smoking and hypertension remains unclear. Initially, smokers may evidence an increase in blood pressure because of the vasoconstriction caused by the nicotine. Chronic smoking is not usually associated with hypertension, although contradictory results have been reported.[14] Smoking cessation may cause an initial slight increase in blood pressure, probably because of weight gain. Women who use estrogen are strongly encouraged to quit smoking. Patients who smoke while receiving antihypertensive agents may require larger dosages of estrogen. Smokeless tobacco is also associated with hypertension, probably because of its high sodium content.[14]

Physical activity

Physical fitness clearly has a role in the prevention and control of hypertension. One large epidemiologic study of Harvard alumni shows an increased incidence of hypertension associated with lack of exercise or exercise levels insufficient to produce positive cardiovascular effects.[46] Blair et al. showed that persons with low physical fitness levels have a relatively increased risk of 1.5% for the development of hypertension when compared with highly fit individuals.[34]

The benefits of exercise include an increase in endorphins, which contribute to one's sense of well-being, and an increase in high-density lipoproteins, which protect against cardiovascular illness. Thus exercise is imperative for patients at risk for hypertension. Also, exercise is one of the best-known stress management strategies. Exercise has been shown to be beneficial in preventing and controlling hypertension through weight reduction, decreased peripheral resistance, and decreased body fat.[8]

Pathophysiology

Primary hypertension

The pathophysiology of primary hypertension remains unknown. Factors involved in the development and regulation of blood pressure are illustrated in Figure 31-2. Systemic arterial blood pressure is determined by cardiac output and peripheral vascular resistance. Therefore a rise in arterial blood pressure reflects an alteration of blood flow in the vascular compartment mediated by changes in cardiac output or alterations in vascular resistance. Mechanisms affecting this rise in blood pressure include a physiologic complex process involving the nervous, renal, and endocrine systems.

Research has shown that hypertension occurs when a greater than normal pressure is required for the kidney to excrete salt and water. Over time, adaptive mechanisms elevate pressure until the level is reached that is required to facilitate normal salt and water excretion. One mechanism may involve a maladaptive response to excessive salt ingestion. As shown in Figure 31-2, varied pathologic responses lead to an increase in intracellular sodium and subsequently increased intracellular calcium.

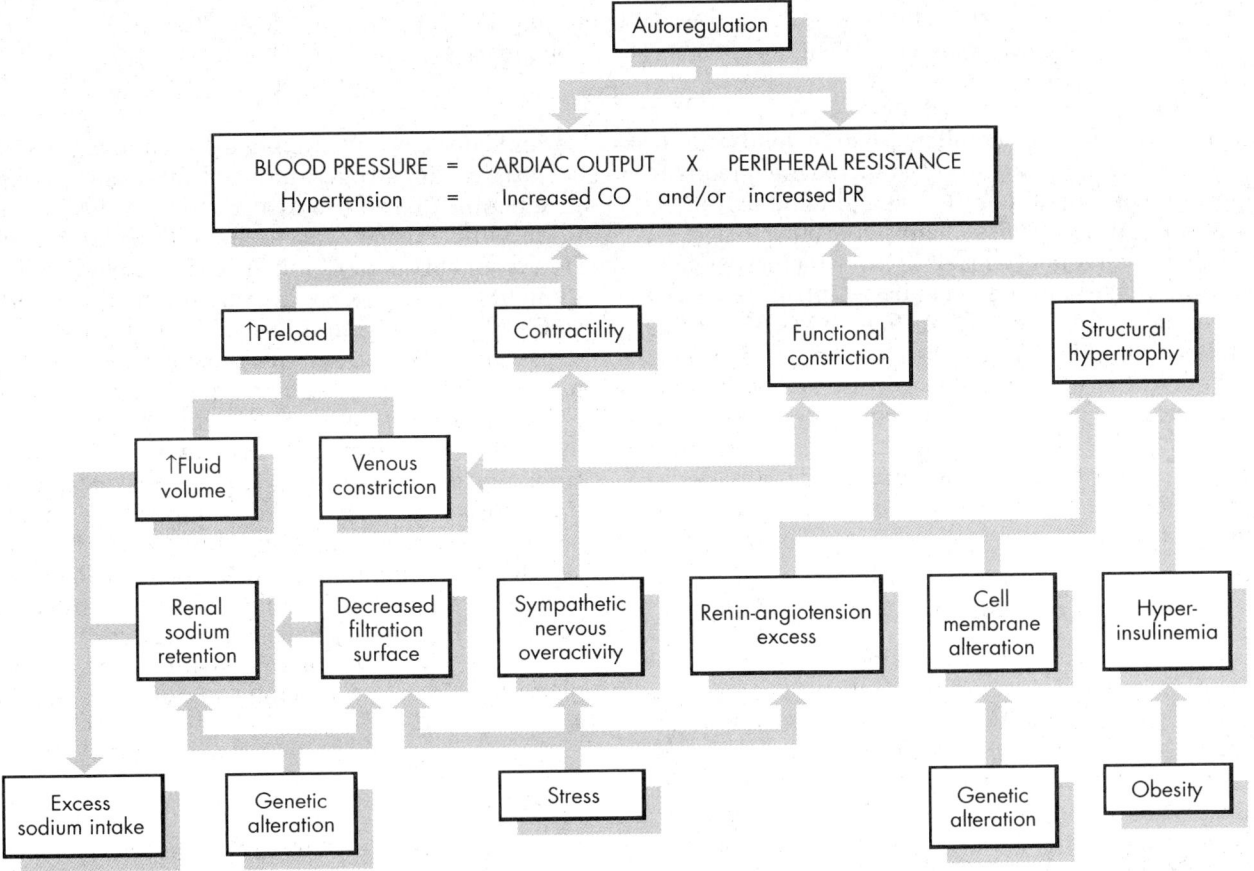

FIGURE 31-2   Factors involved in blood pressure control. (From Kaplan NM: *Clinical hypertension,* ed 5, Baltimore, 1990, The Williams & Wilkins Co.)

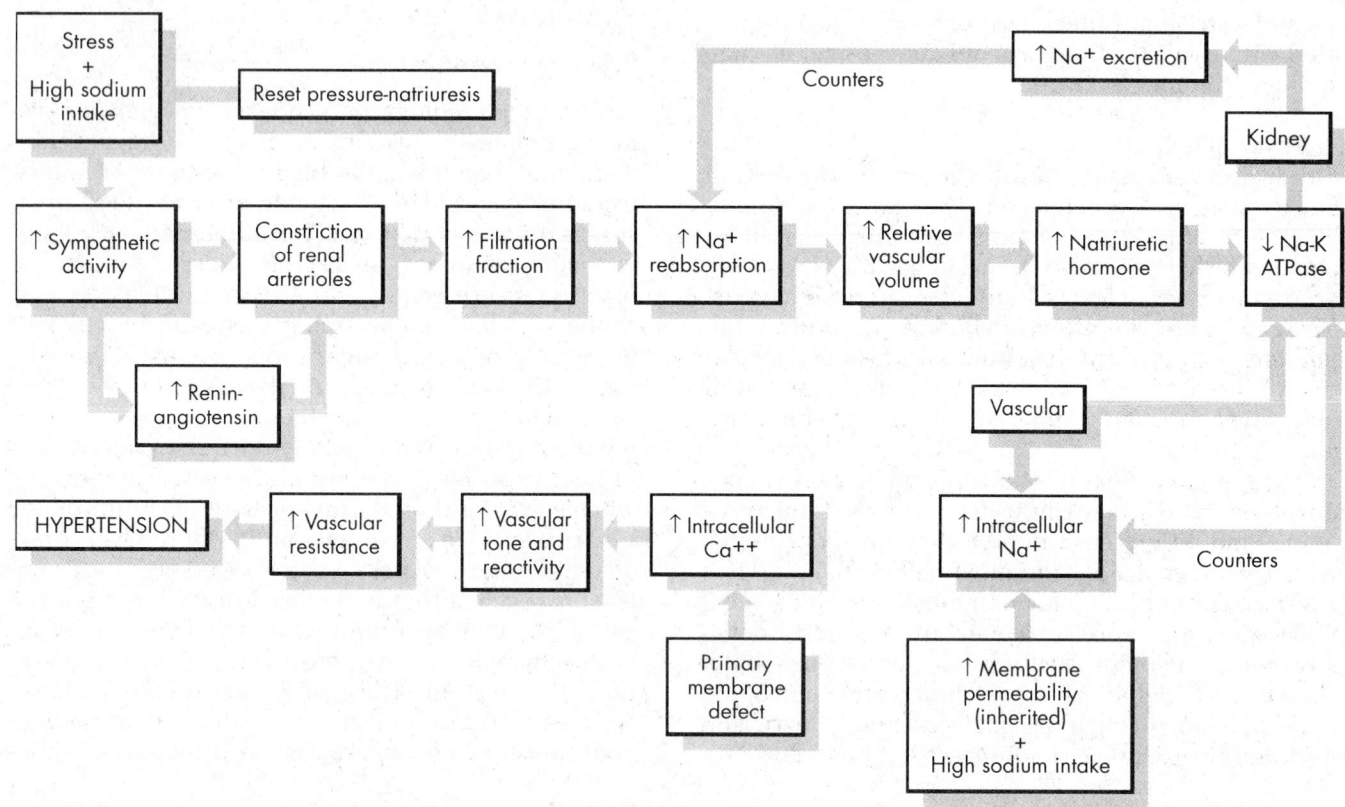

FIGURE 31-3 Pathogenesis of primary hypertension. (From Kaplan NM: *Clinical hypertension,* ed 5, Baltimore, 1990, The Williams & Wilkins Co.)

The increase in intracellular calcium leads to increased vascular tone and resistance, which leads to hypertension. This theory is strengthened by the efficacy of the newest class of antihypertensive agents, the calcium channel blockers. Other factors such as genetics, obesity, and stress may contribute to the development of hypertension (Figure 31-3). Various metabolic and genetic factors may directly increase peripheral vascular resistance by structural hypertrophy of the arterial wall. Chronic stress contributes to hypertension by increases in cardiac output and peripheral resistance mediated by increases in norepinephrine caused by sympathetic nervous system overreactivity.

Secondary hypertension

In cases of secondary hypertension where there are known metabolic or anatomic disturbances, the pathophysiology ultimately depends on the factors in Figure 31-2. For example, renal vascular hypertension, the significant stenosis of a renal artery, can lead to diminished blood flow and subsequent ischemia to that same kidney. This ischemia activates the renin-angiotensin system, which increases peripheral vascular resistance and increases blood pressure. The state of estrogen excess (in pregnant patients and patients taking birth control pills) is associated with estrogen-induced increases in hepatic production of renin substrate. However, most patients with estrogen excess do not develop hypertension from subsequent angiotensin activation. This is thought to be due to concurrent increases in vasodilatory prostaglandins. The recent use of aspirin in pregnancy-induced hypertension suggests a defect in vasodilatory prostaglandins.[2] A variety of endocrine disorders including Cushing's syndrome and hyperaldosteronism are associated with hypertension, probably caused by excessive sodium retention. Patients with pheochromocytoma have increased vascular resistance from direct effects of increased catecholamines. Regardless of the etiology of hypertension, the primacy of the equation BP = CO × PVR (blood pressure equals cardiac output times peripheral vascular resistance) in the pathophysiology of hypertension cannot be overemphasized.

Complications

Untreated hypertension greatly increases the risk for stroke, ischemic heart disease, and renal and cardiac failure. However, therapy with medications also carries undesirable effects such as glucose intolerance and lipid elevations that may increase risk for coronary artery disease. The efficacy and side effects of therapy must be weighed against the complication of untreated hypertension, especially for mild hypertension. The most common complications of untreated hypertension are strokes, premature cardiovascular disease, accelerated atherosclerosis, retinal damage, left ventricular hypertrophy, and renal damage. Stroke, which affects 500,000 victims yearly in the United States, is usually due to lacunar infarcts and hemorrhages.

Premature cardiovascular disease results from untreated or uncontrolled hypertension. This accelerated vascular disease, although unproven, probably occurs by three interrelated mechanisms: exaggerated pulsatile flow, endothelial denudation, and resultant smooth muscle cell replication.[14]

Hypertension may accelerate atherosclerosis. Injury to the arterial wall, thickening and narrowing of vessels, aneurysms in cerebral arterioles, and hemorrhages, as well as thrombus formation, complicate the formation of vascular lesions found in hypertension. These lesions rupture or become occlusive, causing the infarction or ischemic heart disease commonly associated with hypertension.

Chronic compensation for high blood pressure levels results in hypertrophy of the left ventricle. With hypertrophy a compensatory mechanism for increased workload demand, an increased myocardial oxygen demand or need, develops. Over time, the "compensatory mechanism" fails, and coronary insufficiency, decreased myocardial contractility, and congestive heart failure ensue. Left ventricular hypertrophy is associated with an increased risk for sudden death. Detection via a fourth heart sound, electrocardiogram (ECG) changes of a tall T wave and an abnormal P wave indicative of left atrial enlargement, or a diminished ejection fraction predicts a risk for a cardiovascular insult. Negative inotropic agents and after-load reducing agents are commonly recommended to treat hypertension complicated with left ventricular hypertrophy.[3] Thus the level of blood pressure and status of the complications influence how the hypertensive patient is treated.

Finally, renal damage is a major complication of hypertension. This slow and asymptomatic process may not be demonstrable until considerable damage has been done. Hypertension-induced arteriolar nephrosclerosis may be the end result of such injury to the kidneys. Moreover, hypertension can accelerate the course of other renal diseases such as diabetic nephrosclerosis.

Clinical Manifestations

Hypertension is known as the "silent killer," since it has no overt manifestations that can be easily detected. This asymptomatic condition continues until organ damage has been established. Headaches, although commonly regarded as a sign or symptom of hypertension, have not been validated as such but may be associated with nocturnal hypoxia caused by sleep apnea.[13] Headaches appear to be more common among obese and anxiety hypertensive patients. Other associated problems such as epistaxis, dizziness, and fainting are not always symptomatic of hypertension.

Therapeutic Management

Treatment of hypertension in the 1990s is directed beyond just lowering blood pressure. Treatment to date has resulted in a dramatic reduction in mortality from stroke but to a lesser degree in mortality related to coronary artery diseases. Treatment considers the relationship of hypertension to arteriosclerotic heart disease. Drug therapy is considered for its impact on organ perfusion, minimizing the spectrum of cardiovascular risk factors, and the quality of life. Nonpharmacologic measures are directed to prevention, adjunct therapy, and control.

Associated risks and benefits are always best considered before instituting a therapeutic regimen. Convincing evidence exists for the use of antihypertensive agents in lowering the incidence of stroke, congestive heart failure, and progressive renal insufficiency. However, coronary artery disease may actually be worsened by antihypertensives that elevate the serum lipoproteins.[17]

Pharmacologic modalities

Stepped care approach

Traditionally the **stepped care approach** (Figure 31-4), as recommended by the National Committee on Hypertension, has been the standard regimen for the treatment of individuals having a diastolic blood pressure greater than 90 mm Hg despite close observation over several months. Underlying the use of the stepped care approach are the following premises:

1. More success in blood pressure control may be obtained by using low doses of medications with differing therapeutic actions.
2. Intolerable side effects may be avoided by using small doses of several medications rather than a large dose of one medication.
3. The progression to the next step in this approach is required only if the present step is not successful in lowering the blood pressure.

The pharmacologic management of hypertension is directed at lowering or controlling blood pressure with the least amount of medication. In the past, medications have been the major mode of therapy. Greater emphasis is now being placed on nonphar-

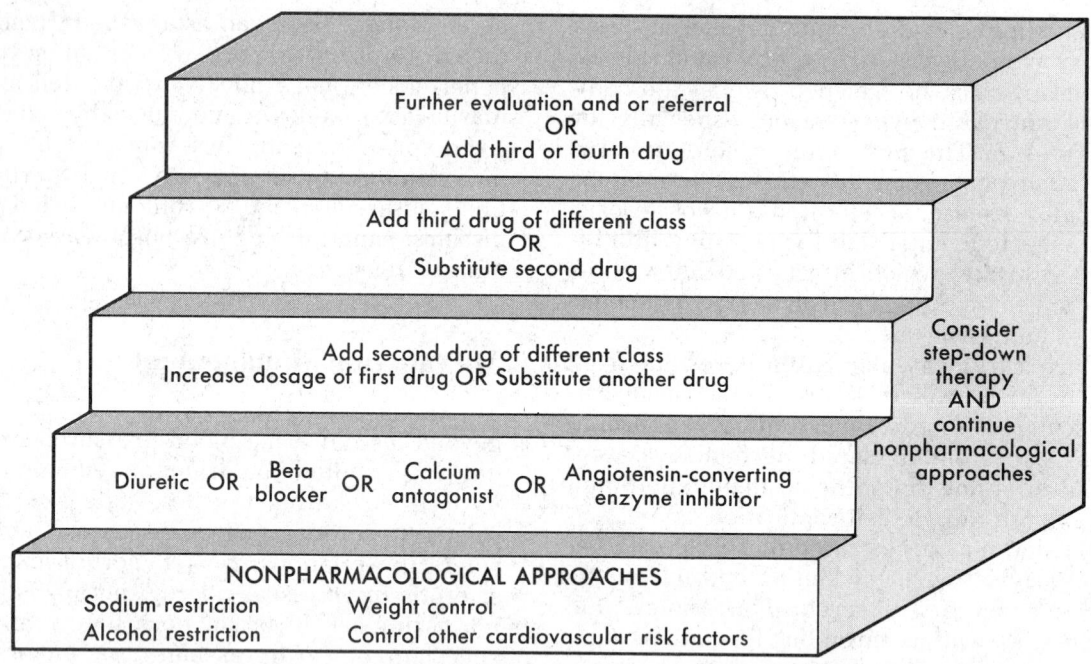

FIGURE 31-4 Stepped care approach. (From Joint National Committee on Detection, Evaluation, and Treatment of High Blood Pressure: The 1988 report of the Joint National Committee on Detection, Evaluation, and Treatment of High Blood Pressure, *Arch Intern Med* 148:1023, 1988.)

macologic approaches by the National Committee on Hypertension.[12]

Antihypertensive agents

Two large categories of drugs are used to treat hypertension: those acting on the kidneys (e.g., furosemide [Lasix]) and those that affect the cardiovascular system (e.g., beta blockers). Antihypertensive agents are classified into five groups: diuretics, adrenergic inhibitors, vasodilators, angiotensin-converting enzyme (ACE) inhibitors, and calcium antagonists. Nurses need to know the specific side effects, precautions (Table 31-1), and drug interactions (see box on p. 733) of the major classifications of drugs.

Diuretics are essential ion transport inhibitors that prevent the reabsorption of bicarbonate, sodium, and chloride. The four classifications of diuretics are thiazides, carbonic anhydrase inhibitors, loop diuretics (see box), and potassium-sparing diuretics.

Thiazide diuretics have been the mainstay of antihypertensive therapy for the last 30 years. These drugs are associated with the significant side effects of hypokalemia, hyperuricemia, hyperglycemia, hyperlipidemia, orthostatic hypotension, and sexual impotence. Diuretics reduce arterial pressure and cardiac output by decreasing vascular resistance.

In some countries the first line of treatment for hypertension is beta blockers. Beta-adrenergic blocking agents have been effective in the treatment of both hypertension and angina. These drugs have a tendency to decrease high-density lipoproteins and increase triglycerides.

Vasodilators tend to decrease peripheral vascular resistance leading to a decrease in left ventricular hypertrophy (positive impact) and stimulation of the sympathetic nervous system (negative impact). These are potent drugs, especially minoxidil, that may precipitate angina and orthostatic hypotension if not carefully monitored. They are used in emergency situations involving severe hypertension but only with extreme caution, since orthostatic hypotension may occur, especially in elderly persons.

Angiotensin-converting enzyme (ACE) inhibitors decrease left ventricular hypertrophy and increase

CLINICAL ALERT

Patients receiving loop diuretics (e.g., furosemide [Lasix]) need to have their potassium levels monitored and supplement their diet with high potassium foods (e.g., bananas, parsley, tea, prunes).

TABLE 31-1   Pharmacology Summary: Antihypertensives

Classification	Benefits/effects	Side effects	Precautions

Diuretics (oral, intravenous)	Old standard for hypertension
	Decreased fluid volume
	Inexpensive
	Effective (especially in blacks and elderly)
	Used in severe hypertension
		Hypokalemia, hyperuricemia, glucose intolerance, hypercholesterolemia, hypertriglyceridemia, sexual dysfunction, weakness; hyperkalemia (potassium-sparing diuretics); gynecomastia, mastodynia, and sexual dysfunction	May be ineffective in renal failure; hypokalemia increases digitalis toxicity; hyperuricemia may precipitate acute gout; may cause an increase in blood levels of lithium patients
			Be aware of lethargy, nocturia, impotence, and social inconvenience of these drugs
			  Take last pill by 6 PM
			  Monitor blood pressure
			  Have patient sit before standing
			  Monitor weight
			  Drink six to eight glasses of water daily
			  Check K^+ levels
			  Have patient restrict Na^+ intake
			  Have patient adhere to high K^+ diet; use K^+ supplement
			  Diabetics may require increase in daily insulin
			Gout patients may need higher doses of drugs to reduce serum uric acid
			Listen for chief complaint: muscle weakness, cramps, dizziness, fatigue, loss of appetite
			Check serum creatinine levels and BUN for renal functioning
			Danger of renal calculi

Adrenergic inhibitors (oral, intravenous)	Potent antihypertensive Effective in young and older ischemic heart disease Decreased Ca^{++} cellular influx Decreased left ventricular hypertrophy	"First dose" syncope, orthostatic hypotension, weakness, and palpitations (tachyphylaxis) Bronchospasm Asthma, nausea, fatigue, dizziness, and headache Peripheral vascular insufficiency Bradycardia, lethargy, insomnia, bizarre dreams, sexual dysfunction, hypertriglyceridemia, decreased high-density lipoprotein cholesterol (except for pindolol and acebutolol), cold extremities, wheezing	Use cautiously in elderly patients because of orthostatic hypotension; needs slow titration Note rash, taste disturbance, and cough Contraindicated in cardiac failure, chronic obstructive pulmonary disease, sick sinus syndrome, and heart block (greater than first degree); use with caution in patients with diabetes Should not be used in patients with asthma, congestive failure Report changes in cardiac heart rate, rhythm, and blood pressure Advise patient not to discontinue abruptly without conversing with physician, rebound hypertension may occur with abrupt discontinuance, particularly with prior administration of high doses or with continuation of concomitant beta-blocker therapy May cause liver damage and positive Coombs' test result Check laboratory results for high-density lipoprotein and triglyceride levels Contraindicated in patients with history of mental depression; use with caution in patients with history of peptic ulcer

Continued.

TABLE 31-1   Pharmacology Summary: Antihypertensives—cont'd

Classification	Benefits/effects	Side effects	Precautions
Vasodilators	Decreased peripheral vascular resistance	Headache, tachycardia, fluid retention, orthostatic hypotension Positive antinuclear antibody (without other changes) Hypertrichosis, ascites (rare)	May precipitate angina in patients with coronary artery disease (CAD) Practically no side effects Monitor blood pressure; have patient sit before standing Lupus syndrome may occur (rare at recommended doses) May cause or aggravate pleural and pericardial effusions
Angiotensin-converting enzyme (ACE) inhibitors (oral, intravenous)	Multiple sites of action Limited side effects Decreased left ventricular hypertrophy Increased renal flow Drug of choice with diabetes mellitus Blunt undesirable effects of diuretics Quality of life	Rash and dysgeusia (rare at recommended doses) Cough, angioneurotic edema	Can cause reversible, acute renal failure in patients with bilateral renal arterial stenosis; neutropenia may occur in patients with autoimmune collagen disorders, and proteinuria (rare at recommended doses); listen for patient complaint of loss of taste or appetite Observe for skin rash and swelling; report Ask patient if awakened at night by coughing Check laboratory values for K^+, BUN, serum creatinine
Calcium antagonists	Low incidence of side effects Effective in cardiac cases (antianginal, Printzmetal) Improved peripheral vascular disease Effective in blacks and elderly patients Decreased peripheral resistance	Headache, hypotension, dizziness, and edema Can aggravate cardiac condition Nausea, edema, constipation	Use with caution in patient with congestive heart failure; contraindicated in first- and second degree blocks; pump failure Monitor heart rate Monitor blood pressure Advise patient to swallow, not chew up pill; advise whether pill is to be taken with or without food

Modified by permission from Joint National Committee of Detection, Evaluation and Treatment of High Blood Pressure: The 1988 report of the Joint National Committee on Detection, Evaluation, and Treatment of High Blood Pressure, *Arch Intern Med,* 148:1023, 1988.

renal flow. ACE inhibitors are effective in reducing blood pressure independently or in combination with diuretics that do not have the adverse effects seen with other antihypertensive agents. To some extent, ACE inhibitors prevent the undesirable effects of diuretics.[30] However, orthostatic hypotension with the first dose is common. The use of ACE inhibitors in the treatment of mild to moderate hypertension is thought to improve the quality of life. Minimal to rare side effects such as cough, rashes, angioedema, and taste disturbances can occur.

Calcium antagonists, or calcium channel blockers, are potent arterial vasodilators, especially useful in older patients and those with low renin levels.[4]

These drugs act to reduce an enhanced calcium influx, which can be brought about by altered smooth muscle cation handling and increased intracellular concentrations of free calcium. Calcium channel blockers decrease peripheral vascular resistance, increase blood flow to the major organs, and decrease blood pressure. They are becoming widely used in the treatment of hypertension and angina.

Life-style modifications

The nonpharmacologic control of essential hypertension is not new. What is different is the preventive vs. curative emphasis and the use of life-style

DRUG INTERACTIONS IN ANTIHYPERTENSIVE THERAPY

Diuretics

Diuretics can raise lithium blood levels by enhancing proximal tubular reabsorption of lithium.

Nonsteroidal anti-inflammatory agents, including aspirin, may antagonize antihypertensive and natriuretic effectiveness of diuretics.

ACE inhibitors magnify potassium-sparing effects of triamterene, amiloride, or spironolactone.

ACE inhibitors blunt hypokalemia induced by thiazide diuretics.

Sympatholytic agents

Guanethidine monosulfate and guanadrel sulfate: ephedrine and amphetamine displace guanethidine and guanadrel from storage vesicles. Tricyclic antidepressants inhibit uptake of guanethidine and guanadrel into these vesicles. Cocaine may inhibit neuronal pump that actively transports guanethidine and guanadrel into nerve endings. These actions may reduce antihypertensive effects of guanethidine and guanadrel.

Hypertension can occur with concomitant therapy with phenothiazines or sympathomimetic amines.

Monoamine oxidase inhibitors may prevent degradation and metabolism of released norepinephrine produced by tyramine-containing food and may thereby cause hypertension.

Tricyclic antidepressant drugs may reduce effects of clonidine and guanabenz.

Beta blockers

Cimetidine may reduce bioavailability of beta blockers metabolized primarily by liver by inducing hepatic oxidative enzymes. Hydralazine, by reducing hepatic blood flow, may increase plasma concentration of beta blockers.

Cholesterol-binding resins (i.e., cholestyramine and colestipol) may reduce plasma levels of propranolol hydrochloride.

Beta blockers may reduce plasma clearance of drugs metabolized by liver (e.g., lidocaine, chlorpromazine, coumarin).

Combinations of calcium channel blockers and beta blockers may promote negative inotropic effects on failing myocardium.

Combinations of beta blockers and reserpine may cause marked bradycardia and syncope.

ACE inhibitors

Nonsteroidal anti-inflammatory drugs, including aspirin, may magnify potassium-retaining effects of ACE inhibitors.

Calcium antagonists

Combinations of calcium antagonists with guanidine may induce hypotension, particularly in patients with idiopathic hypertrophic subaortic stenosis.

Calcium antagonists may induce increases in plasma digoxin levels.

Cimetidine may increase blood levels of nifedipine.

From Joint National Committee on Detection, Evaluation, and Treatment of High Blood Pressure: The 1988 report of the Joint National Committee on Detection, Evaluation, and Treatment of High Blood Pressure, *Arch Intern Med* 148:1023, 1988. Copyright 1988, American Medical Association.

changes for 3 to 6 months for mild hypertension. Kaplan stresses that "nondrug therapies may provide enough antihypertensive effect to lower blood pressure to a safe level without the need for antihypertensive drugs."[38]

According to Kaplan, the nonpharmacologic therapies advocated are (1) weight reduction if one's body weight is excessive; (2) dietary sodium restriction to 2 g/day (88 mmol/day); (3) alcohol limitation to 1 oz/day, as contained in two usual portions of wine, beer, or spirits; (4) regular aerobic exercise; (5) dietary potassium intake increase; (6) calcium and magnesium supplementation; (7) more dietary fiber and less saturated fat; and (8) some type of relaxation therapy.[14] The evidence for benefit is considerably stronger for the first four modalities.

Weight reduction

Weight loss usually entails a total behavior change involving metabolic rate, emotional state, value structure, perception of and attitudes toward food, self-concept, and one's locus of control. The assistance of groups such as Weight Watchers, which provide the necessary social support, education, motivation, counseling, and instruction in behavioral modification, may be helpful (see Chapter 16).

Sodium restriction

Limiting processed foods, added salt, and foods preserved with sodium (canned foods, carbonated drinks, juices, and cereals) constitutes only a few of the easily modifiable diet changes that individuals can make to lower their sodium consumption. The preference for salt may be lost as early as 2 weeks following diet modifications. It is important to know the sodium content in foods. Reading food labels is imperative. Many fast food institutions provide the nutrient content of their products as do labels on

LIFE-STYLE MODIFICATIONS FOR HYPERTENSION

- Lose weight, if patient is more than 10% above ideal weight.
- Limit alcohol intake to no more than 1 oz of ethanol (i.e., 2 oz of liquor, 8 oz of wine, 24 oz of beer) per day.
- Get regular aerobic exercise (e.g., a 30- to 45-minute brisk walk) three to five times per week.
- Cut sodium intake from the average 150 mmol/L (150 mEq/L) to less than 100 mmol/L (100 mEq/L) per day (less than 2.3 g of sodium or 6 g of sodium chloride).
- Include the recommended daily allowances of potassium, calcium, and magnesium in the diet.
- Stop smoking.
- Reduce dietary saturated fat and cholesterol.

From the Joint National Committee on Detection, Evaluation, and Treatment of High Blood Pressure (JNC): *Evaluation and treatment of high blood pressure,* Washington, DC, 1992, National Institutes of Health.

drinks (e.g., 58 mg/oz), cereals (e.g., 220 mg/oz), and canned and frozen foods. Sodium chloride may be the significant culprit associated with blood pressure elevation; thus knowing whether the sodium on a particular food is sodium chloride, sodium bicarbonate, or another sodium derivative is important.

Alcohol consumption

The 1988 "Report of the Joint National Committee on Detection, Evaluation, and Treatment of High Blood Pressure" specifies restricting one's alcohol consumption to no more than 30 mL (1 oz) of ethanol daily; that is, 60 mL (2 oz) of 100-proof whiskey or 240 mL (8 oz) of wine or 720 mL (24 oz) of beer.[11]

Anger modulation

Anger modulation consists of cognitive reappraisal, social skills training, social support, and exercise. Cognitive reappraisal involves rethinking of the situation that prompted a feeling of anger through the use of self statements. For example, changing the statement, "I'd like to slap you" to "I won't waste my energy. It's not worth it." Social skills training is a combination of behavioral techniques such as assertiveness training, problem-solving/decision-making sessions, and relaxation training. The use of behavioral techniques has been shown to be effective for some individuals as a nonpharmacologic approach. Changing perceptions and attitudes about a situation and directing one's energy into a constructive activity such as exercise may have a positive impact on one's health status.

Stress management involves modifying the "hot reactor" response of instant anger and hostility. Deep chest breathing can be effective in controlling stressful situations. Patel and Marmot showed a positive effect of relaxation on blood pressure.[20] This approach can serve as an adjunct to medication or a nonpharmacologic approach for mild hypertension. The five steps to relaxation (comfortable position, slow rhythmic chest breathing, deep concentration, repetitive sound, and tension release) can be practiced at home or at the office. Other forms of relaxation such as yoga, meditation, and biofeedback can also be helpful in controlling hypertension.

NURSING MANAGEMENT OF THE PATIENT WITH HYPERTENSION
Assessment

The detection, screening, and follow-up of patients with hypertension commonly rest with the nurse. The appropriate focuses of the nursing history, examination, and laboratory analysis are indicated in the box on p. 735. The nurse may conduct the initial history and physical examination of the patient in the primary care setting.

The blood pressure reading is the sole determinant of hypertension and should be measured three consecutive times before making a diagnosis of hypertension. Having one's blood pressure measured is a critical event in light of the lifetime implications. Thus every effort should be made to eliminate errors. Sources of error in taking blood pressure measurements are noted in the box on p. 736.

Six criteria have been established by the Joint National Committee on Detection, Evaluation, and Treatment of Hypertension to ensure accurate blood pressure measurement.[12] These techniques are as follows:

1. Patients should be seated with their arm bared, supported, and positioned at heart level. They should not have smoked or ingested caffeine within 30 minutes of measurement.
2. Measurement should begin after 5 minutes of quiet rest.
3. The appropriate cuff size must be used to ensure an accurate measurement. The rubber bladder should encircle at least two thirds of the arm. Several sizes of cuffs should be available.
4. Measurements should be taken with a mercury sphygmomanometer, a recently calibrated aneroid manometer, or a validated electronic device.
5. Both the systolic and diastolic blood pressures should be recorded. The disappearance of sound (phase V) should be used for the diastolic reading.

NURSING ASSESSMENT FOR HYPERTENSION

Blood pressure Lying   Day 1 _____   Day 2_____   Day 3 _____
              Standing
Asymptomatic _____
Associated complaints: Headache _____   Blurred vision_____
              Vertigo _____   Nocturnal frequency_____
              Flushed face _____   Pedal edema_____
              Epistaxis _____
Concomitant diseases: Heart disease _____   Visual disturbances_____
              Renal disease _____   Sleep disorders_____
              Endocrine/diabetes _____
Risk factor profile: Age _____   Gender_____   Ethnic group_____
           Occupation _____
           Life-style: Alcohol_____
                 Cigarettes: Number/day_____for_____years
                 Exercise_____30-40 min 3-4×/week
                 Personality type _____
Family history: Hypertension _____
           Cardiovascular (strokes)_____
           Renal _____
History of blood pressure changes
   Knowledge of blood pressure level
   Last reading: Date_____   Time _____
   Diagnosis_____
Nutritional history (24-hour recall)_____
   Na$^+$ _____   Ca$^+$ _____   Weight_____   Height_____
   Anthropometric measures_____
Pharmacologic history
   Name _____   Drugs (over-the-counter)
   Amount_____   Allergy medicines
   Frequency_____   Diet medicines
   Side effects_____   Cold medicines
   Length taken_____   Steroids
                            Other (please name) _____

Teaching/learning needs
   Knowledge _____
   Behavior change skills_____
   Dietary _____
   Exercise_____
Attitudes, beliefs, feelings about hypertension_____
Physical examination and laboratory analysis
   K$^+$ _____   Na$^+$ _____
   Hematocrit, hemoglobin_____
   Urinalysis_____   BUN _____   Creatinine_____
   Cholesterol: HDL_____   LDL _____   Triglycerides_____
   Glucose level _____
   ECG_____
Therapeutic effect (outcome measures)
   Quality of life   Cost
   Functional status   Adherence
   Sexual history   Satisfaction

ERRORS IN MEASURING BLOOD PRESSURE

Instrument error

Inaccurate sphygmomanometer

Inaccurate cuff size (child vs. adult; obese vs. thin)

Observer error

Inadequate rest period before measurement and anxiety possibly caused by the "white coat phenomenon"

Inaccurate readings: missing auscultatory gap, confusion about muffling, dysrhythmias

Improper position: bladder not centered over artery, arm not at heart level, or arm without support

Failure to take three readings at three different visits

Failure to control extraneous factors: talking, bladder distension, pain, or recent eating, smoking, medications, or exertion

Unconscious prejudice about reading patient expects to hear

6. Two or more readings should be averaged. If the first two readings differ by more than 5 mm Hg, additional readings should be obtained.

Korotkoff in 1905 defined the five phases of blood pressure commonly referred to today. These phases are as follows: phase I is the initial tapping sound heard for at least two consecutive beats and referred to as the systolic pressure. Phase II is the auscultatory gap where sounds may become swishing, creating a period of turbulent sounds as much as 40 mg Hg, especially in hypertensive individuals. Phase III is the resuming of sounds. Phase IV is where sounds become muffled, and phase V is the complete cessation of sounds or the diastolic pressure in adults.[13]

The critical thinking guide (Figure 31-5) helps the nurse decide how to manage the patient's care based on the Joint National Commission's recommended protocol for specific blood pressure levels. Although the hypertensive patient is usually asymptomatic, the nurse should inquire about associated complaints as well as concomitant diseases related to hypertension.

Assessment of the patient's risk factors helps the nurse identify the patient's risk for developing hypertension (Table 31-2). The nurse can use this information to help the patient make decisions about interventions to decrease the risk. For example, a nutritional history identifies eating habits, such as caloric or sodium intake, related to hypertension. Weight and skin fold, or anthropometric measures, help to determine the body mass index or percent-

TABLE 31-2   Risk Assessment for Hypertension

	Low risk	Moderate risk	High risk
Family history	No		Yes
Sex	Female below 60 years	Male below 35 years	Female below 60 years
			Male above 60 years
Age	Below 35 years	Below 35 years	Above 60 years
Ethnic group	White		Black
Stress and attitude		Personality A	Personality A
		Personality E	Personality E
Occupation			Air traffic controller
			Secretary
Life-style habits	Nonsmoker	Moderate smoker	Heavy smoker
	Moderate alcohol	No alcohol	Heavy alcohol
	Adequate physical activity	Little physical activity	No physical activity
Nutrition			
Sodium	1 to 2 g Na$^+$ daily	2 g Na$^+$ daily	Above 4 g Na$^+$ daily
Calcium	800 to 1000 mg daily	325 to 500 mg daily	Below 325 mg daily
Weight	Normal weight	Less than 20% overweight	More than 20% overweight

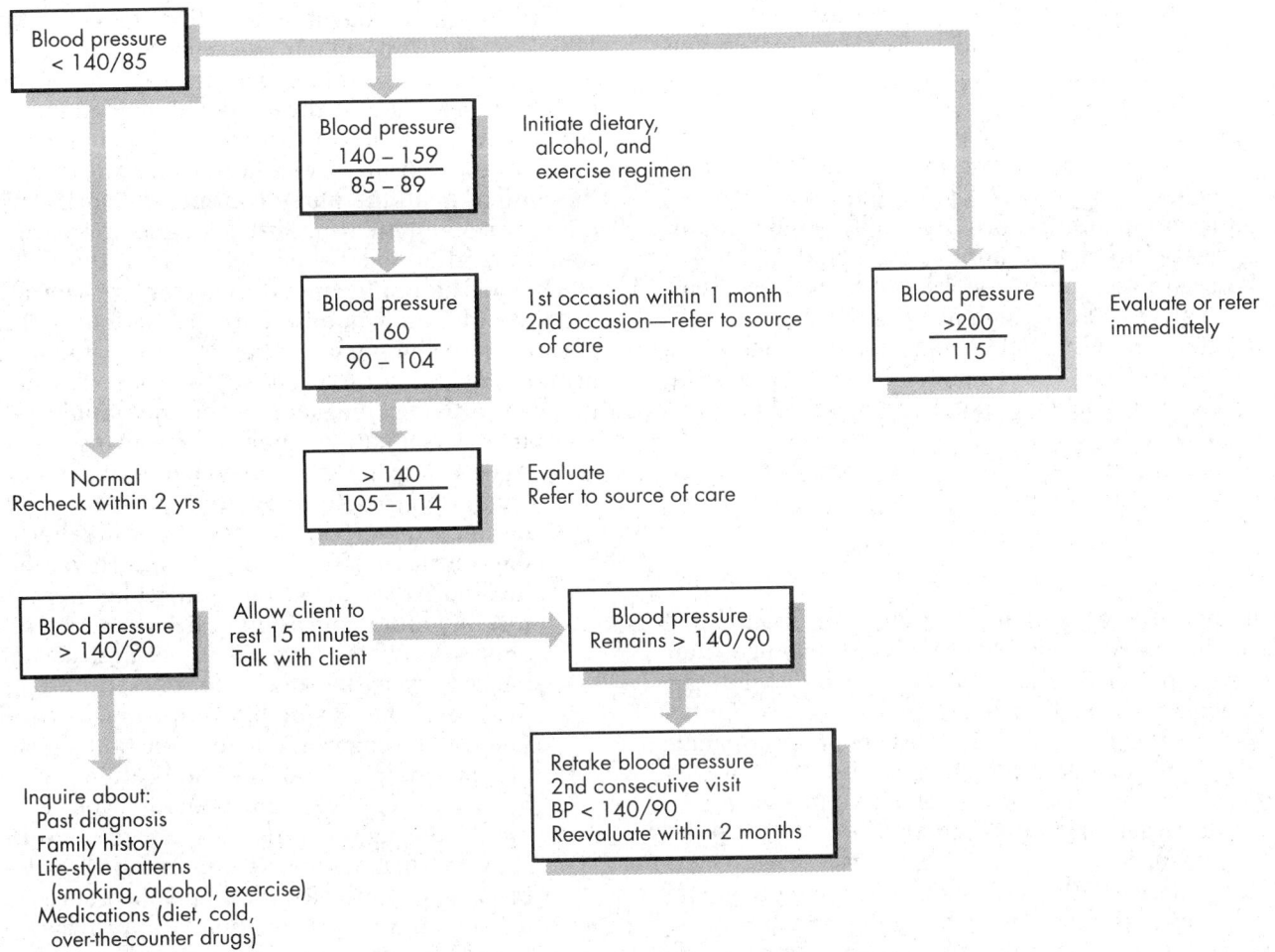

FIGURE 31-5   Critical Thinking Guide: hypertension.

age of fat of the body. Since obesity is an independent risk factor for hypertension, these outcome measures are critical.

The patient's pharmacologic history is evaluated during the initial examination. Patients may need to be assisted in knowing the name of the drug, the amount, frequency of taking the drug, and side effects. Any side effects and the length of time patients have been taking the medicine need to be noted. Also, it is important to note over-the-counter drugs and other medications the patient takes. Follow-up examination may assist to evaluate the effectiveness or outcome measure of both pharmacologic and non-pharmacologic regimens. These outcome measures also consider the cost, quality of life, sexual problems, adherence, and satisfaction with the treatment.

The physical examination gives further validation of what is suspected. Other findings, specifically cardiovascular changes, may indicate complications of hypertension such as left ventricular hypertrophy,

congestive heart failure, arteriolar nicking, and papilledema. In addition, laboratory assessments give the nurse clues of complications of other primary body systems that may be associated with hypertension.

It is important to listen to a patient's feelings about being hypertensive, changes for the patient and family, and potential needs for follow-up. A follow-up assessment to determine the effectiveness of the therapeutic regimen and the presence of side effects of medications is part of the nursing assessment. The nurse assesses for patient problems regarding quality of life, adherence, economics, sexual functioning, and satisfaction with therapy.

Nursing Diagnosis

Depending on the initial or follow-up assessment of the patient with hypertension, common diagnoses include the following:

Altered health maintenance related to lack of

knowledge and skills for hypertension control such as lack of physical activity, lack of relations

Noncompliance related to side effects and cost of medications

Knowledge deficit related to lack of prior experience with disease process and treatment protocols

Altered nutrition: more than body requirements, related to high sodium, calorie, and fat intake

Altered tissue perfusion related to increased vascular resistance, high nicotine intake, etc.

Ineffective individual coping related to perceived limitations of being labeled hypertensive or inability to believe that life-style modifications are needed

High risk for sexual dysfunction related to medication side effects

Planning

Nursing interventions are directed toward helping patients control their blood pressure, change their life-style patterns, and enhance their independence and control through self-care measures in conjunction with the prescribed medical regimen. Specific goals might include the following:

Modification of life-style behaviors to lessen risk for target organ damage or to lower the blood pressure

Compliance with medication regimen without significant side effects or economic constraints

Being knowledgeable about hypertension, the therapeutic regimen, potential risks and side effects of the pharmacologic measures, and the use of nonpharmacologic measures

Diet with recommended levels of calcium, sodium, calories, and reduced cholesterol

Recognition of side effects and ability to take appropriate steps to deal with them

Verbalization of fears and anxieties about hypertension using appropriate stress management strategies to control them

Establishment and maintenance of an adequate level of exercise

Implementation

Nurses help patients develop the skills needed or refer patients to groups that can foster behavioral changes. Also, the nurse encourages the patient to assume an active role in therapy through contracting or voicing intentions to make appropriate changes. Patients are given opportunities to explore, problem solve, and make responsible decisions; the nurse guides them in these endeavors. Nurses need to discover any barriers to adherence before they instruct patients to modify their life-style.

Restoring a sense of control is important and can be encouraged by having the patient take responsibility for recording blood pressure daily or weekly and monitoring the number and type of health protective behaviors and the medication regimen prescribed. A self-monitoring record for documentation may be appropriate. Telephone calls and cards to the patient from the nurse continue to clarify information, convey a caring attitude, and increase the commitment and active participation of the patient.

The decision to begin antihypertensive therapy is usually a lifetime commitment for a patient. It is imperative that the nurse, as patient advocate and educator, answer the patient's questions thoroughly before the patient engages in therapy. Subjects for the nurse to evaluate include the following:

1. Age: young people have higher renin levels compared to older individuals, and the cardiac output is inversely related to age (higher cardiac output in younger patients). Also, older individuals may have left ventricular hypertrophy and other concomitant diseases such as diabetes mellitus, lung diseases, and coronary heart disease that may interact with the pharmacologic therapy in different ways. The nurse needs to be cognizant of and constantly observing for side effects of the medications.

2. Weight: excessive weight tends to occur with increasing age. Losing this weight has been shown to be an effective nonpharmacologic approach to decreasing blood pressure. The nurse can support and make appropriate referrals for the patient who wishes to join a weight reduction group.

3. Level of blood pressure: mild hypertension may be treated nonpharmacologically initially or with less potent medications; severe hypertension requires more aggressive treatment. Nurses play a major role in teaching nonpharmacologic hypertension reduction skills to patients.

4. Sex: impotence is known to be a major side effect of some diuretics; therefore some men may be less likely to comply with the prescribed regimen. Nurses need to conduct a sexual assessment and determine the reasons patients do not comply with the prescribed treatment plan.

The nurse can easily initiate several nonpharmacologic interventions including reduction of dietary fat, calories, cholesterol, sodium, and alcohol; exercise to promote fitness; stress management; and smoking cessation.

For patients to make informed decisions regarding their care, they may need help from nurses in considering the issues regarding quality of life, economics, mortality and morbidity, and adherence.

Quality of life is defined as the fulfillment of goals in a normal life. This concept is perceived differently

NURSING CARE PLAN   *The Patient with Hypertension*

Nursing diagnosis/ Expected outcomes	Interventions	Rationale
Knowledge deficit related to lack of prior experience with disease process and treatment protocols • *Patient will be able to explain causes, risk factors, treatment, and complications of hypertension*	Teach patient about what hypertension is; risk factors, causes, treatment approaches, long-term complications, life-style modifications, relationship of treatment to control of complications	Knowledge of the disease process can help patients make informed decisions about treatment choices and life-style modifications
Altered health maintenance related to lack of knowledge and skills for hypertension control • *Patient will be able to explain reasons for prescribed treatments and demonstrate correct skills for medication administration and taking own blood pressure*	Teach patient how to take own blood pressure Help patient obtain necessary equipment Teach patient reasons for use of each treatment and medication Teach patient how each medication is taken Help patient plan medication schedule consistent with daily activities Teach nonpharmacologic measures to control hypertension (e.g., exercise, stress management, smoking cessation)	Monitoring one's own blood pressure promotes self-care and involvement in health care; convenience and accessibility will encourage patient participation in changing health behaviors When patients have requisite knowledge and skills they will have more confidence in carrying out necessary treatments Patient will be more willing to follow a treatment plan that is tailored to life-style and routines and involves the least amount of change
Noncompliance related to side effects and costs of medications • *Patient will take medication as prescribed* • *Patient will notify health care provider of problems with administration*	Teach patient expected side effects of medications Teach patient which side effects to report to health care provider Teach patient about measures to prevent side effects (e.g., potassium supplements) Refer patient to appropriate social services for financial assistance	Patients are more likely to adopt new health behaviors when they have the necessary knowledge, skills, and resources to make decisions
Altered nutrition: more than body requirements related to high sodium, calorie, and fat intake • *Patient and family will select foods consistent with dietary plan to control calorie, sodium, and fat intake* • *Patient will maintain desired body weight*	Provide sample meal plans and food guides Teach patient relationship of calorie, sodium, and fat intake to control of blood pressure and complications Help patient set realistic weight loss goals (e.g., 1 or 2 lb/wk) Refer patient and family to weight control support groups	Including family members and organized support groups can help patient make changes in eating habits Realistic goals will help patient maintain motivation in changing eating habits
Ineffective individual coping related to perceived limitations and life-style changes • *Patient will be able to demonstrate coping skills to support life-style changes*	Help patient identify support system among family, friends, co-workers, and health care providers Allow patient time to verbalize concerns about diagnosis and treatment Help patient identify personal strengths Help patient learn new stress management skills (e.g., exercise, assertiveness training, meditation, relaxation)	Talking to a concerned listener can help patient with problem solving and anxiety reduction Identifying strengths can help patient in building a positive self-image Learning new skills for stress management can add to feeling of self-control

ETHICAL ISSUES

What kind of support should the nurse offer a patient who decides to refuse treatment for hypertension because it may make him impotent? because it does make him impotent?

RESEARCH BRIEF

Schmieder RE et al: Antihypertensive therapy: to stop or not to stop, *JAMA* 265:1566-1571, March 27, 1991.

Discontinuance of antihypertensive therapy is not generally considered. This meta-analysis of 19 studies gave evidence that a relatively small group of patients who may benefit from discontinuance were those patients who had made major life-style changes such as weight loss or reduced sodium and alcohol consumption, at the time of medication discontinuance. Patients with severe hypertension and combination therapy did not consistently maintain normal blood pressure after discontinuance of their medication. It is reasonable to assume that mild hypertensives, most especially women who make major life-style changes and receive estrogen replacement, may be able to delay or lessen their medication regimen. More studies need to be conducted in this area.

THERAPEUTIC COMMUNICATION GUIDE

The Patient with Hypertension

1. Acknowledge patient's anger through reflection and clarify the nurse's role and purpose.

Example: Patient: "Look Ms. Carter, I came to the hospital to see the doctor, not some nurse. I'll talk to the doctor about my medications."

Nurse: "Ms. Jones, I think you are upset about seeing me today instead of your doctor. Dr. Solomon has requested I speak with you about your medication regimen. Would you like to talk about this?"

2. Reflect message, enlist patient's cooperation, offer an alternative.

Example: Patient: "No, I want to see my doctor. He's the only one who knows about me and is qualified to treat me."

Nurse: "I know you expected to see Dr. Solomon. He and I work together as a team. It would really help the doctor and me to treat you if we could talk about your medication. Otherwise, I can schedule a meeting in 2 weeks with Dr. Solomon."

---

by each individual and has become very significant to the hypertensive patient because of the known adverse effects of antihypertensive agents. In the case of hypertension, therapy is initiated to prevent the complications of an asymptomatic illness. However, the therapy itself can cause substantial ill effects (depression, sexual dysfunction, hypokalemia). Thus patient's perception of quality of life may be evaluated when assessing compliance and reporting to a physician who chooses one medication over another and to justify treating or not treating mild or borderline hypertension. Adherence rates may be strongly associated with a patient's perception of a change in the quality of life after having been placed on a specific therapeutic regimen.[39]

Adherence or compliance is the extent to which an individual's actual behavior coincides with the prescribed behavior. Adherence rates vary, but the lack of adherence is particularly evident in the case of antihypertensive agents, in which side effects are often blamed for such low rates of adherence. Other factors that may affect adherence relate to the provider/patient relationship and the psychosocial and demographic characteristics of the patient.[5,43]

In addition to monitoring for side effects of the drugs, nurses will make direct (urine assay, blood chemistry) and indirect (self-reports, pill counts, refills, appointment keeping) assessments of compliance/adherence. Nurses can enhance compliance/adherence through reminders, contracts, self-monitoring records, tailoring interviews to the patient's needs, reinforcement, use of support systems, and making home visits. Active patient involvement is an essential requirement of increasing adherence.

PATIENT EDUCATION GUIDE

Hypertension

Health protective behaviors and hypertension

Directions: Health protective behaviors are activities that may lessen or help prevent or control hypertension. You may contract with your health care provider to begin at least one weekly.

1. Exercise (one of the best protective behaviors for all illnesses)
   a. Walk at least 2 miles four times weekly, attaining 75% of target heart rate
   b. Swimming, jogging, and aerobic exercise of any type are also acceptable (Target heart rate = 220 − Age × 0.75)
2. Nutrition:
   a. Avoid sodium and maintain calcium, potassium, magnesium; eat fresh or frozen rather than canned foods (e.g., oranges, bananas, broccoli, collards)
   b. Restrict sodium intake to no more than 2 g daily
   c. Maintain adequate calcium intake of at least 1000 mg daily (e.g., yogurt, calcium supplement)*
   d. Maintain adequate potassium intake of at least 40 mEq or 1585 mg daily (parsley, tea, and fresh fruits)
   e. Maintain adequate magnesium intake of at least 375 mg daily

f. Avoid pork (especially cured) and fast foods
g. Drink no more than two cups of caffeinated coffee daily (use decaffeinated)
h. Drink no more than one carbonated drink daily (use 100% lemon juice instead to promote a natural diuresis)
3. Relaxation
   a. Build resistance to stress through exercise, relaxation, and nutrition
   b. AAABC: *A*void stress, *A*lter stress, *A*ccept stress, *B*uild resistance to stress, *C*hange perception of stress*
   c. Sleep 7 to 8 hours nightly
   d. Practice one stress reduction technique daily for approximately 20 minutes (e.g., yoga, meditation, progressive relaxation, exercise)
   e. Ventilate: gain a support person to whom you can express your feelings
4. Habits (substitute constructive for nonconstructive behaviors)
   a. Avoid or quit smoking*
   b. Take no more than 2 oz whiskey, 8 oz wine, or 24 oz beer daily*
   c. Maintain appropriate weight for age, sex, body frame*

From Kirkpatrick MK: Self-care guide for hypertension risk reduction, *AAOHN* 35:254, 1987.
*Very important.

The less complicated the regimen, the more likely adherence will be attained. An effective way to improve adherence is through the use of an in-hospital or in-clinic educational program.[9]

Teaching/learning skills are imperative in that the nurse can assist the patient to gain the knowledge, skills, and life-style changes essential to any therapeutic regimen. This self-care approach gives the nurse an opportunity to make a difference in the outcome of the therapeutic regimens. Also, by determining the attitudes and feelings that the patient has about hypertension, the nurse gains clues about the patient's level of motivation to adhere to the therapeutic regimen (see patient education guide).

Evaluation

Attaining an appropriate blood pressure with a minimum of side effects is the primary goal that will prevent complications. Other outcome measures such as the patient's satisfaction and quality of life are im-

portant, since this illness extends over a lifetime. Demonstrating knowledge of one's condition, medications, and necessary life-style changes is inadequate, since the patient must make the actual behavioral changes to prevent or control hypertension. Thus evaluation of behavioral changes from destructive to constructive behaviors is essential. Nurses evaluate the outcome of the educational interventions based not on knowledge change but on change in the number of health protective behaviors and risk reduction behaviors practiced and the control of blood pressure within acceptable limits.

Documentation

Documentation of care for the patient with hypertension relies on the accurate recording of blood pressure. Implementing measures to avoid errors is imperative. Documentation of adherence as evidenced by the blood pressure reading, weight change, 24-hour dietary history, cholesterol level, pill count, and self-monitoring record can serve as objective evidence of adherence. Goal setting by the patient can help in evaluating progress toward specific outcomes and may be more significant than the objective evidence.

Another area for documentation relates to the learning needs of and knowledge gained by the patient but, more important, to the patient's behavior changes. Documentation of carrying out the plan and evaluation of the effectiveness of the teaching are integral parts of the nursing care plan. A self-reported record can be monitored so the nurse can help identify areas of difficulty in attaining a specific goal and the actual behavioral or life-style change.

Ongoing Care

The responsibility for continual monitoring for the remainder of the hypertensive patient's life is shared by the patient, nurse, and physician. Continued assessments are made monthly, biannually, or annually depending on difficulties and patient experiences.

Classifications of blood pressure and follow-up criteria have been specified by the 1988 National Committee on Detection, Evaluation, and Treatment of High Blood Pressure (Table 31-3). Both first and second follow-up visits are specified. The nursing interventions have also been specified for each blood pressure level.

Patient education is an ongoing role assumed by the nurse. This educational responsibility entails frequently updating the patient regarding educational materials and community resources. The nurse fosters patient independence and increased self-care. Assessing for complications is done throughout the life span of the patient.

CRITICAL THINKING QUESTIONS

1 Briefly describe the differences between primary and secondary hypertension.
2 Which type is the most common, and what are the signs and symptoms?
3 Describe the benefits and risks of engaging in an antihypertensive regimen.

TABLE 31-3   First-Occasion Measurement of Blood Pressure

Range (mm Hg), category*		Recommended follow-up†	Nursing interventions
DIASTOLIC			
Below 85	Normal blood pressure	Recheck within 2 years	Teach patient what blood pressure is
85 to 89	High normal blood pressure	Recheck within 1 year	Introduce patient to health protective behavior checklist
90 to 104	Mild hypertension	Confirm within 2 months	Institute nonpharmacologic measures, referring patient to weight reduction, exercise, or other appropriate group(s)
105 to 114	Moderate hypertension	Evaluate or refer promptly to source of care (within 2 weeks)	
115 or higher	Severe hypertension	Evaluate or refer immediately to source of care	Monitor blood pressure and adherence to therapeutic regimen
SYSTOLIC WHEN DIASTOLIC IS BELOW 90			
Below 140	Normal blood pressure	Recheck within 2 years	
140 to 159	Borderline isolated systolic hypertension	Confirm promptly (within 2 months)	Reinstitute health protective behavior checklist
160 or higher	Isolated systolic hypertension	Evaluate or refer promptly to source of care (within 2 weeks)	

Used with permission from *Arch Intern Med,* May 1988.
*A classification of borderline isolated systolic hypertension (systolic 140 to 159 mm Hg) or isolated systolic hypertension (systolic above 160 mm Hg) takes precedence over a classification of high normal blood pressure (diastolic 85 to 89 mm Hg) when both occur in the same person. A classification of high normal blood pressure (diastolic 85 to 89 mm Hg) takes precedence over a classification of normal blood pressure (systolic below 140 mm Hg) when both occur in the same person.
†If recommendations for follow-up of diastolic and systolic blood pressures are different for those aged 18 years or older, the shorter recommended time period supersedes, and a referral supersedes a recheck recommendation.

4 Which nonpharmacologic interventions might the nurse initiate appropriate to the patient's condition?

5 What risk factors does the nurse assess when interviewing a hypertensive patient?

6 Define white coat, resistant, and isolated systolic hypertension.

7 What are the major complications of hypertension?

8 Identify two classifications other than diuretic drugs used in the treatment of hypertension, and describe what they do.

9 Describe the role of nutrition in the development of hypertension.

10 List at least four controversies or issues that surround hypertension and its treatment.

11 List three studies that have particular relevance to the present knowledge of hypertension.

12 What is meant by the self-care, nonpharmacologic approaches to hypertension? Specify two times when these may be particularly useful.

13 List three specific behaviors that hypertensive patients should exhibit.

14 Through what three strategies can adherence be enhanced?

15 What outcome measures are necessary for evaluating a patient with hypertension?

16 Around which five major areas does a teaching plan for a hypertensive patient center?

17 What effect does the health care provider have on the accuracy of blood pressure measures?

18 Why should diuretics be administered in the morning?

19 What are health protective behaviors? What health protective behaviors can a patient do to lessen risk of developing hypertension or as an adjunct to a therapeutic regimen?

20 What are five questions to consider when teaching a patient about hypertension?

21 Describe how hypertension develops based on the formula HBP = CO × PR.

22 What skills are important for the nurse to possess when teaching the use of nonpharmacologic approaches to blood pressure control?

RESOURCES

1 American Heart Association Literature
"About High Blood Pressure"
"About High Blood Pressure in Children"
"About Your Heart and High Blood Pressure"
"Buying and Caring for Home Blood Pressure Equipment"
"High Blood Pressure"
"High Blood Pressure Fact Sheet"
"High Blood Pressure in Teenagers"
"How You Can Help Your Doctor Treat High Blood Pressure"

National organizations associated with hypertension

1 National High Blood Pressure Committee National Institutes of Health, Bethesda, MD 20814 (301) 951-3269

2 National High Blood Pressure Education Program Health and Human Resources, Washington, DC

BIBLIOGRAPHY

Current

1. Atinkugbe OO: World epidemiology of hypertension in blacks, *J Clin Hyperten* 3:15, 1987.
2. Benigni A: Effect of low-dose aspirin on fetal and maternal generation of thromboxane by platelets in women at risk for pregnancy induced hypertension, *N Engl J Med* 321(6):357-362, 1989.
3. Borhani NO: Left ventricular hypertrophy, arrhythmias and sudden death in systematic hypertension, *Am J Cardiol* 60(17):13I-18I, 1987.
4. Buhler FR, Kiowski W: Calcium antagonist in hypertension, *J Clin Hyperten* 5(suppl 3):3, 1987.
5. Cameron R, Best JA: Promotion adherence to health behavior change in recent findings from behavioral research, *Patient Educ Counseling* 10:139, 1987.
6. Crump WJ: Nonpharmacologic treatment of hypertension: implementing lifestyle changes, *Fam Pract Recert* 13(10):46-50, 1989.
7. Department of Health and Human Services: *Healthy people 2000*, Washington, DC, 1990, US Government Printing Office.
8. Francis KT: The role of endorphins in exercise: a review of current knowledge, *J Ortho Sports Phys Therapy* 4(3):169, 1990.
9. Gonzalez-Fernadez RA et al: Usefulness of a systematic hypertension in-hospital educational program, *Am J Cardiol* 65(20):1384-1386, 1990.
10. Hall JE: Abnormal pressure natriuresis: a cause or a consequence of hypertension? *Hypertension* 15(6, pt 1):547-559, 1990.
11. Johnson EH: The relationship of anger expression to health problems among black Americans in a national survey, *J Behav Med* 10(2):103-116, 1987.
12. Joint National Committee on Detection, Evaluation, and Treatment of High Blood Pressure: The 1988 report of the Joint National Committee on Detection, Evaluation, and Treatment of High Blood Pressure, *Arch Intern Med* 148:1023, 1988.
13. Jolly A: Taking blood pressure, *Nurs Times* 87(15):40-43, 1991.
14. Kaplan NM: *Clinical hypertension*, ed 5, Baltimore, 1990, The Williams & Wilkins Co.
15. Lee TL, Goldman L, co-editors: Measuring pressure around the clock, *Harvard Heart Letter* 2(8):2, 1992.
16. Lifton RP et al: A chimaeric II beta-hydroxylase/aldosterone synthage gene causes glucocorticoid-remediable aldosteronism and human hypertension, *Nature* 355:262-265, Jan 16, 1992.

17. Lindholm LH: Cardiovascular risk factors and their interactions in hypertensives, *J Hyperten* (Suppl) 9(3):s3-6, 1991.

18. Mason DT: Antihypertension therapy and the concept of total cardiovascular protection, *Am J Cardiol* 60:29E, 1987.

19. Pappas G et al: Hypertension prevalence and the status of awareness, treatment, and control in the Hispanic Health and Nutrition Examination Survey (HHNANES), 1982-84, *Am J Pub Health* 80(12):1431-1436, 1990.

20. Patel C, Marmot M: Stress management, blood pressure and quality of life, *J Hyperten* 5(suppl 1):521, 1987.

21. Powers M, Jalowiec A: Profile of the well-controlled, well-adjusted hypertensive patient, *Nurs Res* 3612:106, 1987.

22. Reisin E: Sodium and obesity in the pathogenesis of hypertension, *Am J Hyperten* 3(2):164-167, 1990.

23. Rocella EJ: Progress of and lessons learned from the National Blood Pressure Education Program, *Patient Educ Counseling* 6(3):103-4, 1984.

24. Russell M: Alcohol drinking patterns and blood pressure, *Am J Pub Health* 81(4):452, 1991.

25. Ryan CL, Pappas RA: Prenatal exposure to antiadrenergic antihypertensive drugs: effects on neurobehavioral development and the behavioral consequences of enriched rearing, *Neurotoxicology Teratology* 12(4):359-365, 1990.

26. Simopoulos AP: The relationship between diet and hypertension, *Compr Ther* 16(5):25-30, 1990.

27. Stamler J et al: Cardiac status after four years in a trial on nutritional therapy for high blood pressure, *Arch Intern Med* 149(3):661-665, 1989.

28. Surgeon General's Report on Nutrition: *Nutrition.* Department of Health and Human Services publication, Washington, DC, 1988, US Government Printing Office.

29. Schron EB: The systolic hypertension in the elderly program: implications for nursing practice and research, *Prog Cardiovasc Nurs* 4(4):138-45, 1989.

30. Weinberger MH: Sodium chloride and blood pressure, *N Engl J Med* 317:1084, 1987.

31. Whelton A: Ambulatory monitoring of blood pressure, *Hosp Pract* 26(suppl 2):13-19, 1991.

Classic

32. Alexander F: Emotional factors of essential hypertension: presentation of tentative hypothesis, *Psychiatr Med* 1:173, 1939.

33. Baum C et al: Drug use in the United States in 1981, *JAMA* 251:1293, 1985.

34. Blair SN et al: Physical fitness and incidence of hypertension in healthy normotensive men and women, *JAMA* 252:487, 1984.

35. Gentry WD et al: Habitual anger-coping styles. I. Effect on mean blood pressure and risk for essential hypertension, *Psychosom Med* 44:195, 1982.

36. Havlik RJ, Fenleick M: Epidemiology and genetics of hypertension, *Am J Epidemiol* 4(suppl 111):121, 1983.

37. Haynes SG, Feinleib M: Women, work, and coronary heart disease: prospective findings from the Framingham heart study, *Am J Pub Health* 70:133, 1980.

38. Kaplan NM: Non-drug treatment of hypertension, *Ann Intern Med* 102:359, 1985.

39. Kaplan NM: *Clinical hypertension,* ed 4, Baltimore, 1986, The Williams & Wilkins Co.

40. Lawrence L, McLemore T: *1981 summary: national ambulatory medical care survey: advance data.* DHHS Pub No (PHS) 83-1250, Washington, DC, 1983, National Center for Health Statistics.

41. Levine S, Croog SH: Quality of life and patient's response to treatment, *J Cardiovasc Pharmacol* 7:S132, 1985.

42. McCarron DA et al: Blood pressure and nutrient intake in the United States, *Science* 224:1392, 1984.

43. McCord MA: Compliance: self-care or compromise, *Top Clin Nurse* 7:1, 1986.

44. Multiple Risk Factor Intervention Trial Research Group: MRFIT: risk factor changes and mortality results, *JAMA* 248:1465, 1982.

45. National Center for Health Statistics: *Health and nutrition examination survey I (HANES I and II).* DHEW Pub (1979), PHS 79-1658 (1977), (HRA) 77-1310, Washington, DC, Department of Health, Education and Welfare.

46. Paffenbarger RS: Physical activity and incidence of hypertension in college alumni, *N Engl J Med* 117:245, 1983.

47. Ploeg H et al: The role of anger in hypertension, *Psychotherapeutics* 43:186, 1985.

48. Strasser T, Ganten D: *Mild hypertension: from drug trials to practice,* New York, 1986, Raven Press.

49. Whitehead WE et al: Anxiety and anger in hypertension, *J Psychosom Res* 21:383, 1977.

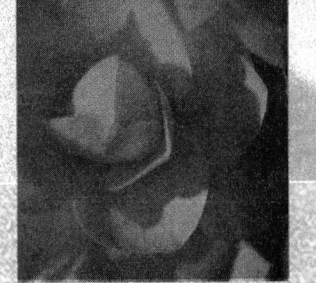

CHAPTER THIRTY-TWO

Nursing Management of Adults with Venous or Lymphatic Disorders

LEARNING OBJECTIVES

1 Identify common disorders of the venous system.
2 Recognize clinical manifestations in the individual with chronic venous insufficiency.
3 Discuss nursing diagnoses commonly associated with venous insufficiency.
4 Discuss nursing interventions appropriate in venous insufficiency.
5 Describe the nursing management for a patient having medical or surgical treatment for varicose veins.
6 Identify risk factors associated with the development of deep-vein thrombosis (DVT) and/or pulmonary embolus (PE).
7 Relate principles of nursing management to the care of the patient receiving anticoagulants.
8 Recognize the signs and symptoms of complications of anticoagulation, including heparin-induced thrombocytopenia and warfarin skin necrosis.
9 Discuss the clinical manifestations of DVT and PE and their sequelae.
10 Discuss the clinical manifestations of the patient with lymphatic disorders.
11 Identify patient risk factors for complications in lymphatic disorders.
12 Relate principles of nursing management to the care of patients with lymphatic disease.

EFFECTS of gravity on the body are very evident in the veins of the legs. Venous disease is divided into acute and chronic conditions. The acute conditions are life-threatening, and the chronic ones are lifetime aggravations. One can look upon varicose veins as hemorrhoids of the legs; both are venous conditions secondary to a human's ability to move in the upright position. Individuals can have any combination of vascular diseases in one limb. Chronic venous stasis and chronic lymphedema are frequently concurrent entities. It is not unusual to find absent arterial pulses in a leg plagued by venous stasis, since both arterial and venous disease are more common in the elderly patient. The treatment of patients with combinations of arterial and venous disorders becomes more complex because the treatment of one problem often compromises the treatment of the other. Patients with chronic venous or lymphatic disease require a great deal of information. The burden of care rests with them. They must be made aware that the battle against these diseases is lifelong.

VARICOSE VEINS
Definition

Varicose veins are superficial veins that are dilated and tortuous as a result of nonfunctional valves or venous hypertension. They appear just under the skin as bulbous, often corkscrewed vessels. Varicose veins are either primary or secondary, with the distinction between the two diagnoses being critical to planning treatment strategies. Primary varicose veins are those that develop from faulty venous architecture, and secondary varicose veins occur as a result of injury to the venous system.

Etiology/Epidemiology

In the United States 15% to 20% of all adults have varicose veins. Seventh in a health survey of chronic diseases, varicose veins are approximately nine times as common as arterial disease in the United States. More women than men are affected. Many situations contribute to the development of varicose veins. Jobs that require prolonged standing are conducive to varicose veins. Obesity increases the probability of development as a result of external compression of the main veins in the pelvis. Pregnancy, with uterine compression of the pelvic veins and increased venous pressure in the legs, is a contributing factor. Heredity may have some role in varicose veins, with a weakened vein wall structure being the primary culprit. Other factors include trauma, abdominal tumors, and Klippel-Trenaunay syndrome (rare). Spider veins or the larger reticular veins are not varicose veins. They are more superficial and may appear as starbursts or fine red or blue lines in

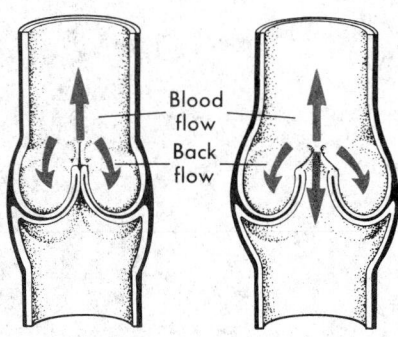

FIGURE 32-1   Venous valve incompetence causing reflux of blood in varicose veins.

the skin. They are not harmful but may cause mild discomfort such as aching. Spider veins may be a result of heredity or injury.

Pathophysiology

There are two types of varicose veins—primary and secondary. Primary varicosities are the most common and occur in the superficial veins with no components of deep-vein abnormality. These tend to occur early in life or following pregnancy or trauma. Primary varicosities are a result of incompetent valves of the superficial venous system. An increase in hydrostatic pressure from the long column of blood extending from the inferior vena cava to the saphenous vein causes the blood to reflux (go backward) through the incompetent (nonfunctioning) valve to the area of the next competent valve (Figure 32-1). At this place it stops and the vein dilates. Side branches of the saphenous vein above the competent valve become dilated, and the branches may not be capable of withstanding this increase in pressure. Over time, they stay dilated when the patient is standing erect. Trauma over a competent valve may render it nonfunctional, and dilation may continue. Incompetency of the valves in the perforating veins connecting the superficial and deep venous systems also occurs. Pregnancy or any condition that increases intraabdominal pressure raises the pressure in the column of blood, and the back force on the vein increases, causing an increased incidence of varicose veins. In addition, hormonal changes in pregnancy decrease the compliance of the vein wall.

Secondary varicose veins are a result of an earlier episode of deep venous thrombosis or incompetence of the deep vein or the perforator system (Figure 32-2). After these occur the blood cannot return via the deep system of veins (or part of it), and the blood is shunted to the superficial veins, resulting in dilation. Long-term presence of secondary varicosities can result in postphlebitic syndrome.

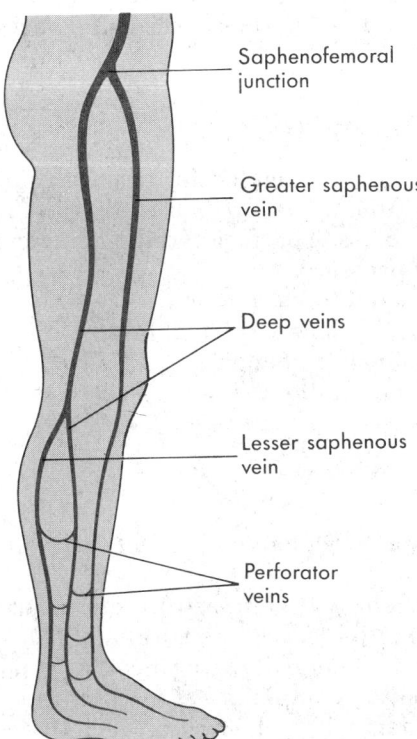

FIGURE 32-2   The deep and the superficial veins drain the lower extremity. The two systems are connected by perforator veins in ladder-like fashion so that the blood will be shunted into the deep system if it is competent and if the superficial veins are compressed. Likewise, if the deep system is blocked by old phlebitic injury, the blood will be shunted to the superficial system if the perforator valves are incompetent.

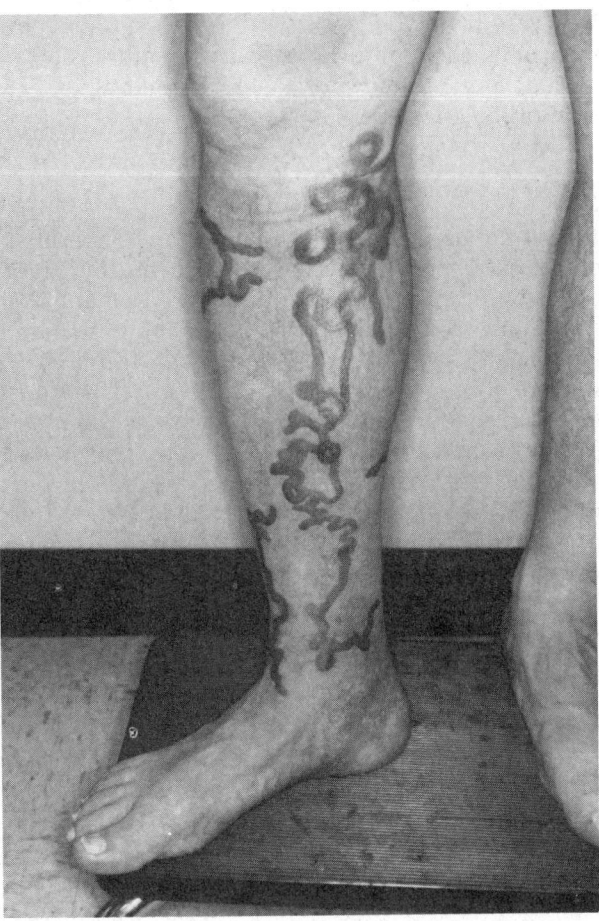

FIGURE 32-3   A patient with varicose veins marked for surgery. Note the tortuous nature of the veins.

Clinical Manifestations

Clinical manifestations vary with the number and severity of the varicosities as well as whether the varicosities are primary or secondary. Some symptoms are common to both. Complaints may vary from distress over the cosmetic appearance of the leg to edema and severe pain. Varicose veins may be merely dilated or may appear bulbous and corkscrewed. In mild, symptomatic cases, the patient complains of heaviness, aching, and edema after prolonged standing. Occasionally, itching occurs. These symptoms are generally relieved by elevating the feet. Itching and edema disappear overnight. In secondary varicose veins the pain may come on in shorter periods, and edema may occur soon after rising. Postphlebitic changes may also be present and will be discussed under that section. Bleeding may occur spontaneously from a varicosity or secondary to trauma, and the patient may be fearful of recurring episodes.

Therapeutic Management

Medical management

Treatment is aimed at decreasing the venous pressure in the legs. Elevating the feet when sitting or lying, increasing the calf pump action of the leg by walking to assist venous return, wearing support hose, and avoiding prolonged sitting or standing all help attain this goal. Weight-reduction advice is important if obesity is a contributing factor. The patient is advised not to cross the legs at the knee for long periods because it impedes venous return.

Sclerotherapy is a nonsurgical treatment of varicose and spider veins. Treatment is appropriate in patients with unsightly or symptomatic veins and in whom the valves at the saphenofemoral junction are competent. A sclerosing agent (chemical irritant) is injected in the vein. Types of medications used include hypertonic saline, Sotradecol (sodium tetradecyl sulfate), aethoxysclerol, and hyperosmolar salt-sugar solution. Following injections, some form of compression is used for a specific time. Compression may vary from an elastic wrap to full-support pantyhose at 30 to 40 mm Hg pressure. Compression time varies from 24 hours to weeks, depending on physician preference.

Surgical management

Increased use of veins for peripheral arterial and coronary artery bypass has decreased the incidence of stripping of an asymptomatic greater and lesser saphenous vein. The dilated and nonfunctional vein cannot be used for bypass and is still frequently removed. Vein ligation and/or stripping is an outpatient procedure. Before surgery the veins are marked while the patient is standing. This is necessary because once the patient is recumbent on the operating table, the veins flatten and disappear (Figure 32-3). Incompetent perforators are also marked.

During surgery the incompetent veins are either ligated (tied off) or stripped (removed). Multiple small incisions allow easy access to the vein. Closure of the incisions may be with steristrips, sutures, or staples. These are removed in 5 to 10 days, depending upon location of the incisions and surgeon preference. After surgery, the leg is dressed with a compression dressing from foot to groin, or a prescription surgical support hose is applied. The purpose of this compression is to decrease oozing or hematoma formation. Compression is maintained for 3 to 5 days. Ambulation is allowed immediately after surgery and is encouraged.

NURSING MANAGEMENT OF THE PATIENT WITH VARICOSE VEINS

Assessment

History taking includes patient and occupational history as well as family history of varicose veins, any trauma to the leg, history of pregnancies, and any history of phlebitis. Questions regarding family history of clotting problems identify the patient at risk for congenital coagulation disorders (such as antithrombin III and protein C or S deficiencies) and identify the person who may have secondary varices. Identification of behaviors that place the patient at risk for discomfort or complications from varicosities is essential. Alteration of these behaviors is incorporated in planning.

Physical assessment is performed with the patient standing, and veins are inspected from the groin to the foot. The ankle area is examined for skin changes, and the calves are measured to determine any difference in circumference. Assessment of edema and the results of examination are recorded. The time of the examination is important to record because symptoms of secondary varicosities tend to occur earlier in the day. Any discussion of difficul-

ties with body image because of the varicosities is explored.

Nursing Diagnosis

Nursing diagnoses related to varicose veins may include:

Impaired tissue perfusion related to increased venous pressure

Pain related to tissue edema

Knowledge deficit related to treatment options and life-style changes

Alteration in body image related to unsightly veins

Planning

Interventions are planned to meet the following outcomes:

The patient will demonstrate and practice measures to increase venous return

Pain and edema will be reduced as evidenced by decreased complaints of discomfort

The patient will verbalize knowledge of treatment options and necessary life-style changes

Implementation

Rationale for compression of varicose veins is explained to the patient. Diagrams may be helpful to illustrate anatomy and illustrate the rationale of treatment. If prescription hose are ordered, demonstrating the application and removal of the hose is helpful (Figure 32-4, A). If the patient has poor hand strength or arthritis, the nurse explains that there are commercially available devices ("butlers") that may help (Figure 32-4, B). These devices do not require strength to apply the stockings.

For the patient undergoing sclerotherapy, written instructions are helpful. The nurse explains activity restrictions and comfort measures to postoperative patients. Instructions vary from surgeon to surgeon but may include frequent ambulation, elevation of the legs above the heart if the ankles become edematous, and avoidance of tub baths. Showers are generally permitted after 24 to 48 hours. Elevation of the extremity is helpful for the first 24 hours after these procedures, and vigorous activity should be avoided. Some surgeons may restrict heavy lifting (more than 25 lb) but this is not universal.

It is important that patients are aware that there will be scars and ecchymoses following surgery. The areas of discoloration may take several weeks to fade, but warm baths (once permitted) assist in softening the incisions and relieve the discomfort. After injections, the areas treated may be firm, tender, and discolored. Most of this resolves in a few weeks, but some residual brown staining may persist. Patients who have sclerotherapy must be made aware that they may need to return periodically for more injections in other areas.

Evaluation

Evaluation of the therapeutic treatment is done at the follow-up visit. The incisions/injection areas are examined and healing noted. Any additional areas that may need to be injected are recorded. Small clots in injected dermal varicosities may be removed with an 18-gauge needle. This is done by puncturing the vein and "rolling" the clot out of the vein through the puncture. Patient awareness of risk factor modification and restrictions on activity must be assessed at this visit. The necessity for further follow-up will be emphasized and the patient evaluated for knowledge. Encourage the patient to continue wearing support hose of some type and elevate the legs whenever possible.

SUPERFICIAL THROMBOPHLEBITIS
Definition

Thrombophlebitis is the presence of a clot in the vein with accompanying inflammation. There are two types that will be discussed, superficial phlebitis and deep-vein thrombosis. **Superficial thrombophlebitis** is a clot in a superficial vein with inflammation of that vein. It is not normally a result of an infective process. It is a fairly common and seldom serious problem. It usually affects the superficial veins in the extremities.

Etiology/Epidemiology

Superficial phlebitis occurs spontaneously, or secondary to some form of trauma. Trauma can be from an intravenous (IV) line, injection of irritating solutions (such as potassium or antibiotics), or a blow to the vein or varicosity. Intravenous drug abusers often have superficial phlebitis. Dehydration may contribute to development of superficial phlebitis secondary to increased blood viscosity.

Approximately 125,000 cases of this condition are reported yearly in the United States. It is more common in older patients and three times more common in women than in men. Patients who have recurrent bouts of superficial thrombophlebitis, especially at a young age, are evaluated for inherited coagulation disorders.

Clinical Manifestations

A patient may first voice complaints of discomfort in a specific vein. Physical examination may reveal warmth, redness, tenderness, and swelling. It may be possible to palpate the vein as a cord for some distance around the tenderness. As long as the area is superficial and distant from the groin (saphenofemoral junction), clinical assessment only is needed, and no intervention may be necessary. If the area is close to the groin, evaluation to rule out deep venous thrombosis is necessary, and that evaluation is discussed on p. 751.

In some cases, infection may be present. Suppurative thrombophlebitis may be evident as pus at the IV site and signs of general sepsis. Suppurative thrombophlebitis is usually a more systemic problem and not related to benign superficial thrombophlebitis.

Therapeutic Management

If there is an obvious cause for the patient's phlebitis, such as an IV line, it must be removed. Otherwise, treatment is symptomatic and supportive. Comfort measures such as warm soaks, elevation of the affected part, and nonsteroidal antiinflammatory agents may be given. Some patients may benefit from elastic support over the area. Antibiotics are not generally ordered. The patient must be assessed in a few days to be certain that the phlebitis is subsiding. Patients with coagulation disorders may require more aggressive treatment.

NURSING MANAGEMENT OF THE PATIENT WITH SUPERFICIAL THROMBOPHLEBITIS
Assessment

The patient is often the first to identify a local problem as discomfort in the area. Nursing assessment includes inspection of the skin for redness, swelling, heat, and boundaries of pain. Redness will follow the course of the vein. If the area is close to the groin, the physician is notified.

Nursing Diagnosis

Diagnoses for the patient with superficial thrombophlebitis include:
   Pain related to an inflammatory process
   High risk for anxiety related to fear that the clot will break loose and go to the lungs
   High risk for infection

Planning

Nursing care is planned to achieve the following outcomes:
   Pain will be decreased
   The patient will verbalize understanding that this type of clot does not usually migrate

Redness, heat, and swelling in the area will be reduced or eliminated

Implementation

The nurse provides comfort measures such as warm moist soaks to the affected part. Assistance in elevating the area is given. If ordered, pain medication or nonsteroidal antiinflammatory drugs may be ad-

TABLE 32-1   DVT Predisposing Factors

Factors	Examples
Immobilization	Paralysis
	Operating room time >2 hr
	Bedridden or chairbound
	Long plane or car rides
Disease processes	Sepsis
	Hematologic disorders
	Malignancy
	Congestive heart failure
	Myocardial infarction
Pressure	Obesity
	Pregnancy
	Tumor
Trauma	Fractures
	Venipuncture
Clotting dysfunction	Antithrombin III deficiency
	Proteins C and S deficiency
	Disorders of plasminogen activators
	Anticardiolipin disorders
	Abrupt heparin withdrawal
Surgical procedures	Orthopedic (hip pinning)
	Neurologic (craniotomy)
	Urologic (transurethral resection)
	Gynecologic (hysterectomy)
Other	Dehydration
	Advancing age
	Prior thrombosis or thromboembolic event
	Oral contraceptives/hormone replacement

ministered. Outpatients who are self-medicating are advised to take these medications with food and not to take more than the prescribed dosage. They are also warned to advise their physician of any increase in the number of affected veins, any chest pain, or shortness of breath. If the patient has involvement of the lower extremities, modified bed rest may help. Once symptoms decrease, activity is then encouraged to assist with venous return.

Nursing measures specific for preventing the development of this problem include elevation of the legs when patients are sitting, aseptic technique when inserting IV lines, changing IV sites according to hospital protocol, avoiding administration of irritating substances in small veins, and cautious use of restraints in the elderly. Multiple IV sticks in the same vein are avoided, and a central line is used if long-term access is needed.

DEEP-VEIN THROMBOSIS
Definition

Deep-vein thrombosis (DVT) is a clot in a deep vein. This most often occurs in the lower extremities, but it may also occur in the upper extremities and the pelvis. The most serious are those in the upper thigh and the iliac veins. Ninety-eight percent of DVTs are in the lower extremities, and only 2% occur in the upper extremities. Superficial thrombophlebitis may extend into a deep vein, especially in the area of the saphenofemoral junction.

Etiology/Epidemiology

Approximately 50,000 to 60,000 people in the United States die each year from pulmonary emboli that originate from DVT. Many more cases of DVT are treated each year. DVT is a major health problem, and primary prevention is an important goal of nursing. Many patients in all areas of the hospital and outpatient settings are at risk for DVT (Table 32-1). Approximately 10% to 30% of all general and orthopedic patients over the age of 40 experience DVT. The nurse must be aware of those patients whose medical condition puts them at risk and must implement plans to decrease the risks.

Pathophysiology

In 1846, Virchow identified three factors necessary for development of deep-vein thrombosis: stasis of blood, trauma to the vessel (endothelial damage), and hypercoagulability. Current research indicates that a decrease in venous return in the legs (stasis) is the primary factor leading to the development of DVT.

Venous stasis occurs during bed rest, general anesthesia, hypotension, intraoperative positioning, dehydration, episodes of hypovolemia, and in the presence of a leg cast. The absence of calf-muscle action (pump) during anesthesia may be the precipitating cause of development of calf thrombi during major surgical procedures. The longer the period of stasis (e.g., bed rest, anesthesia, cast time) the more likely venous thrombosis will occur. Forward, or return flow, of venous blood depends almost entirely upon muscle action in the calf. On rare occasions, stasis can be caused by the external compression of a vein.

Trauma to a vein can cause endothelial damage with resultant aggregation of platelets and fibrin and formation of a clot. Fibrinolytic activity is decreased with endothelial damage. Damage can occur from manipulative injury of a vein, a blow, puncture, or the introduction of irritating solutions in a vein. The increase of subclavian vein thrombosis in the past few years seems directly related to increased use of the vein for central venous access.

Hypercoagulability is hard to quantify except in certain circumstances. In many patients the alteration in the clotting cascade is not measurable. Changes in blood components such as those in polycythemia rubra vera are rare. Dehydration, use of oral contraceptives, smoking, abrupt withdrawal of anticoagulants, and anemia can contribute to an increasingly coagulable state. Some experts believe that an increased rate of coagulation occurs in areas of stasis. One theory to explain this finding is that the decrease of fibrinolytic activity in the leg-vein endothelium decreases the body's ability to lyse small clots and increases the likelihood of clots originating in the small veins of the legs. In addition, as one ages these calf veins dilate and increase the likelihood of blood pooling.

Venous thrombosis can occur in any vein in the body, but it is most common in the veins of the legs. These thrombi may extend to include the entire length of the vein, or the tip or tail of the clot can detach and travel to the lungs. When a thrombus travels, it is called an embolus; one that travels to the lungs is called a pulmonary embolus.

Clinical Manifestations

Approximately half of all patients with DVT have no obvious signs or symptoms. The degree of symptomatology is sometimes related to the size and location of the thrombus and the amount of collateral circulation. The most common physical indication of DVT is the presence of unilateral edema in an extremity. Edema may be mild or severe.

Onset of symptoms may be very subtle with a slight elevation of temperature and calf pain. Palpation of the calf muscle is more likely to elicit pain than the time-honored Homans' sign (dorsiflexion of

the foot). Homans' sign is accurate less than one third of the time. Other signs of DVT include dilation of the superficial veins complaints of warmth in the calf, and extremity "heaviness." In severe ileofemoral thrombosis, a rare condition known as phlegmasia cerulea dolens may occur with venous outflow occlusion, resulting in a rise in arterial pressure. Subsequently, arterial flow is obstructed and tissue death is imminent. These events are rapid and begin with acute pain and a bluish cast to the skin of the leg. It is a life- and limb-threatening condition.

Noninvasive venous duplex imaging (ultrasound) may be used to diagnose DVT. If the test is equivocal or if the hospital facility does not have the capability for the test, then venography may be performed. Venography has the disadvantage of introducing a contrast medium to which the patient may be allergic.

Therapeutic Management

Prevention

A combination therapy for preventing DVT is most effective. Heparin, immediate mobility, sequential compression devices, support hose, and elevating the foot of the bed all contribute to prophylaxis. Patients should be adequately hydrated, and blood volume should be within normal if possible. During long operative procedures not involving the legs, intermittent sequential compression devices may be used to facilitate blood return in the legs. Some surgeons prefer compression stockings (TEDS), but research does not support their effectiveness. If extended bed rest is prescribed for the patient, leg exercises (unless contraindicated) are helpful in assisting with venous return. Deep breathing exercises are also helpful.

Prophylactic anticoagulant therapy is ideal for patients who will be immobilized for some time. Preoperatively, 5000 units of subcutaneous heparin are given 2 hours before surgery and every 12 hours thereafter until the patient is ambulatory. Intravenous dextran can be given immediately preoperatively and once or twice a day postoperatively for its antithrombotic effect. It seems less effective than heparin. Aspirin has been shown to be ineffective in altering the coagulation cascade enough to prevent clotting.

Immobilization

Once a DVT has been diagnosed, bed rest is prescribed for the patient. The purpose of bed rest is to decrease the possibility of the clot breaking loose and becoming an embolus. Elevation of the affected part decreases swelling and aids venous return.

TABLE 32-2   Pharmacology Summary: Anticoagulant Drugs

	Heparin	Coumarin derivatives
Mechanism of action	Direct—inactivates factors IX, X, XI, and XII	Indirect—interferes with liver synthesis of vitamin K; depresses synthesis of factors X, IX, VII, and prothrombin
Route of administration	IV, SC	Oral
Onset of action	IV—immediate; SC—20 to 60 min	24 to 48 hr
Duration of action	Less than 4 hr	2 to 5 days
Distribution in body	Highly protein bound	Highly protein bound
Laboratory test for dosage control	Activated partial thromboplastin time (APTT)	Prothrombin time (PT)
Antidote	Protamine sulfate	Vitamin K, whole blood, plasma
Adverse reaction	Bleeding	Bleeding

Modified from McKenry LM, Salerno E: *Mosby's pharmacology in nursing,* ed 18, St. Louis 1991, Mosby–Year Book.

Anticoagulant therapy

The primary means of clot control is the use of anticoagulants. These drugs do not dissolve clots but keep them from extending; they block the formation or activation of several of the clotting factors.

Initially the patient will receive heparin. Intravenously, this is generally given with an initial IV bolus, followed by a set continuous rate per hour. Occasionally heparin is given intermittently IV. The effectiveness of the therapy is gauged by the partial thromboplastin time (PTT). The clot becomes adherent to the vein wall after 1 week, at which time it is safe to discontinue the heparin.

In earlier years, coumarin derivatives were begun a few days before discharge so that they were effective before heparin was discontinued. Frequently, the patient was not at a therapeutic value at the planned discharge time, and discharge was delayed. In the current atmosphere of rapid discharge, many physicians initiate coumarin drugs the day following initiation of heparin therapy. In this way the therapeutic level will be achieved more quickly. Effectiveness is judged by the prothrombin time (PT), deheparinized PT, or the international normalized ratio (INR) test. The patient takes coumarin drugs for 3 to 6 months after a DVT. The exception is the pregnant patient or a patient with a sensitivity to coumarin drugs. Pregnant or drug-sensitive patients may receive subcutaneous heparin for the duration of the pregnancy or for 3 to 6 months. Table 32-2 summarizes a comparison of the two main groups of anticoagulant agents used in clinical practice.

Thrombolytic therapy

Thrombolytic therapy (primarily streptokinase and urokinase and, recently, tissue plasminogen activator [TPA]) is used to dissolve clots. TPA is used less than urokinase and streptokinase partially because of its enormous expense. Because thrombolytic therapy dissolves both undesired clots and therapeutic clots, it cannot be used immediately after surgery or with a history of recent intracranial bleeding or bleeding ulcer. Thrombolytic drugs (lytic agents) are usually reserved for patients with massive DVT. Lysis is frequently accomplished in 1 or 2 days.

Thrombolytic agents are given systemically as well as locally. The greatest risk for patients receiving lytic agents is bleeding. The patient is evaluated regularly for any signs of bleeding and serial laboratory tests to evaluate the coagulation cascade performed. The patients do not receive any intramuscular injections. If a patient has received streptokinase within the previous 6 months it will not be repeated, and recent streptococcal infection indicates the need to use urokinase (because the patient will have antibodies against the streptococcus). Heparin and coumarin drugs are given following lytic therapy.

Compression stockings

Once the patient is ambulatory, the patient's leg will be measured for a below-the-knee prescription elastic **compression stocking**, p. 753 (Sigvaris, Medi, or Jobst types). Custom or prescription hose come in a variety of sizes and can be ordered to fit any size. The purpose of the stocking is to prevent the long-term sequelae occurring in the ankle and lower leg. (See chronic venous disease, p. 758.) Thigh-high stockings are not ordered because the patients commonly choose not to wear them. They are difficult to put on, difficult to hold up, and constricting behind the knee when the knee is bent.

PATIENT EDUCATION GUIDE   *Taking Oral Anticoagulants*

The nurse instructs the patient to:
  Take anticoagulant at same time each day
  Change dose *only* if directed by physician
  Wear identification stating that anticoagulants are
    being used
  Avoid other medications unless ordered by physician
  Do not take aspirin or ibuprofen
  Avoid multivitamins containing vitamin K
  Use soft toothbrush
  Use electric razor
  If cut, apply pressure 5 to 10 minutes
  Avoid dietary changes
  Intake of green vegetables should be consistent
  Avoid alcohol unless approved by physician
  Inform other physician/dentist about anticoagulant
    therapy

Women, if pregnant, notify physician
Report the following to physician:
  Any bleeding that does not stop
  Nosebleeds
  Red or pink-tinged urine
  Red or black bowel movement
  Faintness or weakness
  Headaches
  Stomach pain
  Skin rash
  Any other skin changes
The effect of this medication is determined by a
  blood test; it is necessary to be monitored by a phy-
  sician when taking this medication

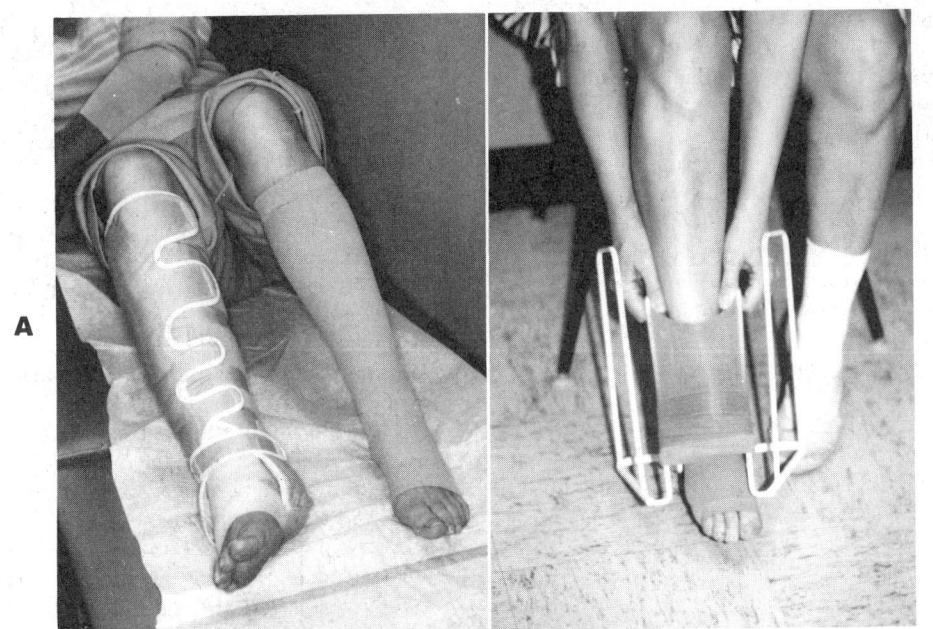

FIGURE 32-4   Below-the-knee compression stockings. **A,** Knee-length support hose
(left leg) and inflatable air boot (right leg) to assist venous return. **B,** Assist device
for patients to put on support hose.

Surgical management

Thrombectomy was routine some years ago. Rethrombosis of the vessel caused the operation to fall into disuse. It is rarely used unless venous obstruction compromises arterial flow.

NURSING MANAGEMENT OF THE PATIENT WITH DEEP-VEIN THROMBOSIS

Assessment

Obtaining a thorough history is essential. The time of onset of mild pain is important to document. Any history of injury, prolonged immobility, dehydration, or previous clot is obtained. Physical assessment includes determining the degree of edema in the leg, measuring the circumference of both legs, and comparing/recording the measurement, noting changes in skin color and temperature and areas of pain. Palpate and record peripheral pulses for a baseline, and to detect any changes that might occur with increasing edema. Since a primary complication of DVT is pulmonary embolism, questions about shortness of breath, chest pain, or tachycardia are important. If the patient is receiving anticoagulant therapy, assessment for complications is important. The patient and family must be knowledgeable about the disease process and anticoagulant therapy.

Nursing Diagnosis

Nursing diagnoses for the patient with DVT include:
Pain related to tissue edema and obstructed blood flow
Increased risk for bleeding related to anticoagulation
Knowledge deficit related to lack of information about prevention and treatment of DVT

Planning

Nursing care for the patient with a DVT is planned to achieve the following:
Pain and edema will be relieved as evidenced by decreased complaints of discomfort; redness

---

LEGAL ISSUES *Nursing Malpractice Case Source: Belmon (LA. 19xx)*

Alice Belmon was admitted through the emergency room (ER) to the intensive care unit (ICU) with a diagnosis of possible pulmonary embolism. In the ER she received an IV bolus of 7500 U of heparin. She received heparin by continuous IV drip in the ICU, totaling 2000 U per hour. The ICU nurse observed Mrs. Belmon throughout the night, taking her blood pressure (BP) regularly. At 5 AM a medical technician took a blood sample from the patient's right arm. At 7:30 AM the arm began to hurt and showed swelling and discoloration. Mrs. Belmon and her husband complained to the ICU nurse about her arm.

Here were the notations from the record of what happened:

5 AM Med. tech. in, blood drawn
7:30 AM BP 125/70
9:30 AM Pt. c/o pain, upper arm seems swollen slightly
10 AM BP 130/70
11 AM BP 128/68
11:50 AM Pt c/o pain, MD called

At noon the patient's physician arrived and discovered a large hematoma on the upper right arm underneath the BP cuff. The patient's arm was wrapped and elevated, and the physician ordered the heparin therapy be decreased by one half. At 2 PM the physician ordered the heparin therapy discontinued.

In this case the hospital was sued for the nurse's negligence under the principle of *respondeat superior*. The allegation the plaintiff presented was that the nurse's inaction permitted the patient's injury to reach serious proportions before a physician was called and that the nurse failed to recognize and respond properly to signs of hemorrhage.

The plaintiff presented an expert nurse witness who testified the nurse's duty of care to the patient increased as the PTT value increased. The hospital/defendant argued this was improper testimony, because it exceeded the nurse's expertise and invaded the physician's field of practice. The court did not accept this argument, stating that the expert nurse's testimony was proper, because it stated the nursing standard of care at issue. In addition, the court said even if the expert nurse's opinion was discarded, there was other medical testimony to support a finding of liability. In particular, the plaintiff had also presented a physician expert who testified that the patient experienced "blood pressure cuff trauma" and that the nurse should have properly investigated the patient's complaint of pain by looking under the BP cuff.

The hospital was found liable for the nurse's negligence. The nurse breached a standard of care, which led to and was the proximate cause of the patient's injuries, including pain, suffering, and longer hospital stay in the amount of $58,000.

and erythema will be absent or decreased

Bleeding will not occur or will be easily controlled

Patient will not experience a pulmonary embolism

The patient and family will verbalize knowledge to prevent further clots and side effects of anticoagulant therapy

Implementation

Bed rest is prescribed for several days. Patients with pain or edema may have difficulty cooperating with the activity restriction. The nurse needs to teach the patient and family the importance of bed rest to decrease the possibility of pulmonary embolism. The patient is reassured that the activity restriction is temporary. The entire affected limb must be elevated. Placing 4- to 6-inch blocks under the foot of the bed elevates the legs without the pressure of the knee gatch on the popliteal fossa. Placing pillows under the legs is futile. Pillows slip off of the bed or slide up to the knee, where pressure is applied and venous return is slowed.

As the patient's activity increases, the nurse teaches the patient to avoid sitting with the legs dependent and to avoid standing or sitting in any one position for too long. Elastic compression stockings should be worn as ordered, and instructions are given on their application. The skin is inspected at regular intervals with the stockings off to assess for skin breakdown or areas of pressure.

Anticoagulant therapy

When administering low-dose prophylactic heparin subcutaneously, the nurse uses a 25- or 27-gauge needle to reduce tissue trauma. To decrease the possibility of hematoma formation, the injection site should not be rubbed. The abdomen, lateral thighs, and the soft pad over the scapula are the preferred sites, and some research indicates that the drug should be administered away from any incisions. If the patient is learning to administer his or her own heparin, careful instructions are given. A chart to record sites may be helpful in rotating the areas.

Patients receiving heparin must be monitored for side effects. Fall precautions are taken, and the patient is told to shave with an electric razor. All personnel should be aware that the patient is undergoing anticoagulant therapy and that additional time is needed for pressure after venipuncture. The results of the laboratory tests determine dosage, and these are called in a timely fashion. An anticoagulant flowsheet is available in some facilities and is extremely helpful in assessing effectiveness and monitoring changes in results.

Patients taking anticoagulants are given verbal and written instructions at discharge on their medications and the side effects. The nurse arranges for an appointment for the patient to obtain a PT at regular intervals. For patients who are recovering from a major illness, this may mean using visiting nurses for a short time. Medicare will generally cover the cost of a skilled-nurse visit to assess compliance with medical routine and side effects of drug therapy and to draw a PT.

The patient needs to know what situations to avoid to prevent recurrence of a thrombus. Prolonged immobility in a plane or car is restricted. Emphasize to the patient to walk about every 1 or 2 hours for a few minutes. Encourage fluid intake, since volume deficit predisposes the patient to clot formation.

Evaluation

Evaluation of treatment effectiveness and nursing interventions is measured by a decrease in signs and symptoms. Decreased pain and decreased swelling are important measurements. In addition, the absence of side effects of anticoagulant therapy indicate teaching effectiveness.

Ongoing Care

It is important for patients to understand that they have endured a serious illness. In addition, they have an increased risk of developing DVT again and a significant risk of progressing to chronic venous insufficiency (postphlebitic syndrome). External compression stockings may assist with the return of venous blood and decrease venous hypertension at the ankles. This may mean a lifelong commitment to stockings and may require much enforcement. If patients believe that noncompliance may result in disability and ulcer formation, they may be more compliant about wearing the stockings.

PULMONARY EMBOLISM
Definition

A **pulmonary embolus (PE)** is a clot (thrombus) that has broken loose from its original site and traveled to lodge in the pulmonary artery. Generally, the clot is actually the free-floating tail of a clot that breaks off. Rare causes are air embolus, or fat emboli that originate from air entry or fat entry into the venous system, especially in trauma. For the purpose of this discussion, PE will indicate blood clot.

Etiology/Epidemiology

Conservative estimates place the death rate from pulmonary embolism in the United States at 50,000 to 100,000 per year. A significant number of terminally ill patients expire without autopsy, and of those a large portion expire from pulmonary embolism. The frequency of fatal pulmonary embolism in elective general surgery is approximately 0.8%, while patients undergoing emergency surgery for hip fracture may experience a 1% to 4% fatality rate. Pulmonary embolism occurs in 10% to 40% of patients with DVT. Even if a patient has no obvious risk factors, research has shown that DVT occurs approximately 10% of the time with a 1% incidence of pulmonary embolism. In a patient with three or more known risk factors for DVT, the rate jumps to 50% for DVT and 8% for PE. The clinical signs of DVT are not necessary for the development of PE. Often PE is the first indication of a clotting problem.

Pathophysiology

A majority of PEs are from a DVT in the lower extremities. Seventy-five percent of patients studied after a PE had a documented clot in the lower extremities. Large, obstructing venous thrombi in the thigh and pelvis are responsible for 90% of all PEs. Far less common are clots from the right side of the heart, the vena cava, or the upper extremities. When a clot breaks loose, it travels through the venous circulation, through the right side of the heart, and into the pulmonary artery. As it moves through the heart it is frequently broken into smaller pieces and may lodge in several areas.

The physiologic changes that occur after a large clot blocks a pulmonary artery are complex. A major reduction in the diameter of the pulmonary artery or its branches occurs with a large clot, and this diameter reduction decreases pulmonary blood flow. Platelet degradation, which occurs at the time of the PE, causes a release of serotonin, prostaglandin, histamine, and thromboxane, resulting in constriction of both the bronchi and pulmonary arterioles. When the arterioles are blocked, oxygen continues to enter the alveoli, but the oxygen does not reach the bloodstream. The patient becomes hypoxemic and ceases to produce surfactant in the alveoli. The alveoli collapse as a result of a lack of surfactant. Deoxygenated blood returns to the heart around the collapsed alveoli and increases the load on functional alveoli and vessels. Increased pressure in these vessels (pulmonary hypertension) causes the right side of the heart to work harder. If the lung area that is nonfunctional is large, there is a significant decrease in cardiac output as well as pulmonary perfusion and ventilation. The end result may be cardiopulmonary arrest.

Clinical Manifestations

PE commonly has no warning signs. The symptoms are related to the size of the clot as well as to the patient's own cardiac and pulmonary reserve. More than 80% of all patients develop sudden and severe chest pain, dyspnea, and tachypnea. Other symptoms include hemoptysis, pleural friction rub, cardiac gallop, cyanosis, diaphoresis, tachycardia, restlessness, pupillary dilation, anxiety, and cough. In massive PE (when more than 50% of the pulmonary artery flow is stopped) signs may include cardiac decompensation, dysrhythmia, hypotension, and cyanosis. The electrocardiogram findings may show evidence of right-ventricular strain and arrhythmias. Arterial blood gas values are a helpful diagnostic adjunct, but a normal Po_2 does not rule out a PE. A low Po_2 in a patient with one previously in normal range is helpful to assess the degree of hypoxia.

Diagnosis is based upon a ventilation/perfusion lung scan (VQ scan) and/or a pulmonary arteriogram. VQ scans, when perfectly normal, can rule out PE with a high degree of accuracy. However, an abnormal scan is not always consistent with PE. In cases where a scan is equivocal, the pulmonary arteriogram is the choice of diagnostics. It is extremely accurate, but exposes the patient to the risk of contrast reaction.

Therapeutic Management

Approximately 10% of all patients with PE die within an hour despite adequate treatment. The success of therapy in the other 90% depends upon rapid, accurate diagnosis and treatment. Supportive measures to maintain circulatory function are followed with immediate administration of anticoagulants. The purpose of heparin is to prevent extension of the clot or recurrent episodes. Support measures include oxygen administration, intubation if necessary, correction of dysrhythmias, and pain relief. In hypotension, in the absence of pulmonary congestion, a fluid challenge is given.

Anticoagulant therapy

If possible, obtain a baseline PTT, platelet count, and prothrombin time before initiating therapy. However, do not let laboratory tests delay heparin administration. Heparin is given in a bolus of 10,000 to 20,000 units when PE is suspected. If it is ordered, do not wait for all of the diagnostic tests to be completed. The heparin stops the thrombotic process and may be life-saving. If the tests are negative, the patient can have the heparin reversed, though this is seldom necessary. After the initial bolus, heparin is generally administered at 1000 U/hr IV and is adjusted according to the results of the PTT. Therapeutic levels are 1.5 to 2 times normal. Heparin is continued for 7 to 10 days. Oral anticoagulants are started soon after the heparin and continued for 3 to 6 months.

Thrombolytic therapy

In cases of massive PE, thrombolytic therapy is used to rapidly dissolve the clot and thereby relieve the load on the heart. Research is still being conducted on the efficacy of this treatment. Results of early studies showed significant lysis of clot but no reduction in mortality rates. Others show a reduction in post-PE pulmonary hypertension. Urokinase or streptokinase can be given in large doses peripherally or via a pulmonary artery catheter used in pulmonary arteriography. This method also allows reangiography at intervals to assess clot lysis. When lytic agents are given peripherally, the results of clot lysis are followed by serial VQ scan.

Surgical intervention

Pulmonary embolectomy

Pulmonary embolectomy is reserved for those patients who are hemodynamically unstable despite optimum therapy 1 hour after massive PE. It is considered a life-saving option only. Originally this was an open procedure; recently, however, pulmonary embolectomy catheters have been developed that use suction to remove the embolus. This is performed in the angiography suite.

Vena cava interruption

If anticoagulation therapy must be interrupted for some reason, or if the patient has recurrent emboli on adequate anticoagulation, then the patient needs a method to prevent further emboli from traveling to the lungs. This is called **vena caval interruption.** Several methods are available. Early treatment called for an open surgical method in which a clip was placed across the inferior vena cava. This involved an abdominal incision in a critically ill patient. This is seldom used today unless there is no access for other methods.

In the 1960s, the Mobbin-Uddin filter was developed to allow return of venous blood through the vena cava but not to allow large clots to travel to the lungs. Disadvantages of this filter were that it tended to migrate and occasionally would thrombose. Redesign of the filter resulted in one (e.g., Kimray-Greenfield filter) that can be inserted percutaneously through the jugular or the femoral vein and one that seldom migrates (Figure 32-5). It is effective in preventing clots from traveling to the lungs. The incision is very small, and nursing care is similar to care for the patient who has had an arteriogram. These patients may still be given very low-dose coumarin drugs, unless contraindicated, for the

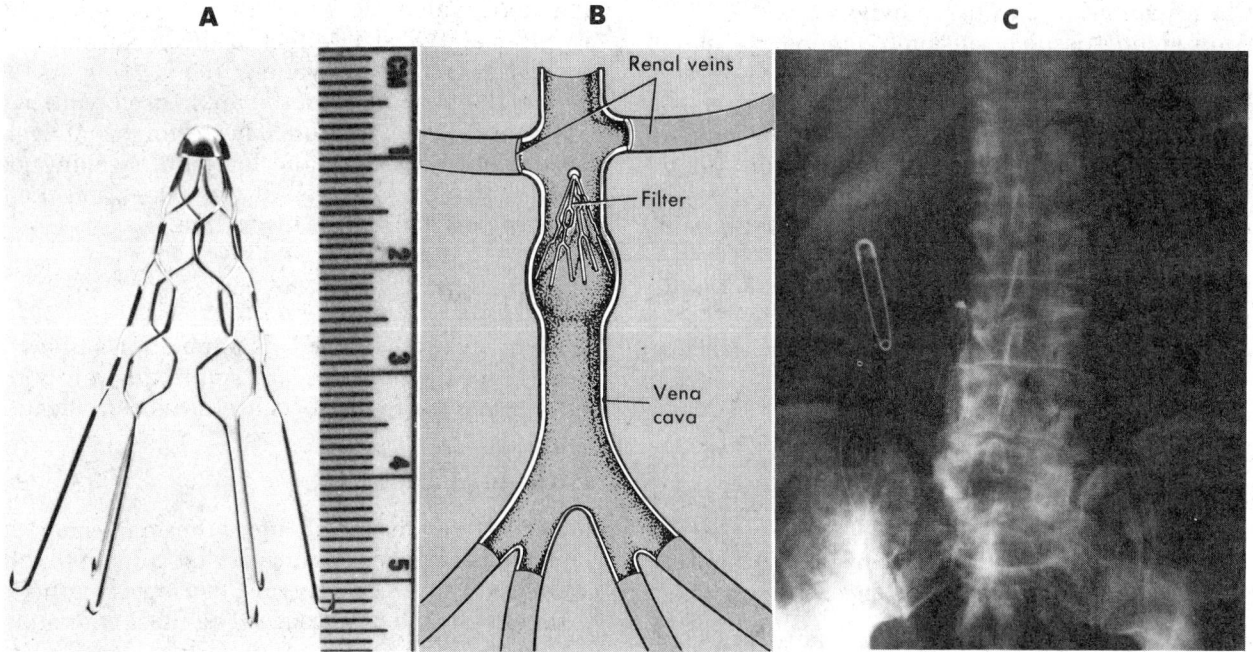

FIGURE 32-5   **A,** Greenfield vena cava filter. **B,** Greenfield filter is placed in the inferior vena cava just below the renal veins. **C,** X-ray film showing Greenfield filter in inferior vena cava. The safety pin is external and was used as a marker for filter insertion. (**A** from Davis JH et al: *Clinical surgery,* St Louis, 1987, Mosby–Year Book.)

rest of their lives to prevent recurrent DVT. In addition, patients will be advised to wear prescription compression stockings for the rest of their lives. The filters remain in the patient for life. Rarely, these filters clot off but do not need replacement.

Other percutaneous methods of vena cava interruption have been developed in the 1980s and are in use in some locations. The bird's-nest filter consists of a mesh of four wires that wind around and have hooks to attach into the vena cava. Migration has occurred with this device. Two recently released devices include the Nitinol and the Venatech filters.

NURSING MANAGEMENT OF THE PATIENT WITH PULMONARY EMBOLISM
Assessment

The nurse assesses the patient for risk factors for DVT and PE. If the patient has one or more risk factors, the nurse should be extremely diligent in observing for any signs of DVT or PE and in implementing all preventive measures mentioned earlier. If the patient exhibits any of the signs of PE such as tachypnea, tachycardia, or a generalized restlessness, the nurse should be highly suspicious. Oxygen should be started, and the physician should be alerted (Figure 32-6).

Nursing Diagnosis

Nursing diagnoses for the patient with PE include:
   Chest pain related to tissue hypoxemia
   Altered lung-tissue perfusion (pulmonary) related to obstruction of blood flow
   Impaired gas exchange related to ineffective breathing patterns, reflex bronchoconstriction, and partial or complete obstruction of pulmonary arterial blood flow
   Ineffective breathing patterns related to fear, anxiety, chest pain, and hypoxia
   High risk for injury related to side effects of anticoagulation
   Anxiety related to dyspnea, chest pain, lack of knowledge, and threat of death

Planning

Nursing care is planned to achieve the following outcomes:
   The patient experiences relief from pain and effective gas exchange as evidenced by improved ABGs
   The patient verbalizes knowledge of the physiologic event
   There will be no fall in hemoglobin and hematocrit; no transfusions will be necessary
   The patient will suffer no ill effects from anticoagulation

Implementation

Nursing care centers on prevention of DVT. These measures include promoting mobility; suggesting the patient do passive exercises while immobile; implementing physician-ordered interventions such as low-dose heparin, alternate compression devices, or compression hose; and teaching the patient to reduce risks. Patient teaching includes the following:
   • Do not sit or cross legs for prolonged periods
   • Do not wear constrictive clothing
   • If traveling, exercise at least every 2 hours
   • Know the classic signs of PE

Nursing measures to facilitate gas exchange include administering oxygen as ordered and promoting coughing and deep breathing exercises. In addition, morphine or other narcotics are administered to relieve chest pain and assist with breathing. A heparin IV is administered to halt the clotting cascade.

CHRONIC VENOUS INSUFFICIENCY
Definition/Etiology

Deep venous thrombosis is responsible for approximately 90% of the development of **chronic venous insufficiency** or postphlebitic syndrome. It is estimated that 10% of all patients with DVT develop postphlebitic syndrome. The syndrome is a result of deep venous incompetence from valve damage during a DVT. The clot dissolves and leaves behind nonfunctional valves. It is the greatest cause of morbidity after a DVT. The effect of this syndrome is that the entire weight of venous blood from the right atrium down rests upon the ankle area, with resultant venous hypertension. The term chronic venous insufficiency refers to the leg pain, swelling, dark-brown skin discoloration at the ankle, and the dermatitis with or without ulceration.

Epidemiology

An estimated 5% of the U.S. population suffers from postphlebitic syndrome, and approximately 200,000 working days are lost because of its complications.

Pathophysiology

In chronic venous insufficiency the venous blood column transmits the pressure of that column to the ankle area. There are several theories as to the long-term effect of this pressure. The most common theory involves the final areas of backflow and pressure, which are the veins and the skin venules. These become dilated; as the venules dilate, the interendothelial pores in the vessels themselves dilate with subsequent leaking of fluid into the tissue. Studies of this fluid reveal a high level of fibrinogen as op-

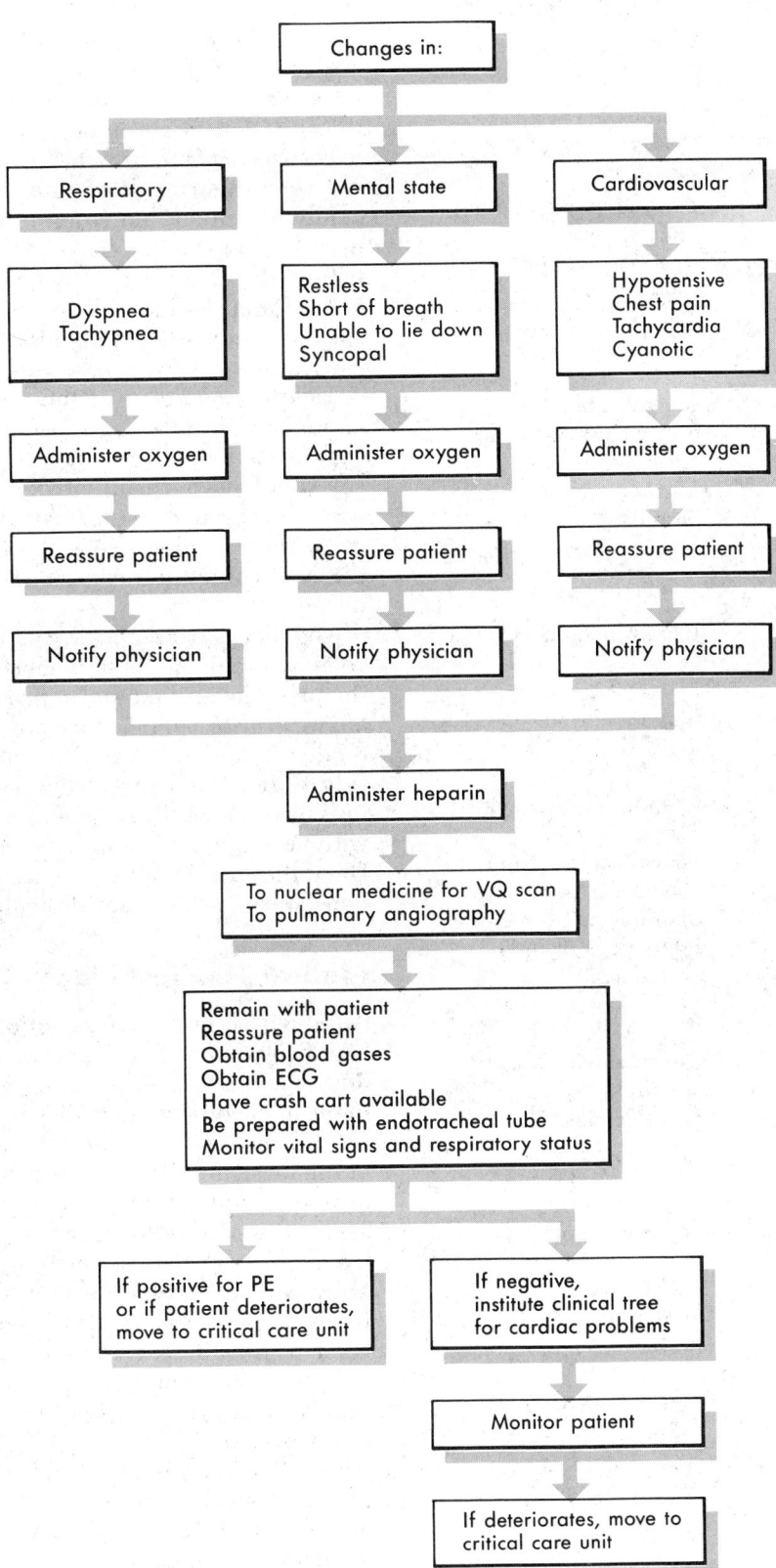

FIGURE 32-6   Critical Thinking Guide: pulmonary embolism.

TABLE 32-3   A Comparison of Arterial and Venous Ulcers

Arterial	Venous
LOCATION	
Tips of toes	Around medial malleolus
Heels	
Over phalangeal heads	Pretibial/laterotibial
Over metatarsal heads	
Points of trauma	
ULCER CHARACTERISTICS	
Well-demarcated border	Irregular borders
Eschar	Soft yellow necrosis
Pale base	Granulating base
No edema	Marked edema
May be dry	Drainage
PAIN	
Sharp or burning	Usually aching
PULSES	
Absent	May be normal
SURROUNDING TISSUE	
Pallor on elevation	Cyanotic when dependent
Dependent rubor	
Cool temperature	Brown color around lower leg
Smooth shiny skin	Skin normal to warm
	Edematous or indurated skin
ULCER TREATMENT	
Eschar—keep dry	Debridement (may be by dressing)
Open, clean—keep dry	Leg elevation
	Support dressing (Unna or elastic wrap, hydrocolloid elastic wrap)
SURGICAL TREATMENT	
Revascularization	Skin graft
Debridement	Perforator vein ligation
Amputation	Venous valve transplant

posed to the lymphatic fluid found in a leg not affected by venous hypertension. Further laboratory research suggests that venous ulceration develops as a result of the combination of venous hypertension, increased capillary permeability to fibrinogen, and the fact that fibrin deposited outside of a capillary decreases oxygen flow to the tissue.

Other theories of venous ulcer development include inadequate nutrition of the area secondary to pressure on the capillaries by the edema. Some attribute the changes to a high venous pressure diverting oxygenated blood from the skin, resulting in tissue ischemia and stagnation of the blood, which causes the area to receive inadequate nutrition.

Ulcerations occur at the ankle level because the edema and loss of tissue occur at the point of greatest gravitational force (the ankle). The brownish discoloration is a result of deposits of hemosiderin, which occur because of extravasation of red blood cells; the red blood cells then break down, leaving the iron-containing component of the cell, hemosiderin.

Leg ulcers from chronic venous stasis usually develop around the sites of perforator veins, such as the pretibial and medial supramalleolar areas of the ankle. A true venous stasis ulcer begins as a small, tender inflamed area. With any slight trauma, the skin breaks, and the ulcer is the resultant relief of pressure under the tissue. In many cases, trauma without much edema may be the precipitating event. Once the skin has lost its integrity in an area of venous stasis, it becomes difficult to restore.

Clinical Manifestations

Although clinical manifestations of chronic venous insufficiency are many and include many stages before ulcerations, ulcerations are a major development in chronic venous disease. The ankle area appears brownish, and there is some degree of edema of the lower leg. The skin may be indurated and may have a "woody" feel to it as a result of liposclerosis. There may be many areas of thin skin or old scars from previous ulcerations. The skin may be dry and scaly with a chronic dermatitis—stasis dermatitis. Itching may be severe. The lower leg may be a dusky color from venous engorgement.

Ulcerations vary from very small to those that nearly girdle the ankle. The ulcer border is generally irregular. The ulcer itself is usually shallow with bright, beefy, granulated tissue. If the ulcer has been present for some time, there may be soft-tissue necrosis at the base. This may appear yellow-green and have a stringy consistency. Patients may complain of pain in the leg, especially in the ulcers. Swelling, itching, and pain may be improved by elevating and supporting the legs. Table 32-3 compares venous and arterial ulcers.

must continue to practice good support of the affected leg. If support is discontinued, the skin may break down once more. Patients must understand that their disease is controlled, not "cured."

NURSING MANAGEMENT OF THE PATIENT WITH CHRONIC VENOUS INSUFFICIENCY

The nursing assessment, diagnoses, and planning are combinations of those for patients with varicose veins and those with venous thrombosis. To summarize, patients wear prescription support stockings for the rest of their lives whenever they are up out of bed. The stockings are replaced every 3 to 6 months even if they show no signs of wear. Compression effectiveness is lost after that time. Stockings are worn morning to night, and legs are elevated at night.

Skin care of the feet and legs is critical. The skin is kept clean and well lubricated. Over-the-counter products are avoided as are lotions containing alcohol. Trauma is avoided if at all possible. The patient should remind the health care provider to examine the feet and ankles at each visit, even if that is not the reason for the visit.

If the patient maintains intact skin and supportive stockings and has a minimum of edema, the education efforts will have been a success. The patient must know that this is a lifetime problem and should visit the health care provider every 3 to 6 months even if there is no current problem.

LYMPHEDEMA
Definition

Lymphedema is a condition caused by impaired drainage of lymph fluid. The failure of this transportation of fluid causes an accumulation of protein, an increase in interstitial osmotic pressure, and a movement of fluid to the interstitial space. The result is swelling of an extremity.

Pathophysiology

Lymph is collected from the intercellular fluid and transported via lymphatic vessels to the lymph glands and on to the lymphatic ducts. In the superficial lymphatics, this flow may be blocked or reduced because of a decrease in the actual number of vessels, obstruction or a lack of valves in the lymphatic vessels. The leakage of lymphatic fluid into the subcutaneous tissue results in fibrosis and inflammation.

Primary, or idiopathic, lymphedema has no demonstrable cause. It is further divided into three types by time of onset: congenital, which may occur at birth or during early childhood as a result of ab-

the toes to just below the knee [...] with an elastic wrap. The disadvantages to this dressing are discomfort and the fact that the odor is often overwhelming when the drainage leaks through.

Hydrocolloid dressings provide cover for the ulcer and decrease leakage. Newer elastic compression bandages also come impregnated with hydrocolloid (Duoderm). The advantages of this dressing are that it does not have to be rewrapped like a traditional elastic wrap, the impregnated material keeps the skin from drying out, and it provides uniform flexible pressure to the leg.

Surgical management

Surgical treatment for venous ulcers consists of treatment of the ulcer and the cause of the ulcer. Treatment of the ulcer includes debridement, excision, and skin grafting. Treatment of the cause includes removal of the veins with incompetent valves. Valve transplantation has been performed in some facilities but is not widely used. In severe cases of venous obstruction that is causing venous hypertension, a venous bypass going from saphenous vein to saphenous vein (much as a femoral-femoral bypass works in arteries only for return blood) is sometimes used.

Once the ulcer or skin graft is healed, the patient

sence of lymphatic vessels; precox, which occurs from puberty until age 30; and tarda, which occurs after the age 30. Congenital lymphedema represents less than 10% of primary lymphedema. Lymphedema precox is the most common type of primary lymphedema and is three times more common in women than in men. This condition occurs when there are some functioning lymphatics present at birth, but not enough as the individual grows.

Secondary, or acquired, lymphedema is caused by obstruction of the lymphatic channels. Causes of the obstructions may be external pressure from malignancies, traumatic injury, removal or disruption of lymphatics from surgery (mastectomy or groin dissection), or radiation. In countries where parasitic infections are common, filariasis is commonly the cause of lymphedema.

Clinical Manifestations

In primary lymphedema, the left leg seems to be affected most often. Edema generally begins first, at the ankle level and the patient complains of limb heaviness. Many times the feet are not affected, and the skin seems to "fold" over the feet. Once the foot is affected, the edema occurs in the forefoot, and the foot is humped (Figure 32-7). As edema ascends, the limb becomes more trunklike. The skin becomes pinkish-red and has a puckered, pitted appearance. Once the subcutaneous tissue is involved, the tissue becomes fibrotic and lacks elasticity. It was once believed that lymphedema did not "pit" like dependent edema; however, the lack of indentation is due to the fibrosis and not the cause of the edema. Skin ulcerations found in venous disease are uncommon in lymphedema. However, odor problems and fungal infections in the "creases" of skin are common.

FIGURE 32-7 Severe lymphedema in a 45-year-old Caucasian female. Note the "humping" of the feet and the puckered texture of the skin from the fibrotic changes in the subcutaneous tissue.

Therapeutic Management

Treatment is aimed at preserving and improving skin quality, softening the subcutaneous tissue, treating or preventing cellulitis and lymphangitis, and reducing limb size and weight. In addition, cosmetic improvement is a desired outcome. Nonsurgical management includes skin care with persistent, frequent applications of water-based skin lotion. Nondrying soaps are used. Antifungal powders are applied daily between toes and in appropriate creases, if ordered.

Pharmacologic control of the condition may include long-term prophylactic antibiotics such as penicillin or erythromycin to prevent severe cellulitis or lymphangitis. Some patients are also given a stock amount to begin at the first sign of infection. Coumarin derivatives are given in some centers, not for venous thrombosis prophylaxis, but for the effect of softening subcutaneous tissues. Standard instruc-

tions on complications of coumarin derivatives are given.

External pneumatic compression is used to promote flow through the lymphatics by increasing the interstitial pressure. A single-compartment compression device that disperses the edema both distally and proximally does not work as well as one with a sequential inflation cycle. This cycle provides a distal-to-proximal milking action that is necessary to move fluid. Results may be impressive after initial therapy, but the patient must be on a long-term maintenance program. Custom stockings are worn in the day, and lymphatic compression may be used all evening or night.

Surgical intervention is performed on only a small number of patients. Reducing the size of a limb is generally the indication. Two types of operations are done—one to improve function and one to debulk. Lymphatic-to-lymphatic bypasses for patients with obstructive primary lymphatic edema are used with limited success. Debulking procedures attempt to remove large amounts of subcutaneous tissue and the overlying skin. This reduces the size of the limb.

NURSING MANAGEMENT OF THE PATIENT WITH LYMPHEDEMA

Assessment

A focused assessment for the patient with lymphedema includes determining the onset of the symptoms and the reason for seeking medical/nursing intervention. In the absence of infection, the usual reason for seeking health care is the size or cosmetic appearance of the limb. Assessment of patient commitment to therapy, patient knowledge of the difficulties of therapy, and physical ability to perform daily treatments such as pneumatic compression is important. Questions on injuries, frequency of infections, and self-treatment of skin problems give insight into the patient's self-care abilities. Problems with self-image are addressed, and the conditions of the legs are dealt with nonjudgmentally.

Physical assessment includes the entire affected limb and a comparison with the nonaffected limb, if applicable. Skin color, condition, presence of wounds, odor, infections in the creases, and presence of pulses (if detectable through the edema) are important to document. Measuring of calf, ankle, and feet may provide helpful information.

Nursing Diagnosis

High risk for infection related to moist skin between skin folds

Alteration in body image related to massive enlargement of the limbs and possible odor of skin

Knowledge deficit related to pathophysiology of lymphedema

Planning

Nursing care is planned to achieve the following outcomes:

The patient will have intact skin free from organism growth

The patient will verbalize understanding of the need to follow care plan instructions to reduce size of the limb

The patient will verbalize knowledge of the causes of lymphedema

Implementation

If the patient is to use elastic wraps alternating with pneumatic compression, he or she must be taught how to wrap the elastic compression so that it is even and tight. Rewrapping is done every 8 hours. Elevation of the limb with a foam wedge is more ef-

fective at night than using pillows, because pillows compress and slip. If the patient is unable to wrap the compression, a family member or friend must be taught. Emotional support is essential for the patient and family. This is especially true if the patient is an adolescent, concerned with not appearing different from peers. Time must be spent listening to the emotional concerns of the patient and to help the patient planning activities that do not compromise health. Emphasizing that lymphedema include normal activities may increase the self-esteem of the patient. Fitting compression therapy in time frames with realistic expectations is arranging for professional foot care (physician, practitioner, or reliable podiatrist) at a convenient is conducive to patient compliance.

Evaluation

Evaluation of the treatment is the decrease (or lack of increase) in the size of the limb, patient satisfaction, and the absence of injury. The patient should report to the provider on a regular basis. Emotional support for positive results is important during visits.

CRITICAL THINKING QUESTIONS

1 What is the cause and treatment of thrombophlebitis?

2 What is deep-vein thrombosis (DVT), and how does it differ from thrombophlebitis? What three factors are necessary for thrombosis to occur? How can the nurse assess for DVT?

3 What should the nurse teach the patient taking oral anticoagulants?

4 What is the most serious complication of DVT, and how may the patient prevent it?

5 What is phlegmasia? Clinical manifestations? What is thrombolytic therapy? What is its greatest risk? Nursing implications?

6 What are the classic signs of pulmonary embolism? What procedures are used when heparin therapy is contraindicated?

7 What are varicose veins? What is the nursing management after surgical removal or sclerotherapy?

8 What is the nursing management for a patient with chronic venous insufficiency? Venous ulcers?

9 What is lymphedema and how is it manifested? How does external pneumatic compression work? Nursing management?

BIBLIOGRAPHY

Current

1. Baldwin DR: Heparin-induced thrombocytopenia, *J Intraven Nurs* 12(6):378, 1990.
2. Battery PM, Salam AA: Venous gangrene associated with heparin-induced thrombocytopenia, *Surgery* 97(5):618, 1985.
3. Browse NL: The etiology of venous ulceration, *World J Surg* 10:938, 1986.
4. Browse NL: The diagnosis and management of primary lymphedema, *J Vasc Surg* 3(1):181, 1986.
5. Cole MS, Minifee PK, Wolma FJ: Coumarin necrosis—a review of the literature, *Surgery* 103(3):271, 1988.
6. Consensus Conference: Prevention of venous thrombosis and pulmonary emboli, *JAMA* 256(6):744, 1986.
7. Dann C: Treatment of varicose and spider veins with injection therapy, *J Vasc Nurs* 8(5):9, 1990.
8. DeWeese MS: Nonoperative treatment of acute superficial thrombophlebitis and deep femoral venous thrombosis. In Ernst CB, Stanley JC, editors: *Current therapy in vascular surgery II,* Philadelphia, 1991, BC Decker.
9. Dixon MB, Bergan JJ: Lymphedema. In Fahey VA, editor: *Vascular nursing,* Philadelphia, 1988, WB Saunders.
10. Erban SB, Kinman JL, Schwartz S: Routine use of the prothrombin and partial thromboplastin times, *JAMA* 262(17):2428, 1989.
11. Foldes MS et al: Standing versus supine positioning in venous reflux evaluation, *J Vasc Tech* 15:321, 1991.
12. Geelhoed GW, Burkitt DP: Varicose veins: a reappraisal from a global perspective, *S Med J* 84(9):1131, 1991.
13. Graor RA et al: Comparison of cost effectiveness of streptokinase and urokinase in the treatment of deep venous thrombosis, *Ann Vasc Surg* 1(5):524, 1987.
14. Greenfield LJ: Percutaneous devices for vena cava filtration. In Ernst CB, Stanley JC, editors: *Current therapy in vascular surgery II,* Philadelphia, 1991, BC Decker.
15. Holcomb S: Pulmonary embolism—preventing a disaster, *RN* September:52, 1991.
16. Karp D: Venous ulceration: assessment, healing prediction and treatment, *J Soc Periph Vasc Nurs* 5:14, 1987.
17. Kornblit P et al: Anticoagulation therapy: patient management and evaluation of an outpatient clinic, *Nurse Pract* 18(8):21, 1990.
18. Moser KM: Pulmonary embolism; your challenge is prevention, *J Resp Dis* 10(10):83, 1989.
19. Nunnelee JD: Medications used in vascular patients. In Fahey VA, editor: *Vascular nursing,* Philadelphia, 1988, WB Saunders.
20. O'Donnell TF: Management of primary lymphedema. In Ernst CB, Stanley JC, editors: *Current therapy in vascular surgery II,* Philadelphia, 1988, BC Decker.
21. *Prevention of venous thrombosis and pulmonary embolism,* NIH Consensus Development Conference Statement, 6, 2.NSDHHS, Public Health Service, NIH, Bethesda, Md, 1987.
22. Seabrook GR et al: An outpatient anticoagulation protocol managed by a vascular nurse clinician, *Am J Surg* 160:501, 1990.
23. Silver D: An overview of venous thromboembolism prophylaxis, *Am J Surg* 161:537, 1991.
24. Wheeler HB, Anderson FA: Prophylaxis against venous thromboembolism in surgical patients, *Am J Surg* 161:507, 1991.
25. Westblom TU, Marienfeld RD: Prolonged hospitalization because of inappropriate delay of warfarin therapy in deep venous thrombosis, *S Med J* 78:1164, 1985.

Classic

26. Bell WR, Meek AG: Guidelines for the use of thrombolytic agents, *N Engl J Med* 301:1266, 1979.
27. Coon WW: Anticoagulant therapy. In Sasahara AA, editor: Symposium on deep venous thrombosis, *Am J Surg* 150(4A):44, 1984.
28. Cranley JJ, Canos AJ, Sull WJ: The diagnosis of deep venous thrombosis: fallibility of clinical signs and symptoms, *Arch Surg* 111:34, 1976.
29. Dodd H, Cockett FB: *The pathology and surgery of the veins of the lower limb,* Edinburgh, 1976, Churchill Livingstone.
30. Doyle JE: The intracaval filter: new nursing challenge, *RN* 4:38, 1980.
31. Kakkar VV et al: Efficacy of low doses of heparin in prevention of deep vein thrombosis after major surgery, *Lancet* 2:101, 1972.
32. Nicolaides AN, Fernandes J, Pollock AV: Intermittent sequential pneumatic compression of the legs in the prevention of venous stasis and postoperative deep venous thrombosis, *Surgery* 87:69, 1980.
33. Porter JM: Massive deep vein thrombosis of the lower extremities, *Curr Ther* 233, 1980.
34. Salzman EW: Heparin therapy in venous thromboembolism. In Bergan JJ, Yao JS, editors: *Venous problems,* Chicago, 1980, Mosby–Year Book.
35. Wolfe WG, Sabiston DC: *Pulmonary embolism: major problems in clinical surgery* (Vol 25), Philadelphia, 1980, WB Saunders.

UNIT VIII

Cardiac System

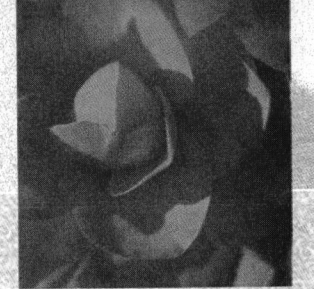

CHAPTER THIRTY-THREE

Nursing Assessment of the Cardiac System

LEARNING OBJECTIVES

1 Describe the basic structures and functions of the cardiac system.
2 Understand the cardiac cycle.
3 Obtain relevant subjective information from the patient who has a cardiac alteration.
4 Using correct technique, examine the patient to obtain appropriate objective information about the cardiac system.
5 Differentiate abnormal from normal subjective and objective findings related to the cardiac system.
6 Describe procedures and tests related to disorders of the cardiac system.
7 Describe patient care and preparation related to diagnostic tests of the cardiac system.

KEY TERMS

afterload, p. 773
atrioventricular valves, p. 770
blood lipids, p. 787
cardiac catheterization, p. 784
cardiac cycle, p. 771
cardiac output, p. 773
diastole, p. 770
echocardiography, p. 781
isovolumetric contraction period, p. 771

isovolumetric relaxation period, p. 772
murmurs, p. 779
myocardium, p. 768
pericardial sac, p. 768
preload, p. 773
semilunar valves, p. 771
stroke volume, p. 773
systole, p. 770

THE CARDIAC SYSTEM, along with the vascular, blood, and lymphatic systems, maintains homeostasis (a constant environment) around the cells. This environment is provided by the interstitial fluid, which is in dynamic equilibrium with the fluid in the capillaries. The capillaries serve as the functional units of the cardiovascular system, with the heart acting as the system's pump. The peripheral blood vessels and lymphatic system provide conduction for the transport mediums of blood and lymph.

The focus of the cardiac assessment is to determine whether the heart and great vessels (the precordia) are intact and functional. The cardiac examination is conducted in conjunction with an assessment of the peripheral vascular and respiratory systems. Factors capable of compromising the integrity of the cardiac system must be identified during the assessment.

ANATOMY AND PHYSIOLOGY
Structural Description

The heart lies in the mediastinum close to the points of attachment of ribs 2 through 6 on the left side (Figure 33-1). It rests on thoracic vertebrae T5 through T8 and can be compressed to circulate blood by depressing the lower portion of the sternum as is done during cardiopulmonary resuscitation.

The heart is enclosed and supported by the **pericardial sac,** which is composed of strong white fibrous connective tissue and lined with epithelium. It prevents the heart from overfilling during short periods of overload, and its serous fluid provides lubrication to prevent friction during the cardiac cycle.

The heart muscle **(myocardium)** receives its blood supply from the right and left coronary arteries, which branch from the aorta just behind the flaps of the semilunar valves (Figure 33-2). These arteries circle the heart on its outer surface and anastomose on the posterior surface. The left coronary artery branches to form the anterior interventricular artery, which supplies the anterior portion of both ventricles, and the circumflex artery, which supplies the left atrium and ventricle. The right coronary artery divides to form the posterior interventricular artery, which supplies the posterior portion of both ventricles, and the marginal artery, which supplies the walls of the right atrium and ventricle. The blood returns to the right atrium from the myocardial capillaries via the great and middle cardiac veins and the coronary sinus.

The heart acts as two separate pumps, each made up of one atria and one ventricle. Although both sides of the heart pump the same volume of blood, the left ventricle is considerably stronger than the right ventricle and has much thicker muscle, because it pumps blood into the systemic circulation against pressures approximately five times higher than those the right ventricle encounters in the pulmonary circulation. In cross section the left ventricle is round, and it forces the right ventricle to take up a crescent shape.

Cardiac muscle differs from skeletal muscle in that an action potential generated in either the atria or the ventricles passes to all the muscle fibers of the atria or ventricles because they branch and interconnect into a single unit or syncytium. Thus all the atrial or ventricular muscle fibers contract as if they were one large fiber. The atrial and ventricular muscle fibers only interconnect via the atrioventricular (AV) node.

The Heart's Action Potential

An electrical and a mechanical change must occur before a heartbeat or a pulse is palpable. First, an action potential must reach each part of the myocardium to release calcium into the sarcoplasm, and second, the calcium must stimulate the actin and myosin to contract. Generating the action potential, which stimulates the heart to contract, does not require nervous innervation. The heart possesses in-

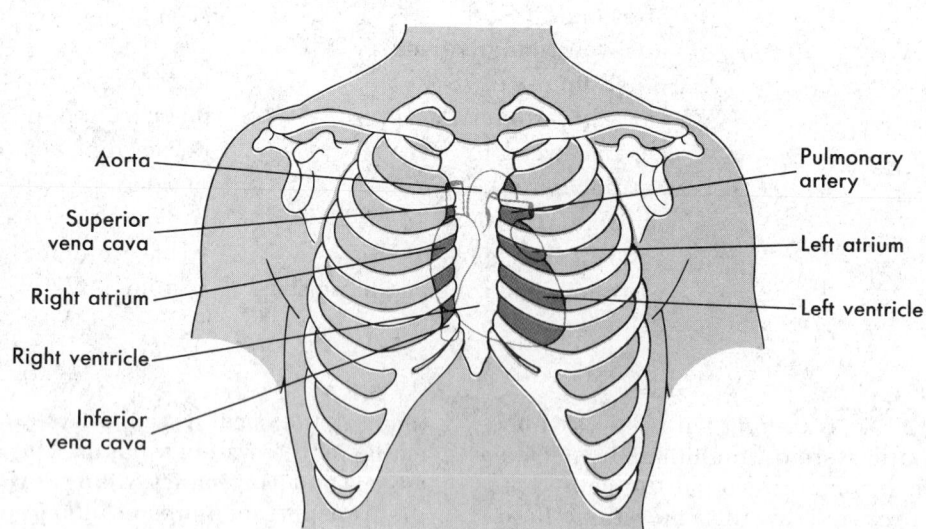

FIGURE 33-1   Anatomic position of heart.

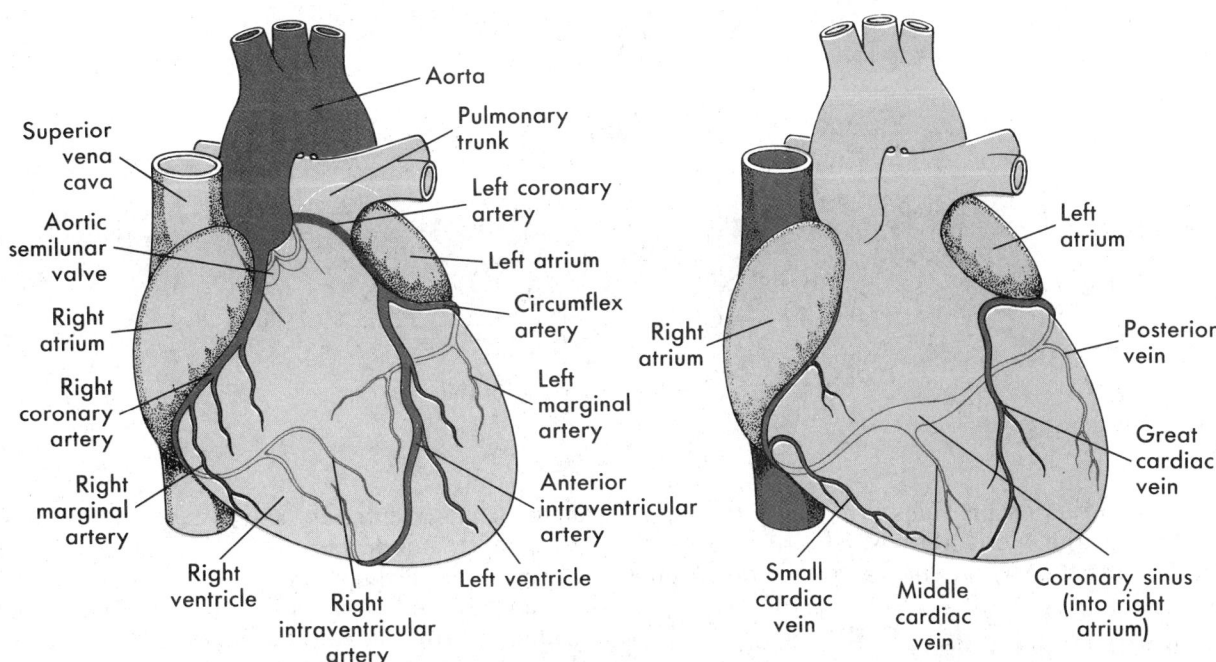

FIGURE 33-2   Anterior and posterior surfaces of heart, illustrating location and distribution of principal coronary vessels.

trinsic pacemakers that depolarize regularly and generate action potentials. The pacemaker with the fastest depolarization rate provides the stimulus for the contraction. Normally this is the sinoatrial (SA) node, which lies in the right atrium close to the great veins. If the SA node is not functioning, the atrioventricular (AV) node will act as a pacemaker, although it will pace the heart at a slower rate. Other areas of the heart may also depolarize and generate additional action potentials and stimulate the ventricle muscle to contract at the wrong time. However, this only occurs where the ventricle is damaged or when normal tissue is irritated by substances such as medications or caffeine. A detailed discussion of electrophysiology of the heart is explained in Chapter 34.

The action potential is conducted at a much faster rate along special myocardial muscle fibers that lie just under the endothelium. This allows the action potential to reach all parts of both ventricles earlier, and a stronger more efficient contraction (heartbeat) is produced, because it is better coordinated. The chemical events responsible for the cardiac action potential and the release of cardiac ions from the sarcoplasmic reticulum are similar to those of skeletal muscle fibers (see Unit XIII). However, the stimulation of cardiac (and smooth) muscle contraction also involves additional calcium entering the cardiac fibers from the extracellular compartment through slow calcium channels (i.e., after the fast entry of sodium into cardiac fibers produces depolar-

ization and the release of calcium from the sarcoplasmic reticulum, sodium and calcium continue to enter the fibers through "slow" calcium channels). This influx of calcium through slow channels produces a plateau on the action potential, which lasts approximately 100 to 200 ms and increases the force and *duration* of the cardiac contraction (Figure 33-3). (Drugs that block the influx of calcium through the slow calcium channels reduce both the rate and strength of the heart's contraction and cause smooth muscle relaxation.) At the end of the plateau the diffusion of potassium out of the muscle fibers restores the resting potential. Movement of the cardiac action potential can be detected at the surface of the body by an ECG. The contraction produced after the action potential can be monitored indirectly by listening for heart sounds or palpating the pulse.

Cardiac muscle is sensitive to the plasma concentrations of sodium, potassium, calcium, and magnesium. Elevation of extracellular potassium or sodium and a deficiency of calcium cause cardiac dysrhythmia and weakness, whereas an excess of extracellular calcium causes excessively strong contractions. Fortunately the blood concentrations of these ions are well controlled, and these untoward effects are unlikely. (Low sodium concentrations may occur with water intoxication and can cause cardiac muscle fibrillation and death.)

The calcium released by the action potential causes the actin and myosin to slide closer together and shorten the myocardial fibers or produce ten-

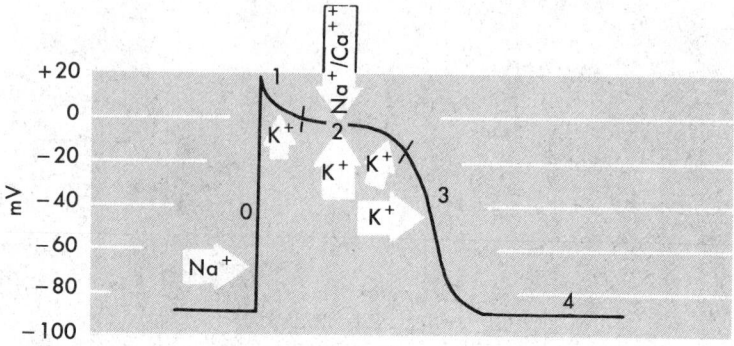

FIGURE 33-3   Action potential.

sion. This contraction provides the energy to pump blood through the blood vessels. The heart valves ensure that the blood flows in the correct direction.

Function of Heart Valves

The function of the valves that lie at the entrance and exit of the ventricle is to ensure that blood travels in only one direction (i.e., from the ventricle, to the arteries, then the arterioles, the capillaries, the venules, the veins, the atrium of the opposite side of the heart, and so on). The valves open easily and do not obstruct the filling of the ventricles or the movement of blood into the arteries. However, blood beginning to move in the opposite direction closes the valves and prevents blood flowing from the ventricles into the atria or from the arteries back into the ventricles. The closing of these two sets of valves causes vibrations and turbulence, which can

be heard as a "lub dub" sound. The lub sound is the first heart sound, and the dub sound is the second heart sound. If the valves are constricted (stenosed) or if they leak (incompetent), additional sounds, called murmurs, will be heard. The contraction **(systole)** of ventricles lasts from the beginning of the first heart sound to the beginning of the second sound. The relaxation of the ventricles **(diastole)** lasts from the beginning of the second heart sound until the beginning of the first heart sound.

The bicuspid (mitral) valve in the left ventricle and the tricuspid valve in the right ventricle shut and prevent blood from flowing into the atria when the ventricles begin to contract (Figure 33-4). These **atrioventricular valves** are tethered to the papillary muscles of the myocardium by chordae tendineae. The chordae tendineae prevent the cusps from being pushed back into the atria and leaking during systole, and the papillary muscles, which contract when

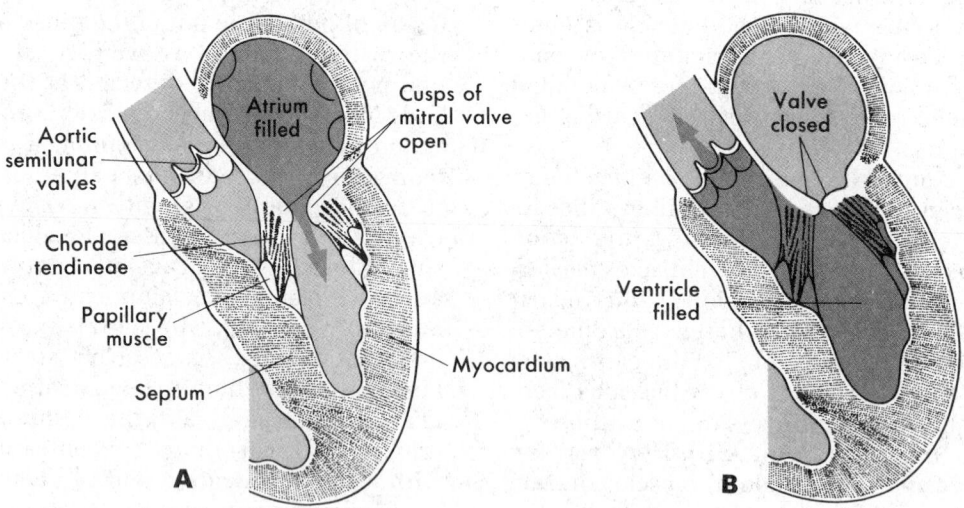

FIGURE 33-4   Action of cuspid valves. **A,** When valves are open, blood passes freely from atria to ventricles. **B,** Filling of ventricles closes valves and prevents backflow of blood into atria when ventricles contract.

the ventricle contracts, tighten the chordae tendineae and make this action more efficient when the dimensions of the heart are reduced during systole.

The aortic and pulmonary **semilunar valves** are each made up of three half-moon–shaped flaps that are pushed flat against the artery wall by the blood that leaves the heart during systole. However, when diastole begins and the ventricle relaxes, the higher pressure of blood in the aorta and pulmonary arteries causes blood to begin to flow backward into the ventricle. This blood pushes the semilunar valves away from the arterial wall, and the flaps completely close the arteries.

Cardiac Cycle

The **cardiac cycle** includes all the activities occurring in the heart during one contraction and the subsequent period of relaxation. The length of the cardiac cycle is usually referred to as the R-R interval, because the peak of the R wave is clearly defined on the ECG, and measuring the time elapsing from one R wave to the next provides the most accurate method of timing a cardiac cycle.

The cardiac cycle is presented graphically for the left side of the heart in Figure 33-5, which shows the interrelationship of aortic, atrial, and ventricular pressures; aortic blood flow; ventricular volume; the heart sounds (phonocardiogram); and the ECG at any point during the cycle. It is presented graphically in Figure 33-6.

The ventricles fill with blood from the great veins. Then atrial depolarization, which produces the P wave of the ECG, stimulates the atria to contract. This causes a small increase in the volume and pressure of blood in the ventricle, which can be seen to start at the end of the P wave. During ventricular depolarization, which produces the QRS complex, the ventricle begins to contract, the AV valves close, and the vibrations produce the first heart sound. Diastole ends and systole begins with the closing of the AV valves.

Between the closing of the AV valves and the opening of the semilunar valves the pressure in the ventricle rises rapidly, but the blood is not able to leave the ventricle, because both sets of valves are closed. Therefore the volume of blood in the ventricle remains constant during this interval, which is referred to as the **isovolumetric contraction period.** Because the myocardial fibers are not able to shorten, much of the energy of their contraction is stored in the elastic elements of the ventricle walls, and this stored energy ejects the blood, extremely rapidly, when the ventricular pressure rises above the pressure in the aorta. The violence of the ejection can be seen in the speed with which ventricular volume falls and arterial flow rises as soon as the semilunar valves open.

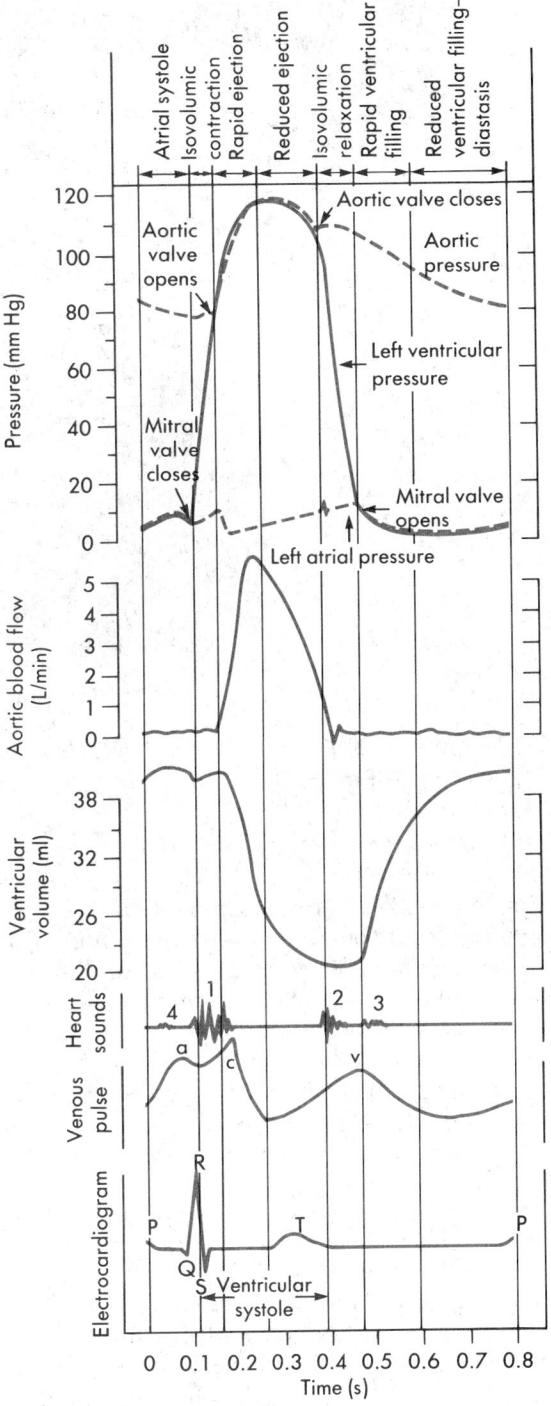

FIGURE 33-5   Cardiac cycle. Left atrial, aortic, and left flow; ventricular volume; heart sounds; venous pulse; and ECG for complete cardiac cycle. (From Berne R, Levy M: *Physiology,* ed 3, St Louis, 1992, Mosby–Year Book.)

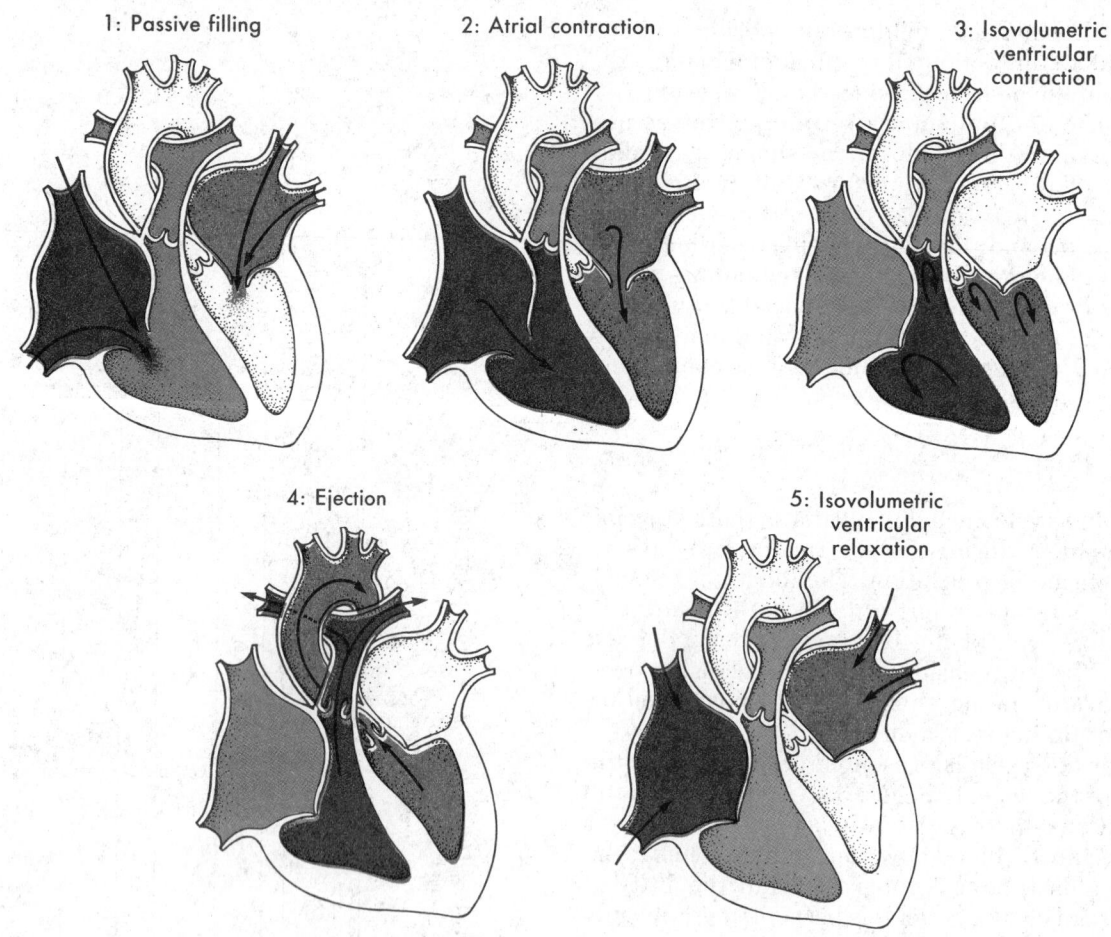

1: Passive filling

2: Atrial contraction

3: Isovolumetric
ventricular
contraction

4: Ejection

5: Isovolumetric
ventricular
relaxation

FIGURE 33-6   Heart during five phases of cardiac cycle. Arrows indicate direction
of blood flow.

The ventricle remains contracted until it begins to repolarize. Ventricular relaxation coincides with the beginning of the T wave of the ECG and is responsible for the fall in ventricular and arterial pressure, which causes aortic blood to reverse momentarily and close the semilunar valves. This produces a deflection (incisura) in the aortic pressure curve and the audible vibrations of the closing of the semilunar valves. Systole ends and diastole begins with the second heart sound.

Once again both sets of valves are closed, but now the ventricles relax and ventricular pressure falls rapidly while the volume of blood in the ventricle remains constant. This period is called the **isovolumetric relaxation period,** and again the walls are under elastic tension. However, this time the volume of blood is small and the ventricle fibers are not able to lengthen as they relax. This again stores elastic energy, and when the AV valves open, the ventricles expand quickly and blood is sucked in from the veins by the negative pressure generated during isovolumetric relaxation. This can be seen in the speed with which ventricular volume rises when the cuspid valves open. During the later portion of diastole, ventricular volume rises slowly and arterial pressure falls.

The oxygen supply to the heart muscle varies with the time in the cardiac cycle. When the ventricle muscle is contracting, particularly during the isovolumetric contraction period, the tension developed in the myocardium forces blood out of the blood vessels that supply it with oxygen and nutrients, and the myocardium develops an oxygen deficit. This oxygen deficit can only be repaid during diastole. This is particularly important at fast heart rates, because the actual time available for diastole shortens significantly as heart rate increases: diastole takes up approximately 70% of each minute at heart rates of 60 beats/min, 50% at heart rates of 120 beats/min, and 33% at heart rates of 180 beats/min. Therefore the risk of cardiac hypoxia (e.g., angina, myocardial infarction) is much greater at high heart rates, not only because the time available to deliver oxygen is reduced, but also because ventricular filling time is reduced and because the heart works less efficiently. As heart rate increases, it requires more oxygen each minute to eject a constant volume of blood. Very high heart rates must always be treated as an emergency.

The actual work done by the heart is related to the volume of blood ejected. The volume ejected by one ventricle in one beat is called the **stroke volume,** and the volume ejected in 1 minute is called the **cardiac output.** Cardiac output is equal to the stroke volume multiplied by heart rate, and it is adjusted from minute to minute by controlling these two factors so the heart is able to meet the varied demands made on it.

Control of Stroke Volume and Heart Rate

Stroke volume and heart rate are continually controlled and adjusted so the heart pumps the exact volume of blood that returns to it. This volume is in turn controlled by the metabolic needs of the tissues, because blood flow through each tissue is controlled by the tissue's own oxygen consumption. Therefore the tissues control venous return and hence the cardiac output. A state of shock results when the heart, for whatever reason, is not able to provide adequate flow to maintain the homeostasis of the tissues.

Several mechanisms control stroke volume and heart rate to ensure the heart pumps all the blood that returns to it. If the mechanism is a property of the heart muscle itself and does not require nervous or endocrine stimulation, it is referred to as an intrinsic mechanism. If the mechanism requires nervous or endocrine stimulation, it is referred to as an extrinsic mechanism.

Intrinsic mechanisms

Like skeletal muscle, cardiac muscle contracts more efficiently when it is stretched (preloaded) before it contracts. The force determining cardiac **preload** (and thus the volume of blood in the ventricle at the end of diastole [end-diastolic volume]) is the pressure in the great veins that supply the atria. Within normal limits, increases in end-diastolic volume produce significant increases in the force of the cardiac contraction. When the myocardium contracts more forcibly, it empties more completely, and stroke volume is increased. End-diastolic volume is normally at its maximum when the individual is lying down, it decreases slightly when the person stands up, and it will again become maximum with moderate activity. End-diastolic volume changes are small from minute to minute.

Cardiac **afterload** is provided by the pressure in the arteries against which the heart must eject its blood. Whenever arterial pressure rises, more of the heart's energy is applied to increasing ventricular

pressure and the amount of blood ejected declines initially. However, over the next few beats, venous pressure and end-diastolic volume increase until stroke volume again equals venous return. If the heart is chronically stressed over weeks or months by high venous return or by having to pump against abnormally high arterial pressures, end-diastolic volume increases beyond normal levels because the pericardial sac gradually increases in size. In addition, when arterial pressure is chronically elevated, ventricular wall thickness also increases.

An enlarged heart is a sign of a chronically overworked or failing heart. The enlargement increases the strength of the contraction and compensates for the extra load or the failure so the heart is able to pump all the blood returning to it. However, the individual may have no symptoms to indicate that the heart is using its reserve capacity. This is appropriate for an athlete, where the hypertrophy is physiologic, but not for an individual at rest. In this case the enlargement is pathologic. It is possible for the heart to enlarge until the myocardial fibers are stretched to the point that further increases in end-diastolic volume reduce the ability of the heart to pump all the blood that comes to it. Then a vicious cycle sets in whereby a further increase in end-diastolic volume results in a smaller stroke volume, and the development of heart failure accelerates.

Extrinsic mechanisms

Stimulation by the sympathetic nervous system and the hormone epinephrine are the most important extrinsic factors that increase stroke volume. They produce an increase in the strength of the myocardial contraction and increase the stroke volume ejected for any given end-diastolic volume. This extrinsic mechanism is particularly important during exercise and stressful events. For example, after the stress of a major hemorrhage, reduced venous return leads to reduced end-diastolic volume, which in turn leads to weaker contractions and reduced stroke volume. To compensate for the weaker contractions, sympathetic stimulation increases the contractility of the myocardium and allows the heart to maintain its stroke volume despite the reduced end-diastolic volume.

Heart rate appears to be controlled primarily by extrinsic mechanisms, and changing heart rate is a more powerful way to control cardiac output than changing stroke volume. Reflexes with their integrating centers in the medulla oblongata control heart rate. Sympathetic stimulation increases the heart rate generated by the SA node when a fall in aortic or carotid arterial pressure is detected by stretch receptors in the aortic arch or the carotid sinuses. This reflex ensures that arterial pressure is adequate to supply the heart and brain with blood.

GERIATRIC CONSIDERATIONS

Physiologic Changes in the Cardiac System

Like other organs, the heart experiences a reduction in its elastic properties with increased age. This reduces the potential energy stored during isometric contraction and relaxation and thus reduces the velocity of ventricular ejection and filling. From 20 to 80 years of age, cardiac output declines and total peripheral resistance increases by approximately 1%, perhaps because of a decrease in lean body mass that accompanies aging.

The heart is vulnerable to injury caused by infections, environmental pollutants, and deleterious lifestyle choices. It cannot function without an adequate vascular system, and its work is increased by the presence of arteriosclerosis. It is seriously injured by ischemia, and its orderly functioning is upset by myocardial infarctions, which can destroy the sinoatrial pacemaker, reduce the heart's pumping ability, and cause valvular incompetence. However, these problems are not normal components of aging despite the fact that an individual's risk of experiencing them increases markedly with age.

POTENTIAL SYMPTOMS RELATED TO CARDIAC DISORDERS

Ascites (increase in girth or swelling in abdomen)
Abdominal pain (caused by hepatomegaly secondary to congestive heart failure [CHF])
Chest pain
Chest tightness
Clubbing
Cyanosis
Diaphoresis
Dyspnea at rest
Dyspnea on exertion (DOE)
Edema or swelling in lower extremities
Fatigue, weakness, or change in activity tolerance
Hemoptysis
Indigestion
Orthopnea
Palpitations
Paroxysmal nocturnal dyspnea (PND)
Syncopal episodes or "falling out" spells
Unexplained weight gain
Unexplained joint pain (may be related to rheumatic fever)

When an increase in arterial pressure is detected by stretch receptors in the carotid sinuses and aortic arch, another reflex activates parasympathetic efferents to the SA node and decreases the heart rate generated by the SA node. This prevents excessively high arterial pressures, which over time damage the brain, kidneys, and other organs. In addition to integrating these reflexes, the cardiac control centers in the medulla are affected by the activities of other regions of the brain. For example, they are stimulated by the pons when respiration is under stress, by the hypothalamus during emotional stimulation, by the thalamus during intense sensory stimulation such as pain, and by the cerebral cortex as a result of thinking and other conscious activities.

Heart as Part of Endocrine System

In addition to its contractile function, the right atrium also acts as an endocrine gland by secreting atrial natriuretic hormone when its walls are stretched by high central venous pressures. The actions of this hormone increase sodium and water loss through the kidney, inhibit the actions of antidiuretic hormone, and inhibit the feeling of thirst. Also, right atrial stretch receptor stimulation serves to inhibit the release of antidiuretic hormone when central venous pressure or volume rises. When central venous volume is reduced below normal, this inhibition is removed and antidiuretic hormone is released.

ASSESSMENT
Subjective

A focused health history for a patient with a suspected or previously diagnosed cardiac disorder requires the nurse to use knowledge of pathophysiology to guide questioning in an appropriate and complete manner. An appropriately detailed patient history may be as diagnostically significant as laboratory or ECG findings. A patient may experience more than one disease entity at a time, such as hypertension, angina (ischemic cardiac pain), and diabetes mellitus.

Specific dimensions of the cardiac system are used to delineate positive findings and include onset, duration, frequency, alleviating factors, aggravating factors, precipitating events, location, quality, quantity, associated symptoms, and chronology of events. The box above lists potential symptoms to review with the patient. The absence of symptoms does not guarantee the absence of heart disease, and the presence and magnitude of symptoms do not necessarily parallel the seriousness of the heart disease. Not all angina presents as chest pain. Some patients will deny chest pain and discomfort but complain of "indigestion" that is associated with difficulty breathing (dyspnea) and diaphoresis and is relieved with rest. Ischemia may also be felt in the jaw, hard palate, cheek, and deep in the ear canal. In addition to specific symptoms, ask the patient about previous myocardial infarctions (heart attacks), a past diagnosis of hypertension, previous heart surgery, a history of rheumatic fever or rheumatic heart disease, a history of murmurs, previous ECG or other cardiovascular tests, and any history of cerebral vascular accident (CVA) or transient ischemic attacks (TIAs). Also inquire as to any previous diagnosis of dysrhythmia.

Other appropriate history to explore includes major adult illnesses, hospitalizations, surgeries, injuries or accidents, immunizations, current medications, allergies, and habits. Current medications include all prescription medications (including oral contraceptives) as well as any over-the-counter medications especially antacids and cold or sinus remedies. Sinus or cold remedies may contain ephedrine, which may raise blood pressure. Symptoms of indigestion may actually be of cardiac origin rather than gastrointestinal. If possible, determine the prescribing physician and the condition for which the medication was prescribed. Ask when the patient began taking medication, what dosage, frequency of medication (i.e., once per day, twice per day, four times per day), and level of compliance. Habits include alcohol consumption, tobacco use, use of recreational or illicit drugs, caffeine consumption, and exercise. Some clinicians also include use of seat belts.

Some clinicians include a risk assessment. This encompasses some information already specified such as alcohol consumption, tobacco use, and exercise patterns. In addition, noting level of stress the patient experiences daily, any support systems, and dietary habits is appropriate. Another risk factor is a positive family history of cardiac disease.

Family history that is relevant to the cardiac system includes hypertension, stroke, myocardial infarction (MI), sudden death of young or middle-aged relatives, chest pain, past cardiovascular tests, diabetes mellitus (DM), and obesity.

COMPONENTS OF THE CARDIOVASCULAR EXAMINATION

Inspection
Symmetry
Visible pulsations
Lifts/heaves
Palpation
General (be methodical)
Specific: thrills, apical impulse
Percussion
Very limited value
Was used to determine borders of cardiac dullness
Auscultation
  Auscultatory areas
    Aortic: second right intercostal space at sternal border
    Pulmonic: second left intercostal space at sternal border
    Erb's: third left intercostal space at sternal border
    Tricuspid: fourth left intercostal space at sternal border
    Mitral: fifth left intercostal space at midclavicular line
  Listen carefully and systematically in each auscultatory area with the bell and diaphragm
  Bell: low pitch
  Diaphragm: higher pitch
  Listen at areas of radiation if appropriate
    Carotids
    Axillae

Sounds
  S_1: beginning of systole; mitral and tricuspid valves close; note single sound vs. split
  S_2: beginning of diastole; aortic and pulmonic valves close; note single sound vs. split (physiologic vs. pathologic)
  S_3: may be normal or abnormal (ventricular gallop)
  S_4: may be normal or abnormal (atrial gallop)
  Summation gallop: sound of S_1, S_2, S_3, and S_4 with fusing of S_3 and S_4
  Pericardial friction rub: squeaky leather, scratchy
  Opening snap: mitral valve stenosis
  Ejection clicks: semilunar valves
  Mid-to-late systolic clicks: mitral prolapse
  Murmurs: intensity, frequency (pitch), timing and duration, location and radiation, quality, pattern, and type (functional or innocent)
Jugular venous pressure

Objective

The patient with a known or suspected cardiac disorder requires more than an examination of the precordium. Some patients have more complex symptom involvement than others. Systems the nurse may evaluate include integumentary, cardiovascular, respiratory, gastrointestinal, and peripheral vascular (see the box on p. 775 for components of the cardiovascular examination). General assessment is included for any patient and refers to the examiner's overall impression of the patient's state of health.

General assessment

General assessment includes vital signs, height, and weight. Note facial expression, apparent age relative to chronological age, nutritional status, general appearance, and stature. Any obvious abnormalities or assistive devices are also noted. In addition, record whether the patient appears to be comfortable or in distress.

Integumentary

Inspect and palpate the skin noting temperature, color, moisture, turgor, integrity, and lesions. Note

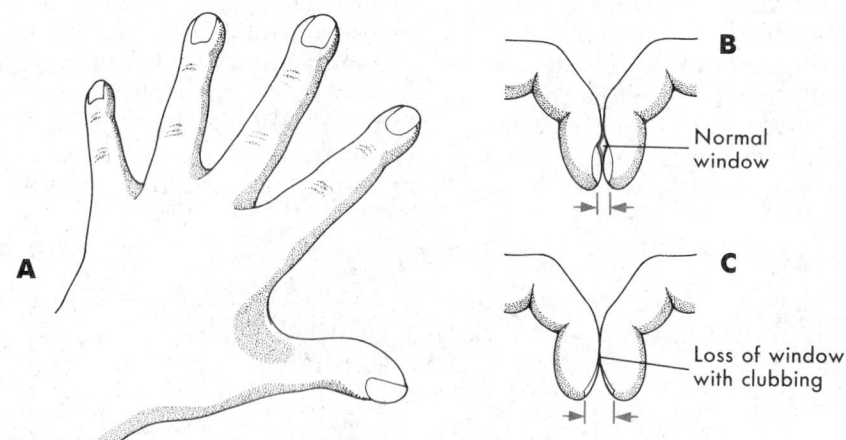

FIGURE 33-7   Comparison of normal nails to clubbing. **A,** Nail beds are convex, and, **B,** normally a diamond shape is formed by them, as compared to, **C,** clubbing, where this diamond shape does not appear.

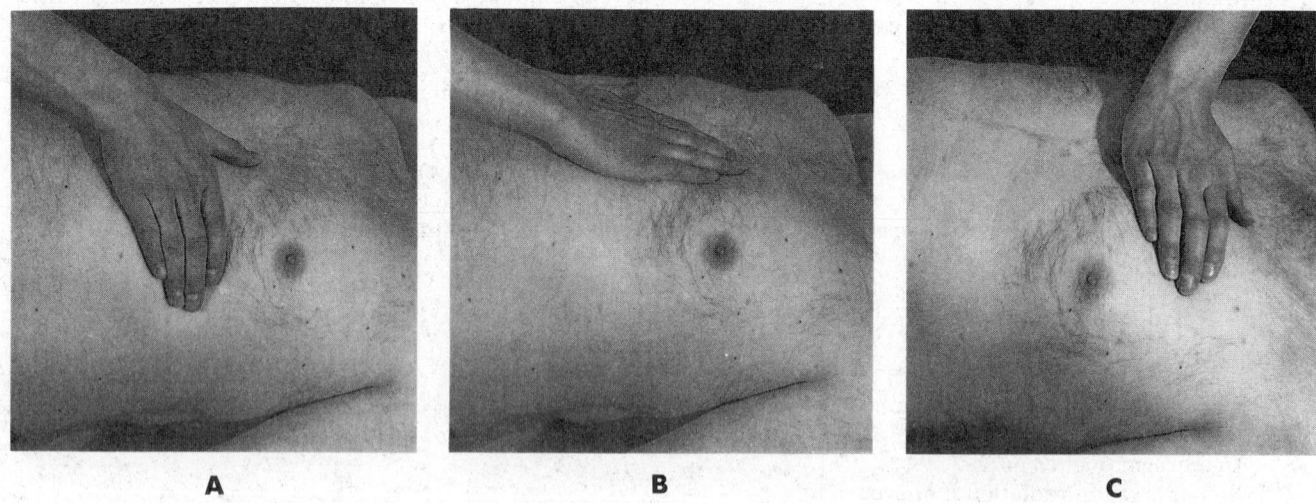

FIGURE 33-8   Sequence for palpation of precordium. **A,** Apex. **B,** Left sternal border. **C,** Base. (From Seidel HM et al: *Mosby's guide to physical examination,* ed 2, St Louis, 1991, Mosby–Year Book.)

PROCEDURE FOR AUSCULTATING THE HEART

Adopt a routine for the various positions the patient is asked to assume, although you should be prepared to alter the sequence if the patient's condition requires it. Instruct the patient when to breathe normally and when to hold the breath in expiration and inspiration. Listen carefully for each heart sound, especially while the respirations are momentarily suspended. The following sequence is suggested:

1. Patient sitting up and leaning slightly forward and, preferably, in expiration: listen in all five areas (Fig. 33-10, *A*). This is the best position to hear relatively high-pitched murmurs with the stethoscope diaphragm.
2. Patient supine: listen in all five areas (Fig. 33-10, *B*).
3. Patient left lateral recumbent: listen in all five areas. This is the best position to hear the low-pitched filling sounds in diastole with the stethoscope bell (Fig. 33-10, *C*).
4. Other positions depend on your findings. Patient right lateral recumbent: this is best position for evaluating right rotated heart or dextrocardia. Listen in all five areas.

From Seidel HM et al: *Mosby's guide to physical examination,* ed 2, St Louis, 1991, Mosby–Year Book, Inc.

nail color, thickness, curvature, clubbing (Figure 33-7), and texture (surface changes).

Cardiovascular

Inspect the precordium, noting symmetry, visible pulsations, lifts or heaves, and retractions. Palpate

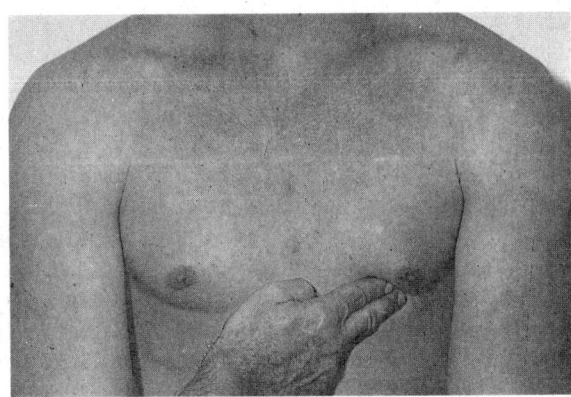

FIGURE 33-9   Palpation of apical impulse. (From Seidel HM et al: *Mosby's guide to physical examination,* ed 2, St Louis, 1991, Mosby–Year Book.)

the precordium generally in a methodic manner (Figure 33-8). Follow general palpation with palpation specifically to note thrills and the apical impulse. Thrills are vibrations associated with grade IV to VI murmurs and have been likened to palpating over the larynx of a purring cat. Note the location of any thrills on the precordium. Determine the location and size of the apical impulse. The apical impulse is generally located in the fifth left intercostal space at the midclavicular line. Normally, it is faint, short, and less than 2 cm in diameter. The apical impulse, previously referred to as the point of maximal impulse, may be shifted laterally in pregnancy and in left ventricular hypertrophy. The apical impulse may not be palpable in obese patients (Figure 33-9).

Percussion of the precordium is of limited value. In past times it was used to determine borders of cardiac dullness. Cardiac size is obviously now de-

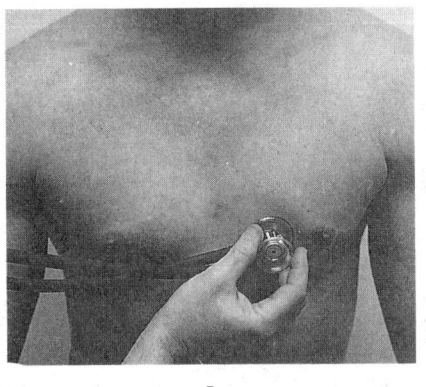

A

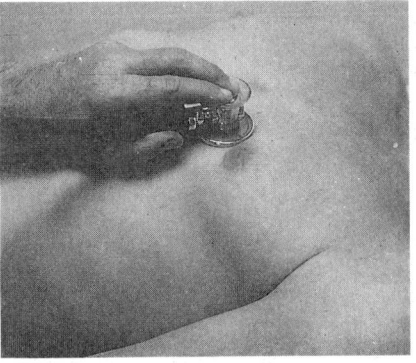

B

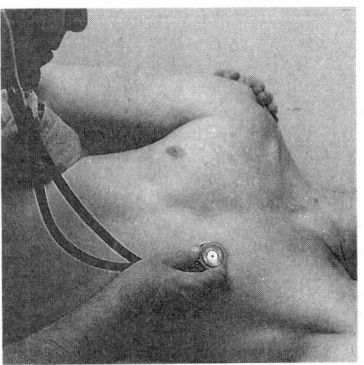

C

FIGURE 33-10   Sequence of patient positions for auscultation. **A,** Sitting up, leaning slightly forward. **B,** Supine. **C,** Left lateral recumbent. (From Seidel HM et al: *Mosby's guide to physical examination,* ed 2, St Louis, 1991, Mosby–Year Book.)

termined much more accurately by chest radiography.

Auscultation of the precordium should be done in a methodic, systematic manner using the bell and the diaphragm in each of the auscultatory areas (see the box on p. 777). Examine the patient in the sitting, supine, and left lateral recumbent positions (Figure 33-10). The bell is used to listen to low-pitched sounds, and the diaphragm is used to listen to high-pitched sounds.

The examiner would do well to "inch" the stethoscope along the precordium beginning at the second right intercostal space at the sternal border and continuing through the fifth left intercostal space at the midclavicular line. If appropriate, listen to areas of potential radiation, the axillae, and the carotids (Figure 33-11).

When auscultating the precordium, note the presence or absence of the following heart sounds: S_1, S_2, S_3, S_4, pericardial friction rubs, and murmurs. The first heart sound, S_1, is created by the closure of the mitral and tricuspid valves at the beginning of systole and is best heard at the apex with the diaphragm of the stethoscope. Although events in the left side of the heart slightly precede those on the right side, closure of the mitral and tricuspid valves is usually heard as a single sound. However, at times, a normal physiologic split of S_1 may be audible at the lower left sternal border (tricuspid area). Splitting of S_1 is more commonly abnormal than normal (Figure 33-12).

The second heart sound, S_2, is created by closure of the aortic and pulmonic valves at the beginning of diastole and is best heard at the base. Because of earlier depolarization of the left side of the heart, a normal physiologic split of S_2 may be heard at the second left intercostal space, especially during inspiration (see Figure 33-12). Abnormal splitting of S_2 (wide, fixed, or paradoxic) may be heard in expiration with the patient in the supine and upright positions.

The third heart sound, S_3, is a low-frequency sound immediately following S_2 that may be physiologic in children and young adults. A physiologic S_3 is associated with conditions that increase the velocity of ventricular expansion such as tachycardia secondary to nervousness or exercise. Prevalence of a physiologic S_3 decreases with age. The exact mechanism for generation of S_3 is unknown, but it is associated with the period of rapid ventricular expansion just after the AV valves open in early diastole. A pathologic S_3 is sometimes known as a ventricular gallop and may be associated with poor left ventricular function and congestive heart failure. The third heart sound is best auscultated at the apex in the left lateral position with the bell of the stethoscope (see Figure 33-12).

The fourth heart sound, S_4, is also a low-frequency sound. It immediately precedes S_1. The exact mechanism of sound production is unknown, but it is thought to be generated by a strong atrial contraction although produced in the ventricle. The fourth heart sound is associated with conditions in which the ventricle is "stiffer" than normal; that is, the ventricle has decreased distensibility or compliance such as in ischemia or chronic hypertension. Atrial contraction must be present for production of an S_4. Thus S_4 is also sometimes known as an atrial gallop. It is best heard at the apex with the bell of the stethoscope with the patient in the left lateral

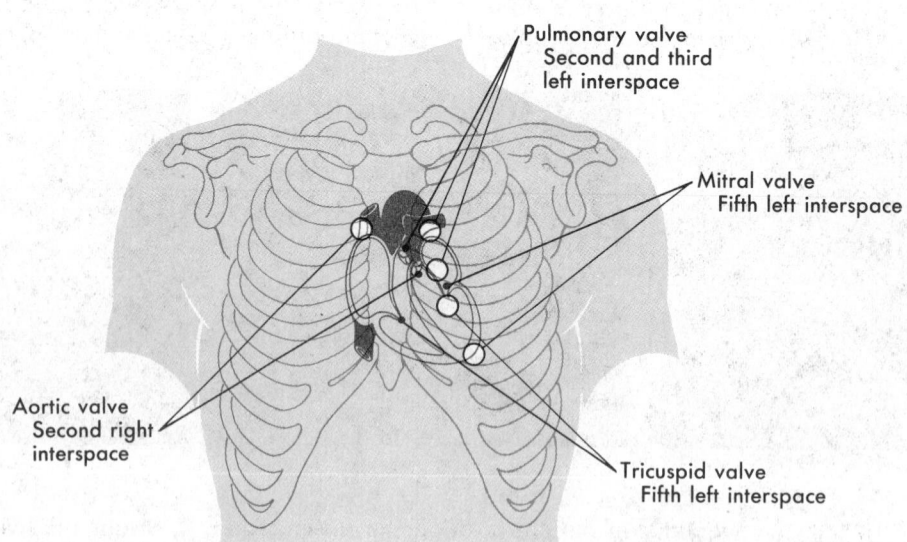

FIGURE 33-11 Areas for auscultation of heart.

position. Maneuvers that increase venous return, such as leg raising, increase the intensity of the sound and cause it to occur earlier, further separating it from S_1 (see Figure 33-12).

A summation gallop is a gallop consisting of both S_3 and S_4. It is audible in the presence of delayed atrioventricular conduction time or tachycardia. The sound of the two gallops fuses, and the resulting sound has been compared with the sound of a horse cantering on a dirt track. A summation gallop is best heard with the bell of the stethoscope and the patient in the left lateral or supine position (see Figure 33-12).

A pericardial friction rub is a high-pitched, leathery, or scratchy sound best heard with the patient leaning forward, holding his or her breath after expiration. The pericardial friction rub may have three components when the heart has the greatest excursions in the pericardial sac: atrial systole, ventricular contraction, and during rapid early diastolic filling. Generally, the first two components are heard.

Normal cardiac valves open noiselessly. Diseased valves may be thickened or rough, which causes the valve to produce an opening and/or closing sound of clicks or snaps. Valvular stenosis produces an opening snap (mitral valve stenosis), ejection click (semilunar valves), or mid-to-late systolic clicks (mitral valve prolapse).

Murmurs occur because of turbulence of blood flow. This turbulence may be caused by (1) a high flow rate through a normal or abnormal orifice; (2) a forward flow through a constricted or irregular orifice or into a dilated vessel or chamber; or (3) a backward or regurgitant flow through an incompetent valve, septal defect, or patent ductus arteriosus. Murmurs are evaluated in terms of intensity, frequency (pitch), timing, duration, location and radiation, quality, and pattern.

Intensity of a murmur may be affected by obesity, emphysema, the presence of significant pericardial or pleural effusion, or a thin, asthenic body habitus. Intensity is graded on a scale from I to VI. See the box below for grading criteria. Frequency or pitch of a murmur is related to the velocity of blood flow and may be described as high, medium, or low. Timing and duration refer to when in the cardiac cycle the murmur occurs and how long it is audible. For example, a murmur may be systolic, occurring between S_1 and S_2, or diastolic, occurring between S_2 and S_1. It may be classified as a holosystolic murmur, or it may only be heard through part of systole and be labeled a midsystolic or late systolic murmur. Location and radiation are determined by site of origin, intensity, direction of blood flow, and physical characteristics of the chest. A murmur may be best heard at the left sternal border with radiation to the left axillae. Quality of a murmur may be described as musical, harsh, blowing, or rumbling. The pattern

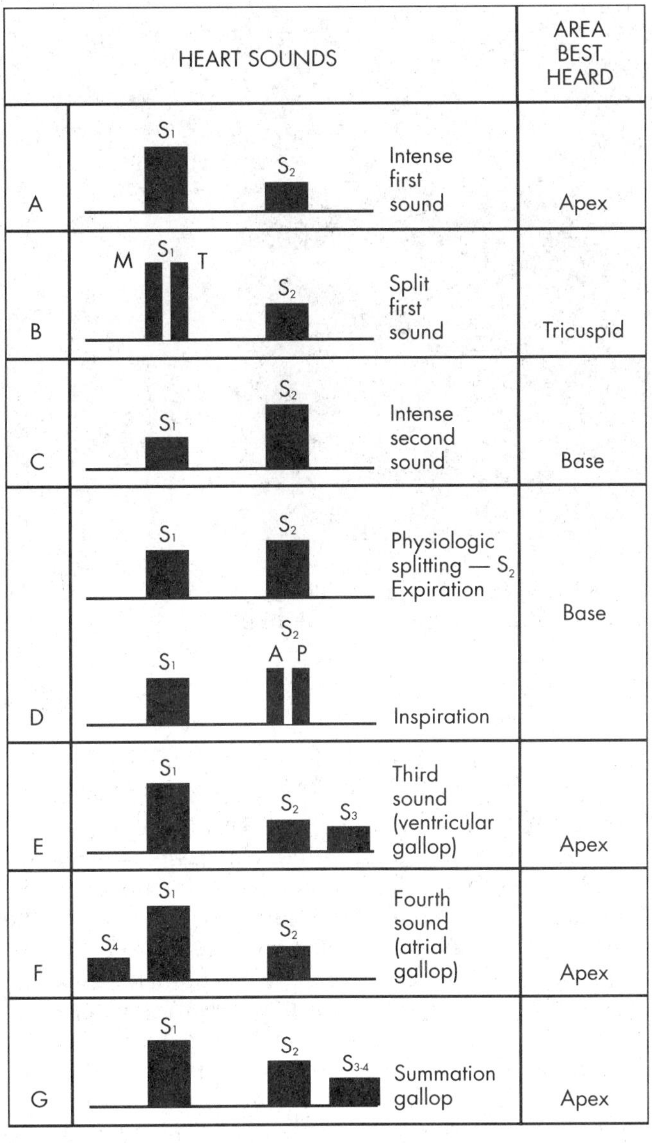

HEART SOUNDS			AREA BEST HEARD
A	S_1 S_2	Intense first sound	Apex
B	M S_1 T S_2	Split first sound	Tricuspid
C	S_1 S_2	Intense second sound	Base
D	S_1 S_2 Physiologic splitting — S_2 Expiration; S_1 S_2 A P Inspiration		Base
E	S_1 S_2 S_3	Third sound (ventricular gallop)	Apex
F	S_4 S_1 S_2	Fourth sound (atrial gallop)	Apex
G	S_1 S_2 S_{3-4}	Summation gallop	Apex

FIGURE 33-12   Normal heart sounds.

GRADING INTENSITY OF A MURMUR

Grade I	Barely audible in a quiet room
Grade II	Quiet but clearly audible
Grade III	Moderately loud
Grade IV	Loud; associated with a thrill
Grade V	Very loud, audible with stethoscope partially off chest; thrill easily palpable
Grade VI	Very loud, audible with stethoscope off chest; palpable thrill

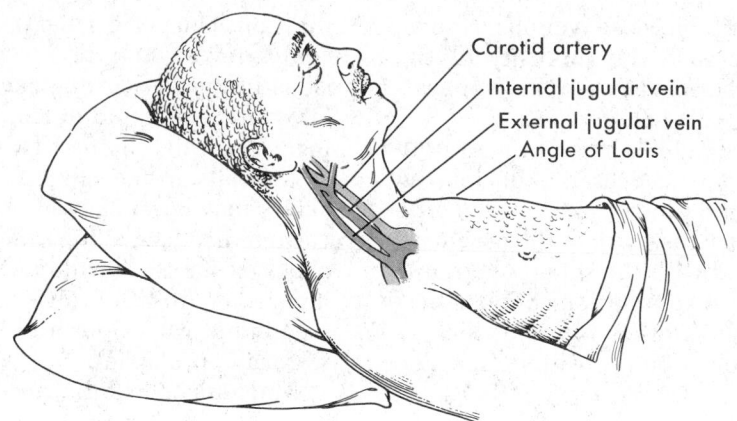

FIGURE 33-13 Inspection of jugular venous pressure.

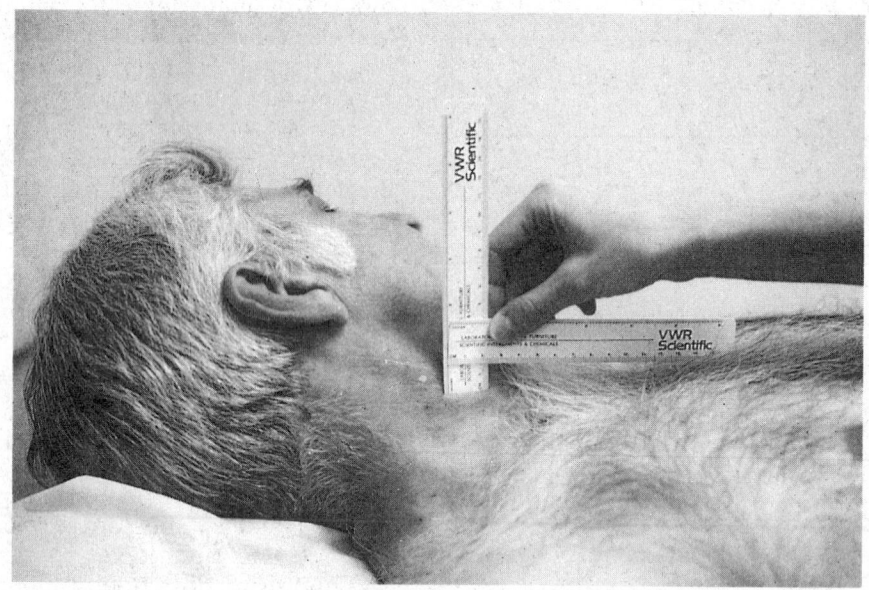

FIGURE 33-14 Measuring jugular venous pressure. (From Seidel HM et al: *Mosby's guide to physical examination,* ed 2, St Louis, 1991, Mosby–Year Book.)

of a murmur may be described as crescendo (increasing in intensity) or decrescendo (decreasing in intensity). Some murmurs are described as being crescendo-decrescendo, meaning they increase in intensity and then decrease in intensity.

Some murmurs are functional or "innocent." These murmurs radiate poorly, change significantly with change in position, are never holosystolic, and are rarely associated with a thrill. In general, these murmurs are not loud except in a state of increased cardiac output such as fever or severe anemia.

Jugular venous pressure is evaluated with the patient at a 45-degree angle using tangential lighting. Palpate the carotid artery. Do not palpate bilateral

carotid arteries simultaneously, because carotid massage could occur, resulting in a slowing of the pulse and a drop in blood pressure. Inspect the neck for the external jugular veins, which lie superficially above the clavicle. The internal jugular lies between the carotid and external jugular (Figure 33-13). Using the angle of Louis as a reference or zero line, bring a straight edge from the angle of Louis to the neck (Figure 33-14). Drop a centimeter ruler from the highest level of internal jugular venous pulsation to the level of the line from the angle of Louis as denoted by the straight edge. A measurement of 2 cm or less above the angle of Louis is considered normal.

Respiratory

Inspect the thorax, noting symmetry, configuration, and pattern of respirations, including depth, regularity, and ease of respirations. Palpate the thorax for tenderness and masses. Percuss the throat generally for quality and symmetry. Auscultate the thorax, noting breath sounds and any adventitious sounds such as crackles (rales), wheezes (rhonchi), or pleural friction rubs. A patient with congestive heart failure may potentially have bilateral rales posteriorly to the scapula. (See Chapter 25 for a complete discussion of respiratory assessment.)

Gastrointestinal

Inspect the abdomen for lesions, scars, striae, visible peristalsis, symmetry, and contour. Auscultate the abdomen for presence of bowel sounds and vascular sounds. Percuss the abdomen generally for tone and specifically to note liver span in the right midclavicular line. Also percuss the spleen to determine size. Palpate the abdomen lightly and then more deeply, noting muscle tone, tenderness, and the presence or absence of any masses. Palpate deeply to identify liver and spleen borders. If splenomegaly is noted on percussion, palpate gently to avoid rupture of the spleen. Hepatomegaly may be noted on percussion and palpation in the patient with congestive heart failure.

Peripheral vascular

Inspect the extremities, noting symmetry, obvious edema, color, pigmentation changes, hair presence and distribution, clubbing, ulcerations, varicosities, rashes, and scars. Palpate the extremities, noting temperature, calf tenderness, palpable cord, and Homan's sign. Palpate pulses, noting presence or absence, amplitude, symmetry, rate, and rhythm. (See Chapter 29 for a more complete discussion of assessment of the peripheral vascular system.)

DIAGNOSTIC AND LABORATORY TESTS
Holter Monitor

Holter monitoring (ambulatory monitoring) is a noninvasive, accurate method for evaluating subtle changes in cardiac rhythm that may not be seen in random electrocardiograms. It is indicated for patients with a history of presyncope, syncope, palpitations, congestive failure, or possible pacemaker failure or for patients beginning a new drug treatment program. During the monitoring period (usually a 24-hour period), the patient wears a small, lightweight, ECG cassette tape recorder that is connected to electrodes placed on the chest and that is carried in a shoulder strap or special belt. Patient-activated monitors are worn for 5 to 7 days and are activated when the patient experiences symptoms. The patient is instructed to engage in normal activity patterns and to keep a journal related to symptoms; taking medications; walking, eating, urinating, defecating, and sexual activities; and emotional upsets. Microcomputers are used to analyze the tapes at the end of the recording period, and cardiac irregularities, if present, are correlated with the activities recorded in the patient's journal.

Routine Chest X-Ray Study

A routine chest x-ray study can depict heart contours, size, changes in individual chambers, placement in chest, and configuration. Since the dynamic aspects of the heart are not depicted, signs of severe organic disease can be missed, but the test is particularly useful in detecting enlargement or displacement of the heart. Patient preparation has been discussed in Chapter 27.

Echocardiography

Echocardiography is a common, noninvasive procedure that uses ultrasonography in diagnosing hypertrophic and related cardiomyopathies, congenital heart disease, and intracardiac masses or clots. Echocardiography is the definitive test in the diagnosis of mitral stenosis, mitral valve disorders, and atrial tumors. In echocardiography, gel is applied to the chest wall, and a transducer is moved over an acoustic window (an area free of bone and lung tissue). Echoes from high-frequency sound waves are used to locate the movements and dimensions of cardiac structures. Four techniques of echocardiography are commonly employed. M-mode (motion-mode) echocardiography involves use of a stationary, pencillike ultrasound beam that is especially useful in delineating the precise motion of intracardiac structures. Two-dimensional (cross-sectional) echocardiography uses a fan-shaped view or sector scan to provide a two-dimensional image of the spatial relationships of cardiac structures. Doppler echocardiography is used to evaluate the direction and pattern of blood flow within the heart. These images can be superimposed on M-mode and two-dimensional images (real time two-dimensional Doppler flow imaging) to provide particularly useful information in the diagnosis of congenital heart disease. In transesophageal echocardiography, the patient swallows a small transducer. Ultrasound waves pass through less tissue and thereby overcome a limitation of standard echocardiography. Contrast echocardiography, which uses a contrast medium, complements the other forms of cardiac ultrasound and is also a valuable adjunct in the diagnosis of cardiac abnormalities. Echocardiography is also per-

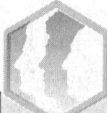

GERIATRIC CONSIDERATIONS

Cardiac Assessment

General approach

Allow more time than for younger adult

Articulate clearly; the elderly patient may be hearing impaired

Impaired sight, comprehension, or mobility may result in less than optimum cooperation

Provide clear, concise instructions

History collection

Interviewer may need to use fewer open-ended questions and provide some specific choices; for example, "Is your chest pain sharp, dull, stabbing, or just a heaviness?"

Interviewer may need to repeat questions

Be alert for answers that do not appear appropriate; the patient may not have understood the question correctly because of impaired hearing or impaired comprehension

Myocardial ischemia may frequently present "silently" without typical anginal pain; therefore think of isch

emia when the patient complains of shortness of breath or increasing activity intolerance

Physical assessment

The physical examination itself is not different, but the approach needs to be altered such that the appropriate information is assessed without undue discomfort or embarrassment for the elder

Environment with minimal noise, distractions, and interruption

Systolic murmurs are very common

Dysrhythmias are prevalent and may be poorly tolerated in the elderly patient because of decreased reserve capacity

Apical impulse may be more difficult to locate because of the increased anteroposterior diameter of the thorax

A fourth heart sound (S_4) may be commonly auscultated in the geriatric patient because of decreased ventricular compliance

---

formed using high-dose dipyridamole (Persantine). This particular variation is more accurate than standard echocardiography and has greater specificity in the evaluation of coronary artery disease in women. Little special preparation is necessary for echocardiography except to explain the procedure to the patient and to prepare the patient for the possibility of being asked to hold his or her breath or to inhale and exhale slowly. The patient is reassured that the test produces no discomfort.

Computed Tomography

Computed tomography (CT) is sensitive to fine variances in body tissue and is useful in evaluating left ventricular wall motion, cardiac tumors, myocardial infarction, pericardial effusion, aortic aneurysm, and aortic dissection. Little special preparation of the patient is necessary unless a contrast medium is used. For a more detailed description of CT, see Chapter 44. This procedure has not achieved widespread use in cardiac imaging, because of the popularity of echocardiography.

Nuclear Cardiology

Radioactive tracer techniques are being used with increasing frequency in cardiovascular diagnosis.

Small amounts of radioactive material are injected intravenously, and a variety of tracers and recording techniques are used to record radioactivity in the heart. The nurse explains the procedure to the patient and provides reassurance that the amount of radioactive material is minimal. The radionucleotide will be excreted from the body in 6 to 24 hours and will not affect family, visitors, or staff. The nurse makes clear that radioactive material will be injected and that its movement will be recorded with a special camera that passes repeatedly over the patient. Since ECG electrodes may be applied, the patient is instructed to wear loose clothing or a gown that allows easy access to the chest. The nurse obtains a signed consent if it is required and instructs the patient in fluid or food restrictions if necessary.

Radionuclide angiography

Radionuclide angiography (multiple gated radioisotope scan; multigated acquisition; MUGA; gated equilibrium heart scan) is useful in the evaluation of left ventricular function, motion of the heart wall, and ejection fraction and in the detection of intracardiac shunts. A short-lived tracer such as technetium 99m is used during *first pass imaging*, when rapid sequential images of the size, shape, and sequence of filling of the various cardiac chambers are made. The radioisotope is tagged in vivo to red blood cells or albumin before injection. This prevents rapid exit of the radioisotope from the vascular pool and permits a more prolonged blood study of the heart. The ECG provides a gate or physiologic marker of end-diastole and end-systole pressures. Multiple images obtained throughout the cardiac cycle are synchronized or gated with the ECG. Synchronization enables comparison of the volume of blood pumped during one ventricular contraction with the total volume in the left ventricle. This comparison, which is known as the ejection fraction, is a sensitive and critical indicator of ventricular function. Radionuclide angiography can be combined with exercise to further evaluate cardiac function. A drop in ejection fraction is abnormal and clearly indicates ventricular dysfunction. No dietary restrictions are necessary before the test, and no preparation is necessary other than that outlined under the general guidelines.

Myocardial perfusion scan

Myocardial perfusion scan (thallium imaging) involves injection of a radioactive tracer (thallium 201; ^{201}Tl), which substitutes for ionic potassium. Unlike radionuclide angiography, thallium 201 does not stay in the bloodstream but accumulates in the myocardium in areas where blood flow is adequate and myocardial cells are viable. When areas are inadequately perfused, the accumulation of thallium 201 is decreased. These areas are termed *cold spots* on a scan. Myocardial perfusion scanning enables indirect evidence of coronary artery narrowing or obstruction and detection and location of myocardial infarctions.

Perfusion scanning can also be combined with exercise testing or exercise electrocardiography to assess changes in the coronary blood flow during exercise (thallium stress testing). Injection of thallium and scanning during performance of aerobic exercises and following aerobic exercises enable evaluation of areas that are adequately perfused at rest and ischemic under stress. Ischemic areas accumulate the tracer normally under restful conditions but lack uptake during exercise. The persistence of low intake during rest and exercise signals infarction.

The nurse explains the procedure for the scan to the patient and instructs the patient to avoid oral ingestion for 3 hours before the test. If thallium stress testing is being performed, the nurse encourages the patient to report any subjective symptoms of distress or discomfort that may occur during exercise.

Technetium 99m pyrophosphate imaging

Technetium 99m pyrophosphate imaging (pyrophosphate scan) is of particular value in imaging acute myocardial infarctions. It is also used in the evaluation of right ventricular infarcts and reinfarcts. False-positive results may occur with abnormal blood pooling, ventricular aneurysms, or metastatic carcinoma. In this test the tracer or radioisotope is injected intravenously and will accumulate in areas where there is damaged or infarcted myocardial tissue *(hot spots)*. Although imaging can be done between 16 hours and 7 days after initial symptoms, peak accuracy is obtained at 48 hours. The patient is instructed to avoid smoking and caffeine or alcoholic beverages for 3 hours before the test. The procedure takes 45 to 60 minutes to complete.

Cardiac positron emission tomography scan

Positron emission tomography (cardiac PET scan; cardiac emission computed tomography [cardiac ECT scan]; cardiac emission CT scan) is a relatively noninvasive and increasingly popular test that uses radioactive tracers and nuclear imaging. The cardiac PET scan provides precise information about surviving tissue and about areas that are deprived of blood flow. It is used to evaluate narrowing of the coronary arteries, collateral circulation throughout the heart's secondary vessels, patency of bypass grafts, and size and location of dead tissue and as a first step in bypasses and angioplasties.

During the scan the patient receives an intravenous dose of an isotope. The areas of positron-emitting isotope concentration are measured, and images are detected and reconstructed using tomographic techniques.

The nurse explains the procedure to the patient. The procedure will vary with the isotope being used. If rubidium 82 is used, the patient is given an intravenous injection of dipyridamole (Persantine), which causes rapid vasodilation and simulates the stress of exercise. The patient is asked to squeeze a handgrip as isotope concentrations are measured. The test takes approximately 50 minutes. Since a history of asthma, significant coronary artery disease, or allergic reactions may be a contraindication for the procedure the nurse collects a thorough health history before the test. If nitrogen 13 ammonia is used, dipyridamole is injected and the patient is required to use a treadmill or stationary bicycle. This procedure lasts 3 hours. A third isotope, fluorodeoxyglucose (FDG), is used to differentiate infarcted myocardium from viable myocardium while the heart is at rest.

If dipyridamole is being used, the nurse encourages the patient to report headache, lightheadedness, nausea, or chest discomfort, because intravenous aminophylline can be given to relieve these symptoms. The patient is instructed to avoid caffeine for 18 hours before the test if dipyridamole is being used and to avoid smoking for 4 hours before the test. The patient is to have nothing orally except for medications with water from 10 P.M. the evening before the test. If the patient is taking antihypertensives, diuretics, calcium channel blockers, aminophylline, nitrates, or insulin the nurse checks with the physician, because dosages of these medications may be withheld or adjusted. A signed consent must be obtained for the procedure. Following the test the patient is encouraged to drink fluids to promote excretion of the radioactive substance.

Magnetic Resonance Imaging

Magnetic resonance imaging (MRI) is a noninvasive procedure that aids in the diagnosis and detection of thoracic aortic aneurysm and in evaluating coronary artery disease, pericardial disease, and cardiac masses. During MRI the patient's body is enclosed within a huge electromagnet that irradiates hydrogen nuclei with a short magnetic pulse. When irradiation ceases, the nuclei realign and the radio frequency pulses caused by the activity are picked up by sensitive receivers. Computers analyze the signals and are able to produce cross-sectional (tomographic) images with high contrast of soft tissue. MRI cannot be used in the presence of metal and cannot be used for patients on life-support systems, with pacemakers, or with aneurysm clips. Metal implants such as heart valves and surgical clips can be moved during the procedure. If the patient has a dental filling or bridge that contains ferrous material, odd oral sensations may be experienced.

The nurse explains the procedure and that the patient will hear a variety of noises similar to a soft drum and then like a muffled jackhammer as the radio waves are manipulated. The noises are not usually unbearably loud, but the patient can wear earplugs if desired. The patient lies on a moving pallet that enters a cylinder containing a magnet, so the nurse needs to make personnel operating the MRI aware if the patient has claustrophobic tendencies. The nurse also needs to consult with the personnel operating the MRI if the patient is on intravenous infusion, since some drip regulators are affected by the MRI. No food or fluid restrictions are necessary for the test. All jewelry, hair clips, and clothing with metal fasteners are removed before the test. The patient is encouraged to void, because the test may take 1 hour or more.

Invasive Procedures

Cardiac catheterization

Cardiac catheterization involves passing a catheter into the right or left side of the heart and is the definitive test for obtaining information about cardiac disorders. It can be used to evaluate intracardiac pressures and oxygen levels in specific areas of the heart, as well as cardiac output. Use of a contrast medium enables visualization of the cardiac chambers. Because of the risks involved, the procedure may be contraindicated in patients who would refuse surgery if such intervention were warranted or in patients who have allergies to iodine contrast media and have not received preventive treatment (prednisone and diphenhydramine [Benadryl]).

During right-sided cardiac catheterization, a catheter is inserted through an arm vein (basilic or cephalic) or a leg vein (femoral vein) into the vena cava and then into the right atrium and right ventricle. The catheter is advanced further, into the pulmonary artery, where it is lodged or wedged in position (pulmonary wedge position) and can be used to measure pressures. During left-sided cardiac catheterization, a catheter is inserted into the basilic or femoral artery and advanced up through the aorta, across the aortic valve, and into the left ventricle. A cutdown, or percutaneous, technique may be used with either the right-sided or the left-sided approach.

Selective coronary arteriography is often performed in conjunction with cardiac catheterization and is used to identify lesions and obstructions in the coronary artery. Selective coronary arteriography is performed using a left-sided approach so the catheter is advanced into the aorta and then into the openings of the coronary arteries. Dye is injected through the catheter, and x-ray films are taken. Complications of cardiac catheterization include looping, kinking, or breaking of the catheter; dysrhythmias; allergic reaction to the contrast medium; arterial thrombosis; myocardial infarction; infection; and hemorrhage at the insertion site.

Patient preparation

The patient should be informed of the procedure and risks. The nurse assesses the patient for allergies to iodine or other contrast dyes and shellfish. The patient is instructed to fast for 6 hours before the procedure. Medications may be taken with sips of water. The nurse describes the sensations the patient will likely experience, such as palpitations as the catheter touches the ventricles; a warm, flushed feeling as the dye is injected; a tingling, numb feeling in the arm if the brachial artery is used for access; and coughing as the catheter is passed into the pulmonary artery. The patient is told that it will be necessary to remain still on a movable table in a dark room. The patient needs to remain awake to follow directions such as taking a deep breath and holding it during injection of the dye and to report chest, neck, or jaw discomfort. The nurse provides emotional and psychologic support and an opportunity for the patient to verbalize concerns. A written, informed consent must be obtained for the procedure. The nurse needs to check if insulin and diuretics are to be withheld the morning of the procedure and to administer preprocedure medications, if ordered, after the patient has voided. Baseline vital signs are obtained, and the quality and location of peripheral pulses are recorded.

Postprocedure care

The nurse monitors vital signs and assesses peripheral pulses every 15 minutes for 2 to 4 hours or according to agency protocols. The extremity in which the catheter was placed is immobilized in a straight position for 6 to 12 hours to prevent hemorrhage and hematoma formation at the insertion site. The nurse instructs the patient to apply pressure to the insertion site before coughing or sneezing. The nurse assesses the immobilized extremity for color, temperature, and signs of ischemia (numbness, tingling, pain, diminished or absent peripheral pulses, and loss of function) and encourages the patient to report symptoms of ischemia, chest pain, dizziness, dyspnea, or warmth in the groin area (this may signal bleeding if a femoral route has been used). Fluids are encouraged for 24 hours to replace lost fluids and to flush the contrast medium. The patient is instructed to avoid bending, squatting, and lifting for 24 hours. If a cutdown technique was used, sutures are removed 5 or 6 days after the procedure.

Cardiac biopsy

Cardiac biopsy is a specialized form of cardiac catheterization. A biopsy is obtained from the apex or septum in either ventricle and is examined for the effect of cardiotoxic drugs and for evidence of rejection of a transplanted heart, active inflammatory carditis, tumors, storage disorders, and primary myocardial disease. Since a tissue sample is removed, the patient must be observed carefully for signs of cardiac perforation, such as chest pain, hypotension, or dyspnea. Patient preparation is similar to that for cardiac catheterization.

Pericardiocentesis

Pericardiocentesis involves the removal of fluid from the pericardial sac for diagnostic or therapeutic purposes. Fluid samples assist in the diagnosis of infective pericarditis, hemopericardium, tumors, systemic lupus erythematosus, and rheumatoid arthritis.

Patient preparation

The nurse explains that the test removes fluid from around the heart for analysis (or to relieve pressure). The patient is told that a local anesthetic will be injected before the needle is inserted and is re-

---

TABLE 33-1   Blood Studies

Determination	Diagnostic value in cardiac assessment
Complete blood cell count (CBC)	Indicates oxygen-carrying capacity of blood; increased hemoglobin levels may occur with congestive heart failure
White blood cell count (WBC)	Increased in patients with bacterial endocarditis, myocardial infarction, and Dressler's syndrome
Erythrocyte sedimentation rate (ESR)	Increased with myocardial infarction, bacterial endocarditis, and Dressler's syndrome; decreased with congestive heart failure
Electrolytes	Decreased potassium and magnesium levels with congestive heart failure; abnormalities occur with drug therapy; monitoring of electrolytes will decrease problems with drug therapies
Antistreptolysin O (ASO)	Evaluates serologic response to streptolysin O, an enzyme produced by group A beta-hemolytic streptococci; reference range: less than 166 Todd units; increased with acute rheumatic fever
Venereal Disease Research Laboratory (VDRL) test	Positive VDRL may be evidence of syphilitic heart disease
Prothrombin time (PT) and partial thromboplastin time (PTT)	Values useful in monitoring anticoagulant therapy, which is instituted in patients with congestive heart failure
Blood cultures	Crucial test to diagnose bacterial endocarditis
Arterial blood gases (ABGs)	Abnormalities of ABGs common in patients with myocardial infarction or congestive heart failure

assured that no actual pain should be felt but that a feeling of pressure might be experienced as the needle is inserted. The nurse tells the patient that he or she will be in a semisitting position during the procedure and that ECG electrodes will be attached.

A signed consent must be obtained. The nurse establishes an intravenous line and reports any evidence of a bleeding disorder to the physician. Sedation is administered if ordered.

Postprocedure care

The patient's vital signs and ECG patterns are monitored every 15 minutes in decreasing frequency. The nurse assesses for respiratory or cardiac distress.

Blood/Serum Tests

Blood studies

Numerous blood studies contribute information about the status of the cardiovascular system. Table 33-1 summarizes these tests and their diagnostic values. A more complete discussion of the hematologic tests is given in Chapter 37 and of blood gases in Chapter 12.

Cardiac enzymes

Enzymes are proteins that act as catalysts in chemical reactions and are found in all cells. Each cell type has its own enzymes. With infarction and tissue necrosis, the permeability of cell membranes increases, allowing the enzymes to leak into the bloodstream. The pattern and timing of changes in blood levels of enzymes and isoenzymes are useful in diagnosing myocardial infarction. (Table 33-2 summarizes these patterns.)

Three isoenzymes of creatine phosphokinase (CPK) have been identified. CK-BB is present in brain and nervous tissue. CK-MM is found in skeletal and cardiac muscle, and CK-MB is found primarily in cardiac muscle. The pattern of total creatine kinase (CK) and CK-MB values is especially significant in establishing the diagnosis of myocardial infarction. CK levels are also elevated with trauma, intramuscular infections, severe coughing, shock, vigorous exercise, and pulmonary infarction. CK levels are decreased with halothane, alcohol, and lithium.

Five isoenzymes of lactic dehydrogenase (LDH) have been identified. LDH_1 and LDH_2 are found in red blood cells, the renal cortex, and cardiac muscle; LDH_3 is found in the thyroid, lymph nodes, spleen, adrenal glands, and lungs; and LDH_4 and LDH_5 are found in kidney, liver, and skeletal muscle. LDH_1 and LDH_2 are increased with myocardial infarction and hemolytic anemias; and LDH_4 and LDH_5 are increased with congestive heart failure, liver disease, and acute glomerulonephritis. When LDH_1 values surpass those of LDH_2 (LDH flip), myocardial damage may be present.

The identification of isoenzymes of CK and LDH has made other enzyme tests obsolete.

Myoglobin

Myoglobin is a small protein that is found in cardiac and muscle tissue. Serum myoglobin levels are sensitive, early indicators of myocardial infarction, but they are not as specific as CK isoenzyme determinations (ISDs), since muscle injury or disease will also cause elevations in myoglobin levels. Normal reference range is 30 to 90 ng/mL.

Blood lipids

Blood levels are useful in determining a patient's risk for coronary artery disease. Determination of

TABLE 33-2   Serum Enzyme Activity After Myocardial Infarction

Enzyme	Normal values*	Patterns of activity afterward
Creatine kinase (CK; creatine phosphokinase [CPK])	Male: 55-170 U/L (55-170 U/L) Female: 30-135 U/L (30-135 U/L)	CK-MB and total CK rise 3-5 hours after infarction; CK-MB and total CK levels peak at 18-36 hours after infarction; levels return to normal in 3-6 days
Lactic dehydrogenase (LDH)	LDH_1: 18.1-29% of total LDH_2: 29.4-37% of total LDH_3: 18.8-26% of total LDH_4: 9.2-16.5% of total LDH_5: 5.3-13.4% of total LDH_2 > LDH_1	Rise begins in LDH levels 12 hours after infarction; LDH_1 > LDH_2 levels 12-24 hours after infarction; peak LDH levels found 48-72 hours after infarction; LDH levels return to normal in 6-8 hours

*SI values given in parentheses.

total cholesterol levels is not sufficient for the assessment of coronary risk, since high-density lipoproteins (HDLs) are associated with a low risk for cardiac disease, and low-density lipoproteins (LDLs) are associated with a high risk for cardiac disease. Through electrophoresis, lipoproteins (**blood lipids** bound to protein) have been separated into groups:

Chylomicrons—primarily composed of ingested triglycerides

Very low-density lipoproteins (VLDLs)—primarily endogenous triglycerides

Low-density lipoproteins (LDLs)—50% cholesterol with moderate amounts of phospholipids

High-density lipoproteins (HDLs)—approximately 50% protein; may serve a protective function; transport cholesterol back to liver from the periphery

Normal reference range (SI units)* is as follows:

Total cholesterol
  20-39 years old
    Male: 124-270 mg/dL
    Female: 122-242 mg/dL
  40-59 years old
    Male: 151-277 mg/dL
    Female: 147-300 mg/dL
  60-69 years old
    Male: 158-276 mg/dL
    Female: 171-303 mg/dL
  70+ years old
    Male: 144-265 mg/dL
    Female: 173-280mg/dL
  (recommended adult levels in terms of coronary artery disease: < 200 mg/dL)

Triglycerides
  20-39 years old
    Male: 44-321 mg/dL (0.50-3.62 mmol/L)
    Female: 36-266 mg/dL (0.41-3.01 mmol/L)
  40-59 years old
    Male: 55-320 mg/dL (0.62-3.61 mmol/L)
    Female: 45-262 mg/dL (0.51-2.96 mmol/L)
  60+ years old
    Male: 55-291 mg/dL (0.62-3.29 mmol/L)
    Female: 56-240 mg/dL (0.63-2.71 mmol/L)
  (recommended adult levels—Male: 40-160 mg/dL [0.45-1.81 mmol/L]; female: 35-135 mg/dL [0.40-152 mmol/L])

LDL cholesterol
  20-39 years old
    Male: 66-189 mg/dL (1.71-4.90 mmol/L)
    Female: 57-172 mg/dL (1.48-4.45 mmol/L)
  40-59 years old
    Male: 87-203 mg/dL (2.25-5.26 mmol/L)
    Female: 74-210 mg/dL (1.92-5.44 mmol/L)
  60+ years old
    Male: 83-210 mg/dL (2.15-5.44 mmol/L)

Female: 100-224 mg/dL (2.59-5.80 mmol/L)
(recommended adult levels: < 130 mg/dL [< 3.37 mmol/L])

HDL cholesterol
  20-39 years old
    Male: 28-63 mg/dL (0.72-1.63 mmol/L)
    Female: 33-83 mg/dL (0.85-2.15 mmol/L)
  40-59 years old
    Male: 27-71 mg/dL (0.70-1.84 mmol/L)
    Female: 34-92 mg/dL (0.88-2.38 mmol/L)
  60+ years old
    Male: 30-75 mg/dL (0.78-1.94 mmol/L)
    Female: 38-96 mg/dL (0.98-2.48 mmol/L)

TABLE 33-3   Serum Values for Therapeutic and Nontherapeutic Agents

Agent	Therapeutic range	Toxic level
Acetaminophen (Tylenol)	4.5-25 µg/mL	> 120 µg/mL
Aspirin (ASA)	15-30 µg/dL	> 30 mg/dL
Carbamazepine (Tegretol)	3-9 g/mL	> 10 g/mL
Chlordiazepoxide (Librium; Relaxil)	0.1-3 µg/mL	> 3 µg/mL
Clonazepam (Klonopin)	3-50 ng/mL	?
Desipramine (Norpramin, Pertofrane)	20-160 ng/mL	> 1000 ng/mL
Diazepam (Valium)	105-1540 ng/mL	> 3000 ng/mL
Digitoxin	20-35 ng/mL	> 40 ng/mL
Disopyramide (Norpace)	2-4 µg/mL	> 6 µg/mL
Doxepin (Adapin, Sinequan)	100-240 ng/mL	> 1000 ng/mL
Iron	60-200 µg/dL	> 500 µg/dL
Lead	30 µg/dL	> 50-80 µg/dL
Lidocaine	1 µg/mL	> 6 µg/mL
Lithium carbonate (Lithane)	0.6-1.4 mEq/L	> 1.5 mEq/L
Mexiletine (Mexitil)	0.5-2 µg/mL	> 3 µg/mL
Phenobarbital (Luminal)	10-25 µg/mL	> 25 µg/mL
Phenytoin (Dilantin)	10-18 µg/mL	> 18 µg/mL
Primidone	5-12 µg/mL	> 15 µg/mL
Procainamide (Pronestyl)	4-8 µg/mL	> 10 µg/mL

*SI values given in parentheses.

Patient preparation

The nurse explains to the patient that the test evaluates the types and amounts of fats in the body. The patient is instructed to eat a normal diet for 3 to 7 days and then to fast for 12 to 14 hours before the test. The patient is told several blood samples may be required before a complete evaluation can be made, since lipoprotein levels vary from day to day. Since glucose levels are increased after a myocardial infarction, samples should not be drawn for days to weeks after an infarction, if blood glucose measurements are to be made.

Measurement of drug levels

Drug levels of cardiac medications are measured to determine if therapeutic ranges have been reached or maintained and to determine if toxicity is present. Therapeutic and toxic levels (Table 33-3) provide a guide for decision making and are considered with the cardiac condition and clinical status of the patient.

CRITICAL THINKING QUESTIONS

1 How is the heart stimulated to contract?

2 Describe the mechanisms that control heart rate.

3 Develop at least three questions to ask patients regarding risk factors for heart impairment.

4 Discuss possible psychosocial concerns of patients with cardiac alterations.

5 Design a logical plan for assessing the precordium of a patient in cardiac distress, setting priorities of assessment to allow for immediate intervention if indicated.

6 Describe the pretest and posttest care for a patient undergoing cardiac catheterization.

7 Using lay terms, describe the procedure of radionuclide angiography.

BIBLIOGRAPHY

Current

1. Bates B et al: *A guide to physical examination and history taking,* ed 5, New York, 1991, JB Lippincott Co.
2. Bowers A, Thompson J: *Clinical manual of health assessment,* ed 3, St Louis, 1988, Mosby–Year Book, Inc.
3. Burrell, LO: *Adult nursing in hospital and community setting,* Norwalk, 1992, Appleton & Lange.
4. Dennis, JW, Greisler HP: Noninvasive cardiac monitoring, *Nurs Clin North Am* 22(1):111-120, 1987.
5. Gallo JJ et al: *Handbook of geriatric assessment,* Rockville, Md, 1988, Aspen Publishers.
6. Gordon M: *Manual of nursing diagnosis,* New York, 1987, McGraw-Hill, Inc.
7. Kane RL et al: *Essentials of clinical geriatrics,* ed 2, New York, 1989, McGraw-Hill, Inc.
8. Kenny RA: *Physiology of aging: a synopsis,* Chicago, 1992, Year Book Medical Publishers, Inc.
9. Malasanos L et al: *Health assessment,* ed 4, St Louis, 1990, Mosby–Year Book, Inc.
10. McDonagh A: Getting your patient ready for a nuclear scan, *Nurs 91* 21(2):53-57, 1991.
11. Murray R, Zentner S: *Nursing assessment and health promotion through the life span,* Englewood Cliffs, NJ, 1989, Prentice-Hall.
12. Rossi L, Leary E: Evaluating the patient with coronary artery disease, *Nurs Clin North Am* 27(1):171-188, 1992.
13. Schultz SJ, Foley CR: Preparing your patient for a cardiac PET scan, *Nurs 91* 21(9):63-64, 1991.
14. Seidel HM et al: *Mosby's guide to physical examination,* ed 2, St Louis, 1991, Mosby–Year Book, Inc.
15. Swartz MH: *Textbook of physical diagnosis,* Philadelphia, 1989, WB Saunders Co.

Classic

16. ANA Division on Medical-Surgical Nursing Practice & AHA Council on Cardiovascular Nursing: *Standards of cardiovascular nursing practice,* Kansas City, Mo, 1981, American Nurses' Association.
17. Bloch B, Hunter M: Teaching physiological assessment of black persons, *Nurse Educ* 6(1):24, 1981.
18. Block G, Nolan J: *Health assessment for professional nursing: a developmental approach,* New York, 1986, Appleton-Century-Crofts.
19. Carnevali DL, Patrick M: *Nursing management for the elderly,* 1986, JB Lippincott.
20. Carotenuto R, Bullock J: *Physical assessment of the gerontologic client,* Philadelphia, 1981, FA Davis Co.
21. Fields W, McGinn-Campbell K: *Introduction to health assessment,* Reston, Va, 1983, Reston Publishing Co, Inc.
22. Guzzeta CE, Dossey BM: *Cardiovascular nursing,* St Louis, 1984, Mosby–Year Book, Inc.
23. Price S, Wilson L: *Pathophysiology,* New York, 1986, McGraw-Hill, Inc.
24. Prior JA, Silberstein JS, Stang J: *Physical diagnosis: the history and examination of the patient,* ed 6, St Louis, 1981, Mosby–Year Book, Inc.

CHAPTER THIRTY-FOUR

Nursing Management of Adults with Common Complications of Cardiac Disease

LEARNING OBJECTIVES

1 Describe the properties of cardiac muscle and conduction tissue that influence heart rate and rhythm.

2 Identify common cardiac dysrhythmias through assessment of the electrocardiogram.

3 Describe appropriate nursing care for the patient experiencing dysrhythmias.

4 Choose nursing interventions appropriate to the care of patients with pacemakers.

5 Describe the pathophysiologic and compensatory mechanisms of heart failure.

6 Describe the major clinical signs and symptoms of heart failure.

7 Explain the rationale for treatment options designed to restore the balance between myocardial oxygen supply and demand.

8 Discuss nursing interventions appropriate to the care of patients experiencing heart failure.

9 Explain each step involved in the application of basic life support techniques.

10 Differentiate between defibrillation and cardioversion with respect to the physiologic effects and expected clinical outcomes of each intervention.

THE HEART is vulnerable to the effect of both diseases and their treatment that may ultimately impair cardiac rhythm, conduction, and mechanics. The physiologic consequences of these disturbances and their treatment will influence the choice of nursing interventions.

Heart rhythm, rate, and contractile strength are regulated by four basic properties (or qualities) inherent in cardiac tissue.

PROPERTIES OF CARDIAC TISSUE

Cardiac cells that demonstrate the first electrical property, **automaticity,** are potential pacemakers. The sinoatrial (SA) node is the dominant pacemaker, initiating impulses at rates usually between 60 to 100 impulses/min. Cells in the atrioventricular (AV) junction and Purkinje system in the ventricles are capable of assuming pacemaker control under abnormal conditions. These subsidiary, or escape, pacemakers (also called latent pacemakers) initiate impulses at slower rates and are normally overshadowed by the faster sinus pacemaker.

Under abnormal conditions, the usually dormant subsidiary pacemakers can pace the heart at slower rates. In contrast, the subsidiary pacemakers may discharge rapidly when automaticity is enhanced, thus *overriding* the healthy sinus node and producing a fast cardiac rhythm.

Cardiac cells that *do not* demonstrate automaticity are nonautomatic working (muscle) cells. Nonautomatic cells, unlike pacemaker cells, are normally unable to initiate an electrical impulse and must be stimulated before they will respond. Under abnormal conditions, nonautomatic cells can become automatic, thus producing abnormal—or **ectopic** —beats.

Disturbances in automaticity are commonly caused by clinical conditions such as myocardial ischemia, electrolyte imbalances, acid-base disturbances, drug effects, and more. The result is a change in heart rate or the production of ectopic beats.

Excitability refers to the cell's ability to respond to the electrical impulse. After it has been stimulated, the cell must have sufficient time to recover before it can respond to the next stimulus. Refractory periods represent the time intervals following electrical stimulation when cardiac cells exhibit varying levels of responsiveness, or excitability.

Conductivity refers to a cell's ability to transmit the electrical impulse. Conduction from cell to cell is contingent on the kind of tissue conducting the impulse (e.g., conduction down the bundle branches and through cardiac muscle is rapid, whereas conduction through the AV node is slow) and the clinical condition of the tissue (e.g., conduction may be enhanced or depressed by drugs, ischemia, and trauma).

Contractility refers to the ability of cardiac fibers to contract, or shorten, in response to an electrical stimulus. It represents the mechanical property of cardiac muscle. Contractility can be significantly impaired by clinical conditions such as myocardial infarction (MI), drug therapy, and electrolyte disturbances. Depressed contractility results in reduced stroke volume (the volume of blood ejected from the heart with each contraction) and inadequate oxygen delivery to the tissues.

Pathway of Current Flow

Cardiac muscle is arranged in two functional groups composed of atrial and ventricular muscle. They are physically separated by muscular and fibrous tissue, the septa, and electrically connected via specialized conduction tissue, the AV junction complex and the bundle branches. Stimulation of a single cell within a functional group results in stimulation of all cells within the group. This phenomenon, called the *"all-or-none" principle,* results in the coordinated contraction of the entire atrial muscle group followed by the coordinated contraction of the entire ventricular muscle group.

The electrical impulse emerging from the SA node in the right atrium is conducted first to the atria via preferential conduction pathways, the interatrial tract to the left atrium (Bachmann's bundle) and the internodal tracts (anterior, middle, and posterior) within the right atrium. Stimulation of the atria produces the P wave on the electrocardiogram (ECG) and results in a coordinated mechanical contraction (atrial systole). After a brief delay at the AV node to allow the atria sufficient time to squeeze additional blood into the ventricles (atrial kick), the impulse travels to the bundle of His, down the left and right bundle branches, and finally terminates in the Purkinje system penetrating ventricular muscle. The resulting electrical stimulation of the ventricles pro-

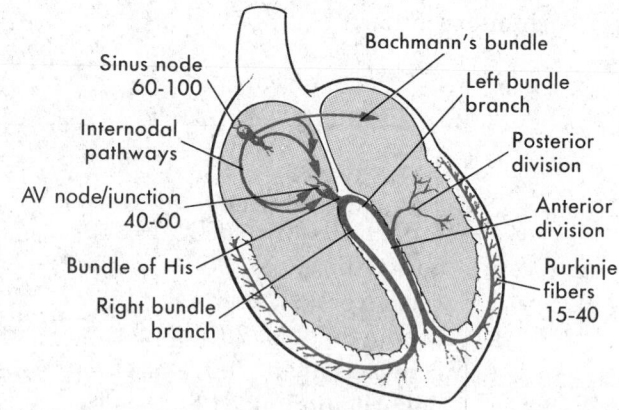

FIGURE 34-1   The electrical conduction system with the rates of the potential pacemakers.

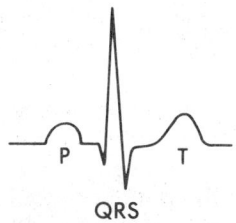

FIGURE 34-2 Major waveforms on the ECG. The P wave and QRS complex represent stimulation of the atria and ventricles, respectively; the T wave represents electrical recovery of the ventricles.

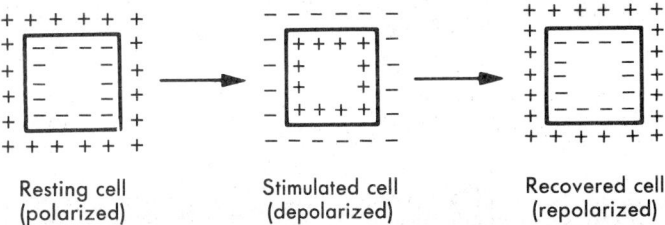

FIGURE 34-3   Changes in cell charge during depolarization and repolarization. The interior of a resting cell is electronegative. Depolarization (stimulation) shifts interior voltage to positive. Repolarization (recovery) returns the voltage to negative.

duces the QRS complex on the ECG and results in coordinated ventricular contraction (ventricular systole). (See Figure 34-1 for an illustration of the electrical conduction system.)

The major waveforms inscribed on the ECG—the P wave, QRS complex, and T wave (Figure 34-2)—are produced as a result of electrical activity in cardiac tissue (an expression of automaticity, excitability, and conductivity). Mechanical pumping, an expression of contractility, follows electrical stimulation of heart muscle.

Electrical events are assessed on the ECG, whereas mechanical events are assessed clinically (e.g., via the pulse, blood pressure, and heart sounds). Under abnormal conditions an electrical event may not result in a mechanical response. When electrical activity is *not* associated with mechanical pumping, a life-threatening emergency known as electromechanical dissociation (EMD) exists. EMD is associated with conditions such as hypovolemia, hypoxemia, tamponade, extreme acidosis, and tension pneumothorax.

Generation of an Action Potential

Stimulation of a cell by an electrical impulse causes a shift in the location of electrically charged particles called ions found inside and outside the cell. Positively charged cations include sodium (Na^+), potassium (K^+), and calcium (Ca^{++}). Negatively-charged anions include chloride (Cl^-), proteins (PRO^-), and phosphates ($HPO^=_4$). As these major ions move into and out of the cell in response to electrical stimulation, the cell's voltage changes (Figure 34-3).

When an electrical impulse stimulates a resting muscle cell, the permeability of the cell membrane is altered, allowing sodium ions to move across the cell wall, causing **depolarization.** Sodium rushes to the inside of the cell, converting its charge from negative (at rest) to positive. Depolarization is followed by a period of electrical recovery called **repolarization** when the balance of cations and anions is reestablished in anticipation of the next impulse. Repo-

larization—restoration of resting negativity—is accomplished by the sodium-potassium (Na-K) pump, as well as by diffusion of potassium to the outside of the cell. It is also during repolarization that the calcium required for mechanical contraction enters the cell.

This depolarization/repolarization sequence is called the action potential. It represents the shift of ions across the cell membrane and the change in voltage (or cell charge) associated with electrical stimulation and recovery. Each "phase" of the action potential correlates with a major ion shift and with selected waveforms on the ECG (waveforms will be described in the section on ECG assessment).

Resting cell

The major ions sodium and potassium are present both inside and outside the cardiac cell, but sodium is highly concentrated on the outside of the resting cell (one that has recovered from a prior stimulus), whereas potassium is highly concentrated on the inside of a cell.

Phases of the Action Potential

Nonautomatic or working cells

The action potential recorded from a ventricular muscle cell (Figure 34-4) reveals that the inside of a resting, or polarized, cell is electronegative at approximately -90 mV. Stimulation of the cell by an impulse suddenly reduces cellular membrane permeability to potassium and enhances membrane permeability to sodium (permeability to these two ions is usually just the opposite). Sodium rushes to the interior of the cell through pathways, or gates, called *fast channels,* making the cell electropositive during *Phase 0* (depolarization). Working cells are sometimes called "fast cells" because depolarization is mediated by entry of sodium through fast channels. As positive sodium ions enter the cell, its interior voltage becomes more and more positive, or

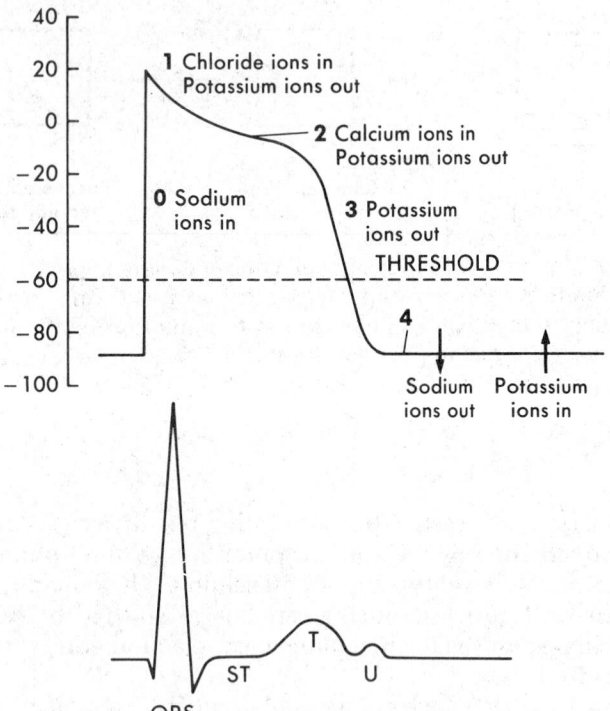

FIGURE 34-4 The action potential recorded from a ventricular muscle cell. Phase 0 corresponds to the QRS recorded on the ECG. Phase 2 corresponds to the ST segment. Phase 3 corresponds to the T wave.

closer to zero. If a critical membrane potential called threshold is reached (usually about −60 mV to −80 mV), the action potential will be propagated; if not, no electrical response will occur until the cell is stimulated by the next cardiac impulse. When the cells's interior voltage approaches −30 mV to −40 mV, slower secondary gates, called *slow channels,* open to allow entry of calcium into the cell; these gates stay open well into electrical recovery (repolarization). In response to a depolarizing stimulus, fast channels open and close quickly to allow rapid sodium entry into the cell; slow channels stay open longer and allow a more prolonged influx of calcium into the cell. Depolarization of working atrial cells produces the P wave on the ECG, whereas depolarization of ventricular cells produces the QRS complex.

Phases 1, 2, and 3 of the action potential represent electrical recovery (repolarization) when the cell's original electronegativity is restored. *Phase 1* represents early repolarization when the fast sodium channels close, effectively preventing further sodium entry. In addition, potassium begins to leave the cell, and a small amount of chloride (−) enters the cell, resulting in a loss of part of the electropositivity achieved during depolarization. *Phase 2* of

electrical recovery represents continued entry of calcium (+) into the cell through the slow channels that are still open. During Phase 2, a plateau is created on the action potential curve as a result of a relative balance between entry and exit of positively charged ions (calcium enters, potassium leaves). It is during Phase 2 that calcium-mediated mechanical contraction (or systole) occurs. Phase 2 correlates with the ST segment observed following the QRS on the ECG. *Phase 3* repolarization finds the slow channels closed, preventing further calcium entry. This phase primarily reflects rapid potassium exodus from the cell as electronegativity is restored. It is correlated with the T wave on the ECG. *Phase 4* finds the cell electronegative again, but the concentration gradient between potassium and sodium is reversed (sodium inside and potassium outside). The Na-K pump restores the proper concentration gradient by actively pumping potassium into the cell and sodium out of the cell.

During repolarization of the cardiac cell, the positive interior voltage generated by depolarization returns to negative resting levels. As the cell's voltage becomes increasingly negative, some of the channels that control the entry of sodium and calcium into the cell (the fast and slow channels) may open in response to a stimulus, thus initiating ectopic beats.

Automatic or pacemaker cells

Automatic cells—the pacemaker cells that normally exhibit the property of automaticity—do not require a separate stimulus to depolarize. Though several potential pacemakers exist in the heart, this discussion focuses on the dominant *sinus* pacemaker only. The action potential recorded from a pacemaker cell (Figure 34-5) exhibits the same phases as the action potential recorded from a working cell, but there is no correlation with waveforms on the ECG. Pacemaker cells are sometimes called "slow cells" because depolarization is mediated by entry of calcium through slow channels. Repolarization proceeds through recovery phases 1, 2, and 3 until resting electronegativity is restored during phase 4.

The phases of the action potential—like the waveforms on the ECG—can be altered by clinical pathologic conditions and by a host of drugs.

Refractory periods

Refractory periods are times during the cardiac cycle when stimulation of a cell may or may not produce a response depending on the cell's voltage (cardiac cells must achieve a certain interior electronegativity before they can respond). The presence of refractory periods helps ensure adequate time for diastolic filling before mechanical systole. Refractory periods correlate with the phases of the action

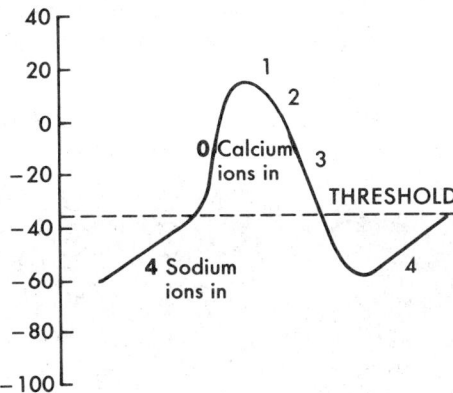

FIGURE 34-5 The action potential recorded from a pacemaker cell. Pacemaker cells depolarize spontaneously and are not dependent on an outside stimulus. Note the loss of resting electronegativity as positive sodium ions leak into the cell during phase 4 (slow diastolic depolarization). When threshold is reached, calcium enters during the Phase 0 depolarization.

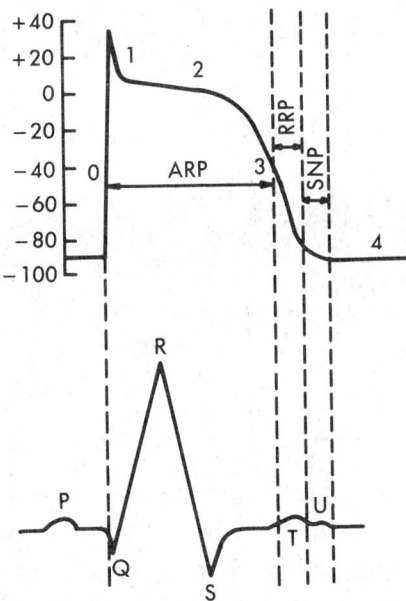

FIGURE 34-6 Refractory periods. Note the correlation between refractory periods, phases of the action potential, and ECG waveforms.

potential and with certain waveforms recorded on the surface ECG (Figure 34-6).

The absolute refractory period (ARP), or effective refractory period, begins when working myocardial cells are depolarized and ends during repolarization. Further electrical stimulation during the ARP will not produce a response because cells are unresponsive to stimuli of any magnitude (in other words, they are not excitable). The ARP can be correlated with the action potential: The ARP begins with Phase 0 depolarization (when the cell's voltage suddenly shifts from negative to positive) and ends during Phase 3 repolarization (when the cell's voltage begins returning to negative). On the surface ECG, the ARP corresponds to the time measured from the beginning of the QRS to the early portion of the T wave.

The relative refractory period (RRP) occurs during repolarization of working ventricular cells when excitability has been partially restored. Cell voltage is becoming increasingly negative, but the cells have not completely repolarized. A stimulus of sufficient magnitude delivered during the RRP may produce a chaotic response if cell voltage has decreased enough to open either fast sodium channels or slow calcium channels. The RRP can be correlated with most of Phase 3 repolarization on the action potential and with most of the T wave on the surface ECG. The R-on-T phenomenon refers to delivery of a stimulus during the vulnerable period that coincides with the peak of the T wave, and it may result in production of a life-threatening rhythm.

The supernormal period (SNP) represents a brief period during repolarization when a weak stimulus can produce a response. Recovery is nearly com-

plete, and cell voltage is *almost* at resting levels once more. But because voltage is relatively close to threshold levels, a weak stimulus delivered during the SNP can produce a response. The SNP corresponds to the terminal portion of Phase 3 repolarization of the action potential and to the u wave that may be observed following the T wave on the ECG.

ASSESSING THE ELECTROCARDIOGRAM

The **electrocardiogram** (or ECG) is a graphic representation of the electrical forces produced by the heart. As the electrical impulse travels from its pacemaker source through the cardiac muscle, representative waveforms are written on the surface ECG. The ECG is an essential diagnostic tool that can reveal valuable clinical information about the status of the cardiovascular system, as well as other body systems. It can provide useful information about metabolic status, fluid and electrolyte balance, and the effects of various therapeutic interventions (e.g., drugs, fluids, and mechanical supports).

12-Lead System

A lead is an electrical system that senses the magnitude and direction of current flow in the heart. A standard ECG records different views of cardiac electrical activity utilizing 12 distinct lead configurations. Some lead configurations consist of both a pos-

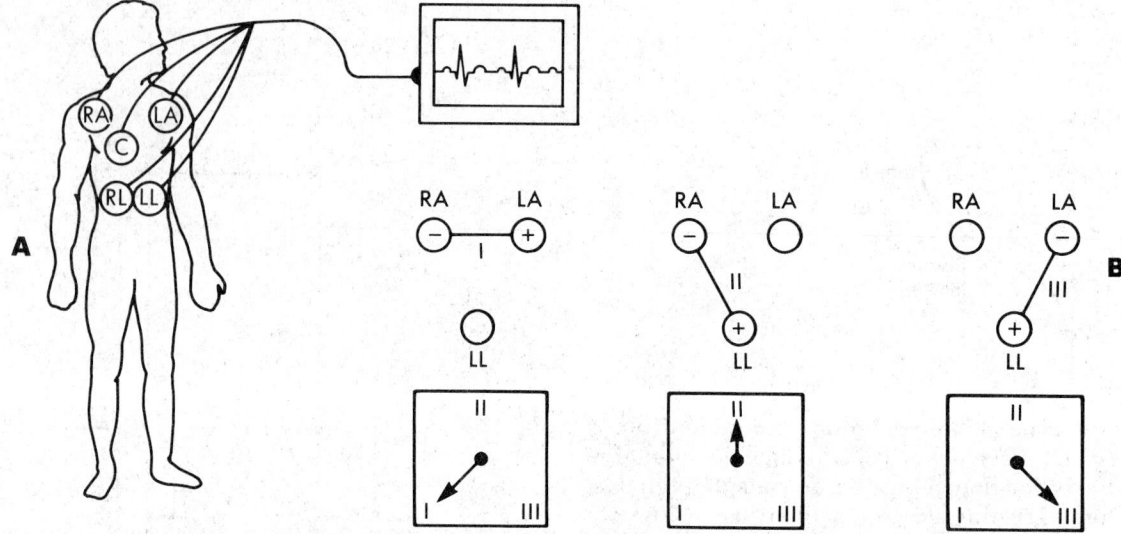

FIGURE 34-7   **A,** Schematic of bedside monitoring. Electrodes are normally placed on the left arm *(LA),* right arm *(RA),* left leg *(LL),* right leg *(RL),* and one of six locations on the chest wall *(C).* The RL electrode serves as a ground. **B,** Choosing leads. Adjusting the lead selector switch will automatically program the electrodes to be positive or negative depending on the lead chosen.

RESEARCH BRIEF

Drew BJ, Ide B, Sparacino PSA: Accuracy of bedside electrocardiographic monitoring: a report on current practices of critical care nurses, *Heart Lung* 20(6): 597, 1991.

The accuracy of monitoring data influences the diagnosis and choice of treatment for many dysrhythmias. The purpose of this study was to determine which leads nurses select for continuous monitoring (was the best lead selected?) and the accuracy of lead placement. A random sample of 1000 staff nurses working in adult critical care and telemetry units received a monitoring questionnaire, and 302 nurses (30%) returned it. Of the nurses who routinely used single-channel monitors (capable of recording one lead), 63% demonstrated incorrect technique for obtaining their lead of choice (most often lead II). Of the nurses who used dual-channel monitors (capable of recording at least two leads simultaneously), 87% demonstrated incorrect techniques; this group preferred lead II and either V_I or MCL_1. In both groups electrode placement was the major problem, especially with chest leads. The authors suggest that more time should be spent educating nurses about the basics of ECG monitoring.

itive and a negative electrode (bipolar leads), while others use only a positive electrode and an electronically created central reference point (unipolar leads). Each lead looks at cardiac electrical activity from a unique perspective.

To record electrical activity in the heart, electrodes are placed in designated positions on the body surface and are connected by a recording cable to either a bedside monitor or an ECG machine (see Figure 34-7 and box on continuous monitoring). Lead selection and electrode placement influence the accuracy of monitoring data (see Research Brief at left).

A standard ECG is composed of six limb leads and six chest leads that are derived in different "planes of reference," imaginary two-dimensional reference points for recording electrical activity.

Limb leads are derived in the imaginary frontal plane that bisects the body, separating it front to back (Figure 34-8). Electrodes placed on the borders of the frontal plane form standard leads I, II, and III and augmented leads aV_R, aV_L, and aV_F. Limb leads I, II, and III are called bipolar, because they compare the electrical potentials generated between two electrodes (one positive and one negative) placed on the body surface at points equally distant from the heart. Limb leads aV_R, aV_L, and aV_F are called unipolar, because they compare electrical potentials generated between the positive electrode (posi-

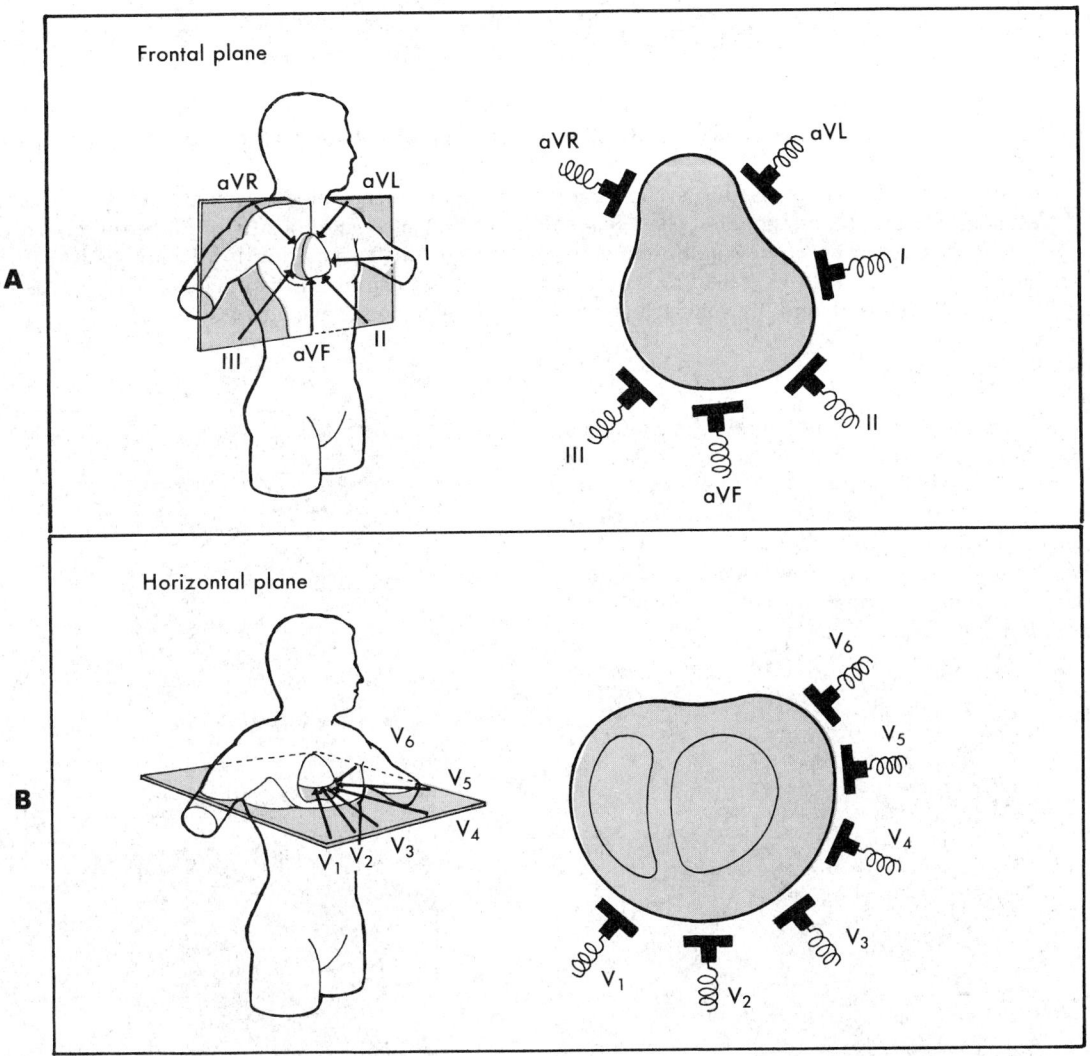

FIGURE 34-8   Planes of reference. **A,** The frontal plane. **B,** The horizontal plane.

tioned at a point distant from the heart) and a reference point.

Chest leads (precordial leads) are derived in the imaginary horizontal plane that bisects the body, separating it top to bottom. Electrodes placed on the borders of the horizontal plane form chest leads V_1 through V_6. Though limb electrodes remain stationary during ECG monitoring, the chest electrode (the positive electrode) must be moved to a designated position on the outer chest wall to record electrical activity from different precordial sites. Chest leads V_1 through V_6 are unipolar leads, because they compare electrical potentials between the positive electrode (positioned close to the heart) and a reference point.

Each lead sees the flow of electrical current in the heart in relation to the lead's axis. The axis of a lead refers to an imaginary line drawn between the positive and negative electrodes of a bipolar lead or between the positive electrode and the reference point of a unipolar lead (Figure 34-9). Current flowing parallel to a lead's axis will yield the tallest positive or negative deflection on the ECG, whereas current flowing perpendicular to it will yield the smallest, or most equiphasic (equally positive and negative) deflection. Note that when current flows somewhere "in between"—neither parallel nor perpendicular to a lead's axis—the amplitude of the waveform varies between the tallest and the smallest possible.

The concept of lead axis is related to the "rule of current flow" (Figure 34-10) which states that:
- Current flowing toward the positive end of a lead produces a predominantly positive (or upward) deflection on the ECG.
- Current flowing away from the positive end of a lead produces a predominantly negative (or downward) deflection on the ECG.

CONTINUOUS MONITORING

A 5-electrode system (see Figure 34-7) can display any lead, and some systems can display two or more leads at the same time. A three-electrode system can display limb leads I, II, and III and modified chest leads (called MCL leads) that closely approximate conventional V leads. There is no single best lead for continuous monitoring, but leads II and V_1 (or MCL$_1$) are commonly used.

To monitor lead II or lead V_1 (using a 5-electrode system):

To display lead II, place the four limb electrodes as shown in Figure 34-7, and set the lead selector switch on lead II. To display lead V_1, set the lead selector switch on V (or C), and place the chest electrode in the V_1 position; there is no need to move the limb electrodes. Any V lead may be displayed by moving the chest electrode to the desired position, as illustrated below.

To monitor lead MCL$_1$ or MCL$_6$ (using a 3-electrode system):

Set the lead selector switch on lead I (this makes the LA electrode positive). Place the LA electrode (+) in the V_1 position to display lead MCL$_1$ or in the V_6 position to display lead MCL$_6$. Place the other electrodes as shown.

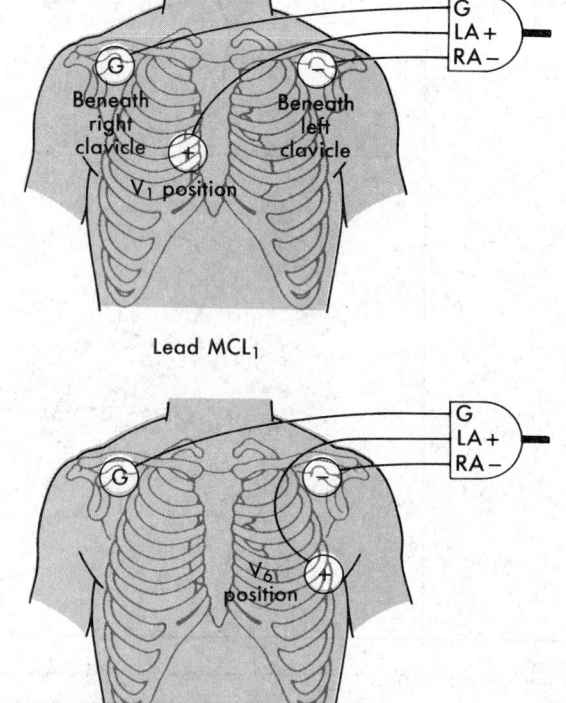

Lead MCL$_1$

Lead MCL$_6$

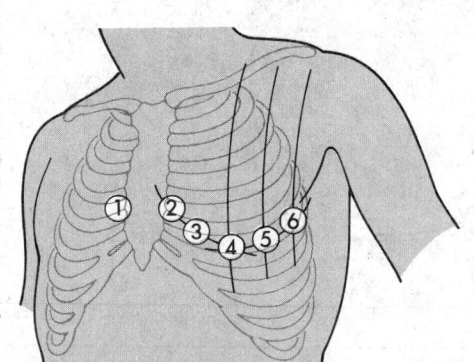

The concepts of lead axis and current flow are incorporated into the following example: Current flow in the normal adult heart parallels the axis of lead II and spreads toward lead II's positive end. Thus waveforms recorded from lead II will be taller compared with other leads (because current flows parallel to the lead's axis) and positive (because the current flows toward the positive end of lead II).

The average direction of current flow in the normal adult heart—known as the *cardiac axis* as opposed to the lead's axis—is down and to the left as viewed in the frontal plane. Current flows "down" because the wave of depolarization spreads from the sinus node (oriented superiorly) to the ventricles (oriented inferiorly). Current flows "left" because

the average current flow is pulled toward the greater muscle mass of the left ventricle. When viewed in the horizontal plane, the cardiac axis is pulled toward the back because the larger left ventricular muscle mass is oriented posteriorly (Figure 34-11).

Assessment Parameters

ECG tracing

The ECG tracing is recorded on special graph paper composed of intersecting horizontal and vertical lines that form a grid. The lines on the grid display large squares (formed by dark lines) and small squares (formed by light lines). Each large square is composed of five small squares horizontally and ver-

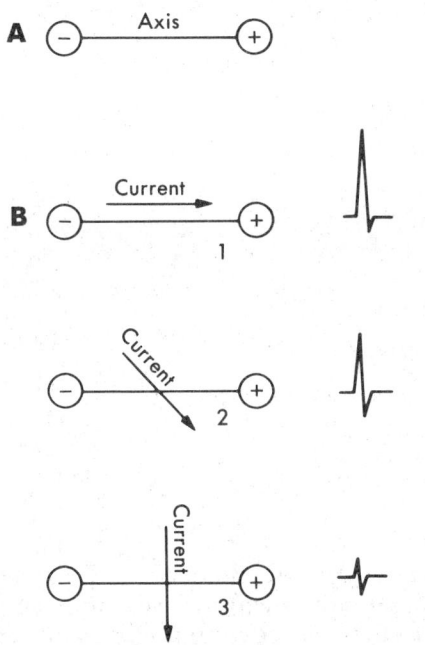

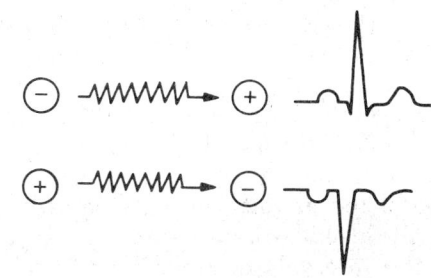

FIGURE 34-10   Rule of current flow. Current flowing toward the positive end of a lead writes a positive deflection on the ECG, while current flowing toward the negative end writes a negative deflection.

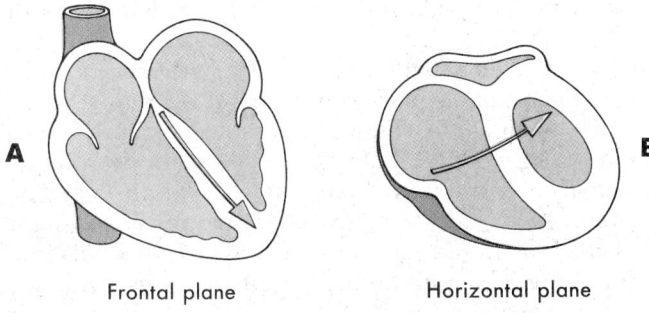

FIGURE 34-9   **A,** Lead axis. An imaginary line drawn between the two ends of a lead forms its axis. **B,** Waveform voltage (amplitude) in relation to lead axis. The waveform is tallest when current flows parallel to a lead's axis *(1)* and is smallest when current flows perpendicular to it *(3)*. Voltage is somewhere in between when current flows neither parallel nor perpendicular to a lead *(2)*.

FIGURE 34-11   The cardiac axis. **A,** Current flows down and to the left as viewed in the frontal plane. **B,** Current flows toward the back as viewed in the horizontal plane.

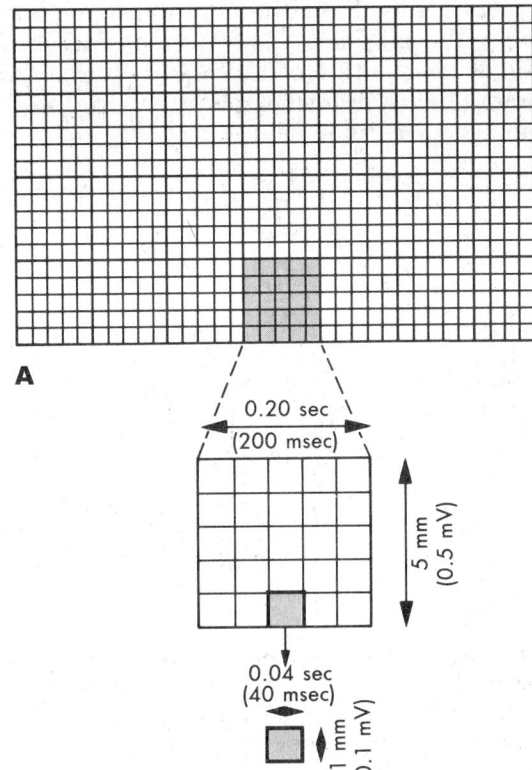

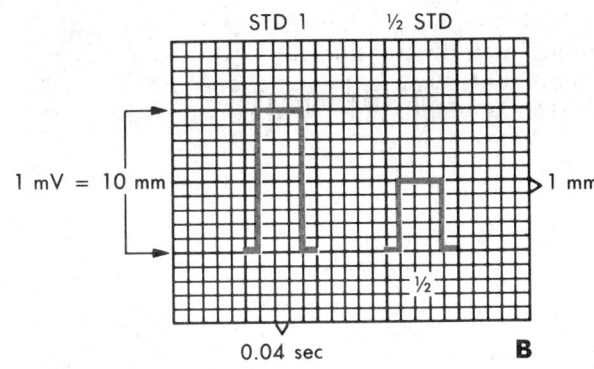

FIGURE 34-12   **A,** Horizontal increments on the ECG paper represent units of time. Vertical increments represent voltage. **B,** Standardization. A standard 1 mV signal deflects the writing arm 10 mm (STD 1). Decreasing the standardization will shrink large complexes; at ½ STD a 0.5 mV signal deflects the writing arm 5 mm. Standardization can also be doubled to enlarge small complexes; a 2 mV signal (STD 2) will deflect the writing arm 20 mm (not shown).

tically that are used to assess rate, intervals, and voltage changes. When the ECG machine is recording, the paper rolls under the writing arm at a speed of 25 mm/second. The deflections of the writing arm above and below the baseline inscribe the characteristic ECG waveforms on the moving paper.

Horizontal increments on ECG paper represent units of time used to determine heart rate and to measure the intervals between waveforms (Figure 34-12). Each small square represents 0.04 seconds across, whereas each large square represents 0.2 seconds across ($5 \times 0.04'' = 0.2''$). Five large squares across represent 1 second ($5 \times 0.2'' = 1''$). The top of the ECG graph paper is marked with either a dot or a vertical line representing either 2-second or 3-second intervals for use in rapid calculations of rate.

Vertical increments on the ECG represent voltage. Each small square represents 0.1 mV (or 1 mm), while each large square represents 0.5 mV (or 5 mm). The height of the QRS deflection, or voltage, reveals information about the size of the cardiac chamber. In addition, the presence of ST segment displacement either above or below the baseline (measured in millimeters) often provides evidence of myocardial injury.

Waveforms

The **P wave** represents depolarization of the atria and normally precedes the QRS complex (Figure 34-13). Its shape and deflection in relation to the baseline will vary according to the lead and the clinical state of the heart. It should be gently rounded without peaking or notching (indicative of atrial chamber enlargement), and its height should not exceed 2 to 3 mm in any lead. The P wave is normally pos-

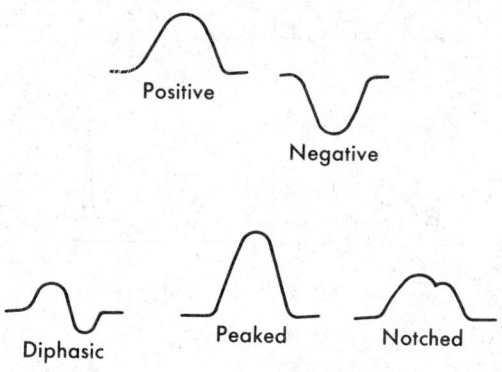

FIGURE 34-13   P waves

itive (deflected above the baseline) in leads II, III, and aV_F, negative in lead aV_R, and may be diphasic (half up and half down) in leads III and V_1. The low voltage waveform representing atrial repolarization (the T_P wave) is usually buried in the QRS and therefore not visible on the ECG.

The **QRS complex** represents depolarization of the ventricles and normally follows the P wave. Its shape and deflection in relation to the baseline will also vary from lead to lead and will reflect the status of electrical conduction in the ventricles. The waveforms that comprise a QRS complex can be labeled, and many different waveform sequences are possible (Figure 34-14), but they all represent the same thing—ventricular depolarization. The amplitude of the QRS, or the total deflection above and below the baseline, may vary considerably, but it usually does not exceed 25 mm. Voltage of less than 5 mm implies diffuse coronary disease, widespread damage, or cardiac failure.

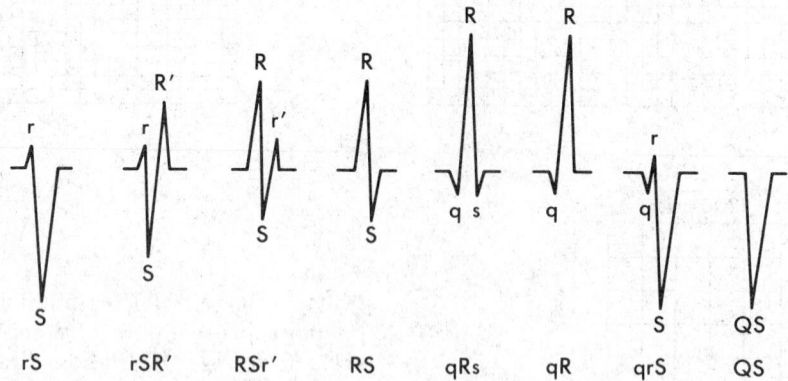

FIGURE 34-14   QRS complexes and labeling: Q wave = the first negative deflection preceding an R wave; R wave = the first positive deflection; S wave = the negative deflection following an R wave; R′ wave = the second positive deflection; S′ wave = the negative deflection following an R′ wave; QS wave = a totally negative deflection.

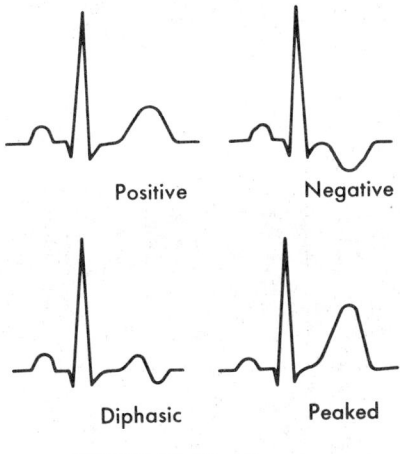

FIGURE 34-15   T waves.

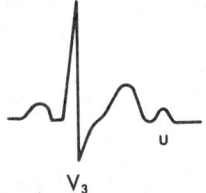

FIGURE 34-16   u wave.

The **T wave** represents repolarization of the ventricles. It follows the QRS complex and is usually slightly rounded and asymmetric without pointing or notching (Figure 34-15). The T wave is normally upright in leads I and II and in left chest leads, negative in lead aV_R, and variable in other leads. The T wave is usually not analyzed to determine cardiac rhythm, but its assessment can reveal additional information about the clinical status of the heart; for example, a tall peaked T wave is associated with hyperkalemia (e.g., caused by renal failure or potassium replacement therapy), whereas an inverted T wave is often associated with myocardial injury.

The **u wave** is a small waveform (looks somewhat like a small P wave) that may be observed following the T wave (Figure 34-16). It is normally oriented in the same direction as the T wave and is more easily visible in chest leads. The source of the u wave is unclear, and like the T wave, it is not analyzed to determine cardiac rhythm. The u wave may be more conspicuous when hypokalemia is present, and its polarity may be reversed in the presence of coronary artery disease, myocardial ischemia, valvular dysfunction, and left ventricular overload.

Intervals

The intervals between waveforms are analyzed to determine if conduction in the heart is normal and to assess the influence of drugs, electrolyte disturbances, and the like, on the heart (Figure 34-17).

The **PR interval** is measured from the beginning of the P wave to the beginning of the QRS complex. It represents the time it takes for the electrical impulse to travel from the SA node to the Purkinje fibers in the ventricles. The PR interval normally does not exceed 0.20 seconds in the adult, ranging from 0.12 to 0.20 seconds. It may be prolonged by factors such as AV nodal ischemia, drug effects (e.g., digitalis preparations), and excessive vagal tone; it may

be shortened by factors such as increased rate, drug effect (e.g., from atropine), congenital heart disease, and cardiac dysrhythmias.

The **QRS interval** is measured from the beginning of the QRS to the end of the QRS. (NOTE: The end of the QRS can be identified by locating the J point, that point marking the beginning of the ST segment.) The QRS interval represents the time required for the electrical impulse to depolarize both ventricles (normally from endocardium to epicardium). Since the impulse descends down both bundle branches essentially at the same time, depolarization of the left and right ventricles should occur almost simultaneously. The resulting QRS interval should reflect this normal sequence of depolarization and should measure less than 0.10 seconds in the adult (the normal range is from 0.08 to 0.10 seconds). It should be noted that QRS width may not be identical in all leads, because each lead sees current flow from a different perspective. A QRS interval that exceeds the upper limit of normal reflects abnormal intraventricular conduction. A wide QRS suggests the presence of clinical conditions such as chamber enlargement, ectopic rhythms, pacemaker rhythms, or altered conduction within the bundle branches.

The **ST segment** is measured from the end of the QRS (at the J point, if visible) to the beginning of the T wave. It is recorded early during ventricular repolarization. The ST segment is normally isoelectric (neither above nor below the baseline), but it can be displaced by clinical conditions such as myocardial ischemia-injury, aneurysm, and drug effects. ST segment displacement should be evaluated in accordance with the clinical setting in which it appears.

The **QT interval** is measured from the beginning of the QRS complex to the end of the T wave. It represents the time required to completely depolarize and repolarize the ventricles. The QT interval is influenced by factors such as age, gender, and heart rate. The QT interval can be affected by a host of factors, including selected drugs and electrolyte imbalances.

The **R-R interval** reflects the regularity of the heart rhythm and is measured from one QRS to the next. Any consistent landmark within the QRS (i.e., every R wave) may be used to determine the R-R interval.

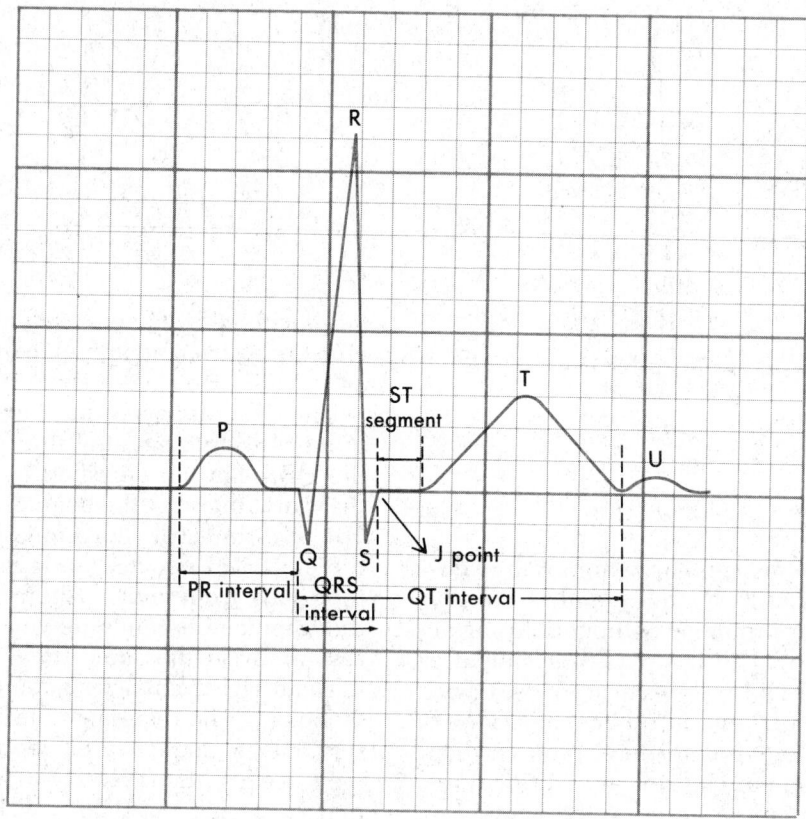

FIGURE 34-17   Intervals.

SYSTEMATIC ASSESSMENT OF A RHYTHM STRIP

P wave—Present or absent? Before the QRS or after the QRS? Any relationship between the P wave and the QRS?

PR interval—Normal, short, or prolonged?

QRS—Narrow or wide?

Rate—Fast or slow? Calculate atrial and ventricular rates; unless otherwise stated, "rate" means ventricular rate.

R-R interval—Regular or irregular?

Ectopic beats—Present or absent? Atrial, junctional, or ventricular?

The final step—Is the patient tolerating the rate and rhythm?

Calculating Heart Rate

Heart rate (HR) most often refers to ventricular rate, so expressions of rate generally reflect ventricular activity. It is also appropriate to determine atrial rate, particularly when assessing atrial rhythm disturbances. Calculation of ventricular rate is determined using the QRS complex as a guide, whereas calculation of atrial rate is determined using the P wave. There are three methods for calculation of HR, and each one is acceptable, though the first method is superior to the others when the ventricular rhythm is irregular (see box on p. 801).

Assessing the Rhythm Strip

Analysis of a rhythm strip requires systematic assessment of major waveforms and intervals, HR, the relationship between waveforms, and the occurrence of abnormal beats. Yet it must be appreciated that ECG assessment merely reflects electrical activity. The nurse must also assess *the patient* to appreciate the physiologic and mechanical consequences of alterations in cardiac rhythm and rate (see box at left).

If the patient is continuously monitored, the nurse should document rhythm strip examples that illus-

6-Second rule

The 6-second rule is the easiest and fastest method for determining HR. Because it provides a good approximation of heart rate, the 6-second rule can be used when rhythms are irregular, as well as when they are regular.

Step 1—Count the number of QRS complexes in 6 seconds. Use the dots or vertical lines at the top of the graph paper to assist you; remember that they are spaced at either 2-second or 3-second intervals.

Step 2—Multiply by 10 to find heart rate for 1 minute.

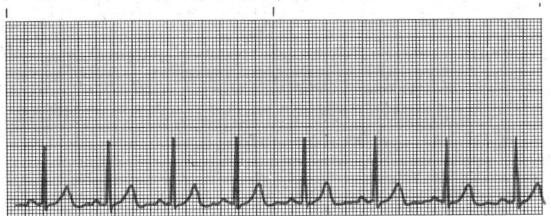

The 6-second rule: Rate = 80 beats/min; rhythm regular.

1500 rule

The 1500 rule is the most accurate method for determining heart rate, but it is most appropriately used when rhythms are regular.

Step 1—Count the number of small squares between two consecutive complexes. Use the R wave or Q wave of each QRS as a guide.

Step 2—Divide this number into 1500. (Why 1500? There are 1500 small squares in 1 minute [1500 × 0.04″ = 60″].)

R-to-R rule

The R-to-R rule represents a variation on the 1500 rule. This method provides another way to quickly assess rate without having to perform complicated calculations. It should be utilized only when rhythms are regular.

Step 1—Find a QRS that falls on a dark line; this QRS will become your reference point.

Step 2—Begin counting to the right to determine HR:

• If the next QRS falls on the first dark line, the HR will be 300. Why? According to the 1500 rule: 1500 ÷ 5 = 300.

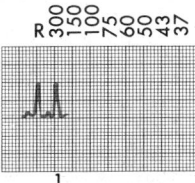

• If the next QRS falls on the second dark line, the HR will be 150. Why? According to the 1500 rule: 1500 ÷ 10 = 150.

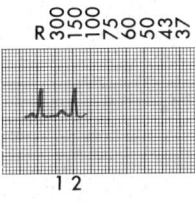

• If the next QRS falls on the third dark line, the HR will be 100. Why? According to the 1500 rule: 1500 ÷ 15 = 100. As you count from your reference point to a QRS falling on a dark line, a pattern emerges: From the reference point to the first dark line, HR = 300, to the second dark line, HR = 150, to the third dark line, HR = 100. As HR decreases further, the pattern continues.

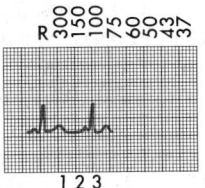

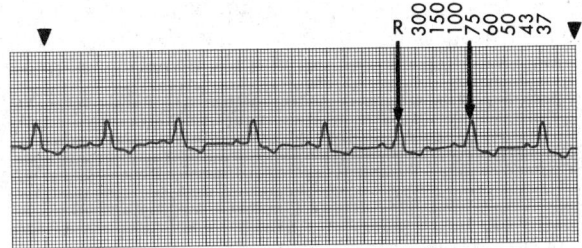

Calculating HR using the R-R rule. Rate = 75 beats/min. The first QRS after the reference point falls on the fourth dark line to the right where the rate equals 75 beats/min (300-150-100-75).

Step 3—What if the next QRS after the reference point does *not* fall on a dark line? Some additional calculations must be made to accurately determine HR (see example in figure below).

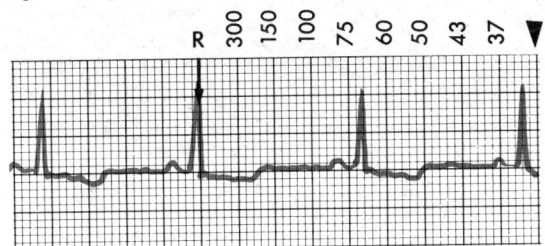

• Find the reference point. Start counting to the next QRS. Because it does *not* fall on a dark line, you must determine the range of HR. For example: If the next QRS falls between the fourth and fifth dark line to the right of the reference point, the HR ranges between 75 and 60.

• To determine how much each small square between 75 and 60 is worth: Subtract the low rate from the high rate (75 − 60 = 15). Divide this number by 5 (15 ÷ 5 = 3): Each small square changes the HR by 3.

• Does this work? If the HR ranges between 75 and 60, then based on our calculations, each small square is worth 3. Therefore, if the QRS falls 1 small square to the right of the dark line corresponding to "75," the rate is 72 beats/min (or 75 − 3). If it falls 2 small squares to the right of "75," the rate is 69 beats/min (or 75 − 6).

trate ectopic beats or rhythms. Each rhythm strip should be labeled with the patient's name, the date and time, and the lead used.

Dysrhythmias

A **dysrhythmia** is a disturbance in heart rate or rhythm. Dysrhythmias—whether in the form of isolated ectopic beats or sustained rhythms—are caused by disturbances in automaticity, conductivity, or (more commonly) both. Tachydysrhythmias are fast rhythms produced as a result of enhanced automaticity or altered conductivity. Bradydysrhythmias are slow rhythms produced as a result of depressed automaticity or altered conductivity. Both fast and slow rates can result in decreased cardiac output and coronary artery perfusion, but fast rates also increase myocardial oxygen demand, and slow rates set the stage for so-called breakthrough dysrhythmias.

SUPRAVENTRICULAR DYSRHYTHMIAS

Supraventricular dysrhythmias are rhythm disturbances that originate above the ventricles. They may include isolated ectopic beats or sustained rhythms arising from the sinus node, the atria, or the AV junction. Though often less ominous than their ventricular counterparts, supraventricular rhythm disturbances can nonetheless result in frequent ectopic beats or excessive changes in rate that produce detrimental clinical effects.

Careful analysis of the waveform produced by atrial depolarization is essential when assessing supraventricular rhythm disturbances. The clinician should examine lead II, because it usually displays atrial waveforms more prominently than other leads. An acceptable alternative is lead V_1 (or its variant MCL_1).

Because supraventricular dysrhythmias originate above the ventricles, conduction of the impulse within the ventricles is normally undisturbed, resulting in a normal, narrow QRS on the ECG. The appearance of abnormal, or wide, QRS complexes reflects altered conduction within the ventricles, which is often associated with either changes in HR or intraventricular conduction defects.

Sinus Rhythm and Variants

Sinus rhythm

Sinus rhythm represents the normal rhythm produced by the dominant sinus pacemaker. The sinus node initiates an electrical impulse that rapidly depolarizes the atria and is conducted into the ventricles after a brief delay at the AV node. Since discharge of the sinus node is not recorded on the surface ECG, the appearance of normal P waves provides presumptive evidence of the rhythm's sinus origin. Unless intraventricular conduction is disturbed, the resulting width of the QRS complex will be within normal limits. Sinus rhythm may be described as regular sinus rhythm or normal sinus rhythm (Figure 34-18).

ECG criteria
1. One P wave before each QRS, in the same position in relation to the QRS.
2. All P waves look alike (same morphology); the P wave is upright in leads I and II, inverted in lead aV_R, and diphasic (deflected above and below the baseline) in lead V_1.
3. Atrial and ventricular rates are identical.
4. Rate is between 60 to 100 beats/min.
5. R-R interval is regular.

GERIATRIC CONSIDERATIONS

Dysrhythmias in the Older Adult

Older adults are susceptible to a number of cardiac dysrhythmias and conduction disturbances. Atrial fibrillation is a common dysrhythmia in the elderly. Many older adults with atrial fibrillation will experience palpitations, fatigue, and fainting. The risk of systemic arterial embolization increases in the older adult with atrial fibrillation.

Sick sinus syndrome is another dysrhythmia that develops frequently in the elderly. This dysrhythmia is associated with abrupt changes in heart rate from bradycardia to tachycardia. The older adult with sick sinus syndrome will experience confusion, syncope, weakness, palpitations, or dizziness. These manifestations can result in falls and potential injury. Pacemaker insertion is a common intervention for this dysrhythmia to control the dysrhythmia and reduce the risk of injury from falls.

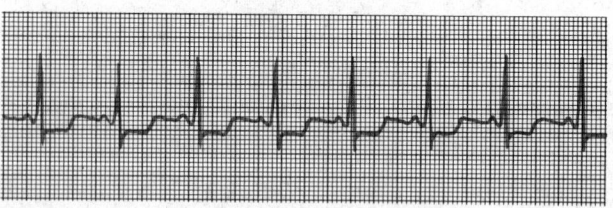

FIGURE 34-18   Sinus rhythm. Note depressed ST segment.

6. QRS is narrow unless conduction in the ventricles is disturbed.
7. PR interval is within normal limits unless conduction through the AV node is disturbed.

Sinus tachycardia

Sinus tachycardia describes a sinus rhythm with a ventricular rate of 100 beats/min or more produced in response to enhanced automaticity in the sinus node (Figure 34-19). Sinus tachycardia may reflect a physiologic demand for increased oxygen associated with a wide variety of normal situations. For example, exercise commonly increases oxygen requirements by tenfold or more. Other factors associated with sinus tachycardia include emotional stress, pain, fever, the ingestion of stimulants (e.g., coffee and tea), and drug therapy with agents that accelerate HR. Still other stressors linked to sinus tachycardia include anemia, thyrotoxicosis, pulmonary embolus, pericarditis, hypovolemia, and heart failure. The nurse must be aware that whereas sinus tachycardia may not reflect a serious underlying disturbance, even slight increases in heart rate may prove detrimental to the patient with a diseased heart. Tachycardia, whether it originates above the ventricles or from within the ventricles, can result in poorly tolerated physiologic responses. As heart rate gradually increases, diastolic filling time in the ventricles is shortened, resulting in reduced ventricular ejection volumes, as well as compromised coronary artery perfusion and production of anginal pain. Furthermore, an increased heart rate is accompanied by an increase in myocardial work and oxygen demand.

ECG criteria
All the criteria for sinus rhythm are met except for one: rate exceeds 100 beats/min, most commonly falling in the range of 100 to 150 beats/min.

Therapeutic management
The decision to treat sinus tachycardia is guided by its cause and accompanying symptoms. In other words, "treat the patient, not the ECG." Often sinus tachycardia will subside spontaneously as its underlying cause (e.g., anxiety or hypovolemia) is treated

and resolved. If rapid rates are clearly detrimental to cardiac function, judicious slowing of heart rate may be indicated. Pharmacologic management of sinus tachycardia may include drugs that exert negative chronotropic (or rate slowing) effects, such as beta-blockers (e.g., propranolol), calcium channel blockers (e.g., verapamil), and parasympathetic agonists (e.g., digitalis preparations). An additional technique to control heart rate includes vagal maneuvers (e.g., carotid sinus massage and Valsalva maneuvers) that may temporarily decrease rate by exerting parasympathetic effects.

Sinus bradycardia

Sinus bradycardia describes a sinus rhythm with a rate of 60 beats/min or less produced in response to depressed automaticity in the sinus node (Figure 34-20). It represents a slowing of the HR that often accompanies sleep and may appear in response to myocardial ischemia, vagal stimulation, electrolyte imbalances such as hyperkalemia, heart blocks, and drug therapy with agents that exert negative chronotropic effects. Slow rates can result in detrimental decreases in cardiac output when present in hearts unable to compensate with increased stroke volume. On the other hand, sinus bradycardia *may* prove beneficial to the distressed heart, because the accompanying increase in diastolic filling time results in enhanced stroke volume and coronary perfusion. Slow rates are also associated with the appearance of breakthrough dysrhythmias that may include dangerous ventricular ectopy (discussed in depth later) and escape beats. When sinus discharge slows significantly, a previously dormant subsidiary pacemaker may escape and fire to pace the heart until the sinus node is able to resume pacemaker control. The appearance of escape beats represents an intrinsic electrical backup that should not be suppressed with antidysrhythmic drugs. A more prudent response is cautious acceleration of the underlying sinus rate with a pharmacologic agent such as atropine.

ECG criteria
All the criteria for sinus rhythm are met except for one: rate is 60 beats/min or slower.

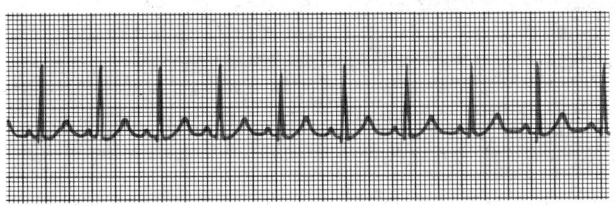

FIGURE 34-19 Sinus tachycardia. HR = 107 beats/min.

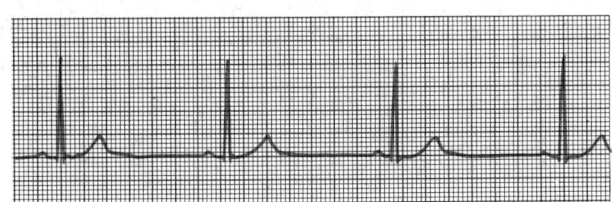

FIGURE 34-20 Sinus bradycardia. HR = 41 beats/min.

Therapeutic management

Therapeutic management of sinus bradycardia is guided by its etiologic factors and symptomatology. A patient who is warm and dry, perfusing, and pain-free is usually not treated. However, the patient who is symptomatic—hypotensive, weak, or experiencing anginal pain—is treated with pharmacologic agents designed to increase heart rate. These agents include drugs that exert positive chronotropic effects, such as the parasympathetic blocking agent atropine. The nurse must appreciate that acceleration of heart rate can have a deleterious effect on cardiac function as a result of the increase in myocardial oxygen demand, reduced stroke volume, and compromised coronary perfusion associated with fast rates.

Sinus arrhythmia

Sinus arrhythmia describes a benign cardiac rhythm disturbance characterized by alternate speeding up and slowing down of the heart rate (Figure 34-21). Sinus arrhythmia most often reflects the vagal effect of respiration and is quite common in children. It is usually not associated with the production of rate-related symptomatology.

ECG criteria

All the criteria for sinus rhythm are met except for one: the R-R interval is irregular. By definition, sinus arrhythmia exists when the difference between the longest R-R interval and the shortest R-R interval equals 0.12 seconds or more.

Therapeutic management

Because clinical signs and symptoms occur infrequently, therapeutic interventions are usually not indicated.

Atrial Dysrhythmias

Atrial dysrhythmias represent disturbances in electrical activity arising from within the atria that result in the generation of premature beats, as well as a variety of abnormal rhythms.

Premature atrial complex

Premature atrial complexes (PACs) describe ectopic impulses that arise from within atrial tissue (Figure 34-22). They are also referred to as atrial premature beats (APBs). PACs are early beats that interrupt the regularity of the basic underlying rhythm and may or may not produce symptoms depending on the frequency with which they occur. Though PACs are often relatively benign rhythm disturbances, they may represent evidence of developing heart failure and may signal the onset of more clinically significant rhythm disturbances such as atrial fibrillation. PACs can occur in normal hearts, but they are more often associated with a variety of pathologic conditions, including myocardial ischemia, infection, and inflammatory processes. PACs can appear in conjunction with stress situations, as well as in association with the consumption of caffeine or tobacco products.

PACs are identified on the ECG because they interrupt the regularity of the underlying rhythm. The ectopic impulse firing from within the atria is responsible for prematurely depolarizing the atria, causing the resulting P wave (P′) to appear earlier than expected on the ECG. Most of the time the ectopic impulse is conducted normally through the AV node and down the bundle branches resulting in a narrow QRS. Occasionally the ectopic impulse is not conducted into the ventricles, because both conduction pathways (the bundle branches) are refractory, and no associated QRS is observed following the premature P wave. This phenomenon—referred to as a blocked, or nonconducted, PAC—represents one of the most common reasons for a pause on the ECG. At other times the premature impulse will be conducted abnormally in the ventricles as a result of differing responsiveness of the bundle branches. The descending impulse arriving earlier than expected in the ventricles finds that one bundle branch has not yet recovered from the previous depolarization. Conduction of the impulse in the ventricles proceeds abnormally, or aberrantly, resulting in production of a QRS that looks different from the others.

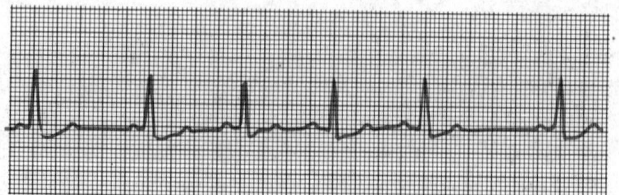

FIGURE 34-21   Sinus arrhythmia. Note the variability in the R-R interval.

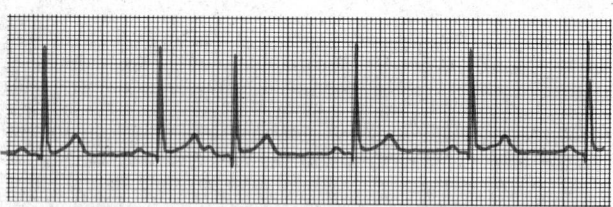

FIGURE 34-22   Premature atrial complexes. The third beat is a PAC; conduction in the ventricles is normal.

ECG criteria

1. The ectopic P wave (P') is early, or premature. If significantly premature, the ectopic P wave may distort the T wave of the preceding beat.
2. The contour of the early P wave will appear different from the normal sinus P waves. As with any ECG analysis, comparing waveforms in more than one lead may be helpful.
3. The morphology of the associated QRS will appear the same as the morphology of the normal QRS as long as conduction in the ventricles is normal. If conduction of the early impulse in the ventricles is abnormal, the ectopic QRS will assume a different shape (PAC conducted with aberration). If conduction in the ventricles is absent, no QRS will be observed after the early P wave (blocked PAC).
4. The P'R interval is often prolonged, but it may also be normal when compared with the other beats. The length of the P'R interval reflects the ability of the AV node to conduct the premature impulse.
5. The R-R interval will be irregular.

Therapeutic management

If underlying disease is absent, treatment of PACs is usually unnecessary. In the presence of disease, however, therapeutic management decisions should be considered in relation to the specific underlying pathologic condition, because successful resolution of the cause (i.e., heart failure) may eliminate the dysrhythmia. The appearance of clinically significant symptoms, such as anginal pain, may reflect adverse physiologic effects associated with the alterations in heart rate and stroke volume that accompany PACs. Premature beats act like fast rates because, like fast rates, they result in reduced diastolic filling time, reduced stroke volume (reduced systolic ejection), and compromised coronary artery perfusion. Elimination of PACs can be accomplished utilizing antidysrhythmic drugs (e.g., quinidine and procainamide) that are designed to suppress the formation of ectopic foci in the atria.

Atrial tachycardia

Atrial tachycardia describes an ectopic supraventricular rhythm with a ventricular rate ranging from 140 to 250 beats/min (Figure 34-23). It may occur in normal hearts but is more likely in the setting of digitalis toxicity or in the presence of excessive catecholamine levels. Furthermore, the development of atrial tachycardia has been linked to electrolyte disturbances, ischemia, and myocardial stretch.

Atrial tachycardia is a rapid ectopic atrial dysrhythmia often associated with altered conduction through the AV node. It commonly occurs as a sustained rhythm, particularly when digitalis is impli-

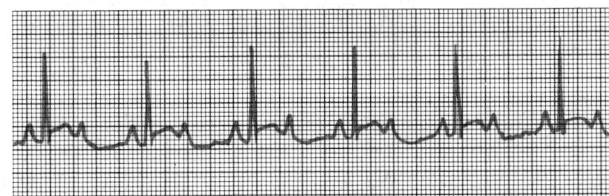

FIGURE 34-23   Atrial tachycardia as a result of digitalis toxicity. AT with 2:1 AV conduction. Every other atrial impulse is blocked from reaching the ventricles. The atrial rate is 136 beats/min; the ventricular rate is 68 beats/min.

cated, but in isolated instances it may appear in short bursts, or paroxysms, that begin and end abruptly (paroxysmal atrial tachycardia or PAT).

When the atrial rate accelerates in ectopic atrial tachycardia, the AV node blocks impulses in an attempt to prevent the rapid ventricular rate that would result from conduction of every impulse. Thus the atrial rate exceeds the ventricular rate as a result of the triaging efforts of the AV node (atrial tachycardia "with block"). Moreover, conduction through the AV node may be altered further by the depressant effects of digitalis preparations.

ECG criteria

1. Ectopic P waves (P' waves) look alike and may closely resemble sinus P waves; variable P' morphologies may also appear.
2. The atrial rate ranges from 140 to 250 beats/min.
3. The ventricular rate is commonly half the atrial rate as a result of digitalis-induced block within the AV node, but atrial and ventricular rates will be identical if 1:1 conduction is present.
4. Every other P' wave is followed by a QRS when 2:1 conduction is present. At faster rates, the P' wave may distort the T wave of the preceding beat. An isoelectric interval should be apparent between P' waves, but at rapid rates, this too may be obscured.
5. The P'-P' interval may be slightly irregular.
6. P'R interval is short (a function of fast rate).
7. The QRS is narrow unless intraventricular conduction is disturbed.

Therapeutic management

Atrial tachycardia may not produce symptoms if it occurs in short, infrequent bursts. Resolution of the underlying cause may prevent a recurrence. If digitalis preparations are implicated, withdrawal of the offending drug is indicated. Since hypokalemia aggravates the electrical derangements associated with overdigitalization, potassium replacement may represent a prudent therapeutic option. Artificial cardiac pacing may be indicated as an electrical backup.

Paroxysmal supraventricular tachycardia

Paroxysmal supraventricular tachycardia (PSVT) is an umbrella term applicable to a pair of rhythm disturbances characterized by rapid atrial rates and altered conduction. Unlike ectopic atrial tachycardia, PSVT reflects abnormal conduction either within the AV node or along an accessory conduction pathway (or bridge) into the ventricles. In both forms of PSVT the initiating event is a premature beat.

AV nodal reentry

One form of PSVT is called AV nodal reentry (see Figure 34-24, A). This unique disturbance reflects altered conduction along dual pathways (one fast, the other slow) found within the AV node. A premature impulse conducted into the ventricles via the slow pathway reenters the atria via the fast pathway, resulting in nearly simultaneous depolarization of both atria and ventricles. The tachycardia will persist as long as the impulse is able to reexcite both cardiac chambers by traveling forward into the ventricles via one AV nodal pathway and back up into the atria via the other AV nodal pathway.

The initiating premature beat is usually conducted with a prolonged P'R interval followed by a narrow QRS. Subsequent beats reveal the same narrow QRS closely followed by a P' wave barely visible in the terminal portion of the QRS; more commonly, the P' wave is buried within the QRS.

AV nodal reentry is often a benign, self-limiting disturbance easily abolished with vagal maneuvers such as carotid sinus massage. When recurrent or refractory to therapeutic interventions, it can produce clinically significant rate-related symptomatology. Drug therapy with digitalis, verapamil, procainamide, quinidine, or adenosine may be required to successfully interrupt conduction within the AV node. Surgical intervention may also be considered for refractory tachycardias.

Circus movement tachycardia

The other form of PSVT, called circus movement tachycardia (CMT) (see Figure 34-24, B), is a disturbance closely associated with the Wolff-Parkinson-White (WPW) syndrome. WPW syndrome involves altered conduction of supraventricular impulses along a congenital pathway (or bridge) into the ventricles. In CMT a premature beat is conducted normally through the AV node into the ventricles and reenters the atria via the accessory pathway. A self-perpetuating "circus movement" is established between the two chambers, resulting in rapid sequential stimulation of ventricles and atria.

The initiating premature beat is usually con-

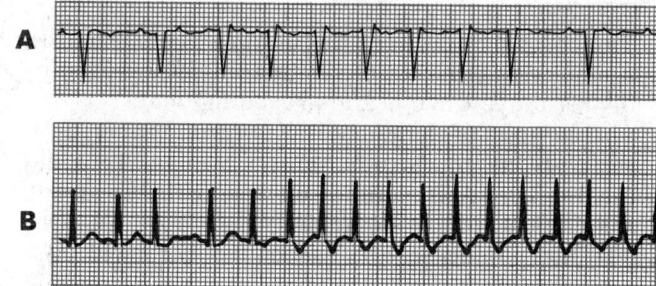

FIGURE 34-24   Paroxysmal supraventricular tachycardia. **A,** AV nodal reentry. **B,** Circus movement tachycardia.

ducted with a normal P'R interval and narrow QRS. Subsequent beats may write a similar QRS pattern followed by a clearly visible P' wave; ventricular aberrancy is common.

CMT can degenerate into atrial fibrillation with exceedingly rapid ventricular rates or it can degenerate into fatal ventricular fibrillation. A definitive diagnosis of CMT requires electrophysiologic testing, while therapeutic options include drug therapy (e.g., adenosine) and surgical interruption of the accessory pathway with techniques such as radio frequency catheter ablation.

Atrial flutter

Atrial flutter describes an ectopic supraventricular dysrhythmia characterized by uniform, rapid contraction of the atria (Figure 34-25). It usually occurs in diseased hearts (e.g., in association with coronary artery disease, pulmonary embolism, and valvular disease), but both paroxysmal and chronic atrial flutter may occasionally appear in normal hearts. The atrial rate accelerates markedly to rates ranging from 250 to 350 beats/min. Instead of producing a normal P wave on the ECG, atrial depolarization yields a contiguous pattern of sawtooth waveforms called flutter waves (F waves). The AV node selectively blocks some of these impulses from entering the ventricles to prevent the excessively fast ventricular rates that would result from conduction of every impulse. The result of the AV node's triaging efforts is a slower ventricular response that reflects intermittent conduction. Despite AV node protection, hemodynamic deterioration may still result if rapid ventricular rates are present. Rarely, every impulse is conducted into the ventricles (1:1 conduction) resulting in excessively fast rates approaching 300 beats/min and requiring immediate therapeutic intervention. When ventricular rates are rapid enough to render identification of F waves difficult, the vagal, or rate slowing, effects of carotid sinus massage

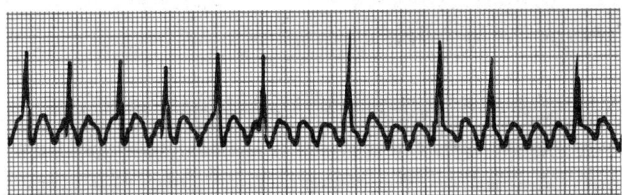

FIGURE 34-25   Atrial flutter. Atrial flutter with variable conduction; note the irregularity of the R-R interval and the sawtooth baseline.

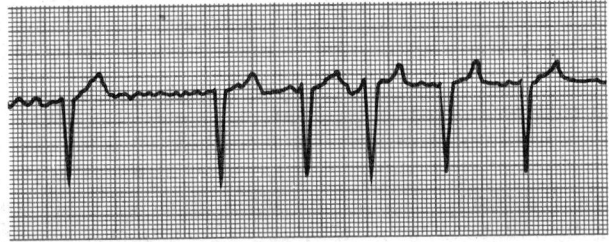

FIGURE 34-26   Atrial fibrillation. Atrial fibrillation with a characteristically irregular ventricular response. Note the uneven, wavy baseline.

may increase block at the AV node, temporarily unmasking the F waves. When carotid massage, which should be performed by a physician, is terminated, accelerated AV conduction resumes and so does the rapid ventricular response.

ECG criteria

1. No P waves (therefore no PR interval).
2. Identical F waves appear continuously on the baseline (easily counted and no isoelectric line between them); F waves assume a sawtooth or picket-fence appearance best seen in lead II. Some F waves may be partially obscured by the QRS.
3. Atrial rate between 250 to 350 beats/min; the atria characteristically flutter at approximately 300 beats/min.
4. Ventricular rate slower than the atrial rate (reflects block at the AV node).
5. R-R interval will be regular if the AV node blocks impulses in a repeating pattern or if all impulses are conducted through the AV node into the ventricles (1:1 conduction). Conduction ratios in atrial flutter are usually even, reflecting conduction of every second or every fourth impulse (2:1 or 4:1 conduction). The R-R interval will be irregular (variable conduction) if the AV node conducts impulses into the ventricles at irregular intervals.
6. QRS will be narrow if intraventricular conduction is normal; QRS will be wide if conduction in the ventricles is abnormal.

Therapeutic management

Therapy for the patient experiencing atrial flutter is designed to convert the rhythm to normal sinus or to decrease the ventricular response when conduction through the AV node is enhanced. Both pharmacologic and electrical therapies can be selected. Digitalis alone may restore sinus rhythm, but commonly conversion to sinus rhythm is facilitated by administration of agents such as quinidine or procainamide (to slow the flutter rate) along with digitalis (to slow the ventricular rate by increasing conduction block at the AV node). If excessive ventric-

ular rates produce a symptomatic drop in cardiac output, calcium channel blocking agents may successfully slow the rate by increasing block at the AV node, but they may be unable to restore sinus rhythm. Cardioversion may be the treatment of choice if the clinical situation is acute, as in the setting of an acute MI, and is associated with untoward clinical symptoms. Atrial flutter can often be converted to sinus rhythm via synchronized cardioversion at lower energy levels (50 J to start) than those required to terminate ventricular dysrhythmias. The nurse should be aware that cardioversion may be dangerous, or even contraindicated, in the presence of digitalis, because the digitalized heart is sensitive to electroshock. Even low energy levels may induce ventricular fibrillation, so caution is warranted if cardioversion is attempted. Rapid atrial pacing may be indicated for atrial flutter resistant to drugs or when cardioversion is not advisable.

Atrial fibrillation

Atrial fibrillation describes a dysrhythmia characterized by chaotic electrical activity in the atria, resulting in uncoordinated mechanical activity (Figure 34-26). More common than atrial flutter, atrial fibrillation is usually associated with organic heart disease (mitral stenosis, cardiomyopathy, pericarditis, and acute MI) but may also appear in normal hearts (idiopathic).

In this rhythm disturbance, the atrial rate becomes so rapid that depolarization is no longer uniform, and a well-defined P wave cannot be identified on the ECG. Instead, small, poorly defined waveforms (f waves) are observed occurring at rates of 350 beats/min or more. Conduction to the ventricles is variable, because the AV node is unable to conduct the multiple impulses bombarding it, allowing only a random number to pass through. When describing atrial fibrillation (and atrial flutter as well), it is important to note the ventricular response, because it can be markedly varied. Since depolarization of the atria is uncoordinated, mechanical contraction is also not coordinated. The atria merely quiver instead of contracting as a unit. The result is a loss of the synchronous atrial contractions normally responsible for about 20% of ventricular stroke volume (the atrial kick). Sluggish blood flow within the atria sets the stage for the formation of mural thrombi that can dislodge and travel to the brain, pulmonary circulation, or periphery.

ECG criteria

1. No P waves (atrial depolarization is not coordinated); since the P wave is absent, no PR interval exists.
2. f waves on the baseline (cannot be counted easily); f waves may appear coarse and easily recognizable or they may appear so fine that they are difficult to identify.
3. R-R interval characteristically irregular.
4. QRS is narrow if conduction within the ventricles is normal; if a conduction disturbance is present, the QRS may be wide and abnormally shaped.

Therapeutic management

Like other disturbances in rate or rhythm, atrial fibrillation may resolve spontaneously when its underlying cause is corrected. However, atrial fibrillation is often treated with a combination of drugs designed to suppress the formation of ectopic impulses in the atria (quinidine or procainamide) and to depress conduction through the AV node (digitalis), thus slowing the rate. If the ventricular response to atrial fibrillation is fast enough to produce a symptomatic drop in cardiac output, short-term therapy with a calcium channel blocking agent (verapamil) or beta-blocker (esmolol) may be indicated to slow the rate. If drug therapy is ineffective or if hemodynamic deterioration is apparent, cardioversion may be performed, but it should be avoided if excessive digitalis is on board. The digitalized heart is extremely sensitive to electroshock and may fibrillate in response to cardioversion. Unless cardioversion is required as an emergency intervention, it should be preceded by anticoagulation in patients at risk for embolic complications, such as those with mitral stenosis or cardiomegaly.

Junctional Dysrhythmias

Junctional dysrhythmias may represent abnormal automaticity in the AV junction, or they may appear as a manifestation of digitalis toxicity. Junctional rhythms can represent protective escape mechanisms that appear in response to depression of the higher sinus pacemaker as a result of digitalis, myocardial ischemia, and excessive vagal tone. Junctional dysrhythmias may occur in normal hearts and are relatively uncommon when compared with the frequency of atrial and ventricular disturbances.

Premature junctional complex

Premature junctional complexes (PJCs) describe ectopic impulses that arise from within the AV junction (Figure 34-27). Like PACs, PJCs are early beats that interrupt the regularity of the underlying rhythm and may or may not produce symptoms depending on the frequency with which they occur. They are produced in response to conditions that enhance automaticity in the AV junction, such as myocardial ischemia and hypokalemia, but they are also linked to digitalis toxicity. PJCs usually are not associated with acute clinical symptoms, though loss of the atrial kick could result in the symptoms of low cardiac output if PJCs occur frequently.

PJCs are recognized on the ECG because they appear earlier than expected in the cardiac cycle. The electrical impulse emerging from the AV junction commonly travels in a reverse direction (retrograde) to depolarize the atria (assuming that penetration into the atria is possible), producing a P' wave that is inverted (negative) in lead II. The impulse also travels forward (anterograde) to depolarize the ventricles, producing an upright (positive) QRS in lead II. Analysis of the P' wave in relation to the QRS provides presumptive evidence regarding the speed of impulse conduction. If the P' wave appears just before the QRS, depolarization of the atria must have occurred before ventricular depolarization. If the P' wave is not visible (hidden within the QRS), depolarization of both atria and ventricles must have occurred essentially at the same time. If the P' wave appears just after the QRS, atrial depolarization is assumed to have occurred after ventricular depolarization.

ECG criteria

1. The ectopic QRS is early.
2. If visible, the P' wave may appear slightly before or slightly after the QRS.
3. The P' wave will be inverted in leads II, III and aV$_F$.
4. If the P' wave precedes the QRS, the P'R interval will be abnormally short (often less than 0.12 second).

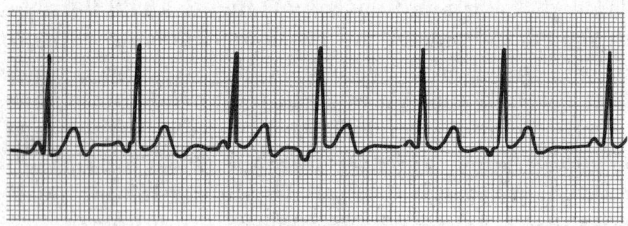

FIGURE 34-27 Premature junctional complexes. The second, fourth, and sixth beats are PJCs. The P' wave preceding each beat is inverted.

5. The ectopic QRS will look like the normal QRS complexes unless conduction in the ventricles is disturbed; the QRS should be upright (positive) in lead II.
6. The R-R interval will be irregular.

Therapeutic management

Because PJCs are not usually associated with production of acute clinical symptoms, specific treatment appropriately focuses on determining the underlying cause of the ectopic beats. When PJCs result from digitalis excess, reduction of digitalis dosage, coupled with appropriate potassium replacement, may successfully abolish ectopic activity in the AV junction.

Junctional escape rhythm

Junctional escape rhythm represents a passive escape mechanism originating in the AV junction in response to depression of the higher (and faster) sinus pacemaker (Figure 34-28). This may occur in association with acute MI, sinus node disease, electrolyte disturbances, and drug depression, and is occasionally observed accompanying sinus bradycardia in well-trained athletes. If the dominant sinus pacemaker is depressed, the normally dormant pacemaker in the AV junction can escape to assume pacemaker control at its inherent rate of approximately 40 to 60 beats/min. Firing of this subsidiary pacemaker results in the conduction patterns described for PJCs. Conduction proceeds from the AV junction in both a retrograde direction to produce the P' wave and in an anterograde direction into the ventricles to produce the QRS.

ECG criteria

1. The ventricular rate is between 40-60 beats/min.
2. The R-R interval is regular.
3. The P' wave may appear before or after the QRS, or it may be hidden within the QRS; the P' wave will be inverted in lead II.
4. The QRS will be narrow if conduction in the ventricles is normal and wide if conduction is abnormal.

5. The QRS will look like the QRS produced by the sinus pacemaker.

Therapeutic management

One of the primary goals in the therapeutic management of junctional escape rhythm is to determine why the sinus node lost pacemaker control of the heart. A brief episode commonly requires no specific treatment unless the slow rate results in a symptomatic fall in cardiac output associated with loss of the atrial kick. Interventions for the symptomatic patient reflect efforts to revive the higher sinus pacemaker with drugs such as atropine, or they may be designed to provide artificial pacemaker control when drugs are ineffective or when sinus dysfunction is thought to be permanent. Suppression of a junctional escape rhythm should never be attempted, because this rhythm represents a *protective* electrical backup system.

Junctional tachycardia

Junctional tachycardia describes an ectopic rhythm originating in the AV junction that results either from enhanced automaticity or from the effects of digitalis toxicity (Figure 34-29). In junctional tachycardia, the normally dormant AV junctional pacemaker usurps control from the higher sinus pacemaker. In addition to the often-implicated drug digitalis, a host of factors including MI, acute rheumatic fever, and manipulation during open heart surgical procedures are associated with junctional tachycardia.

ECG criteria

All the criteria for junctional rhythm are met except for one: rate exceeds 100 beats/min. Though confusing and not precisely correct with respect to the accepted definition of tachycardia (rate greater than 100 beats/min), various descriptions have been assigned to junctional tachycardia that reflect its faster-than-normal rate. Some clinicians refer to a sustained junctional rhythm exceeding about 60 beats/min (the upper limit of the inherent junctional escape pacemaker) as junctional tachycardia,

II

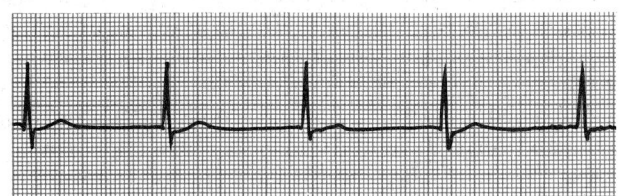

FIGURE 34-28   Junctional escape rhythm. The P' wave is buried within the QRS; conduction in the ventricles is normal. HR = 50 beats/min.

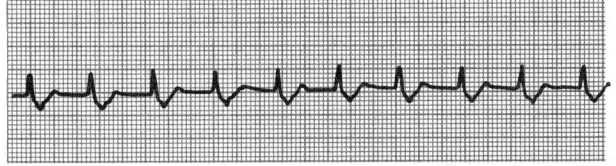

FIGURE 34-29   Junctional tachycardia. HR = 110 beats/min. Note the retrograde P waves observed in lead II.

though a more accurate description would be "accelerated junctional rhythm."

Therapeutic management

Therapy for the patient experiencing junctional tachycardia is directed toward investigation of the underlying cause and slowing of the rate if a symptomatic fall in cardiac output is present. Junctional tachycardia may subside spontaneously when its underlying cause is eliminated. Vagal maneuvers, including carotid sinus pressure and gagging, may abruptly terminate the dysrhythmia. Junctional tachycardia resulting from digitalis intoxication responds best to withdrawal of the drug and perhaps to administration of Dilantin. Cardioversion, if required as a therapeutic alternative for the symptomatic patient, should be approached with caution as a result of the digitalized heart's sensitivity to electroshock.

NURSING MANAGEMENT OF THE PATIENT EXPERIENCING A SUPRAVENTRICULAR DYSRHYTHMIA

Assessment

The patient is assessed to determine if alterations in heart rate are producing a symptomatic fall in cardiac output. Alterations in diastolic filling time associated with fast rates, as well as loss of the atrial kick associated with some atrial and junctional dysrhythmias, can result in a decreased cardiac output. Slow rates can be equally detrimental to the patient with a diseased heart because of the heart's inability to maintain adequate cardiac output by increasing stroke volume.

The nurse should assess blood pressure and apical heart rate, pulse volume, peripheral perfusion, skin color and temperature, presence of jugular venous distention, urinary output, and sensorium. The nurse should ask whether the patient has experienced episodes of dizziness, lightheadedness, or weakness. If the patient's ECG is continuously monitored, the ECG is assessed for the presence of dysrhythmia accompanied by alterations in HR, breakthrough dysrhythmia, escape beats, and heart blocks. Is the patient experiencing dyspnea? The patient's breathing pattern should be observed and all lung fields auscultated for the presence of fluid. Is the patient experiencing pain? The patient should be questioned directly and observed closely for nonverbal cues that may indicate the presence of pain, such as contorted facial expression and body posturing.

Nursing Diagnosis

Nursing diagnoses that may be applicable to the patient experiencing a supraventricular dysrhythmia include:

Activity intolerance related to alterations in heart rate (too fast or too slow) and diminished stroke volume

Altered peripheral tissue perfusion related to tachycardia or embolic complications

Decreased cardiac output related to alterations in heart rate and loss of the atrial kick

Knowledge deficit (disease process, medications, treatment plan) related to lack of information

Planning

The list below describes desired patient outcomes related to the suggested nursing diagnoses.

Activity tolerance is increased as evidenced by increased ability to engage in normal activities of daily living without experiencing dizziness, fatigue, dyspnea, or pain; return of blood pressure and pulse rate to resting levels within 3 minutes after termination of activity

Peripheral perfusion is adequate as evidenced by warm, dry skin without cyanosis; peripheral pulses present with good pulse volume

Cardiac output is adequate as evidenced by acceptable, stable vital signs and invasive hemodynamic indicators such as cardiac output; lungs clear to auscultation, normal breathing pattern; adequate urinary output

Knowledge level is increased as evidenced by ability to verbalize increased knowledge about health status, treatment plans, and health maintenance behaviors

Implementation

The nurse should investigate to determine possible causes of the dysrhythmia. MI is associated with multiple rhythm disturbances that may be caused by tissue hypoxia or may reflect the mechanical complications of infarct, such as heart failure. Inferior (or diaphragmatic) wall MI is often associated with sinus bradycardia and junctional escape rhythm, whereas anterior wall MI is often accompanied by sinus tachycardia and PACs, especially in the presence of developing heart failure. Pain, anxiety, fever, and stimulants such as caffeine and tobacco are associated with fast rates.

Serum electrolyte levels and drug levels are monitored as appropriate. Electrolyte disturbances may be associated with alterations in rate and rhythm.

Myocardial function is supported through nursing interventions designed to decrease myocardial work. Physical care activities are spaced to minimize myocardial oxygen demand and to avoid subjecting the patient to periods of excessive physical demand without sufficient rest breaks. A quiet and stress-free environment is provided, and therapeutic options, such as the addition of soft music to the patient's environment, are supplied if feasible and desirable.

The patient is monitored closely to detect the occurrence of side effects related to therapeutic interventions. The nurse should be familiar with the particular side effects related to the patient's drug regimen. If the patient is receiving either a negative or a positive chronotropic drug, HR trends are monitored. If the patient is receiving a digitalis preparation such as Lanoxin, the nurse should observe the ECG for the development of new rhythm disturbances.

If the patient is receiving an agent such as quinidine, procainamide, or disopyramide, the nurse should examine the QRS complex carefully, because these agents tend to depress intraventricular conduction resulting in a widened QRS. If the patient is receiving quinidine, the nurse should be alert for GI distress and syncopal episodes (the latter could be caused by quinidine-induced ventricular tachycardia). If procainamide is used, the nurse should be aware that hypotension and a syndrome resembling systemic lupus erythematosus may develop. If the patient is receiving propranolol, the nurse monitors respiratory status closely, especially if pulmonary disease is present. Propranolol is a nonselective beta-blocking agent that blocks both beta$_1$ effects in the heart and beta$_2$ effects in the lung and may cause worsening of pulmonary symptoms. If multiple pharmacologic agents are included in the therapeutic regimen, the nurse considers that their effects may be both cumulative and additive. Because impaired metabolic function is common in the elderly, the nurse should be especially vigilant when assessing these patients.

If the patient is hemodynamically unstable as a result of rapid rates, the nurse should be prepared to assist with cardioversion and should obtain a baseline 12-lead ECG if time permits. After the procedure, the nurse monitors the patient for the appearance of symptoms such as altered peripheral perfusion, chest pain, and shortness of breath that may be associated with embolic complications. Mural thrombi formed in the presence of sluggish blood flow (e.g., during atrial fibrillation) can dislodge and travel to the brain, lungs, or periphery if coordinated mechanical contraction is suddenly restored. Frequent assessment of vital signs is warranted, particularly during the first few hours after a cardioversion attempt. If cardioversion is performed in the presence of digitalis, the nurse should be prepared to defibrillate the patient immediately if electroshock results in ventricular fibrillation.

The nurse assesses the ECG for the appearance of breakthrough dysrhythmias, such as ventricular ectopy and escape beats, when slow rates are present. Atropine should be readily available. Intravenous (IV) access should be established in case atropine must be quickly administered.

The nurse assesses the ECG for the development of additional rhythm disturbances. PACs occurring with increasing frequency may precede atrial flutter or atrial fibrillation. The appearance of junctional dysrhythmias, such as junctional escape rhythm, may suggest a pathologic condition in the sinus node.

Evaluation

Evaluation of the patient experiencing a supraventricular dysrhythmia will likely focus on whether drug therapy successfully controls the dysrhythmia and its accompanying symptoms. For example, atrial flutter is often associated with a rapid HR that can produce symptoms of decreased cardiac output. Evaluation will determine if drug therapy or cardioversion has slowed the rate and abolished the symptoms. The nurse will evaluate the patient's hemodynamic stability through assessment of heart rate, peripheral perfusion, and complaints of shortness of breath and anginal pain.

Documentation

The medical record should reflect trends in the patient's clinical status, such as HR, blood pressure, and fluid balance, as well as the appearance of new dysrhythmia. Ongoing assessment data and patient responses to therapeutic interventions, especially those related to stat or prn drug therapy, should be carefully documented. If the patient is continuously monitored, a rhythm strip labeled with the patient's name, the date and time, and the monitoring lead should be placed in the record at the beginning of each shift and whenever a significant change in status is observed. In addition, the plan for patient/family teaching should be recorded so that all care providers will know what information should be communicated to the patient.

Ongoing Care

Ongoing care for the patient experiencing a supraventricular dysrhythmia is primarily concerned with maintenance of the treatment plan after discharge from the hospital. The nurse should formulate a discharge plan that addresses components of home care, including medication administration, exercise, and nutrition. The plan should focus on the importance of promptly reporting symptoms including palpitations, anginal pain, dyspnea, unusual fatigue or weakness, dizziness, visual disturbances, and GI upsets to the physician. These symptoms could reflect worsening of the dysrhythmia, the appearance of a new disturbance, or side effects of drug therapy, so the patient should be aware of their significance.

Discharge planning involves teaching both the patient and his family or significant others about the treatment plan. If the patient is confused or exhibits any sort of altered mentation, compliance with a self-administered drug regimen may be unrealistic. Home care follow-up through a home health agency should be strongly considered for any patient who is elderly or debilitated or whose support systems in the home are either absent or inadequate.

VENTRICULAR DYSRHYTHMIAS

Ventricular dysrhythmias are rhythm disturbances that originate within the ventricles. Like their supraventricular counterparts, ventricular dysrhythmias may include isolated ectopic beats, paroxysms (bursts) of ectopy, or sustained rhythms. Ventricular dysrhythmias are caused by alterations in automaticity, conductivity, or both. They are clearly more dangerous and clinically significant than most supraventricular dysrhythmias.

The clinician should examine lead V_1 (or its variant MCL_1) when assessing the ECG, because V_1 provides the best information. Furthermore, examination of V_1 can help differentiate between intraventricular conduction defects (bundle branch blocks) and ectopic rhythms (ventricular tachycardia).

Premature Ventricular Complex

Premature ventricular complexes (PVCs) describe ectopic impulses that arise from within the ventricles (Figure 34-30). PVCs are also referred to as ventricular premature beats (VPBs). Like PACs and PJCs, PVCs are early beats that interrupt the regularity of the underlying rhythm and may or may not produce symptoms depending on their frequency. PVCs are often found in normal hearts and may represent a marker for underlying heart disease, but their occurrence is more likely in the setting of organic heart disease, myocardial ischemia, and electrolyte disturbances. Additional factors implicated in the genesis of PVCs include anxiety, caffeine, exercise, and excessive intake of alcohol. Selected therapeutic interventions may also be responsible for the production of PVCs. For example, certain pharmacologic agents (i.e., dopamine, isoproterenol, and amiodarone) are said to be proarrhythmic, which means that they are capable of producing dysrhythmias. Moreover, when foreign objects such as pacing catheters and flow-directed pulmonary artery catheters are inserted into an ischemic heart, the mechanical stimulation of the sensitive endocardium can result in ventricular ectopy. The success of relatively new therapeutic interventions such as recanalization, which is restoration of blood flow via balloon dilation or thrombolytic therapy, is partly determined by the appearance of PVCs reflecting restoration of blood flow to previously ischemic muscle. Thus ventricular ectopy, while obviously unde-

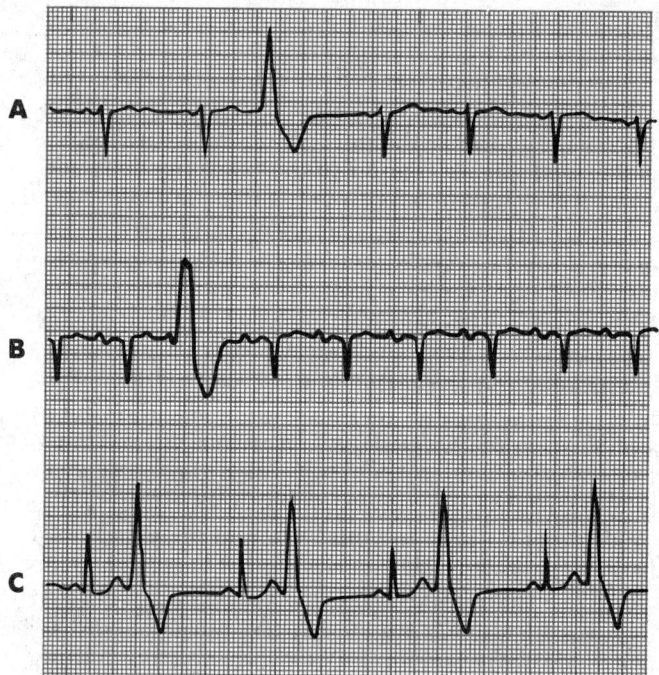

FIGURE 34-30   Premature ventricular complexes. **A,** The third beat is a PVC. It appears earlier than expected and is shaped differently from the normal beats. **B,** End-diastolic PVC. The P wave that precedes the PVC comes on time. **C,** Sinus rhythm with ventricular bigeminy. Every second beat is a PVC.

sirable in the majority of circumstances, may nevertheless provide evidence that therapeutic goals have been achieved.

PVCs are identified on the ECG because they interrupt the regularity of the basic underlying rhythm and usually assume a somewhat wide and "bizarre" shape. The ectopic ventricular impulse prematurely depolarizes the ventricles producing a wide QRS that reflects sequential (rather than simultaneous) depolarization of the ventricles. Though the ectopic QRS commonly occurs without an associated P wave, it is followed immediately by a P′ wave if the ectopic impulse is conducted backward through the AV node to depolarize the atria. If retrograde spread of the impulse stops before it reaches the atria, the resulting pause observed on the ECG is called "fully compensatory" and reflects undisturbed sinus discharge. However, if the impulse penetrates the atria to prematurely depolarize the sinus node, the pause will be "less than fully compensatory," indicating that the sinus node has been reset.

Characteristics

PVCs reflect a variety of characteristics that describe their origin, their timing within the cardiac cycle, and their relationship to other beats.

PVCs arising from the same focus will assume the same shape and should be described as uniform or unifocal. If they arise either from different foci or from the same focus but are conducted in different directions, their shapes will be variable, and they should be described as multiform. The alternative description, multifocal, although perhaps not as precise a term, will also suffice.

PVCs often occur singly, but when uniform or multiform PVCs occur consecutively, or in pairs, they are described as coupled (or occurring in couplets).

One of the most clinically significant characteristics of ventricular ectopic impulses reflects their timing within the cardiac cycle. When an ectopic impulse is significantly premature, it may cause impairment of both electrical and mechanical activity in the heart. The earlier the impulse fires, the more likely it is that it will encroach on the T wave of the preceding beat during the vulnerable period of electrical recovery. The danger here lies in the risk of the R-on-T phenomenon that can produce ventricular tachycardia or ventricular fibrillation. Furthermore, significantly premature beats are associated with impaired hemodynamics as a result of shortened diastolic filling time in the ventricles. Clinical symptoms, such as the sensation of skipped beats, palpitations, and anginal pain, can result from significantly premature beats that frequently occur.

Uniform PVCs can occur in repeating patterns known as *bigeminy* (PVCs occurring every other beat), *trigeminy* (PVCs occurring every third beat), or *quadrigeminy* (PVCs occurring every fourth beat). Unfortunately, these terms can be confusing. For example, by definition trigeminy means "a grouping of three" in any combination. So trigeminy could mean one ectopic beat and two normal beats (the most commonly accepted definition), or it could mean two ectopic beats and one normal beat. The term quadrigeminy is likewise open to differences in interpretation. To eliminate some of the confusion over terminology, the clinician is encouraged to describe the basic underlying rhythm first, followed by a description of the ectopic activity and its frequency: "sinus rhythm . . . with ventricular trigeminy . . . PVCs occurring 8 times/minute."

PVCs that appear to be "sandwiched" between two normal beats are called interpolated. They are often significantly premature ectopic beats that barely disturb the regularity of the underlying rhythm.

ECG criteria
1. The QRS is early, or premature.
2. The QRS is wider than the normal beats.
3. The QRS is shaped differently from the normal beats.
4. The QRS is usually not preceded by a P wave. The

QRS may be followed immediately by a P′ wave if conduction spreads into the atria (ventriculoatrial conduction). Occasionally an ectopic QRS that is only slightly premature will be preceded by a non-premature P wave (end-diastolic PVC).

5. The QRS is followed by a compensatory pause that ends when the underlying rhythm resumes. The length of the pause provides presumptive evidence about the ectopic beat's influence on normal sinus discharge. If the ectopic impulse penetrates into the atria to prematurely depolarize the sinus node, the pause will be less than fully compensatory, because the sinus node was reset. If sinus node discharge is not disturbed by the ectopic impulse, the pause will be fully compensatory. Assessment of the compensatory pause requires measurement of the distance between three consecutive normal beats (two full cardiac cycles). This interval is compared with the distance between three consecutive beats when the second beat represents the ectopic. If the latter measurement (two cycles inclusive of the ectopic) equals the former (two normal cycles), the pause is "fully compensatory" and indicates that sinus node discharge was not disturbed. If the latter measurement is less than two full cardiac cycles, the pause is "less than fully compensatory" and indicates that the sinus node was reset by ectopic depolarization.

Therapeutic management
The decision to treat PVCs should be guided by the clinical setting in which they occur and the hemodynamic alterations they produce. Many protocols are available to help the clinician decide whether to treat PVCs. These guidelines include: PVCs encroaching on the T wave (increased risk of the R-on-T phenomenon); impaired hemodynamics (hypotension, anginal pain); more than 5 or 6 PVCs per minute; and PVCs that are multiform or occurring in couplets or bursts.

Once the decision has been made to treat PVCs, the clinician has a variety of pharmacologic agents from which to choose. The most common drug used to treat PVCs is lidocaine (Xylocaine). Given intravenously, lidocaine is fairly effective and nontoxic. Lidocaine may produce undesirable side effects, including visual disturbances, headache, trembling, seizures, and respiratory depression. Lidocaine should initially be given as an IV bolus (1 to 1.5 mg/kg body weight) followed by a maintenance infusion (usually 2 to 4 mg/min) titrated to response. Additional drugs that may be effective in abolishing ventricular ectopic beats are procainamide, quinidine, propranolol, disopyramide, bretylium, moricizine, magnesium, and amiodarone (because of its potential toxicity, this drug is reserved for use in selected situations only). Because the response to drug therapy is highly individual, these drugs may be administered alone or in combinations. Dosages of all antidysrhythmic agents should be reduced when hepatic or renal function is impaired, as is often the case with elderly patients. A final drug not to be overlooked in the therapeutic regimen is oxygen. Its administration may help enhance myocardial oxygenation and ultimately decrease the frequency of ectopic activity in the ventricles.

Ventricular Tachycardia

Ventricular tachycardia (VT) describes a series of three or more PVCs occurring at a rate of 100/min or more (Figure 34-31). The basic causes of PVCs apply to VT as well, but clinical conditions such as ventricular aneurysm, cardiomyopathy, and prolongation of the QT interval have also been associated with the development of VT. The physiologic derangements accompanying VT are a reflection of hemodynamic deterioration brought on by the accelerated rate and associated drop in cardiac output. The clinical picture is not unlike what should be anticipated in the presence of any fast rate, but with this particular dysrhythmia, symptomatology tends to be acute in the majority of circumstances. Though an occasional patient will be asymptomatic in the presence of VT, most exhibit a symptomatic drop in cardiac output (hypotensive, faint or absent peripheral pulses, weakness, complaints of anginal pain) that often precedes a loss of consciousness.

VT is identified on the ECG because it is a fast rate distinguished by wide, abnormally shaped QRS complexes. It may occur without preceding "warning" dysrhythmias. If the onset of the dysrhythmia is recorded, one may observe that it results from a stray PVC falling by chance on the apex of a T wave. The VT produced can occur in bursts or may persist, perhaps degenerating eventually into the chaotic, and fatal, pattern known as ventricular fibrillation.

ECG criteria
All the criteria for PVCs are met, with the following additions:

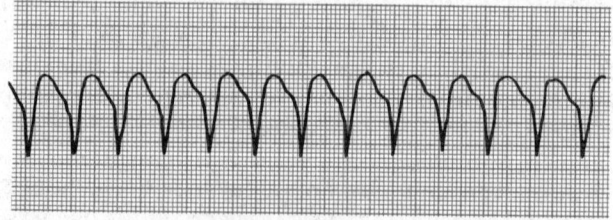

FIGURE 34-31 Ventricular tachycardia. VT at 150 beats/min. Note the regularity of the rhythm.

1. Three or more PVCs occur in a row.
2. HR 100 beats/min or more, often ranging from 110 to 250 beats/min.
3. Uniform (ectopic impulses are shaped the same and are easily distinguished).
4. R-R interval almost precisely regular.
5. Dissociated P waves (P waves may be visible sporadically but they bear no relationship to the ectopic QRS complexes). A retrograde P' wave appearing consistently indicates intact ventriculoatrial conduction, but the rapidity of the rate often makes identification difficult.

Therapeutic management
Treatment for VT is designed to reverse the hemodynamic derangements produced by a dysrhythmia rapid enough to cause a critical drop in cardiac output and made worse by the associated loss of the atrial kick. Besides the reduced forward stroke volume that accompanies a sustained VT, an additional problem is that of congestive heart failure. At rapid rates the ventricle is unable to fill efficiently or to eject volume efficiently. Eventually blood "backs up" into the pulmonary circuit resulting in pulmonary congestion and edema.

Treatment decisions regarding when and how to treat VT should again be guided by the clinical setting and the patient's tolerance of the dysrhythmia. Initial assessment of the patient should focus on whether the VT produces a pulse. If the pulse is absent, VT should be treated as though it were ventricular fibrillation. If the pulse is present, the patient should be further assessed to determine the stability in the presence of the fast rate. If the patient is stable (conscious, pain-free, normotensive), administration of oxygen and insertion of an IV access may be followed by antidysrhythmic therapy to depress the ectopic focus. Lidocaine remains the drug of choice, especially in the setting of acute myocardial ischemia, but other agents (e.g., procainamide) may be chosen if the response to lidocaine is unsatisfactory. If VT persists despite drug therapy in the stable patient, low-energy (i.e., 100 J to start) **cardioversion** (synchronized electroshock) is indicated after administration of adequate sedation. If the patient with a pulse is unstable (hypotensive, complaining of pain, in heart failure, or unconscious), **defibrillation** (unsynchronized electroshock) is the most appropriate initial response. IV access, oxygenation, and sedation should precede attempts to shock the patient only if these maneuvers can be accomplished quickly and if they will not worsen the situation (e.g., administration of sedation to a severely hypotensive patient may cause an additional drop in pressure). Antidysrhythmic therapy is begun after attempts are made to electrically restore a normal rhythm. Lidocaine, bretylium, and procainamide are the usual agents selected, though quinidine and disopyramide are also used.

Long-term management

The interventions described above commonly terminate VT in the acute setting. However, persistent VT often reflects resistance to both conventional drug therapy and attempts to electrically convert the rhythm. Patients who suffer from either sustained or repeated bouts of VT are at particular risk considering the often unpredictable nature of the dysrhythmia. These individuals may require more aggressive therapy, including the use of diagnostic procedures, such as endocardial or epicardial mapping, the application of experimental antidysrhythmic drug therapy, or surgical procedures designed to abolish, control, or physically excise the irritable focus in the ventricles (e.g., via cryosurgery, endocardial ablation, use of the automatic internal cardioverter-defibrillator, or aneurysmectomy).

The **automatic internal cardioverter-defibrillator (AICD)** is a fully implantable device designed to detect and terminate episodes of VT and ventricular fibrillation (VF). The AICD represents a viable therapeutic option for patients who have experienced a non–infarct-related episode of hemodynamically unstable VT or who are unresponsive to conventional (or experimental) drug therapy. The system functions much like a pacemaker in that it detects a rhythm abnormality and delivers an electrical signal to terminate it. A pulse generator is implanted within a subcutaneous pocket created in the abdominal wall (Figure 34-32). Leads that act as transmission lines for sensing electrical activity and for delivering the shock are threaded from the generator into the heart or are sewn to the heart muscle. When the AICD recognizes VT or VF, the pulse generator delivers a low-energy shock directly to the heart muscle via one of the leads (usually a patch lead). If the dysrhythmia is terminated after the initial shock, the unit will resume its sensing function; if not, the AICD will deliver up to three additional shocks in an attempt to restore a normal rhythm. Fortunately, most patients respond to the first shock.

Torsade de pointes

Torsade de pointes represents a unique form of VT associated with prolongation of the QT interval (Figure 34-33). Though its exact mechanism is unknown, alterations in repolarization that are reflected in the QT interval may set the stage for this dysrhythmia. Torsade de pointes—which means "twisting points" in French—is characterized on the ECG by alternating polarity of the ectopic QRS. The course of Torsade de pointes is variable; it may terminate spontaneously or degenerate into VF. The association between antidysrhythmic agents that prolong repolarization (quinidine, procainamide, and disopyramide) and the appearance of Torsade de pointes is strong enough to warrant close inspection of QT trends when these agents are administered.

Ventricular Fibrillation

Ventricular fibrillation (VF) represents total disorganization of electrical and mechanical activity in

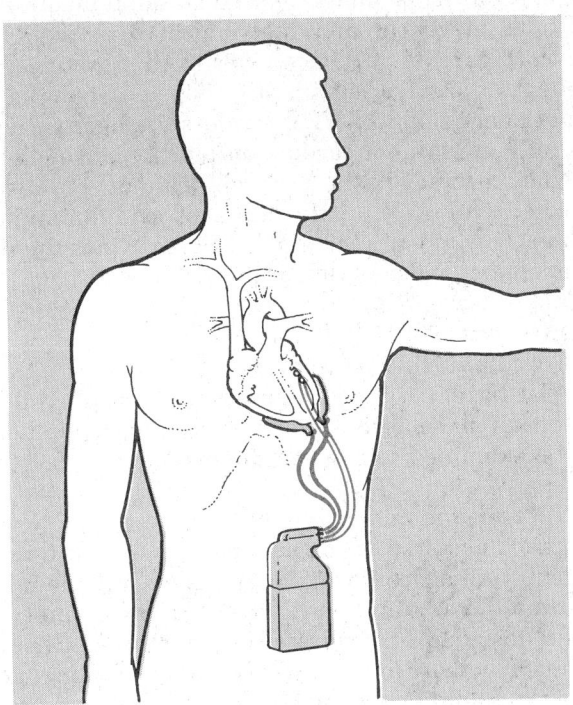

FIGURE 34-32 The automatic internal cardioverter defibrillator (AICD). The pulse generator is implanted within a pocket created in the abdominal wall. Rate sensing electrodes and patch electrodes form a bridge between the generator and the heart.

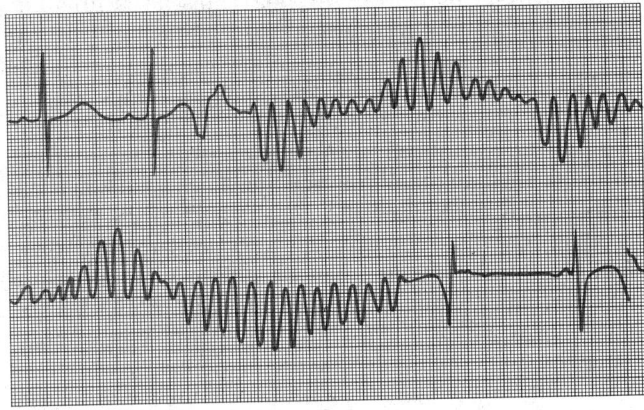

FIGURE 34-33   Torsade de pointes. This variation of VT is characterized by alternating polarity of the ectopic QRS. Note that in this example the first few QRS complexes are negative, but their polarity subsequently swings back and forth between positive and negative until the episode of Torsade de pointes terminates. Torsade de pointes is associated with conditions that prolong the QT interval.

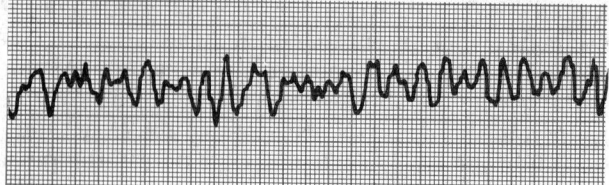

FIGURE 34-34   Coarse ventricular fibrillation.

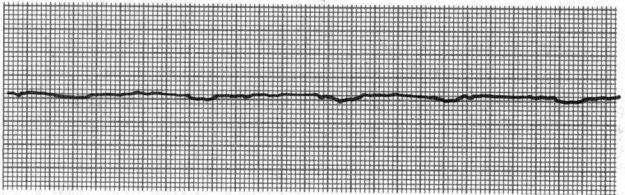

FIGURE 34-35   Ventricular asystole. No identifiable waveforms are present. Because asystole may resemble fine ventricular fibrillation, the clinician is encouraged to examine the rhythm in additional leads to confirm the diagnosis.

the heart (Figure 34-34). Depolarization is chaotic, rendering the heart unable to contract in a coordinated fashion. Instead, the heart quivers uncontrollably in the chest and is incapable of generating a cardiac output. If allowed to continue, VF will prove fatal. The causes of VF are the same as those described for other ventricular dysrhythmias (i.e., myocardial ischemia, electrolyte disturbances, drug effects), and it may represent the terminal event in a variety of illnesses. But VF may also represent an unfortunate outcome of treatment. For example, surgical manipulation of the heart, the use of powerful anesthetics, drug toxicity, current leakage from improperly grounded equipment, and incorrect cardioversion technique can result in VF. Obviously VF is not always preventable, but it should never result from operator error or inattention to the risks inherent in today's high-tech environment.

ECG criteria
1. No identifiable waveforms (no P wave, no QRS, no T wave).
2. Uneven, irregular baseline composed of undulating waveforms of variable amplitude.
3. Waveforms may appear coarse or fine. Coarse waveforms are more likely to appear early during the course of VF, whereas fine waveforms tend to appear after the heart has been fibrillating for several minutes.

Therapeutic management
VF is associated with the clinical picture of cardiac arrest. Pulses, blood pressure, and respirations are absent, and seizures may occur. Loss of consciousness is inevitable. Treatment of VF (and VT without a pulse) should be aggressive and begun without delay. If clinical cardiac arrest is observed in an unmonitored patient, cardiopulmonary resuscitation (CPR) should be initiated and continued until ECG monitoring is available to confirm the presence of VF. If the onset of VF is witnessed in a monitored patient, delivery of a precordial thump is appropriate. If this maneuver fails to terminate VF, immediate defibrillation is indicated. As soon as VF is confirmed in a previously unmonitored patient, defibrillation remains the most appropriate response. High energy levels will likely be required to terminate VF,

so an initial shock of no less than 200 J is recommended, followed by higher energy shocks if conversion to a normal rhythm does not occur. If conversion is not accomplished after three consecutive attempts, CPR must be initiated. Pharmacologic support with agents such as epinephrine, bretylium, and lidocaine is indicated along with measures such as intubation to establish oxygenation and an IV access. The use of sodium bicarbonate is reserved for arrest situations that last several minutes or more, and dosages should ideally be guided by arterial blood-gas reports.

Ventricular Asystole

Ventricular asystole represents a situation of clinical cardiac arrest characterized by the total absence of both electrical and mechanical activity in the heart (Figure 34-35). In contrast to VF, asystole (also known as cardiac standstill) reflects a completely quiet heart, and like VF it renders the heart incapable of generating a cardiac output. Because clinical cardiac arrest exists, asystole cannot be distinguished from VF on the basis of symptomatology alone. The appearance of the ECG provides the only confirming evidence of asystole.

ECG criteria
1. No identifiable waveforms.
2. Flat baseline. Because fine VF can also exhibit a nearly flat baseline, more than one lead should be examined to confirm the presence of asystole.

Therapeutic management
Ventricular asystole, or standstill, must be treated quickly and aggressively. Supportive CPR should be instituted without delay. Pharmacologic interventions designed to generate and support electromechanical activity in the heart should be administered as soon as either a central or peripheral venous access is established. Drugs such as atropine and epinephrine can be administered either IV or via the endotracheal tube if venous access is delayed. Arti-

ficial cardiac pacing may be required if these therapeutic attempts fail to establish a cardiac output. Unfortunately, asystole may persist despite prompt and vigorous treatment.

NURSING MANAGEMENT OF THE PATIENT EXPERIENCING A VENTRICULAR DYSRHYTHMIA

Assessment

Assessment parameters for the patient experiencing a ventricular dysrhythmia are essentially the same as those for the patient experiencing a supraventricular disturbance.

The nurse assesses the patient to determine if alterations in heart rate and rhythm are producing a symptomatic fall in cardiac output. The patient experiencing VF or ventricular asystole will be in clinical cardiac arrest and will not exhibit a pulse, blood pressure, or respirations. On the other hand, the patient experiencing VT with a pulse may or may not be symptomatic. The symptomatic patient will be hypotensive and may complain of chest pain. Peripheral perfusion will be poor, and the patient may quickly lapse into unconsciousness, often within a minute. The patient experiencing PVCs may be symptomatic as a function of the frequency of the PVCs and their hemodynamic effects. The nurse assesses the patient for hypotension, altered sensorium, and pulmonary congestion, as well as for complaints of chest pain, skipped beats, or palpitations.

Nursing Diagnosis

The nursing diagnoses for the patient experiencing a ventricular dysrhythmia are similar to those previously described, but a few additional diagnoses may also be appropriate. These include:

   Activity intolerance related to tachycardia and diminished cardiac output

   Altered cerebral and peripheral tissue perfusion related to diminished cardiac output

   Decreased cardiac output related to alterations in HR and diminished stroke volume

   Fear related to risk of fatal dysrhythmic event (VF or asystole)

   Knowledge deficit (disease process, medications, treatment plan)

   High risk for injury related to risk for syncopal episodes and to side effects of pharmacologic agents

Planning

The following list describes desired patient outcomes related to the suggested nursing diagnoses for the patient experiencing a ventricular dysrhythmia.

   Activity tolerance is increased as evidenced by increased ability to engage in normal activities of daily living without experiencing dizziness, fatigue, dyspnea, or pain

   Cerebral perfusion is adequate as evidenced by appropriate level of consciousness and sensorium; peripheral perfusion is adequate as evidenced by warm, dry skin without cyanosis; peripheral pulses present with good pulse volume

   Cardiac output is adequate (see previous explanation)

   Fear is diminished as evidenced by stable heart rate and blood pressure; dry skin; stable speech patterns; calm, constructive verbal expression; relaxed body posturing

   Knowledge level is increased (see previous explanation)

   Patient remains free of bodily injury

Implementation

The nurse investigates to determine the possible causes of the dysrhythmia. Is the patient hypoxemic? Ischemia, especially in the setting of acute MI, is responsible for multiple ventricular dysrhythmias. Are electrolyte disturbances present? The nurse should pay particular attention to potassium levels, because ventricular dysrhythmias are often associated with hypokalemia. Is the patient receiving digitalis or any other proarrhythmic drug? Are QT levels prolonged? Is the patient receiving a drug such as quinidine that is expected to lengthen the QT interval? The nurse should be alert for ECG cues that may warn of impending Torsade de pointes. Does the patient have a documented ventricular aneurysm? VT commonly occurs in association with this condition. Is the patient undergoing invasive procedures such as cardiac catheterization or insertion of a transvenous pacing catheter or flow-directed pulmonary artery catheter? Endocardial stimulation can result in ventricular dysrhythmias. Has a recanalization procedure been performed within the last few hours? Restoration of myocardial blood flow can result in PVCs.

The nurse should make sure that lidocaine is readily available in case rapid administration becomes necessary. It should be available in bolus form for quick IV injection. An IV access should be available, and an infusion pump should be on standby for controlled administration of continuous antidysrhythmic infusions.

If antidysrhythmic drugs are administered, the nurse assesses the patient for the appearance of drug-related side effects.

The nurse assesses the ECG frequently to detect the development of additional or more serious rhythm disturbances.

Evaluation

The patient will be assessed for hemodynamic stability, as well as for a decrease in ectopy. In addition, the results of pharmacologic and electrical intervention, such as defibrillation and cardioversion, will be evaluated primarily through assessment of the ECG. Ambulatory monitoring, also known as Holter monitoring, may be prescribed to assess the frequency of ectopy, as well as the efficacy of drug therapy. Holter monitoring may be done either before discharge from the hospital or on an outpatient basis.

Documentation

Accurate documentation assumes greater significance when a ventricular dysrhythmia is present. The potential for significant clinical deterioration makes timely assessment of patient status a paramount concern. Documentation of a rhythm strip, especially one that shows new dysrhythmia or the onset of a life-threatening dysrhythmia, is helpful. Likewise, notification of the physician and subsequent documentation of orders are important clinical and legal considerations.

Ongoing Care

As a result of the danger inherent in ventricular ectopy, the discharge plan must focus heavily on patient teaching. Faithful adherence to the prescribed medical regimen and prompt reporting of untoward symptoms must be strongly emphasized. The patient should understand the importance of follow-up visits to the physician so that drug therapy can be appropriately adjusted. If unconventional interventions, such as the AICD or special pacemakers, are used to treat ventricular dysrhythmias, the patient must be informed of essential information about the treatment.

ATRIOVENTRICULAR BLOCKS

Atrioventricular blocks (AVBs) represent disturbed conduction of the electrical impulse between the atria and the ventricles. Depressed impulse transmission results in cardiac rhythms that reflect either prolonged, intermittent, or absent conduction. AVBs are described according to their location within the electrical conduction system and according to their behavior (also known as the "degree" of block).

AVBs may be produced in association with myocardial ischemia, excessive vagal tone, electrolyte imbalances, and drug effects. Less common causes include compression of conduction tissue (caused by tumors or resulting from surgical manipulation), inflammation of cardiac tissue, and fibrosis of the electrical conduction system.

Symptoms associated with AVBs are variable. Their occurrence relates primarily to overall HR and resultant cardiac output. Treatment is designed to enhance conduction from atria to ventricles or to support the ventricular rate.

Analysis of the P wave's relationship to the QRS is the most critical factor in ECG assessment of AVBs. Therefore a lead revealing prominent P waves should be chosen, and lead II probably best fits that criterion.

First-Degree Atrioventricular Block

First-degree AVB reflects a conduction disturbance between the sinus node and the ventricle characterized by consistently *prolonged* conduction through the AV node (Figure 34-36). Causes of first-degree AVB include inferior wall MI, the effects of drugs that alter conduction through the AV node (such as digitalis and verapamil), and excessive vagal tone. This conduction disturbance may also be a normal variant. It rarely produces symptoms, but first-degree AVB accompanying a slow underlying sinus rate may result in symptoms associated with the slow rate.

First-degree AVB is identified on the ECG through analysis of the PR interval accompanying the underlying sinus rhythm. It will be consistently prolonged, exceeding the upper limit of normal in an adult (>0.20 seconds). The clinician is encouraged to describe the basic underlying rhythm first, followed by any qualifications referring to the presence of AVB; for example, "sinus rhythm . . . with first-degree AVB" or "sinus bradycardia . . . with first-degree AVB."

ECG criteria
1. PR interval is greater than 0.20 seconds.
2. Prolongation of the PR interval is consistent; it does not vary from beat to beat.
3. Every sinus impulse is conducted into the ventricles (1:1 conduction).

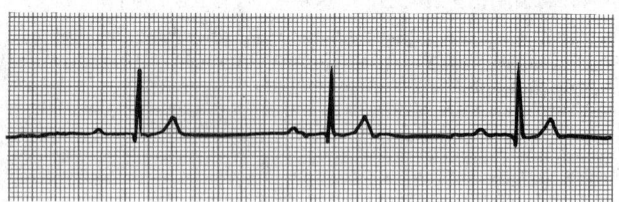

FIGURE 34-36 Sinus bradycardia with first-degree AVB; PR = 0.36 seconds.

Therapeutic management

First-degree AVB rarely produces symptoms, so specific treatment is usually unnecessary. It is essential, however, to assess the progression of first-degree AVB to detect excessive disturbances in AV node conduction caused by drug therapy or worsening of disease. Agents such as digitalis are expected to cause prolongation of the PR interval, so first-degree AVB is not surprising during digitalis therapy. However, as administration of digitalis continues, the PR interval may reflect extreme conduction delay at the AV node. The PR interval may lengthen even beyond 0.40 seconds in unusual circumstances. If depressed AV conduction is associated with toxic drug levels, clinical symptoms (such as GI upset or confusion) and the development of additional ECG clues are likely to occur. In this circumstance, elimination of the offending drug will probably eradicate both the symptoms and the additional ECG derangements without necessitating further intervention.

Second-Degree Atrioventricular Block

Second-degree AVB describes a conduction disturbance characterized by *intermittent* conduction between atria and ventricles. Although the majority of impulses are conducted into the ventricles, occasional impulses are either unable to pass through the AV node or, once past the node, are prevented from reaching the ventricles. Thus the conduction disturbance implicated in second-degree AVB may be confined to the AV node, or it may be found in the bundle branch system. Consequently, the two forms of second-degree AVB described below are differentiated according to the location of the primary disturbance. Type I block, generally a reflection of disturbed conduction within the AV node, is referred to as "proximal" block, because it occurs above the bundle of His. Type II block, on the other hand, is described as "distal," because it usually reflects a conduction abnormality below the bundle of His.

Type I block

Type I block (Figure 34-37)—also known as the Wenckebach phenomenon or Mobitz type I block—usually reflects a transient conduction disturbance at the level of the AV node caused by inferior wall MI, drug effects, or increased vagal tone. It may occasionally occur as a normal variant in athletes and may appear chronically in patients experiencing ischemic heart disease. Type I block is distinguished on the ECG by progressive prolongation of the PR interval until a beat is nonconducted, or "dropped." A P wave will appear on time, but it will not be followed by a QRS, because the impulse arrives during the refractory period of the the AV node and can-

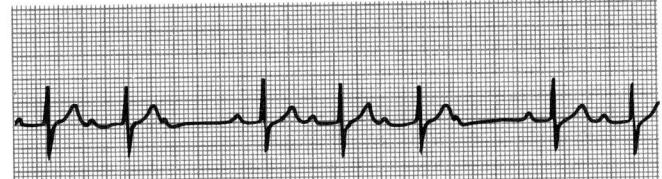

FIGURE 34-37   Second-degree AVB, type I. Characteristic "group beating" is observed in the middle of this rhythm strip. Conduction within the ventricles is normal (QRS is narrow). Note the progressive prolongation of the PR interval until a beat is dropped (the P wave after the second and fifth QRS is not conducted into the ventricles).

not be conducted into the ventricles. Since this disturbance is commonly confined to the AV node, conduction within the ventricles remains normal, as does the resulting QRS.

ECG criteria

1. Group beating (the pause following the dropped beat causes grouping of subsequent beats).
2. Progressive prolongation of the PR interval until a beat is dropped. The PR interval of the first beat in a group may be normal, but it is more often prolonged. Regardless of the length of the initial PR interval, all subsequent PR intervals will gradually lengthen until eventually a P wave appearing on schedule will not be followed by a QRS. The next beat (the first in the next group) will be conducted with the original, shorter PR interval. Subsequent PR intervals will lengthen as before until a beat is dropped.
3. P-P interval is regular.
4. The overall R-R interval is irregular (as a result of the dropped beat); the R-R interval within a group of beats progressively shortens as the PR intervals lengthen.
5. QRS interval is normal unless conduction is also disturbed in the ventricles.

Therapeutic management

Symptoms rarely appear unless type I block is associated with a reduced cardiac output caused by a slow underlying sinus rate or frequent dropped beats. Therefore specific therapy is often not indicated. The ECG should be observed, however, for the development of additional conduction disturbances, such as complete heart block. If treatment of type I block is required, it most often focuses on eradicating the underlying cause (e.g., withholding offending drugs) and supporting ventricular rate if the patient either does not tolerate a slow rate or if additional conduction disturbances appear likely.

Acceleration of heart rate with atropine may be indicated, but it must be used with caution, particularly in the setting of acute MI. Increased rates are often associated with detrimental increases in myocardial oxygen demand that can extend an infarction. Occasionally, artificial cardiac pacing may be required to support the ventricular rate when drug therapy is ineffective or when a symptomatic block is considered permanent.

Type II block

Type II block—also known as Mobitz type II block (Figure 34-38)—reflects disturbed conduction at the level of the bundle branches commonly resulting from myocardial ischemia caused by anterior wall MI or fibrosis of the electrical conduction system. Type II block, less common but potentially more lethal than type I block, also reflects intermittent conduction between atria and ventricles. Occasional impulses fail to depolarize the ventricles because of unpredictable block in the bundle branch system. Type II block is distinguished on the ECG by constant PR intervals, wider-than-normal QRS complexes, and occasional dropped beats. In this form of block, two of the three available fascicles, or pathways, in the bundle branch system are blocked as a result of a pathologic condition, leaving only one potential pathway available for conduction of the descending sinus impulse. The majority of sinus impulses are conducted into the ventricles without difficulty, though the QRS will be wider than normal, because intraventricular conduction is abnormal. The PR interval of the conducted beats will be constant, or fixed, because conduction through the AV node is undisturbed. Occasionally, the only remaining pathway for conduction of the impulse to the ventricles will block off, rendering the impulse incapable of reaching the ventricles. This is known as an intermittent trifascicular block. The ECG will reveal a P wave that comes on time but is not followed by a QRS (the dropped beat). The pathway usually unblocks quickly so that conduction to the ventricles

will resume. Dropped beats that occur rarely are not associated with production of specific symptoms, but when they appear frequently, a symptomatic drop in cardiac output may be observed. While both type I and type II block may be precursors to complete heart block, type II block is clearly the more serious of the two. Complete heart block that develops suddenly in the presence of type II block is generally accompanied by a slow ventricular escape pacemaker. Unfortunately this "last resort" escape pacemaker is notoriously unreliable, so type II block can quickly deteriorate into ventricular asystole.

ECG criteria
1. PR interval is constant (usually normal but may be prolonged).
2. P-P interval is regular.
3. R-R interval is irregular (as a result of the dropped beat); the R-R interval within a group of beats is regular.
4. The QRS is wide (as a result of disturbed conduction in the ventricles).
5. The P wave associated with the dropped beat comes on time but is not followed by a QRS.

Therapeutic management
Like Wenckebach phenomenon, type II block rarely produces clinical symptoms unless the underlying rate is slow or the nonconducted beats are frequent. The danger in type II block lies primarily in its potential to produce either complete heart block or ventricular asystole. It is impossible to predict when or if trifascicular block, or complete block, will develop as a permanent consequence of this comparatively uncommon kind of intraventricular conduction defect. The few treatment options that are available focus on support of the underlying rate with drugs such as atropine and long-term artificial cardiac pacing.

Third-Degree Atrioventricular Block

Third-degree AVB (also known as complete heart block) represents *absent* conduction between atria and ventricles (Figure 34-39). Disturbances in conduction either at the AV node or within the bundle branches may be caused by myocardial ischemia or necrosis, drug toxicity, electrolyte disturbances, excessive vagal tone, and degenerative heart disease. Symptoms produced in association with complete AVB reflect alterations in rate and loss of the atrial kick.

Third-degree AVB is identified on the ECG because no relationship exists between the P waves and the QRS complexes, resulting in slow ventricular rates that produce the symptoms of low cardiac output. If the AV node is totally unable to conduct impulses into the ventricles, a subsidiary (escape)

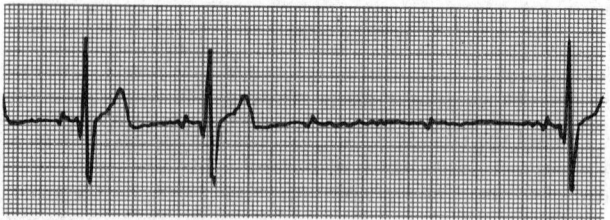

FIGURE 34-38 Second-degree AVB, type II. The PR interval of all conducted beats is fixed; the P wave comes on time; the QRS is wide because of disturbed conduction in the ventricles. Strip shows a two-beat pause on the ECG as a result of dropped beats.

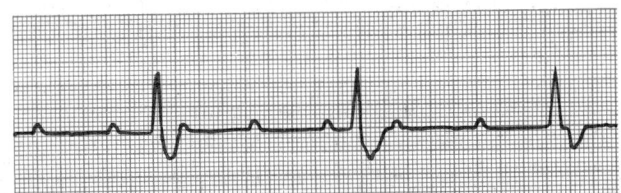

FIGURE 34-39   Third-degree AVB. The P-P intervals are nearly regular; the R-R intervals are regular. The rates are different. No relationship exists between P waves and QRS complexes. Sinus rhythm with third-degree AVB. The atrial rate = 94 beats/min; the ventricular rate = 35 beats/min. This example represents complete block with an idioventricular pacemaker. The QRS is wide, and the rate is within the range of a ventricular escape pacemaker (15 to 40 beats/min).

pacemaker located below the level of the block (i.e., below the AV node) must fire to stimulate the heart. The AV junctional pacemaker usually assumes this role, driving the heart at its inherent rate of 40 to 60 beats/min and producing a narrow QRS. On the other hand, if the bundle branch system is totally unable to conduct impulses into the ventricles, an escape pacemaker located below the level of the block must fire to stimulate the heart. In this situation, a ventricular escape pacemaker drives the heart at its slow inherent rate of 15 to 40 beats/min and produces a wide QRS. In each of these circumstances, the sinus node continues to fire, causing the P waves of atrial depolarization to appear in a regular pattern on the ECG. However, when conduction from atria to ventricles is completely absent, separate pacemakers drive the upper and lower cardiac chambers independently. This condition—independent beating between atria and ventricles—represents an example of AV dissociation (the atria and ventricles are dissociated from one another). The resulting cardiac output can be affected as a consequence of the inherently slow rates of the escape pacemakers, as well as from loss of the atrial kick.

ECG criteria

1. P-P interval is regular.
2. R-R interval is regular.
3. Atrial and ventricular rates are different; the atrial rate is usually faster than the ventricular rate.
4. No relationship exists between the P waves and the QRS complexes.
5. If complete block exists at the AV node, an "idiojunctional" pacemaker will produce narrow QRS complexes at 40 to 60 beats/min. If complete block exists within the bundle branches, an "idioventricular" pacemaker will produce wide QRS complexes at 15 to 40 beats/min.

Therapeutic management

Complete heart block is likely to produce symptoms such as dizziness, hypotension, and syncope if the escape pacemaker drives the heart at slow rates. The associated loss of the atrial contribution to cardiac output can compound these symptoms. Management of third-degree AVB supports the ventricular rate and enhances conduction.

If the conduction disturbance in complete block results from AV node depression, pharmacologic agents that accelerate conduction through the node (e.g., atropine) may be given. If this is unsuccessful and the patient exhibits symptoms, short-term therapy with isoproterenol or temporary artificial cardiac pacing may be indicated. If the conduction disturbance is confined to the bundle branch system, an attempt may be made to accelerate the ventricular rate with atropine, though this parasympathetic blocking agent may be ineffective against an idioventricular rhythm (parasympathetic blockers exert their effects at the sinus node and the AV node and generally do not influence the ventricles). Though an isoproterenol infusion can be administered to increase the ventricular rate in acute situations, caution must be exercised whenever this agent is administered. The acceleration of rate associated with isoproterenol often comes at great cost in terms of myocardial oxygen demand. Artificial cardiac pacing may represent a more definitive approach to therapy.

NURSING MANAGEMENT OF THE PATIENT EXPERIENCING DISTURBED AV CONDUCTION
Assessment

Assessment parameters for the patient experiencing disturbed AV conduction are similar to those utilized in the assessment of dysrhythmias. The special points of interest are explained below.

The patient is assessed to determine if alterations in rate as a result of dropped beats or escape pacemakers are producing a symptomatic fall in cardiac output. Third-degree AVB is associated with slow rates and loss of the atrial contribution to cardiac output. Heart rate, blood pressure, pulse volume, skin color and temperature, and sensorium are assessed. Pacemaker therapy may be indicated if the patient is complaining of weakness, dizziness, lightheadedness, or pain, or if syncopal episodes have occurred.

Nursing Diagnosis

Selected diagnoses assume increased significance when heart block is present. These include:

Altered thought processes related to altered cerebral perfusion or to drug therapy

Activity intolerance related to diminished cardiac output

Decreased cardiac output related to slow heart rate or diminished stroke volume

High risk for injury related to risk for syncopal episodes

Planning

Outcomes and goals for the patient experiencing disturbed AV conduction include:

Orientation to person, place, and time is maintained as evidenced by ability to verbalize appropriate responses to questions, ability to conduct meaningful conversation, and ability to interact appropriately with others

Activity tolerance is increased (see previous explanation)

Cardiac output is adequate (see the first explanation)

Patient remains free of bodily injury

Implementation

Treatment priorities focus on maintenance of an acceptable heart rate.

The cause of the conduction disturbance is determined. Has the patient experienced an MI? Inferior wall MI is often associated with the development of first-degree AVB, second-degree AVB type I, and third-degree AVB with an idiojunctional pacemaker. Anterior wall MI is often associated with the development of second-degree AVB type II, and third-degree AVB with an idioventricular pacemaker. Is the patient receiving drugs that depress conduction through the AV node? Digitalis and calcium channel blocking agents, such as verapamil, can cause altered conduction through the AV node. The nurse should be aware that calcium channel blockers can increase serum concentrations of digitalis when given together, thereby increasing the risk of digitalis-related heart block. Serum digoxin levels are monitored, as appropriate. Mechanical manipulation and tissue edema may have affected the electrical conduction system if the patient has recently undergone a surgical procedure.

Emergency equipment and drugs should be readily available in case critically slow rates require emergency intervention. This equipment includes items required for emergency cardiac pacing. A cardioverter with transcutaneous pacing capabilities should be available. Temporary pacing can also be initiated using transthoracic pacing kits or transvenous pacing wires connected to a battery-powered pulse generator. A functioning IV access should be available in case rapid administration of IV drugs, such as atropine, is required. Infusion pumps should be available for controlled infusion of potent rate-supporting drugs. The nurse should be prepared to initiate CPR if ventricular asystole develops. Second-degree AVB type II and third-degree AVB can progress to asystole without warning.

The nurse should monitor the ECG for the progression of block and be prepared to intervene if necessary. The PR interval is inspected carefully to detect evidence of worsening AV conduction; close attention is paid to the relationship between P waves and QRS complexes. The nurse keeps the physician informed of the trends noted in AV conduction, especially when digitalis is on board, and reports any sudden changes in AV conduction. The nurse should be prepared to initiate rate-supporting drug therapy and assist with pacemaker insertion as required. First-degree AVB may progress to second-degree AVB type I or to third-degree AVB. Second-degree AVB types I and II may progress to complete AVB or to ventricular asystole. Second-degree AVB type I may subside spontaneously when its cause is removed. Symptoms will vary according to the ventricular rate associated with a conduction disturbance.

Evaluation

The focus of evaluation will be on the outcomes of pharmacologic and pacing interventions designed to maintain an acceptable HR and improve AV conduction. Clinical assessment parameters, as well as the ECG, will be evaluated to determine the success of therapy. In addition, the patient will be evaluated with respect to his or her ability to conduct activities of daily living without experiencing the signs and symptoms of decreased cardiac output.

Documentation

Documentation should provide information about the progression of heart block, associated symptomatology, and patient responses to therapeutic interventions. As with any rhythm disturbance, an ECG example of AV block should be recorded in the medical record at least once a shift and whenever a significant change occurs. As always, any unusual event, such as an episode of confusion or syncope, should be documented and promptly reported.

Ongoing Care

The discharge plan should focus on preventing injury and teaching the signs and symptoms of worsening block. Syncopal episodes can occur if the heart block progresses suddenly or if pacemaker failure occurs in a pacemaker-dependent patient. Falls and related injury may result. The nurse should teach the patient about symptoms that must be reported to a physician, including weakness, dizziness, lethargy, increased activity intolerance, shortness of breath, and syncope.

PACEMAKERS

A pacemaker is an electronic device that delivers a controlled electrical stimulus to the heart through electrodes that are placed in contact with heart muscle. Pacemakers are designed to provide an artificial electrical signal when the heart's intrinsic electrical system is faltering. The major indication for the use of pacemakers is when the heart rate is too slow. Pacemakers may be employed as short-term electrical backups whenever an actual or potential decrease in the heart rate is possible. Therefore temporary pacing is appropriate during emergency situations associated with critical rate reductions, as protection in the presence of transient heart blocks, after cardiac surgery, and during recovery from the effects of drug toxicity. Permanent pacing is indicated when advanced AVB, degenerative disease, myocardial necrosis, or other pathologic conditions (e.g., sick sinus syndrome) result in an actual or potential symptomatic decrease in the heart rate. A few sophisticated pacing systems respond to *fast* rates rather than slow rates. They are equipped with a special "antitachycardia" feature that detects an accelerated rate and delivers a timed electrical signal to interrupt the rhythm, thereby slowing the rate.

Common Components

All pacemaker systems contain two basic components, the pulse generator and the pacemaker catheter. The *pulse generator* contains the energy source that powers the pacemaker. It also contains circuits required for sensing intrinsic electrical signals, timing the release of the artificial signal, and modulating current output. The pacing catheter operates as a two-way transmission line between the pulse generator and the heart. It not only delivers the electrical signal to the heart but also transmits information about natural electrical activity back to the pulse generator for processing.

Temporary pulse generators

Temporary pulse generators (Figure 34-40) are external units powered by removable batteries requiring periodic replacement. These generators are constructed for use in pacing either a single cardiac chamber or both chambers sequentially (single versus dual chamber pacing). Temporary pulse generators are operator-controlled in the sense that all pacing parameters are controlled through adjustment of dials located on the face of the units. The generator is interfaced with the pacing catheter via

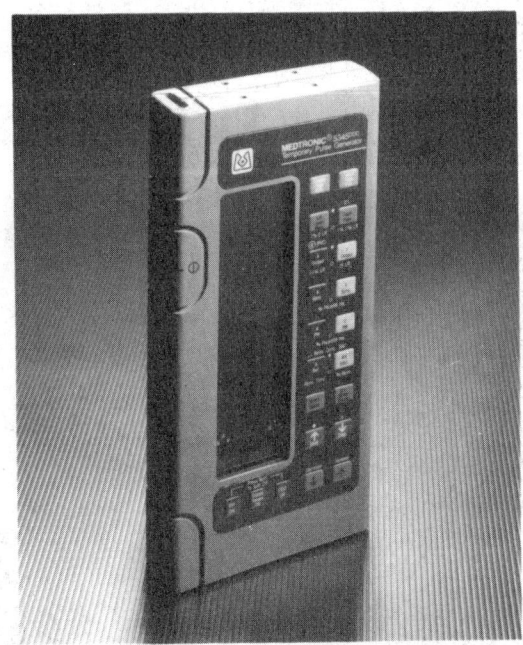

FIGURE 34-40   Temporary pulse generator. (Courtesy Medtronic, Inc.)

electrically insulated terminals located on the generator. Though temporary pulse generators are manufactured by several companies, they all retain the same basic features, including an on/off control, pace/sense indicator, and sometimes a battery test feature. The clinician can dictate parameters such as firing rate, voltage output, and system sensitivity simply by adjusting the dials.

Permanent pulse generators

Permanent pulse generators (Figure 34-41) are small, lightweight, surgically implanted units commonly powered by lithium batteries that are expected to last between 3 and 15 years. Nuclear-powered pacemakers with an expected battery life of 10 to 20 years are also available, but their use has been limited in part as a result of restrictions mandated by the federal government. Permanent generators are hermetically sealed and encased in a titanium housing to isolate their circuits from the biologic environment. Like temporary units, they may be configured for either single or dual chamber use. Unlike their external counterparts, permanent units are programmed with respect to firing rate, voltage output, and sensitivity during the operative procedure.

Insertion

Temporary pacing is accomplished using either the transvenous, transthoracic, or transcutaneous ap-

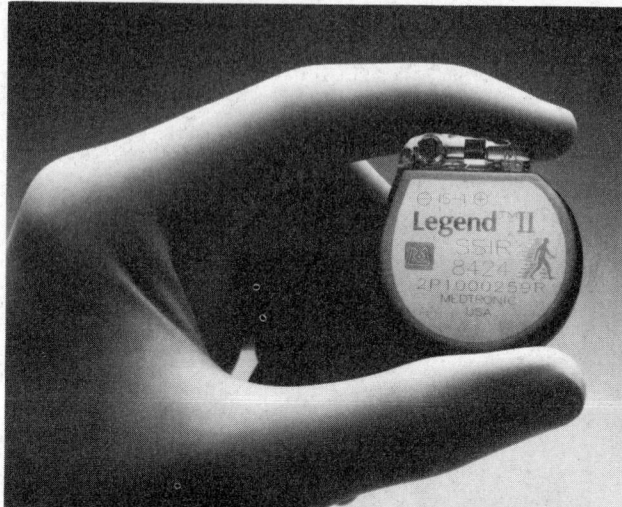

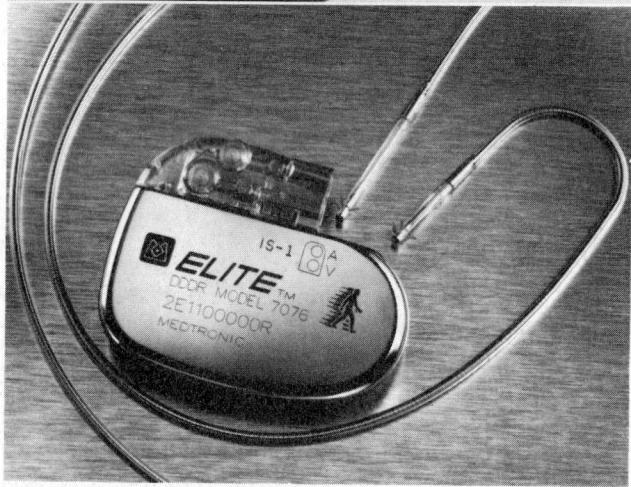

FIGURE 34-41 Permanent pulse generators. Implantable units are thin, lightweight, and relatively unobtrusive once implanted beneath the skin. (Courtesy Medtronic, Inc.)

proach. Transvenous pacing catheters are guided (ideally under fluoroscopy) into the right side of the heart through a percutaneous introducer inserted through the subclavian, external jugular, antecubital, or femoral vein (Figure 34-42). After contact is made with the wall of the heart, the two external pins on the pacing catheter (one is marked negative, or distal; the other represents the positive lead, but may be unmarked) are inserted into the corresponding terminals (marked negative and positive) usually located at the top of the pulse generator. Pacing parameters are set by manipulating the generator controls.

Transcutaneous pacing resembles defibrillation in that the electrical stimulus is delivered through the chest wall to produce a response. This mode of emergency pacing requires the use of surface pacing electrodes applied to the outer chest wall and connected to an external pacing unit via pacing cables. Delivery of an electrical stimulus through the chest wall should cause depolarization of the heart and subsequent mechanical contraction.

Permanent pacing requires an operative procedure with attendant surgical risk. The most common, and least hazardous, approach is the transvenous approach utilized for endocardial pacing (Figure 34-43). The procedure is generally done with the patient under local anesthesia in a cardiac catheterization laboratory. The pulse generator is implanted into a subcutaneous pocket created beneath the clavicle. The pacing catheter is guided into the right side of the heart through the cephalic, subclavian, or jugular vein. The catheter and generator are connected, pacing parameters are set, and the wound is closed (antibiotic irrigation before wound closure has significantly lowered the incidence of postoperative infection).

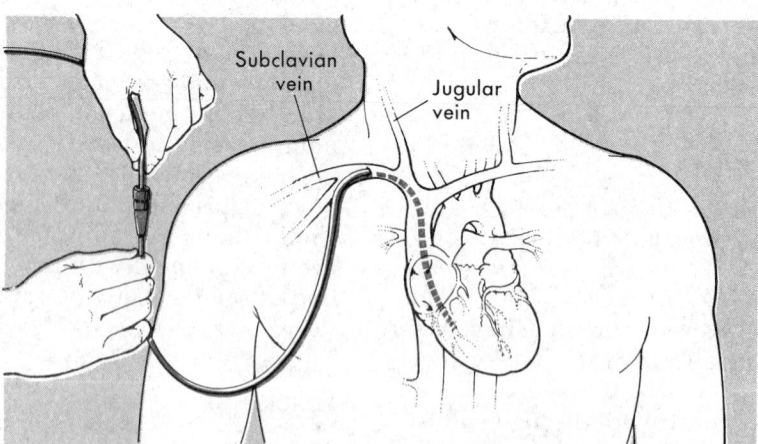

FIGURE 34-42 Insertion of a temporary endocardial pacing catheter using an introducer. A cut-down may also be performed to obtain venous access.

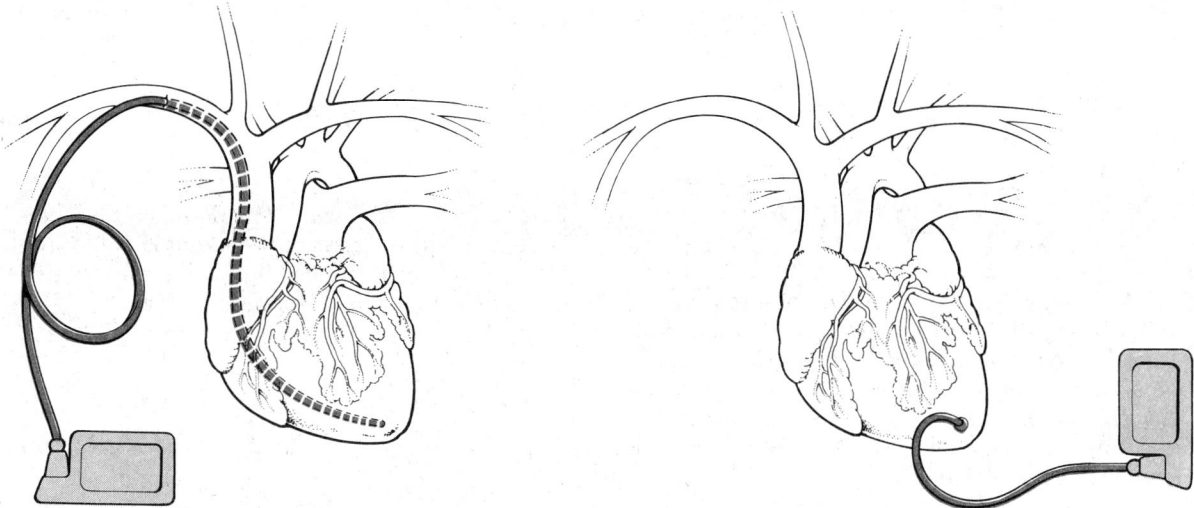

FIGURE 34-43   Permanent endocardial versus epicardial pacing. Endocardial catheters are positioned within the RV apex, while epicardial catheters are attached to the outer surface of the LV.

Epicardial pacing involves a clearly more invasive operative procedure performed with the patient under either local or (more commonly) general anesthesia, depending on the surgical approach used. The transthoracic approach requires thoracotomy (includes interruption of the pleura) and is done using a general anesthetic. The transmediastinal approach can be performed with the patient under local anesthesia and does not involve interruption of the pleura. In either case, a subcutaneous pocket to house the permanent pacemaker generator is created in the abdominal wall. The catheter is attached at one end to the epicardial surface of the heart, and the other end is inserted into the receptacle on the pulse generator. The pacing parameters are set, the pocket is irrigated, and the wound is closed.

Basic Pacing Parameters

Pacemaker functions can be analyzed with respect to two primary factors, release of the electrical signal from the pacemaker generator and the heart's response to it. Release of the stimulus is influenced by programmed instructions that regulate the pacing system's sensitivity, the strength of the electrical output signal created by the pulse generator, and timing of the output signal. Response to the stimulus is influenced by the clinical state of the heart, the site of stimulus delivery, and additional pacemaker instructions that tell it how to respond to intrinsic cardiac signals.

Stimulus release

Sensitivity refers to the pacing system's ability to process intrinsic voltage signals, the natural electrical activity of the heart. This is important, because modern pacemakers are instructed to fire either "on demand" or "in sync" with an intrinsic ECG signal, and they must be able to sense electrical activity to accomplish these tasks. Sensitivity is ultimately influenced by the configuration of the pacing system and the settings on the pulse generator. Pacing systems may be bipolar or unipolar.

The main difference between unipolar and bipolar systems is their sensitivity, so each system is selected for use in different clinical circumstances. Unipolar systems are highly sensitive to intracardiac electrical activity, which makes them ideally suited for permanent pacing. An occasionally troublesome characteristic of unipolar systems, however, is their sensitivity to extracardiac signals such as skeletal muscle tremors. This extra sensitivity could prove detrimental if muscle activity is interpreted as cardiac activity, resulting in inhibition of pacing. Bipolar systems, on the other hand, are far less sensitive to both intracardiac and extracardiac signals, but their ability to process intrinsic cardiac signals is normally quite adequate and appropriate to meet the requirements of temporary pacing.

Sensitivity is not only a function of the pacing system configuration (i.e., unipolar versus bipolar). The ability of the system to process incoming electrical signals can also be controlled on a temporary generator by adjusting the sensitivity, or mV, dial located on the face of the unit (Figure 34-44). Setting the dial to its lowest numeric setting (all the way to the right, or on "full demand") makes the system maximally sensitive, giving it the ability to process low voltage cardiac signals. Conversely, moving the dial to its highest numeric setting (all the way to the left, or on "asynchronous" or "fixed rate") essentially

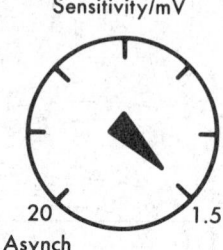

Sensitivity/mV

20
Asynch
1.5

FIGURE 34-44 Adjusting the sensitivity of a temporary pacemaker. When the sensitivity/mV dial is turned all the way to the right (to demand), the system is maximally sensitive. When it is turned all the way to the left (to asynchronous, or fixed rate), the sensing circuits are blinded and the pacemaker will fire without regard to intrinsic electrical activity.

blinds the system, so that it will be unable to process even large cardiac signals.

The strength of the output signal reflects the voltage released by the pulse generator each time the pacemaker fires. The output signal is measured in milliamperes, or mA, and represents a pacing parameter that can be adjusted on temporary pulse generators or set during an operative procedure. When the output signal is released, a sharp narrow deflection called a stimulus artifact, or pacing spike, is written on the ECG. The pacing spike immediately precedes the electrical response (depolarization). The size of the pacing spike is influenced by the configuration of the pacing system; bipolar systems produce small spikes, whereas unipolar systems produce large spikes.

The timing of the output signal reflects a portion of the pacing system's instructions about when to release the electrical stimulus. The period between a natural event to the first paced event is called the escape interval (Figure 34-45). It represents a type of electrical backup, not unlike the escape beats previously discussed, designed to provide an *artificial* cardiac stimulus when the dominant pacemakers fail. Another programmed interval called the automatic interval (also called the pulse interval) represents the time between consecutive paced events. In permanent pacing systems, an escape interval slightly longer than the automatic interval can be programmed into the pacemaker's instructions. Theoretically, the longer the pacemaker waits before firing after sensing a natural beat, the more likely it is that the sinus node will fire and retain pacemaker control. This feature, called hysteresis, is an optional programmable feature of questionable benefit. The unwary clinician, failing to recognize the presence of hysteresis, can easily diagnose pacemaker malfunction where none exists.

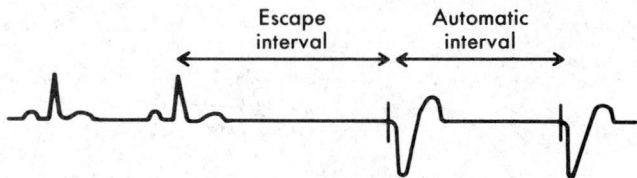

Escape interval   Automatic interval

FIGURE 34-45 Intervals. The distance between a natural event and the first paced event is called the escape interval. The distance between consecutive paced events is called the automatic interval.

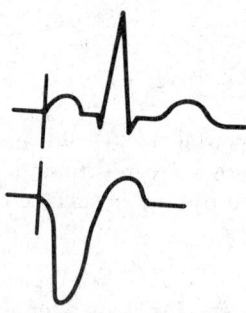

FIGURE 34-46 Stimulus release and response (capture). Release of the stimulus into the atrium produces a stimulus artifact, or pacing spike, followed by a P wave. Release of the stimulus into the ventricle produces a spike followed by a wide QRS. The QRS is wide because depolarization of the ventricles is sequential.

Stimulus response

Stimulus response (Figure 34-46) refers to the heart's response to the electrical signal transmitted from the pulse generator. As previously noted, stimulus response is influenced by the clinical state of the heart, the site of impulse delivery, and additional instructions that tell the pacemaker how to respond to intrinsic electrical activity.

Threshold represents the smallest amount of electrical stimulation required to elicit a response. Threshold is influenced by clinical conditions (such as electrolyte abnormalities, drug effects, and myocardial ischemia) that affect the ability of the heart to respond to an electrical signal. The voltage output of the pacemaker (the mA) must be set to equal or exceed threshold, or the heart will not depolarize in response to the artificial stimulus. During the first few weeks after insertion of a pacemaker catheter, fibrosis at the catheter tip causes the threshold to rise. The pacemaker's voltage output is normally set higher than the original stimulation threshold (measured during the insertion procedure) to compensate for the expected rise in threshold that accompanies lead maturation.

Capture implies depolarization of the heart in response to the electrical stimulus. Capture is assumed when the pacing artifact (or spike) is immediately followed by either a wide QRS (if the stimulus is delivered in the ventricle) or a P wave (if the stimulus is delivered in the atrium). Capture is an electrical phenomenon that can be assessed on the ECG. The mechanical response to depolarization must be clinically assessed.

The mode of response describes additional instructions that tell the pacemaker what signals it should fire in response to and how long it should wait before firing. The asynchronous, or fixed-rate, mode instructs the pacemaker to fire at a continuous, preset rate without regard for intrinsic electrical activity. Fixed-rate firing does not require sensing. Firing only when needed—when intrinsic electrical activity is absent—is known as the demand, or inhibited, mode of response. Demand pacing is the most common programmable mode of pacing. An additional mode of response that may be incorporated into the pacemaker's instructions is called the triggered, or synchronous, pacing mode. The pacemaker is asked to sense an electrical event, wait a preset time interval, and fire. Many of the more sophisticated dual-chamber pacing systems combine the features of demand and triggered pacing to produce a sequential response. Stimuli are delivered through two pacing catheters to produce a response in both chambers.

The ICHD code

The ICHD code represents a simple shorthand method for describing a wide variety of pacing systems. Originally developed in 1974 by the Inter-Society Commission for Heart Disease as a three-letter coding system, the ICHD code was expanded in the early 1980s to a more descriptive five-letter system appropriate for identification of the multiple sophisticated pacing units in use today (Table 34-1).

The first letter in the ICHD code represents the *chamber paced.* If the ventricle is paced the code letter is a "V"; if the atrium is paced the code letter is an "A." If both atrium and ventricle are paced the designation is a "D" (for double, or dual). The second letter in the ICHD code represents the *chamber sensed,* and the identical designations are used (V, A, or D). In addition, if sensing is not present, the code "O" (for none) is used. The third letter in the ICHD code represents the *mode of response.* If the pacemaker fires in response to an electrical signal, the code "T" (for triggered) is used. If firing is inhibited by an electrical signal, the code is "I" (for inhibited, or demand). If the response is asynchronous (or fixed rate) the code is "O" (for continuous). If both inhibition and triggering are present, the code is "D" (for double, or dual).

Today's pacemakers are capable of responding to diverse instructions that are easily appreciated in light of the simple three-letter ICHD code.

TABLE 34-1   ICHD Codes

Chamber(s) paced	Chamber(s) sensed	Mode of responses (sensing function)	Programmable functions	Special tachydysrhythmia functions
1974				
V = Ventricle	V = Ventricle	T = Triggered		
A = Atrium	A = Atrium	I = Inhibited (demand)		
D = Double (dual)	D = Double (dual)	O = None (continuous)		
	O = None			
1981				
V = Ventricle	V = Ventricle	T = Triggered	P = Programmable	B = Bursts
A = Atrium	A = Atrium	I = Inhibited (demand)	M = Multiprogrammable	N = Normal rate competition (dual demand)
D = Double (dual)	D = Double (dual)	D = Double (dual function: T and I)	O = None (permanent pacemakers only)	S = Scanning
	O = None	O = None (continuous)		E = External
		R = Reverse		

From Vinsant-Crawford MO, Spence MI: *Commonsense approach to coronary care,* ed 5, St Louis, 1989, Mosby–Year Book.

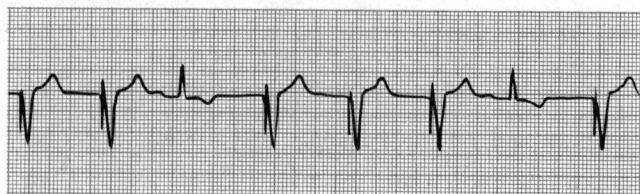

FIGURE 34-47 Ventricular (VVI) pacing. The pacing spike is delivered into the ventricle only if electrical activity is absent. The third and seventh beats represent intrinsic activity that is sensed by the pacemaker, thus inhibiting its output until the programmed escape interval has passed.

Systems configured for VVI pacing remain the most common type in use today. Both pacing and sensing occur in the ventricle (the first and second letters = V). This *demand* pacemaker is looking for ventricular activity and will pace in the ventricle if no QRS is sensed. If intrinsic electrical activity is sensed in the ventricle, the VVI pacemaker will respond by shutting down (the third letter = I, for inhibited). VVI pacemakers fire only when needed and function like escape rhythms in that they never allow the HR to fall below a preset rate (Figure 34-47).

Other pacing systems are the DVI and the DDD.

Physiologic Pacemakers

Physiologic pacemakers represent a generation of pacemakers designed to preserve AV synchrony—the normal sequence of electrical activation in the heart. Normal AV synchrony (atrial depolarization followed by ventricular depolarization) preserves the atrial contribution to cardiac output (the atrial kick) and is recognized on the ECG as a P wave followed by a QRS. Unfortunately, the most common pacing system in use, the single chamber VVI pacemaker, is "nonphysiologic" and unable to maintain AV synchrony, because it fires in response to ventricular events without regard for atrial events. Though the usual mechanical response to ventricular pacing preserves the major share of cardiac output, the VVI pacemaker fails to generate the approximately 20% of cardiac output provided by atrial contraction. In other words, the VVI pacemaker cannot simulate natural AV synchrony by putting a P wave in front of a QRS.

The loss of normal sequential activation of the cardiac chambers is associated with a set of clinical signs and symptoms known as the **pacemaker syndrome.** Patients experiencing a drop in cardiac output in response to VVI pacing may complain of fatigue, weakness, dizziness, lack of energy, or exhaustion. If reprogramming the pacemaker does not

eliminate, or at least greatly reduce, the frequency and intensity of these symptoms, many physicians will consider replacing a single chamber unit with a physiologic dual chamber pacemaker.

The latest generation of physiologic pacemakers reflects a qualitative leap in pacemaker technology. These new units incorporate sensing of selected biologic parameters into their impressive repertoire of features, thereby instructing the pacemaker to adjust its rate in accordance with physiologic demands such as skeletal muscle vibrations (this is known as rate-responsive pacing).

Pacemaker Malfunctions

Pacemaker malfunctions can usually be traced to either component failure, battery failure, or problems at the electrode-to-myocardium interface. Because these malfunctions are described as disturbances in sensing, firing, and capturing, the clinician must be able to assess alterations in these parameters to identify pacing problems.

Sensing represents the pacemaker's ability to "see" electrical activity in the heart. Appropriate sensing is usually assessed with respect to the various pacing intervals programmed into the pacemaker's instructions (e.g., the escape and automatic intervals). Firing reflects release of the electrical signal and is represented on the ECG by the stimulus artifact, or pacing spike. Capturing represents the heart's electrical response to the artificial stimulus and is reflected on the ECG by the appearance of a wide QRS following the pacing spike (assuming ventricular pacing).

Sensing disturbances

Disturbances in sensing occur when the pacemaker fails to "see" intrinsic electrical activity in the heart resulting in inappropriate timing of the pacemaker stimulus. One kind of sensing disturbance results when a temporary pacemaker is instructed to fire at "fixed-rate" (the sensitivity control is set all the way to the left, or on "async"), effectively disabling the sensing circuit. Dialing the sensitivity control all the way to the right (to full demand) will correct this problem. On the other hand, the sensing circuit can be temporarily or permanently blinded as a result of high-energy defibrillation currents. The only reasonable ways to avoid this problem are to avoid the area of the pacemaker generator when placing the defibrillator paddles on the chest (if feasible, anteroposterior paddle placement is recommended) and using the lowest energy levels appropriate to the situation.

Undersensing (Figure 34-48) reflects failure to sense intrinsic electrical activity (e.g., QRS complexes) that should have been sensed. Paced beats

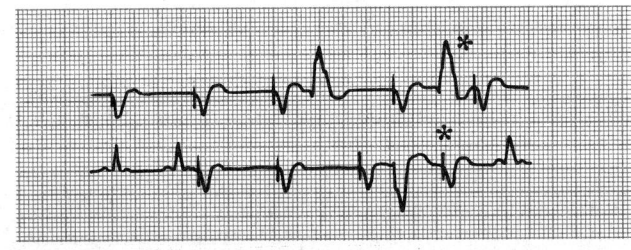

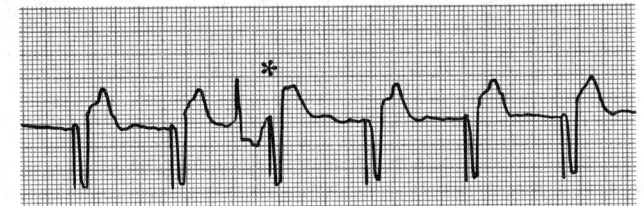

FIGURE 34-48   Failure to sense (undersensing). **A,** Some intrinsic beats are not sensed, resulting in firing earlier than expected. **B,** The third QRS (intrinsic) is not sensed, causing the pacemaker to fire too early.

appear earlier than expected on the ECG and may result in dangerous competition. The cause of undersensing may lie in the configuration of the system itself. For example, bipolar systems are less sensitive than their unipolar counterparts, so they may be unable to sense low-voltage cardiac signals. To solve an undersensing problem, the sensitivity setting on a temporary generator can be increased (unless it is already maximal), or the system can be changed to a unipolar one, which requires disabling the positive electrode on a bipolar catheter and creating another one on the body surface. If dangerous competition develops in the presence of undersensing, the unit should be shut off.

Oversensing reflects inappropriate sensing of cardiac signals, such as tall T waves, thereby inhibiting current output. Paced beats do not appear when they should. The extreme sensitivity of a unipolar pacing system may result in oversensing; reconfiguring the system for less sensitive bipolar pacing may be appropriate. Adjusting the sensitivity control on a demand pacemaker to a position somewhere between demand and fixed rate may decrease the sensitivity enough to solve the problem.

In addition, inappropriate sensing of muscle potentials rather than intracardiac potentials (more common with unipolar pacing) can result in inhibition of current output (this is known as myopotential inhibition). Placing a magnet directly over a permanent pulse generator will convert a demand unit to a fixed rate unit, essentially blinding the overly sensitive sensing circuit. Long-term resolution of sensing problems encountered during permanent pacing will require reprogramming of the pacemaker's sensitivity.

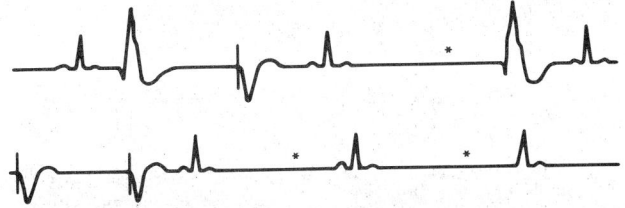

FIGURE 34-49   Failure to fire. The pacemaker does not fire as expected following the fourth, ninth, and tenth beats. No spike appears on the ECG.

Electromagnetic interference from sources such as overhead transmission lines, welding equipment, older model microwave ovens, and electrocautery devices can also result in inhibition of the output signal. Crosstalk, a problem unique to dual chamber systems, involves inappropriate sensing of an electrical signal from one chamber by a catheter in another chamber, resulting in inhibition of pacer output.

Firing disturbances

Firing disturbances occur when the pacemaker fails to release its stimulus when expected (Figure 34-49). When sensing is intact, a pacing spike does not appear when it should, perhaps resulting in symptomatic slow rates. The causes of "failure to fire" include battery failure, fracture of the pacing catheter, and a disconnection somewhere in the system.

Capturing disturbances

Capturing disturbances occur when the heart does not respond to the electrical stimulus (Figure 34-50). When both sensing and firing are intact, the ECG reveals a pacing spike delivered on time but not followed by a wide QRS (or a P wave if the stimulus is delivered in the atrium). "Failure to capture" represents one of the most common pacemaker malfunctions observed in the clinical setting. It most often results from faulty catheter position as a result of migration of the catheter to an area of higher threshold or loss of contact with the heart muscle. Increasing the current output (or mA) on a temporary pulse generator may produce adequate capture, but the pacing catheter may need to be repositioned if it has lost contact with the heart. Sometimes, if the patient lies on the left side, gravity will allow the pacing catheter to float downward until it touches the wall of the heart. If loss of capture occurs in a permanent pacing system, the pacemaker must be reprogrammed or the lead must be repositioned, depending on the cause of the problem. In any case, an overpenetrated chest x-ray examination should be performed for close analysis of catheter position within the heart.

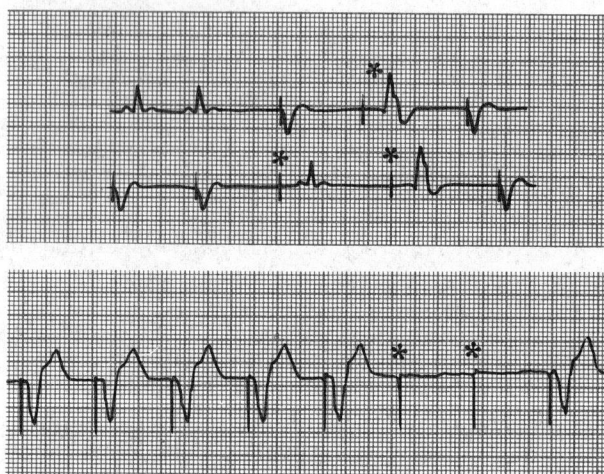

FIGURE 34-50   Failure to capture. Sensing and firing are intact. Occasionally the pacing spike is not followed by a wide QRS.

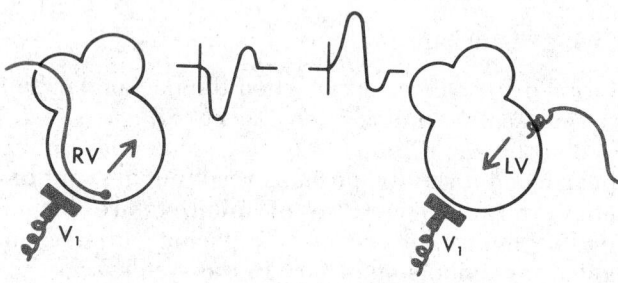

FIGURE 34-51   RV versus LV pacing. It is suggested that the clinician use lead V_1 to assess pacemaker rhythms. RV pacing will produce a spike followed by a wide and negative QRS. LV pacing will produce a spike followed by a wide and positive QRS.

A related capturing problem may reflect perforation of the cardiac wall by endocardial pacing catheters. The thin right ventricular wall can be punctured by a stiff catheter resulting in diaphragmatic stimulation (and annoying hiccups) at a rate equal to the pacemaker firing rate. Tamponade is rare unless the patient is anticoagulated. Extracardiac stimulation is alleviated by withdrawing the catheter into the right ventricle. Rarely, a stiff catheter can puncture the intraventricular septum causing paced beats to assume a different shape on the ECG.

The clinician is encouraged to monitor pacemaker patients in the right-sided precordial lead V_1 so that changes in catheter position can be easily detected (Figure 34-51). If an endocardial pacing catheter is firing as expected in the right ventricle, the pacing spike should be followed by a wide and negative QRS (the right ventricle will be depolarized ahead of the left ventricle, or, from right to left; V_1 will see

the depolarization current moving away from its positive end). If the catheter perforates the septum resulting in delivery of the stimulus in the left ventricle, V_1 will record a wide and positive QRS following the spike (the left ventricle will be depolarized before the right ventricle, or, from left to right; V_1 will see the depolarization current moving toward its positive end). Septal perforation usually causes no significant problems to the patient, but the physician will have to withdraw the catheter through the self-sealing septum to its original right ventricular location.

NURSING MANAGEMENT OF THE PATIENT WITH AN ARTIFICIAL PACEMAKER
Assessment

Assessment of the patient with an artificial pacemaker is primarily concerned with the effects of HR on maintenance of an adequate cardiac output. Parameters including HR, blood pressure, peripheral perfusion, and sensorium should be assessed along with the ECG.

Nursing Diagnosis

Nursing diagnoses for the patient with an artificial pacemaker reflect concerns related to vital organ perfusion, activities of daily living, safety, knowledge level, and emotional state. These include:

Activity intolerance related to the pacemaker syndrome

Altered peripheral tissue perfusion related to presence of a temporary pacing catheter in a peripheral vessel

Anxiety related to the need for lifelong artificial cardiac pacing

Decreased cardiac output related to loss of the atrial kick associated with nonphysiologic pacing

Knowledge deficit (pacemaker function, need for follow-up care, situations/devices to avoid, pulse-taking technique)

High risk for injury related to risk for syncopal episodes associated with pacemaker failure

Planning

The goals of therapy for patients with pacemakers generally focus on maintaining an adequate HR and returning the patient to a normal life-style. Goals for the patient include:

Activity tolerance is increased as evidenced by no complaints of fatigue, weakness, dizziness, or exhaustion associated with VVI pacing

Peripheral perfusion is adequate as evidenced by

good skin color, temperature, and pulses distal to the catheter insertion site

Anxiety is diminished as evidenced by ability to verbalize recognition of anxiety; decrease in physical and behavioral symptoms such as hyperventilation, muscle tension, and change in sleeping pattern

Cardiac output is adequate as evidenced by acceptable, stable vital signs, especially heart rate; adequate peripheral perfusion; normal sensorium

Knowledge level is increased as evidenced by ability to verbalize the rationale for pacing, the treatment plan, and the need for follow-up care; ability to explain the procedure for taking a radial pulse and to demonstrate same

Patient remains free of bodily injury

Implementation

Interventions prescribed for the patient with an artificial pacemaker focus on maintenance of appropriate pacemaker function, safety, and patient teaching.

Appropriate teaching regarding preoperative and postoperative concerns should be provided. The nurse addresses "need to know" and "want to know" information in simple terms, without flooding the patient with a jumble of technical facts that may not be understood. The patient is asked what he or she wants to know about the pacemaker and the insertion procedure.

Regarding temporary pacing, the patient will need to know why the pacemaker is necessary, how it works, and that nothing will be felt when the pacemaker is working. The nurse explains what can be expected during the insertion procedure: that the procedure will usually last only a few minutes, that the insertion site will be anesthetized, and what the patient is likely to see in the cardiac catheterization laboratory. The patient is instructed about postinsertion physical activity. If the catheter is inserted into the antecubital or femoral vein, the patient should avoid excessive movement of the extremity to prevent dislodging the catheter. If a femoral approach is used, a soft restraint may be placed on the ankle as a "reminder" to the patient not to bend the leg. A bridging cable, or pacemaker "extension cord," can be used to prevent traction on the pacemaker catheter. The patient is informed that most people experience no postinsertion discomfort other than that associated with activity restrictions.

Regarding permanent pacing, the patient should be given instruction in the same points previously listed. The endocardial pacing procedure should take about an hour, local anesthesia is used so the patient will be awake, a large dressing will be applied over the wound, and postinsertion discomfort

is usually minimal and easily treated with a mild analgesic. The patient is instructed about postoperative activity. The arm on the operative side should not be raised above shoulder height for approximately 48 hours after surgery, but some physicians will extend this period.

If epicardial pacing is accomplished via thoracotomy, a general anesthetic will be used, and the procedure will take longer. A chest tube will be inserted, and discomfort will result from the chest tube as well as from the wound. Adequate turning, coughing, and deep breathing will be encouraged to prevent the development of postoperative atelectasis and pneumonia.

The patient is protected from injury as a result of faulty or improperly grounded equipment. Current leakage can cause VF, particularly in the patient with a temporary pacemaker. Electrical beds are acceptable if they are grounded. Temporary pacemaker generators are protected by using a cover over the face of the unit to protect it from spills and accidental manipulation of the controls. All exposed metal is insulated. Most temporary systems are well insulated and require no further protection, but any exposed metal should be insulated with a rubber glove. For example, if the metal tips on the pins of temporary pacing catheters are evident after insertion into the terminals on the pulse generator, the nurse should slip the unit into a rubber glove, making sure that the glove contains no powder. Exposed surgical wires should be protected by a dressing.

The ECG is assessed for the presence of pacemaker malfunction. Failure to sense, failure to fire, and failure to capture may result in inappropriate pacing; the stimulus may be delivered too early or not at all, or the heart may not respond to it. The nurse reports all cases of suspected malfunction to the physician and requests an order for an overpenetrated chest x-ray to confirm catheter position and integrity. The nurse should be prepared to institute CPR if pacemaker failure results in asystole. Emergency drugs and equipment should be readily available. The nurse documents ECG examples of suspected malfunction and marks the patient's name, the date, the time, and the lead on every strip. If *failure to sense* is present in a temporary system, the sensitivity setting on the pacemaker generator is increased unless it is already maximal. If *failure to fire* is present in a temporary system, the pacemaker batteries are inspected, because they may need to be changed. Temporary generators should be marked with the date of each battery change. The nurse confirms that all connections are tight. If *failure to capture* is present in a temporary system, the current output on the pacemaker is increased; the nurse might also try repositioning the patient on the left side.

The patient is assessed for the presence of complications associated with pacing. The nurse looks for evidence of *perforation* of either the right ventricle or the septum. Hiccups are associated with diaphragmatic pacing; tamponade may result if anticoagulants are on board. Change in the polarity of the paced QRS is associated with septal perforation. The ECG is evaluated for evidence of pacemaker-induced dysrhythmias. Insertion of a pacing catheter into a sensitive ventricle can result in ventricular ectopy. Lidocaine should be readily available. The wound is assessed for signs of infection. Redness, swelling, tenderness, presence of exudate, and temperature elevation may indicate infection. The nurse should use good handwashing technique before caring for any wound. Sterile technique should be used when redressing a temporary catheter insertion site.

The patient is assessed for evidence of the pacemaker syndrome. VVI pacemakers are associated with fatigue and weakness when ventricular pacing is present. Reprogramming may be required. The nurse should report untoward symptoms to the physician.

Evaluation

Evaluation of patient responses to pacemaker therapy will include assessment of heart rate and whether the pacemaker is functioning as programmed. As always, hemodynamic stability, as well as the ECG, will be evaluated. Other patient responses that should be assessed include activity tolerance and whether symptoms associated with the pacemaker syndrome are present during pacing.

Documentation

Documentation is critically important, especially during the early phase after insertion of a pacemaker. ECG rhythm strip examples should be documented at least once a shift and whenever a suspected pacemaker malfunction is observed. Each strip should be labeled with the date, time, and lead. All nursing interventions undertaken to support pacemaker function when a malfunction is present, such as manipulation of the mA on a temporary pacemaker generator, should be recorded. Clinical assessment parameters, including vital signs, peripheral perfusion, wound status, and sensorium, should be entered into the medical record so that trends can be accurately evaluated. The teaching plan developed for the patient should also be documented to ensure consistency.

Ongoing Care

Ongoing care for the patient with a pacemaker focuses heavily on discharge planning, an integral component of long-term therapeutic management.

Teaching should include essential information about how the pacemaker works, how long it will last, sensations experienced during pacing (contrary to common belief, pacemaker firing produces no sensation), and the importance of follow-up visits.

Additional information should focus on adherence to medication and activity protocols, the need to carry pacemaker information and to wear a medic alert ID, and potentially hazardous situations to avoid. Each pacemaker manufacturer can provide a list of devices that should be avoided (e.g., older model microwave ovens). The patient should be instructed to move away from any device that may be causing untoward symptoms such as dizziness or lightheadedness.

The nurse teaches the patient how and when to take a radial pulse. The pulse should be taken at the same time each day and if symptoms such as dizziness or weakness develop. The patient should be able to demonstrate the pulse-taking skill before discharge from the hospital. The patient should also be taught to promptly report unusual symptoms to the physician, including a pulse rate below the minimal pacing rate.

CONGESTIVE HEART FAILURE
Definition/Etiology

Congestive heart failure (CHF) represents the inability of the heart to pump enough blood to meet tissue requirements for oxygen, resulting in a discrepancy between myocardial oxygen supply and demand. It can result from any clinical situation that alters myocardial performance. Ischemic heart disease, MI, cardiomyopathy, valvular heart disease, septal defects, and hypertension rank among the primary pathologic conditions associated with acute and chronic forms of heart failure. Each of these clinical conditions represents an alteration in either muscle contractility, vascular tone, or internal volume load. CHF can also be caused by therapeutic interventions such as drug therapy and fluid replacement therapy. The increased incidence of heart failure in the elderly is most often associated with an age-related decline in cardiac function. Ischemic heart disease, hypertension, and degenerative calcification of the cardiac valves are major causes of CHF in the older adult. Regardless of the cause, however, the nurse must be able to recognize the classic signs and symptoms of heart failure, understand the body's response to it, and appreciate the rationale behind prescribed therapeutic interventions.

Pathophysiology

When the heart is subjected to situations of acute or chronic stress, adequate tissue oxygenation is preserved by intrinsic compensatory mechanisms.

Compensatory mechanisms represent automatic tissue and organ responses to altered cardiac pumping. The signs and symptoms of heart failure in large measure reflect the work of compensatory mechanisms as they attempt to maintain vital organ perfusion. The degree of heart failure, ranging from mild CHF to cardiogenic shock, is an indication of how successful the compensatory mechanisms are at preserving tissue oxygenation.

Myocardial performance

Depressed cardiac pumping is associated with alterations in one or more of the variables that determine cardiac output.

Contractility

Contractility represents the ability of a muscle fiber to contract, or shorten. It reflects the degree of "stretch" inherent in muscle fibers. The more a fiber is stretched, the more forcefully it will recoil, much like a new rubber band. Myocardial fibers stretch in response to blood volume entering the chambers during diastolic filling; they shorten again when blood is ejected during systolic contraction. Ischemic muscle fibers lose much of their elastic recoil, forcing healthy fibers to work harder in an effort to maintain an adequate cardiac output.

Contractility is not measured directly. Instead, it is assessed indirectly by measuring cardiac output and other hemodynamic parameters.

Heart rate

Heart rate varies according to physiologic demands for oxygen and as a result of diseases and their treatments. In the normal heart physiologic demands for oxygen are met by increasing HR. Blood is ejected from the heart more efficiently, and cardiac output increases. A depressed heart does not respond in the same way. The weakened heart is unable to pump extra volume so stroke volume is compromised. Furthermore, increased HR shortens diastolic filling time, compromising SV and coronary perfusion even more.

Afterload

Afterload is the resistance that the ventricle must pump against with each contraction. Afterload is primarily a reflection of vascular tone, but it is also a reflection of the stress or tension generated in the ventricular wall during systolic contraction. When afterload increases, the ventricle works harder to pump blood into a constricted vascular bed. Cardiac muscle mass enlarges over time so the heart can generate the higher pressures required to overcome greater vascular resistance. The healthy heart can tolerate the increased work, but the diseased heart cannot. Stroke volume falls because the compromised heart is unable to pump hard enough to overcome increased afterload.

Afterload for the left ventricle (called "systemic vascular resistance," or SVR) reflects resistance or tone in the systemic vessels. Afterload for the right ventricle (called "pulmonary vascular resistance," or PVR) reflects resistance in the pulmonary vessels. Both SVR and PVR are derived parameters calculated from data gathered during hemodynamic monitoring.

Preload

Preload is primarily a reflection of the pressure exerted by blood volume in the ventricle at the end of diastolic filling. Preload is often called "filling pressure." When preload increases in the healthy heart, the extra volume load imposes maximal stretch on myocardial fibers, resulting in enhanced SV and cardiac output. The diseased heart is unable to handle increased preload efficiently. Since contractility is depressed, the diseased heart ejects reduced stroke volumes, trapping blood in the heart. The extra volume load overstretches ischemic fibers, causing chamber dilation.

Preload for the left ventricle is reflected in the pulmonary capillary wedge pressure (PCWP) or the left atrial pressure (LAP). PCWP is an indirect estimation of left ventricular filling pressure that is measured using a flow-directed pulmonary artery catheter. LAP is also a reflection of LV filling pressure, and it is measured using a left atrial catheter. Both kinds of hemodynamic monitoring are confined to the critical care setting.

Left versus right ventricular failure

Left ventricular failure (LVF) reflects impaired ejection of blood from the left ventricle (Figure 34-52). MI (usually left ventricular infarction) and systemic hypertension are specifically associated with LVF. The inability of the left ventricle to pump blood efficiently results in forward failure and compromises the delivery of oxygenated blood to the tissues, causing tissue hypoxia. Backward failure represents the congestive component of LVF. Blood dams up in the left side of the heart because it cannot be pumped efficiently; increasing left ventricular pressures are transmitted to the left atrium and the pulmonary vascular bed, and the lungs become congested with fluid. Stiff, noncompliant lungs increase the work of breathing and produce many of the clinical signs of LVF, such as shortness of breath. If left untreated, left-sided failure will eventually result in right-sided heart failure as the retrograde transmission of increasing pressures eventually reaches the right side of the heart.

Right ventricular failure (RVF) reflects impaired ejection of blood from the right ventricle (Figure 34-53). Pulmonary hypertension and right ventricular MI are commonly associated with right-sided failure. RVF can occur separately from LVF, but its appear-

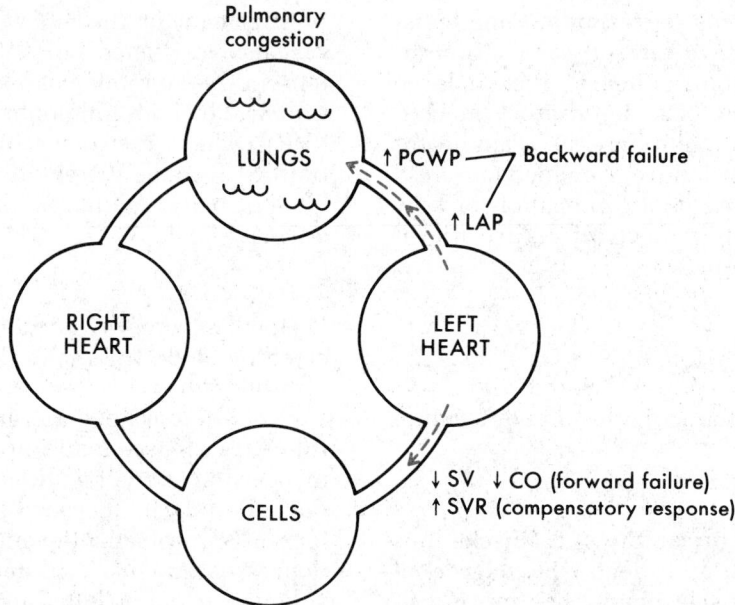

FIGURE 34-52 Left ventricular failure. Decreased SV and CO reflect forward failure; increased SVR represents a compensatory response. Increased PCWP/LAP and pulmonary congestion reflect backward failure.

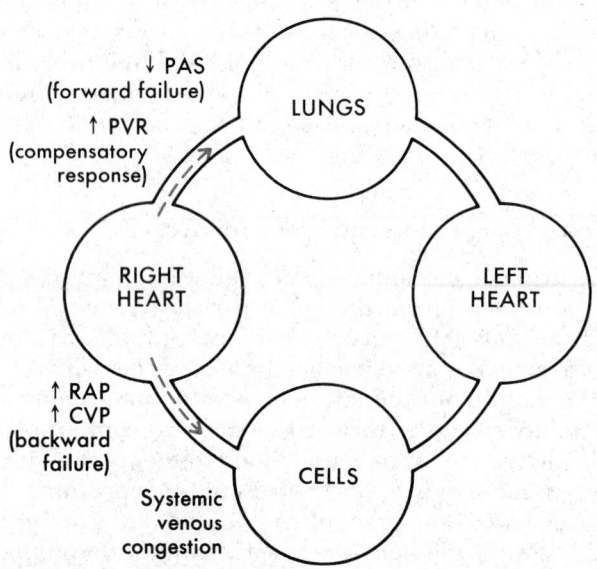

FIGURE 34-53 Right ventricular failure. Decreased PA systolic pressure reflects forward failure; increased PVR represents a compensatory response. Increased RAP/CVP and systemic venous congestion reflect backward failure.

ance is more often a consequence of left-sided failure. Forward failure of the right ventricle alone implies reduced right ventricular ejection of blood flow and compromised left ventricular filling. Diminished left ventricular preload ultimately results in reduced left ventricular stroke volume and a falling cardiac output. Failure to eject blood from the right ventricle also results in damming of blood in the right side of the heart (backward failure) with eventual transmission of increasing right-sided pressures into systemic venous circulation, thereby producing other clinical signs (e.g., peripheral edema and jugular venous distension).

Parameters measured *distal* to the failed ventricle reflect reduced systolic ejection of blood (reduced stroke volume and cardiac output) (forward failure).

Parameters measured *proximal* to the failed ventricle reflect the congestive component of heart failure (rising proximal pressures) (backward failure).

Clinical Manifestations

The signs and symptoms of heart failure reflect the status of intrinsic compensatory mechanisms and vary according to the degree of failure. Mild left ventricular dysfunction responsive to activity restriction, dietary control, and drug therapy is usually classified as congestive heart failure (CHF). The onset of CHF may be acute, but it often progresses over months or years, causing chronic disability. When left ventricular function suddenly deteriorates, resulting in acute clinical symptoms associated with pulmonary congestion and altered hemodynamics, the description *cardiogenic pulmonary edema* is assigned. Episodes of pulmonary edema are usually responsive to aggressive interventions that may include pharmacological and mechanical therapies. Table 34-2 compares the manifestations of RVF,

TABLE 34-2   Clinical Manifestations of Heart Failure

Type	Manifestation
Right ventricular failure	Elevated central venous pressure (CVP)
	Hypotension, tachycardia
	Distended neck veins,
	Hepatic congestion/ enlargement
	Peripheral edema
	Crackles, tachypnea
	Lethargy, easy fatigability
Left ventricular failure	Elevated LA or pulmonary capillary wedge pressure (PCWP) (ICU)
	Hypotension, tachycardia
	Peripheral hypoperfusion
	Crackles, tachypnea
	Pulmonary congestion/edema
	Signs and symptoms of RVF
	S_3
	Weight gain
	Cardiomegaly
Pulmonary edema	Respiratory distress
	Increased distribution of crackles
	Cough and increased secretions with blood-tinged, frothy sputum
	Bulging neck veins
	Pallor, cyanosis
	Diaphoresis
	Apprehension, restlessness
	Tachycardia
	PCWP > 25 to 30 mm Hg (ICU)

LVF, and pulmonary edema. The label *cardiogenic shock* implies the most devastating form of heart failure. It commonly occurs in association with extensive left ventricular MI and results in production of critical derangements in hemodynamics. Normal compensatory mechanisms are unable to restore the balance between myocardial oxygen supply and demand. A vicious cycle is established in which mechanisms designed to preserve vital organ perfusion actually interfere with it. Cardiogenic shock is uniformly fatal if left untreated. Despite prompt and aggressive treatment, cardiogenic shock is associated with a mortality often exceeding 80%.

Physiologic responses to heart failure involve the cardiovascular, pulmonary, renal, endocrine, and neurological systems (see box on p. 836).

Cardiovascular responses

When stroke volume (SV) and cardiac output (CO) begin to fall, the sympathetic nervous system mediates release of the catecholamines epinephrine and norepinephrine, resulting in one of the first compensatory responses, tachycardia. The heart beats faster in an attempt to preserve adequate tissue oxygenation, but rapid rates increase myocardial demands for oxygen and may compromise both SV and coronary artery perfusion. Associated myocardial ischemia may precipitate a variety of cardiac dysrhythmias, including PVCs.

Arterial pulse pressure narrows. (Pressure = flow × resistance.) When blood flow diminishes (reduced SV and CO), mean arterial pressure (MAP) is maintained through catecholamine-mediated increases in vascular resistance. Hypotension results when this compensatory mechanism fails.

LVF results in reduced forward flow, or SV. (CO = HR × SV.) Cardiac output will fall to less than the normal 4 to 8 L/minute when diminished SV cannot be compensated by increases in HR. Pulse volume is poor; pulses are weak and thready.

LVF causes damming of blood in the left side of the heart. If pulmonary artery pressure monitoring is available (refer to Chapter 13), pulmonary capillary wedge pressure (PCWP) (a reflection of left ventricular preload, or filling pressure) will usually exceed normal levels (8 to 12 mm Hg), often approaching 25 to 30 mm Hg. LVF is sometimes associated with normal or low filling pressures, and this alters the therapeutic approach.

RVF results in reduced ejection of blood into the pulmonary artery (PA). If PA pressure monitoring is available, PA systolic pressures will decrease, while PA diastolic pressures will increase (narrow pulse pressure represents a compensatory response). Rising pressures proximal to the failing right ventricle will reflect the congestive component of RVF. Right atrial pressures (mm Hg) or central venous pressures (cm H_2O) will rise as the volume load in the right side of the heart increases.

Rising right-sided pressures (right atrial pressures or central venous pressures) are poor indicators of left ventricular function. Elevated left-sided heart pressures transmitted into the pulmonary vascular bed are accompanied by compensatory responses that cushion the right side of the heart from rising pressures. The pulmonary vascular bed, normally a low pressure, low volume circuit, is very compliant and can expand or contract to accommodate extremes of blood volume. Thus right-sided heart pressures will not begin to increase until the pulmonary vascular system's ability to protect the right side of the heart is overwhelmed by the rising pressures it seeks to deflect.

Sluggish forward flow, which is expected when

PHYSIOLOGIC RESPONSES TO HEART FAILURE

Cardiovascular responses

Tachycardia
Narrow pulse pressure
Hypotension
↓ CO
Poor pulse volume
Pulses weak, thready
↑ PCWP/left atrial pressure (LVF)
↑ Right atrial pressure/CVP (RVF)
Jugular venous distention, edema
Hepatomegaly
S_3, S_4
Cyanosis
↓ Svo_2

Neurologic responses

Drowsiness
Lethargy
Confusion
Coma
↓ Level of consciousness

Pulmonary responses

Dyspnea, orthopnea, nocturnal dyspnea
Coughing
Hemoptysis
Crackles, rhonchi (wheezes)
$Pao_2 < Pao_2$

Endocrine and renal responses

↓ Glomerular filtration rate
↓ Urinary output
↑ Aldosterone
Sodium, water retention
↑ Antidiuretic hormone

Miscellaneous responses

Activity intolerance
Fatigue

---

the heart does not pump efficiently, can set the stage for the formation of mural thrombi. Increasing preload results in stretch of ischemic fibers, and atrial dysrhythmias such as atrial fibrillation often result, thus adding to the risk of stasis-related mural thrombi.

RVF is associated with systemic venous congestion caused by retrograde transmission of elevated vascular pressures from the right side of the heart into the peripheral vascular bed. Jugular venous distention (JVD; also described as "neck vein distention"), peripheral edema (especially in dependent areas), and hepatomegaly are commonly observed when fluid volume is sequestered in the periphery.

Heart sounds reflect altered ventricular compliance, or resistance to filling. When heart failure is not severe, the ventricles will fill adequately during the initial rapid filling stage of diastole, but they will be unable to accept the last bit of volume squeezed from the atria during atrial systole (the atrial kick). Altered compliance produces the S_4 gallop, a filling sound heard best at the end of ventricular diastole or just before mitral and tricuspid valve closure produces the first heart sound (S_1). As the heart continues to fail, impaired systolic ejection coupled with damming of blood in the chambers reduces ventricular compliance even during initial diastolic filling. Thus severe LVF produces the S_3 gallop, an early filling sound heard best at the beginning of ventricular

diastole just after closure of the aortic and pulmonic valves produces the second heart sound (S_2).

Continuous measurement of systemic venous oxygen saturation (Svo_2) indirectly reflects the heart's response to tissue oxygen demands. Increased tissue demands for oxygen are met primarily by increasing cardiac output. If the failing pump cannot increase CO, the second compensatory response is to extract more oxygen from the available supply. Normally the tissues use only a portion of the oxygen delivered to them, returning the rest to the heart for reoxygenation. It is this "venous oxygen reserve" that is tapped when the heart cannot increase CO enough to meet increased tissue demands for oxygen.

Svo_2 (the percentage of oxygen bound to hemoglobin in venous blood returning to the right side of the heart) is about 60% to 75%. When increased tissue demands for oxygen are satisfied by an increase in CO, Svo_2 remains within normal limits, because the venous oxygen reserve is untapped. When the heart is unable to increase CO, however, as in severe heart failure, extra oxygen is pulled from the venous oxygen reserve, and Svo_2 falls.

Skin pallor, sometimes coupled with peripheral cyanosis, represents compensatory vasoconstriction in nonessential areas as the body shunts blood to vital organs. Central cyanosis, a bluish discoloration of mucous membranes, is visible in advanced heart failure and appears in association with either low levels of hemoglobin, situations of acidosis, or alterations in oxygen transport in the lung, which may be caused by the accumulation of fluid in the alveoli.

Pulmonary responses

LVF results in pulmonary congestion when blood volume is not ejected efficiently during ventricular systole. The buildup of pressure in the left ventricle is transmitted backward until the pressure wave reaches the lungs. Increased pulmonary vascular pressures cause fluid leakage from the vascular space into the interstitial space (interstitial edema) and eventually into alveolar airspace, thereby compromising gas exchange. Alveolar congestion causes subjective complaints related to the increased work of breathing imposed by stiff, noncompliant lungs; feelings of dyspnea, orthopnea, and nocturnal dyspnea are not uncommon and are often accompanied by extreme anxiety, productive coughing, and hemoptysis. Auscultation of the lungs reveals the presence of fluid in the airways. Crackles (formerly called rales) are abnormal sounds produced by air passing over fluid in the small airways. Since fluid collects in dependent areas, crackles are commonly auscultated over the bases of the lung. Progressive accumulation of fluid in lung tissue will result in auscultation of crackles over larger regions of the lung. Rhonchi (wheezes) are abnormal sounds produced by air passing over fluid in the larger airways. These sounds are harsher than crackles and are heard over the bronchi when pulmonary exudates obstruct airflow. Arterial blood gases reflect alterations in gas transport in the lung.

Renal and endocrine responses

Decreased arterial blood flow through the kidneys reduces the glomerular filtration rate and causes the release of renin from the juxtaglomerular apparatus. Renin initiates an endocrine cascade that results in production of angiotensin II, a potent vasoconstrictor that stimulates the release of aldosterone from the adrenal cortex. Aldosterone causes retention of sodium and water, compounding the problem of volume overload. When circulating volume is retained, urinary output drops.

Rising osmotic pressures, caused by high levels of serum sodium, and reduced CO stimulate the release of antidiuretic hormone (ADH) from the posterior pituitary. Renal absorption of free water is enhanced, thus placing additional strain on the heart.

Atrial natriuretic factor (a peptide released from atrial tissue) promotes the renal excretion of sodium, blocks adrenal production of aldosterone, and inhibits endogenous vasoconstrictors (e.g., norepinephrine). Atrial natriuretic factor may assist in the regulation of salt and water by facilitating better renal flow and promoting diuresis.

Neurologic responses

Sensorium changes accompany poor oxygenation and altered cerebral perfusion. Various degrees of drowsiness, lethargy, confusion, and coma may be observed in association with heart failure.

Therapeutic Management

The therapeutic management of heart failure (Table 34-3) is based on a simple premise: restore the balance between myocardial oxygen supply and demand, and optimize hemodynamics. Measures designed to enhance the available oxygen supply and to decrease the work of the heart can often control or eliminate the clinical symptoms that accompany heart failure.

Heart failure is associated with depressed contractility, increased rate, increased afterload, and in-

TABLE 34-3   Therapeutic Options in Heart Failure

	Refers to	To increase	To decrease
Contractility	Stretch	+ Inotropic agents	− Inotropic agents
Heart rate	Rate	+ Chronotropic agents	− Chronotropic agents
Afterload	Vascular tone	Vasoconstrictors	Vasodilators
			Intraaortic balloon pump
Preload	Volume	Volume replacement	Vasodilators
			Diuretics
			Position
			Phlebotomy

creased preload. Each of these derangements puts a strain on the weakened heart and hinders its ability to respond to increased tissue demands for oxygen. Treatment is designed to decrease the work of the heart through support of contractility and restoration of rate, afterload, and preload to acceptable levels.

Increasing oxygen supply

Oxygen therapy

When oxygen transport in the lungs is impaired, additional oxygen coupled with measures to support cardiopulmonary function can facilitate adequate tissue oxygenation.

- In nonacute situations oxygen is often delivered at 2 to 6 L/minute via a nasal cannula.
- The use of alternative oxygen delivery systems, such as a simple face mask or non-rebreather mask, should be guided by analysis of arterial blood gases.
- Mechanical ventilation may be required if arterial blood gases reveal acute hypoventilation and acid/base imbalances (e.g., respiratory acidosis). The cautious addition of positive end-expiratory pressure (PEEP) may enhance oxygen transport in the lungs, but cardiac output will be impaired by this maneuver.

Vasodilating drugs

Vasodilators can improve oxygenation to ischemic areas of the heart, thereby improving myocardial performance.

Decreasing oxygen demand

Drug therapy: Positive inotropic agents
Digitalis preparations

Digitalis slows the HR and enhances contractility. Reduction in HR may be beneficial because diastolic filling time is prolonged, resulting in improved diastolic filling, enhanced SV, and better coronary perfusion. Digitalis also augments contractility, so it is a mainstay in the treatment of chronic heart failure. The positive inotropic effects of digitalis may prove dangerous in the *acute* setting, however. The increase in myocardial oxygen demand that accompanies stronger contractions is usually an undesirable result of therapy. For this reason digitalis is used sparingly, if at all, in the setting of acute ventricular failure. When digitalis is given, a carefully calculated loading dose (the "digitalizing dose") is administered, followed by a reduced maintenance dosage given once daily or in divided doses.

Dopamine or dobutamine

Both of these agents exert beta-adrenergic effects on the heart that can augment contractility; dopamine

GERIATRIC CONSIDERATIONS

Digitalis Therapy for the Older Adult

The older adult is at risk for developing side effects from digitalis because of decreased lean body mass and impaired glomerular filtration. The myocardium of the older adult tends to be more sensitive to digitalis. The drug can cause dysrhythmias in the elderly such as ventricular premature complexes, atrial tachycardia, and heart block. For these reasons the older adult may benefit from lower doses of digitalis. The nurse will need to monitor heart rate and rhythm more carefully in these patients.

also has alpha-adrenergic effects at high doses. The use of dopamine or dobutamine is confined to the critical care setting where hemodynamic monitoring is available.

Isoproterenol

Isoproterenol is a pure beta-adrenergic stimulator that enhances contractility, increases rate, and vasodilates peripheral vessels. Though isoproterenol exerts positive inotropic effects, it must be used with great caution. The increase in oxygen demand that accompanies the faster HR may negate any beneficial effect on cardiac pumping derived from isoproterenol. The drug must be given in the critical care setting.

Amrinone. Amrinone enhances contractility and has potent vasodilating properties (decreases afterload). It is given in the critical care setting.

Drug therapy: Negative chronotropic agents

Reduction in HR to acceptable levels should be accompanied by decreased myocardial oxygen demand, longer diastolic filling time, enhanced forward stroke volume, and augmented coronary artery perfusion.

Digitalis

Digitalis exerts desirable rate-slowing effects, but its positive inotropic actions may create an unwanted increase in myocardial oxygen demand.

Beta-blockers

Beta-blockers (e.g., propranolol) slow HR but may also depress contractility, so their use is also not without risk. Beta-blockers should be avoided in patients experiencing severe LVF, bradycardia, or AVB.

Calcium channel blockers

Verapamil is the drug of choice for short-term slowing of HR when rate-mediated clinical symptoms are present.

Reducing afterload and preload

Drug therapy

Afterload is reduced by drugs that primarily dilate arteries, the resistance vessels, while preload is reduced by drugs that primarily dilate veins, the capacitance vessels. Though vasodilators can affect afterload, preload, or both, one effect often predominates. Commonly called "unloading agents," vasodilators reduce vascular resistance, trap volume in the periphery, and ultimately reduce cardiac work.

- Nitrates (e.g., nitroglycerin, sodium nitroprusside, and isosorbide dinitrate). Nitroglycerin is given via sublingual, aerosol, transdermal, and IV routes. IV administration is undertaken in the critical care setting for the purpose of unloading the heart. NTG is primarily a venodilator and a useful agent for preload reduction. Nitroprusside sodium is given via IV infusion titrated to response. It is a potent drug given for its ability to dilate arteries, thus reducing afterload (systemic vascular resistance) and lowering blood pressure. Isosorbide dinitrate is a nitrate given orally or sublingually to unload the heart through reduction of preload.

Other drugs with vasodilating capabilities include calcium channel blockers (e.g., nifedipine and diltiazem), alpha-adrenergic blockers (e.g., prazosin), angiotensin-converting enzyme (ACE) inhibitors (e.g., captopril and enalapril), and morphine.

Diuretics (e.g., furosemide and ethacrynic acid) are commonly prescribed in combination with vasodilators in the treatment of heart failure. Furosemide, a loop diuretic, is responsible for preload reduction through inhibition of sodium reabsorption in the kidneys (reduces circulating volume) and venodilation (reduces venous return). Furosemide is the usual drug of choice in the management of heart failure; administration of ethacrynic acid, also a loop diuretic, is a potent alternative when the response to furosemide is unsatisfactory.

Diastolic augmentation

Intraaortic balloon pumping (IABP) represents a technique of internal counterpulsation designed to reduce the work of the heart. It is confined to the critical care setting and is reserved for the treatment of severe LVF.

Other interventions

Oral and IV intake is often restricted to reduce preload. Occasionally patients experiencing heart failure as a result of acute MI exhibit normal or low filling pressures. These patients require volume loading sufficient to maintain a PCWP at about 16 to 18 mm Hg, clearly higher than normal. The ischemic ventricle requires a high filling pressure to exert maximal stretch on myocardial fibers with a resultant increase in forward stroke volume and cardiac output.

Dietary sodium is restricted to prevent accumulation of excess volume, thereby reducing preload.

Semi-Fowler's or high Fowler's position reduces preload by inhibiting venous return to the heart.

Continuous arteriovenous hemofiltration (CAVH), also called "ultrafiltration," is a procedure designed to remove plasma water from the blood to reduce circulating volume. Arterial blood driven by the patient's own blood pressure flows through an extracorporeal hemofilter where controlled amounts of water and dissolved solutes are removed; remaining blood components are returned to venous circulation. CAVH is undertaken in the critical care setting where close monitoring is available.

Ventricular assist devices (VADs) are designed to assist the failing heart by assuming a portion of ventricular work. VADs can be used to support the left ventricle (LVAD), the right ventricle (RVAD), or both (BiVAD). Blood is diverted from the heart to a pump and is returned to circulation via a cannula placed in a vessel distal to the failing ventricle (e.g., in the aorta). VADs are used to treat cardiogenic shock and are confined to the critical care setting.

Surgical interventions undertaken to correct an underlying abnormality may include coronary artery bypass grafting (CABG) or repair of a structural defect (e.g., perforated septum or valve abnormality). Transplantation represents a viable alternative for selected patients whose heart failure is unresponsive to conventional therapeutic interventions.

NURSING MANAGEMENT OF THE PATIENT WITH CONGESTIVE HEART FAILURE

Assessment

The patient experiencing heart failure should be assessed carefully not only for the *presence* of failure but also for the *progression* of failure. The diagnosis of heart failure is based on analysis of the history, physical examination, and the results of diagnostic tests. Obviously, the acute onset of heart failure is more likely in the setting of MI and sudden structural failure, such as septal perforation or valve dysfunction. Heart failure, however, can also begin insidiously and develop slowly, resulting in progressive worsening of symptoms and requiring increasingly aggressive therapeutic interventions (see Figure 34-54, critical thinking guide for the patient with pulmonary edema).

The physical examination reflects the conse-

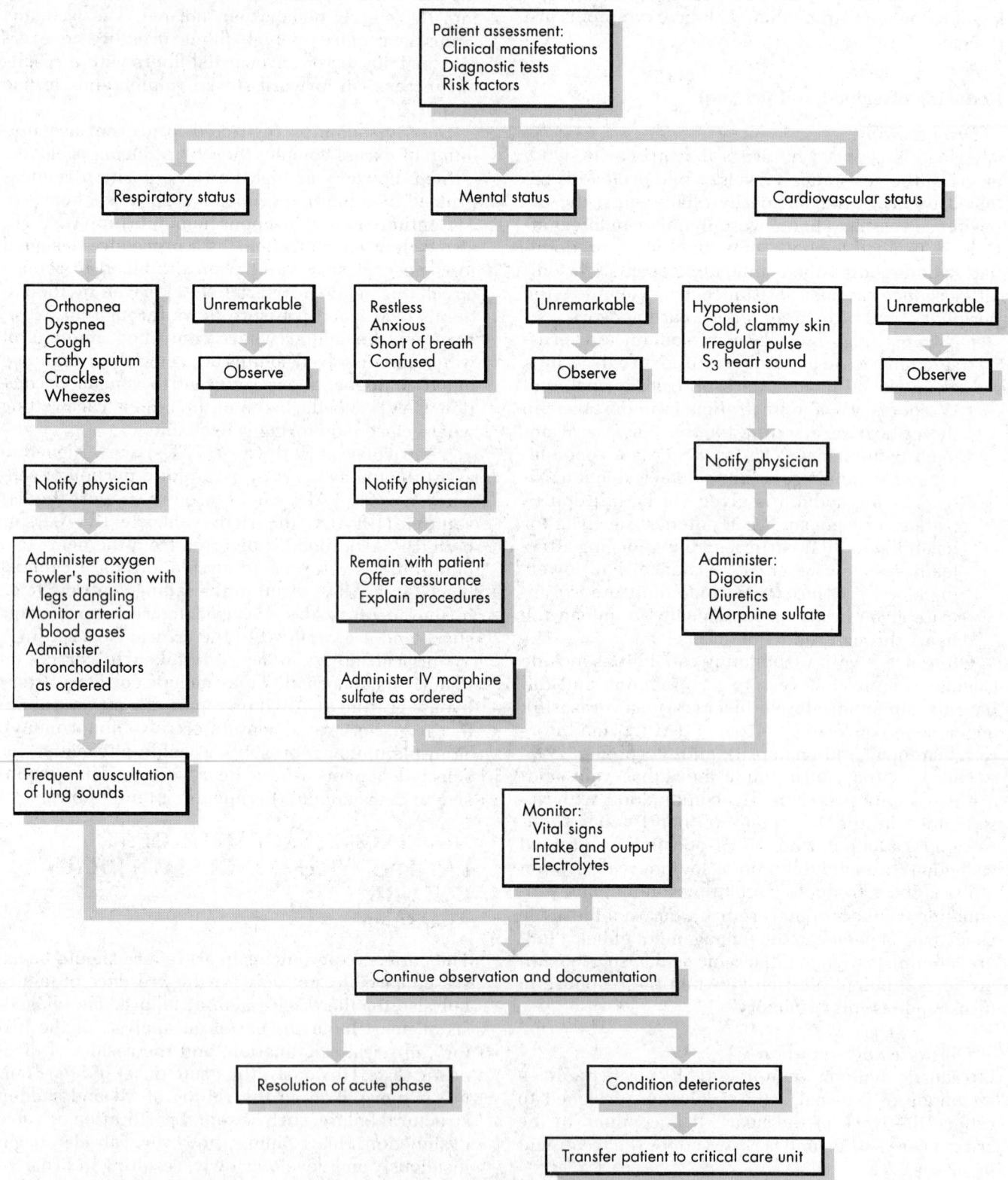

FIGURE 34-54 Critical Thinking Guide: the patient with pulmonary edema.

quences of altered hemodynamics caused by failure of the left or right ventricle, or both (biventricular failure). Tachycardia, atrial dysrhythmias, and abnormal heart sounds (e.g., S_4 and S_3 gallops) are common. Failure of the left ventricle is associated with an elevated PCWP, reduced cardiac output, and pulmonary congestion. Elevated right atrial pressure/central venous pressure accompanied by jugular venous distention, liver engorgement, and dependent edema are common if RVF is present. Swelling around the ankles may progress toward the trunk, involving the limbs and genitals; sacral edema is often apparent when the patient has been sitting for a time. Edema associated with heart failure is typically soft and pitting; the skin overlying swollen tissue often appears shiny and may weep if pressure is applied. Increase in abdominal girth and total body weight are additional clinical indicators of the fluid retention common in heart failure. Hypotension and low urinary output are typically present. Auscultation of lung fields reveals crackles and rhonchi; coughing and complaints of breathing difficulties are common. Restful sleep may only be possible in the sitting position or with the aid of extra pillows. Activity intolerance accompanied by extreme fatigue, anxiety, and effort angina commonly complicate the clinical picture. The patient experiencing chronic heart failure may appear malnourished as a result of compression of the stomach by an enlarged liver (inhibits adequate nutritional intake). Heart failure may impair the overall quality of life to the extent that withdrawal, depression, and the inability to cope interfere with activities of daily living.

Nursing Diagnosis

Nursing diagnoses related to the patient in heart failure will primarily reflect manifestations of impaired cardiac performance, alterations in life-style, lack of knowledge, and emotional dysfunction. They include the following:

Decreased cardiac output related to mechanical dysfunction and dysrhythmias

Impaired gas exchange related to decreased cardiac output and fluid overload

Fluid volume excess related to impaired cardiac pumping and renal retention of sodium and water

Altered cerebral tissue perfusion related to low cardiac output and impaired gas exchange

Altered renal tissue perfusion related to low cardiac output

Altered patterns of urinary elimination related to diuretic management

Activity intolerance related to orthostasis, fatigue, and shortness of breath as a result of decreased cardiac contractility

Anxiety related to lack of adequate oxygenation, fear of death, hopelessness, and powerlessness

Sleep pattern disturbance related to nocturnal dyspnea and alteration in sleep/wake cycle

Sexual dysfunction related to impaired cardiac performance and medications

Personal identity disturbance related to cachexia, loss of role in workplace/home, and chronic fatigue

Knowledge deficit (medications, diet)

Planning

Patient outcomes are geared toward maximizing myocardial performance and helping the patient with emotional adjustments and changes in lifestyle. Goals for the patient include:

Cardiac output is maximized as evidenced by acceptable blood pressure and pulse; lack of dysrhythmia; warm, pink skin; acceptable cardiac output, if measured; adequate urinary output; alert and oriented.

Gas exchange is improved as evidenced by lack of reported dyspnea, comfortable respirations; skin pink without evidence of central or peripheral cyanosis; lungs clear to auscultation; improved activity tolerance

Excess volume is reduced as evidenced by loss of water weight; reduced abdominal girth; intake less than output; reduced swelling in dependent areas.

Mental acuity and awareness are restored as evidenced by orientation to time, place, and person; intact memory; ability to communicate clearly and logically; ability to understand directions

Renal blood flow is improved as evidenced by adequate fluid balance; adequate blood pressure without hypotensive episodes; normal laboratory values (blood urea nitrogen, creatinine).

Pattern of urination is acceptable as evidenced by ability to sleep at night with fewer interruptions for urination

Activity level is restored and maintained as evidenced by fewer complaints of fatigue; ability to verbalize limitations and activities to avoid

Anxiety is reduced as evidenced by willingness to communicate concerns; presence of family/friend supports; fewer complaints of shortness of breath and other somatic symptoms; ability to modify life-style and adjust to same

Sleeping pattern is acceptable as evidenced by ability to sleep without experiencing nocturnal dyspnea; ability to enjoy uninterrupted sleep

Feelings of intimacy and sexual adequacy are restored as evidenced by verbalization of same

Personal identity and self-concept are restored as

evidenced by ability to verbalize increased self-esteem

Knowledge level is adequate as evidenced by ability to verbalize treatment plan, including information about disease, diet, and medications

Implementation

The nurse should monitor hemodynamic trends so that progression of disease and the response to therapeutic interventions can be appropriately evaluated. Blood pressure and pulse represent basic hemodynamic indicators. The presence of jugular venous distention and peripheral edema provides indirect hemodynamic information. Assessment of invasive hemodynamic monitoring data measured in the critical care area provides additional information about cardiac function. Right atrial pressure and central venous pressure represent right ventricular preload but are poor indicators of left ventricular function. PCWP and left atrial pressure represent left ventricular preload and, in the absence of mitral valve disease, are usually accurate indicators of left ventricular function. CO and Svo_2 data reflect the two primary compensatory mechanisms designed to preserve tissue oxygenation.

Fluid volume status is monitored closely. Fluid retention is a common manifestation of heart failure. The damaged heart cannot pump intravascular volume efficiently, so fluid intake is often restricted. The nurse should maintain accurate intake and output records and consider *all* fluids in the assessment of intake and output. Intake should include oral fluids, IV solutions, and intravenous piggyback (IVPB) solutions. Output should include urine, emesis, and drainage.

When appropriate, the nurse concentrates IV admixtures to reduce the volume of solution infused. For example, dopamine infusions are often mixed using 200 mg of dopamine in 500 ml D_5W (concentration equals 400 µg/mL). By mixing 400 mg of dopamine in 250 ml D_5W, the concentration quadruples (to 1600 µg/ml). By infusing one fourth the volume of the more concentrated solution (e.g., infusing 1 mL of concentrated solution as opposed to 4 mL of dilute solution) the same dosage (1600 µg) will be delivered in far less volume. Intake from IV fluids can be significantly reduced by concentrating admixtures. The nurse should always check with the physician and pharmacist before altering any admixture.

If not contraindicated, oral drugs are administered with meals so that extra intake of fluids will be not be required.

Lung fields are auscultated for the presence of abnormal sounds such as crackles and rhonchi. The nurse should listen over anterior, posterior, and lateral fields with the patient in the sitting position.

Weight is recorded daily and trends are noted that indicate weight gain or loss in response to fluid retention or therapeutic intervention. Mechanical ventilation can increase body water through humidification of inspired gases and by stimulating the secretion of ADH. Abdominal girth is measured to detect hepatomegaly or ascites.

Dietary sodium is restricted as ordered. The nurse should consult the dietitian to learn which foods and beverages contain large amounts of sodium. Some commercial salt substitutes contain large amounts of potassium. If the patient is receiving a potassium-sparing agent, such as spironolactone, the accumulation of potassium from multiple sources, such as diet and drugs, can result in hyperkalemia. High levels of potassium are detrimental to the patient with impaired renal function.

Activities are scheduled to allow for adequate rest periods. Patients experiencing heart failure typically experience varying levels of activity intolerance. Activity control can help balance oxygen supply and demand. The nurse should avoid bunching nursing tasks merely to expedite care delivery.

Measures are provided to ease breathing. Pulmonary congestion often makes breathing difficult, thus provoking anxiety and fear. The nurse should make sure that the patient is not slumped in bed. When this occurs, lung expansion is limited, thereby contributing to poor oxygenation and difficulty breathing. The patient is placed in high Fowler's position to decrease venous return to the heart and to facilitate adequate lung expansion. It may be helpful to sit the patient upright, place a pillow at his back at about shoulder height, and position an overbed table directly in front of him. Extra pillows are provided so the patient may lean forward onto them for support. All siderails should be up and the patient's call bell within easy reach. Supplemental oxygen should always be available.

The nurse monitors the patient's electrolyte status closely, paying particular attention to potassium and sodium levels. Diuretics can deplete serum potassium and aggravate the toxic effects of digitalis. This problem tends to be more significant in elderly patients, because both their hepatic and cardiac function tends to be suboptimal.

CLINICAL ALERT

If the patient is at risk for developing acute heart failure, a functional IV access should be available in case IV drug therapy is required.

Drug effects are closely monitored. Therapy with multiple agents can produce both additive and cumulative effects. Digitalis has negative chronotropic effects, so caution should be used if this agent is given with drugs that exert the same effect (e.g., propranolol and verapamil). Drugs such as verapamil, quinidine, and amiodarone can increase serum digitalis levels. Beta-blockers (e.g., propranolol) exert negative inotropic effects, so caution should be used if they are given with agents that also depress contractility (e.g., calcium channel blockers and antidysrhythmics). Nitrate drugs (e.g., NTG) vasodilate, so caution should be used if they are given with agents that produce a similar effect (e.g., calcium channel blockers). Level of consciousness (LOC) may be a manifestation of either poor cerebral perfusion or drug effects.

The nurse monitors the patient for embolic complications associated with forced inactivity or dysrhythmias. Bed rest predisposes the patient to clot formation in the deep veins as a result of stasis of flow. Dysrhythmias, commonly atrial fibrillation, also represent stasis of flow and can set the stage for clot formation in the cardiac chambers. The patient should be assessed for complaints of sudden chest pain, shortness of breath, and tachycardia.

Evaluation

Evaluation of the patient in heart failure should focus on responses to treatment with special emphasis on cardiopulmonary function. The ability to perform activities of daily living, as well as the patient's emotional state, should also be noted during evaluation.

Documentation

Documentation of trends is important when the diagnosis is heart failure. The nurse must be vigilant in documenting clinical assessment parameters that indicate the progression of the pathologic condition, because left ventricular failure often results in right ventricular failure. Responses to interventions also must be recorded so decisions to alter the therapeutic approach can be made appropriately.

Ongoing Care

Ongoing care should focus on creation of a discharge plan that addresses the need for patient/family teaching and periodic follow-up. The teaching plan should include information about medication administration, fluid restriction, and activity. The patient should be encouraged to report any untoward symptoms that could indicate either worsening of disease or side effects of medications. These symptoms include shortness of breath, nocturnal dyspnea, productive coughing, ankle edema, anginal pain, palpitations, and extreme fatigue. Sodium and fluid restrictions should be explained, and a list describing the sodium content of various foods should be provided. A dietitian should be consulted to help the patient cope with any drastic changes in eating patterns created by these restrictions. The patient's ability to perform normal activities should also be evaluated.

CARDIOPULMONARY RESUSCITATION

Before discussing the techniques of cardiopulmonary resuscitation (CPR), it is important to recognize circumstances in which emergency intervention may be required. What clues alert the clinician to anticipate clinical deterioration? There are some clinical conditions in which CPR is most likely to be needed, and these include life-threatening derangements of electrical and mechanical cardiac function. For example:

- The patient experiencing significant disturbances in cardiac rhythm or conduction: PVCs can degenerate into VT or VF; second-degree AVB type II and third-degree AVB can degenerate into ventricular asystole without warning
- The patient experiencing a symptomatic drop in CO as a result of mechanical failure of the heart: depressed pump function often precedes disturbances in rate, rhythm, and conduction

Basic Life Support

CPR represents the most elemental form of resuscitation. Its success hinges on the prompt application of basic techniques that are simple to learn and easy to apply. CPR can be attempted in any setting by any trained individual present. It is clear that the quicker CPR is begun, the greater the victim's chance for survival. The ABCs of CPR stand for *Airway*, *Breathing*, and *Circulation*. The steps of CPR described below are applicable to *adult* victims only. The decision to apply basic life support is based first and foremost on assessment. The rescuer's first priority should be to determine unresponsiveness *before* intervening (see box, pp. 848 and 849).

Airway

After unresponsiveness has been established, the rescuer should open the victim's airway. Airway represents the first real hands-on intervention in the ABCs of CPR. The tongue can occlude the airway in an unconscious victim, so the head tilt−chin lift maneuver is recommended to lift the tongue from the back of the throat, thereby reestablishing the airway.

NURSING CARE PLAN   *Congestive Heart Failure*

Nursing diagnosis/ Expected outcomes	Interventions	Rationale
Decreased CO related to mechanical dysfunction and dysrhythmias •*Maximize cardiac output* •*Pink color* •*Warm skin* •*Absence of orthostasis* •*Blood pressure is within acceptable range* •*Tachycardia is controlled* •*Cardiac output is improved, if measured* •*Dysrhythmic events are suppressed as much as possible* •*Alert mental state*	Monitor vital signs q4h or prn Monitor for irregular HR, tachycardia Administer antidysrhythmics, vasodilators, as ordered Provide rest, as necessary Have patient change position slowly, to avoid dizziness	Low blood pressure, tachycardia may indicate low CO Ectopy, tachycardia lower CO Vasodilators, antidysrhythmics promote cardiac efficiency Rest reduces cardiac work Changing positions slowly allows blood pressure and pulse to accommodate to gravitational stress
Impaired gas exchange related to decreased CO and fluid overload •*Improved gas exchange* •*Comfortable respirations* •*Pink color* •*Pink nailbeds* •*Clear lungs* •*Reduction in episodes of shortness of breath* •*Improved activity tolerance* •*Ability to sleep without dyspnea*	Assess for evidence of hypoxia: restlessness, tachycardia, angina Auscultate lungs q4h Provide oxygen therapy, as ordered Elevate head of bed, or provide pillows or chair to aid breathing Advise patient to avoid strenuous activity, or separate taxing activities Administer diuretics, as ordered	Respiratory/cardiac effort increases with hypoxia Crackles, rhonchi indicate impaired gas exchange Oxygen therapy enhances oxygen supply in blood Semi-Fowler's position provides better mechanics for breathing Separating activities reduces frequency, intensity of dyspneic episodes Diuretics reduce fluid overload by increasing water loss by kidneys
Fluid volume excess related to impaired cardiac pumping, renal retention of sodium and water •*Excess fluid volume is reduced* •*Loss of water weight with stabilization as "dry" weight is approached* •*Reduced abdominal girth from fluid accumulation* •*Intake ≤ output* •*Reduced swelling in dependent areas*	Daily weights Daily intake/output Measure abdominal girth, at umbilicus level, daily Record relative amount of edema in extremities (1+ to 4+) daily Elevate lower extremities while sitting Limit salt intake to 2 to 3 g daily, or as ordered Counsel patient on salt restriction	Weight gain over 24 hr may be fluid weight Intake exceeding output increases risk for fluid overload Peripheral and abdominal edema indicate fluid deposition in extracellular compartment Elevating legs promotes extracellular fluid shift to vascular space, diuretics act to reduce circulating volume Salt reduction decreases fluid retention Patient understanding may aid diet compliance
Altered cerebral tissue perfusion related to low CO and impaired gas exchange •*Restoration and maintenance of mental acuity and awareness* •*Awareness of current events, surroundings* •*Intact memory* •*Communicates logically, clearly* •*Understands directions*	Observe mental status constantly Keep shades open in day Keep calendar/clock in view Administer therapy to maximize CO, as ordered Provide family/friend stimulation	Subtle behavior changes may indicate perfusion problems Constant reorientation prevents confusion in certain patients Impaired cardiac output, oxygen exchange reduces cerebral acuity Allowing visits stimulates patient's mental state

NURSING CARE PLAN   *Congestive Heart Failure—cont'd*

Nursing diagnosis/ Expected outcomes	Interventions	Rationale
Altered renal tissue perfusion related to low CO • *Renal blood flow is improved* • *Balanced intake/output* • *Blood urea nitrogen (BUN), creatinine, electrolytes within normal limits* • *Adequate blood pressure* • *Absence of hypotensive episodes*	Monitor fluid intake and output, increasing urinary output volume Maintain adequate blood pressure, renal blood flow, by administering fluids, medications, as ordered Avoid inducing hypotension by administering two blood pressure-lowering agents concurrently Administer diuretics, as ordered	Intake/output, BUN, creatinine, electrolytes indicate renal function Dramatic hypotension may induce acute renal failure Antihypertensive drugs may lower blood pressure excessively Diuretics reduce fluid overload
Altered pattern of urinary elimination related to diuretic management • *Urination pattern is acceptable to patient* • *Patient can sleep at night with fewer interruptions for urination*	Administer diuretics in early morning, if ordered qd For bid administration, give second dose late afternoon to avoid nighttime urination	Diuretic administration may cause frequency and nocturia
Activity intolerance related to orthostasis, fatigue, shortness of breath, as a result of impaired cardiac performance • *Restoration, maintenance of activity level* • *Fatigue is lessened* • *Patient understands limitations* • *Patient can avoid symptoms induced by certain activities*	Assess activity needs in home, workplace, recreation Explain reasons for limits Assess for orthostasis when patient stands, ambulates Maintain moderate, supervised activity in hospital Allow periods of rest Alleviate breathlessness by adjusting behavior	Usual activity may be limited by symptoms Certain activity level is desirable, but activity that exacerbates shortness of breath/fatigue should be curtailed Rest alleviates fatigue Patient should be aware of unsuitable activities (e.g., climbing stairs, driving)
Sleep pattern disturbance related to nocturnal dyspnea, and alteration in sleep/wake cycle • *Sleeping pattern is acceptable* • *Adequate rest periods at night, with relief of dyspnea* • *Increase in solid sleep time* • *Respiratory status does not interfere with sleep*	Provide pillows to aid breathing Limit daily napping Provide periods of daily activity Administer sleep medications, if ordered	Semi-Fowler's position improves mechanics of breathing Napping in daytime may reduce nighttime requirement Daily activity routines help tire patient for sleep Sleep medications should be given if other alternatives fail to provide quality sleep
Sexual dysfunction related to impaired cardiac performance and medications • *Restore feelings of intimacy, adequacy*	Allow verbalization about loss of libido, impotence Counsel about specific changes—ejaculation, altered erection Explore alternate methods of sexual expression	Feelings of failure may contribute to feelings of inadequacy Education about illness, medications helps patient understand new limitations Formulates new avenues for expression of intimacy with partner
Personal identity disturbance related to cachexia, loss of role in workplace/home, and fatigue • *Personal identity and self-concept is restored* • *Increase in self-esteem*	Explore methods of continuing to work Discuss home activity limitations Assess home environment for hazards (e.g., steps, bath)	Disturbances in personal identity result from new symptoms and limitations; setting and achieving realistic goals reestablishes self-esteem
Knowledge deficit (disease, medications, diet) • *Knowledge level is adequate* • *Improved awareness about disease, medications, diet* • *Greater patient/family understanding about disease, medications, diet*	Assess knowledge of disease, medications, diet Educate patient/family on importance of compliance Educate about rationale for diet/medications Review potential side effects of medications Review management of complications (syncope) Invite feedback about material	Establishes baseline knowledge for planning nursing intervention Knowledge of disease process and treatments may enhance compliance Safety Promotes communication, understanding

Breathing

Breathing represents the next intervention in the ABCs of CPR. Cessation of breathing is caused by a variety of conditions, including neurologic pathologic conditions (e.g., tumors and injuries to the head and spine), cardiovascular disease (e.g., associated with ventricular dysrhythmias), and drug effects (e.g., overdose of narcotics).

If breathing is absent, the next step in CPR involves rescue breathing. The rescuer delivers ventilations to the victim in an attempt to provide sufficient oxygen to sustain life. Exhaled air contains roughly 16% oxygen, obviously not the desired amount, but enough to suffice for a short time. Airway obstruction renders delivery of the initial breaths impossible and will require maneuvers to relieve the obstruction before rescue breathing can be performed successfully (airway obstruction will be addressed later).

Circulation

Circulation represents the last step in the ABCs of CPR. Absent circulation, like absent breathing, can result from a host of conditions that result in clinical cardiac arrest. Absence of circulation is easily determined with proper assessment, but the *cause*

LEGAL ISSUES: *Do Not Resuscitate Orders*

Do not resuscitate (DNR) orders are commonly understood to mean withholding CPR in specific cases of cardiac arrest. Nurses have long realized and struggled with the fact that DNR does not mean the same thing to all health care providers. In many institutions, there is a new understanding that DNR is not a treatment plan, but a boundary or framework for care. To be effective, DNR orders should clearly spell out for each patient specific conditions and the interventions that should or should not be used in each case.

The practice of not writing a DNR order is unacceptable. Also unacceptable is the "slow code" order given verbally by some physicians. Until the physician writes a DNR order, the patient is considered a full code. The nurse should arrange a conference with the patient and/or family and the health care providers to determine what options are available and what the patient or the family desires. The order should then be documented fully in the medical record, showing the patient's condition, the rationale for the order, and the process used in its formulation. Some facilities have even more specific requirements in their policies that the medical-surgical nurse should follow. Above all, the patient, family, and all health care providers should realize that a DNR order does not mean the patient is abandoned or that an inferior standard of care is used. Comfort measures and pain control are important components of care that should be spelled out at the same time a DNR order is considered or written.

DNR orders are sometimes difficult for health care providers to write or implement. Taught to preserve life, the nurse or physician may feel he or she has somehow failed if asked to write or care for a DNR patient. Fortunately, most professionals realize that death is a natural and unavoidable part of life and that patients deserve the same respect and high standard of care as they die as they do in getting well.

Above all, nurses must remember that every competent adult has the right to refuse treatment, even life-sustaining procedures such as CPR. The patient's informed consent should be obtained by the physician who will write the order, and should be documented in the medical record. Or, if unable to consent and no advance directive has been executed, the patient's family should be consulted and their participation sought and documented. The patient's incapacity to participate must also be documented to reflect the rationale for involving the family. In some states, the law may require two physicians' opinions that the patient lacks capacity to consent, or may have specific requirements for a surrogate or guardian making the decisions.

DNR orders must be reviewed periodically, but especially if the patient's condition changes or new knowledge about the patient's condition becomes available. Frequent review of the DNR order helps reassure staff that they are not abandoning the patient, and that the care being provided best meets the patient's needs.

A DNR order is acceptable then if:
- the order is documented in the written medical record
- the order spells out the exact treatments or interventions to be withheld
- patients, when they are able, and families participate in the decision and give informed consent
- the decision not to resuscitate is discussed with all involved caregivers, particularly the nurses
- the order is periodically reviewed
- staff realize that the order is not equivalent to medical or psychologic abandonment of patients.

From Youngner S: Do-not-resuscitate orders: no longer a secret, but still a problem, *Hastings Cent Rep* 17(1):24, 1987; and Wandel JC: Moral outrage and moral discourse in nurse-physician collaboration, *J Prof Nursing* 7(6):351-363, 1991.

of an arrest—whether VF or ventricular asystole—cannot be differentiated without cardiac monitoring. Both dysrhythmias produce identical clinical symptoms (absence of pulse, blood pressure, and breathing). In either case, external chest compression will be required.

A single rescuer can coordinate external chest compressions with rescue breathing by following a simple pattern: 2 rescue breaths are delivered after each sequence of 15 chest compressions (15:2 ratio). The victim is assessed for return of the pulse after 1 minute of CPR (4 cycles of 15 compressions alternating with 2 ventilations) and every few minutes thereafter.

Airway Obstruction

The victim of airway obstruction may require all the techniques just described, because lack of oxygen inevitably results in cardiopulmonary arrest. Until the offending object is removed from the airway, attempts to deliver rescue breaths and chest compressions are futile.

Clinical manifestations

The most common cause of airway obstruction in the conscious adult is food, often a large piece of meat. The victim will frantically attempt to expel the offending object by coughing vigorously. If the airway is totally obstructed, air exchange is impossible, and the victim will be unable to speak, cough, or breathe. He will likely clutch his throat, the "universal distress signal" for choking. Immediate intervention is required or lack of oxygen will quickly result in death. If the airway is only *partially* obstructed, some degree of air exchange is still possible. If the victim is able to cough forcefully (partial obstruction with good air exchange), the rescuer should not interfere with his efforts. A partial airway obstruction, however, may block the airway enough to prevent effective coughing. A weak cough associated with high-pitched inspiratory sounds reflects a partial obstruction with poor air exchange and, like total obstruction, requires immediate intervention.

The most common cause of airway obstruction in the unconscious adult is the tongue. When the

THERAPEUTIC COMMUNICATION GUIDE

Cardiac Arrest

Nursing management

Assess family's knowledge regarding cardiac arrest.

Example:	*Nurse:*	"Ms. Rowland, your husband suffered a cardiac arrest 2 hours ago. What do you know about his condition?"
	Family:	"I know that all of a sudden his eyes rolled back in his head and he passed out. Next thing I knew, all these people rushed in and hit him. They did something to him and he went into a spasm. Now he's on a machine to help him breathe, but he won't talk to me. Will he be all right?"

Intervention

Provide information and help family gain a realistic understanding of the situation. Offer help and positive reassurance. Allow the patient to identify with a staff member who is responsible for their loved one.

Example:	*Nurse:*	"Ms. Rowland, your husband is on a ventilator that helps him breathe, and a machine to monitor his heartbeat. We are trying to help him all we can, but it's too early to know if he'll be okay. I'll keep coming back to let you know what is happening and to answer your questions. I know how frightening this must be."
	Family:	"Yes, he's all I have in this world. I don't know what I'll do if anything happens to him."

Provide support, yet recognize the family's need for privacy.

Example:	*Nurse:*	"That must be a scary feeling. Would you like to visit your husband? I can go with you or provide you time alone with your husband."
	Family:	"No, I just can't look at him like that yet."

Provide support.

Example:	*Nurse:*	"Do you have a friend or relative I could call for you who might help you?"
	Family:	"No one, just my friends at Bible study."

Explore alternative resources.

Example:	*Nurse:*	"Would you like for me to call one of these friends or perhaps our hospital chaplain? He's very good at helping people who have sick family members."
	Family:	"Yes, I think I need someone who might pray with me."

STEPS IN CARDIOPULMONARY RESUSCITATION

Step 1: Establish unresponsiveness

Place the victim in a supine position

Gently shake the victim's shoulder and shout, "Are you okay?"

Call for help; if someone responds outside of the hospital setting, direct him or her to activate the EMS system (911); if alone, activate the EMS system personally

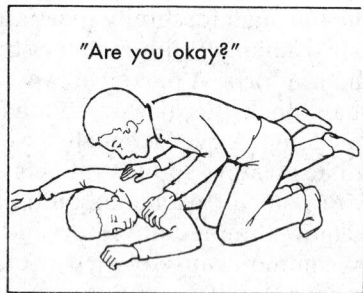

"Are you okay?"

Step 2: Establish the airway

Use the head tilt–chin lift maneuver

* Kneel close to the victim; place the heel of one hand on the victim's forehead; place the first few fingers of your other hand on the bony prominence of the chin, being careful to avoid pressing on the soft tissues under the chin; lift the chin to establish the airway

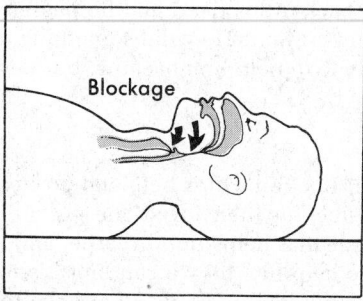

Blockage

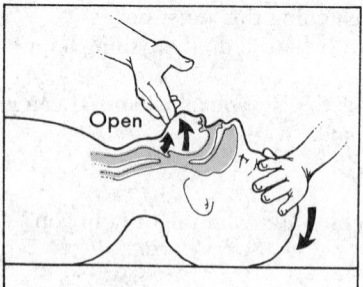

Open

Step 3: Assess for breathlessness

Look, listen, and feel for 3 to 5 seconds

* With the airway open, position your face close to the victim's; look for the chest to rise, listen for air escaping from the mouth, and feel the escape of air against your cheek

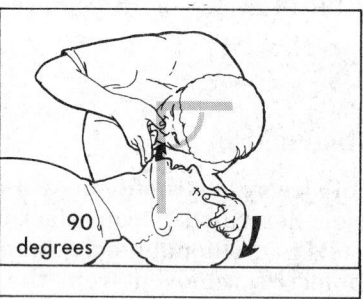

90 degrees

Step 4: Rescue breathing

If the victim is not breathing, maintain the airway with the head tilt/chin lift maneuver, and deliver two full breaths

* Take a deep breath
* Place your mouth over the victim's mouth using gentle pressure to form a tight seal; pinch the victim's nose to prevent escape of air

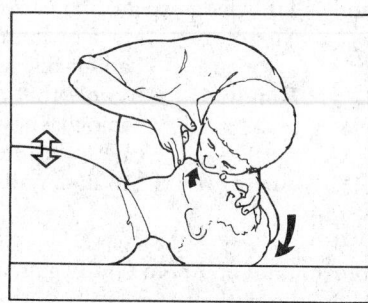

* Deliver two full breaths; each ventilation should last about 1½ to 2 seconds and should be of sufficient volume for the chest to rise; allow the victim to exhale completely after each breath
* If the first breath does not go in, the airway may have been positioned incorrectly; gently place the victim's head in the "neutral" position (no head tilt) and reestablish the airway; reattempt to ventilate; be sure to give two full breaths. If repositioning the head tilt does not facilitate delivery of rescue breaths, airway obstruction is present; additional interventions will be required before the rescuer can proceed with ventilations (see description of the Heimlich maneuver)

Illustrations redrawn from and used with permission of the American Heart Association, Instructor's manual for basic life support.

STEPS IN CARDIOPULMONARY RESUSCITATION—cont'd

Step 5: Assess pulselessness

Assess the carotid pulse for 5 to 10 seconds

- Place two fingers lightly over the carotid artery on the side of the victim closest to the rescuer; press gently

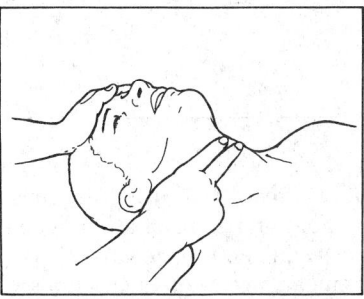

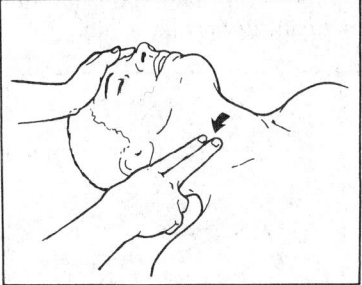

Step 6: Deliver external chest compressions

Deliver 15 chest compressions at a rate of 80 to 100/minute

Make sure the victim is on a firm surface

- Place a cardiac board under the victim's torso if one is available
- Find the proper hand position for chest compressions; run the middle finger of the hand nearest the victim's foot (the "foot hand") along the rib margin until the xiphoid process ("the notch") is felt; place the index finger next to the middle finger; place the heel of the other hand (the "head hand") onto the sternum next to the index finger of the foot hand

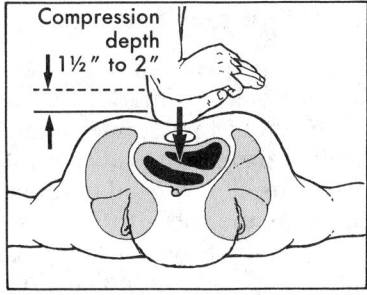

- Place the foot hand over the head hand; interlace the fingers to keep them from touching the chest wall during compressions
- The rescuer should kneel directly over the victim with his elbows locked; external compressions should be delivered to a depth of 1½ to 2 inches in the adult; compressions should be delivered using a smooth downward thrust, allowing the sternum to return to its original position after each compression; jerking, stabbing, and bouncing should be avoided

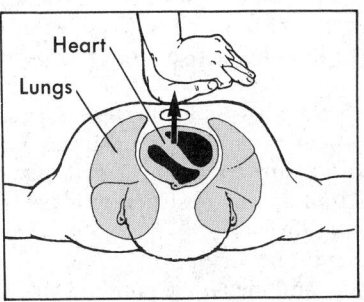

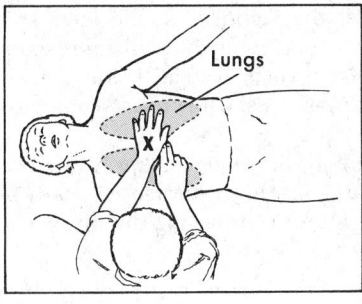

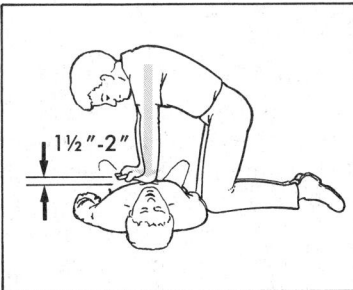

Continue CPR by alternating chest compressions and ventilations in a 15:2 ratio. Assess for return of the carotid pulse every few minutes.

HEIMLICH MANEUVER

Conscious adult victim

Ask victim, "Are you choking?"

Stand behind the victim and wrap your arms around his waist; make a fist with one hand and place the thumb side against the victim's abdomen in the midline; be careful to place your fist below the xiphoid process and above the umbilicus; grasp your wrist with your other hand

Deliver inward and upward thrusts to relieve the obstruction; continue until the object is expelled or until the victim loses consciousness

Unconscious adult victim

Determine unresponsiveness; call for help; if someone responds, direct him or her to activate the EMS system (911); if alone, activate the EMS system personally

Open the airway; assess for breathlessness

Attempt rescue breathing: if unsuccessful, reposition the head tilt and try again; if still unsuccessful, assume that an airway obstruction is present

Apply manual thrusts

- Kneel astride the victim
- Locate the umbilicus and xiphoid process; manual (abdominal) thrusts will be delivered between these two landmarks; abdominal thrusts should be avoided if the victim is in the later stages of pregnancy or is extremely obese; the rescuer should deliver chest thrusts instead using the same position and landmarks used for chest compressions during CPR
- Interlocking your fingers, apply 5 inward and upward thrusts; these thrusts should be delivered with the intent of relieving the obstruction

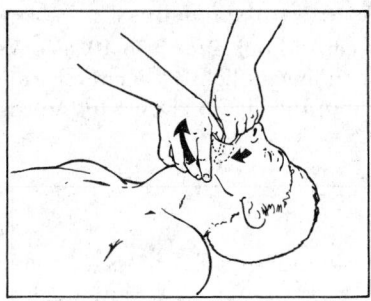

Return to the victim's head; using the tongue-jaw lift, inspect the mouth for signs of the offending object; if the object is visible and retrievable, remove it; if not, perform a finger sweep of the victim's mouth (this maneuver should only be used in unconscious adults); attempt to ventilate; if air does not go in, reposition the head tilt and try again.

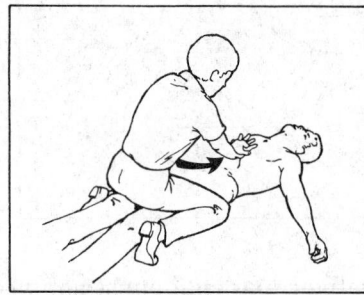

Resume application of the Heimlich maneuver until the object has been expelled; if the victim is not breathing, ventilate twice; assess the victim for pulselessness, and administer CPR as required

---

tongue falls back in the throat the airway can be occluded enough to prevent airflow into and out of the lungs. The obstruction may be relieved simply by establishing the airway using the head tilt–chin lift maneuver. The presence of breathing indicates that further interventions are unnecessary, but absence of breathing obviously warrants additional action. Attempts to deliver rescue breaths will fail despite repositioning the head tilt if a foreign object (such as a piece of food) obstructs the airway.

Therapeutic management

The most effective method to relieve an airway obstruction as a result of a foreign object is the Heimlich maneuver, a series of manual thrusts delivered with enough force to dislodge the offending object from the airway (see box above).

Emergency Response Team

Cardiopulmonary arrest in the hospital setting commonly results in a "code" situation. A team of nurses, physicians, and support personnel combine the techniques of basic life support with the more sophisticated interventions of advanced life support in an attempt to stabilize the victim of arrest. Obviously, codes can occur anywhere at any time. Nurses should be prepared to respond to situations of arrest whenever and wherever they may occur. In a code situation someone from the team is usually required to do the following:

DEFIBRILLATION AND CARDIOVERSION

Defibrillation and cardioversion are forms of electrical countershock designed to slow rapid cardiac rhythms. Electrical currents (measured in "watt-seconds" or "joules") are delivered to the heart through metal electrodes placed on the outer chest wall. The goal is to completely depolarize the heart so that the sinus node can resume its normal pacemaker role.

Defibrillation currents are not timed to coincide with any specific ECG waveform. Defibrillation ("unsynchronized countershock") is used to terminate life-threatening dysrhythmias such as VF and pulseless VT. Cardioversion currents are electronically synchronized with the R wave of the QRS; the machine is instructed to sense the R wave, wait for a brief interval, and fire into the QRS complex. Delivery of the stimulus is timed to avoid the T wave. Cardioversion ("synchronized countershock") is usually used to slow rapid supraventricular dysrhythmias.

Procedure

Administer IV sedation as appropriate
Connect the machine to a power source

Lower the siderails

Apply conductive paste to the paddle electrodes; acceptable alternatives are commercially prepared gel pads (also known as defib pads) or saline-soaked gauze pads (usually 4 × 4s)If cardioversion is required, set the machine on "SYNC" and look for a marker on each QRS

Place the paddles on the chest wall in the anterior-anterior (or transverse) position (along the long axis of the heart) or anterior-posterior position

Charge the machine to the desired energy level

Recheck the cardiac rhythm

Make sure that no one is touching the bed or the patient; state "clear"

Deliver the countershock

Observe for the return of an acceptable cardiac rhythm; always check the pulse after each defibrillation attempt to assess the return of mechanical pumping; if the dysrhythmia persists, recharge the machine to the voltage ordered and deliver a second countershock; repeat as directed

---

- Manage the airway (physician, respiratory therapist, or nurse)
- Perform chest compressions (physician or nurse)
- Administer drugs and fluids (physician or nurse)
- Establish IV access (physician or nurse)
- Perform defibrillation or cardioversion (physician or nurse) (see box above)
- Document all activities (nurse or designee)
- Miscellaneous: run ECG machine, act as a runner to obtain additional supplies, control traffic (nurse or designee)

Pharmacologic interventions

Selected drugs are commonly used in an emergency to eliminate or control dysrhythmias, control heart rate, and enhance myocardial perfusion pressure during CPR (see box on p. 852).

NURSING MANAGEMENT OF THE PATIENT REQUIRING RESUSCITATION

Preparation is the key to successful resuscitation. Recognizing situations likely to deteriorate and preparing ahead of time to respond to emergencies will increase the chance for a successful outcome. Basic CPR techniques should be practiced so that they can be performed perfectly and without hesitation. The nurse should know where emergency equipment is located and how to use each item. The nurse should become familiar with common "code drugs," including indications for use, dosages, administration guidelines, and side effects.

The nurse should learn to anticipate clinical deterioration before overt signs and symptoms are apparent. For example, if the patient has been experiencing breathing difficulties, it is reasonable to assume that he may need an artificial airway or rescue breathing. An oropharyngeal airway is placed at the bedside, and the patient is monitored for deterioration. If mouth-to-mask ventilation is an option in the clinical setting, the nurse should practice using this airway adjunct. The nurse should know where and how to obtain it quickly, and where and how to obtain supplemental oxygen and the equipment needed for intubation of the trachea and suctioning. The suction apparatus should be in working order.

If the patient has been experiencing potentially life-threatening cardiac dysrhythmias (e.g., multiformed PVCs or episodes of VT), the nurse should be prepared for sudden progression to VF. If a defibrillator with quick-look paddles is available in the clinical setting, the nurse should practice obtaining the ECG with this device and be prepared to defibrillate the patient (if allowed) and to administer antidysrhythmic drugs such as lidocaine and

DRUGS COMMONLY USED IN A CODE

Lidocaine (Xylocaine)—For treatment of ventricular dysrhythmias (PVCs, VT, VF); given via IV bolus and followed by a maintenance infusion titrated to response

Bretylium (Bretylol)—For treatment of ventricular dysrhythmias unresponsive to lidocaine (PVCs, VT, VF); given via undiluted IV bolus (for VF), IVPB infusion, or continuous IV infusion

Procainamide (Pronestyl)—For treatment of ventricular dysrhythmias unresponsive to lidocaine (PVCs, VT); given via slow IV bolus, IVPB, or maintenance infusion

Epinephrine (Adrenalin)—Given to increase coronary perfusion pressure during CPR; given via IV bolus or endotracheal route when IV access is delayed

Atropine—Given to increase HR in situations of symptomatic bradycardia (e.g., asystole, sinus bradycardia, atrioventricular block); administered via IV bolus or the endotracheal route when IV access is delayed

Adenosine (Adenocard)—Given via IV bolus to slow HR in situations of symptomatic supraventricular tachycardia

Magnesium—For treatment of refractory VT/VF and Torsade de pointes; given via slow IV bolus, IVPB, or infusion

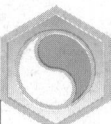

ETHICAL ISSUES

Should a patient's circulatory and respiratory functions be continued artificially after the patient has died in order to maintain tissue oxygenation until the organs can be removed for transplantation?

tored to detect the lingering depressant effects of sedative drugs. Safety precautions (e.g., siderails up) are maintained until these effects have diminished.

If elective cardioversion is attempted, the procedure should be discussed with the patient. The nurse should explain that the procedure will deliver a "signal" to the heart telling it to slow down, thereby relieving many uncomfortable symptoms. The patient is assured that he or she will be asleep during the cardioversion and will not feel the "signal." The nurse explains that the blood pressure, pulse, and respirations will be monitored frequently for a few hours after the procedure as a precaution.

The patient has a right to privacy. Emergencies are usually accompanied by frenzied activity and considerable noise, and the victim's privacy is often sacrificed. The nurse should make an effort to maintain the patient's dignity by closing the door or drawing the curtains around the bed. The nurse should also avoid unnecessarily exposing the patient. Because a code often draws curious bystanders who play no role in the resuscitation, the nurse should try to remove these people from the immediate area.

A professional atmosphere should be maintained during and after a code. The very nature of an emergency commonly causes emotions and tensions to surface in inappropriate ways. Jokes and comments that are neither evidence of indifference nor intentionally disrespectful may be overheard by others. Remember that the victim may be able to hear everything that is being said and may be able to relate these things to the caregiver when the experience is over. The nurse should consider the painful reality that his or her touch or words could be someone's last memory, so a concerted effort should be made to provide comfort along with clinical expertise.

The patient's family will require considerable emotional support both during and after a resuscitation. When possible, the nurse should keep the family informed of the code's progress. There is perhaps nothing so emotionally draining as anxiously waiting for what seems like an eternity without knowing the fate of a loved one. As much emotional support as possible is provided after the resuscitation. If the outcome is positive, the nurse should prepare the family for whatever they may encounter when they visit their loved one for the first time. If the outcome is negative, the family is allowed the

bretylium. If the patient has had high-grade AVB (e.g., third-degree AVB with an idioventricular pacemaker), the nurse should be prepared for the sudden onset of ventricular asystole and anticipate the need for CPR and emergency pacing.

Successful defibrillation and cardioversion require advance planning and close patient follow-up. The patient should have a stable IV line for administration of emergency drugs. Additional emergency equipment (e.g., airway, bag-valve-mask device, drugs) should be available in case postresuscitation dysrhythmias or hypoventilation require additional interventions. The digitalized patient may fibrillate in response to high-energy currents, therefore the lowest energy level possible should be used if digitalis is on board.

After successful countershock, the patient is observed for evidence of peripheral embolization. The nurse continues to monitor the ECG closely for the appearance of new dysrhythmias or the reappearance of old ones. The patient's vital signs are moni-

time and privacy to express their grief. The nurse should be available to the family. The use of cliches should be avoided, but sympathy should be expressed honestly and directly.

CRITICAL THINKING QUESTIONS

1 Briefly describe the three methods used to calculate heart rate using an ECG rhythm strip. Which method(s) should be used when the cardiac rhythm is irregular?

2 Describe the major ECG characteristics of the following cardiac rhythms:

    Sinus rhythm
    Sinus tachycardia
    Sinus bradycardia
    Sinus arrhythmia
    Premature atrial complexes
    Atrial tachycardia
    Paroxysmal supraventricular tachycardia
    Atrial flutter
    Atrial fibrillation
    Premature junctional complexes
    Junctional escape rhythm
    Junctional tachycardia
    Premature ventricular complexes
    Ventricular tachycardia
    Ventricular fibrillation
    Ventricular asystole

3 Describe nursing interventions appropriate to the care of patients experiencing dysrhythmias.

4 Which dysrhythmias are life-threatening? Why?

5 Describe nursing interventions that are appropriate to the care of patients experiencing heart blocks.

6 Describe nursing interventions appropriate to the care of patients experiencing each pacemaker malfunction.

7 Differentiate between physiologic effects of "forward" and "backward" failure on each side of the heart. Which component reflects compromised pumping? Which reflects congestion?

8 Discuss three cardiovascular and three pulmonary responses associated with heart failure. How are these responses assessed clinically?

9 What do the ABCs of CPR represent?

10 What is the Heimlich maneuver? Why is it effective?

11 Describe the procedure for defibrillation and cardioversion.

12 Identify the most common indications for use of each of the following emergency drugs: epinephrine, atropine, and lidocaine. Which of these can be given via the endotracheal route?

BIBLIOGRAPHY

Current

1. Abou-Awdi N, Ragsdale D: High-tech help for failing hearts, *RN* 54(5): 42, 1991.
2. American Heart Association: *Textbook of advanced cardiac life support*, ed 2, Dallas, 1990, American Heart Association.
3. Appel-Hardin S: The role of the critical care nurse in noninvasive temporary pacing, *Crit Care Nurse* 12(3): 10, 1992.
4. Barbiere CC, Liberatore K: Automated external defibrillators: an update of additions to the ACLS algorithms, *Crit Care Nurse* June: 17, 1992.
5. Barden C, Lee R: Update on ventricular assist devices, *AACN Clin Issues Crit Care Nurs* 1(1): 13, 1990.
6. Bartz C: Pharmacologic augmentation of cardiac output following cardiac arrest, *Crit Care Nurs Q* 10(4): 43, 1988.
7. Britt J: What to do when your patient codes, *Nurs '90* 20(1): 42, 1990.
8. Brown KR, Jacobson S: *Mastering dysrhythmias: a problem-solving guide*, Philadelphia, 1988, FA Davis Co.
9. Callahan ML: High-dose epinephrine therapy and other advances in treating cardiac arrest, *West J Med* 152:697, 1990.
10. Conover MB: *Understanding electrocardiography: arrhythmias and the 12-lead ECG*, ed 5, St Louis, 1988, Mosby–Year Book.
11. Curran CC, Mathewson M: Use of cardiac glycosides in the critically ill, *Crit Care Nurse* 7(6): 31, 1987.
12. Darovic GO: *Hemodynamic monitoring: invasive and noninvasive clinical application*, Philadelphia, 1987, WB Saunders Co.
13. DeBorde R, Aarons D, Biggs M: The automated implantable cardioverter, *AACN Clin Issues Crit Care Nurs* 2(1): 170, 1991.
14. Drew BJ: Cardiac rhythm responses. (I) An important phenomenon for nursing practice, science, and research, *Heart Lung* 18(1): 8, 1989.
15. Drew BJ: Cardiac rhythm responses. (II) Review of 22 years of nursing research, *Heart Lung* 18(2): 184, 1989.
16. Drew BJ, Ide B, Sparacino PSA: Accuracy of bedside electrocardiographic monitoring: a report on current practices of critical care nurses, *Heart Lung* 20(6): 597, 1991.
17. Dubin D: *Rapid interpretation of EKG's*, ed 4, Philadelphia, 1989, WB Saunders.
18. Dunn SL: Moricizine hydrochloride (Ethmozine®), *Crit Care Nurse* 12(4): 61, 1992.
18a. Emergency Cardiac Care Committee and Subcommittees, American Heart Association: Guidelines for cardiopulmonary resuscitation and emergency cardiac care, I: introduction, *JAMA* 268:2184-2241, 1992.
19. Finkelmeier NE: Pacemaker technology: an overview, *AACN Clin Issues Crit Care Nurs* 2(1): 99, 1991.
20. Gillman PH: Continuous measurement of cardiac output: a milestone in hemodynamic monitoring, *Focus Crit Care* 19(2): 155, 1992.
21. Goe MR, Massey TH: Assessment of neurologic damage: creatinine kinase-BB assay after cardiac arrest, *Heart Lung* 17(3): 247, 1988.
22. Guzzetta CE, Dossey BM: *Cardiovascular nursing: assessment and intervention*, St Louis, 1992, Mosby–Year Book.

23. Halfman-Franey M, Coburn C: Techniques in cardiac care: lasers, stents, and atherectomy devices, *AACN Clin Issues Crit Care Nurs* 1(1): 87, 1990.
24. Jones S, Bagg AM: L-E-A-D drugs for cardiac arrest, *Nurs '88* 18(1): 34, 1988.
25. Jost P: The role of antidysrhythmics in cardiac arrest, *Crit Care Nurs Q* 10(4): 63, 1988.
26. Kelleher RM: Cardiac drugs: new inotropes, *Crit Care Nurs Clin North Am* 1(2): 391, 1989.
27. Kennedy GT: Acute congestive heart failure: pharmacologic intervention, *Crit Care Nurs Clin North Am* 4(2): 365, 1992.
28. Kern LS, editor: *Cardiac critical care nursing,* Rockville, Md, 1988, Aspen Publishers.
29. Lefor N, Cardello FP, Felicetta JV: Recognizing and treating torsade de pointes, *Crit Care Nurse* June: 23, 1992.
30. Lepley-Frey D: Dysrhythmias and blood pressure changes associated with thrombolysis, *Heart Lung* 20(4): 335, 1991.
31. Marriott HJL: *Practical electrocardiography,* ed 8, Baltimore, 1988, Williams & Wilkins.
32. Menza MA, Stern TA, Cassem NH: Treatment of anxiety associated with electrophysiologic studies, *Heart Lung* 17(5): 555, 1988.
33. Miracle VA: Coronary atherectomy, *Crit Care Nurse* 12(3): 41, 1992.
34. Morton HS: Rate-responsive cardiac pacemakers, *AACN Clin Issues Crit Care Nurs* 2(1): 140, 1990.
35. Moser SA, Crawford D, Thomas A: Caring for patients with implantable cardioverter defibrillators, *Crit Care Nurse* 8(2): 52, 1988.
36. Mulford E: Nursing perspectives for the patient receiving postoperative ventricular assistance in the critical care unit, *Heart Lung* 16(3): 246, 1987.
37. Mutnick AH, Fecitt S, Rogers B: Cardiac drugs: inotropic and chronotropic agents, *Nurs '87* 17(10): 58, 1987.
38. Opie LH, editor: *Drugs for the heart,* ed 3, Philadelphia, 1991, WB Saunders.
39. Powers MZ, Powers RJ: ECG lead placement and configuration, *Crit Care Nurse* 9(3): 78, 1989.
40. Roach A: Adenosine-Adenocard®: a new intravenous antiarrhythmic agent for supraventricular tachycardia, *Crit Care Nurse* 11(7): 78, 1991.
41. Roden DM: Magnesium treatment of ventricular dysrhythmias, *Am J Cardiol,* 63: 43G, 1989.
42. Ruzevich SA, Swartz MT, Pennington DG: Nursing care of the patient with a pneumatic ventricular assist device, *Heart Lung* 17(4): 399, 1988.
43. Schactman M, Greene J: Signal-averaged electrocardiography: a new technique for determining which patients may be at risk for sudden death, *Focus Crit Care* 18(3): 202, 1991.
44. Stevens LL, Redd RM: Bedside electrophysiology study, *Crit Care Nurse* 7(4): 36, 1987.

45. Stevens LL, Redd RM, Buckingham TA: Ventricular burst pacing: an alternative to electric countershock for terminating ventricular arrhythmias, *Crit Care Nurse* 9(3): 38, 1989.

46. Valladares BK, Lemberg L: Problem solving for complications with the AICD, *Heart Lung* 16(1): 105, 1987.

47. Vinsant-Crawford MO, Spence MI: *Commonsense approach to coronary care: a program*, ed 5, St Louis, 1989, Mosby–Year Book.

48. Waggoner PC: Transcutaneous cardiac pacing, *AACN Clin Issues Crit Care Nurs* 2(1): 118, 1991.

49. Weiner B: Second generation antidysrhythmic agents, *Crit Care Nurs Clin North Am* 1(2): 417, 1989.

50. Whipple JK et al: Selected vasoactive drugs: A readily available chart reference, *Crit Care Nurse* 12(3): 23, 1992.

Classic

51. Bognolo DA: *Practical approach to physiologic cardiac pacing*, Tarpon Springs, Fla, 1983, Tampa Tracings.

52. Chung EK: *Electrocardiography: practical applications with vectorial principles*, ed 3, Norwalk, CT, 1985, Appleton & Lange.

53. Corbett KM, Lynch LC: Professional nursing issues in the administration of investigational antiarrhythmic medications, *Heart Lung* 13(4): 395, 1984.

54. Goldman MJ: *Principles of clinical electrocardiography*, ed 7, Los Altos, Ca, 1970, Lange Medical Books.

55. Guyton AC: *Textbook of medical physiology*, ed 7, Philadelphia, 1986, WB Saunders.

56. Hasegawa EAJ: The endotracheal use of emergency drugs, *Heart Lung* 15(1): 60, 1986.

57. Kernicki JG, Weiler KM: *Electrocardiography for nurses: physiological correlates*, New York, 1981, John Wiley & Sons.

58. Lipman BS, Massie E, Kleiger RE: *Clinical scalar electrocardiography*, ed 6, Chicago, 1972, Mosby–Year Book.

59. Little RC: *Physiology of the heart and circulation*, ed 3, Chicago, 1985, Mosby–Year Book.

60. Miller MJ: *Pathophysiology: principles of disease*, Philadelphia, 1983, WB Saunders.

61. Touloukian JE: Calcium channel blocking agents: physiologic basis of nursing intervention, *Heart Lung* 14(4): 342, 1985.

62. Walraven G: *Basic arrhythmias*, ed 2, Englewood Cliffs, NJ, 1986, Prentice-Hall (Brady).

63. White KM: Completing the hemodynamic picture: SvO_2, *Heart Lung* 14(3): 272, 1985.

64. Zschoche DA, editor: *Comprehensive review of critical care*, ed 3, St Louis, 1986, Mosby–Year Book.

CHAPTER THIRTY-FIVE

Nursing Management of Adults with Disorders of the Coronary Arteries, Myocardium, or Pericardium

LEARNING OBJECTIVES

1 Describe the pathophysiology of coronary artery disease.

2 Discuss the alterations in life-style the patient should make to reduce the risk factors associated with coronary artery disease.

3 Indicate the teaching interventions for the patient with angina pectoris.

4 Describe the nursing management during the acute and rehabilitative stages for the patient who has experienced a myocardial infarction.

5 List the patient teaching objectives in preparation for discharge of the patient with myocardial infarction.

6 Differentiate pericarditis, pericardial effusion, and cardiac tamponade as to clinical manifestations and therapeutic and nursing management.

7 Compare dilated, hypertrophic, and restrictive cardiomyopathy as to etiology, pathophysiology, and therapeutic and nursing management.

8 Describe the types of cardiac surgery and the preoperative and postoperative nursing management for the patient undergoing cardiac surgery.

CARDIOVASCULAR DISEASE remains the leading cause of death in the United States. Despite advances in treatment, research, and education of the public, cardiovascular disease continues to cost billions of dollars per year.

The major category of cardiovascular disease is coronary artery disease (CAD). Many patients with CAD are limited in their life-styles and daily care activities because of ischemia of the myocardium.

Early prevention and education are the key to reducing the human and financial costs related to the mortality and morbidity of CAD. Nurses provide care for patients with CAD in all sectors of the health care field and must be knowledgeable in providing the necessary preventive and management interventions to their patients.

CORONARY ARTERY DISEASE
Definition

Coronary artery disease (CAD) is a progressive obstruction of blood flow through one or more of the coronary arteries. This decreased blood flow deprives the myocardium of an adequate supply of oxygenated blood.

Etiology/Epidemiology

CAD accounted for 497,850 deaths (52.6% of all deaths) in the United States in 1989.[4] Approximately 6 million people have a history of angina pectoris, myocardial infarction, or both. Although men continue to have a higher incidence of myocardial infarctions caused by CAD, women, particularly black women, over 65 years of age, are twice as likely to die within a few weeks after sustaining a myocardial infarction. Because of its insidious onset, the incidence of atherosclerosis increases with age. The disease progresses for many years before symptoms develop; therefore emphasis has been placed on the identification and reduction of risk factors. Risk factors are categorized into those that are uncontrollable and those that are controllable, depending on the person's ability to influence their occurrence. The major risk factors are hyperlipidemia, hypertension, cigarette smoking, family history, obesity, inactivity, diabetes mellitus, and stress.

Uncontrollable risk factors

In men the incidence of CAD increases steadily with age. In women the incidence rises sharply after menopause, but in both sexes it increases with age. The correlation of CAD with age may result from the length of exposure to one or more of the other risk factors since it is not a direct result of the aging process. A history of CAD in blood-related family members has been associated with an increased risk of fatal myocardial infarctions. The mechanism for this correlation is presently unknown. Ethnic background may contribute to the risk factors of CAD through its relationship to other risk factors or variabilities in life-style. For example, the incidence of hypertension is significantly higher in the black population than in the white, and Japanese men living in Japan have a lower incidence of CAD than Japanese-American men.

Controllable risk factors

Overwhelming evidence exists that elevated serum lipid levels, primarily cholesterol and triglycerides, increase the incidence of CAD. In particular, elevated total serum cholesterol and low-density lipoprotein (LDL) cholesterol are associated with increasing risk. High-density lipoproteins (HDLs), which have a higher concentration of protein rather that cholesterol, appear to have some protective effects against the development of atherosclerosis. Elevated blood pressure in excess of 160/90 mm Hg is a major factor in the incidence of CAD, including stroke and heart failure. Hypertension associated with the presence of other risk factors significantly increases the risk of CAD.

Cigarette smoking is among the three greatest risk factors associated with CAD in both men and women. Its impact on both the incidence of CAD and mortality from CAD is related to the number of cigarettes smoked per day, duration of smoking, age the person began smoking, and the pattern of inhaling. The chief effects of cigarette smoking on the cardiovascular system are cardiac stimulation and peripheral vasoconstriction, which contribute to anginal symptoms. Platelet aggregation may be enhanced by cigarette smoking, since nicotine

GERIATRIC CONSIDERATIONS

The Aging Heart

Aging changes that occur in the heart result in an increase in the thickness and rigidity of the cardiac valves, widening and decreased elasticity of the aorta, and an increase in connective tissue in the conduction system. These changes cause increased time necessary for left ventricular ejection of blood, delayed cardiac conduction, and decreased myocardial contractility. The elderly person may not be able to achieve adequate increases in heart rate or cardiac output during situations that require increased blood flow such as exercise, fever, or emotional stress.

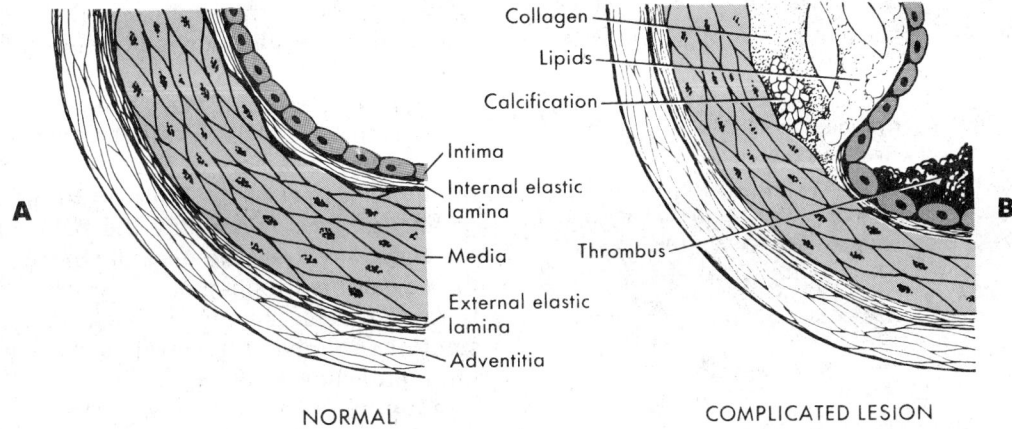

FIGURE 35-1   Atherosclerotic lesion. **A,** Normal cross section of artery. **B,** Advanced atherosclerotic lesion with thrombus formation.

stimulates catecholamine secretion. The risk of death from CAD is reduced within a few years after smoking cessation and may reach that of a nonsmoker within 10 years.

Other risk factors include diabetes mellitus, obesity, physical inactivity, and emotional stress.

Pathophysiology

For patients with CAD, atherosclerosis remains the leading cause of obstruction to flow in coronary arteries, the pathogenesis of which remains unknown. **Atherosclerosis** is characterized by a proliferation of smooth muscle cells and accumulation of lipids in the intima, or innermost layer of the artery. The lesions seen in atherosclerosis consist of three morphologic types: the fatty streak, the fibrous plaque, and the complicated lesion (Figure 35-1).

The fatty streak consists of lipid deposits within the intima. Increased blood levels of low-density lipoproteins (LDLs) irritate and damage the inner layer of the coronary artery. LDLs enter the damaged vessel lining, accumulating with macrophages to form foam cells. These foam cells cluster under the endothelial lining of the coronary artery, creating a bulge in the artery called a fatty streak. Smooth muscle cells from the media, or middle layer of the coronary artery, grow and engulf the fatty streak, creating a fibrous plaque that stimulates calcium deposits. This process results in the calcification and disruption of the lumen of the coronary artery. The clinical symptoms of myocardial ischemia or infarction occur when blood flow past the obstructed coronary lumen is inadequate or when the plaque ruptures or bleeds or a thrombus forms at the site of the lesion.

When a coronary artery is partially occluded, enlargement of other coronary arteries or the growth of new small arterioles may develop to maintain ad-equate blood flow to the myocardium. This is known as **collateral circulation** (Figure 35-2).

Clinical Manifestations

Absence of clinical symptoms depends on the maintenance of a delicate balance between myocardial oxygen supply and myocardial oxygen demand. If oxygen supply or blood flow to the myocardium diminishes below the oxygen needs of the myocardial cells, the cells can experience either reversible injury (ischemia) or irreversible destruction of that tis-

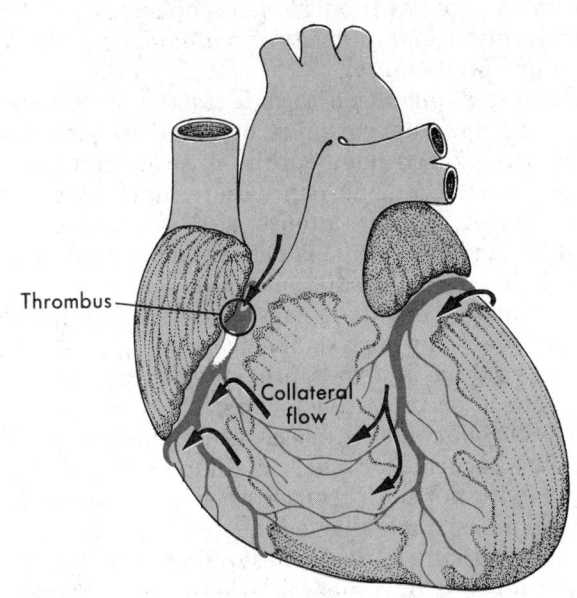

FIGURE 35-2   Collateral/coronary circulation. Thrombus or atherosclerotic lesion can obstruct blood flow through major coronary vessel. Intertributary communication allows flow to be reestablished distal to area of occlusion.

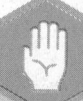

CLINICAL ALERT

In elderly persons, dyspnea may be the major initial complaint of myocardial ischemia although chest pain remains the presenting symptom in over 80% of the population. Coexistence of other medical diseases, such as pulmonary diseases or gastrointestinal disorders, may mask or confound the symptoms.

sue area (infarction). During ischemia varying degrees of cell damage occur, manifested by chest pain. These cells heal once the blood supply to the affected area of the heart is restored. If blood supply is not restored, infarction or death of the cells occurs. Factors that can diminish oxygen supply include thrombus formation, hypotension, anemia, hypoxemia, and coronary artery spasm. Increased oxygen demand, including exercise, strong emotion, hyperthyroidism, and diastolic hypertension, can also cause an imbalance between myocardial oxygen demand and supply.

The majority of patients with myocardial ischemia or infarction develop chest pain or **angina pectoris.** This pain occurs when the lumen of the coronary artery is narrowed by 75%.

Stable angina pectoris occurs when physical exertion or emotional stress causes an increase in myocardial oxygen demand beyond the ability of the coronary arteries to increase blood supply. The onset, duration, and intensity of symptoms in stable angina are predictable.

Unstable angina pectoris is known as preinfarction angina. The coronary arteries are unable to meet the oxygen needs of the myocardium even at rest. Unstable angina pain occurs more frequently, lasts longer, is more intense, and is not relieved by rest or medications. This pain is considered to be a precursor to myocardial infarction.

Intractable angina is chest pain that is refractory to interventions such as medications or rest. *Prinzmetal's angina* is severe, prolonged chest pain in the absence of precipitating factors. The apparent etiology is coronary artery spasm. The ischemic episodes follow a recurrent, cyclic, circadian pattern and may occur with normal coronary arteries. *Nocturnal angina* is chest pain that occurs only at night. *Silent ischemia* occurs without chest pain and is diagnosed when there is documented evidence of ischemia to the myocardium on electrocardiogram (ECG) or exercise stress test.

The presenting chest pain may range from mild to severe. The patient may describe it as heavy, squeezing, pressing, burning, crushing, choking, or aching. The pain may appear suddenly or gradually. The majority of patients experience pain behind the upper or middle third of the sternum. When asked to point to the site of pain, the patient may make a fist over the site of pain, called a positive Levine sign. The pain may radiate to the left shoulder and down the inner aspect of the left arm to the elbow, wrist, or fingers. Less commonly the pain may radiate to the right shoulder, the neck, or the jaw. The patient may describe a feeling of weakness or numbness in the wrist, arms, hands, or back. Pain may be transient or prolonged; however, it is usually sudden in onset and short in duration. Typically an attack lasts 1 to 5 minutes after removing the precipitating factor. The precipitating factor may be specific for a given individual, but any activity that increases myocardial oxygen demand (exercise, exposure to heat or cold, a heavy meal, mental tension, or sexual intercourse) may precipitate an attack in a susceptible individual.

Symptoms that may occur with anginal pain include dyspnea, tachycardia, palpitations, nausea, vomiting, fatigue, diaphoresis, pallor, weakness, syncope, apprehension, or a sense of impending doom.

Physical examination

The physical examination between episodes of angina may be normal and therefore not diagnostic. Physical findings during an anginal attack may include tachycardia, increased or decreased blood pressure, dysrhythmias, ST segment and T wave ECG changes, apprehension, diaphoresis, and pallor.

An ECG between episodes of angina may be normal, or it may show evidence of organic heart disease. An ECG tracing obtained during an anginal attack may document the ischemic event. ST segment changes and symmetrically inverted T waves occur if ischemia is present. ECG stress testing of patients with CAD may cause myocardial ischemia during the procedure as demonstrated by a depression of the ST segment and T wave inversion on ECG. This ischemia may also precipitate chest pain and associated symptoms.

When thallium 210, a radioisotope, is injected intravenously into the patient with CAD, scanning during exercise shows regions of ischemia or poor perfusion that appear as "cold spots" where the myocardial muscle has not taken up the isotope. Images taken after a period of rest show a reversal of ischemia where the reperfused myocardium takes up the isotope. Radionuclide ventriculography or gated blood pool scanning is performed during rest and exercise to visualize ventricular wall motion abnormalities that may occur from damage to the myocardium and to estimate the patient's ejection fraction.

Cardiac catheterization

Cardiac catheterization or coronary angiography is a procedure in which a catheter is floated into an artery and dye is injected to visualize blood flow through the coronary arteries. It can determine the presence, location, and extent of lesions in the coronary arteries. During cardiac catheterization, abnormalities in the pressures in each of the cardiac chambers and inflow and outflow tracts can also be determined. Injection of dye into the ventricles allows visualization of the motion abnormalities of the ventricular walls that may occur after injury to the myocardium.

Laboratory studies

No specific laboratory tests diagnose CAD. However, laboratory studies will determine the presence and extent of risk factors, namely, cholesterol, LDL, HDL, triglycerides, serum glucose, and uric acid. Most drugs are metabolized by the liver and excreted by the kidneys; therefore an assessment of renal and liver function is necessary. Creatine kinase (CK) and isoenzymes may be drawn to rule out myocardial infarction.

Therapeutic Management

Therapeutic management of the patient with CAD focuses on relieving acute attacks of angina, preventing further attacks, and preventing the progression of CAD. To achieve these goals, therapies must reduce the work load of the heart to decrease oxygen demand, improve oxygen supply by increasing blood flow to the heart muscle, and reduce the risk factors associated with CAD.

Pharmacologic intervention

Three major classes of antianginal medications are used to decrease myocardial oxygen demand and increase oxygen supply. They are nitrates, beta-adrenergic blockers, and calcium channel blockers. Medications are also available to help reduce circulating blood cholesterol levels.

Nitrates

Nitrate therapy causes a generalized vasodilation throughout the body. Nitrates reduce venous return to the heart, thereby lowering filling pressure in the left ventricle (preload). They reduce blood pressure, which decreases afterload, decreasing myocardial oxygen demand. Nitrates also dilate coronary arteries, increasing oxygen supply. By decreasing myocardial oxygen requirements and increasing oxygen supply, the balance between supply and demand is optimized. Nitrates can be administered by various routes. Nitroglycerin is the most common nitrate used. Short-acting nitrates are administered sublin-

gually or intravenously to relieve acute anginal attacks. Long-acting nitrates are administered orally or in the form of topical pastes or patches to prevent anginal attacks (Table 35-1). The side effects of nitrates are a result of their vasodilator properties and include headaches, hypotension, and syncope. Skin reactions can occur with transdermal preparations. Patients receiving long-term therapy should not abruptly discontinue the use of nitrates. Nitrate withdrawal syndrome has been documented in cardiac patients. The symptoms include angina, myocardial infarction, and sudden death on sudden cessation of nitrates. Recent research has also documented the development of nitrate tolerance with long-acting nitrates. Continued research is being conducted on the effects of increasing dosages and nitroglycerin-free periods of several hours to prevent this tolerance.

Beta blockers

Beta-adrenergic blockers inhibit circulating catecholamines from stimulating beta-receptor sites. "Nonselective" beta blockers inhibit both $beta_1$ and $beta_2$ receptors. They reduce heart rate and myocardial contractility and conductivity, thereby reducing myocardial oxygen demand. Blockade of the $beta_2$ receptors results in bronchoconstriction, coronary vasoconstriction, and peripheral vascular constriction. This effect can cause bronchospasm in patients with underlying obstructive lung disease. Examples of nonselective beta blockers include propranolol (Inderal), nadolol (Corgard), timolol maleate (Blocadren), and pindolol (Visken). "Cardioselective" beta blockers affect only the heart and can be used safely in patients with lung disease. They include atenolol (Tenormin) and metaprolol (Lopressor).

Side effects of beta blockers include bradycardia, cardiac failure, fatigue, weakness, hallucinations, nightmares, impotence, and depression. Beta blockers are used with caution in patients who are prone to coronary artery spasm because of their vasoconstrictor effects.

Calcium channel blockers

Calcium channel blockers inhibit the movement of calcium across the cell membranes within the heart muscle, conduction system, and vascular smooth muscle. By blocking the influx of calcium, these agents reduce cardiac muscle force and therefore contractility, reduce pacemaker activity and slow the heart rate, and relax vascular smooth muscle causing vasodilation. Their overall effects cause a decrease in myocardial oxygen demand and an increase in coronary blood supply. Examples of calcium channel blockers include verapamil (Isoptin, Calan), diltiazem (Cardizem), and nifedipine (Procardia). Combination drug therapy of two or more of these medications may be used to control anginal

TABLE 35-1 Pharmacology Summary: Medications for Coronary Artery Disease

Medication	Average dose	Side effects	Nursing interventions
NITRATES			
Nitroglycerin	Loading dose: 0.15-0.6 mg	Headache	1. Monitor response to medications (relief of anginal symptoms, blood pressure, and pulse rate and rhythm) before and after each sublingual dose
Sublingual	(1/400-1/100 grain); repeat	Flushing	
Oral (sustained release)	every 3-5 min twice	Dizziness	
Loading dose	1.3-6.5 mg q6-8h	Weakness	
Maintenance dose	2.6-9 mg q8-12h	Postural hypotension	
Topical paste	½-2 inches q6-8h	Tachycardia	2. Headaches tend to decrease or disappear as tolerance develops
Transdermal patch	5-20 mg q24h	Palpitations	
Intravenous	10-300 µg/min	Nausea	
Isosorbide dinitrate		Skin reactions	3. Patient should carry medications at all times and take sublingually at first sign of anginal attack (tablet should be placed under tongue until completely absorbed); patient should sit or lie down after taking medication; may repeat dose for two doses; if no relief, call physician or emergency phone number
Oral tablets	5-300 mg q3-4h	(transdermal systems)	
Sustained release	20-40 mg q6-12h		

4. Patient to keep record of number of tablets taken with each pain episode to monitor for changes in pain relief

5. Medication stored in its original container, tightly closed, with cotton packing removed; medication kept in cool, dry place and replaced every 6 mo after opening

6. Long-acting nitrates taken regularly

7. Oral tablets taken on an empty stomach ½ hr before meals or 1-2 hr after meals and should be swallowed whole; chewable tablets chewed thoroughly before swallowing

8. Ointments applied using glove or paper provided for measuring in thin layer to nonhairy area; do not rub in; all ointments removed from previous site before applying new dose; rotate sites to avoid skin irritations

Medication	Average dose	Side effects	Nursing interventions
			9. IV preparations must be mixed in nonabsorbable container and administered via nonabsorbable tubing, since drug can be absorbed by regular plastic bags and tubing and is sensitive to light
			10. IV form is initiated at 5-10 μg/min and increased in 5 μg/min increments until pain relief is achieved without compromising blood pressure
			11. Monitor patient closely during cessation of therapy, because pulmonary edema may occur in patients with poor left ventricular function
BETA BLOCKER Propranolol	Starting dose: 10-20 mg q6-8 h; may be increased at 7- to 10-day intervals	Fatigue Lethargy Hallucinations Depression Bradycardia Hypotension Congestive heart failure Bronchospasm Blood dyscrasias Hypoglycemia Nightmares Impotence	1. Nonselective beta blockers contraindicated in patients with bronchial asthma, since they block vasodilatory effects of $beta_2$ receptors; in patients with sinus bradycardia and greater than first-degree atrioventricular block, since they block cardiac $beta_1$ receptors
			2. Administer cautiously in patients with heart failure, chronic bronchitis, asthma, emphysema, or renal or hepatic insufficiency
			3. Check apical pulse before administering; if less than 50, notify physician
			4. Monitor for bronchospasm and hypoglycemia
			5. Teach patients to take their pulse and to inform physician if it goes below 50 beats/min
			6. Do not discontinue medication abruptly since serious withdrawal symptoms may occur
			7. Beta blockers will mask common signs of shock, hypoglycemia, and hyperthyroidism

TABLE 35-1   Pharmacology Summary: Medications for Coronary Artery Disease—cont'd

Medication	Average dose	Side effects	Nursing interventions
			8. Propranolol: administer PO with meals; IV administration: monitor blood pressure, cardiac rate and rhythm; vasopressors may be required to treat hypotension
CALCIUM CHANNEL BLOCKERS Verapamil Nifedipine	Starting dose: 80 mg PO q6-8h; may be increased at weekly intervals; maximum dose: 480 mg daily Starting dose: 10 mg PO q8h; range: 10-20 mg q6-8h; maximum dose: 180 mg/day; during acute pain, capsule can be punctured and fluid squirted under tongue	Dizziness Postural hypotension Fatigue Headache Syncope Palpitations Peripheral edema Bradycardia Constipation (verapamil) Diarrhea (nifedipine) Hypokalemia	1. Administer with caution in patients with congestive heart failure and elderly patients 2. Monitor blood pressure for postural hypotension 3. Patient should swallow tablets or capsules whole 4. Store medications at room temperature, away from heat and light 5. Patient may take sublingual nitroglycerin to abort acute anginal attack 6. May cause constipation; advise patient to drink plenty of fluids and eat high-fiber foods, fruits, and vegetables 7. Patient should take medications 1 hr before meals or 2 hr after 8. If dizziness occurs, inform patient to rise slowly from lying to sitting to standing position to decrease orthostatic hypotension
Diltiazem	Starting dose: 10 mg PO q8h; range: 10-20 mg q6-8h; maximum dose: 360 mg daily		
ANTILIPIDS BILE ACID SEQUESTRANTS Cholestyramine Colestipol	Two packets, scoops, or bars bid or tid	Constipation Bloating Nausea Flatulence Malabsorption of vitamins or other drugs	1. Powder must be mixed in liquid or pureed sauce such as applesauce 2. Available in candy bar form, which is more expensive; can be used for convenience when not at home 3. Dosing can be increased over several weeks to decrease side effects 4. May cause constipation; advise patient to drink plenty of fluids and eat high-fiber foods, fruits, and vegetables

TABLE 35-1   Pharmacology Summary: Medications for Coronary Artery Disease—cont'd

Medication	Average dose	Side effects	Nursing interventions
			5. Evaluate its effect on absorption of other drugs (e.g., digoxin, warfarin, thyroxine, and beta blockers) 6. Instruct patients to take other medications 1 hr before or 2-4 hr after taking bile acid sequestrants 7. Instruct patients to take 30 min before meals
Nicotinic Acid (Niacin)	500 mg to 3 g tid	Elevated levels of liver function tests Hyperuricemia Hyperglycemia Flu syndrome Blurred vision Gastrointestinal upset Flushing Itching	1. Instruct patients to take with meals 2. Obtain baseline liver function tests and glucose and uric acid levels and monitor at frequent intervals 3. Explain importance of increasing dose gradually
Lovastatin	20-80 mg/day	Elevated levels of liver function tests Fatigue Insomnia	1. Liver function tests must be monitored frequently during first 15 mo of therapy and intermittently thereafter 2. Encourage patients to take with meals

symptoms. This approach can help offset potential side effects of one class of drugs or act synergistically to optimize oxygen supply.

Antilipid medications

Antilipid medications decrease blood cholesterol and/or triglyceride levels in patients with elevated levels. Because of antilipids' side effects, they are reserved for patients after careful consideration of the benefits of other therapeutic alternatives, such as a low cholesterol diet, weight reduction, exercise, smoking cessation, and treatment of hypertension. Examples of antilipid medications include cholestyramine, colestipol, niacin, and lovastatin.

Aspirin

In patients with angina, both the number of platelets and their activity are increased in the arterial circulation and may participate in the progression of

CAD. Aspirin suppresses platelet aggregation by blocking a specific step in the prostaglandin pathway. Incidence of death and MI in those people with CAD has been shown to decrease with a daily low dose of aspirin.

Life-style modification

Other medical therapeutic management is directed at modifying the patient's life-style to reduce risk factors. Behavioral changes and alterations in life-style are difficult to achieve and may require a long period for success. Some individuals may benefit from the support and structure provided by group activities (e.g., Weight Watchers, smoking cessation groups, stress management workshops, and cardiac rehabilitation or exercise programs). Information about these programs, people to contact, and telephone numbers should be provided to patients.

Percutaneous transluminal angioplasty

Percutaneous transluminal angioplasty (PTCA) is a procedure used to dilate coronary arteries that are obstructed by atherosclerotic plaque. The procedure is performed in a cardiac catheterization laboratory where a balloon-tipped catheter is introduced via a femoral or brachial artery into a coronary artery containing a noncalcified atheromatous lesion. The balloon is inflated, causing fracturing and splitting of the plaque and stretching of the arterial wall. This results in an increase in the diameter of the coronary artery, improving blood flow distal to the lesion. Repeated inflations and deflations may be performed until satisfactory results are visualized during dye injections into the coronary artery (Figure 35-3).

PTCA is indicated for the relief of myocardial ischemia caused by CAD in patients who meet the following criteria:

1. Stable angina of less than a 1-year history or unstable angina of less than a 6-month history
2. Coronary lesions that are proximal and non-calcified
3. Acceptable candidates for coronary artery bypass graft surgery and who have consented to surgery in the event of complications
4. Those patients experiencing an evolving myo-

cardial infarction (may be used in combination with thrombolytic therapy) or those who have occluded coronary bypass grafts

PTCA is contraindicated in patients who have severe left main coronary artery disease, who have severe left ventricular dysfunction, or who are not candidates for surgery since coronary occlusion, arterial dissection, myocardial infarction, and coronary artery spasm are complications that may require immediate coronary artery bypass surgery. Restenosis of the coronary artery can occur abruptly or within a few years after a patient has undergone PTCA.

Innovations in treatment of CAD

Intracoronary stents

Intracoronary stenting refers to mechanically supporting the arterial vessel wall after balloon angioplasty, using a prosthetic device known as a stent. These devices are primarily made of surgical stainless steel and range between 15 to 30 mm in length and 3 to 5 mm in diameter after expansion. A number of stent designs are under investigation. Each exhibits a unique configuration and varies in the mechanism by which it is deployed within the coronary vessel (Figure 35-4).

After a balloon angioplasty has been performed on a compressible coronary atheroma, a balloon catheter with a stent crimped over it is guided to the site. The stent is deployed in the coronary artery by inflating the balloon, allowing for stent expansion, and then deflating the balloon. The stent remains in the vessel as the catheter is removed. Stent placement may prevent abrupt closure of the vessel after PTCA and may improve long-term patency of the coronary vessel. Because of the thrombogenic nature of the stent, anticoagulation and antiplatelet therapy is necessary indefinitely to prevent local thrombus formation on the stainless steel stent.

Laser angioplasty

Laser angioplasty refers to a technique in which a percutaneously inserted flexible fiberoptic catheter is introduced into the coronary vessel. Laser light is emitted from the catheter to vaporize the plaque from the obstructed arterial vessel. Laser angioplasty can be performed as a primary therapy or in combination with a PTCA. This technique may minimize damage to the vessel intima since it does not create the fracturing and stretching of PTCA, and it may open more effectively diseased vessels by removing the plaque rather than redistributing it. Research is investigating its ability to prevent abrupt closure and long-term stenosis. It may also be proven effective with calcified or total occlusions of coronary arteries. Depending on the type of laser system used, this procedure can cause adjacent tissue damage or arterial vessel perforation.

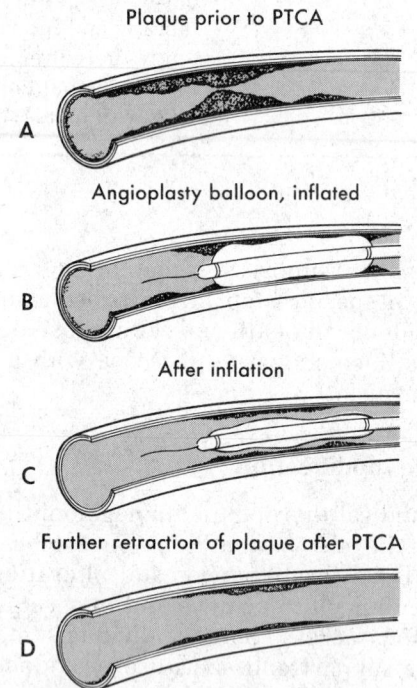

Plaque prior to PTCA

A

Angioplasty balloon, inflated

B

After inflation

C

Further retraction of plaque after PTCA

D

FIGURE 35-3 Percutaneous transluminal coronary angioplasty (PTCA). **A,** Plaque before PTCA. **B,** Inflation of angioplasty balloon. **C,** Plaque after PTCA. **D,** Six months after PTCA, plaque has retracted even further.

Atherectomy

Atherectomy is a procedure in which a catheter device is inserted percutaneously via the femoral or brachial artery into a coronary artery to remove the atheroma. Two major techniques for plaque removal are presently under clinical investigation.

One technique uses a "shaving and retrieval" approach where plaque is shaved from the atheroma and deposited in a small "cup" in the catheter. Once the cup is full, the catheter is removed and the cup emptied. The procedure can be repeated until adequate vessel diameter is achieved (Figure 35-5).

The transluminal extraction catheter is the second technique used in atherectomies. This device consists of a motorized cutting head at the distal tip of a hollow catheter. The cutting head rotates extremely rapidly to pulverize plaque into small fragments that are removed from the coronary artery by applying gentle suction through the catheter.

Atherectomies may in the future open diseased coronary vessels more effectively, especially in patients who have calcified lesions not amenable to PTCA.

Coronary artery bypass graft surgery

Coronary artery bypass graft surgery (CABG) is a surgical revascularization procedure used to increase coronary blood flow distal to occlusive coro-

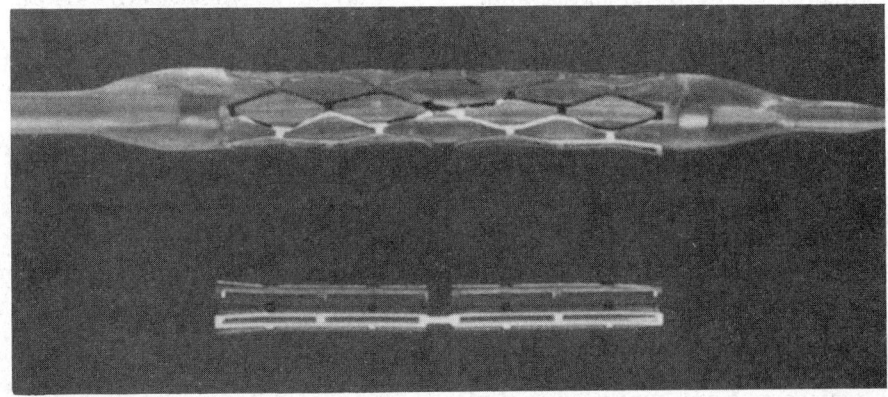

FIGURE 35-4   Palmaz coronary stent. (Courtesy Richard Schatz, MD, and Johnson & Johnson.)

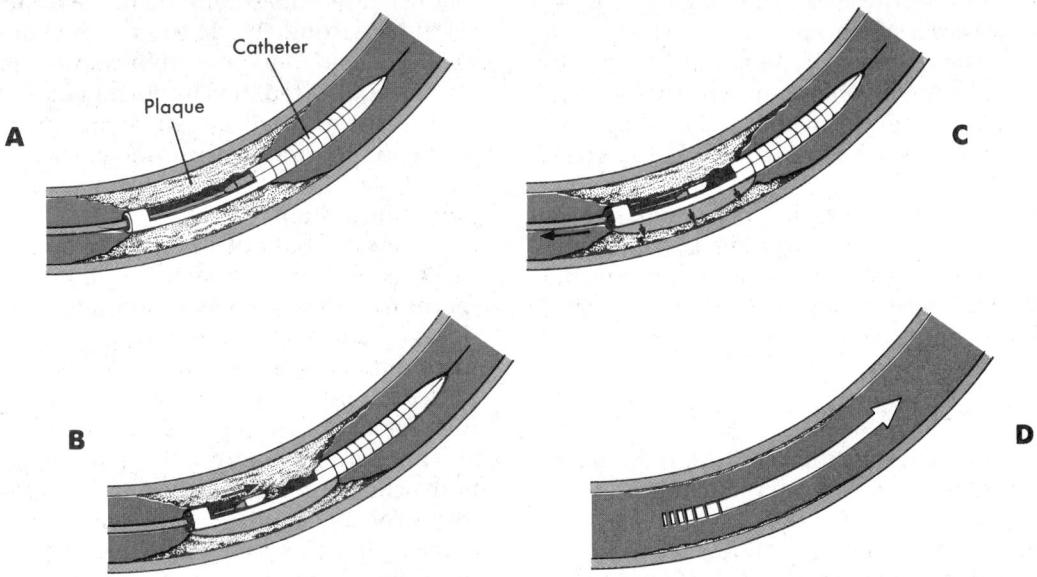

FIGURE 35-5   **A,** Transluminal extraction catheter is inserted into coronary artery. **B,** Motorized cutting head rotates and pulverizes plaque into small fragments. **C,** Fragments are removed through catheter via gentle suction. **D,** Artery is cleared.

nary lesions. The main goals of surgery are to relieve symptoms and improve the quality of the patient's life. The surgery does not cure atherosclerosis. The patient must still reduce or modify controllable risk factors to retard the underlying disease progression. (See discussion of cardiac surgery, p. 900.)

NURSING MANAGEMENT OF THE PATIENT WITH CORONARY ARTERY DISEASE

Assessment

The assessment process must be modified for the patient experiencing an acute anginal attack to include rapid and perhaps lifesaving measures. For the patient with a chronic history of CAD, the assessment includes a description of anginal pain: frequency, location, duration, intensity, radiation, and precipitating and alleviating factors. Ask about associated symptoms such as diaphoresis, syncope, nausea, vomiting, palpitations, or shortness of breath.

A careful history of the stable patient provides data on past medical and family history. Data regarding presence of risk factors can assist the nurse in planning a program to assist the patient in reducing those factors that may be controlled. Assess the patient and family's knowledge of the disease and determine the patient's present tolerance for activity. Important to the success of any care plan is the nurse's identification of the patient and family's anxiety levels and their ability to use appropriate coping mechanisms.

Between anginal attacks, the patient may not have any apparent evidence of CAD. Assessment of the patient during an anginal episode can provide objective data that may substantiate the diagnosis, however. The nurse assesses the patient for changes in blood pressure, heart rate, rhythm, and ECG readings, as well as accompanying symptoms such as pallor, diaphoresis, vomiting, syncope, and anxiety. Ask the patient about precipitating factors to the chest pain.

The nurse reviews the results of diagnostic procedures to determine the extent of the CAD and the risk of experiencing a myocardial infarction. Results of laboratory tests are reviewed to determine the presence and extent of risk factors.

Nursing Diagnosis

Based on the information gathered during the nursing history, nursing diagnoses may include the following:

Pain (acute) related to myocardial ischemia
Anxiety (severe) related to pain and fear of death
Knowledge deficit about disease process, therapies, and methods for avoiding complications
High risk for decreased cardiac output related to myocardial ischemia or side effects of medications

Planning

Individualized goals are identified for each patient. General goals may include the following:

Patient will relate the underlying causes of CAD to the presence of anginal symptoms
Patient will describe risk factors for CAD
Patient will identify precipitating/alleviating factors for angina
Patient will verbalize the names, dosages, actions, and side effects of medications
Patient will describe actions to take in the event of chest pain
Patient will avoid factors/events that precipitate an anginal attack
Patient will pace activities and provide for periods of rest
Patient will practice relaxation techniques
Patient will plan to participate in a regular exercise program
Patient will modify controllable risk factors
Patient will continue medical follow-up as instructed
Patient will identify signs and symptoms that warrant immediate medical attention
Patient will identify physician's telephone number and ambulance service to obtain emergency care

Implementation

Initially, interventions should be implemented to relieve pain and anxiety and provide concrete directions for pain control and accomplishing diagnostic testing. Attempts should be made to provide a quiet, restful environment. The nurse explains the purpose and expected outcomes of invasive studies and therapies as indicated. It is important at this stage to provide answers to all questions in concrete terminology and provide reassurance, since the patient's anxiety level may impair ability to learn more complex information.

While the patient is in the hospital, the nurse is responsible for administering the medications and monitoring for beneficial and adverse effects. Drug dosages and combinations may need frequent adjustments before a suitable regimen is found for the patient. Table 35-1 summarizes nursing responsibilities for each group of medications.

The nurse monitors the patient for verbal and nonverbal cues of pain, as well as for clinical evidence of ischemia. A decrease in blood pressure, changes in heart rate or rhythm, ECG changes, restlessness, or diaphoresis may indicate an alteration in cardiac output related to ischemia. Medications to alleviate ischemia must be administered promptly to restore the balance between myocardial oxygen supply and demand.

As the patient adjusts to the diagnosis of CAD and

NURSING CARE PLAN *The Patient with Acute Angina*

Nursing diagnosis/ Expected outcome	Interventions	Rationale
Pain (acute) related to myocardial ischemia • *Patient will verbalize relief of chest pain*	Instruct patient experiencing chest pain to stop activity and return to bed or chair to rest	Resting reduces oxygen requirements of myocardium
	Determine intensity of anginal pain: ask patient to compare present pain to other experiences of pain on a scale of 1 (lowest) to 10 (highest)	Assists in determining objective evaluation of subjective symptom
	Observe for other signs and symptoms: diaphoresis, shortness of breath, protective body posture, dusky coloring, changes in level of consciousness	Associated symptoms help validate cause of pain as cardiac in origin
	Ask patient to report symptoms of nausea, syncope, or palpitations	Subjective feelings that may accompany pathophysiologic changes during angina
	Administer oxygen at 2 to 4 L/min via nasal cannula or face mask; administer antianginal medications such as nitroglycerin sublingually, as prescribed	Oxygen and antianginal medication administration helps to increase myocardial oxygen supply
	Obtain blood pressure, apical heart rate and rhythm, and respiratory rate; monitor vital signs every 15 minutes until pain subsides and then every 2 to 4 hours	Myocardial ischemia can impair the heart's functioning, decreasing blood pressure and increasing heart rate; patients are also at risk for dysrhythmias
	Obtain a 12-lead ECG	The 12-lead ECG can document presence and location of myocardial ischemia and/or infarction
	Notify physician if patient's chest pain is not relieved after three doses of sublingual nitroglycerin	More aggressive therapy may be required
	Constantly monitor for relief of chest pain	Pain relief may be inadequate with initial efforts and may require morphine sulfate or intravenous nitroglycerin therapy
	Evaluate patient's chest pain to determine if it has increased in severity, frequency, or duration or if it is becoming less responsive to treatment	These data are imperative in recognizing whether patient's chest pain is progressing from stable angina to unstable angina
Anxiety (severe) related to pain and fear of death • *Patient will verbalize reduced anxiety*	Stay with patient during episodes of pain	Presence of another person while experiencing chest pain is often very reassuring
	Assure patient that you will remain with him or her until chest pain is relieved	Patients frequently experience sense of impending doom or death
	Administer antianxiety medications as prescribed	Reduction of catecholamine stimulation can decrease myocardial oxygen demand and potential for dysrhythmias
	Discuss with patient importance of reducing anxiety; offer measures (e.g., relaxation techniques, imagery) to facilitate this and mechanisms to measure their success	

anxiety is controlled, it is imperative to begin patient education and consistently reinforce the information in order for the patient to begin planning for life-style changes and effective medication administration before discharge. A summary of patient teaching is provided below. The nurse can use diagrams of the heart or booklets from the American Heart Association to provide information on CAD. Explore with the patient the presence of risk factors and precipitating events or factors for angina. The patient may need assistance in developing ways to avoid or control these events, if possible, or may need to take a dose of nitroglycerin prophylactically before engaging in activities that cause pain. The patient may need to pace activities or schedule rest periods during the day. Discuss with the patient actions

to take should pain occur. Written and oral instructions about all medications, names, dosages, actions, and side effects should be provided for the patient. Special considerations for each medication are given in Table 35-1.

The patient must understand that the therapeutic interventions relieve the symptoms of angina but do not cure or arrest the disease process. Discuss with the patient individual risk factors and ways to reduce or modify the controllable factors in an attempt to reduce or slow the progress of the CAD. Written materials regarding CAD, diet, self-care activities, and medications can be provided to reinforce instruction after discharge.

If it is a repeat admission for the patient with CAD, it is important to identify specific areas of lack

---

 **PATIENT EDUCATION GUIDE** *Coronary Artery Disease*

Objective: Patient will demonstrate behaviors that reduce the risks and complications of CAD.
1. Prevention and control of anginal pain
   a. Relate basis for anginal symptoms to the underlying causes of CAD.
   b. Identify precipitating/alleviating factors for angina.
   c. Discuss life-style changes that will eliminate precipitating factors, such as getting up earlier to allow for a slower pace during the day.
   d. Describe actions to take when anginal pain occurs: rest, take antianginal medications, notify physician/emergency services if pain is unrelieved after 15 minutes.
   e. Identify signs and symptoms that warrant immediate medical attention, that is, unrelieved pain, changes in intensity or duration, alleviating factors, or associated symptoms.
2. Risk factors
   a. Avoid smoking; identify measures to assist this, such as American Cancer Society or smoking cessation groups.
   b. Practice appropriate methods of relaxation daily.
   c. Follow low-cholesterol, low-sodium diet as prescribed.
      (1) Eat foods containing unsaturated fats and complex carbohydrates rather than foods high in saturated fat and cholesterol.
      (2) Consult dietitian.
      (3) Offer appropriate cookbooks (American Heart Association) for planning and preparing meals.
   d. Maintain ideal weight for body build, size, and gender.
   e. Maintain a regular exercise program three to five times per week, such as walking, swimming, or other aerobic exercise, within cardiac limitations. Avoid isometric exercises, such as weight lifting.
   f. Pace activities to allow for rest periods.
   g. Control associated health problems with physician coverage: hypertension, hypercholesterolemia, diabetes mellitus.
3. Avoidance of activities that may increase myocardial oxygen demand.
   a. Avoid excessive caffeine intake, which may increase heart rate and increase myocardial oxygen demand.
   b. Avoid activities known to cause anginal pain: extremes of temperature, stress, straining, sudden exertion, high altitudes.
   c. Refrain from physical activity after meals.
   d. Avoid alcohol, or drink alcohol in moderation.
4. Medications
   a. Take medications as prescribed.
   b. Do not stop medications, skip doses, or make up forgotten doses without physician's approval.
   c. Report any side effects, changes in anginal symptoms, or undesirable effects to the physician.
   d. Avoid diet pills, nasal decongestants, and all over-the-counter medications that increase heart rate without first consulting the physician.

of knowledge, specific changes that have occurred in life-style and symptomatology, or inabilities to modify risk factors or comply with the therapeutic regimen. This information allows the nurse to individualize the nursing care plan to the specific needs of the patient and family.

Evaluation

Ongoing evaluation during hospitalization allows the nurse to modify interventions to meet the individual patient's needs before discharge. To reduce the incidence of pain, the patient should be able to identify and avoid those activities that precipitate it. The patient should be able to describe what to do when an anginal attack occurs as well as the criteria for calling the physician. Before discharge the patient should exhibit a stable blood pressure, heart rate, and rhythm, indicating stable hemodynamic parameters. Reduced anxiety in the patient and family will be evidenced by their verbalization as well as by their ability to pay attention and learn information, ask questions, and demonstrate realistic comprehension of their situation. With the nurse the patient should devise a concrete plan for pain control, risk factor modification, activity regimen, and medication administration within the structure of the patient's usual daily home or work schedule.

Documentation

Key points in documentation for the patient with CAD are risk factor profile; nature of chest pain, including quality, severity (i.e., level of pain on scale of 1 to 10), location and radiation, duration, precipitating and alleviating factors, and associated symptoms; response to interventions, pharmacologic and other; and level of ability to meet learning objectives.

Ongoing Care

The patient must be able to effectively manage the therapeutic regimen. The nurse is responsible for

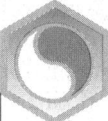

ETHICAL ISSUES

- How should a nurse respond to a patient who is clearly having a myocardial infarction but whose advance directive states that she does not want to receive CPR? What if the patient is unconscious? What if the patient is conscious?
- Are there situations in which an advance directive should not be honored?

providing the patient with the information needed to perform knowledgeable self-care including risk factor modification, avoidance of precipitating factors, and medication administration. If the patient is elderly or lives alone, a community health nursing referral may be helpful in making changes. Ongoing medical follow-up is essential to evaluate the success of these measures in controlling the patient's symptoms, identify progression of the disease, and monitor for complications.

MYOCARDIAL INFARCTION
Definition

Myocardial infarction (MI) is an acute process in which myocardial tissue experiences a severe and prolonged decrease in oxygen supply because of a disruption or deficiency in coronary blood flow causing necrosis or "death" of the tissue. It is commonly referred to as a "heart attack."

Etiology/Epidemiology

Estimates suggest that of the more than 6 million Americans with CAD, 1.5 million people will suffer an MI each year. During the acute phase of an MI, mortality is approximately 25%.[4] Acute coronary thrombosis, or clotting of an atherosclerotic coronary artery, is the "culprit" in 90% of MIs. Usually the coronary vessel is already at least 75% occluded as a result of CAD.

Other conditions that can precipitate an MI include coronary artery spasm, coronary artery embolism, inflammatory processes of the coronary artery, hypoxia, anemia, prolonged hypotension, and cocaine abuse. Patients with significant CAD may also sustain an MI in the absence of thrombosis when excessive oxygen demand is placed on the myocardium, such as severe exertion or stress.

Pathophysiology

Thrombosis of an atherosclerosed coronary artery occurs when the plaque in the vessel ruptures, allowing coronary blood to enter the lesion and clot (Figure 35-6). The initial thrombus activates the aggregation of platelets and stimulates the coagulation cascade. The thrombus can occlude the coronary artery and interrupt blood flow to the distal portion causing ischemia and necrosis to the nonperfused myocardial tissue. Myocardial cellular damage begins subendocardially where the tissue is supplied by the most distal branches of the coronary artery (Figure 35-7). The damage can continue and extend through to the epicardium. Necrosis of the affected area occurs within approximately 6 hours. The necrotic area is surrounded by a zone of reversible ischemic tissue. At this point there are three zones

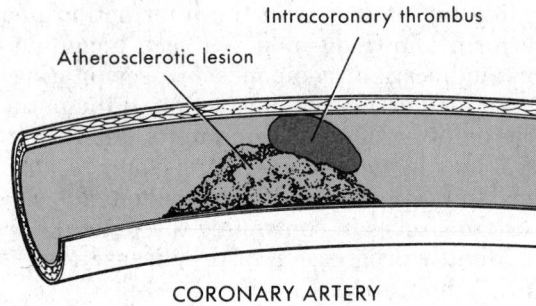

FIGURE 35-6 Coronary atherosclerosis complicated by thrombosis. Obstruction of coronary artery blood flow leads to MI.

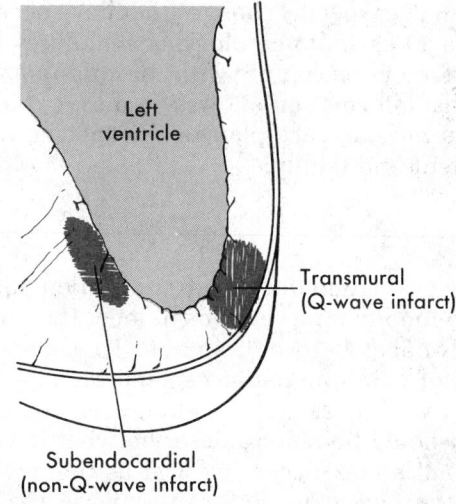

FIGURE 35-7 Subendocardial MI involves death (necrosis) of subendocardial layer, whereas transmural MI involves death of entire thickness of myocardial tissue (endocardium, myocardium, and epicardium).

CLINICAL ALERT

Delay in seeking medical assistance at the onset of an MI increases mortality and morbidity. Public education and accessible emergency medical services are key variables in reducing the large number of individuals who die within the first hour of the onset of symptoms.

of cellular changes: an area of injury, an area of ischemia, and an area of infarction. The ischemic and injured tissue can heal when appropriate treatment is provided, whereas the infarcted necrotic tissue damage is permanent. The necrotic area becomes infiltrated with white blood cells. During this time a mural thrombus can form over the affected region within the cardiac chamber. Degradation of the necrotic tissue occurs during the first week after an MI, thinning the myocardial wall. By 4 weeks after necrosis, granulation occurs, eventually developing into a tough white fibrous scar. This entire process may take up to 3 months to complete.

The damaging effect of this decreased blood supply to the myocardium depends on multiple variables. Size of the damaged area, location of the infarct, and presence of collateral circulation are important factors.

Size of an infarct refers to the amount of tissue damaged during an acute event. It is the most important factor in determining the extent of mechanical contractile failure. Damage to myocardial tissue may be limited to the subendocardial tissue (non–Q wave infarction), or it may involve the entire thickness of the heart muscle (Q wave infarction) (Figure 35-7). Left ventricular contractility in the affected area may exhibit **hypokinesis** (reduced

movement), **dyskinesis** (outward movement), or **akinesis** (absent movement). Changes in muscle wall contractility can decrease the cardiac stroke volume and place the patient at risk for heart failure.

The anatomic location of the MI depends on the coronary artery occluded (Table 35-2). Anterior wall MIs are frequently accompanied by heart failure and may produce some degree of heart block. Inferoposterior MIs can cause sinus node block, atrial dysrhythmias, or varying degrees of heart block.

The damaging effects of decreased blood supply to the myocardium may be limited by the presence of collateral circulation. Persons with good collateral circulation can experience a 100% occlusion of a coronary artery without suffering an MI.

Clinical Manifestations

Chest pain

The patient with an MI usually comes to the hospital with chest pain related to myocardial ischemia. The chest pain is often reported as severe, crushing, squeezing, stabbing, or burning and lasts longer than 15 to 30 minutes. It is usually substernal and can radiate to the neck, jaw, and left arm, hand, and shoulder. It is not relieved by rest or nitroglycerin. The pain may be epigastric and mistaken for gastrointestinal disorders, such as indigestion or the flu. Less commonly, the pain may radiate to the right arm or intrascapular region, or it may not be any more severe than a typical anginal attack.

Patients may also present with a wide variety of associated symptoms, including diaphoresis, pallor,

TABLE 35-2   Location of MI and Structures Affected by Coronary Artery Occlusion

Coronary artery	Location of MI	Structures/functions affected
Left main	70% of left ventricle	
Left anterior descending	Anterior MI	Anterior wall of left ventricle, anterior septum, papillary muscle, bundle of His, bundle branches
Left circumflex	Lateral MI	Lateral or inferoposterior wall of left ventricle
Right coronary artery	Inferoposterior MI, right ventricular MI	Inferoposterior wall of left ventricle, right ventricle, inferior septum, papillary muscle, AV node

nausea and vomiting, weakness, palpitations, or disorientation.

Most patients with an MI appear anxious or distressed or have a sense of impending doom. Vital signs are variable even without complications. Initially the heart rate may be rapid (100 to 120 beats/min) and the blood pressure elevated as a result of pain, anxiety, and sympathetic stimulation. However, the heart rate may be slow and the blood pressure low if parasympathetic (vagal) activity predominates. The respiratory rate is often increased until pain and anxiety are relieved. Fever up to 38.3° C (101° F) and a mild leukocytosis develop over the first day or two because of myocardial necrosis, which usually resolves within 1 week.

In the absence of complications the heart and lung examination is essentially normal. The heart sounds may be muffled, however, and a fourth heart sound (S_4) can be auscultated in the presence of decreased left ventricular compliance. When left ventricular failure is present, heart examination will reveal a third heart sound (S_3) on auscultation and crackles will be heard over the lung fields. Jugular venous distention may be present if right-sided heart failure occurs.

Diagnostic studies

The diagnosis of MI is based primarily on the patient history combined with 12-lead ECG analysis and elevated cardiac enzymes.

When myocardial cells are injured, the cell membranes lose their integrity and intracellular enzymes are released. The extent of cardiac enzyme elevation is relative to infarct size. The different enzymes enter the circulation at varying intervals and are characterized by a rise, a peak, and a return to normal levels (Table 35-3).

Lactic dehydrogenase (LDH) has two isoenzymes that are specific to myocardial tissue: LDH_1 and LDH_2. Normally LDH_2 is greater than LDH_1, but within 8 to 24 hours of heart muscle damage, these isoenzymes become "flipped" and LDH_1 exceeds LDH_2.

Serial readings of the 12-lead ECG provide information about the size, location, evolution, and resolution of the ischemia, injury, and infarction occurring in the heart muscle. ECG changes generally occur within 2 to 12 hours of the event but occasionally may take 72 to 96 hours to be manifested. The 12-lead ECG shows changes in the leads facing the area of MI (Figure 35-8). In transmural MI, ST segment elevation appears first, followed by T wave inversion and the development of abnormal Q waves. In subendocardial MI there is usually ST segment

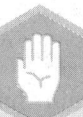 CLINICAL ALERT

Some patients do not experience chest pain, especially elderly persons or patients with diabetes mellitus, and initially exhibit symptoms of decreased cardiac output, such as shortness of breath, changes in sensorium, or syncope. A "silent" MI, which may be unrecognized and nonfatal, is one in which there are no signs or symptoms.

TABLE 35-3 Enzyme Circulation at Varying Intervals

Enzyme	Rise	Peak	Return to normal
Creatine kinase	4 to 8 hours	12 to 24 hours	3 to 5 days
CK-MB	2 to 4 hours	12 to 20 hours	72 hours
Lactic dehydrogenase	24 hours	3 to 6 days	8 to 14 days

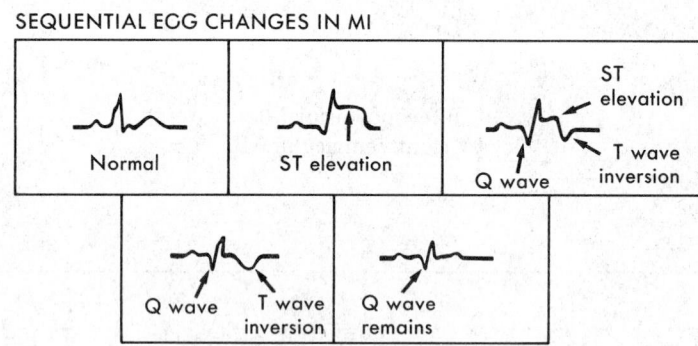

SEQUENTIAL ECG CHANGES IN MI

(in leads facing the area of MI)

FIGURE 35-8. Sequential ECG changes occurring in MI are shown. ECG leads that reflect location of MI are as follows:

Location of MI	Leads with ECG changes
Anterior	V_1 to V_4
Interior	II, III, AVF
Lateral	V_5, V_6, I, AVL

depression with T wave changes but no abnormal Q waves, hence the term non–Q wave infarction. As ischemia and injury resolve, the ST segment and T wave changes return to normal. In transmural infarctions the Q wave remains.

Nuclear cardiac imaging using injected radionuclide tracers may be performed to assess for perfusion and ventricular function. Thallium perfusion scans can detect size and location of myocardial ischemia and infarction. Radionuclide ventriculography and radionuclide angiography (RNA) can help to assess the significance of MI on ventricular performance. Positron emission tomography (PET) can be performed after an MI to differentiate the extent of irreversible damage or necrotic tissue from areas of reversible or ischemic damage. Echocardiography is an important imaging modality for determining abnormal ventricular contraction of a damaged myocardium.

Therapeutic Management

The goals of therapy are to prevent the extension of the infarct size and prevent complications. To limit the infarct size, early restoration of coronary blood flow must occur and an improved balance between oxygen supply and demand must be established. To best recognize and treat complications, patients are generally admitted to a cardiac care unit (CCU) for several days for close observation and management.

Pharmacologic therapy

Medical management to control pain and limit infarct size includes the use of oxygen, nitrates, morphine, beta blockers, angiotensin converting enzyme (ACE) inhibitors, and rest (Table 35-4). Nurses must prepare for administration of these therapies in their order of priority until the goals of pain management and prevention of complications are achieved. Medications for the patient with coronary artery disease are summarized in Table 35-1.

Oxygen administration is initiated immediately at 2 to 4 L/min via nasal cannula or face mask to improve oxygenation to ischemic heart muscle. Nitroglycerin (intravenous, sublingual, or in paste form) is administered for its coronary and peripheral vasodilating effects, improving myocardial oxygenation

TABLE 35-4   Pharmacology Summary: Myocardial Infarction Medications

Medication	Usual dosage	Effect	Side effects	Nursing implications
Angiotensin-converting enzyme (ACE) inhibitors (enalapril)	IV bolus: 1.25 mg over at least 5 min PO: 2.5-5 mg/day	Vasodilation: reduces myocardial oxygen demands Reduces release of aldosterone and decreases sodium and water reabsorption in kidneys	Hypotension Dizziness Nausea Diarrhea Hyponatremia	Monitor for orthostatic hypotension Supervise ambulation initially to ensure patient safety Monitor intake and output and daily weights to determine fluid loss; ascertain changes in electrolyte values
Aspirin	80-325 mg/day	Decreases platelet adhesion and decreases risk of myocardial thrombosis	Bleeding Gastrointestinal distress	Stress importance of observing for symptoms of gastrointestinal bleeding (black stools, persistent gastrointestinal distress) May take with meals
Digoxin	PO, IV loading dose: 0.5-1.5 mg divided over 24 hr; maintenance dose: 0.125-0.5 mg daily; doses may need to be decreased in elderly persons	Increases force of contraction Reduces heart rate by decreasing sympathetic stimulation	Bradycardia Hypotension Weakness Fatigue Toxicity: anorexia, nausea, visual green halos	Take apical pulse for 1 full minute before administration and notify physician if < 60; check K+ levels before administration; hypokalemia increases risk of toxicity Monitor serum levels (0.9-2 ng/mL is therapeutic)
Heparin	Dose adjusted to maintain PTT at one and one half to two times control value	Decreases thrombin production and reduces coronary artery reocclusion	Bleeding	Assess for overt or occult bleeding: bruising, guaiac-positive body fluids Can be reversed with protamine Place on bleeding precautions: avoid trauma; use soft toothbrush; use only electric razor; no rectal temperatures
Furosemide	IV: 20-40 mg given over 2 min PO: 40-80 mg every 12 hr; dose may be increased depending on response	Promotes diuresis by inhibiting sodium and chloride reabsorption in kidneys	Orthostatic hypotension Volume depletion Hypokalemia Hypocalcemia Hypomagnesemia	Monitor intake and output and daily weights to determine fluid loss; ascertain changes in electrolyte values Administer IV doses slowly: may cause transient or permanent deafness

Continued.

TABLE 35-4	Pharmacology Summary: Myocardial Infarction Medications—cont'd			
Medication	**Usual dosage**	**Effect**	**Side effects**	**Nursing implications**
Lidocaine	IV: 1 mg/kg, repeat with 0.5 mg/kg after 5-10 min (maximum dose = 3 mg/kg) Maintenance drip: 1 - 4 mg/min	Suppresses ventricular ectopy by decreasing excitability	Confusion Anxiety Numbness Twitching Convulsions Hypotension Tinnitus	Document baseline blood pressure, heart rate, ECG tracing, and lung sounds; repeat assessment every hour or with changes in dosage Titrate drip to control dysrhythmias
Morphine	IV: 4-8 mg initially, followed by 2-8 mg every 5 to 15 min until pain is relieved	Reduces anxiety Promotes analgesia Dilates peripheral arteries and veins	Hypotension Respiratory depression Nausea and vomiting Constipation	Monitor blood pressure and respiratory rate every 5-15 min; hold further doses if respiratory rate is less than 12/min or hypotension occurs If patient's condition allows, place patient in supine position to treat hypotension May be reversed with naloxone if respiratory depression occurs

and decreasing myocardial work by reducing afterload. Morphine, 2 to 8 mg, is frequently given as a bolus intravenously every 5 to 15 minutes as an analgesic, sedative, and peripheral vasodilator to relieve pain and anxiety and decrease the work load of the heart. Beta blockers can be administered to protect the heart from the effects of sympathetic stimulation, especially if the patient is tachycardic or hypertensive. ACE inhibition (enalapril) has been shown to improve survival in patients with mild to moderate heart failure after MI. ACE inhibitors not only dilate the peripheral vasculature but also suppress the neurohormonal responses of renin-angiotensin, vasopressin, and norepinephrine, decreasing myocardial work load and oxygen demand.

Thrombolytic agents

The use of thrombolytic agents early in the course of MI can restore blood flow and salvage injured myocardium in certain patients. **Thrombolytic agents** accelerate the natural fibrinolytic process by activating plasminogen. Plasminogen generates plasmin, an enzyme that dissolves clots. Successful coronary artery thrombolysis with subsequent reperfusion of the myocardium results in decreased infarct size, improved left ventricular function, and increased survival.

Each of the thrombolytic agents differs slightly in its mode of action, its length of hypocoagulability, and whether it acts systemically or is specific to a formed clot (Table 35-5). Some agents are manufactured synthetically and can cause an allergic reaction, exhibited by fever, rash, hypotension, or less commonly, bronchospasm. It is recommended that patients receiving these antigenic agents be premedicated with steroids and antihistamines. Therapy should be started within 4 to 6 hours of onset of infarction, but research is presently investigating its efficacy over longer periods of time. The most significant complications of treatment with all of these agents are bleeding and stroke. To prevent acute coronary reocclusion, which most frequently occurs within the first 24 hours after thrombolytic administration, most patients are given intravenous heparin and subsequently placed on aspirin/dipyridamole therapy for its anti−platelet-aggregating effect.

TABLE 35-5   Pharmacology Summary: Thrombolytic Agents

Agent	Antigenic	Half-life/length of activity	Clot specificity
Streptokinase	Yes	20 min; can persist for 18-24 hr	Poor; activation occurs throughout system
Tissue plasminogen activator (t-PA)	No; recombinant human protease	5 min	Clot specific; remains inactive until it encounters clot
Anisoylated plasminogen-streptokinase activator complex (APSAC)	Yes	90 min; can persist for 24-48 hr	Poor

Surgical Management

Percutaneous transluminal coronary angioplasty

PTCA is the mechanical dilation of a coronary artery with a balloon-tipped catheter. In patients with acute MI, PTCA can be used to open the occluded coronary artery as a primary treatment or after thrombolytic therapy fails to achieve reperfusion. Patients who are to undergo PTCA should also be candidates for coronary artery bypass surgery in the event of complications.

Coronary artery bypass graft surgery

Surgical revascularization with a coronary artery bypass graft can be performed within 4 to 6 hours of the onset of acute MI in order to limit infarct size. Patients whose infarct continues to evolve in size or who develop coronary occlusion during cardiac catheterization, coronary arteriography, or PTCA are also candidates for immediate coronary bypass surgery.

Complications

Dysrhythmias

Rhythm disturbances occur in most patients experiencing an MI, frequently within the first hour. Therefore patients are placed on continuous ECG monitoring to assess for dysrhythmias. After sinus tachycardia subsides with the alleviation of the stress response, sinus bradycardia becomes the most common dysrhythmia noted because of increased activity of the parasympathetic nervous system. This may be accompanied by hypotension. Conduction disturbances such as varying degrees of heart block may be caused by ischemic injury to the conduction system, depending on the involved coronary artery.

Supraventricular tachycardias such as atrial tachycardia, atrial flutter, or atrial fibrillation can be initiated by sympathetic nervous system stimulation, distention of the atria secondary to heart failure, or less commonly, as a result of ischemic injury to the atria. Ventricular dysrhythmias including premature ventricular contractions (PVCs), ventricular tachycardia, and ventricular fibrillation are also seen after acute MI.

Dysrhythmias are treated pharmacologically when their presence causes hypotension, causes decreased oxygen supply to the myocardium, or places the patient at risk for developing life-threatening rhythms, such as ventricular tachycardia and fibrillation. Lidocaine is the drug of choice in treating the ventricular dysrhythmias. It is first administered as an intravenous bolus of 1 mg/kg followed by a maintenance infusion of 1 to 4 mg/min. If sympathetic stimulation is thought to be contributing to the frequency of PVCs, the patient may receive a beta-adrenergic blocking agent, such as propranolol, to reduce their occurrence. Life-threatening rhythms are treated with defibrillation if medications do not alleviate them. Atropine or temporary pacemaker insertion may be required for bradycardias and heart blocks.

Congestive heart failure/cardiogenic shock

Cardiac failure, which causes the signs and symptoms of congestive heart failure (CHF), may occur in varying degrees in patients after an MI. Decreased cardiac output caused by damage to the heart muscle underlies many of the complications of MI. This is usually caused by left ventricular damage or dysfunction and, although not as common, by right ventricular failure, which can occur after right ventricular infarction.

The presence and severity of the signs and symp-

THROMBOLYTICS FOR MYOCARDIAL INFARCTION

Patient selection

1. Acute MI symptoms present for less than 6 hours
2. ECG evidence of MI

Contraindications

1. Bleeding or bleeding disorders, such as hemophilia or thrombocytopenia
2. History of cerebrovascular accident with residual symptoms or other intracranial disorders, such as cerebral aneurysm, intracranial neoplasm, or surgery
3. Severe uncontrolled hypertension

Used with caution

1. Recent major surgery, pregnancy or delivery, trauma, gastrointestinal/genitourinary bleeding, recent cardiopulmonary resuscitation (CPR)

Patient management

1. At risk for bleeding related to altered hemostasis:
   a. Assess nervous system status for signs of intracranial hemorrhage, such as headache, changes in level of consciousness, muscle weakness.
   b. Assess blood pressure and heart rate for signs of possible concealed hemorrhage, such as gastrointestinal bleeding, recognizing signs and symptoms of potential side effects of thrombolytic agents and effects of MI that may decrease blood pressure and increase heart rate.
   c. Monitor for signs of bleeding from puncture sites, gastrointestinal/genitourinary systems, gums, body fluids. Apply pressure to surface bleeding sites; most common is the site of catheter insertion.
   d. Implement bleeding precautions: minimize puncture sites; careful patient handling; use electric razors only; no rectal temperatures.
   e. Monitor partial thromboplastin time (PTT) and complete blood counts; PTT should be maintained at 1½ to 2 times normal for adequate anticoagulation.
   f. Be prepared to administer blood or fresh frozen plasma if significant bleeding occurs.
2. At risk for chest pain related to reocclusion:
   a. Monitor chest pain, ECG findings (usually ST segment elevation), cardiac enzymes, and cardiac dysrhythmias.
   b. Maintain anticoagulant and antiplatelet therapy.
   c. Treat ischemic signs and symptoms as would treat an angina attack or MI; reocclusion occurs most frequently in first 24 hours after treatment.

toms of CHF depend on the size and location of the damaged myocardium. CHF can occur when 20% to 35% of the left ventricle is damaged. The blood pressure and heart rate may be maintained despite the presence of CHF after an MI by the body's activation of the sympathetic nervous system, fluid retention by the kidneys, and increased oxygen extraction to the tissues. As these compensatory mechanisms become inadequate, signs and symptoms of heart failure will occur. When over 40% of the myocardium is damaged, cardiogenic shock ensues. In cardiogenic shock the severely damaged left ventricle cannot maintain systemic perfusion. The patient becomes hypotensive, tachycardic, oliguric, hypoxic, and obtunded.

The goals of treatment for heart failure are to reduce the myocardial work load by reducing circulating blood volume and improving myocardial contractility.

Structural changes

Myocardial rupture of acutely infarcted tissue can involve the papillary muscles, the interventricular septum, or the free wall of the ventricle. The incidence of myocardial rupture is greater in elderly patients. With rupture of a papillary muscle the valve leaflets of the affected valve become incompetent and regurgitation or back flow of blood causes decreased cardiac output and shock. Shock occurs with rupture of the septum caused by blood moving from the left ventricle back into the right ventricle rather than out the aorta, called left to right shunting, thereby decreasing the output from the left ventricle. Rupture of the free wall of the ventricle allows blood to accumulate in the pericardial sac and usually leads to death from cardiac tamponade.

Immediate treatment of these acute complications is imperative to prevent death. Early recognition and stabilization with inotropic drug therapy such as dopamine or dobutamine and intra-aortic balloon pump support are necessary to maintain the patient while preparing for emergency surgery.

Ventricular aneurysm is a less life-threatening structural change that can occur after MI. The damaged myocardial wall is thinned and can become stretched to form a noncontractile outpouching. Blood can become trapped in the outpouching, decreasing cardiac output and causing heart failure. Ischemia from decreased cardiac output and coronary blood flow can produce ventricular dysrhythmias and angina. Control of dysrhythmias and surgical aneurysmectomy can be successful in treating this complication.

Pericarditis

Contact of the pericardium with the damaged myocardial tissue may cause pericarditis in the first several days after infarct or less commonly, in

Dressler's syndrome occurring several weeks after infarct. The patient usually complains of chest pain that worsens on inspiration and is relieved by sitting up. It may be accompanied by fever, generalized malaise, and a pericardial friction rub. Medication to relieve pain and inflammation, such as aspirin and nonsteroidal anti-inflammatory drugs, is successful in treating these patients.

Postinfarction angina

Postinfarction angina with or without extension of the infarct may complicate an MI. If the pain is caused by an increasing size of infarcted myocardium, it adversely affects recovery. Revascularization procedures may be required to prevent further myocardial damage.

Thromboembolic events

The incidence of thromboembolic complications has decreased as a result of early mobilization. However, emboli may occur from deep-vein thrombosis or left ventricular thrombi, especially in the patient with heart failure or prolonged bed rest.

NURSING MANAGEMENT OF THE PATIENT WITH MYOCARDIAL INFARCTION

Assessment

The nursing history for a patient experiencing an MI includes detailed information regarding the patient's chest pain. Ask the patient to describe the pain and compare it with pain experienced in the past. The description of pain includes onset, duration, location, radiation, precipitating and aggravating factors, and associated symptoms. Elicit from the patient how these symptoms differ from previous anginal symptoms.

A risk factor profile is obtained as in CAD to identify teaching needs. The history also includes information regarding prior health status such as current medications, allergies, recent surgeries or trauma, presence of ulcers, and drug and alcohol use. This information is helpful in determining contraindications for thrombolytic therapy. A psychosocial history is obtained regarding the patient and family's responses to illness and hospitalization, support systems, coping mechanisms, and potential caregivers.

Physical assessment of the patient with an MI includes blood pressure, heart rate, rhythm and heart sounds, respiratory rate and breath sounds, and temperature. Assessments should be performed every 15 minutes to 1 hour to promptly detect any changes or complications. A 12-lead ECG is documented immediately and with any subsequent reports of chest pain. Continuous ECG monitoring is initiated to determine changes in heart rate or rhythm.

The patient's mentation is observed, since it is a sensitive indicator of decreased cerebral perfusion caused by decreased cardiac output. Observation of the skin is also important, since pallor and diaphoresis may also indicate a falling cardiac output. The periphery is assessed for pulses, temperature, and the presence of edema. A decreased urinary output and increased specific gravity may be early indicators of cardiogenic shock. Patients who have received thrombolytics or anticoagulants are observed for signs of bleeding, such as gingival and puncture site bleeding, guaiac-positive stool and emesis, or hematuria. Patients who have undergone PTCA are assessed for hematoma formation or bleeding from the catheter insertion site, for changes in peripheral pulses in the involved extremity, and for chest pain, which may indicate abrupt closure of the coronary artery.

Laboratory data are monitored for abnormalities. These include cardiac enzymes, electrolytes, blood gases, blood counts, clotting studies, chemistries, and lipid and drug levels.

Invasive hemodynamic monitoring, including arterial and pulmonary artery catheters, may be used to monitor acutely ill patients for signs of cardiac failure.

Nursing Diagnosis

Nursing assessment data collected from patients with an MI usually indicate the following nursing diagnoses:

Pain (acute) related to myocardial ischemia

Anxiety (severe) related to pain, fear of death, and hospital environment

High risk for decreased cardiac output related to impaired left ventricular contractility, dysrhythmias, or complications

Activity intolerance related to decreased cardiac output

Knowledge deficit about the disease process and therapeutic regimen

Another possible nursing diagnosis for the patient after PTCA is as follows:

High risk for fluid volume deficit secondary to bleeding caused by anticoagulation and thrombolytic therapy

Planning

Priorities for nursing care include those interventions that will achieve relief and prevention of chest pain, hemodynamic stability, psychologic comfort, and adherence to a self-care program.

Expected outcomes for the patient with an MI include the following:

Relief of chest pain

Verbalization of fears, concerns, and questions

Reduction of anxiety

Adequate cardiac output as demonstrated by no

NURSING CARE PLAN   *The Patient with Myocardial Infarction*

Nursing diagnosis/ Expected outcome	Interventions	Rationale
High risk for decreased cardiac output related to impaired left ventricular contractility, dysrhythmias, or complications • *Patient will exhibit hemodynamic stability as evidenced by vital signs within patient's normal range; no dysrhythmias; no change in heart sounds; clear breath sounds; urine output greater than 30 mL/hr; warm, dry skin; no changes in mentation*	Monitor blood pressure every 1 to 2 hours or as prescribed; evaluate pulse pressure for pulsus paradoxus or pulsus alternans	Hypertension can increase myocardial work while hypotension can decrease coronary artery perfusion; a decreased pulse pressure (the difference between systolic and diastolic pressures) may be seen after an MI and is an early indicator of decreased cardiac output Clinical indicator for complication of cardiac tamponade Clinical indicator for complication of left ventricular failure
	Monitor apical and radial heart rate and rhythm every 1 to 2 hours or as prescribed	Discrepancies in apical and radial heart rates can indicate presence of ventricular dysrhythmias
	Record and document an ECG rhythm strip every 4 hours	Dysrhythmias will decrease cardiac output
	Evaluate respiratory rate and breath sounds every 2 to 4 hours	Shortness of breath and crackles can indicate left ventricular failure, pulmonary edema, or pulmonary embolus
	Note presence of jugular venous dististention	
	Evaluate heart sounds for changes or additional heart sounds	S_3 may indicate ventricular failure; S_4 is commonly heard as a result of blood hitting stiffened ventricular wall; friction rub may result from pericarditis; murmurs may be caused by valvular regurgitation because of valve or papillary muscle dysfunction
	Assess skin color, temperature, and peripheral pulses	Provides an indication of adequacy of peripheral perfusion
	Assess for presence of peripheral edema in periorbital and sacral areas if patient is on bed rest; in ankles and tibial regions of legs if patient is ambulatory	Occurs in presence of ventricular failure
	Be alert for changes in level of consciousness, restlessness, or confusion	Change in level of consciousness is one of the first signs of decreased cardiac output
	Monitor temperature every 4 hours or as indicated	Most patients develop low-grade fever because of tissue necrosis
	Monitor intake, output, and urine specific gravity	Decrease in urine output with increase in specific gravity can reflect decrease in renal perfusion
	Assist patient to rise slowly from supine position; encourage patient to sit on side of bed with feet on floor before getting out of bed	Reduces orthostatic hypotension
	Instruct patient not to cross legs while in bed or sitting	Decreases perfusion in lower extremities, which increases risk of thrombus formation
	Administer medications as prescribed	Increases myocardial oxygen supply while decreasing oxygen demand

hypotension (systolic blood pressure greater than 90 mm Hg); breath sounds clear, no crackles; urine output greater than 30 mL/hr; skin warm and dry; good peripheral pulses; normal mentation; heart rate and rhythm within normal parameters for patient's baseline
- Verbalization of knowledge of disease process and therapeutic regimen
- Performance of activities of daily living (ADL) without pain or fatigue

Implementation

On admission the patient is immediately placed on bed rest with a cardiac monitor and oxygen via nasal cannula or face mask at 2 to 4 L/min. A series of 12-lead ECGs is begun to establish the site of infarction and presence of changes representing ischemia and infarction or the presence of dysrhythmias. An intravenous line is established to provide a route for the administration of medications, such as nitroglycerin, morphine, or antidysrhythmics. Intramuscular injections are avoided to prevent elevation of muscle enzymes and because intravenous medications are more rapidly and better absorbed. The monitor alarms are set to notify the nurse of changes in the ECG rate and rhythm, and emergency equipment is available and functioning properly.

The patient is instructed to tell the nurse if any chest pain or shortness of breath occurs. Any change in the patient's condition must be promptly reported to the physician. Some hospitals have "standing orders" that permit the nurse to initiate therapy in the absence of a physician. An example of a standing order is to "administer 1 mg/kg lidocaine IV bolus for sustained ventricular tachycardia."

Some institutions have cardiac teams who assess the patient's condition for appropriateness of immediate thrombolytic therapy. If the patient is a candidate, thrombolytics will be administered immediately. During and after administration, patients must be monitored continuously for bleeding, vital sign changes, ECG changes, level of consciousness, and relief of pain.

Emotional support

Interventions to lessen the psychologic impact of MI on the patient and family are continuously provided. The patient and family are encouraged to express their feelings, concerns, and questions. Causes of anxiety in patients and families vary and may include pain, hospitalization, changes in role and self-image, alterations in daily living or work patterns, and financial concerns. The nurse addresses concerns that are specific to the patient and family in order to relieve anxiety. The nurse offers reinforcement, reassurance, and repetition of information as

THERAPEUTIC COMMUNICATION GUIDE

Myocardial Infarction Patient

Assessment

Assess threat of illness to person's self-esteem and sense of identity.

Example	*Patient:*	"I feel like I'm never going to be normal again. I'm not sure I'll ever be a man again after this heart attack."
	Nurse:	"Mr. Sullivan, please tell me how you think your heart attack will affect your life."

Intervention

Clarify patient's concerns through restatement.

Example	*Patient:*	"Well, I have a friend who had a heart attack, and he couldn't work full time anymore. He was tired and stressed, and he lost interest in sex. Now he and his wife argue a lot."
	Nurse:	"Are you afraid that you won't be able to hold down a job or have sex with your wife?"

Accept feelings of anger.

Example	*Patient:*	"Yes. (Several profane statements) heart attack. It's not my fault I had a heart attack."
	Nurse:	"Mr. Sullivan, it's okay for you to feel upset. Most patients are able to resume their normal lives again, depending on the extent of damage. You can talk with your doctor about returning to work. I can help you find answers to your concerns."

often as necessary. The patient and family's level of understanding is often decreased because of psychologic and physiologic stress.

Other emotional responses to MI include denial, anger, and depression. Acceptance of these responses as normal immediately after an MI is important. The nurse tries to help the patient cope with these feelings by active listening, reflecting, and guiding the patient. A referral for counseling may be indicated when the patient's own coping mechanisms and support systems are not successful in working through these responses.

Activity

Initial activity restrictions generally include bed rest with bedside commode privileges for the first 24 to 48 hours. The patient is allowed to feed himself or herself and assist with the bed bath. No isometric activity, such as straining, is allowed. Stool softeners are ordered to help prevent straining and constipation. While the patient is on bed rest, encourage active range of motion, such as plantar flexion and dorsiflexion of the feet and knee bends to prevent venous stasis, which can lead to thrombus formation. Activity progresses to chair sitting, limited ambulation around the room by day 3 or 4, and then hall ambulation. Activity progression with an emphasis on self-care provides positive reinforcement for the patient.

The level of activity appropriate for each stage of recovery is measured by the amount of energy used for that activity and is expressed in metabolic equivalents (METs). At rest a person uses 3.5 mL of oxygen/kg/min, or 1 MET. Self-care activities range from 1 to 3 METs and are considered very light activities (Table 35-6). To decrease oxygen demands on the heart, in-hospital activity is frequently kept in the very light range with the exception of the use of the commode. Provide the patient with options for quiet diversional activities such as reading, listening to music, puzzles, or crafts to provide mental diversions and promote coping with inactivity.

Activity progression is based on the patient's physiologic response. Activity tolerance is determined using criteria such as the following:
- Heart rate increase less than 20 beats/min
- No decrease in systolic blood pressure
- No chest pain, dyspnea, or extreme fatigue
- No dysrhythmias

As long as the criteria are met, activity progression continues. The nurse teaches the patient to be aware of adverse symptoms and to stop activity if they occur.

Diet

A low-cholesterol, salt-restricted (2 g, 4 g, or no salt added) diet is recommended. Caffeine (coffee, tea, colas) should be avoided, since it increases cardiac work. If nausea and vomiting are present, the diet is limited to liquids, and antiemetics are given.

TABLE 35-6   MET* Levels of Various Activities

Very light activity (1 to 3 METs)	Light activity (3 to 5 METs)	Moderate activity (5 to 8 METs)	Heavy activity (8 to 10 METs)
Eating	Commode (3.6)	Stair climbing (4 to 8)	Carrying loads upstairs
Dressing	Bedpan (4.7)	Snow shoveling	Snow shoveling (wet)
Bathing	Housework	Carpentry (2 to 7)	Moving heavy objects (>75 lb)
Driving	Stair climbing (one flight)	Jogging 5 mph	Cross-country skiing
Cooking	Sexual activity (orgasm 4 to 6)	Singles tennis	Handball
Walking ≤2 mph	Raking leaves	Downhill skiing	Jumping rope
Bowling	Walking ≤4 mph	Swimming	
Golfing (cart)	Lifting <30 lb	Skating	
	Gardening (3 to 8)	Basketball	
	Calisthenics	Lawn mowing (hand)	
	Social dancing		
	Cycling <8 mph		
	Lawn mowing (power)		

*1 MET (metabolic equivalent) is the amount of energy used at rest, or 3.5 mL O_2/kg/min.

Patient education

As soon as possible the nurse begins preparing the patient and family for discharge. The nurse provides both verbal and written information about the disease process, medications, and activity (see "Patient Education Guide"). Patient teaching should also include information about risk factor modification and diet restrictions. The patient and family are instructed about problems that should be reported to a health care provider. Throughout the teaching process the nurse encourages the patient and family to ask questions.

Evaluation

The patient's response to care is evaluated in terms of progress toward goal achievement. The patient must be free of chest pain and hemodynamically stable for at least several days before discharge. A patient with an uncomplicated MI may be discharged in 6 to 10 days. Medications may need to be adjusted, or further testing, such as exercise testing, and treatments may be necessary to meet these goals. When complications occur, progress will be slowed and goals may need to be changed. For example, a patient with a ventricular aneurysm may

---

PATIENT EDUCATION GUIDE *Myocardial Infarction*

During the acute phase, limit patient teaching to simple, concrete explanations and directions since the patient's comprehension and retention of information will be limited because of anxiety, pain, and narcotic analgesic administration. As soon as feasible, however, the patient and family should begin preparation for discharge. Both verbal and written instruction is provided so that the patient and family can ask questions during hospitalization and have reference material at home to reinforce teaching.

Objective: Patient will regain maximal independent functioning within the limitations of disease.

1. Understanding of cardiac condition
   a. Explain basic cardiac anatomy and physiology.
   b. Describe in simple terms the differences among coronary artery disease, angina, and myocardial infarction.
   c. Discuss how the heart heals following an MI.
2. Chest pain management
   a. Stop activity and rest.
   b. Take nitroglycerin sublingually every 5 minutes for three doses.
   c. If not relieved, call physician or go immediately to the emergency room.
   d. Avoid activities that have been identified as precipitating pain (see patient education guide on CAD).
3. Activity
   a. Identify the basic principles of activity progression.
      (1) Increase activity levels gradually.
      (2) Stop activity if chest pain, shortness of breath, dizziness, or extreme fatigue occurs.
      (3) Avoid lifting heavy objects, isometric activities, straining, or pushing.
      (4) Ensure adequate sleep with daily rest periods.
      (5) Avoid extremes in temperature.
      (6) Avoid tension and stressful activities.

     (7) Eat several small meals per day rather than two or three large meals.
   b. Describe activity regimen and progression.
      (1) Discuss with physician the amount, type, and frequency of daily activities.
      (2) Identify time intervals to progress activities, such as work, driving, aerobic exercise, and lifting.
      (3) Determine pulse rate before and after activity to identify acceptable increases in heart rate.
      (4) Resume sexual relations with physician recommendation and when able to climb two flights of stairs without developing chest pain or shortness of breath; avoid sexual activity with unfamiliar partner, after eating a heavy meal, after drinking alcohol, or when tired.
4. Medications
   a. State purpose, dose, and side effects of each drug.
   b. Design a routine within daily structure when medications will be remembered.
5. Risk factors (see patient education guide on CAD)
6. Diet
   a. Consult dietitian to review and reinforce prescribed diet (low fat, low sodium).
   b. Ensure that primary caregiver has diet instructions.
7. Signs and symptoms to report to the physician
   a. Chest pain or pressure that is not relieved in 15 minutes with nitroglycerin and rest.
   b. Increased shortness of breath.
   c. Increased swelling of feet and ankles.
   d. Rapid weight gain (i.e., 2 to 4 pounds in 1 day).
   e. Unusual fatigue.
   f. Dizziness or fainting.
   g. Palpitations or unusually fast or slow heartbeat.
   h. Side effects of medications.

experience sustained dysrhythmias, or a patient with heart failure may experience sustained dyspnea.

For optimal activity progression, the patient should be able to perform self-care activities such as bathing and dressing. If stairs are present in the home, stair climbing (3.5 to 4 METs) should be a goal and should be performed in the hospital under monitored conditions. A low-intensity exercise test is frequently done before discharge to help evaluate the patient's activity tolerance and often gives the patient needed confidence in his or her abilities.

Psychologic comfort is evaluated by the patient's verbal and nonverbal cues. Patient and family verbalization of fears and concerns is important. However, if the patient states lack of nervousness but experiences sleeplessness and anorexia, further exploration of emotional status is necessary. Another example of difficulties identified during evaluation is the unresolved denial of some patients. They may be psychologically comfortable, but denial puts them at high risk for noncompliance with the necessary lifestyle changes.

Documentation

Key points in documentation for the patient with an MI are risk factor profile; ongoing monitoring for signs and symptoms of complications, particularly the occurrence of changes in vital signs, chest pain, or dyspnea; response to pharmacologic therapy for symptom management; activity tolerance; and level of understanding related to learning objectives.

Ongoing Care

Once the patient is discharged from the hospital, the overall prognosis is good for MI patients without left ventricular dysfunction, continued ischemia as evidenced by further episodes of chest pain, or activity intolerance. The focus of ongoing care is on the patient's opportunity to follow healthy living patterns with improved well-being. Many patients with uncomplicated MIs actually feel better after their convalescence and changed life-style than before their MI. Most patients return to work within 8 to 12 weeks. Delays in return to work tend to be psychosocial in nature rather than physical in uncomplicated MIs.

Cardiac rehabilitation

Cardiac rehabilitation is a comprehensive program to help the cardiac patient achieve and maintain optimal health and well-being. For the MI patient the rehabilitation process begins with hospitalization and continues indefinitely (Table 35-7). Cardiac rehabilitation may be accomplished through a struc-

TABLE 35-7   Cardiac Rehabilitation

Phase	Focus
Inpatient	Education
	Low-level activity
	Discharge preparation
Convalescent	Education
	Exercise conditioning
	Risk factor reduction
	Positive psychologic outlook
	Resumption of role performance
Long-term	Maximal improvement/maintenance of cardiovascular fitness and risk factor control

tured hospital-based program or implemented by the patient with follow-up by hospital personnel. Risk factor reduction, cardiovascular fitness, and psychologic well-being are lifetime goals. The components of rehabilitation include education, counseling, activity progression, and medical therapy. A team approach is optimal involving the nurses, physicians, dietitians, psychologist, physical therapist, and vocational specialists.

Education
The overall purpose of ongoing education is to provide the patient with a sound basis for following health care management recommendations and for coping with MI. Knowledge is only a first step; the patient must use that knowledge to pursue a healthy life-style. Hospital teaching is supplemented and reinforced after discharge to improve the patient's ability to make necessary life-style changes. Once the patient is home, educational support is provided through reading materials, telephone and office follow-up, and referral to group activities or organizations such as the local chapter of the American Heart Association. The patient is encouraged to write down questions as they arise so they will not be forgotten during follow-up visits. Risk factor reduction, such as behavior modification for stress, smoking, or dieting, may also be supported through these methods.

Counseling
It is typical for the patient to have "post-MI" or "homecoming" depression or anxiety as a result of

fatigue, worry, alteration in self-concept, and unwelcome restrictions. Reassurance, physical conditioning, and education usually relieve this short-term situational depression. Group rehabilitation programs can foster a positive psychologic outlook. However, psychotherapy may be necessary if the depression is severe or prolonged. The patient's family may also experience emotional stress such as fear, frustration, or guilt. They should be encouraged to discuss their feelings, and they should be reassured these stresses will decrease as the patient recovers. It is not unusual for family members to be overprotective of the patient, but they should be sensitized to the fact that this is usually an unnecessary strain on both the patient and themselves. Education helps the family have realistic expectations about home care management. Families should be encouraged to be supportive of the life-style changes necessary for the patient but not made to feel responsible for the success of their implementation.

Activity progression

A major concern of newly discharged patients is activity progression. The patient can immediately resume light household tasks and leisure activities such as cooking. Several rest periods throughout the day are encouraged until the patient is free of the normal fatigue experienced after MI. This fatigue is most often not a result of decreased cardiac performance, but a result of the deconditioning effects of reduced muscle activity during hospitalization. A gradual increase in activity is important to recondition the muscles and prevent excessive cardiac demand. The patient should be taught to avoid isometric activity such as lifting, pushing, or straining. Isometric activity causes a sudden increase in muscular tension and vascular resistance, placing an excessive strain on the heart.

Exercise programs are the mainstay of improving and maintaining cardiovascular fitness. An individualized "exercise prescription" describes the recommended exercise in regard to type (such as walking, treadmill, cycling), intensity, frequency, and duration. Intensity, or how hard the patient should work, is usually based on a target heart rate derived from an exercise stress test. The patient's perceived exertion may also be used as an intensity gauge. Frequency is important, since regular exercise is necessary to achieve conditioning. Duration must include a warm-up and cool-down period. The exercise prescription is updated frequently as the patient progresses and tolerates higher work loads.

During the first weeks of reconditioning and myocardial healing, the patient is prescribed limited low-intensity exercise such as walking. At approximately 6 weeks after MI, aerobic training is begun to achieve exercise conditioning. A maximal, symptom-limited exercise stress test is usually per-

RESEARCH BRIEF

Hilgenberg C et al: Changes in family patterns six months after a myocardial infarction, *J Cardiovasc Nurs* 6(2):46-56, 1992.

Changes in patients', spouses', and children's life patterns 3 and 6 months after a patient experienced a myocardial infarction were investigated in this descriptive study. A convenience sample of 15 patients who had experienced an MI were interviewed using an interview guide. The broad categories of changes that emerged from the data analysis consisted of changes in family and social activities, emotions, and personal life-style habits. Patients, spouses, and children reported a continued decrease in family and social activities, an increase in worries and fears about the future, and a continued struggle with changes in diet and smoking habits. A positive change that was noted 6 months after discharge was an increase in feelings of family closeness. More than half the patients and families also described continued feelings of overprotectiveness 6 months after the patient had experienced an MI. These findings have implications for family teaching, discharge planning, and home health care. The focus of teaching during hospitalization and at discharge should help patients and families anticipate stressful situations and make provisions for dealing with them. The changes experienced by families suggest that they also should be included in the patient's rehabilitation plan. The nurse can also help to emphasize the positive aspects of recovery.

formed at this point. The patient performs at least 30 minutes of continuous, isotonic, rhythmic exercise such as cycling, brisk walking, or jogging at least three to five times per week. Patients with poor left ventricular function or other complications of MI usually stay with low-intensity exercise and gradually increase duration rather than intensity. Patients should be taught to "listen to their bodies." Increasing shortness of breath or chest pain during exercise is an indication to stop and rest. It is important for patients to be aware of what symptoms to report to their physician such as changes in chest pain or an increase in shortness of breath. For all patients, changes in pharmacologic therapy may be necessary if symptoms develop during activity progression. For example, the patient may need to take a sublingual nitroglycerin tablet before exercising.

Exercise programs may be supervised or unsupervised. Low-risk patients can progress well in a self-monitored program such as a walking program. Supervised programs may be recommended, especially for patients with left ventricular dysfunction or dysrhythmias. Supervised programs allow nurses or physicians to closely monitor for complications, activity intolerance, and noncompliance. Rehabilitation in the group setting also provides for increased psychologic support, reassurance, and motivation.

Sexual activity

Resumption of sexual activity may be an anxiety-producing aspect of activity progression for both the patient and partner. A frank discussion with clear information regarding sexual activity guidelines is helpful. Sex requires the same amount of energy as climbing two flights of stairs (4 to 6 METs during orgasm), which can be used as a guideline for when it is safe to resume sexual activity (usually 4 to 8 weeks after an MI). Some medications may adversely affect sexual desire or ability and should be brought to the attention of the physician.

Medical therapy

Antianginal medications such as nitroglycerin used after MI are necessary for symptom control and improving the balance between myocardial oxygen supply and demand. In addition, the use of beta blockers such as propranolol and aspirin has been shown to decrease the risk of another MI (secondary prevention). Aggressive ongoing care results in positive patient outcomes. Quality of life is enhanced through physical and psychologic recovery, improvement in functional abilities, and secondary prevention through risk factor reduction and medical therapy.

PERICARDITIS
Definition

Pericarditis refers to an inflammation of the pericardium, the membrane surrounding the heart.

Etiology/Epidemiology

Pericarditis may be caused by a variety of etiologic factors. The pericardium may be either primarily affected or secondarily affected, and the onset can vary from insidious to abrupt. Some instances are benign, self-limited, and managed without hospitalization, whereas others involve hemodynamic instability that can progress rapidly to death. The prognosis depends on the underlying cause and the occurrence of complications such as cardiac tamponade or pericardial constriction.

Although the most common cause of pericarditis is idiopathic, there are a variety of other causes, which can be classified as infectious, noninfectious, or autoimmune (Table 35-8). *Infectious* causes include viral (influenza, coxsackievirus), bacterial, tuberculous, fungal, or parasitic etiologic factors. *Noninfectious* causes are acute MI, trauma, severe chronic anemia, thoracic irradiation, myxedema, and aortic aneurysm with leakage into the pericardial sac. Any cancer in the chest, such as lymphomas or Hodgkin's disease, may lead to pericarditis. Causes of *autoimmune* pericarditis include postmyocardial infarction (Dressler's) syndrome, which generally occurs within 1 to 4 weeks after infarction; postpericardotomy syndrome (including pacemaker implantation); rheumatic disease; and rheumatic fever. Collagen vascular diseases, such as systemic lupus erythematosus, can also lead to pericarditis. Drugs that can cause pericarditis include procainamide, hydralazine, and phenytoin.

Pathophysiology

In pericarditis the two layers of the pericardium are inflamed and roughened. An inflammation of the pericardium may be acute or chronic, depending on the rate, severity, and duration of symptoms. Acute pericarditis may be classified as fibrinous (dry or inflammatory) or effusive, and it usually lasts less than

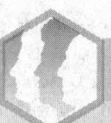

GERIATRIC CONSIDERATIONS

The Elderly Patient with Acute Myocardial Infarction

The principles of diagnosis and treatment of the elderly patient with acute MI are the same as those of younger patients, but a few general factors need to be considered. Retrospective studies indicate that patients over 65 to 70 years of age may be at higher risk of complications after an MI possibly because of the aging process of all the body's systems. The nurse must be especially vigilant in evaluating and reporting changes in assessment parameters that may indicate complications. Medications such as morphine, lidocaine, and digitalis may need to be administered at lower doses. Beta-adrenergic blocking agents, such as propranolol, may require higher doses in elderly patients to obtain therapeutic effects because of the decreased number of sympathetic receptors. The elderly patient who has led a sedentary life may require a slower activity progression. Supervised cardiac rehabilitation programs are recommended for elderly patients, especially those who have any signs or symptoms of complications, in order that they may be physically monitored during their exercise regimen. Risk factor modification, including smoking cessation and control of hypertension and hyperglycemia, is considered beneficial in reducing future risk of MI, whereas extensive dietary modifications may be unrealistic and of less certain short-term benefit in the elderly patient.

TABLE 35-8	Etiology of Pericarditis	
Infectious	**Noninfectious**	**Autoimmune**
Virus	Acute myocardial infarction	Dressler's syndrome
Bacteria	Trauma	Postpericardiotomy syndrome
Tuberculous	Uremia	
Fungus	Severe chronic anemia	
Parasite	Thoracic irradiation	Rheumatic disease
	Myxedema	Systemic lupus erythematosus
	Aortic aneurysm	Drugs
	Neoplasm	

6 weeks. In acute fibrinous pericarditis, localized or generalized deposits of fibrin cause the pericardium to become rigid and unable to stretch. The prognosis of acute pericarditis depends on the underlying cause, but it is generally good unless constriction occurs.

In cases of fibrosis, constriction of the stiffened pericardium decreases cardiac compliance, increasing the pressure around the heart (constrictive pericarditis). The pressure may impede cardiac filling. When less blood fills the heart, less is ejected and cardiac output decreases.

Chronic pericarditis is usually the result of a recurrence of a preexisting condition, such as uremia or systemic lupus erythematosus, and rarely represents reinfection by an organism. Chronic forms generally last between 6 weeks and 6 months but may last longer. The prognosis of chronic pericarditis greatly depends on the ability to treat the associated preexisting condition. Both acute and chronic pericarditis can lead to severe cardiac compromise depending on how rapid, how severe, and how persistent the symptoms are.

Complications

The pericardial sac normally contains 10 to 20 mL of pericardial fluid. This thin, clear, lymphlike fluid serves as a lubricant allowing the heart to move freely without friction within the pericardial sac. The fluid that normally drains into the mediastinal lymph channels may be increased in pericarditis. This is referred to as **pericardial effusion.** If exudate accompanying acute pericarditis is present, it may be serous, purulent, or hemorrhagic. As exudate accumulates in the pericardial space, there is decreased cardiac compliance and distensibility and increased pressure around the heart, which can lead to cardiac tamponade.

Cardiac tamponade is an accumulation of pericardial fluid that restricts cardiac filling and output. If left untreated, cardiac tamponade can lead to cardiac arrest. Cardiac tamponade occurs when accumulated fluid in the pericardial cavity restricts diastolic filling. In chronic states up to 1000 mL of pericardial fluid can accumulate in the pericardium before hemodynamic compromise occurs. On the other hand, in acute states, cardiac tamponade may occur if as little as 100 to 250 mL of fluid accumulates rapidly, causing an acute onset of symptoms.

Clinical Manifestations

Pericardial pain

The most common presenting complaint of patients with pericarditis is pain. Pericardial pain varies from mild to severe. Differentiation must be made between the pain of pericarditis and that of diseased coronary arteries, such as angina or an acute MI, dissecting aortic aneurysm, and pulmonary embolism. The pain is usually sharp and persistent, resembling that of pleuritic pain. The pain often arises suddenly and usually starts retrosternally and radiates to the neck, shoulders, back, and arms. It may radiate to the trapezius ridge, the area between the shoulder and the root of the neck. This usually occurs on the left side but sometimes is bilateral or on the right side. Unlike anginal pain, pericardial pain is exacerbated by inspirations and body movements. It usually increases with deep inspiration, coughing and swallowing, or movement of the chest as a result of increased friction of inflamed tissue with surrounding structures. It also commonly increases when the patient is lying flat and decreases or resolves when the patient is sitting up and leaning forward.

Pericardial friction rub

The pericardial friction rub is the most definitive physical sign of pericarditis because it indicates the presence of pericardial inflammation. Rubs can be described as grating, scraping, squeaking, scratching, or crunching and result from the movement between the roughened surface of the two pericardial layers. They are best heard with the diaphragm of the stethoscope, and although they may be heard anywhere over the precordium, they are frequently best heard over the left sternal border from the second through fifth intercostal spaces. Friction rubs are often transient and may vary according to position or at different times of day or during the course of the disease. The amplitude may increase or decrease with inspiration or expiration.

Dyspnea

Dyspnea is the third classic sign of pericarditis. Dyspnea is usually the result of compression of the bronchi and lung parenchyma by a distended pericardium or by decreased cardiac output, resulting in rapid, shallow breaths rather than full, relaxed breaths. In addition, dyspnea is also associated with precordial pain, which causes the perceived need to splint the chest to prevent the pain. If the dyspnea is caused by a distended pericardium, a sitting position in which the patient is leaning slightly forward causes the accumulated pericardial fluid to move from the inferior surface of the heart to the anterior surface and often provides relief.

Pericardial effusion

If pericardial effusion is present, the patient may exhibit additional symptoms. Smaller effusions produce subtle signs, whereas larger effusions produce pronounced signs. Signs associated with distention of the pericardial sac are dyspnea, diminished heart sounds, a mild or absent friction rub, and increasing anxiety and restlessness. Whether pericardial effusion is acute or chronic, as the fluid accumulation increases, hypotension and a narrowing of the pulse pressure develop. The body compensates for the hypotension and poor cardiac output with a tachycardia. If the condition continues, further hemodynamic decompensation may occur.

In cases of a rapid accumulation of fluid and a decreasing cardiac output, other signs may develop. Cardiac compression results in elevated cardiac filling pressures. High cardiac pressures are revealed by an elevated central venous pressure (CVP) and jugular venous distention (JVD). These signs reflect right-sided heart failure. Left-sided heart failure may ensue and is reflected by a reduced cardiac output and pulmonary congestion.

Cardiac tamponade

Rapid accumulation of fluid in cardiac tamponade produces more marked signs and symptoms of reduced cardiac output. The classic triad of cardiac tamponade signs is hypotension, muffled heart sounds, and an elevated JVD. Pulsus paradoxus is a more sophisticated but key indicator as well. **Pulsus paradoxus** is an abnormally large (greater than 10 mm Hg) fall in systolic blood pressure on inspiration. Although systolic pressure normally decreases during inspiration, a normal change in systolic pressure is less than 10 mm Hg. Pulsus paradoxus is an exaggerated decrease in arterial systolic pressure during inspiration. A change of more than 10 mm Hg is clinically significant for altered pressures.

Signs and symptoms of reduced cardiac output, such as hypotension, oliguria, thready pulses, and peripheral cyanosis, will also be evident. As fluid collects in the pericardial sac, heart sounds may also become muffled or sound distant. Systemic manifestations of pericarditis include fever, chills, diaphoresis, fatigue, malaise, weight loss, ECG changes such as ST segment elevation and PR segment depression, and dysrhythmias, especially sinus tachycardia.

Diagnostic tests

Several diagnostic studies are used to evaluate pericarditis. The echocardiogram is the single most useful test in detecting pericardial effusion. An echocardiogram outlines the cardiac chamber borders and can detect as little as 20 mL of fluid by showing an "echo-free" space between the ventricular wall and the pericardium. It can also show functional cardiac changes associated with cardiac tamponade. Occasionally a thickened, calcified pericardium can be identified in constrictive pericarditis.

Chest x-ray studies may be useful in the evaluation of pericardial effusion and cardiac tamponade. In mild cases of acute pericarditis the chest radiograph is normal, but when a significant pericardial effusion exists, the cardiac silhouette will be enlarged. Chest x-ray studies can also be helpful in establishing the etiology of tuberculous pericarditis. ECGs, although not diagnostic, may reveal changes produced by pericarditis. Common findings include changes in wave configuration (ST segment elevation and PR segment depression), low-voltage QRS complexes, and dysrhythmias such as sinus tachycardia.

Therapeutic Management

The objectives of treatment focus on determining the cause of the problem, controlling symptoms, managing related systemic disorders, and monitoring for the complication of cardiac tamponade. The initial approach depends on the acuity of the symptoms and the presence of cardiac tamponade.

In acute pericarditis a known etiologic disease process or agent is treated; for example, antibiotics are given for a specific organism. Supportive relief is provided for fever, pain, and anxiety. Nonsteroidal anti-inflammatory agents such as ibuprofen, indomethacin, or aspirin are prescribed to reduce inflammation, which then decreases the pain. For continued or more severe symptoms, corticosteroids may be considered. Because of their major side effects of fluid retention, gastrointestinal irritation, and immunosuppression, corticosteroids are only used if more conservative therapy fails to relieve the symptoms. Systemic conditions such as uremic pericarditis are usually treated with hemodialysis. Lupus erythematosus responds to steroids and antimetabolite drugs.

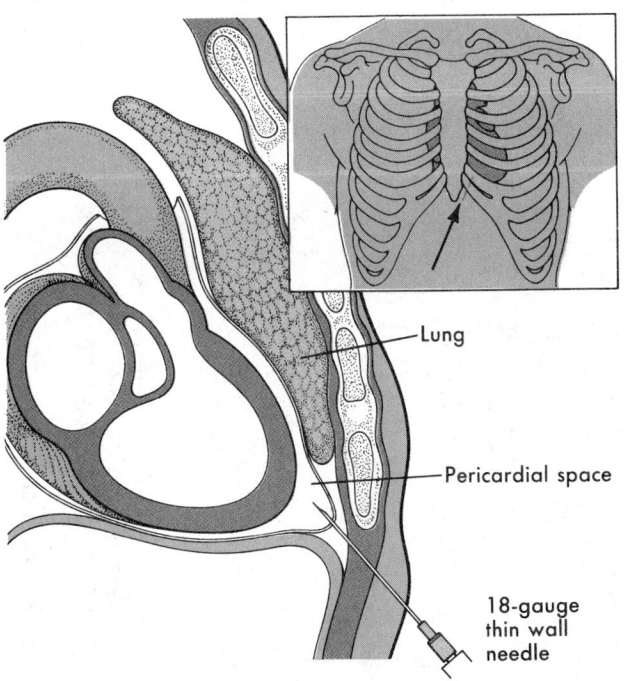

FIGURE 35-9 Pericardiocentesis using subxiphoid route of pericardial aspiration. The 18-gauge needle is introduced at 30- to 40-degree angle. When pericardial fluid is readily aspirated, pericardium has been entered.

Cardiac tamponade requires urgent therapy to prevent cardiac arrest. The definitive treatment is pericardial drainage, either by pericardiocentesis (Figure 35-9) or by surgical drainage. During pericardiocentesis a needle is introduced into the subxyphoid area and the pericardial fluid is aspirated to relieve the compression. If a needle aspiration is performed, fluid is usually sent to the laboratory for culture. To maintain hemodynamic stability before a drainage procedure, intravenous normal saline, blood, or inotropic agents, such as dopamine or dobutamine, can be used. If hemodynamic compromise is caused by cardiac tamponade, successful pericardiocentesis will result in a dramatic improvement in the patient's condition.

Chronic pericarditis, in a mild constrictive form, may be treated with digitalis, diuretics, and a low-sodium diet to improve cardiac output. A pericardial window may be required to treat a pericardial effusion. A pericardial window is a partial removal of the pericardium to allow excess pericardial fluid to drain into the pleural space. In more severe forms of constrictive pericarditis or in recurrent pericarditis, a pericardiectomy, or removal of the pericardium, may be necessary to permit adequate filling and contraction of the heart.

NURSING MANAGEMENT OF THE PATIENT WITH PERICARDITIS
Assessment

A complete history is necessary to identify possible causes of pericarditis. Pertinent information includes any history of upper respiratory tract infections, systemic or chronic disease, recent invasive testing, surgery, dental work, and the patient's nutritional status, as well as current medications. While obtaining the history, the nurse can also assess for systemic manifestations such as diaphoresis, chills, fever, fatigue, and weight loss. Patient/family interaction, level of understanding, and anxiety are also assessed at this time.

The signs and symptoms of pericarditis need to be evaluated, particularly precordial pain, pericardial friction rub, and dyspnea. The assessment of precordial pain includes information such as location, radiation, duration, quality, severity, timing, and aggravating and alleviating factors such as position change. Nonverbal cues are noted as well. Pericardial friction rubs, the most commonly found diagnostic sign, should be evaluated for location, effect of position changes, and quality of sound. Dyspnea is assessed in terms of respiratory rate and depth, its association with pain and anxiety, and any precipitating or alleviating factors such as position change (e.g., leaning forward).

The second major area of assessment focuses on the two major complications surrounding pericarditis: pericardial effusion and cardiac tamponade. Initially a baseline assessment of the following parameters is needed to evaluate a pericardial effusion: dyspnea, diminished heart sounds, and a friction rub. If a large amount of pericardial fluid has accumulated, signs of reduced cardiac output may be present. Signs and symptoms include those associated with decreased cerebral perfusion, such as restlessness, confusion, and irritability. The blood pressure and pulse must be assessed every 1 to 4 hours, depending on the patient's condition, for hypotension, a narrowed pulse pressure, and tachycardia. Other signs of a low cardiac output, such as oliguria, peripheral cyanosis, and thready pulse, may also be present. A worsening of any of the signs associated with a pericardial effusion may indicate increasing fluid accumulation and cardiac compression reflecting cardiac tamponade.

The assessment for cardiac tamponade includes monitoring of all the previously mentioned parameters every 1 to 4 hours as well as periodic assessment for a pulsus paradoxus. To measure a pulsus paradoxus the patient breathes normally. The blood pressure cuff is applied and inflated to 20 mm Hg above the patient's systolic blood pressure and then slowly deflated. The nurse notes when Korotkoff's sounds are heard during expiration. The cuff is then

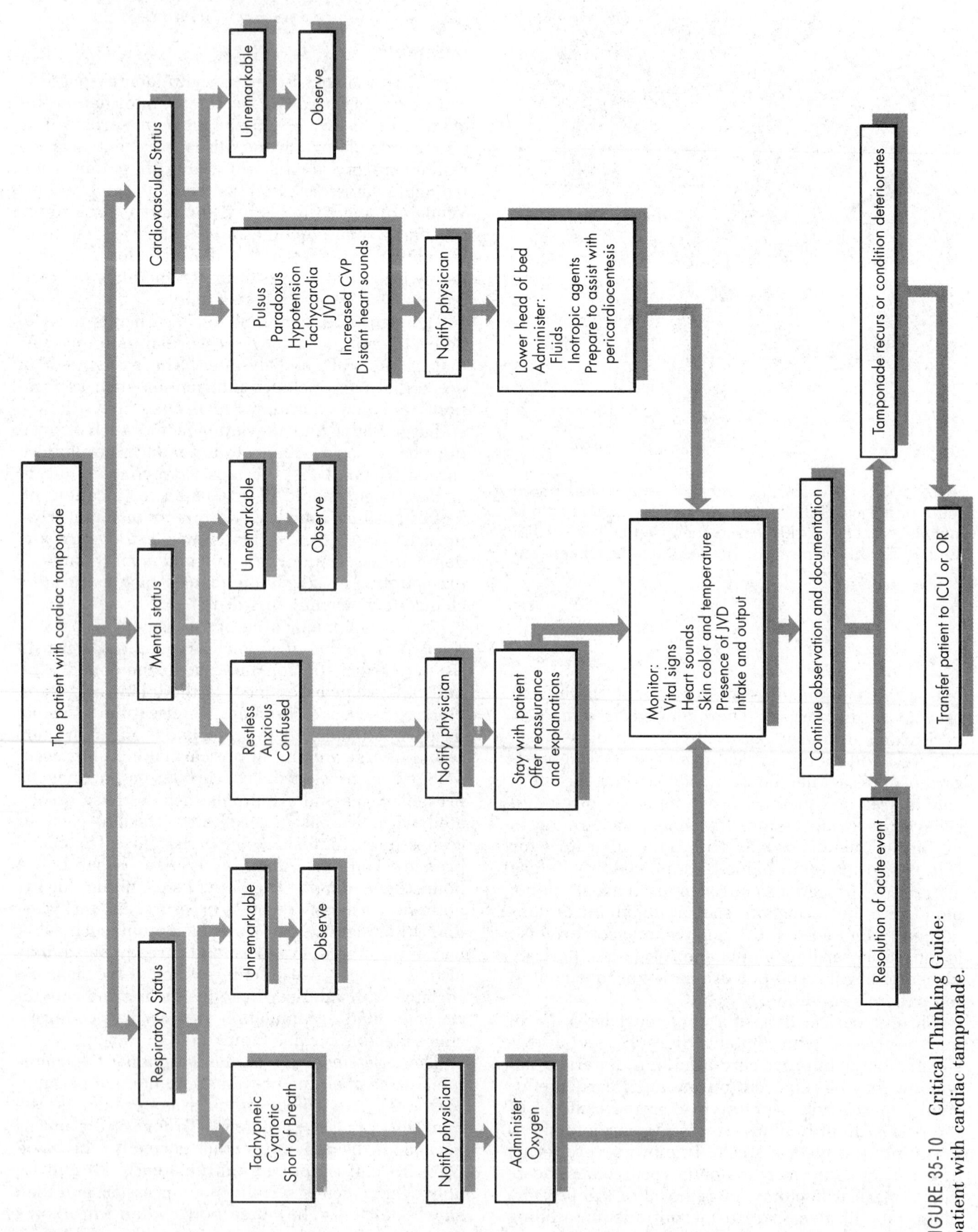

FIGURE 35-10 Critical Thinking Guide: patient with cardiac tamponade.

deflated until Korotkoff's sounds are heard regardless of the phase of respiration. The mm Hg difference represents the millimeters of paradoxus. If a central venous catheter is inserted, the nurse assesses for elevation. A normal CVP is 3 to 15 mm H_2O. A CVP of more than 20 mm Hg indicates possible tamponade. The nurse's assessment of the classic signs of cardiac tamponade (hypotension, a pulsus paradoxus, and an elevated CVP) is now complete and needs to be correlated with the other signs of a poor cardiac output (Figure 35-10).

Blood studies are monitored for abnormalities. Some typical findings with pericarditis and which indicate an infection or inflammation include a normal or slightly elevated white blood cell count (WBC) and erythrocyte sedimentation rate (ESR). A slight elevation of cardiac enzymes reflects some myocardial muscle damage. Last, all laboratory data reflecting a potential underlying disorder are monitored, such as the blood urea nitrogen (BUN) in cases of uremic pericarditis, tuberculin skin tests in cases of tuberculosis, blood cultures in cases of bacterial infection, the antinuclear antibody test in cases of myxedema, and neoplastic studies in cases of cancer. If a pericardiocentesis or surgical drainage is performed, a culture of the fluid is done to detect an infectious cause. If surgery is required, pericardial tissue may be obtained by biopsy to aid in defining the abnormal process.

Nursing Diagnosis

Nursing diagnoses for the patient with pericarditis may include the following:

Pain (severe) related to pericardial inflammation

High risk for decreased cardiac output related to diminished left ventricular filling caused by decreased cardiac compliance, pericardial effusion, cardiac tamponade, or dysrhythmias

Knowledge deficit regarding discharge regimen

Planning

Specific patient goals are determined based on the acuity or chronicity of the condition as well as the severity and threat to the patient's physical and psychologic being. General goals may include the following:

Patient verbalizes there is no pain, and nonverbal cues indicate relaxation and comfort

Patient will not have signs of pericardial effusion or cardiac tamponade (i.e., dyspnea, diminished heart sounds, hypotension, pulsus paradoxus > 10 mm Hg)

Patient and family will describe the course of pericarditis, signs and symptoms, and information needed for home care (i.e., medication administration, avoiding exposure to respiratory tract infections, and when to contact the physician)

Implementation

Whether the pericarditis is acute or chronic, pain control is an important nursing focus. Instructing the patient to lean forward over a bedside table will position the heart away from the irritated nerve fibers. Nonsteroidal anti-inflammatory agents such as ibuprofen or indomethacin are often given to help control the pain and inflammation. These medications are best given in divided doses and after meals to prevent gastrointestinal irritation. In addition, analgesics such as codeine may be necessary. Relaxation exercises may decrease anxiety associated with pain. Patients should be helped with the basic needs such as bathing, mouth care, and elimination since excessive activity may aggravate pericardial inflammation and pain. Bed rest should be maintained until the pain and fever subside. Emphasizing that the pain will decrease as the disease process resolves may allow patients to monitor their own progress. Monitor the patient for signs and symptoms of decreased cardiac output. Cardiac tamponade requires prompt intervention to preserve adequate tissue perfusion. Oxygen may be administered to maximize oxygenation to the tissues during the low cardiac output state. Normal saline, blood, and inotropic agents such as dopamine or dobutamine are given to increase cardiac output. Finally, the patient may need to be prepared for procedures such as pericardiocentesis or surgical repair to relieve the cardiac compression. Teaching should be implemented as the patient's condition permits. Explaining the operative procedure and postoperative routine may reduce anxiety and aid in compliance.

Reducing the patient's anxiety is a major focus in caring for the patient with pericarditis. Explain the course of the disease as well as the signs and symptoms of pericarditis. Stress the importance of reporting new symptoms to the physician. Promoting a positive attitude may decrease anxiety and enhance self-image. Patients and families are encouraged to report any stressors of the illness to enhance coping and the identification of new problems. Support effective coping mechanisms and teach relaxation techniques and imagery to decrease anxiety and enhance progress toward recovery.

Plans for home care and rehabilitation begin as soon as the patient's physical condition and psychologic condition permit. Family members are included in the planning and educational sessions whenever possible. Teaching includes the course of pericarditis and the signs and symptoms as well as instructions to notify the physician of any changes in the patient's signs and symptoms. Medication instruction includes the actions, dosages, contraindi-

NURSING CARE PLAN *The Patient with Pericarditis*

Nursing diagnosis/ Expected outcome	Interventions	Rationale
High risk for decreased cardiac output related to diminished left ventricular filling caused by decreased cardiac compliance, pericardial effusion, cardiac tamponade, or dysrhythmias • *Patient will maintain vital signs, urine output, and level of consciousness within his or her normal limits*	Monitor blood pressure, heart rate and rhythm, and respiratory rate and depth every 15 minutes to 1 hour; identify signs of dyspnea	Initial symptoms of cardiac compromise will be manifested by tachycardia and minor decrease in systolic blood pressure
	Assess for increased muffling of heart sounds Assess for presence of pulsus paradoxus or JVD	Fluid accumulation in pericardium will make heart sounds "muffled" As fluid accumulates in pericardium, pressure in heart increases and elevates pressures backward into venous circulation
	Evaluate the patient for other signs and symptoms of decreased cardiac output: decreased urine output, cyanosis, restlessness, thready pulses Be conscious of other complications of pericarditis (dysrhythmias and congestive heart failure) by evaluating ECG, presence of peripheral edema, and presence of adventitious breath sounds	
	Be prepared for emergency interventions if necessary, such as pericardiocentesis	Rapid accumulation of fluid in pericardium can cause rapid decompensation of patient's hemodynamic status and lead to death

cations, side effects, and actions to take to decrease side effects, such as taking anti-inflammatory agents after meals. The patient and family are instructed to avoid exposure to upper respiratory tract infections and to report cold or flu symptoms promptly to the physician. Stress the importance of rest and avoiding fatigue as well as the need for follow-up appointments and laboratory tests to monitor the resolution of the disease.

Evaluation

The effectiveness of nursing interventions is evaluated through ongoing assessment. Successful interventions will help the patient control or eliminate pain and get adequate amounts of rest and sleep. The patient's vital signs will be stable, peripheral pulses will be baseline, and the patient will be without chills or malaise. The patient will not exhibit signs of a low cardiac output such as exertional dyspnea, a decreasing pulse pressure, an elevated CVP, hypotension, tachycardia, or a pulsus paradoxus. The patient and family will verbalize an understanding of pericarditis, any needed tests or procedures, medication therapy, follow-up appointments, and the importance of adequate amounts of rest.

Documentation

Documentation of care for the patient with pericarditis involves accurately recording the assessment data, interventions, and patient teaching. Detailed documentation of ongoing assessment is essential since many parameters when analyzed concurrently may indicate a progression from uncomplicated pericarditis to tamponade or a low cardiac output state.

Ongoing Care

Once the patient with pericarditis is discharged from the hospital, the overall prognosis varies, but patients with acute pericarditis that has resolved will experience no life-style changes. Patients with chronic pericarditis will require careful ongoing medical follow-up. These patients should be aware of the relationship between their underlying condition and the resulting pericardial inflammation and constriction. They should be able to describe any worsening of signs and symptoms and the importance of contacting the physician. The importance of adhering to a long-term medication regimen, where applicable, should be emphasized. Patients with chronic forms of pericarditis need ongoing follow-up appointments for physical examination, laboratory tests, and possible surgical intervention. Stress the importance of wearing a Medic Alert bracelet because of the potential for recurrent cardiac compromise.

Cardiomyopathy

Cardiomyopathy refers to structural and functional changes of the myocardium. Three distinct groups exist: dilated cardiomyopathy, hypertrophic cardiomyopathy, and restrictive cardiomyopathy. Because of their variability in etiology, manifestations, and treatment, each group is discussed separately.

DILATED (CONGESTIVE) CARDIOMYOPATHY
Definition

Dilated cardiomyopathy (DCM) is a disorder of the myocardium characterized by impaired contractility and pumping ability. Its striking features are cardiomegaly, slight hypertrophy, and dilation of both ventricles.

Etiology/Epidemiology

Dilated cardiomyopathy, formerly known as congestive cardiomyopathy, is the most prevalent of the cardiomyopathies. It is distributed throughout all age groups, with the majority of cases in the elderly population. The course of the disease consists of a progressive deterioration of the myocardium with three fourths of patients dying within 5 years after symptom onset. The cause of DCM is usually unknown, but many diseases of the heart muscle can produce the clinical manifestations of DCM. The precipitating factors include chronic alcohol ingestion, immunologic disorders, long-term uncontrolled hypertension, pregnancy, and a variety of chemical and physical agents that may have toxic effects on the myocardium.

Pathophysiology

In dilated cardiomyopathy the contractile function of the myocardial fibrils is impaired. The heart enlarges with dilation of the chambers of both ventricles. To compensate for the compromised ability to contract, the myocardium hypertrophies. The poor contractile state allows blood to remain in the left ventricle after contraction. Excessive volume in the left ventricle at the end of systole increases the pressure back to the left atrium and subsequently, the pulmonary circulation. Fluid accumulation in the pulmonary system can leak into the interstitium of the lung causing pulmonary edema. As the disease progresses, further backup occurs in the right ventricle and eventually into the venous system, producing symptoms of both left-sided and right-sided heart failure.

A low cardiac output reduces blood flow to the myocardium, producing ischemic angina and dysrhythmias. The sympathetic nervous system can maintain adequate cardiac output for a time by increasing heart rate in the presence of a limited ability to increase contractility. Additional stresses or disease can initiate a cycle of decompensation. That is, any factor, such as fever, exertion, or dysrhythmias, that puts more stress on the heart can further decrease cardiac output. This decreases renal perfusion, resulting in sodium and water retention. This added fluid volume load puts additional stress on the heart and further compromises its ability to pump blood.

Clinical Manifestations

The signs and symptoms of DCM depend on the progression of the disease. Manifestations generally reflect first evidence of left ventricular failure and then later both left and right ventricular failure. The diagnosis of DCM rests primarily on the assessment findings and pertinent data from the person's health history. Patients initially exhibit exertional dyspnea that later progresses to dyspnea at rest. They frequently complain of a nocturnal, dry cough. Chest pain may be caused by decreased coronary perfusion secondary to left ventricular failure. Signs and symptoms of congestive heart failure and pulmonary edema occur with biventricular failure. Frequent atrial and ventricular ectopic beats and various forms of tachycardia are common dysrhythmias accompanying DCM.

The most helpful diagnostic tests are the chest radiograph and the echocardiogram. The chest radiograph reveals cardiac enlargement, pulmonary venous engorgement, and interstitial edema characteristic of heart failure. An echocardiogram can assess cardiac chamber size and ventricular function. The characteristic dilated and poorly contracting left ventricle of congestive cardiomyopathy can be visualized using this test. The ECG, although not specific, may reveal clues as to the cause of heart failure. Cardiomyopathy can produce conduction delays, which are indicated by a widened QRS or prolonged PR interval.

Therapeutic Management

There are many degrees of heart failure, and the patient's stage of failure will determine the selection of therapeutic interventions. Therapy is directed toward identifying and treating precipitating factors, reducing the work load of the heart, improving the force and efficiency of contraction, and treating the symptoms and complications of DCM.

Physiologically, myocardial work load is reduced by physical and emotional rest, which can reduce heart rate, relieve dyspnea, and promote diuresis. For patients with limited functional ability, in whom any amount of activity precipitates symptoms, partial or complete bed rest and oxygen administration can reduce the work of the heart. Diuretics such as aldactone or furosemide may improve the symptoms of congestive heart failure, whereas vasodilator therapy (enalapril, hydralazine, and nitrates) can improve cardiac output by reducing afterload. Recent research suggests the use of beta blockers such as propranolol or atenolol may be helpful in treating patients. Cardiac output tends to decrease in patients with DCM when tachycardia occurs, causing lower filling pressures, because of the heart's inability to compensate with increased contractility. Beta blockers can reduce the sympathetic response of increased heart rate as well as reduce myocardial oxygen demand.

In patients with large dilated atria or ventricles, mural thrombi can form. Anticoagulants are often administered to prevent the formation of clots. Antidysrhythmic medications such as procainamide or quinidine are commonly prescribed for ventricular dysrhythmias.

Complete blood counts, electrolytes, and renal profile tests must be monitored during medication therapy with particular attention given to creatinine, sodium, and potassium levels. Commonly, potassium supplements are necessary when diuretics are administered. Serum sodium may be low, but fluid restriction may alleviate this problem. Serum creatinine must be monitored as an indicator of renal function. Altered glucose tolerance is common with the administration of diuretics, beta blockers, and some vasodilators; therefore glucose levels should be monitored.

Heart transplantation provides an alternative for the patient who is chronically ill with heart failure and who fails to respond to conventional therapy. The implications of major surgery, other organ damage, and long-term immunosuppressive therapy must be considered. This approach involves dramatic psychologic events and requires considerable family and social support. The decision for heart transplantation is made only after extensive evaluation and assessment.

HYPERTROPHIC CARDIOMYOPATHY
Definition

Hypertrophic cardiomyopathy (HCM) is a disorder of the myocardium characterized by left ventricular hypertrophy and hypercontractility, particularly in the interventricular septum.

Etiology/Epidemiology

Hypertrophic cardiomyopathy is primarily genetically transmitted by an autosomal dominant gene. The dysfunction of the myocardium may be manifested in the young adult with the onset and progression of symptoms most commonly occurring in persons 30 to 50 years of age. Small children and adolescents diagnosed with HCM may be symptomatic with bradydysrhythmias and syncope. Elderly patients may present with many of the morphologic and clinical features of HCM, which may be a result of the aging changes in the heart.

Pathophysiology

In HCM the structure of the myocardium is disrupted by patches of disorganized myocardial fibers and myocardial fibrosis producing ventricular stiffness and hypertrophy, particularly in the septal region. This results in a change in the shape, size, and distensibility of the left ventricular chamber. The stiffness of the myocardium impairs the ventricles' ability to relax during diastole, reducing diastolic filling. The lack of distensibility also does not allow the left ventricle to increase the amount of filling during normal hemodynamic changes, for example, increased blood flow return to the heart during exercise.

The hypertrophied left ventricle becomes hypercontractile and rapidly ejects more blood than usual with each beat. This hyperdynamic contraction can complete ejection of blood during the first half of systole, rather than using the entire systolic cycle as seen in healthy hearts. This can cause the anterior leaflet of the mitral valve to meet with the hypertrophied septum, obstructing aortic outflow during systole and reducing cardiac output. The obstruction is exacerbated by the increased contractile state. When exercise or some other event further increases contractility, evidence of marked obstruction of the narrowed outflow tract occurs.

Cardiac ischemia can occur in HCM by mechanisms that are yet to be fully understood.[10] One potential mechanism is the increased oxygen demand of the enlarged muscle mass of the hypertrophied ventricle. An enlarged muscle mass coupled with an increased diastolic pressure may compress the small coronary vessels, thus limiting blood flow.

Fibrosis also affects the conduction system in patients with HCM. There are documented instances of both decreased and accelerated conduction in the atrioventricular node and bundle of His, increasing the risk of tachydysrhythmias. The myocardial disarray also increases the incidence of spontaneous ventricular tachycardia and fibrillation in this patient population.

Clinical Manifestations

Patients with the diagnosis of hypertrophic cardiomyopathy may manifest abnormal signs and symptoms. Their presence depends on the extent and severity of the disease, its rate of progression, and the age of the patient. Patients with "obstructive" HCM, in which blood flow is blocked at the end of systole, frequently exhibit more symptoms than patients with "nonobstructive" HCM.

The primary manifestations of HCM are dyspnea, fatigue, chest pain, syncope, and palpitations. Dyspnea is caused by "backward congestion," and fatigue is caused by reduced "forward flow" or decreased cardiac output. As the disease progresses, more marked evidence of backward congestion occurs, essentially presenting a picture of CHF.

Chest pain, dysrhythmias, palpitations, and restlessness are manifestations of reduced oxygen delivery to the myocardium. These symptoms occur more often during exercise, although they may also occur at rest. Supraventricular or ventricular tachycardias may result in dizziness, syncope, and even sudden death. Supraventricular tachycardias, such as atrial fibrillation and junctional tachycardia, may precipitate or exacerbate CHF, because they compromise the "atrial kick" (20% to 30% of the cardiac output), the blood the atrium ejects into the ventricle during atrial systole. Patients with HCM may depend on the "atrial kick" to maintain adequate left ventricular filling and therefore adequate cardiac output.

The chest radiograph shows enlargement of the left atrium and ventricle and may reveal pulmonary edema. The ECG shows hypertrophy of the left ventricle, left atrial enlargement, and Q waves from septal fibrosis. The ECG pattern may mimic changes seen after a myocardial infarction. Dysrhythmias may be present. The echocardiogram confirms increased thickness of the left ventricular septum with poor motion and abnormal motion of the mitral valve. The cardiac output may be high, normal, or low. Cardiac catheterization can detect the pressure gradients between the left ventricle and the ascending aorta that frequently accompany HCM and indicate whether "obstruction" is present.

Therapeutic Management

The therapeutic goals focus on improving cardiac function and preventing complications in an effort to relieve and prevent symptoms and avoid death. Beta-adrenergic blocking agents, such as propranolol, are prescribed to reduce the force of contraction, helping to relieve outflow obstruction and decrease myocardial oxygen demand. These agents also reduce the catecholamine-induced increases in heart rate, particularly after exercise and with stress. This effect can also reduce anginal episodes. However, since these agents can reduce contractility, they may worsen evidence of CHF; in this case, a calcium channel blocking agent such as verapamil or nifedipine may be chosen.

Antidysrhythmic therapy is implemented to prevent dysrhythmias and reduce the risk of sudden death. Procainamide or quinidine may be prescribed. Amiodarone has been shown to be effective in suppressing dysrhythmias without adversely affecting ventricular function when procainamide or quinidine is not successful.[14] Implantable cardioverter defibrillator devices may be required to control lethal dysrhythmias in some patients.

Patients experiencing atrial fibrillation are treated with cardioversion or atrioventricular sequential pacing to avoid CHF. If CHF develops, digitalis and diuretics may be administered but with caution. These medications can enhance the signs and symptoms of HCM because of digitalis's ability to increase contractility in an already hypercontractile myocardium. Because of the risk of mobilizing clots that have formed in the dilated atria, anticoagulation therapy is begun before cardioversion, and it is continued if atrial fibrillation persists.

The patient is encouraged to avoid situations that may provoke symptoms, such as exercise, prolonged standing, or performing the Valsalva maneuver during activities such as lifting, straining, or isotonic exercise. The symptoms can be relieved by having the patient squat or lie down and raise his or her legs to increase left ventricular filling and therefore cardiac output.

If medical management provides insufficient relief of symptoms, surgery, known as a ventricular myotomy and myectomy, may be indicated to excise a section of the hypertrophied septum below the aortic cusp. Occasionally a simultaneous mitral valve replacement is performed if significant mitral valve dysfunction is present.

RESTRICTIVE CARDIOMYOPATHY
Definition

Restrictive cardiomyopathy is an infiltrative process that causes fibrosis and thickening of the heart muscle.

Etiology/Epidemiology

A variety of pathologic processes may result in restrictive cardiomyopathy. Some causes include endomyocardial fibrosis, amyloidosis, and sarcoidosis. Other disorders that produce this picture are glycogen storage diseases and hemochromatosis (excess iron deposits). Restrictive cardiomyopathy is the least common of the cardiomyopathies seen in the Western world.

Pathophysiology

In restrictive cardiomyopathy, fibrotic infiltrations into the myocardium, endocardium, and subendocardium cause the ventricles to lose their ability to stretch. Thus the heart cannot completely fill and cardiac output falls. CHF and mild ventricular hypertrophy develop. Dilation of the atria occurs and allows thrombi to form on the walls of the atrial appendages. If restrictive cardiomyopathy is caused by other systemic disorders, associated pathologic conditions will also be manifested.

Clinical Manifestations

Early evidence of restrictive cardiomyopathy includes shortness of breath, fatigue, exercise intolerance, and weakness. Later signs include neck vein distention, peripheral edema, and ascites such as are seen in CHF. Atrial fibrillation may be present as a result of the atrial enlargement. Severe restrictive cardiomyopathy is similar to chronic constrictive pericarditis. The echocardiogram may reveal thickening of the left ventricular wall. Endomyocardial biopsy, CT scanning, and magnetic resonance imaging help to determine cellular infiltrates and differentiate this disease from constrictive pericarditis.

Therapeutic Management

No specific therapy for restrictive cardiomyopathy exists, so the focus is on symptomatic relief. CHF is controlled by using digitalis, diuretics, sodium restriction, and vasodilators. Anticoagulants may be prescribed to reduce the risk of mural thrombus formation and embolization. Rest and activity restriction may be prescribed to help reduce the cardiac work load. Patients with endocardial fibrosis may require surgical removal of the fibrous myocardial tissue and replacement of affected valves.

NURSING MANAGEMENT OF THE PATIENT WITH CARDIOMYOPATHY
Assessment

Assessment of the patient with cardiomyopathy begins with the nursing admission interview and history. Factors contributing to the development of current symptoms are investigated, such as ischemic events, exposure to toxins, viral infection, recent travel, or family history of cardiac disease. Duration and severity of the patient's symptoms are evaluated. Ask the patient about symptoms of shortness of breath, fatigue, dyspnea on exertion, palpitations, or syncope. Question the patient regarding chest pain, including the nature, frequency, and duration of pain. Ask about the quality, radiation, associated symptoms, and precipitating and alleviating factors. Consideration of the patient's current medication regimen is necessary to completely assess how well the patient's symptoms are being controlled.

Perhaps most important is the assessment of quality of life. Establishing which activities the patient can perform without symptom development and noting those that evoke fatigue, dyspnea, palpitations, or chest pain are essential components of the nursing assessment. In addition, ask how often the patient awakens during the night and the apparent reasons. The number of pillows needed for comfortable sleep and recent changes in this routine are assessed. Ventricular dysrhythmias associated with HCM may be life threatening; ask the patient about syncopal episodes or sudden death experiences.

The admission interview and history taking also enable the nurse to assess the patient's mental status. Since the acutely ill patient may not be able to provide detailed information because of dyspnea or fatigue, the assessment may need to be performed over several limited conversations. At the same time, orientation, absence or presence of somnolence, and anxiety level are observed. This initial evaluation provides the basis for assessing any changes in mental status that may occur. Frequent reassessment of the patient's mental status can reveal subtle changes in orientation, reflecting increasing cardiac manifestations.

Important aspects of assessment include the heart rate and rhythm. The heart rhythm may be irregular if underlying atrial fibrillation, heart block, or frequent ectopy exists. A Holter monitor (worn for 24 hours) can reveal the frequency and nature of irregular heartbeats. Runs of ventricular tachycardia may correlate with patient complaints of dizziness.

Simultaneous assessment of apical and radial pulses (pulse deficit) reflects whether each heartbeat is perfusing and provides an estimate of the number of ventricular ectopic beats occurring per minute. The right and left radial pulses are also assessed for equality. Peripheral circulation can be evaluated by the warmth and color of the skin.

The blood pressure and heart rate are determined with the patient supine, with the patient sitting, and after 5 minutes of standing when feasible. This will be a true reflection of orthostatic hypotension. If the patient becomes dizzy on standing, he or she should immediately be placed supine. When the patient is stable, vital signs may be recorded every 4 hours; they are assessed more frequently during the administration of certain medications such as beta-blocking agents or calcium channel blockers and when symptoms worsen.

Auscultation may reveal evidence of heart failure, including an S_3 or S_4 gallop or murmur. Observation of JVD is associated with CHF or hypervolemia.

Assessment of respiratory rate and quality may reveal respiratory distress resulting from cardiac compromise. The lungs are auscultated for adventitious sounds such as crackles, wheezes, or diminished breath sounds. Some patients have chronic bibasilar crackles and remain asymptomatic. On the other hand, coarse crackles one half of the way up the lung fields frequently require intervention with diuretics. Other evidence of respiratory distress includes mouth breathing, orthopnea, dyspnea, nasal flaring, intercostal or supraclavicular retractions, and tachypnea. Anxiety, central cyanosis (oral mucous membranes), and ashen color are signs of hypoxia seen in the patient with CHF from cardiomyopathy. Patients in extreme distress are highly anxious and agitated.

Peripheral venous congestion, or dependent edema, is a common finding in CHF as a result of volume overload and sodium and water retention. Peripheral edema may be present in trace amounts or pitting, estimated from 1+ to 4+. The location and amount of edema are recorded daily. Dependent edema occurs in the parts of the body that are lowest. It is often seen in the ankles and feet and increases at the end of the day, after the patient ambulates. If the patient is on bed rest, it is seen in the sacrum, scrotum, and posterior malleoli. The abdomen may also be distended as a result of edema or ascites from the increased hepatic pressure that can occur in CHF. Weights should be taken daily at the same time of the day as an important parameter of water retention. Generally, an increase in weight over 24 hours indicates significant fluid retention. Sodium intake is also assessed by diet recall when managing the patient with heart failure since a high-sodium intake can cause fluid retention by the kidneys.

Assess the patient and family's knowledge of the disease, diet, and medications. Family members who can or do assist the patient are included in the discussion. Specific knowledge of these areas is explored to define strengths and weaknesses.

Nursing Diagnosis

The diagnoses below may be used in the development of a care plan for the patient. Depending on the severity of the symptoms, flexibility must be used in specific cases.

Activity intolerance related to fatigue, shortness of breath, and changes in cardiac contractility

Decreased cardiac output related to changes in cardiac contractility and dysrhythmias

Impaired gas exchange related to decreased cardiac output and interstitial pulmonary edema

Altered (cerebral) tissue perfusion related to decreased cardiac output and decreased cerebral perfusion

Pain related to myocardial ischemia and dysrhythmias

Anxiety related to lack of adequate oxygenation or fear of death and feelings of hopelessness

Knowledge deficit (patient/family) related to disease process, medications, activity restrictions

Sleep pattern disturbances related to dyspnea

Planning

Goals for the patient must be tailored to meet the needs of the individual, considering the type of cardiomyopathy and the age, social setting, and severity of illness of the patient. Goals for the patient include the following:

Patient can tolerate mild activity and build activity into each day

Cardiac output is maintained as demonstrated by blood pressure, heart rate, and urine output within patient's normal limits

Respirations are comfortable, and breath sounds are clear

Patient is oriented

Patient verbalizes absence of chest pain

Anxiety is channeled constructively, with reduction in stress

Before discharge, the patient and family state information necessary for compliance with discharge regimen related to activity management, diet, medications, and follow-up care

Patient meets perceived sleep needs

Implementation

The nursing interventions for patients with cardiomyopathy include those for congestive heart failure, as well as the prevention, detection, and management of problems that occur as a result of the underlying pathophysiology, such as dysrhythmias and chest pain. Providing patient education regarding the disease process, medications, control of signs and symptoms, and other therapeutic modalities is an important consideration.

Vital signs are monitored at least every 4 hours for changes in blood pressure, heart rate and rhythm, and adventitious heart sounds. ECG tracings are analyzed and documented every 4 hours or with a change in rhythm for patients who are on a cardiac monitor. Respiratory rate, rhythm, and breath sounds are assessed every 4 hours, noting the use of accessory muscles or other signs of respiratory distress. If the patient is experiencing signs and symptoms of CHF, he or she may obtain respiratory relief when the head of the bed is elevated 30 to 45 degrees or when sitting in a chair. Supplemental oxygen is administered via nasal cannula or face mask. Peripheral pulses and skin temperature are evaluated every 4 to 8 hours to determine adequacy of peripheral perfusion. During patient interactions, observe the patient for signs and symptoms of decreased cerebral perfusion, such as restlessness, lethargy, or disorientation.

Changes in vital signs may reflect a deterioration of the heart's function, requiring reassessment of the patient's circulatory status, notification of the physician, and alteration in the therapeutic regimen as needed. For example, if the patient is receiving beta-blocking agents and calcium channel blockers, administration may need to be staggered to minimize their synergistic effects on vascular tone. In this instance the patient should also be encouraged to move slowly when changing position to avoid dizziness.

Adequate, frequent rest periods reduce cardiac work. Rest and activity should be alternated to avoid undue fatigue. Activity improves oxygen delivery to the periphery while maintaining function of intact myocardial tissue. Mild activity, particularly walking, improves circulation and maintains muscle mass. Such exercise also improves the quality of sleep at night.

If syncope occurs in the patient with HCM, sit the patient immediately with legs raised or have the patient squat to reduce the effects of obstruction and relieve symptoms. The nurse should stress the use of mild exercise and review the measures mentioned above to alleviate syncope should it occur. Since syncope can occur with the Valsalva maneuver, the patient's safety at the time of bowel movements is assessed, and suggestions for safety precautions, such as handrails in the bathroom, are provided. Constipation is avoided through the use of stool softeners. Certain medications such as vasodilators and inotropic agents (i.e., dopamine, dobutamine) should be avoided in patients with HCM, because they lower preload and afterload and increase the risk of obstruction in this patient population.

Patients experiencing CHF are at risk for fluid retention or, if they are receiving diuretics such as aldactone or furosemide, for volume depletion. Accurate daily weights and intake and output measurements are used to evaluate fluid balance. Daily weights, measured on the same scale, at the same time of day, and in the same amount of clothes are the best indication of fluid gain or loss over 24 hours. Diuretics are administered as ordered, and salt intake is limited to 2 to 3 g daily to prevent water retention. Overdiuresis should be avoided, since this reduces blood flow to the kidneys and causes a more severe orthostasis and hypotension. Diuretics are not administered at night to avoid interrupting the patient's sleep. Once-a-day diuretics are administered in the morning; twice-a-day diuretics are administered in the morning and afternoon.

Dysrhythmias may occur as a result of the CHF or the underlying pathologic changes in the heart. Atrial fibrillation is common in the patient with CHF or HCM. If the patient is hemodynamically unstable, synchronized cardioversion may be required. The nurse carefully reviews the rationale for and nature of the procedure and then supports the patient before, during, and after the procedure. For sustained atrial fibrillation, especially with an enlarged atrium, digitalis is used to control the rate of the ventricular response. If oral anticoagulation is prescribed, inform the patient regarding bleeding precautions. Patients with HCM frequently experience ventricular dysrhythmias such as premature ventricular contractions or ventricular tachycardia, which may or may not cause symptoms. Antidysrhythmic therapy with procainamide, quinidine, or amiodarone may be indicated. Administer amiodarone with food to minimize gastrointestinal distress. Patients should be taught to take their pulse and report irregularities to their physician. Corneal microdeposits are one side effect of amiodarone, and patients are instructed to have an eye examination twice each year. Also encourage these patients to use sunscreen and wear sunglasses when out-of-doors to avoid a photosensitivity reaction from this drug. When antidysrhythmic therapy is unsuccessful in suppressing ventricular dysrhythmias in the patient with HCM, an implantable cardioverter defibrillator (ICD) device may be recommended. Important teaching considerations include its purpose, method of implantation, discharge sequence, what to do when the device discharges, and follow-up care.

During episodes of chest pain, the frequency, duration, quality, radiation, and predisposing factors are determined and recorded. Rest or nitroglycerin is administered, and the degree of pain relief is determined. Vital signs are taken frequently during and after the anginal episode until the pain is relieved and the vital signs are stable.

Since restrictive cardiomyopathy can be caused by an infection, and the patient's temperature tends to be elevated early in the disease, the temperature is taken frequently during this period. If the temperature is elevated, antipyretics are administered. In addition, agents specific for the infection are administered, such as antibiotics or antiparasitic agents. Since infection and fever increase body fluid loss through diaphoresis, careful monitoring of fluid intake and output, skin turgor, and the turgor of the patient's mucous membranes provides a guide to the patient's needs for supplemental fluids.

For patients having trouble sleeping as a result of orthopnea, the head of the bed is elevated and pillows are used for elevation and support. If despite these measures sleeping is still a problem, a sleep medication is considered.

An assessment of the patient and family's level of understanding of the patient's condition and therapeutic regimen provides the basis for teaching. To prepare the patient for discharge and improve compliance with the therapeutic regimen in and out of the hospital, the nature and rationale for interventions are discussed on an ongoing basis. A special focus is given to diet, medications, and activity guidelines. The patient is taught the medications, dosages, and side effects. If fluid restriction has been prescribed, review with the patient and family its rationale and its impact on daily oral intake. When the nurse invites questions, unclear areas can be clarified.

Patients with hypertrophic cardiomyopathy must be aware of activities that will provoke symptoms of orthostasis or chest pain. The nurse teaches the patient that raising the heart rate through exercise may lead to syncope. The patient should understand that squatting or lying down with legs elevated will relieve dizziness. The nurse teaches the patient to hold onto stable objects for support while walking. Strenuous bowel movements may also promote syncope, and the nurse must instruct the patient in dietary and fluid measure to avoid constipation and to avoid straining during bowel movements. The patient is taught to report increases in frequency of syncopal attacks to the physician, particularly if diuretic therapy is part of medical management, since overdiuresis may induce syncope. Reviewing factors that precipitate chest pain with the patient will help identify activities to avoid. Encourage patients to carry a copy of their most recent 12-lead ECG in their wallet or purse. Their ECG pattern frequently mimics that of a patient experiencing an MI. Knowledge of the patient's previous ECG tracing will prevent possible misinterpretation by health care providers un-

familiar with this disorder. Patients with hypertrophic cardiomyopathy and their families should understand the need for CPR training of family members because of the risk of sudden death in this patient population. The nurse should recommend a facility for CPR instruction and ensure that family members know how to activate emergency medical services in their area. Accurate assessment of the pulse is demonstrated to family members by the nurse, to teach the differentiation of syncope and cardiac arrest.

Patient and family fears and anxiety limit their cooperation and compliance with therapeutic regimen. The patient is often fearful about the prognosis, as well as death; or the patient may be anxious about altered roles and activity limitations at home or at work. The patient and family are encouraged to verbalize these concerns; the nurse provides appropriate information, guidance, encouragement, and support. When appropriate, the nurse helps the patient in identifying new roles at work or at home.

If the patient has been identified as a candidate for heart transplantation, the nurse can discuss with the patient the future challenges that lie ahead as well as the potential for a lengthy wait until a donor is found. During this process the nurse maintains a positive and hopeful attitude with the patient and family.

Documentation

Documentation of care for the patient with cardiomyopathy primarily involves accurate recording of assessment data and interventions as well as validation of patient teaching. The recording of frequent thorough physical assessments is essential while the treatment plan is being established to determine the patient's response and quickly identify complications. The patient's activity levels and those activities that precipitate symptoms should be documented. The patient's record should contain accurate and detailed documentation of those measures that are successful in reducing symptoms or that assist the patient in coping with the physical limitations of the disease. Since self-care is the foundation of therapy, the patient's record should contain a description of the verbal and written instructions the patient and family received regarding the disease process, treatment plan, prescribed medications, and side effects.

Ongoing Care

Regardless of the treatment used, it is impossible to guarantee whether a patient will remain stable with an adequate cardiac output. Careful ongoing medical follow-up is essential, and patients are evaluated at least every 6 months for progression of the disease or the need for changes in the therapeutic regimen. It is important that patients be knowledgeable about the symptoms that indicate deterioration and who to contact if they have an increase in shortness of breath, fatigue, syncope, or pain. The nurse assumes primary responsibility for patient and family education concerning diet, activity, medications, and other necessary care. The nurse plays an essential part in preparing the patient to successfully manage the disease and to know when to seek help.

• • •

CARDIAC SURGERY

Cardiac surgery may be performed to promote optimal cardiac function for many cardiac disorders. For coronary artery obstruction of greater than 75%, vessel bypass improves myocardial blood flow and relieves symptoms. In the setting of marked valvular stenosis or incompetence, valvular repair or replacement significantly improves the flow of blood through the heart. Congenital anatomic heart defects such as coarctation of the aorta and atrial or ventricular septal defects can be managed using palliative or corrective surgery. Special resection techniques are employed for certain dysrhythmias such as atrial and ventricular tachydysrhythmias, tumors, and ventricular aneurysms. When ischemic heart disease or cardiomyopathy results in severe heart failure, cardiac transplantation is considered. The postoperative care for a patient having a transplant is similar to that required for other types of cardiac surgery but also includes immunosuppressive therapy to prevent rejection of the foreign tissue. Each of these procedures commonly requires the use of temporary cardiopulmonary bypass, in which blood is diverted from the heart and lungs and is oxygenated and circulated via a machine (**cardiopulmonary bypass [CPB] machine**).

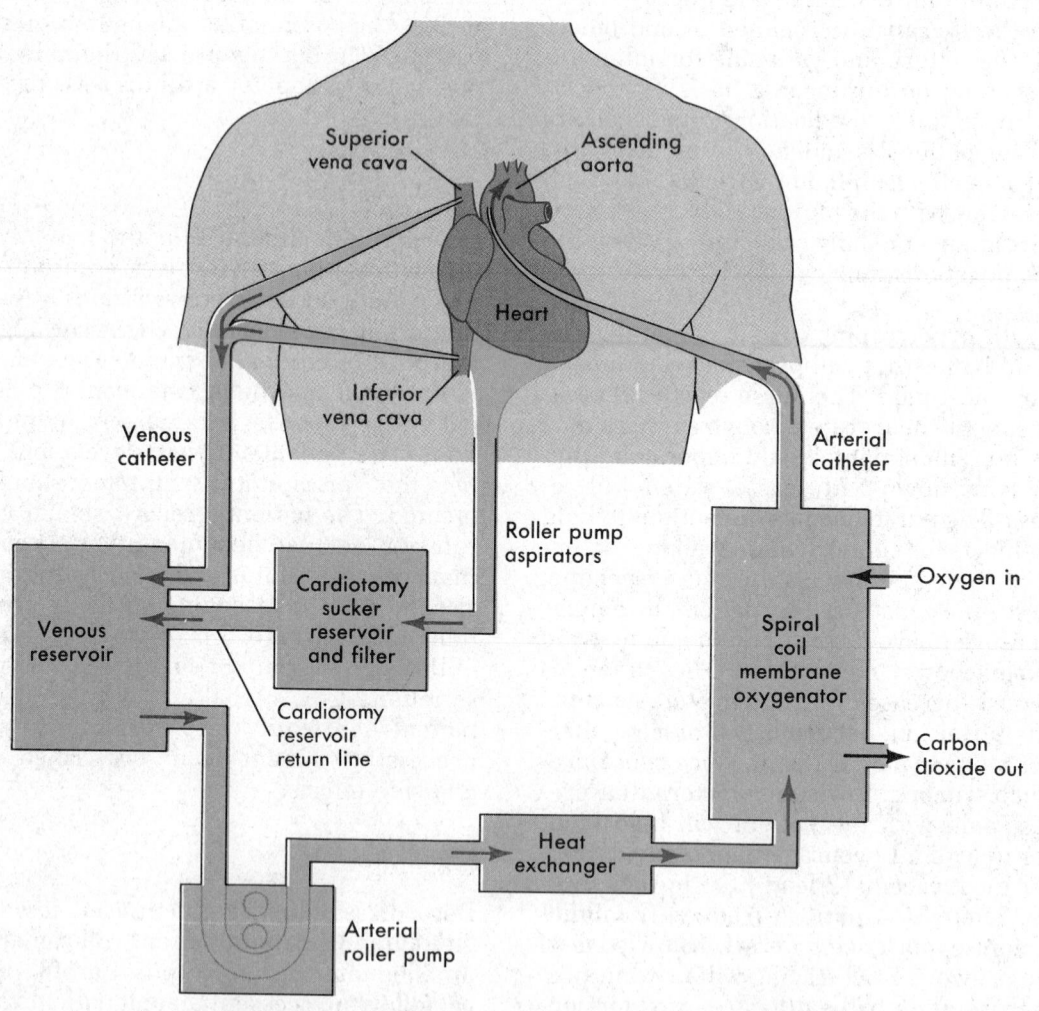

FIGURE 35-11 · Setup for cardiopulmonary bypass (CPB).

Cardiopulmonary Bypass

Use of the CPB machine allows for adequate perfusion to the patient and for a dry, bloodless surgical field that enhances visualization of the heart (Figure 35-11). During surgery, blood is removed from the body through a cannula or tube inserted into the right atrium or vena cava and routed to the CPB machine. This machine has an oxygenator that oxygenates the blood and removes carbon dioxide. The heat exchanger in the machine allows for cooling or heating of the blood. Cooling the patient's body temperature to 28° to 32° C (82.4° to 89.6° F) during surgery decreases the body's metabolism and need for oxygen. A pump and filter keeps the blood moving through the patient's system while filtering it before reinfusion. Blood is then returned to the body through a cannula in the ascending aorta or femoral artery to maintain systemic perfusion of the patient.

Since thrombi can occur at many points along the circuit, anticoagulation with heparin is employed during the procedure. The patient's blood is hemodiluted with crystalloid solution to decrease viscosity (thickness of the blood), decrease hemolysis (destruction of red blood cells), minimize peripheral and pulmonary vascular resistance, and decrease the need for blood administration.

Types of Surgery

When cardiac surgery is performed for coronary artery obstruction, a coronary artery bypass graft (CABG) is used. The graft is placed to bypass the obstructive lesion in the coronary artery or arteries. Saphenous vein grafts use a long segment of the saphenous vein from the leg. Before the vein is inserted, its direction is reversed because of the direction of the venous valves. One end is anastomosed to the coronary artery distal to the occlusion, and the proximal end is anastomosed to the ascending aorta. The internal mammary artery (IMA) may also be used as a bypass graft. The IMA is dissected from the surrounding chest wall, its branches ligated, and the distal end anastomosed to the coronary artery beyond the obstruction. Multiple grafts may be performed in patients with multiple vessel disease.

Placement of a CABG distal to a stenotic lesion provides additional blood flow and therefore oxygen to the area of the myocardium that is fed by the artery. This results in a reduction of anginal symptoms and ischemia. Such a bypass can prevent an MI and consequently prolong a patient's life but does not cure the underlying coronary artery disease.

In considering the need for CABG surgery an evaluation of the patient's symptoms and the extent of the CAD is needed. Typical testing includes chest radiographs, electrocardiography, stress testing, blood serum analysis of cardiac enzymes, cardiac catheterization, coronary angiography, echocardiography, nuclear cardiac studies, and phonocardiography. During coronary angiography the severity of obstruction, distal runoff, number of diseased vessels, and collateral blood flow are visualized. Distal runoff refers to the sufficiency of coronary blood flow through the distal branches of a coronary artery. Good blood flow beyond the obstruction is crucial to the success of a bypass graft in supplying the myocardium with the desired increase in blood flow. Other factors that are considered are preexisting damage to the myocardium from an MI and overall risk factors such as age, diabetes mellitus, and other organ diseases.

Congenital heart defects such as atrial or ventricular septal defects may be repaired or reconstructed with heart surgery. Ventricular aneurysms may be surgically resected or septal tissue may be removed (myectomy) in patients with HCM who experience obstruction to the outflow of blood as a result of their disease.

Surgical Preparation

In the surgical suite, several intravenous lines and an arterial line are inserted into the patient. The arterial line is used for continuous monitoring of the blood pressure and for frequent arterial blood gas determinations. A pulmonary artery catheter is inserted to indirectly monitor pressures in the left side of the heart. Alternatively, a left atrial line may be placed during surgery to directly measure left side of the heart pressures. Continuous ECG monitoring during surgery permits detection of ischemic changes and dysrhythmias. Finally, a Foley catheter is placed to measure urine output and indirectly measure renal perfusion. A nasogastric tube is placed to prevent gastric distention.

A light anesthetic is generally administered, and the patient is intubated and placed on mechanical ventilation. The patient is then fully anesthetized, and an extensive skin preparation is performed on the cardiac incision site, where chest tubes will be placed, and, if appropriate, where the saphenous vein bypass graft or grafts will be harvested if the patient is undergoing a coronary artery bypass graft.

The surgical procedure usually requires a midsternal incision where the sternum is cut vertically with a saw and retracted to visualize the surgical field. Frequently a cold cardioplegia solution is applied into and around the heart to produce further local cooling and minimize myocardial oxygen consumption. A solution containing high amounts of potassium is injected into the aorta near the heart to obtain cardiac arrest to allow surgery to take place on an immobile heart.

Postoperative Stabilization

Once surgery is completed, the blood is warmed and the heart is defibrillated to reinitiate sinus rhythm. After the patient's temperature and hemodynamic status return to normal, the cardiopulmonary bypass cannulas are removed and the patient is given protamine to reverse the anticoagulation effects of heparin. Pacemaker wires may be attached to the epicardium and then brought out through a separate incision on the chest wall. They can be used to manage conduction abnormalities or dysrhythmias that may occur in the early postoperative period. Mediastinal chest tubes are placed to permit postoperative drainage of residual blood in the operative field, which could cause tamponade or infection. If the pleural cavity was opened, then a pleural chest tube is placed to maintain lung expansion. Finally, the sternum is closed with strong suturing material.

Some patients who have damaged left ventricles may be unable to maintain an adequate blood pressure while being weaned from CPB. In this case they can be placed on the **intra-aortic balloon pump (IABP)** (Figure 35-12) to help their heart's pumping action until the heart has a chance to recover from the stress of surgery. The IABP may also be used in selected patients in the critical care setting who have angina refractory to pharmacologic therapy such as nitroglycerin or after MI complicated by heart failure.

The IABP catheter is inserted percutaneously into a femoral artery and positioned in the descending thoracic aorta. The balloon catheter is attached externally to an electric console that times the inflation and deflation of the balloon in synchrony with the cardiac cycle. The balloon inflates during diastole, increasing diastolic aortic pressures, which increases blood flow back toward the aortic valve, increasing coronary artery perfusion. The balloon deflates during ventricular systole causing a temporary decrease in aortic resistance, which helps to decrease the work load of the heart. Clinically, the increase in coronary artery perfusion and decrease in the work load of the heart improve the balance between cardiac oxygen supply and demand. Use of the IABP can improve cardiac functioning while the heart heals postoperatively, as demonstrated by an increased cardiac output, an increased urinary output, a decrease in left ventricular filling pressures, and an overall improvement in the patient's clinical picture.

Complications

The following complications of cardiac surgery include those relating to CPB or the surgical procedure itself.

Hypothermia. The patient is cooled to 28° to 32°

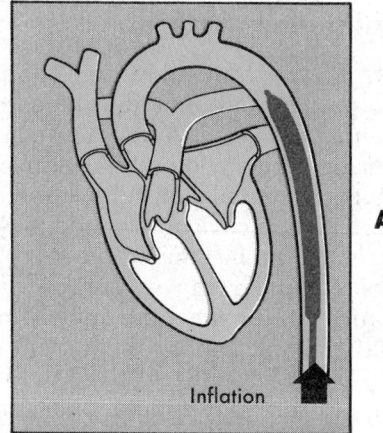

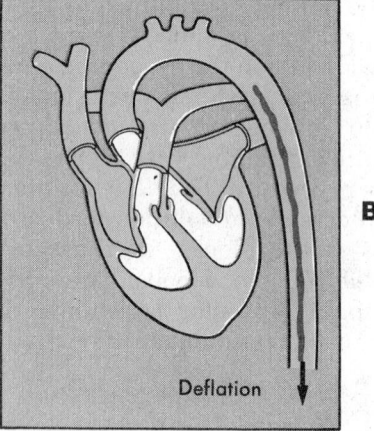

FIGURE 35-12   Intra-aortic balloon pump. **A,** Inflation: aortic pressure is increased, and blood volume is displaced. Desired effects of inflation are (1) coronary blood flow is potentially increased; (2) perfusion is augmented to aortic arch and distal systemic circulation; and (3) coronary collateral circulation is potentially increased. **B,** Desired effects of deflation are (1) reduction of aortic end-diastolic pressure reduces afterload; (2) systole following balloon inflation should be lower than unassisted systole; (3) myocardial oxygen consumption (MVO_2) is decreased; (4) cardiac output is increased; and (5) reduction in peak systolic pressure reduces left to right shunting in ventricular septal defects and regurgitant blood flow in mitral insufficiency. (From Quaal SL: *Comprehensive intra-aortic balloon pumping,* St Louis, 1984, Mosby–Year Book.)

C. Rewarming does not occur uniformly in all organs; tissues with a higher blood flow warm more quickly. This effect can produce shock or dysrhythmias during the warming process.

Coagulation. Heparinization is used throughout CPB and is reversed by protamine at the end of surgery. Since protamine is metabolized more quickly than heparin, a heparin "rebound" can occur, requiring additional protamine. Additional alterations in the coagulation system are produced because clotting factors are damaged during CPB and hypothermia also alters the patient's clotting process.

Damage to blood components. Blood components are damaged by contact with the tubing surfaces and compression by the roller pumps. Platelets are affected to the greatest degree, followed by other plasma proteins, red blood cells, white blood cells, and certain clotting factors. Damage to plasma antibodies and leukocytes impairs the patient's immune response.

Fluid balance: hemodilution. The CPB machine is primed with a crystalloid solution, such as normal saline, producing hemodilution. This improves flow in the microcirculation, reduces the risk of embolic complications, and reduces the need for blood administration. However, hemodilution increases extracellular water and interstitial fluid, which will need to be mobilized postoperatively. Such a postoperative diuresis can produce marked fluid and electrolyte shifts.

Electrolyte shifts. Potassium balance and to some extent sodium, calcium, and magnesium balance are altered by hemodilution and postoperative diuresis.

Microemboli. The use of microfilters and hemodilution has reduced the incidence of microemboli, but they still can occur.

Reduced lung compliance. During CPB the lungs are inactive and surfactant production is decreased. This can make the lungs stiff (decreased compliance) and increase the work of breathing.

• • •

Complications may also occur that are not specific to the CPB machine.

Hemorrhage. Untoward bleeding can occur after cardiac surgery. Hemorrhage may be caused by inadequate surgical hemostasis, prolonged cardiopulmonary bypass time, which damages platelets, or the administration of large amounts of stored bank blood that does not contain coagulation factors.

Low cardiac output state. A low cardiac output state is caused by cardiac tamponade; it is one of the most worrisome complications and can occur if the chest tubes do not adequately drain the surgical site or become clotted. A low cardiac output state may also result from dysrhythmias.

Thrombotic/embolic complications. Peripheral arterial occlusion caused by embolism can occur and is most commonly seen in patients who have underlying atherosclerosis, atrial dysrhythmias, and mechanical valves. Possible venous complications include phlebothrombosis or thrombophlebitis. Embolization of blood clots to the lung can occur, producing evidence of a pulmonary embolus.

Postpericardiotomy syndrome. Postpericardiotomy syndrome is thought to represent an immune response directed against the epicardium. It is identified by the presence of fever, pericarditis, and pleuritic-type pain occurring more than 1 week after cardiac surgery.

Respiratory complications. The cardiac patient is at risk for several postoperative respiratory problems. During surgery the lungs are partially collapsed to keep them out of the operative field. This promotes alveolar collapse and postoperative atelectasis. The function of gas exchange is assumed by the CPB machine. Patients with cardiac dysfunction often experience some degree of pulmonary edema, which decreases surfactant production and promotes alveolar collapse. A pneumothorax may occur during surgery, and a hemothorax can develop soon after surgery if the chest is not adequately drained with chest tubes. Once a pneumothorax or a hemothorax is detected, a chest tube may be needed. Other complications include a pleural effusion, bronchial aspiration, pulmonary edema, and noncardiogenic pulmonary edema (adult respiratory distress syndrome).

Fever/infection. The most common source of fever in the early postoperative period (3 to 5 days) is a pulmonary infection, often associated with atelectasis that begins intraoperatively. Occasionally a urinary tract infection or bacteremia causes fever during this period. A wound infection can become manifest several (5 to 10) days postoperatively. Any wound site can be affected, such as sternal, thoracic, leg, or chest tube sites. Fevers that occur 7 to 10 days postoperatively may be associated with an infected fluid collection. Fevers after this period are often associated with endocarditis or infection of a prosthetic valve or graft.

Renal complications. A postoperative hypovolemia and low cardiac output can produce renal dysfunction postoperatively.

Gastrointestinal complications. Gastric distention sometimes occurs in the early postoperative period. It results from air swallowed during intubation and from the stress of surgery.

Central nervous system complications. Patients often demonstrate abnormal behavior postoperatively, including confusion, irritability, disorientation, memory lapses, bizarre acting, and even episodes of hallucinations. Contributing factors include sleep deprivation, the psychologic and physical stress of surgery, atherosclerotic insufficiency, and sometimes embolization of particulate matter or air during CPB.

NURSING MANAGEMENT FOR THE PATIENT UNDERGOING CARDIAC SURGERY

Assessment

The nurse assesses for a broad range of signs and symptoms. A thorough history is essential and includes data about specific patient symptoms, how they have changed or progressed over time, and what treatment has been undertaken. The results of previous diagnostic studies, such as cardiac catheterization, help define the extent of the patient's problems. The nurse inquires about underlying cardiac problems that might reveal the presence of coronary artery, congenital heart, or valvular disease, and occasionally ventricular aneurysm or septal defect. When coronary artery disease exists, the presence of one or more risk factors is common, including hypertension, glucose intolerance/diabetes mellitus, hyperlipidemia, cigarette smoking, obesity, a sedentary life-style, and advanced age. An evaluation into the presence of a family history of any of the aforementioned risk factors also correlates with the presence of CAD. Evaluation of the presence and nature of anginal symptoms is an essential component of the preoperative and postoperative assessment of the patient. Other evidence of myocardial ischemia, such as dysrhythmias or palpitations, is also considered.

A key component of the nursing assessment is the level of cardiac function. Compromised cardiac performance may be reflected by activity intolerance or easy fatigability, hypotension, tachycardia, abnormal pulse (such as irregular rhythm, pulsus alternans, and weak pulse), and evidence of diminished peripheral circulation (such as pallor, duskiness, cyanosis, cool skin temperature, and diaphoresis). An altered level of consciousness may result from decreased cerebral perfusion. In addition, cardiac compromise may be manifested by evidence of venous distention, including dependent edema, distention of neck veins, sacral edema, ascites, and hepatomegaly. Auscultation of heart sounds may reveal a murmur or S_3 or S_4 gallop.

An assessment of the patient and family's level of anxiety and identification of specific concerns permit appropriate support. Investigation into patient and family roles, how they have been altered, and problems with activities of daily living (ADL) helps focus the efforts of the nurse and other members of the health team. Finally, an evaluation of the patient and family's knowledge regarding the planned therapeutic regimen helps define areas for patient and family teaching. Information regarding fears about surgery and its outcome, previous experiences with surgery, and experiences of other family members or friends with heart disease provides direction for support of the patient and family.

Nursing Diagnosis

Multiple nursing diagnoses may be appropriate for the patient undergoing cardiac surgery, depending on the severity and extent of the disease process and the surgery performed. Common diagnoses include the following:

Anxiety (patient/family) related to the cardiac disease, hospitalization, medical therapy employed, altered activity level, impending major surgery and its associated risks, altered family roles, separation from family members, and possible altered job roles

Knowledge deficit regarding perioperative procedures and experience, discharge regimen

Decreased cardiac output related to cardiac tamponade, MI, CHF, dysrhythmias, and rejection (in the patient undergoing heart transplant)

High risk for impaired gas exchange related to hypoventilation, accumulation of secretions, pulmonary edema, fluid volume overload, and immobility

Pain related to the incision, chest discomfort associated with chest tube irritation of surrounding tissue, tissue trauma caused by surgery, wound infection, or anxiety

High risk for altered thought processes related to CPB machine, embolization, sedation, medications, sensory overload or deprivation, immobility

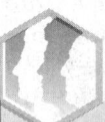

GERIATRIC CONSIDERATIONS

Risk Factors and Complications of Cardiac Surgery

The elderly patient population tends to have a higher incidence of risk factors such as stroke, diabetes mellitus, renal dysfunction, and hypertension. A careful assessment of the general condition of these patients is important in determining aspects of their care. Underlying problems must be resolved before surgery, and risk factors must be analyzed for their impact on complications such as respiratory complications, changes in level of consciousness, renal failure, and decreased cardiac output.

The increased mortality and morbidity associated with complications of cardiac surgery in the elderly patient population require that key factors be considered in their care. Respiratory compromise is a major problem postoperatively, and patients should be weaned from mechanical ventilation as soon as possible, followed by aggressive coughing and deep breathing exercises and use of the incentive spirometer. Adequate rest and nutrition are important in supporting the resources of the elderly patient during the recovery process. Avoiding excessive sedation and providing a normal environment outside the intensive care unit (ICU) help to reduce postoperative confusion, which can frequently occur in this patient population.

Certain nursing diagnoses are more common in the intensive care unit (ICU). Diagnoses common to the ICU are as follows:

High risk for fluid volume deficit related to hypovolemia from inadequate fluid volume replacement, rapid rewarming

High risk for fluid volume excess related to cardiopulmonary bypass followed by inadequate diuresis, preexisting CHF, or overaggressive volume replacement

Ineffective airway clearance related to immobility, discomfort, decreased compliance, or effects of anesthesia

High risk for infection related to pulmonary secretions, presence of a surgical wound, urinary tract catheter, or other tubes and catheters

Planning

Expected outcomes will relate to the severity of cardiac disease, symptoms being experienced, and the nature of the surgery performed. Goal priority depends on the severity of the threat to the patient's physical and psychologic integrity. General goals might include the following:

Patient and family verbalize a reduction in anxiety with provision of information, explanations, and encouragement

Patient and family demonstrate knowledge of disease process, purpose of hospitalization, surgery planned, preoperative and postoperative management, and expected outcomes

Patient demonstrates adequate cardiac output as evidenced by blood pressure, heart rate and rhythm within patient's baseline parameters; urine output greater than 30 mL/hr; no JVD or peripheral edema

Patient will maintain adequate gas exchange as evidenced by respiratory rate and rhythm and arterial blood gas measurements within limits normal for the patient; clear breath sounds

Patient will obtain relief of pain

Patient is alert and oriented to time, place, and person and returns to preoperative neurologic status

Before discharge patient and family accurately describe dietary and activity guidelines, medications, and special care activities (e.g., suture line care) if appropriate

Implementation

The nurse caring for the patient undergoing heart surgery needs to consider each patient's medical and social history and clinical condition to appropriately individualize care. It is important to consider the nature of the underlying heart condition, how long it has existed, other underlying disease conditions, and the anticipated surgical procedure. An estimation of the extent of cardiac impairment can be made by determining the patient's limitations in lifestyle.

Investigation into the occurrence of previous cardiopulmonary events and presence of certain risk factors will help the nurse be alert to the occurrence of certain postoperative complications. Events that put the patient at higher risk for postoperative complications include MI, blood clotting abnormalities, pulmonary emboli, bacterial endocarditis, and risk factors such as smoking and high blood pressure.

In establishing an individualized care plan the prehospital medical regimen, medications, and other therapeutic measures are considered. Some alteration in the previous therapeutic regimen, as well as diet and activity levels, may be necessary after hospitalization. The rationale for these changes and their role in the preoperative preparation need to be carefully explained to the patient and family.

An initial and ongoing assessment of the patient and family's level of anxiety permits delivery of appropriate support. Investigation into their concerns regarding risks of surgery and its outcome illuminates specific areas that can be addressed and clarified. Assessment of their understanding of the disease process and need for surgery provides a basis for teaching. In collaboration with the physician, information is provided regarding the relationship of the disease process and the rationale for various therapeutic interventions, medications, and need for surgery. Providing such support and information can significantly reduce the patient and family's anxiety. In addition, an informed patient can maximally participate in self-care.

Patients are generally hospitalized 1 day before surgery. Patient teaching is an important component of nursing interventions for the patient undergoing heart surgery to facilitate recuperation and prevent complications. The day before surgery is not an optimal time to perform teaching since patients may be extremely anxious and unable to retain the information. Therefore a system should be devised to provide the patient with necessary instructions before admission, either in the physician's office or through a preadmission visit to the hospital.

Postoperative management

In the early postoperative period (i.e., during the first 24 to 48 hours), patients are cared for in the intensive care unit. In this environment hemodynamic monitoring provides continuous information regarding the patient's cardiovascular status and indicates the need for intervention. An arterial line provides constant feedback about the blood pressure. This provides information necessary for adjustment of fluids, diuretics, and essential inotropic/va-

NURSING CARE PLAN   *The Patient Undergoing Cardiac Surgery*

Nursing diagnosis/ *Expected outcome*	Interventions	Rationale
High risk for decreased cardiac output related to dysrhythmias, hemorrhage, decreased contractility, complications, or rejection (in heart transplant patient) • *Patient will maintain adequate cardiac output as evidenced by vital signs, cardiac pressures, and cardiac output within patient's baseline range; no bleeding; skin warm and dry; urine output greater than 30 mL/hr; and electrolyte levels normal*	Monitor the following parameters every 1 to 2 hours and analyze for trends: blood pressure, heart rate and rhythm, heart sounds, and cardiac output (when available)	Isolated measurements are not diagnostic; trends in measurements assist in detecting presence and cause of altered cardiac output; decrease in blood pressure, increase in heart rate, irregular heart rhythm, additional heart sounds, or a decrease in cardiac output indicates complications causing decreased cardiac output
	Assess and record every 1 to 2 hours or as prescribed urine output, color and temperature of extremities, peripheral pulses, capillary refill time, and neurologic status	These parameters reflect adequacy of cardiac output
	Assess for symptoms of hypoxia: restlessness, confusion, dyspnea, hypotension, tachycardia	Hypoxia can be created by inadequate cardiac output
	Assess for signs and symptoms of complications:	
	Cardiac tamponade: elevated CVP, JVD, decreased pulse pressure, pulsus paradoxus (> 10 mm Hg), and large amounts of chest tube drainage, if applicable	Cardiac tamponade can occur as result of blood or fluid accumulation in pericardial sac
	Dysrhythmias: irregular pulse, decreased blood pressure, ECG abnormalities	Increased incidence of dysrhythmias occurs perioperatively and between second and fifth postoperative days
	MI: obtain and assess 12-lead ECG, enzymes, and isoenzymes daily (see discussion of MI, p. 874)	Perioperative MIs are difficult to determine because of elevations in enzymes and ECG changes that normally occur after heart surgery
	CHF: elevated CVP, JVD, crackles, dependent edema, decreased blood pressure, decreased urine output (see discussion of CHF in Chapter 36)	Preexisting left ventricular dysfunction and a wide range of perioperative and postoperative factors can place patient at risk for CHF
	Notify physician of any changes in patient status or signs and symptoms of complications	Prompt intervention imperative to maintain or promote hemodynamic stability
	Implement measures to treat cause of decreased cardiac output as prescribed (i.e., blood and blood products if bleeding; isotonic infusions if hypovolemic; antidysrhythmic agents; vasopressor/inotropic medications)	Cause of decreased cardiac output determines treatment measure

NURSING CARE PLAN   *The Patient Undergoing Cardiac Surgery—cont'd*

Nursing diagnosis/ Expected outcome	Interventions	Rationale
At risk for impaired gas exchange related to alveolar capillary membrane changes, immobility, effects of anesthesia, or hypoventilation • *Patient will maintain adequate gas exchange as evidenced by respiratory rate and rhythm and arterial blood gas measurements within limits normal for individual, and clear breath sounds*	**Rejection of cardiac transplant** Assess and monitor for fever, peripheral edema, general malaise, shortness of breath, and new S_3 gallop Administer immunosuppressant medications as prescribed Monitor BUN/creatinine and cyclosporine levels Note results of endomyocardial biopsy if performed Provide ventilatory support with mechanical ventilation for first 24 hours postoperatively	Reflects signs of rejection Promotes compatibility of host and donor heart Low levels may indicate inadequate cyclosporine therapy or predispose patient to rejection Endomyocardial biopsy is helpful in diagnosing infection and rejection Provides airway in event of emergencies, such as cardiac arrest; provides effective ventilation and oxygenation and reduces work load of heart
	After extubation Assess for respiratory rate, rhythm, and depth every 2 to 4 hours Analyze arterial blood gas results as they are performed Auscultate breath sounds every 2 to 4 hours or as indicated Turn patient side to side while on bed rest; ambulate as soon as possible Encourage patient to use incentive spirometer every 2 hours Assist patient in deep breathing and coughing exercises every 2 to 4 hours Involve family in assisting patient to perform respiratory exercises Administer analgesics such as acetaminophen (Tylenol) with codeine or meperidine (Demerol) if indicated before respiratory care Instruct patient in splinting chest incision with pillow during respiratory exercises	Anesthesia, sedation, and pain may depress respirations; monitoring these parameters permits early detection of ineffective gas exchange Provides data about changes in oxygenation and ventilation Crackles and wheezes may be present if patient is not adequately ventilating lungs; diminished breath sounds may indicate fluid accumulation in alveoli or atelectasis Activity and ambulation promote respiratory excursion and improve lung function Promotes lung expansion and reduces risk of atelectasis Mobilizes secretions and promotes airway clearance Family can be an excellent reinforcer and motivator for patient Pain can decrease patient's willingness or ability to take deep breaths and cough Helps reduce pain and discomfort

PATIENT EDUCATION GUIDE   *The Patient Undergoing Cardiac Surgery*

1. Preoperative preparation
   a. Shower using germicidal soap
   b. Skin shaved in operative area
   c. Nothing to eat or drink after midnight the night before surgery
   d. Tests that may need to be performed before surgery if they have not already been completed (i.e., ECG, echocardiogram, chest x-ray film, exercise testing, pulmonary function tests, cardiac catheterization)
   e. Visits from various members of the surgical team such as surgeon and anesthesiologist
   f. Pain and sleep medications
   g. Smoking cessation
2. Immediately before surgery
   a. Administer medications such as a sedative, an anticholinergic agent, and a narcotic analgesic
   b. Inform about the appearance and expectations in operating room
      (1) Cold room with many people
      (2) Intravenous line will be started
      (3) Other catheters inserted
   c. Identify where the family can wait during surgery
3. Immediate postoperative period
   a. Environment: what to expect in the ICU, namely, equipment, personnel, invasive lines, tubes, and catheters (intravenous lines, endotracheal tube, ventilator, pacemaker wires, arterial catheter, pulmonary artery catheter, chest tubes, urinary catheter)
   b. Sensations the patient may feel: drowsy, unable to talk because of the presence of the endotracheal tube, chest and back discomfort, feel the need to void from the urinary catheter, the noise
   c. Diet: nothing to eat or drink for the first 24 hours, then clear liquids as tolerated
   d. Routine care: suctioning, dressing changes, turning and position changes, constant monitoring
   e. Method of communication while intubated
   f. Activities: leg and arm exercises, bed rest
   g. Family expectations: surgeon's visit, ICU visiting hours, how to communicate with the patient, how to receive ongoing status reports
4. Recuperation
   a. When tubes, lines, and equipment will be removed
   b. Transfer from the ICU
   c. Coughing and deep breathing exercises and use of the incentive spirometer
      (1) How to perform them
      (2) Frequency
      (3) Measures to decrease pain and discomfort
   d. Activities
      (1) When to get out of bed
      (2) Ambulation: frequency and duration
      (3) Bathing/showering and self-care activities
   e. Pain management
   f. Family involvement
      (1) Visiting hours
      (2) Assistance with breathing exercises and ambulation
      (3) Acceptance of possible changes in mentation

sopressor agents such as dopamine, dobutamine, norepinephrine, or nitroglycerin, if they are needed. Inotropic/vasopressor agents are frequently used to maintain a blood pressure adequate for brain perfusion, to prevent cardiac ischemia, and to decrease the risk of renal failure. A catheter in the pulmonary artery provides pressure readings of the pulmonary artery diastolic and systolic pressures and the pulmonary capillary wedge pressure, and a catheter in the left atrium provides left atrial pressure readings. These measurements approximate the filling pressures on the left side of the heart and provide the most precise information regarding the left ventricular response to fluids, inotropic/vasopressor medications, and diuretics. These catheters are removed when the patient is hemodynamically stable with an adequate cardiac output, which is normally the first or second postoperative day.

A Foley catheter drains the patient's bladder of urine and is measured hourly. The balance of fluid intake and output from all sources and assessment of daily weights assist in evaluating the patient's fluid status to determine the adequacy of diuresis and signs of hypovolemia or hypervolemia.

Drainage of residual blood from the operative area is made possible by the placement of chest tubes. Bloody drainage should not exceed 200 mL/hr for the first 2 to 6 hours and should steadily decrease so that by the second or third postoperative day the drainage becomes serous and stops. The tubes are then removed.

Pleural chest tubes are placed if the type of surgery required that the pleural cavity be opened; they remove air from the pleural space. These tubes are removed when there is no more air bubbling out through the tube and the pleural and pulmonary tissues have sealed over. This usually occurs on the second or third postoperative day.

The patient is maintained on artificial mechanical ventilation until the effects of anesthesia have worn off and the patient's arterial blood gases and pulmonary function tests indicate the patient can be extubated. The patient must demonstrate the ability to take deep breaths spontaneously and expectorate secretions before the endotracheal tube can be removed, usually the first or second postoperative day.

A careful ongoing evaluation of cardiac performance helps ensure adequate cardiac output and early detection of problems. Electrical instability may develop postoperatively, particularly tachycardia and ectopic beats. Tachydysrhythmias such as supraventricular tachycardia, atrial flutter, or atrial fibrillation may be treated pharmacologically with verapamil, digoxin, propranolol, procainamide, or esmolol. Ventricular ectopic beats or rhythms may be treated with lidocaine, procainamide, or bretylium. Cardioversion or defibrillation may be necessary to control tachydysrhythmias that do not respond to pharmacologic treatment. The correction of causal factors for the dysrhythmia, such as hypoxemia, electrolyte imbalance, or fluid overload or depletion, is important in resolving and preventing the recurrence of the dysrhythmia.

Electrolytes are monitored frequently during the postoperative period to determine abnormalities, especially of potassium, sodium, calcium, and magnesium. If extremely high or low levels of these electrolytes are not treated promptly, the patient may experience significant complications, such as weakness, confusion, convulsions, or dysrhythmias.

Prophylactic antibiotics are generally recommended for all cardiac surgery patients. They are begun before surgery and continued through the first 48 hours or until major intravenous lines, chest tubes, and other catheters have been removed. The patient's temperature is monitored every hour to identify possible infections or, later in the postoperative period, signs of postpericardiotomy syndrome. If fever is present, all incisions and wounds are cultured to determine the presence of infection. Sputum and urine samples are also cultured, and antibiotics are adjusted based on the results of the cultures and sensitivity. If symptoms of postpericardiotomy syndrome are present (i.e., malaise, pericardial effusion, pericardial friction rub, pericardial pain), anti-inflammatory agents are prescribed.

A mild anticoagulant effect is produced in many patients undergoing CABG surgery by the use of low-dose aspirin or aspirin and dipyridamole. The drugs help promote graft patency by inhibiting platelet aggregation. In patients with a history of emboli, particularly in the presence of atrial fibrillation or valvular disease, a stronger anticoagulant, such as warfarin sodium (Coumadin), is considered. Mechanical prosthetic valves also require warfarin sodium; for porcine valves, mild or no anticoagulation is employed.

After 1 to 3 days of ICU care, the patient is transferred to an intermediate care unit or general care area. There is a gradually increasing level of independence in ADL over an average of 7 to 10 days until discharge. A summary of nursing responsibilities for maintaining cardiac output and adequate ventilation is presented in the nursing care plan for the patient undergoing heart surgery.

After transfer out of the ICU the focus of nursing actions is to monitor for signs and symptoms of complications as well as assist the patient and family in the recuperation phase and prepare them for discharge.

Fluids and diet

Daily weights and fluid intake and output are checked to detect any retention of body water. The patient's weight should return to the preoperative level. If the weight remains high, the patient may have had inadequate diuresis after surgery. This may be accompanied by continued peripheral edema, JVD, and pulmonary crackles and wheezes. Occasionally fluid restriction and diuretics are employed, especially if marked CHF or hypertension is present.

Sips of water are followed by clear and then full fluids. Once the patient can tolerate solid foods, a full diet is started, which may be regular or special, such as diabetic or low sodium and low cholesterol. If the prescribed diet is new to the patient and family, careful education will prepare them to continue it on discharge.

Activity

Early mobilization is encouraged after surgery to optimize pulmonary function and promote cardiovascular fitness. By the third or fourth postoperative day, most patients are able to ambulate with limited assistance. If incisional pain limits the patient's ability to ambulate, analgesics such as acetaminophen should be administered 30 minutes before the activity. The patient's activity gradually progresses during hospitalization. By the time of discharge, most patients can walk in the hallways several times each day. Modifications in the activity progression are made for individuals experiencing complications such as heart failure or pericarditis in the postoperative period. Before discharge, guidelines for a reasonable activity level are provided based on the patient's disease process and surgical outcome.

Pulmonary function is optimized with the use of the incentive spirometer and deep breathing and coughing exercises every 2 hours postoperatively. The patient should be taught how to splint the sternal incision with a pillow during these exercises to reduce the incidence of pain that makes the patient less likely to comply with this important activity. Analgesics provided before respiratory exercises will help the patient be comfortable during their implementation.

Comfort

Patients may not verbalize the occurrence of pain because of fear of narcotic addiction or cultural background; it is essential for the nurse to observe and listen to the patient for verbal and nonverbal clues regarding pain. Patients may experience incisional pain or a more diffuse feeling of discomfort from the interruption of nerve endings during surgery or the irritation caused by the presence of a chest catheter. These types of pain must be differentiated from anginal pain. Many patients experience back pain along the spinal column because of rib retraction during surgery.

Analgesics such as acetaminophen (Tylenol) with codeine, meperidine (Demerol), or morphine may be prescribed to control pain. The patient should be encouraged to use these measures to allow for adequate rest and comfort during ambulation, respiratory exercises, and participation in self-care.

Postoperatively, psychologic difficulties may be devastating; they occur for several reasons. Dependence on life-support systems and the often radical change in the patient's role in the family, work, or social activities may give rise to depression and a feeling of futility, which require support and encouragement to counteract. Sleep deprivation, anxiety, disorientation to day and night, and sensory overload contribute to abnormal responses such as restlessness, disorientation, or depression. Careful patient and family preoperative preparation, shorter CPB times, and briefer stays in the ICU help reduce but do not eliminate these problems. Measures that reduce the stress that may cause these psychologic changes include providing for uninterrupted periods of sleep, encouraging sleep at night with short naps during the day, frequently calling the person by name, orienting the patient to time and place, and providing explanations tailored to the patient's readiness.

Patient education

Appropriate instruction and guidance are provided throughout the hospital stay. An assessment of risk factors provides the basis for instruction regarding modification. An assessment of the patient's knowledge of appropriate dietary habits provides the basis for recommendations regarding prudent dietary guidelines. In general, a low cholesterol, low to moderate sodium diet is recommended.

Medications are carefully reviewed as well, including name, purpose, dosage, possible side effects, and selected precautions. Finally the plan for follow-up care is described. This might include visits with the surgeon, cardiologist, or clinical nurse specialist. In collaboration with the social worker, information is provided about appropriate community resources, and assistance in obtaining them is provided as needed. Organizations specifically designed to assist the patient after cardiac surgery include local chapters of "Mended Hearts," cardiofitness programs, and other community organizations designed to help patients with such physical needs.

Cardiac transplantation

Cardiac transplantation is considered for patients experiencing refractory heart failure (not responding to medications, modification of risk factors, and in some cases previous surgeries). The postoperative care of the cardiac transplant patient is the same as that for other cardiac surgery patients, except it also includes immunosuppression. Some centers maintain full reverse isolation precautions, whereas others use modified precautions. The nurse needs to remember that this patient has a new, healthy heart and is less likely than other cardiac surgical patients to suffer the complications of MI, heart failure, or dysrhythmias. The patient will not experience angina, because the new heart has no nerve connections. Surgical complications such as hemorrhage or tamponade may occur. The endotracheal tube and all other invasive tubes and lines used postoperatively are removed as soon as possible to prevent infections, since the patient is medically immunosuppressed.

Cardiac transplant patients are usually euphoric immediately after surgery. They have survived the wait for a donor heart and the surgery and are filled with hopes and plans for the future. They ambulate early and eagerly, restricted only by their degree of physical debility caused by the preoperative illness. They often go home 7 to 10 days after surgery.

The immunosuppressive drug of choice in most centers is cyclosporine. It provides excellent immunosuppression in most patients but does not decrease the WBC. The patient is less susceptible to infection than with other agents. Rejection occurs less often and with slower onset than with former drug regimens, allowing early detection of most rejection episodes through endomyocardial biopsy. Side effects seen in most patients include mild-to-moderate renal compromise, hypertension, hirsutism, a burning sensation in the feet, and tearing of the eyes.

Patients are carefully monitored for signs of infection or rejection while hospitalized. Cultures are done routinely and at the first sign of infection. Most patients have several endomyocardial biopsies in the first month and at decreasing intervals after that. Usually between 15 and 20 biopsies are done in the first year.

Treatment for rejection usually consists of a boost

in oral steroids. This increase can be done at home if the patient has been discharged. A repeat biopsy after 5 to 7 days will generally show resolving rejection. Persistent rejections usually require hospitalization, stronger steroid therapy, and antithymocyte preparations.

Discharge readiness involves the patient's understanding of routine clinic or office visits, medication self-administration, and signs and symptoms to recognize and report to the health care team.

The patient who has undergone cardiac transplantation is monitored carefully for months to years at the transplant center. Some centers return the patient to the referring physician for routine health care. Other centers assume responsibility for all aspects of the transplant patient's care in perpetuity.

Evaluation

The effectiveness of nursing interventions is evaluated through ongoing assessments. Successful interventions will help the patient maintain an adequate cardiac output without discomfort or pain. The patient's vital signs will be stable, and peripheral pulses will be baseline. The ECG and laboratory results will return to baseline. The patient will be without signs of a low cardiac output (i.e., hypotension, tachycardia, lethargy, easy fatigability, and myocardial ischemia) or signs of CHF (i.e., crackles, wheezes, tachypnea, exertional dyspnea, edema, or hepatomegaly).

The patient will be without untoward effects of surgery, such as dysrhythmias, diminished perfusion to the various body systems, respiratory distress, electrolyte imbalance, infection, and disorientation. The patient and family will verbalize an understanding of the residual cardiac disease/dysfunction; any needed tests, procedures, and medications; and the rehabilitation program. The patient will show a reduction in anxiety and a knowledge of when to contact the physician or nurse and come in for follow-up appointments. Most important, the patient will demonstrate knowledge of the disease process, the surgical outcome, and the rehabilitation plan. The patient describes medications, how to take them, and their side effects, as well as the signs that indicate the need for medical assistance. Finally, the nurse looks for evidence that the patient and family feel in control of the situation and are able to appropriately problem solve.

Documentation

Documentation of care for the patient undergoing cardiac surgery primarily involves accurate recording of assessment data before and after surgery and the interventions employed to meet the nursing care goals. If complications arise, the assessment data, in-terventions, and the patient's response to them should be documented in detail. Validation of patient teaching and level of understanding regarding the learning objectives is important in preparing the patient and family for discharge. The patient's response to surgery and the rehabilitation program is carefully evaluated and recorded. Since self-care is the foundation of treatment, the verbal and written instructions that the patient has received regarding the disease process, treatment plan, prescribed medications, and side effects should be documented.

Ongoing Care

Careful ongoing medical follow-up is essential to promoting self-care, identification of complications, and tailoring the patient's treatment to individual needs. The nurse assumes primary responsibility for patient and family education concerning activity, medications, diet, and selected interventions (e.g., wound care, pacemaker care). Mobilization of assistance from the community support agencies may be appropriate, depending on the needs of the patient and family. The nurse plays an essential part in preparing the patient to effectively balance the desire to lead as full a life as possible with the sustained effects of cardiac disease.

Emotions

The patient should be assured that it is normal to have a letdown or depressed feeling and to cry easily. Some patients experience an impairment of memory or concentration. These complaints usually subside in 4 to 6 weeks.

Discomfort and pain

The patient can be reassured that discomfort from the incision is common and the incision area may be numb for several weeks or months after the operation. Soreness may be worse if the weather is very hot, cold, or rainy. The patient may notice that the incision becomes more bothersome when he or she has been doing more activities than usual. The physician may instruct the patient to use acetaminophen to help ease the pain. Exercise by raising and lowering the arms may help relieve discomfort.

Activities

The normal recovery of the body takes 4 to 6 weeks. It takes this much time for the sternum to completely heal and muscles to be reconditioned with activity. During this time the patient may notice a slight clicking or movement of the breast bone during breathing or turning. This is because the sternum is slightly unstable; the movement should disappear in 4 to 12 weeks. Activities begin gradually with walking, which helps recondition the muscles. "Light" household activities such as clearing the table and dusting are recommended. Rest periods should be interspersed throughout the day, with at least two rest periods of 20 to 30 minutes each day during the first or second week at home. Adequate rest at night (8 to 10 hours of sleep) also helps provide the energy required for daytime activities.

Because the sternum remains unstable for several weeks, lifting objects of 10 pounds or more, such as children, briefcases, suitcases, or groceries, or opening stuck windows or heavy doors is to be avoided. Activities that are extremely tiring or cause discomfort are also avoided. Similarly, recreational activities are resumed gradually, beginning with "lighter" activities such as playing cards, photography, painting, needlework, and attending movies. More rigorous exercises (e.g., tennis, swimming, jogging, golf) are resumed after consulting the physician at the 4- to 6-week checkup.

The patient is encouraged to resume sex when feeling good and well rested. Many clinicians use the guideline of the patient's ability to walk two blocks or climb two flights of stairs without dyspnea as a gross index indicating sufficient energy to engage in sex. Sex should be avoided when the patient feels tense or tired or after a heavy meal.

Stair climbing requires more energy, and the patient is encouraged to proceed slowly and stop if tired, short of breath, or dizzy. The day's activities should be organized to reduce the frequency of stair climbing.

Driving a car should be avoided for the first 4 to 6 weeks after surgery. If an accident occurs, the patient's chest could hit the steering wheel and if the sternum is still unstable, it would not protect the patient's heart against injury. In addition, reaction time is slowed by weakness, fatigue, or medications. Similarly, riding bicycles, motorcycles, lawn mowers, tractors, and horses should be avoided during this period. Riding in a car is permitted, but it should include a stop every 1 to 2 hours to walk around, which will improve circulation in the legs and prevent swelling.

Occupation

Usually the decision regarding returning to work is made at the 4- to 6-week follow-up visit. The decision depends on the type of work, demands of the particular job, the patient's level of physical stamina, and other information obtained from the checkup, such as the need to modify medications or continuing tiredness. Major changes in work or plans for retirement should be avoided until recovery is complete.

Ongoing care for altering risk factors and ensuring safety with medication administration is the same as for the patient with CAD. Evaluation of compliance will provide direction for the need for additional intervention.

CRITICAL THINKING QUESTIONS

1 Describe how atherosclerosis affects the coronary arteries and what alterations in lifestyle should be made to reduce the risk factors associated with atherosclerosis.

2 What factors may precipitate an anginal attack? What teaching is necessary to help the patient reduce anginal attacks? slow down the disease process? prevent complications?

3 What clinical manifestations and diagnostic criteria would be exhibited by a patient experiencing an MI? What complications would the nurse be assessing for after an MI? What signs and symptoms would be seen for each of the complications?

4 Compare the drug therapy used in the treatment of angina and myocardial infarction. What are the nursing implications? patient teaching implications?

5 What guidelines are used for the patient who has had an MI for progressing in activity levels?

6 What are the teaching objectives for the patient being discharged after an MI? What are the ongoing care issues?

7 What are the causes of pericarditis? What clinical signs would indicate pericarditis, pericardial effusion, and cardiac tamponade?

8 What is the medical management and nursing management for a patient with pericarditis, pericardial effusion, and cardiac tamponade?

9 How do restrictive, hypertrophic, and dilated cardiomyopathy differ in etiology and pathophysiology? What are the differences in medical treatment and nursing management?

10 What are the different types of procedures performed during cardiac surgery? What complications can occur after heart surgery?

11 Describe the preoperative teaching objectives for the patient undergoing heart surgery.

12 What are the postoperative and ongoing nursing issues for the patient undergoing heart surgery?

RESOURCES

Books and publications

1 *Eating to lower your high blood cholesterol* (National Institutes of Health Publication 89-

2920; 1989). National Cholesterol Education Program and National Heart, Lung, and Blood Institute, Department of Health and Human Services Bethesda, MD 20892

2 *Facts about blood cholesterol* (National Institutes of Health Publication 90-2696; 1990) National Heart, Lung and Blood Institute, Department of Health and Human Services Bethesda, MD 20892

3 *So you have high blood cholesterol* (National Institutes of Health Publication 87-2922; 1987) National Cholesterol Education Program and National Heart, Lung, and Blood Institute, Department of Health and Human Services Bethesda, MD 20892

4 *The healthy heart book for women* (National Institutes of Health Publication 87-2720) National Institutes of Health, Office of Medical Applications of Research Building 1, Room 216 Bethesda, MD 20892

Organizations

5 American Heart Association 7320 Greenville Avenue Dallas, TX 75231

6 National Cholesterol Education Program National Heart, Lung, and Blood Institute (NHLBI) National Institutes of Health 9000 Rockville Pike Bethesda, MD 20892

BIBLIOGRAPHY

1. Abrams J: Nitrates for acute MI and in post-MI patients, *Cardiology*, pp 37-44, 97, May 1991.
2. Alfaro-LeFevre R et al: *Drug handbook: a nursing process approach*, Redwood City, Calif, 1992, Addison-Wesley Nursing.
3. Alspach JG: The cost of cardiovascular disease: a life every 32 seconds, *Crit Care Nurs* 11(2):8, 1991.
4. American Heart Association: *1992 heart and stroke facts*, Dallas, 1992, The Association.
5. Anardi DM: Assessment of right heart function, *J Cardiovasc Nurs* 6(1):12-33, 1991.
6. Ardire L: IV NTG: monitoring vital signs hourly versus every two hours, *Crit Care Nurs* 10(9):52-56, 1990.
7. Artinian NT: Stress experience of spouses of patients having coronary artery bypass during hospitalization and 6 weeks after discharge, *Heart Lung* 20(1):52-59, 1991.
8. Bailey SR, editor: Status of percutaneous transluminal coronary angioplasty, *Curr Probl Cardiol* 15(12):723-804, 1990.
9. Barbiere CC: Cardiac tamponade: diagnosis and emergency intervention, *Crit Care Nurs* 10(4):20-22, 1990.
10. Baroldi G et al, editors: *Advances in cardiomyopathies*, Berlin, 1990, Springer-Verlag.
11. Bousquet GL: Congestive heart failure: a review of non-pharmacologic therapies, *J Cardiovasc Nurs* 4(3):35-46, 1990.
12. Boykoff SL: Strategies for sexual counseling of patients following a myocardial infarction, *Dimen Crit Care Nurs* 8(6):368-373, 1989.
13. Brady PK: Cardiac assessment tool, *Crit Care Nurs* 9(4):71-81, 1989.
14. Braunwald E, editor: *Heart disease: a textbook of cardiovascular medicine*, Philadelphia, 1992, WB Saunders Co.
15. Budny J, Anderson-Drevs K: IV inotropic agents: dopamine, dobutamine, and amrinone, *Crit Care Nurs* 10(2):54-62, 1990.
16. Bumann R, Speltz M: Decreased cardiac output: a nursing diagnosis, *Dimen Crit Care Nurs* 8(1):6-15, 1989.
17. Buse SM, Pieper B: Impact of cardiac transplantation on the spouse's life, *Heart Lung* 19(6):641-648, 1990.
18. Caroselli-Cervan C: Modifying stress in cardiovascular patients: nursing intervention, *J Adv Med Surg Nurs* 1(4):11-20, 1989.
19. Chyun D et al: Silent myocardial ischemia, *Focus Crit Care* 18(4):295-306, 1991.
20. Conover M: Inferior-wall myocardial infarction, *Crit Care Nurs* 8(7):20-22, 1988.
21. Conover M: Infero-posterolateral myocardial infarction, *Crit Care Nurs* 9(5):24-25, 1989.
22. Cupples SA: Effects of timing and reinforcement of preoperative education on knowledge and recovery of patients having coronary artery bypass graft surgery, *Heart Lung* 20(6):654-660, 1991.
23. Daily EK: Clinical management of patients receiving thrombolytic therapy, *Heart Lung* 20(5):552-565, 1991.
24. Dennis KE et al: Beta-blocker therapy: identification and management of side effects, *Heart Lung* 20(5):459-456, 1991.
25. Doenges ME, Moorhouse MF: *Application of nursing process and nursing diagnosis: an interactive text*, Philadelphia, 1992, FA Davis Co.
26. Dracup K: Treatment-seeking behavior among those with signs and symptoms of acute myocardial infarction, *Heart Lung* 20(5):570-575, 1991.
27. Emde KL, Searle LD: Current practices with thrombolytic therapy, *J Cardiovasc Nurs* 4(1):11-21, 1989.
28. Farrell EM et al, editors: *Advances in the diagnosis and treatment of coronary artery disease*, Boston, 1990, Blackwell Scientific Publications.
29. Fleury JD: Wellness motivation in cardiac rehabilitation, *Heart Lung* 20(1):3-8, 1991.
30. Folta A, Metzger BL: Exercise and functional capacity after myocardial infarction, *Image J Nurs Sch* 21(4):215-219, 1989.
31. Frasure-Smith N: In-hospital symptoms of psychological stress as predictors of long-term outcome after myocardial infarction in men, *Am J Cardiol* 67(2):121-127, 1991.
32. Fukuda N: Outcome standards for the client with chronic congestive heart failure, *J Cardiovasc Nurs* 4(3):59-70, 1990.
33. Furst E, editor: Cardiovascular technology, *J Cardiovasc Nurs* 6(2):36-42, 1992.
34. Gallo JA, Todd BA: Mediastinitis after cardiac surgery, *Crit Care Nurs* 10(6):64-68, 1990.
35. Gerber RM: Coronary artery disease in the elderly, *J Cardiovasc Nurs* 4(4):23-34, 1990.
36. Gibson RK: Beta-receptor regulation: dynamics of density and function throughout the cardiac cycle, *J Cardiovasc Nurs* 5(4):49-56, 1991.
37. Gift AG, Bolgiano CS, Cunningham J: Sensations during chest tube removal, *Heart Lung* 20(2):131-137, 1991.
38. Good LP, Gentzler RD: Coronary atherectomy, *AORN J* 53(1):32-39, 1991.
39. Grady KL, Costanzo-Nordin MR: Myocarditis: review of a clinical enigma, *Heart Lung* 18(2):347-354, 1989.

40. Grines CL: Current thrombolytic options for myocardial infarction, *Prim Cardiol* 17(1):62-68, 1991.

41. Halfman-Franey M, Coburn C: Techniques in cardiac care: lasers, stents, and atherectomy devices, *AACN Clin Issues Crit Care Nurs* 1(1):87-109, 1990.

42. Halfman-Franey M et al: Using stents in the coronary circulation: nursing perspectives, *Focus Crit Care* 18(2):132-142, 1991.

43. Hanisch PJ: Identification and treatment of acute myocardial infarction by electrocardiographic site classification, *Focus Crit Care* 18(6):480-488, 1991.

44. Hilgenberg C et al: Changes in family patterns six months after a myocardial infarction, *J Cardiovasc Nurs* 6(2):46-56, 1992.

45. Hurst JW, editor: *The heart*, ed 7, New York, 1989, McGraw-Hill Co.

46. Julian DG, editor: *Current status of clinical cardiology*, Boston, 1990, Kluwer Academic Publishers.

47. Kalman JM: Nitrate tolerance: a new look at an old problem, *Focus Crit Care* 17(5):407-409, 1990.

48. Karlick BA et al: Learning needs of patients with angina: an extension study, *J Cardiovasc Nurs* 4(2):70-82, 1990.

49. Keckeisen ME, Nyamathi AM: Coping and adjustment to illness in the acute myocardial infarction patient, *J Cardiovasc Nurs* 5(1):25-33, 1990.

50. Kris-Etherton PM et al, editors: *Cardiovascular disease: nutrition for prevention and treatment*, Dallas, 1990, The American Dietetic Association.

51. Lange SS et al: Infection control practices in cardiac transplant recipients, *Heart Lung* 21(2):101-105, 1992.

52. Lewis PS: Clinical implications of non-Q-wave (subendocardial) myocardial infarctions, *Focus* 19(1):29-33, 1992.

53. Liehr P et al: Effect of venous support on edema and leg pain in patients after coronary artery bypass graft surgery, *Heart Lung* 21(1):6-11, 1992.

54. Linden B: Unit-based phase I cardiac rehabilitation program for patients with myocardial infarction, *Focus* 17(1):15-19, 1990.

55. Lindsay C, Jennrich JA, Biemolt M: Programmed instruction booklet for cardiac rehabilitation teaching, *Heart Lung* 20(6):648-653, 1991.

56. Litzenberger R et al: Nursing grand rounds, *J Cardiovasc Nurs* 5(2):58-66, 1991.

57. Luchi RJ, editor: *Clinical geriatric cardiology*, Edinburgh, 1989, Churchill Livingstone.

58. Mahon PM: Orthoclone OKT3 and cardiac transplantation: an overview, *Crit Care Nurs* 11(8):42-50, 1991.

59. Marik PE: Myocardial infarction prognostic scoring system, *Heart Lung* 20(1):16-19, 1991.

60. Maze SS, Adolph RJ: Myocarditis: unresolved issues in diagnosis and treatment, *Clin Cardiol* 13:69-79, 1990.

61. McMillan JY et al: Right ventricular infarction, *Focus Crit Care* 18(2):158-163, 1991.

62. Medich C et al: Psychophysiologic control mechanisms in ischemic heart disease: the mind-heart connection, *J Cardiovasc Nurs* 5(4):10-26, 1991.

63. Miller SP et al: Regimen compliance two years after myocardial infarction, *Nurs Res* 39(6):333-336, 1990.

64. Misinski M: Myocardial reperfusion injury, *Crit Care Nurs Clin North Am* 2(4):651-662, 1990.

65. Moore HS: Preventing coronary artery reocclusion following t-PA, *Crit Care Nurs* 10(10):52-58, 1990.

66. Murphy MC et al: Education of patients undergoing coronary angioplasty: factors affecting learning during a structured educational program, *Heart Lung* 18(1):36-45, 1989.

67. Nagelhout JJ: Pharmacologic treatment of heart failure, *Nurs Clin North Am* 26(2):401-415, 1991.

68. Paul SC et al: Early recognition of critical stenosis high in the left anterior descending coronary artery, *Heart Lung* 19(1):27-30, 1990.

69. Peterson KJ: Competency-based orientation program for cardiovascular surgery unit. II, *Crit Care Nurs* 11(3):17-19, 1991.

70. Pierce JD, Piazza D, Naftel DC: Effects of two chest tube clearance protocols on drainage in patients after myocardial revascularization surgery, *Heart Lung* 20(2):125-130, 1991.

71. Pitts P et al: The thrombolysis and angioplasty in myocardial infarction (TAMI) trial: review and nursing implications, *Prog Cardiovasc Nurs* 5(2):65-72, 1990.

72. Robertson D et al: Relationships among health beliefs, self-efficacy, and exercise adherence in patients with coronary artery disease, *Heart Lung* 21(1):56-63, 1992.

73. Ross AM: Role of angioplasty in myocardial infarction management strategies: a review, *Heart Lung* 19(6):604-607, 1990.

74. Rountree WD et al: The HEMOPUMP cardiac assist system: nursing care of the patient, *Crit Care Nurs* 11(4):46-57, 1991.

75. Schigoda MG, Hook ML: "Take heart . . .": developing support sessions for families of acutely ill cardiac patients, *AACN Clin Issues Crit Care Nurs* 2(2):299-301, 1991.

76. Shanfield SB: Return to work after an acute myocardial infarction: a review, *Heart Lung* 19(2):109-117, 1990.

77. Shoulders-Odom B: Managing the challenge of IABP therapy, *Crit Care Nurs* 11(2):60-76, 1991.

78. Smith A: Case example: cardiac tamponade after coronary bypass, *Am J Nurs* 91(4):69-70, 1991.

79. Stanley R: Drug therapy of heart failure, *J Cardiovasc Nurs* 4(3):17-34, 1990.

80. Stoy D: Pharmacotherapy for hypercholesterolemia: guidelines and nursing perspectives, *J Cardiovasc Nurs* 5(2):34-43, 1991.

81. Stradtman JC, Ballenger MJ: Nursing implications in sternal and mediastinal infection after open heart surgery, *Focus* 16(3):178-183, 1989.

82. Suddarth DS, editor: *The Lippincott manual of nursing practice*, ed 5, Philadelphia, 1991, JB Lippincott Co.

83. Sulzbach LM, Lansdowne LM: Temporary atrial pacing after cardiac surgery, *Focus* 18(1):65-74, 1991.

84. Tack BB, Gilliss CL: Nurse-monitored cardiac recovery: a description of the first 8 weeks, *Heart Lung* 19(5):491-499, 1990.

85. Thadani U: Nitrate tolerance: what are the best strategies to avoid it? *Choices Cardiology* 5(2):68-70, 1991.

86. Turk M: Acute pericarditis in the post-myocardial infarction patient, *Crit Care Nurs Q* 12(3):34-38, 1989.

87. Underhill SL et al, editors: *Cardiac nursing*, ed 2, Philadelphia, 1989, JB Lippincott Co.

88. Urban N: Hemodynamic clinical profiles, *AACN Clin Issues Crit Care Nurs* 1(1):119-130, 1990.

89. Vaska PL: Biventricular assist devices, *Crit Care Nurs* 11(8):52-60, 1991.

90. Willetts K: Assessing cardiac pain, *Nurs Times* 85(47):52-54, 1989.

91. Wingate S: Acute effects of exercise on the cardiovascular system, *J Cardiovasc Nurs* 5(4):27-38, 1991.

92. Wingate S: Women and coronary heart disease: implication for the critical care setting, *Focus Crit Care* 18(3):212-220, 1991.

93. Wright SM: Pathophysiology of congestive heart failure, *J Cardiovasc Nurs* 4(3):1-16, 1990.

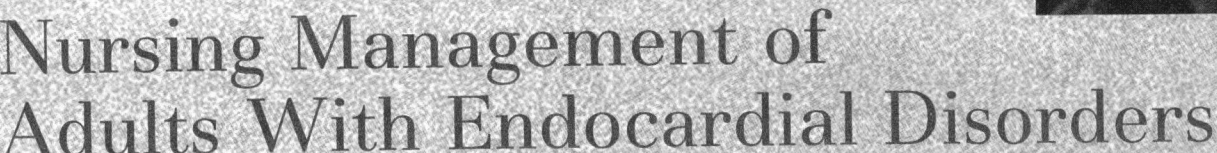

CHAPTER THIRTY-SIX

Nursing Management of Adults With Endocardial Disorders

LEARNING OBJECTIVES

1 Discuss the high-risk patient population, high-risk procedures, and preventive therapy for infective endocarditis.
2 Correlate the hemodynamic alterations with the clinical manifestations and major complications of each valvular disorder.
3 Discuss the medical and surgical management of patients with valvular disease.
4 Describe the assessment findings, nursing diagnoses, expected outcomes, and nursing interventions for patients with valvular disorders.
5 Identify patient and family learning needs for preventive therapy and discharge planning needs.

DISORDERS OF THE ENDOCARDIUM affect the endothelium and the valves of the heart. When a person experiences a cardiac valve disorder, the blood flow through the cardiac chambers is affected and the pressures of the heart and pulmonary vascular system are altered. Although many valvular disorders originate in childhood, signs and symptoms may not become apparent until adulthood.

INFECTIVE ENDOCARDITIS
Definition

Infective endocarditis is an infection of the endocardial layer of the heart. Infections most commonly occur on the valve leaflets but may also invade the lining of the heart chambers/or the lining of the large arteries.

Etiology/Epidemiology

The predisposing factors associated with infective endocarditis are varied and include prosthetic valve surgery, previous episodes of endocarditis, congenital heart disease, rheumatic heart disease, hypertrophic cardiomyopathy, and mitral valve prolapse with valvular regurgitation. Causes affecting the right side of the heart are intravenous drug use and long-term placement of intravascular devices, such as intravenous catheters, dialysis shunts, and pacemakers. Persons who are immunosuppressed are also at higher risk for infective endocarditis.

The incidence of endocarditis has decreased dramatically in the past 20 years as a result of increased awareness of risk factors, effective antibiotic therapy, and antibiotic prophylaxis in susceptible individuals. The proportion of elderly patients with endocarditis has increased because of delays in diagnosis, decreased immunologic responses to infection, and a higher incidence of medical procedures such as prosthetic heart valves and intravenous lines and catheters.

The infecting organisms vary with the predisposing variables and the patient population. The infecting organisms and their most common routes of introduction in the patient are summarized in Table 36-1. Culture-negative endocarditis can occur in patients with preexisting valve disease when they are treated with antibiotics ineffective against the invading organism.

Infective endocarditis can be classified as subacute or acute depending on its severity and progression. Subacute endocarditis progresses over several weeks to months with vague and nonspecific symptoms. Acute endocarditis occurs over days to weeks and is characterized by symptoms of congestive heart failure and systemic involvement. Acute endocarditis may convert to subacute disease, whereas subacute endocarditis may suddenly have serious complications reflective of acute disease.

Pathophysiology

Several mechanisms are thought to contribute to the development of infective endocarditis. Turbulent blood flow resulting from either damaged endothelium or a valvular disease allows a sterile platelet-fibrin thrombus to form on the endothelium or valve. An infecting organism may be introduced and grow on the thrombus during a transient bacteremia resulting from an invasive procedure such as surgery, bronchoscopy, or laparoscopy; indwelling catheters such as pacemakers or venous access devices; skin or wound infections; or urinary tract infections to name a few. These thrombi provide a medium for infection should bacteria enter the circulation. The bacteria clump and adhere to the thrombotic le-

TABLE 36-1   Infecting Organisms for Endocarditis

Infecting organisms	Routes of introduction
Streptococcus	Dental procedures, such as cleaning or extractions
Staphylococcus	Upper respiratory procedures, such as bronchoscopy
Enterococcus	Gastrointestinal and genitourinary surgery and procedures, such as urinary catheterization or cystoscopy
Staphylococcus aureus and *epidermidis*	Intravenous drug use Cardiac surgery
Gram-negative bacilli *Pseudomonas* *Enterobacter* *Serratia*	Intravenous drug use Prosthetic cardiac valves
Fungus *Candida* *Aspergillus*	Prosthetic cardiac valves Intravenous drug use

sions, which support bacterial growth (Figure 36-1). The clumped bacteria on the platelet-fibrin thrombi are called **vegetations.** The vegetation is composed of three layers: (1) the outer layer contains the infecting microorganisms and fibrin, forming a protective covering over the other layers; (2) the middle layer contains microorganisms; and (3) the inner layer contains fibrin, platelets, red blood cells, neutrophils, lymphocytes, and elastin. The microorganisms lying deep in the vegetation are somewhat protected from the patient's immune system and from antimicrobial therapy, making effective treatment more difficult to achieve.

When the infection involves a valve, growth of the vegetations thins and destroys the valve tissue and results in valvular dysfunction. When not treated, the vegetations can invade the endocardial and adjacent myocardial tissue, resulting in impaired pumping efficiency of the heart. The greater the pumping inefficiency, the more likely the patient will experience signs and symptoms of congestive heart failure. Dysrhythmias may occur when infection spreads from the valves to the intraventricular septum or myocardium. Fragments of friable vegetative lesions can break off and enter the circulation as emboli. Lesions from the left atrium or ventricle can embolize to the brain, extremities, renal arteries, coronary arteries, or splenic arteries. Lesions from

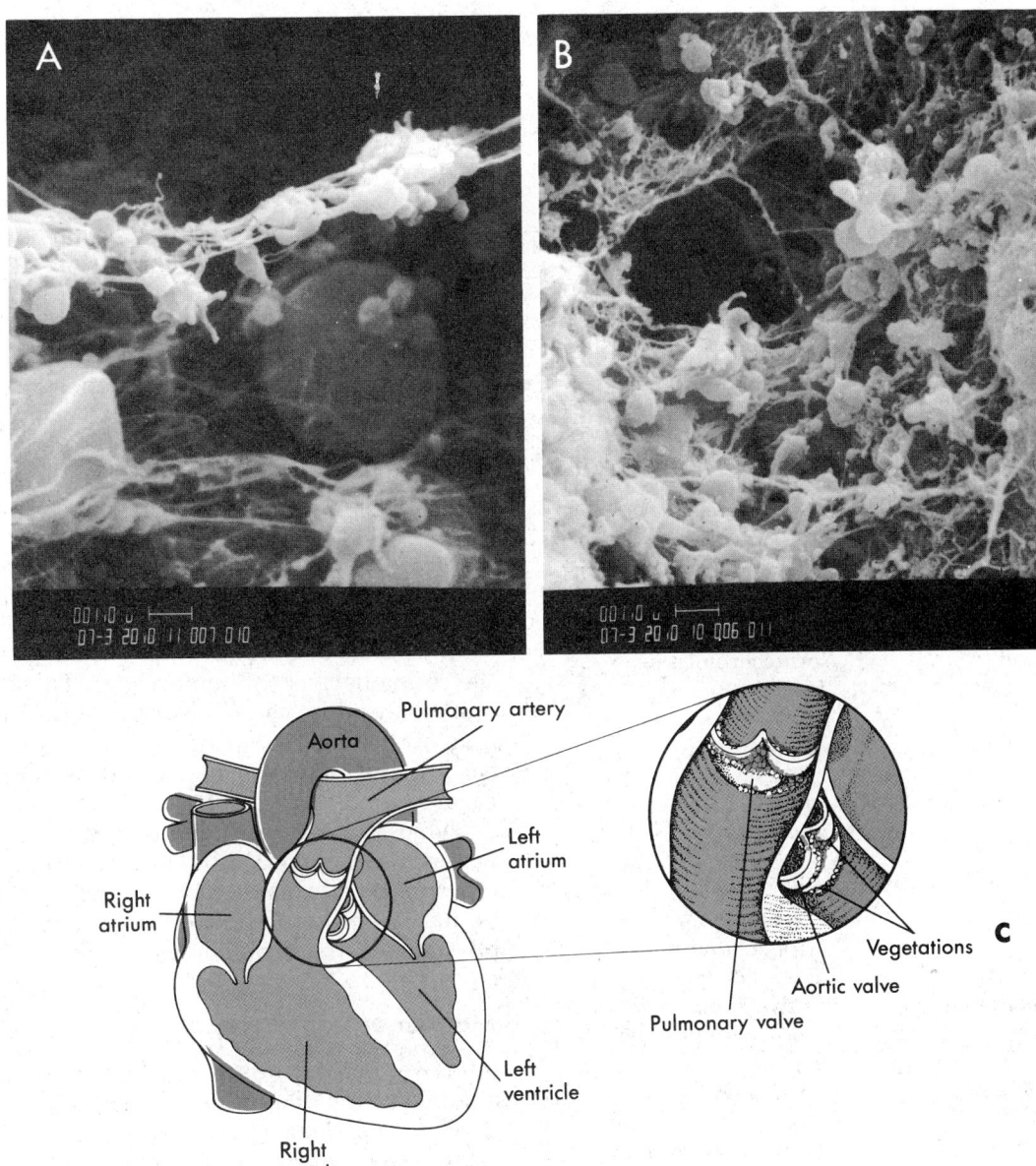

FIGURE 36-1   Scanning electron micrographs of cardiac vegetations (× 5100). **A,** Nonbacterial thrombotic vegetation with fibrin stands and platelets. **B,** Infected vegetation with streptococci enmeshed in fibrin-platelet matrix. **C,** Development of vegetations in endocarditis. (**A** and **B** from Wright AJ, Wilson WR: Experimental animal endocarditis, *Mayo Clin Proc* 57:10-14, 1982. By permission Mayo Foundation.)

the right atrium or ventricle may embolize to the pulmonary circulation.

Clinical Manifestations

Endocarditis is often difficult to diagnose. The subacute form may mimic almost any systemic disease such as the flu, depending on the nature of the infecting organism, the site of the vegetation, and the complications that develop. Patients with endocarditis often manifest symptoms of systemic infection, such as fatigue, malaise, anorexia, weight loss, headache, fever, chills, and sweating. Acute endocarditis can cause signs and symptoms of a systemic infection with temperature elevations up to 103° F (39.5° C) and shaking chills. Cardiac assessment will usually reveal a murmur or a change in an existing murmur.

Assessment findings of embolization depend on the location of embolization. Cerebral embolization is reflected in changes in level of consciousness or nervous system deficits such as hemiparesis or aphasia. Pulmonary embolization causes respiratory distress, cough, hemoptysis, pleuritic pain, or dyspnea. Embolization of a coronary artery may cause a myocardial infarction accompanied by acute chest pain, palpitations, or signs of heart failure. Splenic infarction from emboli can cause pain in the upper left quadrant that can radiate to the left shoulder. It may also produce abdominal rigidity. Hematuria, flank pain, or decreased urine output may be caused by embolization to the renal artery.

Peripheral manifestations can also occur. Vascular occlusion may be manifested by numbness and tingling or loss of pulses in an affected extremity. Tiny emboli to the skin or inflammation of small vessels can produce **Osler nodes,** typically on the pads of the fingers and toes. These are painful, erythematous, papular nodules, 0.5 to 1.5 cm in diameter. They tend to appear in groups and may disappear in hours or in a day. Janeway lesions are small, erythematous, macular, papular lesions, 1 to 4 mm in diameter. They appear on the fingertips, palms, soles, or plantar surfaces and are usually not tender.

A vascular manifestation of endocarditis is petechiae, which are flat, red lesions that appear in groups; they fade within a few days and occur in up to 50% of patients. They most commonly appear around the conjunctiva, mucous membranes, wrists, ankles, neck, and clavicles because of microembolization of small blood vessels. Microemboli can cause splinter hemorrhages of the nail beds. These are single or multiple small hemorrhages located in the distal one third of the fingernails, resembling small splinters of wood. Roth's spots can appear in the retina because of hemorrhage. These areas contain a pale white center near the optic fundus. Clubbing of the fingers may occur in long-standing endocarditis but may also be caused by the underlying cardiac condition.

Table 36-2 lists common laboratory and diagnostic tests for endocarditis. Arteriography, radioisotope imaging scans, or cardiac catheterization may be necessary for more precise definition of pathophysiologic/structural changes.

TABLE 36-2   Laboratory and Diagnostic Tests for Endocarditis

Test	Finding in endocarditis
COMMON LABORATORY TESTS	
Blood cultures	Bacteria present
Red blood cell count	Normochromic, normocytic anemia (60%-70%)
Leukocyte count	Elevated levels in acute form
Erythocyte sedimentation rate	Usually elevated level
LESS COMMON LABORATORY TESTS	
Platelet count	Thrombotic thrombocytopenia purpura–like syndrome
Teichnoic acid antibody test	Positive in *Staphylococcus aureus* infection
Immunoglobulins G and M	Elevated levels
Urine and microanalysis	Albuminuria, pyuria, casts, hematuria, uremia (immunologic reaction affecting kidneys)
Blood (serum)	Immune complexes and rheumatoid factor may be present in serum, along with decreased complement (immunologic reaction)
DIAGNOSTIC TESTS	
Electrocardiography	Conduction or rhythm disturbance and myocardial ischemic changes (uncommon)
Echocardiography	Will reveal large valvular lesions

Therapeutic Management

Infective endocarditis is managed medically by the administration of antibiotics. The antibiotic must be given in sufficient doses over a long enough period of time to eradicate the infecting organism because the layers of vegetation tend to protect the organism. Parenteral antibiotic therapy is started promptly and continues for 4 to 6 weeks. The antibiotic chosen depends on sensitivity studies of the infecting organism. Penicillin is usually the drug of choice for bacterial infections, but numerous antimicrobial regimens are currently in use. Amphotericin B is often required for fungal infections. After adequate antimicrobial therapy is begun, the patient's sense of well-being should return, appetite should improve, and the patient should be afebrile. Temperature is monitored daily as one indication of the effectiveness of therapy. Supportive therapy includes bed rest, antipyretics, and analgesics. Once the patient recovers from the infection, seriously damaged valves may require surgical replacement, depending on the severity of the patient's symptoms. Valve damage may result in stenosis or regurgitation of the affected valve.

For persons at risk for developing endocarditis, the American Heart Association (AHA) recommends a prophylactic regimen of antibiotics before, during, and after invasive procedures to prevent occurrence.[13] The current AHA guidelines specify specific antibiotic regimens for various procedures that increase the likelihood of introducing organisms systemically into patients at risk. For example, before dental, oral, or upper respiratory tract procedures, patients at risk for developing the disease should receive 3.0 g of amoxicillin 1 hour before the procedure and 1.5 g after the initial dose.

NURSING MANAGEMENT OF THE PATIENT WITH INFECTIVE ENDOCARDITIS

Assessment

The history includes all previously diagnosed conditions, including rheumatic, congenital, and syphilitic heart disease, prosthetic cardiac valves or patches, frequent self-injections (narcotics or diabetic medication), and previously diagnosed endocarditis. Information is obtained regarding a possible port of entry, including recent dental treatment, surgical procedures, or instrumentation involving the upper respiratory tract, genitourinary tract, or lower gastrointestinal tract.

Further history questions are asked, and a physical assessment is performed to detect any abnormal signs and symptoms, including the following:

1. Infection: fever, diaphoresis/chills/rigors, anorexia, weight loss, malaise, headache, arthralgias or myalgias
2. Heart failure: peripheral edema, shortness of breath, jugular venous distention, adventitious breath sounds, such as crackles or wheezes
3. Myocardial infarction: chest pain, diaphoresis, palpitations
4. Other cardiac complications: pericarditis, pericardial friction rub, cardiac tamponade
5. Embolization: stroke, cough, hemoptysis, cold and painful extremities, flank pain, hematuria, petechiae, Osler nodes, Janeway lesions, splinter hemorrhages

During the interview the patient is asked whether

CLINICAL ALERT

Patients at risk for developing infective endocarditis should be placed on a prophylactic antibiotic regimen before, during, and after any invasive procedure, including dental cleaning and extraction, catheterizations, and pulmonary diagnostic studies.

he or she has had problems previously, such as complaints of shortness of breath, fatigue, changes in activity levels, or chest pain. In addition, the patient and family's perception of and reaction to the diagnosis and requirements of therapy are considered. Questions regarding the patient's knowledge of and compliance with prophylactic antibiotic therapy will delineate some of the learning needs of the patient and family.

Nursing Diagnosis

The nursing care associated with endocarditis is common to that for related disorders of the endocardium. Diagnoses common in the endocarditis patient include the following:

Alteration in comfort related to symptoms of fever

High risk for decreased cardiac output related to mechanical changes in the heart valves

High risk for altered cardiopulmonary, cerebral, and peripheral perfusion related to thromboembolus

Anxiety related to limited knowledge of disease

High risk for activity intolerance related to increased oxygen requirements, alteration in cardiac output, or heart failure

Knowledge deficit related to therapeutic management of the disease and its prevention

Planning

Goals for the patient with endocarditis include the following:

Patient will maintain a temperature within normal limits for the patient

Patient will verbalize a feeling of comfort

Patient will maintain hemodynamic stability within patient's normal limits

Patient will maintain adequate tissue perfusion as evidenced by no changes in level of consciousness, no dyspnea, no changes in peripheral pulses, and an adequate urine output

Patient will be able to cope with anxiety

Patient will be able to perform activities of daily living with minimal assistance

Patient will be able to describe the cause, treatment, and preventive measures of the disease

Implementation

During the acute phase of infection, the patient may have symptoms such as fever, chills, diaphoresis, and arthralgias. Nursing care to minimize the patient's discomfort during this period includes the following:

Avoiding prolonged exposure of the patient to avoid chills

PATIENT EDUCATION GUIDE *Infective Endocarditis*

Objective: The patient and family will be able to identify how to prevent endocarditis and the signs and symptoms of complications that require notification of the nurse or physician

1. Discuss measures to prevent the occurrence or recurrence of endocarditis, including the following:
   a. Identification of the procedures that require prophylactic antibiotic therapy
   b. Discussion of the importance of compliance with medication regimen when receiving antibiotic therapy
   c. Notification of the nurse or physician in the event of any signs and symptoms of infection (fever, malaise, anorexia, headache)
   d. Notification of all physicians, including dentists, regarding need for prophylaxis
   e. Description of the signs and symptoms of complications; nurse or physician should be notified immediately if there is evidence of myocardial infarction, increasing episodes of dyspnea, feelings of dizziness or blackouts (syncope), lapses in memory or changes in level of consciousness, and irregular or rapid pulse; if chest pain occurs with other symptoms of myocardial infarction or stroke, patient is instructed to go to the nearest emergency room
2. Instruct the patient to carry an antibiotic prophylaxis medication card in his or her wallet

3. Advise the patient and family to keep emergency numbers near the telephone, including the local ambulance service.
4. Instruct the patient and family regarding medications and their importance, including the following:
   a. Review each medication with the patient and family and provide any written information available
   b. Include instructions on drug name, indications, dosage, administration schedule, and any special instructions for administration (e.g., take before or after meals)
   c. Explain adverse side effects and actions to take if these occur
   d. General medication instructions should include the following:
      (1) Do not change the dosage without consulting the physician
      (2) If an adverse reaction occurs or is suspected, the drug should not be taken and the physician should be notified
      (3) Do not skip doses
      (4) Do not stop any medications abruptly without first consulting the physician
5. Emphasize to the patient the importance of good oral hygiene, including the following:
   a. Maintenance of good oral hygiene with regular tooth brushing and flossing
   b. Visits to the dentist regularly
   c. Avoidance of overzealous dental hygiene measures such as water pressure cleaning devices or brushing until gums bleed

Using cooling measures, such as tepid sponge bath or cooling blanket if prescribed

Administering antipyretics as ordered and monitoring the patient's response

Maintaining adequate hydration by encouraging oral intake within any fluid restrictions

Administering antibiotic and monitoring for allergic reactions

No specific measures prevent the occurrence of embolization of vegetative growths, but the nurse assesses the patient for signs and symptoms such as changes in level of consciousness, hemoptysis, dyspnea, decreased urine output or hematuria, a decrease in the volume of peripheral pulses, or the presence and location of pain. (See also the patient education guide above.)

Evaluation

Evaluation includes continued monitoring of the patient's temperature and identification of the signs and symptoms of infection and its resolution. Blood cultures should show no growth of organisms. In addition, congestive heart failure and signs or symptoms of pulmonary manifestations should be resolved.

Documentation

The nurse documents the patient's signs and symptoms and their resolution as the patient responds to antibiotic therapy. If complications occur, their signs and symptoms are noted as well as their response to treatment. Documentation reflects the patient's ability to describe how to prevent the recurrence of endocarditis and the importance of prophylactic antibiotic therapy.

Ongoing Care

Relapses may occur in a small percentage of patients following treatment; therefore follow-up cultures are obtained every 1 to 2 weeks for up to 6 weeks, and the patient's temperature is monitored. All health care personnel are notified before any invasive procedures, such as dental surgery or urinary diagnostic procedures, because prophylactic antibiotic therapy may be instituted.

Valvular Disorders

Valvular disorders occur when the valves of the heart are unable to open completely (stenosis) or to close completely (regurgitation or insufficiency). These dysfunctions lead to abnormal pressures within the chambers of the heart. Disorders are categorized by the valve involved (mitral, aortic, tricuspid, or pulmonic), the nature of the problem (stenosis or regurgitation), and the degree of dysfunction that results.

MITRAL STENOSIS
Definition

Mitral stenosis is a fibrotic thickening that results in fusion of the mitral valve leaflets and chordae tendineae. The thickened leaflets interfere with valve opening, thus obstructing blood flow through the valve to the left ventricle.

Etiology/Epidemiology

The majority of patients with mitral stenosis are women, and the most common cause of mitral stenosis is rheumatic fever. Other less common pathologic conditions that may cause mitral stenosis are calcium accumulation, thrombus formation, and bacterial vegetation. Another cause is atrial myxoma, which is a primary cardiac neoplasm in the left atrium resembling a thrombus.

Pathophysiology

Normally, during ventricular diastole, blood flows through the mitral valve and the openings between the chordae tendineae, which form secondary orifices for blood flow. When mitral stenosis occurs, the leaflets become fused, thus decreasing the orifice size. Also, the chordae tendineae become fibrous

and shorten, producing closure of the secondary orifices. It becomes more difficult to eject blood through the smaller orifice, and the end-diastolic left atrial blood volume increases. Normally the pressures in the left atrium and left ventricle equalize when the mitral valve is open during diastole. In mitral stenosis, with an increased atrial blood volume there is an associated rise in left atrial pressure, creating a pressure difference between the left atrium and left ventricle.

A prolonged rise in left atrial pressure causes left atrial hypertrophy and dilation, and hyperplasia of the pulmonary arterioles. Eventually, the high pressures in the left atrium create a backward flow resulting in elevated pressure in the pulmonary veins, capillaries, and arteries. Continued elevation of left atrial pressure in pulmonary vessels produces pulmonary hypertension and right ventricular hypertrophy (Figure 36-2).

The increased blood volume and pressure in the pulmonary capillaries may result in the "leak" of plasma and plasma proteins from the capillary bed into the interstitium of the lung, which cannot all be absorbed. As the rate of fluid "leakage" exceeds the rate of lymphatic drainage of the lung tissue, pulmonary edema occurs.

The degree of mitral stenosis determines the reduction in cardiac output. Patients with mild to moderate stenosis are usually able to maintain a normal cardiac output at rest but have problems with exercise. Exercise tends to raise the cardiac output in normal individuals, but with the obstruction to blood flow and an enlarged left atrium, the cardiac output fails to increase and may actually be reduced. Additionally, the tachycardia that is associated with physical exertion further lowers the cardiac output by decreasing left ventricular diastolic filling time.

Right-sided heart failure may occur with the backward flow of blood. Heart failure can be exacerbated by atrial dysrhythmias, particularly atrial fibrillation, which frequently arises because of the abnormal stretch on the muscle fibers in the atrium. This may further reduce left ventricular filling and cardiac output because of the loss of the amount of blood provided by the "atrial kick." In later stages of severe disease, left ventricular failure may result from increased left atrial blood volume and decreased left ventricular filling.

Clinical Manifestations

The size of the opening of the mitral valve determines the acuity of symptoms; many patients remain asymptomatic for some time. Symptoms may appear gradually or abruptly. A gradual onset is more common, because mitral stenosis usually develops over a period of approximately 20 years. However, a

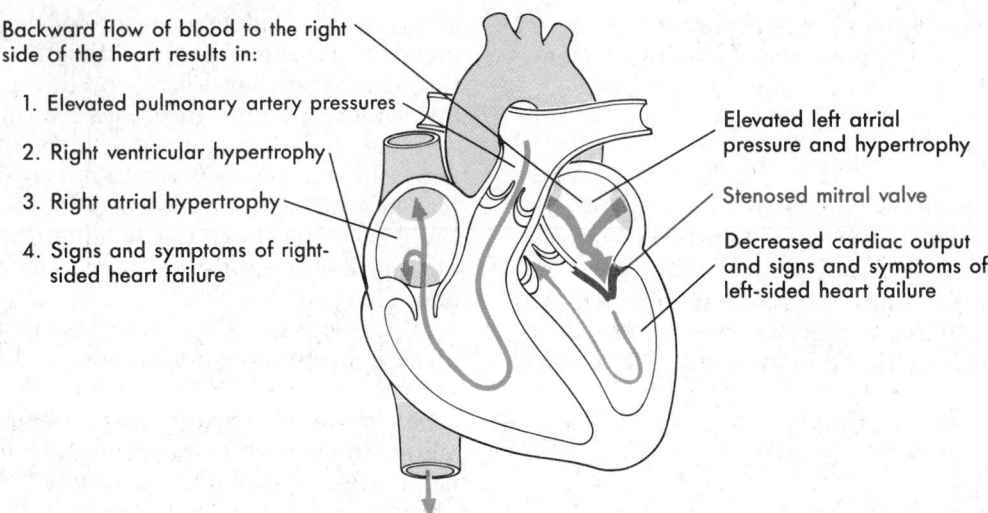

Backward flow of blood to the right side of the heart results in:

1. Elevated pulmonary artery pressures

2. Right ventricular hypertrophy

3. Right atrial hypertrophy

4. Signs and symptoms of right-sided heart failure

Elevated left atrial pressure and hypertrophy

Stenosed mitral valve

Decreased cardiac output and signs and symptoms of left-sided heart failure

FIGURE 36-2   Effects of mitral stenosis.

rapid progression of the disease can occur over 2 to 5 years.

The most frequent complaint is dyspnea, resulting from pulmonary venous hypertension. Even if the patient is asymptomatic at rest, dyspnea frequently occurs with an increased venous return. This can be precipitated by exercise, fever, emotional stress, recumbent positions, or pregnancy. This increase in venous return is unable to pass through the stenotic valve, and right atrial pressures rise. Other initial symptoms that patients may demonstrate include fatigue and weakness, although the patient's blood pressure is not usually affected until late in the disease progression.

As the orifice opening becomes progressively smaller, obstruction to flow can occur at rest. Signs and symptoms of pulmonary edema that may occur include shortness of breath, orthopnea, and paroxysmal nocturnal dyspnea. Dyspnea and hemoptysis may be precipitated with minimal exertion.

Cardiac symptoms associated with right-sided failure can occur with severe mitral stenosis and are demonstrated by fatigue, weakness, peripheral edema, jugular venous distention, hepatomegaly, and abdominal discomfort or distension. Signs and symptoms of left-sided failure include hypotension, fatigue, dizziness, and signs of decreased perfusion such as decreased urine output and weak peripheral pulses. Abnormal heart sounds can usually be auscultated in mitral stenosis and typically include a low-pitched diastolic murmur best heard at the apex and an opening snap of the mitral valve. Atrial fibrillation can occur as a result of left atrial dilation. This further decreases left ventricular filling and leads to pooling of blood in the left atrium, which places the patient at risk for thrombus formation and embolization. An echocardiogram can illustrate

the low flow through the mitral valve, and cardiac catheterization delineates the degree of pressure gradient caused by mitral stenosis.

MITRAL REGURGITATION
Definition

Mitral regurgitation is created by any abnormality of the mitral valve that results in blood leaking backward from the left ventricle to the left atrium.

Etiology/Epidemiology

Chronic mitral regurgitation, also known as mitral insufficiency, is often seen with mitral stenosis. Rheumatic heart disease is the predominant cause, but several other causes of mitral regurgitation include the following:

1. Coronary artery disease and acute myocardial infarction
2. Infective endocarditis
3. Leakage through a prosthetic valve
4. Mitral valve prolapse
5. Any condition causing left ventricular dilation with associated enlargement of the ventricle and displacement of the papillary muscles and distortion of the valve leaflets
6. Associated connective tissue disorders (e.g., amyloidosis, ankylosing spondylitis)

Acute mitral regurgitation is associated with rupture of chordae tendineae, papillary muscle rupture, and mitral valve leaflet perforation. Chordae tendineae rupture may result from infective endocarditis, mitral valve prolapse, trauma, and less commonly spontaneous rupture. The most common cause of papillary muscle rupture is acute myocardial infarction.

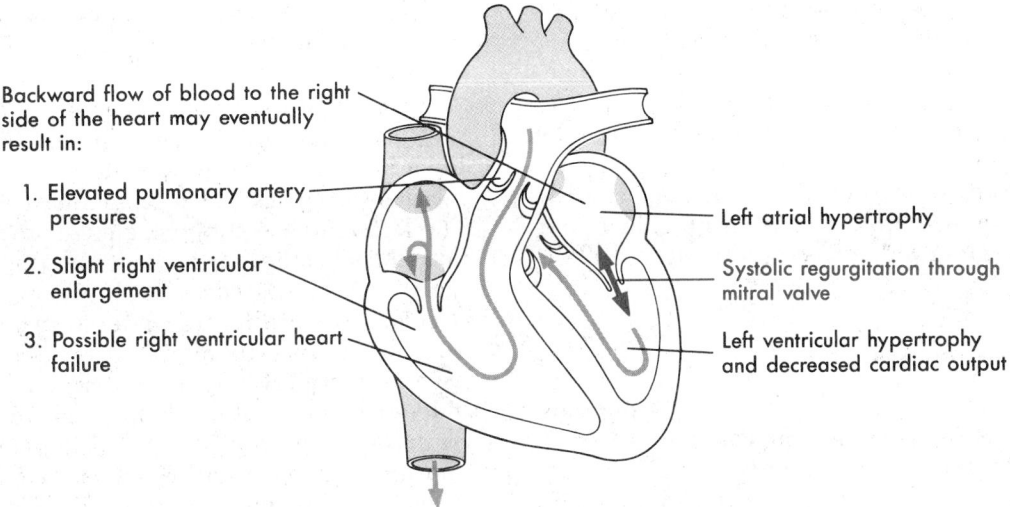

Backward flow of blood to the right side of the heart may eventually result in:

1. Elevated pulmonary artery pressures

2. Slight right ventricular enlargement

3. Possible right ventricular heart failure

Left atrial hypertrophy

Systolic regurgitation through mitral valve

Left ventricular hypertrophy and decreased cardiac output

FIGURE 36-3   Effects of mitral regurgitation.

Pathophysiology

In mitral regurgitation, blood from the left ventricle is shunted back through the mitral orifice to the left atrium during ventricular systole. The left ventricular output is therefore divided between the system (forward flow) and regurgitating into the left atrium (backward flow). The amount of forward flow depends on the severity of the insufficient valve and the degree of resistance to "forward" flow (afterload). In response, both the left atrial myocardium and the left ventricular myocardium gradually dilate and hypertrophy to compensate for the additional workload. Progressive left ventricular hypertrophy and atrial fibrillation from a dilated left atrium may lead to a reduction in cardiac output (Figure 36-3). Usually left ventricular failure develops slowly in chronic mitral regurgitation, but in acute mitral regurgitation the acute rise in left atrial pressure produces rapid heart failure, pulmonary edema, and shock.

Clinical Manifestations

Mitral insufficiency usually progresses slowly and may therefore not produce symptoms for many years. Initial symptoms are fatigue, exertional dyspnea, and palpitations. Pulmonary edema and hemoptysis are not as common as they are in mitral stenosis. Right ventricular failure is a late sign of chronic mitral insufficiency. The adventitious heart sound of mitral regurgitation is a high-pitched, blowing systolic murmur best heard at the apex. In acute mitral regurgitation, hypertrophy and dilation do not have time to develop. An acute event, such as rupture of the chordae tendineae or papillary muscles, causes rapid onset of left atrial and left ventricular

overload, pulmonary hypertension, pulmonary edema, and left ventricular failure. Electrocardiogram (ECG) findings in mitral regurgitation often demonstrate left ventricular hypertrophy. If left ventricular enlargement and left atrial enlargement are present, these may be visualized on both chest x-ray and the echocardiogram. The degree of disease progression is more completely defined by the findings from cardiac catheterization and left ventricular angiography.

MITRAL VALVE PROLAPSE
Definition

Mitral valve prolapse results from abnormalities in the valve leaflets, chordae tendineae, and papillary muscles. Varying degrees of incompetence and incomplete valve closure occur. Other names for mitral valve prolapse include billowing or floppy mitral valve syndrome and Barlow's syndrome.

Etiology/Epidemiology

This disease occurs in 4% to 7% of the adult population, more commonly in women, and may be inherited as an autosomal dominant gene. In many patients the disease is benign, and they remain asymptomatic and undiagnosed. Etiologic factors vary and include infective endocarditis, coronary artery disease, myocarditis, cardiomyopathy, and cardiac trauma, among others.

Pathophysiology

In mitral valve prolapse, cells proliferate in the middle layer of the valve, causing the leaflet to enlarge.

The leaflet prolapses into the left atrium during ventricular systole and does not seal the valve opening sufficiently. Varying degrees of valve incompetence will be present, depending on the extent of disease. Tissue changes in the valve annulus such as annular calcification and structural enlargement or abnormal distensibility of the mitral valve leaflets contribute to valvular incompetence. If valvular incompetence becomes marked, mitral regurgitation will develop.

Clinical Manifestations

Most patients have no complaints or symptoms. Symptomatic patients commonly complain of atypical chest pain not associated with exertion nor relieved by rest or nitroglycerine. Dysrhythmias may cause palpitations or a reduction in cardiac output, resulting in angina, fatigue, dizziness, lightheadedness, chest tightness, and syncope. Dyspnea without exertion accompanied by anxiety may occur unexpectedly. A midsystolic click may be heard. It is caused by a sudden tensing of the mitral valve leaflet as it reaches its limit and prolapses into the left atrium during systole. In addition, a late systolic murmur may be heard. The clicks and murmur may be elicited or accentuated by postural changes or isometric exercises that increase venous return.

AORTIC STENOSIS
Definition

Aortic stenosis is a stiffening or fusion of the valve leaflets, resulting from calcification that produces a narrowed valve opening.

Etiology/Epidemiology

Aortic stenosis results from calcification associated with different conditions and is most common in men. The following are some common etiologic factors:

Less than 30 years old	Congenital malformations
Between 30 and 70 years old	Congenital malformations or rheumatic heart disease
More than 70 years old	Congenital malformations, rheumatic heart disease, degenerative disease, calcification with age; may be associated with mitral stenosis

Pathophysiology

Rheumatic heart disease causes thickening and fibrosis of the leaflets, ending in calcification of the valve. In conditions other than rheumatic fever, aortic stenosis is caused by turbulent blood flow through an abnormal valve resulting in leaflet damage, fibrosis, and calcification.

Aortic stenosis usually progresses over years. As the valve opening decreases in size, the pressures in the left ventricle increase and the left ventricle must increase its work to eject adequate blood volume. The left ventricle compensates for the resistance to flow through the aortic valve by gradually increasing the thickness of the wall, causing the left ventricular myocardium to undergo hypertrophy without dilating the chamber. Aortic stenosis is usually asymptomatic as long as ventricular hypertrophy is able to compensate and maintain cardiac output. Symptoms develop when calcification progresses and the compensation becomes inadequate.

The left atrium also plays an important role in compensation to maintain the cardiac output. The left atrium increases its force of contraction (atrial kick) to increase the left ventricular end-diastolic volume. This elevation in left atrial pressure eventually causes enlargement of the left atrium. An increasing left ventricular end-diastolic volume or pressure (preload) increases the end-diastolic length of the left ventricular muscle fibers, increasing the force of contraction. By increasing the left ventricular force of contraction, stroke volume increases, augmenting cardiac output. Aortic stenosis will increase the severity of any underlying mitral regurgitation because the increased left ventricular pressures enhance the backflow of blood through an incompetent mitral valve. When the atrial kick is lost, as in atrial fibrillation or atrioventricular dissociation, a reduction of cardiac output occurs that may result in a rapid progression of symptoms of right-sided failure.

Late in the course of the disease, less blood is ejected out of the left ventricle during systole. The increase in blood volume in the left ventricle can cause left ventricular dilation. Following left ventricular dilation, ejection fraction, stroke volume, and cardiac output decrease. Angina may result from poor coronary perfusion, low systemic diastolic pressure, and high left ventricular end-diastolic pressure. The effects of aortic stenosis are shown in Figure 36-4. Complications associated with severe aortic stenosis include left- and right-sided heart failure, atrial fibrillation, mitral or tricuspid regurgitation, myocardial ischemia with angina, and sudden death.

Clinical Manifestations

In patients with congenital bicuspid aortic valves, calcification and subsequent development of symptoms may not appear until after 40 years of age. The presentation of symptoms partly depends on the degree of calcification. Calcification may occur rapidly

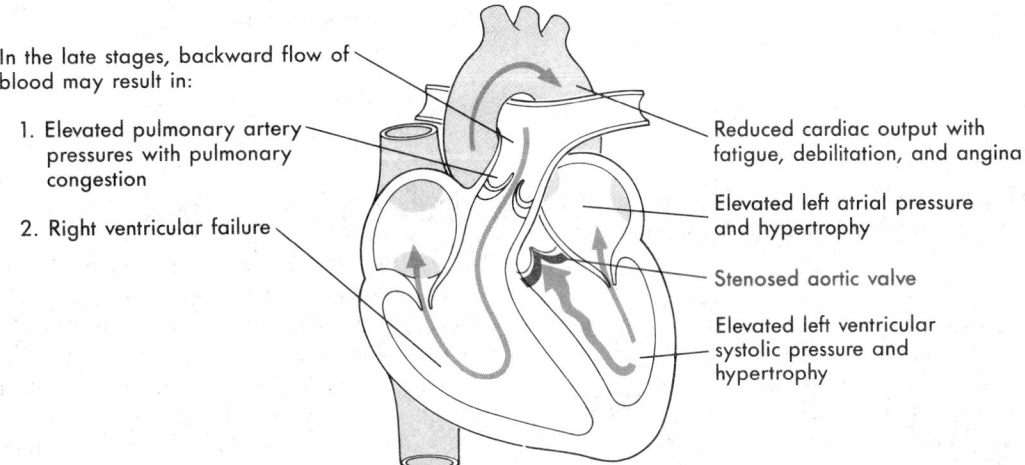

In the late stages, backward flow of blood may result in:

1. Elevated pulmonary artery pressures with pulmonary congestion

2. Right ventricular failure

Reduced cardiac output with fatigue, debilitation, and angina

Elevated left atrial pressure and hypertrophy

Stenosed aortic valve

Elevated left ventricular systolic pressure and hypertrophy

FIGURE 36-4   Effects of aortic stenosis.

in the degenerative form or more slowly, as in the congenital form. The cardiac output and stroke volume may be maintained within normal limits while resting but fail to increase during exercise, resulting in exertional dyspnea. During exercise there is normally an increased heart rate and resultant increase in cardiac output. Patients with a fixed cardiac output from aortic stenosis are unable to increase the cardiac output, resulting in angina because of the decreased blood flow to the coronary arteries and syncope from the decreased blood pressure. Exertional syncope may be caused by a reduction in arterial pressure from vasodilation in exercising muscles, combined with a fixed cardiac output. The symptoms in the later stages of the disease are those seen in left- and right-sided heart failure and include the following:

1. Paroxysmal nocturnal dyspnea, orthopnea, exertional dyspnea
2. Fatigue, debilitation
3. Signs and symptoms of congestive heart failure and pulmonary edema
4. Angina

Systemic arterial pressure usually remains normal until the late stage in which stroke volume is decreased. This causes systolic pressure to fall along with or without a narrowing of the pulse pressure. A systolic thrill can be palpated at the base of the heart, in the jugular notch, and along the carotid arteries during expiration with the patient leaning forward. If the patient is positioned lying on the left side, a double apical pulse can be palpated.

An aortic ejection click and a crescendo-decrescendo murmur can be heard on auscultation. This murmur is caused by the flow of blood being forced through the stenotic opening. It is heard best at the base of the heart in the second intercostal space to the right of the sternum and travels upward to the jugular notch and along the carotid arteries. The murmur can be heard beginning after the first heart sound with intensity increasing toward the middle of systolic ejection and then decreasing until the aortic valve closes. The aortic ejection sound is heard immediately after S_1 and is followed by the murmur.

A ventricular gallop (third heart sound) can occur when left ventricular dilation and failure develop. The presence of an atrial gallop (fourth heart sound) indicates left ventricular hypertrophy. When heart failure and pulmonary venous hypertension occur, crackles in the lungs can be heard.

A regular rhythm with changes produced by left ventricular hypertrophy is present on the ECG. Large S waves in the right precordial leads and large R waves in the left precordial lead, along with depression of the ST segment and inversion of the T waves, are common ECG changes. First-degree heart block and left bundle branch block may sometimes be present. The chest x-ray film may show left ventricular enlargement and pulmonary congestion in later stages of the disease. An echocardiogram may reveal the regurgitation, ventricular hypertrophy and thickening, decreased mobility, and calcification of the valve cusps.

AORTIC REGURGITATION
Definition

Aortic regurgitation is a condition in which blood is ejected forward into the aorta but also regurgitates backward into the left ventricle because of an incompetent, "leaky" aortic valve.

Etiology/Epidemiology

Causes include rheumatic heart disease, infective endocarditis, trauma, rheumatoid arthritis, dissecting aortic aneurysm, chronic hypertension, and congenital bicuspid valves. Aortic regurgitation is also associated with connective tissue diseases, such as Marfan's syndrome or myxomatous valvular degeneration.

Pathophysiology

In the early stages of chronic aortic regurgitation, diastolic regurgitation causes an increase in left ventricular volume. With this increased volume and increased left ventricular end-diastolic pressure, contractility increases to improve stroke volume and maintain cardiac output. Over time, this causes dilation and hypertrophy of the left ventricle. When the left ventricle can no longer compensate for the increased filling pressure, stroke volume will fall and the cardiac output will decrease, manifested by signs of left ventricular failure.

As aortic regurgitation progresses, left atrial pressure increases, pulmonary congestion and hypertension subsequently develop, and then right-sided failure may develop (Figure 36-5). Peripheral vasodilation may help compensate by reducing afterload or the pressure the left ventricle must eject against, which improves forward flow and reduces the regurgitant volume. As in aortic stenosis, low diastolic pressures decrease coronary perfusion, resulting in a decreased supply of oxygen to the myocardium. This may precipitate myocardial ischemia and angina.

Acute aortic regurgitation, most commonly caused by infective endocarditis or trauma, does not have the opportunity to adapt to volume and pressure changes. The left ventricle cannot accommodate the volume of blood from both regurgitation and the left atrium, and decompensation with signs of left ventricular failure occurs rapidly.

Clinical Manifestations

The clinical signs and symptoms of acute vs chronic aortic regurgitation vary. Patients with chronic aortic regurgitation may undergo left ventricular hypertrophy for many years with minimal or no symptoms. The chief complaints when symptoms do develop are exertional dyspnea, orthopnea, paroxysmal nocturnal dyspnea, and fatigue. Patients with severe aortic regurgitation may complain of an unpleasant awareness of heartbeat and palpitations. Patients frequently exhibit visible arterial neck pulsations and prominent neck vein pulsations. Nocturnal chest pain with diaphoresis may also occur. Typically in compensated aortic regurgitation the systolic blood pressure will be elevated with an abnormally low diastolic pressure.

The patient with chronic aortic regurgitation will develop left ventricular failure gradually, reveal an enlarged left ventricle on chest x-ray film, and demonstrate left ventricular hypertrophy. ECG changes will reflect the left ventricular hypertrophy. A diastolic murmur may be present, best heard at the second right intercostal space and radiating to the left sternal border. It is described as a high-pitched decrescendo murmur. An echocardiogram can reveal the regurgitation abnormalities across the valve and the abnormal wall motion of the left ventricle. As left ventricular failure progresses, symptoms of right-sided failure such as peripheral edema, ascites, and congestive hepatomegaly develop. The patient with

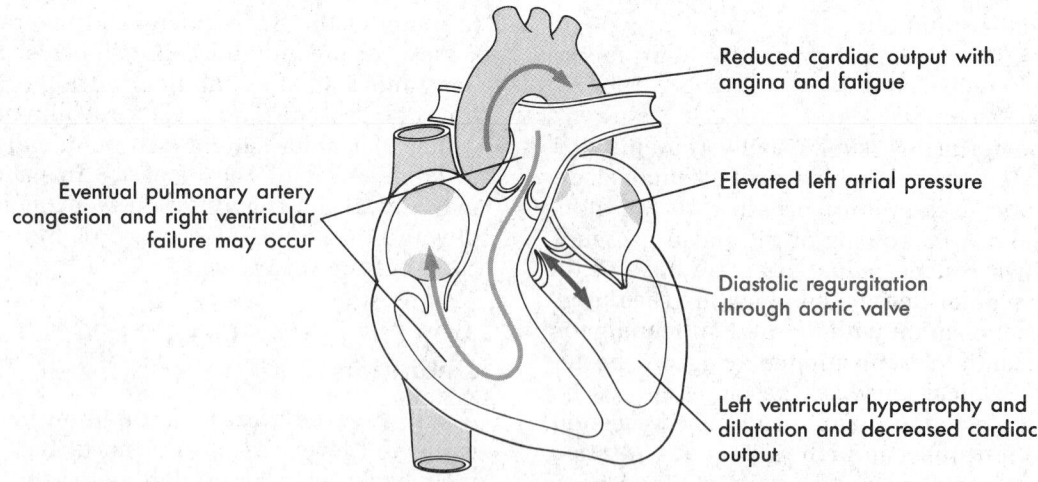

Reduced cardiac output with angina and fatigue

Eventual pulmonary artery congestion and right ventricular failure may occur

Elevated left atrial pressure

Diastolic regurgitation through aortic valve

Left ventricular hypertrophy and dilatation and decreased cardiac output

FIGURE 36-5 Effects of aortic regurgitation.

acute aortic regurgitation will have significant left ventricular dysfunction quickly, with tachycardia, peripheral vasoconstriction, cyanosis, and possibly symptoms of pulmonary congestion and edema.

TRICUSPID STENOSIS
Definition

Tricuspid stenosis is restriction of the tricuspid valve orifice because of commissural fusion and fibrosis. Chordae tendineae thickening and shortening may also occur.

Etiology/Epidemiology

Tricuspid stenosis is not a common valvular lesion. It is most commonly caused by rheumatic fever, often occurring in conjunction with disease of the mitral or aortic valve. The most common group of patients with this condition is women with mitral stenosis who have a history of rheumatic fever. Less frequently, tricuspid stenosis may result from infective endocarditis or congenital fusion of valve cusps. Commonly, patients with tricuspid stenosis also have some degree of tricuspid regurgitation.

Pathophysiology

In tricuspid stenosis the pressure in the right atrium is increased because of difficulty ejecting blood through the narrowed orifice into the right ventricle, causing a diastolic pressure gradient across the valve between the right atrium and right ventricle. It increases during inspiration and decreases during expiration. The central venous pressure or right atrial pressure increases, thus reducing cardiac output. This can eventually result in systemic venous congestion, ascites, and edema. Figure 36-6 illustrates the effects of tricuspid stenosis.

Clinical Manifestations

The signs and symptoms are related to the severity of the stenosis and the compliance of the right atrium. They are typically not evident for many years and, when they occur, are frequently associated with those symptoms caused by mitral and aortic disease.

One symptom that occurs with tricuspid stenosis is increased fatigue secondary to diminished cardiac output. In the late stage, symptoms of right-sided failure occur such as jugular venous distention, hepatomegaly, peripheral edema, and ascites. If the patient is in a sinus rhythm, the ECG will show tall, peaked P waves without the ECG findings of right ventricular hypertrophy. Atrial fibrillation may occur late in the disease. Visible pulsations of neck veins may also be present, causing a fluttering sensation. Murmurs similar to those of rheumatic mitral disease, but occurring before the mitral valve, are heard on auscultation, such as the high-pitched diastolic murmur along the left sternal border. In tricuspid stenosis the chest x-ray film often will reveal right atrial enlargement and a prominent superior vena cava shadow. Echocardiography can show valve motion abnormalities and the enlargement of the right atrium and superior vena cava.

TRICUSPID REGURGITATION
Definition

Tricuspid regurgitation involves an incompetent tricuspid valve that allows blood to flow backward from the right ventricle into the right atrium.

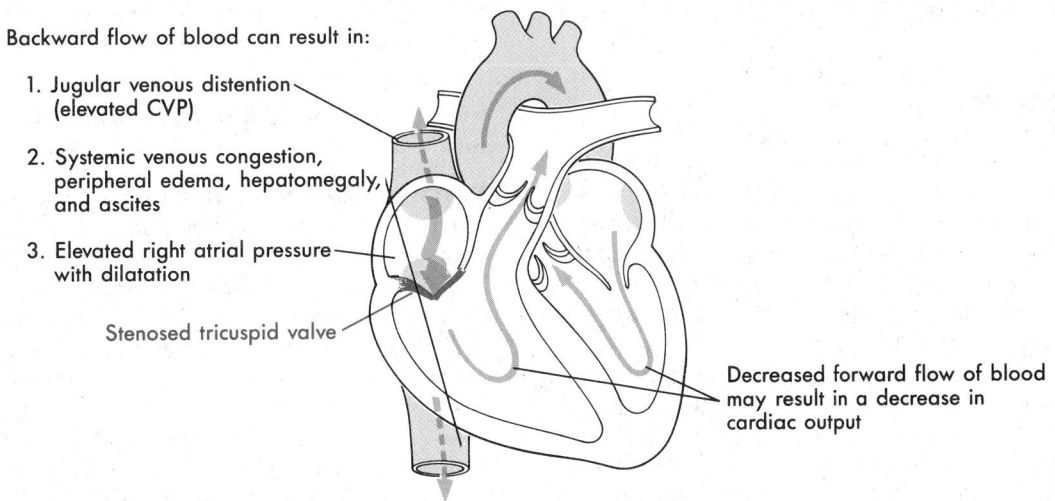

Backward flow of blood can result in:

1. Jugular venous distention (elevated CVP)

2. Systemic venous congestion, peripheral edema, hepatomegaly, and ascites

3. Elevated right atrial pressure with dilatation

Stenosed tricuspid valve

Decreased forward flow of blood may result in a decrease in cardiac output

FIGURE 36-6   Effects of tricuspid stenosis.

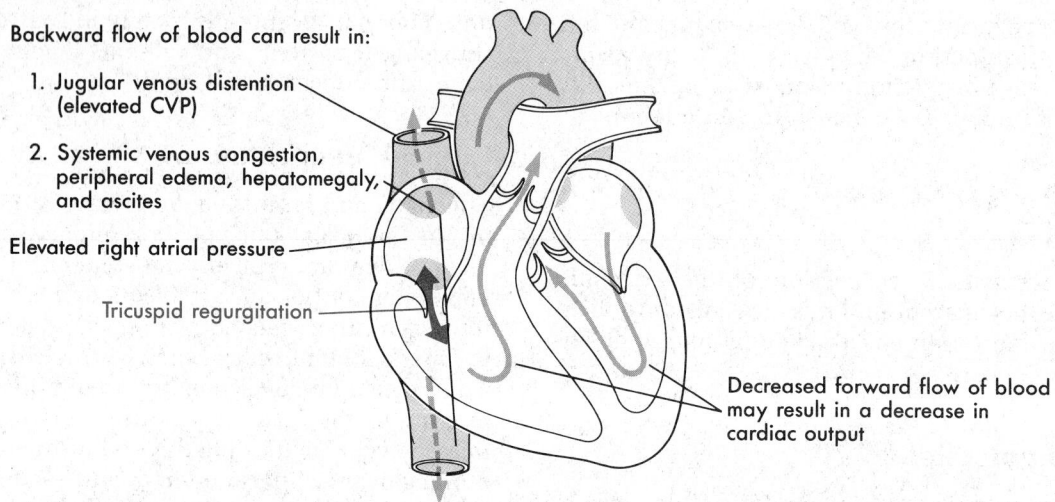

Backward flow of blood can result in:

1. Jugular venous distention (elevated CVP)

2. Systemic venous congestion, peripheral edema, hepatomegaly, and ascites

Elevated right atrial pressure

Tricuspid regurgitation

Decreased forward flow of blood may result in a decrease in cardiac output

FIGURE 36-7   Effects of tricuspid regurgitation.

Etiology/Epidemiology

Tricuspid regurgitation is uncommon but may result from a primary cause, such as infective endocarditis, rheumatic fever, or a congenital malformation. Right ventricular failure and dilation may indirectly produce tricuspid regurgitation.

Pathophysiology

Blood in the right ventricle regurgitates into the right atrium during systole, with a resultant increase in right atrial pressure. The increase in right atrial pressure raises the central venous pressure, the pressure in the superior and inferior venae cavae and in the hepatic veins. The workload of the right ventricle increases, because only part of the blood volume is ejected into the pulmonary artery. Ultimately right ventricular hypertrophy and dilation occur, and the heart eventually decompensates to right-sided failure and a decreased cardiac output (Figure 36-7).

Clinical Manifestations

Systemic venous congestion and reduced cardiac output produce the following symptoms: distended neck veins, peripheral edema, weakness and fatigue, marked hepatomegaly and ascites, positive hepatojugular reflux, and systolic pulsations of the liver. The chest x-ray film usually reveals right atrial and right ventricular dilation.

Atrial fibrillation is a frequent finding in tricuspid regurgitation, and diastolic overload of the right ventricle can result in right bundle branch block. On auscultation a blowing pansystolic murmur is heard on inspiration and decreases during expiration or during Valsalva's maneuver. This murmur is heard best along the left sternal border in the fourth or fifth intercostal space.

Therapeutic Management

The focus of management of the patient with valvular disease is twofold: medical management of the signs and symptoms of heart failure and treatment of the underlying cause of the valvular dysfunction.

Antibiotic therapy

The first consideration in the treatment of valvular disease is always prevention. Antibiotic prophylaxis for patients undergoing certain invasive procedures is administered to prevent the occurrence or recurrence of infective endocarditis. Antibiotics are administered to patients with all types of valvular disease, including mitral valve prolapse, and patients with a history of endocarditis, in accordance with AHA guidelines (see p. 919).

Sodium restriction, diuretic therapy, and inotropic agents

Symptoms caused by pulmonary congestion and ventricular dysfunction, particularly in patients with mitral stenosis, mitral regurgitation, and tricuspid stenosis, can be partially relieved by sodium restriction and administration of diuretics to reduce preload. The degree of sodium restriction required depends on the presence and severity of signs of pulmonary congestion and heart failure, such as orthopnea, dyspnea on exertion, crackles, and peripheral edema. The goal of sodium restriction is to reduce the blood volume. If sodium restriction does not adequately control symptoms, a diuretic such as furosemide or hydrochlorothiazide may be helpful. Inotropic agents such as digitalis may also be useful in improving contractility, decreasing left ventricular end-diastolic pressures (preload), and reducing heart failure. In acute situations the patient may require intravenous inotropic agents such as dopamine or dobutamine.

Activity restriction

Valvular disease will affect the physical activity level of patients in varying degrees. Strenuous activity can precipitate pulmonary symptoms and should be avoided for symptomatic patients. Individuals in the early stages of mitral stenosis and chronic mitral regurgitation should be counseled regarding occupational and recreational activities. Realistic physical activities should be encouraged with adequate rest and avoidance of undue physiologic stress. Patients with acute or severe mitral, aortic, or tricuspid regurgitation may require strict activity restrictions or bed rest during the initial phase of aggressive treatment to control left ventricular failure, myocardial ischemia, or pulmonary edema. Patients with aortic stenosis may remain asymptomatic for quite some time and do not require any restriction. However, patients with chronic aortic stenosis and those complaining of angina may have to limit their activities.

Vasodilator and antianginal therapy

In patients with pulmonary congestion, vasodilator therapy with nitroglycerine, amyl nitrate, or nifedipine helps to reduce preload and improve ventricular ejection secondary to reduction of afterload. The reduced afterload also improves forward flow of blood in patients with aortic and mitral regurgitation by reducing the resistance against which the heart must pump, thereby improving cardiac output. Patients with myocardial ischemia in aortic stenosis and aortic regurgitation may develop left ventricular failure and subsequent myocardial infarction. Nitrates improve perfusion of the coronary arteries and reduce oxygen consumption and ischemic episodes. Myocardial ischemia in tricuspid regurgitation is associated with right ventricular infarction.

Antidysrhythmic therapy

Dysrhythmias are a common complication related to valvular disease. The medical management often requires concomitant drug therapy. See Chapter 34 for a detailed discussion of treatment of dysrhythmias.

Patients with aortic stenosis, mitral stenosis, mitral regurgitation, and mitral valve prolapse are especially at risk for developing atrial fibrillation. Hemodynamic compromise may occur with these patients secondary to the loss of filling volume from the

"atrial kick." If patients become symptomatic, initial therapy is directed toward reducing the ventricular rate with verapamil and digoxin. Attempts are then made to convert the rhythm to normal sinus rhythm with a supraventricular antidysrhythmic therapy such as procainamide or quinidine. If this therapy does not achieve normal sinus rhythm, elective synchronized countershock may be required. Atrial fibrillation places these patients at high risk for thromboembolic complications, and they may be therefore placed on anticoagulation therapy.

Patients with mitral valve prolapse more commonly complain of palpitations and uncomplicated episodes of irregular or rapid heart rhythms, for which drug therapy is not recommended. However if patients with mitral valve prolapse are persistently symptomatic, treatment with a beta-adrenergic blocking agent may be helpful in controlling symptoms.

Surgical management

The goal of surgery is to repair or replace the diseased valve in an attempt to relieve symptoms and improve the patient's functional abilities.

The following factors are included when considering surgical intervention:
1. Degree of disease, physical limitations, and presence of symptoms
2. Risk factors (age, sex, prior operations, other diseases)
3. Mortality risk
4. Potential for valve-related complications (bleeding, hemorrhage, thromboembolic episodes)
5. Potential complications of cardiac surgery (shock, dysrhythmias, renal failure, stroke, respiratory failure)
6. Type of surgical procedure

Mitral valve

When physical symptoms of mitral valve disease limit the patient's normal activities or cardiac decompensation occurs despite maximum medical therapy, surgical intervention may be indicated. Surgery for mitral valve disease is palliative, not curative. Surgery ameliorates some signs and symptoms but does not resolve all abnormalities; future surgery may also be necessary. Types of procedures include percutaneous balloon mitral valvuloplasty, commissurotomy (valvulotomy), valve replacement, surgical valvuloplasty, or annuloplasty.

A **commissurotomy** can be performed as an open or closed heart surgical procedure, in which the stenosed valve leaflets are surgically separated (Figure 36-8). An open commissurotomy is usually done through the sternum or right anterolateral thorax, and a cardiopulmonary bypass machine is used. The

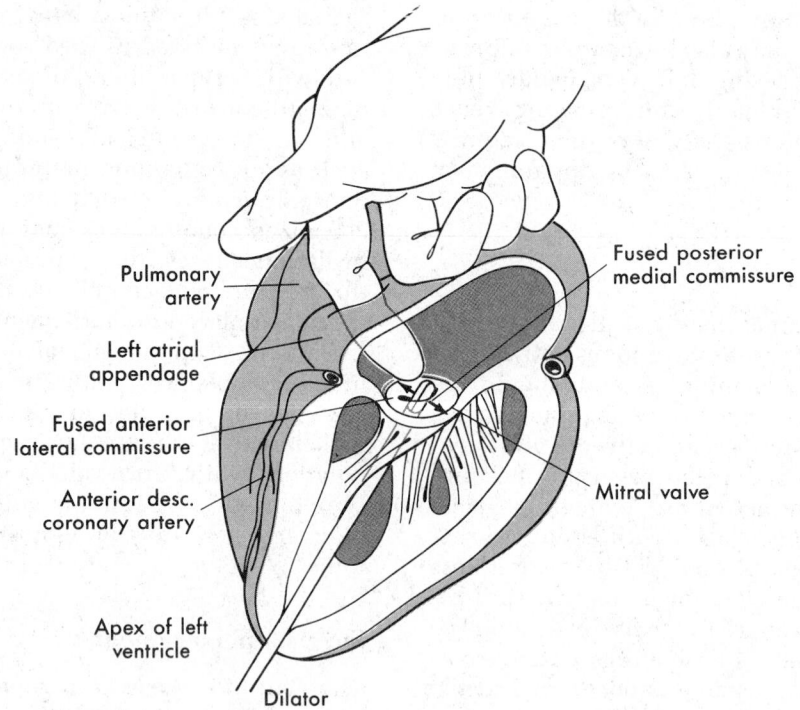

Pulmonary artery

Left atrial appendage

Fused anterior lateral commissure

Anterior desc. coronary artery

Apex of left ventricle

Dilator

Fused posterior medial commissure

Mitral valve

FIGURE 36-8   Technique of closed mitral commissurotomy using mitral dilating instrument.

left atrium is surgically incised, and the fused commissure is cautiously incised. A closed commissurotomy, where the operation is performed through the left posterior thorax, does not require the cardiopulmonary bypass machine. This may be the treatment of choice for patients whose preoperative evaluation has revealed no gross calcification, no significant fusion and shortening of chordae tendineae, no atrial thrombus, and no significant mitral regurgitation. In the closed procedure a small incision is made in the pericardium anterior to the phrenic nerve, and the opening of the commissures is done by digital (using the index finger) or mechanical (using a dilator) manipulation. Advantages of the open procedure are that there are fewer thrombotic and embolic complications, fewer tears, and less chance of hemorrhage, since it allows direct visualization of the mitral valve and surgical field.

Open surgical **valvuloplasty** (reconstruction of the incompetent mitral valve) is indicated for treatment of mitral regurgitation not responding to optimal medical therapy and is usually done for repair of cusp perforations seen with infective endocarditis and for repair of ruptured chordae. Repair is becoming more frequent than replacement, especially for high-risk patients. One advantage of valvuloplasty is that the thromboembolic rate without anticoagulation therapy is lower than that with grafts and prosthetic valves.

Annuloplasty, or repair of the annulus, is done for a small number of patients who have an enlarged valvular annulus and intact leaflets. This surgical procedure involves tightening the annulus with a purse-string suture or a rigid or flexible annular ring.

Mitral valve replacement is considered when the valve is so stenotic and calcified that a valvulotomy would not achieve long-term relief of the obstruction or repair would not adequately decrease regurgitation. The surgery may also be performed on an emergency basis when rupture of the papillary muscle or chordae tendineae is present.

Aortic valve

The aortic valve is not amenable to reconstruction, and surgical replacement is not indicated in the absence of clinical symptoms. The percutaneous balloon aortic valvuloplasty for aortic stenosis is demonstrating effectiveness in patients who are high-risk surgical candidates, including elderly patients, patients with previous myocardial infarction, or patients with depressed left ventricular function. Surgery is usually performed for patients with severe aortic stenosis and regurgitation, who are generally symptomatic.

There is evidence that aortic valve replacement for aortic stenosis can prolong life and improve symptoms. Several factors need to be considered in the decision to perform surgery. Predictors of increased risk for a first aortic valve replacement include advanced age (more than 70 years old), endocarditis, and the number of coronary vessels obstructed by greater than 70%. These risk factors are evaluated, recognizing the patient's severity of stenosis and present and potential loss of left ventricular function. Mortality is higher for patients more than 70 years old, when performed with a concurrent coronary artery bypass surgery, or in emergency situations.

When the aortic regurgitation is moderate in severity, the decision to operate is more controversial and many patients with aortic regurgitation may be treated medically. Valve replacement for aortic regurgitation should be performed before a decrease in left ventricular function becomes irreversible.

Tricuspid valve

Tricuspid disease occurs infrequently in the absence of mitral/aortic valve disease. Therefore intraoperative evaluation of the tricuspid valve after mitral or aortic valve correction helps direct the need for further intervention with the tricuspid valve. Reparative surgery such as commissurotomy or annuloplasty is usually considered before valve replacement, but if, after correction of the mitral and aortic valves, there are still significant pressure gradients because of the tricuspid valve, valve replacement may be indicated. However, tricuspid valve replacement has a greater risk of mortality than does mitral or aortic valve replacement. Considerations regarding the decision for surgery are the same as for mitral valve repair.

Prosthetic heart valves

Prosthetic heart valves may be mechanical or biologic. Mechanical heart valves are constructed of synthetic materials such as stainless steel and special plastics. Biologic heart valves are taken from animals or human organ donors. All prosthetic heart valves, whether mechanical or biologic, have certain similarities. All heart valves when open should exert minimal obstruction to blood flow and should close completely (Figure 36-9). The valve should not change its shape or wear out during the expected lifetime of the patient. The valve should not cause hemolysis of red blood cells or generate significant audible noises.

There are currently two mechanical prosthetic heart valve designs in use, the caged-ball valve, such as the Starr-Edwards (Figure 36-10,A), and the tilting-disk valve (Figure 36-10,C), such as the St. Jude Medical heart valve. The caged-ball valve has a ring that is covered with a cloth surface suitable for suturing the valve in the annulus. It does carry a significant risk of thromboembolism and requires

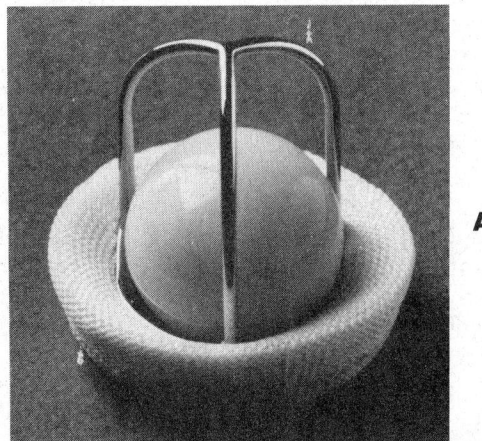
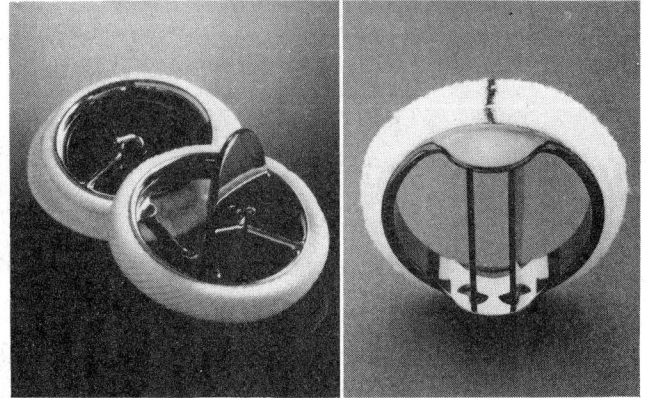

FIGURE 36-10 **A,** Starr-Edwards prosthetic valve. **B,** Medtronic Hall prosthetic valve. **C,** St. Jude Medical heart valve. (**B** courtesy of Medtronic, Minneapolis, Minn. **C** courtesy of St. Jude Medical Inc., St. Paul, Minn. From Kinney MR et al: *Comprehensive cardiac care,* ed 7, St Louis, 1991, Mosby–Year Book, Inc.)

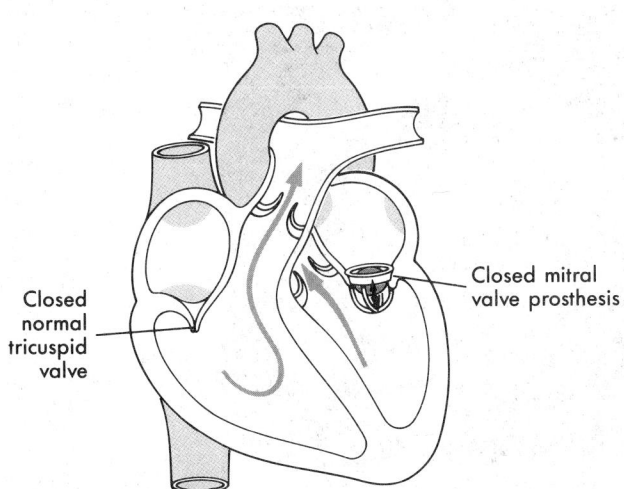

FIGURE 36-9 Prosthetic valve in mitral orifice, illustrating function during systole.

that patients remain on anticoagulation after its implantation. Tilting-disk valves were developed in an attempt to reduce the bulky nature of the caged-ball valve. Their orifice is larger than that of the caged-ball valve, and the semicentral flow of blood allows minimal gradients across the mechanical valve. The incidence of thromboembolism is less than with caged-ball valves, but it can still occur, thus requiring oral anticoagulation indefinitely.

Biologic tissue valves can be either xenograft or homograft and are used to avoid the thrombogenic tendency of prosthetic mechanical valves. Xenografts are derived from animal cardiac tissue, either porcine or bovine heart valves. Porcine valves provide a greater range of available sizes suitable for humans than bovine valves (Figure 36-11). The bovine pericardial xenograft has leaflets made of the pericardium taken from 16- to 18-month-old calves, which may limit their use in some patients where valve size is a consideration. These valves may be used in patients in whom anticoagulation is not desirable, such as women of childbearing age; young, athletic patients; or patients with a history of peptic ulcer or liver disease. A major drawback of the porcine valves is the tendency toward tissue degeneration, stiffening of the leaflets, and calcification that can occur after 5 years, with subsequent impairment of the valvular function. Homografts are human heart valves harvested from cadaver donors. Although the performance of the homografts is near ideal, their use has been limited because of their limited availability, duration of viability before implantation (cryopreservation is presently the preferred method of preservation), and the tendency for early calcification.

Percutaneous balloon valvuloplasty (nonsurgical)

Percutaneous balloon valvuloplasty is a relatively new procedure; its use is indicated in patients with significant valvular stenosis for whom medical therapy provides insufficient relief of symptoms. The procedure has been used most often in elderly patients who are too high risk to undergo surgery and may be an alternative for younger patients with rheumatic heart disease who do not wish to undergo surgery. The procedure is contraindicated in patients with significant mitral or aortic regurgitation and in the presence of left atrial thrombus because of possible septum perforation. The advantage of this procedure is that it is performed in the cardiac catheterization laboratory and does not require anesthesia.

Valvuloplasty has similarities to other procedures performed in the catheterization laboratory. A preprocedure medication, such as diazepam or midazolam (Versed), is given to help the patient relax, and heparin is frequently administered to prevent thromboembolus. A thermodilution catheter is inserted to measure right-sided heart and pulmonary artery pressures and cardiac output.

For aortic stenosis a left-sided heart catheter is advanced using fluoroscopy and pressure readings to determine location. The balloon-dilating catheter is then advanced over the guide wire, and the balloon is inflated across the stenosed valve. Initially an indentation of the balloon can be visualized because of the stenosis. A gradual decrease in the amount of indentation signifies a lessening of the amount of stenosis. Successive inflations with larger balloons may be necessary to achieve acceptable orifice size and

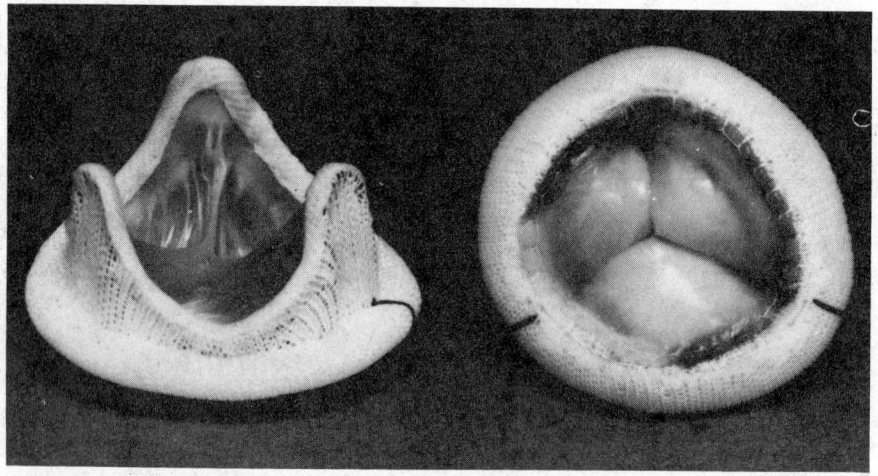

FIGURE 36-11   Carpentier-Edwards porcine valve, mitral position. (From Kinney MR, Packa DR, Dunbar SB: *AACN's clinical reference for critical-care nursing,* ed 2, St Louis, 1988, Mosby–Year Book, Inc.)

a decrease in the pressure gradients across the valve.

In mitral stenosis the procedure is done via a right-sided heart catheterization. The balloon dilation catheter is advanced through a puncture in the interatrial septum to the left atrium, and the dilation is performed across the mitral valve.

Valvuloplasty is associated with decreased risks and shorter hospitalization, but the results are more often temporary, requiring repeat valvuloplasty. In addition, a potential complication is valvular regurgitation or perforation of heart structures that may then require surgery.

NURSING MANAGEMENT OF THE PATIENT WITH VALVULAR DISORDERS

Assessment

The history includes a family history to identify diseases that can affect cardiac function and put the patient at risk for valvular disease. Pertinent information includes prior illnesses, particularly episodes of rheumatic fever or endocarditis. The dates related to this information should also be obtained. The patient is questioned regarding signs related to valvular disease and symptoms of its complications. The interview includes questions to identify which of the following symptoms the patient has experienced:

1. Fatigue
2. Chest pain (if present, pattern, quality, intensity, duration, and treatment)
3. Palpitations
4. Cough, dyspnea, orthopnea, paroxysmal nocturnal dyspnea
5. Decreased activity tolerance
6. Episodes of peripheral swelling
7. Increased abdominal girth
8. Episodes of loss of consciousness or memory lapses
9. Difficulty sleeping and use of sleeping aids
10. Episodes of syncope, dizziness

Fatigue and activity tolerance are particularly significant in patients with mitral valve disease, and a thorough assessment is done to establish a baseline capacity for activities of daily living and ambulation. This is important in developing rehabilitation plans.

Assess the patient and family's understanding of the disease to identify teaching needs. The patient and family's response to the disease and their related anxiety will influence their ability to cope with the illness. The family systems assessment is important in determining how much and what kind of support will be needed and to begin to identify resources for the future.

The patient's response to current cardiac medications is assessed to detect their effectiveness and any potential adverse effects related to the patient's complaints. Once the interview is completed, the objective data are obtained (Table 36-3).

Assessment of blood pressure, heart rate and rhythm, respiratory rate, depth, and breath sounds can provide the nurse with early indicators of complications of heart failure, atrial fibrillation, and progression of valvular dysfunction. Presence of increased body weight, peripheral edema, distended neck veins, or ascites should alert the nurse to the presence or progression of heart failure. The nurse should auscultate for extra heart sounds or changes in murmurs to establish the extent of valvular disease and monitor for its progression.

Routine tests to confirm the diagnosis of valvular disease include electrocardiogram, chest x-ray, echocardiogram, Doppler phonocardiogram, and radionuclide scanning. Less common tests may include a cardiac pulse tracing and a jugular venous tracing.

Patients may require cardiac catheterization to obtain a definitive diagnosis of valvular disease and an estimation of the severity of valvular disease. This is only performed in symptomatic patients when treatment decisions need to be made (such as surgery or valvuloplasty) or the degree of disease progression needs to be determined. The catheterization definitively identifies the involved valve or valves and estimates the degree of stenosis or regurgitation by measuring pressure gradients. Also, right-sided and left-sided heart pressures, ejection fraction, and left ventricular function are determined.

TABLE 36-3 Objective Data and Related Complications

Objective data	Related complications
Systolic blood pressure less than 90 mm Hg or 30 mm Hg below baseline	Heart failure, dysrhythmias, myocardial ischemia/infarction
Irregular pulse	Atrial fibrillation Ventricular ectopy
Pulse greater than 100 beats/min	Atrial fibrillation SVT
Distended neck veins, ankle edema, or ascites	Right-sided heart failure
Crackles or wheezing	Pulmonary venous congestion, heart failure progressing to pulmonary edema
Increased body weight	Heart failure, pulmonary edema

Nursing Diagnosis

Multiple nursing diagnoses may be appropriate for the patient with valvular disease and depend on the severity and extent of the disease process. Common diagnoses include the following:

Decreased cardiac output related to valve disease obstructing flow of blood or allowing backward flow of blood, heart failure, myocardial ischemia, papillary muscle dysfunction or rupture, or dysrhythmias

Altered tissue perfusion (cardiopulmonary, cerebral, peripheral) related to decreased blood pressure and cardiac output, venous pooling, emboli, dysrhythmias

Impaired gas exchange related to pulmonary congestion and edema

Activity intolerance related to fatigue, shortness of breath, and dyspnea

Anxiety related to diagnosis, symptoms, limitations, treatments, outcomes, and lack of knowledge

Knowledge deficit related to therapeutic management of disease, events during hospitalization, and the rehabilitation period

Patients who undergo valvular surgery will have a hospital course and needs similar to the patient undergoing cardiac surgery (see Chapter 35), but postoperatively, depending on the type of valve implanted, they may also require long-term anticoagulation. In this case the following nursing diagnosis would be important:

High risk for injury related to anticoagulation therapy

Planning

Goals for the patient with valvular disease include the following:

Patient will maintain hemodynamic parameters within normal limits for that patient; patient will remain free of signs and symptoms of heart failure, myocardial infarction, pulmonary edema, and dysrhythmias

Patient will maintain adequate peripheral perfusion as evidenced by warm, pink skin and adequate peripheral pulses

Patient will maintain baseline neurologic status without signs and symptoms of decreased cerebral perfusion

Patient will not experience angina or signs or symptoms of myocardial ischemia or infarction (see Chapter 35)

Patient will be adequately oxygenated as evidenced by PaO_2 within normal limits for patient and absence of dyspnea, tachypnea, cyanosis, and crackles

Patient will be able to increase tolerance to previous levels of daily activities

Patient will express reduced anxiety

Patient will be able to describe treatment plan and the care requirements during hospitalization and after discharge

Patient will have no evidence of bleeding

Implementation

Decreased cardiac output

The primary focus of nursing actions is to monitor for signs and symptoms of decreased cardiac output and the etiologic factors or complications. Routine monitoring of the medical or ambulatory patient helps to ensure hemodynamic stability. Included are measurements of blood pressure, pulse, respirations, ECG, and breath sounds. This assessment should be done with each office visit or at least every 8 hours in the hospital setting.

Other parameters reflecting cardiac output and circulatory function to be monitored are intake and output, urine specific gravity, level of consciousness and mental status, and skin color and temperature. Assess for signs and symptoms of cardiac failure such as the presence of jugular venous distention, peripheral edema, and adventitious heart sounds. The patient's physiologic response to activity should be closely monitored. Activities should be planned to minimize the cardiac workload and oxygen requirements and to ensure adequate sleep cycles. Positioning the patient in semi-Fowler's can reduce venous return to decrease preload. Sodium and fluid intake may be restricted to prevent additional workload on the heart. In addition, serum electrolyte levels should be monitored, because alterations in serum potassium may aggravate dysrhythmias or potentiate the action or adverse effects of certain drugs, such as digoxin.

Patients requiring intravenous inotropic support to maintain their cardiac output need continuous monitoring of pulmonary artery pressures and serial measurements of all other vital signs, including direct cardiac output measurements using a pulmonary artery catheter. The patient's response to drug therapy should be documented hourly, noting the occurrence of potential adverse effects.

Altered cardiopulmonary, cerebral, and peripheral tissue perfusion

Nursing actions for altered cardiopulmonary tissue perfusion include assisting the patient to identify stressful events that precipitate angina and planning patient care activities to prevent angina. The patient must be taught how to accurately describe the pain, including pattern, quality, intensity, and duration. The patient's response during anginal episodes must be clearly documented in the patient record, including activity precipitating the event, vital signs, and description of the pain. Nitrate therapy may be used to alleviate chest pain and decrease preload. For a more in-depth explanation of the management and interventions for patients receiving antianginal therapy refer to Chapter 35.

Patients with a history of atrial fibrillation or endocarditis (blood clot formations on vegetation) are at greater risk for cerebral emboli. Preventive measures focus on optimizing the cardiac output to enhance perfusion and prevent the stasis of blood and potential formation of clots. Administration of anticoagulants to patients in atrial fibrillation may be helpful in preventing embolism.

Monitoring for abnormal findings of cerebral tissue perfusion includes evaluating for the following signs and symptoms:

1. Alteration in mental status, level of consciousness, orientation, behavior pattern, memory
2. Weakness of extremities, either transient or permanent
3. Seizure activity
4. Dysphagia, aphasia, visual loss

Preventive measures to support tissue perfusion to the periphery include the following:

1. Application of antithromboembolic stockings or sequential compression device to postoperative patients and to patients requiring bed rest
2. Passive and active range of motion (ROM) exercises at least three times per day
3. Repositioning of patients on bed rest every 2 hours
4. Encouraging early ambulation as tolerated and ordered
5. Instructions to patient to do the following:
   a. Keep feet elevated when out of bed if not contraindicated by condition
   b. Do not cross legs or ankles
   c. Avoid straining or Valsalva's maneuver (may dislodge thrombi)

During therapy the patient's peripheral vascular status is evaluated against the baseline assessment data for changes and detection of abnormalities, including peripheral pulse checks, skin color and temperature, and extremity strength. These are monitored during office examinations, at least daily during medical treatment, and frequently in the postoperative phase.

Impaired gas exchange

Nursing actions include monitoring for signs and symptoms of pulmonary congestion, edema, or embolism, such as changes in respiratory rate and depth, breath sounds, heart rate, and skin color. Dyspnea is a common complaint in valvular disease. If pulmonary edema or congestive heart failure occurs, immediate intervention may be necessary (see "Clinical Alert"). The patient should be put in a

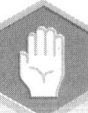

CLINICAL ALERT

Patients who experience pulmonary edema with severe shortness of breath require prompt intervention. Place the patient in high Fowler's position with legs dangling over the side of the bed. Medications may be required to improve oxygenation, reduce preload, and optimize the pumping action of the heart, such as oxygen, morphine, furosemide (Lasix), and digoxin.

semi-Fowler's or high Fowler's position to decrease venous return and facilitate respirations. Supplemental oxygen is administered as needed. Morphine sulfate may be administered intravenously to decrease preload and reduce anxiety. Digoxin will optimize the cardiac output to also reduce the amount of backflow of blood to the pulmonary circulation. Diuretics such as furosemide may also be required to decrease preload and resolve pulmonary edema. Coughing and deep breathing exercises help maintain adequate oxygenation.

Activity intolerance

Actual sustained activity intolerance is usually associated with complaints of dyspnea, which occurs in the presence of heart failure. Patients need to identify their usual activities of daily living and when they become fatigued. Patients with severe preoperative limitation of activity will require greater assistance with self-care. Encourage the patient to determine when activities should be scheduled. At the same time, assist the patient in recognizing limitations to prevent undue cardiac stress or the precipitation of complications such as dysrhythmias or heart failure. Rest periods are scheduled between activities to optimize the patient's level of self-care.

The patient's response to activity should be monitored and documented by the nurse. Assess the patient's heart rate after activity and determine the length of time it takes to return to baseline as one indicator of the patient's cardiac reserve. The patient's perception of the activity intolerance is important in promoting self-care and self-esteem. Objective assessment of blood pressure, pulse, respirations, and signs of fatigue is also considered. Physical activities, activities of daily living, and self-care are increased gradually as the patient's tolerance increases.

Anxiety

Most people, whether in the community or in the hospital, are anxious about heart disease; their knowledge deficit related to the disease, tests, or surgery; their fear of dying/complications with surgery; and their uncertainty regarding their future. Patients experiencing shortness of breath from pulmonary edema exhibit high levels of anxiety. Emotional support and encouraging the verbalization of patient and family expectations and fears are crucial. An assessment of the patient and family's understanding of the therapeutic regimen provides a basis for an individualized plan of instruction. Determine the patient's ability to use appropriate coping methods. In addition to providing reassurance and comfort, the nurse may help the patient explore techniques, such as guided imagery, relaxation techniques, music therapy, and other forms of comfort or distraction.

Knowledge deficit

Patients requiring any treatment need to understand what preparation is done, what medications will be administered, any potential related problems, and what postprocedure care entails. This information is based on the hospital standards for these procedures (e.g., cardiac catheterization). Patients undergoing valvular surgery should receive additional information regarding the surgery. This information helps the patient provide self-care and also allays fears regarding surgery and improves compliance with the postoperative regimen. See the preoperative teaching guide for the patient undergoing cardiac surgery (Chapter 35). Before discharge the patient should have a complete understanding of medications, activities to avoid, self-care, and signs and symptoms to report to the physician. Patients who are discharged on anticoagulation therapy must be knowledgeable in bleeding precautions such as use of only electric razors, avoiding contact sports, oral hygiene, and methods to stop bleeding if it occurs. Patients should be aware that certain foods and medications can inhibit or potentiate the effects of anticoagulants and the importance of return visits to the physician to monitor the level of anticoagulation. Knowledge of diet, rest, and exercise will help to optimize the patient's health within the cardiac limitations.

Evaluation

Ongoing patient assessment helps the nurse evaluate the effectiveness of interventions. A successful treatment plan helps the patient maintain an adequate cardiac output and thus sustain daily activities and normal body function (including perfusion to vital organs), maintain adequate oxygenation and airway clearance, and be alert and oriented so that prior levels of self-care may be maintained or resumed. The patient should not show signs of de-

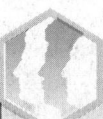

GERIATRIC CONSIDERATIONS

Valvular Disease

Special considerations for the geriatric patient focus on monitoring for adverse effects of medications, activity intolerance, and nutritional needs. The elderly patient population also tends to have a higher incidence of co-morbidities such as hypertension, coronary artery disease, and hepatic and renal insufficiency. Risk factors must be analyzed for their impact on complications and nursing interventions.

Responses to medications may vary, depending on the ability of the patient's renal or hepatic system to metabolize different agents and on the normal aging changes of the patient. The nurse must be alert for signs and symptoms of drug-related complications and report these immediately. Some older patients may require reduced dosages for drugs excreted by the kidneys or liver in the presence of renal or hepatic dysfunction. Because of the decreased number of adrenergic receptors in the aging process, some medications require increased doses to be effective, such as beta-adrenergic blocking agents.

The geriatric patient who has been sedentary may require more assistance with activities of daily living and may become fatigued more easily. Patients should be allowed to set their own goals based on how they feel. A home health referral may be necessary for the patient who is being discharged with limited resources available to assist at home.

Another area that may require support is meeting nutritional requirements. The elderly patient may eat less and need smaller and more frequent meals. If the patient is hospitalized, a dietary consultation may be necessary to help the patient maintain usual eating patterns.

creased cardiac output or altered tissue perfusion, including decreased blood pressure, abnormal heart rate, angina, decreased urine output, or altered levels of consciousness. The patient should not have fatigue, dyspnea, shortness of breath, or the presence of crackles when carrying out necessary activities of daily living. The patient's anxiety level should not interfere with ability to participate in the care plan and activities of daily living. The patient should demonstrate knowledge of the disease process, the therapy employed, the medications prescribed, and their side effects, as well as the signs indicating the need for medical assistance. Finally, the nurse should look for evidence that the patient and family feel in control of their situation and are able to solve problems appropriately.

Documentation

Documentation of care for the patient with endocardial/valvular disease primarily involves accurate recording of assessment data, interventions, and the patient's response and validation of patient and family teaching. The recording of thorough physical assessments is essential while the treatment plan is being established, including the patient's response to treatment. For the surgically treated patient the record should reflect an accurate and detailed description of the preoperative and postoperative care delivered and the response, including patient and family teaching. Assessment of progress toward achieving self-care and the related patient and family teaching must be documented regularly. The patient should receive both verbal and written instructions about the disease process, treatment plan, and medications.

Ongoing Care

The goal of cardiac rehabilitation in this patient population is to achieve and maintain optimal cardiac conditioning, avoid progression of the disease, prevent complications, and control cardiac risk factors. Individuals are started on an exercise program while in the hospital. The patient is observed and assisted by the nurse or physical therapist to evaluate tolerance for continued activity at home. The importance of avoiding or modifying activity after meals, with stress, or in extremes of temperature should be explained to both the patient and family. Additionally, activities or clothing that promote circulatory stasis should be avoided (e.g., tight stockings, crossing legs). See Chapter 35 for cardiac rehabilitation.

Preventive measures should be discussed with the patient and family to prevent recurrence of illness, complications, and rehospitalization. This includes teaching regarding measures to prevent endocarditis, review of potential indications of complications, and actions to be taken should problems arise. The patient's diet, medications, and follow-up visits with the surgeon and cardiologist should be discussed.

Patients who have had a valve replacement will be receiving anticoagulation therapy, potentially indefinitely. Periodic blood tests are necessary to ascertain if the dosage is adequate in controlling the potential for thromboembolism. The nurse emphasizes the importance of this ongoing care with the patient and family, particularly given the risks of long-term anticoagulation.

CRITICAL THINKING QUESTIONS

1 Who is at risk for developing infective endocarditis? What procedures increase patients' risk of developing infective endocarditis? What are the recommendations for preventing infective endocarditis in the high-risk population?

2 For each valvular disorder (mitral, aortic, and tricuspid stenosis and regurgitation) describe how changes in cardiac and pulmonary pressures are created. What signs and symptoms develop as a result of these changes?

3 What is the medical management of the patient experiencing heart failure? What are the nursing implications of this medical management?

4 Describe the surgical interventions available for patients with valvular disorders. How does postoperative nursing management of these patients differ from management of other cardiac surgery patients (see Chapter 35)?

5 Describe the major nursing diagnoses, expected outcomes, and nursing interventions for the patient with valvular disease. What can the nurse do to promote cardiac output, improve gas exchange, optimize physical activities, and prevent complications?

6 What should the nurse include in postoperative teaching? discharge teaching?

BIBLIOGRAPHY

1. Antunes MF: Mitral valvuloplasty for rheumatic heart disease, *Semin Thorac Cardiovasc Surg* 1(2):164-175, 1989.
2. Barden C et al: Balloon aortic valvuloplasty: nursing care implications, *Crit Care Nurse* 10(6):22-28, 86, 1990.
3. Bertorini TE, Gelfand M: Neurological complications of bacterial endocarditis, *Comp Ther* 16(12):47-55, 1990.
4. Birrer RB, Karl M, Volpe S: Infective endocarditis, *J Fam Pract* 24(3):289-295, 1987.
5. Bisno AL et al: Antimicrobial treatment of infective endocarditis due to viridans Streptococci, Enterococci, and Staphylococci, *JAMA* 261(10):1471-1477, 1989.
6. Bumann R, Speltz M: Decreased cardiac output: a nursing diagnosis, *Dimen Crit Care* 8(1):6-15, 1989.
7. Burden LL, Rodgers JC: Endocarditis: when bacteria invade the heart, *RN* 51(12):38-46, 1988.
8. Burger AJ et al: The role of two-dimensional echocardiography in the diagnosis of ineffective endocarditis, *Angiology* 42(7):552-560, 1991.
9. Cassally MG: Antibiotic prophylaxis for infective endocarditis, *Todays FDA* 3(6):3c, 7c, 1991.
10. Chan JC, Bisno AL: Rheumatic fever and rheumatic heart disease, *Pract Cardiol* 17(4):25-42, 1991.
11. Child JS: Infective endocarditis: risks and prophylaxis, *J Am Coll Cardiol* 18(2):337-338, 1991.
12. Dalen JE: Valvular heart disease, infected valves and prosthetic heart valves, *Am J Cardiol* 65(6):29c-31c, 1990.
13. Daljani AS et al: Prevention of bacterial endocarditis: recommendations by the American Heart Association, *JAMA* 264(22):2919-2922, 1990.
14. Delaney KA: Endocarditis in the emergency department, *Ann Emerg Med* 20(4):405-414, 1991.
15. Douglas PS: Rheumatic heart disease and other valvular disorders in women, *Cardiovasc Clin* 19(3):259-265, 1989.
16. Friedlander AH, Yoshikawa TT: Pathogenesis, manage-

ment, and prevention of infective endocarditis in the elderly dental patient, *Oral Surg Oral Med Oral Pathol* 69(2):177-181, 1990.

17. Fukuda N: Outcome standards for the client with chronic congestive heart failure, *J Cardiovasc Nurs* 4(3):59-70, 1990.

18. Gantz NM: Geriatric endocarditis: avoiding the trend toward mismanagement, *Geriatrics* 46(4):66-68, 1991.

19. Giuliani ER et al: *Cardiology: fundamentals and practice,* ed 2, St Louis, 1991, Mosby–Year Book, Inc.

20. Gray IR: Rational approaches to the treatment of culture-negative infective endocarditis, *Drugs* 41(5):729-736, 1991.

21. Hurst JW, *Current therapy in cardiovascular disease,* ed 3, Philadelphia, 1991, BC Decker Inc.

22. Karp RB: Role of surgery in infective endocarditis, *Cardiovasc Clin* 17(3):141-162, 1987.

23. Keys TF: Diagnosis and management of infective endocarditis, *Cleveland Clin J Med* 57(6):558-562, 1990.

24. Kinney MR et al: *Comprehensive cardiac care,* ed 7, St Louis, 1991, Mosby–Year Book, Inc.

25. Miller LC: Rheumatic fever and rheumatic heart disease, *Curr Opin Rheumatol* 1(3):257-261, 1989.

26. Nord CE, Heimdahl A: Cardiovascular infections: bacterial endocarditis of oral origin. Pathogenesis and prophylaxis, *J Clin Periodontol* 17(7, pt 2):494-496, 1990.

27. Rafalowski M: Cardiac valve replacement: the homograft, *Focus Crit Care* 17(2):111-114, 1990.

28. Robbins MJ, Eisenberg ES, Frishman WH: Infective endocarditis: a pathophysiologic approach to therapy, *Cardiol Clin* 5(4):545-562, 1987.

29. Sandor GKB, Vasilakos SS, Vasilakos JS: Mitral valve prolapse: a review of the syndrome with emphasis on current antibiotic prophylaxis, *J Can Dent Assoc* 57(4):321-325, 1991.

30. Schakenbach LH: Physiologic dynamics of acquired valvular heart disease, *J Cardiovasc Nurs* 1(3):1-17, 1987.

31. Seifert PC: Surgery for acquired valvular heart disease, *J Cardiovasc Nurs* 1(3):26-40, 1987.

32. Suddarth DS: *The Lippincott manual of nursing practice,* Philadelphia, 1991, JB Lippincott Co.

33. Trausch PA: Infective endocarditis: nursing care and prevention, *Prog Cardiovasc Nurs* 3(2):45-53, 1988.

34. Williams PM, Epstein JB: American Heart Association updates recommendations for prevention of infective endocarditis, *J Can Dent Assoc* 57(6):494-495, 1991.

35. Wingate S, editor: *Cardiac nursing: a clinical management and patient care resource,* Rockville, Md, 1991, Aspen Publishers, Inc.

36. Wright SM: Pathophysiology of congestive heart failure, *J Cardiovasc Nurs* 4(3):1-16, 1990.

UNIT IX

Hematologic and Immune Systems

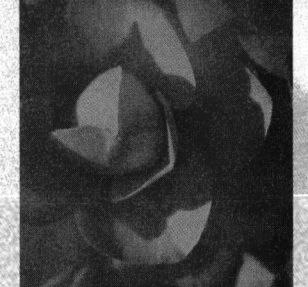

CHAPTER THIRTY-SEVEN

Nursing Assessment of the Hematologic System

LEARNING OBJECTIVES

1 Know the basic components of the blood and the functions of each.
2 Obtain relevant subjective information from the patient who has a hematologic alteration.
3 Using correct technique, examine the patient to obtain appropriate objective information about the hematologic system.
4 Differentiate in relation to the hematologic system abnormal from normal subjective and objective findings.
5 Describe tests related to the diagnosis and detection of disorders of the hematologic system.
6 Discuss patient preparation and care involved in administering tests that diagnose hematologic disorders.

KEY TERMS

AN UNDERSTANDING of the hematologic system requires a knowledge of the blood's composition and the functions of its various constituents. Approximately 55% of the blood volume is made up of plasma and 45% of cells. Three types of cells are found in the blood, and these have specialized functions: (1) the erythrocytes carry oxygen; (2) the platelets prevent loss of blood through breaks in blood vessel walls; and (3) the leukocytes provide protection against infectious agents, other foreign substances that manage to enter the body, and defective tissue.

ANATOMY AND PHYSIOLOGY
Blood Plasma

Plasma is a pale yellow liquid consisting of water and dissolved solutes. Blood proteins form the largest portion of the plasma solutes (Table 37-1). All the albumin, fibrinogen, and 60% to 80% of the glob-

941

TABLE 37-1 Composition of Blood Plasma

Components	Percentage
Water	90%
Solutes	10%
Proteins	6%-8%
Albumin	55% of protein
Globulins	38% of protein
Fibrinogen	7% of protein
Other substances	2%-4%
Organic	
Cholesterol	
Glucose	
Amino acids	
Triglycerides	
Urea, uric acid	
Lactic acid	
Hormones	
Enzymes	
Inorganic ions	
Sodium, chloride, bicarbonate, potassium, calcium, etc.	

ulins are formed and secreted by the liver. The remaining globulins are the immunoglobulins (gamma globulins) secreted by the lymphatic system.

The liver and body cells obtain the amino acids they require to synthesize protein from the blood by active transport or by facilitated diffusion. When the blood levels of amino acids rise, the liver and other body tissues serve as storage reservoirs. When the blood level of the various amino acids falls, protein is catabolized and the resulting amino acids enter the blood. However, the liver is responsible for the homeostasis of the amino acid concentration of the blood. It prevents amino acid concentrations from rising to toxic levels, and when the protein storage potential of the body is exceeded it converts excess amino acids to urea and carbohydrate.

Although the level of amino acids in the blood is only 35 to 65 mg/dL this amount is adequate to move protein back and forth between the liver and tissues, because the amino acids have a high rate of turnover. The obligatory degradation of protein amounts to approximately 20 to 30 g/day even during starvation. When blood proteins are being lost at an unusually high rate, as during kidney disease or following a major burn, the liver is able to replace up to an additional 50 g/day. A fall in blood protein is one of the strongest stimulants for new liver cell growth.

The blood proteins, particularly albumin, are responsible for the colloid osmotic pressure of the blood and thus affect the tendency to form edema (see Chapter 12). Other blood proteins serve:

1. As a reservoir for lipid-soluble hormones
2. To maintain the stability of the micelles that carry blood lipids
3. As substrates for enzymic action, for example, angiotensinogen and the blood clotting factors
4. As enzymes and proenzymes
5. As antibodies and other chemicals of the immune system

Erythrocytes

The percentage of the blood volume made up of cells is called the hematocrit and is made up almost entirely of **erythrocytes** (red cells). Erythrocytes are the most plentiful of the blood cells. There are between 4.5 and 5.5 million/mm^3, which amounts to a total of approximately 30 trillion erythrocytes for each adult. They have no nucleus, are disk shaped with a relatively large surface area, and are narrower in the center of the disk (Figure 37-1). The chief function of erythrocytes is to enclose the 12 to 16 g of hemoglobin per 100 mL of blood needed for respiration. It is important that hemoglobin remains within cells because its molecule is small enough to filter into the nephrons, and, in large amounts, it tends to block them and produce kidney failure.

Erythrocytes are about the same size as the diameter of the smallest capillaries but are sufficiently flexible to move through them. In some genetic conditions, such as sickle cell anemia, the chemical structure of the hemoglobin is defective and reduces the flexibility of the erythrocytes.

Erythrocytes are produced in the adult in the red bone marrow of the ribs and sternum, the vertebrae, and the proximal ends of the long bones; in the fetus and young child they are produced in all the bone marrow and in the spleen. Their production is controlled by the renal hormone, *erythropoietin,* that is secreted in increased amounts when the partial pressure of oxygen in the blood is less than a critical amount. They are produced by mitosis from hemocytoblasts and lose their nuclei and much of their cytoplasmic reticulum at a late stage of their development while they are still in the bone marrow. When they first enter the blood, some of their cytoplasmic reticulum is still visible and they are called reticulocytes. A higher-than-normal number (0.5% to 1.5%) of reticulocytes in the blood is an indication that the rate of erythrocyte production is elevated, while a lower-than-normal number indicates that the rate is depressed (Figure 37-2).

Erythrocytes survive in the circulation for approximately 105 to 120 days. As they age, their outer membrane deteriorates and they are detected and

RED BLOOD CELLS   PLATELETS

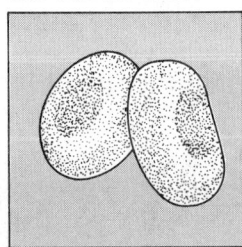
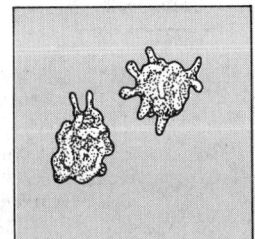

WHITE BLOOD CELLS (LEUKOCYTES)
Granular leukocytes

Basophil   Neutrophil   Eosinophil

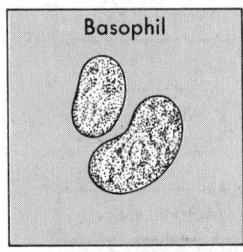
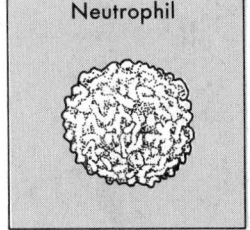
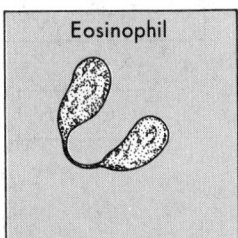

Nongranular leukocytes

Lymphocyte   Monocyte

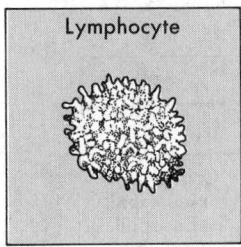
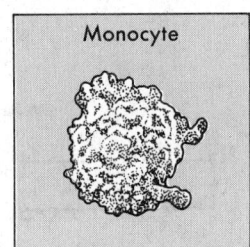

FIGURE 37-1 Human blood cells.

removed by large macrophages in the sinusoids of the liver, the spleen, and in the bone marrow. The iron from the hemoglobin is stored as ferritin; the pigment bilirubin is excreted in bile.

Platelets

Platelets are not true cells. They have no nucleus, are ovoid or spindle shaped, and are formed by the segmentation and shedding of the cytoplasm of large megakaryocytes in the bone marrow. When they come into contact with a foreign surface or with a damaged blood vessel wall, they stick to it and to each other and can spread to cover a surface several hundred times the size of their own initial surface area. They prevent blood loss (1) by sticking together to block small breaks in blood vessels and capillaries; (2) by secreting chemicals, such as prostaglandins, that cause the broken vessel to constrict and partially close the hole; and (3) by initiating coagulation of the blood (clot formation).

Blood **coagulation** is the conversion of plasma from a colloid to a gel (Figure 37-3). It must make this conversion swiftly when required to prevent blood loss but must not change inside normal blood vessels, because this inhibits blood flow to the tissues. For this reason, coagulation of the blood is controlled by a series of reactions involving at least 13 different factors (Table 37-2). The basic mechanism includes four steps and four of the 13 factors:

1. Thromboplastin is released from either damaged tissue (extrinsic activation) or from platelets (intrinsic activation) when they stick to each other or to damaged blood vessel walls.
2. The enzyme thrombin is produced from the blood protein prothrombin. This reaction is activated by the thromboplastin, released in step 1, and by calcium ions that act as a catalyst.
3. Fibrin is produced from the blood protein fibrinogen. This reaction is activated by the thrombin produced by step 2.
4. The long strands of fibrin become entangled

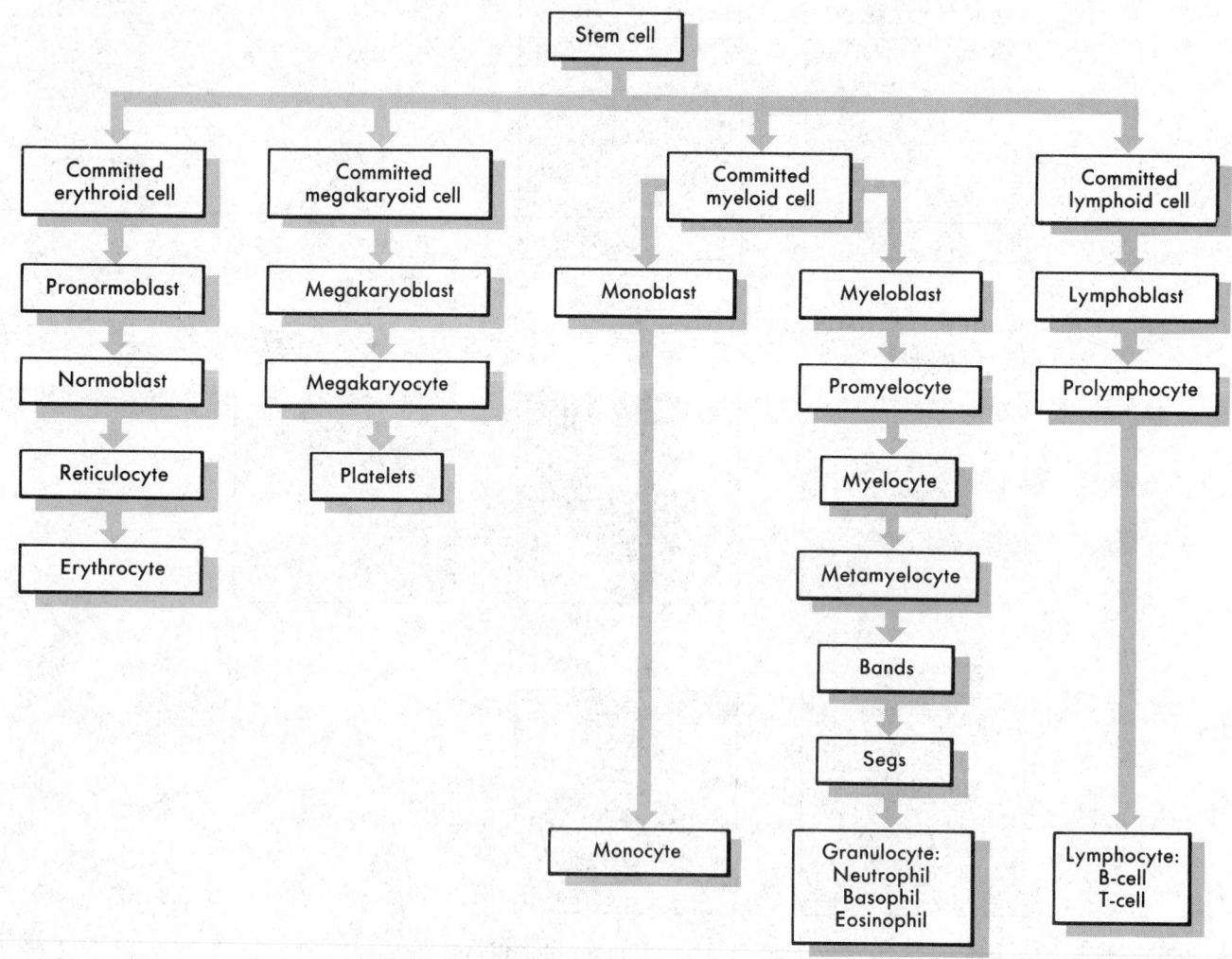

FIGURE 37-2   Formation and maturation of blood cells. All circulating blood cells originate from a common stem cell.

and turn the blood or plasma into a gel. The clot is red if erythrocytes are trapped in the fibrin mesh and yellow if none are trapped. The clot is yellow when plasma coagulates or when a clot forms slowly as blood flows past the clot quickly. If plasma is stirred while the coagulation reaction is occurring, the strands of fibrin can be removed from the plasma to produce serum (plasma without the clotting chemicals).

The remaining nine coagulation factors accelerate the clotting mechanism. For example, once the clotting mechanism has begun, thrombin activates factor V, which, in turn, accelerates the conversion of prothrombin to thrombin and has a cascade like effect on the clotting process.

Several factors oppose intravascular clot formation:

1. Antithrombins (such as heparin) that either inhibit thrombin formation or inactivate it to prevent fibrin formation

2. Substances that impair the liver's use of vitamin K and thus reduce liver synthesis of prothrombin and factors VII, IX, and X
3. Fibrinolysins that dissolve intravascular clots when they form

In addition to the chemicals that activate or oppose clotting, physical factors are important. Clot formation is accelerated by:

1. Rough surfaces in the lumen of blood vessels or surfaces associated with wounds because they activate platelet aggregation.
2. Slow or sluggish blood flow, because clotting chemicals that may be formed in a particular area are not washed away and diluted and therefore may reach levels high enough to trigger the clotting reactions in that area. Once started, clots tend to grow in size because the platelets trapped in the clot release additional thromboplastin, and the slow blood flow around the clot allows its concentration to rise.

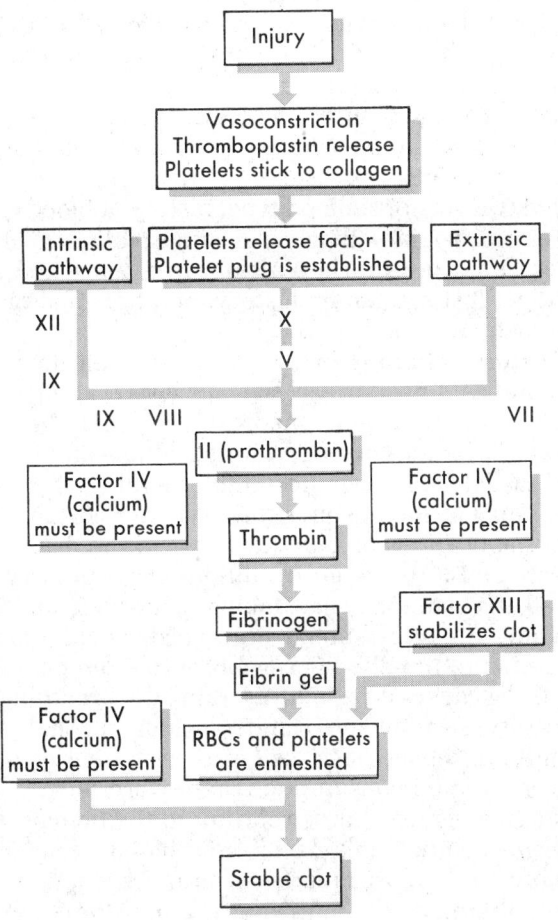

FIGURE 37-3 Pathway of coagulation.

TABLE 37-2 Coagulation Factors—Nomenclature and Synonyms

Factor	Common synonyms(s)
Factor I	Fibrinogen
Factor II	Prothrombin
Factor III	Thromboplastin
	Thrombokinase
Factor IV	Calcium
Factor V	Proaccelerin
	Labile factor
Factor VI (now obsolete)	None in use
Factor VII	Serum prothrombin conversion accelerator (SPCA)
Factor VIII	Antihemophilic globulin (AHG) Antihemophilic factor (AHF)
Factor IX	Plasma thromboplastin component (PTC), Christmas factor
Factor X	Stuart factor
Factor XI	Plasma thromboplastin antecedent (PTA)
Factor XII	Hageman factor
Factor XIII	Fibrin-stabilizing factor

From Thibodeau GA: *Anthony's textbook of anatomy and physiology*, ed 13, St Louis, 1990, Mosby–Year Book.

Leukocytes

Leukocytes (white blood cells) protect the body against disease. They are classified into granulocytes and agranulocytes depending on the presence or absence of granules in their cytoplasm. The granulocytes are further classified into neutrophils, basophils, and eosinophils depending on their ability to take up stain. The proportion of the various leukocytes in the blood is given in Table 37-3.

Neutrophils, basophils, eosinophils, monocytes, and a small proportion of lymphocytes are produced in the bone marrow. In the adult, most of the lymphocytes are produced in the lymph nodes and spleen.

The leukocytes are able to squeeze through small pores in capillary walls by diapedesis. This is made easier because the nuclei of the large leukocytes are lobed and can change shape to fit through small pores. By ameboid movement, leukocytes are able to circulate through the various tissues, search out and ingest microorganisms and other harmful particles, and prevent them from reaching the blood-

TABLE 37-3 Proportions of Cells in the Blood

Cells	Proportion
Erythrocytes (red blood cells)	
Hematocrit	42%-45% of blood volume
Count	4.5-5.5 million/mm^3
Platelets	
Count	150,000-350,000/mm^3
Leukocytes (white blood cells)	
Total count	5000-9000/mm^3
Granulocytes	
Neutrophils	65%-75% of all leukocytes
Eosinophils	2%-5% of all leukocytes
Basophils	0.5%-1% of all leukocytes
Agranulocytes	
Lymphocytes	20%-25 of all leukocytes
Monocytes	3%-8% of all leukocytes

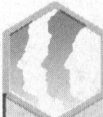

GERIATRIC CONSIDERATIONS

Physiologic Changes in the Hematologic System

The morphology of blood cells and the composition of plasma change slightly with age. There is a small decline in plasma albumin and colloid osmotic pressure, a small increase in the plasma globulins, and a more significant increase in fibrinogen concentration in a proportion of the population as they age.

However, it should be noted that any marked change in the composition or physical properties of blood usually indicates the presence of disease. For example, anemia, which is more prevalent in the elderly, may be a sign of cancer, poor digestive function, poor nutrition, or inadequate exercise.

stream and spreading throughout the body. They provide the second and third lines of defense designed to protect the body against infectious disease and damaged or abnormal tissue cells.

ASSESSMENT
Subjective

A focused health history for a patient with a suspected or previously diagnosed hematologic problem requires the nurse to use knowledge of pathophysiology to guide questioning in an appropriate and complete manner. Hematologic disorders may manifest in a variety of vague symptoms or may be an incidental finding during an examination for an unrelated reason. For example, a patient may be evaluated because of complaints such as fatigue, weight loss, joint pain, lethargy, and anorexia. Conversely, anemia may be an incidental finding when blood work is done as part of a routine preoperative workup.

An adequate system-specific history for any patient includes a review of related systems and delineation of any positive findings (symptoms the patient complains of) through exploring various dimensions. Determination of these appropriate related systems is guided by the nurse's knowledge base of pathophysiology and treatment. Specific dimensions used to delineate positive findings include onset, duration, frequency, alleviating factors, aggravating factors, precipitating events, location, quality, quantity, associated symptoms, and chronology of events. Noting any significant negatives (symptoms the patient denies) is important because it allows other clinicians to know specifically what the inter-

viewer asked. To record "no problems" does not communicate which symptoms the patient denied. The box on p. 947 provides a list of potential symptoms to review with the patient.

In addition to specific symptoms, ask the patient about previous exposure to radiation, previous blood transfusions, blood type, history of blood clots, or any previously diagnosed abnormality of blood cells. Other appropriate history to explore includes medical history, family history, and personal or social history.

History generally includes: major adult illnesses, hospitalizations, surgeries, injuries/accidents, immunizations, current medications, allergies, and habits. When recording hospitalizations and/or surgeries, determine the hospital, attending physician, and dates of the hospital stay. When recording current medications include the name of the drug, who prescribed it, for what condition it was prescribed, when the patient began taking it, dosage, and frequency. Allergies should be recorded with careful attention to the allergic response. Ask the patient if anything causes a rash, hives, difficulty breathing, or difficulty swallowing. Habits include alcohol consumption, tobacco use, use of recreational or illicit drugs, caffeine consumption, and exercise.

Family history that is relevant to the hematologic system includes anemia or "low blood," leukemia, lymphoma, thalassemia (seen in black populations, and patients from Southeast Asia and the Mediterranean), sickle-cell anemia or sickle-cell trait, multiple myeloma, hemolytic jaundice, or hemophilia. A positive finding should include the disease as well as the individual's relationship to the patient (for example, Hodgkin's disease, paternal uncle).

Objective

Based on the history obtained and knowledge of pathophysiology, the nurse determines the appropriate systems to be assessed. Some patients will have more complex symptom involvement than others, and therefore assessment needs may vary from patient to patient. Systems the nurse may incorporate in objective evaluation include integumentary, oropharyngeal cavity, lymphatic, cardiovascular, respiratory, gastrointestinal, musculoskeletal, urinary, and neurologic. General assessment is significant in every patient and refers to the examiner's overall impression of the patient's state of health. The box on p. 948 includes potential objective findings that may be noted on examination of a patient with a hematologic disorder.

Oropharyngeal cavity

Examine the patient's oropharynx using a light and tongue blade and wearing gloves. Observe the oral

POTENTIAL SYMPTOMS IN HEMATOLOGIC DISORDERS

General

- Fever
- Night sweats
- Unexplained weight loss
- Loss of appetite (anorexia)
- Lethargy
- Easy fatigability
- Malaise

Integumentary

- Easy bruising (ecchymosis)
- Excessive bleeding from cuts
- Itching (pruritus)
- Brittle, ridged nails
- Change in shape of nails

Oropharynx

- Gingival hypertrophy
- Gingival bleeding
- Fissuring of the lips
- Dryness and scaling of the lips
- Sore tongue
- Sore throat

Lymphatic

- Tender, swollen nodes (may also use terms such as kernel or lump)

Cardiopulmonary

- Difficulty breathing (dyspnea)
- Shortness of breath (SOB)
- Chest pain
- Cough
- Bloody sputum (hemoptysis)

Gastrointestinal

- Bloody emesis (hematemesis)
- Melena (blood in feces)
- Abdominal pain
- Abdominal fullness
- Early satiety
- Bright-red bleeding per rectum (BRBPR)
- Constipation

Genitourinary

- Excessive bleeding during menses (menorrhagia)
- Bloody urine (hematuria)
- Painful urination (dysuria)
- Urgency and frequency
- Scanty urine (oliguria)

Musculoskeletal

- Bone pain
- Joint pain (arthralgias)
- Swollen, erythematous joints
- Muscle aches and pains (myalgias)

Neurologic

- Headache
- Blurred vision
- Change in mental status
- Change in level of consciousness

and buccal mucosa noting moisture, color, and the presence of any lesions. Observe the gums for hypertrophy, bleeding, or the presence of any lesions. Inspect the posterior pharynx for the presence or absence of tonsils, exudate, lesions, and noting color. A patient with acute myelomonocytic or monocytic leukemia may have gingival hypertrophy as a result of massive infiltration of gingiva with leukemic cells. A patient receiving warfarin therapy may have gingival bleeding.

Lymphatic

Palpate for enlarged lymph nodes in the following areas: preauricular, postauricular, submental, submaxillary, tonsillar, occipital, anterior cervical chain (internal jugular chain and anterior superficial chain), posterior cervical chain (spinal nerve chain and posterior superficial cervical), supraclavicular, infraclavicular (subclavian), epitrochlear, inguinal, and popliteal (Figure 37-4). When palpating lymph nodes in the neck, it is helpful to have the patient's neck slightly flexed (Figure 37-5, A and B). Axillary nodes are palpated with the patient sitting up or lying down. It is important to provide support for the arm being examined. With the arm supported and relaxed at the patient's side, palpate the axillae medially toward the chest wall, laterally toward the arm being examined, anteriorly, and posteriorly (Figure 37-6). The inguinal nodes (groin) are palpated with the patient in a supine position. Palpation of the popliteal nodes (popliteal fossa) is facilitated by having the knee flexed.

Note location, size, contour, mobility, tenderness, and consistency (i.e. firm vs. hard) of any palpable nodes. Palpate nodes using the dorsal surfaces of the fingers (finger pads) and moving fingers in a gentle circular motion. Using too much pressure on palpa-

POTENTIAL OBJECTIVE FINDINGS IN HEMATOLOGIC DISORDERS

General
- Weight change
- Fever
- Tachypnea
- Tachycardia
- Hypotension
- Ill appearing
- Cachectic

Integumentary
- Alopecia
- Areas of hyperpigmentation
- Spoon nails
- Pallor
- Ecchymoses
- Petechiae
- Purpura
- Xeroderma

Oropharyngeal cavity
- Gingival hypertrophy
- Gingival bleeding
- Mucosal ulcerations
- Xerostomia
- Cheilosis

Lymphatic
- Lymphadenopathy

Cardiovascular
- Tachycardia
- Ventricular gallop (S3)
- Atrial gallop (S4)
- Irregular rhythm (auscultation or ECG)
- Arrhythmia (ECG)

Respiratory
- Tachypnea
- Cough
- Hemoptysis
- Rales (crackles)
- Decreased breath sounds

Gastrointestinal
- Abdomen tender to palpation
- Marked decrease in general areas of tympany
- Hepatosplenomegaly
- Guaiac-positive stool
- Hematemesis

Genitourinary
- Turbid urine
- Hematuria
- Oliguria (this would be noted over time)
- Vaginal bleeding
- Vaginal discharge

Musculoskeletal
- Decreased range of motion of a particular joint
- "Hot" joint; increased local temperature, erythematous, tender
- Unilateral, non-pitting edema of an extremity

Neurologic
- Decreased or absent deep tendon reflexes (DTRs)
- Impaired mental status
- Decreased sensory function
- Cranial nerve palsies
- Decreased or impaired peripheral sensation

---

tion could possibly prevent the determination of the presence of lymphadenopathy. A patient who has Hodgkin's disease or a patient who has a non-Hodgkin's lymphoma may have one or many enlarged lymph nodes. Lymph nodes may also be enlarged and are usually tender if an infection is present.

Musculoskeletal

Inspect the joints for color and swelling. Palpate the joints for tenderness, crepitations, edema, and temperature change. Observe active range of motion (ROM) if desired. A patient with hemophilia may bleed into a joint (hemarthrosis), resulting in edema, pain, tenderness, inflammation, and decreased ROM. (See Chapter 56 for a complete discussion of musculoskeletal assessment.)

Urinary

Examine the urine for evidence of bleeding (hematuria) using a Multistix. Patients receiving warfarin therapy may develop hematuria and patients receiving some antineoplastic agents may develop hemorrhagic cystitis. Please refer to Chapter 15 for further details regarding cancer chemotherapy side effects. (See Chapter 41 for a complete discussion of urinary assessment.)

Neurologic

The complete neurologic examination comprises evaluation of several areas including cranial nerves, cerebellar function, sensory function, motor function, mental status, and reflexes. Generally, the neurologic examination will not be done in its entirety.

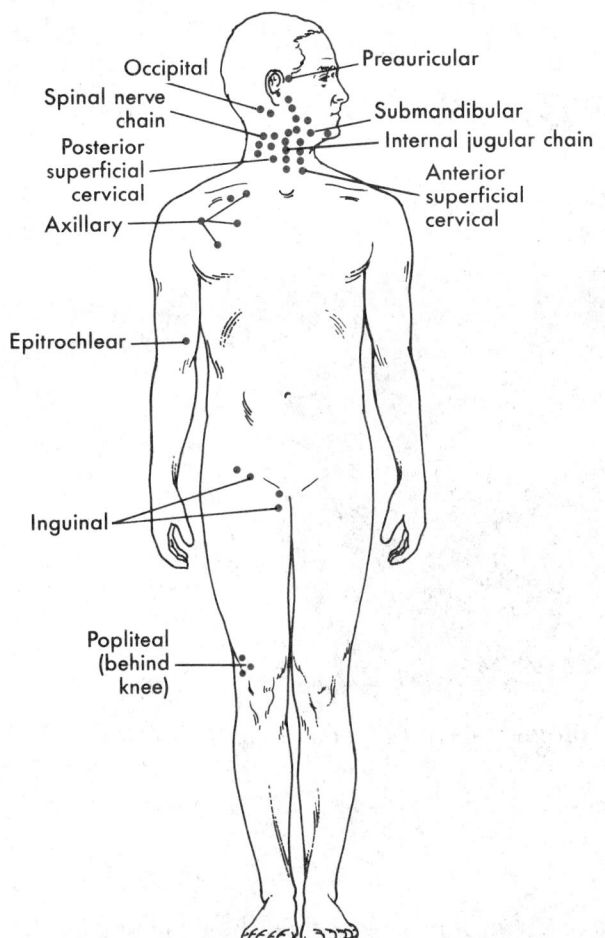

FIGURE 37-4 Lymph nodes to assess during physical examination.

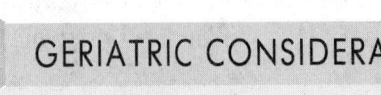

GERIATRIC CONSIDERATIONS

Hematologic Assessment

General approach
- Allow more time than for a younger adult
- Articulate clearly; the geriatric patient may be hearing impaired
- Impaired sight, comprehension, or mobility may result in less than optimum cooperation
- Provide clear, concise instructions

History collection
- Be alert for answers that do not appear appropriate; the patient may not have understood the question correctly because of impaired hearing or impaired comprehension
- Some questions may need to be repeated in a different manner

Physical assessment
- The physical examination itself is not different, but the approach needs to be altered such that the appropriate information is assessed without undue discomfort or embarrassment for the patient
- Maintain an environment with minimal noise, distractions, and interruption
- Anemia may be common in the elderly population, but it is not a normal physiologic response to aging
- B_{12} and folate should be evaluated in the presence of dementia

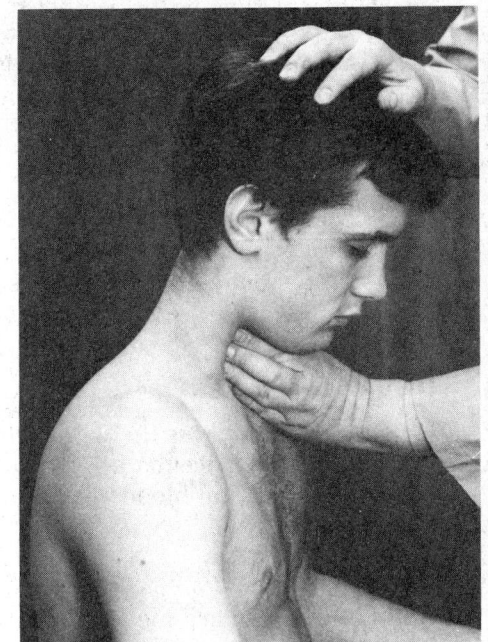
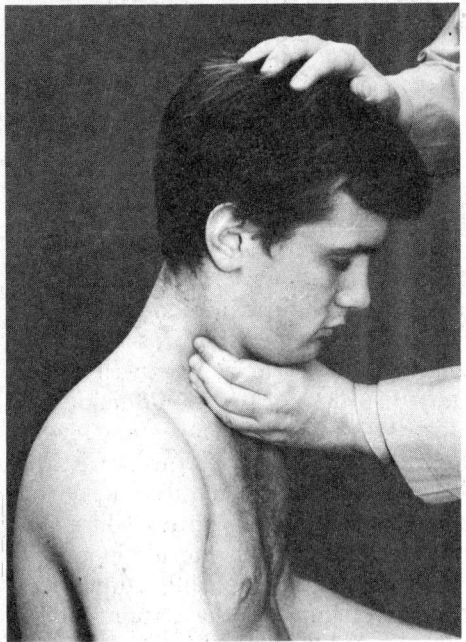

FIGURE 37-5 **A,** Palpation of the anterior cervical chain, and **B,** posterior cervical chain. (From Malasanos L et al: *Health assessment,* ed 3, St Louis, 1986, Mosby–Year Book.)

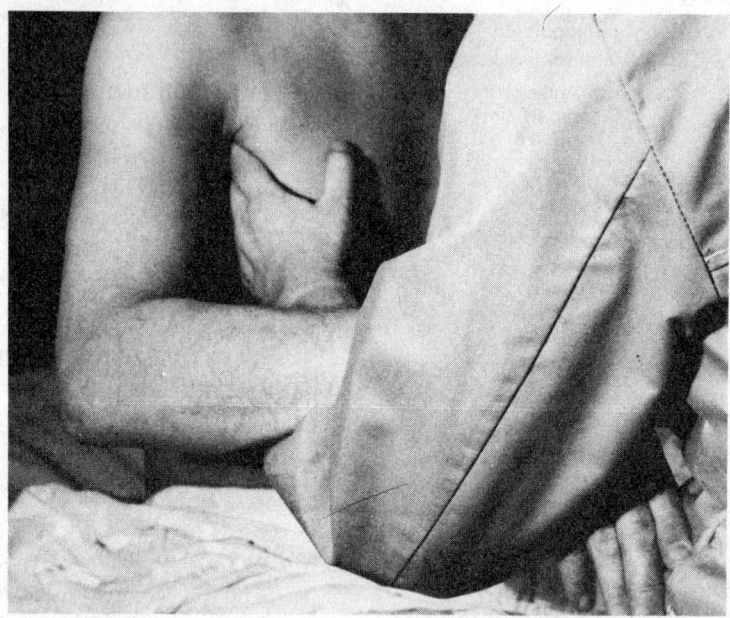

FIGURE 37-6 Palpation of the axillary nodes. (From Malasanos L et al: *Health assessment,* ed 3, St Louis, 1986, Mosby–Year Book.)

Rather, the nurse will determine the component or components that are relevant to the individual disease and patient. Different disease processes have different neurologic manifestations. The patient may experience cranial nerve palsies in acute leukemia, change in level of consciousness or change in mental status as a result of a hemorrhagic CVA secondary to warfarin therapy, or change in sensory function as a result of neurotoxicity secondary to antineoplastic chemotherapy. (Please refer to Chapter 44 for a complete discussion of neurologic assessment.)

DIAGNOSTIC AND LABORATORY TESTS
Complete Blood Count

The **complete blood count (CBC)** is an important part of routine screening and hospital admission. It involves several tests, each of which assesses the three major cells formed in the bone marrow. The CBC detects many disorders of the hematologic system and provides data for the diagnosis and evaluation of disorders in other body systems. A CBC includes red and white cell counts, hematocrit, hemoglobin, erythrocyte indices, differential white cell count, and examination of the peripheral blood cells (Table 37-4). No special patient preparation is required other than explaining to the patient that a blood sample will be taken from the hand or arm and that the sample will be evaluated for the presence of infection or anemia in the body. A limb that is receiving intravenous fluid should not be used, because this results in hemodilution.

Red blood cell count

The red blood cell count or erythrocyte count is a determination of the number of red blood cells in a microliter of venous or capillary blood. The red blood cell count is not in itself always sufficient to determine the adequacy of red cell function, so it is frequently considered in conjunction with hemoglobin, hematocrit, and red cell indices.

Hemoglobin

Hemoglobin is the oxygen-carrying pigment, the main component of red blood cells, and is reported in g/dL.

Hematocrit

Hematocrit compares the volume of red blood cells to the volume of plasma and is measured as a percentage of the total blood volume.

Red cell indices

Red cell indices are measurements of the size and hemoglobin content of erythrocytes. The mean corpuscular volume or mean cell volume (MCV), mean corpuscular hemoglobin or mean cell hemoglobin

TABLE 37-4   Complete Blood Count Studies

Determination	Reference range (SI values)	Clinical significance
Red blood cell (RBC) count	18-44y, M: 4.3-5.7 × 10^6 cells/µL (4.3-5.7 × 10^{12} cells/L) F: 3.8-5.1 × 10^6 cells/µL (3.8-5.7 × 10^{12} cells/L) 45-64y, M: 4.2-5.6 × 10^6 cells/µL (4.2-5.6 × 10^{12} cells/L) F: 3.8-5.3 × 10^6 cells/µL (3.8-5.3 × 10^{12} cells/L) 65 +y, M: 3.8-5.8 × 10^6 cells/µL (3.8-5.8 × 10^{12} cells/L) F: 3.8-5.2 × 10^6 cells/µL (3.8-5.2 × 10^{12} cells/L)	Increased with dehydration, polycythemia at high altitudes, and with hypoxia caused by cardiac or respiratory disorders Temporary increases occur with strong emotions or a cold shower Decreased with anemias, leukemias, and hypothyroidism
Hemoglobin (Hb), Total	18-44y, M: 13.2-17.3 g/dL (132-173 g/L) F: 11.7-15.5 g/dL (117-155 g/L) 45-64y, M: 13.1-17.2 g/dL (131-172 g/L) F: 11.7-16.0 g/dL (117-160 g/L) 65 + y, M: 12.6-17.4 g/dL (126-174 g/L) F: 11.7-16.1 g/dL (117-161 g/L)	Increased with chronic obstructive pulmonary disease (COPD), high altitudes, and polycythemia Decreases indicate anemia; also decreased with severe hemorrhage
Hematocrit (Hct)	V RBCs /V whole blood × 100 18-44y, M: 39-49 (0.39-0.49) F: 35-45 (0.35-0.45) 45-64y, M: 39-50 (0.39-0.50) F: 35-47 (0.35-0.47) 65 +y, M: 37-51 (0.37-0.51) F: 35-47 (0.35-0.47)	Increased with severe burns, shock, severe dehydration, and polycythemia vera Decreased with severe blood loss and leukemia Decreases establish presence and severity of anemias
Red cell indices Mean corpuscular volume (MCV)	fL 18-44y, M: 80-99 F: 81-100 45-64y, M: 81-101 F: 81-101 65+ y, M/F: 81-103	Increased with folic acid deficiency, vitamin B_{12} deficiency, cirrhosis, aplastic anemia, smoking, and alcohol consumption Large number of reticulocytes will elevate MCV values Decreased with chronic iron deficiency, thalassemias, and anemia of chronic disease Helps identify anemias as normocytic, microcytic, or macrocytic
Mean corpuscular hemoglobin (MCH)	27-35 pg/cell	Low MCH indicated microcytosis or hypochromia High MCH indicates macrocytosis
Mean corpuscular hemoglobin concentration (MCHC)	31-37 g Hb/dL RBCs (310-370 g Hb/L RBCs)	Low MCHC indicates hypochromia; found with chronic iron deficiency and anemia of chronic disease High MCHC found with spherocytosis
White blood cell count (WBC)	4.5-11.0 × 10^3/µL (4.5-11 × 10^6/L)	Increased with infectious diseases (usually of bacterial origin), and with trauma, surgery, or acute leukemia Decreased by toxic agents with aplastic anemia, agranulocytosis, and acute chronic leukemias
Differential WBC count Segmented neutrophils	*Mean %* 56-70	Increased neutrophils are found with a number of bacterial infections, inflammatory but noninfectious diseases (collagen disorders, rheumatic fever, pancreatitis), and with malignancies; also increased with burns, crushing injuries, diabetic acidosis, and infarctions

Continued.

TABLE 37-4   Complete Blood Count Studies—cont'd

Determination	Reference range (SI values)	Clinical significance
Bands	3-5	Increased bands found with severe stress on bone marrow or severe bacterial disease.
Lymphocytes	21-35	Marked increases in lymphocytes occur with chronic lymphocytic leukemia and infectious diseases; mild increases with chronic infections; decreases occur with lupus erythematosus and Hodgkin's disease
Monocytes	4-6	Increased monocytes found with chronic inflammatory conditions
Eosinophils	1-4	Increased eosinophils found with allergic and parasitic disorders
Basophils	0-0.3	Increased basophils are uncommon and are found with myelofibrosis; blast (primitive white cell) forms may indicate acute leukemia

(MCH), and mean corpuscular hemoglobin concentration or mean cell hemoglobin concentration (MCHC) are included in red cell indices. The indices are valuable in the diagnosis of various anemias.

White blood cell count

A white blood cell count is a determination of the number of white blood cells or leukocytes/unit volume in a sample of venous blood. It is possible for the white blood cell count to remain within normal limits despite a marked shift in one type of leukocyte. Variations are normal within given ranges of the white cell and may not be significant as long as the differential count and peripheral blood smear are normal.

Differential WBC count

An examination of a stained slide of peripheral blood allows estimations of the size, shape, and structure of individual WBCs. The peripheral smear is examined closely for abnormal lymphocytes and monocytes, immature WBCs, abnormal granulations in the *leukocyte*, hypersegmentation, atypical lymphosis, and shifts in the numbers of each type of cell. A differential count is expressed in percentages, and an increase in the percentage of one type of cell is accompanied by a decrease in another type of cell. Detailed evaluation of the white cell distribution and morphology helps diagnose specific infections.

An important concept related to neutrophil counts is a *shift to the left*. With acute bacterial disease or acute stress on the bone marrow, early elements in the granulocytic series (bands) are released to meet increased demand. The existence of many immature cells is referred to as a "shift to the left."

Peripheral smear

The peripheral smear often accompanies the differential WBC count and permits examination of the size, shape, and structure of individual RBCs and platelets (Table 37-5). This information is useful in *differentiating* various forms of anemias and blood dyscrasias.

Laboratory Tests for Leukemias and Anemias

In addition to the complete blood count, a number of other tests should be performed that are useful in determining the specific classification of leukemia or anemia being experienced by the patient (Table 37-6).

Bone marrow aspiration

Bone marrow aspiration is a valuable diagnostic procedure used in the diagnosis of blood dyscrasias and multiple myeloma, and in differentiating chronic iron deficiency anemia from the anemia of chronic disease. The procedure involves removal of cells from the bone marrow, a site of active hematopoie-

TABLE 37-5   Terms Associated with Erythrocytes

Terms	Description
Acanthocytes	Small, spheric erythrocytes with fingerlike projections; found with liver disease
Anisocytosis	Erythrocytes of variable size, found with anemias
"Burr" cells (echinocytes)	Normal erythrocytes with uniform projections of a triangular shape; may be seen with uremia or polycythemia
"Helmet" cells (chistocytes)	Helmet-shaped, spiral, triangular erythrocytes; found in hemolytic anemias and uremia
Hyperchromic	Erythrocytes with more than normal color because of high hemoglobin content; associated with congenital spherocytosis
Hypochromic	Pale erythrocytes caused by low hemoglobin content; suggestive of chronic iron deficiency
Macrocytic	Abnormally large erythrocytes; found with macrocytic anemias (e.g., pernicious anemia and folic acid deficiency anemia)
Microcytic	Abnormally small erythrocytes; indicative of microcytic anemias (e.g., iron deficiency anemia and thalassemia major)
Sickle cell	Crescent-shaped erythrocytes caused by presence of abnormal hemoglobin; indicative of sickle cell anemia
Spherocyte	Small, round erythrocytes without a central clear area; associated with congenital spherocytosis and some hemolytic diseases (e.g., ABO incompatibility)
Target cell	Thin erythrocytes with small amount of central hemoglobin; associated with hemoglobin C disease and chronic liver disease
Teardrop cell	Tear-shaped erythrocytes; found with myeloid metaplasia and metastatic malignancy of the bone marrow

sis. Marrow cells are examined for maturational abnormalities.

The most common sites for bone marrow sampling are the posterior iliac crests, although the anterior iliac crests and sternum may also be used. Bone marrow cells may be removed by aspiration or bone marrow biopsy. The cells are removed, smeared on slides, allowed to air dry, and are then taken to the laboratory.

Patient preparation

The patient is told that a small sample of bone marrow will be taken so that blood cells can be examined. The nurse reassures the patient that the area will be anesthetized although pressure and some pain may be experienced as the needle enters the bone, and bone marrow is aspirated. A signed consent and baseline vital signs are obtained. The nurse then checks coagulation tests before the procedure and administers sedation if ordered.

Procedure

The patient is positioned according to the site being used. The nurse meticulously cleanses and then drapes the site. The physician anesthetizes the site (either the sternum or iliac crests) and inserts a specially designed needle with a firm, turning motion. The stylus is removed and a sample of bone marrow is removed. The patient is supported during aspiration, because suction often produces moderate to acute pain that subsides when suction is discontinued. The nurse applies firm pressure following removal of the needle to control bleeding. Failure to promptly stop bleeding can lead to a hematoma, which can cause the patient discomfort for days. If a biopsy is performed, a small incision is made, and a core biopsy instrument is used.

Postprocedural care

The nurse observes the dressing site for bleeding, tenderness, and erythema and checks vital signs frequently for signs of bleeding and infection. The patient will likely experience soreness at the site if a biopsy was performed.

Schilling test

The **Schilling test** is the definitive test for pernicious anemia although it is also useful in detecting hypothyroidism, sprue, and liver disease. The test measures the absorption of radioactive vitamin B_{12}, before and after parenteral injection of the intrinsic factor, by examination of the urinary excretion of vitamin B_{12}.

TABLE 37-6   Laboratory Tests for Anemias and Leukemias

Determination	Reference range (SI values)	Purpose/description
Transferrin saturation	30%-50%	Evaluates the percentage of total iron-binding protein saturated with iron
		Saturation of <30% is indicative of chronic iron deficiency anemia or anemia of chronic disease
		Saturation of >30% is indicative of hemolytic and sideroblastic anemias or iron overload
Serum ferritin	Iron deficiency 0-12 ng/mL (0-4.8 nmol/L)	Most sensitive test for detecting iron deficiency anemia; level of serum ferritin is directly related to the amount of stored iron
		Patients with chronic iron deficiency anemias have decreased levels, and patients with megaloblastic and hemolytic anemias have increased levels
Serum folic acid	>3.3 ng (>7.3 nmol/L)	Folic acid (folate) is a water-soluble vitamin that is required for DNA synthesis and hematopoiesis
		Decreased with megaloblastic anemia, malabsorption syndromes, pregnancy, hyperthyroidism, and certain drugs
		Increased with hepatic disorders and chronic myelocytic leukemia
Serum folate	30-16 ng/mL (7-36 nmol/L)	Folate deficiency is the most common vitamin deficiency
		Reduced levels occur in alcoholism, malnutrition, liver disease, vitamin B deficiency, vitamin B deficiency anemia, hemolytic anemias, pregnancy, and in the elderly
		Increased with distal small bowel disease and vegetarian diets
Serum iron	50-150 µg/dL (10-27 nmol/L)	Test measures iron that is bound to transferrin, a transport protein
		Decreased levels occur with inadequate amounts of iron and transferrins decreased with iron deficiency anemia, rheumatoid-collagen disorders, and sprue
		Increased with hemolytic anemia, acute hepatitis, and thalassemia major
		Patient must fast 8 hours before test
Serum total iron-binding capacity (TIBC)	300-400 µg/dL	Estimates amount of transferrin available to bind with and transport iron
		Normally, 30% of binding sites of transferrin are occupied
		Increased levels occur with iron deficiency anemia, alcoholism, and acute hepatitis
		Decreased with hypoproteinemia and iron overload conditions
Vitamin B_{12} assay	205-876 pg/mL (150-674 pmol/L)	Vitamin B_{12} is important for folic acid metabolism and therefore for DNA synthesis and hematopoiesis; stored in liver
		Increased with hepatic disease and chronic myelocytic leukemia

TABLE 37-6   Laboratory Tests for Anemias and Leukemias—cont'd

Determination	Reference range (SI values)	Purpose/description
Reticulocyte count test	0.5%-1.5% (number fraction of cells: 0.005-0.015)	Decreased with inadequate absorption and dietary intake Measures the responsiveness and adequacy of bone marrow production Reticulocytes are immature RBCs, and the reticulocyte count will rise following blood loss or during therapy for particular kinds of anemia if the bone marrow is responsive Expressed as a percentage of mature RBCs
Urine for Bence Jones protein	No Bence Jones protein detected	A 50-mL specimen of uncontaminated urine is collected and examined for Bence Jones protein Commonly found in patients with multiple myeloma

Plasma proteins	Adult:
	  Ambulatory 6.4-8.3 g/dL (64-83 g/L)
	  Recumbent 6.0-7.8 g/dL (60 to 78 g/L)
	Older adult (60 +): Lower by ~ 0.2 g/dL (~ 2.0 g/L)
		Plasma proteins are involved in clotting and maintain the osmotic pressure of the blood
		Increased total protein levels occur with multiple myeloma, monocytic leukemia
		Decreased with Hodgkin's, liver disease, severe burns, and hemorrhage
		Increased with multiple myeloma and dehydration

	Albumin 3.5-5 g/dL (35-50 g/L)	Decreased with Hodgkin's, hypogammaglobulinemia, and renal and liver disorders
	Globulin 2.3-3.5 g/dL (23-35 g/L)	Increased with multiple myeloma, Hodgkin's, SLE, and collagen disorders Decreased with renal and liver disorders and in some blood disorders

Patient preparation

The patient is told that the test measures the body's ability to absorb vitamin B_{12}. The nurse instructs the patient to avoid oral intake for 8 to 12 hours before the first stage of the test. The procedure for the 24-hour collection of urine is then explained.

Procedure

In the first stage (without intrinsic factor) the patient collects and discards a urine specimen. A 24-hour urine collection is started. The patient is given an oral dose of vitamin B_{12} tagged with radioactive cobalt and 1 to 2 hours later an IM injection of nonradioactive B_{12}. If the intrinsic factor is present, the oral dose is absorbed and large amounts of radioactive vitamin B_{12} are found in the urine. If less than 8% of the original dose of radioactive B_{12} is excreted, stage two of the test is indicated.

The procedure for the second stage (with intrinsic factor) is similar to the first stage, except that the patient receives intrinsic factor with the radioactive dose of vitamin B_{12}. After receiving the intrinsic factor, patients with pernicious anemia will excrete normal amounts of the radioactive dose in the urine.

Gastric analysis

Gastric analysis is useful in detecting pernicious anemia. In pernicious anemia, the gastric secretions are minimal, and the pH remains elevated, even after injection of histamine. Gastric analysis involves analysis of gastric juices before and after injection of histamine or betazole hydrochloride, which will stimulate maximal stomach acid production. To obtain the gastric samples, a nasogastric tube is inserted, and the entire gastric contents are aspirated every 15 minutes.

Patient preparation

The test is explained to the patient. The nurse in-

TABLE 37-7   Laboratory Tests for Hemolytic Disorders

Determination	Reference range (SI values)	Purpose/description
Serum haptoglobin	60-270 mg/dL (0.6-2.7 g/L)	Haptoglobins are transport proteins that bind to free hemoglobin to conserve body iron; hemoglobin is released during red blood cell destruction and binds to haptoglobins Haptoglobin levels are decreased with megaloblastic anemia and liver disease (haptoglobins are produced in the liver) and increased with burns, tissue destruction, and severe infection
Hemoglobin electrophoresis	HgA: 95% HgA$_2$: 2%-3% HgF: <1% HgS and C absent	Hemoglobin electrophoresis is useful in distinguishing the different types of hemoglobin present in cells and separates normal types from abnormal ones; relative percentages of each type are also determined Useful in diagnosing sickle cell anemia (HDS), mild hemolytic anemia (HgC), and thalassemias (Hg A$_2$; HgF)
Osmotic fragility	Increased if hemolysis occurs in over 0.5% NaCl; decreased if hemolysis is incomplete in 0.30% NaCl	Osmotic fragility measures the ability of a cell to hold extra water; at a certain volume, a red blood cell becomes a sphere and can admit no more water before lysis occurs; a cell that is already spheric will admit less water before lysis occurs Most useful test in congenital spherocytosis and useful in detecting hemolytic anemia
RBC enzyme assays (erythrocyte enzymes)	Glucose-6-phosphate dehydrogenase G-6PD 5-15 U/gHb (5-15 U/g) Pyruvate kinase 13-17 U/gHb (13-17 U/g)	Many forms of hemolytic anemia are associated with deficiencies in specific erythrocyte enzymes Test aids in differential diagnosis of hemolytic anemias
RBC survival time		RBC survival time is an expensive and lengthy test that involves tagging RBCs with a radioactive isotope, reinjecting them into the patient, and withdrawing a series of blood samples over a 30-day period to count the isotopes Detects decreased RBC survival, as found in hemolysis

structs the patient to fast after midnight the day of the test and to avoid smoking. Anticholinergic medications should not be taken before the test.

Procedural care
The patient is observed for symptoms of overdose (flushing, vomiting, intense headache, dyspnea, drop in blood pressure, and shock) following the injection of histamine. The nurse administers epinephrine, if needed, to counteract symptoms.

Laboratory Tests for Hemolytic Disorders

Hemolysis refers to the premature destruction of red blood cells. Determination of the presence of hemolysis depends on identification of compensatory red blood cell production and increased destruction of erythrocytes. Tests, such as the reticulocyte count, peripheral blood smear, and bone marrow aspiration, aid in detection of hemolysis and compensatory mechanisms. Other tests useful in detecting hemolytic disorders are described in Table 37-7.

TABLE 37-8   Laboratory Tests for Bleeding Disorders

Determination	Reference range (SI values)	Purpose/description
Platelet count	150,000-400,000/µL (0.15-2.4$10^{12}$/L)	Platelets (thrombocytes) are tiny, disk-shaped cells that largely control hemostasis and help form the hemostatic plug; when the platelet count drops, bleeding time is prolonged because of the platelet-deficient clotting process; platelets are visible on blood smears Thrombocytosis (increased platelets) is found in polycythemia, essential thrombocytosis, hemorrhage, and malignant lymphoma Decreased platelet counts occur with acute leukemia, thrombocytopenic purpura, and aplastic anemia
Bleeding time	3.4 ± 1.3 min (204 ± 78 sec)	Evaluates length of time a small incision or puncture wound bleeds; a blood pressure cuff is wrapped on the arm and inflated to 40 mm Hg, the forearm is cleansed and incised, and the blood is blotted with filter paper every 30 sec until bleeding stops Prolonged bleeding occurs with severe thrombocytopenia, defects in platelet function, von Willebrand's disease, and aspirin ingestion; if bleeding lasts longer than 15 min, apply direct pressure and call a physician
Partial thromboplastin (PTT) or **activated partial thromboplastin time (APTT)**	25-38 sec	Assesses the intrinsic and common pathways of the coagulation process by measuring factors I, II, V, VIII, IX, X, XI, XII (see Figure 39-3) Sensitive to the effects of heparin; not as sensitive to abnormalities in prothrombin as PT (*APTT* is a sensitive and shortened variation of PTT, in which activators are added to the PTT reagent)
Prothrombin time (PT; pro time)	11-15 sec	Assesses extrinsic pathway of coagulation by measurement of factors II, VIII, IX, X; the test measures the length of time required for fibrin clot to form after tissue extract and calcium ions are added to citrated plasma PT will be prolonged with coumarin administration, vitamin K deficiencies, and factors V, VII, or X deficiencies; various drugs will prolong or shorten PT Abnormalities in both PTT and PT may be indicative of disseminated intravascular coagulation (DIC)
Thrombin time	Control: ±5 sec	Evaluates the adequacy of thrombin and abnormalities in the fibrinogen/fibrin stage of coagulation; measures time required for plasma to clot after addition of thrombin

Continued.

TABLE 37-8   Laboratory Tests for Bleeding Disorders—cont'd

Determination	Reference range (SI values)	Purpose/description
		Prolonged with disseminated intravascular coagulation, hepatic disease, multiple myeloma, and hypofibrinogenimia
Prothrombin consumption time (PCT; serum prothrombin time; two-stage prothrombin time)	Complete after 20 sec Abnormal <20 sec	PCT evaluates the rate and amount of prothrombin activation in residual serum after clotting in the standard PT test; it indirectly measures the capacity of platelets and intrinsic clotting factors to generate thromboplastin; if the platelets or factors are abnormal, there will be more residual prothrombin, and clotting time for the PCT specimen will be shortened
Platelet aggregation	Full response to ADP, epinephrine, and collagen	Measures the ability of platelets to clump when mixed with known aggregation agents (adenosine diphosphate [ADP], epinephrine, collagen, ristocetin) Decreased platelet adhesiveness occurs with von Willebrand's disease, uremia, severe anemia, and multiple myeloma Patient fasts 8 hours before the test and should avoid aspirin products for 14 days
Fibrinogen level	200-400 mg/dL (2.00-4.99 g/L)	Measures fibrinogen levels in plasma Increased fibrinogen levels (with burns, surgery, nephrosis) indicate enhancement of fibrin formation, making the patient susceptible to clot formation Decreased fibrinogen levels (with liver disease, disseminated intravascular coagulation, congenital deficiencies) predispose patient to bleeding
Fibrinogen degradation products (FDP; fibrin split products, FSP)		Evaluates the extent of fibrinolysis accomplished by the fibrinolytic system A high level of fibrin degradation products indicates increased fibrinolysis, found with disseminated intravascular coagulation and primary fibrinolytic disorders
Antithrombin III (AT III)	Plasma: 21-30 mg/dL (210-300 mg/L) Serum: 17-25 mg/dl (170-250 mg/L)	AT III, a plasma protein, is a natural inhibitor of the coagulation sequence; AT III is a cofactor of heparin, as both interfere with thrombin activation; effective heparin therapy requires AT III concentrations greater than 60% of normal Stress situations such as pregnancy, trauma, or infections reduce AT III levels; reduced AT III levels also occur with congenital abnormalities, disseminated intravascular coagulation, cardiovascular disorders, and oral contraceptives; if AT III concentrations fall below 50% of normal, the patient is at significant risk for thromboembolic disorders Increased concentrations occur with menstruation, acute hepatitis, renal transplant, and vitamin K deficiency

TABLE 37-8   Laboratory Tests for Bleeding Disorders—cont'd

Determination	Reference range (SI values)	Purpose/description
Coagulation factor assays	Factor II: 60%-150% of normal (60-150 μmol/L) Factor V: 60%-150% of normal (60-150 μmol/L) Factor VII: 65%-135% of normal (65-135 μmol/L) Factor VIII: 60%-145% of normal (60-145 μmol/L) Factor IX: 60%-140% of normal (60-140 μmol/L) Factor X: 60%-130% of normal (60-130 μmol/L) Factor XI: 65%-135% of normal (65-135 μmol/L) Factor XII: 65%-150% of normal (65-135 μmol/L)	Assays of the intrinsic factor (VIII, IX, XI, XII) and extrinsic factor (II, V, VII, and X) coagulation systems are useful in determining specific factor deficiencies in coagulation and in monitoring the effects of anticoagulant therapy If PT and APTT are abnormal, the assay is useful in determining deficiencies in factors II, V, or X If PT is abnormal and APTT is not, factor VII may be deficient Deficiencies in factors VIII, IX, XI, and XII may be present when PT is normal and APTT is not

TABLE 37-9   Laboratory Tests for Gammopathies

Determination	Reference range	Purpose/description

Protein electrophoresis	% of total protein
	Albumin 52-68%
	Globulin
	  Alpha-1: 2-5
	  Alpha-2: 7-13
	  Beta 8-14
	  Gamma 12-22
		Immunoelectrophoresis is a relatively simple but expensive procedure that identifies monoclonal proteins such as IgM, IgA, IgG, IgE
		Ordinary protein electrophoresis is performed with the passage of an electrical current through serum containing gel, causing the immunoglobulins and other serum proteins to separate, then antiserum is added to the gel and reacts with specific serum proteins, allowing identification of the immunoglobulins and other proteins
		The test is useful in identifying hypoglobulinemia and hyperglobulinemia, as well as nonimmunologic diseases with high immunoglobulin levels (cirrhosis and nephrosis hepatitis)
		Fasting is required for 8 hours before the test; water and medications may be taken

Direct Coombs' (direct antiglobulin test)	Normal: negative Positive: 1+ to 4+	Detects autoantibodies against RBCs; Coombs' serum is derived from rabbit serum, and, when mixed and incubated with human serum, antibodies from the Coombs' serum will attach to any antibody coating the human RBCs Agglutination will result from the attachment and is a positive result Lack of agglutination is normal The test is useful in differentiating between acquired immunologic hemolytic anemias (globulins on the RBCs) and nonimmunologically mediated hemolytic anemia and in the early diagnosis of hemolytic transfusion reactions

Laboratory Tests for Bleeding Disorders

When bleeding is suspected or encountered, the diagnostic process begins with a CBC and platelet count. Results of these tests are used to establish the need for other tests for bleeding disorders (Table 37-8).

Laboratory Tests for Gammopathies

In addition to the specific tests outlined in Table 37-9, a bone marrow aspiration is useful in confirming the diagnosis of gammopathies (a group of immunologic disorders in which neoplastic cells secrete immunoglobulins) through detection of atypical plasmacytosis.

Erythrocyte Sedimentation Rate

Erythrocyte sedimentation rate is a common, although nonspecific, screening procedure that measures the rate at which RBCs settle out in well-mixed venous blood. Red cell volume, surface area, density, and surface change affect aggregation. Plasma proteins, especially fibrinogen and globulin, encourage aggregation.

The erythrocyte sedimentation rate will often rise significantly in widespread autoimmune or infectious diseases that cause inflammation. Age and sex affect values (men under 50 years: <15 mm/hr; men over 50 years: <20 mm/hr; women under 50 years: <20 mm/hr; women over 50 years: <30 mm/hr).

C-Reactive Protein (CRP)

C-reactive protein is an abnormal protein produced in the liver in response to an acute inflammatory process or tissue destruction. CRP appears in the blood within 6 to 10 hours after inflammatory process or tissue destruction, making CRP an earlier indicator of inflammation than the ESR. CRP levels rise during bacterial but not viral infections and are useful in monitoring the acute phases of rheumatoid arthritis, rheumatoid fever, cancer, Burkitt's lymphoma, cancer, and inflammatory bowel disease, systemic lupus erythematosus, bacterial infection, and myocardial infection. Oral contraceptives may cause false positive results. Fasting (except for water) is necessary for 4 to 12 hours before collection of the specimen.

CRITICAL THINKING QUESTIONS

1 Name the different types of blood cells and describe their functions.
2 How does the blood coagulate?
3 Design at least three questions to ask patients about health care habits in relation to bleeding.
4 Describe an effective approach in examining a painful joint.
5 What laboratory determinations are usually considered part of the complete blood count?
6 What laboratory tests are useful in the detection and diagnosis of leukemia?

BIBLIOGRAPHY

Current

1. Baird SB et al: *Cancer nursing: a comprehensive textbook,* Philadelphia, 1991, WB Saunders.
2. Burrell LO: *Adult nursing in hospital and community settings,* Norwalk, 1992, Appleton & Lange.
3. DeGowin RL: *DeGowin and DeGowin's bedside diagnostic examination,* ed 5, New York, 1987, MacMillan Publishing.
4. Kenny RA: *Physiology of aging: a synopsis,* St Louis, 1992, Mosby–Year Book.
5. Lefever Kee J: *Handbook of laboratory and diagnostic tests with nursing implications,* Norwalk, 1990, Appleton & Lange.
6. Malasanos L et al: *Health assessment,* ed 4, St Louis, 1990, Mosby–Year Book.
7. Murray R, Zentner S: *Nursing assessment and health promotion through the life span,* Englewood Cliffs, New Jersey, 1989, Prentice-Hall.
8. Norris MK: Lab test tips: Evaluating C-reactive protein levels, *Nurs 92* 22:5, 1992.
9. Norris MK: Lab test tips: Evaluating prothrombin time, *Nurs 91* 21:11, 1991.
10. Otto SE: *Oncology nursing,* St Louis, 1991, Mosby–Year Book.
11. Seidel HM et al: *Mosby's guide to physical examination,* ed 2, St Louis, 1991, Mosby–Year Book.
12. Swartz MH: *Textbook of physical diagnosis,* Philadelphia, 1989, WB Saunders.
13. Tilkian SM, Conover MB, Tilkian AG: *Clinical implications of laboratory tests,* St Louis, 1987, Mosby–Year Book.

Classic

14. King RC: Exploring the neck and lymphatics, *RN* June:49-99, 1982.
15. Price S, Wilson L: *Pathophysiology,* New York, 1986, McGraw-Hill.
16. Prior JA, Silberstein JS, Stang J: *Physical diagnosis: the history and examination of the patient,* St Louis, 1981, Mosby–Year Book.

CHAPTER THIRTY-EIGHT

Nursing Management of Adults with Hematologic Disorders

LEARNING OBJECTIVES

1 Correlate the pathophysiology of patients with common hematologic disorders with their typical clinical manifestations.

2 Discuss the options for therapeutic management of patients with disorders of the hematologic system.

3 Apply the nursing process to the care of patients with disorders of the hematologic system.

4 Discuss the nursing implications associated with medications used to treat hematologic disorders.

5 Develop patient education guides for patients with common disorders of the hematologic system.

6 Discuss the psychosocial implications of the symptoms associated with hematologic disorders.

7 Identify potential complications of hematologic disorders, and describe appropriate nursing assessment and intervention strategies.

8 Discuss nursing implications for continuity of care for patients with hematologic disorders.

KEY TERMS

HEMATOLOGIC DISORDERS can be complex and challenging. Assessments of patients with varied signs and symptoms depend on sound knowledge and clinical practice. The patient and family are affected physiologically, psychologically, and spiritually and need nursing intervention for their responses. The stages of disease range from acute to chronic. The following overview presents the nursing implications of acute and chronic care for three major categories of hematologic disorders: disorders of red blood cells (RBCs), white blood cells (WBCs), and coagulation.

Disorders of Red Blood Cells

Disorders of the red blood cell can be categorized as **erythrocytopenia** (a condition of too few) and **erythrocytosis** (a condition of too many). Erythrocytopenia, namely the anemias, is examined first, followed by a discussion of polycythemia vera, a condition of erythrocytosis. **Anemia** is a deficiency of RBCs as reflected in decreased hemoglobin level, decreased hematocrit, and decreased RBC count. Red blood cells of normal size are **normocytic,** and those with normal hemoglobin levels are **normochromic.** Thus small RBCs with low hemoglobin are termed **microcytic, hypochromic,** and large RBCs with normal hemoglobin are **macrocytic,** normochromic. Anemias are most clearly classified into two kinds: (1) those caused primarily by impaired formation of viable red cells and (2) those caused primarily by increased loss or destruction of red cells. Anemia can be further categorized in several

different ways, for example, by morphology, physiology, or etiology (Table 38-1).

APLASTIC ANEMIA
Definition

Aplastic anemia is a decrease in the number of circulating RBCs caused by bone marrow malfunction. Persons with aplastic anemia are usually pancytopenic; that is, all three major blood elements (red cells, white cells, and platelets) from the bone marrow are reduced or absent.

Etiology/Epidemiology

The cause may be unknown or may be the result of injury to stem cells in the bone marrow from drugs, irradiation, viruses, toxins, or congenital defects. Agents that have been implicated include anticonvulsants (diphenylhydantoin), antimicrobials (chloramphenicol), antithyroids, cytotoxic agents, hypoglycemic agents, phenothiazines, hair dyes, benzene, and insecticides.

Pathophysiology

Bone marrow cellularity is reduced, leading to anemia, neutropenia, or **thrombocytopenia** (a decrease in the number of circulating platelets). Blood cell production by the bone marrow depends on the presence of stem cells, which have two functions: (1) to proliferate cells identical to themselves and (2) to differentiate or mature into functional cells (red cell, white cell, or platelet). As a result, patients develop erythrocytopenia (anemia), **leukopenia** (a decrease

TABLE 38-1   Classification of Erythropoietic Disorders

Category	Functional defect	Marrow morphology	Red cell morphology	Common causes
Aplastic anemias	Disturbed stem cell kinetics	Hypoplastic	Normocytic or macrocytic, normochromic	Chemicals, radiation, renal insufficiency, carcinomatosis, idiopathic
Megaloblastic anemias	Impaired DNA synthesis	Hyperplastic, megaloblastic	Macrocytic, normochromic	Vitamin B_{12} deficiency, folate deficiency
Hypochromic anemias	Impaired hemoglobin synthesis	Hyperplastic, deficient hemoglobinization	Microcytic, hypochromic	Iron deficiency, anemia of chronic disease, thalassemias, sideroblastic disorders

From Jandl JH: Introduction to erythropoiesis, *Medicine* 43:615, 1964.

in the number of circulating white blood cells), and thrombocytopenia.

Clinical Manifestations

The clinical diagnosis of aplastic anemia is usually based on the gradual development of symptoms. Fatigue and pallor of the skin and mucous membranes are characteristic signs, and dyspnea on exertion may be present. Infections may occur with leukopenia and bleeding with the thrombocytopenia. Laboratory values reflect pancytopenia, and the reticulocyte count is low. Definitive diagnosis is made through a bone marrow biopsy showing hypocellularity. The anemia is usually normochromic and normocytic.

Therapeutic Management

The primary treatment is removal of the causative agent, if known. Transfusion therapy, in which the specific blood components are transfused (RBCs, platelets, WBCs), supports the patient until he or she spontaneously recovers or responds to treatment. Treatment may include glucocorticoids and androgens, but modest benefits do not outweigh dangerous side effects.[13] Antibiotics are recommended for infection and fever. If the patient has an HLA-identical donor, then bone marrow transplantation is the treatment of choice. Cyclophosphamide and antithymocyte globulin increase hemopoiesis. Granuloycte-macrophage colony-stimulating factor (GM-CSF), an immunoaugmentor, is used as biologic response modifier treatment for aplastic anemia.[26]

IRON DEFICIENCY ANEMIA
Definition

Iron deficiency anemia is a condition in which red blood cells contain decreased levels of hemoglobin. The poorly hemoglobinized erythrocytes are pale with only a rim of hemoglobin. The erythrocytes are microcytic and hypochromic.

Etiology/Epidemiology

The most common cause of iron deficiency anemia is excessive iron loss. In adults, the most common source is chronic intestinal or uterine bleeding; however, iron deficiency anemia can also be caused by bleeding from gastric or duodenal ulcers, esophageal varices, hiatal hernia, colonic diverticula, and tumors. Menstrual blood losses and blood losses related to pregnancy are common causes of iron deficiency anemia in young adult women. Rarely, excessive losses occur through microhemorrhages into lung tissue or from intestinal parasites. Even without excessive blood loss, this deficiency can also re-

---

HEMATOPOIETIC GROWTH FACTORS

Definition: Increase blood cell counts by stimulating growth, differentiation, and survival of hematopoietic cells.
Types: Colony-stimulating factors (CSFs)—stimulate white blood cell production; certain types stimulate all classes of myeloid precursors.
   Interleukins (e.g., IL-3)—enhance the effects of other hemataopoietins.
   Erythropoietin—stimulates red blood cell production.
Clinical indications: Bone marrow failure or damage
   chemotherapy
   radiation therapy
   aplastic anemia
   bone marrow transplantation
Hematopoietic neoplasms
   leukemias
   multiple myeloma
   lymphomas
   myelodysplastic syndrome
Infectious diseases
   sepsis

---

sult when the body's demand for iron exceeds its absorption, which commonly occurs in infants, young adolescents, and pregnant women. Less commonly, iron deficiency anemia results from malabsorption of iron caused by diseases such as celiac disease and sprue. Subtotal gastrectomy may lead to iron deficiency caused by achlorhydria (loss of hydrochloric acid), occult bleeding, and decreased iron in postgastrectomy diets. Deficiency caused by poor dietary intake is rare in middle-aged adults. See the box on p. 964.

Pathophysiology

Deficient iron caused by loss or excess demand leads to red blood cells with lower levels of hemoglobin and eventually decreases the actual number of red blood cells. The average adult body contains approximately 4 g of iron. Three grams are in hemoglobin, 0.5 to 1 g in iron stores in the liver and bone marrow, and the rest in certain tissues and enzyme systems. Average daily loss of iron is approximately 1 to 1.5 mg, which is easily replaced if a normal diet is eaten. Excessive blood loss, however, disrupts this balance, and diet alone cannot compensate.

Clinical Manifestations

The symptoms of iron deficiency anemia are fatigue, weakness, and shortness of breath. Symptoms typi-

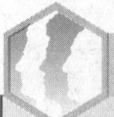

Iron Deficiency Anemia

Iron deficiency anemia and the anemia of chronic disease are the most common anemias found in the elderly population. Iron deficiency anemia can be caused by several conditions. Although occult blood loss is the most common cause, deficient diet is a major consideration. Achlorhydria is a cause that exists in 30% to 40% of older adults.

In the elderly, it is not uncommon to see signs and symptoms of iron deficiency anemia appear at higher hemoglobin levels than in younger adults. Mild to moderate anemia may also produce confusional states or aggravate existing dementia. A misdiagnosis of dementia is commonly made without appropriate laboratory documentation. It is not uncommon to find a vitamin B deficiency occurring concomitantly with an iron deficiency in the elderly.

Causes of Dietary-Related Iron-Deficiency Anemia in the Elderly

Income below levels to buy adequate food
Inability to prepare food or purchase food because of physical disability
Eating foods low in dietary iron
Anorexia (may be due to grief or loneliness)
New or ill-fitting dentures
Dislike of cooking and eating alone
Poor nutrition due to alcoholism

cal of heart failure may also occur. Peculiar to iron deficiency anemia are gastrointestinal symptoms, such as glossitis (manifested by inflammation and soreness of the tongue), and pagophagia (the desire to eat ice, clays, or starches). The signs include pallor and tachycardia. Fingernails may be fragile and assume the shape of the head of a spoon with a central depression and raised borders (koilonychia). Mucous membranes may be inflamed (stomatitis), and lips may be reddened with cracking at the angles (cheilosis). In the peripheral blood the morphology of RBCs is characterized by microcytosis and hypochromia, and serum iron levels are low (< 50 µg/dL). Bone marrow examination reveals mild erythroid hyperplasia with a decreased myeloid/erythroid cell ratio.

Therapeutic Management

Iron salts such as ferrous sulfate are administered to diagnose iron deficiency. If iron deficiency anemia is present, oral iron will increase the reticulocyte count 7% to 10% 5 to 10 days after therapy is initiated. The hematocrit should rise 5% to 15% in 3 weeks and the hemoglobin 2 to 5 g/dL. So that the body can incorporate 100 mg of iron per day, 900 mg should be administered per day. Iron is administered orally or by injection. Ascorbic acid has been shown to enhance iron absorption. Food sources of iron include meat, fish, poultry, eggs, green leafy vegetables, whole grains, and dried beans.

ANEMIA ASSOCIATED WITH CHRONIC DISEASE
Definition

Anemia of chronic disease is a moderately severe anemia and is often normochromic and normocytic but may be hypochromic and occasionally microcytic. It is characterized by low serum iron, low total iron-binding capacity, normal or low transferrin saturation, and normal or elevated ferritin levels.

Etiology/Epidemiology

The anemia of chronic disease is extremely common and is associated with conditions such as infection, inflammatory disease, disseminated cancer, tissue necrosis, or chronic renal failure. The bone marrow is morphologically normal and is filled with reticuloendothelial iron, but the RBC production index is either decreased or not increased proportionately to the severity of the anemia.

Pathophysiology

The factors responsible for the decreased bone marrow function are not known. Reticulum cell hyperplasia may contribute to a reduction in red cell life span. There seems to be a basic, unexplained disturbance in the mobilization of iron from marrow reticuloendothelial cells. In chronic diseases, it may be that iron and transferrin are taken up by reticuloendothelial cells, which would account for the decreased plasma levels. In anemia caused by chronic disease it may be that insufficient amounts of erythropoietin are produced (e.g., with chronic renal failure).

Clinical Manifestations

The signs and symptoms are similar to those of other anemias. The serum iron is low, as it is in iron deficiency anemia. The total iron-binding capacity is decreased (as opposed to increased in iron deficiency anemia). Serum ferritin is increased (as opposed to decreased in iron deficiency anemia). Bone marrow examination shows that reticuloendothelial iron is adequate. The anemia develops slowly, is well tolerated, and may not require treatment.

Therapeutic Management

Anemia associated with chronic disease rarely responds to treatment of therapeutic amounts of iron, as iron deficiency anemia does. The hematocrit is usually 25% to 30%. If treatment is indicated, packed red cells are given.

HEMOLYTIC ANEMIA
Definition

Anemia may be caused by increased red cell breakdown or hemolysis. Although erythrocyte destruction occurs in practically every disease, in hemolytic anemia the erythrocyte survival is shortened to less than 15 to 20 days.

Etiology/Epidemiology

Hemolytic anemia may be drug-induced or caused by an autoimmune disorder. Drugs that have been associated with hemolytic anemia are methyldopa (Aldomet) and high-dose penicillin. In an autoimmune disorder, an antibody develops that is directed against an antigen on the individual's own erythrocytes. Other causes include transfusion reactions, mechanical factors (e.g., friction with abnormal cardiac valves), and chemical toxins.

Pathophysiology

The antibody develops against an antigen on the red cells. The antibody-coated red cells are destroyed by the reticuloendothelial cells, especially in the spleen. The autoimmune disorder may be caused by lymphocytic lymphomas or chronic lymphocytic leukemia, or it may be idiopathic. Normally, red cells are destroyed in the reticuloendothelial system, especially in the spleen, without a release of hemoglobin. However, if hemolysis is severe, hemoglobin will appear in the plasma and urine.

Clinical Manifestations/Therapeutic Management

The manifestations that occur in other anemias may not be present. Family history may include evidence of jaundice, anemia, or splenomegaly and indicate an hereditary cause. Jaundice may be seen in patients with hemolytic anemia caused by transfusion reactions, an autoimmune disorder, or inherited erythrocyte defects. Splenomegaly may result from excessive red cell breakdown. Hemoglobin present in the plasma or urine indicates hemolysis. Diagnosis can be made by presence of erythrocytopenia with an elevated reticulocyte count. In autoimmune disorders, however, an antiglobin or Coombs' test must be used to detect the antibody. Corticosteroids

help approximately 50% of patients. For those not improved, splenectomy is indicated. Transfusions are dangerous because the antibodies act on the donor cells, too.

SICKLE CELL ANEMIA
Definition/Etiology

Sickle cell anemia is a disorder of abnormal hemoglobin also termed hemoglobinopathy, in which one or both of the polypeptide chains are abnormal. The hemoglobin type is Hgb S instead of Hgb A. Sickle cell anemia is a genetic disorder that is homozygous recessive. It occurs predominantly in blacks. Approximately one of every 10 black Americans has sickle cell trait and about one out of every 500 has sickle cell anemia.[50]

Pathophysiology

The erythrocytes in sickle cell anemia contain more Hgb S than Hgb A. The Hgb S causes the RBCs to assume a sickle, or crescent, shape when exposed to decreased oxygen tension (Figure 38-1). Hypoxia can occur in high altitudes, from strenuous exercise,

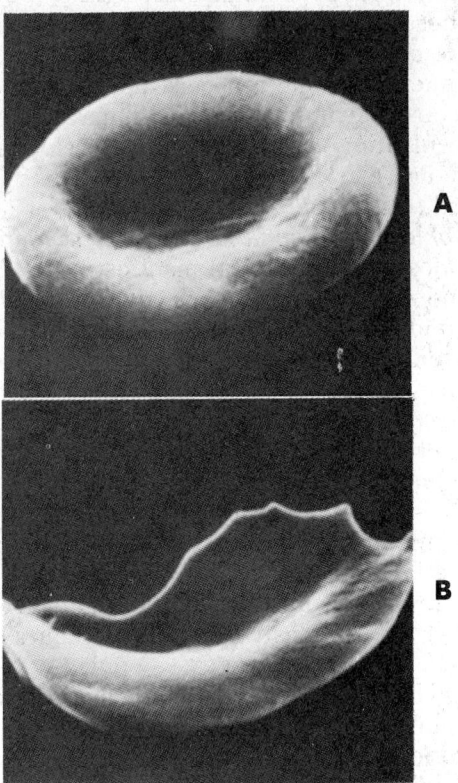

FIGURE 38-1   **A,** Normal red blood cell. **B,** Sickled red blood cell. (From Miale JB: *Laboratory medicine: hematology,* ed 6, 1982, Mosby–Year Book.)

or with compromised oxygenation (e.g., during anesthesia). Sickling can also occur with acidosis or when the blood viscosity is increased as in dehydration. The sickled cells are unable to move through the microcirculation and, therefore, occlude the blood flow. The obstruction can result in tissue and organ infarction and thrombosis (e.g., in the brain, kidneys, bone marrow, and spleen).

Clinical Manifestations

Joint pains occur as a result of infarction and necrosis of tissue caused by local obstruction of microcirculation during sickling episodes. This crisis or pain episode can also include swelling and limitation of movement of the joint. Vascular occlusion may occur in the abdomen, spleen, myocardium, kidney, liver, or brain. Clinical manifestations to be alert for are pallor or lethargy. These signs may signal an impending crisis. The thrombosis may result in chronic leg ulcers, especially around the ankles; bone infarction with pain; and splenic infarction, causing autosplenectomy and hyposplenism. Infarctions of vital tissues may damage the heart, liver, central nervous system, and lung. Sickling and infarction may occur in the renal medulla and produce hematuria and inability to concentrate urine. Symptoms of hemolytic anemia and an increased tendency to develop infections may be present.

There are various types of sickle cell anemia. *Sickle cell trait (HbSA):* Individuals with HbSA are not anemic. Their red cells do not hemolyze, and they are asymptomatic. They may have difficulty concentrating urine and may develop hematuria. They are at risk for splenic infarctions if compromised (e.g., under anesthesia).

Sickle cell anemia (HbSS): These patients have the most severe clinical manifestations. They have splenomegaly that develops with repeated thromboses and autosplenectomy. They develop bilirubin gallstones due to red cell hemolysis. Other complications include leg ulcers, bony abnormalities (aseptic necrosis), priapism, maternal and fetal morbidity and mortality, congestive heart failure, pulmonary infarction, and neurologic defects, including convulsions and paralysis. Sickle cell crisis occurs spontaneously or with infection. The pain is severe in the bones, joints, back, and abdomen. The temperature and white blood cell counts are elevated. The crisis may last from several hours to several days.

Sickle cell thalassemia (HbS-thal): Patients have two abnormal alleles, one for sickle cell hemoglobin and one for thalassemia. These patients have a variable course; the disorder is discussed in the section on thalassemias.

Sickle cell-n-hemoglobin C (HbSC) disease: These individuals carry two abnormal B-alleles, hemoglo-

bin S and hemoglobin C. Many of the signs and symptoms are similar to sickle cell anemia, but the prognosis for a long life is better.

Therapeutic Management

Persons with mild HbS syndromes do not require treatment. In persons with high concentrations of sickle hemoglobin and frequent painful crises, treatment is required. Therapy includes rest, hydration, oxygen, analgesics for pain, and treatment of infections. Treatment can include local application of heat for comfort in joint pain. Those undergoing major surgery or pregnancy may need partial RBC exchange transfusion. Folic acid replacement is given due to the increased folic acid requirement. Genetic counseling is indicated (see patient education guide).

PATIENT EDUCATION GUIDE
Sickle Cell Anemia

Objective: To provide comfort and avoid complications.

Precursors of pain episodes

Patient may appear pale and lethargic
Strenuous physical exercise
Infection
Dehydration

Management of pain episodes

Heat application to joints
Analgesics
Rest
Hydration

Fever

A low-grade fever may occur for several days associated with pain onset
Temperature elevations may indicate an infection and warrant notifying the physician

Assess for complications

Tissue and organ necrosis can occur as a result of vaso-occlusion by sickled cells; signs may include: joint pain, leg ulcers (especially medial malleolus), renal problems, abdominal pain, visual problems

Family counseling

Community resources
Genetic concerns—sickle cell trait

BLOOD LOSS ANEMIA
Definition

Blood loss anemia is a condition in which there is loss of red cells externally or to an internal extravascular site. A decrease in RBCs causes anemia. The average adult has an approximate total blood volume of 6000 mL and can tolerate a loss of up to 500 mL. If the loss approaches 1000 mL, acute complications may occur such as hypovolemia and hypotension.

Pathophysiology

The cause of the blood loss may be either acute or chronic. In acute blood loss, the causes may be hemorrhage from trauma to vessels or internal hemorrhage, which may occur, for example, with trauma or as a complication of surgery. Chronic blood loss may have causes such as gastrointestinal bleeding from ulceration, menstrual bleeding, and complications of pregnancy.

Clinical Manifestations

Signs and symptoms of acute blood loss include those seen with hypovolemia, e.g., weakness, cool moist skin, hypotension, tachycardia, and, eventually, shock. Decreased hemoglobin and hematocrit levels will be evident after the blood loss. The severity of clinical manifestations correlates with the severity and rapidity of acute blood loss. Chronic blood loss will be associated with the usual signs of anemia.

Therapeutic Management

Treating acute blood loss involves treating the cause of loss. The patient must be stabilized by replacing the lost blood volume to maintain blood pressure. RBCs and plasma can be replaced by transfusions. Anemia from chronic blood loss is treated by iron supplements.

MEGALOBLASTIC ANEMIA
Definition/Etiology

Megaloblastic anemia is characterized by macrocytic red cells. The bone marrow contains large erythroid precursors with immature nuclei and mature, hemoglobin-containing cytoplasm (megaloblasts). The two main categories of megaloblastic anemia are deficiencies in vitamin B_{12} and deficiencies in folic acid. The defective DNA synthesis that underlies megaloblastic anemia is caused by a vitamin B_{12} or a folic acid deficiency. In a minority of patients the secondary causes are diseases such as leukemia.

Pathophysiology

Defective DNA synthesis leads to ineffective erythropoiesis that results in death of erythroid cells before release from the marrow and early destruction of circulating erythrocytes. It is not clear how deficiencies in vitamin B_{12} or folic acid lead to defective DNA synthesis or how defective DNA synthesis results in premature cell death. The premature cell death may result from unbalanced cell maturation. Vitamin B_{12} deficiency is almost always caused by malabsorption. Vitamin B_{12} normally binds with a glycoprotein, called intrinsic factor (IF), that is secreted by parietal cells in the stomach. The IF-B_{12} complex is absorbed in the ileum, where the IF is removed. Vitamin B_{12} is transferred to the liver via the plasma. The most common disease associated with vitamin B_{12} malabsorption is **pernicious anemia,** which is caused by a failure to secrete adequate amounts of IF.

In addition to lack of intrinsic factor, other common causes of vitamin B_{12} deficiency are poor absorption of vitamin B_{12} or inadequate dietary intake. Uncommon causes include cancer, folate deficiency, drugs, pregnancy, severe chronic pancreatitis, thyroid disease, and congenital and malabsorption syndromes.[53] Malabsorption syndromes can include overproduction of intestinal bacteria that prevents vitamin B_{12} absorption. Therefore the deficiency may be caused by a failure to secrete the IF (pernicious anemia) or a lack of vitamin B_{12} absorption or intake.

Folates (folic acid) participate in many reactions, especially those involving the synthesis of purines, pyrimidines, and DNA. Insufficiency of folates impairs DNA synthesis and leads to megaloblastosis. Folate deficiency occurs as a result of dietary deficiency. Poverty, alcoholism, improper food preparation (prolonged cooking), or simply an improper diet may cause this deficiency. In alcoholics, in addition to decreased folate intake, there is also impaired hepatic storage of folates. Folate deficiency may also occur as a result of malabsorption syndromes such as sprue, subtotal gastrectomy, resection of the jejunum, and infiltration of the small intestine by lymphoma, leukemia, amyloidosis, or Whipple's disease. Folate deficiency has been associated with scleroderma and diabetes mellitus.

Antifols, drugs that inhibit folic acid metabolism, result in folate deficiency. The antifols include methotrexate (cancer chemotherapy), pyrimethamine (antimalarial), triamterene (diuretic), pentamidine (antiparasite drug), and trimethoprim (treats urinary tract infection). Anticonvulsants and oral contraceptives have been found to interfere with folic acid absorption. Folic acid deficiency may also be a result of an increased demand, for example, in pregnancy.

Clinical Manifestations

Megaloblastic anemia is suspected with a peripheral blood smear for anemia that shows macrocytosis. Low serum folate or vitamin B_{12} levels may be the diagnostic sign. Persons with severe folic acid deficiency may have glossitis and diarrhea. Persons with pernicious anemia may have weakness, shortness of breath, and skin that has a lemon yellow pallor. The tongue may be sore, pale, and smooth. There may be gastrointestinal symptoms of abdominal pain, diarrhea, nausea, and vomiting. In addition, there may be neurologic symptoms such as numbness and tingling of the extremities, muscle weakness, and loss of position sense.

Diagnosis is made with a bone marrow sample showing giant myeloid forms of megaloblasts. Laboratory studies such as measurement of serum B_{12} and folate levels and gastric analysis will confirm etiology. Gastric analysis will show decreased hydrochloric acid and elevated pH in pernicious anemia. If vitamin B_{12} deficiency is suspected, a Schilling test should be done. The Schilling test detects the lack of IF and is positive in pernicious anemia.

Therapeutic Management

Therapy for vitamin B_{12} deficiency is vitamin B_{12} replacement therapy. Vitamin B_{12} is usually administered by intramuscular or deep subcutaneous injection. Initial treatment includes daily injections and once symptoms have subsided, monthly maintenance therapy begins. Patients with pernicious anemia require maintenance injections for the remainder of their lives to prevent irreversible neurologic damage.

Folate deficiency requires folic acid replacement therapy. If the cause of the megaloblastic anemia is the administration of antifols, for example, the therapy would involve discontinuation of the antimetabolite. Folic acid is usually administered orally. The range of the usual therapeutic dose is 0.25-1.0 mg daily.

THALASSEMIAS
Definition/Etiology

In thalassemia, a genetic disorder, synthesis of one of the globin chains (beta) of hemoglobin is decreased, which consequently decreases the synthesis of whole hemoglobin. However, the other globin chain is unaffected and eventually accumulates in the erythrocyte. This situation results in decreased RBC production and a chronic hemolytic anemia. Thalassemias are a group of inherited disorders of hemoglobin synthesis. The disorder, also known as Cooley's anemia, is mainly found in persons of Mediterranean and Asian descent.

Pathophysiology

Beta-thalassemia, the most common type, is usually caused by mRNA abnormalities that cause reduced or absent beta-globin chain production. Prenatal diagnosis is possible through gene-mapping techniques.[53]

Clinical Manifestations

Four clinical types of beta-thalassemia—thalassemia major, thalassemia intermedia, thalassemia trait, and thalassemia minima—have been identified. Thalassemia major is the most severe type, usually recognized in the first years of life. Signs and symptoms include small body size, poor weight gain, progressive severe anemia (4 to 6 g/dL), jaundice, chronic leg ulcers, and mongoloid facies. Long bones are thin, and fractures may occur. Physical and mental development is delayed. Hepatosplenomegaly and infections occur. Bone marrow examination reveals erythroid hyperplasia, and megaloblastic changes may be present with folate deficiency. Iron overload, because of transfusions, may occur and lead to iron deposition in the tissues, such as in the myocardium, and to organ failure. Persons with thalassemia intermedia condition have abnormalities similar to those of persons with thalassemia major, but have only moderate anemia. They live with chronic disease into adult life. Persons with thalassemia trait have mild or no anemia. Diagnosis is made by family studies or by examination of peripheral blood. Thalassemia minima cannot be detected clinically and is determined by genetic studies.

Therapeutic Management

If the anemia is severe, blood transfusion therapy is indicated. Hemoglobin is kept at least at 5 to 6 g/dL. The low level requires fewer transfusions and therefore less of an iron load. Persons with a higher hematocrit develop more normally, grow faster, and exhibit fewer complications. However, these patients still do not survive beyond the second decade of life. Splenectomy may decrease the transfusion requirement, but increased incidence of severe infections may occur after the operation. Transfusions do lead to an increased load of iron. Iron-chelating agents such as deferoxamine or diethylenetriamine pentaacetic acid (DTPA) may be given peritoneally or subcutaneously to decrease the level of iron in the blood.[53] Folic acid replacement is recommended because of the ineffective erythropoiesis. Transfusions and folic acid therapy are needed only for individuals with thalassemia major. Genetic counseling may help couples in their family planning decisions.

POLYCYTHEMIA VERA
Definition/Etiology

Polycythemia vera is characterized by erythrocytosis. The elevated red cell mass leads to hyperviscosity and vascular distention; stasis may occur, leading to thromboembolic or hemorrhagic complications. The etiology by which the stem cells become autonomous and proliferative is unknown. Polycythemia vera is mainly seen in middle-aged or elderly men and in European Jews.

Pathophysiology/Clinical Manifestations

Red cell production is increased by autonomous proliferation of the erythroid stem cells in the bone marrow. The increased red cell mass causes hyperviscosity, vascular distention, and stasis. Symptoms, such as pounding headache, dizziness, angina, visual disturbances, paresthesias, and ringing in the ears, occur because of hyperviscosity. Thrombocytosis and erythema may cause thrombosis. Hemorrhage may occur because of defective platelets or thrombocythemia (refer to the discussion of disorders of coagulation). Other signs include itching, gastrointestinal symptoms (e.g., peptic ulcers), and splenomegaly caused by extramedullary hemopoiesis. A peripheral blood smear will contain increased red blood cells that are microcytic and hypochromic. Granulocytosis, thrombocytosis, and basophilia are commonly present. The bone marrow is hypercellular with loss of fat spaces. Hyperuricemia may be present.

Therapeutic Management

For patients with little or no clinical discomfort, the treatment is phlebotomy (the removal of blood at regular intervals). For patients with clinical symptoms, myelosuppressive therapy is indicated to decrease production of red blood cells. Radiophosphorus may be administered in the form of sodium phosphate. Alkylating drugs may be used for 1 to 3 weeks, then tapered to maintenance therapy. Hydroxyurea has been prescribed also. Systemic symptoms such as pruritus may be relieved by antihistamines or phenothiazines. Uric acid elevations are treated with allopurinol. Polycythemia must be recognized before surgery and the hematocrit reduced to normal to avoid perioperative mortality.

NURSING MANAGEMENT OF THE PATIENT WITH A RED BLOOD CELL DISORDER
Assessment

Symptoms of anemia (roughly in order of appearance in an increasingly anemic patient) include pal-

GERIATRIC CONSIDERATIONS

Assessment for Megaloblastic Anemia

Because such a large number of elderly are affected by a vitamin B_{12} deficiency, causing megaloblastic anemia, it is important to assess the elderly in this area. This is particularly important since this deficiency may not be diagnosed because older adults frequently attribute signs to age and do not seek medical assistance. The signs and symptoms include:

Weakness
Sore and beefy tongue
Apathy mixed with irritability
Loss of appetite
Pallor
Numbness and tingling peripherally
Vertigo
Dyspnea on exertion
Jaundiced sclera
Wakefulness
Paranoia

lor, fatigue, rapid pulse, shortness of breath, irritability, difficulty in concentrating, headache, dizziness, nausea, and decreased appetite. In addition, menstrual irregularities, loss of libido or potency, heart murmurs, angina pectoris, heart failure, and coma may occur. The nurse assesses the patient's activity tolerance and listens for complaints of general malaise. Assessment of dietary intake should be done. A family history is obtained for genetic disease (e.g., sickle cell) or for a history of exposure to drugs or toxins (e.g., aplastic anemia). Signs of bleeding should be assessed to determine anemia from blood loss (hematemesis, hematuria, melena, menorrhagia). Physical assessment should include inspection of the nailbeds for blanching, pallor, and spoon-shaped nails. Assess the mucous membranes, the skin for pallor, jaundice, purpura, or petechiae, and the tongue for redness or atrophy of papillae. Palpate the abdomen for masses, ascites, and splenomegaly. Assess the patient neurologically for paresthesias.

Nursing Diagnosis

Nursing diagnoses associated with red blood cell disorders include:

Activity intolerance related to decreased hemoglobin and imbalance between oxygen supply and demand
Knowledge deficit related to new information regarding disease and treatment

NURSING CARE PLAN *Patient with Aplastic Anemia*

Nursing diagnosis/ Expected outcomes	Interventions	Rationale
Altered protective mechanisms related to immunosuppression and immunomodulation as evidenced by anemia, leukopenia, thrombocytopenia, fever, and chills • *Patient is protected from infection, hemorrhage, and injury* • *Complications detected early* • *Comfort maintained* • *Patient knowledge regarding management*	Teach measures to prevent infection Teach patient to conserve energy (schedule activities after periods of rest) Teach/provide patient comfort measures for fever, chills Encourage patient to maintain rest and nutrition Reinforce safety to prevent injury and bleeding Maintain environmental and personal cleanliness	When the body's protective mechanisms are decreased, additional measures must be instituted to provide protection and prevent harm.
Anxiety related to knowledge deficit of investigative protocol and uncertain prognosis • *Anxiety will be experienced at a minimal level*	Monitor level of anxiety Determine what is troubling the patient Maintain calm attitude Teach about drug, action, side effects Explore coping mechanisms, and support existing strategies Teach coping strategies (e.g., relaxation)	High levels of anxiety interfere with learning and effective coping

Anxiety related to threat to health status

Self-care deficit related to weakness in managing care

Altered health maintenance related to new health practices and behaviors

High risk for trauma (falling) related to weakness, dizziness

Altered tissue perfusion (peripheral) related to vasoocclussive episodes

Ineffective family coping: compromised related to genetic family planning decisions

Altered nutrition: less than body requirements related to malabsorption or inadequate intake of vitamins, minerals (B_{12}, folic acid, iron)

Pain related to decreased circulation to body parts associated with sickling of RBCs

Altered sexuality patterns related to decreased libido, decreased potency, and fatigue

High risk for infection related to myelosuppression, immunosuppression.

Planning

For the patient with a red blood cell disorder the nurse plans interventions to achieve the following outcomes:

The patient will complete desired activities without fatigue.

Infection or injury will not occur.

The patient and family will plan meals that include nutrients to support erythropoiesis.

The patient and family will make appropriate decisions about modifying health practices and family planning.

Laboratory values for hemoglobin, hematocrit, and red blood cell count will be within normal limits.

The nurse may develop additional outcomes to guide the plan of care based on a patient's specific red cell disorder. For example, an outcome for the patient with sickle cell anemia would be relief of pain. The care for a patient with aplastic anemia is summarized in the Nursing Care Plan above.

Implementation

The nurse helps the patient learn to alternate periods of activity with periods of rest. The nurse can help the patient assign priorities to activities. The patient decides what daily activities are most important. Based on these priorities, the patient will feel a sense of accomplishment when desired activities

TABLE 38-2 Food Sources of Iron, Folic Acid, and Vitamin B₁₂

Nutrient	Source
Iron	Organ meats: liver, kidney, heart, and tongue
	Muscle meats, especially dark meat from poultry
	Eggs
	Shellfish
	Whole-grain breads and cereals
	Iron-enriched or -fortified breads and cereal
	Dark green vegetables: spinach, Swiss chard, kale, greens (dandelion, beet, and turnip)
	Dried fruits: apricots, dates, figs, prunes, and raisins
	Legumes and nuts
	Iron cookware
Folic acid	Green leafy vegetables
	Asparagus, broccoli
	Organ meats: liver and kidney
	Whole-grain breads and cereals
	Enriched and fortified breads and cereals
Vitamin B₁₂	Organ meats: liver and kidney
	Muscle meats
	Milk and cheese
	Eggs

PATIENT EDUCATION GUIDE
Iron Administration

Iron preparations supplement iron stores. Dosages are determined by the elemental iron content of the preparation. Iron supplements may be contraindicated in peptic ulcer disease. Side effects include gastrointestinal upset (nausea, vomiting), constipation or diarrhea, and green to black stools. Elixir may stain teeth.

Administer iron with or after meals to avoid gastric upset. Do not administer with antacids.

If a dose is missed, continue with schedule. Do not double a dose.

Iron may interfere with absorption of oral tetracycline antibiotics. Do not take within 2 hours of each other.

Dilute liquid iron preparations in juice or water, and administer with a straw to avoid staining of teeth.

Drink juice (preferably orange juice) to promote absorption.

Check for constipation or diarrhea. Record color (iron turns stools green to black) and amount of stool.

Iron is toxic and caution must be taken to store iron preparations out of a child's reach.

---

are completed without fatigue. Learning to include frequent rest periods helps the patient adapt to the imbalance between tissue oxygen demand and oxygen supply.

The patient and family also need to learn about food selection and meal planning to support red blood cell formation. The nurse can provide the patient and family with lists of foods high in iron, folic acid, and vitamin B₁₂. Table 38-2 lists food sources of these nutrients. The nurse should encourage the patient and family to read food labels to identify foods that have been enriched or fortified with these vitamins and minerals. The use of unlined iron cookware also contributes to the patient's overall iron intake. The nurse may make a referral to a dietitian to assist the patient and family in food selection and meal planning.

The patient who takes vitamin and mineral supplements needs to learn about the proper administration and expected side effects of these medications. If the patient experiences gastric upset with oral iron supplements, the nurse instructs the patient to take them with food. The patient needs to be aware of the changes in bowel movements that occur with supplemental iron therapy. The feces may turn a dark greenish-black.

For the patient who receives intramuscular injections of iron, the nurse uses a Z-track method of administration. This method of injection decreases the leakage of the iron solution along the needle track into the subcutaneous tissue. The dorsogluteal site in the upper outer quadrant of the buttocks is the preferred site for injection.

Steps in the Z-track method include:
- Use one needle to withdraw the medication into the syringe
- Change needles—use a new one for injection to avoid leakage of drug
- Draw 0.5 mL of air into syringe before injecting medication
- Retract the skin laterally before inserting the needle
- Inject the medication and then the 0.5 mL of air to prevent drug leakage
- Withdraw the needle
- Release the skin

Patients with genetic red blood cell disorders will need support in making decisions about childbearing. The patient and family may need help in working through feelings of anger and grief. The nurse can make a referral to a family counseling therapist to help the family develop appropriate coping skills. A genetic counselor can help the family understand the probabilities of siblings and offspring developing the same or related red blood cell disorders.

Evaluation

Changes in laboratory values will provide information about the success of nursing interventions. The values for hemoglobin, hematocrit, and red blood cell count should be within normal limits for the patient. The patient should have fewer subjective reports of fatigue, dyspnea, or pain with activity.

Documentation

Documentation includes assessment findings, especially noting symptoms such as pallor, fatigue, shortness of breath, and change in vital signs. The nurse records the status of the patient's activity level. All patient and family teaching about diet and drug therapy is documented, along with the patient's and family's response. Referrals for counseling are also documented.

Ongoing Care

Persons are told how to manage symptoms, when to report signs to the physician, and generally how to care for themselves. Routine outpatient visits for laboratory tests, prescription refills, and information are sufficient to ensure that a normal life can continue. Home care and long-term care are necessary with the late complications of anemia such as vasoocclusion or infarction. The ultimate goal of assessing an individual's personal values, support networks, and the home setting, in light of the identified needs, is continuity of care. Continuity of care enables individuals to regain or maintain optimum health and maximize their personal resources and level of independence. This goal is achieved through coordination of various disciplines as the patient makes the transition from ambulatory to home to long-term care.[51]

The patient and family may benefit from periodic contacts with the nurse as they adjust to the course of the disease and its management. The patient may need support to continue with drug therapy. The nurse can make home visits or phone calls to provide support. The patient needs to learn about preventing and managing crises that exacerbate the disease process.

The nurse assesses the status of the home environment, including equipment and resources. If it is determined that the household members need assistance, the nurse collaborates with them to establish a safe environment. The strategies include removal of environmental hazards, provision of equipment (e.g., bathtub rails), and arrangement for home health services or community assistance (e.g., financial or transportation).

Disorders of White Blood Cells

LEUKEMIAS

Leukemia is a group of malignant diseases of the bone marrow, and is characterized by an unregulated proliferation of cells of hematopoietic origin. Although the term "leukemia" literally means "white blood," the disease can occur in any of the bone marrow cellular lines, including the white blood cell line, the red blood cell line, or the platelet line. It also can occur at any stage of blood cell development. In healthy bone marrow, a variety of regulatory mechanisms interact to ensure that normal blood cell maturation and proliferation occur (see Fig. 37-2.)

In leukemia, it is thought that a single stem cell (or clone) undergoes a malignant change. It then proliferates and begins to replace normal cellular elements. This process causes the patient to experience anemia, thrombocytopenia, and leukopenia. Eventually, the normal cellular elements die out, and the malignant leukemia cells remain. Leukemic cells may leave the bone marrow and infiltrate the reticuloendothial system, including lymph nodes, liver, and spleen. Additionally, the cells may invade any other body tissue, such as the central nervous system, gastrointestinal tract, testes, skin, and gingiva. The clinical manifestations of leukemia are the result of bone marrow failure, organ/tissue infiltration, and immunologic abnormalities.

The classifications of leukemia are acute and chronic. The acute leukemias are characterized by an overgrowth of very immature (often termed "undifferentiated" or "poorly differentiated") cells in the bone marrow. These cells are called blast cells. The acute leukemias are further subdivided into lymphoid or myeloid, depending on which specific white blood cell type is involved. Table 38-3 summarizes the French-American-British (FAB) classification system currently used for the wide variety of acute leukemias. The chronic leukemias are characterized by abnormal growth of more mature, or "well differentiated" cells. They, too, are subdivided as myelogenous or lymphocytic, depending on which specific white blood cell type is involved.

As a group, the leukemias represent about 10% of all cancers.[19] Approximately 28,000 new cases will occur in the United States each year; more than

TABLE 38-3   Acute Leukemia Classification

Classification		Predominant marrow cellular characteristics
ACUTE MYELOCYTIC LEUKEMIAS		
M-1	Myeloblastic leukemia without maturation	Blasts are ≥ 90% nonerythroid cells
M-2	Myeloblastic leukemia with maturation	Blasts are 30% to 89% nonerythroid
M-3	Promyelocytic leukemia	Promyelocytes
M-4	Myelomonocytic leukemia	Mixture of monocytes and myeloblasts
M-5	Monocytic leukemia	> 80% monocytes
M-6	Erythroleukemia	Erythroblasts
M-7	Megakaryoblastic leukemia	Megakaryoblasts
ACUTE LYMPHOCYTIC LEUKEMIAS		
L-1	Lymphoblastic leukemia, predominantly childhood	Small lymphoblasts
L-2	Lymphoblastic leukemia, adult	Large lymphoblasts, heterogeneous in size
L-3	Lymphoma-like leukemia (Burkitt type)	Large lymphoblasts, homogeneous in size

18,000 deaths from leukemia will occur annually. Overall, lymphoid and myeloid subtypes are seen with virtually the same frequency. Although often thought of as a childhood disease, leukemia annually strikes many more adults (greater than 25,000) than children (less than 3,000).[1]

The cause of leukemia in humans is unknown. Many factors, however, have been linked to its development. The factors appear to cause chromosomal abnormalities, which may precipitate the dis-ease. Although viruses in particular have undergone close scrutiny in animal studies, there is no conclusive evidence that human leukemia is a viral disease. In most persons with leukemia, no potential etiologic agent can be identified at all. Table 38-4 summarizes potential factors linked with the development of leukemia.

The four most common types of leukemia are acute myelogenous leukemia (AML), acute lymphocytic leukemia (ALL), chronic myelogenous leukemia (CML), and chronic lymphocytic leukemia (CLL). A group of "preleukemic" states, termed the myelodysplastic syndromes, have recently been identified as a variety of myeloproliferative disorders that most often arise in the elderly population (see box on p. 974).

TABLE 38-4   Leukemia: Predisposing Agents

Classification	Examples
Genetic abnormalities	Down's syndrome
	Fanconi's anemia
	Bloom's syndrome
	Wiskott-Aldrich's syndrome
	Klinefelter's syndrome
Ionizing radiation	Therapeutic radiation
	Atomic radiation
Chemicals and drugs	Benzene
	^{32}P (phosphorus radioisotope)
	Alkylating chemotherapeutic agents
	Immunosuppressive agents
	Chloramphenicol
	Phenylbutazone
Viral infection	Human T cell leukemia viruses

ACUTE MYELOGENOUS LEUKEMIA
Definition

Acute myelogenous leukemia (AML) is a subtype of leukemia characterized by an uncontrolled overgrowth of very primitive cells from the myeloid stem cell line (see Figure 37-2). Often AML is preceded by a hematologic disorder, such as anemia (of unknown etiology), or a variety of "preleukemic" changes in the bone marrow.

Etiology/Epidemiology

Ninety percent of all cases of AML occur in adults, with an incidence of approximately 6,500 new cases a year.[1] The incidence increases with age; over half of all patients are older than 60 years. Of all the dif-

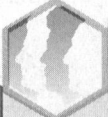

Myelodysplastic Syndromes

The myelodysplastic syndromes (MDS) are a group of malignant hematologic disorders characterized by ineffective hematopoiesis and blood cytopenias.[37] The etiology is unknown in most cases, although a history of ionizing radiation or previous cytotoxic drug therapy is associated with the disease. Myelodysplastic syndrome is primarily a disease of the elderly, with an incidence that increases steadily with each decade over the age of 50. The overall evidence of MDS is impossible to determine because many patients who present with acute myelogenous leukemia may have actually first had the disorder, which then progressed to leukemia.

Five subtypes of myelodysplastic syndrome have been identified, ranging from "refractory anemia" (least severe) to "refractory anemia with excessive blasts in transformation" (most severe). The accepted standard therapy is supportive care (transfusions and antibiotics); clinical trials investigating the potential for chemotherapy and biotherapy are in progress. Unfortunately, the syndrome is extremely resistant to treatment and carries a uniformly poor prognosis. The length of time between diagnosis and death varies greatly due to the many different subtypes and different responses to therapy.

ferent types of leukemia, AML is most closely linked to the suspected etiologic factors outlined in Table 38-3.

Pathophysiology

The malignant cell in AML is the very immature myeloblast cell of the white blood cell line. As with all leukemias, the malignant myeloblast cell proliferates and crowds out other normal components of a patient's bone marrow. Diagnosis is made when a bone marrow aspiration and biopsy reveal an overgrowth of very immature cells of the myeloblast cell line. These "blast" cells may also be detected in the blood stream when a CBC is done. Patterns in blood counts vary greatly among patients. General trends include a normocytic, normochromic anemia (hemoglobin less than 10 g/dL), and thrombocytopenia (platelet count less than 150,000/mm^3). White blood cell counts may be low, normal, or high. The key white cell factor to examine is the maturity of the circulating and marrow elements. Patients with

AML will have predominantly blastic, or immature, white cells. Another tool used to diagnose and classify the disorder is that of cytogenetic studies. These are studies designed to detect chromosome abnormalities in the leukemic cells. Abnormalities could include chromosome deletions, additions, inversions, or translocations of pieces of genetic material between two chromosomes. Cytogenetic studies are also used to predict response of the leukemia to treatment and disease prognosis.

Clinical Manifestations

Clinical manifestations of bone marrow dysfunction include recurrent infections, general malaise and fatigue, and unexplained bleeding; such as easy bruising, bleeding gums, or unusually heavy menses. Physical examination will show pallor and evidence of spontaneous hemorrhage, such as petechiae and ecchymoses. Lymph nodes and the spleen may be enlarged, but usually not remarkably so. Leukemic cells may infiltrate the gingiva and rectal areas, giving rise to tissue hypertrophy. Manifestations of local or systemic infection appear. Bone pain is caused by the presence of rapidly proliferating cells in the marrow.

Therapeutic Management

Acute myelogenous leukemia is difficult to treat successfully. The initial therapeutic goal is to eradicate the leukemic clone in the marrow so that normal elements can repopulate. The initial goal is complete remission—defined as reduction of blasts to less than 5% in the marrow, restoration of normal RBC, WBC, and platelet counts, and eradication of extramedullary disease. This treatment approach is called remission induction. High doses of combinations of toxic chemotherapeutic agents are used. Currently, cytarabine and anthracycline antibiotics form the mainstay of treatment. Table 38-5 summarizes the standard chemotherapeutic approaches for all four major types of leukemia.

Additional chemotherapy must follow to destroy any remaining leukemia cells, a process called consolidation. Typically consolidation consists of repeated courses of the same drugs used for induction therapy, but dose levels are often greater. Maintenance therapy then follows; usually, a variety of different drugs at lower doses are administered. The goal of maintenance is to prevent the leukemic cells from reappearing. Use of maintenance chemotherapy is controversial; many treatment centers do not utilize this stage, because its value is not yet well proven. The final stage is intensification, in which intensive chemotherapy is administered 6 to 12 months after remission is achieved. The entire course of treatment for AML may last 2 to 3 years.

TABLE 38-5 Pharmacology Summary: Chemotherapy for Leukemia

Drug	Route	Side effects and toxicities	Leukemia
Amsacrine	IV	Myelosuppression, mild nausea, vomiting, stomatitis, alopecia, phlebitis	AML, ALL
5-Azacytidine	IV	Nausea, vomiting, diarrhea, myelosuppression, hypotension (caused by rapid infusion), fever, neurologic toxicity, hyperglycemia reactions	AML
Busulfan	PO	Myelosuppression, amenorrhea; long-term: pulmonary fibrosis, muscle wasting, skin hyperpigmentation, Addison-like syndrome	CML
Cytarabine	IV, IT, SC	Myelosuppression, nausea, vomiting, diarrhea, fever, hepatotoxicity, central nervous system toxicity (high doses)	AML
Chlorambucil	PO	Myelosuppression, minimal anorexia, nausea, vomiting	CLL
Cyclophosphamide	PO, IV	Myelosuppression, hemorrhagic cystitis, nausea, vomiting, alopecia, cardiotoxicity (high doses)	CLL, ALL
Daunorubicin*	IV	Myelosuppression, nausea, vomiting, abdominal pain, alopecia, stomatitis, fever, skin rash, cardiomyopathy	AML, ALL
Doxorubicin*	IV	Myelosuppression, alopecia, cardiomyopathy, stomatitis, nausea, vomiting	AML, ALL
Etoposide	IV	Myelosuppression, nausea, alopecia, anaphylaxis, hypotension (caused by rapid infusion)	AML
Fludarabine	IV	Myelosuppression, neurotoxicity at higher doses, nausea, vomiting, diarrhea, stomatitis, skin rash	CLL
Hydroxyurea	PO	Myelosuppression, nausea, vomiting, stomatitis	CML
Asparaginase	IM, IV	Anaphylaxis, chills, fever, skin rash, pancreatitis, nausea, vomiting, anorexia, hyperglycemia, hepatotoxicity, coagulopathies	ALL
Mercaptopurine	PO	Myelosuppression, hepatotoxicity, mucositis, nausea, vomiting, diarrhea, rash	ALL, CML
Methotrexate	PO, IV, IT	Myelosuppression, stomatitis, alopecia, nausea, vomiting, diarrhea, enteritis, hepatotoxicity, renal toxicity	ALL, AML
Mitoxantrone	IV	Myelosuppression, phlebitis, nausea, vomiting, diarrhea, mucositis, hepatotoxicity, alopecia	AML
Prednisone	PO	Cushingoid symptoms, sodium retention, immunosuppression, diabetes, nausea, vomiting, gastric irritation, retarded growth in children	ALL, CLL
Thioguanine	PO	Myelosuppression, nausea, vomiting, anorexia, hepatotoxicity	AML
Vincristine*	IV	Neurotoxicity (peripheral, deep tendon, central nerve palsy, autonomic effects such as constipation, ileus, urinary retention), alopecia, mild myelosuppression, nausea, vomiting	ALL

*Vesicant agents. Infiltration into soft tissue may cause severe damage and result in necrosis, cellulitis, and pain.

Bone marrow transplant is the other important treatment modality for AML. Both autologous and allogeneic approaches are used. Although mortality from infection or graft versus host disease is a significant problem, survival rates continue to improve. Best results occur in an allogeneic transplant in the young adult. Overall, the 2- to 5-year disease-free survival is approximately 50%, a clear advantage over chemotherapy alone.[19] Unfortunately, allogeneic transplant is limited by the patient's age and availability of compatible donors.

Although disease remission can be achieved in up to 75% of cases, relapse will eventually occur in most cases.[35] Overall, only about 20% to 25% of adults with AML experience a 5-year remission. The primary cause of death is overwhelming infection, caused by either the disease or the treatment. Supportive therapy in the form of transfusions and antibiotics is applied rigorously to sustain patients during prolonged periods of myelosuppression.

ACUTE LYMPHOCYTIC LEUKEMIA
Definition/Etiology

Acute lymphocytic leukemia (ALL), the predominant childhood leukemia, is characterized by a prolifera-

ETHICAL ISSUES

- Should patients for whom all treatments have failed be offered a phase I drug* trial?
- What constitutes informed consent in a phase I clinical trial? Is it different from informed consent obtained in non-research procedures?
- Is it ethical for the nurse who cares for a patient to recruit that patient into a clinical trial in which the nurse is involved?

*A phase I drug is an experimental drug given to patients for the purpose of determining side effects. The drug is not given with a therapeutic goal.

tion of primitive lymphocyte white blood cell precursors, termed lymphoblasts.

The peak incidence occurs in children between 2 and 10 years of age; an additional rise in frequency occurs from middle age and onward. Given that ALL comprises about 20% of all cases of adult leukemia, approximately 5000 new cases arise each year.[1,19] Of the etiologic factors noted in Table 38-4, radiation exposure and genetic abnormalities have been specifically linked to ALL.[19]

Pathophysiology

The malignant cell in ALL is the very immature lymphoblast cell of the white blood cell line. As with other leukemias, the malignant lymphoblast leukemia cells crowd out the normal elements of the bone marrow. A bone marrow aspiration and biopsy will reveal an overgrowth of these lymphoblastic cells. Blood studies reveal an increased white blood cell count (**leukocytosis**) in two thirds of the cases; often the total count will exceed 100,000/mm^3.[19] Thrombocytopenia and anemia will also be present. As in AML, the immature blast cells may leave the bone marrow and can be detected in the peripheral circulation. Blast cells may subsequently infiltrate the central nervous system. Patients may also exhibit chromosomal abnormalities in the malignant cells. Immunologic and morphologic studies are also used to identify which of the three subtypes of acute lymphocytic leukemia is present (see Table 38-3 for subtypes).

Clinical Manifestations

Clinical symptoms are similar to those of AML. Problems related to anemia, thrombocytopenia, and leukopenia predominate. Additionally, bone pain caused by rapid proliferation of cells in the marrow, lymphadenopathy, and marked hepatosplenomegaly

are common. Patients may also complain of fatigue, malaise, a tendency to bruise easily, and sweating. If the patient has central nervous system involvement, clinical manifestations may include cranial nerve palsies, headache, nausea and vomiting, or seizures. Unlike AML, ALL usually has a rapid onset of only a few weeks before diagnosis. A preleukemic syndrome does not occur.

Therapeutic Management

As in AML, treatment is aimed at eradicating the leukemia with chemotherapy or bone marrow transplant. Chemotherapy usually consists of a combination of vincristine, prednisone, and an anthracycline drug (daunorubicin or doxorubicin), given over repeated courses (see Table 38-5). This approach usually yields a 35% long-term (5-year) survival rate.[11] Other approaches, including the use of very high doses of other antileukemia drugs, are currently under study. Allogeneic bone marrow transplant can be curative in some patients,[2] but is an option for few patients due to either age restrictions or unavailability of a compatible donor (see also section on bone marrow transplant). Because the central nervous system is a potential site for relapse of disease, most treatment plans include prophylactic treatments, such as instillation of intrathecal chemotherapy or cranial radiation. These approaches are also used when CNS involvement is documented.

Tumor lysis syndrome is a major complication of chemotherapy in ALL. This syndrome refers to a group of metabolic complications that include hyperkalemia, hypocalcemia, hyperphosphatemia, and hyperuricemia. Patients who have extremely high white blood cell counts are at risk because rapidly proliferating lymphoid cells are extremely sensitive to chemotherapy. As cells are lysed, they release their contents into the bloodstream, resulting in numerous imbalances. Table 38-6 summarizes the clinical manifestations of tumor lysis syndrome. Treatment begins with vigorous IV hydration in order to promote urinary excretion of the metabolic byproducts of the cell lysis. Allopurinol is given to reduce serum uric acid, a substance that can crystallize in the kidneys and cause renal failure. Excretion of uric acid is also facilitated by maintaining a urine pH of 7 or greater through administration of oral or intravenous sodium bicarbonate. Additional approaches may be used to correct electrolyte imbalances.

CHRONIC MYELOGENOUS LEUKEMIA
Definition/Etiology

As opposed to acute myelogenous leukemia, chronic myelogenous leukemia (CML) is characterized by an abnormal proliferation of more mature, or well-differentiated, white blood cells of the myeloid cell

TABLE 38-6 Tumor Lysis Syndrome

Abnormality	Manifestation
Hyperkalemia	Confusion, weakness, numbness or tingling, bradycardia
	Electrocardiogram: tall T waves and prolonged PR, QRS, and ST segments
	Dysrhythmias, hyperactive reflexes, abdominal and muscle cramps, nausea, diarrhea
Hyperphosphatemia	Usually asymptomatic
Hypocalcemia	Numbness, tingling, irritability, muscle cramps, seizures, positive Chvostek's sign, tetany
	Electrocardiogram: lengthened QT interval
Hyperuricemia	Uric acid crystalluria, renal tubular obstruction, acute renal failure

line (see Figure 37-2). Although the etiology is unknown in most cases, both ionizing radiation and chemical exposure are known causative agents. Chronic myelogenous leukemia comprises about 20% of all leukemias; peak age of onset is 50 to 60 years, with a slight predominance of males over females.[19]

Pathophysiology

CML has the unique distinction of being the first malignancy ever associated with a known chromosome aberration. This abberation, known as the Philadelphia chromosome (Ph1), involves a translocation of genetic material between chromosomes 9 and 22. The Ph1 chromosome occurs in 95% of cases and is seen in both bone marrow and circulating blood cells.[19] Although the cause of this abnormality is unknown, the presence of the Ph1 chromosome is associated with a better prognosis than occurs when the chromosome is absent.

Chronic myelogenous leukemia is also unique from the other leukemias in that it may occur in three phases. Onset tends to be much more insidious than that of the acute leukemias. When the patient presents in the first phase, known as the "chronic" phase, bone marrow studies reveal myelocytic leukemia cells that mature normally and function fairly normally. A CBC will reflect an increased white blood cell count (often greater than 100,000). Unlike AML, which is characterized by a

predominance of blast cells, CML will manifest white blood cells at all levels of maturity. The patient will likely be anemic due to impaired red cell production in the marrow. The platelet count is often elevated; this may be due to an excess of platelet precursor cells in the bone marrow in the chronic stage of the disease.

The average time frame for the chronic phase is three years; most patients then experience an "acceleration" stage in which the disease progresses to a more aggressive form. In this stage, symptoms worsen as the bone marrow begins to produce more cells that are increasingly less mature. Within several weeks or months, the third stage, "blast crisis," occurs. At this point, CML resembles acute leukemia in that the patient experiences a rapid rise in blast cells and bone marrow failure. Laboratory findings also include thrombocytopenia and anemia. The white blood cell count may be 500,000/mm^3 or higher and may result in leukostasis lesions, which are vascular blockages due to "clumps" of large numbers of leukemic cells. These lesions can cause widespread organ damage throughout the body.

Clinical Manifestations

Although some patients may be asymptomatic at time of diagnosis in the chronic phase, most exhibit clinical symptoms such as fatigue, malaise, splenomegaly, weight loss, increased sweating, and bone pain. Most of these symptoms are due to the hypermetabolic state that supports the rapid expansion of the white blood cell count. When the patient moves into the accelerated phase, the symptoms recur and worsen due to progression of bone marrow involvement. At this point, the patient will experience fever, infections, and increased bruising or bleeding. Lymphadenopathy may also occur, due to infiltration of lymph nodes by leukemia cells. In the blast phase, symptoms experienced in the accelerated phase continue to worsen.

Therapeutic Management

Treatment in the chronic phase is typically conservative. Attempts are made to control the disease with oral chemotherapy, such as hydroxyurea or busulfan. Intensive, high doses of chemotherapy and bone marrow transplantation are also used for patients. Bone marrow transplantation is a potentially curative treatment,[29] but, again, due to age constraints and donor constraints, allogeneic bone marrow transplantation is not an option for most patients. Clinical studies continue for both allogeneic and autologous approaches to bone marrow transplantation in the CML population.

Alpha interferon is a biologic response modifier, produced by recombinant DNA technology. Although currently approved by the FDA only for use in hairy cell leukemia (an extremely rare form of lymphocytic leukemia), it has also shown promise in the treatment of chronic myelogenous leukemia, multiple myeloma, and lymphocytic lymphomas. Alpha interferon is used in CML and can prolong the chronic phase to 5 years or longer.[31] Although its action differs from that of chemotherapy, interferon has an antiproliferative effect on these diseases.[32] Side effects of treatment may include myelosuppression, a flu-like syndrome, fatigue, hyperglycemia, nausea, diarrhea, and proteinuria.

CHRONIC LYMPHOCYTIC LEUKEMIA
Definition/Etiology

As opposed to ALL, chronic lymphocytic leukemia (CLL) is characterized by a proliferation of more mature cells from the lymphocyte white blood cell line. CLL is characterized by an accumulation of dysfunctional lymphocytes in the bloodstream and other body tissues. As with the other forms of leukemia, the etiology is largely unknown. It is not associated with chemical or radiation exposure, but may be linked to immunodeficiency disorders such as Wiskott-Aldrich syndrome, ataxia telangectasia, and chronic immunosuppression following organ transplantation.[19] CLL is a disease of adults and has the best prognosis of the four major types of leukemia. It occurs much more frequently in men than women, and is primarily seen in people over 50 years of age. Approximately 8,200 new cases arise each year.[1]

Pathophysiology

The key pathophysiologic activity in CLL is the unexplained proliferation of relatively mature lymphocytes. The lymphocyte count may be as high as 1,000,000/mm^3 on diagnosis. Bone marrow studies will show a proliferation of the lymphocyte white cell line; some crowding of the red blood cell and platelet lines may result in anemia or thrombocytopenia. The lymphocytes produced will appear normal, but are not fully mature and thus are unable to produce immunoglobulins (proteins responsible for antibody production). Blood, bone marrow, and lymph nodes may be crowded with these large quantities of white blood cells.

Clinical Manifestations

Many persons are diagnosed with CLL in the course of routine workups for surgery or other medical problems. If symptoms are present, they generally consist of vague complaints of fatigue or malaise. Lymphadenopathy and splenomegaly may be present. Skin infiltrates of leukemia cells may occur,

along with rashes and lesions. Because lymphocytes are primarily involved, the patient has a diminished ability to produce antibodies and may have recurrent infections.

Therapeutic Management

Overall survival is variable. In early stages, median survival ranges from 10 to 12½ years; in advanced stages, survival is approximately 18 months.[14] Indeed, many persons succumb to other diseases of old age before clinical manifestations become troublesome. Treatment presents a dilemma because of the increased age of the population. Many patients do well without treatment for years, whereas side effects due to a more aggressive approach could cause a premature death. Thus, a more conservative approach is usually chosen. Asymptomatic patients are often not treated; onset of symptoms (such as lymphadenopathy) warrants administration of oral chemotherapy such as chlorambucil. Radiation to the areas of lymphocyte infiltration (such as lymph nodes) also provides local palliation. As the disease progresses, increasing bone marrow failure occurs with accompanying symptoms. Treatment usually includes intravenous administration of chemotherapy, such as fludarabine or others. Once the disease is refractory to treatment, death is usually a result of overwhelming infection.

NEUTROPENIA
Definition/Etiology

The term **neutropenia** refers to a decrease in the number of circulating neutrophils in a person's bloodstream. This condition can arise due to a wide variety of causes. For example, the leukemia and lymphoma disease processes can cause failure of the bone marrow to produce sufficient neutrophils. Also, any cancer patient who receives treatments that are toxic to the bone marrow will experience transient periods of neutropenia after treatment (see Chapter 15). However, there are also several noncancer-related causes of neutropenia. Many drugs can cause neutropenia. The mechanisms of action vary, and may include direct suppression of bone marrow cells, or drug-induced development of antibodies against blood cells. Table 38-7 summarizes a variety of substances known to induce neutropenia.

Clinical Manifestations

Patients who are neutropenic are at risk for infection; thus, clinical symptoms of this syndrome are usually associated with an active infectious process. Patients may present with fever, chills, malaise, and other symptoms that depend on the specific site of infection (e.g., sore throat, dysuria).

TABLE 38-7   Drugs Associated with Neutropenia

Classification	Examples
Antibiotics	Penicillin derivatives, cephalosporins
Antiepileptics	Phenytoin, carbamazepine
Antiinflammatories and antiarthritics	Phenylbutazone, oxyphenbutazone, indomethacin, colchicine, gold salts
Antithyroids	Propylthiouracil, methimazole, carbimazole
Phenothiazines	Chlorpromazine, prochlorperazine, promazine
Sulfonamides	Trimethoprim-sulfamethoxazole, sulfasalazine

Therapeutic Management

Treatment of drug-induced neutropenia involves stopping the offending drug; the neutrophil count usually begins to rise within a few days. Time to full recovery varies greatly depending on the drug involved and individual patient response.

LYMPHOMAS

Lymphomas are a group of malignancies occurring in the lymphoreticular system. Lymphocytes originate from stem cells in the bone marrow. The stem cell has the potential to follow various paths of differentiation. Those cells in the path of lymphocytes can further differentiate to a T lymphocyte or a B lymphocyte. Lymphocytes are responsible for the immunologic defense. The humoral immunity is provided through the B cells and the cellular immunity through the T cells. The term lymphoma includes a number of diseases that have variable manifestations, treatments, and prognoses, depending on the lymphocyte type and stage of differentiation. Lymphomas are discussed under two main classifications: Hodgkin's disease, and non-Hodgkin's lymphomas.

HODGKIN'S DISEASE

Definition

Hodgkin's disease is characterized by enlargement of the lymph nodes. Debate continues as to the specific cell origin, but the presence of the Reed-Sternberg cell is diagnostic.

Etiology/Epidemiology

The etiology is unknown in Hodgkin's disease. Infectious etiology has been investigated, especially regarding viruses such as the oncovirus and the Epstein-Barr virus. Increased incidences of Hodgkin's disease have been reported in certain groups of persons with close contact. However, a viral etiology has not been isolated independent of genetic or environmental factors.

Hodgkin's disease constitutes 1% of all cancers and 14% of malignant lymphomas. It is estimated that there are 7400 new cases a year with approximately 1500 deaths.[1] The incidence of the disease is greater in men than women, and men have a worse prognosis. The age-incidence curve is bimodal. There is a peak early in life, in the second and third decades, and a peak later in life, in the sixth and seventh decades. The two peaks in incidence have been suggested as two separate diseases. The first incidence peak suggests a viral etiology.

Pathophysiology

The cell of origin has not been confirmed, but may be from a B-lymphocyte, T-lymphocyte, or macrophage/reticulum cell line.[9] Immune deficiency, especially cellular, is characteristic of Hodgkin's disease and places persons at risk for infections, especially herpes zoster and *Pneumocystis carinii*. The histopathologic classification system used in Hodgkin's disease is from the work of Lukes and Butler.[49] The classification involves four types of cells:

Nodular sclerosis—This type (50% of the total), is characterized by the lymph node being divided into nodules by sclerosing bands of collagen.

Lymphocyte-predominant—This type (approximately 5% of the total), is characterized by abundant lymphocytes with few Reed-Sternberg cells and has a good prognosis.

Lymphocyte-depleted—This type (approximately 5% of the total), is characterized by few lymphocytes and a large number of Reed-Sternberg cells and has a poor prognosis.

Mixed cellularity—This type (approximately 40% of the total), has a histology intermediate between lymphocyte-predominant and lymphocyte-depleted and a moderate number of Reed-Sternberg cells.

Clinical Manifestations

The most common sign is one or more enlarged lymph nodes. The lymph node is painless, firm, rubbery, and freely movable. In addition, one third of individuals have symptoms of fever, night sweats, and weight loss. Individuals may also have pruritus and complain of pain in the enlarged nodes after al-

ANN ARBOR STAGING CLASSIFICATION FOR HODGKIN'S DISEASE

Stage I Involvement of a single lymph node region (I) or a single extra-lymphatic organ or site (I_E*)

Stage II Involvement of two or more lymph node regions on the same side of the diaphragm (II) or localized involvement of an extralymphatic organ or site (II_E)

Stage III Involvement of lymph node regions on both sides of the diaphragm (III) or localized involvement of an extralymphatic organ or site (III_E) or spleen (III_{IS}) or both (III_{SE})

Stage IV Diffuse or disseminated involvement of one or more extralymphatic organs with or without associated lymph node involvement. The involved extralymphatic site should be identified by symbols used for pathologic staging:
H+ = hepatic   P+ = pleura
L+ = lung   O+ = osseous
M+ = marrow   D+ = dermal

A and B systems—Each stage is subdivided into A and B categories. B is for those with certain general symptoms, and A is for those without. B symptoms include unexplained weight loss of more than 10% of body weight in the 6 months previous to admission, unexplained fever with temperatures above 38 C °, and night sweats.

* E, Extralymphatic organ or site; S, spleen.

cohol ingestion. Lymph node biopsy confirms the diagnosis. The disease process is anatomically classified or staged to facilitate communication and plan treatment. The four-stage Ann Arbor system (1971) is used (see box). Staging is done clinically by assessing lymphadenopathy and anatomically through lymphangiogram, laparotomy, or roentgenographic studies and computerized tomography scans.

Therapeutic Management

Treatment is directed by the stage of the disease. In general, radiation therapy is used against the localized forms (stage I and II), and chemotherapy is used against the generalized forms (stages III and IV). For care of the individual receiving radiotherapy and chemotherapy, see Chapter 15. For individuals with stage III and IV, chemotherapy is the treatment of choice. The MOPP (mustargen, oncovin, procarbazine, and prednisone) protocol may be indicated (Table 38-8) or ABVD (adriamycin, bleomycin, vinblastine, DTIC). Combination chemotherapy and radiotherapy has been used. Additional chemotherapy protocols may be used, depending on patient response. The prognosis is steadily improving. Bone marrow transplantation and biologic response modifiers are treatment options. Seventy-five percent of people are cured of Hodgkin's and survive at least ten years.

NON-HODGKIN'S LYMPHOMA
Definition

Non-Hodgkin's lymphoma (NHL) is a malignancy of the lymphocyte. Most NHLs are derived from B lymphocytes and their subpopulations (e.g., nodular or follicular) at the proliferative site of the B cell system. Diffuse, well-differentiated lymphomas relate to the secretory site of the B cell system. In the elderly, the non-Hodgkin's lymphomas are predominantly B cell tumors. Non-Hodgkin's lymphomas can be derived from the T lymphocytes and result in malignant skin disease such as mycosis fungoides or Sézary syndrome. Non-Hodgkin's lymphoma is beginning to be characterized as a neoplasm of the immune system.[12]

Etiology/Epidemiology

A viral etiology has been suggested, especially certain types such as Burkitt's lymphoma. A herpeslike virus is implicated, but a causal relationship has not been established. There is an association of NHL with immunosuppressed states (immunosuppressive therapy for organ transplants, acquired immunodeficiency syndrome [AIDS]). Recent theories involve the function of the immune suppressor cell or activation of oncogenic viruses. There is a risk seen in persons with autoimmune disorders, such as Sjörgen's syndrome. Non-Hodgkin's lymphoma is more common than Hodgkin's disease. The estimated number of new cases is 41,000 for 1992 with 19,400 deaths.[1] The incidence is greater in men, and the age incidence is later in life (over 60 years). Incidence rates have increased 123% since 1950 primarily due to increases in older persons.[12]

Pathophysiology

The malignant cell in NHL is the lymphocyte at some stage in its development. Lymphocytes proliferate and then invade and debilitate various organs, especially the bone marrow. The most widely used classification system has been that of Rappaport. In the classification known as the Working Formulation, tumors are divided into low, intermediate, and

TABLE 38-8   Chemotherapeutic Agents for Hodgkin's Disease

Drug	Route	Side effects
Mechlorathemine (nitrogen mustard)	IV	Bone marrow suppression, nausea, vomiting, vesicant properties, risk to reproductive capacity
Oncovin (vincristine)	IV	Neuropathy, constipation, alopecia, nausea, vomiting, vesicant properties
Procarbazine	PO	Bone marrow suppression, nausea, vomiting, central nervous system depression, arthralgia, myalgia, drug interactions
Prednisone	PO	Cushingoid syndrome, fluid and electrolyte disturbances, diabetes, gastrointestinal disturbances, decreased immunity

high-grade lymphomas. In each area there are categories by histologic, anatomic, and immunomorphic characteristics. These systems are useful in directing treatment choices because they predict the biologic and clinical behavior of the disease. Currently other classification systems are being examined.[7]

Clinical Manifestations

Signs and symptoms are similar to those of Hodgkin's disease except for the following generalizations:

1. Early involvement of oropharyngeal lymphoid tissue, skin, gastrointestinal tract, and bone is somewhat more common in NHL. Unsuspected bone marrow involvement has also been demonstrated much more frequently.
2. Initial intraabdominal manifestations are relatively common (over one in three), as compared with Hodgkin's disease.
3. Leukemia transformation with high peripheral lymphocyte counts occurs in about 13% of lymphocytic lymphomas.
4. Increased susceptibility to bacterial, viral, and fungal infections is seen but in NHL it is associated with hypogammoglobulinemia and poor humoral antibody responses. (In Hodgkin's disease it is associated with impaired cellular immunity.)
5. Autoimmune anemia with positive antiglobulin (Coombs) tests occurs more commonly.

The staging system for NHL is the same as for Hodgkin's disease (see box on p. 980). The prognosis is influenced more by histologic subtype than by anatomic extent of disease, as in Hodgkin's disease. Diagnosis is made by lymph node biopsy.

Therapeutic Management

Radiation therapy may be indicated for localized disease. However, most patients will receive chemotherapy as the primary treatment. The choice of drugs is based on histology, stage, age, and functional status. A protocol used widely is CHOP (cyclophosphamide, doxorubicin, oncovin, prednisone). Bleomycin may be added to this regimen (Table 38-9). In addition, bone marrow transplantation may be indicated. Clinical testing of immune agents, such as tumor necrosis factor (TNF) is currently being done. Tissue necrosis factor has direct cell toxicity and

TABLE 38-9   Chemotherapeutic Agents for Non-Hodgkin's Lymphoma

Drug	Route	Side effects
Cyclophosphamide	IV	Bone marrow suppression, nausea, vomiting, hemorrhagic cystitis
Hydroxydaunomycin (doxorubicin)	IV	Bone marrow suppression, nausea, vomiting, stomatitis, alopecia, vesicant, cardiotoxicity
Oncovin (vincristine)	IV	Neuropathy, constipation, alopecia, nausea, vomiting, vesicant
Prednisone	PO	Cushingoid syndrome, fluid and electrolyte disturbances, diabetes, gastrointestinal disturbances, decreased immunity

also stimulates the immune system.[25] Interferon is currently being investigated as a treatment option.[26] Elderly patients have difficulty tolerating the aggressive chemotherapy regimens. This population is increasing and new approaches are being examined.[12]

MULTIPLE MYELOMA
Definition

Multiple myeloma is a neoplastic proliferation of plasma cells, characterized by lytic bone lesions, anemia, and homogeneous serum or urinary globulin elevation. It is a malignancy of the plasma cell, which is the mature cell of the B-lymphocyte origin.

Etiology/Epidemiology

No specific etiology has been established. The role of immunoglobulins in the plasma cell suggests that neoplastic cell proliferation may be the result of an inappropriate response to an initial antigenic stimulus. Viruslike particles have been seen in human and mouse plasma cell tumors, but no causal relationship has been established. Approximately 12,500 new cases and 9200 deaths are estimated for 1992.[1] Multiple myeloma accounts for 1% of the hematologic malignancies. The disease is more common in blacks than in whites. It is the most common lymphoreticular neoplasm in nonwhites and the third most common in whites. Multiple myeloma occurs mainly in middle-aged to elderly patients. The peak age incidence is 60 years old. The incidence is approximately equal in men and women under 60 years old, but over that age the male/female ratio is about 2:1.

Pathophysiology

In multiple myeloma, plasma cells that have undergone a malignant transformation proliferate. The transformed plasma cells produce a homogeneous immunoglobulin called the M-protein. The M-protein is produced in excessive amounts and is incapable of effective antibody production. Criteria for staging have been developed based on M-protein production, hemoglobin, calcium, and bone lesions.[28]

Clinical Manifestations

The symptoms of multiple myeloma are a result of the neoplastic plasma cells within the bone and abnormal proteins throughout the body. The signs and symptoms include bone pain, hypercalcemia, anemia, and renal failure. Serum and urine protein electrophoresis can make the definitive diagnosis.[28]

The bone pain is caused by the plasma cells producing osteoclast-activating factors that lead to osteolysis, severe bone pain, and pathologic fractures. The thoracic and lumbar vertebrae are most commonly involved, but the ribs, skull, pelvis, and proximal long bones may be affected as well. X-ray films show multiple "punched-out" osteolytic lesions and diffuse osteoporosis. The increased number of plasma cells in the bone marrow results in mild to moderate normochromic, normocytic anemia caused by crowding of the marrow. The degree of anemia depends on the percentage of plasma cells in the marrow. The anemia is also caused by the decreased survival of red blood cells coated with the M-protein. Bleeding may occur because of the M-protein coating on the platelets. Leukopenia and thrombocytopenia also occur as a result of the disease or chemotherapy. Proteinuria with the Bence Jones protein occurs and may lead to precipitates in the tubules.

Renal insufficiency may also be caused by hypercalcemia present as a result of bone destruction or by amyloid deposits present as a result of the reaction between the M-protein and tissue polysaccharides. Amyloid deposits may cause a carpal tunnel syndrome.

One of the consequences of multiple myeloma is infection. Infections occur because of deficient antibody production and because of the granulocytopenia caused by bone marrow infiltration by abnormal plasma cells. There may be a hyperviscosity syndrome present that manifests itself in circulatory impairment caused by occlusion of small blood vessels. The blood vessels affected may be in the extremities, retina, or cerebrum. Plasma exchange may be done to remove the excess components in the blood (see plasmapheresis section).

Therapeutic Management

Chemotherapy consisting of alkylating drugs alone or with prednisone is the treatment of choice for patients with multiple myeloma (progressive and symptomatic). The most commonly used alkylator is phenylalanine mustard (also known as L-PAM or melphalan). Chemotherapeutic agents used in treatment are listed in Table 38-10. Bone marrow transplantation is a treatment option.

NURSING MANAGEMENT OF THE PATIENT WITH A WHITE BLOOD CELL DISORDER
Assessment

Assessment focuses on a thorough history and physical examination, with an emphasis on checking for past or present illnesses that may indicate a WBC disorder. Be sure to note previous exposure to chemicals, and obtain a medication history. Nutritional status, current life-style, and age-related

TABLE 38-10   Chemotherapeutic Agents for Multiple Myeloma

Drug	Route	Side effects
Melphalan	PO	Bone marrow suppression
	IV	Vesicant
Prednisone	PO	Cushingoid syndrome, fluid and electrolyte disturbances, diabetes, gastrointestinal disturbances, decreased immunity
Oncovin (vincristine)	IV	Neuropathy, constipation, alopecia, nausea, vomiting, vesicant
Doxorubicin	IV	Bone marrow suppression, vesicant, nausea and vomiting, stomatitis, alopecia, cardiotoxicity
Dexamethasone	PO	Cushingoid syndrome
	IV	Depression, euphoria, fluid and electrolyte imbalances, depressed immunity

changes should all be reviewed. If infection is or has been a problem, determine sites and fever patterns.

A systems approach to the physical examination is used. Pay careful attention to any potential signs of infection or manifestation of organ dysfunction related to WBC infiltration. Generalized assessment findings may include fever, enlarged lymph nodes, weight loss, bone and joint pain, pruritus, abnormal bleeding, malaise, night sweats, anorexia, and splenomegaly. Cough, pleuritic pain, rales, sputum production, or pleural rub may indicate respiratory infection. Oropharyngeal changes are common in WBC disorders. Typical alterations include gingival hypertrophy, oral lesions, ulcerations, and sore throat. When assessing the gastrointestinal system, assess for abdominal pain or fullness, nausea, increased abdominal girth, diarrhea, perianal lesions, and rectal abscesses. Be alert for both tachycardia and hypotension, potential indicators for sepsis.

Cutaneous lesions, rash, exudate, ulceration, or pruritus may be present. WBC infiltration into the nervous system can be accompanied by headaches, cranial nerve impairment, and sensorimotor changes specific to the area of the brain involved. Also note paresthesias or confusion. When assessing mental status, be sure to solicit input from family or friends, because they are often the first to notice subtle changes. Changes in the genitourinary system include cloudy, foul-smelling urine, dysuria, vaginal or penile discharge, pruritus or burning, and menorrhagia.

Also note the person's level of growth and development, support systems, methods for coping, spiritual state, and self-concept. Onset of WBC malignancy in particular may quickly and often permanently disrupt all previous patterns of interacting and coping. Especially note the person's current knowledge base about the disease, diagnostic

When WBCs are deficient in numbers or dysfunctional, the patient may not exhibit the classic signs and symptoms of infection (e.g., pus, drainage, swelling, heat, pain, erythema). Neutrophils normally comprise the vast majority of the WBC differential and are most responsible for the typical inflammatory response. Thus, in the presence of neutropenia, the patient may develop an overwhelming infection while exhibiting few clinical indicators. If a neutropenic patient develops a fever of ≥38.5° C, infection should be strongly suspected, regardless of absence of other manifestations.

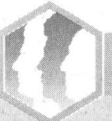

GERIATRIC CONSIDERATIONS

Multiple Myeloma

When an elderly patient has bone pain, there is a tendency to think of osteoporosis or degenerative joint disease as the most likely cause of the pain. The older adult may ignore the pain and consider it to be "the aches and pains of old age." The nurse carefully questions the older adult for symptoms of bone or joint pain and makes appropriate referrals for follow-up investigation and diagnosis of other causes such as multiple myeloma.

workup, or treatment, ability to learn, and learning styles. Successful prevention and management of infectious complications will depend, in part, on the patient's ability to learn about the disease and master requisite self-care measures.

Nursing Diagnosis

The primary nursing diagnosis for the individual with a WBC disorder is high risk for infection related to WBC deficiency or dysfunction. Associated nursing diagnoses also include:

Pain related to rapid proliferation of leukemic cells, bony lytic lesions, tumor pressure, peripheral neuropathies, or infectious lesions

Ineffective coping (individual or family) related to impact of malignant disease, disruption of lifestyle, roles, and self-concept.

Impaired gas exchange related to pneumonia, pleural effusions, drug toxicity, radiation fibrosis

Anticipatory grieving related to potential for death

Altered growth and development related to illness and hospitalizations

Knowledge deficit related to disease and treatment

Altered oral mucous membranes related to drug toxicities or infection

Altered thought processes related to cerebral leukostasis lesions, hypercalcemia, hypoxia, increased intracranial pressure

Impaired tissue integrity related to infectious lesions, malignant lesions, radiation therapy, chemotherapy toxicity

Altered (cardiopulmonary, renal, cerebral) tissue perfusion related to sepsis

Planning

The plan of care is developed with the following goals in mind: The patient will remain free of infection or will exhibit resolution or control of infectious episodes. Also, the patient or caregiver will identify or demonstrate measures to prevent or control infection, as well as verbalize and report indications of infection.

Implementation

Most of the interventions for the patient with white blood cell disorders are related to the patient's risk for infection. The nurse carefully monitors the patient's vital signs for indications of infection. When the patient has an elevated temperature, the nurse obtains specimens for culture. Specimens of urine, blood, sputum, and any obvious wound drainage will be collected and sent to the laboratory. If neurologic

symptoms are present, cerebrospinal fluid may be collected by spinal tap for culture. Antimicrobial drugs are used when infection is present. It is important for the nurse to administer these drugs on time. If a dose is delayed, serum drug levels will decrease and lead to rapid overgrowth of the microorganism or increased drug resistance.

In addition to treating existing infections, the nurse implements interventions to decrease the patient's exposure to pathogens. Handwashing and universal precautions are of major importance for the patient with white blood cell dysfunction. If hospitalization is required for the patient, the nurse arranges for a private room to decrease the patient's exposure to additional pathogens. Skin integrity is maintained with attention to bathing and the use of emollients to prevent the skin from drying and cracking. The nurse encourages the patient to use a soft toothbrush and nonabrasive toothpaste for oral hygiene. If changes in the oral mucosa occur such as redness, pain, or ulcerations, the nurse alters the interventions for oral care (see Chapter 15).

Preventing other sources of infection includes interventions such as pulmonary hygiene, administration of stool softeners or antidiarrheals to decrease trauma to gastrointestinal mucosa, adequate fluid in-

TABLE 38-11   Nursing Intervention Summary: Multiple Myeloma

Intervention	Rationale
Hydration	Hypercalcemia can lead to renal failure; dehydration can be lethal; do *not* keep a patient NPO
Prevention of infection	Persons are susceptible to infections, especially pneumonia; infections are leading cause of death
Ambulation	Immobility can lead to further bone destruction, increased hypercalcemia, and pneumonia
Pain relief	Pain can immobilize a person and cause undue suffering
Safety	Bone fractures can occur as a result of bone destruction; care in touching patient may avoid fractures
Provide independence	Loss of control over mobility, comfort occur; disease may be out of control; pain and side effects of treatment; allow decision making and participation in procedures through choices and patient teaching

take to promote urine output, and avoiding the use of suppositories and catheters. When invasive catheters or intravenous lines are necessary, the nurse implements agency policies for the care of those lines to prevent infection.

A summary of interventions specifically for the patient with multiple myeloma is presented in Table 38-11. Also refer to the Nursing Care Plan on p. 986.

Evaluation

Successful patient response to the plan will be indicated by prevention of infection or resolution of infectious episodes. The patient should demonstrate normal body temperature and absence of inflammation, purulent drainage, tenderness, and redness. Laboratory and x-ray findings will return to or remain within normal limits. The patient or caregiver will be able to demonstrate or verbalize measures to prevent infection. In the profoundly leukopenic (WBC<100) patient, infections will likely occur in spite of meticulous care. A positive outcome in this case is the prompt detection and quick intervention to avoid potentially overwhelming sepsis.

Documentation

The nurse documents findings from the history and physical, with emphasis on indications of infection. The patient's response to interventions and indications that infection is resolving or worsening are included as part of documentation. When the patient/family is learning to administer chemotherapy in the home, documentation of each teaching episode is critical. The nurse documents topics taught, teaching materials used, and the patient's/family's verbal understanding or return demonstration of skills, reflecting any barriers to learning and plans to overcome those barriers.

Ongoing Care

Successful patient adaptation to a WBC disorder depends on a thorough understanding of the disease and its treatment. A patient's life quite literally rests on his or her ability to detect infection and promptly seek assistance. Many disorders require the administration of chemotherapeutic agents, many of which can be given in an ambulatory setting. The implications for thorough patient education become even greater. Many regimens require intensive patient participation in the home setting. Patients may be required to closely monitor intake and output, maintain vigorous hydration, self-administer antiemetics, and monitor urine pH, to name a few. Family support and understanding of the regimens is vital for success. Occasionally, a patient may be eligible to

mix and administer his or her own chemotherapy in the home setting. Patient/family education then must include drug-reconstitution techniques, precautions for handling cytotoxic agents, drug-administering techniques, intravenous catheter care, and guidelines for monitoring early and late side effects. In some cases many patients can master drug administration via small-volume administration pumps as well. If the patient prefers home administration but is unable to self-administer, many private agencies are available to provide this complete service. Opting for home administration provides a new avenue for decreasing the disruption that intensive and repetitive chemotherapy protocols cause the patient.

The unpredictable nature of WBC disorders leads to significant disruptions in daily patterns of living. The course of illness is frequently punctuated by acute episodes of life-threatening complications, such as sepsis or hemorrhage. Moreover, once the disease is controlled, persons then live with the continuous stress of potential recurrence. Repeated relapses and remissions may create a "roller-coaster" of emotions as the patient and family attempt to cope. Although cure is becoming more common in this area of cancer, the concept of "survivorship" becomes an accompanying theme. Intensive radiotherapy and chemotherapy can predispose patients to secondary complications many years after treatment. Significant renal impairment, cardiomyopathy, pulmonary fibrosis, and development of second malignancies are but a few complications. Clearly, successful long-term care requires a health care team skilled in the treatment of biologic, psychologic, and social sequelae of the diseases and associated treatments.

Disorders of Coagulation

THROMBOCYTOPENIA
Definition/Etiology

Thrombocytopenia is defined as a decrease in the number of circulating platelets. Although a wide range of etiologic factors can cause thrombocytopenia, these factors can be broadly categorized as follows: (1) decreased production of platelets in the bone marrow, (2) sequestration of circulating platelets by the spleen, and (3) abnormal destruction of circulating platelets.

Pathophysiology

A decrease in production of platelets indicates that the bone marrow is unable to effectively engage in thrombopoiesis.

Many factors can cause impairment of bone mar-

NURSING CARE PLAN *Patient with Leukemia*

Nursing diagnosis/ Expected outcomes	Interventions	Rationale
High risk for infection related to leukopenia •*Patient will remain free of infection* •*Patient will exhibit resolution or control of infection* •*Patient or caregiver will identify measures to prevent or control infection* •*Patient or caregiver will verbalize and report signs and symptoms of infection*	Inspect all body sites for infection at least daily; NOTE: report fever, sore throat, pus formation, chills, cough, burning with urination, redness, swelling, tenderness, pain, pain with defecation Monitor vital signs	Continual efforts must be made to identify potential site. Fever may be the only indication of infection in the patient because of lack of inflammatory response Fever accompanied by hypotension and tachycardia heralds septic shock. In early shock, blood pressure may be normal or slightly increased due to compensatory mechanisms
	Monitor WBC counts and culture reports	Decreasing WBC count is inversely proportional to risk and severity of infections; appropriateness of antibiotic therapy can be determined by positive culture reports
	Obtain cultures as ordered	Fever of unknown origin is much more difficult to treat due to risk of administering antibiotics that are not effective for the infecting organism.
	Administer antimicrobials on time as ordered	Delay may result in rapid overgrowth of organisms
	Promote and maintain hygiene integrity of skin and mucous membranes	These barriers provide the frontline of defense against infection
	Use aseptic technique in patient care treatments	Asepsis decreases exposure to microbes

	Teach the patient and family:
	  Role of the WBC in prevention
	  Effects of treatment on marrow function and immune system
	  Necessity of avoiding crowds/ patients with infections while WBC count <1,000
	  Technique for taking temperature and reading thermometer
	  Personal hygiene measures
	  Signs and symptoms of infection
		The patient can significantly reduce risk of infection, and if infection occurs can reduce complications by promptly reporting signs of infection

High risk for injury related to thrombocytopenia •*Patient will be free from bleeding* •*Patient will exhibit resolution or control of bleeding episodes* •*Patient or caregiver will demonstrate measures to prevent or control bleeding*	Monitor platelet counts Assess for bleeding Institute bleeding precautions Infuse platelets as prescribed Teach patient measures to prevent or control bleeding	Spontaneous hemorrhage may occur with platelet count <20,000 Protective measures can prevent further occurrences

From Division of Nursing Standards of Patient Care, The University of Texas M.D. Anderson Cancer Center, Houston.

NURSING CARE PLAN *Patient with Leukemia—cont'd*

Nursing diagnosis/ Expected outcomes	Interventions	Rationale
Impairment of mucous membrane integrity: stomatitis, related to chemotherapy, leukemia infiltrates, myelosuppression • *Patient will be free from stomatitis* • *Patient will exhibit resolution or control of stomatitis* • *Patient will demonstrate oral hygiene regimen* • *Patient or caregiver will verbalize symptoms to report* Activity intolerance related to anemia • *Patient will demonstrate self-care measures within functional capacity*	Assess oral cavity: note color, moisture, and presence and description of lesions Assess for signs of infection Implement oral hygiene regimen: salt rinses, dilute peroxide rinses, use of soft toothbrush or sponge-tipped applicator Encourage bland, nonirritating diet Use artificial saliva and lip lubricants for comfort Teach patient oral hygiene regimen, symptoms to report Monitor hemoglobin and hematocrit Assess for signs and symptoms of anemia Assess ability to perform self-care Promote frequent rest periods, and provide assistive devices to decrease energy expenditure Transfuse red blood cells as ordered Teach patient signs of anemia and measures to conserve energy	Oral impairment of mucous membranes provides portal for infection to enter; pain from stomatitis may significantly impact toxicity, nutritional intake Maximizing self-care measures will promote retention of self-esteem Transfusions can significantly reduce symptoms

Knowledge deficit related to diagnosis and treatment
 	
• *Patient demonstrates knowledge related to diagnosis of leukemia and prescribed treatments*
	Determine patient/caregiver learning needs and levels of knowledge related to leukemia disease process and prescribed therapy
	Assess patient/caregiver for barriers to learning related to:
	  Physical deficiencies/dysfunctions
	  Psychologic deficiencies/ dysfunctions (e.g., assess readiness to learn)
	  Verbal deficiencies/dysfunctions
	Provide written materials to reinforce teaching
	Initiate referrals to other health team members if necessary
	Repeat information as frequently as needed
	Evaluate response to teaching
	Teach signs/symptoms of disease process and side effects of treatment modalities
	Inform patient of resources available for health care, both in hospital and at home
	Teach symptoms that should be reported to a nurse or physician (e.g., elevated temperature, bleeding, nausea/vomiting, pain, drainage)
	Teach importance of proper nutrition and hydration
		An understanding of the disease and treatment will facilitate safe self-care

row function. Toxic drugs and chemicals, irradiation, and infection (including HIV infection) can all reduce ability to manufacture all types of blood cells, including platelets. A variety of neoplastic disorders such as leukemia, lymphoma, and metastatic cancer may also decrease platelet production. Disseminated tuberculosis and chronic alcohol abuse will also exert a similar suppressive effect on the marrow.

The second etiologic category is splenic sequestration of platelets. Splenomegaly, regardless of the cause, may lead to a thrombocytopenia because a shift in platelet availability occurs. Platelets circulate more slowly through an enlarged spleen, thus allowing more prolonged contact and subsequent adhesion to blood vessel walls. Although adequate numbers of platelets are produced by the bone marrow, a massively enlarged spleen may hold up to 90% of the total platelet mass.[33] Normally, only one third of the total platelet pool is found in the spleen.

The third etiologic category, abnormal destruction of platelets, causes thrombocytopenia when the rate of platelet destruction exceeds the rate of bone marrow production. Platelets can be destroyed by either immune or nonimmune processes. Immune destruction usually occurs when anti-platelet antibodies are produced in the body. This syndrome is termed idiopathic (immune) thrombocytopenic purpura. In this case, production of antiplatelet antibodies may be stimulated by bacterial infection, viral infection, chronic inflammatory disease (e.g., ulcerative colitis), leukemia, lymphoma, systemic lupus erythematosus, and HIV infection.[5] A variety of drugs may also stimulate an immune-modulated thrombocytopenia. The box summarizes common drugs implicated in thrombocytopenias.

Premature destruction of platelets can also be caused by nonimmune processes. Accelerated consumption of circulating platelets may be triggered by disseminated intravascular coagulation (DIC) [see section on DIC] or thrombotic thrombocytopenic purpura (TTP). TTP is a syndrome of abnormal platelet aggregation in the microvasculature. In other words, circulating platelets are stimulated to form clots; the clots cause ischemic damage and infarction in virtually any tissue or organ, although the central nervous system is particularly vulnerable. TTP is also accompanied by severe hemolytic anemia.

Although many theories have been suggested to explain the pathophysiology of TTP, this disorder is probably caused by the development of a substance that stimulates platelet aggregation.[20] Hemolysis of red blood cells may then be triggered as the cells attempt to flow through areas that are occluded by platelet plugs. Suggested stimulants that cause TTP include infection, pregnancy, immune disorders, HIV infection, and chemotherapy.[20]

DRUGS THAT MAY CONTRIBUTE TO THROMBOCYTOPENIA

Nonsteroidal antiinflammatory agents

Aspirin	Naproxen
Ibuprofen	Oxyphenbutazone
Indomethacin	Phenylbutazone

Antibiotics

Penicillins	Sulfonamides
Rifampicin	

Cinchona alkaloids

Quinine	Quinidine

Miscellaneous

Acetaminophen	Gold salts
Chlorothiazide	Heparin
Cimetidine	Heroin
Digitalis derivatives	Morphine
Diphenylhydantoin	Valproic acid
Furosemide	

Clinical Manifestations

Clinical manifestations of thrombocytopenia are all related to varying degrees of bleeding. The severity of signs and symptoms correlates with the platelet count. As the level drops below 150,000, the risk for bleeding from mucous membranes and into cutaneous sites and internal organs increases. Significant risk for serious bleeding occurs once the count is below 20,000. Clinical manifestations may include spontaneous petechiae and ecchymoses, prolonged bleeding from sites of invasive procedures, epistaxis, gingival bleeding, and gastrointestinal and genitourinary bleeding. Symptoms of organ dysfunction caused by bleeding are site specific. The central nervous system is at particular risk; indications may range from headache, confusion, disorientation, and visual changes to coma and death caused by massive hemorrhage.

Therapeutic Management

Management begins with a thorough history and physical examination. Bleeding tendencies, potential for genetic disorders, underlying immune disorders, recurrent infections or transfusions, and exposure to drugs and toxins must all be explored. Physical examination centers on signs and symptoms of bleeding and splenic size. Laboratory tests can then further pinpoint potential etiologic factors. Platelet count, bleeding time, complete blood count, and bone marrow aspiration and biopsy should be obtained. Platelet-associated immunoglobulin G (IgG) may be ordered if an immune-modulated mechanism is suspected.

Once the etiology is identified, treatment can be determined. Thrombocytopenia caused by decreased production of platelets in the bone marrow is treated by identifying and treating the underlying cause of the bone marrow dysfunction. For example, control of a malignancy, or recovery of marrow from the effects of chemotherapeutic drugs should allow for normalization of a platelet count. This approach is quite successful, provided the cancer is responsive to available treatments. Transfusion of donor platelets supports the patient during periods of extreme thrombocytopenia (platelet count less than 20,000) until the bone marrow can recover.

Thrombocytopenia secondary to splenomegaly is best reduced by treating the cause of the enlarged spleen. Splenic irradiation may provide some relief, especially in leukemia and lymphoma. Although unusual, splenectomy may be indicated if the surgical risk is acceptable, the spleen is the principal cause of the thrombocytopenia, and symptoms cannot be otherwise medically controlled. Short-term complications of splenectomy include infection, bleeding, and thromboembolism; a long-term effect is potential for overwhelming infection.[33]

Thrombocytopenia due to ITP is treated by a variety of approaches. If the precipitant can be identified, treatment or discontinuation of the precipitant may be sufficient treatment. For example, if the ITP is caused by a bacterial infection, control of that infection via antibiotic therapy is desirable. Likewise, if a medication such as quinidine is causing the ITP, discontinuation of the drug and substitution of another appropriate antiarrhythmic is the correct approach. In this case, the thrombocytopenia usually resolves within days.[33] Glucocorticosteroids are also used to treat many immune-modulated thrombocytopenias. This approach increases the platelet count by decreasing the antiplatelet antibody production; however, this approach may take from several days to several weeks to take effect. Plasmapheresis and plasma exchange have been used with some success in the treatment of both ITP and TTP. This technique physically extracts the circulating immune complexes. In TTP, treatment may need to be administered for a period of 3 to 4 weeks before a complete response is seen.[20]

High dose intravenous immunoglobulin (IVIG) therapy shows much promise for the treatment of ITP. The mechanism of action appears to be interference with cell receptors that are responsible for destroying platelets. Approximately 50% of patients will respond to high dose IVIG (1 g/kg/day IV infusion for 2 to 3 days followed by a maintenance dose every 3 to 4 weeks).[23] The major risk associated with IVIG is anaphylaxis. Patients are typically premedi-

cated with diphenhydramine and acetaminophen; resuscitation equipment should also be close by. Patients must be monitored closely for headache, chills, fever, nausea, restlessness, flushing, abdominal pain, joint pain, wheezing, shortness of breath, and changes in vital signs. Treatment of anaphylaxis follows standard resuscitation principles.

THROMBOCYTOSIS
Definition/Etiology

An increased number of circulating platelets is termed **thrombocytosis.** Platelet counts may go as high as several million and cause problems of thrombosis and bleeding. Thrombocytosis is categorized as reactive or essential. Reactive elevations are caused by a hyperactive bone marrow response in other conditions such as malignancies, inflammation, hemolysis, splenectomy, hemorrhage, or iron deficiency. An essential thrombocytosis is a type of myeloproliferative syndrome and is often termed essential or autonomous thrombocythemia. Abnormal platelet structure and function occur accompanied by extremely high platelet counts, massive thrombosis, and significant bleeding.[44]

Clinical Manifestations

Clinical manifestations of bleeding are similar to those of thrombocytopenia and are caused by the platelets' inability to function normally. Problems of disseminated thrombosis may occur in both the venous and arterial systems and manifest as erythema, cyanosis, or pregangrenous changes.[13]

Therapeutic Management

Management is based on control of the underlying cause. Thrombocythemia can be treated with myelosuppressive drugs, such as busulfan or hydroxyurea. Plasmapheresis to reduce the platelet mass and antiplatelet drugs (such as aspirin) may also be helpful.

HEMOPHILIA
Definition

Hemophilia is an inherited disorder of the clotting mechanism. It is estimated that approximately 20,000 persons in the United States have hemophilia.[18] Two major types exist: hemophilia A (classic), which is the most common type, and hemophilia B, also known as Christmas disease.

Etiology/Epidemiology

Hemophilia A represents 85% of the total incidence. It is a deficiency of factor VIII activity, which may

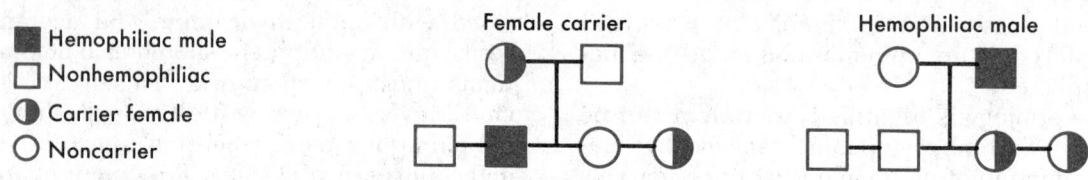

■ Hemophiliac male
□ Nonhemophiliac
◑ Carrier female
○ Noncarrier

Female carrier   Hemophiliac male

FIGURE 38-2   Inheritance patterns in hemophilia.

occur in varying degrees. Hemophilia B is characterized by a deficiency in factor IX activity. Both have indistinguishable patterns of genetic transmission and clinical manifestations. Hemophilia is an X-linked recessive disorder and therefore occurs almost exclusively in males (Figure 38-2). Female carriers can transmit the defective chromosome to both sons and daughters. Sons who inherit the gene develop hemophilia; daughters who inherit the gene become carriers. Genetic transformation does occur spontaneously independently of family history and accounts for as many as one-third of all cases.[18] The resultant clotting disorder results from defective or diminished factor VIII (or IX) production. Etiology remains unknown.

Clinical classification stems from the severity of inactivity:[53]

- Severe hemophilia—clotting factor activity < 1% of normal
- Moderate hemophilia—clotting factor activity is 1% to 5% of normal
- Mild hemophilia—clotting factor activity > 5% of normal

The severity of bleeding directly correlates with the degree of coagulant inactivity. Thus patients with severe hemophilia tend to experience both spontaneous bleeding and severe bleeding with trauma. Conversely, patients with mild hemophilia may only experience excessive bleeding with trauma or surgical procedures.[18]

Clinical Manifestations

Spontaneous bleeding episodes throughout life occur in severe hemophilia. Areas of mechanical stress or trauma are particularly at risk and include musculoskeletal sites (such as joints) and skin. Excessive bleeding after circumcision typically warrants suspicion of hemophilia. **Hemarthrosis,** or bleeding into a joint space, is a hallmark of severe disease and usually occurs in the knees, ankles, and elbows. Pain, swelling, redness, and fever accompany hemarthrosis. Over time, repeated episodes lead to joint destruction and loss of motion. Hematomas also develop and may cause tissue damage and neuropathies from decreased blood flow. In moderate or mild hemophilia, abnormal bleeding more characteristically occurs after dental or surgical proce-

dures. Although hemarthroses can develop, they rarely lead to the crippling, destructive process that characterizes severe hemophilia.

Before the appearance of the HIV virus, the average life span of the person with hemophilia was near normal.[3] Although estimates of prevalence of HIV in the hemophiliac population vary widely, the majority of severe hemophiliacs who had received clotting factor concentrates before 1984 are seropositive for HIV.[8] Now, with the development of methods to heat inactivate the virus, the risk of contracting HIV from clotting factor concentrates is almost nil.

Therapeutic Management

Although a careful family history is indicated in the presence of severe, spontaneous bleeding, laboratory testing will confirm the diagnosis. Quantitative assays for factors VIII and IX will determine the type and severity of disease. Deficiency of factor IX denotes hemophilia B; factor VIII deficiency must be further explored to differentiate between hemophilia A and von Willebrand's disease, an inherited vascular disorder of factor VIII secretion. Coagulation profiles reveal a normal platelet count, bleeding time, and prothrombin time (PT). The activated partial thromboplastin time (APTT) will be prolonged.

The immediate focus of medical therapy is to halt the bleeding. Transfusion of clotting factor concentrates is the mainstay of treatment. Two different products that are both made from human plasma can be used. One, cryoprecipitate, is a clotting factor concentrate rich in factor VIII. Its use is waning due to the risk, albeit small, of viral disease transmission. Additionally, home administration of cryoprecipitate is difficult because of the need to store it at low temperatures. The second human-derived product, factor VIII concentrates, is most typically used. A wide variety of products of this type are available, and are all freeze-dried concentrates of factor VIII prepared from pooled plasma from thousands of donors. These products are specially treated to inactivate any viral contamination (such as HIV or hepatitis viruses). Factor IX concentrates are also available and prepared in a similar fashion.

Because human plasma products still carry a very slight risk of infection transmission and require availability of human donors, scientists have used genetic engineering to manufacture factor VIII. This product, termed "recombinant factor VIII," is potentially advantageous because of viral safety, unlimited supply, and lower cost.[18] Recombinant factor VIII should soon become commercially available for widespread use.

Desmopressin (DDAVP) is the treatment of choice in mild hemophilia.[18] This drug is a synthetic analog of the human antidiuretic hormone, vasopressin. It acts by causing an increase in factor VIII release from storage sites in the body. Desmopressin is often administered prophylactically to mild hemophiliacs who require surgery or dental extractions. The recommended dose is 0.3 μg/kg/dose, given IV.[17] Because desmopressin is a potent antidiuretic, the patient's fluid balance and electrolytes must be monitored closely postoperatively. Although rare, hyponatremia and water overload leading to convulsions can occur.[17]

Other supportive care measures include pain management, surgical correction of musculoskeletal complications (e.g., synovectomy, joint debridement, arthroplasty), and genetic counseling. Implications for patient/family teaching include factor replacement in the home setting, management of bleeding, and impact on growth and development of both the individual and family.

DISSEMINATED INTRAVASCULAR COAGULATION
Definition

Disseminated intravascular coagulation (DIC) is an acquired syndrome of clotting cascade overstimulation. Not a disease unto itself, DIC may be triggered by a wide variety of underlying pathologic processes. DIC is also termed consumption coagulopathy, defibrination syndrome, and intravascular coagulation with fibrinolysis.

Etiology/Epidemiology

The incidence of DIC remains unknown because of the varying degrees of clinical severity. Etiologic factors, however, have been well identified; the box summarizes the most common factors. Obstetric complications liberate tissue factor into the maternal bloodstream in a number of ways. A classic example is that of abruptio placentae (premature detachment of the placenta). Placental tissue and amniotic fluid are rich in substances that provide strong stimuli for the clotting cascade. Many neoplastic disorders are also known for their ability to overstimulate coagulation by releasing procoagulant factors. Initiation of chemotherapy or radiation therapy may accelerate DIC as cells are destroyed and factors released at an even faster rate.

PRECIPITATING CAUSES OF DIC

A. Obstetric
1. Abruptio placentae
2. Retained dead fetus
3. Amniotic fluid embolism
4. Retained placenta
5. Toxemia
6. Hydatidiform mole
7. Acute fatty liver of pregnancy

B. Neoplastic
1. Carcinomas
2. Acute leukemias
3. Giant cavernous hemangioma
4. Adenocarcinomas
5. Sarcomas
6. Polycythemia vera
7. Pheochromocytoma

C. Hematologic
1. Blood transfusion reaction
2. Sickle cell crisis
3. Thalassemia major

D. Trauma
1. Burns
2. Multiple injury
3. Transplant rejection
4. Surgery—particularly if extracorporeal circulation was used
5. Heat stroke
6. Fat emboli
7. Snake bite
8. Aspirin poisoning

E. Other
1. Acute infectious process/sepsis
2. Hepatitis
3. Glomerulonephritis
4. Purpura
5. Cirrhosis
6. Shock
7. Necrotizing enterocolitis
8. Systemic lupus erythematosis
9. Anaphylaxis

From Young LM: DIC: The insidious killer. *Crit Care Nurs* 10(9):27, 1990.

Localized vascular impairment, such as in a dissecting aortic aneurysm or giant hemangioma, causes endothelial damage or abnormalities that precipitate rapid consumption of clotting factors and platelets.

Although almost every type of infectious agent has

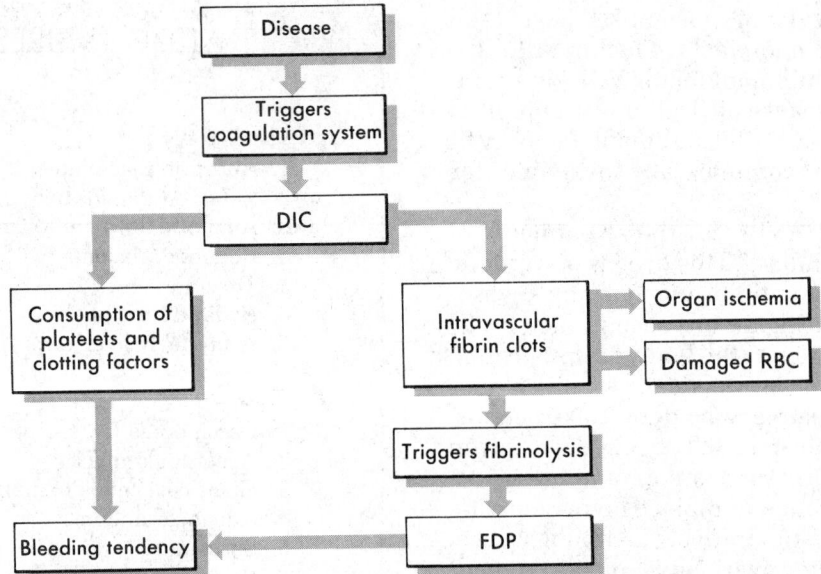

FIGURE 38-3 Disseminated intravascular coagulation. Rapid consumption of clotting factors by multiple microemboli predisposes the patient to bleeding problems. (Used with permission from Griffin JP: *Hematology and immunology: concepts for nursing,* Norwalk, Conn, 1986, Appleton & Lange.)

been implicated in the development of DIC, gram-negative bacteremia is probably the most common cause. Release of endotoxins in disseminated sepsis leads to widespread vascular damage, stimulation of factor XII, and platelet destruction.

Pathophysiology

In DIC, the pace of the clotting cascade is rapidly accelerated to the point of exhaustion. Precipitants of the syndrome abnormally stimulate the production of thrombin, with a resultant rapid conversion of fibrinogen to fibrin threads. Subsequent dissemination (of the threads) throughout the bloodstream then leads to aggregation of platelets and formation of multiple, microscopic emboli. The fibrinolytic system is activated in an attempt to lyse the emboli, causing a reactive rise in fibrin split products (FSPs). Although the disseminated emboli disrupt blood flow via capillary infarcts, the patient will also have problems with bleeding. Formation of multiple microemboli requires the rapid overconsumption of clotting factors and platelets (Figure 38-3). Thus the patient cannot form a stable clot even in response to only minimal trauma, because of inadequate reserves of these key ingredients. In short, the demand for clotting factors exceeds the supply, and hemorrhage results.

Clinical Manifestations

Disseminated thrombosis and bleeding form the basis for clinical symptoms (see Table 38-12). In acute DIC, clinical problems tend to develop rapidly, becoming evident within a few hours to a day. Bleeding may be mild at first but can soon progress to multisite, serious hemorrhage. Prolonged oozing from sites of minor trauma, such as venipuncture, is often the first indication of DIC. Wounds and invasive catheter sites may ooze spontaneously. Patients with DIC typically bleed from at least three unrelated sites; the patient with ecchymoses, hematuria, and hematemesis is an example of this phenomenon.[38]

Thrombosis occurs less commonly than bleeding but causes serious damage nevertheless. Systems most often affected by circulating microemboli are the cardiac, pulmonary, renal, and central nervous systems.[38] Resultant organ ischemia and dysfunction may be caused by a combined effect of infarcts and bleeding.

Therapeutic Management

Diagnostic findings are summarized in Table 38-13. Test results that measure raw materials necessary for normal coagulation, such as clotting factors, platelets, and fibrinogen, tend to be decreased because of rapid consumption. Decreased circulating clotting factors also cause prolonged values for prothrombin time (PT), partial thromboplastin time (PTT), and thrombin time (TT). Fibrin split products (FSP) rise because of plasmin-activated destruction of circulating emboli.

Schistocytes (red blood cell fragments) may be detected when a complete blood count is done. These reflect the cell lysis that may occur as circu-

TABLE 38-12   Clinical Manifestations of DIC

System	Characteristics
General	Fever, hypotension, acidosis, proteinuria
Skin/mucous membranes	Petechiae, purpura, ecchymoses, hematomas, acral cyanosis, conjunctival hemorrhage, bleeding from puncture and wound sites, epistaxis, bleeding gums
Gastrointestinal	Hematemesis, abdominal pain, abdominal distention, guaiac-positive stools, melena
Central nervous system	Headache, vertigo, decrease in level of consciousness, disorientation, irritability, sensorimotor changes, visual changes
Pulmonary	Hypoxia, tachypnea, hemoptysis, rales, cyanosis
Genitourinary	Hematuria, oliguria, vaginal bleeding

From Volker DL: Challenge of disseminated intravascular coagulation, *Dimens Oncol Nurs* 5(2):28, 1991.

TABLE 38-13   DIC Diagnostic Findings

Test	Finding
Prothrombin time	Increased
Partial thromboplastin time	Increased
Thrombin time	Increased
Fibrinogen	Decreased
Platelets	Decreased
Fibrin split products	Increased
D dimer	Increased
Schistocytes	Present
Reticulocytosis	Present

Adapted from Volker DL: Challenge of disseminated intravascular coagulation, *Dimens Oncol Nurs* 5(2):28, 1991.

lating red blood cells attempt to squeeze through the meshwork of fibrin threads. Reticulocytes (immature red blood cells) may also be seen. This represents a reaction by the bone marrow to increase the production of red cells prior to full maturation. A newer diagnostic test, D dimer, is often used in conjunction with the other tests to confirm the diagnosis of DIC. D dimer is a type of fibrin split product that is generated by clot lysis. No single test is particularly diagnostic for DIC; relative trends must be evaluated in conjunction with clinical findings. In subacute or chronic DIC, all laboratory values may be near normal because of the body's ability to compensate by rapidly replacing clotting components.

Treatment is fourfold, including treatment of the precipitating cause, blood component and factor replacement, therapy to control emboli formation, and antifibrinolytic agents. Therapy for the underlying cause is paramount; all other measures are futile unless the precipitant is removed or controlled. Specific treatment depends on the primary disease, i.e., antibiotics for gram-negative sepsis, chemotherapy for leukemia, and so forth. Transfusion therapy consists of platelets and packed red blood cells to replace those consumed or lost and cryoprecipitate or fresh-frozen plasma to replenish clotting factor levels. Heparin therapy will block the subsequent formation of microemboli by inhibiting thrombin activ-

ity. It has no effect, however, on existing clots. The goal underlying the administration of heparin is to stop the rapid overproduction of microemboli and thus allow for reperfusion of vital organs and replenishment of clotting factor supplies. The major hazard is an increased risk of hemorrhage. In rare instances, the fourth approach, antifibrinolytic therapy, may be necessary. Epsilon-aminocaproic acid (EACA) inhibits plasmin activity, thus disrupting fibrinolysis. The rationale for EACA is to prevent bleeding by protecting therapeutic clots and to prevent accumulation of FSPs. Disseminated thrombosis is a major hazard of antifibrinolytic therapy; thus it is typically begun only after emboli formation has been controlled by heparin. Mortality in DIC varies because of the vast numbers of precipitants and the varying degrees of severity. Death is usually a result of either uncontrolled hemorrhage or irreversible end organ damage or both.

VITAMIN K DEFICIENCY
Definition

Vitamin K deficiencies are disorders of either intake or absorption of vitamin K. Vitamin K is a fat-soluble vitamin necessary for the formation of several clotting factors. Thus, vitamin K disorders or deficiencies may result in coagulation defects. Both dietary intake and bacterial synthesis in the gastrointestinal tract provide body stores of vitamin K. Leafy, green vegetables, cheese, bacon, liver, butter, and coffee are a few food sources rich in vitamin K. Bacteria, such as *Bacteroides* and *Peptostreptococcus,* found in normal gut flora also synthesize the vitamin. Absorption takes place in the small intestine.[54]

Etiology

Vitamin K deficiency usually occurs as a result of insufficient dietary intake, malabsorption, or drug interactions. Malnutrition and parenteral nutrition without concurrent vitamin K supplementation are major causes of insufficient intake. Additionally, newborns require supplementation because of the time lag before bacterial colonization of the gut. Disorders that interfere with fat absorption will impair vitamin K absorption as well. Examples include obstructive jaundice, sprue, inflammatory bowel disease, chronic diarrhea, and pancreatitis.[54] Certain drug interactions induce a vitamin K deficiency. Antibiotics (especially cephalosporins) suppress normal gastrointestinal flora, resulting in a decrease in microbial production of vitamin K. Antibiotic therapy coupled with either poor dietary intake or a malabsorption syndrome is the most common setting for a vitamin K deficiency to occur.[54] Coumadin anticoagulant therapy may also be a precipitant, because this therapy inhibits vitamin K function.[24]

Pathophysiology

Regardless of etiology, the result of this deficiency is impaired generation of thrombin because of a deficiency in production of vitamin K-dependent clotting factors.

Clinical Manifestations

Bleeding from varying sites may occur, depending on the severity and type of deficiency present. Gastrointestinal hemorrhage is the most common manifestation, with hemarthrosis and bleeding after dental procedures the least likely events.[54]

Therapeutic Management

Vitamin K deficiency results in the following laboratory profile of a prolonged PT, prolonged PTT, and normal thrombin time. Ultimately, confirmation of the diagnosis may come only after the successful administration of a vitamin K supplement. Subsequent correction of laboratory values and clinical manifestations will then occur. Vitamin K may be administered both orally and parenterally. Intravenous vitamin K (Aquamephyton) is administered as a one time 10 to 15 mg dose. Or, oral daily doses of 100 to 150 mg may be given until the prothrombin time normalizes. In the event of serious bleeding, fresh-frozen plasma can be infused so that vitamin K-dependent clotting factors can be rapidly replaced.

NURSING MANAGEMENT OF THE PATIENT WITH A COAGULATION DISORDER
Assessment

Assessment of the patient with a coagulation disorder begins with a careful history to determine po-

tential precipitants and patterns of bleeding. Complaints of easy bruising and prolonged or unusual bleeding are noted by the nurse. Because bleeding problems in adults are often caused by drug effects on coagulation, the nurse inquires about any family history of bleeding, and obtains a medication profile for medications that interfere with platelet function, such as nonsteroidal antiinflammatory agents containing aspirin or phenylakanoic acid.[53]

Physical assessment focuses on manifestations of abnormal bleeding and clotting. Changes in skin and mucous membranes include petechia, purpura, acrocyanosis, conjunctival hemorrhage, bleeding from puncture and wound sites, hematomas, epistaxis, and bleeding gums. Hematemesis, abdominal pain, abdominal distention or fullness, guaiac-positive stools, and melena may all indicate gastrointestinal bleeding. Central nervous system changes are particularly important, because bleeding may progress rapidly. Symptoms resemble those of a patient suffering a transient ischemic attack (TIA) or stroke. The presence of headache, vertigo, decrease in level of consciousness, disorientation, irritability, sensorimotor changes, or visual changes are of major importance. Signs of pulmonary bleeding include tachypnea, dyspnea, hemoptysis, rales, and cyanosis. Genitourinary bleeding may be evidenced by hematuria, oliguria, vaginal bleeding, bladder distention, or inability to void.

Nursing Diagnosis

The primary nursing diagnosis for the person with a bleeding disorder is high risk for injury related to a coagulopathy. Other nursing diagnoses include
   Ineffective airway clearance related to bleeding from oronasopharynx
   Decreased cardiac output related to hemorrhage-induced hypovolemia
   Impaired gas exchange related to pulmonary bleeding
   Altered growth and development related to illness and hospitalizations
   Knowledge deficit related to disease and treatment
   Impaired physical mobility related to joint damage induced by hemarthrosis
   Altered tissue perfusion (systemic) related to ischemia and necrosis induced by microemboli and decreased circulating blood volume

Planning

The plan of care is developed with the following goals in mind: the patient will remain free from bleeding, or will exhibit resolution or control of bleeding episodes. An associated goal is that the patient/caregiver can demonstrate knowledge related to the prevention and control of bleeding.

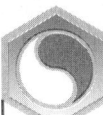

ETHICAL ISSUES

- How should a nurse respond when a man who is hemorrhaging begs her not to administer blood to him because he fears everlasting damnation according to religious beliefs that forbid receiving transfusions?
- What if this same patient discussed his beliefs with the nurse prior to any acute bleeding episode?
- What if this patient were a pregnant woman?

PATIENT EDUCATION GUIDE
Coagulation Disorders

Teach to recognize and report signs and symptoms of bleeding
Bleeding gums, nose
Bruising or petechiae
Blood in urine, stool, or emesis
Excessive bleeding after trauma
Change in mental status
Teach protective measures
Maintain safe environment
Avoid trauma and excessive or vigorous activity or exercise
Avoid medications containing aspirin
Bleeding precautions if indicated
Teach information regarding the nature of the specific disorder and treatment

Implementation

Interventions for the patient with a coagulation disorder include reviewing the laboratory data, noting abnormalities in platelet count, bleeding time, hemoglobin, hematocrit, red blood cell count, and the coagulation profile. Fluid intake and output are monitored, noting the appearance of urine and frequency of voiding. Bladder distention may indicate urethral obstruction by clots. Bladder irrigation via three-way Foley catheter may be ordered. Orthostatic changes in blood pressure may be the earliest indication of a fluid volume deficit. The nurse monitors vital signs for clinical manifestations of hypovolemia. Blood products and other intravenous fluids may be administered to maintain circulatory volume. When the patient is receiving platelets or other clotting factors, the nurse carefully monitors the patient for signs of transfusion reactions (see Table 38-16).

If gastrointestinal bleeding is present, cool lavage via nasogastric tube may be indicated. Antacids, antiemetics, and stool softeners may be administered to decrease trauma to the gastrointestinal mucosa that can cause bleeding. If pulmonary bleeding is present, the nurse maintains a patent airway and notifies the physician immediately. The patient is positioned to prevent aspiration and gently suctioned using a soft catheter. The nurse administers oxygen and assists with intubation. If vaginal bleeding is present, the nurse records the number of sanitary pads soiled by the patient and provides perineal care as needed. It is important to notify the physician immediately of any indications of central nervous system bleeding. The nurse monitors neurologic signs and raises the head of the bed to decrease intracranial pressure. The nurse maintains a patent intravenous line and administers steroids, diuretics, and anticonvulsants as ordered.

If oral bleeding is present, the nurse institutes cool saline rinses. If the source of bleeding is identified, direct pressure is applied to the area with moistened gauze. Topical thrombin is applied as ordered. The patient is placed on bleeding precautions. Skin integrity is promoted with use of emollients, an egg-crate or water mattress, or other assistive devices. It is important to maintain a safe environment to avoid traumatic injury to the patient.

The nurse provides the patient or caregiver with information on self-care measures, such as teaching how to recognize signs and symptoms of bleeding (see patient education guide).

Evaluation

Successful patient response to the plan will be indicated by prevention of bleeding or resolution of hemorrhagic episodes. Laboratory values will return to or remain within normal limits. The patient/caregiver will be able to demonstrate or verbalize measures to prevent and control bleeding.

Documentation

Document the findings of the history and physical examination with special note of indications of bleeding. Include the patient's response to your interventions and evidence of resolution of bleeding. The patient and family will likely need to learn to administer clotting replacement therapy at home. Document teaching sessions, including topics taught, teaching materials used, and evidence of learning. Documentation of return demonstrations of critical skills is essential.

Ongoing Care

Even though most coagulation disorders are short-term, singular events, chronic disorders such as he-

CLINICAL ALERT

Bleeding precautions are indicated for the patient with a severe coagulation disorder. Suggested measures include:

Prolonged direct pressure at venipuncture and invasive procedure sites

No intramuscular injections

No vaginal tampons or suppositories

No rectal suppositories or enemas

Oral hygiene with soft, sponge-tipped applicators

No straight-edged razors; electric razors only

Extreme caution during manicure or pedicure

Avoidance of aspirin-containing substances

mophilia require patient and family adaptation to a wide spectrum of potential problems. Comprehensive hemophilia programs developed in the 1970s have indeed served as models for success in continuity of care. These state and federally funded programs call for a multidisciplinary team approach to ambulatory care of the hemophilia patient and family. They assist in the management of the many medical, dental, vocational, and emotional problems that accompany the disease. Such an approach has resulted in significant decreases in time lost from school or work, number and length of hospital admissions, and total health care costs. Improvement in quality of life is the ultimate goal.

Regardless of the mechanisms of care, several key components must be included in the ambulatory care setting. Instruction in home administration of factor clotting replacement therapy is vital. The ability to administer replacement therapy promptly at home results in less damage related to bleeding and fosters a greater sense of well-being because of increased control and less disruption of family activities. Programs should also include counseling services for both the patient and family. Because hemophilia is a genetic disease passed by the mother, maternal feelings of guilt, fear, anxiety, and overprotectiveness may prevail. Siblings may become resentful of the attention and disruption that accompany a chronic illness. The patient will need assistance coping with self-administration of replacement factor, activity limitations, chronic pain, and potentially long absences from work or school. Ideally, vocational counseling should be available as well. Genetic counseling may become necessary if the parents wish to have more children. Support groups, such as those provided by chapters of the National Hemophilia Foundation, may also be suggested.

Special Treatment Considerations

TRANSFUSION THERAPY

Most patients with hematologic disorders undergo transfusion therapy during the course of illness. Although fraught with potential hazards, transfusion therapy is a safe, effective means of replacing deficient or dysfunctional blood components.

Donors and Donation

Blood banks depend on donors as the source of blood products for the patients. Meticulous screening techniques are employed to avoid potential complications to the donor to ensure a safe blood supply for the public. A brief health history and vital sign check are obtained before donation. The history focuses on detection of any diseases that could be transmitted via the donated blood and on medical conditions that could endanger the donor if he or she were to donate. Specific criteria for blood donor eligibility is summarized in the box. Adverse reactions during donation are unusual but may occur. A slight reaction is defined as a shocklike syndrome without loss of consciousness. The donor may feel dizzy, diaphoretic, or nauseous. Hyperventilation may be present. This may progress to a moderate reaction, in which loss of consciousness may occur. In a severe reaction, seizure activity, cyanosis, and incontinence are likely. Although vasovagal mechanisms caused by a reduction in circulating blood volume may precipitate a reaction, psychologic factors, such as anxiety, are strongly implicated. The donor may also experience a hematoma at the venipuncture site.

Processing

Once the donation is completed, processing of the blood begins. Serologic testing includes ABO group, Rh type, antibody screening, syphilis serology, and determination of hepatitis B surface antigens and human immunodeficiency virus antigens.

The four blood groups in the ABO system of blood typing are A, B, AB, and O. The system is based on the presence (or absence) of antigens (A and B) in red-cell surface membranes and antibodies (anti-A and anti-B) in the serum. For example, a person with type A blood has A surface antigens and anti-B antibodies. Table 38-14 summarizes the characteristics of each type. Persons with type O are known as "universal donors" because their red cells have no antigens that could interact with antibodies in the recipient's blood. Conversely, type AB persons are termed "universal recipients" because their blood contains no antibodies that interact with antigens on red cells from donated blood. After serologic test-

WHO CAN DONATE BLOOD?

Before giving blood, potential donors are given the information they need to decide whether they are eligible, based on the regularly updated criteria established by the FDA and the American Association of Blood Banks. Blood-collection staff review these donor requirements with potential donors. Nonregulated eligibility factors may vary slightly among blood centers but, in general, donors must be at least 17 years old, in good health, and must weigh at least 110 pounds. In many blood centers, people over 65 years can also donate if they are in good health.

Some conditions may warrant temporary deferral from donation, such as colds, flu, and therapy with certain drugs, but the following groups are **permanently** ineligible as homologous blood donors:

- People who have AIDS or symptoms of AIDS or who have ever tested positive for AIDS or for the AIDS virus.
- Men who have had sex with another man since 1977—even just one time.
- Men and women who have ever taken illegal drugs by needle—even just one time.
- Men and women who have had sex with a prostitute in the last 12 months.
- People who have had sex with anyone described above.
- People who have ever had hepatitis.
- People who have a history of certain types of cancer (other than minor skin cancer).
- People who have hemophilia or who have received clotting-factor concentrates.

From National Blood Resource Education Program's Nursing Education Working Group: Transfusion nursing: Trends and practices for the '90s, *Am J Nurs* 91(6):51, 1991.

ing, the blood may then be separated into various components. Table 38-15 summarizes the characteristics of each component and indications for use.

Administration

Although each agency has its own procedure for transfusing blood components, certain key steps must be consistently followed. Proper identification of both the blood product and the recipient must be validated by at least two registered nurses. In addition to verifying patient identification by checking the hospital wristband, the nurse must ask the patient to spell his name. The blood component bag label, compatibility tag, and patient's medical record must all be checked to verify correct component, ABO and Rh type and compatibility, and expiration date. Clarify any discrepancy noted. The patient's vi-

TABLE 38-14   Blood Types

Blood type	Red cell antigens	Antibodies
A	A	Anti-B
B	B	Anti-A
AB	A,B	None
O	None	Anti-A, Anti-B

tal signs should be noted before, during, and after the transfusion is completed. Throughout the procedure, pay particular attention to symptoms of an adverse reaction. Be sure to document the date, time, venipuncture site, amount and type of component transfused, and your assessments.

Transfusion Reactions

During the transfusion, pay particular attention to symptoms of an adverse reaction. Potential transfusion reactions, including symptoms, treatment, and prevention are summarized in Table 38-16. Although adverse reactions are unusual, the nurse must recognize and respond to them immediately. Management of a transfusion reaction is summarized in the box on p. 1002.

Infection Risk

If a blood donor has active infection at the time of donation, it is possible for that infection to be subsequently transmitted to the recipient of the blood product. The two major infections of concern are human immunodeficiency (HIV) and hepatitis.

In order to ensure a safe blood supply, donors are meticulously screened for signs and symptoms of infection, or history of high risk behaviors (unsafe sex, intravenous drug use). Additionally, the Food and Drug Administration (FDA) requires that all donated blood be tested for the presence of antibody to HIV, and hepatitis B surface antigen (HBsAg). Many blood centers also test for the presence of other antibodies for infections such as hepatitis C (anti-HCV) and T-cell lymphotrophic virus, type I (anti-HTLV-I).[21] These testing and screening procedures provide a very safe blood supply in the United States. There remains, however, a slight risk of infection transmission because of the difference in time between infection and development of antibodies. Theoretically, a donor could donate blood while actively infected, but before antibodies to that infection had been developed. The risk for HIV infection from transfusion of screened blood is approximately 1 in every 60,000 units, which is about a 0.0017% incidence.[22]

| TABLE 38-15 | Blood Component Summary | |

Product	Description	Storage (°C)
Whole blood	All the components of 450 mL donor blood plus the anticoagulant	1-6
Red blood cells	CPD, CPDA-1: whole blood with 200-250 mL plasma removed; final volume is ~300 mL, Hct <80% AS: whole blood with most plasma removed and 100 mL preservative added; final volume is ~350 mL, Hct 55-65%	1-6
Red blood cells, leukocytes removed	RBCs modified by centrifugation, washing, or filtration to remove >70% leukocytes while retaining >70% of the original RBCs	1-6
Red blood cells, washed	RBCs washed with normal saline to remove non-red-cell elements; RBC loss (often 20%), plasma removal (up to 99%), WBC reduction (up to 85%) varies with methodology	1-6
Platelets	>5.5 × 10^{10} platelets in 40-70 mL plasma (20-24° storage) or 20-30 mL plasma (1-6° storage); may contain trace-0.5 mL RBCs, ~10^8 WBCs, and hemostatic levels of coagulation factors	1-6 with no agitation 20-24 with agitation
Fresh frozen plasma (FFP)	200-250 mL plasma plus anticoagulant frozen within 6 hr of collection; contains ~200 units of all plasma clotting factors and 200-400 mg fibrinogen	Frozen: <−18 Thawed: 1-6
Cryoprecipitated AHF	A concentration of 80-120 units Factor VIII, 40-70% von Willebrand factor, and 20-30% Factor XIII present in original unit; 150-250 mg fibrinogen, ~55 mg fibronectin in <15 mL plasma	Frozen: <−18 Thawed: 20-24
Albumin; plasma protein fraction (PPF)	Albumin: 5% or 25% protein solution; ~96% albumin and 4% globulins PPF: 5% solution; 83% albumin, 17% α/β globulins All 3 products have Na content ~145 mEq/L	2-8 Room temperature
Immune serum globulin	ISG:concentrated solution containing 16 g/dL protein (95-98% IgG, 1-2% IgM and IgA) IVIG: 5 g/dL protein solution	2-8
Factor VIII concentrate	Lyophilized concentrate of factor VIII, activity units are on label; may also contain some fibrinogen and von Willebrand factor	2-8 Room temperature

Abbreviations: RBCs, red blood cells; WBCs, white blood cells; HES, hydroxyethyl starch; ITP, idiopathic thrombocytopenia purpura; ISG, immune serum globulin; IVIG, intravenous immunoglobulin; TTP, thrombotic thrombocytopenic purpura; IV, intravenous; IM, intramuscular.
From Calhoun L: Blood product preparation and administration. In Petz LD, Swisher SN, editors: *Clinical practice of transfusion medicine*, ed 2, New York, 1989, Churchill Livingstone.

Indications	Dose	Handling comments
Symptomatic anemia with acute volume deficits; massive transfusions/exchange transfusions	As needed for replacement:1 unit will increase Hct 3%	Can be infused as fast as patient tolerates
Symptomatic anemia not treatable with diet/medication; decreased plasma volume is ideal for patients with chronic anemia, volume change intolerance, and renal and liver disease	Same as whole blood	Allow 10 min preparation time if packed just before issue; infuse within 4 hrs or as patient tolerates
Symptomatic anemia plus history of repeated nonhemolytic febrile transfusion reactions; may be useful to prevent HLA alloimmunization	Same as whole blood	Allow 15-60 min if prepared just before issue; if prepared at bedside, use special designated filter
Symptomatic anemia plus history of repeated allergic or febrile transfusion reactions; paroxysmal nocturnal hemoglobinuria	Same as whole blood	Allow 20-30 min preparation time
Bleeding related to thrombocytopenia or platelet dysfunction, low or rapidly dropping platelet counts	Hemostatic dose: 1 bag/10 kg body weight: 1 bag will increase platelet count 5,000-10,000/μl	Allow 10-20 min to pool, 10-60 min to prepare as leukocyte-poor or volume-reduced; infuse 5 mL/min or as patient tolerates
Bleeding related to coagulation factor deficiencies where specific concentrates are not available or are contraindicated; coumarin drug reversal; TTP	Hemostatic dose: 10 mL/kg body weight; 15 mL/kg may be indicated for initial loading dose	Allow 15-30 min to thaw; infuse 5-10 mL/min or as patient tolerates
To control bleeding associated with hemophilia A, von Willebrand's disease, uremia, and factor XIII and fibrinogen deficiencies; fibronectin replacement; fibrin glue to stop topical bleeding or to remove renal calculi	Dose is calculated on plasma volume; 8-10 bags supply 2 g fibrinogen (hemostatic dose)	Consider alternative therapies; allow 5-10 min to thaw, 15 min to pool; transfuse 5-10 mL/min or as patient tolerates
Large, acute colloid losses occurring with severe burns or hypovolemic shock; blood pressure support during hypotensive episodes; not indicated for nutritional hypoproteinemia	Shock: determined by patient's condition and response Burns: as needed to maintain protein level of 5.2 g/dL	No filter required; PPF infusion can precipitate severe hypotensive episodes; do not infuse intra-arterially or >10 mL/min; PPF has been reported to cause hemolysis when mixed with older RBCs
ISG: prophylactic passive immunity for immuno-incompetent patients or those at risk of disease IVIG: same as above, for patients requiring high-dose therapy or those who cannot tolerate IM injection	Congenital deficiencies: ISG—0.7 mL/kg/mo IVIG—100 mg/kg/mo Hyperimmune products for specific diseases: as manufacturer recommends ITP: 1-2 g IVIG/kg as needed	No filter required; must be given via proper route: ISG—IM IVIG—IV
To control bleeding in severe hemophilia A	As needed: 1 unit/kg will increase activity level 2%; larger loading dose required	Must be filtered; reconstitute per manufacturer's directions; give IV and use plastic syringe

TABLE 38-16   Transfusion Reactions

Reaction	Cause	Clinical manifestations	Management	Prevention
ACUTE HEMOLYTIC	Infusion of ABO-incompatible whole blood, red blood cells, or components containing 10 mL or more of red blood cells. Antibodies in the recipient's plasma attach to antigens on transfused red blood cells causing red-blood-cell destruction.	Chills, fever, low back pain, flushing, tachycardia, tachypnea, hypotension, vascular collapse, hemoglobinuria, hemoglobinemia, bleeding, acute renal failure, shock, cardiac arrest, death.	Treat shock. Draw blood samples for serologic testing. To avoid hemolysis from the procedure, use a new venipuncture (not an existing central line) and avoid small-gauge needles. Send urine specimen to the laboratory. Maintain BP with IV colloid solutions. Give diuretics as prescribed to maintain urine flow. Insert indwelling catheter or measure voided amounts to monitor hourly urine output. Dialysis may be required if renal failure occurs. Do not transfuse additional red-blood-cell-containing components until the transfusion service has provided newly crossmatched units.	Meticulously verify and document patient identification from sample collection to component infusion.
FEBRILE, NONHEMOLYTIC (MOST COMMON)	Sensitization to donor's white blood cells, platelets, or plasma proteins.	Sudden chills and fever (rise in temperature of greater than 1°C [2°F]), headache, flushing, anxiety, muscle pain.	Give antipyretics as prescribed. Do not give aspirin to thrombocytopenic patients. *Do not restart transfusion.*	Consider leukocyte-poor blood products (filtered, washed, or frozen).
MILD ALLERGIC	Sensitivity to foreign plasma proteins.	Flushing, itching, urticaria (hives).	Give antihistamines as directed. If symptoms are mild and transient, restart transfusion slowly. Do not restart transfusion if fever or pulmonary symptoms develop.	Treat prophylactically with antihistamines.

From the National Blood Resource Education Program's *Transfusion Therapy Guidelines for Nurses,* 1990.

TABLE 38-16	Transfusion Reactions—cont'd			
Reaction	**Cause**	**Clinical manifestations**	**Management**	**Prevention**
ANAPHYLACTIC	Infusion of IgA proteins to IgA-deficient recipient who has developed IgA antibody.	Anxiety, urticaria, wheezing, tightness and pain in chest, difficulty swallowing, progressing to cyanosis, shock, and possible cardiac arrest.	Initiate CPR if indicated. Have epinephrine ready for injection (0.4 mL of a 1:1,000 solution subcutaneously or 0.1 mL of 1:1,000 solution diluted to 10 mL with saline for IV use). *Do not restart transfusion.*	Transfuse extensively washed red blood cell products from which all plasma has been removed. Alternatively, use blood from IgA-deficient donor.
CIRCULATORY OVERLOAD	Fluid administered faster than the circulation can accommodate.	Cough, dyspnea, pulmonary congestion (rales), headache, hypertension, tachycardia, distended neck veins.	Place patient upright with his feet in a dependent position. Administer prescribed diuretics, oxygen, morphine. Phlebotomy may be indicated.	Adjust transfusion volume and flow rate based on patient's size and clinical status. Have transfusion service divide unit into smaller aliquots for better spacing of fluid input.
SEPSIS	Transfusion of contaminated blood components.	Rapid onset of chills, high fever, vomiting, diarrhea, and marked hypotension and shock.	Obtain culture of patient's blood and send bag with remaining blood to transfusion service for further study. Treat septicemia as directed—antibiotics, IV fluids, vasopressors, steroids.	Collect, process, store, and transfuse blood products according to blood banking standards and infuse within 4 hours of the starting time.

Although much debate about infection transmission centers on AIDS, the risk for hepatitis transmission actually is much higher than the HIV virus. Death from hepatitis B infection is quite rare, but does occur. Prior to availability of hepatitis C screening tests, about 1% to 2% of units transfused in the United States led to non-A, non-B hepatitis.[10] Now that testing is available, the incidence is expected to drop.

Plasmapheresis

Apheresis is the process of separating whole blood into its major components: plasma, platelets, red blood cells, and white blood cells. One of the components can then be removed and the rest returned to the donor. Leukapheresis is the process of removing white blood cells, red blood pheresis removes red blood cells, platelet pheresis removes platelets, and plasmapheresis removes plasma. The removed component can be used for transfusion to recipients who need the components (e.g., transfuse platelets for persons with bone marrow failure and platelet concentration below 20,000/mm^3). Another reason for apheresis is to remove components from a patient not necessarily to donate to another but to alleviate an abnormal excess in the patient. For example, in polycythemia vera or in sickle cell anemia, the patient may need red cell pheresis. In leukemia, leukapheresis may be indicated.

Plasmapheresis may involve removing multiple liters of plasma that contain abnormal substances and then replacing an equal volume of plasmalike solutions (e.g., fresh-frozen plasma or a mixture of normal saline and albumin). Hematologic diseases that can be treated by plasmapheresis are hemolytic anemia and multiple myeloma. Other diseases that may be treated by plasmapheresis include Goodpasture's

MANAGEMENT OF TRANSFUSION REACTIONS

When a patient exhibits signs or symptoms of a potential blood transfusion reaction:

1. Discontinue the transfusion immediately and begin a slow infusion of normal saline to maintain patency of the IV line. Recheck the name and blood group on the donor unit with the patient's name and blood group.
2. Reassure the patient and family.
3. Obtain the patient's vital signs and assess the severity of the reaction.
4. Remain at the bedside.
5. Contact the physician immediately and relay assessment findings, including vital signs, untoward signs and symptoms observed, blood component infused, and amount of blood infused.
6. Physician orders may include further infusion therapy (fluid and infusion rate), and drug therapy, such as epinephrine, steroids, diphenhydramine, etc.).
7. Discontinue the blood transfusion by taking down the bag, administration set, any attached IV solution tubing or fluid, and cap the system with a sterile cap.
8. If specified IV solution is ordered, infuse with new IV tubing.
9. Notify the blood bank and initiate appropriate documentation.
10. Facilitate drawing of blood specimens as ordered.
11. Continue close observation of the patient.
12. Obtain first voided urine specimen (if blood has hemolized, hemoglobinuria may be present).
13. Arrange for a second urine specimen to be obtained 24 hours after the first specimen.

DOCUMENT: all events prior to, during, and after the transfusion reaction is detected (i.e., signs and symptoms observed, vital signs, notification of the physician and blood bank, nursing actions, etc.) in the patient's medical record. Include when the 24-hour post-transfusion period is to elapse. Document date and time that the blood product was discontinued.

From Blood Transfusion Reaction Procedure, Division of Nursing, The University of Texas M. D. Anderson Cancer Center, Houston, Texas, 1992.

syndrome, myasthenia gravis, renal transplant rejection syndrome, systemic lupus erythematosus, rheumatoid arthritis, Waldenström's macroglobulinemia, biliary cirrhosis, hyperlipidemia, and familial hypercholesterolemia. Usual treatments last 1 to

2 hours daily or every other day until desired results are achieved.

The patient requires monitoring during and after the treatment for response. Parameters that may be monitored include hemoglobin, hematocrit, prothrombin time, activated partial thromboplastin time, fibrinogen, potassium, calcium, albumin, complement, and immune complexes. Nursing management involves monitoring signs and symptoms of bleeding, hypotension, electrolyte imbalance, fluid overload, and infection. The person's coping response must be supported and also the coping response of the family.

Documentation

Documentation of the treatment should include the blood component removed and the amount, replacements given, the amount given, and the person's responses to the treatment. Responses include the vital signs and signs and symptoms that may be noted that indicate how the treatment was tolerated.

BONE MARROW TRANSPLANT
Definition/Etiology

Bone marrow transplantation is an increasingly accepted treatment option. It is most commonly used with patients who have leukemia, aplastic anemia, and immunodeficiency disorders. Innovations and successes have resulted in a wider applicability to patient populations that can benefit from this treatment option (e.g., patients with lymphoma, multiple myeloma, and selected cases of solid tumors, such as breast cancer). Indications include the need to bolster and rescue the immune cells to allow high doses of chemotherapy and/or radiation therapy and to hasten recovery after prolonged pancytopenia. Another indication is the need to replace diseased marrow.[30]

A bone marrow transplant is the intravenous infusion of bone marrow cells from a donor to the patient (recipient). The purpose is to replace or stimulate a nonfunctioning bone marrow. Three types of BMT are autologous, syngeneic, and allogeneic.

In an **autologous transplant,** patients receive their own bone marrow cells to recover from the bone marrow suppression of high-dose chemotherapy or radiation treatment. The patient's bone marrow cells are harvested through bone marrow aspirations before chemotherapy, treated with chemotherapy if necessary, frozen, and stored for the reinfusion that will take place following the chemotherapy and radiation treatments. The patient is the donor and recipient.

Syngeneic transplants are those in which the donor and recipient are identical twins and are genetically identical. An **allogeneic transplant** involves a donor who is not genetically identical to the recipient. However, histocompatibility typing is done with the human leukocyte antigen (HLA) to determine a genotypical match for donor and recipient. Mixed lymphocyte culture (MLC) establishes compatibility by determining a nonreactive state between the donor's and recipient's lymphocytes. Research is being conducted on bone marrow transplants using unrelated donors.

Therapeutic Management

The procedure consists of three stages: treatment with chemotherapy or total body irradiation, infusion of the bone marrow cells, and recovery, or engraftment. In the first stage, the patient's bone marrow that is either diseased or nonfunctional is destroyed by high-dose chemotherapy, alone or in combination with total body irradiation (TBI). TBI is necessary at times in addition to chemotherapy to ensure destruction of malignant cells that may find sanctuary in the central nervous system, for example, and escape the effects of chemotherapy. TBI destroys bone marrow cells and provides an empty space for the new marrow to implant. This process is called cytoreduction.

The second stage is infusion of the bone marrow cells. The bone marrow cells are injected intravenously over a period of 20 to 30 minutes. The patient can be premedicated to control possible side effects such as chills and flushing. A side effect of autologous transplants that the patient may experience is the taste and smell of the preservative added to the bone marrow. The smell and taste may be like garlic, tomato juice, or oysters. Patients may report nausea, vomiting, and headache during infusion.

The third stage of bone marrow transplant is recovery or engraftment. Engraftment of the bone marrow stem cell usually occurs in 1 to 2 weeks, as evidenced by the presence of hemopoietic elements in the bone marrow. In 3 to 4 weeks, the peripheral blood counts begin to rise. Hematologic normalization occurs in 2 to 3 months. The patient is hospitalized during this time in either a laminar airflow (germ-free) unit or a private hospital room with or without reverse isolation.

Complications from the transplant can include infection, bleeding, stomatitis, nutritional deficits, disease relapse, or graft rejection. A major complication is graft versus host disease (GVHD). GVHD occurs when donor T lymphocytes are introduced into an immunologically incompetent host. The T lymphocytes proliferate and attack the host cells that they recognize as foreign. The donor T lymphocytes may come from the donor bone marrow in allogeneic transplants. Although primarily seen in allogeneic recipients, this complication may occur in any immunocompromised patient who receives a blood

transfusion. To avoid this, blood transfusions for bone marrow recipients in general must be irradiated to prevent lymphocyte proliferation.

Acute GVHD is a syndrome of dermatitis, hepatitis, and enteritis. Treatment includes cyclosporin A, methotrexate and steroids, and antithymocyte globulin. Prevention of GVHD includes HLA typing, use of methotrexate or cyclosporin A, irradiation of blood products, and elimination of T cells from the donor's marrow before infusion.

Results of bone marrow transplantation may significantly improve as treatment measures are developed to prevent major complications such as infection and bleeding. One of these measures is the use of colony-stimulating factors to stimulate certain types of white blood cell production. CSFs can be used to stimulate multipotential stem cells which will result in clinical benefit through production of WBCs and also RBCs and platelets.[26]

Another approach to prevent complications after BMT is immune globulin administration. Intravenous immune globulin provides temporary protection against infection by conveying passive immunity.[34]

RESEARCH BRIEF

Larson PJ et al: Comparison of perceived symptoms of patients undergoing bone marrow transplant and the nurses caring for them, *Oncol Nurs Forum* 20(1):81, 1993.

This study was designed to determine the symptoms of patients undergoing bone marrow transplant (BMT) and to determine the perceived distress from the symptoms from the perspective of the nurse and the patient. Measurements were done at four time periods: within 48 hours of BMT day one (T_1); day 7-10 post BMT (T_2); day 20-23 post BMT (T_3); and day 30-34 post BMT (T_4). The sample included 30 adult patients and 28 nurses assigned to care for these patients. Three instruments were used: Symptom Distress Scale, Profile of Mood States, and Karnofsky Performance Status. Significant differences in perception of distress were noted at T_1, with patients perceiving significantly more distress than the nurses. Differences in perception of distress were noted at the other time periods, but the differences were not significant.

The implications for nursing practice are the importance of nurses exploring the perceived symptom distress of patients undergoing BMT so that distress can be adequately managed.

NURSING MANAGEMENT OF THE PATIENT WITH BONE MARROW TRANSPLANT

Nursing care is complex, and the impact on patient and family is significant. Nursing management includes the side effects of anemia, leukopenia, and thrombocytopenia. (Please refer to the specific sections of the chapter.) Nursing management must include emotional support for the patient and family experiencing a bone marrow transplant. Nursing diagnoses include:

Altered protection related to decreased immune function

Knowledge deficit of treatment and side effects related to lack of exposure

Anxiety related to change in health status

High risk for infection related to leukopenia

High risk for injury (bleeding) related to thrombocytopenia

Activity intolerance related to anemia

Altered nutrition: less than body requirements related to nausea, vomiting, anorexia, taste distortion

Impaired skin integrity related to dermatitis of GVHD

Altered oral mucous membrane related to stomatitis of GVHD

Diarrhea related to enteritis of GVHD

Social isolation related to restrictions on ability to interact with others

Ineffective family and individual coping related to situational crisis

CRITICAL THINKING QUESTIONS

1 What patient teaching is appropriate for patients receiving iron therapy?
2 What components should be included in a nursing history and assessment for anemia?
3 List two common nursing diagnoses appropriate for most patients with anemia.
4 Explain the nursing implications for continuity of care for the patient with anemia.
5 Discuss nursing implications in the care of the patient with multiple myeloma.
6 Discuss nursing management of the person receiving a bone marrow transplant.
7 How does the leukemic disease process lead to problems of anemia, thrombocytopenia, and leukopenia?
8 What components should be included in a nursing history and assessment with a white blood cell disorder?
9 List three common nursing diagnoses associated with WBC disorders.
10 What nursing strategies should be used to decrease incidence of infection in patients with white blood cell disorders?
11 Why won't the leukopenic patient necessarily exhibit the classic signs and symptoms of infection?
12 What teaching is appropriate for the patient with a white blood cell disorder?
13 What supportive care measures could be used to improve comfort for the hemophiliac patient (and family)?
14 What components should be included in a nursing history and assessment with a coagulation disorder?
15 List three potential nursing diagnoses associated with coagulation disorders.
16 List five nursing interventions included in bleeding precautions.
17 What nursing strategies could be used to improve patient comfort in the presence of active bleeding?
18 How would you evaluate the effectiveness of the care for patients who are at risk for bleeding?
19 What are measures that promote continuity of care for the patient (and family) with a coagulation disorder?
20 What are the three types of bone marrow transplant?

RESOURCES

1 THE LEUKEMIA SOCIETY OF AMERICA, INC. 733 Third Avenue New York, NY 10017
Sponsors research; provides patient financial aid; conducts public and professional educational programs; publishes public and professional educational materials.

2 AMERICAN ASSOCIATION OF BLOOD BANKS 1117 North 19th Street, Suite 600 Arlington, VA 22209
Formulates and publishes standards for transfusion therapy.

3 NATIONAL ASSOCIATION FOR SICKLE CELL DISEASE, INC. (NASCD) 4221 Wilshire Blvd., Suite 360 Los Angeles, CA 90010

4 THE NATIONAL HEMOPHILIA FOUNDATION SOHO Building, Suite 406 110 Greene St. New York, NY 10012

5 APLASTIC ANEMIA FOUNDATION PO Box 22689 Baltimore, MD 21203

BIBLIOGRAPHY

Current

1. American Cancer Society: *Cancer facts and figures—1992,* Atlanta, GA, 1992, American Cancer Society, Inc.

2. Arlin ZA, et al: "Quality" remissions: A new target of induction therapy in acute leukemia and the next step in developing curative treatment, *Semin Hematol* 28(3)Suppl 4:44, 1991.

3. Blanchette VS, Vick S, Gafni A: Available clotting concentrates: a cost-effectiveness analysis. In Westphal RG, Smith DM, editors: *Treatment of hemophilia and von Willebrand's disease: new developments*, Arlington, Va, 1989, American Association of Blood Banks.

4. Brown BA: *Hematology principles and procedures*, ed 5, Philadelphia, 1988, Lea & Febiger.

5. Bussel JB, Schreiber AD: Immune thrombocytopenic purpura, neonatal alloimmune thrombocytopenia, and post-transfusion purpura. In Hoffman R et al, editors: *Hematology: basic principles and practice*, New York, 1991, Churchill Livingstone.

6. Cook MB: Multiple myeloma. In Groenwald SL et al, editors: *Cancer nursing: principles and practice*, ed 2, Boston, 1990, Jones & Bartlett Publishers.

7. DeVita VT et al: Lymphocytic lymphomas. In DeVita VT, Hellman S, Rosenberg SA, editors: *Cancer: principles and practice of oncology*, ed 3, vol 2, Philadelphia, 1989, JB Lippincott Co.

8. Eyster ME: Natural history and transmission of hemophilia-associated human immunodeficiency virus (HIV) infections. In Hilgartner M, Pochedly C, editors: *Hemophilia in the child and adult*, ed 3, New York, 1989, Raven Press, Ltd.

9. Hellman S, Jaffe ES, DeVita VT: Hodgkin's disease. In DeVita VT, Hellman S, Rosenberg SA, editors: *Cancer: principles and practice of oncology*, ed 3, vol 2, Philadelphia, 1989, JB Lippincott Co.

10. Heymann SJ et al: How safe is safe enough? New infections and the U.S. blood supply, *Ann Intern Med* 117:612, 1992.

11. Hoelzer D: High-dose chemotherapy in adult acute lymphoblastic leukemia, *Semin Hematol* 28(3) Suppl 4:84, 1991.

12. Holleb AI, Fink OJ, Murphy GP: *Clinical oncology*, Atlanta, 1991, American Cancer Society, Inc.

13. Jandl JH: *Blood: textbook of hematology*, Boston, 1987, Little, Brown & Co.

14. Keating MJ et al: Fludarabine: a new agent with marked cytoreductive activity in untreated chronic lymphocytic leukemia, *J Clin Oncol* 9:44, 1991.

15. Kim MJ, McFarland GK, McLane AM: *Pocket guide to nursing diagnoses*, ed 4, St Louis, 1991, Mosby–Year Book.

16. Kurzrock R et al: Hematopoietic growth factors in bone marrow failure states, *Ca Bull* 43(3):215, 1991.

17. Lusher JM: Management of hemophilia. In Westphal RG, Smith DM, editors: *Treatment of hemophilia and von Willebrand's disease: new developments*, Arlington, Va, 1989, American Association of Blood Banks.

18. Lusher JM, Warrier I: Hemophilia A, *Hematol/Oncol Clin N Amer* 6(5):1021, 1992.

19. Mitus AJ, Rosenthal DS: Adult leukemias. In Holleb AI, Fink DJ, Murphy GP, editors: *American Cancer Society textbook of clinical oncology*, Atlanta, GA, 1991, American Cancer Society, Inc.

20. Moake JL: Thrombotic thrombocytopenic purpura and the hemolytic-uremic syndrome. In Hoffman R et al, editors: *Basic principles and practice*, New York, 1991, Churchill Livingstone.

21. National Blood Resource Education Program's Nursing Education Working Group: Transfusion nursing: trends and practices for the '90s, *Am J Nurs* 91(6):42, 1991.

22. Nelson K et al: Transmission of retroviruses from sero-negative donors by transfusion during cardiac surgery, *Ann Intern Med* 117:554, 1992.

23. Parsons LP, Klopovich PM: Immune globulin therapy, *Semin Oncol Nurs* 6(2):136, 1990.

24. Rapaport SI: *Introduction to hematology*, ed 2, Philadelphia, 1987, JB Lippincott Co.

25. Robeschon T: Phase II trial of TNF in lymphoma commences, *Oncol Biotechnol News* 2(2):21, 1988.

26. Robinson WA: Clinical use of colony-stimulating factors, *Mediguide to Oncol* 8(3):11, 1988.

27. Roth MS, Foon KA: Biotherapy with interferon in hematologic malignancies, *Oncol Nurs Forum*, 14(6)(suppl 16):1987.

28. Salmon SE, Cassady JR: Plasma cell neoplasms. In DeVita VT, Hellman S, Rosenberg SA, editors: *Cancer: principles and practice of oncology*, ed 3, vol 2, Philadelphia, 1989, JB Lippincott Co.

29. Snyder DAS, McGlave PB: Treatment of chronic myelogenous leukemia with bone marrow transplantation, *Hematol/Oncol Clin North Am* 4(3):335, 1990.

30. Strohl RA: Autologous bone marrow transplantation: an overview, *Nurs Acum* 3(3):3, 1991.

31. Talpaz J et al: Interferon-alpha produces sustained cytogenetic responses in chronic myelogenous leukemia, *Ann Intern Med* 114:532, 1991.

32. Terebelo HR: Alpha interferon: perspectives in the biotherapy of chronic myelogenous leukemia, *Oncol Nurs Forum* 18:5, 1991.

33. Trimble MS, Warkentin TE, Kelton JG: Thrombocytopenia due to platelet destruction and hypersplenism. In Hoffman R, et al, editors: *Hematology: basic principles and practice*, New York, 1991, Churchill Livingstone.

34. Volker DL: Research trends in bone marrow transplantation, *Nurs Acum* 3(3):2, 1991.

35. Wujcik D: Options for postremission therapy in acute leukemia, *Semin Oncol Nurs* 6(1):25, 1990.

36. Yarbro CH: Lymphomas. In Groenwald SL et al, editors: *Cancer nursing: principles and practice*, ed 2, Boston, 1990, Jones & Bartlett Publishing.

37. Yeomans AC, Harle MT: Myelodysplastic syndromes, *Semin Oncol Nurs* 6:9, 1990.

Classic

38. Bick RL: *Disorders of hemostasis and thrombosis*, New York, 1985, Thieme, Inc.

39. Burnside IM: *Nursing and the aged*, ed 2, New York, 1981, McGraw-Hill.

40. Dune BG, Salmon SE: A clinical staging system for multiple myeloma, *Cancer* 36:842, 1975.

41. Ellerhorst-Ryan J: Complications of the myeloproliferative system: Infection and sepsis, *Semin Oncol Nurs* 1:244, 1985.

42. Ford EJ, Fuller LM, Hagemeister FB: *Hodgkin's disease and non-Hodgkin's lymphoma*, New York, 1984, Raven Press.

43. Griffin JP: Hematology and immunology concepts for nursing, Norwalk, Conn, 1986, Appleton-Century-Crofts.

44. Handin RI: Hemorrhagic disorders. II. Platelets and purpura. In Beck WS, editor: *Hematology*, ed 4, Cambridge, Mass, 1985, The MIT Press.

45. Jandl JH: Introduction to a symposium on the mechanism of disorders of erythropoiesis, *Medicine* 43:615, 1964.

46. Lacher MJ: Hodgkin's disease: historical perspective, current status, and future directions, *CA* 35:88, 1985.

47. Lopez J, Hausz M: Therapeutic apheresis, *Am J Nurs* 82(10):1572, 1982.

48. Lukes RJ et al: Report of the nomenclature committee, *Cancer Res* 26:1311, 1966.

49. Lukes RJ, Butler JJ: The pathology and nomenclature of Hodgkin's disease, *Cancer Res* 26:1063, 1966.

50. McFarlane J: Sickle cell disorders, *Am J Nurs* 77(12):1948, 1977.

51. McClelland E, Kelly K, Buckwater KC: *Continuity of care: advancing the concepts of discharge planning*, Orlando, Fla, 1985, Grune & Stratton.

52. Megliola B: Multiple myeloma, *Canc Nurs:* 209, June 1980.

53. Reich PR: *Hematology: physiopathologic basis for clinical practice*, ed 2, Boston, 1984, Little, Brown & Co.

54. Savage D, Lindenbaum J: Clinical and experimental vitamin K deficiency. In Lindenbaum J, editor: *Nutrition in hematology*, New York, 1983, Churchill Livingstone.

55. Shackelford P: Multiple myeloma, *Orthop Nurs* 4(5):61, 1985.

56. Ultmann JE, Jacobs RH: The non-Hodgkin's lymphomas, *CA* 35:66, 1985.

CHAPTER THIRTY-NINE

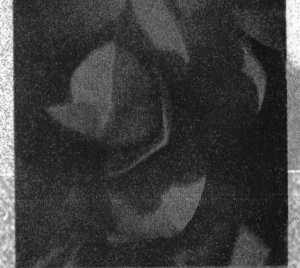

Function of the Immune System

LEARNING OBJECTIVES

1 Identify the essential components of the immune system.

2 Describe the role of antigens in differentiating "self" from "nonself" in immune responses.

3 Compare and contrast the functions of immunologic tissues and cells.

4 Characterize agents and events that can stimulate immune activity.

5 Differentiate between the nonspecific and specific immune response in terms of the purpose and cells involved.

6 Describe the phases in the nonspecific immune response.

7 Describe the role of T4 cells as coordinators of the specific immune response.

8 Differentiate between resolution, regeneration, and replacement in tissue repair following an immune response.

9 Identify factors that alter the function of the immune system.

10 State measures appropriate for use in assessing a patient's immune function.

KEY TERMS

antibodies, p. 1017

antigens, p. 1008

B cells, p. 1010

cell-mediated immunity (CMI), p. 1014

human leukocyte antigens (HLAs), p. 1008

immunocompetence, p. 1008

immunoglobulin, p. 1016

inflammation, p. 1012

interferons, p. 1014

interleukin-1 (IL-1), p. 1014

interleukin-2 (IL-2), p. 1015

lymphocytes, p. 1010

macrophages, p. 1010

memory cells, p. 1016

natural killer cells, p. 1015

nonspecific immune response, p. 1008

phagocytosis, p. 1009

plasma cells, p. 1016

specific immune response, p. 1008

T cells, p. 1010

HUMAN GROWTH and development are marked by continual encounters with agents potentially injurious to biologic integrity. Our world is filled with microorganisms that lie dormant, waiting for an opportunity to grow and multiply in the receptive environment of the human body. Without adequate defenses, individuals would be highly vulnerable to thousands of agents that cause disease and death.

THE BODY'S DEFENSES

The defense system of the body, called the immune system, is made up of all the physiologic mechanisms that allow the body not only to recognize proteins as abnormal or foreign, but also to eliminate or neutralize them (see box).

The skin serves as the major protective mechanism against invasion of microbes. Inside the body, the leukocytes or white blood cells (WBCs) control and eliminate invading pathogens or tissue damage. There are two levels of responses by the immune system: the **nonspecific immune response** (inflammation) begins immediately, using neutrophils and macrophages to eliminate the organism as soon as possible. The inflammatory response is backed up by the **specific immune response** that primarily involves lymphocytes programmed to recognize and respond to particular antigens. When the immune system is intact and functioning effectively, it is referred to as a state of **immunocompetence.** The essential components of immunocompetence are listed in the box below.

Antigens

Central to the effective function of the immune system is its ability to recognize and distinguish between "self" and "nonself." WBCs interact with other cells by examining protein markers on the surface of the cell membranes. These protein markers are called **antigens,** and they serve to identify a cell as self or nonself, just as flags identify different countries. Every nucleated cell in the body has surface antigens; these markers tell the immune system,

"This is *your* cell." In addition, other antigens identify each particular type of cell (e.g., muscle, skin, heart).

Human leukocyte antigens

The first group of self antigens was found on human leukocytes; thus they were named **human leukocyte antigens (HLAs).** Although we now know that these markers occur on all cells, not just WBCs, self antigens on cells continue to be called HLAs. HLAs on cells are inherited as part of genetic makeup; sites on chromosome 6 are the source of thousands of HLA markers that collectively are called the major histocompatibility complex. HLAs are the means by which the body differentiates self and nonself, enabling the body to recognize invading organisms and abnormal tumor cells that arise within the body. In addition, they determine the success of organ transplantation. When a person receives an organ transplant, histocompatibility antigens are matched between the donor and recipient to minimize rejection.

White blood cell response to antigens

WBCs circulating in the body detect anything with a nonself antigen and attack it. The antigen fits into receptors on the WBC membrane like a key fits into a lock, stimulating a destructive response. Actual destruction occurs through lysis, phagocytosis, isolation, or neutralization of toxins (see box).

When injury occurs, more WBCs from the blood and lymphoid tissues are recruited to the area, a process called chemotaxis. Leukocytosis, or a WBC count higher than normal, is one way of measuring the severity of an infection. At the same time the bone marrow is stimulated to produce more WBCs; this can be seen in laboratory tests that show an increase in immature WBCs (commonly referred to as a "shift to the left").

ROLE OF THE IMMUNE SYSTEM

Destroy, control, or eliminate invading organisms and other nonself antigens

Manage tissue damage

Eliminate old or damaged cells

Destroy abnormal cells in body (immune surveillance)

ESSENTIAL COMPONENTS OF IMMUNOCOMPETENCE

Bone marrow capable of producing effective WBCs

Adequate numbers of functioning, mature WBCs

Functioning lymphoid tissue that stimulates maturation and differentiation of lymphocytes

Collections of WBCs in lymphoid tissues that provide an opportunity for close interactions among the cells, blood, and lymph, for the recognition of nonself antigens

Adequate amounts of chemical mediators to stimulate and augment WBC activity

MECHANISMS OF DESTRUCTION OF ORGANISMS

Lysis: direct killing by enzymes, called lysozymes, in WBC

Phagocytosis: movement of cell membrane around organism, engulfing it. Once inside the WBC, lysozymes destroy it. Enhanced by *opsonins,* substances that coat nonself antigens, making them more attractive to phagocyte.

Isolation: used against viruses. Receptors on nearby cells are blocked, preventing spread of virus. Infected cell is then destroyed by lysis or phagocytosis.

Neutralization: toxins produced by organisms or venom secreted by snakes or insects is bound by antibodies and becomes unable to cause cell damage.

CATEGORIES OF WHITE BLOOD CELLS

Myeloid stem cell produces:
   Granulocytes
      Neutrophils
         Mast cells
         Basophils
      Eosinophils
   Monocytes
      Macrophages
Lymphoid stem cell produces:
   T-lymphocytes
      Helper/T4 cells
      Suppressor/T8 cells
      Natural killer cells
      Cytotoxic T cells
   B-lymphocytes
      Plasma cells
      Memory cells

TISSUES OF THE IMMUNE SYSTEM
Physical Barriers

Skin and mucous membranes

The body's best defense mechanism is the skin, which serves as a significant physical barrier between internal organs and the external environment. The skin is able to regenerate and heals rapidly after infection or injury to maintain an effective barrier against organisms. In addition, chemicals are secreted by the sweat, lacrimal, and sebaceous glands that destroy microbes that come in contact with the skin. The skin is assisted by mucous membranes that line all parts of the body open to the air. The mucus traps and holds foreign particles of any kind so they can be eliminated or destroyed.

Normal bacterial flora

Millions of bacteria inhabit the skin, body orifices, and most of the gastrointestinal tract, serving as a significant part of the body's protective mechanisms. Without these normal flora, the body would be at considerably greater risk for infection.

The relationship between the human body and normal bacterial flora is one of mutual benefit, a relationship termed commensalism. The human body is "infected" in a technical sense, but no disease occurs because the normal flora are controlled by the immune system. In turn, the normal flora inhibit the growth of pathogenic organisms and therefore protect the body against disease. Several mechanisms may be involved in this protection. Normal flora may (1) consume all available nutrients, (2) create an environmental pH unsuited for pathogens, or (3) directly inhibit pathogen growth or pathogens' attachment to epithelial cells. High doses of antibiotics destroy the normal bacterial flora, resulting in an overgrowth of fungal organisms that lead to diarrhea and vaginal infections.[10]

Bone Marrow

The active cells of the immune system are the leukocytes. Almost all WBCs are produced by two "parent" cells (called stem cells) in the bone marrow. There are two stem cell lines: the *myeloid stem cells* produce the granulocytes and monocytes; and the *lymphoid stem cells* produce the two types of lymphocytes, B cells and T cells (see box).

Granulocytes

The largest number of WBCs in the body are granulocytes. There are two primary classes of granulocytes: neutrophils and eosinophils. The primary role of granulocytes is played during inflammation as they ingest and destroy microorganisms and release chemical mediators that enhance and prolong the inflammatory response.

Neutrophils

Neutrophils make up 50% to 70% of all circulating WBCs and are the most important WBCs in the nonspecific immune response. Neutrophils act through phagocytosis and the stimulation of other WBCs. Approximately 100 billion neutrophils enter and leave the bloodstream to settle in tissues daily; this number increases greatly during an acute infection.[1] If an inadequate number of neutrophils is present (neutropenia), the body is in immediate danger from infection by common organisms such as staphylococci and Gram-negative bacteria.

Basophils are a small subdivision of circulating neutrophils. Although less than 1% of the total WBCs, basophils play an important part in phagocytosis, chemotaxis, and the release of vasoactive mediators during the inflammatory response.

Mast cells are a special group of noncirculating neutrophils. Mast cells are located primarily at sites where the environment and body interact, such as the lungs, gastrointestinal tract, skin, and mucous membranes. Many of the chemical mediators involved in the inflammatory response are released by mast cells.

Eosinophils

The primary granulocytes responsible for allergic reactions and the destruction of parasitic organisms are eosinophils. These cells comprise only 1% to 3% of the WBCs in the bloodstream, but huge numbers are found in reservoirs in the bone marrow and connective tissue, available to act and release important chemical mediators as needed.

Monocytes/macrophages

The second major group of cells produced by the myeloid stem cell, monocytes, also plays a vital role as phagocytes. Monocytes that have left the blood circulation and settled in tissues are called **macrophages.** The lymph nodes, alveoli, spleen, tonsils, and liver contain significant numbers of macrophages, which act as filters for circulating blood. Macrophages in the liver are called *Kupffer's cells.* The monocyte/macrophage network of fixed and moving cells used to be called the reticuloendothelial system.

Receptors for antigens on monocytes and macrophages are nonspecific; they recognize all foreign antigens and can respond quickly during inflammation. Recognition of foreign proteins is aided by opsonins, substances that coat the antigen, making it more "attractive" to the phagocytic cells. Macrophages also release chemical mediators necessary for regulation of immune activity and process antigens to activate B- and T-lymphocytes for the specific immune response.[1]

Lymphocytes

Lymphocytes make up 20% to 40% of the circulating WBCs. Unlike neutrophils and macrophages, they are antigen specific, or able to respond only to certain antigens rather than to any nonself markers. Their ability to recognize and respond to nonself antigens develops as they mature and differentiate in lymphoid tissue.

T cells are lymphocytes that mature and differentiate in the thymus gland. There are several subsets to T-lymphocytes: T4 or helper T cells, T8 or suppressor T cells, natural killer cells, and cytotoxic T cells. **B cells** are lymphocytes that do *not* mature in the thymus. B cells have two subsets: memory cells, which maintain long-term responses to specific antigens, and plasma cells, which produce the immunoglobulins commonly called antibodies.

Lymphoid Tissue

The thymus, spleen, lymph nodes, and mucosal tissues in the gastrointestinal and respiratory tracts containing lymphocytes and macrophages are collectively referred to as lymphoid tissue. These tissues are the sites at which lymphocytes mature, differentiate, and develop their ability to recognize nonself antigens. In addition, they serve as reservoirs from which additional WBCs may be obtained to fight off an invading pathogen or as sites to which organisms are brought for destruction.

Thymus

The thymus, a flat, two-lobed organ lying below the thyroid and behind the sternum, is largest during childhood and begins to atrophy at puberty. The thymus produces most lymphocytes during fetal life and childhood. In later life, chemicals in the thymus stimulate T-lymphocyte differentiation, the change from an immature lymphocyte to a mature, active T cell that responds to one specific foreign antigen.[15]

Spleen

The spleen, which lies in the upper abdomen, contains large numbers of macrophages and B-lymphocytes. It has both immunologic and nonimmunologic functions. Blood traveling through the spleen is filtered to remove old blood cells, abnormal cells, and cell debris. In addition, macrophages in the spleen process foreign antigens to activate B- and T-lymphocytes.[7] People whose spleen is removed because of abdominal trauma are at increased risk for developing systemic infections because of the lack of these macrophage and lymphocyte activities.

Lymphatic system

The lymphatic system is a vessel system in the body's tissues that interacts with the bloodstream to maintain fluid balance through the conservation of plasma proteins. It is also an essential part of the immune system. The lymph nodes positioned within the system filter the lymphatic fluid and trap organisms, preventing them from reaching the general circulation.

Lymph node channels are lined with phagocytic macrophages that destroy both organisms and abnormal cells, including cancerous and precancerous cells, thus providing a major defense against the establishment or spread of malignant tumors. Lymph nodes also are involved in the proliferation of lymphocytes and store, remove, or add T and B cells to the blood depending on the body's needs. When an infection is present in the body, the lymph nodes frequently become swollen (lymphadenopathy) because of their increased activity.

Mucosal lymphoid tissue

The tonsils, appendix, and Peyer's patches, which lie in the submucosa of the small intestine, make up the major portion of the gut-associated lymphoid tissue (GALT). Composed primarily of B cells, the GALT controls pathogens in the gastrointestinal tract and prevents them from entering the general circulation. Similar to the GALT is the bronchus-associated lymphoid tissue (BALT), which lies along the bronchi of the lungs. The BALT and the alveolar macrophages destroy organisms that enter the body through the respiratory system.[7] All of the tissues of the immune system work together to produce an effective system that recognizes antigenic markers as foreign to the self and destroys or neutralizes the offending agent, protecting the body from infection (see box). When one or more parts of the immune system is nonfunctional, the body is at increased risk for infection.

STIMULATION OF IMMUNE ACTIVITY

The immune system is activated not only when WBCs encounter a foreign antigen, but also when cells are damaged. The environment in which we live is full of potential harm from microorganisms, trauma, or the damage provoked by lack of oxygen.

Living organisms injure tissues through infection. As long as the microbe is present in the body it has the potential to reproduce itself and cause damage. Mechanical trauma breaches the protective barrier of the skin or destroys the tissue itself. Although minor breaks in skin integrity are handled with ease unless they become infected, surgery and crushing injuries increase the risk of pathogen invasion. Other injuries are only apparent when they disrupt tissue function. Thus someone whose chest has struck the steering wheel during an automobile accident may have no overt signs of injury; however, contusions and inflammation in the lung may interfere significantly with respiratory function.

The body responds to the sound waves producing noise as if they were a mechanical force. Noise is measured in decibels, and the ear is particularly sensitive to high decibel levels from any source. Prolonged exposure to loud machinery, engines, or even music produces inflammatory changes in the ear causing reversible or irreversible hearing loss.

Extreme changes in temperature also can injure tissue and activate the body's defense system. The depth of the damage from burns determines the extent to which blood flow and cell function are disrupted. Electrical injuries result not only from heat, but also from disruption of the normal electrical impulses in the heart and brain. Extreme cold produces vasoconstriction; the resulting decrease in blood flow may produce ischemic injury. The tissues of the fingers, toes, and face are particularly susceptible to the formation of ice crystals, a condition commonly known as frostbite.

Ionizing radiation (x rays) disrupts the deoxyribonucleic acid (DNA) within the cell, damaging essential proteins. Radiation can cause immediate cell death, impaired cell reproduction, or changes in DNA activity that can produce abnormal or mutated cells. These cells are seen by the WBCs as nonself, initiating an immune response.

TISSUES OF THE IMMUNE SYSTEM

Physical barriers

Skin/mucous membranes
Normal bacterial flora
  Gastrointestinal tract
  Vagina
  Respiratory tract
Chemicals
  Sweat, tears
  Sebaceous glands
  Hydrochloric acid in stomach

Bone marrow

White blood cells

Lymphoid tissue

Thymus
Spleen
Lymphatic system
Mucosal tissue
  GALT
    Tonsils
    Appendix
    Peyer's patches
  BALT

Many chemicals also cause cell and tissue damage. Some chemicals such as strong acids or bases are corrosive and immediately destroy cells with which they come in contact. Other chemicals disrupt the cell membrane, intracellular structures, or metabolic processes. Environmental pollution with chemicals may set up chronic inflammatory responses in the body. Although chemicals are essential in the treatment of disease, drugs or their by-products have adverse effects on many organs within the body.

Ischemia refers to a state in which the oxygen supply for cell metabolism is inadequate; as a result the cell dies. Any condition that decreases cardiac output, inhibits flow through the blood vessels, or interferes with adequate oxygenation of blood can cause ischemia. As a result, ischemic injury is one of the most common stimuli for the inflammatory response.

NONSPECIFIC IMMUNE RESPONSE

When any injury occurs from an organism, trauma, or ischemia, the body's first reaction is a stereotyped, nonspecific response commonly known as local **inflammation**. The inflammatory response does not require previous exposure to the invading organism; it occurs under any condition that disrupts homeostasis. Thus the same response occurs when people bang their thumb with a hammer, get a cold, or have surgery.

Frequently inflammation is thought of as bad by health care providers because it is one of the major components of multiple disease states. Any disease that has an "itis" ending (e.g., appendicitis, pericarditis, bronchitis) indicates that an inflammatory process is present. Inflammation also may be associated with infection and, as described in Chapter 40, causes the damage in autoimmune disorders. However, it is a vital part of our defense system. Individuals who are unable to mount an inflammatory response are at increased risk from organisms easily handled by those with an intact immune system. In addition, inflammation is a signal to nurses that injury has taken place.

Purpose

Inflammation serves to (1) localize the damage or the invading organism, (2) control reproduction of the organism, and (3) clear the area of debris so that healing may occur. The local inflammatory response is the result of several steps involving blood vessels, chemical mediators, and WBCs (see box above).

Cardinal Signs

The inflammatory response produces four cardinal signs: rubor (redness), calor (heat), tumor (swell-

---

STAGES IN NONSPECIFIC IMMUNE RESPONSE

1. Traumatic injury, invasion of organism, or presence of nonself antigen
2. Vasodilation of microvessels increasing blood flow
3. Increased vascular permeability
4. Movement of fluid and plasma proteins out of capillaries and into tissues
5. Emigration of neutrophils and later monocytes and natural killer cells out of capillaries and into tissues
6. Release of chemical mediators from WBCs and tissue
   a. Histamine: promotes steps 2 to 4
   b. Kinins: induce steps 2 to 5
   c. Complement: amplifies steps 2 to 5; acts as opsonin
   d. Arachidonic acid metabolites
      (1) Leukotrienes B4, C4, D4, E4: promote steps 2 to 6
      (2) Prostaglandins: promote steps 2 to 4
   e. Interleukin-1 (from macrophages): acts as communicator between cells; stimulates B and T cell response
7. Chemotaxis, bringing additional WBCs to site
8. Destruction of organism
9. Tissue repair

---

ing), and dolor (pain), that provide the basis for assessing the extent of the inflammatory response. Rubor, calor, tumor, and dolor are words derived from Latin and remind us that these signs of inflammation have been recognized for centuries. Figure 39-1 displays the vascular, cellular, and chemical events involved in inflammation.

Vascular Activity

Vasodilation

When traumatic injury or invasion of a foreign agent occurs, the body's first response is vasodilation of the small blood vessels, producing an increase in blood flow to the area and rubor. The blood that comes to the area is drawn from the body's core and therefore has a higher temperature than the peripheral tissue, producing warmth.

Increased vascular permeability

After vasodilation the epithelial cells of the blood vessel wall separate, increasing the permeability of

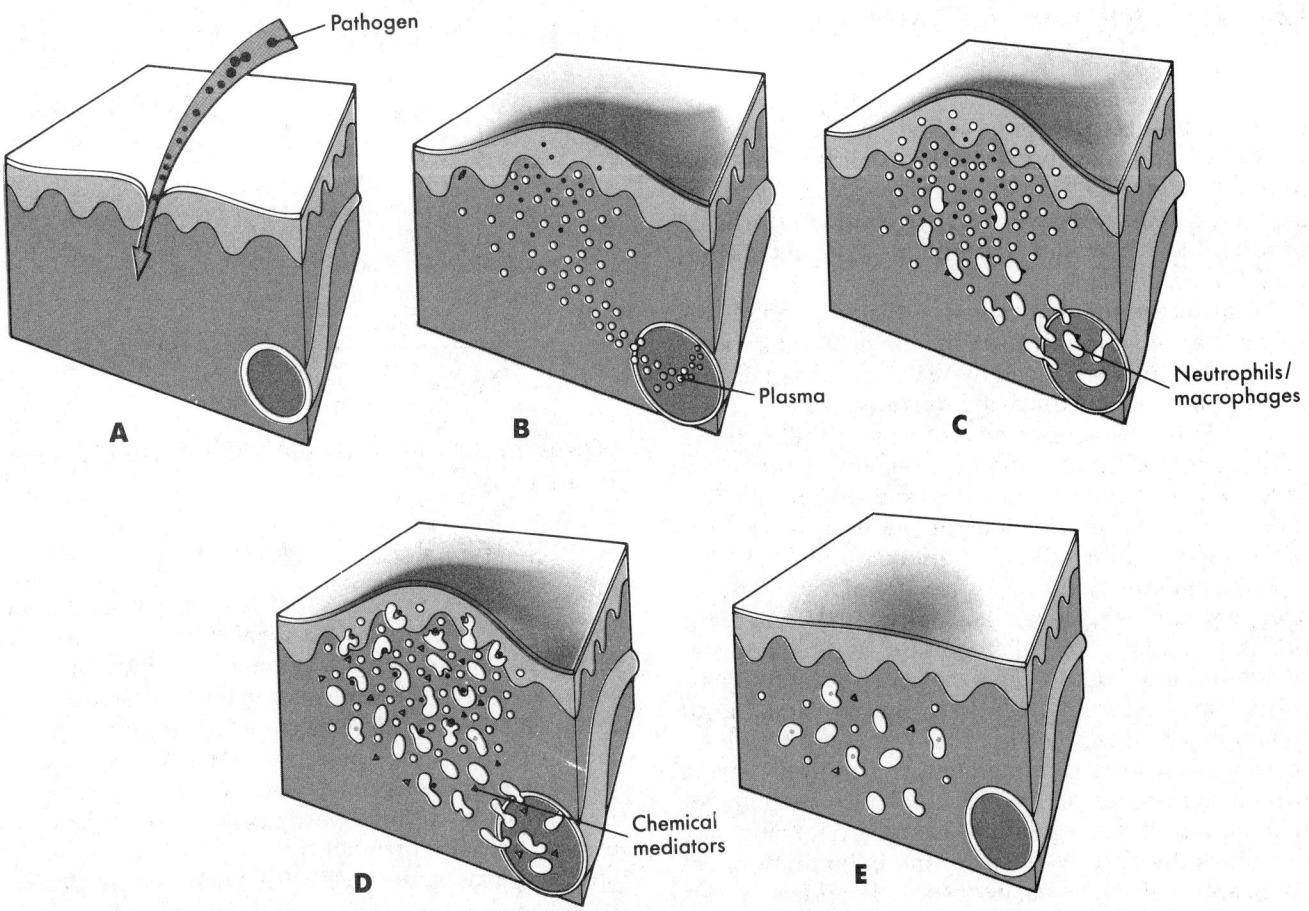

FIGURE 39-1   Mechanisms involved in inflammation. **A,** Cell injury occurs because of pathogen entry. **B,** Local blood vessels dilate and increase permeability, promoting loss of fluid into tissues. Area becomes red, warm, and swollen. **C,** Neutrophils and macrophages move into tissues for phagocytosis and lysis of pathogen. **D,** Release of chemical mediators stimulates chemotaxis, bringing more cells to site. **E,** Phagocytosis has occurred, vasculature begins to return to normal, and repair of damaged tissues can begin.

the vascular wall. First plasma moves out of the capillaries into the tissues, which dilutes any noxious substance and produces swelling in the area. The movement of fluid out of the vessel is aided by *increased hydrostatic pressure* that has been created by the increased blood flow within the capillary and by *decreased oncotic pressure* created by plasma proteins also leaving the bloodstream (see Chapter 12). Treatment of an inflamed area often involves elevating the affected part because it decreases hydrostatic pressure and therefore reduces movement of fluid into the tissues.

Initially inflammatory fluid (exudate) is clear, but later it becomes cloudy because of the presence of cell debris. For example, during a head cold, the nasal drainage is clear at first and later becomes opaque. Purulent exudate, or pus, is composed of WBCs, tissue debris, and dead organisms. As the fluid accumulates, it presses on local nerve endings

and causes pain; it may also fill the spaces in a joint, promoting loss of function.

Cellular Activity

In response to the presence of a foreign antigen, neutrophils and monocytes quickly leave the bloodstream to get to the site of injury. Both types of cells attempt to destroy the organism through phagocytosis or direct lysis. They also release chemical mediators that augment the initial steps of inflammation and promote chemotaxis, the process by which additional WBCs are brought to the area to ensure an adequate defense. Although they are not WBCs, platelets also play a role in the inflammatory response. Platelets aggregate or clump at the site of injury and release chemical mediators to assist the inflammatory process and lay the groundwork for repair.

Chemical Mediators and Cytokines

Chemical mediators are vital to maintaining and increasing the inflammatory process. Histamine, serotonin, and kinins induce vasodilation, capillary permeability, and movement of neutrophils to the site of injury. Kinins also activate the neuronal pain receptors, which, along with the extra fluid in the area, produce the pain that accompanies the inflammation.

Many of the mediators active during immune responses are cytokines, proteins, or proteinlike substances that are produced by WBCs to stimulate the activity of other leukocytes. **Interleukin-1** (IL-1) is a cytokine released by macrophages that allows WBCs to "talk" to one another, regulating the activity of cells in both inflammation and the specific immune response as needed. In addition, IL-1 produces the systemic effects of inflammation.

Prostaglandins and leukotrienes are arachidonic acid metabolites, local hormones that augment the initial stages of inflammation. It is the prostaglandins and leukotrienes that are inhibited by aspirin, corticosteroids, and the nonsteroidal, antiinflammatory drugs used in the treatment of inflammatory disorders. Complement, a group of plasma proteins, plays an extremely vital role in both inflammation and coagulation. Complement not only magnifies the first five steps of the inflammatory response, but also acts as an opsonin for phagocytosis and mediates antigen-antibody reactions in the specific immune response.

Interferons (IFNs) are released by WBCs when the invading organism is a virus. Alpha, beta, and gamma interferons inhibit the reproduction of viruses inside the body's cells. They bind to the cell membrane and stimulate the production of enzymes that block the synthesis of proteins required by the virus for replication. In addition, IFNs prevent the spread of viruses to neighboring cells. Interferons also inhibit the growth of certain tumors and participate in the specific immune response.[11]

Systemic Effects of Inflammation

When macrophages release IL-1 during a prolonged inflammatory response, it has systemic as well as local effects (see box). The most common systemic indicator of inflammation is fever, generally defined as a temperature greater than 38.1° C. IL-1 also causes increased production and release of WBCs by the bone marrow, indicated by leukocytosis and an increase in immature WBCs in the serum. In addition, IL-1 enhances maturation and differentiation of lymphocytes, increases the release of other chemical mediators, and decreases blood levels of iron by changing the uptake or release of iron in the liver or spleen. Bacteria require iron to reproduce; lack

---

SYSTEMIC EFFECTS OF INFLAMMATION

Fever
Increased production and release of WBCs
Increased proliferation of lymphocytes
Increased release of chemical mediators
Decreased blood levels of iron

---

of iron in the blood inhibits the growth of bacteria in the body.[11]

SPECIFIC IMMUNE RESPONSE

When the local inflammatory response is inadequate to cope with organisms or foreign antigens, the specific immune response is required. The way in which antigens enter the body determines the site of the initial specific immune response. Lymph nodes control organisms that penetrate the skin; the spleen controls pathogens that enter the bloodstream; and the mucosal lymphoid tissue controls organisms that attack the body through the gastrointestinal and respiratory tracts. Because WBCs continually circulate between the bloodstream and lymphoid tissues, immune responses that begin at one site can quickly spread throughout the body to destroy organisms that escape local control.

The specific immune response, also called **cell-mediated immunity** (CMI), involves mature lymphocytes that have been programmed to eliminate specific antigens. Unlike neutrophils and macrophages, T- and B-lymphocytes must mature, differentiate, and become activated before they can react to nonself antigens.

Lymphocyte Activation

Activation of lymphocytes depends on (1) recognition of an antigen as nonself and (2) stimulation by IL-1. Lymphocyte recognition of a nonself antigen requires a macrophage activity called "antigen processing and presenting." Because macrophages have a sophisticated ability to distinguish self from nonself, they react to all foreign antigens. Macrophages then process the nonself antigen so that a lymphocyte can recognize it.

The macrophage first attaches to the foreign antigen using receptors on its cell membrane. After phagocytosis, lysozymes within the macrophage break up the antigen. A few fragments of the marker are carried to the outer surface of macrophage cell membrane where they are displayed next to a self

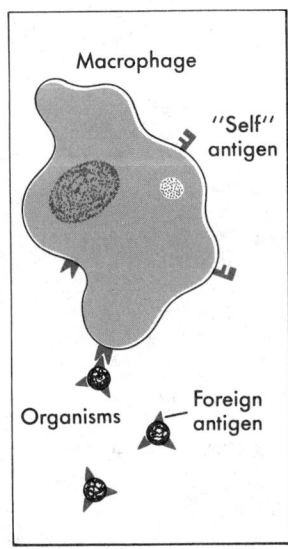 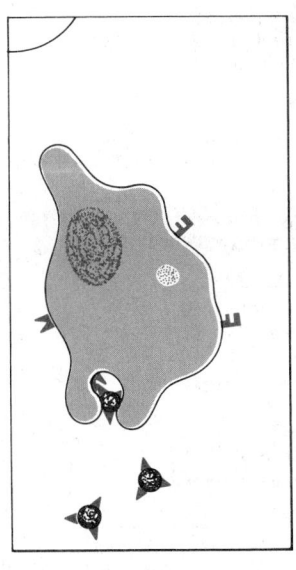 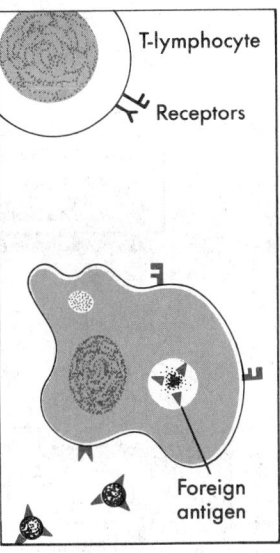 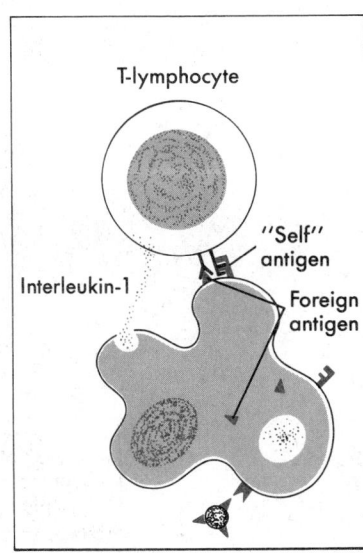

A. Recognition   B. Phagocytosis   C. Digestion   D. Display

FIGURE 39-2   Macrophage processing and presenting. Macrophages are able to recognize any foreign antigen. **A,** Through phagocytosis, they take in antigen and, **B,** digest it. **C,** Part of it is then placed on surface of cell membrane next to an HLA, or self antigen, **D.** Most B-lymphocytes and T-lymphocytes require this process and stimulation by interleukin-1 (secreted by macrophages) to respond to foreign antigens.

antigen (Figure 39-2). Only when the piece of foreign antigen is placed right next to a self antigen are T cells able to recognize it as nonself. At the same time, macrophages secrete IL-1, which completes the activation process.[5]

T Cell–Mediated Immunity

T4 cells

The T4/helper T cell subset of T-lymphocytes controls the specific immune response. T4 cells migrate from the bone marrow to the thymus, where they mature, differentiate, and learn to recognize specific foreign antigens that have been processed by a nearby macrophage. After they are activated, the T4 receptor sites can bind to nonself antigens and initiate a broad spectrum of defensive activities (Figure 39-3). **Interleukin-2** (IL-2) and gamma interferon are the major chemical mediators coordinating these activities.

Interleukin-2

One of the most important mediators in the specific immune response, IL-2 acts as a communicator that allows lymphocytes to "talk" to one another and produce an adequate response to the threat imposed by an organism. As shown in Figure 39-3, IL-2 has a wide variety of roles essential to the specific immune

response. All of the activities are directed at controlling and eliminating the specific organism or nonself antigen that triggered T cell activation.

Gamma interferon

When the invading antigen is a virus, gamma interferon plays a dominant role. The interferon prevents replication of the virus inside a cell, protects nearby cells from viral invasion, and increases the number and activity of available macrophages. Macrophages stimulated by gamma interferon are called "angry macrophages" because of their increased phagocytic activity.

Cytotoxic T cells and natural killer cells

Both cytotoxic T cells and **natural killer (NK) cells** are unique subsets of T-lymphocytes that do not require macrophage assistance to recognize, attack, and destroy organisms rapidly. Many researchers believe that NK cells play an important role in immune surveillance against the abnormal cells of benign and malignant tumors.[6]

T8-lymphocytes

T8-lymphocytes are also called suppressor T cells because they inhibit T4 cell activity, usually after 7 to 10 days. Their goal is to prevent excessive cyto-

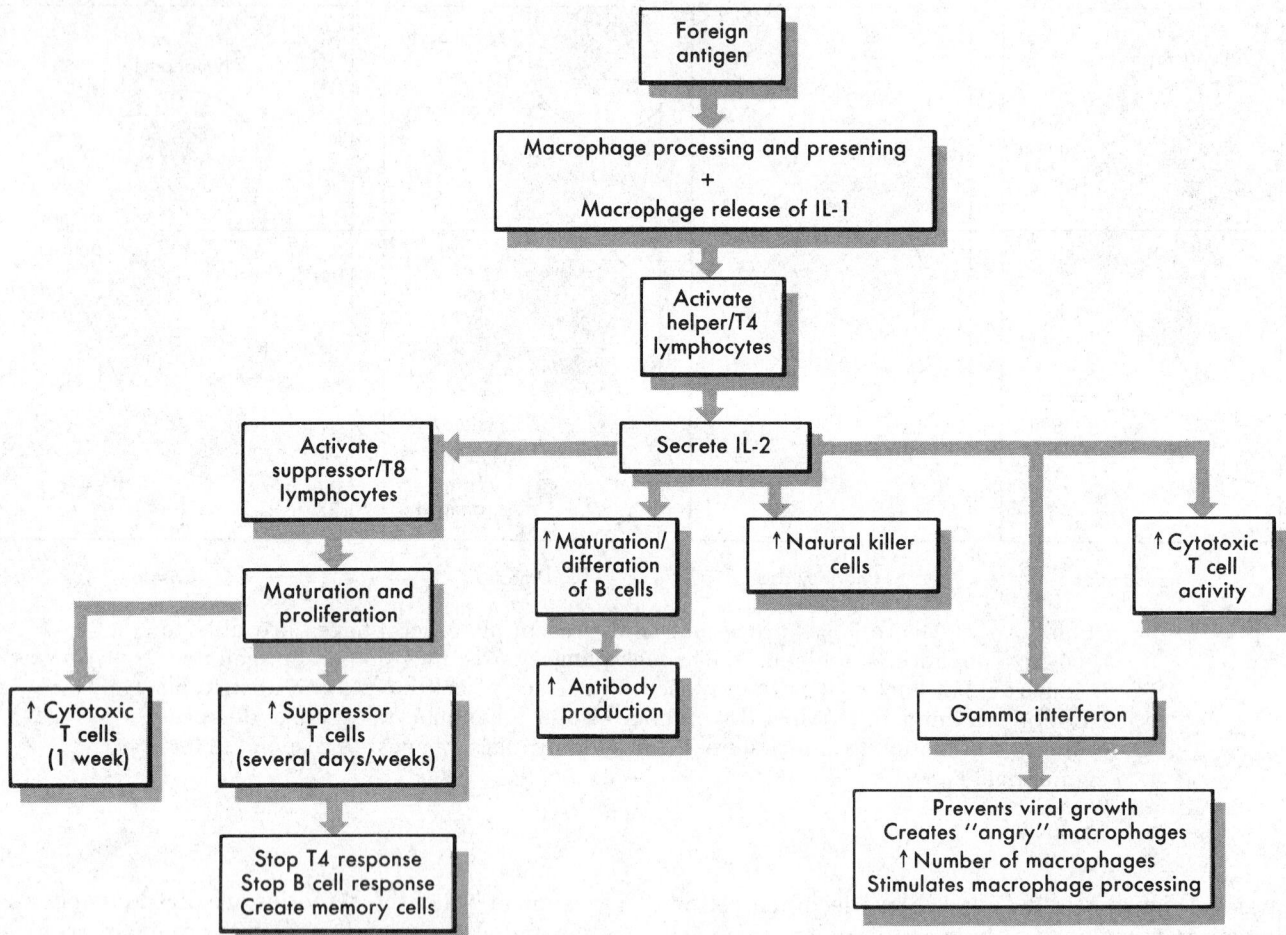

FIGURE 39-3   Specific immune response. Macrophages process nonself antigen and secrete interleukin-1 to activate T4-lymphocytes, which act in coordinator role. T4 cells release interleukin-2, stimulating cytotoxic T cells, natural killer cells, B cell production of antibodies, and gamma interferon to destroy organism initiating response. T8 cells activated by interleukin-2 moderate response to prevent excessive tissue damage and promote production of memory cells, which initiate a rapid response if organism is encountered at a later time.

toxic activity that might damage the body rather than defend it. T8 cells also help maintain recognition of self antigens and prevent WBCs from attacking normal body tissues. In addition, T8-lymphocytes stimulate the production of B memory cells to provide a rapid defense against specific organisms when they are encountered again.

B Cell–Mediated Immunity

When a foreign agent invades the body, B-lymphocytes can be activated by three methods: (1) macrophage processing of the antigenic marker, (2) IL-2 stimulation, or (3) direct contact with a specific antigen to which it has been previously sensitized.[5] After B-lymphocytes are produced in

the bone marrow, they mature and differentiate in the spleen and other unknown sites. Unlike T-lymphocytes, some B cells are capable of recognizing and attacking foreign antigens without macrophage help. Scientists are unclear how this independent activation occurs but believe it may be the result of close interaction between immature B cells and the blood flow through various lymphoid tissues.

During the initial exposure to an organism, B cells differentiate into either **plasma cells** or **memory cells.** Plasma cells produce antigen-specific antibodies or **immunoglobulins**. Memory cells store information about nonself antigens for future reference. As a result the body is able to mount an immediate defense with antibodies the next time that antigen is present. Because there is one specific antibody for

TABLE 39-1 Classes of Immunoglobulins

Immuno-globulin	Definition/role
IgG	Accounts for 75% of all immunoglobulins
	Antiviral, antibacterial, antitoxin activities
	Protects newborns by crossing placental barrier
	Acts as an opsonin and stimulates complement
	May be used in temporary prophylaxis against hepatitis
IgA	Primary antibody in body secretions and mucosa
	Blocks uptake of nonantigens by cells
	Inhibits toxin activity, allergic reactions
	Limits inflammatory response
IgM	Primary antibody in ABO blood types; develops without nonself antigen stimulation
	Most efficient stimulant for complement activity
IgE	Attaches to mast cells and mediates hypersensitivity reactions
	Stimulates release of chemicals, producing local anaphylaxis
IgD	Present in tiny amounts only; unclear role
	May help stimulate B cell differentiation

each specific antigen, thousands of immunoglobulins are produced, providing us with resistance to common microorganisms.

The activities of plasma cells and memory cells are mediated primarily through the complement system of plasma proteins. Each time immunoglobulins interact with or destroy an organism or nonself antigen, complement is involved. This process can be measured in the laboratory by the complement fixation test, which evaluates the amount of antigen-antibody activity in the body during an infection.

Immunoglobulin activity

Antibodies destroy or control antigens in a variety of ways. They may (1) link with the antigen, forming a precipitate that is highly vulnerable to phagocytosis; (2) directly lyse or kill the organism; (3) cause antigens to clump together (agglutination) and become inactive; (4) neutralize toxins produced by

bacteria; (5) prevent antigens from adhering to cells; (6) opsonize antigens to promote phagocytosis; or (7) stimulate activity of the complement protein system. Immunoglobulins have been grouped into five major classes (A, D, E, G, and M) whose activities are described in Table 39-1.[5]

Transplant Rejection

In the past 20 years, transplantation of organs from one person to another has become a clinical commonplace. However, because the donor organs contain nonself antigens, significant efforts must be made to eliminate an immune response by the recipient. Rejection of transplanted organs is primarily due to the reaction of T-lymphocytes, although macrophages and B cells are also involved. Preoperative evaluation has significantly improved the success rate of organ transplant by matching blood types, matching histocompatibility antigens on tissues (called HLA typing), and assessing for the presence of preformed antibodies to the donor HLA antigens. All recipients, however, must remain on cyclosporine or other immunosuppressive drugs to prevent rejection.

Assessment of Immune Responses

Assessment of immunologic defenses is based on an examination of laboratory studies performed on the patient's blood and an assessment of the clinical signs and symptoms of inflammation and infection. In addition, careful listening may yield valuable data indicating problems with immune function, including infections that occur frequently, are slow to resolve, and spread to other locations.

The WBC count with differential (Table 39-2) is the most common and useful diagnostic and assessment tool, since it provides information about the number of different types of WBCs in the blood. Serial total WBC counts are used to diagnose an immune disorder and to assess both the severity of an infection and the effectiveness of drug therapy. Generally the total WBC count begins to drop within 48 hours after the administration of anti-infective agents. Absolute neutrophil counts are used as one clinical indicator of immunocompetence. With an absolute neutrophil count less than $500/mm^3$ a patient is considered neutropenic and requires protective isolation. An increase in immature neutrophils (called segs or bands) indicates that the body's need for the phagocytic cells has outstripped the available supply of mature cells and immature cells are being released from the bone marrow. In addition, following cancer chemotherapy immature neutrophil levels are observed closely to assess the return of bone marrow production of leukocytes.

Recent advances in technology over the past few

TABLE 39-2   White Blood Cell Count with Differential

Cell type	Normal range	Increased	Decreased
Total WBC	5000-10,000/mm³	Infection Tissue damage Inflammation WBC malignancy	Bone marrow depression (drugs/disease) Nutritional deficiency Overwhelming infection Agranulocytosis
Differential neutrophils	1500-7500/mm³ (55-70% of total)	Inflammatory disorders Myelocytic leukemias Trauma Cushing's syndrome Ketoacidosis	Overwhelming bacterial infections Bone marrow depression (prescribed drugs or radiation) Addison's disease Hepatitis, influenza, other viral infections
Immature neutrophils Bands; segs	< 5% of total (40-80% of total)	Overwhelming infection Need for additional phagocytic cells	
Basophils	0.5-1% of total	Polycythemia vera	Allergic reactions Hyperthyroidism
Eosinophils	< 6% of total	Allergic reactions Parasitic infections Autoimmune disorders	Adrenal hyperactivity
Monocytes	100-800/mm³ (1-12% of total)	Chronic inflammatory disorders Infectious mononucleosis Parasitic infections	Bone marrow depression (especially from corticosteroids)
Lymphocytes	1000-5000/mm³ (15-40% of total)	Chronic bacterial infection Lymphocytic leukemia Infectious mononucleosis Viral infections	Bone marrow depression (prescribed drugs or radiation) Sepsis Lupus erythematosus Immunodeficiency disorders

Modified from Pagana KD, Pagana TJ: *Diagnostic and laboratory test reference,* St Louis, 1992, Mosby—Year Book, Inc.

years have provided the means to measure lymphocyte subsets and chemical mediators, an advantage in patients with various immunodeficiency disorders. In addition, serum levels of IgG, IgA, IgM, IgE, and IgD can now be measured. These provide data useful in diagnosing and treating patients with hypersensitivity disorders, autoimmune diseases such as rheumatoid arthritis and systemic lupus erythematosus, immunodeficient states, and chronic infections caused by viruses and bacteria.

FACTORS THAT INFLUENCE IMMUNE FUNCTION

Over the past 20 years, as researchers have been able to identify the physiologic mechanisms involved in specific and nonspecific immune responses, they have also become aware of factors that impair immune function. Evidence has begun to accumulate demonstrating a significant interrelationship among the function of the immune system, age, gender, nutritional status, therapeutic treatment modalities,

TABLE 39-3   Physiologic Changes in Elderly Persons Affecting Immune Function

Changes	Consequences	Changes	Consequences
SKIN		**GENITOURINARY SYSTEM**	
Decreased elasticity	More easily torn/ traumatized, permitting organisms to enter body	Decrease in mucosal barrier	Decreased bladder emptying
		Greater opportunity for microbe growth	Increased entry of organisms
RESPIRATORY SYSTEM		**CARDIOVASCULAR SYSTEM**	
Decreased effectiveness of cilia	Ineffective removal of inhaled organisms	Decrease in cardiac output/increased peripheral resistance	Decreased oxygen delivery to tissues, increasing risk of ischemic injury
Decrease in elastic recoil and decreased tidal volume while supine	Decreased alveolar ventilation causing collapse of alveoli (atelectasis)	Fragile capillaries	Increased risk of damage causing decreased oxygen/nutrient supply to tissues
	Decrease in macrophage function		
	Impaired gas exchange	**IMMUNOLOGIC TISSUES**	
	Lower blood oxygen levels	Smaller thymus gland	Decreased T cell maturation/ differentiation
Reduced muscle strength	Increased work of breathing	White blood cells	Decreased recognition of nonself
Impaired cough/gag reflexes	Decreased ability to remove particles and organisms		Increased production of autoantibodies
	Increased risk of aspiration		
GASTROINTESTINAL TRACT			
Decreased HCl secretion	Decreased destruction of organisms		
Decreased motility	Ineffective removal of organisms		

the central and autonomic nervous systems, and the stress response. Although the exact mechanisms by which these factors influence immunocompetence is not yet entirely clear, consistent measurable effects have been demonstrated in both the laboratory and clinical settings.

Age

The immune system displays dramatic changes with increased age that decrease the effectiveness of the general physical barriers and the activation of WBCs.[3,9,14,16] Consequently, elderly persons have an increased susceptibility to infection and a diminished capacity to destroy organisms. Table 39-3 lists physiologic changes in elderly persons and their im-

munologic consequences. (See also the geriatric considerations box.)

Sex

The role of sex in immunocompetence can be seen in the widespread discrepancies that exist between the life span of males and females in both animals and humans. Animal studies have shown that females reject tumors and grafts more readily than males and that they have macrophages with greater phagocytic ability. The differences have been related to the presence of estrogen in females. However, women in one study had better responses to vaccination than men, even though they were past menopause.[13]

GERIATRIC CONSIDERATIONS

Physiologic Changes in the Immune System

The important role of the protective physical barriers is highlighted in elderly persons; changes in these barriers enable microorganisms to enter and establish themselves in the body. Once organisms have gained entrance to the body, cellular changes associated with aging result in a decreased responsiveness to foreign antigens. In addition, the declining ability to differentiate self from nonself increases the risk of autoimmune disorders.

Nurses need to be aware of the situational factors commonly seen in aged persons that increase the risk of infection. Disorders that increase immobility are common. As a result, elderly individuals face the hazards of immobility that increase susceptibility to infection: decreased alveolar ventilation and atelectasis; decreased cardiac output and obstruction of blood flow at pressure points (heels, sacrum, elbows) promoting ischemic injury and the development of decubitus ulcers; and decreased gastrointestinal motility. In addition, antibiotics given to combat common respiratory and urinary tract infections destroy normal gastrointestinal flora and promote growth of pathogenic organisms.

Older persons are more likely to have chronic diseases and therefore to be hospitalized more frequently. Institutionalized elderly persons undergoing invasive diagnostic or therapeutic procedures such as nasogastric tubes, tracheal intubation, indwelling urinary catheters, intravascular lines, and surgery can be infected by organisms no longer blocked by physical barriers. Consequently, ongoing nursing assessment of the signs of inflammation and infection, particularly around indwelling catheters, is vital.

Nutritional Status

Nutritional status is also known to have an impact on immune function.[3,4,9] Protein-calorie malnutrition is the most prevalent cause of immunodeficiency in the world and has been associated with impaired physical barriers, decreased inflammatory responses, and abnormal lymphocyte function. The anatomic and chemical barriers of the immune system are affected primarily by the lack of vitamins A, B, and C as well as inadequate protein and zinc.

Nutrients are required to maintain normal mucous membranes (vitamins A and B); intracellular activity and tissue stability (vitamin C); wound healing, thymus activity, and T cell activity (protein and zinc); and intact skin. Protein-calorie malnutrition is also associated with a lack of iron-binding proteins such as transferrin and lactoferrin. These proteins, found in blood, tears, saliva, and other body fluids, prevent bacteria from using the iron they need for reproduction in the body.

When infection or serious injury is present, the problem of malnutrition is compounded by the body's metabolic responses. Anabolic and catabolic activities occur simultaneously, but the catabolism of muscle protein frequently dominates, promoting muscle wasting, negative nitrogen balance, and the use of amino acids to meet increased energy needs through gluconeogenesis. The production of all the active components of the immune system (phagocytes, antibodies, lymphocytes, and chemical mediators) requires adequate sources of cellular energy and protein synthesis; without these, every aspect of an individual's resistance is impaired. Nurses can assess the patient's nutritional status best by obtaining a careful diet history for an average 24-hour period, gathering information about any recent weight loss, checking serum albumin levels, and obtaining serial weights during hospitalization.

Stressors

During the past 15 years scientists have become interested in examining the interactions among the psychologic, neurologic, endocrine, and immune systems, a field called psychoneuroimmunology. The idea that phenomena that affect the mind may also be related to changes in physiologic functions and increase an individual's susceptibility to disease or alter the progression of an illness goes back to ancient times. However, it was not until the last decade that this assumption has gained empiric support.

A stressor is generally defined as any situation psychologically or biologically perceived to be threatening to a person's well-being. Stressors produce the biochemical changes in the body known as the stress response. Two of the earliest events recognized as part of the stress response were increased activation of the sympathetic nervous system and the adrenal glands. Elevated levels of glucocorticoids (released by the adrenal cortex) and catecholamines (released by the sympathetic nervous system and adrenal medulla) have been shown to alter many activities in both the nonspecific and specific immune responses.

Specific stressors that have been studied include lack of sleep, academic examinations, bereavement, marital disruption, caring for a chronically ill individual, and unemployment. Each of these has been shown to diminish the activity of one or more types of WBCs. Currently psychoneuroimmunologic research is focusing on whether this decreased immune cell function, which can be demonstrated in

RESEARCH BRIEF

Cohen S, Tyrrell DA, Smith AP: Psychologic stress and susceptibility to the common cold, *N Engl J Med* 325(9):606-612, 1991.

"Stress causes colds" is a common saying, but it is one that has had no scientific basis until recently. British scientists recruited 394 healthy adults, 18 to 54 years old, to examine the relationship between stress and respiratory infections. Subjects were questioned about stressful life events during the past year, current levels of stress, and emotional states before being given nose drops containing respiratory viruses. Subjects were placed in quarantine for 2 days before and 7 days after exposure to the virus and were monitored for signs and symptoms of upper respiratory infection.

A significant relationship between infection and stress levels was demonstrated; 38% of the subjects developed colds, and the rate of infection increased as subjects' stress levels increased. Important demographic variables were controlled and had no effect on the relationship. This study provides a basis for additional studies relating stressors to immune function.

---

the laboratory, also results in an increased susceptibility to infectious organisms in the individuals involved.[2,8]

Therapeutic Modalities

Drugs that have a direct or indirect impact on the immune system are commonly used in patient care (Table 39-4). All drugs have the possibility of causing hypersensitivity reactions, producing clinical signs ranging from hives to circulatory shock (see Chapter 40). In addition, some drugs such as corticosteroids and immunosuppressants are used specifically to inhibit both the inflammatory and specific immune response in patients with chronic inflammatory conditions and autoimmune disorders. However, at the same time these drugs reduce the patient's ability to resist organisms so nurses must observe patients closely for signs of skin, gastrointestinal, respiratory, or urinary tract infections.

Recipients of bone marrow, renal, or other organ transplants are deliberately given immunosuppressive therapy such as cyclosporine, azathioprine, and/or corticosteroids to reduce the risk of rejection. Although the HLA antigens of donated organs are similar or identical to those of the recipient, use of drugs for the suppression of lymphocytes is still

TABLE 39-4 Pharmacology Summary: Drugs Affecting Immune Function

Drug	Effect
Immunosuppressants	Inhibit production of WBCs by bone marrow
Anti-inflammatory agents	
Corticosteroids	Block arachidonic acid metabolites (leukotrienes/prostaglandins)
Aspirin/salicylates	Decrease macrophage activity
Nonsteroidal anti-inflammatory drugs (NSAIDS)	Inhibit IL-1 and IL-2 production
	Lyse T, B, and natural killer cells
	Inhibit interferon production
Sympathomimetics	Decrease chemotaxis
	Inhibit WBC response to antigens
	Alter antibody production
	Decrease lysozyme activity
	Decrease WBC reproduction
Anti-infectives	
All oral antibiotics	Destroy normal bacterial flora
	Increased risk of allergic reactions
Tetracyclines/sulfonamides	Inhibit chemotaxis
	Inhibit activation of lymphocytes
Chloramphenicol	Depress WBC production
Phenytoin (Dilantin)	Lymph node hyperplasia
	Inhibits effects of corticosteroids
Antidysrhythmics	
Procainamide (Pronestyl)	Decreased production of WBCs
	Production of antinuclear antibodies (SLE-like syndrome)
Propranolol (Inderal)	Inflammation of airways
ALL DRUGS	Possible type I hypersensitivity reactions

essential to prevent a cell-mediated immune response to nonself antigens on the transplanted organ.

Ionizing radiation is commonly used in the treatment of some cancers because of its ability to inhibit cancerous cell reproduction. However, WBC production also is affected since a high percentage of these cells, like malignant cells, are constantly in the active phase of cell division. As a result, patients being treated for cancer often experience bone marrow depression and a significant drop in the number of circulating WBCs (leukopenia).

Individuals with leukopenia or depressed WBC function usually develop infections in those areas open to the external environment: the lungs, urinary tract, and gastrointestinal tract. In addition, when the body's defenses have been severely compromised, opportunistic infections (from organisms normally controlled easily by the body) can be life-threatening. Thus hospitalized patients receiving immunosuppressive therapy must be monitored closely and, when necessary, placed in isolation to reduce the threat of infection.

CRITICAL THINKING QUESTIONS

1 What are the essential components of the immune system?

2 How do the various tissues and cells of the immune system provide protection against nonself?

3 Give examples of different agents and events that can stimulate an immune response.

4 What are the primary differences between a nonspecific and a specific immune response?

5 What is the sequence of events in a nonspecific immune response?

6 How do age and nutritional status affect the function of the immune system?

BIBLIOGRAPHY

Current

1. Broide DH: Inflammatory cells: structure and function. In Stites DP, Terr AI, editors: *Basic and clinical immunology,* ed 7, Norwalk, Conn, 1991, Appleton & Lange.
2. Cohen S et al: Psychological stress and susceptibility to the common cold, *N Engl J Med* 325:606, 1991.
3. Dubey DP, Yunis EJ: Aging and nutritional effects on immune functions in humans. In Stites DP, Terr AI, editors: *Basic and clinical immunology,* ed 7, Norwalk, Conn, 1991, Appleton & Lange.
4. Good RA, Lorenz E: Nutrition, immunity, aging and cancer, *Nutr Rev* 46:62, 1988.
5. Goodman JW: The immune response and immunoglobulin structure and function. In Stites DP, Terr AI, editors: *Basic and clinical immunology,* ed 7, Norwalk, Conn, 1991, Appleton & Lange.
6. Herberman RB et al: Lymphokine-activated killer cell activity, *Immunol Today* 8:178, 1987.
7. Kamani NR, Douglas SD: Structure and development of the immune system. In Stites DP, Terr AI, editors: *Basic and clinical immunology,* ed 7, Norwalk, Conn, 1991, Appleton & Lange.
8. Kiecolt-Glaser JK, Glaser R: Stress and immune function in humans. In Ader R, Felton DL, Cohen, N, editors: *Psychoneuroimmunology,* ed 2, San Diego, 1991, Academic Press, Inc.
9. Lipschitz DA: Nutrition, aging and the immunohematopoietic system, *Clin Geriatr Med* 3:319, 1987.
10. Mills J, Drutz DJ: Mechanisms of immunity to infection. In Stites DP, Terr AI, editors: *Basic and clinical immunology,* ed 7, Norwalk, Conn, 1991, Appleton & Lange.
11. Oppenheim JJ et al: Cytokines. In Stites DP, Terr AI, editors: *Basic and clinical immunology,* ed 7, Norwalk, Conn, 1991, Appleton & Lange.
12. Pagana KD, Pagana TJ: *Diagnostic and laboratory test reference,* St Louis, 1992, Mosby–Year Book, Inc.
13. Roghmann KJ et al: Immune response of elderly adults to *Pneumococcus:* variations by age, sex and functional impairment, *J Gerontol* 42:265, 1987.
14. Saltzman RL, Peterson PK: Immunodeficiency of the elderly, *Rev Infect Dis* 9:127, 1987.
15. von Boehmer H: The developmental biology of T lymphocytes, *Ann Rev Immunol* 6:309, 1988.

Classic

16. Wekser ME: The senescence of the immune system, *Semin Immunol* 16:53, 1986.

CHAPTER FORTY

Nursing Management of Adults with Immune Disorders

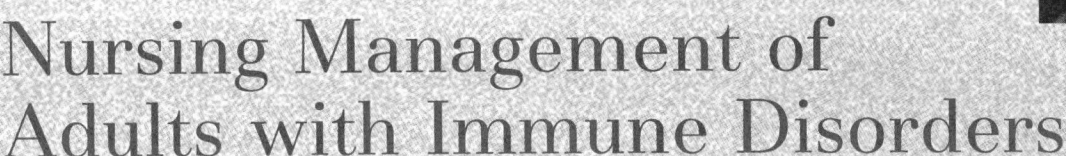

LEARNING OBJECTIVES

1 Identify common causes of immunodeficient states.
2 Develop a nursing care plan for the neutropenic patient.
3 Explain the possible influence of social mores on the nursing care of HIV-infected patients.
4 Describe the source and significance of opportunistic infections in the patient with AIDS.
5 Identify available resources for individuals with HIV disease.
6 Implement the nursing process with patients with AIDS.
7 Describe common theories underlying autoimmune disorders.
8 Identify the nursing needs of patients with SLE.
9 Differentiate among type I, type II, type III, and type IV hypersensitivity reactions.
10 State the precautions needed in providing blood products and new drugs to patients with a history of allergic reactions.

KEY TERMS

acquired immune deficiency syndrome (AIDS), p. 1032
AIDS-related complex (ARC), p. 1032
anaphylaxis, p. 1046
antinuclear antibodies (ANAs), p. 1043
autoantibodies (AABs), p. 1041
autoantigens (AAgs), p. 1041
biologic response modifiers, p. 1026

human immunodeficiency virus (HIV), p. 1029
hypersensitivity, p. 1045
Kaposi's sarcoma, p. 1034
retroviruses, p. 1030
serum sickness, p. 1047
urticaria, p. 1046

IMMUNODEFICIENCY REFERS to the inability of the immune system to control or destroy invading pathogens causing tissue damage. Immunodeficient or immunocompromised states result when one or more of the active components of the immune system described in Chapter 39 are not present or are inhibited.

Etiology/Pathophysiology

Immunodeficient states can arise from genetic disorders, chronic diseases, infections, nutritional deficiencies, and treatment regimens used for cancer and organ transplant (Table 40-1). In the United States the most common causes of immunodeficiency are chemotherapy agents or radiation used to treat cancers, immunosuppressive drug regimens used with chronic diseases or following organ transplantation, malignancies of the immune system, and infection with the human immunodeficiency virus (HIV).

Chemotherapy and radiation

The goal of most cancer chemotherapeutic agents and radiation treatments is to destroy malignant cells in the process of mitosis. Because chemotherapy and radiation have their greatest effect on sites in which new cells are being produced rapidly, white blood cell (WBC) production in the bone marrow is severely inhibited. For example, in the patient with leukemia, chemotherapy destroys both malignant and normal WBCs, severely reducing the patient's immune response. The rapidly dividing cells of the gastric mucosa also are destroyed, increasing the opportunity for organisms to enter the bloodstream and cause infections.

Immunosuppressive drugs used to manage chronic diseases and organ transplantation (Table 40-2) have a less dramatic effect on the patient. The goal is to inhibit the immune response, thus decreasing inflammation or tissue rejection, while maintaining an immune system capable of defending itself against most organisms. Nevertheless, the risk of infection is always present.

In patients receiving cancer chemotherapy, immunodeficiency is a temporary state. If drugs can control the infections until normal immune function returns, the patients will no longer be at risk. However, the patient who has received a transplanted organ must continue immunosuppressive drug therapy that balances the risk of infection against the risk of rejection.

Diseases and infections

Cancers of the immune system have a direct adverse effect on the lymphoid tissues and/or the production

TABLE 40-1 Acquired Immunodeficient States	
Disorder	**Immunologic defect**
Myelogenous leukemia	Decreased granulocytes, particularly neutrophils
	Reduced phagocytosis of pathogens
Lymphocytic leukemia	Decreased T and B cell numbers
Lymphoma	Decreased specific immune response
Multiple myeloma	Decreased number of B cells
	Decreased antibody activity
Hepatic cirrhosis	Inhibited WBC proliferation
Splenectomy	Reduced filtration of organisms in blood and their destruction by lymphocytes and macrophages
Chronic renal failure	Decreased neutrophil movement
Diabetes mellitus	Unclear; decreased lysis of bacteria
Protein calorie malnutrition; radiation	Decreased production and maturation of WBCs
Alcohol and drug abuse	Unclear; decreased lymphocyte and macrophage activity
Immunosuppressive drugs; cancer chemotherapy	Decreased production/function of WBCs
Viral infections (CMV, EBV, rubeola, HIV)	Inhibited T-lymphocytes; may reduce other WBC functions
Genetic disorders	Inadequate production/function of chemical mediators, WBCs, or antibodies

Modified from Stites DP, Terr AI, editors: *Basic and clinical immunology,* ed 7, Norwalk, Conn, 1991, Appleton & Lange.

of effective WBCs. Depending on the disease state, these patients display varying degrees of immunodeficiency. There also are several infectious organisms that directly inhibit the immune system. Currently, the human immunodeficiency virus (HIV) is the most well-known infection. Other organisms

TABLE 40-2   Immunosuppressive Drugs

Drug	Action	Effects
Corticosteroids	Decrease circulating lymphocytes and monocytes Decrease phagocytosis Inhibit macrophage activity	Block acute inflammatory response/exacerbations Inhibit immune response in autoimmune disease
Cytotoxic drugs (e.g., azathioprine, cyclophosphamide, methotrexate)	Destroy WBCs, particularly lymphocytes, but also other rapidly dividing cells of bone marrow and gastrointestinal tract	Inhibit immune response in rheumatoid disorders
Cyclosporine	Specifically inhibits T_4/helper lymphocytes; no effect on bone marrow function	Inhibits rejection of transplanted organs
Antilymphocyte antibodies	Impair T cell function	Inhibit rejection of transplanted organs Treat graft vs. host (GVH) reactions

suppressing immune function include the rubeola virus, which causes measles, cytomegalovirus (CMV), and the Epstein-Barr virus (EBV), which causes mononucleosis.[13]

Protein calorie malnutrition

Adequate nutrition is essential for the production of effective WBCs and the activity of the thymus and lymph nodes. Patients with severe malnutrition are immunodeficient as a result of decreased maturation of T cells in the thymus and impaired macrophage and neutrophil activity (see Chapter 39).

Clinical Manifestations

The primary indicator of immunodeficient states is a decrease in the number of WBCs or their chemical mediators in blood. Although a significant decrease in any WBC is important, the risk of infection in the clinical setting is usually measured by the number of neutrophils in the blood, the absolute neutrophil count (ANC). If the ANC is less than $1000/mm^3$, the patient is considered at risk for infection; if the ANC is less than 500, the patient is considered neutropenic and will develop an infection.

The types of infections these patients acquire vary, to some extent, because of the specific immunologic defect. However, these distinctions are not absolute. For example, patients who have received chemotherapy to treat leukemia are at high risk for bacterial infections not only because their neutrophils have been destroyed, but also because the rap-idly dividing cells lining the gastrointestinal tract have been destroyed, enabling organisms to enter the bloodstream. In contrast, HIV-infected patients are more likely to succumb to infections normally controlled by lymphocytes. Table 40-3 lists common infections associated with specific immunologic disorders (see Chapter 11 for the mechanisms of infection).

Therapeutic Management

The goals in managing the immunodeficient patient are to prevent and treat infection. The care of these patients is collaborative, since both nurses and physicians monitor for signs of infection as well as for the side effects of anti-infective drug therapy, particularly adverse effects on the kidney, liver, red blood cells (RBCs), or platelets.

Anti-infective drug therapy provides the basis for medical treatment. For many of these drugs, blood levels (peaks and troughs) are measured after the third dose to ensure that therapeutic levels are being maintained. The nursing staff is responsible for arranging the times at which blood is drawn, for example, just before the drug's administration for a trough level and ½ to 1 hour after the drug has been infused for a peak level.

The specific drug used to treat the patient is determined after the causative organism has been identified through a culture and sensitivity study performed in the laboratory on blood, urine, stool, sputum, and wound specimens. Specimens are cultured, or grown, and anti-infective drugs added to assess their capacity to kill the pathogen. Specimens

TABLE 40-3   Susceptibility to Organisms in Immunodeficient States[43,52]

Disorder/treatment	Deficit	Organisms

Acute myelocytic leukemia/ cyclophosphamide	Loss of neutrophil and macrophage phagocytosis	Staphylococci
		Gram-negative bacteria
		   Escherichia coli
		   Pseudomonas
		   Klebsiella
		Fungi

Chronic lymphocytic leukemia/ antimetabolite agents, high-dose corticosteroids	Lack of normal lymphocytes Decreased WBC production Low number of antibodies	Streptococci, pneumococci *Haemophilus influenzae* *Neisseria meningococcus* Gram-negative bacteria
HIV infection, Hodgkin's disease/cyclosporine	Reduced number of lymphocytes, mono-cytes, and macrophages	Mycobacteria Protozoa Viruses Fungi Gram-positive bacteria *Nocardia*
Splenectomy	Decreased phagocytosis by macrophages Decreased B cell production/reserve	Streptococci, pneumococci *Haemophilus influenzae* *Klebsiella* Staphylococci Meningococci

are obtained for culture and sensitivity whenever the patient has a fever or other signs of infection described in Chapter 11.

In addition, drugs also may be given to stimulate the immune system, treat deficits, or provide chemical mediators the immune system is unable to produce. **Biologic response modifiers** are drugs created in the laboratory, using a process called recombinant deoxyribonucleic acid (DNA). DNA from active immune proteins acquired from animals is combined with DNA from the same protein obtained from humans. This process allows laboratories to produce large quantities of essential substances, replacing or supplementing immunologic agents that are missing in the patient.[33] Table 40-4 lists the biologic response modifiers currently used to treat immunodeficient states.

Because of the large number of medications required by the acutely ill immunodeficient patient, nurses must obtain information about drug compatibilities from a pharmacist and document these on the medication administration record to prevent adverse interactions. Scheduling medications is often difficult when the patient is receiving not only several drugs, but also frequent blood products. Using a notebook to keep a permanent record of interactions among commonly administered drugs can save considerable time for the nursing staff.

NURSING MANAGEMENT OF THE IMMUNODEFICIENT PATIENT
Assessment

Continual assessment of the degree to which the patient is at risk for infection and the early presence of infection is the framework around which the nursing management of the severely immunodeficient patient is built. Particularly if the patient is neutropenic, all efforts must be made to minimize the patient's exposure to pathogens. As a result, at least once per shift the nurse carries out the specific physical assessments outlined in Table 40-5.

The nurse also assesses the patient's baseline nutritional status, emotional state, normal coping mechanisms, and social supports. Helping the patient cope with life-threatening situations and maintaining adequate nutritional intake require teamwork among the nursing staff, the patient's support system, and members of the nutritional support service.

Nursing Diagnosis

Several diagnoses are appropriate to the patient with significant immunodeficiency:

High risk for infection related to an inadequate immunologic defense system

TABLE 40-4 Biologic Response Modifiers Used for Immunodeficient Patients

Biologic response modifier	Action
Granulocyte-macrophage colony stimulating factor (GM-CSF [Filgrastim])	Stimulates production and maturation of granulocytes
Immune globulin (gamma globulin/Gamimune)	Treats deficit of immunoglobulin G (IgG); increases strength of specific immune response
Alpha-interferon	Prevents growth and replication of viruses directly Increases cytotoxic ability of natural killer cells
Interleukin-2	Stimulates production and activity of B cells, T cells, and natural killer cells
Erythropoietin (epoetin alpha)	Stimulates the production and maturation of red blood cells in bone marrow

TABLE 40-5 Assessment for Immunodeficiency

System	Parameters
Respiratory system	Cough (productive or nonproductive) Change in sputum amount, color, smell, consistency Change in breath sounds Dyspnea
Skin/mucous membranes	Inflammation (redness, heat, swelling, pain) Petechiae or bruising Drainage Skin tears, ulceration
Eyes	Redness Itching Drainage
Genitourinary	Frequency/urgency/pain with urination Blood, mucus, or sediment in urine Change in urine color or odor Vaginal drainage
Gastrointestinal tract	Oral inflammation or ulcers Nausea/vomiting Change in consistency, frequency of stool Blood in stool
Systemic	Temperature change (>38.5° C or <37° C) Chills Restlessness, irritability Increased pulse (>10%) Decreased blood pressure (>10%)

Acute pain related to presence of oral ulcers (may be manifested by self-reports or a refusal to eat or swallow medications)

Alteration in nutrition: less than body requirements, related to nausea, stomatitis, anorexia, or fatigue (may be manifested by decrease in weight, low serum albumin, loss of muscle mass)

Social isolation related to requirements for protection against infection (may be manifested by flat affect, withdrawal, hostility, and preoccupation)

Anticipatory grieving related to perceived possibility of death (may be manifested by withdrawal, guilt, anger, changes in sleep patterns, and self-reports)

Anxiety related to lack of understanding of treatment regimen (often manifested by self-report, hypervigilance, information seeking, and signs of sympathetic nervous system stimulation)

Decisional conflicts related to participation in various treatment regimens (may be manifested by self-reports, delay in making decisions, and information seeking)

Fatigue related to reduction in tissue oxygenation caused by destruction of RBCs by chemotherapy (may be manifested by expressions of continued lack of energy and inability to perform normal daily activities)

Planning

Immunodeficient patients are admitted to the hospital when they have a severe infection or when they are at risk for becoming neutropenic. Patients who are neutropenic on admission or are expected to become neutropenic after chemotherapeutic treatment should be placed in a private room immediately, and visitors should be limited to those most important to the patient. To minimize exposure to pathogens, the patient's nurse should not be assigned to other patients with active infections, particularly infections spread by respiratory droplets.

Implementation

Reducing risk of infection

Infection control manuals in each institution provide guidelines for implementing the protective isolation required by neutropenic patients. The importance of careful hand washing by anyone entering the patient's room cannot be overemphasized as a preventive measure. Also, anyone with an upper respiratory infection should wear a mask or avoid going into the room entirely.

A fever may be the patient's first sign of infection and therefore often serves as a signal for obtaining specimens for culture and sensitivity studies. However, protocols for the use of antipyretics differ once the pathogen has been identified and treatment started. Thus planned responses to the presence of a fever, including plans for obtaining cultures, should be clearly established with the physician when the patient first becomes neutropenic.

Respiratory infections are one of the major threats to the immunodeficient patient. The risk of respiratory infections is reduced by ambulating the patient around the room or maintaining a regular regimen for turning, coughing, and deep breathing exercises. Family members often like to assume some responsibility for the pulmonary toilet so that they can be more involved in the patient's care.

To reduce the possibility of other infections, the nurse should avoid invasive procedures such as injections, bladder catheterizations, enemas, rectal suppositories, rectal temperatures, or the use of vaginal tampons or suppositories. A central venous line is usually inserted to eliminate the need for invasive blood draws and peripheral intravenous lines. The nurse must adhere closely to the hospital's policy for central and peripheral line care.

As part of discharge planning, patients need education about avoiding large crowds or friends who are ill, taking their medications, and maintaining a healthy life-style. These patients should see their health care provider regularly and receive annual vaccinations against influenza as well as other protective vaccines such as pneumococcal polysaccharide vaccine (Pneumovax) as needed. Pneumovax is particularly important for patients who have had a splenectomy and lack B-lymphocyte reserves.

Oral hygiene

The mouth provides an ideal environment for pathogen growth and is a common site for infection in im-

TABLE 40-6 Characteristics of Common Oral Infections

Infection	Characteristic
Candida albicans	Whitish patches; localized or extensive
Herpes simplex	Painful clusters of small vesicles
Gram-positive bacteria	Dry, brownish yellow, raised vesicles
Gram-negative bacteria	Moist, white, raised, painful, nonpurulent ulcers
Pseudomonas	Yellowish, dry, painless ulcers with necrotic core surrounded by red halo

munodeficient patients. Table 40-6 lists the signs and symptoms of common oral infections. Drug therapy specific to the type of infection is started as soon as any signs of infection appear, since these organisms can spread to the bloodstream, causing septicemia.

Patients' teeth should be cleaned with a soft toothbrush after each meal and before sleep. If the patient's platelet count is below 50,000/mm^3, a sponge brush is used to clean teeth and gums at least three times each day. In addition, patients should rinse their mouths with saline every 3 hours or if they vomit. Chlorhexidine mouthwash may be ordered twice daily after cleaning to minimize gingivitis. Topical solutions such as 2% viscous lidocaine may be used before oral care if it causes pain. Ice chips and iced fluids also may provide some pain relief, but systemic pain medications are often necessary.

Skin care

Personal hygiene often becomes difficult for acutely ill patients because of severe chills (rigor), extreme fatigue, and discomfort in moving. Consequently, helping the patient bathe with antimicrobial soap becomes a nursing priority, and the patient's perineum must be cleaned with soap and water after each voiding or bowel movement. Powerful antibiotics destroy normal intestinal flora and can produce an overgrowth of fungi that cause skin infections in the groin, under pendulous breasts, or in the abdominal folds of obese patients. Vigorous early treatment with nystatin or another antifungal cream can reduce the risk of serious excoriation in these areas.

Nutrition

Most of the disorders causing neutropenia involve factors that interfere with adequate nutrition. Loss of appetite (anorexia), altered taste sensation, stomatitis, fatigue, nausea, and diarrhea make it difficult for the patient to eat. The nurse can encourage family members to bring familiar food from home and provide the patient with several small, frequent, high-protein, high-calorie meals during the day. Spicy and greasy foods should be avoided, and no liquids should be taken with meals. Rest periods should be provided before meals, and, when possible, meals should be separated from any medication or activity that tends to make the patient nauseated. Although most patients develop infections from organisms already in the body (e.g., *E. coli*), raw vegetables, fresh fruits, and flowers are usually not permitted, since they could contain organisms capable of causing infection. Some institutions allow fruit if it is washed first, but others mandate peeling the fruit before it enters the patient's room. Often the patient is placed on total parenteral nutrition (TPN) to maintain adequate nutrition. Although a change in body weight is the best indicator of nutritional status, serum albumin levels also should be checked, since protein is essential for the production of new WBCs.

Psychosocial needs

Many patients and their families are quite knowledgeable about the dangers of severe immunodeficiency. As a result, they may demonstrate a high level of anxiety on admission and have many questions. Also, they often have internal conflicts about the type and amount of treatment they want and need an opportunity to talk with a nurse who can help them explore their options. Finally, patients may begin grieving if the hospital admission reawakens the possibility of their death. In the midst of the many tasks required in the care of the neutropenic patient, nurses must take time to provide emotional support. Often, when these patients have been discharged, their letters to the hospital indicate that these opportunities to talk about feelings are what they valued most in their nursing care.

Evaluation/Documentation

Documentation of the patient's status on admission is essential for ongoing evaluation of nursing care. Actual and potential problems need to be addressed in the patient's chart in a concise, problem-oriented manner so that the effectiveness of interventions can be assessed. Signs of infection, changes in lesions of the skin or mucous membranes, and factors interfering with nutritional intake are particularly impor-tant to document. Discharge plans should also be included to ensure a smooth progression from hospital to home.

HUMAN IMMUNODEFICIENCY VIRUS DISEASE
Definition

HIV disease is a chronic viral infection of human immunodeficiency virus (HIV) that is associated with progressive deterioration of the immune system, particularly T_4/CD_4 cells, which results in the development of severe opportunistic infections. Opportunistic infections are caused by organisms that are commonly present in our environment and that cause disease only when there is immunosuppression. The spectrum of HIV disease ranges from asymptomatic HIV infection to acquired immune deficiency syndrome (AIDS).[12,22]

Etiology/Epidemiology

Human immunodeficiency virus (HIV) is the etiologic agent of HIV disease.[9,12,22,42] The first reported cases of HIV disease (in particular AIDS) were in mid-1980. HIV was first identified in 1983. Diagnostic testing for HIV infection began in 1985.

The three methods of HIV transmission are (1) intimate sexual contact; (2) the parenteral route, that is, exposure to contaminated blood, including blood products, transfusions, occupational exposure, and sharing used needles; and (3) perinatally or across the placenta, that is, infected woman to fetus or exposure in utero, during birth, or to infant via breast feeding.[1,10,11]

The World Health Organization (WHO) estimates that there are 8 to 10 million HIV-infected persons in the world, with 1.5 to 2 million of these in the United States. During 1992, 47,106 cases of AIDS were reported to the Centers for Disease Control (CDC).[11] As of December 1992, there were 245,472 reported cases of AIDS in the United States.[11] The case-fatality rate from July to December 1992 was 88.7%.[11] The cumulative case-fatality rate from 1981 to September 1992 was 66.5%.[11] Epidemiologic data suggest that 50% of HIV-infected persons will develop AIDS 10 to 12 years after becoming infected. Currently in the United States the ratio of male to female AIDS cases is 8:1, whereas in Africa the ratio is 1:1.[12,23]

The majority of people with AIDS or HIV infection in the United States are homosexual/bisexual men or intravenous drug users; however, transmission is increasing in heterosexuals, especially in black and Hispanic communities. Heterosexual transmission has increased the rate of HIV infection in women and infants. The risk of HIV transmission by occupational exposure is estimated as 0.3% or 1 in 250 incidents.[40]

Pathophysiology

HIV infects helper T-lymphocytes (T_4/CD_4 cells), B-lymphocytes, macrophages, promyelocytes, fibroblasts, and epidermal Langerhan's cells. T-lymphocytes and macrophages control an important aspect of the immune system, cell-mediated immunity. Cell-mediated immunity protects the body against viruses, bacteria, fungi, and parasites that are not controlled by antibodies and neutrophils. These pathogens (e.g., herpes simplex, *Mycobacterium tuberculosis*) are often controlled by cell-mediated immunity but not eliminated from the body. When cell-mediated immunity weakens, latent infections may reactivate to cause the opportunistic infections of HIV disease (i.e., pulmonary tuberculosis). In addition, some pathogens in the environment, which most immunocompetent persons easily resist (e.g., *Candida*), become infectious (i.e., opportunistic infections). Symptoms of HIV disease manifest when latent infections reactivate or there is recent exposure to opportunistic infections.[22]

HIV is a retrovirus that carries its genetic code as ribonucleic acid (RNA). There are two related retroviruses, HIV-1 and HIV-2, which can cause HIV disease. Unlike other RNA viruses, **retroviruses** replicate by first transcribing their genetic code into double-stranded deoxyribonucleic acid (DNA) of the host cell. HIV has a unique enzyme, reverse transcriptase (RT), which enables HIV to reverse the usual flow (DNA to RNA) of genetic information. The conversion of genetic code (RNA to DNA) allows HIV to reproduce and become specific to the host.[12,22]

HIV infects the T_4/CD_4 cells by binding to the outer viral coat of the host's T_4/CD_4 cell. After the binding, HIV integrates into the host cell. Viral RT converts the viral RNA to double-stranded DNA. This DNA is then integrated into the host cell chromosomes. The infected host cell can then spread the virus through production of infectious cells or by fusion with uninfected cells.[22]

T_4/CD_4 lymphocytes begin to decline in both number and function as a result of cell lysis. When the normal number (600 to 1200/mm³ blood) of T_4/CD_4 cells is reduced to below 200, the risk of opportunistic infections is greatest.[22] Some patients remain healthy despite low numbers of CD_4 cells. Others have systemic symptoms such as fever, fatigue, diarrhea, or weight loss as the number of T_4/CD_4 cells decreases.[12]

In addition to its impact on lymphocytes, HIV can infect bone marrow cells causing anemia, low neutrophil counts, and in some patients, platelet counts low enough (< 20,000/mm³) to cause bleeding. B-lymphocytes are stimulated to divide massively, causing swollen lymph nodes (lymphadenopathy), and to overproduce antibodies (hyperglobulinemia). Another immunologic problem related to hyperglobulinemia is an increased tendency for drug allergy, which commonly interferes with treatment of infections.

Clinical Manifestations

The incubation period of HIV disease may be prolonged and varies from 1 to 10 or more years.[22,23] The spectrum of HIV disease consists of four stages: primary or acute HIV infection, asymptomatic HIV infection, mild symptomatic HIV disease, and advanced HIV disease (Figure 40-1). The CDC has a group classification system for HIV infection according to clinical conditions and T_4/CD_4 cell counts (see box).[12] Patients do not necessarily progress from one stage or group to the next; the first presenting stage may be advanced HIV disease. The CDC has expanded the case definition for advanced HIV disease or AIDS (see box).[12]

Primary or acute HIV infection resembles flulike or mononucleosis-like viral syndrome (fever, chills, sore throat, myalgia, arthralgia, diarrhea, malaise, and rash) and can occur within 2 to 4 weeks after exposure. Asymptomatic HIV-infected individuals

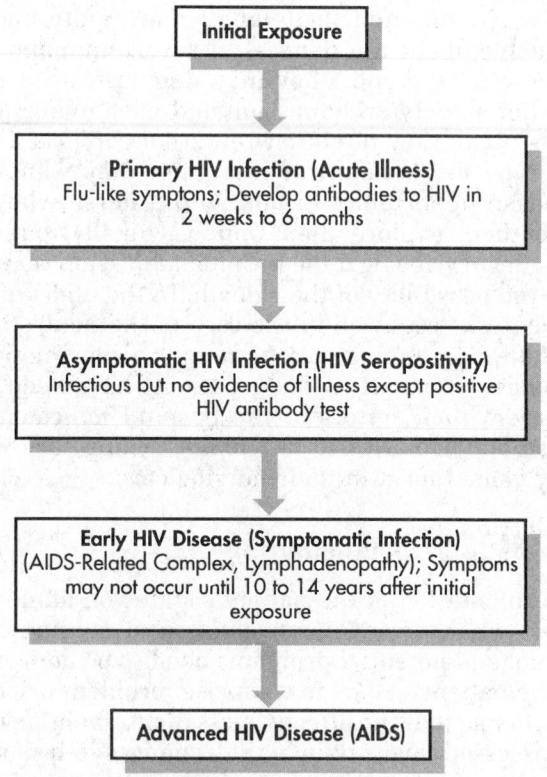

SPECTRUM OF HIV DISEASE

Initial Exposure

↓

Primary HIV Infection (Acute Illness)
Flu-like symptons; Develop antibodies to HIV in 2 weeks to 6 months

↓

Asymptomatic HIV Infection (HIV Seropositivity)
Infectious but no evidence of illness except positive HIV antibody test

↓

Early HIV Disease (Symptomatic Infection)
(AIDS-Related Complex, Lymphadenopathy); Symptoms may not occur until 10 to 14 years after initial exposure

↓

Advanced HIV Disease (AIDS)

FIGURE 40-1 Spectrum of HIV disease.

CLASSIFICATION SYSTEM FOR HIV INFECTION

T_4/CD_4 categories*

Category 1: $\geq$ 500 cells/μL
Category 2: 200-499 cells/μL
Category 3: < 200 cells/μL

Clinical categories

Category A

Categories B and C have not occurred
Asymptomatic HIV infection
Persistent generalized lymphadenopathy
Acute (primary) HIV infection

Category B

Category C has not occurred
Conditions attributed to HIV infection or indicative of
   a deficient cell-mediated immune system
Conditions considered by physician to have a clinical
   course or require management that is complicated by
   HIV infection

Examples of Category B conditions include but are not
   limited to the following:
   Bacillary angiomatosis
   Candidiasis, oropharyngeal (thrush)
   Candidiasis, vulvovaginal
   Cervical dysplasia
   Constitutional symptoms such as fever or diarrhea
      for more than 1 month
   Oral hairy leukoplakia
   Herpes zoster
   Idiopathic thrombocytopenic purpura
   Listeriosis
   Pelvic inflammatory disease
   Peripheral neuropathy

Category C

All clinical conditions listed as advanced HIV disease
   or AIDS (Once in category C, the person remains in
   this category.)

From Centers for Disease Control (CDC): 1993 Revised classification system for HIV infection and expanded surveillance case definition for AIDS among adolescents and adults, *MMWR* 41 (RR-17):1, 1993.
*The lowest accurate T_4/CD_4 cell count should be used for the classification process.

AIDS CASE DEFINITION

The AIDS surveillance case definition for adults has been expanded to include persons with T_4/CD_4 lymphocyte counts below 200 cells/μL or T_4/CD_4 percentage below 14 or with previous clinical conditions in the 1987 AIDS case definition, with the inclusion of pulmonary tuberculosis (MTB), recurrent pneumonia, and invasive cervical cancer. The following are the AIDS-defining illnesses according to the CDC guidelines:
   Candidiasis of esophagus, trachea, bronchi, and lungs
   Cervical cancer, invasive
   Coccidioidomycosis, disseminated or extrapulmonary
   Cryptococcosis outside of lungs
   Cryptosporidial diarrhea for over 1 month
   Cytomegalovirus disease or retinitis (with loss of vision)
   Encephalopathy, HIV related
   Herpes simplex causing skin ulcers for over 1 month, pneumonia, bronchitis, or esophagitis

Histoplasmosis, disseminated or extrapulmonary
Isosporiasis, chronic diarrhea for over 1 month
   Kaposi's sarcoma in patients less than 60 years of age
   Lymphoma, Burkitt's
   Lymphoma, immunoblastic
   Lymphoma of brain
   Mycobacterium avium-intracellulare or *M. kansasii,* disseminated or extrapulmonary
   Mycobacterium tuberculosis, any site (pulmonary or extrapulmonary)
   Mycobacterium, other species, disseminated or extrapulmonary
   Pneumocystis carinii pneumonia
   Pneumonia, recurrent
   Progressive multifocal leukoencephalopathy (PML)
   Salmonella septicemia, recurrent
   Toxoplasmic encephalitis
   Wasting syndrome caused by HIV

generally appear well. Laboratory evaluation, however, reveals an insidious decline in T_4/CD_4 cell counts, which may decrease from normal to 500 cells/mm^3 without development of signs or symptoms. Constitutional symptoms such as fever, weight loss, diarrhea, night sweats, and fatigue characterize mild symptomatic HIV disease. Other sentinel manifestations of this stage are oral thrush, seborrhea, psoriasis, molluscum contagiosum, xeroderma, pruritus, hairy leukoplakia, idiopathic thrombocytopenic purpura, hypocholesterolemia, herpes zoster, and generalized lymphadenopathy. Presence of any of these symptoms may signal progression to advanced HIV disease. **AIDS-related complex (ARC)** is within the mild symptomatic HIV disease stage. ARC is diagnosed in an HIV-infected person presenting with two constitutional signs and symptoms and two laboratory abnormalities associated with HIV but who does not meet an AIDS definition. ARC is also referred to as early HIV disease. **Acquired immune deficiency syndrome (AIDS)** is also known as advanced or late HIV disease. Advanced HIV disease is characterized by severe immunosuppression. Life-threatening opportunistic infections and malignancies, as well as severe wasting syndrome and HIV-related encephalopathy, can occur in the absence of other reasons.[12,26,42]

A major and possibly first sign of HIV complications is the AIDS dementia complex, also known as HIV encephalopathy. HIV dementia can be caused by direct HIV infection macrophages in the central nervous system (CNS) that cause demyelination. It is currently believed that 70% to 90% of the patients with advanced HIV disease may have AIDS dementia complex. Signs and symptoms of AIDS dementia complex may be very subtle or severe. They include cognitive, motor, or behavior changes. Cognitive changes may involve loss of concentration, forgetfulness, confusion, or slowed mental processes. Motor is exemplified by loss of balance or coordination, leg weakening, and deterioration in handwriting. Behavioral symptoms may be apathy, withdrawal, dysphoric mood, depression, psychosis, behavior regression, and violence. Depending on the area of the brain affected, headaches, seizures, or loss of sight may occur. Medical management of AIDS dementia complex consists of treating the primary HIV infection.[28] Other CNS symptoms caused by opportunistic infections improve when the opportunistic infection is treated.

Diagnosis of HIV infection is made by detecting antibodies to HIV in the blood using enzyme-linked immunosorbent assay (ELISA) confirmed by the more sensitive and specific Western blot test.[12] The confirmatory Western blot test should be positive before patients are informed of their test results. Pre-HIV and post-HIV test counseling should accompany all HIV testing. Other detection methods for HIV infection are polymerase chain reaction, p24 antigen, immunofluorescence, and viral culture.

Therapeutic Management

A variety of approaches to treating HIV infection are under study. At present there are three U.S. Food and Drug Administration (FDA) approved antiretroviral (anti-HIV) agents: zidovudine, dideoxyinosine, and dideoxycytidine. Zidovudine (ZDV, AZT) is currently indicated for all HIV-infected adults, symptomatic or asymptomatic, with CD_4 cell counts below 500 cells/mm^3. AZT inhibits the action of reverse transcriptase and slows the rate of disease progression. Early initiation of AZT is associated with better tolerance. The standard dosage of AZT is 500 mg/day (100 mg every 4 hours for five doses). Side effects of AZT are bone marrow suppression (anemia and neutropenia), nausea, malaise, fatigue, and headache. Dose reduction for side effects is preferred to interruption of treatment. Dideoxyinosine is approved for adults with symptomatic HIV infection who are intolerant or failed AZT therapy. The most serious side effects of dideoxyinosine are pancreatitis and peripheral neuropathy. Dideoxcytidine is presently the third-line antiviral agent with similar side effects to dideoxyinosine.[3,12,22]

SPECIFIC OPPORTUNISTIC INFECTIONS AND MALIGNANCIES
Protozoal Infections
Pneumocystis carinii pneumonia

Pneumocystis carinii pneumonia, whose etiologic agent is *Pneumocystis carinii,* is the most common opportunistic infection that occurs in adults with T_4/CD_4 cells of less than 200/mm^3 or less than 20% of total lymphocytes.[12,22] Symptoms are persistent, nonproductive cough; shortness of breath; hypoxia; fever; and shallow respirations. Therapeutic management consists of trimethoprim-sulfamethoxazole, trimethoprim-dapsone, or pentamidine (Table 40-7). Adjunctive corticosteroid therapy is beneficial for moderate-to-severe *Pneumocystis carinii* pneumonia. Several other drugs and regimens are under investigation.

Toxoplasmosis

Toxoplasmosis, whose etiologic agent is *Toxoplasma gondii,* is a leading cause of encephalitis. Toxoplasmosis usually represents reactivation of previous infection. Common symptoms are fever, headache, altered mental state, focal neurologic deficits (motor and sensory), and seizures. Therapeutic management is sulfadiazine, pyrimethamine, and folinic acid. Continued suppressive therapy is essential.

TABLE 40-7 Drugs for Opportunistic Infections

Drugs	Nursing considerations
ANTIVIRAL	
Acyclovir/ganciclovir	Infuse slowly—at least over 1 hour
	Make sure patient is well hydrated
	Monitor complete blood count for bone marrow depression
	Causes increased sedation and bone marrow depression if given with AZT
Foscarnet	Monitor serum blood urea nitrogen (BUN) and creatinine; increased risk of renal damage if given with other nephrotoxic drugs
ANTIFUNGAL	
Amphotericin B	Infuse slowly over 6-hour period
	Never dilute with normal saline; use D_5W
	Monitor for hypersensitivity reactions and phlebitis at intravenous site
	Causes *significant* hypokalemia; patients must receive intravenous potassium replacement
Fluconazole/ketoconazole	Monitor for renal or hepatic damage; check for interactions with other drugs
Flucytosine	Have patient take capsules over 15-minute period to reduce gastrointestinal upset
Nystatin	*Solution* ("swish and swallow"): have patient rinse mouth thoroughly before using and hold in mouth for several minutes; can be frozen into popsicle to increase oral retention for treating severe oral ulcers
	Cream or powder: wash skin well before application; apply after each episode of diarrhea if excoriation is present
Clotrimazole lozenges	Risk of noncompliance is high; if patient does not readily take them in hospital, talk to physician about substituting another drug
ANTIPROTOZOAN	
Trimethoprim-sulfamethoxazole (Bactrim)/sulfadiazine	Ensure patient takes tablets with full glass of water; monitor intake and output carefully
Pentamidine	Aerosol form can only be used with special nebulizer
	Do not stay in room while patient is receiving treatment; may cause irritation to skin and airways
	Never mix with saline; use sterile water
	Monitor for multiple adverse effects including hypotension, hypoglycemia, bone marrow depression, liver or kidney damage
ANTIMYCOBACTERIAL	
Amikacin	Aminoglycoside; must be separated by at least 1 hour from any intravenous penicillin dose
	Flush intravenous tubing well or use separate tubing
	Obtain peak and trough blood levels after third dose

Cryptosporidiosis

Cryptosporidiosis, whose etiologic agent is *Cryptosporidium,* principally infects the intestines, biliary ducts, gallbladder, and respiratory tract. Symptoms are profuse watery diarrhea (1 to 10 L/day), abdominal cramping and bloating, lactose intolerance, vomiting, and anorexia. There is no proven therapy, although several drugs are being tried. Supportive management consists of vigorous fluid and electrolyte replacement and nutritional support.

Fungal Infections

Candidiasis

Candida albicans is the etiologic agent of candidiasis (thrush), *Candida* esophagitis, or pneumonia. Symptoms consist of dysphagia and odynophagia. Disseminated disease can occur. Therapeutic agents are nystatin, clotrimazole, or ketoconazole for thrush. Amphotericin B or fluconazole is the drug of choice for disseminated or resistant infections.

Cryptococcosis

Cryptococcosis, whose etiologic agent is *Cryptococcus neoformans,* usually presents as cryptococcal meningitis. Cryptococcosis can present as skin infection, disseminated infection, or pneumonia. Cryptococcal meningitis presents as fever, headache of gradual onset, nausea, vomiting, photophobia, and signs of meningitis. Therapeutic management consists of amphotericin B or fluconazole. Continued suppressive therapy is essential.

Histoplasmosis

Histoplasmosis, whose etiologic agent is *Histoplasma capsulatum,* presents nonspecifically as fever, chills, weight loss, fatigue, abdominal pain, hepatosplenomegaly, and lymphadenopathy. Histoplasmosis can involve the lungs and skin. Therapeutic management consists of amphotericin B or fluconazole. Continued suppressive therapy is essential.

Bacterial Infections

Mycobacterium avium-intracellulare complex

Mycobacterium avium-intracellulare usually presents as bacteremia and can infect the lungs, liver, spleen, lymph nodes, and bone marrow. About 50% of persons with advanced HIV disease experience *Mycobacterium avium-intracellulare* infection. Symptoms generally include fatigue, night sweats, fever, weight loss, and lymphadenopathy. There are several therapeutic possibilities including three- or five-drug combinations with amikacin, ethambutol, ciprofloxacin, clofazimine, rifampin, rifabutine, azithromycin, and ciprofloxacin.

Mycobacterium tuberculosis

Mycobacterium tuberculosis (MTB) occurs in 50% of persons with advanced HIV disease. Presenting symptoms are fever, malaise, weight loss, and productive cough. MTB can disseminate. The CDC recommends HIV testing in all persons with tuberculosis and tuberculin skin testing in all persons with HIV infection. Patients with suspected MTB should be placed on respiratory isolation. Therapeutic management consists of a two- to four-drug regimen of isoniazid, rifampin, pyrazinamide, ethambutol, or streptomycin.

Viral Infections

Herpes simplex virus

Herpes simplex virus (HSV) infection can present as non-self-limiting, painful, mucocutaneous or skin eruptions (vesicular bullous lesions). With HIV dis-ease the lesions may be persistent, may be severe, and may involve multiple sites. Therapeutic management consists of acyclovir (Zovirax). Acyclovir prophylaxis in doses of 400 to 1000 mg/day may alleviate frequent recurrences, and intravenous administration may be necessary.

Varicella-zoster virus

Varicella-zoster virus, a herpes virus, causes shingles. Shingles presents as painful vesicular lesions usually along a single dermatome on one side of the body. In HIV infection, multidermatome varicella-zoster virus can occur. Shingles is treated with acyclovir (Zovirax). Intravenous acyclovir administration may be necessary.

Cytomegalovirus

Cytomegalovirus (CMV), a herpes virus, infects the retina, intestines, or liver. The lungs and CNS can be involved. Symptoms of CMV retinitis include blurred vision, floaters, and decreased visual fields. CMV colitis presents as profuse diarrhea. Ganciclovir and foscarnet are used for acute and chronic treatment of CMV infection.

Malignancies

Kaposi's sarcoma

Kaposi's sarcoma is the most common tumor associated with HIV disease. Kaposi's sarcoma is a vascular hyperplasia. Kaposi's sarcoma lesions appear on the skin, oral cavity (gums and palate), lungs, and intestines. Kaposi's sarcoma is a nodular, palpable, usually painless lesion. Large lesions can be painful, especially on the legs and feet (Figure 40-2). Color of the lesion varies with skin color and can be dark red, purple, or black. Therapeutic management consists of surgical excision, cryotherapy, radiation, or chemotherapeutic agents (doxorubicin/bleomycin/vincristine or bleomycin/vincristine).

NURSING MANAGEMENT OF THE PATIENT WITH HIV DISEASE
Assessment

HIV-infected patients may present with several opportunistic infections at the same time. The nurse must be knowledgeable about the clinical presentation of opportunistic infections to accurately assess an HIV-infected patient. Assessment of HIV complications is a collaborative process involving the physician, nurse, and patient. The patient must also be knowledgeable of the signs and symptoms of opportunistic infections. The duration and characteristics of presenting symptoms should be noted in relation-

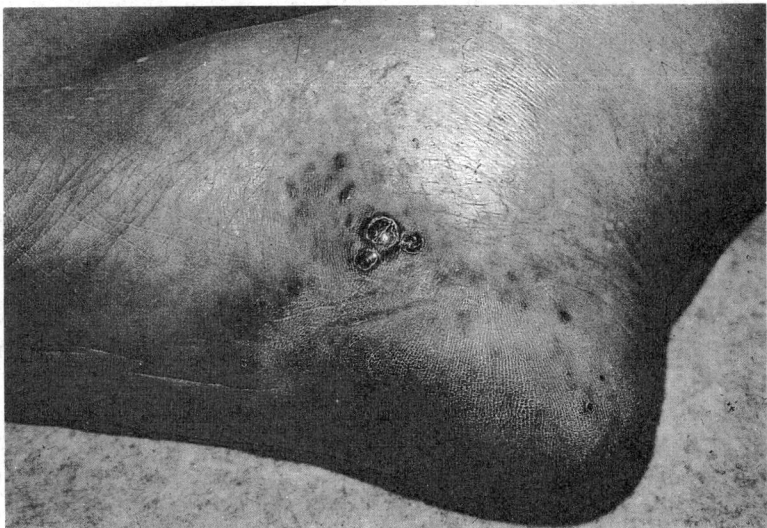

FIGURE 40-2 Kaposi's sarcoma: purple lesions on foot. (From Habif TP: *Clinical dermatology: a color guide to diagnosis and therapy,* St Louis, 1985, Mosby–Year Book, Inc.)

ship to the individual's sexual orientation, risk behaviors, and social and medical history.

The nurse must take a complete history, including psychosocial, medication, medical, and surgical areas. Social history includes sexual history (see Chapter 69), use of mood-affecting drugs and route of administration, travel within the last 10 years, and present and past residence. The nurse should assess current or previous use of prescribed and nonprescribed medications, dose, frequency, route, and side effects. It is important to check for allergies, especially to antibiotics. The patient should specify the type of allergic reaction experienced. A detailed medical history of all major illnesses and childhood diseases should be obtained. The nurse assesses the type, date, and conditions surrounding surgical intervention. A psychosocial history includes support system, present and past coping mechanisms, and fears. Patients' physical symptoms are commonly complicated by their emotional responses, depression, anger, fear, and guilt. Mental status evaluates cognitive (memory, concentration, orientation), behavioral (apathy, depression, agitation, psychosis, hallucinations), and motor (strength, coordination, incontinence, seizures) areas. Activities of daily living assess current level of function.

Physical examination begins with vital signs. Frequent weights are suggested to assess weight loss and fluid balance. Orthostatic measurements of heart rate and blood pressure should be taken if hypovolemia or autonomic neuropathy is suspected. The skin is inspected for lesions, tumors, itching, dryness, redness, rashes, lumps, color changes, bruises, and changes in hair or nails. A tuberculin skin test with controls is used to assess tuberculosis exposure and anergy. Lymph nodes are palpated for size, tenderness, texture, moveability, and symmetry. Eyes are examined for baseline acuity, utilizing pupillary reaction, visual fields, and ophthalmoscopic examination. Tinnitus and hearing loss should be assessed. Inspect for symptoms of sinusitis, rhinitis, and nosebleeds. The oral cavity is inspected for

GERIATRIC CONSIDERATIONS

HIV Disease

- Approximately 4% of the AIDS cases in 1992 were in persons 65 years or older.
- Sexual activity continues past 65 years of age.
- HIV infection should be considered in the differential diagnosis of all persons presenting with symptoms indicative of immunosuppression.
- Assessment of past medical and surgical history should include a history of past blood/blood product transfusions.
- Diagnosis of AIDS dementia complex may be difficult because of other organic processes associated with aging.
- Opportunistic infections may be reactivation of previous infections rather than primary infections.
- Medications used to treat common opportunistic infections may precipitate side effects earlier in elderly persons.
- Elderly persons have a higher risk for fluid and electrolyte imbalances.

ulcers, vesicles, plaques, tumors, nodules, gingivitis, and bleeding gums. Assess for symptoms of dysphagia, odynophagia, and changes in taste.

Auscultate respiratory rate, breath sounds, heart rate, and murmurs. The abdomen is auscultated for bowel sounds and palpated for tenderness, masses, and size of liver and spleen. Assess bowel habits: cramping, bloating, and nausea suggest gastric or small bowel involvement (consider infection with *Cryptosporidium, Isospora belli,* or *Giardia*); hematochezia implies large bowel inflammation (CMV, *Shigella, Chlamydia,* or *Campylobacter*); and rectal urgency indicates inflammation of rectal mucosa or proctitis (*Shigella, Chlamydia,* anorectal herpes).

Male genitals are inspected for signs of sexually transmitted diseases (STDs); foreskin is retracted and examined; and testicles are palpated for lumps, induration, tenderness, and swelling. Female genitals are inspected internally and externally for signs of STDs and vaginitis. Any discharges, in males and females, should be smeared and cultured. Anus and rectum should be visually and digitally examined for discharges, fissures, proctitis, abscesses, traumatic tears, and STD lesions.

Muscles, bones, and joints are examined for strength, muscle mass, and pain.

Nursing Diagnosis

Nursing diagnoses for patients with HIV disease include the following:

High risk for infection related to low CD_4 cell counts, neutropenia, or impaired skin integrity

Alterations in temperature: hyperthermia, related to infectious processes or drug reactions

High risk for fluid volume deficit related to profuse diarrhea, vomiting, or hyperthermia

Alterations in nutrition: less than body requirements, related to anorexia, nausea, vomiting, or diarrhea

Alterations in elimination: diarrhea, related to infectious processes, supplemental nutrition

Alterations in elimination: constipation, related to narcotics, decreased mobility, decreased fluid intake

Impaired gas exchange related to opportunistic infections

Alterations in skin integrity related to poor nutrition, STDs, immobility, or skin contact with excretions

Alterations in sexual patterns related to safer sex, change in self-concept, or physical limitations

Alterations in self-concept related to changes in body image, multiple losses of roles, depression, fear, or anxiety

Alterations in thought processes: confusion, related to opportunistic CNS infections, CNS malignancies, or dementia

Planning

Nursing goals for the patient with HIV disease are as follows:

The patient will be free of infections

The patient will have temperature within normal limits

The patient will maintain a positive fluid balance

The patient will maintain adequate caloric intake and balanced diet

The patient will maintain normal bowel function

The patient will experience relief of dyspnea, air hunger, weakness; demonstrate effective coughing

The patient will maintain skin integrity without ulceration or breakdown

The patient will practice safer sex; identify change in sexual role

The patient will verbalize feelings, perceptions of self; practice alternative strategies for coping

The patient will be oriented to person, place, and time; function optimally in environment

Implementation

HIV disease may affect every system of the body and every aspect of a person's life. The nurse has the op-

---

SAFER SEX PRACTICES[41]

Safe
Abstinence
Fantasy, voyeurism
Using own sex toys
Hugging
Body massage
Social (dry) kissing
Frottage (body rubbing)
Masturbation

Moderately safe
French (wet) kissing
Anal intercourse with condoms
Vaginal intercourse with condoms
Fellatio interruptus (oral sex without ejaculation)
Cunnilingus (oral-vaginal sex)
"Water sports" (urine contact)

Unsafe
Anal intercourse without condom
Vaginal intercourse without condom
"Fisting" (insertion of fist into rectum)
Fellatio with ejaculation in mouth
"Rimming" (oral-anal contact)
Blood contact
Urine ingestion

PATIENT EDUCATION GUIDE   *Condom Application*

1. Only latex condoms should be used. Condoms made of natural skin have pores large enough to allow viruses to pass through. Condoms should only be used once. Always check the expiration date on the condom package. Condoms should not be exposed to petroleum products such as petrolatum (Vaseline) or baby oil, extreme light, or heat to prevent degradation.
2. Laboratory studies have shown that 5% nonoxynol-9 is effective in killing HIV and preventing other sexually transmitted diseases.
3. Inspect condom for holes and tears when it is removed from the package.
4. For adequate protection the condom should be on the erect penis before entry into the partner.

5. The reservoir of the condom should be held to squeeze out the air as the condom is rolled onto the penis to be safe. If the condom does not have a reservoir, ½ inch of condom should be held to provide space for the ejaculate.
6. When rolling the condom onto the penis, the head of the penis is held.
7. After ejaculation the condom should be removed while the penis is erect. When removing the penis from the partner, the penis and condom should be held to prevent slippage of the condom into the partner or leakage of semen.
8. Condom use can be eroticized by using colorful or flavored condoms. Condom use can be more exciting if the partner places the condom on the penis. Unlubricated condoms with nonoxynol-9 inside the condom should be used with oral sex.

---

portunity to influence the patient's experience with HIV by educating patients, families, and colleagues. Factual information should be presented in written form with verbal reinforcement.

Confidential HIV antibody testing should be encouraged in individuals with risk factors. People at risk for HIV infection who know their HIV antibody status can protect themselves, if negative, and their sexual or intravenous drug-sharing partners from infection, if positive (see boxes on safer sex practices and condom application). Infected people may desire referral to an institution that participates in clinical trial protocols for HIV disease.

Patients and families confronting a catastrophic illness with many attached stigmas require extensive emotional support. Many symptoms of HIV disease negatively affect the person's self-image and can result in isolation. Patients with HIV disease face many unique physical, psychologic, and socioeconomic problems. Profound fatigue interferes with work and recreation; the symptoms of CNS involvement are frightening to patients and their loved ones; and the unpredictable waxing and waning of symptoms is frustrating and disruptive. Housing, employment, and insurance discrimination is illegal but has occurred as a result of stigmatization. The nurse advocates for patients with employers, families, significant others, and friends and provides referrals to community support agencies (state and local AIDS projects, Mothers of AIDS Patients, etc.), antidiscrimination attorneys, social services agencies (welfare, etc.), and health care providers with HIV disease expertise. Confidentiality is a special responsi-

RESEARCH BRIEF

Longo MB et al: Identifying major concerns of persons with acquired immunodeficiency syndrome: a replication, *Clin Nurse Specialist* 4:21-26, 1990.

A semistructured interview was used to identify the physical and psychologic concerns considered most important by HIV-infected individuals. Data were collected from 34 subjects (mean age 33.6 years), the majority of whom were white, homosexual, professional males. Average time since diagnosis was 8 months. Five primary areas of concern were identified: uncertainty about the future, desire to maintain physical and psychologic health, social unacceptability, fatigue, and weight loss.

Uncertainty was manifested by the grieving process and reduced by expressing their feelings. Most respondents used coping strategies to increase control to maintain health, but some subjects exhibited denial and excessive reliance on alternative therapies. Subjects reported feeling stigmatized; lack of acceptance was demonstrated not only by the general public, but also by health care providers. For over 40%, fatigue and weight loss were the major physical problems, both of which are amenable to nursing interventions.

LEGAL ISSUES   *AIDS and Discrimination*

On August 5, 1986 the Department of Health and Human Services (DHHS), Office of Civil Rights, completed its investigation of a complaint filed by a nurse in North Carolina, who said that he had been placed on involuntary leave of absence, without pay, on May 20, 1984, by the hospital-employer, based on the perception that he was handicapped because he had developed AIDS. The nurse also alleged that his employer failed to provide reasonable job accommodations for his perceived handicap, violating §504 of the Rehabilitation Act of 1973. This federal law applies to any program or activity receiving federal financial assistance. The nurse's employer was a 777-bed, nonprofit facility that received federal funds through Medicare and Medicaid.

In May 1984 the nurse was concerned about sight loss, fatigue, and a recent needle stick he had experienced while giving an injection to a patient who had been exposed to the virus responsible for AIDS. The nurse requested that he be examined by the hospital's chief of epidemiology. Based on this examination the doctor determined that the nurse suffered from symptoms of AIDS. The hospital removed the nurse from his position and would not assign him to any other job despite two medical opinions that the nurse could be placed safely in another job in the hospital not involving direct patient contact and a third medical opinion advising continued employment with appropriate precautions, such as the use of gloves.

The nurse filed a complaint with the Department of Health and Human Services, Office of Civil Rights, which is the federal agency responsible for investigating violations of civil rights under federal law. The Office of Civil Rights completed its investigation on August 5, 1986. It conducted an on-site visit to the hospital, reviewed relevant documents, and interviewed hospital personnel and others knowledgeable about the issues in the case. In a written memorandum letter to the hospital, the Office of Civil Rights charged that the nurse's employer had illegally discriminated against the nurse because he had developed AIDS.

The Office of Civil Rights stated that although the hospital's initial decision to place the nurse on a leave of absence may have been appropriate, its refusal to reevaluate the nurse's employment abilities was illegal. The hospital discriminatorily denied the nurse individualized consideration for possible reemployment.

The Office of Civil Rights asked the hospital to voluntarily comply, within 1 month, and required that the hospital submit to the Office of Civil Rights a corrective action plan including the following:

1. The hospital must establish an infectious disease control policy applicable to its employees who have AIDS or who have symptoms consistent with a possibility of developing AIDS that is protective of employees' rights.
2. The policy must include provisions for continued employment or transfer to another appropriate position where such transfers are feasible.
3. Decisions regarding employment should be made on the basis of individual circumstances, taking into account the available medical and scientific evidence at the time of the decision.

Although the nurse had, unfortunately, died since filing the complaint, the Office of Civil Rights stated that the hospital's policy must nevertheless be applied retroactively to the nurse with any appropriate relief, such as back pay or benefits, being provided. The Office of Civil Rights also required that the hospital provide assurances that it will follow its infectious disease control policy in all subsequent applicable cases.

This action by the Office of Civil Rights is significant because it sets a precedent, demonstrating that nurses who develop AIDS as a result of a work accident may be able to continue employment as long as they are able. Employers must individually evaluate job possibilities in light of a nurse's capabilities, according to medical condition and health status. An employer cannot arbitrarily decide that all nurses who develop AIDS from an accidental needle stick will be terminated from employment.

The Americans with Disabilities Act of 1990 (ADA) provides further protection for a nurse in this type of situation. The ADA specifically prohibits discrimination against persons with AIDS in all areas of employment and public accommodations and services, among others. Nurses who have AIDS or are HIV seropositive should seek legal counsel for any situation involving discrimination.

From Department of Health & Human Services, Office of Civil Rights, Region IV, Complaint Number 04-84-3096, Memorandum Letter (August 5, 1986); Pear: U.S. files first AIDS discrimination charge, *New York Times,* August 9, 1986, page 1, column 4; Rehabilitation Act of 1973, 29 U.S.C. §794 and regulations, 45 C.F.R. 84; Americans with Disabilities Act of 1990 42 § U.S.C. 12010.

UNIVERSAL PRECAUTIONS

Since medical history and examination cannot reliably identify all patients infected with HIV or other blood-borne pathogens, blood and body fluid precautions should be consistently used for *all* patients. This approach, previously recommended by CDC and referred to as universal blood and body fluid precautions or universal precautions, should be used in the care of *all* patients. Universal precautions apply to blood, semen, vaginal secretions, cerebrospinal fluid, synovial fluid, pleural fluid, peritoneal fluid, pericardial fluid, amniotic fluid, and any body fluids containing visible blood. Universal precautions do not apply to feces, nasal secretions, sputum, sweat, tears, urine, and vomitus unless they contain visible blood.

1. All health care workers should routinely use appropriate barrier precautions to prevent skin and mucous membrane exposure when contact with blood or other body fluids of any patient is anticipated. Gloves should be worn for touching blood and body fluids, mucous membranes, or nonintact skin of all patients, for handling items or surfaces soiled with blood or body fluids, and for performing venipuncture and other vascular access procedures. Gloves should be changed after contact with each patient. Masks and protective eye wear or face shields should be worn during procedures that are likely to generate droplets of blood or other body fluids to prevent exposure of mucous membranes of the mouth, nose, and eyes.

2. Hands and other skin surfaces should be washed immediately and thoroughly if contaminated with blood or other body fluids. Hands should be washed immediately after gloves are removed.

3. All health care workers should take precautions to prevent injuries caused by needles, scalpels, and other sharp instruments or devices during procedures; when cleaning used instruments; during disposal of used needles; and when handling sharp instruments after procedures. To prevent needle-stick injuries, needles should not be recapped, purposely bent or broken by hand, removed from disposable syringes, or otherwise manipulated by hand. After they are used, disposable syringes, needles, scalpel blades, and other sharp items should be placed in puncture-resistant containers for disposal; the puncture-resistant containers should be located as close as practical to the use area. Large-bore reusable needles should be placed in a puncture-resistant container for transport to the reprocessing area.

4. Although saliva has *not* been implicated in HIV transmission, to minimize the need for emergency mouth-to-mouth resuscitation, mouthpieces, resuscitation bags, or other ventilation devices with one-way valves should be available for use in areas in which the need for resuscitation is predictable.

5. Health care workers who have exudative lesions or weeping dermatitis should refrain from all direct patient care and from handling patient-care equipment until the condition resolves.

6. Pregnant health care workers are not known to be at greater risk of contracting HIV infection than health care workers who are not pregnant; however, if a health care worker develops HIV infection during pregnancy, the infant is at risk of infection resulting from perinatal transmission. Because of this risk, pregnant health care workers should be especially familiar with and strictly adhere to precautions to minimize the risk of HIV transmission.

Implementation of universal blood and body fluid precautions for all patients eliminates the need for use of the isolation category of "blood and body fluid precautions" previously recommended by the CDC for patients known or suspected to be infected with blood-borne pathogens. Isolation precautions (e.g., enteric, acid fast bacillus) should be used as necessary if associated conditions, such as infectious diarrhea or tuberculosis, are diagnosed or suspected.

---

bility of nurses who care for HIV-infected persons because of the nature of HIV transmission in groups (homosexual or bisexual contact or intravenous drug use). The practice of risk behaviors exposes a person to HIV infection, not membership in a risk group.

Blood and body fluid precautions (universal precautions) must be observed from the first contact with *all* patients (see box). Personal protective equipment (gown, gloves, goggles/face shield, and mask) should be used with direct patient care activities. Care must be taken to dispose of contaminated dressings and needles correctly. All reusable equipment for patient care must follow strict sterilization and disinfection guidelines.[40]

Myalgia, myositis, and arthralgia are concurrent symptoms with HIV disease. Aching muscles and joints need very careful handling. Lifting and turning should be done as gently as possible. Use of equipment such as hydraulic lifts, rollers, and lifting and turning sheets will ease the process for the patient in pain.

Several of the opportunistic infections such as herpes zoster and peripheral neuropathy are very painful. Care must be exercised when the patient has herpes zoster to avoid abrading blister surfaces. Gloves are worn when applying medications to infected surfaces, and gentle touch must be used. Teeth are cleaned with a soft bristle brush or thick cotton swabs to avoid irritating the gums or oral lesions.

Diarrhea is one of the symptoms most often present with advanced HIV disease. The diet is high in protein and calories and low in bulk to help reduce the number of stools. Assess what foods increase or decrease diarrhea, and change or modify diet as needed. Vigorous fluid replacement should be anticipated. Medications prescribed by the physician for diarrhea are administered on time. Emollient creams should be applied to the anal area to protect the skin from the effects of stools. Frequent weights are encouraged. Continually assess the fluid and electrolyte balance of the AIDS patient who is experiencing prolonged diarrhea. Daily weights are necessary if diarrhea is severe. Fluids, juices, and electrolyte solutions should be administered by whatever route the patient is able to receive them. If the patient's mouth is inflamed, soothing, cool drinks can be used. Weight loss is one of the usual symptoms of advanced HIV disease. The patient must have high-protein, high-calorie, low-residue meals. Preferably small frequent feedings can be provided to help avoid further weight loss. Encourage patients to drink between meals, so more food can be eaten at mealtime. Calm, comfortable surroundings for dining, with a pleasing and appetizing arrangement of food items, will encourage the patient to eat adequate amounts.

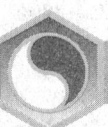

ETHICAL ISSUES

- Should nurses who care for AIDS patients be subject to periodic testing for HIV infection?
- Should an HIV-positive nurse be removed from direct patient care? confined to care of AIDS patients? prevented from practicing nursing at all? If the nurse continues, should patients be informed of the nurse's HIV status?
- Should nurses respect the confidentiality of an AIDS patient who asks them not to disclose the diagnosis to family or friends?
- Should AIDS patients be allowed to subject themselves to greater risks from experimental therapy than patients whose prognosis is not as serious? Can patients who are desperate for a cure rationally evaluate the risks of unproven treatment?
- Should all health care workers be tested for HIV? Should such testing be mandatory?

Fatigue is constant; however, exercise is needed. It is important to give needed exercise, passive exercise if necessary, while avoiding an increase in the patient's feelings of fatigue. As the person's strength returns, it is important to increase exercise to tolerance.

There may be disfigurement by Kaposi's sarcoma, ecchymoses, loss of hair, loss of weight, or other body changes. It is important to help the patient cope with the changes in body image that accompany HIV disease. Gentleness, an attitude of caring, and a calm, unhurried, accepting approach will help. If the nurse displays disgust or avoids these patients, their sense of self-respect can be impaired even further.

If the patient is receiving an investigational drug, the nurse is responsible for educating the patient on the drug administration protocol and reporting all effects and side effects according to protocol. All other medications should also be administered carefully, and observations for therapeutic effectiveness and side effects should be assessed. The nurse should assess all medications being taken by the patient, prescription and nonprescription. The nurse should assist the patient in developing reminders for timing and dosage of medication administration.

Care of the advanced HIV disease patient's family members and significant others is as important as care of the patient. In some cases a family member or significant other may also be infected with HIV. It is especially important to be caring and accepting of an individual's significant others no matter what the sexual orientation.

Nurses may have to confront their personal beliefs regarding sexuality, sexual orientation, and drug use to therapeutically interact. If steps are not taken to come to terms with life-styles that differ from the conventional norm, caring for HIV-infected patients is likely to be difficult for the nurse and, in turn, devastating for the patient and family.

Anger may be common with HIV-infected patients. Anger directed inside, for having placed one's self at risk, occurs often. Anger is also common when HIV infection is the result of a contaminated transfusion or occupational exposure. Anger at the medical establishment for having no cure is quite common. Nurses need to be able to see their patient's anger for what it is, namely, a reaction to vulnerability, frustration at helplessness, and the hopelessness of a cure. The nurse needs emotional stamina and an objective yet caring manner when patients, families, and significant others are exhibiting anger.

Because of the devastation caused by progression of HIV disease nurses and other health care workers, not to mention those who give care at home, are especially vulnerable to burnout. With little hope for recovery come feelings of futility, depression, and helplessness in the patient and hopelessness in the caretaker. Persons who care for chronically ill and aged people have developed networks and group support systems to help in caring for themselves.

Evaluation

The nurse evaluates whether the patient has avoided transmission to others, uses barrier precautions correctly, and complies with medical care and follow-up. The nurse should determine whether the patient has assisted partners to seek and receive treatment. The nurse evaluates the patient's immune status, functional level, and response to treatment for opportunistic infections. Each nursing diagnosis should be evaluated.

Documentation

The nurse documents both developing opportunistic infections and responses to medical and nursing interventions. Current symptoms, nursing plans, sexual practices, and emotional state should be documented. Compliance and reasons for noncompliance are documented. Reporting of communicable diseases to local and state regulatory organizations may be required.

Ongoing Care

Continue education about the disease process and possible medical and nursing interventions. Encourage the patient to be an active member of the management team. Encourage active participation in decision making, planning for care, and advance directives. Provide verbal and written instructions. Reinforce safer sex. Provide emotional support to the patient and significant others. There is no reason why persons with HIV infection cannot share living quarters with others, as long as basic hygiene is practiced (see box).

AUTOIMMUNE DISORDERS
Definition

Autoimmunity defines a state in which the normal tolerance and acceptance of self-antigens disappear. As a result the antigens on the cells of a person's body are seen by the immune system as foreign or nonself, stimulating an immune response that causes tissue damage and disruption of normal function. Self-antigens that trigger an immune response are called **autoantigens (AAgs);** antibodies that are formed against them are called **autoantibodies (AABs).**

Many of the diseases for which the etiology has been called idiopathic, that is, unknown, are now recognized to be the result of autoimmune processes

---

SELF-CARE TO REDUCE RISK OF OPPORTUNISTIC INFECTIONS

The following measures will reduce the risk of opportunistic infections in the immunosuppressed person and the risk of transmitting HIV infection:

1. Care should be taken not to exchange or touch body fluids of another person, particularly blood, semen, and vaginal secretions. Avoid sharing razors.
2. Bathe regularly using a mild soap, and rinse well. For dry skin, use lotions or creams. Take showers rather than baths, especially if there is foot or skin fungus present.
3. Practice good hand washing: wash hands after using the bathroom and before eating and cooking, preferably with liquid soap.
4. Keep hands away from eyes, nose, and mouth.
5. Maintain good dental hygiene by brushing teeth with a soft toothbrush. Avoid sharing toothbrushes. Hydrogen peroxide can be used as a mouthwash (1 part hydrogen peroxide to 9 parts water).
6. Keep fingernails and toenails clean and cut to prevent fungal infections or transmission of organisms from soil.
7. Visitors with respiratory infections should wear masks and/or cover mouth when coughing or sneezing. Avoid crowds.
8. Use sitz baths and witch hazel wipes or other soothing lotions for irritation of rectum or vagina.
9. Maintain a balanced diet with daily vitamin supplements.

(Table 40-8). More than 25 diseases are currently believed to have an autoimmune pathogenesis. Although scientists have not established one concept to explain the development of all autoimmune disorders, several probable pathologic mechanisms have been described.

Tolerance of self-antigens

To understand why autoimmune diseases develop, one must understand *tolerance* of self-antigens, that is, the mechanisms that prevent the immune system from reacting to the antigenic self-markers on all body cells under normal conditions. Several theories exist to explain the concept of tolerance. One theory hypothesizes that during fetal life, continual interaction between the antigens on fetal tissues and circulating T and B cells makes these lymphocytes tolerant of the body's antigens. Other theories postulate that AABs are produced but that their activ-

TABLE 40-8 Pathology of Common Autoimmune Disorders

Disorder	Pathologic mechanism
Myasthenia gravis	AAB destruction of acetylcholine receptors prevents normal transmission of impulses at myoneural junction
Insulin-dependent diabetes mellitus	AAB destruction of isles of Langerhans that produce insulin; possible AABs against insulin or insulin receptors on tissue cells
Graves' disease	AABs against thyroid antigens stimulate thyroid cell proliferation and function
Inflammatory bowel disease	AABs attack antigens on epithelial cells of gastrointestinal tract, causing ulceration
Rheumatoid arthritis	AABs to IgG create immune complexes that deposit in sinovium, producing inflammation; increased activation of complement
Pernicious anemia	AABs destroy parietal cells in gastric mucosa, resulting in lack of hydrochloric acid and intrinsic factor; these inhibit absorption of vitamin B_{12}

ity is blocked by T_8/suppressor lymphocytes or a chemical mediator, preventing them from initiating an immune response. Laboratory research has shown that the lack of T_8 cells produces spontaneous B and T cell activity against self-antigens. Because cell antigens are very diverse, it may be that these mechanisms work together to ensure that tolerance of self is maintained. Thus if one mechanism were ineffective, another would be available to accomplish the task.

Theories of Autoimmunity

The basic premise behind all theories of autoimmunity is the loss of tolerance of self-antigens. As a result of some change, self-antigens appear as nonself. Cytotoxic T cells or AABs attack them, creating an inflammatory response that impairs normal function of the tissue involved in loss of tolerance and may be genetically susceptible to change, damage to self-antigens, and abnormalities in immune responses that promote perpetuation of initial reactions. The major theories currently being tested are described below.[47]

Changes in AAgs/mimicry

One theory of autoimmune disease proposes that bacterial or viral damage changes the shape of self-antigens so that they appear to be nonself, triggering an immune response. A similar theory suggests that part of the molecular structure of many nonself antigens is almost identical to certain self-antigens. As a result, when a pathogen initiates an immune response, the WBCs attack both the antigens on the organism and self-antigens that have a similar structure. For example, rheumatic fever is an autoimmune disorder that follows a beta-streptococcal in-

fection. The cells of the heart have surface antigens that are either damaged by the bacteria or are similar to antigens on the bacteria. In either case these AAgs are seen as foreign by B-lymphocyte plasma cells, which create both antibodies to destroy the streptococcal organism and AABs to attack the cardiac AAgs.

Additional support for these theories is found in autoimmune responses to drugs. For example, alpha methyldopa (Aldomet) can cause hemolytic anemia by binding to antigens on the surface of RBCs, changing their shape and stimulating their destruction by AABs.

Impaired regulation

The ability of T_8-lymphocytes to recognize other WBCs is part of the regulatory system controlling the strength and duration of an immune response. However, according to one theory of autoimmune disease, this regulatory system becomes either overactive or inactive. In overactive states, AABs attack both the antibody fighting the organism and the receptor site on the cell to which the organism has linked. In inactive states the normal inflammatory response is permitted to go unchecked. Both of these changes in regulation promote tissue damage.

Sequestered antigens

Another theory of autoimmune disease is based on the proposal that some of the body's cell antigens are segregated or hidden from blood and lymph during fetal development. As a result, no tolerance can be acquired. If these self-antigens are released into blood or lymph because of trauma or surgery, they are seen as nonself and AABs form against them. Researchers have been able to demonstrate the production of AABs against lens protein released following eye injuries and against sperm following a vasectomy, when the vas deferens is blocked and sperm are released into the body. However, there is disagreement as to whether the AAgs from a lens or sperm are released in large enough quantity to produce an ongoing autoimmune response.

SYSTEMIC LUPUS ERYTHEMATOSUS
Definition

Systemic lupus erythematosus (SLE) is a chronic, progressive inflammatory disease of multiple organ systems caused by AABs that attack AAgs on the membranes and nuclei of cells in all parts of the body. The disease is characterized by a "butterfly" rash over the cheekbones, joint pain, fatigue, the presence of antinuclear antibodies in the blood, and signs of specific organ system dysfunction (Figure 40-3). The term *lupus* (wolf) is derived from the similarity between the facial rash and the shading on a wolf's muzzle.

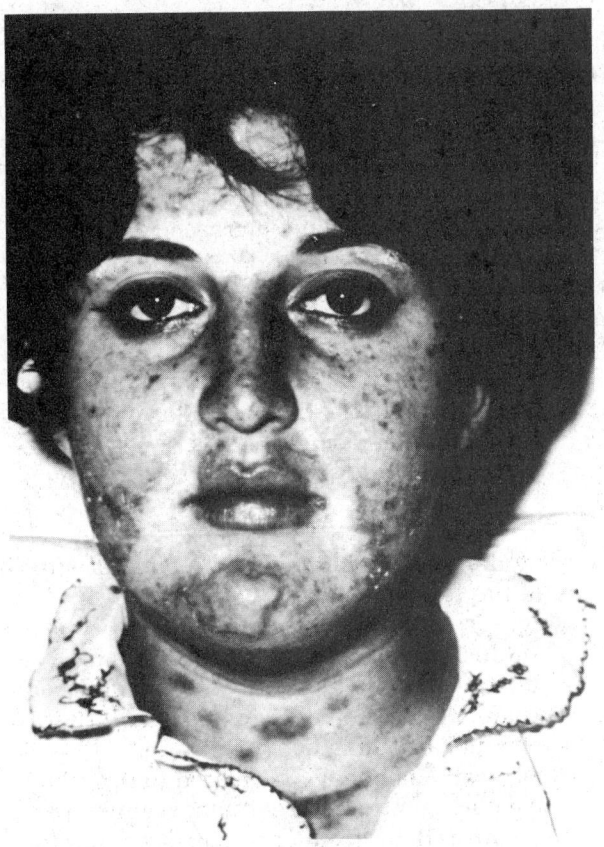

FIGURE 40-3   Rash seen with systemic lupus erythematosus. Widespread, discrete lesions are present on face and neck. Typical peeling is noted on chin and cheeks. (From the Arthritis Foundation, New York, copyright 1972.)

Etiology

The inflammatory process that damages organ systems in SLE is the result of both hyperactivity of the immune system and autoimmune activity. No one specific reason for these abnormal changes has been identified. However, inherited defects in the regulation of immune activity and environmental stimuli such as viral or bacterial infections, drugs, food, and ultraviolet light have been related to the disease. The incidence of SLE is relatively low. It usually appears between 13 and 40 years of age, is far more common in females than males, and occurs most often in African Americans, Asian Americans, and certain native American tribes. A lupuslike disorder can be triggered as a side effect of several drugs, including procainamide, hydralazine, phenytoin, quinidine, chlorpromazine, and isoniazid. The symptoms usually disappear when the drug is stopped.[47]

Pathophysiology

In SLE, genetic defects or environmental factors stimulate production of autoreactive B-lymphocytes. These B cells produce AABs known as **antinuclear antibodies (ANAs),** because they attack the nuclei of cells, and other AABs that attack the cell membranes of RBCS, WBCs, and platelets, as well as active particles inside the cell such as lysosomes, mitochondria, and RNA. Neutrophils containing the nucleus of another cell they have destroyed are called LE cells and are considered diagnostic for SLE.

The AABs stimulate an inflammatory response that can involve tissues throughout the body. The severity of the disease depends on the degree of inflammation, since normal function is disrupted by destruction of the cells. Patients with SLE have periods of exacerbations and remissions depending on AAB activity.

Clinical Manifestations

Eleven criteria for SLE have been established (see box). Patients demonstrating four or more of these criteria are given the diagnosis of SLE. However, because of the variable nature of the disease, patients may have only one or two signs and symptoms when they are first seen by a physician. The most common initial findings are vague (e.g., fatigue, arthritis, fever, and anemia), making SLE difficult to diagnose. The sign most often associated with SLE, a butterfly rash across the cheekbones that gets worse when exposed to sunlight, occurs in about 60% of the patients. Other common clinical signs include lymphadenopathy, renal dysfunction, personality disorders, purpura (small hemorrhages in the skin and mucous membranes), vasculitis, and inflammation of

CLINICAL MANIFESTATIONS OF SLE[47]

Red rash over cheekbones (malar rash)

Disk-shaped, raised, scaly rash (discoid rash)

Photosensitive rashes

Oral ulcers

Arthritis of two or more peripheral joints

Pleuritis or pericarditis (pleural inflammation)

Renal dysfunction (proteinuria or presence of cells)

Neurologic dysfunction (seizures or psychoses)

Hematologic disorder (anemia, leukopenia, thrombocytopenia)

Immunologic disorders (presence of LE cells or anti-DNA antibodies)

Antinuclear antibodies present in blood

serosal membranes (pleura, pericardium, peritoneum). Blood tests reveal the presence of LE cells, ANAs, antibodies against blood cells and clotting factors, and abnormally low levels of hematologic cells.[47]

Therapeutic Management

Drug therapy is the primary method used to manage SLE. Treatment is focused on reducing the effects of inflammation on organ systems through the use of corticosteroids. Although high doses of corticosteroids are used to manage exacerbations, the goal is to maintain the patient on fairly low (e.g., 15 to 20 mg) doses of prednisone every other day during remission. Alternate-day therapy reduces the appearance of side effects and reduces the possibility of suppressing normal adrenal production of corticosteroids. Prolonged high-dose therapy increases the risk of significant side effects, including infection from depression of WBC activity, hyperglycemia, osteoporosis caused by disruption of protein and calcium metabolism, and cataracts.

Immunosuppressive drugs such as cyclophosphamide (Cytoxan) and azathioprine (Imuran) may be used in conjunction with steroids to moderate the inflammatory damage to the kidneys. Table 40-2 describes the action and effects of common immunosuppressive drugs. Dosages are based on a balance between the drugs' beneficial effects and the increased risk of infection. During an exacerbation, drug therapy is augmented by *plasmapheresis*, a process that separates elements within the blood. Plasmapheresis removes the circulating AABs, thus directly removing the agent causing the inflammatory damage.

Patients with major organ involvement are monitored closely to ensure that the maintenance regimen of corticosteroids is adequately controlling renal, CNS, cardiac, and hematologic damage. Additional drugs are used to minimize the synergistic effects of steroids with other disorders, such as hypertension, that cause additional renal damage. Although high doses of phenytoin (Dilantin) have been associated with a lupuslike syndrome, it does not appear to have adverse effects on the patient diagnosed with SLE and is used if the patient begins to have seizures.

Symptoms related to non-life-threatening aspects of the disease are treated with as little medication as possible. Nonsteroidal anti-inflammatory drugs (NSAIDs) are useful for reducing the pain associated with arthritis, pericarditis, or pleuritis and for controlling fevers, one of the systemic manifestations of inflammation. Antimalarial drugs have proven beneficial in treating skin rashes.

NURSING MANAGEMENT OF THE PATIENT WITH SYSTEMIC LUPUS ERYTHEMATOSUS

Assessment

Most patients with SLE are admitted to the hospital because of an infection or an acute exacerbation resulting in severe renal or CNS problems. As a result the nurse's primary focus is on the collaborative care issues such as monitoring fluid and electrolyte balance, neurologic or psychiatric changes, and responses to antibiotic and increased corticosteroid therapy. However, patients also require a careful assessment of those aspects of the disease most amenable to independent nursing interventions, such as fatigue, pain, and skin rashes, and the extent to which these have interfered with normal life activities. These assessments are also the primary focus in the ambulatory setting.

Nursing Diagnosis

Nursing diagnoses common to the patient with SLE include the following:

Fatigue related to chronic inflammatory process and to decreased oxygenation of tissues as a result of anemia (manifested by expressions of continued lack of energy and inability to perform normal daily activities)

Health-seeking behaviors related to desire for active participation in treatment regimen (may be manifested by frequent requests for information or support services)

Pain related to inflammation of joints, muscles, and serosal membranes (may be manifested by self-reports, hesitation in movement, facial tension or grimacing, and careful positioning)

Body image disturbance related to presence of butterfly rash (may be manifested by use of makeup, dark glasses, self-reports)

Fluid volume excess related to decreasing renal function (may be manifested by decreased urinary output, dependent edema, and increased weight)

Altered thought processes related to inflammation of cells in the cerebral cortex (often manifested by inappropriate behavior, difficulty solving problems, and poor judgment)

High risk for injury: trauma, related to seizures

High risk for infection related to inflammatory destruction of leukocytes and corticosteroid suppression of immune function

Planning

Therapeutic goals are set after discussions have indicated what is most important to the patient. Because the risk for noncompliance to a complex treatment regimen increases when patients have not participated in the decision-making process, the nurse must ensure that the patient is fully involved. Writing out the objectives for treatment and the patient's role in meeting these objectives can be very helpful for both nurse and patient.

Implementation

Almost all individuals with SLE will feel chronically exhausted and unable to carry out the activities they want to do. This problem is frequently the patient's most pressing concern and therefore becomes a major focus for nursing activities. The goal for each patient is to be able to carry out the activities required for his or her role in a family and at work. A detailed record of the patient's fatigue during a 24-hour day enables the nurse to help the individual plan a schedule that combines activities with adequate rest. Most patients will require at least 9 hours of sleep at night and a nap during the day. A conference with the patient's employer may be necessary to determine if lunch or break periods can be used for naps. During an exacerbation, when the disease is more active, additional rest is needed. The care plan should reflect a balance of rest periods and progressive exercise to maintain muscle tone.

Pain relief also is a high priority for SLE patients since 90% of them have arthritis or arthralgia. In the hospital the nurse can assess pain levels by having patients rate their pain on a 0- to 10-point scale before and after administering pain medications to monitor the effectiveness of the current regimen. On an outpatient basis, if the current pain control prescription does not appear to be working, patients can keep a diary between appointments, noting the severity of the pain, medication taken, and degree of relief. Patients may need teaching about the benefits of taking pain medications on a regular basis or just before activity.

Patients are not usually admitted to the hospital unless they are experiencing an acute exacerbation of symptoms. During this period they may develop acute inflammation of the kidney or brain, requiring close supervision. The nurse should monitor the patient's level of orientation closely to determine the need for restraints and implement seizure precautions for patients with any signs of CNS irritation. Equally important is the need to detect early signs of fluid retention through daily weights and documentation comparing fluid intake to urinary output. In addition, as their dosage of corticosteroids is increased to manage the exacerbation, patients become immunocompromised and may require protection from nosocomial infections.

Hospitalization may provide an opportunity for patients to talk realistically about the impact of the disease on their life-style. Because SLE strikes a younger population, the need for rest, avoiding sunlight, and adhering to a renal diet can interfere with career and family plans and create problems with patients' self-image. These problems are aggravated by the weight gain and other adverse side effects from corticosteroid therapy. Patients who lack understanding may view remissions as "cures" and reduce their adherence to the treatment regimen. Time spent talking with patients about the impact of their disease can promote acceptance and increase compliance to treatment.

Evaluation/Documentation

The effectiveness of nursing interventions can be evaluated best by patients, whose reports of fatigue and pain should diminish. The nurse also assesses the patients' responses to teaching about the disease and treatment regimen and their degree of interest in participating in their therapy.

Because nurses spend more time with the patient than physicians, it is vital to document the patient's physical and psychologic status each day so that changes requiring physician intervention can be noted and responded to. Also, clarity is of primary importance whenever a nurse is communicating about pain, fatigue, or other subjective data, as well as changes in the patient's neurologic state.

ALLERGIC IMMUNE REACTIONS
Definition

Allergic or **hypersensitivity** disorders are a broad range of inflammatory conditions caused by a special group of antigens called allergens, common substances found in the environment. In a hypersensitivity state the body responds to these normal sub-

TABLE 40-9 Hypersensitivity Reactions

Type	Reaction
Type I	Immediate reactions: IgE-mediated local or systemic anaphylaxis; atopic disorders
Type II	Cytotoxic reactions: IgG- and/or IgM-mediated destruction of cells; drug and transfusion reactions
Type III	Immune complex reactions: IgM- or IgG-mediated formation of antigen-antibody complexes; serum sickness; Arthus reactions
Type IV	Cell-mediated reactions: mediated by sensitized T cells; allergic contact dermatitis; delayed hypersensitivity reactions

stances with an exaggerated response. Any agent capable of inducing an immune response is a potential allergen. Natural chemicals, particularly proteins, are most likely to stimulate a reaction mediated by antibodies; other compounds more frequently cause a T cell–mediated response. In addition, eosinophilic WBCs are frequently associated with allergic reactions; elevated levels of eosinophils in the WBC count are used in the clinical setting as one indication of an allergic process. The presence of an allergic reaction requires sensitization, or prior exposure to the allergen during which T cells are activated or antibodies produced. A second contact with the allergen then triggers inflammation. Allergens may be inhaled (e.g., pollen), ingested (e.g., chocolate, shellfish, or other food), or injected (drugs). Hypersensitivity reactions are generally classified into four categories based on the immunologic cells involved. Table 40-9 highlights the four categories of hypersensitivity reactions.

Etiology/Pathophysiology

Type I hypersensitivity

Type I allergic reactions are called local or systemic **anaphylaxis,** because they occur very rapidly. IgE antibodies serve as the primary mediator. Mast cells in the body, especially those in the mucosa, skin, bronchial smooth muscle, and vascular endothelium, have specific receptors on their surface for IgE to which the antibody attaches, sensitizing them to certain allergens. An individual's first exposure to an allergen increases serum levels of IgE, which binds to the mast cells, sensitizing them. When the allergen is encountered again, granules within the sensitized mast cells release the chemical mediators of inflammation. These mediators, such as histamine, kinins, and leukotrienes, produce an instantaneous localized or systemic inflammatory response. Many local type I reactions are atopic (inherited).[49]

Local anaphylactic responses

Local anaphylaxis may be displayed in several ways. In allergic rhinitis, inflammation of the nasal mucosa produces increased mucus and sneezing, often accompanied by swollen red eyes after exposure to pollens or animal dander. Other common responses are **urticaria** or hives, raised red swollen wheals on the skin, and angioneurotic edema (accumulation of fluid in the skin of the eyelids, lips, and hands) caused by the release of chemical mediators by mast cells in the walls of superficial blood vessels. The reversible bronchial constriction of asthma is also a local anaphylactic reaction. Allergies to certain foods (e.g., shellfish, chocolate, peanuts, milk) provoke local responses in the gastrointestinal tract where IgE antibodies attach to mast cells in the intestinal mucosa, causing diarrhea.

Often contact between the allergen and IgE antibodies on mast cells is facilitated when an infection or inflammatory response from another source increases the permeability of the bronchial or gastric mucosa. This mechanism explains how asthmatic attacks may be triggered by upper respiratory infections. Although they are annoying, local anaphylactic reactions are rarely dangerous, except in asthma, because the inflammatory response is limited.

Systemic anaphylactic responses

In contrast, systemic anaphylactic responses are life threatening and can result in death. Systemic anaphylaxis occurs when the allergen, absorbed into the blood either directly or through the mucosal lining of the respiratory or gastrointestinal tract, stimulates a massive release of histamine and other chemical mediators throughout the entire body. The result is dramatic. Constriction of bronchiole smooth muscle produces wheezing and severe respiratory distress, while vasodilation and the increased permeability of small blood vessels in the body cause edema and a drop in blood pressure. The edema can be life threatening if it affects the larynx, because little room is available for swelling without obstructing air flow into the lungs.

If vasodilation and loss of plasma fluid are extensive, the blood pressure may fall significantly, producing the clinical condition of shock, in which the circulatory system fails to deliver necessary oxygen and nutrients to body tissues. Consequently, the brain and other vital organs do not receive blood flow adequate for normal function and the patient may die. Anaphylactic shock most commonly occurs as the result of an allergy to a drug (e.g., penicillin), to the contrast media commonly used in diagnostic tests of vascular patency (e.g., cerebral and coronary artery angiograms), or to insect venom.

Histamine and other chemicals stimulate receptors on the skin, producing the hives that may be one of the first signs of anaphylaxis. Histamine also stimulates the parietal cells of the stomach, which secrete hydrochloric acid and smooth muscle cells in the gastrointestinal tract. The increased acidity and muscle contraction produce the nausea, vomiting, and diarrhea that may accompany or precede a systemic anaphylactic reaction.[49]

Type II hypersensitivity

Type II allergic reactions or cytotoxic reactions are mediated by IgG and/or IgM that reacts to the allergen. The antigen and antibody link on circulating erythrocytes, leukocytes, and platelets and cause lysis of these cells by activation of complement. Two common examples of type II allergic reactions are blood transfusion reactions and some types of drug reactions.

Hemolytic transfusion reactions occur because of blood type incompatibilities. The surface of erythrocytes contains many antigens that are the result of our genetic inheritance. These antigenic markers are classified into the common blood groups A, B, and AB; type O erythrocytes have no surface antigens. The antibodies that develop against blood type antigens are unique in that they develop genetically shortly after birth rather than after exposure to a specific erythrocyte antigen. Consequently, if a patient with type A blood is given type B blood, antibodies are already present to attack the donor RBCs and destroy them.

Type O blood is referred to as the universal donor, because it has no antigens against which antibodies can be created. In contrast, individuals with type AB blood are universal recipients, because they do not develop antibodies to either A or B antigens. Careful screening by laboratory personnel and nurses administering blood has significantly minimized the risk of hemolytic transfusion reactions. The signs of hemolytic reactions include fever and chills, a drop in blood pressure, flank pain, and the presence of RBC fragments or hemoglobin in the urine.

Allergic reactions also can occur because non-RBC antigens or antibodies present in the donor's blood react with the recipient's immune system. The response may be limited to a febrile reaction, defined as an elevation in temperature of more than 1° C. Febrile reactions are most common in patients who have received multiple transfusions and can be treated with antipyretics. Other common signs of mild transfusion reactions include urticaria and hematuria (from RBC fragments in the urine). Antihis-

tamines such as diphenhydramine hydrochloride (Benadryl) are effective treatment for the urticaria, although corticosteroids may be required. Occasionally severe problems occur, including bronchospasm and noncardiogenic pulmonary edema, that require intensive interventions. Patients with a history of transfusion reactions usually receive blood products that have been "washed" to remove surface antigens on blood cells or leukocyte-poor blood from which many of the WBCs have been removed to decrease the number of donor antibodies present.

Type II drug reactions result when drug-antibody-complement complexes attach to a circulating blood cell, resulting in the target cell's death. Allergies to a drug depend on the pharmacologic makeup of a drug or on its activity inside the body. Drugs and their active by-products are haptens, substances that are not immunogenic by themselves but that can react with antibodies as the result of binding with a carrier protein. The binding process somehow changes the antigenic marker of the protein; as a result, antibodies see a nonself antigen and react to it, activating complement and the inflammatory response.

Type III hypersensitivity

In a type III reaction, or immune complex reaction, IgM or IgG antibodies in the bloodstream bind with antigens to form immune complexes. These complexes attach to the wall of blood vessels, activating complement and producing a localized inflammatory response. **Serum sickness,** which is caused by antitoxins derived from horses or other animals to treat rabies, diphtheria, tetanus, or snake bites, is one type of type III hypersensitivity. The antigens in the animal serum stimulate the production of antibodies, which bind to form inflammatory complexes. The penicillin cephalosporin and sulfonamide antibiotics also can cause mild serum sickness reactions. Signs and symptoms of serum sickness (i.e., fever, muscle and joint pain, pruritus, urticaria, and lymphadenopathy) begin 7 to 14 days following administration of the drug or antitoxin and resolve in a few weeks.[49]

Another type III allergic response is the Arthus reaction in which the antibody-antigen reaction forms a local necrotic lesion. Arthus reactions occur rarely in humans but are part of the inflammatory response causing tissue damage in immunologic disorders such as systemic lupus erythematosus, rheumatoid arthritis, and glomerulonephritis.[49]

Type IV hypersensitivity

Sensitized T cells, rather than antibodies, are responsible for causing type IV hypersensitivity reactions. Allergic contact dermatitis, the most common immunologic disease encountered by dermatologists, may be induced by many substances. The most common agents are poison ivy, the rubber compounds used in elastic materials, and nickel compounds used in costume jewelry. All of these substances combine with skin proteins, changing them into nonself skin antigens that are attacked by T cells. Clinically, contact dermatitis is called eczema, a skin condition characterized by areas of acute erythema (redness), edema, and scaling. Other examples of type IV hypersensitivity are various forms of chronic pneumonitis or alveolitis such as "farmer's lung" caused by inhaled organic dusts in individuals who work closely with animals.

Delayed hypersensitivity, or skin testing, which is based on the type IV reaction, is a useful clinical tool for assessing hypersensitivity reactions and exposure to pathogens. For example, to determine exposure to tuberculosis, the tuberculosis bacillus is injected intradermally. If the individual has had previous contact with the bacillus, the area becomes red and swollen within about 2 days. Patch testing also is commonly used to check for agents thought to be responsible for contact dermatitis or respiratory allergies. The suspicious agent is applied to the skin and covered with an occlusive dressing for 24 to 48 hours, after which the area is examined for the presence of an inflammatory response. Finally, patients suspected of anergy may be tested with sensitizing agents, which react with and change skin self-antigens. Individuals who do not react to new antigens may have an impaired immune response and require protection against infection.

NURSING MANAGEMENT OF THE PATIENT WITH ALLERGIC IMMUNE REACTIONS

Assessment

The first step in assessing a patient for a possible allergic reaction is completion of a comprehensive nursing history on admission. Patients with one allergy are at risk for the development of others. Thus, if the patient reports any allergic episodes, the nurse needs to document clearly both the allergen and the response. In addition, whenever patients are given blood or a drug for the first time, they must be observed for an allergic reaction.

Nursing Diagnosis

Two primary nursing diagnoses are appropriate for the patient at risk for hypersensitivity reactions:
High risk for injury related to allergic reactions
Health-seeking behavior related to knowledge of allergens and treatment regimens

Planning

By anticipating the patient's course of illness, nurses can raise their own awareness of periods of increased risk and share their plans to minimize these with the patient. At the same time the nurse can determine the most effective teaching strategies to help patients reduce their risk for allergic reactions outside the hospital.

Implementation

Blood transfusions and new drugs present the two most common dangers for the patient with a history of allergic reactions. Clear warnings should be placed on the patient's hospital record and medication administration record indicating the patient's allergic history. Some institutions keep a small kit containing essential equipment on the emergency cart where it can be reached immediately if a serious anaphylactic response occurs.

Transfusion reactions

Early signs and symptoms of transfusion reactions include urticaria, chills, fever, headache, low back pain, and wheezing; these usually occur within 20 minutes after the transfusion is started. Consequently, it is the nurse's responsibility to observe the patient closely during this period. If the individual has a history of allergic reactions, antihistamines may be given before the transfusions. The fever and shaking chills (rigors) observed in some patients cause significant discomfort and require treatment with antipyretics and narcotic or nonnarcotic pain medications. To reduce the possibility of a transfusion reaction, these patients are generally given washed and leukocyte-poor blood.

The nurse must always be aware that in highly sensitive patients, anaphylactic shock may occur, requiring the administration of drugs to support the circulatory system, reduce bronchial obstruction, and prevent death. Normal saline is always hung with the blood so that an alternative solution is available for immediate use if an allergic reaction occurs. In addition, diphenhydramine (Benadryl) or one of the corticosteroid drugs (hydrocortisone, prednisone) must be readily available. These act against the histamine released during the allergic response, inhibiting its dangerous vascular and bronchial effects.

Drug reactions

Drugs can also present a significant danger to patients with a history of allergies. Thus observation for signs of drug reactions must be a consistent part of the daily assessment of each patient. In particular, nurses must be alert for any type of skin rash, the most common sign of a drug reaction. The record of any patient who develops a skin rash should be assessed for new medications. The nurse also must be alert for anaphylactic reactions; these may be mild or severe depending on the extent to which the individual was sensitized during the drug's first administration.

Drug reactions often cause damage to blood cells. Cytotoxic RBC reactions (hemolytic anemia) can limit oxygen-carrying capacity, producing fatigue and weakness; destroyed RBCs will also appear in the urine, making it pink or dark. Thrombocytopenia (decreased platelet numbers) must be considered if the patient shows signs of delayed clotting, such as bleeding from the gums or injection sites, increased menstrual flow, heme-positive urine, or guaiac-positive stools. These assessments can be verified by checking blood cell counts through laboratory values. In addition, immune complex formation may produce delayed responses characterized by fever, urticaria, swollen lymph nodes, myalgia, arthralgia, and edema of the face and hands.

Occasionally hypersensitivity reactions to drugs produce damage to the kidneys or liver. These organs are responsible for the metabolism of many drugs. Their enzymatic action on drugs may produce active metabolites that interact with the organ tissue, forming new antigens that provoke antibody responses. Routine assessment of laboratory results for changes in BUN, creatinine, AST, or lactic dehydrogenase (LDH) levels (indications of reduced renal and liver function) is essential.

Health-seeking behaviors

Patients with a history of allergies or clinical disorders that have an allergic component (e.g., asthma) usually have a desire to learn how to identify potential allergens. This may require skin testing by a clinical immunologist or allergist. Common allergens are injected intradermally or placed on the skin with patches, and the degree of inflammatory response is noted after 24 to 48 hours. If the patient is reactive to a broad spectrum of allergens that interfere with normal activities of daily living, a treatment called desensitization may be used to modify the hyperactivity. Desensitization involves administering repeated injections of dilute solutions containing the specific allergen. Researchers believe that the injections increase the level of IgG, which blocks the binding of IgE to specific receptor sites on mast cells, preventing the release of histamine and other chemical mediators of inflammation. Desensitization seems to be most effective in patients with respiratory system hyperactivity.

Patients also need to know exactly what substances cause their hypersensitivity reactions and the clinical signs and symptoms of an allergic response. Patients with respiratory allergies often are not aware of the large number of agents in their environment that can stimulate a hyperactive response. If they are allergic to any inhaled substance, they need to avoid all aerosol sprays such as hair spray and household cleansers. Exposure to animal dander and dust mite allergens can be minimized by avoiding "dust catchers" in the house, ensuring that all bedding is washed frequently, eliminating or frequently vacuuming rugs and draperies, and not keeping pets. Learning that a beloved dog or cat is the source of their respiratory allergies may be difficult for patients, and they often choose to tolerate the symptoms rather than give up their pet.

Avoiding foods that produce allergies is often easier than eliminating respiratory allergens. Patients need to remember, however, to ask about the content of casseroles or snacks served at someone else's home. Infants who are allergic to certain foods may also have hypersensitivity reactions to others; new foods need to be introduced slowly and separately to identify allergens.

Patients receiving drugs with a known potential for allergic reactions need to be taught to observe for manifestations of the reaction. The appearance of urticaria, a rash, or feelings of chest tightness may indicate a type I anaphylactic response. Chronic weakness or fatigue, frequent bruising or bleeding gums, or signs of infection may indicate type II damage to RBCs, platelets, or WBCs, respectively.

Patients also need to be taught about the adverse effects of medications used to treat allergic symptoms. Antihistamines, the most commonly prescribed drugs, may produce dry mouth, difficulty voiding, and thick bronchial secretions. Sucking on sugar-free hard candy, frequent mouth care, voiding before taking the medication, increasing fluid intake, and using a humidifier may help minimize discomfort. Antihistamines also increase the effects of sympathomimetic drugs, nonprescription cold medications, and alcohol or other central nervous system depressants. Ensuring that patients know the names and effects of all medications they are taking is particularly important to prevent drug interactions.

Evaluation

The effectiveness of patient education can only be judged over time. Patients who adhere to recommendations for changes in life-style will generally have fewer allergic symptoms and will decrease their risk for infections. All hypersensitivity reactions promote the inflammatory response, which in turn provides an opportunity for microorganisms to gain entry into the body.

Documentation

The nurse must be careful to document the specifics of any type of hypersensitivity reaction. Skin eruptions (e.g., rashes or urticaria), respiratory wheezes, changes in blood pressure or heart rate, and subjective data obtained from the patient must be clearly described to assist in the diagnosis and to compare to any later reactions.

CRITICAL THINKING QUESTIONS

1 Explain the key nursing interventions for a patient who is immunodeficient.
2 Compare and contrast the following stages of HIV disease: primary or acute HIV infection, asymptomatic HIV infection, mild symptomatic HIV disease, and advanced HIV disease.
3 Describe the clinical manifestations of advanced HIV disease.
4 Discuss the psychologic factors that might complicate your care of a patient with HIV disease.
5 Describe the important patient care needs that should be addressed in a care plan for a patient with HIV disease.
6 How does an autoimmune disorder develop?
7 What are the clinical manifestations associated with SLE?
8 Give an example of each of the four types of hypersensitivity reactions.
9 What teaching is required for a patient with an allergic reaction?

RESOURCES

1 AMERICAN FOUNDATION FOR AIDS RESEARCH (AMFAR)
5900 Wilshire Blvd.
Second Floor—East Satellite
Los Angeles, CA 90036
(213) 857-5900
2 CENTERS FOR DISEASE CONTROL
AIDS Information Office
1600 Clifton Rd., NE
Atlanta, GA 30333
(404) 639-3311
3 GAY MEN'S HEALTH CRISIS (GMHC)
129 West 20th St.
New York, NY 10011
(212) 807-6655
4 NATIONAL AIDS HOTLINE
(24 hr/day)
1-800-342-2437
1-800-344-7432 (Spanish)
1-800-AIDS-TTY (for the hearing-impaired persons)
5 NATIONAL AIDS INFORMATION CLEARINGHOUSE
P.O. Box 6003
Rockville, MD 20850
1-800-458-5231
6 NATIONAL ASSOCIATION OF PEOPLE WITH AIDS (NAPWA)
2025 I St., NW
Suite 415
Washington, DC 20006

BIBLIOGRAPHY

Current

1. American Nurses' Association: *Nursing and the human immunodeficiency virus: a guide for nursing's response to AIDS*, Kansas City, Mo, 1988, The Association.
2. Ammann AJ: Mechanisms of immunodeficiency. In Stites DP, Terr AI, editors: *Basic and clinical immunology*, ed 7, Norwalk, Conn, 1991, Appleton & Lange.
3. Anastasi JK, Rivera JL: Nursing considerations in administering ddI and ddC, *AIDS Patient Care* (1), 1991.
4. Blanchet KD: *AIDS: a health care management response*, Rockville, Md, 1988, Aspen.
5. Brew BJ et al: The neurological features of early and "latent" human immunodeficiency virus infection, *Aust NZ J Med* 19:700-704, 1989.
6. Brown SE et al: Kaposi's sarcoma, *Med Clin North Am* 76(1):235-252, 1992.
7. Canning EU: Protozoan infections: *Toxoplasma gondii, Trans R Soc Trop Med Hyg Suppl* 84:19-23, 1990.
8. Centers for Disease Control: *Facts about AIDS*, Washington, DC, 1987, US Government Printing Office.
9. Centers for Disease Control: Human immunodeficiency virus infections in the United States: a review of current knowledge, *MMWR* 36(suppl S-6), 1987.
10. Centers for Disease Control: Recommendation for prevention of HIV transmission in health-care settings, *MMWR* 36(2S), 1987.
11. Centers for Disease Control: *HIV/AIDS surveillance report*, Atlanta, Oct 1992, US Government Printing Office, pp 1-18.
12. Centers for Disease Control: 1993 Revised classification for HIV infection and expanded surveillance case definition for AIDS among adolescents and adults, *MMWR* 41(RR-17), 1992.
13. Chiu J et al: Treatment of disseminated *Mycobacterium avium* complex infection in AIDS with amikacin, ethambutol, rifampin, and ciprofloxacin, *Ann Intern Med* 113:358-361, 1990.
14. Chuang HT et al: Psychosocial distress and well-being among gay and bisexual men with human immunodeficiency virus infection, *Am J Psych* 146:876-880, 1989.
15. Cotton D: Case watch, *AIDS Clin Care* 3(3):17, 1991.
16. Crowe S, Mills J: Infections of the immune system. In Stites DP, Terr AI, editors: *Basic and clinical immunology*, ed 7, Norwalk, Conn, 1991, Appleton & Lange.
17. Daar ES, Meyer RD: Bacterial and fungal infections, *Med Clin North Am* 76(1):173-204, 1992.
18. Damrosch S et al: Critical care nurses' attitudes toward, concerns about, and knowledge of the acquired immunodeficiency syndrome, *Heart Lung* 19:395-400, 1990.

19. *Disseminated MAI in persons with AIDS: questions and answers,* Princeton, NJ, 1990, The Liposome Co, Inc.
20. Douglas RG: Herpes simplex virus infections. In Wyngaarden JB et al, editors: *Cecil textbook of medicine,* ed 19, Philadelphia, 1992, WB Saunders Co.
21. Finberg H: The social dimensions of AIDS, *Sci Am* 259:128, 1988.
22. Flaskerud JH, Ungvarski PJ: *AIDS/HIV infection: a reference guide for nursing professionals,* ed 2, Philadelphia, 1992, WB Saunders Co.
23. Gee G, Moran T: *AIDS: concepts in nursing practice,* Baltimore, 1988, The Williams & Wilkins Co.
24. Gellin BG, Soave R: Coccidian infections in AIDS, *Med Clin North Am* 76(1):205-234, 1992.
25. Gold JWM: HIV-1 infection: diagnosis and management, *Med Clin North Am* 76(1):1-18, 1992.
26. Grady C: AIDS, *Nurs Clin North Am* 23(4), 1988.
27. Haseltine WA, Wong-Staal F: The molecular biology of the AIDS virus, *Sci Am* 259:52, 1988.
28. Hilton G: AIDS dementia, *J Neurosci Nurs* 22(1):24-29, 1989.
29. Hirschel B et al: A controlled study of inhaled pentamidine for primary prevention of *Pneumocystis carinii* pneumonia, *N Engl J Med* 324:1079, 1991.
30. Holmes KK, Motulsky AG: *AIDS: a guide for the primary physician,* Seattle, 1988, University of Washington Press.
31. Hopp JW, Rogers EA: *AIDS and the allied health professions,* Philadelphia, 1989, FA Davis Co.
32. Hoyt MJ, Staats A: Wasting and malnutrition in patients with HIV/AIDS, *J Assoc Nurses AIDS Care* 2(3):16-26, 1991.
33. Jaffe HS, Sherwin HS: Immunomodulators. In Stites DP, Terr AI, editors: *Basic and clinical immunology,* ed 7, Norwalk, Conn, 1991, Appleton & Lange.
34. Karch AM: *Handbook of drugs and the nursing process,* ed 2, Philadelphia, 1992, JB Lippincott Co.
35. Kaslow RA, Francis DP: *The epidemiology of AIDS,* New York, 1989, Oxford University Press.
36. Kiecolt-Glaser JK, Glaser R: Stress and immune function in humans. In Ader R et al, editors: *Psychoneuroimmunology,* ed 2, San Diego, 1991, Academic Press, Inc.
37. Leoung G, Mills J: *Opportunistic infections in patients with the acquired immunodeficiency syndrome,* New York, 1989, Marcel Dekker, Inc.
38. Longo MB et al: Identifying major concerns of persons with acquired immunodeficiency syndrome: a replication, *Clin Nurse Spec* 4:21-26, 1990.
39. *Management of HIV disease: treatment team workshop handbook,* New York, 1991, World Health Communications, Inc.
40. Porche DJ: Universal precautions. In Nichols RL et al, editors: *Decision making in surgical sepsis,* Philadelphia, 1991, BC Decker.
41. Porche DJ et al: HIV counseling and testing: a primer for health care professionals, *AIDS Patient Care* 6(3):130-133, 1992.
42. Redfield RR, Burke DS: HIV infection: the clinical picture, *Sci Am* 259:90-98, 1988.
43. Ryan JL: Bacterial diseases. In Stites DP, Terr AI, editors: *Basic and clinical immunology,* ed 7, Norwalk, Conn, 1991, Appleton & Lange.
44. Sande MA: Guidelines for initiation of ZDV therapy in early HIV disease. In Sande MA, Volberding PA, editors: *The medical management of AIDS,* ed 2, Philadelphia, 1990, WB Saunders Co.
45. Sande MA, Volberding PA: Medical management of AIDS, *Infect Dis Clin North Am* 2(2), 1988.
46. Schilts R: *And the band played on: people, politics, and the AIDS epidemic,* New York, 1987, St Martin's Press Inc.
47. Steinberg AD: Systemic lupus erythematosus. In Wyngaarden JB et al, editors: *Cecil textbook of medicine,* ed 19, Philadelphia, 1992, WB Saunders Co.
48. Swanson B et al: Dementia and depression in persons with AIDS: causes and care, *J Psychosoc Nurs* 28(10):33-39, 1990.
49. Terr AI: Anaphylaxis and urticaria and immune complex allergic diseases. In Stites DP, Terr AI, editors: *Basic and clinical immunology,* ed 7, Norwalk, Conn, 1991, Appleton & Lange.
50. Young LS, Inderlied CB: *Mycobacterium avium* complex infections, *AIDS Patient Care* 4:10-18, 1990.
51. White DA, Zaman MK: Pulmonary disease, *Med Clin North Am* 76(1):19-44, 1992.
52. Winkelstein A: Immunosuppressive therapy. In Stites DP, Terr AI, editors: *Basic and clinical immunology,* ed 7, Norwalk, Conn, 1991, Appleton & Lange.
53. Wolff PH, Colletti M: AIDS: getting past the diagnosis and on to discharge planning, *Crit Care Nurse* 6(4):76-81, 1986.

Classic

54. American Nurses' Association Committee on Ethics: *Statement regarding risk v. responsibility in providing nursing care,* Kansas City, Mo, 1986, The Association.
55. Klug RM: AIDS beyond the hospital, *Am J Nurs* 86:1015-1021, 1986.

UNIT X

Renal and Urinary Systems

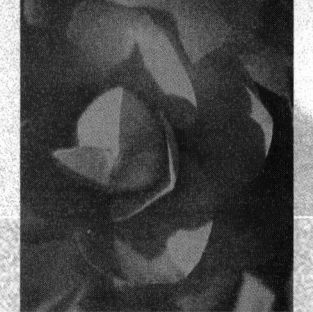

CHAPTER FORTY-ONE

Nursing Assessment of the Renal and Urinary Systems

LEARNING OBJECTIVES

1 Describe the basic structures and functions of the renal and urinary systems.
2 Obtain relevant subjective information from the patient who has a renal/urinary alteration.
3 Using correct technique, examine the patient to obtain appropriate objective information about the renal and urinary systems.
4 Differentiate in relation to the renal and urinary systems abnormal from normal subjective and objective findings.
5 Describe tests and procedures used in the diagnosis of renal and urinary disorders.
6 Describe patient preparation and care related to diagnostic tests of the renal and urinary system.

KEY TERMS

THE RENAL AND URINARY SYSTEMS are assessed in conjunction with an examination of the gastrointestinal and reproductive systems. Since abdominal pain—often the major complaint of the individual with a renal/urinary alteration—has many possible causes, an adept assessment is needed to distinguish the specific source of the symptom.

Factors that compromise the integrity of the renal and urinary systems include reproductive alterations (e.g., masses resulting in pressure), infections (stemming from diminished physical mobility or decreased oral liquid intake), and illnesses or conditions such as diabetes mellitus or hypotension. Repeated infection may lead to the formation of renal calculi. Diabetes mellitus can result in renal nephropathy and progress to renal failure. The focus of the renal and urinary assessment is to determine whether the systems' structures are intact and functional.

ANATOMY AND PHYSIOLOGY

Renal System

Structural description

The two kidneys are attached by connective tissue and an extensive fat pad to the dorsal wall of the abdominal cavity. They lie outside the parietal layer of the peritoneum, level with the last thoracic vertebra and the first three lumbar vertebrae. The renal arteries, veins, nerves, lymph vessels, and ureters all enter or leave the kidney on the medial surface in the indented region called the hilum.

The basic structure of the right kidney can be seen in coronal section in Figure 41-1. The kidneys are enclosed by a strong, white fibrous connective tissue membrane called the renal capsule. The outer layer of the kidney is called the cortex. When cut, it has a granular appearance because of knobby renal corpuscles and convoluted tubules. The cortex surrounds the medulla, which has a fibrous appearance resulting from the loops of Henle and collecting ducts of the nephron that lie parallel to each other in the radial plane. The medulla is organized into pyramids with columns separating them. The renal pelvis is found medially in the region of the hilum. It is hollow and collects urine as it passes out of the collecting ducts and delivers it to the ureter.

The **nephrons** are the functional units of the kidneys. The structure of a typical nephron can be seen in Figure 41-2. The different regions of the nephron are Bowman's capsule, the proximal and distal convoluted tubules, and the loop of Henle. The nephrons empty into collecting ducts.

Each nephron has its own blood supply (Figure 41-2). Blood is delivered by the afferent arteriole to the spherical knot of capillaries called the glomerulus that lies in the cup of the Bowman's capsule. From the glomerulus, the blood collects into the efferent arteriole, which delivers it to the peritubular capillaries. They follow the course of the nephron, looping into the medulla and back to the cortex, and supply the venules that direct the blood back to the general circulation.

One area of the afferent arteriole is joined to an area of the distal convoluted tubule to form the juxtaglomerular apparatus that monitors and controls the function of the nephron.

Functions of nephrons and collecting ducts

Each region of the nephron is modified to carry out particular functions: filtration, reabsorption, and secretion. However, if anything interferes with the

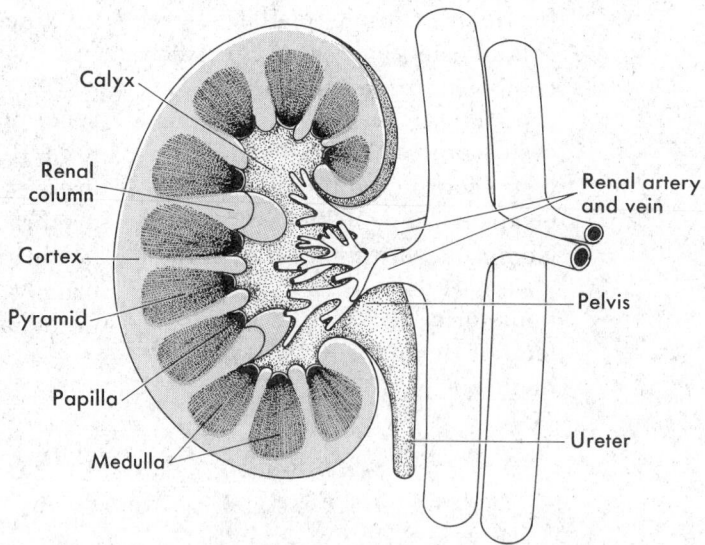

FIGURE 41-1   Cross section of the kidney.

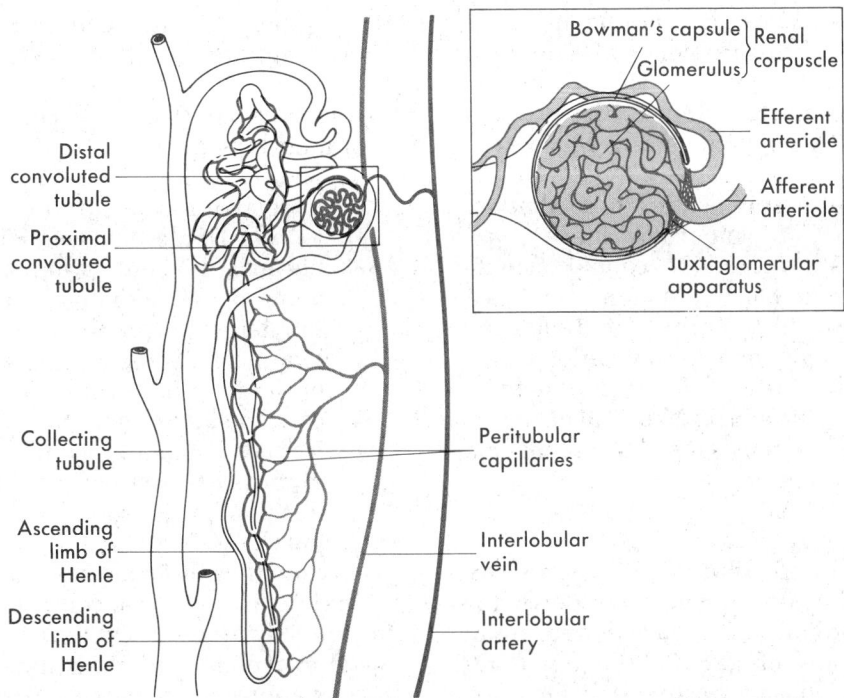

FIGURE 41-2   The nephron unit with its blood vessels. Blood flows through nephron vessels as follows: interlobular artery → afferent arteriole → glomerulus → efferent arteriole → peritubular capillaries (around the tubules) → venules → interlobular vein.

production of filtrate, the nephrons cannot maintain homeostasis because they can only purify the blood if sufficient filtrate passes through their tubules.

Normally the nephrons process approximately 180 L/day of filtrate and are able to reabsorb all its essential constituents because they have considerable reserve reabsorptive capacity. However, there is an upper limit to the quantity of each solute that can be actively reabsorbed. This is called the transport maximum, and it is expressed as the maximum amount that can be completely reabsorbed in 1 minute. For example, the transport maximum of glucose is 225 mg/min. This is normally reached when the blood glucose concentration is 180 mg/dL. When the concentration rises above this, glucose begins to escape into the urine.

Filtration is a function of the Bowman's capsules, whereas reabsorption and secretion are functions of the tubules and the collecting ducts.

Bowman's capsule
Glomerular filtration rate (GFR) is the term used to describe the amount of fluid filtering into all the nephrons in 1 minute. GFR is normally approximately 125 mL/min (i.e., 20% of the plasma passing through the glomerular capillaries).

Composition of the filtrate depends on the structure and integrity of two layers of epithelium and the layer of basement membrane between them. The epithelial cells of the glomerular capillaries retain plasma protein and cells but allow smaller substances to enter the nephron easily. Protein in the urine is one of the first signs that the glomerular membrane is damaged because it indicates that unusually large amounts of protein have escaped across the glomerular membrane into the tubule. Where the membrane is more seriously damaged, even red blood cells may enter the nephron. However, they are not seen as blood because the cells are hemolyzed by the concentration and dilution of the filtrate as it passes through the nephron. Instead, the hemoglobin gives the urine a dark color.

The amount of filtrate formed depends on the balance between the blood pressure and the colloid osmotic pressure in the glomerular capillaries.

Blood pressure is the force that drives filtrate out of the glomerulus into the cup-shaped **Bowman's capsule,** and therefore filtration is reduced during hypotension or vasoconstriction of the afferent arteriole (i.e., during the strong sympathetic stimulation that accompanies and follows traumatic events, such as surgery, hemorrhage, accidents, and cardiovascular shock). Monitoring urine production is one way to determine if kidney function has returned to normal following the sympathetic inhibition generated by such a traumatic event. Blood pressure is so important for kidney function that the nephrons have their own blood pressure control system: low blood pressure in the afferent arteriole activates the renin-angiotensin hormone system of the juxtaglomerular apparatus. This system returns blood pressure to normal.

Colloid osmotic pressure is the force that opposes the formation of glomerular filtrate, and therefore conditions that reduce colloid osmotic pressure (i.e., reduced blood albumin concentration) tend to increase the quantity of fluid filtering into the tubule. Blood albumin concentration is normally kept constant by the liver. However, it may fall for short periods when fluid intake is high or for longer periods when albumin is lost during renal disease or severe starvation.

Proximal convoluted tubule

The **proximal convoluted tubule** reabsorbs approximately 65% of the filtrate entering from Bowman's capsule. Solutes (sodium ions, glucose, and amino acids) are actively transported out of the lumen into the interstitial fluid. These reabsorbed solutes produce an osmotic pressure gradient that attracts the water to follow them. This osmotic attraction is strengthened by the increase in the colloid osmotic pressure created in the blood of the efferent arteriole by the formation of the glomerular filtrate. This reabsorption is obligatory (i.e., the active transport enzymes always work at their maximum potential, and they are not affected by hormones or by the nervous system).

Hydrogen ions are actively secreted in exchange for sodium ions, and they convert the bicarbonate ions in the tubule to carbon dioxide and water, which are able to diffuse into the interstitial fluid easily. The electronegative chloride and phosphate ions are reabsorbed because they are attracted to the interstitial fluid by the electropositive actively transported sodium ions. Other small substances are reabsorbed passively (e.g., urea diffuses across the wall as a result of the concentration gradient caused by the reabsorption of water).

The small amount of protein and other large molecules that succeed in crossing the Bowman's capsule are reabsorbed by pinocytosis.

Loop of Henle

The proximal convoluted tubule passes the unabsorbed filtrate into the descending limb of the **loop of Henle.** This limb is very permeable to water and electrolytes. Approximately 20% to 25% of the glomerular filtrate is reabsorbed by the tubular cells of the ascending limb of the loop of Henle, and most of this reabsorption is obligatory.

In addition to reabsorbing filtrate, the loop of Henle generates a very high concentration of sodium chloride in the medulla, especially in the region of the papilla. This high concentration is an essential component in controlling the homeostasis of water, because it allows the kidney to concentrate urine. The high concentration is achieved by a countercurrent mechanism:

1. Sodium chloride is transported out of the filtrate as it moves up the *ascending* limb of the loop of Henle, but water is not able to follow because this limb is impermeable to water.
2. Some of the sodium chloride enters the peritubular capillaries and is removed from the kidney, but some reenters the *descending* limb of the loop of Henle, making the filtrate more concentrated than the blood it was derived from. Over time, this process increases the osmotic pressure in the capillaries and tubules of the papillary region of the kidney, until it is four times stronger than that of the blood in the afferent arteriole.

In contrast to the concentration of the papilla, the filtrate leaving the ascending limb and entering the distal convoluted tubule is dilute. Its osmotic pressure is approximately one third that of the blood in the afferent arteriole.

Distal convoluted tubule

Approximately 10% to 15% of the glomerular filtrate normally remains to enter the **distal convoluted tubule** from the loop of Henle. It is still a considerable amount (27 L/day), and most of it must be reabsorbed to maintain the fluid balance of the body. Normally only 1% of the glomerular filtrate is excreted as urine. Unlike the obligatory reabsorption of the rest of the nephron, reabsorption of this region is facilitated by intrinsic and extrinsic mechanisms that adjust excretion to maintain the homeostasis of the plasma water, electrolytes, and pH.

The distal convoluted tubule is impermeable to water, unless it is made permeable by antidiuretic hormone (ADH).

Collecting ducts

Filtrate flows from the distal convoluted tubules into the collecting ducts, which are also impermeable to water unless stimulated by ADH. In the presence of ADH, water is attracted into the medulla from the filtrate by a high concentration of salt, and the urine is concentrated. In the absence of ADH, the filtrate is unchanged and the urine very dilute.

Control of renal function

The homeostatic functions of the kidneys can be divided into the homeostasis of water, electrolytes, and pH. However, whenever additional water is excreted or retained, the osmolarity of body fluids is affected; and while the maintenance of normal body fluid volume is extremely important because of its effect upon blood pressure, the homeostasis of the osmotic pressure of body fluids is also important because neurons and muscle cells are extremely sensitive to any changes. Therefore, whenever reabsorption of sodium is increased, it will be followed rapidly by increased reabsorption of water. The following is a summary of the renal mechanisms to maintain fluid, electrolyte, and pH balance. For additional information, see Chapter 12.

Homeostasis of water

The homeostasis of water is maintained in part by antidiuretic hormone (ADH), which is secreted whenever osmoreceptors in the hypothalamus are stimulated by an increase in the osmotic pressure of body fluids, or atrial receptors are stimulated by a significant fall in venous blood volume. ADH is produced by neurons in the hypothalamus and secreted from their axons, which terminate in the posterior lobe of the pituitary gland. These neurons are inhibited by a decrease in osmotic pressure and by afferent impulses from right atrial stretch receptors.

After it is secreted, ADH combines with receptors on the cell membrane of the cells of the distal convoluted tubules and collecting ducts, where it increases the permeability of the ducts to water. This results in water being reabsorbed by osmosis because the tubule and ducts contain hypotonic filtrate and pass through the isotonic and hypertonic regions of the cortex and medulla. Thus filtrate and urine are concentrated, interstitial fluid is diluted, and water is conserved. The return of interstitial osmotic pressure and blood volume to their normal set points inhibits further secretion of ADH.

This mechanism is extremely effective and it maintains plasma volume and osmotic pressure constant even though fluid intakes are extremely variable. Individuals lacking ADH, or those whose collecting ducts are insensitive to it (diabetes insipidus), can only produce dilute urine, and they have difficulty drinking sufficient water to maintain the homeostasis of their blood volume, pressure, and electrolytes.

Homeostasis of electrolytes

Electrolytes are molecules that dissociate into electrically charged particles. The major positively charged electrolytes (cations) of plasma and interstitial fluid are sodium and potassium. The major negatively charged electrolytes (anions) of the blood are chloride and bicarbonate. The concentration of these electrolytes in the intracellular fluid is very different from their concentration in interstitial fluid. Tissue cells maintain this difference by taking the ions that they require from interstitial fluid and excreting the ions that they do not require into it. The homeostasis of interstitial fluid electrolytes is an extremely important function of the kidney.

The mechanisms that control the homeostasis of sodium are very efficient and are able to reabsorb most of the sodium from the filtrate. Intrinsic mechanisms include all the local tissue mechanisms that do not require nerve or hormone stimulation to adjust to changes in load. For example, the amount of sodium reabsorbed in exchange for hydrogen ions increases during an acidosis, and the amount of sodium reabsorption in exchange for hydrogen ions and potassium increases whenever excessively large amounts of sodium enter the distal tubule convoluted tubule. This does not normally deplete potassium, which is plentiful in a balanced diet. However, chronic use of diuretics that reduce the obligatory sodium transport enzymes of the proximal tubule and the loop of Henle significantly increases the amount of sodium entering the distal convoluted tubule, and they may cause cellular potassium reserves to decline.

Extrinsic mechanisms are mechanisms that involve the nervous system or by hormones, and, for sodium, they are necessarily complex because the homeostasis of sodium cannot be separated from the homeostasis of water, blood volume, or blood pressure. Sodium provides much of the osmotic pressure of interstitial fluid, and therefore, because ADH keeps this osmotic pressure constant, it also maintains its sodium concentration. However, because ADH alters the amount of water that is reabsorbed, it alters blood volume and pressure, which must also be kept constant.

At least two extrinsic mechanisms modify renal function to keep blood volume and pressure within the normal range. They do so by controlling the rate at which sodium is reabsorbed by the distal convoluted tubule. The renin-angiotensin system increases it by increasing sodium reabsorption, and atrial natriuretic hormone decreases it, decreasing sodium reabsorption. The changes in osmolarity that these hormones produce modify the release of ADH until blood volume and pressure return to normal.

The renin-angiotensin system acts to raise blood pressure whenever it falls because the enzyme renin is secreted by cells of the juxtaglomerular apparatus whenever they are stimulated by the sympathetic nervous system or by a fall in afferent arteriole blood pressure. Renin initiates a cascade of reactions by splitting angiotensin I from a plasma globulin precursor, angiotensinogen. Angiotensin I is rapidly converted to angiotensin II as it passes through the lungs. Angiotensin II is converted to angiotensin III in the adrenal cortex to stimulate the production and secretion of aldosterone (a mineral corticoid hormone). A few hours after aldosterone combines with receptors in the distal convoluted tubule, extra sodium is reabsorbed and potassium is secreted. The sodium increases interstitial osmotic pressure and thus increases the secretion of antidiuretic hormone, so that plasma volume and blood pressure increase and exert a negative feedback on further renin secretion.

Atrial natriuretic hormone acts to reduce blood pressure whenever blood volume increases. It is secreted by cells of the atrial wall when they are stretched because of an increase in venous volume. It reduces the reabsorption of sodium by the kidney tubules, and consequently, extra sodium is excreted, interstitial fluid osmotic pressure falls, and the secretion of ADH is reduced, so that extra water is also lost and blood volume is reduced. This in turn reduces venous volume and lowers cardiac output and arterial blood pressure. It also reduces the tension in the atrial wall and exerts a negative feedback upon the continued secretion of the atrial natriuretic hormone. ADH and angiotensin II also have vasoconstrictor effects and stimulate thirst. Atrial natriuretic hormone is a vasodilator and also inhibits thirst and the secretion of ADH.

The homeostasis of potassium is also extremely important, despite its low concentration in interstitial fluid. Deviations have potent effects upon nerve and muscle activity. Most of the body's potassium is found within cells, and since more potassium is normally eaten than the body requires, a surplus usually exists. This is excreted in exchange for sodium by the distal convoluted tubule. However, if plasma potassium rises, a slight increase is sufficient to stimulate the adrenal cortical cells directly to secrete aldosterone, which increases potassium secretion into the tubule.

Chloride ions are reabsorbed by the proximal convoluted tubules, either by the electropositive attraction of the actively transported cations or by active transport mechanisms in the loop of Henle.

Bicarbonate is reabsorbed throughout the kidney tubules as a result of the secretion of hydrogen ions in exchange for sodium. The secreted hydrogen ions combine with bicarbonate in the filtrate to produce carbon dioxide, which then diffuses rapidly into the interstitial fluid, where the reaction is reversed to produce bicarbonate to neutralize the reabsorbed sodium, and produce more hydrogen ions for secretion. This reaction is speeded up by the enzyme carbonic anhydrase, which a number of diuretics inhibit to produce their effect.

The renal homeostasis of calcium and phosphate is reviewed in Chapter 59.

Caution should be taken in interpreting the results of blood tests that measure the concentration of substances like potassium that are found predominantly in the cells, or calcium that is found predominantly in the skeleton. The amount of potassium in the cells may be below normal, and bones may have lost significant amounts of calcium, and yet their blood concentrations will be within the normal range as a result of extremely efficient homeostatic mechanisms.

Homeostasis of blood acidity (pH)

Acids are substances that dissociate to produce hydrogen ions, which can be measured as pH units. To maintain the homeostasis of pH, many buffer systems exist inside and outside the cells. These buffers maintain pH by combining with surplus hydrogen ions or releasing hydrogen ions to maintain their concentration in body fluids within narrow limits. This is necessary because enzyme function is very sensitive to changes in pH. The kidney functions to excrete unwanted metabolic acids and reabsorb the bases of these buffer systems. Normally the pH of venous blood is 7.35 as a result of the carbon dioxide produced by metabolism, and it is 7.45 in arterial blood because this carbon dioxide was eliminated as the blood passed through the lungs.

Carbonic acid and sodium bicarbonate form the most important buffer for neutralizing strong acids in plasma and interstitial fluid. This buffer is in equilibrium with all the other body buffers and is especially useful because its two constituents can be controlled simply: the concentration of carbonic acid can be rapidly controlled by using the respiratory system to adjust the concentration of carbon dioxide, and the concentration of sodium bicarbonate can be controlled by the kidneys.

The normal pH of plasma and interstitial fluid is maintained by keeping the ratio of the concentrations of sodium bicarbonate to carbon dioxide at 20:1. This is true regardless of the absolute amount of sodium bicarbonate in the plasma. The total amount of sodium bicarbonate in the blood may vary with different disease conditions, but as long as the respiratory system maintains the 20:1 ratio by adjusting the concentration of carbonic acid, the pH of the plasma and thus of the other body buffers will be in the normal range.

Similarly, the concentration of carbonic acid may change as a result of respiratory disease, but as long as the kidneys maintain the 20:1 ratio by adjusting the plasma concentration of sodium bicarbonate, the pH of the plasma will be in the normal range.

The homeostasis of plasma pH involves three steps when metabolic acids enter the blood:

1. Strong acids are neutralized by plasma sodium bicarbonate in a reaction that produces carbonic acid and the sodium salt of the strong acid. This reaction succeeds in converting the dissociated and highly damaging hydrogen ions of the strong acid to the associated and less damaging hydrogen ions of carbonic acid. However, it upsets the 20:1 ratio by increasing plasma carbonic acid and decreasing plasma sodium bicarbonate. This upset is rapidly corrected.

2. The extra carbonic acid rapidly dissociates into water and carbon dioxide that immediately stimulates the respiratory system so that it is exhaled until the 20:1 ratio of bicarbonate to carbon dioxide is restored.

3. When the sodium salt of the strong acid enters the nephron along with the other electrolytes, its sodium is actively reabsorbed in exchange for hydrogen ions split from interstitial fluid carbonic acid, or potassium. In the tubule lumen, the secreted hydrogen ions reconstitute the original strong acid, which is promptly neutralized by ammonia that diffuses from the tubule cells as required. Normally most of the blood sodium bicarbonate used to neutralize strong acids is reabsorbed, and the acid is excreted as its ammonium or potassium salt. However, if large amounts of metabolic acid are produced, some sodium will remain attached to the acid and be lost in urine.

Other renal functions

In addition to the homeostasis of water, electrolytes, and pH, the kidney is important in the excretion of water-soluble waste products and other substances that are not required by the body. A minimum of 25 to 30 g of **urea** are formed each day in the liver from the amines removed from surplus amino acids. This urea is excreted by the kidneys along with other nitrogenous wastes such as uric acid, ammonia, and creatinine. The kidney also plays a role in the transamination and homeostasis of blood amino acids.

Substances that are excreted in urine can be thought of as having been cleared from the blood. **Renal plasma clearance** is the volume (milliliter) of plasma that contains the amount of the substance excreted by the kidneys in 1 minute. For example, the renal clearance of urea is normally approximately 75 mL. GFR is estimated by determining the renal plasma clearance of inulin, while renal blood flow is determined by the renal plasma clearance of para-aminohippuric acid (PAH).

Bacterial toxins and water-soluble drugs are excreted by the kidney. Although drugs and other substances in the body are inactivated for excretion mainly by the liver, some inactivation is carried out by the kidney.

The kidney is the most important route for the excretion of water-soluble drugs and drug metabolites. They are excreted:
1. Because they are not actively reabsorbed
2. Because they are actively secreted
3. By a combination of both these processes

In addition to its excretion and homeostatic functions, the kidney also serves as an endocrine gland. It secretes renin and erythropoietin and plays a role in the production of 1,25-dihydroxycholecalciferol.

Changes in renal function in the older adult

Kidney function is immature at birth, and the newborn lacks the ability to concentrate urine and is inefficient in handling electrolytes. No new nephrons

GERIATRIC CONSIDERATIONS

Physiologic Changes in the Renal/Urinary Systems

Renal function begins to decline at approximately 30 years of age as a result of a slow loss of nephrons and a decrease in enzymatic and metabolic activity of the tubular cells. Kidney weight decreases by approximately 30% by 80 years of age. Although they take a longer time to return the system to its stable state, the kidneys are normally able to cope with the demands made upon them because they are decreased by the age-related reduction in lean body mass and metabolic activity that also accompanies aging. Problems develop when the decline in renal function is exacerbated by reduced renal blood supply, infections, allergic reactions and environmental toxins, and when the kidneys cannot eliminate drugs at a satisfactory rate.

The function of the lower urinary tract is normally well-maintained in elderly individuals. However, in some individuals, urine storage and elimination may be impaired by problems related to surrounding structures. For example, enlargement of the prostate gland may impede micturition in males and childbearing and relaxation of the pelvic floor muscles increase the risk of urinary incontinence for women.

Kenny RA: *Physiology of aging: a synopsis.* St Louis, 1992, Mosby–Year Book.

are formed in the kidneys after the fetal period; however, the nephrons and kidneys continue to grow in size until maturity. As the adult grows older, renal weight, blood flow, and glomerular filtration decline, especially after 50 years of age. These changes are most obvious when they are standardized to body surface area. Normally, as the individual ages, the kidney is still able to maintain the homeostasis of the plasma constituents but it is slower to respond to changes in load.

When one kidney ceases to function, the remaining kidney is capable of considerable compensatory hypertrophy because there are a large number of reserve nephrons that can enlarge and increase their function. However, the number of reserve nephrons declines with age, and consequently hypertrophy is also reduced in the older individual.

Urinary System

Structural description

The urinary system is made of a pair of ureters, the urinary bladder, and the urethra (Figure 41-3).

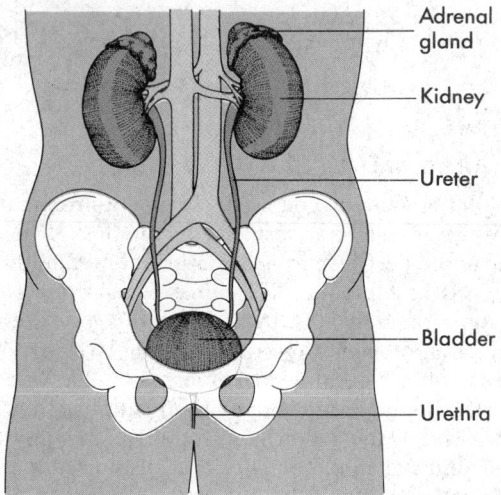

FIGURE 41-3   Location of urinary system organs.

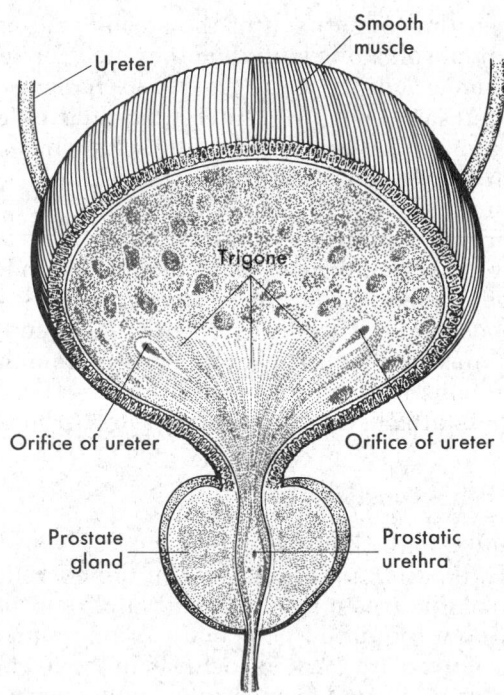

FIGURE 41-4   Cross section of male urinary bladder showing urethra.

The **ureters** begin at the renal pelvis and end in the trigone region on the inferior dorsal surface of the bladder. They are made of an inner layer of transitional epithelium, two layers of muscle (circular and longitudinal smooth muscle), and an outer fibrous layer. Urine is propelled actively along the ureters by peristalsis.

The bladder lies between the pubic symphysis and the rectum in men. In women it lies between the pubic symphysis and the uterus and vagina. When empty it takes up a conical shape, and as it fills it becomes ovoid. It is made of four layers, the innermost layer being transitional epithelium that is supported by a submuscosal layer and changes in thickness as it adjusts to the volume of the bladder. The three layers of smooth muscle of the bladder together are referred to as the detrusor muscle. Only the upper surface of the bladder is covered by a serous layer of peritoneum. The trigone, ureters, and blood vessels of the bladder are innervated by sympathetic fibers of the T-12 to L-2 spinal nerves. Two sphincters surround the neck of the bladder. The detrusor muscle and the internal sphincter are innervated by parasympathetic fibers of the sacral S-2 to S-4 spinal nerves, and the external sphincter (made of voluntary skeletal muscle fibers) is innervated by motor neurons of the pudendal nerve.

Micturition (urination) is the reflex action of emptying the bladder. It is initiated when increased tension is detected by stretch receptors in the bladder wall. The reflex center lies in the cord in the sacral region (S-2 to S-4). Parasympathetic impulses cause the detrusor muscle to contract and the internal sphincter to relax. In the baby, micturition is involuntary. In the adult it will not occur unless the voluntary external sphincter is relaxed via fibers of the pudendal nerve.

The **urethra** is the tube that carries the urine from the bladder to the exterior. It is short (2.5 to 4 cm) in the woman and only carries urine. It is longer in the man (18 to 20 cm), passes through the prostate gland (Figure 41-4) and penis, and also carries semen during ejaculation.

ASSESSMENT
Subjective Assessment

Differing renal/urinary disorders will manifest through a variety of symptoms as well as signs. Patients may experience alterations in renal function secondary to other processes such as trauma, inadequate perfusion secondary to hypotension, renal toxicities secondary to chemotherapeutic agents, or patients may experience primary renal/urologic alterations such as renal calculi or urinary tract infections (UTIs).

The box on p. 1063 provides a list of potential symptoms to review with the patient. In addition to specific symptoms, ask the patient about any history of renal calculi, renal failure, frequent or chronic UTIs, nephrotic syndrome, nephritis, bleeding disorders (hemophilia), hemolytic disease (hemolytic-uremic syndrome), sickle-cell disease, AIDS, diabetes mellitus, congestive heart failure, hypertension, cancer, or previous tests or procedures (intravenous pyelogram [IVP], sonogram or ultrasound, cystoure-

POTENTIAL SYMPTOMS RELATED TO RENAL DISORDERS

Amenorrhea
Anuria (no urine production)
Dyspnea
Dysuria (painful or difficult urination)
Edema
Fatigue
Fever
Flank pain
Frequency
Hematuria
Incontinence
Nausea and vomiting
Nocturia (excessive urination at night)
Oliguria (decreased urine production in relation to fluid intake)
Polyuria (excessive production of urine)
Pruritus
Rash
Suprapubic pain
Urgency (feeling the urge to void but voiding only a small amount with each attempt)
Weight gain

throgram, cystoscopy, etc.) related to kidney or bladder function.

Determination of the appropriate related systems to review is guided by the nurse's knowledge of pathophysiology, treatment, and associated symptoms determined in delineating the renal symptoms. For example, the patient may complain of bloody urine **(hematuria)**. Because gross hematuria may be associated with trauma, urinary tract infection, renal or bladder cancer, cancer chemotherapeutic agents, or renal calculi, the nurse's questioning is guided by the associated symptoms and medical history. If the patient gives a history of severe, colicky pain initially beginning in the flank and moving anteriorly and possibly into the labia or scrotum, renal calculi should be suspected. If the patient is female, gives a history of urgency, frequency, burning, and recent sexual intercourse, a urinary tract infection should be considered. If the patient gives a history of leukemia and being treated with cyclophosphamide, hemorrhagic cystitis secondary to the cyclophosphamide should be strongly considered. If the patient is a male in his fifties and complaining of gross hematuria, the possibility renal or bladder cancer should be considered.

Other appropriate history to explore includes major adult illnesses, hospitalizations, surgeries, injuries or accidents, immunizations, current medications, allergies, and habits. Hematuria may be associated with warfarin therapy. Nonsteroidal antiinflammatory drugs may result in diminished renal function in some patients.

Family history that is relevant to renal system includes renal calculi, polycystic disease, renal agenesis, renal or bladder cancer, bleeding disorders (hemophilia), hemolytic disease (hemolytic-uremic syndrome), sickle-cell disease, nephritis, and renal tubular necrosis. A positive finding should include the disorder as well as the individual's relationship to the patient, (e.g., renal calculi, grandfather; polycystic disease, sister). Family history usually includes grandparents, parents, aunts, uncles, siblings, spouse, and children.

Objective Assessment

Physical examination of the renal system is usually included in the examination of the abdomen. In addition, measuring intake and output may also be helpful. Assessment of the male and female genital systems may be indicated. This examination is discussed in detail in Chapter 68. General assessment is included for any patient and refers to the examiner's overall impression of the patient's state of health.

General assessment

General assessment includes height, weight, vital signs, apparent age as relative to chronologic age, nutritional status, general appearance, and stature. Any obvious abnormalities or assistive devices also should be noted. Record whether the patient appears to be comfortable or in distress. Daily weights and frequent blood pressure checks may be useful in some patients.

Integumentary system

Inspect and palpate the skin, noting warmth, color, moisture, turgor, lesions, and vascularity. Note any rashes, describing color, texture, and location. Observe for peripheral and periorbital edema.

Cardiovascular system

Observe the precordium for any heaves, lifts, or pulsations. Palpate the precordium for thrills and apical impulse. Auscultate the precordium with the bell and the diaphragm noting the rate, rhythm, the first heart sound (S1), the second heart sound (S2), any gallops (S3,S4), murmurs, or other extra sounds. (See Chapter 33 for a more complete discussion of cardiovascular assessment.)

Respiratory system

Inspect the thorax noting symmetry, configuration, and pattern of respirations, including depth, regularity, and ease of respirations. Palpate the thorax for tenderness and masses. Percuss the thorax generally for quality and symmetry. Auscultate the thorax, noting breath sounds and any adventitious sounds such as crackles (rales), wheezes (rhonchi), or pleural friction rubs (see Chapter 25 for a complete discussion of respiratory assessment).

Abdomen

Inspect the abdomen noting scars, striae, dilated veins, umbilicus, contour, and symmetry. Also observe for peristaltic waves and pulsations. Auscultate the abdomen for bowel sounds, bruits, and venous hums. Next, percuss the abdomen generally noting percussion tones throughout all four quadrants. After general percussion, begin percussion of specific organs. (Percussion of specific organs is described in more detail in Chapter 63.) Specific organs to be percussed include the liver, spleen, and potentially, the bladder. The stomach may be percussed by noting the gastric air bubble. The bladder is percussed as suprapubic dullness only when full.

Costovertebral angle tenderness (CVAT) is tested by fist percussion, is usually done while examining the posterior thorax, and is usually written in the abdominal portion of the documentation or SOAP note. Fist percussion may be done either directly or indirectly. The patient should not perceive the percussion as painful unless a renal disorder such as pyelonephritis or renal calculi exists. If you suspect such a renal disorder and have been given a history of CVAT, do not perform fist percussion. To perform fist percussion for CVAT, have the patient seated. Place the palmar surface of your nondominant hand

flat over the costovertebral angle (Figure 41-5). With the ulnar surface of the fist of your dominant hand, strike the dorsal surface of the nondominant hand. Evaluate for CVAT bilaterally (Figure 41-6).

Palpation of the abdomen is first done generally and then more specifically for specific organs as well as any masses. Begin with light palpation. If the patient is unable to relax, have the patient flex his or her knees. This facilitates relaxation of the abdominal musculature. Following light palpation, begin deep palpation, noting any tenderness or masses. Palpate for liver, spleen, and kidney borders.

Palpate for the right kidney with the patient in the supine position. Standing at the patient's right side, slide your left hand under the patient's right flank with the palmar surface up. Using your left hand, try to displace the right kidney anteriorly. With your right hand on the patient's abdomen just inferior to the costal margin, attempt to "capture" the right kidney on deep inspiration as shown in Figure 41-7. A normal right kidney may be palpable in a thin, relaxed patient.

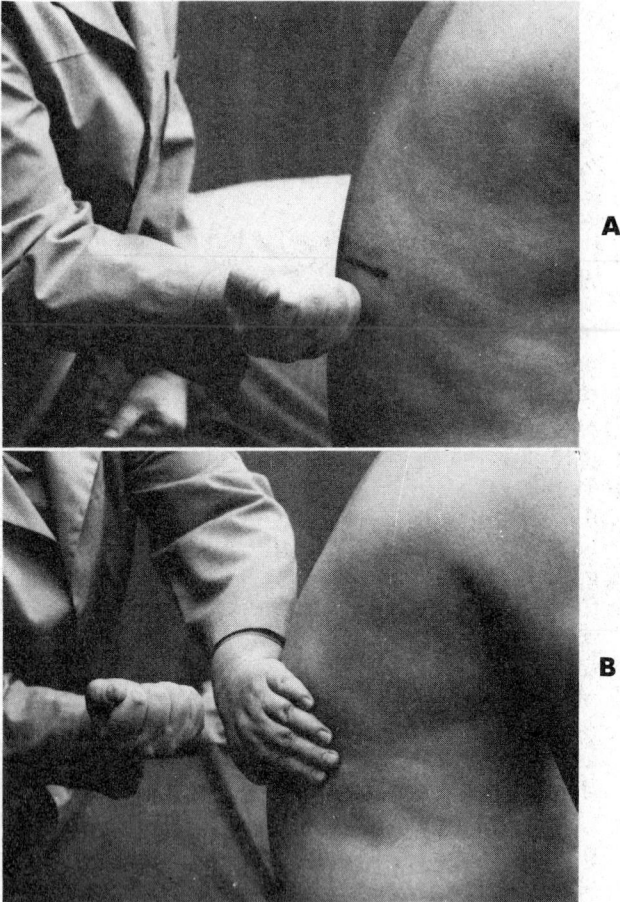

FIGURE 41-6   Percussion for CVAT, **A,** direct, **B,** indirect. (From Malasanos L et al: *Health assessment,* ed 4, St Louis, 1990, Mosby–Year Book.)

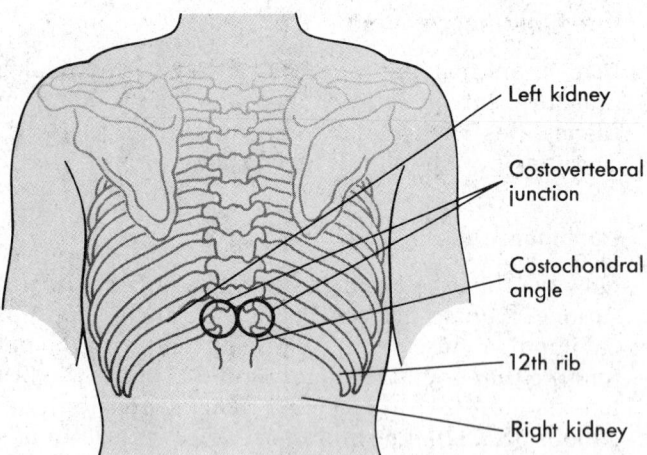

FIGURE 41-5   Location of the costovertebral angle.

Labels in Figure 41-5:
- Left kidney
- Costovertebral junction
- Costochondral angle
- 12th rib
- Right kidney

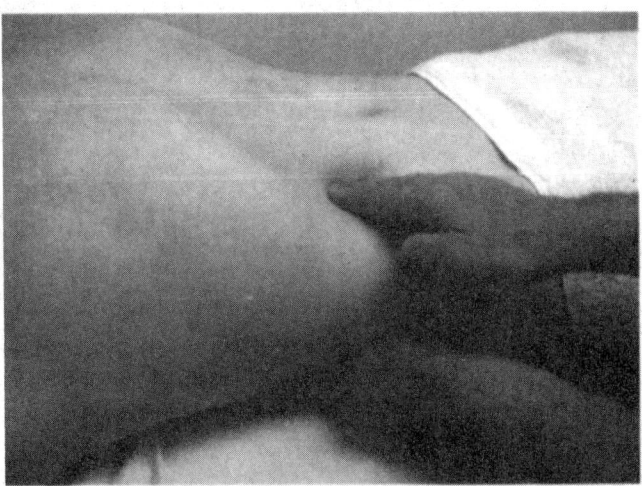

FIGURE 41-7   Palpation of the left kidney. (From Seidel H et al: *Mosby's guide to physical examination*, ed 2, St Louis, 1991, Mosby–Year Book.)

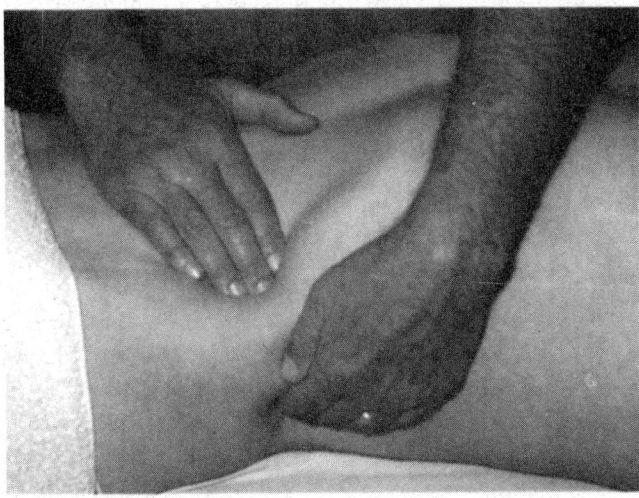

FIGURE 41-8   Palpation of the right kidney. (From Seidel H et al: *Mosby's guide to physical examination*, ed 2, St Louis, 1991, Mosby–Year Book.)

To palpate the left kidney, reach across the patient and place your left hand under the patient's left costovertebral angle. Place your right hand over the patient's left costal margin. Instruct the patient to take a deep breath. Palpate deeply on the patient's deep inspiration. The normal left kidney is generally not palpable because of its retroperitoneal location (Figure 41-8).

Male genitalia

Urethritis (inflammation of the urethra) in the male begins with symptoms of dysuria. The cause can be

GERIATRIC CONSIDERATIONS

Renal/Urinary Assessment

General approach

- allow more time than for a younger adult
- articulate clearly; the geriatric patient may be hearing impaired
- impaired sight, comprehension, or mobility may result in less than optimum cooperation
- provide clear, concise instructions

History collection

- may need to repeat questions
- be alert for answers that do not appear appropriate; the patient may not have understood the question correctly because of impaired hearing or impaired comprehension
- new onset incontinence may be a manifestation of UTI

Physical assessment

- the physical examination itself is not different, but the approach needs to be altered such that the appropriate information is assessed without undue discomfort or embarrassment for the patient
- maintain an environment with minimal noise, distractions, and interruption
- the GFR decreases with age
- creatinine clearance decreases with age

related to (but not limited to) a sexually transmitted disease (STD) such as chlamydia. The urethra should be assessed and a urethral culture performed. Prostatitis and benign prostatic hyperplasia can also include urinary complaints such as hesitancy, change in size of the urinary stream, and difficulty in beginning the stream. The prostate should be examined when these symptoms are present. The male genitalia examination is discussed in detail in Chapter 68.

Female genitalia

When a female complains of dysuria, examination of the external genitalia may be useful to determine if any external inflammation is apparent. If the dysuria is reported as external or exacerbated as the urine flows across the perineum and there is an increased or abnormal vaginal discharge, vaginitis may be the etiologic agent. Symptoms suggesting vaginitis necessitate a pelvic exam with cervical cultures for chlamydia and gonorrhea and examination of the discharge for candida, trichomonas, or bacte-

TABLE 41-1 Findings of Urinalysis

Elements	Normal findings (SI values)	Abnormal findings
GENERAL EXAMINATION		
Color	Pale yellow to deep gold	Variations in color may occur with various medications
		Color varies with the concentration of the urine
		Brown or black coloration is a serious sign
Odor	Aromatic	Fetid odor common in infection
		Fruity odor found with diabetes mellitus, starvation, or dehydration
		Other changes occur with medications, such as paraldehyde, vitamins, and antibiotics
Appearance	Clear	Turbidity may reflect renal infection
Specific gravity	1.001-1.025	Higher specific gravity indicates concentrated urine
		Specific gravity is increased by radiopaque contrast media, albumin, dextran, and in dehydration, CHF, and liver failure.
		Low specific gravity indicates dilute urine and may occur with diabetes insipidus, acute tubular necrosis, or salt-restricted diets
pH	5.0-8.0	Alkaline pH occurs with urinary tract infection, metabolic or respiratory alkalosis, a diet high in fruits and vegetables, or administration of sodium bicarbonate and potassium citrate
		Acidic pH occurs with metabolic or respiratory acidosis, pyrexia, starvation, phenylketonuria, a diet high in protein, and administration of ascorbic acid and methenamine
Protein	Negative to trace	Protein may be indicative of glomerulonephritis, preeclampsia in pregnant woman, or multiple myeloma
		The dipstick method may not detect significant proteinuria in very dilute urine or myeloma
Glucose	None	Glucose may appear under normal conditions, as a result of ingestion of a high-carbohydrate meal, stress, pregnancy, or ingestion of a wide variety of medications, such as corticosteroids, lithium carbonate, aspirin, and thiazide derivatives
		Glucose may be indicative of diabetes that is not well controlled, CNS disorders, Cushing's syndrome, infection, and intravenous administration of dextrose-containing fluids
		Glucose levels may be tested using dipsticks such as Tes-Tape, Clinistix, and Clinitest. Pregnancy, ascorbic acid, keflin, and streptomycin may produce a false-positive reaction in Clinitest
Ketones	None	Ketones may be indicative of poorly controlled diabetes, dehydration, starvation, or excessive ingestion of aspirin
Occult blood	Negative	Hemoglobulinuria is indicative of hemolytic anemia, drug ingestion (arsenic, coumadin), toxins, or transfusion reactions
		A positive result may also occur if myoglobin (a muscle pigment) is present; it also occurs with muscle infarction, trauma, burns, and convulsions
Leukocyte esterase	Negative	A positive reaction indicates presence of neutrophils and the presence of a urinary tract infection
		False-positive results can occur if sample is contaminated with vaginal secretions
		False-negative results can occur in the presence of high levels of protein or ascorbic acid in the urine, test performed using a dipstick method

TABLE 41-1   Findings of Urinalysis—cont'd

Elements	Normal findings (SI values)	Abnormal findings
Nitrite	Negative	Positive reaction indicates presence of bacteria in the urine False-negative results may occur with freshly voided random urine specimens and if yeasts or gram-positive bacteria are present Test is performed with the dipstick method

MICROSCOPIC EXAMINATION

Elements	Normal findings (SI values)	Abnormal findings
WBCs	0-5/hpf (high-power field)	Increased WBCs may indicate upper or lower urinary tract infection
RBCs	0-5/hpf	Increased RBCs are indicative of microscopic hematuria, which may occur with stones, tumor, or acute glomerulonephritis
Casts	Negative, or occasional hyaline crystals	Hyaline casts or clumps of protein are found with concentrated urine and are not indicative of renal disease unless they occur in excessive numbers White blood cell casts indicate pyelonephritis Red blood cell casts occur with glomerulonephritis, vascular disorders, collagen disorders, subacute bacterial endocarditis, and renal infarction; the presence of these casts is indicative of serious disease and should be thoroughly investigated Phosphate and calcium oxalate crystals occur with hyperparathyroidism or malabsorption Urate crystals occur with high serum acid levels (gout)

rial vaginitis. The female genitalia assessment is discussed in detail in Chapter 68.

DIAGNOSTIC AND LABORATORY TESTS
Urinalysis

Urinalysis (UA; routine UA) is an important routine screening test that gives information about the status of the renal and urinary tracts and the total body system (Table 41-1). The test involves collection of a random sample of at least 15 mL (0.5 oz) of urine. A first-voided morning specimen is preferred. Female patients should be instructed to clean external genitals before voiding, because the specimen should be free of vaginal discharge and feces. The specimen is sent to the laboratory or refrigerated if it must be kept longer than 1 hour. If left standing at room temperature for 5 hours, the specimen will not be suitable for culture; erythrocytes will decompose, and casts will disintegrate. Nurses can obtain immediate information on ketones, pH, protein, glucose, and blood by using a Multistix reagent strip. The strip should only be taken from a bottle that is tightly sealed. The nurse must check the expiration date on the bottle and manufacturer's instructions before using the strip. Containers in which reagent strips, tablets, or tapes are stored must be tightly sealed and kept in a dry place otherwise results may be incorrect. Precise timing and comparison of color changes against the color chart on the bottle are essential to ensure accuracy.

Urine Culture

The urine culture remains a standard procedure for diagnosing urinary tract infections. A test of the antimicrobial sensitivity of identified organisms is usually ordered. Newer methods help identify positive specimens more accurately and rapidly. For example, photometry detects significant bacterial changes by alterations in light transmission through innoculated media. Broluminescence identifies bacteriuria through the detection of bacterial adenosine triphosphate. Other rapid automated methods such as carbon 14 labeling and microcalorimetry are currently in development.

A colony count of less than 10,000 bacterial units/ml of urine is not significant, and a count of

10,000 to 100,000 is inconclusive. A count of 100,000 is considered a positive culture and is indicative of pyelonephritis if accompanied by fever and flank pain. A positive culture that is accompanied by dysuria, frequency, and urgency is indicative of cystitis. A positive culture that is not accompanied by symptoms may indicate contamination of the specimen during collection or chronic low-grade pyelonephritis. The presence of more than two organisms or of vaginal or skin organisms is suggestive of contamination.

Patient preparation

The patient is told that the test detects urinary tract infection and that proper collection is necessary for useful results. The nurse ensures that the patient has a sterile container, is aware that only the outside of the container is to be touched, and that the container should be held in such a way that it does not contact legs, genitalia, or clothing. The patient is instructed in proper cleansing techniques. Women should separate the labia and clean from front to back, using at least three sponges impregnated with cleansing solution. Men need to retract the foreskin and cleanse with at least three cleansing sponges. The patient is directed to start voiding, wash the distal urethra, stop, and then continue voiding into the cup. Female patients are told that they will need to lean forward slightly so that urine flows directly downward without touching the skin. Specimens for urine culture may also be collected through catheterization or directly from an indwelling catheter. A urine-collecting bag is not an appropriate source of urine for culture.

The nurse records the patient's current antibiotic history on the laboratory requisition and takes the urine sample immediately to the laboratory. If transport is delayed, the specimen must be refrigerated unless collected for cytomegalovirus (refrigeration destroys the virus).

Composite Urine Collections

Composite urine specimens are collected over 2 to 24 hours and are used to measure or examine specific components, such as electrolytes, 17-ketosteroids, and creatinine (Table 41-2). The patient is instructed to void and discard the urine. NOTE: the time of voiding is recorded, since this is the start of the test. All subsequent voidings are saved in a collection container. At the end of the designated period, the nurse instructs the patient to void and add the specimen to the container.

TABLE 41-2   Composite Urine Collections

Determination	Reference range (SI values)	Minimal quantity required	Clinical significance
Aldosterone	Normal salt intake: 100-200 mEq/day (100-200 mmol/day) −3-19 µf/24 hr (8.3-52.7 nmol/24 hr) Low salt intake: 10 mEq/day (10 nmol/day) −20-80µg/24 hr (55.4-230 nmol/24 hr)	24 hr	Increased with primary aldosteronism and secondary aldosteronism (resulting from malignant hypertension, congestive heart failure, and cirrhosis) Decreased with Addison's disease, high sodium intake, hypokalemia, and pregnancy
Amylase	24-76 units/mL (24-76 arb unit)		Increased with acute pancreatitis
Calcium	300 mg/day or less (7.5 mmol/day or less)		Increased with hyperparathyroidism Decreased with hypoparathyroidism or vitamin D deficiency

TABLE 41-2   Composite Urine Collections—cont'd

Determination	Reference range (SI values)	Minimal quantity required	Clinical significance
Catecholamines	Epinephrine: under 20 μg/day (<109 nmol/day) Norepinephrine: under 100 μg/day (<590 nmol/day)	24 hr	Increased with pheo-chromocytoma
Chorionic gonadotropin (pregnancy test)	Negative		Positive with pregnancy or hydatidiform mole
Copper	0-100 μg/day (0-1.6 μmol/day)	24 hr	Increased with cirrhosis or nephrosis
Coproporphyrin	50-250 μg/day (80-380 nmol/day)	24 hr	Increased with poliomyelitis or porphyria hepatica
Creatine	M: <40 mg/day (<0.30 nmol/day) F: <80 mg/day (<0.61 nmol/day)	24 hr	Increases with fever, pregnancy, or carcinoma of liver
Creatinine clearance	<40 y M: 90-139 mL/min/1.73 m^3 (0.87-1.34 mL/s/m^2) F: 80-125 mL/min/1.73 m^3 (0.77-1.20 mL/s/m^2) From the 4th decade on, values decrease 6.5 mL/min/1.73 m^3 (0.06 mL/s/m^2)	2, 12, or 24 hr	Increases with *Salmonella* infections or tetanus Decreased when glomerular filtration rate impaired, accompanied by increase in plasma levels Decreased with anemia, leukemia, or muscle atrophy
Cystine or cysteine	0 <38.1 mg/day (<317 μmol/day)	10 mL 24 hr	Increased with cystinuria
Hemoglobin; myoglobin	Negative		Increased with transfusion of incompatible blood, extensive burns, or crushing trauma to muscles
5-Hydroxyindoleacetic acid	2-6 mg/day (10.4-31.2 μmol/day)	24 hr	Increased with carcinoid tumors
Lead	<80 mg/L (<0.39 μmol/L)	24 hr	Increased with lead poisoning
Osmolality	50-1400 mOsm/kg 300-900 mmol/kg (with usual daily fluid intake)	Random 24 hr	Decreased urine osmolality and increased serum osmolality with diabetes insipidus Increased with oliguric states secondary to hypovolemia
Phosphorus (inorganic)	Varies with intake; average 1 g/day (32 nmol/day)	24 hr	Increased with fever, rickets, or tuberculosis Decreased with acute infections or nephritis

Continued.

TABLE 41-2   Composite Urine Collections—cont'd

Determination	Reference range (SI values)	Minimal quantity required	Clinical significance
Porphobilinogen	0	24 hr	Increased with acute porphyria or liver disease
Protein (quantitative)	1-14 mg/dL (10-140 mg/L)	24 hr	Increased with hematuria, fever, cardiac failure, or nephritis
Sodium	40-220 mEq/L (40-220 mmol/L)	24 hr	Decreased with vomiting, diarrhea, and prerenal failure

Steroids
17-ketosteroids

	(mg/day)		*(µmol/day)*			
Age	M	F	M	F		
20 yr	6-21	4-16	21-73	14-56	24 hr	Increased with adrenal hyperplasia or Cushing's syndrome
30 yr	8-26	4-14	28-90	14-49		
50 yr	5-18	3-9	17-62	10-31		
70 yr	2-10	1-7	7-35	3-24		Decreased with Addison's disease and hypertension

Determination	Reference range (SI values)	Minimal quantity required	Clinical significance
17-hydroxysteroids	3-8 mg/day (8-22 µmol/day)	24 hr	Increased with Cushing's syndrome Decreased with Addison's disease
Sugar, quantitative glucose	0.5 g/d (<2.78 µmol/day)	24 hr	Increased with diabetes mellitus
Urea clearance	12-20 g/day (0.42-0.71 mol/day) Blood urea nitrogen (BUN) should be determined during the urine collection period	24 hr	Increased during excessive protein catabolism Decreased with impaired kidney function
Urine volume	Adult, M: 800-1800 mL/24hr F: 600-1600 mL/24hr >60 y: 250-2400 mL/24hr		Increased with diabetes insipidus, acquired renal disease, mannitol infusion, infusion of contrast media, adrenal insufficiency, protein insufficiency, after menstruation, and some drugs Decreased with dehydration, blood loss, shock, CHF, cirrhosis, renal calculi, and renal failure
Urobilinogen	Up to 1.0 Ehrlich unit (to 1.0 arb unit)	2 hr	Increased with liver disease Decreased with diarrhea or renal insufficiency
Uroporphyrins	<50 µg/day (<60 nmol/day)	24 hr	Increased with porphyria
Vanillylmandelic acid (VMA)	2-7 mg/day (10.1-35.4 µmol/day)	24 hr	Increased with pheochromocytoma

Creatinine Clearance

Creatinine clearance is a common accurate measure of the GFR. Creatinine, the nonprotein waste product of skeletal muscle, is normally excreted by the kidneys. Impaired glomerular filtration will result in a rise in serum creatinine levels and a drop in the creatinine clearance rate. Increases in the creatinine clearance rate are not usually clinically significant. Because of smaller muscle mass (the source of circulating creatinine), women will have a lower creatinine clearance rate (74-130 mL/min) than men (82-162 mL/min). Accurate timing and complete collection, as well as refrigeration of the composite urine specimen, are essential. A 24-hour urine specimen is usually collected, although 2-, 6-, or 12-hour specimens may also be obtained. Serum creatinine is drawn at any time during the collection period since serum creatinine levels will remain fairly constant over a 24-hour period.

Patient preparation

The patient is told that the test for creatinine clearance measures kidney function and that, before taking it, a regular or usual diet may be eaten, although excessive ingestion of meats should be avoided before and during the test. The nurse determines if the patient is on medications such as furosemide, L-dopa, gentamicin, or thiazide derivatives that will influence test results; the nurse also encourages the patient to avoid strenuous exercise during the test period. The details of a composite urine collection are explained to the patient.

Use of Radioisotopes for Renal Clearance

The GFR can be determined by measuring iodine-125 in the urine and plasma, following subcutaneous injection of iothalamate labeled with iodine-125. Iodine-125 enters the tubules by proximal tubular secretion and glomerular filtration. The patient is informed that the test helps determine the functioning of the kidney and that no dietary restrictions are involved.

Serum Collections

A number of serum tests are useful in evaluating the function of the renal and urinary system (Table 41-3) and the status of electrolyte regulation.

Diagnostic Imaging

Routine x-ray studies of kidneys, ureters, and bladder

A flat plate of the abdomen and pelvis is useful in delineating the size, shape, and location of the kidneys and aids in the diagnosis of calculi, tumors, and malformations of the kidney. The patient is told that the test outlines the structure of the kidneys. No special preparation is usually necessary although a laxative or enema may be prescribed to clear the bowels for better visualization. The test is contraindicated during pregnancy.

Excretory urogram

Excretory urogram (intravenous pyelogram; IVP) is a radiographic procedure that provides visualization of the entire urinary tract and is useful in the diagnosis of bladder abnormalities, renal tumors and cysts, renal trauma, retroperitoneal tumors, and ureteral obstruction.

The test involves intravenous injection of a contrast dye. Multiple x-ray films are taken after injection of the dye. A final post-void film is taken to check for bladder emptying. A timed sequence IVP may also be ordered in which x-ray films are taken every 5 minutes following injection of the dye. This variation of the IVP is useful in detecting unilateral kidney disease but is not totally reliable in ruling out renal artery stenosis. The test takes approximately 45 minutes.

Patient preparation

The patient is told that the test permits visualization of the entire renal system. The procedure is explained and reassurance is provided that efforts will be made to maintain comfort while the patient remains in the supine position. The nurse checks the patient's history for sensitivity to shellfish and iodine dyes, congestive heart failure, diabetes mellitus, hyperthyroidism, asthma, hay fever, and hypertension. The patient's hydration level is assessed, since severe dehydration may precipitate nephrotoxicity. The patient is told that flushing, warmth, and a salty taste may be experienced during injection of the dye, but the effects are temporary. The nurse tells the patient that fasting is necessary 8 hours before the test to produce moderate dehydration and better concentration of the dye and that a liberal fluid intake is desired following the test, to flush out the dye.

An enema or cathartic is administered, as ordered, the evening before the test to prevent films from being obscured by feces and gas. The nurse also obtains an informed consent. Since retained barium can obscure the kidneys, tests involving barium should be scheduled after an IVP.

Renal angiography

Renal angiography visualizes the renal blood vessels and is useful in the diagnosis of renal artery stenosis, extra or missing renal vessels, renovascular hypertension, and renal masses. During the procedure, the patient is placed in a supine position and a cath-

TABLE 41-3   Blood Chemistry Values

Determination	Reference range (SI values)		Clinical significance
	ng/dl	*nmol/L*	
Aldosterone	Supine: 3-10	0.08-0.28	Increased as a result of increased renin activity and with congestive heart failure, nephrotic syndrome, or hypovolemia
	Upright:		
	F: 5-30	0.14-0.83	
	M: 6-22	0.17-0.61	
	(Values based on an average sodium diet 100 mEq/day [100 mmol/day])		Decreased with heparin administration
Blood urea nitrogen (BUN)	8-25 mg/dL (2.9-8.9 mmol/L)		Increased with impaired glomerular filtration, excessive protein intake, or trauma
Calcium, total	8.4-10.2 mg/dL (2.10-2.55 mmol/L) >60 y: 8.8-10.0 mg/dL (2.20-2.50 mmol/L)		Increased with hyperparathyroidism or nephritis with uremia
			Decreased with diarrhea, nephrosis, chronic renal failure or hypoparathyroidism
Creatinine	Adult *mg/dL* *μmol/L*		Increased when glomerular filtration impaired; not a sensitive indicator of early renal disease
	M: 0.6-1.2 53.0-106.0		
	F: 0.5-1.1 44.0-97.0		
Osmolality	275-295 mOsm/kg H_2O (275-295 mmol/kg H_2O) >60 y: 280-301 mOsm/kg H_2O (280-301 mmol/kg H_2O)		Increased with dehydration
Potassium	3.5-5.0 mEq/L (3.5-5.0 mmol/L)		Increased with anuria, oliguria, or Addison's disease
			Decreased with diabetic acidosis, diarrhea, or vomiting
Renin (RIA; PRA)	Normal diet:		Increased with nephrotic syndrome, chronic renal failure, malignant hypertension, renal artery stenosis, congestive heart failure, hemorrhage, or Addison's disease
	Supine: 1.6 ± 1.5 ngAI/mL/hr		
	1.6 ± 1.5 μg AI		
	Upright: 4.5 ± 2.9 ngAI/mL/hr		
	(4h) 4.5 ± 2.9 μgAI		
	Low sodium diet:		Decreased with primary aldosteronism, increased salt intake, or licorice ingestion
	Supine: 3.2 ± 1.1 ngAI/mL/hr		
	3.2 ± 1.1 μgAI		
	Upright: 9.3 ± 4.3 ngAI/mL/hr		
	(4h) 9.3 ± 4.3 μgAI*		
	(*AI, Angiotensin I)		
	Specimen is collected in a chilled syringe prepared with anticoagulant, placed on ice, and taken immediately to laboratory)		
Sodium	135-145 mEq/L (135-145 mmol/L)		Increased with nephritis or pyloric obstruction
			Decreased with Addison's disease or myxedema

eter is inserted through the femoral artery, up the aorta to the level of the renal arteries. A contrast dye is inserted while rapid x-ray filming is performed. Smaller amounts of contrast media are necessary if digital subtraction angiography is performed.

Patient preparation

The nurse explains the procedure and tells the patient that the test allows visualization of blood vessels in the renal system, usually under local anesthesia. The patient may be instructed to fast after midnight; some angiographers prefer that the patient maintain a diet of clear fluids for 6 to 8 hours before the procedure to avoid hemoconcentration and possible subsequent occlusion. The nurse checks for sensitivity to foods or contrast dyes containing iodine and determines if the patient is on anticoagulant therapy.

An informed consent is obtained. The nurse administers an enema or cathartic the evening before, if ordered. Baseline vital signs and peripheral pulses are established, and the peripheral pulse distal to the catheter insertion site is marked. The patient is required to void before the procedure, and the nurse administers sedation, if ordered.

Postprocedure care

Bed rest is prescribed for the patient for 8 to 12 hours and the patient is nonambulatory for a total of 24 hours following the procedure. Peripheral pulses, capillary filling, and vital signs are checked every 15 minutes for 2 hours and then hourly, or in accordance with agency protocol, and these are compared with the baseline data that were obtained. The nurse observes the puncture site for bleeding and monitors the urinary output.

Renal scans

Renal scans are useful in monitoring rejection of a transplanted kidney and in the detection of tumors, abscesses, cysts, renal vascular disease, and trauma. A radioactive isotope such as ^{99m}Tc-DTPA, ^{99m}Tc DMSA, or glucoheptonate is injected intravenously, and the radioactivity over each kidney is measured with a gamma camera or a probe. The amount of radioactivity rises rapidly and then declines as the radioactive tracer leaves the kidneys, resulting in a characteristic curve. Various patterns in the curve are associated with specific conditions. A double isotope technique may be ordered in which a second isotope is used to obtain a series of studies, followed by static images made 4 hours later when the renal system is free of radionucleotides. The test takes approximately 1½ hours.

Patient preparation

The patient is informed that the test enables evaluation of kidney function and is reassured that the amount of radioactivity is minimal and that the radioactive material is completely excreted within 24 hours. The nurse instructs the patient to remain still during scanning, which is usually done with the patient in a prone position. No dietary restrictions are required. A signed consent is obtained.

Computed tomography for evaluation of kidneys

Computed tomography provides excellent visualization of the kidney and has the advantage over ultra-sound in its ability to distinguish more subtle differences in tissue density. It is particularly useful in differentiating benign cysts from malignant cysts and in detecting kidney tumors, suprarenal masses, hydronephrosis, and retroperitoneal bleeding from the kidney (see Chapter 44 for a more detailed description of the procedure). The nurse informs the patient that the test provides visualization of the kidneys and that it will be necessary to lie supine on an x-ray table while a scanner rotates around the patient's body. The nurse prepares the patient for the noise that the scanner makes. The patient must remove all metallic objects before scanning.

Renal ultrasonography

Renal ultrasonography is particularly useful in differentiating renal cysts from solid tumors, detecting renal calculi, and identifying obstructions. The procedure can be safely used with patients who have renal failure since there is no special preparation required. A small transducer is passed over the patient's back. Sound waves are passed into the body structures, and images are recorded as the waves are reflected back. Those waves are interpreted by a computer and presented in picture form. The nurse informs the patient that deep breathing may be required during the procedure, which takes about 30 minutes.

Special Procedures

Cystoscopy

Cystoscopy provides direct visualization with a cystoscope (Figure 41-9) of the bladder wall and urethra and is useful in detecting tumors, inflammation, structural irregularities, and enlargement of adjacent structures such as the prostate. During this procedure, a tissue biopsy can be obtained and small renal calculi can be removed from the bladder. Cystoscopy is contraindicated in the presence of acute urinary tract infection and with severe prostatic obstruction. A **retrograde pyelography** may be performed in conjunction with a cystoscopy, during which catheters are directed into the right or left ureters. Urine samples are collected and a contrast medium is injected through the catheters to outline the renal collecting system. Retrograde pyelography is useful in the diagnosis of ureteral obstruction.

Cystography or cystogram involves instillation of a solution containing radiopaque dye into the bladder via a cystoscope or catheter. To obtain a voiding cystogram the catheter is clamped and x-ray films are taken as the patient micturates. For a cystourethrogram, dye is instilled into the urethra and bladder, and for a urethrogram, a radiopaque substance is placed into the urethra as x-ray films are

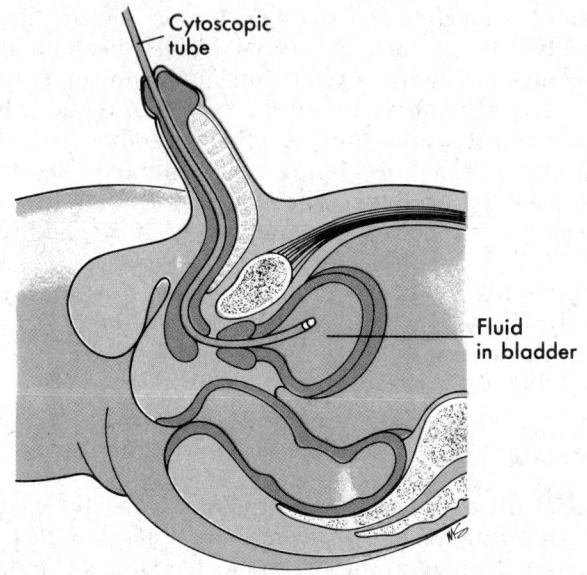

FIGURE 41-9 Cystoscopic examination of the male bladder.

taken. Cystography is useful in detecting vesicoureteral reflux, bladder tumors, diverticula, fistulas, and prostatic enlargement and is indicated with recurrent urinary tract infections.

Patient preparation

The patient is told that the procedure enables close visualization of the urinary collecting system and takes 30 minutes to 1 hour. The patient is reassured that he or she will be adequately draped while in a lithotomy position, and the nurse encourages verbalization of the patient's concerns. If a general anesthetic is to be given, the patient is told that fasting is necessary after midnight before the procedure and that intravenous fluids may be started to ensure adequate flow of urine. If a local anesthetic is used, a full fluid breakfast may be taken before the procedure. The nurse instructs the patient in deep breathing techniques that will alleviate sensations of pressure or burning during the procedure. The nurse checks for a history of sensitivity to foods or contrast media containing iodine and determines urinary voiding patterns and baseline vital signs. A signed consent is obtained from the patient, and preprocedure sedatives are administered, if ordered.

Postprocedure care

The nurse monitors vital signs as indicated by the procedure and agency policy. The patient is reassured that pink-tinged urine and burning on voiding are expected for a day or two following the procedure. An increased fluid intake, application of heat to the lower abdomen, administration of mild anal-

gesics, and sitz baths will relieve discomfort. The patient is advised to avoid alcoholic beverages for 2 days after the test.

Gross hematuria, pain, bladder distention, fever, and tachycardia may indicate complications such as bladder perforation, urinary retention, infection, and dysrhythmias and should be monitored and reported. For each test the nurse prepares the patient by explaining the procedure and, if ordered, discontinues drugs such as urinary spasmolytics or anticholinergics that may affect test data. Following the procedure, the nurse helps the patient to relieve mild symptoms of dysuria, hematuria, and urinary frequency with sitz baths, warm tub baths, and an increased fluid intake.

Renal biopsy

Renal biopsy involves a skin (percutaneous) biopsy through needle insertion into the lower lobe of the kidney. Renal tissue is obtained and examined to determine the type and progression of renal disease. Renal biopsy is the most important definitive test for final diagnosis of intrinsic renal disease. An IVP or ultrasound is usually done before the biopsy. Needle insertion is often guided by fluoroscopy or scanning.

Patient preparation

The patient is told that the test helps diagnose kidney disorders. The nurse informs the patient that a prone position is necessary during the procedure and reassures the patient that a local anesthetic will be given. The patient is instructed to restrict food and fluids 8 hours before the test. During the procedure the patient may be asked to hold his or her breath as the needle is inserted and will be asked to remain very still.

The nurse checks the patient's history for bleeding disorders. The results of coagulation studies are noted, and the nurse ensures that the patient is typed and crossmatched for blood, if ordered. A signed consent is obtained and a mild sedative is administered, if ordered.

Postprocedure care

The patient is usually instructed to lie still for 4 to 12 hours and vital signs are taken every 15 minutes for 4 hours, every 30 minutes for 4 hours, every hour for 4 hours, and every 4 hours for 24 hours. The biopsy site is checked frequently for bleeding, and voidings are checked for gross and microscopic hematuria. The nurse encourages a liberal fluid intake to diminish the possibility of colic and blood clotting. The patient is cautioned to avoid strenuous or jarring activities for a few days and to report flank pain, fever, hematuria, or burning on voiding.

Urodynamic studies

Urodynamic studies are used in the evaluation of abnormalities in micturition. Urodynamics involves the use of cystometry (cystometrogram), uroflowmetry, electromyography, and urethral pressure profile in various combinations.

During cystometry, a catheter that is connected to a cystometer is passed into the bladder. The cystometer records related pressure and volume as the bladder is filled with sterile water, normal saline solution, or carbon dioxide and during voiding. The patient is asked to report when the first sensation of filling is experienced, which is usually between 150 and 200 mL, and when the feeling of fullness is reached, usually around 300 mL. The data gained from the test are useful in planning effective times to stimulate voiding or to schedule intermittent catheterization and in evaluating interstitial cystitis. A signed consent is necessary for the procedure, and the nurse asks the patient to void immediately before the test.

Uroflowmetry records the flow rate of the urinary stream. For this procedure, the patient sits in a special commode chair and pushes a button when urination begins and after it ends. A uroflowmeter, which is contained in a funnel into which the patient voids, measures flow rate, continuous flow, and intermittent flow. Flow rates vary with age, gender, and volume voided. For patients ages 14 to 45 years, the average flow rate is 21 mL/sec for males and 18 mL/sec for females. Patients ages 46 to 65 average 12 mL/sec for males and 15 mL/sec for females. Patients ages 66 to 80 average 9 mL/sec for males and 10 mL/sec for females. Increased flow rates occur with reduced urethral resistance and decreased flow rates with outflow obstruction or hypotonia of the detrusor muscle. The nurse instructs the patient not to urinate for several hours before the test. The patient is also instructed to increase fluid intake before the test because a voiding of 200 mL or more is necessary for accurate results. Assure the patient that voiding will be allowed in whatever position is comfortable and that privacy will be maintained during the test. The test takes 10 to 15 minutes to complete.

Electromyography records the electrical activity in striated muscles during micturition and assists in evaluating neuromuscular coordination of bladder activity. Electrical activity is measured through placement of skin or needle electrodes in periurethral or perineal areas or through electrodes in an anal plug. The patient is asked to alternately tighten and relax the external urinary sphincter during recording. The test is particularly valuable in evaluating the cause of incontinence. The nurse prepares the patient by explaining the purpose of the test and the type and placement of electrodes that will be used.

A urethral pressure profile evaluates the activity of smooth muscle surrounding the urethra and is useful in detecting strictures and excessive muscle tone related to retention. During this test, a catheter is inserted through which carbon dioxide or water is infused. The catheter is slowly and automatically withdrawn while the resistance exerted by the urethral wall is recorded.

CRITICAL THINKING QUESTIONS

1 What is the glomerular filtration rate and what factors influence the production of glomerular filtrate?

2 Design at least three questions to discretely ask patients about voiding symptoms.

3 Distinguish between the meaning of dull versus tympanic sounds elicited by percussion over the urinary bladder area.

4 Discuss patient preparation and posttest care for intravenous pyelography, retrograde pyelography, and cystoscopy.

5 Explain the procedure for collecting composite urine specimens, as it might be explained to a patient.

BIBLIOGRAPHY

Current

1. Bates et al: *A guide to physical examination and history-taking,* ed 5, New York, 1991, JB Lippincott.
2. Burrell LO: *Adult nursing in hospital and community settings,* Norwalk, 1992, Appleton & Lange.
3. Foley RN, Barrett BJ, Parfrey PS: Toxic nephropathy, *The Royal College of Physicians and Surgeons of Canada Annals* 25:1, 1992.
4. Gallo JJ et al: *Handbook of geriatric assessment,* Rockville, Maryland, 1988, Aspen Publishers.
5. Gordon M: *Manual of nursing diagnosis,* New York, 1987, McGraw-Hill.
6. Kane RL et al: *Essentials of clinical geriatrics,* ed 2, New York, 1989, McGraw-Hill.
7. Karram M, Parsons CL: Interstitial cystitis: advances in evaluation and treatment, *Illustrat Med* 1:4, 1991.
8. Kenny RA: *Physiology of aging: a synopsis,* St Louis, 1992, Mosby–Year Book.
9. LeFever Kee J: *Handbook of laboratory and diagnostic tests with nursing implications,* Norwalk, 1990, Appleton & Lange.
10. Malasanos L et al: *Health assessment,* ed 4, St Louis, 1990, Mosby–Year Book.
11. Murray R, Zentner S: *Nursing assessment and health promotion through the life span,* Englewood Cliffs, NJ, 1989, Prentice-Hall.
12. Nurse's ready reference: *Diagnostic tests,* Springhouse, 1991, Springhouse Corporation.
13. Seidel HM et al: *Mosby's guide to physical examination,* ed 2, St Louis, 1991, Mosby–Year Book.

14. Shafer M et al: Urinary leukocyte esterase screening for asymptomatic chlamydial and gonococcal infections in males, *JAMA* 262:18, 1989.

15. Swartz MH: *Textbook of physical diagnosis*, Philadelphia, 1989, WB Saunders.

16. Thelan LA, Davie JK, Urden LD: *Textbook of critical care nursing: diagnosis and management*, St Louis, 1990, Mosby–Year Book.

17. Tilkian SM, Conover MB, Tilkian AG: *Clinical implications of laboratory tests*, St Louis, 1987, Mosby–Year Book.

18. Woodhandler S et al: Dipstick urinalysis screening of asymptomatic adults for urinary tract disorders, *JAMA* 262:9, 1989.

Classic

19. Bloch B, Hunter M: Teaching physiological assessment of black persons, *Nurse Educat* 6(1):24, 1981.

20. Block G, Nolan J: *Health assessment for professional nursing: a developmental approach,* New York, 1986, Appleton-Century-Crofts.

21. Bowers A, Thompson J: *Clinical manual of health assessment,* St Louis, 1984, Mosby–Year Book.

22. Carnevali DL, Patrick M: *Nursing management for the elderly,* Philadelphia, 1986, JB Lippincott.

23. Carotenuto R, Bullock J: *Physical assessment of the gerontologic client,* Philadelphia, 1981, FA Davis.

24. Fields W, McGinn-Campbell K: *Introduction to health assessment,* Reston, Va, 1983, Reston Publishing Company.

25. Mundy AR, Stephenson TP, Wein AJ: *Urodynamics: principles, practice and application,* Edinburgh, 1984, Churchill Livingstone.

26. Price S, Wilson L: *Pathophysiology,* New York, 1986, McGraw-Hill.

27. Prior JA, Silberstein JS, Stang J: *Physical diagnosis: the history and examination of the patient,* St Louis, 1981, Mosby–Year Book.

CHAPTER FORTY-TWO

Nursing Management of Adults with Renal Disorders

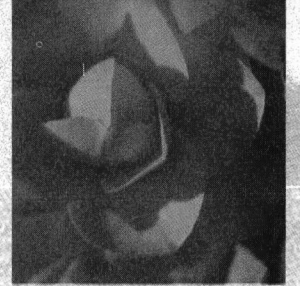

LEARNING OBJECTIVES

1 Apply the nursing process to the management of patients with renal disorders.
2 Discuss ongoing health maintenance for patients with renal disorders.
3 Identify factors that may contribute to the development of renal disorders.
4 Compare acute and chronic renal failure.
5 Compare the etiology and clinical presentation of prerenal, intrarenal, and postrenal acute renal failure.
6 Compare the oliguric and diuretic phases of acute renal failure.
7 List effects of renal dysfunction on the major body systems.
8 Explain the uremic syndrome.
9 Differentiate among hemodialysis, peritoneal dialysis, and hemofiltration.
10 Describe nursing interventions for patients undergoing hemodialysis, peritoneal dialysis, and hemofiltration.

KEY TERMS

acute renal failure (ARF), p. 1096
anuria, p. 1099
azotemia, p. 1098
chronic renal failure (CRF), p. 1096
dialysis, p. 1107
end-stage renal disease, p. 1102
hemodialysis, p. 1109

hemofiltration, p. 1112
hydronephrosis, p. 1089
nephrolithiasis, p. 1089
nephrotic syndrome, p. 1084
oliguria, p. 1096
uremic frost, p. 1104
uremic syndrome, p. 1100

RENAL DISORDERS can be caused by a variety of problems including injury, infection, compromised renal perfusion, vascular and structural abnormalities, and nephrotoxic substances. Renal disorders may also occur because of another disease process such as hypertension or diabetes mellitus. Renal disorders may cause a range of alterations from mild discomfort and dysfunction to profound alterations in control of fluids and electrolytes, which can result in death.

1077

PRERENAL DISORDERS

Definition

Prerenal vascular disorders are those that impair renal perfusion. The kidneys are normally perfused by 25% of the cardiac output; therefore any changes in renal perfusion can significantly alter renal function. Decreased renal perfusion is secondary to impaired cardiac output, hypotension, dehydration, or shock. Renal vascular disease may result because of thrombosis, stenosis, or occlusion of the vascular bed or vascular changes caused by other diseases such as diabetes mellitus or hypertension.

Arterial problems include the following:

1. Embolic occlusion: total or partial occlusion of the renal artery caused by thrombus embolization
2. Renal artery stenosis: partial occlusion of one or both of the renal arteries and their branches because of atherosclerotic narrowing or fibromuscular dysplasia[30]
3. Diabetic nephropathy: accelerated atherosclerotic changes in patients with diabetes mellitus
4. Nephrosclerosis: sclerosis of the small arteries and arterioles of the kidney, leading to diminished blood flow and patchy areas of necrosis of the renal parenchyma

Venous problems include unilateral or bilateral renal vein thrombosis, thrombosis caused by trauma, abscess, tumor, surgery near the renal hilus, nephrotic syndrome, or membranous glomerulonephritis.[11]

Etiology/Epidemiology

Progressive vascular impairment caused by atherosclerosis or fibromuscular dysplasia accounts for 90% of all renal artery disease.[13] Atherosclerosis primarily affects the proximal third of the artery. It is found more often in men than in women. Fibromuscular dysplasia affects women four to five times more often than men. The exact etiology of fibromuscular dysplasia is unknown, but it causes alternating areas of stenosis and dilation within the artery, causing a "string-of-beads" appearance on arteriogram.[13]

Renal artery stenosis accounts for about 5% of all cases of hypertension. When hypertension develops abruptly, renal artery stenosis is considered to be a major factor, especially in patients under 20 and over 50 years of age and also in patients with no family history of hypertension.

Essential hypertension, which primarily affects patients between the ages of 30 and 50 years, is a major precipitating factor in renal disease. It has been estimated that approximately 10% of these individuals will go on to develop severe renal damage, and approximately 1% will eventually develop end-stage renal failure.[16]

Approximately 30% to 40% of patients with type I insulin-dependent diabetes develop end-stage renal disease. Patients with diabetes who have had the disease longer than 10 years usually demonstrate some impairment in renal function.

Renal vein thrombosis is the primary dysfunction of the renal vein. Venous stasis is the most important factor leading to thrombus formation. Stasis may result from reduced blood flow in low cardiac output states, immobility, or impairment in venous return. Renal vein thrombosis is also seen in patients with diabetic nephropathy, collagen vascular disease, hypercoagulable states, trauma, tumors, pregnancy, use of oral contraceptives, and nephrotic syndrome.

Pathophysiology

The kidneys normally receive about 20% to 25% of the cardiac output. Any major reduction in renal blood flow because of vascular impairment or abnormality will result in renal parenchymal ischemia and eventual atrophy. The decrease in renal perfusion triggers the renin-angiotensin-aldosterone system. The end result is systemic hypertension. When both kidneys are involved, renal failure will occur. Collateral circulation may help preserve renal function for a few weeks. In a total occlusion, infarction and tissue necrosis are evident about 2 hours after the insult.[17]

Clinical Manifestations

Mild to moderate stimulation of the renin-angiotensin-aldosterone system leads to compensatory responses that help maintain renal blood flow; however, large quantities of angiotensin II may compromise renal blood flow because of afferent arteriole vasoconstriction. The patient who has a gradual reduction in renal blood flow may experience very few symptoms. The clinical manifestations of diabetic nephropathy and nephrosclerosis are the same as those of chronic renal failure (CRF), such as edema and hypertension. The major symptom of renal artery stenosis is hypertension. If the obstruction to renal blood flow is acute, as in an embolus, the patient may complain of flank pain over the affected kidney or abdominal pain. In addition, the patient may have a fever. Atrial fibrillation may be noted as the source of embolization.

Other clinical manifestations include unequal kidney size and arteriographic changes. The arteriogram will demonstrate a narrowed lumen and diminished blood flow distal to the area of renal artery stenosis. The urinalysis may be normal immediately after an acute obstruction, but later it will increase the specific gravity and the color may appear more concentrated. Microscopically, it will demonstrate casts and cellular debris. Blood chemistries may show elevated aspartate aminotransferase and lactic dehydrogenase secondary to tissue hypoxia.

Therapeutic Management

Restoration of blood flow and prevention of ischemia may be accomplished by surgical revascularization of the kidney. Surgery may also reverse symptoms of renovascular hypertension. The type of surgical procedure varies but may involve an aortorenal bypass graft or anastomosis between the kidney and another major artery, usually the splenic artery. If an aortorenal bypass is performed, the patient may experience an exacerbation of hypertension during the first 48 hours postoperatively. The exact cause is unknown, but it may be from a variety of factors, including severe pain, systemic vasoconstriction as a result of anesthesia and intraoperative hypothermia, or increased renin secretion caused by surgical manipulation of the kidney and cross clamping of the aorta.[13]

If the patient is not a good candidate for surgery, percutaneous, transluminal renal angioplasty may be considered. A special ballooned catheter is inserted to position the balloon at the site of the obstructing lesion. The balloon is inflated, and the lesion is compressed. If the procedure is not successful, then an endarterectomy may be performed, with subsequent anticoagulant or antiplatelet therapy. A surgical thrombectomy may be performed for renal vein thrombosis. Some patients who have experienced severe renal ischemia or necrosis may require a nephrectomy if enough damage has occurred or, in selected cases, if one kidney is responsible for high renin production.

Pharmacologic management involves the use of anticoagulants and antihypertensive agents. Early detection of hypertension and aggressive antihypertensive therapy have been shown to improve the prognosis for patients with benign nephrosclerosis.[11] Anticoagulant therapy is important in the management of patients with renal vein thrombosis because of a high incidence of pulmonary emboli. Intravenous streptokinase, urokinase, or tissue plasminogen activator may be used to lyse an occlusive clot.

NURSING MANAGEMENT OF THE PATIENT WITH PRERENAL DISORDERS
Assessment

Nursing assessment of patients with prerenal vascular disorders includes measurement of blood pressure, since hypertension and hypotension are major precipitating factors in renal disease. The patient is assessed for associated symptoms of hypertension such as headache, dizziness, chest pain, epistaxis, or palpitations.

If the patient describes a history of hypertensive disease, the nurse further assesses for hypertension control. Has the patient been on a fluid or salt-restricted diet? What medications were prescribed? Determine whether the patient has complied with the therapeutic regimen. For example, has the blood pressure been maintained within reasonable limits, or has it steadily increased over time? Has the patient gained weight? Weight gain could indicate fluid retention, which would elevate the blood pressure. The nurse also notes the ethnicity of the patient, since there is a high incidence of hypertensive disease in black populations.

If an acute vascular obstruction is present, the patient may complain of flank pain over the affected kidney, or the pain may be described as abdominal. The nurse assesses for evidence of fever, which may be seen during acute embolic obstructions. The nurse also notes any irregularity in the pulse, since atrial fibrillation may be the source of emboli.

The nurse obtains a history of recent surgery or trauma that could precipitate renal thrombosis. Venous stasis, which could result from prolonged immobilization or dehydration, is an important factor leading to potential thrombus formation. Additionally, assessment includes a history of other disorders that could lead to prerenal disease. As stated earlier, approximately 30% to 40% of patients with type I insulin-dependent diabetes develop end-stage renal disease because of alterations in the basement membrane and changes in the microvasculature.

Nursing Diagnosis

Nursing diagnoses for patients with prerenal vascular disorders include the following:

Fluid volume excess: actual or potential, related to decreased renal blood flow

Alteration in health maintenance related to knowledge deficit about dietary restrictions

Altered renal tissue perfusion related to vascular changes of renal blood supply

High risk for sexual dysfunction related to pharmacologic treatment

Body image disturbance related to weight gain and edema

Pain, acute, related to obstructed renal artery

Planning

Patient outcomes vary according to the diagnosis and may include the following:

The patient will describe the disease process and measures to control hypertension

The patient will follow fluid and dietary restrictions to maintain a desired weight

The patient will establish control of blood pressure within prescribed limits

The patient will demonstrate the ability to monitor blood pressure and pulse

The patient will use methods to prevent injury to self while receiving anticoagulation therapy

The patient will discuss any problems with sexual dysfunction related to administration of antihypertensive medications

Implementation

The nurse helps the patient document hypertension by monitoring the patient's blood pressure and pulse. The nurse assesses for dysrhythmias when measuring vital signs and administers antidysrhythmic medications as ordered. Patients are instructed how to monitor their own pulse and blood pressure. Blood pressure is controlled through pharmacologic intervention and dietary management. The nurse begins discussion of dietary alterations, keeping the patient's normal diet and cultural preferences in mind. The patient may be placed on a low-sodium diet. Fluid intake may need to be restricted as well. If diuretics are included in the therapeutic plan, then potassium supplements may be required; however, patients with renal dysfunction often have associated hyperkalemia, so careful monitoring is essential. The nurse and dietitian play a vital role in helping the patient develop meal plans that incorporate the recommended dietary and fluid restrictions.

If the patient is receiving anticoagulant therapy, nursing care is taken to minimize the risk of bleeding. Injections are avoided. The nurse monitors for evidence of bleeding such as hematuria or bleeding gums. Coagulation studies are monitored closely. Intravenous heparin and thrombolytic agents are administered by using a controlled infusion pump. Stress to the patient that medication must be taken on a daily basis to avoid further complications of hypertension. Referral to a therapist may be necessary if sexual dysfunction becomes a major problem.

Nursing measures such as meticulous hand washing and aseptic technique are used to protect the patient from infection and injury. Indwelling urinary catheters carry a high risk of infection and are to be avoided if possible. Explore strategies to promote rest and relaxation with the patient and family. Stress reduction can help decrease blood pressure in some patients.

Evaluation

Nursing interventions related to controlling hypertension are successful when the systolic and diastolic blood pressures approach normal ranges. Comfort and stress reduction are evidenced by relaxed facial expressions and body movements. The patient or family member can monitor and evaluate blood pressure changes. Dietary modifications and fluid restrictions are evaluated based on how well the patient tolerates the meals. The patient is able to describe meal plans that incorporate dietary restrictions and cultural preferences. The coagulation laboratory test results should reflect attainment of therapeutic levels of anticoagulation, which are indicated by a prothrombin time that is prolonged 1½ to 2½ times the control.[14] Within these parameters no excessive bleeding is expected. If the patient undergoes renovascular surgery or nephrectomy, adequate recovery will be evidenced by maintenance of vital signs, absence of infection or complications, and a return toward normal renal function.

Documentation

Documentation of care for the patient with prerenal vascular disease involves measuring vital signs, weight, and fluid intake and output. The patient's unique responses to therapeutic interventions are included. It is important to document anticoagulation therapy and laboratory data. A flow sheet is useful because it is easier to monitor developments.

Ongoing Care

The patient who recovers from renovascular surgery or nephrectomy is monitored for control of blood pressure and body weight on an ongoing basis. The patient or a family member must demonstrate the ability to correctly monitor blood pressure and weight and to describe strategies for maintaining the blood pressure within prescribed ranges. Fluid and dietary restrictions may be required for the rest of the patient's life. If renal failure develops, dialysis or transplantation may be necessary. Home dialysis may be an option for these patients.

Inflammatory, Infectious, and Congenital Renal Disorders

POLYCYSTIC KIDNEY DISEASE
Definition

Polycystic kidney disease is a congenital disorder in which cysts form within the nephrons (Figure 42-1). In adults this autosomal dominant disorder generally manifests itself at about 40 years of age.

Etiology/Epidemiology

Polycystic kidney disease affects men and women equally. It often affects more than one family mem-

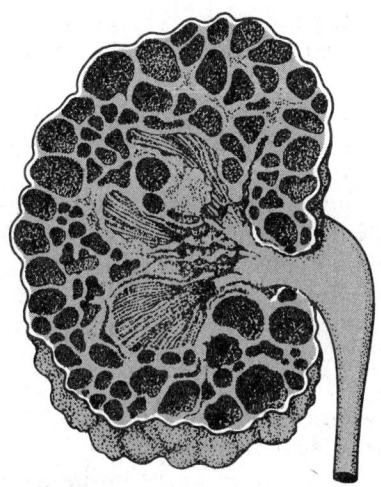

FIGURE 42-1   Polycystic kidney disease.

ber and recurs in successive generations. The symptoms appear at similar chronologic ages from one generation to the next. A family history of polycystic kidney disease or less specific renal disease is reported in 75% to 80% of cases.[31] Although symptoms generally appear at about 40 years of age, they may occur as early as 20 years or as late as 80 years. Ultrasound may demonstrate the presence of cysts years before symptoms develop. The disease usually affects both kidneys and may also be associated with cystic diseases of other organs such as the pancreas, spleen, testis, ovary, lung, thyroid, and uterus. Approximately 30% of patients with polycystic kidney disease also have hepatic cysts.[31] Polycystic kidney disease is also associated with aneurysms of the cerebral arteries. Adult polycystic disease is the third most common cause of end-stage renal disease and is found in up to 12% of patients receiving dialysis or renal transplantation.[15]

Pathophysiology

Multiple cysts resembling grape clusters form within the nephrons. These thin-walled cysts are filled with fluid and may contain pus or blood. The kidney enlarges up to two or three times its normal size as the cysts expand, thus compressing intrarenal and extrarenal structures. The cysts may rupture and become infected, leading to the production of scar tissue that reduces the number of functional nephrons. The eventual outcome is renal failure. Uremia usually develops within 16 years of onset of symptoms.

Clinical Manifestations

Common findings are abdominal or flank pain that may be colicky in nature. Hematuria is present in about 50% of cases, because bleeding into the cysts occurs. Hypertension is also common, because the kidneys lose their ability to regulate sodium. Two thirds of patients with polycystic kidney disease have palpable masses over the kidneys with depression of abdominal tissue. Light palpation is done to prevent potential pain and bleeding. Recurrent urinary tract infections are common. The patient may initially have Gram-negative sepsis.[17] Uremia, which develops slowly over the years, is controlled by fluid and dietary restrictions and eventual dialysis or transplantation.

Therapeutic Management

No specific treatment exists for polycystic kidney disease. Treatment is aimed at the relief of pain and other symptoms of the disease. Heat and analgesics may relieve some of the discomfort caused by the enlarging kidneys. If the patient bleeds, discontinue heat and place the patient on bed rest. If bleeding is significant, transfusions may be necessary. Severe bleeding may necessitate segmental renal artery embolization or even complete or partial nephrectomy. Hypertension is treated vigorously with antihypertensive agents, diuretics, and fluid and dietary modifications. Since infections are common, antibiotics are often prescribed. Patients with polycystic kidney disease may respond poorly to conventional antibiotic therapy; therefore nephrectomy may be required to gain infection control. As the disease progresses, dialysis may be required.

INTERSTITIAL NEPHRITIS
Definition

The term *interstitial nephritis* is assigned to a category of renal diseases associated with inflammation of the cells in the spaces between the renal tubules.

Etiology/Epidemiology

There are many causes of inflammation, ranging from infection or irritation to hypersensitivity reactions. These include analgesic abuse, especially with phenacetin, aspirin, and acetaminophen; immunologic disorders; heavy metal toxicity; vascular and collagen diseases; radiation injury; hyperuricemia; hypercalcemia; and hypokalemia.[13] Many drugs have been associated with a hypersensitivity reaction that occurs in the renal interstitium, especially methicillin, other synthetic penicillins, and sulfonamides. Drugs less commonly associated with this disease are the cephalosporins, thiazides, furosemide, allopurinol, phenytoin, and cimetidine.[32]

Pathophysiology

Interstitial nephritis is characterized by interstitial edema, cellular infiltration, and interstitial fibrosis leading to atrophy of the tubular cells. The disease progresses causing fibrosis of Bowman's capsule and involvement of the glomeruli.[13]

Clinical Manifestations

Early signs of interstitial nephritis are tubular changes that are disproportionate to changes in glomerular filtration rate (GFR). The kidneys are unable to concentrate the urine. Damaged tubules are ineffective in reabsorption of sodium, glucose, uric acid, phosphates, amino acids, and bicarbonate. Urine sediment is a common finding. Proteinuria may be present but is less severe than in other forms of renal disease with glomerular membrane dysfunction.[13] The disease can manifest with minimal functional loss and abnormal urinary findings, or it may manifest as acute oliguric renal failure that requires dialysis. Symptoms may include fever, skin rash, eosinophilia, or acute oliguria. Gross hematuria occasionally may be seen.[13] Hypertension is a common finding in acute oliguric renal failure.

Therapeutic Management

Treatment may include the use of steroids to reduce the inflammatory process and hasten recovery. If the disease is drug induced, improvement will be seen with discontinuation of the drug. Recovery may take up to several months and may be incomplete. The patient is instructed about drug sensitivities and cautioned to prevent recurrent episodes. Skin testing may help identify hypersensitivity to related drugs. The patient in acute oliguric renal failure is managed with dialysis. In chronic interstitial disease, alterations in renal structure make it indistinguishable from chronic pyelonephritis.[13] Therefore management of the two diseases is similar.

GLOMERULONEPHRITIS
Definition

Glomerulonephritis is a term that describes a variety of diseases that result in inflammation of the glomeruli of both kidneys. It is generally the result of an antigen-antibody reaction and is thus termed an immunologic disease. It occurs in both acute or chronic forms.

Etiology/Epidemiology

Acute glomerulonephritis occurs in two forms: postinfectious and infectious. Of the two, postinfectious glomerulonephritis is the most common. It is caused by a group A beta-hemolytic streptococcal infection elsewhere in the body. The disease typically occurs 2 to 3 weeks after a throat infection (tonsillitis or strep throat) or a skin infection (impetigo).

Postinfectious glomerulonephritis is primarily a disease of children and young adults. About 50% of adults will fully recover.[16] The rest will go on to develop chronic glomerulonephritis. Of all the individuals who develop acute postinfectious glomerulonephritis, approximately 1% to 2% will develop end-stage renal failure.[16] Dialysis or transplantation will be required in these individuals. Glomerulonephritis may also be caused by a variety of disorders including immune diseases such as lupus erythematosus, hypertension, diabetes mellitus, and disseminated intravascular coagulopathy (DIC).

Acute infectious glomerulonephritis is also caused by an infection elsewhere in the body. However, the renal insult occurs within only a few days of the original bacterial, viral, or parasitic infection. Chronic glomerulonephritis may occur after the acute disease, but more often there is no evidence of a previous infection. This may be the result of such a mild antigen-antibody reaction that it is overlooked.

Pathophysiology

Acute glomerulonephritis results from an antigen-antibody reaction that produces swelling and death of capillary cells within the glomerular tissue. An immune reaction activates the inflammatory response with release of lysosomal enzymes that attack the glomerular basement membrane. Damage to the glomerular basement membrane allows protein and red blood cells to penetrate through it. Increased production of endothelial cells lining the glomerulus and infiltration by leukocytes lead to a thickening of the glomerular filtration membrane, resulting in scarring. This loss of filtration surface decreases glomerular filtration rate (GFR), resulting in oliguria and fluid and electrolyte retention. The patient becomes edematous and azotemic. The kidneys become swollen and congested.

In chronic glomerulonephritis the kidneys atrophy and become severely contracted as the glomeruli and tubules are chronically destroyed. The kidneys may atrophy to as little as one fifth their normal size. Bands of scar tissue form, causing a roughened, irregular surface to the kidneys. There is progressive scarring of the glomeruli and tubules. Branches of the renal artery may become thickened. Chronic glomerulonephritis leads to end-stage renal failure.

Clinical Manifestations

Symptoms of acute glomerulonephritis may develop suddenly, or the disease may be so mild that it is initially detected by routine urinalysis. In the severe forms the patient has fever, chills, weakness, nausea, and vomiting. A typical finding is generalized and periorbital edema. Abdominal or flank pain may be present because of the congestion of the kidneys. A decrease in GFR results in oliguria, fluid overload, and hypertension. Fluid overload may be evidenced by pulmonary congestion, jugular venous distention, ascites, and symptoms of congestive heart failure. Retinal edema may cause a reduction in visual acuity.

Cardinal findings in the urinalysis are gross proteinuria and hematuria. The specific gravity will be elevated, and the urine may appear dark and smoky, the color of cola. Renal damage is also evidenced by an elevation of serum blood urea nitrogen (BUN) and creatinine. Other diagnostic findings are an elevated antistreptolysin O titer in acute glomerulonephritis caused by antibodies from a recent streptococcal infection. The serum complement level is usually low in chronic glomerulonephritis, indicative of a streptococcal infection months previous.[13]

The patient with acute glomerulonephritis may quickly develop uremia; however, most recover within 4 weeks. Hematuria and proteinuria may persist for several months. If full recovery does not occur after 2 years, the patient will most likely be classified as having the chronic disease.

Chronic glomerulonephritis generally produces insidious manifestations. The patient may be unaware that there is a problem. Hypertension and abnormal findings in the urinalysis such as the presence of red blood cells and protein may be detected during a routine physical examination. The patient may complain of headache, especially in the morning. Other symptoms include general fatigue or weakness, blurring of vision, and dyspnea on exertion.

Dyspnea and edema are the most common initial symptoms in elderly persons. Few older patients have hematuria. A history of sore throat with *Streptococcus* cultures may lead the practitioner to conclude that the symptoms represent only an upper respiratory infection rather than renal involvement as well. In addition, a reduction in renal function in elderly persons may be seen when there is volume depletion, hypotension, or impaired renal perfusion from other causes. The nursing home resident or cerebrovascular accident (CVA) patient who does not have ready access to water may experience dehydration with resulting azotemia.

Clinical manifestations of CRF may be observed. Once the disease is diagnosed, the patient faces a variable course. Good health may be maintained for up to 30 years, or end-stage renal failure may develop within only 1 to 2 years.

Therapeutic Management

Acute glomerulonephritis is treated vigorously. Patients with the poststreptococcal form of the disease are treated with penicillin, which may be continued prophylactically for several months after the acute phase of the illness to protect against recurrence of the disease. Bed rest is maintained during the acute phase until clinical signs of nephritis have resolved. Activity during this time may increase proteinuria and hematuria.

Hypertension and fluid overload are managed by restricting sodium and fluid intake. Other dietary modifications include reduction of protein to reduce nitrogen retention and elevation of the BUN. A diet high in carbohydrates will provide energy and spare protein catabolism. Potassium will be restricted if the patient becomes hyperkalemic.

Pharmacologic management may include the use of diuretics and antihypertensive agents to control the fluid overload and hypertension. Steroids and cytotoxic agents may be ordered to suppress the immune system, reduce antibody formation, and suppress the glomerular inflammatory response. Anticoagulants may be used to reduce nonimmunologic mediators of glomerular damage.[19] Additionally, plasmapheresis may be useful in removing immune complexes or antiglomerular basement antibodies. Plasmapheresis is usually used in conjunction with immunosuppressive therapy.[13]

Dietary management and fluid control are essential to the patient with chronic glomerulonephritis. Treatment for uremic symptoms is the same as that for the patient with CRF. The patient is encouraged to maintain optimal health and prevent infections. Bed rest is ordered if there is an exacerbation of symptoms such as hematuria, edema, or hypertension. Treatment at this time is similar to that for acute glomerulonephritis. Dialysis is often begun before uremic symptoms become severe.

PYELONEPHRITIS
Definition

Pyelonephritis is a bacterial infection of the renal pelvis, calices, and parenchyma. It is one of the more common diseases of the kidney and usually occurs because of an ascending urinary tract infection.

Etiology/Epidemiology

Pyelonephritis is commonly caused by a bladder infection. Fecal bacteria such as *Escherichia coli,* *Klebsiella,* or *Proteus* gain access to the urinary tract from the perineum. Approximately 90% of the cases of acute pyelonephritis occur in women. Women are at higher risk than men for this disease because of the short length of the female urethra as compared with the male urethra. The lower urinary tract infection itself may be asymptomatic. Pyelonephritis may also be caused by reflux of urine into the ureters during urination because of an incompetent ureterovesical valve. Other causes include any condition in which there is obstruction to urine flow such as prostatic hypertrophy or renal calculi. Diabetic patients and spinal cord–injured patients who develop autonomic neuropathy with subsequent bladder atony are at increased risk for the development of acute or chronic pyelonephritis. Bacterial invasion during urethral instrumentation such as catheterization or cystoscopy also predisposes the patient to infection. Patients who are at higher risk for urinary tract infections and pyelonephritis include pregnant women, people with diabetes, men over 50 years of age with prostatitis, elderly persons, and patients who are immunosuppressed. Pyelonephritis may be acute or chronic. It has been estimated that the original diagnosis in approximately one third of all patients with CRF was pyelonephritis.[15]

Pathophysiology

After the bacteria reach the kidney, they begin to multiply. The infection causes an inflammatory exudate that accumulates in the interstitium. Focal abscesses develop that are scattered throughout the kidney. The glomerular capillaries are usually spared. The inflammatory process may eventually lead to atrophy and destruction of the renal tubules. Chronic pyelonephritis usually results from recurrent bouts of the acute form. The kidneys eventually become scarred and contracted. Renal failure results.

Clinical Manifestations

Acute pyelonephritis may be present without any symptoms, or the patient may have acute flank pain, fever, chills, nausea, and vomiting. The patient may complain of urgency, dysuria, and a cloudy, foul-smelling urine. Typically, the patient appears acutely ill. The pain may radiate down the ureter or toward the epigastrium. Pain may be constant, or it may be colicky in nature if renal calculi are present. Marked tenderness is evident with percussion or deep palpation over the costovertebral angle. Urinalysis reveals bacteria, white blood cells, and white cell casts. Hematuria may be present. The clinical features of chronic pyelonephritis may be quite vague. Diagnosis may be made during routine examination with a finding of proteinuria, hypertension, or symptoms of chronic renal failure.

Therapeutic Management

A urine culture is obtained to identify the causative organism so that appropriate antibiotic therapy can begin. A broad-spectrum antibiotic will be used until the organism is isolated. Repeat cultures are done to determine whether the infection has been resolved. Antipyretics may be given to control the fever and discomfort. If not contraindicated, increas-

ing the fluid intake will help relieve dysuria. Juices such as cranberry, plum, and prune leave an acid ash in the urine that may help inhibit bacteriuria.[33] However, this may not be achievable since the actual juice concentration is quite low in many commercially available brands. Medications such as vitamin C may help to acidify the urine. Additionally, an acid-ash diet may be of some benefit. Antispasmodics may be used to relieve bladder spasm. Chronic pyelonephritis is monitored by ongoing evaluation of urine cultures and serum BUN and creatinine levels. Infection, if present, is treated with the appropriate antibiotic. CRF may result.

NEPHROTIC SYNDROME
Definition

The **nephrotic syndrome** describes a variety of symptoms that accompany any condition that seriously impairs the glomerular capillary membrane, resulting in increased permeability to protein. Hallmarks of this syndrome are increased excretion of protein in the urine, decreased serum albumin levels, increased serum lipids, and edema.

Etiology/Epidemiology

Any glomerular disease may cause nephrotic syndrome, although the primary cause is membranous nephropathy in adults and lipoid nephrosis in children.[32] Membranous nephropathy is a chronic immune complex disease. Its cause is unknown, but it usually develops in young and middle-aged adults and is more common in men than in women.[32] Approximately a 10% incidence of adult membranous nephropathy is associated with neoplasms. The tumor may be diagnosed only months after the onset of proteinuria. Finding a tumor when this pathologic condition is exhibited in an older adult may lead to early diagnosis of cancer and subsequent remission of proteinuria.[24] Glomerulonephritis and diabetic nephropathy are also common causes of the disease. Numerous other conditions that may lead to the disease include diabetes, sickle cell disease, pregnancy, renal vein thrombosis, amyloidosis, hepatitis B, congestive heart failure, systemic lupus erythematosus, and allergic reactions from drugs, pollen, and insect bites. Drugs that most commonly cause the nephrotic syndrome are penicillamine, trimethadione, gold, heroin, mercury, probenecid, and nonsteroidal anti-inflammatory agents.[32] It is estimated that approximately 50% to 75% of adults who develop this syndrome will progress to renal failure within 5 years.[16]

Pathophysiology

The nephrotic syndrome is characterized by a derangement in the cells of the glomerular basement membrane, resulting in increased capillary membrane permeability. Proteins are lost in the urine, lowering the plasma colloidal osmotic pressure. The loss of protein impairs the liver's ability to synthesize albumin, resulting in a decreased plasma oncotic pressure. As the vascular hydrostatic fluid pressure exceeds the serum oncotic pressure, the ability to reabsorb fluid into the vascular system becomes impaired, leading to excess fluid in the interstitial spaces. The result is generalized edema. This third spacing of fluid lowers the overall circulating volume, causing stimulation of the renin-angiotensin-aldosterone system. Sodium and fluid retention further compounds the edema.

Because the serum albumin level is low, the high−molecular weight lipoproteins remain in the blood, resulting in hyperlipidemia.[15] Some of the smaller lipoproteins are lost in the urine, causing the urine to appear foamy.

Clinical Manifestations

The nephrotic syndrome is manifested by edema, proteinuria (greater than 3.5 g in a 24-hour urine collection), hyperlipidemia, and decreased serum albumin levels (hypoalbuminemia). One of the earliest symptoms is periorbital edema that is noticed especially in the morning. There is a gradual progression to generalized pitting edema. Anemia is a common finding, depending on the degree of renal impairment. The skin may take on a characteristic waxy pallor that is caused more by edema than by anemia. Other symptoms may include anorexia, nausea, diarrhea, lethargy, and fatigue. The movement of fluid out of the vascular compartment as a result of the reduced plasma oncotic pressure may lead to ascites and pleural effusions. Urine output may be normal or markedly altered, with oliguria and weight gain. Women generally experience amenorrhea or abnormal menses. Men have decreased sperm production. Hypertension or hypotension may be present, depending on the primary renal disease and the effective circulating volume.

Therapeutic Management

Treatment is aimed at controlling the symptoms and treating the underlying disease. Corticosteroids such as prednisone may be used to control the inflammation and glomerular damage. Cytotoxic agents may be used as an alternative to steroid therapy.

Controlling edema is a critical aspect of therapeutic management. A diet high in protein may help restore the body's normal plasma oncotic pressure, thus ameliorating edema. Daily protein intake may be as much as 150 g.[13] Sufficient calories must be included so that protein will not be used for energy. Dietary modifications may include salt restriction; however, this is a controversial issue among clinicians. Fluids are restricted based on the patient's symptoms. Diuretic therapy may be continued on a long-term basis, so the patient must be monitored for hypokalemia. Potassium-sparing diuretics may be used. Bed rest may be ordered to promote diuresis when the edema is severe. Careful monitoring of fluid intake and output along with daily measurements of weight and abdominal girth will help the clinician determine whether weight loss is caused by diuresis or protein loss. If the patient is hypotensive because of intravascular volume depletion, plasma volume expanders such as plasma or 25% albumin may be used.

Edematous tissue is particularly susceptible to injury. Specific attention to skin care is required to prevent breakdown. Therapy is also aimed at prevention of infection, since body defenses are impaired by protein loss, renal impairment, and immunosuppressive therapy.

A high incidence of renal vein thrombosis is associated with nephrotic syndrome. Because of this, long-term anticoagulation may be prescribed.[13] The patient receiving anticoagulation therapy must be protected from injury and monitored for bleeding.

RENAL TUBERCULOSIS
Definition

Renal tuberculosis is caused by the organism *Mycobacterium tuberculosis* and is rarely a primary lesion. The organism usually spreads from the lungs to the kidneys by way of the bloodstream.

Etiology/Epidemiology

The infecting organism, *Mycobacterium tuberculosis*, gains access to the kidneys through the bloodstream. After infecting the kidneys the organism may be carried down the ureters into the bladder, causing it to become infected also. The onset of infection usually occurs 5 to 8 years after the primary pulmonary infection; however, once the organism reaches the kidneys, it may lie dormant for several years. Renal tuberculosis is more common in men than in women, and it generally affects people between the ages of 20 and 40 years.[16] It is estimated that approximately 4% to 5% of patients with primary pulmonary tuberculosis will also develop renal tuberculosis.[32] The prognosis is very good, and the disease is arrested in up to 98% of patients who are treated.[32]

Pathophysiology

Once the organism reaches the kidney, it causes slow destruction of the renal cortex or medulla. Destruction of tissue occurs throughout the kidney, with eventual erosion into a calix at the tip of a papilla with progressive ulceration into the renal pelvis.[13] From the renal pelvis it can spread to all areas of the urinary tract. Left untreated, the infection will form large, caseating masses that join together to destroy renal tissue. The kidney will appear "moth eaten" on x-ray examination.[13] As the organism spreads throughout the lower genitourinary tract, it results in fibrosis and stricture formation. The descending route of infection may affect the epididymis and prostate in men, leading to reduced reproductive function.

Clinical Manifestations

Clinical symptoms are often nonspecific. The patient may complain of general malaise, loss of appetite, unexplained weight loss, night sweats, and intermittent fever. If the original pulmonary lesion is already well healed, diagnosis may be difficult. Once the infection spreads to the bladder, the patient has symptoms similar to those of cystitis: pain, dysuria, and urinary frequency. Flank pain, hematuria, and pyuria are common findings. Normally, pyuria is found in urine that is alkaline; however, in renal tuberculosis, the pyuria is found in urine that is acid.[2]

Therapeutic Management

Prevention of renal tuberculosis is aimed at early detection and treatment of pulmonary tuberculosis. Treatment of renal tuberculosis is based on chemotherapy. Medications commonly used include a combination of rifampin, ethambutol, isoniazid, cycloserine, pyridoxine, streptomycin, and sodium para-aminosalicylate. These medications are generally given in a single daily dose; however, they may be divided if side effects occur. Chemotherapy is usually effective in 4 to 6 months, but some physicians continue treatment for a minimum of 2 years. Urine cultures are collected on at least three successive mornings. The tubercle bacilli shed intermittently; therefore from 3 to 12 negative cultures must be obtained to determine absence of disease. It is important to remember that the urine of patients with active renal tuberculosis is infectious. Special precautions such as wearing gloves and flushing the toilet three times are necessary when handling and disposing of the urine. Surgery is generally reserved for patients who have developed ureteral strictures and require urinary diversion. Other indications for surgery include nephrectomy for an extensively damaged kidney, renal malignancy, hemorrhage, or uncontrollable pain or hypertension. Patients require follow-up urine cultures every 6 months during treatment and then annually for up to 10 years to detect signs of reactivation. If a relapse occurs, chemotherapy is reinstituted.

RENAL ABSCESS
Definition

A renal abscess is an infection within the kidney. It may involve single or multiple sites of bacterial infection. A perinephric abscess is an abscess in the fatty tissue of the kidney.

Etiology/Epidemiology

Renal abscess formation may arise as a result of any infection of the kidney, such as pyelonephritis, or from spread of infection through the bloodstream to the kidney. The infection may spread from adjacent areas of involvement such as appendicitis or diverticulitis. Renal abscesses are most common in patients with a history of pyelonephritis, chronic obstruction, or renal calculi.[30]

Pathophysiology

Abscess formation is the result of a localized bacterial infection that is characterized by a collection of pus within solid tissue. Pus contains white blood cells, bacteria, and necrotic tissue.

Clinical Manifestations

The patient with a renal abscess is seriously ill and may become septic. Symptoms, often acute in onset, include fever, chills, and flank or abdominal tenderness or pain. The pain is constant and may resemble renal colic.[13] Because the collection of pus is within the kidney and does not extend into the urinary collecting system, the urine is sterile. This helps differentiate an abscess from pyelonephritis. Patients may also have weakness, weight loss, and anorexia.

Therapeutic Management

The treatment for renal abscess is similar to that for pyelonephritis. Aggressive antibiotic therapy is instituted. A needle aspiration of the abscess is useful in culturing the organism. The abscess may require surgical incision and drainage. The drainage may be profuse, requiring frequent dressing changes. A drain will be left in place until drainage stops.

NURSING MANAGEMENT OF THE PATIENT WITH INFLAMMATORY, INFECTIOUS, AND CONGENITAL RENAL DISORDERS
Assessment

A thorough history is essential for the nursing assessment of patients with inflammatory, infectious, and congenital renal disorders. This includes a complete symptom analysis, a family history for renal disease, and assessment for recent exposure to allergens as a source of possible inflammatory process and for symptoms that could indicate alterations in renal function, such as changes in patterns of elimination. A weight gain could indicate renal dysfunction. Nursing observations include the tongue and mucous membranes for swelling caused by overhydration or inflammation or for dryness caused by fever from infection. Skin turgor is assessed for level of hydration. Generalized edema could indicate a change in renal function. Thorough auscultation of the heart and lungs for signs of congestive heart failure may indicate fluid overload from renal dysfunction. Other findings may include presence of an S_3 gallop, jugular venous distention, rales, or complaints of dyspnea.

It is important that the nurse assess for signs of infection, such as fever, malaise, tachycardia, pain, or swelling. Additionally, the urine is observed for changes in color or odor that could indicate infection. Hematuria may be present. Pain, burning, or itching during urination, as well as flank or abdominal pain, is also a significant assessment finding.

The nurse observes for gastrointestinal symptoms such as nausea, vomiting, or complaints of anorexia that could indicate infection or uremia.

Nursing Diagnosis

Nursing diagnoses for patients with inflammatory, infectious, and congenital renal disorders include the following:

Altered patterns of urinary elimination related to infection, pain, or urgency

Fluid volume excess related to renal disease or inflammatory process

Fluid volume deficit related to renal disease, fever, or infection

Pain, acute, related to infection or inflammation

Altered nutrition: less than body requirements, related to anorexia and dietary restrictions

High risk for impaired skin integrity related to pruritus

Activity intolerance related to infection, pain, or fever

Alteration in health maintenance related to knowledge deficit about disease process and treatment plan

High risk for altered body temperature related to infection

Body image disturbance related to chronic disease or loss of body function

Anxiety or fear related to outcome of illness

The etiologic factor for each diagnosis depends on the underlying disorder.

Planning

Outcome criteria for the patient with inflammatory, infectious, and congenital renal disorders include the following:

The patient will reestablish and maintain a normal pattern of urinary elimination

The patient will not experience dysuria

The patient will ingest a sufficient well-balanced diet to achieve or maintain a desired weight

The patient will describe meal plans that incorporate fluid and dietary modifications

The patient will describe the disease process briefly and the strategies to prevent recurrence or complications

The patient will plan for sufficient rest and activity

Implementation

The nurse carefully monitors fluid intake and output of patients with renal disorders. Therapeutic interventions are based on the 24-hour intake and output record and daily weight measurements. Fluid restrictions are calculated and spread out across the various shifts. Use of ice chips or spraying the mouth with water may alleviate thirst. Intravenous fluids may be administered by using controlled infusion pumps.

Nursing care is aimed at helping the patient with activities of daily living to conserve energy and provide periods of rest. The administration of antipyretic and analgesic drugs helps to control fever and pain. The nurse administers the appropriate drugs as ordered to treat the infection and inflammation. The patient requires additional protection from infection or injury because the immune system is already compromised. Meticulous hand washing is essential.

The nurse needs to discuss dietary modifications with the patient and family, especially the food preparer. Many patients will require lifelong adjustments in their diets. Palatable and attractive meals can help maintain optimal nutrition. The nurse can provide lists of what foods should be included or excluded in the diet. Consultation with the dietitian is recommended. Most diets require many carbohydrates to provide calories and prevent protein catabolism.

One of the most important aspects of nursing care is patient teaching. Each patient must be assessed for potential knowledge deficit. Teaching is directed at the level of the learner and the learner's concerns. The patient must be able to understand what caused the renal dysfunction and describe measures that prevent exacerbations or complications of the disease. The patient and family must become familiar

NURSING CARE PLAN   *Patient with Glomerulonephritis*

Nursing diagnosis/ Expected outcome	Interventions	Rationale
Fluid volume excess related to renal disease/inflammatory process • *Blood pressure will stabilize within normal limits* • *Patient will not exhibit edema*	Assess blood pressure and vital signs every 4 hours Weigh daily Maintain strict fluid intake and output Monitor skin turgor, mucous membranes, and presence of edema Check for presence of jugular venous distention Auscultate breath sounds every 4 hours Maintain fluid restriction as ordered Help patient plan a sodium-restricted diet Administer diuretics as ordered (monitor for hypokalemia) Administer antihypertensive drugs as ordered	Elevation of blood pressure and weight indicate fluid retention; daily weight measurements provide ongoing assessment of overall fluid balance; presence of rales indicates pulmonary congestion from fluid overload; diet low in sodium and restricted in fluids will help relieve fluid overload and hypertension; diuretics may be ordered for symptoms of acute fluid overload; antihypertensive drugs are usually reserved for patients who cannot be controlled by dietary and fluid restrictions

Impaired physical mobility related to prolonged bed rest
 	
• *Patient will tolerate bed rest without undue stress*
• *Patient can verbalize rationale for prolonged bed rest*
• *Patient does not experience negative outcomes of prolonged bed rest (e.g., pressure sores)*
	Help patient maintain bed rest; provide rationale for prolonged bed rest even when feeling well
	Help patient with diversionary activities
	Prevent complications of prolonged bed rest:
	    Turn frequently
	    Use of pressure mattress
	    Range-of-motion exercises
	    Massage skin, especially bony parts
		Bed rest is a major part of therapy during acute phase of illness; bed rest helps promote tissue healing and diuresis; diuresis usually begins 1 to 2 weeks after onset of therapy; bed rest is maintained as long as clinical signs of nephritis are present; bed rest will be reinstituted if patient demonstrates hematuria or elevation of BUN; frequent turning, massage, and range-of-motion exercises will prevent complications of prolonged bed rest

Altered nutrition: less than body requirements, related to anorexia and dietary restrictions • *Patient will ingest sufficient nutrients to provide adequate calories* • *Patient is able to demonstrate meal planning that incorporates dietary restrictions*	Provide diet high in carbohydrates, low in protein, and low in sodium Restrict fluid intake as ordered Have family bring in favorite foods that are within dietary limits	Proteins are restricted to prevent elevation of BUN; sodium- and fluid-restricted diet will help prevent fluid retention and edema; carbohydrates will provide sufficient calories and prevent breakdown of body's protein stores leading to muscle wasting; family interventions with favorite foods that are within diet restrictions will enhance patient compliance with diet
Impaired respiratory pattern related to fluid overload and prolonged bed rest • *Patient will remain free of pulmonary complications of bed rest such as atelectasis* • *Patient does not exhibit rales* • *Patient breathes easily and does not exhibit dyspnea*	Elevate head of bed 30 degrees Turn, cough, deep breathe every 2 to 4 hours Auscultate breath sounds every 4 hours Incentive spirometry as indicated	Pulmonary exercises will help prevent retention of secretions and development of atelectasis; upright position enhances ventilation

with all medications that are prescribed, and the patient must refrain from using over-the-counter drugs unless first approved by the physician. Instructing the patient in medications, diet, and long-term follow-up is an essential nursing activity. It is important to provide instruction in the prevention of urinary tract infections. Female patients must be instructed in the proper method of wiping from front to back after elimination to prevent fecal contamination of the perineal area. Use of cotton underwear or panties with a cotton crotch helps keep the area dry and prevents infections. Emptying the bladder every 3 to 4 hours during the day and once at night may help prevent infections caused by residual urine. Fruit juices that leave an acid ash in the urine, such as cranberry or prune juice, may help; however, commercial fruit juice or fruit drink preparations may not contain a high enough actual juice content to be of value. Patients with congenital disorders may require genetic counseling.

Evaluation

Nursing interventions are evaluated by monitoring patient outcomes. Does the patient state that he or she is free from pain? The patient should appear comfortable, with relaxed expressions. Normal vital signs and temperature are evidence of control of infection. Urine cultures should be negative. Each patient outcome is evaluated based on realistic, yet optimal, goals. The nursing care plan is adjusted accordingly.

Documentation

It is important to document day-to-day changes in blood pressure, temperature, intake and output of fluids, and weight. The patient's unique response to therapy is included. A description of the characteristics of the urine and the pattern of elimination is important in monitoring and assessing the disease process.

Ongoing Care

Rehabilitation

Recovery from infectious or inflammatory diseases of the kidney may take a long time. Patients may be taking medications for several weeks or even for the rest of their lives. Patients should be monitored on an ongoing basis for the possibility of recurrent infections or flare-up of the inflammatory process. Patients who require long-term steroid therapy must be assessed for evidence of cushingoid features and altered body image, infection, gastrointestinal irritation, and fluid retention. Care should be taken to prevent infection in the immunosuppressed patient. Fatigue and discomfort may tax the patient's men-

tal health. The patient will benefit from emotional and physical support during this phase.

Long-term care

The patient with renal dysfunction may develop CRF. Dialysis or transplantation may be necessary. Patients with congenital disorders will be monitored on a lifelong basis. Genetic counseling may be helpful for family planning. Patients with renal tuberculosis must have annual urine cultures for 10 years after treatment to monitor for potential reinfection.

Home care

Home dialysis is one option for patients who develop CRF. Maintenance of optimal health will retard exacerbations of symptoms or complications of the disease. Family and social support services may help in planning for care and maintenance of the home. Such factors as child care, meals, housework, and transportation to the health care facility need to be addressed.

Renal Obstruction

The outflow of urine may be obstructed anywhere along the urinary tract from the urinary calices to the urethra. Hydronephrosis and renal calculi are two obstructive disorders that often occur. Also, benign or malignant neoplasms may lead to obstruction. **Hydronephrosis** is the dilation of the renal pelvis and calices caused by an obstruction of normal urine flow. It may occur in one or both kidneys. Renal calculi **(nephrolithiasis)** are stones that form in the kidney. Renal neoplasms are tumors that usually compress, rather than invade, the renal parenchyma.

HYDRONEPHROSIS
Etiology/Epidemiology

Hydronephrosis results from any condition or structural abnormality that causes urinary tract obstruction. Obstruction in a single ureter will affect only one kidney. If the obstruction is in the bladder or urethra, then both kidneys will be involved. The obstruction may be caused by inflammation, tumor, scar tissue, calculi, or a kink in the ureter. In adults the primary causes are renal calculi and abdominal neoplasms.[32] In the elderly man prostatic hypertrophy may be a cause.

Pathophysiology

When the flow of urine is obstructed, the fluid pressure backs up into the kidney, causing dilation of the renal pelvis. Barotrauma (pressure trauma) eventually has adverse effects on the kidney. If the pressure is not too high, the kidney may dilate with no obvious loss of renal function. However, higher pressures cause irreversible destruction of the nephrons. Renal failure results from hydronephrosis of both kidneys. Additionally, urinary stasis predisposes the patient to pyelonephritis.[13] As a compensatory mechanism, some urine can flow back up the renal tubules into the veins and lymphatics. The unaffected kidney then takes on increased elimination of waste products but, as a consequence, begins to hypertrophy.[16] The hypertrophied kidney may be able to function as adequately as both kidneys did before the obstruction.[16]

Clinical Manifestations

The symptoms of hydronephrosis are proportionate to the degree and rapidity of renal dilation. If hydronephrosis develops slowly, the patient may experience little pain or change in urine output. However, if both kidneys are involved, urine output will drastically decrease or be altogether absent. Pain is caused by stretching of the tissues and compression of adjacent structures. There may be dull flank pain, or the pain may be colicky in nature if the obstruction is caused by a stone. The pain may radiate to the genitals and thighs because of the increased peristaltic action of the smooth muscles of the ureter in an attempt to force urine past the obstruction.[16] Nausea and vomiting may be caused by the intense pain, or they may occur as the dilated kidney begins to press on the stomach. Symptoms of uremia such as nausea and vomiting are seen if renal failure occurs. If the bladder is dilated as a result of urethral obstruction, the patient may complain of feeling the need to void but being unable to do so. The bladder may feel distended on palpation.

Therapeutic Management

Treatment is aimed at relieving the obstruction and preventing infection. A urethral catheter may relieve a lower obstruction. However, obstructions higher in the urinary tract may require surgical intervention. A drainage tube may be inserted above the obstruction to drain the urine. A nephrostomy tube may be inserted into the renal pelvis to drain urine and relieve pressure. It may be inserted percutaneously with the patient under local anesthesia or in an open surgical procedure with the patient under general anesthesia. It is important to never clamp or irrigate a nephrostomy tube unless specifically ordered by the physician. No more than 5 mL of irrigant should be inserted into the tube because of the small size of the renal pelvis. The tubing must be kept free of kinks and in a dependent drainage position. Pain re-

lief is mandatory. Analgesics and antispasmodics are commonly used together. As the obstruction is relieved and the urine is drained, the patient may then experience a syndrome called postobstructive diuresis. The sudden release of pressure and trapped urine may lead to a reflexive diuresis and potential fluid depletion. Careful monitoring of intake and output and vital signs will alert the practitioner to this condition.

RENAL CALCULI
Etiology/Epidemiology

Renal calculi (nephrolithiasis) are a relatively common problem, especially in men. It is estimated that approximately 14% of men will develop a stone by the age of 70 years.[13] Prostatic hypertrophy may contribute to this by creating stasis of urine. The concentration of stone-forming material in the urine may be increased as a result of various systemic diseases and dehydration.[26] Stones occur more frequently in whites than in blacks and can occur in several members of a family. There is also a high incidence of recurrence. Of the patients who experience a renal calculus, 40% can expect a second calculus within 2 years, and 80% can expect recurrence at some point. The rate of occurrence in the United States is 1.6 per 1000 people.[13] More than 200,000 people per year are admitted to hospitals in the United States with a diagnosis of renal calculi.[19] Many people pass stones without even being aware of it.

In the United States, regional differences exist in the rate of occurrence. The Southeast and Southwest have the highest incidence, with the Midwest being next highest.[11] Dehydration may be a factor in stone formation, since stones are more prevalent in the hot summer months. It has been postulated that heavy exercise without proper hydration could predispose a patient to stone formation. The majority of patients with stones range in age from 20 to 55 years.[17]

The kidneys normally excrete substances that are highly insoluble. Certain factors such as diet, presence of infection, or certain medications can increase the tendency for crystallization of these substances around an organic matrix such as pus, blood, tumors, or tissue.

No one theory can account for all stone formation. There are three major theories: (1) the saturation theory, (2) the deficiency of stone formation inhibitors theory, and (3) the matrix theory. The saturation theory states that stones are formed in an environment where the urine is supersaturated with stone components. These stone components include calcium salts, uric acid, cystine, and struvite (magnesium ammonium phosphate). Certain substances such as citrate have been found to chelate and inhibit crystal aggregation. The stone inhibitor theory states that stones are more prone to form in patients deficient in these substances. The matrix theory states that certain organic materials such as muco-proteins act as a nidus for stone formation. Crystal-lites are deposited and trapped, forming a matrix around the mucoproteins.[17] Excessive mucoprotein production may be found in certain individuals and families, predisposing them to stone formation. The largest number of stones (70% to 85%) contain cal-cium as calcium oxalate, calcium phosphate, or a combination of the two.[11] Any factor that promotes increased calcium levels in the urine and blood can predispose the patient to stone formation.

Pathophysiology

Most renal stones contain calcium. Anything that leads to hypercalciuria may predispose the patient to renal stones. An increased amount of calcium may be found in the urine of patients who have condi-tions in which there is an increased rate of bone re-absorption. These conditions include immobility, hy-perparathyroidism, Paget's disease of the bone, and osteolysis caused by malignant tumors of the breast, prostate, and lung.[13] Other factors favoring hyper-calciuria include renal tubular acidosis in which there is impaired renal tubular absorption of filtered calcium and an increased dietary intake of milk or alkali. Certain drugs have been associated with hy-percalciuria. These include ACTH, furosemide (Lasix), vitamin D, excessive thyroid hormone, am-monium chloride, and acetazolaminde. (Figure 42-2 illustrates common sites of stone formation.)

Calcium oxalate stones are the most common type of renal stone and may be related to diet. They are most common in regions where cereals compose a major portion of the diet and least common in dairy farming regions.[13] Oxalate stones are also found in patients with inflammatory bowel disease and resec-tions of the small bowel. These patients tend to ab-sorb more oxalate. Vitamin A deficiency may also in-crease oxalate stone formation.

Uric acid, the end product of purine metabolism, may be the source for stone formation. Uric acid stones are found in patients who have a high dietary intake of purine-rich foods such as herring, sardines, and yeast. They are also found in about 25% of pa-tients with primary gout and in 50% of patients with secondary gout.[13] Uric acid crystals may also absorb some of the normal urinary crystal inhibitors, thus linking hyperuricuria with calcium stone formation as well. Both regional enteritis and ulcerative colitis can precipitate the formation of uric acid stones be-cause of the associated fluid loss and bicarbonate ion loss leading to metabolic acidosis.

Magnesium ammonium phosphate (struvite) stones are caused by the urea-splitting action of cer-

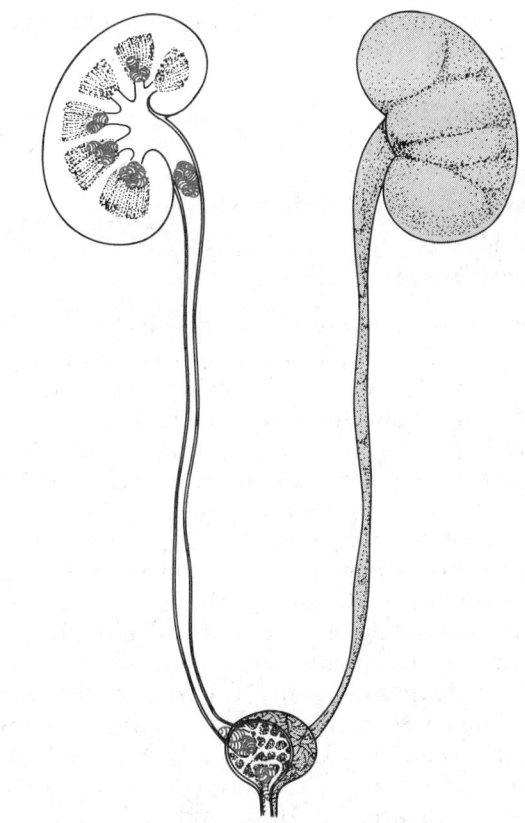

FIGURE 42-2   Most common locations of renal calculus formation.

tain bacteria, usually *Proteus*. *Proteus* bacteria con-tain the enzyme urease, which splits urea into two ammonia molecules, raising the urine pH. This al-kaline environment favors the precipitation of phos-phate crystals. Struvite stones may be called staghorn stones, for they take on the shape of stag antlers. Staghorn calculi are associated with infec-tion, and abscess formation is common. The calculi can erode into the perinephric space. In addition, the bacteria are difficult to destroy because the hard stone forms around the bacteria, protecting them from antibiotic therapy.[13]

Cystine stones are rare and are caused by a ge-netic defect of the renal transport of cystine. Xan-thine stones are also rare and are caused by a he-reditary condition in which there is a xanthine oxi-dase deficiency. Xanthine stones precipitate in acid urine.

Urinary pH influences stone formation. Alkaline urine is associated with infection and struvite stones. Acid urine is associated with uric acid and cystine calculi. Calcium phosphate calculi will dissolve in acidic urine, whereas calcium oxalate stones are not affected by urinary pH.

Calculus formation may be enhanced when there

is scar formation as a result of infection or surgery of the urinary tract or when urinary stasis or cystallization is already present.[30] Recurrent calculi formation may be prevented by promoting adequate fluid intake throughout the day to dilute and decrease the concentration of stone-forming substances and prevent urinary stasis.

Clinical Manifestations

Clinical manifestations of renal calculi depend on their site of formation. If the stone is in the kidney itself, the pain may be dull, aching, and constant in nature. This pain is located in the costovertebral angle and is a result of hydronephrosis caused by obstruction by the stone. Sometimes staghorn calculi are "silent," causing no problem until they become infected. As the stone begins to move down the ureter, the character of the pain changes. It is usually severe and colicky in nature. Renal colic originates deep in the lumbar region and radiates anteriorly and downward toward the bladder in women and toward the testicle in men.[2] Gastrointestinal symptoms of nausea, vomiting, diarrhea, and abdominal pain may accompany the pain and are a result of the anatomic proximity of the kidneys to the stomach, pancreas, and large intestines and to the pain reflex itself.

Ureteral colic is generally excruciating in nature. The pain radiates downward toward the genitals and thighs as the stone moves down the ureter. The pain usually accompanies a desire to void, but little urine is excreted. Gross or microscopic hematuria may be present because of the trauma and abrasive action of the stone.

Intermittent pain usually indicates that the stone is moving. It has been hypothesized that the ureter proximal to the stone dilates, thus allowing urine and the stone to pass. The obstruction is momentarily relieved until the stone lodges in another area of the ureter, causing more pain. The colicky nature of the pain subsides by the time the stone reaches the bladder. Stones in the bladder produce symptoms of irritation and may be associated with infection, hematuria, and fever. The pain associated with renal calculi may be so severe that the patient exhibits mild shock with pale, moist skin. The pain may be resistant to narcotic intervention.

The patient may pass the stone. It is important to strain all urine, so that stone formation can be analyzed and appropriate therapy instituted. The pH of the urine is sometimes tested with nitrazine paper.

Therapeutic Management

The primary goals of management are to relieve pain, eliminate the stones, and prevent recurrence. Narcotics and antispasmodics may be used to relieve the pain. Warm, moist packs to the area or hot baths may offer some relief. Antiemetics may relieve nausea and vomiting. The patient who is able to take oral fluids should be encouraged to do so. Forcing fluids can help pass the stone along, since the hydrostatic pressure built up behind the stone will help in its passage. Fluid intake should be at least 3000 mL/day, either orally or by intravenous administration. A high fluid intake around-the-clock dilutes the crystalloids and enhances stone passage. Stones may be as small as a grain of sand or gravel, or they may be quite large, requiring surgical removal. Stones that are passed are analyzed for composition so that specific strategies to prevent further calculi can be developed.

Dietary management may help prevent certain types of stones. A reduction in dietary calcium and phosphorus may be required. Thiazide diuretics have been noted to increase calcium reabsorption and may be prescribed for patients with calcium calculi. Intake of vitamin D and vitamin D–enriched foods may be restricted to prevent parathyroid hormone production. Patients with oxalate stones should avoid foods high in oxalate such as tea, instant coffee, cola drinks, beer, rhubarb, beans, asparagus, spinach, cabbage, chocolate, citrus fruits, apples, grapes, cranberries, peanuts, and peanut butter. Large doses of vitamin C may help increase oxalate excretion in the urine.[13]

Patients who form uric acid calculi should be placed on a low-purine diet. The intake of fish and meat, especially organ meats, should be restricted. Medications such as allopurinol (Zyloprim) help decrease the formation of uric acid and thus stone formation. Dietary modifications may also help adjust the urinary pH so that stone formation is inhibited. The urine may be alkalinized by increasing the intake of bicarbonate, or it may be acidified by drinking cranberry, plum, or prune juice.[19] Commercial preparations of fruit juices may not contain enough pure fruit juice to be of value.

Struvite calculi are associated with infection and are treated with appropriate antibiotics and acidification of the urine. In addition to antibiotics, acetohydroxamic acid (AHA) may be used. AHA has been shown to inhibit the chemical reaction caused by persistent bacteria and is useful in preventing struvite stone formation.[11]

Surgical intervention may be required in about 10% of patients with renal calculi who do not respond to other forms of therapy. Stones may be removed in a variety of ways (Figure 42-3). A percutaneous nephroscopy may be performed. The stone may be crushed and removed using alligator forceps, or it may be irrigated and flushed through. In a procedure known as coagulum pyelolithotomy, a solution of thrombin, fibrinogen, and calcium chloride is instilled into the renal pelvis. The solution coagu-

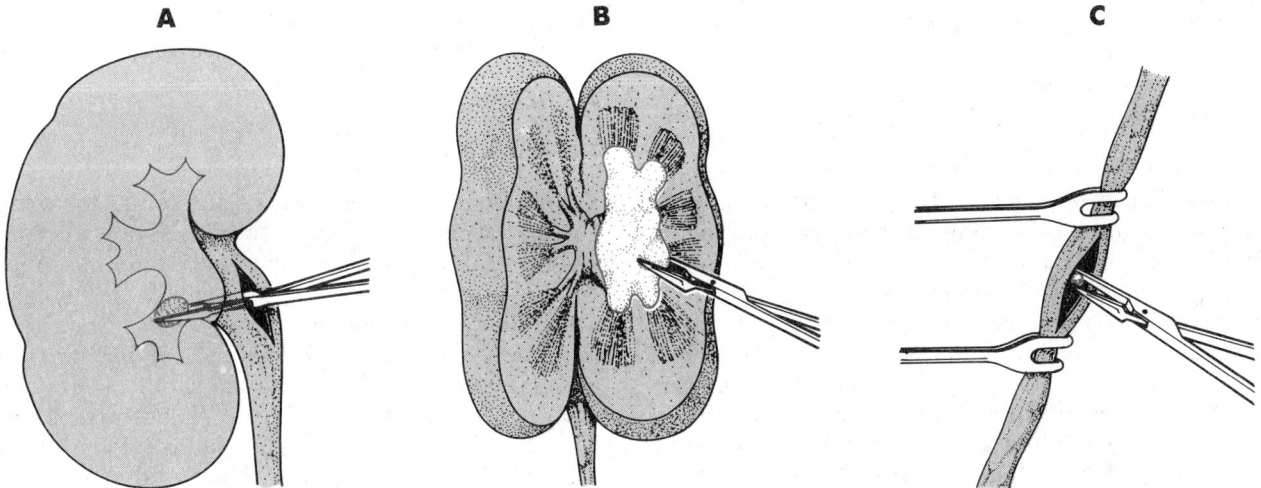

FIGURE 42-3   Location and methods of removing renal calculi from upper urinary tract. **A,** Pyelolithotomy, or removal of stone through renal pelvis. **B,** Nephrolithotomy, or removal of staghorn calculus from renal parenchyma (kidney split). **C,** Ureterolithotomy, or removal of stone from ureter.

lates around the stone into a thick gel that can be removed by forceps.[13]

Large stones can be broken up into smaller fragments. An ultrasound probe can be inserted through a nephrostomy tube, and ultrasonic waves can be used to break up the stone. Smaller pieces can then be removed or flushed through. In a similar method an electrical discharge (electrohydraulic lithotripsy) is used. After extraction of the stone, the percutaneous nephrostomy tube is left in place to maintain patency of the ureter.

The kidney itself can also be incised for stone removal (nephrolithotomy). A pyelolithotomy is removal of stones from the renal pelvis, and a ureterolithotomy is removal of stones from the ureter. If the kidney is severely damaged, a nephrectomy may be necessary. Struvite calculi are most often associated with necessity for kidney removal.

A nonsurgical procedure for stone removal is extracorporeal shock wave lithotripsy (ESWL) (Figure 42-4). In this procedure the patient is placed under local or general anesthesia in a water bath. An epidural block is sometimes used. Multiple shock waves are aimed directly at the stone, using fluoroscopy for stone visualization. Up to 1500 or more shocks may be required to shatter the stone. The shock waves cause some discomfort but do not harm surrounding tissue. The shock waves are synchronized to the patient's electrocardiogram (ECG) so dysrhythmias do not occur. In certain cases, such as very large stones, the physician may insert a ureteral stent via cystoscopy before ESWL. The stent pushes the stone from the narrow lumen of the ureter back up into

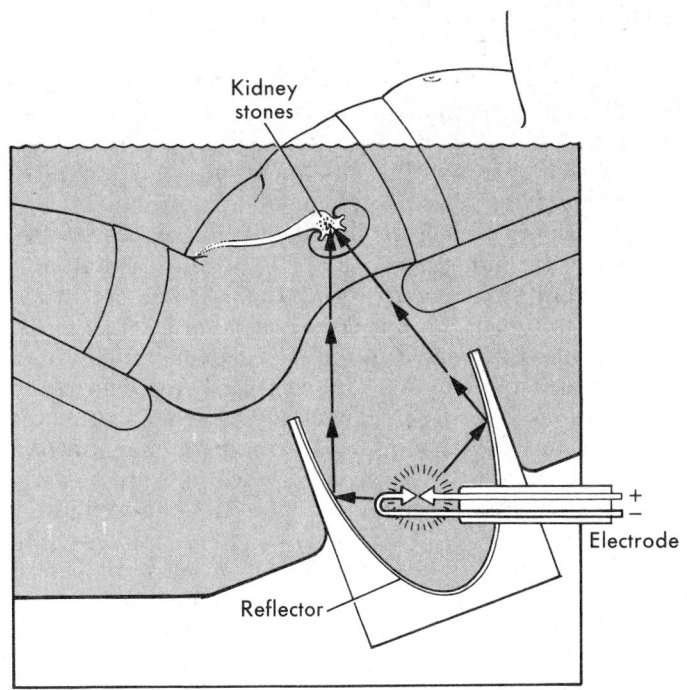

FIGURE 42-4   Extracorporeal lithotripsy. With patient seated in a tub of water, shock waves are aimed at stone. Shock waves break stone into smaller particles that can be eliminated in urine.

the renal pelvis. This in itself helps to decrease some of the pain. After ESWL the stone fragments pass down the stent (which acts as a conduit), thereby eliminating the pain of renal colic. The stent is later removed.

Laser lithotripsy has recently been used to cause fragmentation of particularly large or resistant stones. If the stone is located in the ureter itself, passage of a ureteroscope to direct the laser beam to the proper location may be necessary.

Since ESWL is a nonsurgical procedure, it is usually performed as an outpatient procedure. The stone fragments may take up to 6 weeks or more to pass. Patients are encouraged to increase their fluid intake to 3 to 4 L/24 hr and to strain all urine during this time. Although complications are rare, the patient is monitored for potential hemorrhage. As the patient passes the stone fragments, he or she may experience renal colic. This is controlled by analgesics and use of antispasmodics.

An alternative to surgery is percutaneous nephrostomy and infusion of chemolytic solutions to dissolve the stone. The irrigating solution leaves the system through the ureter or the nephrostomy tube. Postoperative care for any of these procedures involves monitoring the vital signs and observing the patient for evidence of bleeding. Drainage tubes must be monitored for patency and amount of drainage.

RENAL NEOPLASM
Etiology/Epidemiology

Primary renal tumors may arise from the renal capsule, parenchyma, connective tissue, or fatty tissue. However, most renal tumors are the result of metastases from another site, most often the lung. Renal metastasis has been found in approximately 20% of patients who have died from lung cancer.[32] Because the kidneys receive 25% of the cardiac output, they have high exposure to malignant cells traveling in the circulation from other parts of the body.

Approximately 85% of all primary renal neoplasms are malignant and commonly metastasize to the lungs, liver, bone, brain, or the other kidney. At the time of diagnosis it is estimated that approximately 25% to 50% of patients will have metastatic disease.[2] Renal cancer accounts for approximately 1% to 3% of all malignancies.[32] Renal cell carcinomas account for 85% to 90% of primary malignant renal neoplasms; another 5% to 10% arise in the collecting system; and 3% are sarcomas, arising from connective tissue.[32]

Benign renal neoplasms are rare and generally do not cause notable clinical manifestations of renal disease.[32] Renal cell carcinoma occurs more often in men than in women and is most often seen in people from 60 to 70 years of age. Renal cell tumors occur more commonly in smokers than in nonsmokers.[32]

Pathophysiology

With benign renal neoplasms, adenomas form in the cortical area of the renal tubules. They are small, usually only 2 to 3 cm in size. Adenomas appear yellow-gray and are encapsulated. These benign tumors may represent an early stage of renal carcinoma and are found in 7% to 22% of all kidneys examined at autopsy.[32] Renal fibroma is associated with tuberous sclerosis that is characterized by lesions in the cerebral cortex causing epilepsy or mental retardation.[32] Of patients with tuberous sclerosis, 80% have renal fibroma.[2] In patients without tuberous sclerosis, renal fibroma is found most often in women between 30 and 50 years of age.[32] Renal fibromas may cause pain and bleeding.

Malignant renal neoplasms account for up to 90% of all renal neoplasms. Controversy exists, but it is thought that they originate in the upper cortical pole from the convoluted tubules.[2] The tumor is usually unilateral.[32] Renal cell carcinomas are quite vascular and composed of a variety of cell types. They appear bright yellow to gray-white and range in size from 3 to 15 cm.[2] These tumors usually remain within the renal capsule, causing compression of adjacent structures, leading to ischemia, necrosis, and hemorrhage.[32] As the tumor grows it may invade the collecting system or renal vein, thus gaining access to the vena cava and heart. Metastasis most often occurs in the lungs, liver, lymph nodes, and bones.[32]

Clinical Manifestations

Renal neoplasms cause a classic triad of clinical manifestations: (1) hematuria, (2) flank pain, and (3) palpable abdominal mass. This triad of symptoms does not occur in all patients, and when it does, it usually occurs late in the disease.[2] Many renal tumors cause no symptoms but may be found on routine physical examination as a palpable mass. The most common symptom of renal neoplasm is painless hematuria; 60% to 90% of patients will have hematuria, either intermittent and microscopic or gross.[32] Other clinical manifestations of renal tumors include the general symptoms of a malignancy such as weight loss and fatigue. Certain benign tumors may also cause hypertension because of increased renin secretion by the kidney.[32]

Therapeutic Management

Therapeutic management is aimed at surgical removal of the tumor before it can metastasize. The prognosis for survival is very poor (only 1 to 2 years) once the tumor has metastasized.[32] However, if metastasis has not occurred, the survival rate is 5 years for 50% to 70% of patients, with a 20-year survival rate for 5% to 33% of patients.[2] The preferred method of treatment is a radical nephrectomy. This includes removal of the kidney, tumor, adrenal gland, lymph nodes, and surrounding fat and fascia.[2] Adjunct radiation or chemotherapy may also be used.

NURSING MANAGEMENT OF THE PATIENT WITH RENAL OBSTRUCTION

Assessment

Nursing assessment for patients with renal obstruction may pose a challenge, since the patient may be in acute pain. The nurse will assess for changes in patterns of elimination and complaints of pain. Passage of a calculus through the urinary tract causes severe pain that is usually spasmodic. The patient may describe the pain as dull or as 9 or 10 on a scale of 1 to 10. The pain may be felt in the flank or abdominal area, or the pain may extend into the vulva or testes as it moves down the ureter. The nurse observes the patient for nonverbal evidence of pain such as facial grimacing or guarding of the abdomen.

An essential aspect of nursing assessment and ongoing care is to filter the urine and observe for the passage of stones. The stones may appear as large as pebbles or as fine as sand. Testing the urine for pH and for evidence of hematuria provides useful diagnostic data. A thorough dietary assessment is an important nursing function, because many types of stones have a dietary component. A family history for renal calculi is also an important assessment factor. The nurse may note that the patient becomes nauseated and may even vomit during painful spasms. If infection is also present, the patient may have fever and chills.

Nursing Diagnosis

Nursing diagnoses in patients with problems of renal obstruction include the following:

Altered patterns of urinary elimination related to obstructive process
Pain, acute, related to obstruction of the ureter
High risk for infection related to urinary stasis
Knowledge deficit related to lack of knowledge about fluid intake and dietary restrictions
High risk for fluid volume excess related to renal obstruction
Activity intolerance related to pain or infection
Anxiety or fear related to pain or lack of knowledge

Planning

Outcome criteria include the following:

The patient will pass the stone as evidenced by capture in urinary filter
The patient will remain free of infection as evidenced by absence of fever and negative urine cultures
The patient will not experience pain as evidenced by relaxed body posture and facial expression
The patient will ingest up to 3 L of fluids per day to help in stone passage and help prevent further stone formation
The patient will describe dietary modifications that will help prevent stone formation
The patient will be able to describe the disease process, treatment, and medications and can describe measures to prevent complications
The patient will exercise regularly, especially walking, to prevent stone formation
The patient will respond to urge to void and empty bladder at least every 3 hours to prevent stasis

Implementation

The patient is encouraged to increase intake of fluids to help dilute crystal formation and create a hydrostatic force behind the obstruction that will encourage forward movement of the stone. Nursing care is focused on fluid and dietary management and prevention of stone formation. The patient is encouraged to respond to the urge to void in order to flush the bladder and prevent stasis. The nurse helps the patient and family modify diet and meal plans specific to the composition of the stone.

Analgesics and antispasmodics are administered by the nurse in conjunction with one another to promote maximum pain relief. Warm baths or warm compresses to the area may help.

All urine must be strained through a filter or several layers of gauze. It is essential that the stones be recovered and sent to the laboratory for analysis, because the type of stone dictates the specific therapy and also the methods used to prevent further stone formation.

Postoperative care

The patient who undergoes surgical treatment for stone or tumor removal is treated in a similar manner to any surgical patient. A critical nursing measure is maintenance of the patency of drainage tubes and nephrostomy and ureterostomy tubes. Dressings are observed for potential leakage of urine around the drainage tube, which could promote skin breakdown or bacterial invasion. Any odor of urine from the dressing is reported. Postoperative drainage may initially be blood tinged but usually clears within 24 hours. The quantity and the composition of fluid output are measured and recorded. Drainage tubes are not clamped or irrigated unless specifically ordered by the physician and using strict aseptic technique. Clamping a nephrostomy tube could precipitate acute pyelonephritis. No more than 5 to 10 mL of irrigant is inserted into a nephrostomy tube because of the small size of the renal pelvis. Larger quantities of irrigant could cause hydronephrosis or damage surrounding tissues.

Evaluation

Patient outcomes are evaluated on an ongoing basis. Pain control is evidenced not only by statements made by the patient, but also by evidence of relaxed body posture and facial expression. Dietary management is evaluated by adherence to the diet and ability to describe meal plans that are specific to dietary restrictions. Absence of infection is based on negative urine cultures and absence of fever. Stone passage is evaluated by the presence of sand, gravel, or stone capture in the urine filter. Each aspect of care is evaluated independently, with the nursing care plan adjusted accordingly.

Documentation

The nurse documents the onset, location, quality, character, and duration of pain, because these are extremely important in assessing the degree of obstruction. It is also important that the nurse document evidence of stone passage as the stone is captured in the urine filter. Additionally, the nurse must monitor and document vital signs, fluid intake and output, urine specific gravity and pH, and weight.

Ongoing Care

Renal obstruction caused by calculus formation is a commonly recurring problem. It is important that the nurse instruct patients and their families about the etiologic factors of stone formation and methods used to retard it. Instruction is given regarding dietary management and the use of medications. The nurse must instruct the patient to increase fluid intake, void frequently, and exercise regularly. Since some obstructive diseases are familial, family counseling is important.

Renal Failure

Definition

Acute renal failure (ARF) is a reversible syndrome caused by the abrupt deterioration of renal function, resulting in the accumulation of metabolites and other substances that are normally excreted from the body. It is associated with **oliguria** (urine output less than 400 mL/24 hr) or nonoliguria (urine output greater than 800 mL/24 hr). Approximately 40% to 50% of the cases caused by acute tubular necrosis are nonoliguric.[3] Other terms used synonymously with ARF are acute tubular necrosis, renal parenchymal failure, acute tubulointerstitial nephritis, reversible intrinsic renal failure, and vasomotor nephropathy. **Chronic renal failure (CRF)** differs from ARF in that the disease constitutes a progressive destruction of the renal structures over time that is irreversible. In end-stage renal disease the kidneys are often atrophied and filled with scar tissue.

Etiology/Epidemiology

Renal failure represents the kidneys' inability to remove waste products from the body or to perform regulatory functions. This results in impaired fluid and electrolyte balance, acid-base disturbance, and impaired endocrine and metabolic function. Renal failure may occur as a result of a variety of causes, including ischemia, infection, nephrotoxicity, hypertension, glomerulonephritis, vascular disorders, trauma, or obstruction, or as a result of other diseases such as diabetes mellitus or lupus erythematosus.

Each year an estimated 42,000 Americans die of irreversible kidney failure.[2] The incidence of ARF is 20 to 40 cases per 1 million population per year.[32] It is estimated that approximately 50% of all hospitalized patients develop ARF. Mortality approaches 50%. These statistics reflect the increasing number of critically ill patients seen in acute care hospitals today and the increasing elderly population.[16] Elderly persons are particularly at risk because atrophy of the nephrons occurs as a normal component of the aging process. When damage occurs, elderly persons have decreased renal reserves. Others at risk for developing ARF are those who have vascular diseases such as diabetes, hypertension, and atherosclerosis and those who have underlying intrinsic renal disease. Because CRF is a progressively destructive disease, it produces more degenerative changes than does ARF.

ACUTE RENAL FAILURE
Definition

Causes of ARF are categorized into prerenal, intrarenal, and postrenal. Prerenal causes interfere with renal perfusion; intrarenal causes are those that damage the renal parenchyma; and postrenal causes are those that obstruct the urinary tract anywhere from the tubules to the urethral meatus (see box, p. 1097).

ACUTE RENAL FAILURE

Prerenal

Hypovolemia related to
   Dehydration
   Hemorrhage
   Fluid losses via the gastrointestinal system (i.e., diarrhea, vomiting, gastric suction)
   Fluid lost to third spacing (i.e., ascites, burns)
   Excessive diuresis
Decreased cardiac output related to
   Myocardial infarction
   Congestive heart failure
   Dysrhythmias
Decreased renal perfusion related to
   Increased vascular resistance
   Vascular obstruction
   Interruption of renal blood flow caused by surgery and other causes

Intrarenal

Sequelae to prolonged prerenal disease
Nephrotoxins
   Aminoglycocides
   Heavy metals
   Solvents
   Radiographic dyes
   Sulfonamides
Intratubular obstruction
   Uric acid crystals
   Calculi
   Hemolytic reactions
   Rhabdomyolysis
Infections
   Glomerulonephritis
   Acute interstitial nephritis
   Acute pyelonephritis
Renal injury
   Blunt or penetrating trauma
Vascular lesions

Postrenal

Ureteral obstruction
   Calculi
   Tumors
Bladder outlet obstruction
   Strictures
   Calculi
   Prostatic hypertrophy

Two major mechanisms are responsible for the oliguria of ARF: (1) ischemia of renal cells caused by decreased blood volume, as in hypovolemia, or redistribution of blood flow away from the kidneys, as in shock, and (2) nephrotoxicity. Other clinical conditions that result in renal failure include trauma, burns, sepsis, the administration of mismatched blood, and severe muscle injury. Approximately two thirds of the cases of ARF are caused by a sudden episode of renal ischemia. As renal perfusion decreases, oxygen and other nutrients are not available for cellular metabolism. The result is renal ischemia or necrosis. Cellular damage may occur in as little as 30 minutes or as long as several hours after the initial insult.

Prerenal conditions

Prerenal causes are those that impair renal perfusion without causing tubular damage. Conditions that lead to renal hypoperfusion include circulatory volume depletion as in hemorrhage, burns, or excessive gastrointestinal losses such as vomiting, nasogastric suction, or diarrhea; volume shifts as in ascites; decreased cardiac output as in myocardial infarction, cardiac tamponade, or dysrhythmias; vascular obstruction as in renal stenosis or thrombosis; and increased vascular resistance as in hepatorenal syndrome or when the patient is under anesthetic.

Intrarenal conditions

Intrarenal conditions are those that lead to interstitial, glomerular, or tubular damage. A major cause of intrarenal disease is the sequelae of prolonged prerenal disease. Other causes include infection such as glomerulonephritis and nephrotoxic substances such as heavy metals, certain antibiotics (gentamycin, kanamycin, tetracycline, penicillin), and contrast media used during diagnostic studies (see box on p. 1098). Additionally, intrarenal obstructions resulting from hemolytic reactions or myoglobinuria may cause intrarenal disease.

Postrenal conditions

Obstructions caused by stones, prostatic hypertrophy, or tumors are examples of conditions that may lead to postrenal disease.

Pathophysiology

Because the kidneys receive 20% to 25% of the cardiac output, they are sensitive to changes in their blood supply. As stated earlier, two thirds of the cases of ARF are caused by a sudden ischemic event. When renal blood flow is diminished, the basic driving force for filtration is also diminished. In addition, the kidneys are deprived of oxygen and other vital nutrients for cellular metabolism. The kidneys have a tremendous ability to adapt to loss of functioning nephrons and are able to maintain fluid and electrolyte balance with only 25% of the nephrons functional.[16] A normal healthy adult needs a urine output of approximately 400 mL/24 hr to excrete the

SUBSTANCES THAT PRODUCE NEPHROTOXIC INJURY TO THE KIDNEYS

Antibiotics
Gentamicin
Tobramycin
Amikacin
Amphotericin
Polymyxin B
Colistin
Neomycin
Kanamycin

Chemicals
Ethylene glycol
Mercuric chloride
Carbon tetrachloride
Lead
Arsenic
Methanol

Radiographic contrast agents
IVP dye

Drug-induced acute interstitial nephritis
Penicillins
Cephalosporins
Nonsteroidal anti-inflammatory agents
Sulfonamides
Rifampicin
Tetracyclines
Furosemide (Lasix)
Thiazides
Phenytoin (Dilantin)

drostatic pressure by dilation of the afferent arteriole and constriction of the efferent arteriole. This acts to increase the flow of blood into the glomerular capillary bed while retarding blood flow out of it. The net result is an increase in pressure and GFR. This adaptive response is limited and is compromised if these arterioles are affected by vascular disease such as diabetes or chronic hypertension. As stated earlier, these individuals are at increased risk for the development of ARF in times of renal hypoperfusion.

The second adaptive response by the kidneys is the activation of the renin-angiotensin-aldosterone system. Activation of this system stimulates peripheral vasoconstriction, which in itself acts to increase perfusion pressure. Activation of this system also causes aldosterone to be secreted, which results in sodium and water reabsorption and potassium excretion. Reabsorption of sodium and water acts to improve the overall intravascular volume, thus improving perfusion to the kidneys as well as other organs. Sodium reabsorption leads to an increased plasma osmolality, which in turn stimulates the hypothalamic osmoreceptors to release antidiuretic hormone (ADH). ADH enhances water reabsorption from the distal tubules, thus increasing intravascular volume and renal perfusion. ARF develops when the limits of these adaptive responses are overwhelmed.

The pathogenesis of ARF is not completely understood. Several hypotheses have been proposed. The back leak theory purports that glomerular filtrate backs up through damaged tubules into the peritubular circulation, leading to chemical or morphologic changes in the basement membrane of the glomerular capillary.[13] In experimental models, tubular damage was demonstrated after the administration of nephrotoxic substances.

Another theory is that the tubules become obstructed with cellular and protein debris. The resulting elevated intratubular pressure then opposes filtration pressure until filtration stops. Vascular theories relate to renal hypoperfusion resulting in cell death and tubular necrosis.

Phases of Acute Renal Failure

The course of ARF is divided into four phases: the onset, the oliguric phase, the diuretic phase, and the recovery phase. The first stage, or onset, is the initial phase of insult or injury. This stage is important because immediate intervention may result in reversal or prevention of further renal dysfunction.

During the oliguric phase, which lasts from 8 to 14 days, urine output is greatly reduced (less than 400 mL/24 hr). The normal aging process is accompanied by some loss of the ability of nephrons to concentrate the urine, so the older person may develop

body's waste products. In ARF diminished glomerular filtration results in the accumulation of waste products within the body. Regardless of the volume of urine excreted, the patient with ARF will experience rising levels of serum creatinine and BUN as a result of impaired glomerular filtration of waste products. This abnormally high level of nitrogenous wastes in the blood is termed **azotemia.**

The kidneys require a minimal mean arterial pressure of 60 to 70 mm Hg to prevent renal hypoperfusion. In times of hypoperfusion the kidneys activate two major adaptive responses: autoregulation and the release of renin. The renal vascular system is unique. The glomerular capillary bed, unlike others, is situated between two arterioles, and resistance to blood flow can be increased or decreased at either end, altering the glomerular hydrostatic pressure. Autoregulation maintains glomerular hy-

dysfunction at higher urine outputs (600 to 700 mL/24 hr). The degree of azotemia that develops during this phase largely depends on the urine output and the degree of protein breakdown that is taking place. Controversy exists over whether nonoliguric renal failure is an entity in and of itself or whether it is a phase of oliguric ARF. Nonoliguric renal failure occurs predominantly after nephrotoxic antibiotic administration. It may also occur with burns, anesthesia, and traumatic injury.[23] Nonoliguric renal failure is usually associated with less morbidity and mortality than the oliguric form. This may be because of the lesser degree and shorter duration of azotemia.

The diuretic phase of ARF usually lasts about 10 days, marking the recovery of the nephrons and their ability to excrete urine. Diuresis generally occurs before complete recovery of the nephrons, so the patient remains azotemic.

The recovery phase indicates improvement of renal function and may last up to 6 months. Last to recover is the ability to concentrate urine. Often there is some residual impairment of renal function.

Clinical Manifestations

Clinical manifestations of ARF may not appear until 1 week after the initial insult. When clinical manifestations do occur, they occur abruptly, with the patient appearing critically ill. The disruption in regulation of fluids, electrolytes, and waste products affects every system.

Oliguric phase

The most common symptom of ARF is a reduction in the expected urine output. During the oliguric phase urine output is less than 400 mL/24 hr. Some patients exhibit **anuria** (urine output less than 50 mL/24 hr), although this is rare. Patients with nonoliguric ARF may excrete as much as 2 L/day. The oliguric phase lasts 8 to 14 days, with a poorer prognosis associated with the length of time that oliguria is present. The specific gravity of the urine is low and fixed (1.010 compared with 1.025), and the urine osmolality approaches that of the patient's serum, or about 300 mOsm/L.[16]

During this phase metabolic waste products accumulate in the blood. Plasma creatinine levels increase approximately 1 mg/dL/day, and the BUN level increases approximately 20 mg/dL/day (Table 42-1).[7] The patient becomes acidotic as urinary excretion of the acid end products of metabolism decreases. Kussmaul's respirations reflect the lungs' attempt to blow off excess carbon dioxide gas to compensate for the metabolic acidosis.

Oliguria leads to fluid retention with edema formation and hypertension. A weight gain of 1 kg is equivalent to a fluid gain of 1 L. Fluid overload may precipitate congestive heart failure and pulmonary edema.

Decreased excretion of potassium in the urine and increased release of potassium from the cells because of acidosis lead to hyperkalemia. The effects of hyperkalemia can be seen in the ECG as tall,

TABLE 42-1 Laboratory Test Changes in Acute Renal Failure

Finding	Prerenal	Intrarenal	Postrenal
BLOOD VALUE			
BUN	Increases	Increases	Increases
Creatinine	Normal	Increases	Increases
BUN/creatinine ratio	20:1 or greater (increased)	10:1 or less (not increased because both values elevated)	Normal to slightly increased
URINE VALUE			
Urea	Decreases	Decreases	Decreases
Creatinine	≈normal	Decreases	Decreases
Specific gravity	1.020 or more (increased)	Fixed and may be high	Variable
Volume	Oliguria	Nonoliguria or oliguria	Oliguria/polyuria Anuria
Osmolality	400 mOsm or more (increases)	250 to 350 mOsm (low and fixed, similar to plasma osmolality)	Variable: increases or similar to plasma osmolality

peaked T waves, a loss of P waves, and a broadening of the QRS complex, as well as ectopy. Severe hyperkalemia (greater than 6.5 mEq/L) can result in cardiac arrest. Hyperkalemia is less common in nonoliguric ARF, because the kidneys retain some ability to excrete potassium in the urine.

Renal wasting of sodium may occur in ARF. Renal wasting of sodium and hemodilution can result in hyponatremia. The effects of hyponatremia include neurologic irritability such as headache, confusion, seizure, and coma. These neurologic manifestations may also be the result of the accumulation of uremic toxins on the central nervous system.

If ARF persists for more than a few days, nearly all patients will develop some degree of anemia. This is the result of decreased erythropoietin production by the damaged kidneys and the toxic effects of uremia on the hematopoietic system. The accumulation of urea causes decreased platelet adhesiveness and a decreased life span of red blood cells. Symptoms of anemia include fatigue, weakness, shortness of breath, and tachycardia.

The accumulation of waste products in the blood leads to a variety of symptoms known as the **uremic syndrome.** Symptoms include nausea, vomiting, anorexia, diarrhea, hiccoughs, and the neurologic symptoms previously mentioned. Urea is also irritating to the pericardial membrane and can lead to uremic pericarditis and potential tamponade. Uremia compromises both the humoral and cellular immune systems, thus placing the patient with ARF at increased risk for infection.

Diuretic phase

The diuretic phase of ARF develops about 14 days after the initial insult and lasts about 10 days. It is characterized by an increase in urine output of more than 1000 mL/24 hr. This increase in urine output indicates the return of some renal function; however, the BUN and creatinine levels continue to rise during the first few days of diuresis. Urea and other waste products of metabolism act as an osmotic diuretic. Together, this can lead to dehydration and potential death. During this phase 25% of deaths caused by ARF occur. For those who survive, laboratory values eventually begin to return toward normal. Wide fluctuations of fluid and electrolyte balance occur during this phase, and the patient may still require dialysis.

Recovery phase

Recovery continues for up to 12 months. Usually the patient is left with some residual impairment in renal function (Table 42-2).

Therapeutic Management

As with any disease, the primary goal is prevention. It is extremely important to maintain adequate hydration and renal perfusion in patients who are at high risk for the development of ARF. These include elderly persons, surgical patients, any patient who is hemodynamically unstable, and those receiving nephrotoxic drugs or large doses of radiologic contrast dye. Improving blood flow to the kidneys

TABLE 42-2 Comparison of Oliguric and Diuretic Phases of Acute Renal Failure

Physiologic effect	Findings	Symptoms
OLIGURIC PHASE		
Inability to excrete metabolic wastes	Increased serum: Urea nitrogen Creatinine	Nausea Vomiting Drowsiness Confusion Coma Gastrointestinal bleeding Asterixis Pericarditis
Inability to regulate electrolytes	Hyperkalemia Hyponatremia Acidosis	Nausea Vomiting Cardiac dysrhythmias Kussmaul's breathing Drowsiness Confusion Coma
Inability to excrete fluid loads	Fluid overload Hypervolemia	Edema Congestive heart failure Pulmonary edema Hypertension
DIURETIC PHASE		
Increased production of urine	Hypovolemia Loss of sodium Loss of potassium	Urinary output up to 4 to 5 L/day Postural hypotension Tachycardia
Slowly increasing excretion of metabolic wastes	High BUN initially BUN gradually returns to baseline	Improving mental alertness and activity

through the use of intravenous fluids and medications may be all that is necessary in the treatment of prerenal disorders. For example, if the origin of prerenal disease is decreased cardiac output caused by dysrhythmias or impaired contractility of the heart, then the treatment should be aimed at improving cardiac function through the use of cardiac glycosides or antidysrhythmics. The heart should be treated to restore adequate perfusion to the kidneys. The physician may order a bolus of intravenous fluids to be given as a fluid challenge to effect an increase in GFR and thus urine output. Mannitol, an osmotic diuretic, may be given to increase intravascular volume and perfusion to the kidneys. Loop diuretics such as furosemide, bumetanide (Bumex), or ethacrynic acid may be used selectively in these patients. Use of diuretic therapy within 4 to 8 hours of onset may change the oliguric form of ARF to the nonoliguric form, which may have a better prognosis.[13]

Oliguric phase

Therapeutic management during the oliguric phase is aimed at controlling fluid and electrolyte imbalance, acid-base disorders, and the effects of uremia while also preventing infection and maintaining adequate nutrition.

Fluid intake and output are monitored closely, as are other parameters of fluid balance such as central venous pressure (CVP), pulmonary artery wedge pressure (PAWP), and daily weight. Once fluid balance has been restored, fluids are usually replaced at a rate of 400 to 600 mL/day to replace the usual insensible losses from respiration and perspiration, plus some fraction of the previous day's urine output. Fluid and electrolyte losses from vomitus, gastric drainage, or diarrhea must also be accounted for.

Fluid overload resulting from oliguria may cause a dilutional hyponatremia. Intervention is therefore aimed at control of fluid balance. Impaired renal excretion of phosphates can be controlled through the oral administration of phosphate binding gels such as aluminum hydroxide (Amphojel), so excess phosphates can then be excreted in the feces. By maintaining a normal serum phosphate level, alterations in serum calcium levels can be avoided.

Hyperkalemia (see box) can be life threatening and must be treated. If the potassium level remains below 6 mEq/L, the patient can be treated by conservative methods such as dietary restriction or through the use of cation exchange resins such as sodium polystrene sulfonate (Kayexalate) given orally or as an enema to facilitate excretion of potassium through the gastrointestinal tract. Sorbitol, an osmotic cathartic, is given with sodium polystrene sulfonate to prevent impaction and to eliminate the so-

---

TREATMENT FOR HYPERKALEMIA

Cation exchange resins (e.g., Kayexalate) by mouth or rectum

Intravenous calcium gluconate or calcium chloride, 5 to 10 mL of a 10% solution to antagonize cardiac depressant effects

Sodium bicarbonate 1 or 2 ampules intravenously to correct acidosis and move potassium back into cells

Regular insulin in 250 to 500 mL of 10% dextrose intravenously, 10 to 15 units, over 30 to 60 minutes to shift potassium back into cells

Diuretic therapy to cause potassium excretion in the urine

Dialysis to reestablish electrolyte balance and correct acidosis

---

dium released by the exchange resins. As the serum potassium approaches 6.5 mEq/L, ECG changes may be noted and indicate the need for more aggressive therapy. Emergency measures to reduce the cardiotoxic effects of severe hyperkalemia include the intravenous administration of various drugs including 50% glucose and regular insulin, sodium bicarbonate, and calcium gluconate. See Chapter 12 for a discussion of hyperkalemia.

Metabolic acidosis results from decreased renal excretion of fixed acids and from impaired regulation of bicarbonate and potassium. Respiratory efforts at buffering the metabolic acidosis through hyperventilation and excretion of carbon dioxide may be insufficient, and dialysis may be required to control the acidemia.

A reduction in metabolic wastes can be enhanced through dietary control. A diet low in protein but high in fats and carbohydrates can provide energy and spare the body's protein stores, thus decreasing the production of nonprotein nitrogen wastes. Urea is recycled by the body to synthesize amino acids for protein building and tissue repair, even though protein intake is minimal.[16] The diet will also be restricted in sodium and potassium.

Gastrointestinal disturbances such as nausea and vomiting that result from uremia are best controlled with dialysis. Antiemetics seem to offer minimal relief from symptoms. If oral intake is insufficient to meet the body's requirements, then parenteral nutrition or tube feedings may be required. Intralipid infusions can also be given as a dietary supplement to provide a good source of nonprotein calories. The major goal of dietary management is to decrease catabolism of body protein and prevent ketosis from the breakdown of body fat.

A significant number of patients, particularly elderly ones, with ARF die because of secondary infections. Meticulous aseptic technique is critical, as is protection from other patients who have infectious diseases. Indwelling Foley catheters are avoided because of the great potential for introducing infectious organisms. The patient is monitored carefully for evidence of infection, such as fever, swelling, redness, pain, or leukocytosis. Aggressive antibiotic therapy is warranted, keeping in mind that the kidney is the route of excretion for many drugs.

Uremic pericarditis may occur in many of these patients. Symptoms include pleuritic pain, which may be relieved by assuming the upright position, a pericardial friction rub, tachycardia, and fever. Treatment is aimed at decreasing inflammation through the use of steroids or nonsteroidal antiinflammatory agents. If the patient is hemodynamically compromised, pericardiocentesis or pericardiectomy may be required.[13]

If dialysis becomes necessary, the clinical situation will determine which type of dialysis is most appropriate. The goals of dialysis are to reestablish fluid and electrolyte balance, correct acidosis, and control symptomatic uremia.

Diuretic phase

The patient recovering from ARF will enter the diuretic phase within a few days to weeks after the initial insult. Although an increase in urine output signals that some nephrons are healing, the kidneys are not yet healed. Tubular function remains altered as evidenced by the large amounts of sodium and potassium lost in the urine. The BUN and creatinine continue to rise during the first few days of diuresis and actually act as an osmotic diuretic. Dehydration may occur; therefore fluids and electrolytes may need to be replaced in the later phases of diuresis. Dialysis may still be required to clear the uremic toxins and maintain optimal fluid balance.

CHRONIC RENAL FAILURE
Definition/Etiology

Chronic renal failure (CRF) results from a variety of disorders and is characterized by progressive, irreversible damage to the nephrons and glomeruli. Recurrent kidney infections or vascular damage from diabetes or hypertension can lead to scarring of the renal tissue and are but a few of the potential causes of CRF. It may also result from unresolved ARF. For a more detailed list see the box above. Renal damage may be diffuse or limited to only one kidney. The renal parenchyma is primarily affected. Regardless of the cause, the result is gradually decreasing GFR, tubular function, and reabsorptive capability, lead-

CAUSES OF CHRONIC RENAL FAILURE

Infections	Hyperoxaluria
Pyelonephritis	Obstruction
Tuberculosis	Prostatic hypertrophy
Hereditary and congenital etiology	Calculi
Polycystic disease	Tumor
Medullary cystic disease	Stenosis
Renal hypoplasia	Congenital abnormalities
Glomerular disease	Immunologic etiology
Glomerulonephritis	Diabetes mellitus
Nephrotic syndrome	Goodpasture's syndrome
Tubular diseases	Vascular etiology
Renal tubular acidosis	Sickle cell anemia
Chronic electrolyte imbalances	Hypertension
Collagen diseases	Thrombosis
Scleroderma	Renal infarction
Systemic lupus erythematosus	Cancer
Polyarteritis nodosa	Radiation nephritis
Metabolic diseases	Nephrotoxin induced
Amyloidosis	

ing to dysfunction in fluid and electrolyte control, acid-base disturbance, and systemic problems. Generally, a gradual progression toward uremia occurs. Dialysis becomes necessary as renal function diminishes.

The pathogenesis of CRF or **end-stage renal disease** is characterized by progressive, irreversible destruction of the nephron. As renal function declines, the end products of protein metabolism accumulate in the blood (azotemia). The intact nephron hypothesis postulates that some nephrons remain intact, whereas others are progressively destroyed. The intact nephrons maximize their function as they adapt to the increased requirement to filter the solute load. This adaptive response maintains renal function until about three fourths of the nephrons are destroyed. However, as they hypertrophy, they begin to lose their ability to concentrate the urine adequately. As a consequence, a large volume of dilute urine is excreted, predisposing the patient to fluid depletion. One of the earliest signs of renal failure is isosthenuria-polyuria with excretion of urine that is almost isotonic with plasma, that is, about 300 mOsm/L.[2] The tubules also begin to lose their ability to reabsorb electrolytes. This may lead to renal "salt wasting" and intensify the polyuria. As the disease progresses and the body is unable to rid itself of waste products through the kidneys, clinical uremia results. Eventually, the fluid and chemical imbalances in the body begin to affect other body systems.

Clinical Manifestations

The patient tends to retain sodium and water, resulting in a "waterlogged" state. This is evidenced by edema, hypertension, and potential congestive heart failure and pulmonary edema. Activation of the renin-angiotensin-aldosterone system may aggravate the fluid imbalance and hypertension. Certain patients tend to lose salt, resulting in water loss and hypovolemia. Nausea, vomiting, and diarrhea may also worsen the fluid and electrolyte imbalance.

The most common electrolyte imbalances occur with sodium, chloride, potassium, calcium, magnesium, and phosphorus. The patient with CRF can no longer regulate sodium excretion. Hyponatremia may be the result of salt wasting, diarrhea, or vomiting. Hypernatremia results from decreased renal excretion.

Potassium is excreted mainly by the kidneys; however, hyperkalemia does not usually develop until late in the course of the disease as long as water balance and metabolic acidosis are controlled. Hyperkalemia is characteristic of end-stage renal disease. Problems associated with hyperkalemia include depression of the contractile force of the myocardium and ECG changes.

Calcium and phosphorus are present in inverse relationship to one another in the plasma. In CRF the kidneys are no longer able to adequately excrete phosphorus in the urine by buffering the hydrogen ion. As the serum phosphorus level rises, the plasma ionized calcium level decreases, stimulating the release of parathyroid hormone. In turn, this stimulates the mobilization of calcium and phosphorus from the bones, resulting in renal osteodystrophy with loss of the supporting structural matrix. This condition has sometimes been called renal rickets in children. Renal osteodystrophy may also be aggravated as a result of chronic metabolic acidosis and the attempt to use bone salts to buffer the acidosis. With the aid of parathyroid hormone, the kidneys normally metabolize vitamin D to 1,25-dihydroxycholecalciferol, the most potent form necessary for adequate gastrointestinal absorption of calcium. In chronic renal failure the secondary hyperparathyroidism that results from calcium/phosphorus imbalances also results in altered metabolism of vitamin D.

In end-stage renal disease, magnesium ingestion may cause phosphorus levels to become elevated and potentially can lead to cardiac or pulmonary arrest.

Metabolic acidosis is a hallmark of renal disease.

The diseased kidneys are unable to excrete metabolic acids and to conserve bicarbonate. Generally, the decreased excretion of hydrogen ions is proportionate to the decrease in GFR.[3]

Metabolic changes in renal failure are also evidenced by the retention of metabolic waste products such as BUN and creatinine. Carbohydrate intolerance results from impaired peripheral insulin use. The half-life of insulin is prolonged in renal failure; however, this is usually not clinically significant. An almost universal finding in CRF is the elevated triglyceride level causing type IV hyperlipidemia. This is thought to be caused by increased production of lipids by the liver in response to the elevated serum glucose and insulin levels and a reduction in the assimilation of lipids in the peripheral tissues.[13]

The hematopoietic system is also affected by CRF. One of the functions of the kidney is to produce erythropoietin, which stimulates the production of red blood cells by the bone marrow. Depressed secretion of erythropoietin leads to anemia. Other factors that contribute to the anemia include (1) the accumulation of circulating toxins that further suppress bone marrow red cell production; (2) secondary hyperparathyroidism that stimulates fibrous tissue or osteitis fibrosis, taking up space in the bone marrow and decreasing red blood cell production; (3) a shortened life span of red blood cells because of the toxic effects of urea; and (4) bleeding tendencies (caused by decreased platelet adhesiveness as a result of the effects of urea), leading to purpura and the potential for stress ulceration and gastrointestinal bleeding.[3]

Neurologic complications such as headache, fatigue, irritability, and depression resulting from CRF usually develop slowly. Uremic neurologic disorders may be categorized as uremic encephalopathy and peripheral neuropathy.

Uremic encephalopathy affects the central nervous system in ways similar to other toxic or metabolic disorders. The first signs are usually a reduction in alertness and awareness. Afterward, inattention, loss of recent memory, and perceptual errors in identifying persons and objects may occur.[17] In terminal stages the patient may become delirious or comatose. These effects on the central nervous system are thought to be caused by the accumulation of uremic toxins, a deficiency in ionized calcium in the spinal fluid with retention of potassium and phosphates, hypertensive episodes, and altered fluid states.[3]

Symptoms of peripheral neuropathy occur early in uremia. It more commonly affects the lower extremities and involves both motor and sensory functions, causing burning sensations and numbness in the legs and feet. The symptoms are usually symmetric. A common disturbance involving the peripheral nerves of the legs and feet is present in 40% of patients with uremia.[3] It causes deep crawling, itching, prickling sensations that are usually more intense at night. Moving the legs about brings some relief, hence the name "restless legs syndrome." Even in the absence of peripheral neuropathy, evidence of autonomic dysfunction such as hypotension or impotence may occur.[3]

The most common gastrointestinal disturbances seen in uremia are nausea, vomiting, anorexia, and hiccoughs. The breakdown of salivary urea to ammonia causes uremic fetor, or breath that has the odor of urine. This leads to a metallic taste in the mouth that further depresses the patient's appetite. The patient's breath may smell fishy, fetid, or ammoniac. The cause of nausea and vomiting is unclear but may be related to the production of ammonia, a gastric irritant, as urea is decomposed by the intestinal flora. In addition, parathyroid hormone increases gastric acid secretion. This, along with increased bleeding tendencies as a result of platelet dysfunction, may contribute to the gastrointestinal disturbances. Of those patients with uremia, 40% to 60% have gastritis or peptic ulcer disease.[3] Stomatitis with buccal mucosa ulceration is common. Constipation is often a problem, resulting from fluid restriction, decreased activity, and the use of phosphate-binding agents.

As mentioned earlier, CRF leads to fluid imbalance, hypertension, and congestive heart failure. Also, the buildup of uremic toxins can lead to pericarditis in as many as 50% of patients with CRF. Symptoms of pericarditis include pain, a pericardial friction rub, fever, and tachycardia. A different kind of pericarditis is seen in patients on dialysis and is believed to be caused by the effects of stress, infection, or heparinization.[17] Pericarditis may progress to pericardial effusion and cardiac tamponade. It is possible that 50% to 65% of deaths occurring during CRF result from cardiovascular complications.[13]

Atherosclerosis is accelerated in CRF because of altered lipid and carbohydrate metabolism, hyperparathyroidism, and impaired fibrinolysis leading to the development of microemboli.[13] Vascular calcifications may be seen in the ankles, heart, abdominal aorta, pelvis, feet, hands, and wrists.

CRF leads to several integumentary changes. Secondary hyperparathyroidism and calcium deposits in the skin lead to severe pruritus. In advanced stages of renal failure, pruritus is aggravated by the appearance of **uremic frost**—urate crystals that are excreted through the skin in an attempt to rid the body of waste products. Continued scratching of the skin may lead to skin excoriation. Bleeding tendencies caused by platelet dysfunction may lead to petechiae, purpura, and increased bruising.

The color of the skin changes, in part because of the pallor of anemia and the yellowish hue imparted by retained urechrome pigments. Color changes oc-

cur in the nail beds as well. They may be seen as a dark band just behind the leading edge of the nail, with a white band behind that. This is known as Terry's nails.[17] Another nail pattern is the appearance of red bands known as Muehrcke's lines.[13] Nails are thin and brittle. The hair is also brittle and tends to fall out.

The effects of CRF on the respiratory system can be seen as pulmonary edema from fluid overload; pleuritis, especially when pericarditis develops; and a compensatory increase in the respiratory rate as the lungs attempt to blow off more carbon dioxide to compensate for the metabolic acidosis.

There is a reduction in estrogen and testosterone leading to amenorrhea, infertility, a decrease in testicular size, and male impotence. Men and women both report a decrease in libido. This may be the result of both physiologic and psychologic factors. Sexual dysfunction may be a source of great emotional distress for the patient and partner.

Table 42-3 summarizes the various effects of renal failure on the body systems.

Therapeutic Management

Therapeutic management of CRF is directed at conservative measures that help control or relieve symptoms or more aggressive interventions such as dialysis, hemofiltration, and transplantation. Conservative therapeutic measures are aimed at relieving symptoms of fluid and electrolyte imbalance, providing optimal dietary control, and addressing the disturbances that occur among the various body systems, so the patient can maintain an optimal quality of life.

Fluid imbalances are one of the earliest signs of renal failure. Most patients retain sodium and water and therefore have symptoms of fluid overload such as hypertension, congestive heart failure, and edema; however, certain patients are unable to conserve sodium in their urine, and this salt wasting leads to dehydration. Treatment is aimed at maintaining the patient in a normovolemic, normotensive state. Symptoms of fluid overload are managed through sodium and fluid restrictions and the use of diuretics and antihypertensive drugs. Stringent regulation of fluids is usually not necessary until later in the disease. Thiazide diuretics may be used early in the disease to facilitate water excretion but become ineffective when the GFR is less than 20 mL/min, at which time loop diuretics such as furosemide (Lasix) may be used. A variety of antihypertensive drugs may be used, including beta-adrenergic antagonists such as propranolol, which may decrease renin release.[11]

Electrolyte imbalances such as hyperkalemia must be treated to prevent cardiac dysrhythmias and potential cardiac arrest. Dietary restrictions

TABLE 42-3   Effects of Renal Failure on Various Body Systems

Body system	Causes	Signs/symptoms	Assessment parameters
Hematopoietic	Suppression of red blood cell production Decreased survival time of red blood cells Loss of blood through bleeding Loss of blood during dialysis Mild thrombocytopenia Decreased activity of platelets	Anemia Leukocytosis Defects in platelet function Thrombocytopenia	Hematocrit Hemoglobin Platelet count Observe for bruising, hematemesis, melena
Cardiovascular	Fluid overload Renin-angiotensin mechanism Fluid overload, anemia Chronic hypertension Calcification of soft tissues Uremic toxins in pericardial fluid Fibrin formation on epicardium	Hypervolemia Hypertension Tachycardia Dysrhythmias Congestive heart failure Pericarditis	Vital signs Body weight ECG Heart sounds Monitor electrolytes Assess for pain
Gastrointestinal	Change in platelet activity Serum uremic toxins Electrolyte imbalances Urea converted to ammonia by saliva	Anorexia Nausea and vomiting Gastrointestinal bleeding Abdominal distention Diarrhea Constipation Uremic fetor (halitosis)	Monitor intake and output Hematocrit Hemoglobin Guaiac test all stools Assess quality of stools Assess for abdominal pain
Neurologic	Uremic toxins Electrolyte imbalances Cerebral swelling resulting from fluid shifting	Lethargy, confusion Convulsions Stupor, coma Sleep disturbances Unusual behavior Asterixis Muscle irritability	Level of orientation Level of consciousness Reflexes EEG Electrolyte levels
Skeletal	Decreased calcium absorption Decreased phosphate excretion	Osteodystrophy Renal rickets Joint pain	Serum phosphorus Serum calcium Assess for joint pain
Skin	Anemia Pigment retained Decreased size of sweat glands Decreased activity of oil glands Dry skin; phosphate deposits	Pallor Pigmentation Pruritus Ecchymosis Excoriation Uremic frost	Observe for bruising Assess color of skin Assess integrity of skin Observe for scratching
Genitourinary	Damaged nephrons	Decreased urine output Decreased urine specific gravity Proteinuria Casts and cells in urine Decreased urine sodium	Monitor intake and output Serum creatinine BUN Serum electrolytes Urine specific gravity Urine electrolytes

may suffice early in the disease, as long as urine output is at least 1 L/day. Patients are reminded that many salt substitutes contain potassium chloride and must be avoided. When serum potassium measurements approach critical levels, drug therapy or dialysis is instituted. (Refer to the discussion under ARF.)

When the kidneys fail, phosphate excretion is impaired and hyperphosphatemia results. Since phosphate and calcium are present in inverse proportions in the plasma the resultant hypocalcemia causes stimulation of the parathyroid hormone to effect calcium and phosphorus demineralization of bone. This vicious cycle of hyperphosphatemia, parathyroid stimulation, and bone demineralization leads to renal osteodystrophy and potential secondary hyperparathyroidism. Therapeutic management is aimed at maintaining an acceptable phosphate level so these problems can be avoided. One method of treatment is the administration of aluminum hydroxide gels with meals. These preparations bind phosphorus in the intestine, allowing for fecal excretion. Since these preparations can be constipating, they should be given with a stool softener. The continued use of aluminum hydroxide gels can lead to excessive absorption of aluminum, which can cause aluminum bone disease (osteomalacia) and possibly aluminum encephalopathy. Therefore calcium carbonate is now being used as a substitute for aluminum-containing preparations, forming relatively insoluble complexes with dietary phosphates that are excreted in the stool.[11]

Supplemental calcium and the active form of vitamin D, calcitriol, may be given to treat hypocalcemia that persists in spite of controlled phosphate levels. The diseased kidney is unable to metabolize vitamin D to its active form, leading to poor absorption of calcium from the intestinal tract. It is important to lower the phosphate level before administering either vitamin D or calcium preparations, because if both calcium and phosphate levels are elevated, they may precipitate in soft tissue. If the renal bone disease remains severe, as evidenced by bone scan, a subtotal parathyroidectomy may be performed. This will decrease the secretion of parathyroid hormone and resultant bone demineralization.

Metabolic acidosis is generally controlled through dietary management and dialysis. Patients with CRF adjust to lower-than-normal serum bicarbonate levels and do not become acutely symptomatic until serum bicarbonate levels drop to 15 or 16 mEq/L. At that time bicarbonate may need to be given or the patient may need dialysis. Restriction of dietary protein intake can significantly reduce the nitrogenous waste products of metabolism. Studies now indicate that maintaining a daily protein intake below 50 g may slow the progression of renal failure.[29] Proteins included in the diet must be of high biologic value,

such as eggs, milk, poultry, and meat. This allows more efficient use of essential amino acids with less nitrogenous waste. Protein restriction also limits acid, phosphorus, and potassium accumulation. As noted under the discussion of dietary management for ARF, a diet high in carbohydrates and fats provides sufficient calories to ensure that catabolism is reduced or prevented. As uremia progresses, nausea and vomiting occur. Dietary intake may be insufficient, and the patient may be placed on enteral diets or parenteral nutrition.

Patients who require dialysis can increase their protein intake. Protein intake can be increased to 1 to 1.5 g/kg of ideal body weight for patients on hemodialysis. Guidelines for those patients on peritoneal dialysis are increased to 1.5 to 2 g/kg of ideal body weight, since large amounts of albumin are lost in the peritoneal dialysate.[11]

Water-soluble vitamin supplements may be ordered since low-protein diets are usually deficient in these. These vitamins include folic acid, pyridoxine, vitamin B complex, and ascorbic acid. If the patient has an existing coagulopathy, vitamin K may be included.

Anemia associated with CRF is the result of a variety of causes including decreased erythropoiesis, a decreased life span of red blood cells, increased platelet fragility, and a tendency for gastrointestinal bleeding caused by uremia. Hematocrit levels of 16% to 22% are common in these individuals. Supplemental folic acid or iron preparations are usually included in the management of these patients. Oral iron preparations should not be given at the same time as antacids, since they act to decrease the absorption of iron from the gastrointestinal tract. Androgen therapy (testosterone propionate, nandrolone decanoate, and fluoxymesterone) has been helpful in stimulating red blood cell production in some patients. However, the side effects of long-term use of these preparations include hirsutism, voice changes, and acne in women and increased muscle bulk, improved sexual function, and priapism in men.[11] Human recombinant erythropoietin, or epoetin alfa (Epogen), has recently become available as a result of advances in recombinant DNA technology. Patients with chronic renal failure who exhibit low hematocrits (less than 30%) can benefit from intravenous or subcutaneous injections three times per week. Clinical improvement is generally not seen for 2 to 6 weeks after initiation of therapy. The most common adverse effect has been the development or aggravation of hypertension. This is caused in part by hemodynamic changes as the hematocrit increases and also by an increase in platelets that may increase clotting tendencies. Because excessively rapid rises in hematocrit and seizures may be correlated, patients are cautioned to avoid activities such as driving or operating heavy machinery during the initiation of therapy. An increase in clotting tendency may mandate adjustments to heparin therapy during dialysis treatment to prevent clotting in the lines.

Blood transfusions are generally avoided unless the patient exhibits acute symptoms such as dyspnea, tachycardia, palpitations, or extreme fatigue. If transfusions are given often, the patient's own hypoxic stimulus to produce red blood cells is reduced, and the incidence of transfusion hepatitis increases. When transfusions are given, the use of packed cells will decrease the fluid intake, and the use of washed cells will possibly reduce the incidence of hepatitis and antigen-antibody buildup. Until recently transfusions were avoided because they were thought to compromise successful organ transplantation by sensitization of histocompatibility antigens. The use of pretransplant transfusion is highly controversial. However, transfusions are sometimes being used in selected patients in the pretransplant stage to decrease rejection episodes and enhance kidney survival in the recipient.[13]

Problems with the integumentary system include dry skin, pruritus, and purpura. Some relief of pruritus may be afforded by the use of topical ointments or lotions. Ultraviolet B light therapy may be useful. Dialysis has been an effective means of controlling pruritus in many people but in some cases can exacerbate the pruritus.

Since most drugs are excreted totally or partially by the kidneys, dosages must be adjusted to prevent toxicity in the patient with renal disease. Nephrotoxic drugs such as antibiotics and radiographic dyes must be used with caution. Although dialysis does not affect serum levels of digoxin, it does affect the serum potassium by lowering it. The potential for digitalis toxicity in the presence of hypokalemia is enhanced by dialysis and requires monitoring.

Dialysis

Dialysis is the process of moving fluid and particles from one fluid compartment to another across a semipermeable membrane. Clinically, dialysis is the mechanical process of removing waste products of protein metabolism, maintaining fluid and electrolyte balance, and restoring acid-base balance in patients with compromised renal function. Thus the dialysis machine becomes an artificial kidney (Figure 42-5).

The three basic types of dialysis are hemodialysis, peritoneal dialysis, and continuous hemofiltration. In all types of dialysis the patient's blood is one of the two fluid compartments. In peritoneal dialysis the patient's peritoneal cavity becomes the fluid-filled compartment with the peritoneum acting as the semipermeable membrane. Table 42-4 compares the various types of dialysis.

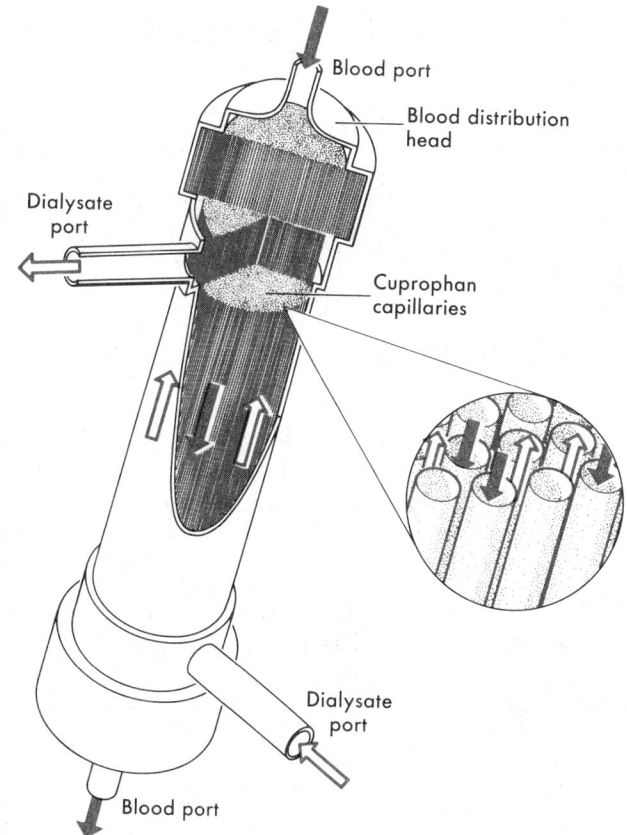

FIGURE 42-5   Hollow fiber dialyzer. Blood enters top of dialyzer and flows through thousands of tiny, hollow, threadlike fibers (cellophane capillaries), which function as a semipermeable membrane. Blood exits at bottom of dialyzer. Dialysate enters at bottom of dialyzer, flows upward around hollow fibers, and exits at top of dialyzer. Blood and dialysate flow countercurrent to each other. Arrows indicate direction of blood and dialysate flow.

Dialysis may be used in the acute phase of renal failure, or it may be used to maintain life in the patient with CRF until such time as a transplant becomes available. Dialysis may also be used to treat accidental or intentional poisonings as a means of clearing drugs or toxins from the body. The clinical status of the patient and the urgency of need for treatment will be considered when determining the method of dialysis to be used. The method of treatment should be part of a comprehensive holistic approach to health care. Today the patient can choose from a variety of dialysis methods, including in-hospital, in-center, or in-home treatments.

Dialysis is based on the principles of diffusion, osmosis, and filtration (Figure 42-6). Diffusion involves the movement of particles (ions) from an area of high concentration to an area of low concentration. Diffusion during dialysis results in the movement of electrolytes, urea, creatinine, and uric acid from the

TABLE 42-4   Comparison of Methods of Dialysis

	Hemodialysis	Peritoneal dialysis	Continuous hemofiltration
Speed	Rapid—3 to 8 hours per treatment	Slow—may do hourly runs initially and then variable or continuous runs	Slow—continuous removal of fluid and electrolytes
Advantages	Rapid correction of fluid and electrolyte problems	Advantageous for patients who cannot tolerate rapid changes in fluids and electrolytes; does not cause blood loss; immediately usable for dialysis	Advantageous for patients who cannot tolerate rapid changes in fluids and electrolytes; does not cause blood loss; immediately usable for dialysis
Disadvantages	May cause rapid shifts of fluid and electrolytes, leading to disequilibrium syndrome; vascular access required; potential blood loss; potential hepatitis B; graft or fistula must "mature" before that type of vascular access site is usable	Slower correction of fluid and electrolyte problems; requires surgical placement of peritoneal catheter; potential peritonitis; potential bowel or bladder perforation; potential exit site and tunnel infections	Requires vascular access; filter may rupture or disconnect, causing blood loss
Vascular access	Required	Not required; therefore useful for patients with vascular problems; peritoneal access required	Arterial and venous access required
Protein loss	Does not result in protein loss	Protein lost in dialysate (to 1 g/L)	Does not result in protein loss
Heparinization	Required: systemic or regional	Little or none required	Heparinization of filter tubing required; minimal systemic heparinization
Cost	Expensive	Manual—fairly expensive Automated—expensive	Filters are costly
Equipment	Complex	Manual—simple Automated—complex	Simple

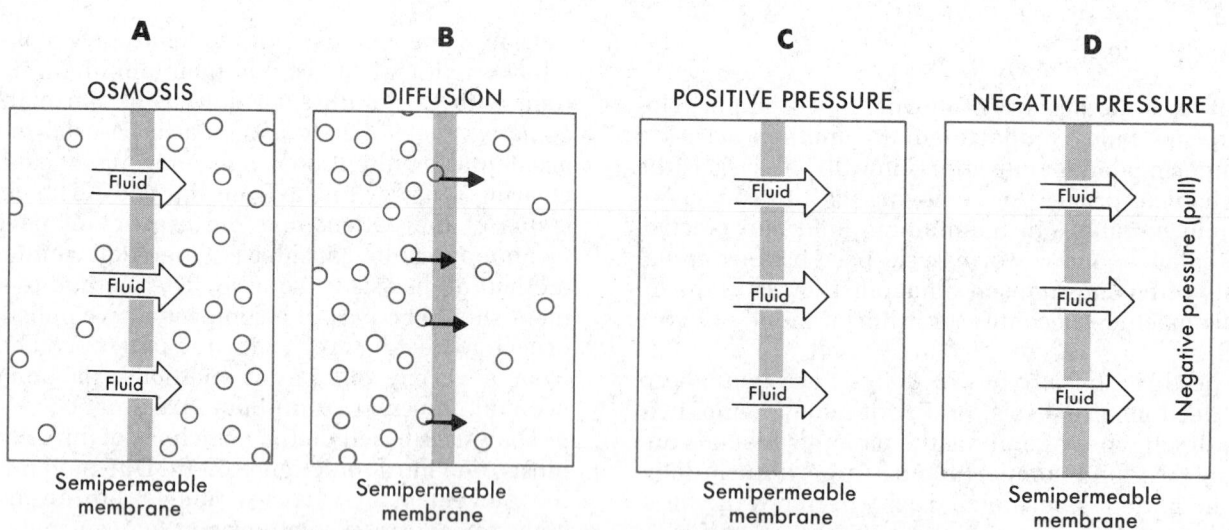

FIGURE 42-6   Principles of dialysis. **A**, Osmosis; **B**, diffusion; **C**, ultrafiltration: positive pressure; **D**, ultrafiltration: negative pressure.

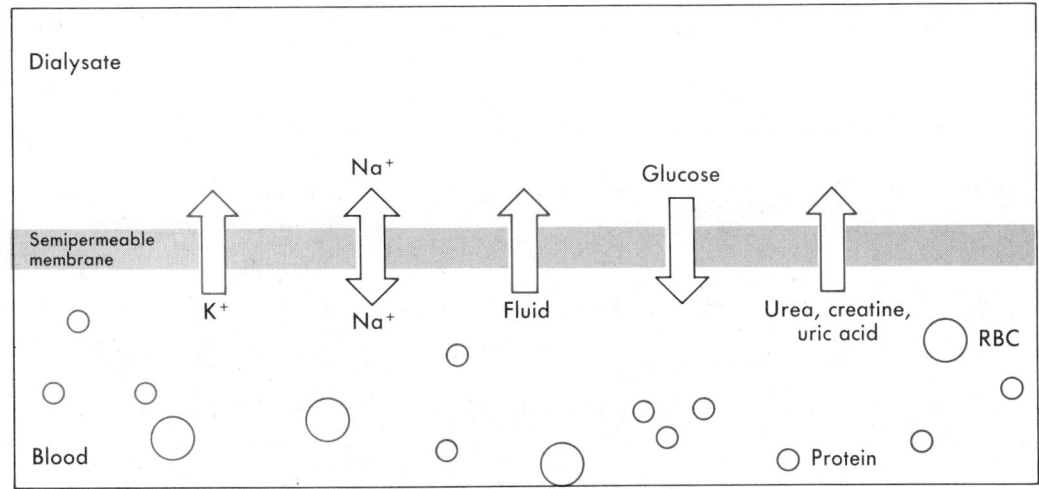

FIGURE 42-7   Dialysis: net movement of fluid and particles by osmosis and diffusion.

patient's blood into the dialysate solution. Red blood cells and protein molecules are too large to pass through the pores of the semipermeable membrane and therefore are not lost from the blood into the dialysate. Osmosis involves the movement of water across a semipermeable membrane from an area of lesser to an area of greater concentration of particles. The dialysate solution contains dextrose, which makes its particle concentration greater than the patient's blood; thus excess fluid moves from the patient into the dialysate (Figure 42-7). The greater the concentration of glucose in the dialysate, the greater the osmotic gradient to enhance fluid loss from the patient into the dialysate. For example, dialysate solution containing 4.25% glucose will pull more fluid off than will dialysate solution containing 1.5% glucose. Filtration involves the movement of fluid across a semipermeable membrane as a result of an artificially induced pressure gradient. During hemodialysis the dialysis machine produces this pressure gradient, which results in more efficient movement of fluid than does osmosis. In continuous arteriovenous hemofiltration, it is the patient's own pressure system that provides the pressure gradient for ultrafiltration.

Dialysis is begun when conservative therapeutic management proves to be insufficient in controlling the uremic symptoms in patients with CRF or when acute interventions are required, as in ARF or drug overdose. One guideline is to start dialysis when the GFR is less than 5 to 10 mL/min.[11] Another is to keep the BUN below 80 to 100 mg/dL and the serum creatinine below 8 to 10 mg/dL.[15] Immediate dialysis is needed to control pulmonary edema, hyperkalemia, or other life-threatening sequelae of renal failure.

Hemodialysis

In simple terms, **hemodialysis** involves removing "unfiltered" blood from the patient; filtering out electrolytes, urea, creatinine, and so on through the dialysis process; and returning the "filtered" blood back to the patient. To remove and return the blood, vascular access is required. A variety of methods for vascular access may be used: cannulation of a large vessel (femoral or subclavian) and insertion of two single-lumen catheters or one large double-lumen catheter (vas-cath), surgical creation of an internal arteriovenous fistula or graft, or surgical creation of an external arteriovenous shunt (Figure 42-8). Besides vascular access, hemodialysis requires anticoagulation of the blood while it is outside the body and being filtered in the dialyzer. Hemodialysis may also incorporate the use of a mechanical pump that generates artificial pressure gradients across which fluid is filtered. Hemodialysis is the most efficient form of dialysis because of the rapidity of the process.

Percutaneous femoral or subclavian catheterization can be done quickly, but these catheters are generally only for short-term use. Complications include infection, embolization, clotting, and hemorrhage. If two single-lumen catheters are used, one is inserted low in the femoral vein for blood removal and the second one is inserted higher in the vein for blood return. If one double-lumen catheter is used, the lower lumen is designated the "arterial" end for blood removal, whereas the upper lumen is designated the "venous" end for blood return.

An internal arteriovenous fistula is created surgically by anastomosing an artery to a vein. The higher arterial pressure system feeding directly into a vein causes dilation and venous engorgement. The arteriovenous fistula is not available for immediate ac-

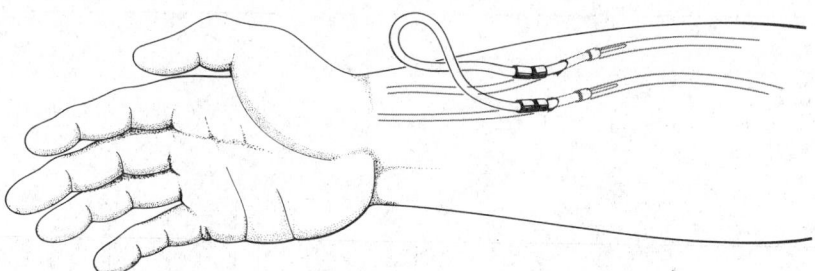

FIGURE 42-8   External arteriovenous shunt.

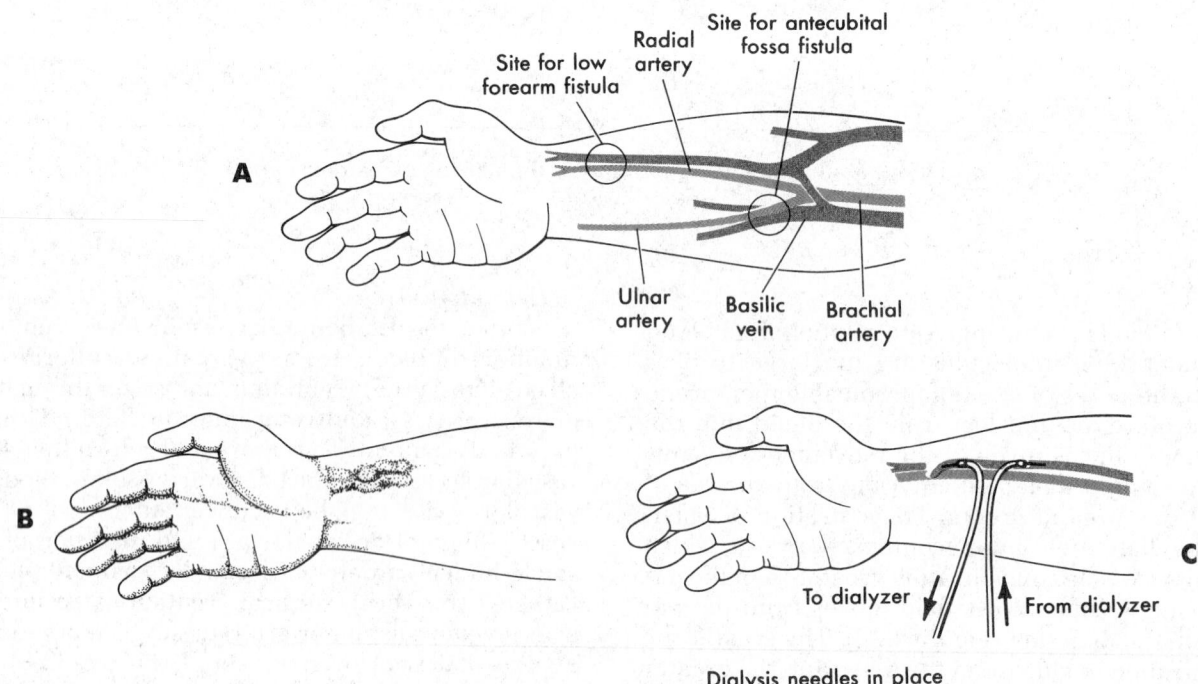

FIGURE 42-9   Internal arteriovenous fistula. **A,** Types of fistula construction. **B,** Appearance of arm with fistula. **C,** Dialysis needles in place.

cess; however, after 2 to 6 weeks, during which time the fistula "matures," the engorged vein can be punctured using large-bore needles. One needle is placed in the prominent vein, and a pump pulls the arterialized blood from the vein to the dialyzer. Blood is returned by way of a needle further up the same vein or a needle in a different vein (Figure 42-9).

An arteriovenous graft is a synthetic or vessel implant anastomosed between an artery and a vein that can be cannulated with large-bore needles for dialysis. Both the fistula and the graft have similar potential problems: thrombosis, hemorrhage, infection, aneurysm, and swelling or ischemia of the hand caused by "arterial-steal" syndrome, in which arterial perfusion to the hand suffers because too much

blood is diverted into the vein. Because both the graft and the fistula are internalized, they have the least incidence of infection for vascular access methods.

The external arteriovenous shunt requires the surgical implantation of two Silastic cannulas into an artery and a vein of the leg or arm. The ends of the two cannulas are tunneled subcutaneously to skin exit sites 2 to 4 cm from the vessel tips. Between dialyses the two cannulas are connected by means of a Teflon connector, forming a U-shaped shunt on the surface. When dialysis occurs, the connection is removed and the shunt entered. Blood is removed from the arterial cannula, pumped through the dialyzer, and returned to the venous cannula. When dialysis is complete, the two cannulas are reconnected together. Potential complications with use of the shunt are infection, hemorrhage, thrombus, ischemia, and accidental or intentional disconnection of the connecting U piece leading to exsanguination. Infection and thrombi formation are the most common complications of shunts, which make the estimated time of use of this access route only about 8 to 10 months. Because of this, external shunts are rarely used today.

Because the shunt, fistula, and graft are vascular access sites necessary for dialysis, care needs to be taken to prevent compromised blood flow to the area. The patient is instructed not to wear tight or constrictive clothing and not to sleep with his or her head on an arm. Signs are posted at the head of the patient's bed to alert health care personnel against taking blood pressures or performing venipunctures on the involved extremity. The access site is inspected for evidence of infection, and strict aseptic technique is used. The nurse must palpate for a thrill or auscultate for a bruit at the access site and notify the physician immediately if a change indicates potential thrombus formation or clotting of the access site.

Hemodialysis is a complex procedure that requires special education of the nursing staff. A variety of hemodialysis systems are in use: coil (rarely used), flat (parallel) plate, and hollow fiber. The flat plate and hollow fiber dialyzers use the balance of two hydrostatic pressure systems to control the rate and amount of fluid removal: a positive pressure system in the blood compartment and a negative pressure system in the dialysate compartment.

No matter which type of dialysis system is used, the process is the same. Within the dialysis machine, blood and dialysate compartments are separated by a semipermeable membrane. Blood is removed from the arterial end of the vascular access device, pumped through the machine at a rate of 100 to 300 mL/min, and returned to the body through the venous access. The dialysate bath is warmed to body temperature and pumped into the machine in the opposite direction of the blood at a rate of 300 to 900 mL/min. Heparin may be added to the blood at the arterial end to prevent clotting while in the machine. If the patient is at risk for bleeding, protamine sulfate, a heparin antagonist, may be added to the venous end as the blood reenters the body, or it may be given as a single dose at completion of dialysis.

The dialysate bath is specifically formulated to the patient's unique needs. For example, additional glucose may be added to the bath to create an increased osmotic gradient enhancing water removal, or dialysate with a higher-than-usual potassium concentration may be used in the patient receiving digitalis to prevent hypokalemia and potential digitalis toxicity. If the patient is extremely acidotic, sodium bi-

carbonate or sodium acetate may be added to the bath. This will diffuse into the patient's blood where it will be metabolized by the body to bicarbonate ions that can help buffer the acidosis. Thus by manipulating both the concentration of the dialysate and the hydrostatic pressures on either side of the semipermeable membrane, hemodialysis can affect the removal of fluid and waste products from the body and the addition of substances to the body that are specific to the unique needs of each patient.

Patients in ARF may require daily hemodialysis; however, hemodialysis usually lasts 3 to 5 hours and is performed three times per week. The patient with CRF may choose to be treated at a hemodialysis center or may opt for home care if a family member or friend can be trained in the procedure. About 15% of patients today use home hemodialysis.[11]

Advantages to home hemodialysis include the psychologic benefits of self-care and freedom in dialysis scheduling. A recent technologic development is the production of a portable, wearable artificial kidney that is about the size of an attache case. The dialysate is made at home by mixing a concentrated solution of dialysate with water that has been treated by a deionizing filtrating cartridge that can be directly attached to a bathroom or kitchen faucet.[11] It is currently available to only a limited patient population but offers yet another choice for patients receiving long-term hemodialysis. The portable machine allows mobility during dialysis, whereas conventional hemodialysis requires the patient to remain in a bed or recliner chair during the procedure. Most patients choose to watch television or read during dialysis.

Many patients think that they are going to feel better immediately after dialysis, but in fact that is not usually the case. Most patients experience some minor discomforts that subside after several hours. They usually feel best the day after dialysis. There are many reasons why the patient may not feel his or her best immediately after dialysis. One of the complications of the first few dialyses is the disequilibrium syndrome. This develops as a result of rapid changes in the composition of the extracellular fluid. Solutes such as urea and sodium are removed from the blood faster than from the cerebrospinal fluid and the brain.[11] The resulting higher osmotic gradient in the brain cells causes fluid to be pulled into them. This leads to cerebral edema and symptoms of nausea, vomiting, headache, restlessness, confusion, and occasionally seizures. The rapid changes in osmolality may also lead to muscle cramping and potential hypotension. Treatment is aimed at slowing the rate of dialysis and infusing mannitol or some other hypertonic solution to draw fluid from the swollen brain cells back into the circulation. Severe cases of disequilibrium syndrome are generally seen in patients whose blood chemistries were very high before dialysis; however, this process may occur to some degree in patients during each dialysis and helps explain why they do not feel their best immediately after dialysis. Hypotension and shock may result from the sudden removal of vascular volume. To avoid this, vital signs are monitored frequently and adjustments are made to the dialysis filtration rate. Additionally, rapid-acting antihypertensive drugs are usually withheld the morning of dialysis until the procedure is completed. Other drugs such as nitrates and sedatives may precipitate hypotensive episodes. The physician and nurse must carefully review medication schedules with patients to prevent such complications.

Other complications of dialysis include muscle cramping from sudden electrolyte changes, potential loss of blood, sepsis, hepatitis, and dialysis encephalopathy. Dialysis encephalopathy may be a result of aluminum toxicity. It is a progressive neurologic impairment characterized by speech disturbances, dementia, myoclonic seizures, and muscle incoordination. Aluminum toxicity occurs as a result of aluminum in the water sources used in the dialysate bath, the ingestion of aluminum-containing antacids to control phosphate levels, and the kidneys' decreased ability to excrete aluminum. Water purification systems and new phosphate-binding antacids are being studied.

Continuous hemofiltration

Continuous arteriovenous hemofiltration (CAVH) is a method of treatment for acute or chronic renal failure. It is a technology that uses the patient's own arteriovenous blood pressure gradient for filtration. The procedure is depicted in Figure 42-10. As with hemodialysis, vascular access by cannulation of a large artery and vein is required. The connection lines and filter are primed with heparinized saline solution. Unlike hemodialysis, there is no special dialysis machine. Blood flow begins at the arterial site, passes through the tubing to the filter, and returns by the venous line, all under the influence of the patient's own blood pressure. The key to this technology is the use of a highly permeable, hollow-fiber filter that measures only 12.5 cm by 4.5 cm (e.g., Amicon Diafilter 20).[36] This special filter removes plasma water and all unbound substances with a molecular weight between 500 and 10,000 daltons, producing an "ultrafiltrate."[36] The ultrafiltrate is passed on to a graduated measuring device that is positioned at the side of the bed as would be any other drainage device. A mean arterial pressure of 60 mm Hg or greater is required to produce a pressure gradient great enough to produce the ultrafiltrate. An external pump may be used to augment the rate of filtration.

Hemofiltration of micromolecules is based on the principle of convection, which is that some elements

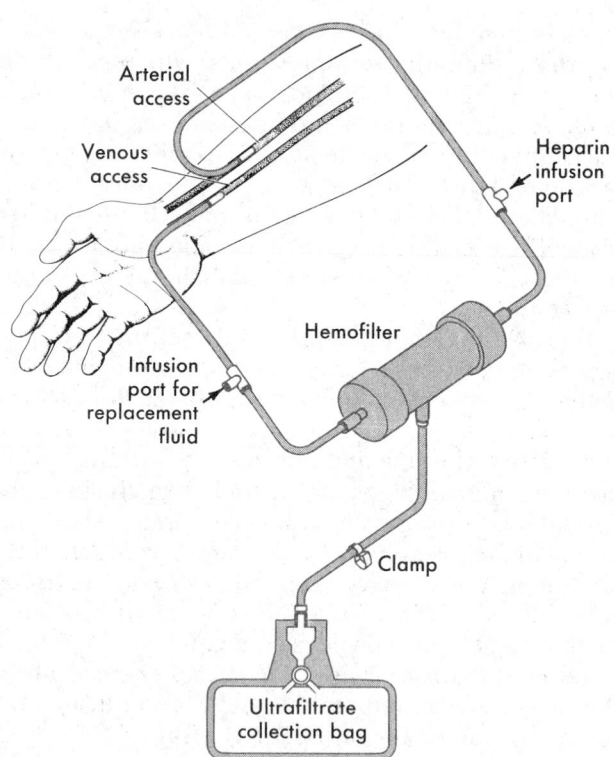

FIGURE 42-10   Continuous arteriovenous hemofiltration.

in plasma water are conveyed across a semipermeable membrane as a result of differences in hydrostatic pressure in the system.[36] Any elements larger than 10,000 daltons are retained by the filter; thus albumin, other proteins, and protein-bound substances such as certain drugs are not lost but are returned to the patient. Intermediate-sized elements such as glucose and certain vitamins are removed by convection based on the time it takes for the patient's blood to clear the filter. Therefore in low-flow states these substances may be cleared from the patient's system. Creatinine is not removed by hemofiltration as well as by hemodialysis. Hemofiltration is not as effective as dialysis in treating renal failure.

Since hemofiltration is continuous, it is not associated with the rapid fluid and electrolyte shifts seen in intermittent hemodialysis and may be well suited for patients who are hemodynamically unstable, such as patients with congestive heart failure who are resistant to diuretic therapy, or for infusing parenteral nutrition or multiple intravenous drug therapies in patients who are on fluid restrictions. The use of CAVH is limited to special care units since the patient requires close monitoring of vital signs and fluid and electrolyte balance.

Filterable solutes are removed in direct proportion to the volume of plasma water; small amounts

LEGAL ISSUES   *Refusing to Dialyze a Patient*

In this case the nurse was an at-will employee (she had no employment contract) who had been employed 11 years, with the last 3 years being in the kidney dialysis unit. During 1982 the nurse was periodically assigned by her supervisor to dialyze a double-amputee patient with many health problems. On two occasions the nurse had to cease treatment because the patient suffered cardiac arrest and severe internal hemorrhaging during the dialysis procedure.

After this the nurse was again scheduled to dialyze the same patient. She informed her head nurse that she had moral, medical, and philosophic objections to performing this procedure on this patient, because he was terminally ill and the procedure was causing the patient additional complications. The head nurse granted the nurse's request for reassignment.

The next time the same assignment was made the nurse refused again, but this time the supervisor refused to reassign the nurse. The nurse requested a meeting with the treating physician who told her that the patient's family wanted the patient kept alive through dialysis and that the patient would not survive without it. The nurse continued to refuse to perform the treatment, and the hospital fired her after asking her to reconsider, which she refused to do.

The nurse brought a lawsuit against the hospital for wrongful discharge from her job, stating that the hospital was not justified in firing her and that such termination of employment was a violation of public policy. The issue before the court was whether there is a public policy articulated in the nurse's code of ethics (the evidence presented by the nurse to substantiate her refusal) that would permit a member of the nursing profession to refuse to participate in a patient's treatment because it is against her conscience.

The trial court granted summary judgment to the hospital and stated the following:

> The nurses' code of ethics is a personal, moral judgment and permits the nurse to have personal, moral judgment, but it does not rise to public policy in the face of the general public policies that patients must be cared for in hospitals and patients must be treated basically by doctors and doctor's orders must be carried out.

The nurse argued that the summary judgment should not have been granted, because her refusal to dialyze the patient was justified as a matter of law by her adherence to the Code for Nurses. The court discussed the role of professional codes of ethics as sources of public policy in at-will employment cases. For the court to hold that an employer has violated public policy by firing an employee (in essence holding that there is a public policy exception to the at-will employment doctrine), there must be a clear mandate of public policy. The court stated that whole statutes and judicial opinions contain public policy and that a professional code of ethics may contain an expression of public policy, but not all such sources express a clear mandate of public policy.

The court stated that a code of ethics designed to serve only the interests of a profession would not be sufficient; public policy benefits the entire public and cannot be contained in a document that defines a standard of conduct beneficial only to the individual nurse.

Important to the court's analysis was the fact that the nurse never referred to her obligations according to her code of ethics when she told the head nurse she would not care for the patient. In fact, the nurse told the head nurse she was motivated by her own personal morals. Additionally, the court noted that the patient and family had requested that dialysis be continued and that patients have a fundamental right to expect that medical treatment will not be terminated against their will. The court noted that this basic policy clearly outweighs any policy favoring the right of the nurse to refuse to participate in treatments that the nurse personally believes threatens human dignity:

> The position asserted by the nurse serves only the individual and the nurse's profession, while leaving the public to wonder when and whether they will receive nursing care. Moreover, as the hospital argues, it would be a virtual impossibility to administer a hospital if each nurse or member of the administrative staff refused to carry out his or her duties based upon a personal private belief concerning the right to live . . .

The court concluded, "By refusing to perform the procedure she (the nurse) may have eased her own conscience, but she neither benefited the society-at-large, the patient, nor the patient's family."

Sources: *Warthen v. Toms River Comm. Mem. Hosp.*, 488 A.2d 229 (N.J.Super. A.D. 1985); American Nurses Association: *Code for nurses with interpretive statements*, 1985.

of plasma water being removed result in small amounts of filterable solutes being removed. This results in an unchanged concentration of microsolutes left in the patient's blood. To lower the concentration of solutes in the patient's blood, removed plasma must be replaced with a solution that is free of the undesired solute. For example, a sodium-free solution would be infused in the patient who is hypernatremic. The need for intravenous fluid replacement therapy is titrated according to the ultrafiltration rate required to control weight and fluid reduction. It is recommended that patients on CAVH be weighed once every shift. The need for replacement therapy adds to the overall cost of CAVH. As much as 24 to 36 L of intravenous fluid replacement may be necessary in a 24-hour period.

CAVH may be continued for up to 30 to 40 days, but the hemofilter may have to be changed every 12 to 48 hours because of clotting or changes in filtration efficiency.[36] The ultrafiltrate that is formed is clear and yellow. If it becomes bloody or blood tinged, this may indicate a rupture of the filter membrane and necessitate a change of filter.

Peritoneal dialysis

Peritoneal dialysis (see box) may be used for therapeutic management of both chronic and acute renal failure. In this form of dialysis the patient's perito-

PROCEDURE FOR PERITONEAL DIALYSIS

Procedure	Rationale

Check physician's order for dialysis
   Composition of dialysate, especially concentration of glucose
   Add drugs such as heparin or sodium bicarbonate as ordered
   Check timing of "runs" (i.e., hourly or otherwise)
	The higher the glucose concentration, the greater the osmotic pressure to pull fluid into dialysate; additional medications may be ordered by physician to correct electrolyte or acid-base imbalances; runs of dialysis may be ordered hourly or at other intervals

Warm dialysate to body temperature	Enhances vasodilation, clearances, and patient comfort; prevents heat loss; dialysate should be warmed using dry heat such as a warming cabinet, heating pad, microwave oven, or incubator; warming dialysate in a warm water bath increases risk of peritonitis; even though dried, when inverted to spike bottle or bag, some water may run down to opening and contaminate spike on dialysate tubing as it enters bottle; can be removed carefully
Prime dialysis infusion apparatus, clamp off tubing, and aseptically connect to peritoneal catheter	Tubing must be primed to prevent air entering peritoneal space; procedure requires strict aseptic technique to prevent infection at catheter site or peritonitis
Hang bottle or bag of dialysate on an intravenous pole, open clamp, and allow dialysate to infuse rapidly; reclamp	Dialysate infuses by gravity flow; infusion generally takes about 10 minutes; a slowed infusion may be caused by catheter obstruction
Allow dialysate to "dwell" within peritoneal space for 30 to 40 minutes or as ordered	Dialysis takes place during this time
Observe patient for signs of discomfort, changes in vital signs, or respiratory distress	Many patients experience abdominal fullness during dwell phase; respiratory difficulty may be caused by pressure on diaphragm; any change in vital signs because of fluid and electrolyte shifts must be managed accordingly
Place drainage bag in gravity-dependent position; open clamp on drainage tubing and allow dialysate to drain out	Drainage usually takes about 20 to 30 minutes; effluent should be odorless; color may be clear or yellow; fluid will appear slightly frothy because of presence of proteins
Measure output; maintain a running total of amount in, amount out, and difference	Goal of dialysis is to remove fluid and metabolites; patient should achieve a negative fluid balance with dialysis
Repeat steps of infusion, dwell, and drainage as ordered	Dialysis will be maintained as ordered

neal membrane becomes the surface across which dialysis takes place. A peritoneal catheter is surgically implanted between the two surfaces of peritoneum: one surface of the peritoneum lines the abdominal cavity, whereas the other covers the abdominal viscera. Dialysate is infused into the peritoneal space; allowed to "dwell," or equilibrate, inside the body while diffusion, filtration, and osmosis occur between the patient's blood and the dialysate; and then is drained from the peritoneal space.

The catheter may be inserted at the bedside with a trocar, but it is usually inserted during surgery under direct visualization. Catheters vary, but one version is about 25 cm long and has one or two Dacron cuffs that are located at the subcutaneous and peritoneal ends (Figure 42-11). The cuffs help to secure the catheter in place and seal out organisms that may track down the catheter from the insertion site.[11] The peritoneal end of the catheter contains many holes through which dialysate is infused and drained. Externally, the catheter is attached to a sterile dialysis system that is composed of the dialysate bag and connecting tubing. Initially after insertion, the catheter is usually irrigated with heparinized dialysate to clear any blood and fibrin from the system. Some physicians order that peritoneal dialysis take place immediately after catheter insertion, whereas others wait 5 to 7 days for wound healing to take place before dialysis begins. Complications of catheter insertion include infection, perforation of the bowel or bladder, and bleeding. Brown-tinged returns suggest bowel perforation, which is usually accompanied by severe pain and diarrhea. Yellow-tinged returns suggest possible bladder perforation.

Controversy exists over what constitutes a contraindication to peritoneal dialysis. Some clinicians say there are no contraindications, whereas others state that peritoneal dialysis is contraindicated in patients with abdominal adhesions, infections, or a history of multiple abdominal surgeries; obese patients with large abdominal wall and fat deposits; and those with chronic back problems, chronic obstructive pulmonary disease (COPD), or advanced peripheral vascular disease. Peritoneal dialysis offers an alternative method to hemodialysis for those patients with poor vascular access, those who are hemodynamically unstable, those awaiting maturation of a fistula or graft, diabetic patients who suffer complications such as exacerbation of vision loss during hemodialysis, and those patients who simply prefer this method for personal or religious reasons. Peritoneal dialysis has demonstrated efficacy and safety in the geriatric patient, often in spite of preexisting cardiovascular disease. The elderly patient does not incur the risks of heparinization and dramatic fluid shifts seen with hemodialysis.[24]

The three basic types of peritoneal dialysis are intermittent peritoneal dialysis, continuous ambulatory peritoneal dialysis, and cyclic continuous peri-

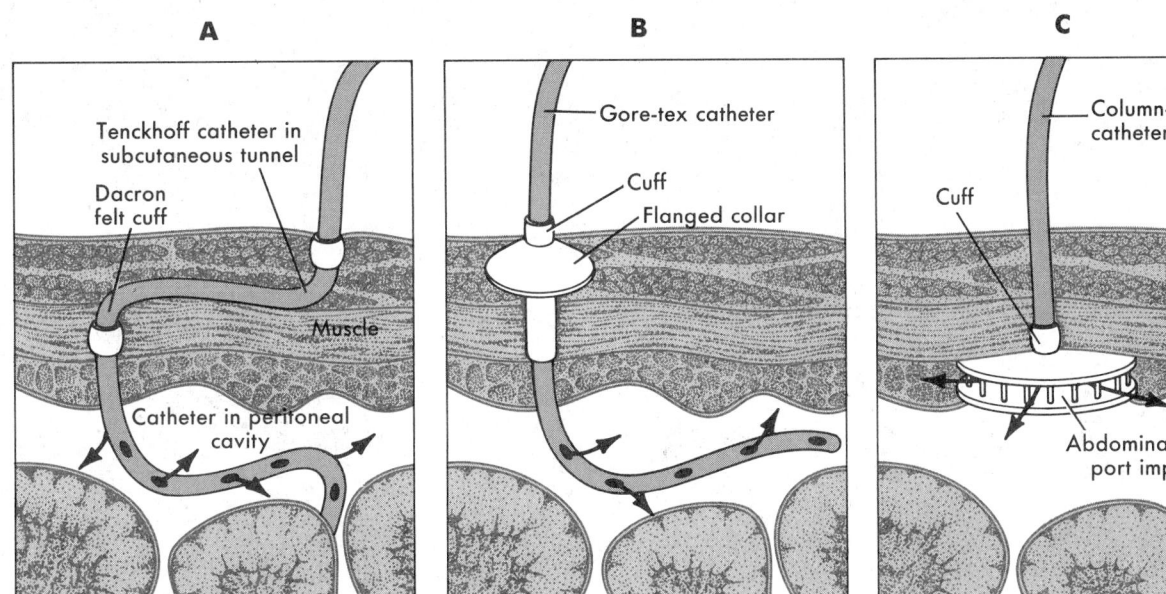

FIGURE 42-11   Three types of peritoneal dialysis catheters. **A,** Tenckhoff catheter has two Dacron felt cuffs that hold catheter in place and prevent dialysate leakage and bacterial invasion. Subcutaneous tunnel also helps prevent infection. **B,** Gore-tex catheter with Dacron cuff above flanged collar. **C,** Column-disk catheter has cuff and large abdominal entry port implant.

toneal dialysis. No matter which type is used, the process is similar. Fluid removal during dialysis depends on the osmotic gradient offered by the glucose concentration in the dialysate. Commercial solutions are available in 1 to 2 L bags of 1.5%, 2.5%, and 4.25% glucose. The electrolyte composition is similar to plasma. As with hemodialysis, substances may be added to the dialysate, depending on the individual patient's needs. Heparin is almost always added to prevent clot formation within the catheter. Diabetics may add insulin to their dialysate solution. The solution is warmed to body temperature for patient comfort, to prevent hypothermia, and to increase peritoneal clearance. The dialysate is infused, allowed to dwell, and then drained. The amount of dwell time differs among the three types of peritoneal dialysis. Equilibrium usually occurs within 15 to 30 minutes with the maximum exchange occurring in the first few minutes. Therefore the dialysate is usually left to dwell for 20 to 30 minutes when using manual dialysis or for 10 to 20 minutes when an automatic timed cycler is used.

In intermittent peritoneal dialysis the patient dialyzes three to five times per week for about 8 to 12 hours per treatment. This is usually done while the patient sleeps. Automated cycling equipment controls the inflow and drain time of the dialysate to and from the peritoneal space.

In continuous ambulatory peritoneal dialysis the patient manually infuses and drains the dialysate four or five times daily with the dwell time ranging from 4 to 8 hours each time. For example, the patient may infuse 2 L of dialysate at 7 AM. Once the dialysate is infused (it usually takes about 10 minutes), the patient clamps the tubing, rolls up the empty bag, and conceals it in the clothing, such as in a pocket or in pantyhose. The patient then engages in normal daily activities. At noon the patient may initiate another cycle. The patient places the empty bag in a dependent position, opens the clamp, and allows the solution to drain. It takes about 10 to 20 minutes for the peritoneal cavity to drain. The tubing is then reclamped, the bag disconnected and discarded, and a new run of dialysis begun (Figure 42-12). Typically, the patient on continuous ambulatory peritoneal dialysis infuses four runs during the day and one 8-hour run during the night.

Advantages to using this system are that the patient requires no special equipment, it can be carried out during normal activities with little interruption, and most importantly, the continuous process most closely approximates normal renal function. Because of this, the patient has fewer fluid and dietary restrictions, and homeostasis may be maintained more easily.

Cyclic continuous peritoneal dialysis is a combination of intermittent peritoneal dialysis at night and continuous ambulatory peritoneal dialysis during the day.[11] Using this system, three or four runs are made at night using an automatic cycling machine. The final run leaves 2 L that remain within the peritoneal space during the day and is drained out when first reattached to the automatic cycling machine at night. With this system the incidence of infection is reduced since the system is opened only twice each day, once in the morning to disconnect

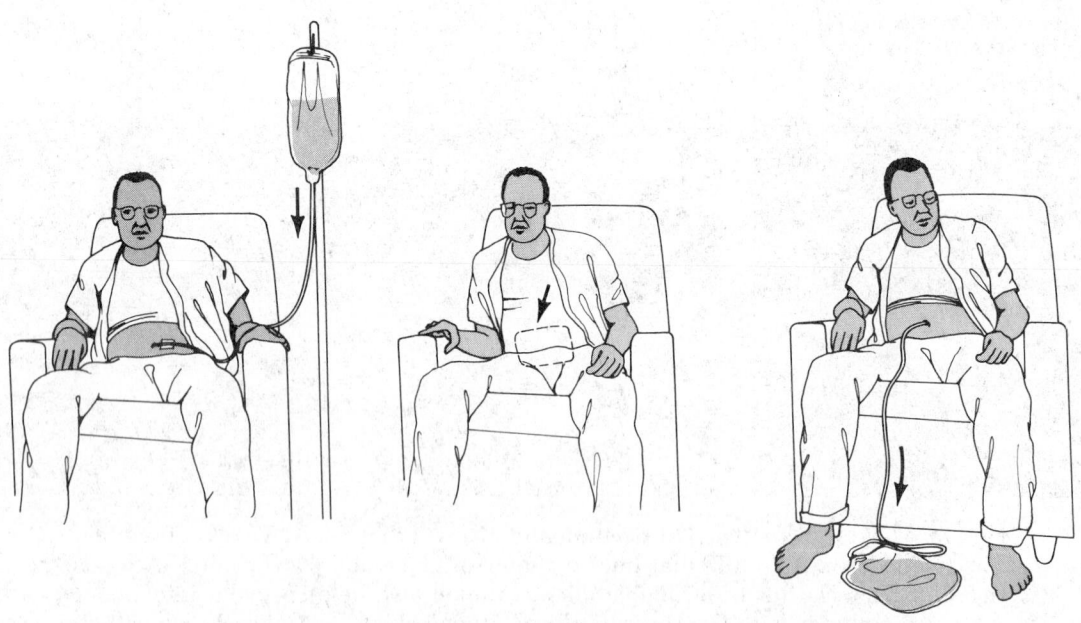

FIGURE 42-12   Patient at home with peritoneal dialysis.

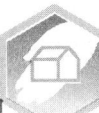

HOME CARE GUIDE   *Peritoneal Dialysis*

There are primarily two types of home peritoneal dialysis. The first is continuous ambulatory peritoneal dialysis. This type of dialysis involves 24-hour dialysis in which fluid is instilled into the peritoneal cavity, allowed to remain for a period of 4 to 6 hours, and then drained out of the peritoneal cavity. This procedure uses a special plastic container and connecting devices that are designed to be attached to a special catheter, surgically implanted through the skin into the peritoneal cavity.

The second type is continuous cycler peritoneal dialysis. This type of dialysis is designed to be used at home while the patient sleeps and is an 8- to 10-hour process. The cycler machine is connected to the implanted catheter, and it continuously fills and drains the dialysate from the abdominal cavity.

These two types of dialysis work on the same principle. Dialyzing solution is infused into the peritoneal cavity, it is left in the cavity where the peritoneum is able to act as a dialyzing membrane, and wastes pass across it into the solution in the cavity. After a specified time the solution is drained from the cavity and new solution instilled.

Because of the complex and long-term nature of the process, dialysis patients are usually referred to a dialysis center where they receive specialized education, special dialysate solution, follow-up care, and monitoring.

Short-Term Goals

By the time of discharge:
   The patient will understand the procedures needed to carry out home peritoneal dialysis and demonstrate these before discharge
   The patient will understand the physiology of peritoneal dialysis
   The patient will understand diet and fluid restrictions
   All equipment and supplies will be available for the procedure

Long-Term Goals

The patient will be able to carry out the procedure without complications
The procedure will be incorporated into the patient's life-style with the least amount of restrictions possible

Nursing Assessment

Health management pattern—The patient or caregiver must be able to understand the procedure and the need for meticulous cleanliness to prevent peritonitis and have a place to do the exchanges

Nutrition-metabolic pattern—Because continuous dialysis regulates the patient's fluid balance and metabolic environment on a 24-hour basis, the patient may be able to eat a normal diet and have only modest fluid restrictions

Elimination—Elimination of fluid and wastes is done through the dialysate

Activity and exercise—There are no restrictions on activities because of the peritoneal dialysis, but activities should be discussed with the patient's physician

Sexuality-reproductive pattern—Many persons on dialysis continue to have an active sexual life; in some cases peritoneal dialysis may result in increased sexual activity, because the person is less tired or irritable; some persons have diminished sexual desire because of the kidney disease; dialysis affects each person differently, so concerns about sexuality must be addressed individually

Planning

Planning for discharge of a patient who will be receiving home peritoneal dialysis should be done in collaboration with staff from a dialysis center
The patient must be instructed in the procedure for the continuous peritoneal dialysis:
   In a clean environment, using sterile technique, a plastic bag of sterile dialysate is attached to the catheter that enters the peritoneal cavity
   The bag is raised to shoulder level or higher
   The roller clamp on the tubing from the bag is opened, allowing the dialysate solution to run into the peritoneal cavity; gravity pulls the solution into the abdominal cavity
   Once the plastic bag is empty, the roller clamp is closed, and the bag is rolled up and placed under the clothing or in a carrying pouch; this part of the procedure takes 7 to 10 minutes
   The patient can then go about normal activities with the dialysate solution in the peritoneal cavity
When the specified time is up, usually 4 or 6 hours during the day and every 8 hours at night, the patient unrolls the plastic bag and lowers it to a level below the abdominal cavity; then the roller clamp is opened, allowing gravity to drain the fluid out of the abdominal cavity back into the original bag; this may take 20 to 35 minutes
   The bag and used dialysate solution are discarded
   A new bag of solution is attached, and the process is started over; each "exchange," which includes the time it takes to drain the solution from the abdominal cavity, attach a new bag using sterile technique, and fill the abdominal cavity, may take 30 to 45 minutes

Continued.

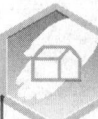

HOME CARE GUIDE   *Peritoneal Dialysis—cont'd*

Instructions in the signs and symptoms of peritonitis and fluid and electrolyte balance should also be given

Monitoring the patient's fluid and electrolyte balance must be done on an ongoing basis; the patient is taught to monitor fluid status by recording daily weight and blood pressure and glucose concentration of dialysate readings; there may be some electrolyte restrictions such as sodium, potassium, or phosphorus

Dietary restrictions and requirements must be compatible with the orders of the physician; the patient may need protein supplements because of the loss of protein through dialysis

Patients who will be using continuous cycler peritoneal dialysis will need instruction about the cycler machine that will be used in the home; the machine is usually set to run 8 to 10 hours while the patient sleeps; this machine is set up with enough dialysate to accommodate the number of prescribed exchanges; the catheter is attached to the tubing, and the dialysate is continuously cycled into and out of the peritoneal cavity throughout the night until all the exchanges have been completed

Implementation

When the patient is ready for discharge, all instructions given for care must be verified

The patient must be instructed where to get follow-up medical care, where to get dialysis supplies, and who to contact in case of an emergency; in the case of an older patient and older caregiver, a referral to an agency may be necessary

Documentation

The hospital staff nurse must document all activities related to patient education, ability to demonstrate and manage the procedure independently, and the ability of the patient to tolerate the procedure

If a dialysis center nurse is doing the teaching, this must also be documented; if the nurse is an employee of the hospital, he or she should document in the patient's medical record; if the nurse is from a freestanding dialysis center, the staff nurse must document that teaching is being done, the name and phone number of the nurse doing the teaching, and the phone number of the dialysis center

Patients with other health care needs may require a referral to a home care agency to continue to provide skilled nursing care after discharge; this also should be included in the discharge note

---

and once in the evening to reconnect to the automatic cycler.

Hourly manual runs of peritoneal dialysis may be required for the patient in ARF; however, hemodialysis is usually the treatment of choice in that situation.

Complications of peritoneal dialysis include peritonitis, obstruction to flow, abdominal pain, bleeding, electrolyte disorders, dysrhythmias, and respiratory distress.

Peritonitis is a major concern. Abdominal pain, fever, rebound tenderness, and a cloudy fluid return with presence of white blood cells support the diagnosis of peritonitis. Diarrhea, vomiting, and abdominal distention may also be present. Antibiotics can be added to the dialysate and infused directly into the peritoneal space. The patient may also require systemic antibiotic therapy. If the patient does not respond to therapy, the catheter may have to be removed and the patient placed on hemodialysis.

Infection of the catheter site is commonly caused by *Staphylococcus aureus* and *Staphylococcus epidermidis*. Antibiotic therapy is indicated. If the infection progresses down the catheter producing a subcutaneous tunnel infection, an abscess may form,

necessitating catheter removal and drainage. With proper care a catheter should last 18 months or longer. Daily catheter care involves cleansing around the site with an antiseptic solution, assessing for evidence of infection such as redness or exudate, and applying a dry sterile dressing.

Transplantation

Renal transplantation involves the surgical implantation of a human kidney from one person to another. Advances in tissue matching and immunosuppressive therapy have made transplantation a viable alternative for treatment of CRF. The renal transplant, or allograft, may be from a living donor or a cadaver donor. Living donors provide about 25% to 35% of the allografts, with cadaver donors providing the rest. Current survival rates 1 year after transplantation are 80% to 90% for related donor transplants and 70% to 90% for cadaver donor transplants.[16] Successful transplantation restores renal function; therefore the recipient no longer depends on dialysis.

The Uniform Anatomical Gift Act provides one mechanism for people to donate their organs when

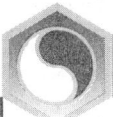

ETHICAL ISSUES

- Should a mentally retarded sibling be allowed to donate a kidney to a brother?
- If a dying patient has a signed organ donation card and consent to donation repeated in his or her advance directive, what should the nurse do? What if the family refuses to allow the donation?

they die. Once the donor kidneys have been removed, they can be preserved and transported as necessary. One way of preserving kidneys for up to 36 hours is to flush them with an electrolyte solution and pack them in cold or hypothermic storage units for transport. Another method is to use a kidney preservation pump. This machine pumps a cold electrolyte-albumin solution through the renal artery, thus decreasing the kidney's metabolic rate and allowing a preservation time of up to 72 hours. Both living and cadaveric donors must have good renal function, no evidence of infection, and no significant systemic health problem such as diabetes, hypertension, or malignancy outside the central nervous system.

In living related donors, studies have shown that the renal blood flow and GFR of the one remaining kidney have been able to increase up to 70% to 80% of the preoperative values when both kidneys were functioning. Additionally, the 24-hour creatinine clearance level can recover up to 87% of preoperative values within 6 years after surgery.[13]

Renal transplants are now performed on high-risk patients. These include patients with diabetes or previous malignancies and those who are very young or very old. Contraindications to transplantation still include chronic respiratory disease, active infection, or disseminated malignancies. Patients with extensive vascular disease, liver disease, or psychologic disorders are considered carefully. The hepatitis B carrier state is not a contraindication for transplantation, but it may negatively affect the outcome.[11]

The major requirement for successful renal transplantation is histocompatibility between the donor organ and the recipient. ABO blood group antigens and human leukocyte antigens (HLA) are important determinants of histocompatibility. Although pretransplant donor-specific blood transfusions are highly controversial, recent evidence has shown that they reduce the incidence of posttransplant rejection and increase graft survival.[11,13] The exact mechanism of action is not fully understood, but it seems that presensitization to the donor's tissue within the last few months before transplantation not only has a positive effect on graft survival, but also can iden-

tify those recipients who would respond in a negative manner to the donated organ. Potential cadaveric recipients also benefit from pretransplant blood transfusions that are matched for red blood cell types but are taken from random donors.[11]

Before organ transplantation the recipient must be in the best state of health possible at that time. The patient is usually dialyzed within 24 hours before transplantation to correct any fluid and electrolyte imbalances that exist. The recipient is also given immunosuppressive drug therapy to suppress the body's immunologic defense mechanism and to ameliorate posttransplant rejection episodes.

The surgical procedure for transplantation involves positioning the donor kidney extraperitoneally in the iliac fossa. The iliac fossa is the chosen site because of the ease of exposing the iliac blood vessels and the natural bony protection afforded to the transplanted kidney. The renal artery is anastomosed to the recipient's internal iliac (hypogastric) artery. The renal vein is anastomosed to the external iliac vein. The donor kidney's ureter is then implanted into the recipient's bladder. Diuresis usually begins immediately but may be delayed for a few days in some cases. Dialysis may be necessary postoperatively until adequate renal function is obtained.

Whenever possible, the recipient's own kidneys are left intact. It is believed that they are still physiologically active as far as certain endocrine and metabolic functions are concerned and thus add to the overall well-being of the patient. They may help to maintain erythropoietin synthesis, blood pressure control, and prostaglandin synthesis and metabolism.[16] Pretransplant nephrectomy may be required in cases where the recipient's native kidneys are infected or are the cause of significant hypertension.

The major postoperative complication is transplant rejection. Immunosuppressive drug therapy usually consists of azathioprine (Imuran) and corticosteroids. Azathioprine inhibits deoxyribonucleic acid (DNA) and ribonucleic acid (RNA) synthesis, thus suppressing antibody formation. Corticosteroids act by decreasing antibody production and inhibiting antibody-antigen complex formation. In addition, they prevent leukocyte infiltration of the graft.[16] Cyclosporine (Sandimmune) was approved by the U.S. Food and Drug Administration in 1983 for use in organ transplantation. This drug specifically inhibits antibody production that can lead to graft rejection but does not cause bone marrow suppression or alter the body's normal inflammatory response. Because of its specificity, cyclosporine has greatly enhanced graft survival even in patients at increased risk for rejection. Polyclonal antibody preparations such as antilymphocytic globulin and antithymocytic globulin may be used during periods of acute rejection. Monoclonal antibody preparations have gained recent attention in the treatment of acute rejection episodes.

NURSING MANAGEMENT OF THE PATIENT WITH RENAL FAILURE
Assessment

Nursing assessment of the patient in renal failure involves a multisystem approach, incorporating both subjective and objective data analysis. Vital to any patient assessment is a thorough history including a previous medical history, use of medications, family history, and a thorough assessment of current signs and symptoms. Certain chronic diseases such as diabetes mellitus and lupus erythematosus may lead to renal failure. Familial disorders such as renal stones or polycystic renal disease are also important assessment data.

Since inadequate renal perfusion is a major factor in renal failure, the nurse assesses for past or current problems that could lead to renal hypoperfusion. For example, a hypotensive episode would decrease renal perfusion. Hypotension can be a result of a variety of causes including cardiac disorders such as congestive heart failure, myocardial infarction, or dysrhythmias. Hypotension may also be a result of inadequate circulating volume because of fluid depletion from dehydration or blood loss. Volume depletion may result from excessive fluid losses from vomiting, nasogastric suction, or diarrhea. Certain medications, especially diuretics and those used to treat hypertension, can cause a hypotensive episode. Anaphylactic reactions to blood transfusions, drugs, foods, or insect bites are also important assessment data.

Patients with a history of vascular disorders such as peripheral vascular disease or hypertension are also at risk for development of renal disease.

The nurse must document a thorough medication history because many drugs can be nephrotoxic. Additionally, the patient is assessed for compliance with the therapeutic regimen. Omission of prescribed antihypertensive medications or drugs used to control cardiac rhythm or otherwise improve cardiac performance may precipitate renal failure. Also, the patient is assessed for use of over-the-counter drugs since many contain sodium, potassium, or agents that could alter blood pressure. Ask if the patient uses a salt substitute since many brands contain potassium.

The patient is assessed for abdominal trauma or recent surgery. Both blunt and penetrating trauma may cause renal failure resulting from organ injury, bleeding, or infection. Women are also assessed for a history of toxemia of pregnancy or recent abortion.

Infections from any source can lead to fever with fluid loss and dehydration. Also, sepsis can cause vasodilation with resulting hypotension.

Each of the major body systems is assessed for evidence of renal disease. Cardiovascular assessment includes measurement of blood pressure because both hypertension and hypotension can precipitate renal dysfunction. Cardiac dysrhythmias can compromise cardiac output and therefore renal perfusion. Febrile states can lead to dehydration. Presence of an S_3 or S_4 gallop could indicate congestive heart failure or hypertensive disease, respectively. Presence of a pericardial friction rub could indicate uremic pericarditis. An overall assessment of fluid balance can be done by looking at the mucous membranes. Are they moist or dry? What is the skin turgor? Does the patient evidence edema? Bounding pulses could indicate fluid overload. Presence of jugular venous distention indicates a higher than normal right atrial filling pressure. This could be caused by fluid overload or cardiac dysfunction.

The integumentary system is assessed for color. Pallor could indicate anemia from decreased erythropoietin production by the kidneys. Excretion of urochrome pigment through the skin will cause a pale yellow hue to the skin. Pruritus, purpura, or uremic frost may indicate renal failure. Uremia causes color changes in the nail beds as well. The nurse will assess for the presence of Terry's nails, a dark band just behind the leading edge of the nail followed by a white band, or the appearance of red bands in the nails known as Muehrcke's lines. The patient may also report brittle hair and nails.

Respiratory assessment is essential. Renal failure leads to fluid overload that can cause a "wet lung." Rales would indicate fluid at the alveolar level. Rhonchi would indicate secretions in the larger airways because of poor clearance. Patients who are debilitated may be too weak to effectively clear secretions from their airways. If the patient is in metabolic acidosis from renal failure, the appropriate compensatory response by the lungs would be to increase minute ventilation in an attempt to blow off carbon dioxide and buffer the acidic serum pH. The patient who is in acute fluid overload may present with pulmonary edema. Lung sounds will be very wet, and the patient may have frothy sputum production.

The genitourinary system assessment includes information regarding patterns of elimination. Has urine output been increasing or decreasing? Has the color of the urine become darker? This could be evidence of very concentrated urine or the presence of blood in the urine. Is the urine clear or cloudy? Presence of renal casts or cellular debris resulting from changes in renal filtration will alter the clarity of the urine. If infection is present, white blood cells will cause the urine to become cloudy. Frothy urine can indicate protein in the urine.

Assessment of the gastrointestinal system may also provide the nurse with important information about the renal system. The patient may be nauseated or vomit because of uremia. The patient may be anorexic. Uremic patients may complain of a metallic taste or uremic fetor, a smell of ammonia to the breath. A careful nursing assessment of the patient's dietary habits is important. Has there been weight loss or gain? Does the patient understand and follow dietary restrictions?

In the neurologic assessment, findings might include a change in level of consciousness. Does the family report changes in the patient's mentation? Confusion, restlessness, or drowsiness may indicate uremia. Symptoms of peripheral neuropathy are present early in uremia, so many patients complain of burning, itching, or tingling, especially in the lower extremities. If the patient is hypocalcemic, tremors or seizure activity might be evident.

The nurse also assesses for existing access sites for dialysis. Shunts, fistulas, or grafts are auscultated for presence of a bruit and palpated for evidence of a thrill. The extremity distal to the vascular access site is assessed for evidence of adequate circulation such as pulse, warmth, and sensation. If a peritoneal catheter is in place, the abdomen is assessed for evidence of potential infection such as redness, heat, or pain. The nurse must obtain information about the dialysis schedule and determine when the patient was last dialyzed.

If laboratory data are available, the nurse monitors for elevations in the BUN, creatinine, and potassium levels that could indicate renal failure. Metabolic acidosis is another common finding. The ECG is assessed for changes such as peaked T waves or a widening of the QRS segment that are consistent with hyperkalemia.

Nursing Diagnosis

Nursing diagnoses for patients with renal failure may include the following:

Altered patterns of urinary elimination related to dehydration

Fluid volume excess: actual or potential, related to decreased urine output or dietary and fluid restrictions

Anxiety or fear related to outcome of illness or stress of hospitalization

Altered health maintenance related to lack of knowledge, new or complex treatment

Impaired home maintenance management related to chronic debilitating disease, lack of support system, lack of knowledge, or insufficient finances

High risk for injury related to increased susceptibility to bleeding, fatigue, stress, or pathologic fractures

High risk for altered respiratory function related to fluid overload and fatigue

Altered nutrition: less than body requirements, related to anorexia

Impaired skin integrity related to pruritus

High risk for infection related to renal failure or compromised immune system

Activity intolerance related to renal failure, anemia, chronic fatigue, or peripheral neuropathy

Hopelessness or powerlessness related to chronic illness

Body image disturbance related to chronic disease or loss of body function

Knowledge deficit related to disease process, treatment plan, or follow-up care

Sensory-perceptual alterations related to fluid and electrolyte alterations

Sexual dysfunction related to fatigue, decreased libido, or impotence

Sleep pattern disturbance related to hospitalization or uremia

Altered thought processes related to depression or anxiety

Noncompliance related to complex, prolonged therapy

Planning

Outcome criteria for the patient in renal failure are related to the stage and severity of the disease. Ultimate goals are to restore the patient to a realistic level of wellness and to prevent further deterioration in health status, both physical and psychologic. Patient outcomes might include the following:

The patient will maintain blood pressure, heart rate, and rhythm within desired limits

The patient will reestablish and maintain a "dry" weight

The patient will adhere to fluid and dietary restrictions

The patient will ingest sufficient calories to spare protein breakdown

The patient will maintain skin integrity

The patient will use measures to protect shunt, fistula, graft, or peritoneal catheter site

The patient will demonstrate an understanding of the disease process and therapeutic regimen

The patient will state measures to prevent potential complications of the disease process

The patient will describe the rationale for use of medications and treatments and can describe potential side effects

The patient will obtain sufficient rest and sleep to make participation in normal activities of daily living possible without undue stress or fatigue

The patient will maintain optimal dialysis regimen as indicated

The patient will maintain effective coping patterns

The patient will describe a plan for ongoing health maintenance

The patient will remain free of infections

The patient will maintain a functional role within the family

Implementation

Fluid intake

Careful monitoring of intake and output is critical in the care of patients with renal failure. The physician will prescribe therapeutic interventions based on the 24-hour intake/output record and the daily body weight measurement. When the patient is critically ill, as in ARF, the nurse will record intake and output on an hourly basis. Controlled infusion pumps are used for all parenteral fluids so that absolute control of intake is maintained. If the patient is ordered to have nothing by mouth, then care is taken to provide mouth care. If the patient is allowed oral fluids, the 24-hour restricted volume is spread out among the various nursing shifts so the patient is not denied fluids during any one shift. Use of ice chips or spraying the mouth with water may help alleviate the problem of thirst. Use of lip ointments may help as well.

The nurse assesses the overall fluid status of the patient at least every 4 hours by monitoring vital signs, examining for jugular venous distention or edema, and observing mucous membranes. It is also important to assess heart and lung sounds for the presence of an S_3 or rales that would indicate fluid overload. Edema is generally first noted in dependent portions of the body such as the feet and ankles, the sacrum, and the dependent lung fields. Intravascular monitoring lines may be used when caring for the critically ill patient in order to assess hemodynamic pressures and fluid status. As the patient recovers from ARF and enters the diuretic phase, care must be taken to prevent dehydration as evidenced by weight loss, poor skin turgor, tachycardia, hypotension, dry mucous membranes, and complaints of thirst.

Dietary intake

Uremia is usually accompanied by nausea, anorexia, and an unpleasant taste in the mouth. This creates a challenge in the nutritional management of patients with renal failure. Many patients experience more nausea and vomiting in the morning; therefore serving a light breakfast in the morning and larger meals later in the day may help the patient maintain optimal nutrition.[15] Also, nausea and vomiting are more prevalent during dialysis in patients who eat within 1 hour before treatment. Dietary management is usually aimed at restricting protein, sodium, and potassium. The diet may be high in calories and essential amino acids with at least 100 g of carbohydrate per day.[10] As with any patient, pleasant surroundings and an attractively presented meal will enhance compliance with dietary restrictions and promote optimal nutrition. It has been observed that a combination of hyperalimentation and daily dialysis may promote a rapid recovery in the patient with ARF. However, meticulous care must be taken to prevent infection in these patients. They must also be monitored carefully for electrolyte imbalance and fluid overload.

Comfort/rest

The patient in renal failure often exhibits fatigue. This is caused not only by the accompanying anemia, but also by disruptions in sleep patterns. It has recently been observed that patients with CRF suffer from sleep disturbances, especially during the night before dialysis. This may be due in part to anxiety and in part to high levels of circulating uremic toxins. Nursing care should be aimed at helping the patient with activities of daily living to conserve energy and to provide periods of noninterrupted rest and sleep. Posting "Do not disturb, patient sleeping" signs may help.

Prevention of infection and injury

The patient with renal failure is particularly susceptible to infection as a result of a compromised immune system and diminished inflammatory response. Therefore it is vital that care is taken to prevent infection. Urinary catheters carry a high risk of infection and are avoided if possible. If a catheter is required, meticulous aseptic technique is used. Since the skin provides the first barrier to invasion of organisms, care must be taken to prevent injury and breakdown. Lubricating the skin with emollients may help prevent the patient from scratching and further irritating the skin. Edematous areas and bony prominences are most prone to breakdown. Frequent positioning and use of pressure mattresses are important aspects of care. The nurse cares for vascular access sites with strict aseptic technique and is alert to early signs of infection. The uremic patient may be confused. Care must be taken to prevent the patient from self-injury. The bed is kept in a low position, and siderails are raised if appropriate. Frequent orientation to surroundings is helpful.

Psychologic care

Patients in renal failure require both psychologic and physiologic care. The patient in acute failure needs frequent reassurance that care is being taken to return kidney function to normal. The patient may be frightened by the environment of a critical care unit. Careful explanations are important to the psychologic well-being of the patient and family. The patient with CRF is faced with a life-threatening disease and an uncertain future. The patient is chronically challenged with modifications in life-style, diet, and body image. Role changes may occur within the family. For example, the wife may become the breadwinner for the family if the husband can no longer work. CRF leads to alterations in sexual function that may create a threat to the integrity of the marriage and family unit. Sexual counseling may be appropriate. Chronic fatigue adds to the psychologic stress of this disease. The patient may become depressed, and concern over quality of life may bring on suicidal thoughts.

The nurse has an important role in helping the patient and family discuss their feelings and concerns in a therapeutic manner. The nurse can help the patient and family assume responsibility for managing the treatment plan. Promoting self-control and active participation in the treatment plan maximizes compliance and feelings of self-worth.

Patient teaching

An important aspect of any nursing care plan is patient teaching. All patient teaching is based on sound learning theory. The nurse must assess for patient readiness to learn and develop instructional strategies that can be individualized. Previous and ongoing learning must always be evaluated. The patient with a chronic disease not only must learn about the disease and its manifestations, but also must be able to state what types of behaviors or activities will aggravate it. It is important that patients be knowledgeable about their prescribed medications, because they may be receiving multiple drug therapies. Patients and their families must be cautioned about the patient using over-the-counter drugs without first checking with the physician. Many over-the-counter drugs are high in sodium content. Certain drugs such as nasal sprays may contain vasoactive substances that could aggravate a preexisting hypertension. Both the patient and family are instructed about how to monitor for patency of the vascular access site and how to identify signs and symptoms of complications. Because of changes in level of consciousness as a result of uremia, the patient may not be able to comprehend instruction. Actively involving the family in all aspects of patient teaching is necessary.

Preoperative care

The goal of preoperative management is to restore the physiologic and metabolic state of the patient with end-stage renal disease to optimal levels. This may involve dialysis. Meticulous attention must be paid to identifying and treating any areas of infection before surgery and subsequent initiation of immunosuppressive therapy. As with any patient, preoperative teaching is mandatory. Patients who are well informed about the surgery and postoperative course tend to have fewer complications and a shorter postoperative recovery time.

Postoperative care

The renal transplant patient is cared for in a manner similar to any surgical patient. Vital signs are monitored frequently, and the patient is assessed for excessive wound drainage. These patients, however, are immunosuppressed and may be placed in protective isolation. Meticulous hand washing is observed. Careful monitoring of fluid and electrolyte levels is essential, since dialysis may still be required after transplantation until the graft begins to function adequately. Additionally, the patient is assessed for signs and symptoms of graft rejection, including a change in urine output, edema, fever, pain or tenderness over the graft site, weight gain, an increase in blood pressure, or an elevated white blood cell or lymphocyte count.

Evaluation

All patients are evaluated on an ongoing basis for the effectiveness of therapeutic interventions. Patient outcomes are evaluated, and the individualized care plan is adjusted accordingly. Nursing interventions are effective if the patient reestablishes and maintains a stable "dry" weight and maintains the blood pressure within desired limits. Patients on dialysis will use measures to protect their dialysis access site. A successful nursing care plan will help the patient maintain dietary and fluid restrictions. It is important the patient demonstrate knowledge of the disease process and be able to describe measures that will optimize health status and help him or her remain free of infection. Finally, the patient is able to describe the rationale for use of medications and continued medical follow-up.

Documentation

A specific care plan is generated that reflects the unique needs of each patient. A vital aspect of documentation in the care of the patient with renal failure is the record of fluid intake/output, daily weight, and vital signs. Much of the care and many of the specific therapeutic interventions are based on these data. It is also imperative the nurse maintain accurate records of the patient's ongoing physical assessment findings and responses to therapeutic interventions. Finally, the nurse may be required to document vital signs, fluid intake/output, laboratory values, and medications on a dialysis or transplantation flow sheet.

Ongoing Care

Rehabilitation

The patient who recovers from ARF may not experience normal renal function for up to 1 year after the insult. The last function that returns to normal is that of concentration of urine. Until that time the patient will have to be monitored on an ongoing basis. Fluid and dietary restrictions may still be required. The patient will require physiologic and psychologic support until complete recovery is attained. These patients must be knowledgeable about the precipitating factor that caused acute failure so that they can guard against further insults. Additionally, any underlying health problem must be treated, monitored, and evaluated on an ongoing basis so that another bout of ARF can be avoided.

Long-term care

Patients with CRF face a lifetime of illness and uncertainty. They must be observed on an outpatient basis for the rest of their lives. As the disease progresses the patient may begin to question quality of life. Ongoing psychologic and physiologic support is mandatory. The strain on emotional and financial resources becomes problematic. The patient and family must be supported through this time. Effective coping strategies need to be identified and maximized. The optimal care plan will be structured around the unique wants and needs of the patient and family.

Home care

Home dialysis is one alternative for the patient with CRF. This affords the patient optimal control over health and minimizes reliance on the health care team. Patients who opt for this form of therapy are encouraged and supported in their decision. The patient and family must always be able to make informed decisions regarding ongoing therapeutic management. The patient who opts for home care must be helped to adjust the home environment and life-style to meet the needs of required care. Home health care nurses may provide the necessary assessment, diagnosis, intervention, and evaluation required for the patient on home care. If the patient opts to deny treatment, the patient will be afforded the dignity of dying at home, in a hospice, or in a hospital.

The patient in end-stage renal disease is critically ill. If the patient does not opt for dialysis or a transplant does not become available, death will occur. The signs and symptoms of end-stage renal disease are those mentioned under CRF. The symptoms, however, are grossly apparent and debilitating. For example, the patient will be severely anemic, acidotic, and dyspneic. Neurologically, the patient may be somnolent or comatose. Fluid and electrolyte alterations will be maximized. The patient will show evidence of severe uremia such as skin color changes, bleeding tendencies, uremic frost, and nausea and vomiting. It is important for nurses to understand that patients with a chronic debilitating disease may wish to deny further treatment rather than live a life that does not provide the quality they desire. Patients and their families are supported in their decisions.

CLINICAL THINKING QUESTIONS

1 What would be an appropriate home care plan for a patient on continuous ambulatory peritoneal dialysis?
2 List at least five possible causes of prerenal disease, and develop at least two nursing interventions specific to each.
3 Compare and contrast hemodialysis and peritoneal dialysis on at least five criteria.
4 List eight drugs that can be nephrotoxic.
5 Discuss at least one systemic effect that chronic renal failure has on each of the following systems: cardiovascular, respiratory, genitourinary, gastrointestinal, neurologic, integumentary, and hematopoietic.
6 Develop a low-purine meal plan appropriate to patients who form uric acid renal calculi.
7 Develop a patient teaching plan specific to the prevention of recurrent urinary tract infections.
8 Compare and contrast the oliguric and diuretic phases of ARF on at least five criteria.
9 Identify five signs or symptoms of pyelonephritis, and describe appropriate nursing interventions for each.
10 Describe at least five clinical manifestations of the uremic syndrome, and develop two nursing interventions appropriate to each.
11 How would you evaluate your nursing interventions for a patient with renal neoplasm?
12 What community resources are available to help family members and patients with CRF?

RESOURCES

1 AMERICAN KIDNEY FUND
7315 Wisconsin Ave., 203 E
Bethesda, MD 20014

2 AMERICAN NEPHROLOGY NURSES ASSOCIATION
North Woodbury Rd., Box 56
Pitman, NJ 08071

3 AMERICAN SOCIETY OF NEPHROLOGY
6900 Grove Rd.
Thorofare, NJ 08086

4 NATIONAL ASSOCIATION OF PATIENTS ON HEMODIALYSIS AND TRANSPLANTATION
505 Northern Blvd.
Great Neck, NY 11021

5 NATIONAL KIDNEY FOUNDATION
2 Park Ave.
New York, NY 10006

BIBLIOGRAPHY

Current

1. Baumann T: Minimum urine collection periods for accurate determination of creatinine clearance in critically ill patients, *Clin Pharm* 6:393, 1987.
2. Brunner LS, Suddarth DM: *Textbook of medical-surgical nursing*, ed 7, Philadelphia, 1992, JB Lippincott Co.
3. Bullock BL, Rosendahl PP: *Pathophysiology: adaptations and alterations in functions*, ed 3, Philadelphia, 1992, JB Lippincott Co.
4. Carpenito L: *Nursing diagnosis, application to clinical practice*, ed 3, Philadelphia, 1989, JB Lippincott Co.
5. Corbett JV: *Laboratory tests and diagnostic procedures with nursing diagnoses*, ed 3, Norwalk, Conn, 1992, Appleton & Lange.
6. Harkonew S, Kjellstrand C: *Exacerbation of diabetic renal failure following intravenous pyelography. Abstracts of American Society of Nephrology annual meeting*, Washington, DC, 1989, The Society.
7. Holloway NM: *Nursing the critically ill adult*, ed 3, Menlo Park, Calif, 1988, Addison-Wesley Publishing Co Inc.
8. Ignatavicius D, Bayne M: *Medical-surgical nursing: a nursing process approach*, Philadelphia, 1991, WB Saunders Co.
9. Keating S, Kelman G: *Home health care nursing: concepts and practice*, Philadelphia, 1988, JB Lippincott Co.
10. Kinney MR et al: *AACN's clinical reference for critical-care nursing*, New York, 1988, McGraw-Hill Inc.
11. Lewis SM, Collier IC: *Medical-surgical nursing: assessment and management of clinical problems*, ed 3, St Louis, 1992, Mosby–Year Book, Inc.
12. Long BC, Phipps WJ, editors: *Essentials of medical-surgical nursing: a nursing process approach*, ed 3, St Louis, 1993, Mosby–Year Book, Inc.
13. Luckmann J, Sorensen K: *Medical-surgical nursing: a psychophysiologic approach*, ed 3, Philadelphia, 1987, WB Saunders Co.
14. McKenry LM, Salerno E: *Mosby's pharmacology in nursing*, ed 18, St Louis, 1992, Mosby–Year Book, Inc.
15. Patrick M et al: *Medical-surgical nursing: pathophysiological concepts*, ed 2, Philadelphia, 1991, JB Lippincott Co.
16. Phipps WJ et al, editors: *Medical-surgical nursing: concepts and clinical practice*, ed 4, St Louis, 1991, Mosby–Year Book, Inc.
17. Porth C: *Pathophysiology: concepts of altered health states*, ed 3, Philadelphia, 1990, JB Lippincott Co.
18. Price S, Wilson L: *Pathophysiology: clinical concepts of disease processes*, ed 4, St. Louis, 1992, Mosby–Year Book, Inc.
19. Swearingen P: *Manual of nursing therapeutics*, ed 2, St Louis, 1990, Mosby–Year Book, Inc.
20. Swearingen PL et al, editors: *Manual of critical care: applying nursing diagnosis to adult critical illness*, ed 2, St Louis, 1992, Mosby–Year Book, Inc.
21. Thompson JM et al: *Clinical nursing*, ed 3, St Louis, 1993, Mosby–Year Book, Inc.

Classic

22. Binkley L: Keeping up with peritoneal dialysis, *Am J Nurs* 84:729, 1984.
23. Brezis M et al: Acute renal failure. In Brenner BM, Rector FC, editors: *The kidney*, ed 3, Philadelphia, 1986, Ardmore.
24. Cali TJ: Renal disease. In Covington TR, Walker JI: *Current geriatric therapy*, Philadelphia, 1984, WB Saunders Co.
25. Carnevali D, Patrick M: *Nursing management for the elderly*, ed 2, Philadelphia, 1986, JB Lippincott Co.
26. Eliopoulos C: *Health assessment of the older adult*, Menlo Park, Calif, 1984, Addison-Wesley Publishing Co Inc.
27. Fishbein EI: Renal disease in the elderly. In Rossman I: *Clinical geriatrics*, Philadelphia, 1986, JB Lippincott Co.
28. Harter H, Martin K: Acute renal failure: classification, education, and clinical consequences, *Postgrad Med* 72:175, 1982.
29. Hirsch D: Limited-protein diet: a means of delaying the progression of chronic renal disease? *Can Med Assoc J* 132:913, 1985.
30. Kneisl CR, Ames SW: *Adult health nursing: a biopsychosocial approach*, Reading, Mass, 1986, Addison-Wesley Publishing Co Inc.
31. Metheny N: Renal stones and urinary pH, *Am J Nurs* 82:1372, 1982.
32. Richard C: *Comprehensive nephrology nursing*, Boston, 1986, Little, Brown & Co Inc.
33. Sobota A: Inhibition of bacterial adherence by cranberry juice: potential use for the treatment of urinary tract infections, *J Urol* 131:1013, 1984.
34. Ulrich S et al: *Nursing care planning guides: a nursing diagnosis approach*, Philadelphia, 1986, WB Saunders Co.
35. Van Den Berg CJ: Clinical evaluation of renal lithiasis, *Geriatrics* 34:35, 1979.
36. Winkelman C: Hemofiltration: a new technique in critical care nursing, *Heart Lung* 265-271, 1985.

CHAPTER FORTY-THREE

Nursing Management of Adults with Urinary Tract Disorders

LEARNING OBJECTIVES

1 Describe the pathophysiology, clinical manifestations, and therapeutic management of the different types of incontinence.
2 Develop a nursing care plan for the incontinent patient.
3 Identify nursing interventions to promote urinary continence in the older adult.
4 State the pathophysiology and clinical manifestations associated with urinary retention.
5 Outline the nursing management required for urinary retention.
6 Discuss the common causes and management of urinary tract infections.
7 Identify the clinical manifestations of urinary tract infections in the older adult.
8 Develop a teaching plan that would help prevent a recurrence of a urinary tract infection.
9 Identify the major causes of urinary obstruction.

KEY TERMS

WHEN AN ALTERATION in the pattern of urinary elimination occurs, many individuals are embarrassed to discuss the problem with anyone, including a health care provider. This makes a sensitive nursing assessment of the area of urinary elimination vital, since information needs to be elicited in such a way that will not inhibit the responses of the person. The nurse needs to be aware of social attitudes about excretion held by the individual and the support system on which the patient depends. In knowing this, a plan of care can be devised to fit the individual's needs. Subsequently, implementation and evaluation of the intervention take place.

URINARY INCONTINENCE
Definition

Urinary incontinence is the involuntary loss of urine from the lower urinary tract. It often produces a social or hygienic problem. There is a wide continuum in the amount of incontinence a person may experience. It may range from continuous loss of urine associated with fecal incontinence to a slight trickle while exercising.

Etiology/Epidemiology

Estimates of incontinence reveal that over 12 million Americans may be incontinent. It is the second most common reason given for institutionalization of an older person.[16] Twenty-six percent of women between the ages of 30 and 59 report having urinary incontinence at some time.[14] Incontinence is a common cause of loss of independent life-style. The fear of embarrassment when incontinence occurs can be so great that it causes limitation of social activities and social interactions, which leads to increased social isolation. Incontinence, costly in both time and resources, is estimated to be two and one half times the expense of continent patient care.[26] This includes clothing/linen changes, laundering, cleaning, absorbent materials, treatment of skin breakdown, supplies, and nursing time. A prevalent and debilitating condition, incontinence is most common among the elderly. The noninstitutionalized elderly are believed to suffer from incontinence at a rate of 15% to 30% while approximately 50% of nursing home residents experience incontinence.[6]

Pathophysiology

The bladder is a collapsible muscular bag lined with mucous membrane that stores urine. A variety of mechanisms may be present in incontinence. As the bladder reaches capacity, the pressure makes it more difficult to control the urge for micturition, and leaking may occur. Factors such as medication, tumors, strictures, and prostatic enlargement may affect the detrusor muscle causing the bladder to become overdistended with leakage of urine.[6] Administration of anticholinergic agents may result in urinary retention with urinary frequency and overflow incontinence. In addition, environmental and psychologic inhibitors can be causative factors in certain types of incontinence. For example, difficulty in reaching the toilet in a timely fashion may increase the incidence of urinary incontinence. The physiologic effects of incontinence are skin breakdown and urinary tract infection. These occur in almost one half of incontinent patients.[26]

Urinary incontinence is separated into two categories, acute and persistent (established) incontinence.[9,17] Differentiating these two categories helps the health care provider plan a comprehensive approach to this complex health problem.

Acute (transient) incontinence

Acute incontinence is a temporary condition that may be associated with an acute illness or infection, psychologic disorders such as depression, fecal impactions, and certain medications. Both prescription and nonprescription pharmaceuticals with anticholinergic properties (antihistamines, antidepressants, anti-Parkinsonism agents) may cause transient urinary incontinence. In the older adult immobility, environmental changes, mental confusion, and metabolic changes that accompany an acute illness or infection can bring on acute incontinence. Once the cause is addressed and treated, the incontinence will resolve on its own.

Symptomatic urinary tract infections (UTIs) can cause acute incontinence. The stretch receptors in the bladder become sensitized leading to frequency, urgency, and dysuria. An appropriate antibiotic such as trimethoprim-sulfamethoxazole (Septra, Bactrim) can help relieve the problem.

Psychogenic incontinence is occasionally seen in adults with underlying emotional disturbances. Individuals in depressive states become so withdrawn and apathetic that seeking an appropriate site to empty the bladder becomes unfeasible. This may also be identified as functional incontinence.

Both prescription and nonprescription drugs often have side effects that affect bladder function. Common offenders are diuretics and central nervous system (CNS) depressants. Diuretics are commonly used in the management of hypertension and edematous conditions. The result of their therapeutic effect is diuresis, or a loss of body water, through increased urination. When mental alertness or physical ability is altered, this induced diuresis may overwhelm bladder capacity and result in incontinence. CNS depressants diminish awareness and sensation. The patient may experience a lack of interest in his/her surroundings along with a decrease in psychic

DRUGS CAPABLE OF INDUCING INCONTINENCE

Opioids
Sedatives
Hypnotics
Anticholinergics
Alpha-adrenergic antagonists
Diuretics—furosemide (Lasix)
Antispasmodics
Antidepressants—amitriptyline, imipramine
Antiparkinsonian agents—levodopa
Antidysrhythmics—digoxin
Antihistamines
Antipsychotic agents—haloperidol (Haldol)
Antihypertensives—methyldopa, propranolol, hydralazine
Anesthetics—spinal anesthetics
Alcohol
Caffeine

and motor activities. Other drugs that can cause incontinence are listed in the box above.

Fecal impaction causes an increase in rectal distention. This distention can obstruct urinary outflow. Overflow incontinence is often the result. If the impaction is removed, continence is restored.

Persistent (established) incontinence

Persistent incontinence is that which continues even after an acute illness has been resolved or the patient has ceased taking a possibly offending drug. The five classifications of persistent incontinence, recommended by the North American Nursing Diagnosis Association (1988), are stress, urge, reflex, total, and functional incontinence.

Stress incontinence, the involuntary loss of urine during coughing, sneezing, laughing, or other physical activities that increase abdominal pressure, occurs more often in women than men. Weakening of the pelvic muscles that support the bladder following childbirth is one reason for stress incontinence. It may also occur in men following transurethral resection of the prostate (TURP) (see Chapter 71). Urge incontinence, the involuntary loss of urine associated with an abrupt and strong desire to void, occurs frequently in the older adult if the patient cannot get to the toilet soon enough after perceiving the urge to urinate. It is the most common type of urinary incontinence in the elderly. Overflow incontinence is the frequent to constant leaking of urine because the patient is unable to sense bladder fullness. It may be associated with urinary retention.

However, this is often the result of a neurologic defect of the spinal cord that affects the contractility of the detrusor muscle. Functional incontinence is not an organic defect of the lower urinary tract. Rather it is the result of impaired mobility, depression, confusion, chronic organic brain syndrome (COBS), or when environmental barriers inhibit elimination. The patient may forget how to locate the bathroom or be unable to communicate the need to void.

Causes of persistent incontinence are summarized in Table 43-1. These disorders may occur alone or can exist simultaneously in the same person.

Clinical Manifestations

Incontinence may be present with a wide degree of severity. Stress incontinence involves an involuntary loss of urine when an increase in intraabdominal pressure occurs (i.e., laughing, coughing, sneezing, or exercising). Urge incontinence is characterized by the involuntary loss of urine associated with frequency and urgency. In reflex incontinence, there is a loss of urine without awareness at regular intervals. A constant flow of urine at unpredictable intervals is specific to total incontinence. Functional incontinence is the loss of urine before reaching an acceptable receptacle.

Measurement of post-void residual volume (PVR) is recommended for all patients with urinary incontinence. Catheterization or ultrasound assessment of the bladder is performed several minutes after the patient voids. A PVR less than 50 mL is considered adequate bladder emptying while more than 200 mL is considered inadequate emptying.[14,22] Urodynamic studies help determine the cause and extent of the incontinence. These studies include electromyography of sphincter activity, uroflowmetry, rectal pressure, cystometry, and urethral pressure measurement. The patient voids into a device attached to a pressure transducer and a computer measures the amount voided, the maximum and average flow rates, and the total time of voiding.[25] A urinalysis, urine culture and sensitivity, blood urea nitrogen (BUN), serum creatinine, and creatinine clearance are needed to evaluate renal/urinary function. Urine cytology is used to rule out malignancy.

Geriatric considerations

Changes in the urinary system as one ages predispose the elderly to incontinence. Consequently, patients and nursing staff expect that urinary incontinence is an unavoidable consequence of aging. This is a misconception; not all deficits in functioning are attributable to the aging process. Infections and medication are just two of the correctable causes for incontinence in the elderly.

TABLE 43-1   Causes of Persistent Urinary Incontinence

Classification	Definition	Etiology	Treatment
Stress incontinence (pelvic relaxation incontinence, urethral sphincter incontinence)	Involuntary loss of urine with increased intraabdominal pressure (e.g., coughing, laughing, or lifting)	Multiple pregnancies Obesity Menopause Prostatectomy surgery (TURP) Low estrogen level	Pelvic floor exercises (Kegel exercises) Weight reduction for obesity Bladder neck suspension surgery Topical or oral replacement of estrogen Containing garments, condom catheters Alpha-adrenergic agonists Intravaginal electrical stimulation Artificial stimulation

Urge incontinence (unstable bladder, detrusor hyperreflexic bladder, uninhibited bladder)	Loss of a large volume of urine preceded by only a brief urgency to void; urgency, frequency, bladder spasms, and nocturia are common characteristics	CNS damage
		  Cerebrovascular accident (CVA)
		  Dementia
		  Parkinson's disease
		  Alzheimer's disease
		Bladder irritation
		  Chronic UTI
		  Atrophic vaginitis
		  Cancer of the bladder
		  Tumor
		  Kidney stones
		  Radiation
		Bladder outlet obstruction
		  Benign prostatic hyperplasia (BPH)
		Decreased bladder capacity
		Others
		  High intake of alcohol, caffeine, fluids
		Idiopathic
			Treat the primary cause
			Anticholinergic or antispasmotic medications
			Bladder retraining programs
			Biofeedback
			Intravaginal electrical stimulation
			Containing garments and condom catheters

Reflex incontinence (upper motor neuron lesion)	Involuntary loss of urine that is not preceded by a warning to void; urination occurs at predictable intervals without the awareness of filling or urge to void	Lesions above S-2 level of the spinal cord (spinal cord injury, CVA, Parkinson's disease)	Treat the primary cause Intermittent self-catheterization Alpha-adrenergic blockers (internal sphincter) Baclofen, diazepam, dantrolene (external sphincter) Surgical urinary sphincter
Total incontinence	Continuous leakage of urine at unpredictable times without distention; characterized by nocturia and lack of filling awareness	Neurologic damage Trauma Fistula Congenital anomalies Sphincter damage (i.e., genitourinary [GU] surgery)	Treat primary cause Containment garments Catheter—external or indwelling Artificial urinary sphincter

TABLE 43-1	Causes of Persistent Urinary Incontinence—cont'd		
Classification	**Definition**	**Etiology**	**Treatment**
Functional incontinence	Involuntary leakage of urine in socially unacceptable circumstances; individual possesses an intact bladder and sphincter function; loss of urine occurs before reaching an appropriate site to empty the bladder	Impaired sensory, cognitive, or mobility functions Environmental barriers Alzheimer's disease Confusional states Mental retardation Locomotor deficits Iatrogenic caused by drug therapy	Bladder training program Containing garments Environmental alterations Catheters—external or indwelling

Incontinence disrupts lives as elders voluntarily isolate themselves from social activities because of embarrassment and fear of accidents or odor. Nursing's role then is to assist the elderly in finding ways to correct or manage the incontinence.

Bladder volume normally averages between 400 and 600 mL of urine with micturition volume usually 200 to 400 mL.[16] As people age there is a decrease in bladder capacity and diminished muscle tone of the bladder, pelvic muscles and sphincter. These factors may lead to nocturia, frequency, urgency, and contribute to stress or urge incontinence. Ebersole and Hess (1990) indicate that nocturia occurs in 64% of the elderly population. The reflex that initiates contraction of the bladder muscles and relaxation of the internal sphincter to produce micturation is delayed as one ages.[7] The effect of vasopressin, a hormone that produces an antidiuretic action, decreases with aging, a possible contributor to incontinence.[1] Male patients may experience hesitancy, dribbling, nocturia, and/or difficulty in initiating urination as the prostate gland enlarges.

Many of the medications that the elderly take such as sedatives, tranquilizers, and hypnotics produce drowsiness or confusion that facilitates incontinence by dulling the transmission of the desire to micturate. In addition, diuretics may contribute to incontinence by increasing output. Incontinence, most prevalent among institutionalized elders, also occurs among community-based elders. Often the elderly cope with incontinence by treating the results rather than the cause. Restricting fluid, using absorbent pads, and withdrawal from activities are just some of the coping mechanisms utilized.

Therapeutic Management

Surgical interventions

Multiple operative procedures are available for urinary incontinence. Transvaginal or transabdominal suspension of the bladder neck has proven 80% to 95% successful after 1 year in patients with stress incontinence.[16] Prostatectomy is performed in men who have incontinence or retention from benign prostatic hyperplasia. Implantation of an artificial sphincter corrects incontinence as a result of sphincter dysfunction in 70% to 90% of these patients.[6] A urethral sling restores continence by passing a ribbon of fascia or a synthetic material below the urethra to raise and squeeze the urethra.[6] Fascial slings are favored over synthetic slings because of a lower rate of severe complications. This provides correction in 80% of selected patients. Bladder reconstruction with bowel segments is performed to increase bladder capacity. Detrusor overactivity that does not respond to pharmacologic or behavioral therapy is treated surgically by augmentation cystoplasty. Individual circumstances determined by urodynamic testing will determine the procedure suitable for each individual patient.

Artificial urinary sphincter

The sphincter device is a prosthesis consisting of an inflatable cuff, a reservoir, and a control pump (Figure 43-1). Placement of an artificial sphincter is the most commonly used surgical procedure for the treatment of male urethral insufficiency.[22] The artificial sphincter has also been used for females with intrinsic sphincter deficiency. During the operative procedure, a hydraulically activated cuff is placed around either the bladder neck or bulbous urethra. The balloon is placed intraabdominally, acting as a reservoir for the cuff fluid during urination. The pump is implanted in the testicles of a man and the labia of a woman. When there is a need to void, the patient squeezes the pump. A radiopaque isotonic solution is shifted from the cuff into the balloon. Emptying the cuff releases the pressure around the urethra, allowing urine to flow. After the bladder is emptied, the fluid automatically fills the cuff, thereby constricting the urethra.

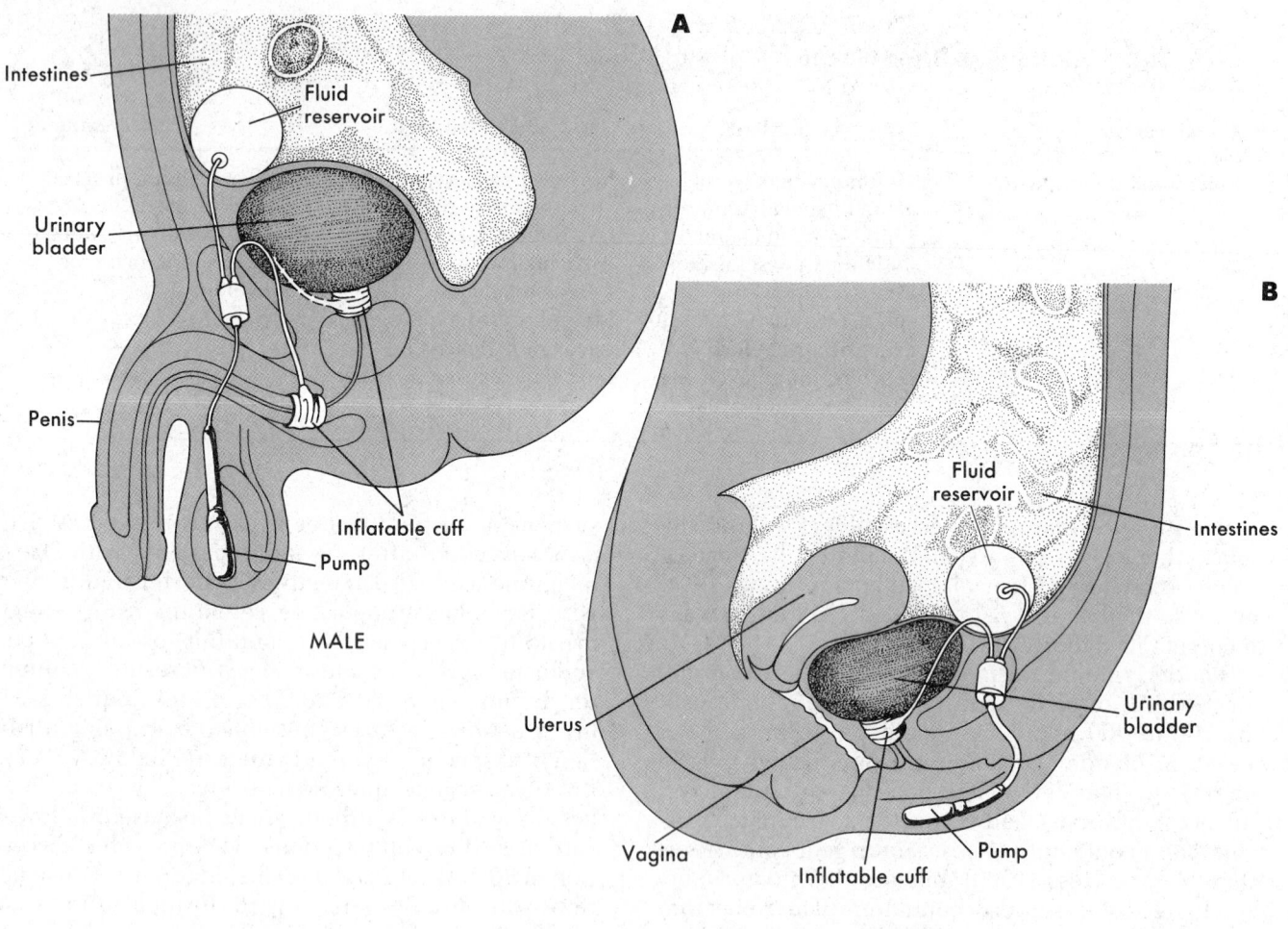

FIGURE 43-1   Artificial urinary sphincters. **A,** Male, **B,** female.

Vesicourethral suspension

Severe stress incontinence can be corrected by bladder suspension. The operative goal is to return the urethra to a well-supported position and restore the closure of the bladder outlet. The Marshall-Marchetti-Krantz procedure is done using the extraperitoneal abdominal approach. The bladder neck and urethra are suspended to the posterior surface of the pubis. The modified Pereyra bladder neck suspension is another way of correcting female stress incontinence without necessitating open pelvic surgery. A vaginal dissection and small suprapubic incision are used to access the bladder and urethra for suspension.

Transurethral Teflon injections

Teflon injections are mainly used in patients who have damage to the sphincter muscles (i.e., prostate surgery or suspension surgery). Polytetrafluorethylene (PTFE) or collagen may also be utilized for periurethral bulking injections. Teflon paste is injected into the surrounding tissues of the urethra to increase the urethral resistance. This causes a swelling of the tissue, narrowing the urethra enough for sphincter control. A fiberoptic cystourethroscope is used to pass the syringe transurethrally to make the injection. The procedure may have to be repeated several times to achieve the desired effect.

Pharmacologic interventions

Drug therapy can help the incontinent patient in certain circumstances. If the diagnostic workup reveals detrusor overactivity, smooth muscle relaxants such as flavoxate (Urispas), oxybutynin (Ditropan), propantheline (Pro-Banthine), and dicyclomine (Bentyl) can be used to decrease detrusor contractility by direct action on the bladder. The feeling of urgency may be diminished but the patient must be monitored for symptoms of retention. These drugs exert mild anticholinergic side effects such as dry eyes, dry mouth, constipation, and increased intraocular pressure in narrow-angle glaucoma. Anticholinergics such as propantheline (Pro-Banthine) delay, decrease, or inhibit detrusor contractions and may improve bladder capacity. Anticholinergic effects are more pronounced in these drugs. Imipramine (Tofranil) and doxepin (Adapin, Sinequan) are tricyclic antidepressants that exhibit both anticholinergic and direct relaxant effects on the detrusor muscle in addition to contraction of the bladder outlet. Side effects include hypotension, sedation, fatigue, dizziness, and insomnia. Although flavoxate is commonly used to control incontinence, randomized, controlled studies of its efficacy for incontinence have not demonstrated a significant benefit.[22]

Phenylephrine, ephedrine (Marax), pseudoephedrine (Sudafed), phenylpropanolamine (PPA) in sustained-release form, and bethanechol (Urecholine) stimulate the alpha-sympathetic nervous system to increase bladder neck tone and detrusor activity. Control of stress incontinence has shown improvement in studies of the effectiveness of PPA.[22]

Beta-blocking agents inhibit the beta receptors to the urethral sphincter mechanism. Propranolol (Inderal) is one beta-adrenergic blocker that has been suggested to improve urinary control. Current studies do not support the use of this drug in treatment of stress incontinence and it is not recommended for treatment of incontinence at this time.[22] Calcium channel blockers such as verapamil (Calan) and nifedipine (Procardia) have a depressant effect on the bladder and have been used in urge incontinence. Because of the rate of side effects, these agents are not recommended for general use for the treatment of detrusor overactivity.[22]

For incontinence related to UTI, an antibiotic appropriate for the specific organism should be prescribed. This therapy is based on the urine culture and sensitivity.

Both topical and oral administration of estrogen therapy may help the postmenopausal woman with a urethral deficiency caused by an estrogen deficit. Although the exact mechanism of action is unknown, it is thought estrogen may increase vascularity and tone of urethral muscle. Estrogen is also thought to increase bladder outlet resistance and decrease stress incontinence in the woman who has atrophic vaginitis associated with stress or urge incontinence.

NURSING MANAGEMENT OF THE PATIENT WITH URINARY INCONTINENCE

Assessment

When assessing for urinary incontinence, the nurse elicits specific information from the patient. Questions such as "Do you ever lose urine (water) when you don't want to?", "Do you have difficulty holding your urine?", and "Do you ever wear a pad or other device to stay dry?" are helpful in eliciting the type of information needed. The nurse asks the patient for a detailed voiding history, including the time, place, amount, stimulus, awareness of urine passage related to urination, subsequent incontinence, the type of incontinence, and management. Any burning, itching, or feeling of pressure is noted. Fluid intake pattern, including caffeine-containing or other diuretic fluids, is assessed. The nurse also asks the patient about any previous surgeries (genitourinary surgeries) and any drugs the patient has taken, paying particular attention to sedatives, hypnotics, anticholinergics, diuretics, and antidepressants. A history of precipitating factors, which includes a history of stroke, Parkinson's disease, cystocele, rectocele, uterine prolapse, neurologic disease, delirium, or dementia should be part of the assessment, too. Other associated symptoms the nurse should explore include polyuria, nocturia, dysuria, urgency associated with the involuntary loss of urine, and confusion. The nurse also assesses the patient's bowel pattern since stool adds pressure to a weak bladder. Any vaginal discharge is noted. A social history of the patient's environmental alterations and accessibility to toilet facilities is obtained. Assessment of toilet access both during the day and at night, adequacy of bathroom lighting, need for grab bars in the bathroom, and the need for mobility aids are just some of the areas that should be addressed.

The nurse compiles a record of measurable data that includes a description of the amount and characteristics (odor, color, sediment, clarity) of the urine. Hydration status will be assessed as dehydration concentrates urine and can lead to bladder irritation. Palpation of the lower abdomen will reveal retention that may cause overflow incontinence. The nurse will gather any data regarding a rectal impaction or rectal mass. An altered mental status examination and any evidence of physiologic factors contributing to incontinence (i.e., spinal cord injury) will also be noted.

Nursing Diagnosis

Based on the clinical manifestations, the data analysis will reveal a nursing diagnosis of actual or high risk for altered patterns of urinary elimination related to stress incontinence, urge incontinence, reflex incontinence, total incontinence, or functional incontinence. Other nursing diagnoses related to incontinence include:

Impaired skin integrity related to skin irritation by urine

Body image disturbance related to the fear of being incontinent in public

Toileting self-care deficit related to the inability

to reach an appropriate receptacle or to carry out proper toilet hygiene

Social isolation related to the fear of being incontinent in public or around friends

Knowledge deficit of the various methods of treating incontinence

Impaired home maintenance management related to the inability to manage the incontinence at home

Planning

The expected outcomes based on the above findings include:

Patient will decrease or alleviate incontinent episodes

Patient will establish a bladder routine

Patient will maintain skin integrity

Patient will engage in activities that increase promotion of self-worth and dignity

Patient will perform self-care activities of toilet hygiene to be free of urinary odor

Patient will modify the environment to decrease episodes of incontinence

Patient will reestablish social networks

Patient will demonstrate an increased knowledge of incontinent garments, bladder training, Kegel exercises, and catheters (indwelling or external)

Implementation

Supportive measures

The nurse's attitude is supportive rather than judgmental. The nurse must ensure that the toilet or its substitutes (bedpan, urinal, commode chair) are readily available. The patient is assisted in a timely fashion to the toilet in response to a signal that indicates the need to void. With physical or cognitive impairment, a protocol of bladder training that ensures regular toileting may alleviate incontinence. The skin is kept clean and dry. The nurse monitors for incontinent episodes often. The skin is not left in contact with urine-contaminated linens, gowns, or absorbent pads/garments. The skin is cleansed with warm, soapy water and gently dried. A protective layer of petrolatum jelly or A & D ointment may aid in preventing skin breakdown.

Pelvic floor exercises (Kegel)

If the evaluation reveals stress incontinence, the first action taken toward the resolution of symptoms should be pelvic floor exercises (see Chapter 70). These exercises are used to strengthen perineal and sphincter muscle control. The first week the patient is instructed to tighten the pubococcygeal muscle,

GERIATRIC CONSIDERATIONS

Incontinence

1. Assess toileting facilities
   - height of the toilet, availability of lift, or grasp bars
   - physical barriers such as obstructions, poor lighting
   - room large enough to accommodate walker or other assistive devices
   - toilet readily accessible, on same floor?
2. Can clothing be easily manipulated or removed as needed?
3. Can elder position self to void?
4. Remind or cue elder to go to the toilet (after meals, before bedtime)
5. Encourage fluid during the day, limit fluid after evening meal.
6. Assess the effect being incontinent has on social activities, mood, self-esteem, personal relationships.
7. Assess for conditions such as vaginitis, cystocyle or rectocele, uterine prolapse that may contribute to urinary incontinence.

hold it for at least 3 to 5 seconds, and then relax. The nurse may need to insert two gloved fingers in the vagina. Ideally the fingers will override when the patient squeezes the muscles. This contraction needs to be extended to 20 seconds over time. These sets can be performed when sitting, standing, or lying. The patient needs to work up to performing 80 sets throughout the day.[9] Most patients with adequate musculature learn to be continent within 6 to 8 weeks.

A new type of aid for treating incontinence involves cones with increasing weights that are inserted in the vagina to train muscles in Kegel exercises. The weighted cone is inserted vaginally and retained for up to 15 minutes by contracting the pelvic muscles. This procedure is performed twice daily.[22]

Bladder training

The goal of bladder training is to establish habits of elimination. The patient is taught to void at regular intervals with attempts to lengthen the interval between voidings. This type of program is useful when the patient is incontinent because of cerebral clouding or confusion. It is also useful with urge incontinence.

To start, the patient is given a measured amount of fluid regularly throughout the day totaling 2000 to

3000 mL/day (assuming this is not contraindicated by other medical problems). The patient is taken to the toilet 30 minutes after the fluids are consumed and asked to attempt to void. It may be helpful to massage the bladder or have the patient rock back and forth on the toilet to aid in voiding. The schedule is usually set at 2-hour intervals throughout a 24-hour day. Gradually the 2-hour interval is lengthened as control is gained. The plan must be consistently implemented to be successful. Staff participation through case conferences increases the awareness of toileting patterns and increases staff compliance with the plan.[23]

Fluids may be limited or withheld in the evening, usually after dinner, to avoid nocturia, but only if the 3000 mL fluid intake has been achieved. Positive reinforcement is given when continence has been maintained, and a neutral response is given for incontinence episodes.

Bladder retraining for the patient with urge incontinence involves assisting the patient to suppress the urge until elimination is possible. The goal is to urinate no oftener than every 4 hours. The patient is instructed to use relaxation techniques if it has been less than 2½ hours since the last voiding. The patient is encouraged to breathe slowly, deeply, and to concentrate on breathing until the urge diminishes. After the urge is suppressed, the patient should wait 5 minutes and then void whether the urge exists then or not. The interval between suppression and voiding is gradually lengthened. This patient is instructed not to go to the bathroom before the urge is felt. Furthermore, the patient is told not to run to the bathroom.

Another alternative, habit training, is to schedule the voiding times similarly to the person's normal voiding pattern. For example, schedule voiding before and after meals, on arising, and before retiring. There is no attempt to postpone or restrict voiding. The key to a successful regimen is regularity.

Biofeedback

Biofeedback is the use of a machine to provide visual or audio reply in response to changes in the human body. Recently biofeedback has been used in conjunction with Kegel exercises to treat stress incontinence. A perineometer is inserted in the vagina of a woman or anus of a man. The perineometer senses muscle activity and displays the results on a computer screen or display gauge. This feedback lets the patient know whether the correct muscles are being contracted and also the intensity of the pressure being used. This gives the user direct feedback concerning progress with the exercises. Behavioral conditioning with a bell pad has resulted in bladder behavior changes.[13] An auditory signal, such as a bell or buzzer, sounds to indicate inappropriate

voiding, which is then followed by corrective verbal feedback. The advantages of biofeedback techniques are that there are no side effects and they do not prevent any future alternative therapies.

Mechanical devices

Penile clamps for men are temporarily used with intrinsic sphincter deficiency. The clamps are released at 3-hour intervals to empty the bladder. Complications include penile and urethral erosion, penile edema, pain, and obstruction.[13] Pessaries for women are devices that are introduced into the vagina to temporarily reduce pelvic prolapse and relieve symptoms of pelvic relaxation in women with or without urinary incontinence. Although studies regarding their effectiveness in reducing incontinence are not reported, they may provide an alternative to frail elderly who are not candidates for other therapies.[13]

Containing (incontinence) garments

Multiple incontinence products (shields, undergarments, combination pad-pant systems, diaperlike garments, and bed pans) are on the market in many shapes and sizes. Disposable garments have the advantage of ease and availability without the cleanup, but they have the disadvantage of being costly. Reusable products are available that are less costly. The individual needs to be assessed on the basis of amount and frequency of urine lost before a product is recommended. A major factor determining success with any containment garment is fit. This is especially important at the legs, where leakage may occur. Containing garments are recommended for use only after everything else is tried and is unsuccessful.

Urinary drainage devices

External urinary drainage devices are available for both men and women. These catheters should be removed and cleaned daily. Close monitoring for skin irritation, meatal edema, and breakdown, as well as UTI and fungal skin infections, is essential. Intermittent catheterization may be utilized in persons with overflow incontinence secondary to an inoperable obstruction, an underactive detrusor, or detrusor hyperreflexia. Indwelling catheters are the last resort for incontinence and should be viewed only as a stopgap method until other methods can be implemented.

Psychologic support

Because of incontinence, the person limits social activities and social interactions. This limitation leads to increased social isolation related to the fear of embarrassment when incontinence occurs. Many people become reclusive, unable to cope with the problem in public; this is a common reason for loss of an independent life-style. Sometimes the underlying cause of incontinence may not be correctable, but with the available products, the situation is far from hopeless. Organizations have been formed that help the incontinent person cope (see resource list). These support groups help the individual deal with the embarrassment and lowered self-image that are often associated with incontinence.

Patient education

Written instructions and directions will be needed in the following areas:

The importance of adequate fluid intake of 2000 to 3000 mL/day; limit intake after supper; avoid intake of caffeinated beverages such as coffee, tea, or cola, as well as alcohol since they produce a diuretic effect

Instructions on all medications, including the dosage, purpose, route, frequency of administration, and side effects; take diuretics in the morning to prevent nocturia; limit use of sedatives/hypnotics since they dull the sensation to urinate

Care of external drainage devices

Maintenance of perineal skin care

Instructions on Kegel exercises

Availability of incontinent garments

Schedule for bladder training; empty the bladder completely before and after meals, upon arising, and before retiring at night; urinate every 2 hours during the day and every 4 hours at night (may need to use alarm clock). Urinate when the urge arises and never ignore it; stay on the toilet for several minutes after voiding to ensure complete emptying of the bladder

Prevention of constipation by the inclusion of bran and other fiber in the diet (prophylactic stool softeners or bulk laxatives are used if diet alone is ineffective)

Indication for seeking medical care

Maintenance of urine acidity (decrease the risk of UTI)

Removal of obstacles in the path to the toilet

Evaluation

The nurse evaluates how well the patient has regained voluntary control of urine (if control is possible) and how the patient manages incontinence environmentally, socially, and physically. The nurse evaluates prevention of skin breakdown in the patient (through the efforts of the patient or the family member caring for the patient) and performance

by the patient of self-care activities of toilet hygiene. The nurse also evaluates the patient's demonstration of a working knowledge of incontinent garments, bladder training, Kegel exercises, and catheters (indwelling or external) as appropriate.

Documentation

Key points to document are the urinary pattern, including amount, number of times voided, character of the urine (odor, color, clarity), and whether there were episodes of nocturia or dysuria; precipitating factors associated with the incontinence (laughing, coughing); and whether there was an awareness of the sensation to void. The condition of the skin is also noted. The patient's ability to perform Kegel exercises, toilet hygiene, and utilize incontinent garments are further areas for documentation.

Ongoing Care

Rehabilitation

A major goal of rehabilitation is helping the patient manage the incontinence at home. To ensure continuity of care, local community health agencies may be contacted to evaluate the home. Environmental modifications may be needed to ensure independent living. It may be necessary to install handgrips in the bathroom, arrange furniture to facilitate access to the toilet, or obtain a commode chair. The community health nurse will reinforce the patient education, discuss how to obtain needed supplies and equipment, and provide information on available support services. The nurse will continue to help the family learn about bladder training and offer suggestions as needed. Follow-up is necessary at 6 weeks to reinforce therapy and teaching.

Long-term care

Unfortunately, the second most common reason for institutionalization of an older person is incontinence. Families often conclude that incontinence in an elderly relative makes caring for them at home impossible. If the decision is made to transfer the patient to a long-term care facility, the nurse should discuss the activities of daily living (ADL) sheet with the receiving agency. This helps the staff provide continuity of care. The ADL sheet states the patient's goals and the program that has been implemented.

Home care

The management of urinary incontinence at home is a family project. Protective pads must be used to protect beds and furniture. If the patient is in a confused state, the caregiver needs to be instructed on the use of protective pads, briefs, and external drainage devices. The maintenance of the integrity of the skin is vital. Skin breakdown occurs quickly, so daily inspection, personal hygiene, and prompt intervention when the skin integrity is broken are musts.

URINARY RETENTION
Definition

Urinary retention is the inadequate emptying of the bladder resulting in a large residue of urine or urinary stasis. Stasis of urine promotes bacterial growth. The stagnant urine contributes to UTIs and stone formation if left untreated.

Etiology/Epidemiology

Factors contributing to urinary retention are detrusor function deficit or an obstruction at or below the bladder outlet. Bladder outlet obstruction is the most commonly occurring factor. It is associated with benign prostatic hyperplasia (see Chapter 71), urethral stricture, urethral distortion, vesical neck contracture, and carcinoma of the prostate.

Impaired detrusor function is seen in myelomeningocele, spina bifida occulta, diabetic neuropathy, tumors, and sacral spinal cord injury. These diseases cause neurologic impact on the sacral micturition cord, resulting in retention.

Other factors that can contribute to urinary retention are life-style, surgery, and pharmacologic side effects. Chronic overdistention is seen in certain professions where time is not taken to void. The "nurse's bladder" is a common term used when the nurse, because of a busy schedule, does not take time to urinate. This practice can cause serious damage to the bladder and should be avoided. Medications often have side effects that result in urine retention. Common offenders are sedatives, antihistamines, opioids, and anesthetics. Calcium-channel blockers, such as verapamil (Calan) and nifedipine (Procardia), also have been associated with urinary retention. Anticholinergics such as ditropan may promote retention.

Pathophysiology

Urinary retention occurs when high urethral pressure exceeds bladder pressure and prevents micturition. If left untreated, the bladder becomes distended and higher intraabdominal pressure causes involuntary loss of urine. Overflow incontinence results when maximum bladder capacity is reached.

Clinical Manifestations

Suprapubic pain is the key symptom experienced in acute urinary retention. This distinguishes it from anuria or oliguria. Other common findings are a poor stream of urine, hesitancy, straining, frequency, nocturia, and dribbling after urination. There may be the sensation of bladder fullness. Palpation of the lower abdomen (suprapubic area) will reveal a hard round mound that resembles a grapefruit and will elicit a complaint of pain from the patient. Catheterization will reveal an increased residual urine.

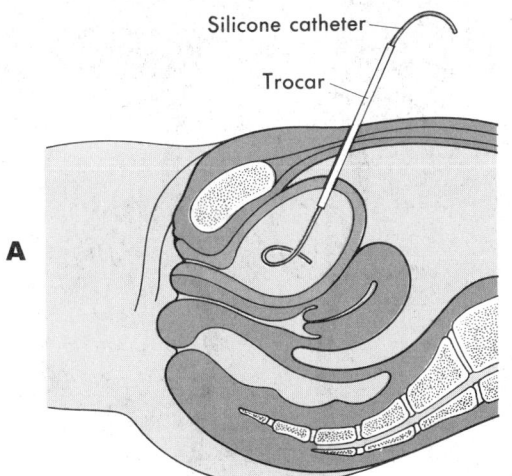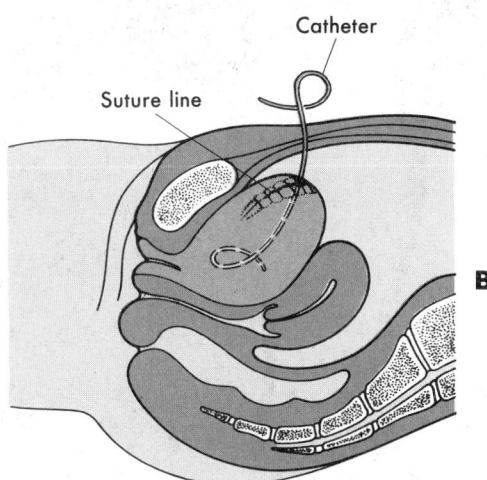

FIGURE 43-2   **A,** Percutaneous suprapubic cystostomy in which a silicone catheter is inserted into the bladder. A trocar is used to puncture the abdominal wall and serves as a guide for catheter insertion. Once the catheter is in place, the trocar is removed. **B,** Open suprapubic cystostomy in which the catheter is placed in the bladder through a surgical incision above the symphysis pubis.

Therapeutic Management

Catheterization

Catheterization, the process by which a tube (catheter) is inserted into a cavity such as the urinary bladder, may be necessary to establish urinary drainage. The bladder, the ureters, or the renal pelvises may be drained via catheters. The process of catheterization allows for the introduction of microorganisms into the urinary tract. By traumatizing delicate urethral and bladder mucosa during instrumentation, the stage is set for microorganisms to proliferate. Catheterization, therefore, must remain a solution of last resort because of the high incidence of urinary tract infection that occurs as a result of instrumentation.

Urinary catheterization is used to provide relief from urinary retention or stasis that may be a result of obstruction from stones, edema, or strictures. In addition, the inability to void, for example postoperatively, or neurologic conditions causing paralysis may also cause retention that will necessitate catheterization. Other reasons for assisted urinary drainage include precise measurement of urinary output in critically ill patients, introduction of medication into the bladder, and measurement of residual urine after voiding. Finally, when surgical repair of the urinary tract or surrounding area will result in edema or when bladder decompression (emptying) is needed, catheterization is utilized.

Suprapubic catheterization is one means of urinary drainage (Figure 43-2). Although most often inserted in surgery, the catheter can be inserted at the bedside with the use of a local anesthetic. The physician either makes a small abdominal wall incision above the pubis or uses a trocar to insert the catheter. Once inserted, the catheter is then sutured in place to prevent dislodgment, covered with a sterile split dressing, and connected to a closed drainage system. This type of catheter is used when the urethral route is obstructed, after gynecologic or urinary tract surgery, or after pelvic fractures.

The advantages of a suprapubic catheter are its low rate of urinary tact infections (UTIs), increased comfort, and convenience of evaluating the patient's voiding status. Voiding can be assessed with the catheter clamped but still in place for use if necessary. The disadvantages of the catheter are its tendency for poor drainage because of obstruction (small lumen). Sediment, clots, and tube kinkage are common occurrences that need to be monitored.

To assess readiness for removal, the catheter is clamped for several hours after which the patient attempts to void. The tube is then unclamped and residual urine measured. There should be less than 100 mL in residual on two separate occasions.

Ureteral catheters are inserted into one or both ureters via the urethra and bladder or by insertion through the abdominal wall (Figure 43-3). Each catheter's urine volume is recorded separately. The pa-

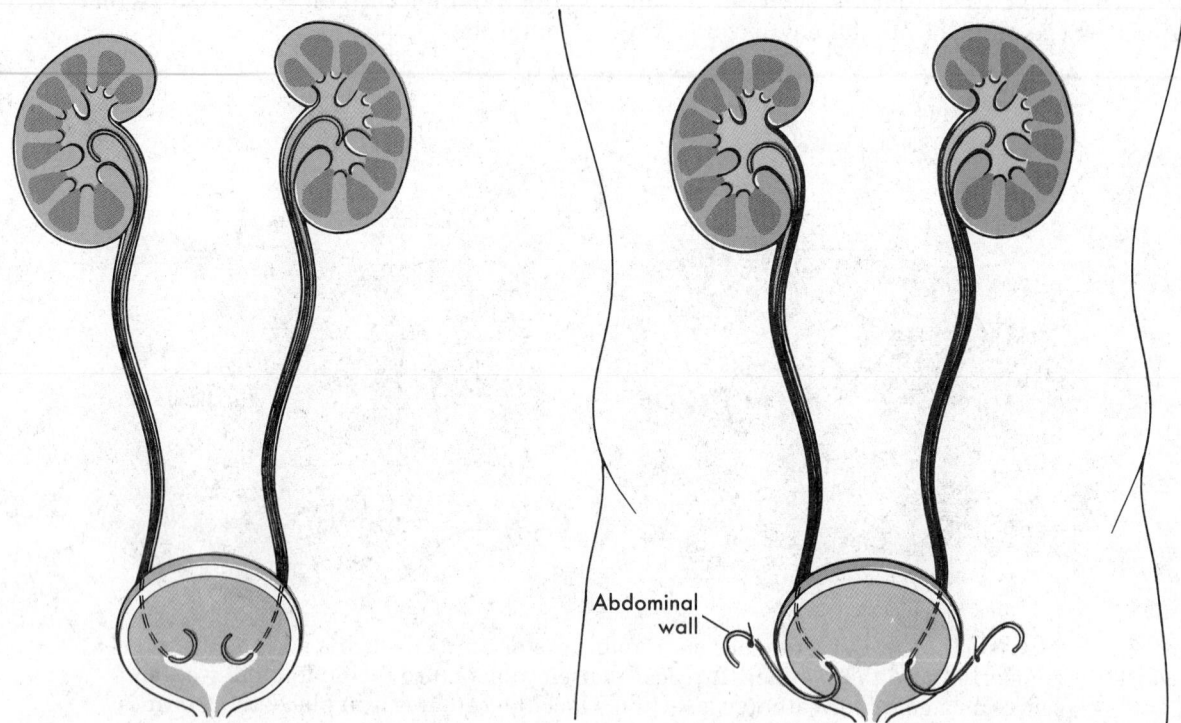

Abdominal wall

FIGURE 43-3   Ureteral catheters.

tient is placed on bed rest to prevent dislodgment of the catheter. The nurse must never clamp ureteral catheters since they drain urine from the renal pelvis. Because the renal pelvis holds a maximum of 3 to 5 mL of urine, renal damage will occur rapidly if urine flow is obstructed. The physician is notified immediately of any decrease in output from ureteral catheters.

Nephrostomy tubes are usually a temporary method of bypassing the ureters and draining urine directly from the renal pelvis. The care of nephrostomy tubes is similar to that of ureteral catheters. If the physician orders irrigation of the nephrostomy tube, no more than 3 mL of sterile saline should be used as irrigant. Any more than 3 mL could result in damage to the kidney. Associated problems include infection and stone formation.

Urethral catheterization is used to promote urinary drainage and relieve urinary retention. Catheterization should be used only when necessary and discontinued as soon as possible. Either a straight catheter (in and out) or an indwelling catheter (Foley) may be used depending on the cause of the retention (Figure 43-4). Adult catheters range in size from 14 to 22 French, with 14 to 18 French in females and 16 to 20 French in males most commonly employed. It is essential to choose the proper size catheter, one just smaller than the meatus. Too small a catheter may result in obstruction of output by clots or mucus plugs. Too large a catheter may cause tissue trauma or erosion from pressure.

An indwelling catheter that permits continuous drainage is a double lumen tube with an inflatable balloon near the end. After the catheter is sufficiently inserted into the bladder, the balloon is inflated with sterile water to ensure the catheter remains in place. A catheter with a 5 mL balloon is most often used. The 30 mL balloon, frequently used for maintaining hemostasis by application of pressure on bleeders, is used following a transurethral resection of the prostate (TURP) (Figure 43-5).

The catheter is inserted via the urethra, past the internal sphincter, and into the bladder. The balloon is then inflated and the catheter connected to a closed drainage system. Strict aseptic technique is vital for prevention of a urinary tract infection (see box on p. 1140 on do's and do nots of catheter care).

Adequate lighting via a gooseneck lamp is preferable when inserting a catheter. The meatus is cleansed with an antiseptic solution such as povidone-iodine (betadine). The catheter, lubricated with a water-soluble jelly, is gently advanced through the urethra and into the bladder until urine starts to flow. With male patients, an enlarged prostate gland may inhibit passage of the catheter. If resistance is met, have the patient take a deep breath to relax the muscles and continue passage. If resistance continues, cease catheterization to prevent traumatizing tissues and notify the physician.

The balloon is inflated once the catheter is inserted far enough into the bladder to prevent urethral trauma. The catheter is taped securely on the upper thigh or lower abdomen in males to decrease the penoscrotal angle and lower the risk of urethral ulceration from the pressure of the catheter (Figure 43-6). In females the catheter is taped to the inner

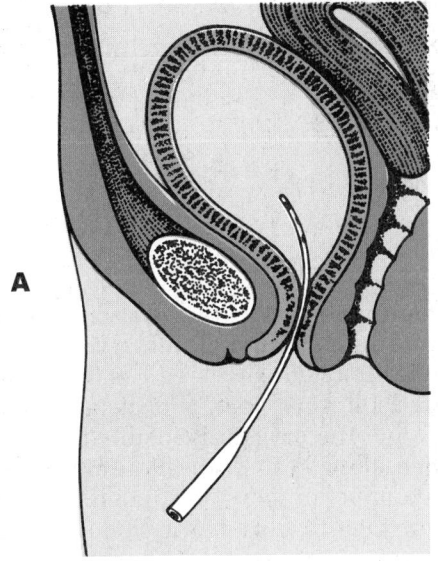 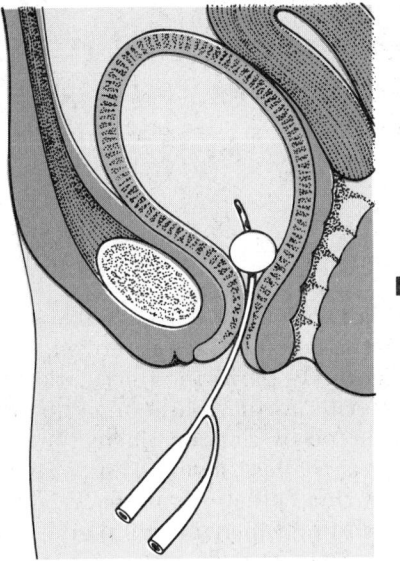

FIGURE 43-4   **A,** Indwelling Foley catheter inserted into the urinary bladder. **B,** Balloon inflated to prevent the catheter from slipping.

CATHETER CARE

Do:

Do maintain strict sterile technique when handling the closed drainage system

Do empty the GU bag every 8 hours to decrease bacterial growth

Do use latex gloves when draining the system to protect the nurse from contamination

Do keep the drainage bag below the level of the bladder to prevent reflux of contaminated urine back into the bladder and infecting the urinary tract

Do tape the catheter securely to prevent traction on the urinary meatus

Do clean the perineum, catheter junction, and urinary meatus with soap and warm water twice a day

Do monitor and document the output, color, and characteristics of urine

Do increase fluid intake with consideration of the patient's cardiac limits to flush the bladder of bacterial contaminants

Do not:

Do not open the closed drainage system except to empty the bag. This prevents bacterial contamination

Do not permit urine to collect in the tubing since unobstructed flow prevents infection

Do not contaminate the drainage spout when emptying the bag

Do not allow dependent loops or kinks in the tubing as this inhibits proper drainage by requiring the urine to travel against gravity to empty into the bag

Do not allow the patient to lie on the tubing as this will obstruct the drainage

Do not allow the collection bag to rest on the floor because of possible contamination

Do not irrigate the catheter without an order since this may introduce microorganisms

Do not put lotion or powder near the catheter/meatal junction

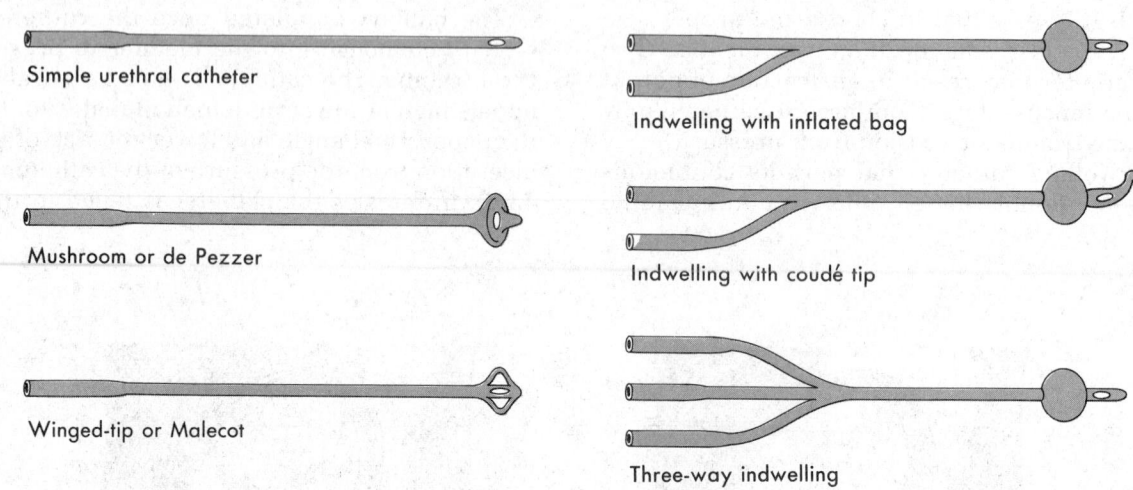

FIGURE 43-5   Commonly used catheters.

aspect of the thigh with extra length to prevent traction on the meatus when the leg is moved.

While not routinely performed, irrigation of the catheter with sterile normal saline may be ordered when it is obstructed by clots or mucus plugs. Typically the patient is restless, sweaty, and says he has to void even though a catheter is in place. The urine output is scant and a grapefruit size bladder is palpable. Manually irrigating the catheter expresses large clots and restores the patency of the catheter. Manual irrigation may be accomplished without in-

terrupting the system by drawing up 30 to 50 mL of normal saline into a 60 mL syringe with a 20-gauge needle attached. The needle is then inserted into the latex aspiration port, the distal tubing is pinched shut, and the irrigant is instilled. The normal saline is then allowed to drain naturally by gravity via the system. Suction may be applied gently by aspirating the syringe to dislodge a clot. The nurse must remember to subtract the irrigant from the urinary drainage when computing true urine output.

It is not necessary to open the closed drainage system to obtain a urine specimen. Cleanse the aspiration port and puncture it with a 20 to 21 gauge needle and 5 mL syringe and withdraw urine (Figure 43-7).

When it is anticipated that frequent irrigation will be necessary, a 3-way indwelling catheter is utilized. This system employs a 3-lumen catheter: one lumen drains urine, one lumen instills irrigant, and one lumen holds the water to inflate the balloon (Figure 43-8). This type catheter is used most commonly following transurethral resection of the prostate or bladder/urethral trauma. Sterile normal saline irrigant is administered at a rapid rate to decrease the chance of clotting if the drainage is bloody.

Because catheterization carries with it the increased risk of nosocomial infection, the nurse must be diligent in utilizing interventions to prevent infection. If an infection is suspected (cloudy urine, foul odor, chills, hematuria, elevated temperature), a urinalysis and/or culture and sensitivity are or-

dered. Sensitive specific antibiotics are administered and usually include sulfisoxazole (Gantrisin), nitrofurantoin (Furadantin), or sulfamethoxazole-trimethoprim (Bactrim, Septra).

Traditionally nurses have accepted that when removing a large amount of urine at one time, rapid decompression of the bladder could result in hematuria or syncope. That practice, however, has not been supported by research. There have been several studies that indicate completely emptying a distended bladder without clamping midway through emptying is safe for the patient.[3,5]

When an indwelling catheter is removed, the nurse will encourage fluid intake within safe patient limits and will monitor the first voided specimen for

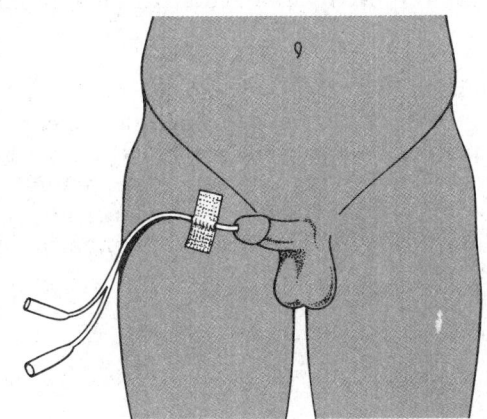

FIGURE 43-6   Taping of catheter in male patient.

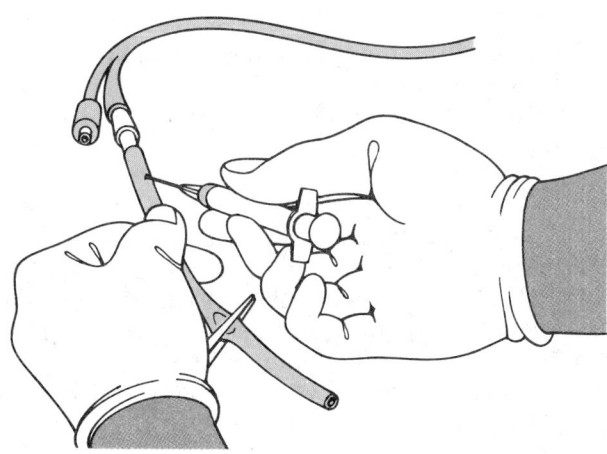

FIGURE 43-7   Obtaining a urine sample from a closed urinary drainage system.

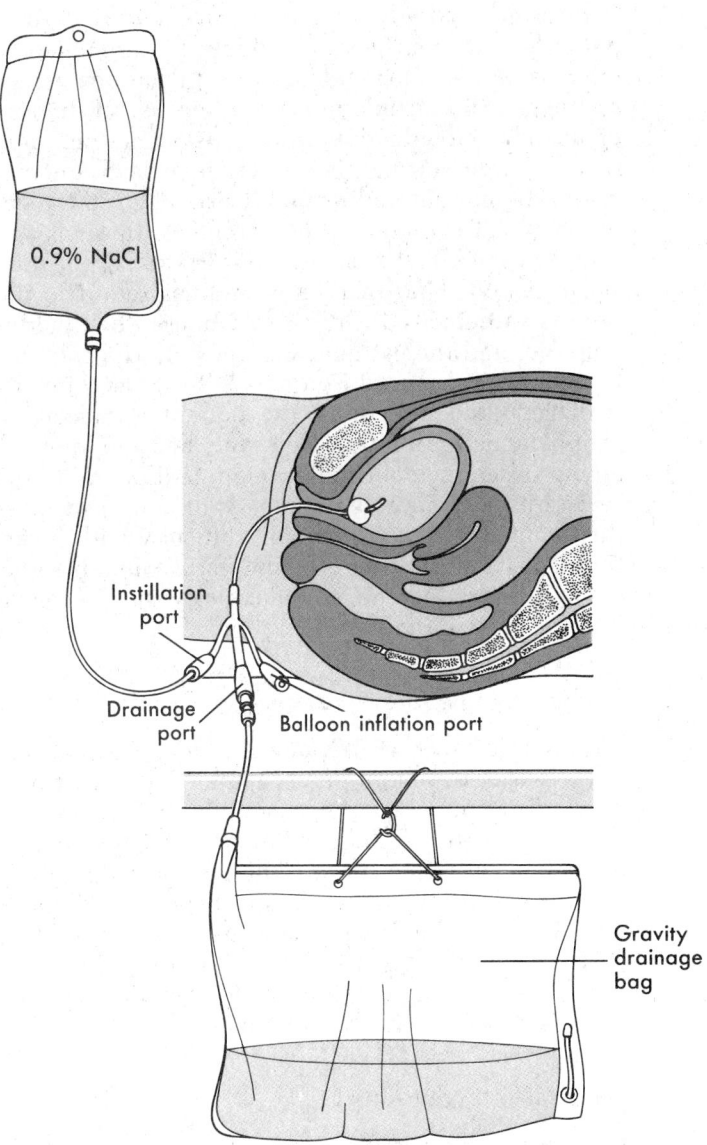

FIGURE 43-8   Closed urinary drainage system with three-way catheter.

time interval and volume. If the patient has not voided within 4 to 6 hours, retention is suspected. If the patient is only voiding small amounts frequently, then retention with overflow is suspected. In either case, if the bladder is not emptied, the patient is re-catheterized.

Catheterization is often the causative agent in UTI in the elderly. Because of incontinence (see previous discussion), a catheter may be inserted to prevent skin breakdown. Elderly patients, however, often do not exhibit the typical signs and symptoms (frequency, dysuria) of a urinary tract infection. Monitoring for signs or symptoms plus meticulous catheter care are essential for these patients. Catheters employed in chronic use may need changing periodically. Furthermore, confused patients must be prevented from pulling out the catheter when the balloon is inflated since this will traumatize tissues.

Intermittent catheterization is frequently used in patients with neurogenic bladder (e.g., spinal cord injuries or neurologic disorders). In the acute care setting, sterile technique is used because of the risk of nosocomial infection from cross-contamination. In the home setting clean technique is frequently used. The patient and/or family are taught the technique of self-catheterization as well as the signs and symptoms of UTI that require notification of the physician. Good handwashing is emphasized. The patient is catheterized every 3 to 5 hours, the bladder emptied, and the catheter is removed. The catheter is cleaned and stored in a plastic bag. Occasionally with repeated infections, the patient is placed on prophylactic antibiotics. However, because there is an increased incidence of development of antibiotic-resistant bacteria, this practice is discouraged. Urethritis, urinary tract infection, difficulty with insertion, urethral stricture, epididymitis, and bladder stone are among the complications that occur in 20% of these patients.[14]

Pharmacologic interventions

Cholinergics such as bethanechol and neostigmine may be used to stimulate bladder contractions. These drugs increase detrusor tone and activity. At no time are they to be used during the presence of a mechanical obstruction. If the urinary retention is caused by an infection, the appropriate antibiotics will be used. Analgesics such as phenazopyridine HCl (Pyridium) may also be necessary for pain relief. A combination antibacterial/urinary analgesic such as Azo Gantrisin may be used.

Surgical interventions

If an obstruction is the cause of retention, surgical intervention may be necessary. The primary focus will be to remove the obstruction or dilate the ure-thra if a stricture exists. Urethral dilation is the procedure used for urethral strictures. Metal sounds, bougies, or woven filiforms and followers are used periodically for dilation.

NURSING MANAGEMENT OF THE PATIENT WITH URINARY RETENTION
Assessment

Profound suprapubic pain with a change in voiding pattern is seen in acute urinary retention. Restlessness, diaphoresis, and a change in mental status (especially in the older adult) are also seen. Inspection of the abdomen will show an abdominal profile in which the lower third of the abdomen is distended. Percussion over a fluid-filled bladder will elicit a kettle drum quality. Light palpation will reveal a distended bladder and often increased discomfort. Patterns displayed are inability to void, constant dribbling, or voiding at frequent intervals with only 25 to 50 mL at a time (retention with overflow). A postvoid residual volume upon in and out catheterization of 100 mL or more indicates retention.

Nursing Diagnosis

Urinary retention related to high urethral pressure is the primary nursing diagnosis. Other nursing diagnoses related to urinary retention include:

Knowledge deficit of the technique of self-catheterization related to unfamiliarity of technique

High risk for infection related to urethral catheterization

Planning

The expected outcomes based on the above findings include:

Patient will reestablish previous voiding pattern

Patient will empty the bladder completely when voiding

Patient will demonstrate the technique of intermittent self-catheterization

Patient will exhibit no signs or symptoms of a UTI

Implementation

Initial nursing intervention to promote relief of urinary retention is to provide privacy and to let the patient assume a normal sitting or standing position. Increased intraabdominal pressure (if not contraindicated) may help. The male patient will find it easier to evacuate the bladder in a standing position (unless contraindicated). Turning on the faucet, so the patient can hear the sound of running water, may help the patient relax the bladder sphincter. Placing the feet in warm water or pouring warm water over the perineum often facilitates urination. Measure the amount of water first to ensure calculating an accurate urine output.

Catheterization may be prescribed to relieve the urinary retention. If chronic retention exists, intermittent self-catheterization may need to be taught. A schedule of every 4 hours will be planned to prevent bladder distention. Proper technique must be taught to prevent the occurrence of a UTI (see box on p. 1146). Written instructions and directions for the patient will be needed in the following areas:

Indicators that would necessitate seeking medical care, including signs of urinary retention or UTI

Instructions on all medications, including dosage, purpose, route, frequency of administration, and side effects

Care of an indwelling catheter or self-catheterization technique if applicable

Evaluation

The nurse evaluates whether the patient can regain previous voiding pattern and demonstrate the technique of intermittent self-catheterization.

Documentation

The nurse documents the findings from the physical examination and any change in voiding pattern, including the amount voided (if any), frequency, character of the urine, and complaints of suprapubic pain. Procedures (i.e., catheterizations after voiding to evaluate the residual urine) should be documented. The nurse should also document nursing measures taken to facilitate urination, the effectiveness of these measures, and patient education provided and the patient's response to it.

URINARY TRACT INFECTIONS
Definition

Urinary tract infection (UTI) is an all-inclusive term referring to a bacterial infection or inflammation located at any segment along the urinary tract. An inflammation, or infection, of the lower urinary tract involves the bladder (cystitis) and urethra (urethritis). Bacteriuria is the presence of bacteria in the urine.

Etiology/Epidemiology

The majority of UTIs are ascending infections arising from bowel contaminants. For this reason, bacterial infections (cystitis) occur more commonly in women because of the proximity of the urethra to the vagina and rectum. Contamination from the vagina and rectum in a female because of poor hygienic practice is a common occurrence. The long urethra

and the presence of bacteriocidal prostatic secretions in males protect them in some degree from UTI.

The most common ascending organism is *Escherichia coli* (approximately 85% to 90%). Other common gram-negative bacterial infections are *Klebsiella pneumoniae*, *Proteus mirabilis*, *Enterobacter aerogenes*, and *Pseudomonas aeruginosa*. In urethritis, *Chlamydia trachomatis* and *Neisseria gonorrhoeae* are common bacterial invaders.

Descending infections originate systemically and are carried from the kidneys down the urethra. *Pseudomonas aeruginosa, Staphylococcus epidermidis, Staphylococcus aureus*, alpha-hemolytic streptococci, and beta-hemolytic streptococci are common descending pathogens.

Persons at a high risk for UTIs are those with diabetes, women who are pregnant or postpartum, older men with prostatitis (diminished bactericidal properties of prostatic fluid), immunosuppressed or catheterized patients, and patients with a neurologic disease. Low fluid intake or excessive fluid loss predisposes to UTI.

Aging also puts an older person at risk because of the increase in chronic diseases (i.e., diabetes mellitus and gout), lower estrogen levels in women, and declining function of the immune system. UTI and bacteriuria are five times more frequent in the 70- to 80-year-old population than for those between the ages of 20 and 40.[20] In addition, the bacteria found in institutionalized elderly are often more resistant to antibiotics. Factors such as perineal soiling, fecal incontinence, loss of estrogen protection in women, bladder dysfunction, prostatic enlargement, loss of protective prostatic secretions in men, and changes in acid-base balance put the elderly at risk for UTIs.

Instrumentation increases the risk of UTI. Urethral flora may be pushed into the bladder during these procedures. Urethral catheterizations, cystoscopy, and operative procedures on the bladder and kidneys put a person in jeopardy of contracting a UTI.

Urine flow flushes out bacteria along the urinary tract; therefore, conditions of urinary stasis place the patient at risk for UTI. An obstruction along the urinary tract, trauma, inability to completely empty the bladder, and urethrovesical reflux (reflux of urine from the urethra after voiding) are high risk conditions for UTI. Constant surveillance is needed when these factors exist.

Pathophysiology

When pathogens invade the urinary tract, multiple changes occur with micturition. The bladder becomes irritated and develops an ineffective filling capacity. This irritation decreases the anti-adherence

GERIATRIC CONSIDERATIONS

Urinary Tract Infection

The elderly patient commonly presents a different clinical picture as many UTIs in the elderly are asymptomatic.

The institutionalized elder often does not display the typical signs of UTI because of multiple diagnoses or chronic indwelling catheters. Malaise, anorexia, and low-grade fever may be the early symptoms of UTI in this population.

Symptomatic UTIs (e.g., cystitis) may initially exhibit urinary frequency, nocturia, urgency, and dysuria; features that are difficult to interpret because they commonly occur in the elderly in the absence of infection as the result of underlying bladder abnormalities, especially neurogenic bladder dysfunction. Confusion and incontinence often herald a UTI in the older person, but just as often, these symptoms go unnoticed.[2]

effects of the mucosa and allows bacteria to colonize. As filling capacity is altered, the bladder loses its elasticity. As the inflammation progresses, a moderate stretching of the bladder develops in which urinary frequency and urgency develop.

Urinary tenesmus is a common complaint. It is described as small voidings accompanied by the persistent desire to urinate.

If the pathogens spread to the bladder neck and urethra, painful urination (**dysuria**) may develop. Gross blood in the urine (**hematuria**) may be seen in some cases.

Urethral inflammation may be caused by a chemical irritant. Common offenders are perfumed feminine hygiene products, sanitary napkins, spermicidal jellies, and bubble bath.

Clinical Manifestations

Clinical signs of cystitis are frequency, urgency, burning, and dysuria with the possible complaint of nocturia. Suprapubic and low back pain are commonly described by the patient. Bladder spasms may be present. The patient has bacteriuria with the urine cloudy and foul-smelling. In severe cases hematuria will be present. Fever may or may not be present.

A clean-catch midstream urine collection is used to diagnose lower UTIs. Good technique is imperative for the culture and sensitivity tests. The presence of greater than 100,000/mL bacterial count is presumptive evidence of UTI. If 3 or more bacterial organisms are cultured from a sample, contamination of the urine collection is suspected. A Gram

stain may be used as a preliminary screen while waiting for the urine culture and sensitivity to return.

Urethritis in a man will be manifested by a purulent or whitish-mucoid discharge with dysuria, frequency, and urgency. In a woman, urethritis has the signs and symptoms of an acute bladder infection.

Therapeutic Management

Based on the urine culture and sensitivity, antibiotic therapy specific for the microorganism is the treatment of choice for an initial infection. Those with uncomplicated infections may be given tetracycline, ampicillin or amoxicillin, ciprofloxacin, cotrimoxazole, or sulfonamides. The usual course of therapy is 7 to 10 days (see Table 43-2).

Phenazopyridine (pyridium) is often given to relieve the burning associated with a UTI. Patients should be informed that this drug will turn the urine red-orange.

Persistent infections may require more aggressive therapy. Long-term, low-dosage antibiotic therapy with sulfamethoxazole-trimethoprim (Bactrim, Septra) is often prescribed to be taken at bedtime or after intercourse.

The use of urine-acidifiers is another therapeutic approach, although research is inconclusive concerning their benefits. Acidifying the urine discourages bacterial multiplication. Drinking cranberry juice (although not supported by research) and eating an acid-ash diet are two approaches to lowering the pH of the urine. Foods included in the acid-ash diet are meats, eggs, nuts, cheese, and whole grains. Foods to be avoided are milk, citrus fruits, and juices which have an alkalinizing effect on urine. In addition, the physician may order vitamin C as a acidifying agent, although there have been some reports that implicate high doses of vitamin C with the development of kidney stones.

NURSING MANAGEMENT OF THE PATIENT WITH A URINARY TRACT INFECTION
Assessment

When obtaining a history from a person with a possible UTI, a detailed voiding history is obtained. Does the person void at the first urge or is the urge chronically ignored? Delaying urination leads to urinary stasis and the development of a UTI. The nurse also asks about diet; a high consumption of sugar in the diet promotes UTI. The nurse asks the patient about contraception and sexual activity. Multiple partners increase the chance of UTI, and contraceptive foams and jellies can irritate the urethra. Other possible irritants include feminine hygiene sprays, bubble bath, and perfumed products. Any history of

TABLE 43-2   Pharmacology Summary: Urinary Tract Infection Drugs

Drugs	Nursing considerations
ANTIBIOTICS	
Ampicillin	Take on an empty stomach 1 hour before or 2 hours after meals with a full glass of water
Amoxicillin	Take without regard to meals
Cephlalosporins	
Ciprofloxacin (Cipro)	Do not give with antacids containing aluminum or magnesium (decreases bacterial effectiveness)
	Prevent alkaline urine since it renders the drug less soluble and promotes crystalluria
	Monitor for theophylline toxicity since theophylline clearance is lowered
Sulfonamides	Do not give with PABA (decreases therapeutic effect) or methanamine (requires an acid urine)
Sulfacytine (Renoquid)	
Sulfamethoxazole (Gantanol)	Needs an alkaline urine to achieve maximum effectiveness
Sulfamethoxazole and trimethoprim (Bactrim, Septra)	Administer with a full glass of water; needs fluids to produce at least 1 L of urine daily
Sulfisoxazole (Gantrisin)	Do not administer with antacids because of decreased absorption
URINARY TRACT ANTISEPTICS	
Cinoxacin (Cinobac)	Avoid bright sunlight; wear sunglasses because of photophobia
Methanamine mandelate (Mandelamine)	Maintain acidic urine
Nalidixic acid (NegGram)	Avoid sunlight due to photosensitivity
Nitrofurantoin (Furandantin, Macrodantin)	Advise of possible brown urine
	Give with food or milk to minimize gastric irritation
URINARY TRACT ANALGESICS	
Phenazopyridine (Pyridium)	Advise of red/orange urine

previous UTIs is noted. The nurse should ask about associated symptoms including frequency, dysuria, urgency, nocturia, and bladder spasms. Precipitating factors, which include a history of diabetes, gout, prostatitis, menopause, neurologic disease, and poor hygiene, are noted as well.

Data collected by the nurse will include the amount, frequency, and characteristics of the urine; a urinalysis positive for red blood cells, bacteria, white blood cells, and an alkaline pH; and a positive urine culture of greater than 100,000 colonies/mm of urine on a clean-catch specimen.

Nursing Diagnosis

Based on the clinical manifestations, the data analysis will reveal an actual or high risk primary nursing diagnosis of alteration in comfort: pain related to dysuria, frequency, and urgency. Other nursing diagnoses related to a UTI include:

Altered patterns of urinary elimination related to urgency, frequency, dysuria, and/or nocturia

Knowledge deficit: methods of preventing UTI related to recurrence of a UTI

Planning

The expected outcomes based on the above findings include:

Patient will verbalize relief of pain

Patient will resume normal voiding patterns for the individual without frequency, urgency, or dysuria

Patient will verbalize an understanding of the disease process, methods of prevention, and follow-up instructions

Implementation

The discomfort associated with a UTI is relieved soon after antibiotic therapy is started. Sitz baths may also help relieve the pain or itching in the perineum that may accompany a UTI. Avoid catheterization if possible, but if deemed necessary then maintain an unobstructed flow of urine. Force fluids to flush the bladder. Education focuses on preventing the recurrence of a UTI. Both written and verbal instruction are provided to patients (see Patient Education Guide).

PATIENT EDUCATION GUIDE   *Urinary Tract Infection*

Drink 2500 to 3000 mL to flush bacteria from the urinary tract

Avoid tea, coffee, carbonated drinks, and alcohol because of bladder irritation

Void at first urge and do not delay urination; void at least every 3 hours during waking hours and completely empty the bladder

Maintain acidic urine by methamine, sodium biphosphate, vitamin C, and/or an acid-ash diet

Monitor urine pH with a dipstick

Recognize the symptoms of UTI (painful urination, urinary odor, frequency, urgency, burning urination) and seek immediate medical attention

Take antibiotics as scheduled; do not stop taking when symptoms subside; take the full course to ensure the complete eradication of the infection

Specifically for Women

Use proper hygienic measures—wipe from front to back and clean thoroughly after defecation

Refrain from using bubble bath, perfumed sanitary pads, strong or perfumed soaps, feminine vaginal hygiene sprays, or bath powders in the perineal area

Use an alternative method of contraception if chronic infection occurs with the use of a diaphragm and/or spermicidal jelly or cream

Urinate before and immediately after sexual intercourse

Avoid trauma to the urethra by using a position during intercourse that minimizes pressure on the anterior vagina

Avoid nylon underwear and wear only cotton undergarments to decrease the warm, moist environment; wear loose clothing to decrease perineal moisture

Shower, rather than take a tub bath, to prevent introduction of bacteria

Utilize oral/topical estrogen if hormone depletion is contributing to UTI

Evaluation

The patient will verbalize a decrease in the pain and an absence of burning, frequency, and dysuria; void clear, odorless, yellow urine; and verbalize an understanding of the disease process, methods of prevention, and follow-up instruction.

Documentation

Key areas to document are the character of the urine (note the odor, clarity, and appearance of sediment or blood), fluid intake and output; patient education provided and the patient's response to it; and factors relating to the pain, such as location, intensity, duration, and precipitating or alleviating factors.

Ongoing Care

If recurrent UTIs occur, the patient can monitor the urine at home with the use of a dipslide (Microstix, Multistix). A diary can also be kept to help discover possible contributing factors.

URINARY TRACT OBSTRUCTION
Definition

Urinary tract obstruction is the complete or partial blockage of urine flow at any segment of the urinary tract. Common locations are the urethral meatus,

the bladder neck, and the ureteropelvic and ureterovesical junctions. The site and the extent of the obstruction will determine the presenting signs and symptoms.

Etiology/Epidemiology

There are four major causes of obstruction in the lower urinary tract: urethral strictures, **urolithiasis** (calculi), cancer of the bladder (see later in chapter), and benign prostatic hyperplasia (BPH). (For a complete discussion of BPH, see Chapter 71; for a complete discussion of urolithiasis, see renal calculi in Chapter 42.) Other causes are meatal stenosis, blood clots, fibrosis, tumors, and phimosis.

Pathophysiology

When an obstruction occurs, urine cannot effectively pass the blocked area; urine is then retained. Hydrostatic pressure builds, resulting in bladder distention with urinary stasis. This stagnant urine promotes bacterial growth. If the pressure is not relieved, the structures behind the obstruction dilate. In the bladder the detrusor muscle hypertrophies with trabeculae and diverticula formation. The increased pressure causes ureteral changes including elongation, fibrosis, and a tortuous shape. Gradually hydronephrosis (distention of renal pelvis and calices) occurs. The condition will progress to affect both kidneys, leading to renal failure if untreated.

Clinical Manifestations

Because of bladder distention during the initial phase of a lower urinary tract obstruction, the signs and symptoms of lower abdominal tenderness and a palpable bladder above the symphysis pubis occur. There will be little or no urinary output depending on the extent of the obstruction. Many symptoms of obstruction are similar to urinary retention. With the development of a UTI, clinical manifestations will include frequency, dysuria, and urgency. As the upper urinary tract becomes involved, pain and tenderness over the costovertebral angle develop. If a stone is present, excruciating colicky flank pain with diaphoresis, hypotension, and hematuria will appear. Nausea and vomiting may accompany obstruction.

Therapeutic Management

The goal of medical therapy is to reestablish urinary flow and treat the cause of the obstruction. To relieve the urinary retention, instrumentation is necessary. A urethral catheter will be inserted by the physician to drain the urine. If the catheter cannot

TABLE 43-3   Medical Interventions for Urinary Obstructions

Obstruction	Intervention
Benign prostatic hyperplasia	Transurethral prostatectomy
	Suprapubic transvesical prostatectomy
	Retropubic extravesical prostatectomy
Urolithiasis	Ureterolithotomy
	Pyelolithotomy
	Nephrolithotomy
	Litholapaxy
	Transcutaneous shock wave lithotripsy
Urinary stricture	Gradual dilation of stricture with metal sounds or bougies
Cancer of the bladder	Chemotherapy (early)
	Surgical removal of the bladder with possible urinary diversion

pass the obstruction, a suprapubic cystostomy will be performed. Medical interventions to relieve the obstruction will be directed toward the cause (Table 43-3). Drug therapy will be directed toward pain control, the management of spasms, and treatment of UTIs. Opioids, antispasmodics, and antibiotics are examples of the drug classifications used.

NURSING MANAGEMENT OF THE PATIENT WITH A URINARY TRACT OBSTRUCTION
Assessment

The nurse should elicit information from the patient concerning a detailed voiding history, including a change in voiding pattern, dysuria (burning), straining to start voiding, dribbling, hematuria, hesitancy, incontinence, nocturia, and enuresis. The nurse asks the patient to describe the pain, noting character, intensity, and location. Any history of renal calculi, BPH, UTI, urethral strictures, neoplasms, trauma, or congenital anomalies should be noted. Bladder tenderness may be present. Pertinent information related to a lower urinary tract obstruction includes urinary output and frequency, palpation revealing a palpable bladder, and percussion eliciting a "kettle drum" sound over the bladder.

Nursing Diagnosis

From the assessment data, actual or potential nursing diagnoses are determined. Actual or high risk nursing diagnoses include:
- Pain related to the urinary obstruction
- Altered patterns of urinary elimination related to the specific type of obstruction
- Ineffective individual coping related to knowledge deficit of the disease process

Planning

The expected outcomes based on the above findings include:
- Patient will verbalize relief or control of the pain
- Patient will resume the pattern of urinary elimination present before the obstruction
- Patient will verbalize an understanding of the disease process, symptoms of an obstruction, home care, and follow-up instructions

Implementation

The implementation of the care plan for the person with a lower urinary tract obstruction will be specific for the underlying cause. (See the specific cause of the obstruction for detailed care-urethral stricture, BPH, renal calculi, and cancer of the bladder.)

Evaluation

The patient will experience pain relief or control; the urinary pattern present before the obstruction will be regained; and the patient will demonstrate a working knowledge of the disease process, interventions, home care, and follow-up instructions.

Documentation

Key areas to document are voiding pattern, character of the urine, results of straining the urine, fluid intake and output, a pain description, and patient education and patient response.

BLADDER/URETHRA TRAUMA
Definition

Bladder and urethral trauma is that damage that occurs to either the bladder or urethra when force is applied to the urinary structures.

Etiology/Epidemiology

The majority of traumatic injuries to the bladder occur when blunt force is applied to the lower abdomen with contusion and rupture being the most common consequences. Injury such as this frequently results from motor vehicle accidents. Contact sports as well as stabbings and shootings may also result in damage to the lower urinary tract structures. Contusion occurs with either direct force or as a result of the damage generated by the close passage of a high-velocity missile such as a bullet. Seat belts have been implicated in both bladder rupture and bladder contusion. Bladder rupture is classified as extraperitoneal bladder trauma, which accounts for 80% of injuries with the remaining 20% being intraperitoneal (Figure 43-9).[24]

Pathophysiology

A full bladder is most vulnerable to injury since the force is transmitted through the abdomen to the bladder and ultimately pushes the urine to exert pressure on the weakest area of the bladder, the dome (Figure 43-10). With an intraperitoneal rupture such as this, urine is released into the peritoneal cavity causing irritation and contamination of abdominal tissues. Paralytic ileus and, more seriously, peritonitis may develop. A fractured pelvis may produce an extraperitoneal injury when either the rami or pubis punctures the bladder. Although peritonitis is not an attendant complication with extraperitoneal injury, blood loss or escape of urine may occur. When severe pelvic fractures are accompanied by bladder rupture, the mortality rate is high.[11] Urethral injury from blunt force is rare since the pelvic ring provides protection. However, gunshots, stabbings, and instrumentation of the urethra have been associated with urethral trauma.

Clinical Manifestations

Gross hematuria is usually always present in bladder trauma. Other common findings with either bladder or urethral trauma include low abdominal pain, inability to urinate, or a decrease in urinary output, abdominal distention, hypogastric tenderness, visible blood at the urethral meatus, and abnormal position of the prostate on rectal exam in male patients. Signs of peritonitis may develop. Bladder or urethral damage is suspected with pelvic fractures or perineal or scrotal hematoma. Although early signs of urethral damage may not be apparent, bleeding from the urethra without micturition should be investigated. In addition, swelling and tenderness of scrotal or perineal tissues may result from eccyhmosis, urine leakage, or local bleeding.

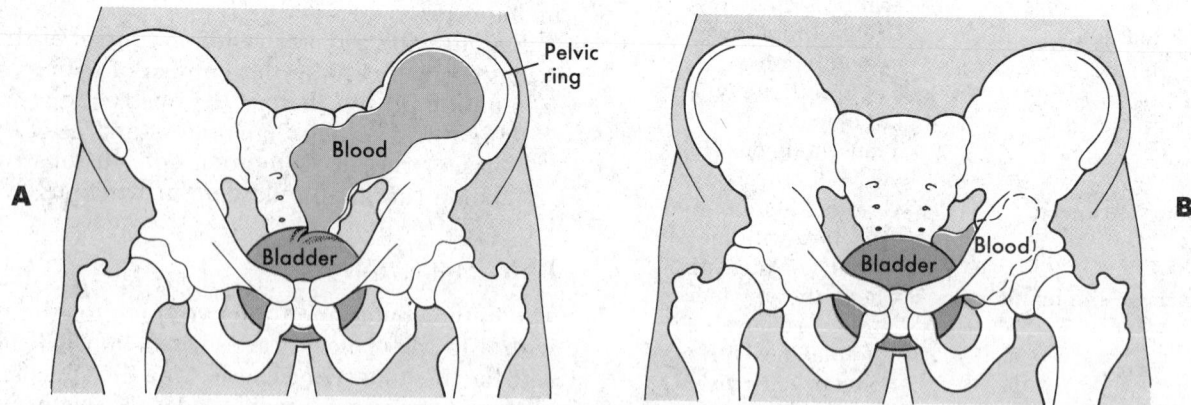

FIGURE 43-9   Traumatic bladder rupture. **A,** Intraperitoneal. **B,** Extraperitoneal.

Therapeutic Management

A CT scan, excretory urogram, and cytoscopy are frequently done to diagnose lower urinary tract damage. Hemoglobin and hematocrit are monitored to determine blood loss. Contusions of the lower urinary tract are normally treated with bed rest and an indwelling catheter. Bladder rupture requires surgical repair of the bladder followed by bladder decompression to prevent bladder distention and pressure on the sutures during the recovery phase. Bladder decompression is accomplished in males with a suprapubic catheter and with a urethral catheter in females. Bladder drainage is continued for 10 to 14 days to ensure wound healing of the sutured bladder mucosa.[24] A drain is usually placed in the perivesical space (area around the bladder). Medical treatment generally includes parenteral fluids, analgesics, and antibiotics.

A retrograde urethrogram should be performed if urethral damage is suspected. A urethral catheter is usually contraindicated with laceration until repair is accomplished. Some physicians complete an early surgical correction of the urethral damage while others wait several weeks to allow the tissue time to heal on its own. Early repair tends to favor later development of stricture or impotence in about 50% of patients.[19] In either case urinary drainage must be accomplished through a urethral catheter or suprapubic cystotomy.

NURSING MANAGEMENT OF THE PATIENT WITH BLADDER OR URETHRAL TRAUMA

Assessment

The history should include the type of force applied to the lower urinary tract. Secondary survey should involve palpation of the abdomen for distention, tenderness, or rigidity as well as investigation of symptoms of blood loss such as alteration of vital signs and a decrease in hematocrit and hemoglobin. Low volume output, hematuria, bleeding visualized at the urinary meatus, and lower abdominal pain will alert the nurse to suspect lower urinary tract injury. Ecchymosis over the lower abdomen, scrotum, and perineum are further red flags to the nurse suspecting internal trauma to the area.

Nursing Diagnosis

Applicable nursing diagnoses for the patient with bladder/urethral trauma include:
- Altered pattern of urinary elimination related to trauma and the presence of urethral/suprapubic catheterization
- Pain related to trauma
- Alteration in tissue perfusion related to hypovolemia
- High risk for infection related to intraabdominal leakage of urine, penetrating objects, and/or surgical incision

Planning

Expected patient outcomes include the following:
- Patient will produce clear yellow urine that is negative for red blood cells
- Patient will demonstrate balanced intake and output
- Patient will demonstrate patent catheter
- Patient will experience no difficulty voiding following catheter removal
- Patient will report a decrease in pain
- Patient will demonstrate stable vital signs
- Patient will exhibit no frank signs of bleeding
- Patient will exhibit no elevation in WBC

Implementation

Nursing interventions for the patient with lower urinary tract injury focus on maintenance of adequate urinary output. Intake and output are monitored closely, including the characteristics of the urinary output. Meticulous catheter care is performed twice a day (see p. 1140). The nurse must ensure the patency of the catheter. Prescribed analgesics are administered as needed. Alterations in vital signs and a dropping hemoglobin and hematocrit are reported to the physician. Antibiotics are often ordered on a prophylactic basis.

Evaluation

Ongoing patient evaluation is essential and will include monitoring the quantity and quality of urinary

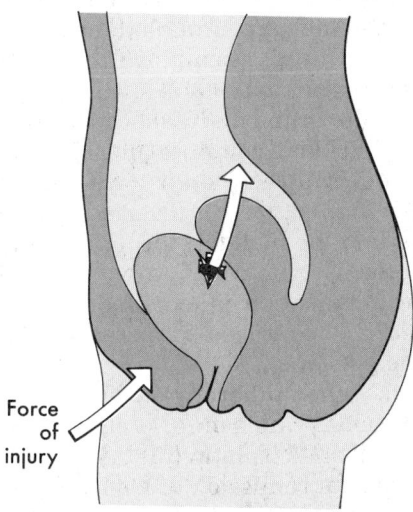

FIGURE 43-10   Traumatic rupture of bladder dome.

output. Pain control is evidenced by statements rendered by the patient as well as by the patient's relaxed body posture. Prevention of hypovolemia is evaluated by maintenance of normal vital signs, normal hemoglobin and hematocrit, and no obvious bleeding. Absence of infection is based upon absence of fever and normal WBC. The nursing care plan is then modified based upon the evaluation.

Documentation

Documentation includes recording of intake and output and the character of the urine output. The location, intensity, and character of pain must be documented as well as the patient's response to pain relief interventions. Any eccyhmosis or distention is also noted.

Ongoing Care

After the catheter and/or drains are removed, adequate urinary output must be maintained. Since strictures, incontinence, or impotence may occur following urethral trauma, discharge teaching should include the importance to the patient regarding reporting any abnormalities even after discharge.

TUMORS OF THE BLADDER
Definition

Bladder cancer is an abnormal formation of tissue within the bladder lumen and progressive infiltration of the bladder wall. Bladder cancer is the most commonly occurring malignancy of the urinary tract.

Etiology/Epidemiology

Cancer of the bladder occurs more often in men than women (2:1 ratio) and accounts for 2% of all cancer deaths in the United States.[8] The age group most commonly affected is 50 to 70 years of age. Cigarette smoking and tobacco tar are associated with a high incidence of bladder neoplasms.[8] Exposure to aniline dyes, rubber, textiles, and packing materials is also implicated in the development of bladder cancer. There is generally a prolonged delay between exposure and tumor development. Other possible causes are chronic cystitis, ingestion of large amounts of phenacetin, pelvic radiation, bladder calculus disease, and chronic schistosomiasis. There has been some suggestion of an association between coffee drinking and bladder cancer but the relationship is uncertain. It is also unclear what link there is between bladder cancer and the artificial sweeteners saccharin and sodium cyclamate.[12]

Pathophysiology

The majority of cancers are papillomatous growths within the bladder. Transitional cell carcinoma is the most common type of bladder tumor (85%). True squamous cell and glandular cancer may also occur, with some tumors undifferentiated. Staging is determined by the depth of tumor penetration into the bladder wall (see Chapter 15 for information on the TNM tumor classification system). Metastases spread along lymphatic and hematogenous routes, with regional lymph nodes, liver, lung, and bones being common sites. Diagnostic studies include urinalysis, which may demonstrate microscopic hematuria when blood is not apparent. An intravenous pyelogram may be used as an early yet inconclusive diagnostic measure. DNA ploidy by cytology and flow cytometry are used in screening high risk patients.[8] Excretory urogram evaluates bladder filling. Pelvic CT scan may be used in staging. Bimanual assessment under anesthesia aids in clinical classification. Cystoscopy with biopsy is definitive in diagnosing.

Clinical Manifestations

Hematuria is the presenting sign in 75% of patients with bladder cancer. Painless hematuria, either microscopic or gross, often occurs intermittently. Frequency, burning, bladder irritability, dysuria, and pyuria are present in about one third of patients and progress in severity with time.

Therapeutic Management

Patients with carcinoma in situ, a malignancy that has yet to invade underlying tissue, have the best prognosis for 5-year survival (80%) when treated by cystectomy, lymph node dissection and radiation.[21] With invasive carcinoma the survival rate drops dramatically.

Chemotherapy

Both topical and systemic chemotherapy may be given in the management of bladder cancer. Topical chemotherapy (intravesical) involves instilling a high concentration of antineoplastic agent (thiotepa, bleomycin, doxorubicin, 5-fluorouracil, mitomycin C, or BCG-bacillus Calmette-Guerin) into the bladder to come in direct contact with the neoplastic cells. A urethral catheter is inserted. The medication is instilled into the bladder, the fluid is retained, and the catheter is removed. After approximately 2 hours, the medication is expelled via voiding, and the patient is encouraged to increase fluids to facilitate the expulsion.

Systemic chemotherapy using methotrexate (Amethopterin), vinblastine (Velban), doxorubicin (Adriamycin), and cisplatin (Platinol) have been successful in partial remission of transitional cell carcinoma. Thus far the most effective agent in treating bladder cancer has been cisplatin.[8] Other agents used are 5-fluorouracil (5-FU), cyclophosphamide

(Cytoxan), and mitomycin-C (Mutamycin). MVAC (Methotrexate, Vinblastine, Adriamycin, Cisplatin) regimen is currently under investigation.

Radiation therapy

Radiation therapy is seldom used alone due to the low survival rates and the complications from radiation damage. Rather radiation is used with radical cystectomy or in combination with cisplatin (a radio-potentiator). The best results are obtained with radiation and surgery. Radiation therapy may be given internally or externally, and it is administered preoperatively to retard tumor growth, as well as postoperatively. In advanced stages radiation may be used palliatively to control pain and bleeding.

Surgical management

For simple papillomas, transurethral resection or fulguration (tissue destruction by electrical current) may be performed. Recurrence is common, so cytology and cystoscopy should be performed every 3 months for 2 years and then every 6 months for an additional 3 years. Because these papillomas can also grow along ureters and even in the collecting system at the top of the ureters, some centers recommend cystoscopy every 3 months with retrograde pyelograms every 6 months for one year; cystoscopy with retrograde pyelogram every 6 months for the second year and then cystoscopy with retrograde pyelogram once a year thereafter. If during any of these procedures another papilloma is found, the patient is placed back onto the 3-month rotation and the cycle starts over.

Used to treat superficial bladder cancers, the NT: Yag laser, can be repeated numerous times if there is recurrence. Single large lesions, especially those located on the dome or lateral wall of the bladder, may be treated with segmental resection (partial cystectomy) of the bladder. If the tumor is invasive, multifocal, or involves the trigone, a simple **cystectomy** (bladder removal) or radical cystectomy with permanent urinary diversion will be necessary. A radical cystectomy involves removal of the bladder and urethra and pelvic lymph node dissection. In men, removal of the prostate and seminal vesicles, and in women, removal of the uterus, fallopian tubes, ovaries, and anterior vagina are also done.

Urinary diversions

Urinary diversions supply an alternate pathway for urine elimination when the normal route through the bladder is impassable or restricted (Table 43-4). Although most commonly performed in patients who have required a partial or total cystectomy as a result of bladder cancer, urinary diversions may be done in patients with strictures, congenital anomalies, neurogenic bladder, chronic UTI with declining renal function, or trauma to the ureters, bladder, or urethra.

There are two main types of urinary diversion: incontinent and continent. Incontinent diversion includes the ileal conduit, cutaneous ureterostomy, ureterosigmoidostomy, and nephrostomy. The disadvantages of these type diversions center around the fact that urine flow is constant and an external collection device is required permanently. Continent diversion includes the Kock's pouch, Mainze reservoirs, Indiana pouches, continent vesicostomy, and the Camey procedure. Although there is no consensus as to the ideal means of diversion, the ileal con-

---

TABLE 43-4   Urinary Diversion

Type	Characteristics	Particulars
Ileal conduit	Abdominal stoma; ureters are anastomosed to an isolated section of the terminal ileum, then brought to the abdomen, forming an ileostomy	Ostomy appliance needed; drains only urine
Ureterosigmoidostomy	Urine is diverted into the colon and excreted out the rectum by implanting the ureters to a segment of the ileum and anastomosing them to the sigmoid colon	Rectal tube may be necessary; monitor for electrolyte imbalance
Cutaneous ureterostomy	Detaching the ureter from the bladder and bringing it through the abdominal wall and through the skin	Urinary appliance needed; ureteral dilation may be necessary to maintain patency
Nephrostomy	Placement of a ureteral catheter that enters the kidney and exits at the flank	Urostomy appliance or collection system necessary; do not irrigate or clamp tube

duit remains the most commonly performed diversion.

Incontinent diversions

With the **ileal conduit** the ureters are transplanted to a 4- to 6-inch resected segment of the ileum or sigmoid colon while the bowel ends are anastomosed to provide an intact intestine (Figure 43-11, *A*). The mesentery is allowed to remain connected in order to maintain perfusion and tissue viability to the isolated segment. The proximal end of the ileal loop is sutured closed and the distal end is brought out onto the abdominal wall in the form of a stoma. There is no reservoir, therefore, continuous urine flow occurs. This is an involved surgical procedure with increased postoperative complications over simple cutaneous ureterostomy. On the other hand, the stoma is larger and easier to manage than the ureterostomy stoma. Complications associated with the ileal conduit are obstruction, urine leakage, stomal changes such as stenosis, prolapse or gangrene, wound infection, skin irritation, encrustation around the stoma, odor, pyelonephritis, renal calculi, and electrolyte imbalances such as hyperchloremic acidosis.

Cutaneous ureterostomy, a less extensive procedure, is used for high risk patients. One or both ureters are transplanted from the bladder and brought out through the skin to form one or two stomas (Figure 43-11, *B*). This procedure is successful on chronically dilated ureters. In addition, since the intestine is not involved, there is little risk of peritonitis, intestinal complications, or electrolyte imbalances. Because of continuous urine flow, a collection bag is applied. A transureteroureterostomy (Figure 43-11, *C*) results in one stoma (one ureter is anastomosed into the other ureter), whereas a bilateral ureterostomy produces two stomas. Because of the small, flush stomas created, frequent skin irritations and strictures occur. Ureteral dilation may be necessary to maintain patency.

A **ureterosigmoidostomy** is an internal urinary

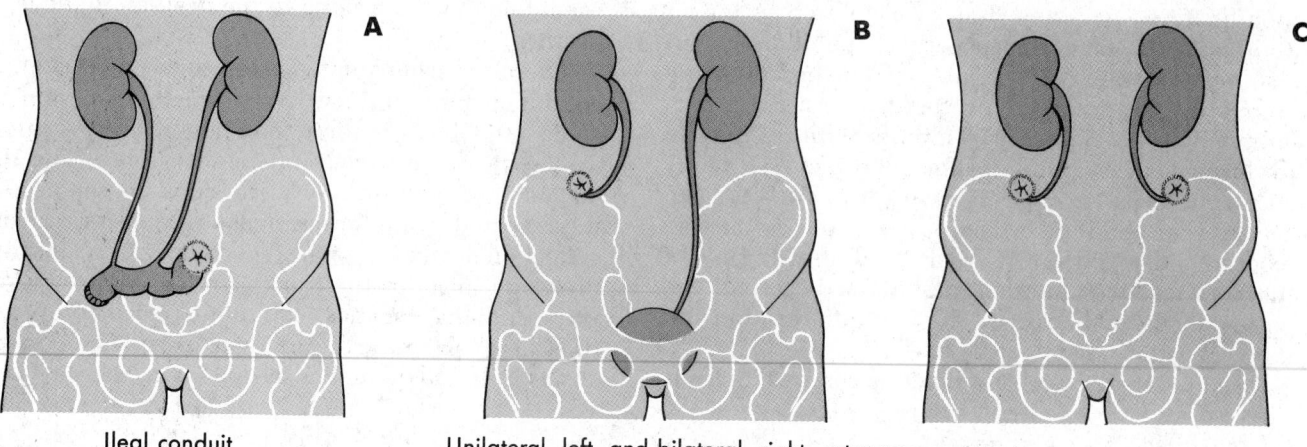

A   B   C

Ileal conduit   Unilateral, left, and bilateral, right, cutaneous ureterostomy

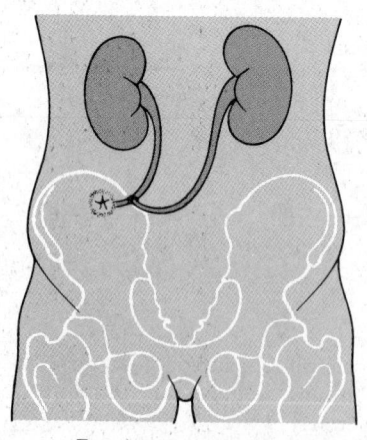
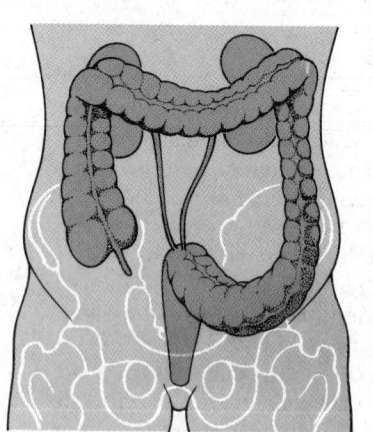
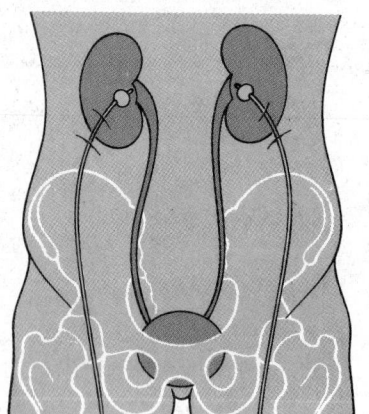

D   E   F

Transureterostomy   Ureterosigmoidostomy   Nephrostomy

FIGURE 43-11   Incontinent urinary diversions.

diversion that redirects urine through the colon and then out the rectum (Figure 43-11, *D*). The ureters are anastomosed to a nonrefluxing segment of the sigmoid colon. This detour into the colon causes two major complications: metabolic disorders (hyperchloremic acidosis) and pyelonephritis. To be a candidate for this procedure the patient must have a competent anal sphincter since urine excretion will occur from the rectum permanently. The drainage from the rectum will have the consistency of watery diarrhea. This can result in acidosis and electrolyte imbalances involving potassium, chloride, and magnesium. Pyelonephritis occurs as a result of reflux of bacteria from the colon. Adenocarcinoma may develop over time as the colonic mucosa is irritated by the exposure to urine.

A nephrostomy is the insertion of a catheter into the renal pelvis (Figure 43-11, *E*). It may be done percutaneously or by using a flank incision. This procedure is usually done palliatively because of the high risk of infection and stone formation (see nephrostomy tubes elsewhere in this chapter).

Continent diversions

Kock's pouch, a continent ileal urinary reservoir, is created by transplanting the ureters to a 2-foot-long dissected segment of the terminal ileum that remains attached to the highly vascular mesentery to maintain perfusion.[10] This segment of bowel is fashioned into a pouch (reservoir) inside the patient's abdomen (Figure 43-12, *A*). A nipplelike one-way valve is created at both ends to prevent urinary reflux and leakage. One end of the pouch is attached to the abdominal wall creating a stoma. To drain the reservoir, a catheter is inserted through the stoma and nipple valve and urine is drained every 2 to 3 hours. This procedure is advantageous since an external collection bag is unnecessary. It is also safer for the kidneys since a valve is formed that prevents urine reflux. Disadvantages include the possibility of leakage and difficulty in catheterizing the stoma.

A variation of the Kock's pouch involves attaching the distal end of the pouch to the patient's urethra so the patient can void almost normally (Figure 43-12, *B*). Women are not candidates for this pro-

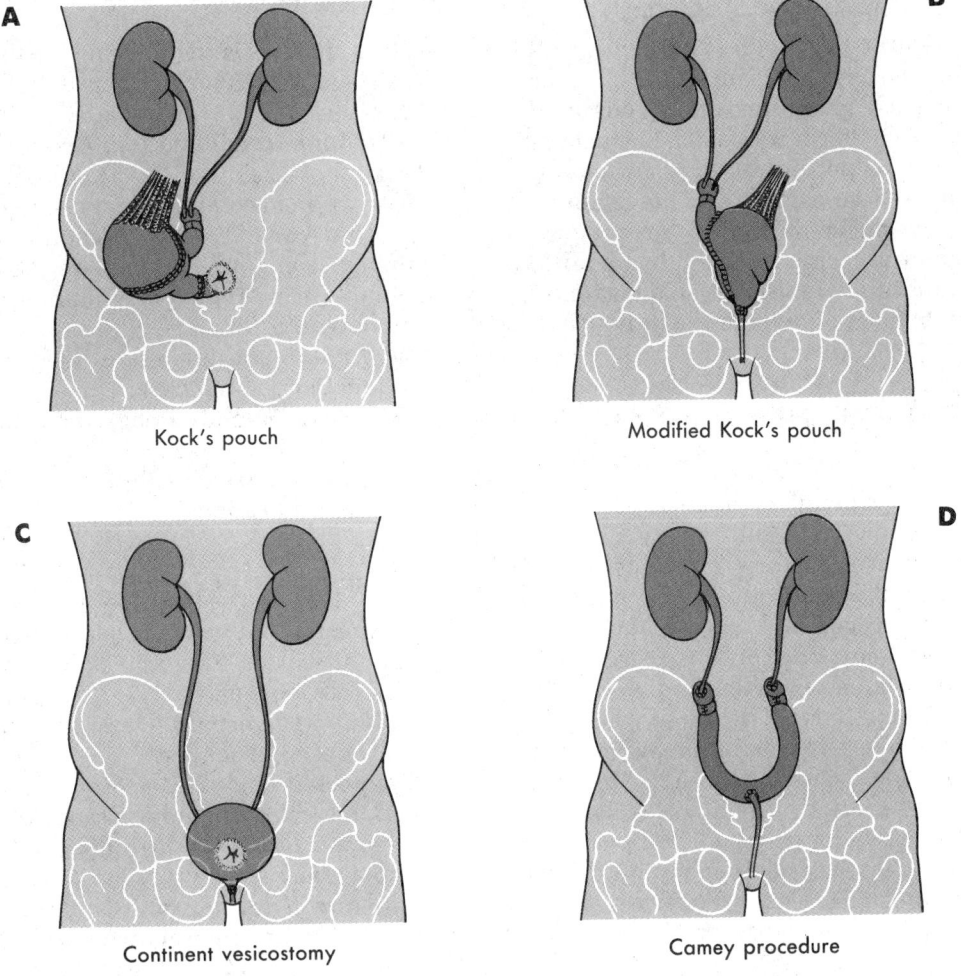

FIGURE 43-12 Continent urinary diversions.

cedure because their urethras are too short. In addition, the patient's urethra must appear to be free of malignancy. Cancer patients who have this procedure are at greater risk of recurrence of cancer within two years because the urethra is susceptible when there is bladder cancer.[10] Although still a relatively new procedure, there seems to be a great deal of success when used in selected patients.

The Mainze reservoir is another variation of the Kock's pouch that is created from the ileum and cecum. The ureters are implanted through the wall of the colon into the pouch. The stoma is then created either above the pubis or in the umbilicus.

The Indiana reservoir creates an artificial bladder from the terminal ileus, ascending colon, and cecum. The stoma may be placed either on the abdomen, the vaginal wall, or anastomosed to the urethra.

With a continent vesicostomy the urethra is sutured closed (Figure 43-12, C). The anterior bladder wall is attached to the abdominal wall and a flush stoma is created. A valve is created surgically that prevents urine leakage at the stoma. The bladder is then emptied periodically by self-catheterization. This procedure is performed most often in cases of neurogenic bladder.

The Camey procedure involves creating an artificial bladder from 40 cm of ileum, shaping it into a "U" and attaching the apex to the urethra.[18] The ureters are anastomosed to the proximal ends of the loop (Figure 43-12, D), permitting near-normal voiding. This procedure is performed only on male patients. There must be no evidence of malignancy at or near the urethra and confirmation during surgery that the malignancy was organ-confined. In addition, the mesentery must allow tension-free anastomosis, otherwise another form of diversion will be used.

NURSING MANAGEMENT OF THE PATIENT WITH BLADDER CANCER
Assessment

The nurse will obtain a detailed voiding history, noting a history of chronic UTIs and previous bladder tumors. A detailed drug history, inquiring specifically about the use of Phenacetin is also obtained. The nurse will note precipitating factors including a history of cigarette smoking or excessive coffee drinking and associated symptoms such as frequency, dysuria, and urgency. The nurse will obtain a social history and a description of the patient's environment and evaluate whether there has been exposure to chemical carcinogens in the workplace. The nurse also assesses for any pain the patient is experiencing, especially low back pain, and the patient's response to analgesics. Preoperatively the nurse assesses the knowledge of the patient and

family regarding the planned procedure and how it will affect excretory function. If a stoma is planned, preoperative teaching will include information about the stoma. The nurse will also explore the patient's feelings about the procedure's effects on body image and sexual function. Additional data collected by the nurse include the amount and character of the urine, evidence of a palpable pelvic mass, a urinalysis positive for red blood cells, and a cytology report detecting abnormal cells. If output is decreased, palpation of the lower abdomen may be necessary to detect bladder distention and retention.

Nursing Diagnosis
Preoperative

Based on data analysis, the nursing diagnoses would be:

Knowledge deficit related to perioperative events and self-care postoperatively

Anxiety related to the effects of the procedure and anticipatory grieving

Postoperative

Nursing diagnoses include the customary postoperative diagnoses (refer to Chapter 24). Diagnoses specific to bladder cancer include:

Alteration in elimination: Urinary related to surgical diversion

Alteration in comfort: Pain related to surgical procedure or effects of chemotherapy

High risk for infection related to surgical procedure, urine reflux, or immunosuppression from chemotherapy

High risk for altered skin integrity related to inadequate stoma care

High risk for body image disturbance related to changes in self-concept

High risk for sexual dysfunction related to anatomic alterations

Planning

The expected outcomes preoperatively are:

Patient will verbalize an understanding of perioperative events

Patient will verbalize less anxiety regarding the proposed procedure

The expected outcomes postoperatively are:

Patient will participate in care of stoma and collection device or in management of continent diversion

Patient will develop daily routine to accommodate urinary diversion management

Patient will demonstrate increasing independence in self-care

Patient will report adequate pain control

Patient will exhibit proper hygiene

Patient will develop no wound infection

Patient will develop no UTI

Patient will develop no systemic infection

Patient will verbalize actions to prevent/treat skin excoriation

Patient will demonstrate a pink, moist stoma and intact peristomal skin

Patient will verbalize acceptance of urinary diversion and accompanying changes

Patient will resume normal ADLs and returns to near-normal life-style

Patient will verbalize concerns regarding sexual functioning

Patient will verbalize alternate positions for intercourse

Patient will identify alternative methods of sexual expression

Implementation

Preoperative

Assessment of the patient's knowledge base guides the nurse in developing a teaching plan. Teaching prior to surgery includes routine operative instructions including turn, cough, deep breathe, and calf muscle exercises. Specific instructions include a description of the procedure, appearance, location, and care of a stoma and appliance if applicable. The patient is instructed regarding a general anesthetic. If the procedure includes manipulation of the intestines, then the patient is prepared for the likelihood of a nasogastric tube.

The teaching plan includes the social aspects of living with a stoma, or the aspects of training that may be necessary for some type of continent diversions. When there is an internal reservoir created that is connected to the urethra, muscle exercises are performed to prevent dribbling. A visit from a successful ostomy patient might be helpful at this point.

Changes in sexual functioning are also discussed preoperatively, including loss of ejaculation, and possible impotence in men, as well as possible painful intercourse in women if the vaginal wall is significantly disrupted.

The bowel is prepared prior to surgery to reduce the risk of infection from intestinal flora. A low residue diet is begun 2 days before surgery, with a clear liquid diet ordered the day before surgery. Laxatives, cleansing enemas, bowel preps (e.g., Golytely), and antimicrobials such as neomycin and kanamycin for bowel cleansing are administered preoperatively.

Postoperative

Nursing interventions center around maintenance of adequate urinary output. Careful intake and output are maintained. The volume should be assessed hourly. If it falls below 30 mL/hour, the physician must be notified since there may be obstruction or leakage. Often stents (hollow tubes) are placed in the ureters to ensure drainage until the swelling subsides. The patient can expect them to remain in place between 1 and 2 weeks. The urine flow from each stent is measured and recorded individually. Any decrease in output is reported immediately.

The patient is encouraged to take in between 2500 mL and 3000 mL of fluid daily to flush the urinary tract and decrease the risk of infection. With diversions that utilize segments of the bowel, a great deal of intestinal mucus in the urine is expected immediately postoperatively. For this reason high fluid intake also serves to decrease the accumulation of mucus. The nurse will expect a little blood-tinged urine in the immediate postoperative period, but should report bloody urine.

Drainage tubes are often inserted into the abdomen to remove fluid that may accumulate from surgical trauma. These are monitored for bleeding. The dressings are changed using aseptic technique when they become damp.

The stoma is monitored for bleeding. Any change in color from the normal pink/red to dark purple implies impaired vascular supply and is immediately reported to the physician.

Electrolyte imbalance may occur when urine comes in contact with bowel mucosa. With the ureterosigmoidostomy the urine evacuated from the bowel simulates diarrhea with its attendant complications. The nurse will monitor serum electrolytes as ordered. Sodium chloride intake is reduced to prevent hyperchloremic acidosis while potassium intake is increased via foods and medication since potassium is lost when the patient experiences acidosis.

Pain is managed by use of opioid analgesics, heat application, and position changes. Any sudden increase in pain is reported to the physician as this may signal obstruction or leakage.

The patient may have a nasogastric tube to prevent stress on the suture line for the first 3 to 5 days after surgery. The nurse will ensure patency of the tube through normal saline irrigations as ordered. Early ambulation will promote peristalsis. The presence of bowel sounds and passing of flatus and stool signal the return of peristalsis. These cues indicate the advisability of removing the tube. Stool softeners are frequently ordered prophylactically to prevent constipation and stress on the suture line.

Aseptic technique is used when changing dressings and when manipulating collection devices. These devices should be drained at least every 8 hours to prevent urine from standing in the bag or being reintroduced into the stoma. Likewise, initially continent diversions require emptying every 2 hours to prevent collection of stagnant urine, reflux, and pressure on the suture line. The interval between emptying will gradually increase to about every 2 to 4 hours depending upon the volume of the reservoir. The patient is taught to recognize vague abdominal discomfort as the cue to empty the reservoir. The nurse is alert to fever, flank pain, abdominal pain, and cloudy, foul-smelling urine as symptomatic of UTI. To decrease bacterial growth, ensure the urine is acidic by administration of an acid-ash diet after peristalsis resumes and diet is reinstated. In addition, the nurse monitors for signs and symptoms of peritonitis that may occur with either urine or bowel leaks.

The patient is taught good hygienic practice that includes the proper care of reusable bags (see Chapter 66 for further information about ostomy care). Use of a straight drainage system connected to gravity drainage at night or when in bed decreases the risk of infection with incontinent diversions.

The stoma and the skin adjacent to it are inspected for adequate circulation as well as irritation. There should be no tight binders over the stoma. Any retraction of the stoma is reported since this may indicate stenosis. The stoma is not sensitive to touch but the skin around it may be irritated by urine or the appliance. The position of the appliance is observed for accurate fit. If urine comes in contact with the skin, the area is cleansed with warm soapy water and patted dry. Karaya powder may be helpful in preventing skin breakdown. Alkaline urine is irritating to the skin and will cause encrustations, therefore maintain an acidic urine. The collection device must fit snugly around the stoma to prevent leakage. Frequent emptying of the collection bag will aid in eliminating odor. A consultation with an enterostomal therapist is usually beneficial for the patient with a stoma.

Encourage the patient to share feelings about body changes. The patient may have fears about the cancer and its progression. Be willing to listen. Encourage a gradual resumption in ADLs. Discuss with the patient adjustments in social activities since they may have to be planned around the need to eliminate. Encourage the patient to vent feelings of frustration, anger, embarrassment, or isolation. Assist the patient in viewing the stoma.

The nurse provides accurate information to the patient and significant other regarding sexual activity. Different positions may be necessary to accommodate an appliance. The collection bag should be emptied prior to sexual intercourse. If an erection is impossible, then the nurse will advise the patient to discuss the possibility of a penile implant with the physician.

Chemotherapy

Intravesicular chemotherapy is introduced directly into the bladder where it remains for approximately 2 hours. During this time the patient is reminded to roll from side to side often so that all areas of the bladder wall come in contact with the medication. Although thiotepa may cause myelosuppression, mitomycin C rarely does since it is poorly absorbed. It does, however, irritate the bladder and may cause rashes on genitals and palms.[21]

Patients receiving systemic chemotherapy are monitored for infection since they become immunosuppressed and leukopenic. Neupogen has proven effective in quickly elevating a depressed WBC. Thrombocytopenia is another common adverse reaction and may result in bleeding. The nurse assesses for bleeding gums, hematuria, and melena. The patient is instructed to use a soft cloth to clean the teeth. Anemia causes fatigue that is unrelenting. The patient is reminded to take rest breaks, naps, and not to overextend.

Should stomatitis (ulceration of the buccal mucosa) occur, spicy, acid, and salty foods are restricted. In addition, sucralfate (Carafate) dissolved or swished in the mouth has provided some relief. Ondansetron hydrochloride (Zofran) has proven effective in controlling the nausea and vomiting associated with chemotherapy.

Intravenous fluids administered before cisplatin (Patinol) aid in decreasing the risk of renal toxicity.[21] The BUN, creatinine, and uric acid levels are monitored for increases that may be associated with renal toxicity.

Since cisplatin causes ototoxicity, baseline hearing is evaluated. Any report of tinnitus should be investigated. Vinblastine (Velban) may cause neurotoxicity. Instruct the patient to report tingling, numbness, or pain in the extremities. Doxorubicin (Adriamycin) causes cardiotoxicity. Shortness of breath, tachycardia, chest pain, or peripheral edema is reported to the physician.

Both vinblastine (Velban) and doxorubicin (Adriamycin) are vesicants, meaning they will cause tissue necrosis if they extravasate (leak out of the vein). Any patient receiving a vesicant is instructed to notify the nurse immediately if there is pain or swelling at the IV site. Should extravasation occur, notify the physician and follow the institution's policy and procedure (additional information about chemotherapy and radiation therapy can be found in Chapter 15).

Evaluation

Preoperatively the nurse will evaluate the patient's understanding of the planned perioperative events and the patient's anxiety regarding the events. Postoperatively the patient will regain an effective means of urine evacuation, including demonstrating stoma care or continent diversion care. The patient will verbalize comfort and indicate those methods that are most helpful. The patient will not develop an infection of any kind. Furthermore, the patient will demonstrate acceptance of life-style changes and accompanying modifications in sexual functioning.

Documentation

Documentation should reflect voiding pattern and the character of the urine, intake and output, and any symptoms of UTI. Nursing measures directed at pain management and their effectiveness are noted. Patient self-care abilities are documented. Further documentation also includes education provided for the patient with a urinary diversion and coping mechanisms that help the patient in dealing with changes in body image and sexuality as well as the implications of a diagnosis of cancer.

Ongoing Care

The patient is advised that the stoma will probably shrink within 2 months and the faceplate size for the stoma appliance may need to be changed to maintain the proper fit. If mucus remains thick enough to clog the urinary appliance outlet, suggest that the patient drink at least three liters of fluid/day. Instruct the patient to report chronic thick mucus since this may indicate infection. The nurse will instruct the patient in intermittent self-catheterization prior to discharge. The nurse refers the patient to a local ostomy club for support. Information about where to obtain supplies should be covered prior to discharge. The patient is advised of the symptoms of obstruction/infection and the actions to take. The patient needs a phone number to call should there be difficulty with any aspect of care in the home setting.

Because of the high incidence of malignancy recurrence, the need for follow-up care must be emphasized. Names and phone numbers of support groups and counselors are made available to help the person deal with the diagnosis of cancer. The signs and symptoms of recurrence or progression are reviewed with the patient so intervention can take place quickly if needed.

CRITICAL THINKING QUESTIONS

1 What are the four types of urinary incontinence?
2 Develop a bladder training program for an incontinent patient.
3 List the clinical manifestations of acute urinary retention.
4 What interventions should be taken to establish urinary drainage in a patient with urinary retention?
5 Describe the common causes of a UTI.
6 What behaviors are necessary to prevent recurrence of a UTI?
7 How do strictures and cancer of the bladder contribute to a urinary obstruction?

RESOURCES

Publications and support groups
1 Information regarding incontinence and treatment. Send stamped, self-addressed envelope:
The Continent Program
University of Rochester
Monroe Community Hospital
435 E. Henrietta Road
Rochester, New York 14620
Phone: 716-274-7560
2 Quarterly newsletter and audiocassettes. For a small fee a Resource Guide of Continence Aids and Services can be obtained.
HIP
PO Box 544
Union, SC 29379
Phone: 803-579-7900
3 Continence Restored, Inc. (a HIP chapter) has nationwide support groups. Send self-addressed envelope:
Continence Restored, Inc.
785 Park Avenue
New York, NY 10021
4 Quarterly newsletter on continence called The Informer. Film/videos, publications, and audiocassettes dealing with continence are also available. Send self-addressed stamped envelope:
The Simon Foundation for Continence
PO Box 835-M
Wilmette, IL 60091
Phone: 800-23-SIMON
5 Information on a bladder training program:
Alliance for Aging Research
2021 K Street, N.W.
Suite 305
Washington, DC 20006

6 Guidelines are available in formats suitable for health care practitioners, the scientific community, educators, and consumers from the Urinary Incontinence Guideline Panel, US Department of Health and Human Services, Public Health Service, Agency for Health Care Policy and Research.

Urinary Incontinence in Adults: Clinical Practice Guideline. AHCPR Pub. No. 92-0038. Rockville, MD: Agency for Health Care Policy and Research, Public Health Service, US Department of Health and Human Services, March 1992.

Urinary Incontinence in Adults: Quick Reference Guide for Clinicians. AHCPR Pub. No. 92-0041. Rockville, MD: Agency for Health Care Policy and Research, Public Health Service US Department of Health and Human Services, March 1992.

Urinary Incontinence in Adults: A Patient's Guide: AHCPR Pub. No. 92-0040. Rockville, MD: Agency for Health Care Policy and Research, Public Health Service, US Department of Health and Human Services, March 1992
Contact:
Agency for Health Care Policy and Research
Publications Clearinghouse
P.O. Box 8547
Silver Spring, MD 20907
Phone: 800-358-9295 or 301-495-3453f

BIBLIOGRAPHY

1. Anderson GP: A fresh look at assessing the elderly, *RN* 52(6):28, 1989.
2. Bently D: Infectious diseases. In Rossman I, editor: *Clinical geriatrics,* Philadelphia, 1986, JB Lippincott.
3. Bristoll SL et al, The mythical danger of rapid urinary drainage, *Am J Nurs,* 89(3):344, 1989.
4. Clark JB, Queener SF, Karb VB: *Pharmacological basis of nursing practice,* ed 3, St. Louis, 1990, Mosby–Year Book.
5. Dodds P, Hans AL: Distended urinary bladder drainage practices among hospital nurses, *Appl Nurs Res* 3(2):68, 1990.
6. Ebersole P, Hess P, editors: *Toward healthy aging: human needs and nursing responses,* ed 3, St Louis, 1990, Mosby–Year Book.
7. Farrell J: *Nursing care of the older person,* Philadelphia, 1990, Lippincott.
8. Frank IN, Graham, SD, Nabors WL: Urologic and male genital cancers. In Holleb AI, Fink DJ, Murphy GP, editors *American Cancer Society textbook of clinical oncology,* Atlanta, 1991, American Cancer Society.
9. Goldsmith J: Scientist wins one for women, *Sigma Theta Tau International Re. ections* 17(4):8, 1992.
10. Greig BJ: A new option for cystectomy patients, *RN* 53(9):34, 1990.
11. Hill, MG: Intra-abdominal trauma. In Howell E, Widra L, Hill MG, editor *Comprehensive trauma nursing: theory and practice,* Glenview, Ill, 1988, Scott, Foresman, & Co.
12. National Cancer Institute: *Cancer of the bladder research report,* 1990, US Department of Health & Human Services.
13. McCormick KA et al: Urinary incontinence: an augmented approach, *J Gerontol Nurs* 18(3):3, 1992.
14. McCormick KA et al: Clinical guidelines: urinary incontinence in adults, *Am J Nurs* 92(10):75, 1992.
15. McKenry LM, Salerno E: *Mosby's pharmacology in nursing,* ed 17, St. Louis, 1989, Mosby–Year Book.
16. Newman DK et al: Restoring urinary continence, *Am J Nurs* 91(1):28, 1991.
17. Orzeck S, Ouslander J: Urinary incontinence: an overview of causes and treatment, *J Enterostomal Therapy* 14(1):20, 1987.
18. Rauscher J, Farber RD, Parra RO: Camey procedure: a continent urinary diversion technique, *AORN* 54(1):34, 1991.
19. Ruhl JM: Pelvic trauma, *RN* 54(7):50, 1991.
20. Stolley JM, Buckwalter KC: Nosocomial infections, *J Gerontol Nurs* 17(9):30, 1991.
21. Tootla J, Easterling AD: Current options in bladder cancer management, *RN* 55(4):42, 1992.
22. Urinary Incontinence Guideline Panel: *Urinary incontinence in adults: clinical practice guideline,* Pub No. 92-0038, Rockville, Md, 1992, Agency for Health Care Policy and Research, Public Health Service, US Department of Health & Human Services.
23. Warkentin R: Implementation of a urinary continence program, *J Gerontol Nurs* 18(1):31, 1992.
24. White KM, Kenner CV: Abdominal trauma. In Dossey BM, Guezzetta CE, Kenner CV, editors: *Critical care nursing: body, mind, spirit,* ed 3, Philadelphia, 1992, JB Lippincott.
25. Wozniak-Petrofsky J: Treating older men's most common problem, *RN* 54(7):32, 1991.
26. Yu LC et al: Urinary incontinence: Nursing home staff reaction toward residents, *J Gerontol Nurs* 17(11):34, 1991.

UNIT XI

Neurologic System

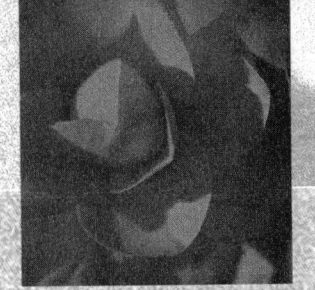

CHAPTER FORTY-FOUR

Nursing Assessment of the Neurologic System

LEARNING OBJECTIVES

1 Understand the basic anatomic structure of the neurologic system.
2 Outline the manner in which information is carried to and relayed from the central nervous system.
3 Describe the difference between stereotyped and voluntary responses.
4 Obtain relevant subjective information from the patient who has a neurologic alteration.
5 Using correct technique, examine the patient to obtain appropriate objective information about the neurologic system.
6 Differentiate abnormal from normal subjective and objective findings related to the neurologic system.
7 Describe procedures and tests used in the diagnosis and detection of disorders of the neurologic system.
8 Discuss the preparation and care of patients undergoing diagnostic tests of the neurologic system.

KEY TERMS

acetylcholine, p. 1165
adaptation, p. 1163
autonomic nervous system, p. 1165
brain scan, p. 1196
brainstem, p. 1173
cerebellum, p. 1173
cerebrospinal fluid, p. 1175
cerebrum, p. 1175
computed tomography, p. 1193
cranial nerves, p. 1163

diencephalon, p. 1173
echoencephalography, p. 1197
electroencephalography, p. 1196
electromyography, p. 1197
evoked potential studies, p. 1197
ganglia, p. 1165
limbic system, p. 1175
lumbar puncture, p. 1190
magnetic resonance imaging, p. 1196
medulla oblongata, p. 1174
meninges, p. 1175
myelography, p. 1194

nerve impulse, p. 1165
neurons, p. 1163
neurotransmitter, p. 1165
norepinephrine, p. 1165
receptors, p. 1162
reflex, p. 1172
resting potential, p. 1165
reticular activating system, p. 1175
spinal cord, p. 1169
spinal nerves, p. 1163
stereognosis, p. 1187
ventricles, p. 1175

THE NEUROLOGIC SYSTEM functions to sense changes in the external and internal environments of the individual, to carry information about these changes to the central nervous system, and to carry to the tissues the commands required to perform a response. These tasks are the responsibility of the sensory receptors and nerves of the peripheral nervous system and the projection tracts of the central nervous system. The response to environmental changes is planned and integrated by the central nervous system, the spinal cord, and the brain.

The assessment of the neurologic system includes an examination of the patient's mental status, speech patterns, cranial nerve function, proprioception, balance and coordination, reflexes, and sensory perception. Also important is an appraisal of psychosocial functioning. A review of the musculoskeletal system is an inseparable part of the neurologic assessment. Muscle mass, tone, and strength and range of motion are primary concerns for patients reporting neurologic alterations. Throughout the assessment, the nurse must take care to relate assumptions about the cause of neurologic dysfunction to the patient's developmental stage.

ANATOMY AND PHYSIOLOGY
Detecting Changes in Internal and External Environment

A wide variety of physical and chemical changes in the internal and external environment of the body are detected by specialized structures called **receptors** and converted into nerve impulses. The number of nerve impulses generated per second (frequency) is directly related to the strength of the change detected by the receptor. The magnitude of a change is perceived by the brain, which evaluates the frequency of nerve impulses and the number of sensory neurons activated by the change. Receptors are widely distributed throughout most of the body. However, their distribution is not uniform; for example, the skin, which is important in monitoring the external environment, has a wide range of different receptors, and they are particularly plentiful in its most sensitive areas. Conversely, the brain lacks receptors and is insensitive, although its blood vessel walls and meninges possess receptors and are sensitive to pain.

TABLE 44-1 Classification of Receptors by Location and Structure

Types	Locations	General senses
CLASSIFICATION BY LOCATION		
Superficial receptors	At or near surface of body; in skin and mucosa	Touch, pressure, heat, cold, and pain
Deep receptors (proprioceptors)	In muscles, tendons, and joints	Proprioception (sense of position and movement) Vibration, deep pressure, deep pain
Internal receptors (visceroceptors)	In viscera and in blood vessel walls	Usually no sensations result from stimulation of internal receptors; exceptions: hunger, nausea, and pain from certain stimuli (notably distention and some chemicals)
CLASSIFICATION BY STRUCTURE		
Meissner's corpuscles	Skin (in papillae of dermis); numerous in fingertips and lips	Fine touch, vibration
Ruffini's corpuscles	Skin (dermal layer) and subcutaneous tissue of fingers	Touch, pressure
Pacinian corpuscles	Subcutaneous, submucous, and subserous tissues, around joints, in mammary glands and external genitalia of both sexes	Pressure, vibration
Krause's end-bulbs	Skin (dermal layer), subcutaneous tissue, mucosa of lips and eyelids, external genitalia	Touch
Golgi tendon receptors	Near junction of tendons and muscles	Subconscious muscle sense
Muscle spindles	Skeletal muscles	Subconscious muscle sense

Adapted from Thibodeau GA: *Anthony's textbook of anatomy and physiology*, ed 13, St Louis, 1990, Mosby–Year Book, Inc.

Receptors are very specific in that they are sensitive to only one kind of stimulus: photoreceptors are sensitive to only light energy; mechanoreceptors to mechanical stresses that deform them; cold thermoreceptors to a decrease in temperature; and chemoreceptors to one particular chemical.

The response of receptors to their physical change shows adaptation. **Adaptation** means that the frequency of the nerve impulses created declines over a period of time even though the strength of the stimulus remains constant. Consequently, receptors provide only relative information about a change that has occurred. They do not provide absolute information. Pain receptors do not show adaptation.

The structure of receptors varies markedly. The large specialized receptor organs—the eye and ear—are reviewed in Unit XII. The names, structure, and senses detected by the other important receptors are provided in Table 44-1 and Figure 44-1.

Carrying Sensory Information to and Motor Information from Central Nervous System

Sensory information is carried to the central nervous system, and motor commands are carried from the central nervous system, by nerve impulses traveling along the fibers of specialized cells called **neurons.** These fibers are collected together in bundles that are named according to their origin: **spinal nerves** originate in the spinal cord, **cranial nerves** originate in the cranium, and nerve tracts lie entirely within the central nervous system.

Structure of neurons

The neuron cell body contains a nucleus that controls the function of the neuron, and Nissl bodies and neurofibrils that are important in producing chemi-

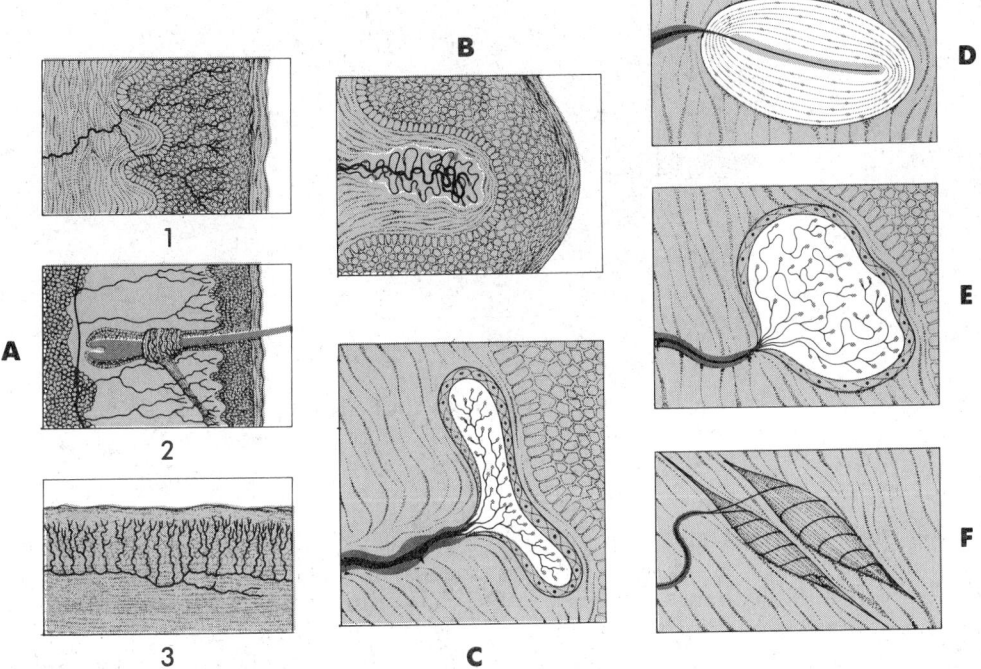

FIGURE 44-1   **A,** Free nerve endings: *1,* in dermis of skin; *2,* surrounding, in linear and circular fashion, root of hair follicle; *3,* in cornea. **B,** Meissner's corpuscle (tactile corpuscle) in skin papilla, an encapsulated nerve ending found in hairless portions of skin. Meissner's corpuscles mediate sensation of touch. **C,** Ruffini's corpuscle, a skin receptor that probably mediates touch, rather than hearing, as formerly thought. **D,** Pacinian corpuscle, an encapsulated nerve ending widely distributed in subcutaneous tissue; mediates sensation of pressure. **E,** Krause's endbulb, an encapsulated nerve ending; may mediate sensation of cold, but evidence indicates that it is not the only type of receptor for cold. **F,** Muscle spindle, sensitive to state of muscle contraction and to degree to which it is stretched.

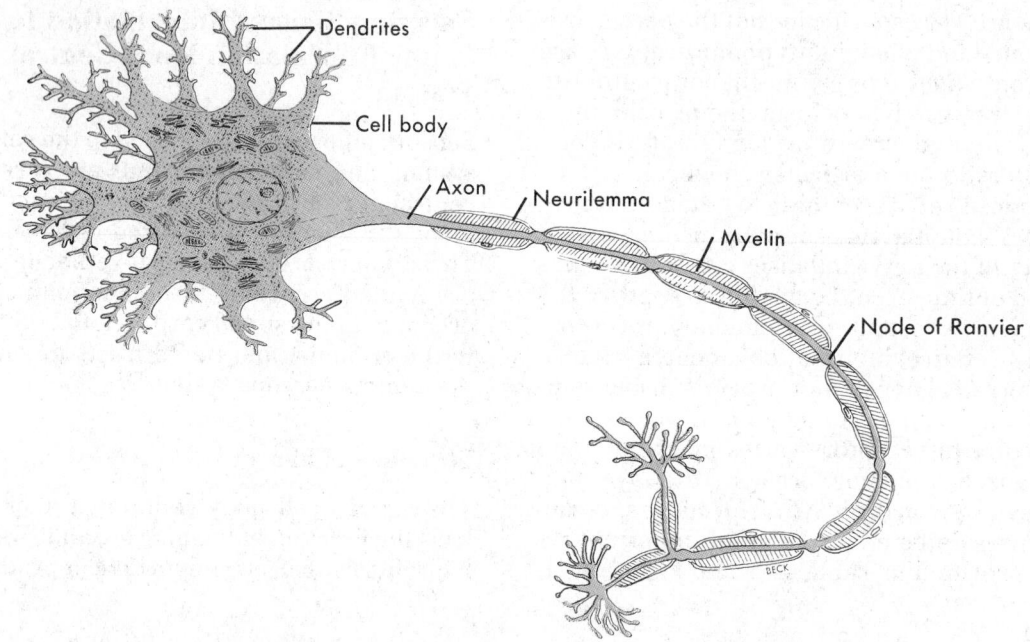

FIGURE 44-2   Structure of neurons. (From Thibodeau GA: *Anthony's textbook of anatomy and physiology,* ed 13, St Louis, 1990, Mosby–Year Book, Inc.)

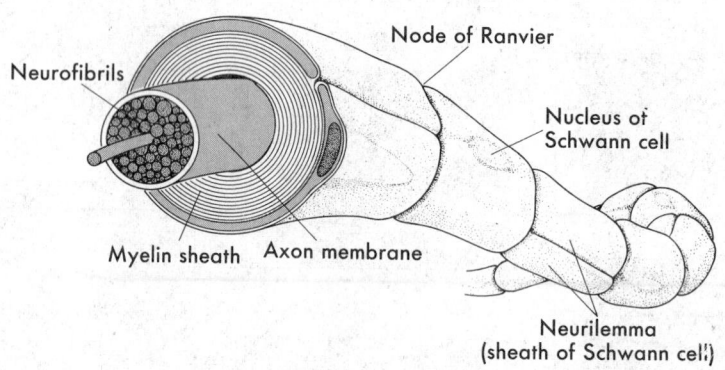

FIGURE 44-3   Nerve fiber and coverings.

cals and organizing their transport along the nerve fibers.

The neuron dendron and dendrites are extensions of the cell body that carry information to it, whereas the axon and its branches are extensions that carry information away from the cell body and secrete neurotransmitter (Figure 44-2). Dendrons and axons can be very long and in the periphery are protected and insulated by specialized cells called Schwann's cells. Schwann's cells may enclose several small-diameter, slow-conducting (C) fibers or may be wrapped many times around a single, large-diameter, fast-conducting (A) fiber. In this latter case the fiber is covered by multiple layers of Schwann's cell membrane for most of its length and

is only exposed at the junctions between Schwann's cells, called nodes of Ranvier (Figure 44-3). This Schwann's cell sheath is composed of phospholipid and is called the neurilemma. It gives nerves and nerve tracts their white color and must be healthy for the nerve fibers to survive. *Neurons do not reproduce after the neonatal period.* If an axon or dendron is damaged, it will die and be slowly replaced but only if the neurilemma is intact and the cell body does not die also. If large numbers of the neurons die, the resulting muscle paralysis or lack of sensation is obvious. In the central nervous system the myelin sheath is produced and maintained by cells called oligodendrocytes.

The cells that carry sensory impulses to the central nervous system are sensory, or afferent, neurons. The cells that carry motor impulses from the central nervous system are motor, or efferent, neurons. Afferent neurons are described as unipolar because the axon and dendron are both attached to the same pole of the cell body. Their cell bodies are found collected together in the dorsal root ganglia outside the spinal cord within the vertebral foramen. **Ganglia** are collections of cell bodies that form swellings in nerves or nerve roots outside the central nervous system. Efferent neurons are called multipolar because they have many projections on their cell body (see Figure 44-2). They are found throughout the nervous system. However, the cell bodies of the efferent skeletal muscle motor neurons always lie in the ventral horns of the spinal cord; the cell bodies of the first of the two efferent motor neurons of the autonomic nervous system lie either in the brain or in the ventral horns of the spinal cord; and the cell bodies of the second efferent neuron lie in peripheral ganglia.

Function of neurons

The function of a neuron is to transmit information by generating nerve impulses, conducting them from one end of the neuron to the other, and stimulating or inhibiting the activities of the cells that they supply by secreting neurotransmitter.

Resting neurons maintain a marked difference in electric potential **(resting potential)** across the nerve cell membrane by the activity of the Na-K ATPase enzymes of the cell membrane. The resting potential provides the neuron with the potential energy to produce nerve impulses at a very high frequency, rather like a battery provides the potential energy to create a high-frequency series of sparks. A **nerve impulse** is an extremely rapid reversal of the resting potential (depolarization) and its recovery (repolarization). Nerve impulses are generated when the neuron is stimulated by a chemical or physical stimulus.

Nerve impulses spread over the nerve cell membrane in all possible directions from their source, but only the axon terminals are able to secrete **neurotransmitter** in response to the impulses. After it is secreted, the neurotransmitter diffuses across the narrow space, or synapse, between the axon and another neuron, or a skeletal muscle fiber, smooth muscle fiber, or glandular cell. The transmitter then binds to receptors on the second cell membrane and alters this cell's resting potential. Inhibitory neurotransmitters produce an increase in a cell's resting potential, and excitatory neurotransmitters produce a decrease in the resting potential. If the summated effect of a number of different neurons decreases the resting potential to a critical level, then a nerve impulse is generated in the second cell.

In order to allow the second cell to recover its resting state, enzymes rapidly destroy the neurotransmitter, or it is reabsorbed into the neuron. **Acetylcholine,** the neurotransmitter at most synapses in the peripheral nervous system (which includes both somatic and autonomic systems), is destroyed by acetylcholine esterase. Receptors stimulated by acetylcholine are called cholinergic receptors and are classified as either nicotinic or muscarinic. **Norepinephrine,** the neurotransmitter of most postganglionic sympathetic neurons, is inactivated by being reabsorbed into the neuron or by being destroyed by catechol-O-methyl transferase in the peripheral nervous system or monoamine oxidase in the central nervous system. Adrenergic receptors, classified as $alpha_1$, $alpha_2$, $beta_1$, or $beta_2$, are selectively stimulated by norepinephrine, by the hormone epinephrine secreted by the adrenal medulla, and by other related neurotransmitters that are collectively called catecholamines. The effects of activation of the sympathetic nervous system are strengthened by epinephrine and weakened by activation of the parasympathetic nervous system. The effects of the parasympathetic and sympathetic systems of the **autonomic nervous system** are listed in Table 44-2.

Acetylcholine and norepinephrine are the chief neurotransmitters of the periphery. Many more transmitters are used by the central nervous system. Some of these are listed in Table 44-3 and Figure 44-4.

Structure and function of spinal nerves, cranial nerves, and nerve tracts

Nerve impulses are conducted between the periphery and the central nervous system by spinal and cranial nerves. The spinal and cranial nerves are made up of the neuron axons and dendrons, Schwann's cells, and the connective tissue sheaths that surround and support the nerves. The spinal nerves, their origin, and the parts of the body that they supply are listed in Table 44-4. With the exception of the intercostal nerves, spinal nerves originate in plexi, which mix the neurons of several spinal segments. The cranial nerves, their origins, and their most important functions are listed in Table 44-5. The origins of the various spinal and cranial nerves in the skin can be mapped out, and the mapped areas (dermatomes) are shown in Figure 44-5.

Nerve impulses traveling between the spinal cord and the brain are carried by the nerve tracts that lie in the white matter of the spinal cord and the brain itself. The sensory pathways originating in one side of the body cross over to the opposite side, either where they enter the spinal cord or at the level of the medulla. Similarly, the motor pathways originating in one hemisphere of the brain cross over to

TABLE 44-2 Autonomic Functions

Visceral effector	Effect of sympathetic stimulation	Effect of parasympathetic stimulation
HEART	Increased rate and strength of heart-beat (beta receptors)	Decreased rate and strength of heartbeat
SMOOTH MUSCLE OF BLOOD VESSELS		
Skin blood vessels	Constriction (alpha receptors)	No parasympathetic fibers
Skeletal muscle blood vessels	Dilation (beta receptors)	No parasympathetic fibers
Coronary blood vessels	Dilation (beta receptors)	No parasympathetic fibers
Abdominal blood vessels	Constriction (alpha receptors)	No parasympathetic fibers
Blood vessels of external genitalia	Ejaculation (contraction of smooth muscle in male ducts, e.g., epididymis and vas deferens)	Dilation of blood vessels causing erection in male
SMOOTH MUSCLE OF HOLLOW ORGANS AND SPHINCTERS		
Bronchi	Dilation (beta receptors)	Constriction
Digestive tract, except sphincters	Decreased peristalsis (beta receptors)	Increased peristalsis
Sphincters of digestive tract	Contraction (alpha receptors)	Relaxation
Urinary bladder	Relaxation (beta receptors)	Contraction
Urinary sphincters	Contraction (alpha receptors)	Relaxation
Eye		
Iris	Contraction of radial muscle; dilated pupil	Contraction of circular muscle; constricted pupil
Ciliary	Relaxation; accommodates for far vision	Contraction; accommodates for near vision
Hairs (pilomotor muscles)	Contraction produces goose pimples, or piloerection (alpha receptors)	No parasympathetic fibers
GLANDS		
Sweat	Increased sweat (neurotransmitter, acetylcholine)	No parasympathetic fibers
Digestive (salivary, gastric, etc.)	Decreased secretion of saliva; not known for others	Increased secretion of saliva
Pancreas, including islets	Decreased secretion	Increased secretion of pancreatic juice and insulin
Liver	Increased glycogenolysis (beta receptors); increased blood sugar level	No parasympathetic fibers
Adrenal medulla*	Increased epinephrine secretion	No parasympathetic fibers

From Thibodeau GA: *Anthony's textbook of anatomy and physiology,* ed 13, St Louis, 1990, Mosby–Year Book, Inc.
NOTE: Norepinephrine primarily affects alpha receptors; epinephrine affects both alpha and beta receptors. Hence their effects differ.
*Sympathetic preganglionic axons terminate in contact with secreting cells of the adrenal medulla. Thus the adrenal medulla functions, to quote someone's descriptive phrase, as a "giant sympathetic postganglionic neuron."

TABLE 44-3 Neurotransmitters of Central Nervous System

Type	Name	Region	Predominant effect
Cholinergic	Acetylcholine	Pyramidal cells, basal ganglia	Excitatory
Amine	Norepinephrine	Brainstem, pons, hypothalamus	Excitatory
	Dopamine	Brainstem	Inhibitory
	Serotonin	Brainstem	Inhibitory
Amino acids	Gamma-aminobutyric acid	Spinal cord, cerebellum, basal ganglia	Inhibitory
	Glycine	Spinal cord	Inhibitory
Peptides	Beta endorphins	Spinal cord	Excitatory
	Enkephalins	Limbic system, thalamus	
	Substance P	Pain fibers in spinal cord	Excitatory

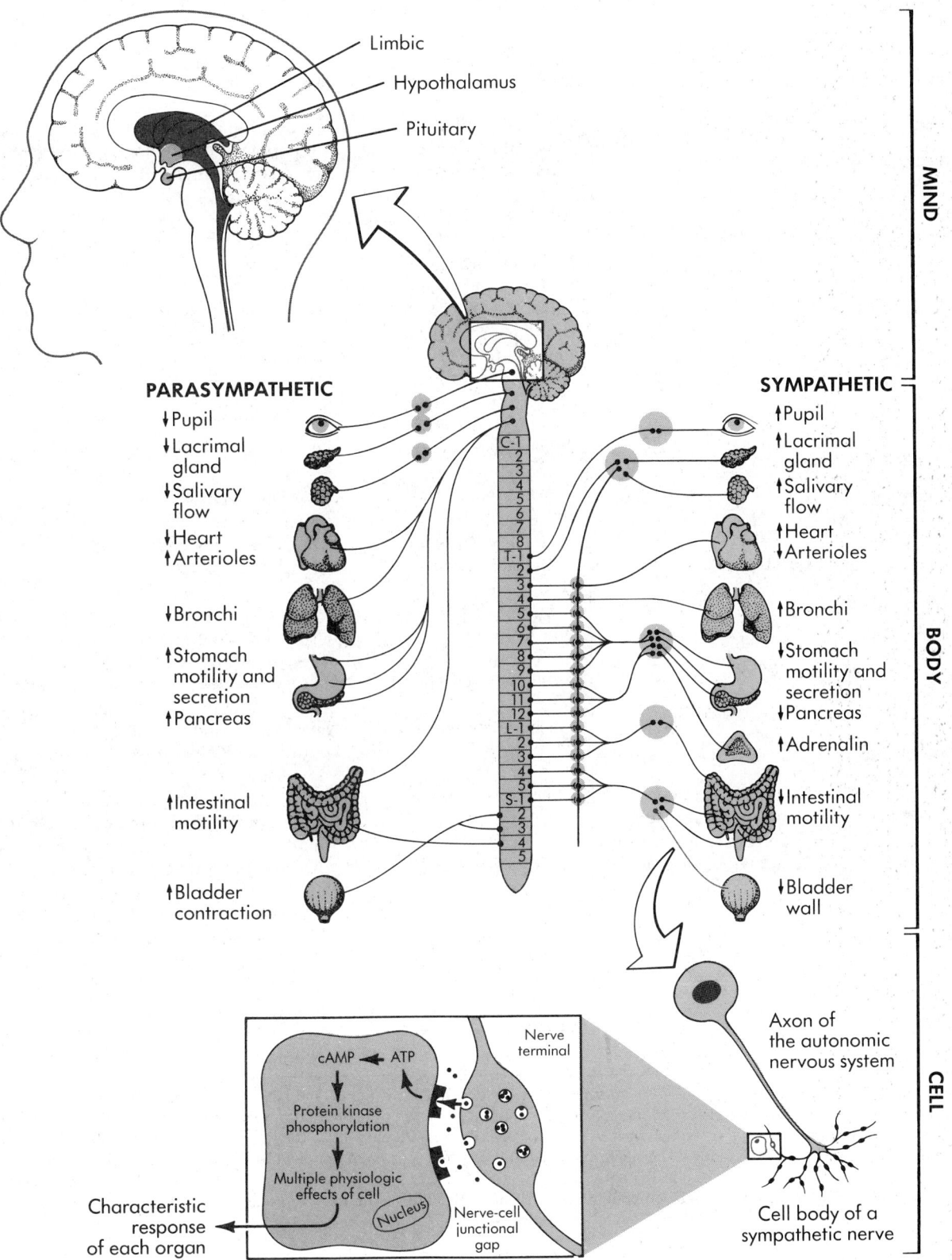

FIGURE 44-4   Autonomic nervous system and its two branches (sympathetic and parasympathetic) down to cellular level.

TABLE 44-4   Spinal Nerves and Peripheral Branches

Spinal nerves	Plexuses formed from anterior rami	Spinal nerve branches from plexuses	Parts supplied
Cervical 1 2 3 4	Cervical plexus	Lesser occipital Great auricular Cutaneous nerve of neck Anterior supraclavicular Middle supraclavicular Posterior supraclavicular Branches to muscles	Sensory to back of head, front of neck, and upper part of shoulder: motor to numerous neck muscles
		Phrenic (branches from cervical nerves before formation of plexus; most of its fibers from fourth cervical nerve)	Diaphragm
Cervical 5 6 7 8 Thoracic (or dorsal) 1 2	Brachial plexus	Suprascapular and dorsoscapular	Superficial muscles* of scapula
		Thoracic nerves, medial and lateral branches	Pectoralis major and minor
		Long thoracic nerve	Serratus anterior
		Thoracodorsal	Latissimus dorsi
		Subscapular	Subscapular and teres major muscles
		Axillary (circumflex)	Deltoid and teres minor muscles and skin over deltoid
		Musculocutaneous	Muscles of front of arm (biceps brachii, coracobrachialis, brachialis), skin on outer side of forearm
3 4 5 6 7 8 9 10 11 12	No plexus formed; branches run directly to intercostal muscles and skin of thorax	Ulnar	Flexor carpi ulnaris and part of flexor digitorum profundus; some of muscles of hand; sensory to medial side of hand, little finger, and medial half of fourth finger
		Median	Rest of muscles of front of forearm and hand; sensory to skin of palmar surface of thumb, index, and middle fingers
		Radial	Triceps muscle and muscles of back of forearm; sensory to skin of back of forearm and hand
		Medial cutaneous	Sensory to inner surface of arm and forearm

From Thibodeau GA: *Anthony's textbook of anatomy and physiology,* ed 13, St Louis, 1990, Mosby–Year Book, Inc.
*Although nerves to muscles are considered motor, they do contain some sensory fibers that transmit proprioceptive impulses.
†Sensory fibers from the tibial and peroneal nerves unite to form the *medial cutaneous* (or sural) *nerve* that supplies the calf of the leg and the lateral surface of the foot. In the thigh the tibial and common peroneal nerves are usually enclosed in a single sheath to form the *sciatic nerve,* the largest nerve in the body with a width of approximately ¾ inch. About two thirds of the way down the posterior part of the thigh, it divides into its component parts. Branches of the sciatic nerve extend into the hamstring muscles.

TABLE 44-4   Spinal Nerves and Peripheral Branches—cont'd

Spinal nerves	Plexuses formed from anterior rami	Spinal nerve branches from plexuses	Parts supplied
Lumbar 1 2 3 4 5 Sacral 1 2 3 4 5 Coccygeal 1	Lumbosacral	Iliohypogastric	Sensory to anterior abdominal wall
		Ilioinguinal	Sensory to anterior abdominal wall and external genitalia; motor muscles of abdominal wall
		Genitofemoral	Sensory to skin of external genitalia and inguinal region
		Lateral cutaneous of thigh	Sensory to outer side of thigh
		Femoral	Motor to quadriceps, sartorius, and iliacus muscles; sensory to front of thigh and medial side of lower leg (saphenous nerve)
		Obturator	Motor to adductor muscles of thigh
		Tibial† (medial popliteal)	Motor to muscles of calf of leg; sensory to skin of calf of leg and sole of foot
		Common peroneal (lateral popliteal)	Motor to evertors and dorsiflexors of foot; sensory to lateral surface of leg and dorsal surface of foot
		Nerves to hamstring muscles	Motor to muscles of back of thigh
		Gluteal nerves, superior and inferior	Motor to buttock muscles and tensor fasciae latae
		Posterior cutaneous nerve	Sensory to skin of buttocks, posterior surface of thigh, and leg
		Pudendal nerve	Motor to perineal muscles; sensory to skin of perineum

the opposite side. Thus one side of the brain receives information from, and controls, the opposite side of the body. The name, function, location in the spinal cord, origin, and termination of some important ascending and descending tracts are listed in Table 44-6. Figure 44-6 shows their location in the spinal cord.

Planning a Response to Sensory Stimulation

The responses of the central nervous system to sensory stimulation are of two main types. The first type (reflexes) are involuntary, stereotyped responses that are always the same for a particular stimulus. They are preprogrammed and produced by fixed circuits of neurons in the spinal cord and less complex regions of the brain. The second type of responses are the result of thinking and are voluntary and unpredictable. They are planned by the cerebrum and are not preprogrammed. However, they are affected by the brain's own interpretation and memory of

previous life experiences, and they may be learned with repetition.

Planning and Integrating Involuntary, Stereotyped Responses
Spinal cord

Structure
The **spinal cord** is an oval cylinder that lies in the vertebral foramen and extends from the first cervical to the first lumbar vertebra (Figure 44-5). Although the cord itself stops at the level of the first lumbar vertebra, the lumbar and sacral nerves form the cauda equina and remain in the vertebral foramen until they exit at the appropriate level of the spinal column. The cord is protected by meninges, adipose tissue, and blood vessels.

Figure 44-6 shows a cross section of the spinal cord. In the center is a small spinal canal surrounded by a butterfly-shaped area of gray matter. The gray matter is made up of nerve cell bodies, neuroglia, and synapses. The surrounding white matter is made

TABLE 44-5 Cranial Nerves

Nerve*	Sensory fibers†			Motor fibers†			Functions#
	Receptors	Cell bodies	Terminatio	Cell bodies	Termination		
1. Olfactory	Nasal mucosa	Nasal mucosa	Olfactory bulbs (new relay of neurons to olfactory cortex)				Sense of smell
2. Optic	Retina	Retina	Nucleus in thalamus (lateral geniculate body); some fibers terminate in superior colliculus of midbrain				Vision
3. Oculomotor	External eye muscles except superior oblique and lateral rectus	?	?	Midbrain (oculomotor nucleus and Edinger-Westphal nucleus)	External eye muscles except superior oblique and lateral rectus; fibers from Edinger-Westphal nucleus terminate in ciliary ganglion and then to ciliary and iris muscles		Eye movements, regulation of size of pupil, accommodation, proprioception (muscle sense)
4. Trochlear	Superior oblique	?	?	Midbrain	Superior oblique muscle of eye		Eye movements, proprioception
5. Trigeminal	Skin and mucosa of head, teeth	Gasserian ganglion	Pons (sensory nucleus)	Pons (motor nucleus)	Muscles of mastication		Sensations of head and face, chewing movements, muscle sense
6. Abducens	Lateral rectus	?	?	Pons	Lateral rectus muscle of eye		Abduction of eye, proprioception
7. Facial	Taste buds of anterior two thirds of tongue	Geniculate ganglion	Medulla (nucleus solitarius)	Pons	Superficial muscles of face and scalp		Facial expressions, secretion of saliva, taste
8. Acoustic a. Vestibular branch	Semicircular canals and vestibule (utricle and saccule)	Vestibular ganglion	Pons and medulla (vestibular nuclei)				Balance or equilibrium sense

Nerve	Receptors (location)	Ganglion	Termination (sensory)	Origin (motor)	Structures supplied	Function
b. Cochlear or auditory branch	*Organ of Corti in cochlear duct*	*Spiral ganglion*	*Pons and medulla (cochlear nuclei)*			*Hearing*
9. Glossopharyngeal	*Pharynx; taste buds and other receptors of posterior third of tongue*	*Jugular and petrous ganglia*	*Medulla (nucleus solitarius)*	**Medulla (nucleus ambiguus)**	**Muscles of pharynx**	*Taste and other sensations of tongue, swallowing movements, secretion of saliva, aid in reflex control of blood pressure and respiration*
	Carotid sinus and carotid body	*Jugular and petrous ganglia*	*Medulla (respiratory and vasomotor centers)*	**Medulla at junction of pons (nucleus salivatorius)**	**Otic ganglion and then to parotid gland**	
10. Vagus	*Pharynx, larynx, carotid body, and thoracic and abdominal viscera*	*Jugular and nodose ganglia*	*Medulla (nucleus solitarius), pons (nucleus of fifth cranial nerve)*	**Medulla (dorsal motor nucleus)**	**Ganglia of vagal plexus and then to muscles of pharynx, larynx, and thoracic and abdominal viscera**	*Sensations and movements of organs supplied; for example, slows heart, increases peristalsis, and contracts muscles for voice production*
11. Spinal accessory	?	?	?	**Medulla (dorsal motor nucleus of vagus and nucleus ambiguus)**	**Muscles of thoracic and abdominal viscera, pharynx, and larynx**	
				Anterior gray column of first five or six cervical segments of spinal cord	**Trapezius and sternocleidomastoid muscle**	*Shoulder movements, turning movements of head, movements of viscera, voice production, proprioception?*
12. Hypoglossal	?	?	?	**Medulla (hypoglossal nucleus)**	**Muscles of tongue**	*Tongue movements, proprioception?*

From Thibodeau GA: *Anthony's textbook of anatomy and physiology*, ed 13, St Louis, 1990, Mosby–Year Book, Inc.

*The first letters of the words in the following sentence are the first letters of the names of the cranial nerves. Many generations of anatomy students have used this sentence as an aid to memorizing these names. It is "On Old Olympus Tiny Tops, A Finn and German Viewed Some Hops." (There are several slightly differing versions of this mnemonic.)

†Italics indicate sensory fibers and functions. Boldface type indicates motor fibers and functions.

‡An aid for remembering the general function of each cranial nerve is the following 12-word saying: "Some say marry money but my brothers say bad businesses marry money." Words beginning with S indicate sensory function. Words beginning with M indicate motor function. Words beginning with B indicate both sensory and motor functions. For example, the first, second, and eighth words in the saying start with S, which indicates that the first, second, and eighth cranial nerves perform sensory functions.

up of the axons and neuroglia of the ascending and descending nerve tracts.

Functions

The spinal cord has two important functions. One is to carry sensory information to, and motor information from, the brain. The second is to provide neuron and synapse networks to produce involuntary, stereotyped responses (reflexes) to sensory stimulation, and to control the ease with which afferent pain impulses pass through the spinal cord "pain gate" to reach the brain.

A **reflex** is a protective, stereotyped response to a change in the frequency and pattern of sensory nerve impulses reaching the spinal cord; for example, the response to touching a painfully hot object is to withdraw the hand. The integration of the motor responses of spinal reflexes occurs entirely in the spinal cord, and the brain is informed of the sensation that initiated the reflex while the response is occurring. The simplest reflexes are stretch reflexes, which involve only a sensory neuron, a motor neuron, and the synapse between them. Having only one synapse (i.e., no interneurons) allows the stretch re-

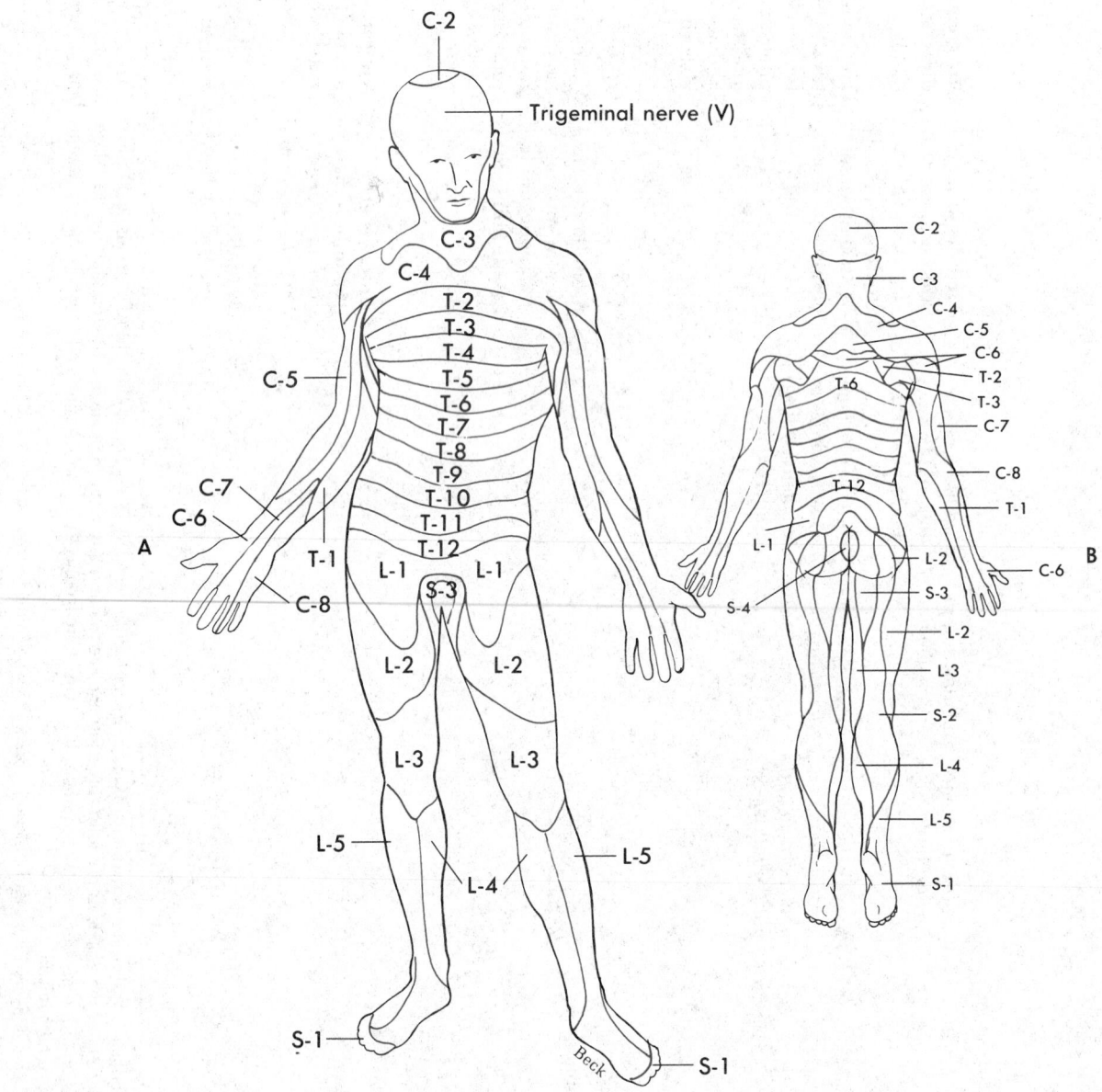

FIGURE 44-5 A, Segmental distribution of spinal nerves to front of body. *C,* Cervical segments; *T,* thoracic segments; *L,* lumbar segments; *S,* sacral segments. **B,** Segmental distribution of spinal nerves to back of body. (From Thibodeau GA: *Anthony's textbook of anatomy and physiology,* ed 13, St Louis, 1990, Mosby–Year Book, Inc.)

TABLE 44-6   Spinal Pathways

Pathways	Function
ASCENDING	
Spinothalamic	
Lateral	Pain and temperature
Anterior	Light touch, pressure, tickle, and itch sensation
Medial lemniscal system	Proprioception, two-point discrimination, pressure, and vibration
Spinocerebellar	Proprioception to cerebellum
Spino-olivary	Proprioception relating to balance
Spinotectal	Tactile stimulation causing visual reflexes
Spinoreticular	Tactile stimulation arousing consciousness
DESCENDING	
Pyramidal	Muscle tone and skill movement, especially of hands
Corticospinal	Movements, especially of hands
Corticobulbar	Facial movements
Extrapyramidal	Pathways involved in unconscious general body movements
Rubrospinal	
Vestibulospinal	
Reticulospinal	

From Seeley R et al: *Anatomy and physiology,* St Louis, 1992, Mosby–Year Book, Inc.

flex to quickly adjust the posture setting of the muscle fibers surrounding the muscle spindle receptors when they are stretched unexpectedly. It is the interneurons that allow the spinal cord to integrate extremely complex activities involving many spinal segments and both sides of the body.

Although the brain is not a necessary part of the circuits integrating these complex reflexes, it does influence the ease with which sensory stimulation is able to activate reflexes, because it provides tonic excitatory and inhibitory nerve impulses via the descending tracts. The predominant influence of the brain is excitatory; that is, facilitates reflex action. Reflexes are lost after the spinal cord is cut because the facilitatory impulses no longer reach the reflex centers. This lack of reflexes is referred to as spinal shock.

The pain gate is a complex integrated circuit that controls the ease with which pain impulses reach the brain. Pain is discussed in Chapter 14.

Brainstem, cerebellum, and diencephalon

Structure

The brainstem, cerebellum, and diencephalon form the more primitive areas of the brain (Figure 44-7). The **brainstem,** which includes the medulla oblongata, pons, and midbrain, begins at the foramen magnum and connects with the cerebellum and the diencephalon. The large pyramidal tracts lie on the anterior surface of the medulla oblongata. The **cerebellum** is located on the posterior surface of the brainstem, inferior to the cerebrum. The white matter of the cerebellum, which is called the arbor vitae, is made up of tracts connecting the cerebellum with other areas of the brain. The arbor vitae is surrounded by the gray matter of the cerebellar cortex. The **diencephalon** includes the hypothalamus and thalamus and connects with the cerebrum. It lies between the sphenoid bone and the third ventricle.

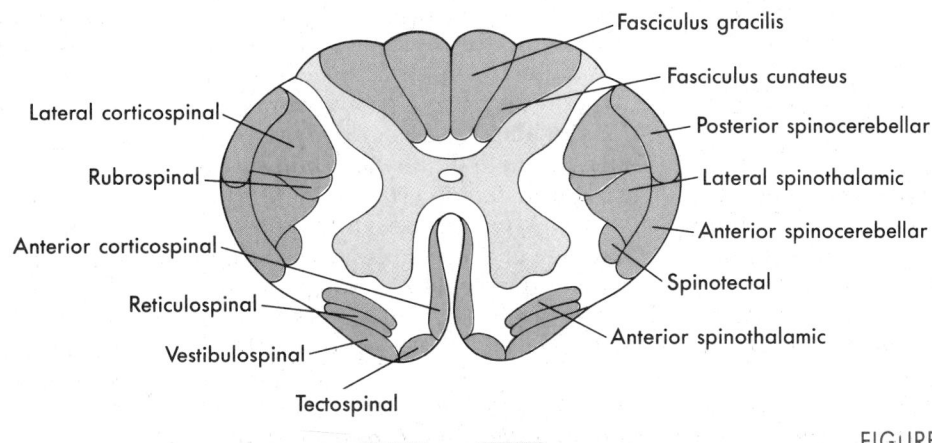

Fasciculus gracilis
Fasciculus cunateus
Posterior spinocerebellar
Lateral spinothalamic
Anterior spinocerebellar
Spinotectal
Anterior spinothalamic

Lateral corticospinal
Rubrospinal
Anterior corticospinal
Reticulospinal
Vestibulospinal
Tectospinal

Descending fibers   Ascending fibers

FIGURE 44-6   Cross section of spinal cord depicting pathways.

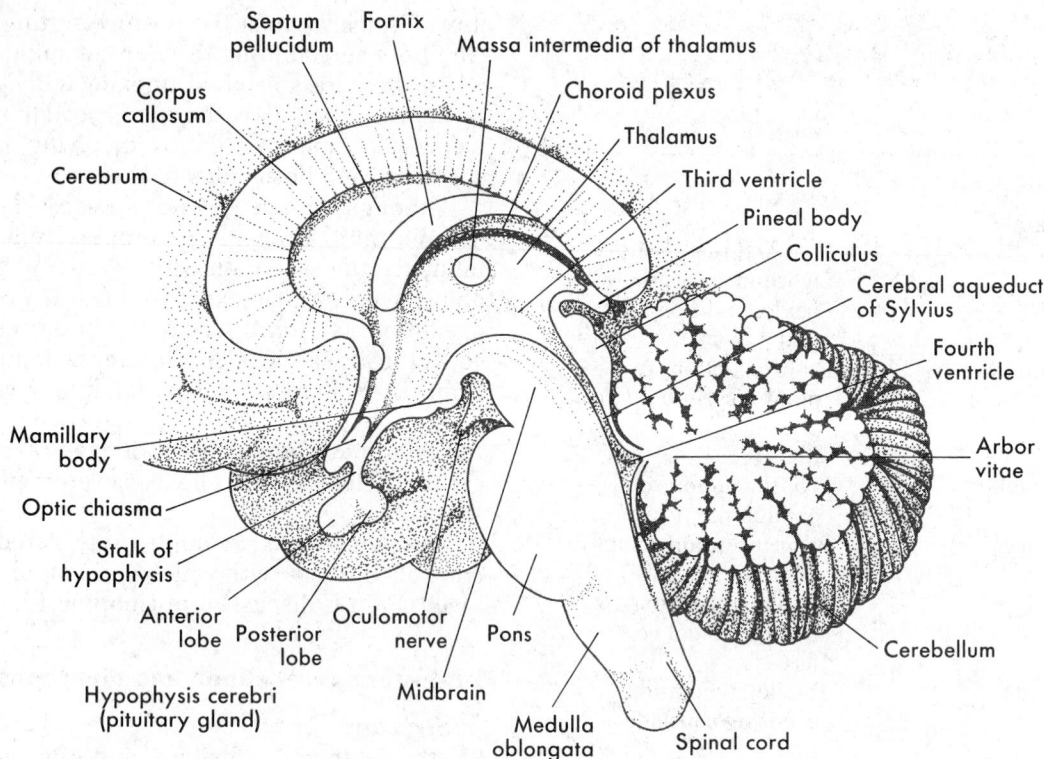

FIGURE 44-7   Sagittal section through midline of brain showing structures around third ventricle.

Functions

The functions of the brain are carried out by collections of neurons and synapses that are referred to as nuclei when they lie deep in the brain tissue and as cortex when they lie on the surface of the brain.

The **medulla oblongata** contains reflex centers responsible for controlling balance, the rate and strength of the heartbeat, the rate and depth of respiration, the diameter of blood vessels, sneezing, coughing, swallowing, and vomiting. The pons contains nuclei responsible for respiration. The midbrain contains nuclei for pupillary reflexes and eye movements. In addition, all the tracts projecting to the periphery and ascending to the higher brain regions and to the cerebellum pass through the brainstem.

Although the initiation of skeletal muscle contractions is a function of the cerebrum, the cerebellum plays an essential synergistic role by modifying the force of contraction of the muscles primarily responsible for the movement and the relaxation of the muscles opposing the movement. This role is essential to produce smooth coordinated movement of the correct intensity. For example, the cerebellum ensures that the right tension is used to pick up an egg so that it is not crushed or dropped. Another vital reflex function of the cerebellum is to detect loss of balance by interpreting sensory input from the eyes, vestibular apparatus, and somatic proprioreceptors. Having detected loss of balance, the cerebellum acts rapidly to restore it by modifying muscle contraction. Damage to the cerebellum does not result in paralysis but in such things as ataxia and hypotonia, muscle incoordination, drooling, and tremors.

The functions of the hypothalamus include organizing the responses of the autonomic nervous system that are an essential part of the emotions, and organizing the secretion of hormones that regulate the adenohypophysis or are secreted by the neurohypophysis. The hypothalamus also is responsible for the homeostasis of body temperature, the osmolarity of body fluids, and hunger and satiety.

The thalamus crudely identifies some of the sensory nerve impulses that it receives, controls the number of these sensory nerve impulses that reach the cerebral cortex, and determines to which parts of the brain they will be relayed. The crucial role the thalamus plays in organizing the conscious activity of the cerebrum is often ignored. It determines which part of the cerebrum is active at any particular time and thus is crucial in all conscious activity, in emotions, and in thinking.

Planning and Integrating Voluntary, Unpredictable Responses

The planning and integration of the voluntary, unpredictable responses of the nervous system are functions of the nuclei and cortex of the cerebrum when they are stimulated by the thalamus.

Cerebrum

Structure

The **cerebrum** is divided into the right and left hemispheres by the deep longitudinal fissure. Cerebral lobes are named according to the cranial bones that they lie against (Figure 44-8). The surface area of the gray matter making up the outer layer of the cerebrum is increased by many gyri (ridges) and the sulci (folds) tucked between them. Beneath the cortex the white matter is made up of a variety of tracts connecting the various lobes of the cerebral cortex with each other and with other areas of the central nervous system. The two cerebral hemispheres are connected by the corpus callosum. The gray matter of the basal ganglia, which includes the corpus striatum, the caudate nucleus, and the lentiform nucleus, lies beneath the white matter of the cerebrum, in close proximity to the thalamus (Figure 44-9).

Nuclei in various areas of the brain that function together are called systems. For example, the **limbic system** is made up of a series of nuclei and tracts that form a ring around the brainstem and includes part of the cerebral cortex and the amygdala, hippocampus, and septal nuclei. The **reticular activating system** includes parts of the spinal cord, pons, midbrain, hypothalamus, and thalamus.

The cerebral cortex and the rest of the central nervous system are supported and protected by the meninges, the ventricles and spinal canal, and the cerebrospinal fluid. The **meninges** are composed of three layers and the spaces between: the first layer is the pia, which is attached to the nervous tissue; the second is the arachnoid layer; and the third is the dura, which is attached to the periosteum of the cranium. The **ventricles** are four large, fluid-filled chambers in the brain. The first and second ventricles (lateral ventricles) lie in the cerebral hemispheres, the third ventricle lies above the thalamus, and the fourth ventricle lies between the cerebellum and the medulla and pons. **Cerebrospinal fluid** fills the ventricles, the subarachnoid space, and the central canal of the spinal cord. It is secreted by the choroid plexi in the roof of the ventricles and circulates through the ventricles to the subarachnoid layer of the meninges, where it is reabsorbed. Needles can be inserted into the subarachnoid space between lumbar vertebrae 3 and 4, or 4 and 5, to monitor the pressure and composition of cerebrospinal fluid or into the epidural space to instill a local anesthetic.

The blood supply to the brain is supplied by the right and left internal carotid and the right and left vertebral arteries. These four arteries supply an arterial anastomosis called the circle of Willis. This anastomosis allows blood to reach all the major arteries supplying the different divisions of the brain even when blood flow through one of the four source arteries is deficient. However, low pressure in any

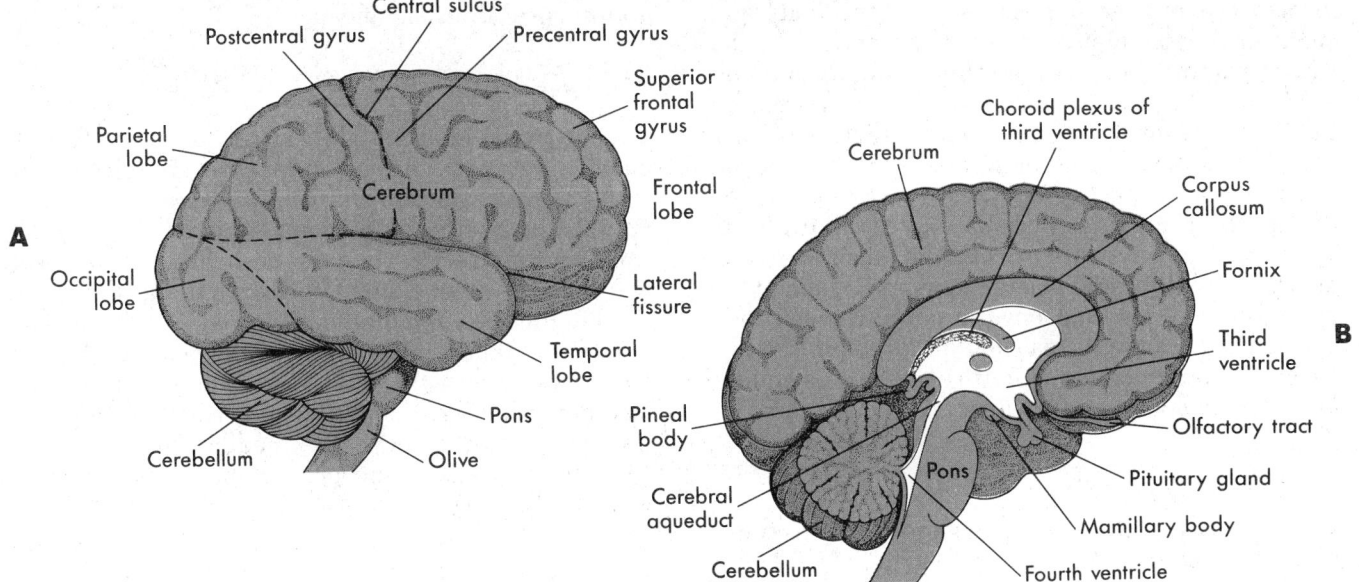

FIGURE 44-8   Right hemisphere of cerebrum. **A,** Lateral surface. **B,** Medial surface.

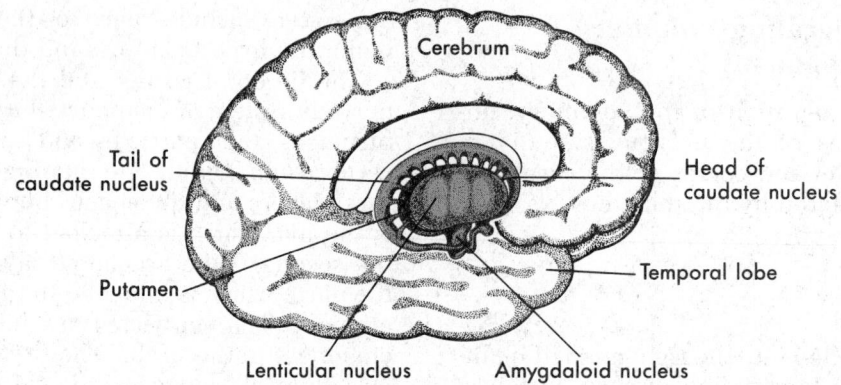

FIGURE 44-9   Basal ganglia (or cerebral nuclei) within cerebral hemisphere. Main basal ganglia are caudate nucleus, putamen, and pallidum.

artery within the cranium will reduce blood flow and place brain tissue farthest from the supplying artery at risk of hypoxia and death. High pressure also puts the brain tissue at risk because hypertension may cause an aneurysm or vessel rupture and hemorrhage, which compress brain tissue and cause hypoxia and death.

Functions

The aspects of planning and integration carried out by the cerebral cortex vary from area to area. However, all the areas are closely interrelated. The cerebrum is the region of the brain most associated with the characteristics that set humans apart from other mammals, characteristics such as the ability to learn complex tasks, thinking, imagination, language, calculation, and planning for the future.

Each hemisphere of the brain receives sensory information from the opposite side of the body and controls the skeletal muscles of the opposite side. However, both sides of the brain communicate and are involved in most activities. To reduce the potential confusion of having two control centers (one in each hemisphere), each hemisphere specializes and has priority for particular types of activity. For example, the right side specializes in the individual's perception of physical environment, such as space, art, nonverbal communication, and music, and in the perception of spiritual environment. The left side specializes in analysis, calculation, problem solving, verbal communication, interpretation of symbols, language, reading, and writing.

Language and speech

Thoughts are generated throughout the cerebrum and interpreted in Wernicke's area (in the left hemisphere), which synchronizes the muscles of speech through Broca's area of the frontal lobe. The left hemisphere is dominant for interpretation and speech in 95% of individuals, and damage to this hemisphere can leave the individual unable to communicate or interpret thoughts. Music, which is interpreted by the right hemisphere, may provide a way for the health care professional to communicate with and soothe the troubled minds of these individuals.

Sensory perception and interpretation

Sensory perception depends on the activity of the primary sensory areas of the cerebral cortex. However, understanding the significance of what is perceived depends on the surrounding secondary sensory areas or association areas (Figure 44-10). The primary areas function from the time of birth, but the function of the association areas develops as the individual experiences various sensations and learns to interpret their significance.

Muscle control

Voluntary skeletal muscle control starts in the primary motor area of the frontal lobe of the cerebral cortex (Figure 44-10). One neuron carries the nerve impulses directly to the ventral horn of the spinal cord and indirectly, via axon branches, to the basal ganglia and cerebellum to ensure that all the associated muscles function appropriately. The nerve impulses taking the direct route are carried by the pyramidal tracts; those taking the indirect route are carried by the extrapyramidal tracts. Damage to the pyramidal tracts above the medulla oblongata results in paralysis or incoordination on the opposite side of the body.

Emotion

Emotions such as anger, fear, pleasure, sorrow, sexual feelings, love, and hate are generated by the lim-

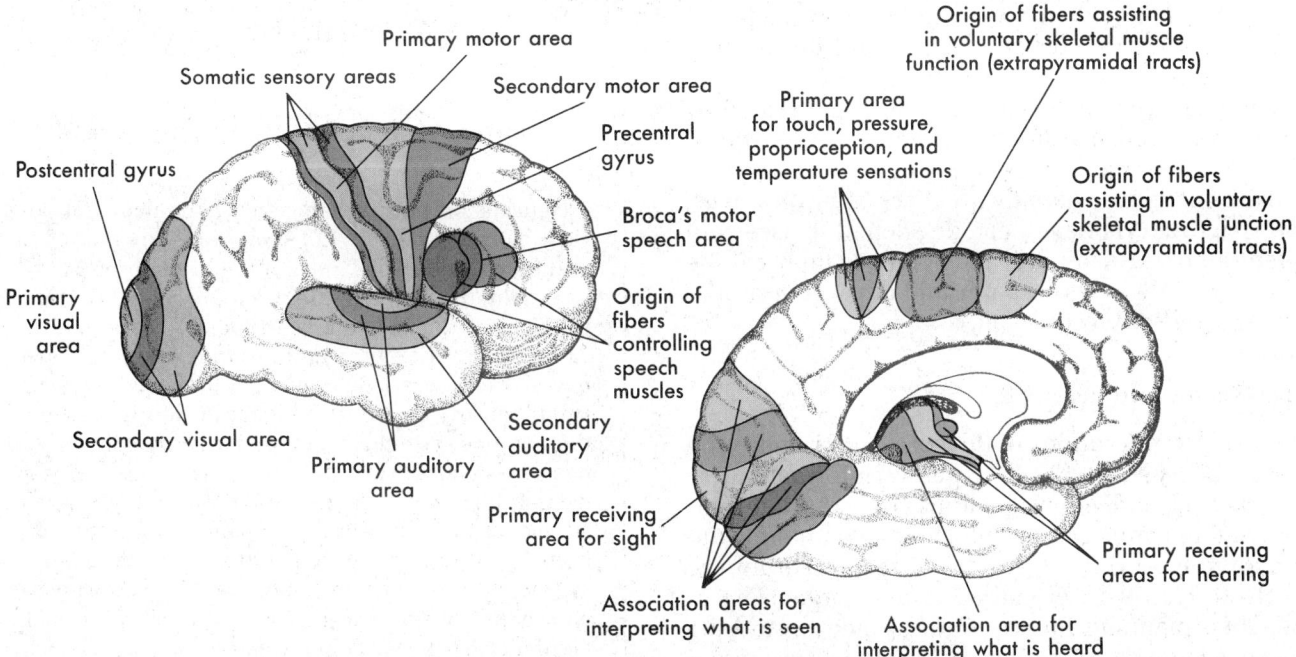

FIGURE 44-10   Map of human cortex with corresponding functions.

bic system. The limbic system generates emotions in response to stimuli from the cerebral cortex and the thalamus and in turn stimulates specific nuclei in the hypothalamus to produce the affective responses associated with each emotion. Affective responses produced by the autonomic nervous system, such as increased heart rate and blushing, are sensed by the cerebral cortex and add to the perception of the emotion. Emotions are sensed as pleasant or unpleasant, and they form one of the most important drives controlling memory, learning, and behavior.

Consciousness of self

Consciousness, or awareness of one's self and one's environment, relies on the active function of the cerebral cortex. This is maintained by continuous stimulation of the cerebral cortex by nerve impulses from a series of nuclei in the brainstem that together are called the reticular activating system (RAS) (Figure 44-11). The RAS (1) keeps the cerebrum active by relaying impulses received from the sensory neurons of the periphery to the cerebrum, (2) receives stimulation from the cerebrum, (3) generates facilitatory and inhibitory impulses to the reflex centers and pain gates of the spinal cord, (4) is responsible for rapidly alerting the cerebral cortex to sudden changes in the internal and external environment, and (5) is responsible for initiating and terminating sleep.

Sleep is associated with lack of consciousness and

with inhibition of the perception of sensory stimuli. It differs from coma because sleeping individuals can be roused. Sleep can be delayed voluntarily by deliberately increasing sensory stimulation by, for example, washing in cold water or increasing muscle activity. Normally, two types of sleep alternate: deep sleep, which is associated with reduced metabolic rate and no memory of dreams, and rapid eye movement sleep (REM), which is associated with active dreaming and an increase in heart rate and metabolism. Preventing REM sleep for prolonged periods results in irritability and abnormal or even psychotic behavior. REM sleep is essential for the well-

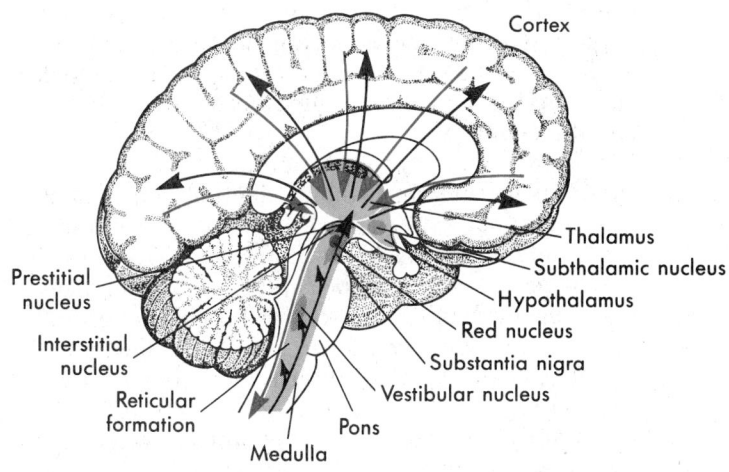

FIGURE 44-11   Reticular activating system.

being of the individual. Even during deep sleep and coma the cerebral cortex is active, and this activity can be monitored with an electroencephalograph, which measures the electrical changes generated by the nerve impulses directly under the electrodes. The electrical changes are called brain waves. Death of the brain is associated with a lack of brain waves, and strict criteria have been developed to ascertain when the brain-dead individual, whose body can be kept alive only by a ventilator and intravenous feeding, may be said to be dead.

Analysis and thought

The analytic operations of the cerebrum require the brain to focus on specific types of information, to separate out individual qualities from the information, and to compare new information with information already stored. All regions of the cerebrum are involved. However, organization and sequencing of thoughts, planning for the future, and considering the consequences of actions before they are carried out are functions of the frontal lobes. The individual with damage to the frontal lobes is easily distracted and has little ambition or concern for the implications of his or her actions. Using words to integrate sensory information and to analyze thoughts is a function of an area of the posterosuperior temporal gyrus of the dominant hemisphere called Wernicke's area (see Figure 44-10). Damage to Wernicke's area results in the inability of the person to interpret thoughts, to read, or to speak.

Memory

Memories are stored in all regions of the cerebral cortex in special neuronal circuits that are permanently changed by an activity or experience. These memory traces (engrams) may include the muscle control sequences necessary to perform complex movements, or they may include sensory recall of events experienced in the past. Events are most likely to be remembered if they are associated with strong emotion. When the emotional factor is lacking, information to be remembered must be repeated frequently.

There are three types of memory:
1. *Sensory memory* allows fleeting recall of an event just experienced. It is not stored and is available for up to 1 second. However, in this brief interval it can be rapidly scanned and significant details selected for further action.
2. Primary, or *short-term, memory* allows fleeting recall of bits of information such as a few words or numbers. It is not stored and is instantly available for a few words or seconds. However, primary memory has limited capacity, and a second bit of information will replace the first so that the first is no longer available.

GERIATRIC CONSIDERATIONS

Physiologic Changes in the Neurologic System

Neurons do not reproduce after the neonatal period. During a normal life span, approximately 3% of the body's neurons die and the brain loses 7% of its weight, the majority after 65 years of age. To compensate for this loss the ventricles increase in size. Although reaction time and the time taken to learn new material are longer and the threshold for activating sensory receptors is higher in elderly persons, the nervous system remains remarkably efficient in healthy seniors. However, because it has an extremely high metabolic rate and little energy reserve storage capacity it is easily damaged by a reduction in its blood supply. Consequently, as the circulatory system ages and becomes inefficient, it predisposes elderly persons to a greater risk of cerebrovascular accidents (strokes). Other changes that develop in the nervous system as age advances become apparent when critical areas of the central nervous system are affected; for example, a noticeable loss of motor control, memory loss, or an inability to carry out normal daily activities may be caused by lipofuscin pigment deposited in neuron cell bodies, a decline in the concentration of certain neurotransmitters, or neurofibrillar tangles and plaques.

3. *Long-term memory* is information that is stored in the brain for hours, days, or years and, except for deeply ingrained memories, long-term memories must be searched for before they can be recalled. The limbic system is essential in generating emotion, and the hippocampus plays an important role in consolidating primary memories into long-term memories. Consolidation requires from 5 to 60 minutes, and events that inhibit brain activity, such as concussion or deep anesthesia, can block consolidation so that events just before the concussion or anesthesia are not remembered.

Rehearsal and codifying potentiate storage of information in long-term memory. Rehearsal is recalling memories already stored. Codifying is comparing new information with information already stored in long-term memory. It allows the new information to be stored in association with similar or contrasting information. Both processes make it easier to locate and recall the information at a later date.

ASSESSMENT
Subjective

Patients may experience alterations in neurologic functioning secondary to other processes such as

POTENTIAL SYMPTOMS RELATED TO NEUROLOGIC DISORDERS

Seizures, fits, or convulsions
Headache
Loss of consciousness
Numbness, tingling
Vertigo
Tic
Tremor
Aphasia
Changes in memory
Changes in personality or behavior
Disorientation
Hallucinations
Paresis
Paralysis

metastatic disease or infectious disease, or they may experience primary neurologic alterations such as a cerebrovascular accident or seizure disorder.

The box above lists potential symptoms to review with the patient. In addition to specific symptoms, ask the patient about any history of head trauma, spinal cord injury, cerebrovascular accident, meningitis, aneurysm, hypertension, or circulatory problems. If the patient's chief complaint is related to memory loss, ask about sleep patterns, appetite, weight loss, history of depression, and any previous or current psychiatric care.

Determination of the appropriate related systems to review is guided by the nurse's knowledge of pathophysiology, treatment, and symptoms associated with the neurologic symptoms delineated. For example, the patient may complain of headache. Because headache may be associated with fever, increased intracranial pressure, hypertension, stress, or visual impairment or strain or may simply be vascular in origin, the nurse's questioning is guided by the associated symptoms. If the patient states onset was sudden, sharp, severe, unilateral, precipitated by flashing lights, associated with nausea and photophobia, aggravated by noise, and alleviated minimally with lying down in a darkened quiet room, knowledge of pathophysiology guides the nurse to explore migraine headache further rather than fever and infectious disease. If the patient complains of headache that is dull, is worse in the morning and, in fact, wakens the patient, is not precipitated by any event, is not aggravated by any event, and is minimally alleviated with some "borrowed" narcotics, and the patient notes a somewhat recent onset of diplopia, the nurse will further explore the concept of increased intracranial pressure secondary to a

space-occupying lesion, rather than a migraine headache.

Family history that is relevant to the neurologic system includes epilepsy or seizure disorder, headaches, Alzheimer's disease, Huntington's chorea, thyroid disease, diabetes mellitus, cerebrovascular accident, or hypertension. A positive finding should include the disorder as well as the individual's relationship to the patient (e.g., Huntington's chorea, father; Alzheimer's disease, maternal grandmother).

Objective

Physical examination of the neurologic system consists of assessment of cerebral function, cranial nerve function, cerebellar function, motor function, sensory function, and reflexes. Some patients will have more complex symptom involvement than others, and therefore assessment needs may vary from patient to patient. The box on p. 1180 outlines the screening neurologic examination.

Cerebral function

General assessment of cerebral function is accomplished through mental status evaluation. Mental status evaluation consists of appearance and behavior, speech and language skills, mood, thought processes and content, and cognitive abilities. Evaluation of mental status begins when first meeting the patient while conducting the interview.

Observation of appearance includes the patient's dress, grooming, and personal hygiene. Compare the patient's dress with the typical dress of the average individual of the same age and sex at the same time of year. Note if the patient is clean and neat or unkempt and disheveled. An inpatient will be clothed in a hospital gown, but in the outpatient setting, observation of the patient's dress may be very helpful. When observing the patient's behavior, note if the patient is agitated, excessively irritable, or cooperative as well as whether the patient's verbal and nonverbal responses are congruent.

Observations regarding speech and language skills include articulation, fluency, comprehension, coherence, and aphasia. If the patient articulates poorly, determine if any particular sounds are especially affected. Fluency refers to the patient's ability to speak smoothly, with appropriate inflections, and at an appropriate rate.

Mood refers to the patient's overall, pervasive feelings. One approach is to ask the patient about his or her spirits in general. Ask if the mood has been labile or steady. Note any indications of depression. If the patient acknowledges depression, gently question further to determine if the patient has had any thoughts of suicide.

Evaluation of thought processes includes observations of the patient's patterns of thinking. Is the pa-

SCREENING NEUROLOGIC EXAMINATION

Assessment of cerebral function: mental status

Appearance and behavior
Speech and language
Mood
Thought processes and content
Cognitive abilities (frequently tested via Folstein's Mini-Mental Status Exam)

Assessment of cranial nerve function

CN I (olfactory): generally not tested
CN·II (optic): visual acuity and visual fields
CN III (oculomotor): eye movement, lid movement, pupillary response to light and accommodation
CN IV (trochlear): eye movement
CN V (trigeminal): sensory and motor
CN VI (abducens): eye movement
CN VII (facial): sensory and motor
CN VIII (acoustic): vestibular function and hearing
CN IX (glossopharyngeal): sensory and motor
CN X (vagus): sensory and motor
CN XI (spinal accessory): motor
CN XII (hypoglossal): motor; innervates muscles that move tongue

Assessment of cerebellar function

Finger to nose to finger
Romberg's test
Rapid alternating movements
Gait: relaxed walking, tandem, heel walking, toe walking
Heel down shin

Assessment of motor function

Muscle strength, tone, size
Fasciculations, tremors

Assessment of sensory function

Pain
Light touch
Position sense
Vibration
Stereognosis
Graphesthesia
Point localization
Extinction

Assessment of reflexes

Deep tendon reflexes: brachioradialis, biceps, triceps, patellar, Achilles
Superficial reflexes: abdominal and cremasteric

RESEARCH BRIEF

Segatore M, Way C: The Glasgow Coma Scale: time for change, *Heart Lung* 21:548, 1992.

This study reviewed the reliability and validity of the Glasgow Coma Scale for the brain-injured adult. The researchers proposed that the psychometric properties of the scale are weak, because it fails to provide clear definitions of levels of consciousness and behavioral indicators for consciousness, sufficient rationale for scoring, and comprehensive sets of operational indicators for monitoring levels of consciousness and predicting outcomes.

Although the Glasgow Coma Scale may be a reliable and valid predictor of coma outcome, it is not a reliable and valid measure for monitoring change in levels of consciousness or predicting outcome for patients with middle range scores on the tool. The researchers conclude that practitioners who rely on the Glasgow scale should critically analyze its comparative value and seriously consider the respective merits of alternative scales.

tient able to answer questions logically? Note any consistent need to repeat words or phrases. Thought content refers to what the patient thinks about. Note any delusions, anxieties, phobias, or obsessive/compulsive thoughts or behaviors.

Cognitive abilities include level of consciousness, abstract reasoning, arithmetic calculations, writing ability, memory, and judgment. A widely used tool to assess only cognitive abilities is Folstein's Mini-Mental Status Exam (Figure 44-12). This tool is frequently used in the clinical setting because the results are reproducible. The Glasgow Coma Scale may also be used to rate the patient's state of consciousness. This scale allows for evaluation of eye opening response, verbal response, and motor response (see box on p. 1182).

Cranial nerve function

Testing of cranial nerve I (olfactory) is generally not done unless the patient complains of a loss of smell. When CN I is tested, a familiar but not strongly aromatic odor is applied to one nostril while the other nostril is occluded. With eyes closed, the patient is asked to identify the odor.

Patient _____
Examiner _____
Date _____

"MINI-MENTAL STATE"

Maximum Score	Score	
		ORIENTATION
5	( )	What is the (year) (season) (date) (day) (month)?
5	( )	Where are we: (state) (county) (town) (hospital) (floor).
		REGISTRATION
3	( )	Name 3 objects: 1 second to say each. Then ask the patient all 3 after you have said them. Give 1 point for each correct answer. Then repeat them until the patient learns all 3. Count trials and record. Trials
		ATTENTION AND CALCULATION
5	( )	Serial 7's. 1 point for each correct. Stop after 5 answers. Alternatively spell "world" backwards.
		RECALL
3	( )	Ask for the 3 objects repeated above. Give 1 point for each correct.
		LANGUAGE
9	( )	Name a pencil, and watch (2 points)

Repeat the following "No ifs, ands or buts" (1 point)
Follow a 3-stage command:
"Take a paper in your right hand, fold it in half, and put it on the floor"
(3 points)
Read and obey the following:
CLOSE YOUR EYES (1 point)
Write a sentence (1 point)
Copy design (1 point)
_____ Total score
ASSESS level of consciousness along a continuum_____
                                          Alert   Drowsy   Stupor   Coma

INSTRUCTIONS FOR ADMINISTRATION OF MINI-MENTAL STATE EXAMINATION

ORIENTATION
(1) Ask for the date. Then ask specifically for parts omitted, e.g., "Can you also tell me what season it is?" One point for each correct.
(2) Ask in turn "Can you tell me the name of this hospital?" (town, county, etc.). One point for each correct.

REGISTRATION
Ask the patient if you may test his or her memory. Then say the name of 3 unrelated objects, clearly and slowly, about one second for each. After you have said 3, ask patient to repeat them. The first repetition determines the score (0-3) but keep saying them until patient can repeat all 3, up to 6 trials. If the patient does not eventually learn all 3, recall cannot be meaningfully tested.

ATTENTION AND CALCULATION
Ask the patient to begin with 100 and count backwards by 7. Stop after 5 subtractions (93, 86, 79, 72, 65). Score the total number of correct answers.
If the patient cannot or will not perform this task, ask him or her to spell the word "world" backwards. The score is the number of letters in correct order (e.g. dlrow=5, dlorw=3).

RECALL
Ask the patient if he or she can recall the 3 words you previously asked patient to remember. Score 0-3.

LANGUAGE
Naming: Show the patient a wrist watch and ask what it is. Repeat for pencil. Score 0-2.
Repetition: Ask the patient to repeat the sentence after you. Allow only one trial. Score 0-1
3-Stage command: Give the patient a piece of plain blank paper and repeat the command. Score 1 point for each part correctly executed.
Reading: On a blank piece of paper print the sentence "Close your eyes", in letters large enough for the patient to see clearly. Ask patient to read it and do what it says. Score 1 point only if patient actually closes eyes.
Writing: Give the patient a blank piece of paper and ask patient to write a sentence for you. Do not dictate a sentence, it is to be written spontaneously. It must contain a subject and verb to be sensible. Correct grammar and punctuation are not necessary.
Copying: On a clean piece of paper, draw intersecting pentagons, each side about 1 in. and ask to copy it exactly as it is. All 10 angles must be present and 2 must intersect to score 1 point. Tremor and rotation are ignored.
Estimate the patient's level of sensorium along a continuum, from alert on the left to coma on the right.

FIGURE 44-12 Mini-Mental Status Exam, a standardized screening tool of mental status. Score greater than 20 is acceptable. Score of 20 or less is found in patients with dementia, delirium, schizophrenia, or an affective disorder. (Reprinted with permission from Folstein MF et al: "Mini-mental state": a practical method for grading the cognitive state of patients for the clinician, *J Psychiatr Res* 12:189, 1975. Copyright 1975, Pergamon Press, Ltd.)

GLASGOW COMA SCALE*

Best eye opening response	Spontaneously	4
	To speech	3
(record "C" if eyes closed by swelling)	To pain	2
	No response	1
Best motor response to painful stimuli	Obeys verbal command	6
	Localizes pain	5
(record best upper limb response)	Flexion-withdrawal	4
	Flexion abnormal†	3
The examiner applies pressure to the sternum with the knuckle.	Extension abnormal‡	2
	No response	1
Best verbal response	Oriented × 3	5
	Conversation confused	4
(record "E" if endotracheal tube in place, "T" if tracheostomy tube in place)	Speech inappropriate	3
	Sounds incomprehensible	2
	No response	1

NOTE: The Glasgow Coma Scale also correlates well with survival and cognitive outcome. Patients with low scores (3, 4) have a high mortality and poor prognosis for cognitive recovery, whereas patients with high scores (greater than 8) have a good prognosis for recovery.
*Eye + Motor + Verbal = 3 to 15.
†Abnormal flexion—decorticate.
‡Abnormal extension—decerebrate.

Testing of cranial nerve II (optic) is discussed in Chapter 52. Testing includes visual acuity and visual fields. Cranial nerves III, IV, and VI are also discussed in Chapter 52. These nerves are tested through extraocular movements, pupillary response to light and accommodation, observation of lid movement, and the cover/uncover test.

Cranial nerve V (trigeminal) performs both sensory and motor functions. To evaluate sensory function of the trigeminal nerve, evaluate pain (sharp vs. dull) and light touch sensation on the face and anterior scalp and, if the patient is comatose, evaluate the corneal reflex (Figure 44-13). The motor function of the trigeminal nerve is innervation of the muscles of mastication. To evaluate the motor function of this nerve, instruct the patient to clench the teeth. Palpate the jaws bilaterally, noting muscle tone and symmetry (Figures 44-14 and 44-15).

Cranial nerve VII (facial) also performs both sensory and motor functions. The sensory function is taste on the anterior two thirds of the tongue and is not evaluated unless the patient is complaining of a loss of taste. Motor function includes innervation of facial muscles. Testing of the facial nerve is accomplished through instructing the patient to smile, frown, wrinkle the forehead, puff out cheeks, and show teeth while observing for symmetry of movements.

Cranial nerve VIII (acoustic) is responsible for hearing and balance. The auditory branch may be tested through audiometry, or, more commonly, through evaluation of gross hearing as well as the Weber and Rinne tests (see Chapter 54). Vestibular function testing is not routinely done.

Cranial nerves IX and X (glossopharyngeal and vagus) are tested together. The sensory component of the glossopharyngeal nerve, taste on the posterior one third of the tongue, is not tested unless the patient has a complaint regarding taste. Motor function of the vagus and glossopharyngeal nerves is tested by observing the patient swallowing and speaking, by eliciting the gag reflex, and by observing the soft palate rising on phonation with the uvula remaining midline.

Cranial nerve XI (spinal accessory) is evaluated by examination of the sternocleidomastoid and trapezius muscles. To evaluate sternocleidomastoid function, position the patient facing you. Place your hand on one side of the patient's head and instruct the patient to turn the head in that direction while you provide resistance. Repeat this procedure on the contralateral side (Figure 44-16). The trapezius muscles are evaluated by placing your hands on the patient's shoulders and instructing the patient to shrug as you provide resistance. In evaluating both muscle groups, note symmetry of strength (Figure 44-17).

Cranial nerve XII (hypoglossal) innervates the muscles that are responsible for movement of the tongue. Instruct the patient to stick out the tongue and move it from side to side. The tongue should protrude midline. Any deviation of the tongue to one side is abnormal. Table 44-7 summarizes testing for all of the cranial nerves.

Cerebellar function

Cerebellar function may be evaluated through several tests, including finger to nose to finger, Romberg's test, rapid alternating movements, observation of gait (relaxed walking, tandem, toe walking, and heel walking), and heel down shin. To perform the finger to nose to finger test, begin with clear instructions. With the patient seated on the examining table or on the bed, stand in front of the patient. Hold your index finger at approximately arm's length from the patient. Instruct the patient to touch your index finger with his or her finger and then touch his or her nose with the same finger. Explain that you will be moving your index finger to various

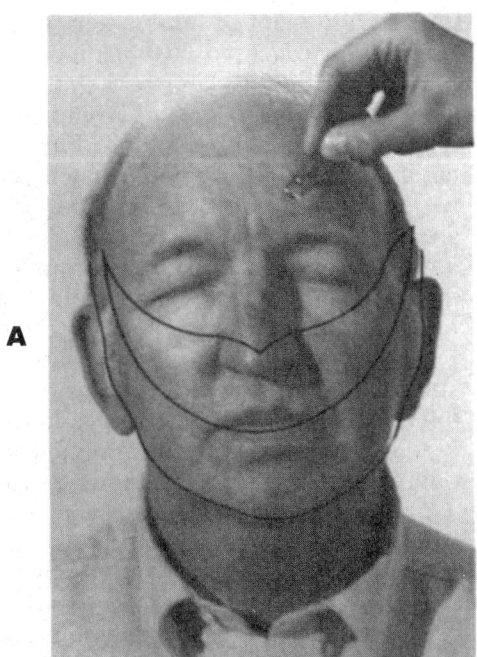
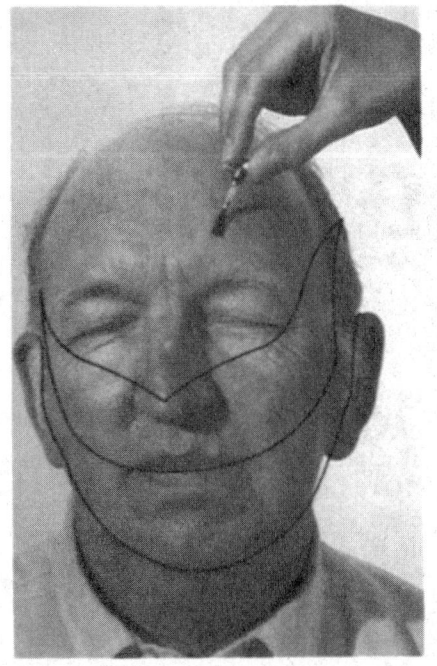

FIGURE 44-13   Examination of trigeminal cranial nerve. Touch each side of face at scalp, cheek, and chin areas alternatively, using no predictable pattern with, **A,** point and rounded edge of paper clip and, **B,** brush. Ask patient to discriminate between sensations. (From Seidel HM et al: *Mosby's guide to physical examination,* ed 2, St Louis, 1991, Mosby–Year Book, Inc.)

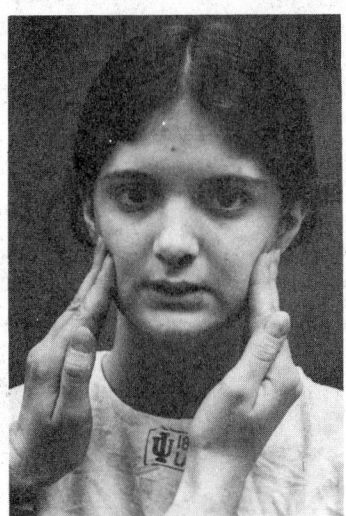

FIGURE 44-14   Palpation of masseter muscles to test CN V. (From Malasanos L: *Health assessment,* ed 4, St Louis, 1990, Mosby–Year Book, Inc.)

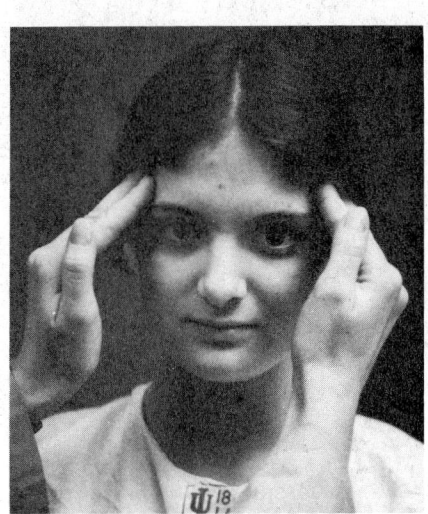

FIGURE 44-15   Palpation of temporal muscles to test CN V. (From Malasanos L: *Health assessment,* ed 4, St Louis, 1990, Mosby–Year Book, Inc.)

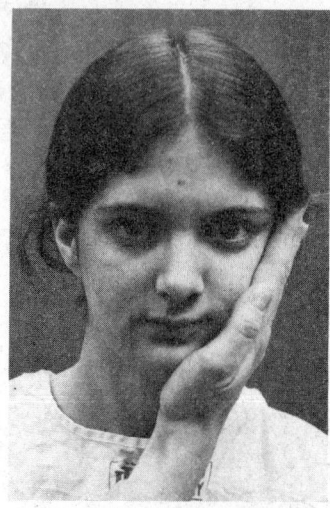

FIGURE 44-16 Assessment of sternocleidomastoid muscle (CN IX). (From Malasanos L: *Health assessment,* ed 4, St Louis, 1990, Mosby–Year Book, Inc.)

positions in front of him or her. The patient should repetitively touch your index finger and then his or her nose as rapidly, smoothly, and accurately as possible. After moving your index finger to several different places, keep your index finger at the same location and have the patient touch your index finger two or three times at this same location. Then instruct the patient to close the eyes and touch your index finger. Observe for coordination, overshooting, or past pointing (dysmetria). Past pointing may be associated with cerebellar dysfunction.

To perform Romberg's test, instruct the patient to stand with feet together and arms at sides (Figure 44-18). Maintenance of this position requires intact cerebellar and vestibular function as well as adequate muscle strength of lower extremities. Place yourself in a position to prevent the patient from falling should he or she become unsteady. Instruct the patient to stand with eyes open and then with eyes closed. Some slight swaying is expected with eyes closed. If the patient demonstrates loss of bal-

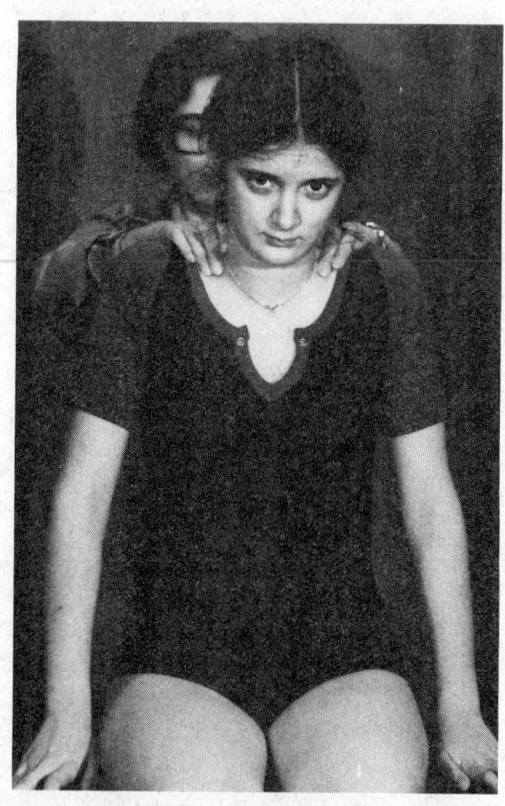

FIGURE 44-17   Assessment of trapezius muscle (CN IX). Patient shrugs shoulders against resistance of examiner's hands. (From Malasanos L: *Health assessment,* ed 4, St Louis, 1990, Mosby–Year Book, Inc.)

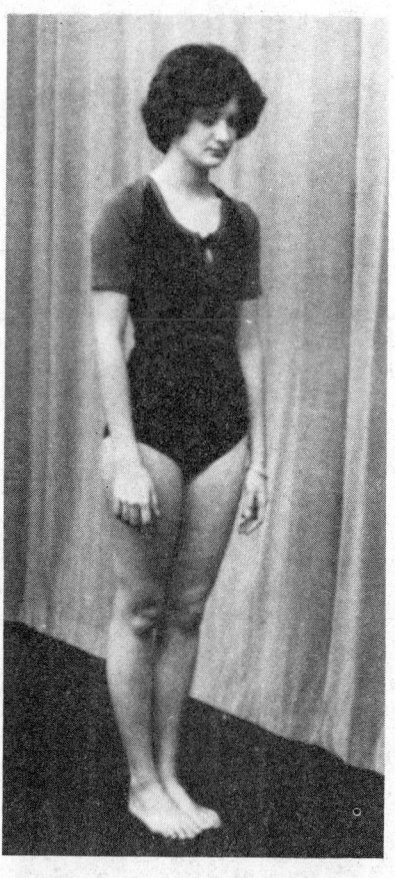

FIGURE 44-18   Romberg's test. Patient should be able to stand with eyes closed and feet together without swaying for approximately 5 seconds. (From Malasanos L: *Health assessment,* ed 4, St Louis, 1990, Mosby–Year Book, Inc.)

TABLE 44-7   Cranial Nerve Examination

Cranial nerve	Procedure
CN I (olfactory)	Test ability to identify familiar aromatic odors, one naris at a time with eyes closed.
CN II (optic)	Test vision with Snellen chart and Rosenbaum near vision chart.
	Perform ophthalmoscopic examination of fundi.
	Test visual fields by confrontation and extinction of vision.
CN III, IV, and VI (oculomotor, trochlear, and abducens)	Inspect eyelids for drooping.
	Inspect pupils' size for equality and their direct and consensual response to light and accommodation.
CN V (trigeminal)	Inspect face for muscle atrophy and tremors.
	Palpate jaw muscles for tone and strength when patient clenches teeth.
	Test superficial pain and touch sensation in each branch. (Test temperature sensation if there are unexpected findings to pain or touch.)
	Test corneal reflex.
CN VII (facial)	Inspect symmetry of facial features with various expressions (smile, frown, puffed cheeks, wrinkled forehead, etc.).
	Test ability to identify sweet and salty tastes on each side of tongue.
CN VIII (acoustic)	Test sense of hearing with whisper screening tests or by audiometry.
	Compare bone and air conduction of sound.
	Test for lateralization of sound.
CN IX (glossopharyngeal)	Test ability to identify sour and bitter tastes.
	Test gag reflex and ability to swallow.
CN X (vagus)	Inspect palate and uvula for symmetry with speech sounds and gag reflex.
	Observe for swallowing difficulty.
	Evaluate quality of gutteral speech sounds (presence of nasal or hoarse quality to voice).
CN XI (spinal accessory)	Test trapezius muscle strength (shrug shoulders against resistance).
	Test sternocleidomastoid muscle strength (turn head to each side against resistance).
CN XII (hypoglossal)	Inspect tongue in mouth and while protruded for symmetry, tremors, and atrophy.
	Inspect tongue movement toward nose and chin.
	Test tongue strength with index finger when tongue is pressed against cheek.
	Evaluate quality of lingual speech sounds (l, t, d, n).

From Seidel HM et al: *Mosby's guide to physical examination,* ed 2, St Louis, 1991, Mosby–Year Book, Inc.

ance with the eyes closed (positive Romberg's sign), a disorder of proprioception is suspected. The patient with a proprioceptive disorder is able to maintain balance with the eyes open by using visual cues. In a cerebellar or vestibular disorder, visual cues do not effect a difference in ability to maintain balance. Thus the patient sways with eyes open as well as closed (see the box on p. 1186).

Rapid alternating movements are evaluated with the patient sitting on the examining table or bed. Instruct the patient to place his or her hands, palms down, on the thighs and then to alternately supinate and pronate the hands as rapidly as possible. The inability to perform rapid alternating movements is known as dysdiadochokinesia and indicates cerebellar dysfunction.

Observe the patient's relaxed walking gait. Instruct the patient to walk several feet across the room. Alternatively, observe the patient walking from the waiting area to the examining room when in an outpatient department or from the bed to the bathroom when in an inpatient environment. Note the patient's posture and upper extremity movements. Posture should be upright, and arms should be close to the body and swing gently. The components of gait are stance and swing. During the stance phase the foot is on the ground, and during the swing phase the foot is moving forward. Generally, most individuals can walk with feet approximately 2 to 4 inches apart and with a step length of approximately 15 inches. If the width of the base exceeds 2 to 4 inches, suspect some pathologic condition such as cerebellar dysfunction. Some disorders have characteristic gait disturbances such as Parkinson's disease (see Chapter 46).

Tandem gait may demonstrate balance problems and is evaluated by instructing the patient to walk heel to toe as when walking a straight line. Gener-

DISORDERS OF CEREBELLUM, POSTERIOR COLUMNS, AND VESTIBULAR NEURONS

Cerebellar dysfunction

Ataxia not made worse in darkness or with eyes closed
Clumsiness
Poor coordination
Decomposition of movement
Dysmetria
Dysdiadochokinesia
Scanning speech
Hypotonia
Asthenia
Tremor
Nystagmus

Posterior column dysfunction

Ataxia made worse in darkness or with eyes closed
Positive Romberg's sign
Inability to recognize limb position
Astereognosis
Loss of two-point discrimination
Loss of vibratory sensation

Vestibular dysfunction

Nystagmus
Nausea
Vomiting
Ataxia

From Malasanos L et al: *Health assessment*, ed 4, St Louis, 1990, Mosby–Year Book, Inc.

ally, patients should be able to demonstrate a tandem gait through the fifth decade. Other testing for balance and muscle strength includes heel walking and toe walking. In addition to balance, heel walking demonstrates strength of the tibialis anterior muscle, and toe walking demonstrates strength of the gastrocnemius and soleus muscles. Patients should generally be able to demonstrate heel and toe walking through the seventh decade. Another test of cerebellar function is heel down shin. While the patient is seated with legs dangling or lying in bed, instruct the patient to take one heel and place it on the contralateral leg just inferior to the patella. Have the patient move the heel down the shin and repeat with the other heel. In a cerebellar disorder the patient is unable to maintain the heel on the shin.

Motor function

Motor function is evaluated for muscle strength, tone, size, and fasciculations or tremors. Disorders of motor function occur in such degenerative diseases as amyotrophic lateral sclerosis (Lou Gehrig's disease) or muscular dystrophy. Motor function testing is discussed in Chapter 56.

An additional test that is usually combined with Romberg's test is the test for pronator drift. Rather than instructing the patient to stand with hands at sides for Romberg's test, instruct the patient to stand with arms horizontally forward, palms up, and eyes closed. Weakness of the extremity will result in the hand slowly drifting downward and pronating.

When assessing the patient's grips, remember to cross your arms so as to offer your left hand to the patient's left hand and your right hand to the patient's right hand. Ask the patient to grasp your index and middle fingers. Try to withdraw your fingers from the patient's grasp.

Sensory function

Sensory function is evaluated through several tests, including pain, light touch, position sense, vibration, stereognosis, graphesthesia, point localization, and extinction. Pain and temperature both travel along the lateral spinothalamic tract. Therefore only pain is tested. If the patient has difficulty with discrimination of pain, temperature may then be tested. Light touch travels along the anterior spinothalamic tract, whereas position sense and vibration travel along the posterior column.

To test pain use a sterile needle and demonstrate sharp and dull with the patient's eyes open. Then, with the patient's eyes shut, instruct the patient to tell you if he or she feels a sharp or dull sensation each time you touch the sterile needle to the patient. A safety pin may be used if it is disposed of immediately after use with a patient. Because sensory deficits usually begin distally and progress proximally, it is acceptable to test sensation on only the hands and feet unless sensory loss is reported in the history. If no sensory loss is determined, there is no need to test the more proximal areas of the body. Touch the patient with the sharp and dull ends but do not use any predictable pattern such as sharp, dull, sharp, dull. If the patient can only discern dull, a sensory deficit is present.

Light touch is evaluated using a cotton ball. Light touch may be combined with point localization by instructing the patient to point to each area he or she feels the light touch or state exactly where the sensation is felt (e.g., left shin). Again, work from most distal to more proximal with the patient's eyes shut (Figure 44-19).

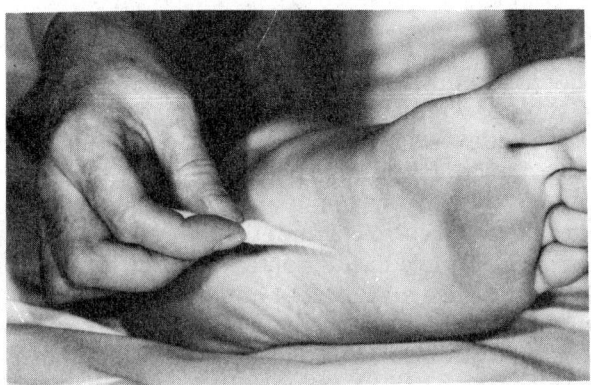

FIGURE 44-19   Evaluation of light touch. (From Malasanos L: *Health assessment,* ed 4, St Louis, 1990, Mosby–Year Book, Inc.)

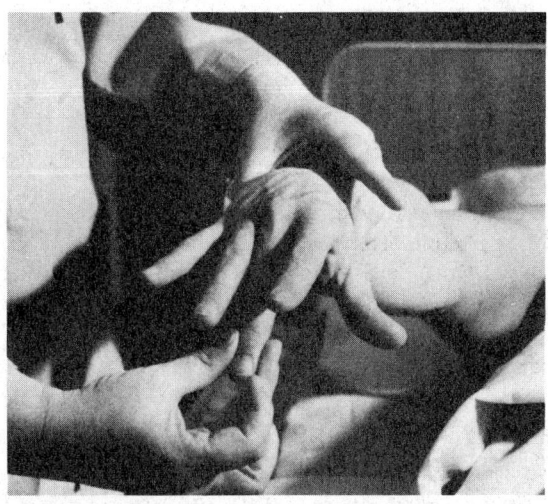

FIGURE 44-20   Evaluation of position sense—finger. (From Malasanos L: *Health assessment,* ed 4, St Louis, 1990, Mosby–Year Book, Inc.)

Vibration is evaluated using a 128 or 256 cycles per second (cps) or Hertz (Hz) tuning fork. Vibration sense is also tested distally over joints, usually at the ankles and wrists or great toe and fingers. With the patient's eyes closed, tap the tuning fork and place it on the area chosen to test (e.g., medial or lateral malleolus). Place your nondominant hand on the other side of the area being tested (e.g., ankle, wrist, great toe, or finger) so as to feel the vibration. Instruct the patient to tell you initially when the vibration is felt and, second, when the vibration is no longer felt. You should feel the vibration through the patient's joint for approximately the same period of time as the patient feels the vibration. If a deficit is present, move more proximal and retest.

Position sense is evaluated by using the great toe and the thumb. With the patient's eyes open, demonstrate and instruct the patient regarding position of the great toe and thumb. Holding the digit with your fingers on either side, move the digit up, saying "this is up," and then move the digit down, saying "this is down." After this demonstration, have the patient close the eyes and tell you if the digit is up or down (Figure 44-20).

Stereognosis is the ability to discern an object placed in the hand without looking at it. With the patient's eyes closed, place a familiar object such as a quarter or a key in the patient's palm. Have the patient grasp the object in his or her palm and tell you what it is.

Graphesthesia is the ability to discern a letter or number "written" or traced onto the palmar surface of the hand. With the patient's eyes closed, trace a letter or number on the patient's hand and have the patient identify what was traced. When performing this test, be sure the letter or number is traced or "written" facing the patient (Figure 44-21).

Point localization is the ability to determine where on the body one has been touched. Although

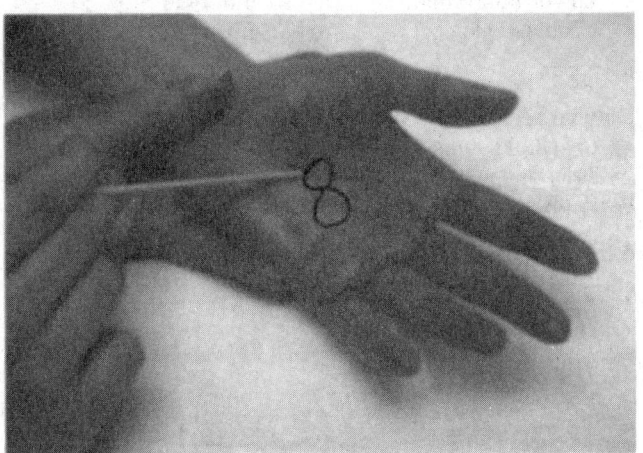

FIGURE 44-21   Test for graphesthesia. (From Seidel HM et al: *Mosby's guide to physical examination,* ed 2, St Louis, 1991, Mosby–Year Book, Inc.)

this is a sensory test in and of itself, it may be incorporated with testing for light touch as discussed earlier.

Extinction is the ability to determine when one or both sides of the body are being touched. For this test have the patient close the eyes and tell you where he or she feels you touch. Place your hands on corresponding areas of the patient's body (e.g., each upper arm, each lower leg). If the patient only feels you touching on one side, a lesion of the sensory cortex should be considered.

TABLE 44-8   Deep Tendon Reflex Scores

Grade	Response
0	No response
1+	Sluggish or diminished
2+	Active or expected response
3+	More brisk than expected, slightly hyperactive
4+	Brisk, hyperactive, with intermittent or transient clonus

TABLE 44-9   Superficial and Deep Tendon Reflexes and Corresponding Spine Segmental Level

Reflex	Spinal level
SUPERFICIAL	
Upper abdominal	T7, T8, and T9
Lower abdominal	T10 and T11
Cremasteric	T12, L1, and L2
DEEP	
Biceps	C5 and C6
Brachioradialis	C5 and C6
Triceps	C6, C7, and C8
Patellar	L2, L3, and L4
Achilles	S1 and S2
Plantar	L4, L5, S1, and S2

Reflexes

Testing of reflexes may include deep tendon reflexes (DTRs) as well as superficial reflexes. DTRs are stretch reflexes and require the muscles being tested to be relaxed. Inability to relax the muscles may prevent the reflex from being elicited. When assessing reflexes, observe for symmetry and strength of response. DTRs are graded on a scale of 0 to 4 (Table 44-8 and Figure 44-22). It is important to determine whether a reflex is absent vs. not elicited because of inability to relax the muscle. The DTRs that are routinely tested are brachioradialis, biceps, triceps, patellar, and Achilles. The brachioradialis and biceps DTRs assess the nerves at roots C5 and C6. The triceps DTR evaluates the nerves at roots C6, C7, and C8. The patellar DTR evaluates the nerves at roots L2, L3, and L4. The Achilles DTR assesses the nerves at roots S1 and S2 (Table 44-9). The reflexes may be evaluated with the patient either sitting or supine.

When testing DTRs, hold the reflex hammer loosely in your dominant hand. Keeping your wrist relaxed, swing the hammer gently to tap the appropriate tendon. Use the nondominant hand to support the joint or extremity being tested.

To test the brachioradialis, the patient's arm is resting in a relaxed position with the forearm semipronated on the patient's lap or supported by you. Using the reflex hammer, tap the arm approximately 2 inches proximal to the radial styloid. Observe the forearm for supination and flexion (Figure 44-23).

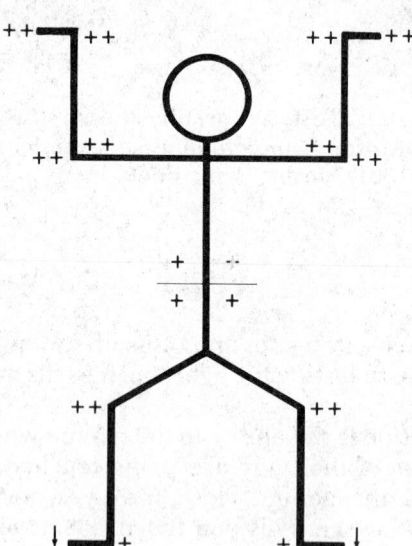

FIGURE 44-22   Stick figure drawing for recording reflexes. (From Malasanos L: *Health assessment,* ed 4, St Louis, 1990, Mosby–Year Book, Inc.)

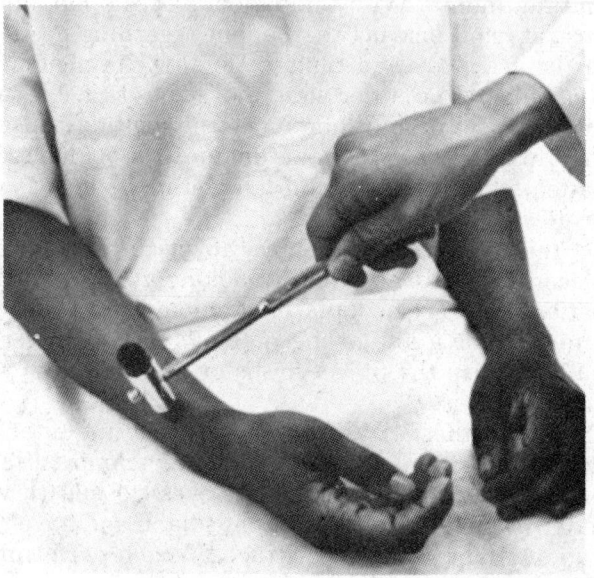

FIGURE 44-23   Elicitation of brachioradialis reflex in sitting position. (From Malasanos L: *Health assessment,* ed 4, St Louis, 1990, Mosby–Year Book, Inc.)

To test the biceps, position the patient's arm flexed at the elbow. Place your nondominant thumb firmly on the biceps tendon in the antecubital fossa. Strike your thumb with the reflex hammer. Observe and palpate the patient's arm for flexion at the antecubital fossa and contraction of the biceps tendon (Figure 44-24).

When testing the triceps, position the patient's arm as shown in Figure 44-25. Using the reflex hammer, strike the triceps tendon immediately proximal to the elbow. Observe for extension of the elbow caused by contraction of the triceps tendon.

The patellar reflex is also known as the knee jerk reflex. With the patient dangling his or her legs over the side of the bed or examining table, tap the pa-tellar tendon and observe for extension of the lower leg as the patellar tendon contracts. Some clinicians prefer to hold the anterior aspect of the patient's thigh just proximal to the patella so as to palpate contraction of the quadriceps (Figure 44-26).

The Achilles reflex, also known as the ankle jerk, is tested by having the patient dangle the feet over the side of the bed or examining table. Using your nondominant hand, partially dorsiflex the patient's foot. Tap the Achilles tendon with the reflex hammer. Observe and palpate for plantar flexion of the foot (Figure 44-27).

Testing for Babinski's reflex, an abnormal reflex, is generally done after the Achilles reflex. To test for Babinski's, firmly stroke the plantar surface of the patient's foot with the tip of the handle of the reflex hammer. Begin at the patient's heel, and move laterally and distally toward the ball of the foot and then along the ball of the foot medially (Figure 44-28). Dorsiflexion of the great toe frequently accompanied by fanning of the other toes is a positive Babinski's sign and may indicate an upper motor neuron lesion (Figures 44-29 and 44-30).

Testing for ankle clonus is usually done on completion of assessing DTRs, especially if the reflexes are hyperactive. Supporting the knee in a partially flexed position, sharply dorsiflex the foot. Observe for rhythmic involuntary dorsiflexion and plantar flexion oscillating movements known as clonus. Clonus may be associated with upper motoneuron disorders.

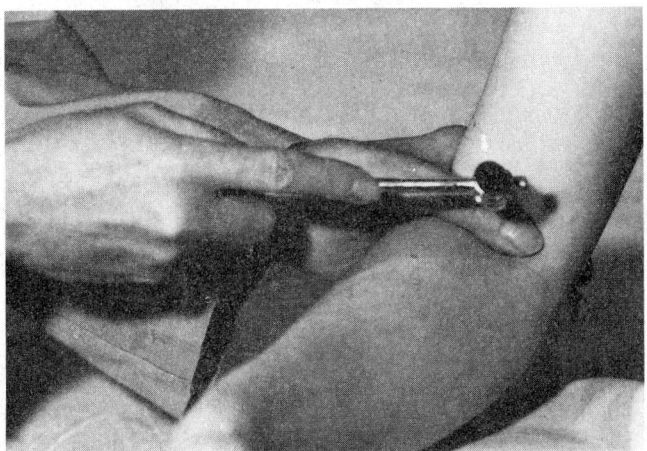

FIGURE 44-24   Elicitation of biceps reflex. (From Malasanos L: *Health assessment*, ed 4, St Louis, 1990, Mosby–Year Book, Inc.)

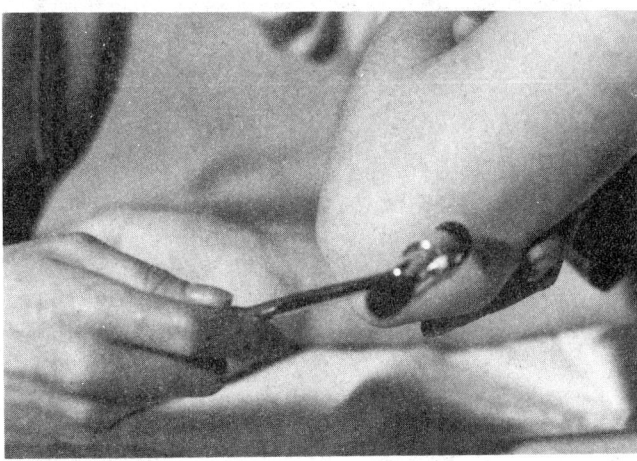

FIGURE 44-25   Elicitation of triceps reflex. (From Malasanos L: *Health assessment*, ed 4, St Louis, 1990, Mosby–Year Book, Inc.)

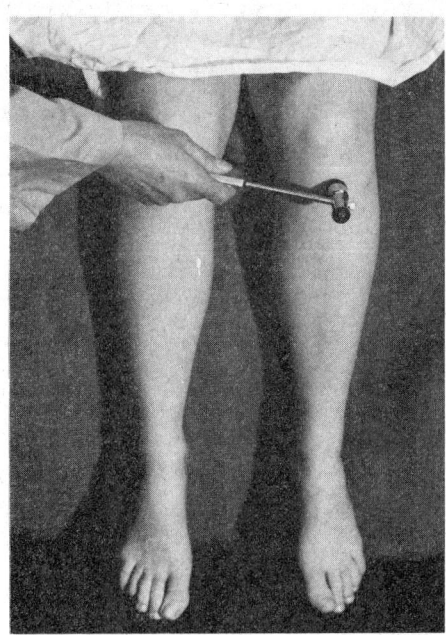

FIGURE 44-26   Elicitation of patellar reflex. (From Malasanos L: *Health assessment*, ed 4, St Louis, 1990, Mosby–Year Book, Inc.)

Superficial reflexes include the superficial abdominal reflexes and the cremasteric reflex. Because the cremasteric reflex is generally not tested, only the abdominal reflexes will be discussed here. To test the superficial abdominal reflexes, the patient should be relaxed, lying supine with the abdomen exposed. Quickly stroke the abdomen in each of the four quadrants from areas superior and inferior to the umbilicus toward the umbilicus. Observe the abdomen for contraction of the abdominal muscles and deviation of the umbilicus toward the stimulus (Figure 44-31).

DIAGNOSTIC AND LABORATORY TESTS
Lumbar Puncture

The **lumbar puncture** (spinal tap, spinal puncture) is a relatively common diagnostic test that is carried out on patients with neurologic signs and symptoms and those with leukemia. The procedure involves insertion of a needle into the subarachnoid space any-

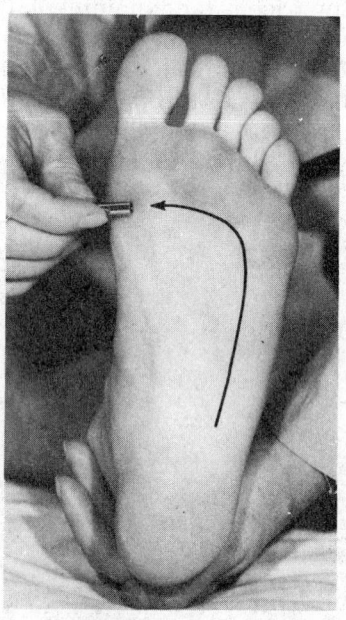

FIGURE 44-28 Elicitation of plantar reflex. (From Malasanos L: *Health assessment,* ed 4, St Louis, 1990, Mosby–Year Book, Inc.)

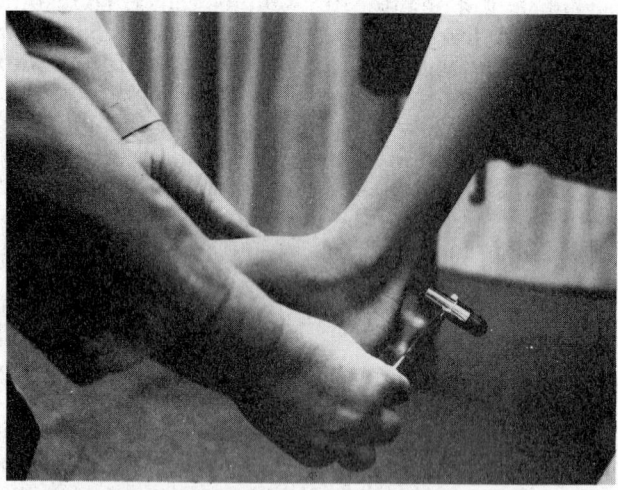

FIGURE 44-27 Elicitation of Achilles reflex. (From Malasanos L: *Health assessment,* ed 4, St Louis, 1990, Mosby–Year Book, Inc.)

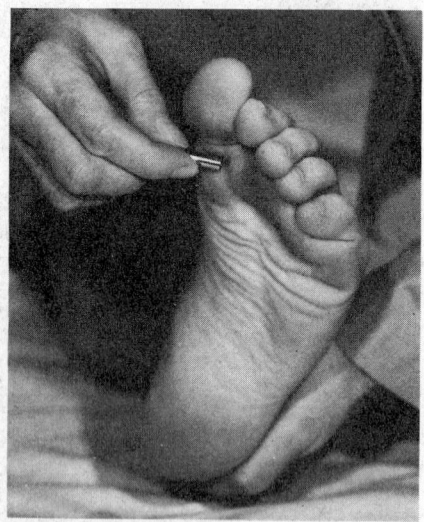

FIGURE 44-29 Normal response (negative Babinski's reflex) to plantar stimulation. (From Malasanos L: *Health assessment,* ed 4, St Louis, 1990, Mosby–Year Book, Inc.)

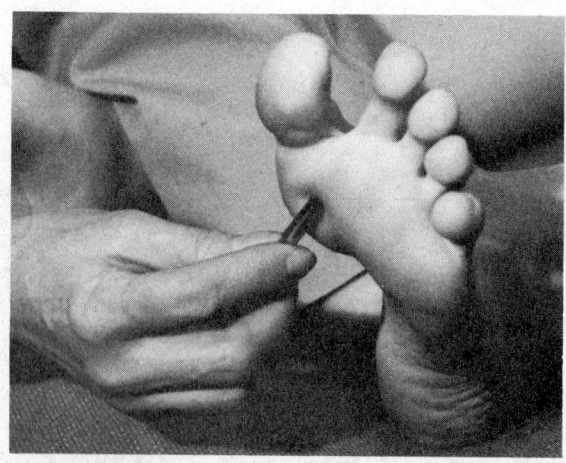

FIGURE 44-30 Abnormal response (positive Babinski's reflex) to plantar stimulation. (From Malasanos L: *Health assessment,* ed 4, St Louis, 1990, Mosby–Year Book, Inc.)

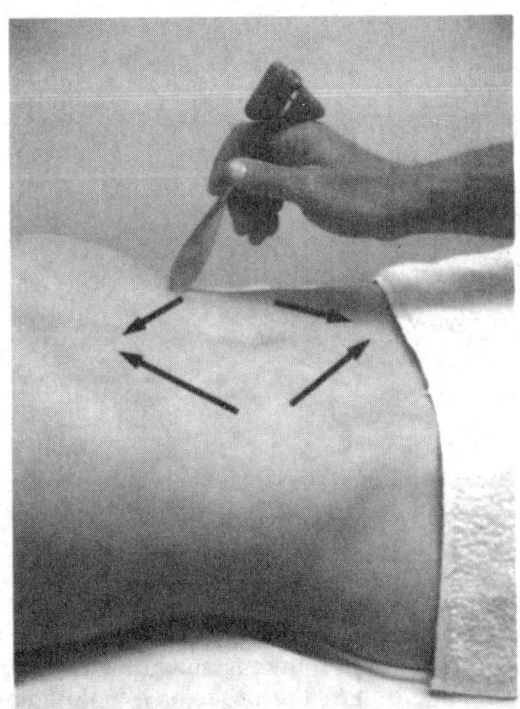

FIGURE 44-31 Examination of superficial abdominal reflexes. (From Seidel HM et al: *Mosby's guide to physical examination*, ed 2, St Louis, 1991, Mosby–Year Book, Inc.)

where between L2 and S1 and is performed for a variety of therapeutic or diagnostic purposes. Therapeutic purposes include withdrawal of pus and blood from the subarachnoid space, withdrawal of cerebrospinal fluid (CSF) to reduce intracranial pressure in some instances, and administration of spinal anesthesia or other drugs. Diagnostically, a lumbar puncture enables the removal of a small amount of CSF for examination and for measurement of CSF pressure. Measurement of CSF pressure helps detect an obstruction to the flow of CSF. Examination of the fluid aids in the diagnosis of bacterial or fungal meningitis, herpes simplex encephalitis, tumors, brain abscesses, neurosyphilis, and chronic CNS infections. Examination of the fluid may be indicated if a brain hemorrhage is suspected and a CT scan is inconclusive. A lumbar puncture should not be performed if there is evidence of greatly increased intracranial pressure, such as papilledema.

Patient preparation

The nurse describes the procedure to the patient and explains that a small amount of fluid will be withdrawn from the lower spine for the purposes of analysis. No dietary or fluid restrictions are required before the test. The nurse emphasizes the need for full cooperation during the test and the need for bed rest following the test. The patient is told that the test will take approximately 15 to 60 minutes.

A signed consent is obtained from the patient. The nurse advises the physician if the patient is very anxious, because the physician may order a sedative before the procedure.

GERIATRIC CONSIDERATIONS

Neurologic Assessment

General approach

Allow more time than for a younger adult

Articulate clearly; the geriatric patient may be hearing impaired

Impaired sight, comprehension, or mobility may result in less than optimum cooperation

Provide clear, concise instructions

History collection

May need to use fewer open-ended questions and provide some choices; for example, "Is your headache sharp, dull, pounding, or throbbing?"

May need to repeat questions

Be alert for answers that do not appear appropriate; the patient may not have understood the question correctly because of impaired hearing or comprehension

Physical assessment

The physical examination itself is not different, but the approach needs to be altered such that the appropriate information is assessed without undue discomfort or embarrassment for the patient

Maintain an environment with minimal noise, distractions, and interruptions

Geriatric patients may have a decreased vibratory sensation (especially in the lower extremities), less brisk DTRs, and decreased muscle mass as well as strength

Geriatric patients may have an increased incidence of impaired mental status that is not readily noticeable to the casual observer

If mental status appears to be impaired, consider exploring the existence of depression

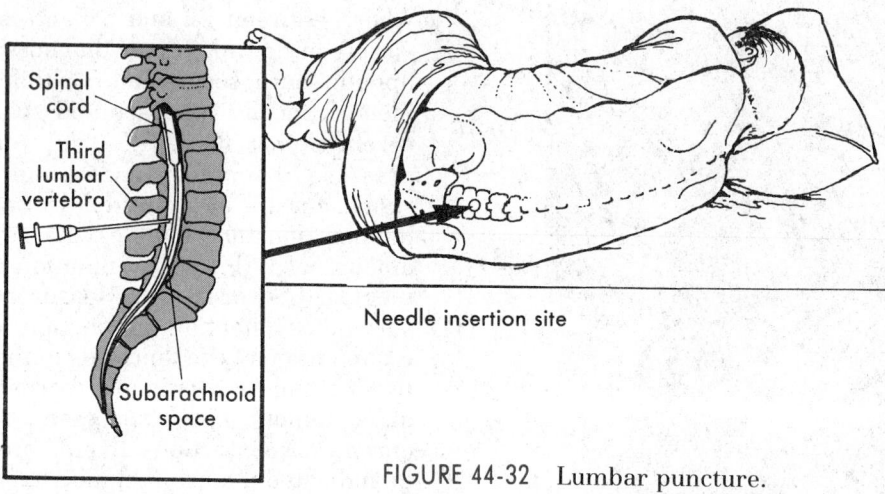

Spinal cord

Third lumbar vertebra

Subarachnoid space

Needle insertion site

FIGURE 44-32   Lumbar puncture.

Procedure

The patient is encouraged to empty the bowel and bladder and is assisted into a fetal position at the edge of the bed, with knees drawn up to the chest (Figure 44-32). This position allows full flexion of the spine and wider spaces between the vertebrae. The nurse places a pillow between the patient's legs to prevent the upper leg from rolling forward and a small pillow under the patient's head to support the spine in a horizontal position. If this position cannot be tolerated, the nurse asks the patient to sit up and to extend the chest and head toward the knees. Regardless of position, the patient must remain still and may need reminders and encouragement to do so. The nurse provides support throughout the procedure and monitors the patient's neurologic and respiratory status.

After injection of a local anesthetic, the physician inserts a spinal needle. A sterile manometer is attached to the needle at this point so that pressure readings may be taken. Readings may be misleadingly high if the patient is still tightly flexed because intra-abdominal pressure will remain high. Samples of CSF are collected in three labeled tubes for protein and glucose determinations, blood cell counts, and culture (Table 44-10). The patient may experience some mild burning as the local anesthetic is injected and a feeling of pressure or brief, flitting pains as the spinal needle is inserted.

Postprocedure care

For 1 hour following the procedure the patient assumes a prone position, if able, with a pillow under the abdomen to increase intra-abdominal pressure. This position retards leakage of CSF. The patient then remains flat in bed for 6 to 24 hours depending on the physician's orders and the patient's status. Turning from side to side is permissible, and some physicians allow a 30-degree elevation of the head. A liberal fluid intake is encouraged to replace CSF removed during the procedure, unless contraindicated by the patient's condition. The nurse checks the puncture site for swelling, redness, and drainage and assesses the patient's ability to void and to move the extremities. The patient is observed for further signs of complications such as neck stiffness, irritability, decreasing levels of consciousness, and altered vital signs. A common sequela of a lumbar puncture is a postlumbar headache, which can appear from a few hours to several days following the procedure. It is a throbbing bifrontal or occipital headache that worsens as the patient sits or stands upright and is caused by leakage of the CSF. A postpuncture headache can be alleviated by bed rest in a quiet, darkened room and analgesics.

Queckenstedt's Test

If blockage in the subarachnoid space is suspected, Queckenstedt's test is performed. The jugular veins are simultaneously occluded for 10 seconds, using either manual pressure or a medium-sized blood pressure cuff inflated to 10 mm Hg. The increase in CSF pressure is noted. Normally, the CSF fluid pressure will increase from 150 to 400 mm H_2O within 10 seconds after jugular occlusion and return to normal within 10 seconds after release of the obstruction. This test is very dangerous if increased intracranial pressure is present because the brain may herniate.

Neuroradiologic Examinations

Skull and spinal roentgenograms

Skull x-ray studies may be ordered as part of a routine neurologic workup and are extremely useful in studying increased cranial pressure and abnormali-

TABLE 44-10   CSF Findings

Determination	Conventional value (SI value)	Abnormal value	Implications
Pressure	60 to 180 mm H_2O	Increased	Acute bacterial tuberculosis or viral meningitis
			Subarachnoid hemorrhage, cerebral thrombosis
			Brain tumor
		Decreased (below 100 mm H_2O)	Subarachnoid obstruction above puncture site
			CSF leak
			Severe dehydration
Appearance	Clear, colorless	Bloody	Cerebral hemorrhage into subarachnoid space
			Traumatic tap
		Cloudy to turbid	Infection (elevated WBC or protein, microorganisms)
		Brown, orange, yellow	Elevated protein
			RBC breakdown
Cell count	0 to 5 mononuclear cells/ mm^2	Increased	Acute infection, abscess
			Chronic illness (such as multiple sclerosis)
			Tumor
			Infarction
	No RBCs	RBCs	Hemorrhage
			Traumatic tap
Culture and sensitivity	No organisms present	Organisms	Infection
Protein	20 to 45 mg/dL (0.20 to 0.45 g/L)	Increased	Infection
			Tumor
			Multiple sclerosis, neurosyphilis or degenerative spinal or brain disease
			Hemorrhage
		Decreased	Rapid production of CSF
Glucose	40 to 70 mg/dL (2.22 to 3.89 mmol/L)	Increased	Diabetes mellitus, diabetic coma
			Uremia
		Decreased	Acute meningitis
			Neoplasm
Chloride	120 to 130 mEq/L (120 to 130 mmol/L)	Decreased	Meningeal infection, tubercular meningitis
Lactic dehydrogenase (LDH)	2 to 7.2 U/mL (33.3-120 nmol·sec^{-1}L)	Increased	Infection or inflammation
Cytology	No malignant cells	Malignant cells	Neoplasm
VDRL	Negative	Positive	Neurosyphilis

ties of the base of the skull and of the cranial vault. Skull x-ray films are more useful than routine CT scans in the diagnosis of pituitary tumors. The procedure causes no discomfort. Patients are instructed to remove glasses, dentures, metal objects, and jewelry before the x-ray examination.

Spinal x-ray films are useful in the evaluation of fracture, bone erosion, and obstruction of the vertebral canal. They are frequently used to evaluate the cause of low back pain, especially when the patient reports pain radiating down one or both legs.

Computed tomography

Computed tomography (CT scan, computed axial tomography) is one of the most effective methods of studying the brain and can eliminate the need for more painful, invasive procedures such as cerebral angiography and pneumoencephalography. Using a minimal amount of radiation exposure, the brain can be visualized through cross-sectional images or slices of various layers of the head. The CT scanner is particularly sensitive to variances in tissue density and provides more specific views of bone and tissue than conventional x-ray studies. CT, which may use contrast enhancement, is useful in detecting tumors, hemorrhage, hematomas, ventricular enlargement, and cortical atrophy. It is also gaining use in the diagnosis of spinal disorders such as herniated disks and intraspinal tumors.

Patient preparation

The patient is informed that the test enables assessment of the head (or of the spine). The nurse tells the patient that the test causes no discomfort but that it is absolutely necessary to be motionless during the procedure. Although the patient can breathe normally, even talking will cause artifacts on the images. The patient is positioned on an x-ray table while a scanner rotates around the head. If the patient is receiving a scan of the head, the head is cradled on a water-filled chamber. The scanner will make clicking noises as it moves, but the patient will not feel the movement. Foods and liquids need not be restricted before the test unless contrast enhancement is anticipated. If contrast enhancement is scheduled, the patient must avoid oral intake for 4 hours before the procedure, because the iodine dye may cause nausea. The nurse tells the patient that the dye is administered through a peripheral intravenous line and that the patient may experience a warm, flushed feeling or a salty taste as the dye is injected. If a dye is to be used, the nurse must determine if the patient has a sensitivity to shellfish, iodine, or contrast media. The physician is informed of sensitivities, because prophylactic medication or omission of contrast enhancement may be warranted.

The patient must remove wigs, hairpins, clips, and jewelry before the test. If the patient is restless or apprehensive, the nurse notifies the physician, who may order a sedative.

Procedure

A series of images is taken before the contrast medium is administered. A peripheral intravenous line will be started for administration of the dye, after which the scanning process is repeated. The entire test takes 30 to 60 minutes.

Postprocedure care

The patient is told to resume a usual diet and all usual activities. If a contrast medium was used, the patient should increase fluid intake, because the dye will cause diuresis. The nurse must remain alert for allergic reactions to the dye, although these usually manifest within about 2 minutes after dye administration.

Myelography

Myelography involves x-ray visualization of the spinal subarachnoid space following injection of a contrast medium or air into the subarachnoid space. Because myelography is useful for visualizing obstructions within the spinal canal, it is particularly useful in diagnosing herniated intravertebral disks and spinal tumors.

Patient preparation

The patient is told that the procedure will be performed in the x-ray department and that the patient will be tilted into up-down positions after injection of the dye so that the flow of dye in the spinal canal can be observed. Positioning and sensations during the injection of the dye are the same as for a lumbar puncture. The patient will need to restrict food and fluids 4 to 8 hours before the procedure. The nurse checks the patient's history for sensitivity to iodine or dyes, chronic alcoholism, multiple sclerosis, severe cardiovascular disease, and epilepsy. If water-soluble dye (Amipaque) is used, phenothiazines should be discontinued for 48 hours before the test and should not be resumed until the dye has been absorbed. The patient is informed that the procedure takes about 45 minutes.

An informed consent is required. The patient will need to remove jewelry and metal objects from the test area. Pretest medications may be administered to relax the patient.

Procedure

Following positioning, a lumbar puncture is performed, and a small amount of CSF is removed. Dye or air is injected into the spinal canal. The type of dye that is used will guide the procedure and postprocedural care. If an oil-based dye (Pantopaque) is used, the dye must be aspirated at the completion of visualization, and the patient's head is elevated above the level of the spine to prevent the dye from traveling upward and causing meningeal irritation. If Amipaque is used, it is not removed, because it will be absorbed.

Postprocedure care

If an oil-based dye has been used, the patient must be kept flat for several hours. Headache is relatively common following the procedure, but neck stiffness (especially on flexion) and pain should be reported, because they may signal meningeal irritation. The patient is monitored for allergic reactions such as confusion, dizziness, tremors, and hallucinations. If a water-soluble dye is used, the patient is kept semirecumbent with the head elevated 30 to 60 degrees for the first 24 hours to prevent seizures and must lie quietly to decrease the possibility of headache. If air is used, the patient is positioned for several hours with the head lower than the trunk. Vital signs and ability to void are carefully monitored, and the patient is encouraged to drink extra fluids. Usual diet and activities may be resumed the day following the test if no complications occur.

Pneumoencephalography

Pneumoencephalography has been made almost obsolete as a result of the availability of the CT scan. The test involves introduction of air into the subarachnoid space and ventricular system through a lumbar puncture and is useful in studying degenerative diseases and hydrocephalus. The preparation and procedure are similar to those for a lumbar puncture and myelography. The patient is informed that he or she will feel the inserted air rising and experience a sloshing noise as it circulates through the ventricles. Following the procedure, the patient will be on bed rest for 24 to 48 hours and should turn from side to side at least every 2 hours to hasten absorption of the air. After 48 hours the head of the bed is progressively elevated. Nausea and headache, which frequently accompany pneumoencephalography, can be alleviated by lowering the head of the bed. In the immediate period following the procedure, vital and neurologic signs must be monitored every 15 minutes for 2 hours, then hourly for 4 hours, and then every 4 hours for 24 hours or according to agency protocol.

Cerebral angiography

Cerebral angiography involves the diffusion of a contrast medium into the cerebral arterial system and is useful in determining the causes of strokes, headaches, seizures, or motor weakness. The closed method involves injection of dye indirectly into the carotid or cerebral vessels via the femoral (the most commonly used site), brachial, or axillary arteries. The open method involves surgical exposure of the internal carotid artery before injection of the dye. Following injection of the contrast medium, rapid sequential films are taken as the dye is followed through the cerebral circulation.

Patient preparation

The nurse tells the patient that the test shows circulation of blood in the brain and takes 1 to 2 hours. The patient must remain still on the radiographic table, because head movement will interfere with accurate interpretation of the radiographs. A hot, burning sensation and flushing may be experienced, especially if the dye is injected into the external carotid system. The nurse assesses the patient's his-

tory for sensitivity to iodine, seafood, or contrast media and for anticoagulant therapy. If anticoagulants are not ordered discontinued, the nurse must be alert to the possibility of severe bleeding. The nurse evaluates the patient's vital signs, level of consciousness, pupil responses, facial symmetry, strength and motion of the extremities, and distal pulses. The patient is instructed to fast for 6 to 10 hours before the test. Some angiographers prefer that the fluid intake is maintained to prevent hemoconcentration and possible vessel occlusion. An informed consent is required. The patient needs to remove jewelry, hairpins, dentures, and hearing aids before the procedure. The nurse administers an anticholinergic and sedative before the procedure if ordered.

Postprocedure care

The nurse maintains the patient on bed rest for 12 to 24 hours and monitors vital signs, distal pulses, and neurologic status every 15 minutes for the first 2 hours, then every hour for 4 hours, and then every 4 hours in the first 24 hours (or according to agency protocol). If the carotid artery was used, the nurse assesses for dysphagia, respiratory distress, and arterial spasms that produce the symptoms of transient ischemic attacks. If the brachial approach was used, the nurse immobilizes the arm for 12 hours and avoids taking blood pressure readings in that arm. If the femoral approach was used, the affected leg is maintained in a straight position. The nurse checks the puncture site for bleeding, redness, and swelling. Pressure is applied to the site if bleeding occurs.

Digital subtraction angiography

Digital subtraction angiography (DSA; digital vascular imaging; digital subtraction fluorography), a relatively new method of radiographically studying blood vessels, is used when the area of study is blocked by bone. Digital subtraction angiography is particularly useful in the evaluation of patients who are having brain surgery involving vasculature or tumors. During digital subtraction angiography an image of the target area is taken before injection of contrast dye (mask image) that is compared with an image taken after injection of the dye (contrast image). The pictures are digitized, stored, and compared in a computer that subtracts anything that is common between the mask and contrast images. The result is an enhanced image of high contrast that can be recorded on videotapes, disks, or x-ray film. Intravenous digital subtraction angiography is sometimes preferred over routine angiography, because it uses less radiation, it is less invasive, and there is less possibility of serious complications. It requires a cooperative patient who has good cardiac output and who can lie still on command.

Patient preparation

The nurse explains that the test gives information about blood vessels and that the patient will have to lie on a special hard table. An intravenous line will be started, and then a catheter will be inserted into the desired vein. The patient may experience a pinching sensation as the catheter is inserted. The injection of the dye may produce a transient warm sensation and a metallic taste. The patient will need to refrain from all motion, including swallowing, as the dye is injected and images are taken. A variety of clicks and noises will be heard as the equipment moves about. The procedure takes 20 to 45 minutes.

The nurse determines if the patient is to fast or if clear fluids are allowed and instructs the patient appropriately. The nurse checks the patient's history for allergies to seafood, iodine, or contrast media.

Postprocedure care

Once the films have been taken, the catheter is removed and a small bandage is applied. The patient is allowed to walk away from the table and is instructed to avoid vigorous use of the limb in which the dye was injected for 24 hours. The nurse instructs the patient to drink large amounts of fluid to promote excretion of the dye. If intra-arterial digital subtraction angiography has been performed the postprocedure care is similar to that for conventional arteriography.

Brain scan

A **brain scan** is a relatively safe, painless procedure that is useful in detecting intracranial lesions such as neoplasms, brain abscess, cerebral hemorrhage, acute infarction, and arteriovenous malformation. It is particularly useful in identifying subdural hematomas and also in determining brain death. The patient is given an intravenous injection of a radionucleotide (usually technetium 99m pertechnetate), and then the radioactivity is traced with a gamma scintillation camera or a scanner, which converts the rays into images displayed on an oscilloscope screen. The test is based on the principle that the radionucleotide can penetrate only a disrupted blood-brain barrier and therefore will collect where there is abnormal cerebral tissue.

Patient preparation

The patient is informed that the test will visualize the brain and be performed in the nuclear medicine department. The nurse reassures the patient that the radioactive material will be excreted within 24 hours and poses no danger. The patient is told that some burning at the injection site after administration of the technetium may be felt, but that the test is painless otherwise. The nurse explains that a scanning machine will move back and forth around the patient's head and that it will make some noise. The patient is told to remove jewelry and metal from the x-ray field. The nurse ensures that a potassium chloride capsule is administered to the patient, as ordered, before injection of the radionucleotide. The potassium chloride prevents excessive uptake of the technetium by the choroid plexus.

The injection site is checked for the presence of hematoma following the procedure, and warm soaks are applied if needed.

Magnetic resonance imaging

Magnetic resonance imaging (MRI) uses an immense electromagnet to detect radio frequency pulses from the alignment of hydrogen protons in the magnetic field. Computers pick up the electromagnetic echo and produce images with high contrast of soft tissue. This technique provides excellent visualization of tissue without the use of contrast media or ionizing radiation. MRI does not visualize bone, and so soft tissue adjacent to bone is readily viewed. It is particularly useful in visualizing lesions that have not been detected by CT scans, such as brainstem tumors, brain abscess, and encephalitis. Because it is so sensitive to tissue variations, it is able to delineate white from gray matter and may potentially help localize lesions in white matter, as in multiple sclerosis. It cannot be used for patients on pacemakers, since MRI may deactivate the pacemaker. If a patient has an intravenous infusion with a drip regulator, the nurse must check with MRI personnel, because some regulators are affected by the MRI.

Patient preparation

The patient is informed that the test is painless and requires no dye or radiation and no dietary restrictions. The nurse informs the patient that MRI may damage credit cards and watches and that jewelry and hair clips cause artifacts; these objects should be removed before the test. If the patient has dental work that contains ferrous material, the nurse reassures the patient that an odd sensation experienced in these areas is normal. The nurse checks the patient's history for evidence of surgical or orthopedic clips and heart valves, because MRI may displace these. The patient is prepared for the beating noise of the MRI machine and is reassured that earplugs will be supplied if the noise is uncomfortable.

Electroencephalography

Electroencephalography (EEG) amplifies and records the electrical activity of the brain ("brain waves") through the attachment of 14 to 21 electrodes to the scalp. It is useful and economical in screening for brain tumors and subdural hematomas and is indicated in almost all patients who have unexplained confusion, loss of consciousness, or first seizures. It is also useful in providing supporting evidence for the establishment of brain death. The presence of slowed activity, spikes, or asymmetric rhythms suggests abnormalities.

The nurse reassures the patient that EEG is not a form of shock therapy and that it cannot read the mind. The patient is informed that the procedure is painless and requires no dietary restrictions other than avoidance of cola, tea, and coffee on the morning of the test, because these produce a stimulating effect. Patients may benefit from less sleep the night before the test, because they will be more likely to rest during the study. Hair should be washed the evening before the study and gels, hair sprays, and lotions avoided. The patient is told that movement must be minimal because even opening the eyes will alter the EEG recording but that opportunities to move will be given if desired. Medications are usually not withheld before the test. The patient is informed that the test will take 45 minutes to 2 hours.

If sleep EEG is ordered, as may be done when certain seizure disorders are suspected, the patient must remain awake the night before the test. A sedative such as chloral hydrate is ordered to promote sleep during the test.

Procedure

The patient is placed in a reclining or a supine position. Electrodes are applied to the scalp with electrode paste in a uniform pattern. The patient then lies in the quiet, darkened room with eyes closed. Movements such as blinking, swallowing, and talking are noted since these may produce artifacts on the recording. After the recording the electrodes and paste are removed.

Evoked potential studies

Evoked potential studies (external stimuli, or "activating," procedures) may be performed during the EEG. Changes and responses evoked by these stimuli are detected with computers that extract the signal, display it on an oscilloscope, and store the data. Evoked brain potentials are useful in patients with suspected multiple sclerosis or suspected tumors of the brainstem or of the eighth cranial nerve.

1. Visual evoked responses (VER, VEP). A strobe light is flashed over the patient's face with eyes opened and closed. A response may also be achieved through retinal stimulation or checkerboard patterns. VER is useful as an aid in determining multiple sclerosis and other neurologic disorders.
2. Somatosensory evoked potentials (SEP). A peripheral sensory nerve is repeatedly stimulated with a mild electrical shock. This test is useful in evaluating the neurologic activity that can be conducted through a spinal cord lesion.
3. Auditory brainstem evoked potentials (ABEP). Patients are exposed to clicking noises or tone bursts through earphones. ABEP aids in detecting early posterior loss and tumors.

Echoencephalography

In **echoencephalography** (brain echogram, ultrasound of the brain), a sound transducer/receiver, placed against the skull, transmits and receives sound waves. Sound waves that are received are converted to electrical impulses and displayed on an oscilloscope. The test is useful in determining the position of the brain's midline structures, particularly of the third ventricle. The procedure has been largely supplanted by CT scanning.

Patient preparation

The nurse reassures the patient that the procedure is painless. The patient is informed that a gel will be applied to the head to aid in transmission of sound waves. All objects should be removed from the hair. The study takes approximately 10 minutes.

Electromyography

Electromyography (EMG) involves insertion of needle electrodes into selected skeletal muscles to evaluate changes in the electrical potential of the muscles and of nerves leading to them. Electrical potentials are shown on an oscilloscope and amplified by loud speaker, so that muscle activity can be both seen and heard. The test is useful in evaluating suspected lumbar or cervical disk disease, myasthenia gravis, muscular dystrophies, motoneuron disease, and polymyositis.

Patient preparation

The patient is reassured that the needle will not electrocute him or her and that he or she will experience sensations similar to an injection as the needles are inserted. An informed consent is obtained. No special preparation is required.

Procedure

The patient will be positioned in accordance with the muscle being examined. An electrode will be inserted into the muscle, and the patient will be asked to first relax the muscle and then to progressively contract it. The muscle waves will be studied for their number and form.

Nerve conduction velocities

Nerve conduction velocities are often performed in conjunction with EMG. They measure the speed with which electrical impulses are transmitted along sensory or motor nerves. The nerve is stimulated electrically through the overlying skin, and the response is recorded on an electrode placed over a supplied muscle. The time between response and stimulation is recorded on an oscilloscope. Velocities will be slower in individuals with polyneuritis, with poorly controlled diabetes, or on long-term renal dialysis. The patient may experience discomfort, spasm, or a tightening sensation as the nerve is stimulated.

Cerebrovascular Flow Tests

Noninvasive cerebrovascular flow tests are useful in identifying patients who are at risk for stroke because of embolic or thromboembolic areas in the internal carotid system. Three tests are commonly performed as part of this assessment.

Oculoplethysmography and oculopneumoplethysmography

In oculoplethysmography a local anesthetic is applied to the eyes, and fluid-filled contact lenses are applied. Pulsations of the fluid in cups represent pulsatile flow in the ophthalmic artery, the first branch of the internal carotid artery. Narrowing of the internal carotid artery will produce changes in volume and in the pulse wave. Tracings of the pulse waves are compared with pulse waves in the right earlobe, which reflect external carotid pulses. The pulse waves in the earlobe, which are picked up through small photoelectric cells, are used for reference. In oculopneumoplethysmography, which is considered more accurate, air-filled transducers are applied to each sclera, and negative pressure is applied. With the application of the pressure, the pulses disappear. The point at which they reappear enables estimation of systolic pressure in the ophthalmic artery.

Carotid phonangiography

In carotid phonangiography, special microphones are placed over areas of bruits, usually in the carotid arteries. The sound is picked up on an oscilloscope and photographed. The test is useful for estimating the amount and location of stenosis but is not useful in diagnosing severe carotid stenosis. No special preparation is necessary.

Ultrasound arteriography

The anatomy of arteries can be demonstrated through the use of the Doppler imaging instrument, which provides a static image of the outline of a vessel wall, and the B-mode ultrasonic scanner, which provides dynamic images of the vessel wall. Ultrasound arteriography is useful in diagnosing total occlusion of an internal carotid artery and in the noninvasive evaluation of patients with a history of transient ischemic attacks, strokes, claudication, and asymptomatic bruits. It is painless and safe, and the patient should be informed that he or she will have to remove all clothing over the site to be examined. The patient will be supine during the procedure.

CRITICAL THINKING QUESTIONS

1 Describe the path a nerve impulse takes in the following situations:
  a. Bringing about a simple rectus femoris stretch reflex
  b. Smelling and identifying a smoky odor
2 Design at least three pertinent questions to ask a witness to an accident regarding an unconscious patient brought into the emergency room.
3 Describe an effective approach to examining the pupils of a restless, disoriented patient with brain damage.
4 Discuss potential etiologic factors to consider when a patient reports severe headache.
5 Differentiate between CT and a brain scan.
6 Explain electroencephalography as it might be explained to a patient.

BIBLIOGRAPHY

Current

1. Bates B et al: *A guide to physical examination and history-taking,* ed 5, New York, 1991, JB Lippincott Co.
2. Bowers A, Thompson J: *Clinical manual of health assessment,* ed 3, St Louis, 1988, Mosby–Year Book, Inc.
3. Burrell LO: *Adult nursing in hospital and community settings,* Norwalk, Conn, 1992, Appleton & Lange.
4. Cacayorin ED et al: Headache in the athlete and radiographic evaluation, *Clin Sport Med* 6:4, 1987.
5. Cacayorin ED et al: Lumbar and thoracic spine pain in the athlete: radiographic evaluation, *Clin Sports Med* 6:4, 1987.
6. Gallo JJ et al: *Handbook of geriatric assessment,* Rockville, Md, 1988, Aspen Publishers, Inc.
7. Goldberg S: *The four-minute neurologic exam,* Miami, 1989, MedMaster, Inc.
8. Gordon M: *Manual of nursing diagnosis,* New York, 1987, McGraw-Hill Book Co.
9. Hickey JV: *The clinical practice of neurological and neurosurgical nursing,* Philadelphia, 1992, JB Lippincott Co.
10. Hunt AH: Digital subtraction angiography: patient preparation and care, *J Neurosci Nurs* 19:4, 1987.
11. Kane RL et al: *Essentials of clinical geriatrics,* ed 2, New York, 1989, McGraw-Hill Book Co.
12. Kenny RA: *Physiology of aging: a synopsis,* Chicago, 1992, Year Book Medical Publishers, Inc.
13. Lee K, Kucharczyk W: Magnetic resonance imaging of the brain and spine, *Med Series* 3:36, Aug 1989.
14. LeFever Kee J: *Handbook of laboratory and diagnostic*

tests with nursing implications, Norwalk, Conn, 1990, Appleton & Lange.

15. Malasanos L et al: *Health assessment,* ed 4, St Louis, 1990, Mosby–Year Book, Inc.
16. McDonagh A: Getting your patient ready for a nuclear scan, *Nurs 91* 21:2, 1991.
17. Murray R, Zentner S: *Nursing assessment and health promotion through the life span,* Englewood Cliffs, NJ, 1989, Prentice-Hall.
18. *Nurse's ready reference: diagnostic tests,* Springhouse, Pa, 1991, Springhouse Corp.
19. Pagana KD, Pagana TJ: *Diagnostic testing and nursing implications,* St Louis, 1990, Mosby–Year Book, Inc.
20. Seeley R et al: *Anatomy and physiology,* St Louis, 1992, Mosby–Year Book, Inc.
21. Seidel HM et al: *Mosby's guide to physical examination,* ed 2, St Louis, 1991, Mosby–Year Book, Inc.
22. Swartz MH: *Textbook of physical diagnosis,* Philadelphia, 1989, WB Saunders Co.

Classic

23. Bloch B, Hunter M: Teaching physiological assessment of black persons, *Nurs Educ* 6(1):24, 1981.
24. Block G, Nolan J: *Health assessment for professional nursing: a developmental approach,* New York, 1986, Appleton-Century-Crofts.
25. Carotenuto R, Bullock J: *Physical assessment of the gerontologic client,* Philadelphia, 1981, FA Davis.
26. Fields W, McGinn-Campbell K: *Introduction to health assessment,* Reston, Va, 1983, Reston Publishing Co, Inc.
27. Folstein MF et al: "Mini-mental state": a practical method for grading the cognitive state of patients for the clinician, *Psychiatr Res* 12:189-198, 1975.
28. Pfeiffer E: A short portable mental status questionnaire for the assessment of organic brain deficit in elderly patients, *J Am Geriatr Soc* 23:441, 1975.
29. Price S, Wilson L: *Pathophysiology,* New York, 1986, McGraw-Hill Book Co.
30. Prior JA et al: *Physical diagnosis: the history and examination of the patient,* ed 6, St Louis, 1981, Mosby–Year Book, Inc.
31. Teasdale G, Jennett B: Assessment of coma and impaired consciousness: practical scale, *Lancet* 2:81, 1974.

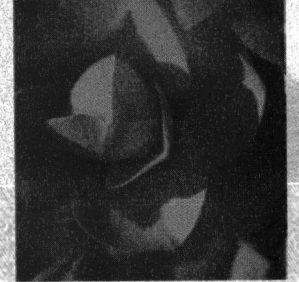

CHAPTER FORTY-FIVE

Nursing Management of Adults with Common Neurologic Problems

LEARNING OBJECTIVES

1 Define the relevant terms associated with the common neurologic problems of altered level of consciousness, increased intracranial pressure, seizure, and headache.
2 Describe the etiologic factors for, pathophysiologic conditions of, clinical manifestations associated with, and therapeutic management for common neurologic problems.
3 Describe the types of seizure and the types of headache.
4 Discuss the nursing management including assessment, nursing diagnosis, planning, implementation, evaluation, and documentation for common neurologic problems.
5 Discuss the ongoing nursing management related to long-term care, home care, or rehabilitation for common neurologic problems.

KEY TERMS

clonic phase, p. 1224
coma, p. 1202
convulsion, p. 1222
decerebration, p. 1205
decortication, p. 1205
epilepsy, p. 1222
headache, p. 1234
herniation syndrome, p. 1214
increased intracranial pressure (ICP), p. 1214

oculocephalic reflexes (doll's eyes), p. 1203
seizure, p. 1222
status epilepticus, p. 1224
stupor, p. 1202
tonic-clonic seizures, p. 1225
tonic phase, p. 1223

CERTAIN NEUROLOGIC problems exist or have the potential to develop when the brain is affected by a pathologic condition regardless of the cause of that condition. These common problems include development of a coma state, increased intracranial pressure, seizure, or headache.

ALTERED LEVEL OF CONSCIOUSNESS
Definition

Consciousness is a state of awareness of self, environment, and one's response to that environment. To be fully conscious means that the individual appropriately responds to the external stimuli. An altered level of consciousness represents a decrease in this full state of awareness and response to environmental stimuli (e.g. sounds).

Etiology/Epidemiology

Etiologic factors that may cause an altered arousal state of acute onset are structural, metabolic, or psychogenic. Structural causes are classified according to original location of the pathologic condition—supratentorial lesions and infratentorial (subtentorial) lesions as well as extradural, subdural, and intraparenchymal. Etiologic factors are also categorized by the type of pathologic process, such as infection.

Pathophysiology

Awakeness (arousal) is mediated by brainstem centers of the ascending reticular activating system (ARAS). A decreased level of awakeness can be caused by either a reduction in cerebral metabolism or a reduction in cerebral blood flow. Central nervous system pathology may directly destroy the diencephalon-midbrain-pontine reticular formation and its pathways, or it may indirectly destroy these structures by compression.

Clinical Manifestations

Changes in level of consciousness, breathing patterns, pupillary responses, ocular positioning and reflexes, and motor responses may indicate the location of the brain injury and how extensive the injury is.

Level of consciousness

Level of consciousness is the most critical index of central nervous system dysfunction. Changes in level of consciousness can indicate clinical improvement or deterioration. The Glasgow Coma Scale (see Chapter 44) and other tools may be used to assess level of consciousness. With confusion the ability to think rapidly and clearly is lost. Judgment and decision making are impaired. Disorientation specifically results from memory dysfunction. Disorientation to time occurs first; next, disorientation to place; and then disorientation to person.

Lethargy indicates a more severe cerebral hemisphere dysfunction and is demonstrated by limited spontaneous movement and speech. The patient is easily aroused with normal speech or touch. When aroused, the patient may or may not be oriented. Lethargy is commonly seen in metabolic causes of coma, for example, with a high fever.

Obtundation involves a mild to moderate loss of arousability with a limited ability to respond to the

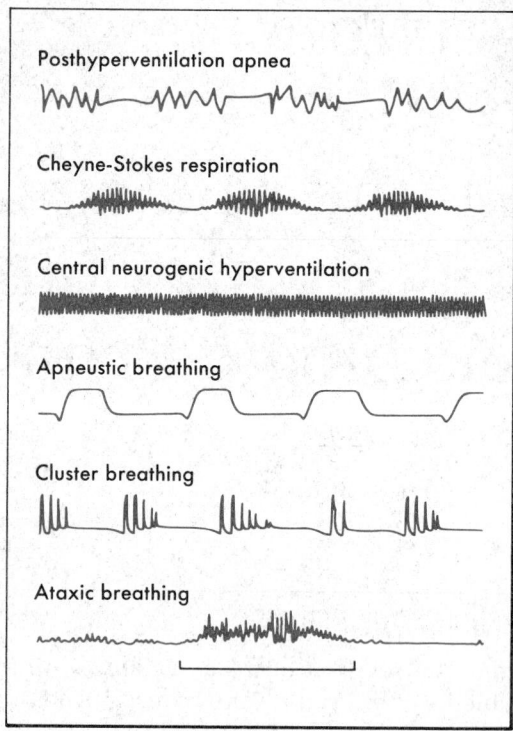

FIGURE 45-1 Breathing patterns at different levels of consciousness.

environment. The patient falls asleep unless verbally and tactilely stimulated. Questions are answered with minimal responses when the patient is aroused. This individual falls asleep while being bathed or as the nurse tries to administer medications.

Stupor is a condition of deep sleep or unresponsiveness. The patient is very difficult to arouse and may have only limited motor withdrawal or grabbing.

Coma is a state of no motor or verbal response to the external environment or to any stimuli such as deep pain or suctioning. There is no arousal to any stimulus.

Pattern of breathing

Rate, rhythm, and pattern of breathing are important indicators of level of brain dysfunction (Table 45-1 and Figure 45-1).

Pupillary changes

Anatomically, brainstem areas controlling arousal are adjacent to areas controlling pupils. Pupillary changes are a valuable guide to the present level of brainstem dysfunction (Table 45-2 and Figure 45-2). Drugs, ischemia, and hypothermia may affect pupils.

TABLE 45-1   Patterns of Breathing

Breathing	Description	Location of injury
HEMISPHERIC BREATHING PATTERNS		
Normal	After a period of hyperventilation that lowers the arterial carbon dioxide (P_{CO_2}), the individual continues to breathe regularly but with a reduced depth	
Posthyperventilation apnea (PHVA)	Respirations stop after hyperventilation has lowered the P_{CO_2} level below normal; rhythmic breathing returns when the P_{CO_2} level returns to normal	Associated with diffuse bilateral metabolic or structural disease of the cerebrum
Cheyne-Stokes respirations (CSR)	The breathing pattern has a smooth increase (crescendo) in the rate and depth of breathing (hyperpnea), which peaks and is followed by a gradual smooth decrease (decrescendo) in the rate and depth of breathing to the point of apnea when the cycle repeats itself; the hyperpneic phase lasts longer than the apneic phase	Bilateral dysfunction of the deep cerebral or diencephalic structures, seen with supratentorial injury and metabolically induced coma states
BRAINSTEM BREATHING PATTERNS		
Central neurogenic hyperventilation (CNH)	A sustained, deep, rapid, but regular pattern (hyperpnea) with a decreased P_{CO_2} and a corresponding increase in pH and increased P_{O_2}	May result from central nervous system damage or disease that involves the midbrain and upper pons; seen following increased intracranial pressure and blunt head trauma
Apneusis	A prolonged inspiratory cramp (a pause at full inspiration) occurs; a common variant of this is a brief end-inspiratory pause of 2 or 3 seconds, often alternating with an end-expiratory pause	Indicates damage to the respiratory control mechanism located at the pontine level; most commonly associated with pontine infarction, but documented with hypoglycemia, anoxia, and meningitis
Cluster breathing	A cluster of breaths having a disordered sequence with irregular pauses between breaths	Dysfunction in the lower pontine and high medullary areas
Ataxic breathing	Completely irregular breathing with random shallow and deep breaths and irregular pauses; often the rate is slow	Originates from a primary dysfunction of the medullary neurons controlling breathing
Gasping breathing pattern	A pattern of deep "all-or-none" breaths accompanied by a slow respiratory rate	Indicative of a failing medullary respiratory center

From McCance K, Huether S: *Pathophysiology: the biologic basis for disease in adults and children*, St Louis, 1990, Mosby–Year Book.

Oculomotor responses

Eye position and oculomotor responses are controlled by brainstem and higher brain centers. Eye position, eye movements, and oculomotor responses may be used to assess the level of brain function (Figure 45-3).

With cortical dysfunction or disruption of the efferent pathway many changes occur in both spontaneous and reflexive eye movements. Roving eye movements may be present because cortical gaze centers no longer inhibit these brainstem-generated eye movements. With an injury that depresses cortical gaze center function, the eyes and often the entire head will deviate or appear to look toward the side of the injured hemisphere. If the injury stimulates the neurons of the cortical gaze center, the eyes and the entire head will deviate away from the injured hemisphere. **Oculocephalic reflexes** *(doll's eyes)* are no longer inhibited by frontal gaze centers, leaving the patient's gaze fixed straight ahead regardless of head position. This change is called pos-

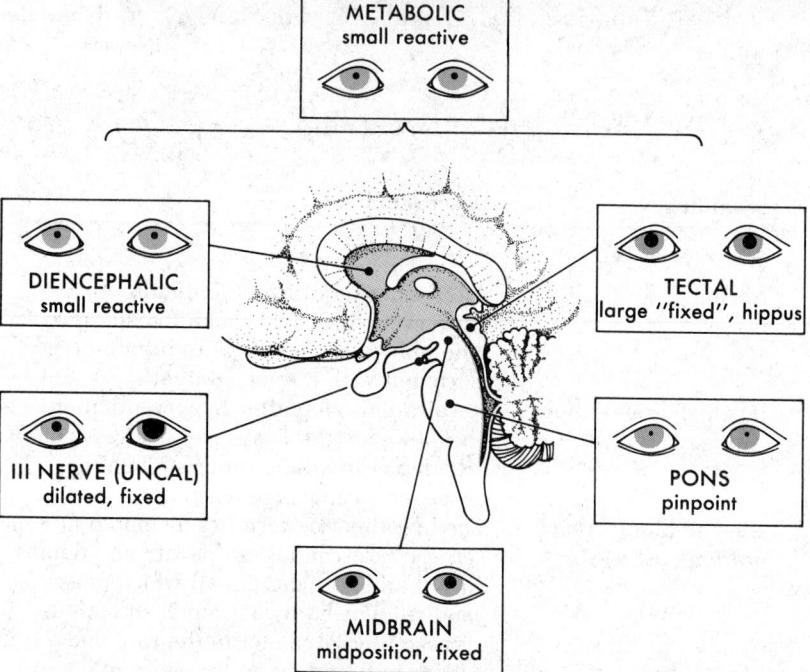

FIGURE 45-2 Pupils at different levels of consciousness.

TABLE 45-2 **Pupillary Changes**

Pupillary change	Location and pathogenesis
Small (under 4 mm in diameter) reactive pupils Regularly shaped	Cerebral dysfunction, especially of metabolic origin Bilateral diencephalon dysfunction caused by sustained increased intracranial pressure
Irregularly shaped	Often found in encephalopathy, multiple sclerosis, and vascular disease including diabetes mellitus
Midposition (4 to 5 mm in diameter or slightly larger, 5 to 6 mm in diameter), round, regular, but light-fixed pupil that spontaneously fluctuates in size	Damage to dorsal tectum or pretectum of the midbrain interrupts the pupillary light pathways, but the accommodation pathways remain intact Hippus, alternating slight constriction and slight dilation of the pupils creating the impression that the pupils are bouncing, may be found
Dilated, fixed pupil	Anoxia Atropine, scopolamine (large concentration)
Midposition (4 to 5 mm in diameter), pupils fixed to light (may be slightly irregular or unequal)	Sympathetic and parasympathetic pathways that control pupil size and response in the midbrain are damaged most commonly by herniation, but may be produced by tumors, hemorrhages, anoxia, and infarcts Drug effect: glutethimide (Doriden), atropine, scopolamine (large concentration)
Dilated, fixed pupil with extraocular paralysis (usually bilateral)	Interruption of the oculomotor (cranial nerve III) tract between the nucleus and its point of exit from the brain
Sluggish-responding pupil that is gradually dilating (unilateral initially)	Temporal lobe herniation compressing the ipsilateral oculomotor nerve against the posterior communicating artery or tentorial notch as it passes through the tentorial notch en route to innervate the eye
Small pinpoint pupils	Dysfunction in the pons interrupts the descending sympathetic pathway Opiate effect In the absence of drugs, this is highly suggestive of a pontine hemorrhage

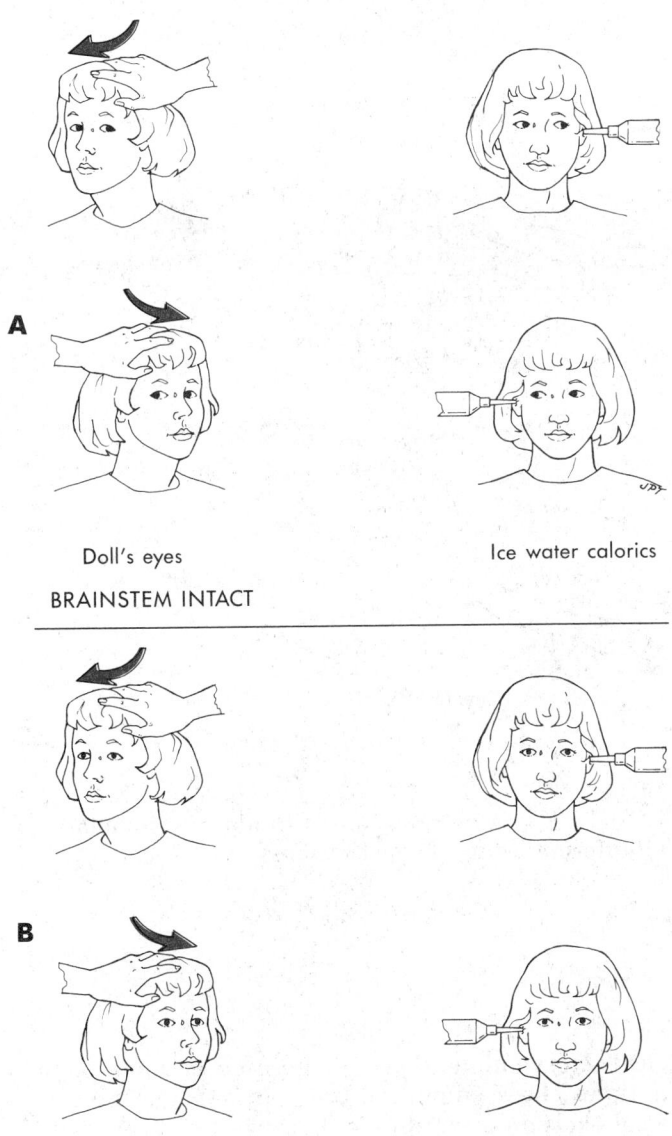

Doll's eyes

Ice water calorics

BRAINSTEM INTACT

Doll's eyes

Ice water calorics

BRAINSTEM NOT INTACT

FIGURE 45-3   Ocular reflexes at different levels of consciousness. **A,** Response when brainstem is intact; eyes move in opposite direction of head movement. Nystagmus is present with ice water calorics. **B,** Response when brainstem is not intact; gaze remains fixed in direction of head movement. Nystagmus is not present with ice water calorics.

itive doll's eyes. Nystagmus is no longer induced by caloric stimulation.

Mesencephalon dysfunction is associated with the loss of roving eye movements. The eyes become immobile and directed ahead. Oculovestibular reflexes become inconsistent and abnormal. Loss of spontaneous blinking occurs with pontine dysfunction.

Motor responses

Motor responses contribute to identifying the level of brain dysfunction and the hemisphere that is maximally damaged. The pattern of response is described as (1) appropriate, that is, purposeful—a defensive or withdrawal movement to noxious stimuli; (2) inappropriate (nonpurposeful)—generalized motor movement, grimacing, or groaning; or (3) not present (no motor response) (Figure 45-4).

Decortication, or decorticate rigidity, is an abnormal motor response that occurs with an injury that involves primarily cortical damage with less severe hemispheric dysfunction. The patient slowly develops flexion of the arm, wrist, and fingers with adduction in the upper extremity. The lower-extremity motor response is characterized by extension, internal hip rotation, and plantar flexion.

Decerebration, extensor response in the upper and lower extremities, is associated with severe hemispheric damage. The patient develops decerebrate rigidity with hyperextension of the spine and clenching of the teeth. Extension, adduction, and hyperpronation occur in the upper extremities. The lower extremities are held in extension. In acute brain injury, shivering and hyperpnea may be present.

The patient with pontine level dysfunction has tensor responses in the upper extremities accompanied by flexion in the lower extremities. A flaccid state with little or no motor response to stimuli is characteristic of damage to the lower pons and upper mesencephalon.

Therapeutic Management

Emergency management

Oxygenation and circulation must be maintained. Oxygen is given to maintain a Po_2 at greater than 100 mm Hg. Circulation is supported with intravenous fluid volume expansion, infusion of vasoactive agents, and dysrhythmia control. The person is usually treated for hypoglycemia by administering 50 mL of $D_{50}W$ intravenously. Wernicke encephalopathy is treated by administering 50 to 100 mg of thiamine intravenously as soon as blood studies are drawn. Seizure activity is treated usually with 5 to 10 mg of diazepam (Valium) or 2 to 4 mg of lorazepam (Ativan) intravenously, then administration of 500 mg to 1 g of phenytoin (Dilantin) intravenously but slowly (less than 50 mg per minute). If the intracranial pressure is high, hyperventilation and osmotic diuresis with mannitol may be used. If there is systemic infection, treatment with a broad spectrum antibiotic is initiated as soon as blood cultures are drawn. If an acid-base imbalance occurs the imbalance is treated with drugs such as bicarbonate or acetazolamide (Diamox) or control of ven-

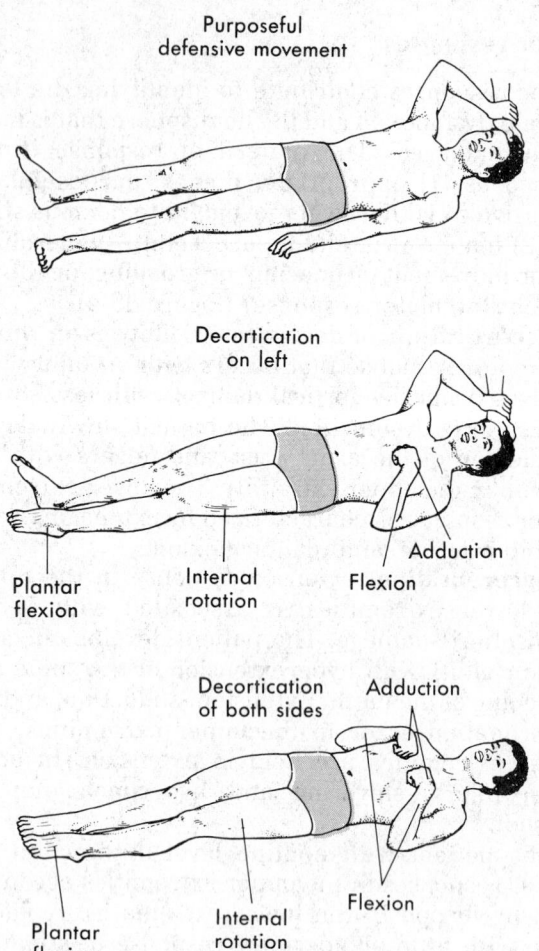

Purposeful defensive movement

Decortication on left

Plantar flexion Internal rotation Flexion Adduction

Decortication of both sides Adduction

Plantar flexion Internal rotation Flexion

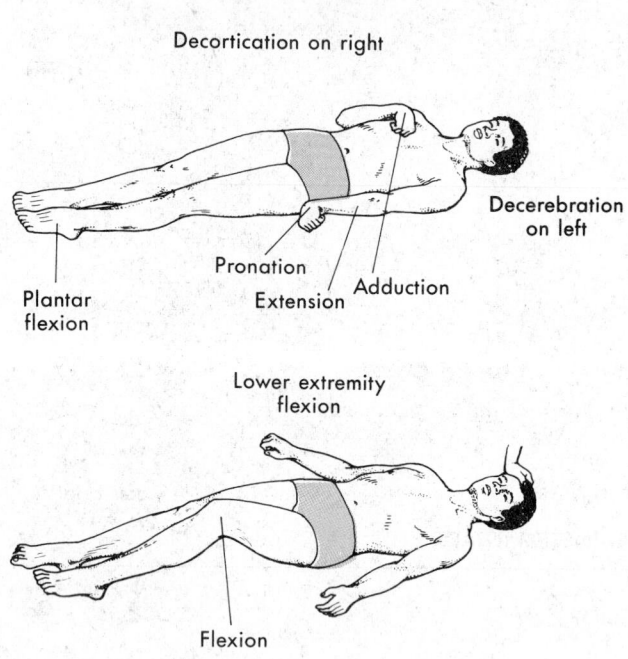

Decortication on right

Decerebration on left

Plantar flexion Pronation Extension Adduction

Lower extremity flexion

Flexion

FIGURE 45-4 Motor responses to noxious stimulation at different levels of consciousness.

tilation. When drug overdose is suspected, antidotes such as naloxone may be administered to reverse certain effects of some sedative drugs with anticholinergic properties. Agitation is treated with environmental control. A minor or major tranquilizer may be used, occasionally haloperidol (Haldol) in very low doses. In patients who have lost corneal reflexes and closure of the eyes, measures to protect the eyes are taken using ophthalmic ointment and closing the eyelid by taping or using a corneal bandage.

Surgical management

Altered consciousness states caused by epidural and subdural hematomas may require immediate surgical evacuation. Other masses (hemorrhage, primary or metastatic tumors, cerebral abscess, or infarcts) may be initially managed nonsurgically by treating the increased intracranial pressure. Surgical decompression or partial or total resection of primary brain tumors, radiation therapy, chemotherapy for some primary and secondary brain tumors, and surgical clipping of cerebral aneurysms are other sur-

gical interventions that may be used at some point in time. The treatment of brain abscess may be surgical excision or antibiotic therapy.

In altered consciousness states caused by infratentorial lesions, large hematomas of the cerebellum or in the subdural space, and cerebellar infarcts are surgically evacuated (decompressed) and infarcted tissues are resected. Intraparenchymal lesions of the brainstem do not usually respond to surgery. Conservative medical management is used to control intracranial pressure.

Metabolic encephalopathies such as drug overdose, hypoglycemia, metabolic acidosis, hyperosmolar states, hypoxia, bacterial meningitis or endocarditis, and severe electrolyte imbalance are treated with appropriate therapy.

NURSING MANAGEMENT OF THE PATIENT WITH AN ALTERED LEVEL OF CONSCIOUSNESS
Assessment

The nurse collects information from the patient, if possible, and also from the family and relevant others about the patient's mentation and awakeness. The nurse asks how the symptoms developed over time. This may be difficult since the patient or family may not remember small changes in the patient or activities of daily living. Changes in work habits, daily routines, decision-making ability, lack of initiative, distractibility, and mood should be noted too. The nurse also asks about changes in sleep-wakefulness patterns, including lethargy and inability to stay awake.

The mental status examination should include assessment of the patient's attention span, language ability, and general appearance. Assessment of level of consciousness should focus on patterns of breathing, pupillary responses, eye movements, and motor responses. Blood pressure, pulse, and temperature are also taken.

Assess skin integrity in the person with decreased consciousness. Pressure points could already be developing or decubiti may already be present. The cornea are checked for lesions. Corneal ulcerations may be developing because the lids are not fully closed. The bladder is palpated for fullness. Bladder distention may be present. The lungs are auscultated. Aspiration may have occurred and atelectasis may be present.

The nurse reassesses the patient's neurologic status on an ongoing basis. In the critically ill, unstable patient (that is, the patient with increased intracranial pressure), this nursing reevaluation may take place every hour or more frequently. With seriously ill patients and potentially unstable patients, this reassessment may take place every 2 to 4 hours. For the stable patient, reevaluation may take place every 6 to 8 hours in an acute care setting.

Cardiac status may be continuously evaluated or reassessed whenever neurologic status is reevaluated. Pulmonary status is observed including respiratory rate, pattern, and lung sounds, usually as frequently as neurologic status is checked. Less frequent pulmonary reassessment may include blood gases and pulmonary artery pressures if a pulmonary artery catheter is in place. Laboratory data such as electrolytes, BUN, and hematologic studies are monitored by the nurse daily, sometimes more frequently, for critically ill patients.

Skin integrity and corneal integrity are reassessed with each position change and each time eye care is provided. Renal and bladder status may be reassessed hourly in critically ill patients via intake and output measurement. Bladder status is monitored less frequently in stable patients with urinary catheters or external catheters, usually every 4 to 8 hours. Bowel status is monitored daily or more frequently if the patient has diarrhea.

The nurse reassesses the family members with each contact, reevaluating their anxiety levels, coping methods, levels of understanding, and physio-

logic status. Their progression in terms of crisis, grieving, and possibly adapting to chronic illness is also monitored.

Nursing Diagnosis

Nursing diagnoses relevant to coma in addition to the primary nursing diagnosis of altered level of consciousness include:

Ineffective breathing pattern related to deep coma

Ineffective airway clearance related to loss of protective reflexes

Impaired gas exchange related to aspiration, atelectasis

Cardiac output decreased related to brainstem dysfunction

High risk for altered body temperature related to hypothalamic dysfunction

High risk for injury related to decreased consciousness

Impaired physical mobility related to decreased consciousness

Self-care deficit: bathing/hygiene, dressing/grooming, toileting related to decreased consciousness

Altered nutrition: less than body requirements related to decreased intake

Urinary incontinence related to loss of inhibition of voiding reflex

Bowel incontinence related to loss of inhibition of bowel evacuation reflexes; high risk for constipation related to immobility; high risk for diarrhea related to tube feedings

Impaired or at high risk for impaired skin integrity related to immobility and/or inadequate nutrition

Impaired tissue integrity: high risk for corneal ulceration related to loss of blink reflex

Impaired tissue integrity: high risk for oral and nasal mucosa ulceration related to impaired self-care

Sensory/perceptual alteration related to decreased consciousness

Anxiety related to impaired cognitive functions as consciousness decreases into coma or increases out of coma

Planning

Outcome criteria relevant to the patient in coma are:

Sufficient oxygenation as evidenced by normal breath sounds, tidal volume, and Po$_2$

Airways are clear as evidenced by normal breath sounds and blood gases

Normal cardiac output as evidenced by normal heart rate, blood pressure and mean arterial pressure (MAP); palpable peripheral pulses, warm extremities, and adequate urine output

Normal or prescribed body temperature

No injuries or related incidences

Potential for normal mobility maintained as evidenced by proper alignment, full range of joint motion, no contractures, no extremity edema

Self-care needs met as evidenced by clean, dressed patient; mouth, nose, ears clean; clean, groomed hair and nails trimmed and clean

Adequate nutrition maintained as evidenced by normal body weight; positive nitrogen balance; and normal BUN, serum albumin, and serum protein

Hygiene and toileting needs met as evidenced by dry clothing and unsoiled undergarments; dry and unsoiled bedding; intact, clean, dry skin; and normal bowel pattern

Skin healing or remains intact as evidenced by no signs of infection, and wound clean and dry; or no areas of broken skin and no reddened areas

Corneas intact as evidenced by no redness, no watering, no eye pain, and no ulceration

Oral and nasal mucosa intact as evidenced by no ulcerations or lesions, no odors, and nose and mouth clean

Progression to a higher level of responsiveness as evidenced by higher Glasgow coma scale, stabilized and normal blood pressure, normal pulse pressure, normal heart rate, normal sinus rhythm, higher or normal breathing pattern, normal respiratory rate, stabilized and normal temperature, pupils equal and reactive, higher level of oculomotor reflexes, higher-level postures

Patient is calm as evidenced by quiet appearance and comfortable attitude

When brain death has occurred, the nursing goal is to provide as the patient would have wished, to the best of the nurse's knowledge, an atmosphere for a dignified death.

The nursing goals for the family are to promote the use of adaptive coping methods and the mobilization of support systems and to facilitate family/patient interaction.

Implementation

Prevention of secondary brain injury requires the nurse to constantly reevaluate the patient's neurologic status to detect decreases in level of brain function. When a decreasing level of brain function is detected, the nurse initiates treatment measures prescribed by the physician, and notifies the physician.

The nursing care includes measures to maintain or restore the skin, oral mucosa, and corneal integrity. Nursing interventions also focus on pulmonary hygiene; positioning, alignment, and range of motion; a bladder and bowel program; a fluid replacement plan; and a nutritional support plan. The nurse

preserves the patient's dignity by maintaining the patient's privacy, pulling the curtains to prevent exposure during therapeutic and care interventions, dressing the patient and keeping the patient covered; talking to the patient, explaining what is being done even when the patient does not respond; speaking about the patient in a way that conveys he or she is thought of as a person, not a thing; and demonstrating care and concern in voice, touch, and other behaviors.

The nurse shows the family and significant others how to interact with the unconscious patient by role-modeling the behaviors of talking to and touching the patient. The nurse gradually involves the family members in the care of the patient, teaching them to bathe, groom, turn, and carry out range-of-motion exercises and coma stimulation protocols.

Evaluation

The nurse monitors the effectiveness of the therapeutic medical and nursing measures. If the therapeutic goals are being achieved, the measures are maintained. If the goals are not being achieved, the therapeutic measures are manipulated until the goals are being achieved.

Documentation

The nurse carefully documents the initial neurologic assessment and the ongoing neurologic assessment (Figure 45-5). Additionally, cardiac, pulmonary, skin, eye, bladder, and bowel initial and ongoing assessments are documented. All pertinent data related to expected outcomes as given in the care plan are recorded.

Nursing diagnoses, goals, and plans of care are documented. Diagnostic tests and the patient's response to them should be noted in the patient's health care record. The nurse documents therapeutic medical and nursing interventions and the patient's responses to these interventions. Additionally document assessment and presence of any untoward effects of interventions.

The nurse documents the interventions taken in behalf of the family members and documents the teaching done to increase the family members' understanding of the situation and ability to participate in the care. The nurse documents referrals made in the patient's or family members' interest.

Ongoing Care

Rehabilitation

The major concern in coma rehabilitation is increasing the patient's level of responsiveness. A coma stimulation program is the foundation of this reha-

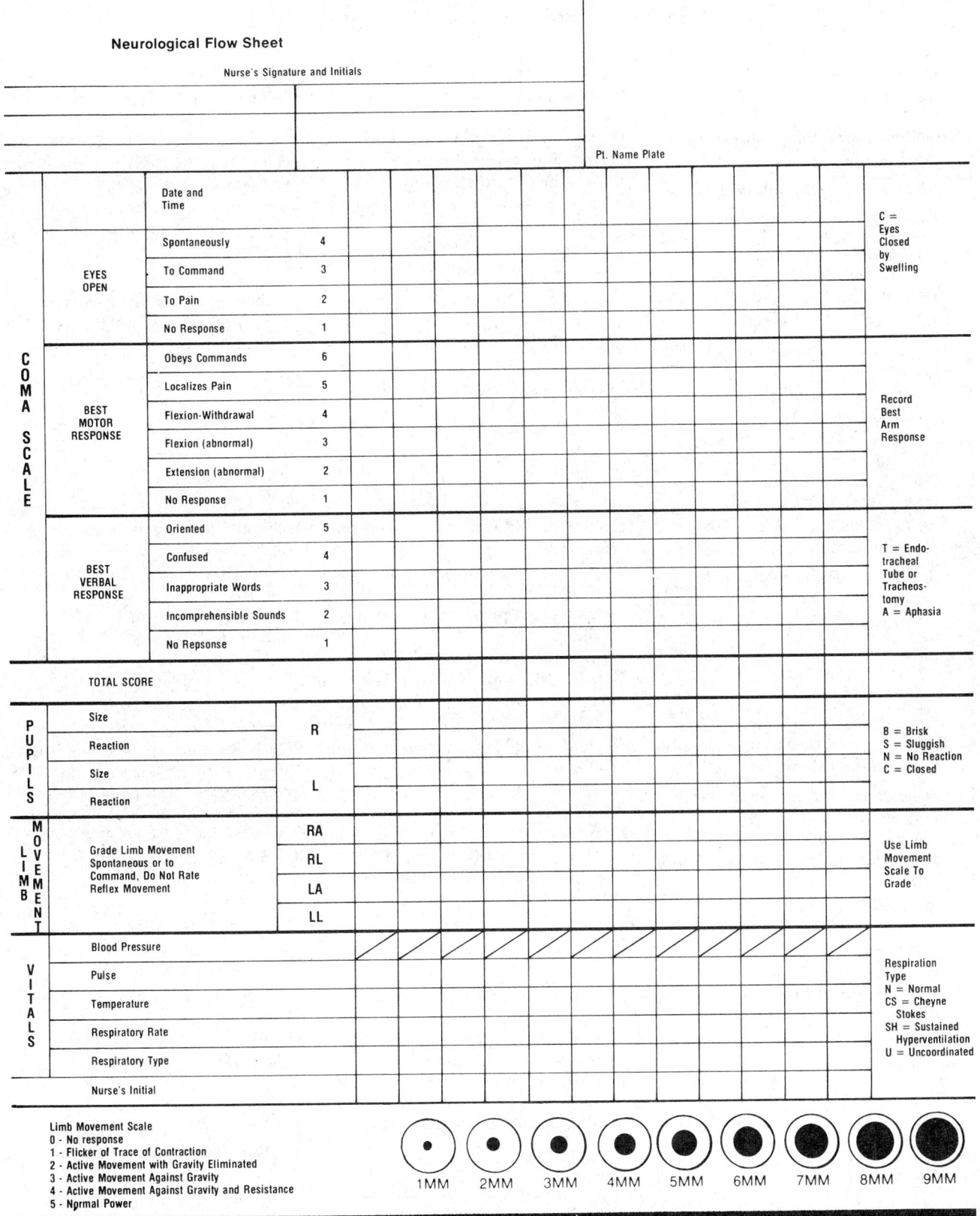

Neurological Flow Sheet

Nurse's Signature and Initials

Pt. Name Plate

COMA SCALE		Date and Time	
	EYES OPEN	Spontaneously	4
		To Command	3
		To Pain	2
		No Response	1
	BEST MOTOR RESPONSE	Obeys Commands	6
		Localizes Pain	5
		Flexion-Withdrawal	4
		Flexion (abnormal)	3
		Extension (abnormal)	2
		No Response	1
	BEST VERBAL RESPONSE	Oriented	5
		Confused	4
		Inappropriate Words	3
		Incomprehensible Sounds	2
		No Repsonse	1
	TOTAL SCORE		

C = Eyes Closed by Swelling

Record Best Arm Response

T = Endotracheal Tube or Tracheostomy
A = Aphasia

PUPILS	Size	R
	Reaction	
	Size	L
	Reaction	

B = Brisk
S = Sluggish
N = No Reaction
C = Closed

LIMB MOVEMENT	Grade Limb Movement Spontaneous or to Command, Do Not Rate Reflex Movement	RA
		RL
		LA
		LL

Use Limb Movement Scale To Grade

VITALS	Blood Pressure
	Pulse
	Temperature
	Respiratory Rate
	Respiratory Type
Nurse's Initial	

Respiration Type
N = Normal
CS = Cheyne Stokes
SH = Sustained Hyperventilation
U = Uncoordinated

Limb Movement Scale
0 - No response
1 - Flicker of Trace of Contraction
2 - Active Movement with Gravity Eliminated
3 - Active Movement Against Gravity
4 - Active Movement Against Gravity and Resistance
5 - Normal Power

1MM   2MM   3MM   4MM   5MM   6MM   7MM   8MM   9MM

FIGURE 45-5   Neurologic flow sheet. (From St. Francis Medical Center, LaCrosse, Wis.)

NURSING CARE PLAN   *Patient in Coma*

Nursing diagnosis/ Expected outcome	Interventions	Rationale
Ineffective breathing pattern related to deep coma • *Sufficient oxygenation as evidenced by:* *Normal breath sounds* *tidal volume > 500 mL* *Po$_2$ 80-100 mm Hg*	Document and report changes in breathing pattern. Elevate head of bed. Position patient to allow maximum ventilation. (Also see measures to decrease increased intracranial pressure.)	Breathing pattern changes are associated with increased intracranial pressure. Interventions are directed at controlling increased intracranial pressure.
Ineffective airway clearance related to loss of protective reflexes • *Airways are clear as evidenced by:* *normal breath sounds* *blood gases normal:* *Po$_2$ 80-100 mm Hg* *Pco$_2$ 35-45 mm Hg* *pH 7.35-7.45* *Hco$_2$ 22 mEq-26 mEq* *O$_2$ sat 94%-100%*	Hold patient NPO and provide mouth care q4h. Suction PRN, no more than 15 seconds. Provide tracheostomy care q4h, if present.	Swallowing and cough reflexes are often impaired with decreased consciousness.
Impaired gas exchange related to aspiration, atelectasis • *Sufficient oxygenation as evidenced by normal or prescribed blood gases (see normal values above)*	Document and report impaired gas exchange. Turn q2h, cough, and deep breathe if possible q2h. Provide chest physiotherapy as prescribed. Provide oxygen as prescribed. Hyperventilate patient with 100% oxygen for 60 sec before and after suctioning and q1-2h.	Ischemia of brain tissues may result in increased pulmonary vasculature resistance causing an ARDS syndrome. Immobility and aspiration further impair gas exchange.
Cardiac output decreased related to brain stem dysfunction • *Normal cardiac output as evidenced by:* *heart rate 80-100/min* *blood pressure 60-90/100-140 mm Hg* *MAP 60-80 mm Hg* *palpable peripheral pulses* *warm extremities* *urine output > 30-50 mL/hr*	Document and report rate, rhythm, ECG, pressure, and cardiac output changes. Administer medications as prescribed. Elevate head of bed if possible. Prevent Valsalva maneuver.	Acute brain injury including brainstem injuries are associated with rate, rhythm, and ECG changes. Blood pressure and cardiac output changes are affected by flat positioning and immobility.
High risk for altered body temperature related to hypothalamic dysfunction • *Normal or prescribed body temperature (98.6° F, 37° C).*	Document and report temperature changes. Keep dry and lightly covered. Sponge with tepid water. Use hypothermia blanket as prescribed.	Acute brain injuries often impair hypothalamic function. Infection may also contribute to temperature changes.
High risk for injury related to decreased consciousness • *No injuries or incidences occurred.*	Position bed in low position with siderails up. Pad siderails if patient is agitated. Restrain patient if removing tubes/ equipment or trying to get out of bed.	Safety is a major concern when consciousness is decreased.

Nursing diagnosis/ *Expected outcome*	Interventions	Rationale
Impaired physical mobility related to decreased consciousness • *Potential for normal mobility maintained as evidenced by:* *proper alignment* *full range of motion of joints* *no contractures* *no extremity edema*	Provide passive range of motion q2-4h. Sit up in bed or place in chair tid/qid. Maintain proper body alignment, reposition q2h. Position to prevent dependency edema. Apply splints as prescribed to prevent footdrop, wristdrop, and improper alignment.	With decreased consciousness, normal posture, alignment, and movement are lost and may be replaced with abnormal posturing, alignment, and movement because of central nervous system injury.
Self-care deficit: bathing/hygience, dressing/grooming, toileting related to decreased consciousness • *Self-care needs are met as evidenced by:* *clean, dressed patient; mouth, nose, ears clean; clean, groomed hair; nails trimmed and clean*	Provide bathing, grooming, dressing. Provide mouth care, nose care, and ear care. Wash hair weekly. Cut and file fingernails and toenails.	Ability self-care is lost with decreased consciousness, but basic human needs must still be met.
Altered nutrition: less than body requirements related to decreased consciousness • *Adequate nutrition maintained as evidenced by:* *normal body weight maintained* *positive nitrogen balance* *BUN 8-25 mg/dL* *serum albumin 6%-8%* *serum protein 55% of protein*	Document and report weight changes. Maintain calorie count and hydration. Administer feedings as prescribed.	Normal food and fluid intake requires alertness, yet nutritional need must be met; this is done by alternate means.
Altered patterns of urinary elimination: incontinence related to loss of inhibition of voiding reflex • *Hygiene and toileting needs met as evidenced by:* *dry clothing* *dry bedding* *intact, clean and dry skin*	Record intake and output. Insert catheter using sterile technique and maintain patent closed drainage; prevent kinking of tubing. Secure catheter to patient and to bed. Prevent reflux drainage of urine from collection bag. Provide catheter care q8h. Discontinue Foley catheter as soon as intake and output not needed, use diaper or condom catheter.	An accurate intake and output record is needed to identify complications early; therefore it may be necessary to maintain an indwelling Foley catheter initially; the indwelling catheter should be removed as soon as intake and output precision is not needed; bladder will reflexly empty and risk of infection will be reduced.
Bowel elimination: incontinence related to loss of inhibition of bowel evacuation reflexes; high risk for constipation related to immobility; high risk for diarrhea related to tube feedings • *Hygiene and toileting needs are met as evidenced by:* *unsoiled undergarments* *unsoiled bedding* *clean, unsoiled patient* *normal bowel pattern maintained*	Document and record bowel movements. Initiate bowel program including administration of stool softeners and suppositories. Adjust feeding consistency and volume to control diarrhea; administer antidiarrheal medication as prescribed.	Bowel will reflexly empty with a simple bowel program, and constipation from immobility can be easily avoided with such a program. Diarrhea from tube feedings can be controlled with changes in formula and use of medication.

Continued.

NURSING CARE PLAN *Patient in Coma—cont'd*

Nursing diagnosis/ Expected outcome	Interventions	Rationale
Impaired or at high risk for impaired skin integrity related to immobility and/or inadequate nutrition •*Skin healing or remains intact as evidenced by:* *no signs of infection* *wounds clean and dry* *or* *no areas of broken skin* *no reddened areas*	Position to keep patient off injured tissues. Massage pressure points. Provide wound care as prescribed. Place on an alternating pressure or special mattress. <div align="center">or</div>Provide skin care q2-4h. Turn and reposition q2h; keep heels off bed. Provide clean, dry, wrinkle-free sheets. Prevent dependency edema and venous stasis. Moisturize dry skin with lotion, use emollient.	The described nursing interventions promote healing of damaged skin. Skin is not made to continuously bear weight. These measures promote maintaining the health of skin, making it more resistant to injury and minimizing weight-bearing time.
Impaired tissue integrity: high risk for corneal ulceration related to loss of blink reflex •*Corneas intact as evidenced by:* *no redness* *no watering* *no eye pain evidenced by rubbing eyes* *no ulceration*	Cleanse eyes with normal saline at least q8h, instill methylcellulose eye drops q4h. Use protective eye shields if eyes remain open.	These measures promote health of cornea and prevent injury.
Impaired tissue integrity: high risk for oral and nasal mucosa ulceration related to impaired self-care •*Oral and nasal mucosa intact as evidenced by:* *no ulcerations or lesions* *no odors* *nose clean* *mouth clean*	Cleanse nose with normal saline at least qd. With endotracheal tube or NG tube in place, remove tape and clean skin qd, reapply tape on other skin. Moisturize lips with ointment.	These measures promote health of oral and nasal mucosa.
Sensory/perceptual alteration related to decreased consciousness •*No injuries or incidences occurred.* •*Progression to a higher level of responsiveness as evidenced by:* *higher Glasgow Coma Scale score* *stabilized and normal blood pressure (60-90/100-140 mm Hg)* *normal pulse pressure* *normal heart rate (60-100/min)* *normal sinus rhythm* *higher breathing pattern (ataxic → apneusis → central neurogenic hyperventilation → Cheynes-Stokes → posthyperventilation apnea)*	Provide stimulation and interaction, talk to and touch patient. Encourage family to talk to and touch patient. Provide visual, auditory, and tactile stimuli; institute a coma stimulation program.	The degree of perception of stimuli is unclear, but stimulation is essential to maintain CNS integrity and function; these measures are designed to provide such stimulation.

NURSING CARE PLAN   *Patient in Coma—cont'd*

Nursing diagnosis/ Expected outcome	Interventions	Rationale
normal respiratory rate (12-20/ min) normal breathing pattern (eupnea) stabilized and normal temperature pupils equal and reactive higher-level oculomotor reflexes (absent ice water calorics → normal ice water calorics → normal doll's eyes → eyes open to stimuli → eyes open and following commands and stimuli) higher level postures (flaccid, no responses → flexion lower extremities → decerebration → decortication → defensive movements to stimuli → purposeful, intentional movement)		
Anxiety related to impaired cognitive functions as consciousness decreases into coma or increases out of coma • *Patient is calm as evidenced by: quiet appearance comfortable attitude*	Provide as quiet an environment as possible. Talk softly, calmly, caringly; move slowly. Reassure. Tell patient what you are doing. Use gentle, caring touch, stroke, hold hand.	The environment and the injury are stressors eliciting anxiety, perhaps outright fear; the measures are designed to counteract the stressors.

bilitation. The purpose of the coma stimulation program is to increase responsiveness. The rationale is that coma is a state of decreased responsiveness to the environment related to sensory deprivation. Coma rehabilitation is therefore built on a stimulation-oriented program. Intersensory stimulation is used. The coma stimulation plan begins with the most primitive sensory system (tactile) and moves through stimulation of each successively higher system (vestibular, olfactory, gustatory, auditory, and visual) until a failed or inappropriate response is observed. As appropriate responsiveness is restored, the coma stimulation program is extended to the next higher sensory system.

Another concern of rehabilitation is helping the patient attain the best possible state of physical health. This includes preventing deconditioning. In rehabilitation the patient is placed on a skin and eye care regimen that maintains the skin and cornea intact (or returns and maintains the skin and cornea intact). A bowel regimen is established and a bladder program is initiated. If possible, the patient is made free of an indwelling urinary catheter by use of intermittent catheterization, external catheter, or bladder evacuation schedule. If making the patient

catheter free is not possible, a bladder care program is established to minimize the risk of infection. In rehabilitation, nurses are primarily responsible for skin, bladder, and bowel care.

A passive range-of-motion exercise program and positioning regimen are established. Splints and other assistive devices may be employed. If the patient becomes able, an active exercise program is planned and implemented. Pulmonary hygiene is emphasized. If the patient requires ventilatory support or oxygen therapy, a weaning program may be initiated when appropriate. An appropriate nutritional plan must be established, and a safe, efficient method of delivery must be established.

Family members are helped through the stages of grieving and adaptation to chronic illness. Referrals for the necessary support services for the family, both in and outside of the rehabilitation setting, are made.

Long-term care

The patient with a prolonged alteration in consciousness may change over time. Patients in some coma states reestablish the sleep-awake cycle; there are times that the patient is awake with eyes open but with no apparent ability to interact meaningfully with the environment. The nurse in the long-term care setting prepares the staff and family for this possible change. The care plan is modified, especially in terms of the coma stimulation program. The program is implemented during periods of wakefulness.

The nurse in the long-term care setting may be principally responsible for preparing the family to take the patient home. Family coping patterns are assessed. The family members are taught all aspects of nursing care and allowed to practice the care elements before the patient's discharge from the long-term care setting. The nurse may need to make social services and nursing referrals to help the family members obtain the resources and assistance needed to take the patient home. The family members are also taught to recognize early signs and symptoms of secondary problems such as a beginning decubitus or the development of diarrhea or constipation, how to modify the care to treat these problems, and how to identify problems that require contacting the physician or rehospitalization.

Home care

The nurse in the home setting prepares the family members for possible changes in level of awakeness and establishment of a sleep-awake cycle. The family members are taught how to alter the coma stimulation program if this occurs. They are also helped with altering their responses to the patient with this change in level of consciousness. Caregiver fatigue is a major concern for the nurse in the home care setting. The nurse often works to prevent or treat this phenomenon by encouraging the primary caregiver to remain attentive to his or her own physical, psychologic, and social health.

INCREASED INTRACRANIAL PRESSURE
Definition

Increased intracranial pressure (ICP) is defined as intracranial pressure greater than 15 mm Hg or 180 cm H_2O. When a patient's compensatory mechanisms fail this is referred to as intracranial hypertension and represents a potentially life-threatening situation. Intracranial hypertension is defined as a sustained intracranial pressure of 15 mm Hg or greater.

Etiology/Epidemiology

Intracranial hypertension may result from (1) an increase in intracranial content as occurs in tumor growth, abscess development, hematoma, hemorrhage, or edema; (2) an increased cerebral blood volume such as occurs in hypercapnea, hypoxemia, vasodilation, obstruction of venous outflow, and increased intrathoracic pressure; or (3) increased cerebrospinal fluid volume from positioning, increased formation, decreased reabsorption, or hydrocephalus.

Pathophysiology

The Monro-Kellie hypothesis states that the cranial vault is filled with brain tissue, blood, and cerebrospinal fluid. Intracranial pressure rises with any further increase in any one of these.

Cerebral Edema and Brain Swelling

Cerebral edema is an increase in the fluid content of brain tissue. After brain insult from trauma, infection, tumor, hemorrhage, ischemia, infarct, or hypoxia, cerebral edema occurs. There is an increase in extracellular or intracellular tissue volume of the brain. Four types of cerebral edema—vasogenic, cytotoxic, ischemic, and interstitial—are described in Table 45-3. Brain swelling is an increase in cerebral blood volume. Brain swelling is a major mechanism operating early in acute brain injury.

Herniation syndrome

When increased intracranial pressure is greater in one compartment of the cranial vault and not evenly distributed throughout the other vault compartments, a **herniation syndrome** occurs. In the last stage of intracranial hypertension, brain tissue shifts (herniates) from the compartment of greater pressure to a compartment of lesser pressure. With this shift in brain tissue the herniating brain tissue's blood supply is compromised, causing further ischemia and hypoxia in the herniating tissues. The herniated brain tissues exert pressure on the brain tissue in the compartment, impairing that tissue's blood supply. Small hemorrhages often develop in the involved brain tissue. Obstructive hydrocephalus may develop. The herniation process markedly and rapidly increases intracranial pressure. Mean systolic arterial pressure soon equals intracranial pressure, and cerebral blood flow ceases at this point.

Herniation syndromes are classified into two categories—supratentorial and infratentorial herniation syndromes—based on whether the herniating tissue is above or below the tentorium. Supratentorial herniation syndromes are further classified into three types—uncal (temporal lobe, lateral transtentorial) herniation, central (transtentorial) herniation, and cingulate gyrus herniation—based on what brain tissue is herniating (Figure 45-6).

TABLE 45-3   Classification of Brain Edemas

Variable	Vasogenic	Cellular (cytotoxic)	Interstitial (hydrostatic)	Ischemic
Pathogenesis	Break in blood-brain barrier (BBB) with increased capillary permeability	Disturbance of cellular metabolism with cellular swelling	Increased CSF or BP; increased hydrostatic pressure forces fluid into ISF	Initially cellular swelling, then secondary increased capillary permeability
Location of edema	Chiefly white matter	Gray and white matter	Interstitial (perivascular and periventricular white)	Gray and white
Composition of edema fluid	Water, sodium, and plasma proteins	Water and sodium	Water and sodium	Water, sodium, then plasma protein
BBB	Disrupted	Intact (initially)	Intact	Initially intact, then disrupted
ECF volume	Increased	Decreased	Increased	Decreased, then increased
Treatment:				
Steroids	Beneficial in tumors and abscesses	Ineffective	Uncertain effectiveness	Equivocal
Osmotherapy	Reduces brain volume acutely in normal brain only	Reduces brain volume acutely in hypoosmolality	Rarely useful	?
Acetazolamide	Dubious	Dubious	Minor usefulness	Dubious
Hyperventilation	Useful	Useful	Useful	Useful
Clinical disorders	Tumors, abscesses, infarcts, trauma, hemorrhage, infarction, lead encephalopathy, ischemia	Hypoxia, hypoosmolality, disequilibrium syndrome, Reye's syndrome, ischemia, purulent meningitis	Obstructive hydrocephalus, pseudotumor cerebri (?), purulent meningitis, acute brain swelling	Infarction

From *The New England Journal of Medicine.* In Fishman, RA: *Brain edema,* 273:706, 1975.

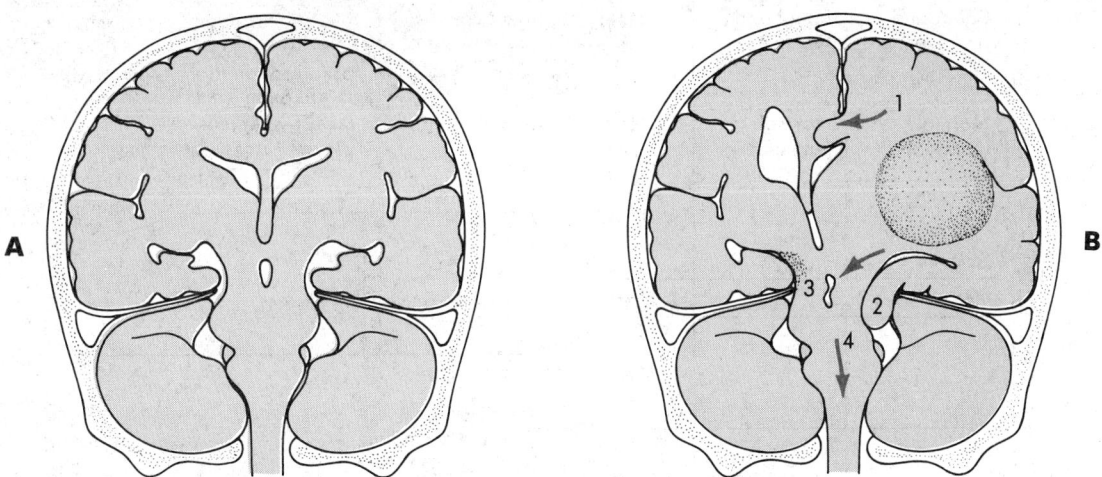

FIGURE 45-6   Herniation syndromes depicted. Intracranial shifts from supratentorial lesions. **A,** Normal location of structures. **B,** Various herniation syndromes are demonstrated. *1,* Cingulate gyrus is herniating under falx cerebri. *2,* Temporal lobe is herniating downward through tentorial notch. *3.* Compression of contralateral cerebral peduncle is seen. *4.* Downward displacement of brainstem through tentorial notch is a central herniation syndrome.

Clinical Manifestations

Clinical manifestations in early intracranial hypertension are subtle (Figure 45-7) and may often be transient, lasting for only a few minutes in some cases. These early clinical manifestations include episodes of confusion, drowsiness, and slight pupillary and breathing changes (stage 2). Clinical manifestations of later intracranial hypertension include decreasing levels of consciousness, a widened pulse pressure, and bradycardia in stage 3. Cheyne-Stokes respiratory pattern or a central neurogenic hyperventilation respiratory pattern, and sluggish and dilating pupils appear in stage 4.

Therapeutic Management

Intracranial pressure monitoring is used to detect changes in intracranial pressure. Intracranial devices that provide a measurement of the intracranial pressure may be placed in a ventricle, in the subarachnoid or subdural spaces, extradurally, or intraparenchymally. Changes in intracranial pressure are transmitted to a transducer, where they are converted from a mechanical impulse to an electrical impulse. This electrical impulse is then displayed on an oscilloscope, graph paper, or both.

Intracranial pressure monitoring can be done via numerous monitoring modes—an intraventricular catheter; a subarachnoid bolt, screw, or subdural cup catheter; an epidural fiberoptic, pneumatic, or telemetric probe; or a brain-tissue pressure monitor (Figure 45-8). Noninvasive techniques for ICP monitoring using evoked potentials are currently being explored.

Techniques used to reduce intracranial pressure include hyperventilation to produce vasoconstriction, thus decreasing cerebral blood volume, and administration of hyperosmolar agents to decrease the water content of the brain. Mannitol in a 20% solution at 1.5 to 2 g/kg may be used when the blood-brain barrier is intact to reduce water content of the brain.

Furosemide (Lasix), 40 to 120 mg IV, or acetazolamide (Diamox) works selectively on injured brain cells to reduce edema.

Corticosteroids (steroids) are given intravenously every 6 hours in cases of brain tumor and certain other extracerebral mass lesions to decrease the cerebral edema. Some authorities advocate barbitu-

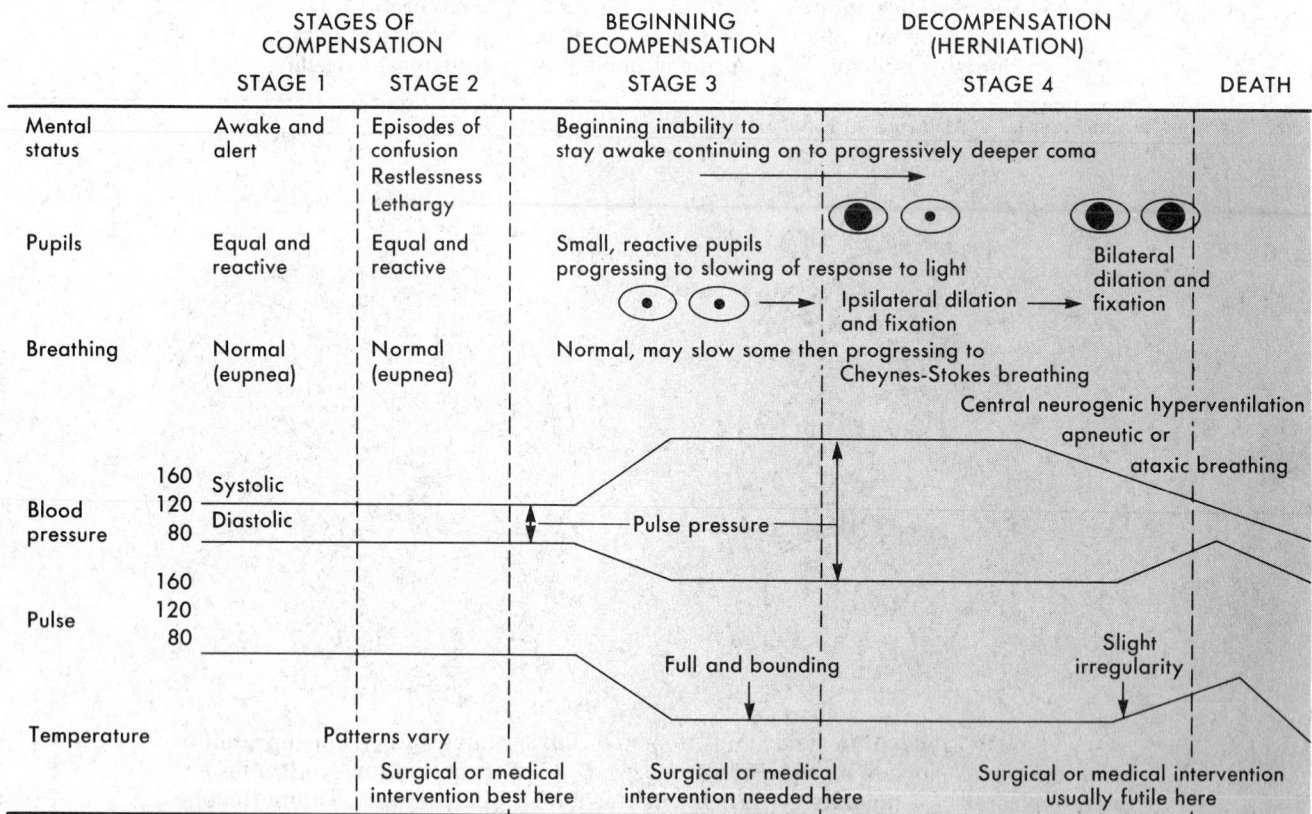

FIGURE 45-7   Clinical correlates of compensated and uncompensated phases of intracranial hypertension.

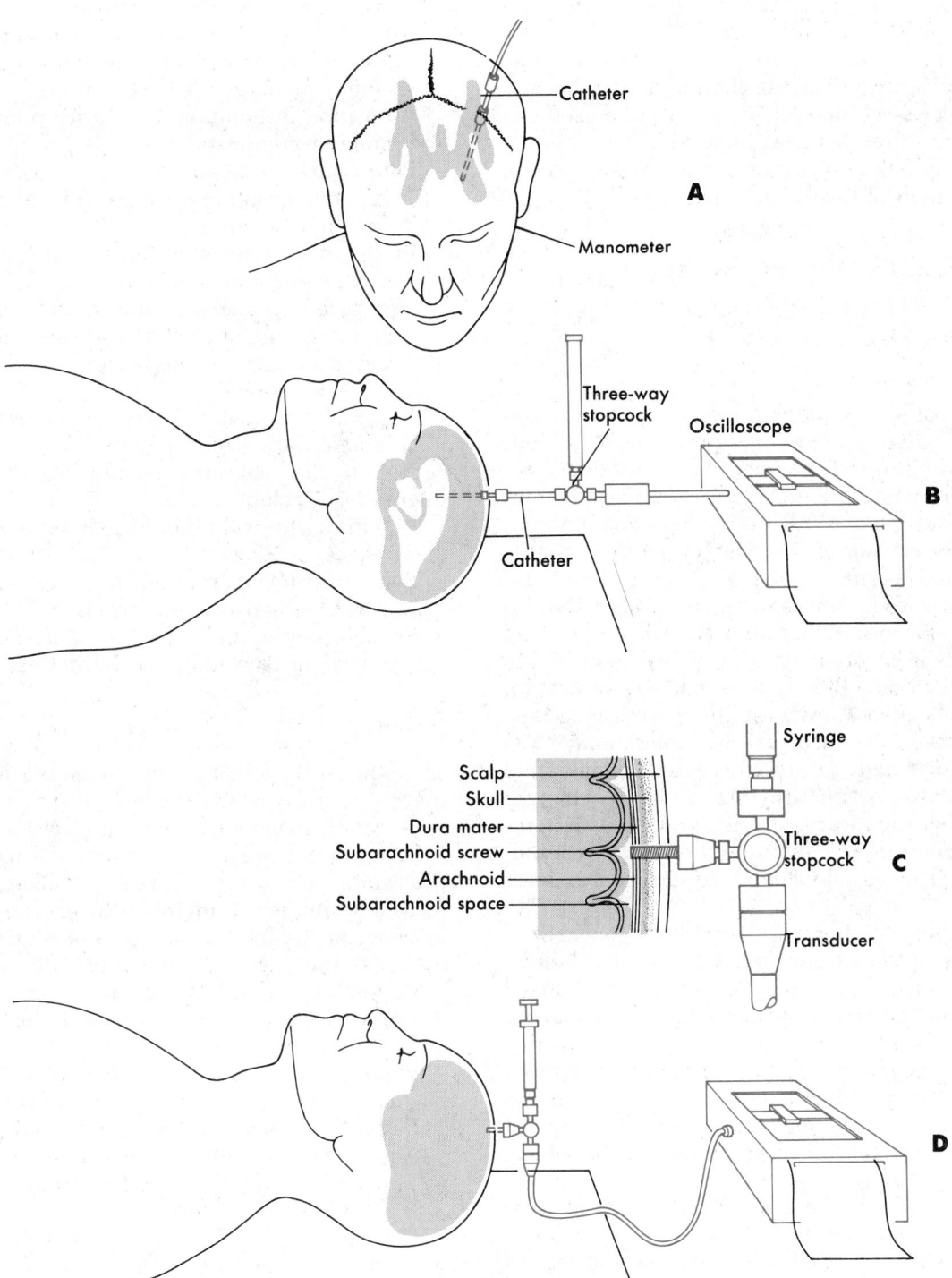

FIGURE 45-8   Increased pressure monitoring. **A,** Overhead view of catheter placement. **B,** Side view of catheter placement. **C,** Subarachnoid or hollow screw. **D,** Monitor connected.

rate anesthesia to decrease metabolic rate in treating severe intracranial hypertension. Thiopental (up to 30 mg/kg by titrated IV infusion) or pentobarbital (3 to 5 mg/kg IV initially, followed by IV infusion to keep a blood level of 2.5 to 3.5 mg/dL) may be administered to accomplish this. Neuromuscular blockade to control decerebration and hypothermia to reduce cerebral blood flow may also be used.

Ventricular drainage may be used. Surgical interventions may be pursued to provide decompression or debridement of necrotic tissues.

NURSING MANAGEMENT OF THE PATIENT WITH INCREASED INTRACRANIAL PRESSURE

Assessment

With the conscious patient, behavior, affect and mood, immediate memory, recent memory (including orientation to self, person, place, and time), remote memory, ability to abstract, and judgment should be assessed. With the unconscious patient, level of consciousness, respiratory pattern, pupils and eye movements, motor responses, and vital signs are assessed. Ventilatory status is assessed. Increasing hypoventilation, cyanosis, tachycardia, and restlessness are noted. Physical assessment of the lungs is indicated. Blood gases and O_2 saturation should be checked. Cardiac status is assessed. Many brain injuries produce dysrhythmias and ECG changes unrelated to the increased intracranial pressure. Pulse, cardiac rhythm, and ECG changes are assessed. Blood pressure is assessed as is temperature. Fluid intake and output are closely monitored. Electrolytes and fluids are checked at least daily.

In compiling the health history, both generalized and focal symptoms associated with increased intracranial pressure are noted by the nurse. Generalized symptoms of increased intracranial pressure are a generalized headache, often worse in the morning on rising, unexplained projectile vomiting without nausea, lethargy, mental dullness, or drowsiness. Focal symptoms that may arise from the cerebral edema are weakness, sensory impairment (visual, auditory, or tactile), and apraxia or clumsiness.

Physical findings suggestive of increased intracranial pressure that the nurse notes are the generalized finding of decreased consciousness and the focal findings of paresis or paralysis of the face, arm, or leg, sensory (tactile, visual, or auditory) impairment, and ataxia. Changing respiratory patterns, pupillary changes, increasing systolic blood pressure (widening pulse pressure), and bradycardia are late (stage 3 and stage 4) signs of intracranial hypertension where compensation has failed and herniation is impending or taking place.

Nursing Diagnosis

Nursing diagnoses include:
  Altered cerebral tissue perfusion
  Altered level of cognitive function or decreased level of responsiveness related to ischemia or compression
  Alteration in emotional integrity related to ischemia or compression
  Pain related to headache
  Ineffective breathing pattern related to compression and ischemia
  Ineffective airway clearance related to impaired swallowing and cough reflexes
  Decreased cardiac output related to compression and ischemia of cardiac and vasomotor centers (or secondary to compensatory mechanisms in the early stages)
  High risk for injury related to decreased cognitive function or seizure activity
Nursing diagnoses specifically related to cerebral edema may include:
  Impaired physical mobility related to paresis, paralysis, or ataxia
  Self-care deficit related to paresis, paralysis, ataxia, or sensory impairments
  Sensory/perceptual alterations related to impaired visual, tactile, or auditory sensation

Planning

The goal of nursing care when increased intracranial pressure exists is to promote the reduction of cerebral edema and increased intracranial pressure. When it is not possible to reduce the increased intracranial pressure, the nursing goal is to prevent further secondary brain injury by preventing further increase of the intracranial pressure during performance of nursing care. Outcome criteria are:
  Patient experiences no sustained rises in intracranial pressure during interventions, monitoring activities, or care activities
  Patient maintains current level of brain function or progresses to higher levels of brain function
  Patient eventually will have a normal intracranial pressure as evidenced by pressure reading or absence of clinical manifestations of increased intracranial pressure
Other nursing goals for the patient with increased intracranial pressure include:
To reduce headache
To prevent seizure activity and injuries including those from deconditioning (hazards of immobility)
To maintain vital functions for the patient when they are unable to do so
Outcome criteria for these goals are:
Patient reports the head pain is under control or

patient is quiet, not reaching for and rubbing head or pulling at head dressings

Patient is free from seizure

Patient is free from injury

Patient's vital functions (blood pressure, pulse, and respiration) are within normal limits

Implementation

To promote venous drainage from the cranial vault, the head of the bed is elevated to 30 degrees or higher during acute ICP elevations. The nurse determines that nothing is snug around the patient's neck (e.g., clothing, oxygen tubing, endotracheal tube tape, or dressing) to impede venous drainage into the jugular veins. The neck is also maintained in a neutral position. All neck flexion, extension, and rotation when turning is avoided as is extreme hip flexion (greater than 90 degrees) to prevent impeding of venous drainage from the cranial vault. The patient is log rolled. The conscious patient is taught how to maintain the head in a neutral position and how to avoid extreme hip flexion.

To promote the reduction of the cerebral edema and thus the intracranial pressure, the nurse administers corticosteroids such as dexamethasone (Decadron) and osmotic diuretics such as mannitol (Osmitrol) as ordered. To maintain the desired decreased vascular volume, the nurse monitors fluid input, establishes a fluid plan, and carefully regulates IVs to the prescribed amount. Body weight may be measured daily. If the patient is conscious, the patient and family should be taught about the fluid restriction, the fluid plan, and how to monitor the IVs.

The nurse helps the patient avoid activities that raise intracranial pressure. Any activity that causes the patient to perform a Valsalva maneuver, such as lifting, straining to void or to evacuate the bowel, coughing, sneezing, gagging, or blowing the nose, increases intracranial pressure. The nurse is careful with postural drainage and suctioning. Suctioning is done only when needed, not on a routine basis. The patient is hyperoxygenated with 100% oxygen for 1 minute before suctioning, between suctions, and following suctioning. Suctioning is done rapidly, never more than 15 seconds per catheter insertion. The number of catheter insertions should be kept to a minimum. All nursing interventions are spaced out over as long a time as possible to provide periods of no procedural contact so that the intracranial pressure has a chance to return to baseline. Even during the night hours activities are spaced rather than compressed to allow a period for uninterrupted sleep. Control of the pressure is more important than the undisturbed sleep period. REM sleep has been shown to increase intracranial pressure. Therefore avoid other activities that may increase intracranial pressure during REM sleep. Do not awaken the patient, since this may further elevate intracranial pressure.

Noxious stimuli such as pain, loud noises, or a plugged urinary catheter with resulting spasms increase intracranial pressure and should be minimized.

Dim lights. Limit painful procedures. Avoid tension on any tapes. Avoid unnecessary neurologic testing using noxious stimuli. Allow no isometric activity including posturing or pushing against a footboard. Minimize activities that stimulate posturing since these, as well as shivering, are isometric activities. Only essential activities are done. Routine bed baths, linen changes, and similar procedures are not done until the intracranial pressure is reduced or stabilized. Regulate tube feedings to avoid high gastric residuals.

The conscious patient is taught to either breathe out during activities that can possibly elicit a Valsalva maneuver or to avoid that particular activity. The nurse institutes a regimen of stool softeners and fiber in the patient's diet to prevent constipation. Enemas are avoided because they produce cramping and the tendency to perform the Valsalva maneuver. The patient is moved in bed by the nurse. The nurse should not ask the patient to help or to pull up in bed unless the patient has been taught to breathe out while doing so. Isometric, active, and active-resistance exercises are avoided since again patients may use the Valsalva maneuver when performing them. Only range-of-motion exercises are instituted until the intracranial pressure is under control. Deep breathing, coughing, and postural drainage are done carefully. Vigorousness and time length are reduced. Postural drainage positioning is modified to avoid placing the head in a downward or flat position.

Fear and anxiety cause the intracranial pressure to rise. Nursing activities must be directed at reducing fear and alleviating anxiety by keeping the patient comfortable and informed, allowing time for the patient to express feelings, and creating a caring environment. Emotionally charged conversation at the bedside is not permitted since this has been documented to increase intracranial pressure.

Nursing interventions to reduce the increased intracranial pressure include providing a caring touch by the nurse and family members; soft, gentle, calm verbal conversation from the nurse and family members; therapeutic touching if the nurse has been so trained; and soft, relaxing music, and gentle massage.

Brain hypoxia and hypercapnia need to be prevented or minimized. The nurse maintains a patent airway, administers oxygen as ordered, and takes measures to improve ventilation. The unconscious patient is positioned so that the lungs may maximally expand, that is, positioned on the back or slightly to one side with the arms supported off the chest wall so they are not pressing against the patient. The patient is turned frequently. Postural drainage with mild cupping and clapping may be carried out as ordered, but the patient is not positioned with the head dependent in order not to increase intracranial pressure. Ventilatory support is often required. The patient using a ventilator should be sighed or an Ambu-bag should be used a few minutes every hour to ensure full expansion of the lungs while receiving ventilatory support. A PO_2 greater than 85 mm Hg is desired.

The nurse administers antidysrhythmic drugs as ordered or as established by critical care area protocols. The nurse administers appropriate antihypertensive or hypertensive medications as ordered.

Because fever increases the brain cells' requirements for oxygen and glucose and demands increased blood be delivered into the cranial vault, temperature elevations are treated promptly and aggressively. The nurse administers antipyretic medications as ordered. A cool environment is created, and the patient is covered with only a light sheet or blanket. In case of very high fever the patient is covered with only enough clothing to preserve modesty and dignity. If the fever is resistant to the above measures, a cooling system such as alcohol rubs, brisk tepid water sponging, ice packs, or a hypothermia blanket is instituted. The nurse guards against shivering, since this would likely increase intracranial pressure.

Preventing seizure activity is extremely important. Seizing markedly elevates intracranial pressure and uses tremendous quantities of oxygen and glucose. The nurse administers the prescribed antiseizure medications. If the patient does experience a seizure, seizure precautions are instituted. The conscious patient and family members are taught about the nature of seizure activity after injury, the signs and symptoms to look for, the medications being given to control seizure activity, and the side effects of the medication.

Careful thought must be given to restraining the patient with increased intracranial pressure. If the patient fights against the restraints, this will increase the intracranial pressure. Having a family member or sitter remain with the patient may be a better choice under the circumstances. Prevention of injury also includes protecting the patient from aspiration if the decrease in consciousness is severe enough to put the individual at risk. Aspiration precautions are instituted. The normal position for improved venous drainage will minimize the aspiration potential.

The nurse helps the conscious patient reduce head pain. Positioning, analgesic medications, cold compresses, reduction of environmental stimuli, and comfort measures such as massage and relaxation are provided. With the unconscious patient who is restless and pulling at the head region, ice and massage may help to reduce the pain.

When an intracranial pressure monitoring device is present, the nurse must consider risk factors, minimize the number of risk factors that are present, and maintain strict aseptic technique. Risk factors associated with ICP monitor-related infections are (1) diagnosis of intracranial hemorrhage with intraventricular hemorrhage, open head trauma, neurosurgical procedures, intracranial hypertension (ICP >20 mm Hg) and older age; (2) physical environment and insertion techniques that include burr hole larger than necessary, placement of device without aseptic technique and devices that penetrate the meninges; and (3) maintenance and care of monitor that includes length of monitoring more than 3 to 5 days, irrigation of ICP monitoring system and open system.

With a ventricular drainage system in place, the nurse maintains the drainage setup at the prescribed level above the insertion point, and maintains the bed in the prescribed position as well as maintaining strict aseptic techniques.

Evaluation

Evaluation of the patient with intracranial hypertension is one of the most critically important aspects of nursing care for such a patient. The patient's neurologic, pulmonary, and cardiac status are continuously reassessed in the critically ill patient.

Blood pressure is continuously monitored when unstable or when vasopressor agents are being given. Pulse oximetry may be used for continuous noninvasive monitoring of oxygen saturation; otherwise blood gases are reassessed at least several times a shift. *Use only stimuli needed and at specified intervals for neurologic assessment.*

Therapeutic interventions are maintained or changed based on this ongoing reevaluation of the interventions' impact on intracranial pressure.

Outcome criteria are:

During interventions, monitoring activities, or care activities, no sustained rises in intracranial pressure as evidenced by

    Normal ICP (<15 mm Hg)
    Absence of A (plateau) waves
    Absence of B waves
    CPP >70 mm Hg
    MAP 60-160 mm Hg
    PO >70 mm Hg

Normal ICP as evidenced by

    ICP 0 to 15 mm Hg (180 mm Hg)
    Awakeness and alertness
    Equal and reactive pupils
    Eupnea
    Blood pressure 60-90/80-120 mm Hg
    Pulse rate 60-100/min

Normothermia (98.6° F, 37° C)
Normal DTR
No headache
No nausea and vomiting
No paresis or paralysis
No sensory impairment
No nuchal rigidity
Stable or progressively higher level of brain function as evidenced by
    Stable or higher score on GCS
    Stable or increasing level of consciousness
Head pain under control as evidenced by
    Patient resting quietly
    Patient not reaching for dressing
    Patient not rubbing head
    Patient not pulling at head dressing
Seizure free as evidenced by
    No abnormal motor activity
    No seizure focus on EEG
    No sustained rise in ICP
Insertion site free of infection as evidenced by
    Normothermia
    Clean line insertion site

Any patient with intracranial hypertension is reevaluated hourly or every 2 hours if not more frequently. Patients with compensated increased intracranial pressure may be assessed every 4 to 8 hours.

In all patients the nurse monitors the therapeutic effectiveness of all medical interventions including the drugs. Additionally, the nurse observes for untoward effects of the medical interventions and for drug side effects. When the patient is receiving corticosteroids, the nurse checks stool, vomitus, and gastric content for blood and monitors hematocrit and hemoglobin. The nurse carefully checks for the slightest indications of infection at puncture sites or IV sites. Urine is observed for signs of infection, and the lungs are auscultated for any signs of congestion. When the patient is receiving osmotic diuretics, the nurse monitors intake and output, urine specific gravity (or urine osmolality), and serum electrolytes.

Documentation

Because of the seriousness of increased intracranial pressure, documentation by the nurse must be frequent and detailed. Document the presence of both generalized manifestations—generalized headache, projectile vomiting without nausea, lethargy, mental dullness, or drowsiness—and focal manifestations—weakness, sensory impairment or ataxia (clumsiness)—of increased intracranial pressure. Document type and duration of the stimulus required to initiate the response. Document respiratory rate, depth, and pattern; cranial nerve alterations; increased, decreased, or absent DTRs; response or movement to stimuli; rate and quality of peripheral pulses, blood pressure, mean arterial pressure and pulse pressure; and body temperature.

Document blood gases and ventilatory status noting hypoventilation, cyanosis, tachycardia, and restlessness. Document cardiac status noting pulse rate, blood pressure, rhythm, and ECG changes. Temperature is recorded. Intake and output, osmolality and/or electrolytes are noted. Body weight is documented. Many hospitals develop neurologic assessment checklists to facilitate this detailed and frequent charting. Many times the checklists have to be supplemented, especially regarding cardiac monitoring.

Nursing diagnoses, goals, and plans of care, including activity schedule and fluid plans, are documented. Diagnostic tests and the patient's response to them should be noted in the patient's health care record. The nurse documents therapeutic medical and nursing interventions and the patient's responses. Document assessment for and presence of untoward effects of medical interventions and drug side effects. Record laboratory and other test results.

Ongoing Care

Increased intracranial pressure is generally viewed as an acute care phenomenon, but recently some patients have been transferred so rapidly from acute care settings to extended care and rehabilitation facilities or to home, that patients with still unresolved brain edema and increased intracranial pressure are now being seen by nurses in ongoing care settings. Edema from trauma, infarction, and hemorrhage may take several weeks to resolve. Patients with brain tumors may also be seen, as they have in the past, by nurses in ongoing care settings.

Rehabilitation

Nurses collect information about the presence of edema and the degree of increased intracranial pressure in patients transferred from acute care settings with recent brain insults (days to 2 or 3 weeks). This may mean looking at the CT scan, checking for papilledema, and contacting the referring physician. The patient with unresolved edema and increased intracranial pressure is placed on more frequent checks of vital signs with neurologic assessments. The nurse institutes the same nursing interventions to control intracranial pressure as were used in the acute care settings and helps the patient and family maintain the control measures they have been using. Care is taken not to implement an increased fluid intake protocol until the brain edema and increased intracranial pressure is resolved. Therapy protocols are adjusted to be less aggressive and demanding until the edema clears. The nurse reassesses the patient's neurologic status during and after each new therapeutic intervention.

Long-term care

In long-term care facilities the nurse may collect information about the presence of cerebral edema and increased intracranial pressure in patients with brain tumors and in patients with recent acute brain insults. If edema or increased intracranial pressure is present, the patient's neurologic status is checked along with vital signs, often more frequently than with the ordinary routine. The nurse continues the nursing interventions implemented in the acute care setting to control intracranial pressure. The patient and family require ongoing education about the medical and nursing care.

Home care

In the home, the nurse is predominantly faced with teaching the patient and family members the knowledge and skills required in the home setting. Teach how to assess the neurologic status of the patient and how to judge the appropriate frequency of these assessments. The family members are taught what findings require notification of the nurse or physician and what measures can be used to control edema and increased intracranial pressure. Patient teaching in regard to medications includes the importance of not discontinuing drug therapy abruptly. The nurse may need to help the family acquire and use equipment such as a turning sheet or commode chair that prevents the patient from eliciting a Valsalva maneuver. Teach the patient and family members how to establish a fluid plan, maintain the prescribed fluid intake, and measures to control head pain.

The nurse helps the family members provide safety for the patient in the home environment. This may involve alterations in the physical environment such as rearrangement of furniture in the bedroom, providing a call system for the patient, or arranging with family and friends to visit while the primary caregiver must be out of the home. If the patient is recovering from an acute brain injury, the nurse helps the patient and family understand how brain edema and increased intracranial pressure resolve, so they can plan a gradual increase in activity and exertion.

Patients with benign intracranial pressure and their family members are taught how to control the intracranial pressure with medications and fluid plans. Teach patients and family members how to recognize the need to return to the clinic or emergency room for a therapeutic lumbar puncture to reduce the intracranial pressure and relieve the headache.

SEIZURES
Definition

A **seizure** is a sudden, explosive, disorderly discharge of cerebral neurons (Figure 45-9) characterized by a sudden, transient alteration in brain function. The clinical manifestations usually involve an alteration in level of consciousness and motor, sensory, autonomic, or psychic symptoms. Seizures are a syndrome not a specific disease entity. **Convulsion** is the term that describes the clonic-tonic (jerky, contract-relax) movement associated with some seizures.

Etiology/Epidemiology

Causes

Seizure disorder may result from a variety of disease processes, genetics, or changes in the neuron's environment. Disease processes that may cause a seizure disorder are presented in the box below. One way to group the causes of seizures is to divide them according to (1) those originating from cerebral lesions, (2) those originating from biochemical disorders, (3) those following cerebral trauma (posttraumatic), and (4) those resulting from idiopathic **epilepsy.** The causes of recurrent seizure activity are different across the various age groups.

Seizure activity may be precipitated by a variety of factors. Hypoglycemia, fatigue or lack of sleep, emotional or physical stress, febrile illness, large amounts of water ingestion, constipation, use of stimulant drugs, withdrawal from depressant drugs including alcohol, and hyperventilation (respiratory alkalosis) have the potential to alter the neuron's cellular environment and initiate seizure activity. Some environmental stimuli such as blinking lights, a poorly adjusted television screen, loud noises, certain music, certain odors, or merely being startled can trigger seizure activity. Women may have in-

CAUSES OF SEIZURE

Metabolic defects
Congenital malformation
Genetic defect (genetic epilepsy)
Perinatal injury
Postnatal trauma
Myoclonic syndromes
Myoclonic epilepsy
Infection
Brain tumor
Vascular disease

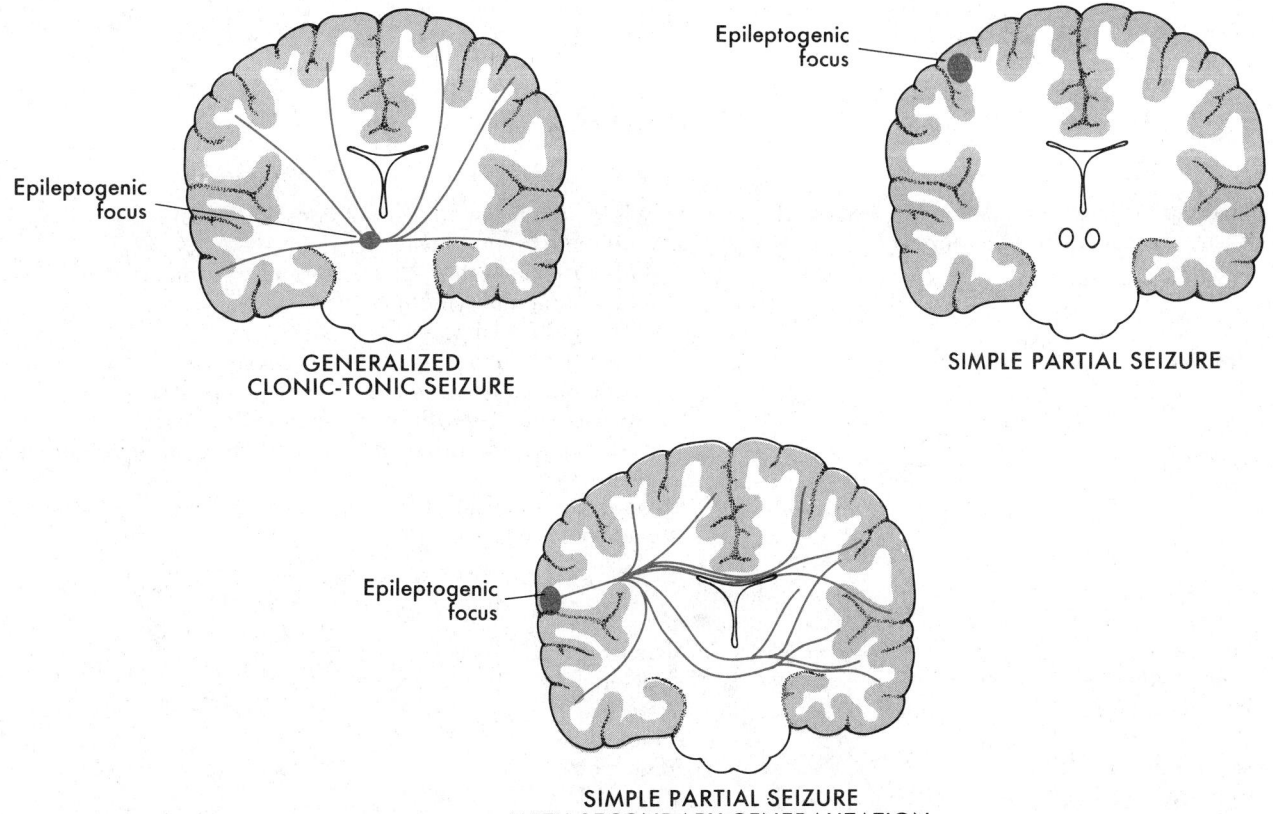

GENERALIZED
CLONIC-TONIC SEIZURE

SIMPLE PARTIAL SEIZURE

SIMPLE PARTIAL SEIZURE
WITH SECONDARY GENERALIZATION

FIGURE 45-9   Schematic representation of electric discharge spread with different types of seizures.

creased seizure activity immediately before or during menses.

Classification

The international classification of epileptic seizures offers a uniform, consistent system worldwide. Table 45-4 gives both the international classification terms and the traditional terms still used by many health care professionals.

Generalized seizures often do not have a local (focal) onset since they originate from a subcortical or deeper brain focus. Generalized seizures involve neurons bilaterally, with the patient's consciousness always impaired or lost. Partial seizures have a local onset because they usually originate from cortical brain tissue, a superficial focus. Partial seizures only involve neurons on a unilateral basis, consciousness is usually maintained as long as the seizure activity is limited to one hemisphere. Partial seizures may spread (generalize) to involve neurons of the other hemisphere and deeper brain nuclei. If this secondary generalization occurs, consciousness is lost at that point of generalization.

Pathophysiology

The neurons that discharge spontaneously to produce the seizure activity are called the epileptogenic focus. These neurons are hypersensitive and may even remain in a partially depolarized state continuously. The cell membranes of such neurons appear to be more permeable, making the cells more responsive to hyperthermia, hypoxia, hypoglycemia, hyponatremia, repeated sensory stimulation, and certain sleep phases. Epileptogenic foci are sensitive to acetylcholine and slower at degrading it.

Tonic phase

In a seizure the firing of involved epileptogenic neurons becomes increasingly greater in frequency and amplitude. The epileptogenic discharge spreads to adjacent normal neurons and then spreads via white matter tracts connecting the two hemispheres to the contralateral cortex and via projection pathways to the subcortical areas including the basal ganglia, thalamus, and brainstem. Subcortical spread is manifested as the **tonic phase** of the seizure. Subcortical spread of the seizure activity is associated with

TABLE 45-4   Seizure Classifications

Traditional terminology	International classification
	PARTIAL SEIZURES (SEIZURES BEGINNING LOCALLY)

Focal motor; jacksonian seizures (occasionally become secondarily generalized)	Simple (without impairment of consciousness)
	  With motor symptoms
	  With special sensory or somatosensory symptoms
	  With autonomic symptoms
	  With psychic symptoms

Temporal lobe or psychomotor seizures	Complex (with impairment of consciousness)
	  Simple partial onset followed by impairment of consciousness)—with or without automatisms
	  Impaired consciousness at onset—with or without automatisms
	Secondarily generalized (partial onset evolving to generalized tonic-clonic seizures)

	GENERALIZED SEIZURES (BILATERALLY SYMMETRIC AND WITHOUT LOCAL ONSET)
Petit mal	Absences
Minor motor	Myoclonic
Limited grand mal	Clonic
	Tonic
Grand mal	Tonic-clonic
Drop attacks	Absences
	Infantile spasms
	UNCLASSIFIED SEIZURES (BECAUSE OF INCOMPLETE DATA) **STATUS EPILEPTICUS (PROLONGED PARTIAL OR GENERALIZED SEIZURES WITHOUT RECOVERY BETWEEN ATTACKS)**

From Rothner AD, editor: *Recent developments in the treatment of epilepsy,* Philadelphia, 1983, Borland-Coogan Associates, (© Abbott Laboratories, Chicago).

loss of responsiveness. Autonomic nervous system clinical manifestations such as pupillary dilation may emerge at this point. Apnea may be present for a few seconds. The excitation is further projected downward to the spinal cord neurons via the corticospinal and reticulospinal pathways.

Clonic phase

The **clonic phase** of the seizure begins as inhibitory neurons in the cortex, anterior thalamus, and basal ganglia begin to inhibit the cortical excitation. This attempted inhibition of the seizure activity results in an interruption in the seizure discharge producing an intermittent contraction–relaxation pattern of muscle. Gradually the clonic activity becomes more and more infrequent and finally ceases. At this point the epileptogenic neurons are exhausted.

Metabolic changes

For seizure activity to be maintained requires a 250% increase in ATP and a 60% increase in cerebral oxygen consumption. Cerebral blood flow undergoes a 250% increase during the seizure activity but glucose and oxygen at the neuronal level are depleted. Lactate accumulates in the brain tissues. Secondary hypoxia, acidosis, and lactate accumulation may further alter the brain chemistry and result in progressive brain tissue injury and destruction. Cellular exhaustion and cell destruction are consequences of prolonged seizure activity.

Status epilepticus

Status epilepticus is the occurrence of multiple sequential seizures before the patient fully regains consciousness after the preceding seizure. Because of the resulting cerebral anoxia, the situation is a medical emergency. A postictal state is still present when the next seizure occurs. Most commonly status epilepticus arises from abrupt discontinuation of anticonvulsant medications. Status may occur in untreated or inadequately treated patients with a seizure disorder. The patient in status may suffer aspiration, mental retardation, dementia, other brain damage, and ultimately death.

Clinical Manifestations

Tonic-clonic seizures or grand mal seizures are the most commonly observed type of seizure activity and are one form of generalized seizure (see Table 45-5). Although the tonic-clonic seizure may be preceded by a prodromal period, in the majority the seizure begins without warning. Tonic-clonic seizures characteristically begin with a sudden loss of consciousness and generalized tonic muscle contractions. The person then falls to the ground. The body stiffens in an opisthotonos position with the legs and usually the arms extended. The jaws snap shut. A shrill cry may be heard at this point because of air being forcefully exhaled through closed vocal cords as the thoracic muscles initially contract. The bladder, and less commonly the bowel, may evacuate. The person is apneic with ensuing cyanosis. The pupils are dilated and unresponsive to light. This tonic phase lasts less than 1 minute, an average of 15 seconds.

The clonic phase of the seizure is characterized by violent, rhythmic muscular contractions accompanied by strenuous hyperventilation. The face is contorted. The eyes roll. There is excessive salivation resulting in frothing from the mouth. The person sweats profusely. The pulse is very rapid. The clonic jerking subsides by slowing in frequency and losing strength (amplitude) over a period of 30 seconds.

Tonic-clonic seizures last from 2 to 5 minutes at most. After the clonic phase, the person is unresponsive for about 5 minutes. The extremities are limp. Breathing is quiet. The pupils begin to respond to light. When the person awakens, the individual is usually confused and disoriented and may complain of a headache, muscle aching, and fatigue. There is no memory of the seizure.

Therapeutic Management

Prevention of seizures is the dominant therapeutic goal. Medical care for persons with seizures focuses on three areas—diagnostic evaluation and treatment, seizure care, and follow-up care. Emphasis is on physical wellness, elimination of precipitating factors, and reduction of drug side effects.

For diagnostic evaluation the most critical aspect

in making the diagnosis of the seizure disorder and establishing the cause is the health history. The physical examination and routine blood and urine laboratory tests such as blood glucose, serum calcium, BUN, urine sodium, and creatinine clearance supplement the health history. An array of systemic diseases known to have a seizure disorder as a clinical manifestation are evaluated in this manner. Skull x-ray films, CT scan, MRI, and cerebrospinal fluid examination are useful in examining the array of neurologic diseases associated with seizures. The electroencephalogram is useful in assessing the type of seizure and may help to determine its focus. Video monitoring is playing an increasingly important role in seizure assessment. Using portable EEG devices may be useful for some patients.

Once the diagnosis is made, the underlying medical, surgical or neurologic problem is corrected if possible. Thus the major medical method of treating a seizure disorder is to correct or control the cause when possible. If correction is not possible, the major means of therapeutic management is the judicious administration of antiseizure medications and elimination of precipitating factors. With a first unprovoked seizure and no risk factors for another seizure, many physicians do not recommend a medication regimen. With risk factors present or after a second unprovoked seizure, a medication regimen is prescribed. The medical therapeutic goal is eradication (complete suppression) of seizure activity without producing intolerable drug side effects. Other medical therapies may include prescription of a ketogenic diet and biofeedback. Seizure surgery is indicated for a resectable seizure focus or in some intractable seizure states and because of recent advances is increasingly used.

Seizure care involves protection of the patient during the seizure and termination of the major motor seizure. Diazepam (Valium) 10 mg or lorazepam (Ativan) 2 to 4 mg IV push is generally given for this purpose. If the patient has not previously taken antiseizure medication or does not have a therapeutic blood level, phenytoin (Dilantin), usually 500 mg, is given IV drip or push. The pharmacologic management for seizures is presented in Table 45-6.

Follow-up care promotes physical wellness. Oral health must be promoted also because of antiseizure drug side effects. Additionally, psychologic, social, educational, and vocational counseling are often appropriate for the patient and family.

NURSING MANAGEMENT OF THE PATIENT WITH SEIZURES
Assessment

The nurse asks if the patient experiences any prodromal symptoms, dizziness, or numbness. The nurse collects data on the sensory and motor mani-

TABLE 45-5   Clinical Manifestations Related to Seizure Types

Type	Clinical manifestations	Site

I. PARTIAL SEIZURES
  A. Simple
    1. With motor symptoms:
      a. Without Jacksonian march (focal motor seizure—the motor movements do not extend into adjacent areas)
	Motor activity is usually clonic.
	Motor movement elicited by the seizure activity depends on the anatomic-physiologic portion of the irritated cortex but motor seizures most often begin in the face and hands.
	Focal seizures begin with slow, repetitive jerking of the body part, which increases in strength and rate over a period of 5 to 15 seconds.
	The seizure can cease spontaneously, with a gradual decrease in clonic movement
		Primary motor area

b. With Jacksonian march (Jacksonian seizure—the seizure activity spreads in an orderly fashion to adjacent areas)	Seizure activity spreads to adjacent areas after the initial clonic movement increases; motor movements, for example, would begin in the fingers of one side and spread to the hand, wrist, forearm, arm, face, and finally the lower extremity on the same side of the body. After spreading, the jerking movements in all areas would spontaneously stop.	Primary motor area
c. Adversive seizure	Turning movement of hand and eyes to the side opposite the irritative focus. Often associated with contractions of the trunk and extremities. May remain local or develop into a generalized seizure.	Frontal lobe anterior to the primary motor area
2. With special sensory or somatosensory symptoms (focal sensory seizure); less common than focal motor seizures; any age may be affected	Sensory experience is subjective and confined to the primary sensory modalities (somesthetic, visual, auditory-vestibular, or olfactory). If sensory seizure begins on the hand area of the sensory cortex, the patient experiences numbness, tingling, or "pins and needles" phenomena. Other sensory experiences include burning, a crawling sensation, or a feeling of movement of the body part. Most frequent areas affected include lips, fingers, and toes. May remain local or develop into a generalized seizure.	Sensory cortex Postcentral gyrus (parietal lobe) with involvement of the primary sensory area
B. Complex (temporary lobe or psychomotor seizure) 1. Simple partial onset followed by impairment of consciousness—with or without automatisms; common seizures found in both children and adults but in most persons occurs before the age of 20	The person is able to interact with the environment with purposeful, although inappropriate, movements; although the body muscles stiffen, the person does not fall and may even continue the complex activity in which he or she was involved, such as driving; the person may appear "wide eyed." A wide variety of sensory experiences precede the automatism and include illusions, hallucinations, and primitive visceral, olfactory, and gustatory sensations.	Temporal lobe and its connections

TABLE 45-5 Clinical Manifestations Related to Seizure Types—cont'd

Type	Clinical manifestations	Site
	Most characteristic event of a temporal lobe seizure is the automatism; common examples of automatism are lip-smacking, chewing, facial grimacing, swallowing movements, and patting, picking, or rubbing oneself or one's clothing. Temporal lobe seizures generally last from 1 to 4 minutes and are followed by several minutes of postictal confusion.	
2. Impaired consciousness at onset—with or without automatisms	See above, under Simple Partial Onset.	
C. Secondarily generalized	Unconsciousness appears. General symptoms are produced.	
II. GENERALIZED SEIZURES		
A. Myoclonic (minor major seizure)	Characterized by sudden, uncontrollable jerking movements of one or more extremities or the entire body. Seizures usually occur in the morning. Usually momentary loss of consciousness followed by postictal confusion. Person often violently flung to the ground so that injury is a real possibility. Myoclonic seizures can occur in clusters. If the frequency and amplitude of the seizures are severe, mental retardation can result.	Multifocal
B. Clonic	Characterized by repetitive clonic jerks of constant amplitude and diminishing frequency.	
C. Tonic (affects infants and children)	Loss of postural tone without evidence of clonicity, with flexion of the upper limbs and extension of the lower limbs. Child assumes an abnormal posture for seconds or minutes without losing consciousness.	
D. Tonic-clonic (grand mal seizure) (affects both children and adults)	A prodromal period of irritability and tension may precede a tonic-clonic seizure by several hours or days; however, in majority of persons, seizures begin without warnings. Characteristically tonic-clonic seizures begin with a sudden loss of consciousness and generalized tonic muscle contractions; the person falls to the ground and the body stiffens in an opisthotonos position with legs and, usually, arms extended; the jaw snaps shut; a shrill cry may be heard due to forceful exhalation of air through the closed vocal cords as the thoracic muscles initially contract; the bladder and, less often, the bowel may evacuate; during the tonic phase, the person is apneic with subsequent cyanosis; pupils are dilated and unresponsive to light. The tonic phase lasts less than 1 minute (average 15 seconds).	Multifocal

Modified from McCance KL, Huether SE: *Pathophysiology: the biological basis for disease in adults and children* St Louis, 1990, Mosby–Year Book.

Continued.

TABLE 45-5   Clinical Manifestations Related to Seizure Types—cont'd

Type	Clinical manifestations	Site
	The clonic phase is characterized by violent, rhythmic, muscular contractions accompanied by strenuous hyperventilation; the face is contorted; the eyes roll, and there is excessive salivation with frothing from the mouth; profuse sweating, and a rapid pulse are evident.	
	The clonic jerking subsides in frequency and amplitude over a period of about 30 seconds.	
	The tonic-clonic seizure lasts from 2 to 5 minutes.	
	After the clonic phase, the person is in a stupor or coma for about 5 minutes; the extremities are limp; breathing is quiet; and the pupils begin to respond to light.	
	When the person awakens, he or she may be confused and disoriented, complains of headache, muscle aching, and fatigue.	
	There is no recollection of the attack.	
	Tonic-clonic seizures may occur at any time of the day or night, whether the person is awake or asleep.	
	The frequency of recurrence may vary from hours, weeks, months, or years.	
E. Atonic (drop attack, akinetic seizure)	Characterized by sudden loss of postural muscle tone.	Multifocal

festations noted by the patient or observers during the seizure including eye movements, body or extremity movement, or changes in consciousness. Information on the presence of urinary or fecal incontinence is collected as well as data on how long the seizures last. A description of the postictal state is obtained from the patient or observers. Data on the age of onset, frequency, duration, and severity are collected.

Assess for the presence of any precipitating factors such as fatigue, hypoglycemia, or flashing lights. The patient's history related to seizures and the family history related to the presence of a seizure disorder in other family members are noted. Social history related to alcohol use and drug use is collected. Information on the current medical regimen and the past medical regimen is noted.

The nurse conducts a physical examination of the nervous system noting changes in mental status, cranial nerve function, muscular tone or strength, primary or cortical sensations, abnormal reflexes, gait, and cerebellar function. Any seizure activity that occurs during the history assessment and physical examination is noted.

If a seizure is witnessed, the nurse notes the onsetting clinical manifestations, especially the initial manifestations (e.g., which way the eyes or the head turns). The progression of seizure activity is carefully noted as is the duration of the seizure. Level of consciousness and pupil size and gaze are checked during the seizure. Incontinence of urine and feces is noted. The postictal state is also assessed. The patient is checked for injury including tongue and mouth damage. As the patient regains consciousness, mental status and muscular strength are assessed.

Nursing Diagnosis

Nursing diagnoses relevant to the seizure (ictal) phase are:

Alteration in consciousness related to seizure activity

High risk for injury related to altered consciousness and/or clonic-tonic motor activity

High risk for aspiration related to ineffective airway clearance

Ineffective airway clearance related to clonic-tonic motor activity

Sensory/perceptual alterations related to aura and impaired neuronal function

Impaired physical mobility related to altered con-

TABLE 45-6 Pharmacology Summary: Drugs Used for Seizures

Drug	Clinical use	Route/daily dose	Nursing implications
HYDANTOINS			
Phenytoin (Dilantin)	Tonic-clonic Complex partial Status epilepticus	PO: 300-400 mg IV: 10/15 mg/kg	Not given fast, max 50 mg/min; watch cardiac status; may be used in combination with phenobarbital or primidone; because of gingival hyperplasia, oral hygiene and, regular dental care; drug must be withdrawn gradually, not abruptly stopped; watch for signs of toxicity—nystagmus, ataxia, sedation, diplopia.
BARBITURATES			
Phenobarbital (Luminal)	Tonic-clonic Simple and complex partial Status epilepticus	PO: 50-100 mg bid/tid IV: 200-320 mg, repeat q6h	Observe for drowsiness; sedation and cognitive impairment are serious drawbacks to use and compliance; less expensive; must be withdrawn gradually
Primidone (Mysoline)	Tonic-clonic Simple and complex partial	PO:100-125 mg hs, gradually	Same as for phenobarbital
BENZODIAZEPINES			
Diazepam	Status epilepticus	IV: 5-10 mg, repeat in 10-15 minutes to 30 mg	Given slowly; considered drug of choice for status epilepticus but give only in large vein; have ventilatory support available; effectiveness is short-lived.
Clonazepam (Klonopin)	Absence Myoclonus	PO: up to 0.5 mg tid, increasing q3 days to 20 mg daily	Generally used for persons who have failed to respond to ethosuximide or valproic acid; may become tolerant to drug in a few months.
Lorazepam (Ativan)	Status epilepticus	IV: 2-4 mg	Similar to diazepam
SUCCINIMIDES			
Ethosuximide (Zarontin)	Absence	PO: 500 mg daily, with 250 mg increase q4-7 days to optimum effect	Generally no side effects; lacks significant drug interactions; should be gradually withdrawn; monitor clinical response to drug, not blood levels.
OTHER			
Carbamazepine (Tegretol)	Tonic-clonic Complex partial	PO: 200 mg bid, increased 200 mg weekly to 800-1200 mg daily in divided doses	Increases GABA adjunct to phenytoin, phenobarbital, or primidone; watch CBC; watch pulmonary and cardiac status; initially may experience sedation, ataxia, nausea, and vomiting; more expensive than phenobarbital.
Valproic acid (Depakene)	Absence Tonic-clonic Complex partial Myoclonic	PO: 15 mg/kg/qd initially, weekly increase 10 mg/kg/qd to 60 mg/kg/qd max	Monitor liver function; observe for GI distress, tremor, alopecia, and weight gain; effective for all generalized seizures, so good to use if more than one type of seizure exists.

sciousness and/or clonic-tonic motor activity

Impaired skin integrity related to clonic-tonic motor activity or fall

Urinary incontinence related to altered consciousness

Bowel incontinence related to altered consciousness

Nursing diagnoses related to the postictal phase are:

High risk for injury related to altered cognitive function

Alteration in consciousness related to seizure activity

Altered thought processes: confusion related to seizure activity

Impaired physical mobility related to postictal fatigue or Todd's paralysis

Nursing diagnoses relevant to the interictal phase are:

Altered oral mucous membrane related to phenytoin therapy

Bowel incontinence related to antiseizure medication

Altered thought processes related to antiseizure medications and knowledge deficit

Anxiety and fear related to seizure activity

Ineffective individual coping related to presence of seizure disorder

Self-esteem disturbance related to anxiety, fear, and social stigma

Noncompliance related to therapeutic regimen

Altered parenting or ineffective family coping related to presence of seizure disorder

Social isolation related to anxiety, fear, ineffective coping, and social stigma

Knowledge deficit related to therapeutic regimens, control of side effects, coping strategies, social and vocational implications

Planning

During a seizure and during the postictal phase, the primary nursing goal is to promote seizure control and protect the patient from both physical and psychologic injury.

For the patient whose seizure disorder cannot be cured the nursing goals are extended to include helping the patient and family live with the seizure disorder and minimizing the impact of the seizures on their lives.

Implementation

Seizure care

During a seizure the nurse protects the patient from injury and remains with the patient. If an aura occurs, the nurse helps the patient lie down. If a seizure with unconsciousness occurs without warning,

the nurse attempts to prevent or break the fall. The patient is placed on the bed or floor. Constricting clothing about the neck is loosened. All objects in the immediate environment that could cause injury are removed. The patient's head is protected from injury by placing a pillow under it or placing the head in the nurse's lap if possible. An open airway is maintained by placing the patient's head in a lateral position to allow drainage of secretions. (It may not be possible to accomplish this action until the seizure stops.) Objects such as tongue blades are *not* placed in the mouth during seizure activity. The patient is covered if possible to prevent undue physical exposure. When the seizure stops, the patient may be placed on the side to facilitate drainage from the mouth. The occurrence is handled with minimum attention and disruption.

The postictal status of the patients vary depending on the type of seizure and the intensity of seizure activity. Full cognitive function is rapidly regained in most partial seizures and in absence attacks. As the patient regains consciousness, the patient's attention (immediate recall), recent memory (orientation), and remote memory and ability to abstract are assessed. The nurse reorients the patient. If cognition is intact, the patient may go about his or her activities. If cognition is not intact, a quiet environment is provided, and the patient is allowed to rest until the postictal phase abates. Reassess the patient every 30 minutes. The nurse should be reassuring and supportive allowing the patient to express fears, anxiety, frustration, and other feelings being experienced.

With generalized clonic-tonic seizures, the postictal state persists longer. With intense seizure activity of long duration, the patient may be extremely fatigued and cognitively impaired for several hours or more. Move the patient to a quiet place to sleep or rest until recovered. The nurse assesses the pa-

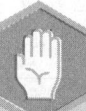

CLINICAL ALERT

Do not leave the patient during a seizure.

If the patient experiences an aura, have the patient lie down.

Attempt to prevent or break the patient's fall if a seizure with unconsciousness occurs without warning.

Place the patient on the floor or on a bed.

Maintain an open airway by placing the patient's head in a lateral position; do not insert objects such as tongue blades.

tient every 30 minutes to an hour until full cognition returns or bedtime arrives.

Occasionally patients experience Todd's paralysis postictally, which gradually resolves. The patient needs to be at rest until the paralysis resolves and may need reassurance that the motor loss will go away shortly.

During absence seizures and partial seizures, protective measures are instituted as required by the nature of the seizure. It is most important not to be overrestrictive or overprotective. The nurse protects the patient from undue exposure and embarrassment and provides reassurance and support to the patient.

Family members may also need support and information during and after the seizure.

Status epilepticus

If the patient begins to experience a second seizure before recovering from the preceding one, the physician is notified immediately. This may be the beginning of status epilepticus and would be a medical emergency. In status epilepticus, the nurse provides supportive care and administers the prescribed drugs, usually sodium phenobarbital, phenytoin (Dilantin), lorazepam (Ativan) and diazepam (Valium) in a two- or three-drug combination, usually intravenously. Oxygen is given via nasal route. Sometimes an airway device must be placed while the patient is between seizures, and suctioning is required between seizures. Hydration needs to be maintained via an intravenous route, and glucose needs to be part of the IV solution. Full seizure precautions are instituted. If the patient's temperature becomes elevated, external cooling methods must be instituted. See Figure 45-10 for clinical decision-making steps in care of the status epilepticus patient.

Seizure precautions

The nurse institutes seizure precautions if the patient has had a recent seizure that involved loss of consciousness or potential for injury. Full seizure precautions include bed rest with padded siderails in a raised position, suction machine at the bedside, diazepam (Valium) 10 mg or lorazepam (Ativan) 2 to 4 mg at the bedside, and sometimes oxygen. If the person never has breathing problems during the seizure, then suction and oxygen are not needed at the bedside. If the person has seizures only at night, then bed rest and siderails during the day are not necessary. Seizure precautions are not initiated for persons whose seizure disorder is controlled with medication or who had a seizure disorder in the remote past. This serves only to stigmatize and embarrass the person.

Patient and family education

When the patient is hospitalized for a seizure workup, the nurse teaches the patient and family members about the diagnostic workup. When a diagnosis is made, the nurse reinforces the physician's information and teaches the patient and family members about the cause of the seizure, possible precipitating factors, and therapeutic management protocols.

The nurse must help the patient and family members assume responsibility for the management of the seizure disorder. The patient and family members are taught about the antiseizure drug(s)–drug actions, side effects and how to control them, toxic effects and what to look for and report immediately to the physician (such as anemia and ataxia), dosage and administration schedule, and when additional amounts of antiseizure medications may be necessary. The patient and family members are taught why taking other drugs, whether prescription, over-the-counter, or street drugs, along with antiseizure drugs is dangerous. They are informed how stimulant drugs including caffeine may cause a seizure to "break through" and depressant drugs including alcohol may cause the patient to accidentally overdose. They need to understand that sudden stopping of a depressant drug may cause breakthrough seizure. The patient and family members are encouraged to consult the pharmacist and physician before taking any other medication or drugs.

The nurse teaches the patient and family how hypoglycemia, fatigue, exhaustion, hormonal changes, illness, overhydration, and other factors can precipitate seizure activity. The nurse emphasizes promotion of physical wellness, which includes a dietary regimen that prevents hypoglycemia and a rest and activity schedule that prevents undue fatigue and exhaustion. Types of activities need to be in concert with the level of seizure control. A regular bowel regimen often needs to be instituted since antiseizure medications often interfere with normal bowel function and elimination. The nurse teaches the patient about the impact of antiseizure medications on teeth and gums and how to care for the mouth. The importance of ongoing dental care is emphasized.

Compliance with the therapeutic regimen may become a predominant issue. The patient and family members also need help to understand the rationale for life-style changes such as the restriction against driving motor vehicles, operating heavy equipment, and using potentially dangerous equipment, and the need to refrain from swimming and possibly tub bathing until the patient is seizure free for a specified time. This period is often 1 to 2 years depending on state regulation for licensing purposes. These life-style losses must be grieved for before the patient and family can progress onward with their adaptation to this chronic disability.

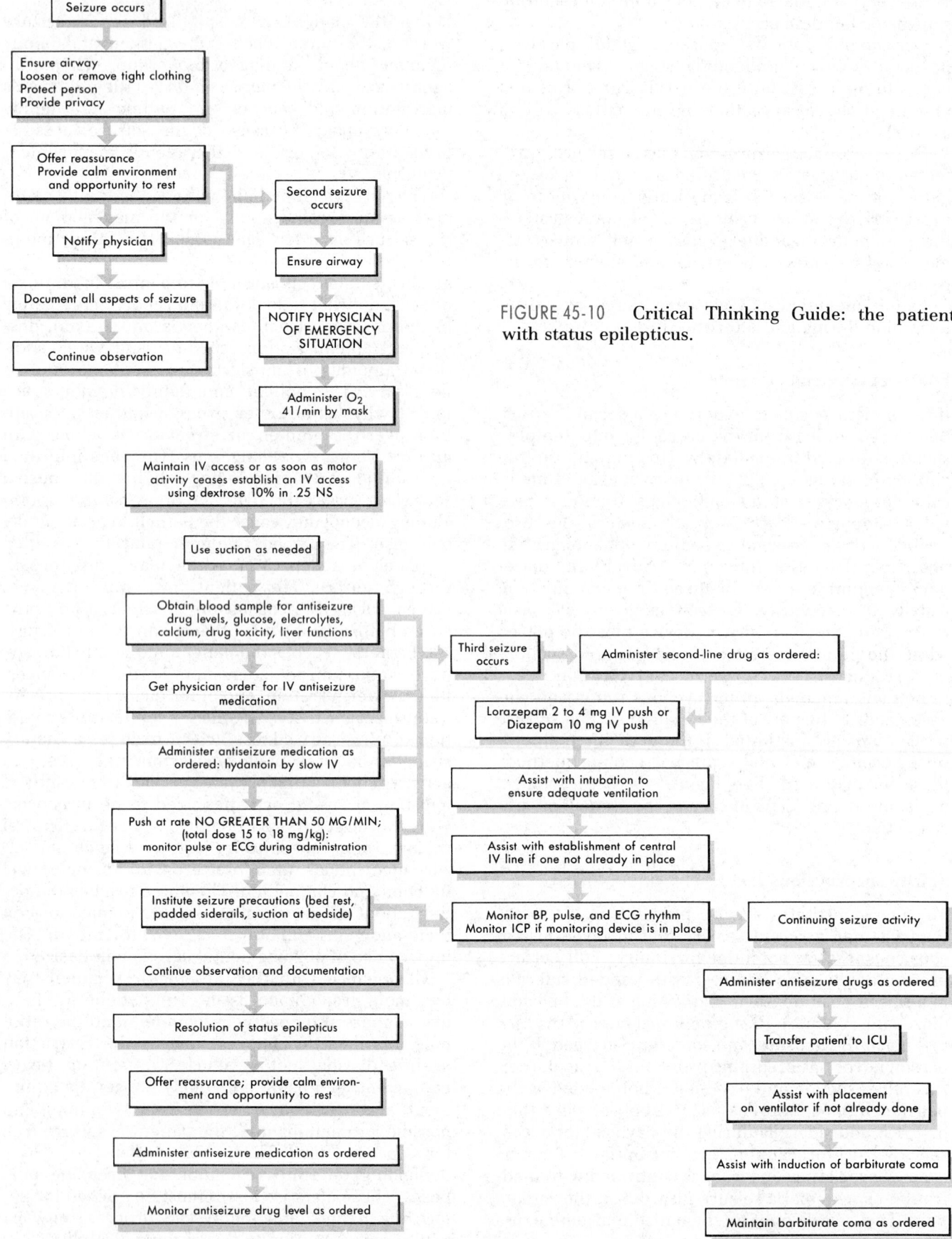

FIGURE 45-10   Critical Thinking Guide: the patient with status epilepticus.

The patient and family members need help gaining insight into their own feelings and behaviors. The nurse encourages the patient and family members to participate in structured groups of people confronted with a similar situation. The nurse provides the name and address of the local and national Epilepsy Foundation.

If the epilepsy is one of the hereditary epilepsies such as myoclonic epilepsy, the nurse supports the patient seeking genetic counseling.

Evaluation

During hospitalization in an acute care setting the nurse monitors the effectiveness of the therapeutic regimen, particularly noting the blood levels of antiseizure medications and the seizure control achieved. The patient is also observed for signs of drug side effects and toxic effects of the antiseizure medication(s). Short-term outcome criteria are:

Therapeutic management regimen maintained as evidenced by therapeutic antiseizure levels and decreased intensity and frequency of seizures

Freedom from seizure as evidenced by no seizure activity

The patient's and family members' responses to the diagnostic workup, the diagnosis, and the therapeutic regimen prescribed are evaluated. The nurse continuously reevaluates the patient's and family's level of learning of the information and skills needed to manage the seizure disorder. Long-term outcome criteria include:

Knowledge deficit needs met as evidenced by
  ability to explain diagnostic and therapeutic measures
  ability to identify special needs
  ability to develop a therapeutic management regimen that fits life-style
Effective coping as evidenced by
  ability to accept the responses of those who witness a seizure
  ability to work to help other persons understand seizures and any measures they may need to implement during a seizure
  pursuit of academic and/or career options limited only by the specific functional limitations of the individual
  ability to develop realistic current and long-term plans for continued personal development psychologically, socially, recreationally, economically, educationally, and vocationally
Acceptance of the seizure disorder as evidenced by exhibition of activities and developmentally appropriate behaviors and tasks

During status epilepticus the nurse monitors the patient's temperature, blood pressure, pulse, blood gases, electrolytes, intake and output, and drug levels.

Documentation

The nurse documents the history and physical assessment findings, particularly related to seizure history and to any observed seizure activity. Record prodromal symptoms experienced, sensory and motor manifestations during the seizure, state of consciousness during the seizure, presence or absence of urinary or fecal incontinence, length of seizure, and postictal manifestations.

Documentation of information that contributes to the differential diagnosis and localization is notably important.

Document presence of any precipitating factors such as fatigue, hypoglycemia, menses, or flashing lights; past history of seizures, family history of seizures; substance abuse, and current and past medication regimens.

The nurse may be the only health-related professional to witness the seizure. In such an instance, record onsetting clinical manifestations; how the seizure progressed, whether generalized or localized, and the type of movement and duration of the seizure; level of consciousness, pupil size and gaze during the seizure and presence of urinary or fecal incontinence. During the postictal period, document the patient's level of cognition—awakeness, ability to concentrate (immediate recall), recent memory, and remote memory. Note the type and extent of injury sustained during the seizure. Also note the presence and location of paralysis following the seizure and its duration.

When status epilepticus is present, the nurse documents the patient's temperature, blood pressure, pulse, blood gases, electrolytes, intake and output, and drug levels.

Nursing diagnoses, goals, and plans of care are documented. Diagnostic tests and the patient's response to them are placed in the patient's health record. The nurse documents, in particular, response to medical therapy and nursing interventions related to seizure control. Side effects and toxic effects of antiseizure medications are noted in the patient's health record. Blood levels of antiseizure medications are recorded.

The patient's and family members' responses to the diagnosis and treatment are documented. All teaching interventions specifying the information and skills taught are placed in the record. Referrals are documented.

Ongoing Care

Long-term care

In long-term care the nurse may maintain control of the seizure management to a much greater extent than in the home care situation. In the long-term care setting the nurse may administer the antiseizure medications, control the use of other medications, and be able to impose compliance related to diet, rest and activity, and use of alcohol and nicotine. If this is the case, the nurse institutes all the health promoting actions discussed in the section of therapeutic management. Institute a bowel regimen. Oral hygiene receives special emphasis due to drug side effects. The nurse sees that the patient receives dental care on a regular basis as well. The nurse alters the drug route with physician approval if the patient becomes unable to take the medication by mouth, such as in the case of nausea and vomiting. The nurse also recognizes when the patient may be at risk for breakthrough seizures, such as with a temperature elevation, and notifies the physician.

Home care

The nurse in the home care setting helps the patient and family come to terms with living with a seizure disorder. Coping with a seizure disorder is difficult and it takes work. The nurse works to reduce the factors that cause noncompliance with the therapeutic regimen. The patient needs to learn stress reduction techniques, relaxation exercises, imaging, or different ways of responding to stressors.

Help institute a medication regimen to help routinely remind the patient to take the medication. With the nurse's help the patient identifies daily habits or rituals to associate with taking the medication.

Patients and their family members often have misconceptions about seizures and their therapeutic regimens. Education is an ongoing responsibility of the nurse. Patients living with a seizure disorder and also their families need anticipatory guidance about changes to expect and how development needs will be influenced by the seizure disorder.

Rehabilitation

The rehabilitation of a patient with a seizure disorder often needs to focus on the learning of skills, not just the skills of seizure management, but social skills and independent living skills. Many patients with seizures, because of societal stigma and discrimination and overrestrictiveness and overprotectiveness on the part of family members and health care providers, can become socially disabled. The nurse can intervene by finding or initiating or possibly, in some cases, conducting skills training groups, mood management classes, human relationship classes, and sexuality classes. Likewise many patients with seizures have not learned independent living skills. Again, the nurse intervenes by teaching the patient to perform these independent living skills such as grocery shopping, cooking, cleaning, and paying bills. Rehabilitation also involves voca-

tional training, whether it is an initial vocational pursuit or retraining in another field where the seizure disorder is not an issue.

HEADACHE

Headaches are one of the most common neurologic complaints. The majority of headaches are mild, not of a serious nature, and can be relieved by using a mild analgesic. A small percent of headaches, however, are indicative of a serious pathologic condition and may require opioids before relief is obtained.

Definition

Headache may be defined as pain located in the upper regions of the head from the orbits to the suboccipital area.

Pain from intracranial structures above the tentorium is referred to the anterior portion of the head. Pain from the intracranial structures below the tentorium is referred to the occipital and suboccipital regions.

Etiology/Epidemiology

Headaches have been classified in different ways. In 1988 a new classification was published (Table 45-7).

Migraine

Migraine headaches tend to have their onset during adolescence or in the second decade of life, although childhood migraine does occur and initial attacks may be seen in the 30-years-of-age group. These headaches tend to decrease in the late 50s and early 60s, presumably because of cranial blood vessel sclerosis.

The frequency of attacks is highly variable, but rarely occurs more than once, at most twice, a week. Vascular headaches are rarely a daily occurrence with the exception of cluster headaches.

Migraine is a familial disorder characterized by periodic, usually unilateral, throbbing headache that begins in childhood, adolescence, or young adulthood and recurs with decreasing frequency in later life. Of the general population, 3% to 5% experience migraines. Migraine is more common in women than in men in a 2:1 ratio.

Tension-type headache

Tension-type (pressure, psychomotor) headache is the most common form of headache. These headaches are more common in women and are more likely to occur in middle age. Headaches may be a direct result of stress, anxiety, or depression with associated tension.

TABLE 45-7   Headache Classifications

1. Migraine
   Migraine without aura
   Migraine with aura
   Ophthalmoplegic migraine
   Retinal migraine
   Childhood periodic syndromes that may be
      precursors to or associated with migraine
2. Tension-type headache
   Episodic tension-type headache
   Chronic tension-type headache
3. Cluster headache and chronic paroxysmal
   hemicrania
   Cluster headache
   Chronic paroxysmal hemicrania
4. Miscellaneous headache unassociated with
   structural lesion
5. Headache associated with head trauma
   Acute post-traumatic headache
   Chronic post-traumatic headache
6. Headache associated with vascular disorders
   Acute ischemic cerebrovascular disease
   Intracranial hematoma
   Subarachnoid hemorrhage
   Unruptured vascular malformation
   Arteritis
   Carotid or vertebral artery pain
   Venous thrombosis
   Arterial hypertension
7. Headache associated with nonvascular intra-
   cranial disorder
   High cerebrospinal fluid pressure
   Low cerebrospinal fluid pressure

Intracranial infection
Intracranial sarcoidosis and other noninfec-
   tious inflammatory diseases
Intracranial neoplasm

8. Headache associated with substances or their
   withdrawal
9. Headache associated with noncephalic infection
   Viral infection
   Bacterial infection
   Headache related to other infection
10. Headache associated with metabolic disorder
    Hypoxia
    Hypercapnia
    Mixed hypoxia and hypercapnia
    Hypoglycemia
    Dialysis
    Headache related to other metabolic abnor-
       mality
11. Headache or facial pain associated with disor-
    der of cranium, neck, eyes, ears, nose, sinuses,
    teeth, mouth, or other facial or cranial struc-
    tures
12. Cranial neuralgias, nerve-trunk pain and deaf-
    ferentation pain
    Persistent pain of cranial nerve origin
    Trigeminal neuralgia
    Glossopharyngeal neuralgia
    Occipital neuralgia
    Central causes of head and facial pain
13. Headache not classifiable

Cluster headache

Cluster headaches typically involve unilateral orbital, supraorbital, and/or temporal pain lasting
from 15 minutes or so to several hours. They may
occur from several times a day to once every other
day. Attacks occur in a series lasting for weeks to
months (cluster periods) with remission periods
lasting months to years, although some persons have
chronic headaches. Often accompanying symptoms
include conjunctival injection, lacrimation, nasal
congestion, rhinorrhea, facial sweating, miosis, and
ptosis. Often the pain is extreme. Cluster headaches
occur more commonly in men than women with an
age of onset between 20 and 40 years.

Other types of headaches

Headaches occur with systemic infections and are
usually associated with fever, various metabolic ab-

normalities such as hypoglycemia and hypoxia, and
circulatory insufficiency. The headache is usually
generalized and has a strong throbbing quality.

When increased intracranial pressure is present,
the headache is a generalized dull ache and the localization of the injury cannot be reliably based on
the location of the headache. In the absence of increased intracranial pressure, unilateral headache is
indicative of the side where the pathologic condition
is located. Headache is one of the first symptoms of
a posterior fossa mass, whereas headache is often
absent in a supratentorial mass.

Headaches may result also from faulty posture
(malalignment of neck, head, and shoulder girdle) or
degenerative neck disease. Osteoarthritis and other
degenerative diseases affecting the cervical spine
(e.g., cervical spondylosis and degenerative disk disease) often result in diffuse occipital pain that may
radiate bitemporally.

Pathophysiology

Most of the scalp and facial structures are pain sensitive including the arteries, muscles, orbital structures, mucous membranes, skin, subcutaneous tissue, eye and ear structures, nasal cavity, sinuses, and teeth. Any stretching (traction), dilation, inflammation, or pressure (compression) of the pain-sensitive structures of the cranial vault, scalp, and face will produce headache.

The pathophysiologic mechanism of most spontaneous cranial pain is one of the following:

Traction on or dilation of intracranial arteries and distention of extracranial arteries

Traction on or displacement of large intracranial veins or the dural envelopes in which they lie

Compression or traction on or inflammation of sensory cranial or spinal nerves

Voluntary or involuntary spasm and possibly interstitial inflammation of cranial or cervical muscles

Meningeal irritation or raised intracranial pressure[39]

Clinical Manifestations

The manifestations of a headache vary by type. Table 45-8 compares the differences in the signs and symptoms of the various types of headaches.

Therapeutic Management

Initially the physician seeks to diagnose the type of headache. This is done by taking a complete history and conducting a physical examination with emphasis on the neurologic examination and blood pressure. A CT scan or MRI scan may be done to rule out a bleed or mass such as a tumor or abscess. A dynamic brain scan, in which images are obtained at regular intervals, may be used to rule out an arteriovenous malformation in suspicious cases. A lumbar puncture may be performed if inflammation is the suspected etiology.

In migraine, therapy is directed at two goals: (1) to control the current episode and (2) to reduce the frequency and severity of the migraine attacks. Vasoconstriction is believed to lessen the attack. Pressure over the temporal arteries and common carotid and external carotid artery compression sometimes provides pain relief. Cold applied to the painful area may help. Inhalation of 100% oxygen produces vasoconstriction. Inhalation of amyl nitrate during the aura has been shown to prevent the attack. See Table 45-9 for a summary of drugs used to treat headaches.

In tension-type headaches butalbital (Fiorinal) is often the analgesic of choice. Opioid medications should be avoided. Opioid addiction becomes a serious threat to patients with severe recurrent mus-

---

TABLE 45-8   Differential Diagnosis of Headaches

Manifestations	Migraine and cluster headaches	Tension-type headache	Headache associated with increased intracranial pressure	Headache associated with disorders of the head and face
Laterality	Usually unilateral onset	Usually bilateral	Unilateral or bilateral	Unilateral or bilateral
Severity	Severe	Mild to severe	Usually mild	Mild to severe
Throbbing	Present at onset	Usually absent at onset, but may be present during peak	Usually absent	Usually absent
Change with head position	Severe	Mild	Moderate	Mild
Time course	Acute	Subacute to chronic	Subacute to chronic	Acute to subacute
Gastrointestinal disturbance	Severe	Absent or mild	Moderate	Absent
Visual disturbance	Present	Absent	May be present	Absent
Tenderness	Mild over extracranial vessels	Severe in suboccipital and temporalis muscles	Absent	Present in sinusitis
Focal neurologic signs	May be present	Absent	May be present	Absent
Stiff neck	Absent	Mild	Mild to severe	Absent

Modified from Heilman KM, Watson RT, Greer M: *Handbook for differential diagnosis of neurologic signs and symptoms,* New York, 1977, Appleton-Century-Crofts.

TABLE 45-9   Pharmacology Summary: Drugs Used for Headaches

Drug	Clinical use	Route/dosage	Nursing implications
SYMPTOMATIC TREATMENT			
Nonopioid analgesics			Used for mild headaches
Aspirin	Migraine Tension headache	PO: 0.6 g	Take with food or full glass of water to minimize GI side effects; watch for signs of salicylism—tinnitus, dizziness, sweating; increased bleeding or as a result decreased platelet aggregation
Acetaminophen (Datril, Panadol, Tylenol)	Migraine Tension headache	PO: 325-625 mg	Lifelong high use may produce renal impairment
Ibuprofen (Motrin)	Tension headache	PO: 400 mg q4-6h	Take with food or full glass of water to minimize GI side effects; increased bleeding
Analgesic combination			
Butalbital (Fiorinal)	Tension headache	PO: 2 tablets	Used for severe headaches once headache is established; used rarely when dealing with chronic headache because of tolerance or physiologic dependence; watch for constipation
Opioid analgesics			
Codeine sulfate	Migraine Cluster headache	PO, SQ, IM: 30 mg	
Meperidine (Demerol)	Migraine Cluster headache	PO, IM: 50 mg	Monitor respirations, pulse, and blood pressure; warn person about drowsiness
Muscle relaxants	Tension headache		
Antiemetic	Migraine	PO, PR: 25 mg	Relieves nausea and vomiting; provides relaxation
Promethazine (Phenergan)	Cluster headache	IM: 12.5-25 mg	
Alpha-adrenergic blockers			Most effective treatment for migraine; has a cumulative effect, watch for ergotism—numbness, tingling, coldness of hands; use cautiously and as ordered; contraindicated in diabetes mellitus, sepsis, hypertension, peripheral and coronary artery disease, and pregnancy; rebound headache may occur if drug taken for 2 days or if dosage exceeds recommendation

Continued.

TABLE 45-9 Pharmacology Summary: Drugs Used for Headaches—cont'd

Drug	Clinical use	Route/dosage	Nursing implications
Ergotamine tartrate (Gynergen)	Migraine	PO, sublingual: 2 tablets, repeat in ½ hr	Max dose 6 to 8 mg within 1 day
		PR: 2-4 mg, repeat 2 mg in ½ hr	Max dose 10 to 15 mg in 1 week
		SQ, IM: 0.25 mg-0.5 mg, repeat in ½ hr	Max dose 1 mg
	Cluster headache	PO: 3 mg hs	Used as a prophylactic treatment; a single dose at bedtime is used
		IM: 1 mg hs	
Ergotamine (1 mg) with caffeine (100 mg) (Cafergot)	Migraine Cluster headache	PO: 2 tablets, repeat in ½ hr	Max dose 6 tablets; do not take late in the day
Ergotamine (0.3 mg), phenobarbital (20 mg), and belladonna (0.1 mg)	Migraine Cluster headache	PO: 1 tablet bid/tid for a few weeks	May be used prophylactically; associated with dryness of mouth and drowsiness
			Watch for signs of glaucoma; contraindicated in persons with glaucoma
Steroids			
Dexamethasone (Decadron)	Migraine	PO: 2-8 mg	
Corticotropin (ATCH)	Migraine	PO: 40 U/day	Used in persons with refractory migraine and to terminate status migrainosis; used in cluster at high dose if ergotamines are ineffective
Prednisone	Migraine	PO: 45mg/day for 3 to 4 wk	

PROPHYLACTIC TREATMENT

Beta-adrenergic blockers

Drug	Clinical use	Route/dosage	Nursing implications
Propranolol (Inderal)	Migraine Cluster headache	PO: 20 mg tid, can be gradually increased to 240 mg daily	Monitor pulse, blood pressure; side effects include fatigue, insomnia, and nausea

Serotonin antagonists

Drug	Clinical use	Route/dosage	Nursing implications
Methysergide maleate (Sansert)	Migraine Cluster headache	PO: 2-6 mg qd PO: 3-9 mg qd	Has serious pulmonary, cardiac, and renal side effects; to control, discontinue after 5 months; report immediately to physician urinary tract obstruction, dysuria, back pain, peripheral vascular insufficiency, cold, numb or painful extremities, dyspnea, chest pain, or decreased pulse

Antidepressants

Drug	Clinical use	Route/dosage	Nursing implications
Amitriptyline (Elavil)	Migraine Tension headache	PO: 50-75 mg qd	May experience dizziness, drowsiness, dry mouth, or weight gain
Imipramine (Tofranil)	Migraine	PO: 100 mg qd	
Doxepin (Sinequan)	Tension headache	PO: 25-50 mg qd	

TABLE 45-9   **Pharmacology Summary: Drugs Used for Headaches—cont'd**

Drug	Clinical use	Route/dosage	Nursing implications
Platelet antagonists			
Aspirin	Migraine	PO: 1300 mg qd in 2 to 4 doses	See above
Sulfinpyrazone (Anturane)	Migraine	PO: 200-400 mg qd initially, up to 200-800 mg qd	
Dipyridamole (Persantine)	Migraine	PO: 75-100 mg qd	Used in conjunction with aspirin
Monoamine oxidase inhibitor			
Phenelzine (Nardil)	Cluster headache	PO: 3-6 mg qd	Used in persons who cannot tolerate methysergide maleate
Calcium channel blockers			
Nifedipine (Procardia)	Migraine Cluster headache	PO: 10 mg tid initially, 10-20 mg tid	May decrease frequency and severity of migraine
Verapamil (Calan, Isoptin)	Migraine Cluster headache	PO: 80-120 mg tid initially, 240-480 mg tid	
Other			
Lithium carbonate	Used occasionally in cluster headache	PO: 900-1200 mg qd	Used when ergotamine, methysergide maleate, or prednisone is not successful

cular contraction headaches. A large group of these patients have a long record of emergency room visits for intramuscular injections to relieve the headaches. If anxiety is a predominant feature, mild tranquilization and a calm environment may help. If depression is predominant, an antidepressant such as amitriptyline (Elavil) or a psychic energizer such as imipramine (Tofranil) may be prescribed. Heat, massage, and muscle relaxation exercises are also useful. If muscular contraction headaches become severely disabling, biofeedback, behavioral modification, and psychiatric counseling may be recommended.

With degenerative neck disease heat, massage, a cervical collar, and antiinflammatory drugs are used. Indomethacin (Indocin) and phenylbutazone (Butazolidin) are often prescribed. Muscle relaxants may be tried.

With nonrecurrent headaches the medical goal is to remove the underlying disease or functional disturbance and to control the pain. Analgesia is used to control the pain while definitive treatment is initiated where possible.

With the postlumbar puncture headache, recumbency flat in bed affords relief. Use of a small gauge needle when performing the lumbar puncture helps to minimize leakage of cerebrospinal fluid, thereby reducing the intensity and duration of the headache.

In the case of the hypertensive headache, correction of the hypertension will alleviate the headache. Many physicians use an antihypertensive with a muscle relaxant such as diazepam (Valium) 5 mg bid, meprobamate (Miltown, Equanil) 200 mg tid, and chlordiazepoxide (Librium) 5 mg tid. Another regimen used when the patient is experiencing a morning headache is one capsule of sodium nitrite (30 mg), caffeine sodium benzoate (5 g), and acetophenetidin (6 g) or the caffeine in a cup of strong black coffee with acetylsalicylic acid. In the case of hypertensive encephalopathy (which is a medical emergency), the blood pressure must be lowered rapidly before the cerebral edema becomes irreversible.

In brain tumors, corticosteroids are used in gradually increasing dosages to control the cerebral edema and thus the head pain. With larger tumors and more cerebral edema, diuretics may be used to supplement the corticosteroids.

NURSING MANAGEMENT OF THE PATIENT WITH HEADACHES
Assessment

Nursing assessment related to headache should include the following:

1. Nature of pain—deep or superficial, severe or

mild, throbbing or aching, constant or intermittent
2. Location—focal or generalized, unilateral or bilateral, frontal or occipital
3. Incidence—frequency of attack, periodic or regular in appearance, age of onset
4. Duration and usual course of headache
5. Presence of associated ocular, neurologic, or systemic manifestations
6. Factors that may precipitate the headache (such as anxiety, changes in posture, ingestion of alcohol or medication)
7. Factors that aggravate the headache
8. Factors or agents that can be identified as providing relief
9. How incapacitating the head pain is

The nurse also assesses the presence and degree of nausea and vomiting, hydration status, and nutritional status. Patients with debilitating head pain may become very diaphoretic, further complicating the dehydration. A skin assessment also may be indicated. The presence and degree of anxiety and depression are assessed. The nurse investigates the influence the head pain is having on the patient's activities of daily living, role functions, and life-style as well as its influence on the family. The patient's and family's pattern of coping with the headache is also explored.

The nurse investigates possible abuse of ergots if a patient with frequent migraines or cluster headaches is found to have cold, pale, or even cyanotic extremities and experiences numbness and tingling sensations, especially of the hands and feet, without other supporting evidence for the existence of peripheral vascular disease.

Nursing Diagnosis

The predominant nursing diagnosis related to headache is pain. Etiologies for this nursing diagnosis are listed in Table 45-7. Other nursing diagnoses relevant to the aural symptoms in migraine and associated clinical manifestations may include:

Sensory/perceptual alterations: visual, tactile related to vasoconstriction
Altered thought processes related to pain, medication
Impaired physical mobility related to pain
Fluid volume deficit related to nausea and vomiting
Altered nutrition: less than body requirements related to nausea and vomiting
Self-care deficit related to nausea, vomiting, and pain
Anxiety related to pain, nausea, and vomiting
Sleep pattern disturbance related to pain, nausea, vomiting, and medication

Additional nursing diagnoses for the patient with headaches may include the following:

Knowledge deficit related to etiology, therapeutic regimens, control of side effects
Altered role performance related to pain and medication side effects
Ineffective individual coping related to potential or actual headache pain
Noncompliance related to therapeutic medication regimen

Planning

In the acute care setting the major immediate nursing goals for the patient with head pain are:

To control the head pain
To reduce the associated problems of nausea and vomiting
To reduce the patient's anxiety level

If the patient is acutely ill, additional goals include the following:

To restore fluid volume and electrolyte balance
To restore nutritional status

When the above goals have been met, long-term goals are set including:

To be in control of the head pain and associated symptoms
To reduce the influence of the head pain on activities of daily living, role functions, and life-style
To be in control of the anxiety
To reduce stressors or change personal responses to stressors

Long-term goals focus on the patient learning more effective coping strategies to deal with the head pain or situations that may help produce head pain.

Implementation

The patient admitted to an acute care setting because of head pain is initially placed on bed rest in a quiet, minimally stimulating environment. Lights, noise, activity, and visitors are minimized.

The pain, nausea, and vomiting should next be addressed by obtaining and giving appropriate pain and antinausea medications by the appropriate route. If nausea or vomiting is present, the patient is generally kept NPO until the nausea and vomiting subside.

Application of cold and massage may be instituted by the nurse while the patient is being reassured that all the measures taken will begin to provide relief, and the patient is further helped to relax.

If sleep is induced within the hospital setting, the patient's degree of nausea and vomiting determines whether the drug is given orally or intramuscularly.

Frequent assessment of the level of consciousness is then critical to ensure that the patient is not oversedated. The success of this therapy is totally a nursing responsibility since the medication must be held when the patient becomes unresponsive to loud calling or moderate shaking, yet administered before the patient becomes awake and alert.

If nausea and vomiting are present or the patient is placed NPO, dehydration can become a major nursing concern. Intravenous therapy can be helpful, although this is not always considered by the physician. If the patient is hospitalized, consideration should be given to this intervention.

In stress-related or depression-related tension-type headaches, nursing care is primarily concerned with providing reassurance and attention in addition to the above described nursing actions. Someone showing concern, empathy, and willingness to listen must accompany administration of analgesia. Some patients are relieved to find that the headache is not life-threatening and will respond positively to having the nature of the headache explained. Others refuse to even consider the possibility that the headache stems from anxiety or depression. The majority of patients with tension-type headaches lack full insight into the cause of the headache but respond to attention and concern. Often if given the opportunity, they will ventilate some of their feelings. This may provide the nurse with direction to help the patient begin to identify how to reduce stressors in the environment or how to begin to respond differently to stressors that cannot be eliminated.

The nursing care for the patient with both a migraine and tension-type headache is a combination of the nursing interventions for each type of headache. The patient must be helped to relax and verbalize but first must have pain relief from appropriate medication.

Nursing care for individuals with a nonrecurrent vascular headache should include administration of analgesia, provision of rest, maintenance of hydration, and nursing measures appropriate to eliminating the causative factors.

In headaches associated with intracranial tumors, nursing interventions are directed at providing relief of the head pain through analgesia, but the predominant nursing concern is preventing any increase in intracranial pressure that occurs (1) with any activity eliciting a Valsalva maneuver, (2) with any compression that occludes the venous drainage from the head, and (3) with level or Trendelenburg positioning of the head (see nursing care interventions under increased intracranial pressure).

In a patient whose headache is caused by hypertensive encephalopathy, vital signs must be monitored closely, and the patient's neurologic status frequently checked. If the headache recurs, the blood pressure should be checked immediately. If the hypertension precipitates a subarachnoid hemorrhage, the headache will become more intense and more prostrating.

Evaluation

The nurse evaluates the effectiveness of the therapeutic medical and nursing interventions in reducing the head pain and associated symptoms. If the nursing goals are being achieved, the regimen is continued until the head pain ceases or is at least back in the patient's control. If the regimen is not achieving the nursing goals, the medication or medical therapy should be manipulated until the desired results are obtained. The nurse monitors the patient's level of anxiety as the therapeutic interventions are put in place. If the anxiety level is not abating, further assessment as to why is needed. The anxiety source then needs to be eliminated, or the patient needs to be taught how to respond differently by using stress reduction strategies or relaxation exercises. An antianxiety agent (mild tranquilizer) may need to be prescribed. The nurse also evaluates the success of the rehydration and restoration of nutritional status until these goals are achieved. The outcome criteria are:

Pain control as evidenced by:
   Decrease in pain intensity score
   Report of decreased pain intensity
Nausea and vomiting control as evidenced by
   Report of decreased pain nausea
   Absence of vomiting
Normovolemia as evidenced by:
   Normal electrolytes
   Urinary output > 50 mL/hr
   Stable weight (less than 2 kg change from baseline)
Anxiety control as evidenced by:
   Report of decreased anxiety
   Decreased anxiety score
   Appearance of resting quietly

The nurse also evaluates the patient's learning of the knowledge and skills needed to manage the headache if it should recur. Learning to manage a recurring headache or to change one's response to stressors takes time and practice along with support and reinforcement from the nurse.

Long-term outcome criteria need to be individualized based on the cause of the head pain. They may include the following:

Pain control as evidenced by:
   Reduced episodes of head pain
   Ability to abort onset of head pain
   Ability to prevent nausea and vomiting
   Report of ability to control head pain
   Report of less anxiety about head pain episodes

Documentation

The nurse needs to document the assessment findings including nature of pain, location, frequency, duration and usual course, presence of associated manifestations, factors that aggravate headache, factors or agents that provide relief, and degree of incapacitation. Document the presence and degree of nausea and vomiting, amount of food and fluid taken in the last 24 hours, skin turgor and urine output, and presence and degree of diaphoresis. Additionally the nurse documents any positive or negative findings that may help the physician in the differential diagnosis such as blood pressure or flushed facies. The presence and degree of anxiety and/or depression are recorded. The nurse documents the influence of the headache on activities of daily living, role functions, and life-style as well as its impact on family and patterns of coping by the family. Nursing diagnoses, goals, and plans of care are always documented. The nurse then must document responses to the therapeutic medical and nursing interventions related to head pain control, nausea and vomiting control, and anxiety control. All teaching interventions with the information given and the skills taught are documented. The patient's ability to use the information or skill are is documented. Diagnostic tests and the patient's response to them are noted in the patient's health care record.

Ongoing Care

Long-term care/home care

The nurse may need to help the patient keep a headache diary for the physician to help with diagnosis or treatment (see box at right). The patient may also need to identify potential precipitating factors in the diet or the environment. Coffee, tea, cola, cheeses, chocolate, red wine or other alcoholic beverages, monosodium glutamate (often found in Chinese foods), cured meats, pickled herring, chicken livers, and canned figs have all been implicated in some patients with migraine. Bright lights, fatigue, fever, stress, and decreased estrogen, such as that experienced before the onset of menses or when taking the last birth control pills of the month, have induced migraine attacks in some patients.

The method of administration of the ergotamine preparation is critically important when providing nursing care to the patient who experiences migraines and when teaching the patient how to control the headaches. With Cafergot one or two tablets (as ordered) are taken immediately with the onset of the aural symptoms or the migraine. The dose is repeated every 30 minutes until the symptoms or the headache subside or until 6 mg of ergotamine is taken. More than 6 mg of ergotamine tartrate within 24 hours may result in ergot poisoning (ergotism).

EXAMPLE OF A HEADACHE DIARY

Location
Where is the pain?
Is the pain on one side or both sides?
Does the site of the pain move during the course of the headache?
Are your shoulders and neck involved?

Onset
Did the headache onset gradually or suddenly?
What were you doing when the head pain started?
Were there any warning signs before the pain onset?
Do you have any idea what might have caused the headache to start?
Is there anything unusual or stressful going on in your life?

Duration of Headache
Date and time of onset:
    Day of week:
Date and time headache stopped:
    Day of week:

Nature of Headache
What makes the headache worse?
What makes the headache better?
Are there any other symptoms associated with headache?

Other
Women

When did your last period begin?
When do expect your next period?
What symptoms do you experience with your periods?

Men and Women

Other comments you think are relevant.

A primary nursing responsibility is to reinforce the information the physician gives to help the patient with migraine understand and respect the drugs that are prescribed and recognize the possible consequences of drug abuse.

The nurse can reinforce this drug information while assessing the patient's management of the migraine and while reassessing the degree of migraine control afforded.

Rehabilitation

Formal rehabilitation for head pain is sometimes necessary when the patient has developed a chronic pain syndrome that is producing total disruption of the patient's and family's lives or problems with substance abuse of either pain medications, ergots, or alcohol. In these instances, the patient may need to be referred to an inpatient chronic pain facility or outpatient chronic pain clinic and placed under chronic pain management protocols.

CRITICAL THINKING QUESTIONS

1 Describe the clinical features of the various levels of consciousness.

2 How do breathing patterns, pupillary and motor responses, and ocular positioning and reflexes relate to levels of brain function?

3 How does the nurse prevent deconditioning and promote safety for the patient with an altered level of consciousness?

4 Relate the compensatory mechanisms for increased intracranial pressure to the therapeutic interventions used to decrease intracranial pressure.

5 What is the progression of clinical manifestations as intracranial pressure increases?

6 Describe the nursing interventions to reduce intracranial pressure.

7 Compare the clinical manifestations of generalized seizures and partial seizures.

8 Why is status epilepticus a medical emergency?

9 What is included in a teaching plan for a patient with seizures?

10 How do etiologic mechanisms that produce headaches relate to therapeutic strategies prescribed?

11 What is included in the nursing assessment of a patient with a headache?

RESOURCES

1 EPILEPSY FOUNDATION OF AMERICA Local Chapter of Epilepsy Foundation of America

2 VOCATIONAL REHABILITATION SERVICES

3 MENTAL HEALTH DEPARTMENT

4 SOCIAL SERVICES FOR MEDICAID, SSI

5 ADMINISTRATION OF DEVELOPMENT DISABILITIES Hubert H. Humphrey Building, Room 340 E. 200 Independence Ave., SW Washington, DC 20201

BIBLIOGRAPHY

Current

1. Andrus C: Intracranial pressure: dynamics and nursing management, *J Neurosci Nurs* 23:85, 1991.
2. Bes A et al: Classification and diagnostic criteria for head-ache disorders, cranial neuralgias and facial pain, *Cephalalgia* 8 (Suppl 7):9, 1988.
3. Cammermeyer M, Appeldorn C: *Core curriculum for neuroscience nurses*, Chicago, 1990, AANN.
4. Campbell VC: Effects of controlled hyperoxygenation and endotracheal suctioning on intracranial pressure in head-injured adults, *App Nurs Res* 4:138, 1991.
5. Daroff RB: New headache classification, *Neurology* 38:1138, 1988.
6. Dettbarn CL, Davidson LS: Pulmonary complications in the patient with acute head injury: neurologic pulmonary edema, *Heart Lung* 18:583, 1989.
7. Diamond S, Medina JL: Headaches, *Clinical Symposia* 41:2, 1989.
8. Dodson WE et al: Are you up-to-date on seizures? *Patient Care* 25:162, 1991.
9. Drummond BL: Preventing increased intracranial pressure: nursing care can make the difference, *Foc Crit Care* 17:116, 1990.
10. Engel JR: *Seizures and epilepsy*, Philadelphia, 1989, FA Davis.
11. Gallagher RM: Headache diagnosis and treatment, *A Am Acad Nurse Prac* 3:3, 1991.
12. Gasser PA: Creating a headache diary, *A Am Acad Nurse Prac* 3:53, 1991.
13. Germon K: Interpretation of ICP waves to determine intracranial compliance, *J Neurosci Nurs* 20:344, 1988.
14. Gilliam EE: Intracranial hypertension advances in intracranial pressure monitoring, *Crit Care Nurs Clin North Am* 2(1):21, 1990.
15. Grant JS: Altered level of consciousness: validity of a nursing diagnosis, *J Neurosci Nurs* 22:250, 1990.
16. Hall LT: Recovery from coma that results as a complication of cardiac arrest followed by cardiopulmonary bypass, *Heart Lung* 18:559, 1989.
17. Hendrickson SL: Intracranial pressure changes and family presence, *J Neuro Nurs* 19:14, 1987.
18. Hickey J: *The clinical practice of neurologic and neurosurgical nursing*, Philadelphia, 1992, JB Lippincott.
19. Hickman KM et al: Intracranial pressure monitoring: review of risk factors associated with infection, *Heart Lung* 19:84, 1990.
20. Hoff JT, Betz AL: *Intracranial pressure* VII, New York, 1989, Springer-Verlag.
21. Jess LW: Assessing your patient for increased ICP, *Nursing '87* 17(6):34, 1987.
22. Johnson SM et al: Effects of conversation on intracranial pressure in comatose patients, *Heart Lung* 18:56, 1989.
23. Latham CLP: Intracranial pressure monitoring part I: physiologic principles, *Crit Care Nurse* 7:40, 1987.
24. Lechtenberg R: *Seizure recognition and treatment*, New York, 1990, Churchill Livingstone.
25. Luchka S: Working with ICP monitors, *RN* 54(4):34, 1991.
26. March K et al: Effects of backrest position on intracranial and cerebral perfusion pressures, *J Neurosci Nurs* 22: 375, 1990.
27. Marshall SB et al: *Neuroscience critical care pathophysiology and patient management*, Philadelphia, 1990, WB Saunders.
28. McCance KL, Huether SE: *Pathophysiology: the biological basis for disease in adults and children*, St Louis, 1990, Mosby–Year Book.
29. North B, Reilly P: *Raised intracranial pressure: a clinical guide*, Oxford, 1990, Heinemann Medical Books.
30. O'Brien K: Managing the seizure patient, *Nursing '91* 21(1):63, 1991.

31. Parson LC, Kidd PS: Neurologic nursing research, *Annual Rev Nurs Res* 7:3, 1989.
32. Rauch ME et al: Validation of risk factors for the nursing diagnosis decreased intracranial adaptive capacity, *J Neurosci Nurs* 22:173, 1990.
33. Rise FC: *The management of headache*, New York, 1988, Raven Press.
34. Ropper AH, Martin JB: Coma and other disorders of consciousness. In Wilson JD et al, *Harrison's principles of internal medicine*, ed 12, New York, 1991, McGraw-Hill Book Co.
35. Sisson R: Effects of auditory stimuli on comatose patients with head injury, *Heart Lung* 19:373, 1990.
36. Walleck CA: Intracranial hypertension: interventions and outcomes, *Crit Care Nurs Quart* 10(1):45, 1987.
37. Whitney CM: New headache classification: implications for neuroscience nurses, *J Neurosci Nurs* 22:385, 1990.
38. Whitney CM, Daroff RB: An approach to migraine, *J Neurosci Nurs* 20:284, 1988.

Classic

39. Adams RD, Victor M: *Principles of neurology*, New York, 1985, McGraw-Hill Book Co.
40. Allen N: Prognostic indicators in coma, *Heart Lung* 8:1075, 1979.
41. Fishman RA: Brain edema, *N Engl J Med* 293:708, 1975.
42. Plum F, Posner F: *Diagnosis of stupor and coma*, Philadelphia, 1982, FA Davis.
43. Powner DJ et al: Brain death certification: a review, *Crit Care Med* 5:230, 1977.
44. Shapiro HM: Intracranial hypertension, *Anesthesiology* 43:445, 1975.
45. Spielman G: Coma: a clinical review, *Heart Lung* 10:700, 1981.
46. Walker AE: An appraisal of the criteria of cerebral death, *JAMA* 237:982, 1977.

CHAPTER FORTY-SIX

Nursing Management of Adults with Degenerative Disorders

LEARNING OBJECTIVES

1 Identify the physiologic and psychosocial principles underlying the medical and nursing regimens for the patient with a degenerative neurologic disorder.

2 Intervene effectively to support positive coping mechanisms used by the patient and family.

3 Provide patient and family education on diet, exercise, medications, and complications associated with degenerative diseases.

4 Support the patient's need for independence and safety.

5 Implement the nursing process for a patient and family with a degenerative neurologic disorder.

6 Identify changes in nursing interventions that occur as the patient moves from the initial to late stages of a degenerative disease.

7 Provide information about local and national resources for patients and families.

KEY TERMS

agnosia, p. 1250
Alzheimer's disease, p. 1246
amyotrophic lateral sclerosis (ALS), p. 1262
apraxia, p. 1250
bradykinesia, p. 1255
chorea, p. 1260

dementia, p. 1246
dyskinesia, p. 1258
Huntington's disease, p. 1260
Parkinson's disease, p. 1254
rigidity, p. 1255
syringomyelia, p. 1262

DEGENERATIVE NEUROLOGIC diseases include all illnesses in which the neuronal tissue and its supporting structures are destroyed. Continuous exposure to a pathologic process has been suggested as the underlying mechanism that severely affects some neurons and spares others. The most common illnesses include Alzheimer's disease, parkinsonism, Huntington's disease, syringomyelia, and amyotrophic lateral sclerosis.

Several explanations for the degenerative process have been given. The most popular current hypotheses point to environmental toxins, immunologic and viral processes, genetic protein defects, and endogenous factors such as premature aging. Recent advances in understanding nerve cell growth, regeneration, and transplantation of cellular tissue have exciting implications for neuronal tissue cell regeneration.

This discussion has been grouped according to the site of the principal pathologic change to simply describe the common clinical manifestations and anatomic correlates. The major categories are cerebrum, basal ganglia, and spinal cord.

Degenerative Disorders of the Cerebrum

Disorders of cerebral function affect the most vital human processes: thinking, creating, conversing, feeling, and moving.

ALZHEIMER'S DISEASE
Definition

Alzheimer's disease is the most common cause of **dementia,** a term used to describe a diffuse progressive loss of mental function because of an organic disturbance. Dementia can be differentiated from confusion—which affects attention and the speed, clarity, and amount of mental activity, and delirium—which consists of short-lived disorientation, restlessness, hyperirritability, fear, and hallucinations.[30]

Etiology/Epidemiology

The National Institute of Aging, Washington, DC, places the incidence of severe dementia at 50 per 100,000, with a prevalence of 250 per 100,000. It is estimated that some 1 million persons are affected. Alzheimer's disease accounts for 50% to 60% of cases of dementia. Other causes of intellectual deterioration and their frequency are described in Table 46-1.

The familial incidence of Alzheimer's disease ranges from 5% to more than 40% and often conforms to an autosomal dominant pattern.[7] Patients with Alzheimer's disease and Down's syndrome share similar pathologic changes in the brain, in addition to the gene defect identified in familial cases on chromosome 21. The gene that codes beta-amyloid precursor protein (β-APP) is also located on chromosome 21. β-APP is found in abnormally high concentrations in the brain of Alzheimer patients. It is believed that the build-up of amyloid, the development of the neurofibrillary tangles, and the changes in neurons such as decreased dendritic arborization contribute to the progressive intellectual decline seen in Alzheimer's disease. Senile plaques and neurofibrillary tangles have been linked to excess levels of aluminum, although this finding may be the result of nerve cell death. Loss of neuronal plasticity, along with abnormalities in protein oxidation and phosphorylation, have been reported and

TABLE 46-1 Potential Causes and Incidence of Dementia

Causes	Incidence (%)
UNTREATABLE, PROGRESSIVE DISORDERS	
Alzheimer's disease	50-60
Vascular disease	
Multiple infarct dementia	10-20
Infections	
Creutzfeldt-Jakob disease	1-5
Acquired immune deficiency syndrome	1
Degenerative disorders	
Pick's disease	1
Huntington's disease	1
Parkinsonism and other basal ganglion disorders	1-5
POTENTIALLY TREATABLE DISORDERS	
Neurosyphilis	<1
Drugs and toxins	
Alcohol, reserpine, opiates, barbiturates, bromides	1-5
Nutritional disorders	
Wernicke-Korsakoff syndrome	1-5
Niacin, folate, and vitamin B_{12} deficiencies	1
Metabolic disorders	
Cushing's syndrome, dialysis dementia, thyroid and hepatic disorders	1-5
Head injury and post-traumatic brain disorders	1-5
Normal pressure hydrocephalus	1-5
Intracranial masses such as tumors, subdural hematoma, brain abscess	1-5
Depression	1-5

Modified from Katzman R: Dementia. In Asbury A, McKhann G, McDonald W: *Diseases of the nervous system*, Philadelphia, 1992, Ardmore Medical.

may have implications for future treatment.[18] However, the exact cause of Alzheimer's disease is unknown.

Pathophysiology

Selective vulnerability of specific nerve cell populations has been identified in Alzheimer's disease. Typical pathologic changes associated with Alzheimer's disease involve neuron cell death and disruption of the neurotransmitter circuits, particularly

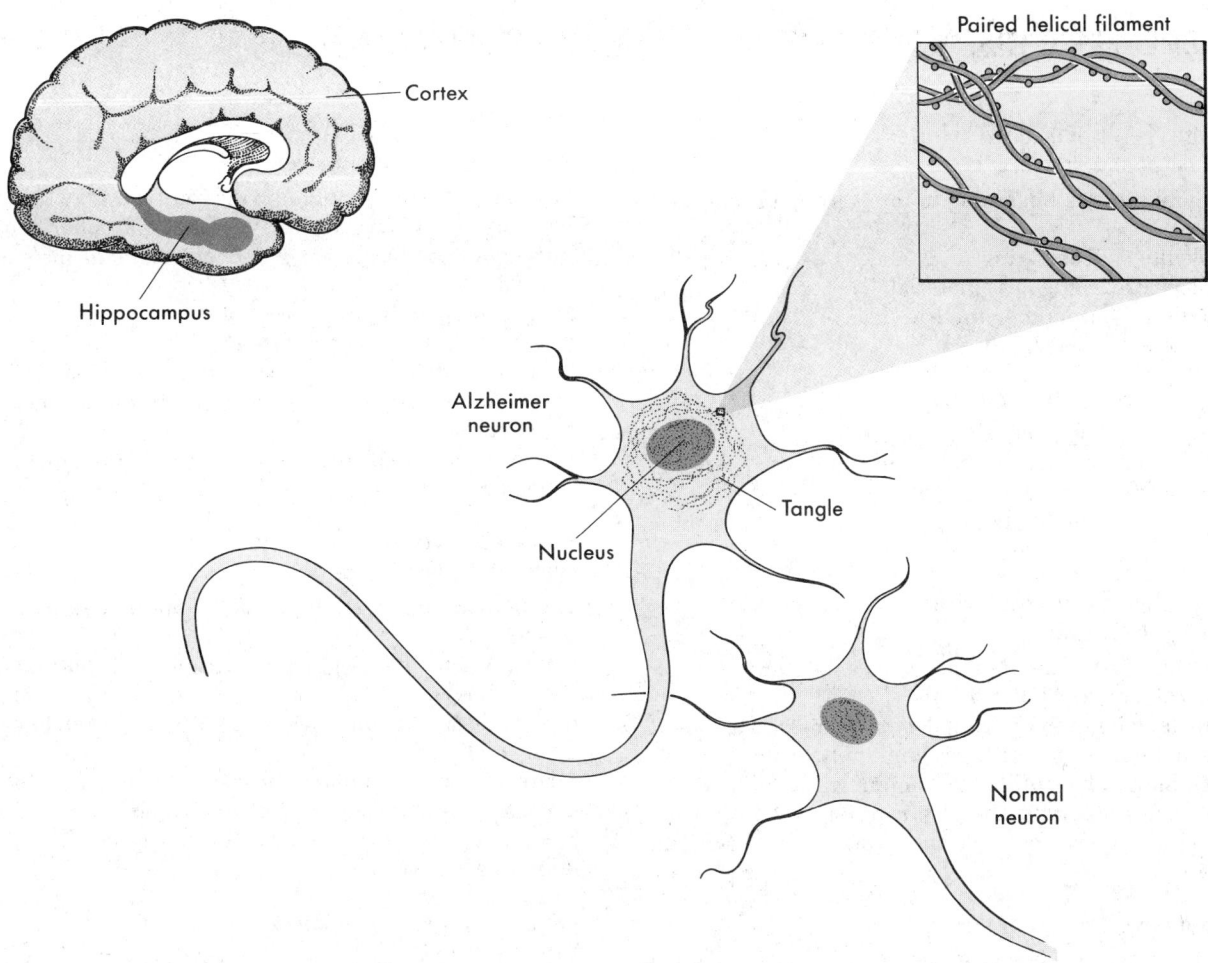

FIGURE 46-1   Common pathologic findings in Alzheimer's disease.

cholinergic neurons and the enzyme system. The most common pathologic findings are cerebral atrophy, senile plaques, and neurofibrillary tangles (see Figure 46-1). These changes are found primarily in the frontal (90% cell loss) and temporal (50% cell loss) cortex when compared with age-matched controls. The hippocampus, amygdala, brainstem nuclei, nucleus basalis, and locus ceruleus show similar changes both in cellular composition and neurotransmitter loss. The exact significance of these findings is unclear. The hippocampus is known to play a role in information processing, acquisition of new memories, and retrieval of information. The amygdala may contribute to the emotional, motivational, and associative abnormalities that occur. Dysphasia, apraxia, and visuospatial abnormalities correlate with defects in the temporoparietal area.[2]

Clinical Manifestations

Alzheimer's disease rarely develops before age 40. In the early stage, memory loss and carelessness in dress and conduct are noticed. Often performance on the job suffers and family tasks and responsibilities are neglected. As the disease progresses, the individual experiences speech problems, including slurring and difficulty in finding words, followed by nonsense talkativeness to a reduction in speech output to use of a few isolated words and phrases. Later, complete disorientation, restlessness, wandering, and failure to recognize friends and family occur.

The disease affects movement, leading to difficulty in ambulation, falling, generalized stiffness, and rigidity. In the final stages, the patient is bed bound and develops spastic paralysis and contractures. Pathologic reflexes can be elicited in persons with Alzheimer's disease, including snout, suck, root, and grasp reflexes in the middle to late stages. The duration of illness ranges from 1½ to 15 years; the average length of illness is 5 to 7 years. The stages of illness are described in the box on p. 1248. Evidence suggests that Alzheimer's disease (AD) may differ from patient to patient in the progressive

ALZHEIMER'S DISEASE: STAGES AND FAMILY STRESS RESPONSES

Stage 1—Early confusion
Observable behaviors

Forgetfulness is beginning to interfere with daily routine

Difficulty concentrating

Difficulty learning new material

Good days outnumber the bad days

Loss of empathy for others

Family expressions of stress

Where are your dirty clothes (or towels)?

When will you sort through your mail?

When will you balance the checkbook?

You seem to be in a fog today

Am I going out of my mind?

Stage 2—Late confusion
Observable behaviors

Gets lost easily in unfamiliar places

Recent memory shows decline

Forgets appointments, i.e., doctor, hair-dressers, etc.

Losing interest in world or community events

Beginning to have difficulty shopping

May refuse to admit anything is different

Covers behavior by accusing others—especially the family

Family expressions of stress

Where have you been? It has been 3 hours since you left to get groceries.

We don't have any electricity. Have you paid the bill?

This is the third dentist appointment you have missed.

We always watch the evening news before we eat, remember?

You forgot to bring home the ingredients I needed the most.

Why would I steal your dentures?

Either you are confused or I am going out of my mind.

Why do you feel the children are neglecting us? They were here on the weekend.

Stage 3—Early dementia
Observable behaviors

Goods days are less frequent

Confusion causes person to eat too much or too little food

Forgets names of grandchildren and friends

More easily frustrated

Difficulty following sequenced tasks, such as cooking a meal

Frequent repetition of particular subjects or stories

Has trouble word finding

May wander

Family expressions of stress

I would rather go shopping with you than play bridge.

You can't be hungry again. We just ate an hour ago.

How could you forget our grandson's name is the same as yours?

I can't do anything to please you.

You burned the oatmeal, again!

If I hear that story one more time, I will scream.

The Golden Gate Bridge used to be in San Francisco, remember?

Where have you been? I have searched the neighborhood for you.

Stage 4—Middle dementia
Observable behaviors

The person no longer can be alone and needs supervision

Difficulty with bathing; cannot accomplish bath alone or refuses

In the middle of a task question: "What are we doing?"

Easily distracted

Made anxious if too many things are happening at once

Outbursts of fear, anger, and frustration

Sleep patterns change—may mix nights and days

Follows caregiver around constantly

Family expressions of stress

Who said these were the golden years?

I don't have a moment of peace.

Another word for bath is fight.

I just told you 2 minutes ago, we are making cookies.

You never follow my directions.

You are just plain stubborn.

I am exhausted. I need sleep even if you don't. Come to bed.

I have a shadow everywhere I go. Good thing there is a lock on the bathroom door.

Stage 5—Middle-middle dementia
Observable behaviors

Needs assistance in everything he or she does

Words no longer identified with their meaning

Difficulty in walking, rising from a chair, and standing

Poor judgment in where to put body parts as in sitting

Incontinence of urine and sometimes stool

Language becomes more incomprehensible

Family expressions of stress

I never knew someone could be this tired and still be awake.

If you don't behave, I'll put you in a nursing home. Is that what you want?

Stages of Alzheimer's disease and observable behaviors from Blondin M: *Alzheimer disease stages,* Alzheimer's Information and Support Service, 517 N Segoe Road, Madison, Wis, 1988.

ALZHEIMER'S DISEASE: STAGES AND FAMILY STRESS RESPONSES—cont'd

I don't want to be a burden to our friends or family.

I am tired and weak all over. This ache in my lower back never goes away.

I don't have time to see a doctor for myself.

What came over me? My anger scared me. If I had pushed harder he might have fallen and broken something.

I have tried using diapers but I still find messes in unusual places.

I feel like no one understands me.

Why do I feel like crying all the time?

I cannot afford to put her in the nursing home.

Stage 6—Late stage of dementia
Observable behaviors

Person must be fed

Incontinent

Communicates nonverbally all the time

Susceptible to pneumonia and complications as a result of immobility

Family expressions of stress

I worry because he has lost so much weight. Every bite is a struggle.

People with AD are like overgrown babies.

When the nursing home uses up all our money, what will I live on?

I wish I knew if she knows who I am.

I am not sure my visit to the nursing home makes a difference.

This AD is not living, it is existing.

He is the shell of the person I used to know.

---

nature of the symptoms. The patient who develops AD in middle age and has aphasia usually develops a more rapidly progressive course.

The characteristic history of insidious onset and steady progression can be elicited during the history and patient biography. Often a family member is needed to corroborate the history. The physical examination, along with laboratory tests, will give the diagnosis further support. Potentially treatable causes of dementia (Table 46-1) are ruled out by computed tomographic (CT) or magnetic resonance imaging (MRI) scans, lumbar puncture, and serum tests. CT or MRI scans eliminate possibilities such as vascular or space-occupying lesions. The presence of cerebral atrophy can be seen in normal aging and is not a definitive finding. Recent studies with positron emission tomography (PET) confirm that there is widespread hypometabolism.[18] Cisternography may be necessary to exclude normal pressure hydrocephalus, if CT scans reveal enlarged ventricles. Lumbar puncture is needed to exclude meningeal processes such as syphilis. Blood tests such as the Venereal Disease Research Laboratories (VDRL) test, thyroid function screening, serum chemistry levels, B_{12} levels, liver function tests, and blood cell counts help exclude other treatable conditions. Other tests include chest and skull films, electroencephalography, and neuropsychologic screening tests. The definitive diagnosis can only be made by observing pathologic changes in the brain at autopsy.

Therapeutic Management

Care of the patient with Alzheimer's disease is primarily symptomatic and supportive. The patient and family will require a close relationship with care providers to monitor symptoms and develop strategies to cope with the progressive nature of the illness. Symptoms such as depression and sleep disorders are carefully evaluated at each visit. Pharmacotherapy for these disorders is one of the few treatment options available. Medications for constipation and attention to skin care and home equipment (e.g., wheelchairs, the bedside commode, an alternating pressure mattress, and a hospital bed) should be provided to ease the caregiver burden when the patient becomes immobile.

Supportive care consists of counseling, planning, and education that includes the patient and family. The anticipated stages of illness should be outlined and the symptoms explained. Supportive techniques to decrease stress and reduce the family burden should be discussed. Specific diets and exercise have shown no benefit in halting the disease process, but should be kept at consistent levels to prevent further complications. Day treatment and respite for spouses is an important aspect of care. Support groups for families are available in many communities. Long-term care is usually necessary in the final stages of the illness.

Drugs such as lecithin, tacine/THA, arecoline, and physostigmine have been studied in an attempt to compensate for the loss of neurotransmitters but have shown no benefit. Clinical trials with nimopidine, a calcium channel blocker, and L-deprenyl, a MAO-B and antioxidant, have been identified as having potential positive treatment effects.[13] Surgical procedures such as ventricular shunting have not prevented further symptom progression.

NURSING MANAGEMENT OF THE PATIENT WITH ALZHEIMER'S DISEASE
Assessment

Assessment of the patient will vary depending on the setting or the stage of the illness. If the patient requires hospitalization, it is usually for an acute episode of a problem unrelated to dementia. Treatment of a medical-surgical condition, a fall, or pneumonia are the most common. The diagnosis and ongoing care of the patient with Alzheimer's disease is often conducted in the outpatient unit.

The nurse must determine the patient's stage of illness. The mental status examination, including attention span, memory, orientation, intellectual ability, abstract thinking, judgment, and language ability, should be interwoven throughout the interview to reduce threat or embarrassment. The presence of **apraxia** (inability to perform voluntary acts) and **agnosia** (inability to recognize stimuli) is noted. The results of more in-depth neuropsychologic testing may also provide information for a data base. Motor ability and the ability to perform self-care tasks such as bathing, dressing, feeding, and toileting are recorded. The nurse uses the family's input to document information about the history and the patient's home routines. The presence of constipation and other health problems is discussed. Other aspects of the physical assessment include measures related to nutritional status, such as appetite, weight, and swallowing ability. Examination of the skin and recording of sleep habits are included.

The family's response to the patient's care needs and ability to plan for future needs should be ascertained. The family's understanding of the progression of Alzheimer's disease, informative resources, and long-term care needs are important parts of the assessment.

Nursing Diagnosis

Nursing diagnoses related to the stages of illness include the following:

Impaired verbal communication related to memory loss, expressive and receptive language disorder, and reduced attention span

Altered thought processes related to short-term memory loss and reduced ability to tolerate frustration

Self-care deficit related to apraxia, reduced attention span, fatigue, memory loss, and impaired planning ability

Altered nutrition: less than body requirements related to dysphagia and difficulty handling complex tasks

High risk for injury related to unsteady gait, reduced memory and judgment, apraxia, and fatigue

Sleep pattern disturbance related to fragmentation of diurnal rhythms and sleep-cycle disturbances

Ineffective family coping related to isolation and lack of knowledge, resources, and support

Knowledge deficit related to the patient and family's need to learn information about the illness and new methods of interaction

Planning

In determining the goals for a patient with Alzheimer's disease, it is important to know the stage of illness (see box on p. 1248). Setting short-term goals helps prevent overwhelming family resources and provides an immediate sense of achievement. Appropriate goals include the following:

Patient uses an effective two-way communication system to meet needs appropriate for the stage of illness

Patient demonstrates thinking processes that are consistent with the stage of illness

Patient participates as well as possible in normal activities, such as hygiene, meals, toileting, and dressing

Patient ingests sufficient nutrients to maintain weight and has sufficient energy to accomplish daily activities

Patient lives in a safe environment that fosters cognitive and functional abilities

Patient achieves adequate rest and does not experience undue fatigue

Family explains coping strategies to deal with the physical and mental stress of caring for a person with Alzheimer's disease

Patient (to the best of his or her abilities) and family demonstrate an understanding of the illness and treatment efforts

Implementation

The treatment plan is dictated by the stage of illness and disease manifestations. The essential feature of care is a creative approach to maintaining functional independence for as long as possible while dealing with change and loss of motor and intellectual abilities. In the early stages of illness, avoiding fatigue, overstimulation, and relying on routines to keep the patient active seem to provide support.[9] Mnemonic devices such as calendars, clocks, posted schedules, and notebooks with specific references seem to enhance memory. Familiar surroundings and people are a source of constant reassurance. Changing circumstances and schedules should be attempted slowly.

Providing simple explanations and allowing sufficient time for verbalization reduce frustration in communication. Relaying one idea or question in a sentence of 3 to 5 words is helpful. The patient may respond more readily to voice tone, gestures, or facial expression than content. Using nonverbal forms of communication, touch, and good listening skills are all necessary for the nurse to communicate effectively with these patients. Communication problems may cause bowel and bladder difficulties because the patient may not communicate toileting needs or remember where the bathroom is.

Catastrophic reactions can occur in stages 2 and 3 when the patient becomes frustrated, anxious, depressed, angry, or uncooperative. Recognizing that fatigue and schedule changes can induce catastrophic reactions will allow caregivers to manage the environment and prevent dysfunctional behavior. The schedule is kept routine and simple. Environmental changes should be minimal.

Monitoring weight, dysphagia, and diet help meet nutritional needs; however, avoid forcing meals or mealtimes. Meals provided in calm surroundings without distractions are helpful. Early in the disease, patients may have increased activity and eat larger quantities of food. Later, as the patient forgets how to chew and swallow, assistance at meals may become necessary.

Sleep problems and falls are common in confused patients. Fatigue, pain, toileting needs, darkness, fear, and isolation are factors in the development of sleeplessness and increased agitation at night, also called sundowning. Methods to reduce these problems include assessment of contributing factors, avoiding fatigue, arranging for someone to stay with the patient, and ensuring a safe environment.[23] Sedatives are avoided if possible because some further alter rapid eye movement sleep cycles. Falling or injury as a result of gait changes and altered sensory perception may become worse at night when poor vision and lighting contribute to confusion. Nursing problems and interventions are detailed further in the discussion on the care plan.

An estimated two thirds of patients with Alzheimer's disease live at home with the family as primary care providers. Research has pointed to the extensive burden this disease places on caregivers. Chronic fatigue, anger, and depression have been reported in 87% of caregivers.[9] Many families are afraid to leave the patient alone and assist the patient in daily activities. Teaching the family such basics as bathing, assisted feeding, and toileting may be helpful in the late stages of the illness.[20] Reviewing the daily routine for sources of stress that can be alleviated may avoid problems.

Evaluation

A successful plan of care enables the patient and family to cope with the stresses of the illness and the impact of hospitalization. Continual assessment allows the nurse to evaluate plans designed to maintain an effective communication system, participate in meeting self-care needs, maintain a stable body weight, avoid injury, and promote adequate rest. Family members will evidence behaviors that show that they are coping with the patient's illness and verbalize an understanding of the disease process and treatment plan.

Documentation

The nurse documents the patient's reactions to stressors if the patterns can be altered. Records of elimination and intake are helpful to monitor weight loss and constipation. Sleep records and behaviorally based flowsheets can provide information to develop interventions that reduce sleep and dysfunctional behavior-related problems. Documentation of family teaching is essential to promote continuity. The patient's response to pharmacotherapy for sleep, dysfunctional behavior, and depression are recorded as well.

Ongoing Care

In the final stages of Alzheimer's disease many families are forced to choose nursing home placement because of the burden of care. Some communities have specialized long-term care units for Alzheimer's patients. The decision for nursing home placement is difficult and is almost always made late in the course of the illness, although planning in anticipation of its need should occur 1 to 2 years in advance.

Home care

Early in the illness education regarding course of illness and activities is necessary. Outpatient nurses, nurse educators with the local Alzheimer's disease chapter, and members of support groups are helpful to families as they cope in the early stages of illness. Later, adult day health (ADH) services are also helpful in the confused and early dementia patient (stages 2, 3, and 4). Care at home is enhanced by the support of nursing and home care aides to assist the family in everyday tasks. Nurses in ADH settings and community health nurses and social workers can provide support and information regarding home care and nursing home placement. The nursing care plan (see box) should be individualized to each patient and reviewed with home care aides at frequent intervals.

NURSING CARE PLAN   *Patient with Alzheimer's Disease*

Nursing Diagnosis/ Expected Outcome	Interventions	Rationale
Impaired verbal communication related to memory loss, expressive and receptive language disorder, and reduced attention span • *Effective two-way communication system meets patient's needs throughout stages of illness*	Enhance verbal communication by slow, calm approach; reducing unnecessary and uninformative background noise; and speaking slowly and simply Use yes/no questions when possible; state facts and be clear Give patient ample time to respond (1 to 2 min), then repeat question	Soothing environment and approach allow patients to pay attention to speaker, not background With reduced memory and attention span, patient needs clarity and brevity to increase chances of responding Increases possibility of response
Altered thought processes related to short-term memory loss and reduced ability to tolerate frustration • *Existing abilities are strengthened and optimal behavior patterns maintained to achieve highest level of independent function possible*	Provide orientation cues in environment (e.g., clock, calendar, easily read labels with name and place) Signal meals by chimes, bedtime by dimming lights or music; mark room and belongings with similar symbol or color Provide orienting information in normal conversations Promote old associations from past, discussing past events and familiar objects, photos from home Develop routines and post daily schedule that has flexibility to accommodate needs	Cues make use of remaining skills to promote reality Appropriate physical cues enhance orientation and environmental stability Verbal reminders can reduce stress of recalling information, yet continuous reminders of memory loss may increase anxiety and frustration Makes use of remaining cognitive abilities and promotes sense of individuality Consistency reduces environmental demands that can increase dysfunctional behavior patterns
Self-care deficit related to apraxia, reduced attention span, fatigue, memory loss, and impaired planning ability • *Develop plans that meet self-care needs yet provide for patient dignity and independence*	Break down tasks into individual steps; give specific instructions with each step If patient is uncooperative, leave and try later; allow sufficient time for tasks Plan fatiguing activities in morning	Simple consistent routine reduce stress and promotes automatic responses; patient's planning ability is often impaired, making supervision necessary Rushing and forcing activity increase stress Cooperation is enhanced when patient is rested
Altered nutrition: less than body requirements related to dysphagia and difficulty handling complex tasks • *Sufficient nutrients will be ingested to maintain weight and energy to accomplish activities*	Allow self-feeding and use of hands; patient may need to be fed in later stages Provide verbal and nonverbal cues at mealtimes; for example, place utensils in patient's hand, ring chimes to announce mealtime Provide for privacy and restful surroundings during meals; allow sufficient time Assist with selection of well-balanced meals that have adequate calories, fiber, and fluids	Fosters independence Automatic performance of tasks reduces stress of focusing on task Soothing environment reduces stress; patient's attention span is reduced by competing stimuli Poor planning and memory impair patient's ability to select balanced diet; choices can increase frustration

NURSING CARE PLAN   *Patient with Alzheimer's Disease—cont'd*

Nursing Diagnosis/ Expected Outcome	Interventions	Rationale
	If patient is agitated, delay meal or provide snacks that can be easily handled	Forcing behavior never works if patient is agitated
	Avoid caffeine and alcoholic beverages	Stimulants can increase agitation
High risk for injury related to unsteady gait, reduced memory and judgment, apraxia, and fatigue	Reduce environmental hazards: clear hallways of clutter, remove breakable and dangerous objects, and keep bed in low position, locked in place	Poor judgment, communication, and gait disturbance make patient prone to injury; environmental support and modifications are key interventions
• Patient will be protected in a safe environment that fosters existing cognitive and functional abilities	If wandering is a problem, reduce access to dangerous areas (bathroom, medication area); lock exits; label clothing; use identification bracelet	Patient may not be able to identify self or home; wandering may be effective tension release for some, expression of boredom and anxiety for others
	Dress should be appropriate to environment (coat if chilly) and fit properly (shoes, clothing) to prevent trips and slips	Confusion and poor planning and judgment may cause wandering and carelessness with dress
	If falls are a problem, patient may need bedside alarm; staff may need to place mattress on floor, make frequent rounds, and continue to assess for further risks	Safety is the primary objective
	Use restraint only when injury is unavoidable; present restraints calmly, explain need frequently and fully to patient and family	Restraints increase agitation; reduced attention span and memory make frequent explanations mandatory
	Have someone stay with patient if agitated	Patient may not communicate needs, but may act impulsively, adding to risk of injury
	Teach family techniques to protect patient in home environment; lock up medications; restrict use of stove, matches, and cigarettes; remove clutter and rugs that cause falls; assess driving ability	Keep the environment consistent with patient's abilities; too much or too little restriction or support can increase problems or frustrate limited abilities
Sleep pattern disturbance related to fragmentation of diurnal rhythms and sleep-cycle disturbances	Encourage daily rest period	Fosters routine that minimizes stress and dysfunctional behaviors
• Patient has adequate rest and does not experience undue fatigue or injury	Provide morning nap or rest period if reduced rapid-eye-movement sleep is suspected	Morning naps simulate rapid-eye-movement sleep, loss of which can increase restlessness
	Provide afternoon nap or rest period if end-of-day fatigue occurs	Fatigue increases agitation and anxious behaviors; institutions should accommodate reduced sleep requirement of elderly
	Develop bedtime routine, reviewing day's activities and other cues such as brushing teeth or donning sleep clothes	Routine helps automatic functioning
	Avoid strenuous activity late in day	Excess activity can increase agitation and fatigue

Continued.

NURSING CARE PLAN   *Patient with Alzheimer's Disease—cont'd*

Nursing Diagnosis/ Expected Outcome	Interventions	Rationale

Ineffective family coping related to isolation and lack of knowledge, resources, and support
 	
• *Family expresses positive coping strategies to deal with physical and mental stresses of caring for their loved one as illness progresses*
	Provide time for family to vent frustration, fear, and anxiety
	Give family factual information about methods that enhance patient care:
	  Use of consistent routine
	  Environmental and safety supports
	  Modified social activity
	  Avoidance of fatigue and overstimulation
	  Basic techniques for activities of daily living and body mechanics
	Introduce family to community resources early; encourage family to share their burdens with other members, professionals, and home care personnel
	Encourage family to plan for their future needs; financial and estate planning, nursing home applications, and hospice
	Reinforce teaching efforts
		Emotional support and validation of this experience enhance coping
		Problem solving and factual information to reduce demands and frustration help maintain patient in home
		
		Fatigue and increased sensory stimuli increase patient agitation
		
		Arrange respite care early in illness to incorporate it into routine
		
		Late in course of illness family may be overwhelmed by demands of caregiver role and unable to make realistic decisions

Degenerative Diseases of the Basal Ganglia

Degenerative diseases that affect the basal ganglia are of two types: those associated with reduced movement and those associated with excessive movement.

PARKINSON'S DISEASE
Definition

Parkinson's disease, or parkinsonism, is defined by the presence of specific motor dysfunctions that include resting tremor, bradykinesia, rigidity, and loss of postural reflexes. These findings reflect a syndrome of nerve cell loss in the basal ganglia and related neuronal groups, as well as neurotransmitter deficiencies.

Etiology/Epidemiology

The incidence of Parkinson's disease is 20 per 100,000, with a prevalence of 187 per 100,000. This disease is believed to affect up to 1% of the population over age 50. The symptoms begin between ages 40 and 70, with peak onset at age 60. It is rarely seen before age 30. Men are affected slightly more frequently than are women. Morbidity is normal for age since the advent of levodopa therapy.

Genetic and viral factors have not been clearly delineated in the etiology of parkinsonism. Endogenous factors are believed to be responsible, because dopamine-containing neurons are progressively lost with age and are increasingly vulnerable to toxins. The study of environmental toxins, such as the "designer drug" MPTP, has led to new avenues of therapy. The neurotoxicity of MPTP can be blocked by monoamine oxidase (MAO) inhibitors. Current research focuses on the toxicity of naturally occurring oxidants, free radicals, and endogenous defects in enzyme systems.[6] Trials with the MAO inhibitor drug selegiline (Eldapryl) slow the course of parkinsonism and are an important application of this research.[15]

Pathophysiology

Understanding the extrapyramidal motor system, particularly the neurotransmitter connections between the substantia nigra and the basal ganglia

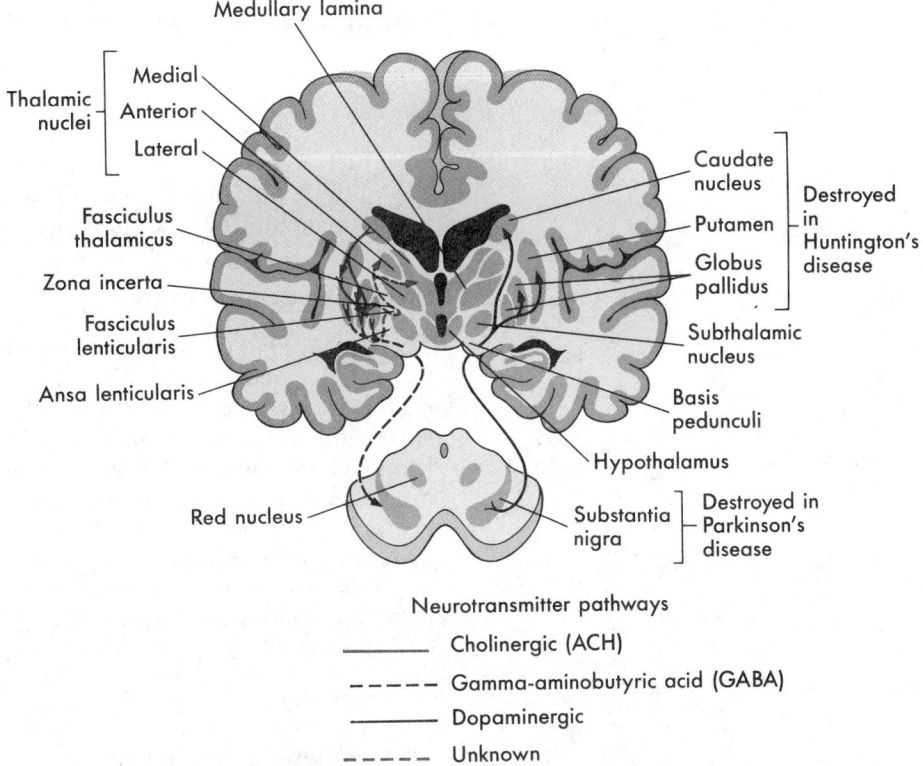

Medullary lamina

Thalamic nuclei
- Medial
- Anterior
- Lateral

Fasciculus thalamicus

Zona incerta

Fasciculus lenticularis

Ansa lenticularis

Red nucleus

Caudate nucleus
Putamen
Globus pallidus

Destroyed in Huntington's disease

Subthalamic nucleus

Basis pedunculi

Hypothalamus

Substantia nigra

Destroyed in Parkinson's disease

Neurotransmitter pathways

——— Cholinergic (ACH)

– – – – Gamma-aminobutyric acid (GABA)

——— Dopaminergic

– – – – Unknown

FIGURE 46-2   Common pathologic findings in parkinsonism.

(corpus striatum), has led to knowledge of the pathophysiologic defect in parkinsonism (see Figure 46-2). This system integrates the activity of many structures to control the performance of motor function, posture, muscle tone, coordination, and automatic movements. The neurotransmitters dopamine, acetylcholine (ACh), and gamma-aminobutyric acid are found in the corpus striatum of the basal ganglia.

The pathologic process of parkinsonism consists of a loss of the pigmented cells in the substantia nigra and depletion of the monoamine neurotransmitter dopamine. Reduced dopamine input from the substantia nigra to the corpus striatum leads to loss of the inhibitory modulation of dopamine on the striatum and increased dominance of ACh (solid line in Figure 46-2). ACh has an excitatory effect on the neuron. The imbalance between dopamine and ACh results in increased tonic activity of the alpha-motor neurons, which produces resistance to passive stretch, rigidity, and bradykinesia. It has been calculated that the dopamine level in the striatum must be reduced to 20% of normal before symptoms of parkinsonism develop.[6]

Clinical Manifestations

The characteristic motor symptoms of parkinsonism are the presence of one or more of the following: ri-

gidity, bradykinesia, resting tremor, and loss of postural reflexes. **Rigidity,** an intense muscular stiffness, is present in all directions of passive range of motion and active movement. The resistance encountered with rigidity resembles that found when bending a lead pipe, and a "cogwheel" halting character when tremor is present.

Bradykinesia, or slowness of body movement, has many facets and is believed to be the most difficult symptom to treat. It affects many automatic or stereotypical behaviors such as blinking, swallowing, changes in facial expression, and arm swing and can progress to total akinesia, or lack of movement. With more complex activities, including accomplishing two tasks at once (such as talking and walking), akinesia may occur.

Tremor usually occurs in the distal part of the extremities and is present at rest and diminished with active movement. Loss of postural reflexes, including loss of the postural righting reflex, is another clinical manifestation of parkinsonism. When patients are moved from their center of gravity, they are easily propelled backward (retropulsion) or forward (propulsion). This reflex loss, coupled with the flexed postural deformity seen in parkinsonism, often results in the shuffling "festination" gait in which the patient moves faster to keep the center of gravity balanced.[15]

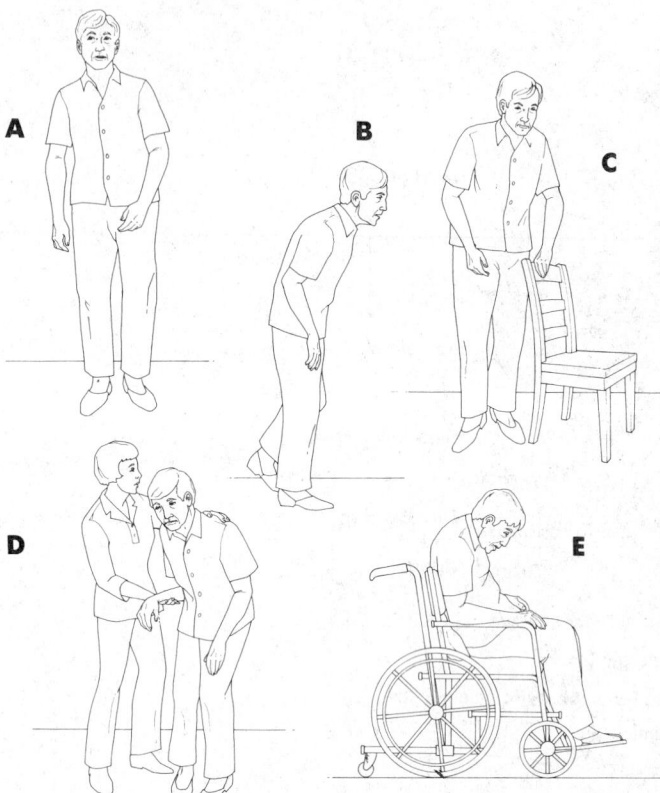

FIGURE 46-3 Stages of parkinsonism. **A,** Flexion of affected arm. Patient leans toward the unaffected side. **B,** Slow shuffling gait. **C,** Patient has increased difficulty walking and looks for sources of support to prevent falls. **D,** Further progression of weakness. Patient requires assistance from another person for ambulation. **E,** Profound disability. Patient may be confined to a wheelchair because of increasing weakness.

The illness begins slowly and may go unnoticed until tremor appears. The five stages of the illness are shown in Figure 46-3. Parkinsonism initially involves only one side of the body, then later progresses to involve both sides. Diminished cognitive functioning, with bradyphrenia (slowness of thinking), memory impairment, and visuospatial imperceptions may occur. Other manifestations include drooling; dysphagia; rapid, slurred, or soft speech; constipation; and urinary frequency. Depression has been identified in more than 40% of patients and dementia in 15%. Anxiety disorders also commonly increase with age.

The diagnosis is based on the clinical features. The history, electroencephalogram, CT or MRI scans, and serum tests (serum copper/ceruloplasmin, complete blood cell and differential counts, and serum chemistry analyses) are helpful in identifying treatable causes of the symptoms.

Therapeutic Management

The most effective symptomatic treatment for parkinsonism continues to be anticholinergics and dopaminergic and dopamine-agonist preparations. Attention to diet and exercise are necessary to keep the patient healthy. Detection of other chronic illnesses which affect life quality is also important.

Protective drug therapy

The use of selegiline (Eldepryl) as protective therapy for the neurons involved in Parkinson's disease (PD) is the second revolution in PD therapy. The first revolution was the use of L-dopa.[15] Treatment with Eldepryl can be started as soon as the diagnosis is made. There is rarely a need for symptomatic therapy at this point (see below). Use of Eldepryl has delayed the time until L-dopa is needed by 50%. There are few side effects to Eldepryl (see Table 46-2). However, when the symptoms interfere with ADL and lead to disability, symptomatic therapy is initiated.

Symptomatic drug therapy

The patient may receive anticholinergics and amantadine (Symmetrel) when the symptoms are mild. The anticholinergics have potential side effects, such as urinary retention, memory impairment, disorientation, and hallucinations, which makes them difficult to use in older patients. The anticholinergics reduce symptoms by approximately 20%. Amantadine induces the release of dopamine from storage sites, serving as an indirect dopamine-agonist, and has some weak anticholinergic effects.

The next most commonly used medications are the dopaminergics: levodopa (L-dopa) and carbidopa/levodopa (Sinemet). L-dopa has been associated with many side effects and has largely been replaced by the use of carbidopa/levodopa. Levodopa, the dopamine precursor, can cross the blood-brain barrier, whereas dopamine cannot. Once in the brain it is metabolized into dopamine, which is then picked up by the receptors in the striatum. Carbidopa has alleviated the severe side effects of dopamine (hypotension, gastrointestinal [GI] upset) by blocking its peripheral degradation.

Direct-acting dopamine agonists, such as bromocriptine mesylate (Parlodel), and more recently pergolide, have been clinically tested. These drugs mimic the effects of dopamine at the striatal receptors. The side effects are the same as those for L-dopa preparations. Some clinicians advocate adding bromocriptine mesylate early in the treatment phase before using carbidopa/levodopa. Table 46-2 includes the common drugs, dosages, and side effects used in the management of parkinsonism.

TABLE 46-2 Pharmacology Summary: Parkinson's Disease Symptomatic and Protective Therapy

Drugs	Total dosage*	Side effects	Nursing actions
PROTECTIVE THERAPY			
Selegiline hydrochloride (Eldepryl)	5 mg 1-2 times/day	Do not exceed 10 mg/day. SE: orthostatic hypotension, other CNS, CV, GI + GU problems, dystonia, headache, pain, sexual dysfunction, rashes	Patient and family teaching regarding actions and side effects. Explain dosage and stress not to exceed prescribed amount. Teach to rise slowly from lying and sitting position to reduce hypotensive effects.
SYMPTOMATIC THERAPY ANTICHOLINERGICS			
Benztropine (Cogentin) Biperiden (Akineton) Trihexyphenidyl (Artane) Ethopropazine (Parsidol)	0.5-4 mg, 1-2 times/day 2-8 mg, 3-4 times/day 1-4 mg, 3-4 times/day 30-50 mg, 3-5 times/day	Similar for all anticholinergics: dry mouth, mydriasis, blurry vision, constipation, urinary retention, confusion, mental impairment	Suggest mouth care, increased fluids, sugarless gum and lozenges. Review side effects to report: urinary retention, reduced visual acuity, confusion, heat prostration. Review methods to reduce constipation (fluids/fiber in diet), orthostatic hypotension (rising slowly). Caution the patient never to discontinue the medication suddenly because toxic effects can occur. Advise the patient to have yearly ophthalmic examinations to detect glaucoma.
DOPAMINERGICS			
Levodopa (L-dopa)	500 mg-5 g, 3-5 times/day	Nausea, hypotension	Teach patients to recognize side effects and signs of underdosage and overdosage of medication. Do not discontinue the drug suddenly.
Carbidopa/ levodopa (Sinemet)	10/100, 215/250, 25/100 3-7 times/day	Psychiatric symptoms, hypokinesia, hyperkinesia. Most side effects are dose-related	
DOPAMINE AGONISTS			
Bromocriptine (Parlodel)	2.5-7.5 mg, 2-5 times/day	Similar to L-dopa (i.e., CNS, CV, GI, and CTU problems), more expensive	Report all untoward symptoms.
PERGOLIDE MESYLATE			
(Permax)	3 mg/day (gradually increased)	Similar to L-dopa (nausea, hypotension)	Report all symptoms. • Take medication with food. • Change position slowly.
OTHER			
Amantadine (Symmetrel)	50-100 mg, 2 times/day	Similar to L-dopa (see above) Lower extremity edema Protects from influenza Insomnia if taken in evening	Report all symptoms. Patient teaching: • Avoid sudden position changes. • Do not discontinue suddenly. • Take medication with food.

Modified from Snyder M, editor: *A guide to neurological and neurosurgical nursing*, New York, 1983, John Wiley & Sons.
*Divided dose, individualized.

After long-term use of dopaminergics (>5 years) and with the progression of parkinsonism, the patient responds less predictably to drug therapy. Adverse reactions such as dyskinesias or hallucinations may increase at previously effective dosages. Another problem with dopaminergics is the "wearing off" effect. Mobility declines before the next dose is due. This problem is corrected by more frequent dosing, selegiline, and controlled-relapse L-dopa preparations. Intravenous infusions and duodenal instillation have reduced fluctuations but are impractical for long-term treatment. The "on-off" response is another unpredictable adverse effect in parkinsonism. It is considered to be an exaggerated response to the dopaminergic agents; the patient may have "on" periods of normal ability interrupted by "off" times of total immobility. The "on" periods also may be complicated by involuntary movements called **dyskinesias.** The result is daily fluctuation of symptoms and severe frustration with their unpredictability.[6]

Drug holidays are used periodically to restore receptor sensitivity and responsiveness to dopaminergic drugs. During a drug holiday the patient is weaned from the drugs for up to 10 days, and the drugs may then be reinstituted at lower doses.[27]

Supportive care

Attention to diet and exercise are important to maintain strength and energy levels. Some reports have recommended a daytime low-protein diet and an evening high-protein diet to improve levodopa uptake to the brain during the day.[17] Levodopa competes with other amino acids for entry to the central nervous system at the blood-brain barrier. Because the brain accepts a limited number of amino acids over a certain period, reduced protein intake minimizes amino acid competition with levodopa for central nervous system uptake.

Speech therapy, physical therapy, and occupational therapy consultations are indicated for those who have progressive disease and whose symptoms do not respond to therapy. Many patients benefit from the continued reinforcement and creative approaches to problems that these consultations bring.

Stereotaxic thalamotomy to decrease tremor is used in some medical centers. Transplantation of adrenal and fetal substantia nigra cells into the brain to increase brain catecholamines has been attempted but is without clear and consistent therapeutic benefit.[6]

NURSING MANAGEMENT OF THE PATIENT WITH PARKINSON'S DISEASE
Assessment

Assessment begins with a thorough review of the patient's knowledge of the illness, medication regimen, and response to treatment. The nurse inquires about patterns of mobility and fluctuations with medication, for example, the amount of time per waking hour the patient is mobile.

Physical assessment includes the motor system, functional ability, and activities of daily living. When performing a motor assessment the nurse asks when the patient took the last dose of medication because the motor response can vary from dose to dose. The motor assessment is individualized to the patient but should minimally involve testing strength, tone, gait, coordination, speech, and functional ability (e.g., rising from a chair, walking a specified distance, timing the performance of activities). The presence of tremor and involuntary movements should be noted. Review of nutritional status, weight, and swallowing ability is important for those who are severely affected. Sexual functioning is included in the assessment because of the frequent problems in this area. How the patient and family are functioning can be assessed by reviewing family activities, communication, and decision making. Assessment of the home environment often helps detect concerns about safety and equipment needs. The patient's cognitive function and emotional state are assessed routinely.

Nursing Diagnosis

The typical nursing diagnoses applicable to patients with parkinsonism, like many of the degenerative diseases, depend on the stage of illness. The severity ranges from minimal symptoms to total immobilization. Diagnoses unique to the patient with parkinsonism include the following:

Self-care deficit related to slowness of movement and muscular rigidity

High risk for injury related to postural instability and muscular rigidity

Impaired verbal communication related to slowness of movement

Altered nutrition: less than body requirements related to poor oropharyngeal muscle control and coordination

Knowledge deficit related to the complexity of and fluctuations in the treatment regimen

Ineffective coping related to a fluctuation in symptoms and the progressive nature of the illness

Planning

The general goal is to maximize the patient's potential and reduce the isolation that can occur with a chronic immobilizing illness. Goals appropriate for the patient with parkinsonism include the following:

Patient performs and directs self-care

Patient maintains normal mobility and does not sustain physical injury

Patient maintains effective communication and social activities

Patient's weight remains in the range acceptable for height and age, and intake is adequate to maintain the desired energy level for normal activity

Patient verbalizes medication effects and controls his own medication schedule

Patient and family demonstrate knowledge of the illness and treatment and coping strategies that enhance family functioning

Implementation

The patient with parkinsonism may require hospitalization for changing and adjusting the medication regimen and during drug holidays. Otherwise, the only other indication for hospitalization is for surgery or treatment of coincidental illness. The care priorities should reflect assessment of medication effects and supportive care while the patient is dependent.

General care of the patient with parkinsonism begins with establishing a similar routine to that used at home for performing basic self-care tasks. During periods of immobility, the patient may need assistance during meals, bathing, dressing, and toileting. Attention to hygiene is essential. The patient may drool excessively, have poor oral hygiene, and have sweaty, oily skin, necessitating daily baths, shampoos, and oral care after meals. Safety during bathing is improved by well-placed grab bars, a bath bench, nonskid appliques, using a small amount of water, and completely emptying the tub before attempting to exit. Dressing is facilitated by using large zippers, snaps or Velcro closures, and rubber-soled, low-heeled, well-fitting shoes. As improvements occur, the patient is encouraged to plan the day and perform these activities in a reasonable time.

In this daily routine, extra opportunities to walk with the assistance of the nurse or family members are planned to compensate for reduced activity. Rigidity is worsened by staying in one position for prolonged periods and may increase discomfort. If bed rest has been prescribed, active and passive range of motion should be planned at least 3 times a day. This is also a good opportunity to teach the patient and family range of motion and other exercises to reduce muscular stiffness.

When the patient has been inactive for any period or has increasing periods of stiffness and shuffling gait, preventing falls is an important aspect of care. The nurse teaches the patient techniques that emphasize voluntary motor control over activities, for example, taking large marching steps to an unvoiced count, practicing walking by stepping over imaginary lines, and rocking side-to-side to initiate leg movement.[5] Patient education should include exercises to improve posture, such as standing against a wall, with shoulders, buttocks, and heels touching the wall. Relaxation techniques that take muscle groups through maximal extension and flexion while the patient listens to a preprogrammed tape have been used to reduce stiffness and anxiety associated with off periods.

Problems related to communication are addressed by several approaches: encouraging the patient to take deep breaths before initiating a conversation, using gestures in place of words, and using diaphragmatic breathing.[27] The nurse should be patient during conversations because many patients are slow to respond. The rigidity in facial expression often belies the patient's true feelings; the nurse should be careful not to assume a lack of emotional responsiveness. If the patient shows evidence of memory impairment, the care plan is amended accordingly.

The degree of speech impairment alerts the nurse to the potential for a similar degree of swallowing difficulty, since similar musculature is involved. These problems are usually most apparent during off periods. Meals are planned with few distractions to enhance concentration. Foods should be easy to chew; thickened liquids and semisolids are easier to swallow than clear fluids. The patient always eats in the upright position. Reflex coughing to protect against aspiration of food and fluids may be reduced in the patient with parkinsonism. Suction should be available. A Yankeur suction catheter may be helpful to those patients with profuse secretions, drooling, and difficulty swallowing who can perform their own suctioning. Weight is routinely measured to monitor nutritional status. Constipation related to slow GI motility is best countered by maintaining maximal mobility, drinking at least 6 to 8 8-ounce glasses of fluid a day, and taking supplemental roughage such as bran or psyllium.

The nurse advises the patient and family of the medication effects, including the peak and duration of action and all side effects (Table 46-2). Dopaminergic drugs are given on an empty stomach $\frac{1}{2}$ to 1 hour before meals to facilitate increased absorption. The dietary distribution of protein includes high-protein foods in the evening to enhance drug uptake during the day. The spacing of medications is in response to the patient's activity schedule. If the patient experiences fluctuations or side effects, a home diary or bedside flowsheet helps to record drug responsiveness.

Evaluation

A successful nursing treatment plan will result in a patient who is in control of the medication regimen and other aspects of care. The patient and family should show evidence of understanding the illness and treatment plan. The patient will maintain normal weight and all self-care activities. The patient will participate in an exercise program tailored to his or her needs.

Documentation

Flowsheets are used at home or in the hospital to document response to medications, particularly during periods of medication adjustment and drug holidays. This information is often an excellent method to reinforce medication teaching. All patient drug, exercise, and diet teaching is documented. Specific problems with sleep, constipation, memory impairment, and depression are recorded.

Ongoing Care

Patients with parkinsonism require frequent contact with health care providers to manage the medication and treatment regimen. Phone calls are often helpful to monitor changes in status and response to medications with knowledgeable patients. The more informed the patient and family are, the more likely they are to cope positively with a progressive illness such as parkinsonism. Long-term planning is essential. Typical parkinsonism does not statistically alter the duration of life but it does affect life quality. Remaining active is important. Working on hobbies, walking regularly, participating in community-sponsored exercise programs and peer support groups, and socializing regularly should be continued at the patient's pre-illness level. Long-term care is only necessary for those with severe dementia, immobility, and limited resources.

HUNTINGTON'S DISEASE
Definition

Huntington's disease is a genetic disorder characterized by increased involuntary movements, progressive intellectual decline, and personality and mood changes. Autosomal dominant inheritance is the rule; each child of an affected parent has a 50% risk of inheriting the illness.

Etiology/Epidemiology

The incidence of Huntington's disease is 0.5 cases per 100,000, and the prevalence is 5 per 100,000. An estimated 25,000 persons in the United States are affected by the clinical symptoms; 125,000 are believed to be at risk for inheriting the disease.[19] The etiologic factors for the selective vulnerability and degeneration of certain neurons are unknown. Defects in the cell membrane and the presence of toxic neuronal proteins that interfere with cell metabolism (excitotoxins) are under investigation. Studies implicating glutamate, aspartate, and quinolinic acid are promising. Initial symptoms usually appear dur-

RESEARCH BRIEF

Hurwitz A: The benefit of a home exercise regimen for ambulatory Parkinson's disease patients, *J Neurosci Nurs* 21(3):180, 1989.

This study assessed the impact of a weekly home exercise program administered by senior nursing students over 1 year. In this case control study, 15 patients were assigned to the control group and 14 to the experimental group. Patients in the experimental group showed improvement in recent memory, nausea, incontinence, sucking from a straw, and eating habits. All patients in the experimental group were positive about the intervention and the experience with the nursing students.

ing early middle age. The average age of onset is 38 years; however, symptoms can appear at any age.

Pathophysiology

Huntington's disease is characterized by selective neuronal deterioration and neurotransmitter abnormalities in the basal ganglia, particularly the corpus striatum (caudate nucleus and putamen) and globus pallidus. Normally, a balance exists between the dopamine, ACH, and gamma-aminobutyric (GABA) pathways in the basal ganglia. These pathways integrate the performance of motor and mental tasks. In Huntington's disease the dopamine pathway becomes overactive. The resulting hyperexcitability is expressed as abnormal involuntary movements of the extremities, such as **chorea.** The movement disorder associated with Huntington's disease appears to be the mirror image to that seen in parkinsonism. Persons with Huntington's disease (see Figure 46-2) have heightened sensitivity to dopamine, whereas persons with parkinsonism have dopamine depletion. This ties in with the clinical observation that administration of L-dopa increases chorea and that antipsychotics (e.g., phenothiazines), which block dopamine, usually decrease chorea. The defects in Huntington's disease are a presumed consequence of the autosomal dominant genetic abnormality. Recombinant DNA techniques and genetic linkage studies have located the abnormal gene on the short arm of chromosome 4.

Clinical Manifestations

The presenting symptoms consist of impairment in motor, cognitive, and behavioral function. Early symptoms include restlessness, forgetfulness, clumsiness, falls, balance and coordination problems, and altered speech and handwriting. The motor symptoms are often more readily acknowledged than the involuntary movement, emotional, and intellectual problems.

The motor signs include involuntary hyperkinetic movements, such as chorea and dystonic posture, that affect the extremities, torso, face, oropharynx, and respiratory muscles. The parkinsonian signs of bradykinesia and rigidity may be present in some cases. The patient progresses through stages of hyperkinetic, choreic movements to slower dystonic movements. Speech lacks resonance and articulation because of the hyperkinetic movements. Swallowing is slow and uncoordinated in later stages. Problems with imbalance, rigidity, and weakness lead to a bedfast state. In the final stages, anarthria, aspiration, and immobility result; the patient may die from these complications.

The mental problems affect performance skills more than verbal skills. The patient has a reduced capacity for organization, planning, and sequencing of behavior. Early in the course of the disease the individual has difficulty learning new information and, to a lesser extent, recalling remote events. Impairments such as aphasia, agnosia, or apraxia do not occur. In advanced Huntington's disease, patients are often communicative, insightful, and aware, despite deficits in articulation and cognition.

Behavioral manifestations include personality changes and eccentricities, as well as affective disorders, such as depression and psychoses. Personality changes range from apathy to extroversion. The major affective disorders, unipolar and bipolar depression (50%), are more common than acute psychosis (10%). The risk for suicide is greater than that seen in the normal population because of the presence of psychiatric disorders, recognition of problems, and progressive physical decline.

Therapeutic Management

Care is primarily supportive, emphasizing information about the illness, genetic counseling, planning for future needs, psychologic support, and prevention of complications related to increasing disability. Therapies that slow the neuronal degeneration or replace the neurotransmitter deficiency have been unsuccessful in halting the progressive nature of the symptoms.

Medications are available to treat emotional symptoms such as depression and psychosis. Tricyclic antidepressants are frequently used successfully to treat depression. Antidopaminergic drugs such as the phenothiazines have been used for treating both psychosis and choreic movements. Phenothiazines may be used only for disabling symptoms and for brief periods at minimal doses to achieve an effect.

Genetic counseling using nondirective and supportive techniques is mandatory for those affected by this autosomal dominant illness. Studies show that genetic counseling has been effective in reducing gene frequency in families with a history of Huntington's disease. Fully disclosing the presence of the illness to the family is difficult, and most patients benefit from the services of a multidisciplinary clinic dedicated to the care of this specialized disease.

Consultations with speech therapists, physical therapists, and dietitians can provide information that benefits the patient and should be incorporated in the care plan. Assisting the patient and family with psychosocial concerns, dealing with social service agencies, and managing day-to-day routines are the mainstays of care.

NURSING MANAGEMENT OF THE PATIENT WITH HUNTINGTON'S DISEASE

The nursing care plans appropriate for the patient with Huntington's disease are similar to those for patients with Alzheimer's disease and parkinsonism in regard to the cognitive and behavioral deficits. Supportive care is designed to make maximal use of the patient's abilities, prevent complications, and promote patient and family knowledge and coping with the illness.

Establishing a daily schedule that the patient believes meets his or her needs is often helpful. The nurse fosters independence in meeting activities of daily living and allows sufficient time for the patient to complete agreed-on tasks. For example, shaving can be a problem, but using an electric razor may help. Mouth care after meals is essential and can be facilitated by an electric toothbrush. Clothing should be lightweight and loose fitting. Tennis shoes with a Velcro closure are suggested. Using the shower instead of the tub for bathing is necessary for patients with mobility impairment. The environment should be safe and support the patient's abilities. Handrails, a shower chair, and a raised toilet seat make bathing and toileting easier. If involuntary movements are a threat to safety, padded siderails, placing the mattress on the floor, and wearing a helmet help protect the patient. Maintaining mobility is fostered by a regular exercise regimen that might include daily walks, bicycling, range of motion (active and passive) exercise, isometric exercise, and relaxation techniques. The involuntary movements are absent during sleep. Laying in an extended position reduces flexion deformities.

Maintaining ideal body weight can be a challenge. Foods may need to be prepared in bite-sized amounts. Finger foods, plates with adhesive bottoms, covered cups, and straws may be needed so those patients with severe involuntary movements can maintain their independence. Choking on food and fluids becomes a problem later in the illness. Foods that form a soft bolus (casseroles, puddings) are most easily chewed and swallowed. Mealtime should be free of distractions; however, the patient may need a companion to help monitor intake and prevent aspiration during meals.

Communication may be impaired, particularly articulation. Adequate time should be allowed for responses, and questions should be short and direct. Word boards are introduced early in the course of the disease to develop skills that may be hard to learn in later stages. Outside hobbies, contact with friends, and pastimes provide stimulation and maintain the patient's quality of life. The family may need support to deal with the unpredictable nature of the symptoms. Changes related to illness that might be amenable to treatment are differentiated from those which are not.

Degenerative Disorders of the Spinal Cord

SYRINGOMYELIA
Definition

Syringomyelia produces a chronic progressive condition of sensory defects, muscular weakness, atrophy, and spasticity associated with cavitation and gliosis in the spinal cord and medulla.

Etiology/Epidemiology

The incidence is 0.4 per 100,000, with a prevalence of 7 per 100,000. The etiologic factors are unknown. A developmental anomaly causing abnormal pressure changes and an imbalance in posterior fossa development has been suggested by the frequent association with other congenital anomalies. Other etiologic factors include spinal arachnoiditis after meningeal infections and dilation of the spinal canal associated with vascular lesions, tumors, and trauma.

Pathophysiology

The syrinx is a fluid-filled cavity in the spinal cord. Cavities in the anterior commissure disrupt the pain and temperature fibers as they cross in the spinal cord before ascending to the cortex, giving rise to dissociated sensory loss. The process can extend to the anterior and posterior horn cells, nerve root, and white matter, causing destruction or displacement of the motor, sensory, and autonomic nerve fibers. The cavity can be localized to one side or run the entire length of the cord. The cervical and lumbar areas are most commonly affected. When the cavity extends above the cervical level to the medulla and pons it is called *syringobulbia*.

Clinical Manifestations

The onset of symptoms begins in the third to fifth decade. The presenting symptoms are usually confined to one extremity and consist of muscle atrophy, weakness, and loss of pain sensation. The classic finding is dissociated sensory loss: loss of pain and temperature sensation with preservation of sensation to light touch. With cervical cavitation, sensory loss occurs in a capelike distribution over the shoulders and neck. Associated findings include absence of reflexes, painless burns, Charcot joints, and joint pain in the affected limb. Scoliosis and chest wall atrophy on the affected side eventually occur.

The course of illness is that of gradually increasing weakness, with periodic plateaus of stability. As the cavity size increases, spasticity, ataxia, increased sensory deficits (reduced vibration and position sense), and bowel and bladder incontinence occur.

The major diagnostic problem is eliminating treatable conditions such as spinal cord tumor. CT and myelography should be performed in patients with rapidly progressive symptoms.

Therapeutic Management

Care is aimed at maximizing the patient's abilities and preventing complications. The extent of functional limitation is assessed to determine if further modifications are necessary to improve the patient's life-style. When the patient has difficulty with activities of daily living, referrals to physical and occupational therapy are indicated. Preventing complications such as pressure sores and contractures is essential. Assessment of the home and occupational setting to determine if modifications are necessary is extremely helpful. Some patients with inadequate social supports may require long-term care, but this can be avoided with careful planning. Surgical decompression of the spinal cord has been attempted for those patients who experience severe worsening of symptoms. The results have been equivocal in experienced hands and are not effective in changing longstanding symptoms.[31]

AMYOTROPHIC LATERAL SCLEROSIS
Definition

Amyotrophic lateral sclerosis (ALS), progressive spinal muscular atrophy, and progressive bulbar palsy are illnesses that involve progressive degeneration of the motor neurons in the anterior horn cell (AHC) of the spinal cord, brainstem, and motor cortex. This causes progressive muscular weakness, atrophy, and corticospinal tract abnormalities.

Etiology/Epidemiology

The most common and well-known motor neuron disease is ALS, also called *Lou Gehrig's disease.* The incidence of ALS is 2 cases per 100,000 with a prevalence of 6 cases per 100,000.[26] Symptoms of the disease appear between the ages of 40 and 70; the mean age at onset is 56. The course of the illness lasts from 2 to 6 years. It is often rapidly progressive, with death occurring in 3 years in 50% of patients and in 90% within 6 years. Approximately 10% of patients have a prolonged course lasting 10 years or more.

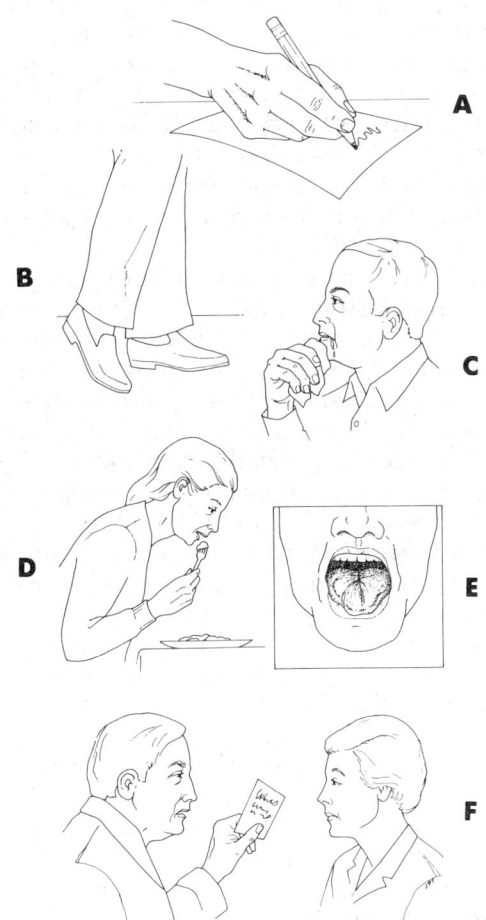

FIGURE 46-4   Clinical manifestations of motor neuron disease. **A,** Patient has decreased fine motor movement. Note the prominent metacarpal bones because of muscle atrophy. **B,** Slow dragging gait. Patient tires easily with walking. **C,** Drooling is caused by impaired swallowing and decreased muscle tone. **D,** Patient has difficulty chewing because of muscle weakness. **E,** Fasciculations of tongue. **F,** Patient has difficulty talking and may communicate better in writing.

The etiology of ALS remains obscure. Research has not supported infectious etiologic factors. New research findings suggest a genetic etiology for ALS. Premature aging because of an accumulation of abnormal DNA is a popular hypothesis. Diverse factors such as abnormal metal, mineral, DNA repair and nucleic acid metabolism, toxins (cycad, excitotoxins), and abnormal glutamate metabolism are believed to precipitate the premature neuronal degeneration. Autoimmune disease is suggested by the presence of antibodies to ganglioside, but they may be a result of secondary damage to the AHC. New treatments with nerve growth factors (CNTF, IGF-1) may shed light on the etiology of ALS.[14]

Pathophysiology

The pathologic process is similar in all three forms of motor neuron disease: loss and degeneration of the upper motor neurons (the cranial nerve motor nuclei, Betz cells, and pyramidal neurons in the motor cortex), and the lower motor neurons (anterior horn cells of the spinal cord) (see Chapter 44). Both upper and lower motor neuron damage causes muscle weakness. Patients with upper motor neuron signs have widespread degeneration of the corticospinal tracts, the nerves that conduct impulses from the cortex to the spinal cord. This leads to a loss of neuronal inhibition to the lower motor neuron, which leads to spasticity and an increase in muscle stretch reflexes. Lower motor neuron lesions affect the anterior horn cell, which innervates between 50 and 2000 muscle fibers through its peripheral extension, the axon. As the motor nuclei in the anterior horn cells die, the axonal connections, which conduct electrical impulses from the spinal cord to muscle, degenerate. This decreased muscle innervation results in muscular weakness, atrophy, and fasciculations.

Clinical Manifestations

The initial symptom is a mild clumsiness, usually in the distal portion of one extremity. The patient may complain of tripping and drag one leg when the lower extremities are involved. Upper extremity weakness causes difficulty grasping objects and any task requiring fine movement. Muscle wasting and fasciculations in the affected extremity may not be immediately noticed by the patient. Muscle cramps and stiffness are a frequent complaint. Approximately 25% initially have bulbar symptoms; otolaryngologists or speech therapists are often consulted first. Over time the weakness, wasting, fasciculations, and muscle stiffness progress to involve all of the muscles in the body. The patterns by which the disease progresses vary (Figure 46-4).

On examination, muscle weakness parallels the

atrophy in the affected extremity. The distal portion of the extremity is usually more involved than the proximal musculature. When the upper extremities are involved, the shoulder girdle can become stiff and immobilized as the hands lose function. Reflexes may be absent in the most affected extremity, but are usually hyperactive if upper motor neuron involvement is apparent. Ankle clonus and the Babinski sign may be present in the lower extremities. The tongue may be atrophied and show fasciculations. Facial weakness, drooling, and the inability to manage secretions are evident. The gag reflex may be diminished and choking occurs frequently. Speech disorders include difficulty articulating (dysarthria) and a forced, nasal tone, which later progresses to a complete inability to communicate verbally (anarthria). Mentation and intellectual function are usually normal. Pseudobulbar palsy, manifested by inappropriate weeping or laughing to emotional stimuli, is caused by the illness, not the patient's emotional reactions.

Finally, involvement of the respiratory muscles, the diaphragm and intercostal muscles, leads to respiratory failure. The ocular muscles and bowel and bladder sphincters are rarely involved. Autonomic and sexual functions are preserved. Sensory function remains intact, and patients do not develop pressure sores despite the debilitated state.

The diagnosis is made by history and physical examination. Laboratory studies such as electromyography and muscle biopsy demonstrate the presence of widespread denervation. Pulmonary function tests performed with the patient in supine and sitting positions document respiratory involvement.[24] Blood tests to exclude thyroid disease and heavy metal intoxication are indicated. MRI and lumbar puncture exclude other causes of muscle weakness. Most tests can be completed on an outpatient basis.

Therapeutic Management

Care of the patient with ALS is primarily supportive; no treatments are available to halt the progressive weakness. Antiviral agents, steroids, plasma exchange, and thyrotropin-releasing hormone therapy have all been tried without demonstrable change in muscle function. This does not mean that the illness is untreatable. Current clinical trials with nerve growth factors—insulin-like growth factors (IGF-1) and ciliary neurotrophic factor (CNTF)—are based on positive response with animal models. These drugs are hoped to potentially slow the rapid deterioration and enhance nerve survival. Also, trials with drugs to block glutamate (excitotoxins) and reduce oxidant-stress (Eldapryl) are underway. Immune suppressants have also been given on an experimental basis.

Symptomatic management becomes necessary when the weakness progresses. Many of the symptoms are amenable to pharmacotherapy, surgical procedures, technologic devices to replace lost abilities, and, most important, psychosocial support. A physical therapist may be consulted to provide guidelines for exercise and the use of braces and assistive devices. The shoulder often becomes immobile and painful; twice daily full range of motion exercises should be started before signs of a "frozen" shoulder occur. If foot-drop is present, the use of a posterior plastic splint can provide support and prevent falls. A cervical collar is helpful to support weak neck muscles. A cane or crutches will provide stability, but both depend on upper extremity function. Occupational therapists can design feeding utensils or hand splints when fine motor movement in the upper extremity is impaired.

Muscle relaxants, such as diazepam (Valium) and baclofen (Lioresal), are available to treat spasticity if it interferes with hygiene or functional ability. Many patients complain of increased weakness with these drugs, however. Swallowing problems are first manifested by difficulty managing secretions and drooling. Anticholinergics and antihistamines are often prescribed to control profuse secretions. Some patients only use them before socializing because of bothersome side effects.

Speech therapists can assist in devising a workable communication system, be it lipreading, word boards, or computer-driven devices. For the patient who cannot communicate, computerized systems activated by eye blink are a new development. These systems range from inexpensive word processing systems to complex, rapid-paced, computer-driven programs. These programs can be hooked up to a voice synthesizer. An example is ALS patient and physicist Steven Hawking's computer and synthesizer seen in the book and movie "A Short History of Time."

Respiratory care is essential throughout the illness. Pulmonary function studies (i.e., FVC and NIF) should be performed during each outpatient visit. Pulmonary exercises such as deep breathing, incentive spirometry, and the use of an intermittent positive pressure breathing machine should be considered. Respiratory tract infections necessitate aggressive treatment with antibiotics when associated with fever and a change in sputum color and consistency. Influenza vaccine and pneumococcal pneumonia vaccine should be routinely administered. Drugs that increase breathing capacity, such as aminophylline, have been used. Respiratory failure is usually the major cause of death. Abrupt deterioration can occur in patients with previously reduced, but adequate, pulmonary function. Blood gases are usually normal until late. Oximetry and capnography, both non-invasive methods to monitor Po_2 + Pco_2 are helpful in the acute setting. For this reason, respiratory failure needs to be anticipated and plans for ventilatory support discussed in advance (see Chapter 26).

NURSING MANAGEMENT OF THE PATIENT WITH AMYOTROPHIC LATERAL SCLEROSIS

Assessment

The nurse assesses the patient's understanding of the illness and the effect it has on functional ability. The presenting symptoms and response to treatment are documented. Respiratory and nutritional problems require further investigation. The nurse determines whether the person needs special home routines for performing activities of daily living or overcoming self-care deficits. It is often difficult for these patients to leave the protected environment of the home when their routine is well established. Awareness of the patient's plans to use ventilatory support if respiratory failure occurs is mandatory.

Physical assessment encompasses motor strength, gait, and functional ability (performance of activities of daily living, getting up from a chair, arms over head, hand grip, walking on heels and toes), as well as the presence of atrophy, fasciculations, and hyperreflexia. Bulbar function tests measure gag response, tongue movement, swallowing, chewing, the presence of choking, and weight loss. The patient's ability to communicate is assessed by asking the patient to read aloud, noting the presence of hoarseness and nasal or slurred speech. Respiratory function tests include forced vital capacity, coughing, and counting aloud in a single breath.

The patient's emotional and psychosocial adjustment to the illness should be assessed. Assessment of individual coping includes congruence of verbalizations and body language, accurate appraisal of the situation, successful management of symptoms, and normalization of role function. Observation of successful use of assistive devices such as walkers, wheelchairs, a suction machine, and communication aids is documented. The individual's caregiver should be interviewed to determine sources of stress, an understanding of the illness, and present coping patterns.[5,24]

Nursing Diagnosis

Nursing diagnoses appropriate for the patient with ALS depend on the stage of illness and progression of symptoms. They include the following:

Self-care deficit related to motor weakness caused by anterior horn cell dysfunction

Altered nutrition: less than body requirements related to dysphagia and bulbar weakness

Ineffective breathing pattern related to intercos-

tal and diaphragmatic muscle weakness and bulbar weakness

Impaired verbal communication related to bulbar weakness

Altered family and individual coping related to the progressive nature of the illness and the disruption of life-style

Planning

The general goal is to maintain the patient's abilities and assist with adaptation to reduced levels of function as deterioration occurs. Prevention of emergencies such as aspiration, respiratory insufficiency, and falls is also extremely important. As the illness progresses, counseling the patient about decisions regarding extraordinary means of life support is a goal for nursing care. Other goals include the following:

Patient remains active and directs care to the best of his or her potential

Patient ingests sufficient calories and fluids to maintain energy and prevent severe weight loss

Patient remains active and has adequate respiratory capacity

Patient uses a meaningful communication system

Patient and family feel supported and in control of situations that involve a change in previous patterns

Implementation

Care of the ALS patient reflects the stage and severity of the illness. General care includes support of self-care abilities, comfort care, and preventing complications. Teaching the patient and family to anticipate and manage symptoms in an illness that has a progressive downward trajectory is a major part of nursing care and requires providing continuous psychologic support.

Support of the patient's self-care abilities can be facilitated by allowing the patient to determine the daily schedule. The nurse should allow sufficient time for the patient to accomplish tasks and evaluate the need for assistive devices such as built-up eating utensils, clothing adaptations, and an electric toothbrush. Occupational therapists can help devise ways to use the patient's existing ability to complete activities of daily living.

Exercise in the daily routine enables patients to maintain mobility and the ability to perform self-care activities. As ambulation becomes more difficult, the use of a walker and wheelchair may be beneficial for safety and stability. When the patient cannot move an extremity through a full range of motion voluntarily, the nurse performs passive range of motion exercises several times a day to promote comfort. Heel cord stretching exercises at bedtime may prevent night cramps. Massage, skin care, turning, and positioning at least every 2 hours are extremely important for the immobilized patient.

If the patient is severely dysphagic, preventing aspiration and weight loss is critical. Swallowing is assessed frequently. The patient should be given a sufficient amount of time to eat; semisoft foods are easier to swallow and require less chewing. Oral hygiene is a must after each meal. Suction should be available for those who have persistent drooling and dysphagia.

The patient and family need to be involved in plans that relate to treatment of respiratory failure. The nurse assists in plans for support of ventilation. The nurse is responsible for teaching the family techniques that prevent complications, such as the Heimlich maneuver, use of the suction machine and incentive spirometer, intermittent positive pressure breathing, and chest percussion and drainage. If the patient requires a gastrostomy or tracheostomy, the nurse will need to prepare the patient and family for home management (see Chapters 16 and 26).

Open communication and providing opportunities for social interaction will enhance the patient and family's adjustment and coping with this illness. The communication system used at home should be adopted by the staff. If there is none, the speech therapist works with the family, patient, and staff to devise a workable system. Computer-driven systems, electronic spellers, word boards, and lipreading have been used with success.

The patient and family must be given opportunities to verbalize their feelings of frustration, powerlessness, and anxiety. Establishing a supportive relationship is a key aspect of nursing care. Maintaining independence, social activities, and participation in previous role-related activities should be encouraged.

Patient education is summarized in the box below.

Evaluation

Effective care plans enable patients to direct their own care, make choices, and be in control of their lives. Patients should show evidence of managing their symptoms and anticipating changes to prevent or plan for a crisis. With proper education, they will demonstrate an understanding of adaptive equipment, as well as exercise, dietary, and respiratory interventions used to manage ALS.

PATIENT EDUCATION GUIDE   *Patient with Amyotrophic Lateral Sclerosis*

Exercise

Do range of motion exercises for all joints at least twice a day.

Maintain the upright position, standing, and perform frequent position changes to prevent stiffness and promote bony integrity.

Participate in an exercise program that is suited to self-interests and abilities: swimming, walking, riding an exercise bike, or maintaining activities of daily living for some patients. Avoid fatigue.

Pulmonary care

Use incentive spirometry or inspiratory resistance devices daily.

Know how to treat upper respiratory tract infections (with fluids, decongestants, and pulmonary care) and when to call a professional).

Diet

Maintain ideal body weight.

Eat three meals a day, balanced from the major food groups and including foods high in fiber.

If swallowing is a problem (patients with ALS), have small frequent meals and snacks and avoid liquids that increase secretions (milk-based products).

Bowel routine

Take at least 6 to 8 8-ounce glasses of liquid a day. Avoid caffeinated liquids because of their diuretic effects.

If fiber-containing foods (fruits and vegetables) are difficult to chew, take supplements containing psyllium.

Rest and comfort

Maintain a comfortable position and do range of motion exercises before bedtime to reduce cramps and enhance sleep.

Use a water bed with an alternating pressure or egg-crate mattress when turning in bed is difficult.

Elevate the legs when resting to reduce lower extremity edema.

Planning

Have emergency phone numbers and contacts posted near the phone.

Discuss emergency plans with caregivers in advance.

Continue all health maintenance plans, dentist visits, visual examinations, and preventive health behaviors (e.g., Pap smears, breast examinations, and flu shots).

Documentation

All teaching is recorded. Flowsheets to document strength, respiratory status, and weight help record responses to interventions longitudinally. Communication of the care plan to home care agencies is essential to provide continuity of care. The patient's wishes for ventilatory support are recorded and periodically reevaluated.

Ongoing Care

Most patients remain at home throughout the course of their illness, but require ongoing medical and nursing visits to monitor symptoms. Home visits are helpful to assess the need for environmental adaptation and family functioning. Ramps, bathroom remodeling, or moving the bedroom to the first floor may be needed if the patient can no longer climb stairs. The nurse encourages normal social activities. Information about patient manuals and local patient and family support groups are available from the ALS Society.

When the illness advances to the terminal stages, the family may need assistance in arranging for respite or hospice services. If ventilatory support is needed, the patient and family will require an extensive amount of education and support. Admission to the hospital is often necessary to stabilize the patient and to coordinate home care services.

CRITICAL THINKING QUESTIONS

1 List three nursing assessments essential to the care of the patient with degenerative diseases.
2 List four nursing diagnoses common to all patients with degenerative neurologic diseases.
3 Identify interventions aimed at preventing common complications, including contractures, thrombophlebitis, atelectasis, decubitus ulcers, and constipation.
4 Construct guidelines for home care after hospitalization, including diet, activities of daily living, exercise, and medications for patients and families coping with each of the degenerative diseases.
5 Describe circumstances under which the patient should be permitted independence and those under which the nurse should intervene to maintain patient safety.
6 State guidelines for determining the need for genetic counseling for patients and families coping with a degenerative disorder.
7 Describe the characteristics of successful patient and family adjustment to degenerative neurologic disease.

RESOURCES

1 ALZHEIMER'S DISEASE AND RELATED DISORDERS ASSOCIATION 70 East Lake St. Chicago, IL 60601
2 THE AMERICAN PARKINSON'S DISEASE ASSOCIATION 47 East 50th St. New York, NY 10022
3 AMYOTROPHIC LATERAL SCLEROSIS ASSOCIATION 15300 Ventura Blvd. Sherman Oaks, CA 91403
4 HEREDITARY DISEASE FOUNDATION 606 Wilshire Blvd. Suite 504 Santa Monica, CA 90401
5 HUNTINGTON'S DISEASE SOCIETY OF AMERICA 140 West 22nd St. 6th Floor New York, NY 10018

BIBLIOGRAPHY

Current

1. Beck C, Heacock P: Nursing interventions for patients with Alzheimer's dementia, *Nurs Clin North Am* 23(1):95, 1988.
2. Burne E, Buckwalter K: Pathophysiology and etiology of Alzheimer's dementia, *Nurs Clin North Am* 23(1):11, 1988.
3. Christensen R: Progressive supranuclear palsy: nursing care implications, *J Neurosci Nurs* 20:296, 1988.
4. Delgago J, Billo J: Care of the patient with Parkinson's disease: surgical and nursing interventions, *J Neurosci Nurs* 20:142, 1988.
5. Donohoe K, Miller C, Craig B: Chronic alterations in mobility. In Mitchell P et al: *AANN's neuroscience nursing: phenomena and practice*, East Norwalk, Conn, 1988, Appleton & Lange.
6. Fahn S: Parkinson's disease and other basal ganglion disorders. In Asbury A, McKhann G, McDonald W: *Diseases of the nervous system*, Philadelphia, 1992, WB Saunders.
7. Fitch N, Becker R, Heller A: The inheritance of Alzheimer's disease: a new interpretation, *Ann Neurol* 23:14, 1988.
8. Grossman D: Wilson's disease: a genetic disorder of copper metabolism, *J Neurosci Nurs* 19:216, 1988.
9. Hall G: Care of the Alzheimer's patient living at home, *Nurs Clin North Am* 23(1):31, 1988.
10. Harding A: Hereditary ataxias and related disorders. In Asbury A, McKhann G, McDonald W: *Diseases of the nervous system*, Philadelphia, 1992, WB Saunders.
11. Hurwitz, A: The benefit of a home exercise regimen for ambulatory Parkinson's disease patients, *J Neurosci Nurs* 21(3):180, 1989.
12. Jackson L: A predictive test for Huntington's disease, *J Neurosci Nurs* 19:244, 1987.
13. Katzman R: Dementia. In Asbury A, McKhann G, McDonald W: *Diseases of the nervous system*, Philadelphia, 1992, WB Saunders.
14. Kuncl R et al: Motor neuron diseases. In Asbury A, McKhann, G McDonald W: *Diseases of the nervous system*, Philadelphia, 1992, WB Saunders.
15. Lieberman A: Emerging perspectives in Parkinson's disease, *Neurology* 42(suppl 4):5, 1992.

16. Mitchell P et al: *AANN's neuroscience nursing: phenomena and practice,* East Norwalk, Conn, 1988, Appleton & Lange.
17. Pincus JH, Barup KM: Influence of dietary protein on motor fluctuations in Parkinson's disease, *Arch Neurol* 44:270, 1987.
18. Selkoe DJ: Aging brain—aging mind, *Sci Am* 267(3):135, 1992.
19. Shoulson I: Huntington's disease. In Asbury A, McKhann G, McDonald W: *Diseases of the nervous system,* Philadelphia, 1992, WB Saunders.
20. Stevenson JP: Family stress related to home care of Alzheimer's disease patients and implications for support, *J Neurosci Nurs* 22(3):179, 1990.
21. Stone N: Amyotrophic lateral sclerosis: a challenge for constant adaptation, *J Neurosci Nurs* 19:166, 1987.
22. Wahlquist G: Evaluation and primary management of spasticity, *Nurse Pract* 12(3):27, 1987.

Classic

23. Campbell E, Williams M, Mlynarczyk S: After the fall: confusion, *AJN* 86(2):151, 1986.
24. Goldbaltt, D et al: *Managing ALS manuals* (I-V), Sherman Oaks, Calif, 1983, ALS Association.
25. Hickey J: *The clinical practice of neurological and neurosurgical nursing,* ed 2, Philadelphia, 1986, JB Lippincott.
26. Kurtzke JF: Neuroepidemiology, *Ann Neurol* 16:265, 1984.
27. Lannon M et al: Comprehensive care of the patient with Parkinson's disease, *J Neurosci Nurs* 18:121, 1986.
28. Mulder D, editor: *The diagnosis and treatment of amyotrophic lateral sclerosis,* Boston, 1980, Houghton Mifflin.
29. Siegel G et al: *Basic neurochemistry,* ed 3, Boston, 1985, Little, Brown & Co.
30. Snyder M, editor: *A guide to neurological and neurosurgical nursing,* New York, 1983, John Wiley & Sons.
31. Walton J: *Brain: diseases of the nervous system,* ed 9, New York, 1986, Oxford University Press.

CHAPTER FORTY-SEVEN

Nursing Management of Adults with Cerebrovascular Disorders

LEARNING OBJECTIVES

1 Describe the incidence and social impact of cerebrovascular disorders.
2 Identify the major risk factors for developing cerebrovascular disorders.
3 Differentiate between ischemic and hemorrhagic cerebrovascular disorders.
4 Differentiate the pathophysiology and clinical manifestations of transient ischemic attack (TIA), completed stroke, and subarachnoid hemorrhage (SAH).
5 Differentiate the signs and symptoms of persons with right and left hemispheric stroke.
6 Discuss major medications and surgical procedures that may be used to treat cerebrovascular disorders.
7 Relate principles of nursing management to the care of a patient in the acute stage of stroke.
8 Relate principles of nursing management to the care of the stroke patient in the rehabilitative stage.
9 Differentiate between the traditional and neurodevelopmental (Bobath) approaches in the care and retraining of stroke patients.
10 Identify essential elements for family teaching and preparation for home care of the stroke patient.
11 Identify long-term needs in the rehabilitation of the elderly stroke patient.

KEY TERMS

BRAIN CELLS depend on a continuous blood supply to provide oxygen and nutrients and to remove the end products of metabolism. Inadequate oxygen delivery to part of the brain causes focal or discrete areas of ischemia and tissue hypoxia. Ischemia ultimately leads to necrosis (cell death), or infarction, of the brain tissue. Disruption of the blood supply to the brain results in signs and symptoms of loss of function in the affected area. These neurologic deficits may range from mild to severe, depending on the location and extent of injury to the brain. Many patients recover completely but have varying degrees of disability.

Cerebrovascular disorders is an umbrella term that encompasses all of the disorders that cause ischemia and disruption of the blood supply that can result in neurologic deficits. The deficits resulting from cerebrovascular disorders place a great responsibility on the nurse caring for these patients because of the complex care required and the psychologic stress imposed on both patient and family. Optimal management of these patients is multidisciplinary, with cooperation among various disciplines contributing to total patient care.

CEREBROVASCULAR DISORDERS
Definition

Cerebrovascular disorders include all of the disease states that cause interruption in the blood supply to or within the brain. Examples of these are embolism, thrombosis, and intracerebral and subarachnoid hemorrhages (SAHs). The actual disruption of the blood supply to a part of the brain resulting in ischemia and tissue death of that area of the brain and corresponding neurologic deficits is a cerebrovascular accident (CVA), or **stroke.**

Etiology/Epidemiology

CVA is the third leading cause of death and a major health problem in the United States. Each year 500,000 Americans suffer a stroke, and an estimated 150,000 of these people die from the damage inflicted.[3,12] There are currently over 2 million stroke survivors facing long-term disability and financial burden.[3,12] The cost of care and loss of earnings as a result of stroke have been estimated at $7.5 to $11.2 billion per year.[14]

Despite these alarming figures, the rate of death from stroke has steadily declined over the past decade.[9,36] This improvement is attributable in part to better identification and control of hypertension, a major risk factor; improved diagnosis and treatment of transient ischemic attacks (TIAs); better intervention during the acute phase of stroke; and changes in general attitude toward health, such as sounder diets, exercise, and less cigarette smoking.[9,12,36]

RISK FACTORS ASSOCIATED WITH STROKE

Hypertension (systolic blood pressure greater than 160 mm Hg; diastolic blood pressure greater than 90 mm Hg)
Arteriosclerotic heart disease
Diabetes mellitus
Hyperlipidemia
Obesity
Smoking
Increased blood viscosity (e.g., polycythemia)
Dehydration
Sickle cell anemia
Family history of vascular disease
Sedentary life-style
Cardiac disorders (e.g., cardiac dysrhythmia, congestive heart failure)
Chronic obstructive pulmonary disease

High blood pressure, or hypertension, is the major risk factor for all types of stroke, but control of hypertension can decrease the incidence of stroke.[12,54,55,62] In addition to hypertension, other risk factors for stroke are age, a transient ischemic attack, a prior stroke, and atrial fibrillation.[54-56] The box above lists common risk factors associated with stroke.

CVAs can occur in relatively young adults and children but are seen most often in middle-aged to older people. At present three fourths of all CVAs occur in elderly persons.[10] In fact, the probability of stroke increases steadily with age, from 5.9% at 50 to 59 years to 22.3% at 80 to 84 years for men and 3% to 23% over the same age range for women.[56]

CVA is generally categorized by its cause (Table 47-1). An ischemic CVA results from inadequate blood flow, which causes cerebral infarction, such as with cerebral thrombosis, embolism, or systemic reduction of blood pressure. The most common cause of thrombosis of arteries to the brain is atherosclerosis, which causes progressive narrowing of major cerebral arteries. Elderly persons are particularly prone to atherosclerosis, with a steep rise in the prevalence of arteriosclerotic plaques between 65 to 74 years of age and 75 to 84 years of age, with stabilization in the subsequent decade.[48] Cerebral thrombosis may also be caused by other disorders, such as arterial dissection, fibromuscular dysplasia, drugs, sickle cell disease, and arteritis.[12]

A hemorrhagic CVA is caused by rupture of a blood vessel within the brain. This includes both bleeding into the brain parenchyma (intracerebral

TABLE 47-1	Etiologic Classification of CVA

Classification	Causes
Ischemic	Thrombosis
	Embolism
	Reduced blood flow
Hemorrhagic	Intracerebral hemorrhage
	Subarachnoid hemorrhage

hemorrhage) and bleeding into the subarachnoid space (subarachnoid hemorrhage).[12]

Pathophysiology

Ischemic cerebrovascular accident

When ischemia has been severe enough to produce cerebral infarction, several cellular changes occur, but they vary according to the age of the patient, the location and rapidity of infarct, the adequacy of collateral arteries, and the presence of concurrent complications. With ischemia a vicious cycle of metabolic and electrical changes and edema in the brain causes progressive and irreversible cell death. With large infarcts intracranial pressure may increase enough to cause displacement of brain tissue and herniation.[9]

Lacunar brain infarction refers to small, deep infarcts resulting from occlusion of penetrating branches of larger cerebral arteries.[9] Lacunae are actually small holes within the brain, most commonly in the basal ganglion. Hypertension is present in almost all patients with lacunar infarcts, and this type of stroke seems to occur more frequently in diabetic patients. Lacunar infarcts cause more specific syndromes than infarcts in larger vessels. Pure motor hemiparesis (such as weakness of the face, arm, and leg, and dysarthria) and a pure hemisensory stroke (with complete or partial sensory loss involving the face, arm, and leg) are examples of common lacunar syndromes.

Multiple lacunar infarcts over time can lead to a condition known as multi-infarct dementia. This is a stepwise deterioration in higher mental capacities as a result of multiple small infarcts.[9]

Cerebral emboli consist of fibrin-platelet material; platelets; or fragments from clots, thrombosis, or atheromas. Cardiac sources of emboli are by far the most common cause of cerebral embolization, although emboli may also arise from the carotid arteries, cerebral arteries, and the aorta. Emboli tend to lodge in the distal parts of the middle and posterior cerebral arteries, usually next to the cortex. Patients diagnosed with recent myocardial infarction, subacute bacterial endocarditis, atrial fibrillation, and valvular heart disease are at high risk for developing an embolic stroke.

Elderly persons are particularly vulnerable to stroke when atrial fibrillation is present.[55] Intracardiac thrombi tend to form in the poorly contracting left atrium. Embolic stroke may occur after cardioversion or natural transition from atrial fibrillation to normal sinus rhythm. Mural thrombi typically form after acute myocardial infarction and may migrate to the brain, usually during the first to third weeks after the occurrence of the infarct.

Infarction by embolism can progress to a hemorrhagic stroke. The embolus undergoes lysis, allowing blood to flow from the artery into the surrounding ischemic tissue.

Hemorrhagic cerebrovascular accident

Hemorrhagic CVA is caused by rupture of a blood vessel, usually a sudden event with severe neurologic impairment. Hemorrhagic stroke results in damage or destruction of neurons in the area of hemorrhage and can cause rapid increased intracranial pressure. Signs of increased intracranial pressure include changes in the following: level of consciousness, motor and sensory function, pupil size and reactivity, eye movements, and vital signs.[35] These are described in detail in Chapter 45.

Intracerebral hemorrhage

Intracerebral hemorrhage occurs most often in older adults with poorly controlled hypertension. Hypertensive hemorrhage proceeds from the small, penetrating vessels of the brain that have been damaged by hypertension. Consequently, hypertensive hemorrhage occurs most often in the basal ganglia, thalamus, cerebellum, and brainstem.[36] Intracerebral hemorrhage may also be the result of anticoagulant therapy, bleeding disorders, and trauma. Prognosis depends on age, lesion location, size, and the rapidity with which the hemorrhage produces brain shift and distortion.[36] The expanding lesion can greatly affect adjacent brain tissue and cause an increase in intracranial pressure and the signs and symptoms associated with it.

Subarachnoid hemorrhage

Subarachnoid hemorrhage (SAH) is most commonly caused by rupture of intracranial aneurysms. SAH may also occur as a result of intracerebral hemorrhage that bleeds into the subarachnoid space. Rupture of an aneurysm usually occurs with activity. Blood moves under high pressure from the vessel into the subarachnoid space. The blood spreads and causes irritation of underlying cortex and other vessels. Bleeding is stopped by clot formation, which is broken down and absorbed within 3 weeks.

A cerebral **aneurysm** is a localized dilation in cerebral blood vessels of congenital, traumatic, arteriosclerotic, or septic origin. The distribution of congenital aneurysms is 80% in the anterior circulation and 15% in the posterior circulation of the brain.[12,62]

Saccular (berry) aneurysms are the most common type. Saccular aneurysms are round or berry shaped, have a neck, and are usually located at or near the circle of Willis (Figure 47-1).[20] Berry aneurysms are the result of a congenital weakness in the media that allows the intima to bulge, particularly at arterial bifurcations where the muscular layer is incomplete.[62] Some researchers believe that berry aneurysms are remnants of embryonic vessels that normally would have become larger intracranial vessels. This type of aneurysm usually enlarges until it ultimately ruptures.[62]

Giant aneurysms are similar to berry aneurysms except that they are larger (greater than 25 mm in diameter).[20] Giant aneurysms are less likely to rupture as a result of atherosclerosis that develops on the walls. These aneurysms tend to calcify and form thrombi within, which causes a decrease in circulating blood in the aneurysm.[62] Giant aneurysms act as space-occupying lesions, pressing on adjacent structures and causing neurologic deficits.

Fusiform aneurysms, related to atherosclerotic disease, appear as a ballooning of the artery without a neck. Degenerative changes occur in the vessel wall, and cholesterol is deposited in the intimal layer. Fusiform aneurysms are most often found on the internal carotid and basilar arteries. These aneurysms rarely rupture and cause SAH.[20]

Traumatic aneurysms result from injury to the artery that weakens the arterial wall. Traumatic aneurysms commonly arise along the fracture line of a basilar skull fracture.

Septic aneurysms are rare and result from a septic embolus from acute or subacute bacterial endocarditis. The emboli lodge in the lumen of the artery, causing the arterial wall to weaken and dilate.

Complications of SAH can be rebleeding, cerebral edema, and hydrocephalus, as well as other intracranial and extracranial complications.[26]

Cerebral vasospasm, another serious complication of ruptured aneurysm, is caused by blood in the subarachnoid space. Vasospasm is a localized contraction of the artery that alters the blood flow and cerebral perfusion. If this occurs, it is usually between the fourth and twelfth days after the initial bleeding and further damages the already compromised brain.[23,28] By causing infarction, vasospasm may threaten the recovery of the patient. Vasospasm is thought to result from the release of serotonin and catecholamines from the breakdown of blood, causing vasoconstriction.

Arteriovenous malformation (AVM) in the brain is a congenital cluster of direct communications between arteries and veins that enlarges gradually over time. AVM, which causes about 10% of intracranial hemorrhage, can often be surgically removed before hemorrhage occurs. AVM may bleed into both the brain parenchyma and the subarachnoid space. A history of seizures and headaches in a young normotensive patient favors the diagnosis of an AVM.[62]

Clinical Manifestations

The signs and symptoms of a CVA are classified by the time course involved. This does not reflect the underlying etiologic factors or pathophysiologic conditions. CVAs are generally classified in the following manner: (1) transient ischemic attack; (2) reversible ischemic neurologic deficit; (3) stroke in evolution status; and (4) completed stroke.[9]

Transient ischemic attacks

A **transient ischemic attack (TIA)** should be regarded as a warning of impending stroke. TIA is a localized ischemic event that produces temporary neurologic deficits.[9,30,36] TIAs occur most commonly in those over 65 years of age.[30] Clinical manifesta-

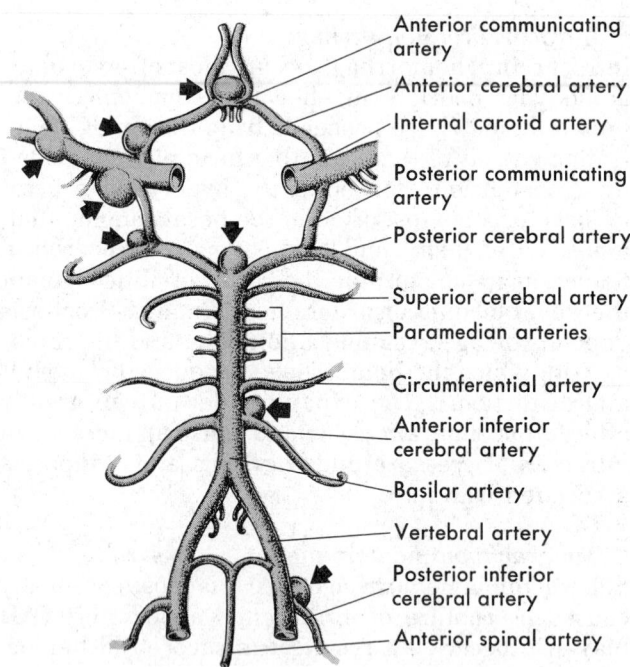

Anterior communicating artery

Anterior cerebral artery

Internal carotid artery

Posterior communicating artery

Posterior cerebral artery

Superior cerebral artery

Paramedian arteries

Circumferential artery

Anterior inferior cerebral artery

Basilar artery

Vertebral artery

Posterior inferior cerebral artery

Anterior spinal artery

FIGURE 47-1   Common sites of berry aneurysms. Size of aneurysm is directly proportional to frequency of occurrence at a particular site.

tions of a TIA depend on the area of the brain affected. A TIA of the carotid system will result in weakness or aphasia. A TIA in the vertebral-basilar system will result in impairment of the cranial nerves or drop attacks.[63] An individual who experiences a drop attack falls to the floor for no apparent reason. These deficits develop suddenly and usually disappear within minutes or hours but may continue for 24 hours. Normal neurologic functioning returns as the episode resolves.[9]

TIAs are caused by cerebrovascular disease, such as atherosclerosis. They also can be caused by microemboli from atherosclerotic plaque; from extracranial vessels, such as an external carotid artery; or from other materials such as cholesterol fragments. Additionally thrombotic narrowing of arteries as a result of cerebral atherosclerosis leads to thrombotic embolization to distal vessels.

Reversible ischemic neurologic deficit

Reversible ischemic neurologic deficit (RIND) is similar to TIA except that the neurologic deficits persist longer than 24 hours (usually 24 to 48 hours).[9,12] Some clinicians believe that RIND is a period of persistent ischemia without actual infarction, whereas others believe that RIND is really submaximal infarction, despite complete recovery. Functional recovery is essentially total, but the risk of subsequent infarction is much greater than with TIA.

Stroke in evolution

Stroke in evolution is a pattern of increasing neurologic deficit occurring over a period of hours or days; it is also referred to as a **progressing stroke.**[8,11] Clinical worsening is estimated to occur in 20% to 35% of stroke patients within the first 7 days after onset of symptoms.[9] Patients report feeling extremely frightened and desperate while a stroke is in evolution.[16]

Completed stroke

Completed stroke is stabilization of the patient's physical condition with persistence of the neurologic deficit.[9]

Right and left cerebrovascular accidents

The clinical manifestations of CVA in the areas of motor, perception, and behavior are often classified as right or left CVA. A right CVA refers to a lesion on the right side of the brain, which results in left hemiplegia. The right hemisphere is considered specialized in sensory-perceptual and visual-spatial processing and awareness of body space, whereas the left hemisphere is dominant for language. Defec-

tive perception of one half of the body and the surrounding space may inhibit the functional rehabilitation of hemiplegic patients. Patients with right hemisphere dysfunction tend to exhibit greater deficits in functional skills than those with left hemisphere dysfunction. This holds true both on admission as well as on discharge from rehabilitation settings.[43]

The patient with a right hemispheric stroke may be alert and oriented to time and place. These signs of apparent wellness result in the nurse considering the patient to be less disabled than is the case. However, impulsive actions and confusion in carrying out activities may be very much a problem for these patients as a result of perceptual and spatial disabilities.[21] Anosognosia may occur in a right CVA as well. In **anosognosia** the patient denies the affected side of the body. The patient may neglect the affected side (often creating a safety hazard as a result of potential injuries), or the patient may state that the paralyzed arm or leg belongs to someone else.[21]

The patient with left hemispheric damage tends to be more cautious. Strokes involving the left hemisphere commonly leave the patient with impaired verbal communication, as demonstrated by aphasia or dysarthria. Table 47-2 summarizes the motor, behavioral, and perceptual impairments of the left- and right-sided CVA. Behaviors common to both right and left hemispheric damage include weakness or paralysis, visual changes, memory loss, early fatigue, and emotional liability.[21]

Aphasia

Aphasia is the impairment of the ability to formulate or interpret language symbols.[9] Aphasia may involve comprehension of spoken language, verbal expression, repetition, naming, oral reading, reading comprehension, and written expression.

TABLE 47-2 Impairments with Cerebrovascular Accidents

	Left lesion	Right lesion
Motor deficits	Right-sided weakness	Left-sided weakness
Behavior	Cautious Plodding Careful	Impatient Impulsive Lack of insight
Perceptions	Receptive aphasia	Problems with spatial relationships Left neglect

The term aphasia is often used interchangeably with the term dysphasia. By definition, dysphasia is impairment of the comprehension or production of verbal or written language. Aphasia generally involves exclusive loss of the comprehension or production of verbal or written language.[57]

Aphasia may be classified in various ways. One approach has been to classify aphasia on a neuroanatomic basis. Other approaches include classifying aphasia as expressive aphasia (motor or Broca's aphasia), receptive aphasia (sensory or Wernicke's aphasia), and expressive-receptive aphasia (mixed or global aphasia).[57]

Aphasia may also be categorized as fluent or nonfluent. Fluent aphasias include Wernicke's (receptive) aphasia, conduction aphasia, amnesic aphasia, and transcortical aphasia. Nonfluent aphasias include Broca's (expressive) aphasia and global aphasia.

Nonfluent aphasia results from a lesion in the area of the third frontal gyrus of the cerebral cortex in the left hemisphere, near the region of the motor cortex. This type of aphasia includes difficulty in selecting, organizing, and initiating motor speech, resulting in a hesitant, slow, labored speech.[57] The patient often struggles visibly, using facial grimaces and hand gestures in trying to communicate. Telegraphic speech may be present, demonstrated by a manner of speaking in which small parts of speech and the ends of nouns and verbs are omitted.[57] Thus speech is sparse, labored, or limited to short phrases or single words. A single word, however, often conveys much information.

In fluent aphasia, several types of speech may be at a normal or rapid rate, with grammar and rhythm intact, so that the speech sounds almost normal. The content of the speech, however, is affected in this receptive, or sensory, type of aphasia. Auditory comprehension and auditory feedback are impaired; persons with fluent aphasia are not able to monitor their speaking. These patients, for example, are unable to correct their speech because they are not aware of their mistakes. Wernicke's aphasia is a type of fluent aphasia because the area of damage is in the left hemisphere in the posterior part of the left superior temporal convolution, known as Wernicke's area. Another characteristic of this type of aphasia is the use of literal paraphasia, or the substitution of a syllable, word, or group of sounds. Patients with Wernicke's aphasia substitute incorrect sounds (such as "dork" for "fork"). Verbal paraphasia occurs when a word is substituted for another (such as "table" for "chair"). Such patients are less disturbed by their disabilities because they are not really aware of their speech impairments. Circumlocution, a rambling type of speech, is also characteristic.[9] The patient substitutes descriptions of

words when a particular substantive word is not able to be used.

In anemic aphasia the patient has fluent, rhythmic speech, but the patient's problem is in correctly naming objects or places, often defining or describing in circumlocutory speech what he or she is unable to name. These patients are readily frustrated by their disability, because they are aware of their errors in the use of names.

Conduction aphasia is also known as central aphasia.[9] Persons with conduction aphasia have difficulty repeating words spoken by another, and their speech is characterized by literal paraphasias with intact comprehension.

Global aphasia is a condition in which a person has few language skills as a result of extensive damage to the left hemisphere. The speech is nonfluent and is associated with poor comprehension and limited ability to name objects or repeat words.[57]

Other stroke patients may have intact language comprehension and appropriate language in speaking, but they may have dysarthria. In this condition the musculature used in speaking is paralyzed, weak, or uncoordinated. Speech is slurred and un-

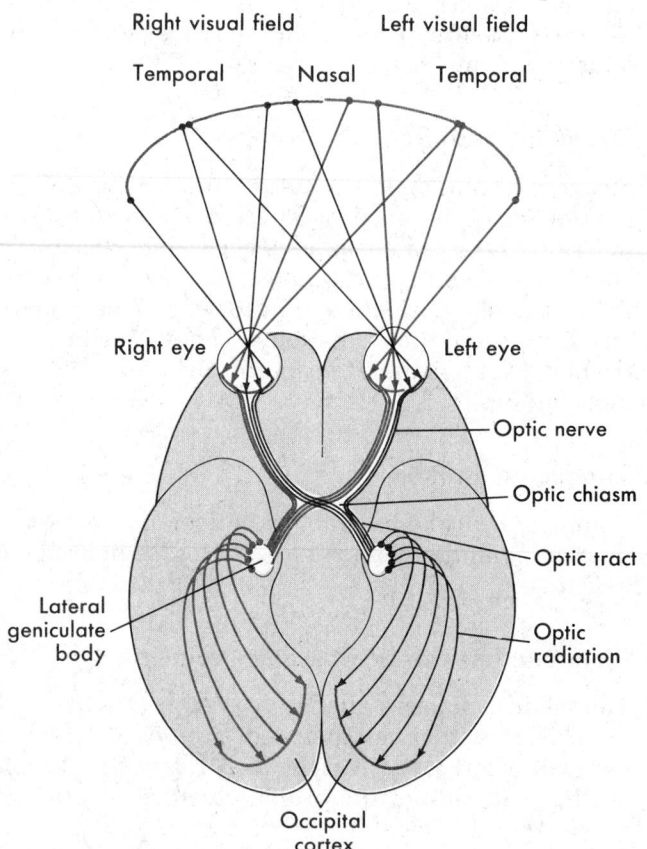

Right visual field   Left visual field

Temporal   Nasal   Temporal

Right eye   Left eye

Optic nerve

Optic chiasm

Optic tract

Lateral
geniculate
body

Optic
radiation

Occipital
cortex

FIGURE 47-2   Visual pathway.

clear, and there are problems in phonation and articulation. Weakness, slowness, incoordination, or other alterations in muscle tone characterize this speech problem. Dysarthria may occur singly or in combination with aphasia.

Visual changes

Visual field deficits interfere with perception and negatively affect the stroke patient's performance of activities of daily living (ADL). Homonymous hemianopsia is the most common type of visual field defect in stroke. It is caused by damage to the optic tract posterior to the optic chiasm and results in loss of vision in the temporal field of one eye and the nasal field of the other eye, causing a half blindness[9,62] (Figure 47-2).

Arterial occlusion

Ischemia in certain cerebral arteries produces various syndromes depending on which cerebral artery is involved and the location of the occlusion. The arterial circulation to the brain is divided into the anterior portion (those arteries fed by the carotid arteries) and the posterior portion (those arteries fed by the vertebral arteries).[9] Table 47-3 lists the major cerebral arteries and the corresponding signs and symptoms of occlusion. Figure 47-3 shows the major cerebral vessels.

The pathologic condition of the extracranial carotid artery is often detected by signs and symptoms related to ischemia. A diffuse, localized, bilateral or unilateral carotid bruit is predictive of moderate to severe atherosclerosis in the extracranial carotid system 85% of the time.[29]

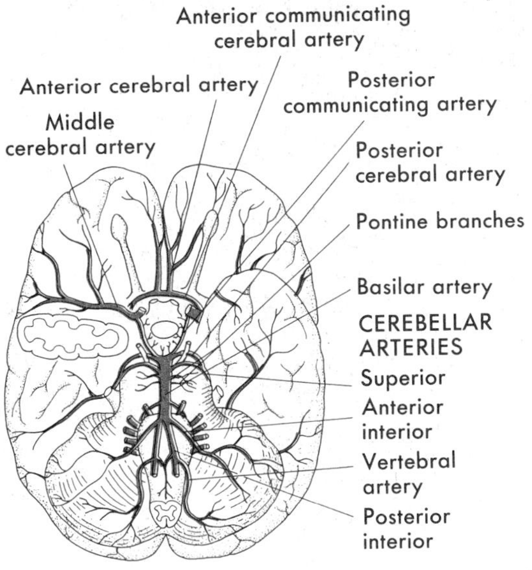

Another important finding related to carotid artery ischemia is transient monocular visual loss, termed amaurosis fugax.[2] Lasting from a few seconds to a few minutes, this event causes sensations of darkening, graying, clouding, or fogging of vision. The visual loss most commonly begins in the upper visual field and may progress to the entire visual field. Because of the risk of a TIA, stroke, or blindness a workup for an episode of amaurosis fugax should be undertaken without delay.[2]

Middle cerebral artery syndrome varies with the level of occlusion. Symptoms of large middle cerebral artery territory involvement include contralateral hemiparesis and hemianesthesia, homonymous hemianopsia, anosognosia, and aphasia.[9]

Occlusion of the anterior cerebral artery may cause urinary incontinence, contralateral motor and sensory loss in the leg, and apraxia.[9] Posterior cerebral artery occlusion can result in contralateral homonymous hemianopsia, memory loss, contralateral hemiparesis, and hemisensory loss and dyslexia. Vertebrobasilar artery syndrome may include ataxia, contralateral hemiplegia and sensory loss, abnormal eye movements, hemianopsia, vertigo, ataxia, and loss of consciousness.[9,37]

Cerebral aneurysms

Aneurysms may become apparent before or after rupture. Unruptured aneurysms can be detected incidentally by causing symptoms of cranial nerve compression, seizures, or hydrocephalus.[50] Aneurysms of the internal carotid artery or the posterior communicating artery may cause oculomotor nerve palsy by compressing cranial nerve III. Compression of the optic nerve at the optic chiasm causes bitemporal hemianopsia (tunnel vision). Patients are more likely to present after a hemorrhage secondary to a ruptured aneurysm. Severe headache (often described by patients as "the worst of my life") is the most common symptom.[50] Transient loss of consciousness, vomiting, neck pain, photophobia, and low-grade fever are other symptoms associated with SAH. Nuchal rigidity, altered sensorium, focal neurologic deficits, seizures, and coma are more vivid signs that occur with increased bleeding from the ruptured aneurysm. See Table 47-4 for clinical grading of aneurysms. Lumbar puncture is contraindicated in the case of increased intracranial pressure and is usually not needed if CT or MRI is available. If lumbar puncture is performed, the specimen may appear grossly bloody. A number of patients with SAH or intracerebral hemorrhage have used cocaine. Cocaine is a potent vasoconstrictor and causes hypertension and elevated pulse.[34]

FIGURE 47-3   Cerebral arteries at base of brain.

Anterior communicating cerebral artery

Anterior cerebral artery

Middle cerebral artery

Posterior communicating artery

Posterior cerebral artery

Pontine branches

Basilar artery

CEREBELLAR ARTERIES

Superior

Anterior interior

Vertebral artery

Posterior interior

TABLE 47-3   Clinical Syndromes of Arterial Occlusion

Artery	Structures supplied	Associated dysfunction
Internal carotid artery	Eyes Basal nuclei Hypothalamus Frontal lobe Parietal lobe Temporal lobe	Contralateral hemiplegia Transient monocular blindness Aphasia
Anterior cerebral artery	Medial surface of frontal lobe Medial surface of parietal lobe Corpus callosum	Perseveration Contralateral monoplegia Contralateral hemiplegia or hemiparesis (leg more affected than arm) Gegenhalten Urinary incontinence Gait apraxia Confusion
Middle cerebral artery	Putamen Head of caudate nucleus Globus pallidus Genu Posterior limb of internal capsule	Contralateral hemiparesis (arm and face more affected than leg) Contralateral hemiplegia Apraxia Cerebral gaze palsy Dysarthria-anarthria Hemianopsia All types of aphasias Hemisensory loss of spatial neglect
Posterior cerebral artery	Posterior limb of internal capsule Thalamus Wall of third ventricle Portions of optic chiasm and optic tract	Contralateral hemiplegia Cerebellar ataxia Ipsilateral III nerve paresis Contralateral hemiballismus Intention tremors Dystonia
Vertebrobasilar system	Portions of temporal lobe Occipital lobe Thalamus Midbrain Pons Medulla oblongata Inner ear Upper portion of spinal cord	Dysarthria Dysphagia Diplopia Facial palsy and numbness Oculomotor paralysis Ptosis Nystagmus Ataxias Ipsilateral tongue paralysis Tremors of extremities Vertigo Dysphonia Headache Vomiting Limb weakness (unilateral, bilateral, alternating) Altered consciousness

TABLE 47-4   Clinical Grading of Aneurysms

Grade	Condition
1	Alert without neurologic deficit and with or without signs of meningeal irritation (minimal bleed)
2	Drowsy, without significant deficit (mild bleed)
3	Drowsy and confused with minimal deficit (moderate bleed)
4	Major neurologic deficit and generally deteriorating, possibly result of intracerebral clot (moderate to severe bleed)
5	Moribund, or nearly so, with vegetative disturbance and extension rigidity (severe bleed)

Modified from Botterell EH et al: Hypothermia in the surgical treatment of ruptured intracranial aneurysm, *Neuroscience* 15:4, 1958.

Indications of spontaneous intracerebral hemorrhage are a sudden onset of headache and confusion, followed by rapid neurologic deterioration. Signs and symptoms of intracerebral hemorrhage depend on the location of the hemorrhage. Diagnosis is based on history of hypertension, physical findings, coagulation studies, CT, angiography, and lumbar puncture.

Diagnosis of Cerebrovascular Accident

Diagnosis of CVA is determined by observation of clinical signs and is confirmed with specific diagnostic tools to estimate the extent and location of infarcted areas and hemorrhage. The diagnostic tests used are cranial computed tomography (CT), magnetic resonance imaging (MRI), magnetic resonance angiography (MRA), digital subtraction arteriography (DSA), and single photon emission computerized tomography (SPECT).[33] See Table 47-5. Assessment of neurologic signs is essential, not only in diagnosis, but also in planning appropriate care for the patient in both the acute and rehabilitative phases (see Chapter 44).

Therapeutic Management

When TIA occurs, secondary prevention of stroke is often attempted. Controversy continues, however, regarding whether medical treatment of TIA affects mortality. Two types of medical treatment are used to interfere with intra-arterial clot formation: (1) chronic anticoagulation with oral anticoagulants and (2) platelet inhibition with aspirin, dipyridamole (Persantine), or ticlopidine (Ticlid).[9,25] In addition, part of the regimen includes correcting risk factors that predispose the patient to another TIA. For example, the obese patient would be placed on a calorie-restricted diet, and the person with hypertension would be treated with an antihypertensive agent.

Drug therapy

Pharmacologic treatment of the patient with a stroke is centered on decreasing or preventing extension of the stroke and minimizing permanent damage. Early treatment for acute ischemic stroke is essential.[5] Table 47-6 summarizes pharmacologic therapy for stroke along with desired effects.

Anticoagulants are used in selected patients with stroke to interfere with fibrin formation and throm-

TABLE 47-5   Diagnostic Test Results with Stroke

Test	Results
Computed tomography (CT)	Important in differentiating between hemorrhagic and nonhemorrhagic strokes; increase in density is characteristic of hemorrhage; low density is characteristic of infarction; shift of intracranial contents may be detected
Lumbar puncture	Intracerebral hemorrhage: bloody (<1000 RBCs); elevated pressure >200 cm H_2O Subarachnoid hemorrhage: grossly bloody (>25000 RBCs); xanthrochromic 4 to 6 hours after bleed; elevated pressure >200 cm H_2O; increased WBCs; increased protein count; decreased glucose level
Electroencephalogram	Abnormal with large vessel disease
Arteriography	Identifies aneurysms, AVM, carotid artery stenosis, ulcerated carotid plaques
Oculoplethysmography	Delay in pulse arrival, showing obstruction of flow in internal carotid artery
Doppler imaging	Reverse flow direction of supraorbital artery with carotid artery stenosis

TABLE 47-6   Pharmacology Summary: Drugs for Stroke

Drug	Dosage	Desired effect
SUBARACHNOID HEMORRHAGE		
Phenobarbital	100-200 mg daily; divided doses	Antihypertensive Sedative Anticonvulsant
Chlorothiazide (Diuril)	250 mg bid or tid	Antihypertensive
Hydrochlorothiazide (Hydrodiuril)	25-50 mg 1 or 2 times daily	Antihypertensive
Furosemide (Lasix)	40-80 mg IV	Diuretic Antihypertensive
Propranolol (Inderal)	10-30 mg PO tid or qid; 1-3 mg IV	Antihypertensive
Methyldopa (Aldomet)	250-500 mg IV q6h	Antihypertensive
Diazoxide (Hyperstat)	5 mg/kg IV	Hypertensive crisis
Diazepam (Valium)	2-10 mg PO bid to qid	Sedative
Docusate sodium (Colace)	300 mg daily; divided doses	Stool softener
Aminocaproic acid (Amicar)	30-36 g/day IV	Antifibrinolytic
Dexamethasone	6-10 mg IV q6h	Antiedema; decreases intracranial pressure
Glycerol	1 g/kg PO q6h	Antiedema
Isoproterenol (Isuprel)	0.5-5 μg/min IV	Questionable effects in controlling vasospasm; lidocaine controls cardiac irritability
Lidocaine	Concurrent administration (1-4 mg/min)	
Dopamine	Up to 7 μg/kg/min	Increases blood pressure to increase mean arterial pressure, which, in some cases, improves cerebral blood flow through small vessels
Albumin 5%	2 to 4 mL/min	Volume expanders to assist cerebral perfusion
Nitroglycerin	50 mg/250 mL D_5W infused at 5 μg/kg/min	Controls/prevents vasospasm; increases cerebral perfusion
Neosynephrine		Neosynephrine instituted if hypotension occurs
CEREBROVASCULAR OCCLUSIVE DISEASE		
Anticoagulant therapy		
Heparin	IV bolus (loading dose): 5000-10,000 units Continuous IV: 1000-2000/hr	Anticoagulation: prevents conversion of prothrombin to thrombin
Coumadin	Loading dose: 4-60 mg Maintenance: 5-10 mg	Anticoagulation: alters synthesis of clotting factors II, VII, IX, and X
Antiplatelet therapy		
Aspirin	300 mg/day	Inhibits platelet aggregation
Dipyridamole (Persantine)	50 mg PO tid	Inhibits platelet aggregation
Others		
Dexamethasone	IV loading dose: 10 mg, followed by 4 mg IV q4-6h	Antiedema
Glycerol	1 g/kg PO q6h	Antiedema

bus propagation.[17,54] Patients with cerebral emboli that have likely arisen from the heart are clearly candidates for heparin therapy.[17,52] Anticoagulant therapy is of no value in a large completed thrombotic stroke and may be detrimental by actually stimulating hemorrhage. Patients receiving anticoagulation therapy have a 1% to 2% rate of heparin-induced thrombocytopenia with thromboembolic complications, including stroke.[6] Anticoagulant therapy has been used for patients with stroke in evolution; RIND; recent TIA (especially if multiple); and cardioembolic stroke. Lifetime anticoagulation with coumadin may be required for long-term risk patients, such as those with chronic atrial fibrillation.[55]

Platelet antiaggregants including aspirin, dipyridamole, and ticlopidine are the most beneficial in preventing stroke.[9,25] The theory behind this therapy is that by inhibiting platelet function there will be less chance of thrombi developing, especially in the tortuous, stenotic cerebral vessels.[9] Aspirin prevents the synthesis of prostaglandins and thromboxane, thereby decreasing platelet aggregation. Dipyridamole also inhibits platelet aggregation, and ticlopidine inhibits platelet aggregation, prolongs bleeding time, and blocks platelet release action.[9]

In acute stroke, protecting the brain from further damage by maintaining cerebral blood flow is important. Systemic blood pressure must be managed appropriately, because a precipitous increase or decrease in systemic blood pressure may increase infarct size. This is because systemic blood pressure directly affects cerebral blood flow. A wide variety of antihypertensive drugs may be used to maintain the blood pressure within normal range. Nimodipine is a calcium channel antagonist that has been used effectively in acute ischemic stroke to improve cerebral blood flow around infarcts.[4] Vasopressors such as dopamine also may at times be useful in maintaining cerebral blood.[54] Another important way to protect the brain from further damage is to prevent seizure activity. Seizures occur in approximately 4% of patients with stroke and TIA.[36] Seizures tend to occur within 48 hours of the stroke onset.[36] Control of seizure activity is important, because it increases blood pressure and oxygen demand on the brain cells. Anticonvulsants such as phenobarbital are effective in preventing seizures and act also as antihypertensive agents. Stool softeners are effective in preventing the patient from straining to defecate and preventing a Valsalva maneuver.

Controlling cerebral edema resulting from stroke is a complicated issue. Because of the increased risk of infection, gastrointestinal bleeding, and hyperglycemia, steroids are not routinely used in acute ischemic stroke.[52] Mannitol may be of some use in controlling vasogenic edema in hemorrhagic stroke. For the patient with an SAH related to a ruptured aneurysm, corticosteroids such as dexamethasone and methyprednisolone are used at times to control edema. Also in SAH, antifibrinolytic agents, such as aminocaproic acid (Amicar), are sometimes used to prevent rebleeding. Hypervolemic hemodilution is used to augment cerebral blood flow and control vasospasm after aneurysmal clipping in a SAH. The most widely used pharmacologic agent in this therapy is 5% albumin.[9]

Surgical management

Restoration of blood flow by surgical revascularization after cerebral infarction may be accomplished by direct thrombectomy or embolectomy of neck vessels or large intracranial arteries. Carotid endarterectomy is a type of secondary prevention in which the underlying pathologic condition (atherosclerotic plaque) is removed to prevent an initial or recurrent stroke (Figure 47-4). This procedure is also used as a surgical therapy in selected patients experiencing TIAs caused by carotid artery stenosis. This surgery is clearly effective for patients with a 70% or greater narrowing of their arteries.[42] The effectiveness of carotid endarterectomy in stroke prevention is still under investigation for patients with a 30% to 69% narrowing of the carotid artery.[42]

Complications following carotid endarterectomy include hemorrhage at the operative site and neurologic complications. Respiratory crisis can result from hematoma pressing against the trachea. Cranial nerve dysfunction may occur as a result of retraction during surgery. Occasional mortality from carotid endarterectomy is usually related to myocardial infarction and only rarely to stroke.

Secondary prevention to avoid more brain damage may also be attempted by maintaining adequate perfusion to marginally ischemic areas and by reducing edema formation.[9] Extracranial-intracranial bypass (EC-IC bypass) is sometimes performed to augment cerebral blood circulation. Superficial middle temporal artery to middle cerebral artery bypass grafting (STA-MCA) is the most common type of bypass performed. STA-MCA has been used in selected patients when carotid and cerebral occlusive diseases are not amenable to direct surgical procedures. In selected cases and experienced hands, this bypass surgery has diminished the incidence of TIAs and stroke, but its precise role has not yet been established.[9,36]

The surgeon makes the STA-MCA bypass incision approximately 1 cm anterior and superior to the ear and exposes the donor vessel. A craniectomy is performed, and the dura is opened. The surgeon locates a branch of the middle cerebral artery; then the donor vessel (STA) is transposed intracranially and anastomosed to the recipient artery (MCA) (Figure

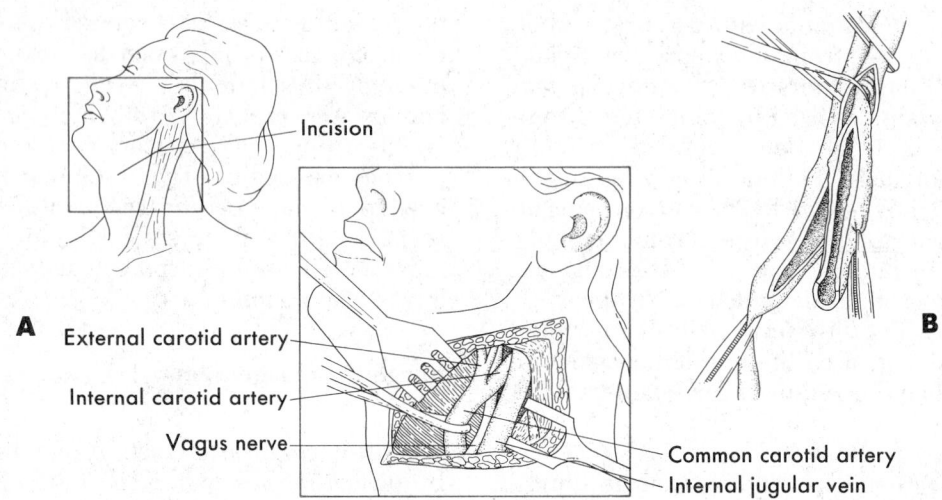

FIGURE 47-4   **A,** Incision site and exposure of carotid bifurcation area. **B,** Carotid endarterectomy.

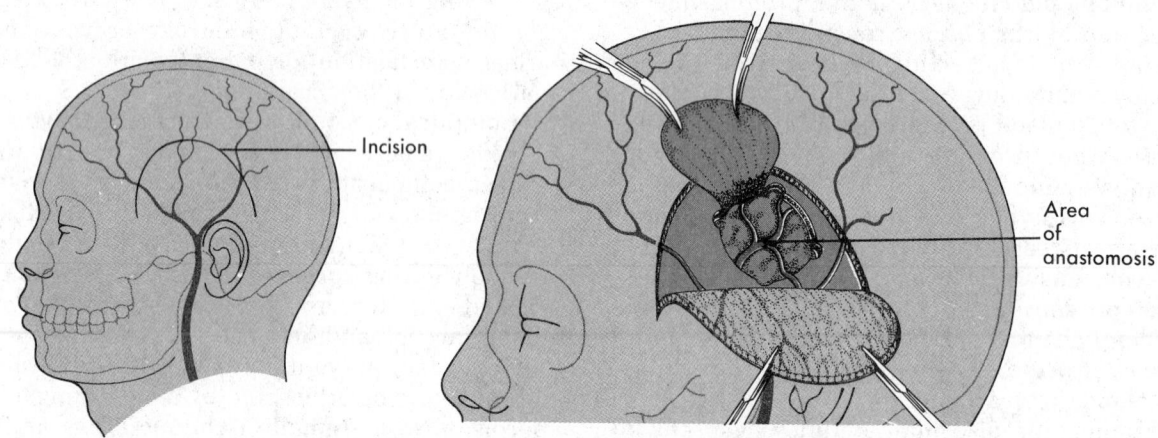

FIGURE 47-5   Intracranial-extracranial anastomosis showing connection of superficial temporal artery to branch of middle cerebral artery.

47-5). Complications of this surgical procedure include spasm of the vessels, loss of patency of the anastomosis, and hemorrhage.

A complication of cerebellar infarction and hemorrhage is brain swelling, which can progress to coma and death. Various lifesaving surgical procedures are used to relieve the pressure caused by the swollen brain. When swelling of the infarcted cerebellum occurs in stroke, surgical decompression of the posterior fossa may be used. If a large intracra-

nial hematoma is present, a craniotomy may be used to remove the clot and thus provide pressure relief.[9] Right hemispheric cerebral infarction with severe edema has been successfully treated with hemicraniectomy.[13]

When an unruptured aneurysm is diagnosed surgical excision may cure the condition without any residual neurologic deficit. Thus the ideal procedure is to eliminate the aneurysm surgically by clipping it at the neck of the sac, preserving the normal vasculature. When an aneurysm has ruptured, there is controversy about the timing of surgery; some physicians prefer operating within the first 7 days, whereas others prefer to wait 7 to 14 days until the patient's neurologic status has stabilized.[1,23,26] Surgery prevents the aneurysm from rebleeding by placement of an aneurysm clip.[23] A rebleed is a complication of a ruptured aneurysm that occurs 5 to 7 days following a rupture when dissolution of the clot begins.

Arteriovenous malformation is also amenable to surgical treatment. Surgical treatment consists of excision of the lesion after all feeder vessels are eliminated, either by coagulation and cutting or by clipping and coagulation.[38] Transarterial embolization can also be used in conjunction with surgery or as a primary treatment modality.[62] A number of embolic agents and delivery techniques are currently used for these procedures.[62] A stereotaxic radiosurgery using the cobalt gamma unit, commonly referred to as the gamma knife, may also be an option for selected AVMs that are small, deep, and not as accessible to surgery or embolization.[41]

NURSING MANAGEMENT OF THE CVA PATIENT IN THE ACUTE CARE PHASE
Assessment

Neurologic assessment findings depend on the area of the brain injury. The patient's level of consciousness may range from alert and oriented, to barely arousable, to coma. The Glasgow scale is sometimes useful in measuring level of consciousness. The nurse should ask questions to measure orientation to person, place, and time. The patient's ability to follow simple commands is assessed. Recent or remote memory, attention span, perception, and orientation are commonly disturbed by stroke. Assessment of level of consciousness is presented in Chapter 45.

Blood in the subarachnoid space produces meningeal irritation. Assessment for meningeal irritation includes headache as well as Brudzinski's sign and Kernig's sign.[12] A positive Brudzinski's sign is flexion of the hip and knee on flexion of the patient's neck toward the chest. Kernig's sign is positive when the patient is unable to extend the leg after flexion of the hip and knee. Other signs of meningeal irritation are headache, nuchal rigidity, low-grade fever, irritability, restlessness, and seizures.

Assessment for signs of increased intracranial pressure is paramount (see Chapter 45), because intracranial pressure may rise as a result of hemorrhage or edema.

The nurse should determine the extent of involvement of the cranial nerves. It is important to assess for visual changes such as blurred or double vision. Visual field cuts such as homonymous hemianopsia

or monocular blindness may be present. Cranial nerves V, VII, IX, X, and XII are evaluated because they are important for swallowing and speech.[9]

Motor function is examined for hemiparesis or hemiplegia. Muscle strength and tone are assessed, including whether there has been a change (e.g., worsening or fluctuation) or whether there is a difference between extremities (e.g., right vs. left, and upper vs. lower). Muscle tone is assessed for rigidity, spasticity, clonus, and flaccidity.[9]

Sensation and perception are commonly decreased. The patient's ability to detect temperature extremes and pain often is diminished. Also, assessment of headache pain is important, since it may be a sign of rebleeding.

The nurse must observe for signs of seizures and hydrocephalus, which are complications of hemorrhage (see Chapter 45). Vital signs must also be monitored closely. Alterations in blood pressure, heart rate, respiratory rate, and temperature are common and may signal or be the cause of severe complications.

Vasospasm is another complication of ruptured aneurysm for which the nurse must monitor the patient closely. Vasospasm may become apparent as a new neurologic deficit, usually after the fourth day of initial bleeding.[26] The slightest change in the neurologic status of the patient, such as drowsiness, aphasia, or newly developed pronator drift, may be an indication of new cerebral ischemia. Vasospasm may cause infarction of previously uninvolved brain.

Nursing Diagnosis

Nursing diagnoses in the acute stage after stroke include the following:

  Ineffective airway clearance related to inability to handle secretions
  Altered cerebral tissue perfusion related to pathophysiologic changes that decrease blood flow
  Altered physical mobility related to decreased muscle strength, tone, balance, or coordination
  Fluid volume deficit related to decreased ability to ingest fluids
  Ineffective individual coping related to feelings of grief, loss, and discomfort
  High risk for injury related to impaired mobility and risk of seizures
  Impaired verbal communication related to altered expression, comprehension, or a combination of the two
  Knowledge deficit related to stroke care, expected outcomes, and community resources

Planning

Expected outcomes for the stroke patient during the acute phase include the following:

Airway patent and patient free of aspiration
Maintains adequate cerebral tissue perfusion
Remains free of contractures and subluxations
Maintains fluid and electrolyte balance
Verbalizes anxious feelings and effectively copes with feelings
Remains free of injury; environment safe
Communicates needs effectively
Knowledgeable regarding procedures, expected outcomes, and community resources

Implementation

Early care of the patient requires simultaneous assessment and treatment as a result of the complexity and acuteness of the situation. The concept of intensive early care for patients after a stroke is controversial, because the value in terms of improved outcome has not been demonstrated.[27] Despite this, acute stroke units with more intensive nursing care as well as electrocardiographic (ECG) and respiratory monitoring capabilities have become more common. The major goal in the acute phase after stroke is to maintain or restore cerebral perfusion to preserve viable and partially damaged brain tissue. This goal requires actions related to reducing intracranial pressure associated with edema and ischemia and monitoring the patient closely to detect signs of increased intracranial pressure. Maintaining blood pressure and providing hydration are important interventions at this time. The nurse is also concerned with preserving function by maintaining joint mobility, promoting muscle function, and preventing secondary complications such as pressure sores, contractures, and pneumonia. Early mobilization and activation of patients with stroke are beneficial for long-term functioning. Maintaining a positive nutritional status and preserving or striving to restore normal bowel and bladder elimination patterns are other important nursing goals during the acute period.

The major complications during hospitalization for stroke care are infections such as urinary tract infection and pneumonia; thrombophlebitis; limb, musculoskeletal, and nerve lesions; cerebral edema; progression of the infarct; seizures; and depression.[12] In the acute stage the nurse is also concerned with educating the patient and family regarding the stroke and what can be expected in each stage. Increased age and loss of consciousness have been cited as the most important predictors of mortality associated with stroke. Laterality (i.e., left-sided vs. right-sided cerebral damage) has not been a factor in influencing eventual outcome.

Airway clearance

Ineffective airway clearance may be caused by hemiparesis and immobility, and in this case, nursing interventions focus on helping the patient cough and deep breathe using incentive spirometry and providing chest physical therapy. These interventions are performed to maintain a patent airway and ensure adequate ventilation. If the patient experiences loss of consciousness and inability to clear secretions, then nursing interventions include using an airway, humidity, changes in positioning, and suctioning. If alterations in neuromuscular control of swallowing or the cough and gag reflex are factors causing ineffective airway clearance, then positioning to promote airway clearance is indicated. Patients are turned on their sides rather than to a supine position to promote drainage of oral secretions. Pooling of oral secretions in the oropharynx may increase the likelihood of respiratory infection. In some cases an airway or tracheostomy may be needed to prevent aspiration, maintain a patent airway, and remove secretions by suctioning.[38]

Cerebral perfusion

To limit or avoid progression of neurologic deficits, nursing interventions are concerned with prevention of events that increase or decrease cerebral blood flow to abnormal levels. For example, decreased cerebral blood flow in an acute stroke patient is undesirable because it leads to further ischemia, edema, and progressive neurologic dysfunction. Events that can cause decreased cerebral blood flow are a decrease in systemic blood pressure accompanied by a loss of autoregulation; hypertension, which increases cerebrovascular resistance in the presence of arteriolar disease; a decrease in P_{CO_2}; vasospasm; or cerebral edema.[28] Increases in cerebral blood flow above the patient's normal level may further increase cerebral edema, intracranial pressure, or the risk of bleeding. Events that can increase cerebral blood flow are a decrease in P_{O_2}, an increase in P_{CO_2}, hyperthermia, severe anemia, or a decrease in venous return or cerebrovascular resistance.

Nursing interventions are concerned with maintaining blood pressure at the patient's high normal level to avoid sudden changes in blood pressure that might alter cerebral blood flow. This requires close monitoring of the blood pressure, precise administration of antihypertensive or diuretic drugs, and accurate observation of the effects of the drugs. In addition, bed rest is indicated in the initial period after a stroke, with restrictions on head-of-the-bed elevation. If the goal is to maintain adequate perfusion, as with a patient with thrombosis, then the bed may be flat. In the case of hemorrhage the head of the bed may be elevated to decrease intracranial pressure.[9]

Avoiding neck and hip flexion and teaching the patient to avoid isometric movements are other measures taken to reduce intracranial pressure. Isometric movements are those that increase intrathoracic pressure and interfere with venous return from the brain to the heart. These cause the patient to hold breaths and keep the chest fixed while straining. Straining on defecation and doing the Valsalva maneuver when pulling up in bed are examples of isometric movements to be avoided by these patients.

Monitoring of drugs used to maintain normal blood flow, such as antihypertensives, anticoagulants, sedatives, hyperosmolar agents, calcium channel blockers, and vasopressors, is also an important nursing responsibility for preventing further neurologic deterioration. Ongoing neurologic assessment to detect important changes is mandatory. A decreased level of consciousness and decreased or increased blood pressure should be reported to the physician immediately for proper management.

In the case of ruptured intracranial aneurysm, the physician sometimes orders SAH precautions for the patient. These include placing the patient in a quiet, darkened room to reduce stress and excitement. Usually, no television or radio is allowed. No smoking is permitted in the room, especially by the patient, to avoid any abrupt change in systemic arterial pressure that could precipitate rebleeding. Bed rest is essential, usually with the head of the bed elevated and the neck in straight alignment to help promote venous return.[28] Visitors are restricted to immediate family only. Neurologic signs are monitored at least hourly with particular attention to pupil size, motor strength, level of consciousness, speech, and orientation. Some clinical settings use a sign saying "aneurysm precautions" or "SAH precautions" to warn health care professionals and visitors of the need for a quiet environment and caution in moving or observing the patient. Vigorous coughing and suctioning are avoided to prevent increased intracranial pressure. Nothing is to be administered to the patient by rectum to prevent rectal stimulation, and temperature should be taken orally with an electronic thermometer. The box below summarizes the precautions to be taken with these patients.

SAH OR ANEURYSM PRECAUTIONS

Quiet dark environment
No television, radio, or telephone calls
No smoking
Restricted visitors
Bed rest
Oral temperatures
Frequent neurologic checks

Anticonvulsants often are prescribed to minimize the chance of a seizure. Sedation with phenobarbital or analgesia with codeine is often indicated to counteract restlessness. Stool softeners are also necessary to avoid straining, especially if the patient is receiving codeine. Antihypertensive agents may be needed, but vital signs must be monitored very closely to prevent hypotension. In the event of increasing intracranial pressure, steroids or hyperosmolar diuretics, such as mannitol, may also be prescribed. Antipyretics are important in controlling temperature elevations.

Neurologic deterioration may occur with ruptured aneurysm as a result of rebleeding, vasospasm, delayed cerebral ischemia, hydrocephalus, or other complications such as a subdural hematoma or seizures.[26] Since early surgery for clipping of the aneurysm has reduced the rate of rebleeding the most significant complication has become vasospasm.[23,28] Vasospasm usually occurs between the fourth and twelfth days after the initial hemorrhage and either resolves gradually over several days or progresses to coma and death within hours or days. Hypervolemia hemodilution is an important treatment for maintaining or improving cerebral blood flow.[8] Hydrocephalus results from hemorrhage into the ventricles, requiring emergency ventriculostomy. Hydrocephalus may also result from blockage of the subarachnoid pathways and interference with the reabsorption of cerebrospinal fluid by the blood in the subarachnoid space.

Altered physical mobility

Most stroke patients suffer an alteration in physical mobility. Early care focuses on preserving intact function, restoring impaired function, preventing complications such as contractures, deep venous thromboses, or subluxations and educating both the patient and family. Early use of the Bobath techniques focuses care on involvement of the affected side; facilitation of normal tone, posture, and movement; and development of more normal function.[46] Detailed explanations show how nurses can apply the principles in routine nursing care.[45,46] Bobath principles provide nurses with a means to maximize the stroke patient's potential and influence functional outcome.[46]

Fluid balance

Fluid and electrolyte imbalance may be caused by alterations in consciousness or dysphagia that affects intake of fluids and nutrients. Monitoring urine specific gravity, blood chemistries, and serum osmolarity; maintaining accurate intake and output records; and observing for clinical signs and symptoms of fluid and electrolyte imbalance are some interventions indicated for this area of patient care.

Areas of particular concern are nitrogen and calcium balance.[38]

Hyponatremia and hypernatremia commonly occur after rupture of an aneurysm.[38] Hypokalemia may develop as a result of diuretic and steroid therapy. Potassium must be replaced if the patient's level is below 3.5 mEq. Severe fluid restriction should be avoided, since it exacerbates the tendency for hyperatremia and hyperviscous blood. Conversely, fluid volume excess can occur; therefore the patient should be carefully monitored for peripheral edema, tachycardia, distended neck veins, and respiratory rales.[28]

Ineffective coping

Fear of another stroke and depression about physical condition contribute to the patient's emotional reaction to stroke.[15,16] After a stroke the patient may experience an exaggerated form of previous personality, so assessment of past coping patterns may be helpful. To enhance the patient's self-esteem and to overcome feelings of hopelessness and powerlessness, help the patient set goals and offer praise when they are met. Help the patient in identifying effective coping responses and others that may be used. Socialization may provide added support. Help the patient work through feelings of anger and denial, and encourage a realistic attitude of hope as a way of dealing with feelings of helplessness. Interdisciplinary stroke family support and education programs can provide basic education and support for patients and families as they adjust to the crisis of stroke.[31]

High risk for injury

The patient is at high risk for injury during a seizure. If seizure occurs, support and protect the patient, especially the head, from injury. If the patient is out of bed, lower the patient to the floor. If the patient is in bed, provide protection from hard siderails by placing pillows along them. If possible, turn the patient's head to the side. After the seizure, assess vital signs and neurologic status, and maintain an open airway by turning the patient to the side, suctioning, and administering oxygen as needed (see Chapter 45).

Secondary to the diagnoses of altered physical mobility and sensory-perceptual deficits the stroke patient is at risk for injury from falls. Maintain the bed in the low position, and keep the siderails up. Place the nurse call light within the patient's reach. This is especially important for the patient with neurologic deficits such as hemiplegia. If the patient is able to get out of bed, keep the environment as clutter free as possible. Remind the patient with a visual defect to compensate for the impairment. Place objects that the visually impaired patient may need

within the patient's view. The patient will have a much easier time attending to the health team members involved in his or her care if the bed is situated so the door to the patient's room can be visualized. Patients who are in a room where the door is within their area of visual deficit have a much more difficult time keeping up with what is going on around them.

Impaired verbal communication

Some stroke patients may experience an alteration in communication in the form of a speech and language disorder. The communication disorder is further complicated by other cognitive deficits that may be present, such as impairment of auditory and visual memory, visual perception, logical reasoning and judgment, motivation, and the ability to think abstractly. In addition, emotional reactions to the motor and sensory losses resulting from stroke can affect communication ability. Impaired verbal communication requires prompt attention so that a patient with a stroke does not become more anxious and isolated as a result of a lack of comprehensive or expressive abilities. There is a need even during the acute period to establish a means of communication, even if it consists only of talking to the patient, whether alert or not, to create a communicating environment. The use of touch and gestures, and the use of slow, careful movements around the patient to create a calm atmosphere are means of dealing with patients who have impaired verbal communication after a stroke. It is important to convey a feeling of wishing to communicate with the patient, even when the patient does not respond or responds inappropriately. Spontaneous recovery, or at least considerable improvement, may occur in the first 3 to 4 months after a stroke, so it is difficult to make a prognosis of speech recovery at this early stage after stroke.

Assessment of neurologic and psychologic status of the patient will help the nurse identify other problems that may affect speech rehabilitation. To assess spontaneous speech the nurse should listen to the person during a conversation and note fluency, rhythm, melody, articulation, phrase length, paraphasia, and word content.[58] Often the patient will have a combination of fluent and nonfluent speech.[57] To determine the patient's ability to comprehend spoken language, the nurse should give simple, one-step directions such as "pick up the spoon" while being careful to avoid giving clues to the patient by pointing or mimicking the expected action. If the patient is able to follow one-step directions, then the nurse can give two-step and three-step directions to determine the patient's level of understanding. Asking the patient some "yes" and "no" questions, being careful not to give cues by nodding or changing facial expressions, is another way to determine the patient's comprehension. To test repetition ask the person to repeat grammatical phrases such as "no ifs, and, or buts."[58] It is important to remember that syndromes often overlap in any single patient, depending on the type of cerebrovascular disruption and damage.

The nurse can determine the patient's comprehension of written language by assessing whether the patient can follow simple commands that are printed in large script. The nurse can also determine the patient's ability to name objects, repeat a series such as the days of the week, and write a sentence.[58]

Interventions to promote communication include creating an environment that is stimulating to the auditory senses. Acceptance of any attempts at speech is important in encouraging the patient to continue to try to use verbal communication. Providing a comfortable and caring environment, while accepting limited speaking abilities, fosters a communicating atmosphere. Speech therapy should begin soon after the stroke occurs. The speech therapist can suggest ways to work with the patient most effectively during nursing care to enhance speech.[9] Speech therapy sessions initially may be short and directed toward assisting the patient in communicating essential needs. Important images, such as a glass of water, a bedpan, or food, can be used in a book form, so that the patient can point to specific items that are needed if unable to communicate these needs verbally. In the early stage after stroke, the patient is better able to grasp what is being said if the nurse speaks slowly and uses short phrases, but not in exaggerated tones.[58] Simple words, short sentences, demonstration with gestures, and written communication can be helpful. Praising the patient when communication is improved or satisfactory is important. Avoid excessive correction of patients' speech, as well as any attempt to force them to use language properly. Otherwise, patients' speaking attempts become frustrating and stressful, and they become hesitant to continue trying. Nurses should not overtire the patient by expecting that speech exercises be done, especially when the patient is already working intensely in speech sessions with a therapist. This can best be managed by frequent consultation and conferences with the speech therapist as well as with other persons on the interdisciplinary team.

Other general guidelines to help nurses work with patients with altered communication as a result of aphasia include listening to and waiting for the patient to attempt to communicate, without finishing sentences for the patient. Avoid the inclination to speak or shout loudly in attempting to make the patient understand; this is frustrating rather than helpful. Gently but honestly inform the patient when unable to understand the patient's speaking. Avoid pressuring or tiring the patient (aphasia worsens if the patient is fatigued, anxious, or upset), and talk to the patient in an adult manner. A quiet environment is helpful for one-to-one communication.[58]

When working with patients who have dysarthria, the nurse can be helpful by asking the patient to take time in speaking and to exaggerate the words. Tongue and lip exercises may be prescribed to strengthen muscles for speech. If the patient is severely dysarthric, it may be necessary to provide an alternate means of expressing immediate needs, such as a communication board for the patient to use to point to needed items or a sophisticated computer-augmented communication system.[37]

Knowledge deficit

During the acute stage, patient education is directed toward answering questions from the patient and family regarding the cause of the stroke, expected outcome, purpose of interventions and treatments, the basis for the patient's behavior and physical changes, and what is expected of the patient and family. Initially the family is concerned whether the patient will survive the stroke. They are vulnerable and need interdisciplinary counseling and emotional support to handle the subsequent events and behavioral and physical changes and limitations involving the stroke patient.[31]

It is important at this time to advise patients of resources available to them, including referrals to social service agencies, rehabilitation settings, home care, and support groups, such as stroke clubs sponsored by the American Heart Association or local hospital or community agencies.

Evaluation

The nurse must continuously evaluate interventions used and alter them to reach the patient's goals. An effective nursing care plan in conjunction with medical care will help the patient in maintaining adequate cerebral tissue perfusion. Nursing care must also help the patient in maintaining an open airway and effective breath exchange and help the patient in adapting to perceptual and sensory changes. This should help keep the patient free from injury. The nurse should help minimize frustration as a result of communication disorders and ensure that adequate methods of communication are established. Finally, the nurse must evaluate the patient's ability to cope with depression, anxiety, and feelings of helplessness.

Documentation

Accurate documentation is extremely important during the acute phase of stroke. Vascular and neurologic status can vary by the minute. Monitoring and documenting these changes, however small, may be lifesaving. Without documentation, trends in neurologic assessments and vital signs may go undetected. Documentation of nursing interventions and medical treatment is also important in evaluating the care plan and the patient's response to care.

NURSING MANAGEMENT OF THE PATIENT WITH CEREBROVASCULAR ACCIDENT IN THE REHABILITATION PHASE

Early rehabilitation in stroke care has been documented as resulting in better recovery for stroke patients. Rather than assuming that earlier rehabilitation is always better, however, rehabilitation programs should be planned according to the capacities and needs of individual patients.[7,43] For example, the outcome for patients with bilateral cerebral dysfunction is less favorable than for patients with involvement of one hemisphere. Patients with left-sided difficulties exhibit greater difficulties in functional skills than patients with right-sided difficulties on admission and at discharge from rehabilitation.[43] Also, the functional gains of stroke patients with coronary artery disease are limited.[49] There is generally some spontaneous improvement as cerebral edema subsides. Active rehabilitation usually does not begin until the patient is medically stable. The most dramatic changes in functional gains generally occur within the first 6 months after onset of the stroke, yet a gradual period of functional recovery can last from 3 months to 2 years.[54] Rehabilitation attempts to reduce the impairments and disability in stroke and to restore and develop physical and psychologic functioning.

The aims of rehabilitation are (1) improvement of motor, speech, cognitive, and other impaired functions; (2) mental and social readaptation of patients to restore functional autonomy, social activity, and interpersonal relationships; and (3) where possible, a return to activities of daily living (ADL). Rehabilitation is intended to assist in and accelerate the recovery of impaired functions.[54] The basic principles of rehabilitation include the following: (1) carefully select the patient; (2) begin early; (3) be systematic; (4) build up in stages; and (5) include the types of rehabilitation treatment specific to the deficit.[54]

Assessment

Assessment in neurorehabilitation is ongoing. Components of assessment must include a thorough past health and vocational, educational, and psychosocial history. Physical assessment of all systems must be done initially and on an ongoing basis. Assessment of the patient's functional abilities should include mobility, ADL, elimination, and communication. Mobility assessment includes evaluation of the patient's ability to move about in bed, sitting and standing balance, walking, and transfers. Evaluation of ADL consists of the patient's ability to carry out dressing, grooming, toileting, bathing, eating, and drinking. Elimination assessment consists of evaluating continence for both bowel and bladder. The patient's ability to communicate is assessed by evaluating his or her conversation as to intelligibility and appropriateness; ability to read and write is also assessed. Cognitive assessment is based on nursing observations during rehabilitation. Formal cognitive function testing is performed by neuropsychologists.

Several tools are available to measure functional abilities and changes over time for individuals who are physically disabled, such as after stroke. The Barthel index includes 15 self-care, sphincter control, and mobility items, with the total score ranging from 0 (total dependence) to 100 (complete independence). The modified Barthel index of ADL is a reliable measure for assessing stable (i.e., fixed deficits) stroke patients.[60]

The PULSES profile is a scale consisting of six components that reflect levels of independence in ADL. The acronym consists of physical condition, upper limb function, lower limb functions, sensory components, excretory functions, and support factors.[60]

The Functional Independent Measure (FIM) is yet another scale used to evaluate progress in stroke rehabilitation. This scale was designed to measure disability regardless of the underlying pathologic condition and to be reliable regardless of the clinical background of the user.[22,59] The six domains of measurement in the FIM are self-care, sphincter control, mobility, locomotion, communication, and social cognition. A seven-point scale that ranges from complete dependence (1) to complete independence (7) is used to score these six domains. The box on p. 1287 lists the FIM and its components.

Regardless of which scale is used, the nurse documents the patient's behavior and ability, noting consistency of performance, degree of performance, and attitudes and behaviors affecting performance ability. Mutual goal setting, in which the patient is an active participant on a multidisciplinary team, rather than a passive recipient of care, is a basic principle of rehabilitation. Having the patient assume responsibility for self-care to the optimal level possible is the goal of rehabilitation nursing.

A stroke is a devastating event not only for the patient but also for the family and significant others. It is important to involve families routinely in stroke rehabilitation. Since the patient is an inseparable part of the family system, rehabilitation efforts should consider how the stroke affects other individuals in the household. Adherence to treatment is difficult for the stroke patient with cognitive, perceptual, or physical deficits and mood changes. Adherence also is affected by the presence or absence of

FUNCTIONAL INDEPENDENCE MEASURE

Self-care
Eating
Grooming
Bathing
Dressing: upper body
Dressing: lower body
Toileting

Sphincter control
Bladder management
Bowel management

Mobility (transfers)
Bed, chair, wheelchair
Toilet
Tub, shower

Locomotion
Walk/wheelchair
Stairs

Communication
Comprehension
Expression

Social cognition
Social interaction
Problem solving
Memory

adequate family functioning. Vocational loss, emotional reactions, role changes, and altered communication are some of the problems that reportedly change the family system.[18] Family support improves patients' motivation, so family involvement in the rehabilitation process is essential for optimal progress.

Nursing Diagnosis

Nursing diagnoses appropriate in the rehabilitative phase after stroke include the following:

Impaired physical mobility related to specific neurologic deficits

Self-care deficit related to immobility and altered sensory perception

Altered patterns of urinary elimination (incontinence) related to loss of conscious inhibition by central nervous system damage

Bowel incontinence related to loss of conscious inhibition by central nervous system damage

Altered cognitive functioning related to impaired memory and learning

Sensory/perceptual alterations related to neglect, right/left disorientation, homonymous hemianopsia

Altered nutrition: less than body requirements related to dysphagia

Activity intolerance related to muscle weakness

High risk for ineffective individual coping related to difficulty with psychosocial adjustment

Planning

The expected outcomes for the stroke patient during the rehabilitation phase include the following:

Recovers and maintains optimal mobility

Obtains optimal ability to perform ADL

Reestablishes regular bladder routine or has fewer incontinent episodes, better self-esteem, and no skin breakdown

Reestablishes normal bowel routine, maintains self-esteem, and is free of skin breakdown

Demonstrates long-term and short-term memory function and learning ability

Maintains appropriate orientation to the environment and moves about safely

Does not aspirate and is able to swallow well enough to maintain adequate nutritional status

Attains resocialization

Progress in rehabilitation can be inhibited by inadequate bowel and bladder management if incontinence interferes with scheduling of therapy. Other aspects of the rehabilitation program may be delayed because a problem with unpredictable incontinence interferes with skin integrity, carrying out ADL, and resocialization adjustment.[11]

Implementation

Mobility

Affected extremities are usually flaccid initially after stroke, but eventually spasticity develops. In some patients, however, flaccidity that may hamper successful rehabilitation in mobility continues. Hemiplegia results in an abnormal posture, consisting of the following: flexed elbow, wrist, and fingers; pronated forearm with the affected arm held against the body; internally rotated hip with extension and adduction; extended knee; flexed toes; and ankle in plantar flexion with supination and inversion (Figure 47-6). The patient's neck tends to tilt to the affected side, and the shoulder and scapula are pulled down. To prevent contractures and permanent deformities, therapeutic positioning of the patient should incorporate methods to promote normal positioning and to counteract the abnormal posturing usually found in these patients. Flexor muscles, for example, are

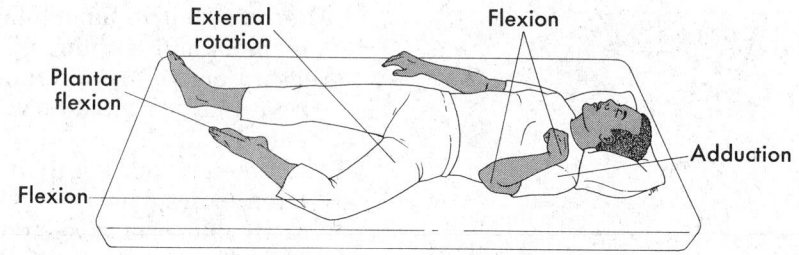

FIGURE 47-6   Common nonfunctional positioning of hemiplegic patient.

stronger than extensors in the upper extremity. Instead of using soft washcloths to position the patient's affected hand, as has been common practice, the nurse uses hard devices, such as a firm cone made of heavy cardboard. Stationary soft devices that provide light tactile cutaneous stimulus to the palmar surface of the hand tend to elicit primitive reflex patterns and palmar grasp reflexes, which prompt flexor hand contractures. Hard devices appear to inhibit hypertonia of the fingers and thus prevent contractures.[61] Frequent turning is also necessary to prevent problems with skin integrity. Edema of the affected arm and hand may occur as a result of changes in circulation and lack of movement. Wearing isotonic gloves and elevating the affected arm on a trough attached to the wheelchair during the day, or on pillows or specially designed devices during the night, are useful interventions to manage problems with edema.

Orthoses are devices attached to the external surface of the body to support a limb or to facilitate motion. Hand splints may be prescribed to prevent contractures and promote extension (Figure 47-7). The nurse is responsible for ensuring that devices are used appropriately and checking for proper wearing times and for any sign of pressure that might cause alterations in skin integrity. When there is inadequate dorsiflexion of the ankle or instability of the ankle, patients may need to wear a short leg brace on the affected extremity. The nurse should teach patients and families the proper use and maintenance of orthoses and prosthetics and safe procedures for transferring the patient.

It is essential to move the patient's joints through the full range of motion at least four times each day and to maintain proper body alignment in the bed or in a chair. When positioning the patient in bed, the use of footboards is discouraged. Footboards tend to increase spasticity in the lower extremities, and the patient often slides down toward the footboard, causing contraction of the limbs.

Stroke patients actively participate in various physical therapies and exercises to strengthen muscles and increase coordination and balance. They also perform stretching exercises and range-of-

motion exercises to prevent contractures, as well as to relearn lost functions such as ambulation. For stroke patients with additional medical problems, such as cardiovascular disease, use of a wheelchair may be the only reasonable means for locomotion if ambulation is unsafe or physically taxing.

There is relative stability of disability (i.e., functional ability) from 6 months through 2 years after stroke.[54] There are two approaches used in retraining patients with a stroke: the traditional approach and the Bobath neurodevelopmental approach.

The traditional nursing approach views the use and treatment of the affected and unaffected sides as separate and unrelated procedures. In this approach the nurse has traditionally approached patient care on the unaffected side, transferred the patient from the unaffected side, and instructed the patient to use the unaffected side in one-handed techniques for self-care. On starting ambulation the patient is usually taught to avoid bearing weight on the paralyzed side. Thus the patient initially is taught to focus mainly on the nonaffected side. In contrast to this approach, the **Bobath technique,** discussed briefly under the acute care section, concentrates on facilitating bilateral functioning so that the affected side also regains mobility. The Bobath neurodevelopmental approach encourages the use of the affected arm and leg and proposes to foster the patient with stroke to restore more normal posture, tone, movement, and function.[45,46] The Bobath technique results in improved quality of gait, balance, and use of the affected arm. In another setting the Bobath technique has shown a higher level of functional gain in patients compared with those receiving traditional care. It is important to introduce Bobath techniques during the acute care stage and continue them throughout the rehabilitation stage of care of the stroke patient.[46]

Bobath techniques have been used primarily by physical and occupational therapists, but they can be easily incorporated into the nursing care of the stroke patient. The focus is on inhibition of abnormal tone through the use of reflex-inhibiting patterns and facilitation of automatic reactions such as righting, equilibrium, and protective extension

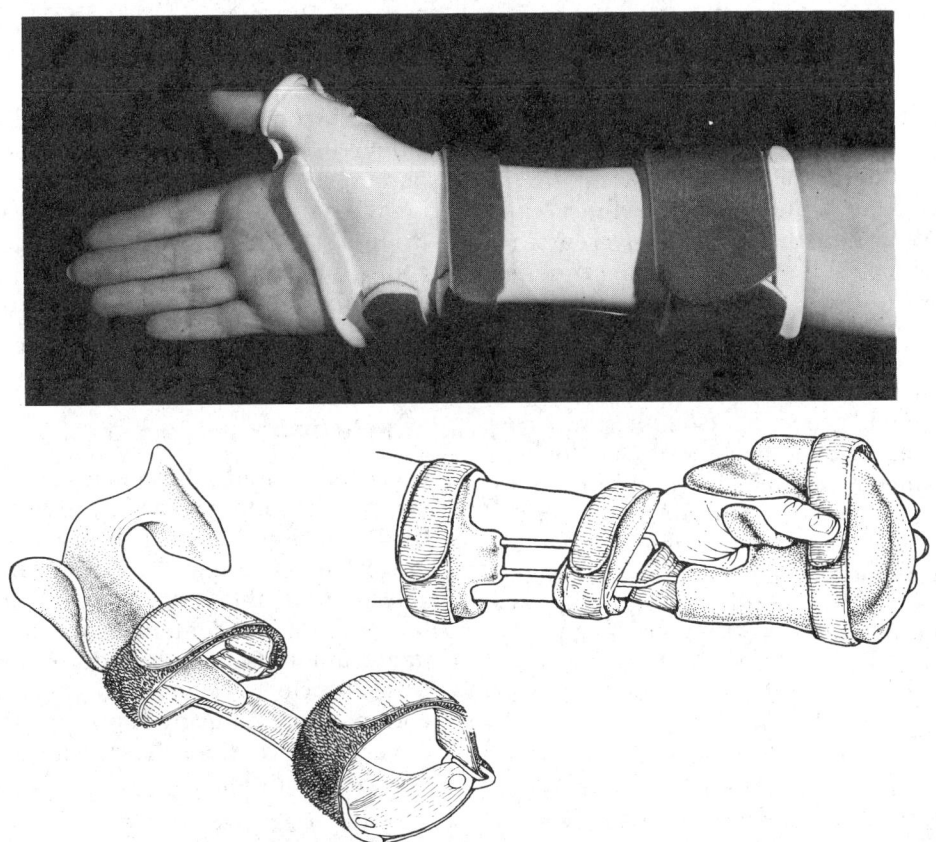

FIGURE 47-7   Hand splints. (From Fess EW, Philips CA: *Hand splinting: principles and methods,* ed 2, St Louis, 1987, Mosby–Year Book.)

through the use of handling and sensory stimulation.[45,46] Establishing reflex postural stability and regaining control over individual movements by breaking up synergistic patterns and by changing treatment during the flaccid stage, spastic stage, and stage of relative recovery are the interventions used in this approach.[46]

In neuromuscular facilitation techniques, bilateral weight bearing, and bilateral weight shifting, the use of reflex-inhibiting patterns and tactile stimulation actions is promoted. There is also emphasis on reducing spasticity and pain and improving balance. Each nurse should know the basic principles of each approach to promote consistency in techniques used in particular clinical settings. For example, it is confusing to the stroke patient for one nurse to use traditional techniques and have the patient lead with the nonaffected side for transferring when another nurse uses the Bobath approach and has the patient lead with the affected side for transferring. Consistency in approach is essential to promote effective learning and avoid confusion.

Although shoulder slings have been almost universally used to support flaccid upper extremities in the past, more discriminate use is now prescribed.

A sling may be helpful in preventing subluxation of the shoulder and may help with balance problems during ambulation. When the affected arm remains flaccid, subluxation of the shoulder may result. As a result of severely paralyzed muscles, the weight of the affected arm can pull the humeral head out of the glenoid cavity in the shoulder joint by stretching the shoulder capsule and shoulder muscles. The nurse needs to reapply suspension slings at regular intervals to ensure that they are providing adequate support and maintaining the hand and arm in the proper position. Some feel slings only keep the arm flexed and increase the likelihood of contracture formation.[9] It may prove more effective to support the affected arm with pillows whenever it in a dependent position.[9] A lapboard attached to a wheelchair or coma chair is helpful in providing arm support for stroke patients who are out of bed.

The stroke patient may progress from a wheelchair to walking on parallel bars to walking with a quad cane that gives a wide, low base of support for lateral instability and weakness.

To correct gait abnormalities such as footdrop during swing, and ankle instability, hemiplegic patients may use ankle-foot orthoses.

Self-care

Training for upper extremity functioning is conducted primarily by the occupational therapist in the usual ADL (i.e., dressing and grooming, bathing and hygiene, feeding) and other self-care activities. Reinforcement of techniques used by the occupational therapist is carried out by nurses on the clinical unit as they help patients in their dressing, grooming, bathing, and hygiene. Following the same sequence and daily routine with ADL is imperative; repetition facilitates learning.[54]

Some assistive devices that can facilitate performance of ADL are one-handed devices for feeding, hygiene, dressing, and grooming. Isotonic gloves can be worn if the affected hand becomes edematous. A trough for the wheelchair can also be used to manage an edematous upper extremity. A lapboard facilitates independence for the wheelchair-bound patient by making equipment and supplies available for ready access. Other adaptive equipment that may be indicated includes a rocker knife, nail brush with suction cup, raised toilet seat, and bathtub seat.

Urinary elimination

During the acute stage the patient with a stroke may require an indwelling catheter because of altered consciousness. The catheter is removed as soon as possible to avoid urinary tract infection. The patient is likely to have a neurogenic bladder of the uninhibited type because of cerebral cortical damage that affects the inhibitory centers or pathways that control the bladder. Urinary frequency, urgency, and reflex voiding are characteristic of bladder functioning in stroke patients.

Interventions to promote appropriate urinary elimination include regularly scheduled emptying of the bladder as determined by the patient's schedule of fluid intake, bladder capacity, and usual voiding patterns. Consistency and adherence to the toileting schedule are mandatory if increasing the length of time between voidings and eliminating episodes of incontinence are to be attained.[9] The nurse helps the patient to the bathroom every 2 hours during the day to avoid incontinence. Several days later, if this program is successful, the nurse lengthens the interval of time between toileting to 3 hours. If the patient is successful in achieving 3 hours between toileting without episodes of incontinence, then the nurse might increase the interval to 4 hours. In addition, the nurse should provide fluid at regular intervals, so that the pattern of intake is consistent with regular toileting patterns. Fluid intake is discontinued after 8 PM so that night incontinence is eliminated or at least limited. Toileting the patient at least twice during the night would probably eliminate incontinence during the night. Again, it is important to emphasize that observation of the patient's voiding patterns and incontinence episodes is essential if the toileting program is to be individualized successfully.

The incontinent patient most likely suffers from embarrassment after urinary incontinence. The nurse preserves self-esteem by immediately changing the patient's wet clothes after an incontinent episode. Incontinence aids are used as necessary until control is obtained. The nurse encourages good grooming and washes, rinses, and dries the area well to prevent skin breakdown.

Bowel elimination

Consistency and adherence to a toileting schedule also apply to managing the problem with neurogenic bowel usually occurring after stroke. Assess former bowel habits so that the nurse can adapt any intervention to facilitate as normal a pattern as possible. Increasing fiber content in the diet, providing adequate amounts of fluid, adding prune juice to the diet, ensuring a regular toileting schedule for bowel elimination, and using suppositories or stool softeners are interventions that the nurse may use to manage this condition.

Cognitive function

Depending on the extent and location of cerebral damage, the patient with a stroke will have varying levels of cognitive function, particularly because there is often a loss of memory for recent events. Learning situations should be held in quiet areas, because the patient is likely to be easily distracted. The stroke patient will have a short attention span, so short sessions are more appropriate than long sessions. Capitalizing on the times of day when the patient is most alert and energetic is also an important measure for the nurse to use in teaching sessions. Breaking tasks into component parts will help keep the patient from becoming overwhelmed or frustrated. Memory aids, such as written directions, printed schedules, cue cards, notebooks with cues and pictures, and checklists are helpful for the patient with memory deficits.

A consistent routine is helpful in reinforcing learning and decreasing confusion. The stroke patient often has a problem with generalizations and the transfer of knowledge, so the nurse should make the setting and equipment as similar to the actual situation as possible when teaching a specific task. It is helpful if each teaching session ends on a positive note and if positive reinforcement and praise of appropriate learning behavior are given to promote motivation.[9] Family members and friends should be included in teaching sessions so that they also follow similar approaches and consistent routines.

Sensory-perceptual function

Perceptual dysfunction results in difficulty in interpreting objects, events, and qualities that stimulate the sensory organs and can interfere with learning and progress in rehabilitation. Body image is often disrupted after stroke. Anosognosia, or unilateral neglect, is one example of a sensory-perceptual deficit.

Interventions to help the patient with anosognosia and integrate the affected extremity into his or her body image include teaching the patient to use the paralyzed arm as a weight, balance an article being used, or do an act with the nonaffected limb. To stimulate awareness of the paralyzed arm, the nurse can touch and rub the affected arm while the patient watches. Reminding the patient to perform activities that force looking at the affected arm or leg also helps to increase the patient's awareness of the affected side.[11]

Apraxia is another disorder in perception that affects motor performance. Apraxia is defined as an inability to carry out motor activities in response to a verbal command in spite of the presence of an intact motor and sensory system and normal comprehension, attention, and coordination.[21] It is often frustrating for the nurse caring for such patients when the patient can carry out certain activities spontaneously but not on command. For example, such patients can automatically brush their teeth when a toothbrush is placed in their hand but cannot brush their teeth on command. Such behaviors may cause the nurse to feel that the patient is being stubborn or noncooperative. The nurse may then erroneously interpret the problem to be a behavioral one when, in fact, the patient is simply unable to carry out the verbal command. The nurse who recognizes the presence of apraxia can better help family and staff understand the problem and intervene by using gestures, cue cards, and pictures or techniques of visual skills rather than verbal skills to cope with this disability.[59] Such patients can often learn effectively through demonstrations and imitation.

Patients with spatial disorders have difficulty in finding position in space, often causing the patient to bump into objects (Figure 47-8). Such patients are unable to find things on top of or behind something, when directed to do so. Techniques in managing the problem of visual field deficits vary, depending on the stage of the person's rehabilitation and the specific goals being sought. Initially it is important to avoid isolating the patient; this causes increasing confusion. For that reason the patient's undisturbed field of vision is the one that the nurse initially tends to support and promote. For example, the patient is approached from the nonaffected side, and items are placed on the unaffected side to aid in finding them and to avoid confusion. The nurse may be the

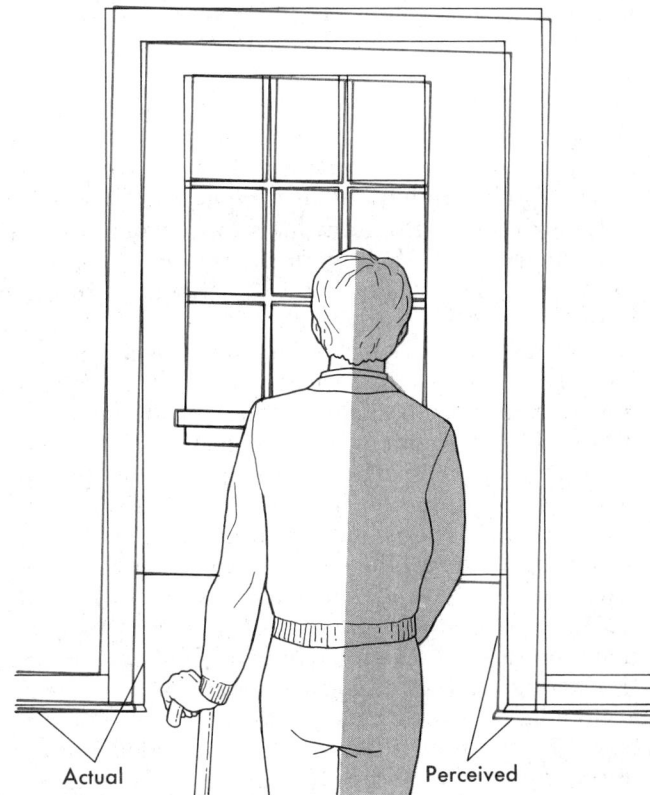

Actual   Perceived

FIGURE 47-8   Spatial-perceptual deficit in hemiplegia.

first person to detect the presence of a visual field deficit when observing a lack of response to environmental stimuli, such as the patient's not responding when approached from the affected side or eating food from only one half of the tray. When the patient is able to understand the presence of the deficit, the nurse begins teaching the patient to compensate by scanning the environment by turning the head and moving the eyes in the direction of the affected visual field.[9] Scanning is an effective technique that improves functioning in mobility and performance of ADL. Scanning is necessary to avoid injury caused by accidentally bumping into or tripping over objects. Patients will often need reminding to do the scanning until it becomes a natural, integrated process. Hemianopsia usually recedes gradually as patients learn to scan effectively.

Impaired swallowing

Swallowing disorders (dysphagia) associated with stroke have been related to muscle weakness, incoordination of muscular function, inadequate cough and gag reflex, attention deficits, perceptual disorders, lethargy, or confusion.[9] Because of the danger of aspiration, the nurse should have suction equipment available if the patient is suspected of having a swallowing problem. The nurse should suspect that persons who have dysarthria also may have swallowing problems, since the same cranial nerves that are involved with speech articulation are used in gag and swallowing reflexes. For some patients, feeding is most appropriately managed with nasogastric or alternate methods temporarily.[39]

Consultation with individuals in the speech therapy department is helpful in determining regimens to facilitate the swallowing reflex. Liquids are generally more difficult to handle than solids. Gagging, sputtering, nasal regurgitation, and aspiration of food may all occur in patients with impaired swallowing. Supervision during mealtimes and provision of a quiet environment to avoid distracting the patient from concentrating on the sequential steps of swallowing are other interventions indicated for these patients. Foods that are stimulating in temperature and texture often help in initiating the swallowing reflex. Loss of sensation or diminished control of oral and facial muscles often results in accumulation of food on the affected side of the mouth. "Pocketing" requires that the nurse check for such accumulation after meals are taken and provide oral hygiene. The patient should be positioned upright during the meal and the chin should be tilted down, small amounts of food should be placed in the intact side of the mouth, and feeding should be discontinued if the patient becomes fatigued.[11]

Monitoring food and fluid intake, appropriate diet planning, socialization to increase appetite and normalize mealtimes, the use of adaptive or assistive equipment, and providing regular oral hygiene are all necessary interventions to ensure an adequate nutritional status.

Activity intolerance

In their enthusiasm for encouraging progress in stroke rehabilitation, individual therapists and nurses may overtax the stroke patient unless endurance and medical status are taken into consideration. Failure to determine a patient's endurance can result in overtaxing the patient and can cause excessive fatigue or even congestive heart failure in vulnerable patients.[49] Myocardial infarction is the leading cause of late mortality among patients with completed stroke. This indicates the importance of awareness of cardiovascular aspects in stroke rehabilitation. The increased energy demands of an active rehabilitation program may inhibit functional skill performance or result in clinical manifestations of coronary artery disease.[49] Since stroke occurs most often in elderly persons, it is important for nurses to be aware of the presence of cardiovascular and other chronic diseases in this population. These diseases may affect the patient's performance and endurance in rehabilitation programs.

The patient with a stroke can sustain a neurologic dysfunction in level of consciousness, mentation, as well as orientation.[11] Deficits can include diminished swallowing or gag reflex, paresis, apraxia, agnosia, right and left disorientation, and neglect or denial of paralyzed extremities.[11] The stroke patient in the rehabilitation phase of care can be compromised by a continued increase in energy demands combined with physical disabilities that negatively influence the ability to meet nutritional needs.[11]

Decreased attention span and distractibility, characteristic of both right and left hemisphere strokes, also affect patients' endurance levels. When patients start new exercises, therapies, or increased wheelchair or ambulation activity, it is important to monitor their vital signs and subjective symptoms before and after the activity to determine patient tolerance. Weakness, pallor or cyanosis, cerebral changes such as increased confusion, incoordination, change in equilibrium, and progressive slowing are other indications of decreased endurance and a need to stop or alter the activity. Monitoring activity tolerance is an area in which the family requires teaching, particularly when the patient is elderly or has cardiovascular problems. Modification of the home setting, for example, may be necessary for the older homemaker with a stroke.

Scheduling the patient's daily activities and therapies is another aspect for consideration in the area of endurance, with a need to identify appropriate rest periods and appropriate scheduling that do not exhaust the patient. The older patient or one with other medical problems or disabilities requires teaching in planning ways to conserve energy for priority tasks. Careful observation of the patient is necessary to identify behaviors and stressors that test or overtax his or her endurance level.

Coping

To effectively intervene with the stroke patient the rehabilitation nurse must first understand the coping process and the nature of a stressful event. The patient and family's coping response to the stroke must be assessed as well as the personal and situational variables that are affecting coping.[9] Utilization of a conceptual model that describes the complex factors involved in the process of coping after stroke may be helpful. The Coping After Stroke Model combines the concepts of loss, cognitive appraisal, adaptive tasks, coping strategies, coping effectiveness, hope, and rehabilitation outcomes to describe a dynamic process that is influenced by feedback from variables in the model.[9] All of the components of the model may change over time during the recovery process.

Families are an important component of the coping process. Family interaction and treatment adherence after stroke have been studied.[18] The characteristics of families who adhere to treatment principles were are follows: (1) they communicate and exchange information clearly and directly; (2) they solve problems effectively; and (3) they report a strong, emotional interest in one another.[18]

Patients with stroke often demonstrate apathy, disinterest, and emotional lability. Depression is often associated with stroke and can be a major factor impeding rehabilitation efforts.[19] Tricyclic antidepressant drugs have been used to alleviate depression and enhance stroke recovery. These agents, however, also cause central nervous system, cardiac, and other anticholinergic side effects, such as sedation, which interfere with rehabilitation efforts.

Evaluation

Patient care conferences are especially important to evaluate progress in the rehabilitation phase. The multidisciplinary team must evaluate interventions used at least once each week and alter them to assist the patient in reaching the rehabilitation goals and preventing secondary complications. An effective nursing plan in conjunction with the team plan will assist the patient in reaching his or her potential in terms of mobility, self-care, elimination, cognitive function, sensory-perceptual function, swallowing, activity intolerance, and coping.

Documentation

Accurate documentation is important during the rehabilitation phase of CVA. Many aspects of care, such as functional status, are documented when the patient is admitted to the rehabilitation unit and on a weekly basis thereafter. Monitoring and documenting changes are essential in evaluating the nursing and team care plan and the patient's response to care.

Ongoing Care

Discharge planning from the hospital or rehabilitation center to the home or long-term care facility must prepare the patient and family for many changes, including those in functional performance, roles in the family, employment, and socialization. Research has shown that elderly patients demonstrate a strong need for information about new med-

ications, dietary changes, modifications in activity, and measures to relieve signs and symptoms associated with the stroke.[40]

Discharge planning for the stroke patient needs to begin at the time of admission. The overall goal is to ensure uninterrupted health care and meet the actual and anticipated needs of the patient. Additional patient-centered goals include (1) active patient and family participation, (2) early identification of high-risk patients or patients with potential discharge planning problems, (3) solid communication among all individuals involved in discharge planning, (4) selection of the most economic and appropriate options, and (5) maintenance of current knowledge of available health care providers, programs, and resources.[9] Three adjuncts to discharge planning are self-medication programs, therapeutic passes, and home visits.[9] All three of these provide opportunities for the patient to practice self-care behaviors and develop problem solving skills before actual discharge.[9]

Many services are available to assist in community reintegration of the stroke patient. These may include home health care services of a nurse, physical or occupational therapist, or home health aide; outpatient medical care; emergency alerting services; meals and transportation; equipment and supplies; stroke clubs and stroke support groups; and organizations providing information and referral.[9] The nurse must be cautious in helping the patient become reintegrated into the community. Routine referrals for increasing socialization commonly are not helpful, unless caregivers respect the patient's past patterns of social interaction. For example, someone with a lifelong pattern of tolerance for isolation may be extremely uncomfortable with the dramatic changes caused by inclusion in a group.

Strong family support is a clearly cited factor influencing progress and improvement after stroke. Family support and education groups have often been initiated in institutions to facilitate family/staff interaction and provide families with a source of peer support.[31,44,47] Sharing ideas about managing home behavior, financial information, effects of brain damage from stroke, and coping strategies are some common topics discussed in these support groups. Support groups are also helpful in guiding families who feel that they are overprotective and overcommitted.

NURSING CARE PLAN   *Patient with Stroke*

Nursing diagnosis/ *Expected outcome*	Interventions	Rationale
Impaired verbal communication related to aphasia • *Patient will regain maximum communication abilities*	Maintain a calm, quiet, and unhurried environment Encourage patient to speak, and praise any attempts to speak Stimulating conversation should occur throughout the day Allow the patient sufficient time to speak; do not interrupt unless the patient is frustrated Do not constantly correct mistakes or mispronunciation Use nonverbal communication such as facial expression, gestures, pointing, or a communication board Education for family and patient to help them understand the speech deficit and to learn how the patient can best be assisted	Distractions are minimized to maximize patient's attention span; extraneous noise competes with conversation; impatience may discourage patient; nonverbal cues supplement auditory comprehension
High risk for fluid volume excess: edema in extremities related to the hemiparesis or hemiplegia • *No edema in dependent areas such as the sacrum or the extremities*	Do not infuse intravenous fluid into the affected side Elevate hemiparetic/hemiplegic extremities above the level of the heart Monitor intake and output accurately to prevent overhydration Use alternating pneumatic boots or thigh-high antiembolic stockings Turn and reposition every 2 hours Weigh patient daily Active and passive range of motion exercises every 4 hours for all extremities	Intravenous fluids collect in affected arm Edema contributes to development of skin breakdown Pneumatic boots or thigh-high stockings prevent pooling of blood in immobile legs Daily weights assess hydration status Range-of-motion exercises improve circulation
High risk for altered nutrition: less than body requirements related to swallowing dysfunction • *Body weight maintained* • *Patient demonstrates ability to handle oral secretions, food, and fluid without aspiration or choking*	Keep head of bed elevated during feedings Monitor serum electrolytes, intake, output, and stools (diarrhea, constipation) Weigh at least weekly Assess gag and swallow reflexes before instituting oral feedings Begin oral intake with sips of water; be sure patient demonstrates ability to handle own secretions first Advance diet as tolerated; soft foods are usually easier to swallow than liquids Observe the patient closely, and remain with patient during meals	Elevating head of bed will prevent aspiration Weekly weights assess nutritional status Prevents aspiration

NURSING CARE PLAN   *Patient with Stroke—cont'd*

Nursing diagnosis/ Expected outcome	Interventions	Rationale
	Place food toward the back of the patient's mouth and on the unaffected side	
	Encourage patient to chew foods thoroughly and slowly on unaffected side of mouth	
	Forward tilting of the head aids swallowing	
	Be sure that food has not accumulated in the affected cheek	
Self-care deficit related to immobility and muscle weakness	Encourage mobilization early (chair, bedside commode)	Early mobilization prevents complications of bed rest
• *Patient is able to move in bed, transfer, ambulate, and perform self-care with increased independence, with or without assistive devices, consistent with physical limitations*		
	Active range-of-motion exercises and passive range-of-motion exercises for all joints, providing good support under joints; do not go beyond the point of pain	Range-of-motion exercises and body alignment, prevent debilitating contractures
	Maintain proper body alignment using pillows, sandbags, trochanter rolls, slings, handrolls, tennis shoes	Too much activity without rest tires the patient and may cause frustration
	Alternate rest with activity	
• *Patient mobile at home and within the community*	Encourage independence with activities patient can perform within functional capacities	Independence increases self-esteem, motivation
	Evaluate sitting tolerance based on blood pressure, sitting balance, and level of fatigue	
	Discuss alternative ways to perform daily activities	
	Patient and family teaching regarding positioning, range-of-motion exercises, transfer techniques, ADL, gait training, and assistive devices	
High risk for injury related to visual impairment	Arrange the environment in a consistent manner	Enhances safety, familiarity
	Position objects within visual field	Items are easier to locate
• *Patient will adapt to visual deficit and move about safely in the environment*	Use good lighting	Scanning compensates for visual deficit
	Teach patient to scan the environment	
Altered family processes	Assess family dynamics, coping strategies, knowledge of disease process, and attitudes	Family participation in care during hospitalization helps the family feel useful, and also teaches them how to care for the patient at home
• *Family will demonstrate ability to care for the member with a mobility deficit*	Create a supportive environment for the family	

Continued.

NURSING CARE PLAN   *Patient with Stroke—cont'd*

Nursing diagnosis/ Expected outcome	Interventions	Rationale
• *Family will verbalize feelings to the nurse and each other* • *Family will verbalize understanding of mobility deficit* • *Family will not feel overprotective or overcommitted*	Include family members in care of the patient when appropriate (feeding, bathing, ambulating) Provide family teaching regarding sick role, mobility deficits, and how to care for the patient at home Assist with family counseling to help in their efforts to cope Consultations with social worker for discharge planning Encourage family to divide duties at home so that one member does not provide all of the care Prepare the family for periods of depression and overdependence by the patient that occur during illness Teach family members to let the patient be as self-sufficient as possible, progressing gradually; to praise patient's efforts and not to be discouraged with failures Have the patient participate in family planning and activities as much as possible	Family participation in care facilitates a healthy family process

CRITICAL THINKING QUESTIONS

1 Discuss the major causes of stroke.
2 Why is close monitoring of the patient with SAH so important when antihypertensive agents are used?
3 What are the three major complications that threaten the recovery of the patient with SAH?
4 Discuss the role of surgery in treatment of SAH—types and timing.
5 During what period after SAH is vasospasm most likely to occur?
6 Consider the typical positioning of the patient who has suffered a stroke, and describe the nursing interventions indicated to promote functional positioning.
7 Differentiate the traditional and neurodevelopmental (Bobath) approaches in the care and retraining of stroke patients.
8 What are four priority nursing diagnoses essential during the acute stage of care of the stroke patient?
9 Describe interventions and rationale for the following nursing diagnosis: impaired physical mobility in a stroke patient during the rehabilitation phase.
10 Develop a standard nursing care plan for an adult patient with a completed stroke with severe residual effects after either a right or left CVA.
11 How would you respond to a person saying that the older stroke patient should not participate in a comprehensive rehabilitation program because it would not be cost effective?
12 Discuss the major teaching required by the family in preparation for the transition to the home.
13 Discuss the impact of stroke on the family, the community, and national resources.

BIBLIOGRAPHY

Current

1. Adams HP: Intracranial operation within seven days of aneurysmal subarachnoid hemorrhage, *Arch Neurol* 45:1065-1069, 1988.
2. Amaurosis Fugax Study Group: Current management of amaurosis fugax, *Stroke* 21(2):201, 1990.
3. American Heart Association: *1989 stroke facts*, Dallas, 1988, The Association.
4. American Nimodipine Study Group: Clinical trial of Nimodipine in acute ischemic stroke, *Stroke* 23(1):3-8, 1992.
5. Barsan WG et al: Early treatment for acute ischemic stroke, *Ann Intern Med* 111(6):449-451, 1989.
6. Becker PS, Miller VT: Heparin-induced thrombocytopenia, *Stroke* 20(11):1449-1459, 1989.
7. Bernspang B et al: Motor and perceptual impairments in acute stroke patients: effects on self-care ability, *Stroke* 18(6):1081-1086, 1987.
8. Bonita R, Ford MA, Stewart AW: Predicting survival after stroke: a three-year followup, *Stroke* 19(6):669-673, 1988.
9. Bronstein KS, Popovich JM, Stewart-Amidei CS: *Promoting stroke recovery*, St Louis, 1991, Mosby–Year Book.
10. Buckwalter KC et al: Increasing communication ability in aphasic/dysarthric patients, *West J Nurs Res* 11(6):736-747, 1989.
11. Buelow JM, Jamieson D: Potential for altered nutritional status in the stroke patient, *Rehab Nurse* 15(5):260-263, 1990.
12. Caplan LR: *Stroke clinical symposia*, West Caldwell, NJ, 1988, Ciba-Geigy Corp.
13. Delashaw JB et al: Treatment of right hemispheric cerebral infarction by hemicraniectomy, *Stroke* 21(6):874-881, 1990.
14. Dombovy ML et al: Disability and use of rehabilitation services following stroke in Rochester, Minnesota, 1975-1979, *Stroke* 18(5):830-836, 1987.
15. Doolittle ND: Stroke recovery: review of the literature and suggestions for future research, *JNN* 20(3):169-173, 1988.
16. Doolittle ND: Clinical ethnography of lacunar stroke: implication for acute care, *JNN* 23(4):235-240, 1991.
17. Estol CJ, Pessin MS: Anticoagulation: is there still a role in atherothrombotic stroke? *Stroke* 21(5):820-824, 1990.
18. Evans RL et al: Family interaction and treatment adherence after stroke, *Arch Phys Med Rehabil* 68(8):513-517, 1987.
19. Finklestein SP, Weintraub RJ, Davar G: Antidepressant drug treatment for poststroke depression: retrospective study, *Arch Phys Med Rehabil* 68(11):772-776, 1987.
20. Fode NC: Subarachnoid hemorrhage from ruptured intracranial aneurysm, *Am J Nurse* 88(5):673-679, 1988.
21. Hahn K: Left vs right, *Nursing*, pp 44-47, 1987.
22. Hamilton BB et al: A uniform national data system for medical rehabilitation. In Fuher MS, editor: *Rehabilitation outcomes: analysis and measurement*, Baltimore, 1987, Paul H. Brooks Publishing Co.
23. Hanley DF, Kirsch JR: Cerebral vasospasm, *Crit Care Rep* 1:80-87, 1989.
24. Hartshorn J, Malloy C: *Acute care nursing in the home*, Philadelphia, 1988, JB Lippincott Co.
25. Hass WK et al: A randomized trial comparing ticlopidine hydrochloride with aspirin for the prevention of stroke in high-risk patients, *N Engl J Med* 321(8):501-507, 1989.
26. Hijdra A et al: Aneurysmal subarachnoid hemorrhage, *Stroke* 18(6):1061, 1987.
27. Hinkle JL: Evolution of the acute stroke unit, *JNN* 24(2):113-116, 1992.
28. Hummel SK: Cerebral vasospasm: current concepts of pathogenesis and treatment, *JNN* 21(4):216-224, 1989.
29. Ingall TJ et al: Predictive value of carotid bruit for carotid atherosclerosis, *Arch Neurol* 46:418-422, 1989.
30. Kane-Carlser PA: Managing patients with TIA's, *Nursing*, pp 34-39, 1992.
31. Kernich CA, Robb G: Development of a stroke family support and education program, *JNN* 20(3):193-197, 1988.
32. Kilpatrick CJ et al: Epileptic seizures in acute stroke, *Arch Neurol* 47:157-160, 1990.
33. Kirkwood JR: *Essentials of neuroimaging*, New York, 1990, Churchill Livingstone.
34. Klonoff DC et al: Stroke associated with cocaine use, *Arch Neurol* 46:989-993, 1989.
35. Leahy NM: Complications in the acute stages of stroke, *Nurs Clin North Am* 26(4):971-983, 1991.
36. Marshall SB et al: *Neuroscience critical care*, Philadelphia, 1990, WB Saunders Co.
37. Mauss-Clum N et al: Locked-in syndrome approach, *JNN* 23(5):273-285, 1991.
38. Mitchell PH et al: *AANN's neuroscience nursing*, Norwalk, Conn, 1988, Appleton & Lange.
39. Mochizuke RM et al: Heparin lock for nighttime intravenous fluid management in a dysphagic patient, *Rehabil Nurse* 15(6):322-324, 1990.
40. Naylor MD, Shaid EC: Content analysis of pre- and postdischarge topics taught to hospitalized elderly by gerontological clinical nurse specialists, *Clin Nurse Specialist* 5(2):111-115, 1991.
41. Neatherlin JS, Brent VA: The Gamma knife: implications for nursing practice and patient education, *JNN* 23(1):71-74, 1991.
42. North American Symptomatic Carotid Endarterectomy Trial Investigators: Clinical alert: benefit of carotid endarterectomy for patients with high-grade stenosis of the internal carotid artery, *Stroke* 22(6):816-817, 1991.
43. Novack TA, Haban G, Satterfield WT: Prediction of stroke rehabilitation outcome from psychologic screening, *Arch Phys Med Rehabil* 68(10):729, 1987.
44. Pasquarella MA: Developing, implementing and evaluating a stroke recovery group, *Rehab Nurse* 15(1):26-29, 1990.
45. Passarella P, Gee Z: Starting right after stroke, *AJN* 87:802-807, 1987.
46. Passarella PM, Lewis N: Nursing application of Bobath principles in stroke care, *J Neurosci Nurse* 19(2):106, 1987.
47. Pierce LL: Stroke support group: a reality, *Rehabil Nurse* 13(4):189, 1988.
48. Pujia A, Rubba P, Spencer MP: Prevalence of extracranial carotid artery disease detectable by echo-doppler in an elderly population, *Stroke* 23(6):818-822, 1992.
49. Roth EJ, Mueller K, Green D: Stroke rehabilitation outcome: impact of coronary artery disease, *Stroke* 19:42-47, 1988.
50. Salibi SS et al: Aneurysmal subarachnoid hemorrhage, *Crit Care Rep* 1:22-38, 1989.
51. Seitz RH et al: Functional changes during acute rehabilitation in patients with stroke, *Phys Ther* 67(11):1685, 1987.
52. Sila CA, Furlan AJ: Drug treatment of stroke, *Drugs* 35:468-476, 1988.

53. Spilker J: Thrombolytic therapy: nursing implications. In Sawaya R, editor: *Fibrinolysis and the central nervous system,* Philadelphia, 1990, Hanley & Belfus.

54. WHO Task Force on Stroke and Other Cerebrovascular Disorders: Stroke: 1989 recommendations on stroke prevention, diagnosis, and therapy, *Stroke* 20(10):1407-1431, 1989.

55. Wolf PA et al: Atrial fibrillation as an independent risk factor for stroke: the Framingham study, *Stroke* 22(8): 983-988, 1991.

56. Wolf PA et al: Probability of stroke: a risk profile from the Framingham study, *Stroke* 22(3):312-318, 1991.

Classic

57. Boss BJ: Dysphasia, dyspraxia, and dysarthria: distinguishing features. I. *J Neurosurg Nurs* 16(3), June 1984.

58. Boss BJ: Dysphasia, dyspraxia, and dysarthria: distinguishing features. II, *J Neurosurg Nurs* 16(4), Aug 1984.

59. Granger CV et al: Advances in functional assessment for medical rehabilitation, *Top Geri Rehab* 1(3):59-74, 1986.

60. Jacelon CS: The Barthel index and other indices of functional ability, *Rehabil Nurse* 11(4):9, 1986.

61. Jamison SL, Dayhoff NE: A hard positioning device to decrease wrist and finger hypertonicity: a sensorimotor approach for the patient with nonprogressive brain damage, *Nurs Res* 29:285, 1980.

62. Netter FH: *The CIBA collection of medical illustrations,* vol 1. *Nervous system. II,* West Caldwell, NJ, 1986, CIBA Pharmaceutical Co.

63. Plum F, Posner JB: *The diagnosis of stupor and coma,* Philadelphia, 1982, FA Davis Co.

CHAPTER FORTY-EIGHT

Nursing Management of Adults with Infectious, Inflammatory, or Autoimmune Disorders

LEARNING OBJECTIVES

1 Apply principles of nursing management to the care of the patient with infectious and autoimmune disorders of the nervous system.
2 Describe the medical and nursing treatment for the patient with infectious and autoimmune disorders of the nervous system and the physiologic principles underlying these treatment modalities.
3 Identify the common complications of infectious and autoimmune disorders of the nervous system.
4 Evaluate the needs of the patient's family for information, emotional support, and planning.
5 Evaluate the home care needs of patients with chronic nervous system disease.

KEY TERMS

brain abscess, p. 1309
bulbar weakness, p. 1321
encephalitis, p. 1310
epidural abscess, p. 1309
Guillain-Barré syndrome (GBS), p. 1320
meningitis, p. 1300

multiple sclerosis (MS), p. 1315
myasthenia gravis (MG), p. 1323
nuchal rigidity, p. 1303
optic neuritis, p. 1316
parameningeal infections, p. 1309
subdural empyema, p. 1309
thymectomy, p. 1325

RESEARCH REGARDING the role of the immune system in the pathogenesis of infectious, inflammatory, and autoimmune diseases that affect the central nervous system (CNS) has led to more specific therapeutic management, including drug treatment. The nursing management involved in the ongoing care and treatment of patients with these illnesses is complex. Many of these diseases are rare, but patients require an extensive amount of nursing care in hospitals and extended care facilities. This chapter discusses the most common infectious diseases, acute meningitis, encephalitis, and the parameningeal suppurative infections. Illnesses with a presumed inflammatory or autoimmune cause, such as multiple sclerosis, myasthenia gravis, and Guillain-Barré syndrome will also be covered, with an emphasis on specific nursing implications.

Infectious and Inflammatory Diseases

The discovery and development of antibiotics has dramatically changed the course of many infectious diseases. For example, in the preantibiotic era, meningitis was almost always fatal. It is unfortunate that antibiotic therapy has not totally eliminated these infections, and mortality has remained relatively unchanged at 14% since 1950. In addition, of those who survive, 50% of adults and 35% of children have significant long-term neurologic sequelae.[16]

The portal of entry for the infectious agent is most commonly blood *(hematogenous)*. The reticuloendothelial cells and the phagocytic activity of the leukocytes usually overcome and clear a mild infection. Certain properties of the infectious agent can inhibit these defenses, cause an alteration in the blood-brain barrier, and allow for the hematogenous spread of the organism.

Another route of infection, direct extension from a source outside the CNS, occurs when the integrity of the skull, meninges, or spinal nerves is altered following trauma, fractures, and neurosurgical procedures. Other routes for direct extension occur because of their proximity to the CNS. The nasopha-ryngeal mucosa is in direct contact with the olfactory nerve fibers, which are bathed in cerebrospinal fluid (CSF). The presence of bacteria and viruses in the nasopharynx has led some investigators to implicate this route in the spread of some bacterial and viral CNS infections.

Finally, some infections can spread from one neuron to another by the mechanism of flow up and down the spinal nerves, called bidirectional axonal transport.

MENINGITIS
Definition

Meningitis is an acute or chronic inflammation of the meningeal membranes and the CSF. Meningitis can affect both the meninges and the ventricles as a result of reflux and free communication throughout the system (Figure 48-1).

Etiology/Epidemiology

Meningitis is fairly common, with an incidence of 15 cases per 100,000 and a prevalence of 5 cases per 100,000. The average length of illness and disability is estimated to be approximately 4 months.[29] There are four main types of meningitis: bacterial, viral,

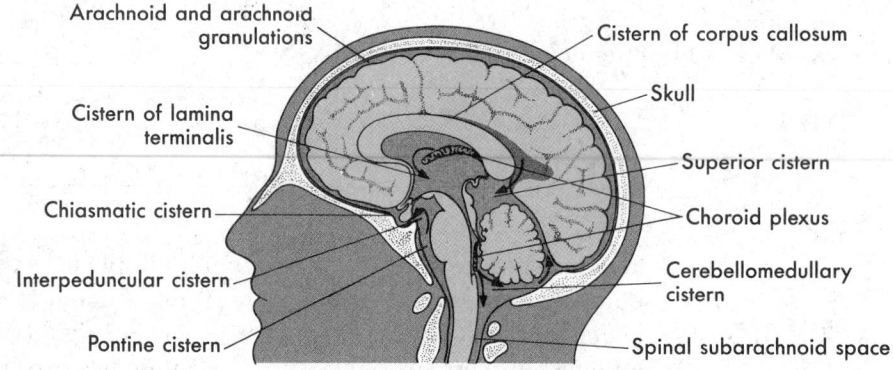

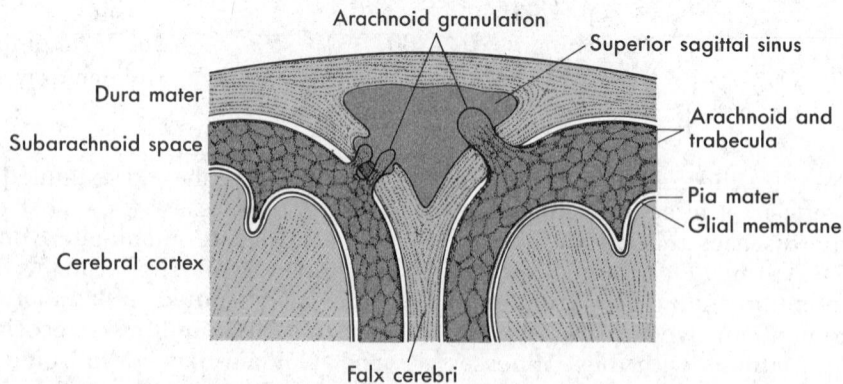

FIGURE 48-1   Cerebrospinal fluid circulation.

TABLE 48-1 Features of Infectious Meningitis

Causative agent	Features
ACUTE BACTERIAL MENINGITIS REQUIRING ANTIBIOTICS	
Haemophilus influenzae	Most common meningitis (48%)
	Rarely seen in adults; 90% < 5 years of age
	In children: follows upper respiratory infection or otitis media
	In adults: follows parameningeal infection, CSF leak, immunodeficiency
	Death rate 3% to 8%; leading cause of acquired mental retardation, 30% to 50% have neurologic sequelae
Neisseria meningitidis (meningococcal)	Common (20%) and rapidly progressive
	Children and young adults most often affected, 90% are < 45 years of age
	Epidemics occur in winter and spring
	50% of those hospitalized die within 24 hours of onset of symptoms
	50% have petechial or purpuric rash
	Common toxic complications: DIC, adrenal infarction, pneumonia, and concurrent infections
Diplococcus pneumoniae (pneumococcal)	Less common (8%) but has severe consequences
	Seen in children, elderly persons, and those with predisposing factors: infections of lungs, ears, and sinuses; splenectomy; alcoholism; sickle cell disease; CSF leak; endocarditis; immunosuppression
	30% to 60% die, some despite antibiotic treatment
	Common neurologic sequelae: deafness, mental retardation
Nosocomial infections (gram negative)	Rarely seen except in hospitalized patients
	Associated with neurosurgery (50%), trauma (30%), entry of CSF, debilitated or immunosuppressed patients
	Onset of fever and low glucose in CSF are helpful in diagnosis
	May need intraventricular reservoir plus systemic therapy
Staphylococci	Associated with infected shunts, brain abscess, sinusitis, endocarditis, and septicemia
Streptococci	Group B seen in endocarditis, cellulitis
ACUTE MENINGITIS NOT REQUIRING ANTIBIOTICS	
Viral meningitis	Common in summer; self-limited illness
	Sequelae or need for hospitalization is rare
CHRONIC AND SUBACUTE MENINGITIS TREATED WITH ANTIMICROBIAL AGENTS	
Mycobacterium tuberculosis	Rare except in areas of endemic primary infection, increased drug resistance and coincidence in AIDS patients
	Active disease found elsewhere in body: lung, bone, or kidney
	Cranial nerve palsies common
	One third of patients die, one third have neurologic sequelae
Treponema pallidum (syphilis)	Meningitis may be asymptomatic (25%) or have typical meningitis symptoms plus cranial nerve palsies, seizures, and increased intracranial pressure
	Lack of treatment results in progressive illness and ultimately neuronal damage with paralysis, seizures, and aphasia
	General paresis (dementia plus the above) and tabes dorsalis (spinal cord involvement) occur 15-20 years after untreated infection
Fungal meningitis (coccidioidomycosis, *Candida, Cryptococcus,* aspergillosis, mucormycosis)	Rare form of chronic meningitis
	More common as nosocomial infection in immunologically impaired hosts
	Coccidioidomycosis is endemic in southwest United States
	Candida, Cryptococcus, aspergillosis are opportunistic and found throughout environment
	Typical symptoms of meningitis (headache, fever, and stiff neck) occur in 50%; focal neurologic deficits suggest mass lesion (microabscess or intravascular process)
Parasitic meningitis (*Toxoplasma gondii, Acanthamoeba*)	Although rare, toxoplasmosis has two presentations
	Congenital: with seizures, mental retardation, and blindness
	Acquired: most patients are immunosuppressed as result of malignancy or autoimmune disease
Rickettsial meningitis	Subacute meningitis
	Rocky Mountain spotted fever is most common form; easily treated and rarely fatal
	Carried by vector (lice, ticks, fleas); has typical rash, few focal neurologic deficits

fungal, and parasitic. Bacterial meningitis and viral meningitis are far more prevalent than fungal meningitis and parasitic meningitis. Approximately one third of cases of acute meningitis are caused by bacteria; the remaining cases are caused by viruses or other agents. Table 48-1 summarizes the characteristic features of most of the meningitis syndromes.

Pathophysiology

Having overcome the host defenses to meningeal invasion, the infectious agent sets up an inflammatory reaction in the meninges and subarachnoid space that also affects the blood vessels, brain cells, and other supporting structures. The initial response to a CNS infection relates to activation of the nonspe-

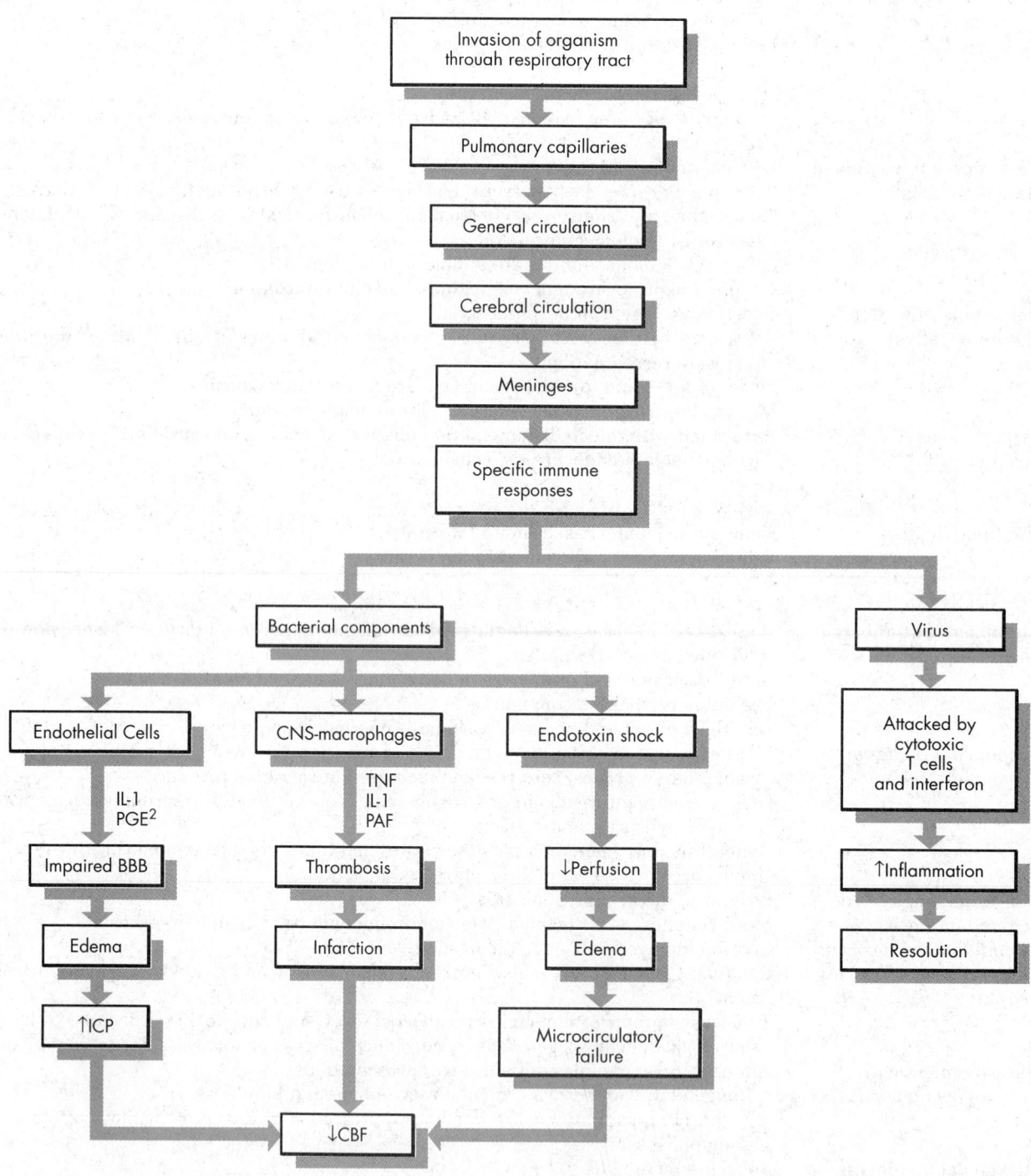

FIGURE 48-2   Pathophysiology of meningitis.

cific immune response. Later, the specific immune response is called on to fight the infection. Figure 48-2 illustrates the pathophysiology of meningitis.

The basic components of the specific immune response—the neutrophils, lymphocytes, complement, and specific antibody—are inadequate or absent in normal CSF. Antibodies in the CSF result from diffusion across the injured blood-brain barrier or by local synthesis by plasma cells. This process is usually a late development and of limited value. For example, in bacterial meningitis the levels of complement and immunoglobulins increase in response to infection but remain below concentrations that enhance bactericidal activity.[16]

As the infectious process continues, exudate increases, fibrin is stimulated, and layers of inflammatory cell exudate develop, creating fibrous adhesions.

One of the most important effects of infection on the CNS is altered permeability of the blood-brain barrier. Because of this alteration, antibiotics can be used to treat the infection. Normally, the only substances to cross the blood-brain barrier are those that are lipid soluble or transported by carrier-facilitated diffusion, a mechanism that moves glucose, amino acids, and ions in and out of cerebral tissue. This accounts for the low concentrations of antibiotics in the CSF and brain tissue when they are used to treat infections in other parts of the body.

Altered vascular permeability also results in cerebral edema. There are several types of edema seen during meningitis: cytotoxic occurs from meningeal exudate, interstitial occurs from reduced CSF outflow, and vasogenic occurs as a result of altered blood-brain barrier.

Complications

Vascular changes are prominent because of the fact that the adventitial layer of the subarachnoid veins is formed by a part of the arachnoid membrane. Thrombosis occurs in the cerebral veins because of the thin walls and slow blood flow. Other vascular changes are intracranial thrombophlebitis and cerebral infarction, which have great significance in terms of functional outcome.

During the course of meningitis, metabolic demand increases because of toxin-related changes, leading to problems in maintaining cerebral perfusion.

Hydrocephalus can be a complication if the exudate blocks outflow of the CSF in the arachnoid or CSF production in the choroid plexus and ependymal cells that line the ventricles. Cellular infiltration and exudate can cause permanent damage to the cranial nerves at the base of the brain. Reduced cerebral blood flow and the toxin-related changes are thought to cause dysfunction of the cortical neurons and account for disorders of consciousness and seizures. These changes can reach a point of irreversibility that results in the late neurologic sequelae to meningitis.

Clinical Manifestations

The classic signs of meningitis are severe headache, fever, stiff neck, and a change in the level of consciousness. The headache reported in meningitis is attributed to stretching of the meningeal membranes because of inflammation in the subarachnoid space. Photophobia may also be a prominent early symptom and is thought to be related to the presence of meningeal inflammation.

Fever may rise to as high as 39.5° C (103° F) and may be accompanied by chills, tachycardia, and tachypnea. Chills are common in pneumococcal meningitis. In chronic meningitis, such as tuberculosis and syphilis, the febrile response is less prominent.

Neck pain and stiffness are often early signs of meningitis. Another term commonly used to describe this finding is **nuchal rigidity.** Further signs of meningeal irritation include Brudzinski's and Kernig's signs, back pain, and opisthotonos. Brudzinski's sign consists of flexion of the hip and knee in response to forward flexion of the neck. Kernig's sign involves the inability to completely extend the legs. Opisthotonos is a severe arching of the neck and back caused by extensor muscle spasm.

Disorders of consciousness, common in meningitis, can range from mild disorientation and decreased concentration to confusion, drowsiness, delirium, and the abrupt onset of coma. These symptoms can result from increased intracranial pressure related to cerebral edema or mechanical obstruction of CSF flow. Other clinical manifestations of meningitis include increased deep tendon reflexes and signs of cranial nerve dysfunction: diplopia, facial weakness, deafness, and pupillary abnormalities. The key diagnostic test used in meningitis is the lumbar puncture. Test results that indicate a bacterial infection of the CSF include cloudy appearance, pressure over 200 mm H_2O, protein over 15 mg/dL, increased white blood cells (PMNs), and reduced glucose level. CSF Gram stain is used to identify bacteria; other stains are used to identify tuberculosis and fungi. Peripheral white blood count (WBC) is usually markedly elevated in bacterial meningitis and mildly elevated in viral meningitis. Serum electrolytes should be checked; hyponatremia caused by inappropriate antidiuretic hormone (ADH) secretion is a common complication. In viral meningitis the CSF is usually clear and the glucose level is normal, although other values may be increased. Viral titers are necessary to confirm the diagnosis.

TABLE 48-2 Pharmacology Summary: Meningitis, Encephalitis, and Parameningeal Disorders

Infection	Medication	Approximate IV dosage
BACTERIAL MENINGITIS		
Haemophilus influenzae	Ceftriaxone	4 g/day (qd or bid)
	Ampicillin	100 mg/kg/day
	Chloramphenicol*	100 mg/kg/day
Meningococcal	Penicillin G	15-24 million U/day (q4h)
	Chloramphenicol*	50-100 mg/kg/day
	Ceftriaxone*	
Pneumococcal	Penicillin G	As above
	Chloramphenicol	50-75 mg/kg/day
	Ceftriaxone*	4 g/day (q6h)
NOSOCOMIAL†		
Staphylococcus	Methicillin	10-12 g/day
Streptococcus group B	Penicillin G	As above
Gram-negative	Gentamycin (IV and/or intrathecal‡)	3-5 mg/kg/day
	Chloramphenicol	50-75 mg/kg/day
Pseudomonas	Third-generation cephalosporin	
	Gentamycin	As above
TUBERCULOUS MENINGITIS	INH	10 mg/kg/day
	Rifampin	600 mg/day
NEUROSYPHILIS	Penicillin G (erythromycin/ tetracycline*)	12-18 million U over 21-24 days
PARAMENINGEAL INFECTIONS†		
Brain abscess	Penicillin G and chloramphenicol (or tetracycline*)	20 million U/day 1-1.5 g q4h
Epidural and subdural empyema	Methicillin/nafcillin and	1.5-2 g q4h
Staphylococcus	chloramphenicol	1-1.5 g q4h
FUNGAL MENINGITIS	Amphotericin B	0.3-0.6 mg/kg/day
	5-Flucytocine	150 mg/kg/day
PARASITIC MENINGITIS		
Toxoplasmosis	Pyrimethamine and sulfadiazine	100 mg loading dose; 25 mg qod 8 g/day bid
Rickettsia	Tetracycline	25 mg/kg/day
ENCEPHALITIS		
Herpes simplex	Vidarabine (Ara-A)	15 mg/kg/day
	Acyclovir	30 mg/kg/day

*If allergic to penicillin.
†Dependent on sensitivity results.
‡Needs ventricular reservoir.

Therapeutic Management

Eradicating the source of infection with antibiotics, treating the discomforting symptoms, and preventing complications are the general goals for managing meningitis. The acute presentation of meningitis is a life-threatening emergency. Patients who are initially seen with progressive symptoms that have been present for less than 24 hours should have a lumbar puncture and antibiotic therapy started within the first 30 minutes of seeking professional assistance.[31] Careful observation in an intensive care unit is essential in most cases. For bacterial meningitis, isolation is maintained for 24 hours after institution of antimicrobial therapy to prevent respiratory transmission of the disease. Meningitis is often a part of the terminal picture in patients with malignancy and other immunosuppressive illnesses, in whom nosocomial infections are frequent. Reverse isolation may be necessary to protect the patient from hospital-acquired infections.

Drug therapy

The initial choice of drug is often determined by the presenting symptoms and the results of the Gram stain of the CSF. Later the results of the CSF culture and sensitivity are used to select the most effective antimicrobial agent. Table 48-2 summarizes the antimicrobial drugs and approximate doses commonly used to treat meningitis. Dosage is often calculated by the patient's age, weight, and renal status.

For chronic meningitis and nosocomial infections, the patient may require prolonged intrathecal and intravenous therapy. When given intravenously or via lumbar intrathecal injection, many antibiotics have poor CSF concentrations. Research demonstrates that in many of the nosocomial and chronic meningitides, optimal treatment requires antibiotic concentrations in the CSF of at least 10 times the minimal bactericidal concentration (MBC) of the antibiotic for the infectious agent.[36] Antibiotics are often given for a prolonged period ranging from 10 weeks to 12 months or until the CSF picture is normal. An Ommaya or a Rickham reservoir is often surgically placed in the ventricles (Figure 48-3). These devices are used to enhance CSF absorption of antibiotics and to maintain treatment over an extended period. Addition of corticosteroids to the acute treatment of bacterial meningitis has been reported. When dexamethasone was administered with or just before antibiotics, there were fewer symptoms (e.g., patient was afebrile sooner) and fewer long-term sequelae such as sensorineural deafness.[16] This is a preliminary finding that requires further study.

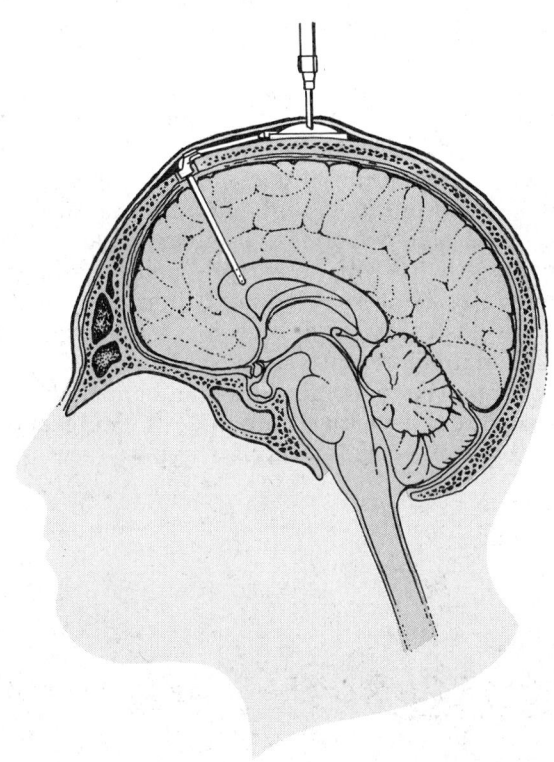

FIGURE 48-3   Ommaya reservoir and placement.

Symptomatic and preventive care

Some degree of fever is beneficial for the protective features of the immune response to occur. However, cellular damage is possible with protracted temperature elevations. Fevers over 39° C (103° F) are usually treated with acetaminophen every 4 hours or as needed. Rapid reduction of fever can cause shivering, which places further metabolic stress on the patient and should be avoided. Chlorpromazine selectively reduces shivering if it becomes a problem. Severe headache can be treated with a mild analgesic, such as codeine. Drugs that impair alertness are avoided, because they may mask signs of increased intracranial pressure.

Prevention of such complications as seizures, increased intracranial pressure, dehydration, and the syndrome of inappropriate antidiuretic hormone (SIADH) secretion is a major feature of therapeutic management. Controlling seizures with appropriate anticonvulsants is mandatory to prevent further cerebral compromise. Many patients will be dehydrated on admission to the hospital because of confusion and the presence of fever, general malaise, and weakness. The patient may forget to drink fluids or be too weak to drink. An effort should be made to balance the presence of dehydration against the danger of increased intracranial pressure potentiated by intravenous overhydration. Increased intracranial pressure is treated with hyperventilation, osmotic diuretics, and corticosteroids. The hypoosmolar state (SIADH) is common in patients with meningitis. The features include confusion, somnolence, and retention of excess free water. An accurate account of intake and output, measuring serum and urinary electrolytes, osmolarity, and urinary specific gravity will detect this complication. It is treated by fluid restriction. Other complications, such as gastrointestinal bleeding, vascular collapse, disseminated intravascular coagulation (DIC), respiratory failure, and aspiration pneumonia, should be anticipated. Preventive therapy for meningeal infections is summarized in the box below.

NURSING MANAGEMENT OF THE PATIENT WITH MENINGITIS
Assessment

The onset and extent of headache, stiff neck, fever, photophobia, and other signs and symptoms should be reviewed. A history of trauma, surgical procedures, and ear, sinus, and mastoid infections should be documented. Exposure to others with epidemic forms of meningitis (*H. in uenzae* and meningococcal meningitis) should be considered in patients at high risk, such as children in day care and military personnel. The presence of other chronic illnesses is a predisposing factor associated with a poor prognosis. CNS infections are commonly seen in immu-

PREVENTIVE THERAPY FOR MENINGEAL INFECTIONS

Meningococcal meningitis
Vaccine
Four vaccines are available:
1. Monovalent serogroup A
2. Monovalent serogroup C
3. Bivalent A-C
4. Quadrivalent A/C/Y/W-135

Indications
1, 2, 3 recommended for use in epidemics of serogroup A and C; 4 used for military personnel and travelers in epidemic areas. Vaccine cannot be used as a substitute for chemoprophylaxis in documented exposures. CDC can assist with determining epidemic status and with vaccine program planning.

Chemoprophylaxis
Rifampin, 600 mg twice daily for adults or 10/mg/kg for 2 days.

Indications
All close family contacts and at-risk populations (military camps and day care). Crowded classrooms (with less than 30 inches distance between chairs) and frequent contact during lunch and breaks are also indications.

Pneumococcal meningitis
Vaccine
The vaccine (Pneumovax) was reformulated in 1983 to include 23 serotypes yet does not prevent all infections. The dose is 0.5 mL IM. Initial treatment lasts 5 years or more; booster injections equivocal.

Indications
All those over 2 years of age who lack splenic function (as a result of surgery or sickle cell disease); diabetic patients; persons with chronic cardiorespiratory, hepatic, and renal disease; immunosuppressed patients; and residents of chronic care facilities.

Chemoprophylaxis
Not recommended.

Haemophilus influenzae vaccine
A new vaccine (ProHIBiT) is indicated for children 18 months to 5 years of age; dosage is 0.5 mL IM given once.

Indications
Children with chronic illnesses and all children over 18 months attending day care. A vaccine to protect those under 2 years of age is under development.

Chemoprophylaxis
Rifampin, 20 mg/kg (up to 600 mg) once each day for 4 days.

Indications
All household contacts should be treated, especially those under 6 years of age. Treatment is advised for those exposed or in close contact, such as in day care centers.

nosuppressed patients. A history of lymphoma, leukemia, renal failure, acquired immune deficiency syndrome (AIDS), and use of immunosuppressants is important to obtain. Other historical information includes recent travel, occupational exposure, and recent insect bites (Lyme disease). The nurse should ask the patient or family members about allergies, particularly to antibiotics.

Physical assessment includes detection of abnormalities in vital signs, such as fever, hypotension, tachycardia, and respiratory failure. Because of the frequency of reduced level of consciousness and the potential for seizure, rectal temperatures should be taken to ensure accurate recording and avoid injury if the patient should bite down on the thermometer.

The neurologic vital signs should be recorded on admission and at frequent intervals usually coinciding with vital signs. This includes assessing level of consciousness, pupil size and reactivity, and motor, sensory, and verbal response. The nurse should record both the type of testing used (e.g., sternal pressure) and the patient's response.

The presence of cranial nerve abnormalities such as signs of extraocular muscle (EOM) paresis, which include diplopia and ptosis, should be investigated. Impaired corneal reflex, pupillary response, facial muscle weakness, deafness, and vertigo are also signs of cranial nerve involvement. Changes in level of consciousness can imply increased intracranial pressure and early brain herniation (see Chapter 45). Changes in the level of consciousness, lethargy, difficulty following commands, incoherent communication, and/or combativeness should be noted because of safety implications.

During the diagnostic phase, in particular during lumbar puncture, the nurse must monitor the patient for changes in headache and neck pain. The nurse should provide comfort measures and give support and information about the diagnostic procedures and the implications of the results.

Nursing Diagnosis

The extent of the infectious process will determine the appropriate application of the nursing diagnoses listed below:

Altered cerebral tissue perfusion related to increased intracranial pressure and the inflammatory process in the meninges

High risk for fluid volume excess/deficit related to altered level of consciousness and the possibility of hypo-osmolar state, dehydration, and other complications

High risk for injury related to seizures and altered intracranial fluid dynamics with resultant motor and cognitive neurologic deficits

Pain related to headache, stiff neck, and general malaise

Self-care deficit related to general incapacity, confusion, pain, and bed rest

Knowledge deficit related to meningitis and the antibiotic treatment protocol

Anxiety related to hospitalization, isolation, and ambiguity of outcome

Planning

Specific goals depend on the health of the patient before the illness and the severity of the meningitis. Outcomes include the following:

Patient will not experience undetected complications, and perfusion of tissues will be maintained

Patient will maintain fluid and electrolyte balance through careful observation and treatment

Patient and family understand the need for interventions and monitoring to protect the patient from injury

Patient will remain comfortable; fever, headache, and stiff neck will be recognized and treated

Patient is able to carry out normal activities, and thought processes will return to preillness state

Patient and family will be knowledgeable about the disease process and treatment measures, including the need for intravenous drug therapy, case finding of carriers, and rehabilitation

Implementation

The patient with meningitis will have multiple problems that seem to need intervention immediately. Aside from assistance with the diagnostic testing, essential nursing care measures include careful monitoring to prevent complications, measures to promote comfort, and rapid institution of antibiotic therapy. The patient and family should receive continued explanations and support throughout the illness.

Preventing complications

Because of the rapid deterioration related to altered cerebral perfusion and fluid volume disturbance, many patients require hemodynamic monitoring of arterial pressure, central venous pressure, intracranial pressure, and heart rate; this is most efficiently provided in the intensive care setting. One of the most dangerous complications is increased intracranial pressure. Further information is presented in Chapter 45.

Fluid volume disturbances will affect cerebral function. Measures that determine hydration status need to be included in the ongoing care plan, including strict intake and output and skin hydration assessment. Fluid restriction should be carefully initiated if ordered by the physician to treat SIADH or prevent increases in intracranial pressure. On the other hand, nursing measures to ensure adequate fluid intake may be necessary if the patient maintains a sustained elevated temperature. Monitoring elimination patterns is important, because constipation, paralytic ileus, urinary retention, and bladder infections are hazards associated with prolonged bed rest. Specific interventions to detect and treat these complications need to be addressed early.

Safety measures, such as seizure precautions, should be instituted on admission and be explained to the patient and family. This often includes padding the siderails and keeping the bed in a low position with the siderails up at all times. The nurse should be aware of appropriate interventions during a seizure and document all observations thoroughly (see Chapter 45).

Maintaining comfort

Avoiding neck and abrupt body movements is helpful while headache and meningeal pain are acute. Careful transfers and turning, as well as gentle repositioning, are of assistance to decrease pain. Gentle range of motion during bathing is of value in preventing complications and providing comfort. A dark, quiet room; limiting visitors; and providing ice caps or a cold cloth on the forehead will be of comfort to the patient with severe headache and photophobia.

General care of the patient with acute meningitis includes directing self-care needs such as bathing, hygiene, positioning, and turning, and maintaining nutrition and elimination as the patient slowly improves. The extent to which the patient can participate in these activities depends on the level of cognitive function. Despite the patient's cognitive deficits, the nurse should carefully explain all procedures and treatments to gain cooperation and allay anxiety. Involving the family in the patient's care allows them to become more aware of the illness and care requirements.

Drug therapy

In acute meningitis, antibiotics are administered parenterally, usually for a 10- to 14-day course. The drugs should be given on a regular schedule to promote consistent levels in the CNS. An intravenous site must be maintained for parenteral infusion the entire time. Removing the intravenous tubing and maintaining the site with a heparin lock, triple-lumen catheter, or Hickman central line may be helpful to maintain the intravenous site in the confused patient. Asking family or volunteers to stay with the patient during the infusion is helpful. Soft restraints should be used only when other measures fail. Sedation should be avoided, because level of consciousness is an important intracranial pressure assessment measure.

Several of the infectious meningitis syndromes are communicable and require treatment for those exposed. The nurse should interview the patient and family in the case of *H. influenzae* and meningococcal meningitis, because close household contacts are treated with antibiotics. The box on p. 1306 includes the current forms of preventive therapy, both for vaccination and chemoprophylaxis.

Evaluation

If therapeutic management and nursing management have been effective, the patient will not experience any complications and will return to normal functioning when discharged. If complications occur, they will be resolved without impairment of the patient's mental or physical functioning.

Documentation

Flowsheets on which to record vital signs, neurologic checks, and fluid balance should be kept at the bedside. The Glasgow Coma Scale (see Chapter 44) has been used in some studies to predict outcome. The nurse will be able to detect changes in level of consciousness with this scale; other supplemental tests of brainstem and motor function should be used to detect brain herniation.[10] Comparisons should be made over time and all significant changes reported. The care plan should include any instructional efforts in preparation for home care.

Ongoing Care

Patients with uncomplicated bacterial meningitis rarely require extensive rehabilitation or home care. With the emphasis on early discharge, some patients will be eligible for home antibiotic therapy if their course remains stable. Patients with viral meningitis rarely require hospitalization. The patient will require a support person to manage household chores and meals for 10 to 14 days or until he or she is able to resume normal activities.

Patients with chronic meningitis, seizures, or permanent deficits such as hemiparesis, sensorineural hearing loss, and aphasia will need rehabilitation and continuous medical follow-up. Some patients can be managed at home, whereas others will benefit from extended care, depending on their level of independent functioning. Long-term care may be necessary for patients with severe dementia and patients who lack a supportive home environment. The nurse is responsible for continuously evaluating the patient's progress with rehabilitation and the ability of the home situation to support the patient's abilities.

PARAMENINGEAL INFECTIONS
Definition

Parameningeal infections share many similar features. **Brain** or spinal **abscess** is a localized collection of exudate that may occur anywhere in the brain or spinal cord parenchyma. Infection developing between the skull or vertebrae and the dura causes **epidural abscess.** Infection between the arachnoid and dura results in **subdural empyema.**

Etiology/Epidemiology

Parameningeal infections are uncommon. The incidence of brain abscess is 1/100,000, and prevalance is 2/100,000.[29] The incidence appears to be the same as in the preantibiotic era, although mortality has been reduced to 40% by early diagnosis. Children and young adults are commonly affected, males twice as often as females. A majority of brain abscesses are located in the cerebrum, with 70% in the frontal and temporal lobes; 30% to 50% of the survivors have neurologic sequelae such as seizures and focal neurologic deficits.

A subdural empyema, although rare, constitutes 13% to 23% of all intracranial infections. Most empyemas are located over the frontal, temporal, and occipital lobes.

Most parameningeal infections are caused by bacteria, although in rare cases fungal and parasitic organisms are cultured. The parameningeal infections commonly arise in direct extension from a source outside the nervous system. This includes bacterial spread from infected sinuses, middle ear, and mastoid or entry from skull trauma and surgical procedures. Epidural abscess is also associated with osteomyelitis of a cranial bone. The second most common etiologic factor is hematogenous spread from lung infections, vascular shunts (congenital heart disease), and chronic infections (pyelonephritis and bacterial endocarditis).

Pathophysiology

A brain abscess evolves in two stages. There is an initial focal area of cerebritis. Bacteria and white cells cluster in this area, with softening, edema, hyperemia, and petechial hemorrhages in the surrounding brain parenchyma. In the encapsulated stage, proliferating fibroblasts in the adjacent capillaries lay down collagen fibers to contain the infectious focus. There is a focal accumulation of pus, varying from a few milliliters to several hundred milliliters surrounded by a fibrous capsule and edema. Subdural empyema and epidural abscess follow a similar course.

Complications

Neuronal injury is caused by tissue displacement as a result of the location and effect of the expanding mass and local edema. If the brain abscess extends to the cortex, meningitis may be a complication. If it extends and ruptures into the ventricles, a catastrophic reaction with brain herniation can develop. In epidural abscess and subdural empyema, cerebral edema also contributes to the mass effect; signs of increased intracranial pressure develop rapidly. A problem associated with the parameningeal infections and occasionally meningitis is intracranial thrombophlebitis.

Clinical Manifestations

The early symptoms associated with cerebral parameningeal infections are nonspecific and similar to meningitis: intermittent fever, headache, confusion, and lethargy. Factors that suggest focal infection include subacute onset (7 to 14 days), history of predisposing infections, unilateral headache, and the presence of focal neurologic signs, such as papilledema. Seizures, hemiparesis, and aphasia are present in up to 50% of cases and depend on the location and size of the lesion. With increasing size of a lesion located in the cerebral hemispheres, the patient exhibits signs of increased intracranial pressure and brain herniation.

The suspicion of the diagnosis is critical because lumbar puncture is contraindicated in cerebral parameningeal infections. With rapid decompression of the mass lesion that can occur during lumbar puncture, brain herniation and death can follow. In addition, lumbar puncture gives little diagnostic information. The spinal fluid is often normal or only exhibits a mild increase in the number of inflammatory cells.

An essential test to localize the lesion is the computed tomography (CT) scan. An abscess will appear as a poorly circumscribed region of decreased density with a thin rim of enhancement if contrast dye is used. CT also can document the presence of cerebral edema. Skull films may reveal the sinusitis, mastoiditis, and osteomyelitis. Angiography may be needed to further identify the lesion if surgery is considered.

Abscess formation in the spinal cord is associated with fever and localized back pain. As the pain intensifies and spreads, progressive weakness, sensory loss, and sphincter incontinence develop rapidly. Myelography is needed to determine the location of the lesion and operative site.

Therapeutic Management

The approach to treatment of subdural empyema and brain and epidural abscess includes administration of antibiotics, surgical decompression, and prevention of complications. Broad-spectrum antibiotics are usually selected for their ability to penetrate the spinal fluid and brain tissue (see Table 48-2). As in meningitis, rapid treatment is associated with a better prognosis, and antibiotics are continued for at least 14 days and up to 6 weeks.

If the abscess produces increased intracranial pressure, urgent operative excision and drainage by craniotomy or burr holes is necessary. The mortality associated with surgical intervention is 25% in the alert or drowsy patient and greater than 50% in the stuporous patient.

Intracranial pressure monitoring and treatment of elevations with osmotic diuretics and hyperventilation are necessary to stabilize the patient before surgery. The use of steroids is controversial as a result of the potential for impeding encapsulation and reduction of antibiotic penetration. Seizures should be controlled with anticonvulsants. Treatment of intracranial thrombophlebitis with anticoagulants is occasionally indicated although the danger of intracranial hemorrhage is high.[25]

Neurologic sequelae to parameningeal infections are more common than in meningitis. Over 40% of patients develop a seizure disorder. In some cases, seizures develop months after recovery. Hemiparesis and other focal deficits may resolve if the process is treated promptly.

NURSING MANAGEMENT OF THE PATIENT WITH PARAMENINGEAL INFECTIONS
Assessment

Assessment proceeds as described in the section on meningitis. The nurse reviews the patient's history for evidence of predisposing factors such as head and neck infections, pneumonia, and previous surgery, as well as unilateral headache. Vital signs are recorded at frequent intervals. Fever can be absent in 40% of patients. Increasing stupor, nausea and vomiting, and other signs that might indicate increased intracranial pressure should be reported immediately. Detection of subtle changes before catastrophic progression requires serial monitoring of those patients at risk.

Implementation

The patient with a parameningeal infection will require similar interventions to those described for meningitis: antibiotic therapy and symptomatic and preventive care. In addition, surgical intervention is required to aspirate, drain, or excise the abscess/empyema.

Of utmost importance is detecting the signs of neurologic deterioration. This calls for continued as-

sessment of neurologic status as previously discussed. Intracranial pressure monitoring has been used to detect intracranial pressure changes. Subdural empyemas and epidural abscess usually require immediate surgical intervention. In the cerebritis stage of brain abscess, antibiotic therapy alone may be attempted with rapid neurosurgical intervention reserved until neurologic deterioration occurs. Standard postoperative care is described in Chapter 49 for the patient following a burr hole and craniotomy.

Antibiotics are started immediately and may be continued for a prolonged period. Antibiotics are given on a consistent schedule to promote adequate levels in the abscess and affected area. Central lines may be used for long-term antibiotic administration, but these require careful management.

Many patients exhibit changes in level of consciousness and memory. They will need close observation and continued reorientation to prevent falls and other threats to their safety. If the patient develops seizures during the course of hospitalization, appropriate observation and care as described in Chapter 45 are in order.

Measures designed to promote comfort for fever, headache, and other toxic manifestations are indicated. General care of the patient includes providing a nutritious diet and helping with self-care activities such as bathing, dressing, and ambulation. Range-of-motion exercises and an active physiotherapy program are begun as soon as possible and are needed to address the needs of the patient with residual neurologic deficit.

ENCEPHALITIS
Definition

Encephalitis is an acute inflammatory disease of the brain that is usually caused by a virus. The encephalitis syndrome is an acute febrile illness with evidence of meningeal involvement. Focal neurologic signs, such as aphasia and seizures, differentiate this syndrome from meningitis.

Etiology/Epidemiology

The incidence of acute encephalitis is 15 cases per 100,000, and the prevalence is 10 cases per 100,000. Encephalitis can occur in epidemics or sporadically. Epidemics of arboviruses are found in the summer, coinciding with an increase in mosquito vectors. Some forms of encephalitis are endemic to certain areas.

There are over 25 types of viral encephalitis; the prognosis depends on the type of viral strain identified. The overall death rate ranges from 5% to 20%. In herpes simplex encephalitis, the death rate ranges from 30% to 70%, and most patients do not

TABLE 48-3 Slow-Virus Infections

Virus	Description	Clinical manifestations	Therapeutic management
CONVENTIONAL VIRUSES			
Subacute sclerosing panencephalitis (SSPE)	Progressive illness, eventually fatal in 6 months to 2 years Rare in those over 18 years Severe demyelination, gliosis, and perivascular inflammation of cerebral white matter and brainstem	Initially—behavioral and personality changes followed by aphasia, intellectual deterioration, seizures, and myoclonus Late—muscular rigidity, pathologic reflexes precede unresponsiveness and decorticate posturing Abnormal electroencephalogram and CSF abnormalities common	Supportive care, maintaining comfort and family support during terminal phases of illness
Progressive multifocal leukoencephalopathy (PML)	Rare disease seen in late adulthood and in those with immune system suppression Rapidly progressive; death within 3 to 6 months Widespread patchy demyelinating lesions in cerebral hemispheres, brainstem, and cerebellum Papovavirus of two serologic types has been identified in brain cells	Clinical course consists of initial hemiparesis, aphasia, ataxia, visual field defects, and dementia that progresses to coma CT scan demonstrates low-density lesions	Supportive care, management of mobility, behavioral problems, and providing comprehensive terminal care
UNCONVENTIONAL VIRUS			
Creutzfeldt-Jakob disease (C-J disease; subacute spongiform encephalitis)	Rapidly progressive, profound dementia occurs in late middle age Reported iatrogenic transmission following corneal transplant, neurosurgical procedures, intracranial electrodes Recipients of human growth hormone have developed C-J 8 to 12 years later Widespread vacuolation of neuron producing a spongy appearance, with neuronal destruction and gliosis of cerebral cortex, cerebellum, and spinal cord Caused by prions (viruslike particles)	Early depressive symptoms followed by hallucinations and impairment of memory and reasoning Later ataxia, reduced visual acuity, myoclonic jerks, stupor, and coma; a striking startle response is a hallmark	Consists of symptomatic and supportive care until patient dies Prevention of transmission to others requires special precautions in handling of body fluids and tissues

fully recover. The incidence of fatality and neurologic sequelae is high in eastern equine encephalitis, in which 90% of patients have residual neurologic deficits. Western equine encephalitis has a milder course and prognosis; only 5% to 10% of these patients have deficits, and most recover.

The most common sporadic encephalitis is that caused by herpes simplex. This type 1 virus is responsible for the adult encephalitis syndrome, although patients who have chronic type 1 infections (cold sores) may not be at increased risk of encephalitis. It is speculated that there are two forms of pathogenesis, one from the virus chronically residing in the host and another from an exogenous infection. There is no seasonality or predilection for herpes simplex encephalitis by age, gender, or socioeconomic status.

Chronic "slow-virus" infections that simulate degenerative disease of the nervous system were originally proposed in the pathogenesis of encephalitis after an epidemic of von Economo disease in 1918 was linked with the development of Parkinson's disease up to 25 years after the initial infection. There are two major types of these rare chronic viral infections; those caused by a conventional virus and those caused by unconventional viruslike particles, called prions. Table 48-3 describes the characteristics of these disorders.

Pathophysiology

Viruses are intracellular parasites that damage the nervous system by destroying selected neuronal cells. Some viruses exhibit neurotropism, a selective affinity of the virus to infect certain types of cells. This is true in rabies and poliomyelitis where the virus attacks the motor neuron and in myxovirus infections where the ependymal cells are affected. Some spread preferentially to selected locations, such as the herpes simplex virus, which involves the frontal and temporal lobes. Evidence of destruction, including intense hemorrhagic lesions in the frontal and temporal lobes, has been observed in herpes simplex encephalitis.

Clinical Manifestations

The clinical manifestations of viral encephalitis include abrupt onset of fever, headache, seizures, and stiff neck. Next, disorders of consciousness occur and lethargy progresses to confusion, stupor, and coma. Focal findings such as hemiparesis, aphasia, increased deep tendon reflexes, Babinski's sign, and cranial nerve abnormalities differentiate this syndrome from meningitis. Seizures are common in all forms of encephalitis and indicate severe neuronal involvement. During convalescence the patient may experience extreme weakness, anorexia, and mental depression. In herpes simplex encephalitis, focal signs point to involvement of portions of the frontal and temporal lobes. These signs include hallucinations, anosmia, periods of bizarre behavior, aphasia, and temporal lobe seizures.

In the epidemic viral encephalitis syndromes, the diagnosis is supported by viral cultures of CSF and the clinical history. Additional cultures of pharynx, rectum, and urine and paired antiviral antibody tests on serum (one early in the course and one during convalescence) provide supportive evidence of a viral infection.

The diagnosis of herpes simplex encephalitis can be made by brain biopsy and rarely from culture of CSF. The electroencephalogram (EEG) is abnormal in 80% of cases with temporal lobe abnormalities. The CT scan is normal up to the first 5 days, with low-density lesions in the temporal lobe coming later. Magnetic resonance imaging (MRI) provides a more specific diagnosis and requires a cooperative patient.

Therapeutic Management

In acute uncomplicated viral encephalitis, supportive and preventive care during the early phase of the illness is the major focus of therapy. Bed rest, a nutritious diet, and sufficient fluid intake are essential to maintain health. Controlling seizures and reducing increased intracranial pressure also are included in the treatment plan. Convalescence is slow and may take weeks. Rehabilitation may be necessary for patients with residual neurologic deficits. Epidemic encephalitis caused by vectors is prevented by destruction of mosquito carriers and protection from bites.

Treatment of herpes simplex encephalitis consists of administration of antiviral drugs and prevention of complications. The most commonly used drugs are vidarabine (Vira-A) and acyclovir (Zovirax). Treatment is instituted as soon as 12 hours after brain biopsy and is continued until the culture confirms the diagnosis. The drugs work by blocking DNA synthesis and viral replication. Acyclovir is less toxic to uninfected brain cells than vidarabine and has fewer side effects. The route of administration for both is by slow intravenous infusion, and the medication is continued for 10 days. The drugs are poorly soluble and require a large fluid volume to administer, which can complicate cerebral edema. The use of antiviral drugs has decreased mortality to 30%.

Osmotic diuretics and corticosteroids are used to control cerebral edema. Cerebral edema and brain herniation resulting in coma and respiratory arrest are the major complications during the first 24 to 72 hours. The most severe sequelae include psychosis and global dementia, seizures, memory disorders, and aphasia.

NURSING MANAGEMENT OF THE PATIENT WITH ENCEPHALITIS

Assessment

A careful history to elicit symptoms and a physical assessment to determine the extent of the intellectual, motor, and sensory deficits are essential. Procedures for monitoring vital signs and to detect changes in intracranial pressure are the same as described for meningitis. If the patient is elderly or has been incapacitated for an extended period, attention is paid to factors that provide information about nutritional status, elimination patterns, self-care abilities, sleep cycle, and safety concerns. The impact of the hospitalization on the family must be investigated as well.

Nursing Diagnosis

Many nursing diagnoses are the same as those previously discussed regarding meningitis. These include altered cerebral tissue perfusion, potential for injury, fluid volume deficit/excess, self-care deficit, knowledge deficit, anxiety, and pain. The previously discussed plans and goals are relevant as well.

Implementation

Many nursing interventions can support the patient with encephalitis. Patients with the potential for recovery require attention to preventing complications that will impede their progress, such as aspiration, skin breakdown, and falls. In self-limiting diseases, such as epidemic encephalitis caused by arboviruses, supportive care, comfort, and safety measures predominate. Interventions for fever, headache, and discomfort are similar to those seen in meningitis.

The nurse may need to spend extra time with the confused patient to gain cooperation. Sedatives are rarely administered. Precautions such as padding the siderails to ensure safety should be instituted. Nutritional support via a nasogastric tube may be necessary to provide an adequate caloric and fluid intake. Bed rest and complete support of the patient's hygienic needs and activities of daily living will be necessary until the patient is alert and active. Supportive physiotherapy and measures to prevent contractures are indicated. Sleep and behavioral disturbances are treated by a consistent schedule of daytime activities to provide diversion and stimulation.

While the patient is receiving antiviral drugs, a careful accounting of the intake and output is necessary. An infusion pump should be used to administer the medications to prevent fluid overload and fluctuations in the plasma concentration of the

---

TABLE 48-4   Other Infectious Syndromes

Syndrome	Description	Clinical manifestations	Therapeutic management
VIRAL SYNDROMES			
Herpes zoster (shingles)	Affects dorsal root ganglia and portions of spinal nerves Caused by DNA virus varicella-zoster (also responsible for chickenpox) Common in elderly, immunosuppressed, and those with malignancies	Malaise, fever, lymphadenopathy, and pain in dermatomal distribution precedes eruption of vesicles by 3 to 4 days Vesicles dry to form crusts in 5 to 10 days; burning, tingling pain will last 1 to 4 weeks and can last after lesions disappear Trunk and face commonly affected; ophthalmic involvement can cause blindness Most recover completely; postherpetic neuralgia is common in aged and can last months	Pain control with aspirin; codeine for severe pain Antiviral agents (vidarabine [Vira-A], acyclovir [Zovirax]) for widespread and ophthalmic involvement Local cleansing, dressing care, and prevention of secondary infection For postherpetic neuralgia: carbamazepine (Tegretol), narcotics, TENS units Antidepressants may be necessary to treat depression that accompanies long-term pain

Continued.

TABLE 48-4 Other Infectious Syndromes—cont'd

Syndrome	Description	Clinical manifestations	Therapeutic management

Poliomyelitis	Now a rare illness following initiation of vaccine program 30 years ago
	Common worldwide in developing nations without mass vaccination programs
	Incidence following vaccination is .02 to .04 cases in 1 million doses
	Highly communicable; fecal-oral route of infection
	Small RNA picornavirus spread via hematogenous and neural paths
	Destruction of anterior horn cells of spinal cord and motor nuclei of pons and medulla
		Classic paralytic polio: rapid development of paralysis, reaches maximum severity 48 hours to 1 week after onset; little progression after temperature has been normal for 48 hours
		Paralytic features predominate (asymmetric paralysis, fasciculations, reduced reflexes, muscle atrophy, bulbar weakness, and respiratory failure) over encephalopathy (fever, headache, and stiff neck)
			Care similar to Guillain-Barré syndrome
			Assessment of increasing muscular weakness, support of ventilatory function, and prevention of complications
			Physical therapy and splinting to prevent deformity useful
			Rarely fatal, many recover completely in 3 to 4 months; exceptions:
			  Postpolio syndrome—delayed increase in muscle weakness years beyond recovery
			  Postpolio survivors—require full- and part-time mechanical ventilation, managed at home; creativity and adaptability have maintained quality of life

BACTERIAL TOXIN

Syndrome	Description	Clinical manifestations	Therapeutic management
Tetanus	Caused by anaerobic spore-forming rod, *Clostridum tetani,* producing exotoxin, tetanospasm Enters through local wound Hematogenous and direct spread via peripheral nerves to CNS Frequently fatal, prevented by immunization Seen in rural areas, migrant workers, narcotic addicts, newborns, and undeveloped countries Exotoxin blocks neuromuscular transmission in neuromuscular junction, spinal cord, and brainstem inhibitory neurons	Incubation period 1 to 30 days Cephalic form affects ocular and facial muscles Generalized tetanus most common (80%); initial sign is trismus (spasm of jaw muscles); then fever, muscle rigidity, and bulbar and extremity paralysis leading to respiratory failure Paroxysms of painful seizurelike spasm in alert patient	General care: administration of immune sera and antibiotics; wound debridement *Passive immunity:* human tetanus immune globulin (TIG) *Active immunity:* tetanus toxoid (Td) To reduce spasm: quiet dark room, sedation, treatments clustered to minimize stimulation Respiratory spasm treated by curare with prior tracheotomy and ventilatory support Prevention strategies of utmost importance: monitoring vaccination by the primary care provider, public information programs to increase consumer awareness and case finding in hospital and emergency department admissions

drugs. Medications to control seizures and signs of increased intracranial pressure are similar to those for patients with meningitis.

OTHER INFECTIOUS DISEASES

Less common but equally important infections of the nervous system are summarized in Table 48-4.

Autoimmune Disorders

MULTIPLE SCLEROSIS
Definition

Multiple sclerosis (MS) is a demyelinating disease that results in destruction of the CNS myelin. MS is the third most common cause of severe disability in people between the ages of 15 and 60 years.

Etiology/Epidemiology

Epidemiologic studies have established a link between prevalence of MS and geographic location. People in areas furthest from the equator carry the highest risk for developing MS, with a prevalence greater than 80/100,000. Countries closest to the equator carry the lowest risk (0 to 5/100,000). Age of onset is from 10 to 50 years, most commonly between 20 and 40 years. MS occurs more commonly in women than in men, with an almost 2:1 ratio, and predominantly in whites.

Although the specific cause of MS remains unknown, it is postulated to be an autoimmune disease, the result of an alteration in the immune response mediated in some way by a viral trigger.[19]

Pathophysiology

Demyelination results in both direct damage to myelin and to the oligodendrocytes—the supportive cells that produce and maintain myelin. Lesions are scattered predominantly throughout white matter, most commonly around the ventricles, but also to a lesser degree in gray matter. There are two distinct types of lesions, acute and chronic. The acute lesion demonstrates an initial inflammatory response characterized by proliferation of lymphocytes, lipid-laden macrophages, and antibody-producing B lymphocytes. Phagocytosis occurs with myelin as the primary target, and subsequent secondary edema surrounds the lesions, extending into undemyelinated areas. Over time, the inflammation subsides, the edema resolves, and a chronic lesion develops, showing little or no evidence of active demyelination. A hard sclerotic plaque then forms.

In the acute lesions and early stages of the illness, demyelinated axons are spared, but conduction is slow and intermittent. In advanced disease, axon destruction results in complete conduction block. Remyelination occurs, but not extensively, and the mechanism is not clearly understood. Remyelination requires several weeks and may be responsible for gradual rather than rapid recovery. Symptoms related to axonal loss cannot be relieved by improved conduction.

Recent research using MRI studies confirms that many plaques are clinically silent. New lesions occurred without clinical exacerbations; this was more common in active progressive disease. This may make MRI useful to test immunologic therapies.

Clinical Manifestations

The presentation of signs and symptoms covers a wide range of CNS dysfunction and reflects the anatomic location of the plaque. Table 48-5 lists the most common clinical manifestations. The severity of the clinical course ranges from a benign course with few impairments to a chronic progressive course that leads to complete paralysis. Two thirds of those patients with MS have exacerbations, followed by nearly complete or complete remission of symptoms. Up to 50% of the patients are ambulatory 25 years after the initial diagnosis. The diagnosis of MS has always been based on clinical evidence (historical report of symptoms, signs of neurologic dysfunction on examination). Making the diagnosis is often a matter of eliminating other diseases that mimic MS. There is still no one single test that confirms the diagnosis of MS (Table 48-6).

Therapeutic Management

There is no one specific treatment for MS. Management goals are aimed at developing a care plan to reduce or alleviate symptoms, prevent complications, and provide continued emotional support.

Drug therapy

Administration of short courses of adrenocorticotrophic hormone (ACTH) or corticosteroids is the most widely accepted method of treatment for acute MS attacks. Steroids do not alter the disease course or reduce the risk and number of future exacerbations. The mechanism of action is presumed to be immunologically based, resulting in reduction of the inflammatory response, restoration of the electrolyte balance, resolution of associated edema, and early improvement in clinical symptoms.

Intramuscular ACTH and oral prednisone administration varies per clinician, but the usual course is short, starting with a high dose (prednisone, 80 to 100 mg/day) and tapering to discontinuation over 2

TABLE 48-5   Multiple Sclerosis Symptoms

Area of dysfunction	Symptoms
Cranial nerve dysfunction	Blurred central vision; faded colors; blind spots (optic neuritis)
	Diplopia
	Dysphagia
	Facial weakness, numbness, pain
Motor dysfunction	Weakness
	Paralysis
	Spasticity
	Abnormal gait
Sensory dysfunction	Paresthesias
	Lhermitte's sign (electric shock–like sensation radiating down spine into extremities)
	Decreased proprioception
	Decreased temperature perception
Cerebellar dysfunction	Dysarthria
	Tremor
	Incoordination
	Ataxia
	Vertigo
Bowel and bladder dysfunction	Fecal urgency, constipation, incontinence
	Urinary frequency, urgency, hesitancy, nocturia, retention, incontinence
Cognitive dysfunction	Decreased short-term memory
	Difficulty learning new information
	Word-finding trouble
	Short attention span
	Decreased concentration
	Mood alterations (depression, euphoria)
Sexual dysfunction	Women: decreased libido, decreased orgasmic ability, decreased genital sensation
	Men: erectile, orgasmic, and ejaculatory dysfunction
Fatigue	Overwhelming weakness not overcome with increased physical effort

TABLE 48-6   Diagnostic Test Results of MS

Test	Result
CSF analysis	Increased protein
	Increased lymphocytes
	Increased IgG
	Presence of oligoclonal bands
	Increased myelin basic protein
Evoked potentials Visual Brainstem Somatosensory	Prolonged impulse conduction
Magnetic resonance imaging	Demonstrates white matter lesions (plaques) of brain, brainstem, and spinal cord
Myelogram, skull and spine x-ray films, CT scan	Rule out other neurologic disease
Urodynamic studies	Abnormalities consistent with neurogenic bladder

to 4 weeks. Methylprednisolone (1g/day) is administered intravenously over 3 to 5 days and followed by a short tapering course of prednisone.

Despite the fact that the etiology of MS remains unknown, major research efforts are focused on treatments that either alter or suppress the immune system response or affect the presumed triggering agent. Clinical trials are in progress to evaluate copolymer I and beta interferon. Both have been tested in exacerbating remitting MS with encouraging results. Patients had fewer exacerbations and less disease progression. They are now being evaluated in larger clinical trials.

Treatment of chronic progressive MS is more controversial. Cyclophosphamide (Cytoxan) in combination with ACTH or methylprednisolone has been shown to be effective in patients with chronic progressive disease who demonstrate a rapid deterioration. It has been used in Europe for over 20 years. The treatment goal is to modify the disease progression, producing a temporary remission lasting from 1 to 3 years. The treatment is not effective in everyone. Patients experience several side effects, and long-term toxicity is not well defined. Cytoxan is administered intravenously on both an inpatient and an outpatient basis. Immunosuppression, characterized by a decrease in the white blood cell count, produces the following side effects: alopecia, anorexia, nausea, and vomiting. The risk of developing an infection (upper respiratory or urinary tract) is increased. Hemorrhagic cystitis may also occur. In addition, the patient experiences side effects associated with steroid therapy.

A meta-analysis of azathioprine (Imuran) treatment noted a slight clinical benefit (a reduced disease relapse and progression rate) that must be weighed against the potential risks of long-term treatment. Plasmapheresis is considered an investigative procedure because of the minimal and transient benefits reported. Total lymphoid irradiation, which reduced WBCs and progressive disability in chronic MS, is also considered experimental. Cyclosporine A demonstrated slightly reduced disability; however, significant renal toxicity makes this unsuitable for ongoing treatment. Several new treatments under development include anti-CD4 or anti-CD8 monoclonal antibodies to inhibit helper or cytotoxic T-cell responses; T-cell vaccination to induce immune tolerance; and interferons with antiviral properties.

Symptomatic management

Management of motor dysfunction requires combined interventions including medication (Table 48-7), physical and occupational therapies, and occasionally surgical intervention. Weakness and spasticity are addressed through a program of progressive resistive and stretching exercises aimed at maintaining and improving muscle strength, joint range of motion, and tone. For bed-bound patients with severe spasticity unresponsive to conservative measures, intrathecal phenol injection may provide temporary relief by promoting comfort and facilitating the administration of nursing care. Because of the associated loss of sensory perception and bowel and bladder function, phenol injection is not indicated in someone who is minimally to moderately impaired. Myelotomy and surgical rhizotomy have been used in rare instances.

Mood alterations are managed with a combination of medication and counseling. Emotional lability is especially responsive to amitriptyline. Cognitive impairment has typically been associated with

TABLE 48-7   Pharmacology Summary: Multiple Sclerosis

Symptom	Medication	Expected benefit	Side effects
Spasticity	Baclofen (Lioresal) Diazepam (Valium) Dantrolene (Dantrium)	Decreased stiffness Decreased spasms Improved mobility and comfort	Weakness Sedation Hepatotoxicity
Tremor	Isoniazid (INH) Propranolol (Inderal) Clonazepam (Klonopin)	Decreased tremor Improved mobility, coordination, function	Hepatotoxicity (INH) Hypotension and cardiac abnormalities (Inderal) Sedation and ataxia (Klonopin)
Bladder dysfunction	Oxybutynin (Ditropan) Propantheline bromide (Pro-Banthine)	Decreased frequency, urgency incontinence, nocturia Improved control	Dry mouth Constipation Blurred vision Urinary hesitancy, retention
Bowel dysfunction	Bulk additives (Metamucil) Stool softeners (Colace) Stimulants (Dulcolax)	Decreased constipation Improved control	Diarrhea
Fatigue	Amantadine (Symmetrel) Pemoline (Cylert)	Improved endurance	Nausea, dizziness, drowsiness, livedo reticularis, insomnia (amantadine) Insomnia (pemoline)
Mood alterations	Tricyclic antidepressants Amitriptyline (Elavil) Imipramine (Tofranil) Desipramine (Norpramine) Fluoxetine (Prozac)	Improved mood Decreased emotional lability	Dry mouth Constipation Urinary hesitancy Sedation Orthostatic hypotension Weight gain Weight loss (fluoxetine)

advanced disease but in fact may occur at any stage of MS and may range from subtle to marked impairment. Neuropsychologic testing is helpful in documenting disability in situations where cognitive impairment is the predominant disability and physical dysfunction is minimal.[34] It is also useful in determining the patient's ability to continue functioning safely in a given occupation and for determining rehabilitation potential.

When attempts at conservative management of dysphagia are ineffective, thorough evaluation by the speech pathologist and radiographic assessment (barium swallow, cine-esophagram) are indicated. The dietician can determine whether minimum daily requirements are being maintained and devise a plan to achieve optimal nutrition. Surgical intervention may be necessary for placement of a feeding tube. Percutaneous endoscopic gastrostomy (PEG) is the method of choice, because it does not carry the risks associated with general anesthesia or major surgery incurred by patients with advanced disease.

NURSING MANAGEMENT OF THE PATIENT WITH MULTIPLE SCLEROSIS
Assessment

Important information to collect includes the history of symptoms, progression of the illness, and the types of treatment received and the response. The nurse should identify additional health problems that may influence neurologic dysfunction. A current and complete medication history is obtained to identify potential side effects that may contribute to symptoms. The nurse determines the patient and family's understanding of the illness and their perceptions about how the resulting problems have affected activities of daily living function, job performance, and family relationships. The sources of stress in daily life should be identified as well as the patient's primary sources of support (both for physical care and emotional support). A screening cognitive assessment may also be indicated. The nurse should identify past and present involvement with community agencies that provide either care or social support.

Physical examination includes thorough assessment of cranial nerve function to determine the presence of visual and swallowing dysfunction, impaired speech, and facial weakness. The patient's gait, posture, muscle strength, and coordination are evaluated to determine the effect of abnormalities on the performance of activities of daily living. The nurse inquires about the presence of fatigue and its triggering factors and determines the effect on function. The nurse ascertains the presence and degree of spasticity and its aggravating and alleviating factors. Sensory perception is assessed and the skin is examined for subsequent signs of trauma or decubitus ulcers.

The presence of bladder dysfunction is determined. Failure-to-store syndrome, caused by detrusor hyperreflexia, is characterized by increased frequency, urgency, urge incontinence, nocturia, and a postvoid residual of less than 100 mL. Failure-to-empty syndrome is caused by detrusor hyporeflexia; symptoms include decreased frequency and urge to void, hesitancy, a feeling of incomplete emptying, incontinence, frequent urinary tract infections, and a postvoid residual volume greater than 100 mL. A third syndrome is detrusor-sphincter dyssynergia—incoordination between contractions of the external urethral sphincter and the detrusor muscle—which results in retention and obstructed outflow. Symptoms are usually the same as for failure-to-empty syndrome. Bowel dysfunction is characterized primarily by constipation, but urgency may also be a problem. Fecal incontinence does occur but more so in advanced disease.[30]

Nursing Diagnosis

Nursing diagnoses relevant to the care of the patient with multiple sclerosis are as follows:

Self-care deficit related to weakness, ataxia, tremor, spasticity, sensory impairment, fatigue

Urinary retention/incontinence related to spinal cord dysfunction, cognitive impairment, decreased functional ability

Constipation related to spinal cord dysfunction, decreased functional ability

Impaired skin integrity related to decreased mobility, spasticity, sensory impairment, incontinence

Altered nutrition: less than body requirements related to dysphagia and motor or sensory deficits

Fatigue related to disease process

Knowledge deficit of disease process related to complex and changing nature of symptoms and treatment regimen

Sexual dysfunction related to mobility and sensory impairments, bowel and bladder dysfunction, medication side effects, cognitive dysfunction and mood alteration, interpersonal issues, maladaptation to illness

Ineffective individual/family coping related to knowledge deficit about disease or treatment regimens, disease course variability, cognitive impairment

Body image/self-esteem disturbance related to decreased mobility, decreased independence, changes in vocational or family roles

Impaired home maintenance management related to progressive nature of illness, lack of knowledge about available services

Planning

Goals for the patient with MS include the following:

Patient will demonstrate maximal safe mobility and independence in activities of daily living using techniques to prevent trauma, conserve energy, and prevent the complications of immobility

Patient will follow a bladder program that reduces irritative symptoms, promotes continence, and prevents associated complications and social isolation

Patient will follow a bowel regimen for regular elimination

Patient will follow a prescribed regimen for treating existing decubitus ulcers and utilize measures to prevent skin breakdown

Patient will follow a balanced diet to meet daily energy requirements

Patient will verbally relate knowledge of the disease process and applicable treatment regimens

Patient will have the knowledge to develop and maintain satisfying sexual function

Patient will utilize knowledge about the disease process to develop effective coping strategies

Patient will have a positive attitude and accept role changes, actively participate in decision making, and maintain satisfying social interactions

Patient will live in a home environment that supports abilities and functional status through continuity of care and appropriate use of community services

Implementation

In general, nursing interventions are devised to (1) maximize and maintain independent function within the limitations of the disease, (2) prevent complications, (3) promote continuity of care in a variety of settings, and (4) provide patient and family education and emotional support.

The patient may experience several levels of self-care deficit during the course of the illness. Allow the patient to keep his or her usual routine. Even though it may take a patient longer to do a task independently, a balance between assisted and independent activities should be achieved and supported.

Failure-to-store syndrome responds to anticholinergic medication. Educate the patient about the expected benefits as well as side effects. Decreasing fluid intake in early evening can reduce nocturia. Large amounts of caffeinated liquids should be avoided. Failure-to-empty syndrome and detrusorsphinctor dyssynergia are managed by intermittent self-catheterization using the clean technique (see Chapter 43). Instruct patients about the identification and prevention of urinary tract infections. Inability to transfer independently, upper extremity tremor, ataxia, weakness, and hip adductor spasticity may interfere with self-catheterization, necessitating assistance from a family member or the use of adaptive equipment (knee spreader, catheter holder). Total incontinence in men, if retention is not a problem, is managed with an external catheter. Indwelling or suprapubic catheters are other alternatives in controlling complete incontinence.

Bowel dysfunction is best managed by establishing a regular routine for elimination. For mild constipation, adherence to a diet high in fiber and fluid (at least 64 oz per day) is often sufficient. Successive addition of bulk formers, stool softeners, and stimulants may be required. Bulk formers can reduce urgency also. To enhance compliance, patients should be aware that change does not occur quickly, and the original plan may require modification.

Maintaining skin integrity in the patient with moderate to severe disability requires vigilance. Nursing management is directed at increasing the patient's awareness and prevention of potential or actual risk factors. Regular changes in position, the use of pressure-relieving devices, routine skin care, successful management of incontinence, and daily assessment of skin integrity are crucial. For treatment of existing decubitus ulcers and prevention of infection, see Chapter 74.

For treatment of altered nutrition, see Chapter 16. Help the patient to identify triggering factors of fatigue and incorporate the management techniques recommended by physical and occupational therapists. Often a more structured plan of activities is needed with the inclusion of rest periods.

Providing patients and families with the information needed to manage the illness is a continuous process. The content of an educational session may include information about disease pathophysiology, signs and symptoms, the diagnostic process, symptomatic therapies, and management of fatigue. For patients with cognitive impairment, creative modification of the teaching and care plans promotes better understanding of care needs, encourages continuity of care, and lessens frustration.

Open communication is promoted, and reassurance that sexual enjoyment can be regained and continued is provided, as well as information about anatomy and sexual function to dispel misconceptions. Continued emotional support is crucial in helping patients and families in coping with the uncertainty of the illness and the multiple losses incurred. The nurse encourages participation in social and recreational activities outside the home, helps in locating appropriate support groups in the community, encourages the patient to adopt an active role in goal planning and decision making about the future, and involves the patient in vocational rehabilitation if appropriate.

Evaluation/Documentation

Determining the effectiveness of nursing interventions is an ongoing process. Assessment of patient progress and revision of the care plan require communication between all health team members. Involvement of the patient and family in the evaluation process fosters their participation in goal setting and care provision and promotes continuity of care. Documentation of all components of the nursing process is critical in providing comprehensive care through several disciplines. The care plan and patient responses to interventions serve as a foundation for continuity of care. With the shift of health care delivery to the outpatient setting, the patient also benefits from written information and instruction about the disease and treatment regimens.

Ongoing Care

In providing ongoing care to the patient with MS in a variety of settings, the nurse is responsible for (1) helping the patient in maintaining an active role in health maintenance, (2) providing patient and family education, (3) facilitating patient and family adaptation through physical and emotional support, and (4) promoting continuity of care.

Hospitalizations are primarily for symptomatic treatment of acute attacks, management of complications, and participation in experimental therapies. As a result, these patients are more disabled. Rehabilitation efforts occur throughout the course of the disease. Whenever there is a significant change in functional level, reassessment and compensatory training need to be initiated. Hospital admissions for complications include management of urosepsis and severe decubitus ulcers, as well as surgical intervention in dysphagia. Infection is the primary cause of premature death of a patient with MS. Hospitalization for intensive immunosuppression therapy with cyclophosphamide (Cytoxan) and ACTH requires specialized nursing care.[35] Nursing interventions are based on a complete assessment and thorough knowledge of the potential side effects of cyclophosphamide and ACTH. Because cyclophosphamide metabolites irritate the bladder mucosa, a daily oral fluid intake of at least 3 L is indicated. This may place additional stress on an already compromised bladder, resulting in increased irritative symptoms. For patients with significant impairment in gait and balance, use of an external catheter or commode at night reduces the risk of falls and activity-related fatigue. If there is a large postvoiding residual, intermittent catheterization should be instituted every 3

to 6 hours. An indwelling catheter is not advised, since there is increased risk of developing a urinary tract infection. Urine is assessed daily for the presence of blood and at the beginning and end of therapy for infection. Reduction of gastrointestinal side effects is achieved through diet modification and regular administration of antiemetics. During the treatment period a temporary decline in the patient's functional and energy levels may occur, necessitating increased assistance with activities of daily living. The institution of physical and occupational therapies helps in maintaining maximum strength and function. Discharge plans should include a community health nurse to administer remaining ACTH injections, monitor for additional side effects caused by medication, and identify infection. Throughout treatment, efforts directed at patient education and emotional support are crucial. The patient should know all side effects of medications (see Table 48-7) and when to report problems (see the patient education guide above). Anticipatory education for the patient and family alleviates the fear of the unknown and encourages family support.

GUILLAIN-BARRÉ SYNDROME
Definition/Etiology

The **Guillain-Barré syndrome (GBS)** is an acquired inflammatory disease that results in demyelination of the peripheral nerves with relative sparing of axons. The patient has a progressive ascending paralysis that is usually reversible. GBS is also called

---

PATIENT EDUCATION GUIDE

Long-term Immunosuppressive Therapy

1. Do not stop medication abruptly.
2. You will have reduced resistance to infection; take precautions, and report fevers and infections.
3. Know side effects of medications and when to report symptoms.
4. Wear a Medic Alert bracelet.
5. Tell your dentist, pharmacist, and other health care providers about all medications.
6. Complete monthly or quarterly blood tests and checkups as requested to monitor and treat side effects (i.e., bone marrow suppression, hepatotoxicity, osteoporosis, cataracts, hypertension, hyperglycemia).
7. Use effective contraception if taking azathioprine (Imuran) or cyclophosphamide (Cytoxan).

acute inflammatory polyradiculoneuropathy (AIP). GBS is an uncommon illness. Incidence figures are 1.6/100,000. Etiologic factors are unknown. An altered immune response directed against a component of myelin in the peripheral nerve is a postulated factor. Precipitating factors include a viral infection in the preceding 1 to 3 weeks in over half of those affected.

Pathophysiology

The pathophysiologic defects seen in GBS are similar to those seen in MS, yet the demyelination is confined to the peripheral nervous system (PNS) and the illness rarely recurs. There are focal and segmental areas of cellular infiltration by macrophages in the motor, sensory, autonomic, and cranial nerve pathways. Macrophages attack normal myelin, producing variable degrees of demyelination and blocked conduction of the nerve impulse to muscle that results in paralysis. In severe cases, destruction of the axon (wallerian degeneration) occurs. It is theorized that GBS is initiated by the cell-mediated immune system and accentuated by humoral immune factors. Evidence of reduced suppressor T cell response and abnormal lymphocyte reactions directed against PNS myelin is consistent with a cell-mediated immune process. Antibodies that destroy PNS myelin have been found in the serum of GBS patients.

Clinical Manifestations

The hallmark of GBS is progressive muscle weakness that develops in a matter of hours or up to 10 days. The distal lower extremities are usually affected first. The patient may fall, develop footdrop, and then be unable to walk. Over time, the proximal muscles of the upper extremities, trunk, and neck are involved. There is a flaccid paralysis with hypotonia and loss of superficial and deep tendon reflexes. The facial nerve is almost always affected causing bilateral facial weakness. **Bulbar weakness,** dysphagia, and dysarthria also occur as a result of cranial nerve involvement. The respiratory muscles and muscles innervated by the cranial nerves are usually affected last. Respiratory muscle paralysis leads to the need for intubation and ventilatory support.

Sensory symptoms such as pain and tingling in the legs and back are common, although there is no evidence of severe sensory loss. Autonomic manifestations include postural hypotension, arterial hypertension, heart block, and tachycardia. Bladder atony requiring temporary catheterization occurs in many cases, yet the sphincters are often spared. The hypoosmolar state (SIADH), bladder infection, embolic phenomenon, and pneumonia are common complications. The patient does not have symptoms such as fever or headache. Cerebral function, level of consciousness, and pupillary response are normal.

The diagnosis is made on clinical grounds, supported by the results of lumbar puncture and electrophysiologic studies. CSF protein level is increased, with either a normal or moderate amount of mononuclear cells present. Electrical studies show a slowing in the motor and sensory nerve conduction velocity. Prognosis for recovery is excellent.

Therapeutic Management

Rapidly progressive acute GBS is now treated with plasma exchange. Controlled trials have demonstrated impressive reductions in ventilator dependency and hospital stay and more rapid return of ambulation and functional ability. The plasma exchange is completed over 4 to 5 days in sessions lasting 2 to 3 hours. Albumin is used to replace the plasma, 200 to 250 mL/kg body weight, exchanged. A new treatment, administration of intravenous immune globulin (IVIg), has been suggested as an equally effective treatment. It is given intravenously for 4 to 5 days at a dose of 0.4 mg/kg body weight per day. Both treatments are expensive and require hospital monitoring. After plasma exchange or IVIg is started, treatment is primarily directed at prevention of complications such as respiratory failure. Respiratory failure should be anticipated: Up to 40% of patients have some detectable respiratory muscle weakness. The patient should be prepared for a tracheostomy, since many require prolonged ventilatory support.

Autonomic symptoms such as bradycardia and heart block are common. Patients are monitored for these complications. If severe bradycardia occurs, atropine or a temporary pacemaker may be needed. Blood pressure fluctuations should be observed and treated cautiously with short-acting agents. SIADH is managed by close attention to fluid balance and fluid restriction. Low-dose heparin is indicated to prevent thrombophlebitis. Antacids are often given to reduce the risk of gastrointestinal bleeding. Nutritional support via a nasogastric tube will be necessary in those patients requiring ventilatory support and with severe dysphagia.

NURSING MANAGEMENT OF THE PATIENT WITH GUILLAIN-BARRÉ SYNDROME

Care of a patient who is completely paralyzed, yet whose sensation and mentation are intact, is one of the greatest challenges to nursing care. Key nursing issues while the patient is acutely paralyzed include respiratory care, communication, self-care, and nutritional support. Preventing injury and complications should be addressed throughout the hospitalization. Care of the patient during plasma exchange is discussed in Chapter 38. Complications to monitor include hypotension, arrhythmias, and vascular access problems. There are few complications reported with IVIg therapy; hypotension, dyspnea, fever, and transient hematuria can occur.

Recognition of respiratory failure and aspiration is essential. The patient requires close observation in the hospital unit and intensive care to detect sudden deterioration. Frequent measurement of forced vital capacity is necessary because changes in arterial blood gas values will be a late occurrence (Figure 48-4). After intubation, preventing atelectasis, pneumonia, and retained secretions through a pulmonary program is the goal of treatment. Tracheostomy care should be routine. Weaning from the ventilator should proceed when forced vital capacity indicates improved respiratory muscle strength. The patient must be free of pulmonary infiltrate and retained secretions, as well as be able to swallow before weaning is attempted. Intermittent mandatory ventilation and increasing intervals off the ventilator are attempted as the patient's total volume and forced vital capacity improve. Oximetry is also of assistance and does not involve the discomfort of frequent needle puncture for arterial blood gases.

Establishing an effective communication system with the intubated patient is vital. The nurse should develop two methods, one for the nurse to be summoned immediately and another to communicate basic needs, answer questions, and, if possible, converse.

The immobility associated with GBS can cause self-care deficit and discomfort. Maintaining the same position for long periods can result in uncomfortable sensations. Range of motion should be completed three to four times each day and is helpful as both a comfort and preventive measure. Some patients may request turning more frequently than every hour. Including the patient in the scheduling of turning helps give a sense of control. The nurse should be alert to the signs of thrombophlebitis and contractures. Splints, high-top sneakers, sand bags, and a correctly placed footboard are used to support the extremities and prevent contractures. Heel and elbow protectors are also indicated if skin breakdown and discomfort become problems.

Preventing eye injury is extremely important. Interventions that protect the eye, such as use of artificial tears hourly during the day and Lacrilube ointment at night, prevent dryness caused by lack of automatic blinking and poor eyelid closure.

Preventing injury caused by autonomic dysfunction is another part of the nursing care plan. As the patient becomes more mobile, the nurse should help the patient slowly change position and avoid postural hypotension.

Nutritional support should be addressed early. A small bore nasogastric feeding tube is placed when the patient is unable to swallow or requires ventilatory support. A balanced liquid diet will be contin-

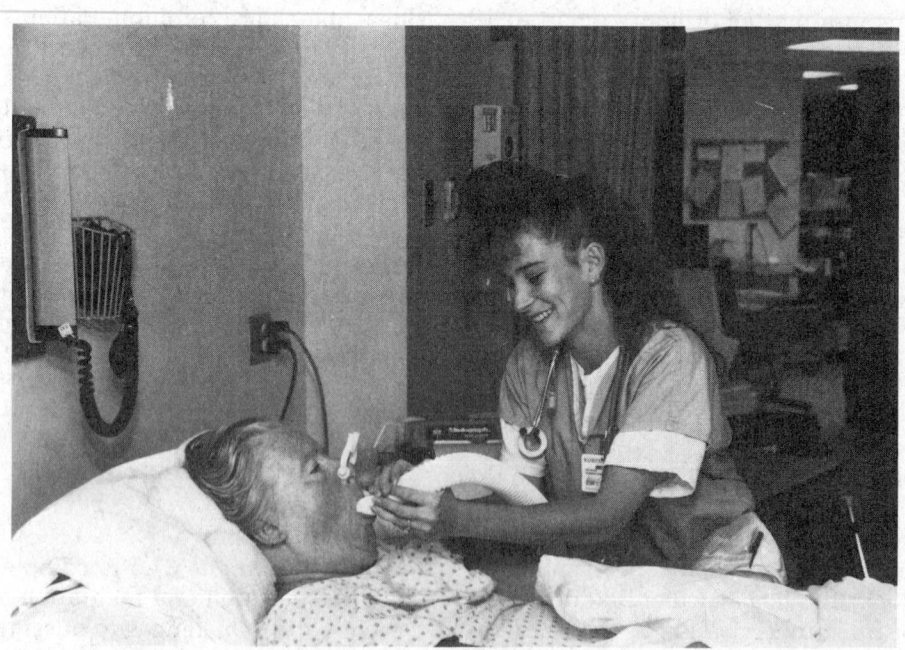

FIGURE 48-4   Bedside assessment of forced vital capacity.

ued until the patient is able to take oral nourishment. Mouth care and skin care around the nasogastric and tracheostomy tubes should be included in the daily regimen to prevent infection and promote comfort.

Problems with urinary elimination and constipation should be considered in the GBS patient. Urine output and specific gravity should be monitored. The patient may require intermittent catheterization for urinary retention. Constipation should be addressed with adequate fluid intake, dietary fiber, stool softeners, and a regular bowel routine. Enemas are avoided if possible to prevent further autonomic problems.

MYASTHENIA GRAVIS
Definition/Etiology

Myasthenia gravis (MG) is characterized by abnormal fatigability of voluntary muscles as a result of a defect in neurotransmission. Patients report diurnal fluctuation in strength. They may feel normal in the morning, but by evening they may be completely immobilized. Rest can improve but not eliminate the symptoms. MG is more common in women than men in a 3:2 ratio. Incidence is estimated to be 5/100,000. From 5% to 7% of patients with MG have other family members affected. There are two age clusters: women are affected between the ages of 10 and 40 years and men between the ages of 50 and 70 years. A congenital MG is commonly discovered during childhood and has different pathophysiologic features. The autoimmune etiology of MG has been accepted since the early 1970s.

Pathophysiology

The defect in MG is located at the neuromuscular junction, specifically the acetylcholine receptor (AChR) (Figure 48-5). The neuromuscular junction is where transmission of the impulse from the nerve to the muscle takes place. The nerve impulse stimulates the release of the neurotransmitter acetylcholine (ACh). ACh diffuses across the synaptic cleft, combines with the AChR on the muscle membrane, and begins the process of muscle contraction. After muscle contraction, ACh is destroyed by the enzyme acetylcholinesterase (AChE) thus terminating impulse transmission.

Patients with MG do not have reduced amounts of ACh available at the neuromuscular junction. The pathologic changes seen in MG consist of electron-microscopic evidence of a reduced number of functioning AChR sites. In addition, the normal folded pattern of the postsynaptic membrane of the muscle end-plate is altered. It is believed that complement and antibodies to AChR cause accelerated destruction and blockade of the AChR. There are more than 400 muscles in the body, and each has numerous AChR sites. There may be 30 to 40 million AChR sites per neuromuscular junction, although only a few may be activated at one time. This accounts for the variability in severity of MG symptoms and response to medications. The enzyme AChE is inhibited by the anticholinesterase drugs used to treat MG, thereby leaving more ACh available to the damaged AChRs.

Several findings support the theory that MG is caused by an autoimmune process: the presence of other autoimmune diseases (lupus erythematosus,

NORMAL NEUROMUSCULAR JUNCTION

MYASTHENIA GRAVIS

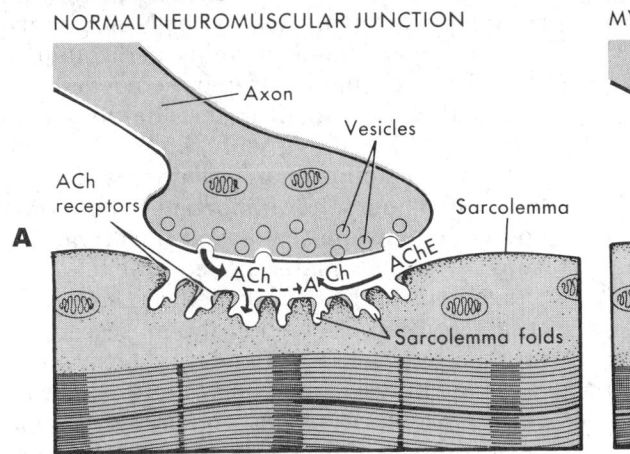
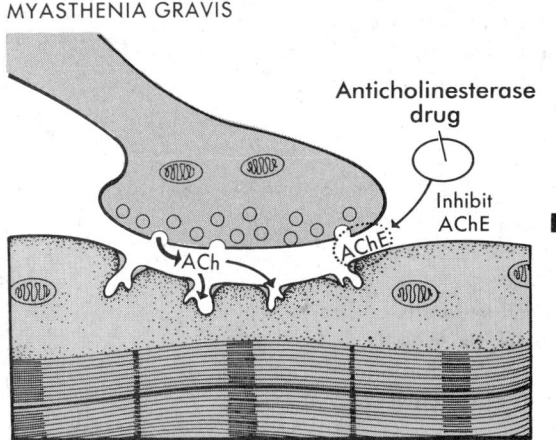

FIGURE 48-5   Anticholinesterase drugs in myasthenia gravis. **A,** Normal neuromuscular junction: acetylcholine (ACh) released from nerve initiates muscle contraction. Acetylcholinesterase (AChE) breaks down ACh, limiting duration of muscle contraction. **B,** In myasthenia gravis, there is a defect in muscle receptors at neuromuscular junction. Anticholinesterase drugs block action of AChE. This effect increases duration of action of ACh, thereby increasing muscle contraction.

thyroid disorders, and rheumatoid arthritis), an association with specific HLA types (HLA-B8), an increased frequency of skeletal muscle and AChR (90%) antibodies, and experimental MG in animals. The role of the thymus gland in the autoimmune process is not fully understood. Thymic abnormalities, such as thymic hyperplasia and tumors, occur in over 80% of MG patients. How these abnormalities relate to the production of antibodies continues to be the subject of intense research.

Clinical Manifestations

The MG patient initially exhibits abnormal fatigue of the voluntary muscles; specifically the ocular, bulbar, respiratory, and limb muscles are involved. Acutely, the patient is unable to sustain repeated muscle contractions. Most patients report early ocular symptoms; after diagnosis, 80% have detectable ocular weakness. Weakness of the ocular muscles produces visual disturbances—ptosis, diplopia, reduced eye closure, and blurry vision. Weakness of the bulbar muscles produces speech and swallowing abnormalities—dysarthria, dysphonia, and dysphagia. The patient may describe progressive difficulty chewing, weight loss, and choking during meals.

SIDE EFFECTS OF ANTICHOLINESTERASE DRUGS (CHOLINERGIC REACTIONS)

Muscarinic
On smooth muscle

Epigastric discomfort
Abdominal cramps
Anorexia
Nausea
Vomiting
Diarrhea
Pupillary miosis
Bronchospasm

On glands

Increased salivation
Cold moist skin
Increased lacrimation
Increased bronchial secretions

Nicotinic
On skeletal muscle

Fasciculations (twitching)
Spasm
Weakness

During prolonged conversations, the patient's speech may become unintelligible. Evidence of facial muscle weakness, difficulty smiling, and neck flexor weakness are also common. The respiratory muscles show a pattern consistent with restrictive lung disease—reduced maximal static pressures and forced vital capacity. Muscle weakness in the limbs must be severe before it can be detected on examination.

An edrophonium (Tensilon) test is often conclusive evidence of MG. Edrophonium is a short-acting anticholinesterase that enhances neurotransmission and results in abrupt, but short-term, improvement of symptoms. The electrocardiogram should be monitored in view of the cardiac effects of the drug. Atropine should be available to treat potential cholinergic side effects. Other tests that support the diagnosis include fatigue on repetitive electrical stimulation of the contracting muscles, high serum AChR antibody titers, and CT evidence of thymus enlargement.

Therapeutic Management

The most common regimens used to treat MG are anticholinesterase, corticosteroid and immunosuppressive drugs, thymectomy, and plasma exchange. Mortality has changed significantly from 30% in the 1950s to 3% in the 1970s as a result of improved diagnosis and treatment and intensive nursing care.

Drug therapy

Early in the course of the disease, patients are managed with anticholinesterase medications: pyridostigmine (Mestinon), neostigmine (Prostigmin), or ambenonium (Mytelase). There is no fixed dosage that relieves the symptoms. Different muscles will respond to the same dose with greater improvement than others. The dose and medication schedule should be the minimal amount needed to provide maximal improvement in the vital muscles of swallowing and breathing with the fewest side effects. The onset of action of an oral dose is 30 minutes and lasts 3 to 4 hours. It is important to note the reduced dosage for intramuscular and intravenous preparations to approximate the equivalent oral dosage. Side effects of the drug, called cholinergic reactions, result from excess ACh at the muscarinic receptors in smooth muscle and glands and nicotinic receptors in skeletal muscle (see box at left). Gastrointestinal symptoms, diarrhea, and abdominal cramps are the most common side effects and are managed by taking a light snack with the medication. Anticholinergics, such as atropine, are used to reduce side effects but may increase the tenacity of secretions and mask deterioration when the drug becomes less effective. Fasciculations and increasing weakness occurring 60 minutes after administration of the drug are signs of toxicity and should be reported immediately. If increasing weakness is coupled with respiratory muscle weakness, a cholinergic crisis can occur.

Patients are usually on a demand schedule when they are at home. Intake of the drug is based on need, and patients are usually advised to take it before meals or strenuous activity. Most hospitalized patients require fixed dosage schedules. The medication must be given *on time,* or the patient may be too weak to swallow it as a result of poor control of the illness. Anticholinesterase medications provide symptomatic improvement for variable periods but do not alter the abnormal immune process. Also, these medications are associated with structural changes at the motor end-plate, which may cause further difficulty with neurotransmission. As the anticholinesterase becomes less effective, some other form of therapy is usually required.

Corticosteroid therapy as a treatment for patients with MG addresses the autoimmune process presumed to perpetuate the illness. ACTH is given intravenously or intramuscularly for 10 days but has largely been replaced by oral prednisone. Two protocols are used. High-dose (50 to 90 mg) daily prednisone is given until there is evidence of symptomatic improvement. The dosage is then changed to an alternate-day regimen at approximately half of the daily dosage. In the second protocol, treatment is initiated by gradually increasing a low starting dose (10 to 20 mg) given early in the morning on alternate days. The medication is increased up to 120 mg (qod) or until symptoms diminish. In both protocols the dosage is then slowly reduced to the lowest that maintains improvement. Most patients improve with this treatment, although maximal benefit may not occur for up to 9 months.

Immunosuppressants, particularly azathioprine, have also been used successfully to treat MG. The dosage is usually 2 to 2.5 mg/kg/day. The onset of improvement is gradual, often over 12 months. The drug must be given continuously to maintain symptomatic improvement; less than 10% of patients are able to discontinue use of the medication. Compared with prednisone, the side effects of azathioprine are less pervasive yet still severe. The potential for mutagenic or teratogenic effects in a young, primarily female population needs to be carefully considered. The risk of acquired malignancy has been suggested but is unknown. Cyclophosphamide (Cytoxan) and cyclosporine have been used on an experimental basis. Intravenous immunoglobulin (IVIg) has been used with success; however, the effects are short lived and the treatment is extremely expensive.

Some patients report improvement in strength when taking oral potassium supplements (20 to 40 mEq/day). Hypokalemia is associated with muscle weakness caused by diarrhea and steroid therapy; however, some patients report subjective improvement in spite of normal serum potassium tests. Ephedrine (25 to 50 mg two to three times per day) has also been prescribed to improve presynaptic release of ACh.

Several drugs have been shown to impair neuromuscular transmission and should be used with caution in the severely weak MG patient (Table 48-8).

Surgical therapy

Thymectomy continues to be associated with improvement in 60% to 87% of cases observed for at least 5 years. Thymectomy is accomplished by a median sternotomy or transcervical procedure. Removal of the complete gland is most easily accomplished by the median sternotomy approach. Preoperative preparation, including corticosteroid-induced remission and plasma exchange, has reduced the incidence of myasthenic crisis after surgery. Anticholinesterase medication is usually tapered before surgery. Patients receiving long-term steroid therapy may require extra "stress" doses to prevent addisonian crisis. The need for ventilatory support after the procedure depends on the degree of respiratory weakness preoperatively and whether muscle relaxants that reduce neuromuscular transmission were given during anesthesia. Postoperatively the patient will have a chest tube in the mediastinum. Pain medication is given as needed with close observation for respiratory depression. Lactated intravenous solutions are usually avoided, since they can increase weakness.

Plasma exchange

Plasma exchange has been used to treat patients in acute MG crisis occurring when patients either do not respond to or relapse during drug and surgical treatment. Electrolytes and clotting factors are checked before and after the procedure. The patient is monitored for changes in MG symptoms, vital signs, and electrolyte abnormalities. Weakness may increase during the treatment as a result of fluctuating levels of anticholinesterase medications. Plasma-bound medications (prednisone, immunosuppressive agents, digitalis, thyroid preparations) are withheld until after the procedure. Venous access sites are protected. Some patients do not respond to plasma exchange; those who do usually improve within 24 hours.[28]

Crisis management

Crisis is characterized by severe generalized weakness and respiratory failure. Crisis occurs most commonly in patients with severe bulbar weakness following stresses such as upper respiratory infections,

TABLE 48-8   Drugs that Impair Neuromuscular Junction Transmission

Antibiotics	Cardiovascular drugs	Antirheumatic drugs	Psychotic drugs	Anticonvulsants	Hormonal agents	Other drugs
Clindamycin	Lidocaine	Chloroquine	Lithium	Phenytoin	ACTH	Lactate
Colistin	Quinidine	D-Penicillamine	Phenothiazines	Trimethadione	Corticosteroids	Curare
Kanamycin	Phenytoin				Thyroid hor-	Narcotics
Lincomycin	Procainamide				mones	Agents
Neomycin	Propranolol				Oral contracep-	producing
Streptomycin	and other				tives	hypokalemia
Tobramycin	beta blockers					
Tetracyclines	Disopyramide					
Gentamicin	Calcium antag-					
Polymyxin B	onists					
Trimethoprim-						
sulfamethox-						
azole						

From Griggs R, Donohoe K: Emergency management of neuromuscular disease. In Henning R, Jackson D, editors: *Handbook of critical care neurology and neurosurgery,* New York, 1985, Prager Publishers.

surgery, and obstetric delivery, as well as in those patients who are recently diagnosed or have symptoms that do not respond to therapy. Crisis has been attributed to disease worsening (myasthenic crisis) and to anticholinesterase overdosage (cholinergic crisis). Cholinergic crisis is less common. In fact, few patients require large doses of anticholinesterases. It is often difficult to differentiate between the two types of crisis. Myasthenic crisis is associated with a positive edrophonium (Tensilon) test; cholinergic crisis is associated with a negative test. The most important principles in the treatment of crisis are recognition of respiratory failure, maintenance of gas exchange, and secretion management. The patient in crisis will need ventilatory support until the illness or precipitating cause is treated.

NURSING MANAGEMENT OF THE PATIENT WITH MYASTHENIA GRAVIS
Assessment

The nurse documents the presence of factors that aggravate MG symptoms, such as infection, stress, and changes in medication regimen. History and initial physical assessment help the nurse determine which of the tests of muscle strength will be of assistance in ongoing patient management of the acutely ill MG patient.

Physical assessment includes tests that detect changes in bulbar function (swallowing, speech), respiratory function, general muscle strength and functional ability, and visual ability. Tests of bulbar function include the gag reflex, rating voice quality,

and observation of swallowing ability using water or saliva alone. These are crucial tests to prevent aspiration. Inadequate nutrition can be a problem in patients with reduced swallowing and chewing ability. Assessment includes review of appetite, eating patterns, likes and dislikes, and previous weight loss and gain. Calculation of ideal body weight is helpful in detecting abnormalities.

Pulmonary function often varies and should be checked frequently. Measuring forced vital capacity is the most commonly used test. To ensure accuracy and consistency, the nurse has the patient sit upright, prevents leakage around the mouthpiece, and uses the same machine for sequential tests. If the patient is taking anticholinesterase medications, note the timing of the test. Other pulmonary assessment measures for the MG patient include (1) estimating counting in one breath, (2) presence of secretions, and (3) subjective sensations of shortness of breath or choking. Patients with MG rarely have significant blood gas abnormalities unless chronic obstructive pulmonary disease or pneumonia is present.

Additional assessment includes identification of subjective and objective measures of muscle strength. The patient may describe weakness after strenuous activity or late in the day. The patient may be unable to perform activities of daily living or ambulate independently. Functional testing provides more information for the nurse to use in the care plan. Functional testing includes measuring in seconds how long the patient can read aloud, keep his or her arms above the head, or hold the head off the bed.

Assessment of the patient and family's knowledge and reaction to the illness is an important part of the psychosocial function. The stress associated with uncertainty and fear about the illness provokes extreme anxiety in the newly diagnosed patient. Many have been thought to have psychiatric problems or be malingerers before the diagnosis. For experienced patients, coping with a chronic changeable illness can severely tax the resources of even the most well-adjusted patient. The stress of exacerbation and hospitalization may recall fears of previous difficult periods. Changes in the patient's sleep patterns, coping responses in the past, and other indicators of anxiety and depression are important to assess.

Nursing Diagnosis

Possible nursing diagnoses for the patient with MG include the following:

Ineffective airway clearance related to muscle weakness and fatigue

Impaired verbal communication related to oropharyngeal muscle weakness or to the need for ventilatory support

Altered nutrition: less than body requirements related to fatigue and weakness of the muscles involved in swallowing and chewing

Self-care deficit related to fluctuations in muscle strength

Activity intolerance related to deconditioning as a result of muscle fatigue and weakness

High risk for injury related to the presence of muscle weakness

Sensory/perceptual alterations (visual) related to muscle weakness causing functional and cosmetic impairment

Knowledge deficit related to the complex nature of the treatment protocols

Ineffective individual/family coping related to the fluctuations and unpredictability of the illness

Planning

Specific outcomes include the following:

Patient maintains effective airway clearance and does not suffer from preventable pulmonary complications

Patient develops effective communication patterns to meet needs

Patient maintains normal body weight and has sufficient energy to meet daily activities

Patient assumes responsibility for and executes all desired activities and role-related functions

Patient is able to obtain sufficient rest and benefit from the treatment program to tolerate an increase in activity

Patient is protected from injury

Patient is able to manage visual impairment so as not to interfere with activity

Patient and family obtain sufficient knowledge about the illness to understand or manage symptoms and participate in the treatment process

Patient and family will verbalize coping methods that demonstrate they are in control of the situation

Implementation

The patient with MG will require close observation throughout the hospitalization to prevent complications. The nurse should initiate measures that promote comfort and continue the process of educating the patient and family about the disease and treatment process.

Crisis management

Airway management is the immediate concern if the patient is in crisis. If crisis is anticipated, the patient's room should be close to the nurses' station to facilitate close observation and rapid response if serious worsening occurs. The nurse should continue to closely monitor pulmonary function tests (forced vital capacity, count) and swallowing ability to prevent respiratory failure and aspiration. Mechanical ventilation may be necessary until plasma exchange or medication therapy induces improvement.

After the airway is established, the nurse must develop a communication system. The patient should be interviewed to document the extent of communication difficulty and to work out a preferred method of communication, such as using a magic slate, paper and pencil, or lip reading. The patient should have a tap bell to indicate critical needs.

The patient may be profoundly weak during crisis and need assistance in all activities—feeding, bathing, toileting, dressing, and getting out of bed. The patient with severe swallowing difficulty may need nutritional support with a nasogastric tube. Monitoring the patient's weight and providing a diet consistent with swallowing ability are helpful. Complications associated with immobility can be prevented by routine nursing interventions such as skin care, range-of-motion exercises, and changing the patient's position every 2 hours. Suctioning, chest percussion, and drainage to prevent pneumonia and eye care to prevent corneal abrasion are also essential aspects of care to prevent injury.

The patient should be involved with all aspects of care, since he or she is alert and aware of surroundings. All procedures must be explained in detail to the patient and family to minimize fear and anxiety. As the patient improves, activity should be gradually increased. The nurse encourages the patient to be responsible for self-care activities and monitors ability perform these tasks safely.

Newly diagnosed patients need to learn how to manage their illness, and increased responsibility is a major form of coping with the powerlessness they may feel in the face of fatigue and weakness. Anxiety, depression, and fear are all commonly experienced by these patients. Providing an environment where the patient can verbalize specific apprehensions can lead the way to avoiding further stress. Continued assessment of the patient's knowledge level, providing written information to reinforce teaching, and introducing the patient to resources in the community, such as the Myasthenia Gravis Foundation, are helpful interventions.

Drug therapy

The nurse is responsible for instructing the patient about the expected effects and side effects of medications. The patient taking anticholinesterases must be informed of when the peak effect and duration of action occur. Comparison with the patient's asymptomatic breathing capacity should be completed to establish a baseline and to gauge the patient's response to therapy. Pulmonary function tests and other assessment measures should be taken at intervals to correspond with the anticholinesterase dosage to establish the patient's lowest point of function. All anticholinesterase medications should be given on time. The patient should be aware of side effects (increasing muscle weakness, excess salivation, and diarrhea) and toxicity (weakness at the peak dose effect) that are signs of cholinergic reactions. Patients who have increased symptoms should keep a diary and be encouraged to maintain communication with providers to titrate the dosage to their symptoms. In addition, the patient should be aware that certain drugs will cause increased weakness and that this information should be shared with other care providers, dentists, pharmacists, and internists.

Thymectomy

The patient should be fully informed about the surgical procedure. Instruction on turning, coughing, and deep breathing should be reviewed before surgery. Leg exercises should be instituted to prevent thromboembolic complications. If anticholinesterase medications are tapered before surgery, the patient needs close observation of symptoms of muscle weakness and treatment of increased bronchial secretions. Pain control should be discussed beforehand. Median sternotomy incisions are painful; chest splinting should be demonstrated preoperatively.

After surgery, respiratory status and vital signs are monitored hourly until stable. Drugs and lactated intravenous solutions that increase muscle weakness should be avoided. The patient should turn, cough, and deep breathe every hour to prevent atelectasis. An incentive spirometer can be used as a method to reinforce deep breathing every hour. A chest tube is usually inserted into the mediastinum and will require observation to document bleeding. As soon as possible, the patient resumes normal diet and activity. If stable, the patient can be discharged to the floor within 24 hours. Plasma exchange may be necessary. Medications should be resumed as soon as possible.

Plasma exchange

Plasma exchange will often induce a prompt yet brief improvement after crisis. The nurse monitors preprocedure and postprocedure vital capacity, swallowing ability, and other functional tests. Anticholinergic medications are administered as ordered, and the patient is monitored closely for cholinergic reactions. Vital signs should be taken at frequent (every ½ to 1 hour) intervals during the procedure, since fluid volume shifts can cause hypotension and dysrhythmias. Electrolytes and clotting factors should be checked before and after the procedure. Venous access sites should be inspected during the procedure and carefully monitored thereafter. The patient should be offered blankets if chilled—a common complaint. Between fluid exchanges, the extremity being used should be gently exercised to decrease discomfort. Fluid and a light meal should be provided as requested.

Evaluation

The outcome is to maintain the highest level of functional ability possible. Most patients are able to live full and normal lives. The patient will exhibit the ability to monitor symptoms. The side effects of medications will be recognized and reported. The successful treatment plan encourages the resumption of all activities, normal weight maintenance, effective communication, and participation in treatment decisions. The patient and family will verbalize sufficient knowledge of the illness and be comfortable with their ability to manage at home.

Documentation

The use of a bedside flow sheet to record respiratory muscle strength and functional ability is necessary to document improvement after crisis. The nurse records the response to preoperative and postoperative teaching. When any new therapy is initiated, the patient will require frequent assessment and documentation of the response. Patients benefit from continued reinforcement of oral and written medication instruction.

Ongoing Care

Although some patients achieve permanent remission, most will require some sort of extended outpatient management. The nurse continually reinforces instructions about medication. Most well-controlled patients independently regulate anticholinesterases and are well aware of side effects of immunosuppressives. The patient should be cautioned about taking over-the-counter medications or any medication that has not been checked with a specialist. The nurse should encourage the patient to consider wearing a Medic Alert identification bracelet. The nurse carefully reviews emergency plans with the patient, since crisis can occur precipitously. Early recognition and treatment of infection and prevention with an annual flu vaccination are encouraged.

All patients who continue to have symptoms need to learn energy conservation techniques to manage household duties and employment and resume normal activity. Exercise programs should not be discouraged in the well-controlled patient if they are carefully designed and gradually implemented.

Family teaching about the illness will promote a better understanding about the patient's fluctuating abilities. Peer support is often helpful to cope with the disease. Local chapters of the Myasthenia Gravis Foundation can be contacted about the availability of support groups, literature, and other resources.

CRITICAL THINKING QUESTIONS

1 List the assessment priorities for the acutely ill patient with an infection of the nervous system.
2 Describe the common techniques used to assess pulmonary status in the patient with Guillain-Barré syndrome and myasthenia gravis.
3 State how therapeutic regimen priorities differ for meningitis, parameningeal infections, and encephalitis.
4 Name the chemoprophylactic drugs and vaccines available to prevent common forms of meningitis.
5 List the purpose and side effects of immunosuppressive drugs used to treat autoimmune disorders.
6 State interventions aimed at preventing common complications of Guillain-Barré syndrome.
7 Discuss ways in which the nurse can involve the family in the care of the patient with an infec-

tious or autoimmune disease of the nervous system.
8 Construct a care plan for home care following discharge of a patient with a chronic autoimmune or infectious disease of the nervous system.

RESOURCES

1 Guillain-Barré Syndrome Foundation International PO Box 262 Wynnewood, PA 19096 (215) 667-0131
2 Myasthenia Gravis Foundation 53 West Jackson Boulevard Suite 660 Chicago, IL 60604 (312) 427-6252 or (800) 541-5454
3 National Multiple Sclerosis Society 733 Third Avenue New York, NY 10017

BIBLIOGRAPHY

Current

1. Adams R, Victor M: *Principles of neurology,* ed 4, New York, 1989, McGraw-Hill.
2. Ashwal S, Tomasi L, Schneider S: Bacterial meningitis in children: pathology and treatment, *Neurology* 42:739-748, 1992.
3. Baringer J: Viral infections. In Asbury A, McKhann G, MacDonald WI: *Diseases of the nervous system,* ed 2, Philadelphia, 1992, WB Saunders Co.
4. Birk K, Smeltzer S, Rudick R: Pregnancy and multiple sclerosis, *Semin Neurol* 8(3):205, 1988.
5. Carter JL, Rodriguez M: Immunosuppressive treatment of multiple sclerosis, *Mayo Clin Proc* 64:664-669, 1989.
6. French Cooperative Study Group: Plasma exchange in Guillain-Barré syndrome: one year follow-up, *Ann Neurol* 32:94, 1992.
7. Johns TR: Long-term corticosteroid treatment of myasthenia gravis, *Ann NY Acad Sci* 505:568, 1987.
8. Johnson RT: Response of the nervous system to infection. In Asbury A, McKhann G, MacDonald WI, editors: *Diseases of the nervous system,* Philadelphia, 1992, WB Saunders Co.
9. Kelly B, Mahon S: Nursing care of the patient with multiple sclerosis, *Rehabil Nurs* 13(5):238, 1988.
10. Mitchell P et al: *AANN's neuroscience nursing: phenomena and practice,* Norwalk, Conn, 1988, Appleton & Lange.
11. Oosterhuis HJGH: Myasthenia gravis and other myasthenic syndromes. In Swash M: *Clinical neurology, II,* Edinburgh, 1991, Churchill-Livingstone.
12. Prendergast V: Bacterial meningitis update, *J Neurosci Nurs* 19(2):95, 1987.
13. Scheinberg L, Holland N: *Multiple sclerosis: a guide for patients and families,* ed 2, New York, 1987, Raven Press.
14. Shapiro R: *Symptomatic management in multiple sclerosis,* New York, 1987, Demos Publications.
15. Thompson AJ, MacDonald WI: Multiple sclerosis and its pathophysiology. In Asbury A, McKhann G, MacDonald WI, editors: *Diseases of the nervous system,* ed 2, Philadelphia, 1992, WB Saunders Co.
16. Tunkel A, Scheld WM: Bacterial infections in adults. In Asbury A, McKhann G, MacDonald WI, editors: *Diseases*

of the nervous system, ed 2, Philadelphia, 1992, WB Saunders Co.

17. Yudkin PL et al: Overview of azathioprine treatment in multiple sclerosis, *Lancet* 338:1051-1055, 1991.

18. Van der Meche FGA et al: Intravenous immune globulin for Guillain-Barré syndrome, *N Engl J Med* 326:1123, 1992.

19. Weiner H, Hafler D: Immunotherapy of multiple sclerosis, *Ann Neurol* 23:211, 1988.

Classic

20. Ahern J, Schwetz K: Comprehensive supportive therapy in multiple sclerosis, *Semin Neurol* 5(2):146, 1985.

21. Anderson SB: Guillain-Barré syndrome: giving the patient control, *J Neurosci Nurs* 24(3):158-162, 1985.

22. Argov Z, Mastaglia FL: Disorders of neurotransmission caused by drugs, *N Engl J Med* 285:773, 1979.

23. Beghi E et al: Encephalitis and aseptic meningitis, Olmsted County, Minnesota, 1950-1981. I. Epidemiology, *Ann Neurol* 16:283, 1984.

24. Eisendrath S et al: Guillain-Barré syndrome: psychosocial aspects of management, *Psychosomatics* 24(5):465, 1983.

25. Greenlee J: Brain abscess, subdural empyema, suppurative infections. In Mandell G, Douglas R, Bennett J: *Principles and practice of infectious disease,* ed 2, New York, 1985, John Wiley & Sons, Inc.

26. Griggs R, Donohoe K: Emergency management of neuromuscular disease. In Henning R, Jackson D, editors: *Handbook of critical care neurology and neurosurgery,* New York, 1985, Praeger Publishers.

27. Grob D, Brunner NG, Namba T: The natural course of myasthenia gravis and the effect of therapeutic measures, *Ann NY Acad Sci* 377:652, 1981.

28. Howard JF: Nonsteroidal immunosuppressive therapy for myasthenia gravis, *Semin Neurol* 2(3):265, 1982.

29. Kurtzke JF: Neuroepidemiology, *Ann Neurol* 16:265, 1984.

30. Maloney F, Burks J, Ringel S, editors: *Interdisciplinary rehabilitation of multiple sclerosis and neuromuscular disorders,* Philadelphia, 1985, JB Lippincott Co.

31. McKee Z, Kaiser A: Acute meningitis. In Mandell G, Douglas R, Bennett J, editors: *Principles and practice of infectious disease,* New York, 1985, John Wiley & Sons, Inc.

32. Noroian E: Myasthenia gravis: a nursing perspective, *J Neurosci Nurs* 18(2):74, 1986.

33. Ropper AH: Management of the Guillain-Barré syndrome. In Ropper AH, Kennedy SK, Zervas NT, editors: *Neurological and neurosurgical intensive care,* Baltimore, 1983, University Park Press.

34. Schiffer R, Slater R: Neuropsychiatric features of multiple sclerosis: recognition and management, *Semin Neurol* 5(2):127, 1985.

35. Schweitzer S: Immunosuppressive treatment of multiple sclerosis, *J Neurosci Nurs* 17(3):256, 1985.

36. Tauber M et al: Antibacterial activity of beta-lactam antibiotics in experimental pneumococcal meningitis, *J Infect Dis* 149:568, 1984.

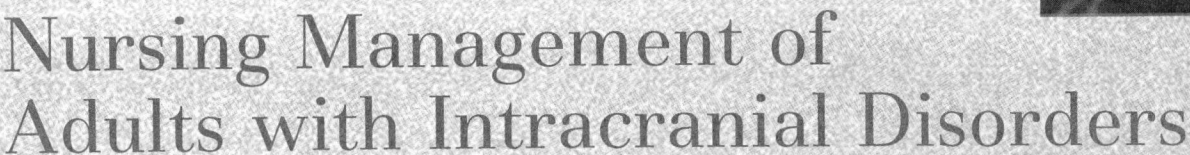

CHAPTER FORTY-NINE

Nursing Management of Adults with Intracranial Disorders

LEARNING OBJECTIVES

1 Differentiate among mild, moderate, and severe head injury.
2 Describe the potential complications following a head injury, including cerebral edema, intracranial bleeding, syndrome of inappropriate secretion of antidiuretic hormone, diabetes insipidus, convulsive disorders, carotid-cavernous fistula, meningitis, and hyperthermia/hypothermia.
3 Discuss the techniques needed to assess level of consciousness in the head-injured patient.
4 Implement a plan of care for the head-injured patient and family.
5 Discuss the necessary components of the discharge plan for the head-injured patient.
6 Identify symptoms associated with the specific location of a brain tumor.
7 Describe the nursing care for a patient after a craniotomy.
8 Describe the nursing care required when the patient is undergoing radiation therapy or chemotherapy for the treatment of a brain tumor.

INTRACRANIAL DISORDERS present a unique challenge to the nurse. Whereas the patient experiences many acute problems, they are often only a prelude to long-term ones. The nurse will devote much time and energy to the care of the individual patient but must also devote comparable time to the family and/or significant others. Intracranial disorders commonly affect the entire family unit. The challenge for the nurse is to assess correctly and intervene when necessary. For example, patients with head injuries require constant nursing assessment, since their status changes quickly. The nurse's astute assessment may mean the difference between life and death. The medical therapy for the patient is specific; but whereas the medical therapy may cure the physical problem, the nurse's responsibility is to work with the patient and family as they experience the human responses to the illness.

HEAD INJURY
Definition

Head injury is a leading cause of disability. As such it presents a condition that any nurse may encounter in a variety of settings. Whether the head-injured victim is a patient in an emergency room, critical care unit, medical-surgical unit, rehabilitation facility, or private home, the basic pathophysiology and nursing care remain the same.

Head injuries occur across the life cycle. Older individuals or individuals on various medical regimens may sustain a head injury during a fall. Particularly in the older person, the signs and symptoms of the injury may not appear for several days or even weeks. Therefore the nurse must be able to accurately assess symptoms as they occur.

Etiology

Almost 90% of nervous system trauma results from damage to the head. Motor vehicle accidents are a leading cause of head injuries, and alcohol abuse is a common causative factor in head injuries.[37]

The total number of head injuries in the United States is estimated at over 2 million each year, with 500,000 serious enough to require hospital admission. The highest incidence is in persons aged 15 to 29 years old, and head injuries are two to three times more likely to occur in males than females. Almost one half of all traumatic head injuries are caused by motor vehicle accidents. Each year approximately 70,000 to 90,000 head-injured individuals experience lifelong loss of function, 5000 will develop epilepsy, and 2000 will live in a persistent vegetative state. The overall cost is near $25 billion each year.[16]

Classifications

There are three major classifications for head injury. **Closed injuries** refer to nonpenetrating injuries in which there is no break in the integrity of the skull, although the basal dura may be torn.[1] **Open,** or penetrating, **injuries** occur when there is a break in the integrity of the barrier (skull, meninges) between the environment and the intracranial vault. Both low-velocity and high-velocity missiles (i.e., bullet, knife) can cause open injuries, and the extent of injury can vary from focal to diffuse. A specific classification or grading system is commonly used to further classify head injuries. This system assists in the proper triage and treatment of individual patients.

With mild head injury (grade I), the patient experiences only a momentary loss of consciousness associated with the injury, and there is no decrease in level of consciousness or the presence of focal neurologic signs on admission to the emergency department. Generally, these patients are not admitted to the hospital unless they experience symptoms such as headache, nausea, vomiting, fever, or leakage of cerebrospinal fluid. On discharge, the family and patient are warned to watch carefully for the presence of any of these signs and return immediately to the hospital if any of them occur.[37]

With grade II head injuries the patient experiences a momentary loss of consciousness and an alteration of neurologic function on admission to the hospital. Examples of this neurologic change include an altered level of consciousness, lethargy, confusion, or hemiparesis. Patients with this grade of injury are hospitalized, generally in an intensive care unit. They may require immediate surgery.

The diagnosis of grade III (severe) head injury is made when the patient is unable to follow simple commands because of a decreased level of consciousness. These patients may exhibit signs of serious neurologic damage, such as dilated pupils and posturing. This is the most serious grade of head injury, and without rapid assessment and intervention, the patient may die.

Pathophysiology

Mechanisms of injury

Acceleration-deceleration injuries occur when the movement of the head follows a straight line. The cerebral tissue is affected by changes in both acceleration and deceleration. This type of injury commonly results from motor vehicle accidents. In a motor vehicle accident the head is moving at the same speed as the vehicle. When the vehicle suddenly stops, the head continues to move (acceleration). As the head hits a stationary object (i.e., windshield)

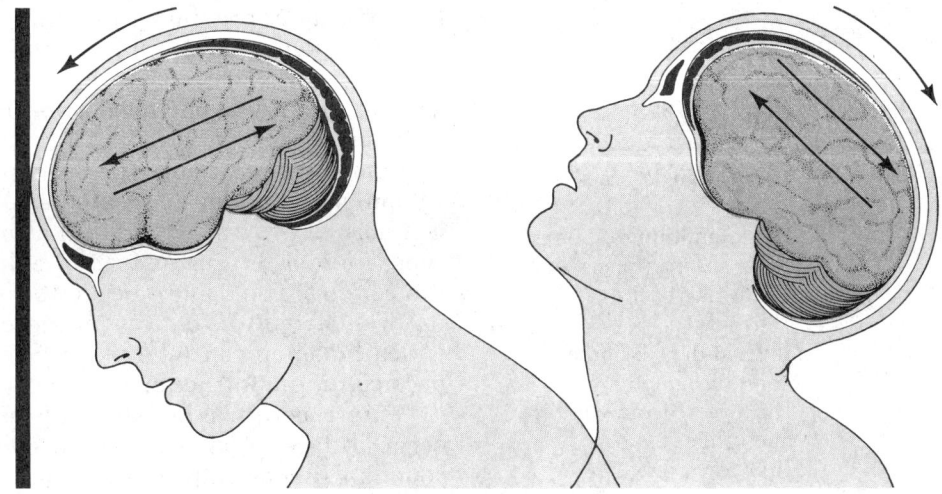

FIGURE 49-1   Coup/contrecoup head injury following blunt trauma.

and stops, the deceleration injury occurs. Injuries to soft tissues on the anterior and posterior walls, as well as friction injuries on the sides of the brain, are common. Often deceleration injuries cause more severe injuries by the effect on the brainstem. **Rotation injuries** occur when the movement of the head results in a rotational force that tears cerebral tissue. This mechanism commonly results in damage to the brainstem.

Another mechanism is the **coup/contrecoup injury.** Coup injuries occur when brain tissue is injured directly below the site of impact. Brain tissue may also then rebound against the surface of the skull on the opposite side of the impact, causing a contrecoup injury. Further, these injuries can be caused by an impact to the head that either stops it while moving (deceleration) or by an object that strikes the head while relatively stationary (acceleration).[51] The mechanisms of this injury are demonstrated in Figure 49-1.

Skull fractures

A skull fracture may also occur in combination with head injury. One of the most common types of fracture is linear, in which there is no displacement of bone. Depressed fractures occur when the outer table of the skull is depressed and may then move to lie beneath the inner table of the adjacent skull. This type of fracture can occur with a closed or open head injury. Finally, basal fractures occur at the base of the skull and then extend into the ear or the orbit of the eye. See Table 49-1 for a further discussion of skull fractures.

Primary and secondary injuries

Primary injuries in the brain may occur in several ways. A **concussion** is caused by a violent shaking of the brain that results in minimal tissue damage. There is generally a temporary change in the level of consciousness with a concussion. A **contusion** is a bruise of the brain tissue itself, caused by a blow with a blunt object.

Secondary injuries include epidural, subdural, and intracerebral hematomas. An epidural hematoma occurs between the dura and skull and is associated with a severe head injury.

An **epidural hematoma** originates from an injury to extracerebral vessels, usually a laceration in the middle meningeal artery or veins. Epidural hematomas account for only 2% of secondary head injuries. They are potentially fatal, since the onset of symptoms is rapid as a result of the bleed, which is usually arterial.

The classic description of an extradural hematoma is that of momentary unconsciousness followed by a lucid period lasting for a few hours or 1 to 2 days. After the lucid period the individual experiences a rapid deterioration in level of consciousness. Other symptoms that may occur include vomiting, hemiparesis, and pupillary changes. Medical treatment is rapid evacuation of the hematoma.

A **subdural hematoma** occurs under the dura and is usually caused by lacerations of the veins crossing the subdural space. Subdural hematomas are commonly divided into three types: acute, subacute, and chronic.

With an acute subdural hematoma, symptoms become apparent within 24 to 72 hours of the head in-

TABLE 49-1   Skull Fractures

Fracture type	Description
Linear (simple)	Line or single crack in skull
Comminuted	Fragmentation of bone into several pieces or multiple fracture lines
Depressed	Inward depression of bone fragments
	Dura may or may not be intact
	Hair, dirt, or other objects may be found within wound
Basal	May be linear, comminuted, or depressed
	Usually arises from extension of linear fracture into base of skull
Anterior fossa (fracture of paranasal sinus)	Symptoms may include rhinorrhea, subconjunctival hemorrhage, periorbital ecchymosis (raccoon's eyes)
Middle fossa (fracture of temporal petrous bone)	Symptoms may include otorrhea, hemotympanum, conductive hearing loss, facial nerve palsy, ecchymosis over mastoid (Battle's sign)

jury. The patient's condition deteriorates rapidly, and then the patient becomes comatose. The brain is unable to compensate for the rapid compression often associated with the severe trauma of an acute subdural hematoma. The most common signs of acute subdural hematomas include headache, drowsiness, and agitation. The ipsilateral (same side as injury) pupil is dilated and may become fixed.

Subacute subdural hematomas are associated with development of symptoms from 3 to 14 days after the injury. Although the prognosis is better than with the acute type, subacute subdural hematoma is associated with a 25% to 35% mortality.[1] The major symptom of subacute subdural hematomas is the failure of a patient to regain consciousness after an injury.

With chronic subdural hematomas, gradual clot formation allows the brain to accommodate. The length of time from injury to symptom development may be months. Even as symptoms develop, they may be subtle and even go unnoticed. The most common symptoms include headache, grogginess, confusion, and seizures.

Elderly people are particularly prone to the development of subdural hematomas. With aging there is a normal process of cerebral atrophy that causes separation of the cortex from the dura. This makes the cerebral veins more prone to rupture and tearing. The atrophy also provides more free space into which bleeding can take place. Symptoms will not occur until the intracranial space is compromised.

An **intracerebral hematoma** is associated with a cerebral laceration that causes edema of the surrounding tissues. Most intracerebral hematomas are related to contusions and therefore tend to occur in the frontal and temporal lobes.[8] Signs and symptoms include headache, decreasing level of consciousness, hemiplegia on the opposite side of the bleed, and a dilated pupil on the same side. Surgical evacuation is the treatment of choice. These hematomas are demonstrated in Figure 49-2.

Progression of tissue injury

Three distinct phases of events occur during a head injury. With the onset of the direct injury there are contusions and lacerations of nerve cells and nerve fibers. On microscopic examination, hemorrhage and destruction of adjacent brain tissue are evident.

After the injury, gradual demyelinization of the affected nerve fibers occurs, resulting in the destruction of neurons. The remaining debris is cleared by circulating microglial cells. Eventually, these microglial cells form a dense scar in the area of injury. At this point the meninges adhere to the injured area of the brain, producing a golden-brown, sunken scar.

The brain responds to the injury in numerous ways. Hemorrhage is one of the most likely and has been described. The hemorrhage occurs from the laceration of cerebral vessels as a result of the shearing force of the movement of the mass.[8] Depending on its location, the hemorrhagic area may exert unequal pressure on the brain. Other responses include ischemia, infarction, fluid imbalances, and cerebral edema.

Potential complications

Potential complications from a head injury include cerebral edema, diabetes insipidus, inappropriate antidiuretic hormone secretion, stress ulcers, and epilepsy.

Cerebral edema

Head injuries can be complicated by **cerebral edema,** which occurs as a result of direct assault to

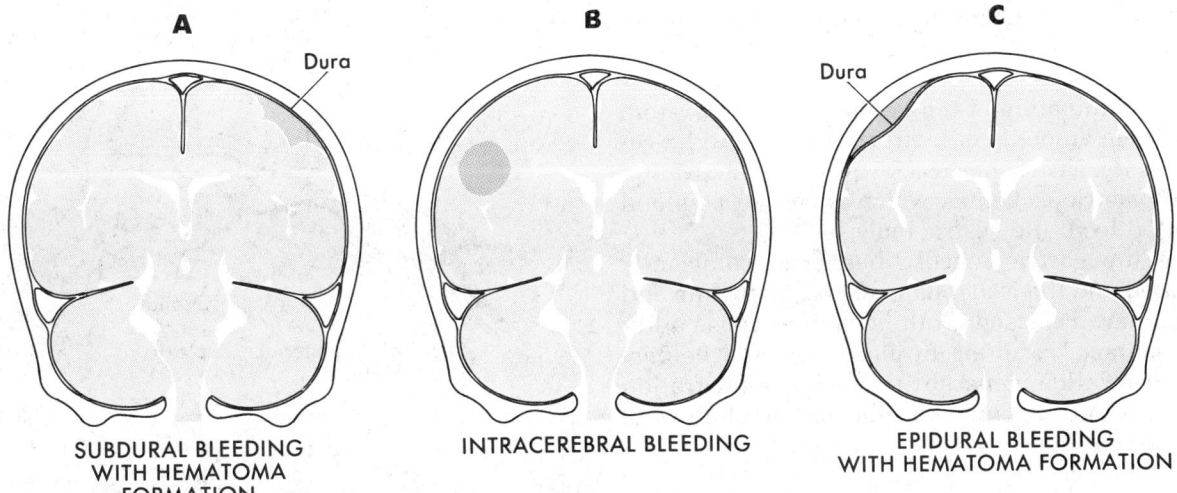

FIGURE 49-2   Types of hematomas. **A,** Subdural bleeding with hematoma formation. **B,** Intracerebral bleeding. **C,** Epidural bleeding with hematoma formation.

brain tissue and secondarily from cerebral ischemia, anoxia, and hypercapnia. There are three specific causes of cerebral edema.

Vasogenic cerebral edema occurs when there is a direct injury to the cells, such as that which occurs secondary to the forces that caused the head injury. Another type of cerebral edema is cytotoxic. In this form, cerebral neurons swell in response to anaerobic metabolism. In cytotoxic edema the cells increase in size, resulting in increased brain volume with a decrease in extracellular space. For the patient with a head injury, it is likely that both mechanisms will be involved in the development of cerebral edema. Ischemic edema quickly follows an ischemic cerebral event. Early ischemic edema is intracellular and is caused by a decrease in available oxygen and metabolic substrates. Without these substances the integrity of the cellular membrane cannot be maintained, and water eventually leaks in and causes the cells to increase in size. If the ischemia continues, then brain cells will die.

Syndrome of inappropriate antidiuretic hormone and diabetes insipidus

A head injury commonly disrupts fluid balance. One of the most common mechanisms for this imbalance is pressure on the hypothalamus caused by edema and, potentially, bleeding. The hypothalamus is unable to function normally, which causes alterations in sodium balance and water balance. In this situation, two conditions are possible: syndrome of inappropriate secretion of antidiuretic hormone (SIADH) and diabetes insipidus (DI). For a detailed discussion, see Chapter 60.

DI results when there is a decrease in the amount of ADH released, which causes an excessive amount of fluid to be excreted through the renal system. The exact mechanism of DI is not well understood but is hypothesized to involve an inability of the osmoreceptors to respond to the normal cues initiated by response to fluid levels. Therefore despite the body's need for ADH, it is not released. Although head injuries may cause DI, it is also caused by direct or indirect damage to the pituitary gland by other conditions, such as tumors.

When DI occurs, the patient's urinary output is increased, and the specific gravity of the urine is decreased. For older patients this loss of fluid can be particularly devastating and can place additional stress on the heart. Major shifts in fluid balance can be difficult for any patient to tolerate.

SIADH involves the release of ADH even when it is not needed—the opposite of DI. Decreased urinary output results from SIADH. One of the most dangerous aspects of this dysfunction is that serum sodium concentrations decrease, usually to below 135 mEq/L. This response is referred to as "dilutional hyponatremia," since the decreased sodium levels are related to the ratio of the sodium to the actual fluid amounts. The more severe the hyponatremia, the greater the effect on cerebral functioning. Hyponatremia may produce serious symptoms such as seizures and coma.

Stress ulcers

Stress ulcers may be a complication from the head injury. The stress (both physical and psychologic) of the injury predisposes the patient to stress ulcers. Steroids are commonly used in the treatment of head injury, and they have been noted to cause gastrointestinal bleeding from ulcers.

Current research suggests that there is a physiologic basis for gastrointestinal hemorrhage caused by head injury. The head injury apparently activates both the parasympathetic and sympathetic nervous systems. Stimulation of the parasympathetic system causes large amounts of hydrochloric acid to be released on the gastric mucosa. Sympathetic activation leads to gastric ischemia, which is caused as blood is shunted from the gastric mucosa.[34]

Once the gastric mucosa has been sufficiently stimulated and the ischemia worsens, histamine and serotonin are released. Both hormones cause additional damage, resulting in ulceration and hemorrhage. Prevention, generally through administration of antacids and histamine-2 blockers, is one of the best interventions.

Convulsive disorders

Convulsive disorders may also be a complication from a head injury. Some suggest that this may occur in as many as 5% of the head-injured population. This problem may be more common with open injuries and laceration of the cortex.[1]

Carotid-cavernous fistula

Carotid-cavernous fistula is a rare but serious complication that may develop as a result of a head injury. The fistula occurs when blood escapes from the carotid artery into the cavernous sinus.[48] This type of bleed is important because the area is surrounded by several cranial nerves, including VI (abducens), III (oculomotor), IV (trochlea), and V (trigeminal).

After the head injury, several pathologic changes occur that promote the development of the fistula. Following the injury, there may be a compromise in the integrity of the cavernous pattern of the carotid artery. This allows for abnormal communication between the high pressure arterial blood and low pressure venous blood. This pressure difference fosters the flow of blood into the cavernous sinus (Figure 49-3).

Carotid-cavernous fistulas often close spontaneously and do not require any direct treatment. If spontaneous closure does not occur, two therapy options exist.

With the first, the internal carotid artery above and below the fistula is ligated. Unfortunately, the artery itself is sacrificed with this treatment.

The second type of therapy is called a balloon occlusion technique and allows for closure of the fistula while the patency of the carotid artery is assured.

This procedure is performed by fluoroscopic examination, either in the x-ray department or operating room. After administration of a general anesthetic, a balloon is inserted and advanced to the approximate site of the fistula. The balloon is then inflated with enough contrast medium to occlude flow. When the exact location of the fistula is found, the balloon is deflated, repositioned, reinflated, and left

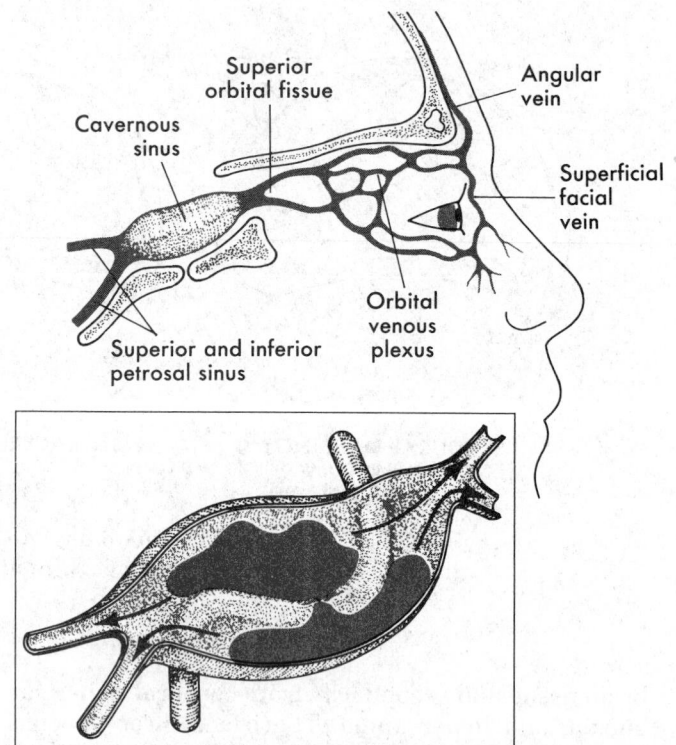

FIGURE 49-3   Carotid-cavernous fistula.

in place (Figure 49-4). This type of therapy will be indicated when the patient experiences symptoms such as a bruit, heard during auscultation over the eye, pulsation of the orbit of the affected eye, exophthalmos and complaints of headache, and visual disturbances.

Meningitis

After a head injury the patient may experience a number of problems related to infection. Meningitis is one of the more common consequences. The head injury causes a disruption in the integrity of the meningeal layer, which promotes the movement of bacteria into the cranial area. Symptoms of meningitis include an elevated temperature and nuchal rigidity (see Chapter 48).

Hyperthermia/hypothermia

Damage or pressure on the hypothalamus after injury can result in significant body temperature change. This change can in turn result in high (hyperthermia) or low (hypothermia) body temperature. The importance of these changes is the effect of the body temperature changes on cerebral metabolism, rather than the body temperature changes themselves.

Hyperthermia is particularly dangerous because it increases the metabolic rate and, in turn, cerebral demand. The higher the body temperature, the more severe the demand on the cerebral tissue. Hyper-

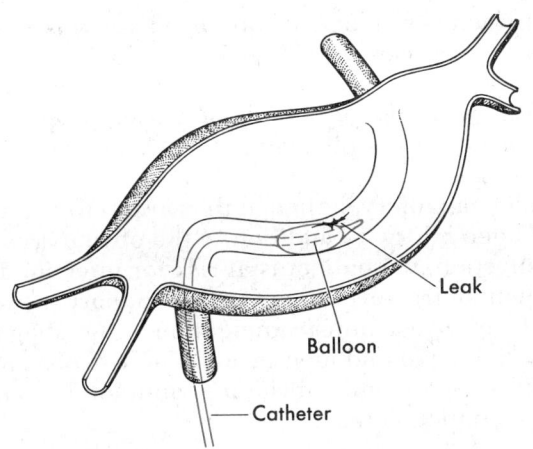

FIGURE 49-4   Balloon treatment for carotid-cavernous fistula.

thermia should be swiftly treated and patient body temperature precisely controlled.

The most common treatment for hyperthermia is the use of the automatic cooling blanket. The goal is to decrease body temperature as quickly as possible without inducing shivering. On occasion, a cooling blanket may not be available. Under those circumstances the patient can be cooled by other means, such as placement of ice bags in areas of major venous circulation.

Throughout the use of cooling, the patient's response to the treatment must be carefully monitored. In particular, changes in vital signs and gastric activity can be expected. The patient's body temperature is lowered gradually, because excessive decreases in body temperature may cause shivering. As the patient shivers, muscle contraction increases, which in turn increases intracranial pressure. This increase in pressure can be dangerous in a compromised patient. If excessive shivering is a problem, then chlorpromazine (Thorazine) may be given to decrease the response.

Hypothermia can similarly result from pressure on the hypothalamus. As body temperature decreases, cerebral metabolism also decreases. In the head-injured patient, hypothermia is preferred to hyperthermia since hypothermia limits demand on the cerebral metabolism. Generally, the patient's body temperature is maintained at around 33° to 34° C.

Clinical Manifestations

The specific clinical manifestations for a head injury depend on the type and location of the injury. The major symptoms are specific to the neurologic system and include a decreased level of consciousness, restlessness, irritability, and confusion. A headache may be reported. Other manifestations include pu-

pillary abnormalities, nausea, vomiting, and vital signs changes. Cases of severe injury may evidence brainstem damage, such as loss of gag or swallowing reflexes. Motor and sensory responses may also be affected.

A number of laboratory studies may be needed to confirm the specifics of the diagnosis. Immediately on admission to the hospital, most patients undergo skull films, which are taken to assist in identifying the location of any fractures. Although a skull series is a helpful diagnostic procedure, not all fractures can be captured on film. Cervical spine films are also completed since there is a high incidence of cervical spine injury associated with head injury. Until this x-ray film is read and cervical injury is ruled out, all head-injured patients are treated as though they have sustained a cervical injury. The patient is always maneuvered carefully, preventing movement of the neck, which may increase the amount of injury. Disregarding this basic principle can result in unnecessary damage and even paralysis. Shortly after the patient is admitted, a computed tomography (CT) scan is ordered to help determine the extent of cerebral injury. CT scans will be repeated throughout the patient's hospitalization in an effort to monitor the patient's progress. In addition to these routine scans, other CT scans are scheduled when there is a major change in the patient's status.

Other diagnostic studies may be ordered but are not routinely indicated for head-injured patients. Lumbar punctures are generally contraindicated following a head injury as a result of the possibility of precipitating a brainstem herniation. However, when there is a suspicion of a complication such as meningitis, a lumbar puncture may be required. On occasion, angiography, CT scan of the brain, and echoencephalograms may be done. However, the results of these tests generally do not add additional information to that provided by the CT scan.[30]

General serum tests including glucose, electrolytes, blood urea nitrogen (BUN), and creatinine level, and complete blood counts (CBCs) and coagulation studies are routinely completed early during the hospitalization. As a result of the high correlation between head injury and accidents involving alcohol and drugs, all patients should be screened for alcohol and drug levels.[37] Throughout the hospitalization, arterial blood gases may be collected to evaluate the arterial oxygenation acid-base balance and carbon dioxide levels. Routine urinalysis should also be completed.

Therapeutic Management

Medical treatment

One of the first medical goals in the treatment of head injury is to lower the intracranial pressure associated with the head injury. Treatment for the increased pressure consists of medical, nursing, and surgical therapies. Medical therapies include drugs, such as mannitol, and steroids. Fluids are monitored closely. In general, patients are maintained on a slightly dehydrated basis to avoid an increase in fluid level, which can exacerbate the increased intracranial pressure. During the early stages of recovery from a head injury, fluid overload can increase the intracranial pressure. Other medical interventions include hyperventilation (which decreases the amount of carbon dioxide, thereby causing cerebral vasoconstriction and decreased intracranial pressure) and drainage of cerebrospinal fluid to decrease pressure (see Chapter 45).

In severe cases of increased intracranial pressure after a head injury, barbiturate coma may be indicated.[8] Surgical management of increased intracranial pressure is often the most definitive. For example, if a hematoma is produced by the injury, then a surgical procedure that includes the introduction of burr holes and subsequent evacuation of the existing hematoma will result in decreased intracranial pressure.

Medical treatment to stabilize any spinal cord injury associated with head injury is essential. As already described, cervical cord injuries commonly occur along with head injuries. All patients are treated as though they have a cervical injury until proven otherwise. Specific medical therapy for cervical and other types of spinal cord injuries is discussed in Chapter 50.

Seizure activity occurs in some patients immediately following the head injury; in others, it may occur many years after the injury. Seizures are probably related to cortical irritation from edema, infection, bleeding, or cellular damage. The incidence of seizures after head injury in patients without prolonged coma is 5%. For patients with depressed skull fractures or penetrating head wounds, the incidence increases to 30% to 50%.[51] For that reason, many patients are given prophylactic anticonvulsants. One of the most commonly used prophylactic anticonvulsants is phenytoin.

Infections may occur with either an open or closed head injury, although they are more common with open injury. In addition to the obvious reasons for infection, the patient is at risk for infection from compound fracture sites, for pulmonary reasons, and from invasive instrumentation. After diagnosis of the infection and identification of its cause, many medical treatments, including antibiotic therapy, can be implemented.

Surgical treatment

Surgical intervention is a common treatment for a head injury. There are two major procedures: burr holes and craniotomy. **Burr holes** refer to holes made in the cranium using a special drill (Figure 49-5, *A*). In the case of the head-injured patient, burr holes are made to evacuate a cerebral clot. Burr holes also may be created before the initiation of a craniotomy.

A **craniotomy** is a surgical opening of the skull to provide access to the brain (Figure 49-5, *B*). This procedure can be used to remove a tumor, aneurysm, or other type of cerebral pathologic condition. In later stages following a head injury, a craniotomy may be needed to evacuate a chronic hematoma that has become gelatinous and therefore inaccessible through the burr hole.

Drug therapy

Steroid therapy has been used for head-injured patients for many years, although periodically there is disagreement regarding the efficacy of steroids.

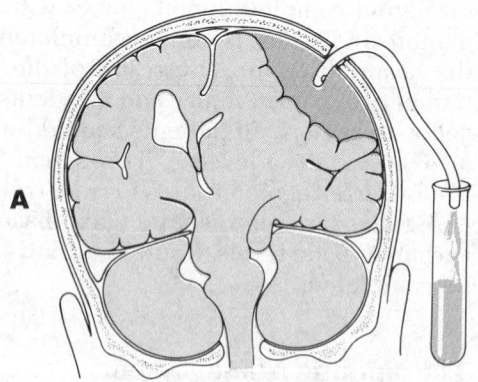 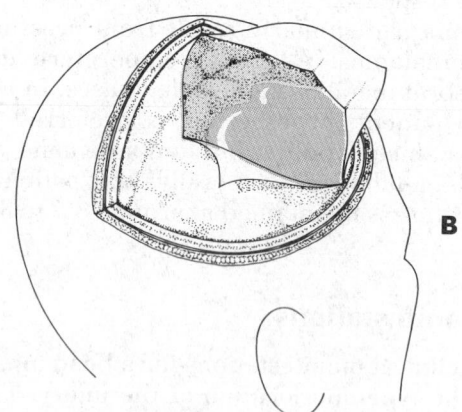

FIGURE 49-5 **A,** Burr hole used to drain subdural hematoma. **B,** Craniotomy used to evacuate large, chronic hematoma.

Following head injury the steroid most commonly selected is dexamethasone (Decadron). The dosage is often calculated based on body size, weight, and renal function. The average loading dose is approximately 10 to 20 mg, followed by maintenance doses of 2 to 6 mg every 4 to 6 hours.

Mannitol is an osmotic diuretic that is also used in the treatment of the head-injured patient. Mannitol is a high-molecular-weight product that pulls fluid from the intravascular to the extravascular space along with the drug. Thus urinary output is increased and intracranial volume is decreased. Since the drug is excreted with the urine, the specific gravity of the urine is quite high.

Antibiotics are used to treat infection in the head-injured patient. In the early stages of treatment the physician will most likely begin therapy with a broad-spectrum antibiotic. As the exact nature of the infection is better understood, the physician orders more specific antibiotics.

Nutritional therapy

Maintenance of nutritional balance is a major goal in the treatment of the head-injured patient. The physical stress of the injury precipitates a period of increased catabolism in the patient. The steroids commonly used in treating the injury also increase catabolism. Without adequate nutritional support, malnutrition from a negative nitrogen balance may occur. As a consequence, the patient may experience muscle wasting, poor wound healing, immunodeficiency, and malabsorption.[41] In an effort to prevent these problems, the patient is started on tube feedings or hyperalimentation as soon as possible.

NURSING MANAGEMENT OF THE PATIENT WITH A HEAD INJURY
Assessment

The first priority of nursing management is to ensure protection of the airway and stabilization of cervical injuries. Next the nurse must establish an assessment baseline, of which one of the basic parameters is determining the patient's level of consciousness. The nurse should continually assess the patient's level of consciousness throughout the recovery period, monitoring for subtle changes, since level of consciousness is the best indicator of intracranial function. In addition to gauging the level of consciousness, the nurse should assess the patient's pupils and evaluate motor responses. The Glasgow Coma Scale (see Chapter 44) establishes objective data about best eye opening response, best verbal response, and best motor response. The patient is given a score reflecting maximal ability in each area.

Pupillary assessment is important not only for noting changes in pupillary response (reactivity:

brisk, normal, or sluggish) and pupillary size, but also for detecting abnormal pupillary response, which indicates brainstem dysfunction. Two pupillary responses that can be used to assess brainstem function include oculocephalic (doll's eyes) and oculovestibular (calorics) (see Chapter 44). Both of these tests are performed only on the unconscious patient. Although the oculocephalic response test can be performed by the nurse, there are two major cautions to consider. First, this test should never be performed on a patient with a cervical cord injury or until a cervical injury has been ruled out because of the risk of paralysis below the level of injury. Second, this procedure can increase intracranial pressure, since extreme turns of the head will interfere with the drainage of blood through the jugular veins.

In assessment of motor function, the nurse monitors for changes such as hemiplegia or decreased movement, checking the patient frequently for both motor and sensory responses. Additional areas to include with assessment of motor function can be found in Chapter 44.

In evaluating for intracranial pressure, the nurse should continually monitor all neurologic signs, particularly those that would indicate the potential for increased intracranial pressure. As a consequence of increased intracranial pressure following a head injury, the patient may experience a herniation of a portion of the brain tissue (see Chapter 45).

Pupillary changes to look for are dilation and slowed reactivity; respiratory changes include abnormal patterns, such as Cheyne-Stokes asthma, central neurogenic hyperventilation, and others, depending on the location of the herniation. Blood pressure changes include an increased systolic pressure along with an unchanged diastolic pressure creating a widening pulse pressure. The pulse rate may also decrease in relation to the blood pressure. Herniation syndromes are serious consequences of increased intracranial pressure that will lead to death for the patient if they are not recognized and promptly treated.

The patient commonly experiences a headache after a head injury. Although nurses tend to be most aware of the presence of pain in an alert patient, there is belief that comatose patients also experience headache. The proposed mechanism for production of headache in these individuals includes cerebral tissue irritation and the accompanying increased intracranial pressure. In addition, many head-injured patients also experience multiple trauma. The nurse must be aware of the likelihood that the patient is suffering from pain from injuries other than the head injury.

After the head injury the associated cerebral irritation and cerebral hypoxia may interfere with normal thought processes. The effects of this change can occur immediately but may also last for many months and sometimes years. Examples of the alterations include confusion and irritability. While beginning to regain physical strength, the patient may become aggressive, with inappropriate verbal or physical responses. The patient's memory may be impaired, and the attention span is often decreased. On a long-term basis the patient's personality may change, sometimes to the extent that families are unable to "recognize" their loved one after the injury.

The patient may temporarily lose the ability to communicate verbally, because of altered levels of consciousness. If the patient is confused or agitated, the verbal responses may be nonsensical or unrelated to the environment. A common example of nonsensical verbal responses is moaning that is not associated with physical stimuli. Cranial nerve damage that makes phonation difficult may also be involved in impaired verbal abilities.

Even a mild head injury can have devastating effects on a family. The reasons for the family's response can vary. For example, if the injury was the result of a motor vehicle accident caused by a drunk driver, then the family may be very angry. If the loved one had been fighting with a family member before the accident, then the response may be a combination of anger and guilt. The injury may also precipitate a change in family roles. An injury to the head of the household or to a single parent may be so devastating that state or federal aid must be sought for the family.

Each family's coping style may be different. Some families have dealt well with previous crises, whereas others may be not be as capable of working through the issues. Therefore an understanding of the family's coping skills is essential.

The nurse can anticipate that the family will participate in the normal steps of grieving, including denial, anger, and eventual acceptance. Many families are unable to deal with any of the long-term consequences of the injury during this early stage. The nurse's responsibility is to gather enough information to determine how both patient and family are adjusting to the changes.

Nursing Diagnosis

Nursing diagnoses for the head-injured patient include the following:

Ineffective airway clearance related to diminished cough reflex

Anxiety related to awakening in unfamiliar environment and impact of injury

Ineffective breathing pattern related to disruption of respiratory center

Pain related to cerebral tissue irritation

Impaired verbal communication related to changes in level of consciousness and impaired phonation

Ineffective family coping related to change in roles and impact of injury

Fluid volume excess related to ADH imbalance

High risk for injury related to impaired sensory and motor function

Impaired physical mobility related to damaged neuromuscular function

Altered nutrition: less than body requirements related to increased catabolism from stress of injury

Sensory/perceptual alterations (visual, auditory, kinesthetic, gustatory, tactile, olfactory) related to cranial nerve dysfunction

Altered thought processes related to cerebral hypoxia and irritation

Altered cerebral tissue perfusion related to interruption of blood flow

Planning

Once the nurse has assessed the head-injured patient and family and formulated appropriate nursing diagnoses, the next step is to develop the individualized nursing care plan. The nurse must recognize that during the acute stages of a head injury, the situation may change quickly. For that reason the nurse must set appropriate outcomes that are concise and achievable. Patient outcomes include the following:

Minimal changes in intracranial pressure

Minimal systemic complications

Minimal loss of control

Participation in self-care activities

Minimal alteration in cerebral tissue perfusion

Implementation

Vital signs and neurologic signs

Constant monitoring of vital signs and neurologic signs is important, but the ability to interpret changes in these signs is critical. The nurse should note any changes in respiratory rate or rhythm, paying particular attention to patterns that include periods of apnea. Specific respiratory changes are generally related to the area of injury and increased intracranial pressure. A description of respiratory patterns can be found in Chapter 45.

Blood pressure and pulse rate should be assessed carefully and frequently. Although small fluctuations in both can be expected, the trend of those fluctuations is more important than their actual values. The nurse should assess for the common signs of increased intracranial pressure, which include a widening pulse pressure (the diastolic pressure remains normal, and the systolic pressure increases). The

RESEARCH BRIEF

Ross AM, Pitts LA, Kobayashi S: Prognosticators of outcome after major head injury in the elderly, *J Neurosci Nurs* 24(2):88-93, 1992.

This prospective study examined the outcomes of elderly (over 65 years of age) patients with major head injuries (severe injuries causing coma [Glasgow Coma Scale ≤8] or injuries causing an intracranial hematoma requiring surgical removal). Glasgow Coma Scale scores on admission and at 72 hours were compared, as were outcomes of patients with elevated intracranial pressure with those of patients with normal intracranial pressure. Overall, this study showed that patients over 65 years have a 25% chance of surviving major head injury and a 13% chance of recovering and maintaining an independent life-style. Patients who were comatose on admission had a 9.5% overall chance of survival and a 4% chance of functioning independently once recovered. All of the survivors had emerged from coma within 72 hours of admission, and all patients died who remained in a coma for the first 72 hours. The authors suggest that in view of these findings, families should be counseled early regarding morbidity and mortality.

Although the results of this study are striking and the number of subjects included (n = 195) is substantial, interpretation is limited since the study involved one institution. The authors also suggest that lack of data on important variables such as early mortality, altering of treatment in accordance with family wishes, and lack of a measurement of brain compliance all limit the interpretation of the results.

pulse can be expected to decrease. The nurse will also monitor for cardiac dysrhythmias, which often accompany bradycardia.

Neurologic assessment should continue on a frequent basis. The specifics to include are level of consciousness and motor, pupillary, and sensory responses. The interval of assessment varies with the acuity of the patient but should be done no less than every 4 hours. Whenever the patient's condition changes, both vital signs and neurologic signs should be evaluated.

Respiratory control

A major goal is to ensure that the patient's airway remains patent at all times. Cerebral tissue is sensitive to any change in oxygenation; therefore the patient will not be able to tolerate even minimal changes in airway patency. Suctioning equipment should be available at all times, including that for oral suctioning. Nasal suctioning may be contraindicated if there is any evidence of a leak of cerebrospinal fluid through the nose. If there is a decrease in respiratory control, it may be necessary to intubate the patient to protect the airway.

The nurse should position the patient with the head of the bed elevated 30 degrees or according to the physician's orders. This will allow for a decrease in intracranial pressure and will also increase the protection of the airway by preventing the patient from aspirating. Congestion or fluid in any of the lung fields should be reported to the physician immediately.

Suctioning in the head-injured patient can be difficult. The nurse should ensure that the patient receives adequate oxygen before, during, and after suctioning, because research has shown that the hypoxia that occurs during suctioning can have negative effects on the individual patient.[2] Strict aseptic technique also should be used throughout suctioning.

When respiratory problems escalate, mechanical ventilation may be necessary. The goal of this therapy, which most commonly takes place in an intensive care unit, is to maintain the patient's normal arterial oxygen level while decreasing the carbon dioxide level to 25 to 35 mm Hg. The patient with chronic respiratory disease (e.g., chronic obstructive pulmonary disease) has very different normal oxygen and carbon dioxide levels during mechanical ventilation so careful monitoring is essential. Decreasing the patient's arterial carbon dioxide level tends to cause vasoconstriction in the cerebral vessels, which in turn decreases intracranial pressure.

Intracranial pressure

Managing intracranial pressure remains an important intervention for the head-injured patient. Refer to Chapter 45 for a complete discussion of relevant nursing care.

Cardiovascular functioning

Head injury may affect a patient's cardiovascular system. Several physiologic mechanisms explain this phenomenon. The heart rhythm is regulated in part by the vasomotor center in the brainstem. Pressure on the vasomotor center may cause cardiac dysrhythmias. The nurse should carefully monitor, assess, and interpret the patient's heart rate and rhythm throughout the time of recovery from the head injury. If available, cardiac monitors should be used. If not, assessment of the apical pulse rate can be effective. The nurse can note irregularities in the patient's heart rhythm more accurately through assessment of the apical pulse rate rather than radial pulse rates, for example.

The prolonged bed rest associated with treatment of the patient with a head injury may result in peripheral circulation impairment. The nurse should assess the patient's peripheral pulse rates daily.

Intake and output

Accurate measurement of intake and output is an important step in assessing fluid balance in the head-injured patient. The goal of the assessment is to determine if the patient is dehydrated or fluid overloaded. Decreased urinary output may indicate impending renal failure or SIADH secretion. Increased output may suggest DI or possibly an early stage of high-output renal failure.

For the head-injured patient the nurse evaluates the patient's intake and output no less often than every 4 hours. In addition to obvious changes in intake and output, the nurse monitors trends in both components.

Pain and restlessness

Controlling pain in the head-injured patient is a challenge. The goal of nursing interventions is to assist the patient in becoming comfortable, without depressing nervous system activity. Drugs traditionally used for pain control, including opiates and sedatives, depress the activities of the nervous system, impair respiration, and increase sleepiness. More important, these drugs may interfere with accurate neurologic assessment. For example, morphine may be effective in decreasing pain, but it also causes pupillary constriction, making an accurate neurologic assessment more difficult.

The drugs most commonly given for pain control in the head-injured patient are acetaminophen or codeine. Small doses are given as infrequently as possible. Before administering any analgesic, the nurse should carefully assess the patient to determine the cause of the pain. Often, pain, particularly headaches, is an indication of increased intracranial pressure that may precede serious complications.

The nurse must not rely totally on drugs for the treatment of pain. Back rubs and careful positioning may help decrease pain. A quiet, darkened environment may be helpful for patients with severe headaches. Other modalities, such as therapeutic touch and guided imagery, also may improve the patient's comfort level.

The patient can also become restless. The nurse must determine why the patient is restless before initiating any treatment. For example, restlessness may be caused by various reasons ranging from cerebral bleeding to urinary retention. If the nurse has investigated these possible causes and found no rea-

son for the restlessness, then the nurse will use nursing interventions, rather than drug therapy, to decrease the patient's restlessness.

The nurse pays close attention to the patient's environment. The room should be as quiet as possible, with lights dimmed. The nurse should remember that, because of the cerebral injury, the patient may not be able to interpret the information presented. Therefore extraneous input in the form of light or noise may be confusing. The nurse can also organize the patient's care in a way that will increase the amount of uninterrupted rest. The goal is to limit activities that increase intracranial pressure. For example, as coordinator of the patient's care, the nurse will be able to plan nursing care around other aspects of the patient's day, including physical therapy, occupational therapy, and physician and family visits. If, in the nurse's judgment, too many daily interruptions are interfering with the patient's ability to rest, the nurse determines which activities are essential.

Seizure activity

Approximately 5% to 10% of head-injured patients develop seizures during the acute stage.[8] For that reason, prophylactic anticonvulsants are commonly given to these patients. The nurse is on the alert for the development of seizures in any head-injured patient. There are many types of seizures, but perhaps the most devastating are tonic-clonic seizures. Seizure precautions, including keeping the bed in the lowest position, with the siderails up, should be observed. (See Chapter 45.)

Infection

Three major areas represent potential sites of infection in a head-injured patient: (1) any compound fracture site, (2) the pulmonary system, and (3) any invasive instrumentation (such as arterial lines or intracranial monitoring lines).

After a head injury, any leakage of fluid from the patient's ear or nose should be tested to determine if it is cerebrospinal fluid. Cerebrospinal fluid has a high glucose content, so the nurse should assess for glucose using a Testape or Dextrostix. If the fluid tests positive for glucose, it is likely to be cerebrospinal fluid. The nurse must exercise caution in ensuring that this fluid is not disturbed until the dura mater (meningeal layer) is sealed. The nurse's primary responsibility is to ensure that the dressing that collects the cerebrospinal fluid is kept dry and intact. The nurse should keep the patient in a position to allow for free drainage of the fluid and caution the patient to avoid excessive movement, since that may produce enough stress to tear the dura. Finally, no cleaning of the ear or cleaning or suctioning of the nose can be allowed, since this is likely to increase the leakage of cerebrospinal fluid.

Family interaction

The family of a head-injured patient undergoes a normal grief process, including denial, anger, depression, and acceptance. Once family members reach the acceptance stage, they are able to work with the nurse to begin facing the long-term consequences of the patient's injury. The length of time needed for the family to progress through these stages varies considerably. The nurse needs to be available to provide support as the family works through the grief process. It may be necessary to refer the family to a psychiatric nurse consultant for assistance.

Research has been conducted into the needs of the family during the acute phase of the patient's injury. A study in 1984[50] looked at the families of patients with acute brain injury.

The study suggests that families have two major needs during the acute phase: the need for information and the need to know that the hospital personnel care about the patient. Being aware of the family's needs enables the nurse to plan effective, realistic care. Supporting the family will help them in supporting their loved one throughout the hospitalization and recovery phase.

Mirr further explored the needs of families by studying their responses during the first two stages of recovery from head injury. Results of Mirr's study indicate that six general factors affect family decisions[27]: personal functioning, relationships, information, uncertain outcomes, environment, and emotions.

Although most researchers have focused on families' psychosocial needs, other researchers have investigated the presence of physiologic responses related to the stress caused by the loved one's illness. Reports suggest that family members may experience duodenal ulcer, heart attack, depression, asthma, and migraine.[15,27] Our current research data base also suggests that the family of a head-injured patient experiences stress, regardless of the degree of injury.[3]

Evaluation

Evaluation is one of the most crucial components of the nursing care plan. The patient's response and family's response to nursing interventions are monitored frequently and the care plan changed accordingly.

The nurse should note the patient's blood pressure, pulse rate, and respiratory effort. The patient should not experience a headache, papilledema, or any signs of decreased level of consciousness. The patient should have stable or improved sensory and motor function. Pupillary size and reactivity should be normal.

The patient should demonstrate no signs of infection. The patient should be afebrile, with minimal leaks of cerebrospinal fluid.

Fluid balance should remain normal, as evidenced by an intake and output that are within balance. The patient will exhibit no signs of fluid overload or dehydration unless being maintained on a slightly dehydrated basis.

The patient will experience minimal seizure activity. If a seizure occurs, the patient is cared for safely. The amount of seizure activity decreases over time.

Both family and patient will begin to demonstrate an early understanding of the causes of the symptoms related to head injury and the resulting responses. The patient and family will verbalize their sense of control as they begin to plan for the future.

Ongoing Care

The acute phase of a head injury is just the beginning of the care needed for both patient and family. Even during early stages of hospitalization, the nurse considers the long-term consequences and determines whether referral to ongoing care providers is needed. The prognosis for head injury is often not clear, and many legal and ethical issues must be considered.[46] Recent studies suggest that the psychosocial consequences of head injury vary considerably among individuals and are at least partially related to severity of injury.[38]

Many other professionals participate in the care of the head-injured patient besides nurses and physicians. Occupational therapists are consulted to assist the patient in several ways during hospitalization. For example, they can involve the patient in activities to decrease the boredom of daily hospitalization. As the patient nears discharge, occupational therapists can assist the patient in making the transition to home. They will be able to help the patient with any splints or other necessary appliances. A major goal of occupational therapy is to enhance the patient's ability to perform activities of daily living.

Physical therapists work with the patient from admission through discharge, and possibly following discharge. The physical therapist participates in determining routine exercise regimens. The goal of physical therapy is to maximize the patient's physical activity abilities.

Behavioral therapies, including behavior modification, have also been used for the head-injured patient. The head-injured patient may expect to experience numerous long-term behavioral changes, ranging from slight aberrations to complex personality changes.[35] Community resources are available to help both the patient and family work through these long-term consequences of a head injury. Agencies dedicated to the care of the head-injured patient are available and utilize numerous behavioral techniques to help the patient in adjusting to the injury.

Rehabilitation

Some practitioners argue that rehabilitation should begin in the intensive care unit. Except in cases of very mild head injuries, the nurse can anticipate that the patient will require some degree of rehabilitation.

The first step is often transfer of the patient to the hospital rehabilitation unit. This unit helps the patient in maintaining independence by helping him or her relearn how to dress, eat, and toilet himself or herself. For the head-injured patient, some cognitive retraining also may begin during this phase.[19] Some patients with head injuries lose aspects of their cognitive abilities and must be retrained to perform even simple tasks. The more severe the injury, the more likely it is that the patient will require extensive rehabilitation.

Patients with severe injuries may be discharged from the rehabilitation unit and admitted to a specifically designated head injury setting. Generally facilities for head-injured patients accept those who are physically stable but require retraining and supervision. Because only a few of these facilities exist, and often patients remain there for several years, the patient's name may be placed on a waiting list. Families need to be aware of these facilities, since both patient and family must be interviewed and "accepted"; the care may be quite costly.

Discharge planning

The type of discharge planning needed is dictated by the extent of injury and eventual placement of the individual patient. The nurse must also recognize the importance of initiating discharge planning as soon as the patient is admitted to the hospital. This approach means the discharge planning takes place at various junctures in the patient's experience, namely, discharge from the emergency department, critical care unit, neuroscience unit, and rehabilitation unit.[14,21]

Despite the variety of times discharge is planned, there are common elements to consider. Discharge planning includes a detailed teaching plan for patient and family. They must understand the origins of the symptoms of the injury and the expected outcomes. They must also understand the therapy and its intended purpose. The patient and family must be able to state the signs and symptoms of complications to report to the physician, including drowsi-

ness, irritability, behavioral changes, headache, and seizures. Specific complications already described, including postconcussion seizures and postconcussion syndrome, also should be reported.

Long-term care

The patient who requires close supervision may need to be admitted to a long-term care facility for some time, ideally one specifically developed for the care of head-injured patients. If such a facility is not available, however, it may be necessary to admit the patient to a more traditional nursing home.

The nurse should ensure that as the patient is discharged to a non–head-injury facility, there is adequate support available in terms of occupational and physical therapy.

To ease the adjustment of patients and families, many institutions have initiated family and individual support groups. These groups provide an opportunity for the patient and family to describe their feelings and to learn about head injury, as well as provide assistance in locating appropriate community and financial assistance.[10,43] The nurse can help the patient and family locate a support group by contacting the National Head Injury Foundation.

Home care

With changes in the prospective payment system, it is increasingly likely for even seriously ill patients to be discharged from the hospital directly to home. There is no reason why the head-injured patient cannot go directly home, assuming that adequate supervision and resources are available.

The first step in planning a patient's discharge to home is to assess the readiness of the family. The nurse is in an excellent position to assess the family's understanding of the illness and judge their ability to provide the care required. Even a patient with only a moderate head injury will require fairly constant supervision. If the family members themselves are unable to provide that supervision, then they must have the financial resources necessary to provide sitters or others.

Once the decision is made to consider placing the patient in a home setting, the in-hospital nurse approaches a home health agency to begin developing the plan for discharge. Physical and occupational therapy consultations should be included in the plan. If necessary, a psychiatric nurse may also be consulted.

If the patient requires a walker, wheelchair, or braces, then some structural changes may be needed in the home. For example, the patient may need a bedroom on the first floor of the house. The nurse should determine the availability of other features, such as accessible bathrooms and doorways.

Perhaps one of the most important interventions in caring for the head-injured patient is to always keep sight of the significance of the event to the patient and family. Even with a minor injury, the lives of both the patient and family will never be the same.[9,33] One of the best ways to become sensitized to this phenomenon is to have patients recount their experiences to help nurses see how care is interpreted.

BRAIN TUMORS
Definition

Brain tumors refer to growths within the intracranial space. These include tumors of the brain tissue itself, the meninges, the pituitary gland, and the blood vessels. Tumors in the intracranial space resulting from metastasis are also included. There is little agreement among authorities as to how to classify tumors. The most commonly used scheme for classifying tumors is based on histology and biologic behavior, or grade of malignancy of the cells.[6,7] Refer to Table 49-2 for a further description of each tumor type.

Etiology

Brain tumors account for nearly 2% of all yearly cancer deaths. Intracranial tumors are found in people of all ages, with peaks occurring in the second half of the first decade and in the fourth and fifth decades. New brain tumors develop in approximately 35,000 adult Americans each year.[6]

The cause of brain tumors is unknown. Some tumors are congenital, whereas others are related to hereditary factors. Intracranial tumors may also metastasize by seeping through the cerebrospinal fluid in the subarachnoid space and ventricles. Some evidence exists that tumors can develop secondary to trauma or infection, but little of the evidence is conclusive.

Metastasis of cancer to the brain is increasing in frequency. Some researchers suggest that neoplastic cells that have been treated in other parts of the body move to the central nervous system, because it is a "safe place." Therefore therapy aimed at protection of the central nervous system, along with treatment of the systemic cancer, may be the most effective.

Pathophysiology

Brain tumors cause symptoms for several reasons, the most common of which include displacement of cerebral tissue, obstruction of cerebrospinal fluid, and potential herniation.

As the tumor grows, edema develops in adjacent tissues. Increased intracranial pressure is the result of tissue destruction. Another result of the compression of tissue is eventual death and destruction of the tissue, which produces signs of focal neurologic damage. As the tumor grows, it may interfere with the normal flow and drainage of cerebrospinal fluid and increase intracranial pressure. If tumor growth is slow, then the development of obstruction will also be slow. Rapid tumor growth, however, results in significant obstruction in flow and drainage of cerebrospinal fluid and rapid deterioration of neurologic function. As the pressure increases, the threat of herniation occurs.

Clinical Manifestations

Approximately 75% of adult brain tumors are located in the cerebrum. There are multiple clinical manifestations related to the presence of a brain tumor. Some develop as a result of the tumor and its growth; others are related to the site of the tumor. See Table 49-3 for further description.

Cranial tumors are also described as "benign" or "malignant." A tumor is designated benign on the basis of the cells that comprise it. In the brain a benign tumor may still be fatal because it is inaccessible and takes up space within the cranial vault. Benign cells may also convert to malignant tissue over time.[3] By the same token, malignant tumors are described on the basis of their histologic makeup.

Headache

Headache is one of the most common symptoms of a tumor. It is believed to be produced by pressure on the pain-sensitive areas of the brain. A common description of a headache associated with a tumor is that the headache occurs at night after retiring, is present on awakening, and may be relieved by midmorning.[47] That the brain tissue drains better through the jugular veins throughout the day as the patient is awake and upright may explain this type of presentation. Thus the headache is relieved as the intracranial pressure decreases through the drainage. Venous drainage is decreased when the patient's head is flat in bed at night, causing the headache to return. Although this is the most common presentation, other types of headaches may also be associated with brain tumors.

Vomiting

The tumor can stimulate the vomiting center in the medulla, producing projectile vomiting without nausea. Vomiting is unrelated to meals and is more common in the morning. This symptom can occur at any time during the course of diagnosis or treatment. The threat of aspiration is particularly important be-

TABLE 49-2 Brain Tumor Classification

Tumor type	Definition
Gliomas	Arise from neuroglia and invade surrounding brain tissue; comprise 40% to 50% of all intracranial tumors
Astrocytoma	
Grade I	Benign tumor; may further differentiate to grade III or IV, particularly with advancing age
Grade II	Cell differentiation less defined than grade I
Glioblastoma multiforme (grades III and IV astrocytoma)	Most malignant form; may develop without previous malignancy or may result from alteration of cells toward malignancy in benign gliomas; rapid growing
Ependymomas grades I to IV	Tumors that develop from ependymal cells lining ventricles
Astroblastoma	Benign
Ependymoblastoma	Malignant, slow-growing tumor that arises from lining of ventricles
Spongioblastoma	Benign glioma that occurs in or near optic nerves or chiasm, hypothalamus, and brainstem
Oligodendrogliomas	Rare, slow-growing tumors that may be encapsulated; may also be present in children
Medulloblastoma	Highly malignant tumor; occurs primarily in children but may also occur in adults; generally found in cerebellum
Meningiomas	Slow-growing tumors that develop from meninges (particularly dura); are generally firm and well encapsulated
Acoustic neuromas	Arise from sheath of Schwann cells found on eighth cranial nerve; may also affect fifth, seventh, ninth, and tenth cranial nerves
Metastatic brain tumors	Tumors that metastasize from other parts of body (lungs, breast, stomach, lower gastrointestinal tract, pancreas, and kidney); comprise 10% of all brain tumors and spread to brain by blood and lymphatic system, usually well differentiated from rest of brain
Pituitary	Tumors arising from one of three cell types—chromophobe, eosinophil, or basophil; generally slow growing and encapsulated
Chromophobic pituitary adenoma	Nonsecreting, space-occupying tumor; most often affects optic chiasm
Basophilic pituitary adenoma	Tumor that secretes adrenocorticotrophic hormone (ACTH); Cushing's syndrome can result
Eosinophilic pituitary adenoma	Secreting tumor that produces growth hormone
Developmental tumors	Tumors that originate as result of maldevelopmental processes in early life
Hemangioblastoma	Slow-growing vascular tumor representing congenital arteriovenous malformation of blood vessels; slow growing; therefore may not produce symptoms for many years
Craniopharyngioma	Solid or cystic tumors that can compress pituitary gland; occur primarily in children
Chordomas	Found in both brain and spinal cord; begin to grow during childhood; symptoms produced during middle age
Teratoma	Rare tumor composed of many types of body tissue, including cartilage, muscle, and intestinal or respiratory epithelium; more common in children than in adults
Von Recklinghausen's disease	Neurofibromatosis of genetic origin; tumors of nervous system and cutaneous system

TABLE 49-3 Symptoms Related to Affected Area of Brain

Area of brain	Symptoms
Frontal lobe	Inappropriate behavior
	Inattentiveness
	Difficulty in concentrating
	Emotional lability
	Loss of self-restraint
	Quiet/flat affect
	Loss of recent memory
	Motor dysfunction
	Slowness
	Hemiparesis
	Hemiplegia
	Possible seizure activity
Parietal lobe	Hyperesthesia
	Paresthesia
	Loss of two-point discrimination
	Astereognosis
	Autopagnosia
	Anosognosia
	Finger agnosia
	Loss of right-left discrimination
	Agraphia
	Acalculia
	Construction apraxia
	Homonymous hemianopsia
	Possible seizure activity
Temporal lobe	Psychomotor seizures
	Aura involving taste or smell
	Lip smacking or chewing
	Swallowing
	Homonymous hemianopsia
	Auditory disturbances
	Aphasia
Occipital lobe	Visual field defects
	Seizures (focal or generalized)
Pituitary and hypothalamus	Visual deficits
	Headache
	Hormonal imbalance
	Hypopituitarism
	Hyperpituitarism
	Thermal control
Brainstem	Dysphagia
	Vomiting
	Ataxia
	Depressed corneal reflex
	Nystagmus
	Corticospinal and sensory tract deficits
	Respiratory control
Cerebellum	Ataxia
	Nystagmus
	Unsteady gait
	Seizures
	Intention tremors

cause the patient is unable to predict the onset of vomiting.

Level of consciousness

Changes in the patient's personality and behavior are often early symptoms of a tumor. Depending on the precise location of the tumor, the patient may exhibit personality changes ranging from anger and hostility to euphoria. The patient also may experience changes in cognition, response time, and memory. As the tumor continues to grow and begins to press on the reticular activating system, the patient may undergo changes in wakefulness and alertness.

Motor and sensory losses

Motor and sensory loss may be among the early symptoms of a tumor. Motor problems include ataxia, unsteady gait, and hemiparesis. Among the sensory problems a patient may have are paresthesias, pain, numbness, and tingling.

Seizures

Tumor growth can lead to a disruption in the normal excitability of the neurons within the brain. About 30% of adults with brain tumors develop seizure activity, which can result in seizures. Many different types of seizures can occur in patients with a brain tumor. Progression in the frequency or severity of the seizures is a good indication of tumor growth.

Seizures generally originate within the gray matter and sometimes the subcortical gray matter of the brain. When seizures are the first symptoms of a brain tumor, the tumor is usually located at the surface of the brain. This means that the tumor has either arisen in the outer surface of the brain or has grown upward from the center of the brain.

Autonomic and vasomotor changes

Pressure on the vasomotor center located in the medulla may cause changes in blood pressure, pulse rate, and respiratory effort. Other potential problems include body temperature variations or hyperhidrosis (excessive sweating), both related to activity within the hypothalamus.

Visual changes

Several visual changes accompany the presence of a tumor. Pressure on the third cranial nerve (oculomotor) leads to diplopia (double vision). Increasing pressure on the optic nerve can result in blindness. Papilledema will be noted on examination of the eye as the intracranial pressure increases. Other visual symptoms including decreased visual acuity and visual field deficits are frequently associated with papilledema.

Therapeutic Management

Management of a patient with a brain tumor depends on the location and size of the tumor and the type of tissue involved. The three major techniques used are surgery, chemotherapy, and radiation therapy.

Surgical Intervention

Craniotomy, a surgical opening of the skull performed to provide access to the patient's brain, is the most common major surgical procedure used in the treatment of brain tumors. Two other major surgical procedures may also be performed. **Craniectomy** refers to the excision of a portion of the skull without replacement. This procedure is sometimes used for decompression when the patient is experi-

encing severe cerebral edema. **Cranioplasty** is a procedure in which a plastic piece is used to restore the integrity of the patient's skull.

Craniotomy

A craniotomy can be performed on a scheduled or emergency basis, as the patient's condition dictates. In general, a bone flap is created by incising the patient's scalp and bone so that the tissue can be turned down. The dura is then incised and the surgery initiated. Once the procedure is completed, the bone flap is replaced, and the patient's muscle and scalp are realigned and sutured (Figure 49-6).

Two main approaches are used for the craniotomy: supratentorial and infratentorial. These two designations use the tentorium (the fold of the dura mater that separates the cerebral cortex from the cerebellum and brainstem) as a landmark. Supratentorial procedures involve the area above the tentorium (including the cerebrum). The supratentorial approach is used to gain access to lesions in the frontal, parietal, temporal, and occipital lobes of the ce-

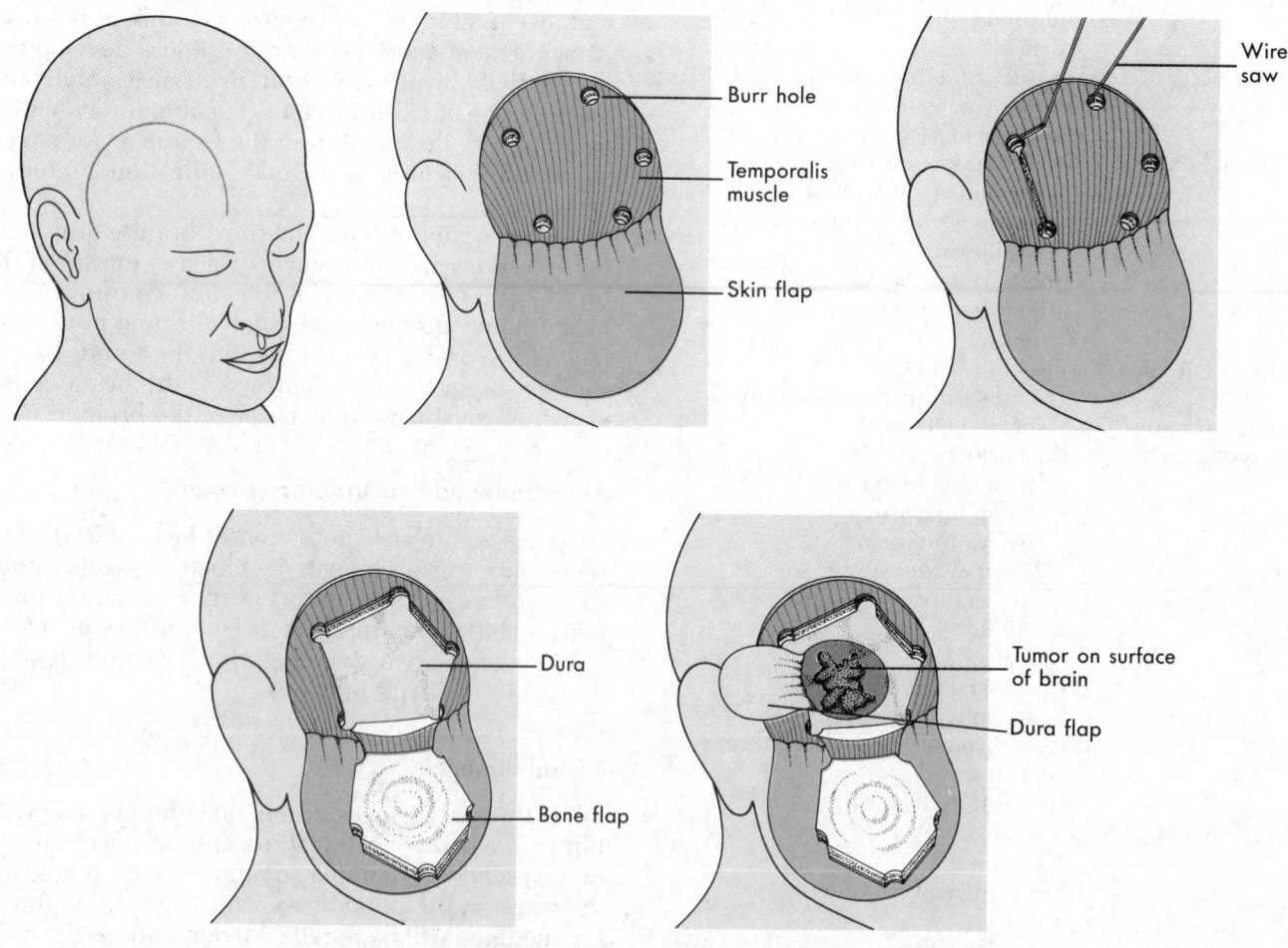

FIGURE 49-6   Stages of a craniotomy.

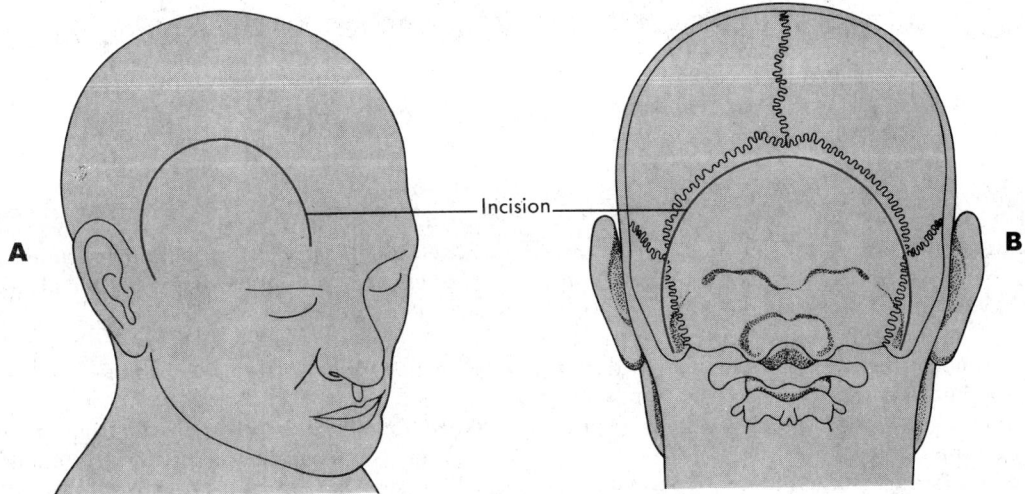

FIGURE 49-7   Surgical approaches to the cranial cavity. **A,** Supratentorial approach. **B,** Infratentorial approach.

rebral hemispheres. Infratentorial procedures involve the area below the tentorium, which includes the brainstem and cerebellum (Figure 49-7).

Although the supratentorial and infratentorial procedures are most commonly used for a craniotomy, advances in other surgical techniques have improved the surgeon's ability to treat specific types of tumors.

Stereotaxic surgery is one of these advances. This type of procedure implies a three-dimensional approach to any anatomically definable point within the brain in relation to a second set of fixed, external reference points.[22] Stereotaxic surgery is directed by CT scan and uses external references on the stereotaxic frame. The lesions within the brain are targeted by the external frame. The major benefits of this procedure are that it allows for accurate approach and it is safe.

One of the major uses of stereotaxic surgery is for tumor biopsy. Other uses include aspiration of colloid cysts, ablative procedures for disorders of the extrapyramidal system, and the implantation of interstitial radiation therapy.[22] Procedures using this technique are generally brief and are performed with the patient under local anesthesia.

The stereotaxic frame is attached to the patient's head on arrival of the patient in the operating room.[22] The frame has three axes that help locate the lesion. Once the lesion is visualized on the CT scan, the coordinates are determined on the stereotaxic frame, and the exact location for the incision is identified.

Laser surgery is one of the newer forms of therapy. The laser has been used to burn tumors and vascular malformations. Tissue destruction caused by the laser is localized; little damage is observed in the tissues adjacent to the tumor. There are several differences with the use of this procedure and traditional types of surgery. The patient loses little blood, since the laser causes coagulation of many of the vessels involved. Lasers are also effective in removing lesions. The long-term effects of laser surgery are not yet known. However, current literature suggests that the procedure is largely a safe one.

Radiosurgery

Over the past 10 years, much progress has been made in the development of procedures that combine different surgical techniques with radiation sources. The goal of radiosurgery is to allow the delivery of a high dose of radiation in a single fraction to a small and well-defined intracranial volume without delivering significant radiation to adjacent normal tissue.[22] This type of procedure is used in the treatment of many types of tumors. Another technique that is offered to patients with small, inoperable benign tumors, vascular abnormalities, or tumors partially removed by past surgery is the gamma knife.[4] This technique is a closed, bloodless operation using high-dose radiation that may obliterate arteriovenous malformation and stop tumor growth through a single dose treatment of cobalt gamma radiation.[29]

Transsphenoidal surgery

Surgical treatment for tumors of the pituitary and hypothalamus is discussed in Chapter 60.

Drug therapy

Chemotherapy

Various chemotherapeutic agents are used in the treatment of brain tumors. The drug selected is

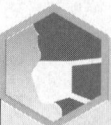

PREOPERATIVE AND POSTOPERATIVE NURSING INTERVENTIONS

Craniotomy

Intervention	Rationale

Intervention

Preoperative care

1. Assist patient through routine medical procedures including blood work (e.g., complete blood count, type, and cross match) and radiologic studies (e.g., chest x-ray film and electrocardiogram).
2. Complete a thorough nursing assessment with particular attention to patient's neurologic status.
3. Assess family's knowledge and response to hospitalization and impending surgery.
4. Complete a thorough assessment of patient's response to hospitalization and impending surgery. Ensure that all of patient's questions have been answered.
5. Provide preoperative teaching tailored to individual needs of patient and family. Include the following:
   a. Type of surgery
   b. Expected outcome
   c. Where patient will be after surgery (surgical ICU, neurosurgical ICU, etc.)
   d. Expected length of surgery
   e. Where family can wait and when surgeon will be available to talk
   f. If possible, give patient and family a tour through the ICU
6. Teach patient deep breathing and leg and foot exercises.

7. Assist patient in washing hair using antibacterial shampoo. Other preparation of head is generally done in operating room.
8. Administer preoperative enema to clear bowels, unless intracranial pressure is elevated.

9. Allow time for patient and family to be together.

Postoperative care

1. Provide a thorough assessment to include the following information about patient:
   a. Age and medical diagnosis
   b. Main signs and symptoms before surgery
   c. Type and length of surgical procedure
   d. Types and amounts of drugs and anesthesia delivered during procedure
   e. Amount of fluid and blood administered during surgery
   f. Reports of any problems during surgery such as hypotension or arrhythmias
   g. Current vital and neurologic signs
   h. Type of head dressing and presence of drains

Rationale

Baseline laboratory and radiologic studies are needed to ensure that patient has no other preexisting medical condition.

Provides basis for future neurologic evaluation.

Need for surgery is frequently frightening to family. Their support will assist patient in adjustment.

All persons have similar responses to surgery. Their recovery will be improved if they understand the situation and can actively participate in their care.

General information will help patient and family to develop a sense of control.

Coughing is avoided in postoperative period, since it may increase intracranial pressure. Patients who are taught to deep breathe and to perform leg and foot exercises will participate more fully after surgery.

Antibacterial shampoo will decrease normal bacterial count and lessen chance of infection.

Clean bowel will decrease patient's tendency to strain. In postoperative period straining is to be avoided since it increases intracranial pressure.

Patients and families need time together to prepare for reality of surgery.

Provides important baseline information that assists in interpretation of any changes in patient status.

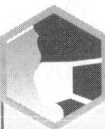

PREOPERATIVE AND POSTOPERATIVE NURSING INTERVENTIONS—cont'd

Intervention	Rationale
2. Develop care plan specific to type of procedure patient has undergone.	Certain aspects of nursing care differ depending on surgical approach used.
Supratentorial Procedures	
a. Elevate head of bed 30 to 45 degrees	Facilitates venous blood return from head.
b. Pillow under head and shoulders can be used, but maintain neck in straight alignment.	Normal alignment facilitates venous return and reduces intracranial pressure.
c. Avoid positioning on operative side (see surgeon's preferences).	Prevents shifting of cranial contents.
d. Monitor for potential cranial nerve dysfunction: (1) II (visual deficits, homonymous hemianopia) (2) III (ptosis) (3) III, IV, VI (deficits in extraocular movement)	Cranial nerves II, III, IV, and VI are most likely to be affected by supratentorial procedures.
Infratentorial Procedures	
a. Head of bed generally remains flat as directed by surgeon, and keep patient off back.	Prevents pressure to neck region and prevents pressure from cerebral contents pressing down on area.
b. Small pillow may be used under head. Keep neck in alignment with head at all times.	Facilitates venous drainage.
c. Monitor for potential cranial nerve dysfunction: (1) III, IV, VI (deficits in extraocular movement) (2) VII (absent corneal reflex weakness, paralysis of facial muscles) (3) VIII (decreased hearing, dizziness, nystagmus) (4) IX, X (diminished gag or swallowing reflex)	Cranial nerves III, IV, VI, VII, VIII, IX, and X are most likely to be affected by infratentorial procedures.
d. Monitor for potential cerebellar dysfunction (ataxia).	
3. Monitor fluid and electrolyte status, particularly sodium, potassium, and calcium.	Surgical manipulation of brain often alters fluid and electrolyte balance. Abnormal serum level of electrolytes may precipitate seizures.
4. Monitor for development of seizure activity.	Some research reports up to a 20% incidence of seizures following surgery.
a. Administer prophylactic anticonvulsants as ordered.	Some studies suggest anticonvulsants will prevent onset of seizures.
5. Carefully monitor body temperature and intervene as needed.	Temperature elevation is most likely caused by blood at operative site or meningeal irritation in subarachnoid space. Fever increases metabolic demand, which may worsen patient's status.
a. Turn and deep breathe every 2 hours.	Assists in removing cause for respiratory infection.
b. Reinforce wet dressings; change as needed when surgeon agrees.	Wet dressings provide medium for growth of bacteria, which can cause cerebral infection.
6. Provide emotional support to patient and family.	Recovery will be improved if patient and family's emotional needs are met.
7. Provide teaching to patient and family.	Patients and family require information to assist them in the many adjustments following surgery.
8. Encourage ambulation.	Early ambulation lessens potential negative effects of immobility.
9. Monitor vital and neurologic signs as needed.	Vital and neurologic signs will be monitored every 15 to 60 minutes immediately following surgery. As patient stabilizes, vital and neurologic signs are checked every 4 hours to determine even minor changes in status.
10. Carefully assess complaints of pain; medicate only when necessary.	Most analgesics make neurologic assessment more difficult since they tend to decrease responsiveness. Their use is frequently contraindicated.

TABLE 49-4   Pharmacology Summary: Chemotherapeutic Agents for Brain Tumors

Drug	Action	Side effects
ALKYLATING AGENTS	Binds to molecules in DNA, preventing cross linking and packing	
Mechlorethamine hydrochloride (Mustargen)	Cytotoxic action is due to cross-linking of DNA and RNA strands and inhibition of protein synthesis	Bone marrow depression Alopecia Jaundice Vertigo Weakness Diarrhea
Carmustine (BCNU)	Major drug used in treatment of brain tumors because it crosses blood-brain barrier	Bone marrow depression Nausea Vomiting Hepatotoxicity Pulmonary fibrosis
Thiotepa (Thiotepa)	Cytotoxic action is due to cross-linking of DNA and RNA strands and inhibition of protein synthesis	Bone marrow depression Nausea Vomiting Headache Anemia Amenorrhea
Lomustine (CCNU)	Interferes with DNA and RNA function; also inhibits DNA synthesis by inhibiting key enzymatic processes	Nausea Vomiting Stomatitis Alopecia Leukopenia
ANTIMETABOLITES	Structurally similar to normal cell products needed for growth and division of cells; interferes with metabolic pathways of dividing cells by blocking DNA synthesis	
Fluorouracil (5-FU)	Activity occurs as result of conversion to active metabolite in tissues and includes inhibition of DNA and RNA synthesis	Bone marrow depression Nausea Vomiting Hepatic toxicity Nephrotic toxicity Stomatitis Alopecia
Floxuridine (FUDR)	Activity occurs as result of activation in tissues and includes inhibition of DNA, and RNA synthesis as result of metabolite	Bone marrow depression Nausea Vomiting Cerebellar ataxia Vertigo Stomatitis Cramps, diarrhea Gastrointestinal bleeding Dermatitis
NATURAL PRODUCTS	Derived from natural products (i.e., plants), but their mechanisms of action are very different	
Vincristine (Oncovin, VCR)	Interferes with microtubule assembly by binding to or crystallizing microtubule proteins necessary for formation of mitotic spindle[25]	Bone marrow depression Areflexia Paresthesia Muscular weakness Peripheral neuritis Paralytic ileus Constipation

TABLE 49-4   Pharmacology Summary: Chemotherapeutic Agents for Brain Tumors—cont'd

Drug	Action	Side effects
Bleomycin (Blenoxane)	Rapidly destroyed by enzymes found in most normal cells but not in cancer cells or lung; believed to inhibit DNA synthesis by scission of DNA strands[25]	Pulmonary fibrosis Skin hyperpigmentation Alopecia Hyperesthesia of scalp and fingers Nail changes
Procarbazine (Matulane)	Exact mechanism of action is unknown; inhibition of DNA, RNA, and protein synthesis has been reported[25]	Bone marrow depression Mental depression Confusion Bleeding Anorexia Stomatitis Alopecia
Methotrexate (MTX, Mexate)	Cytotoxic effect achieved by binding with an enzyme and blocking conversion of folic acid into its active form; blocks DNA synthesis during GI-S interphase of cell cycle	Oral and gastrointestinal ulcers Bone marrow depression Nausea Vomiting Cystitis
Vinblastine (Velban, VLB)	Interferes with microtubule assembly	Alopecia Areflexia Nausea Vomiting

based on the type of tumor, its location, and the patient's response to therapy. The drugs commonly used are shown in Table 49-4. A thorough discussion of chemotherapeutic agents can be found in Chapter 15.

Methods of administration

Chemotherapeutic agents can be given by several techniques, each having specific risks and benefits. Regional chemotherapy is initiated by insertion of a catheter into the carotid artery. This technique allows for direct infusion of the drug, with the potential for producing fewer systemic side effects. Intrathecal injection and intraventricular infusion are additional techniques that may decrease systemic side effects. After a lumbar puncture at the C-4 to L-5 level, a small volume of drug is injected. The intraventricular method of administration uses an Ommaya reservoir (see Figure 48-3) that is surgically implanted and allows for direct instillation of chemotherapy into a lateral ventricle of the brain.[51] Although there are potential problems with this technique (infection), it has been effective in treating many types of brain tumors.

Radiation therapy

The basis for radiation therapy treatment is that tumor cells are more radiosensitive than nontumor cells. Many types of tumors may require radiation therapy. Radiation therapy may be indicated as a primary mode of treatment, for example, when a tumor is not easily accessible by surgery. Radiation therapy may also be used as an adjunct to surgery when some of the tumor remains after the operative procedure. Radiation therapy may also be strictly palliative, used to shrink tumors causing pain or aggravation of symptoms. Whereas in this case the therapy may not prolong life, it is expected to increase the comfort level.

Patients differ in their response to radiation therapy. In some the radiotherapy causes an edema that can increase intracranial pressure. Recurrence of symptoms may be evident in some patients approximately 6 months after the completion of the therapy. The radiation therapy can be the cause, but it may be difficult to differentiate between tumor progression and radiation necrosis.[10]

Interstitial brachytherapy

A specific type of radiation therapy, interstitial brachytherapy, can be used as an adjunct for local control of malignant astrocytomas.[7] With this technique a CT scan is used to identify the exact site of a tumor. High-dose radioactive pellets such as radioactive iodine 125, iridium 192, cesium 177, and radium 226 are implanted directly into the tumor, sparing normal tissue from exposure.[43,45] The course of therapy runs approximately 50 hours, at which time the radioactive material is removed. During the treatment time, several special precautions must be taken. The nurse must be protected from exposure to the radiation, so visits to the patient are limited to less than 15 minutes.[32] Direct nursing care is kept to a minimum, and the patient is encouraged to participate in self-care. During this time the nurse must continue to support the patient and reinforce that the intense isolation will be limited.[32]

Volumetric interstitial hyperthermia

The theory behind volumetric interstitial hyperthermia is that cancer cells are more heat sensitive than normal cells and may incur damage at temperatures not harmful to normal cells.[12] Hyperthermia catheters are percutaneously inserted into the intracranial tumor. Treatments with target tissue temperatures of 105° to 107.6° F are delivered in 3-hour increments every 4 hours. This pattern is continued around the clock until 60 to 72 heated hours are accrued. Up to three cycles are given at 6- to 8-week intervals. Early reports on the efficacy of this therapy are encouraging.[42] Nursing support is essential while the patient undergoes this type of treatment.[13]

Dietary therapy

Nutritional support is an important aspect of the care of the patient with a brain tumor. Specific strategies may be required for those undergoing chemotherapy or radiotherapy. The nausea and vomiting that are commonly associated with both chemotherapy and radiation therapy present special challenges. The dietary requirements for patients with brain tumors are the same as those with cancer of any portion of the body.

Other therapy

Occupational therapy can be useful when the patient needs additional support with activities of daily living. If the tumor affects motor function, then the patient may require assistance with locomotion and other activities requiring motor coordination.

Physical therapy is needed throughout the diagnostic and treatment phases of the tumor. After surgery, physical therapy can help the patient regain strength. If specific areas of deficit exist after resection of the tumor, then the patient can undergo physical therapy to regain full or partial function of those areas.

Behavioral therapy may be needed if the presence of the tumor causes a change in the patient's behavior. Therapies such as behavioral modification may be required for specific patterns of behavior.

NURSING MANAGEMENT OF THE PATIENT WITH A BRAIN TUMOR
Assessment

Several aspects of nursing assessment are needed for all patients with brain tumors. Others are specific to the type of tumor and its location.

The nurse uses the Glasgow Coma Scale to assess the patient's level of consciousness. The patient's response to verbal stimuli and painful stimuli are assessed according to the scale. The nurse should specifically note the trends of the patient's responses.

The nurse should monitor respiratory function, including respiratory rate, airway patency, and the presence of gag, cough, and swallowing reflexes. Specific symptoms related to the portion of the brain affected by the tumor are outlined in Table 49-3.

Families will most likely undergo several emotional stages as the patient's diagnosis is made and treatment initiated. A major nursing responsibility is to assess their responses as the patient progresses through the stages. The nurse notes the amount of information the family has. Providing the family with sufficient information frequently helps allay their fears. The nurse serves as someone with whom members of the family or significant others can verbalize the information that has been provided to them and with whom they can reaffirm the consistency of information provided and received. A complete assessment includes an evaluation of the family's level of anxiety and their ability to cope. As the patient's condition changes, the nurse reassesses these parameters.

Nursing Diagnosis

Multiple nursing diagnoses are appropriate for the patient with a brain tumor. Major diagnoses include the following:

Activity intolerance related to loss of sensory and motor control

Anxiety related to uncertainty of diagnosis and prognosis

Ineffective breathing pattern related to tumor presence in brainstem

Pain related to presence of tumor

Impaired verbal communication related to disruption of speech centers by tumor

Ineffective family coping related to concerns about treatment and prognosis

Fluid volume excess or deficit related to disruption of hormonal regulators by tumor

High risk for injury related to neural deficits

Impaired physical mobility related to sensory and motor dysfunction

Self-care deficit related to loss of motor function

Sensory-perceptual alterations related to presence of tumor

Altered thought processes related to changes in cerebral blood flow

Planning

After assessing the patient and family, the nurse should develop a care plan designed to meet the patient's individual needs. Patient outcomes include the following:

Minimal changes in intracranial pressure

Minimal complications

Minimal loss of control

Implementation

Vital signs

Vital signs and neurologic signs are good indicators of cerebral tissue perfusion. Specific interventions, such as keeping the head of the patient's bed elevated to 30 degrees and maintaining blood flow to the brain, help maintain the patient's cerebral function. The nurse monitors vital signs, including blood pressure, pulse rate, and respiration, at least every 4 hours. In addition to noting changes in values, the nurse also monitors for trends, such as an increased systolic blood pressure or decreased pulse rate. The nurse frequently assesses neurologic signs, such as level of consciousness and motor and pupillary responses. The nurse monitors the patient's temperature carefully. Readings higher than 100.5° F generally are reported to the physician. For patients receiving chemotherapy, temperatures should be taken orally, not rectally, since the thermometer can tear tissues and allow organisms to enter the bloodstream. This can lead to infection and possibly sepsis.

Seizure activity

Seizures can occur at any time while a patient is undergoing the diagnosis or treatment of a brain tumor. Metabolic disorders, hypoxia, and water imbalances can increase the incidence of seizures.

Preoperative nursing care

Preparing the patient for surgery is an important nursing intervention. The nurse should begin with a detailed assessment, paying particular attention to the patient's neurologic status. This assessment forms an important baseline for postoperative comparison. The nurse must also ensure that the patient has had a complete medical history and physical.

The situation is often difficult on the family, so before the patient's surgery, the nurse should assess the family's response. The nurse should determine the family's knowledge and expectations of the procedure, and what their coping abilities are.

One of the most important aspects of preoperative care is to help the patient prepare psychologically for surgery. Past nursing research has indicated that instruction significantly helps decrease the patient's preoperative anxiety. In 1986 Markin[49] conducted a descriptive study on the fears, misconceptions, and concerns of patients scheduled for craniotomy. Patients were asked open-ended questions 2 hours after admission to the hospital. The researchers reported that the top five concerns of patients undergoing a craniotomy include loss of function, return of function, current disability, physician's ability (not the neurosurgeon, but other physicians seen during the course of the illness), and the operation itself. Additional findings from this study were that patients under 50 years of age conveyed more concerns than those over 50 years of age and that the more educated the patient, the more concerns were expressed.

These study results can be directly applied to the care of the patient undergoing surgery. Preoperative teaching includes an understanding of the operative procedure and specifics concerning the potential for loss of function. The nurse uses judgment to determine the amount of information best given to the patient before surgery. Results of the study also emphasize the importance of individualizing all aspects of preoperative assessment.

Intraoperative care

To care for the patient postoperatively the nurse should understand the intraoperative phase. For most routine craniotomies, several events can be expected. Hypotension may be induced during the procedure to slow movement of the vasculature of the brain during the surgery. Hypothermia can also be used to decrease the oxygen consumption in the brain, therefore decreasing its potential for hypoxic response. Hyperventilation, which increases carbon dioxide excretion, causing cerebral vasoconstriction and therefore decreased cerebral blood flow, is also used.

Anesthetic agents can affect the postoperative patient in many ways. Therefore the nurse should be aware of which agents were used and when the last dosage was given before arrival in the unit. Other drugs commonly administered during the intraoperative period include steroids, osmotic diuretics, anticonvulsants, and antibiotics. These drugs may be started in the preoperative period and continued in the postoperative period.

Postoperative care

The nurse assesses the patient for several important parameters following the patient's return to the unit, including the following:

1. Existing signs and symptoms before surgery
2. Type and length of operative procedure
3. Type of anesthetic and other drugs administered during the procedure
4. Amount of fluid and blood received during and immediately after surgery
5. Any problems during surgery, such as uncontrolled hypotension, dysrhythmias, or seizures
6. Current vital signs and neurologic signs
7. The presence of any head dressings and drains

The nurse will also want to determine if the procedure used the supratentorial or infratentorial approach. Supratentorial procedures are the most common. In general, supratentorial motor functioning and sensory functioning are manifested and effected on the side of the body opposite from the hemisphere affected by the tumor. This knowledge assists the nurse in evaluation of symptoms after the surgery.

Infratentorial procedures usually take longer and are more complex than supratentorial procedures for several reasons. The infratentorial region is less accessible, so the patient may be placed in unusual and difficult positions to enable the surgeon to perform the operation. The surgeon works to avoid the many vital structures in the infratentorial area, in particular, the patient's respiratory center and the reticular activating system.

Monitoring these patients after surgery is very important. Commonly, they experience increased intracranial pressure, which can be difficult to control. Compression of areas of the brain in addition to those affected by the tumor often occurs and can produce a range of symptoms that the nurse may not initially expect.[17] The major danger of this surgical approach is damage to or compression of the vital centers within the brainstem or the reticular formation. The nurse can anticipate that recovery from infratentorial procedures takes longer than recovery from supratentorial procedures.

The specifics of the nursing care for patients undergoing surgery are included in the nursing care plan.

Support during chemotherapy or radiation therapy

There are several interventions that can assist the patient who is undergoing chemotherapy or radiation therapy. Both forms of therapy may produce symptoms related to bone marrow depression, such as blood dyscrasias and infection.

Alopecia, or hair loss, can sometimes be slowed, but rarely stopped. New therapies with ice caps have been shown to decrease hair loss from chemotherapy. The patient and family can learn to observe the scalp area on a daily basis. The patient's scalp and hair should be protected as much as possible. Some patients prefer to cover the head with scarfs or hats while hair is being lost.

Blood dyscrasias are very common in radiation therapy patients. The nurse should monitor for symptoms related to bleeding, such as occult blood in secretions, bruising, and signs of petechiae. The oral mucosa is a common site for petechiae. The nursing care plan should include numerous safety measures while bleeding is a possibility.

Infection occurs because the drugs or radiation causes a decrease in the number of white blood cells. The most successful nursing interventions include placing the patient in an environment that provides protection from others and ensuring that all personnel and visitors use good handwashing technique. With a decreased ability to fight infection, the patient should be protected from any potential source of infection.

Evaluation

The nurse should carefully evaluate the response of patient and family to all of the interventions. The patient's vital signs and neurologic signs should be evaluated. The patient should not experience headache, papilledema, or any signs of decreased level of consciousness. The patient's sensory and motor function should remain stable, and pupillary size and reactivity should be normal.

Complications such as seizures, infections, and worsening focal symptoms should be absent. Both patient and family will demonstrate a beginning understanding of the process that is occurring with the brain tumor.

Throughout the process of diagnosis and treatment, the patient and family should be able to participate in decisions concerning care. Patients and family members should verbalize their sense of control in the relationship.

Documentation

The nurse documents the patient's individual behavioral reaction and response to the management of all complications. Examples of important aspects to include are assessment parameters, presence of symptoms related to treatment (nausea, vomiting, diarrhea), and emotional responses. Information concerning the patient's level of anxiety and expression of fear can be beneficial. Documentation includes preoperative and postoperative teaching. A reflection of the family response is also necessary.

Ongoing Care

Rehabilitation

Rehabilitation of the patient following treatment for brain tumor includes an analysis of the resulting cognitive, motor, behavioral, and emotional deficits and an assessment of the patient's prognosis along with the family's coping abilities. Once these assessments have been completed, it is possible to begin plans for rehabilitation.

Discharge planning begins on the patient's admission to the hospital. The presence of a brain tumor may mean that the patient will require placement in a long-term care facility after discharge. If the patient is discharged home, then a number of things must be done to prepare for discharge. The family must be actively involved in planning for discharge. Specific aspects to consider include arrangement of the home environment to meet the individual needs of the patient, which may include redesigning bedrooms and bathrooms to allow access. The effect of discharge of the patient on the family and its normal activities must also be considered.

Long-term care

If necessary the patient may be discharged from the hospital to a long-term care facility. Whether discharge is to a nursing home or a rehabilitation facility, the goal is to provide care while enhancing the patient's independence. It is expected that the patient would be medically stable before being transferred to either type of facility.

While awaiting the patient's transfer to a long-term care facility, the patient and family need time to ask questions and to process information. They can begin to deal with how the "new" environment will differ from their present situation. The nurse is instrumental in helping the patient and family achieve a smooth transition to the new setting.

Another important aspect of long-term care is attention to the behavioral response of both patient and family. As treatment and therapy continue, the nurse anticipates multiple changes in patient and family response. The nurse's responsibility is to note those changes and intervene when appropriate.

Home care

After resection or treatment of the tumor, the patient may be discharged directly home. Other patients may be discharged from a long-term care facility to home. In either event the nursing care considerations are the same. The patient may have some physical limitations, necessitating changes within the structure of the home, such as alterations in stairs or widening of bathroom doors to allow wheelchair access.

The patient and family must fully understand the signs and symptoms of the tumor and also be able to identify symptoms of extension of the tumor. They should be able to discuss the treatment of the tumor and the effects (positive and negative) of this treatment. While preparing for the patient's discharge, the hospital nurse arranges for a consultation with a home health nurse. The home health nurse pays particular attention to the behavioral/emotional responses of both patient and family after the patient has been discharged from the hospital.

✓ NURSING CARE PLAN   *Postoperative Craniotomy*

Nursing diagnosis/ Expected outcome	Interventions	Rationale
High risk for ineffective breathing pattern •*Effective breathing pattern maintained as evidenced by: normal P_{O_2}, P_{CO_2}, and pH; normal breath sounds*	Assess respiratory function (i.e., breath sounds) each shift Encourage coughing every 2-4 hours Position with head of bed elevated 30 degrees; for infratentorial procedures, the head of the bed should remain flat Suction as needed Provide mechanical ventilatory support as needed	Location of the surgical site can interfere with the patient's ability to breathe; positioning, deep breathing, and coughing will help to mobilize secretions
High risk for altered cerebral tissue perfusion •*Cerebral tissue will be adequately perfused as evidenced by: improved or usual level of consciousness; stable vital signs; absence of headache or seizures*	For supratentorial procedures, elevate head of bed to 30 degrees; with patient on back or unoperative side if unconscious. For infratentorial procedures; keep head flat with patient on either side Avoid the precipitating factors of increased intracranial pressure Monitor electrolyte and fluid levels	Cerebral tissue perfusion will be supported by maintaining a normal intracranial pressure

Continued.

NURSING CARE PLAN   *Postoperative Craniotomy—cont'd*

Nursing diagnosis/ Expected outcome	Interventions	Rationale
	Assess neurologic signs every 2-4 hours	
	Avoid isometric muscle contractions (such as shivering)	Isometric contractions increase blood pressure and, subsequently, intracranial pressure
	Maintain strict intake and output	
	Exercise caution in administration of fluids	
High risk for injury related to complications: Intracranial bleeding	Assess at least every 2 hours for level of consciousness and focal neurologic signs	Bleeding is most often demonstrated by deterioration in neurologic status; immediate intervention is indicated
• *Absence of neurologic deterioration*	Report any changes to physician	
Seizures	Continually assess for early signs of seizures	Seizures following a craniotomy probably occur because of an alteration in autoregulation; seizures should be controlled or prevented since they increase intracranial pressure
• *Absence of seizure activity*	Maintain accurate records of seizures	
	Prevent injury to patient during and after seizures	
	Administer anticonvulsants as needed	
Infection	Monitor for signs of a cerebrospinal fluid leak, particularly ear and nose drainage	Infection should be preventable through use of appropriate precautions
• *Absence of infection, particularly meningitis*	Monitor for signs and symptoms of infection	
	Utilize strict aseptic technique	
Cerebrospinal fluid leak	Assess for possible leak:	Cerebrospinal fluid leaks are not uncommon; identification of the leak is a major nursing priority
• *Patient has a decreased risk for cerebrospinal fluid leak*	Presence of glucose in nasal or ear drainage as shown by positive Testape or Dextrostix results	Nursing care should seek to allow the dura to heal by leaving the drainage undisturbed
	Clear halo or a watery, pale ring around bloody or serosanguinous drainage on dressing or pillowcase	
	Complaints of postnasal drip	
	Constant swallowing	
	Discourage patient from blowing or picking nose	
	Maintain a dry, clean dressing; do not disturb healing	
GI bleeding	Monitor for signs of GI bleeding	Antacids and histamine-2 blockers are used to prevent GI bleeding
• *No GI bleeding as evidenced by: no complaints of pain; absence of occult blood in stool and gastric contents; hemoglobin, hematocrit and vital signs within normal limits*	Administer antacids and histamine-2 blockers as appropriate	
	Utilize Salem sump or nasogastric tube as needed	
Diabetes insipidus/SIADH	Maintain input equal to output	Monitoring fluid balance is an important priority; both DI and SIADH can disrupt fluid balance
• *Absence of polyuria and polydipsia*	Monitor vital signs	
• *Urine specific gravity within normal limits*	Observe skin and mucous membranes for evidence of dehydration or overhydration	
• *Urine output in balance with intake*	Monitor osmolarity, electrolytes, BUN, creatinine, and urine specific gravity	

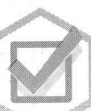

NURSING CARE PLAN   *Postoperative Craniotomy—cont'd*

Nursing diagnosis/ *Expected outcome*	Interventions	Rationale
Ineffective individual coping • *Verbalizes realistic expectations* • *Behaviors reflect ability to cope*	Encourage verbalization of thoughts and feelings Provide adequate time for support of patient and family Develop plans in conjunction with patient and family	With the many changes imposed throughout the surgical process, specific nursing interventions are required to assist patient and family in coping
Pain: headache • *Absence of headache*	Administer analgesics as needed Evaluate patient's response	Headache is often an indication of increased intracranial pressure; analgesics (Tylenol and codeine) can be effective
Knowledge deficit • *Patient will verbalize an under-standing of the disease process and subsequent treatment*	Teach patient and family symptoms to report to physician Instruct in ways to adapt to neuro-logic deficits Initiate referrals to appropriate community agencies	Outcomes are improved with coop-eration of patient and family

CRITICAL THINKING QUESTIONS

1 What are the nursing priorities in the care of the patient with a severe head injury?
2 What symptoms help the nurse in differentiat-ing between diabetes insipidus and syndrome of inappropriate secretion of ADH?
3 How would you interpret a patient's Glasgow Coma Scale score of 7?
4 What information should be available to the family before the patient is discharged?
5 What symptoms would be expected from a frontal lobe tumor? parietal lobe? temporal lobe? occipital lobe?
6 What are the major concerns of a patient who is to undergo a craniotomy?
7 Which diagnostic study is most specific for tu-mors?
8 What specific nursing interventions are appro-priate for the patient following a supratentorial procedure?

RESOURCES

1 AMERICAN ASSOCIATION OF NEURO-SCIENCE NURSES 224 N. Des Plaines Street Suite 601 Chicago, IL 60661
2 THE AMERICAN CANCER SOCIETY National Office 777 Third Avenue New York, NY 10017
3 THE NATIONAL HEAD INJURY FOUNDA-TION Framingham, MA

BIBLIOGRAPHY

Current

1. American Association of Neuroscience Nurses: *Core cur-riculum*, Park Ridge, Il, 1990, The Association.
2. Andrus C: Intracranial pressure: dynamics and nursing management, *J Neurosci Nurs* 23(2):85-92, 1991.
3. Baker J: Family adaptation when one member has a head injury, *J Neurosci Nurs* 22(4):232-237, 1990.
4. Barker E: Brain tumor: frightening diagnosis, nursing challenge, *RN*, pp 46-51, 1990.
5. Becker DP, Gudeman SK: *Textbook of head injury*, Phil-adelphia, 1989, WB Saunders Co.
6. Black P McL: Brain tumors. I, *N Engl J Med* 324(21):1471-1476, 1991.
7. Black P McL: Brain tumors. II, *N Engl J Med* 324(22):1555-1564, 1991.
8. Braakman R: Head injury. In Vinken PJ, Bruyn GW, Kla-wans HL, editors: *Handbook of clinical neurology*, New York, 1990, Elsevier.
9. Caballero D: An open letter to emergency nurses from a survivor of a major head injury, *J Emerg Nurs* 17(4):259-260, 1991.
10. Campbell CH: Needs of relatives and helpfulness of sup-port groups in severe head injury, *Rehab Nurs* 13(6):320-325, 1988.
11. Carpenito LJ: *Nursing diagnosis: application to clinical practice*, Philadelphia, 1992, JB Lippincott Co.
12. Edwards DK, Stupperich TK, Welsh DM: Hyperthermia treatment for malignant brain tumors: nursing manage-ment during therapy, *J Neurosci Nurs* 23(1):34-38, 1991.
13. Edwards DK et al: Volumetric interstitial hyperthermia: role of the critical care nurse, *Focus Crit Care* 18(1):35-50, 1991.
14. Frederick C: Discharge planning for the head-injured patient, *Crit Care Nurs* 11(6):42-45, 1991.

15. Frye B: Head injury and the family: related literature, *Rehab Nurs* 12(3):135-136, 1987.
16. Goldstein M: Traumatic brain injury: a silent epidemic, *Ann Neurol* 27(3):327, 1990.
17. Gordon VL: Recovery from a head injury: a family process, *Pediatr Nurs* 15(2):131-133, 1989.
18. Grinspun D: Teaching families of traumatic brain-injured adults, *Crit Care Nurs* 19(3):61, 1987.
19. Guentz SJ: Cognitive rehabilitation of the head-injured patient, *Crit Care Nurs* 10(3):51, 1987.
20. Hendrickson SL: Intracranial pressure changes and family presence, *J Neurosci Nurs* 19(1):14, 1987.
21. Kozak GS, Yura H: A comparison of teaching methods for ED discharge instruction after head injury, *J Emerg Nurs* 15(1):18-22, 1989.
22. Krause EA et al: Radiosurgery: a nursing perspective, *J Neurosci Nurs* 23(1):24-28, 1991.
23. Lord J, Coleman EA: Chemotherapy for glioblastoma multiforme, *J Neurosci Nurs* 23(1):68-70, 1991.
24. March K et al: Effect of backrest position on intracranial and cerebral perfusion pressures, *J Neurosci Nurs* 22(6):375-381, 1990.
25. Mathewson MK: *Pharmacotherapeutics: a nursing process approach*, Philadelphia, 1991, FA Davis.
26. Miller E, Williams S: Alterations in cerebral perfusion: clinical concept or nursing diagnosis? *J Neurosci Nurs* 19(4):183-190, 1987.
27. Mirr MP: Factors affecting decisions made by family members of patients with severe head injury, *Heart Lung* 20(3):228-235, 1991.
28. Mitchell M: *Neuroscience nursing: a nursing diagnosis approach*, Baltimore, 1989, William & Wilkins.
29. Neatherlin JS, Brent VA: The gamma knife: implications for nursing practice and patient education, *J Neurosci Nurs* 23(1):71-74, 1991.
30. Nikas DL: Critical aspects of head trauma, *Crit Care Nurs Q* 10(1):19, 1987.
31. Parsons LC, Wilson MM: Cerebrovascular status of severe closed head injured patients following passive position changes, *Nurs Res* 33(2):68, 1985.
32. Randall TM, Drake DK, Sewchand W: Neuro-oncology update: radiation safety and nursing care during interstitial brachytherapy, *J Neurosci Nurs* 19(6):315-320, 1987.
33. Siegel T: Six months as a brain injury patient, *Rehab Nurs* 15(5):268-269, 1990.

34. Staller AG: Systemic effects of severe head injury, *Crit Care Nurs Q* 10(1):58, 1987.
35. Stavros MK: Family issues in moderate to severe head injury, *Crit Care Nurs Q* 10(3):73, 1987.
36. Stewart-Amidei C: Alcohol and head injury: a nursing perspective, *Crit Care Nurs Q* 10(1):69, 1987.
37. Stewart-Amidei C: What to do until the neurosurgeon arrives, *J Emerg Nurs* 14(5):296-301, 1988.
38. Tate RL et al: Psychosocial outcome for the survivors of severe blunt head injury: the results from a consecutive series of 100 patients, *J Neurol Neurosurg Psychol* 52:1128-1134, 1989.
39. Ulrich SP, Canale SW, Wendell SA: *Nursing care planning guides*, Philadelphia, 1990, WB Saunders Co.
40. United States Pharmacopeial Conventions: *USP-DI*, 1990, The Convention.
41. Varella LD: Nutrition in the critically ill, *Crit Care Nurs* 9(6):28-29, 32-34, 1989.
42. Welsh DM, Zumwalt CB: Volumetric interstitial hyperthermia: nursing implications for brain tumor treatment, *J Neurosci Nurs* 20(4):229-235, 1988.
43. Williams C, Grove M, Cotter G: Seeding the tumor, *RN*, pp 52-55, 1990.
44. Williams MH: The self-help movement in head injury, *Rehab Nurs* 15(6):311-315, 1990.
45. Willis D: Intracranial astrocytoma: pathology, diagnosis and clinical presentation, *J Neurosci Nurs* 23(1):7-14, 1991.
46. Winslade WJ, Tabaracci JM: Prognosis in head injury: legal and ethical issues, *Crit Care Nurs Q* 10(3):35, 1987.
47. Young HF, Salcman M: Early diagnosis of brain tumors, *Am Fam Physician* 36(1):149, 1987.

Classic
48. Hartshorn JC: Carotid-cavernous fistula, *Focus Crit Care* 12(2):32, 1983.
49. Markin DA: Preoperative concerns of the patient undergoing craniotomy, *J Neurosci Nurs* 18(5):275, 1986.
50. Mathis M: Personal needs of family members of critically ill patients with and without acute brain injury, *J Neurosci Nurs* 16(1):36, 1984.
51. Rudy EB: *Advanced concepts in neuroscience nursing*, St Louis, 1986, Mosby–Year Book.

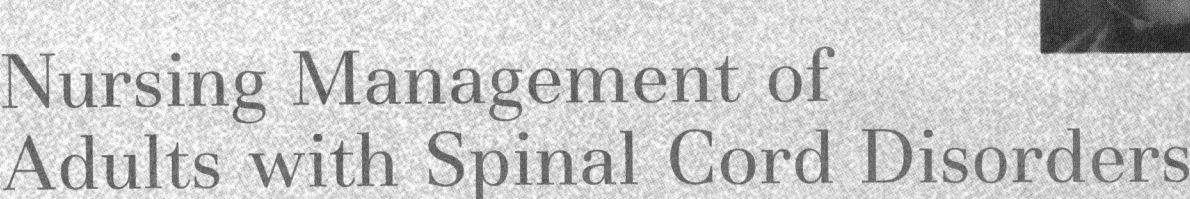

CHAPTER FIFTY

Nursing Management of Adults with Spinal Cord Disorders

LEARNING OBJECTIVES

1 Identify the areas of the spinal cord that are most prone to trauma and explain why.
2 Describe the four major mechanisms of spinal cord trauma.
3 Define the classifications of spinal cord injury and the associated manifestations.
4 Discuss the syndromes of spinal shock and autonomic dysreflexia, and identify the medical and nursing interventions related to these syndromes.
5 Identify five nursing diagnoses associated with spinal cord injury.
6 Identify the major complications of spinal cord injury.
7 List the goals of rehabilitation for the patient with paraplegia and the patient with quadriplegia.
8 Describe the types and clinical manifestations of spinal cord tumors.
9 Describe the various types of medical interventions for spinal cord tumor.
10 Discuss the cause of intervertebral disk disease and the current treatment modalities including preoperative and postoperative care.
11 Develop a care plan for the patient with a spinal cord disorder related to trauma, tumor, or intervertebral disk disease.

KEY TERMS

SPINAL CORD INJURY is a devastating injury that affects the total physiologic, psychologic, and social well-being of the individual. The person with spinal cord injury faces major changes in life-style including compensating for impaired or lost physical function, returning to productive living, reestablishing social contacts, and psychosocial acceptance of injury. The nurse who cares for the patient must understand the physiologic consequences of the injury and the patient's complex psychosocial needs. Initial care focuses on maintaining life and preventing or minimizing complications. Preparing the patient for rehabilitation is an important goal during the acute care phase. Helping the patient adapt to the sequelae of the injury is the focus in the intermediate and rehabilitation phases of care. This chapter also presents care of the patient with spinal tumors and intervertebral disk disease.

SPINAL CORD INJURY
Definition

Spinal cord injuries are classified in several ways: mechanism of injury, level of injury, or lowest segment of normal function in the spinal cord. The American Spinal Injury Association (ASIA) classification system is based on neuromuscular and sensory function (see box below). Spinal cord injuries may be "complete," indicating no impulse traverses the cord below the level of the lesion, or "incomplete," inferring that some impulses are able to travel the cord past the level of the lesion. Incomplete injuries are commonly described in terms of classic syndromes (Brown-Séquard, anterior cord, and central cord) and cauda equina lesions. These lesions are characterized and assessed according to spinal cord tract involvement (Figure 50-1).

With **Brown-Séquard syndrome** the lesion affects only half of the spinal cord function. Voluntary motor tract function is affected below the level of injury on the same side of the lesion, and perception of pain is affected below the level of injury on the opposite side of the lesion (Figure 50-2). With **anterior cord syndrome** the lesion affects anterior aspects of the spinal cord in which voluntary motor and sensory tracts for pain and temperature are located. Clinically these patients exhibit loss of voluntary motor and pain sensation below the level of the lesion; however, proprioception (position sense) is preserved below the level of the lesion (Figure 50-3). With **central cord syndrome** the lesion affects centermost fibers of the spinal cord that are responsible for innervation to the upper extremities and respiratory muscles. Upper extremity function is impaired, whereas lower extremity function is present in variable degrees (Figure 50-4). A **cauda equina lesion** affects peripheral nerves exiting from the tail of the spinal cord. Lesions are associated with vertebral injuries at L2 and below. Reflex arc activity is not restored in these lesions, resulting in flaccid paralysis, bowel and bladder hypoactivity, and sexual dysfunction (Figure 50-5).

Etiology/Epidemiology

The United States has 226,500 spinal cord–injured individuals, and each year 7500 to 8000 new injuries occur.[19] Spinal cord injury most commonly occurs in younger age groups; 60% of spinal cord injuries occur between the ages of 16 and 30 years. The typical victim is a young male (82%) who is injured in a motor vehicle accident. Fifty-seven percent of the victims possess at least a high school education; most either were working or were full-time students at the time of their injury.[1] Medical care costs of spinal cord injury are approximately 4 billion dollars per year. Lost earnings are estimated at 3.4 billion dollars annually.[2] Motor vehicle accidents account for 45% of all injuries, followed by falls (21%), acts of violence (15%),[19] and sports injuries (13%).

Life expectancy of the spinal cord–injured individual has dramatically changed over the last 60 years. During World War I the life expectancy was 6 to 12 months following injury. Over the last decade, improvements in acute care and the management of complications have allowed these patients to live to a nearly normal life expectancy. Factors that affect survival include the level of the lesion, the extent of paralysis, age at the time of injury, and the ability to survive the first year after injury. Most patients (92%) are discharged to the home where they lived before injury.

Many spinal cord injury prevention programs exist in the United States and Canada and are funded by various levels of the government, the insurance industry, and automobile and liquor manufacturers.[31] Preventive information is aimed at all ages, but particularly at adolescents learning to drive, living in high-violence areas, experimenting with drugs and alcohol, and demonstrating high-risk behaviors. Most programs include education to increase the use

---

FRANKEL CLASSIFICATION SYSTEM

A: complete spinal cord lesion
B: preserved sensation only below lesion
C: preserved motor below lesion (nonfunctional)
D: preserved motor below lesion (functional)
E: complete neurologic recovery
Unknown

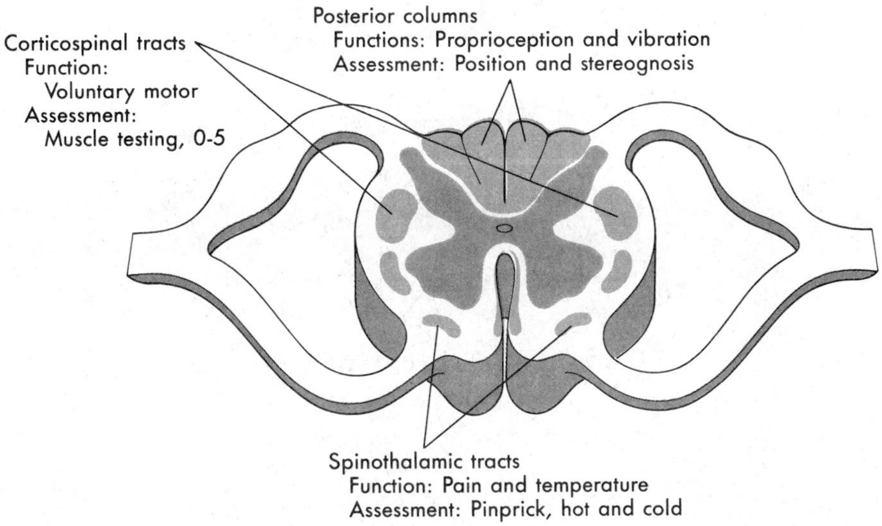

Corticospinal tracts
Function:
   Voluntary motor
Assessment:
   Muscle testing, 0-5

Posterior columns
   Functions: Proprioception and vibration
   Assessment: Position and stereognosis

Spinothalamic tracts
   Function: Pain and temperature
   Assessment: Pinprick, hot and cold

FIGURE 50-1   Function and assessment of specific locations in spinal cord.

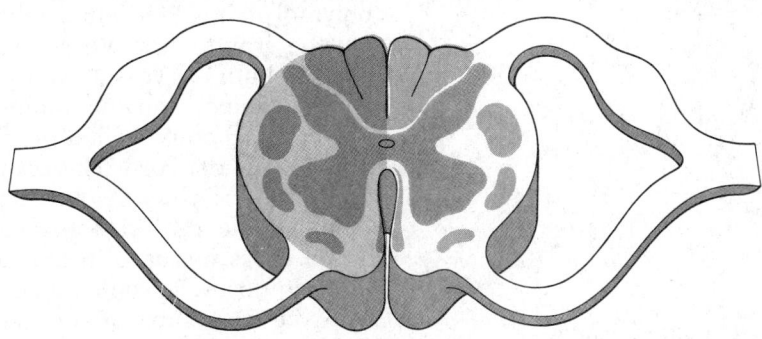

FIGURE 50-2   Brown-Séquard syndrome.

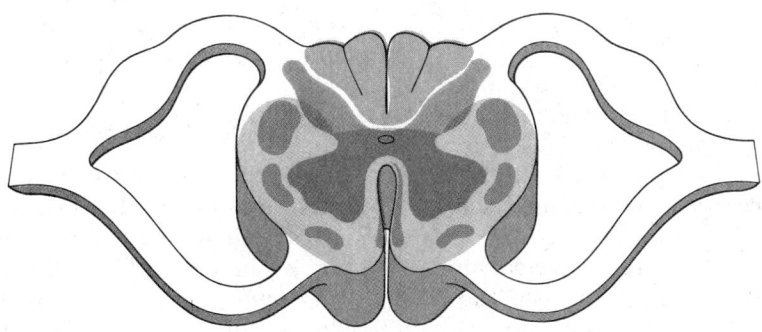

FIGURE 50-3   Anterior cord syndrome.

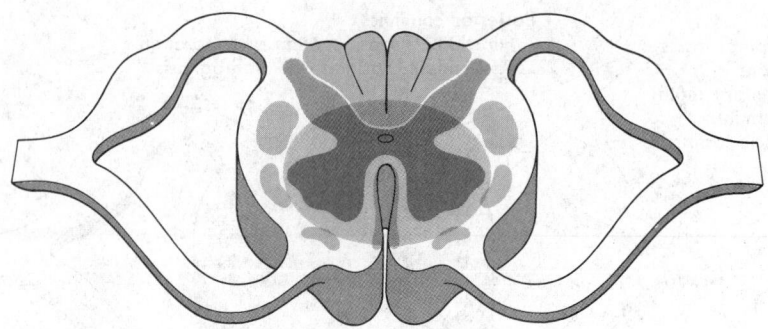

FIGURE 50-4   Central cord syndrome.

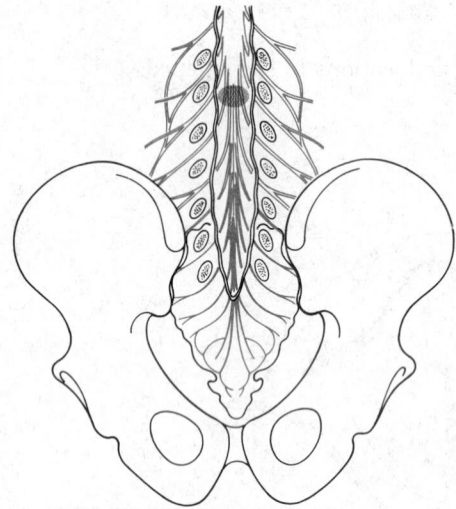

FIGURE 50-5   Cauda equina lesion.

of safety belts and to reduce the use of drugs and alcohol. The compulsory use of seat belts is the single most important measure in reducing the number of deaths and injuries on the road.[31]

Pathophysiology

Spinal cord injury is caused by concussion, contusion, laceration, transection, hemorrhage, or damage to the blood vessels supplying the spinal cord. The major mechanisms of injury are hyperflexion, hyperextension, flexion-rotation, and compression (axial loading) (Figures 50-6 to 50-9). Any level of the spine may be injured; however, cervical and lumbar injuries are most common, because these are the levels associated with the greatest spinal column flexibility and movement. The complete loss of function above C8 is called complete **quadriplegia.** An injury below C8 with preservation of arm function but loss of function in the lower part of the body causes **paraplegia.**

The spinal cord is very tough and is rarely torn or transected by direct trauma. The complete cord dissolution in severe trauma is related to an autodestructive process within the cord. Shortly after the injury, petechial hemorrhages are noted in the central gray matter of the cord. This is followed in 1 to 2 hours by extravasation of red blood cells, fluid, and polymorphonuclear leukocytes that extend throughout the gray matter. Vascular stasis occurs, and the endothelium of vessel walls is damaged. Hemorrhage, edema, and metabolites all act together to produce ischemia, which progresses to necrotic destruction of the cord. The resulting hypoxia reduces the oxygen tension below a level that will meet the metabolic needs of the neurons. Lactate metabolites and a gross increase in norepinephrine are noted; in toxic doses, norepinephrine causes vasospasms, hypoxia, and subsequent necrosis. Unfortunately, the spinal cord has minimal ability to adapt to vasospasm. By 4 hours after the injury, this process has progressed to coagulation necrosis of up to 40% of the gray matter and adjacent white matter.[34]

Because of the hemorrhagic necrosis, the lesion is complete after 48 hours and any function of the nerves in the area or passing through the area is destroyed. Because additional edema will extend the level of injury beyond the immediate level of destruction for 3 to 7 days, the exact extent of injury cannot be determined before that time.

Clinical Manifestations

The permanence of functional loss with spinal cord injury depends on the degree, type, and level of injury. In spinal cord concussion the duration of dysfunction may last 24 to 48 hours with no evidence of permanent neurologic loss of function.[16] In spinal cord compression the function of the spinal cord may be preserved with prompt surgical decompression, if no permanent damage has occurred at the time of the injury. Laceration, severe contusion, and transection will likely result in permanent neurologic dysfunction.

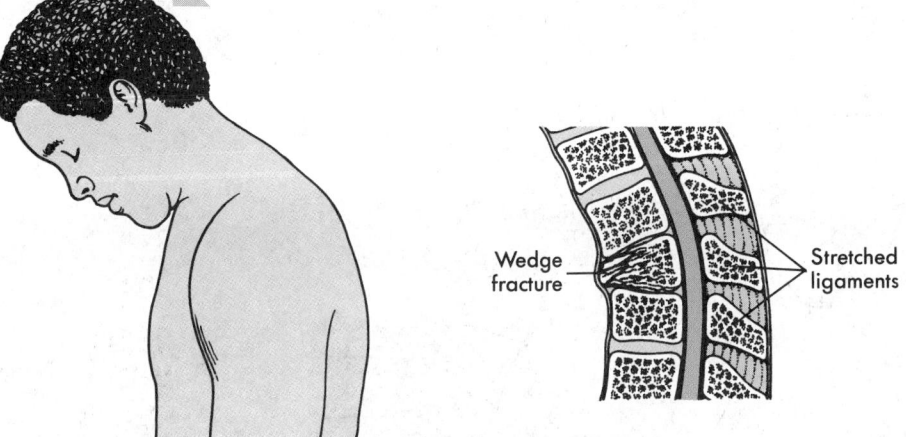

FIGURE 50-6   Spinal cord injury from hyperflexion.

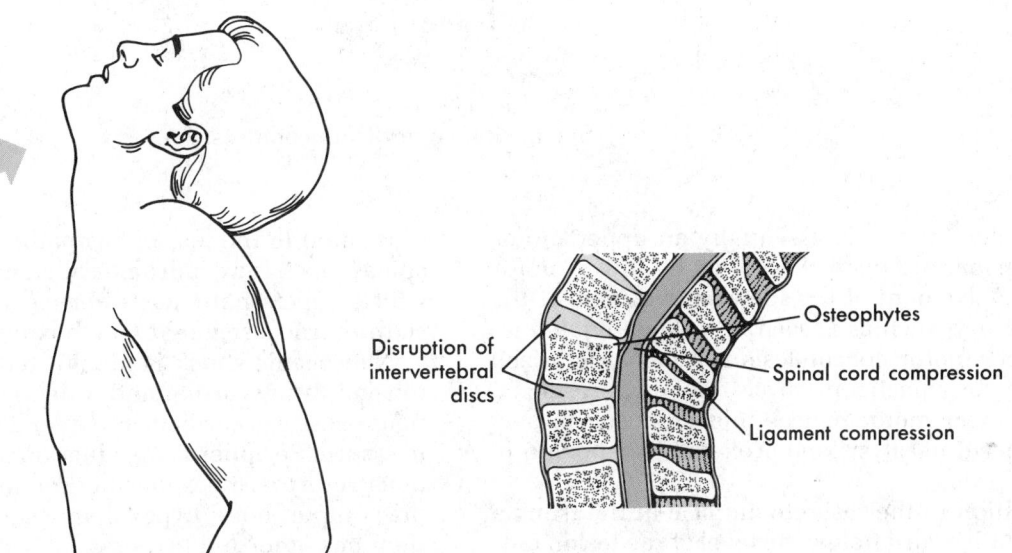

FIGURE 50-7   Spinal cord injury from hyperextension.

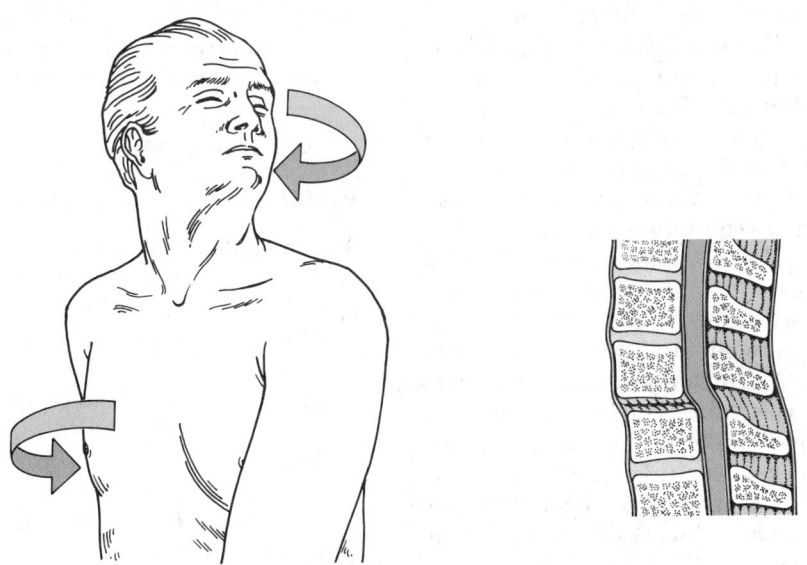

FIGURE 50-8   Spinal cord injury from flexion-rotation.

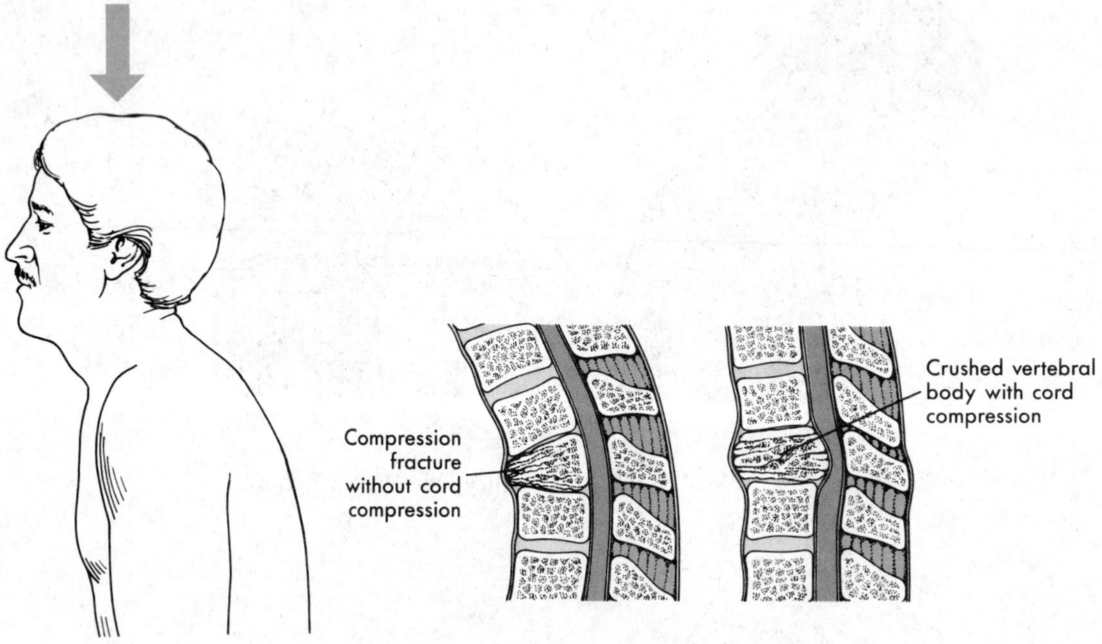

FIGURE 50-9   Spinal cord injury from compression.

Spinal cord injury is essentially an upper motor neuron lesion, although there may be lower motor neuron involvement of the spinal nerve roots at the level of injury, such as is seen in a cauda equina lesion. Upper motor neuron lesions are characterized ultimately by spastic paralysis and hyperreflexia, whereas lower motor neuron injuries result in persistent flaccid paralysis and areflexia (see box on p. 1367).

In addition to the discrete damage at the trauma site, the entire cord below the level of the lesion fails to function, resulting in **spinal shock.** This loss of function below the level of the injury generally occurs immediately after the cord injury. Spinal shock is thought to be caused by the sudden withdrawal of the predominately facilitatory influences of the descending spinal cord tracts complicated by persistent inhibition of extensor reflexes from below the lesion.[7,38] The connections between the brain and spinal cord at and below the level of the lesion are interrupted; so during this shock phase the spinal cord ceases to function. The patient exhibits a flaccid paralysis and loss of sensation below the level of the injury. The intensity of spinal shock varies with the level of the lesion, with the reflexes closest to the injury most severely affected for a greater period of time. The duration of spinal shock varies considerably and may persist for days or weeks after the injury. Indications that spinal shock has dissipated include the return of reflexes (hyperreflexia), muscle spasms, and reflex emptying of the bowel and bladder. When spinal shock has resolved, active rehabilitation can begin.

Related to the loss of sympathetic outflow during spinal shock is a syndrome called **neurogenic shock,** which affects patients suffering injuries above the sixth thoracic segment (see box on p. 1367).

Neurogenic shock is manifested by severe hypotension, bradycardia, and a decrease in central venous pressure, cardiac output, and pulmonary artery pressure. Peripheral vasodilation and decreased venous return are responsible for the decreased cardiac output, not a hypovolemic state, unless the patient has other multitrauma injuries. Poikilothermy, the inability to regulate body temperature, may also be noted during this phase and results in the patient taking on the temperature of the environment. Neurogenic shock is a time-limited process and resolves with supportive treatment to minimize the associated cardiovascular problems.[7]

Therapeutic Management

Prehospital and emergency management

The initial consideration is the recognition of spinal cord injury. The most significant symptoms of acute spinal cord injuries follow:

Motor signs: weakness or paralysis of extremities or trunk muscles

Sensory signs: absence or alteration of sensation of the trunk or extremities

Incontinence: loss of bowel and bladder control

Superficial signs: abrasions, lacerations, or deformities of the spine, neck, or head regions

Pain: tenderness or pain on palpation of the spine or neck

MOTOR NEURON LESIONS

Upper motor neuron area

Includes neurons in the cerebral cortex, thalamus, brainstem, and corticospinal and rubrospinal tracts

Essential for voluntary movement

Activity influenced and modified by the basal ganglia and cerebellum

Dysfunction results in spastic paralysis, loss of voluntary movement, hyperreflexia, and reflexive bowel, bladder, and sexual responses

Lower motor neuron area

Includes the motor neurons of the brainstem, cranial nerves, and anterior horn cells of the spinal cord

Directly innervates skeletal muscles and is essential for muscle contraction

Injury results in flaccid paralysis, areflexia, bowel and bladder hypoactivity, and sexual dysfunction

---

CLINICAL ALERT

Neurogenic Shock

Can be a life-threatening early complication of spinal cord injury, especially in patients with a high thoracic or cervical injury

Is caused by the loss of sympathetic innervation to the heart and peripheral vasomotor centers

Can result in severe bradycardia, dysrhythmias, and significant hypotension

Occurs immediately after injury and may continue for several days to weeks after injury

Symptoms

Heart rate of 40 to 50 beats/min

Systolic blood pressure less than 90 mm Hg

Warm, dry extremities

Loss of reflexes below the level of the lesion

Treatment

Monitor heart rate, blood pressure, mentation, and urine output

Administer intravenous fluids to maintain intravascular volume

Vasopressor support may be required in the intensive care unit if patient does not respond to fluid challenge

Patient Teaching

Patient must understand that this is an expected complication of spinal cord injury and requires frequent evaluation

Reassure patient that symptoms of spinal shock will resolve

In addition to the above signs, any unconscious person who has undergone trauma is considered to have a spinal cord injury until proven otherwise.

The airway, breathing, and cardiovascular status of the patient is evaluated immediately. Airway patency and respirations are evaluated initially. A jaw thrust maneuver is used without hyperextending the neck to establish an airway in any patient with a suspected spinal cord injury. In an unconscious patient a full standard oral airway is inserted. The unconscious patient who does not breathe spontaneously, as determined by auscultation of the lungs, is intubated using a rapid induction anesthetic technique or by blind nasotracheal technique. Arterial blood gases are used as a guide for oxygen application.

It is important to treat hypotension, if present, as quickly as possible to improve tissue perfusion. Judicious use of fluids to expand the total blood volume is appropriate. The use of peripheral vasoconstrictors to raise the systolic blood pressure is also recommended in the intensive care environment. Low doses of dopamine or dobutamine are started and titrated to a mean arterial blood pressure of 80 mm Hg.[12] Atropine is recommended if the pulse drops below 40 beats/min.[14]

Trauma patients commonly have multiple injuries, including intra-abdominal, chest, and long bone trauma. A thorough systems assessment is done to rule out any injury that can cause bleeding leading to hemorrhagic shock. The patient may be incapable of sensing cutaneous or acute pain. The patient may, however, feel visceral sensations of discomfort.

If other injuries are found, prompt surgical intervention is needed to prevent further circulatory compromise. The nurse documents baseline motor movement, strength, and sensory level when caring for the spinal cord–injured patient. Assessment includes testing all major muscle groups and sensory dermatomes, which is detailed later in this chapter. Level of consciousness, memory, and mentation are also assessed on the spinal cord–injured patient to check for possible head injury.

Immobilization

Care must be taken when moving the person. There should be no attempt to flex or rotate the head, neck, or torso. All patients are placed in a neutral position with the head and neck in proper alignment with the body. Generally, a rigid cervical collar is applied to the patient, and the patient is secured on a

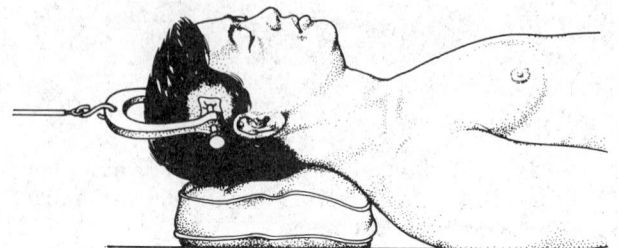

FIGURE 50-10   Gardner-Wells tongs.

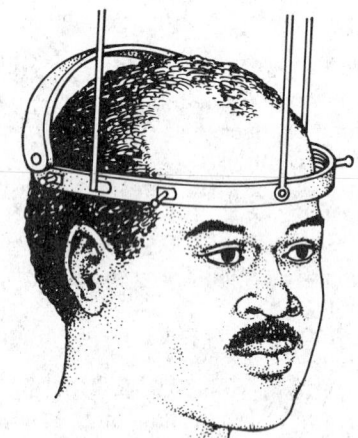

FIGURE 50-11   Halo ring.

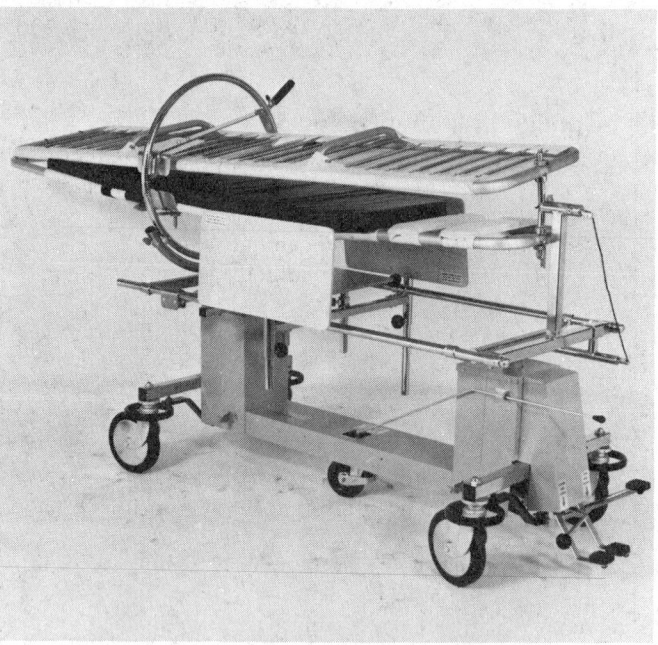

FIGURE 50-12   Stryker frame. (Courtesy Orthopedic Frame Co., Kalamazoo, Mich.)

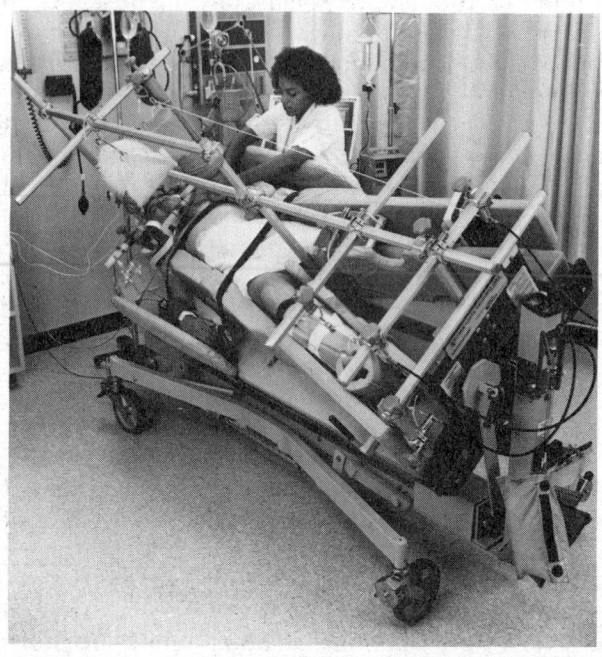

FIGURE 50-13   Kinetic treatment table. (Courtesy Kinetic Concepts, Inc., San Antonio, Texas.)

backboard. Beside a collar, the head is secured to the backboard with tape to prevent movement. Proper immobilization of the neck and the aggressive reestablishment of spinal alignment are essential to the reestablishment of physiologic homeostasis. For cervical injuries, skeletal traction is usually provided by Crutchfield, Gardner-Wells, or some other type of skull tongs or halo ring (Figures 50-10 and 50-11). Traction is provided by attaching a rope to tongs guided over a pulley with weights attached to the end.

Once cervical traction has been applied, the patient is often placed on a special frame or bed for continued management. Stryker frames (Figure 50-12) and the kinetic treatment tables (Figure 50-13) are most commonly used. The **Stryker frame** employs a side-to-side lateral turn on which the patient remains either prone or supine. Caution is used when turning the patient to a prone position. Compression of the diaphragm may result in continued respiratory compromise. The nurse supports weak or paralyzed limbs to prevent the limbs from falling off or out of the frame during the turning process. Patients who exhibit unstable hemodynamic or cardiac parameters may not be able to tolerate a prone position. The kinetic therapy treatment table (Roto-

rest bed) uses a continual side-to-side slow rotation with the patient in constant motion. This bed assists in the prevention of secondary injury in the patient. If properly used, the bed helps prevent pressure sores, respiratory complications, muscle wasting,

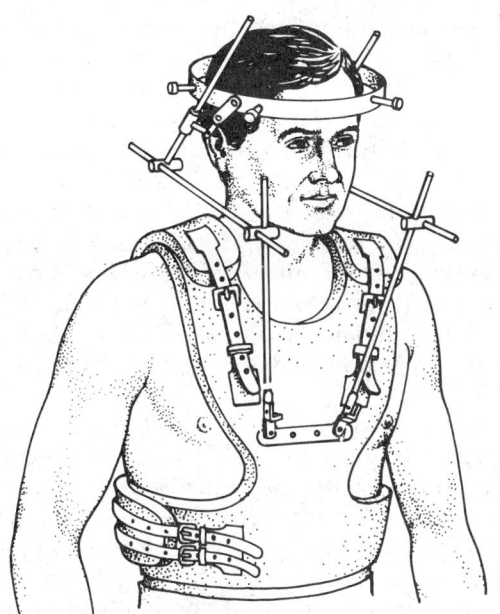

FIGURE 50-14   Halo vest.

bone demineralization, urinary stasis, and renal calculi.[4,37]

Spinal injuries, like any other bony injury, require extended immobilization to promote healing and prevent further disruption at the injured or operative site. One way to maintain cervical immobilization yet facilitate early mobility is placement of the patient in a halo brace (Figure 50-14). A number of halo devices are available, but their basic construction is similar. Four pins are inserted through a ring encircling the patient's head; these pins are advanced through the skin or scalp and secured to the outer table of the skull. Strut bars attach the ring to a plastic vest. The halo vest is applied after cervical injury or surgery when the patient is hemodynamically stable. Once vertebrally stable in a halo brace, the patient can be mobilized as rapidly as tolerated. Most halo braces are now made of graphite and are magnetic resonance imaging (MRI) compatible.

Surgical intervention is indicated for patients who have not attained normal vertebral alignment by traction, if there is bony compression on the cord from a burst fracture, or if vertebral fracture fragments shift their relative positions, resulting in vertebral instability. Anterior and posterior approaches to the spine are employed for optimum decompression and fusion. Bone grafts using autologous or donated bone may be used in addition to wire, rod, or plate instrumentation to support the fracture area and facilitate bone healing. Early surgical stabilization allows for early mobilization of the spinal cord–injured patient.[26]

Pharmacologic therapy

Although somewhat controversial, high-dose corticosteroid treatment of acute spinal cord injury is now recommended.[5] It is hypothesized that high-dose methylprednisolone administered within 8 hours after injury suppresses the breakdown of cellular membranes and secondarily improves blood flow to the ischemic spinal cord. Patients receiving high-dose methylprednisolone within 8 hours after injury are reported to have improved motor and sensation to pinprick and touch 6 weeks and 6 months after treatment. Initially the patient receives an intravenous methylprednisolone bolus of 30 mg/kg of body weight within the first hour of hospitalization. For the next 23 hours the patient receives a maintenance dose of 5.4 mg/kg/h in a continuous infusion. Patients with penetrating trauma should not receive high-dose corticosteroids because of the potential increased risk of infection. During and immediately after the infusion the patient must be observed carefully for untoward effects, such as nausea, vomiting, gastrointestinal bleeding, or steroid psychosis.

Complications

Altered respiratory function is a significant issue for the patient with a cervical or high thoracic injury. If the injury is at or above C3, the patient is likely to be ventilator dependent, with loss of or significant impairment in the ability to maintain independent ventilation. Paralysis of intercostal and abdominal muscles predisposes the patient to ineffective cough ability and retention of secretions. The nurse also considers the potential progressive development of swelling within the cord in anticipation of respiratory complications. In patients with high level lesions, as edema increases, so does the risk of pulmonary compromise from respiratory muscle weakening and fatigue. Respiratory embarrassment may take 24 to 72 hours to manifest. Other complications include urinary tract infection and the development of deep vein thrombosis. The spinal cord–injured patient is also at high risk for development of decubitus ulcer.

NURSING MANAGEMENT OF THE PATIENT WITH SPINAL CORD INJURY: ACUTE PHASE
Assessment

Neurologic assessment of the patient with spinal cord injury focuses on motor and sensory function. Special attention is paid to voluntary motor ability, position and vibratory sense, and pain and temperature perception. All major muscle groups are tested first by asking the patient to move the extremities. If the patient is able to lift each extremity off the

MOTOR SCORE GRADES

> 0 = absent motor activity
> 1 = trace function; evidence of muscle contraction
>   without joint movement
> 2 = motor present with gravity eliminated
> 3 = motor present against gravity
> 4 = motor present against some resistance
> 5 = motor present against full resistance

bed, the examiner then applies a force to each muscle group, which the patient attempts to resist. While the nurse is assessing voluntary motor movement (corticospinal tract function), the patient is asked to flex, extend, abduct, and adduct each extremity (see box above for motor score grades).

Sensory function is assessed by testing either pain or temperature perception (spinothalamic tract function) by specific dermatomes (see Figure 44-5). Painful stimuli are delivered by gentle pinprick with emphasis on the patient's description of the stimuli being sharp or dull. Posterior (dorsal) column function is evaluated by light touch, pressure, or proprioceptive (position sense) testing. A neuromuscular assessment is performed routinely (every 2 to 4 hours initially) and also with changes in traction or whenever the patient is transferred from bed to diagnostic surface, especially if the move necessitates the patient's removal from traction by the physician.

Orthopedic alignment impacts on the neurologic status of the spinal cord–injured patient. Patient injury related to a fracture or instability in the spinal column necessitates evaluating effectiveness and integrity of skeletal traction. Tong insertion sites, maintenance of weights, and system stability are assessed every 8 hours.

Cardiovascular assessment of the spinal cord–injured patient includes heart rate, blood pressure, and a peripheral vascular survey and frequently necessitates continuous hemodynamic monitoring.[25] A Swan-Ganz catheter may be inserted during the neurogenic shock phase to monitor cardiac output and pulmonary artery pressures. This therapy continues until cardiovascular stability is maintained. Cardiac rhythm monitoring is also essential in the acutely injured patient. Auscultation of the heart is important, as is blood work analysis of serum enzyme levels to detect cardiac ischemia.

Assessment of the respiratory system includes respiratory rate, breathing patterns, breath sounds, and pulmonary parameters such as forced vital capacity and negative inspiratory force.[17] Forced vital capacity is a measure of the amount of air expelled by the patient in one forceful exhalation and is measured in liters; negative inspiratory force is a measure of the maximum force a patient generates during inhalation and is measured in pounds per square inch (psi). Additional parameters such as pulse-oximetry oxygen saturation or arterial blood gases are valuable in evaluating respiratory function. Respiratory assessment is performed on admission and then every 2 to 4 hours for the first 72 hours after admission. Respiratory parameters are evaluated independently and also comparatively to identify a significant upward or downward trend in pulmonary reserve.

Physical assessment of the abdomen includes inspection, auscultation, palpation, and percussion. Auscultation for the presence of bowel sounds is necessary to initiate enteral feedings. Since routine assessment parameters such as abdominal pain and tenderness are not valid in the spinal cord–injured patient, measurement of abdominal girth can assist in identification of occult abdominal bleeding or gas. Noting presence of bowel sounds also guides implementation of a bowel program.

Urinary output is a vital assessment feature in the acute care phase, not only for evaluation of renal function, but also for assessing adequacy of kidney perfusion. Following spinal cord injury, the bladder is typically areflexic and flaccid and therefore requires regular emptying for proper management. If frequent assessment of urinary output is necessary, a Foley catheter is inserted; otherwise, intermittent catheterization (every 4 to 6 hours) may be appropriate.

A thorough skin inspection is performed and recorded, including preexisting disruptions in integument. The nurse assesses skeletal traction sites and identifies actual and potential pressure areas.

Nutritional assessment parameters also need to be evaluated.[3] Anthropomorphic measurements are helpful in addition to serum albumin, hemoglobin, hematocrit, and urinary creatinine clearance measurements. Caloric intake is recorded to evaluate nutritional adequacy.

Nursing Diagnosis

During the acute phase of care, nursing diagnoses may include the following:

Altered tissue perfusion: central nervous system, related to spinal instability

Altered cardiac output related to peripheral dilation caused by loss of vasomotor tone

Impaired gas exchange related to muscle fatigue and retained secretions

Ineffective airway clearance related to muscle weakness and poor cough

Impaired physical mobility related to motor paralysis

Alteration in bowel function related to disruption of autonomic innervation

Alteration in urinary elimination related to disruption of reflex and voluntary bladder control

High risk for skin disruption related to immobility and impaired tissue perfusion

High risk for altered nutrition: less than body requirements caused by disruption in gastric motility and increased caloric demands from trauma and stress

Self-care deficit related to paralysis

Knowledge deficit related to spinal cord injury

Powerlessness related to paralysis

Ineffective coping: family and individual, related to trauma, life-style changes, and disability

Alteration in sexual response

Planning

Specific outcome criteria for the acute plan of care include the following:

Progression of neurologic deficit will be identified rapidly

Vertebral column immobility will be maintained

Blood pressure will be within normal limits

Airway will remain patent

Effective bowel elimination will be maintained

Effective urinary elimination will be maintained

Skin will remain intact

Adequate nutrition will be maintained

Self-care needs will be met

Patient will maintain control over at least one aspect of care

Patient/family will verbalize fears and concerns over injury and rehabilitation

Implementation

The nurse's key intervention in ensuring optimum neurologic function is performing, evaluating, and comparing serial motor and sensory assessments. The physician is notified if the patient experiences any disturbance or loss of function in motor or sensory segments. Vertebral immobility and skeletal traction must be maintained on patients with vertebral instability. The nurse ensures that the appropriate weights are applied and effective traction is delivered. The nurse is not responsible for adding or removing weights from the system. The physical hazards and complications of therapeutic immobilization are offset when caring for the patient on a specialty bed, such as a kinetic therapy table or Stryker frame; however, physical mobility remains an important nursing goal.

Joint mobility is preserved with passive range of motion exercises to uninjured upper and lower extremities. The spinal cord–injured patient requires functional splinting, which can be initiated immediately after injury. Patients with wrist paralysis (C5 or above) benefit from application of a tenodesis splint, a device that enables the patient to develop a functional contracture at the wrist, making a grasp possible by passive thumb opposition. Footdrop is prevented by application of high-top sneakers or an orthotic device to support the ankle. Any supportive device is applied and removed every 2 hours to prevent skin complications. Muscle strengthening exercises are also initiated, because atrophy and muscle weakness usually occur during the acute postinjury phase.

Cardiovascular function depends on the degree of neurogenic shock. Initially, continuous electrocardiographic and hemodynamic monitoring of the patient is essential. Intravenous fluid administration is necessary to maintain adequate intravascular fluid volume; however, if neurogenic shock progresses, vasopressor support is instituted. The immobility of the patient superimposed on the injury contributes to poor venous return from the extremities, and dependent edema may be noted. Promoting blood flow through the paralyzed limbs will increase venous return to the heart. Limb elevation, range of motion exercises, antiembolic stockings, and alternating pressure devices may be used to promote venous return and prevent pooling of blood in the periphery. These measures and the administration of subcutaneous heparin are used to prevent deep vein thrombosis.

Maintaining effective ventilation and oxygenation is a key issue on which the nurse must focus. Spinal cord–injured patients frequently require aggressive pulmonary toilet including application and monitoring of supplemental oxygen, humidification, chest physiotherapy, administration of systemic or inhaled bronchodilating agents (aminophylline, isoetharine hydrochloride), and delivery of quad-assist cough. The quad-assist cough is a technique in which the nurse delivers a manual diaphragmatic thrust coordinated with the patient's cough effort. This action supports the diaphragm and simulates abdominal muscle action, assisting to force secretions upward and out. These measures may be required as frequently as every 1 to 2 hours initially and then every 4 hours.

Patients who demonstrate poor oxygenation, decreased ventilation, or respiratory fatigue are electively intubated and supported with mechanical ventilation until they demonstrate weaning ability. Subtle signs of respiratory insufficiency such as a decreased level of consciousness, confusion, restlessness, and increased shallow breathing may be noted but may be attributed to other etiologies, such as associated closed head injury, substance withdrawal, or administration of narcotic or relaxing agents. Tachycardia and vascular changes in the periphery (common patient responses to hypoxia) may *not* be

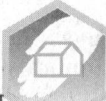

HOME CARE GUIDE   *Intermittent Catheterization*

Intermittent bladder catheterization is a method of draining the urinary bladder by inserting a catheter. Emptying the bladder on an intermittent basis permits a more normal functioning of the bladder, and complete emptying of the bladder eliminates the need for an indwelling catheter and prevents urinary incontinence. The procedure in the home setting is done as a clean technique and can be taught to the patient before discharge.

Short-term goals

By the time of discharge, the patient will:

Be able to do self-catheterization using clean technique.

Have basic knowledge of fluid balance and signs and symptoms of infection.

Understand the importance of personal hygiene, such as washing hands.

Long-term goals

The patient will be able to incorporate intermittent catheterization into the life-style with minimal interruption.

The patient will demonstrate compliance in all aspects of management of bladder emptying to prevent recurrent infection and encourage possible return of function of the bladder.

Nursing assessment

The patient must be assessed for ability to manage the procedure and understand all aspects of care.

The pattern of self-catheterization should be determined, taking into consideration the patient's planned life-style. The patient may need to do the procedure every 4 hours and thus must be near a bathroom suitable for the procedure.

Planning

A. Planning for discharge of a patient who will need to do self-catheterization should be started to allow the patient to practice the procedure three or four times before discharge.

B. Patient education should include the following:

1. Equipment needed includes a catheter and water-soluble lubricant, soap and warm water, cloths for carrying the catheter.

2. A urinal or other large container with measurements marked in ounces to measure the amount of urine is recommended for patients who are doing self-catheterization for residual urine.

3. Hand washing for 5 minutes with soap and warm water must be done before handling the clean catheter.

4. The catheter can be reused several times; thus it must be washed with soap and warm water, drained, and allowed to dry. The catheter can be carried in a clean cloth such as a washcloth.

5. The need for increased fluid intake must be stressed to ensure fluid balance.

6. Scheduling of the procedure and the need for regular self-catheterization should also be stressed, because the patient will not feel bladder distention or the need to void.

7. The signs and symptoms of urinary tract infection are included in teaching. Signs such as cloudy urine or foul-smelling urine or fever may indicate bladder problems. Changes in bowel patterns, such as diarrhea, may also indicate a bladder problem and thus should not be ignored. Bladder discomfort or pain will not be felt by the patient; therefore the other signs and symptoms are important.

C. The following information should be used as a guide for patient teaching:

1. Female catheterization: for an older woman with poor vision this may be a very difficult procedure to perform. The procedure can be done while sitting on the toilet or commode or by placing the open end of the catheter into a urinal. The patient should wash her hands before beginning the procedure.

   a. Lubricate the tip of the catheter.

   b. Wash the perineal area with soap and water.

   c. Wash your hands well with warm soapy water, rinse, and dry.

   d. Take the catheter in one hand 2 to 3 inches from the tip.

   e. Spread the labia apart and insert the catheter into the meatus. This procedure will take practice, and a mirror may help the patient locate the meatus.

   f. Insert the catheter until a flow of urine starts.

   g. When the stream of urine flows, press the lower abdomen to completely empty the bladder.

   h. Remove the catheter slowly.

   i. If necessary, measure the collected urine, and record the amount.

   j. Make other observations such as blood in the urine, foul odor, or increased cloudiness of the urine. Notify the physician of any of these observations.

   k. Clean the catheter, and store for the next use.

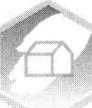

HOME CARE GUIDE *Intermittent Catheterization—cont'd*

2. Male catheterization: This procedure can be done over a toilet or commode or by draining the urine into a urinal. The patient should wash his hands before starting the procedure.
   a. Generously lubricate the tip of the catheter.
   b. Wash the penis well with soap and water.
   c. Wash hands with warm soapy water, rinse, and dry.
   d. Pick up the catheter 2 to 3 inches from the tip.
   e. Insert the catheter into the meatus, and slowly insert the catheter until a flow of urine starts from the end of the catheter.
   f. When the stream slows, gently press on the lower abdomen to empty the bladder.
   g. Remove the catheter slowly.
   h. If necessary, measure the urine, and record the amount.
   i. Make other observations such as blood in the urine, a foul odor, or increased cloudiness. Notify the physician of any of these observations.
   j. Clean the catheter, and store for the next use.

---

seen in the spinal shock phase because of the disruption of sympathetic fibers. The patient must also be observed carefully for signs and symptoms of pulmonary infection in order to initiate appropriate antibiotic therapy.

Genitourinary function is managed initially by ensuring regular bladder emptying via intermittent catheterization or insertion of a Foley or suprapubic catheter. Urine is routinely examined for color, clarity, odor, sediment, or occult or frank blood. Signs of urinary tract infection must be reported promptly to the physician to initiate proper therapy.[15]

In the absence of bowel activity, the patient must be given nothing by mouth. A nasogastric tube is inserted to decompress the stomach, since vomiting will predispose the patient to aspiration and further pulmonary compromise.[15] The patient with a spinal cord injury is at high risk for gastric ulceration, which can be avoided by testing gastric pH and delivering antacids when necessary or on a routine basis. The patient also benefits from continuous or intermittent administration of a histamine-receptor antagonist, such as cimetidine or ranitidine. A bowel program is initiated with the return of intestinal peristalsis as soon as possible after injury. Oral stool softeners and bulking agents are administered routinely. Suppositories are administered daily or on an every-other-day basis to establish regular bowel evacuation. Digital stimulation may also be used to initiate reflex bowel emptying once spinal shock has resolved.

Another nursing care focus is to prevent a disruption in skin integrity. Localized changes from microscopic ischemic changes in capillary blood flow from pressure can be reversed if the pressure is relieved every 2 hours. Regular turning and bridging of bony prominences remain significant in prevention and treatment of pressure sores. Correct positioning of the patient is essential. The patient should be moved carefully to avoid shearing and friction forces. Patients sitting in a wheelchair require weight shifting to redistribute body weight for a short period of time (5 to 10 minutes every 2 hours). Bony prominences that remain reddened even after weight shifting has been performed are at high risk for pressure sore development. Alternate positions are employed to maximize circulation to high-risk areas. Care must be taken to look underneath assistive devices, splints, and supports (including the halo vest) for skin irritation. A flashlight is helpful to identify reddened areas.

Nutrition of the spinal cord–injured patient is addressed as soon as possible after admission. Nutrition can be delivered parenterally if the patient experiences a significant paralytic ileus or requires an endotracheal tube. The enteral route is preferred, and oral or tube feedings are initiated when the patient regains bowel sounds. It is helpful if a professional specializing in swallowing dysfunction evaluates the swallowing function of patients who have tracheostomy tubes, are in halo vests, or are restricted to a supine position. The patient's nutritional status can be evaluated by means of calorie counts, monitoring serum albumin and transferrin levels, and also via urinary creatinine clearance testing, which reveals nitrogen balance. Once enteral nutrition is established, the patient is encouraged to eat high-fiber, high-protein foods to rebuild lost protein stores and enhance motility of wastes through the gut.

The psychologic impact of spinal cord injury is devastating to both the patient and family. Coping responses are quite variable and depend on the patient's previous method of coping, support systems, and ability to understand and process the compli-

cated and permanent nature of spinal cord injury. Powerlessness is one natural response in which nurses can intervene best by establishing a communication pattern with the patient and allowing the patient some choices regarding care. The choices are small at first and may focus on comfort measures or sequencing of care and therapies. Although limited, allowing such seemingly minor choices is the basis on which the patient's senses of self and individuality are rebuilt. It is important at this stage to answer the patient's and family's questions as honestly as possible but not deprive the patient of hope.

Evaluation

Care is evaluated daily. Each expected outcome of care is compared with the actual outcome. The freedom from complications indicates that appropriate care measures have been taken. Preparation of the patient for discharge is a key factor throughout acute care and rehabilitation. Ensuring maximum functionality is also a key evaluation component.

Documentation

It is important to monitor and chart the patient's ability to tolerate and perform activities. Note progress toward the goals of care with specific descriptions of the patient's activity and behavior. Document deviations from the baseline, and notify the physician promptly with this information. Evaluation of the care plan is also clearly documented on a routine basis. Changes in the care plan should be made as needed. Specific schedules for the patient are designed with the patient and documented for all health care team members to see. This not only provides consistency of care for the patient, but also allows the patient some control over activities. Clear discharge documentation regarding the patient's abilities and disabilities is important for the follow-up care to be provided.

Ongoing Care

The spinal cord–injured patient with disability may be discharged from the acute care facility to one of three places: a rehabilitation center, a long-term care center (nursing home), or home. The destination depends on the level of function the patient exhibits, social support systems, and potential to realize rehabilitation goals.

Rehabilitation

Many centers across the United States are dedicated to the rehabilitation of the spinal cord–injured patient. Intensive rehabilitation helps the patient function at the highest level of wellness. Many of the problems identified in the acute phase of care become chronic and continue throughout life, such as bowel and bladder dysfunction and skin issues. Rehabilitation is concerned with refined retraining of the physiologic processes. Braces, electric wheelchairs, and a variety of mechanical apparatuses are used to maximize the functional level of the patient. Goals of rehabilitation are aimed at facilitating patient function in the community.

Long-term care

A few spinal cord–injured patients are not rehabilitation candidates. Usually these are elderly or ventilator-dependent quadriplegic patients. In these cases the patient may be sent to a nursing home for long-term care. It is important that the caregivers at the extended care facility understand the needs of the patient. Sending a copy of the care plan will be helpful for the caregivers. The patient may feel depressed over the decision to send him or her to an extended care facility, so supportive care is essential. Follow-up to the extended care facility may be helpful not only to the caregivers there, but also to the patient and family.

NURSING MANAGEMENT OF THE PATIENT WITH SPINAL CORD INJURY: REHABILITATION PHASE
Assessment

Rehabilitation of the spinal cord–injured patient begins on admission to the health care delivery system; however, once the patient has progressed past the acute phase of the illness, the primary patient care focus is on increasing activity, mobility tolerance, promoting self-care activities, and patient/family education. Mobilization begins as soon as the patient is vertebrally stable; however, it is a gradual process with the spinal cord–injured patient. The head of the patient's bed is elevated slowly, and the patient's vital signs are monitored closely for tolerance to el-

LEGAL ISSUES   *The Americans with Disabilities Act of 1990*

Signed into law July 26, 1990, the Americans with Disabilities Act of 1990 (ADA) has far-reaching implications for medical-surgical nurses and their patients. The primary goal of this act is the eradication of discrimination against disabled persons in all areas of life. ADA complements and vastly extends the scope of the Rehabilitation Act of 1973. Whereas the Rehabilitation Act affected only those businesses receiving federal contracts or monies, ADA affects almost all businesses or services in the United States, whether public or private.

Specific provisions of the act have relevance for nursing practice for the foreseeable future and can be expected to create a revolution in the way disabled persons are treated in our society. In particular, ADA bans discrimination against anyone with an actual disability (an impairment that substantially limits one or more of the major life functions of an individual), a person with a record of such an impairment, a person regarded as having an impairment, or a person who associates with or is related to an individual with an impairment. A number of conditions are covered under this definition, including acquired immune deficiency syndrome (AIDS), cancer, burn victims with scarring, and morbid obesity if it interferes with one or more major activities of daily living.

The basic provision of the act is that no employer with 15 or more employees may discriminate in any area of employment (application, hiring, training, promotion, or discharge) against any qualified person with a disability. Essential functions of a job must be identified, and if the applicant or employee can perform those with reasonable accommodation, the person cannot be denied employment because he or she is disabled. Only if the accommodation causes undue hardship to the business can the applicant be turned down. The definition of undue hardship is limited, and the business must consider many factors before declaring that a hardship exists.

Other provisions of ADA mandate equal access to public transportation, businesses, and services (including movie theaters, stores, health care provider offices and buildings, and parks and recreation areas).

ADA has significance for medical-surgical nurses' practice in several areas. Disabled patients now have better access to jobs and to public places. Nurses involved with discharge planning can urge such patients to become informed about their rights under the act. Medical facilities are not exempt from the act and must be accessible to all disabled persons. Nurses can provide valuable advice and recommendations to administration as the physical facilities are brought into compliance with the law.

Disabled nurses may wish to exercise their rights under the ADA when applying for positions, whether in nursing or another field. The important point to remember is whether or not the nurse can perform the essential functions of the job, either with or without reasonable accommodation. Impaired nurses in treatment for chemical dependency are covered by the provisions of this act. Although state nursing boards and nursing associations are increasingly supportive of nurses who undergo treatment, such nurses still face obstacles to a successful return to practice. ADA bans such discrimination. Similarly, nurses infected with the AIDS virus may not be forced to give up practice but are governed by the guidelines published by the Centers for Disease Control. Employers may not ask questions concerning medical or physical conditions except as part of a new employee physical if it is required of all new employees.

Under this act, nurses may find themselves faced with new requirements for their facilities and their coworkers. Patients should be informed about their rights, and nurses with disabilities can use the act's provisions to help them remain active in their practice and other aspects of their lives.

From The Americans with Disabilities Act of 1990, 42 sU.S.C. 12101.

---

evation. Low blood pressure states with increased elevation are caused by a lack of vasomotor tone to stimuli and result in venous pooling. Once the patient is mobile, musculoskeletal assessment must include evaluation of joint mobility and function, and presence and degree of spasticity. Both factors impact on methods and strategies for rehabilitation.

Heterotopic ossification is a common sequela to spinal cord injury.[9] This is the formation of bony tissue in the muscles and fascia around joints, particularly the hips and knees, but may involve the shoulders as well. Common presentations of this disorder

are fever, inflammation of a joint (with edema), or decreasing range of motion.

Joint mobility and function are assessed by isolating functional joints and asking the patient to move them to the best of his or her ability. The joint is also assessed passively, so that the nurse or therapist identifies the potential joint range. Spasticity occurs after spinal shock has resolved and reflex activity returns. Spasticity is a symptom characterized by hypertonic muscles, increased resistance to motion, hyperactive deep tendon reflexes, and clonus. Muscle spasms can be so severe at times that they

RESEARCH BRIEF

Dunnum L: Life satisfaction and spinal cord injury: a patient perspective, *J Neurosci Nurs* 22(1):43-47, 1990.

Life expectancy of the spinal cord–injured individual has increased because of advances in medical and nursing care and is now comparable to a non-injured individual. The psychologic, physiologic, and economic impacts of spinal cord injury have led to some assumptions about life satisfaction in this population. This study interviewed 31 spinal cord–injured patients and questioned them regarding life satisfaction issues and physical function. Specific satisfaction issues included social contacts, mood, self-concept, meaning, daily activities, health, goals, and finances. Generally, those interviewed expressed at least average satisfaction with all subscales with the exception of goals and finances. Life satisfaction subscales and measures of physical function were correlated. Low correlations were demonstrated with the subscales of goals, mood, and finances, suggesting that the correlation of these factors is minimally related to physical function. Implications for nursing include a variety of patient-focused interventions. The nurse can be instrumental in assisting the patient and family to develop realistic goals during the acute and rehabilitative phases of care. The nurse may also initiate referrals to social service and vocational counselors early to aid in identification of financial resources for these patients. The nurse is in a unique position to listen to and allow adequate time for the spinal cord–injured patient to vent frustrations, provide support, and help the patient feel more positive.

interfere with the mobilization of the patient.

Pain sensations in the spinal cord–injured patient can be difficult to evaluate because of both the physiologic and psychologic responses to trauma. The spinal cord–injured patient may complain of pain at the fracture site, discomfort with muscle spasms, "phantom pain," visceral discomfort, or "burning," shocklike sensations known as **hyperesthesia.** This pain usually results from irritation of the nerve roots; it is quite persistent and can result in complaints of chronic pain. Muscle spasms may also be a consistent source of painful stimuli to the patient. Pain is best assessed qualitatively, by use of a numeric or color scale.

The long-term cardiovascular response to spinal cord injury depends on the level of injury. Patients with spinal cord injury cannot regulate body temper-

ature below the level of the lesion; therefore thermoregulation can be a long-term issue and temperature is assessed every 8 hours.

Patients with lesions at or above T6 are at risk for experiencing a phenomenon called **autonomic dysreflexia** once reflex activity below the level of the lesion returns. This response occurs as a result of a noxious stimulus below the level of the lesion causing visceral reflex activity, such as distended bowel or bladder or cutaneous stimuli. This can be a life-threatening event for the quadriplegic or high-paraplegic patient.[33] A noxious stimulus creates an exaggerated response of the sympathetic nervous system and is beyond the control of higher centers (Figure 50-15).

Respiratory issues remain long-term barriers for the patient to overcome. The higher the level of the lesion, the more likely the patient is to have long-term respiratory needs that range from ventilator dependency to requiring assistance with coughing. Parameters used to assess the patient acutely, such as forced vital capacity and negative inspiratory force, are assessed again in addition to breath sounds and respiratory rate, but with less frequency, depending on the needs of the patient.

The location and completeness of the spinal cord injury determine the extent to which bowel function is altered. When spinal shock resolves, bowel sounds return to normal, but bowel function does not. The level of the patient's injury determines the type of alteration in bowel elimination the patient will experience. The patient who has sustained a cervical or thoracic injury will have a spastic paralysis (upper motor neuron injury) and an inability to feel the urge to defecate; however, the reflex activity for defecation remains intact with loss of voluntary control. With an injury to the peripheral nerve roots in sacral segments such as that seen in cauda equina lesions, the efferent (outgoing) limb of the reflex arc for defecation is destroyed, and anal tone is lost. Fecal retention and oozing of stool through the flaccid sphincter are associated with this type of injury (lower motor neuron damage). Assessment focuses on a history of past elimination patterns, problems, current status of the gastrointestinal tract, sphincter tone, and type of diet the patient tolerates.

Urinary continence also depends on the presence of lower motor or upper motor neuron damage. The patient is assessed for urinary retention, continence, voiding patterns, or ability to void reflexively. Patients who require Foley catheters or any invasive method of bladder emptying are assessed for integrity of the system, urine characteristics, and signs and symptoms of urinary tract infection.

Skin remains a lifelong issue for patients with spinal cord injury. Skin is assessed routinely (at least every 8 hours) for actual or potential disruption sites. Special care must be taken to inspect areas

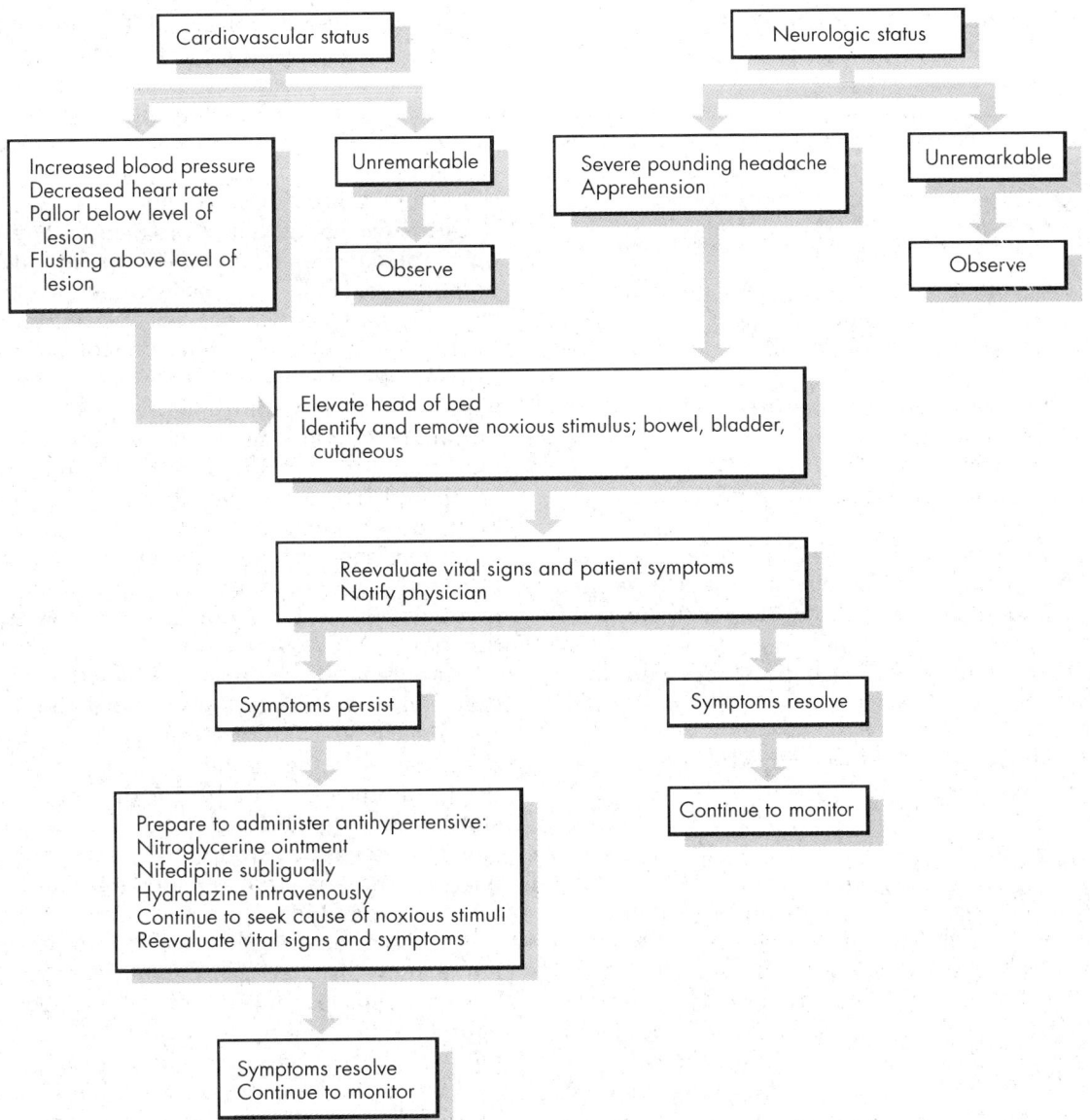

FIGURE 50-15   Critical Thinking Guide: patient with autonomic dysreflexia.

hidden by splints or braces; pressure points at insensate areas are at very high risk for pressure breakdown.

Coping behaviors are identified early in rehabilitative phases and will impact on the patient and family's ability to learn and manage patient care over the long term. Anger and denial are common initial responses by both the patient and family. It is helpful to identify previous adaptive coping mechanisms and support systems.

Nursing Diagnosis

During the rehabilitative phase of care, the following nursing diagnoses may apply:

Impaired physical mobility related to paralysis, muscle spasms, and disuse of joints

Pain related to muscle spasms or disruption of nerve fibers

High risk for impaired skin integrity related to immobility, impaired tissue perfusion, and lack of protective sensation

Ineffective airway clearance related to respiratory muscle weakness/paralysis

Alteration in hemodynamic response to sympathetic stimuli related to autonomic dysfunction

Alteration in bowel elimination related to immobility and loss of voluntary bowel sphincter control

Alteration in urine elimination related to loss of voluntary urinary sphincter control

Self-care deficit related to paralysis

Knowledge deficit related to spinal cord injury

Ineffective individual coping related to injury and long-term changes in life-style

Alteration in sexual expression related to physical changes in sexual function and sensation

Planning

Specific outcome criteria for the care plan include the following:

Optimum joint function and mobility will be maintained

Pain will be relieved or moderated

Skin will remain intact

Airway will remain patent

Blood pressure will remain within normal limits

Adequate nutrition will be maintained

Bowel evacuation will occur at regular intervals

Bladder evacuation will occur at regular intervals

Patient and family will direct/demonstrate self-care skills

Patient and family will verbalize fears and concerns regarding changes in life-style as a result of injury

Sexual concerns will be verbalized in an accepting environment

Implementation

When the patient is orthopedically and hemodynamically stable, the mobilization process begins. Orthopedic stability is usually maintained by some type of external fixation. The patient with a cervical injury may require halo brace immobilization; the patient with a thoracic or lumbar injury may be fitted for a "clamshell" brace, or a body cast may be applied. The nurse initially cares for these devices (see box on Care of the patient in a halo brace). The patient and family are taught all aspects of mobilization, activity, skin inspection, and hygiene before discharge. A teaching plan is developed to ensure that the patient and family are independent and comfortable with these skills by the time of discharge (see home care guide on caring for the individual in a halo brace).

Advancing the mobility of the patient is integral in promoting self-care activities. Initially the head of the bed is elevated slowly with constant monitoring of blood pressure and tolerance to elevation. It is important to anticipate some degree of postural hypotension in the spinal cord−injured patient, and the patient should receive information regarding what to expect and when to alert the nurse. Specific interventions aimed at maintaining the patient's blood pressure during elevation are application of elastic stockings or wraps on the lower extremities and an abdominal binder to decrease venous pooling in the periphery. The patient gradually gains tolerance in changes of body position. If the patient is upright and complains of dizziness, it is necessary to place him or her back in a recumbent position. Initial mobilization efforts are made in reclining wheelchairs that can easily be repositioned to accommodate the patient's positioning requirements.[24]

Transferring the patient to a chair can initially require the coordination of a five-person lift. Once the patient gradually is accustomed to positional changes, one- or two-person transfers are possible for the quadriplegic patient. Paraplegic patients are instructed on independent transfer maneuvers with use of a transfer board. Transfer ability and rehabilitative function again depend on the degree of joint mobility and function. Splinting therapies are continued from the acute care setting, with the "2 hours on−2 hours off" routine. Active range of motion exercises are taught and encouraged by the multidisciplinary team; passive range remains a requirement for joints with no or weak voluntary motor function.

Autonomic dysreflexia is a serious complication that can occur in the spinal cord−injured patient (see Figure 50-15). Once the syndrome is identified, the nurse elevates the head of the patient's bed and then examines the patient for the source of noxious stimuli. The rectum is digitally examined (using a gloved finger lubricated with anesthetic gel) for impaction, and any stool is removed. The Foley catheter is examined for patency, or a catheter is inserted in the bladder to relieve urinary distension. The nurse may also change the patient's position and loosen tight clothing to relieve cutaneous pressure stimuli. When the noxious stimulus is removed, the patient's blood pressure will return to baseline. If the patient's blood pressure remains elevated, the physician is notified immediately, and the patient may require antihypertensive treatment with nitroglycerin ointment (1 to 2 inches to chest wall), sublingual nifedipine (10 mg), or intravenous hydralazine (5 to 10 mg).[9] If symptoms of autonomic dysreflexia are not identified and appropriate action is not taken, the patient is at risk for stroke, myocardial infarction, and death.

Once bowel function returns, the patient is a candidate for a daily bowel program. This consists of stool softeners such as ducosate sodium (100 mg three times per day), a bulk-forming agent once each day, and a daily bisacodyl or glycerin suppository. The suppository is administered routinely 30 minutes after the same meal every day to capitalize on the gastrocolic reflex, which facilitates bowel emptying. In patients with increased anal sphincter tone, digital stimulation (insertion of a lubricated, gloved finger into the anus and performing a circular relaxation of the sphincter) is successful in stimulating large bowel elimination. This is performed about 15

CARE OF PATIENT IN HALO BRACE

Purpose: To provide routine hygiene and assessment to a patient in a halo vest.

Equipment

Towels/washcloths
Peroxide
Normal saline solution
Sterile cotton-tipped applicators

Soap/water
Sterile container
Clean sheepskin liner (if needed)

Nursing Interventions	Rationale
1. Explain routine care and procedure to patient.	Provides basis for patient cooperation and education regarding care while in halo
2. Using proper body mechanics, position patient to perform care. Patient is flat on back to gain access to anterior aspect and side lying for posterior aspect.	Decreases risk of injury to patient; patient is repositioned by grasping shoulders, lower extremities, and posterior portions of vest; patient is *never* lifted, turned, or pulled by strut bars
3. Open one side of vest to visualize desired area.	Maintains vest stability
4. Cleanse skin with soap and water.	
5. Perform visual assessment, noting any reddened or open area.	Identifies any high-risk or broken areas of skin
6. Chest physiotherapy may be performed while patient is on side and vest is open.	Allows greater access to thorax, especially at lower lobes
7. Auscultate breath sounds while vest is open.	Allows for identification of adventitious breath sounds over a greater area
8. Rebuckle vest, and reposition patient.	Maintains vest stability
9. Open alternate side of vest, and repeat hygiene and assessment measures.	
10. Perform pin care every 8 hours.	To prevent crust formation and decrease risk of pin infection
a. Mix 1 oz each of hydrogen peroxide and sterile saline in sterile container.	Half-strength solution used for pin care; solution expires within 24 hours of mixing
b. Dip sterile cotton swab in solution, and cleanse around pin. Repeat if necessary to remove old blood, crusts, or exudate.	Sterile technique used for pin care while patient is hospitalized; use clean swab for each pin site cleansed
c. Rinse with sterile cotton swab soaked in saline only.	Not necessary to apply povidone-iodine (Betadine) or antibacterial ointments at pin sites
d. Note pin integrity to insertion area.	Pin should be set tightly at insertion site; disengaged pin or tenting of skin beneath pin suggests patient is no longer in effective traction and should be reported immediately to the physician
e. Identify any signs and symptoms of localized infection.	Redness, swelling, pain, and exudate are symptoms to be reported to physician

to 30 minutes after the suppository has been administered. Patients with poor anal tone often require manual emptying of the rectum.

Timing the implementation of a bladder program after spinal cord injury remains controversial. Since bladder reflexes are commonly the last reflex activity to return, some physicians believe that the patient should be well into the rehabilitative process before a bladder program is initiated. Others feel that the risk of complication and infection is heightened with long-term Foley catheter use. Therefore

the timing of the bladder program may differ from institution to institution. Once bladder training is in progress, the goal is to simulate normal filling and emptying, which is initially achieved by intermittent catheterization. The patient is generally restricted to 2000 mL of fluid daily to prevent large quantities of urine collecting in the bladder between catheterizations. Initially the patient requires straight catheterization every 4 hours. If urine volumes are noted to be less than 200 mL, the timing should be increased to every 6 hours. If more than 500 mL is obtained,

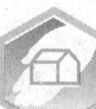

HOME CARE GUIDE   *Caring for Individual in Halo Brace*

Halo immobilization is a commonly used method of cervical fixation. This device maintains traction on and immobilizes the cervical spine while allowing the individual an optimum range of physical mobility. The patient may require halo immobilization for 8 to 12 weeks or longer.

Short-term goals

The patient (or family) will be able to:
Demonstrate pin care and liner change.
Identify high-risk areas for skin irritation.
Explain the purpose of halo immobilization.
Perform hygiene and activities of daily living while in halo brace.
Identify signs and symptoms of pin site infection.
Explain actions in case of emergency.

Long-term goals

The patient will incorporate care of the halo brace into the daily routine with a minimum of disruption.
The patient's cervical spine will remain immobilized to allow for healing of injured or operative site.

Nursing assessment

The patient or family must be assessed for ability to learn and manage the procedure and understand all aspects of care.
The patient's life-style is assessed, and the halo routine is planned within life-style considerations.

Planning

A. Planning for discharge of a patient with a halo brace is initiated when the halo is placed. The patient and family must practice routine care of the brace with supervision and then independently before discharge.
B. Patient education includes the following:
 1. A review of all components of the halo brace and basic maintenance of the suprastructure
 2. Rationale and demonstration of pin site care
 3. Rationale and demonstration of changing the halo vest liner
 4. Discussion of potential areas for skin irritation related to the vest, such as the scapula, rib area, clavicle, and sternum
 5. Demonstration of basic hygiene measures while patient is in halo brace
 6. Demonstration of measures to take in case of emergency, such as choking or cardiac arrest
 7. Rationale of securing a wrench to the body of the halo jacket for emergency use
 8. Discussion of modifications that may be needed for home management, such as:
  a. Restrictions in activity
  b. Comfortable clothing

  c. Sleeping positions
  d. Changes in sexual patterns
C. The following information can be used as a guide for patient teaching.
 1. Checking the suprastructure
  a. Patient is instructed on how to check the screws of the suprastructure. Patient is provided with a wrench for home use to ensure that the screws are at the proper tightness.
  b. Physician is notified if the screws are disengaged.
 2. Performing pin care using clean technique at home
  a. The patient washes hands before cleaning pin sites.
  b. Using a cotton swab, cleanse the pin area with a solution of half peroxide and half saline.
  c. Using a clean applicator, rinse the area with saline. Use a new applicator to cleanse each of the four pin sites.
  d. Inspect each area for redness, pain, drainage, and security of pin to skull.
  e. Notify physician if pin complications occur.
  f. If a pin disengages from the skull, the patient must lie flat and notify the physician immediately.
 3. Changing the vest liner
  a. For any changes of the vest liner, the patient must lie flat before opening the buckled or Velcro sides of the halo vest.
  b. Once the patient is flat, the vest is unbuckled, and the soiled anterior liner is disengaged from the vest.
  c. A clean anterior liner is placed along Velcro guides.
  d. To change the posterior liner, the patient must be either side lying or prone. Any repositioning of the patient necessitates buckling the sides of the vest.
  e. The soiled posterior liner is disengaged from the vest, and a new one is placed along the Velcro guides.
  f. The liners may be sheepskin or acrylic material and can usually be laundered by hand or delicate cycle on machine.
 4. Bathing and grooming: specific suggestions and recommendations regarding bathing and showering may be elicited from the halo brace manufacturer. Before any patient teaching consult the vest literature or company representative regarding recommended practices. General considerations for bathing are as follows:
  a. Make sure skin is clean and dry beneath vest. No lotion or powders are used beneath vest. Take care to keep vest liner dry.

HOME CARE GUIDE   *Caring for Individual in Halo Brace—cont'd*

b. Teach skin inspection while bathing, with specific attention to high-risk areas at bony prominences.

c. The physician is notified if the skin is macerated or broken beneath the vest.

d. Hair washing may be accomplished while wearing the halo brace; however, the patient will likely require assistance.

5. Emergency measures

a. On a practice model, demonstrate rapid release of the two side belts and lifting the anterior portion of the vest for access to the thorax. Demonstrate use of a wrench for removal of anterior vest if necessary. Reinforce that the pins or suprastructure of the vest must not be tightened or loosened routinely with this wrench.

6. Home modifications

a. The patient must be taught to compensate for loss of head and neck movement by using eyes to scan visual area or turning the whole body.

b. Assistive devices may be useful to reach for or pick up objects.

c. The patient's activity is restricted because of altered balance and limited mobility. Operating a vehicle is not recommended. The patient may ride in a vehicle, taking care not to bump the head when entering or exiting the vehicle.

d. The patient may need to buy loose-fitting clothing several sizes larger than normal to accommodate the halo brace structure.

e. Experiment with different positions of comfort for patient relaxation and sleeping. Extra pillows may be useful in achieving comfort.

f. Discuss alternative positions for sexual patterns.

---

fluids are further restricted or the frequency of catheterization is increased. As reflexes continue to return, the bladder may begin to trigger itself with approximately 400 mL of urine and will empty between catheterizations. Initially the patient may be catheterized after a spontaneous void to measure postvoid residual. Cutaneous stimuli, such as tapping on the abdomen, pulling the pubic hair, or stroking the inner thigh may initiate and increase bladder contractions. Medications, such as propantheline bromide to reduce bladder spasticity or bethanecol chloride to increase detrusor tone, may be used. Once bladder training is accomplished, the patient must continue it every 4 hours. The optimum bladder program is one in which the patient is able to rely on reflex voiding techniques throughout the day and intermittent catheterization one or two times per day to measure residual urine. Noncompliance or forgetfulness will result in bladder infections, reflux of urine to the kidney pelvis, and kidney infection.

For the spinal cord–injured patient who cannot achieve reflex voiding patterns, routine "clean" intermittent self-catheterization or long-term Foley insertion is an alternative method of bladder management. In determining which is best, the nurse evaluates the patient and family's willingness and ability to learn these skills. Cost of supplies is also considered. Surgical options may be offered such as electrical stimulation of the detrusor muscle or of spinal segments that innervate detrusor muscle function. Electrical stimulation serves to initiate detrusor contraction and facilitate bladder emptying. Successful bladder management depends on education, patience, and emotional support by the nursing staff and commitment, determination, and responsible actions by the patient.[46] The nurse initiating either a bowel or bladder routine must observe for autonomic dysreflexia in the high-risk patient.

The development of spasticity in the spinal cord–injured patient has both benefits and disadvantages. Some benefits of muscle spasticity are increased muscle tone, decreased venous pooling of blood in the periphery, and abdominal wall tone that assists to support the diaphragm.[9] The patient may actually learn to use spasms to advantage, calling on this reflex activity for support in transfers. The major disadvantages of spasticity are interfering in positioning and mobility, and pain. Treatment of spasticity includes administration of antispasmodics, such as baclofen or diazepam, to minimize severe spasms and allow for the mobilization process to proceed. Some patients develop spasticity refractory to standard treatment measures. Dorsal column stimulators, implantable electrical stimulating devices, can be placed surgically to alleviate spasticity and pain. Clinical trials with baclofen administered intrathecally (within the subarachnoid space) via lumbar catheter are currently underway.

Pain management in the spinal cord–injured patient can be a nursing and medical challenge. Narcotic pain relievers such as meperidine or morphine are initially administered; however, their continued use must be evaluated carefully. Pain resulting from nerve root irritation may be treated with carbamazepine, which is generally an anticonvulsant but has been successful in treating neuralgia. Its mechanism of action as an analgesic is unknown.[16]

Skin integrity is important in both the acute and rehabilitative phases. The patient assumes responsibility for pressure sore prevention as he or she becomes increasingly independent. Nursing interventions aimed at prevention are repositioning or weight shifting at least every 2 hours, keeping the skin clean and dry, and teaching the patient and family to inspect the skin at least daily. The patient and family must learn to recognize reddened pressure areas and identify high-risk areas, such as pressure points of the sacrum, ischium, iliac crests, knees, scapula, and elbows. Patients and families also need to recognize that tight-fitting clothing, especially shoes, may impair circulation to the skin and cause breakdown.

Performance of activities of daily living is taught to the patient and family. For quadriplegics, increased independence is initiated with a variety of assistive devices. One such device, a universal cuff, wraps around the patient's hand and serves to stabilize a variety of items, such as utensils for eating or a toothbrush to assist in completion of basic hygiene. Paraplegics, once rehabilitated, are able to return to independent living. Table 50-1 reviews functional goals in spinal cord injury.

Key to the psychologic adjustment of the patient is the willingness of the nurse or other health care

TABLE 50-1 Functional Goals in Spinal Cord Injury

Spinal cord level	Muscle function	Functional goals
C3 to C4	Neck control Scapular elevators	Manipulate electric wheelchair with mouth stick Limited self-feeding with ball-bearing feeders
C5	Fair to good shoulder control Good elbow flexion	Dress upper trunk Turn self in bed with arm slings Propel wheelchair with hand-rim projections Self-feeding with hand splints Assist getting to and from bed
C6	Good shoulder control Wrist extension Supinators	Transfer from wheelchair to bed and car with or without minimal assistance Self-feeding with tenodesis hands Assist getting to and from commode chair
C7	Weak shoulder depression Weak elbow extension Some hand function	Independent in transfer to bed, car, and toilet Total dressing independence Wheelchair without hand-rim projections Self-feeding with no assistive devices
C8 to T4	Good to normal upper extremity muscle function	Wheelchair to floor and return Wheelchair up and down curb Wheelchair to tub and return
T5 to L2	Partial to good trunk stability	Total wheelchair independence Limited ambulation with bilateral long leg braces and crutches
L3 to L4	All trunk-pelvic stabilizers intact Hip flexors Adductors Quadriceps	Ambulation with short leg braces with or without crutches depending on level
L5	Hip extensors, abductors, knee flexors, ankle control	No equipment needed if plantar flexion enough for push off at end of stance

team member to listen to the patient's concerns. Adaptive coping behaviors are identified and strengthened. The patient and family are encouraged to develop realistic goals within a supportive framework.

Sexual issues may be of prime concern in the spinal cord–injured patient. Sexual function is quite variable, especially in the male, and depends on the level of completeness of the spinal cord injury. The male with a complete high level upper motor neuron lesion may lose functions of psychogenic erection, sensation, and orgasm but may experience reflex erections because of cutaneous stimuli. Maintenance of this erection depends on repeated stimulation of the affected reflex arc, and results may be unpredictable. Several aids are available to the male seeking the ability to maintain erection. Vacuum-principle devices facilitate penile engorgement, thereby producing and maintaining erection. Penile prostheses may be an option for the spinal cord–injured male. Successful results have been experienced with papaverine, a vasodilating agent, which is injected into the spongy erectile tissue of the penis to enhance erection.

The female will likely have loss of sensation below the level of injury but still be able to participate in sexual intercourse. Depending on the level of injury, the woman may require use of a vaginal lubricant. Many times spinal cord–injured patients develop heightened sensitivity in sensate areas, such as the breasts, earlobes, and neck, from which they derive sensual pleasure. High-risk patients (those with injury at T6 and above) must be cautioned to be alert for signs and symptoms of autonomic dysreflexia during sexual encounters.[16] A variety of techniques and positions may be employed for the spinal cord–injured patient and partner to foster intimacy and derive sexual pleasure. Preparation for intercourse may include a bowel and bladder check, disconnecting urinary and drainage devices, oral hygiene, transferring to a bed or other suitable place, positioning, and undressing.

Fertility is another concern of the spinal cord–injured patient. Spinal cord–injured women are generally able to achieve and maintain a pregnancy; therefore contraception, if desired, must be discussed. Male fertility depends on specific dysfunction. The male can experience an inability to ejaculate or retrograde ejaculation. If produced at all, sperm may be decreased in motility. Ejaculation may be artificially elicited by vibratory stimulation to the penis, electroejaculation techniques, or injection of pharmacologic agents (neostigmine or physostigmine). Once produced, the ejaculate will be recovered (by catheter if ejaculation is retrograde) and used for insertion or insemination.[31]

It is important to stress to the spinal cord–injured patient concerned with sexual function that sexuality is more than the act of intercourse. The nurse is alert to clues that the patient wants information or is willing to discuss sexual concerns.

SPINAL CORD TUMORS
Definition/Etiology

Tumors that affect the spinal cord account for only 0.5% to 1% of all neoplasms. These tumors can be classified as extradural (outside the dura), intradural (under or within the dura), and intramedullary (within the spinal cord) (Figure 50-16). **Extradural tumors** arise from the bones of the spine in the ex-

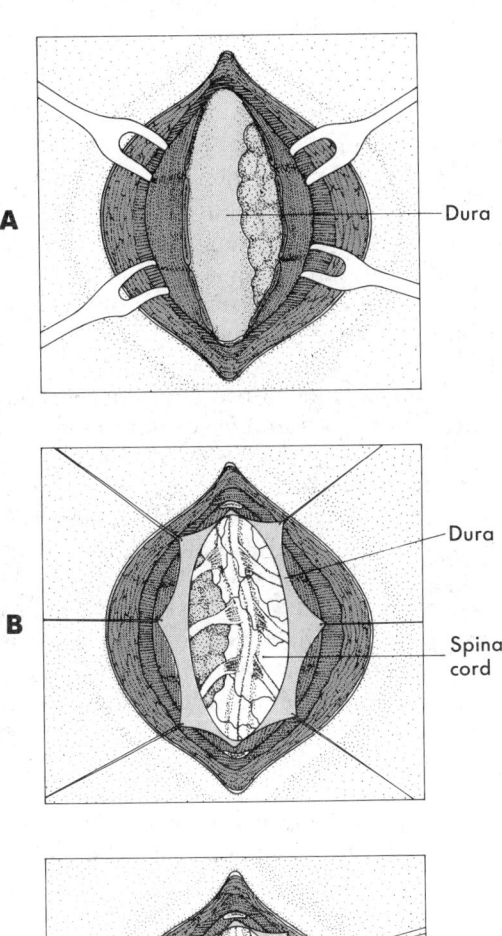

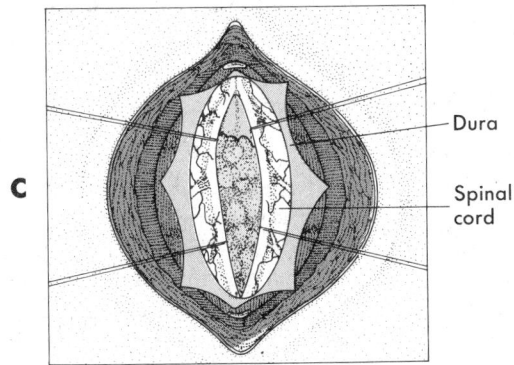

FIGURE 50-16   Spinal cord tumors. **A,** Extradural. **B,** Intradural. **C,** Intramedullary.

TABLE 50-2   Spinal Cord Tumor Classification

Type	Incidence	Treatment	Prognosis
Extradural	20% to 50% of all intraspinal tumors Usually metastatic Usually malignant	Surgical decompression, radiation, and chemotherapy	Poor
Intradural			
Intramedullary (within cord)	Least common—5% to 10%	Radiation therapy is a temporary treatment	Poor
Extramedullary	Most frequent—40% Usually benign	Complete surgical removal; if partial removal, radiation therapy is done	Very good

tradural space or in the paraspinal tissue. Of all intraspinal tumors 20% to 50% are extradural, and most are malignant metastatic lesions.[32] The prognosis is poor with these lesions. **Intradural tumors** are also known as extramedullary lesions. These are the most common spinal cord tumors. Generally these lesions are benign—meningiomas and neurofibromas—and have a good prognosis if the cord has not been damaged by compression. **Intramedullary tumors** are the least common tumor related to the spinal cord, comprising between 5% and 10% of all lesions. Because of their location, the prognosis is poor for recovery from intramedullary lesions.

The cause of intradural and intramedullary lesions is generally unknown. Primary lesions arise from some component of the cord, dura, nerves, or blood vessels. Often these tumors are caused by intraspinal extension from vertebral, neck, thoracic, or abdominal tumors. Metastatic tumors most commonly arise from growths in the breast, thyroid, lung, prostate, and kidney, and most metastatic lesions (90%) are extradural, causing compression on the spinal cord rather than invading it.[32,46] Neurofibromas, meningiomas, gliomas, and hemangiomas are the most common neoplasms (Table 50-2).

Clinical Manifestations

Because many of these tumors are slow growing, their symptoms stem from the mechanical effects of slow compression and irritation of nerve roots, displacement of the cord, or gradual obstruction of the vascular supply. The slowness of the growth does not cause autodestruction as in traumatic lesions; therefore functional restoration is possible when the tumor is removed except with intradural and intramedullary tumors. Complete restoration of spinal cord function may be possible only if spinal cord de-

compression occurs early (within 24 hours of lost function or sooner). Long-standing pressure on the spinal cord is likely to result in permanent disability.

The most common early symptom of a spinal cord tumor outside the cord is back pain with radiations simulating intercostal neuralgia or angina. The location of the pain depends on the level of compression. The pain worsens with activity, coughing, straining, and lying down. Later, sensory disruption is manifested by coldness, numbness, decreased sensation to pinprick, and tingling in one or several extremities, slowly progressing upward until it reaches the level of the lesion. Impaired sensation of pain, temperature, and light touch precedes a deficit in vibration and position sense, which may develop into complete anesthesia. Motor weakness accompanies the sensory disturbances and consists of slowly increasing clumsiness, weakness, and spasticity. Sphincter disturbances are marked by urgency with extreme difficulty initiating voiding. Overflow incontinence may also occur.

Intradural tumor manifestations develop as progressive damage to the spinal tract produces paralysis, sensory loss, and bowel and bladder dysfunction. Pain can be severe as a result of compression of spinal roots.

Extradural tumors are seen early on routine spinal x-ray films, whereas intradural and intramedullary tumors require computed tomography, myelography, or magnetic resonance imaging for diagnosis. Spinal fluid analysis may also reveal tumor cells.

Therapeutic Management

Compression of the spinal cord is an emergency situation requiring immediate treatment. Relief of the ischemia related to the compression is the goal of therapy. Corticosteroids are generally prescribed immediately to relieve tumor-related spinal cord edema. Usually dexamethasone is used, often in large doses (up to 100 mg initially).

Treatment for nearly all spinal cord tumors is surgical removal. The exception is the metastatic tumor that is sensitive to radiation and that has caused only minimal neurologic deficits.[32] In general, tumors of the extradural and extramedullary groups can be completely removed surgically. Intramedullary tumors offer a less favorable prognosis; however, exploration and removal are generally attempted.

The definitive treatment of spinal cord compression is controversial. Surgical decompression followed by radiation therapy is advocated by some investigators, whereas others suggest that radiation therapy alone is just as effective. It is generally conceded that surgical treatment is indicated if one of the following four circumstances exists: (1) the nature of the primary cancer is not known; (2) a relapse occurs following a course of radiation; (3) symptoms progress inexorably during radiation; or (4) the tumor is not known to respond to radiation therapy.[32]

Chemotherapy has been used in combination with radiation therapy to treat malignant lesions, but few drugs appear to be effective against spinal cord tumors.

NURSING MANAGEMENT OF THE PATIENT WITH SPINAL CORD TUMORS
Assessment

The assessment of the patient with spinal cord tumor is generally the same as that outlined for the patient with spinal cord injury. Motor and sensory functions are assessed frequently, and deterioration in status is reported to the physician immediately. A total systems assessment should also be done because respiratory, gastrointestinal, and urinary function may be affected by the loss of spinal cord function.

Nursing Diagnosis

Depending on the amount of neurologic dysfunction the spinal tumor patient exhibits, nursing diagnoses related to spinal cord injury may apply. In addition to the care outlined for the spinal cord–injured patient, other nursing diagnoses to consider include the following:

High risk for injury related to changes in sensation and motor loss

Fear and anxiety related to changes in neurologic status and the diagnosis

Pain related to nerve root compression

Knowledge deficit related to lack of information regarding the disease

Planning

Because of the sudden onset of symptoms the patient is generally not prepared for hospitalization or the diagnosis. The patient should be allowed to express fears related to the loss of motor and sensory function and the prognosis. The patient will need to be protected from self-harm and skin disruption while adapting to sensory dysfunction. Relief of pain is one of the most important goals throughout hospitalization and can pose a nursing challenge.

Implementation

Frequent assessment and documentation of the sensory status of the patient will help in defining areas of altered sensation. Nurses must be sure that the patient understands the loss of sensation and protects himself or herself from injury. Caution should be used when the patient is mobilized to prevent falls. The patient must be turned frequently to relieve any pressure areas, especially in areas of decreased sensation.

Because of the usual sudden onset of symptoms, the patient will be fearful of the loss of function being permanent. The patient must be allowed to express fears. All questions should be answered honestly. The patient must be helped to adapt to disabilities from the neurologic deficits. The nurse should spend time with the patient whenever possible and document the patient's expressions of concern.

The patient is medicated with analgesics as needed and assessed for type, location, radiation, and duration of pain. A change or worsening of patient complaints of pain must be noted and the physician notified promptly, because this may reflect further spinal cord compression. The character of the pain and the effects of analgesia must be documented. A transcutaneous electrical nerve stimulator (TENS) unit, which blocks pain transmission, may be helpful in controlling localized root pain (see Chapter 14).

The nurse spends time with the patient and family, educating them about the type of tumor and incorporating them in the care of the patient.

Evaluation

Surgery is the treatment of choice for patients with spinal cord tumor. Helping the patient adapt to the neurologic deficits following surgery is an important component of the nursing care. Attainment of the goals set during the planning phase should be measured frequently. The patient should be free of skin breakdown or other injury at the time of discharge. Anxiety is allayed by educating the patient and family about the disease and follow-up care needed. Pain should be well controlled or even alleviated by discharge.

Documentation

It is important to accurately document all motor and sensory assessments performed. Deterioration or improvement in neurologic status is noted. The type, location, and duration of pain and the effects of analgesia are carefully documented. The patient's expressions of concern and the interventions employed are included in the care plan to allow for reinforcement of the information by all caregivers. The information regarding diagnosis, prognosis, and adjunct therapy is also included in the care plan so that all caregivers know what the patient and family have been told. Discharge plans are an important part of the care plan.

Ongoing Care
Rehabilitation

Depending on the type of tumor, the patient may not be a candidate for rehabilitation. Generally with total surgical removal, the return of function is good in those patients with extradural or extramedullary lesions. A short course of rehabilitation may be needed for any residual deficits. With patients who have metastatic lesions or intramedullary tumors, which both carry a poor prognosis, rehabilitation may not be indicated. Appropriate referral to home care with hospice help may be needed for those patients with a terminal prognosis.

Home care

Most patients are discharged to home. Outpatient radiation therapy may be carried out for those patients whose tumor is susceptible to treatment by radiation. Outpatient chemotherapy or home chemotherapy may also be indicated. A home care nurse may be needed initially to ensure that all is going well in the home if the patient continues to require skilled nursing. The majority of patients with a spinal cord tumor do well following tumor removal and do not have major neurologic sequelae. The nurse must be prepared to care for these patients as spinal cord–injured patients until the neurologic dysfunction resolves.

INTERVERTEBRAL DISK DISEASE
Definition

The intervertebral disk functions as a shock absorber between vertebrae. It has a gelatinous center (the nucleus pulposus) surrounded by a fibrocartilage ring called the annulus. The disk sits on the body of the vertebra. The disk wall may become weak with age or excessive movement and rupture, allowing the soft gelatin center to exude and compress the nerve root, causing **intervertebral disk**

disease. The disk is also known to degenerate with age or previous trauma to the area. The disk may be ruptured in spinal cord injury.

Although disks are present between all of the vertebrae of the spinal column except the fused sacral vertebrae, the most common sites of disk problems are the cervical and lumbar areas. This occurrence of disk disease is probably related to the amount of motion associated with those areas of the vertebral column. Problems in the lumbar area occur more commonly than problems in the cervical area. Pain in the lumbar region is a common problem, because this area bears most of the weight of the body, is one of the most flexible regions of the spinal column, contains nerve roots that are vulnerable to injury, and has an inherently poor structure.[39] Since the majority of disk problems occur in the lumbar area, this section of the chapter focuses on lumbar disk disease, although rupture of the disk can occur at the cervical and thoracic areas also.

Etiology/Epidemiology

The most common cause of intervertebral disk disease is the normal aging process, which causes a degeneration of the disk. Half of disk herniations are related to trauma from sudden movement or inappropriate movement.[16] Men suffer from disk disease more often than women. Of all disk herniations 90% to 95% occur at the L4 to L5 and the L5 to S1 levels.

Pathophysiology

After 30 years of age the normal aging process causes degenerative changes to occur in the longitudinal ligaments that support the vertebral bodies posteriorly and the annulus fibrosis of the disk. The fraying and tearing of the annulus fibrosis make the disk vulnerable to rupture. The nucleus pulposa can herniate through the weakened cartilage laterally or centrally.

Clinical Manifestations

The most common symptom associated with a ruptured disk is pain. The pain may be sharp (often described as like electricity) and generally follows one nerve (one dermatome). For example, the patient may complain of pain that starts in the low back, going down the buttocks, down the outer part of the thigh, across the knee, and into the large toe. This would describe a nerve compression caused by a ruptured disk between the L4 and L5 vertebrae (the L4 nerve root is affected). The pain is usually associated with some type of activity that causes undue stress on the back, such as bending, or increases pressure within the spinal dura, such as coughing or sneezing. Often symptoms will not appear at the time of injury but develop later as the result of paravertebral muscle spasms.

The diagnosis of the cause of back pain involves an in-depth history of potential causes for the pain. Plain spine radiographs can demonstrate degenerative changes in the vertebral column, congenital abnormalities, or postural changes that will be associated with back pain. Intervertebral disks cannot be seen on plain radiography; therefore an MRI study is the most useful noninvasive diagnostic tool. The myelogram with contrast dye is the best way to diagnose a herniated disk if MRI is not available. The myelogram will show both lateral and central herniation with compression. The myelogram is usually done in conjunction with a computed tomography (CT) scan. Electromyography may be done to assess the function of certain weak muscles to rule out any local muscle degeneration.

Therapeutic Management

Conservative management is often tried as the first therapy to control the pain associated with intervertebral disk disease. The conservative approach to treatment includes complete bed rest for 2 to 6 weeks; avoidance of stress; use of support devices such as a corset, brace, or cervical collar (depending on the level of pain); a firm mattress; and analgesics. Physiotherapy with exercises, cold or hot packs, and diathermy may also be used to help relax the muscle spasms. Rarely, skin traction may be used as an adjunct to bed rest. Pelvic traction for lumbar disk problems or halter traction for cervical disk problems can be used to help ease the muscle spasms. Currently more emphasis is on a supervised, structured exercise program with physical therapy, hydrotherapy, rest, stress reduction, and relaxation.

Medications play an important role in conservative management. Analgesics, muscle relaxants, anti-inflammatory agents, and tranquilizers are all considered for use in the treatment of disk disease. Nonsteroidal anti-inflammatory agents reduce the swelling and irritation of the nerve roots. Phenylbutazone (Butazolidin) and ibuprofen are the most likely agents to be used.[42] Steroids have also been used to reduce inflammation. The steroid of choice is dexamethasone (Decadron). Epidural steroid injections may be performed. The epidural route is usually preferred to the intrathecal route, because root compression most commonly occurs in the epidural space, and spinal headache can be avoided with this technique.[29] Epidural steroids have been shown to decrease pain, speed return of function, and improve objective neurologic signs.

As symptoms subside, activity is gradually increased. Exercises to strengthen the back and abdominal muscles are taught to the patient. The majority of patients treated conservatively will recover. If pain and other symptoms persist following conservative management, surgical intervention is necessary. Many forms of surgical intervention are used to treat disk disease. Patients with central herniations usually require surgery to relieve the compression on the spinal cord. Diskectomy with or without laminectomy is the most commonly performed procedure to relieve disk pressure.

Chemonucleolysis is the injection of chymopapain into the nucleus pulposus of an intravertebral disk. Chymopapain is an enzyme extracted from the papaya plant. When injected into the herniated disk, the enzyme reduces the central disk component by hydrolysis, decreasing the water-binding capacity in the nucleus pulposus and thus the intradiskal pressure.[44] With the pressure removed from the spinal nerve roots, pain is significantly diminished.

Complications have been documented with the use of chymopapain, including anaphylaxis, paraplegia from acute transverse myelitis or cauda equina syndrome, and cerebrovascular bleeding. Other documented problems include diskitis, seizures, Guillain-Barre syndrome, and meningismus. For these reasons and because of improved surgical treatment, little chemonucleosis is done in the United States.

NURSING MANAGEMENT OF THE PATIENT WITH INTERVERTEBRAL DISK DISEASE
Assessment

The assessment of the patient with disk disease includes evaluation of the motor strength and sensory function of the patient. A history of the onset of the pain and a description of the pain including its progress are obtained. The impact of the pain on the patient is important to explore, as well as how the patient manages the pain. If the patient is on complete bed rest, assessment of all body systems is done for the impact of immobility. Postoperatively, ongoing assessment of the motor and sensory status of the patient is important. In addition to the neurologic system function, the assessment focuses on early recognition of complications.

Nursing Diagnosis

Pain related to nerve root compression (preoperatively), muscle spasm (preoperatively or postoperatively), and incisional site (postoperatively) is the most common nursing diagnosis for the patient with a herniated disk. Other nursing diagnoses include the following:

Impaired physical mobility related to pain on movement or therapeutic bed rest

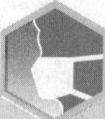

PREOPERATIVE AND POSTOPERATIVE NURSING INTERVENTIONS

Patient with Intervertebral Disk Disease

Nursing Interventions	Rationale

Preoperative

1. Maintain bed rest or activity as ordered by physician. — Provides support or limited activity for the spinal column
2. Assess neurologic function of affected areas. — Identifies any changes in motor and sensory function
3. Maintain proper body alignment of affected areas with cervical pillow or lumbar roll. — Decreases stress on irritated nerves and muscles
4. Assist the patient in log rolling. No turning, twisting, or torquing of the spine is allowed. — Maintains proper body alignment
5. Encourage range of motion exercises. — Maintains muscular and vascular tone
6. Teach coughing and deep breathing measures. — Prevents respiratory complications of immobility
7. Administer muscle relaxants, analgesics, or sedatives as ordered. — Provides comfort and resolution of nerve irritation and inflammation
8. Monitor bowel and bladder patterns. — Prevents complications of bowel and bladder related to immobility or neurologic impairment
9. For lumbar disk, semi-situps, pelvic tilts, and gluteal setting may be taught. — Strengthens abdominal and back muscles

Postoperative

1. Maintain flat bed rest with supportive pillows or devices per physician orders. — Provides support and reduces strain at operative site
2. Monitor and compare serial tests of motor and sensory function, including comparison to preoperative status. — Demonstrates evidence of hemorrhage or other postoperative complications
3. Assist the patient with turns. — Prevents twisting or torquing of the spine
4. Apply elastic hose or pneumatic boots as ordered. — Prevents deep vein thrombosis
5. Encourage range of motion exercise. — Improves circulation and motor tone
6. Have patient perform coughing and deep breathing exercises every 2 hours. — Prevents atelectasis and pneumonia
7. Monitor bowel and bladder function. — Prevents constipation and facilitates bladder emptying; transient voiding problems common after lumbar procedure
8. Observe operative site for swelling, drainage, redness, or poor healing. — Identifies hemorrhage, cerebrospinal fluid drainage, or infection
9. Administer analgesics as ordered. — Provides for patient comfort
10. Initial activity for the lumbar patient includes either lying flat in bed, standing, or walking and may be instituted as soon as the effects of anesthesia dissipate. — Prevents stress and strain on operative site; encourages early mobilization to avoid complications of prolonged bed rest
11. Initial activity for the cervical patient includes gradual elevation of the head of bed with supportive device and ambulation as soon as tolerated. — Provides support to operative site; early ambulation decreases risk for complications of immobility
12. Teach patient regarding proper body mechanics and specific activity instruction. — Educates patient to avoid stress on operative site and prevents further injury

Urinary retention related to immobility or neurologic impairment
Constipation related to nerve root compression
Altered coping responses related to persistent pain/chronic pain syndromes

Planning

The goal of care is to free the patient of pain to allow for normal activity to resume. If the patient can be mobilized with no fear of pain, then altered mobility will not be a problem. The plan should include discharge teaching regarding proper body mechanics and exercises to improve the strength of the back.

Implementation

See the box on preoperative and postoperative nursing interventions for the patient with intervertebral disk disease for a summary of nursing interventions.

Ongoing Care
Rehabilitation

If the patient's symptoms are relieved by conservative therapy, exercise programs need to be maintained. These programs are designed to strengthen weakened back and abdominal muscles. Regular exercise is important to help prevent further problems. If the patient has sustained a nerve root injury, an aggressive physiotherapy program will be needed, along with slings, braces, or splints depending on the involved extremity and the extent of injury. It is possible that even with an aggressive treatment program, the patient may sustain permanent disability.

Home care

Surgery is not always synonymous with relief of symptoms. Pain, weakness, and sensory disturbances may be present for several months after surgery. Home physical therapy may be needed by the patient with a residual neurologic deficit. Continued pain may require additional therapeutic intervention. A disk herniation may also recur at the same level on the same or opposite side or at other levels. Repeated laminectomies on the same patient are not unusual.[17] This points out the need for patient teaching in proper body mechanics and protection from injury. In many instances the recurrence of symptoms is caused by severe degenerative changes and cannot be avoided.

CRITICAL THINKING QUESTIONS

1 Describe the "typical victim" of spinal cord injury.

2 What is the cause of complete spinal cord dissolution in severe trauma?

3 Describe the nursing interventions for the patient exhibiting symptoms of autonomic dysreflexia.

4 How does the growth rate of spinal cord tumors affect the development of related symptoms?

5 What is the major nursing responsibility related to prevention of low back pain?

6 Name three physiologic complications of spinal cord injury, and identify nursing measures aimed at their prevention.

7 What is the importance of a postoperative exercise program for the patient with disk disease?

RESOURCES

1 AMERICAN ASSOCIATION OF SPINAL CORD INJURY NURSES 75-20 Astoria Blvd. Jackson Heights, NY 11370-1178

2 AMERICAN PARALYSIS ASSOCIATION 500 Morris Ave. Springfield, NJ 07081

3 AMERICAN SPINAL INJURY ASSOCIATION Room 619 250 E. Superior St. Chicago, IL 60611

4 NATIONAL HEAD AND SPINAL CORD INJURY PREVENTION PROGRAM 22 South Washington St. Park Ridge, IL 60068

5 NATIONAL SPINAL CORD INJURY ASSOCIATION Suite 2000 600 West Cummings Park Woburn, MA 01801 (800) 962-9629

6 NATIONAL SPINAL CORD INJURY HOTLINE (800) 526-3456; in MD: (800) 638-1733

7 PARALYZED VETERANS OF AMERICA 801 18th St., N.W. Washington, DC 20006

BIBLIOGRAPHY

Current

1. Ablin MS, White RS: Epidemiology, physiopathology and experimental therapeutics of acute spinal cord injury, *Crit Care Clin* 3(3):441, 1987.

2. Acute traumatic spinal cord injury surveillance—United States, 1987, *Morbid Mortal Weekly Rep* 37(18):285, 1988.

3. Blissitt P: Nutrition in acute spinal cord injury, *Crit Care Nurs Clin North Am* 2(3):375, 1990.

4. Borkowski C: A comparison of pulmonary complications in spinal cord-injured patients treated with two modes of spinal immobilization, *J Neurosci Nurs* 21(2):79, 1989.

5. Bracken MB et al: A randomized, controlled trial of methylprednisolone or naloxone in the treatment of acute spinal-cord injury, *N Engl J Med* 322(20):1404, 1990.

6. Buchanan LE, Nawoczenski DA: *Spinal cord injury,* Baltimore, 1987, The Williams & Wilkins Co.

7. Carol MP, Ducker TB: Spinal cord injury and spinal shock syndromes. In Siegel JH, editor: *Trauma emergency surgery and critical care,* New York, 1987, Churchill Livingstone.

8. Chicano LA: Humanistic aspects of sexuality as related to spinal cord injury, *J Neurosci Nurs* 21(6):366, 1989.

9. Dillingham TR: Prevention of complications during acute management of the spinal cord-injured patient: first step in the rehabilitation process, *Crit Care Nurs Q* 11(2):71, 1988.

10. Dunnum L: Life satisfaction and spinal cord injury: the patient perspective, *J Neurosci Nurs* 22(1):45, 1990.

11. Geilser FM, Salcman M: Respiratory system physiology, pathophysiology and management. In Wirth FP,

Ratcheson PA, editors: *Neurosurgical critical care,* Baltimore, 1987, The Williams & Wilkins Co.

12. Gilbert J: Critical care management of the patient with acute spinal cord injury, *Crit Care Clin* 3(3):549, 1987.

13. Goddard LR: Sexuality and spinal cord injury, *J Neurosci Nurs* 20(4):240, 1988.

14. Green BA et al: Spinal cord injury—a systems approach: prevention, emergency medical services and emergency room management, *Crit Care Clin* 3(3):471, 1987.

15. Halm MA: Elimination concerns with acute spinal cord trauma: assessment and nursing interventions, *Crit Care Nurs Clin North Am* 2(3):385, 1990.

16. Hickey JV: *The clinical practice of neurological and neurosurgical nursing,* ed 3, Philadelphia, 1992, JB Lippincott Co.

17. Kocan MJ: Pulmonary considerations in the critical care phase, *Crit Care Nurs Clin North Am* 2(3):369, 1990.

18. Mandzak-McCarron K: Rehabilitation of the patient with spinal cord injury, *Trauma Q* 4(3):45, 1988.

19. National Spinal Cord Injury Statistical Center, University of Alabama at Birmingham: *Spinal cord injury fact sheet,* Birmingham, Ala, 1990, National Spinal Cord Injury Statistical Center (supported in part by Grant No. G008535128 from the National Institute on Disability and Rehabilitation Research, United States Department of Education).

20. Nikas DL: Pathophysiology and nursing interventions in acute spinal cord injury, *Trauma Q* 4(3):23, 1988.

21. Ohman K, Spaniol D: Halo immobilization: discharge planning and patient education, *J Neurosci Nurs* 22(6):351, 1990.

22. Olson B, Ustanko L: Self-care needs of patients in the halo brace, *Orthop Nurs* 9(1):27, 1990.

23. Raney DJ: Malignant spinal cord tumors: a review and case presentation, *J Neurosci Nurs* 23(1):44, 1991.

24. Rhinehart M: Early mobilization in acute spinal cord injury: a collaborative approach, *Crit Care Nurs Clin North Am* 2(3):399, 1990.

25. Schwenker D: Cardiovascular considerations in the critical care phase, *Crit Care Nurs Clin North Am* 2(3):363, 1990.

26. Snowdy AA, Snowdy PH: Stabilization procedures in the patient with acute spinal cord injury, *Crit Care Clin* 3(3):569, 1987.

27. Stelling J: Spinal cord injury. In Howell E et al, editors: *Comprehensive trauma nursing: theory and practice,* Glenview, Ill, 1988, Scott, Foresman & Co.

28. Walleck CA: Nursing management of the client with peripheral and spinal cord problems. In Lewis S, Collier I, editors: *Textbook of medical surgical nursing,* St Louis, 1987, Mosby–Year Book, Inc.

29. Walleck CA: Spinal cord injury. In Cardona VD et al, editors: *Trauma nursing: from resuscitation through rehabilitation,* Philadelphia, 1988, WB Saunders Co.

30. Walleck CA: Neurologic considerations in the critical care phase, *Crit Care Nurs Clin North Am* 2(3):357, 1990.

31. Zejdlik CP: *Management of spinal cord injury,* ed 2, Boston, 1992, Jones and Bartlett, Publishers.

Classic

32. Arsenault L: Metastatic cancer and the nervous system, *Focus Crit Care* 11(6):39, 1984.

33. Bell J, Hannon K: Pathophysiology involved in autonomic dysreflexia, *J Neurosci Nurs* 18(2):86, 1986.

34. Bucy PC, Perot PT: Injury to the spinal cord. In Tower DB, editor: *The nervous system,* vol 2. *The clinical neurosciences,* New York, 1975, Raven Press.

35. Frisbie J, Sasahara AA: Low dose heparin prophylaxis for deep vein thrombosis in acute spinal cord injury patients: a controlled study, *Paraplegia* 19:343, 1981.

36. Green BA et al: A comparative study of steroid therapy in acute experimental spinal cord injury, *Surg Neurol* 13:91, 1980.

37. Green BA et al: Kinetic therapy for spinal cord injury, *Spine* 8:224, 1983.

38. Guttman L: *Spinal cord injuries: comprehensive management and research,* Oxford, England, 1976, Blackwell Scientific Publications.

39. Hejna WA, Sinkors G: Chemonucleolysis of the herniated lumbar disc, *Am Fam Physician* 27(5):97, 1983.

40. King R: Assessment and management of soft tissue pressure. In Martin M et al, editors: *Comprehensive rehabilitation nursing,* New York, 1978, McGraw-Hill Book Co.

41. Lermo DB et al: Massive gastrointestinal hemorrhage and perforation in acute spinal cord injury, *Surg Neurol* 17:186, 1982.

42. Lewinneh GE, Warfield CA: Sciatica and back pain: when to operate? *Hosp Pract* 20:167, 1985.

43. Lloyd LK et al: Initial bladder management in spinal cord injury: does it make a difference? *J Urol* 135:523, 1986.

44. McCagg C: Postoperative management and acute rehabilitation of patients with spinal cord injuries, *Orthop Clin North Am* 17:171, 1986.

45. Richmond T: The patient with a cervical cord injury, *Focus Crit Care* 12:32, 1985.

46. Rudy E: *Advanced neurological and neurosurgical nursing,* St Louis, 1984, Mosby–Year Book, Inc.

47. Solomon J: Sex and the spinal cord injured patient, *J Neurosurg Nurs* 15(3):30, 1986.

48. Tyson GW: Acute care of the spinal cord injured patient, *J Neurosurg Nurs* 15(3):30, 1986.

49. Wahlquist G: Regaining urinary continence through intermittent catheterization, *J Neurosurg Nurs* 12:73, 1980.

50. Warfield CA: Steroids and low back pain, *Hosp Pract* 29:325, 1985.

CHAPTER FIFTY-ONE

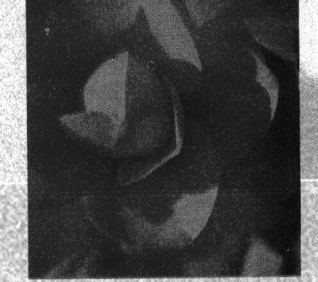

Nursing Management of Adults with Peripheral or Cranial Nerve Disorders

---

LEARNING OBJECTIVES

1 Define the three types of degenerative processes seen in peripheral nerve disease.
2 Describe the six common signs of peripheral nerve disease.
3 Outline the nursing management for patients with trauma of the peripheral nerves.
4 Describe the pathophysiology and clinical manifestations of nutritional polyneuropathies.
5 Discuss the nursing management for patients with nutritional polyneuropathies.
6 Describe the symptoms of neuropathy caused by toxins.
7 Identify the components of a nursing assessment for a patient with toxic neuropathy.
8 Describe the clinical manifestations of Charcot-Marie-Tooth disease.
9 Compare the pathophysiology and clinical manifestations of trigeminal neuralgia and facial nerve paralysis.
10 Discuss the therapeutic management for patients with cranial nerve disorders.

DISORDERS of the peripheral nervous system are one of the most difficult subjects in neurology. The difficulty does not lie in the structure of this system, but rather in the degenerative effect from trauma to the peripheral nervous system. Causes of peripheral nerve disorders include direct trauma, exposure to toxic chemicals, nutritional deficiencies, drugs, diseases, and heredity. These diseases can be difficult to diagnose, and a thorough history and physical assessment are essential for establishing a diagnosis.

Peripheral Nerve Disorders

Pathophysiology

The *peripheral nervous system* includes all neural structures lying outside the spinal cord and brainstem. A nerve is composed of thousands of neurons, and it is the neurons that are affected in peripheral nervous system disorders. Peripheral nerves contain both sensory and motor components. Peripheral nerve disorders lead to alterations in pain, touch, temperature, proprioception, stereognosis, and motor function. When a disease affects the peripheral nervous system, several distinct processes are recognized and may be present in varying combinations in any patient.[1] The three major processes are wallerian degeneration, segmental demyelination, and axonal degeneration. Varying degrees of regeneration occur depending on the type of damage to nerve fibers (Fig. 51-1).

Wallerian degeneration occurs when a nerve fiber (axon) has been severed from its cell body and myelin sheath. Wallerian degeneration is a process that destroys the severed axon stump and moves backward toward the cell body. Cell breakdown and phagocytosis also extend the point of the transection toward the cell body, a process sometimes referred to as *dying back*. Eventually the entire cell disappears, usually over several months. With this type of degeneration, recovery time is prolonged. The axon must first regenerate and reconnect to other tissue before function can resume, extending recovery time from months to years.

Focal degeneration of the myelin sheath with sparing of the axon is called **segmental demyelination.** Recovery of function may be rapid because the intact but denuded axon needs only to become remyelinated. This is in direct contrast with wallerian or axonal degeneration.[1,5]

Degeneration of myelin secondary to axonal disease is called **axonal degeneration,** or medullary-axonic degeneration, and can occur distal to the most proximal site of axonal interruption. This is a more generalized, metabolically determined degeneration, often occurring in polyneuropathies.[1]

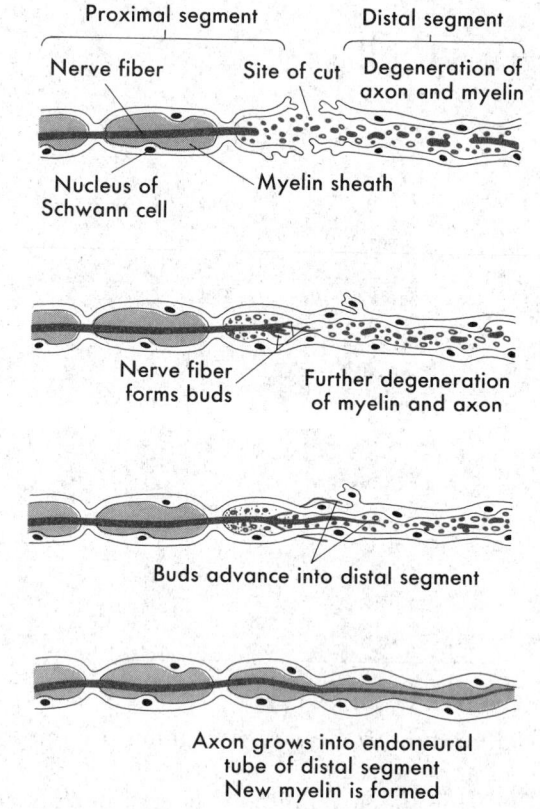

FIGURE 51-1 Changes in nerve fiber that has been cut and then regenerates.

Clinical Manifestations

Temporary weakness or paralysis in an extremity after spinal cord or intracranial surgery may be due to swelling, giving the appearance of permanent damage. With the administration of steroids and over time, strength increases, and no permanent damage is apparent. However, persistent impairment of motor function over days, weeks, or months always signifies segmental demyelination, axonal interruption, or destruction of motor neurons.

Sensation, even more than motor function, is affected in the distal segments of the limbs and more in the legs than the arms. When testing for impaired sensory function, the examiner uses all modalities (touch-pressure, pain and temperature, vibration, and position sense). A variety of responses may be present. Vibration, or more specifically a lack of vibratory sensation, is the most common finding and often the first sign of peripheral neuropathy.

Patients with peripheral nerve disorders can exhibit an ataxic gait. Their motor power is sufficient to propel them, but their lack of position sense (proprioception) causes an unstable gait. The legs and feet are placed on the ground with flinging movements. Intentional tremors of the hands and arms resemble those associated with cerebellar diseases.

Loss of tendon reflexes is another sign of peripheral nerve disease. The degree of loss varies and may change from day to day. Reflexes are often diminished but not absent and are graded by the examiner on a scale of 0 to 5, with 2 being a normal finding.

In many peripheral nervous system disorders, the feet, hands, and spine become deformed, especially when the disease has a childhood onset. The muscle groups responsible for alignment are weakened and unable to provide the support necessary to maintain proper positioning. Denervation atrophy of muscle is the main trophic disturbance resulting from interruption of the motor nerves. Because of decreased sensation, the patient may not notice an injury, which can easily become infected.

Anhidrosis, a lack of sweating, and orthostatic hypotension are among the two most frequent autonomic manifestations of peripheral nerve disorders. Other common symptoms of autonomic paralysis are unreactive pupils, lack of tears and saliva, sexual impotence, and weak bladder and bowel sphincters.

The brachial plexus is created from spinal nerves C5, C6, C7, and C8 and T1 nerve roots. These nerves divide and recombine to form three major trunks: upper C5 and C6), middle (C7), and lower (C8 and T1).[5] The major causes of *brachial plexus injuries* are traction and stretch injuries. Causative factors range from birth trauma to excessive weight applied to limb traction. The degree of severity is related to the nature of the injury. Other causes include complete or partial severance; contusion; compression; electrical, thermal, or radiation injuries; and poor or improper use of crutches. Depending on the type of injury, various degenerative conditions will occur.

Injury to the upper trunk (C5 to C6) of the spinal nerve is known as Duchenne-Erb palsy. A loss of or difficulty in abduction and external rotation of the arm and weak supination and flexion of the forearm are present. The arm hangs at the side, internally rotated and extended at the elbow. Hand function is unaffected. Injury to the middle trunk (C7) affects the triceps. The patient has difficulty extending the forearm and has deficits in sensory function. In lower trunk (C8 and T1) injury the forearm and hand muscle are mainly involved. Paralysis and atrophy of small hand muscles and wrist flexors give the characteristic appearance of a clawhand deformity. Sensory deficit is noted in the medial side of the arm, forearm, and hand.

MEDIAN NERVE INJURY
Definition

Upper extremity injuries of the median nerve originate from C5 to T1 but mainly from C6 nerve roots, where the medial and lateral cords of the brachial plexus meet.

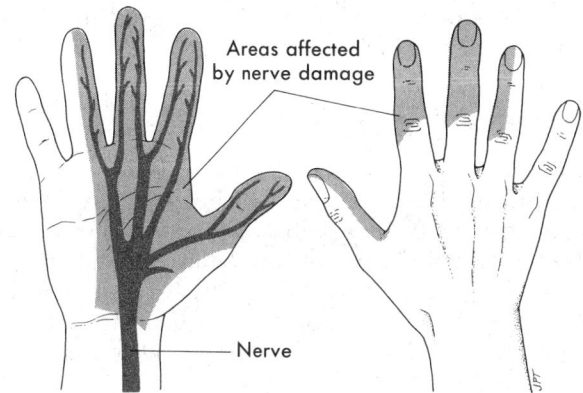

FIGURE 51-2   Median nerve distribution.

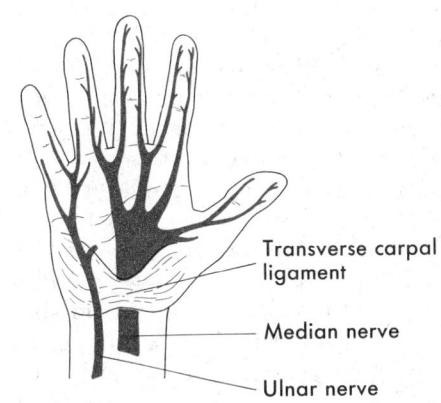

FIGURE 51-3   Carpal tunnel syndrome.

Etiology

Injury to the median nerve can occur from dislocation of the shoulder. However, anywhere along the nerve's pathway, trauma such as lacerations, stab wounds, and gunshot wounds can cause injury. Complete interruption of the median nerve results in inability to pronate the forearm or flex the hand (Figure 51-2). The wrist is the most common location of external injury (Figure 51-3). Compression of the nerve at the wrist is commonly referred to as **carpal tunnel syndrome.** This syndrome often occurs as a result of repeated trauma, but the etiology is unknown. Carpal tunnel syndrome is considered one of the three most common industrial or work-related conditions, resulting from the increasing use of computer-related data processing equipment.[11] Also referred to as repetitive motion syndrome, the twisting or turning of the wrist and fingers may cause compressive symptoms of the median nerve. Carpal tunnel syndrome is more common in women than men. It is also more common in persons with rheumatoid arthritis, menopausal women, and pregnant women in their last trimester.[11] The syndrome may be unilateral or bilateral.

Pathophysiology

Carpal tunnel syndrome is believed to be related to a narrowing of the canal in which the nerve travels. This narrowing causes pain and prompts the patient to seek medical attention. Immediate relief is found with the application of a splint to immobilize the wrist. However, many patients require surgical decompression and regain full, pain-free function of the affected wrist.

Clinical Manifestations

The more common signs and symptoms of median nerve injury include inability to pronate the forearm or flex the hand in a radial fashion, paralysis of flexion of the index finger, weakness of flexion of the remaining fingers, numbness and pain especially at night, and sensory impairment over the radial two thirds of the palmar aspect of the hand. Carpal tunnel syndrome is assessed by testing for *Phalen's sign* and *Tinel's sign*. **Phalen's sign** (Figure 51-4, *A*) is positive for carpal tunnel. The patient is asked to flex the wrist acutely for 1 minute. Numbness and tingling over the distribution of the median nerve, the palmar surface of the thumb, and the index and middle fingers suggest carpal tunnel syndrome. **Tinel's sign** (Figure 51-4, *B*) also suggests carpal tun-

nel syndrome. The nurse lightly percusses the medial nerve at the wrist as it enters the carpal tunnel. A tingling sensation over the distribution of the medial nerve suggests carpal tunnel syndrome.

Therapeutic Management

Conservative therapy is instituted whenever the signs and symptoms are mild or when the etiology dictates a short-term condition (i.e., pregnancy or wrist trauma). Treatment involves splinting of the wrist in a neutral position and resting the hand to prevent mechanical irritation of the nerve. Injection of steroid medication into the flexor tendons in the carpal tunnel may provide some relief, but the effect is usually transient.[12] Analgesics are given for pain relief.

Surgical management

If conservative treatment is unsuccessful, surgery is performed to release the transverse carpal ligament to decompress the median nerve. This procedure should relieve the pain and paresthesias immediately.[12] The surgical technique and type of incision depend on the surgeon. In most institutions today the surgery is performed on an outpatient basis with the patient under local anesthesia. The nurse provides teaching in a limited time period. Information is provided in a succinct manner, concentrating on the key areas necessary for a successful surgical pro-

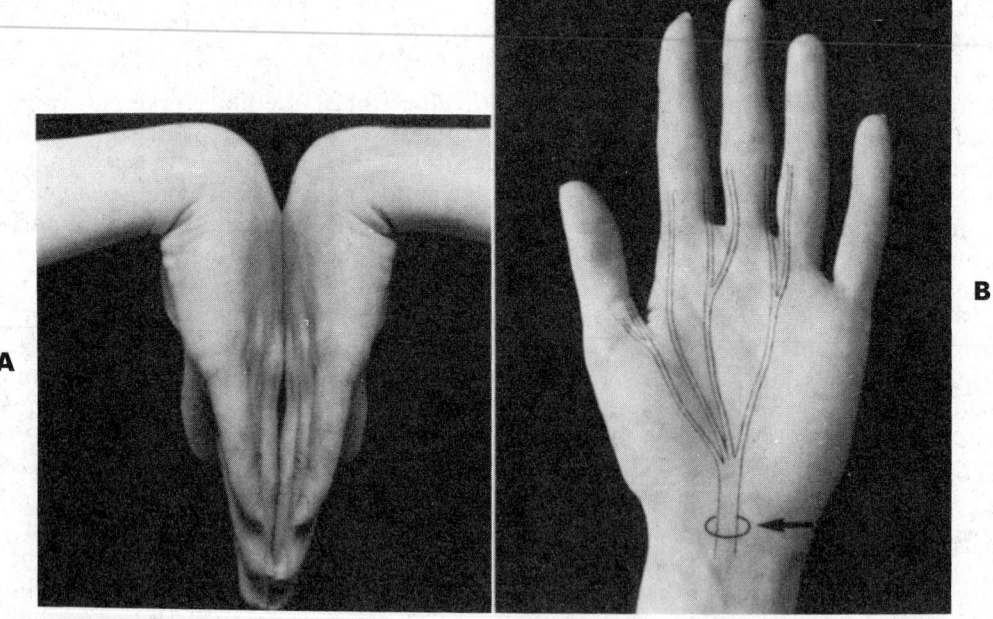

FIGURE 51-4 Assessing carpal tunnel syndrome. **A**, Phalen's test. **B**, Tinel's sign. (From Bates B: *A guide to physical examination and history taking,* ed 5, Philadelphia, 1991, JB Lippincott Co.)

cedure. The areas to concentrate on include the location of the surgery, the position the patient assumes during the procedure, and the personnel in the operating and recovery rooms. A written copy of the instructions is provided before discharge and includes a telephone number for emergencies.

Preoperative teaching is usually instituted in the surgeon's office or the outpatient setting. Depending on the surgeon, preoperative instructions to the patient will include the actual surgical procedure, expected outcome, and preadmission preparation. Included as well are postoperative instructions regarding incisional care, level of activity at home, elevation of the hand and arm for 24 hours, and neurovascular checks every 4 hours for 24 hours. The patient is instructed to note any signs and symptoms of infection or hematoma formation. Written instructions include any appointments and return visits to the surgeon. The patient usually returns to the surgeon's office for follow-up and suture removal in 10 to 14 days.[12]

ULNAR NERVE INJURY
Definition

Upper extremity injuries of the ulnar nerve originate from trauma to C8 and T1 nerve roots.

Etiology/Pathophysiology

Injuries to the ulnar nerve result from elbow fractures or dislocation and from improper positioning during surgery. Complete ulnar paralysis is manifested by a clawhand deformity; wasting of the small muscles permits hyperextension of the fingers at the joints. Because of this deformity, the nerve is stretched in its groove over the ulnar condyle, and its more superficial location renders it vulnerable to compression.

Clinical Manifestations

Clawhand deformity and weakness of flexion of the wrist are among the more common signs and symptoms of ulnar nerve injury. Clawhand deformity is most pronounced in the fourth and fifth fingers because the lumbrical muscles of the second and third fingers, supplied by the medial nerve, counteract the deformity. Sensory loss occurs over the fifth finger, the ulnar aspect of the fourth finger, and the ulnar border of the palm.

RADIAL NERVE INJURY
Definition

Upper extremity injuries of the radial nerve stem from trauma to C6, C7, and C8, but mainly to C7, nerve roots.

Etiology/Pathophysiology

The radial nerve is the termination of the posterior cord of the brachial plexus. It innervates the triceps, brachioradialis, and supinator muscles; the extensor muscles of the wrist and fingers; and the abductor muscle of the thumb. The nerve may become compressed in the axilla by the improper use of crutches. More frequently, the injury is located from a lower point in the arm, where the nerve winds around the humerus. The usual causes are fractures and compressions that occur during sleep.

Clinical Manifestations

Clinical manifestations include paralysis of extension of the elbow and impaired sensation over the posterior aspect of the dorsum of the hand.

FEMORAL NERVE INJURY
Definition

Lower extremity injuries of the femoral nerve originate from trauma to L2, L3, and L4 nerve roots.

Etiology/Pathophysiology

The femoral nerve lies in the pelvis lateral to the femoral artery. It innervates the iliacus and psoas muscles. The femoral nerve carries sensation from the anteromedial surface of the thigh; the posterior division provides the motor innervation to the quadriceps and to the medial side of the leg from the knee to the ankle. The most common cause for femoral nerve injury is a pelvic tumor from injury during pelvic surgery. Femoral neuropathy is also caused by diabetes.[1]

Clinical Manifestations

Clinical manifestations include the following: weakness of extension of the knee, wasting of the quadriceps muscle, absence of the knee-jerk reflex, and sensory loss of the anterolateral thigh.

SCIATIC NERVE INJURY
Definition

Lower extremity injuries of the sciatic nerve originate from trauma to L4, L5, and S3 nerve roots.

Etiology/Pathophysiology

The sciatic nerve supplies motor innervation to the hamstring muscles and all the muscles below the knee; it carries sensory impulses from the posterior aspect of the thigh, the posterior and lateral aspects of the leg, and the entire sole. It may be injured by

CLINICAL ALERT

Proper intramuscular injection technique is imperative to eliminate or decrease the chances of injuring the sciatic nerve. Using correct technique helps prevent accidental injection of the sciatic nerve.

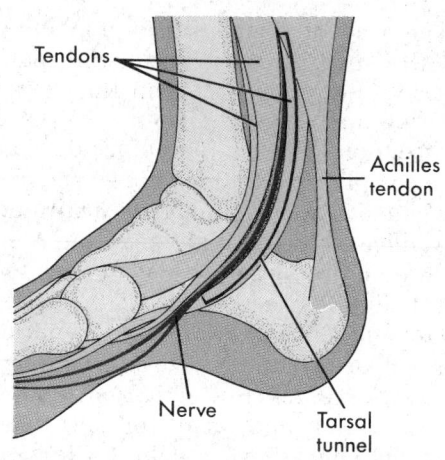

FIGURE 51-5   Locations of tarsal tunnel syndromes.

gunshot wounds, fractures, or injection of medication into the nerve.

Clinical Manifestations

Clinical manifestations include inability to flex the knee, paralysis of muscles below the knee, pain across the buttock and into the thigh, footdrop, and sensory loss in the innervated areas.

COMMON PERONEAL NERVE INJURY
Definition

Lower extremity injuries of the common peroneal nerve originate from trauma to L4 to S3 nerve roots.

Etiology/Pathophysiology

Just above the popliteal fossa the sciatic nerve divides into the tibial nerve and the common peroneal nerve. It then continues around the head of the fibula to the anterior aspect of the leg, leading to the musculocutaneous branch. It is injured from prolonged traction, prolonged application of a tourniquet, or compression at the lateral aspect of the knees during surgery. The application of tight plaster casts and habitual or prolonged crossing of the legs while seated are the most common causes of injury to the common peroneal nerve.

Clinical Manifestations

Clinical manifestations include footdrop and sensory loss of the medial part of the dorsum of the foot and outer aspect of the leg.

TARSAL TUNNEL SYNDROME
Definition

Tarsal tunnel syndrome (Figure 51-5) is a syndrome similar to carpal tunnel syndrome that affects the foot and ankle. The syndrome is divided into two distinct categories. In posterior tarsal tunnel syndrome the distal portion of the posterior tibial nerve is entrapped at the level of the medial malleolus, the

point from which the nerve supplies sensory innervation to the sole of the foot and motor innervation to the intrinsic muscle of the foot.[4] Anterior tarsal tunnel syndrome causes pain and sensory loss in the distal portions of the deep peroneal nerve over the dorsum of the foot. Compression neuropathies secondary to space-occupying lesions such as lipomas, varicose veins, and ganglia of the ankle joint are a few examples of the etiology of this syndrome. Symptoms mimic those of carpel tunnel syndrome and include burning pain with varying degrees of sensory disturbance over the toes and sole of one or both feet. The differential diagnosis includes stress fractures, bursitis, metatarsalgia, and other peripheral neuropathies. Treatment begins conservatively with rest and splinting, followed by steroid injection if pain persists. Surgical intervention permits the freeing up and release of the nerve.

THERAPEUTIC MANAGEMENT OF PERIPHERAL NERVE INJURY

The prognosis for spontaneous recovery for patients with peripheral nerve injuries depends on the type and severity of the injury. Recovery of the upper trunk of the brachial nerve, for instance, is good, although it may be incomplete. Injuries that occurred at birth (Duchenne-Erb palsy) may persist throughout life. As is the case with all brachial nerve injuries, the symptoms are unique; however, the sooner treatment is begun to assist in the recovery of the nerve function, the more likely function will return.

In general, the source of the trauma is attended to first. The injury is treated by first aid initially and surgery if indicated. Attention is then directed to preventing further damage to the nerve. Surgery may be indicated immediately to ascertain the extent of injury. Primary nerve repair is usually performed 3 weeks after injury. However, individual surgeons have their own preferences, and surgery may be delayed for up to 2 months.[5]

Denervated muscle begins to atrophy. This means that when a muscle group does not get impulses to contract or relax, atrophy begins. Measures used to retard atrophy and promote muscle regeneration include electrical stimulation to the muscle and involvement in an active physical therapy program. Additional devices such as leg braces and orthotics to prevent footdrop and wristdrop, massage, whirlpool treatments, and an active exercise program all assist in optimal use of affected limbs.

NURSING MANAGEMENT OF THE PATIENT WITH PERIPHERAL NERVE DISORDER

Assessment

A general physical assessment is performed, with special attention to the motor and sensory components. This baseline assessment can be invaluable as peripheral nerve injuries progress or remain stable. It gives the nurse a sense of direction, either positive or negative, from which function can be determined. A complete neurologic assessment should be performed including sensory and motor assessment. The following points should be addressed during an assessment: gait; voluntary movements, involuntary movements, or lack of movement; reflexes; pain or abnormal sensations, stereognosis, anhidrosis, paralysis, and muscle wasting; and skin breakdown, including infection and poor healing of the affected limb.

Nursing Diagnosis

Nursing diagnoses for patients with peripheral nerve disorders include the following:
  Impaired physical mobility related to motor deficits
  High risk for injury related to sensory and motor deficits
  Pain related to nerve injury
  Self-care deficit related to motor deficits
  Personal identity disturbance related to changes in life-style

Planning

As is the case with all peripheral nerve disorders and injury, it is far better to preserve what function exists than to try to regain lost function. Therefore the nurse concentrates on preventing further injury. The application of braces and casts and their care are discussed in Chapter 57. Helping the patient prepare for the long, arduous rehabilitative plan is an essential responsibility of the nurse. The following goals are included when teaching the patient:
  Patient is knowledgeable about measures to protect self from harm
  Patient copes with changes in body image
  Patient takes protective measures to prevent exposure of the affected extremity to extremes in temperature
  Patient performs activities of daily living whenever possible

Implementation

The nurse educates the patient about safety measures to be taken in the hospital and at home. These include preventing injury from environmental hazards such as scatter rugs, unstable furniture, and hot water settings in the high range. Even though physical changes may occur gradually, body image is often distorted or altered. The patient is reassured that deformities can be minimized using rehabilitative resources such as counseling and patient group interactions.

Evaluation

Evaluating the patient's progress and noting trends in the severity of symptoms are part of a thorough assessment. In reviewing the established plan it is important to assess whether the patient implemented safety precautions. Include documentation of ongoing sensory and motor assessment. The nurse evaluates the plan continually with input from the patient.

Documentation

Documentation is required for evidence that the plan, intervention, and evaluation have been followed and steps have been taken to alter or redirect the plan accordingly. Documenting completion of the plan set by the nurse and the patient or a need to reevaluate the plan is important not only to justify that the plan is being implemented, but also, more importantly, to adequately evaluate the patient's progress.

Ongoing Care

Information necessary for the patient is outlined in the nursing care plan formulated during hospitalization. The work begun in the hospital must be continued at home. Instructions are a vital part of the discharge teaching. Before discharge, the nurse reviews the points listed in the care plan that relate to home care. A home health care agency should be contacted if needed for assessment of the home. This is especially important if the patient lives alone and the nurse questions the safety of the home.

NUTRITIONAL DEFICIENCY NEUROPATHY
Definition/Etiology

Nutritional deficiency neuropathy is a secondary nerve condition. In the Western world the most likely primary causes are alcoholism and anorexia, which are characterized by poor dietary intake of nutrients and weight loss. The most common deficient nutrients are the B complex vitamins (thiamin [B_1], pyridoxine [B_6], and cyanocobalamin [B_{12}]), which help in the production of the myelin sheath.

Pathophysiology/Clinical Manifestations

Deficiency in the B complex vitamins occurs over a period of weeks to months. Axonal degeneration and variable segmental demyelination of the large-diameter axons of the legs cause pain, dysesthesias, paresthesias, and tenderness in muscles surrounding the nerve. The symptoms occur symmetrically and are often transient. Frequently patients report no symptoms, but sensory and motor dysfunction is found on neurologic examination. Transmission of nerve impulses is interrupted by demyelination.

Therapeutic Management

Patients with nutritional deficiency neuropathy are often debilitated by a primary illness, such as alcoholism. The primary problems must be treated first to ensure rehabilitation (see Chapter 21). B complex vitamins, including thiamin (100 mg/day) and cyanocobalamin injections, can be administered to improve the deficiency. A diet high in the B vitamins is also a part of the regimen (see box below). Recovery is slow even if permanent damage has not occurred.[9]

NURSING MANAGEMENT OF THE PATIENT WITH NUTRITIONAL DEFICIENCY NEUROPATHY
Assessment

Assessment begins with a complete dietary history to identify the underlying disease state, such as alcoholism or anorexia. The physical examination includes a thorough neurologic examination, including sensory and motor assessment. The lower limbs are assessed symmetrically for tenderness on squeezing the calf muscles, depressed deep tendon reflexes, and pain or paresthesia. Some patients experience a burning sensation in both the feet and the hands. In advanced cases the examination may reveal footdrop, weakness of the legs because of muscle wasting, and skin changes such as ulcers.

Nursing Diagnosis

Common nursing diagnoses for patients with nutritional deficiency neuropathy include the following:

Sensory/perceptual alterations related to demyelination of long axons

Pain related to axonal degeneration

Altered nutrition: less than body requirements related to the underlying disease state, such as alcoholism

High risk for injury related to diminished or absent sensation

Knowledge deficit related to the disease state and lack of information about nutrition

Planning

Patient goals and their priority reflect the severity of the underlying debilitating disease. The following are general goals:

Patient alters nutrition to include foods rich in vitamin B

Patient obtains information about nutrition and treatment with a vitamin supplement

---

FOODS RICH IN B VITAMINS

Red meats and liver
Whole grain products
Breads
Cereals and wheat germ
Peas and beans
Eggs
Broccoli and spinach
Peanuts and nuts
Tuna
Brewer's yeast

 **CLINICAL ALERT**

B vitamins are water soluble and are rapidly excreted. The target tissues are the heart, liver, kidneys, and peripheral nerves. Normal oral doses range from 1 to 2 mg daily. Because of the fast excretion rate and low body storage activity, B complex vitamins must be taken daily.

Patient reports sensorimotor loss to health professionals

Patient remains free of injury, such as skin ulcers

Implementation

Treatment measures for alcoholism or anorexia are initiated first. The nurse can be instrumental in recovery from these diseases by giving support to the patient and family. The nurse administers the initial vitamin supplement in the form of injections but later may teach the family or patient to administer the medications. The patient and family members will need information and teaching about proper foods to include in the diet. The importance of a balanced diet and vitamin supplements is stressed. The nurse also instructs the patient in foot care to prevent skin breakdown.

Evaluation

Ongoing patient assessment helps the nurse evaluate the effectiveness of the nutritional interventions. The successful treatment plan helps the patient eat a balanced diet rich in vitamin B. The patient will maintain good skin integrity without the sensory system becoming more impaired. The nurse assesses for any change in pain during the follow-up interview.

Documentation

Documentation consists of assessment and history information. Documentation of the sensory and motor assessment of the lower limbs includes findings of paresthesia, pain, or tenderness in the calf muscle. The dietary history includes a 24-hour recall of all foods ingested with an emphasis on foods rich in B vitamins. Recording the amounts of red meats, whole grains, and dark leafy vegetables is important for accurate documentation. Ingestion or injections of vitamin supplements are recorded.

Ongoing Care

Continued nursing care for the patient with nutritional neuropathy usually occurs at the end of hospitalization or in the home setting. The hospital nurse should refer the patient to a home health service for further teaching and possible injection of vitamin supplements. Rehabilitation for these patients includes treatment for the underlying disease state. Physical and emotional support is essential for these patients. Dietary and vitamin supplement needs are monitored by the home health nurse or the clinic nurse, with special attention paid to the skin and sensory assessment on each visit.

TOXIC NEUROPATHY
Definition/Etiology

Peripheral disorders of the nervous system result from exposure to or ingestion of injurious or poisonous substances. These toxic substances are termed exogenous because they have been introduced from outside the body. Toxic agents are subclassified as heavy metals and chemotherapeutic agents. Heavy metals such as lead, arsenic, and mercury cause neuropathies.[1] Toxic chemotherapeutic agents include cisplatin, vincristine, and 5-fluorouracil. Many other chemicals and drugs cause neurologic symptoms; the study of this biochemical problem is termed neurotoxicology.

Neurologic complications from lead poisoning are common in the United States. In adults lead poisoning can occur from breathing fumes of burning batteries, ingestion of lead from pottery cooking utensils, demolition of buildings with lead-painted steel, and home remodeling.

The increasing use of antineoplastic agents has given rise to peripheral neuropathies. It has been reported that 92% of patients receiving cisplatin have symptoms of neuropathy.

Pathophysiology/Clinical Manifestations

Heavy metals and drugs cause peripheral neuropathy by destroying the axonal myelin sheath. The toxic substances are deposited in the nervous system from the high level in the bloodstream. Initially segmental demyelination occurs followed by damage to axons and cells in the spinal cord. The symptoms of heavy metal poisoning appear over 3 to 6 weeks. The initial symptoms are irritability and anorexia, followed by vomiting, clumsiness, and ataxia. Peripheral symptoms occur almost exclusively in adults and involve the upper extremities. The radial nerve is most commonly involved. Wristdrop and fingerdrop may also occur.[1] The peripheral neuropathic side effects of chemotherapeutic agents include paresthesias of the feet and hands and a progressive, symmetric motor/sensory and reflex loss. Cranial nerves and the autonomic nervous system can be affected.[7]

Therapeutic Management

Treatment of lead poisoning involves identifying and removing the source of the lead. Lead in the soft tissues may be mobilized using the chelating agent calcium disodium edetate. The initial dosage of 25 mg/kg of body weight twice daily is gradually increased to 75 mg/kg over 5 days. A second course may be given after a rest period of 3 weeks. Peripheral neuropathy gradually disappears. Treatment for the toxic effects of drugs consists of decreasing or stopping the drug dosage. The symptoms usually disappear over weeks or months. In some patients receiving cisplatin, the symptoms have increased or remained after elimination of the drug.

NURSING MANAGEMENT OF THE PATIENT WITH TOXIC NEUROPATHY
Assessment

A thorough history is taken by the nurse to elicit information about the cause of the toxic neuropathy. Information about the patient's occupation, hobbies, and home may yield clues about the heavy metal contaminant. If the patient has been taking chemotherapy or other drugs, information about the duration, dosage, and use are documented. The physical assessment encompasses a complete neurologic examination with extensive motor and sensory assessment. Findings may include muscle weakness, paresthesia, and possible wristdrop. Pain is a prominent feature in neuropathy from chemotherapeutic agents. Blood levels for the heavy metals sometimes yield concentrations higher than 70 μg/mL, which are considered toxic in adults. Anemia may be found in conjunction with either lead or chemotherapeutic toxic neuropathy. Motor nerve conduction velocities are decreased.[1]

Nursing Diagnosis

Common nursing diagnoses for the patient with a toxic neuropathy follow:

- Knowledge deficit related to peripheral toxic neuropathy
- Sensory/perceptual alteration related to injury to peripheral nerves
- Impaired mobility related to sensory/perceptual loss and muscle weakness
- Pain related to injury to peripheral nerves
- High risk for injury related to sensory/perceptual loss

Planning

Patient goals and their priority reflect the patient's diagnosis and specific toxic chemical neuropathy:

- Patient is knowledgeable about the agents causing the neuropathy and how to eliminate them from his or her environment
- Patient can identify and report sensory/perceptual changes
- Patient performs activities of daily living and maintains physical mobility

- Patient achieves a level of comfort
- Patient remains free of injury

Implementation

Patient education is essential to reduce the risk of further exposure to heavy metals. The nurse must be an active listener and provide information as to the cause and possible treatment. Education is also essential for patients receiving chemotherapeutic agents or drugs and should include information about their possible side effects. The nurse incorporates an assessment regarding the patient's mobility into the care plan. Activities of daily living may become difficult for the patient with decreased mobility. Family members can be involved in the patient's care and new approaches to familiar routines developed. Range-of-motion exercises will keep the unaffected limbs mobile and strong. The patient is also taught to avoid situations that can cause injury or an unsafe environment. The nurse can provide psychologic support for dealing with chronic pain and discomfort while also using interventions such as relaxation, imagery, warmth, and massage.[7]

Evaluation

Ongoing patient sensory and motor assessment of the limbs can determine if interventions are appropriate. Decreased or absent pain indicates the comfort measures have supported the nervous system function. The patient recognizes potential sources of toxic contaminants and eliminates them from the home. Finally, the patient performs activities of daily living to his or her ability level and remains free of injury.

Documentation

Assessment data are recorded on an ongoing basis in the patient's record. The patient's history and possible source of the toxic agent or the dosage of drug received are noted. Patient and family education with teaching materials is kept on record in the patient's chart. Finally, symptoms of toxic neuropathy are reported to the physician so that appropriate treatment can be instituted.

Ongoing Care

A community health referral can be instituted to ensure that initial education about the disease and the source of toxic chemical or drug is reinforced. The home health care nurse can help the patient assess the environment and remove the contaminants. Prevention of further injury to the peripheral nerves can be avoided.

MYELOMATOUS AND CARCINOMATOUS NEUROPATHIES

Definition

Patients who have been diagnosed with cancer or multiple myeloma may have symptoms of a **polyneuropathy.** Affecting mostly the lower extremities, this neuropathy is bilateral and affects mainly the sensorimotor tracts.[1] The cause of paraneoplastic polyneuropathy is unknown. The theories proposed range from an immunologic mechanism to a vitamin deficiency.

Pathophysiology

Just as the etiology of myelomatous and carcinomatous neuropathies is unknown, so is the pathophysiology poorly defined. The purely sensory type of neuropathy involves loss of the dorsal root ganglia, with associated degeneration of the dorsal nerve roots. In the sensorimotor type of neuropathy the symptoms usually cannot be separated from nutritional or metabolic neuropathy.

Clinical Manifestations

A severe weakness and atrophy top the list of patient complaints. Along with ataxia and sensory loss of the limbs, symptoms may advance to the point where the patient is confined to a wheelchair or bed. These symptoms may occur months or even 1 year or more before a small malignant tumor is diagnosed. However, as stated at the outset, this type of peripheral neuropathy is a remote effect of carcinomas and is seen in only a very small percentage of patients.[1]

Therapeutic Management

The prognosis for myelomatous and carcinomatous neuropathies is very poor. Symptoms vary in their severity, with polyneuropathy being the least severe. The patient may die from the tumor within 1 year. Of course, if surgery is feasible, the tumor is removed. Depending on the histologic appearance of the tumor, chemotherapy or radiation can help relieve the symptoms of polyneuropathy. Management of this patient is similar to that of patients with other types of polyneuropathies, as described elsewhere in this chapter. Depending on the type of neuropathy, specific management can be initiated.

CHARCOT-MARIE-TOOTH DISEASE

Definition

In **Charcot-Marie-Tooth disease,** chronic degeneration of peripheral nerves and roots results in distal muscle atrophy. This disease is an inherited autosomal dominant (occasionally recessive) trait.

Etiology/Pathophysiology

Charcot-Marie-Tooth disease was first described in 1886 by Tooth in England and by Charcot and Marie in France. Onset occurs during late childhood or adolescence. Degenerative changes in the nerves result in depletion of the large sensory and motor fibers.

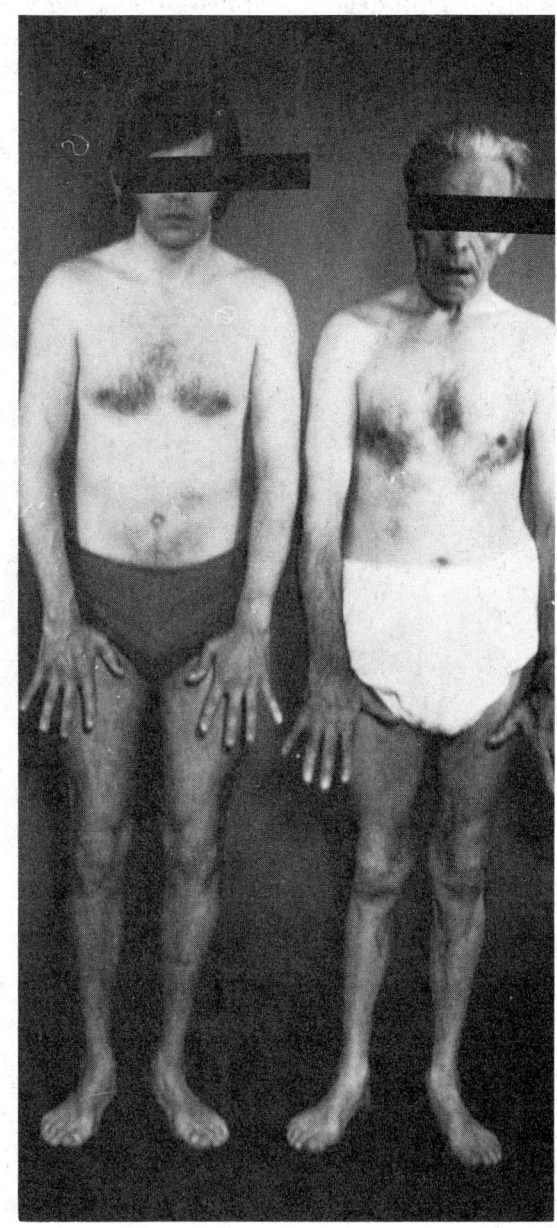

FIGURE 51-6   Charcot-Marie-Tooth disease in two generations: distal wasting is most evident in older patient. (From Perkin DG et al: *Slide atlas of neurology,* London, 1987, Gower Medical Publishing.)

The illness progresses slowly, with periods of stability in symptoms.[1]

Clinical Manifestations

Atrophy begins in the feet and legs and later involves the hands. The characteristic "storklike" legs contribute to the main disability, namely, difficulty in walking (Figure 51-6). As the disease progresses, the hands develop a claw deformity similar to the muscle wasting seen in hands with ulnar nerve deficits (Fig. 51-7). Paresthesias and cramps are always present to some degree. Rarely is the sensory loss severe.

There is no known cure for Charcot-Marie-Tooth disease. Symptomatic treatment is given, however, with attention focused on assisting the patient to ambulate. Treatment involves braces and rehabilitative care.

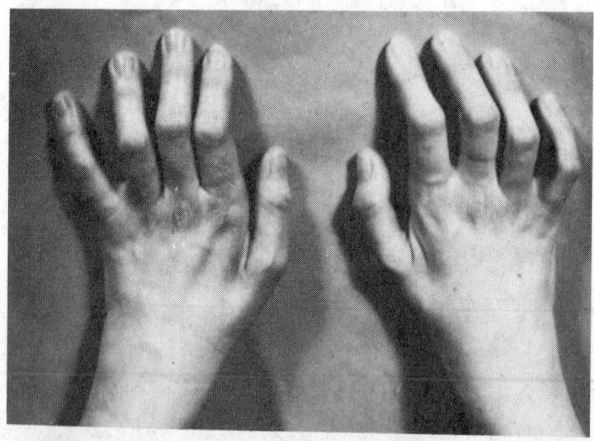
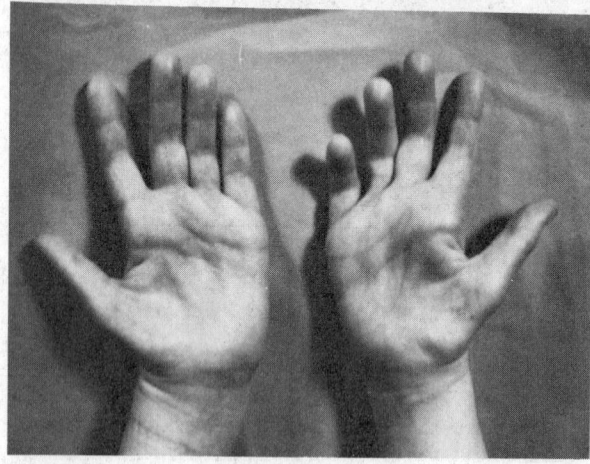

FIGURE 51-7   Charcot-Marie-Tooth disease: wasting of small hand muscles. (From Perkin DG et al: *Slide atlas of neurology,* London, 1987, Gower Medical Publishing.)

NURSING MANAGEMENT OF THE PATIENT WITH CHARCOT-MARIE-TOOTH DISEASE

Assessment

Nursing care is directed to individual symptoms or complaints, again concentrating on the need for ambulation, stability, and pain control. Some patients require leg braces for stability and instruction for the proper positioning and care of braces.

Nursing Diagnosis

Common nursing diagnoses for the patient with Charcot-Marie-Tooth disease include the following:
   Impaired physical mobility related to atrophy
   High risk for injury related to paresthesia
   Pain related to cramping in the extremities

Planning

Patient goals and their priority reflect the severity of symptoms. General goals include the following:
   Patient provides self-care and performs activities of daily living, incorporating needed assistive devices
   Patient remains free of injury
   Patient achieves a level of comfort, especially at night

Implementation

Patient education must involve areas of concern for the patient and the symptoms currently causing deficits, as well as those known symptoms yet to occur. The slow progression of the illness permits adequate time to refer the patient for rehabilitation medicine for instructions and care related to increasing mobility. Assistive devices for the hands are available if the patient requires help with eating and dressing. Cool packs, moist heat, and exercise all play an important role for cramping and paresthesia. The patient is instructed to try several techniques for optimal relief.

Evaluation

Ongoing assessment of the patient's ability to perform activities of daily living must be done. This may be accomplished by the home health care nurse, who should evaluate the home for environmental hazards and recommend removal of hazardous items. Medications prescribed by the physician are evaluated for efficacy and proper administration. Patient education and return demonstration of teaching are performed.

Ongoing Care

The home health nurse can monitor the patient with Charcot-Marie-Tooth disease for extended periods. Incorporating the knowledge that the disease progresses slowly and has periods of stability enables the nurse to provide emotional and physical support for the patient. Periodic checks in the home can provide much needed support.

Cranial Nerve Disorders

TRIGEMINAL NEURALGIA
Definition

Trigeminal neuralgia, a disorder of cranial nerve V, also referred to as tic douloureux, is a syndrome of paroxysmal facial pain that patients describe as the most excruciating ever experienced. Affecting the middle-aged and elderly population almost exclusively, this disorder consists of intense, stabbing, sudden, periodic *(paroxysmal)* pain in the lips, gums, cheek, or chin. A patient suffering from this acute process likens the pain to a thousand burning needles pricking and stabbing, knives cutting and piercing, something searing the flesh, wires that tingle with electrical pain, or a crescendo agony finishing by a burst or explosion as of a firework. The trigeminal nerve is the fifth cranial nerve and is divided into three segments (Figure 51-8). The most common area of pain is the mandibular and maxillary

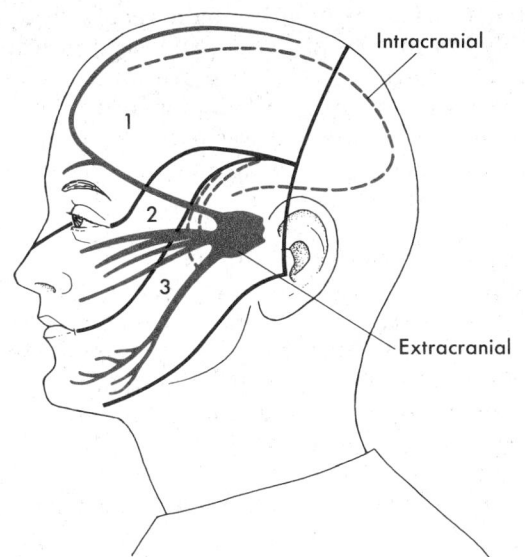

FIGURE 51-8 Major sensory branches of trigeminal nerve and regions supplied by each of sensory divisions of trigeminal nerve.

division. The disorder almost always affects one side of the face, although bilateral cases have been reported. Women are affected three times as often as men, with the onset beginning in the fifth decade.

Etiology/Pathophysiology

Trigeminal neuralgia remains a disorder of unknown etiology, although many theories exist as to the cause. These include a tortuous artery in the posterior fossa of the brain that causes an irritative lesion of the nerve or its root or a tumor (acoustic or trigeminal neuroma, meningioma, or epidermoid cyst) in the cerebellar pontine angle. Some physicians view the disorder as a manifestation of multiple sclerosis when it appears bilaterally in younger adults.

Clinical Manifestations

The pain seldom lasts more than a few seconds to 1 or 2 minutes but may be so intense that the patient winces, hence the name *tic.* The onset of pain can occur at any time during the day or night and may recur several times for weeks at a time.[2] The pain may be initiated by everyday activities such as tooth brushing, hair drying, or drinking a cold beverage. A common characteristic of trigeminal neuralgia is the initiation of pain by stimuli to trigger points in certain areas of the face, lips, or tongue or by movement of these parts. Many patients are so fearful that these activities may provoke a painful event that they often forego activities of daily living in the hope of preventing another pain episode. In addition to the paroxysms, some patients complain of a more or less continuous discomfort and sensitivity of the face. It is important to realize that a light touch or tickle also can provoke a painful event.

Therapeutic Management

Drug therapy

The initial treatment for trigeminal neuralgia is pharmacologic. Conventional therapy using analgesics is ineffective. Anticonvulsant drugs give the patient the best pain relief and are the first mode of treatment for trigeminal neuralgia. Carbamazepine (Tegretol), the drug of choice initially, is effective in 75% of patients. It is believed that the mode of action of carbamazepine decreases the paroxysmal afferent impulses, an action similar to that when this drug is used in the treatment of epilepsy.[5] Carbamazepine is not well tolerated by many patients at the dosage level required for effective management of pain. Therefore the drug should be started at a single dose of 100 mg taken with food and increased

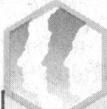

GERIATRIC CONSIDERATIONS

Trigeminal Neuralgia

Trigeminal neuralgia is commonly seen in the fifth decade of life and beyond. Shorter hospitalization dictates astute nursing assessment for home management of the patient following surgery. Frequent home visits to assess pain, eye function, nutrition, and overall hygiene are especially important in this generation of patients.

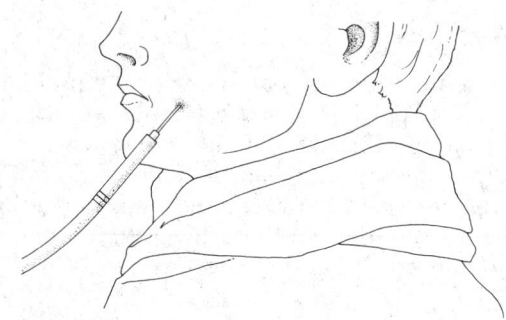

FIGURE 51-9　Percutaneous radiofrequency rhizotomy for relief of pain from trigeminal neuralgia.

gradually to 1200 mg daily. Doses greater than 1200 to 1600 mg provide no additional benefit.

Phenytoin (Dilantin) is another anticonvulsant that is used to treat trigeminal neuralgia. Its mode of action is similar to carbamazepine. The dosage starts at 200 to 400 mg/day. Patients may receive the total dose for the day at one time, or it may be administered throughout the day in divided doses. Carbamazepine and phenytoin have numerous side effects that may not be tolerated by the patient, including gastrointestinal upset, ataxia, skin rash, drowsiness, leukopenia, nystagmus, and gum hypertrophy (with prolonged use).

Surgical management

If drug therapy fails, surgical therapy should be offered to the patient. Surgical therapy can benefit approximately 30% of patients with trigeminal neuralgia that is refractory to medical management.[6] Surgical intervention is categorized as to whether the procedure is major or minor. However, it must be understood that all surgical interventions are major procedures for the patient.

Minor surgical interventions

Of all the minor surgical procedures available for the treatment of trigeminal neuralgia, perhaps the most widely used are radiofrequency gangliolysis and glycerol gangliolysis. Radiofrequency gangliolysis is commonly preferred for elderly persons, because general anesthesia, with all its inherent complications, is not necessary.

Radiofrequency gangliolysis involves heating a percutaneously placed electrode to produce a lesion within the trigeminal ganglion (Figure 51-9). Heat conducted in the trigeminal ganglion disrupts the nerve from sending impulses, thus relieving the pain. Radiofrequency lesions abolish pain in 80% of the patients for 1 year and 60% for 5 years.[2] Many patients experience a sensory loss immediately after the treatment, but this may be transient.

Glycerol gangliolysis involves injecting glycerol into the subarachnoid space surrounding the gasserian ganglion. The treatment was discovered inadvertently by Håkanson[19] in Sweden in the early 1980s. It was originally used as a method to introduce tantalum dust into the trigeminal cistern for localization of the trigeminal ganglion and root.[2] But when the patient's pain had been abolished, Håkanson realized that the glycerol not only provided pain relief, but also did so with little loss of sensory function, an added feature over other therapies. This method proved advantageous in many ways: ease of administration, decreased anesthesia risks, and relatively few experiences of sensory function loss. The latter is especially important in regard to potential side effects such as corneal denervation with secondary keratitis and loss of facial sensation. As many as 89% to 96% of patients can expect complete relief from their pain after glycerol gangliolysis; but within the first 6 months, pain recurs in approximately 7% to 10% of patients. Overall percentages, however, favor the procedure, with long-term follow-up (up to 6 years) demonstrating a 90% to 96% pain-free patient. Some patients may need supplemental drug therapy to enhance the effect derived from the surgery.

Major surgical interventions

Another approach to treating trigeminal neuralgia is the use of microvascular decompression. The patient and the surgeon must concur as to the best possible intervention, taking into consideration the patient's age, general health, and overall chance for a successful outcome, along with the risks of postoperative complications.

Microvascular decompression is performed with the patient under general anesthesia through a posterior fossa craniotomy. The goal of surgery is to separate the offending vessel from its point of contact with the posterior trigeminal root.[6] Keeping the two apart is a piece of Teflon felt or other synthetic material. This permits the nerve to function without being compressed by surrounding vasculature, thereby alleviating the pain. The patient is usually hospitalized for 7 to 10 days. Microvascular decompression is the procedure of choice for younger patients who can tolerate major surgery. Long-term results are promising; adding to the benefit of successfully eliminating pain are minimal sensory loss and its associated complications.

NURSING MANAGEMENT OF THE PATIENT WITH TRIGEMINAL NEURALGIA

Assessment

Subjective data are obtained related to onset, duration, and location of pain.

Nursing Diagnosis

Nursing diagnoses include the following:
   Pain related to nerve irritation
   Altered nutrition: less than body requirements
   Activity intolerance related to pain
   Bathing/hygiene self-care deficit related to pain
   Anxiety related to pain
   Social isolation related to fear of pain attacks, stimulation-free environment

Planning

Goals are set to achieve the following outcome criteria
   Patient identifies causative factors that bring about a painful episode and attempts to decrease or eliminate the factors
   Patient verbalizes adequate nutrition and makes an effort to maintain a balanced diet
   Patient maintains a balanced activity and rest schedule and avoids isolation rationalized as a means of preventing pain recurrence
   Patient is aware of proper oral hygiene and has regular dental checkups

Implementation

For hospitalized patients, medical management has most likely been exhausted and the patient is preparing for surgical intervention. The nursing diagnoses can be appropriate for the surgical patient as well as the patient receiving drug therapy. Pain is often the limiting factor in self-care. The patient continues taking medication while in the hospital to maintain therapeutic blood levels of anticonvulsant. The patient may wish to bring into the hospital comfort measures that have been used at home. A personal pillow or blanket may help allay fears in an unknown environment. These individualized components are incorporated into the nursing care plan.

Patients are often admitted the day of surgery and discharged as soon as possible. Contacting the clinical nutritionist at the time of admission can facilitate the identification of possible nutritional deficiencies related to pain and intolerance to certain food types. The nurse should note the types of foods and temperatures of beverages to be avoided; water pitchers should not have ice. The patient is all too familiar with foods that trigger painful episodes.

Patients often isolate themselves from outside activities for fear of initiating a painful episode. Some patients are housebound and lack contact with friends and family. This life-style should be discouraged. On discharge the patient should be reminded that he or she may now move about without the constant fear of initiating pain. It may take some time for the patient to become comfortable with this idea.

Preoperative care

Care of the patient preoperatively consists of the following:
   Explanation of the surgical procedure and reinforcement of information given to the patient by the surgeon
   Reinforcement of preoperative teaching, allowing the patient to verbalize fears and concerns
   Offering the patient and family a tour of the intensive care unit (if applicable)
   Individualized teaching and care planning, depending on the surgical procedure

Postoperative care

Nursing care after surgery depends on the type of surgical procedure the patient has undergone. After one of the minor surgical procedures, the patient has usually recovered from anesthesia after a brief stay in the recovery room. The nurse continues monitoring the vital and neurologic signs until they have stabilized. The nurse performs neurologic assessments specific to the cranial nerves to adequately assess

 **CLINICAL ALERT**

The patient must be assessed for adequate closing and opening of the eyelid (blinking). The inability to perform this activity can result in corneal irritation and permanent damage. If the patient cannot blink, notify the physician. Administer lubricating eye drops or ointment. In severe cases the eyelid may need to be sutured closed until the ability to blink has returned.

whether the pain has diminished or has been completely eradicated.

Assessment of cranial nerve function, in this case the trigeminal nerve, demonstrates the patient's ability to blink. The inability to blink completely can dry out the eyes and lead to corneal damage. Lubricating eye drops may be necessary to provide comfort and protection of the eye.

Before the patient attempts to drink liquids, the nurse assesses for adequate swallowing ability. The nurse asks the patient to sit upright and try swallowing ice chips, progressing to clear liquids as ordered. Eating solid foods may be painful at first because of the injection site in the cheek. The nurse instructs the patient to avoid (1) hot foods because of decreased sensation and (2) placement of food in the unaffected side of the mouth because of the difficulty in swallowing. The patient, it should be remembered, may hesitate to experiment with unknown foods and liquids, not knowing if the pain will return. New foods and activities are introduced as tolerated.

Postoperative care of the patient after a major surgical procedure is similar to caring for a patient after a craniotomy. As soon as the patient has recovered from anesthesia and is fully awake and neurologically stable, the pain is assessed and compared with the preoperative assessment.

Evaluation

After surgery or during medical management of trigeminal neuralgia, the patient is monitored closely to evaluate the effectiveness of the care plan. The nurse's evaluation focuses on the following points:

- Have the patient and nurse properly identified trigger points that cause the pain of trigeminal neuralgia and taken steps to eliminate these in the patient's day-to-day activities?
- Is the patient maintaining adequate nutrition before and after surgery?
- Are adequate activity and rest being implemented to balance daily activities?
- Does the patient institute proper oral hygiene and provide overall self-care?
- How is the patient coping with the fear of possible recurring pain?
- Has the patient's knowledge of trigeminal neuralgia increased?

Documentation

Documentation is required for evidence that the plan, intervention, and evaluation have been followed and that steps have been taken to alter or redirect the plan if necessary. Vital signs and neurologic assessment are recorded in the medical record. Documenting the difference in the degree or type of

trigeminal pain, the presence or absence of the ability to blink before surgery or medical intervention, or the onset of complications postoperatively is a vital part of nursing care.

Ongoing Care

Instructions are an essential part of discharge teaching. They include mutually agreed-on areas that still need attention, such as adequate performance of oral hygiene. The nurse ensures that the patient is aware of follow-up appointments with the physician and encourages the patient to list questions for the physician. In general, patients with trigeminal neuralgia need minimal care and assistance at home. However, the nurse must evaluate the need for assistance, as well as provide emotional support, by discussing the home situation with the patient and family.

FACIAL NERVE PARALYSIS
Definition

A unilateral facial paralysis of sudden onset, known as **Bell's palsy,** is the most common form of facial nerve paralysis and was named in 1821 after Sir Charles Bell of England. The paralysis affects the motor component of the facial nerve (cranial nerve

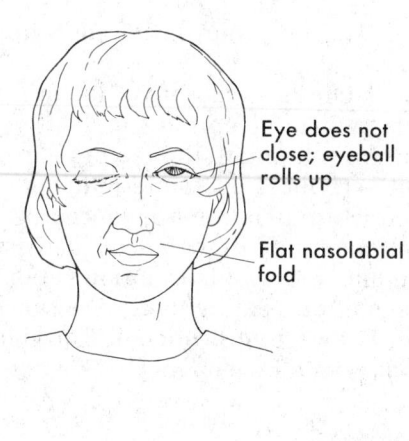

Eye does not close; eyeball rolls up

Flat nasolabial fold

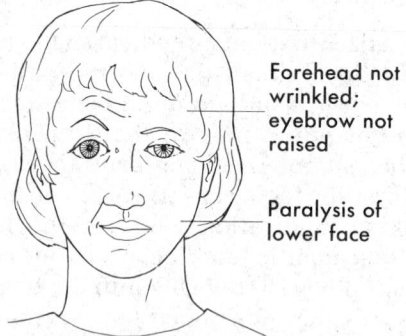

Forehead not wrinkled; eyebrow not raised

Paralysis of lower face

FIGURE 51-10   Clinical manifestations of facial nerve paralysis.

VII), resulting in a characteristic distortion of the face.

Etiology/Epidemiology

Facial nerve paralysis affects approximately 23 out of every 100,000 persons annually. The disorder affects both sexes equally. Onset occurs after 20 years of age but is more common in adults 20 to 60 years old. The side of the face that is affected (and it is only one side) is paralyzed and sags; the patient cannot close the eyelid or mouth; and drooling often occurs (Figure 51-10). The sense of taste is affected on the anterior two thirds of the tongue (Figure 51-11). The etiology is unknown but is attributed to a nondescript change in the actual nerve and not to inflammation, as was commonly presumed.

Pathophysiology

The pathophysiology of Bell's palsy remains, to date, unclear. Inflammation or degeneration of the facial nerve has been addressed as well as a possible viral cause. None of these possibilities have been scientifically proven.

Clinical Manifestations

The onset of the paralysis is acute, with maximal weakness noted by 48 hours. Pain behind the ear may be a symptom, preceded by paralysis by 1 or 2 days. Impairment of taste is noted by almost all patients but rarely persists beyond the second week of paralysis.[1]

About 80% of patients recover fully in weeks or months, with recovery of taste being the first sign. Recovery of taste within the first week signals a good chance for full recovery of motor function. This fa-

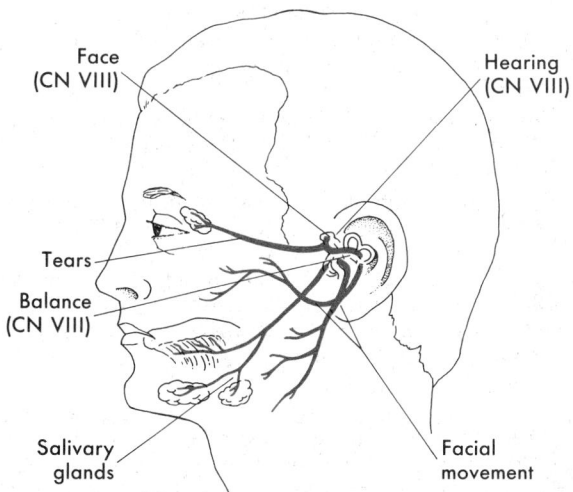

FIGURE 51-11   Areas affected by facial nerve injury.

vorable prognostic sign also holds true if paralysis remains incomplete within the first 5 to 7 days.

Therapeutic Management

The administration of prednisone, 60 to 80 mg/day, given in the first week, may provide some relief of symptoms. This dose should be tapered over the next 5 days. Analgesics help relieve pain associated with the paralysis, as do gentle massage to the affected area and application of warm, moist heat. As muscle tone recovers, facial exercises may expedite full recovery.

Surgery is not recommended for this type of cranial nerve disorder. The process of separating the facial nerve from the facial canal has been suggested, but no evidence proves it is helpful and it may actually be harmful.[2]

NURSING MANAGEMENT OF THE PATIENT WITH FACIAL NERVE PARALYSIS

Assessment

Assessment of the extent and effects of the paralysis is the basis for nursing management of the patient. The assessment includes the ability to blink and chew.

Nursing Diagnosis

Common nursing diagnoses for the patient with facial nerve paralysis include the following:

High risk for injury related to sensory or motor deficits

Alteration in comfort

Altered nutrition: less than body requirements

Body image disturbance related to facial paralysis

Self-esteem disturbance related to facial appearance

Planning/Implementation

Protection of the eye is extremely important when the eyelid does not function normally. When the pa-

CLINICAL ALERT

Prednisone is a powerful steroid. Patients should be instructed about the drug's effect and side effects. The drug should be taken with food or milk. When the therapeutic course has been completed, the patient must be weaned gradually from the drug.

tient cannot blink reflexively, the eye becomes dry and irritated. Lubricating drops used during the day and ointment at night are beneficial. The patient is instructed to manually close the eye several times each day; this provides natural lubrication and stimulates the muscle.

Proper nutrition is compromised in many patients because of their inability to chew foods, drink through a straw, or handle secretions on the affected side.[5] Therefore patients often select foods that are easy to manage yet may be of poor nutritional value. High-caloric drinks such as milk shakes and commercially prepared liquids may add to the overall nutritional intake for the patient. Consulting the clinical nutritionist is helpful in planning a well-balanced meal program. As Hickey[9] describes, eating and drinking in our society are social pleasures and these patients often feel embarrassed eating and drinking in the company of others. Coping mechanisms and adaptation skills are included in the overall teaching plan.

Evaluation/Documentation

A well-prepared care plan with input from the patient and nurse may be revised numerous times throughout a long and difficult hospitalization. The plan is evaluated for completeness, as well as for redirecting care of the patient. Documentation is required for evidence that the plan, interventions, and evaluation have been followed and steps have been taken to alter or redirect the plan accordingly.

Ongoing Care

Information needed by the patient and family is outlined in the nursing care plan formulated while the patient is in the hospital. The patient must carry on with this plan at home. The nurse ensures that the patient is aware of follow-up appointments in the outpatient setting and encourages the patient to list questions for the physician. In general, patients with facial nerve paralysis need minimal care and assistance at home. However, the nurse must evaluate the need by discussing the home situation with the patient and family.

CRITICAL THINKING QUESTIONS

1 What are the three pathophysiologic processes that occur in peripheral nerve disease?

2 Jane Smith is assessed for peripheral nerve disease and is found to have reflex changes, anhidrosis, and sensory impairment. What other three signs of peripheral nerve disease should be included in the assessment?

3 What are the major causes of brachial plexus injuries?

4 Audrey Jones is diagnosed with ulnar nerve injury. Name two appropriate nursing diagnoses.

5 Explain the reason for proper intramuscular technique to prevent peripheral nerve disease.

6 Describe the symptoms of trigeminal neuralgia.

7 John Frazer is being treated with carbamazepine for trigeminal neuralgia. He is experiencing ataxia and drowsiness. What other side effects can he expect with this drug?

8 What medications are often prescribed for patients with trigeminal neuralgia?

9 What are the minor and major surgical interventions for trigeminal neuralgia?

10 Discuss the nursing assessment for trigeminal neuralgia.

11 What factors should be included in the preoperative and postoperative care of patients undergoing surgery for trigeminal neuralgia?

12 Why is it important to administer B complex vitamins on a daily basis?

13 List three causes of toxic neuropathy.

14 Describe the condition of facial nerve paralysis.

15 Why is prednisone the drug of choice to treat facial nerve paralysis?

BIBLIOGRAPHY

Current

1. Adams RD, Victor M: *Principles of neurology,* New York, 1989, McGraw-Hill Book Co.
2. Asbury AK: Diseases of the peripheral nervous system. In Braunwald E et al: *Harrison's principles of internal medicine,* New York, 1987, McGraw-Hill Book Co.
3. Bates B: *A guide to physical assessment, examination and history taking,* ed 5, Philadelphia, 1991, JB Lippincott Co.
4. Burchiel KJ: Percutaneous retrogasserian glycerol rhizolysis in the management of trigeminal neuralgia, *J Neurosurg* 69:361, 1988.
5. Dawson DM et al: Tarsal tunnel syndrome. In Dawson DM, Hallett M, Millender LH: *Entrapment neuropathies,* Boston, 1990, Little, Brown & Co.
6. Devinsky O, Feldman E: *Examination of the cranial nerves and peripheral nerves,* New York, 1988, Churchill Livingstone, Inc.
7. Ellenberg M, Rifkin H: *Diabetes mellitus,* New York, 1983, Medical Examination Publishing Co, Inc.
8. Fromm GH: *The medical and surgical management of trigeminal neuralgia,* Mount Kisco, NY, 1987, Futura Publishing Co, Inc.
9. Hickey J: *The clinical practice of neurological and neurosurgical nursing,* Philadelphia, 1986, JB Lippincott Co.
10. Holden S, Felde G: Nursing care of patients experiencing cisplatin-related peripheral neuropathy, *Oncol Nurs* 14(1):68, 1987.
11. Kirkland J, Williams A: Trigeminal neuralgia: ap-

proaches to nursing care, *J Neurosurg Nurs* 15(3):149, 1983.

12. Lachman T: Clinical aspects of peripheral neuropathy, *Hosp Med* 13(2):84, 1987.

13. Mourad LA: *Orthopedic disorders: Mosby's clinical nursing series,* St Louis, 1991, Mosby–Year Book.

14. Perkins, DG et al: *Slide atlas of neurology,* London, 1987, Gower Medical Publishing.

15. Price M, DeVroom H: A quick and easy guide to neurological assessment, *J Neurosurg Nurs* 17(5):313, 1985.

16. Pyle KL: Carpal tunnel syndrome: case data and nursing implications, *J Neurosurg Nurs* 16(6):292, 1984.

17. Victor M, Martin J: Diseases of the cranial nerves. In Braunwald E et al: *Harrison's principles of internal medicine,* New York, 1987, McGraw-Hill Book Co.

Classic

18. Borges L et al: The anterior tunnel syndrome, *J Neurosurg* 54:89-92, 1981.

19. Hakanson S: Trigeminal neuralgia treated by the injection of glycerol into the trigeminal cistern, *Neurosurgery* 9(6):638, 1981.

20. Tytus JS: General considerations, medical therapy, and minor operative procedures for trigeminal neuralgia. In *Neurological surgery,* Philadelphia, 1982, WB Saunders Co.

UNIT XII

The Eye and Ear

CHAPTER FIFTY-TWO

Nursing Assessment of the Eye

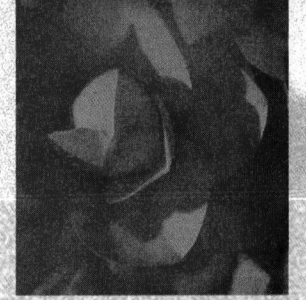

LEARNING OBJECTIVES

1 Know the anatomy of the eye's internal and external structures.
2 Understand the physiologic processes by which visual accommodation, binocular vision, and color perception occur.
3 Obtain relevant subjective information from the patient who has an eye alteration.
4 Using correct technique, examine the patient to obtain appropriate objective information about the eyes.
5 Differentiate abnormal from normal subjective and objective findings related to the eyes.
6 Describe procedures related to the detection and diagnosis of ocular disorders.
7 Describe patient preparation and care for diagnostic tests of the eye.

KEY TERMS

accommodation, p. 1416
aqueous humor, p. 1414
canal of Schlemm, p. 1414
ciliary body, p. 1414
choroid, p. 1414
cones, p. 1415
conjunctiva, p. 1416
electroretinography, p. 1421
fluorescein angiography, p. 1423
iris, p. 1414
lens, p. 1414

nystagmus, p. 1419
palpebral fissure, p. 1420
PERRLA, p. 1420
phoria, p. 1420
ptosis, p. 1420
retina, p. 1414
rods, p. 1415
sclera, p. 1414
tonometry, p. 1422
tropia, p. 1419
vitreous humor, p. 1414

THE EYES are complex, specialized sensory receptors. They are sensitive to light, are shaped much like a camera, and project perfect images of the environment to the cerebral cortex. In addition, the retina modifies and clarifies the outlines of the images to facilitate the central nervous system's interpretation of and reaction to changes in the environment.

Discrepancies in vision can occur at any age—from strabismus and "lazy eye," common conditions of childhood, to the farsightedness (presbyopia) often reported by older adults. Eye alterations may be caused or contributed to by environmental (e.g., smoke or fumes) or psychosocial (e.g., stress) factors. Such discrepancies may also accompany disease. For example, patients with diabetes mellitus are particularly prone to cataracts, glaucoma, and retinopathy.

Throughout the eye assessment, the nurse attempts to establish the cause of visual problems. Precipitating and aggravating factors are recorded, as is prior treatment and the patient's response to it. The nurse notes whether the visual disturbance is unilateral or bilateral.

ANATOMY AND PHYSIOLOGY
The Eyeball

The structure of the eye can be seen in cross section in Figure 52-1. The eye has three layers: the outer layer is the **sclera;** the next is the **choroid;** and the inner layer is the photosensitive **retina.** The lens and its suspensory ligament divide the eye into two chambers. The posterior chamber is filled with a colorless transparent gel called the **vitreous humor,** and the anterior chamber is filled with an aqueous fluid called the **aqueous humor.**

The sclera consists of opaque, extremely tough, white fibrous connective tissue that supports and maintains the shape of the eyeball and also protects it from damage by foreign objects. On the posterior surface of the eye, the sclera is penetrated by the optic nerve, an artery, a vein, and a lymph vessel. The connective tissue fibers of the anterior surface of the sclera are packed tightly to form the transparent cornea, which serves as the window of the eye.

The middle layer of the eye, the choroid layer, is densely packed with blood vessels for the nutrition of the other structures of the eye. It contains a dark pigment that absorbs light and prevents blurring of the image by light reflection within the eyeball. An-

teriorly, the choroid layer is modified to form the iris, the suspensory ligament and the lens, and the ciliary body. A special venous sinus, the **canal of Schlemm,** circles the iris where the iris and the cornea meet.

The **iris** can be seen through the cornea and gives the eye its characteristic color, such as brown, blue, or hazel. The black opening in the middle of the iris is called the pupil. The iris contains two layers of smooth muscle: one with radially directed fibers that contract to dilate the pupil when stimulated by the sympathetic nervous system; and one with circularly directed fibers that contract to constrict the pupil when stimulated by the parasympathetic system. The size of the pupil is adjusted:
1. To protect the retina from being burned by excess light
2. To allow sufficient light into the eye to stimulate the retina under a range of light intensities
3. To improve the depth perception of close-up vision
4. As a part of the "fight or flight" sympathetic response

The **ciliary body** is a ring of smooth muscle behind the iris that contracts to relax the suspensory ligament and reduce the tension that this ligament exerts on the lens. Because the lens is elastic, reducing the tension in the suspensory ligament allows the lens to assume the more spherical shape required for close-up vision. When daydreaming, the ciliary muscle is relaxed and the eye is focused for far vision.

The **lens** converges light so that the image of the object is finely focused on the retina. It is made of layers of epithelial cells, closely packed as the layers of an onion, and organized so that the lens is clear and transparent.

Visual Acuity

Visual acuity refers to the ability to see small objects clearly. It depends upon there being a sufficiently high density of photoreceptors, especially cones in the fovea centralis, and upon the ability of the lens to focus images clearly on the retina. If the eyeball is too long for the power of the lens (myopia, nearsight), only images fairly close to the eyes are well focused. If the eyeball is too short for the power of the lens (hypermetropia, farsight), only images far from the eyes will be focused clearly. Corrective lenses can be prescribed for both conditions: concave for myopia and convex for hypermetropia. If the lens or cornea are not truly symmetric (astigmatism), cylindric lenses can be prescribed to correct the visual problems that this creates.

The retina is the innermost layer of the eyeball. It lines the eyeball posterior to the ciliary body and consists of the following four layers of cells:

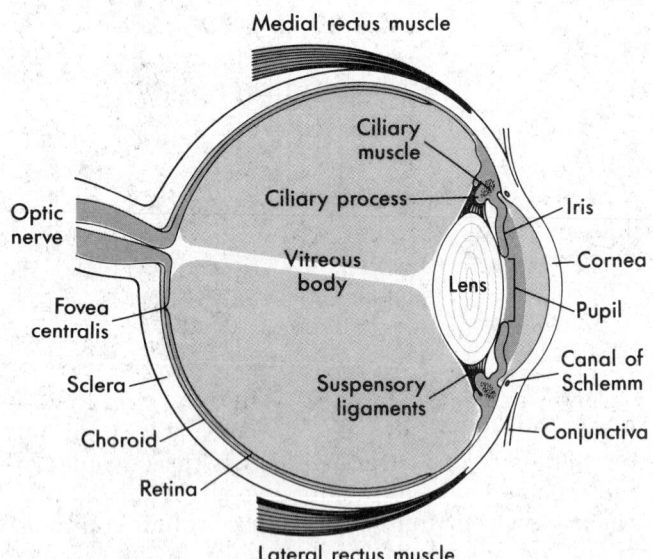

FIGURE 52-1   Cross section of the eye.

1. Pigmented epithelial cells next to the choroid layer
2. Photosensitive cells
3. Bipolar neurons
4. Ganglion neurons that conduct nerve impulses to the brain from the retina

The photoreceptor cells have tips that are either rod-shaped or cone-shaped and are named **rods** and **cones** accordingly. The rods are most prevalent toward the periphery of the retina, and the cones are most prevalent toward the center. Cones are especially prevalent in a circular area called the fovea centralis that lies lateral to the optic disc.

The vitreous humor in the posterior portion of the eye is a transparent gel. It is firm enough to support the internal structures of the eye. The delicate retina, in particular, is supported and held against the choroid layer by the vitreous humor.

The aqueous humor is secreted in the region of the ciliary body and circulates through the suspensory ligament and pupil into the region under the cornea. It filters out of the eyeball into the canal of Schlemm and cleans the eyeball by carrying any particles or debris with it. Anything that increases the amount and pressure of the aqueous humor is dangerous, because high intraocular pressure decreases the blood flow to the retina, which may be permanently damaged. Areas of retina farthest from the supplying arteries are most seriously affected, and high intraocular pressure may cause permanent loss of peripheral vision. This leaves the individual with "tunnel vision." With advancing age, the canal of Schlemm may become partially blocked with debris and intraocular pressure may rise from its normal level of 16 mm Hg to 30 mm Hg or more. This condition is called glaucoma. It is exacerbated by medications that dilate the pupil, because when dilated,

the iris pushes against the canal of Schlemm and may obstruct the flow of aqueous fluid out of the eye.

In addition to the intrinsic smooth muscles of the ciliary body and iris, extrinsic skeletal muscles move the eyes so that the image of the object being examined falls on the fovea centralis of both eyes. There are six sets of extrinsic muscles: the superior, inferior, medial, and lateral rectus muscles, and the superior and inferior oblique muscles (Figure 52-2).

Accessory Structures of the Eye

Approximately 80% of the eyeball lies within the bony depression that forms the orbit of the skull. The remaining 20% is protected by eyelids, eyelashes, eyebrows, and the secretions of the lacrimal glands. The accessory structures of the eye can be seen in Figure 52-3.

The eyebrows jut out and thus protect the eyes from facial blows. The eyelashes, positioned on the outer edge of the eyelids, sweep particles in the air away from the eye. The eyelids are folds of skin that can be moved by skeletal muscles: the levator palpebrae superioris muscles lift the upper lids; the inferior rectus muscles retract the lower lids; and the orbicularis oculi muscles close the eyelids to cover the eyes. Reflex blinking of the eyelids protects the anterior surface of the eye from drying out, because each time the eyelids close, they lubricate the surface of the cornea. This is extremely important, because desiccation produces inflammation and scarring of the cornea and can produce blindness. The eye lubricant, an aqueous, mucoid secretion that contains a bactericidal enzyme, is secreted by the lacrimal glands, which lie in the orbit above the lateral anterior surface of the eye. The lacrimal glands are stimulated to produce abnormal amounts of fluid by substances that irritate the eyes and by strong emotions. The fluid secreted by the lacrimal glands leaves the eyes through two lacrimal papillae above and below the inner canthus and passes into the na-

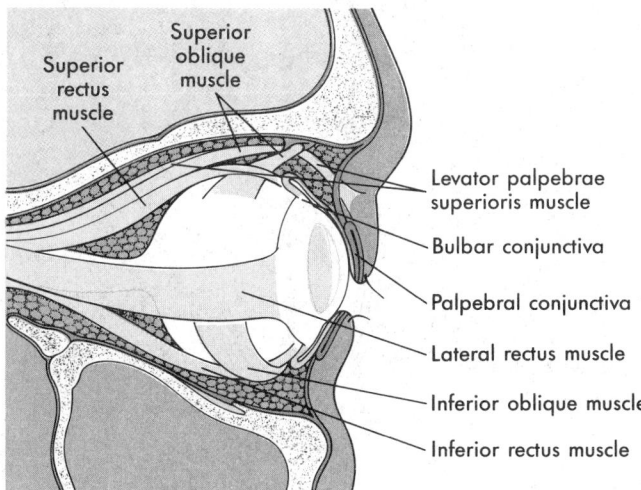

FIGURE 52-2   Eye orbit showing six sets of extrinsic muscles.

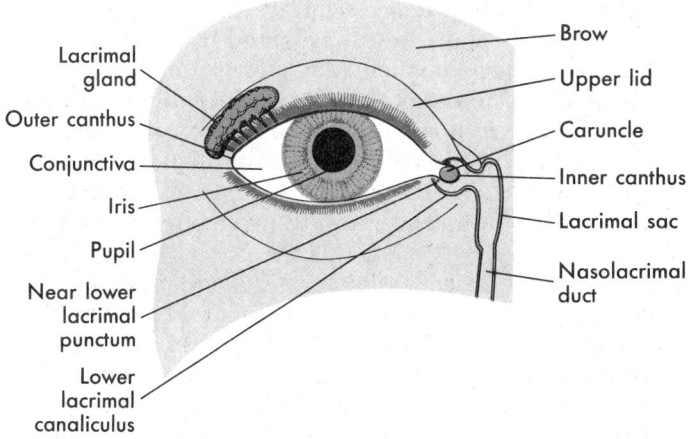

FIGURE 52-3   Visible surface of the eye.

sal cavity through the nasolacrimal duct. This duct provides a route for nasal infections to reach the eyes where they may cause conjunctivitis (pink eye).

The **conjunctiva** is a thin, transparent layer of mucous membrane that covers the anterior surface of the eye (bulbar conjunctiva) and the inner lining of the eyelids (palpebral conjunctiva).

Visual Accommodation

Visual **accommodation** involves the changes necessary for proper vision when the eyes are focused on a near object after they were focused on a far object. These changes are as follows:

1. The eyes converge until the image of the object being observed falls *exactly* on the fovea centralis of both eyes; the act of convergence is largely reflex, but the degree of convergence is also adjusted by the brain to ensure that the images falling on the fovea centralis of both eyes are similar; when the image on the retina of one eye is very indistinct, the brain is unable to make this adjustment and the poor eye will wander slightly; this may happen when a corrective lens is needed for the poor eye. When the eyes are permanently crossed (strabismus) due to muscle weakness or paralysis, the brain will completely ignore the image from one of the eyes to prevent confusion
2. The lens is focused by contracting the ciliary muscles to relax the tension on the lens so that it takes up a more spherical shape, and the images of near objects are clearly focused on the retina
3. The pupil constricts to produce a clearer image on the retina of objects close to the eyes

Physiology of Binocular Vision

Binocular vision allows the brain to determine how far away an object is and gives a three-dimensional quality to what is seen. The images received by the brain from the two eyes differ considerably when the object is close to the eyes and less as the eyes focus on objects farther away. For example, the end of the nose appears to move considerably if viewed by each eye in turn, although a tree on the horizon does not. The brain interprets the distance an object is away from the eyes by evaluating the magnitude of the differences in the images from the two eyes.

The brain also estimates size and distance by evaluating the amount of the retina taken up by the image of familiar objects in the field of vision or by comparing the images of familiar and unfamiliar objects. For example, the size of a rock or a house may be judged according to the height of a person standing beside it.

Comparison of the two images is facilitated by the fact that the images of objects in the right field of vision, which fall on the left side of the eyeball, are both projected to the left side of the brain and vice versa. This makes it easier to respond quickly to what is seen. The right hand, which is controlled by the left cerebrum of the brain, will quickly move to fend off an object approaching from the right, because the image of the approaching object is evaluated by the side of the cerebrum that controls the hand. The neural pathways for vision can be seen in Figure 52-4. Destruction of the left optic tract or the left cerebrum results in blindness in the left side of both eyes and an inability to see the right field of vision. Destruction of the left optic nerve results in a totally blind left eye and vice versa.

Estimates of distance are also made according to the different shades of color in the scene being viewed and in the degree of convergence of the lines making up the various objects. These methods of estimating distance are exploited by artists who create a three-dimensional sense of depth in a two-dimensional painting. For example, the hills farthest from the observer have more gray in them and the shapes of objects are distorted to create a sense of perspective and depth.

Much analysis of the visual image occurs at a subconscious level. Preliminary stereotyped processing of the nerve impulses generated by the photoreceptor is carried out by the retina, and a variety of pat-

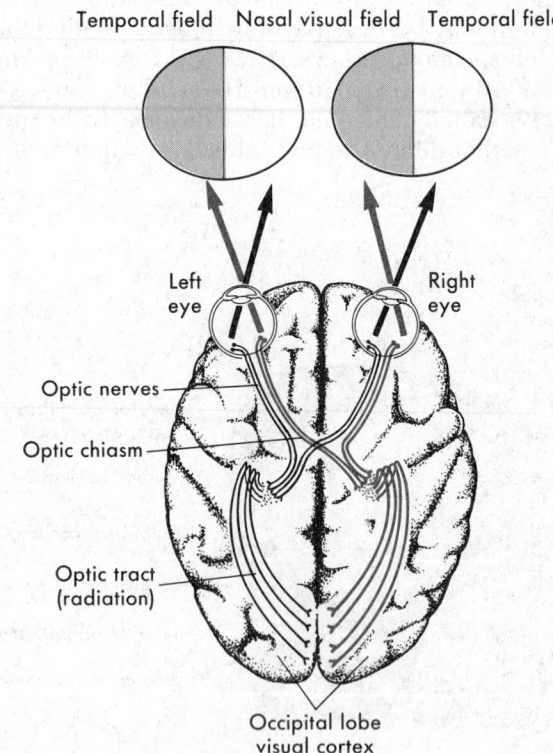

FIGURE 52-4   Neural pathways for vision.

terns are directed toward various subcortical and cortical areas of the brain. For example, the borders of objects and straight lines are highlighted to make them appear clearer and to allow an upset in the body's equilibrium to be detected more easily.

Physiology of Color Vision

The rod photoreceptors are sensitive only to black, white, and shades of gray. They contain rhodopsin, a pigment related to vitamin A, which is dissociated by exposure to light. One of the products of this reaction changes the permeability of the rods and ultimately generates action potentials in the associated ganglion cells. The rods are very sensitive, and bright light rapidly bleaches out the visual pigment. Consequently, the rods do not function in bright light, and they take a few seconds to produce new rhodopsin and become functional after the intensity of the light declines markedly. This is most obvious when the individual enters a dimly lit room after being in a bright hallway, because it takes several seconds in the dim light before the individual can see his or her surroundings. Because rods are found in the periphery and not in the fovea centralis, peripheral vision is much better than detailed vision at low light intensities. Rhodopsin is split by greenish yellow light. Therefore this is seen the best when light intensities are low.

The cones are of three types: red, green, and blue. Each type of cone possesses a pigment that absorbs a specific wavelength of light. Cones are not as sensitive as the rods, and they require higher light intensities than the rods do. They are most plentiful in the fovea centralis, which is the only area where images can be examined in detail. Consequently, cones are used for reading and detailed vision (i.e., the words of a book), and when light levels are low, detail cannot be seen. At night a house number may be seen with our peripheral vision, but when we turn to look at it with our fovea centralis, it disappears.

More colors than red, green, and blue can be seen because the brain interprets other colors from the mix of nerve impulses from the three types of cones (i.e., purple from red and blue, and white when all three types of cones are stimulated).

Color blindness is caused by a complete or relative deficiency of one or more of the three types of cones, most often red or green. The most common form of color blindness is carried by a sex-linked recessive gene.

ASSESSMENT
Subjective

Patients may seek health care for a variety of eye complaints which include red eye, discharge, itching, tearing, or dryness of the eye, loss of vision, diplo-

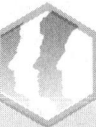

GERIATRIC CONSIDERATIONS

Physiologic Changes in the Eye

After middle age it is considered normal for the elasticity of the lens to decline with age. However, the failure of the lens to rebound and to take up its normal spherical shape in response to relaxation of the suspensory ligament (presbyopia) results in the images of near objects being out of focus. Corrective lenses will usually be required to see close objects clearly at some point after middle age.

Other eye changes are considered to be abnormal. However, the risk of experiencing them increases with age. The lens is susceptible to the formation of opaque chemicals, which may accumulate and become so concentrated that the individual is blind until the opaque lens (cataract) is removed and replaced with an artificial lens. Other conditions may damage the retina: structural changes to the canal of Schlemm may make it harder for the aqueous humor to drain from the eye (glaucoma). This increases the pressure within the eyeball, which reduces blood flow to the retina and damages its photoreceptors, especially those in the peripheral areas. During the last decades of life, deterioration of the vitreous humor may allow the retina to detach and flap about. Like the nervous system itself, the retina is especially susceptible to age-related changes occurring in the circulatory system, so much so that examining the retina with an ophthalmoscope allows the destructive effects of hypertension to be evaluated.

pia (double vision), photophobia, transient or persistent floaters, halos, or eye pain. Eye symptoms may be related to a disorder affecting only the eye, or may be related to a systemic disorder which manifests in a variety of systems.

The box on p. 1418 provides a list of potential symptoms to review with the patient. In addition to specific symptoms, ask the patient about routine eye examinations, date of last eye examination, use of corrective lenses, history of glaucoma or cataracts, any previous eye trauma, previous eye surgery, or any chronic illness such as hypertension, Grave's disease, or diabetes which may affect vision.

Other appropriate history to explore includes major adult illnesses, hospitalizations, surgeries, injuries or accidents, immunizations, current medications, allergies, and habits. Some medications have side effects related to the eyes. For example, corticosteroids can cause cataracts and glaucoma, while phenothiazine tranquilizers can cause retinopathy. The date of last tetanus booster is particularly important if a foreign body is present.

POTENTIAL SYMPTOMS RELATED TO EYE DISORDERS

Blurred vision
Cataracts
Decreased visual acuity
Diplopia
Discharge
Dry eyes
Excessive tearing
Flashes of light
Headaches
Loss of vision
Loss of visual field(s)
Pain
Photophobia (abnormal intolerance to light)
Pruritus (itching)
Ptosis (drooping eyelid)
Red eye
Scotoma (blind spots in visual field)
Tunnel vision (loss of peripheral vision)

ASSESSMENT OF THE EYE

I. Vision: acuity and fields
   • Distant vision (Snellen chart) Cranial Nerve II
   • Near vision (Rosenbaum card) Cranial Nerve II
   • Visual fields (confrontation) Cranial Nerve II
II. Muscle balance and eye movement
   • EOMs—Cranial Nerve III/superior, inferior, and Medial recti and inferior oblique muscles Cranial Nerve IV/ superior oblique muscle Cranial Nerve VI/lateral rectus muscle
   • Cover/uncover test—Cranial Nerves III, IV, VI
   • Corneal light reflex—Cranial Nerves III, IV, VI
   • PERRLA—Cranial Nerve III
III. Extraocular structures
   • Eyebrows, eyelashes, eyelids
   • Lacrimal apparatus
   • Conjunctiva
   • Sclera
   • Cornea
   • Anterior chamber
   • Iris
IV. Internal ophthalmoscopic examination
   • Red reflex
   • Retinal vessels
   • Optic disc (physiologic cup)
   • Macula

Family history related to eye disorders includes glaucoma, use of corrective lenses, cataracts, color blindness, diabetes, or retinoblastoma. A positive finding should include the disorder as well as the individual's relationship to the patient (e.g., glaucoma, mother; color blindness, paternal uncle).

Objective

Examination of the eyes consists of several component parts. In general, begin the assessment with noninvasive testing and observation and finish the assessment with more invasive examination. As with assessment of any other patient, always begin with general assessment. General assessment refers to the examiner's overall impression of the patient's state of health. The box above right outlines the component parts of nursing assessment of the eye.

Assess visual acuity with a Snellen chart or a pocket visual acuity card. If available and appropriate, utilize a standard Snellen chart (see Figure 52-5) having the patient stand 20 feet from the chart. The chart should be in a well-lighted area. Test each eye separately, and then test both eyes together. Instruct the patient to cover one eye using the palm of the hand or an opaque card. Point to a line and have the patient begin reading left to right. If the patient is able to read the entire line with no mistakes, move down to the next line and have the patient read that line. Continue until determining the smallest line in which the patient is able to correctly read more than half the letters. The result is written as a fraction, e.g., 20/200. The top number refers to the distance at which the patient reads the chart. The bottom number refers to the distance at which an individual with "normal" vision could read the line. In the 20/200 example provided above, the patient reads at 20 feet what the "normal" person reads at 200 feet. If the patient misses some of the letters in the smallest line read, record it as the fraction minus the number missed. For example, if the patient correctly reads all but two of the letters on the 20 foot line, record 20/20 −2. Use an illiterate E chart for the illiterate patient (see Figure 52-5). When using the hand-held visual acuity chart (Rosenbaum card), record the number of inches away from the eyes as well as the smallest line read (see Figure 52-6). Usually the hand-held visual acuity chart is held approximately 14 inches away from the eyes. With either approach, test each eye separately as well as both eyes together. If determination of functional vision is the objective, then testing both eyes together is all that is necessary. Remember to have the patient wear whatever lens correction is usually used.

Visual fields may be tested by confrontation. In this test, the examiner's visual fields are assumed to be full or intact. Stand in front of the patient, at eye

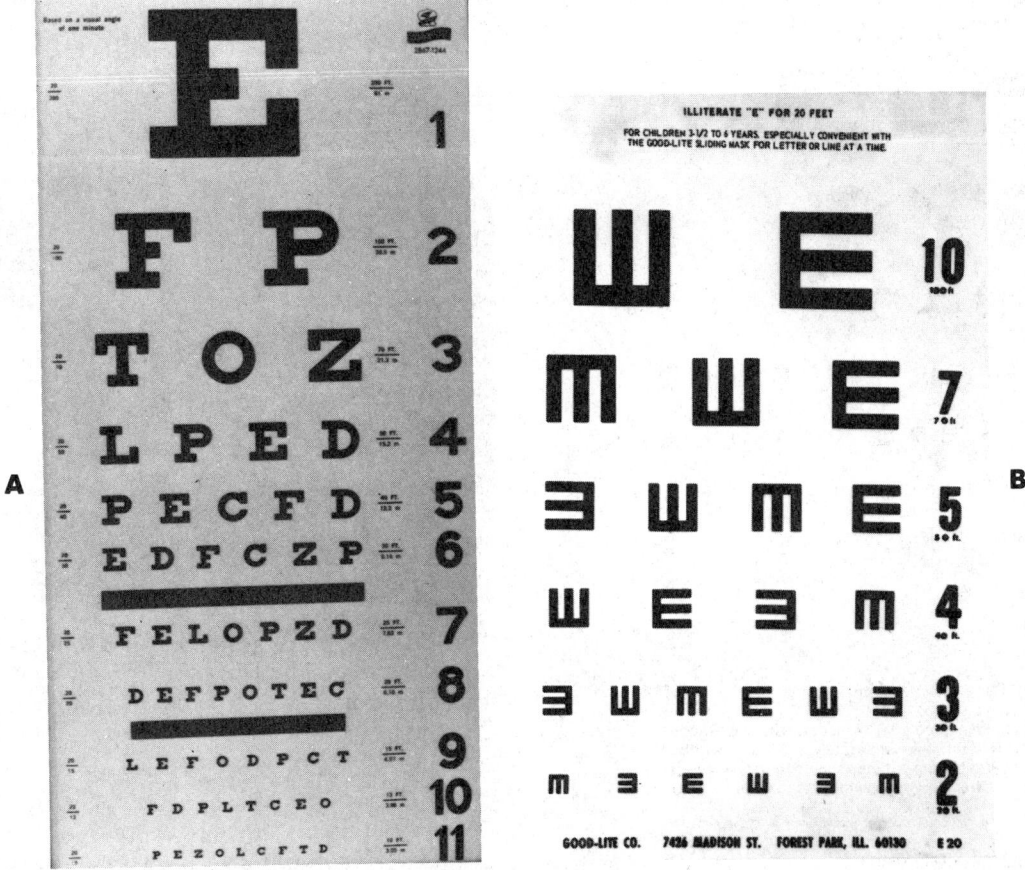

FIGURE 52-5   **A,** Snellen and **B,** E chart for assessment of visual acuity.

level, and instruct the patient to cover one eye using his or her palm or an opaque card. Cover the eye which is directly across from the patient's covered eye. For example, if the patient covers his or her left eye, cover your right eye. An alternative is to simply close the appropriate eye, thus leaving both hands free. Instruct the patient to look straight ahead and to acknowledge the first visualization of the moving fingers or object. Using the contralateral hand and arm, extend your arm midway between you and the patient and bring in your hand wiggling fingers or use a penlight or card from the superior, inferior, and temporal fields of vision. If you are covering your eye with your hand, change hands to evaluate the nasal field of vision (see Figure 52-7). Test both eyes. If the patient's visual fields match those of the examiner, the patient's visual fields are said to be full or intact by confrontation.

Test eye movement and muscle balance. Test extraocular muscles and cranial nerves (CN III—Oculomotor nerve) (superior, inferior, and medial recti and inferior oblique muscles), (CN IV—Trochlear nerve) (superior oblique muscle), and (CN VI—Abducens nerve) (lateral rectus muscle) function

(EOMS) by instructing the patient to look straight ahead and follow your finger's movement without moving his or her head in the direction of your hand. Standing in front of the patient, begin with your finger approximately 10 inches in front of the patient's nose. Move your finger through the patient's six cardinal fields of gaze, coming back to the beginning point between each field of gaze. (See Figure 52-8.) Carefully observe each eye in each field of gaze. Both eyes should move in all six fields of gaze without nystagmus. **Nystagmus** is an involuntary, rapid, rhythmic movement of the eyes in a horizontal, vertical, or rotary fashion. Nystagmus in an extreme lateral gaze is normal.

Muscle balance may also be tested via the cover/uncover test. Instruct the patient to focus on a far object. While the patient is focusing on that object, cover one eye with an opaque card. Observe the uncovered eye for movement. Then remove the cover and observe the just uncovered eye for movement. Repeat the procedure with the other eye. Movement of the uncovered eye is known as a **tropia.** A prefix is added to denote which direction the eye deviates, e.g., esotropia is turning in (nasally) while exotropia

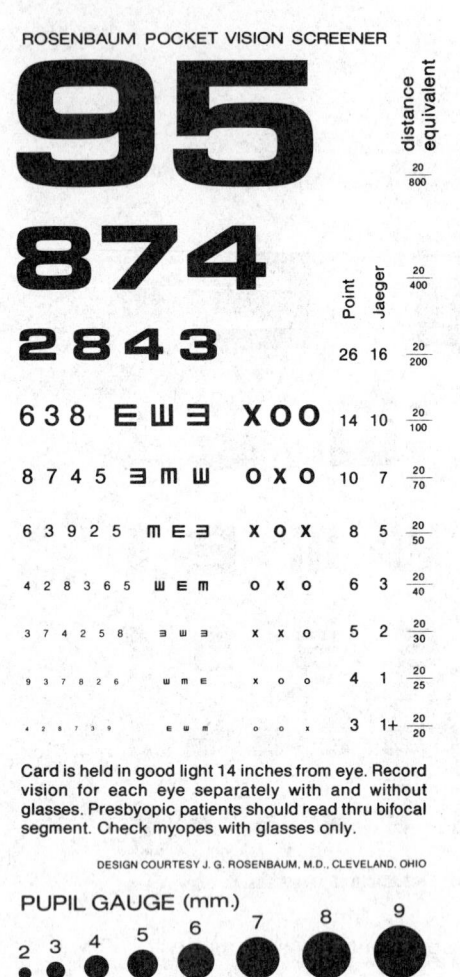

ROSENBAUM POCKET VISION SCREENER

Card is held in good light 14 inches from eye. Record vision for each eye separately with and without glasses. Presbyopic patients should read thru bifocal segment. Check myopes with glasses only.

DESIGN COURTESY J. G. ROSENBAUM, M.D., CLEVELAND, OHIO

PUPIL GAUGE (mm.)

FIGURE 52-6   Handheld Rosenbaum card for assessment of visual acuity. (Reprinted with permission of Cooper Laboratories, San German, Puerto Rico.)

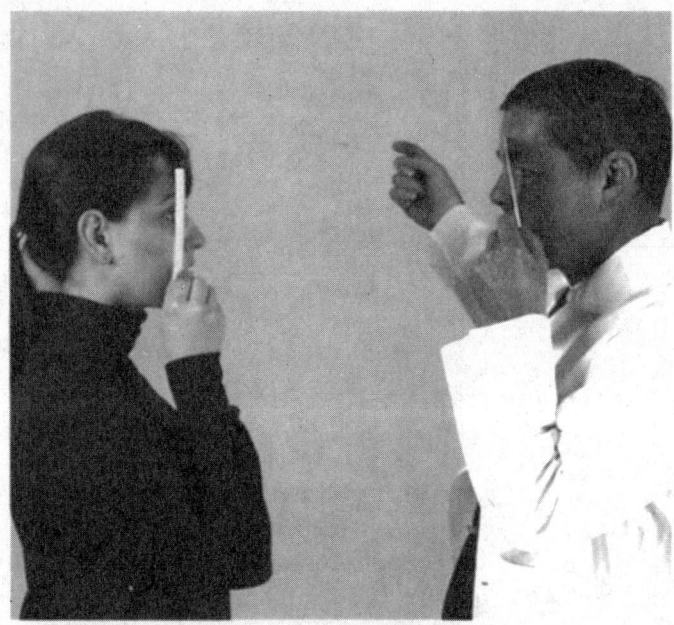

FIGURE 52-7   Assessment of visual fields by confrontation. (From Seidel HM et al: *Mosby's guide to physical examination,* ed 2, St Louis, 1991, Mosby–Year Book.)

is turning out (laterally). Movement of the covered eye is known as a **phoria** and is significant only as a potential for development of a tropia. In general, only a tropia needs to be referred to an ophthalmologist. Repeat the cover/uncover test instructing the patient to focus on a near object.

Another method which may be utilized to evaluate muscle function is the corneal light reflex, also known as Hirschberg's test. This test is not considered to be as reliable as the cover/uncover test. Instruct the patient to look straight ahead. Shine a penlight on the corneas and observe the position of the corneal light reflexes for symmetry. Asymmetry of corneal light reflexes would indicate deviation of an eye and therefore probable muscle imbalance.

Observe the pupils. Note if they are equal, round, and react to light. Pupillary response to light should be both direct and consensual. Instruct the patient to look straight ahead. Shine a penlight from a lat-

eral position in one of the patient's eyes. Observe that eye for pupillary constriction (direct response). Observe the contralateral pupil for constriction (consensual response). Repeat the procedure shining the penlight in the other eye. If the pupils are equal, round, and reactive to light it may be recorded as PERRL. Both pupils should constrict and converge when accommodating from distance vision to near vision. Have the patient focus on a distant object and then on a near object such as your finger approximately 5 inches from the patient's face. The pupils should converge and constrict. These two responses, convergence and constriction, comprise accommodation. Accommodation is written as the A at the end of PERRL: **PERRLA.**

Inspect and palpate extraocular structures. Observe the eyebrows and eyelashes. Note presence and symmetry. Eyelashes should be turned outward. Inturned eyelashes (trichiasis) may cause corneal irritation. Observe the eyelids. Note symmetry, edema, erythema of the lid margins. Have the patient open and close the eyes. When open, the upper lid should cover only the upper margin of the iris. The pupil should not be covered. The distance between the upper lid and the lower lid is known as the **palpebral fissure.** Palpebral fissures should be symmetric. If they are not symmetric, then a **ptosis** may be present (drooping of the upper eyelid). The lacrimal apparatus is not visible for inspection. However, the lacrimal sac is located at the medial canthus of each eye and contains tears. Discharge may

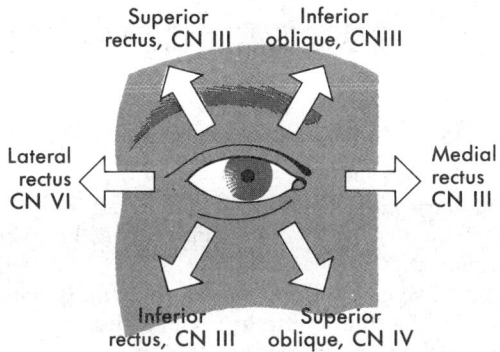

FIGURE 52-8   The six cardinal fields of gaze.

be expressed from the puncta when palpating the lacrimal sac if a blockage is present. Palpate gently on the medial canthus at the lower lid just inside the orbital ring.

Inspect the conjunctiva. Note injection (erythema), exudate, or a cobblestone appearance. Normally, the conjunctiva is referred to as clear. The bulbar conjunctiva covers the sclera, while the palpebral conjunctiva covers the inner portions of the upper and lower lids. To observe the lower palpebral conjunctiva, instruct the patient to look up while you depress the lower lid. Inspection of the upper palpebral conjunctiva is not usually done unless a foreign body is suspected. Instruct the patient to look down while you grasp the upper eyelashes, gently pulling downward and forward. Evert the upper eyelid over a cotton-tipped applicator. To return the lid to its normal position, have the patient look up or blink.

Note any discoloration in the sclera. A blue sclera may be seen in osteogenesis imperfecta. Scleritis is an inflammation of the sclera. This is a rare condition and may be associated with an immune disorder. Inspect the cornea for transparency. There should be no opacities or cloudiness. A whitish line partially surrounding the cornea at its perimeter bilaterally in patients over 40 years of age is probably an arcus senilis. An arcus senilis is composed of lipid deposits and is considered normal in those over age 40. In those under age 40, an arcus senilis may reflect a lipid disorder.

Inspect the anterior chamber for depth and clarity. Shine a light obliquely across the eye. The anterior chamber is the space between the cornea, anteriorly and the iris and lens, posteriorly. Bleeding into the anterior chamber is known as a hyphema and usually results from a traumatic tear of the iris. Inspect the irides for color, shape, and symmetry.

The internal direct ophthalmoscopic examination is not frequently performed by the bedside nurse. This is a skill that requires much practice and therefore develops over time. Thus, it is most often used

by the advanced practitioner. To begin the ophthalmoscopic examination, instruct the patient to look straight ahead. Dim the room lights. Holding the ophthalmoscope in the right hand, use your right eye to examine the patient's right eye. Hold the ophthalmoscope in the left hand, using your left eye to examine the patient's left eye. As the patient is looking straight ahead, look through the ophthalmoscope shining the light onto the patient's pupil approaching the patient from about 15 degrees anterolaterally. Note the presence or absence of the red reflex. Move closer to the patient following the 15-degree line and look for vessels. As you come closer to the patient, you may need to adjust the diopter wheel to bring the vessels into sharper focus. Follow until you see the optic disc, the entrance of the optic nerve into the eye. When visualizing retinal structures with the direct ophthalmoscope, the optic disc will occupy greater than or equal to the entire field of vision seen through the ophthalmoscope. To visualize all the retinal structures move the ophthalmoscope superiorly and inferiorly, nasally and temporally. Arterioles are smaller than veins and will reflect the light. Therefore, they will be seen as brighter than veins. Note any narrowing of the veins or arterioles. Observe the disc margins for clarity. The disc margins should be well defined. Disc margins may be slightly blurred nasally. Otherwise, blurring may be indicative of papilledema. Note disc color and any lesions or exudate. The disc is normally creamy pink or yellow in color. The disc color may be darker in patients of color. Exudate and some lesions may be seen in patients with longstanding diabetes mellitus or hypertension. Move the ophthalmoscope temporally to observe the macula. This is a difficult structure to observe without dilating the pupil. Observation of the macula may be facilitated by instructing the patient to look directly into the light.

DIAGNOSTIC AND LABORATORY TESTS
Electroretinography

Electroretinography is useful in detecting diseases of either the rods or the cones, or both. The procedure evaluates the electrical potential between the cornea and retina. It measures changes in the electrical potential in response to alterations in the wavelength and intensity of light and to the state of adaptation of the eye (whether it is light- or dark-adapted). During the test, electrodes incorporated into contact lenses are applied directly to the eye. Total lack of electrical activity is demonstrated in siderosis bulbi and retinitis pigmentosa. Abnormal activity during dark adaptation is indicative of selective degeneration of the rods, and abnormal activity during light adaptation is indicative of involvement of the cones, as is seen in congenital total color blindness. Electroretinography may be used in conjunction with electro-oculography (EOG), which is used to evaluate retinal functioning and sleep disorders. During electro-oculography skin electrodes are placed on the canthi of the eye and recordings are made of the patient's eye movements and of the electrical potential of the eye in darkness and in light. If the patient is to receive both fluorescein angiography and electro-oculography, the electro-oculography needs to be done first as the eyes are dilated with fluorescein angiography.

Patient preparation

The patient is told that electroretinography will evaluate the response of the eye to darkness and to light. The nurse explains that no dietary restrictions are necessary and that contact lenses will be applied to the eyes following administration of topical anesthetic drops. The patient is told that he or she will fixate on a target and that eye movements must be avoided because these will disrupt the test. The test takes approximately 1 hour.

Tonometry

Tonometry is an integral part of the ocular assessment in adults and involves indirect measurement of intraocular pressure. Tonometry is an effective screen for early detection of glaucoma. As intraocular pressure rises in glaucoma, the eyeball hardens and becomes more resistive to extraocular pressure and flattening. The Schiøtz tonometer and applanation tonometer are used to measure this resistance. Both devices are applied only to an anesthetized cornea. Tonometry should not be performed on a patient with a corneal ulcer or infection unless an extreme circumstance, such as narrow-angle glaucoma, is suspected.

Patient preparation

The patient is informed that the test measures pressure within the eyes and that anesthetic drops will be instilled into the eyes before the procedure to prevent discomfort. The nurse instructs the patient to avoid activity that may raise intraocular pressure during the test, such as coughing, sneezing, or squeezing the eyelids. The patient should loosen restrictive clothing, such as neckties and collars. The nurse asks the patient to remove contact lenses before the test and cautions against reinsertion for 2 hours after the test.

Procedure

The patient is helped to a relaxed position, either sitting with the head back or supine with the head

GERIATRIC CONSIDERATIONS

Eye Assessment

General approach
Allow more time than for a younger adult
Articulate clearly; the elder patient may be hearing impaired
Impaired sight, comprehension, or mobility may result in less than optimum cooperation
Provide clear, concise instructions

History collection
Interviewer may need to use fewer open-ended questions and provide some choices, e.g., "is your eye pain burning, throbbing, or a tenderness of the eye?"
Interviewer may need to repeat questions
Be alert for answers which do not appear appropriate, the patient may not have understood the question correctly due to impaired hearing or impaired comprehension

Physical assessment
The physical examination itself is not different, but the approach needs to be altered so that the appropriate information is assessed without undue discomfort or embarrassment for the elder
Environment with minimal noise, distractions, and interruption
Darkening of the skin around the orbits is associated with aging
The elder has a slower pupillary light reflex, though still equal bilaterally
Decreased tearing
Increased lens thickness and opacity is common and may necessitate better lighting for near vision testing
Arcus senilis is common in patients over 60 years old
Visual acuity may be decreased
Loss of elasticity of the lens is associated with aging and results in presbyopia (farsightedness)

facing upward, and is directed to look at a spot with the eyes wide open. The nurse instills the drops and cautions the patient to not rub the eyes for 15 minutes after the drops are instilled. If applanation tonometry is used, a drop of fluorescein from a fluorescein strip may be applied to the eyes.

Schiötz tonometer
The tonometer is brought in from the side, and the footplate is placed on the cornea without touching the lids, because this may trigger a blink reflex and cause the footplate to move and scratch the cornea.

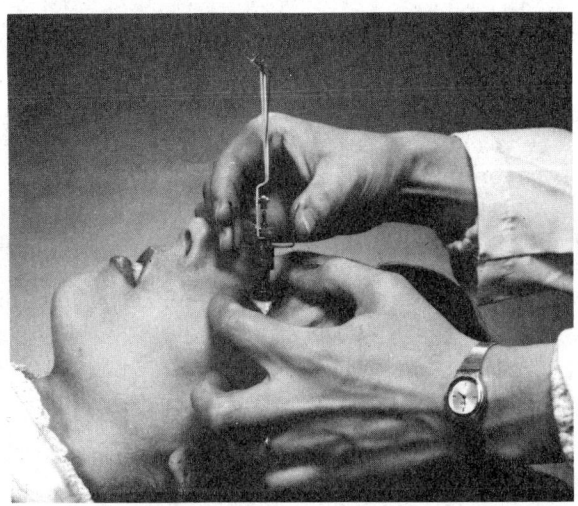

FIGURE 52-9 Screening for intraocular pressure. (From Newell FW: *Ophthalmology: principles and concepts,* ed 6, St Louis, 1986, Mosby–Year Book.)

The tonometer is held steady to avoid corneal abrasion, and a measurement is made as to how deeply the weight depresses the cornea. Normal intraocular pressure is 12 to 22 mm Hg (Figure 52-9).

Applanation tonometer

Applanation tonometry is a more accurate test than indentation tonometry, measured by the Schiötz tonometer. In applanation tonometry, the cornea is flattened while being examined with a slit lamp biomicroscope, and the flattened area is measured. The higher the resistance, the smaller the flattened area.

Intravenous Fluorescein Angiography

Fluorescein angiography records the appearance of blood vessels inside the eye and is useful in evaluating intraocular conditions, such as tumors and retinopathy. After an intravenous injection of sodium fluorescein, a contrast medium, numerous photographs are taken of the fundus using a special camera (fundus camera). The dye and the photographic equipment increase the visibility of the microvascular bed of the retina and choroid, making visualization of the retinal bed possible.

Patient preparation

The patient is told that the test evaluates circulation within the eyes. The nurse informs the patient that eyedrops will be instilled before photographing the eyes and that a dye to increase the visibility of the blood vessels will be injected into an arm or hand. The nurse warns the patient that a yellow discoloration of the skin and urine may occur but that this is a result of the dye and will disappear in 24 to 48 hours. No food or fluid restrictions are necessary before or after the test. If ordered, a patient with glaucoma may have to withhold eyedrops on the day of testing. The nurse checks the patient's history for allergy to contrast dyes and dilating drops. Because the flashing blue light that is used with the camera may produce seizure activity in susceptible individuals, the nurse also checks for a history of epilepsy.

A consent form is obtained if required. The nurse instills mydriatic eyedrops as ordered. At least two instillations are necessary to achieve the maximum mydriasis for clear photographs. The patient should loosen any restrictive clothing around the neck.

Procedure

The patient is seated comfortably in a chair facing the camera with chin in the chin rest and forehead against a bar. The patient is told to keep the eyes wide open, to stare ahead, and to blink normally. Preinjection photographs may be taken, and then dye is injected. The nurse reassures the patient that warmth and nausea, if experienced, are temporary. The patient is observed for signs of an allergic response, such as fainting, hives, suddenly increased salivation, dry mouth, metallic taste, or lightheadedness. A rapid sequence (25 to 30) of photographs is taken as the dye is injected, the needle is removed, and pressure and a dressing are applied to the injection site. Late phase photographs may be taken at 5 and 10 minutes, so the patient is encouraged to sit comfortably and relax between sessions. The various phases of the photography are significant, because the early filling phase during which dye is injected may outline abnormalities, such as microaneurysms and revascularization. The second or arterial filling phase is useful in detecting arterial occlusion. Later phases enable detection of venous occlusion, perhaps associated with dilation and leakage.

Postprocedure care

The patient is cautioned against activities requiring near vision, because vision will be blurred for 40 minutes to 2 hours after instillation of the drops.

Ocular Ultrasonography

Ocular ultrasonography involves the penetration of eye tissues with high-frequency waves. Sound waves, like light waves, pass through some tissues and are reflected by others. Aqueous humor produces no echoes, whereas form tissue masses, such as tumors, and cataractous lenses produce reflection of the sound waves, which is picked up on microfilm and then translated into the electrical impulses displayed on the oscilloscope. Two types of sound waves are used. The A-wave is a single-beam, linear wave that is useful in measuring the axial length of the eye. The B-wave is a radiating wave that yields a two-dimensional, cross-sectional image. The B-scan is used more often to evaluate structures of the eye and to detect abnormalities, because it yields more information, is less likely to miss significant data, and is easier to interpret. Ultrasound is particularly useful in evaluating an eye that is clouded with an opaque medium, such as cataract or hemorrhage, and in measuring the length of the eye and the curvature of the cornea before the insertion of an intraocular lens.

Patient preparation

The nurse explains to the patient that ultrasound evaluates the structures of the eye and that the procedure is painless, safe, and takes about 5 minutes. No food or fluid restrictions are necessary. The patient is told that during the procedure, he or she may be asked to change gaze or to make certain eye movements.

Procedure

During B-scan, a transducer to which water-soluble jelly has been applied is placed on the patient's closed eyelid. For the A-scan, a methylcellulose-filled scleral sheath is placed on the eyelid, and a transducer is placed over the sheath.

Computed Axial Tomography

Orbital computed axial tomography (CT scan) (see Chapter 44) provides three-dimensional visualization of the orbital structures, such as the eye muscles and optic nerve, and enables identification of space-occupying lesions earlier and more accurately than other radiographic techniques. CT scanning in ophthalmology also permits detection of many intracranial lesions outside the eye and eye orbit that may affect vision. Contrast enhancement may be used to help define lesions and to evaluate disorders, such as subdural hematoma, hemangioma, or suspected circulatory disorders.

Patient preparation

The nurse informs the patient that the procedure helps visualize the eyes and their surrounding structures. The patient is told that he or she must lie still on an x-ray table, which is moved into a scanner. The scanner will move around the patient's head and make loud clacking noises. The nurse reassures the patient that the test causes no discomfort and

takes 15 to 30 minutes. No food or fluid restrictions are necessary unless contrast enhancement is scheduled, in which case the patient will fast 4 hours. If contrast enhancement is scheduled, the patient's history is checked for information regarding sensitivity to iodine, shellfish, or contrast dyes. The nurse tells the patient that injection of the dye may cause certain temporary effects, such as flushing, warmth, a salty taste, or nausea and vomiting.

A signed consent is obtained from the patient, and the nurse ensures that all jewelry and metal objects are removed from the x-ray field.

Magnetic Resonance Imaging

Magnetic resonance imaging (MRI) uses an immense electromagnet to detect radio frequencies from the alignment of hydrogen protons in a magnetic field (see Chapter 44 for procedure and patient preparation). The procedure permits excellent visualization of soft tissue and is useful in detecting circulatory abnormalities and tumors of the eye.

CRITICAL THINKING QUESTIONS

1 Describe the three layers of the eye and the functions they serve.
2 How do the accessory structures of the eye serve to protect it?
3 What are the photoreceptor cells, and how do they enable the perception of color?
4 Design at least three questions to ask patients about eye health care habits.
5 Describe an effective approach to examining a painful, edematous, tightly closed eye just after injury.
6 Discuss psychologic factors to consider when a patient must wear an eye prosthesis.
7 Discuss special considerations in regard to eye integrity in adults with chronic systemic conditions, such as diabetes mellitus and cerebral vascular accident.
8 Describe the procedure for intravenous fluorescein angiography as it might be explained to a patient.
9 Discuss tonometry relative to purpose, contraindications, and procedure.

BIBLIOGRAPHY

Current

Burrell LO: *Adult nursing in hospital and community settings,* Norwalk, Conn, 1992, Appleton & Lange.
Gallo JJ et al: *Handbook of geriatric assessment,* Rockville, Maryland, 1988, Aspen Publishers.
Gordon M: Manual of nursing diagnosis, New York, 1987, McGraw-Hill.

Kane RL et al: *Essentials of clinical geriatrics,* ed 2, New York, 1989, McGraw Hill.

Kenny RA: *Physiology of aging: a synopsis,* St. Louis, 1992, Mosby–Year Book.

Leitman MW: *Manual for eye examination and diagnosis,* ed 3, Oradell, New Jersey, Medical Economics Books.

Malasanos L et al: *Health assessment,* ed 4, St. Louis, 1990, Mosby–Year Book.

Nurse's ready reference: diagnostic tests, Springhouse, 1991, Springhouse Corporation.

Seidel HM et al: *Mosby's guide to physical examination,* ed 2, St. Louis, 1991, Mosby–Year Book.

Swartz MH: *Textbook of physical diagnosis,* Philadelphia, 1989, WB Saunders.

Classic

Bloch B, Hunter M: Teaching physiological assessment of black persons, *Nurse Educ* 6(1):24, 1981.

Block G, Nolan J: *Health assessment for professional nursing: a developmental approach,* New York, 1986, Appleton-Century-Crofts.

Bowers A, Thompson J: *Clinical manual of health assessment,* St. Louis, 1984, Mosby–Year Book.

Carotenuto R, Bullock J: *Physical assessment of the gerontologic client,* Philadelphia, 1981, FA Davis Co.

Fields W, McGinn-Campbell K: *Introduction to health assessment,* Reston, Va, 1983, Reston Publishing Company.

Murray R, Zentner S: *Nursing assessment and health promotion through the life span,* ed 4, Englewood Cliffs, NJ, 1989, Prentice Hall.

Prior JA, Silberstein JS, Stang J: *Physical diagnosis: the history and examination of the patient,* St. Louis, 1981, Mosby–Year Book.

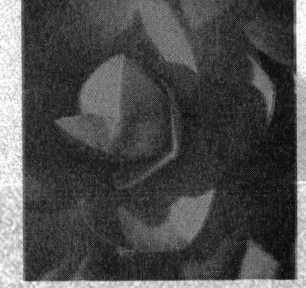

CHAPTER FIFTY-THREE

Nursing Management of Adults with Eye Disorders

LEARNING OBJECTIVES

1 Outline the nursing management for the following eye disorders: disorder of refraction, glaucoma, cataract, retinal degeneration, ocular emergency, retinal detachment, hordeolum, conjunctivitis, trachoma, uveitis, blindness, and diabetic retinopathy.

2 Describe pathophysiology, etiology, incidence, symptoms, and therapeutic management for each of the common eye disorders.

3 Develop a nursing care plan for postoperative care of a patient having cataract surgery.

4 Recognize pertinent observations to document for patients with eye disorders.

5 Identify actions, indications for use, and side effects of medications having mydriatic and miotic properties.

6 Write a teaching plan for a patient with chronic glaucoma.

MANY EYE DISORDERS are preventable. Early detection and treatment of eye injuries or diseases can preserve vision and prevent blindness. The sensory/perceptual alterations that occur with eye disorders and loss of visual acuity can cause varying degrees of disability. Such disability is both physical and psychologic and can limit the patient's ability to perform activities of daily living. Even minor errors of refraction can disrupt an individual's role performance, and loss of vision creates the potential for injury. However, for many people correction of visual changes with glasses or contact lenses threatens their self-concept and body image. The nurse has the responsibility to recognize symptoms and encourage patients to seek medical attention for eye disorders. Nursing interventions for the patient with a visual impairment focus on helping the patient learn new adaptive skills.

DISORDERS OF REFRACTION

The word **refraction** refers to the bending of light rays as they enter the eye. An emmetrope is a person with normal vision. Emmetropia is the refraction of parallel rays of light from a distance of 6 m (20 ft) or more on the macula of the retina. Ametropia is a term used to describe any refractive error. Ametropia occurs when parallel light rays entering the eye are not refracted to focus on the ret-

ina. Four common ametropic disorders are myopia, hyperopia, astigmatism, and presbyopia.

Myopia, commonly referred to as nearsightedness, is caused by the focusing of light rays in front of the retina. Persons with myopia can see near objects clearly but have blurred distant vision (Figure 53-1). Myopia, which has a hereditary tendency, requires a concave lens for correction.

Hyperopia, or farsightedness, is caused by focusing of light rays behind the retina (Figure 53-2). This is the most common refractive error.[51] Blurred close vision with clear distant vision may be the result, although some people have a range where vision is clear (e.g., 4 to 17 ft) but require corrective lenses at 20 ft. Physiologically, the globe or eyeball is too short from front to back to accommodate the power of the lens. The aging process can result in hyperopia, causing decreased visual acuity.[51] Hyperopia is also associated with primary angle closure glaucoma.[37] Difficulty with reading or other close work is a common symptom in all age groups. Hyperopia requires corrective convex lenses only when the eyes will not accommodate for close vision.

Astigmatism is a condition in which parallel light rays do not focus on a point because of irregular surface changes in the cornea. Usually the cornea is a smooth surface.[42] The astigmatic cornea with its irregular surface structure causes light rays to be refracted to focus on two different points and can re-

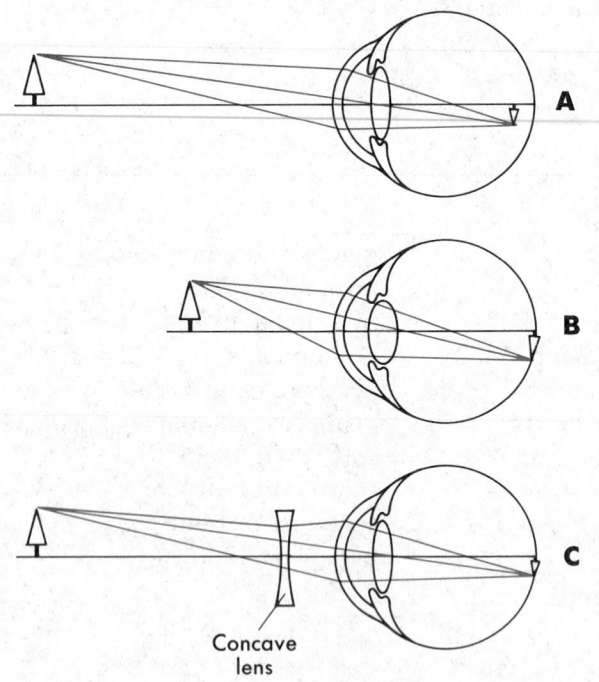

FIGURE 53-1 Myopia. **A,** Without correction, distant objects focus in front of retina. **B,** Near objects are seen clearly. **C,** With correction (concave lens), distant objects are also seen clearly.

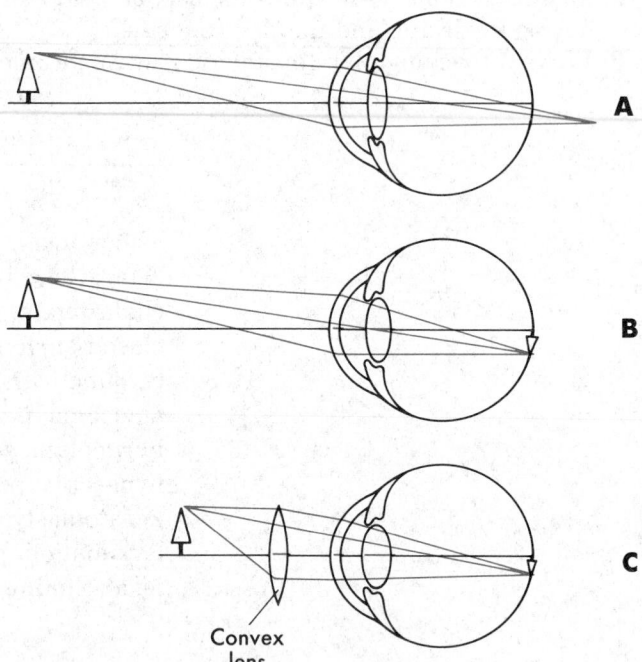

FIGURE 53-2 Hyperopia. **A,** Light rays focus behind retina. **B,** Distant objects may be seen clearly. **C,** With correction (convex lens), near objects are seen more clearly.

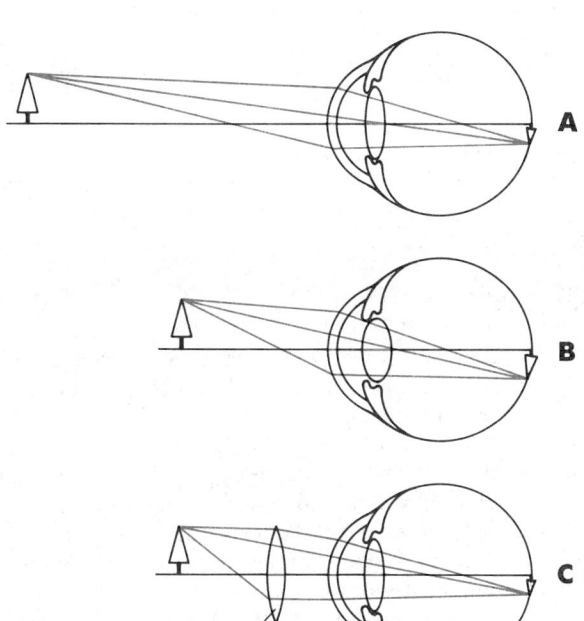

FIGURE 53-3   **A,** Normal vision with distant objects. **B,** Normal accommodation for near vision. **C,** Presbyopia. With aging, accommodation for close vision decreases. Correction with convex lens is needed.

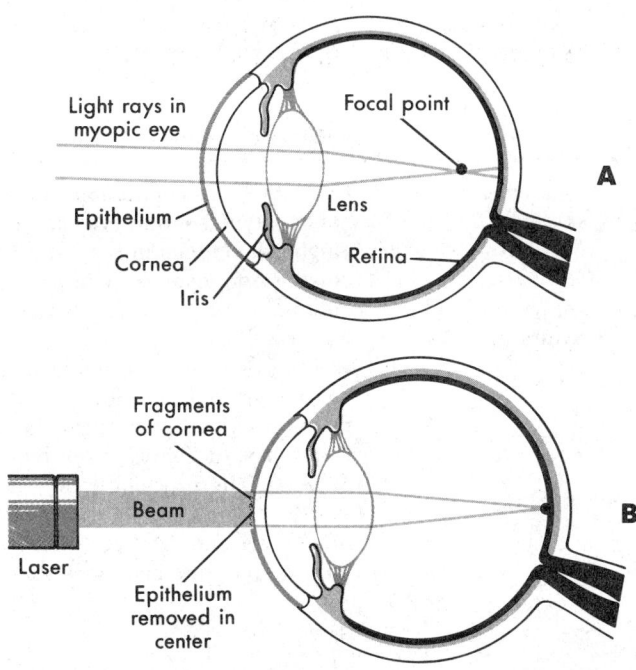

FIGURE 53-4   Photorefractive keratectomy. **A,** Before treatment. **B,** After treatment, outer covering of cornea is flattened, causing light rays to focus on retina.

sult in either myopic or hyperopic astigmatism. Astigmatism can be inherited as an autosomal dominant trait.[23] Astigmatism can also result from injury, inflammation, or corneal surgery. Symptoms occur in varying degrees depending on the irregularity of the curvature in the cornea. Blurred vision and eye discomfort are common complaints.

Presbyopia is caused by the loss of elasticity of the crystalline lens and is associated with the aging process. Changes in the lens, which commonly begin around 40 years of age, cause light rays to be focused behind the retina, resulting in hyperopia (far-sightedness). Hyperopia can cause onset of presbyopia earlier than 40 years, whereas myopic eyes can delay the onset beyond 40 years.[37] Accommodations for close vision are accomplished by lens contraction. Accommodation is the change in convexity of the lens to permit light rays to be refracted to focus on the retina. With aging this ability slows gradually to the age of 55 to 60 years, when the process stabilizes (Figure 53-3). Presbyopia is commonly noticeable around 45 to 50 years of age. It causes difficulty with close vision.[47] People with presbyopia compensate for blurred close vision by holding the object to be viewed further away. This maneuver is an attempt to cause light rays to focus on the retina rather than behind it. As presbyopia progresses, visual acuity for viewing close objects decreases until prescrip-

tive lenses are necessary. Distant vision is unaffected. Complaints of eye strain, mild frontal headache, and feelings of fatigue are common. These symptoms dissipate following eye rest and use of appropriate lenses.

Artificial lenses (eyeglasses and various contact lenses) continue to be the traditional method of managing refractive disorders. Laser therapy is currently being investigated as a new method of treating myopia. The procedure is known as photorefractive keratectomy (PRK) and involves vaporizing part of the cornea with laser light (Figure 53-4). Studies are in progress to determine the safety and effectiveness of PRK.

Glaucoma

Glaucoma is a condition characterized by increased intraocular pressure (IOP) that if unrelieved causes intraocular structural damage. Glaucoma, the sixth leading cause of blindness in the world, is responsible for about 20% of all blindness. The incidence of glaucoma is four to five times higher in African Americans than whites.[30] A national survey revealed the following groups of people to be at high risk: blacks over 40 years, all adults over 60 years, and those with a family history of glaucoma.[27] About 1%

TABLE 53-1 Glaucoma: Open Angle vs. Closed Angle

	Primary open angle	Primary closed angle
Incidence	Commonly affects persons 40 years and above; type seen in majority of persons; higher incidence in blacks; hereditary predisposition, especially in persons with diabetes	Occurs in middle age as lens thickens
Symptoms	Painless	Headache; severe eye pain during attack
	Insidious elevation of IOP at least during part of day up to 30 mm Hg	IOP may rise to 50 to 70 mm Hg; can be higher during acute attack
	Occasional headache (brow aches)	
	Halos around lights caused by corneal edema	Halos around lights caused by corneal edema
	Slow peripheral vision loss	Blurred vision and reduced central vision; edematous eyelids during acute attack
	May affect one eye first; bilateral usually (may affect one eye more than the other)	Lacrimation and photophobia especially during acute attack; nausea and vomiting; one eye affected first with other eye becoming affected later—usually
		Symptoms may be most noticeable in evening and relieved by rest/sleep
		Pupil mid-dilated about 3.5 to 6 mm in diameter during acute attack
		Conjunctional hyperemia during acute attack
Pathology/ structural changes	Narrowing of channels in trabecular meshwork prevents aqueous fluid from draining normally	Shallow anterior angle with lens lying close to trabecular meshwork and blocking drainage of aqueous fluid
Therapeutic treatment	Ocular hypotensive drugs to control IOP Cholinergic agonists Adrenergic agonists Adrenergic blockers Carbonic anhydrase inhibitors Hyperosmotic agents	Miotic medications to pull iris away from anterior angle
	Laser trabeculoplasty	Peripheral iridectomy or laser iridotomy

of people over 40 years have the common form of glaucoma (open angle). Glaucoma and macular degeneration are the major causes of vision loss in elderly persons.[47] Glaucoma is classified as primary or secondary, with primary being more common than secondary. There are three types of primary glaucoma: open angle, closed angle, and congenital. Table 53-1 compares open-angle and closed-angle glaucoma.

PRIMARY OPEN-ANGLE GLAUCOMA
Etiology/Epidemiology

Primary open-angle glaucoma (POAG) is also known as simple, adult primary, and chronic open glaucoma. The most common form of glaucoma, POAG accounts for 90% of the cases of primary glaucoma.[65] The lack of noticeable symptoms by patients can result in severe irreversible vision loss be-

fore medical help is sought. POAG is reported to occur in 2% to 4% of people over 40 years and increases in incidence with age.[22,51] One study showed that POAG was responsible for 19% of blindness among African Americans.[39] A definite hereditary link in all people has been established by extensive research studies. The incidence is greater in persons who have an immediate family member (parent or sibling) who has POAG.[25] Genetically, it may be associated with diabetes. POAG is usually a bilateral condition, but one eye may have more vision loss than the other.

Pathophysiology

Primary open-angle glaucoma occurs when aqueous fluid is not adequately drained from the eye even though there is adequate space for drainage in the anterior chamber. Figure 53-5 shows the anatomic

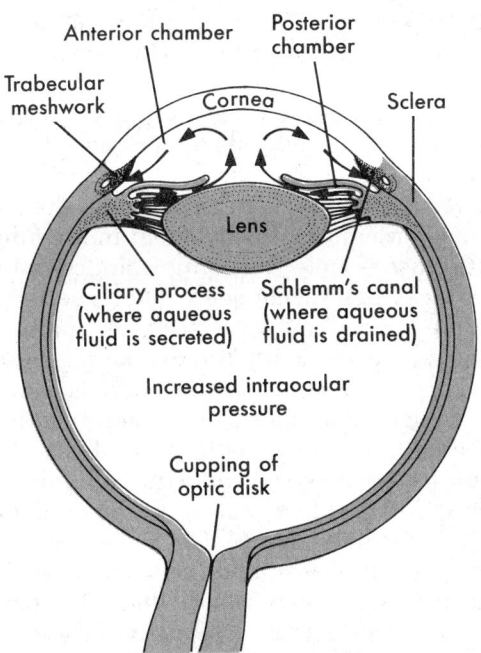

FIGURE 53-5 Open-angle glaucoma. Pathologic changes occur in trabecular meshwork of Schlemm's canal, causing it to totally or partially stop up and prevent drainage of aqueous humor. Result is increased IOP in all directions.

problem causing the obstruction. The exact cause of POAG is unknown. Depending on the degree of blockage of aqueous drainage, there is usually increased IOP at least during part of each day. The pathophysiologic process is much like having a drain that is partially clogged. IOP commonly may be elevated to 30 mm Hg or more. Pressure from elevated IOP causes cupping of the optic disc, which is the weakest and most vulnerable of the intraocular structures. The pressure exerted on the optic nerve causes destruction of nerve fibers in the retina, causing painless visual loss in affected areas. Absolute glaucoma is the term used to describe an eye with total vision loss (no light perception).

Clinical Manifestations

Since the condition is usually symptom free, patients may first note changes in peripheral visual ability. This is followed by progressive loss of peripheral vision. Central vision loss can occur first, but this is rare. Some patients complain of bumping into objects or stumbling. Such symptoms may be attributed to the aging process and prompt many persons to see an optician or optometrist. A routine vision examination reveals ocular changes in the majority of patients with glaucoma. Three signs commonly used to diagnose POAG are elevated IOP, visual field loss, and cupping of the optic disc. When pain oc-

curs with glaucoma, it is usually late in the course of structural changes with an IOP of 40 to 50 mm Hg or higher. More severe pain is characteristic of absolute glaucoma.

Therapeutic Management

The principle of treatment is to maintain IOP at a reduced level to prevent further damage to intraocular structures. Both medical and surgical approaches are used, but surgery is usually done only when medical or laser treatment is unsuccessful. Medications are used to create miosis (constriction of the pupil) and reduce formation of aqueous humor by the ciliary body.

An approach sometimes used to reduce IOP preoperatively is application of a pneumatic eye softener, known as the Honan Intraocular Pressure Reducer (Honan balloon). The reducer can decrease IOP faster than medications and eliminates the side effects of systemic medications. Use of the Honan balloon requires additional education of nurses responsible for its application and the monitoring of patients.[19]

Surgery or laser therapy may be done when medical treatment is not well tolerated and IOP is not controlled. Trabeculectomy is the surgical procedure commonly done. In this procedure a small piece of sclera containing the trabecular network is removed, and an iridectomy is done. This creates a drainage bleb or blister for aqueous fluid to drain under the subconjunctival tissues, bypassing the blocked trabecular meshwork. Postoperatively, the drainage bleb can be seen behind the limbus under the upper lid.

After surgery, IOP should return to normal. Cycloplegic and steroid eye medications will be instilled in the eye until there is no indication of iritis. Antibiotics may also be used. A miotic may be ordered to constrict the pupil and encourage free flow of aqueous fluid for the first few postoperative days. Then a mydriatic medication is used to dilate the pupil and prevent adhesion (synechia) formation. Synechiae are adhesions to the cornea in front (anterior) or to the lens behind (posterior).

An increasingly popular noninvasive treatment for POAG is laser trabeculoplasty. This is done as an outpatient procedure and requires about 30 minutes. Some ophthalmologists divide the treatment into two applications giving 50 small burns per treatment. Patients experience little discomfort during the treatment, and many resume all normal activities within 1 to 2 days including return to work.[65] Topical steroids are sometimes prescribed for a few days postoperatively. Laser therapy is reported to be very successful for many patients.

Following trabeculectomy or laser trabeculoplasty, patients may not need typical glaucoma medications, but they need continued frequent ophthalmic monitoring for signs of recurrence or complications. As with medical treatment, surgery and laser treatment stop further visual loss, but previous vision lost cannot be restored.

CLOSED-ANGLE GLAUCOMA
Definition/Etiology

Closed-angle glaucoma is also referred to as shallow, narrow-angle, primary, or congested glaucoma. More women than men are affected. It is usually not seen before 45 years and is more common at 60 years and over. Persons with hypermetropia are more prone to this type of glaucoma because the angle of the eye may be narrow. Persons who work in dark environments may be subject to it because of long-term pupil dilation resulting in blockage of the angle by the iris. People who have closed-angle glaucoma may have shallow or narrow anterior chambers.

Pathophysiology

In closed-angle glaucoma the iris lies close to the drainage channel and bulges forward against the cornea, creating a mechanical blockage of the trabecular meshwork. The aqueous humor that is attempting to flow through the pupil may push the iris forward, which can result in partial or total pupillary blockage. Figure 53-6 illustrates pupillary blockage. The aqueous humor is trapped, and IOP rises suddenly, sometimes as high as 50 to 70 mm Hg.

Clinical Manifestations

Closed-angle glaucoma can develop gradually with symptoms that appear intermittently for short periods, often in the evening when the pupil dilates. Patients may associate symptoms with stress or fatigue, since they are relieved by sleep when the pupil constricts. Symptoms commonly reported during this early stage are blurred vision, halos or colored rings around white lights, frontal headache, and eye pain. The attack usually starts in one eye, but the pain and stress may precipitate involvement in the other eye.

Acute closed-angle glaucoma is not common, and acute attacks are rarely seen. These patients seek immediate relief for excruciating eye pain. Severe vomiting may accompany the eye pain. The patient may report headache, **photophobia** (sensitivity of the eye to light characterized by squinting, blinking, and turning the head away from the light), and **lacrimation** (the excessive production of tears). Vision is blurred and greatly reduced, to the extent of seeing only hand movements. On ocular examination the eye under the closed lid feels hard. The pupil is fixed, oval in shape, and semidilated. The cornea has a hazy appearance with conjunctival chemosis (excessive edema of conjunctiva), and ciliary injection (engorgement of blood vessels in sclera around the limbus) will be present. The white of the eye appears red.

Therapeutic Management

Treatment involves hospitalization and surgery. Before surgery a combination of medications will be used to control the acute attack. Pilocarpine (2% or 4%) is instilled at 5- to 15-minute intervals for four or five times to create miosis and pull the iris away from the cornea, permitting drainage of the aqueous fluid. A carbonic anhydrase inhibitor such as acetazolamide (Diamox), 500 mg, is given by intravenous push to decrease formation of aqueous fluid. Mannitol is sometimes given intravenously to draw aqueous fluid from the eye by osmosis. Often the other eye is treated with pilocarpine as a prophylactic measure. Analgesics and antiemetics are given when pain and nausea or vomiting persist.

The surgical procedure for correcting the disorder is a peripheral iridectomy (surgical removal of a piece of the iris) or laser iridotomy (incision in the iris to create a hole). The procedure is usually done on the unaffected eye either at the same time or later. Both of these procedures create a hole in the peripheral iris so that aqueous fluid can flow through into the anterior chamber. Since laser iridotomy is noninvasive, patients with documented narrow angles may have prophylactic laser iridotomies performed, preventing an acute attack situation.

SECONDARY GLAUCOMA

Secondary glaucoma may develop when other eye conditions cause structural changes that interrupt

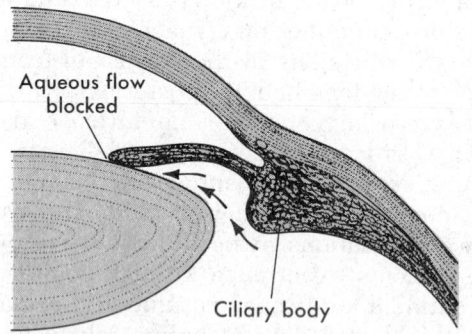

FIGURE 53-6   Closed-angle glaucoma. Pupillary block occurs when pupil dilates and iris clumps against cornea in anterior chamber, preventing outflow of aqueous humor. Resulting amount of increase in IOP depends on whether block is partial or complete.

the drainage of aqueous humor from the eye. Some causes of this type of glaucoma are cataract formation, tumor of the uveal tract or uveitis, hemorrhage into the anterior chamber following trauma or surgery, intraocular surgery such as intracapsular cataract extraction, long-term use of topical steroids, and exophthalmos from thyroid disease.

NURSING MANAGEMENT OF THE PATIENT WITH GLAUCOMA

Assessment

The nurse's assessment of the patient with glaucoma includes the following:

1. Family history of glaucoma (especially in immediate family)
2. History of previous ocular problems
3. Medications being taken (ophthalmic or systemic) and why taken; possible drug interactions should be carefully considered, especially when a patient has medications prescribed by more than one physician (e.g., some of the beta-blocker drugs used for glaucoma can cause a flare-up of allergy symptoms, and they may have an effect on allergy vaccine treatment)
4. Date of last eye examination and measurement of IOP
5. Description of visual problems (such as pain, vision changes, halos around lights, edematous lids or conjunctiva)
6. Visual acuity with and without prescriptive lenses using a standard eye chart and confrontation test (see Chapter 52)
7. Physical assessment, including thorough eye examination (see Chapter 52)
8. Degree to which patient is able to care for self; indications of need for help in the future (what is the effect of the problem on the patient's activities of daily living and life-style)
9. Emotional response to the disorder
10. Resources available for follow-up care (family, significant others, referral agencies); distance from and transportation to follow-up ophthalmic examinations
11. Financial ability to manage cost of long-term therapy

Nursing Diagnosis

Nursing diagnoses for the patient with glaucoma include the following:

Anxiety related to decreased vision and loss of independence

Pain related to increased IOP

High risk for injury related to loss of vision

High risk for infection related to opening between conjunctiva and anterior chamber after trabeculectomy

Sensory/perceptual alterations, visual, related to decreased peripheral vision

High risk for social isolation, related to inability to see well enough to maintain previous activities of work and socialization

Impaired health maintenance related to inability to instill eye drops

Knowledge deficit related to lack of information about measures to reduce IOP

Planning

Nursing care for the patient with glaucoma is planned to achieve the following expected outcomes:

Patient will remain free from injury

Patient will verbalize feelings about visual loss

Patient will demonstrate correct procedure for instilling eye drops

Patient will perform activities of daily living using strategies to adapt to visual loss

Pain will be relieved

Patient will use measures to prevent increased IOP

IOP will be maintained within normal limits

Implementation

To help the patient verbalize feelings about visual loss, the nurse explains that vision lost cannot be regained but further loss can be prevented. The nurse familiarizes the patient with surroundings and explains the anticipated schedule of treatments.

To alleviate the patient's pain, the nurse encourages bed rest with relaxation in a quiet environment. Analgesics or antiemetics are administered, and miosis is maintained with miotic drugs as scheduled. The nurse notifies the physician immediately when pain occurs suddenly and is severe. The nurse administers ordered carbonic anhydrase inhibitors and hyperosmotic drugs when other medications do not reduce IOP. The patient is instructed to turn the head slowly, avoiding sudden, jerky movement. Room lighting is adjusted to a comfortable level, and the patient is instructed to wear shaded glasses when the dressing is removed.

To counteract the high risk for injury, the nurse instructs the patient to scan the full perimetry of surroundings by turning the head from side to side and also explains the importance of using walls, grab bars, and other secure devices to assist with mobilization. The nurse remains with the patient during initial ambulation after surgery and applies an eye shield or other protective eye covering during sleep. Instruct the patient to avoid sleeping on the operative side until advised that it is safe. The nurse may apply glued numbers, rubber bands, or other raised devices to medication containers for identification when the patient's vision is severely impaired. Explain the purpose, action, dosage, time schedule, and side effects of medications to be self-administered. Discuss with the patient activities and habits that may need modification or discontinuation, such as driving an automobile. Instruct the patient to avoid straining at stool by maintaining an intake of six to eight glasses of water per day and a diet high in fiber and bulk; laxatives are recommended when constipation is a problem.

For patients with sensory/perceptual alterations in vision, always introduce yourself on entering the patient's room and speak frequently to the patient with partial or total vision loss. Avoid nonverbal communication, such as facial expressions and body movements that the patient cannot see. Approach the patient from the side of the uninvolved eye. Explain to the patient that adequate lighting (indirect lamp or wall light is preferable to direct lighting) is needed when reading or doing close work. Instruct the patient in the use of aids to assist with independent performance of activities—canes, writing templates for written correspondence, and special insulin syringes for visually impaired diabetic patients. Plan with the patient and family for assistance needed in daily self-care, maintaining as much patient independence as possible. Discuss modifications that can be made in furniture arrangement and location of items at home so patient can do self-care. Modifications needed for the patient to continue work and household responsibilities are also discussed. Inform the patient and family about resources available to help with adjustment to visual impairment, such as use of seeing eye dogs and schools for the blind. To prevent social isolation, the nurse plans with the patient a modified daily schedule with activities of interest when past daily activities or schedule must be changed. The nurse explores with the patient and family how social acquaintances may react to the need to modify past activities and considers realistic alternative social activities. Encourage family and friends to include the patient in family and social events. Discuss with the patient auditory or nonstressful visual diversionary activities (i.e., tape player with headset, talking books) that are appealing and available for use. Encourage the patient to practice a regular exercise program suitable to individual limitations for maintaining physical fitness.

Evaluation

Evaluation of the patient with glaucoma centers around how well patient outcomes are achieved. If the patient comes to the hospital with acute glaucoma, IOP will be relieved and normal vision for that patient will be maintained. If the condition remains chronic, evaluation centers around how well the patient complies with the treatment regimen and how well the patient is coping with changes in life-style.

Documentation

Documentation includes description of visual problems, visual acuity, IOP, and the degree to which the patient complies with ophthalmic monitoring.

Ongoing Care

Teaching and planning for long-term management begin on first contact with the patient and family. Ideally, teaching is done at planned intervals over several days. This provides for clarification of unclear information and for reinforcement of knowledge and assessment of the patient's ability for self-care. However, teaching in this manner is usually not realistic, since many ophthalmic diagnostic and treatment procedures are done on an outpatient basis, on a 1-day admission to a medical center, or with only a few days of hospitalization. Nurses must be knowledgeable of and refer patients to resources in outpatient settings. The written discharge plan communicates and coordinates teaching needs to others who assume responsibility for long-term monitoring and care of the patient (see box on p. 1435).

Resources may be needed for domestic activities, financial assistance, rehabilitation for partial or total blindness, or counseling for emotional adjustment.

GERIATRIC CONSIDERATIONS

Eye drop instillation

Inability to self-administer eye drops correctly is a common problem among older persons because of other conditions such as arthritis and tremors that result in decreased finger dexterity. An alternative method for medication instillation can be accomplished by drilling a hole in the center of a pair of polycarbonate (avoid conventional glass or plastic lenses) eyeglass lenses. The patient places the tip of the dropper through the hole, looks upward, and then squeezes the container. Commercial self-help devices are also available for purchase.[4]

PATIENT EDUCATION GUIDE   *Glaucoma*

1. Explain what glaucoma is and the purpose of treatment. Stress that with proper management, blindness can be prevented, but lost vision cannot be restored. Explain the importance of regular, long-term ocular examinations and be sure the patient has the phone number of his or her ophthalmologist.

2. Provide printed material about prescribed medications including the purpose, action, dosage, schedule, any specific instructions (such as refrigeration), and side effects. Evaluate the patient's (and family's) degree of understanding. Advise patient not to use over-the-counter medications before consulting his or her physician.

3. Discuss with patient how to avoid confusing eye medications when several are being used. Discuss methods of storing eye medications for ease of identification and for avoiding double doses or instillation in the wrong eye. Discuss how to improvise a labeling system.

4. Demonstrate and then observe the patient perform correct technique for instillation of eye medications. Observe a family member perform a return demonstration.

5. Demonstrate and observe a return demonstration by patient or family member of any treatments to be done by self or family such as application of dressings, eye shields, eye irrigation, cold or warm compresses, and insertion/removal of contact lens. Give the patient written, step-by-step directions with illustrations. When impaired central vision is a problem, use large print for written instructions. If supplies are to be purchased by the patient, prepare a written list of items needed.

6. Instruct patient to avoid activities that increase IOP. The most important complication of both medical and surgical therapy, including laser trabeculoplasty, is failure to lower IOP far enough to prevent further visual field loss.[46] Some ways to prevent an increase in IOP include the following:
   a. Advise patient to tie shoelaces by bending knee, raising thigh, and bringing foot within hand reach.
   b. Recommend patient move objects weighing 20 pounds or more by pushing the object on the floor using feet or by using a mechanical dolly.
   c. Instruct patient to use poles or rods with hooks on the end to pick up items (avoid bending).
   d. Advise patient to be alert for steroid-type medications prescribed by other physicians for noneye disorders. Steroids tend to increase IOP, especially in patients with glaucoma.
   e. Tell patient about Medic-Alert and other identification worn to alert health care providers in emergency situations about the eye condition and medications used.
   f. Be specific about what activities may be done to assure patient understanding and obtain compliance.

7. Describe to patient complications to be alert for and measures to avoid them. When a medical term or terms identifying a complication are used, clarify the meaning by describing the signs and symptoms. Tell the patient to seek medical attention for any of the following:
   a. *Upper respiratory infections*—avoid sneezing and coughing, which can increase IOP; avoid crowds of people where respiratory infections can be contracted.
   b. *Retinal detachment*—notify ophthalmologist immediately if sudden painless partial loss of vision (curtain effect) occurs.
   c. *Infection of eye*—seek medical attention for redness, photophobia, lacrimation, and drainage from the eye.
   d. *Blockage of drainage channel*—report to ophthalmologist promptly any eye discomfort, pain, or decreasing visual acuity.
   e. *Cataract formation*—report any change in vision.

8. Review with patient and family a written list of resources available and plan with them how and when to contact selected resources (see end of chapter).

Degenerative Disorders of the Eye—Changes with Aging

All structures of the eye are subject to degenerative disorders. Many of these disorders, some of which are more common than others, occur with aging and cause no noticeable visual defects or complications and do not require treatment. An example that is associated with the aging process is deposits of lipids in scleral layers causing the sclera to change from white to a yellow color (white of eye has a yellowish discoloration). Some other degenerative disorders threaten vision and require medical attention and treatment. Four of these are cataract, retinal degeneration, macular degeneration, and vascular occlusive disease.

CATARACT
Definition

A **cataract** is any opacity of the crystalline lens. By this definition 25% of the population has a cataract, which is one of the six main causes of blindness in the world.[37] Unlike some of the other leading causes of blindness, cataract is not restricted to developing nations and, although not preventable, in the majority of cases can be corrected.

Etiology/Pathophysiology

Senile cataracts, also known as adult-onset cataracts, are the most common cataract, resulting from loss of transparency of the crystalline lens that occurs with aging. The incidence of senile cataracts is steadily increasing, because the population is aging. Breakdown of metabolic processes in the lens is generally the cause. Lens opacities begin to develop after the age of 35 years and grow slowly so that by 70 years approximately 90% of the population has some visual impairment.[22,36] The onset and progression of opacity are individual and variable. A senile cataract may form in the lens nucleus, cortex, or posterior subcapsular region. First the lens appears cloudy, then it takes on a yellow appearance, and it may eventually become brown or black.

Traumatic cataracts, as the term implies, result from some trauma to or about the eye. They develop quite rapidly (commonly within months after a traumatic incident) and usually involve only the eye that was subject to the trauma. Some causes of traumatic cataract formation are blunt trauma, thermal injury, electric shock, and foreign bodies.

Clinical Manifestations

The classic symptom of cataract is painless progressive loss of vision in one or both eyes. Some people also complain of glare from bright lights. Occasionally, pain results when the lens becomes swollen and blocks the normal flow of aqueous fluid, causing an increased IOP. A cataract visibly appears as a white cloud over the lens.

Therapeutic Management

Cataracts are removed surgically when visual impairment interferes with normal daily activities. No known medical treatment can cure or prevent cataract formation. Diagnosis of a cataract can readily be made with an ophthalmoscope as well as by visual observation when the cataract is developed enough to cause marked lens opacity. Detailed evaluation of a cataract is done through microscopic examination using a slit-lamp biomicroscope.

During the developmental stages of centrally lo-cated cataracts, mydriatic medications can be instilled to dilate the pupil and enhance vision through the periphery of the lens.

Cataract surgery to remove a cloudy lens is the most common surgical procedure performed in the United States with 1.2 million operations reported annually.[14] Most operations are done using local anesthesia in an outpatient surgical setting. Mydriatic medications are often instilled preoperatively into the eye so the pupil will be dilated for surgical visualization. Other preoperative preparations may include administration of a relaxant or tranquilizer such as diazepam.[47] Some ophthalmologists prescribe preoperative instillation of cycloplegic (for pupillary dilation and paralysis of the ciliary muscle) and hyperosmolar medications (to lower IOP). A Honan balloon or Wee Bag of Mercury may be applied to the operative eye for 15 to 60 minutes before surgery to decrease IOP.

Two basic surgical approaches are used in cataract surgery. Figure 53-7 illustrates both.[11]

Extracapsular cataract extraction is the procedure of choice for removal of lens contents and leaves the posterior capsule intact.[49] The surgery in-

RESEARCH BRIEF

Smith S: Day care cataract surgery: the patient's perspective, *J Ophthal Nurs Technol* 6(2):50, 1987.

A Canadian study of patients' and family members' perceptions of day-care surgery and their ability to manage at-home care postoperatively was done in a new day-care cataract surgery program. Patients and family members were interviewed on the seventh postoperative day at the clinic where the postoperative check-up was done. During interviews, patients (and family members when possible) were observed for their technique with eye drop instillation and application of an eye shield. All patients and all but two spouses reported satisfaction with the day-care surgery. Implications for nursing practice from study recommendations were as follows:

1. Demonstrate alternative techniques for eye drop instillation by elderly patients and family members who may have hand tremors or poor eyesight.
2. Have the patient or a family member demonstrate eye drop instillation in a normal eye before surgery to evaluate competence and provide positive feedback.
3. Offer preoperative group teaching sessions as a cost-effective way to prepare patients and families for postoperative cataract management at home.

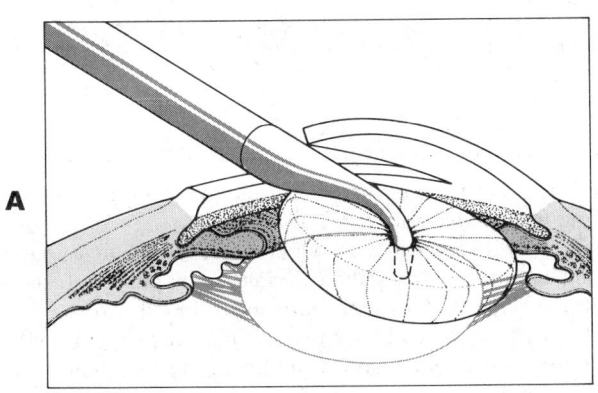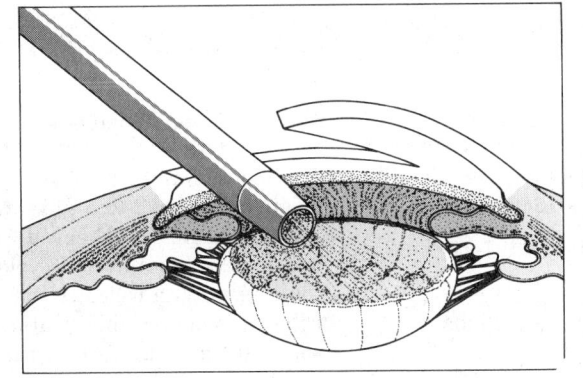

FIGURE 53-7   Cataract extraction. **A,** Intracapsular, when lens and capsule are removed. **B,** Extracapsular, when lens and only anterior part of capsule are removed.

volves removal of the nucleus, cortex, and anterior capsule. Extraction can be done manually or by phacoemulsification. Manual extraction is accomplished by making a series of small incisions in the anterior capsule. Then the anterior capsule and the lens nucleus are removed. Irrigation and aspiration are usually done to remove all lens contents.

Phacoemulsification involves fragmenting lens contents by ultrasonic vibrations and then removing them by irrigation and aspiration.

Rarely, intracapsular cataract extraction is performed to remove the lens contents with the entire intact lens capsule. This is accomplished by use of a cryoprobe (freezing probe). The lens adheres to the frozen probe for removal. Loss of accommodation results in most people so that corrective lenses are needed for near and distant vision. Absence of the lens (aphakia) causes the eye to become hypermetropic.

A peripheral iridectomy may be done as part of the extracapsular or intracapsular cataract extraction procedure. The procedure involves removing one or more small pieces of iris to promote drainage of aqueous fluid from behind the iris to the anterior chamber and the outflow channels. Without iridectomy the vitreous may move forward to fill the pupil and prevent normal flow of aqueous fluid into the anterior chamber, which can result in postoperative glaucoma.

Aphakia (absence of lens of the eye) is corrected by prescriptive glasses, contact lenses, or intraocular lenses. Contact lenses can be used for unilateral or bilateral aphakia and provide a full field of vision. There is about 7% magnification with contacts so that the concern for safety described in the geriatric considerations box is reduced. A disadvantage is that persons with impaired manual dexterity have difficulty manipulating them. When bilateral aphakia is present, it may be difficult to see how to insert the first contact. Permanent corrective glasses and contact lenses are not prescribed until about 3 months postoperatively, because following iridectomy the corneoscleral wound usually requires 10 to 12 weeks to heal completely. During the healing process the curvature of the cornea changes. This curvature affects the focusing ability of the eye and must become stable before permanent lenses can be effectively used. Intraocular implants may be done at the time of cataract removal or later. Because intraocular implants provide normal vision at all times, they are preferred for correction.

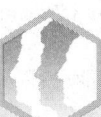 GERIATRIC CONSIDERATIONS

Eyeglass Use

Prescriptive glasses, which are the older, traditional method for correction, are still used but with steadily decreasing frequency. Some older persons who are already accustomed to wearing them may prefer glasses, and, when manual dexterity is a problem such as with arthritis, glasses may be indicated over contact lenses. Although glasses can be used for bilateral aphakia, they have several disadvantages:

1. Only central vision is corrected, and peripheral vision is distorted.
2. There is an approximate 30% magnification of central vision. This requires adjustment to daily activities and safety precautions. Because of the magnification, objects viewed centrally appear distorted, and there is difficulty judging distances such as when driving a car or sitting in a chair.

TABLE 53-2 Complications of Cataract Surgery

Complication	Description and management
Hyphema (free blood in anterior chamber)	Bleeding into anterior chamber postoperatively, bed rest and patching both eyes may be specified for 2 to 5 days during which absorption usually occurs Patients should be observed for signs of increased IOP, which commonly causes sudden ocular pain; miotics and cycloplegics may be prescribed; occasionally paracentesis, sometimes with irrigation of anterior chamber, is done to remove blood
Vitreous prolapse	Prolapse is major complication that can occur from rupture of posterior capsule; vitreous in wound interferes with healing and may cause retinal holes that can lead to retinal detachment; surgical anterior vitrectomy may be performed to remove vitreous from anterior chamber
Intraocular infection	Infection inside postoperative eye can occur despite strictest preventive measures; although rare today, infection is still a feared complication because it is a challenge to eradicate; symptoms are a throbbing or painful eye, which may have external drainage (that can be purulent); medical treatment includes administration of broad-spectrum ophthalmic and systemic antibiotics
Uveitis	Inflammation of any part of uveal tract can result from trauma of surgery and from presence of implanted intraocular lens (eye reacts to foreign body); eye pain, photophobia, and lacrimation are common symptoms; treatment includes topical mydriatics and steroids; sometimes it is necessary to remove intraocular lens implant
Posterior capsule	When posterior capsule is intact following extracapsular cataract extraction, it may cloud up, resulting in decreased vision; treatment is laser therapy or rarely surgical removal of posterior capsule (capsulotomy)

Postoperative complications

The sophistication of current cataract extraction techniques has led to a very low incidence of complications. A general overview of some common postoperative complications is provided in Table 53-2. A critical thinking guide for management of postoperative hemorrhage is shown in Figure 53-8.

NURSING MANAGEMENT OF THE PATIENT WITH CATARACTS
Assessment

Because most cataract surgery is now done exclusively on an outpatient basis, the majority of preparation is also done on an outpatient basis. Ophthalmic assessment is done for both the operative and nonoperative eye. All abnormal findings and visual changes described by the patient are recorded. Some ophthalmologic centers have special forms for recording this information. The patient's general physical condition is assessed to determine the existence of conditions that may affect surgical recovery. Patients are instructed to take a list of the medications with them to the surgical center. Older patients are assessed for a history of anticoagulant therapy used for cardiovascular problems. Ocular power tests will be performed for measurement of an intraocular implant when one is to be done. Power tests identify the axial length of the eye by use of an ultrasound measuring instrument attached to a computer. The measurements are used to calculate the power of the intraocular implant needed following cataract removal. The nurse also assesses the patient's understanding of cataract surgery.

Nursing Diagnosis

The following nursing diagnoses may apply to the patient with a cataract:

Sensory/perceptual alterations related to decreased visual acuity

High risk for injury (falls) related to decreased visual acuity

Impaired health maintenance related to visual changes

Planning

The nursing care for a patient with a cataract is planned to achieve the following outcomes:

The patient will demonstrate adaptive behaviors to changes in visual acuity

The patient will not experience injury or falls

The patient will demonstrate correct techniques for postoperative care such as use of prescrip-

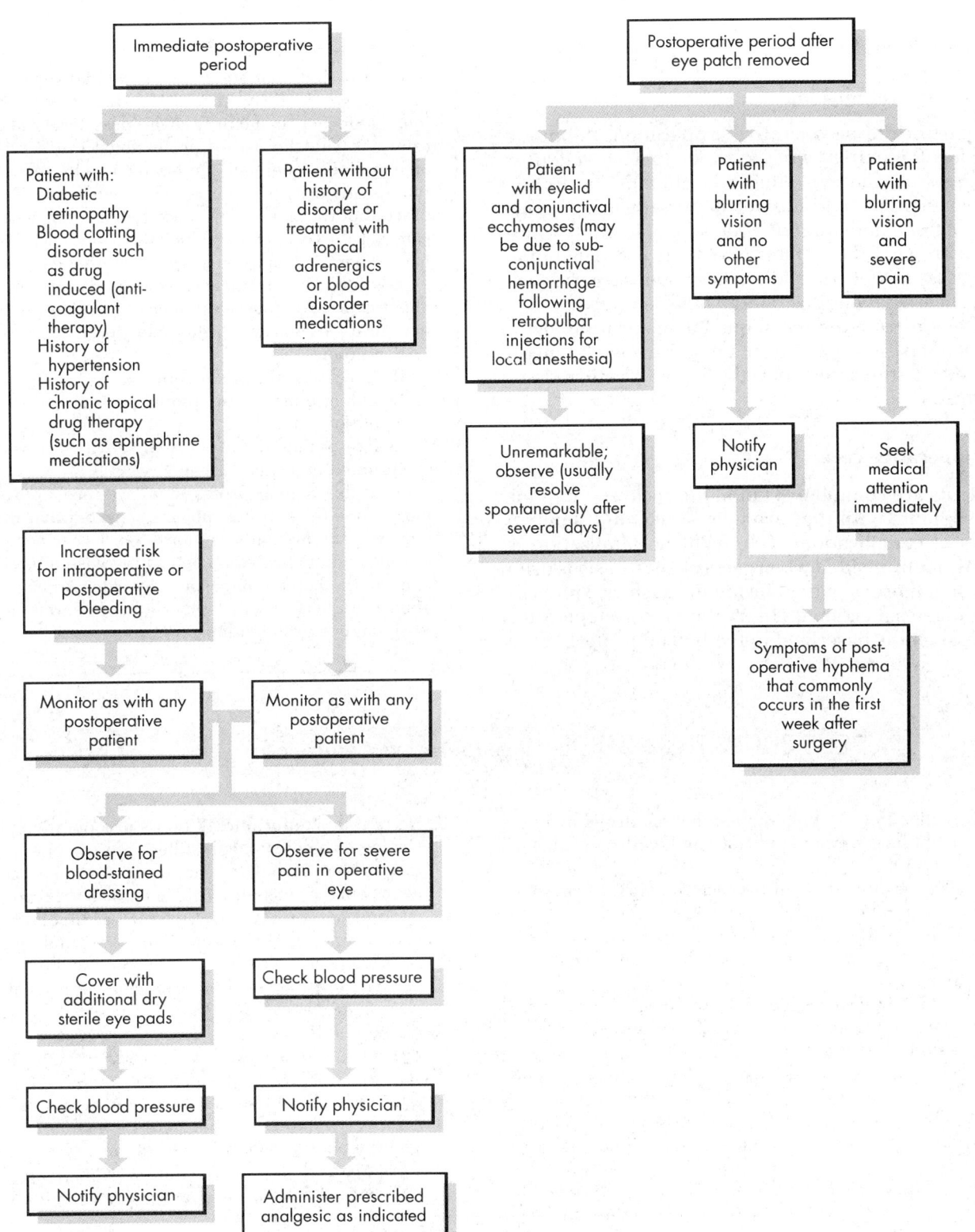

FIGURE 53-8   Critical Thinking Guide: postoperative cataract hemorrhage.

tive lenses, instillation of eye drops, and use of protective eye shields

Implementation

Preoperative teaching

As part of the preoperative preparation, the nurse teaches the patient what to expect before and after surgery (see patient education guide). Clarify any misconceptions and answer questions, using terms the patient understands. Many people think cataracts are growths or films over their eye. The nurse discusses anxiety the patient has about surgery, such as concerns about postoperative vision.

Demonstrate the technique for medication instillation. Have the patient or person who is to instill eye medications postoperatively give a return demonstration.

Postoperative care

Patients are commonly kept in the recovery area for 2 to 3 hours until they are fully awake and show no signs of complications. Overnight hospitalization is occasionally needed when general anesthesia is used or when there is patient instability such as with brittle diabetes. Pertinent observation for postoperative assessment is described in the box on p. 1441. Care

RESEARCH BRIEF

News and announcements: cataract survey reveals knowledge gap, *J Ophthal Nurs Technol* 11(1):33-34, 1992.

A study of 400 men and women aged 60 years and older was funded by Allergan Medical Optics, Irvine, California, to identify awareness levels about cataracts and the use of professional eye services among older Americans. Interview results revealed that the majority of subjects (96%) had heard of cataracts but had inaccurate knowledge about what a cataract is. The majority, including those who had been diagnosed as having a cataract, thought it was a growth or film on the eye. Among misconceptions about cataracts, a large number of the subjects had inaccurate knowledge of the following:

1. Symptoms
2. Risk of surgical complications
3. Length of time before optimal postsurgical vision would be achieved
4. Length of time before normal activities could be resumed following surgery

Regarding regular professional eye care, approximately one third of the subjects reported that their last eye examination was more than 1 year ago.

This study indicates a need to increase efforts to educate the population, especially older Americans, about cataracts and the importance of annual professional eye examinations.

PATIENT EDUCATION GUIDE   *Preoperative Cataract Surgery*

1. Instillation of antibiotic ophthalmic drops or ointment for several days before and on the morning of surgery.
2. Thorough washing of the face the night before and on the morning of surgery with removal of all eye makeup. Mascara that has been worn continually is a good medium for infection if not thoroughly removed.
3. A presurgical scrub around the operative eye with an antiseptic solution such as pHisoHex or povidone-iodine (Betadine) may be done 1 or more days before surgery. Instruct the patient to apply the solution in a circular motion all around the eye with a sterile 4 inch × 4 inch gauze dressing using two to three dressings to complete the scrub and discarding each dressing afterward. The patient should be told that after the antiseptic solution has been on the skin for 1 to 2 minutes, it should be rinsed with sterile dressings moistened with water.
4. A bedtime sedative may be prescribed to take the night before surgery, and, if irregularity is a problem, a laxative may be ordered.
5. No oral intake for 6 to 12 hours preoperatively.
6. Choice of medications instilled into the operative eye on the morning of surgery varies among surgeons but may include a mydriatic such as atropine, cycloplegics, or beta blockers such as timolol maleate (Timoptic). Carbonic anhydrase inhibitors such as acetazolamide (Diamox) may be given orally. Note that mydriatics *should be used with caution by glaucoma patients* because of the resulting pupil dilation.
7. Preoperative analgesics or narcotics may be prescribed to produce relaxation.
8. Eyelashes of the operative eye may be cut before surgery. Eyelashes grow back but slowly.
9. Tell the patient whether local or general anesthesia is planned. The nurse who is unable to answer questions should ask the surgeon or anesthesiologist.
10. Carefully review discharge instructions, ensuring that the patient and significant others understand them.

POSTOPERATIVE EYE ASSESSMENT

1. Position patient in comfortable sitting position and, under good lighting, remove the eye patch (and shield if present). Wash hands thoroughly before and after removing and discarding the eye patch.
2. Determine the patient's visual acuity by holding your hand approximately 12 to 16 inches in front of the patient's eye. If an intraocular implant has not been inserted, patients normally see only blurred hand and finger motions. Tell patients to expect visual distortion until they adjust to wearing aphakic lenses. When an intraocular implant is in place the nurse can share in the patient's joy of greatly improved vision on removal of the first dressing. The nurse should recall that an intraocular implant usually corrects for normal distant vision but that glasses will be needed for reading and other close work.
3. Assess the appearance of the external parts of the eye.*
   a. Note the amount and appearance of any discharge present, such as whether it is clear, viscous, or thick and tenacious. Remove discharge using sterile cotton balls moistened with sterile water. Use each cotton ball once only, and gently wipe the closed lid margin from the inner canthus toward the temple.
   b. Assess the eyelids, conjunctiva, sclera, and position of the eyeball for signs of edema. Some edema of the lids and conjunctiva is normal from the trauma of surgery. This edema should dissi-

pate completely by the third postoperative day.
   c. Observe for redness or discoloration in and about the eye. There will be some redness and bruised-appearing areas about the lids and conjunctiva, caused by bleeding of small vessels during surgery. This should clear by about the third postoperative day. Nurses and physicians in some eye centers record subjective assessment of edema and redness as 1 + (mild), 2 + (moderate), and 3 + (severe).
4. Assess the interior surface of eye structures.
   a. Examine the cornea by shining a penlight or flashlight on it. It should appear round, clear, and smooth. If the cornea has a cloudy appearance with a spotted or scattered appearance of light, increased IOP or infection may be present.
   b. Observe the iris with the light. It should normally appear clear and may quiver if an intraocular implant has not been inserted. It will be difficult if not impossible to visualize the iris when the cornea is cloudy.
   c. Note the size and shape of the pupil using the light. It should appear round in shape. A pear-shaped pupil is an indication of iris prolapse, and an ophthalmologist should be notified immediately. To judge the size and reaction to light of the pupil, consider if mydriatic and cycloplegic eye medications have been instilled.

*Evaluation of the retina requires an ophthalmoscope and advanced assessment skills.

of postoperative cataract patients is described in the nursing care plan.

Evaluation

Evaluation of the patient with cataracts centers on how well the patient is coping with sensory deprivation if the cataract cannot be removed and the effect of surgery if performed. Areas to evaluate include adjustment of the patient to prescription glasses or contact lenses, as well as any inflammation or infection present.

Documentation

During each eye examination the results of the examination, including visual acuity, should be recorded. Patient teaching and compliance with the therapeutic regimen are also essential to documentation. The preoperative and postoperative nursing

interventions shown in the box on p. 1442 serve as a guide for documenting nursing actions.

Ongoing Care

The patient is discharged when fully recovered from the anesthesia. Written discharge instructions are reviewed with the patient and family before discharge (see patient education guide). Some ophthalmologists have patients go to their office the day after surgery for removal of the dressing, evaluation of the operative eye, and instillation of medications. Other surgeons tell patients to remove the dressing for instillation of eye drops between physician visits. In this situation the patient and family should be able to instill eye medications and change the dressing properly before dismissal. Typically the ophthalmologist will change the dressing and assess the eye every 24 hours for the first 4 to 5 days unless the patient lives in a remote area. After 4 or 5 days the

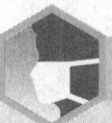

PREOPERATIVE AND POSTOPERATIVE NURSING INTERVENTIONS

Cataracts

Nursing interventions	Rationale

Preoperative

1. Assess patient's knowledge level about what a cataract is, what will be done in surgery, and what the postoperative care will entail.

   Establishes baseline information to use in teaching patient

2. Based on evaluation of no. 1 (above) provide indicated instruction:

   Clarifies misinformation and provides information to ensure compliance

   a. Description of cataract discharge instructions

   Promotes realistic expectations of when improved visual ability should occur

   b. Type of surgery to be done (whether patient will have intraocular lens implant)

   c. Postoperative care

      (1) Demonstrate/return demonstrate instillation of eye medications

      Maintains optimal effects of prescribed medications; understanding purpose of medications promotes patient compliance and prepares patient to report adverse effects to own physician

      (2) Describe and have patient repeat names of eye medications to be instilled and their dosage, actions, and side effects

      (3) Avoid straining, lifting heavy objects, strenuous exercise, and sexual activity until authorized by physician

      Prevents tension and increased IOP on ocular structures

      (4) Instruct to use aseptic technique when caring for eyes (includes hand washing before procedures, proper way to hold medication containers, and correct method to apply eye patch); instruct not to touch eye

      Avoids introducing microorganisms that could cause postsurgical infection

      (5) Instruct to wear an eye shield at night and not to sleep on operative side for prescribed period of time (varies from 3 to 6 weeks usually)

      Prevents pressure or chance of accidental injury to ocular structures

   d. Visual or tactile method to code containers when more than one medication is to be used

   Promotes accuracy with medication identifications

3. Withhold food and fluids for prescribed presurgical time period.

   Prevents nausea and vomiting, which can be induced from medications and anxiety

4. Have patient void.

   Eliminates possibility of discomfort from full bladder during surgical and immediate postoperative periods

5. Have patient remove all makeup and wash face thoroughly.

   Provides clean surrounding field for surgical site

6. Have patient remove shirt or blouse and put on clean surgical top.

7. Perform designated presurgical procedures such as vital signs according to agency protocol.

   Use as baseline data to monitor patient during intraoperative and postoperative period

8. Give prescribed presurgery medications; may include tranquilizer/sedative, ophthalmic antibiotic, cycloplegic, mydriatic, or ocular hypotensive.

   Promote patient relaxation, provide prophylaxis for possible infection, and create dilated pupil with decreased ocular tension

9. Following injection of local anesthetic apply and monitor Honan's balloon (or Wee Bag of Mercury) when prescribed.

   Promotes drainage of aqueous humor and decreases IOP

10. Remove hearing aid when present on same side as operative eye.

    During surgery fluid can drain into ear and could damage apparatus

PREOPERATIVE AND POSTOPERATIVE NURSING INTERVENTIONS—cont'd

Cataracts—cont'd

Nursing interventions	Rationale
Postoperative	
1. Position patient comfortably; can be supine with pillow or head elevated or on unoperative side.	Lying on operative side can increase IOP
2. Monitor as any postsurgical patient (vital signs, etc.) until awake and stable; be alert for postsurgical complications (i.e., complaints of sudden pain in eye and increased pulse rate); notify physician immediately.	Postsurgical bleeding can cause increased IOP, leading to ocular discomfort and agitation; if not relieved eye expulsion can result
3. Give analgesic and/or antiemetic medications when indicated.	Nausea or pain induces increased IOP
4. When patient is awake and oriented, offer oral nourishment used at agency such as juice and a muffin.	Following NPO status, patients can become hypoglycemic
5. When patient is awake and oriented, assist to reinsert hearing aid, if worn, to ear on operative side.	Promotes clear verbal communication between patient and nurse
6. Assist to change from hospital gown into street clothes.	
7. Give and review written discharge instructions (including phone numbers for questions) with patient and family (when possible).	Preparation for discharge and reinforcement of post-surgery self-management

PATIENT EDUCATION GUIDE   *After Cataract Removal*

1. Assess eye medications, dosage, and schedule for instillation along with patient's ability to correctly administer them. Normally, mydriatics (when intraocular lens not present) and cycloplegics are prescribed. Miotics, corticosteroids, antibiotics, and other medications may be ordered on an individual basis.
2. Explain use of analgesics such as ASA or acetaminophen (Tylenol) for eye discomfort. Also explain that regular daily use of ASA has an anticoagulant effect that could influence postoperative bleeding.
3. Advise patient that when tearing or eye drainage occurs, the eye can be cleansed gently with sterile cotton balls and water (inner canthus outward).
4. Tell patient not to rub or place pressure on eyes.
5. Explain that glasses or shaded lenses should be worn to protect the eye during waking hours after eye dressing is removed. Eye shield should be worn for the prescribed time period.
6. Explain what supplies to purchase and where to buy them for daily eye care at home.
7. Caution against lifting objects over 20 pounds, bending, straining at stool, coughing, or any such activities that can increase IOP (for the prescribed period).
8. Explain that showering is usually permissible as long as the eye is shielded and kept dry. Showers are usually advocated because getting in and out of a tub can cause pressure on the eye.
9. Explain that hair can be washed if the head is held backward beauty salon style under the water with no water getting into the eye.
10. Teach patient to practice safety precautions in daily activities to avoid falling, especially when temporary aphakic lenses are worn.
11. Tell patient to report immediately any decrease in vision, pain, or increased discharge to the ophthalmologist.
12. Explain to patient when sexual activity can be resumed (usually 6 to 8 weeks postoperatively).

NURSING CARE PLAN   *Cataract Postoperative Care*

Nursing diagnosis/ Expected outcome	Interventions	Rationale
Sensory perceptual alterations (visual) related to decreased visual acuity • *Visual acuity will be improved so that patient can perform daily activities independently (with or without assistance of prescriptive lenses) upon recovery (4 to 12 weeks postoperatively)*	Introduce self when entering room, and speak frequently with patient Familiarize patient with location of room contents and surroundings preoperatively Encourage use of hand-bars and walls when the patient is ambulating; avoid bumping or injuring eye Explain that vision (with or without corrective lenses) may be distorted Help patient plan daily routine for self-care and household tasks for first 2 postoperative weeks Help patient plan a regular exercise program suitable to limitations Encourage patient to identify diversionary activities of interest that can be done during the recovery period	Inability to visualize surroundings is frustrating Walking in strange surroundings with obscure vision would cause eye or body injury Distance and depth perception is often affected (with or without prescription lenses) Persons (especially elderly who live alone) may need assistance to manage personal care Regular exercise not only promotes physical fitness and prevents problems such as constipation but also promotes a mental sense of well-being Activities such as moderate viewing of television, talking on the phone, listening to tapes, and playing cards help maintain involvement and interest in life and discourage feelings of isolation and loneliness
Impaired tissue integrity (visual) related to surgical procedure • *Eye tissues will heal without complications by 3 months postoperatively*	Instruct patient to report immediately to ophthalmologist any change in the operative eye such as pain, increased drainage, change or decrease in vision, spots before eyes, or a blind spot Teach patient how to care for eye and self daily to promote optimal healing of operative eye: cleaning and dressing eye; installation of medications and action, dosage, and schedule for medication; use of eye shield and dark or protective glasses; safe methods of maintaining daily body hygiene; diet, including adequate fluid and fiber intake; use of mild analgesics for eye discomfort	Patients need to recognize and promptly seek help for signs of complications such as hemorrhage, infection, increased IOP, prolapsed iris, and retinal detachment so problem can be corrected before irreversible damage occurs Promote healing of postoperative eye and prevent complications
Impaired health maintenance related to visual changes • *Patient will adapt to prescriptive lenses or lens implant, with maximum visual acuity possible by 6 months after surgery*	Explain importance of patience and persistence in adjusting to new corrective lenses and lens implants Encourage patient to wear prescriptive glasses for 30 to 60 minutes at first, gradually increasing the length of time	Patients do not adjust immediately to prescriptive lenses (glasses and contacts) Thick, magnifying lenses tend to cause frustration because of feelings of dizziness, headache, and nausea that may result during the adjustment period; when the nonoperative eye has near normal vi-

NURSING CARE PLAN *Cataract Postoperative Care—cont'd*

Nursing diagnosis/ Expected outcome	Interventions	Rationale
		sion, cataract glasses are very difficult to adjust to; a contact lens is indicated if an implant has not been done
	If prescriptive glasses are worn, describe that central vision will be magnified 3 times and that, with absence of peripheral vision, patient should turn head to view the total visual field	The 30% magnification with prescriptive lenses makes objects appear 3 times closer than they actually are
	When an intraocular lens is implanted, explain to patient that prescriptive glasses are often also needed for reading and close work	The healing of the corneoscleral wound takes about 3 months; as wound healing occurs, the curvature of the cornea changes; this affects vision and adaptation to prescriptive lenses
	Reinforce explanation that vision changes as the eye heals and visual stability normally takes 3 or more months	

dressing may be left off during waking hours but the eye shield should be worn when sleeping. Once the dressing is removed, shaded glasses or temporary corrective glasses (if an implant was not done) may be worn.

RETINAL DEGENERATION
Etiology/Pathophysiology

The incidence of retinal degeneration increases with age. The two classifications of degeneration are peripheral and macular.

Peripheral degenerations are important because they may precipitate retinal detachment from formation of a hole in the weakened retina. Degeneration often affects the periphery before affecting the central retina. Many of the degenerative disorders are hereditary and rarely occur.

Retinitis pigmentosa is degeneration of the retinal nerve cells in both eyes. The rod cells are destroyed slowly in the peripheral retina at first, and later the entire retina is affected, resulting in tunnel vision. Tunnel vision means the person can view centrally located objects but misses those located above, below, or to the side. Retinitis pigmentosa is thought to be inherited as a dominant, recessive, or X-linked trait, and sometimes other genetic defects such as deafness and mental retardation will be present. The genetic picture is not clear in all cases. It affects males more than females. The first symptom to appear is usually night blindness **(nyctalopia).** Color vision is affected later and by the time the person reaches 50 or 60 years of age tunnel vision or total blindness results. If the person lives long enough, the macula may be affected, causing total blindness. Progression of symptoms and the end result regarding vision vary considerably. The diagnosis is made with an electroretinogram. There is no known treatment or cure. Persons with a family history should be referred for genetic counseling.

Macular degeneration is also referred to as age-related macular degeneration (ARMD) because it is the most common cause of visual loss in older adults, affecting more than 10 million people over 50 years of age.[32] The incidence of macular degeneration is reported as follows: 1.6% for 52 to 64 years; 11% for 65 to 74 years; and 27.9% for 75 years and over. Central vision for tasks such as reading, driving, and performing detailed eye work is controlled by the macula. Damage or degeneration of the macula causes impairment of central vision but does not affect peripheral vision. The cause of ARMD is unknown, but research done during the last 20 years has shown that environmental factors and artificial lighting can destroy the fragile photoreceptor cells of the retina. There is a hereditary tendency for macular degeneration, and myopia is a predisposing factor.

There are two types of ARMD: dry, or nonexudative, and wet, or exudative. Dry ARMD is the most common type, accounting for 90% of all ARMD. In dry ARMD the pigment epithelium is damaged and retinal photoreceptor cells are lost, which results in loss of the ability to transmit information present in light through the microcircuitry to the optic nerve (loss of photoreceptor ability).

Wet, or exudative, ARMD is much less common, accounting for 10% of ARMD. In wet ARMD a portion of the retinal pigment epithelium becomes detached, causing the exposed detached blood vessels to leak. The leakage may be absorbed, or it may attract neovascular tissue and form a net. If the neovascular tissue hemorrhages, which is common, fibrous tissue is attracted to the area. Subretinal scar formation and atrophy of the overlying retina follow.

Clinical Manifestations/Therapeutic Management

The most common symptom of macular degeneration is blurred central vision, which often occurs suddenly. Patients complain of difficulty with reading and seeing fine detail. Formation of a central **scotoma** (blind spot) occurs in some patients. Other symptoms include visual distortion, usually described as bending or irregularity of straight lines. Some patients note a change in image size with objects appearing smaller than they are (micropsia)

(Figure 53-9). Changes in color perception may also occur.[47] Although macular degeneration can affect only one eye, it is almost always bilateral with severe central vision loss. Peripheral vision is spared, so although affected persons cannot see to read, drive, watch television clearly, or distinguish faces, they do have the ability to walk.

There is no medical or surgical treatment for dry ARMD. Laser photocoagulation has been used in the wet form of ARMD to arrest abnormal growth of blood vessels that cause bleeding followed by scar formation in the retina. Research is currently being done in 15 clinical centers to determine the degree to which laser treatment prevents extension of central vision loss.[33] Other research has shown that vitamin supplements with trace minerals such as zinc may slow the degenerative process. However, patients should consult their physician before taking any vitamin supplement.[32]

Periodic Amsler grid self-testing can be done by patients at home to detect beginning symptoms of ARMD or progression of the problem. The Amsler grid is a box containing vertical and horizontal lines that form 5 mm squares with a black dot in the center of the box (see patient education guide). Grid charts are available from ophthalmologists, offices where ARMD patients are diagnosed and managed.

Type looks blurred

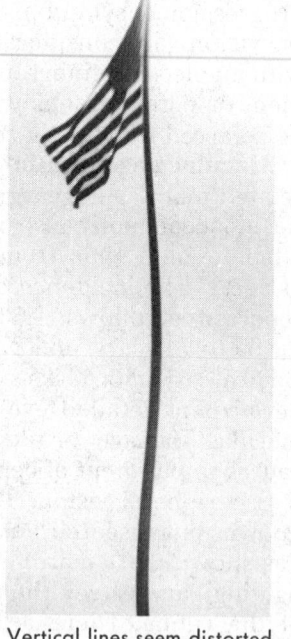

Vertical lines seem distorted

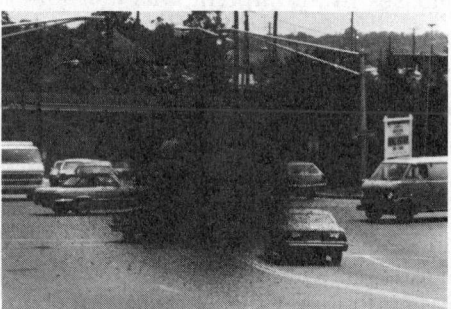

A dark spot at the point of focus

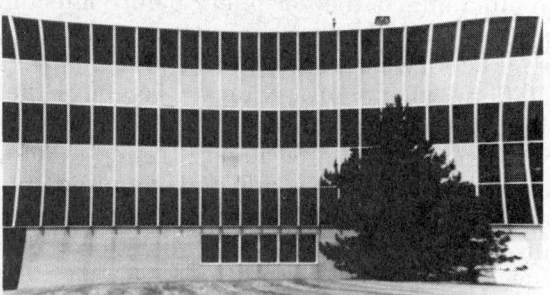

The center looks smaller than the rest of the scene

FIGURE 53-9   Some symptoms of macular degeneration. (Courtesy National Society to Prevent Blindness, Schaumberg, Ill.)

PATIENT EDUCATION GUIDE

Amsler Grid

1. Wear corrective lenses.
2. Test each eye individually; cover the opposite eye.
3. Position the grid about 13 to 14 inches away from the eye being tested, and determine if the black dot is seen. While looking at the dot, note if all four sides of the grid can be seen as straight lines. If blurring or distortion is present, use a pencil and paper to reproduce the appearance of the grid.
4. Take reproduced grid sheets to ophthalmologist for evaluation during regular ophthalmoscopic examinations.[8]

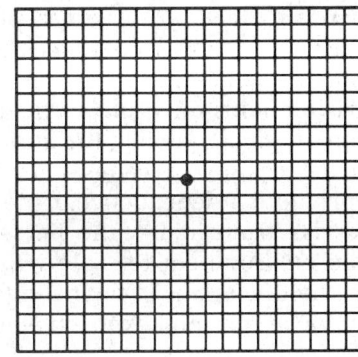

NURSING MANAGEMENT OF THE PATIENT WITH MACULAR RETINAL DEGENERATION

Assessment

The nurse assesses the patient for these characteristic vision changes:

1. Nyctalopia (night blindness)
2. Difficulty differentiating colors
3. Gradual loss of central vision
4. Sudden decrease in central visual ability
5. Blurred central vision
6. Scotoma (blind spot) in central visual field
7. Appearance of visual bending or irregularity of straight lines
8. Presence of micropsia (objects appearing smaller than they are)
9. Involvement of one or both eyes
10. Unaffected peripheral vision
11. History of ocular disease in family
12. History of exposure to environmental and artificial lighting
13. Other ocular problems (such as glaucoma) or systemic disorders (diabetes mellitus, etc.) that could contribute to symptoms
14. Visualization through an ophthalmoscope of drusen (yellow spots) on the macula—dark pigment indicates retinal hemorrhage; white, scar tissue formation
15. Central visual acuity as determined with a Snellen chart
16. Coping styles of patients and families
17. Resources for rehabilitation referral[40,58]

Nursing Diagnosis

Nursing diagnoses for the patient with retinal degeneration may include the following:

High risk for sensory/perceptual alterations (visual)
Impaired physical mobility
High risk for injury
High risk for sensory deprivation
Dysfunctional grieving for loss of vision
Altered role performance
Self-esteem disturbance
Body image disturbance
High risk for social isolation

Planning

Nursing care for the patient with macular degeneration is planned to achieve the following expected outcomes:

Patient will modify daily activities to compensate for visual impairment causing sensory/perceptual alterations
Patient will utilize assistive devices (such as cane, wall security bars) to maintain physical mobility
Patient will remain free from injury
Patient will utilize special resources (such as talking books, audio cassettes) to provide sensory stimulation
Patient will verbalize feelings about visual loss
Patient will utilize resources (such as school for the blind) to assist with alteration of role performance
Patient will participate in appropriate social activities and support groups to maintain self-esteem, positive body image, and discourage social isolation

Implementation

Many of the needed modifications are similar to those for patients with glaucoma:

To compensate for sensory/perceptual alterations, the nurse describes special aids such as magnifying lens and use of remaining peripheral vision fields for central vision loss

To maintain physical mobility, the nurse identifies assistive devices such as canes and wall security bars to promote independence in movement

To reduce risk from injury, the nurse evaluates the home environment for safety hazards and identifies modifications to be made (such as removal of loose rugs and exposed electrical wiring)

To discourage sensory deprivation, the nurse assesses past interests of the patient and guides the patient to select appropriate alternatives. A list of resources avaliable is provided

For dysfunctional grieving, altered role performance, self-esteem disturbance, body image disturbance, and risk for social isolation, review implementation for the patient with glaucoma

VASCULAR OCCLUSIVE DISEASE
Definition/Etiology

Arteries and veins in the eye are subject to occlusion just like vessels in other parts of the body. Vascular occlusive disorders of the eye may not only result in visual loss but also present a threat, since they are usually associated with systemic occlusive disease. Some of the occlusive ocular disorders are (1) branch retinal vein occlusion, (2) central retinal vein occlusion, (3) branch retinal artery occlusion, (4) central retinal artery occlusion, (5) temporal arteritis, and (6) ischemic optic neuropathy. Branch vein occlusion, which is the most common of the retinal disorders, most often occludes the upper temporal branches, causing hemorrhage and edema. Central retinal vein occlusion is strongly associated with systemic cardiovascular disease and is predominate in males. Both branch vein occlusion and central vein occlusion have a peak incidence in the fifth and sixth decades of life. The degree and location of the occlusion in branch vein and central vein occlusion determine whether the visual impairment is peripheral or central. Symptoms of branch vein occlusion usually appear gradually, whereas symptoms of central vein occlusion usually occur suddenly with variable loss of vision. Treatment of both forms of occlusion may include systemic anticoagulant drugs and laser photocoagulation treatments.

Central retinal artery occlusion and branch retinal artery occlusion commonly occur in patients with increased vascular resistance such as internal carotid artery obstruction. Typically, there is a sudden, painless central or peripheral loss of vision in a nondiseased eye. Medical management depends on identifying the cause of the occlusion. Restoration of visual loss depends on restoring circulation within 1 to 2 hours after the occlusion. Treatment may include digital massage of the globe through the eyelid to dislodge a clot, eye paracentesis to lower IOP, measures to create vasodilation, and surgical excision of a clot when its location is identified and it is surgically accessible.[4,8]

Temporal arteritis, also known as giant cell arteritis, is a condition that affects arteries throughout the body. The temporal arteries, which are commonly affected, become tender and thickened, causing symptoms such as pain on chewing and brushing the hair. The eyes are often affected, and permanent, sudden vision loss can occur in one eye because of occlusion of the posterior ciliary arteries. Loss of vision in the other eye may follow without treatment. Treatment involves large doses of systemic steroids and close monitoring of the erythrocyte sedimentation rate, which is usually markedly elevated.[40]

Ischemic optic neuropathy, which results from an infarction in the anterior portion of the optic nerve, causes sudden, painless loss of vision. Typically, patients with this condition are between 55 and 77 years of age and have a history of arteriosclerotic-hypertensive disease. Treatment includes systemic steroids to reduce optic disc edema and prevent atrophy. When atrophy occurs, nothing can be done to reverse the damage and restore some degree of vision.

Therapeutic Management

Medical management of vascular occlusive disorders that affect vision involves not only measures to prevent total irreversible blindness, but also close monitoring of other body systems. Frequent monitoring of vital signs, especially blood pressure, and blood sugar is usually indicated. An important aspect of nursing management of these patients is to teach them the importance of close monitoring of their general health status and to seek prompt medical attention for any symptoms.[4,8]

Nursing management is discussed under blindness (see pp. 1461 and 1462).

DIABETIC RETINOPATHY
Definition

Diabetic retinopathy is a disorder in which pathologic changes occur in the retinal blood vessels.

Epidemiology

All diabetics are at risk of developing vision-threatening disorders, which are common complications of diabetes. These complications include cataract, glaucoma, and diabetic retinopathy. It is estimated that about half of the approximately 14 million people with diabetes in the United States have early signs of diabetic retinopathy. Within this group about 700,000 diabetics have serious retinal disease and approximately 65,000 diabetics progress annually to proliferative retinopathy, which is the most vision-threatening stage of retinopathy. Diabetic retinopathy is a leading cause of blindness among the American population, with about 8000 new cases reported annually.

Although any diabetic can develop diabetic retinopathy, two risk factors identified by researchers help in assessing potential for eye complications. The risk factors are (1) type of diabetic and (2) duration of disease. Type I diabetics are more likely to develop diabetic retinopathy than type II diabetics. Almost all people who have had type I diabetes for 15 or more years have some degree of diabetic retinopathy. Duration of disease is an important risk factor for type II diabetics. The incidence of proliferative retinopathy in type II diabetics who take insulin varies from 2% for persons who have had diabetes for 5 to 10 years to 50% for persons who have had diabetes for 20 or more years.[27]

Pathophysiology

Three stages of diabetic retinopathy have been defined. The earliest (first) stage is background retinopathy. Stage two is preproliferative retinopathy, and stage three is proliferative retinopathy.

In background retinopathy, microaneurysms form on retinal capillary walls. The microaneurysms, which resemble tiny blisters, may leak blood onto the central retina or macula. Leakage from the blood vessels causes edema, and when the edema occurs in the macula, visual acuity and color discrimination are decreased. As the fluid from leaking blood vessels is being absorbed, yellow deposits known as hard exudates begin to collect. Most patients with background retinopathy maintain their independence, but legal blindness can occur.

Preproliferative retinopathy is characterized by cotton wool spots, engorged and irregularly dilated veins, and microvascular shunt formations that bypass vessels. Patients with preproliferative retinopathy are at risk of developing proliferative retinopathy.

Proliferative retinopathy changes begin when new blood vessels start growing into the retina and optic disc as an attempt to increase blood supply to the area. Hypoxia of the retina prompts the formation of new blood vessels, which is known as neovascularization. The newly formed blood vessels are fragile, and they frequently leak blood and protein into the vitreous and retina. New blood vessels may also grow into the vitreous, which can cause a traction effect, resulting in the vitreous detaching from the back of the eye. When vitreous is pulled away, it exerts traction on the retina and retinal detachment can occur. Patients with proliferative retinopathy may lose both central and peripheral vision.[8,28]

The pathologic changes that occur with diabetic retinopathy are believed to be caused by a combination of biochemical, metabolic, and hematologic abnormalities. Biochemical and metabolic changes are influenced by accumulation of excess glucose in the tissues of diabetic patients. Excess glucose is converted to sorbitol, which accumulates in tissues such as the mural cells located along the retinal capillaries. The build-up of sorbitol causes mural cell death.

Hematologic changes that are influenced by loss of mural cells include thickening of retinal capillary walls, formation of microaneurysms, and constriction of retinal blood vessels. The result is sluggishness of blood flow and occlusion of the microcirculatory system within the retina.

Clinical Manifestations/Therapeutic Management

Because there is no pain, blurred vision, ocular inflammation, or other signs, many diabetic patients do not have early symptoms with diabetic retinopathy. Except for some patients who note a decrease in central or color vision because of the presence of macular edema, a large number of diabetic patients do not note visual impairment until the disease has advanced to the proliferative stage. Vision lost in the proliferative stage cannot be restored. The National Eye Health Education Program recommends that diabetic patients have a comprehensive eye examination through dilated pupils at least once each year.[27] Strict control of diabetes during the first 5 years after diagnosis has been shown to reduce the frequency and delay the onset of diabetic retinopathy.[28]

Laser photocoagulation and vitrectomy are the primary methods of management for diabetic retinopathy. Laser photocoagulation involves directing a high-energy beam of light through the pupil onto the retina, causing small burns that seal leaking microaneurysms on the retinal surface. Laser photocoagulation treatment, which is performed in an outpatient clinic setting, has a success rate of approximately 90% for halting continued vision loss from diabetic retinopathy.[27]

Vitrectomy is done to treat long-standing vitreous hemorrhage and traction retinal detachment that occur in the proliferative stage. Vitrectomy involves surgical removal of the vitreous, which is replaced with a basic salt solution or silicon oil. The basic salt solution or silicon oil supports the retina until adequate scarring has occurred to maintain normal retinal positioning. Balanced salt solution or silicon oil used to replace the vitreous is eventually replaced by an aqueous fluid produced by the eye. Vitreous is not replaced naturally by the eye. Air or gas may be inserted at the end of the procedure to hold the retina in place. Laser photocoagulation treatment may be done during vitrectomy to treat bleeding retinal vessels and seal retinal holes.

A scleral buckling procedure may also be performed if a retinal detachment is found. Following vitrectomy, antibiotic ointment is instilled into the eye and a pressure eye patch is applied.

NURSING MANAGEMENT OF THE PATIENT WITH DIABETIC RETINOPATHY

Assessment

Assessment of the patient includes the following:
1. Visual acuity and field: difficulty driving at night is an early symptom of macular edema
2. Changes in color vision
3. Blood pressure: hypertension is a cause of retinal arteriosclerosis, which leads to retinal hypoxia
4. Type (I or II), duration, and degree of control of diabetes
5. Frequency of regular eye examinations through dilated pupils
6. Degree to which patient is able to maintain usual daily activities
7. Resources for follow-up care
8. Financial resources for management of medical monitoring and treatment

Nursing Diagnosis

Nursing diagnoses for the patient with diabetic retinopathy include those listed for macular degeneration and the following:

Noncompliance with having regular eye examinations related to knowledge deficit of how diabetes can cause loss of vision

Self-care deficit related to loss of vision as manifested by inability to maintain activities of daily living

Adjustment, impaired, related to visual impairment as manifested by failure to modify lifestyle and strive for independence consistent with health deficit.[28]

Planning

Nursing care planned for the patient with diabetic retinopathy is directed to achieving the following outcomes:

Patient will have regular eye examinations through dilated pupils by an ophthalmologist (every 6 to 12 months)

Patient will control blood sugar levels by adherence to individually prescribed dietary, medication, and exercise/activity regimen

Patient will utilize measures to control hypertension such as medications, decreased salt intake, and exercise

Patient will modify daily activities to adapt to lost vision

Patient will utilize resources available for the visually impaired

Patient will adhere to scheduled laser photocoagulation treatments as a means of retaining vision not lost

Implementation

Patient education about diabetic retinopathy is essential to prevent noncompliance with having regular eye examinations. Patient education emphasizes the importance of early detection and treatment of diabetic retinopathy. The objective is to preserve sight and prevent blindness. For self-care deficit and impaired adjustment the same interventions discussed in the section on blindness are implemented. The objective is to adapt to the degree of visual impairment and maintain as independent a life-style as possible.

When laser photocoagulation is to be done, inform the patient that eye drops used to dilate the pupil will cause a temporary blurring of vision following the treatment. Advise the patient to wear dark glasses to decrease light sensitivity. Following vitrectomy surgery where balanced salt solution is used to replace the vitreous, the patient is positioned so that the air or gas instilled will float against the retina. Such a position can be accomplished by having the patient lie prone or sit and lay the head face down on a table. The special position must be maintained until the air or gas has absorbed, which requires 4 to 5 days. Special positioning is not necessary when silicon oil is used to replace the vitreous. Results of vitrectomy for vision improvement may not be noticeable until several months following surgery. Such a time period can be emotionally taxing on patients.[8]

Evaluation

The hallmark of measurement is to reduce the percentage of blindness caused from retinopathy among diabetic patients. Nurses have a responsibility to help improve current statistics by educating diabetic patients who are unaware that they are at risk for diabetic retinopathy to obtain regular eye examinations and to adhere to treatment protocols.

Ocular Emergencies

Etiology/Epidemiology

Ocular trauma, also referred to as blinding accidents, is one of the world's six main causes of monocular blindness. In the United States, farm workers are the work group most affected by visual loss. According to the National Society for the Prevention of Blindness approximately 2 to 3 million persons per year receive eye injuries, with 40,000 resulting in permanent blindness.[58] One report states that more than 1000 work-related eye injuries occur daily in the United States. Accurate diagnosis and prompt treatment are essential to prevent blindness.[56]

Four major categories of eye injuries are as follows:

1. Sharp injuries—such injuries occur from foreign bodies (metal, wood, and any environmental material imaginable), automobile accidents, gunshot wounds, scissors, arrows from bow sets, and darts. These injuries can result in penetration of (goes into but not through) and perforation of (goes through) the eye.
2. Blunt trauma—trauma includes blows from fists, projectile objects such as tennis balls, and blows to head or eye in automobile accidents.
3. Chemical injuries—injuries caused by both alkaline and acid vapors, liquids, or solids. Alkaline burns are usually more serious than acid burns because they continue to release hydroxyl ions into the tissues after penetration. This can result in a full-thickness burn. Alkalines are substances with a pH of more than 7.0 and include lime, soda, potash, and ammonia.
4. Heat and radiation—these injuries occur from thermal burns of the body, especially about the head; hot metals (such as from industrial accidents); high electrical voltage such as that carried by high-tension electrical cables or an enormous bolt of lightning; and radiation from infrared, ultraviolet, and x-ray radiation.

Therapeutic Management

Every eye injury should be treated as an emergency. First, a brief but thorough description of the cause of the injury should be obtained. Figure 53-10 is a critical thinking guide for management of ocular emergencies.

First aid and emergency management

When obvious injury of or about the eye has occurred, the nurse must decide how to position the

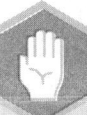

CLINICAL ALERT

Never attempt to remove a penetrating object, such as glass, a sharp piece of steel, or an ice pick, from the eye. This could tear or rupture internal ocular structures, resulting in permanent damage. Encourage the patient to rest as quietly as possible until the ophthalmologist arrives. Reassure the patient and family that medical attention is on the way.

A sedative may be indicated if the patient is agitated or having pain from other injuries. If possible, stay with the patient or ask a family member to stay to help decrease anxiety. Deep scleral and corneal penetrating foreign bodies should be removed in the operating room under strict sterile conditions. When emergency surgery is anticipated, question the patient when he or she last ate or drank anything so that proper anesthesia can be planned. Ask when the last tetanus toxoid was received, and if it has been more than 10 years, arrange for it to be given.

Severe lacerations around the eye or the orbit, a blowout fracture (fracture of the floor of the orbit resulting from a direct blow to the eye), or an evulsion of the eyeball should be covered with a sterile gauze dressing that has been saturated with sterile saline.

patient. Placing the patient in a lying position may increase IOP and intracranial pressure if an accompanying head injury is suspected. A reclining position can cause a penetrating object to advance further into the eye. When any of these conditions are obvious or suspected, place the patient in a sitting position with head support.

Management of injury from foreign bodies

Foreign bodies may get into and be retained in the conjunctiva, in the cornea, or intraocularly (commonly abbreviated IOFB for intraocular foreign body). Management of IOFB is described above.

Conjunctival foreign bodies are common and can usually be easily removed unless embedded. When a foreign body is embedded or suspected of being embedded, a physician should be notified for its removal. Conjunctival foreign bodies are usually dust, loose lashes, or an under-turned lash. Discomfort such as a scratching sensation occurs when foreign bodies lodge under the lower fornix or the upper lid, usually just above the inferior lid margin. The discomfort is caused from lid blinking that rubs the particle against the cornea. Most of these foreign bod-

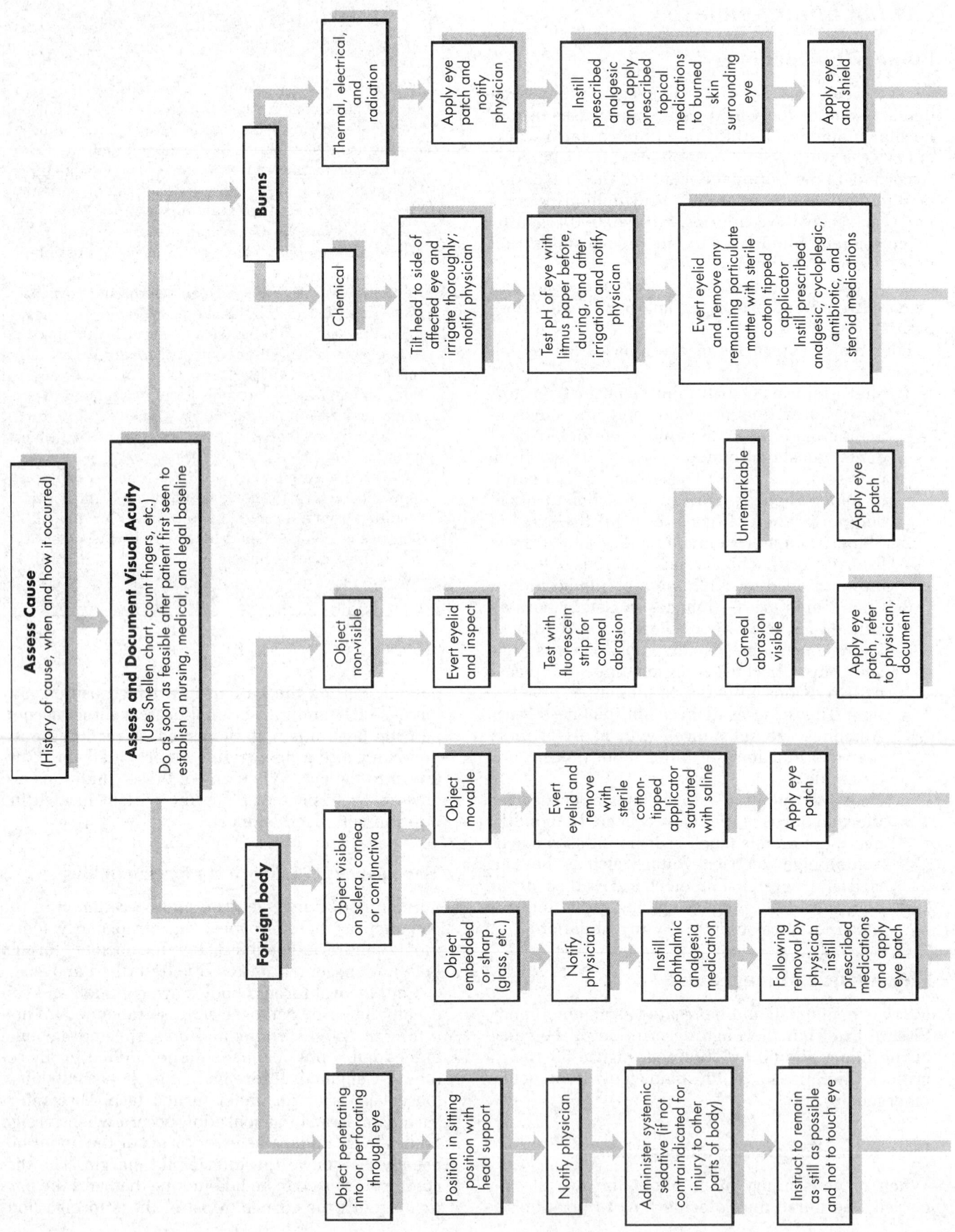

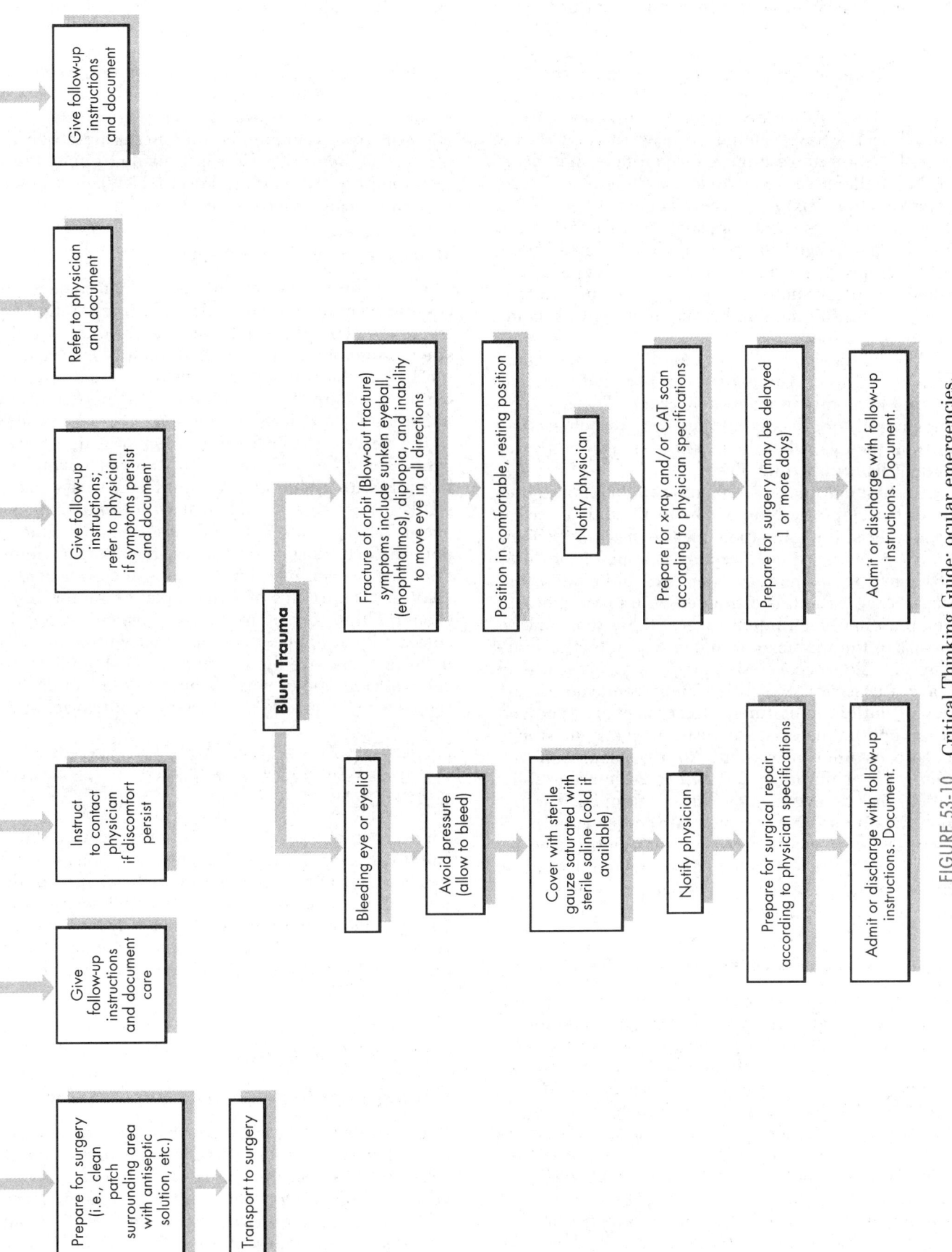

FIGURE 53-10   Critical Thinking Guide: ocular emergencies.

ies are visible with good lighting and can be easily removed. When a foreign body is not embedded the nurse may remove it. The nurse should explain what will be done before proceeding to remove the foreign body. A cotton-tipped applicator stick moistened with sterile saline (or tap water if away from the clinical setting) should be used to remove the particle. Sometimes after a foreign body has been in the conjunctiva for a while, swelling of the conjunctiva (chemosis) may occur. Chemosis usually indicates an allergic reaction, such as from insects or insect parts lodged in the conjunctiva. Lightweight cold compresses can be applied to relieve the edema, and an analgesic can be given for eye discomfort. Antibiotic ophthalmic ointment is commonly prescribed.

Corneal foreign bodies are among the most common eye injuries. The patient complains of pain and tearing and sometimes loss of vision. The eye may appear red, depending on how long the object has been in the eye, what the object is, and whether the patient has rubbed the eye.

Antibiotic drops or ointment is applied and sometimes a cycloplegic drop will be instilled to decrease iridocyclitis (inflammation of the iris and ciliary body). A pressure eye dressing is applied for 24 to 48 hours to promote corneal re-epithelialization. Usually the patient is dismissed with instructions to instill antibiotic ointment several times daily and to report to the physician if undue discomfort or blurring of vision occurs. Metallic foreign objects may leave a rust ring, which is usually removed after 1 day of antibiotic ointment. Rust rings are removed by an ophthalmologist who uses an eye spud, sterile needle, or other instrument. After rust ring removal, the eye is again patched for 12 to 24 hours usually, and antibiotic eye medication is continued. The patient is advised that it is not safe to drive with one eye patched because stereoscopic vision (three dimensionality) is lost. If the patient has to drive, it is best to give him or her eye bandage materials to apply after arriving home.

Complications of corneal foreign bodies

The concern with foreign bodies in the cornea is that complications such as corneal abrasion (denuding of small areas of tissue), corneal erosion, corneal perforation, keratitis (inflammation of the cornea), or degeneration of the cornea can result. A corneal abrasion usually heals with treatment in 24 to 48 hours but can progress to corneal erosion. Corneal erosion is suspected when there is intermittent recurrence of symptoms over a period of weeks or months. Characteristically, the patient describes waking with intense eye pain, photophobia, and tearing because the unstable epithelium has been removed by the upper lid on opening the eye. Symptoms subside during waking hours because adjacent epithelial cells slide over and cover the defect.

Corneal perforation requires surgical repair. Usually the iris herniates into the perforation, resulting in anterior chamber collapse. Serious and untreated corneal injuries can result in keratitis and degeneration of the cornea, which may necessitate keratoplasty. Further discussion is provided about these two conditions (including keratoplasty) in the section on special surgical procedures.

Management of chemical injury

Chemicals in the eye are a medical emergency, necessitating immediate first aid and prompt follow-up treatment. The immediate first aid treatment at the site (commonly industrial) of the injury is irrigation (lavage) of the eye with copious amounts of tap water for a minimum of 5 minutes. As soon as initial irrigation is complete, the person should be rushed to the nearest medical service. On arrival, eye irrigation should be resumed with water or normal saline for 15 to 20 minutes (or until all invasive material is removed) and a pH test with litmus paper is about 7.4. A quick test with litmus paper can be done before, during, and after irrigation to determine the pH and whether the substance was acid or alkaline. If particles of white alkaline material are seen on the cornea or in the fornices, a sterile cotton-tipped applicator moistened with saline can be used to remove them. Unremoved alkaline material will continue to burn through tissue and destroy the cornea, requiring a future corneal transplant.

NURSING MANAGEMENT OF THE PATIENT WITH AN OCULAR EMERGENCY

Ninety percent of eye injuries are preventable.[58] Nurses need to be alert for potential causes of eye injuries and use opportunities to teach preventive measures such as wearing protective safety glasses. Of equal importance is the opportunity for nurses to recognize common hazards that cause ocular trauma and to influence legislation when indicated to protect the public.

Retinal Detachment

Etiology/Epidemiology/Pathophysiology

Retinal detachment is usually a surgical emergency. Retinal detachment is listed as one of the top 12 causes of blindness in the world. Although any age group is subject to retinal detachment, the incidence of occurrence increases after the age of 40 years and peaks between 50 and 60 years.[8] Figure 53-11 illustrates some of the anatomic changes that occur.

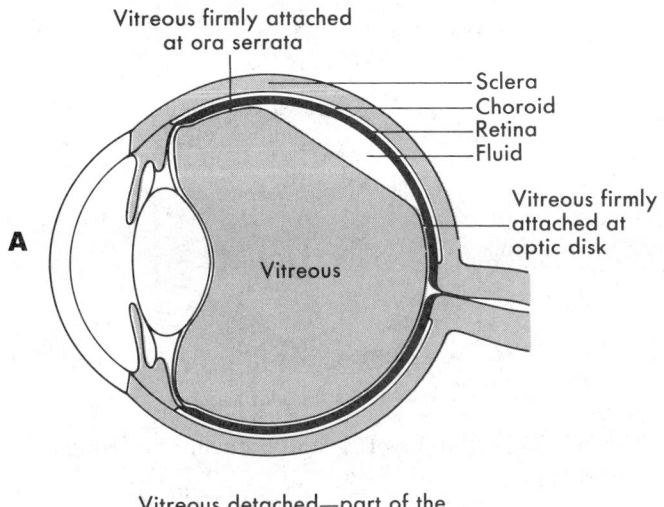

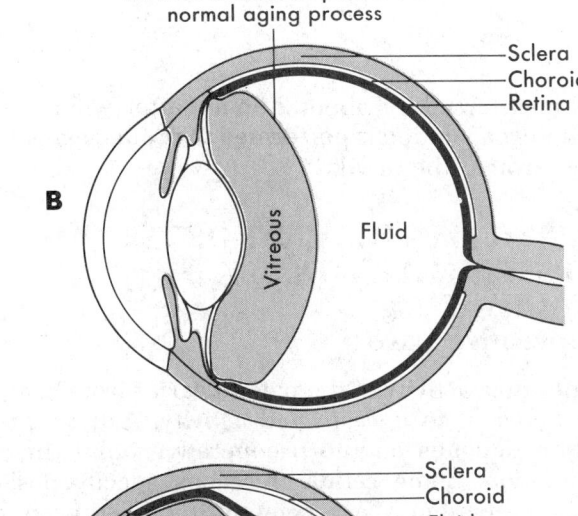

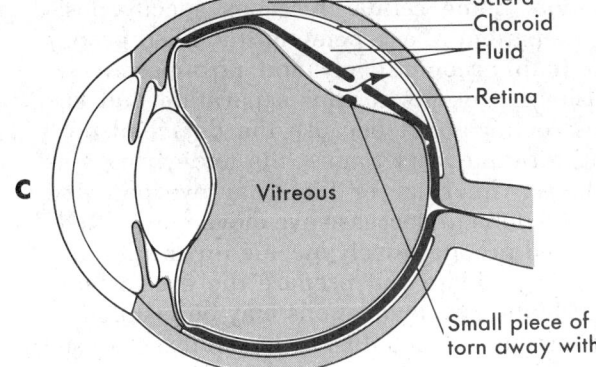

FIGURE 53-11   **A,** Retinal detachment. **B,** Vitreous detached at optic disc. Patient will complain of floaters like spiders. **C,** A hole in retina from choroid. Patient will complain of flashing lights.

Retinal detachments may be classified as either primary or secondary. Primary detachments result when one or more breaks occur in the neural layer, allowing fluid (vitreous) to collect between the neural and pigment layers. Primary detachment is the most common type of retinal detachment. Specific causes include recent or previous trauma (blunt or penetrating), high myopia (as occurs in very near-sighted middle-aged persons), retinal degeneration, and aphakia (i.e., following cataract surgery).

Secondary detachment results when the separation of layers occurs from pulling or pushing (traction) of the pigment layer away from the neural layer. Causes include pressure from intraocular tumors and hemorrhage, scar formation in the vitreous following vitreous hemorrhage, severe hypertension, diabetic retinopathy, toxemia in pregnancy, and retrolental fibroplasia.

Clinical Manifestations

The clinical manifestations of retinal detachment include flashes, described by patients as flashing lights or sparks in the visual field. Some describe them as more commonly seen on arising or entering a darkened room. These flashes are caused by traction on the retina. Floaters are spots or clumps before the eyes that result from thickened particles in the vitreous. When flashes and floaters are reported, the retina should be examined immediately. Flashes and floaters are considered warning signs that may lead to more serious pathologic conditions.

The curtain effect is described as a shade being pulled over part of the vision. This visual field loss or blind spot corresponds to the visual field affected by the separation. The curtain or blind area is opposite the area of separation because the visual field being viewed focuses on the opposite side of the retina. For example, if the lower half of the retina is detached, the visual loss will be in the upper half of the visual field. When the macula is affected, the loss is central. The most common area of separation is the superior temporal region, resulting in inferior nasal field loss. Separation in this area can spread more quickly, endangering the macula. Many patients describe this field loss as occurring suddenly. Although patients with retinal detachment are pain free, they often present with emotional distress sometimes to the point of panic.

Therapeutic Management

Treatment involves hospitalization and usually bed rest during the examination and preoperative period. Surgery is done as soon as possible, especially when the superior retina, representing a threat to the macula, is involved. The purposes of surgery are to return the retina to its original position, seal any breaks, and remove any fluid between the retinal layers. The type of surgery performed varies with the type and degree of the defect (retinal break vs. traction or both) and surgeon preference. Some common surgical approaches that are accomplished from outside the sclera without opening the eye are

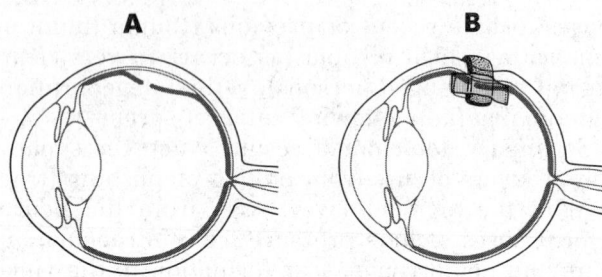

FIGURE 53-12 **A,** Retinal detachment with retinal tear. **B,** Explant scleral buckle in place.

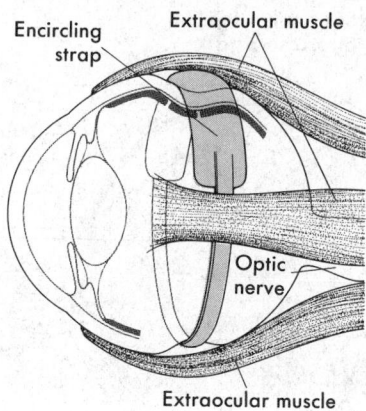

FIGURE 53-13 Repair of retinal detachment using silicone strap.

as follows:

1. Cryotherapy or laser photocoagulation used to seal breaks and holes. The principle is to create an inflammatory reaction to promote healing.
2. Scleral buckling accomplished by suturing a small inert material such as a silicone sponge onto the sclera over the site of the break or hole. The purpose is to create an indentation that reduces the traction on the retina and brings the separated layers of retina together. This surgical approach is used commonly. Figure 53-12 shows an explant scleral buckle.[58]
3. Banding or encirclement, in which a silicone band or strap is placed under the extraocular muscles around the globe. This creates more extensive indentation and is indicated when there is a large area of separation and several breaks or holes. Figure 53-13 illustrates this procedure.[22] When banding or encirclement is done, the fluid between retinal layers (commonly referred to as subretinal fluid) is drained to allow realignment of the layers.

Vitrectomy, which is described in the treatment of diabetic retinopathy, is done to remove blood, vitreoretinal adhesions, or other unwanted material. Laser photocoagulation and scleral buckling may be done in combination with vitrectomy. A bubble of air or gas is instilled at the end of the procedure to provide countertraction to assist the retinal layer to reattach.[40]

Pneumatic retinopexy is a more recent procedure being done to repair primary and secondary retinal detachment. Pneumatic retinal detachment repair, which is done as an out-patient procedure with the patient under topical anesthesia, involves injecting a gas bubble to rest against the retinal break. Following injection of the gas bubble, the patient is positioned so that the gas bubble continues to float against the retinal break, causing flattening of the retinal detachment. Positioning of the patient depends on the area where the detached retina exists. Common positions are prone, side-lying, and sitting with the face down on a table. The special position-

ing is maintained for about 2 hours, after which laser photocoagulation is performed to produce an adhesion around the break.[15]

NURSING MANAGEMENT OF THE PATIENT WITH RETINAL DETACHMENT
Preoperative Care

Preoperative activity of the patient varies from complete bed rest to unrestricted activity. Activity restriction depends on the preoperative ophthalmic examination. Some retinal surgeons specify positioning the patient in a dependent (modified prone) position both preoperatively and postoperatively. This position prevents further separation and encourages reattachment because the detached portion of the retina rests against the underlying epithelial layer. Uniocular or binocular eye patching may also be done to decrease eye movements. Medications used preoperatively include mydriatics and cycloplegics to dilate and prepare the eye for surgery. Antibiotic eye medications may be instilled to prevent infection. A sedative or tranquilizer is usually ordered preoperatively.

Postoperative Care

Postoperative nursing care is the same as for any general surgery patient or patient having eye surgery. Periodic analgesia may be needed during the first few days. Pain and discomfort vary in the operative eye so that the degree of discomfort will determine the medication used and frequency of administration. The eye will be kept dilated for 2 to 6 weeks with regular administration of mydriatics and cycloplegics. Also, an antibiotic and sometimes a steroid may be instilled for a time.

Often a pressure patch is applied after surgery and left for 12 to 24 hours after which it is replaced with an eye dressing. It is common for the lids and conjunctivae to be swollen after surgery. Cold compresses over the eyes may be ordered several times each day to decrease the edema and promote comfort. Most retinal surgeons allow bathroom privileges after recovery from the anesthetic. Progressive ambulation is usual, with dismissal 3 to 5 days after the surgery, unless there are complications. As with any postoperative eye patient, activities that increase IOP should be avoided. Postoperative teaching is the same as that after cataract surgery. When fluid exchange or air/gas bubble instillation is to be done, instruct the patient about postoperative positioning.

Special Surgical Procedures

KERATOPLASTY

Keratoplasty, one of the most common and successful types of transplant surgery, is done by removing damaged corneal tissue and replacing it with corneal tissue from a human donor (live or cadaver). Corneal transplant is indicated when severe visual impairment results from irreversible damage, most commonly following eye injuries. The surgical procedure involves doing one of two types of keratoplasty:

1. Full-thickness graft (penetrating keratoplasty) is the most common surgical procedure and is very successful for patients with opaque, non-vascularized corneas.
2. Partial-thickness graft (lamellar keratoplasty) is seldom done now and is indicated only when the size of the damaged cornea is small and limited to the anterior stroma. Figure 53-14 illustrates a corneal transplant.

NURSING MANAGEMENT OF THE KERATOPLASTY PATIENT
Preoperative Care

Potential corneal tissue for transplant is tested in the eye bank for the HIV virus. Once a donor for corneal transplant has been identified as virus free, the recipient is notified to be ready for admission for surgery. Corneal transplants are elective procedures because of the Food and Drug Administration's approval of K-Sol, the 7-day storage solution. Preoperative preparation of the recipient's eye may include obtaining a culture and sensitivity with conjunctival swabs, instilling antibiotic ophthalmic medication, and cutting the eyelashes. Some ophthalmologists order a medication such as 2% pilocarpine to constrict the pupil before surgery.

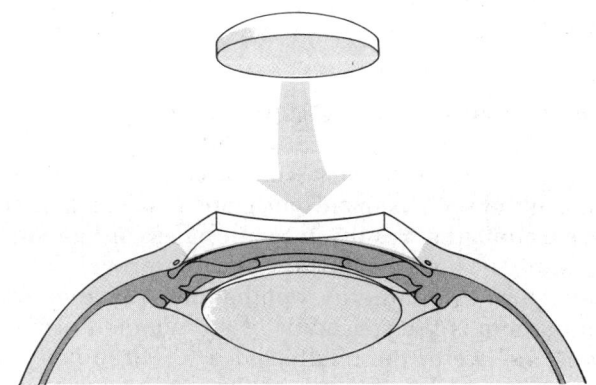

FIGURE 53-14 Penetrating keratoplasty, in which entire clouded cornea is removed and replaced by clear cornea.

Postoperative Care

Whereas patients were hospitalized 5 to 7 days in the past, current legislation specifies discharge on the same day surgery is performed.[7] Immediate postoperative management usually involves quiet bed rest with assistance to the bathroom and pain control measures until the first dressing change (first or second postoperative day). During dressing change the eye is thoroughly inspected as for cataract surgery and suture lines are evaluated. The general rule for all postoperative eye patients is that the patient should not lie on the operative side and should avoid sudden head movement. An eye shield may be worn for about 2 months during sleep. Mydriatic and cycloplegic medications may be instilled to dilate the pupil and discourage formation of adhesions between the iris and cornea. Antibiotic medication is usually instilled because infection is a dreaded complication. Steroid medications may be used to reduce inflammation.

Slow progressive ambulation is usually permitted after the first dressing change. Before discharge, patients and at least one family member or significant other should be skilled in administering medications and inspecting the eye for complications. Any activities that tend to increase IOP such as lifting heavy objects and bending should be avoided. Patients should be told that shaded glasses not only decrease light sensitivity but also prevent injury and the entry of air particles. Crowded environments and smoke-filled atmospheres should be avoided to decrease chances of inflammation and infection.

Sutures are usually left for as long as 6 months. After sutures are removed and complete healing has occurred, prescription glasses or a contact lens will be prescribed. Discharge planning and teaching are generally the same as for post–cataract surgery patients.

REMOVAL OF EYE
Indications for Surgery

Each year an estimated 10,000 persons in the United States have an eye surgically removed.[1] Removal of an eye may be necessary when it is extremely painful, is blind such as in chronic glaucoma, sustains severe trauma that results in sightlessness or has a malignancy or severe infection and for preventing or managing sympathetic ophthalmia. Sympathetic ophthalmia is the spreading of an inflamed process from one eye to the unaffected eye. Three types of surgical procedures are done for eye removal:

1. Enucleation is removal of the eye contents and a small portion of the optic nerve. The conjunctiva, bulbar fascia, and extrinsic muscles remain intact.
2. Evisceration is more extensive than enucleation. All eye contents are removed except for the posterior sclera, which is left to shield the optic nerve from infection that could spread to the brain.
3. Exenteration is the most extensive of the three procedures. The entire orbital contents, lids, and orbital section of the optic nerve are removed. A split skin graft is required to cover the exposed bony orbit. This deforming procedure is necessary when malignant tumors such as basal cell carcinoma threaten to spread.

NURSING MANAGEMENT OF THE PATIENT UNDERGOING EYE REMOVAL

Patients who have experienced severe chronic pain from glaucoma or infection may welcome relief from the pain. On the other hand, patients who must have a traumatized eye removed may be very resistant to the surgery and may require considerable psychologic adjustment. One of the most effective ways to help a patient adjust is to arrange for a person who has undergone the same surgery and recovered with a positive psychologic outlook to visit the patient. Another way to assist with adjustment is to arrange for the ocularist (prosthesis maker) who will make the prosthesis to visit with the patient. Regardless of presurgery psychologic preparation, most patients go through a period of altered body image, low self-esteem, and postoperative grieving.

During enucleation a temporary plastic implant may be inserted to maintain the shape of the eye. A pressure dressing is applied and left in place for several days to discourage hematoma formation and postoperative edema.

Postoperative nursing care includes observing the dressing and reporting any staining or bleeding to the surgeon. Postoperative pain should be minimal. If the patient has severe pain, the nurse should notify the physician immediately. Antibiotic or steroid ointment may be ordered to be instilled in the cul-de-sac once or twice each day. Most patients are discharged from the hospital 4 to 5 days after surgery.

If not done during enucleation, a temporary prosthesis may be inserted about 3 weeks postoperatively, when fitting for a permanent prosthesis is generally done.[2] Nursing care planning includes teaching the patient how to insert, remove, and care for the prosthesis.

Inflammatory and Infectious Disorders

CHALAZION
Definition/Etiology

Chalazion is a sterile granulomatous inflammation or infection of a meibomian gland in the inner upper or lower surface of an eyelid. A chalazion, referred to medically as meibomian or tarsal cyst, results from blockage of sebaceous material in a meibomian gland. The cause is unknown. Given the number of meibomian glands (about 25 in the upper lid and 20 in the lower lid), more than one chalazion can occur at the same time, although this is not common.

Clinical Manifestations

At first, chalazions appear as raised, round, inflamed, and tender areas (same symptoms as internal hordeolum), but over time they increase in size and lose the inflammatory signs. At this point they have the appearance and feel of a hardened cyst. Pressure they exert on the cornea can cause corneal irritation and astigmatism. Discomfort is usually more noticeable when the upper lid is closed. Other symptoms include sensitivity to light, a sensation of tired eyes, and weeping (epiphora). Small chalazions may spontaneously resolve partially or totally. If they do not completely resolve, they may recur within a few months, creating a larger cyst. A chalazion can fibrose and leave a permanent hard nodule.

Therapeutic Management

Application of warm compresses over the affected eyelid for about 15 minutes three to four times per day is a common treatment in the early stages. If accompanying infection is suspected, ophthalmic antibiotic ointments may be used. Analgesic ophthalmic ointments may be used for discomfort, especially at night when the discomfort becomes more noticeable. Some ophthalmologists recommend massaging the lid margins to promote drainage in surrounding glands. In later stages when the chalazion becomes larger, surgical excision is the treatment of choice. The surgery is performed in an outpatient setting with a local anesthetic infiltrated into the lid.

HORDEOLUM
Etiology/Clinical Manifestations

Hordeolum is commonly known as sty. Hordeolum is an infection of the outer superficial lid glands of Zeis or Moll and appears as a raised, reddened, inflamed area that is very tender to touch and contains pus. When the raised area of the hordeolum points toward the skin surface of the lid margin, it is described as external, and when it points toward the skin side or conjunctival surface of the lid margin, it is described as internal. The cause of the infection may be unknown, but infection can occur in persons with lowered resistance, such as those with diabetes mellitus. Usually only one sty on one eyelid occurs, but two or more may appear on both eyes at the same time. Styes are commonly short lived, lasting only a few days whether treated or untreated.

Therapeutic Management

Therapeutic management includes application of warm compresses for 15 minutes four times daily and instillation of an ophthalmic antibiotic ointment to combat the infectious organism and prevent spread of the infection to surrounding lid glands. The warm compresses not only promote comfort but aid in bringing purulent contents to a head, causing rupture with drainage of the contents. If the sty does not rupture spontaneously, it can be incised with a small sterile instrument. Relief from the discomfort is immediate on rupture or incision of the sty and drainage of contents. The person should be told not to press on or squeeze the sty to induce rupture because such pressure could force infectious material into the venous system of the eyelids and face, which can transmit infection to the brain. Persons with repeated sty formation should be encouraged to seek medical attention. Diabetes mellitus can predispose a person to this condition. Any identified precipitating cause of the infection should be treated appropriately.

CONJUNCTIVITIS
Definition

Conjunctivitis is a general term, because there are many causes of inflammation of the conjunctiva. In lay terms it is known as *pink eye*. This inflammation is the most common ophthalmic problem that prompts people to seek medical treatment.[51]

Etiology/Clinical Manifestations

Causes of conjunctivitis include viruses, bacteria, fungi, parasites, toxins, chemicals, allergy, and foreign bodies. Table 53-3 differentiates conjunctivitis according to types, causes, and characteristic features.[8,37,51] The onset is usually sudden with symptoms noticeable on waking. Symptoms include a reddened conjunctiva (hyperemia), serous or mucous discharge from the eye (eyes attempt to wash the irritant out), crusting of eye discharge on lashes and lids causing difficulty in opening eyes on waking, feeling of irritation or grittiness in the eye such as is felt with a foreign body (caused by drying out of the conjunctiva), eye discomfort (often described as a burning sensation), enlarged and tender preauricular lymph nodes, and itching of the eye when the cause is allergy.

Therapeutic Management

Conjunctivitis should be considered highly contagious, and equipment used to examine and treat the eyes should be carefully sterilized. A smear or culture should be obtained before initiating antibiotic therapy. Antibiotic eye drops are usually administered four times per day. Drugs commonly used are erythromycin derivatives, neomycin, or chloramphenicol. When purulent discharge is present, saline eye irrigation or application of warm compresses may be necessary before instilling medication. Systemic antibiotics and corticosteroids are sometimes also administered. Idoxuridine-IDU (Stoxil), adenine arabinoside, and trifluridine may be prescribed for viral infections caused by herpes simplex. Ophthalmic analgesic ointment or drops may be instilled for discomfort, especially at bedtime because discomfort becomes more noticeable when the eyelids are closed. Vasoconstrictor eye medications are sometimes instilled to treat allergic types of conjunctivitis. Visual acuity should be checked to rule out other disorders.

TRACHOMA
Definition/Etiology

Trachoma is caused by the microorganism *Chlamydia trachomatis,* a large virus with characteristics of both a virus and a bacterium. The organism is spread by direct contact with flies, rubbing eyes with contaminated fingers, and sharing infected washcloths, bathing supplies, and bed linens. It is highly contagious, spreads rapidly, and thrives in situations of overcrowding, poor hygiene, and dirty environments. Trachoma is often accompanied by bacterial infection.

The International Agency for Prevention of Blindness states that trachoma is the leading cause of

TABLE 53-3   Conjunctivitis: Causes and Clinical Manifestations

Types	Causes	Characteristic features
Viral infection	Adenovirus, herpes zoster, herpes virus I	Both eyes (OU) affected usually; is infectious and occurs typically in epidemics; spread by respiratory droplets through coughing and sneezing Appears seasonally when upper respiratory infections are prevalent; watery, nonpurulent discharge Preauricular lymph nodes often enlarged Follicles (small, white elevations) appear on conjunctiva Conjunctiva is diffusely red
Bacterial infection	*Staphylococcus* (most common), *Haemophilus* (Koch-Weeks bacillus), *Streptococcus pneumoniae, Moraxella,* and *Neisseria gonorrhoeae* (ophthalmia neonatorum)	Can be unilateral or bilateral; purulent discharge from eye(s); difficulty opening eyes when waking (caused by lashes and lids crusting, sticking together from drainage) Blepharitis (infection of lid margin) may be present Preauricular lymphadenopathy usually not present Edema of eyelids
Toxins and chemicals	Some identified causes are ophthalmic drugs such as atropine, eserine, and pilocarpine; smoke; improper rinsing of contact lenses; ingestion of arsenic and gold; and fumes, such as those from ammonia	History of exposure or contact; symptoms may persist despite treatment; periorbital edema and redness may be present
Allergy	Wide gamut of agents, including animal proteins such as dust, feathers, dandruff; ingested foods; cosmetic makeup	More noticeable during allergy seasons (spring and fall) History of recurrence Itching (pruritus) of eyes; both eyes affected; history of systemic or other allergy; burning sensation in eyes; symptoms worse during waking hours and improve when sleeping

world blindness. As many as 500 million people are said to be afflicted, with 90% to 95% of inhabitants in some regions of the world having trachoma. The incidence appears to be increasing because of rapid population growth in developing countries.

Trachoma is found in the Middle East, North and sub-Saharan Africa, the subcontinent of India, Southeast Asia, Central Australia, Latin America, and in the southwestern United States, especially on Indian reservations. Because trachoma is not as prevalent in the United States today as it was in the past, a limited description is provided here.

Therapeutic Management

Trachoma is both preventable and treatable. Current treatment consists of oral tetracycline or erythromycin for 3 weeks. Because of the side effects that often accompany systemic administration of these antibiotics, the topical route of administration is desirable. Corrective surgery can be done on trachomatous lids that have entropion (turning in of lower lids) and trichiasis (turning in of eyelashes).

UVEITIS
Definition/Etiology

The uvea is the second (vascular) coat of the eye. Interpretation of the term **uveitis** is broad in that it implies inflammation of the uveal tract (iris, ciliary body, and choroid). The inflammation can spread to adjacent connecting structures (retina, vitreous, and optic nerve). Some specific terms to describe the structures inflamed are included in the box on p. 1461.

UVEITIS INFLAMMATION

Iridocyclitis—inflammation of the iris and ciliary body (anterior uvea)

Iritis—inflammation of the iris

Cyclitis—inflammation of the circularly body (intermediate uveitis)

Choroiditis—inflammation of the choroid (posterior uveitis)

Inflammation of adjacent connecting structures includes the following:

Vitreitis—inflammation of the vitreous

Retinitis—inflammation of the retina

Retinochoroiditis—inflammation of the retina and choroid

Inflammation of one part of the uveal tract usually spreads to the other parts, but the degree of inflammation is usually greater in the anterior tract. Uveitis is among those less common disorders that lead to visual disability and loss of vision. Some known causes of the inflammatory response are bacteria, viruses, fungi, allergens, and chemicals. Trauma from surgery or accident can induce uveitis. Anterior uveitis (iris and ciliary body) may result from such systemic diseases as rheumatoid disease, ankylosing spondylitis, and Reiter's disease.

Clinical Manifestations

Common symptoms of anterior uveitis are pain described as inside the eyeball, dull in nature, and preventing sleep; photophobia that is not relieved by wearing shaded lenses; tearing or reflex lacrimation (stimulation of the lacrimal gland branch of the trigeminal nerve from corneal irritation); and blurred vision. Observable signs of anterior uveitis are ciliary injection or a small irregularly shaped pupil. Ciliary injection is engorgement of the episcleral vessels around the limbus. Sometimes the color of the iris changes. Two hallmarks used to diagnose anterior uveitis are flare and cells. Flare is a milklike appearance of the aqueous humor, and cells are inflammatory cell particles that collect on the back part of the cornea.

Complaints that patients commonly verbalize are decreased vision in one eye, variable pain, and mild photophobia. Some patients describe the distortion in vision as floaters. These are caused by opacities in the vitreous and result from the accumulation of inflamed or damaged cells.[36] There are no observable signs with posterior uveitis (choroiditis). Diagnosis is made with an ophthalmoscope or slit-lamp biomicroscope. A fundus lesion may be seen. Inflamed lesions of the choroid may appear as white, gray, or yellow spots with uneven, blurred edges. An inflamed retina will have a white and cloudy appearance. Retinal vasculitis can be seen as an infiltration of cells around vessels and hemorrhages. Edema may be present in the macular or optic nerve region. Continued macular edema can lead to a permanent decrease in vision.[36] Along with ocular examination, various laboratory tests are usually done to identify the systemic disorder causing posterior uveitis.

Therapeutic Management

Medical management of uveitis usually includes instillation of topical mydriatics, antibiotics, steroids, and cycloplegics. Mydriatics are drugs that dilate the pupil and include phenylephrine (Neo-Synephrine, Mydfrin) and hydroxyamphetamine (Paredrine). Cycloplegics cause temporary paralysis of the ciliary muscle, resulting in loss of visual accommodation and a dilated pupil. Some drugs having cycloplegic effects include atropine, cyclopentolate (Cyclogyl), and tropicamide (Mydriacyl). Surgery can create an opening in the sclera to drain aqueous. Anterior uveitis that is untreated or does not respond to treatment can lead to blindness or complications such as glaucoma. After resolution of acute uveitis, frequent reexamination is essential to detect and treat recurrence. When systemic infection is known or suspected to be the cause, an antibiotic specific for the microorganism is given. Surgical procedures such as vitrectomy may be done to remove vitreous opacities that interfere with vision. The patient education guide on p. 1462. includes information to teach the patient with inflammatory or infectious eye disorders.

BLINDNESS
Definition

Blindness occurs in varying degrees. Use of the term blind does not imply total loss of vision or that the person has no light perception. **Legal blindness** is the most widely used definition of blindness in the United States. It is provided by the Internal Revenue Service (IRS) for determination of eligibility for tax deductions. The IRS standard is vision of 20/200 or less in the better eye with the best correction. This means the person cannot read letters smaller than the 20/200 line on the Snellen chart. Legal blindness implies that the person cannot perform work that requires visual ability. The person who is legally blind usually still has some perception of light and movement. Total blindness means absence of all light perception. Low vision is a term that is now being used to refer to legally blind persons or persons with severe vision impairment but who still have some visual ability.[32]

PATIENT EDUCATION GUIDE   *Inflammatory and Infectious Eye Disorders*

Hordeolum and chalazion

1. Emphasize the importance of thorough hand washing before and after touching affected eye or eyes.
2. Instruct patient to adhere to the prescribed regimen for application of warm compresses and ophthalmic medications (antibiotics, analgesics, etc.).
3. Explain importance of not pressing or squeezing a hordeolum.
4. Demonstrate to patient how to massage lid margins to promote normal drainage of unaffected glands.
5. Advise patient to wear shaded glasses for light sensitivity.
6. Describe and document appearance, visual changes, pain, and signs of corneal irritation.

Conjunctivitis

1. Follow steps 1 and 2 for hordeolum and chalazion.
2. Explain to patient when cause is bacterial or viral that family members and others who use the same bath towels or linens are subject to the infection.
3. Instruct patient to use clean washcloths or sterile 4 inch × 4 inch gauze pads one time only for warm compresses to prevent cross contamination or recontamination with infectious agents.
4. Instruct patient not to touch furniture or other objects with tissues used to care for affected eye and to promptly discard tissues in a burnable container.
5. Instruct patient to observe agents touched or ingested that may prompt allergic responses. Advise patient to eliminate exposure to them as much as possible.

6. Stress the importance of follow-up appointments with physician.
7. Teach patient to avoid kissing others on or around the eyes when herpex simplex is present on lips.
8. Advise patient to use prescribed ophthalmic steroids as directed; prolonged use or overuse can cause cataract formation or induce glaucoma.

Uveitis

1. Instruct patient about the side effects of prescribed medications and indicate when to seek medical attention for them.
2. When mydriatics are used, advise patient to practice safety precautions when ambulating and warn that driving is usually restricted.
3. Recommend that patient wear dark lenses for photophobia.
4. Describe what patient can do to discourage increased IOP (bending, straining at stool, lifting heavy objects, etc.)
5. Encourage patient to verbalize anxieties about visual impairment and identify and plan further teaching when lack of information or misinformation is noted.
6. Stress importance of adhering to the medication schedule.
7. Describe eye appearance, lacrimation, visual impairment, appearance of iris or pupil, and pain.

Sensory Deprivation

One special consideration that should be kept in mind by health care providers who assist patients in adapting to macular degeneration, diabetic retinopathy, or any other blinding disorder is that these patients are prime candidates for sensory deprivation. Loss of central vision necessitates changes in many of their former work and diversional activities. Without adequate help and counseling, such persons can become bored, lonely, and frightened. When the cause is macular degeneration, patients need reassurance that their peripheral vision is not threatened and that they will not be totally blind. Usually they can maintain their own self-care in activities of daily living. If geographically accessible, a school for the blind should be recommended to help patients learn techniques for the visually handicapped. Also support and help from another person who has adjusted to visual loss can be helpful. Use of vision aids

such as watches and clocks with raised numbers, telescopic lenses, optical devices such as closed circuit television systems and computer software, special telephones, large print books, and talking books may help persons retain some visual independence. Lighted magnifying lenses may enable them to read documents and other important papers. Businesses that sell low vision aids are located throughout the United States, and some have mail order catalogs. Tell the patient to check with a social service agency to learn about eligibility to register for training and financial assistance with rehabilitation.

Emotional Response

A consideration that should be made when planning nursing care for a blind patient is whether blindness occurred suddenly or slowly. When blindness occurs suddenly, the nurse must allow time for grieving about loss of a valued body function. A sincere attitude of caring and providing needed help with activities of daily living must be balanced with encouragement and direction in learning how to be as independent as possible with the visual handicap. If blindness occurs as result of a slow, progressive disorder, the patient may have partially or totally resolved the emotional response to the loss and may wish to be treated as independently as possible. The newly blind patient's past knowledge of the environment should be emphasized during rehabilitation. An example is explaining that there are 10 steps to walk down to reach a lower floor.

SPECIAL CONSIDERATIONS FOR PATIENTS WITH HIV

The current prominence of acquired immune deficiency syndrome (AIDS) and the awareness that HIV *may be present in tears and on ocular cell walls* as well as in other body fluids have led to the establishment of guidelines for health care professionals published as Universal Precautions by the Centers for Disease Control (CDC) in 1989. In July 1991, the CDC published updated guidelines for prevention of transmission of human immune deficiency virus, hepatitis B virus, and other blood pathogens. These latest guidelines say that universal precautions do not apply to all body fluids including tears unless they contain visible blood. Offices that specialize in provision of eye care and examination procedures continue to follow the initial CDC guidelines for care of instruments, prevention of transmission of the pathogens, and protection of self. The initial guidelines are as follows:

1. Wash hands thoroughly immediately after eye care or examination when there has been contact with tears. Disposable gloves should be worn by a health care professional who has cuts, abrasions, or dermatologic lesions on one or both hands. Gowns, masks, and goggles are recommended during surgery only where there is potential contact with blood, body fluids, and contaminated surgical solutions.
2. Instruments used for external eye care should be cleaned and then cold disinfected for 5 to 10 minutes using one of four methods (described in the following). (After sterilization, the instruments should be rinsed thoroughly in tap water and dried.) The four methods for disinfection are as follows:
   a. 3% H_2O_2 (hydrogen peroxide)—fresh solution
   b. 1:10 dilution of household bleach (0.525% sodium hypochlorite and 5000 parts/million [mg/L] free available chlorine)
   c. 70% ethanol
   d. 70% isopropyl alcohol
3. Contact lenses used in trial fittings should be disinfected after each use. Commercial hydrogen peroxide systems approved for soft lenses can be used to disinfect hard (PMMA), gas-permeable, and soft contact lenses. Other H_2O_2 preparations can discolor lenses because of the preservatives they contain. Most trial hard lenses can also be disinfected with heat methods used for soft lenses (10 minutes at 172° to 176 ° F). The manufacturer of hard lenses should be contacted for directions about safe disinfection.

It has not been shown that HIV infection can be transmitted from contact with eyes or tears. Because transmission is not fully understood, health care professionals should be prudent when having contact with eyes and tears. Patients with AIDS who wear contacts should be instructed to continue use of the lens care regimen recommended by their optical specialist.

Ocular Effects of AIDS

It has been estimated that patients with AIDS will have at least one ocular or neuro-ocular problem during the illness. Ocular effects include eye infection, Kaposi's sarcoma, and cytomegalovirus (CMV) retinopathy. CMV retinopathy, which is the most severe ocular manifestation of AIDS, can lead to full-thickness destruction of the retina and varying degrees of blindness.[4] It is estimated that 20% of patients with AIDS are affected by CMV retinitis. One treatment that has been successful in arresting the progression of CMV retinopathy is intravenous ganciclovir. The serious side effect resulting from this treatment is neutropenia.[4] An alternative approach advocated to avoid this side effect is injection of ganciclovir into the vitreous humor, but currently the only form approved by the FDA is for intravenous use. A study is currently in process to investigate an initial high-dose treatment with ganciclovir and foscarnet for 2 weeks followed by a long-term, low-maintenance dose.[20]

CRITICAL THINKING QUESTIONS

1 Describe the visual changes associated with common errors of eye refraction.
2 Differentiate among the presenting symptoms of primary open-angle and primary closed-angle glaucoma and detached retina.
3 How should a foreign body be removed from the eye?
4 Describe the emergency management of eye injury caused by chemical injury from alkaline and acid substances.
5 What activities increase intraocular pressure?

6 How can the nurse help the patient cope physically and psychologically with blindness? Discuss role changes that may be needed for the blind patient and family.

7 What are the patient teaching implications for the various eye medications used in the therapeutic management of eye disorders?

8 What signs and symptoms in primary closed-angle glaucoma indicate an ophthalmic emergency?

9 What discharge teaching is necessary for the patient after cataract removal?

10 What are the implications for nursing management of the patient with an eye infection?

RESOURCES

1 AMERICAN ASSOCIATION OF OPHTHALMOLOGY 1100 17th St., N.W. Washington, DC 20036

2 AMERICAN FOUNDATION FOR THE BLIND Customer Service Division 15 West 16th St. New York, NY 10011 (800) 232-5463 (information and referral)

3 INDEPENDENT LIVING AIDS, INC. 1500 New Horizons Blvd. Amityville, NY 11701 (800) 262-7827

4 INTERNATIONAL AGENCY FOR THE PREVENTION OF BLINDNESS c/o National Eye Institute National Institutes of Health Bethesda, MD 20205 (301) 496-2234

5 INTERNATIONAL CENTER FOR EPIDEMIOLOGIC AND PREVENTIVE OPHTHALMOLOGY (ICEPO) Wilmer Ophthalmological Institute The Johns Hopkins University 600 North Wolfe St. Baltimore, MD 21205 (301) 955-2770

6 MAP INTERNATIONAL (Medical Assistance Program) P.O. Box 50 Brunswick, GA 31520 (912) 265-6010

7 MAXI AIDS 8630 102nd St. Richmond Hill, NY 11418 (800) 522-6294

8 NATIONAL EYE INSTITUTE National Institutes of Health Building 31, Room 6A25 9000 Rockville Pike Bethesda, MD 20014 (301) 496-2234

9 NATIONAL LIBRARY SERVICE FOR THE BLIND AND PHYSICALLY HANDICAPPED 1291 Taylor St. N.W. Washington, DC 20542

10 NATIONAL SOCIETY TO PREVENT BLINDNESS 79 Madison Ave. New York, NY 10016 (212) 684-3505

11 RECORDING FOR THE BLIND 121 East 58th St. New York, NY 10022

12 VIS—AIDS, INC. 10209 Jamaica Ave. Richmond Hill, NY 11418 (718)847-4734

BIBLIOGRAPHY

Current

1. Albiar E, Holds JB: Hydroxyapatite orbital implants: indications for use and nursing considerations, *J Ophthal Nurs Technol* 11(2):71-76, 1992.
2. Alven MT: Ophthalmic prosthetics: a guide for nurses, *J Ophthal Nurs Technol* 6(6):218, 1987.
3. Artentsen J: A review of complications associated with soft contact lenses, *J Ophthal Nurs Technol* 6(6):230, 1987.
4. Bartlett JD, Jaaanus SD: *Clinical ocular pharmacology,* ed 2, Boston, 1989, Butterworths.
5. Blakeslee S: Using a laser beam, researchers test a new method for correcting myopia, *The New York Times Health,* p B8, Oct 23, 1991.
6. Boyd-Monk, H: Eye trauma in the workplace, *J Ophthal Nurs Technol* 10(3):117-123, 1991.
7. Boyd-Monk H: The river of time: coping with change, *J Ophthal Nurs Technol* 11(1):3-4, 1992 (editorial).
8. Boyd-Monk H, Steinmetz CG: *Nursing care of the eye,* Los Altos, Calif, 1987, Appleton & Lange.
9. Burlew JA: Preventing eye injuries: the nurse's role, *J Am Soc Ophthalmic Regis Nurses* XVI (96):24-28, 1991.
10. Carpenito LJ: *Nursing diagnosis: application to clinical practice,* ed 4, New York, 1992, JB Lippincott Co.
11. Carver JA: Cataract care made plain, *Am J Nurs* 87(5):626, 1987.
12. CDC clarifies universal precautions, *Am J Nurs* 88(10):1322, 1988.
13. Dreizen NG, Stulting RD: Ocular gunpowder injuries, *Am J Ophthalmol* 100(6):852, 1987.
14. Frank A, Werfel N: ECCE with phacoemulsification and flexible IOL implantation, *J Ophthal Nurs Technol* 7(2):62, 1988.
15. Friberg TR, Eller AW: Pneumatic repair of primary and secondary retinal detachments using a binocular indirect ophthalmoscope laser delivery system, *Ophthalmology* 95(2):187, 1988.
16. Goldstein J: Pharmacology of ophthalmic drugs. I, *J Ophthal Nurs Technol* 6(4):146, 1987.
17. Hollins M: *Understanding blindness: an integrative approach,* Hillsdale, NJ, 1989, Lawrence Erlbaum Associates.
18. Holmes P: Modes of entry, *Nurs Times* 84(12):34, 1988.
19. Hunt L: Use of the Honan intraocular pressure reducer, *J Ophthal Nurs Technol* 7(2):59, 1988.
20. Jabs DA: *Studies of the ocular complications of AIDS,* Bethesda, Maryland, Oct 1990, US Department of Health and Human Services.
21. Kim MJ, McFarland GK, McLane AM: *Pocket guide to nursing diagnoses,* ed 3, St Louis, 1989, Mosby–Year Book, Inc.
22. Kirton M, Richardson M: *Ophthalmic nursing,* ed 3, Philadelphia, 1987, Bailliere Tindall.
23. Legro MW: Quality of life and cataracts: a review of patient-centered studies of cataract surgery outcomes, *J Ophthal Nurs Technol* 10(6):260, 1991.
24. Lewis SH, Collier IC: *Medical-surgical nursing: assessment and management of clinical problems,* ed 2, St Louis, 1987, Mosby–Year Book, Inc.
25. Lowe RF, Ritch R: Angle-closure glaucoma. In Ritch R et al, editors: *The glaucomas,* St Louis, 1989, Mosby–Year Book, Inc.
26. Messner RL: Becoming real: the nursing factor in chronic illness, *J Ophthal Nurs Technol* 6(2):66, 1987.
27. National Eye Health Education Program: *Highlights of*

survey results, Bethesda, Md, Dec 1991, National Institutes of Health.

28. National Eye Institute: *Facts about diabetic eye disease,* Bethesda, Md, 1991, National Eye Health Education Program, National Institutes of Health.

29. National Institute for Occupational Safety and Health, Center for Infectious Diseases, Centers for Disease Control: *Guidelines for prevention of transmission of human immunodeficiency virus and hepatitis B virus to health-care and public-safety workers,* Atlanta, 1989, US Department of Health and Human Services.

30. News and announcements: glaucoma five times more common among Blacks, *J Ophthal Nurs Technol* 10(5), 1991.

31. News and announcements: help for legally blind elderly, *J Ophthal Nurs Technol* 10(5):229-230, 1991.

32. News and announcements: help for people with macular degeneration, *J Ophthal Nurs Technol* 10(4), 1991.

33. News and announcements: lasers reduce severe vision loss from macular degeneration, *J Ophthal Nurs Technol* 11(1):35, 1992.

34. Newsletter from Southwestern Eye Center and East Valley Eye Institute: *Macular degeneration: a major cause of loss of central vision,* Mesa, Ariz, 1987, Arizona Eyeways.

35. Pizzarello LD, Haik BG, editors: *Sports ophthalmology,* Springfield, Ill, 1987, Charles C Thomas, Publisher.

36. Rhode SJ, Ginsberg SP: *Ophthalmic technology: a guide for the eye care assistant,* New York, 1987, Raven Press.

37. Schwab L: *Primary eye care in developing nations,* New York, 1987, Oxford University Press.

38. Smiddy WE et al: Cataract extraction after retinal detachment surgery, *Ophthalmology* 95(1):3, 1988.

39. Sommer A et al: Racial differences in the cause-specific prevalence in East Baltimore, *N Engl J Med* 325(2):1412-1417, 1991.

40. Stollery R: *Ophthalmic nursing,* London, 1987, Blackwell Scientific Publications.

41. Tso MOM, editor: *Retinal diseases: biomedical foundations and clinical management,* Philadelphia, 1988, JB Lippincott Co.

42. Wolfe CP: Fundamentals in focus, *J Ophthal Nurs Technol* 6(1):38, 1987.

43. Zavon B, Slater N: A surgical counseling plan for patients undergoing cataract surgery, *J Ophthal Nurs Technol* 7(2):68, 1988.

Classic

44. Antoszyk A et al: Gelatin implants in glaucoma filtering surgery, *Am J Ophthalmol* 101(5):618, 1986.

45. Barraquer J: Immunosuppressive agents in penetrating keratoplasty, *Am J Ophthalmol* 100(1):61, 1985.

46. Beckman H et al: *Symposium on the laser in ophthalmology and glaucoma update,* St Louis, 1985, Mosby–Year Book, Inc.

47. Caird FI, Williamson H, editors: *The eye and its disorders in the elderly,* Bristol, England, 1986, The Stonebridge Press.

48. Coleman D et al: Therapeutic ultrasound in the treatment of glaucoma, *Ophthalmology* 92(3):339, 1985.

49. Emery M, McIntyre J: *Extracapsular cataract surgery,* St Louis, 1983, Mosby–Year Book, Inc.

50. Greemodge LC, Spaeth GL, Traverso CE: Change in appearance of the optic disc associated with lowering of intraocular pressure, *Ophthalmology* 92(7):897, 1985.

51. Jackson CRS, Finlay RD: *The eye in general practice,* New York, 1985, Churchill Livingstone Inc.

52. Keith CG: *Genetics and ophthalmology,* New York, 1978, Churchill Livingstone.

53. Kodadek SM: Working with the chronically ill, *Nurse Pract* 10(3):45, 48, 1985.

54. Lent-Wunderlich E, Ott MJ: Helping your patient through eye surgery, *RN,* 43, June 1986.

55. *Macular degeneration,* New York, 1979, National Society to Prevent Blindness.

56. Mandell R: *Contact lens practice: hard and flexible lenses,* ed 2, Springfield, Ill, 1976, Charles C Thomas, Publisher.

57. March WF: *Practical ophthalmic problems,* St Louis, 1984, Warren H Green Inc.

58. Mellor CM: *Aids for the 80s: what they are and what they do,* New York, 1981, American Foundation for the Blind.

59. Osguthorpe NC: If your patient has contact lenses, *Am J Nurs* 84(10):1255, 1984.

60. Schremp PS: Discharge instructions: providing continuity of care for ophthalmic patients, *J Ophthal Nurs Technol* 4(2):30, 1985.

61. Sheridan E, Patterson HR, Gustafson EA: *Falconer's the drug, the nurse, the patient,* Philadelphia, 1982, WB Saunders Co.

62. Smith JF: The patient having cataract surgery: nursing history and examination, *J Ophthal Nurs Technol* 3(3):124, 1984.

63. Tarrington D: Satisfying hours of care for eye patients, *Nurs Management* 17(9):16, 1986.

64. *Tips for soft contact lens wear and care,* San Jose, 1986, Cooper Vision.

65. Tumulty G, Resler MM: Managing glaucoma using argon laser therapy, *J Ophthal Nurs Technol* 4(1):9, 1985.

66. Urdang L, editor: *Mosby's medical and nursing dictionary,* St Louis, 1983, Mosby–Year Book, Inc.

67. Van Son AR: Managing diabetes at home with blindness or impaired vision. In *Diabetes, vision impairment and blindness,* New York, 1985, American Foundation for the Blind.

68. Vaughan D, Asbury T: *General ophthalmology,* ed 7, Los Altos, Calif, 1974, Lange Medical Books.

CHAPTER FIFTY-FOUR

Nursing Assessment of the Ear

LEARNING OBJECTIVES

1 Know the anatomic structure and general functions of the ear.
2 Understand the process by which the ears sense sound and changes in body position.
3 Obtain relevant subjective information from the patient who has an ear alteration.
4 Using correct technique, examine the patient to obtain appropriate objective information about ear alterations.
5 Differentiate abnormal from normal subjective and objective findings related to the ear.
6 Describe tests related to the diagnoses of otologic disorders.
7 Describe patient care for procedures by which ear disorders are diagnosed.

KEY TERMS

audiometry, p. 1476
caloric test, p. 1477
cochlea, p. 1469
dynamic equilibrium, p. 1470
electronystagmography, p. 1478
eustachian tube, p. 1468
external ear, p. 1467
inner ear, p. 1468
middle ear, p. 1468
past-point test, p. 1477

presbycusis, p. 1467
Rinne's test, p. 1472
Romberg's test, p. 1477
spondee threshold test, p. 1477
static equilibrium, p. 1470
tinnitus, p. 1471
tympanocentesis, p. 1478
vertigo, p. 1471
vestibular apparatus, p. 1470
Weber's test, p. 1472

THE EARS are complex sense organs. They have receptors sensitive to sound and to changes in body position.

During assessment the ears are examined to determine whether they are intact and functional. Because internal ear inflammation is usually related to upper respiratory infection or allergies, the ear assessment includes an examination of the nose, mouth, throat, and local lymphatic system.

Ear alterations occur at all stages of life. Deformities of the ears may be congenital or the result of trauma. Young children commonly have infections of the middle ear (otitis media). Adults may have alterations related to chronic exposure to high noise levels, sensorineural hearing deficits **(presbycusis)**, or conductive hearing deficits.

ANATOMY AND PHYSIOLOGY
Structure and Functions of External and Middle Ear

The ear is divided by its anatomy into three discrete regions: the **external ear,** which is separated from the middle ear by the tympanic membrane; the

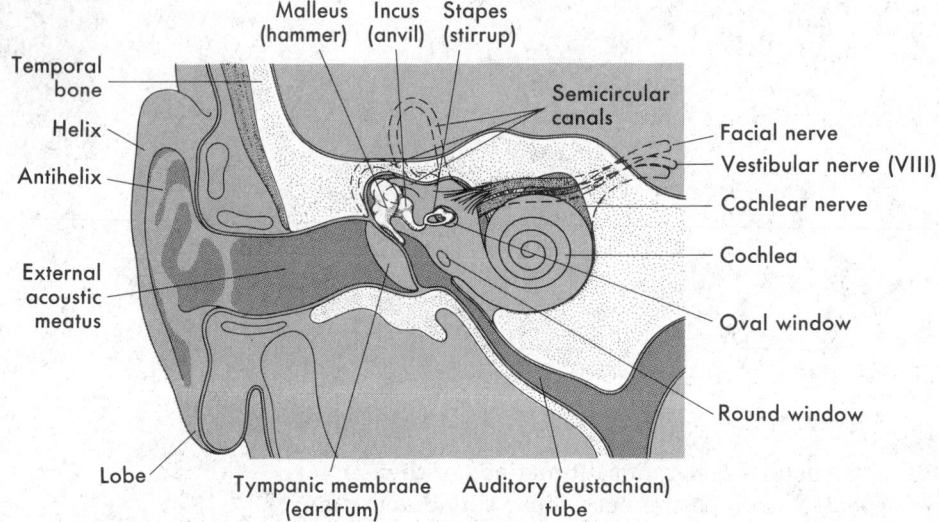

FIGURE 54-1 Components of the ear.

middle ear, which is separated from the inner ear by the oval and round windows; and the **inner ear,** which contains the sensory receptors for sound and equilibrium (Figure 54-1). The external and middle portions of the ear conduct sound waves to the inner ear. The inner ear conducts sound waves to receptors in the cochlea and transduces the mechanical energy of the sound waves and that created by changes in body position to nerve impulses.

The external ear is made up of the auricle, or pinna (Figure 54-2), and the external auditory meatus. The pinna directs sound waves into the auditory meatus (external acoustic meatus), which conducts them through the temporal bone of the skull to the tympanic membrane. To allow the pinna to direct the maximum amount of sound into the external auditory meatus, the tube angles forward and down.

The middle ear is a tiny air-filled cavity containing three small bones (ossicles) called the malleus (hammer), incus (anvil), and stapes (stirrup). The bones are connected by joints and are supported by muscles to form a bridge across the middle ear from the relatively large tympanic membrane to the smaller oval window of the inner ear. The difference in size of the tympanic membrane and the oval window allows the ossicles to magnify small sounds, and thus they make the ear very sensitive. Reflex control of the tension in the muscles of the ossicles reduces this sensitivity for very loud sounds and thus protects the inner ear from mechanical damage.

The **eustachian tube** connects the inner ear with the nasopharynx. When the tube is opened during swallowing, air pressure in the middle ear is equalized with atmospheric pressure and hence with the pressure in the external ear. This is important because when the air pressure in the middle ear is significantly higher or lower than that in the external ear the vibrations of the tympanic membrane are distorted. Unfortunately, the eustachian tube provides a route for nasal and throat infections to spread up into the middle ear or even farther into the mastoid sinuses or the meninges.

Structure and Functions of Inner Ear

The inner ear is composed of a fluid-filled, membranous labyrinth in a similarly shaped, fluid-filled, bony labyrinth. The membranous labyrinth consists of the cochlea and the vestibular apparatus (Figure 54-3). The receptors of the inner ear contain a hairlike structure, and movement of the hair generates a nerve impulse. The tips of the hairs of the organ of Corti are embedded in the tectorial membrane; those of the vestibular apparatus are embedded in

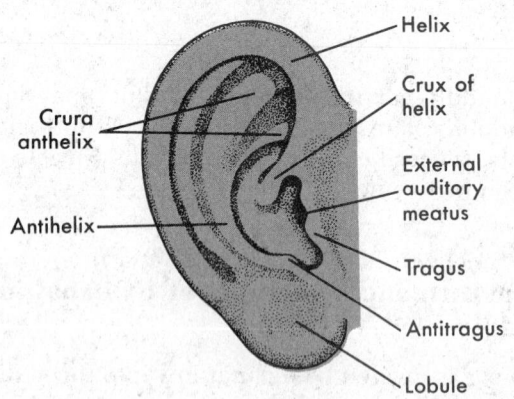

FIGURE 54-2 Structures of the external ear.

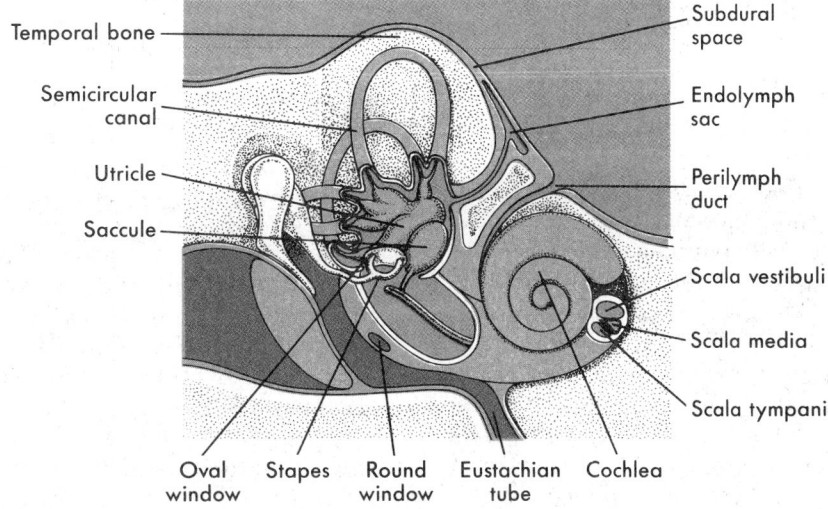

Temporal bone

Semicircular canal

Utricle

Saccule

Subdural space

Endolymph sac

Perilymph duct

Scala vestibuli

Scala media

Scala tympani

Oval window   Stapes   Round window   Eustachian tube   Cochlea

FIGURE 54-3   Bony labyrinth of the inner ear.

a macula or a crista ampullaris. Nerve impulses from the auditory and equilibrium receptors travel from the inner ear to the brain in the acoustic and vestibular branches of cranial nerve VIII.

Cochlea

The bony labyrinth of the **cochlea** consists of a spiral tube that was thought to resemble the interior of a snail's shell. A membranous duct (scala media or cochlear duct) with a triangular cross section lies within the cochlea and opens into the saccule portion of the vestibular apparatus. One side of the cochlear duct is made up of the basilar membrane, the organ of Corti, which contains the receptors for sound, and the tectorial membrane, which is connected to the hairs of the sound receptors. The second side lies against the wall of the bony labyrinth, and the third side is made of Reissner's membrane (Figure 54-4).

Sound is transmitted through air, liquids, and gases by the vibrations of the particles of the substance through which it travels. It cannot travel through a vacuum because there are no particles to bang together and thus propagate the sound from its source. Sound vibrations are often called sound waves, but they should not be confused with electromagnetic waves that transmit, for example, heat, light, radio waves, and x-rays. The pitch of a sound depends on the frequency of the vibrations. Very high-pitched sounds have a high frequency and low-pitched sounds a low frequency. To be audible by the human ear, a sound must be 20 to 20,000 cycles per second (cps). However, the range that can be heard depends on loudness and the efficiency of the

ears of the individual being tested: at low sound intensities, the audible range may be only 500 to 5000 cps, and older individuals' ears are usually far less efficient. Loudness depends on the amplitude (distance the particle moves for each vibration) rather than the frequency, and the quality of the sound (i.e., the squeaking of chalk on a blackboard sounds dif-

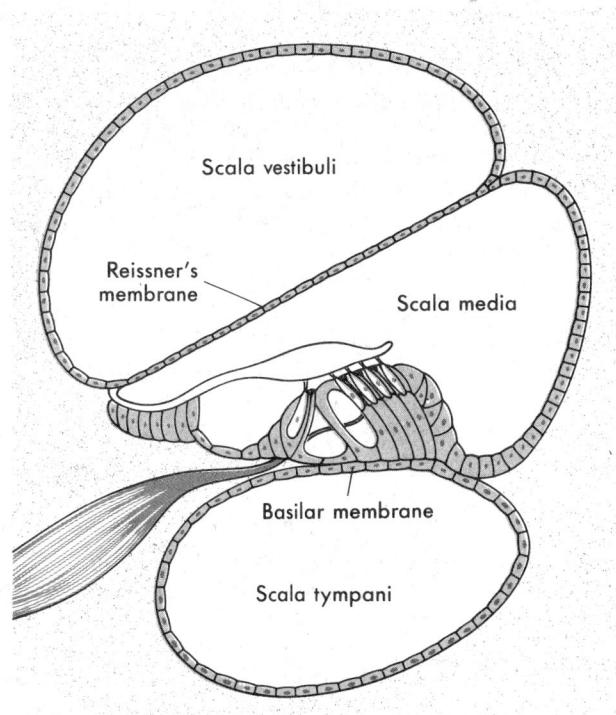

Scala vestibuli

Reissner's membrane

Scala media

Basilar membrane

Scala tympani

FIGURE 54-4   Scala media of cochlea.

ferent from the same pitch played by a violin) depends on overtones that modify the basic form of the vibration. Frequency, amplitude, and the overtones are all faithfully reproduced by the tympanic membrane and transferred to the oval window of the inner ear.

The vibrations are then transferred to the perilymph circulating outside the cochlear duct in the scala vestibuli and the scala tympani. This vibration passes up the scala vestibuli, across the cochlear duct and the organ of Corti, to the scala tympani, and then to the round window. The highest-frequency sound waves, which are also the highest in pitch, cause an area of the tectorial membrane close to the vestibule to vibrate. Lower-frequency sound waves travel proportionately farther up the cochlea and cause other areas of the tectorial membrane to vibrate.

Nerve impulses are generated by sound receptors attached to the vibrating portion of the tectorial membrane, and pitch perception depends on the position of the region of the cochlea that generated the impulses. Loud sounds cause larger deflections of the tectorial membrane and involve more receptors. Very loud sounds may exceed the protective mechanisms of the ear, and the vibrations created in the tectorial membrane may be so great that they permanently damage the hairs of the receptor cells. This is particularly significant for individuals exposed to excessive noise levels at work or who listen to excessively loud music. These individuals may become deaf at an early age.

Deafness may be caused by deficiencies in the external and middle ear structures (conduction deafness). Often this is the result of repeated ear infections or advanced age. Deafness may also be caused by prescribed medications, such as streptomycin, kanamycin, and chloramphenicol.

The sensitivity of the ears is rapidly adjusted by reflexes to be inversely proportional to the level of background noise: the ears are very sensitive during low levels of background noise and less sensitive during high levels. Sensitivity is also decreased during vocalization or coughing. In addition to this type of sensitivity change, the brain can inhibit parts of the cochlea to allow it to decrease the sensitivity of the areas transducing background noises. This helps the individual pick up new sounds in the environment.

The source of sounds can be located because the brain compares and evaluates the slight differences in the sound patterns detected by the two ears. This is made more accurate by turning the head from side to side to determine the direction from which the sound is heard equally well by both ears. In this position the individual is facing the source of the sound.

Vestibular apparatus

The **vestibular apparatus** is made of the membranous saccule, utricle, and semicircular canals, which are surrounded by perilymph and temporal bone (see Figure 54-3). It contains specialized structures designed to detect changes in the body's equilibrium when static (macula) and when moving (crista ampullaris).

The *macula* is a sensory organ on the inside surface of the saccule and the utricle. It consists of receptor cells with hairs similar to those of the organ of Corti. However, the hairs are embedded in a gelatinous layer impregnated with crystals of calcium carbonate. When the position of the head changes with respect to the vertical, each macula is pulled down by gravity and the pattern of nerve impulse generation by the hair receptors changes. The brain determines the position of the head from these impulse patterns (i.e., the head is prone, supine, upright). Other stimuli that make us consciously aware of the position of our head are (1) seeing the angle of the horizon, floor, ceiling, and walls, for example, and (2) feeling pressure on the skin and muscles; we are not usually aware of the usefulness of the maculae. However, they are responsible for reflex adjustments when unexpected changes in the body's static equilibrium occur.

A structure called the *crista ampullaris* lies in the swollen end of each of the semicircular canals. It consists of tufts of receptor cells that have their hairs embedded in a gelatinous mass. The mass is dome shaped and is pushed by movement of the endolymph in the semicircular canals rather than pulled in different directions by gravity. When the body begins to move or change direction, endolymph drags at the crista in the semicircular canals with the greatest fluid displacement, and the brain interprets this as acceleration in the particular direction indicated by the pattern of stimulation received from the three pairs of semicircular canals. Once the endolymph catches up with the body's movement, the cristae are not dragged or pushed and the vestibule sends no particular pattern of nerve impulses. Therefore the brain does not perceive that movement is occurring. (One has little sense of the movement of a plane through the atmosphere unless there is turbulence.) When the body stops moving, the endolymph does not stop. Instead, it pushes the cristae in the direction opposite the initial movement, and this is interpreted by the brain as slowing down.

The **static** and **dynamic equilibrium** receptors in the utricle, saccule, and semicircular canals initiate a number of reflex adjustments to the skeletal muscles, for example:

1. The extrinsic eye muscles produce a rapid eye

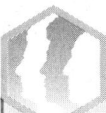

GERIATRIC CONSIDERATIONS

Physiologic Changes in the Ear

Although deafness is considered abnormal, many individuals experience a reduction in their ability to hear after middle age. The older individuals are, the more likely they are to have been exposed to excessively loud sounds or chronic periods of damaging noise, and it is normal for the range of frequencies that can be heard to decline with age. Very loud sounds, which cause excessive vibrations in the organ of Corti, or marginally loud sounds experienced for long periods of time destroy some of the hair cell receptors responsible for transducing the sound waves into nerve impulses. Over a lifetime these destructive effects of environmental noise accumulate and produce progressive, bilateral sensorineural hearing loss (presbycusis). This loss can be partially corrected with a hearing aid but, unfortunately, not as effectively a lenses can correct presbyopia.

Also, during the lifetime, the stapes bone can become encrusted with calcium deposits and adhere to the temporal bone. This reduces its ability to vibrate in response to the vibrations of the tympanic membrane. This type of deafness can be corrected by removing the affected stapes bone and replacing it.

POTENTIAL SYMPTOMS RELATED TO EAR DISORDERS

Decrease in or loss of hearing ability
Discharge (otorrhea)
Ear pain (otalgia)
Ringing, buzzing, or roaring in the ears **(tinnitus)**
Vertigo (illusion of movement, with imagined rotation of one's self [subjective vertigo] or of one's surroundings [objective vertigo]

movement in the direction of the acceleration and a panning movement that allows the eyes to lock onto an object moving past. This reflex activity is called *nystagmus*, and it allows the individual to see objects clearly as they go by.

2. The contraction of skeletal muscles is modified to maintain balance and to alter voluntary movements by the exact amount required to carry out the planned activity during the acceleration.

ASSESSMENT
Subjective

A focused health history for a patient with a suspected or previously diagnosed ear disorder requires the nurse to use knowledge of pathophysiology to guide questioning in an appropriate and complete manner. Patients may have specific complaints such as ear pain (otalgia), or they may simply be at risk because of environmental exposure to loud or continuous noises or use of ototoxic medications.

Complaints related to the ear are relatively few in number. The box above, right identifies specific symptoms to review with the patient. All positive findings (symptoms the patient complains of) should

be delineated through exploration of various dimensions. These dimensions include onset, duration, frequency, alleviating factors, aggravating factors, precipitating events, location, quality, quantity, associated symptoms, and chronology of events. To record "no problems" does not communicate which symptoms the patient denied. In addition to specific symptoms, inquire regarding use of prosthetic devices, exposure to ototoxic medications, noise exposure and use of protective hearing devices, swimming, previous ear disease or surgery, and care habits.

Other appropriate history to explore includes major adult illnesses, hospitalizations, surgeries, injuries or accidents, immunizations, current medications, allergies, and habits. As mentioned above, some medications are ototoxic (e.g., have a deleterious effect on the eighth cranial nerve).

Family history related to ear disorders includes hearing problems or hearing loss and Meniere's disease. A positive finding should include the disorder as well as the individual's relationship to the patient (e.g., hearing loss, father; Meniere's disease, maternal grandmother).

Objective

Ears

Examination of the ear includes inspection, palpation, testing of auditory function (cranial nerve VIII [acoustic nerve]), and otoscopic examination. In general, begin the assessment with noninvasive testing and observation and finish the assessment with more invasive examination (see the box on p. 1472). First, inspect the auricle, noting alignment, symmetry, any obvious abnormalities, or surgical scars. Inspect the external auditory canal, noting discharge, erythema, cerumen (ear wax), or edema. If discharge is present, note color and odor. Next, palpate the auricles, noting tophi, lesions, or masses. Palpate

ASSESSMENT OF THE EAR

Inspection
Auricle
   Alignment
   Abnormalities
   Symmetry
   Surgical scars
External auditory canal
   Discharge (color, odor, clarity)

Palpation
Auricle (tophi, lesions, masses, or tenderness)
Mastoid process (tenderness, erythema, or edema)

Auditory function
Whisper test
Audioscope
Tuning fork tests
   Weber's
   Rinne's

Otoscopic examination
External auditory canal
   Cerumen
   Discharge
   Erythema
   Edema
   Foreign body
   Lesions
Tympanic membrane
   Landmarks
   Color
   Contour (bulging, retracted)

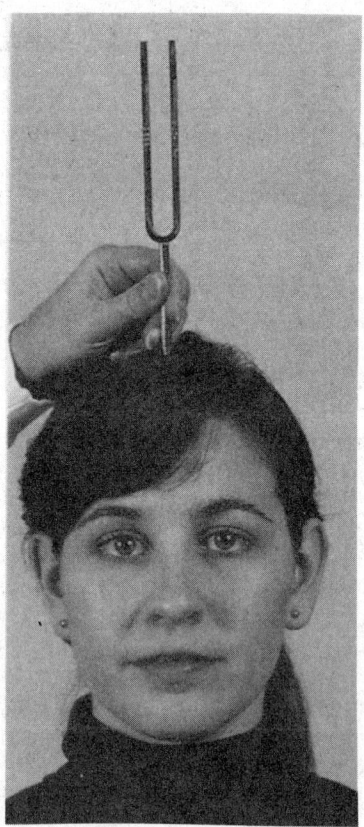

FIGURE 54-5   Weber's test. (From Seidel HM et al: *Mosby's guide to physical examination,* ed 2, St Louis, 1991, Mosby–Year Book, Inc.)

the mastoid process, noting tenderness. Tophi are deposits of sodium urate that may occur in the auricles in gout. Swelling or tenderness over the mastoid process may indicate mastoiditis. Tenderness on palpation of the pinna or tragus is associated with external otitis. Auditory function can be grossly evaluated using the whisper test. Standing behind the patient, occlude one of the patient's ears by pressing in on the tragus. Whisper into the patient's contralateral ear. Have the patient repeat the words whispered. Repeat the procedure with the other ear. Another option is to note that the patient responds appropriately to normal conversational tones.

An audioscope is a hand-held, pocket-sized, screening instrument that can also be used to evaluate hearing acuity. This instrument presents tones at 500, 1000, 2000, and 4000 Hz for 15 seconds each. It is similar in size and shape to an otoscope and must be introduced into the external auditory canal in the same manner as the otoscope.

Another approach in testing cranial nerve VIII (acoustic nerve) involves use of a 512 Hertz (Hz) or cycles per second (cps) tuning fork. Two tuning fork tests should be done: Weber's test and Rinne's test. To perform **Weber's test,** stand in front of the patient and place a vibrating 512 Hz or cps tuning fork in the center of the patient's head or forehead. Ask the patient to tell you if he or she hears the tuning fork. After a positive answer, ask if it is heard better in the left ear, the right ear, or the same in both ears. It is important to provide three choices because patients want to give the "correct" answer. Three choices allows any answer to be "correct" (Figure 54-5). **Rinne's test** is performed by placing a vibrating 512 Hz or cps tuning fork on the mastoid process of one ear. Ask the patient to indicate if he or she hears the tuning fork. After obtaining a positive answer, ask the patient to indicate immediately when he or she stops hearing the tuning fork. Immediately on the patient's indication that he or she no longer hears the tuning fork, move the vibrating tuning fork in front of the external auditory meatus

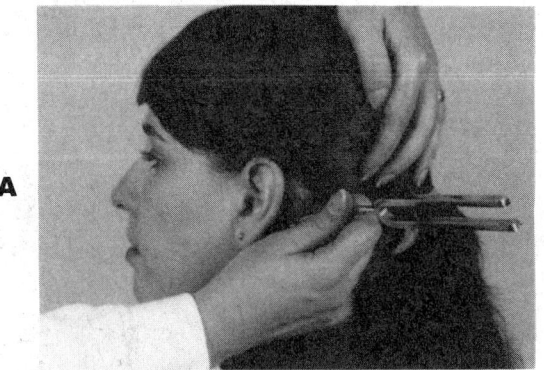
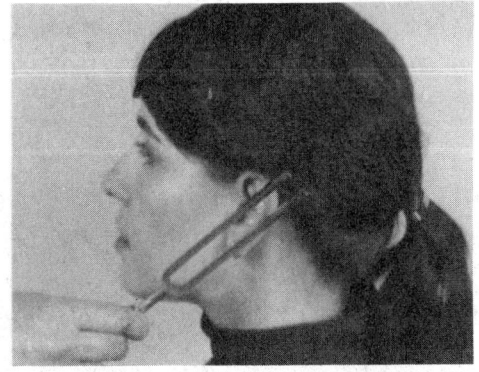

FIGURE 54-6   Rinne's test. (From Seidel HM et al: *Mosby's guide to physical examination*, ed 2, St Louis, 1991, Mosby–Year Book, Inc.)

TABLE 54-1   Interpretation of Tuning Fork Tests

Test	Expected findings	Conductive hearing loss	Sensorineural hearing loss
Weber's	No lateralization but will lateralize to ear occluded by patient	Lateralization to deaf ear unless sensorineural loss	Lateralization to better ear unless conductive loss
Rinne's	Air conduction heard longer than bone conduction by 2:1 ratio *(Rinne's positive)*	Bone conduction heard longer than air conduction in affected ear *(Rinne's negative)*	Air conduction heard longer than bone conduction in affected ear but less than 2:1 ratio

on the same side. Ask the patient if he or she can still hear the tuning fork. Ordinarily, air conduction (AC) is two times greater than bone conduction (BC). If the patient can still hear the tuning fork, the result is recorded as AC > BC (air conduction is greater than bone conduction). Air conduction vs. bone conduction does not need to be specifically timed. Repeat the procedure on the contralateral side (Figure 54-6). Table 54-1 summarizes interpretation of tuning fork tests.

The otoscopic examination is not frequently performed by the bedside nurse. This skill requires practice and therefore develops over time. Thus it is most often used by the advanced practitioner. Select the correct size speculum. The speculum should not be so large as to cause discomfort but should be large enough to allow for adequate light and visualization as well as form a tight seal for the pneumatic examination if desired.

To examine the patient's right ear, hold the otoscope in your right hand. Using your left hand, gently but firmly grasp the auricle, pulling upward and back to straighten the canal (Figure 54-7). Tilt the patient's head toward the opposing shoulder. Gently insert the speculum into the external auditory canal, being careful to note cerumen, discharge, foreign body, erythema, edema, or lesions from the meatus to the tympanic membrane. If discharge or cerumen is present, describe the color, texture, and amount. If you are unable to visualize the tympanic membrane because of the presence of cerumen and the patient is complaining of otalgia, you may need to remove the cerumen with a curette or irrigation (if the tympanic membrane is intact). Next, inspect the tympanic membrane. The healthy tympanic membrane should appear as a pearly gray translucent membrane. Note the presence or absence of landmarks: cone of light (or light reflex), umbo, long handle of the malleus, and short process of the malleus (Figure 54-8). These landmarks are created by the shadows of the middle ear bones reflecting through the tympanic membrane and the convex contour of the tympanic membrane. Also describe color, integrity, and any bulging or retraction. Bulg-

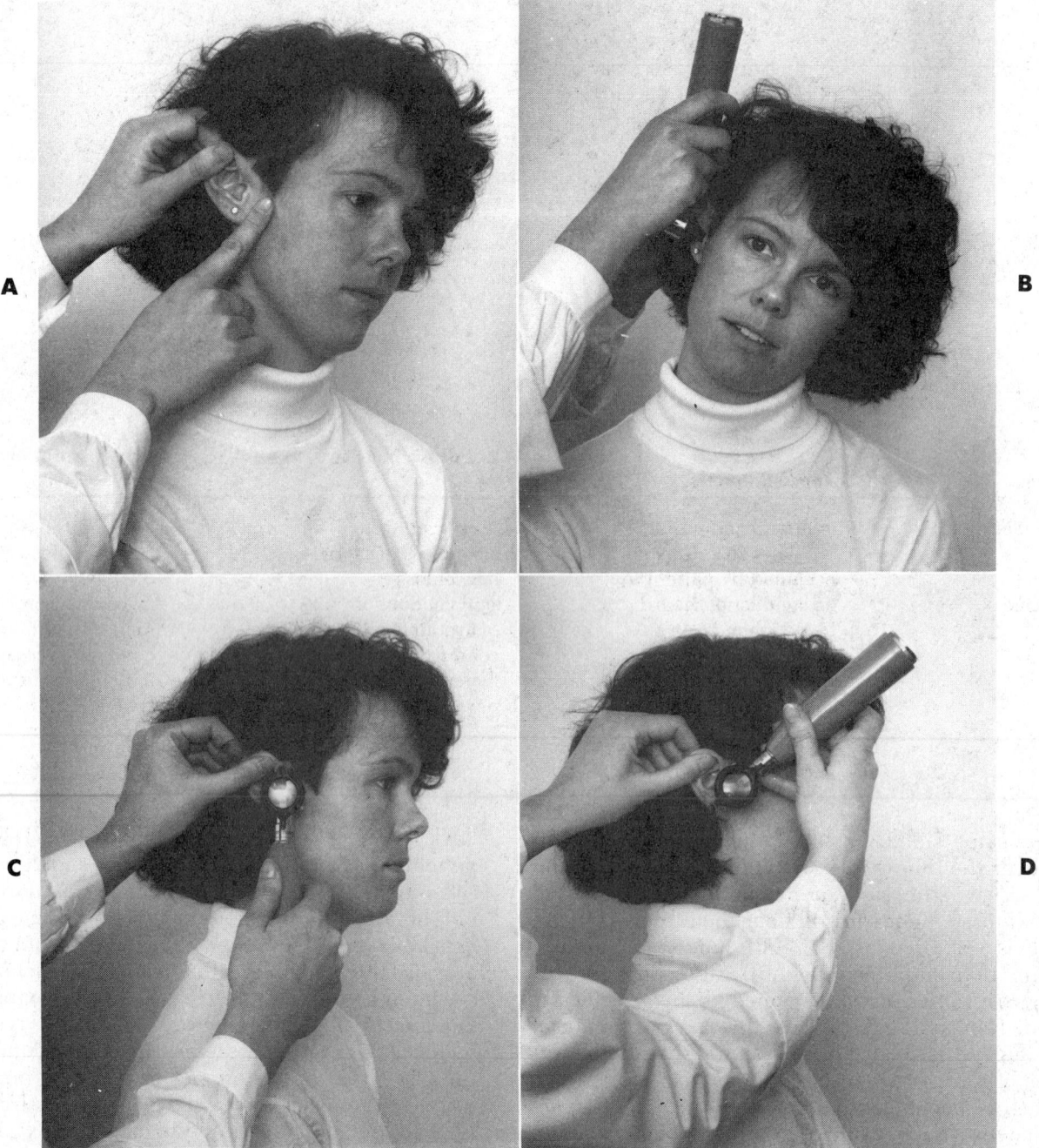

FIGURE 54-7   Otoscopic examination of ear. **A,** Inspection of the meatus. **B,** Patient's head tipped toward opposite shoulder. **C** and **D,** Two ways of holding otoscope. (From Malasanos L et al: *Health assessment,* ed 4, St Louis, 1990, Mosby–Year Book, Inc.)

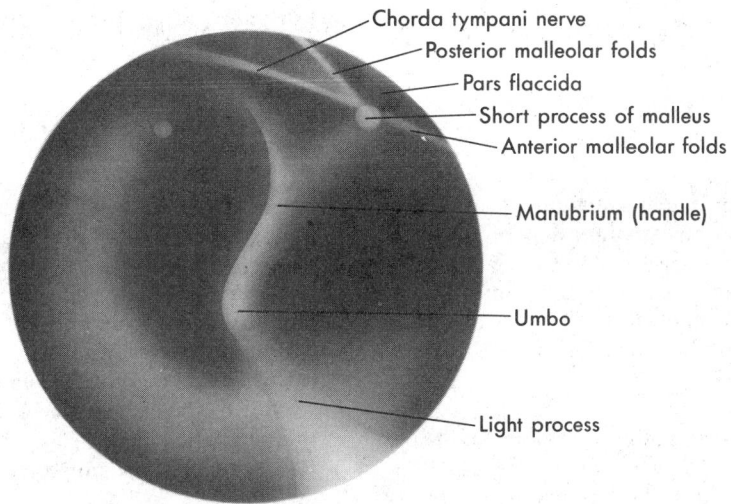

- Chorda tympani nerve
- Posterior malleolar folds
- Pars flaccida
- Short process of malleus
- Anterior malleolar folds
- Manubrium (handle)
- Umbo
- Light process

FIGURE 54-8   Structural landmarks of tympanic membrane.

ing and erythema are associated with otitis media, a middle ear infection.

If there is a question of serous otitis or fluid behind the tympanic membrane in the middle ear cavity, the pneumatic examination is performed. This examination evaluates movement of the tympanic membrane, which is decreased or absent with the presence of fluid in the middle ear. Alternating positive and negative pressure is gently applied into the external auditory canal using either the squeeze bulb or mouthpiece. Observe the movement of the tympanic membrane in and out, indicated by the change in the appearance of the cone of light. Compare movement of the tympanic membranes in both ears. The pneumatic examination is to be used only when a diagnosis cannot be made by otoscopic visualization alone. This examination should not be used in a patient with an acutely inflamed tympanic membrane, because it would be very painful.

Mouth, throat, and temporomandibular joint

In the patient with an ear complaint, examine the oropharynx and temporomandibular joint (TMJ) (Figure 54-9). Inspect the lips, noting symmetry, color, moisture, edema, and surface characteristics. Palpate the TMJ, noting mobility, tenderness, and any crepitation. Inspect the oral/buccal mucosa, tongue, and gingivae. Examine the posterior pharynx, noting color, exudate, and presence or absence of tonsils. If tonsils are present, describe size, color, and any exudate. See Chapter 63 for a more complete description of the examination of the mouth and throat.

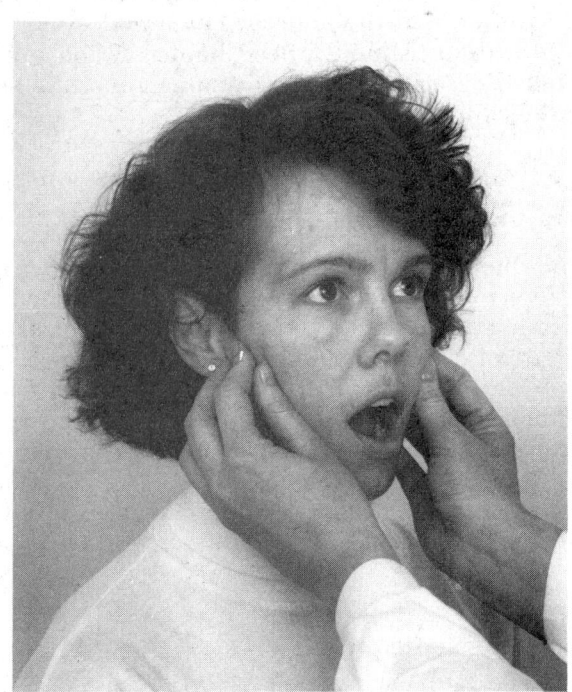

FIGURE 54-9   Palpation of temporomandibular joint. (From Malasanos L et al: *Health assessment,* ed 4, St Louis, 1990, Mosby–Year Book, Inc.)

GERIATRIC CONSIDERATIONS

Ear Assessment

General approach

Allow more time than for a younger adult

Articulate clearly; the geriatric patient may be hearing impaired

Impaired sight, comprehension, or mobility may result in less than optimum cooperation

Provide clear, concise instructions

History collection

May need to use fewer open-ended questions and provide some choices, (e.g., "does your ear hurt the same all of the time, or does it hurt more when you swallow?")

May need to repeat questions

Be alert for answers that do not appear appropriate; the patient may not have understood the question correctly because of impaired hearing or impaired comprehension

Physical assessment

The physical examination itself is not different, but the approach needs to be altered such that the appropriate information is assessed without undue discomfort or embarrassment for the patient

Maintain an environment with minimal noise, distractions, and interruptions

Presbycusis is a common bilaterally symmetric sensorineural loss caused by aging of the inner ear

Conductive hearing loss may be caused by foreign bodies, cerumen, otitis media or externa, or rheumatoid arthritis

Sensorineural and conductive hearing loss may frequently be present simultaneously

If the patient wears a hearing aid, it should be removed and examined

Check the battery by turning up the volume; if the battery is dead, a whistle (feedback) will not be heard

---

Neck and nodes

Palpate the following nodes: preauricular, postauricular, submental, submaxillary, tonsillar, anterior chain, posterior chain, and suboccipital. The preauricular and postauricular nodes may enlarge in otitis externa, and the anterior chain nodes may enlarge with otitis media. See Chapter 37 for a more detailed description of the examination of the head and neck lymph nodes.

DIAGNOSTIC AND LABORATORY TESTS
Audiometric Testing

Audiometry is useful both as a screening tool and in determining the type and degree of hearing loss. The audiometer produces a stimulus that consists of a musical or pure tone. Audiometric testing should be performed in a quiet room that is free of external noises. The patient should be positioned so that the audiometer cannot be seen and instructed to signal when a sound is first heard, even if it is faint and distant. During testing, the patient is exposed to sounds of varying frequency or pitch (hertz [Hz]) and intensity (decibel [dB]).

Screening audiometry

Screening audiometry is a fast, simple test that assists in identifying patients who should be referred for further diagnostic testing. During the test, the patient is presented with frequencies between 125 and 8000 hertz (Hz) to obtain air conduction thresholds and between 250 and 4000 Hz for bone conduction.

During pure tone audiometry, the sound stimulus is presented in varying frequencies and intensities until the thresholds for the various intensities are established. Once earphones are securely placed, testing is begun in the better ear. If no difference between the ears exists, the right ear is tested first. Air conduction testing is begun at 1000 Hz by decreasing intensity in 10 dB decrements until the patient no longer responds. The tone is then increased by 10 dB increments and decreased by 5 dB decrements until the patient responds twice at one level of tone. This is the threshold level, or the lowest decibel level at which hearing occurs. After testing the better or the right ear, the opposite ear is tested.

During bone conduction testing, the earphones are removed and a vibrator is placed on the mastoid process of the right ear. Ascending and descending frequencies are used, as in air conduction testing.

Impedance audiometry

Impedance audiometry is useful in detecting middle ear disorders. With the use of an impedance audiometer, the resistance to the flow of sound is evaluated. At one end of the impedance audiometer is a probe, which is inserted into the external ear canal. This probe has three small tubes. One tube delivers a low tone of varying intensity, one a microphone, and one an air pump. A normal tympanic membrane will yield a low-voltage curve. This test should be performed cautiously in patients with recent middle ear surgery, head trauma, or labyrinthine fistula, and patients should have an otoscopic examination before the test to determine if obstruction is present in the canal.

Tympanometry

Tympanometry makes use of the impedance audiometer to measure the compliance of the tympanic membrane with variations in air pressure in the external canal. It is useful in determining the amount of negative pressure within the middle ear. The normal middle air pressure is $\pm$ 100 daPa, and the shape of the normal tympanogram is smooth. The patient is informed that the test may cause transient vertigo and is told to report nausea or dizziness during the test.

Spondee Threshold Test

The **spondee threshold test** (speech reception threshold, spondaic word threshold) measures the patient's ability to detect and correctly repeat 50% of a set of spondee or two-syllable words presented through earphones. The test is useful in confirming the results of pure tone audiometry and in measuring the degree of hearing loss for speech. The patient is informed that the test measures ability to hear conversational speech and takes about 20 minutes. The nurse explains that the audiologist will present one word at a time in progressively softer volumes and that each word should be repeated as it is heard. One ear is tested at a time.

Word Recognition Tests

Word recognition tests are useful in evaluating the ability to distinguish speech sounds at above-normal levels and in locating auditory tract and central nervous system lesions. The patient is presented with a series of monosyllabic words in a quiet environment. A patient with high-frequency loss will have difficulty hearing consonants in words and will complain of difficulty understanding speech even though it is heard. The patient is informed that the test measures the ability to hear and to understand speech and will assist in determining if a hearing aid would be beneficial. If the patient already wears a hearing aid, the nurse ensures that it is removed before the test. The patient will be in a soundproof booth and will wear earphones. Words will be presented one at a time. The patient is told to repeat each word as it is heard and to guess if unsure.

Romberg's Test

Romberg's test (falling test) is a simple test that is useful in assessing vestibular function in a patient who complains of disequilibrium, dizziness, or nystagmus. The patient is asked to stand with feet together and eyes closed. Normally, minimal swaying can be expected. The examiner should be prepared to support the patient if a fall appears likely.

Past-Point Test

The **past-point test** is another simple test of vestibular function. The patient stands with eyes closed and arms extended while the examiner touches the patient's index fingers. The patient raises the arms over the head and then lowers them to make contact with the examiner's fingers. Normally, the patient should be able to do this.

Caloric Test

The **caloric test** is useful in testing the function of the eighth cranial nerve. The endolymph of the semicircular canals is stimulated by cold (30° C or 86° F) water or warm (44.5° C or 112° F) water that is instilled into the ear. Stimulation with cold water will normally produce rotary nystagmus away from the side of the ear being irrigated. When warm water is instilled, there is rotary nystagmus toward the side of the irrigated ear. If disease of the labyrinth is present, no nystagmus is elicited. The test is contraindicated if the patient has a perforated tympanic membrane (air may be used as a substitute) or if the patient has an acute disease of the labyrinth. An otoscopic examination should be performed before the test to rule out perforation and to determine if the ear canals are full of cerumen, which must be removed before the test.

Patient preparation

The patient is told that the test evaluates the mechanisms that control balance and coordination and that it takes 60 to 90 minutes. The nurse instructs the patient to avoid stimulants, sedatives, tranquilizers, alcohol, and antivertigo drugs 24 to 48 hours before the test and to avoid tobacco, as well as beverages containing caffeine, on the day of the test. A heavy meal should be avoided immediately before the test, since caloric testing may cause nausea. The patient is informed that various positionings of the head and neck may be required.

Procedure

The examiner instructs the patient to report any unusual feeling or discomfort during the test. A towel and an emesis basin are placed beneath the ear during irrigation. The patient is told when irrigation is about to begin so that the sudden stimulation is not startling. Responses to irrigation are timed and recorded.

Electronystagmography Test

Caloric **electronystagmography** (ENG) is a more sophisticated version of the caloric test and is used to assess vestibular function. Electrodes are placed near the patient's eyes, and recordings are made of specific eye movements during irrigation. If horizontal nystagmus is being assessed, an electrode is placed near the outer canthus of each eye. If vertical nystagmus is being evaluated, two electrodes are placed above and below the center of each eye. A ground electrode is placed in midforehead. The skin to which the electrodes is applied is cleansed with alcohol and air dried. Otherwise, preparation is the same as for the caloric test.

X-Ray Examination

Roentgenograms are useful in visualizing the temporal and mastoid bones, the middle and inner ears, and the eustachian tube. The patient is told to remove hairpins and jewelry from the area of visualization.

Culture

Culture of material from the ear is important in the diagnosis and treatment of a variety of localized lesions and abscesses. Diseases of the external ear are commonly associated with skin disorders. Discharges from the external ear are collected using a sterile cotton-tipped or polyester-tipped swab. Sterile swabs should be inserted immediately into transport media and taken to the laboratory.

Tympanocentesis

Tympanocentesis involves the aspiration of middle ear fluid and is commonly done during a myringotomy. Tympanocentesis is indicated if the patient has a history of chronic otitis media with effusions, or complicated otitis media, when it is particularly critical to identify causative organisms. If no fluid is aspirated from the middle ear, the needle used in the aspiration is flushed with 2 to 3 mL of blood culture medium, which is then gram stained and cultured. Discomfort that is caused by fluid pressure in the middle ear will be alleviated by this procedure.

Patient preparation

The patient is informed that the procedure will help determine the cause of middle ear infections. The nurse tells the patient that the head must be kept still during the procedure and that a local anesthetic will be instilled to anesthetize the otic canal. The otic canal is cleansed with cotton swabs and alcohol or benzalkonium chloride before aspiration.

Postprocedure care

Specimens from the ear canal are taken directly to the laboratory. The nurse observes the patient for drainage from the affected ear for 2 to 3 days after the procedure.

CRITICAL THINKING QUESTIONS

1 Describe the roles that the external ear, middle ear, and inner ear play in hearing sounds of different frequencies.
2 Design at least three questions to ask patients about health care habits in relation to the ears.
3 Describe an effective approach to examining a painful ear.
4 Discuss psychologic factors to consider when a patient has an ear deformity.
5 Discuss the nursing implications in examining a patient's ear with the otoscope.
6 Describe how Rinne's and Weber's tests are performed.

BIBLIOGRAPHY

Current

1. Burrell LO: *Adult nursing in hospital and community settings,* Norwalk, Conn, 1992, Appleton & Lange.
2. DeGowin RL: *DeGowin and DeGowin's bedside diagnostic examination,* ed 5, New York, 1987, Macmillan Publishing Co.
3. Gallo JJ et al: *Handbook of geriatric assessment,* Rockville, Md, 1988, Aspen Publishers.
4. Hickey J: *Neurological and neurosurgical nursing,* Philadelphia, 1992, JB Lippincott Co.
5. Kane RL et al: *Essentials of clinical geriatrics,* ed 2, New York, 1989, McGraw-Hill Book Co.
6. Kenny RA: *Physiology of aging: a synopsis,* Chicago, 1992, Yearbook Medical Publishers, Inc.
7. Malasanos L et al: *Health assessment,* ed 4, St Louis, 1990, Mosby–Year Book, Inc.
8. *Nurse's ready reference: diagnostic tests,* Springhouse, Pa, 1991, Springhouse Corporation.
9. Pagana KD, Pagana TJ: *Diagnostic testing and nursing implications,* St Louis, 1990, Mosby–Year Book, Inc.
10. Seidel HM et al: *Mosby's guide to physical examination,* ed 2, St Louis, 1991, Mosby–Year Book, Inc.
11. Swartz MH: *Textbook of physical diagnosis,* Philadelphia, 1989, WB Saunders Co.
12. Thompson JM et al: *Mosby's manual of clinical nursing,* ed 2, St Louis, 1989, Mosby–Year Book, Inc.

Classic

13. Bowers A, Thompson J: *Clinical manual of health assessment,* St Louis, 1984, Mosby–Year Book, Inc.
14. Harkness CK: Clearing the occluded auditory canal, *Pediatr Nurs,* p 24, Jan/Feb 1982.
15. Mechner F: Patient assessment: examination of the ear, *AJN* 75(3):1, 1975.

CHAPTER FIFTY-FIVE

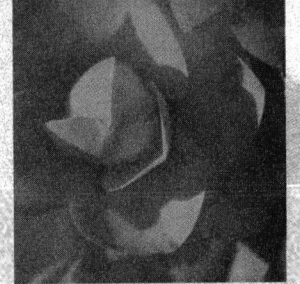

Nursing Management of Adults with Ear Disorders

LEARNING OBJECTIVES

1 Summarize various ways to decrease noise pollution in the home and community.
2 Describe individuals who would benefit from a hearing aid and the importance of choosing and maintaining the aid.
3 Describe the degenerative changes in the ear caused by aging.
4 Describe the various aural hygienic methods used to reduce hearing loss.
5 Perform procedures to keep the ear clean and free of wax or foreign objects.
6 Describe clinical findings and nursing interventions for cholesteatoma and otitis media.
7 Recognize the importance of the symptom of vertigo in inner ear problems.
8 Describe the progress of Ménière's disease and nursing care during the acute and remission stages.
9 Compare the differences in assessing the tympanic membrane and mastoid process and the outer, middle, and inner ears.

KEY TERMS

acoustic neuroma, p. 1499
actinic keratosis, p. 1489
cerumen, p. 1481
cholesteatoma, p. 1494
cochlear implant, p. 1485
conductive hearing loss, p. 1481
external otitis, p. 1488
labyrinthitis, p. 1498
Ménière's disease, p. 1501
myringoplasty, p. 1495

otitis media, p. 1492
otomycosis, p. 1488
otosclerosis, p. 1494
presbycusis, p. 1481
sensorineural hearing loss, p. 1481
swimmer's ear, p. 1488
tinnitus, p. 1485
tympanosclerosis, p. 1493
vestibular neuronitis, p. 1499

FROM BIRTH, people are immersed in sounds that influence their behavior. Sound waves constantly bombard the tympanic membrane and are carried to the acoustic nerve. Background noise helps persons orient themselves and helps keep them alert to their surroundings. Noise also becomes a safety mechanism when an individual hears a warning or a sound indicating danger. Because people communicate through hearing and speaking, hearing plays a significant role in human society. However, many people take their hearing for granted until a problem arises.

CHARACTERISTICS OF NOISE

A person becomes aware of sound when pressure waves in the air hit the tympanic membrane and are relayed through the middle ear to the inner ear and the acoustic nerve. A collection of sounds at different frequencies (measured in hertz [Hz] units) with varying amplitudes (measured in decibels [dB]) usually produces a continuous noise. Noise-induced hearing loss may occur when a person is exposed to 85 dB or more over a period of months or years. The U.S. Department of Labor, Occupational Safety and Health Administration, has set guidelines for noise exposure. The Code of Federal Regulations (CFR 29) 1910.95 states rules and regulations for noise control. An estimated 15 million American workers are currently exposed to hazardous noise on the job. An individual should not be exposed to 90 dB for more than 8 hours each day. Examples of 90 dB noise include heavy street noise and the sound of a power lawn mower or shop tools. An individual working in areas where noise reaches 85 dB or more should wear hearing protectors to prevent noise trauma (Figure 55-1). People are most sensitive to frequencies between 250 and 8000 Hz. A tuning fork used for assessment is middle C, or 256 Hz. Typically, environmental noise ranges between 500 and 2000 Hz. Hearing loss from continuous noise is bilateral.

A sudden impact or acoustic trauma noise is a single-wave noise that usually happens instantaneously, such as an explosion or a gunshot close to the ear. The noise is brief, but the damage can be considerable, even if the person does not perceive the noise as uncomfortably loud. The tympanic membrane may perforate or the ossicles fracture because of the sudden impact noise. This type of hearing loss can be unilateral if the noise is heard on only one side.

Hearing loss from occupational long-term exposure to noise follows a predictable pattern. First, the person notes that immediately after exposure to the sounds, hearing acuity decreases for several minutes to hours. The frequencies involved usually are between 3000 and 6000 Hz, because these are a half octave above the primary frequencies of most envi-

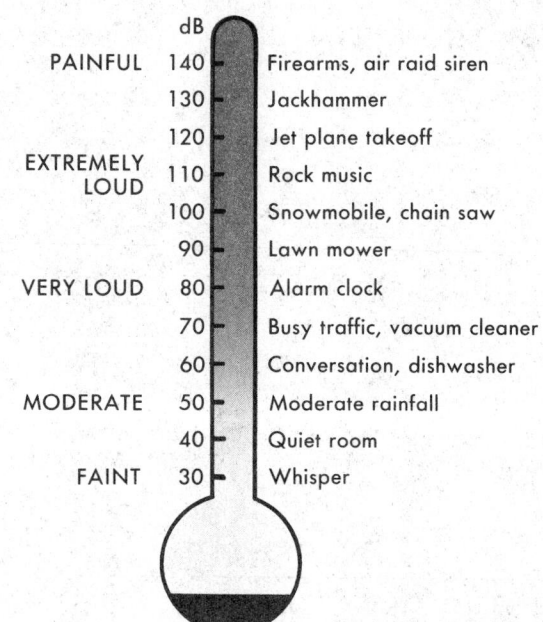

FIGURE 55-1 Average decibels in common types of noise. (Data from the American Speech, Language and Hearing Association.)

ronmental noise. With more exposures to noise, the person notes that hearing does not return to normal but stays at the compromised level. With even more exposure the hearing loss expands to broader frequencies, particularly the low sounds. Finally, the loss is so severe the person cannot hear the normal range of sound. How long it takes noise-induced hearing loss to develop depends on the level of noise exposure, the duration of exposure, and the individual's susceptibility to the noise.

Preventing Noise Damage

Noise damage can be prevented with education, but it persists because of neglect, inadequate control measures, and society's attitude toward noise. The nurse is invaluable in educating patients, families, and staff about loud noises and potential damage. The nurse also must be aware of clues to hearing loss when assessing any patient. Such clues include turning the head to one side, frequently asking that something be repeated, interrupting the conversation, giving inappropriate answers, cupping the ears with the hands, leaning toward the speaker, and talking in an unusually loud voice. Through auditory screening programs in schools and clinics, the nurse can detect early hearing loss, and thus treatment or behavior changes can begin (see the patient education guide).

PATIENT EDUCATION GUIDE   *Noise Prevention*

1. Wear hearing protectors at work when exposure to loud noise is possible. Protectors can be bought at sporting goods stores, at medical supply stores, at hearing clinics, and through audiologists. Various forms of protectors include disposable plugs, reusable plugs, headband plugs, and foam-filled muffs. Plugs should be kept clean and stored in a dry clean place. These protectors should also be worn when working around the home with power tools.
2. Do not sit close to loud music and limit exposure to it.
3. Run only one appliance at a time to decrease the noise level. When buying or replacing appliances, the noise level and decibels generated should be determined.
4. Be cautious when using devices such as headphones and car phones, because loud noises can be generated unexpectedly.
5. Be aware of noise in your community and become an activist to prevent noise if necessary.
6. If a loud noise is anticipated and no protective device is available, cup your hands over the ears.
7. If tinnitus or a decrease in hearing is noted after exposure to loud noise, consult a physician.

HEARING LOSS

Hearing loss, which can be acquired or congenital, is the most common disability in the United States. Twenty-five million Americans suffer some degree of hearing loss; approximately half are over 65 years of age.

Conductive Hearing Loss

Conductive hearing loss refers to the inability to conduct sounds through the external and middle ear (Figure 55-2). Earwax **(cerumen),** an infection, a foreign body in the ear, and trauma are frequent external ear causes of conductive hearing loss. Perforation of the tympanic membrane, sclerosis of bone, a tumor, and fluid in the middle ear also cause conductive hearing loss. If the problem cannot be corrected, a hearing device may improve hearing, since the inner ear and nerve are still functioning.

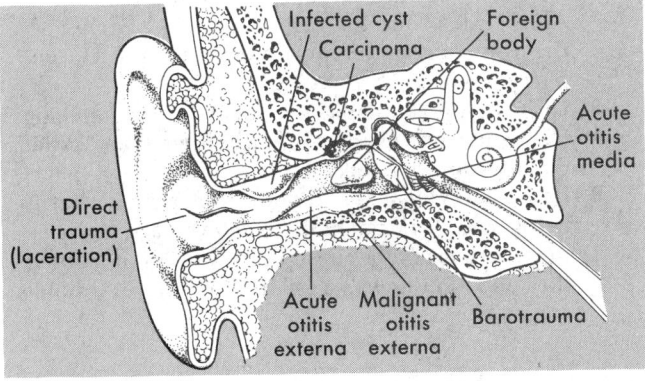

FIGURE 55-2   Disorders that contribute to conductive hearing loss.

Sensorineural Hearing Loss

Sensorineural hearing loss refers to a loss in the sensory or neural components in the inner ear. The loss is in the cochlear or the acoustic branch of the eighth cranial nerve. "Nerve deafness" can be caused by complications from infections (e.g., measles, mumps, meningitis), ototoxic drugs, trauma, neuromas, noise, and the aging process.

Specific types of sensorineural hearing loss include (1) neural hearing loss, which is the loss of hearing originating in the nerve itself; (2) fluctuating hearing loss, which is hearing loss that varies with time; and (3) **presbycusis,** which is hearing loss caused by the aging process.

Aged ear

Presbycusis usually begins in the fifth decade of life with a gradual decline in the ability to hear high-frequency sounds. Between 28% and 50% of people over 65 years of age and 66% of people over 80 years have some hearing impairment. No clinical or audiometric features are found. Structural degenerative changes occur bilaterally in the supporting cells of the organ of Corti, in the neurons in the auditory pathways, and in the elasticity of the basilar membrane of the inner ear. There is atrophy of striae vascularis with impaired endolymph production and degeneration of hair cells in the three semicircular canals. These changes diminish reflex postural control.

As people age, the skin lining the auditory canal becomes thinner and drier. The cerumen-producing glands are affected by this normal change of aging and produce cerumen that is drier. Additionally, sweat gland secretion is diminished all over. Less sweat in the auditory canal results in drier cerumen. As people age, hair in the ears becomes coarser and longer. This helps the cerumen remain in the ear canal until it becomes of sufficient mass and hardness to impair hearing. As the degenerative changes progress, the loss extends to mid- to high-frequency sounds, which leads to impaired hearing of normal speech patterns and sounds.

People with this disorder commonly complain of not understanding what has been said, especially in noisy environments. Since women's voices have a higher pitch than men's, people with presbycusis commonly have more difficulty hearing women's voices. Embarrassed by the inability to hear adequately, a person may exclude himself or herself from group conversations and engage in only one-to-one conversations. At times, decreased hearing may be more socially isolating than blindness. Presbycusis cannot be treated. To maintain or restore a normal life, some elderly individuals must use therapeutic aids such as hearing aids or cochlear implants, which improve communication and prevent social isolation. The box below gives tips on communicating with an older person with a hearing loss. (See the section on social impact of impaired hearing in this chapter for special devices that amplify sound.)

Other Types of Hearing Loss

Another type of hearing loss is mixed hearing loss, which exists when a person has both a conductive and a sensorineural hearing loss. It can be a combination of any of the disorders previously mentioned or of those seen in Figure 55-2. Hearing loss resulting from damage to the brain that has affected the acoustic nerve is said to be a central hearing loss. An example of a central hearing loss would be hearing impaired by a cerebrovascular accident. A hearing loss for which no organic reason can be found is called a functional or psychogenic hearing loss. It may be under voluntary or nonvoluntary control but usually is precipitated by emotional stress. Audiometric testing may be inconclusive and change as the emotional stress fluctuates. Functional or psychogenic hearing loss usually is treated with psychologic counseling. The nurse should display a caring, nonjudgmental attitude toward the patient with a functional hearing loss. If diagnosed as a conversion disorder (hysterical conversion), the deafness is not under voluntary control.

Therapeutic Aids

Standard hearing aids are intricate instruments that amplify sounds. A microphone receives the environmental and speech sounds and converts them to electrical signals, which are amplified to strengthen them. A receiver then converts the signals to sound. The energy source is a small battery.

THERAPEUTIC COMMUNICATION GUIDE

Communicating Better With Older People

Communicating with older people often requires extra time and patience because of physical, psychologic, and social changes of normal aging. Even more effort is needed in nursing homes where 60% to 90% of residents may actually have communication disorders. Speech-language pathologists Martin Shulman of Kean College, Union, New Jersey, and Ellen Mandel of Pace University, Pleasantville, New York, offer these tips for family members and caregivers to make communication with older people easier:

1. Before you begin your conversation, reduce distracting background noises (turn off the radio or television, close the door, move to a quieter place).
2. Begin the conversation with casual topics (the weather, what the person had for lunch). Avoid crucial messages at the beginning.
3. Continue conversation with familiar subjects such as family members and special interests of the person.
4. Stick to a topic for a while. Avoid quick shifts from topic to topic.
5. Keep your sentences and questions short. Rephrase rather than repeat a misunderstood sentence.
6. Give older persons a chance to reminisce. Their memories are important to them.
7. Allow extra time for responding. As people age, they function better at a slower tempo. Do not hurry them.
8. Give the person choices to ease decision making ("Do you want tea or coffee?" rather than "What do you want to drink?").
9. Be an active listener. If you are not sure what is being said, look for hints from eye gaze and gestures. Then take a guess ("Are you talking about the television news? Yes? Tell me more. I didn't see it.").

From the American Speech, Language and Hearing Association, Rockville, Md, 1988.

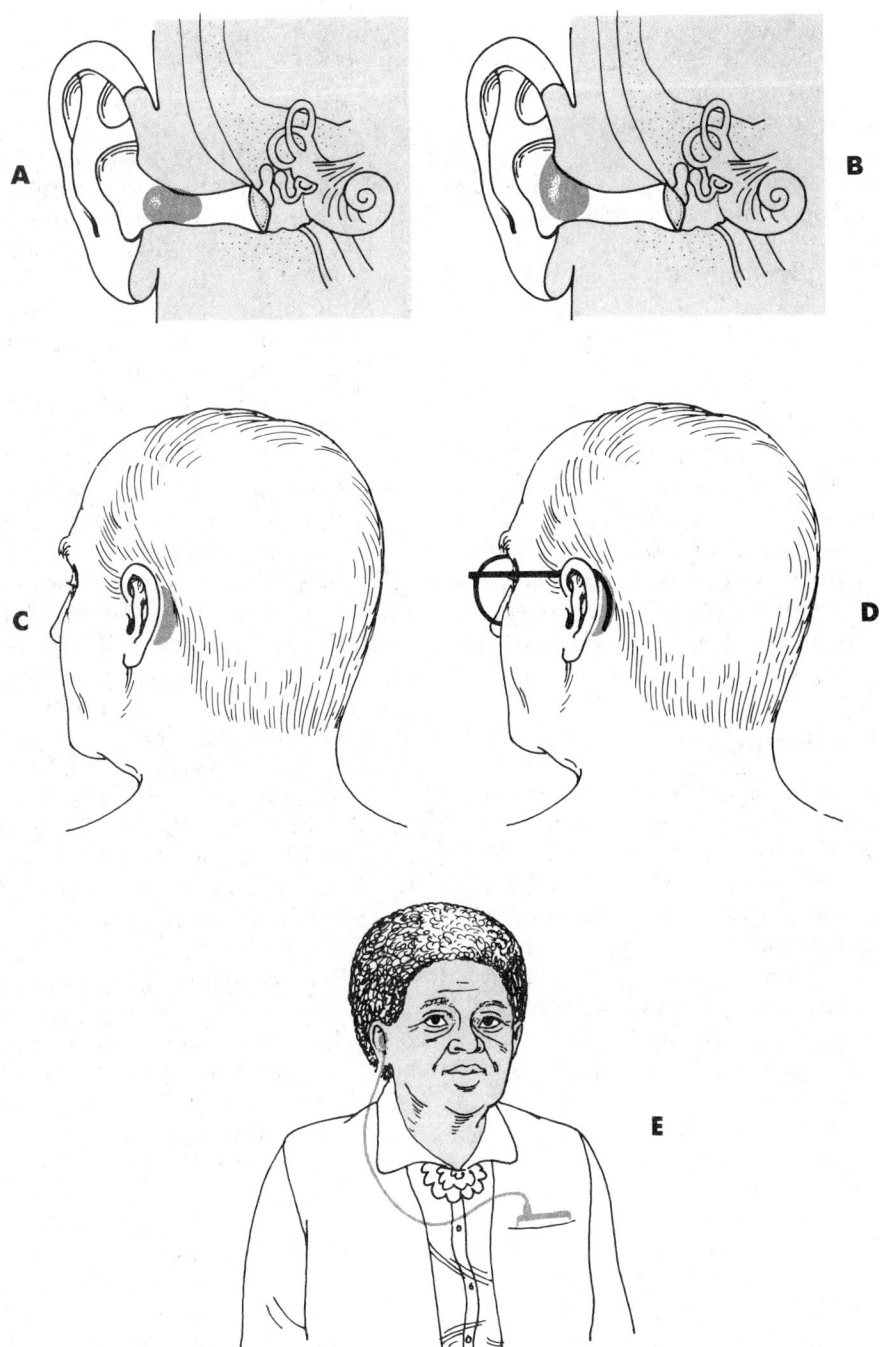

FIGURE 55-3 Types of commonly used hearing aids. **A,** Canal aid: the smallest aid available; self-contained unit that fits into external canal. **B,** In-the-ear aid: larger than canal model; part of device extends outside canal. **C,** Behind-the-ear aid: apparatus contained in case that fits behind ear and is connected to ear mold that fits into external canal. **D,** Eyeglass aid: similar to behind-the-ear model; apparatus contained in eyeglass frame and uses same type of ear mold connection. **E,** Body-worn aid: receiver fits into ear mold connected to hearing aid apparatus by cord; apparatus worn in pocket or special pouch.

There are four common types of hearing aids (Figure 55-3):

1. The in-the-ear aid is small enough for the entire apparatus to fit into the ear. This aid may be preferred, since it is unobtrusive to the wearer and others. A person with a hearing loss of 25 to 55 dB may benefit from an in-the-ear aid.
2. The behind-the-ear or postauricular aid is the most common type of aid worn today. People find the behind-the-ear aid comfortable to wear, and it is helpful for hearing loss of 25 to 80 dB.
3. The all-in-one eyeglass aid is the least used hearing device. It is helpful for hearing loss of 25 to 70 dB.
4. The body-worn aid is used by severely or profoundly deaf persons. The transmitter usually is worn around the neck or connected to clothing. The fitted ear mold is inserted into the external ear and connected to a receiver, which is wired to the transmitter. The wearer cannot hide the receiver and wires but can somewhat conceal the transmitter. The body-worn aid is helpful for hearing loss of 40 to 110 dB.

Therapeutic Management

Before an individual buys a hearing aid, a complete examination should be performed by an otologist (a physician specializing in diseases of the ear) and an audiologist (a person specializing in sound and the mechanisms that produce sound) to determine if hearing will be improved with a hearing aid and the best type for the particular dysfunction. A hearing aid is not guaranteed to restore hearing, and not everyone can tolerate an aid. Most hearing aids pick up environmental noises as well as speech, and these distractions may make it difficult to understand the spoken word, leaving the wearer frustrated. A person may need auditory training to hear sounds clearly through the aid and thus wear an aid successfully. Hearing aids can be individualized to the patient's specific needs.

A new type of hearing aid reduces background noise interference by processing input signals instead of amplifying them. These second-generation aids have special circuits that distinguish low-frequency background noise from high-frequency speech sounds. The background noise is not amplified, so speech sounds are heard more clearly. More analog-digital hybrid and fully digital hearing aids will be available in the future.

NURSING MANAGEMENT OF THE PATIENT WITH A HEARING AID

Before investigating a patient's need for a hearing aid, the nurse should discuss the matter with the patient to find out what is wanted. A standard hearing aid costs between $600 and $1000. Some older individuals may be very comfortable with a quiet environment, and suddenly bombarding that environment with sound may be distressful as well as expensive if the older person does not use the hearing aid.

The person buying a hearing aid is instructed in how to care for it. Nurses must know the general guidelines in caring for a patient with a hearing aid:

1. To gain the patient's attention, the nurse raises a hand or touches the patient. The nurse articulates clearly with light in his or her face and speaks directly to the patient.
2. If the patient's condition allows, the nurse asks the patient to explain how the device is inserted and cleaned, where it is kept when not in use, and how the batteries are changed.
3. If the patient cannot tell the nurse in which ear the aid goes, the nurse should look for the ear bore (hole) in the mold. The bore is inserted into the ear first, so the mold shape indicates the correct ear. The aid should slip easily into the ear canal; it will squeal or not function if the mold is placed incorrectly. The bore should be clean and free of wax.
4. The patient's hospital routine is adapted to safeguard the aid. It is noted on the Kardex or chart that an aid is in use, and nurses are aware that the aid is removed during the night, that it is not allowed to get wet during bathing, and that hospital procedure is followed when the patient has x-ray studies or surgery.
5. Before inserting a hearing aid, the nurse checks to see that it is working. This can be done by closing the battery case and turning the volume to the highest level. The volume control usually is marked from 1 to 4, with 4 being the highest volume. A squealing or whistling noise should be heard. If no noise is heard, a new battery is needed, which should be found in the aid's case. Individuals who use a hearing aid should always have an extra battery. After assuring that the battery is working, the nurse resets the volume control at its original position.
6. After inserting the aid, the nurse asks the patient if he or she can hear. If the answer is no, the wiring and placement are checked. The volume may also need to be turned up.
7. The hearing aid is left in place while the patient is awake except when showering. At night the aid is stored in its case or bag in a safe, dry place.
8. The aid is kept out of direct sunlight and away from high temperatures. Solvents or lubricants are not used on the aid.
9. The aid is cleaned according to the manu-

facturer's instructions. Most detachable ear molds can be washed in warm, soapy water and dried. Plastic tubing can be cleaned with a pipe cleaner.

COCHLEAR IMPLANTS

A **cochlear implant** is used when a person is diagnosed as profoundly deaf and has lost all hearing. All types of cochlear implants have four common features: a microphone for picking up sounds, a microelectronic processor for converting the sound into electrical signals, a transmission system for relaying the signals to the implanted components, and a long, slender electrode that is placed in the cochlea to deliver the electrical stimuli directly to the fibers of the auditory nerve. Figure 55-4 shows the pathways and placement of a cochlear implant.

The electrode is surgically placed through the tympanic membrane, through the round window, and into the organ of Corti. It converts the vibration of the basilar membrane into electrical signals, which travel along the auditory nerve to the brain.

Single-channel and multichannel implants are available. The more channels in the implants, the finer the pitch, tone, and complex sounds that can be heard. The patient hears only the broadest sense of pitch and only at stimulations of a few hundred hertz. Yet even these sounds can be advantageous to the patient, who now may be able to hear the telephone ring, automobiles honk, and voices. Four-channel implants have been found to help people hear or recognize 80% of ordinary conversations. Future models will have finer spatial and temporal control.

NURSING MANAGEMENT OF THE PATIENT WITH A COCHLEAR IMPLANT

Assess the patient for knowledge of the operation and expectations postoperatively, understanding what the patient will be experiencing. Sign language or lipreading may be necessary to communicate with the patient. A booklet is helpful if the patient can read and comprehend. The patient is taught that hearing will not magically begin after the implant and that the implant may help him or her to hear sounds but not spoken words. Family members are included in the teaching and may be able to help the nurse communicate with the patient. The speech therapist or audiologist who will work with the patient after surgery must be present.

Postoperative nursing care includes relieving mild to moderate ear pain or headache with analgesics.

EQUALIZING MIDDLE EAR PRESSURE

A common experience when flying is a "popping" in the ear or temporary decrease in hearing caused by

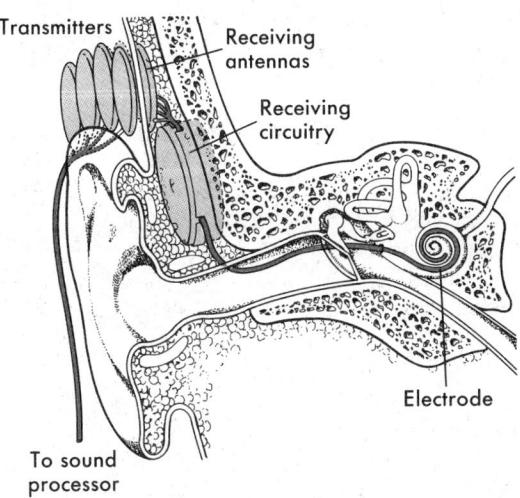

FIGURE 55-4   Cochlear implant.

air trapped in the middle ear. People with allergies may experience this same discomfort. Middle ear pressure can be equalized in several ways, including yawning, chewing gum, or drinking a glass of water, which requires a person to swallow several times in a row. If these methods fail, both nostrils should be held shut with the fingers and the mouth kept closed while gently trying to blow out (Valsalva's maneuver). People with congestion from upper respiratory infections should not use Valsalva's maneuver, because it may introduce the infection into the middle ear.

MONITORING OTOTOXIC DRUGS

Decreased hearing is a side effect of some drugs that damage the cochlea, the vestibule of the ear, or the eighth cranial nerve. When teaching the patient about ototoxic drugs, the nurse should stress that any **tinnitus** (ringing in the ears), dizziness, or hearing loss should be reported to the physician. If the medicine is stopped and hearing does not return to the predrug level, audiometric testing may be indicated.

Several classifications of drugs can cause varying degrees of damage to the vestibular and auditory branches of the eighth cranial nerve, resulting in vertigo, deafness, or disequilibrium. Older people and people with chronic problems appear to be more sensitive to ototoxicity. The vestibular damage may be partially or completely reversed if the medication is discontinued. Often permanent auditory damage occurs even if the medication is stopped. The nurse should caution a patient taking any of the drugs listed in Table 55-1 that any dizziness, loss of balance, tinnitus, or decreased hearing should be reported to the physician.

TABLE 55-1 Ototoxic Substance

Substance	Vestibular loss	Auditory loss
AMINOGLYCOSIDES	X	X
Streptomycin		
Gentamicin		
Tobramycin		
Amikacin		
Neomycin sulfate		
ANTIMYCOBACTE-RIAL DRUGS	X	
Isoniazid		
Cycloserine		
THIAZIDES	X	
Hydrochlorothiazide (Esidrix, Oretic)		
Chlorothiazide (Diuril)		
LOOP DIURETICS	X	
Furosemide (Lasix)		
Bumetanide (Bumex)		
ANTINEOPLASTIC DRUGS	X	X
Cisplatin (Platinol)		
Mechlorethamine (Mustargen)		
Cyclophosphamide (Cytoxan)		
Fluorouracil (5-FU)		
Methotrexate (Mexate, Folex)		
NARCOTICS	X	
Morphine		
Meperidine (Demerol)		
Oxycodone (Percodan)		
Dextropropoxyphene (Darvon)		
NARCOTIC ANTAGONISTS	X	
Nalbuphine (Nubain)		
Pentazocine (Talwin)		

COMMUNICATING WITH THE HEARING-IMPAIRED OR DEAF PERSON

Patients with moderate or profound hearing loss seek medical attention, and a method of communication must be maintained. Being attentive to these patients' special needs ensures that they receive therapeutic care. The following basic points should be kept in mind:

1. Determining that the patient has a hearing loss is the first step in developing a communication plan. Not understanding questions, not jumping at loud noises, and nervousness may indicate that the patient has a hearing loss. The nurse can perform a "finger rub" 1 foot behind each of the patient's ears and observe if the patient can hear the rubbing.
2. The nurse should raise a hand or touch the patient's arm to gain his or her attention. The nurse should speak directly to the patient with the light on his or her face.
3. Only about one third of deaf individuals can lip-read. Chewing gum, covering the mouth, mustaches, and beards may prevent a hearing-impaired person from correctly interpreting words. Overenunciating words does not make lipreading easier and is demeaning to the deaf person. If the patient is lip-reading and appears not to understand the words, the nurse should rephrase and use different words, since some words are easily misunderstood by lipreaders. It is best to speak in a normal manner.
4. Speaking louder to deaf persons does not increase their chances of hearing. Similarly, people wearing hearing aids may have difficulty with clarity of sound when voices are raised. If the patient has a conductive hearing loss, speaking louder and toward the better ear may improve communication. Writing out proper names and any statement that may have been misinterpreted may increase understanding.
5. Because a person cannot hear does not mean that he or she is retarded. Deaf individuals work in all professional areas, including medicine, law, politics, and nursing. Unfortunately, some deaf people do not have the opportunities to obtain the same education as hearing persons.
6. All hearing-impaired people do not communicate the same way. Some lip-read, some sign, some use body gestures, and some write. Pencil and paper should be provided when assessing the manner of communication with a deaf person.
7. Most deaf individuals have vocal cords and can make sounds. Speaking is difficult if the individual has never heard the spoken word. Some deaf people speak very well.

Nursing Diagnosis

Common nursing diagnoses for the deaf individual include the following:

Altered role performance related to decreased communication skills

Anxiety related to decreased or absent hearing

Body image disturbance related to decreased hearing

Fear related to loss of hearing

Hopelessness related to decreased hearing

Impaired social interaction related to decreased hearing

Impaired verbal communication related to hearing loss

Ineffective individual coping related to difficult communication

Ineffective family coping: compromised related to lack of understanding of the hearing impaired person

Knowledge deficit related to ineffective understanding of disease process

Pain related to symptoms or surgical procedure

Personal identity disturbance related to hearing loss

High risk for injury related to loss and equilibrium disturbance

Sensory/perceptual alterations (auditory, kinesthetic) related to loss of equilibrium

Self-esteem disturbance related to loss of equilibrium

Sleep pattern disturbance related to disequilibrium and fear of pain

Social isolation related to decreased communication skills

SOCIAL IMPACT OF IMPAIRED HEARING

Communication is an integral part of society, and when a component of communication, such as hearing, is lost, quality of life changes. Being unable to hear a child sing is regrettable, but being unable to hear a car horn could be disastrous. Individuals with untreated hearing loss show several behavior changes, including social withdrawal, anxiety, frustration, embarrassment, depression, fear, and anger. If the individual has a chronic illness as well as hearing loss, stress is compounded. The nurse may see depression, isolation, or confusion in these individuals.

The goal for individuals with impaired hearing is to have the cause accurately diagnosed, so that appropriate treatment can be implemented. If treatment cannot restore hearing, the individual may need counseling to learn to live with the disability, or the person may need to learn lip-reading or signing. Family members also should be urged to learn the new communication skill, so that effective communication can be restored.

Many assistive listening devices are available to help the hearing-impaired individual. They can be used alone or with a hearing aid to amplify sounds. These devices include alarm clocks with a flashing light or a vibration attachment that is placed under

RESEARCH BRIEF

Fickel V: Acoustic neuroma: postoperative deficits and the role of the neuroscience nurse, *J Neurosci Nurs* 23:1, 1991.

A questionnaire was sent to 541 members of the Acoustic Neuroma Association who had experienced surgery for an acoustic neuroma. Respondents assessed their own acoustic neuroma experience. The most common postoperative deficit reported was unilateral hearing loss: 94% reported total loss, 5% reported partial loss, and 1% had normal hearing. Other postoperative deficits included imbalance (86%), eye-related problems (84%), anxiety-related problems (80%), tinnitus (66%), and headache (34%).

Thirty-seven percent of respondents dissatisfied with the preoperative information stated it was insufficient or inaccurate. Thirty-two percent were dissatisfied with the quality of postoperative information received. Almost half the respondents emphasized that more information was needed in every stage of treatment, namely, preoperative and postoperative. They also requested clearer, less technical language. The nurse can make a difference both preoperatively and postoperatively.

the pillow; a doorbell accessory that vibrates, amplifies sound, or flashes a light; and security systems that flash a light or sound off when tripped. Various devices can increase voice sounds over the telephone, including simple amplifiers in the handset, portable amplifiers that attach to the earpiece, bone conduction receivers, and headset amplifiers. A system can be attached to the phone to alert the individual to the ringing of the phone by amplifying the sound, flashing a light, or turning on a lamp. Headset devices can be attached to the television, radio, or stereo that amplify sound for the hearing-impaired individual but allow a person with normal hearing to enjoy listening at the same time. Other devices available include smoke alarms and baby alert systems. For the completely deaf individual, phone systems are available that can receive, type, and print messages.

Closed-caption television offers another method of communication for the hearing-impaired individual by printing a program's dialogue on the screen. Theaters, concert halls, and meeting rooms frequently are equipped with group listening systems that provide amplified sounds through special receivers. All these devices make listening more enjoyable for the hearing-impaired individual.

External Ear Disorders

INFECTION
Definition/Etiology

Infection, known as **external otitis,** is the most frequently found problem in the external ear. Bacteria or fungi commonly infect the skin in the canal and pinna. Staphylococci are the most common invaders, but other Gram-positive and Gram-negative organisms can cause problems. *Pneumocystis* infections of the external ear have been seen in HIV-positive patients. The ear may be either the primary or secondary site of infection. External otitis can be caused by meticulous cleaning of the ear, which removes the protective earwax and leaves the ear at risk for invading organisms. Inserting such items as hairpins, cotton-tipped swabs, and pencils into the ear can damage the lining of the external ear and lead to infection. Hearing can be affected as a result of blockage of the canal.

Swimmer's ear, or diffuse bacterial external otitis, usually occurs in the summer when moisture is left in the ear after swimming, allowing bacteria to grow in the warm, moist area. Swimmer's ear also can occur in individuals who swim indoors year round. The condition can be acute or chronic. It can be prevented by placing 70% alcohol or an over-the-counter solution for swimmer's ear in the ear immediately after swimming.

Pathophysiology

A localized form of external otitis, called ear canal furuncle or abscess, results when a hair follicle becomes infected, causing an abscess to form (Figure 55-5). If several hair follicles are involved, the abscess is called a carbuncle. Most erupt and drain spontaneously. Individuals with a systemic debilitating disorder such as diabetes could develop a life-threatening malignant otitis externa from a carbuncle. Unchecked, the infection invades the soft tissue around the ear and spreads to the cartilage and temporal bone. **Otomycosis** is caused by a fungus, most commonly *Aspergillus niger* or *Candida albicans*. It commonly is seen after use of topical corticosteroids and antibiotics and occurs more frequently in hot weather. Infection of the auricle (perichondritis) results in necrosis of the cartilage. Treatment is necessary to decrease the destruction of the shape of the pinna.

Clinical Manifestations

Pain and pruritus (itching) are two frequent symptoms of outer ear infection. The ear usually is tender and painful when the pinna is gently tugged, the

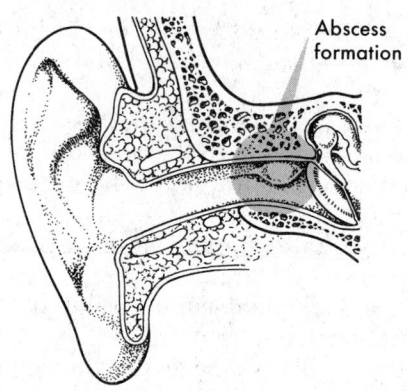

FIGURE 55-5   External otitis.

jaw moved, or an otoscope inserted. The location of the erythematous swelling and desquamation can be seen with the otoscope. The swelling may obscure the tympanic membrane, which should appear normal. In severe cases, cellulitis of the auricle and postauricular lymphadenopathy may develop. If the external canal is completely occluded, conductive hearing loss occurs in the affected ear and the patient will complain of a "blocked" ear. Mild fever may be another symptom, particularly when a furuncle erupts. Whitish yellow drainage can be seen on eruption.

Therapeutic Management

The usual treatment for external otitis is either antibiotic creams or drops instilled directly in the ear canal or a systemic antibiotic taken orally. The ear is inspected and cleaned of debris or dried exudate before medication instillation. If there is considerable swelling, a wick will be needed to instill the medication. Furuncles may be treated with localized heat to promote eruption and drainage. If a furuncle has come to a head but has not erupted, an 18- to 20-gauge sterile needle is used to puncture the furuncle and release the fluid. A local anesthetic such as lidocaine (Xylocaine) may be used to decrease discomfort when draining the furuncle or carbuncle. Short-term systemic antibiotic therapy (4 days) is given when furuncles have been drained in the external ear; prolonged antibiotics (both systemic and local) are given for carbuncles. Patients who develop auricular cellulitis are treated with systemic antibiotics and careful follow-up care.

Analgesics are given in any infectious state when pain is involved. Pain from external otitis may range from mild to severe, and analgesics such an aspirin, acetaminophen, and codeine are used.

External otitis should resolve in several days. If the infection is prolonged, particularly in diabetic or immunodeficient patients, malignant external otitis can develop. In such cases hospitalization with intravenous antibiotic therapy, debridement, and assessment becomes necessary.

Fungal infections are treated with careful cleaning of the ear for several days and a topical antimycotic agent such as nystatin (Nilstat) or clotrimazole (Lotrimin). The antimycotic agent should be used for at least 1 week after the infection has resolved. Analgesics may be given for pain.

NEOPLASTIC CHANGES
Definition

A sebaceous gland cyst is a common benign mass seen in the external ear.

Pathophysiology

In rare cases a cyst develops from a cerumen (earwax) gland. Other benign masses are lipomas, warts, keloids, and infectious polyps that arise from the tympanic membrane. These masses also may begin in the middle ear and protrude through the tympanic membrane into the external ear. Keloids occur at the site of previous trauma and are more common in black populations. **Actinic keratosis,** a precancerous lesion, may be seen in elderly persons, commonly on the auricle. Malignant tumors also can develop, such as basal cell carcinoma on the pinna and squamous cell carcinoma in the ear canal. If not treated, these tumors can invade the underlying tissues and spread to the temporal bone.

Clinical Manifestations

Two frequent findings in the health histories of patients with actinic keratosis or basal cell carcinoma are long-term exposure to the sun and light-colored skin. On assessment, clinical findings of blocked hearing; deep, boring pain on the affected side of the head; ear drainage; or peripheral facial paralysis (a late finding) may indicate a mass in the ear structure.

Therapeutic Management

If the mass is benign, surgical intervention is corrective and usually restorative. In malignancy the prognosis is favorable if the tumor is confined to the cartilaginous canal. If the tumor has invaded surrounding tissues (especially if bone is involved), wide excision, including the temporal bone, and upper neck dissection with skin grafting, followed by deep radiation and/or chemotherapy, usually are the treatments of choice. Treatment of external tumors with invasion can result in ear deformities, which can create a psychologic as well as a functional problem. An

auricular prosthesis may be used more effectively than an auricular reconstruction.

TRAUMA
Etiology

Injuries to the external ear commonly are caused by automobile accidents, blows to the head, burns, foreign bodies introduced into the canal, and extremely cold temperatures. The lack of subcutaneous tissue and the exposed placement of the ears increase the risk for frostbite and burns.

Clinical Manifestations

Lacerations, contusions, hematomas, abrasions, erythema, blistering, and hypertrophy (cauliflower ears) are seen with either sharp or blunt trauma. Conductive hearing loss may accompany any of these injuries if the ear canal is partly or totally blocked. Numbness, pain, and paresthesia of the auricle are common complaints from patients with contusions and hematomas. Lacerations range from minor scratches to deep cuts into the cartilage. Burns can cause extensive erythema, blistering, and destruction of the external ear. Frostbite is seen on the upper outer edges of the pinna; the skin appears whitish yellow, waxy, and cold and hard to the touch.

Therapeutic Management

Of course, prevention is the first step. The nurse can help educate the public on the vulnerability of the ears in cold weather and about hazards of placing foreign objects in the ear. If trauma of the outer ear occurs, the damage is assessed, followed by surgery, debridement, or application of a protective covering. Other more life-threatening problems are usually a priority in a multiple trauma victim; then the outer ear is treated.

NURSING MANAGEMENT OF THE PATIENT WITH EXTERNAL EAR DISORDERS
Assessment

A health history, including onset, duration, and severity of symptoms, is completed by the health team. Pain, loss of hearing, itching, and a sense of fullness in the ear are the most frequent subjective findings.

Often patients with external ear problems visit their physician because they can see the problem. The outer pinna is assessed for the extent of erythema, lacerations, abrasions, drainage, or carcinomas. Manipulating the ear is important in assessing the ear canal. If the patient feels pain when the outer ear is manipulated, the problem usually is in the ear canal and not in the middle ear.

PATIENT EDUCATION GUIDE   *Routine Cleaning of the Ear*

Routine cleaning is simple, because the external canal is self-cleaning. Cerumen lubricates the external ear and helps trap foreign materials that enter, thus acting as a protective device for the auditory canal. If the amount of earwax is inadequate, the ear canal becomes dry and flaky and itches. If this occurs, ear ointments or oils may help. Through the act of chewing, muscles work the cerumen to the outside orifice, where routine washing of the outer ear with soap and water removes the built-up wax. The following procedure produces a clean, healthy ear:

1. Place a wet washcloth over the ear and with the tip of a finger gently cleanse the outermost part of the ear canal.
2. Never insert anything in the ear beyond the area that can be seen from the outside, including hairpins, cotton-tipped applicators, matchsticks, safety pins, toothpicks, paper clips, and fingers, because the tympanic membrane can be perforated or the ear canal scratched.

3. If a person has a history of ear infections, and particularly if the tympanic membrane has been perforated, protection is required when showering, swimming, or diving. Maceration may occur if moisture is introduced into the ear canal. Earplugs or a protective cap (bathing or shower) should be worn. An earplug can be made for showering by rolling a cotton ball into a cylinder, applying petroleum jelly to its surface, and then inserting it into the ear. A hair dryer can be used to dry the external ear, using caution so as not to burn the helix. A few drops of alcohol or an over-the-counter solution for preventing swimmer's ear can help dry the external canal.
4. A person with an upper respiratory infection should not blow his or her nose too hard and should not hold one nostril shut while blowing the other. The nose should be blown gently with both nostrils and the mouth open to decrease pressure and the chance of forcing infected material into the eustachian tubes and middle ear.
5. A physician should be consulted if any growths, pain, tinnitus, or decrease in hearing is suspected or noted during cleaning.

Nursing Diagnosis

Nursing diagnoses that may pertain to problems of the external ear are as follows:

Body image disturbance related to presence of visible lesion

Impaired verbal communication related to hearing loss

Impaired tissue integrity related to type of injury

Knowledge deficit related to lack of information on preventive ear care

Pain related to inflammation of external ear

High risk for injury related to self-cleaning of external ear

Sensory/perceptual alterations (auditory) related to blockage of external ear

Planning

The specific goals for patients with external ear problems are as follows:

Hearing returns to preillness state

Pain decreases or dissipates

Patient can state the symptoms of the problem and knows when to consult physician

Patient can describe and perform any procedures necessary to maintain wellness of the external ear

PATIENT EDUCATION GUIDE

Removing Foreign Bodies

Foreign bodies may be inserted or blown into the ear. Inserted foreign bodies may include food or cleaning materials that were inserted and are unretrievable. Flying insects or debris may be blown into the ear. Removing a foreign body involves the following steps:

1. If vegetable items such as beans become lodged in the ear, mineral oil or water should not be instilled, because the material will swell and possibly damage the canal further. A physician should carefully remove the material using a curette or suction.
2. Insects that fly or crawl into the ear can cause great discomfort. Instilling mineral oil, vegetable oil, or alcohol into the ear usually kills the insect and floats it up to the outside, so it can be retrieved. If the insect is drawn to light, shining a flashlight into the ear may lure it out. An ear forceps is used to remove a tick that attaches in the ear canal.

Patient can describe methods to prevent external ear problems

Implementation

The nurse assesses what the patient knows about ear care and then plans an educational program to cover the patient's knowledge deficits. See the patient education guides for routine cleaning of the ears (including irrigation and instillation) and removal of foreign bodies and cerumen. The patient is taught to wash the hands before and after caring for the ears and between handling each ear if both are treated. No swimming is allowed while an outer ear infection or inflammation exists.

Analgesics often are used to promote comfort in individuals with external ear problems. Depending on the pain and the patient's tolerance of it, mild analgesics, such as aspirin or acetaminophen, or codeine may be indicated. The patient's allergies, intolerances, and other medical conditions play a part in prescribing an analgesic. Heat, incision, and drainage of a furuncle or carbuncle can promote comfort.

Teaching the patient why and how an external ear problem developed increases his or her awareness of how to prevent recurrences. For example, if the patient suffers from swimmer's ear, a simple preventive instillation after swimming decreases the chances of recurrence. Although some problems cannot be prevented, awareness of the symptoms and how they develop alerts the patient to seek medical help before the problem is exacerbated.

Evaluation/Documentation

Since most external ear problems are neither life threatening nor long term, care goals are usually achieved. Healing is evaluated through visualization of the affected area and compliance with medication

---

PATIENT EDUCATION GUIDE   *Removing Cerumen*

Wax blockage is a common problem among children but also occurs in adults. It is essential for visualization to have a clear external canal, so an accurate diagnosis can be made. People with large amounts of hair in their ears or who work in dusty or dirty areas are prone to earwax buildup. The wax can be removed in several ways:

1. If the person has a history of perforated tympanic membranes, instillations and irrigations should not be used. The physician will use a blunt ear curette or a wire curette (commonly called cerumen spoons) to remove the wax (Figure 55-6). The head must be immobilized during this procedure to prevent perforation or injury. If instillation and irrigation are performed and a perforated tympanic membrane is discovered, a systemic antibiotic is administered prophylactically.

2. Individuals prone to cerumen buildup should be taught how to remove earwax safely. A few drops of half-strength hydrogen peroxide are instilled in the ear with a medicine dropper. After 5 minutes the solution is washed out with a medicine dropper or during showering, thus removing the wax with the hydrogen peroxide. This usually is repeated once each week to minimize wax buildup.

3. Commercial ceruminolytics (earwax softeners) such as Auro Ear Drops, Debrox Drops, and Murine Ear Drops and common products such as baby oil, mineral oil, and virgin olive oil can be used to soften earwax. The patient should instill several drops of the solution in the ear at bedtime and then put a cotton plug in the ear to hold the solution in place. In the morning the plug is removed and the outer ear is wiped if excess oil is draining. Some patients may need a twice-daily regimen, in the morning and at bedtime. Most ceruminolytics need 3 to 4 days to soften the wax before removal by irrigation is attempted.

4. An ear syringe or Water-Pik can be used to flush impacted cerumen from the outer ear. The water should be body temperature with either apparatus. The patient sits with a curved (kidney-shaped) basin next to the ear to collect the irrigation fluid. A low-pressure stream of water is directed toward the wall of the canal to avoid triggering the vestibular reflex and causing vertigo, nausea, and vomiting. If the wax is dislodged, the ear is dried with 70% alcohol to prevent maceration and otitis external and then examined for trauma. If the plug is not dislodged, a physician or nurse specializing in ear problems uses a blunt or wire curette to remove the wax. If bleeding occurs, the area is swabbed and an antibiotic instilled to prevent otitis externa.

5. Follow-up is extremely important with patients who have chronic cerumen buildup. The patient is urged not to use cotton swabs to remove wax, because they can push the wax further down the ear canal and increase the risk of impaction. The patient who needs professional cerumen removal should be taught to use one of the earwax softeners previously mentioned several days before the appointment. If a patient is to use the ear syringe at home, directing the flow of water must be fully explained.

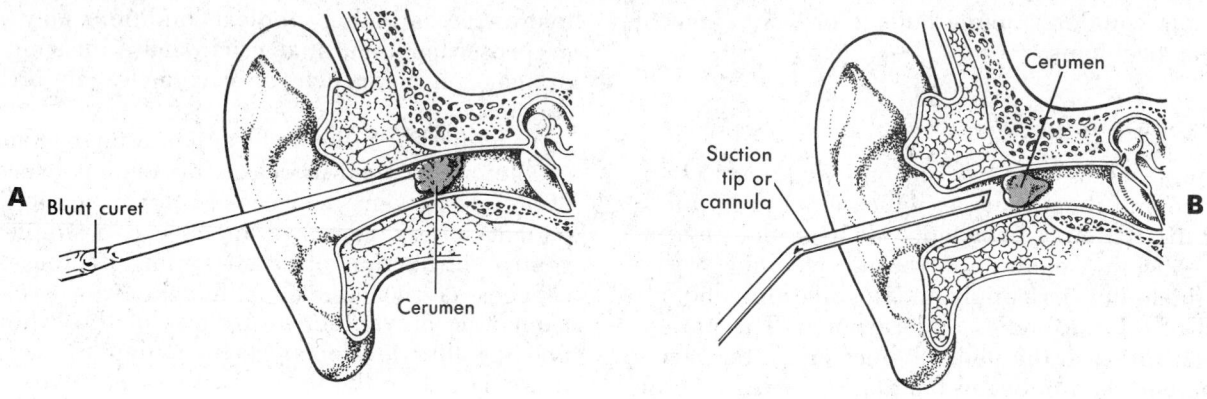

FIGURE 55-6   Removal of cerumen. **A,** With cerumen spoon. **B,** With suction cannula.

regimens. The patient's knowledge is evaluated verbally and reinforced, if necessary, with written materials. Since most patients with external ear problems are seen in the physician's office, presenting symptoms and prescribed effective treatments must be carefully documented. Patient teaching is also documented.

Ongoing Care

Much of the treatment of external ear problems is handled in the home after a visit to the physician's office. Since most of these problems are self-limiting if successfully treated, ongoing care after treatment mainly involves education to prevent recurrence.

Middle Ear, Tympanic Membrane, and Mastoid Disorders

INFECTION
Definition/Etiology

Infection is the most common disease of the middle ear and is known as **otitis media.** Otitis media is the general term for inflammation of the mucous membranes of the middle ear, including all or part of the eustachian tube, mastoid antrum, and mastoid air cells. Since the mucous membranes of the middle ear are continuous with the respiratory tract, an inflammation in the nasal passages, larynx, trachea, or bronchi can travel into the middle ear.

Most cases of otitis media arise from the nasopharynx and affect the middle ear secondarily. Inflammation is a local tissue reaction to injury. The inflamed mucosa becomes thick (edematous) and hyperemic, and a discharge is produced, at first serous and then mucopurulent with desquamation of mucosal epithelium. Hyperemia and edema usually occur in the pharyngeal portion of the eustachian tube, impairing middle ear ventilation. As a result the middle ear is extremely vulnerable to bacterial invasion from the nasopharynx. Otitis media is common in children. It is also seen in adults but frequently goes undetected and untreated, because it often is assumed that a hearing aid is needed without consideration of a treatable problem.

Otitis media without effusion is defined as an inflammation of the middle ear and tympanic mucous membranes without fluid on pneumatic otoscopy. Figure 55-7 gives the different types of middle ear infections. Acute otitis media, often called acute suppurative or purulent otitis media, is a bacterial infection of the middle ear mucous membranes. It frequently is seen bilaterally in children because of their short eustachian tubes, but it usually is seen unilaterally in adults. A full or bulging tympanic membrane is present on pneumatic otoscopy. Acute mastoiditis (inflammation of the mastoid process), which can accompany acute otitis media, is rare when antibiotics are used in treatment, but chronic mastoiditis is still seen. An infection that continues longer than 3 months is labeled chronic otitis media. Fifty-five percent of acute otitis media is caused by pneumococcus and *Haemophilus influenzae.* *Staphylococcus aureus* and streptococcal organisms are also seen as causative agents. Acute otitis media can be a complication of an upper respiratory infection, improper nose blowing, sinusitis, or hypertrophied adenoids.

Otitis media with effusion, sometimes called secretory, nonsuppurative, serous otitis media, or glue ear, is an accumulation of noninfective fluid in the middle ear. It can be further classified as acute (present for less than 3 weeks), subacute (present for 3 weeks to 3 months), or chronic (present for longer than 3 months). Some of the causes of otitis media with effusion are fluid accumulation after an

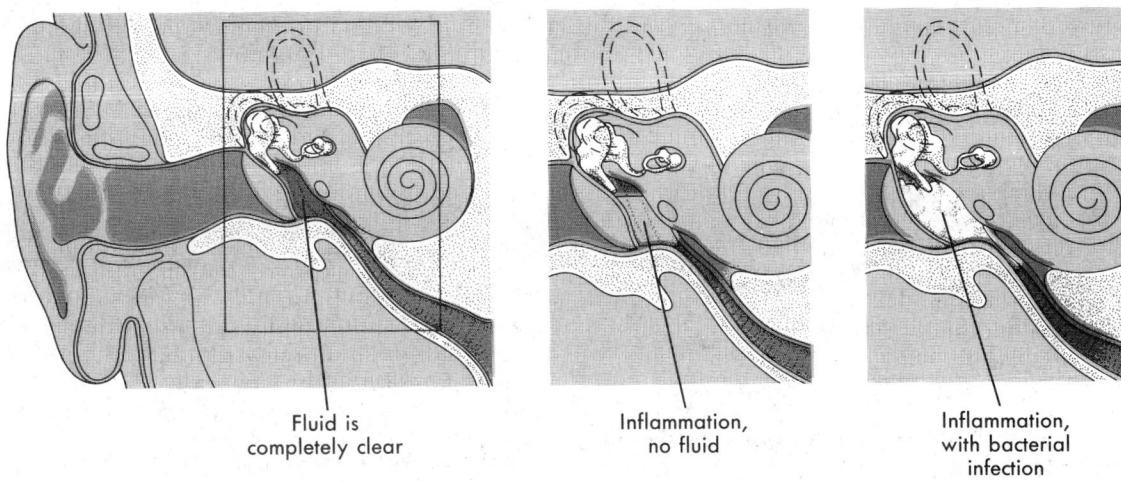

Fluid is
completely clear

Inflammation,
no fluid

Inflammation,
with bacterial
infection

FIGURE 55-7   Types of middle ear infections.

infection, enlarged adenoids, allergies, and mastoid infections.

Clinical Manifestations

Acute otitis media can be self-limiting, depending on the bacterial etiology and the patient's condition. A common scenario is an upper respiratory infection in the recent past followed by a fever, an earache, and a feeling of fullness in the affected ear. With the formation of purulent exudate, there are discomfort, nausea, vomiting, and conductive hearing loss. The otoscopic examination shows a red, bulging, thick, immobile tympanic membrane. If the condition goes untreated, the tympanic membrane may rupture, with purulent drainage from the ear, and the mastoid may become infected. With drainage the patient feels relief of the pressure in the ear and less pain. Deep mastoid tenderness indicates that the infection has spread to the mastoid area. This complication is infrequent when antibiotics are used in treatment. A cholesteatoma (keratinizing squamous epidermal growth) may develop in either the middle ear or mastoid from repeated infections. **Tympanosclerosis,** or hard collagen and calcium deposits on the tympanic membrane, is seen after repeated infections. These deposits also can harden around the middle ear ossicles and contribute to conductive hearing loss.

The clinical picture of otitis media with effusion is less dramatic and may go undetected in adults. There are no signs of an infection and no inflammation. Pneumatic otoscopy shows decreased mobility of the tympanic membrane. The patient may complain of fullness or bubbling in the ear. The patient may be noted to have allergies, to be a mouth breather, or to have a slight conductive hearing loss.

Therapeutic Management

With any type of otitis media or mastoiditis, antibiotic therapy is the treatment of choice. If drainage occurs, culture and sensitivity are done to determine the most effective medication. Amoxicillin is commonly used because of its effectiveness against the pneumococci and *H. influenzae* strains. Penicillin V, erythromycin, cefaclor, and co-trimoxazole (Bactrim, Septra) also are used. Pain is managed with aspirin, acetaminophen, or codeine. Heat applied to the ear may offer some relief.

Paracentesis, or draining of fluid from the middle ear, may be performed with a 2 mL syringe and a short, beveled 10-gauge needle to relieve pressure and fluid in the middle ear. The tympanic membrane is punctured with the needle, and the fluid is drained. With chronic infections the mastoid process and middle ear may be irrigated through an opening in the tympanic membrane, using antibiotic eardrops or powders.

Surgical intervention, through myringotomy with or without tube ventilation, has proven beneficial for otitis media (Figure 55-8). The procedure can be performed in a physician's office, an outpatient surgical care center, or a hospital. General anesthesia may be used, but most adults prefer a topical agent applied directly to the tympanic membrane. An incision is made into the tympanic membrane (myringotomy), and the fluid is allowed to drain out or is removed by suction. A tube can be inserted to allow further drainage until the otitis is cured. The tube may spontaneously extrude in about 3 weeks, or it may be removed by the physician in about 6 weeks or when the otitis has resolved. Occasionally the tube spontaneously extrudes before the otitis has healed, in which case a second tube is inserted to complete drainage.

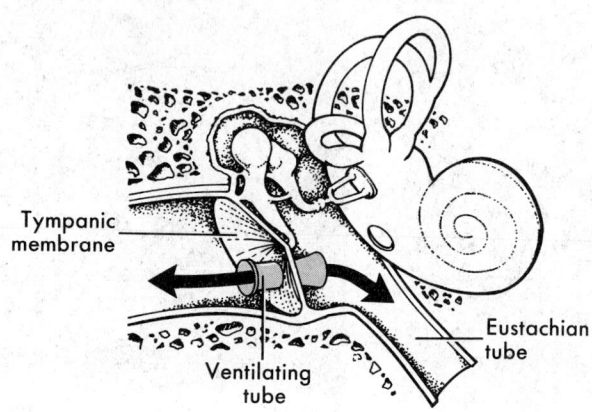

FIGURE 55-8   Surgical intervention for otitis media: insertion of ventilating tube.

CONGENITAL DISORDERS
Definition/Etiology

Defects of the ossicles include malformation of the malleus or incus or fixation of the stapes. Stapes fixation occurs when the annular ligament around the frame of the oval window fails to develop. Other abnormalities include absence of the tympanic cavity or of the bony canal around the facial nerve, an irregular mastoid process, or a malformed tympanic membrane. If a congenital defect is found in the middle ear or mastoid, a defect in the external ear may also be present.

Clinical Manifestations

Congenital defects are found on routine examination or when hearing difficulties develop. The patient should be examined thoroughly to ascertain whether any other congenital problems exist.

Therapeutic Management

Surgical treatment is indicated if congenital defects can be repaired or cosmetically reconstructed. The type of surgery depends on the severity and location of the congenital defect. Complete x-ray studies are done to determine if surgery will increase hearing. A common congenital problem is a deformed or absent ossicle. Fixation of the malleus head or body of the incus occurs congenitally as a result of the lack of suspensory ligament differentiation of the malleus and incus. If this is found, a malleus-stapes assembly prothesis reconstruction is performed; the surgery is called an ossicular chain reconstruction. The usual approach is through the external ear canal to expose the middle ear abnormality. Artificial materials such as polyethylene, Teflon, stainless steel, or bone from the homograft bone bank may be used for

replacement. Commercial bone banks have been established across the United States.

NEOPLASTIC CHANGES
Definition/Etiology

Tumors of the middle ear and mastoid can be benign or malignant. The most common benign growth is the infectious polyp followed by a cholesteatoma. A **cholesteatoma** is a keratinizing squamous epidermal growth that usually begins in the external meatus and extends through a perforated tympanic membrane into the middle ear.

Pathophysiology

A cholesteatoma enlarges by shedding debris into its center. The keratin produced can accumulate and destroy underlying tissue. A cholesteatoma can also begin in the mastoid process, and a secondary infection can develop in the area of the accumulated keratin (Figure 55-9). A rare congenital form of cholesteatoma represents incomplete epithelial rest migration. This is where a small collection of embryonic cells fails to develop properly and is retained in the adult. If left untreated, the growth can erode into the inner ear, temporal bone, middle cranial fossa, and the mastoid process. Malignant growths are uncommon. When they occur, they may be primary or secondary, and they can occur anywhere in the middle ear.

Clinical Manifestations

A cholesteatoma causes conductive hearing loss; painless, fetid, pearly white otorrhea from the secondary infection; and perforation of the tympanic membrane. As the disease progresses, symptoms include facial paralysis and vertigo.

Therapeutic Management

Surgery is the treatment of choice for cholesteatomas. If the tumor has invaded only the middle ear, a myringoplasty with a tympanoplasty is performed. If the cholesteatoma has invaded the mastoid, a myringoplasty and tympanoplasty with mastoidectomy are performed.

DEGENERATIVE CHANGES
Definition/Etiology

Otosclerosis is a hereditary degenerative disorder that involves the formation of new (otosclerotic) bone along the stapes foot plate in the oval window niche. This new bone gradually decreases the stapes' mobility, and a conductive hearing loss occurs.

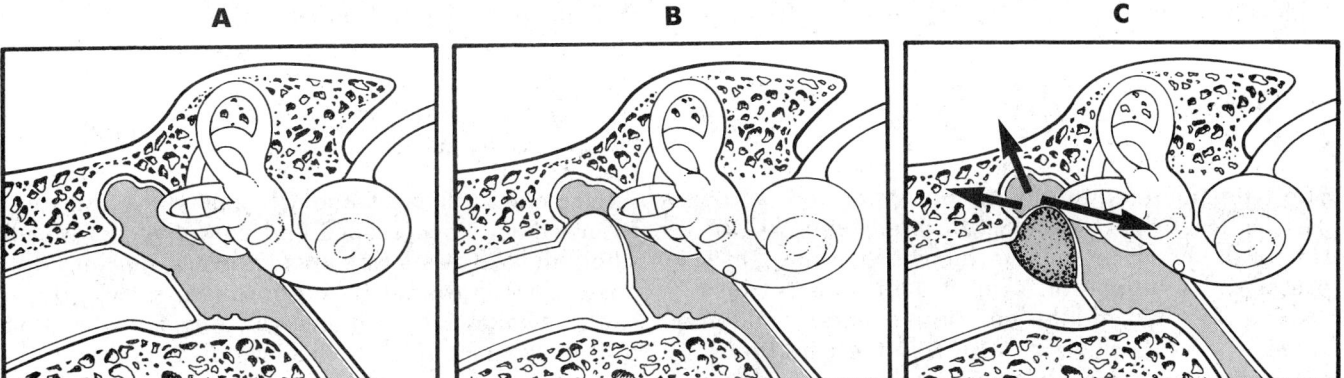

FIGURE 55-9   Development of cholesteatoma as complication of middle ear disorders. Conditions affecting eustachian tube **(A)** interfere with middle ear ventilation, resulting in persistent negative pressure in cavity; superior retraction pockets in tympanic membrane lead to distortion and retraction **(B)**; distorted membrane produces cholesteatoma **(C)**, which can erode into adjacent structures of ear *(arrows).*

Pathophysiology

Tympanosclerosis comprises the sclerotic changes seen in the tympanic membrane and middle ear mucosa as sequelae of middle ear infections. Chalky white plaques are seen on the tympanic membrane, indicating a slowly progressive problem that may result in sclerotic changes in the ossicles later in life. When the ossicles become involved, surgical removal and reconstruction are the treatment of choice.

Clinical Manifestations

Otosclerosis is bilateral in 80% of patients. The formation of new bone begins in the second or third decade of life but does not cause hearing loss until after the fourth decade. Approximately 10% of the population will have this condition. Because of the vascular and bony changes in the middle ear, the tympanic membrane takes on a pinkish orange color (Schwartz's sign). The Rinne test favors bone conduction, whereas the Weber test lateralizes to the ear with the greatest conductive hearing loss. Stapedectomy with replacement of the stapes or use of a hearing aid is the treatment for otosclerosis. Usually a hearing loss of 40 dB will prompt an individual to seek medical attention. Stapedectomy with a stapes prosthesis carries a small risk of permanent sensorineural hearing loss on the affected side. The physician and patient decide together which type of treatment the patient should receive.

Therapeutic Management

A **myringoplasty** is the reconstructive repair of the tympanic membrane perforation. A graft is taken from the temporal muscle behind the ear or from tissue of the external ear. The graft is placed over the tympanum after Gelfoam (which is absorbed) is inserted into the middle ear. The graft may rest on the malleus, on the long process of the incus, or on the head of the stapes, depending on the condition of the middle ear. Cotton balls are placed in the external ear canal.

A tympanoplasty is the surgical removal of the diseased tissue and reconstruction of the middle ear ossicles, if necessary. The incision may be postauricular (behind the ear) or endaural (around the tympanum). Plastic, ceramic, or human bone replacements may be used for reconstruction. A myringoplasty usually is performed with the tympanoplasty.

A mastoidectomy involves incision, drainage, and surgical removal of the mastoid process. A simple mastoidectomy is considered a closed mastoidectomy, because it is done through the ear with a tympanoplasty. A radical mastoidectomy and a modified radical mastoidectomy are considered open mastoidectomies, because they exteriorize the mastoid cavity to the external ear canal. A radical mastoidectomy is performed only when a modified or simple mastoidectomy will not excise the tumor and preserving hearing is a secondary consideration. A radical mastoidectomy and a modified radical mastoidectomy can also be performed with a tympanoplasty.

TRAUMA
Definition/Etiology

The tympanic membrane can be perforated or the ossicles fractured by a blast, a blunt injury to the side of the head, or sudden changes in atmospheric pressure. A temporal skull fracture can cause trauma to the middle and inner ears. Sudden changes in atmospheric pressure in the ears (barotrauma) occur during airplane takeoffs and landings, heavy-weight lifting, and scuba diving. With simple barotrauma such as occurs with airplane flights, the eustachian tube does not ventilate and a negative pressure develops in the middle ear. Pain and conductive hearing loss result. Drinking, swallowing, chewing, and using Valsalva's maneuver (holding the nostrils shut, keeping the mouth closed, and gently trying to blow) are remedies for simple flight barotrauma.

Barotrauma from scuba diving is increasing, since more than 3 million people in the United States pursue the sport each year. Barotrauma is the result of an inability to equalize the air pressure of the ear with the environment. It can occur on descent or ascent. Barotrauma of descent can occur in the external meatus if it is blocked with cerumen or if the diver wears an overly tight wet suit hood or earplugs. In such cases air is trapped in the external ear and is not replaced by water as the diver submerges. As the ambient pressure increases and the pressure in the middle ear equilibrates by way of the eustachian tube, a negative pressure develops in the blocked ear. This can result in edema, hemorrhage, or rupture of the tympanic membrane. The most common type of barotrauma in scuba divers results when the middle ear fails to equalize to the surrounding environment because of an occlusion or dysfunction of the eustachian tube. Pain, edema, and hemorrhage occur and in most cases prevent the diver from descending any farther. If the diver disregards these signals, the tympanic membrane can rupture, causing severe vertigo, nausea, and disorientation; these in turn can cause drowning or cerebral air embolism from overly rapid ascent. Scuba divers are taught to be aware of these dangers. Barotrauma can also occur in springboard divers descending 6 to 8 feet while wearing earplugs.

Clinical Manifestations

Trauma of the middle ear usually causes mild or severe pain. Barotrauma from scuba diving can cause symptoms of fullness of the ears, pain, decreased hearing, vertigo, nausea, disorientation, edema of the affected area, and hemorrhage in the external or middle ear. In severe cases cerebral air embolism from overly rapid ascent can occur.

Therapeutic Management

Management of barotrauma begins with education to prevent its occurrence and compliance with all safety measures specifically for divers. For airplane passengers bothered by barotrauma, sucking hard candy, swallowing, drinking, yawning, chewing, and Valsalva's maneuver may relieve discomfort.

NURSING MANAGEMENT OF THE PATIENT WITH DISORDERS OF MIDDLE EAR, TYMPANIC MEMBRANE, AND MASTOID
Assessment

Data are collected about the presence of pain; its location, onset, duration, and severity; and factors that relieve it. The external ear is assessed for shape, foreign bodies, lacerations, and color. If palpating the external ear causes pain, the problem probably stems from the external ear and not the middle ear or mastoid process. The mastoid process is palpated for tenderness. Pain in this area can be caused by an infection, pressure from a growth, or fluid in the ear.

A loss of hearing may be noted. Frequently, blockage from fluid, growths, or pressure on the tympanic membrane causes conductive hearing loss. Ossicle dysfunction related to sclerosis also causes hearing loss. The nurse can assess for hearing loss by using the Weber and Rinne tests as well as gross hearing evaluations such as the watch or voice test.

An otoscopic examination is performed. The external ear is examined first. Then the ear canal is inspected for wax and irritations using the largest comfortable earpiece; the tympanic membrane is then assessed for color, bulging, bony landmarks, drainage, and light reflexes.

Nursing Diagnosis

Nursing diagnoses that may apply to patients with middle ear and mastoid problems include the following:

Chronic pain related to recurrent infections

Fear (of permanent hearing loss) related to lack of information

Pain related to fluid accumulation in the middle ear

High risk for injury related to impaired equilibrium

Sensory/perceptual alterations (auditory) related to blockage in the middle ear

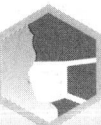

PREOPERATIVE AND POSTOPERATIVE NURSING INTERVENTIONS

Ear Surgery

Preoperative care

1. Relieving fear and increasing understanding of the surgery are two important areas for the nurse to communicate with the patient. Explain the type of anesthesia, whether local or general, to be used.
2. Explain any pain involved in the surgery and whether pain can be expected after surgery. Discuss the use of pain relief medication postoperatively.
3. For any invasive procedure a consent form is signed by the patient and a witness (usually the nurse or physician) (see discussion of informed consent, Chapter 9).
4. The physiologic status of the patient (blood pressure, pulse, respiration, and temperature) is recorded as a baseline for after surgery.
5. If admitted to the hospital for surgery, the patient should be informed of the average stay for his or her type of surgery and what immediate postoperative care will entail.
6. Patients having surgery (such as mastoid) in which bleeding can occur should be told not to take any aspirin or any other medication that prolongs bleeding for at least 1 week before surgery. A single dose of acetylsalicylic acid approximately doubles the bleeding time for 4 to 7 days. The patient who is taking anticoagulants should check with his or her medical physician who should communicate precautions to the surgeon.
7. All patients having ear surgery should understand postoperative home care and precautions if any. The better understanding the patient has of the surgery and postoperative care, the less fear and anxiety will be seen.
8. The patient should understand that surgery will not always correct the impaired hearing.

Postoperative teaching

For minor surgery performed with the patient under local anesthesia, the patient may go home within 1 hour after the surgery is performed. Postoperative teaching and care include the following:

1. Minor pain or discomfort can be expected after even minor surgery. The surgeon generally gives the patient a prescription for pain. Explain how to take the medication or any other intervention before the patient is discharged.
2. If a dressing is applied to the surgical ear, hearing may be decreased in that ear because of the occlusive dressing.
3. The patient's postoperative vital signs should be within the parameters of the presurgical baseline before the patient is allowed to go home.

4. Another person should drive the patient home in case he or she develops vertigo from the manipulation of the ear.
5. If tubes have been inserted, avoid getting water in the ears. This includes showering, washing the hair, and swimming. Usually washing of the hair is delayed for 1 week after surgery. A shower cap or earplug may be worn for prevention. Swimming is avoided until complete healing, removal of tubes, or when physician gives permission.
6. Explain to the patient about bleeding or drainage and when to seek medical advice if they occur. If a cotton plug is prescribed, it should be changed daily. Teacher includes washing the hands before- and after touching the ear to prevent spread of infections.
7. Teach how to blow the nose, namely, by blowing very gently one side at a time for at least 1 week after the surgery. The patient should sneeze or cough with the mouth open. These procedures will cause less pressure in the nasal cavity, with less pressure in the eustachian tube and ear.
8. Explain the need to avoid air travel for a least 1 week after surgery.
9. Arrange for a follow-up appointment to see the physician for assessment after surgery.
10. Depending on the type of surgery done, the patient may return to work within a few days or if work is strenuous in several weeks.

Additional patient teaching and care for patients with general anesthesia include the following:

1. The patient will lie on the *unoperated* side for approximately 4 hours after surgery.
2. Hearing may be decreased because of swelling inside the ear as well as the occlusive dressing.
3. The patient may experience popping or cracking noises in the ears from the trauma of the surgery.
4. The nurse observes for all general postoperative complications associated with general anesthesia.
5. Most pain with ear surgery is minor, but the patient should be instructed to ask for medication when in pain.
6. Teach the patient to report any dizziness or light-headedness after surgery. The most likely time for these occurrences is the first time out of bed after surgery. Patient will require assistance at least the first day after surgery in ambulating to prevent falling. Some patients may experience nystagmus (to and fro movements of the eye that can produce dizziness) if the inner ear was manipulated. Rarely does the dizziness, light-headedness, or nystagmus require medication. Usually the symptoms are self-limiting and pass quickly.

Continued.

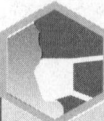

PREOPERATIVE AND POSTOPERATIVE NURSING INTERVENTIONS—cont'd

7. The patient may have adapted to hearing diminished sounds before the surgery was performed, so now postsurgery sounds may be intolerably loud. Explain to the patient that tolerance of normal sounds soon returns.
8. A large bulky dressing is often used following a mastoidectomy and left in place for 5 to 7 days. Teach the patient to leave the dressing on and return to the physician's office for removal.
9. Because of the proximity of the facial nerve (cranial nerve VII) and the middle and inner ear, the nurse needs to assess the patient's face for paralysis, sagging, drooping of the mouth, drooling, or the inability to close the eyelid on the operative side. As soon after surgery as the patient is able he or she should be asked to wrinkle the forehead, stick out the tongue, and show the teeth, all of which will ascertain if the facial nerve has been damaged. If nerve damage is present, further surgery will be done within hours to repair the damaged nerve. If the above symptoms occur several days after surgery, they are probably the result of swelling and will disappear when the swelling decreases.
10. The nurse may administer antiemetics for nausea or vomiting, analgesics for pain, and antibiotics for prevention of infection.

Planning

Specific goals for patients with problems of the middle ear, tympanic membrane, and mastoid process include the following:

Hearing returns to preillness state

Pain decreases or is alleviated

Patient can describe the symptoms of the problem and knows when to consult the physician

Patient can state the rationale and desired outcome of any impending surgery

Patient can describe and perform any procedures necessary to maintain wellness of the middle ear, tympanic membrane, and mastoid process

Patient can describe methods for preventing problems in the middle ear, tympanic membrane, and mastoid process

Implementation

Most problems of the middle ear, tympanic membrane, or mastoid process are treated in the physician's office, clinic, or outpatient surgical facility. When a patient is admitted to the hospital, it is usually because previous treatment was ineffective or because the patient has a number of health risks that need observation during treatment. Surgical interventions may require a stay ranging from overnight to 3 days.

Oral antibiotics and analgesics are prescribed by the physician for infections and pain of the middle ear. Eardrops and ointment may also be prescribed. The patient must understand all instructions related to frequency, amount, and duration of the medication. The nurse demonstrates the correct procedure for instillation of drops or ointment before the patient leaves. The patient or significant other should return the demonstration.

Many times preoperative teaching and care are done immediately before surgery, since the surgery may be performed at the time of initial examination by the physician. The surgery may be very minor and take only a few minutes or be major with the risk of loss of hearing involved. Postoperative care may take only a few minutes or several days. Refer to "Preoperative and Postoperative Nursing Interventions" for specific teaching and care.

Evaluation

The goals of middle ear therapies are to improve hearing, control infection, and improve the quality of life. The nursing interventions are evaluated with the goal for that patient in mind. Patient teaching is also important. For example, the nurse can evaluate patient teaching by observing the patient instill eardrops or successfully perform a procedure. Middle ear infections tend to recur, making it imperative that the patient be taught preventive measures, as well as the signs and symptoms of infection.

Inner Ear Disorders

INFECTION
Definition/Etiology

Labyrinthitis is an infection or inflammation of the inner ear that involves the cochlear and/or vestibular portion of the labyrinth. The infecting agent, either bacterial or viral, can enter the inner ear from the meninges, middle ear, or bloodstream.

Pathophysiology

The two types of acute labyrinthitis are serous and diffuse suppurative labyrinthitis. Serous labyrinthitis usually produces little or no hearing loss. It sometimes follows an overindulgence in alcohol or drug intoxication or is caused by an allergy. It usually is a nonpurulent inflammation showing cellular infiltration with a serous or serofibrinous exudate. Diffuse suppurative labyrinthitis occurs when an acute or chronic otitis media gains entrance to the labyrinth through the round or oval windows or through an erosion of the bony capsule. It also can occur after middle ear or mastoid surgery. In this type of labyrinthitis there is infiltration of polymorphonuclear leukocytes combined with destruction of the soft tissue structures. This causes total, permanent hearing loss. Chronic labyrinthitis can develop after an acute bout of labyrinthitis. The internal ear is filled with granulations that begin to change into fibrous tissue and then calcify as new bone in the labyrinth space. This process takes 6 months to several years and occurs in about 50% of chronic cases. When it occurs, complete deafness results.

Vestibular neuronitis, an inflammation of the auricular nerve, usually is caused by a virus, and no hearing loss results. The condition develops suddenly with the loss of vestibular function.

Clinical Manifestations

The three classical symptoms of labyrinthitis are spontaneous and rotational vertigo, tinnitus, and sensorineural hearing loss. Vertigo or dizziness is manifested when the vestibular structures are involved and causes problems with balance and equilibrium. When tinnitus occurs, the infection is located in the cochlea. Sensorineural hearing loss can be caused by infections in either the cochlear or vestibular structure. Another common symptom is nystagmus toward the affected side or an abnormal jerking, rhythmic, horizontal movement of the eye. The nystagmus is caused by the abnormal current flow in the endolymph fluid. Vertical nystagmus is found with brainstem disease rather than with labyrinthitis. Other symptoms of labyrinthitis include pain, fever, ataxia, nausea, and vomiting. Beginning nerve deafness may accompany labyrinthitis.

Therapeutic Management

The antibiotics mentioned under middle ear infections are used for inner ear infections as well. Viral infections do not respond to antibiotics but fortunately are short lived and run their course in 1 week. Patients are placed on bed rest for 1 to 6 weeks and instructed to avoid turning the head quickly, which should alleviate the vertigo. Mild sedation (e.g., phenobarbital, 32 mg three times per day) may be indicated to help relax the patient. There is no specific medicine for dizziness, but labyrinthine suppressants and antihistamines may help. If the structure or the nerve has been damaged, permanent hearing loss develops. The patient should have a thorough hearing evaluation by an audiologist to determine if a hearing device would improve hearing quality.

NEOPLASTIC DISORDERS
Definition/Etiology

Tumors of the inner ear can be benign or malignant. The most common benign tumor is the **acoustic neuroma** (also called acoustic neurilemoma), which arises from the neurilemmal sheath of the vestibular branch of the eighth cranial nerve. Acoustic neuromas usually are found in the auditory canal or in the area of the cerebellopontine angle. The tumor spreads to the cochlear branch of the eighth cranial nerve and compresses the nerve and adjacent structures. If unchecked such tumors can become life threatening, since they usually invade the facial and trigeminal nerves, the cerebellum, and the brainstem.

Pathophysiology

It is fortunate that malignant tumors arising from the inner ear are rare. Squamous and basal cell carcinoma may occur from the epidermal lining of the inner ear. Another malignant tumor is the glomus jugulare tumor, which is highly vascular and slow growing. Symptoms arise from these tumors after they have grown large enough to impinge on surrounding vital tissue. Without treatment, metastasis to the temporal bone and brain is common because of the proximity of these structures.

Clinical Manifestations

An acoustic neuroma grows slowly, can occur at any age, and usually is unilateral; the cause is unknown. Progressive unilateral sensorineural hearing loss of high-pitched sounds, unilateral tinnitus, and intermittent vertigo are early symptoms. Early diagnosis is important, because the neuroma can compress the facial nerve and arteries in the internal auditory canal. If the tumor expands into the cerebellopontine angle and compresses the fifth and seventh cranial nerves (trigeminal and facial), symptoms include loss of taste in the anterior two thirds of the tongue, absence of the ipsilateral corneal reflex, trigeminal pain, and facial hyperesthesia. If the tumor goes unchecked, nystagmus and ataxia develop. Papilledema, caused by cerebellar pressure, is a late symptom. Most malignant tumors grow quickly, and the symptoms vary depending on the area of the inner ear involved. Unchecked, the tumor spreads to the surrounding area and to the brain. Neuromas are diagnosed through neurologic, audiometric, and vestibular testing. Examination of the cerebrospinal fluid shows increased protein. A computed tomography (CT) scan will show a tumor larger than 2 cm.

Therapeutic Management

Treatment of an acoustic neuroma involves surgical removal if possible. The preferred method is a postauricular incision through the labyrinth, which is destroyed. Hearing loss is permanent in the affected ear. The facial nerve is saved if possible. If the tumor is smaller than 2 cm, gamma knife radiation may be the treatment of choice. A cranial approach may be used if the tumor is large. Steroids or radiation may be used to try to decrease the size of the tumor in patients who cannot withstand surgery or who have inoperable tumors.

MOTION SICKNESS
Definition/Etiology

Since the early 1960s, most researchers have accepted the sensory conflict theory (also called the sensory rearrangement theory) about motion sickness, which is based on the premise that the changing of the velocity/motion information signaled by the vestibular apparatus is different from what the body had expected. The main structures in the inner ear that affect the individual's response to motion are the semicircular canals and the otoliths (concentrations of calcium deposits on the membranous labyrinth of the ear). With motion sickness these structures are disturbed in some way, but exactly how is unknown. A person must have an intact vestibular apparatus to experience motion sickness. Motion sickness affects approximately 90% of the U.S. population at one time or another.

Clinical Manifestations

The signs and symptoms of motion sickness vary but include nausea, vomiting, headache, dizziness, pallor, abdominal cramps, diaphoresis, and yawning. Women are more susceptible than men, and the disorder is uncommon after 50 years of age. For many people the symptoms of motion sickness are severe and recurrent.

Therapeutic Management

For an individual susceptible to motion sickness, prevention is the best recourse. A variety of medications can be used prophylactically, including dimenhydrinate (Dramamine), scopolamine (Transderm-Scop), prochlorperazine (Compazine), promethazine (Phenergan), and meclizine (Antivert, Bonine). The newest device, Transderm-Scop, is a small patch that is worn behind the ear and lasts 3 days. When taking medication prophylactically, the patient should start the drug at least 1 hour before the motion begins. All such drugs have the side effects of drowsiness, dry mouth, blurred vision, headache, decreased alertness, and mood changes. Caution should be taken when driving a motor vehicle and taking any of these drugs.

BAROTRAUMA
Definition/Etiology

Barotrauma of the inner ear can cause rupture of the round or oval window or both, producing a perilymph fistula. The round window is commonly ruptured in diving accidents when an inadequate equilibration of pressure in the middle ear develops. This can occur with sudden excess pressure in the inner ear or with a forceful Valsalva maneuver that suddenly increases the cerebrospinal fluid pressure, exerting pressure on the perilymph and causing an outward explosion of the round window. Barotrauma can also occur when a subluxation of the stapes foot plate occurs as the result of an inward displacement of the eardrum and ossicles. Regardless of the cause of the rupture, leakage of the perilymph can result in permanent cochlear damage and hearing loss if not promptly recognized and treated.

Clinical Manifestations

The classical triad of sensorineural hearing loss, tinnitus, and vertigo comprises the symptoms of inner ear barotrauma. Not all individuals experience the three symptoms; the one most people experience first is vertigo. Other symptoms include a feeling of fullness in the affected ear, nausea, vomiting, disorientation, and ataxia. Weight lifters are also susceptible to rupturing their oval windows. Many people are not aware that they have suffered a hearing loss from barotrauma until their hearing is tested. Many times the degree of hearing loss varies between ears.

Therapeutic Management

The choice of treatment for perilymph fistulas is controversial. Some physicians feel that prompt surgical treatment to repair the rupture in the oval or round window is the treatment of choice. Some otolaryngologists recommend an initial 2- to 3-day trial of bed rest and symptomatic treatment for vertigo to see whether the leak will heal without surgery. Whichever method is chosen, a complete otologic evaluation is done before and after treatment.

MÉNIÈRE'S DISEASE
Definition/Etiology

Ménière's disease is also called idiopathic labyrinthine hydrops or endolymphatic hydrops. The earliest finding in Ménière's disease is dilation of the scala media of the cochlea and the saccule, as evidenced by the stretching of Reissner's membrane. This can lead to herniation and rupture of the membranous labyrinth. Ménière's disease usually develops between 40 and 60 years of age and affects, in varying degrees, 5 of every 100 individuals. The symptoms range from vague and nondebilitating to severe.

Pathophysiology

The dilation is a result of a disturbance in the fluid physiology of the endolymphatic system, but the cause of this disturbance is unknown. It has yet to be determined whether the problem stems from hypersecretion, hypoabsorption, disturbance of the balance between hyposecretion and hypoabsorption, deficit of membrane permeability, alteration of osmotic pressure relationships, allergy, hormonal imbalance, altered carbohydrate metabolism, excess body fatty acids, or mental stress.

Clinical Manifestations

Attacks may be preceded by a feeling of fullness in the ear or by tinnitus. The three characteristic symptoms of Ménière's disease are tinnitus, sensorineural hearing loss on the involved side, and severe vertigo accompanied by nausea and vomiting. The hearing loss may not be detected during an acute attack because of the overriding, loud, roaring tinnitus. The tinnitus may be high or low pitched but is most commonly low pitched. The hearing loss is described as fluctuating with a sensation of fullness.

The patient may require hospitalization during an acute exacerbation of the disease. The vertigo lasts 2 to 4 hours and then subsides, followed by several hours of dizziness and unsteadiness. When the initial attack of vertigo begins, the patient typically feels as if the surroundings are whirling around. This is followed by an episode of light-headedness. The dizziness that follows is felt as light-headedness. The patient is uncoordinated and changes gait when walking. The hearing loss fluctuates, and tinnitus is present. Personality changes such as irritability, depression, and withdrawal are common. The blood pressure, temperature, pulse, and respirations usually are normal. It usually is several weeks before all symptoms subside, leaving a loss of hearing in the involved ear.

After the acute phase, remission occurs, but the symptoms will recur with two or three acute attacks per year. As this pattern of attacks and remissions develops, fewer symptoms occur during the acute phase. This is because of the gradual loss of end-organ responsiveness caused by degeneration of the sensory elements. A complete remission eventually occurs with some degree of hearing loss (varying from slight to complete) and any damage that may have occurred during treatment.

Therapeutic Management

Diagnostic tests are completed to rule out any central nervous system problems and to affirm the diagnosis of Ménière's disease. Audiometric studies such as speech discrimination, tone quality, and loudness determine loss of low-pitched tone. The Bárány caloric test measures vestibular function. An audiologist may perform an electrocochleograph, in which an electrode is passed through the tympanic membrane and sound is measured. A neurologic test and x-rays of the internal ear are indicated to rule out other problems.

Medical intervention during the acute phase includes using atropine or diazepam (Valium) to decrease the autonomic nervous system function, diphenhydramine (Benadryl) for its antihistamine effect, and vasodilators. The patient's safety when walking, sitting, or standing is paramount. The patient needs reassurance that the symptoms will pass and that they are not caused by a cerebral dysfunction.

Management during remission includes any of the following medications: diuretics to decrease the fluid (and thereby decrease pressure in the endolymph), antihistamines, vasodilators (such as nicotinic acid and histamine), vitamins, diazepam (Valium), and meclizine. A low-salt diet (Furstenberg) is prescribed to reduce fluid. Most patients respond to this medical protocol but need to be taught to expect an acute attack at unpredictable times. The major goal in treatment is to preserve the patient's hearing, and careful medical management helps achieve this in most patients with Ménière's disease.

When the medical regimen is not successful, surgical intervention may be necessary to reduce the severe dizziness and vertigo. When involvement is unilateral, labyrinthectomy (surgical removal of the labyrinth) is performed, causing complete loss of cochlear and vestibular function in that ear. Surgical decompression of the endolymphatic sac (endolymphatic-subarachnoid shunt) may be helpful to decrease the pressure on the hair cells in the cochlea and to prevent future sensorineural hearing loss.

NURSING MANAGEMENT OF THE PATIENT WITH DISORDERS OF THE INNER EAR

Assessment

Data are collected about gross hearing, high- and low-pitched hearing loss, and results of the Weber and Rinne tests. A complete physical examination, including a neurologic examination, is necessary to evaluate the patient's symptoms. The physician will order specific diagnostic tests to evaluate inner ear function.

Dizziness is a symptom frequently encountered with inner ear dysfunctions. It may be described as a whirling sensation, light-headedness, imbalance, unsteadiness, or veering to one side when walking. Often it is accompanied by nausea and vomiting. On assessment the nurse may need to interview the family to fully evaluate the effect of the patient's dizziness and any triggering factors. Laboratory tests for sodium, potassium, and glucose levels must be reviewed to ascertain if the dizziness is related to an electrolyte imbalance, dehydration, or diabetes. The nurse must be aware that dizziness may be aggravated by anxiety, fear of the unknown, and depression. The nurse's calm, self-confident, gentle manner helps achieve an accurate assessment of dizziness.

Sensorineural hearing loss is found in approximately 90% of individuals over 65 years of age who have been diagnosed as having a hearing deficit. Such hearing loss has a tremendous impact on the individual's job and social life. Whether through vanity, fear, misinformation, or lack of knowledge, many people do not seek medical attention for their hearing loss. The nurse needs to assess the sensorineural hearing loss through history, physical examination, and audiometry. The Weber and Rinne tests can be done initially, with more refined audiometry tests performed later to determine the exact degree of hearing loss.

The patient may have difficulty pinpointing when the hearing loss began. Many times it is insidious in onset, and other family members note the loss before the patient does. Careful assessment by the nurse should reveal a clear picture of the sensorineural loss.

Nursing Diagnosis

Nursing diagnoses germane to a patient with disorders of the inner ear include the following:

Altered role performance related to impaired equilibrium

Anxiety related to sudden/severe onset of symptoms and unpredictability of attacks

Body image disturbance related to decreased hearing

Fear related to potential permanent hearing loss

Impaired verbal communication related to temporary or permanent hearing loss

Ineffective individual coping related to knowledge deficit

Personal identity disturbance related to hearing loss

High risk for injury related to dizziness

Self-esteem disturbance related to loss of hearing

Sensory/perceptual alteration (auditory) related to sensorineural hearing loss

Social isolation related to sensorineural hearing loss and experiencing an attack in public

Planning

Specific goals include the following:

Patient acknowledges that he or she has a hearing deficit

Patient can describe the signs and symptoms of his or her specific problem and is aware of any triggering mechanisms that aggravate the problem

Patient can state the desired effect of medications and the common side effects

Patient can demonstrate proper use of his or her hearing aid (if appropriate) and states that the aid has enabled him or her to hear more clearly and easily

Implementation

Communication and the use of hearing aids with the hearing-impaired patient were covered at the beginning of this chapter. (Refer to that section for information about working with a hearing-impaired patient.)

Beside hearing aids, aural rehabilitation may include several other modalities. A licensed audiologist may implement auditory training. In auditory training a hearing-impaired patient is exposed to great differences in sound. When the patient has good discrimination of these sounds, the sounds are fine tuned, with less difference between the sounds. The patient relearns to discriminate sounds and can concentrate on the spoken voice (such as when listening to a person). Some patients will be able to discriminate only gross sounds and will never reach the fine-tuned stage.

Emphasize the importance of complying with the prescribed treatment because of the real possibility of hearing loss. When an antibiotic is prescribed, all the medication should be taken, not just the amount required until the patient feels better. Acute problems can become chronic, and then the chances of hearing loss are much greater.

In Ménière's disease, teaching the patient about the disease adds to his or her knowledge and under-

NURSING CARE PLAN   *Ménière's Disease*

Nursing diagnosis/ Expected outcome	Interventions	Rationale
Knowledge deficit related to course and treatment of the symptoms • *The patient can describe the acute and remission phases of the disease and the treatment of symptoms*	Teach the patient not to drink excessive fluids	With the increased volume of endolymph, excessive fluid intake increases the volume even more
	Teach the patient to avoid sodium and foods prepared and served with salt	Excessive sodium in the body retains water, thus increasing the endolymph, which aggravates the symptoms and changes of hearing loss Maintaining a salt-restricted diet should relieve the fullness and pressure felt in the ear and limit future attacks
	Encourage protein in the diet, such as milk, eggs, fish, and poultry	The Furstenberg diet encourages eating protein in these forms
	Help the patient identify any prodromal symptoms that may occur	If the patient knows the prodromal symptoms, injuries can be lessened when they occur; the patient can assume a comfortable position, such as sitting down, and, if driving, the patient can pull over to the side of the road and can begin medication to lessen the dizziness and vertigo
	Encourage the patient to avoid jerking movements	Sudden jerking movements, such as a carnival ride, could precipitate an acute attack
High risk for injury related to dizziness and vertigo • *Patient is safe from injury*	During an acute attack, encourage patient to stay in bed and to keep siderails up, even at home	Safety should be the highest priority for the patient; siderails will remind the patient not to get out of bed without help
	Instruct the patient to call for assistance before ambulating; keep the call light within reach	Dizziness and vertigo cause great difficulty when ambulating; support often is necessary to prevent falling
	Hold the patient securely when ambulating during periods of dizziness	This reassures the patient and provides extra support if weakness occurs
	Administer antivertiginous drugs such as meclizine (Antivert, Bonine), dimenhydrinate (Dramamine), or diphenhydramine (Benadryl) during times of dizziness	Antivertiginous drugs reduce indirect stimulation of the vomiting center and/or reduce dopamine, which acts as a mediator to induce vomiting Antihistamines inhibit tissue edema
	Administer vasodilators with histamine phosphate for vertigo	Vasodilators reduce vasoconstriction and control vasospasms
	Administer diuretics as ordered	Diuretics may be ordered to reduce or decrease production of endolymph; Chlorothiazide (Diuril) is commonly used

Continued.

NURSING CARE PLAN   *Ménière's Disease—cont'd*

Nursing diagnosis/ Expected outcome	Interventions	Rationale
Pain related to dizziness and severe vertigo	Allow patient to assume a comfortable position	Usually a recumbent position with head elevated on one pillow is comfortable
• *Dizziness and vertigo dissipate*	Prevent loud ring and sudden jarring	Loud noises and sudden jarring may precipitate an acute attack; during an attack noises and jarring increase dizziness and vertigo and may cause nausea, vomiting, and headache
	Do not move the patient without telling him or her	Anticipation of movement and allowing the patient to move slowly help prevent increased dizziness and vertigo
	Have emesis basin and protective drape close to patient	Most patients have nausea and vomiting with acute attacks; equipment is ready if needed
Sensory/perceptual alteration (auditory) related to course of disease	Restrict smoking and alcohol	Smoking and alcohol can precipitate an acute attack; they act as vasoconstrictors and can decrease the absorption of endolymph
• *Sensory/perceptual alterations are kept to a minimum*	Restrict fluid and maintain a low-salt diet	See knowledge deficit diagnosis
	Explain any surgical intervention designated by the physician	The membranous labyrinth may need to be removed or destroyed in the future to eliminate severe vertigo
		The patient should understand that hearing is destroyed in the ear undergoing surgery
Social withdrawal related to unpredictability of attacks	Administer antivertiginous and/or vasodilators as prescribed	Drugs administered early may decrease severity of attack
• *Patient will express early symptoms of attacks*	Provide professional counseling services for patient and family	Professional counseling will help patient and family understand the social and emotional aspects of the disease

standing of why treatment is important. The patient should be helped to identify any prodromal symptoms, so he or she can seek help and protect oneself from injury. The patient should know what actions to take at the sudden onset of symptoms. (See the nursing care plan for Ménière's disease for specific nursing management.) If surgery is performed on the inner ear, patient teaching before and after surgery is similar to that for middle ear surgery.

Evaluation

The specific patient goals are evaluated, and if the goals have not been achieved, the need for other or continual interventions must be considered. Hearing acuity is rechecked after treatment if a hearing loss was part of the patient's problem. The patient's ability to describe measures to prevent hearing loss or to conserve hearing should be evaluated.

CRITICAL THINKING QUESTIONS

1 You have been asked to teach a class on ways to decrease noise pollution in the home, hospital, and community. What would you include?

2 As a person ages, hearing quality changes. Describe these changes and what, if anything, can be done about them.

3 What type of hearing-impaired individuals may be helped by a hearing aid? a cochlear implant? How would you teach a patient to keep his or her hearing aid in working order?

4 What similar problems occur in the inner, middle, and outer ear? List various problems that occur only in one particular area of the ear.

5 What procedure or procedures might the nurse use to remove hardened earwax? to remove a foreign body from the ear?

6 What procedure might the nurse use to keep the ear clean (routine cleaning)?

7 What clinical finding and nursing interventions would be used with a patient with a diagnosis of cholesteatoma?

8 What clinical finding and nursing interventions would be used with a patient with a diagnosis of otitis media? otitis media with effusion? otitis media without effusion? acute otitis media?

9 Why is vertigo commonly a symptom of an inner ear problem?

10 What would you teach a patient newly diagnosed with Ménière's disease about home care?

RESOURCES

1 AMERICAN SPEECH, LANGUAGE AND HEARING ASSOCIATION 10801 Rockville Pike Rockville, MD 20852 (301) 897-5700
Operates a hot line under the name the National Association for Hearing and Speech Action. In most states the call is toll free: (800) 638-TALK; however, in Alaska, Hawaii, and Maryland a collect call is necessary: (301) 897-8682. The organization provides information about cochlear implants and where such surgery is performed.

2 AMERICAN TINNITUS ASSOCIATION PO Box 5 Portland, OR 97207 (503) 248-9985
Assists local self-help groups with issues concerning tinnitus.

3 ALEXANDER GRAHAM BELL ASSOCIATION FOR THE DEAF 3417 Volta Place, NW Washington, DC 20007 (202) 337-5220 (voice/TDD)

Has audiovisual materials and a lending library for members and publishes an annual monograph.

4 NATIONAL ASSOCIATION OF THE DEAF 814 Thayer Ave Silver Spring, MD 20910 (301) 587-1788
Has local chapters across the United States; provides information about hearing and offers individual support.

5 NATIONAL HEARING AID SOCIETY HELPLINE 9 AM to 5 PM (800) 368-5779 nationwide; (292) 472-4222 in Washington DC, Maryland, and Virginia
Hot line provides consumer information on hearing aids and names of local dealers.

6 OFFICE OF OCCUPATIONAL MEDICINE Occupational Safety and Health Administration Raymond Kunicki Room N-3653 200 Constitution Ave NW Washington, DC 20210
Office of US government that regulates OSHA's policies.

7 REGISTRY OF INTERPRETERS FOR THE DEAF PO Box 1339 Washington, DC 20013 (301) 588-2406
Provides names of individuals who can interpret for the deaf.

BIBLIOGRAPHY

Current

1. Brinkmann K: Why can't your patient hear you? *RN* 54:1, 1991.
2. Campbell C: Acoustic neuroma: nursing implications related to surgical management, *J Neurosci Nurs* 23:1, 1991.
3. Cassvan A et al: Brainstem auditory evoked potential studies in patient with tinnitus and/or vertigo, *Arch Phys Med Rehabil* 71:8, 1990.
4. Christian E, Dluhy N, O'Nell R: Sounds of silence, *J Gerontol Nurs* 15:11, 1989.
5. Cleveland P, Morris J: Meniere's disease, *RN* 53:8, 1990.
6. Cunningham D, Ganzel T: Hearing aids: how they work and whom they help, *Hosp Med* 27:70, 1991.
7. Erickson R, Yount S: Comparison of tympanic and oral temperatures in surgical patients, *Nurs Res* 40:2, 1991.
8. Ferrara-Love R: A comparison of tympanic and pulmonary artery measures of core temperatures, *J Postanesthesia Nurs* 6:3, 1991.
9. Fickel V: Acoustic neuroma: postoperative deficits and the role of the neuroscience nurse, *J Neurosci Nurs* 23:1, 1991.
10. Glavassevich M, Thomas S, Galloway S: An educational program to improve quality of life for individuals with an acoustic neuroma, *J Neurosci Nurs* 23:4, 1991.
11. Harrison RK: Hearing conservation, *AAOHN J* 37:4, 1989.
12. House J, Schleuning A: Putting a damper on tinnitus, *Patient Care* 25:7, 1991.
13. Morris MK: How to manage tissue donation, *Am J Nurs* 89:10, 1989.

14. Mulrow C: Screening for hearing impairment in the elderly, *Hosp Pract* 26:2A, 1991.
15. Olsen K, Schindles R, Vernick D: Earache in adults: sifting the clues, *Patient Care* 24:6, 1990.
16. Rye S: A confusion of sound, *Nurs Times* 86:37, 1990.
17. Schneiderman H, Garibaldi R: Physical examination of HIV-infected patients: head, neck, eyes, mouth, throat, and lymph nodes, *Consultant* 30:1, 1990.
18. Scura K: Audiological assessment program, *J Gerontol Nurs* 14:10, 1988.
19. Swan I, Tolson D: Facing up to deafness, *Nurs Times* 87:23, 1991.
20. Swan I, Tolson D: Hearing-aid clinics, *Nurs Times* 87:24, 1991.
21. Tolson D: Hearing aids, *Nurs Times* 87:18, 1991.
22. Val Palumbo M: Diving in trouble, *Emerg Med* 21:10, 1989.
23. Val Palumbo M: Hemotympanum with an intact skull, *Emerg Med* 21:5, 1989.
24. Val Palumbo M: Hearing access 2000: increasing awareness of the hearing impaired, *J Gerontol Nurs* 16:9, 1990.
25. Val Palumbo M: Tinnitus, *Patient Care* 25:7, 1991.

UNIT XIII

Musculoskeletal System

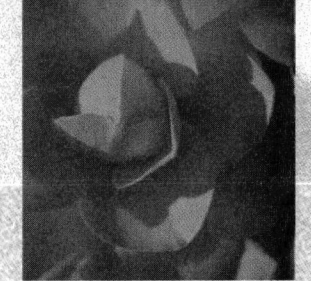

CHAPTER FIFTY-SIX

Nursing Assessment of the Musculoskeletal System

LEARNING OBJECTIVES

1 Know the main structural components of the musculoskeletal system and their functions.
2 Understand the sequence of events that produces muscle contraction and relaxation.
3 Obtain relevant subjective information from the patient who has a musculoskeletal alteration.
4 Using correct technique, examine the patient to obtain appropriate objective information about the musculoskeletal system.
5 Differentiate abnormal from normal subjective and objective findings related to the musculoskeletal system.
6 Describe tests and procedures used in the diagnosis of musculoskeletal disorders.
7 Describe the patient care that is necessary for each of the tests used to diagnose musculoskeletal disorders.

SUPPORT and movement are the main functions of the musculoskeletal system. However, the skeletal system also serves as a reservoir for ions such as calcium, magnesium, and phosphate, and its medullary cavity is the main site for the production of blood cells. The skeletal muscles, in addition to providing the force to move and support the body, close the external orifices of the gastrointestinal and urinary tracts and increase heat production when it is needed for temperature control.

Assessment of the musculoskeletal system primarily involves an examination of functional groups of muscles and joints. A review of other body systems—endocrine, neurologic, peripheral vascular, renal/urinary, and integumentary—is also important, however, because these may influence or reflect musculoskeletal alterations.

ANATOMY AND PHYSIOLOGY
Bones

Structure and function of a typical long bone

Bone is a connective tissue; consequently, it is made up of cells dispersed in a matrix of fibers and protein that is ossified with rock-hard crystals of calcium and magnesium phosphate and carbonate.

Bone stressed predominantly in one direction (e.g., in the shaft of a leg bone) is dense. In **dense bone,** the functional units of the bone, the haversian systems, lie parallel to each other in the direction of the force, and no cavities exist between each haversian system. Dense bone generally forms a cylinder around a large central medullary cavity, or it forms the outermost layer surrounding cancellous bone.

Each haversian system is shaped like a long column that contains a central canal enclosing a blood vessel. The column is made up of concentric cylinders (lamellae) of bone matrix with spider-shaped osteocytes embedded in small cavities (lacunae) between the lamellae (Figure 56-1). The osteocytes have extremely long protoplasmic connections to neighboring cells that pass through microscopic canaliculi in the bone. The canaliculi form the only route by which the cells receive oxygen and nutrition from and excrete waste products to the central canal. The isolation of osteocytes from the blood supply of the central canal is largely responsible for the slow repair of broken bones.

When bone is stressed in many different directions (e.g., at a joint), the forces are borne by *trabeculae* (bony struts) that are also organized in many directions and form a lattice of **cancellous** (spongy) **bone** surrounded by bone marrow (Figure 56-2). Compared with dense bone, a larger volume of cancellous bone is needed for strength; however, cancellous bone is better able to withstand forces applied from many directions. The trabeculae of spongy bone grow as lamellae are laid down around bony spurs and attach themselves to other trabeculae. As with haversian systems, osteocytes embedded between the lamellae of trabeculae receive their nutrition and oxygen by diffusion through the canaliculi. However, in cancellous bone, nutrients and oxygen must diffuse into the trabeculae from the blood vessels of the surrounding bone marrow cavity, because most trabeculae do not contain blood vessels.

Figure 56-2 shows the structure of a typical long bone. Bone growth in length is caused by growth and ossification of epiphyseal cartilage plates at the ends

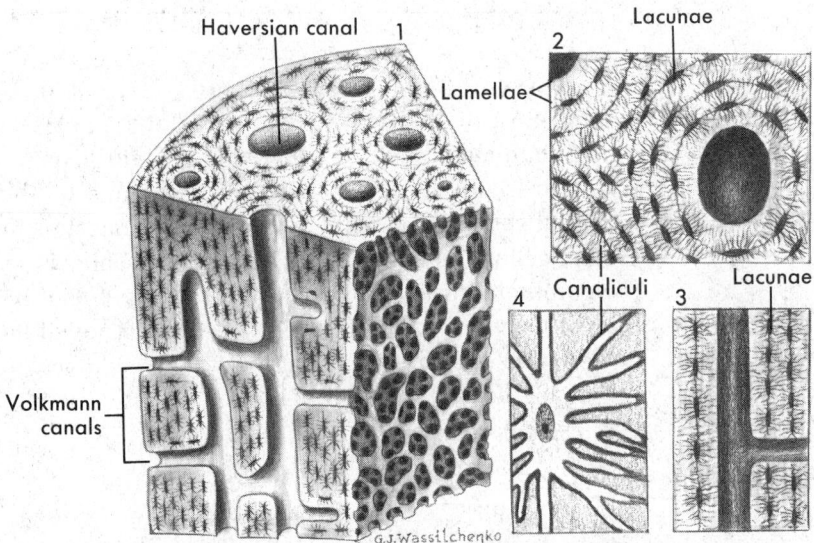

FIGURE 56-1   *1,* Three-dimensional view of compact bone depicting lamellae, lacunae, and canaliculi. *2,* Transverse section. *3,* Longitudinal section of bone with lacunae and canaliculi. *4,* Lacunae occupied by osteocyte.

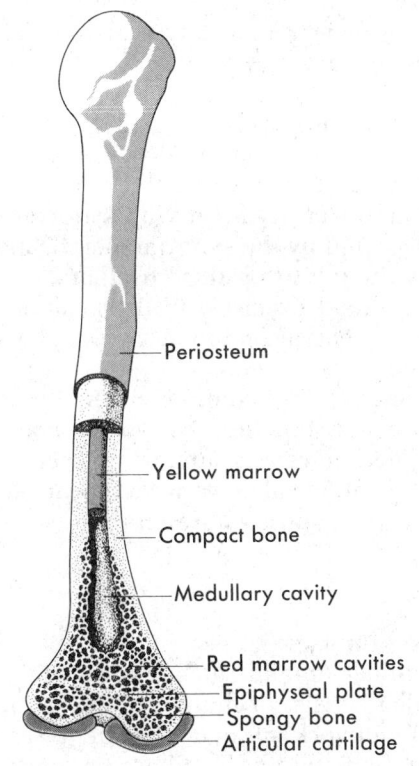

FIGURE 56-2 Cutaway section of long bone.

of bones. This growth ceases between 18 and 25 years of age. However, the plates remain a center of weakness and are often the site of fractures when the ends of the bones are subjected to unusual stresses; for example, the head of the femur may shear off at the epiphyseal plate.

Bone growth in width is produced by osteoblasts on the outer surface of the bones just under the periosteum. Widening of the bones occurs throughout life, although it slows down with age, especially in postmenopausal women. The accompanying absorption of the bone around the marrow cavity by osteoblasts continues throughout life. This absorption prevents bones from becoming too heavy. However, with increasing age, osteoporosis occurs, and the bones are weakened and become susceptible to spontaneous fractures. Often elderly persons fall because a bone breaks rather than the bone breaking as a result of the fall. The deficiency of ovarian hormones increases the rate at which osteoporosis develops in postmenopausal women.

Structure and function of the skeleton

The **axial skeleton** is made up of the cranium, which protects the brain; the vertebrae, whose arches pro-

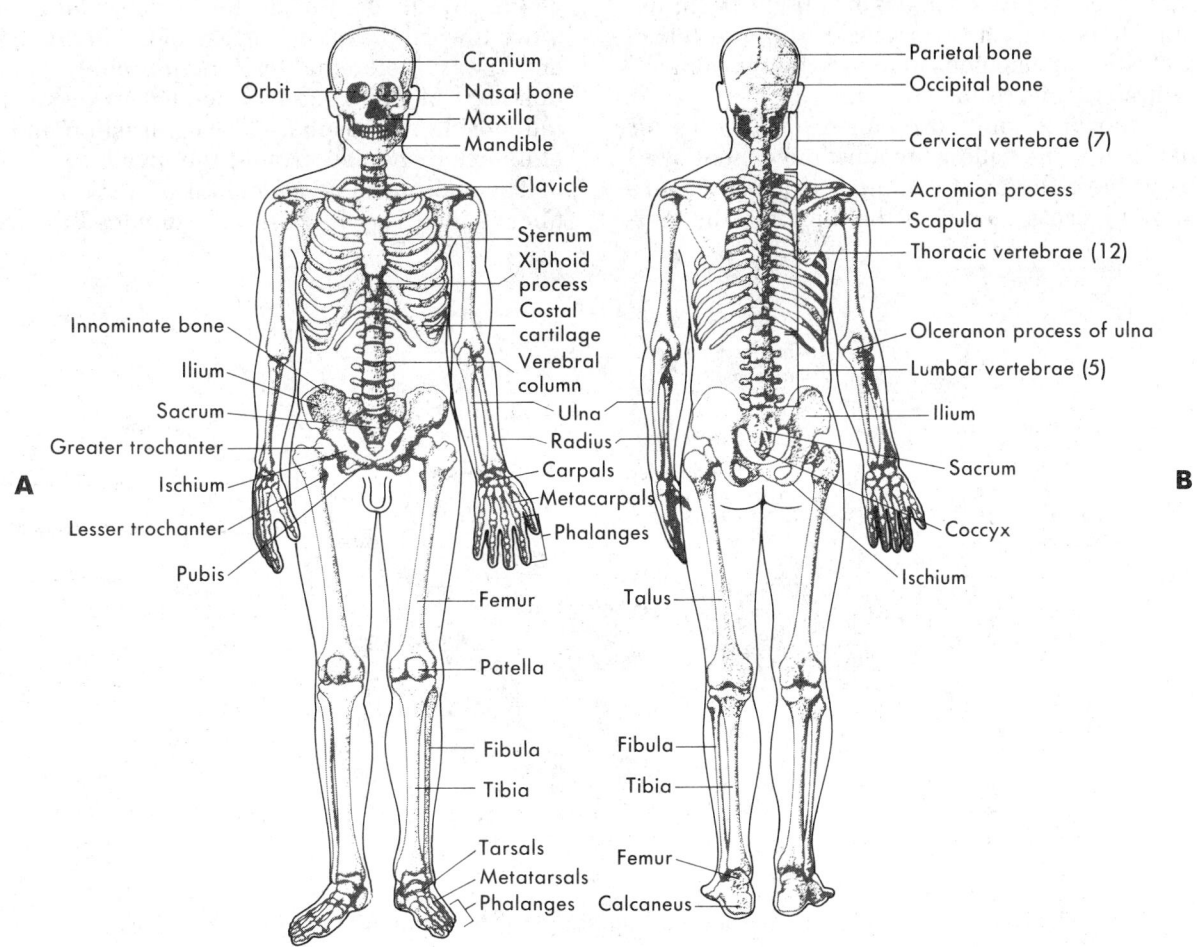

FIGURE 56-3 Skeleton. **A,** Anterior view. **B,** Posterior view.

tect the spinal cord; and the ribs, which, with the vertebrae and sternum, protect the heart and lungs. The vertebral column functions as an axis and contains the center of gravity. Movement of the ribs increases and decreases the volume of the thoracic cavity for respiration (see Unit VI). The **appendicular skeleton** consists of limbs and girdles that transfer the weight of the axial structures to the limbs. The joints necessary for standing, walking, running, and manual dexterity are also part of the appendicular skeleton. Figure 56-3 shows the larger bones of the skeleton.

Joints

Joints are formed where two bones touch each other. They may allow no movement at all, a small amount of movement, or a very large amount of movement.

Fibrous joints, also called synarthroses, are immovable and are found, for example, between the bones of the cranium (sutures), between the distal ends of the radius and ulna, and between the teeth and jaw bones.

Cartilaginous joints, called *amphiarthroses,* allow slight movement. Inelastic cartilaginous joints are found between the two pubic bones (pubic symphysis) and between the vertebrae (intervertebral discs); elastic cartilaginous joints are found connecting the first 10 ribs to the sternum.

Freely movable joints are called *diarthroses,* or synovial joints. They allow the most movement of all joints and have the most complex structure. Figure 56-4 shows a cross section of the hip joint, the larg-

est of the synovial joints. A typical synovial joint has the following composition:

1. Articulating surfaces covered by white, smooth, shiny hyaline cartilage to reduce friction
2. A joint capsule lined with synovial membrane
3. A narrow cavity filled with **synovial fluid** that is secreted by the synovial membrane to lubricate the joint to reduce friction
4. Bones held precisely in the position required for correct articulation by very strong ligaments

If any one of these components malfunctions, the joint does not function correctly. For example, sports injuries may tear supporting ligaments, in arthritis the hyaline cartilage wears away, and in gout abrasive crystals precipitate into the synovial fluid.

Muscles

Structure of muscle fibers

The functional units of muscles are the **muscle fibers,** which consist of many myofibrils enclosed in a special network of endoplasmic (sarcoplasmic) reticulum. Skeletal muscle fibers are multinucleate, and because of the pressure created by contraction of the myofibrils, the nuclei become flattened and move toward the outer surface of the fibers to lie under the sarcolemma (cell membrane). The large numbers of mitochondria needed to produce ATP (adenosine triphosphate) for contraction and relaxation are dispersed around the myofibrils.

The sarcoplasmic reticulum of a skeletal muscle fiber is made up of transverse tubules that are con-

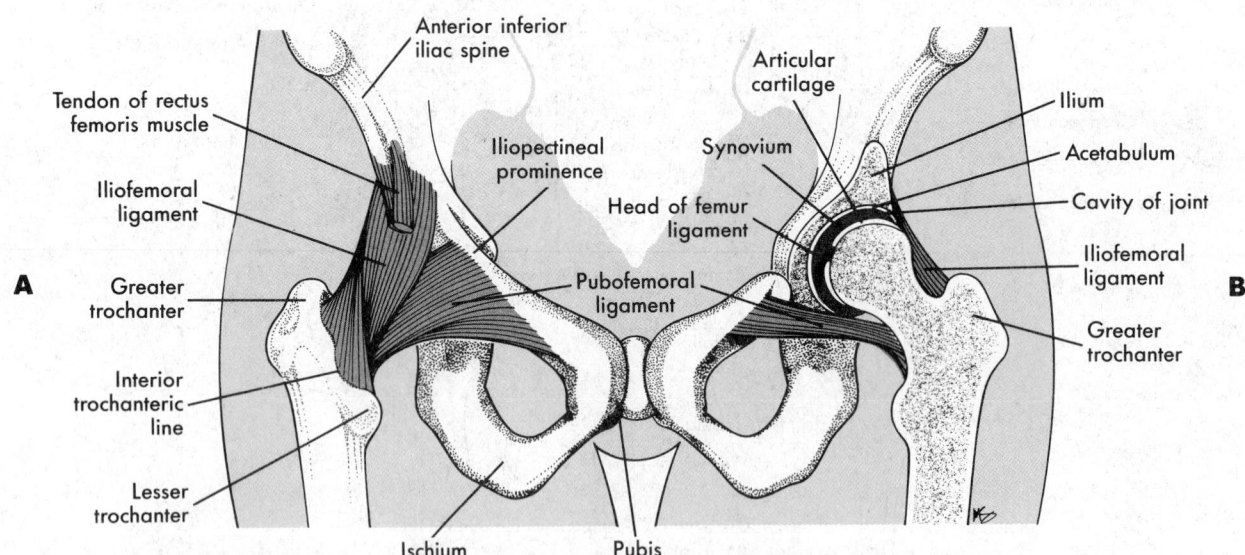

FIGURE 56-4   A, Ligaments surrounding hip joint. **B,** Ligaments holding structures in hip joint.

tinuous with the sarcolemma and sandwiched between sacs of sarcoplasmic reticulum. The transverse tubules lie in close proximity to the actin component of the myofibril and appear as Z lines under the microscope. Myofibrils contain alternating bands of actin and myosin. Under the microscope actin is seen as a light band and myosin as a dark band.

A number of skeletal muscle fibers are controlled by one motor neuron and form a motor unit. Each muscle fiber has an area of contact with its motor neuron, which is called the motor end plate, or neuromuscular junction.

Muscle contraction

The following sequence of events produces muscle contraction and relaxation:
1. A nerve impulse arrives at the motor end plate and causes the release of acetylcholine, which diffuses across the gap and binds to receptors on the sarcolemma.
2. The acetylcholine-receptor combination opens pores in the membrane and initiates a wave of depolarization that spreads rapidly over the fiber surface and into its interior along the transverse tubules.
3. During depolarization, calcium diffuses rapidly into the muscle fiber from the sacs of the sarcoplasmic reticulum close to the transverse tubules.
4. Calcium acts as a catalyst and stimulates actin and myosin in the myofibrils to slide together. The myofibrils contract, shorten, and increase tension in the connective tissue elements of the muscle. If additional calcium enters the fiber as a result of additional motor nerve impulses, actin and myosin contract further, and the muscle fiber continues to shorten or develop tension. Actin and myosin remain contracted as long as calcium is available in the sarcoplasm. Calcium transport across the cell membrane is not an important stimulus for skeletal muscle contraction; therefore cardiac and smooth muscle calcium channel–blocking drugs have little effect on skeletal muscle.
5. After the contraction, calcium is actively pumped out of the sarcoplasm into the sarcoplasmic reticulum. As its concentration around the myofibrils declines, actin is released from myosin and the muscle fiber relaxes.
6. The wave of depolarization is followed by a wave of repolarization, and the muscle membrane returns to its resting potential.

Energy sources for contraction

The immediate source of energy for muscle contraction and relaxation is provided by the conversion of ATP to ADP (adenosine diphosphate). ATP is replenished as follows:
1. ADP is converted to ATP rapidly by the transfer of high-energy phosphate from creatine phosphate.
2. The high energy of creatine phosphate is replenished either by oxidation of pyruvic acid when plenty of oxygen is available or by the conversion of pyruvic acid to lactic acid under anaerobic conditions.
3. The lactic acid produced when oxygen is in short supply diffuses out of the muscle cells rapidly and is carried away by the circulatory system. With poor circulation, lactic acid builds up in the muscles and, with other metabolites, is responsible for the pain of myocardial infarction and intermittent claudication.
4. Approximately 80% of the lactic acid is converted into blood glucose by the liver, which obtains the energy required by oxidizing the remaining 20%. (Only the liver can convert the lactic acid to glucose.)
5. Pyruvic acid in the muscle is produced by the catabolism of muscle glycogen synthesized from glucose obtained from the blood.

Isolated single muscle fibers and complete muscles

In the laboratory a single muscle fiber responds in an "all or none" manner; that is, when stimulated, the fiber either contracts or nothing happens. A muscle fiber cannot show a graded response. However, a complete muscle, which contains many muscle fibers, can show a graded response and produce contractions of different strengths because additional muscle fibers begin to contract as the stimulus intensity is increased.

Laboratory experiments show that a single stimulus produces a single muscle **contraction** (twitch). When repetitive stimuli produce additional contractions before relaxation is complete for the previous contraction, the final contraction is greater than that for a single stimulus. This is called incomplete summation when the individual contractions can be seen and complete summation or tetanic contraction when the individual contractions cannot be seen.

Stronger contractions are produced when the muscle is stretched because the myofibrils do not have to stretch the elastic components to produce an increase in tension or a decrease in length. Similarly, greater tension is produced when the muscle load is increased.

Muscles in the intact individual

The single twitch, incomplete summation, and tetanic contractions of the isolated preparations are not seen in the intact individual because the nervous system never stimulates all the muscle fibers simultaneously. Even when intense muscle contractions are produced in the intact individual, motor units are stimulated at different times and rates to produce a smooth contraction.

Skeletal muscle contractions may be described as follows:

1. *Tonic contraction*—a continual partial contraction produced by a small and constantly changing proportion of the motor units. Some tonic contraction is always present and is necessary for maintaining posture, temperature control, and muscle condition.
2. *Isotonic contraction*—Produces a change in length but not tension. This type of contraction produces movement.
3. *Isometric contraction*—Produces a change in tension but not length.
4. *Fibrillation*—An abnormal fluttering type of contraction in which individual muscle fibers contract asynchronously because of muscle or nerve damage. For example, fibrillation is seen at the cut edge of a skeletal muscle.

Normally the strength of a muscle contraction depends on (1) the initial length of the fibers and their load, because within normal limits the tension that can be generated is proportional to the degree of stretch and the force to be moved; (2) the number of fibers in the muscle activated by the nervous system and the frequency of nerve impulses stimulating the fibers; and (3) the metabolic condition of the muscles. For example, as the muscle is warmed up, muscle contractions improve. (Athletes stretch and exercise gently before a competition to prepare their muscles.) Metabolic condition is affected also by the efficiency with which the circulatory system supplies oxygen and nutrients and removes carbon dioxide and lactic acid.

Skeletal muscles usually are attached to two bones and cross at least one joint. (Some skeletal muscles form sphincters, such as around the external openings of the digestive and urinary tracts; other skeletal muscles connect one bone with the skin, for example, in the cheeks.)

The point of attachment on the bone closest to the trunk is called the *point of origin*; that furthest from the trunk is called the *point of insertion*.

Skeletal muscles act in groups, and the components of the groups serve three functions:

1. Muscles that produce a particular movement or tension are called the *prime movers*.
2. Muscles that oppose the prime movers and relax in a controlled way to assist them are called the *antagonists*.
3. Muscles that contract at the same time as the prime mover to stabilize a part of the body or help the prime mover produce its movement are called *synergists*.

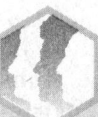

GERIATRIC CONSIDERATIONS

Physiologic Changes in the Musculoskeletal System

Bones become weaker in old age because the rate of new bone formation does not keep up with the rate of bone resorption. This weakening occurs at an earlier age in women than men, because the concentration of their gonadal hormones declines more rapidly and at an earlier age. Thus elderly women have a far greater risk of bone fractures than men. Joint problems, such as osteoarthritis, also increase with age because the joints are particularly susceptible to damage and wear and tear. This is especially true of the articulating cartilage of weight-bearing bones.

Muscle fibers do not reproduce, and muscle function declines with age as muscle metabolism becomes less efficient and muscle fibers are replaced by connective tissue. However, a significant proportion of the decline in muscle function that is seen in elderly persons is due to a lack of exercise. Even at an advanced age, an appropriate increase in movement and exercise improves muscle tone and strength.

Sensory receptors called **muscle spindles** constantly monitor muscle condition, inform the brain, and activate the reflex centers responsible for stretch reflexes. Sensory receptors for balance and sight also stimulate reflexes through the centers responsible for posture and movement so that balance may be restored rapidly when it is upset.

The coordination of muscle groups is complex and involves many tracts and reflex centers in the brain and spinal cord. Muscle coordination can be improved with practice and stored as memory engrams so that it becomes automatic. We are not consciously aware of many of our activities. We are rarely conscious of maintaining posture or of how we walk or run. However, posture and movement do require conscious planning in diseases such as multiple sclerosis and Parkinson's disease.

The names of skeletal muscles often contain information about their location, points of origin and insertion, shape, and function. Figure 56-5 shows some of the superficial muscles of the body.

ASSESSMENT
Subjective

A focused health history for a patient with a suspected or previously diagnosed musculoskeletal disorder requires the nurse to utilize knowledge of pathophysiology to guide questioning in an appropri-

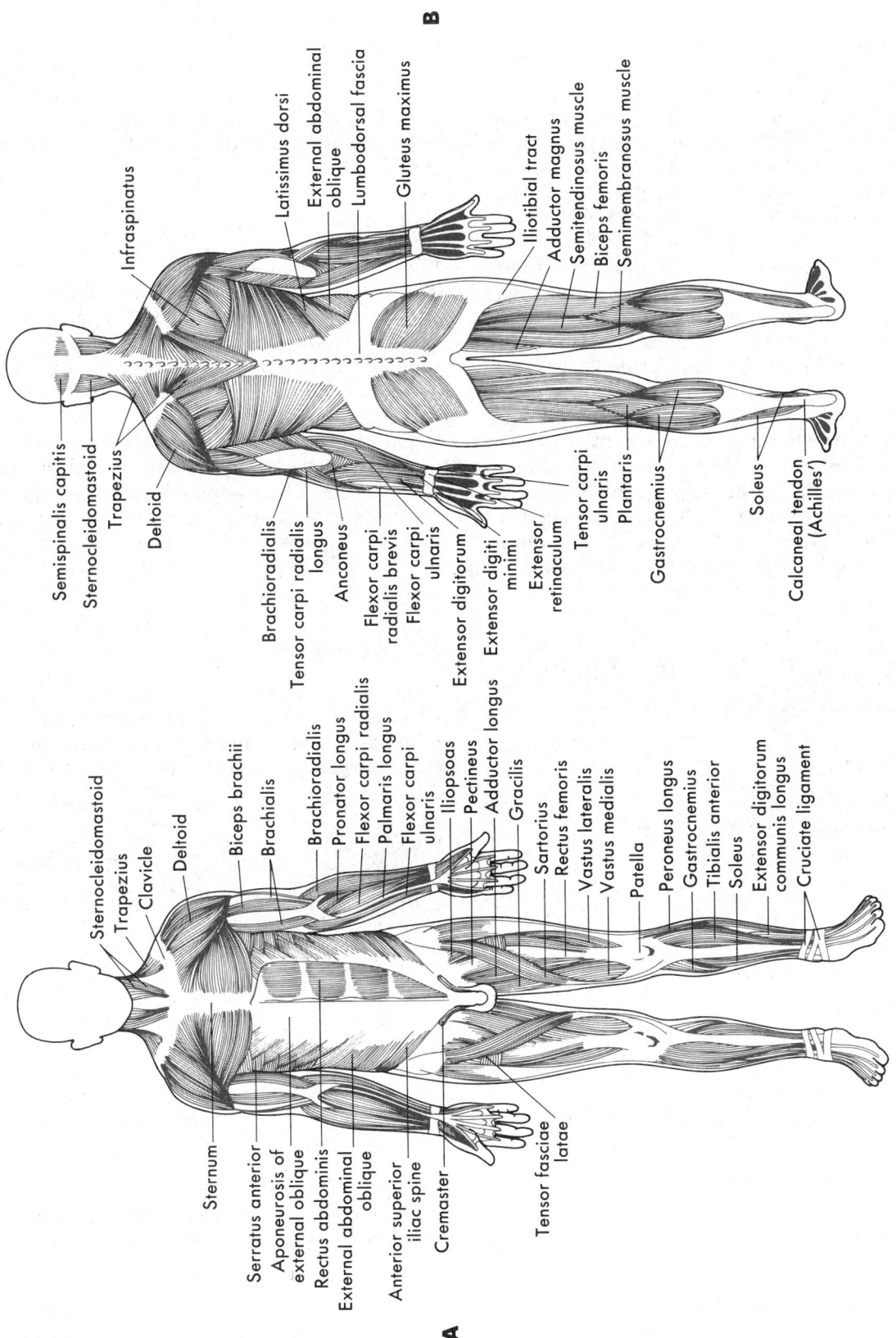

FIGURE 56-5   Superficial muscles of body. **A,** Anterior view. **B,** Posterior view.

ate and complete manner. Patients may experience trauma, pain, or systemic illness related to the musculoskeletal system. Presenting complaints may be of an acute and specific nature, or they may be vague with an insidious onset.

The box below lists potential symptoms to review with the patient. In addition to specific symptoms, ask the patient about previous injury, inciting trauma or injury, mechanism of injury, usual activities or pastimes, and functional limitations as a result of the current problem. Factors such as occupation may relate to the complaint. Laborers would probably have stronger muscles than sedentary workers and therefore be less likely to suffer muscle strain. Laborers would be more susceptible to injury caused by the type of job. Age could also be another factor. Osteoarthritis and osteoporosis are more likely to occur in an adult population greater than 60 years of age. Other appropriate systems to review are identified through determining associated symptoms as well as the various other dimensions of the complaint. Other appropriate history to explore includes major adult illnesses, hospitalizations, surgeries, injuries or accidents, immunizations, current medications, allergies, and habits.

Family history that is relevant to the musculoskeletal system includes back problems, painful joints, curved spine and congenital or other abnormalities of the hip or feet; rheumatoid arthritis or osteoarthritis; osteoporosis, ankylosing spondylitis, and gout. A positive finding should include the disorder as well as the individual's relationship to the patient (e.g., rheumatoid arthritis, maternal aunt; gout, father).

Objective

Physical examination of the musculoskeletal system involves inspection, palpation, range of motion (ROM), muscle strength, and at times specific tests. The box below summarizes the screening musculoskeletal examination. Some patients will have more complex symptom involvement than others, and therefore assessment needs may vary from patient to patient. In the setting of a systemic disorder such as systemic lupus erythematosus (SLE) other systems that may be examined include integumentary, respiratory, and neurologic. General assessment is included for any patient and refers to the examiner's overall impression of the patient's state of health.

General assessment

General assessment includes height, weight, vital signs, apparent age (relative to chronologic age), nutritional status, general appearance, and stature. Any obvious abnormalities or assistive devices

---

POTENTIAL SYMPTOMS RELATED TO MUSCULOSKELETAL DISORDERS

Muscle
Atrophy
Hypertrophy
Pain
Cramping
Weakness

Bones/joints
Inability to bear weight
Pain
Stiffness
Swelling
Redness
Increased local temperature (heat)
Limitation of movement (decreased range of motion [ROM])
Fractures
Clicking, clunking
Locking or catching
Giving way (buckling)

Other
"Pins and needles" or numbness (paresthesias)
Skin changes, such as pale, cyanotic, dusky, butterfly rash

MUSCULOSKELETAL SCREENING EXAMINATION

Inspection
General observation for posture, symmetry, size, gait, involuntary movements, gross deformities

Palpation
Muscle tone, temperature variations, tenderness, masses; tremors, and fasciculations
Joint crepitus, tenderness, and temperature change

Range of motion
Active and passive; spine, neck, shoulder, elbow, wrist, fingers, hip, knee, ankle, toes

Muscle strength
Neck, deltoid, biceps, triceps, wrist/finger musculature, hamstring and quadriceps, ankle/foot musculature

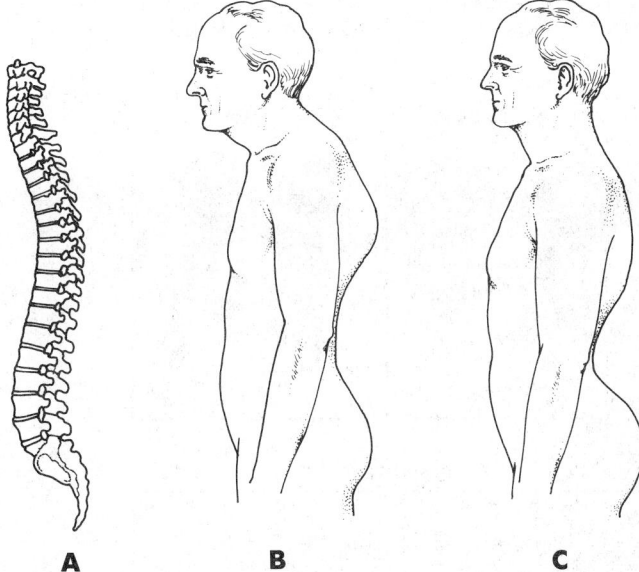

FIGURE 56-6 Spinal curvature. **A,** Normal. **B,** Kyphosis. **C,** Lordosis.

TABLE 56-1 Muscle Strength Grading

Muscle gradations	Description
5—Normal	Complete ROM against gravity, with full resistance
4—Good	Complete ROM against gravity, with some resistance
3—Fair	Complete ROM against gravity
2—Poor	Complete ROM, with gravity eliminated
1—Trace	Evidence of slight contractility; no joint motion
0—None	No evidence of contractility

should also be noted. Also record whether the patient appears to be comfortable or in distress. Inspect and palpate the skin over joints, noting warmth, color, lesions, and vascularity.

Musculoskeletal

Inspect the patient paying careful attention to posture, symmetry, facial expression, patterns of movement (or gait), involuntary movements, and contour or shape of spine. Some common spinal deviations include scoliosis, kyphosis, and lordosis. A laterally deviated spine is known as **scoliosis**, whereas an excessive posterior curvature of the thoracic spine is known as **kyphosis**. An exaggerated kyphosis is known as a gibbus. **Lordosis** is an excessive anterior curvature of the lumbar spine (Figure 56-6).

Follow inspection with palpation. In the setting of an injury or complaint related to a specific body part,

two general considerations are helpful in approaching the patient: (1) support the body part as much as possible to facilitate relaxation of the area to be palpated; and (2) palpate the uninvolved side first. While palpating, note muscle tone, temperature variations, tenderness, masses, **tremors** (involuntary trembling of the body or extremities), and **fasciculations** (small local involuntary muscular contractions). When palpating joints also note the presence or absence of edema or crepitus. **Crepitus** is a dry crackling sound or grating feeling that may occur in joints, skin, or lungs.

Active ROM and passive ROM are used to determine any limitation of movement. Active range of motion (AROM) is performed before passive range of motion (PROM). During AROM, note when and where in the movement the onset of pain occurs and the amount of observable restriction of movement. The purpose of PROM is to determine whether a limitation in ROM is consistent both with and without muscle power. In general, to perform passive testing, put the joint through ROM while the patient is relaxed. During PROM, note limitation of range

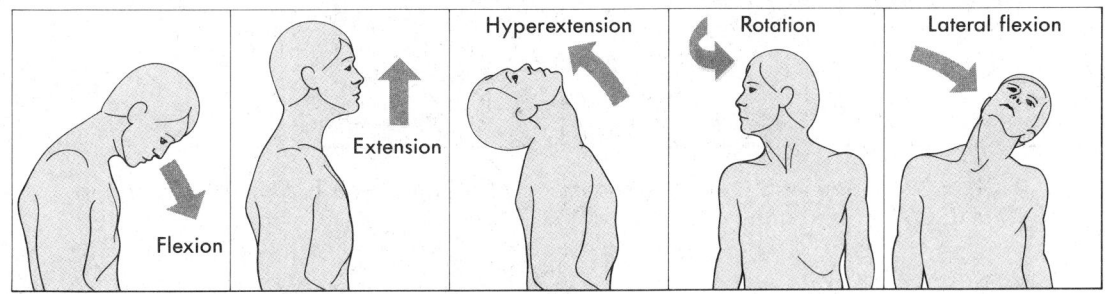

FIGURE 56-7 Neck range of motion.

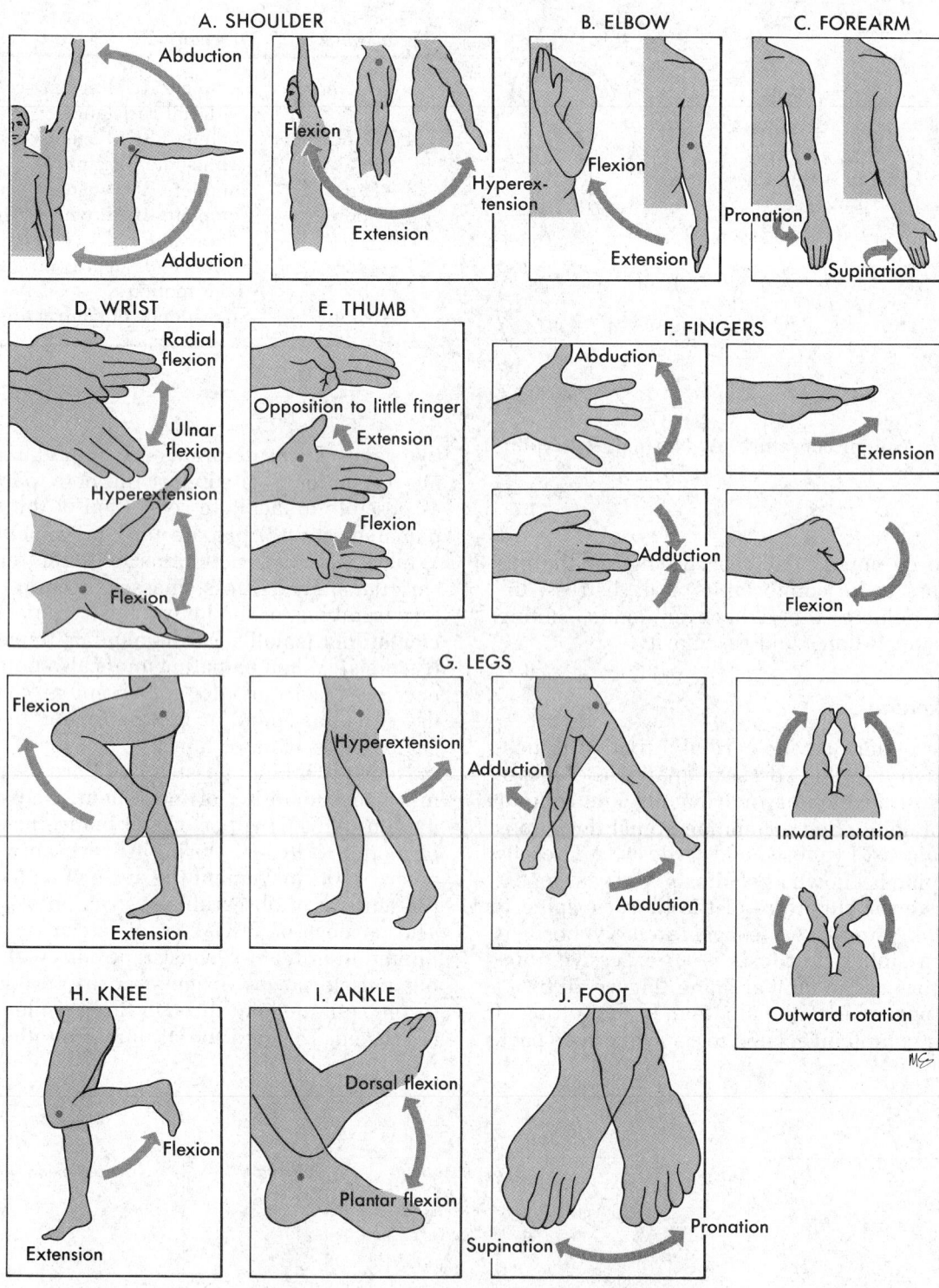

FIGURE 56-8   Range of motion, standards for mobility. **A** to **F,** Upper extremities. **G** to **J,** Lower extremities.

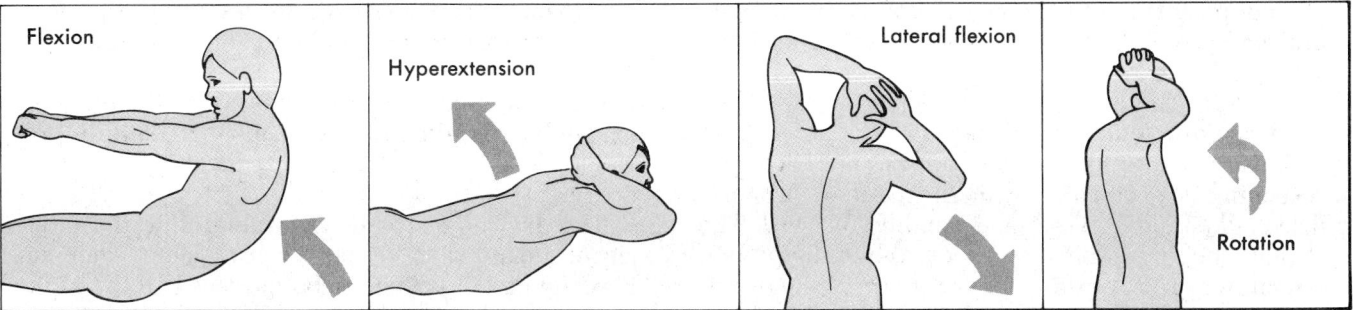

FIGURE 56-9   Waist range of motion.

(hypomobility), excess of range (hypermobility), pain, and quality of movement (e.g., lead pipe, cogwheel). Figures 56-7, 56-8, and 56-9 illustrate ROM of major joints. Muscle strength is usually integrated with ROM testing for the associated joint. Always compare muscle strength bilaterally. Table 56-1 gives a standard grading chart for muscle strength.

Full muscle strength requires complete AROM. Table 56-2 identifies screening muscle strength testing.

Additional tests that may be performed include scoliosis screening, limb measurement, and tests for knee assessment, hip assessment, and wrist assessment. Straight leg raises are also described for the evaluation of low back pain. These tests are gener-

TABLE 56-2   Muscle Strength Screening

Muscles tested	Patient activity	Examiner activity	Muscles tested	Patient activity	Examiner activity
Ocular musculature					
Lids	Close eyes tightly	Attempt to resist closure	Biceps	Flex arm	Pull to extend arm
			Triceps	Extend arm	Push to flex arm
Yoke muscles	Track object in six cardinal positions		Wrist musculature	Extend hand	Push to flex
				Flex hand	Push to extend
Facial musculature	Blow out cheeks	Assess pressure in cheeks with fingertips	Finger muscles	Extend fingers	Push dorsal surface of fingers
				Flex fingers	Push ventral surface of fingers
	Place tongue in cheek	Assess pressure in cheek with fingertips		Spread fingers	Hold fingers together
	Stick out tongue, move it to right and left	Observe strength and coordination of thrust and extension	Hip musculature	In supine position raise extended leg	Push down on leg above knee
Neck muscles	Extend head backward	Push head forward	Hamstring, gluteal, abductor, and adductor muscles of leg	Sit and perform alternate leg crossing	Push in opposite direction of crossing limb
	Flex head forward	Push head backward	Quadriceps	Extend leg	Push to flex leg
	Rotate head in full circle	Observe mobility, coordination	Hamstring	Bend knees to flex leg	Push to extend leg
	Touch shoulders with head	Observe range of motion	Ankle and foot muscle	Bend foot up (dorsiflexion)	Push to plantar flexion
Deltoid	Hold arms upward	Push down on arms		Bend foot down (plantar flexion)	Push to dorsiflexion
			Antigravity	Walk on toes	

ally not performed by the bedside nurse but may be utilized by an industrial nurse or a practitioner in an advanced or extended role.

Musculoskeletal special tests

Scoliosis is a lateral curvature of the spine. Scoliosis screening is performed with the patient, properly disrobed, standing erect and bending forward. The patient should not have on shoes. While the patient is standing erect, observe for symmetry of shoulders, scapulae, and iliac crests and alignment of spinous processes. With the patient bending forward, inspect for symmetry of scapulae, iliac crests, and alignment of spinous processes. Note any rib hump (Figure 56-10).

Leg length is measured from the anterior superior iliac spine to the medial malleolus of the ankle. Leg length may be altered by muscle wasting or obesity. Measuring from the anterior superior iliac spine to the lateral malleolus is less likely to be affected by muscle wasting or obesity. Arm length is measured from the acromion process through the olecranon process to the distal ulnar prominence.

Tests that facilitate evaluation of the knee include bulge sign or ballottement, McMurray's sign, drawer test, and Lachmann's test. The bulge sign or ballottement is used to determine the presence of excess fluid in the knee. Extend the patient's knee. Milk the medial aspect of the patella upward two or three times. Tap the lateral side of the patella. Observe for a bulge of returning fluid to the hollow area medial to the patella.

McMurray's sign is used to determine the presence of a torn meniscus. With the patient supine, flex one knee with the foot flat on the examining table near the buttocks. Internally rotate the patient's leg while extending it. Use your other hand to provide resistance at the medial aspect of the knee (Figure 56-11).

The drawer test is used to determine the integrity of the anterior and posterior cruciate ligaments. Flex the patient's knee to 90 degrees and the hip to 45 degrees. Sit on the patient's foot, placing your hands around the tibia to ensure that the hamstring muscles are relaxed. Draw the tibia forward on the femur. The normal amount of movement that should be present is approximately 6 mm (Figure 56-12).

Lachmann's test is used to indicate injury to the anterior cruciate ligament. With the patient in a supine position stand beside the involved limb. Hold the patient's knee between full extension and 30 degrees of flexion. Stabilize the femur with one hand and move the proximal aspect of the tibia forward with the other hand. A positive sign is indicated by a "mushy" or soft end feel when the tibia is moved forward.

The hip may be assessed using Patrick's test, which is also sometimes called the FABER test. FABER is a mnemonic that stands for flexion, abduction, and external rotation. With the patient lying supine, place the patient's test leg so that the foot of the test leg is on the top of the opposite knee. Slowly lower the test leg in abduction toward the examining table. A negative test is indicated by the test leg

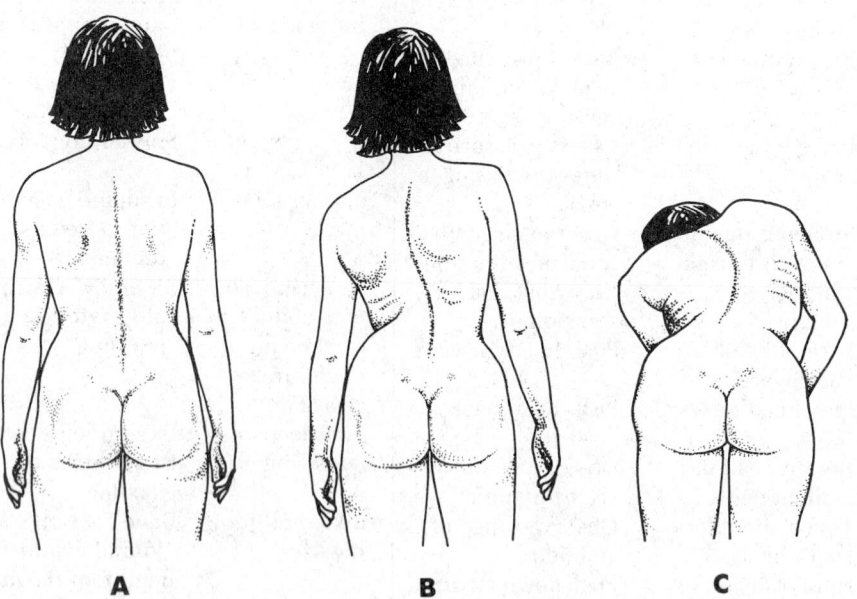

FIGURE 56-10   **A,** Normal spine. **B,** Scoliosis with patient standing. **C,** Scoliosis with patient bending forward.

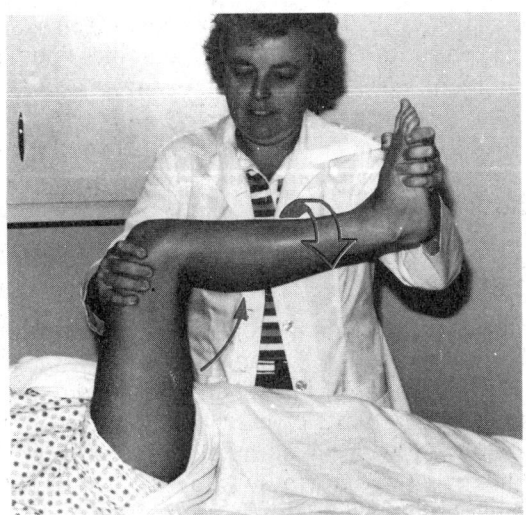

FIGURE 56-11   McMurray test. (From Bowers AC, Thompson JM: *Clinical manual of health assessment,* ed 4, St Louis, 1992, Mosby–Year Book.)

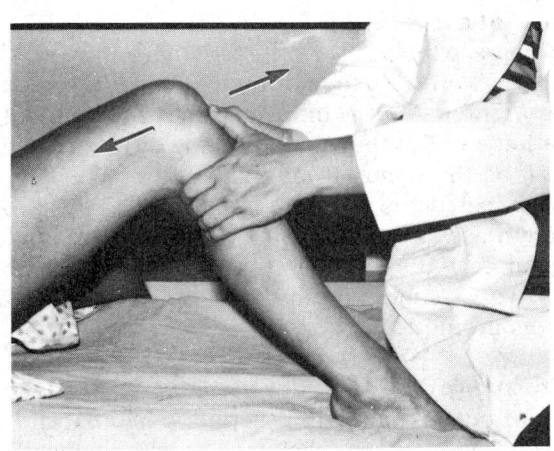

FIGURE 56-12   Drawer test. (From Bowers AC, Thompson JM: *Clinical manual of health assessment,* ed 4, St Louis, 1992, Mosby–Year Book.)

GERIATRIC CONSIDERATIONS

Musculoskeletal Assessment

General approach

Allow more time than for a younger adult

Articulate clearly; the geriatric patient may be hearing impaired

Impaired sight, comprehension, or mobility may result in less than optimum cooperation

Provide clear, concise instructions

History collection

May need to use fewer open-ended questions and provide some choices; for example, "Do your knees feel stiff all day or just in the morning?"

May need to repeat questions

Be alert for answers that do not appear appropriate; the patient may not have understood the question correctly because of impaired hearing or impaired comprehension

Physical assessment

The physical examination itself is not different, but the approach needs to be altered such that the appropriate information is assessed without undue discomfort or embarrassment for the patient

Maintain an environment with minimal noise, distractions, and interruption

Geriatric patients have a decreasing muscle mass

Osteoarthritis, or "wear and tear" arthritis, is common

Osteoporosis becomes more prevalent with increasing age, especially in the thin, white female, and results in a greater susceptibility to fractures

---

falling to the table or being at least parallel with the opposite leg. If the test leg remains above the opposite straight leg, the test is said to be positive. A positive test may indicate iliopsoas spasm or difficulty with the hip joint or the sacroiliac joint.

The wrist may be assessed for Tinel's sign. Tap the patient's wrist on the palmar aspect over the median nerve. If the patient experiences a sensation of tingling or prickling, it is known as Tinel's sign. A positive Tinel's sign is present in carpal tunnel syndrome. Another test is to assess for Phalen's sign. Instruct the patient to maintain palmar flexion for 1 minute. If the patient experiences numbness or tingling (paresthesia) over the palmar surface of the hand, first three fingers, and part of the fourth (ring) finger, Phalen's sign is present.

Straight leg raises are performed to evaluate the presence of disk disease when the patient's complaint is low back pain. Straight leg raises are performed with the patient supine, or distracted leg raises may be performed while the patient is sitting with legs dangling. For standard straight leg raises, have the patient supine. Extend the knee of the side expected to be involved and slowly flex the hip. Normally, the hip can be flexed to approximately 80 degrees without pain. A positive test occurs when the patient reports pain or paresthesias in sciatic distribution on the affected side or bilaterally. A positive test indicates nerve root irritation. To perform distracted leg raises, extend the patient's knee of the leg expected to be involved. Flexion of the hip and extension of the knee stretch lumbar nerve roots. A positive test in indicated by the patient's complaint of pain in the back and "shooting" down the leg (radicular pain).

DIAGNOSTIC AND LABORATORY TESTS
Radiography

Standard radiography

Standard radiographs are commonly used in the diagnosis and evaluation of musculoskeletal disorders because they show structural or functional changes in bones and joints. An anteroposterior (AP) approach allows a one-dimensional view of the area being examined, whereas the lateral approach permits a two-dimensional view.

Patient preparation
The patient is told what areas will be examined and is instructed to remove all jewelry and metal objects.

Myelography

Myelography is an invasive procedure that involves fluoroscopic and radiographic examination of the subarachnoid space after it is defined through injection of a contast medium. The procedure is invaluable in evaluating spinal cord and nerve root lesions and severe scoliosis. Air or contrast dyes may be used for the procedure. Pantopaque (isophendylate) is an oil-based medium that is used when lesions of the upper spine are suspected, and Amipaque (metrizamide) is a newer water-soluble medium that does not need to be removed at the end of the procedure. Amipaque is also less viscous and so flows freely into narrow areas, allowing better differentiation of spinal blockages. A disadvantage of Amipaque is that it may induce seizure activity, and so before the procedure the patient needs to be hydrated and to discontinue medications such as phenothiazines, tricyclic antidepressants, and amphetamines that could lower the seizure threshold. Omnipaque (iohexol) is a recently developed contrast agent that produces less central nervous system toxicity than Amipaque. Air is used as a contrast agent if the patient has a hypersensitivity to iodine or seafood.

Patient preparation
A patient undergoing myelography needs to be instructed to fast before the test to reduce the possibility of vomiting. The nurse informs the patient of the purpose of the test and alerts the patient to the possibility of a transient burning sensation, flushing and warmth, headache, a salty taste, or nausea and vomiting as the dye is injected. The nurse encour-

ages the patient to report other signs of discomfort such as pain down the leg. Premedications and cleansing enemas are given if ordered. Aftercare varies with the medium that has been used (see Chapter 44 for a more detailed discussion of patient preparation and care) and generally includes monitoring of vital and neurologic signs and positioning.

Arthrography

Arthrography involves radiographic visualization of joints after injection of a contrast medium or air or both. Arthrography is useful in visualizing soft tissues such as ligaments or cartilage that are not usually visualized well in standard radiographs. The procedure helps determine the cause of knee or shoulder pain and detect joint derangement and synovial cysts. Complications are rare and include infection at the puncture site or allergic reactions to the contrast medium. The procedure is contraindicated if the patient has joint infection, has active arthritis, has an allergy to the contrast medium, or is pregnant.

Patient preparation
The nurse explains that the test permits visualization of the joint. No food or fluid restrictions are necessary. The patient is informed that the joint will be anesthetized but that some tingling or pressure may be felt as the contrast medium is injected. The patient is instructed to remain still during the procedure, unless directed to walk or move the joint. The nurse determines if the patient has allergies to contrast dyes, seafood, iodine, or local anesthetics and obtains an informed consent.

Procedure
The patient is placed in a supine position, and the area overlying the joint is antiseptically cleansed and anesthetized. A needle is inserted into the joint space, and fluid is aspirated to prevent dilution of the dye. With this needle still in place, the contrast medium is injected. The needle is removed and the joint moved to promote distribution of the dye. Radiographic films are taken of the joint in various positions.

Postprocedure care
Following the procedure an adhesive strip may be applied and the joint wrapped in an elastic bandage. The patient is instructed to leave the bandage in place for several days. The nurse tells the patient to rest the joint for at least 12 hours and to apply ice if swelling occurs. The patient is informed that crepitation may be heard in the joint but will disappear in 1 to 2 days. A mild analgesic may be taken for discomfort.

Bone scan

A bone scan (radioactive bone scan) involves imaging of the skeleton with a scanning camera after intravenous injection of a radioactive tracer such as sodium pertechnetate (^{99m}Tc). The tracer collects at sites of increased metabolism, which appear as "hot spots" on the scan and are detectable much sooner than on radiographs. Nonspecificity is a limitation of the procedure, since areas of nucleotide concentration may reflect increased metabolism related to normal or abnormal bone growth. Bone scanning is of particular value in detecting bone malignancies, occult bone trauma, degenerative bone disorders, and osteomyelitis. Bone scans may also be used to evaluate the body's response to chemotherapy or radiation. Bone scans may be performed in emergencies on lactating or pregnant women using a reduced dose of radioisotope.

Patient preparation
The nurse describes the procedure and explains that the test often picks up abnormalities sooner than ordinary radiographs. The patient is told that the scan detects radiation emitted by the body and that the radioactive tracer is not dangerous. The nurse explains that the radioactive substance is usually excreted in the urine 6 to 12 hours after injection.

The patient is told not to drink large amounts of fluids *before* the test because large volumes of fluid are drunk between injection of the tracer and the scan. These fluids flush tracer from the kidneys that has been picked up by the bone. An informed consent is obtained, and the patient is instructed to remove metal and jewelry. A sedative is administered if necessary.

Procedure
The tracer is injected, and the patient drinks large volumes of fluid. Approximately 1 to 3 hours later, the scanning begins. The patient is instructed to void and then is placed on a scanning table. A scanner moved back and forth over the body translates the images into two-dimensional views on radiographs. The procedure takes 30 to 60 minutes.

Computed tomography

Computed tomography (CT) is highly sensitive to attenuations in tissue density and provides detailed views of bone and tissue. It provides an accurate cross-sectional representation of bony and soft tissue abnormalities without additional manipulation of the patient, an important consideration in cases of severe injury. Radiation exposure is minimal. The patient is placed inside a scanner, and an x-ray tube emits radiation pulses as it moves around the body.

A detector positioned opposite the x-ray tube picks up the pulsations, which are processed by a computer. The computer produces an image that is projected onto a screen. CT scans of the spine are complementary to anteroposterior, lateral, and oblique views obtained through myelography and are useful in detecting herniated disks, spinal stenoses, and tumors.

Patient preparation
The patient is told that the test involves detailed visualization of the spine. The nurse explains that the patient will be placed on a table in the middle of a round piece of x-ray equipment and that it is necessary to remain motionless during the procedure. If a contrast dye is to be used, the patient is told to withhold food and drink for 4 hours before the procedure. The nurse instructs the patient to remove all jewelry and metal objects.

Magnetic resonance imaging

Magnetic resonance imaging (MRI) is a noninvasive procedure that is capable of total imaging of the spine without the use of contrast dyes. MRI is the only diagnostic modality that can demonstrate the demyelinated cord lesions found in multiple sclerosis. It is also useful in detecting tumors, degenerated disks, osteomyelitis, and the Chiari malformation. During MRI the patient is placed inside a large doughnut-shaped electromagnet. The hydrogen nuclei within this field are irradiated with a magnetic pulse, which causes them to be pushed over. When the pulse is removed, the nuclei realign and emit the energy they have absorbed. These electromagnetic echoes are picked up by sensors and are used to produce sensitive images that differentiate solid tissue, fat, blood, and bone.

Patient preparation
The patient is instructed to remove all metal objects, and the nurse notes if the patient has a history of insertion of staples, plates, or other metal appliances. (For a more detailed discussion of patient care, see Chapter 25.)

Biopsy

A biopsy involves removing a piece of bone or tissue for histologic examination. The procedure may be performed with the patient under local or general anesthesia. Samples are obtained through surgical excision (bone, muscle), drill needle (bone), and needle excision (synovial membrane). A biopsy is usually performed after an abnormal or inconclusive bone scan, CT scan, or radiograph and is useful in distinguishing between benign and malignant tumors. **Synovial biopsies** are useful in the differential diagnosis of arthritis and in the diagnosis of systemic lupus erythematosus (SLE), gout, bacterial infections, and rheumatoid arthritis. Muscle biopsies are used in the detection of myopathies.

Patient preparation

The procedure and location of the biopsy are described to the patient. The nurse explains that the biopsy allows close examination of tissue. Patients having excisional biopsies and general anesthetics are instructed to fast 8 hours before the test. Local anesthetics are used for drill and needle biopsies, and fasting is not required. For a patient having a drill biopsy the nurse explains that the patient may experience some discomfort and pressure as the bone drill forces the biopsy specimen from the bone. Patients having a synovial membrane biopsy may experience transient pain as the needle enters the joint. The patient's history is checked for hypersensitivity to anesthetics, and a signed consent is obtained. Sedatives are administered if ordered.

Postprocedure care

The nurse monitors the dressing over the biopsy site for excessive drainage and administers analgesics as ordered. If a synovial membrane biopsy has been performed, the patient is assessed for bleeding into the joint (tenderness and swelling) and instructed to rest the joint for 1 day before resuming regular activity. If a bone biopsy has been performed, the patient is monitored for signs of infection (fever, headache, pain on movement, or tissue redness at the site) for several days following the procedure.

Synovial Fluid Analysis

Synovial fluid is secreted in small amounts into the cavities of most joints. Analysis of synovial fluid (Table 56-3) is useful in detecting noninflammatory, inflammatory, septic, crystal-induced, and hemorrhagic joint disorders and in evaluating the progression of joint disease. Synovial fluid is obtained through arthrocentesis, during which a large needle is inserted into the joint capsule and fluid is aspirated. Anti-inflammatory medications may be injected into the joint capsule during arthrocentesis.

Patient preparation

The nurse explains that the test involves withdrawal of a small amount of fluid from the joint and explains the positioning that the patient will assume. If knee, shoulder, elbow, wrist, or ankle is involved, the patient will be seated or supine; if the hip is involved, the patient will be supine. The nurse explains that the patient may feel a stinging sensation as the local anesthetic is injected and that some discomfort may be felt as the joint capsule is penetrated. The impor-

TABLE 56-3   Findings in Synovial Fluid

Analysis	Results	Implications
Color	Colorless to pale yellow	Normal
	Yellow	Gout, rheumatoid arthritis, osteoarthritis, or tuberculous arthritis
	Bloody	Septic or traumatic arthritis
Clarity	Clear	Normal
	Slightly cloudy	SLE, rheumatic fever, or pseudogout
	Cloudy	Gout, rheumatoid arthritis, tuberculous arthritis
Viscosity	High	Normal; high viscosity also may occur with traumatic arthritis, osteoarthritis, or SLE
	Low	Gout, rheumatoid arthritis, septic arthritis, osteoarthritis, or SLE

tance of keeping the joint still throughout the procedure is emphasized. If synovial fluid values are to be obtained, the patient is instructed to fast for 6 to 12 hours before the procedure. The nurse assesses vital signs and ensures that a written, informed consent is obtained. The procedure takes approximately 10 minutes.

Postprocedure care

The nurse assesses for pain, fever, and swelling in the joint and applies ice to relieve swelling and pain. The pressure dressing is maintained, and the patient is instructed to avoid strenuous use of the joint for a few days. The nurse ensures that the specimen is sent to the laboratory immediately.

Arthroscopy

Arthroscopy involves direct visualization of the interior of a joint using an endoscope inserted through a surgical incision. Arthroscopy is most commonly used to evaluate the knee for meniscus, cartilage, or ligament tears and to diagnosis acute and chronic disorders (Figure 56-13) and is usually performed only after an initial diagnostic workup. Corrective surgery may be performed during arthroscopy using the endoscope. Arthroscopy is often performed with the patient under local anesthesia, using aseptic con-

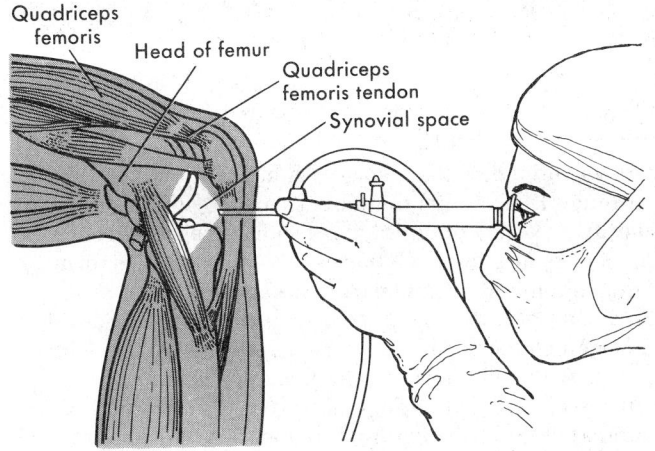

Quadriceps femoris
Head of femur
Quadriceps femoris tendon
Synovial space

FIGURE 56-13   Arthroscopy.

ditions. Complications, which are rare, include infection, hemarthrosis, swelling, or joint injury. The procedure takes 15 to 30 minutes.

Patient preparation

The nurse explains that the patient will be placed on his or her back on an operating table. The limb will be scrubbed and an elastic bandage or tourniquet applied to drain as much blood as possible from the leg. If a local anesthetic is to be used, the patient is told that some transient discomfort may be felt as the drug is injected or as the tourniquet is applied. If spinal or general anesthesia is to be used, the patient is instructed to fast after midnight the day of the procedure; otherwise no food or fluid is restricted. A signed consent is obtained. If crutches are ordered, the nurse teaches the patient the correct crutch gait. Hair is removed 6 inches (15 cm) above and below the knee to prepare for the procedure.

Postprocedure care

The nurse monitors vital signs, the neurovascular status of the affected limb, and the dressing for bleeding. Ice is applied to the affected joint for pain and swelling, and analgesics are administered as ordered. The nurse observes the patient for indications of infection such as fever, swelling, or increased pain or redness at the incision site. The patient is instructed to avoid excessive use of the joint for several days, to elevate the knee while sitting, to avoid twisting the knee, and to return for suture removal in about 7 days.

Electromyography

Electromyography measures and records the electric currents produced by skeletal muscles ("muscle

action potentials"). Small-needle electrodes are inserted into a muscle, and the electrical activity of the muscle is recorded, amplified, and displayed on a screen. The procedure is useful in diagnosing cervical or lumbar disk disease, muscular dystrophy, myasthenia gravis, polymyositis, and motor-neuron disease. No special patient preparation is necessary, although the patient should be told what the procedure entails and that some minor discomfort may be felt as the needle electrodes are inserted. The patient may be required to restrict cigarette smoking or caffeine intake before the test. The procedure takes at least 1 hour.

Laboratory Tests

A number of laboratory tests are useful in the diagnosis and evaluation of musculoskeletal disorders (Table 56-4, p. 1526).

CRITICAL THINKING QUESTIONS

1 Explain the process by which muscle contraction occurs.
2 Describe the different types of normal skeletal muscle contractions.
3 Design three questions to discreetly assess the psychosocial ramifications of musculoskeletal disorders.
4 In what ways might musculoskeletal alterations affect a patient's self-care abilities and independent functioning?
5 Describe musculoskeletal changes related to aging.
6 Your patient seems concerned about having a radioactive substance injected as part of a bone scan. What information can you give the patient about the safety of the radioactive substance?
7 Describe the patient care required before and after arthroscopy.

BIBLIOGRAPHY

Current

1. Bates B et al: *A guide to physical examination and history-taking,* ed 5, New York, 1991, JB Lippincott Co.
2. Cella JH, Watson J: *Nurse's manual of laboratory tests,* Philadelphia, 1989, FA Davis Co.
3. Gallo JJ et al: *Handbook of geriatric assessment,* Rockville, Md, 1988, Aspen Publishers, Inc.
4. Gordon M: *Manual of nursing diagnosis,* New York, 1987, McGraw-Hill, Inc.
5. Kane RL et al: *Essentials of clinical geriatrics,* ed 2, New York, 1989, McGraw-Hill, Inc.
6. Kenny RA: *Physiology of aging: a synopsis,* Chicago, 1992, Year Book Medical Publishers, Inc.
7. Lee K, Kucharczyk W: Magnetic resonance imaging of the brain and spine, *Medicine* 3:36, 1989.

TABLE 56-4   Laboratory Tests for Musculoskeletal Disorders

Determination	Usual reference range	Comments
Anti-DNA binding antibody (anti-DNA)	Negative at 1:10 serum dilution	Detects antibodies that react with native, double-stranded DNA and is the most specific test for SLE
Antinuclear antibodies (ANAs)	Negative for 1:32 serum dilution	Identify presence of antibodies produced against portions of body's own cell nuclei; ANAs sometimes form antigen-antibody complexes that damage tissue, as in SLE; patient's serum is mixed with cell nuclei from rat; if serum contains ANAs, it forms antigen-antibody complexes with cell nuclei; nuclei fluoresce when fluorescein-labeled antihuman serum is added and examined with ultraviolet microscope; false-positive results occur with ingestion of drugs such as procainamide, isoniazid, phenytoin, oral contraceptives, penicillin, and sulfonamides; this is valuable screening test for SLE but is not specific to SLE; elevated ANA titers also occur with viral diseases, with collagen vascular disease, with autoimmune disease, and in normal older adults
Lupus erythematosus cells (LE preparation; LE cell preparation)	No LE cells seen	Patient's blood sample is mixed with laboratory-treated nucleoprotein (ANAs); if ANAs are present, they react with nucleoprotein; test is used to screen for SLE but is less sensitive and reliable than anti-DNA and ANAs
Antistreptolysin O (ASO) tests	Less than 166 Todd units	Measures relative serum concentrations of antibody to streptolysin O, enzyme produced by group A beta-hemolytic streptococci; ASO useful in differentiating between rheumatic fever and rheumatoid arthritis in presence of joint pain and also aids in diagnosis of rheumatic fever and poststreptococcal glomerulonephritis when clinical symptoms are present
HLA-B27 antigen test (human leukocyte antigen B27)	No antigen present	HLA-B27 present with ankylosing spondylitis, Reiter's syndrome, sacroiliitis, and psoriatic arthritis; nucleated cells such as leukocytes, platelets, and most tissue cells contain human leukocyte antigen (HLA) system on surface membranes; these antigens are divided into five series (A, B, C, D, or DR); presence of certain HLAs has been associated with increased susceptibility to some diseases; HLAs also used in matching donor and recipient in organ transplantation and to establish paternity
Rheumatoid factor (RF)	Negative	Detects "renegade" IgG or IgM antibodies; these antibodies, produced by lymphocytes in synovial joints, in turn produce immune complexes, activate complement and destroy tissue; in latex agglutination test, visible clumping of serum with human IgG absorbed onto latex particles indicates presence of RF; test is useful in confirming diagnosis of rheumatoid arthritis and may also be positive in elderly persons
Complement fixation	Total complement: 41-90 U/mL (41-90 kU/mL)	Complement is a collective term for a group of normal serum proteins that destroy and remove foreign materials; in SLE and rheumatoid arthritis, complement is used up in development of antibody-antigen complexes, so serum levels are decreased; serum levels are measured by adding patient's serum to antibody-coated sheep red blood cells; if complement level is normal; 50% of red blood cells are lysed

TABLE 56-4   Laboratory Tests for Musculoskeletal Disorders—cont'd

Determination	Usual reference range	Comments
Uric acid (serum)	Males: 4-8.5 mg/dL (0.24-0.5 mmol/L) Females: 2.7-7.3 mg/dL (0.16-0.43 mmol/L)	Uric acid is end product of purine metabolism; elevated levels occur with gout, chronic renal failure, chronic myeloid leukemia, and polycythemia vera; thiazide diuretics, excessive stress, and high dietary intakes of purine cause increased levels of uric acid
Alkaline phosphatase (ALP)	U/L Age (yr) Males Females 20-24 102 98 25-34 109 100 35-44 122 112 45-54 139 121 55-64 159 132 65-74 161 172 >75 227 199	Experts believe this enzyme is needed for mineralized organic bone matrix, in transport of metabolites across cell membranes, and in transport of lipids; ALP level is elevated with healing fractures, osteomalacia, bone cancers, Paget's disease, rickets, and metastatic liver disease
Calcium (serum)	Total: Adult: 8.4-10.2 mg/dL (2.10-2.55 mmol/L) >65 yr: 8.8-10.0 mg/dL (2.20-2.50 mmol/L)	Gives bone structural strength; bone is primary storage site for calcium; decreased levels are found with bone tumors, acute osteoporosis, osteomalacia, renal disease, and hypoparathyroidism; serum levels are affected by certain drugs (vitamin D, estrogen, cortisone, and antacids) and by radiopaque dyes
Phosphorus (serum)	Adult: 2.7-4.5 mg/dL (0.87-1.45 mmol/L) >65 yr: Males: 2.3-3.7 mg/dL (0.74-1.20 mmol/L Females: 2.8-4.8 mg/dL 0.9-1.32 mmol/L	Directly relates to calcium metabolism; 85% of total body phosphorus is found in bone and 10% in skeletal muscle; elevated levels are found with healing fractures, osteolytic metastatic tumor, chronic renal disease, hypoparathyroidism, and certain drugs (aluminum hydroxide gel [Amphojel], insulin, and epinephrine)
Creatine kinase (CK)	Males: 55-170 U/L at 37° C (55-170 U/L at 37° C) Females: 30-135 U/L at 37° C (30-135 U/L at 37° C)	Activity is greatest in skeletal muscle and myocardium; CK levels are elevated with muscular dystrophy, traumatic injuries, intramuscular injections, surgery, severe coughing, muscle massage, and myocardial infarction

8. LeFever Kee J: *Handbook of laboratory and diagnostic tests with nursing implications,* Philadelphia, 1990, Appleton & Lange.
9. Magee DJ: *Orthopedic physical assessment,* Philadelphia, 1987, WB Saunders Co.
10. Malasanos L et al: *Health assessment,* ed 4, St Louis, 1990, Mosby–Year Book.
11. Mercier LR: *Practical orthopedics,* ed 3, St Louis, 1991, Mosby–Year Book.
12. Murray R, Zentner S: *Nursing assessment and health promotion through the life span,* Englewood Cliffs, NJ, 1989, Prentice-Hall, Inc.
13. *Nurse's ready reference: diagnostic tests,* Springhouse, 1991, Springhouse Corporation.
14. Pagana KD, Pagana TJ: *Diagnostic testing and nursing implications: a case study approach,* St Louis, 1990, Mosby–Year Book.
15. Seidel HM et al: *Mosby's guide to physical examination,* ed 2, St Louis, 1991, Mosby–Year Book.
16. Swartz MH: *Textbook of physical diagnosis,* Philadelphia, 1989, WB Saunders Co.
17. Tilkian SM, Conover MB, Tilkian AG: *Clinical implications of laboratory tests,* St Louis, 1987, Mosby–Year Book.

Classic
18. Block G, Nolan J: *Health assessment for professional nursing: a developmental approach,* New York, 1986, Appleton-Century-Crofts.
19. Bowers A, Thompson J: *Clinical manual of health assessment,* St Louis, 1984, Mosby–Year Book.
20. Bryne CJ et al: *Laboratory tests: implications for nursing care,* Menlo Park, Calif, 1986, Addison-Wesley Publishing Co, Inc.
21. Cacayorin ED, Hochhauser L, Petro GR: Lumbar and thoracic spine pain in the athlete: radiographic evaluation, *Clin Sports Med* 6:4, 1987.
22. Carotenuto R, Bullock J: *Physical assessment of the gerontologic client,* Philadelphia, 1981, FA Davis Co.
23. Fields W, McGinn-Campbell K: *Introduction to health assessment,* Reston, Va, 1983, Reston Publishing Co, Inc.
24. Hoppenfeld S: *Physical examination of the spine and extremities,* Norwalk, 1976, Appleton-Century-Crofts.
25. Malasanos L et al: *Health assessment,* ed 4, St Louis, 1990, Mosby–Year Book.
26. Prior JA, Silberstein JS, Stang JM: *Physical diagnosis: the history and examination of the patient,* ed 6, St Louis, 1981, Mosby–Year Book.
27. Tietz HW, editor: *Textbook of clinical chemistry,* Philadelphia, 1986, WB Saunders Co.

CHAPTER FIFTY-SEVEN

Nursing Management of Adults with Musculoskeletal Trauma

LEARNING OBJECTIVES

1 Explain the nursing management for patients with contusions, strains, sprains, bursitis, epicondylitis, and dislocations.
2 Discuss nursing management of the patient with sports injuries or overuse syndrome.
3 Describe principles of treatment, nursing interventions, and rationales for patients with fractures.
4 Compare the nursing management for a patient with traction to the nursing management of a patient with a cast.
5 Discuss the stages of fracture healing, nonunion, and delayed healing.
6 Identify potential hazards of immobility and complications of musculoskeletal trauma on a patient's health status.
7 Develop a care plan for a patient with an internal fixation device.
8 Identify the therapeutic and nursing management for a patient with a traumatic amputation.
9 Relate the psychologic and physiologic effects of a traumatic amputation.

KEY TERMS

avascular necrosis, p. 1541
Buck's traction, p. 1546
cervical traction, p. 1547
closed fracture, p. 1537
compartment syndrome, p. 1541
external fixation device, p. 1549

fat embolism syndrome (FES), p. 1544
gas gangrene, p. 1542
open fracture, p. 1537
osteomyelitis, p. 1543
phantom pain, p. 1578
Russell's traction, p. 1546

ACCORDING TO THE National Center for Health Statistics, 1 of 10 persons in the United States suffers an acute musculoskeletal injury.[18] These injuries are most commonly contusions, strains, sprains, dislocations, or fractures, with fractures being the most serious. Although fractures result in damage to the skeletal system, injury to the muscular, vascu- lar, and nervous systems also may occur. Since muscles, nerves, ligaments, and bones function together, any injury to one may cause a malfunction of another. Trauma to the musculoskeletal system gener- ally limits the patient's ability to perform activities of daily living. Since musculoskeletal injuries require a long period to heal, many patients need encouragement and support. Factors influencing the time for healing include the age and health status of the patient, the type of injury, and the patient's compliance to the prescribed treatment.

Soft Tissue Trauma

CONTUSION
Definition

A contusion (or bruise) is an injury to soft tissue that results in rupture of the small blood vessels and hemorrhage (ecchymosis) at the trauma site. Contusions are usually caused by trauma from a blunt object and may occur in conjunction with sprains or fractures.

Clinical Manifestations

Clinical manifestations include pain, swelling, and discoloration at the trauma site. This discoloration of the skin may progress from a bruised bluish appearance to brown and then yellow before returning to normal. These skin color changes are the result of the presence of blood in the tissue. The skin color continues to change as blood is absorbed. If the trauma is severe enough to cause a sufficient amount of bleeding and a collection of blood at the site, a hematoma may form.

STRAIN
Definition

A strain is an injury to the muscle as a result of "overstretching," overuse, or excessive stress.[2] When viewed under a microscope, the affected muscle reveals incomplete tears in the muscle tissue. These tears result in bleeding into the muscle with subsequent pain, swelling, and muscle spasms.

Clinical Manifestations

Immediately following a strain, objective symptoms may be absent. The patient may have experienced sudden pain followed by pain on moving the affected part. Discoloration is usually not present unless the patient sustained a contusion or an injury to the soft tissues. If the patient has "overused" the affected part, a complaint of the part "feeling dead" may be voiced. The patient may be unable to participate in exercise or unwilling to move the part because of fear of pain.

SPRAIN
Definition

A sprain is an injury involving the ligamentous structures that surround a joint. This injury may be a tear or stretching of the ligament.

Clinical Manifestations

In addition to ligaments, blood vessels may be injured, resulting in hemorrhage (contusion) to the soft tissue. Usually the patient has rapid swelling at the injury site for the first 2 to 3 hours after injury because of the extravasation of blood within tissues. The degree of pain and swelling may not be directly proportional to the severity of injury. In addition to the sprain, the patient could have a hairline fracture, which may not produce any swelling, although it is usually painful. A mild sprain is present when the ligament is stretched or microscopically torn. Usually the patient has local tenderness and swelling but may be able to move the affected part. A moderate sprain exists when some ligamentous tearing is present. The part is edematous; tenderness and moderate pain on movement are present. A severe sprain is present when the ligament is disrupted, and there is gross joint instability. The patient is unable to flex the joint and is not able to bear weight on the affected part.

Therapeutic Management

If the patient has been involved in an accident, x-ray studies may be obtained to rule out bone injury. Primary treatment for soft tissue injury includes *rest, ice, compression,* and *elevation* (RICE) of the injured part. Immobilization of the injured site is the initial treatment measure, and ice is applied immediately. The application of a cold compress or an ice pack to the site is used to control swelling. Cold therapy promotes vasoconstriction, which decreases swelling. If swelling occurs, the patient experiences pain as a result of the pressure of blood and lymph accumulation on nerve endings. Cold therapy is applied immediately and continued for the first 24 to 36 hours after injury. Some physicians prescribe continuous application of cold compresses, whereas others prescribe an intermittent 20- to 30-minute application every 3 to 4 hours. After the initial 36 hours, moist or dry heat may be prescribed. Application of heat promotes vessel vasodilation and absorption of blood, which enhances tissue repair.

The injured part is elevated above the heart for 24 to 36 hours to promote venous return and decrease edema. In addition, the injured site may be wrapped with an elastic bandage for compression, which will control subsequent bleeding and prevent swelling. This may be continued to prevent or reduce swelling at the site if it has already occurred. The compression bandage not only controls edema but also supports the injured tissue. Muscle relaxants may be administered if the patient is experiencing muscle spasms associated with the injury. The patient may be instructed to keep the affected part at rest. In the case of strains and sprains, rest may be accomplished by use of a splint if the part is an upper extremity or with crutches if it is a lower extremity.

Ready-made splints are available, including the newer types that are inflated with air. For an active athlete a bulky dressing is inconvenient, so a nonrigid dressing, such as taping, that allows early return to activity may be the best choice. The taping procedure protects the joint from additional eversion (turning outward) or inversion (turning inward) stress, but it allows some flexion and mild activity. Early activity prevents muscle atrophy, provides proper organization of collagen fibers during ligament healing, and promotes circulation. Some physicians use braces for treating sprains to the extremities. Braces provide more support than taping and allow the patient more activity than a cast. Braces allow the patient to gradually increase weight-bearing activity as the ligaments heal. Occasionally treatment for a moderate to severe sprain will require casting. If it is determined that a cast is necessary, this may be delayed 2 to 3 days to reduce some of the initial swelling. If a cast is applied before swelling is completed the cast may be too tight, causing damage to the circulatory system and nerve supply. If a cast is applied before swelling is reduced, the cast will become too loose and not provide immobilization as the swelling decreases. Once a cast is removed, a brace may be used to allow limited activity as the ligament heals (see discussion of cast care, p. 1559).

NURSING MANAGEMENT OF THE PATIENT WITH SOFT TISSUE TRAUMA
Assessment

As with any patient who has sustained trauma, the nurse completes an overall assessment. Special attention is directed to the injured part to determine the extent of injury and the soft tissues involved. The nurse assesses the injured site to determine if any other injuries are present. Observations are made for any limitation in activity, pain on movement, and, in the case of contusions, discoloration at the trauma site. In taking a history of the events of the injury, it is important to determine if the joint was involved. An inverted joint or a "cracking" or "snapping" sound heard during the injury may indicate a fracture or tendon injury. Activities and movements that cause pain are included in the assessment. If the injury involves one extremity, it is important for the nurse to examine the unaffected extremity to establish baseline data for comparison.

Nursing Diagnosis

Nursing diagnoses may include the following:
  Acute pain related to tissue damage, swelling, muscle spasm, and/or damage to the ligament

  Impaired physical mobility related to pain, swelling, and/or joint instability

Planning

The nurse plans interventions to achieve the following outcomes:
  Pain will be relieved
  Swelling will be reduced
  Muscle spasms will be relieved
  Weight bearing and mobility will be increased

Implementation

Nursing interventions include applying cold compresses or an ice pack to the site and elevating the affected part. When applying a cold pack to the injury, the nurse places a cloth between the skin and the ice pack. If a cold pack is applied directly to the skin, thermal injury resembling frostbite can occur. The patient is instructed to begin applications of moist or dry heat to the injury after 24 to 36 hours. The nurse applies an elastic (Ace) wrap if indicated. When this bandage is applied, the extremity is wrapped from distal to proximal to prevent trapping blood and causing venous engorgement of the extremity.

For the patient taking muscle relaxants, the nurse teaches the patient and family about any precautions or side effects associated with the medications. The patient may need to limit activities and exercise of the affected part. The nurse instructs the patient and family about proper positioning and elevation of the affected part to alleviate pressure, tension, edema, or further injury. The nurse provides emotional support during episodes of pain, such as informing the patient of pain mechanisms and interventions, acknowledging the patient's pain, and providing the prescribed analgesia.

Nursing interventions for impaired physical mobility include positioning the patient in proper alignment and demonstrating how to maintain position; instituting range-of-motion and strengthening exercises as appropriate after immobilization of the affected part; and encouraging the patient to progress with daily activities, from bed mobility through ambulation with appropriate assistive devices.

Evaluation

Evaluation consists of determining whether pain is under control as evidenced by patient verbalization and ability to move with the use of assistive devices. Before the patient leaves the health care facility, the nurse asks the patient or family member to demonstrate use of assistive devices. In addition, the patient will verbalize a plan for resumption of activities of daily living.

Documentation

The nurse documents the nursing assessment, including location, appearance, and size of any bruising or swelling. Discoloration may not be present until several hours after the trauma. If the patient seeks treatment immediately following an injury, the "bruising effect" may not yet be evident. The nurse records all complaints of pain or discomfort that the patient expresses whether or not discoloration is present. Administration of analgesics and muscle relaxants and their effects are noted. In addition, all instructions given to the patient and evidence of learning are recorded. If assistive or immobilization devices are used, the nurse documents the teaching provided, the patient's ability to use the device, and the individual's subjective and physical responses, especially any fear or fatigue.

Ongoing Care

The patient is told that a hematoma is evidenced by an increase in pain or swelling at the injury site and the patient should return to the health care agency or notify the physician if additional ecchymosis (bluish discoloration related to bleeding into the skin or mucous membranes) occurs. Severe ecchymosis may indicate compartment syndrome rather than an uncomplicated contusion and requires immediate attention (see p. 1541).

The nurse explains to the patient that continued use of a strained muscle will not only delay the repair process but also may cause further damage to the affected muscle. The patient is reminded to keep the affected part immobilized as ordered. The nurse ensures that the patient understands when the bandage can be removed and the correct procedure for its reapplication. The patient is told to return to the health care agency or notify the physician if additional swelling occurs or if muscle spasms become more frequent.

Sprains may take 1 month or longer to heal. The nurse explains the reason for limitation of activities that place additional stress on the injured tissue. The patient is instructed to report any tingling or loss of sensation below the sprain and any increase in swelling or pain.

The nurse advises the patient of the exact time frame for the application of cold packs and when they should be replaced with heat compresses. The nurse demonstrates for the patient how to elevate the affected part above heart level and explains that this is the most effective method of preventing and reducing swelling. The nurse teaches range-of-motion exercises or refers the patient to physical therapy for exercise routines or use of assistive devices.

Several ambulation aids can help the patient become mobile and maintain stability, either with or without weight bearing on an injured lower extremity. The most common are crutches, canes, and walkers. Nursing interventions are formulated to enable the patient to ambulate without injury. The nurse remains near the patient during initial efforts to dangle or ambulate. In this way the nurse can teach the correct use of the device and prevent a fall. If crutches are used, the patient is taught crutch positions, gaits, and maneuvers. With practice the patient should become steadier while using the aid and be able to move about independently without falling.

BURSITIS AND EPICONDYLITIS
Definition

Bursitis is the inflammation of the bursa, a small sac between muscles and joints. Figure 57-1 shows the bursae of the shoulder commonly affected. Epicondylitis, more commonly known as tennis elbow, is the result of damaged tendons of the medial or lateral radial and ulnar epicondyles.

Etiology/Pathophysiology

With bursitis repeated use of or trauma to the joint results in inflammation. Joints commonly affected are the subdeltoid, olecranon, and hip. With epicondylitis the tendons become inflamed with subsequent tissue scarring. Tendon damage follows activities such as tennis or hammering that require excessive pronation and supination of the hand.

Clinical Manifestations

Clinical features of bursitis and epicondylitis are pain, limitation of motion, edema, and erythema. In

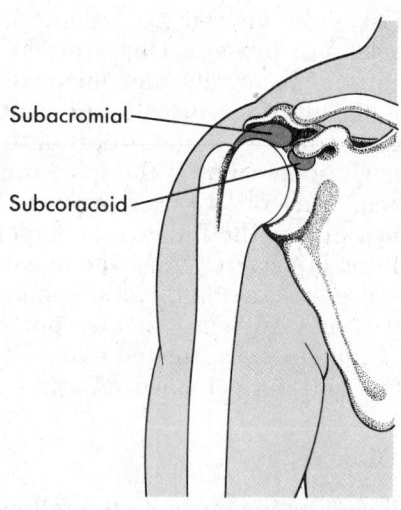

Subacromial

Subcoracoid

FIGURE 57-1   Bursae of shoulder.

addition, with epicondylitis the patient may exhibit decreased grip and strength in the affected arm.

Therapeutic Management

Therapeutic management of bursitis and epicondylitis includes restricting activities of the affected joint for 4 to 6 weeks, cold and moist heat applications, salicylates, nonsteroidal anti-inflammatory drugs (NSAIDs), and corticosteroid injections (see Table 58-4). Medical management may also include splinting with epicondylitis.

NURSING MANAGEMENT OF THE PATIENT WITH BURSITIS AND EPICONDYLITIS

Assessment

Nursing assessment of patients with bursitis and epicondylitis involves noting joint involvement by evaluation of pain, edema, erythema, and limitation of motion. The grasp reflex of both hands is assessed and compared to determine if the weakness is present in the affected extremity with epicondylitis.

Nursing Diagnosis

Nursing diagnoses for these patients include the following:

Acute pain related to tissue/joint damage or swelling

Impaired physical mobility related to pain, swelling, and limitation of motion

Planning

The nurse plans interventions to achieve the following outcomes:

Pain will be relieved
Swelling will be reduced
Mobility will be increased

Implementation

Nursing measures include the application of cold or moist heat compresses to the affected joints to decrease the patient's discomfort and inflammation. Restriction of the involved joint will decrease trauma and promote healing. In addition, prescribed medications such as salicylates, other NSAIDs, and steroids (see Table 58-4) can be administered, with the nurse noting side effects.

As a result of pain with bursitis and epicondylitis, patients restrict use of the inflamed joint. Nurses promote limitation of activities with the affected joint and limited range-of-motion exercises to maintain joint mobility and muscle strength. The use of assistive devices is encouraged to allow maximum use of the joint with minimal discomfort. As with other joint-restrictive disorders, the patient may lose the ability to participate in normal daily and occupational activities. Nursing measures promote self-care activities and encourage maintenance of social and vocational activities to increase self-esteem. Patients are encouraged to verbalize feelings and concerns in regard to their specific musculoskeletal disorder. Written and verbal patient teaching materials are reviewed with the patient. These educational sessions address the inflammatory process associated with epicondylitis and bursitis and their respective treatment regimens.

Evaluation

To determine whether the patient goals are attained, the nurse assesses the patient's use of the involved joint and subjective complaints of pain. Participation in daily activities and the patient's self-esteem are evaluated to determine the effectiveness of nursing interventions. As symptom control is achieved with medications and restricted use of the joint, compliance with the treatment regimen is also examined.

Documentation

The nurse documents the degree of pain and the effectiveness of nursing and pharmacologic measures. In addition, the amount of swelling and limitation in motion is noted. The nurse documents any teaching provided for the patient as well as evidence of patient understanding and compliance.

Ongoing Care

The ongoing care of patients with upper extremity joint impairment requires assessment of the patient's home environment to determine the need for assistive devices to reduce joint inflammation. Range-of-motion exercises are reviewed to prevent reduced joint mobility and strengthen muscles. The patient's use of pain management techniques is continually assessed for effectiveness. If some vocational or recreational activities are restricted as a result of epicondylitis or bursitis, other satisfying activities are identified and encouraged.

Skeletal Trauma

DISLOCATIONS
Definition

A dislocation is the displacement of a bone from its normal position in the joint. A partial displacement between the two bone surfaces of a joint is called a subluxation.

Etiology

Traumatic dislocations occur most frequently in persons under 20 years of age.[18] Congenital or acquired disorders such as congenital hip dislocations and rheumatoid arthritis also cause dislocation.

Pathophysiology

Dislocations in adults are usually the result of a trauma of great force. The force that causes bones to become dislodged, or "out of joint," may also cause significant damage to the joint structure, ligaments, blood vessels, nerves, and adjacent soft tissue. Pressure on blood vessels may result in ischemic paralysis distal to the injury. The femoral head gets much of its blood supply from vessels that emerge from the acetabulum, and when the hip is dislocated, the femoral head may be ripped away from its blood supply with a resultant avascular necrosis[19] (Figure 57-2). This condition occurs when

blood supply is disrupted to the bone. Ischemia develops and can progress to necrosis. For a more complete discussion see p. 1541. Contusion or disruption of the adjacent sciatic nerve can cause permanent, partial, or complete sensory or motor loss in the leg on the side of the dislocation.[28]

Clinical Manifestations

Clinical manifestations include severe pain, change in the length of the extremity because the bone is not in the socket, inability to move the extremity without severe pain, and a change in the contour and shape of the joint.

Therapeutic Management

If the dislocation involves the shoulders, the affected arm is placed in a sling. If the dislocation concerns the hip, the affected leg can be taped to the unaffected leg, or the affected leg can be placed on a firm board or a fracture splint applied. An x-ray film of the affected part is necessary to determine if a fracture is present and to confirm the diagnosis. When the diagnosis of dislocation is established, plans are made for a reduction (i.e., manually placing the bone

CLINICAL ALERT

A dislocation is considered an emergency, since there is a potential for impaired circulation because of the abnormal location of the bone. The affected part is assessed and immobilized immediately so further damage to soft tissue will not occur. An ice pack is applied immediately to minimize swelling at the socket site. Reduction of the dislocation should occur as soon as possible to prevent tissue necrosis and damage to the nerve supply.

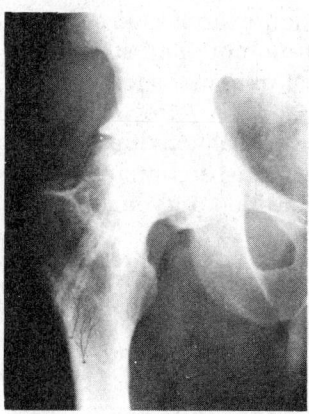

FIGURE 57-2   Avascular necrosis. (From Ferrell J: *Illustrated guide to orthopedic nursing*, Philadelphia, 1986, JB Lippincott Co.)

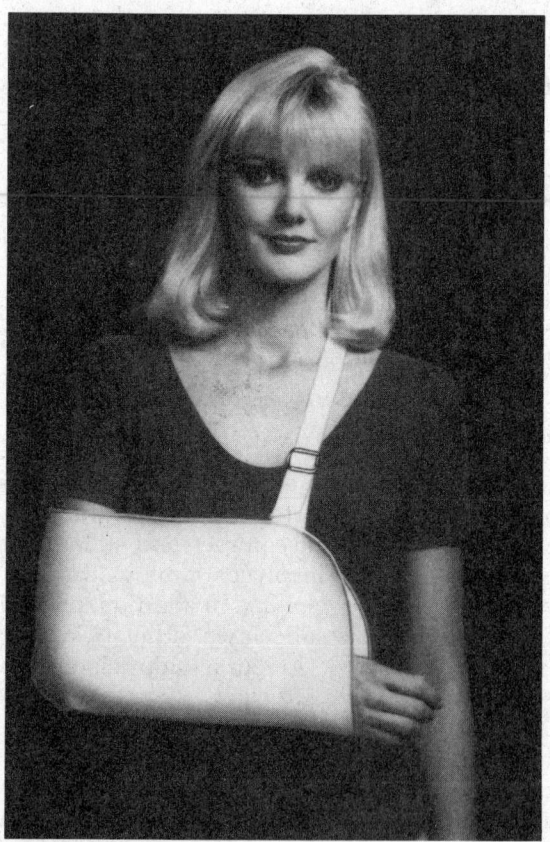

FIGURE 57-3   Sling for shoulder/arm immobilization.

into the joint). Before attempting manual reduction, a sedative is administered intravenously to the patient. General anesthesia with a closed reduction (no incision) may be necessary to reduce the dislocation. For the patient with repeated dislocations of the same joint, an open reduction (surgical incision) with repair of the ligament may be the procedure of choice. After the reduction the area is immobilized to allow for healing of damaged ligaments and tissue. Following reduction the shoulder can usually be immobilized in an arm immobilizer (Figure 57-3) or a splint; the hip may have to be immobilized with skin traction, such as Buck's traction (see p. 1546). Muscle relaxants may be administered to prevent muscle spasm and control the pain.

NURSING MANAGEMENT OF THE PATIENT WITH A DISLOCATION

Assessment

Assessment of the patient with a dislocation both before and immediately following the reduction is very important. Impairment in circulation may occur at either time in the treatment phase. It is imperative that the nurse assesses not only the site of dislocation but also the dependent area distal to the dislocation. The nurse assesses these sites for the 5 P's every 10 to 15 minutes before the reduction and at 30- to 60-minute intervals for the first 12 hours after the reduction. Any signs or symptoms of circulatory or nerve impairment must be reported immediately to the physician.

Assessment of the five P's is an appropriate method to determine neurologic and circulatory status (see box). Pertinent questions and observations confirm and validate each of the five P's. The five P's are as follows:

- **Pain**—progressive pain on movement of the affected part
- **Pallor**—in the affected extremity
- **Paralysis**—inability to move the affected part
- **Paresthesia**—numbness and tingling
- **Pulselessness**—lack of pulse

The nurse continues to assess the affected part and documents the findings at intervals appropriate for the injury. No specific time interval for the assessment is applicable to all injuries. This interval is based on the extent of injury.

Nursing Diagnosis

Nursing diagnoses of the patient with a dislocation include the following:

Pain, acute, related to lack of continuity of bone to joint

Impaired physical mobility related to imposed mechanical restriction, decreased muscle strength, or pain

High risk for altered peripheral tissue perfusion related to interruption of arterial blood flow

Planning

Outcomes for the patient with a dislocation include the following:

Pain relief reported

Restrictions in activity followed as necessary to allow for healing

Neurovascular status within normal limits

Implementation

Nursing interventions for the patient with a dislocation are similar to the care provided the patient with a fracture in the same location as the dislocation. In addition, the care is based on the type of reduction. If the reduction was accomplished by external manipulation, no additional treatment may be necessary except to provide medication for pain relief. If the reduction was accomplished with an incision while the patient was under anesthesia, care is the same as for an open reduction of a fracture. No additional treatment may be necessary except to provide medication for pain relief.

SPORTS INJURIES AND OVERUSE SYNDROME

The main two categories of sports-related injuries are acute injuries and overuse injuries. Acute injuries include fractures, sprains (ligaments), strains, and compartment syndrome. Overuse injuries result from repetitive microtrauma causing inflammation of joints, stress fractures, tendinitis, and bursitis.[32] During growth spurts, soft tissue elongation lags behind long bone growth, and the result is decreased joint flexibility. Other factors that cause overuse syndromes include the following:

- Rotational and angular deformities
- Rapid increase in training intensity
- Improper equipment, especially shoes
- Playing conditions[32]

In the athlete the knee is the most common site of trauma to joints and ligaments and of overuse injury to the extensor mechanism. General symptoms of knee injuries include pain, swelling, popping, clicking, locking, buckling, and joint line tenderness.[9] Symptoms of ligament instability involve knee buckling, whereas tendinitis of the hamstrings causes posterior knee pain with downhill running and the knee "giving out" while stepping down.[32] The diagnosis of ligament injury and tendon rupture is usually made by magnetic resonance imaging (MRI) or arthroscopy, and the treatment is usually surgical repair. After surgery the part may be immobilized in a cast or an immobilizer brace (see p.

ASSESSMENT OF CIRCULATORY AND NEUROLOGIC STATUS

1. *Pain:* usually the patient will report pain to the nurse. Facial grimace and overprotective behaviors indicate pain. Unrelenting or unusual pain as well as pain on passive motion indicates neurovascular impairment. Questions to ask the patient include the following:
   - Tell me about the pain.
   - Is it constant, or does it come at intervals?
   - Is the pain sharp, dull, or throbbing?
   - What activity causes the pain to occur?
   - When you are still, is the pain present?
   - Show me exactly where the pain is located.
2. *Pallor:* inspection of the dependent part below the injury is one of the most effective methods to determine circulation. The skin is assessed to determine the color and capillary filling. Use an unaffected area to determine if the affected area fills as rapidly as the unaffected area. Capillary refill is considered abnormal if it takes longer than 3 seconds.
   - Check to see if the nail beds blanch when pressed.
   - Check to see if there is a rapid return of color when the pressure is released.
   - Compare the affected part with the patient's unaffected part to determine what the color should be.
3. *Paralysis:* have the patient move the fingers or toes on the affected extremity. Since paralysis is the temporary suspension or permanent loss of function, the nurse must encourage and insist that the patient attempt to demonstrate mobility. Excessive swelling may hinder the patient's ability to voluntarily move a part, so the nurse keeps the dependent part at heart level to prevent and reduce swelling.
   - Instruct the patient to move the affected part. This should not involve any weight-bearing or lifting activity; but rather ask the patient to wiggle the toes or the fingers of the affected part.
   - Many patients will immediately say, "I can't do that," when told to move the part. The nurse may need to do passive motion to the part several times at 15- to 30-minute intervals to enhance the blood supply to the part. (Active or passive exercise will cause the cells to demand an increase in oxygen and nutrients to the tissue. Therefore movement will enhance the blood supply to the part and also reduce swelling.) It is imperative that the nurse determines the patient's ability to move the part in order to detect any signs of paralysis.

4. *Paresthesia:* defined as an abnormal sensation that may be described by the patient as numbness, prickling, or tingling. When the patient complains of any of these symptoms, the nurse assesses the part to determine any exterior causes. If there is a cast, an immobilizer, or a bandage, this may be constricting or tight and may create a circulatory impairment. If such a circulatory impairment exists, it is also likely that an impairment to the nerve supply is present. If there is no external cause of impairment the nurse assesses for edema. If edema is present, it is likely that this excess fluid is creating pressure on the nerve supply and thus causing symptoms of paresthesia. When edema is present, the nurse elevates the part above the heart and assesses for the remaining four of the five P's.
   - Many patients, especially those who are reluctant to move the affected part, will frequently report numbness and tingling. The nurse encourages these patients to move the affected part so adequate circulatory and neurologic status is restored.
   - Be alert to the fact that damage to the nerve supply from the injury or from edema may be present when a patient complains of the symptoms of paresthesia. This damage may become permanent without prompt treatment.
5. *Pulselessness:* it is imperative to establish a baseline presence of a pulse in the location of the injury or distal to the injury. This baseline will serve as a guide for the evaluation of the serial pulses taken at intervals after the injury. The peripheral pulse, color, and temperature are assessed on the *unaffected* side to serve as a comparison with the injured part. With circulatory impairment the nurse expects to find a cool to cold skin temperature.

   The lack of a pulse when the pulse had previously been present constitutes an emergency situation. Pulselessness may indicate that the affected part is not being supplied with the necessary oxygen and other nutrients to sustain cellular life. The presence of a pulse does not necessarily constitute adequate circulation. Pulselessness may be one of the last findings in neurovascular deficit. Therefore the nurse manages a diminished pulse in the same manner as pulselessness.

   Routine (at least every hour) pulse checks are imperative during the first 24 to 48 hours after an injury occurred or was treated. When the nurse observes a change in the pulse or the inability to locate a pulse occurs, the injured area is immediately repositioned and reassessed for pulse.

SPORTS INJURIES: EMERGENCY NURSING CARE

- Immediately assess to determine extent of injury. Include interview and visual assessment.
- *Never* move patient until extent of injury is determined.
- Complete five P's of neurovascular assessment for muscle ischemia.
- Immobilize the injured part.
- Apply ice or cooling therapy.
- Elevate the injury above the heart.

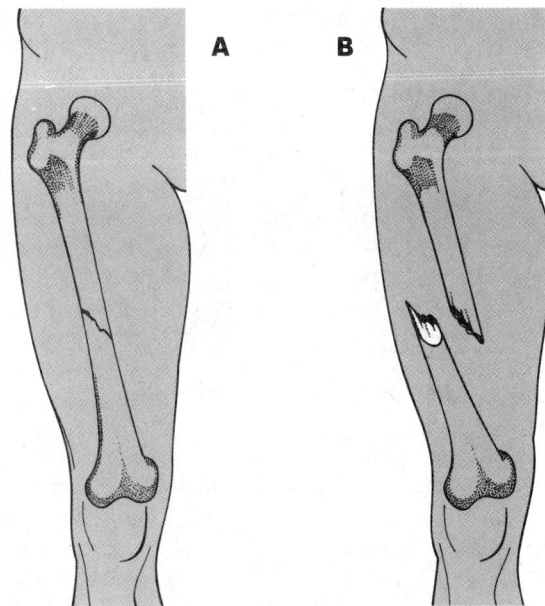

FIGURE 57-4   **A,** Closed fracture. **B,** Open fracture.

1559). Emergency care of the patient with a sports injury is included in the box above. Because the demands and expectations of athletics are greater today, preventive education and rehabilitation of the sports-injured patient are essential.

FRACTURES
Definition

A fracture is a break in the continuity of the bone. This break in continuity may be complete or incomplete, or it may be a bending of the bone.

Etiology

Fractures are rarely life threatening but are life disrupting. A fracture may result in prolonged or permanent disability. Fractures occur most commonly in young males under 24 years of age and in elderly persons. Sports injuries and workplace trauma account for most injuries in the young and middle-aged adult. Osteoporosis is a contributing factor to fractures in the older adult.

Pathophysiology

Most fractures are the result of trauma in the form of excessive stress placed on a bone.[11] Types of stress to the bone include (1) a direct blow to the bone, (2) an indirect twisting motion (torsion) or a severe muscle contraction, and (3) disease, such as cancer. When the bone is diseased, it may "crumble" like dry bread, causing a pathologic fracture. When a fracture occurs, the structural integrity of the bone is disrupted, as well as the vascular system in and to the bone. Fractures are identified based on (1) skin intactness, (2) type, (3) location, and (4) alignment status.

Classification

Broad classification of skin intactness helps determine whether the fracture site is closed or open. A **closed fracture** (Figure 57-4, *A*) exists when there is no break in the skin. This is also referred to as a simple fracture; however, the term *simple fracture* may be misleading. No fracture is "simple" to a patient, because each fracture causes the patient some activity restrictions and limitation. An **open fracture** (Figure 57-4, *B*) or compound fracture exists when the ends of the bone protrude through the skin. It is usually easy to distinguish between open and closed fractures during a visual assessment. However, open fractures in the forearm that occur when the patient catches himself or herself during a fall may retract back into the skin and not be readily evident without closer inspection. The distinction between open and closed is essential, since the open fracture usually requires operative treatment, and both the opening in the skin and the break in the bone are potential sites for infection.

Types of fracture

The type of fracture is based on the direction of the fracture line and the appearance of the fracture. The fracture line depends on the direction of the stress causing the injury and the type of bone involved. The five types (Figure 57-5) are as follows:

1. *Transverse*—across the bone
2. *Oblique*—slanting direction in the bone
3. *Spiral*—around the bone

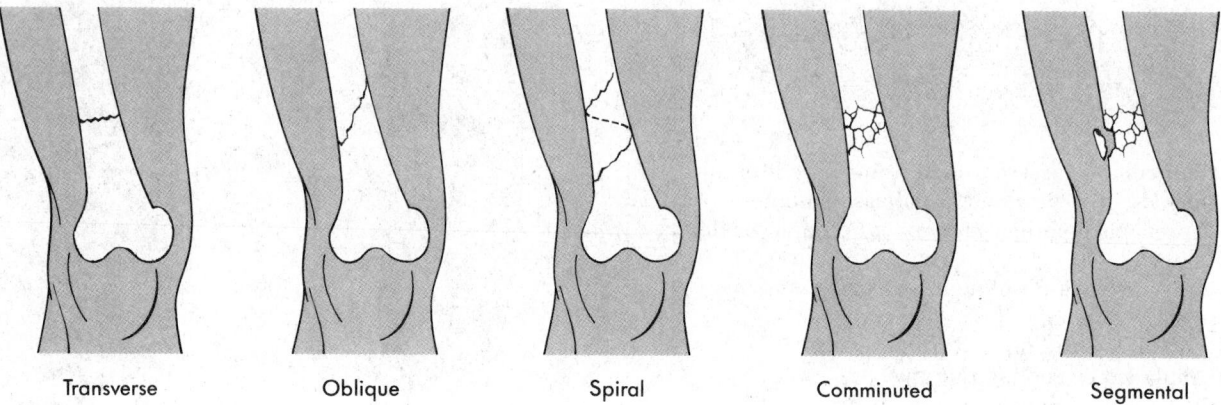

| Transverse | Oblique | Spiral | Comminuted | Segmental |

FIGURE 57-5   Five types of fractures.

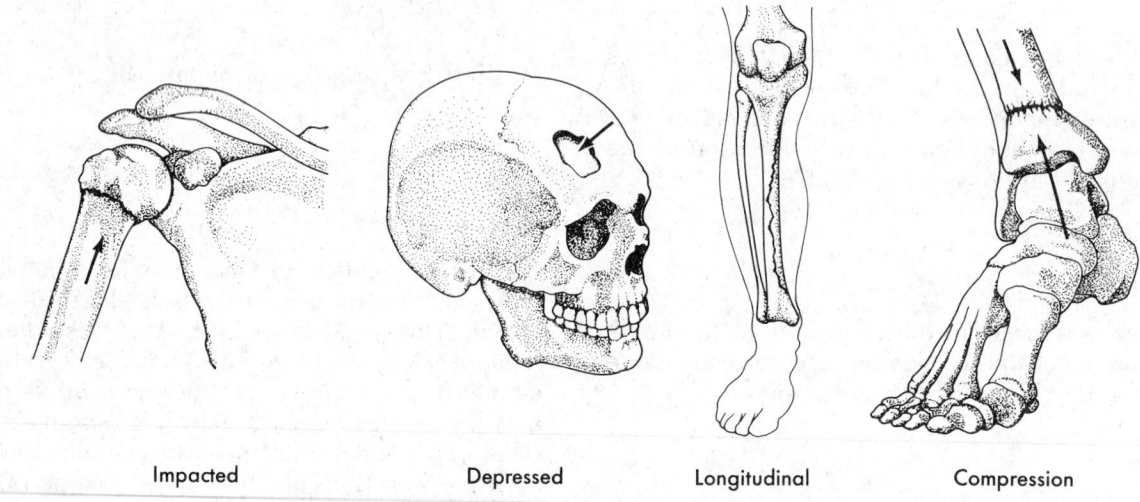

| Impacted | Depressed | Longitudinal | Compression |

FIGURE 57-6   Fractures in relation to bone ends.

4. *Comminuted*—having three or more fragments
5. *Segmental*—having a segment of the bone fractured and detached

Fractures may occur in the diaphysis, or shaft, of a bone. Cancellous or spongy bone, which makes up the long bones of the extremities and short flat bones, is subject to crushing and comminuted fractures. The exterior of a bone and the shafts of long bones are composed of compact or cortical tissue. These bones are likely to sustain transverse, oblique, or spiral fractures. These three directional fractures may be comminuted. Before puberty the epiphysis (broad end of the long bones) is bordered by the epiphyseal plate. Fractures to the epiphyseal growth plate in a child may result in cessation of bone growth with resulting unequal limb lengths.

In addition, the following factors are considered when describing the types of fractures; these terms describe the condition of the fracture in relation to the bone ends[11] (Figure 57-6):

* *Impacted:* the bone ends are pushed into each other under great force.
* *Depressed:* the bone fragments are pushed inward and therefore depressed.
* *Longitudinal:* the fracture is parallel with the bone (i.e., it runs longitudinally rather than horizontally).
* *Compression:* usually describes a bone that is crushed; most often used to refer to the collapse of a vertebra.

Other terms used to distinguish the type of fracture include stress fractures and pathologic fractures. Stress fractures occur from repetitive stress on a bone as in running. Pathologic fractures result from minor stress to a pathologically weakened bone (e.g., osteoporosis or cancer of the bone).

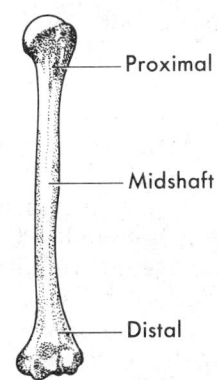

FIGURE 57-7   Location of fractures.

Location

The location of a fracture involving the extremities is usually described as being *proximal* (close to the body), *distal* (away from the body), or *mid shaft* (neither proximal nor distal, but located in the middle portion of the shaft) (Figure 57-7). Fractures of the spine are described according to the vertebra involved (i.e., cervical 4 or C4, lumbar 3 or L3). Fractures of a joint are described according to the location in relation to the joint. The fracture may be intracapsular (within the capsule), extracapsular (outside the capsule), or intra-articular (within the joint). A supracondylar fracture is above the condyle or condyles. This term is commonly used to describe a fracture of the humerus or femur. Avulsion fractures usually occur at a joint. These are the result of a piece of bone being pulled out of the cortex by a tear of a ligamentous attachment. An avulsion fracture of the shoulder occurs when there is avulsion of the greater tuberosity from the humerus at the shoulder.

Alignment status

Alignment status describes the location and positions of the fracture fragments. Several terms are used to describe the alignment status: nondisplacement, displacement, and angulation. The term nondisplacement indicates that bone fragments are aligned at the fracture site. Displacement exists when the two edges of the fracture have moved out of alignment. When this occurs the bone fragments have a zigzag contour. Displacement occurs because of unopposed muscle pull in a fragment. The displacement depends on the causative force and the strength of the surrounding muscle attachments.

Angulation occurs when the edges are positioned but the fragments themselves are out of alignment, so the contour of the bones appears angulated rather than aligned or zigzag. The fracture may be both displaced and angulated. It is important to remember that a fracture can be displaced in at least four directions: (1) sideways, (2) overriding, (3) rotated, and (4) offset.

Clinical Manifestations

The signs and symptoms of a fracture depend on the cause of the fracture and its classification, type of fracture, location, and alignment status. There are both specific and nonspecific signs of a fracture. Swelling at the site of the injury is the first sign. The patient may complain of severe pain at the time of the injury. As the swelling develops and increases, the pain may become more severe. Blood loss in excess of 2 units may occur in femur fractures to the extent that the extremity may swell to twice its normal size. The patient may complain only of tenderness at the site and a loss of function. There also may be a deformity in the bone continuity. This deformity is the most specific sign of a fracture. The other signs are nonspecific, since they may be present when there is a sprain or a strain but not a fracture.

Other signs include discoloration at the site and crepitus. Crepitus is a grating sensation that may be either heard or felt as the bones rub together. If there is an open wound, bleeding may be present. The bone ends may protrude through the open wound. Indications of fractures and their pathologic basis are presented in Table 57-1.

Therapeutic Management

Management of fractures is based on the following principles of treatment:

1. Realignment of bone fragments, known as the reduction of the fracture
2. Maintenance of the realignment by immobilization
3. Restoration of function

These principles do not include any emergency measures that may need to be initiated during the first few minutes or hours after a severe fracture.

Prehospital care

Emergency measures must be instituted before the reduction can be accomplished. Lifethreatening injuries must be managed first. Controlling shock and maintaining an open airway take priority.

Realignment of the fracture at the scene of the injury is not practical and is not attempted, since x-ray studies are necessary to determine the position of the bone fragments. Splinting of the fractured area is essential at the injury scene and must be done before the victim is moved. The orthopedic rule "splint them where they lie" remains the rule today. Splinting immobilizes the part and prevents further injury to the soft tissue and blood supply. The sharp bone fragments may create enough damage for the patient

TABLE 57-1   Signs, Symptoms, and Pathologic Basis of Fractures

Signs and symptoms	Pathologic basis
Swelling	Bleeding into tissue because of extravascular blood at site of injury Soft tissue damage increases degree of swelling
Pain	Accumulation of blood in area surrounding bone, causing pressure on nerve supply
Tenderness	Accumulation of blood in area surrounding bone where nerve supply is found
Loss of functional ability	Related to lack of bone continuity, which must be synchronized with muscles, ligaments, and nerves to function
Deformity	Lack of continuity in bone structure
Discoloration	Bleeding into tissue; may be rupture to a major artery or venous supply
Crepitus	Grating sensation or sound heard when two bones are rubbing together (Do not attempt to elicit.)
Bleeding at site through an open wound	Damage to artery or venous blood supply

to lose a large quantity of blood and cause hemorrhagic shock.

Splinting may prevent or decrease pain because it hinders further motion, which would cause pain. Splinting also lowers the possibility of fat embolism, which is a complication of a fracture of any long bone (see p. 1544). There is less soft tissue damage when the fracture is immobilized. In addition, muscle spasms are managed more easily when the fracture is splinted. Splinting also aids in transporting the patient to the hospital and transporting the patient to and from the x-ray or emergency department.

The type of splint used varies in form (Figure 57-8). The main purpose is to immobilize the part, so any apparatus that accomplishes this is satisfactory. For an upper extremity a sling is best; however, a board applied along the forearm or over a flexed elbow works well. In the absence of a sling or board, the arm can be splinted to the torso. For a lower extremity the ideal method is to place the patient on a stretcher after having placed a firm object under the leg. Lacking a firm object, the nurse can splint the affected leg to the unaffected leg. The ideal method to immobilize a patient suspected of having a cervical fracture is to place a hard cervical collar around the neck. These are usually available in a hospital, but if one is not available at the scene of the injury, towels, sandbags, or rolled clothes can be placed on each side of the neck (for a more complete discussion of cervical spine trauma, see Chapter 50).

After the patient has a splint applied, a neurovascular examination is performed. Since the impact of the injury and the bone fragments can damage the soft tissues and nerves, motor function is tested in the part distal to the fracture. Assessment of the five P's is an appropriate method to test general neurovascular status (see box, p. 1536).

The definitive diagnostic measure to determine the presence of a fracture is an x-ray study. If the patient has sustained multiple trauma, all of the ex-

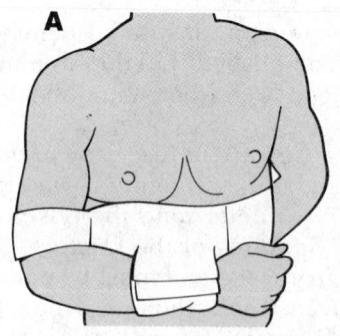 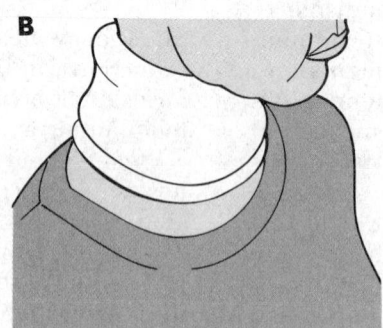 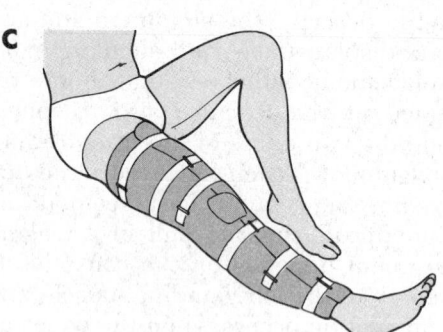

FIGURE 57-8   Examples of splints. **A,** Shoulder immobilizer. **B,** Cervical collar. **C,** Knee immobilizer.

TABLE 57-2   Fracture Complications

Fracture site	Potential complications
Hip	Sciatic nerve damage, avascular necrosis
Pelvis	Profuse bleeding, bladder rupture, or trauma to bladder and bowels
Distal femur	Popliteal artery damage, profuse bleeding
Knee (dislocated or fractured)	Popliteal artery damage, profuse bleeding
Fifth metatarsal	Nerve damage
Proximal fibula	Injury to peroneal nerve

tremities and the trunk are examined to rule out other fractures. After x-ray studies are completed, look for complications or determine if the patient is at risk for complications.

Fracture complications

Some examples of potential complications are shown in Table 57-2. Other complications resulting from fractures include avascular necrosis, compartment syndrome, gas gangrene, osteomyelitis, and fat embolism.

Avascular necrosis (also known as aseptic necrosis) can occur in any bone but most often affects intrascapular fractures (head and neck) of the femur following trauma, causing a decrease in circulation. Avascular necrosis is described as any interference of the blood supply to the particular bone. During trauma the head of the femur may be twisted or dislocated from the hip joint, and this change in alignment disrupts the blood supply.

The process of avascular necrosis may occur over an extended period after the repair of the fracture. The patient may have been discharged from the physician, so the role of the nurse primarily focuses on teaching the patient about the symptoms. Since the disease process may first involve the cartilage, which has no intrinsic blood supply, there may be no early warning symptoms. In the later stages of the disease process, there may be intermittent to constant pain on weight bearing and limitation in the full range of motion of the joint. These two symptoms usually alert the patient to return to the physician. The usual treatment for avascular necrosis is joint replacement with a prosthesis (see Chapter 58).

Compartment syndrome is a progressive degeneration of muscle that results from a severe interruption of blood flow to an area. A rise in pressure within a compartment can eventually occlude the arterial blood supply. Inadequate venous return from the compartment causes edema that can interfere with arterial blood.[38] The first outcomes are muscle ischemia and damage caused by inadequate capillary blood flow.

This process may follow trauma to an extremity or a fracture. The most likely fracture is either an open or a closed fracture of the tibia or a forearm fracture of the radius and ulna. The anterior compartment is primarily involved, and the lateral compartment is the second most commonly involved. Extensive soft tissue damage increases the likelihood of compartment syndrome. Following trauma, fluids accumulate in a closed space, the compartment areas or chambers of muscles, blood vessels, and nerves bound by inelastic fasciae (Figure 57-9). The fascia that surrounds the muscle group or compartment exerts a tourniquet-like effect on the structures within this compartment. Accumulation of fluid causes the pressure within the body compartment to rise.[10] This pressure in turn damages the muscles and nerves. A condition known as Volkmann's ischemic contracture may occur with supracondylar humeral fractures. Hypotension may also place the patient at risk for compartment syndrome, since inadequate arterial perfusion may occur in the presence of only a mild elevation of tissue pressure. For those patients at greatest risk for compartment syndrome, the physician may order compartment pressures be monitored with a slit or wick catheter.

The underlying basis for the damage is too large a volume for a given space. Symptoms of compartment syndrome are pain that is out of proportion to the injury, pain with pressure over the compartment, and pain with passive stretching of the affected muscle group and paresthesia.[36] Recent findings show that diminished to absent pulses are late symptoms of compartment syndrome. Immediate action must be taken to prevent irreversible tissue damage.

Surgical treatment for compartment syndrome may be implemented if nursing measures do not resolve the tissue ischemia. The surgical procedure of decompressive fasciotomy, which involves an opening of the compartment, may be performed. Longitudinal incisions are made through the fascial compartment of the involved extremity. This results in decompression by lowering the compartment pressure. Compartment syndrome may not be detected in patients with life-threatening complications or who are receiving frequent pain medications. This necessitates frequent ongoing assessment and interpretation of findings. The physician may order low—molecular weight dextran to decrease compartment

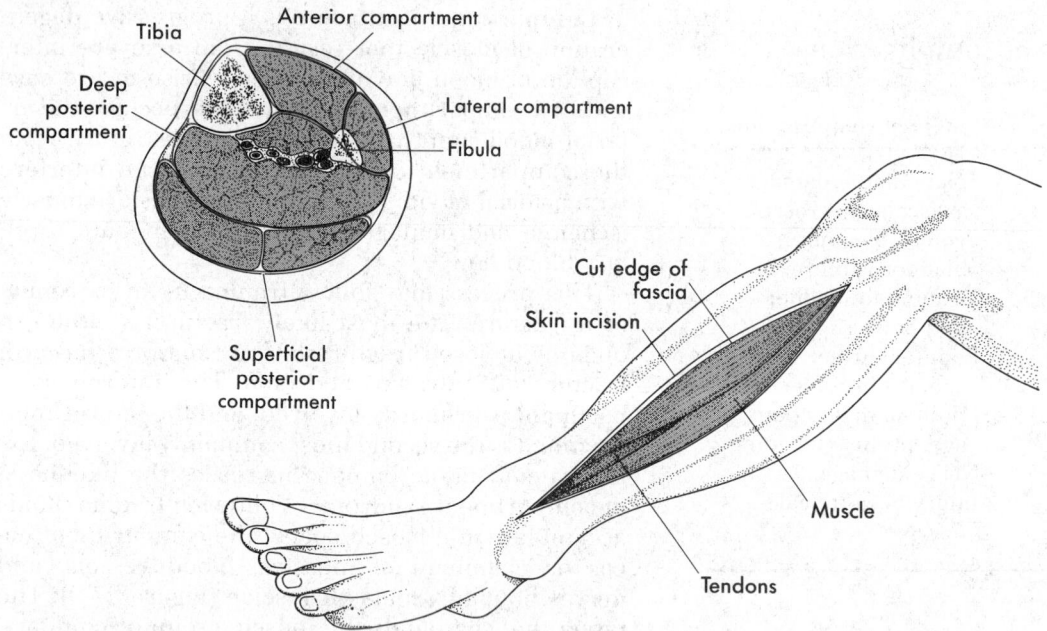

FIGURE 57-9 Compartment syndrome. Often more than one compartment is involved, and anterior compartment is especially vulnerable. Causes include trauma, severe burn, or excessive exercise. A single incision may open more than one compartment.

CLINICAL ALERT

Compartment Syndrome

Hourly neurovascular assessment (the five P's) is essential since permanent tissue damage resulting from ischemia can occur with increased compartment pressure longer than 6 hours. Venous pressure must be relieved to decrease the compartment pressure and lessen ischemia. Venous pressure can be lessened by cutting the cast if present, loosening circumferential dressings, and elevating the limb. The limb will be elevated no more than 5 inches above the heart. Elevations higher than 5 inches impede venous return by interfering with arterial blood flow. Elevation can be correctly accomplished by the use of one or two pillows under the limb for a patient in supine position.[25]

swelling because of its ability to pull interstitial edema back into the vascular space (Figure 57-10).

Gas gangrene is a major consideration when a compound fracture with a relatively small open wound area has occurred. Gas gangrene is caused by the anaerobic Gram-positive saprophytic bacterium *Clostridium welchii* or *Clostridium perfringens,* which grows in deep wounds where there is a decreased supply of oxygen as a result of muscle trauma.[45]

The main role of the nurse is assessment and reporting findings. In the early stage the only symptoms may be that the patient has mental aberration or apprehension. It is imperative that the nurse report any changes in mental status to the physician. The next symptoms may include a chill, an elevation in temperature, a fall in blood pressure, increases in pulse and respiratory rate, and prostration. The wound may be extremely painful, but the initial appearance of the wound may not change.

In the later stage edema and gas bubbles at the wound site may be present, in addition to a profuse drainage with a characteristic fruity odor. This is a fulminating, rapidly progressing toxic infection. Unless the wound is debrided and irrigated with an antiseptic and antibiotics administered, the patient may die. Hyperbaric oxygen therapy is gaining acceptance as a treatment modality. In this therapy the patient is exposed to 100% oxygen under 2 to 2½ atmospheric pressures in a dive chamber for 1 to 2 hours. Oxygen saturation of the tissues is subsequently increased, thereby killing the anaerobic bacteria. Even when these measures are instituted and hyperbaric oxygen is administered, the patient may require an amputation of the affected extremity.

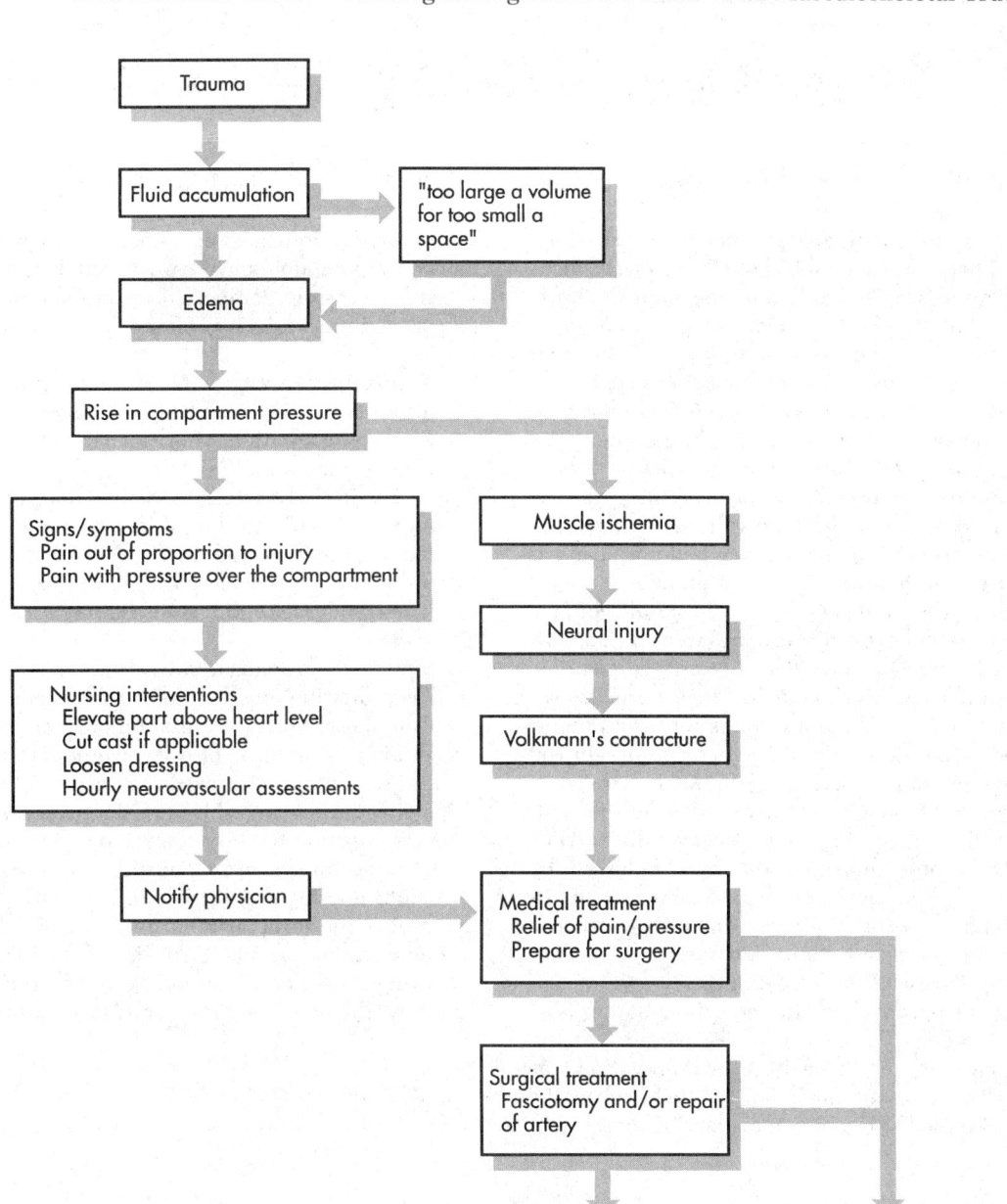

FIGURE 57-10   Critical Thinking Guide: compartment syndrome.

Osteomyelitis is an infection of osseous tissue involving the cortex of the bone and/or marrow. Osteomyelitis can be classified as exogenous (an infection that enters from outside the body) or hematogenous (an infection that results from sites of infection elsewhere in the body). Exogenous osteomyelitis may result from pathogens that enter through an open fracture, penetrating wounds, or surgical procedures. It spreads from soft tissue into surrounding bone.

Any delay in fracture treatment may contribute to the development of osteomyelitis. Patients with long bone fractures, compound fractures, traumatic amputations, fractures with vascular injury or compartment syndrome, or gunshot wounds are candidates for the development of osteomyelitis.

The signs and symptoms of osteomyelitis include low-grade fever, malaise, pain, local tenderness, increased swelling and warmth of the area, and purulent drainage from the sinus tracts.

LEGAL ISSUES   *Negligence*

Dorrence Darling broke his right leg during football practice and was admitted to Charleston Community Memorial Hospital's emergency department. The hospital had 45 beds, was a member of the American Hospital Association, was accredited by the Joint Commission on Accreditation of Hospitals, and was licensed by the state. It had no orthopedic in-house staff, but two orthopedic surgeons were on the consultant staff.

Darling was seen in the emergency department by a private physician who was a general practitioner. The physician set the leg and applied a cast without Stockinette or padding. On previous occasions this physician had been allowed by the hospital to practice orthopedic medicine; his clinical competence had not been reviewed during more than 30 years of practice.

The patient was admitted to the hospital. Nurses' notes indicated that originally the toes were warm with good color, but over 3 days they became edematous, dark blue, and insensitive to touch. There were also repeated notations in the nurses' notes that the patient complained of pain unrelieved by medication. On the second day after admission the doctor notched the cast; on the third day he cut a lengthwise strip in the cast. While cutting the strip, the leg was cut by the Stryker saw. Nurses' notes indicated this was followed by bloody drainage that became purulent and foul smelling. The doctor saw the patient regularly but did not order an orthopedic consultant. The nurses did not notify their supervisor of the situation.

The patient's parents had him moved to another hospital after 2 weeks. There it was discovered that the leg was gangrenous, and a below-knee amputation was necessary. The parents, on behalf of their son, sued Charleston Memorial Hospital and the doctor for negligence.

The result was a landmark decision standing for the following:

1. A corporation, such as a hospital, may be liable if it knows or should have known that an individual physician was not competent to perform the permitted procedures (this is referred to as corporate liability).

2. A hospital could be liable if nurse employees failed to notify medical and hospital administrators when they knew a patient was receiving inadequate medical care from a physician.

3. A hospital that failed to review and monitor treatment rendered to the patient by the physician and failed to enforce the medical staff bylaws requiring attending physicians to obtain medical consultation in certain cases will be held liable for resulting damages.

4. Standards promulgated by the Joint Commission on Accreditation of Hospitals (now called the Joint Commission on Accreditation of Healthcare Organizations), standards of a governmental licensing authority, and provisions of the hospital's medical staff bylaws are admissible as evidence that a jury can consider in a liability suit for damages negligence).

An important legal responsibility of nurses is to notify their nursing supervisor (and similarly the supervisor notify the director and the director notify hospital administration and medical director) of any incompetent, unethical, or illegal behavior observed in patient care by any member of the staff or employee.

Source: The case of Darling v. Charleston Community Memorial Hospital, 211 N.E. 2d 253, cert. denied, 383 U.S. 946 (1966).

Therapeutic management includes early and adequate debridement of open fractures to remove necrotic tissue, which is a site for bacterial growth. Administration of prophylactic antibiotics in patients with open fractures and following surgery to reduce fractures decreases the incidence of posttraumatic osteomyelitis. (For further discussion see Chapter 58.)

Fat embolism syndrome (FES) results when a fracture occurs and fat globules are freed from the bone marrow and from tissue that has sustained damage. It is an acute pulmonary disorder in which changes in the lung are similar to those of adult respiratory distress syndrome (ARDS).

FES is associated with multiple fractures, long bone fractures, and crushing injuries. It is most common in patients with fractures of the femur, pelvis, tibia, or ribs. Fractures that are not promptly and continuously immobilized are at greater risk for FES. In addition, it is seen in postoperative patients who have had a total knee or hip arthroplasty. Bilateral total knee surgery may place the patient at even greater risk of FES.[37]

The exact mechanism for FES is unknown, but two primary theories are generally accepted. The oldest is the mechanical theory, in which there is some trauma that damages the vascular system of the bone, and fat globules in the bone marrow at the fracture site are released into the circulation and become lodged in the lung as they pass through the pulmonary vasculature. Globules will occlude both pulmonary capillaries and small arterioles. The biochemical or physiochemical theory focuses on the stress of trauma that initiates the release of catecholamines. The catecholamines activate lipid from adipose tissue and trigger a loss of chylomicron emulsion stability, resulting in large fat droplets.[21] The fat droplets are converted to free fatty acids that are toxic to the lung.

The foremost pathophysiologic feature is abnormal pulmonary microvascular permeability. There is decreased surfactant production, increased surface tension, decreased lung compliance, and progressive alveolar collapse leading to an intrapulmonary shunt.[21] A defective gas transfer at the alveolar membrane results in hypoxia. Fat and thromboplastin released from the fracture site initiate the clotting mechanism, resulting in platelet aggregation. Acute unexplained anemia may occur as well as hypocalcemia. Hemodilution results from shifts of extravascular fluid into the circulatory system. These pathologic effects result in a defective gas transfer at the arteriolar membrane, causing hypoxia and tissue death.[45] Emboli may also travel to the brain and can cause memory loss, confusion, headache, and an elevation in temperature. Because of this hypoxia from ineffective gas transfer or cerebral emboli, alterations in cognition and level of consciousness may be among the first indications of FES. These typically occur in the first 24 to 72 hours after injury. The appearance of petechiae on the neck, axillae, and upper chest is a classic but late sign of fat embolism that only occurs in about one half the cases of FES.

Altered mental status, confusion, apprehension, agitation, restlessness, lethargy, or delirium alerts the nurse to the possibility of FES. Respiratory manifestations include tachypnea over 30, dyspnea, wheezes, rales, and scattered infiltrates visible on chest x-ray film as a "snowstorm." Arterial blood gases reveal hypoxemia, hypocapnea, and an elevated pH. Additional signs and symptoms are tachycardia greater than 140, pallor, fever, thrombocytopenia with typically less than 150,000 platelets, fat in the urine, escalating serum lipase, and decreasing hemoglobin.

If not detected and treated, fat embolism syndrome can be fatal. Treatment includes oxygen therapy and supportive measures to relieve the symptoms.[25] Oxygen therapy is begun by nasal cannula or Venturi mask. If this is insufficient, mechanical ventilation with positive end-expiratory pressure (PEEP) is initiated. PEEP helps to keep the alveoli open and decrease atelectasis and reduces the pulmonary edema that begins to develop. The physician may order intravenous glucose and/or alcohol. Intravenous glucose is thought to prevent inappropriate fat metabolism, whereas intravenous alcohol is a vasodilator and acts to inhibit lung lipase activity. Par-

CLINICAL ALERT

Clinical Manifestations of Fat Embolism Syndrome

Dyspnea (most predominant symptom)
Restlessness, agitation, confusion, stupor
Tachypnea > 30/min
Tachycardia > 140/min
Fever > 103° F
Petechial skin rash (in 50% to 60% of patients)
Diffuse rales (late symptom)

tial heparinization therapy may be begun to help break down fat globules, decrease platelet aggregation, and promote blood flow; but the nurse must be alert to negative anticoagulant effects such as bleeding. The physician may order low–molecular weight dextran to improve tissue perfusion and expand plasma volume. It alters the surface of erythrocytes and aids in decreasing platelet aggregation. Steroid administration, although controversial, may be used to decrease inflammation and cerebral edema.

Nerve damage is possible with any fracture. It must be remembered that many times an initial x-ray examination does not reveal a fracture. If the patient continues to complain of pain for 8 to 10 days after the injury, a subsequent x-ray examination should be obtained. It is possible that a hairline fracture was undetected on the initial x-ray study but will become visible as healing starts to occur. If the second x-ray study was not done and the fracture treated, the patient could sustain nerve damage from the fracture. If the patient has the symptoms of a fracture but the fracture was not evident on the x-ray study, then a bone scan may be ordered. A bone scan is more sensitive than an x-ray study, and therefore it may reveal even a hairline fracture.

TRACTION

Realignment (reduction) of bone fragments can be accomplished by use of manual traction as prescribed or implemented by a physician. After realignment, immobilization can be accomplished and maintained by (1) traction, (2) casting, or (3) internal fixation. Traction is the application of a pulling force to a part of the body. It is used to align and immobilize fractured bones; to relieve muscle spasms; and to correct flexion contractures, deformities, and dislocations.[31] For traction to be effective, there must also be a pull in the opposite direction (countertraction) by using the weight of the patient's body or by elevating part of the bed.

FIVE PRINCIPLES OF TRACTION

1. Maintain the established line of pull.

Weights will hang freely, not hitting the bed or resting on the floor. The position of the weights is rechecked if the level of the bed is altered. The nurse avoids (1) bumping against the weights when walking near the bed and (2) allowing the weights to sway; both movements can cause pain for the patient in traction. It is preferred that the weights not hang over the patient; if this is necessary, the nurse tapes the ropes so the weights will not fall on the patient.

2. Prevent friction.

Traction rope rests in the groove of the pulley and moves easily. The rope is monitored for fraying. The nurse securely ties the knots in the traction rope and tapes the rope ends well. The rope knots are not lodged against the pulley, because this will interfere with the line of pull. For the same reason the nurse ensures that the pulley, spreader bar, and foot plate do not rest against the foot of the bed.

3. Maintain countertraction.

To provide traction the nurse ensures that countertraction is maintained. If the weight of the patient's body is to provide the countertraction, the body will not interfere with the direction of pull. For instance, the feet of a patient in Buck's traction will not touch the foot of the bed; or if the patient is in cervical traction, the head will not touch the head of the bed.

4. Maintain continuous traction unless ordered otherwise.

The nurse will not remove traction without physician approval. To change the patient's position in bed, the nurse will not lift or adjust the weights if traction is continuous. For intermittent traction the nurse gently places and slowly removes the weights, avoiding jerking or suddenly moving the weights that could jar the patient.

5. Maintain correct body alignment.

The patient will have correct body alignment while lying centered in the bed. The nurse must ensure that the patient does not angle the body or lean off the side of the bed, because the line of traction pull would then be changed or interrupted.

There are three main types of traction: manual, skin, and skeletal traction. Manual traction is a temporary way of applying pull with the hands to a body part. Often this is done in an emergency situation by a person who has been trained to splint an extremity. Manual traction may also be used to reduce or align a fracture before applying traction or a cast or before surgery. Traction is applied either to the skin or soft tissues (skin traction) or directly to the bone (skeletal traction). The pulling force can immobilize fractures, maintain proper alignment, prevent soft tissue injury, and decrease muscle spasm and pain. However, too much force can cause damage to nerves and tissues, and too little can produce painful muscle spasms and impair healing.[23]

Skin traction usually involves the use of belts, halters, boots, or wraps with less than 10 lb and is usually for intermittent use. This traction is contraindicated if the person has a rash or wound in the area to be covered or is allergic to the materials used for wrapping. Because wrapping an area is usually necessary with skin traction, it is not used if the patient has neurovascular problems of the affected extremity, such as paralysis or phlebitis.[45]

Because the skin cannot tolerate heavy pull over long periods without skin breakdown, skeletal traction is usually used when this is required. With skeletal traction, pins, wires, or tongs are used to secure the traction directly into the skeleton of the involved body part.[13]

Both skin and skeletal traction may be applied to the upper and lower extremities and to the cervical and lumbar spine. Nurses need to know the mechanics of traction; however, many agencies have orthopedic technicians to assist with implementation and maintenance of traction.

Although many types of traction exist for different parts of the body, five general principles usually apply for all types of traction (see the box at left).

Lower Extremity Traction

Buck's traction (Figure 57-11, *A*) is probably the most common traction used for reduction and immobilization before surgery for a patient with a fractured hip. It may also be used after surgery to decrease muscle spasms and keep the leg abducted. In addition, Buck's traction may be used to reduce a dislocation, prevent hip flexion contractures, and decrease low back pain. It may be applied unilaterally or bilaterally, depending on the patient's diagnosis. Buck's traction is applied to the lower leg by weights attached by a spreader bar to either (1) a foam boot fastened with Velcro strips or (2) adhesive strips secured with elastic bandage leg wraps.

Russell's traction (Figure 57-11, *B*) looks similar to Buck's traction but also has an upward lift of suspension provided by a sling under the knee or lower

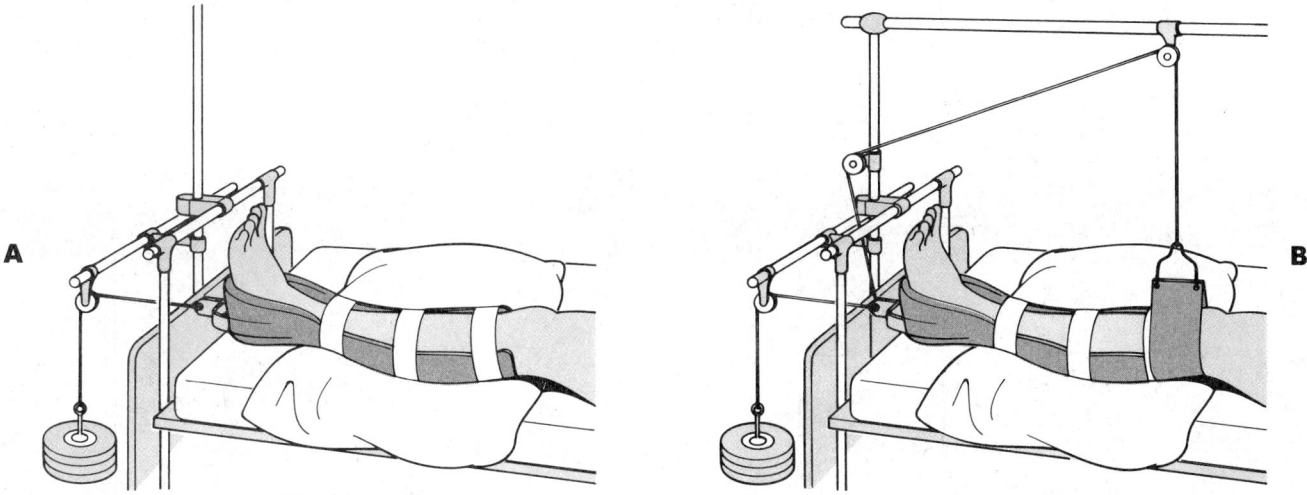

FIGURE 57-11 **A,** Buck's traction. **B,** Russell's traction.

thigh. This suspension allows more movement by the patient without altering the straight line of pull. The result of these two forces creates a pull in line with the femur. Russell's traction is used to reduce and immobilize fractures involving the hip, fractures of the shaft of the femur in adolescents, and certain types of knee injuries.[42]

Upper Extremity Traction

Sidearm traction is used to immobilize a fracture of the humerus and may be applied by either a skin or skeletal approach. There is an outward pull on the upper arm and an upward pull on the forearm. For this reason, two separate setups of adhesive strips and elastic bandage wraps are needed. In addition, if skeletal traction is used, a Kirschner wire is usually inserted through the olecranon[42] (Figure 57-12, *A*). With *overhead 90-90 traction,* there is an upward pull on the upper arm, which is at a 90-degree angle to the body. The elbow is also flexed at a 90-degree angle so that the forearm is suspended in a sling and rests above and across the body. Weight is attached to the sling and to the Kirschner wire that is usually inserted through the olecranon (Figure 57-12, *B*).

Skeletal Traction

Balanced suspension traction provides countertraction by ropes and weights usually connected to pulleys over the head of the bed frame; thus the name balanced suspension skeletal traction, since the suspension is balanced by an equal amount of weight used for countertraction.[25] Balanced suspension traction is used primarily for femoral fractures in adults (Figure 57-13). A Steinmann pin or Kirschner

wire is inserted through the distal end of the femur or through the proximal end of the tibia. A spreader is attached to the protruding ends of the pin or wire, and ropes and weights are applied to the spreader to initiate traction. The traction is maintained by means of a Thomas splint with a Pearson attachment.

Cervical Traction

Skin **cervical traction** is frequently used for patients with sprains or strains to the cervical spine and ruptured cervical disks. It is applied to the cervical spine by a halter with straps under the chin and around the head at the base of the skull. After the halter is placed, the spreader bar and attached weights are connected. The patient may have a small pillow under the head but will rest the back against the bed (Figure 57-14).[42] Skeletal cervical traction to the cervical spine is used to immobilize and reduce fractures of the cervical spine or upper thorax that may injure the spinal cord. This type of traction is always continuous. For further information see Chapter 45.

Pelvic Traction

There are two types of pelvic skin traction: belt and sling. The pelvic belt (Figure 57-15, *A*) is primarily for relief of lower back pain, whereas the pelvic sling is used to treat a pelvic fracture. Pelvic belt traction is applied to the lumbar spine by a pelvic belt with straps attached to weights. It is used to reduce muscle spasms and in the conservative management of low back pain and herniated lumbar disks. This traction may be ordered for continuous use but is more commonly ordered for intermittent periods. However, patient cooperation is crucial to success.

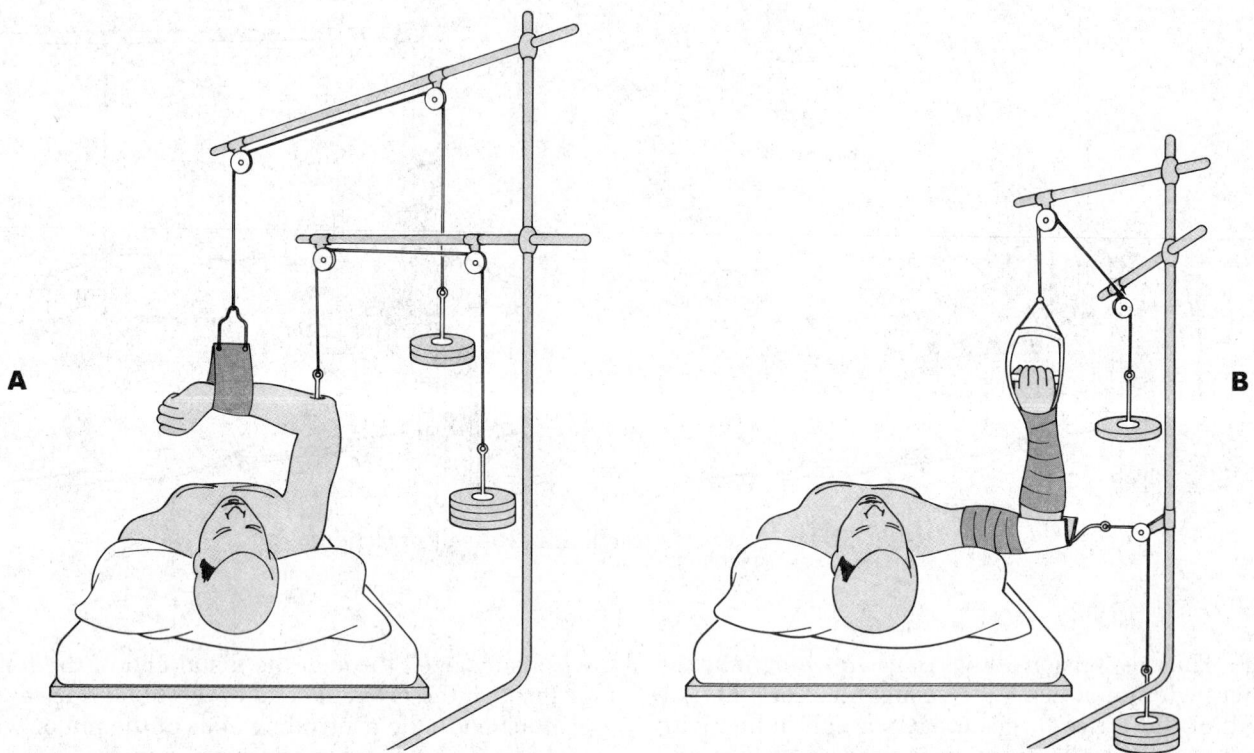

FIGURE 57-12 **A,** Overhead 90-90 traction (skeletal). **B,** Sidearm traction (skin/skeletal).

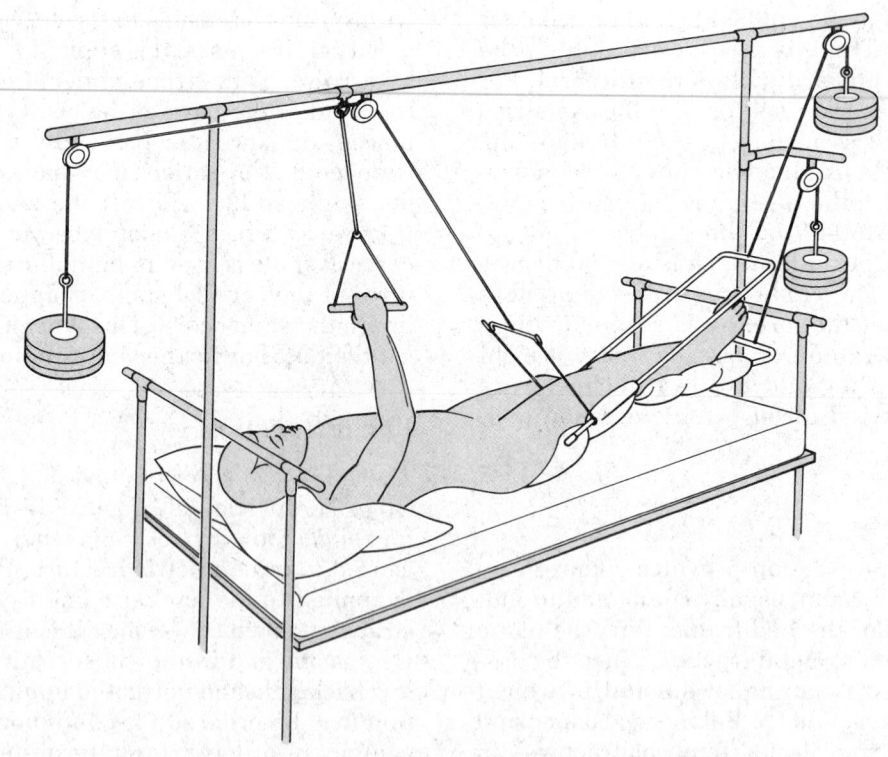

FIGURE 57-13 Balanced suspension traction (skeletal).

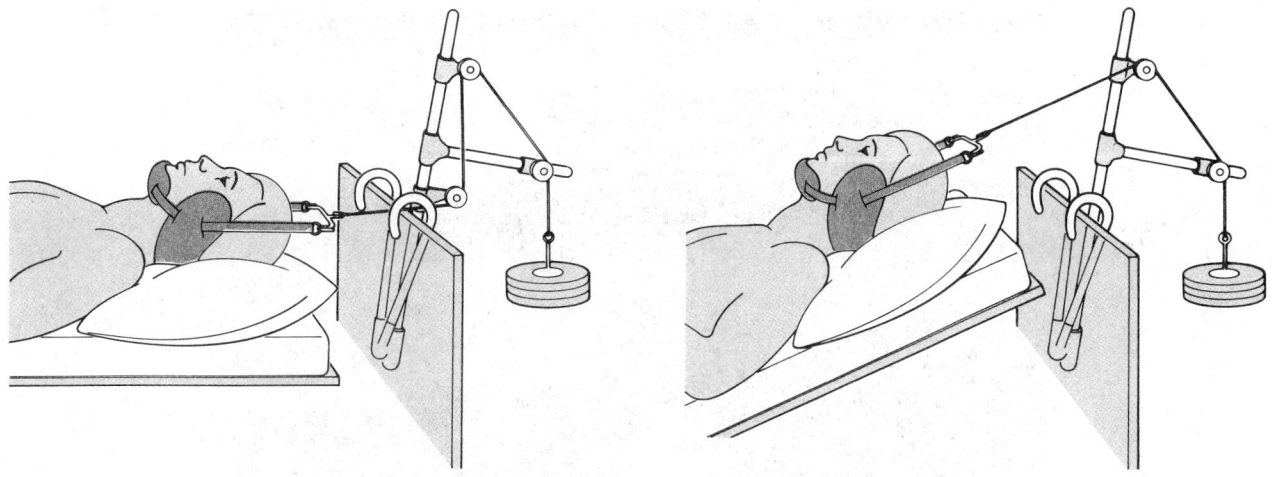

FIGURE 57-14   Cervical halter (skin).

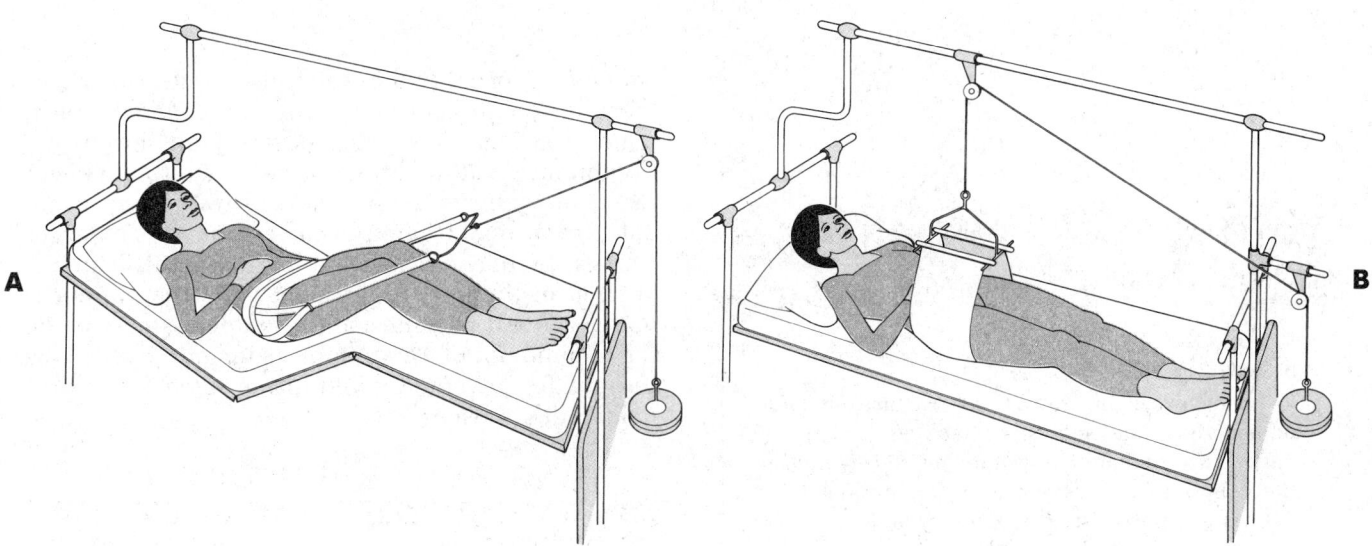

FIGURE 57-15   **A,** Pelvic belt traction (skin). **B,** Pelvic sling (skin).

A pelvic sling (Figure 57-15, *B*) is used continuously to stabilize and immobilize fractures of the pelvis. A large canvas sling attached to weights suspends the patient's buttocks just off the bed. The pelvic sling may also be used to compress the entire pelvis (by applying pressure along each side) if there is a pelvic ring separation. Compression is achieved when the physician repositions the rods from the attached edges of the sling to grooves that are closer together toward the patient's midline.

External Fixation Devices

An **external fixation device** consists of a metal frame that secures pins that are inserted through the bone, above and below the fracture site. In contrast to internal fixation of a fracture with hardware placed within the body, external fixation stabilizes a fracture with hardware visible outside the body. The result is a complicated metal network of pins, rods, and clamps that forms a bilateral frame.[54] The Hoffman device is a common model that has been used successfully since 1970. Other standard models are Universal Day and Portsmouth External fixation bar (Figure 57-16). Indications for use of these devices include complex fractures, such as a compound fracture that has comminuted bone with extensive soft tissue injury or burns. These fractures are often associated with injuries from car or motorcycle accidents and from construction and farm equipment ac-

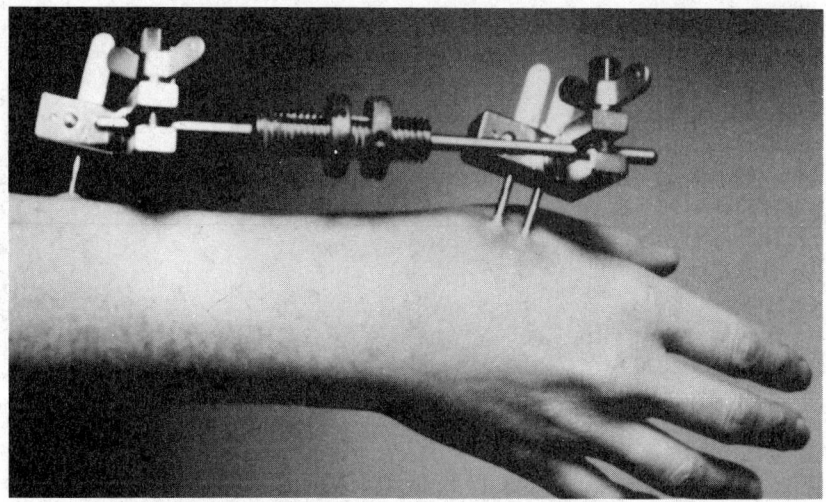

FIGURE 57-16   External fixation device.

cidents. External fixators may be used also where there is nonunion of bones and for leg lengthening, bone grafting, and arthrodesis (joint fusions).[60] Commonly, fixation devices are applied to the lower extremities; however, a variety of frames are available, from small frames for finger fractures to larger frames for pelvic fractures. The external fixator is applied in the operating room while the patient is under general anesthesia. These devices may be on for a minimum of 1 month or as long as 1 year. See the box for advantages and disadvantages of external fixation devices.

NURSING MANAGEMENT OF THE FRACTURE PATIENT IMMOBILIZED BY TRACTION

Assessment

Traction is prescribed to immobilize a body part, so the nurse must assess the effects of traction to prevent the hazards of immobility. Many patients have pain related to muscle spasms or the pull of the traction. The patient is interviewed as well as assessed for objective findings of pain. Objective findings may include restlessness, frequent sighs, and a frown or wrinkled forehead. Before the administration of an analgesic or narcotic, the nurse observes and determines that the traction mechanism is correct. Correcting the traction mechanism or repositioning the patient may alleviate the pain, and thus medication would not be necessary.

Any immobilization may cause the skin to be irritated or torn. This damage may be the result of skin friction or sheet burns (shearing forces). Assess the skin subject to friction at least every 8 hours, especially bony prominences, such as the back of the

---

EXTERNAL FIXATION: ADVANTAGES AND DISADVANTAGES

Advantages

- Provides excellent stability at fracture site, enhancing bone and soft tissue healing
- Particularly valuable in treating a severely injured limb and may possibly prevent amputation
- Allows for more visibility of injury and access for care of traumatized tissue than if a cast were applied
- Permits patient more movement and decreases potential for complications of immobility
- Permits early discharge

Disadvantages

- Pins may become loose or move if patient has excessive movement
- After removal of external fixation device, bone may be weak and there is risk of refracture
- Potential complications
  - Nerve damage related to pin insertion
  - Muscle/vascular entrapment related to pin insertion
  - Cellulitis and osteomyelitis related to infection at pin site
  - Hazards of immobility
  - Edema that interferes with healing
  - Body image disturbance and knowledge deficits

head, scapulae, elbows, coccyx, lateral malleoli, and heels, which may develop decubiti. Assessment of these areas may be done when the patient's position is changed.

Report an elevation in oral temperature of 100° F (37.8° C) to the physician, because this may be an early sign of skin infection. In addition, if the patient develops a skin infection, the pulse and respiration may increase. Assess vital signs every 4 hours while the patient is awake. Also, the nurse assesses areas of skin where traction pull is exerted, such as under a sling or halter. If traction is not continuous, the nurse can remove the appliance and bandages to observe for skin breakdown.

If the patient has traction with an external fixator, the pin sites are assessed at least every 8 hours for signs of infections. These signs include redness, drainage, edema, and warm to hot skin surrounding the pin site.

Because the patient in traction is usually supine, activity is restricted. The nurse assesses the patient for restrictions in range of motion, decreased muscle strength, contractures, and incoordination. In addition, the nurse assesses for changes that signal neurovascular impairment (see five P's). If there is excessive damage to the tissue, compartment syndrome may result.

Nursing Diagnosis

The following nursing diagnoses are relevant for the patient in traction:

High risk for altered peripheral perfusion related to swelling or tight elastic wrap

Pain related to injury, surgery, and confinement in traction

High risk for infection related to pin placement for skeletal traction

Impaired physical mobility related to restriction of traction

High risk for impaired skin integrity related to prolonged use of traction

Knowledge deficit related to traction

High risk for sensory/perceptual alteration related to prolonged immobility

Ineffective individual coping related to injury and traction

High risk for constipation related to immobility

Sleep pattern disturbance related to limited movement because of traction

Planning

The nursing interventions for the patient in traction are planned to meet the following outcomes:

The patient will exhibit no neurovascular deficit

The patient will move without pain

The patient will exhibit no tenderness, redness, swelling, or serosanguineous or purulent drainage at pin sites

The patient will maintain range of motion of joints and muscle tone and strength of extremities

The patient will demonstrate intact skin without redness

The patient will explain the purpose of traction, assist in maintaining traction as ordered, and report complications

The patient will develop no sensory/perceptual alterations

The patient will develop adequate coping responses

The patient will exhibit optimal bowel elimination

The patient will demonstrate optimal rest/sleep patterns

Implementation

Hourly neurovascular assessments are made distal to the fracture site. Any deficits are immediately evaluated and treated (see discussion of compartment syndrome).

Neurologic

When wrapping the elastic bandage for skin traction, the nurse avoids pressure on the outer aspect of the calf just below the knee, because the peroneal nerve lies close to the surface there.[45] This nerve passes around the neck of the fibula on the lateral side of the knee and, if damaged, can lead to footdrop and sensory loss in the lower leg and foot. Patients must be positioned to avoid pressure on this nerve, because it is vulnerable to injury.[20] An early sign of peroneal nerve compression is complaints of tingling on the anterior surface of the leg and dorsum of the foot. In addition, the patient may have difficulty extending the toes. Either of these complaints requires immediate rewrapping of the elastic bandage.

The nurse instructs the patient with 90-90 traction to extend the affected hand frequently. Severe pain in the muscle may indicate compartment syndrome.

Pain

If analgesics are ordered as needed, the nurse teaches the patient to request medication before the pain becomes severe. The patient may require medication for pain 30 minutes before physical therapy and other strenuous activities. By teaching the patient how to apply the five principles of traction, higher levels of comfort may be achieved. Since the patient in traction is unable to turn side to side, other comfort measures include placing a small pillow under the upper left or right torso to promote circulation. In addition, the nurse may provide back care to promote relaxation.

Infection

Regarding infection, the nurse teaches the patient and family not to touch the pin sites with their hands. Also, they are taught to identify the reportable signs and symptoms of infection. The nurse follows physician's orders or hospital protocol for pin site care. General principles include using sterile technique during pin site care and not allowing cross contamination from one pin to another. The pin sites are cleansed with the recommended solution, such as hydrogen peroxide or normal saline. Crusts that may obstruct drainage around pins are removed.[43,47] The nurse works systematically on an extremity, first on one side and then on the other. Pin sites may be covered or uncovered as ordered. An antibiotic, antiseptic solution, or ointment is applied to pin sites according to hospital protocol or physician's order (see Table 57-3).

Nurses have commonly performed pin site care on skeletal traction or external fixator pins. Research studies do not, however, support this practice. No significant difference exists in infection rates between those patients having pin site care and those without.[14] Therefore the nurse only performs pin site care when the physician orders or agency policy dictates.

Altered mobility

To promote patient activity, the nurse encourages the use of an overhead trapeze, if permitted, for lifting, back care, exercise, and linen change. Patient participation in eating and bathing is encouraged. Exercise is also an effective method to prevent muscle weakness. The nurse reminds the patient in skin traction to the lower extremity (Buck's, Russell's) not to turn from the waist down or sit up, because this will interfere with countertraction. However, the patient may lift or tilt the upper body while maintaining a straight line or pull.

With sidearm traction, if the equipment is attached to the bed frame, elevating the head of the bed will not disrupt the traction pull. However, if the frame is attached so that it moves when the bed position changes, the nurse keeps the head of the bed flat. Countertraction can be provided by placing a folded blanket under the mattress near the traction frame.[45]

Because the arm is elevated in 90-90 traction, the patient has less edema. The nurse ensures the patient keeps the involved hand supported in the sling and does not allow it to hang freely.

The nurse gives back care every 4 hours to relieve the constant pressure and associated discomfort, be-

cause no actual turning is allowed. The nurse can provide side-to-side linen change by instructing the patient to grasp the trapeze bar with the unaffected hand. The patient can then bend the leg on the unaffected side and push down with the foot while tilting slightly toward the unaffected side.[45]

Shoulder stiffness may occur with sidearm traction so frequent massage may promote comfort.

Since cervical skin traction is usually ordered intermittently for a specified period, the nurse teaches the patient how to remove and reapply it. This information is especially important for the patient, because there may be the need to remove the halter if vomiting or choking occurs. Any severe headache or pain in the area of the traction is reported.[42]

The patient in pelvic traction is placed in William's position[23] in which the head of the bed and knee gatch are approximately at the same angle (Figure 57-17). This position relieves pressure from the lower back by decreasing the lumbar curve. It also provides countertraction. If traction increases pain to the back or legs, the nurse will report this to the physician. Strict immobilization of the patient in a pelvic sling is required to maintain the traction force.

The elaborate system of balanced suspension skeletal traction may frighten the patient and family. The nurse teaches the patient and family that the traction's main purpose is to provide a sling; this allows the leg to rest comfortably[41] and provides the patient freedom to move without disrupting traction pull or alignment.[45]

By using the overhead trapeze, the patient can lift the shoulders and upper body. This movement allows for change of linen from the top to the bottom of the bed.

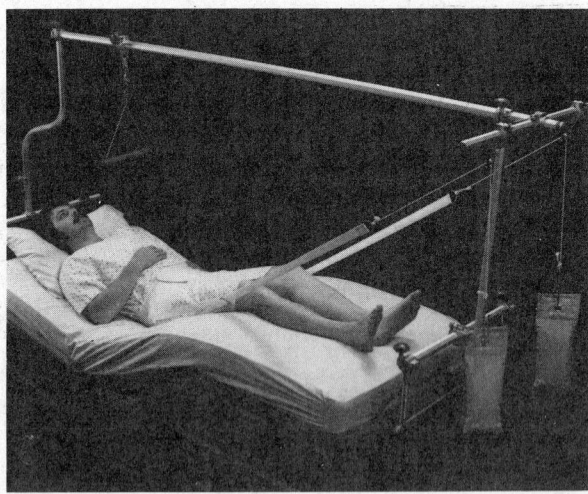

FIGURE 57-17   William's position for pelvic traction.

Range-of-motion exercises (see Chapter 56) are done on the unaffected extremities to maintain muscle strength. Quadriceps and gluteal sets are done to maintain muscle tone for future ambulation. For quadriceps sets the patient is instructed to extend the leg, point the toes upward in a neutral position, and press the knee down into the bed. For gluteal sets the patient is instructed to tense the buttock muscles, hold for 8 to 10 seconds, and then relax. The patient is reminded to perform these exercises in sets of four to six each every 2 hours while awake. Exercise improves circulation and reduces the risk for thrombophlebitis. Calf pumps (ankle rotation, dorsiflexion, and plantar flexion) are performed every 2 hours to promote venous return. Encourage the patient to exercise but also explain to patients any movements that must be avoided.[23]

To prevent contractures the nurse can perform or supervise passive, active, or active-assisted range-of-motion exercises for unaffected extremities. Range-of-motion exercises on the affected extremity are performed only if permitted by the physician. It is crucial that the elderly patient receive early intervention, because permanent functional loss and associated complications of immobility are more likely with this age group.[5]

Skin

To prevent skin breakdown in the traction patient, the nurse places an egg-crate mattress over a firm bed mattress. Sheepskin pads and elbow and heel protectors are applied to areas susceptible to skin breakdown. If prolonged bed rest is anticipated, the patient is placed on an alternating pressure bed or a flotation bed.

Skeletal

The Thomas splint has a sling that supports the thigh, with a ring attached under the upper thigh. The nurse assesses for irritation from the Thomas splint half-ring to the groin, inner thigh, and ischium. The Pearson attachment is connected to the splint at the knee and supports the calf in a position parallel to and above the bed. This splint is positioned so that it does not compress the popliteal space.

Pelvic traction

When applying pelvic traction, the nurse positions the belt around the pelvis and not the waist.[57] The straps are of equal length and parallel to one another and to the patient's thighs. Linens will not rest on the straps (because of the weight), and the straps will clear the bed to allow for a straight line of pull.[45]

The iliac crest is inspected for symptoms of friction rub. The patient is encouraged to wear under-

PATIENT EDUCATION GUIDE
The Patient in Traction

Topics to discuss
- Traction setup and its purpose; principles of traction
- Proper body alignment; positions that are allowed and those to be avoided
- Use of overhead trapeze (if permitted)
- Pin site care
- Prevention of complications of immobility
- Signs/symptoms of neurovascular compromise: pallor, pulselessness, increasing pain on passive movement, paresthesia, and paralysis
- Signs/symptoms of infection in wound or pin site: erythema, swelling, purulent drainage, pain, increased temperature

clothing to prevent further irritation. The nurse can place an abdominal pad under the belt to prevent friction.

The nurse may place a rolled bath blanket under the patient's leg to keep pressure off the heel or a pillow may be used if permitted by the physician. With intermittent pelvic traction, the skin is assessed each shift. If an area of irritation is noted, gently massage the area in order to promote circulation and continue to keep pressure off the affected area.

External fixation

For a summary of nursing interventions see Table 57-3.

Knowledge deficit

The nurse includes the patient and family in establishing specific learning goals for patient teaching. Important areas are knowledge of traction setup, including purpose and principles; use of the overhead trapeze; pin site care; and prevention of complications from immobility, infection, and neurovascular compromise. See the patient education guide for topics to cover with the patient in traction.

Sensory/perceptual alterations

The hospital environment can contribute to sensory/perceptual alterations. Patients in traction are frequently in private rooms, immobilized, recumbent, and exposed to visual and auditory cues that are monotonous and provide little meaningful stimulation.

TABLE 57-3   Nursing Intervention Summary: External Fixation Patient

Potential complication	Nursing management
Nerve damage	Assess five P's.
Muscle/vascular damage	Assess five P's and peripheral pulses when assessing vital signs.
Cellulitis and osteomyelitis	Assess skin around pin sites for tenderness, redness, swelling, and serosanguineous or purulent drainage that occurs after pins have been in place 2 to 3 days. Assess for skin tension at pin sites resulting from pressure of pins on skin. Assess for loosening of pins, which may be associated with infection and increased or purulent drainage; loose pins are less effective in immobilizing the fracture site.[43]
	General pin site care:
	Clean around entry and exit sites with hydrogen peroxide–soaked sterile applicators.
	Remove drainage with dry sterile swabs.
	Leave site uncovered or cover as prescribed by physician.
	Perform pin site care every 8 hours for first 3 days after insertion of external fixator.
	After first 3-day period, drainage is minimal to none. Frequency of pin site care is based on presence of drainage.
	Refer to physician's orders or agency procedure for specific cleaning agents or application of antiseptic ointments.
Hazards of immobility	Determine how restricted patient's activity will be because of external fixator. Patient who is confined to bed in traction will have more limited mobility than patient who can be ambulatory while wearing the device.
	Promote physical mobility by encouraging patient to put weight on extremity as soon after surgery as physician allows.[1] Patient performs range-of-motion exercises to unaffected extremities. Nurse determines physician's plan for other exercises and assists patient in performing them.
Edema that interferes with healing	Prevent edema by elevating affected extremity above level of heart the first few days after surgery. If a leg is involved, elevation can be achieved by balanced suspension traction or by attaching traction ropes to four different points on the external device and tying the ropes to an overhead bed frame. When swelling has subsided, nurse may elevate leg on pillows or raise foot of bed.
Body image disturbance and knowledge deficit	Assess patient's feelings regarding body image and external fixation device. Acceptance of external fixator may be a problem, because metal frame looks like an "erector set" as it extends outward from extremity.[55] Device is also awkward and heavy, which will make affected leg feel different from the other. This change in appearance and weight may cause concern.
	Assess patient and family's knowledge of external fixation device and what their concerns are.
	Prepare patient and family for external fixation by showing them a picture of device. Explain that frame will be visible outside extremity and may be bulky and heavy. Emphasize positive aspects, such as how the device stabilizes the broken bone and that pain usually subsides after early postoperative period.[55]
	Explain how device works, but caution patient not to tamper with nuts and clamps, which could alter bone alignment and impair healing. Grasp external fixator to lift or move extremity rather than lifting the extremity itself.

The nurse must provide communication and stimulation (social, visual, auditory). Orienting aids such as clocks and calendars help to prevent sensory/perceptual alterations. Maintaining the normal sleep/wake pattern is also helpful.

Coping

Traction requires alteration in mobility and therefore interference in life-style. Combined with changes in role, loss of control, and financial pressures, the patient may need assistance from the nurse in developing adaptive coping mechanisms. Often just listening to the patient ventilate concerns relieves stress. Including the patient in planning care and encouraging decision making when possible assist the patient in coping with the changes.

Bowel elimination

To promote optimal bowel elimination the nurse implements measures to eliminate the usual causes of constipation. These include too little exercise, too little dietary bulk, too few liquids, and too little time. For patients in traction for several weeks, increasing exercise may not be feasible so the other causes must be considered. Changes in dietary bulk may be as simple as adding fruit with skin intact or prune juice to the diet. Other patients, especially those without teeth, may require a natural fiber base or psyllium hydrophilic type of daily fiber to promote bowel elimination. Consult the dietitian for menu planning. Privacy for bowel movements enhances elimination. Special efforts to increase the liquid intake are instituted. This would include an accurate measure of intake and the design and implementation of a force fluid schedule.

In addition to the four contributing factors of constipation, certain medications may also contribute to the lack of peristalsis necessary for bowel elimination. These include codeine and other narcotics, belladonna or its derivatives, specific diuretics, iron preparations, and aluminum hydroxide or aluminum phosphate gels. If it is necessary for the patient to receive these medications, stool softeners or laxatives may be necessary to promote optimal bowel elimination.

Sleep

To promote optimal rest and sleep patterns, the nurse assesses the patient's usual rest and sleep patterns. Many patients may sleep or take short frequent "cat naps" during the day, so less sleep may be required at night. A back rub and similar comfort measures before bedtime make conditions conducive to sleep. The development of a sleep plan is helpful to promote optimal rest. The patient can pro-

---

SLEEP PLAN FOR THE TRACTION PATIENT

Outcome: Patient will have optimal rest and sleep patterns.

Interventions

1. Prepare the patient for sleep. This may include the following nightly rituals:
   a. Oral hygiene
   b. Cleaning the face
   c. Soft music
   d. A warm noncaffeinated drink
   e. Reading
2. Control the environment by:
   a. Having no overhead lighting
   b. Dimming the lights in the hall that may frighten the patient when the door is open
   c. Keeping outside noise to a minimum
   d. Organizing nursing activities in 2-hour intervals
   e. Being quick and efficient in providing nursing care or assessments
3. Promote comfort by:
   a. Preparing the patient for sleep and controlling the environment (see above)
   b. Providing medication for pain or sleep as prescribed (If the patient asks for pain and sleep medication at the same time, the pain medication should be given first. By relieving the pain, the patient may be able to sleep.)

---

vide valuable information as to the reasons that the sleep pattern is not adequate. Consider these reasons in the plan (see box).

Patients in traction are subject to sleep disturbances, because the traction prohibits their ability to move freely. Since all persons move during sleep, the patient with traction may be awakened frequently by the traction limitations. Sedatives that induce relaxation or hypnotics that induce sleep may be prescribed. Elderly persons and those with liver disease cannot safely metabolize some sedatives, so nonbarbiturates such as chloral hydrate or flurazepam (Dalmane) may be prescribed. The nonbarbiturates may cause central nervous system depression; however, they have very little effect on the cardiac, respiratory, or gastrointestinal systems. Side effects of nonbarbiturates include muscle relaxation, low blood pressure, cold extremities, fatigue, and a "hangover" effect.[56] If hypnotics are used, they are given early in the night, so their action will be complete before the usual wake-up time. A rule of thumb is not to administer medication to enhance sleep after 2 AM; however, the nurse refers to agency policy related to the time for sleep medications.

Evaluation

The plan is judged effective if circulation, motion, and sensation are maintained distal to the fracture. The effectiveness of analgesia is evaluated 30 minutes after administration by the patient's report of pain relief. The patient is encouraged to discuss the pain experience after the pain has subsided; the nurse can acknowledge the difficulty of the situation.[5]

After receiving analgesics for a few days, management of pain control is evaluated as effective when the patient in traction reports decreased pain, makes fewer requests for pain medication, has fewer pain-associated behaviors, and is better able to focus on other areas of interest. The patient in traction with an infection at the pin sites is expected to have decreased tenderness, redness, swelling, and drainage with treatment. The patient's temperature decreases and remains under 100° F.

The plan is appropriate when the patient remains as active as possible within the restrictions of traction. Full range of motion in unaffected extremities is maintained. Patients who have lost muscle tone and strength will gradually regain them during rehabilitation. The patient's skin is not red nor are there broken areas. If skin breakdown occurred previously, granulation tissue is present and the decubitus becomes smaller as healing occurs.

The nurse evaluates the patient's and family's level of understanding of traction, nursing plans, and teaching (see patient education guide, p. 1553). The patient is not experiencing abnormal sensory/perceptual phenomena; remains oriented to time, person, and place; and exhibits no difficulty in concentration.

The patient is evaluated as coping when the source of the stressors can be identified, when feelings are directly communicated to others in an appropriate manner, and when the patient does not withdraw. Bowel elimination is evaluated as satisfactory when the patient is not preoccupied with it and the frequency of stools meets the patient's need and satisfaction.

The patient is able to rest and sleep for adequate periods. The nurse evaluates the frequency of use of sedatives or hypnotics for sleep to prevent overuse. However, if a patient has been taking medication for rest or sleep at home each night, any attempt to wean the patient from this habit will probably be futile. Hospital environments make it difficult to sleep, so sedatives and hypnotics are usually justified.[56]

For the patient with an external fixator, adjustment to the device is evidenced when the patient looks at it more while care is given. The patient may also talk about feelings and changes in life-style that must be made. The patient begins assuming responsibility for care of the external fixator if possible and is able to report problem areas.

Edema of the affected extremity gradually decreases. Wound healing occurs, and the amount of drainage lessens. The patient performs activities of daily living as allowed and exhibits no problems related to immobility.

Documentation

The nurse documents the type of pain, related pain behaviors, actions taken, and patient response. If the pain is unrelieved, additional actions and patient response are recorded. The nurse documents (1) length of time the patient is in traction (if intermittent), (2) position in bed, (3) status of the traction setup, and (4) patient's response. The nurse documents the assessment of pin sites and reports and notes signs of infection. Vital signs are recorded as well. The nurse documents exercises provided, frequency, and the patient's subjective and physical responses. The nurse records the condition of the patient's skin and measures taken to improve or maintain it. Any signs of redness or skin breakdown are documented along with related nursing interventions and changes in the skin's appearance. The nurse also documents the patient's response to learning by noting the ability to verbalize important points under each area of teaching. Recording the patient's level of orientation and the effectiveness of nursing interventions instituted to prevent sensory deprivation is important. The nurse also assesses and records patient coping and summarizes the theme of the verbalizations, any recommendations made, and changes in coping ability noted over time. Sleep/wake periods are documented as well as the effectiveness of specific nursing interventions to promote sleep. In the case of external fixators, the nurse notes the patient's response to the external fixation device and any related teaching or counseling provided. The nurse documents the degree of swelling and measures taken to relieve it.

Ongoing Care

Most patients will no longer be in traction when discharged. Their needs will depend on their general health, if they are mobile or need the assistance of ambulation aids, and whether they still have pin sites that will need care until healed.

Some hospitals have begun an innovative program to manage the patient in skeletal traction at home.[13] Although visits from a home health nurse are arranged, the family and patient will be more independent in properly maintaining traction and preventing complications. Teaching interventions under the nursing diagnosis of knowledge deficit related to traction become a priority for the patient going home in traction.

Before the discharge of a patient with traction, the nurse tells the caregiver that patients who are confined to bed often feel isolated and may suffer from sensory deprivation. The family or friends are encouraged to make frequent visits in addition to the times they are providing care. The telephone can serve as a source of visitation if the patient has access to it, and, if possible, the patient should have access to the television control. Visitors, the telephone, and the television allow the patient to maintain contact with events outside the home.

CASTING

After realignment of a fracture, a cast may be applied rather than placing the patient in traction. Casting is used as the primary treatment after closed reduction of a fracture. A closed reduction is usually done with the patient under general, regional, or neural block anesthesia and allows for manipulation of the displaced fragments to their normal anatomic alignment.[39] Casts may also be used in conjunction with other techniques such as for fractures of the femur that often require open reduction and internal fixation. The type of cast that is applied is based on the extent and location of the fracture. Casts may be applied to the upper and lower extremities or the trunk. Table 57-4 summarizes fracture sites and the usual types of casts applied.

Cast Materials

Both plaster of paris and synthetic casting material are applied over padding material and Stockinette that cover the affected part. Usually the physician or an orthopedic technician applies the cast; the nurse may be asked to assist.

Traditionally, plaster of paris was the main cast material. However, within the last 10 to 15 years, synthetic cast materials have become increasingly popular. Synthetic casts are made of fiberglass or polyester/cotton knit. There are advantages and disadvantages of each type. Plaster of paris material can be shaped and molded with ease, so it is the material of choice with severely displaced or unstable fractures. The major disadvantage of plaster of paris is that it is slow to dry and is heavier and bulkier than synthetic materials. It is difficult to keep clean and can become weakened or lead to skin breakdown if the cast becomes wet. As plaster of Paris dries, heat is released. To prevent burning the patient and to hasten drying, the cast must be left uncovered while it is still warm. The cast soon becomes cold and damp. If the patient feels cold and clammy because of the wet cast, the nurse can place bedding on all areas of the body not covered by the cast. Even after this initial period, the nurse leaves the cast exposed so that it will dry thoroughly.[64]

The length of drying time of the cast depends on how large and thick it is, humidity, and air temperature. Although some plaster casts may dry completely within 8 to 10 hours, others may require as long as 2 days to dry completely on an extremity and as long as 3 days for a large spica or body cast.[59] Using a blow dryer to dry a plaster cast is rarely necessary and could cause the cast to crack if it dries too rapidly.[45] During the drying period the nurse rests the entire length of the cast on cloth-covered pillows and lifts the cast with the palms of the hands only, with the fingers extended. The nurse assists the patient to turn every 2 to 3 hours so that no area of the cast receives continuous pressure. These measures help avoid indentation of the cast, which could lead to pressure sores on the skin underneath.[45]

Weight bearing during this initial period is impossible if the integrity of the plaster cast is to be maintained. The cast is dry when the plaster is white, shiny, and odorless and when the cast itself is hard and resonant when tapped.[59]

Synthetic casts are recommended for (1) immobilizing nondisplaced fractures with minimal swelling or (2) long-term wear when multiple cast applications are not expected. Synthetic casts harden within minutes and can bear weight within half an hour, because there is no prolonged drying time. Although more expensive than plaster of paris, they are lighter and less bulky, which allows the wearer to resume many normal activities.[52]

These features are especially beneficial for the elderly person, who may be more prone to problems of immobility as a result of restricted activity while the cast dries (as with the plaster cast). Also, the light weight helps the elderly patient maintain better balance and promotes mobility.

The surface of a synthetic cast can be wiped clean with a mild, nonirritating soap and water, because the cast is water resistant. With the physician's permission, the patient can even put it in water, because the cast's strength will be unaffected if it gets wet. (To do this, the lining must be of synthetic material as well.) The major disadvantage is the synthetic cast is not appropriate for full weight-bearing extremities.

Variations in Cast Application

When weight bearing on a casted lower extremity is allowed, a walking heel or cast shoe may be used with either a plaster or synthetic cast. A walking heel is permanently attached to the cast with casting tape, whereas a cast shoe can be put on over the cast and removed at night. Advantages of the cast shoe include less added height to the cast, a more

TABLE 57-4   Fracture Site and Type of Cast or Device

Fracture site	Type of cast or device
Upper extremities	
Metacarpals, carpals, distal radius fracture (also for severe wrist sprains)	Short arm cast extending from below elbow to palm of hand
Stable fractures of elbow joint, distal humerus, radius, and ulna; unstable fracture of carpal bones of hand[59]	Long arm cast including part of hand to upper arm
Thumb fractures	Shorter than a short arm cast but includes hand so thumb is abducted
Humeral fractures	Shoulder spica cast to abduct or extend upper arm; may also use a hanging plaster cast, which is a long arm cast with additional layers of plaster to distract fracture fragments and aid in alignment[39]
Stable, undisplaced humeral fractures	Sling with shoulder immobilizer or functional bracing
Shoulder girdle fractures or dislocation of shoulder	Shoulder spica that abducts shoulder with elbow flexed
Lower extremities	
Stable femoral fractures	Spica cast that extends from thorax and includes affected leg and unaffected leg to mid thigh[53]; may also use a *long leg cast* that extends from mid thigh to base of toes
Stable distal femur fracture and unstable fractures of tibia, fibula, and ankle	Long leg cast
Stable fractures of proximal tibia and distal femur[38]	Long leg cylinder cast
Patellar fractures	Long leg or long leg cylinder cast
Ankle, metatarsals, and distal tibia and fibula fractures	Short leg cast that extends below knee to base of toes
Trunk	
Dorsal and lumbar vertebral fracture, degenerative diseases, and to promote healing of surgical fusions and unstable spinal injuries[59]	Body jacket cast extending from shoulders to below iliac crest and hips
Hip dislocation, hip fractures, and pelvic injuries	Hip spica cast extending from mid chest down trunk with spiral bandage down affected leg(s); may be single hip spica (one leg) or double hip spica (both legs)
Simple fracture of cervical vertebral base[39]	Soft or hard cervical collar
Clavicle fracture	Clavicular strap or figure-of-8 dressing
Dorsal and lumbar vertebral fractures	Lumbosacral brace
Knee surgery, arm surgery, after cast removal, or following sprain	Splints (support extremity without encircling it; most common types are anterior or posterior splints that are wrapped in place with elastic bandage)[59]
Used to treat mid shaft or distal shaft fractures of femur and provides stability of knee joint while allowing for ambulation[60]	Cast brace incorporates brace and cast; cast to upper leg and another cast to lower leg are connected by metal hinge[59]

natural gait, and more protection of the cast against moisture.[62]

If there is a wound under the cast or a suture line that needs observation and possibly a dressing change, the physician may cut out a portion of the cast. This opening is called a window. The cutout portion is saved by the nurse and taped in place over the dressing; otherwise, swelling at the window site can lead to skin necrosis.[59]

When signs and symptoms of neurovascular compromise occur in a casted patient, the cast is bivalved by cutting it lengthwise into two equal parts. It is important that the wadding (padding material) is cut through as well. This is usually done to relieve swelling and to facilitate care. A cast may also be bivalved when a rigid cast is not needed at all times (but can be held together with an elastic bandage and used for support or turning).[45]

NURSING MANAGEMENT OF THE PATIENT IN A CAST

Assessment

Nursing care for the patient with either a plaster or synthetic cast includes neurovascular checks every 30 minutes for the first 4 hours after application, as ordered, and then generally every 4 hours, depending on the patient's condition. The nurse's assessment includes comparisons between the extremity in the cast and the opposite extremity (see discussion of five P's and compartment syndrome).

The nurse looks for any areas of drainage through the cast. It is especially important to report if the drainage is other than the usual bloody drainage that occurs for 2 to 3 days after an open reduction.[45]

To assess movement, the nurse observes whether the patient can fully flex and extend all involved fingers or toes. To test sensation the nurse touches each of the involved fingers or toes while the patient's eyes are closed and asks the patient if each touch can be felt.

The nurse feels the entire cast surface with the palms of the hands at least once per shift to detect any areas of increased heat. Hot areas could indicate infection, skin maceration, or pressure areas under the cast. These findings are reported to the physician immediately. This is especially important if the patient complains of pain or discomfort under the cast.

It is important for the nurse to smell directly the cast edges daily. Usually a cast has a sour smell, but there may be a strong foul odor if the underlying area is infected. The nurse reports this foul odor along with any associated patient complaints.

The nurse listens to the patient describe how the affected area feels and any other complaints the patient has. These complaints are always investigated before medication is given for relief. If a complaint of pain is caused by excess tightness of the cast, medication may mask this crucial warning symptom.

The nurse assesses the patient's balance and coordination with the cast and determines the individual's propensity to injury. Assessment for pain can be accomplished by asking how the person feels. If the patient is having pain, its cause and related pain behaviors, change in vital signs, and emotional impact on the patient are determined.[30] Also assess for sharp cast edges, which could cause pain or skin breakdown. Acceptance of the cast may be a problem, because it is awkward and may interfere with the performance of role-related responsibilities.[5] The nurse needs to assess the patient's feelings regarding body image and wearing of the cast.

Nursing Diagnosis

The following nursing diagnoses are relevant to the patient in a cast:

Altered peripheral tissue perfusion related to the presence of a cast

High risk for injury related to awkwardness and weight of cast

Acute pain related to injury, surgery, and presence of cast

High risk for impaired skin integrity related to presence of cast

---

 **CLINICAL ALERT**

Volkmann's Ischemia

The patient may first complain of severe pain on passive movement of the digits. Later the patient may be unable to move the digits of the affected extremity. There may be an absent distal pulse and pallor as well. These are signs and symptoms of compartment syndrome, which can result from injury or swelling. These symptoms of muscle ischemia can quickly lead to irreversible muscle damage within 6 hours if untreated. In 24 to 48 hours, permanent deformity with scarring, contractures, paralysis, and loss of sensation can occur. Volkmann's contracture of the hand is an example of such a deformity (Figure 57-18).[45]

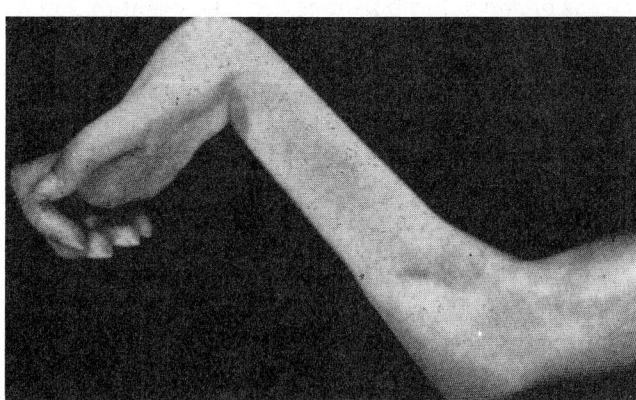

FIGURE 57-18   Volkmann's contracture. (From Farrell J: *Illustrated guide to orthopedic nursing*, ed 2, Philadelphia, 1986, JB Lippincott Co; originally in Boyes: *Bunnell's surgery of the hand*, Philadelphia, JB Lippincott Co.)

Body image disturbance related to cast and restriction in activity

Impaired physical mobility related to cast

Knowledge deficit related to cast care

Planning

The nursing interventions for the patient in a cast are planned to meet the following outcomes:

The patient will demonstrate no increased pain on movement of affected extremity and adequate pulsation, sensation, and color

The patient will remain free of injury while wearing a cast

The patient will verbalize feelings of greater comfort

The patient will maintain intact skin while wearing a cast

The patient will verbalize acceptance of the cast and alter life-style as necessary

The patient will remain free of the complications of immobility

The patient will verbalize proper care of the cast

Implementation

Care of the patient in a cast is directed toward prevention of complications as well as enhancing fracture healing. Major complications include the following:

- Neurovascular compromise, including venous stasis and decreased arterial supply
- Skin maceration[39]
- Compartment syndrome
- Immobility complications

For the first few days after application of the cast, the casted extremity is elevated above the level of the heart to decrease edema. Once swelling decreases, the affected part can be level with the body. Areas of special importance include attention to circulation, safety, comfort, skin care, emotional support, and patient and family education.

Circulation

When the patient is out of bed, the nurse reminds the patient to elevate the involved arm in a sling. When the affected extremity is a leg, it is elevated on a stool; sitting up and standing for long periods are to be avoided. Having the patient move fingers and toes regularly will also increase venous return and decrease edema (see clinical alert).

Safety

Because of the danger of falling, the patient is instructed to walk slowly and avoid uneven areas. If the patient is permitted to shower while wearing an

CLINICAL ALERT

If edema increases under the cast and the five P's of muscle ischemia are present, a medical emergency exists and the nurse should contact the physician immediately. Treatment involves the immediate reduction of pressure, possibly by bivalving the cast or by a surgical procedure called fasciotomy.

external synthetic cast, caution is used when walking on wet surfaces. If crutch walking is ordered, the nurse will walk with the patient initially and after receiving an analgesic.

Comfort

If analgesics are ordered as needed, the nurse must teach the patient in a cast to request medication before the pain becomes severe. Medicating for pain before a strenuous patient activity, such as exercises, may allow the patient to tolerate the activity better.

Skin care

To protect the skin at the cast edge, the nurse can *petal* or *finish* rough cast edges by cutting 2-inch strips of adhesive tape (with ends rounded) in the shape of petals. One end is tucked inside the cast edge, the strip is pulled over the edge, and it is secured on the outside of the cast. (Ensure that the edge inside the cast does not have wrinkles, because this could cause a skin breakdown.) Alcohol applied to fingers can be rubbed on the skin under the cast edges to toughen the skin. Avoid lotion around cast edges, because it can soften skin. Avoid powder, because it can collect under the cast and predispose to skin irritation.

Emotional support

The person wearing a cast may feel demoralized, guilty, silly, or clumsy. If a cast covers considerable body surface, some patients report claustrophobia. The nurse encourages the individual to discuss personal feelings about being in a cast. The nurse prepares the patient for questions asked of him or her regarding the reason for the cast. It may be helpful for the patient to plan a brief explanation of the cause of the injury. Listening to the patient's concerns about how a cast may restrict some activities and problem solving can help the patient adjust to a cast. Including the patient in planning nursing care

TABLE 57-5   Immobility Complications

Complication	Nursing interventions	Rationale
Discomfort	Assess body area involved to determine cause of pain.	May be caused by external factors such as skin pressure or tight cast or dressing
	Complete a neurovascular assessment.	To determine circulatory status; suspect impairment if any of five P's are present
	Question patient about duration and type of discomfort.	Suspect pressure sore or circulatory impairment if patient continues to complain after pain medication is provided
Skin irritation and pressure sores	Wash skin around cast with warm water.	Removes particles of plaster that may break skin
	Place moleskin or gauze pads over rough edges of the cast or traction equipment (half ring of Thomas splint).	Prevents skin irritation
	Assess skin site at point of pain and at any point where pain occurred previously.	Usually patient can pinpoint a specific area when pain is result of a pressure sore; as sore becomes deep (below skin layers) patient will complain of less pain or offer no complaint of pain
Thrombophlebitis	Encourage leg exercises every 2 to 4 hours while patient is in bed. Some physicians order antiembolic stocking, low-dose heparin, sodium warfarin (Coumadin), or aspirin for patients confined to bed.	Prevents coagulation and venous stasis
	Provide adequate fluid intake.	Decreases blood viscosity
	Assess lower extremities for redness, warmth, and positive Homan's sign. Maintain bed rest in presence of these signs and symptoms.	Indicators of thrombophlebitis
Pulmonary emboli	Monitor for sudden chest pain, hypotension, dyspnea, and anxiety. (Calf pain may have occurred earlier but usually disappears before onset of chest pain.)	Indicators of pulmonary emboli
	Assess vital signs for increased pulse and respirations and decreased blood pressure. (If signs are present, prepare to administer oxygen and anticoagulants as ordered.)	
Postural hypotension	Assess for dizziness on standing. If it occurs have patient sit down and assess for drop in blood pressure. Place patient on a tilt table four times daily until blood pressure stabilizes.	Usually related to bed rest and lack of activity and will disappear as activity increases
	If dizziness occurs, it is helpful to force fluids if not contraindicated.	Increases blood volume so hypotension is less likely
Muscle wasting	Consult with physician or physical therapist to determine type and frequency of activity that is permitted.	Within 3 weeks, inactive patients can lose muscle mass unless unaffected muscles are exercised
	Assess amount of liquids and food patient consumes. Allow patient food choices.	Muscle wasting can cause negative nitrogen balance, which causes loss of appetite
	Assist in oral hygiene and hand washing.	Measures to counteract anorexia

and keeping the patient informed of progress may increase his or her feeling of control.

Patient and family teaching

The nurse teaches the patient and family how to perform neurovascular checks and to report any signs and symptoms of muscle ischemia, as well as drainage or unusual odors from the cast. The patient also needs to routinely elevate the extremity to prevent or relieve swelling that can lead to compartment syndrome.[45] The patient is taught how to prevent injury and skin impairment. The patient is instructed not to stick objects under the cast that can scratch the skin or get lost under the cast and cause a pressure sore. The nurse teaches the patient to properly care for the cast and the surrounding skin. Important points are provided in writing (see patient education guides for plaster of paris cast care and synthetic cast care).

Complications of immobility

The patient in a cast is prone to the complications of immobility (Table 57-5).

Evaluation

Successful interventions will reveal a decrease in the patient's edema and no impairment in the neurovascular function of the involved extremity. The patient will demonstrate care in walking and will report an absence of falls. The individual will request fewer analgesics and appear more comfortable. The patient's skin at the cast edges will be intact, and there will be no foul odor or hot spots related to the cast. The patient will have made changes in activities of daily living to accommodate wearing the cast. The patient will return demonstrate cast care, such as elevating the extremity when out of bed. The patient will be independent in performing cast care before hospital discharge and be able to discuss concerns about the cast with others.

Documentation

The nurse documents the appearance of the cast and affected extremity. The nurse documents the neurovascular assessments of the affected extremity, reports the presence of any of the five P's of muscle ischemia, and documents actions taken to relieve them. The patient's ability to move about, safety concerns, and measures taken to improve the situation are noted. The type of pain experienced, related pain behaviors, and actions taken are documented. The nurse needs to evaluate the patient 30 minutes after analgesic administration to determine the medication's effectiveness in providing relief. The

nurse encourages the patient to discuss the pain experience afterward to put the experience into perspective. The condition of the skin at cast edges and associated nursing interventions are documented. In addition, the nurse documents the patient's attitude toward wearing a cast, areas of patient education, and the patient's verbalization of important points. A note is made in the patient's chart if patient education guides or written information is given to the patient.

Ongoing Care

Before individuals wearing casts return home, anticipatory guidance from the nurse is helpful in preventing injuries. Patients are cautioned against too vigorous activity, such as contact sports. Drinking excessive amounts of alcohol is to be avoided because of the danger of falls. The patient or family member will remove throw rugs and clutter on the floor and avoid waxing floors at home. The patient is informed to immediately report a soft, broken, or loose cast to the physician. The cast wearer is instructed when to get the cast changed or removed.

Cast removal

Because cast removal can be frightening, the nurse prepares the patient with sensory and procedural information.[54] Physical sensations and the cause for them are described. As the cast saw vibrates the cast loose the patient may feel heat and vibration, and the skin may be slightly scratched (but will not be

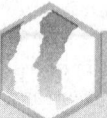

GERIATRIC CONSIDERATIONS

Fracture Rehabilitation

Rehabilitation of the elderly individual with a fracture may be slower than that in the younger adult who has been inactive. Elderly persons may tire more easily and be less steady on their feet. They may have a fear of falling, especially women who were not physically active at a younger age. For those who are afraid of falling, direct physical contact by the nurse (for physical *and* emotional support) can help when patients are beginning something new in their rehabilitation program.[48] It is especially important to determine if elderly patients have any disease or diseases that could interfere with their progress, as well as medications that could alter their perceptions and mobility. The possibility of the elderly individual having delayed reaction times, sensory changes, and difficulty in remembering can also impede performance.

cut). Procedural information is more objective and includes the steps of the cast removal procedure and the appearance of equipment. If the patient is switched from a plaster of Paris to a synthetic cast, the nurse explains the differences in the casts and the care. The nurse provides anticipatory guidance for the time after cast removal. The extremity may feel lighter without the weight of the cast, weaker and smaller from disuse, and scaly from the buildup of old, dead skin. The patient is instructed not to scrub away all the dead skin at once but to apply oil to soften and condition skin and gently wash away old skin over a few days.[59] The nurse teaches the patient any activity restrictions immediately after cast removal. The muscle strength will return gradually (if no muscle injury was involved). The physician instructs the patient on the amount of weight bearing or lifting allowed.[59]

Rehabilitation

Immobilization of a body part by casting, traction, or external fixation allows it to rest and begin healing. Because patients often have been on prolonged bed rest, they may be deconditioned. The rehabilitation program emphasizes the maintenance or return of normal range of motion of joints, prevention of muscle atrophy, and return of normal strength and functional activities.

INTERNAL FIXATION

In addition to traction and casting, the third treatment modality to immobilize a fracture is internal fixation.[33] This is usually accomplished by use of anesthesia and open surgery for the purpose of inserting a nail, screw, or pin with or without a plate at the fracture site. Such devices stay in place for an indefinite period unless the patient has difficulty tolerating the device (Figure 57-19). Previously, surgeons have avoided open reductions with internal fixations (ORIF) because of the possibility of infection. Today, many orthopedic surgeons perform immediate internal fixation with excellent results. Today, antibiotics, antiseptic solutions, and laminar airflow rooms for use during surgery prevent infections.

Intramedullary nailing may be performed in the operating room with the patient under a general or regional anesthesia. This procedure is usually performed for the patient with femoral fractures.[58] An incision is made along the femur at the level of the greater trochanter. A specially designed nail from 12 to 20 mm in diameter and 34 to 48 mm in length is inserted and driven into the cortex well beyond the fracture site. The fracture is reduced just before the insertion so that the bone ends are in correct alignment when the nail is inserted. A large nail is used, since the use of a larger, stronger nail improves the fracture stability and reduces the risk of nail breakage. With subtrochanteric fractures of the femur a nail may be inserted distally and advanced via the intramedullary canal. This patient's incision will be just above and lateral to the knee.

One advantage of the intramedullary nail is that in 2 to 5 days postoperatively the patient is allowed partial weight bearing. The patient may remain in the hospital only 7 to 10 days. The length of stay de-

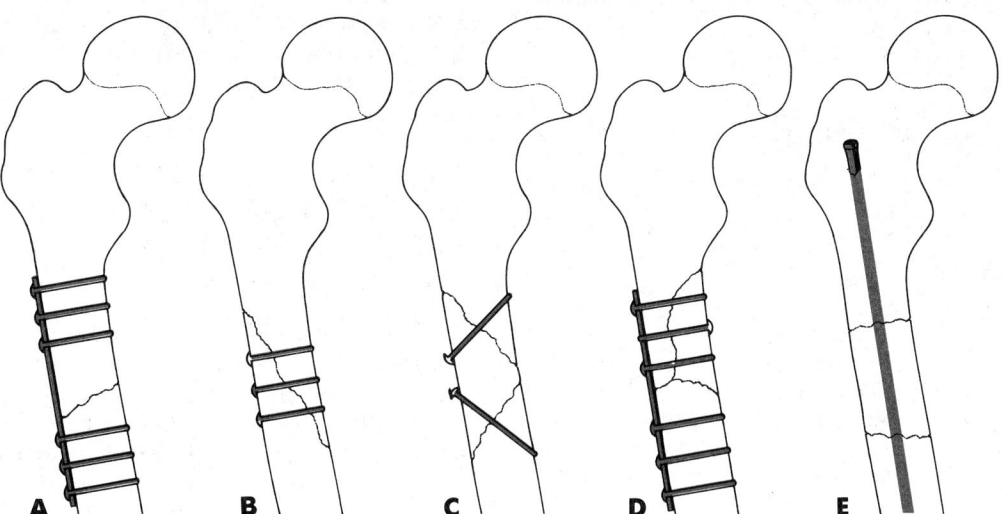

FIGURE 57-19   Techniques of internal fixation. **A,** Plate and six screws for transverse or short oblique fracture. **B,** Screws for long oblique or spiral fracture. **C,** Screws for long butterfly fragment. **D,** Plate and six screws for short butterfly fragment. **E,** Medullary nail for segmental fracture.

pends on the patient's ability for self-care and mobility.

HIP FRACTURES
Etiology

Hip fractures occur in one third of women and one sixth of men older than 65 years of age.[34] Since hip fractures are a common form of trauma in older adults, nursing management of patients with open reduction and internal fixation will be specific for hip fractures. Normal aging problems such as hearing and vision impairment as well as medical problems such as osteoporosis, postural hypotension, or mental status deterioration contribute to falls in elderly persons. Falls frequently are the precipitating factor for loss of mobility and independence in elderly persons. There is a 12% increased mortality for elderly persons in the 4 months following a fracture compared to individuals of the same age who have not had a fracture.[6]

Pathophysiology

There are primarily two types of hip fractures: intracapsular and extracapsular (Figure 57-20). Intracapsular hip fractures include those in the head and neck of the femur, whereas extracapsular hip fractures are those in the intertrochanteric and subtrochanteric regions of the hip (Table 57-6).

When intracapsular fractures occur, there is the risk of disruption of vital blood supply to the head of the femur leading to avascular necrosis. Death of osseous tissue occurs, resulting in pain and limitation of mobility. For this reason replacement of the head and neck of the femur is usually the treatment

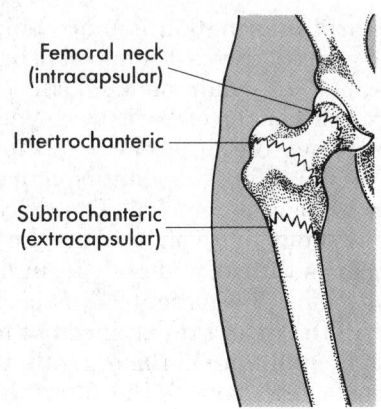

FIGURE 57-20   Types of hip fractures.

Femoral neck (intracapsular)

Intertrochanteric

Subtrochanteric (extracapsular)

of choice. Extracapsular fractures retain adequate blood supply and may be repaired with internal fixation.

Clinical Manifestations

In the patient with a hip fracture, the typical symptoms of fractures are present. In addition to pain and local tenderness, external rotation and shortening of the affected extremity are usually seen.

Therapeutic Management

Intracapsular hip fractures are managed surgically by hemiarthroplasty (replacement of half the joint) or total arthroplasty (replacement of the entire joint) (see Chapter 58). Extracapsular hip fractures are also treated surgically with open reduction and internal fixation. Screws, pins, and plates are most commonly used for internal fixation of these fractures.

NURSING MANAGEMENT OF THE PATIENT WITH OPEN REDUCTION AND INTERNAL FIXATION
Preoperative Assessment

The majority of hip fracture patients are elderly and subject to a variety of chronic health problems such as hypertension, cardiovascular disease, and diabetes mellitus. A careful nursing history must be taken in order to adequately plan nursing care for these individuals. In addition, some patients may require evaluation as to their suitability for anesthesia. Before the surgical procedure of open reduction and internal fixation is done, the fracture site may be temporarily immobilized by (1) traction, (2) a cast, or (3) a splint.

CLINICAL ALERT

High Risk for Falls

Past history of falls

Preexisting cardiovascular disease (decreased cardiac output or cerebral perfusion)

Preexisting neurologic disease (impaired sensorium or sensory deficit)

Preexisting motor deficit (altered locomotion or postural instability)

Hearing or vision impairment

Urinary frequency or urgency (incontinence, benign prostatic hypertrophy)

Specific medications (sedatives, hypnotics, diuretics, analgesics, antihypertensives)

TABLE 57-6   Types of Hip Fractures

	Assessment	Treatment	Complications
Femoral neck (intracapsular)	History of slight trauma Pain in groin and hip Pain with hip movement Usually occurs in women over 60 years Lateral rotation and shortening of leg with minimal deformity	Femoral head replacement with prosthesis, threaded pins Example: Austin Moore prosthesis Occasionally, primary total hip replacement Example: Bipolar, Harris-Galante prosthesis	Avascular necrosis of femoral head Nonunion Pin complications Dislocation of prosthesis
Intertrochanteric (extracapsular)	History of direct trauma over trochanter Severe pain Tenderness over trochanter Usually seen in women 60 to 85 years or in younger women with osteoporosis External rotation and shortening of leg with obvious deformity Loss of hip motion	Open reduction: internal fixation with nail, pin, compression plate with screw Example: Richards compression screw	Shortening of leg Traumatic arthritis Pin migration: bending or breaking of pin Fracture impaction Loss of reduction Delayed union or nonunion of bone
Subtrochanteric (extracapsular)	History of direct trauma of great force Proximal leg pain Usually occurs in women over 60 years External rotation and shortening of leg with some deformity Large hematoma	Open reduction: internal fixation with intramedullary nail, sliding nail plates, and other fixed plates Closed reduction with nail insertion Closed intramedullary device Example: intramedullary nail	Shortening of leg Metal fatigue Lateral displacement of proximal fragment

Modified from Krug B: The hip: nursing fracture patients to full recovery, *RN*, p 57, April 1989.

Nursing Diagnosis

Possible nursing diagnoses are as follows:
  Anxiety related to concerns regarding surgery
  Knowledge deficit related to postoperative care

Planning

Possible outcomes are as follows.
  The patient will verbalize less distress regarding impending surgery
  The patient will verbalize understanding of postoperative care

Implementation

Speaking in a calm, firm, reassuring manner, as well as using short, simple sentences, is appropriate for the management of patient anxiety. The nurse assists the patient in preparing for the surgical experience by providing accurate and factual information regarding what to expect. Positioning, turning, and respiratory and leg exercises are all addressed in a preoperative teaching plan. (See care plan in Chapter 58.)

HIP FRACTURE COMPLICATIONS

Neurovascular complications
   Neurovascular compromise
   Hemorrhage
   Thrombophlebitis
   Avascular necrosis (may occur after discharge
      from the hospital)
Skin and bone impairment
   Wound infection
   Nonunion, delayed union, or pin or device dislo-
      cation
Postanesthesia complications
   Respiratory and circulatory changes
Impaired mobility
   No weight bearing on affected extremity as pre-
      scribed by physician
   Constipation
   Potential for injury
   Postoperative pain
   Body image changes

Evaluation

Nursing interventions have been successful when
the patient expresses a diminished anxiety level,
there is less tremulousness, and muscle tension is
decreased. The teaching plan has been effective
when the patient verbalizes understanding of the instructions provided.

Documentation

The nurse documents any behavior indicative of anxiety and actions taken to alleviate that anxiety. Preoperative teaching and patient understanding are
also noted.

Postoperative Management

Postoperative management for the patient with open
reduction and internal fixation relates to promoting
comfort, preventing postoperative complications,
and enhancing bone and wound healing. Postoperative complications are included in the box.

Evaluation

Evaluation of the care plan consists of determining
if the goals have been met and if the patient problems were adequately solved and potential problems
prevented. The patient with internal fixation will be
hospitalized 5 to 7 days or longer. The length of stay
is based on accomplishment of expected outcomes
and the patient's overall condition.

Documentation

The primary purpose of documentation is to provide
continuity of care. All special equipment (walker,
special mattress) must be documented at least once
each shift. It is especially important to record the patient's noncompliance to any prescribed therapy. It
is important that the nurse attempts to have the patient comply with prescribed treatment, but the
nurse also documents when the patient refuses.

Ongoing Care

Ongoing care may involve rehabilitation treatment
in a long-term care facility or home care. Because
of limitations in mobility the patient may require
some assistance in routine hygiene and health care.[3]
The patient is involved in a period of immobility and
then a period in which active and passive exercises
or therapy is necessary (see p. 1561).

   The outcome of open reduction and internal fixation depends on the patient's adherence to the
therapy. The nurse's primary focus is to know exactly what the prescription regarding activity or immobility is and to verify that the patient is aware of
this prescription. The teaching goal focuses on the
patient's ability to demonstrate the activity to be
performed; the nurse notes the patient's desire and
ability to perform this activity. The nurse allows the
patient time to verbalize concerns regarding immobility. It is very difficult for a patient who has been
accustomed to being active in personal, work, and
recreational life to adjust to some degree of dependency. This feeling of dependency is discussed with
the patient. It helps the patient to know the amount
of time necessary for immobilization.

   For older patients who have other diagnoses,
long-term care may be necessary. If the patient is going to be cared for by the family at home, the nurse
assists in obtaining the necessary equipment or supplies. It is important for the nurse to assess the home
for environmental hazards such as scatter rugs,
which may cause slips or falls, and to promote the
use of safety devices such as bars in the bathroom,
tub, or shower. In addition, thorough teaching may
be necessary so that the family knows how to move
the patient and how to assist the patient to get in
and out of bed. The nurse determines who the primary caregiver will be and assesses the caregiver's
knowledge regarding the patient's needs. A teaching plan is then devised that includes the necessary
information. Lack of knowledge and inadequate
preparation for care at home contribute to the patient's anxiety, insecurity, and nonadherence to the
therapy.[3]

Physical therapy

After musculoskeletal trauma and medical and surgical management, physical therapy may be pre-

NURSING CARE PLAN   *Patient With Postoperative Internal Fixation*

Nursing diagnosis/ Expected outcome	Interventions	Rationale
High risk for peripheral neurovascular dysfunction • *Patient experiences no impairment in neurovascular status*	Assess five P's; record findings and report all abnormal findings to physician; neurovascular checks are completed every 1 to 2 hours as ordered	(See five P's, p. 1536.) Any change may indicate arterial, venous, or nerve compromise; pain may also indicate bleeding at incision site
	Monitor vital signs at least every hour for 4 hours, then every 4 hours for 1 to 3 days, and then according to agency policy; notify physician of changes	After postanesthesia recovery, changes in vital signs may indicate respiratory complications, whereas increased temperature may indicate wound infection
	Consider preoperative vital signs as baseline	Changes immediately after surgery may suggest shock related to blood loss or stress
	Assess surgical drain devices and dressing; record amount and character of drainage; drainage in excess of 100 to 150 mL/hr after first 4 hours is reported to physician	Excessive drainage may suggest active bleeding
	If patient has autologous blood transfusion drainage device, prepare for blood administration according to institution policy	Autotransfusion raises circulatory blood volume without risks of blood-borne disease transmittal
	Monitor results of hemoglobin and hematocrit	Operative and postoperative bleeding into tissue may cause decreased blood values
	Monitor peripheral pulses (popliteal, dorsalis pedis, and posterior tibial); assess presence and character of pulse	Pulses indicate arterial perfusion in extremity
	Apply antiembolism stockings (if ordered); remove stockings for 20 minutes once or twice (refer to procedure) daily and provide skin care	Used to prevent venous stasis and thrombosis
	Apply pneumatic sleeves (sequential compression device) to bilateral extremities (if ordered)	Prevents venous stasis and risk of deep vein thrombosis
	Administer prophylactic low-dose anticoagulant (heparin, sodium warfarin [Coumadin]) as ordered; monitor for bleeding at gums, in urine and stool, and easy bruising	Prevents clot formation
	Monitor prothrombin times (sodium warfarin) and partial thromboplastin times (heparin) and notify physician of abnormalities	Diagnostic tests used to determine anticoagulant dosages
	Assess Homan's sign (passively dorsiflex patient's foot toward tibia), extremity circumference, skin color, and temperature	Pain or tenderness in calf may indicate deep vein thrombosis; sudden increase in extremity circumference, redness (including a streak), and warm to hot skin temperature are additional indicators of thrombophlebitis

Continued.

Nursing diagnosis/ *Expected outcome*	Interventions	Rationale
	Assess respiratory and cardiac status by monitoring breath sounds in all lobes every 4 hours and listening to heart sounds	Changes, including dyspnea, chest pain, and tachycardia, may indicate pulmonary emboli
	If dyspnea, chest pain, tachycardia, orthopnea, and blood-tinged sputum are evident, start oxygen and notify physician	Pulmonary embolism results in inadequate oxygenation secondary to occluded pulmonary vessels; oxygen given to maintain adequate oxygenation
	Monitor comfort level; constant or intermittent pain on weight bearing and limitations in range of motion must be reported to physician (may occur after hospitalization when patient places full weight on extremity)	May indicate avascular necrosis; nurse instructs patient to report these symptoms to physician immediately
High risk for skin and bone integrity impaired, related to surgical intervention • *Patient experiences skin and bone healing*	Monitor vital signs every 4 hours for 1 to 3 days, then according to agency policy; notify physician of changes	Elevated temperature, pulse, and respirations indicate infection
	Assess wound healing and character of any drainage; change dressing as needed using sterile technique; report changes in wound healing to physician, and use ice bags (as prescribed) to incision site; administer antibiotics (as ordered) for at least 48 hours postoperatively	Initially wound drainage may be sanguineous (6 to 8 hours postoperatively), then serosanguineous, then serous, and then clear; changing dressing will prevent maceration of skin and lessen chance of infection; ice bags will prevent swelling, which interferes with tissue healing
	Assess for comfort level and localized incisional pain	Localized pain may be due to infection at site from postoperative hematoma
	Turn patient every 3 hours when on bed rest, and mobilize patient as soon as possible	Continuous pressure results in impaired skin integrity
	Assess weight-bearing ability of affected extremity (may occur after hospitalization, so patient is instructed to report inability to bear weight to physician immediately)	Inability to bear weight may indicate nonunion, delayed union, avascular necrosis, or pin device dislocation
High risk for injury related to post-anesthesia complications • *Patient experiences no complications*	Assess lung and chest sounds	Provides for baseline status and changes
	Promote deep breathing exercises and coughing; may use "blow bottles" or incentive spirometer; reposition every 2 hours	Provides for optional ventilations by prevention of stasis of respiratory secretions
	Monitor body temperature at least every 4 hours	Elevated temperature may indicate chest congestion with infection or postoperative atelectasis

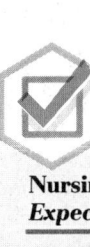
Nursing diagnosis/ Expected outcome	Interventions	Rationale
Physical mobility impaired, related to surgical interventions	Use small pillow between legs	Ensures proper support and body alignment[15]
• *Patient experiences no complications related to immobility*		
	Turn patient side to side in bed every 2 hours; provide overhead trapeze and have patient assist with repositioning	Helps relieve tired muscles and joints, increases circulation, and maintains strength[25]
	Assess ability to ambulate with weight-bearing limitations and assistive device as prescribed	Monitoring patient's progress may suggest need for additional instructions; walkers used immediately after surgery; patients usually progress to use of cane only
	Teach isometric exercises and remind patient to do exercises at least every 4 hours (see quadriceps and gluteal sets, p. 1519)	Provides muscle strength without changing position of joint[25]; increases patient's ability to ambulate with assistive devices
Acute pain related to soft tissue injury from fracture, surgical incision, and insertion of fixation device	Turn or reposition patient every 2 hours	Enhances comfort by relieving pressure
• *Patient will become relatively pain free*[25]		
	Position patient in functional alignment	Diminishes stress on musculoskeletal system[4]
	Reduce sensory overload by modifying environment, which allows patient to relax	Enhances oxygenation and circulation, which relieves pain
	Provide hygiene measures (especially back care) and cleaning after stool or urination	Promotes comfort
	Administer medication as prescribed for pain; medications may be narcotics, NSAIDs (ibuprofen), or muscle relaxants (cyclobenzaprine [Flexeril], carisoprodol [Soma], methocarbamol [Robaxin])	Narcotics relieve pain through decreasing perception of pain; NSAIDs relieve pain through anti-inflammatory effects; muscle relaxants prevent muscle spasms
Body image disturbances related to self-care limitations and uncertain future	Assess patient's self-perception related to limitations imposed by surgery	Provides basis for interventions
• *Patient will regain a positive body image*		
	Allow and encourage as much independence and decision making as possible	Enhances body image and sense of control
	Involve patient/family in discharge planning	Knowledge of what to expect will enhance body image
	Teach patient and family limitations in activity; correct use of ambulation device; and symptoms to report to physician, including fever, pain, and cognitive changes[16]	Allows patient to know what to expect, which enhances body image

scribed. This may include the use of cold, heat, massage, and a variety of exercises.

Cold and heat applications

The usual procedure for a cool therapy system is to place a one-layer dressing over the skin, then the cooling pad, and finally a compression or thick dressing as desired. The usual temperature setting is in the range of 45° to 55° F. Heat is not used over an acutely inflamed area or hematoma or in areas where temperature and pain sensations are altered.[49] In addition, heat is never applied by placing towels, blankets, or bandages in microwave ovens. Uneven heating patterns in the oven can cause hot spots or ignite the material being heated.

Massage

Massage of a body part may relieve abnormal muscle tension by relaxing the muscle and relieving the pain. It is done in a manner that does not cause pain. Deep massage may increase circulation and restore the mobility of soft tissue by lessening the amount of fibrosis that develops in immobilized or injured muscles.[49] Massage also promotes a sense of well-being and gives the patient and nurse time to develop rapport and talk about the patient's concerns. The nurse documents areas massaged and the patient's response.

Exercise

Exercise is an important step toward rehabilitation of the patient with the goals of restoring or maintaining range of motion and strength. It also provides diversion, helps the patient regain self-confidence, and restores a more positive self-image. These exercises are prescribed by the physician, with initial instruction and supervision of the patient by a physical therapist. Types of exercise include isometric, range of motion, isotonic, and isokinetic, based on the type of muscle contraction and movement of the joint.

Isometric exercises

With isometric exercises, muscle tension increases but no movement of adjacent joints is produced. For example, the patient who performs quadriceps setting exercises tightens the anterior thigh muscles in place without moving the knee joint.[45]

Isometric exercises are useful when range of motion is limited by injury or the presence of a cast. They can largely prevent the muscle atrophy that occurs when a fractured extremity is immobilized. Isometric exercises are contraindicated in the person who has severe hypertension or myocardial ischemia, because they constrict the blood vessels and strain the cardiovascular system.[45] The nurse documents specific exercises the patient performs and the response (especially level of fatigue and any complaint of pain).

Range-of-motion exercises

Range-of-motion exercises are used to maintain or increase joint mobility. They can be passive, active-assisted, or active, depending on whether the patient is unable to participate, needs some assistance, or is independent in moving joints. This can be done by the nurse gently putting uninjured joints through their full range of motion as tolerated without pain, at least three times per day. However, the physician's permission is obtained before exercising the joints of the fractured extremity. Functional range of motion is maintained by encouraging the patient to perform activities of daily living as tolerated.[38]

Range-of-motion exercises may be provided by a continuous passive motion machine to an extremity after open reduction and internal fixation of a fracture, after total knee replacement or knee repair, for septic joints, and for arthritis (Figure 57-21). This treatment involves suspension and passive, slow, rotating, or linear movement of the extremity that is provided by a power source.[25] The continuous passive motion machine may be used continuously for days. Benefits of continuous passive motion include improved venous flow, less wound edema and effusion, less need for pain medication, and better range of motion.[44]

The main contraindication to use of continuous passive motion is for those patients who are disoriented and cannot turn the machine off when necessary. The most common complication of using a con-

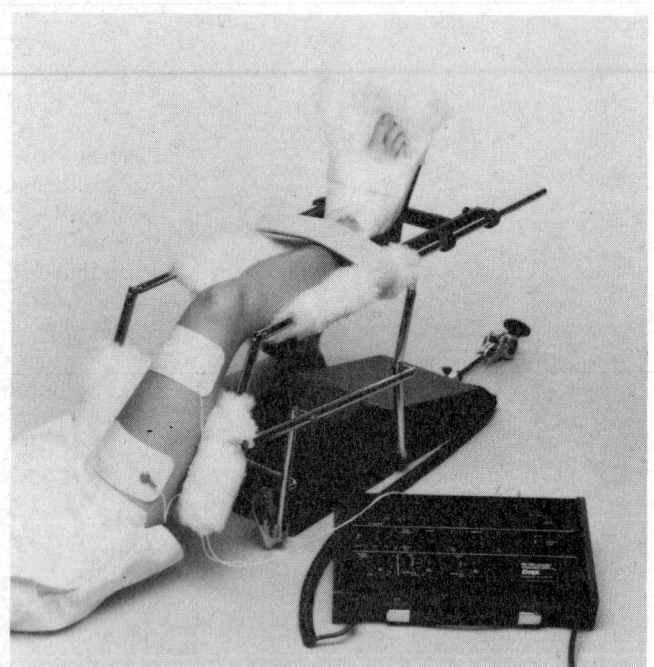

FIGURE 57-21   Continuous passive motion machine (continuous motion therapy device). (Courtesy Empi, Inc., St. Paul.)

tinuous passive motion machine is skin breakdown in the feet, elbows, or groin. The nurse can prevent this by keeping the patient's skin clean, dry, and well protected with pads of sheepskin at points where the equipment may be rubbing the skin.

Isotonic exercises

With isotonic exercises, movement of the muscle is produced and the length of the muscles is changed. For example, if the patient extends and then flexes the arm at the elbow, rhythmic movement of the arm occurs and the muscle lengthens and contracts. Isotonic exercises involve dynamic muscular work that promotes circulation and conditions the cardiovascular system. Because they are aerobic, isotonic exercises cause less muscle fatigue.[51] The nurse documents the exercise, length of time involved, and the patient's response (especially note if the patient is extremely fatigued or complains of chest pain or dizziness). Actions taken related to these complications are noted.

Isokinetic exercises

Isokinetic exercises are usually performed against resistance provided by various isokinetic machines. These machines offer controlled maximum speed of movement and an accommodating resistance that automatically adjusts to always equal the force applied by the patient. The machines are generally located in the physical therapy department, and exercises with them are performed under the physical therapist's supervision. This exercise is recommended to increase strength in muscles after fracture healing is complete.[50,51]

The exercises described may or may not involve movement against resistance. Lifting the weight of the extremity during movement is a type of resistive exercise. The patient works against a fixed resistance (a given amount of weight), and speed of movement varies. The nurse pulls in the opposite direction to the patient's movement or the patient uses antagonistic muscles to produce resistance. For example, if the nurse pushes the patient's foot downward while the patient tries to dorsiflex the foot, the nurse's hand offers resistance against the upward foot movement.

With isokinetic exercises, if the patient moves more slowly than the set speed, there will be no resistance from the system. After reaching the selected speed of movement, the patient cannot go faster. Instead, additional force produced by the patient results in receiving more resistance. In other words, the patient works at a fixed speed with resistance that varies and accommodates.

Active-resistive exercises are generally used to strengthen muscles. Resistive exercises may be permitted by the physician after the affected part is no longer immobilized, but the nurse does *not* perform resistive exercises distal to the fracture until it has completely healed.[61]

Bone healing

After reduction of a fracture and use of one or more of the three methods of immobilization (traction, casting, or internal fixation) the process of healing begins. Restoration of function begins with maintaining the function in the unaffected joints and extremities. Fractures heal faster if adequate circulation is maintained throughout the body. When mechanical factors such as the immobilization of the fracture and ligaments are in place, then the biologic factors are absolutely essential. Function then depends on the biologic process of healing, which always proceeds in an orderly five-stage sequence (see Figure 57-22 and box on p. 1572).

Time for fracture healing

Fracture healing depends on many factors, but in general several weeks, months, or even years are necessary before healing is complete. Fracture healing actually starts with hematoma formation at the time of injury. Stage one usually begins within 10 to 14 days. This time may vary slightly with age as well as with the type of bone involved. Healing time is usually shorter in cancellous (spongy) bones than in compact bones because of the rich blood supply of cancellous bones. Bones that heal slowly (e.g., the humerus, ulna, and tibia) are those with midshaft fractures. Since these bones have less soft tissue surrounding them they have less bleeding, small hematoma formation, and less callus than bones sustaining a metaphyseal fracture.

Delayed healing or delayed union is present when the fracture does not heal in the usual time. It must be remembered that different bones heal at different rates. The bones of the arm may heal in 12 weeks, whereas the femur or tibia may require 24 weeks or twice that amount of time. A greenstick fracture (involves part of the bone thickness, or a bend of the bone) may heal within several weeks, whereas a displaced or comminuted fracture may take several months or up to 2 years to completely heal.

In addition to delayed healing, there may be nonunion (Figure 57-23). This is when healing or union of the bones at the fracture site does not occur even after an extended period (6 to 12 months). There may be excessive bone mobility at the fracture site, and the patient is not able to bear weight on the affected area. Reasons for delayed healing and nonunion are included in the box on p. 1573.[5]

Medical management for both delayed healing and nonunion depend on the cause of the problem. For delayed healing a more complete immobilization may be necessary if the fracture fragments are not

STAGES OF HEALING OF BONE FRACTURES

Stage one: hematoma formation

Stage one begins when the fracture occurs around the fragments and bone marrow. Within the first 24 hours a clot has formed at the injury site. If there is muscle and tissue damage, a massive clot will form that serves as the framework for deposition of new bone cells.

Stage two: cellular proliferation

Stage two involves the proliferation of fibroblasts and new capillaries as the hematoma becomes a fibrin network. On completion of stage two, the hematoma has been replaced by granulation tissue.

Stage three: osteoblast callous formation

As new capillaries and blood vessels form, osteoblasts enter the fibrous area, and the union of the bones becomes firm. The blood supply provides nutrition for building collagen, which begins to incorporate calcium deposits. Depending on the location of the original hematoma, the osteoblasts adjacent to the bone surface form cancellous bone, whereas the osteoblasts more removed from capillary circulation tend to form cartilage.

Stage four: callus ossification

The osteoblasts continue to be the network for new bone formation. The accumulation of new bone at the site is known as the formation of callus. The collagen begins to strengthen as it continues to incorporate calcium deposits. During this stage the fracture ends are knitting together as the final layer of bone is being formed. This stage is referred to as the "union stage," since the bones are uniting.

Stage five: consolidation and remodeling

In the final stage the excess callus is absorbed and the primary cancellous bone is remodeled with compact bone along the lines of stress.

From Thompson J et al: *Clinical nursing,* ed 3, St Louis, 1993, Mosby–Year Book, Inc.

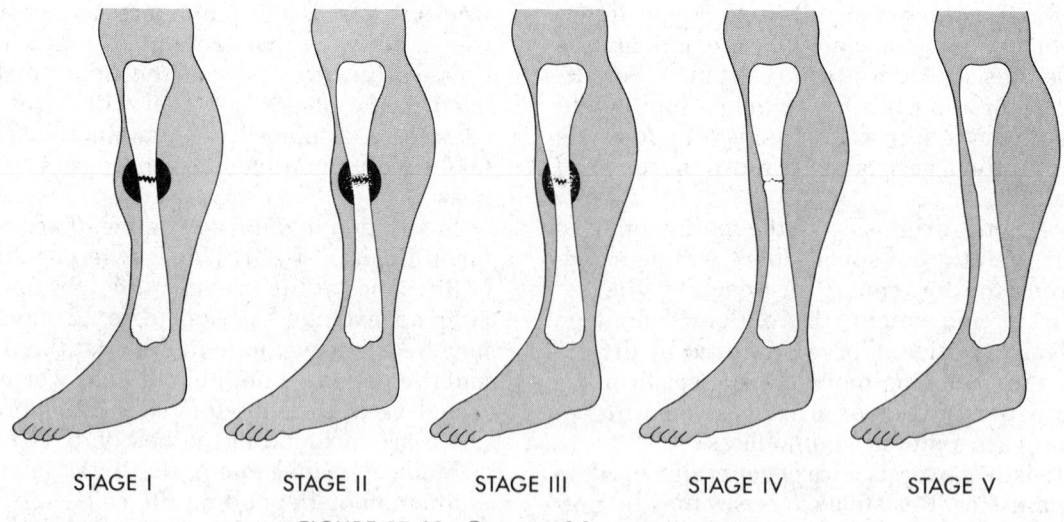

STAGE I   STAGE II   STAGE III   STAGE IV   STAGE V

FIGURE 57-22 Stages of fracture healing.

in alignment, whereas an orthopedic device may be necessary for nonunion. Crutches or a brace may be necessary for an indefinite period. In addition, nonunion may be treated by the use of an electromagnetic stimulator to induce osteogenesis. This stimulator may be either external (placed on opposite sides of the limb at the fracture site) or internal (implanting a stimulator or inserting cathodes)[45] (Figure 57-24). Surgery may be necessary to unite bone fragments or insert a bone graft as well as internal devices such as pins or plates, which may be the treatment of choice.

TRAUMATIC AMPUTATION
Definition

An amputation is a life-changing, devastating injury in most cases. The extent of amputation (single digit as opposed to limb) may not be an accurate indicator of the impact on the individual. For example, the loss of a thumb may necessitate a career change. New microvascular techniques in reimplantation are now making it possible to salvage what otherwise would have resulted in amputation just a few years ago.

Etiology

It is estimated that there are 400,000 amputees in the United States, with 20,000 new amputees per year.[16] Traumatic amputations more commonly occur in the young adult; motor vehicle accidents and occupational accidents account for the major causative factors.

REASONS FOR DELAYED HEALING AND NONUNION OF BONES

Immobilization or fixation of the fracture is not adequate, and there has been excessive movement at the fracture site.

The callus has been dislodged because of repeated attempts to manipulate the fracture.

Circulation is inadequate as a result of the initial injury swelling that impairs blood flow (see discussion of avascular necrosis) or as a result of the reduction process of the fracture.

Infection occurs at the fracture site from an open fracture or from a surgical intervention.

Severe tissue trauma exists at the fracture site (see discussion of compartment syndrome).

Bone fragments separate at the fracture site.

There is a loss of bone from necrosis or excision, or a dislodgement of a bone fragment may interfere with the healing process.

A disease process (e.g., cancer) affects the bone.

There are severe nutritional deficits of protein, calcium, and vitamins.

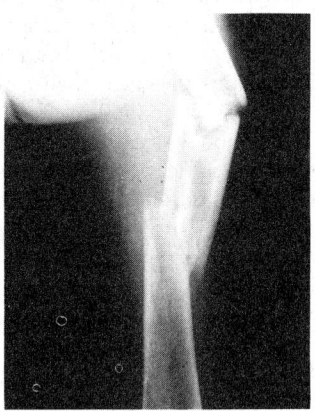

FIGURE 57-23   Nonunion of fracture. (From Ferrell J: *Illustrated guide to orthopedic nursing,* Philadelphia, 1986, JB Lippincott Co.)

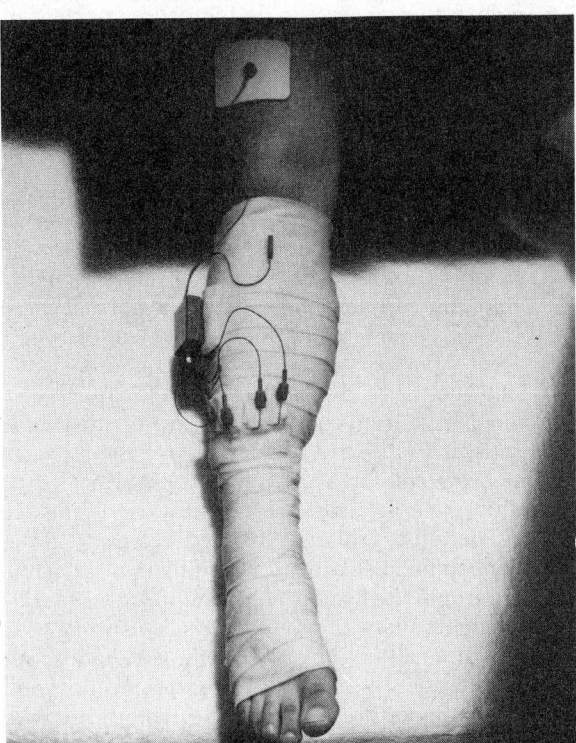

FIGURE 57-24   Bone growth stimulator. (Courtesy Zimmer Co., Warsaw, Ind.)

Pathophysiology

Traumatic amputation may result in a complete amputation when the part is severed from the body and no attaching structures are intact. Incomplete amputation of a part maintains some connecting tissue.[12] Crushing injuries may also necessitate amputation of a body part. The patient who sustains a traumatic amputation resulting from an accident requires emergency action to stop bleeding and emergency surgery to repair the stump.[2]

Under certain conditions, replantation may be attempted. Amputations of the thumb, multiple digits, the palm, wrist, and distal forearm, as well as am-

LEGAL ISSUE· *Amputation and Competency*

A 36-year-old man suffering from a gangrenous condition of both feet as a result of third-degree frostbite was transferred to a Veterans' Administration hospital. Approximately 1 month before seeking medical treatment, he had been living in a station wagon after eviction from his home. He was receiving Social Security benefits based on a mental disability and had a history of psychiatric hospitalizations. In the hospital, physicians recommended amputation of portions of both feet.

The patient refused; relatives declined to be involved. The hospital brought to court the question of the patient's mental competency and asked to be authorized to perform the surgery. The following was evidence in the case:

1. Hospital Chief of Surgery testified that portions of the patient's feet were dead, gangrenous, and mummified; there was localized infection; normal tissue was red and swollen; the dead tissue would not revitalize or heal. Without surgical amputation, the dead tissue would ultimately fall off, leaving exposed bone, which in turn would eventually crack and fall away. The Chief of Surgery testified that in all likelihood there would be a nonhealing stump at least on one foot; that the right foot would not bear weight and would be the source of severe pain; that there was no life-threatening infection, but the failure to amputate would substantially enhance the risk of generalized infection, the development of "wet" gangrene, requiring more serious amputations and possibly leading to death. The Chief of Surgery also testified that the risks of surgery were small; that the patient would have use of one foot and a prosthetic device would be needed for the other.

2. The treating staff psychiatrist and the court-appointed psychiatrist testified, referring to the patient's medical records, including that the patient is a paranoid schizophrenic, manifested generally in his belief that the treating physicians were trying to hurt him, a loosening of thought association, and idiosyncratic thinking. He was intermittently verbally abusive and threatening to staff, interfered with the application of his dressings, and refused intravenous antibiotics and taking of blood samples. For a period he refused to take psychotropic drug medication. During this time he suffered from hallucinations of being attacked by scissors and heard voices of his deceased parents through the radio. The psychiatrists testified that the patient lacked any realistic insight into the nature of his condition or capability of understanding the risks and benefits of surgery or the consequences of his refusal to accept treatment.

3. The patient testified that he knew his feet were hurt and understood what an amputation was but that he was certain that his condition would get better rather than worse and that his feet would be usable. His testimony, the court commented, exhibited a wholly irrational trust in the natural healing of his problem and a belief that his hospitalization and treatment had only been for experimental purposes.

The trial court decided that the patient was mentally incompetent to give or withhold consent to recommended surgery and granted the authorization to perform the amputation. An appeal followed. The appellate court stated that clear and convincing evidence is required in competency determinations: evidence that the patient is incapable of making an informed, rational decision on the basis of the risks and benefits of the surgery and comprehending the seriousness of his condition and the consequences of not having the procedure performed. While the patient knows his feet are hurt and understands what is entailed in an amputation, his psychotic fears and beliefs have resulted in a self-denial of the severity of his condition and the likely and possibly even life-threatening consequences of failing to undergo surgery. The court found that the benefits to be derived from surgery clearly outweighed any risks, despite the possible adverse effects on his mental state if the operation was performed against his will.

The court said the psychiatrist's testimony revealed that it was not the respondent's refusal to consent alone that formed the basis for the opinion expressed but rather the absence of any relation to reality in the reasons the patient gave for refusing. This case differs from cases where a patient, capable of rationally assessing his chances and choices, decides on a fatalistic course for religious or other reasons derived from actual life experiences and whose wishes must be respected despite their conflict with the judgment of the medical professionals.

Source: In the Matter of Harvey U, 501 N.Y.S.2d 920 (A.D. 3rd Dept. 1986).

putations in children, are indicators for attempting replantation.[27]

When replantation is not possible, there may be a limited amount of time to prepare the patient for surgery and the lifetime effects of this procedure. The operative procedure usually is to repair the stump or to stop bleeding from the stump. Much nursing care is necessary to help patients adjust to a life without a particular limb. This section focuses on caring for the patient with a traumatic amputation.

The pathophysiology, operative procedure, and level of amputation are determined by the extent of damaged tissue and the amount of missing tissue. The amputation is performed several inches above the actual site of missing tissue, but this is to ensure that the remaining tissue has a sufficient blood supply, adequate nutrition, and oxygen to survive.

Clinical Manifestations

After a traumatic amputation, the patient may have symptoms of shock related to loss of blood. Some of these wounds may be bleeding profusely, whereas others may have little or no bleeding. The trauma may have sealed off the major blood supply, thereby preventing bleeding. Other patients may present with an incomplete amputation. In addition to bleeding, foreign debris that may cause an infection is present in the wound. If the patient has been on the ground, dirt, grass, or small sticks may be present in the wound. The stump may be smooth, or it may have threads of damaged tissue extending from the site.

Therapeutic Management

Amputated stump

Emergency care for the patient with a traumatic amputation involves controlling bleeding, preventing shock, cleaning the wound, and providing the patient with an explanation of what has occurred and what the medical-surgical plan will be. Before surgical intervention, blood loss is better controlled by direct pressure as opposed to use of a tourniquet since it may contribute to tissue ischemia.

When the severed part is not implantable, the rationale for the surgical procedure and treatment after the traumatic amputation is based on the following principles:
1. The bone is cut shorter than the muscle so that the skin and muscle can be wrapped over the end of the bone.
2. The muscle is cut shorter than the skin so that the skin can be wrapped over the muscle.
3. The incision may be closed with or without a drain or a wound suction in place.

4. Some physicians apply a cast to the stump over the sterile dressing and then a temporary, prefitted prosthesis to the cast. This allows for ambulation as early as the second postoperative day.

A below-knee (BKA) or an above-knee (AKA) amputation may be performed in the case of trauma to the lower extremity. The below-knee amputation offers the patient the advantage of preserving the function and mobility that the knee offers. This type of amputation is preferable for younger persons who will remain physically active because it offers them a more natural gait. Also, the lower the level of amputation, the less energy and balance will be required for walking.

In the upper extremities, including the fingers, the stump is repaired and prepared for a prosthesis at a slightly higher level than the amputation so that healthy tissue is present to facilitate healing. Some stump repairs consist of shaving the bone so that there is a smooth ending, whereas other repairs consist of tissue and bone debridement.

Replantation

Digital replantation has recently been successful at specially equipped centers. The rapid advancements of microsurgical techniques, limb recovery, and preservation methods have contributed significantly to the success of replantation as a viable surgical alternative in the treatment of amputation injuries.[12]

The greater the amount of muscle and nerve tissue involved in the injury, the more difficult it is to predict successful replantation. Amputations above the wrist do not lend themselves as readily to replantation because of the extensive tissue, muscle, nerve, and bone damage that may have occurred in the injury.[12]

The best candidates for replantation surgery are patients with amputation of the palm, wrist, or proximal forearm, because blood vessels in those areas are larger and easier to reattach. Since the thumb is essential for gripping and holding, much effort is made to save it. Lower extremity amputations are usually not considered for replantation, because the patient will be left with legs of different lengths and will lose sensation in the sole of the foot.[26]

The time (ischemia time) that the amputated part is not perfused by circulating blood is crucial in predicting success. During the ischemia time, there is obstruction to the microcirculation; however, large vessels are maintained.

The obstruction is due to aggregation of red blood cells and platelets.[17] Because of the obstruction, tissue necrosis occurs. The time limit for successful replantation is within 6 hours and up to 24 hours with cold ischemia (that period of time that the amputated part is being cooled in accordance with preservation procedures).[12] The success rate depends on several factors. Some of the primary factors are the condition of the stump and the care of the amputated part. The severed part is kept clean (sterile if possible).

Protocols for care of the amputated part vary, but current practice for preservation includes the following procedure:

1. Wrap the amputated part in a cool dry cloth.
2. Moisten the cloth with normal saline or Ringer's lactate solution and, if neither is available, wrap the part(s) in a cloth.
3. Place it in sealed double plastic bags.[12]
4. Place the bag on ice, avoiding direct contact between the ice and the severed part (avoid freezing the part).

General anesthesia is usually used for the procedure. The usual surgical procedure involves irrigating the site with normal saline and antibiotic solutions. Nonviable tissue is then debrided. Bone ends are trimmed for proper alignment and repairs are made to the tendons, grafts, arteries, veins, skin, and nerves as needed.

NURSING MANAGEMENT OF THE PATIENT WITH REPLANTATION
Assessment

The nurse assesses for the condition of the stump, any bleeding, and the length of time the severed part is not perfused. In addition, the patient's feelings regarding the procedure are explored. The nurse avoids giving false hope.

Nursing Diagnosis

A possible nursing diagnosis is as follows:
    Altered peripheral tissue perfusion, arterial, related to venous congestion and arterial insufficiency

Planning

A possible outcome for the patient with replantation is as follows:
    The patient will demonstrate adequate perfusion to the replanted part as evidenced by capillary refill between 3 and 5 seconds, warm skin temperature, and decreased swelling

Implementation

Nursing interventions to promote patient adjustment begin with admission to the emergency department. The goal of preoperative intervention is to reduce the patient's anxiety in preparation for surgery. This can be accomplished with the establishment of trust and rapport. It is essential to prepare the patient in the preoperative and postoperative period by providing explanations for procedures and care.

Educating the family and the patient about the stages of grief for a loss can ease the patient's concerns and assist in adaptation to the loss. Patients with replantations may undergo the stress of loss or changes in their abilities even if the replanted part looks normal.[40]

Other specific nursing interventions depend on the physician's orders. If there are no postoperative complications, the patient is usually discharged 8 to 10 days after surgery. Follow-up dressing changes and site care are continued after discharge. Active exercise may be initiated as early as 2 weeks postoperatively. The major goal of rehabilitation therapy is to return function to the operative site as well as to maintain function in the affected limb.[12] Rehabilitation may include occupational therapy in addition to physical therapy. The nurse is a major impetus in the discharge plan for referral to support networks and other services. These services enhance recovery and minimize barriers to recovery.

Perfusion to the severed part is essential if the area is to remain viable. The nurse elevates the extremity above the heart level. The nurse encourages the patient to avoid caffeine and nicotine to prevent vasospasms. Skin color, capillary refill time, skin turgor, temperature, and evidence of venous or arterial bleeding are assessed, and a pressure dressing or an immobilization splint is applied. Venous congestion is a postoperative complication that has been successfully treated with leech therapy.

Leech therapy

The goal of leech therapy is to promote bleeding in the congested area, facilitating venous outflow during the time that collateral circulation and microvascular knitting develop.[12] This therapy is effective since leech saliva is an anticoagulant, local vasodilator, and local anesthetic.[29,38] These actions help drain tissue engorged with venous blood if thrombosis or inadequate venous drainage is present. Leeches can only be used if there is an intact arterial blood supply.[26]

The regimen for leech therapy is applying the leech for 10 minutes to 2 hours or until the leech is engorged with blood. The usual schedule is intermittent reapplication of the leech at 4- to 8-hour intervals. The time depends on the condition (reestablishment of circulation) of the replanted part. The nurse's role during the leech therapy is to monitor the leech until it is fully distended. In addition, the nurse may be required to remove the leech after therapy is complete.[29] The procedure depends on agency protocol or physician's orders. The patient needs reassurance during the therapy. The leech saliva contains a natural anesthetic, and the replanted part generally lacks sensation in the early recovery period.[12]

Replantation and leech therapy are more often done at a trauma center than at small hospitals. Within the last decade, leeches are being used to prevent complications of microsurgical replantation.

Evaluation

Nursing care directed to replantation is successful when the circulation is maintained to the replanted part. Warm skin temperature, quick capillary refill, and decreasing edema are all indicators that the plan is successful.

Documentation

The nurse documents neurovascular status every 30 to 60 minutes or more often as necessary. Leech therapy is documented as to length of time applied and condition of replanted part before and after leech therapy. The patient's adjustment to the surgery is also noted.

Ongoing Care

Physical therapy to regain mobility in the replanted part will be an ongoing process. The patient is also instructed as to the actions to take should a neurovascular deficit become apparent.

NURSING MANAGEMENT OF THE PATIENT WITH AMPUTATION

Assessment

The immediate nursing assessment includes inspection of the amount of bleeding, the extent of tissue damage, and the exact location of the injury. The nurse may measure the injury site as it relates to the remaining joint. This may also be done by an assessment of the unaffected extremity by measuring the amount of tissue missing at the amputation site on the affected extremity. Additionally, the nurse determines the remaining range of motion for a patient who has sustained an amputation involving a joint. A general head-to-toe assessment is completed to determine if there are other injuries. When patients incur an injury such as an amputation, they often will be so devastated by the appearance of the injury they will completely overlook other injuries of a lesser nature. The nurse assesses the patient's psychologic status. It may be difficult for the patient to accept loss of a body part, so the patient may not have looked at the injury site. The nurse encourages and allows the patient to express fears or concerns regarding the loss. Since accidents are unexpected, the patient may not have yet considered the loss. During the initial assessment, many patients may be in a state of emotional shock and disbelief that the injury has occurred. The patient's psychologic status regarding the injury is determined and documented.

Nursing Diagnosis

Nursing diagnoses depend on the stage of the injury. On first encounter with the patient, the nursing diagnosis may be as follows:

Acute pain related to swelling, muscle spasm, or other musculoskeletal causes

Once the patient realizes the limitations that an amputation presents regarding ambulation, additional nursing diagnoses include the following:

High risk for altered tissue perfusion: arterial, related to blood loss

High risk for infection related to suture line at stump

Impaired physical mobility related to decreased range of motion, imposed activity restriction, imposed mechanical restriction, decreased muscle strength, or pain

Self-care deficit related to impaired physical mobility

High risk for ineffective individual coping related to the loss or injury to a body part, change (perceived or actual) in personal appearance, disruption of role performance, inadequate or unavailable support systems, major recent life changes, inadequate personal resources, and self-concept disturbances[1]

Chronic pain related to phantom limb sensations

Planning

Patient outcomes include the following:

The patient will verbalize that the pain is decreased

The patient will exhibit no signs and symptoms of hypovolemia

The patient will exhibit no signs and symptoms of stump infection

The patient will participate in activities as physical limitations allow and with the required assistive devices (e.g., crutches)

The patient will identify a plan for assistance in provisions of care

The patient will demonstrate coping with body image changes and role change with assistance from others

The patient will verbalize concerns related to phantom pain caused by the amputation

Implementation

The three major concerns for the patient with an amputation are (1) stump care that will be effective in the healing process and that will be effective in the prevention of an infection; (2) exercise that will maintain the tone of the unaffected muscles as well as strengthen those muscle groups that will be used to compensate for the amputation; and (3) psychologic support during the time the patient is grieving for the loss of a body part and during the period when the patient is adapting to the limitations or changes imposed by the amputation.

Effective stump care during the healing process includes keeping the stump elevated so that swelling at the incision site will not occur. This can be done by elevating the foot of the bed. The stump is never elevated in such a way as to cause a contracture at the joint. To prevent a joint contracture, a pillow is not used to elevate the stump after the first 24 hours. The nurse watches for any signs and symptoms of hemorrhage. If excessive bleeding occurs, the nurse has a tourniquet available to apply to the stump. If there is slight bleeding at the incision line, the nurse applies a pressure dressing to the stump site. Usually an elastic bandage is applied to the stump to maintain constant pressure, prevent edema formation, and shape the stump for future prosthesis fitting.

Infection can best be prevented by keeping the site clean and dry. If the patient does not have drainage from the incision, the bandage can be very thin or no bandage may be applied. Some patients prefer a thin dressing to prevent linen from rubbing on the incision and to keep the incision out of the view of themselves and visitors.

The patient must have an exercise program that will "build up" or maintain the muscle groups that will be necessary for crutch walking or for the patient to be fitted with a prosthesis. Some physicians prescribe a program of physical therapy, but it still remains the role of the nurse to ensure that the patient is participating in some exercise routine. Even if the patient is not a candidate for a prosthesis, the nurse ensures that muscle tone is maintained. Otherwise, the patient will be weak, fatigued, and unable to care for daily needs. The old axiom of "what you don't use, you lose" is true of the muscles that are unused while the patient is hospitalized.

The psychologic impact of a traumatic amputation can be devastating for the patient and the family. Nursing interventions affect the adjustment to the loss and the patient's ability to cope.

The phenomenon of **phantom pain** is explained to the patient. Phantom pain is pain in the missing

---

TABLE 57-7 Nursing Intervention Summary: Selected Patient Problems for Patient with Amputation

Patient problem	Nursing interventions
Pain	Position patient to relieve edema and spasms at stump site; when postoperative edema can be controlled, pain in stump is decreased
	Pain medication is administered to relieve phantom pain; remember that pain is real and if it is intense, medication is required
	Handle injured body part smoothly and gently[59]
	Promote sleep and rest by comfort measures and routines that patient uses at home
	Provide support and encouragement during painful episodes and frightening procedures
Impaired physical mobility	Provide passive range-of-motion exercise until patient is able to participate in active range of motion; patient is assisted out of bed as soon as possible to prevent complications of bed rest
	Devise time frame for turning and repositioning patient
	Collaborate with other members of health team in developing or using safe and effective techniques for bed mobility, transfer, and ambulation[59]
Self-care deficit	Provide assistance as needed with care
	Provide sufficient time for patient to participate in self-care
	Allow patient to have input into planning self-care
High risk for ineffective coping	Encourage patient to talk about mechanisms used in past to cope with stress
	Spend time with patient and establish effective patient rapport
	Observe patient to determine coping mechanisms
	Encourage and allow patient to experience grieving process free of guilt[3]
	Listen to what the patient says; are plans realistic based on loss of a body part or is there denial of limitations?
	Communicate nursing observations regarding patient's coping ability to physician and other members of health care team

PATIENT EDUCATION   *Amputation*

Safety measures (lower limb)

Remove or tack down area rugs. If patient is using walker or crutches or has prosthesis, it is dangerous to walk over small area rugs because these rugs will slip and cause patient to fall.

Place rubber pad or safety strips in bathtub. If shower is to be used, have stool installed in shower stall or provide small metal chair in shower.

Appliances to assist in walking or standing are not used in shower.

Upper extremity

Have sleeves of clothes altered to accommodate prosthesis.

Instruct patient on how to place a long sleeve inside of shirt so sleeve will not be likely to be caught in doors or any equipment. This could cause patient to fall.

Care of stump

Inspect stump incision site daily; if there is redness, drainage, blister, or abrasions, physician is notified.

Provide daily care to incision line with mild soap and soft cloth. Pat incision dry. No ointment, antiseptic, or other creams are applied unless patient has been instructed to do so by physician.

Remove bandage at least once each day and whenever it becomes wet or loose. Purpose of bandage is to reduce swelling and to shape stump. Instruct patient in correct method of rewrapping bandage (Figure 57-25).

Use cotton stump sock, and avoid synthetic materials that increase perspiration. Stump sock is kept clean and dry to prevent infection and skin breakdown.

Exercise and activity

Patient continues to practice active range of motion with unaffected extremities.

If patient is using crutches or walker, muscles of upper arms must be developed or muscle ability maintained.

If patient will be using wheelchair, transfer from bed to chair needs to be taught. If patient is using crutches, teach crutch walking.

Reinforce guidelines for amount of rest and exercise from time of discharge until return visit to physician.

Pain

Discuss with patient the concept of phantom pain. Explain to patient that the sensation in the "missing" part may continue for as long as 6 months. Explain that this type of sensation is related to severing of nerves at amputation site.

Encourage patient to talk about phantom pain sensation if present. Remind patient that it is a normal occurrence after amputation of an extremity.

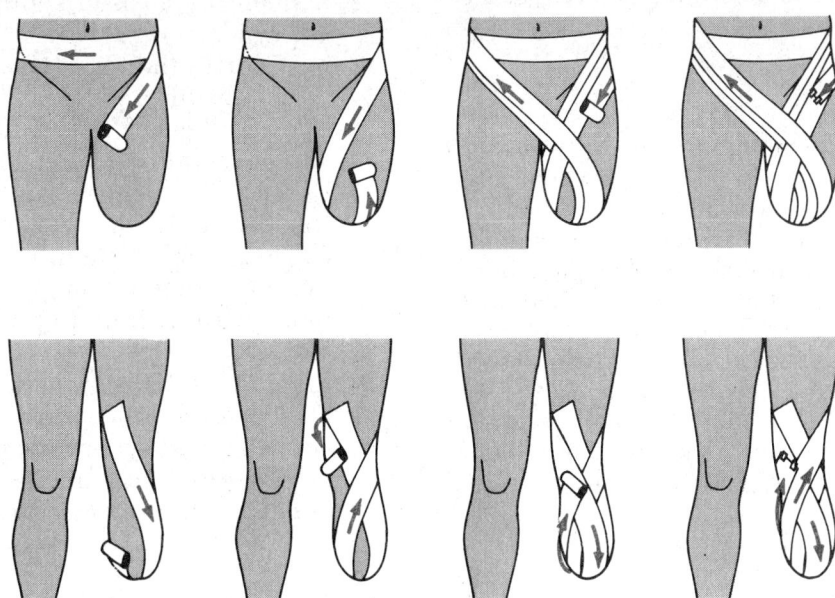

FIGURE 57-25   Correct method to bandage amputation stump. *Top,* It is important to anchor bandage around patient's waist. *Bottom,* Method for bandaging midcalf stump, where bandage need not be anchored around waist.

limb, as though the amputation did not take place. It is important to remember that it is *real pain*. The limb has been severed, but the nerve tracts that register pain in that area still send messages to the brain.[8] Telling patients this will relieve much anxiety, since they may think they are "going crazy" when there is pain in a body part that has been amputated.

Patients with a traumatic amputation are encouraged to talk about the limitations they feel they will have. The nurse may request that other members of the health team provide the patient with some form of therapy (i.e., occupational, recreational, or physical). The patient is also helped to grieve for the missing part in an effort to enhance psychologic adjustment.

Patients are encouraged to consider the impact the amputation will have on their lives. The nurse encourages the patient to face the reality of the amputation and to consider available assistive devices or prostheses if the patient is a candidate. In addition to these three concerns, other specific nursing actions are discussed in Table 57-7 that correlate with selected patient problems.

Evaluation

Evaluation of the care plan focuses on the outcome criteria. Have the nursing interventions allowed the patient to meet these criteria? Since evaluation is an ongoing process, the nurse monitors the patient's progress and revises the nursing diagnoses and expected outcomes as necessary. Progress toward outcome achievement is observed and recorded. Reassessment is necessary to determine progress or lack of progress.

Documentation

Documentation of all steps of the nursing process is important with every patient, but the psychologic assessment stage is of utmost importance when caring for an amputee. Patients who have an amputation experience shifts in their psychologic adaptation to the loss. When they receive permission to ambulate with crutches, they may be optimistic about their progress, but when they attempt crutch walking and realize that it is difficult and tiresome, they may "give up." The recording of assessment findings will assist the nurse to know where the patient is in the adjustment phase and develop an accurate care plan.

It is important to record the condition of the stump, especially if a prosthesis is planned for this patient. Likewise, an accurate recording of the health of the stump may allow signs and symptoms of infection to be treated so the incision line will heal smoothly.

Ongoing Care

Ongoing care for the patient with an amputation may be lengthy. Both the patient and family must be instructed in safety measures that may involve changes in the arrangement of furniture or in the patient's living accommodations. The patient or the caregiver is instructed in the specifics of caring for the stump, the prescribed exercise and activity level of the patient, and measures to reduce pain (see patient education guide).

The patient not fitted with a prosthesis immediately after surgery may be admitted to a rehabilitation unit to be fitted with a prosthesis. The patient is usually treated at the rehabilitation unit until use of the prosthesis is correctly and safely demonstrated.

Many communities have organized amputee support groups that meet on a scheduled basis. These support groups offer the new amputee an opportunity to vent feelings of frustration and anger. If there is a support group in the area, the nurse provides written information about the group to the patient. The patient with an amputation and a successful psychosocial adjustment will be able to incorporate the amputated stump into a revised body image and resolve feelings of loss and grief concerning the loss of the limb.

CRITICAL THINKING QUESTIONS

1 Describe nursing management including RICE for contusions, strains, sprains, bursitis, epicondylitis, and dislocations.

2 Explain the basis of sports injuries and overuse syndrome.

3 Summarize the three treatment methods and rationales for a patient with a fracture.

4 Identify the 5 P's and summarize questions and observations for each one.

5 Describe the eight signs and symptoms of a fracture and explain the pathologic basis of each sign or symptom.

6 Compare the nursing management for patients with traction to that for patients with a cast.

7 Explain the pathologic basis of complications of fractures, including avascular necrosis, compartment syndrome, gas gangrene, osteomyelitis, and fat embolus.

8 What are the stages of fracture healing?

9 Explain the basis of nonunion and delayed healing.

10 What are the hazards of immobility on body systems?

11 What actions should the nurse implement to prevent hazards of immobility?

12 Describe nursing diagnoses, interventions, and rationales for a patient with an internal fixation (hip pinning).

13 Identify the therapeutic management of amputations, digit replantation, and leech therapy.

14 What are the nursing actions for a patient with a traumatic amputation? Include both physiologic and psychologic actions.

BIBLIOGRAPHY

Current

1. American Nurses' Association and National Association for Orthopaedic Nurses: Orthopaedic nursing practice; process and outcome criteria for selected diagnoses, *Orthop Nurse* 6(2):11, 1987.
2. Billings D, Stokes L: *Medical-surgical nursing*, ed 2, St Louis, 1987, Mosby–Year Book, Inc.
3. Broadhurst C: Adjusting to amputation, *Nurs Times* 85(43):55-58, 1989.
4. Brunner LS, Suddarth DS: *Textbook of medical-surgical nursing*, ed 7, Philadelphia, 1992, JB Lippincott Co.
5. Carpenito LJ: *Nursing diagnosis: application to clinical practice*, ed 2, Philadelphia, 1987, JB Lippincott Co.
6. Ebersole P, Hess P: *Toward healthy aging: human needs and nursing response*, ed 3, St Louis, 1990, Mosby–Year Book, Inc.
7. ECRI: Microwave ovens: no blanket approval, *Nurs 89* 7:31, July 1989.
8. Elsenhans VD, Hecht AS: *Musculoskeletal problems. Nurse review: a clinical update system*, Springhouse, Pa, 1990, Springhouse Corporation Book Division.
9. Folcik MA: Meniscal injuries, *Nurs Clin North Am* 26(1):185, 1991.
10. Gamron R: Taking the pressure out of compartment syndrome, *Am J Nurs* 88:1076, 1988.
11. Hansell M: Fractures and the healing process, *Orthop Nurs* 10(3):11, 1991.
12. Higgins RM: Replantation of digits, *Orthop Nurs* 10(3):11, 1991.
13. Hines NA, Bates MS: Discharging the patient in skeletal traction, *Orthop Nurs* 6(4):21, 1987.
14. Jones-Walton P: Clinical standards in skeletal traction pin site care, *Orthop Nurs* 10(2):2-16, 1991.
15. Krug BM: The hip: nursing fracture patients to full recovery, *RN*, p 58, April 1989.
16. Lewis SM, Collier IC: *Medical surgical nursing*, ed 3, St Louis, 1992, Mosby–Year Book, Inc.
17. May J, Littler J: The hand, *Plast Surg* 8:5018-5020, 1990.
18. McCance K, Huether S: *Pathophysiology: the biologic basis for disease in adults and children*, St Louis, 1990, Mosby–Year Book, Inc.
19. Menkes J: Pitfalls in orthopedic trauma. II. The lower extremity, *Emerg Med* 21(6):108, 1989.
20. Miller V, Eden-Kilgour S: Preventing peroneal nerve damage, *Orthop Nurs* 6(4):41, 1987.
21. Mims B: Fat embolism syndrome: a varient of ARDS, *Orthop Nurs* 8(3):22, 1989.
22. Mooney V, Stills M: Continuous passive motion with joint fractures and infections, *Orthop Clin North Am* 18(1):1, 1987.
23. Morris L et al: Nursing the patient in traction, *RN*, p 26, Jan 1988.
24. Morris L et al: Special care for skeletal traction, *RN*, p 26, Feb 1988.
25. Mourad L: *Orthopedic disorders*, St Louis, 1991, Mosby–Year Book, Inc.
26. Mulvey M, Sharma PK: Traumatic amputation, *RN*, pp 26-29, Sept 1991.
27. Neff J, Kidd P: *Trauma nursing: the art and science*, St Louis, 1993, Mosby–Year Book, Inc.
28. Nussman D: Traumatic hip dislocation, *Am J Nurs* 91(11):34, 1991.
29. O'Hara M: Leeching: a modern use for an ancient remedy, *Am J Nurs*, pp 1656-1658, Dec 1988.
30. Olsson G, Parker G: A model approach to pain assessment, *Nurs 87* 17(5):51, 1987.
31. Osborne LJ, DiGiacomo I: Traction: a review with nursing diagnosis and intervention, *Orthop Nurs* 6(4):13, 1987.
32. Perrin JCS et al: Musculoskeletal and soft tissue disorders, *Arch Phys Med Rehabil* 70(5-S):S183-S187, 1989.
33. Practical briefings: internal fixation for open fractures, *Patient Care* 21(4):25, 1987.
34. Ruddy DR: Osteoporosis: overcoming a costly and debilitating disease, *Postgrad Med* 86:151-153, 1989.
35. Salmond SW et al: *Core curriculum for orthopedic nursing*, ed 2, Pitman, NJ, 1991, AJ Janetti.
36. Shirreffs T: Compartment syndrome: an extremity at risk, *Emerg Med* 22(6):103, 107, 110, 1990.
37. Slye DA: Orthopedic complications, *Nurs Clin North Am* 26(1):113-132, 1991.
38. Strangio L: Leeches: when bleeding is exactly what you want, *RN*, pp 31-33, Sept 1991.
39. Swearingen PL: *Manual of nursing therapeutics*, ed 2, St Louis, 1990, Mosby–Year Book, Inc.
40. Wallace B, Herbert C: Managing the psychosocial problems associated with replantation surgery, *Crit Care Nurs Q* 13(1):55-62, June 1990.

Classic

41. Arlington RG: *Internal fixation of the lower extremity: care considerations, assessment and fracture management of the lower extremity*, Pitman, NJ, 1984, National Association of Orthopedic Nursing Monograph.
42. Carini GK, Birmingham JJ: *Traction made manageable: a self-learning module*, New York, 1980, McGraw-Hill Inc.
43. Celeste SM et al: Identifying a standard for pin site care using the quality assurance approach, *Orthop Nurs* 3(4):17, 1984.
44. Coutts RD: Continuous passive motion in the rehabilitation of the total knee patient: its role and effect, *Orthop Rev* 15:126, 1986.
45. Ferrell J: *Illustrated guide to orthopedic nursing*, ed 3, Philadelphia, 1986, JB Lippincott Co.
46. Genge ML: Orthopedic trauma: pelvic fractures, *Orthop Nurs* 5(1):11, 1986.
47. Hoyt NJ: Infections following orthopedic injury, *Orthop Nurs* 5(5):15, 1986.
48. Itoh M, Lee MHN: Rehabilitation for the aged. In Jackson O, editor: *Physical therapy of the geriatric patient*, New York, 1983, Churchill Livingstone, Inc.
49. Kessler RM, Hertling D: *Management of common musculoskeletal disorders: physical therapy principles and methods*, Philadelphia, 1983, Harper & Row Publishers, Inc.
50. Kisner C, Colby LA: *Therapeutic exercise: foundations and techniques*, Philadelphia, 1985, FA Davis Co.
51. Kuprian W: *Physical therapy for sports*, Philadelphia, 1982, WB Saunders Co.

52. Lane PL, Lee MM: New synthetic cast: what nurses need to know, *Orthop Nurs* 1:13, 1982.

53. Lane PL, Lee MN: Special care for special casts, *Nurs 83* 1:50, 1983.

54. McHugh NG et al: Preparatory information: what help and why, *Am J Nurs* 82(5):780, 1982.

55. Miller MC: Nursing care of the patient with external fixation therapy, *Orthop Nurs* 2:11, 1983.

56. Neal M et al: *Nursing care planning guides,* ed 2, Monterey, Calif, 1981, Wadsworth Nurseco, Inc.

57. Nutt RL: Pelvic traction in bed and Buck's traction, *Clin Manage* 3(4):18, 1983.

58. Robinson J, Mary L: A nail-safe method, *Am J Nurs* 85(2):158, 1985.

59. Schoen DCH: *The nursing process in orthopedics,* Norwalk, Conn, 1986, Appleton-Century-Crofts.

60. Seligson D, Pope M: *Concepts in external fixation,* New York, 1982, Grune & Stratton, Inc.

61. Shestack R: *Handbook of physical therapy,* ed 3, New York, 1977, Springer Publishing Co, Inc.

62. *The Zimmer Casting Techniques Handbook,* Charlotte, NC, 1985, Zimmer, Inc.

63. Wassel AC: Sports medicine: acute overuse injuries, *Orthop Nurs* 3(2):29, 1984.

64. Wise LB: A comparison of orthopedic casts: breaking the mold, *Matern Child Nurs J* 11:174, 1986.

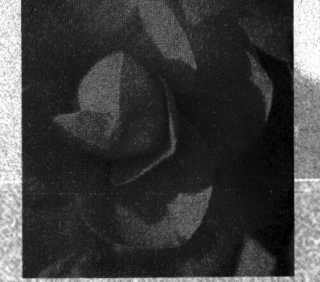

CHAPTER FIFTY-EIGHT

Nursing Management of Adults with Degenerative, Inflammatory, or Autoimmune Musculoskeletal Disorders

LEARNING OBJECTIVES

1 Identify the two classifications of arthritis, giving examples of each type.
2 Identify the effects of at least four major medication groups used to treat arthritis.
3 List five factors contributing to the development of osteoporosis.
4 State the pathophysiology of arthritis, gout, osteoporosis, osteomalacia, osteitis deformans, and muscular dystrophy.
5 State at least two nursing interventions for chronic musculoskeletal disorders in regard to home care management.
6 Identify at least three musculoskeletal disorders significantly affecting the morbidity of the aged adult.
7 Formulate a nursing care plan for patients with arthritis, gout, osteoporosis, osteomalacia, osteitis deformans, and muscular dystrophy.
8 Formulate a nursing care plan for an arthritic patient with a total hip replacement.
9 Apply knowledge of pathophysiology to the nursing care of a patient with osteomyelitis.
10 Identify appropriate nursing care for the patient with low back pain.
11 Outline nursing care for the patient with hallux valgus.

KEY TERMS

MUSCULOSKELETAL DISORDERS are seen often in nursing practice, since they affect persons throughout the life span. These disorders include the arthritic, infectious, periarticular, and metabolic bone diseases. Musculoskeletal disorders may occur during adolescence and early adulthood; however, joint disease more often occurs in men and women over 40 years old and becomes more common with increasing age. Musculoskeletal problems are often chronic, requiring medications, treatments, and surgery to correct or minimize disabilities. Because of the chronicity, the biopsychosocial status of the patient may be affected. It is estimated that 16 million people have a crippling disease that they call "arthritis" and that is severe enough to interfere with their activities of daily living. Arthritis and the rheumatic diseases in general constitute the major cause of disability in the United States.[1]

Arthritis

Arthritis encompasses various diseases involving inflammation and/or degeneration of joints or surrounding structures.[25] More than 100 types of arthritis affect more than 36 million people in the United States.[6]

The cause of arthritis is unknown. Arthritis is often classified in two major categories: noninflammatory and inflammatory (Table 58-1).

The major noninflammatory type of arthritis is osteoarthritis, also known as degenerative arthritis or degenerative joint disease (DJD). Inflammatory arthritis includes rheumatoid arthritis and systemic lupus erythematosus (SLE). Gout is classified as a crystal-induced disease and is the third most common type of arthritis.

OSTEOARTHRITIS
Definition

Osteoarthritis is a slowly progressive, chronic, nonsystemic, noninflammatory disease of primarily weight-bearing joints (Figure 58-1). Osteoarthritis is the most commonly occurring arthritis and may affect any weight-bearing joint.[2] It is more often seen in older adults, so it has been known as a "wear and tear" disease or a "use and abuse" disease. Although the mechanism of primary osteoarthritis is not proven, it is now believed there may be a biochemical process that causes degeneration of cartilage and subchondral bone.

Etiology/Epidemiology

Generally appearing in persons older than 35 years, this degenerative disease has a higher incidence in women over 55 years than in men of the same age group. In persons younger than 55 years there is an equal male/female ratio. There is an increased prevalence of osteoarthritis in Native Americans as opposed to other Americans.[28] Trauma or overuse of joints can lead to osteoarthritis, particularly in the younger person. A genetic defect may be involved in

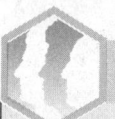

GERIATRIC CONSIDERATIONS

Risk Factors for Musculoskeletal Injury

The bones, joints, and muscles are affected by the aging process. During the aging process there is a loss of bone tissue as a result of changes in the haversian system in compact bones and in bone erosion of the trabeculae in spongy bone. These aging changes cause the bones to have decreased density and decreased strength.

Aging causes the cartilage of the joints to degenerate, which leaves the cartilage rigid, fragile, and less elastic. As a result of the aging process the cartilage becomes more susceptible to break down because of the decrease in the quality and quantity of the proteoglycans in cartilage. Osteoarthritis progresses in three stages: microfractures, bone condensation, and remodeling. With aging the muscle mass atrophies, which leaves the patient with less strength and ability to have full range of movement.

These age changes cause the patient to be more susceptible to injury (fractures, dislocations) from trauma and also susceptible to limitations from degeneration. Age changes may cause the patient to have loss of endurance and strength, limited range of motion, slowed movement, tottering gait, stiff joints, and vulnerability to injury. These changes may start as early as 35 years old and progress steadily until death.[2]

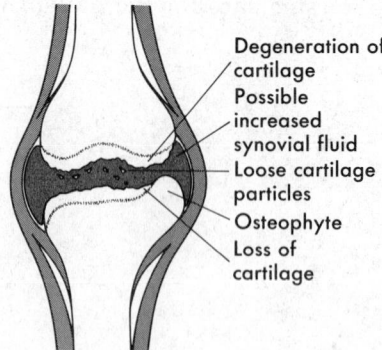

Degeneration of cartilage
Possible increased synovial fluid
Loose cartilage particles
Osteophyte
Loss of cartilage

FIGURE 58-1   Degenerative change in synovial joint.

TABLE 58-1   Characteristics of Arthritis

Diagnostic criteria	Noninflammatory arthritis	Inflammatory arthritis
Synovial membrane inflammation	Absent	Present
Signs and symptoms	Localized	Systemic
Synovial fluid	Normal	Contains blood, coagulation, and fibrin deposits

development of osteoarthritis, especially with Heberden's nodes (bony enlargement of distal interphalangeal joints). The hips and knees are especially vulnerable to osteoarthritis. In addition, the midcervical, midthoracic, and midlumbar areas of the spine are frequently affected.

Osteoarthritis can be divided into primary and secondary forms. The cause of osteoarthritis is unknown; however, aging is the important associated factor. Secondary osteoarthritis can be due to any condition that directly damages the cartilage. In addition, any condition that subjects the joint surfaces or underlying bone to chronic, excessive, or abnormal forces or causes instability in the joint may result in secondary degenerative joint disease.

Risk factors for secondary degenerative disease include trauma, repetitive physical tasks associated with occupation or athletics, joint inflammation, joint instability, neurologic disorders, and congenital or acquired skeletal deformities. In addition, stressors including poor posture and obesity are known risk factors.[6] Current evidence suggests that primary osteoarthritis may be inherited as an autosomal recessive trait.[7] Discovered in 1990, a defective gene in the joint cartilage causes it to repair itself less effectively or to become worn more easily.[6]

JOINTS AFFECTED BY OSTEOARTHRITIS

In order of frequency:
  Distal interphalangeal joint
  First metatarsophalangeal joint
  Knee
  Proximal interphalangeal joint
  Hip
  First metacarpophalangeal joint
  Lumbar spine
  Cervical spine

Pathophysiology

Breakdown of articular cartilage occurs when the enzyme hyaluronidase, a normal component of synovial fluid, attacks the cartilage. Fissuring and irregularity of articular cartilaginous surfaces occur followed by microfractures and separation of cartilage. Over time the smooth articular cartilage becomes rough and cracked. Subchondral bone forms osteophytes (spurs) at joint margins and at attachment sites for ligaments, tendons, and joint capsules. Bits of these spurs or cartilage can move into the synovial fluid, causing pain. As the articular cartilage is damaged, bone ends rub together, causing pain and swelling. Secondary synovitis may occur in late stages.

Clinical Manifestations

In contrast to rheumatoid arthritis, osteoarthritis occurs asymmetrically and usually affects only one or two joints. The osteoarthritic patient may complain of joint deformity, deep aching pain with joint movement, and limitation of mobility. The patient may also complain of transient stiffness, usually lasting less than 15 to 30 minutes, and pain that may be accentuated by use and weight bearing. Pain and immobility vary with the affected joint (see box). The clinician may also note pain and crepitus with passive joint movement. Other physical manifestations include joint enlargement and the appearance of **Heberden's nodes** (Figure 58-2), which are bony proliferations over the distal interphalangeal joint, and **Bouchard's nodes** (Figure 58-3), which are bony knobs over the proximal interphalangeal joint. Later in the disease process, muscle spasms may also occur. In addition, there may be muscle wasting and instability, and as the disease progresses, pain is present even with relief of weight bearing. The diagnosis is usually based on clinical assessment and radiology examinations. There are no diagnostic laboratory studies specific for osteoarthritis. Serum studies for erythrocyte sedimentation rate and complete blood count are usually normal. Rheumatoid factor and antinuclear antibodies are negative. Anal-

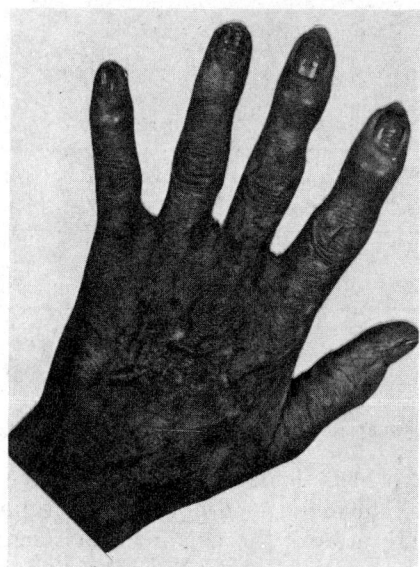

FIGURE 58-2   Osteoarthritis of hand. Note enlargement of distal joints of index, middle, and little fingers (Heberden's nodes). (From Brashear HR, Raney RB: *Handbook of orthopaedic surgery,* ed 10, St Louis, 1986, Mosby–Year Book, Inc.)

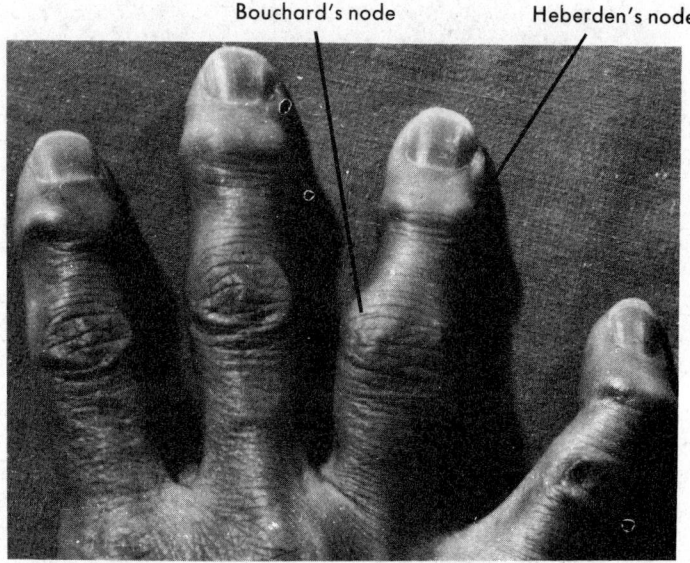

FIGURE 58-3   Bouchard's node. (From Swanson AB: *Flexible implant arthroplasty in the hand and extremities,* St Louis, 1973, Mosby–Year Book, Inc.)

ysis of synovial fluid is essentially normal. These tests are done to rule out diseases such as rheumatoid arthritis. Radiographic studies reveal narrowing of joint spaces secondary to articular cartilage destruction and bony hypertrophy, development of bone spurs and bone cysts, and joint deformity.

Therapeutic Management

Conservative medical treatment for the patient with osteoarthritis includes pain management and maintenance of joint function. Supportive care with the use of assistive devices, nutritional management, physical therapy, and maintenance of mobility and drug therapy are employed. These may be accomplished with the interventions in Table 58-2.[6]

Since osteoarthritis is chronic, it is best for patients to use narcotics only when other analgesics are not effective. The complications associated with osteoarthritis include ankylosis (fusion) of joints, deformity of one or more joints, loss of sensation, and decreased mobility. In cases where crippling occurs or gross joint limitations or continuous pain is present, surgical treatment may be the treatment of choice.

Surgical Management

Joint replacement and other orthopedic surgeries may be performed to improve joint function and alleviate pain. Although fingers, wrists, elbows, an-

kles, and shoulders may be replaced with prostheses, the hips and knees are the most frequently replaced joints. In the past, surgical procedures for osteoarthritis were a treatment for patients who had severe joint pathologic conditions. Today the trend is to use surgery in the early stages so continuous pain and deformities are avoided.

Five categories of surgical procedures may be performed to alleviate pain or correct deformities and restore function:

1. *Arthrodesis:* a surgical fusion of a joint. Most often performed on ankles or wrist, an arthrodesis renders a joint immobile (with an obvious loss of flexibility) but will decrease pain and increase strength. In patients with badly deformed and painful ankles that have become non–weight bearing, an arthrodesis may allow the patient to walk even if the ambulation is awkward and labored. Arthrodesis is also done in adjacent cervical or lumbar segments to relieve pain and increase joint stability.[26]

2. *Osteotomy:* surgical transection of a bone that is done to correct a deformity. The bone is cut and shifted into a preferred alignment. The reset bone then heals in its new position.

3. *Resection:* a surgical procedure for partial removal of degenerated bone; usually done in the wrist or forefoot. This procedure will relieve discomfort and accompanying disability.

4. *Synovectomy:* a surgical procedure to excise a synovial membrane that lines a joint. This surgery usually results in the reduction of pain and swelling. A synovectomy may be performed on the fingers, wrists, or knees to prevent erosions of the bones.

TABLE 58-2   Therapeutic Management of Osteoarthritis

Intervention	Rationale
Intermittent periods of rest	Prevents further stress on joint and delays or prevents progression
Weight reduction	Decreases joint stress
Local moist heat (hydrotherapy)	Provides pain relief and will decrease stiffness
Cold packs	Decreases muscle spasms; may provide anesthetic effect and decrease swelling
Range-of-motion and muscle-strengthening exercise (active, active-assisted, range-of-motion, isotonic, and isometric)	Maintains joint mobility, prevents joint stiffness; also, isometric exercises maintain muscle strength and tone
Analgesics and anti-inflammatory agents	Reduces pain and inflammation
Intra-articular steroids	Provides transient relief of symptoms (not a cure)
Splint and orthotic devices (braces)	Protects joint from excessive strain and used to supplement strength; decreases work load on joint
Assistive devices, (built-up eating utensils, pick-up sticks, and raised toilet seats)	Allow patients to perform activities of daily living with less assistance

RESEARCH BRIEF

Felson D et al: Weight loss reduces the risk for symptomatic knee osteoarthritis in women: the Framingham study, *Ann Intern Med* 116(7):535-539, 1992.

Obesity has been well established as a risk factor for knee osteoarthritis; however, the effect of weight loss on prevention of the disease is unknown. This study investigated the effect of two different aspects of weight: historical weight and more recent change in weight. Sixty-four women who had current symptomatic osteoarthritis were involved in the study. The results suggest that weight change in women occurring in middle or later years affects the risk for subsequent symptomatic knee osteoarthritis. Therefore habitually overweight women can substantially lower their risk for symptomatic osteoarthritis by losing weight. This study found that for those women with a high risk for osteoarthritis caused by elevated baseline body mass index, weight loss also decreased the risk for symptomatic knee osteoarthritis. The findings support an overall conclusion that weight loss reduces the risk for symptomatic knee osteoarthritis in women.

cause of increased gravitational stresses on joints is also considered. The psychologic and sociologic issues to be assessed are body image, vocational and recreational handicaps, sexual adjustment, and family and social roles. Many patients have multijoint involvement and may have constant pain that contributes to depression and fatigue. Family members may also be affected by the patient's attitude.

Nursing Diagnosis

The severity of the osteoarthritis will determine the applicable nursing diagnoses. Nursing diagnoses may include the following:
   Chronic pain related to joint degeneration
   Impaired physical mobility related to restricted joint mobility
   Body image disturbance related to visible body changes
   Knowledge deficit of disease process and treatment regimen

Planning

Goals for patient care are related to age and severity of the osteoarthritis. Expected patient outcomes include the following:
   Pain is managed

5. *Replacement arthroplasty:* a surgical procedure to replace the joint, especially involving the hip, knee, shoulder, elbow, wrist, finger, and ankle. These joint replacements relieve pain, restore motion, or maintain motion.[26]

NURSING MANAGEMENT OF THE PATIENT WITH OSTEOARTHRITIS

Assessment

Nursing assessment of the patient with osteoarthritis addresses the degree of joint involvement. Pain, stiffness, tenderness, symmetry, deformity, nodules, crepitus, and limitation of motion are defining cues for which the nurse assesses. Weight loss attributable to anorexia as a result of pain or obesity as a

Joint range of motion and ambulation are improved

Self-concept is improved

Disease process and treatment regimen can be explained

Implementation

Because osteoarthritis is known as a use and abuse disease, it does affect younger-aged adults as a result of certain types of employment or recreational activities. Nursing care reflects the needs of the patient while considering the unavailability of a cure and the chronicity of the disease. Nursing interventions to decrease joint pain include balancing patient activities with rest. Moist heat applications to the affected joint result in increased comfort. The nurse encourages diversionary activities and promotes the use of imagery and relaxation techniques. Because osteoarthritis is a disease that affects weight-bearing joints, patients are encouraged to maintain ideal body weight. Because many weight-bearing exercises are prohibited, patients tend to gain weight. Many patients eat to distract themselves from their pain. Transcutaneous electrical nerve stimulation (TENS) may also be used to decrease joint pain. A TENS unit is believed to operate on the gate control theory in which stimulation, in this case electrical, of large-diameter nerve fibers closes the gate and inhibits transmission of pain impulses (see Chapter 14). Patients with osteoarthritis often suffer impaired physical mobility. Because of this altered mobility, nursing interventions and the use of assistive devices for joint protection are aimed at the maintenance or improvement of joint mobility (Table 58-3).

TABLE 58-3　Nursing Intervention Summary: Osteoarthritis

Intervention	Rationale	Intervention	Rationale
Heat, moist compresses, whirlpool baths, and ultrasound	Vasodilation	Diversionary activities: humor, exercise, relaxation techniques, imagery, and transcutaneous electric nerve stimulation (TENS)	Gate control theory of pain
	Decreases muscle spasms		
	Decreases edema		Produce endogenous opiates with analgesic potency comparable to morphine
	Decreases joint stiffness		
	Analgesic effect		
	Increases range of motion		
		Alternating rest and activity	Fatigue exacerbates joint pain
Cold packs	Anesthetic effect	Assistive devices	Promote optimal use of restricted joint mobility
	Decreases muscle spasms		
Joint restriction/ immobilization	Decreases weight bearing and gravitational stresses on joints		Decrease weight bearing of joint
Exercises	Range of motion: maintains joint mobility and prevents joint stiffness		Increase self-care ability and esteem
	Quadriceps: increases joint mobility and muscle tone	Body weight within ideal weight range	Decreases weight bearing of joint
	Isotonic: increases joint mobility and muscle tone	Good posture and body mechanics	Promote optimal weight bearing of joints
	Isometric: maintains muscle strength	Verbalization/ventilation	Suppression may hinder optimal physiologic and psychologic functioning
	Recreational: increases muscular endurance	Patient teaching regarding disease process, treatment measures, and plans for follow-up	Knowledge increases self-esteem, patient compliance, and participation

Enlarged joints, pain, and impaired mobility result in an altered body image. The patient and significant others are encouraged to verbalize their fears and concerns about the effects of the disease. Participation in arthritis support groups may have a cathartic effect. Continued engagement in self-care and social and vocational activities is promoted as the disease permits. These activities increase self-esteem.

Patients with osteoarthritis have an established life-style regarding diet, exercise, and social and vocational responsibilities that needs to be considered when planning care. Patient and family education includes use of hot and cold compresses and the importance of optimal nutrition for weight control and maintenance. Although patients are encouraged to remain active, they are instructed to balance their activities with rest. Both written and verbal instructions regarding isometric and isotonic muscle-strengthening exercises are given (see Chapter 57). The nature and chronicity of osteoarthritis are reviewed with the patient, using teaching materials from the Arthritis Foundation. Since successful treatment depends on a specific pharmacologic regimen tailored to the patient, education about the medication's action, dosage, and common side effects is necessary (Table 58-4).

Evaluation

To evaluate the effectiveness of the interventions, the nurse assesses the patient's ability to carry out usual social and vocational roles. Joint range of motion and the ability to ambulate in comparison to previous abilities are evaluated, as well as the patient and family's adjustment and compliance to the treatment regimen.

Documentation

Joint assessment, ambulation, and the patient's subjective complaints regarding pain and joint immobility are documented. The family and patient's responses to the illness and the patient education are also recorded.

Ongoing Care

Since osteoarthritis is a chronic health problem, the patient will require ongoing care, primarily in the home setting. Nurses may coordinate the varied health professionals, including physical and occupational therapists. Arthritic medications and assistive devices are expensive. The limited financial resources of the older patient may be strained, and social services may also be needed. Medications and patient teaching will vary as the joint involvement

intensifies. Periodic nursing assessments are necessary.

RHEUMATOID ARTHRITIS
Definition

Rheumatoid arthritis is a chronic, systemic, progressive inflammatory disease of connective tissue. It is characterized by symmetric inflammation of the lining of the synovial joints (synovitis) with resulting destruction of joints. Although it most commonly involves peripheral joints, it may attack connective tissues throughout the body, including the eyes, lungs, and blood vessels.

Etiology/Epidemiology

Rheumatoid arthritis affects approximately 6.5 million people in the United States.[27] Rheumatoid arthritis is a progressive polyarticular inflammatory arthritis characterized by exacerbations and remissions. It is two to three times more prevalent in women, and the disease manifests itself between the ages of 25 and 55 years.[3] A chronic systemic disease, rheumatoid arthritis results in significant morbidity and chronic disability for women of childbearing age, individuals during their productive work years, and older adults. Although the cause of rheumatoid arthritis is unknown, two etiologies currently being investigated are autoimmune defects and infectious agents,[28] particularly in genetically susceptible individuals.

Pathophysiology

Initially, the joints' synovial lining becomes inflamed, and synovitis occurs secondary to an unknown interval agent. The inflammation process results in increased synovium with pannus (inflammation granulation tissue) formation. Over time pannus destroys cartilage and invades the joint capsule. Later pannus replaced by fibrous connective tissue affects tendons and ligaments, causing joint subluxation (partial dislocation), bony ankylosis (fusion of joints), and consolidation of joints.

Clinical Manifestations

Initially nonspecific complaints of muscle aches, fatigue, anorexia, and weight loss may precede joint inflammation. Clinical manifestations of rheumatoid arthritis are joint pain, warmth, edema, and limitation of motion. Morning stiffness lasting longer than 30 minutes in multiple joints is a positive indicator.[28] An insidious disease, rheumatoid arthritis frequently affects symmetric joints. The most commonly affected areas are the small joints of the hands and wrists (the proximal interphalangeal and

TABLE 58-4   Pharmacology Summary: Agents for Musculoskeletal Disorders

Drugs	Disorders	Dosage	Side effects	Nursing implications
SALICYLATE (ASPIRIN)	Rheumatoid arthritis Osteoarthritis Osteoporosis Osteitis deformans Osteomalacia Bursitis Epicondylitis Low back pain	3.2-6 g/day in divided doses	Gastrointestinal irritation including nausea, vomiting, and abdominal pain Mild liver enzyme elevation Tinnitus (frequent and reversible) Mild salicylism (tinnitus, dizziness, difficulty hearing, vomiting or diarrhea, mental confusion, headache, sweating, hyperventilation)	Therapeutic serum level 150-300 μg/mL before morning dose (after 2-3 weeks of therapy) Take with food or milk or use enteric-coated preparations Monitor for signs of bleeding (bruising) or melena (black stools) Large doses may potentiate peptic ulcer Monitor liver function
NONSTEROIDAL ANTI-INFLAMMATORY DRUGS (NSAIDs)	Rheumatoid arthritis Osteoarthritis Gout Bursitis Epicondylitis Osteitis deformans Osteomalacia Osteoporosis Low back pain	See specific drug	See specific drug	General considerations NSAIDs must be administered for 2 weeks to evaluate efficacy Administer with food, milk, or antacids to decrease gastrointestinal irritation Compliance may be enhanced with once or twice daily dosages Monitor renal and hepatic function Monitor dosage and enhanced side effects in elderly persons Not recommended during pregnancy NSAIDs may mask infections
Diclofenac (Voltaren)	Rheumatoid arthritis Osteoarthritis	150-200 mg/day in divided doses for rheumatoid arthritis 100-150 mg/day in divided doses for osteoarthritis	Gastrointestinal irritation Headache Dizziness	See General considerations

Drug	Uses	Dosage	Side effects	General considerations
Etodolac (Lodine)	Osteoarthritis; Tissue inflammation associated with fractures	600-1200 mg/day in divided doses	Gastrointestinal irritation, particularly dyspepsia	See General considerations
Fenoprofen calcium (Fenoprofen, Nalfon)	Rheumatoid arthritis; Osteoarthritis	300-600 mg three or four times daily	Gastrointestinal irritation; Headache; Genitourinary problems: dysuria, cystitis, hematuria, nephrotic syndrome; Somnolence/drowsiness	Contraindicated with renal disease; Improvement may be noted in a few days but may require 2-3 weeks
Flurbiprofen (Ansaid)	Rheumatoid arthritis; Osteoarthritis	200-300 mg daily in three or four divided doses	Gastrointestinal irritation; Dizziness; Headache	See General considerations
Ibuprofen (Motrin, Advil, Nuprin)	Rheumatoid arthritis; Osteoarthritis; Osteoporosis; Osteitis deformans; Osteomalacia; Epicondylitis	1200-3200 mg/day in three or four divided doses; not to exceed 3200 mg	Gastrointestinal irritation; Hypersensitivity reaction; Rash/dermatitis	Therapeutic responses in a few days to 2 weeks
Indomethacin (Indocin)	Rheumatoid arthritis; Osteoarthritis; Osteoporosis; Bursitis; Gout; Osteitis deformans; Osteomalacia; Epicondylitis	25-50 mg three times daily, not to exceed 200 mg/day, for rheumatoid arthritis and osteoarthritis; 75-150 mg/day in divided doses for bursitis; 50 mg three times daily for gout	Gastrointestinal irritation: Feeling of dissociation (especially in elderly patients); Severe headaches	Contraindicated with active gastric lesions; Use with caution in individuals with depressive disorders, epilepsy, and parkinsonism; Administer with food, milk, or antacids; Adverse effects correlate with dosage, and women may have increased intensity of side effects
Ketoprofen (Orudis)	Rheumatoid arthritis; Osteoarthritis	150-300 mg/day, in divided doses, not to exceed 300 mg/day	Gastrointestinal irritation, particularly dyspepsia; Headache	See General considerations
Meclofenamate (Meclomen)	Rheumatoid arthritis; Osteoarthritis	200-400 mg/day, in three or four divided doses, not to exceed 400 mg/day	Gastrointestinal irritation, particularly dyspepsia; Headache; Rash/dermatitis; Drowsiness/somnolence	Contraindicated in patients with renal disease or active ulceration or inflammation of upper or lower gastrointestinal tract; May administer with food or milk; Improvement in a few days with optimal effects in 2-3 weeks

Continued.

TABLE 58-4 Pharmacology Summary: Agents for Musculoskeletal Disorders—cont'd

Drugs	Disorders	Dosage	Side effects	Nursing implications
Nabumetone (Relafen)	Rheumatoid arthritis Osteoarthritis	1000-2000 mg/day	Gastrointestinal irritation, particularly diarrhea, dyspepsia, and distress/cramps/pain Drowsiness/somnolence	See General considerations
Naproxen (Naprosyn, Anaprox)	Rheumatoid arthritis Osteoarthritis Bursitis Gout Epicondylitis	250-500 mg twice daily for rheumatoid arthritis and osteoarthritis 750 mg initially, then 250 mg three times daily for gout	Gastrointestinal irritation Headache Tinnitus Pulmonary infiltrates Drowsiness/somnolence	Therapeutic effect generally within 2 weeks Monitor hepatic and renal studies
Piroxicam (Feldene)	Rheumatoid arthritis Osteoarthritis Gout Bursitis	20 mg/day	Gastrointestinal irritation Allergic reaction	Assess therapeutic effects at 2 weeks
Sulindac (Clinoril)	Rheumatoid arthritis Osteoarthritis Gout Bursitis Epicondylitis	150-200 mg twice daily, not to exceed 400 mg	Gastrointestinal irritation Rash/dermatitis Hypersensitivity	Do not administer with active gastrointestinal lesions Administer with food Therapeutic response in approximately 1 week for 50% of patients
Tolmetin sodium (Tolectin)	Rheumatoid arthritis Osteoarthritis	300-1800 mg/day in divided doses	Gastrointestinal irritation Tinnitus Headache Anaphylactoid reaction	Take on arising and at bedtime Take with antacids other than sodium bicarbonate; bioavailability affected by milk and food
PYRAZOLINE DERIVATIVES Phenylbutazone (Azolid, Butazolidin)	Rheumatoid arthritis Osteoarthritis Gout Epicondylitis Bursitis'	Initial dose 300-600 mg/day in divided doses; maintenance dose not to exceed 400 mg/day Rheumatoid arthritis and osteoarthritis: 400 mg followed by 100 mg every 4 hours	Gastrointestinal irritation, particularly abdominal discomfort and distress Fluid retention Bone marrow depression Agranulocytosis and aplastic anemia Drowsiness	Trial period of 1 week recommended Use with caution in adults older than 40 years Use only after NSAIDs have proven unsatisfactory Monitor hematologic values Take with food or milk

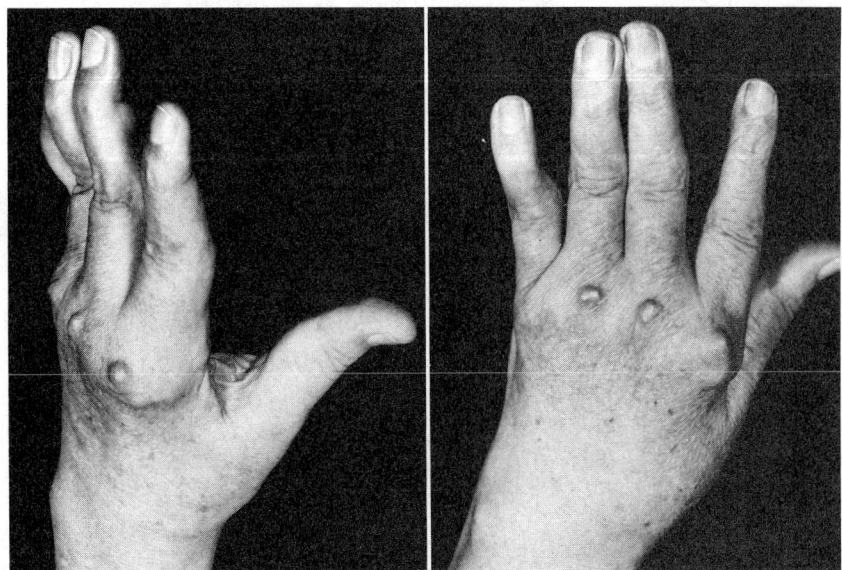

FIGURE 58-4   Swan-neck deformity. (From Brashear HR, Raney RB: *Handbook of orthopaedic surgery,* ed 10, St Louis, 1986, Mosby–Year Book, Inc.)

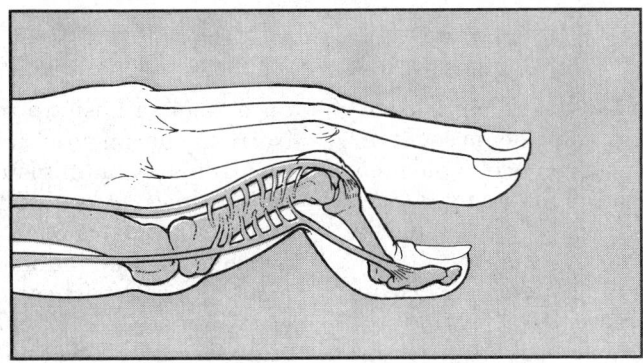

FIGURE 58-5   Boutonnière deformity.

metacarpophalangeal joints) and the feet (the metatarsophalangeal joints). Less commonly, the knee, shoulder, hip, ankle, cervical spine, and jaw may be affected.[28] Firm, nontender subcutaneous nodules occur over bony prominences in approximately 25% of rheumatoid arthritis patients during the later stages of the disease. These nodules, collections of fibroblasts in collagen tissue, include olecranon nodules and cervical nodules. Deformities of the hand include swan-neck deformity (Figure 58-4), or hyperextension of the proximal interphalangeal joints; **boutonnière deformity** (Figure 58-5), or a flexion deformity of the proximal interphalangeal joints; and ulnar drift, in which the fingers drift toward the ulna (Figure 58-6). These deformities result in impaired ability to use the hand in fine or gross motor

activities. Other extra-articular manifestations include synovial cysts, episcleritis (inflammation of the loose connective tissue between the sclera and the conjunctiva), pericarditis, and pulmonary fibrosis.[28] As the disease progresses, patients may have malaise, anorexia, and weight loss secondary to chronic pain and a low-grade fever with inflammation.

A single definitive test for rheumatoid arthritis is not available. Laboratory data generally reveal an elevated erythrocyte sedimentation rate of up to 15 mm/hr in males and 25 mm/hr in females and normochromic or hypochromic anemia.[3] A positive rheumatoid factor, defined as a reactive immunoglobulin M (IgM) molecule (titers greater than 1:80), is present in approximately 80% of the patients.[29] Also, immunoglobulin IgG (normal value of 700 to

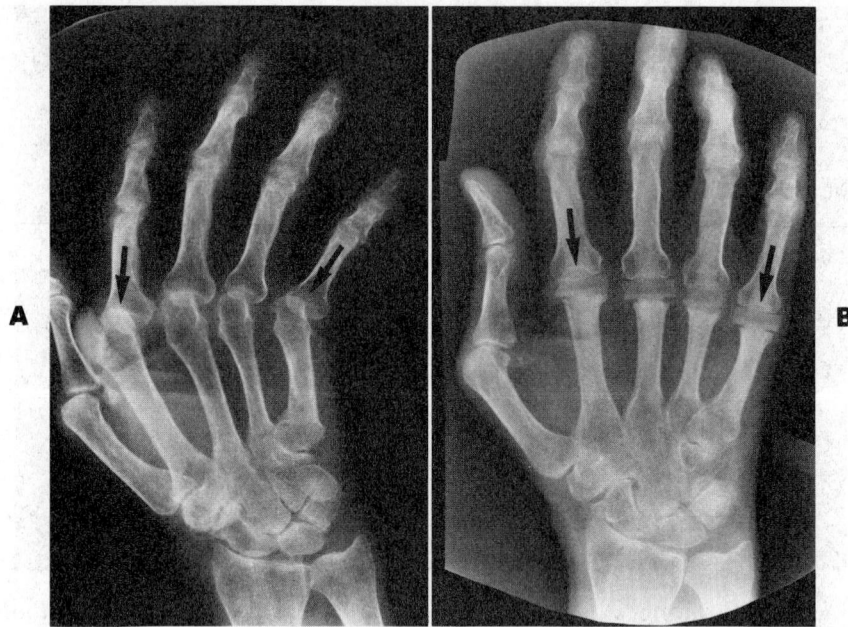

FIGURE 58-6   **A,** Ulnar drift. **B,** Corrected ulnar drift with joint replacement. (From Brashear HR, Raney RB: *Handbook of orthopaedic surgery,* ed 10, St Louis, 1986, Mosby–Year Book, Inc.)

1500 mg/dL) may be elevated with rheumatoid arthritis. Antinuclear antibodies may be present in 60% of patients. Pannus formations are confirmed with synovial biopsy. Synovial fluid analysis frequently reveals inflammatory effusion. Radiologic findings vary, depending on the disease state. Early x-rays indicate soft tissue swelling and osteoporosis, whereas later in the disease process, x-ray findings include joint space narrowing, cartilage destruction, subluxation, deformities, and ankylosis.

Therapeutic Management

Therapeutic management of rheumatoid arthritis strives to provide pain relief, minimize joint destruction, and promote joint function. Treatment to achieve these goals includes warm and cold applications, weight control, and balance between joint use and joint restriction. This limitation may be accomplished with bracing and the use of assistive devices (Figure 58-7). Also, pharmacologic therapy is an important adjunct to the treatment of rheumatoid arthritis (see Table 58-4). Last, surgery may be performed if the above measures do not control the pain or if progressive joint destruction occurs.

Pharmacologic treatment usually begins with salicylate, frequently high doses (8 to 10 tablets daily). Long-term use of these medications may result in gastrointestinal irritation, elevated liver enzymes, and tinnitus. Salicylate serum levels are monitored

on a regular basis to maintain an optimal dosage. Normal therapeutic levels range from 10 to 20 mg/dL before administration of the morning medication dose. Other nonsteroidal anti-inflammatory drugs (NSAIDs) used in the treatment of rheumatoid arthritis include indomethacin, ibuprofen, sulindac, and ketoprofen. These drugs, which may also cause gastrointestinal irritation and fluid retention, are administered for 2 weeks before evaluating the drug's effectiveness.

If the patient's discomfort is not controlled with the NSAIDs, exogenous adrenocorticosteroids may be administered via oral, intramuscular, or intra-articular routes. Pain relief is in direct proportion to drug dose. Common side effects of corticosteroids include Cushing's syndrome, hypertension, gastrointestinal irritation, and impaired immune response.

Antimalarial drugs may also be used for the treatment of rheumatoid arthritis. Hydroxychloroquine is the most commonly used of these drugs. Along with gastrointestinal distress, retinopathy and abnormal extraocular muscle movements are commonly encountered side effects of this therapy. Gold compounds, administered intramuscularly and orally, usually result in a 70% improvement in symptoms. Common side effects of these drugs include stomatitis, pruritus, and skin rashes. Patients receiving gold compounds must be monitored with frequent laboratory tests, including complete blood counts, liver panels, and renal function tests. Penicillamine,

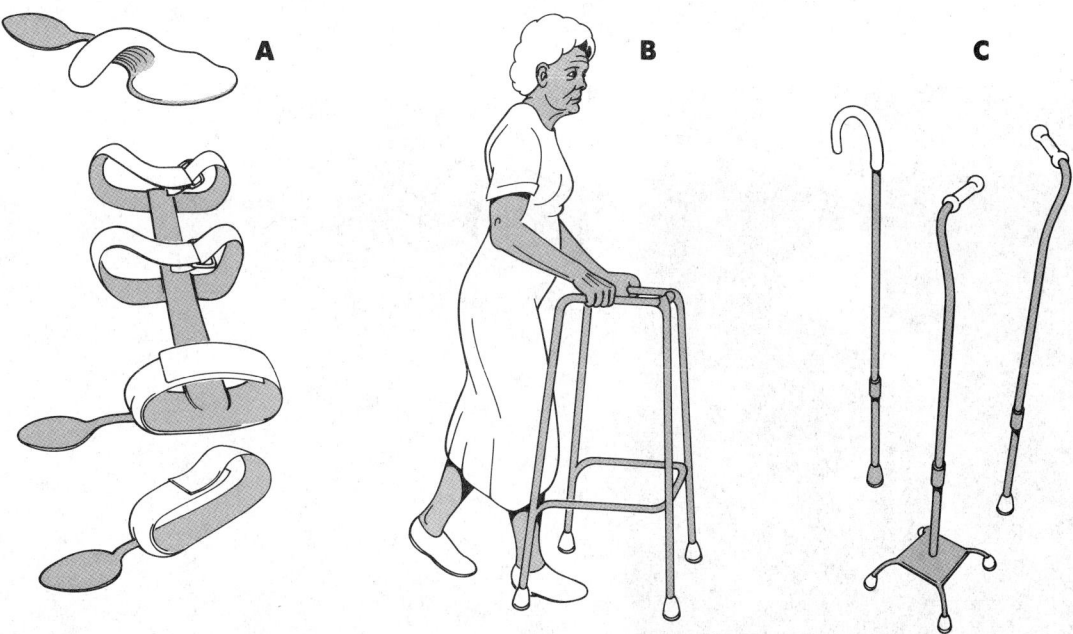

FIGURE 58-7 Assistive devices. **A,** Eating utensils. **B,** Walker. **C,** Single- and quad-foot canes.

a more toxic drug, may be prescribed if pain control has not been established with medications already discussed. Side effects of this drug are gastrointestinal irritation and loss of taste. Finally, the cytotoxic drugs methotrexate, cyclophosphamide, or azathioprine may be used to control the pain and inflammation of rheumatoid arthritis. Side effects of the cytotoxic drugs include cirrhosis and hepatitis. Leukopenia and thrombocytopenia may occur with methotrexate and azathioprine.

Surgical Management

Even with the numerous medications available for arthritis, joint impairment may occur. Joint deformity and degeneration result in impaired physical mobility and chronic pain. Surgical treatment options include synovectomy, arthrodesis, osteotomy, and implant arthroplasty (Table 58-5).

Because of the availability of broad-spectrum antibiotics and the use of antibiotic solutions for irrigation, joint replacements are more frequently performed than previously. Total hip replacement is the most common orthopedic operation performed on older persons and is done over 200,000 times per year as the major surgical treatment for osteoarthritis. Although the hip and knee are the most common and most successful joints replaced, the shoulder, elbow, wrist, finger, and ankle joints may be replaced (Figure 58-8).

Total joint replacement is considered only when

more conservative pharmacologic measures have failed to control pain, joint degeneration, and disability in patients with either rheumatoid arthritis or osteoarthritis. With joint replacement, preoperative instructions are paramount. These instructions include the activity and the limitations that are required postoperatively. Activity may be accomplished with use of a continuous passive motion machine (therapy device; see Chapter 57 for illustra-

TABLE 58-5 Surgical Options for Rheumatoid Arthritis

Procedure	Purpose
Synovectomy: removal of inflamed synovial lining	Relieves pain and increases joint stability and mobility[28]
Arthrodesis: fusion of joint	Decreases joint instability and joint pain[11]
Osteotomy: removal of bone, thus changing weight-bearing surfaces	Relieves pain and increases joint stability[28]
Implant arthroplasty: replacement of joint	Increases joint mobility and stability and decreases pain

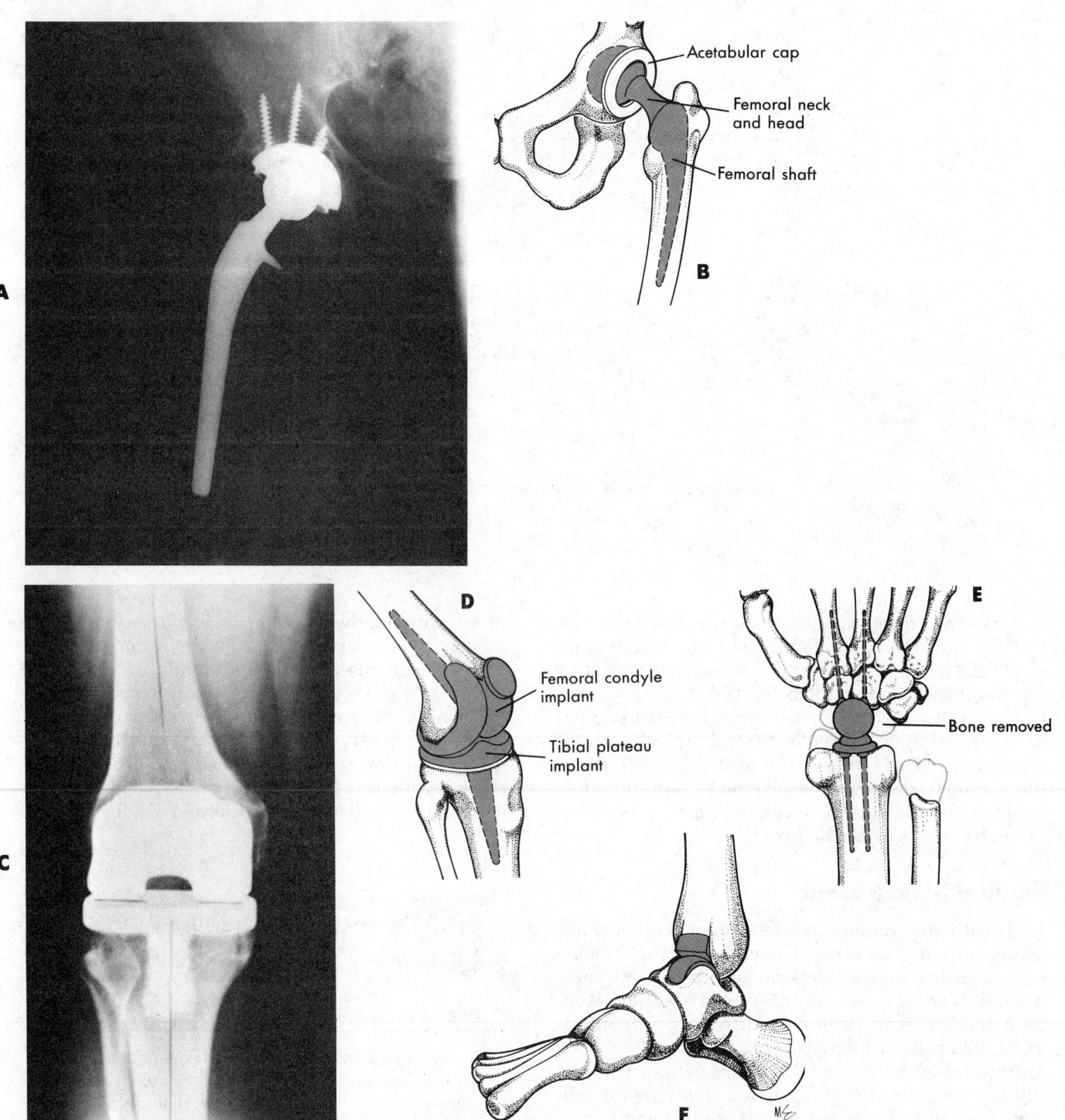

FIGURE 58-8   **A,** Total hip replacement x-ray. **B,** Total hip arthroplasty. **C,** Total knee replacement x-ray. **D,** Total knee arthroplasty. **E,** Total wrist arthroplasty. **F,** Total ankle arthroplasty. (**A** from Thibodeau G, Patton K: *Anatomy and physiology,* ed 2, St Louis, 1993, Mosby–Year Book, Inc. **C** from Brashear HR, Raney RB: *Handbook of orthopaedic surgery,* ed 10, St Louis, 1986, Mosby–Year Book, Inc.)

CONTINUOUS PASSIVE MOTION MACHINE

Keep the leg in a neutral (not internally or externally rotated) position.

Keep the knee at the hinged joint of the machine.

Maintain leg in continuous passive motion for 20 or more hours per day or per physician orders.

Monitor for pressure areas at the knee and the groin.

Follow physician or institution protocol regarding degrees of extension, flexion, and speed.

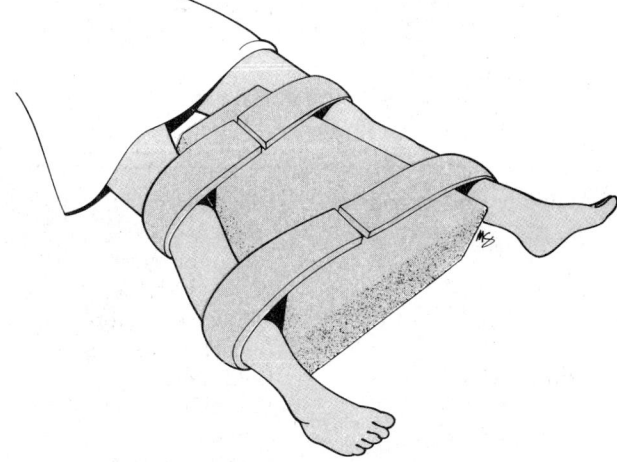

FIGURE 58-9   Abduction pillow used after total hip replacement.

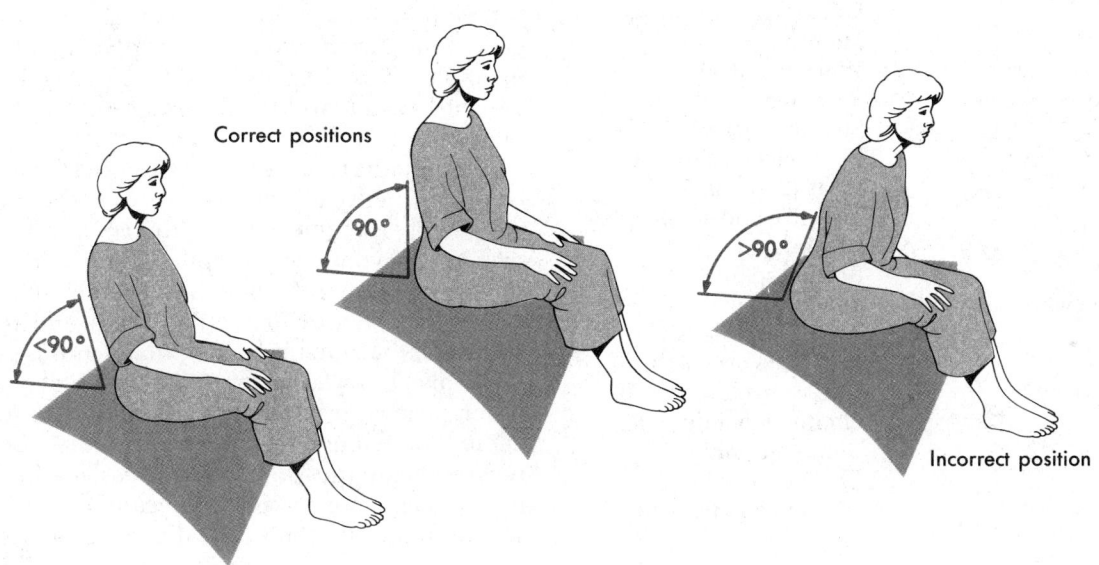

Correct positions

Incorrect position

FIGURE 58-10   Correct and incorrect hip flexion after total hip replacement.

tion). Abduction is maintained with use of an abduction pillow (Figure 58-9). Instructions include site care, dressing changes, and related suction devices. Exercises (isometric and range of motion), positioning (Figure 58-10), use of assistive devices for ambulation, pain relief measures, and general self-care measures for arthritis are taught (Table 58-6).

Patient understanding and compliance to preoperative instructions can prevent the development and progression of postoperative complications including thrombophlebitis, shock, and intense pyramiding pain. The patient needs to know the signs and symptoms of dislocations and the urgency of no-

tifying health care personnel if the symptoms of continued unrelieved pain, inability to extend the joint, and asymmetric length of the extremities occur.

An ongoing high risk exists for the development of wound infection manifested by local erythema and edema, feelings of pressure in the replaced joint site, limited joint mobility, and pain. Infection resistant to treatment may result in temporary or permanent endoprosthesis removal.[11] Therefore prophylactic antibiotics are administered preoperatively and for 5 to 7 days postoperatively.

Hip joint arthroplasty may be accomplished via an incision approximately 8 to 12 inches on the lateral

TABLE 58-6   Self-Care Measures for Arthritis

Area	Self-care measures
Activities and exercise	Balance of rest and activities
	Range-of-motion exercises
	Quadriceps exercises
	Recreational exercise
Pain control	Cold packs
	Warm, moist compresses
	Whirlpool baths and/or ultrasound
	Position changes
	TENS units
	Exercise
	Humor
	Relaxation techniques
	Medication
	Weight control
Home care	Firm bed
	Straight-backed chair
	Elevated chair/toilet seat (3 to 4 inches)
	Assistive and self-help devices
	Resting splints
Psychosocial needs	Role changes
	Vocational needs
	Insurance practices
Sexual issues	Pain control
	Limited mobility
	Joint deformities
	Changes in self-esteem and body image
	Fatigue
Medication	Purpose
	Dosage
	Side effects

or anterolateral thigh. Posterior incisions are used to preserve the muscle, but patients with posterior incisions are more likely to experience hip dislocations. The two basic types of joint protheses are the cemented and porous bone implants. Polymethylmethacrylate is used to cement the joint in place. With the cemented joint a shortened period of immobility is required (approximately 5 days). In contrast, the porous bone implant is press fitted and the patient's healthy bone will "grow" into the endoprosthesis if the blood supply is adequate and healthy bone is present. An endoprosthesis involves an extended period of immobility or assisted mobility with the use of crutches, walkers, or a cane for up to 3 months.

The postoperative course depends on the type of joint prosthesis used and the health status of the patient. Most often, candidates for joint replacements are elderly; thus joint replacement surgery is considered a low-risk, high-benefit operation. The joint replacement will alleviate severe constant pain related to arthritis that is experienced on sitting or walking. In addition, the surgery provides increased mobility that will assist the patient to remain independent.[30]

Following surgery, numerous aspects previously addressed preoperatively are reiterated, including hip abduction, pain management, and prescribed exercise. In addition, follow-up health coordination facilitates the patient's return to a productive lifestyle and minimal pain.

If no complications develop, the patient is able to return to an active life-style within 6 months of surgery. The patient with a hip replacement is a good example of a diagnosis that requires initially no weight bearing and finally progresses to full weight bearing.

When joint replacements were first available and cement (methylmethacrylate) was the method of stabilizing the joint, total hip replacements were avoided in younger patients. Those with an active life-style frequently had a loosening of the joint within 10 years of the replacement and required a second replacement. In fact, many adults were told, "You are too young for a joint replacement." No other surgical treatment was available until they became old enough for a replacement. Because of newer techniques and cementless methods, young patients are more likely to be candidates for a prosthesis. Many patients are disabled before surgery because of joint deterioration and pain. Surgical replacement of the joint allows them to resume an active life-style.

NURSING MANAGEMENT OF THE PATIENT WITH RHEUMATOID ARTHRITIS
Assessment

Nursing assessment includes evaluation of joint inflammation. Inflammation is indicated by limitation of motion, pain, edema, warmth, and erythema. The systemic symptoms of fever, malaise, weight loss, and subcutaneous nodules are noted. In addition, the patient is assessed for recent episodes of stress-related incidents. Rheumatoid arthritis may be induced or exacerbated by stressful events. Some patients report that the symptoms first appear following a time of emotional distress. However, it is not generally thought that this could cause rheumatoid arthritis but rather that it may trigger it. On relief of the stress, patients frequently report a parallel relief of the rheumatoid arthritis symptoms. The nurse also assesses for the effects of rheumatoid arthritis on the patient, including changes in employment ability, recreational limitations, family roles, and alterations in body image.

Nursing Diagnosis

Because rheumatoid arthritis is a multisystem disease, numerous nursing diagnoses are applicable, including the following:

Chronic pain related to joint inflammation

Sleep pattern disturbance related to pain

Activity intolerance related to pain, fatigue, and impaired joint mobility

Self-care deficit related to fatigue and decreased joint mobility

Body image disturbance related to visible joint deformity

Knowledge deficit regarding condition and treatment

Altered health maintenance related to limited joint mobility

Planning

Planning for patient care will depend on the intensity of symptoms and degree of impaired joint mobility. Expected patient outcomes include the following:

Achievement of optimal management of pain

Attainment of and maintenance of optimal sleep pattern

Attainment of highest level of mobility possible within physical restrictions

Engagement in self-care activities and activities of daily living

Maintenance of adequate psychosocial functioning with effective coping mechanisms

Explanation of the disease process, applicability of treatment measures to the patient's condition, and plans for follow-up

Maintenance of optimal level of independence within limits of joint mobility

Implementation

Nursing interventions address pain control and maintenance of joint mobility (Table 58-4). Prescribed pain medications are administered as ordered and the patient observed for side effects. The application of cold packs and warm, moist compresses to inflamed joints approximately 30 minutes before activities decreases joint pain and increases joint mobility. Whirlpool baths or ultrasound and frequent position changes prevent muscle spasms

and contractures and minimize joint stress. Diversionary activities, the use of imagery and relaxation techniques, humor, exercise, and transcutaneous electric nerve stimulation (TENS) relate to the gate control theory of pain. The biostimulation therapy of large fibers blocks the perception of painful stimuli. Transcutaneous electric nerve stimulators send mild electrical impulses to specified areas under the patient's skin and tissue. Diversionary activities produce endogenous opioids that affect the central nervous system with an analgesic potency comparable to morphine. Resting splints and bed rest up to 10 hours each day will decrease weight bearing and gravitational stresses of joints, thereby minimizing pain.

Range-of-motion, quadriceps, isometric, isotonic, and recreational exercises will preserve joint function, prevent stiffness, strengthen key muscle groups, and enhance muscular endurance. A balance of rest and activity will prevent joint fatigue. Good posture and the use of a straight-backed chair with an elevated chair seat of 3 to 4 inches promote optimal weight bearing of joints.

Disturbances in sleep, resulting from chronic pain, may be addressed by administration of pain medications and the application of warm compresses to painful joints approximately 30 minutes before bedtime (see nursing care plan for the patient with rheumatoid arthritis). Other factors promoting sleep include the provision of a quiet environment and a clean, firm, comfortable bed. Strenuous exercises or activity before sleep are discouraged.

Pain, fatigue, and impaired joint mobility also result in activity intolerance. The balance of rest and activities and alternating rest periods in the morning and evening conserve energy and protect impaired joints. The application of moist heat to decrease muscle spasms and pain will also promote activity. During disease exacerbations, activities may have to be limited to prevent joint damage.

Since joint deformities result in physical limitations and an altered body image, it is helpful to encourage verbalization of the impact of this disease on the family. The changes in social and vocational roles experienced by the patient and family are also discussed. To decrease physiologic and psychologic dependence and increase self-esteem, nurses can

PATIENT EDUCATION GUIDE
Quadriceps Exercise

Press down on the bed with the back of your knee
Pull your toes toward the head of the bed
Tighten your thigh muscles

 **NURSING CARE PLAN** *Patient with Rheumatoid Arthritis*

Nursing diagnosis/ Expected outcome	Interventions	Rationale
Chronic pain related to joint inflammation • *Achieves optimal management of pain*	Administer prescribed medications as ordered, observing for side effects	NSAIDs, analgesics, gold compounds, antimalarials, corticosteroids, and chemotherapeutic agents produce pain relief through variety of specific actions to promote rest and comfort
	Administer cold packs to inflamed joints	Cold packs have anesthetic effect and decrease muscle spasm
	Administer warm, moist applications to inflamed joints	Warm moist applications have analgesic effect, relaxing muscles and decreasing joint stiffness and edema
	Encourage diversionary activities	Gate control theory of pain; activation of midbrain cells inhibits transmission of pain
	Encourage position changes	Prevents muscle spasms, decreases potential for contractures, and minimizes stress on joints
	Promote use of imagery and relaxation techniques	Gate control theory of pain; biostimulation therapy
	Administer prescribed medications or cold/heat packs approximately 30 minutes before activities	Acknowledges time of onset for pharmacologic management
	Promote use of resting splints	Support joint in neutral position, decreasing spasm and pain and providing rest
	Assist patient with whirlpool baths and/or ultrasound	Whirlpool baths and/or ultrasound have analgesic effect, relaxing muscles, decreasing joint stiffness and edema, and increasing range of motion
	Encourage bed rest up to 10 hours each day during acute stages using firm footboard	Bed rest decreases weight bearing of joints and pain Footboard decreases footdrop Stress and fatigue exacerbate symptoms
	Investigate use of TENS	Gate control theory of pain; biostimulation therapy of large fibers blocking painful stimuli
	Promote exercise, humor, and relaxation activities	Produces endogenous opioids that affect central nervous system with analgesic potency comparable to morphine
Sleep pattern disturbance related to pain • *Attains and maintains optimal sleep pattern*	Administer medications/heat applications approximately 30 minutes before bedtime	Pain relief, which promotes physical and mental relaxation
	Promote quiet environment	Establishment of sleep environment promotes physical and mental relaxation
	Discourage strenuous exercises or activity immediately before bedtime	Establishment of sleep environment promotes physical and mental relaxation

NURSING CARE PLAN   *Patient with Rheumatoid Arthritis—cont'd*

Nursing diagnosis/ *Expected outcome*	Interventions	Rationale
	Provide clean, comfortable, firm bed	Establishment of sleep environment promotes physical and mental relaxation
	Encourage use of patient teaching materials from Arthritis Foundation	Accurate information
	Discuss chronicity and remission characteristics of disease	Knowledge increases self-esteem and patient compliance and participation
Activity intolerance related to pain, fatigue, and impaired joint mobility	Promote balance of rest and activities	For energy conservation and joint protection
• *Progress to highest level of mobility possible within physical restrictions*		
	Alternate rest periods in morning and evening	For energy conservation and joint protection
	Encourage activities after moist heat application	Decreases muscle spasms and pain, joint stiffness
Self-care deficit related to feeding, bathing, dressing, and toileting	Encourage use of assistive devices	Decreases physiologic and psychologic dependence
• *Demonstrates increased ability to engage in self-care behaviors and activities of daily living*		
Body image disturbance related to joint deformity	Encourage verbalization of disease impact on family and on social and vocational roles of patient and family	Suppression of feelings may adversely affect optimal physiologic and psychologic functioning
• *Maintains adequate psychologic functioning with effective coping mechanisms*		
	Promote self-care activities	Decreases physiologic and psychologic dependence and increases self-esteem
	Explore ways of dealing with changes in roles and image	Reestablishes control, which is related to a person's role
	Promote participation in usual activities and roles as disease allows	Decreases physiologic and psychologic dependence and increases self-esteem
	Promote use of adaptive coping patterns	Use of known adaptive patterns increases self-esteem
	Encourage participation in arthritis support group	Acknowledgment of and talking with other persons with arthritis decrease dependence and increase self-esteem
Knowledge deficit regarding condition and treatment	Teach patient about 1. Medications: action, dosage, frequency, and side effects 2. Hot and cold applications 3. Use and care of splints 4. Balance of rest and activity exercises	Knowledge increases self-esteem and patient compliance and participation
• *Knowledgeable of disease process and applicability of treatment measures to current disease*		

Continued.

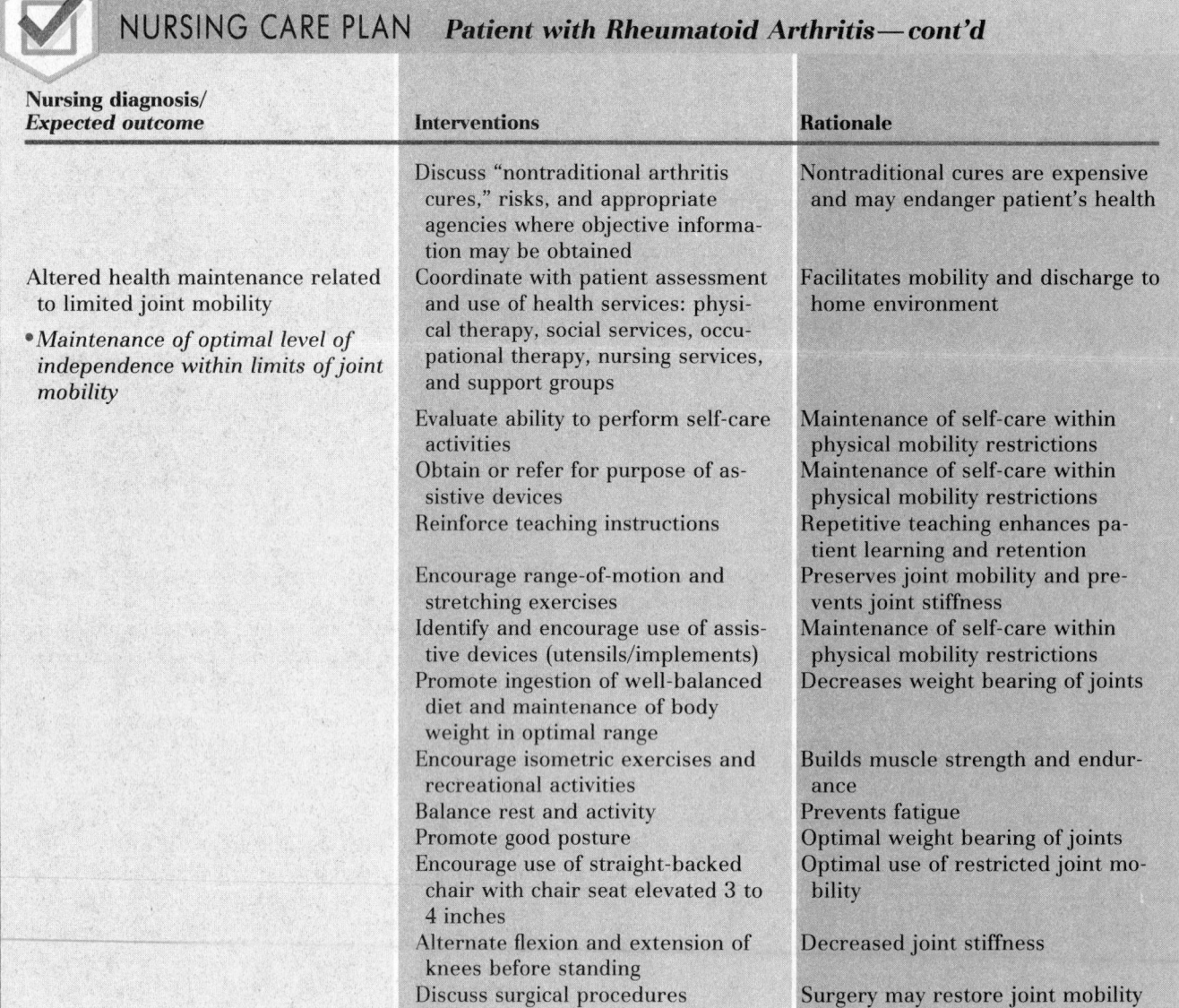

NURSING CARE PLAN *Patient with Rheumatoid Arthritis—cont'd*

Nursing diagnosis/ Expected outcome	Interventions	Rationale
	Discuss "nontraditional arthritis cures," risks, and appropriate agencies where objective information may be obtained	Nontraditional cures are expensive and may endanger patient's health
Altered health maintenance related to limited joint mobility • *Maintenance of optimal level of independence within limits of joint mobility*	Coordinate with patient assessment and use of health services: physical therapy, social services, occupational therapy, nursing services, and support groups	Facilitates mobility and discharge to home environment
	Evaluate ability to perform self-care activities	Maintenance of self-care within physical mobility restrictions
	Obtain or refer for purpose of assistive devices	Maintenance of self-care within physical mobility restrictions
	Reinforce teaching instructions	Repetitive teaching enhances patient learning and retention
	Encourage range-of-motion and stretching exercises	Preserves joint mobility and prevents joint stiffness
	Identify and encourage use of assistive devices (utensils/implements)	Maintenance of self-care within physical mobility restrictions
	Promote ingestion of well-balanced diet and maintenance of body weight in optimal range	Decreases weight bearing of joints
	Encourage isometric exercises and recreational activities	Builds muscle strength and endurance
	Balance rest and activity	Prevents fatigue
	Promote good posture	Optimal weight bearing of joints
	Encourage use of straight-backed chair with chair seat elevated 3 to 4 inches	Optimal use of restricted joint mobility
	Alternate flexion and extension of knees before standing	Decreased joint stiffness
	Discuss surgical procedures	Surgery may restore joint mobility

promote self-care activities and participation in daily activities as the disease process allows. The use of known adaptive coping patterns and participation in arthritis support groups such as those sponsored by the Arthritis Foundation can also increase self-esteem. Patient education includes medications, use of hot and cold compresses, assistive devices, use and care of splints, balancing of rest and activity, exercises, and weight control. Because of the physical changes associated with arthritis and its chronic nature, an issue that may be of concern is the effect of arthritis on sexuality. Patient education also includes discussions of nontraditional arthritis "cures" and their subsequent risks. Limited income for traditional medications places the elderly person at risk for exploitation. However, some home remedies are inexpensive and have a soothing psychologic effect. If the home remedy is harmless, health care providers need not risk alienating themselves from the patient by ridiculing the home remedy.

Evaluation/Documentation

Evaluation of the effectiveness of the nursing care includes joint mobility, pain control, and the ability of the patient to participate in activities and perform self-care skills within physical restrictions. The nurse evaluates the patient's ability to explain the disease process, applicability of treatment measures to the condition, and plans for follow-up in the health care system. The nurse documents the patient's joint mobility, the affected joints, and the impact on vocational and social roles. Patient education regarding home care, in particular the use of medications and self-care, is documented.

Ongoing Care

Home care for the patient with chronic rheumatoid arthritis is an important nursing responsibility. A thorough assessment of the patient's capabilities and limitations allows the nurse to identify assistive devices that would facilitate self-care. Medications and equipment may require significant financial expenditures for patients with limited incomes.

NURSING MANAGEMENT OF THE PATIENT WITH JOINT REPLACEMENT
Assessment

Preoperative assessment specific to the patient undergoing joint replacement (arthroplasty) includes the following: pain intensified by movement, limitation in motion, and protective behaviors such as guarding of shoulders, elbows, or fingers, or limping with hip, knee, or ankle involvement.

Postoperatively the nurse assesses for complications. Shortening of the affected leg, sudden pain, and inability to move the extremity may indicate dislocation of a hip prosthesis. Abnormal positioning of knee, shoulder, or elbow accompanied by pain may also signal dislocation. Infection may be indicated by fever, pain, erythema, and purulent drainage. Neurovascular assessments (5 P's) are performed every 1 to 2 hours in the first 24 hours and every 2 to 4 hours thereafter.

The nurse assesses vital signs, especially pulse and blood pressure, for clues to hypovolemia. Blood loss from drainage collection devices (hemovac, J-Vac, Jackson-Pratt) or on dressings is monitored. Drainage in excess of 150 mL per hour or 500 mL in the first 24 hours is reported to the physician. Hemoglobin and hematocrit as ordered by the physician are monitored for several days postoperatively to further assess for blood-loss anemia. If the patient is using anticoagulant therapy, the nurse observes for bleeding, especially from the nose, gums, and in the stool and urine.

If the patient is using a continuous passive motion (CPM) machine, pressure areas to the groin, knee, and under the straps are assessed. Furthermore, the nurse assesses for a positive Homan's sign, warmth, redness, and swelling that is asymmetric as possible indicators of deep-vein thrombosis.

Nursing Diagnosis

Pain related to surgical procedure, edema, and ineffective pain-relief or comfort measures

High risk for infection related to surgical procedure

High risk altered peripheral perfusion related to edema or blood loss

High risk for injury: dislocation of prosthesis related to improper positioning/movement or infection

Impaired physical mobility related to pain and surgical procedure

High risk for impaired skin integrity related to immobility and therapeutic devices

High risk for altered bowel elimination related to immobility and surgical procedure

Altered health maintenance related to lack of knowledge of surgical procedure and postoperative self-care

Planning

Although the goals for the patient undergoing a joint replacement are influenced by the particular joint being replaced, the following outcomes are generally expected for all such patients:

Pain-relief measures are effective

No evidence of infection such as fever, increased pain, or purulent drainage

No evidence of nerve or circulatory impairment

Absence of joint dislocation

Functional ROM of operated joint

Skin intact without redness

Maintenance of normal bowel pattern

Management of self-care following discharge

Implementation

Preoperatively the nurse provides the patient with information about the surgery and what to expect. Any special equipment that will be used is discussed and demonstrated to the patient. Techniques to reduce the incidence of complications are addressed. This includes measures to prevent dislocation of the prosthesis (see Patient Education Guide), to promote circulation and muscle tone, to prevent hypostatic pneumonia, and to manage pain. The skin is prepped with a germicidal scrub before surgery. The nurse may administer antibiotics immediately before surgery, if ordered.

Initially the patient is often placed on patient-controlled analgesia (PCA) following the surgery. The nurse ensures that the patient knows how to operate the PCA and that the patient is not hesitant to use it because of fears of addiction or overdosage. Since muscle spasms may require the administration of skeletal muscle relaxants, the nurse evaluates the type of pain the patient is experiencing. The nurse further assists the patient in managing pain by frequent position changes and back care.

Strict asepsis in changing dressings and emptying drainage collection devices is used to prevent infec-

NURSING CARE PLAN *Postoperative Care of Patient with Total Hip Arthroplasty*

Nursing diagnosis/ Expected outcome	Interventions	Rationale
Impaired physical mobility related to pain and surgery	Maintain bed rest as ordered	Decreases weight bearing of joint
• *Functional joint mobility*		
	Maintain affected leg in straight position (abducted) using pillows, abduction pillow/brace, or Mar-Mar sling	Prevents prosthetic dislocation
	Maintain use of antiembolism hose, removing every shift to assess skin condition	Decreases venous stasis
	Maintain use of sequential pneumatic hose	Decreases venous stasis
	Promote quadriceps setting exercises, plantar flexion, four times daily	Builds muscle strength and endurance to assist in return to ambulation and prevent circulatory stasis
	Neurovascular checks (5 P's)	Potential for neurovascular impairment and hemorrhage
	Promote ambulation with ambulatory assistive devices, avoiding full weight bearing	Decreases weight bearing of joint
	Promote use of trapeze bar	Increases self-care ability while strengthening muscles of upper extremities
	Administer pain medication approximately 30 minutes before physical therapy	Increases joint mobility
Acute pain related to joint arthroplasty	Assess verbal and nonverbal cues of pain	Individualized responses to pain
• *Minimal pain or pain relief*		
	Administer prescribed medications and observe for side effects (see Table 58-3)	NSAIDs, analgesics, skeletal muscle relaxants, and corticosteroids to produce pain relief through variety of specific actions to promote rest and comfort
	Promote diversionary activities	Gate control theory of pain; activation of midbrain cells inhibits transmissions of pain
	Encourage use of relaxation and imagery technique	Gate control theory of pain; biostimulation therapy
	Position for comfort and frequent changes of position	Increases joint mobility
	Administer prescribed medications approximately 30 minutes before physical therapy	Allows patient to be more active in therapy
High risk for impaired skin integrity related to immobility and incision	Assess incision for erythema, edema, purulent drainage, and warmth	Indications of wound infection
• *Skin remains intact and free of pressure ulcers and infection*		
	Change dressing using aseptic technique as needed, but at least every 2 or 3 days	Prevention of wound infection

Nursing diagnosis/ Expected outcome	Interventions	Rationale
	Turn every 2 hours while maintaining abduction	Prevention of pressure sites
	Assess skin pressure sites every 2 hours	Identify beginning skin breakdown before ulceration
	Utilize special mattress (Geomatt, egg crate, or flotation mattress) and other preventive devices (heel pads, sheepskin pad while in chair)	Prevention of skin breakdown
	Monitor hydration and nutrition status	Prevention of pressure ulcers
	Maintain dry incision line until sutures are removed	Prevention of infection
	Use draw sheet when moving patient	Prevention of shearing forces to skin
	Maintain sheets dry and wrinkle free	Prevention of skin breakdown
Altered health maintenance management related to joint arthroplasty and postoperative flexion restrictions	Coordinate care by varied health professionals: physical therapist, social worker, and home health nurse	Facilitates mobility in hospital and prepares patient for discharge to home
• *Minimal or independent assistance in health care maintenance*	Facilitate ability to perform self-care activities and use self-care devices	Maintenance of self-care within physical mobility restrictions
	Teach patient preoperatively with postoperative reinforcement regarding medications, including actions, dosage, and side effects	Repetitive teaching enhances learning and retention
	Monitor drainage from suction apparatus (Hemovac, Jackson-Pratt, J-Vac) every 2 hours for first 24 hours and every 4 to 8 hours for second 24 hours, and thereafter report excessive amount	Potential for postoperative hemorrhage
	Monitor for positive Homan's sign	Potential for thrombophlebitis
	Assess circulatory and neural status secondary to abductive device or traction	Potential for neurovascular impairment
	Encourage prescribed exercise and repositioning within limitations	Exercise enhances circulation and prevents contractures
Altered peripheral tissue perfusion related to surgery and immobility*	Assess vital signs and surgical dressing	Changes in vital signs or bleeding on dressing may indicate hemorrhage
• *Maintains adequate peripheral tissue perfusion*	Assess circulatory and neural status distal to operative site (see 5 P's of neurovascular status in Chapter 57)	Potential for neurovascular impairment
	Maintain use of antiembolism hose and pneumatic sequential compression hose	Decreases venous stasis

*The remaining three diagnoses are high risk for postoperative complications.

Continued.

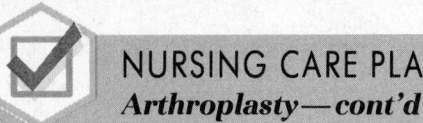

Nursing diagnosis/ Expected outcome	Interventions	Rationale
High risk for infection related to endoprosthesis surgery • *Absence of infection*	Monitor vital signs every 4 hours	Indicates infection
	Monitor amount and character of drainage from incision, and change dressing using aseptic technique	Early detection of infection enhances treatment, whereas aseptic technique prevents introduction of microorganisms
	Monitor for indicators of joint infection such as erythema, local warmth, edema, decreased range of motion, purulent drainage, and fever	Ongoing potential for infection, especially hematogenic
	Monitor nutritional status and hematocrit/hemoglobin	Promotes tissue healing and enhances immune status
Potential complication (dislocation of joint) related to surgery and improper positioning • *Joint will remain in alignment*	Preoperatively, teach patient and significant others and provide postoperative reinforcement regarding the following:	Knowledge increases compliance and participation and decreases postoperative complications related to lack of knowledge; repetitive teaching enhances patient's learning and retention
	Positional restrictions Maintain abduction of affected extremity with pillow or brace	Maintains joint alignment
	Avoid internal rotation, adduction, and hip flexion; no hip flexion permitted greater than 45 to 50 degrees; when sitting, use a tilt-back chair to avoid 90-degree hip flexion; use commode extender or raised toilet seat and avoid chairs that are low to floor; do not cross legs or bend from waist	Prosthesis may press on weakened posterior hip capsule and cause dislocation
	Activity restrictions Maintain partial weight bearing until full weight bearing is permitted by physician; time depends on type of prosthesis	Maintains joint alignment until healing of periarticular tissue around prosthesis has occurred
	Use walker or crutches for ambulation	Prevents excessive strain on tissue around prosthesis
	Use self-care devices such as raised commode and stocking helpers	
	Indicators of infection: wound, respiratory tract, or urinary tract	Temperature elevation, chills, drainage, or redness at incision site, general malaise, or tissue damage indicates possible infection
	Indicators of joint dislocation Shortening of affected extremity Sudden and severe joint pain Limitations of joint function	Early diagnosis of joint dislocation can prevent excessive tissue (soft, nerve, and vascular) damage

*The remaining three diagnoses are high risk for postoperative complications.

PATIENT EDUCATION GUIDE

Discharge Teaching for Total Hip Replacement

Do

Keep legs apart while sitting or lying

Use pillow or blanket between legs as a reminder to keep legs abducted

Sit on a high, firm chair

Use caution when getting in and out of bathtub

Walk with crutches or walker as instructed in physical therapy before discharge

Use elevated toilet seat

Notify physician if operative site becomes reddened or irritated or has any drainage; also if you have pain, swelling, shortening of one leg, or limitation in walking

Advise dentist of prosthesis before dental work so prophylactic antibiotics can be given

Do not

Sit in low, soft chair

Cross legs

Turn hip or knee inward or outward

Participate in sports activities until advised by physician

Bend forward past 90 degrees to put on shoes or socks or to pick things up

Turn in bed without pillow or blanket between legs

tion. The dressing usually remains in place until 2 to 4 days after the operation. After that point, the incision is closely monitored for erythema, drainage, and condition of the incision. The nurse administers prophylactic antibiotics and anticoagulant therapy (aspirin, coumadin, or heparin) as ordered by the physician. To further reduce the risk of deep-vein thrombosis, the physician may order antiembolism hose and a pneumatic sequential compression device (SCD). The nurse removes the hose and compression device every shift to monitor skin condition and to provide skin care. To lessen the risk of clots forming, the nurse does not leave the hose or compression device off for more than 20 to 30 minutes. Calf pumps to promote venous return are encouraged. The nurse monitors for the 5 Ps distal to the surgical site and notifies the physician of any deficits. For lower-extremity arthroplasty, the leg is elevated, and ice may be applied to decrease swelling.

Blood loss occurs perioperatively during the surgical procedure and postoperatively through drainage collection devices. Frequently autologous blood transfusion using a collection device (Solcatrans,

Gish) is used. Each institution develops its own policy surrounding the use of these devices, but generally autotransfusion is performed when there is an excess of 300 mL in 4 hours. Packed red blood cells (PRBC) may also be transfused rather than whole blood to decrease the risk of fluid overload that may occur in the elderly patient.

An abduction pillow is placed between the patient's legs following hip replacement to prevent dislocation. Although dislocation of a total knee replacement does not occur as frequently as that of the hip, when positioning this patient, the knee is not flexed and no pillow is placed beneath the knee itself. A knee immobilizer, splint, or cylinder cast may be used to protect the knee joint. The exception is when the patient is placed in a CPM machine. The shoulder is protected following replacement by use of a shoulder immobilizer.

To maintain or improve muscle strength, exercises are performed specific to the joint replacement. The CPM machine is used primarily with knee surgery patients to prevent adhesions, increase flexion at the knee joint, and decrease pain (see Chapter 57). It is also used with some hip surgery patients to maintain joint mobility and enhance blood flow. The straps are applied loosely to prevent pressure areas. In addition, because of enforced bed rest when using the CPM, the nurse implements measures to prevent pressure areas to the groin (reposition device), promote circulation (calf pumps in opposite extremity), and prevent pulmonary stasis (coughing and deep breathing). The nurse provides back care to the supine patient.

To prevent hypostatic pneumonia, orthostatic hypotension, and skin breakdown, the nurse assists the patient out of bed as soon as possible. For patients with hip replacements a special chair that avoids acute flexion at the hip is used. Patients with knee and ankle replacements may use a regular wheelchair or straight-backed chair. For the patient with either upper- or lower-extremity arthroplasty, it is advisable to avoid low chairs (may dislocate hip prosthesis because of flexion or be difficult to get out of for a shoulder or elbow arthroplasty). Physical therapy is usually started on the first or second postoperative day, beginning with non–weight bearing, progressing to toe touch and standing transfer, and ending with full weight bearing. Physical therapy may use the tilt table, parallel bars, and finally the walker or cane.

The nurse prevents constipation in these patients by administering adequate fluid intake to keep the stool soft and providing diets with fiber. Prune juice or stewed prunes often enhance bowel elimination. The nurse keeps an accurate record of fecal elimination and takes action before constipation develops. Depending upon the patient's normal bowel elimination pattern, in the absence of a bowel movement the nurse consults with the physician regarding administration of stool softeners, laxatives, and enemas, in that order. Initially the patient with lower-extremity joint replacement will require a fracture bedpan for bowel and possibly urinary elimination. Because of its small capacity, the nurse offers it to the patient frequently. An overhead trapeze is helpful when placing the patient on the bedpan or changing linens.

Evaluation/Documentation

Evaluation of the effectiveness of the plan centers around the patient's report of pain relief, the lack of signs and symptoms of complications, intactness of skin integrity, and the ability of the patient to participate in activities and perform self-care skills within the restrictions of the surgical procedure. Treatment measures and their effectiveness are documented. The nurse documents patient teaching and any return demonstrations. Patient education regarding home care is also documented.

Ongoing Care

The patient is instructed to notify the physician if symptoms of infection develop. In addition, the patient is advised to notify the physician before dental procedures or minor surgery for prophylactic antibiotic therapy. Furthermore, if symptoms of disloca-

tion occur, the patient is advised to seek medical assistance. The patient is instructed that if painful ambulation occurs, it may mean loosening of the prosthesis and result in the need for a revision of the joint replacement. The patient is instructed on weight bearing of the affected extremity and any assistive ambulatory device (walker, crutches, cane) recommended. Stair climbing is practiced. Instructions are provided for exercise and activity. The patient is taught specific exercises to perform to maintain muscle strength and joint range of motion. The patient with a porous-coated non-cemented prosthesis may not be allowed full weight bearing for 8 to 12 weeks following surgery. Any environmental modifications to the home are identified (elevated toilet seat, bath/shower seat, extension devices for reaching) and explored. Plans for a return appointment are made, and the importance of keeping the appointment is stressed.

GOUT
Definition

Gout is a monoarticular (arthritis of one joint), asymmetric arthritis characterized by hyperuricemia. Historically, gout has been described as the disease of royalty because of its association with high protein ingestion.[28]

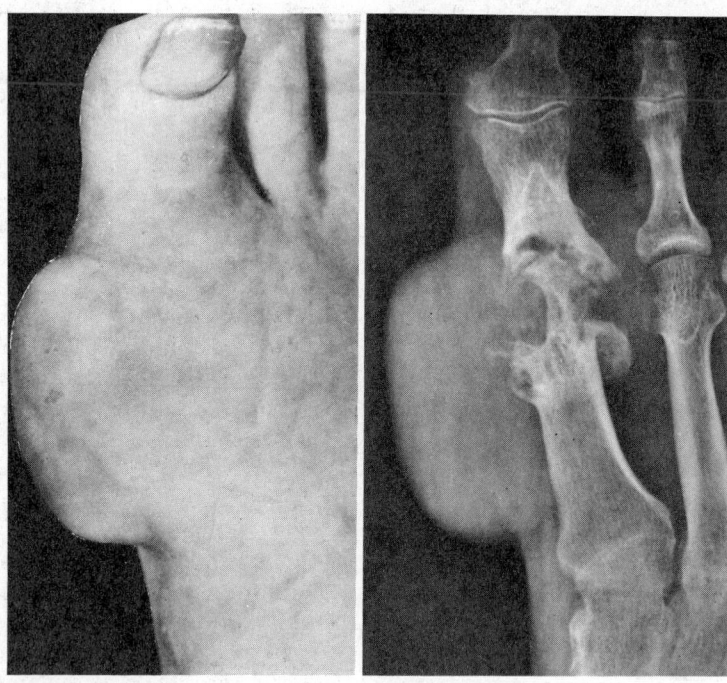

FIGURE 58-11   Gout of long duration. Mass is associated with extensive urate deposits. (From Brashear HR, Raney RB: *Handbook of orthopaedic surgery*, ed 10, St Louis, 1986, Mosby–Year Book, Inc.)

Etiology/Epidemiology

According to the National Center for Health Statistics, gout affects approximately 1.6 million people in the United States.[6] Gout primarily affects men and has a 20:1 sex ratio; the peak incidence occurs from 40 to 60 years of age.[31] Individuals from the higher socioeconomic class are at particular risk because their diets are usually higher in protein. Filipinos from Hawaii and the West Coast of the United States also have a higher incidence of gout.[28] Two etiologic factors are thought to be involved in gout development: (1) a genetic increase in purine metabolism and production and (2) the ingestion of excessive alcohol or a high-purine diet.[28]

Pathophysiology

Abnormal purine metabolism or excessive intake of purine results in the formation of uric acid crystals, an end product of purine metabolism. These crystals precipitate from the body fluid and are deposited in the joints and connective tissue. The deposits are most frequently found in the metatarsophalangeal joint of the great toe. The knee joints, wrists, and proximal interphalangeal joints may also be affected. Joint and tissue inflammation results from the release of lysosomal enzymes.[28]

Chronic gout encompasses joint degeneration and disability related to inflammation and tophaceous deposits in the joint. The patient with chronic gout may also have kidney tubular damage, which can lead to renal stones and renal dysfunction or failure.

Clinical Manifestations

Gout is characterized by tight and reddened skin over the inflamed joint, edema, elevated temperature, and hyperuricemia. In hyperuricemia, serum uric acid levels are above 7.5 mg/dL, which is considered to be diagnostic. According to Kelley et al.,[30] the great toe is affected 90% of the time, followed by other lower extremity joints (Figure 58-11). Upper extremity joints are also susceptible. Acute attacks commonly begin at night and may last from 3 to 7 days. They occur at irregular intervals. The attacks may be precipitated by trauma, diuretics, increased alcohol consumption, or a high-purine diet. The use of diuretics may cause systemic fluid depletion, which results in increased tubular resorption of uric acid crystals. Subsequently serum uric acid is elevated. Systemic manifestations may include fever, renal disease, hypertension, tachycardia, malaise, and tophi. Tophi are nodular formations of uric acid crystals on the ears, fingers, and hands. Renal uric acid stones may also be noted on x-ray examination. Diagnostic studies (elevated serum uric acid levels) and findings for gout include analysis of the inflamed fluid for monosodium urate crystals, elevated sedimentation rate, and the presence of tophi.[7] Radiologic findings in gout may show tophi and soft tissue edema.[28] An association among gout, obesity, and kidney stones composed of uric acid has also been noted. In addition, approximately one third of patients with gout suffer hypertension.[28]

Therapeutic Management

Gout management involves diet therapy, pharmacotherapy (Table 58-7), and joint rest during the acute phase. Dietary management includes restriction of high-purine food and alcohol ingestion and weight control. Foods are avoided that have a high purine content such as meats, organ meats, and yeast products (see box). In addition to food restrictions the patient needs at least 3000 mL of fluid per day to discourage the formation of renal stones. Acute attacks are generally managed with NSAIDs (see Table 58-4). Colchicine may be prescribed during acute attacks and for patients unable to use NSAIDs. Since gout is a chronic disease, cholchicine may be prescribed prophylactically if the patient has two or more attacks per year. Allopurinol or probenecid may be used to prevent future attacks in hyperuricemic patients.[9] During acute attacks the inflamed joint is elevated and the patient is placed on bed rest. Weight bearing intensifies the joint pain and enhances joint deterioration. A bed cradle may be beneficial to relieve pressure from the foot if the toes are affected.

NURSING MANAGEMENT OF THE PATIENT WITH GOUT

Assessment

Nursing assessment of gout includes examination of the joint for pain, tenderness, erythema, limitation of motion, and edema. Systemic involvement is assessed by the presence of a tophus or tophi and low-grade fever. Changes in body image and family and

---

HIGH-PURINE CONTENT FOODS

Meats: poultry
Organ meats: liver, brains, heart, kidney, and sweetbread
Meat extracts: bouillon, meat drippings, and gravy
Fish: sardines, fish roe, anchovies, shrimp, herring
Yeast: all breads containing yeast
Vegetables: asparagus, spinach, and mushrooms

TABLE 58-7   Pharmacology Summary: Uricosurics for Gout

Drug	Dosage	Side effects	Nursing considerations
Probenecid (Benemid)	0.5 g twice daily	Headache, nausea, vomiting, anorexia, urinary frequency	Encourage liberal fluid intake to minimize calculus formation Monitor serum uric acid levels Administer with food or antacids Avoid concurrent use of salicylates (because they decrease uricosuric effect)
Sulfinpyrazone (Anturane)	400 to 800 mg/day	Upper gastrointestinal disturbances (nausea, dyspepsia); reactivation of peptic ulcer disease	Administer with food, milk, or antacids Maintain adequate fluid intake
URIC ACID INHIBITORS			
Allopurinol (Zyloprim)	200 to 600 mg/day	Skin rash, fever, chills, bone marrow depression, gastrointestinal irritation	Monitor liver and renal function in initial month Administer with food Maintain adequate fluid intake Maintain alkaline urine (avoid large doses of vitamin C)
Colchicine	0.5 to 1.8 mg/ day (prophylaxis); 0.5 to 1.2 mg every 1 to 2 hours (acute attack)	Bone marrow depression, aplastic anemia, granulocytopenia, leukopenia, thrombocytopenia, nausea/vomiting, diarrhea, cramps, skin rashes	Monitor complete blood count for blood dyscrasias with long-term use Tell patient to avoid alcohol when taking oral form (increases gastric toxicity and decreases effectiveness of drug) With oral form give with food to decrease gastrointestinal upset Do not give over 12 tablets in 24 hours Give at first sign of impending attack Administer intravenous dose over 2 to 5 minutes Do not give with dextrose 5% or bacteriostatic water (incompatible) Prevent extravasation of intravenous colchicine into surrounding tissue (apply cold compress and give analgesic if this occurs) Do not give more than 4 mg/24 hr intravenously

social roles and modifications in vocational and recreational activities also are considered.

Nursing Diagnosis

Nursing diagnoses applicable to patients with gout primarily address the pain and limitation of motion. Nursing diagnoses can include the following:

Chronic pain related to joint inflammation

Altered nutrition: high risk for more than body requirements related to purine metabolism and alcohol ingestion

Knowledge deficit regarding disease process and treatment regimen

Impaired physical mobility related to restricted joint mobility and inflammation

Planning

Expected patient outcomes generally include the following:

Pain management is achieved

Optimal nutrition is attained

Disease process and treatment regimen can be explained

Joint mobility is improved

Implementation

Nursing care to decrease patient discomfort includes elevation of the affected extremity and avoidance of weight bearing and bed clothing pressure. Cold compresses help anesthetize the inflamed joint. Administering prescribed medications and monitoring side effects are important nursing roles.

Nutritional components of gout management are eating a well-balanced diet, maintaining weight within an ideal range for height and build, and restricting foods high in purine. Nurses promote a fluid intake of 3 L or greater daily and limit alcohol ingestion.[32]

Patient education includes skin care of tophi, the nature and chronicity of the disease, diet, medications, and activity levels. Patients and family members are informed that trauma, high-purine intake, and excessive alcohol ingestion may precipitate gout attacks. Although medications are an important adjunct to dietary measures, patients must also be instructed in the mode of action and side effects of the medications. Because of restricted joint mobility, nurses promote ambulation during asymptomatic periods, elevation of the affected extremity, and range-of-motion exercises (see Table 58-2).

Evaluation/Documentation

Nursing evaluation of the patient with gout includes examination of the joint for inflammation and restricted movement. The nurse evaluates whether the treatment regimen is effective in controlling or maintaining the disease symptoms and whether the patient is complying with the dietary restrictions. An integral component of patient teaching includes documenting the patient's understanding and compliance. Other documentation includes the presence of tophi, intervals between gout attacks, joint assessment, and the occurrence of uric acid kidney stones.

Ongoing Care

Gout, a chronic metabolic disease, requires ongoing care. The focus of home management is the prevention of or decrease in gout attacks. Control is best achieved with adherence to dietary restrictions and the medication regimen.

OSTEOPOROSIS
Definition

Osteoporosis is a reduction in the skeletal bone mass that causes an increased risk of fractures. There are at least three types of osteoporosis: primary, secondary, and senile (Table 58-8). Osteoporosis is a significant cause of morbidity in the older adult. Fractures of osteoporotic bones cause thousands of deaths and much suffering each year. More than most diseases, osteoporosis can generally be prevented or at least minimized. Prevention is focused on adequate calcium intake, moderate exercise, and for some females hormone replacement.[14]

Etiology/Epidemiology

A multifactorial disease, osteoporosis has two major causes, calcium deficiency or lack of absorption and estrogen deficiency. Decreased estrogen levels are secondary to menopause, and hypocalcemia is believed to be a result of chronic inadequate dietary calcium ingestion. Other causative factors include medications such as prolonged steroid usage, cigarette smoking, excessive caffeine ingestion, endocrine disorders, prolonged bed rest, liver disease, alcoholism, and specific malignancies.

Approximately 15 to 20 million Americans are thought to suffer from osteoporosis.[33] The typical person affected by osteoporosis is a thin, sedentary, white, postmenopausal woman. Blacks have denser bones than whites and are at less risk for osteoporosis. It is believed that while both men and women lose bone mineral with age and experience associated fractures, men have greater bone mineral throughout life. Men do not lose bone density as rapidly as women; thus the average 80-year-old woman has lost 50% of her trabecular bone compared to the average man, who has lost less than 20%.[10]

TABLE 58-8   Types of Osteoporosis

Type	Contributing causes
Primary osteoporosis	No identifiable cause
Secondary osteoporosis	Bone loss resulting from endocrine disorders
	Hyperthyroidism
	Hyperparathyroidism
	Diabetes mellitus
	Glucocorticoid excess
	Kidney diseases
	Rheumatoid arthritis
	Pharmacologic therapies
	Corticosteroids
	Heparin
	Anticonvulsants
	Antacids
	Thiazide diuretics
	Thyroid supplements
	Prolonged immobility
	Dietary factors
	Caffeine excess
	Protein excess
	Calcium deficiency
	Other factors
	Liver disease
	Alcoholism
	Genetic factors
	Cigarette smoking
	Malignancies
	Multiple myeloma
	Leukemia
	Lymphoma
Senile osteoporosis (postmenopausal osteoporosis)	Lack of estrogen production

Modified from Graham B, Gleit C: Osteoporosis: a major health problem in postmenopausal women, *Orthop Nurs* 3(6):19, 1984.

Pathophysiology

Osteoporosis is defined as a reduction in bone mass in which bone resorption exceeds bone formation. Bone mass peaks at approximately 35 years and then subsequently begins to decrease. In the perimenopausal period there is increased bone loss. Bone remodeling, or the process of bone breakdown and formation, is a constant process. Lack of stress to the bone causes demineralization of bone. With hypocalcemia, calcium is released from bone to reestablish the normal serum level. After 35 years of age when the bone mass peaks and bones are strongest, bone resorption begins to exceed bone formation, resulting in decreased bone density. Women over 40 years also absorb less calcium from food. Estrogen is thought to decrease bone resorption, decrease renal calcium loss, and increase calcium absorption in the gastrointestinal tract.[30] Estrogen levels decrease with cigarette smoking. Excessive caffeine ingestion is associated with decreased calcium. Calcium absorption from the intestines decreases with age.

Whatever the cause of osteoporosis, it occurs when the remodeling cycle (the process of bone resorption and bone formation) is disrupted. A complete cycle requires approximately 4 months in a normal healthy adult but may require up to 24 months in an adult with osteoporosis. Some hormones and drugs may also contribute to the delay in the cycle by interfering with the rate of resorption and the rate of new bone formation.[14] Large doses of heparin promote bone resorption. This usually resolves when therapy ceases.

Clinical Manifestations

Clinical manifestations of osteoporosis include height loss, dorsal kyphosis, back pain, or fractures. The most common manifestations are pain and bone deformity. Fractures may occur in both compact bone with the affected bone becoming porous and in spongy bone with the trabeculae of the bone becoming thin and sparse. Common sites for fractures include long bones (femurs and humerus), the wrist, and the vertebrae. Vertebral collapse that causes kyphosis (dowager's hunchback) diminishes height[14] (see Figure 56-10). Vertebral crush fractures, most commonly of the twelfth thoracic and first lumbar vertebrae, may result from normal daily activities, such as bending.[30] Other fractures such as those of the distal radius may occur in response to patients extending their hands to protect themselves in a fall. Women suffer from hip fractures two to three times more frequently than men,[34] and minor trauma may result in a fracture of osteoporotic bone. Commonly a fracture of the neck of the femur occurs from normal weight bearing and the patient will fall. The patient may report that he or she fell and broke the hip, whereas the fracture occurred before the fall. Complications of the fracture (fat embolism, hemorrhage, or shock) may prove fatal.[14]

Diagnostic studies of osteoporosis include x-ray findings of porous bone. However, these findings are not definitive until approximately 30% of bone mass is lost.[2] Bone mass changes can also be determined by photon absorptiometry of the wrist and computed tomography to assess the spine.

Therapeutic Management

Management of osteoporosis is aimed at decreasing the process of bone resorption, increasing bone for-

TABLE 58-9   Pharmacology Summary: Osteoporosis and Osteomalacia

Drug	Disorder	Dosage	Side effects	Nursing implications
Vitamin D	Osteomalacia Osteoporosis	Maintain serum calcium at 9 to 10 mg/L	Usually nontoxic if does not exceed physiologic requirement	Dietary intake of vitamin D and calcium must be taken into account Cautious use in patients with renal disease
Calcium	Osteomalacia Osteoporosis	1 to 1.5 g daily elemental calcium Maintain serum calcium at 9 to 10 mg/L	Gastrointestinal irritation Constipation	

mation, and preventing fractures. Treatment measures are postmenopausal estrogen replacement therapy and adequate dietary or supplemental calcium. Recommendations for calcium supplementation are 1000 mg, premenopausal, and 1500 mg, postmenopausal.[34] Studies indicate that the average daily adult calcium intake is 450 to 550 mg. Calcium supplements and vitamin D supplements (Table 58-9) may be prescribed to increase calcium absorption.[32]

Exposure to sunlight produces vitamin D in the body. Patients are reminded, however, of sun exposure risks. Estrogen replacement therapy decreases calcium loss from bones. It should be started within several years following menopause to be effective. Although estrogen replacement therapy is controversial, on the positive side it provides some protection from fractures, especially of the hip, as well as cardiovascular protection. Conversely, this therapy may lead to an increased risk of endometrial cancer, thrombosis, and periodic vaginal bleeding. Thiazide diuretics are being investigated for their effects of decreasing urinary excretion of calcium and increasing bone density. Salicylates and NSAIDs may be given to decrease the associated back pain (see Table 58-4). Moderate weight-bearing exercise stimulates bone formation and maintenance.

Thirty minutes of vigorous aerobic exercise on alternate days is recommended. Excessive exercise that leads to cessation of menstruation in the premenopausal woman is to be avoided, because this may accelerate calcium loss.

Treatment is usually focused on (1) a supplemental dose of calcium for 38% of the mineral composition of bones, (2) sufficient estrogen levels in females since estrogen may help to maintain calcium in bone tissue and counteract the action of the parathyroid hormone that pulls calcium from the bones, and (3) weight-bearing exercises to increase bone mass.[1]

NURSING MANAGEMENT OF THE PATIENT WITH OSTEOPOROSIS
Assessment

Nursing assessment of the osteoporotic patient includes determination of height loss, dorsal kyphosis, presence of back pain, and occurrence of fractures or repeat fractures. Psychosocial issues that should be assessed are changes in body image and limitations in vocational and recreational activities.

Nursing Diagnosis

Pertinent nursing diagnoses for osteoporosis patients include the following:
   Pain (chronic) related to decreased bone mass
   Physical mobility (impaired) related to decreased bone mass and possible fractures
   Nutrition, altered: less than body requirements related to inadequate calcium or vitamin D intake
   Body image disturbance related to body changes and disease process
   Knowledge deficit regarding disease process and treatment regimen

Planning

Nursing care is planned to attain the following patient outcomes:
   Pain management is achieved
   Function is within restricted mobility limitations
   Optimal nutrition is attained or maintained
   Positive self-concept is demonstrated

TABLE 58-10   Calcium in Foods

Food	Calcium (mg)
Tofu (8 oz)	280
Canned salmon with bones (1 oz)	60
Canned sardines with bones (1 oz)	125
Whole milk (8 oz)	290
Low-fat milk (8 oz)	298
Skim milk (8 oz)	300
Yogurt (8 oz)	400
Cottage cheese (8 oz)	170
American cheese (1 oz)	170
Green leafy vegetables (8 oz)	400
Vanilla ice cream (8 oz)	208

Modified from Walker J, Holm K: Osteoporosis: treatment and prevention update, *Geriatr Nurs,* p 142, May/June 1990.

TABLE 58-11   Elemental Calcium in Calcium Supplements

Supplement	Elemental calcium/mg
Calcium gluconate	9%
Calcium lactate	13%
Calcium carbonate	40%

Modified from National Institute of Arthritis and Musculoskeletal and Skin Diseases, National Institutes of Health: Osteoporosis: cause, treatment, prevention. Published in *Orthop Nurs,* p 29, Nov/Dec, 1985.

Disease process and treatment regimen are explained

Implementation

Pain relief measures include administration of salicylates or other NSAIDs and observation for side effects (see Table 58-4). Back bracing or other supportive devices may be used to decrease pain. As with other musculoskeletal diseases, the application of warm compresses facilitates pain relief.

The nurse promotes body mechanics and range-of-motion and moderate weight-bearing exercises. Effective use of the musculoskeletal system with good body mechanics can decrease trauma and subsequent fracture. Exercise, range of motion, and weight bearing will maintain and increase bone formation. Exercises, such as swimming and walking, provide the weight bearing pertinent for bone formation. The establishment of a hazard-free environment will be advantageous to the aged adult with impaired mobility.

Inadequate calcium and vitamin D intake characterize osteoporosis. Dietary changes are implemented, and supplementation may be prescribed (Table 58-10).The nurse encourages the ingestion of a well-balanced diet high in calcium and vitamin D, and wise selection of calcium supplements (Table 58-11). Moderate exposure to sunlight is encouraged to optimize the body's production of vitamin D. Encouraging the patient to dress to decrease the visibility of dorsal kyphosis and to talk about osteoporosis are measures to promote a more positive self-image.

Much information exists regarding osteoporosis and calcium and estrogen therapy. Therefore patient education regarding the disease process and treatment regimen is important. Teaching at the patient's level of comprehension includes the interrelationship of calcium, estrogens, vitamin D, and exercise. The dosage, frequency, and side effects of medications and dietary supplementation of vitamin D and calcium are reviewed with the patient. Patients are advised to take calcium supplements between meals and drink a glass of water when taking the supplement.[34] Because the osteoporotic patient is often aged and fracture prone, the home environment needs to be assessed for hazards and made more safe. In addition, simple first aid for fractures is reviewed with the patient and significant others.

Evaluation/Documentation

The effectiveness of the nursing interventions will be determined by the patient's management of discomfort and the ability to perform self-care skills and to participate in social activities. Compliance with nutritional and pharmacologic therapies is also assessed. Patient teaching is an important aspect of nursing care and is documented. The patient's response and compliance with the dietary changes and supplementation are validated. Subjective comments of the patient regarding pain and the disease limitations are recorded.

Ongoing Care

Osteoporosis is primarily a disease of elderly persons and postmenopausal women. Except for hospitalizations for fractures, particularly hip fractures, the patient with osteoporosis is at home. To prevent fractures the home is evaluated for hazards such as slippery rugs, inadequate lighting, and clutter. Continual assessment of the patient's use of calcium, estrogen, and vitamin D supplementation is another aspect of home care. Participation in weight-bearing activities as a preventive and treatment measure is promoted. Walking is a weight-bearing exercise and is safe if done on a level surface and with correct-fitting support shoes.

OSTEOMALACIA
Definition

Osteomalacia occurs when calcium and phosphorus are not deposited in the bone matrix and the bone does not calcify.

Etiology/Epidemiology

Bone mineralization requires calcium and phosphorus. Calcium is the transport medium for phosphorus, and intestinal calcium absorption is facilitated by vitamin D. With inadequate vitamin D the calcium and phosphorus are not deposited in the bone matrix, resulting in unmineralized bone.[36] People at risk are elderly persons with diets deficient in calcium and limited ultraviolet exposure and adolescents and young adults with inadequate calcium ingestion. Races with increased melanin pigmentation, people receiving chronic anticonvulsant therapy, and people with chronic renal failure are also at risk[30] (see box).

Clinical Manifestations

Adults may experience bone pain that intensifies with activity. Commonly affected bones include the pelvis, lower extremities, spine, and ribs. Demineralized bones are susceptible to minimal trauma fractures. The patient may also complain of tenderness with palpitation and muscle weakness. Tetany may result from hypocalcemia.[2] Laboratory findings for osteomalacia are an elevated plasma alkaline phosphatase. Radiologically, pseudofractures and minute discontinuities in the bone cortex are late manifestations of osteomalacia.[30]

ETIOLOGY OF OSTEOMALACIA[2]

Calcium dietary deficiency
Vitamin D dietary deficiency
Inadequate vitamin D synthesis
    Use of sunscreens
    Limited ultraviolet exposure
    Highly pigmented skin
Intestinal malabsorption of vitamin D
Long-term parenteral nutrition
Mesenchymal tumors
Chronic renal failure
Chronic anticonvulsant therapy

Therapeutic Management

Osteomalacia management depends on the etiologic factors of the vitamin D deficiency. Therapy consists primarily of vitamin D supplementation. Calcium supplementation and ultraviolet irradiation may be adjunct therapies.

NURSING MANAGEMENT OF THE PATIENT WITH OSTEOMALACIA
Assessment

The patient with osteomalacia is assessed for bone pain and tenderness, fractures, bowing of the bones, and muscle weakness. In addition, nurses assess the dietary intake of calcium and phosphorus, ultraviolet exposure, and coexisting diseases. Any factors that could result in vitamin D deficiency are identified.

Nursing Diagnosis

Possible nursing diagnoses for the patient with osteomalacia are as follows:
    High risk for injury related to muscle weakness and falls
    Pain related to bone pathologic condition
    Altered body image related to disease process
    Altered health maintenance related to knowledge deficit regarding disease process and required therapy

Planning

The expected outcomes for the patient with osteomalacia include the following:
    The patient remains free of injury
    Pain is managed or relieved
    Body image is not altered
    The patient exhibits understanding of the disease process and required therapy

Implementation

In an effort to prevent skeletal trauma, nurses promote a safe environment to prevent falls. The home is evaluated for the presence of such hazards as loose rugs and improper lighting. The patient is assisted with ambulation or provided with ambulatory aids. Patients who complain of bone pain and tenderness are given the prescribed analgesics, and the affected areas are splinted to decrease joint stress.

Interventions to increase the patient's self-esteem include encouraging verbalization of concerns and fears regarding osteomalacia. Promoting participation in self-care activities and in vocational and recreational activities also facilitates a more positive body self-image.

Nursing interventions to increase the availability of vitamin D and calcium are necessary. Coordination of care with a nutritionist is needed for in-depth dietary counseling. Because vitamin D is produced by the body in response to ultraviolet light, nurses encourage outdoor activities. Exogenous calcium and vitamin D may be administered if dietary interventions are not effective.

Educational endeavors regarding osteomalacia address the disease nature and the role of pharmacologic and dietary therapy. In addition, the interrelationship between sunlight exposure and vitamin D formation is discussed with the patient and family.

Evaluation/Documentation

The nurse evaluates the safety of the patient's environment and the patient's ability to use ambulatory aids. The patient's management of pain is evaluated and documented. The patient's self-esteem and feelings regarding body image are assessed and documented. The patient's response to and compliance with the treatment plan are also evaluated.

OSTEOMYELITIS
Definition/Etiology

Osteomyelitis, or infection of the bone, can be classified as acute or chronic. The causes of osteomyelitis may be bacterial, fungal, or viral.[2] Causative organisms include *Escherichia coli, Staphylococcus aureus, Proteus, Streptococcus,* and *Pseudomonas aeruginosa.*[18] Acute osteomyelitis is common in children under 12 years of age. It rarely occurs in adults. In chronic osteomyelitis the causative microorganism multiplies in a vascular bone. The three modes of entry for microorganisms to invade bone tissue are the blood, extension of an adjacent infection, and direct entry.[2] In adults the vertebrae are the primary site. Urinary tract infections, hemodialysis, or bacterial endocarditis may be the source of bloodborne infections. Infections that may extend to the bone tissue and cause osteomyelitis include malignancy necrosis, radiation therapy and burns, pressure sores, soft tissue inflammation, and infections secondary to atherosclerosis and diabetes mellitus. Osteomyelitis is often seen in the older adult, since these conditions are associated with aging. Sinus or dental infections may result in skull osteomyelitis. Direct entry of microorganisms may occur with foreign body penetration, fracture, or perioperative contamination.[2]

Pathophysiology

In osteomyelitis the offending organism causes bone tissue inflammation with subsequent erythema, edema, purulence, and increased tissue pressure. This inflammatory process results in bone necrosis and ischemia. Granulation tissue eventually forms beneath the necrotic bone. The granulation tissue is surrounded by new bone tissue that may not revascularize.[18]

Clinical Manifestations

The clinical manifestations of osteomyelitis vary with the etiology. In vertebral osteomyelitis, patients complain of back pain that is worse with movement. Fever may be present. In osteomyelitis resulting from trauma or an extension from an existing infection there is edema, erythema, and local pain and tenderness. This patient may also be afebrile.[2] With osteomyelitis caused by a joint prosthesis the patient may experience a loosening of the prosthesis and pain 3 to 12 months after surgical implantation. The prosthesis may dislocate and require removal. A revision or replacement is often necessary. In the presence of osteomyelitis, surgical intervention may be delayed until the patient has received antibiotic therapy and the causative organism is no longer present. Diagnostic findings with osteomyelitis are leukocytosis and an increased erythrocyte sedimentation rate. Blood cultures should also be obtained to identify the causative organism, although they may be negative.

Therapeutic Management

Therapeutic management depends on the type of osteomyelitis. In vertebral osteomyelitis the infection is treated with parenteral antibiotics for 4 to 6 weeks and bed rest. Antibiotic therapy alone often is not enough for hematogenous, posttraumatic, or tissue infection osteomyelitis. Medical management consists of surgical removal of the necrotic bone and tissue. Antibiotic therapy is continued for 3 to 6 weeks. If the osteomyelitis is a result of a prosthesis, then the prosthesis is removed and antibiotic therapy initiated.[2] If the osteomyelitis exacerbates, a bone graft may be done or amputation of the affected extremity may be required. However, amputation is rarely necessary.

NURSING MANAGEMENT OF THE PATIENT WITH OSTEOMYELITIS
Assessment

Assessment of the patient with osteomyelitis includes factors related to bone tissue involvement. These factors include pain/tenderness, erythema, edema, and increased temperature. In addition, the nurse assesses for predisposing conditions and factors such as diabetes mellitus, atherosclerosis, prosthetic joint implantation, and sinus or dental infections. Since osteomyelitis requires prolonged bed rest and antimicrobial therapy, the psychosocial issues of body image changes and alteration in family and social roles must be assessed.

Nursing Diagnosis

Possible nursing diagnoses for the patient with osteomyelitis include the following:

- Pain related to swelling and tenderness
- Infection related to pathologic process
- Alteration in health maintenance related to bed rest

Planning

The goals for the patient with osteomyelitis include the following:

- Pain is controlled
- Infection resolves
- Complications of bed rest do not occur

Implementation

The patient with osteomyelitis will initially exhibit pain that intensifies with movement. Therefore nursing measures are designed to decrease the pain. Nursing care includes bed rest and splinting of the affected area if feasible to provide support. Prescribed analgesics are administered, and the patient is observed for side effects. Imagery and relaxation techniques may be employed to control discomfort. Osteomyelitis may impair physical mobility. The nurse promotes range-of-motion, isotonic, and isometric exercises to maintain joint flexibility and muscle strength.

Patient education varies with the etiology of the osteomyelitis. Regardless of the etiology, prolonged bed rest and parenteral antibiotic therapy are part of the treatment plan. The nurse discusses the cause and treatment of osteomyelitis with the patient. Questions often arise, such as "how did I get this?" and "why can't I take antibiotics by mouth?" Encouragement and support of the patient and family are also necessary.

Evaluation/Documentation

Management of pain and the efficacy of nursing measures are documented. The nurse monitors for complications of bed rest.

Ongoing Care

Parenteral antibiotic therapy in association with bed rest generally arrests the course of osteomyelitis. Home health nursing is important to the patient receiving intravenous therapy and to assess and eval-

PATIENT EDUCATION GUIDE
Home Antibiotic Therapy for Patient With Osteomyelitis

Medical asepsis
Antibiotics
  Preparation
  Mixture
  Dosage
  Side effects
Site care
  Inspection
  Dressing changes
  Complications
Equipment
  Setup
  Flow rate regulation
  Catheter patency
  Complications
Storage
  Antibiotics
  Equipment
Resources
  "Help" numbers

uate the patient's response to intravenous therapy (see Patient Education Guide). Follow-up medical care, coordination with community agencies, and social services for financial assistance during the prolonged recuperation are other aspects of the ongoing care.

OSTEITIS DEFORMANS
Definition

Osteitis deformans, also known as Paget's disease, is characterized by accelerated bone resorption with resulting cavities in the lamellar bone.[35] Pagetic bone is susceptible to fracture and deformity.

Etiology/Epidemiology

The incidence of osteitis deformans increases with advancing age. It is more common in males than females. A familial connection has been noted among siblings. A high disease incidence has been reported in Great Britain, the United States, Western Europe, and Australia.[35] Whereas the cause of osteitis deformans is unknown, investigations suggest a possible slow viral infection. Evidence supporting this hypothesis is the presence of intranuclear inclusions in the osteoclasts of pagetic bone.[30]

TABLE 58-12   Pharmacology Summary: Osteitis Deformans

Drug	Disorder	Dosage	Side effects	Nursing implications
Calcitonin	Osteitis deformans	50 to 100 I.U. daily	Nausea Flushing Feeling of warmth	Monitor serum alkaline and urinary hydroxyproline excretion Salmon calcitonin hormone approved for use in United States
Plicamycin	Osteitis deformans	15 μg/kg daily for 10 days	Thrombocytopenia Elevated serum glutamic-oxaloacetic transaminase (SGOT), blood urea nitrogen (BUN), and creatinine Anorexia Nausea/vomiting	Contraindicated for patients with impaired bone marrow function Cytotoxic
Etidronate sodium	Osteitis deformans	5 to 10 mg/kg daily for no longer than 6 months	Gastrointestinal irritation Diarrhea Metallic taste or loss of taste Abdominal discomfort	Cautious use with impaired renal function Large doses may result in fracture or osteomalacia Contraindicated with immobilized patients

Modified from Krane SM: Disorders of bone and mineral metabolism. In Braunwald E et al, editors: *Harrison's principles of internal medicine*, ed 11, New York, 1987, McGraw-Hill, Inc; Ross DG: Paget's disease, *Orthop Nurs* 3(3):43, 1984.

Pathophysiology

In Paget's disease, bone resorption is increased with a subsequent increase in bone formation. The bone formation is replaced by dense trabecular bone with decreased vascularity. The end result is a cavity-filled lamellar bone. A characteristic mosaic pattern results from an intermixing of bone.[2]

Clinical Manifestations

Ninety percent of the patients are asymptomatic. Some patients complain of pain in the lower extremities or head, depending on the affected bone tissue.[35] Bones most commonly affected are the skull, lumbar spine, sacrum, pelvis, and femur. Visual and auditory loss and nerve compression may also occur. Pseudofractures, pathologic fractures, and bone deformity may develop. Diagnostic laboratory findings for osteitis deformans include an elevated serum alkaline phosphatase and urinary hydroxyproline excretion. Microfractures, pseudofractures, and a characteristic mosaic pattern in the pagetic bone may be seen on x-ray examination.

Therapeutic Management

Therapeutic management of the patient with osteitis deformans depends on the severity of the pain and bone deformity. Aspirin and NSAIDs are administered for mild to moderate pain. Calcitonin and etidronate sodium may be administered to decrease bone resorption if disease involvement is severe (Table 58-12). The cytotoxic drug plicamycin is used to inhibit bone resorption.[2] Total hip replacement may be performed for debilitating hip involvement.

NURSING MANAGEMENT OF THE PATIENT WITH OSTEITIS DEFORMANS
Assessment

The nurse assesses for pain, complaints of fatigue, and progression of skeletal deformity. Bowlegs, decrease in stature, and enlargement of the skull are just some of the bony defects that may develop. Pathologic fractures often accompany this disorder.

Nursing Diagnosis

Nursing diagnoses for the patient with osteitis deformans include:

Pain related to pathologic fractures

High risk for injury related to bone demineralization

Altered body image related to skeletal deformities

Planning

Expected outcome for the patient with osteitis deformans is as follows:

Patient will be able to explain the treatment program, including pertinent information regarding medications

Implementation

Patient education includes instruction in the nature of the disorder and treatment factors. In addition, patients and families are taught about the medications, including the dosage, indications for use, frequency, and possible side effects. Emphasis is placed on safety factors in the home and basic first aid for injuries or fractures that may occur. Other nursing measures are summarized in Table 58-2.

Ongoing Care

The incidence of osteitis deformans increases with age. Ongoing care of patients addresses the increased potential for injury and fracture as a result of the disease. Safety factors and an assessment of the home environment for hazards are pertinent. First aid and emergency telephone numbers in the event of injury are reviewed with the patient and family. As the disease involvement continues, coordination of care with other health professionals, such as occupational and physical therapists, and social services may be investigated.

LOW BACK PAIN
Definition

Low back pain is a common health problem and a significant cause of morbidity. Millions of dollars are spent each year for treatments, disability costs, and time lost from work. Low back pain is either acute or chronic pain that originates in the low lumbar, lumbosacral, or sacroiliac area of the back. The back is the most likely part of the body to be injured in job-related accidents. Back injuries are as likely to occur in office workers as in physically active workers. Back pain is the leading cause of restricted movement for people under 45 years of age.

Etiology/Epidemiology

Approximately 80% of the population will experience low back pain during their lifetimes. Women may experience back pain beginning in middle age. Men are affected at an earlier age.

Occupations requiring repetitive bending, lifting, or twisting motions or exposure to continuous vibrations may precipitate low back pain. Gymnasts, weight lifters, football linemen, golfers, and tennis players have a higher incidence of low back pain when compared to the general population.

The following spinal abnormalities may contribute to low back pain:

1. Spondylolisthesis: forward slip of affected vertebral body related to inherited anatomic variations
2. Spondylolysis: defect in the pars of the vertebra, most commonly in the fifth lumbar vertebra
3. Ankylosing spondylitis: disorder resulting in progressive fusion of vertebrae
4. Scoliosis: lateral curvature of the spine
5. Kyphosis: round back
6. Lordosis: swayback

Tumors, compression fractures, and infection may also cause low back pain. There may be a link between low back pain and cigarette smoking. It is believed that smoking leads to decreased oxygenation to the disk, which interferes with the repair process and allows for faster degeneration.

Other possible causes include obesity, poor posture and body mechanics, injuries, arthritic inflammation, stress-related tensions, osteomyelitis, and osteoporosis. Disorders of the reproductive and urinary systems may also produce low back pain.

Pathophysiology

The pathophysiology relates to the specific cause. Generally, any condition that puts pressure on the nerves branching out from the spinal cord or vertebral muscles may cause low back pain. Obesity and poor posture and body mechanics overextend muscles, resulting in muscle strain. Emotional upsets can cause muscle spasms. Low back pain from muscle strain is usually worse with activity such as bending or lifting. The pain is localized in the lower back with pain referred to the buttocks and thighs. Nerve root irritation (radiculopathy), on the other hand, may not necessarily be associated with movement and may be worse in the leg than the back and worse at night.

Rheumatoid arthritis and osteoarthritis are painful diseases caused by vertebral inflammation. The low back pain associated with osteomyelitis and osteoporosis relates to the change in the vertebral tissue as a result of the infectious or demineralization process. Injuries may result in muscle strain or damage the vertebral disks with resulting pressure on the spinal nerves.

Clinical Manifestations

Patients with low back pain complain of pain ranging from mild discomfort of a few hours to chronic debilitating pain. Other clinical manifestations may include an altered gait and standing or sitting with a preference for the "good" side over the affected side.

Although not performed as frequently as in the past, a myelogram may be used to determine structural spinal defects. It is an invasive test that requires the use of a radiopaque dye injected into the dural space followed by x-ray films. Computerized tomography (CT) scan and magnetic resonance imaging (MRI) are most commonly used in diagnosing the cause of the low back pain. The CT scan visualizes bone and disk abnormalities in and around the canal. The MRI, in addition to determining structural defects, can visualize soft tissue and define healthy from scar tissue.

Therapeutic Management

Therapeutic management of low back pain ranges from promoting good body mechanics to surgery. Initially the restriction of activities, bed rest, and application of heat and cold may be attempted for pain control. Pelvic traction may be used in an effort to maintain bed rest. Extended bed rest is, however, nontherapeutic. Two days of bed rest are as effective as 7 days and do not result in the complications that 7 days or more of bed rest may cause. Pharmacologic treatment includes salicylates, NSAIDs, and corticosteroids to relieve pain and decrease inflammation (see Table 58-4). Occasionally muscle relaxants are given to decrease muscle spasms. Regardless of the intervention used, there is little difference in the outcome.

Primary treatment for low back pain involves three modalities:
1. Correct poor posture (slouching, rounded shoulders), which results in excess forward curve in the lower back.
2. Participate in exercise to strengthen weak abdominal and back muscles.
3. Lose excess weight, especially a potbelly, which exerts a constant forward pull on the back muscles and further weakens abdominal muscles.

Corsets and braces are often used to immobilize the spine. They may be effective in assisting the patient to ambulate with a minimum of discomfort.

They do not, however, completely immobilize the spine and may lead to further muscle weakness.

Should surgical intervention for herniated nucleus pulposus, also known as herniated disk, be required, a laminectomy, discectomy, or other surgical decompression is performed (see Chapter 50 for further discussion).

NURSING MANAGEMENT OF THE PATIENT WITH LOW BACK PAIN
Assessment

The nurse assesses for the degree, location, and type of pain. Limitations in mobility are also assessed. The following are examples of questions the nurse might ask to elicit this information:
- What were you doing when you first felt the pain?
- Was the onset of pain gradual or sudden?
- What makes the pain better or worse?
- Is leg pain associated with the back pain?
- Is there paresthesia, numbness, or tingling present?

Inspection for asymmetry, kyphosis, lordosis, and scoliosis is performed. The nurse evaluates muscle weakness by having the patient walk on toes and heels, squat, and extend toes. The nurse assesses for nerve irritation or compression by passive straight leg raising and dorsiflexion of the foot. Straight leg raising from a supine position is positive if it elicits leg pain. The nurse also assesses for the patient's understanding of good body mechanics.

Nursing Diagnosis

Nursing diagnoses for low back pain include the following:

Pain related to muscle spasms, inflammation, and the specific physical problem

Altered health maintenance related to knowledge deficit regarding body mechanics, medications, and exercises

LOW BACK PAIN PREVENTION GUIDELINES

Stay physically fit
Avoid or stop smoking
Avoid obesity
Use good body mechanics
Modify environment/workplace
Use common sense (think before acting)
Begin exercising slowly and increase gradually

Planning

Expected outcomes for the patient with low back pain are as follows:

The patient will report a reduction or relief of pain and/or muscle spasms

The patient will demonstrate use of proper body mechanics, medication administration, and exercises

Implementation

Nursing interventions address pain management and maintenance of physical mobility. Measures to control pain include the use of hot and cold compresses, bed rest or limitation of activities, TENS, and the administration of prescribed medications. A bag of frozen peas or crushed ice wrapped in a towel conforms to the shape of the back and provides analgesia as well as helps to decrease swelling. Endogenous opioids are secreted in response to diversionary activities, relaxation techniques, and exercises (see Table 58-3). Patient teaching is an integral part of the nursing care of low back pain. Patient education sessions include a review of proper body mechanics specific to the individual's daily activities, the use of straight-backed chairs, and positioning of the knees higher than the hips when sitting (see box). Use of a firm bed board and weight control to prevent muscle strain are also stressed. Contraindications to be discussed are prolonged standing or sitting, lying prone, and the wearing of high heels. These activities exacerbate back pain. Recreational exercise, such as walking, helps relax and

PATIENT EDUCATION GUIDE
Back Exercises

Back roll

The back roll stretches your back, buttocks, and neck muscles. Lie on your back on the floor, relax, and bring your knees to your chest. Clasp your hands behind your knee and rock back and forth, from your buttocks to your neck. Slowly return to the starting position. Repeat 5 to 10 times.

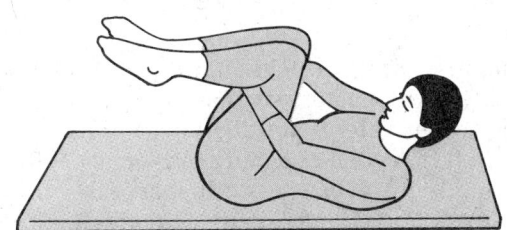

Partial sit-ups

Partial sit-ups strengthen your abdominal muscles. Lie flat on your back on the floor with your knees bent and feet flat on the floor. Tuck in your chin and tighten your abdomen. Slowly raise your head and neck while reaching out with your hands to touch your knees. Hold your knees for a count of five and slowly return to the starting position. Repeat 5 to 10 times.

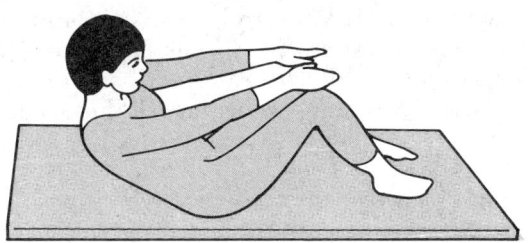

Pelvic tilt

The pelvic tilt strengthens your abdominal and back muscles. Lie flat on your back on the floor with your knees bent and feet flat on the floor. Join your hands behind your head. Firmly tighten your buttock and abdominal muscles, pressing your lower back flat against the floor. Hold for a count of five and relax muscles. Repeat 5 to 10 times.

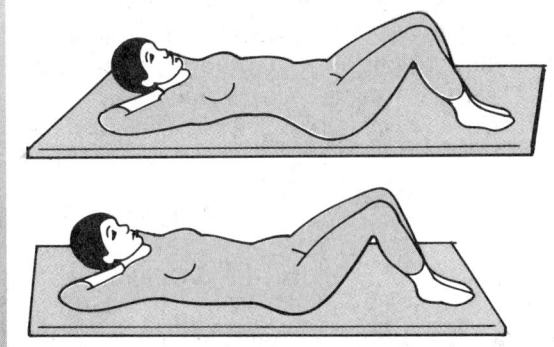

strengthen muscles. Repetition of prescribed back exercises, such as the pelvic tilt, partial sit-ups, and back rolls, will strengthen the muscles that protect the spine and will prevent back strain. Each exercise is done five times and gradually increased to ten times. The patient is told to discontinue any exercise that is painful and to seek professional advice before continuing the exercise (see patient education guide). Instruct the patient to maintain William's position (see Chapter 57 for a diagram of William's position) when lying supine and to place a pillow between the legs when in a side-lying position. This intervention takes the stress off the lower back.

Evaluation/Documentation

The plan is effective when the patient's pain is controlled and the patient develops effective methods of managing continuing pain. The nurse documents the patient's knowledge and use of proper body mechanics and exercises as well as the correct use of medications.

Ongoing Care

Low back pain is often associated with a patient's established life-style. Factors such as poor body mechanics, being overweight, and lack of exercise facilitate low back pain. The ongoing nursing care focuses on the patient's awareness of these issues and how their correction would significantly decrease discomfort and prevent further injury. Other professionals such as physical therapists and vocational rehabilitators may be employed. Physical therapists can assist with exercise and treatment modalities. Vocational rehabilitators offer career counseling if the injury prevents a return to the patient's previous occupation. The nurse coordinates these services.

HALLUX VALGUS
Definition

Hallus valgus, more commonly known as **bunion** (Figure 58-12), is a deformity of the great toe and first metatarsal head. Although not a serious joint problem, hallux valgus is a common, painful foot problem.[24] Hallux valgus occurs more often in women, with female/male ratios ranging from 9:1 to 40:1.[24,26]

Etiology

Etiologic factors implicated in the development of bunions include congenital disorders such as limb bud deficiency in infants, flatfoot deformities, rheumatoid arthritis, and cerebral palsy. Familial tendencies to develop bunions have been noted.[24] A

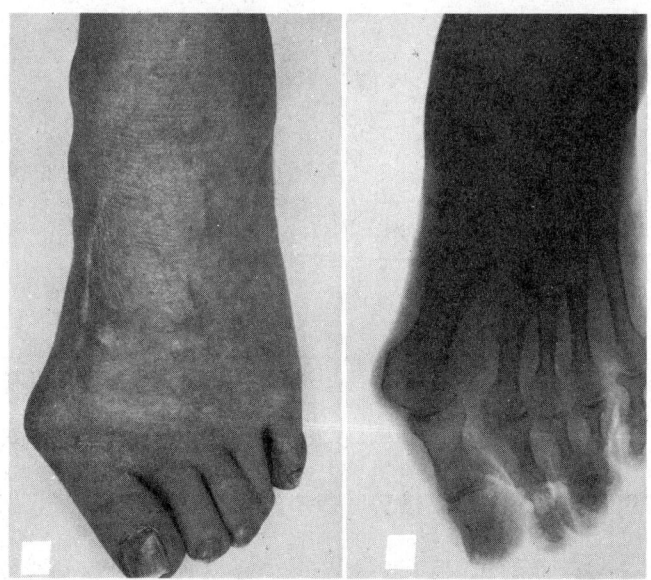

FIGURE 58-12 Hallux deformity. (From Brashear HR, Raney RB: *Handbook of orthopaedic surgery*, ed 10, St Louis, 1986, Mosby–Year Book, Inc.)

common misconception is that ill-fitting shoes result in bunions. Hallux valgus may develop in one or both feet.

Metatarsophalangeal joint heads may vary in shape, making them more susceptible to lateral deviation. The first metatarsophalangeal head may deviate as a result of pronation changes. The patient pushes off with the second and third metatarsal heads rather than the first metatarsophalangeal joint when walking. A bunion will develop as a result of the pressure on the deviated first metatarsophalangeal head.[7,15]

The patient with bunions exhibits corns and calluses, limited joint range of motion, and difficulty with shoes as a result of pain. Discomfort may vary from slight to extreme pain.

Therapeutic Management

Therapeutic management of bunions will range from avoiding pointed, closed-toe shoes to surgical excision of the bunion. Molded shoes, while costly and not cosmetically appealing, are comfortable. If the pain increases and walking becomes difficult, then a bunionectomy may be performed. The length of stay for a bunionectomy depends on the physician, patient, and reimbursement policies. Hospitalization may range from outpatient surgery to a 3- to 5-day stay. Pain is managed with NSAIDs and TENS units. An open-toe, laced, wooden-sole shoe is worn for approximately 1 month, followed by a tennis shoe.

NURSING MANAGEMENT OF THE PATIENT WITH HALLUX VALGUS

Assessment

Nursing assessment of the patient with bunions includes joint deviation, pain, and limitation of joint mobility. The nurse determines how the bunions affect ambulation and the patient's vocational and recreational interests. The patient is also assessed for changes in body image.

Nursing Diagnosis

Nursing diagnoses for the patient with hallux valgus include the following:

Pain (acute) related to joint deformity

Mobility impaired, related to joint deformity

Planning

Expected outcomes for the patient with hallux valgus include the following:

Pain is managed or relieved

Mobility is maintained

Implementation

Nursing interventions to decrease patient discomfort include limited weight bearing during painful periods, the avoidance of poorly fitting shoes, the wearing of shoes conforming to the deformity, and shoe padding in the area of the bunion. To promote joint mobility, nurses advocate range-of-motion exercise. Finding comfortable and attractive shoes for the patient aids in maintaining a positive self-image. If pain is not controlled, surgery may be considered.

Evaluation

To determine the effectiveness of the plan, the nurse evaluates how well the patient is managing the pain and any alteration in mobility.

Documentation

The nurse documents patient reports of pain and the effectiveness of nursing measures to alleviate the pain. Further, a notation is made of any impairment in mobility and the effectiveness of nursing actions to promote joint mobility.

Degenerative Muscle Disease

MUSCULAR DYSTROPHY

Definition

Muscular dystrophy is a group of genetically inherited disorders characterized by progressive weakness and muscle fiber degeneration without neural involvement.

Etiology/Epidemiology

The overall incidence for the muscular dystrophies is 0.7 per 100,000, and the prevalence is 10 per 100,000. Some types are more common than others; Duchenne's dystrophy and myotonic dystrophy account for more than 60% of current cases (Table 58-13). The weakness can appear from 2 years old to adulthood. The rate of progression varies from rapid to slow, and many persons live a normal life span. Although the exact etiology is unknown, a genetic defect is hypothesized as the cause.

Pathophysiology

The most significant finding in muscular dystrophy is skeletal muscle deterioration; however, vital organs such as the cardiac smooth muscles may be affected, leading to serious disability and premature deaths. As the disease progresses, muscles atrophy and form contractures. Muscle fibers degenerate, with fat and connective tissue replacing muscle fibers, which leads to severe muscle weakness.[3] Over time regeneration slows and degeneration dominates.[13]

Clinical Manifestations

The musculoskeletal manifestations are fairly uniform. The patient goes through three definable stages: ambulatory, wheelchair mobility, and bed bound. The illness progresses at variable rates. Generally, muscle weakness is severe, with only mild to moderate muscle atrophy. Most dystrophies preferentially involve the proximal hip and shoulder girdle musculature. This leads to functional difficulties such as raising the arms above the head, rising from a chair, walking, and running. When distal muscles are affected, footdrop and falls are common. Contractures occur when the patient is unable to complete range-of-motion exercises. When the patient is no longer able to stand or walk, scoliosis develops and contractures interfere with comfort.

The diagnosis of muscular dystrophy is made based on serum enzyme measurement, muscle tissue biopsy, and electromyography. The serum creatine phosphokinase (skeletal muscle, CPK-MM) levels are elevated. This elevation is related to the muscle degeneration, which may cause the serum CPK-MM to be elevated 20 to 400 times normal. In long-term, chronic, mild disease, the CPK-MM level may return to normal or near normal.[3] The muscle biopsy indicates muscle tissue degeneration and necrosis of the muscle fibers. Last, electromyography is done to determine nerve conduction and muscle

TABLE 58-13 Types and Characteristics of Muscular Dystrophy

Types	Gender/age of presentation	Manifestations	Associated symptoms	Progression
Duchenne's	Males/3 to 5 years Female carrier with Turner's syndrome	Weakened pelvic muscles Wide stance/waddling gait (Gower's sign) Muscle atrophy (may have enlarged calves) Lordosis Protuberant abdomen Scapular "winging" when arms raised	Contractures; cardiac and respiratory symptoms Nonprogressive mental retardation	Rapid with death in late adolescence from respiratory complications
Becker's	Males/early adolescence Female carrier with Turner's syndrome	Similar to Duchenne's without cardiac manifestations	Crippling disability approximately 25 years after initial symptoms	Slow; near normal life span
Myotonic	Males and females in young adulthood	Myotonia (inability to relax muscles following contractions) Atrophy of hands; forearms and face muscles are affected Late stages: lower leg muscles affected Swan neck (lower part of face narrows and neck curves forward)	Cataracts, cardiac symptoms	Lives into fifth decade and death occurs from cardiac complications
Fascioscapulo-humeral	Males and females from 6 to 30 years	Atrophy and weakness of shoulder, face, and eyes Pelvis affected in late stage		Progresses slowly with normal life span
Limb-girdle (scapulohumeral and pelvifemoral)	Males and females in late childhood and young adulthood	Atrophy and weakness of hip and shoulder muscles		Degenerative changes usually do not progress Normal life span

Modified from Carey KW: *Muscle disorders: nurse review,* Philadelphia, Pa, 1990, Springhouse.

innervation. If this test indicates nerve conduction, neurogenic muscle atrophy is ruled out.

Therapeutic Management

There is currently no cure for muscular dystrophy; therefore therapeutic management focuses on managing the symptoms and delaying the progression of the altered mobility.

NURSING MANAGEMENT OF THE PATIENT WITH MUSCULAR DYSTROPHY

Assessment

The nurse assesses the patient's muscle strength and degree of mobility. The development of any contractures is noted. Cardiovascular and respiratory as-

sessments are done to determine any smooth muscle involvement of the organs.

Nursing Diagnosis

A nursing diagnosis for the patient with muscular dystrophy is as follows:

Altered health maintenance related to muscle weakness and contractures

Planning

The expected outcome for the patient with muscular dystrophy is as follows:

To remain as independent and self-sufficient as possible for as long as possible

Implementation

Currently there is no known drug or therapy that can cure or arrest the progression of muscular dystrophy. Thus nursing interventions are primarily supportive. Anticipation of problems and monitoring progression and adaptation to a reduced level of function are key in preventing complications. Many patients lead long and productive lives with proper management.

When the patient is ambulatory, enhancing self-care abilities and developing an exercise regimen are critical. If the patient cannot perform active exercises, standing and walking opportunities are made available for stretching exercises. Splinting of the arms and legs at night will help to slow the progression of contractures. If the patient falls, a review of the event is necessary to determine possible changes in care, such as the need for a helmet, braces, canes, walkers, or clothing, shoe, and environmental adaptations. If the patient is wheelchair mobile or bed bound, comfort care becomes critical. Many individuals have hip flexion contractures that allow them to be positioned only on their sides. Bolsters, pillows, and frequent repositioning are required to maintain comfort and prevent pressure ulcers. An alternating pressure mattress or water bed may also provide comfort. Frequent skin assessment is necessary to determine evidence of breakdowns. The use of support stockings, passive exercise, and leg elevation may decrease pedal edema for patients in wheelchairs.

Self-care can be facilitated by the use of assistive devices. If the patient has limited hand strength, a pressure-sensitive call bell may be necessary. Placing the patient close to the nurses' station for observation may be considered if pulmonary function and reduced strength prevent the patient from calling for assistance.

If surgery (fasciotomy and tendon lengthening) is considered, it is done to assist the patient in maintaining quality of life. Preoperative and postoperative preparation is essential to prevent complications. Monitoring the respiratory and cardiac status is important to prevent postoperative complications. Early ambulation is essential following surgery because inactivity for 1 day can speed degeneration and weakness.

Nursing care that supports good nutritional practices is essential in that obesity can increase the caregiver burden and risk of injury and cause further respiratory compromise. A diet high in fiber, fluids, and protein will assist in maintaining bladder habits and prevent constipation. Patients and their families also require ongoing emotional support and genetic counseling. As with any chronic disease, maintaining independence is essential to a positive self-esteem and prevention of a helpless and hopeless attitude.

CRITICAL THINKING QUESTIONS

1 Discuss at least two classifications of arthritis and give examples of each classification.
2 Discuss four major medication groups used to treat arthritis.
3 What are the five factors that contribute to the development of osteoporosis?
4 Discuss in detail the pathophysiology of any of the following musculoskeletal disorders: arthritis, osteoporosis, osteomalacia, osteitis deformans, and muscular dystrophy.
5 What are the nursing interventions for patients with chronic musculoskeletal disorders specific to home care management?
6 What are the special implications for the aged adult with rheumatoid arthritis?
7 Formulate a nursing care plan for a patient with a total hip replacement.
8 Discuss the effects of osteomyelitis on the skeletal system.
9 Describe nursing measures for the patient with low back pain.
10 Identify a teaching plan for the patient with hallux valgus.
11 Describe the types of muscular dystrophy.

RESOURCES

1 ARTHRITIS FOUNDATION
1314 Spring Street, NW
Atlanta, GA 30309
2 ARTHRITIS INFORMATION CLEARING-HOUSE
PO Box 9782
Arlington, VA 22209
3 NATIONAL INSTITUTE OF ARTHRITIS AND MUSCULOSKELETAL AND SKIN DISEASES
National Institutes of Health
Bethesda, MD 20892
4 NATIONAL OSTEOPOROSIS FOUNDATION
1625 I Street, NW, Suite 1011
Washington, DC 20006
5 PAGET'S DISEASE FOUNDATION
PO Box 2772
Brooklyn, NY 11202

BIBLIOGRAPHY

Current

1. Blanchard DS: What women can do to protect against osteoporosis, *RN*, pp 61-62, Oct 1990.
2. Braunwald E et al, editors: *Harrison's principles of internal medicine,* ed 11, New York, 1987, McGraw-Hill Book Co.
3. Carey KW: *Muscle disorders: nurse review,* Philadelphia, 1990, Springhouse.
4. Carpenito LJ: *Handbook of nursing diagnosis,* ed 4, New York, 1991, JB Lippincott Co.

5. Decker JL, editor: *Understanding and managing arthritis,* New York, 1987, Avon—The Hearst Corporation.
6. Deutsch P, Sawyer H, editors: *A guide to rehabilitation,* New York, 1987, Times Mirror.
7. Doleysh N: *Arthritis disease: joint inflammation. Nurse review,* Philadelphia, 1990, Springhouse.
8. Dunajcik LM: The hip: when the joint must be replaced, *RN* (4):62, June 1989.
9. Fox IH et al: Management decisions in hyperuricemia, *Patient Care,* p 93, Sept 1986.
10. Holm K, Walker J: Osteoporosis: treatment and prevention update, *Geriatr Nurs* 11(3):141, 1990.
11. Hough D et al: Patient education for total hip replacement, *Nurs Management* 22(3):801, 1991.
12. Lewis CB, Knortz KA: *Orthopedic assessment and treatment of the geriatric patient,* St Louis, 1993, Mosby—Year Book, Inc.
13. Lewis J: How to help your patients with muscular dystrophy, *Nurs 91,* p 32, June 1991.
14. McCance KL, Huether SE: *Pathophysiology: the biologic basis for disease in adults and children,* St Louis, 1990, Mosby—Year Book, Inc.
15. Mourad L: *Orthopedic disorders,* St Louis, 1991, Mosby—Year Book, Inc.
16. O'Toole M, editor: *Encyclopedia and dictionary of medicine, nursing, and allied health,* ed 5, Philadelphia, 1992, WB Saunders Co.
17. Pagana KD, Pagana TJ: *Mosby's diagnostic and laboratory test reference,* St Louis, 1992, Mosby—Year Book, Inc.
18. Pozzi M, Peck N: An option for the patient with chronic osteomyelitis: home intravenous therapy, *Orthop Nurs* 5(5):9, 1986.
19. Resnick D, Niwayama G: *Diagnosis of bone and joint disorders,* ed 2, Philadelphia, 1987, WB Saunders Co.
20. Sands JK: *Clinical manual of medical surgical nursing,* ed 2, St Louis, 1991, Mosby—Year Book, Inc.
21. Swearingen PL: *Manual of nursing therapeutics,* ed 2, St Louis, 1990, Mosby—Year Book, Inc.
22. Thompson JM et al: *Mosby's clinical nursing,* ed 3, St Louis, 1993, Mosby—Year Book, Inc.
23. Urrows ST et al: Profiles in osteoporosis, *Am J Nurs,* p 33, Dec 1991.

Classic
24. Bartell L: Bunionectomies, *Orthop Nurs* 4(1):21, 1985.
25. Beeson PB, McDermott W, editors: *Cecil-Loeb textbook of medicine,* ed 16, Philadelphia, 1982, WB Saunders Co.
26. Berger MR: Bunions: an overview, *Orthop Nurs* 5:17, 1984.
27. Gleit CG, Graham BA: The role of calcium and estrogen in osteoporosis, *Orthop Nurs* 4(3):13, 1985.
28. Hawley D, editor: Symposium on arthritis and related rheumatic diseases, *Nurs Clin North Am* 19(4):565, 1984.
29. Hilt N, Cogburn S: *Manual of orthopedics,* St Louis, 1980, Mosby—Year Book, Inc.
30. Kelley WN et al, editors: *Textbook of rheumatology,* ed 2, Philadelphia, 1985, WB Saunders Co.
31. Koerner ME, Dickinson GR: Adult arthritis, *Am J Nurs,* p 253, Feb 1983.
32. Liddel D: An in depth look at osteoporosis, *Orthop Nurs* 4(3):23, 1985.
33. Meisel AD, Bullough PG, editors: *Atlas of osteoarthritis,* Philadelphia, 1984, Grover Medical.
34. National Institutes of Health: Osteoporosis: cause, treatment, prevention, *Orthop Nurs,* p 29, Nov/Dec 1985.
35. Ross D: Paget's disease, *Orthop Nurs* 3(4):47, 1984.
36. Stacy-Spencer E: Osteomalacia, *Orthop Nurs* 3(4):47, 1984.

UNIT XIV

Endocrine System

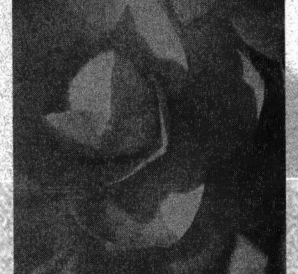

CHAPTER FIFTY-NINE

Nursing Assessment of the Endocrine System

LEARNING OBJECTIVES

1 Know the basic anatomic components of the endocrine system.
2 Describe the manner in which the hormones secreted by the endocrine glands regulate body functions.
3 Obtain relevant subjective information from patients who have selected endocrine system alterations.
4 Using correct technique, examine patients with selected endocrine system alterations and obtain appropriate objective information.
5 Differentiate abnormal from normal subjective and objective findings related to the selected aspects of the endocrine system.
6 Describe tests and procedures that are used in the diagnosis of endocrine system disorders.
7 Describe the patient care that is required for each of the tests and procedures used to diagnose endocrine system dysfunction.

KEY TERMS

corticotropin (ACTH), p. 1632
corticotropin releasing hormone (ACTH-RH), p. 1632
cortisol, p. 1632
exophthalmos, p. 1635
glucagon, p. 1633
glucocorticoid, p. 1632
glycosylated hemoglobin, p. 1652

growth hormone, p. 1631
insulin, p. 1633
melatonin, p. 1631
parathyroid hormone (PTH), p. 1633
thyrotropin (TSH), p. 1633
thyrotropin releasing hormone (TSH-RH), p. 1633

THE ENDOCRINE SYSTEM, with the nervous system, plays an essential part in regulating and integrating the functions of the body. The major endocrine glands include the pituitary (hypophysis), thyroid, parathyroids, adrenals, isles (islets) of Langerhans in the pancreas, and the gonads. Other endocrine glands are the pineal and the thymus (Figure 59-1). Most hormones, the chemical messengers of the endocrine system, diffuse through the interstitial fluid and are carried by the circulatory system from the endocrine glands to their target cells.

In addition to those hormones that are carried by the circulatory system, paracrine hormones act on cells close to their source before reaching the circu-

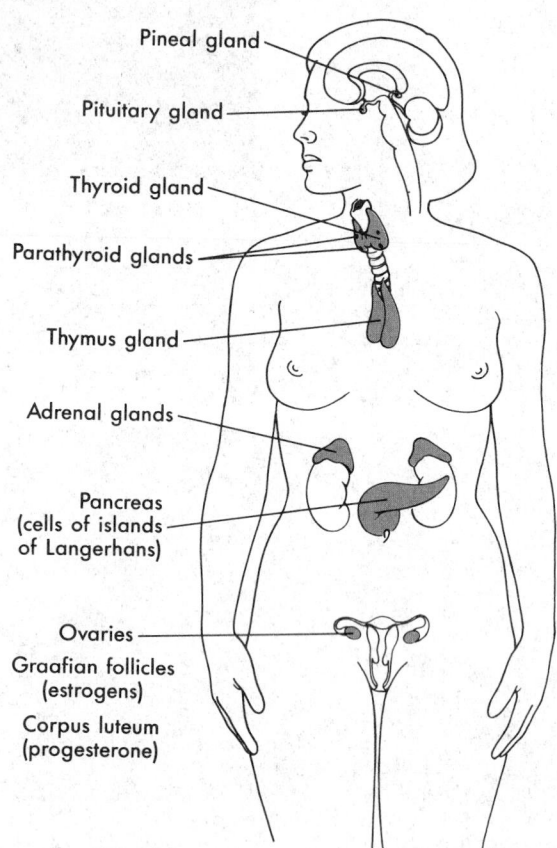

FIGURE 59-1   Location of endocrine glands.

Pineal gland
Pituitary gland
Thyroid gland
Parathyroid glands
Thymus gland
Adrenal glands
Pancreas
(cells of islands
of Langerhans)
Ovaries
Graafian follicles
(estrogens)
Corpus luteum
(progesterone)

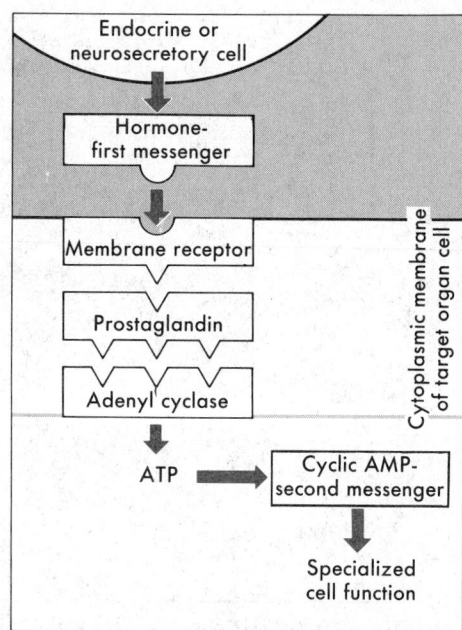

FIGURE 59-2   Mechanism of hormone action.

Endocrine or
neurosecretory cell
Hormone-
first messenger
Membrane receptor
Prostaglandin
Adenyl cyclase
Cytoplasmic membrane
of target organ cell
ATP
Cyclic AMP-
second messenger
Specialized
cell function

latory system. Other substances, such as prostaglandins, act as modulators, enhancing or reducing the effect that the hormones have on their target cells.

Endocrine system alterations occur at all stages of life. Dysfunction may be hereditary, congenital, or caused by trauma, environmental factors, or unknown etiology. Older adults develop fibrosis of the thyroid gland, pancreas, and possibly other endocrine glands. The endocrine glands of older adults may also be impaired because of the effects of arteriosclerosis.

The assessment focuses on whether the endocrine system is intact and functional. Throughout the examination the nurse notes pertinent negative as well as positive cues and seeks clues to the etiology of any reported or observed discrepancy. Reported precipitating and aggravating factors are also important in establishing the cause of endocrine system alterations.

ANATOMY AND PHYSIOLOGY
Mechanism of Hormone Action

Hormones act by changing the metabolism of the target cells in one of two ways—(1) by altering the permeability of the cell membrane to nutrients or

(2) by altering the rate of synthesis, activation, or inhibition of enzymes. In the latter a series of reactions is involved, and this often includes "second messengers," such as cyclic adenosine monophosphate (cAMP) (Figure 59-2), phosphatidylinositol, calcium ions, and calmodulin. Hormone action can be enhanced or diminished, because each reaction of the series has the potential to be speeded up or slowed down by other hormones or modulator substances in the cell. Hormone action may also be diminished by "down regulation," when the presence of high levels of a hormone reduces both the number of active receptors of that hormone on the cell membrane and their ability to bind the hormone.

For convenience, hormones can be divided into three categories according to the way in which the endocrine glands that secrete them are controlled by the nervous system:

1. Category one hormones are secreted by the neurohypophysis (posterior lobe of the pituitary gland), the adrenal medulla, and the pineal gland, which are part of the nervous system and are directly controlled by it.
2. Category two hormones are secreted by the adenohypophysis (anterior lobe of the pituitary gland), which is indirectly controlled by the nervous system through the hypothalamic hormones carried to it by the hypothalamohypophyseal portal system. The hormones of the adenohypophysis in turn control the secretion of certain hormones of glands such as the adrenal cortex, the thyroid gland, and the gonads (Figure 59-3).

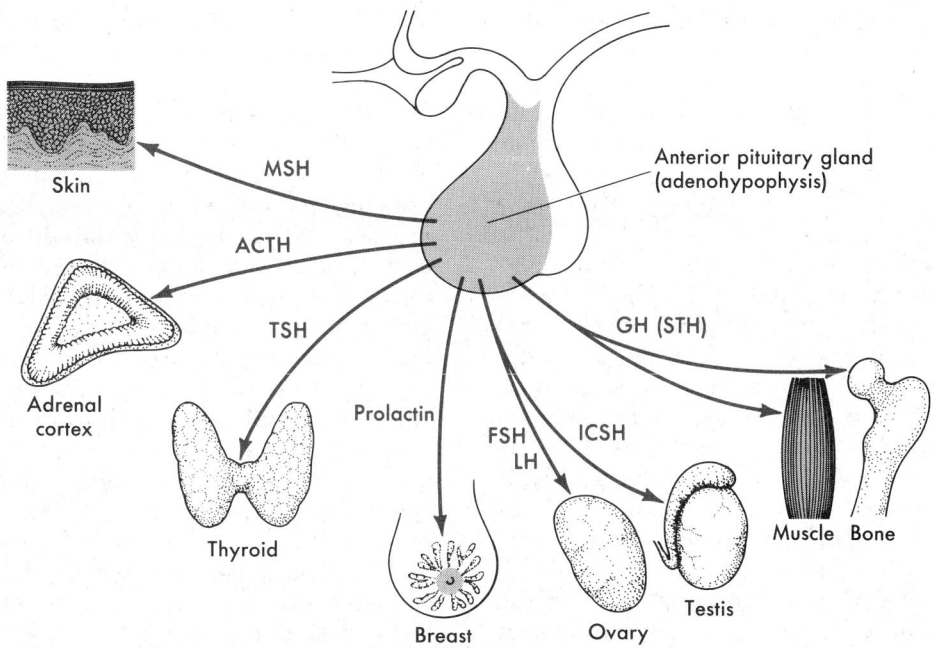

FIGURE 59-3   Target organs of adenohypophyseal hormones.

3. Category three hormones are secreted by the pancreas, the parathyroids, the C cells of the thyroid gland, and the aldosterone-secreting cells of the adrenal cortex, which are primarily controlled, not by the nervous system, but by the concentration of specific chemicals (e.g., calcium ions, glucose, and angiotensin II) in the interstitial fluid.

Hormones Secreted by Nervous System

The hormones of the posterior lobe of the pituitary gland and adrenal medulla are discussed elsewhere in this text: oxytocin with the reproductive system, antidiuretic hormone with the renal system, and epinephrine and norepinephrine with the nervous system. The pineal gland secretes melatonin.

Melatonin

Melatonin modulates the function of a wide range of metabolic activities to ensure that their timing is synchronized with the environmental light cycle. Blood concentrations are highest during the hours of darkness, and this serves to adapt the neuroendocrine system to daily and seasonal light rhythms. Melatonin has also been found to impede cell replication and enhance immune system function, and thus using melatonin or its antagonists may have important implications for health care in the future.

Hormones Indirectly Controlled by Nervous System

Growth hormone

Control of growth hormone

Growth hormone (GH) production by the adenohypophysis is dually controlled by two hypothalamic hormones: somatostatin, an inhibitor, and somatocrinin, a stimulator. The effect of this dual control is that GH is secreted in pulsatile surges. Its secretion is *increased* (1) during deep sleep and (2) by exercise, starvation, and stresses, such as trauma and hypoglycemia; and its secretion is *decreased* by hyperglycemia.

Mechanism of growth hormone action

GH is a protein that binds to receptors on the outer membrane of its target cells. It affects a wide range of cells directly and also indirectly through somatomedin, which is produced by the liver in response to GH stimulation. Somatomedins are essential for growth as is seen in Laron dwarfs, who, although they have high GH levels, do not grow because they lack the ability to synthesize somatomedins. Similarly, when the production of somatomedins is reduced during prolonged starvation, growth is impaired, and this has the advantage of conserving energy.

Directly, or indirectly through the somatomedins, GH stimulates cell growth by increasing the uptake of amino acids, which in turn stimulate the synthesis of new protein. In addition, GH provides the energy required for this synthesis by increasing the availability of fatty acids. In doing so it spares glucose, and blood glucose concentration may increase.

Cortisol

Control of cortisol

Cortisol is secreted by the fasciculata cells of the adrenal cortex when they are stimulated by **corticotropin (ACTH),** which is secreted by the adenohypophysis. In turn, ACTH secretion is stimulated by **corticotropin releasing hormone (ACTH-RH)** secreted by the hypothalamus.

Except when the individual is under high levels of stress, the secretion of both ACTH and ACTH-RH is inhibited by increases in the concentration of cortisol in the interstitial fluid of the adenohypophysis and hypothalamus. This inhibition by cortisol of the hormones controlling its release is an example of negative feedback (Figure 59-4). Stress-related stimulation of cortisol and ACTH by ACTH-RH, such as occurs during anesthesia, surgery, trauma, or psychologic upset, overrides the normal feedback control of the pituitary gland by cortisol.

Mechanism of cortisol action

In the circulatory system much of the cortisol is carried bound to a blood protein and is active only when it is released. Unbound cortisol is lipid soluble and therefore can enter cells easily and bind to its receptors located in the nucleus and cytoplasm.

Cortisol has many important effects on a wide range of body cells, but it is classified as a **glucocorticoid** hormone because a major effect is the conversion of protein to carbohydrate. Cortisol increases the destruction (catabolism) of body protein and the transportation of the resulting amino acids to the liver, where they are converted to glucose and glycogen. It also accelerates the mobilization of fats from adipose tissue and the use made of them for energy. Both of these effects increase the blood sugar level and are an important part of the body's reaction to fasting between meals. Cortisol is also required for proper functioning of muscle—deficiency causes muscle weakness, easy fatigability, and hypotension. It is important for cell membrane stability, wound healing, and the normal inflammatory response to tissue damage.

Because the effects of cortisol vary markedly with concentration, it is important to distinguish between the effects of normal concentrations of cortisol as listed above and of excessive concentrations, such as are produced by medication or disease. With excessive concentrations of cortisol, the catabolic effects on the peripheral tissues are exaggerated and cell growth and reproduction are inhibited. This results in impaired wound healing, a reduction in the inflammatory response, atrophy of the immune system, muscle weakness, and premature osteoporosis.

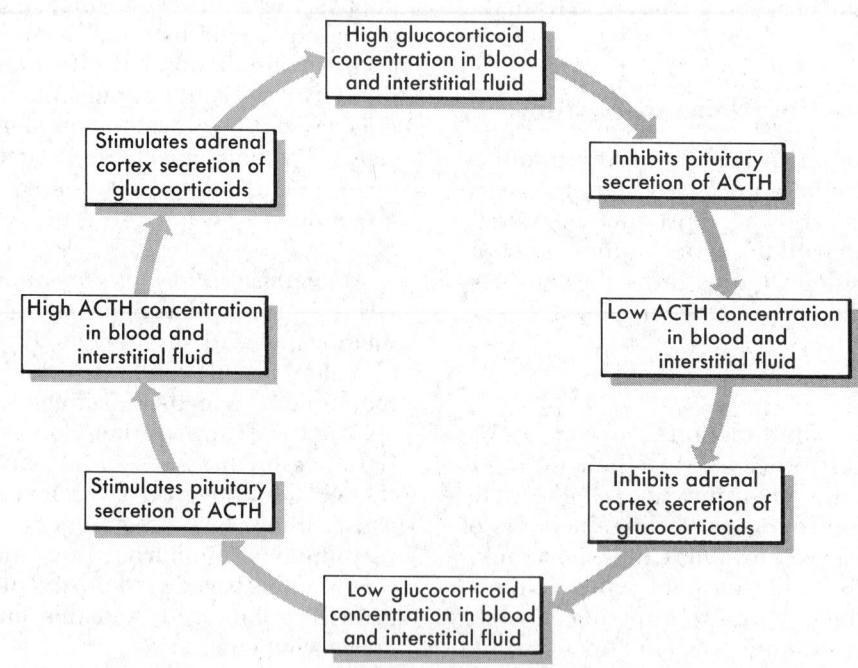

FIGURE 59-4   Negative feedback.

Thus the individual with excessively high concentrations of cortisol has a greater risk of infections, cancer, and ulceration of wounds.

Excessive concentrations of cortisol in the blood, such as are produced by prolonged glucocorticoid medication or adrenal disease, cause excessive negative feedback inhibition of the hypothalamic and adenohypophyseal secretion of ACTH-RH and ACTH. In the absence of ACTH, the adrenal cortices atrophy because the cells cannot maintain their normal metabolism. Therefore adrenal insufficiency develops when the medication is discontinued unless care is taken to reduce it gradually and to monitor the function of the adenohypophysis and the adrenal glands. Complete recovery from chronic suppression of the hypothalamohypophyseal-adrenocortical system may take 12 months or longer.

Thyroid hormones

Control of thyroid hormones

The thyroid hormones are secreted by the follicular cells of the thyroid when they are stimulated by **thyrotropin (TSH),** which is secreted by the adenohypophysis. In turn, TSH is stimulated by **thyrotropin releasing hormone (TSH-RH),** secreted by the hypothalamus, and is inhibited by somatostatin and dopamine. The secretion of both TSH and TSH-RH is inhibited by high levels of the thyroid hormones in the interstitial fluid of the adenohypophysis and hypothalamus (negative feedback).

TSH stimulates the thyroid gland to secrete the thyroid hormones that are stored in large follicles bound to thyroglobulin and stimulates all aspects of the metabolism, growth, vascularization, and function of the thyroid gland—particularly the active transport of iodine into the follicular cells and the synthesis of the thyroid hormones and thyroglobulin.

Mechanism of thyroid hormone action

Two thyroid hormones are secreted by the thyroid gland—tetraiodothyronine (T_4) and triiodothyronine (T_3). In the circulatory system they are carried bound to a blood protein and are active only when they are released. They are lipid soluble and therefore can enter cells easily and bind to their receptors located in the nucleus and cytoplasm.

The thyroid hormones increase the metabolism and energy requirements of all body cells and accentuate these effects by stimulating the sympathetic nervous system. T_3 is more potent than T_4, and normally T_4 is converted to T_3 in peripheral cells. However, this conversion and the stimulation of metabolism that it produces are reduced during severe illness, trauma, fasting, carbohydrate deprivation, and glucocorticoid treatment.

Hormones Controlled by Chemical Concentration

Hormones controlled by calcium concentration

The **parathyroid hormone (PTH)** is secreted by the small, oval parathyroid glands when the concentration of calcium ions falls. All the actions of PTH serve to increase this concentration—it stimulates the reabsorption of calcium from the bones, and it also stimulates the production by the kidney of 1,25-dihydroxycholecalciferol, the active form of vitamin D, which increases the absorption of calcium from the lumen of the digestive system and the reabsorption of calcium by the kidney tubules. The increased concentration of calcium that results removes the stimulus for the continued secretion of PTH.

The concentration of calcium ions in interstitial fluid is precisely maintained between 4.5 and 5.0 mEq/L. If the concentration falls below this level, cell function is seriously impaired because calcium is a catalyst for innumerable chemical reactions. If it rises above this level, calcium crystals are deposited in the bones and tissues.

Calcitonin is produced by the parafollicular C cells of the thyroid gland when they are stimulated by gastrin (a gastrointestinal hormone associated with the digestion of food) and by marked increases in calcium ion concentration. By inhibiting the reabsorption of bone, calcitonin allows bone formation to predominate.

The importance of calcitonin in normal blood calcium control is unclear because its effects on calcium metabolism are transitory, are not essential for survival, and are carried out more effectively by 1,25-dihydroxycholecalciferol, the active form of vitamin D, which is also involved in bone deposition.

Hormones controlled by glucose concentration

Insulin is secreted by the beta cells of the islets of Langerhans of the pancreas when blood sugar and, to a lesser extent, blood amino acid levels rise. Its secretion is stopped by negative feedback when the glucose concentration falls to or below normal.

Most of the cells of the body can use glucose only in the presence of insulin. Exceptions are endothelium, erythrocytes, and cells in the brain, kidney tubules, intestinal mucosa, and islets of Langerhans. Insulin stimulates the facilitated diffusion of glucose into the cells of the sensitive tissues and increases the activity of the enzymes responsible for the synthesis of glycogen, protein, and fat. These actions of insulin promote the utilization and storage of nutrients after a meal.

Glucagon is secreted by the alpha cells of the islets of Langerhans in response to a fall in the concentration of glucose or fatty acids in the interstitial fluid or in response to a rise in amino acid concen-

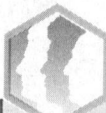

GERIATRIC CONSIDERATIONS

Physiologic Changes in the Endocrine System

With the exception of the ovarian hormones and to a lesser extent testicular hormones, and the changes that occur in the concentration of parathyroid hormones, the endocrine system normally functions well in elderly persons despite some changes in concentration. Blood levels of the anterior pituitary hormones (prolactin, TSH, and ACTH) are well maintained, but nocturnal pulses of growth hormone decline in individuals who have a decline in slow wave sleep. Blood thyroid and glucocorticoid concentrations are well maintained.

Blood insulin is in the normal range, but frequently glucose tolerance decreases with age. However, this may not be a function of age. It may be due to genetic predisposition of some individuals in the population to adult-onset diabetes and obesity, both associated with resistance to insulin. The renin-angiotensin system is less sensitive in older individuals.

The endocrine system is part of the total body coordinating system; however, it is unclear whether the endocrine system plays a key role in the aging process. It is not known whether the changes in the system are a cause of aging or are just due to some other age-related effect.

---

tration. Glucagon primarily affects the liver, where it stimulates the breakdown of fat and glycogen and the production of glucose from protein. Its secretion is stopped by negative feedback when the glucose concentration rises to or above normal.

The blood glucose concentration is maintained between 70 and 115 mg/dL. Minor increases are not harmful, and only one hormone, insulin, lowers blood glucose concentration. However, the consequences of a deficiency of glucose are life threatening. Glucose is the chief energy source for the brain, which can use ketone bodies for energy only after a long period of starvation. Consequently, it is essential that blood glucose be maintained, because below approximately 50 to 60 mg/dL, symptoms progress rapidly from irritability to fainting, convulsions, coma, and brain death.

To provide a safety factor, several hormones are responsible for raising blood sugar levels. These include GH, cortisol, and epinephrine.

ASSESSMENT
Subjective

A focused health history for a patient with a suspected or previously diagnosed endocrine problem requires the nurse to use knowledge of pathophysiology to guide questioning in an appropriate and complete manner. This is especially important to remember because endocrine disorders may present through diverse symptoms in a variety of body systems. Also, patients may not spontaneously report symptoms that can be elicited through directed questioning. The box on p. 1635 lists potential symptoms that should be reviewed with the patient. Any positive findings should be further evaluated by determining onset, frequency, duration, alleviating or aggravating factors, chronology of events, associated symptoms, precipitating factors, quantity or intensity of the symptom, and location (when appropriate). For example, Ms. Wang may complain of being unpleasantly aware of her heart beating rapidly (palpitations). The nurse would then discuss this positive finding with Ms. Wang using the above dimensions to determine that the palpitations first began approximately 2 months ago, lasted about 1 minute, and only occurred once or twice each week. Since that time, she notes that the palpitations have begun to occur more frequently and now experiences palpitations at least once each day. The duration of each episode has increased from about 1 minute to approximately 3 or 4 minutes. Nothing seems to cause the palpitations (precipitating factors) or make them better or worse (alleviating or aggravating factors). Ms. Wang reports that the palpitations may occur at any time of day and appear unrelated to activity level. Thus the nurse gains a much more complete perspective regarding the palpitations.

Relevant family history includes history of goiter, hypothyroidism, hyperthyroidism, autoimmune disease, diabetes, hypoglycemia, gestational diabetes, or Addison's disease.

Objective

Because endocrine disorders may manifest in a variety of body systems, the nurse needs to assess more than one body system. These systems may include integumentary, head and face, neck, cardiovascular, gastrointestinal, neurologic, genitourinary, and musculoskeletal. General assessment is significant in every patient and refers to the examiner's overall impression of the patient's state of health.

General assessment

Vital signs are always of value. Also note weight, facial expression, apparent age (relative to chrono-

POTENTIAL SYMPTOMS IN ENDOCRINE DISORDERS

General

Easy fatigability
Lethargy
Increased sleep requirement
Difficulty sleeping with frequent wakenings
Cold intolerance
Heat intolerance
Weight loss with increased appetite
Weight gain

Skin, hair, and nails

Dry, scaly skin
Patches of increased or decreased pigmentation
Hair loss (alopecia)
Coarse hair
Brittle nails

Head and face

Puffy face
Puffy eyelids
Red eyes
Change in appearance of eyes
Voice change: lower
Enlarging neck

Cardiovascular

Palpitations (conscious awareness of increased or forceful heartbeat)

Gastrointestinal

Constipation
Increased frequency of bowel movements
Polyphagia (excessive ingestion of food)
Dysphagia (difficulty in swallowing)
Polydipsia (excessive thirst)

Neurologic

Tremors
"Nervousness" or jitteriness
Memory loss
Depression (in elderly persons)
Decreased sensation in hands and feet

Genitourinary

Amenorrhea (no menses)
Menorrhagia (excessive or prolonged menses)
Oligomenorrhea (decrease in frequency of menses)
Polyuria (increased amount of urine)

Musculoskeletal

Muscle aching and weakness

---

logic age), nutritional status, general appearance, and stature. Note whether the patient appears to be comfortable or in distress.

Skin, hair, and nails

The skin is assessed for integrity, lesions, warmth, moisture, hair distribution, color, pigmentation, and turgor. Hair is assessed for presence, distribution pattern, texture, quantity, and quality. Nails are assessed for growth, curvature, adhesion, color, thickness, and clubbing.

Head and face

Observe the patient's head and face, noting symmetry and presence or absence of **exophthalmos** (abnormal protrusion of the eye from the orbit). Observe the patient opening and closing the eyes to determine the presence or absence of lid lag (eye and eyelid do not move together; lid lags behind eye in moving from an upward gaze to a downward gaze) or stare. Also note palpebral fissures (distance between the upper lid and the lower lid) and presence or absence of periorbital edema or generalized facial edema.

Neck

First observe the neck for symmetry, and note whether the trachea is midline or deviated. Palpate the neck to determine size, shape, consistency, and tenderness of the thyroid. Facilitate examination of the thyroid by providing a glass of water for the patient and by positioning the patient to relax the sternocleidomastoid muscle. Approach the patient anteriorly or posteriorly using a gentle touch. Have the patient take a sip of water and hold it until instructed to swallow. In the anterior approach, stand in front of the patient and gently place the pads of the first two fingers on the lower portion of the patient's neck. Locate the cricoid. The thyroid isthmus is located just below the cricoid (Figure 59-5). Displacing the thyroid slightly to the patient's right with your right hand, palpate the right lobe with your left hand as the patient swallows. Then, displacing the thyroid slightly to the patient's left, palpate the left lobe with your right hand as the patient swallows again.

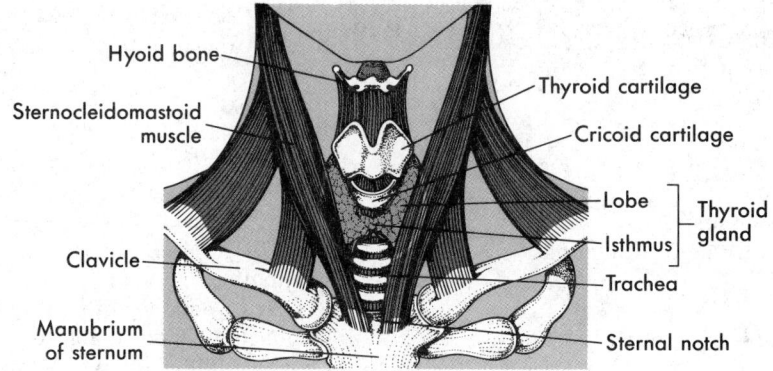

Hyoid bone

Sternocleidomastoid muscle

Clavicle

Manubrium of sternum

Thyroid cartilage

Cricoid cartilage

Lobe
Isthmus   } Thyroid gland

Trachea

Sternal notch

FIGURE 59-5   Landmarks of thyroid.

In the posterior approach, stand behind the patient and gently place your hands on the lower portion of the patient's neck with the pads of your fingers on the patient's trachea. Move your hands laterally to rest your fingers on either side. Displace the thyroid to each side, and palpate each lobe as the patient swallows. Some examiners advocate having the patient turn the head slightly toward the side being examined as well as slightly flexing the neck (Figures 59-6 and 59-7).

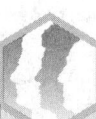

GERIATRIC CONSIDERATIONS

Endocrine Assessment

GENERAL APPROACH
- Allow more time than for a younger adult
- Articulate clearly; the geriatric patient may be hearing impaired
- Impaired sight, comprehension, or mobility may result in less than optimum cooperation
- Provide clear, concise instructions

HISTORY COLLECTION
- Be alert for answers that do not appear appropriate; the patient may not have understood the question correctly due to impaired hearing or impaired comprehension
- Some questions may need to be rephrased

PHYSICAL ASSESSMENT
- The physical examination itself is not different, but the approach needs to be altered such that the appropriate information is assessed without undue discomfort or embarrassment for the patient
- Maintain an enviroment with minimal noise, distractions, and interruption
- Thyroid hormone levels should always be assessesdistractions, and interuption
- Glucose to tolerance increases with age

Heart

Observe the anterior part of the chest for any heaves or thrusts. Palpate the anterior part of the chest for thrills and the apical impulse. Auscultate the precordium, noting the rate, rhythm, the first heart sound (S_1), and the second heart sound (S_2) as well as any extra sounds. (See Chapter 33 for a complete description of the examination of the heart.)

Extremities

Observe the extremities, noting skin and nail changes as above. To facilitate observation of fine tremors, have the patient extend the hands, palmar side down, with fingers extended and abducted. Place a piece of paper on the patient's hands, and note any movement of the paper.

Neurologic

A change in mental status may be a reflection of hypothyroidism, particularly in an elderly patient. Tools are available to facilitate rapid evaluation of mental status such as Folstein's Mini Mental Status Exam or the Short Portable Mental Status Questionnaire. Both of these tools evaluate cognitive function only. Emotional status may be evaluated through the use of a specific tool or in a more informal manner. (See Chapter 44 for a complete discussion of mental status assessment.)

Deep tendon reflexes may change as a result of endocrine imbalance. Therefore testing the deep tendon reflexes (DTRs) is appropriate. These include biceps, triceps, brachioradialis, patellar, and Achilles. Also note the presence or absence of ankle clonus. (See Chapter 44 for a complete discussion of neurologic assessment.)

Vibratory sensation may be decreased. Evaluate the patient's vibratory sensation using a 128 cps or 256 cps tuning fork. (See Chapter 44 for a complete discussion of neurologic assessment.)

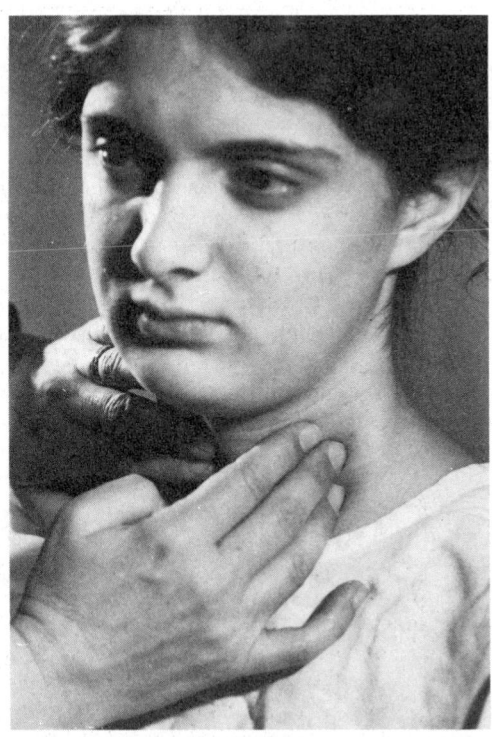

FIGURE 59-6 Anterior approach to thyroid examination. (From Malasanos L et al: *Health assessment,* ed 3, St Louis, 1986, Mosby–Year Book, Inc.)

DIAGNOSTIC AND LABORATORY TESTS
Thyroid Function Tests

Laboratory tests

A number of laboratory tests are useful in evaluating the functioning of thyroid gland (Table 59-1).

Thyroid scan

A thyroid scan (thyroid scintiscan) involves evaluation of the thyroid gland by a scintillation camera or scintiscanner after administration of a radioisotope of iodine or technetium. Areas of hyperactivity in the thyroid will show as gray or black regions or as "hot spots" (Figure 59-8), whereas areas of hypoactivity will show as white or light gray regions. In a normal scan the uptake of the radioisotope is uniform. The scan is useful in evaluating the size, structure, and function of the thyroid gland, in conjunction with other studies of thyroid function.

Patient preparation
The patient is told that this test evaluates the functioning and structure of the thyroid. The nurse reassures the patient that the level of radioactive medication is not dangerous to the patient or to others and determines if the patient has received radiographic contrast agents within the past 3 months, since these may invalidate the scan. If ordered by the physician, the patient is instructed to discontinue medications containing iodine (iodized salt, cough syrups, multivitamins, Lugol's solution) for 14 days before the test and to discontinue thyroid medications 4 to 6 weeks before the scan. The patient is told to fast from midnight before administration of

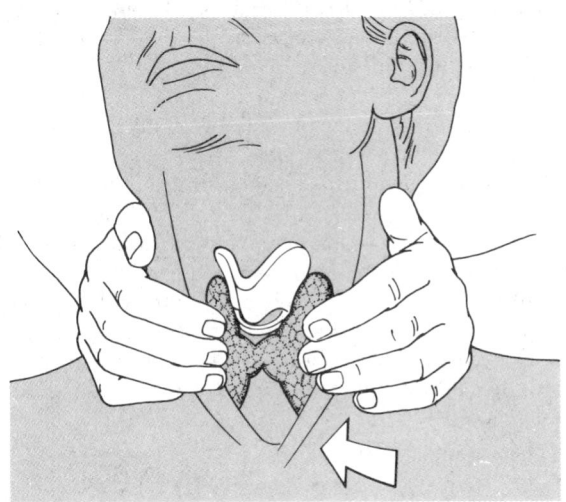

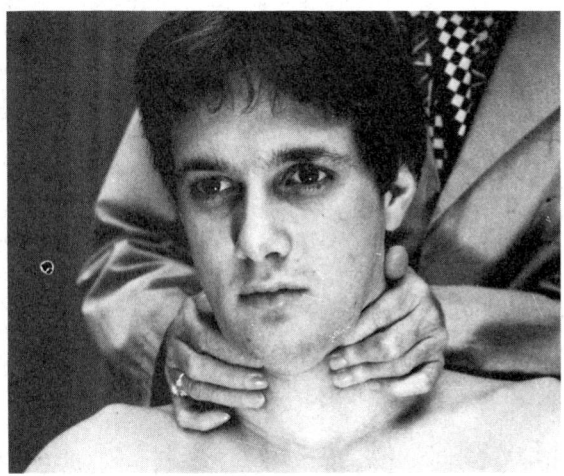

FIGURE 59-7 Posterior approach to thyroid examination. (*Right,* from Malasanos L et al: *Health assessment,* ed 3, St Louis, 1986, Mosby–Year Book, Inc.)

TABLE 59-1   Laboratory Thyroid Function Tests

Test	Normal reference range (SI units)	Discussion of test
Thyroxine, serum (T_4; thyroxine, total)	Radioimmunoassay (RIA) Adult: 5-12 µg/dL (65-155 nmol/L) Male > 60 years: 5.0-10 µg/dL (65-129 nmol/L) Female > 60 years: 5.5-10.5 µg/dL (71-135 nmol/L)	This test measures total serum level of thyroxine and is useful as a basic screening tool for thyroid disease and in monitoring response to treatment. Thyroxine levels are affected by abnormal levels of thyroid-binding globulin (TBG). Any increase in TBG (as in pregnancy or in patients taking oral contraceptives) will cause elevated levels of T_4 and must be considered when interpreting T_4 results. Drugs such as heparin, lithium, and salicylates (in high doses) decrease T_4 levels. T_4 levels are increased with hyperthyroidism and decreased with hypothyroidism. Radioactive materials such as ^{131}I may interfere if serum for T_4 is collected within 2 to 3 days of ^{131}I administration.
Triiodothyronine, serum; triiodothyronine radioimmunoassay, serum (T_3; T_3-RIA)	120-195 ng/dL (1.85-3.00 nmol/L) Male > 60 years: 105-175 ng/dL (1.62-2.69 nmol/L) Female > 60 years: 1.08-2.05 ng/dL (1.66-3.16 nmol/L)	This test measures total (bound and free) serum content of T_3 through radioimmunoassay. Estrogens will increase T_3 levels, whereas heparin, lithium, and salicylates (high doses) will decrease T_3 levels. T_3 levels generally rise and fall in tandem with T_4 levels. However, in T_3 toxicosis only T_3 levels rise. T_3 toxicosis occurs with Graves' disease and toxic nodular goiter.
Triiodothyronine resin uptake; triiodothyronine uptake (T_3RU; T_3U)	Adult: 24-34% uptake (24-34 AU) Male > 60 years: 24-32% uptake (24-32 AU) Female > 60 years: 22-32% uptake (22-32 AU)	T_3RU indirectly measures binding capacity of thyroid-binding globulin (TBG) in patient's serum and is useful in confirming an elevated T_4. Radioactive T_3 and hormone-binding resin are added to patient's serum. When TBG levels are decreased, increased amounts of radioactive T_3 bind to the special resin. Steroids and phenytoin cause increased T_3RU levels; oral contraceptives and salicylates (high doses) cause decreased levels. T_3RU levels are increased with hyperthyroidism, protein malnutrition, and nephrotic syndrome and decreased with hypothyroidism, pregnancy, acute intermittent porphyria, and acute hepatitis.
Free thyroxine assay (FT_4; thyroxine, free)	0.9-2.3 ng/dL (12-30 pmol/L)	This assay measures T_4 present in serum in a free state. Free T_4 and T_3 affect cellular metabolism, and it is the free hormone that determines clinical status. FT_4 is useful in diagnosis of hyperthyroid and hypothyroid states and in monitoring therapy. FT_4 is the most reliable assessment in evaluation of decreased T_4 levels in seriously ill patients.
Free thyroxine index (FTI)	1-4	FTI provides an indirect measurement of FT_4 in blood. The index is obtained from serum T_4 multiplied by TT_3U ratio. FTI is more reliable than a decreased T_4 in hypothyroidism and may be decreased in severe nonthyroidal illness.
Thyroid-stimulating hormone assay, serum (TSH)	Adult: < 10 µU/mL (< 10 mu/L) Male > 60 years: 2.0-7.3 µU/mL (2.0-7.3 mU/L) Female > 60 years: 2.0-16.8 µU/mL (2.0-16.8 mU/L)	This assay measures TSH levels. TSH assay is most useful single test in diagnosis of primary hypothyroidism and helps differentiate primary from secondary or tertiary hypothyroidism. Elevated levels are found with primary hypothyroidism, after ^{131}I therapy, and with iodine deficiency goiter. Decreased levels are found with secondary hypothyroidism, thyroid hormone therapy, hyperthyroidism, and euthyroid sick state.

TABLE 59-1   Laboratory Thyroid Function Tests—cont'd

Test	Normal reference range (SI units)	Discussion of test
Thyrotropin-releasing hormone test; thyrotropin-releasing factor test (TRH; TRF)	Negative (normal degree of TSH elevation after injection of TRH)	This test involves IV injection of TSH, which directly stimulates pituitary to release TSH and prolactin. A venous blood sample is taken for baseline TSH and prolactin levels, and then TRH, 500 μg, is administered. After 20 to 30 minutes, a second blood sample is drawn for serum TSH levels. Nurse warns patient that nausea, urinary urgency, and flushing may be experienced after administration of hormone but that these effects are temporary. TRH is most reliable test for diagnosis of hyperthyroidism in presence of abnormal serum FT_1 and T_3 levels. (Excessive circulating T_3 and T_4 levels suppress TSH levels so that levels are either not increased or increased only slightly.) Positive test (abnormally low TSH response) confirms TSH suppression by T_4 in treatment of thyroid cancers.
Radioactive iodine uptake (RAIU)	3-20% absorbed by thyroid gland after 6 hours; 15-35% absorbed by thyroid gland after 24 hours	RAIU test measures ability of thyroid gland to trap and retain iodine. A small dose of radioactive iodine (^{131}I or ^{123}I) is given orally to patient, and a gamma-ray detector determines amount of radioactive iodine that has been taken up by gland after 6 and 24 hours. Patient is instructed to fast 8 hours before test and 1 hour after administration of radioiodine capsule or liquid. Nurse tells patient to return to laboratory after 6 and 24 hours. This test should not be performed during pregnancy and should precede tests using contrast media. Low uptake levels are found with (1) elevated T_3 and T_4 levels, (2) subacute thyroiditis, (3) iodine overload, and (4) intake of thyroid hormones. Elevated levels are found with hyperthyroidism, early Hashimoto's thyroiditis, or goiter.
Thyroglobulin level	3-42 ng/mL (3-42 μg/L)	Thyroglobulin is useful in monitoring for recurrence of thyroid carcinoma and in monitoring response to therapy. It is not specific enough to be used in definitive diagnosis of thyroid carcinoma. Thyroglobulin is a glycoprotein that contains T_3 and T_4. Thyroglobulin is produced by follicular cells and is released into bloodstream with carcinoma, active thyrotoxicosis, and thyroiditis.
Thyroid microsomal antibodies	Negative	Positive results indicate Hashimoto's disease.

the ^{123}I or ^{131}I. If ^{123}I is used, the patient will fast for an additional 45 minutes after ingestion of the oral isotope, and the scan will be performed in 24 hours. If technetium is used, it is administered intravenously 30 minutes before the scan and fasting is not required.

Just before the scan, the nurse instructs the patient to remove all jewelry, metal objects, and dentures, because these may interfere with visualization.

Thyroid ultrasonography

Thyroid ultrasonography (thyroid echogram) involves noninvasive evaluation of the thyroid gland. Ultrasonic pulses are directed at the thyroid gland, and the echoes are reflected back, to be displayed on an oscilloscope. This procedure can be used safely with a pregnant patient, since no radioactivity is involved. Thyroid ultrasonography is useful in differentiating between a cyst and a tumor. If a tumor is suspected, ultrasonography is followed with

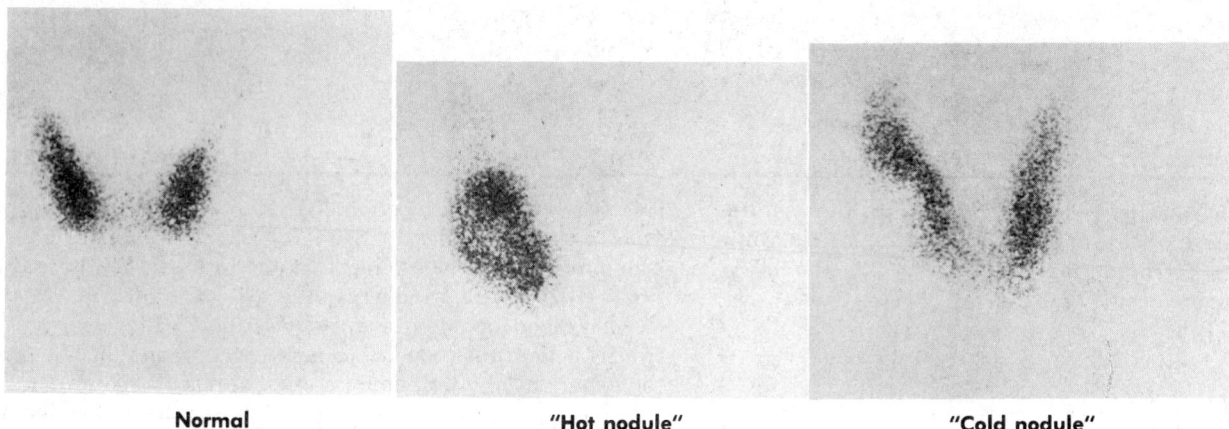

Normal   **"Hot nodule"**   **"Cold nodule"**

FIGURE 59-8   Normal and abnormal thyroid scans. (From Tilkian SM et al: *Clinical implications of laboratory tests,* ed 4, St Louis, 1987, Mosby—Year Book, Inc.)

a fine needle aspiration or biopsy. During the procedure, which takes about 30 minutes, the patient's neck is in a hyperextended position and is coated with a water-soluble jelly. No special patient preparation is necessary for ultrasonography.

Thyroid biopsy

Thyroid tissue for biopsy is obtained through surgical excision with the patient under general anesthesia or fine needle aspiration with the patient under local anesthesia. Fine needle aspiration involves removal of a small amount of thyroid tissue with a 21-gauge needle inserted directly into the thyroid nodule. When sampling is complete, the negative pressure generated during aspiration is released, the needle is withdrawn, and the cells are forced onto a slide. The test enables (1) cytologic evaluation of thyroid nodules, (2) cytologic diagnosis of benign lesions, such as cysts or colloid goiter, and (3) diagnosis of malignant lesions. The primary complications of biopsy are bleeding and respiratory difficulties caused by hematoma and edema. The nurse instructs the patient to fast if a general anesthetic is anticipated and checks for hypersensitivity to anesthetic agents. The patient is told that the test enables close examination of thyroid tissue and that he or she will be in a supine position with a pillow under the shoulders and neck hyperextended. If a local anesthetic is being used some pressure may be felt as the sample is taken. The nurse advises the patient that a sore throat is possible following sampling. A signed consent is necessary for the procedure.

Parathyroid Function Tests

Laboratory tests

Abnormalities in serum calcium and serum phosphorus levels are often the initial clue to parathyroid dysfunction. However, a number of other laboratory determinations are also useful in evaluating the function of the parathyroid glands (Table 59-2).

Skeletal roentgenograms

Roentgenograms of the skeleton are useful in evaluation of fractures and deformities produced by demineralization caused by excessive PTH. The patient is instructed to remove all jewelry and metal objects from the x-ray field before examination.

Adrenal Function Tests

Clinical laboratory tests

A number of blood and urine tests (Table 59-3) are useful in evaluating the function of the adrenal glands, and they aid in the diagnosis of disorders of the adrenal gland.

Computed tomography

Computed tomography (CT scan) of the adrenals is useful in detecting small tumors and in detecting bilateral enlargement caused by pituitary hyperactivity or ectopic ACTH syndrome. The CT scan is discussed in greater detail in Chapter 44.

Adrenal arteriography

Adrenal arteriography (adrenal angiography) is useful in detecting benign and malignant tumors of the adrenals (such as pheochromocytoma and carcinoma) and bilateral adrenal hyperplasia. The adrenal gland and its arterial system are visualized through injection of a radiopaque dye into the adrenal artery (the remainder of the procedure is similar to renal angiography, described in Chapter 41).

Text continued on p. 1647.

TABLE 59-2   Laboratory Determination of Parathyroid Function

Test	Normal reference range (SI units)	Discussion of test
Calcium, serum	Adult: 8.4-10.2 mg/dL (2.10-2.55 mmol/L) > 65 years: 8.8-10.0 mg/dL (2.20-2.50 mmol/L)	Approximately 90% of calcium in body is stored in bones and 50% is ionized and physiologically active. Calcium levels are increased (hypercalcemia) with hyperparathyroidism, parathyroid tumors, adrenal insufficiency, prolonged immobilization, multiple fractures, metastatic carcinoma, or excessive ingestion of calcium (milk products and alkaline antacids increase serum calcium levels). Decreased levels (hypocalcemia) are found with hypoparathyroidism, total parathyroidectomy, Cushing's syndrome, peritonitis, renal failure, and certain drugs (cortisone, insulin, or phenytoin). A sample for determination of serum calcium should not be drawn until 24 hours after injecting a radiopaque material.
Phosphorus, serum	Adult: 2.7-4.5 mg/dL (0.87-1.45 mmol/L) Male > 65 years: 2.3-3.7 mg/dL (0.74-1.20 mmol/L) Female > 65 years: 2.8-4.8 mg/dL (0.9-1.32 mmol/L)	Phosphorus is involved in metabolic processes and is found in all tissues. Of total body phosphorus, 85% is found in bone. Elevated serum phosphorus levels (hyperphosphatemia) are found with hypoparathyroidism, hyperthyroidism, healing fractures, severe muscle injury, or chronic glomerular disease. Decreased serum phosphorus levels occur with hyperparathyroidism, adult osteomalacia, chronic use of antacids containing aluminum hydroxide, and malabsorption syndromes.
Chloride-phosphate ratio (C/P)	30:1	To obtain C/P ratio, serum chloride value is divided by serum phosphorus value. Test is not useful when serum calcium is normal or in chronic renal failure. It is useful, however, in identifying primary hyperparathyroidism. In primary hypoparathyroidism, C/P ratio is > 33.
Parathyroid hormone assay (PTH; parathyroid hormone, serum)	Values vary with laboratory and are interpreted with serum calcium values Intact PTH: 10-65 pg/mL (10-65 ng/L) N-terminal fraction: 8-24 pg/mL (8-24 ng/L)	This test measures serum levels of PTH. PTH is only hormone secreted by parathyroid. Testing is done by radioimmunoassay. Serum calcium levels are usually obtained when PTH specimen is drawn. Patient fasts from midnight before test. Collection of sample may vary with laboratory procedures. Some laboratories require collection of specimen in a plastic, iced syringe. Increased levels are found with hyperparathyroidism and decreased levels with hypoparathyroidism or sarcoidosis.
Adenosine 3',5' monophosphate assay, urine (cyclic AMP or cAMP)	After IV infusion of PTH—tenfold to twentyfold increase in cAMP	PTH causes cAMP to be produced in renal tubules. cAMP influences rate of protein synthesis within cells. Patient receives 15-minute IV infusion of PTH, after which a 3- to 4-hour urine specimen is collected in a bottle, placed on ice, and taken immediately to laboratory. Failure to respond to PTH stimulation, as indicated by normal excretion of cAMP, is found with pseudohypoparathyroidism. This test is contraindicated in patients with hypercalcemia, because infusion of PTH further increases calcium levels, and in patients receiving digitalis.
Glucosteroid suppression (cortisone administration test; Dent's test)		This test is used to evaluate cause of hypercalcemia but is rarely used today because PTH assays are easily performed. Baseline calcium values are determined, and then patient receives high doses of cortisone for 7 to 10 days. Serum calcium determination is repeated after 10 days. In patients with hyperparathyroidism, calcium levels will not be lowered. In patients with hyperparathyroidism related to other causes (bone metastasis or sarcoidosis), serum calcium level will be lowered.

TABLE 59-3   Clinical Laboratory Tests for Adrenal Function

Test	Description and usual reference range (SI units)	Nursing responsibilities
Cortex plasma cortisol	Plasma cortisol is ordered for patients with suspected adrenal dysfunction, but stimulation and suppression tests are usually required to confirm diagnosis. ACTH stimulation causes release of cortisol, a potent glucosteroid. Normally, cortisol levels are highest in morning and lowest in evening. Loss of diurnal variation is an early sign of adrenal hyperfunction. Total cortisol is measured by three basic assay techniques. Radioimmunoassay measures cortisol; fluorometric assay measures cortisol and compound S; and competitive protein-binding assay measures cortisol, cortisone, compound S, progesterone, and 17-hydroxyprogesterone. Knowledge of method is important in some clinical situations. Pregnancy and oral contraceptives falsely increase cortisol levels. Increased levels are found with carcinoma of adrenal gland, stress, obesity, diabetic acidosis, hyperthyroidism, and severe depression. Decreased levels are found with Addison's disease, ACTH deficiency, and hypothyroidism. Reference range—8 AM (0800 hr): 8-19 μg/dL (0.22-0.52 μmol/L) 4 PM (1600 hr): 4-11 μg/dL (0.11-0.30 μmol/L)	Nurse assesses patient for signs of emotional or physiologic stress and reports this to physician. Nurse instructs patient to assume relaxed, recumbent position 30 minutes before sampling.
Urine-free cortisol (cortisol, urine)	Urine-free cortisol is a more useful test than plasma cortisol and is especially useful in diagnosis of adrenocortical hyperfunction. Stress and adrenal tumors also cause increased levels of urine cortisol. Reference range—24-108 μg/24 hr	Nurse instructs patient to avoid stressful situations. Patient voids and discards first specimen and then saves all subsequent specimens for 24 hours in jug labeled with patient's name. Patient voids at end of 24-hour period and saves this specimen. Contamination with stool or toilet paper is to be avoided.

17-Hydroxycorticosteroids urinary assay; 17-ketosteroids urinary assay (17-OHCS; 17-KS)	Urine assays of 17-OHCS and 17-KS are not considered reliable for screening Cushing's syndrome because of high incidence of false-positive and false-negative results. Elevated levels are found with Cushing's syndrome, adrenal cancer, extreme stress, obesity, and hyperthyroidism. Decreased levels are found with Addison's disease, hypogonadism, and hypopituitarism.
	Reference range for 17-KS in urine
	  Male: 8-25 mg/24 hr
	  Female: 5-15 mg/24 hr
	  Elderly: 4-8 mg/24 hr
	Reference range for 17-OHCS/24 hr urine
	  Male: 3-10 mg/day (8.3-27.6 μmol/day)
	  Female: 2-8 mg/day (5.5-22.1 μmol/day)
		Nurse instructs patient to withhold chlorpromazine and meprobamate 3 days before test (if drugs are not withheld, notify laboratory) and to restrict coffee intake before and during collection. Nurse explains to patient the details of 24-hour collection (see urine free cortisol). Specimen must be refrigerated or kept on ice.

TABLE 59-3 Clinical Laboratory Tests for Adrenal Function—cont'd

Test	Description and usual reference range (SI units)	Nursing responsibilities
ACTH, serum	This test evaluates anterior pituitary function and is particularly useful in diagnosis of Cushing's syndrome and Addison's disease. Serum ACTH level is high with Addison's disease. In Cushing's syndrome, caused by a pituitary adenoma, ACTH levels are normal or slightly increased; and in Cushing's syndrome caused by an adrenal tumor, levels are decreased and diurnal variation is absent. Reference range—15-70 pg/mL (3.3-15.4 pmol/L)	Nurse instructs patient to fast 12 to 48 hours before test and to avoid corticosteroids, estrogens, lithium carbonate, alcohol, and amphetamines, as ordered. Strenuous physical activity is avoided for 12 hours before test. A fasting sample is drawn between 8 and 10 AM (0800 and 1000 hr) in a chilled heparinized syringe and placed on ice.
Single-dose dexamethasone suppression test (ACTH suppression test)	This test is especially useful in diagnosis of Cushing's syndrome, since failure to suppress cortisol production is suggestive of Cushing's syndrome (false-positive results occur in obese, chronically ill, and severely depressed patients). Patient is given an oral dose of dexamethasone (Decadron) at 11 PM (2300 hr), which suppresses cortisol production so that morning peak of plasma cortisol does not occur. Reference range for serum cortisol—< 5 μ/dL (138 nmol/L)	Nurse administers 1 to 2 mg of dexamethasone and ensures collection of a blood sample for serum cortisol at 8 AM (0800 hr). Patient is encouraged to have a good sleep after administration of dexamethasone.
Standard dexamethasone suppression test (low-dose and high-dose tests)	This test is useful in confirming Cushing's syndrome and in differentiating Cushing's syndrome from other types of hypercortisolism. Glucosteroids determine amount of ACTH released, which in turn determines amount of steroid produced. Patients are either given low or high doses of dexamethasone, and response is measured through urine 17-OHCS and free cortisol levels, and serum cortisol values. Patients with Cushing's syndrome or Cushing's disease will fail to show suppression with low doses of dexamethasone but will show suppression with high doses. Patients with adrenal carcinoma will not show suppression in either case. Low-dose reference range for urinary 17-OHCS—< 4 mg/24 hr (8.3 μmol/dL) For urinary free cortisol—< 20 μg (552 nmol/24 hr) High-dose reference range for urinary 17-OHCS—50% or less of basal value	Test is described and patient is instructed to discontinue all medications 24 to 48 hours before it. Nurse explains to patient how to collect a 24-hour urine specimen (see urine free cortisol). On day before test, a specimen is collected for plasma cortisol at 8 AM (0800 hr), and a 24-hour urine for 17-OHCS is also collected to determine baseline values. Low-dose test: nurse administers 0.5 mg dexamethasone q6h × 8 doses. A 24-hour urine for 17-OHCS and urinary cortisol is collected on first and second days of test. At 8 AM (0800 hr) of second day, nurse collects a specimen for plasma cortisol. High-dose test: nurse administers 2 mg dexamethasone q6h × 8 doses and collects 24-hour urine specimen.

Continued.

TABLE 59-3 Clinical Laboratory Tests for Adrenal Function—cont'd

Test	Description and usual reference range (SI units)	Nursing responsibilities
ACTH stimulation test (modified Thorn; ACTH infusion; provocative ACTH)	This test evaluates stimulation of adrenal cortex after injection of ACTH. Normally, 17-OHCS and cortisol levels are twice those of baseline levels during 8-hour infusion test. No response occurs with Addison's disease, and patients with pituitary or hypothalamic insufficiency have an intermediate response. ACTH stimulation is contraindicated in pregnancy and in patients who have had previous adverse reactions. Smoking, obesity, steroid medications, lithium carbonate, estrogens, and amphetamines affect test results. Reference range for rapid test—serum cortisol: 2 × baseline Reference range for 24-hour test (8-hour infusion test)— 　17-OHCS: 2 to 5 × baseline 　Plasma cortisol: 25-50 μg/dL (0.7-1.4 μmol/L	Rapid screening test: a blood sample for baseline measurement of plasma cortisol is collected. Nurse administers a synthetic ACTH analog (cosyntropin [Cortrosyn]) IV or IM. Specimens for serum cortisol are collected after 30 and 60 minutes. 8-hour infusion test (24-hour test): test is explained to patient, who is told how to collect a 24-hour urine specimen (see urine free cortisol). Nurse collects a baseline 24-hour urine specimen for 17-OHCS. The day of test, 25 units of cosyntropiun in 500 mL of normal saline is administered over 8 hours. Nurse collects a 24-hour urine specimen for 17-OHCS after commencement of infusion.
Corticotropin releasing factor in ACTH stimulation; corticotropin releasing hormone in ACTH stimulation (CRF; CRH)	CRF causes release of ACTH from pituitary, which is followed by cortisol secretion from adrenal glands. Plasma cortisol response to CRF is more reproducible than that to ACTH because of short half-life of ACTH. CRF in ACTH stimulation is useful in identifying adrenal insufficiency. Decreased cortisol levels may be found with hypopituitarism. Reference range—serum cortisol levels rise at least 10 mg/dL (0.28 mol/L) 30 to 60 minutes after administration of CFR	Nurse instructs patient to withhold glucosteroids for at least 1 month before study if ordered. Patient receives an IV injection of CRF, after which blood samples for serum cortisol are drawn. Nurse reassures patient that mild dyspnea and facial flushing after injection of CRF are transitory, although it may take up to 1 hour for these effects to disappear.
Metyrapone test (metyrapone pituitary reserve test)	This test measures reserve capacity of pituitary to release ACTH. Metyrapone blocks conversion of compounds (11-deoxycortisol) to cortisol. A decline in cortisol levels normally stimulates pituitary to secrete more ACTH. Because cortisol production is blocked, ACTH stimulation causes an increase in precursor compound S, and urinary 17-OHCS levels rise sharply. Pregnancy, hypothyroidism, and drugs (phenytoin and chlorpromazine) will suppress this response. Patients in whom adrenal or pituitary insufficiency is suspected should be observed closely for nausea, vomiting, tachycardia, diaphoresis, or muscle weakness (addisonian crisis). Reference range for 24-hour metyrapone test—17-OCHS: 2 to 4 × baseline Reference range for overnight test—compound S levels: 7200 nmol/L	24-hour metyrapone test: patient is told why test is conducted and is taught how to collect a 24-hour urine specimen. Nurse collects baseline 24-hour urine for 17-OHCS before test. Metyrapone is administered orally every 4 hours for 24 hours. Two 24-hour urine specimens are collected during and after administration of 17-OHCS. Overnight test: metyrapone is administered at 11 PM (2300 hr) with a snack to decrease nausea. Nurse collects blood sample for compound S and cortisol levels at 8 AM (0800 hr) the following morning.

TABLE 59-3   Clinical Laboratory Tests for Adrenal Function—cont'd

Test	Description and usual reference range (SI units)	Nursing responsibilities
Aldosterone assay, plasma and urine	This test measures aldosterone levels and is useful in diagnosis of aldosterone-producing adrenal adenoma and adrenal hyperplasia. Aldosterone is instrumental in sodium and potassium homeostasis and in regulation of blood pressure and volume. Hydralazine, diazoxide, diuretics, and nitroprusside increase aldosterone levels. Reference range for urine excretion /24 hr— 5-19 µg/day (14-53 nmol/day) Reference range for plasma (morning samples on ad lib sodium intake)— Supine: 3-10 ng/dL (0.08-0.27 nmol/L) Upright: 5-30 ng/dL (0.14-0.83 nmol/L)	Sample for serum aldosterone is drawn before patient arises in morning, and another sample 4 hours later, with patient in standing position. For urine, nurse collects 24-hour urine specimen (see urine free cortisol).
18-Hydroxycorticosterone (18-OHB)	18-OHB is considered immediate precursor of aldosterone biosynthesis. Measurement of plasma 18-OHB is not commonly performed. Blood for plasma 18-OHB may be drawn during posture study, which differentiates between two major causes of primary aldosteronism. In patients with bilateral idiopathic hyperaldosteronism (IPA), aldosterone levels will rise normally with upright posture, and recumbent 18-OHB levels will be 100 ng/dL. In patients with unilateral aldosterone-producing adenomas (APAs), aldosterone levels will not rise normally with upright posture, and recumbent 18-OHB levels will be 100 ng/dL	Nurse instructs patient undergoing posture studies to have a generous daily salt intake (150 mEq of sodium/day). On morning of test, blood samples are collected at 8 AM (0800 hr) after overnight recumbency and at 12 noon (1200 hr) after 4 hours of ambulation. These samples are drawn to measure aldosterone, cortisol, plasma renin activity, potassium, and 18-OHB.
Plasma renin activity (PRA)	Renin, an enzyme secreted by kidney, is first stage of renin-angiotensin-aldosterone cycle that maintains fluid volume, sodium-potassium balance, and blood pressure. This test is useful in screening for hypertension of renal origin and in identifying primary aldosteronism. Increased levels occur with adrenal hypofunction, end-stage renal disease, and hypertension. Decreased levels occur with primary aldosteronism and Cushing's syndrome. Reference range for diet with normal sodium intake (3 g/day)— Supine: 1.6 ± 1.5 ng Al/mL/hr (1.6 ± 1.5 µg Al) Upright: 4.5 ± 2.9 ng Al/mL/hr (4.5 ± 2.9 ng Al/mL/hr Reference range for sodium-restricted diet— Supine: 3.2 ± 1.1 ng Al/mL/hr (3.2 ± 1.1 µg Al) Upright: 9.3 ± 4.3 ng Al/mL hr (9.3 ± 4.3 µ Al)	Nurse instructs patient to maintain normal intake of sodium and to avoid taking antihypertensives, licorice, vasodilators, and oral contraceptives for 2 to 4 weeks before test. If patient is on sodium-restricted test, patient receives a diuretic and is instructed to limit sodium intake for 3 days. Patient must maintain either a recumbent or an upright position for 2 hours before test. Samples may be drawn from a peripheral site or during renal vein catheterization. If renal vein catheterization is performed, nurse provides care as for renal angiography.

Continued.

TABLE 59-3   Clinical Laboratory Tests for Adrenal Function—cont'd

Test	Description and usual reference range (SI units)	Nursing responsibilities

Furosemide test for renin release	This test is a less cumbersome test than the PRA and also screens for renin abnormalities.
	Reference range—
	  Whites: > 1.0 ng/mL/hr
	  Blacks: > 0.5 ng/mL/hr
		Nurse administers 60 mg of furosemide (Lasix) orally in morning. Patient is instructed to maintain an upright position for 5 hours, and then blood for renin assay is collected in a cold tube. Nurse monitors the patient for hypokalemia (patients with primary aldosteronism tend to develop hypokalemia).

Catecholamines, plasma	This test is useful in ruling out pheochromocytoma in patients with hypertension and in identifying ganglioneuroma and neuroblastoma. Elevated plasma levels require further confirmation by urinalysis. Catecholamines (epinephrine, norepinephrine, and dopamine) are produced by brain, sympathetic nerve endings; and adrenal medulla. Catecholamine levels are volatile and are influenced by many drugs, stress, smoking, diet, posture, and diurnal variations.
	Supine
	  Epinephrine: < 110 pg/mL (< 601 pmol/L)
	  Norepinephrine: 70-750 pg/mL (0.41-4.43 pmol/L)
	Standing
	  Epinephrine: < 140 pg/mL (< 764 pmol/L)
	  Norepinephrine: 200-1700 pg/mL (1.18-10.05 pmol/L)
	Dopamine (no postural change): < 30 pg/mL (< 196 mol/L)
		Nurse explains to patient that this test helps to determine if symptoms are related to hormonal secretion. Patient is asked to strictly follow all instructions because catecholamine levels are readily influenced. Nurse tells patient to avoid over-the-counter remedies for 2 weeks; to avoid amine-rich foods (bananas, avocados, cheese, coffee, tea, cocoa) for 48 hours; to avoid smoking; and to fast for 10 to 12 hours. Patient is instructed to assume a relaxed and recumbent position for 45 to 60 minutes before collection of first blood sample. Then patient must stand for 10 minutes before collection of second blood samples. Both samples are collected in chilled tubes containing ethylenediamine tetra-acetic acid (EDTA).

Catecholamines, urine	Urine catecholamines are useful in diagnosis of pheochromocytoma, neuroblastoma, and ganglioneuroma. Although a 24-hour urine collection is preferred because of volatile nature of catecholamine levels, a random specimen may be collected after a hypertensive episode.
	Reference range for catecholamines, fluorometric—< 280 μg/day (1655 nmol/day)
	Reference range for catecholamines—
	  Fractionated norepinephrine: 0-100 μg/day (< 590 nmol/day)
	  Epinephrine: 0-15 μg/day (0-81.9 nmol/day)
	  Dopamine: 65-400 μg/day (425-2610 nmol/day)
	  Total: <135 μg/day (< 730 nmol/L)
		Nurse explains that test measures hormone levels that may influence symptoms. Patient is told that no dietary restrictions are necessary, although stress and vigorous activity should be avoided during collection period. Nurse assesses patient's medication history and determines with physician which medications should be withheld. Patient is taught how to collect 24-hour urine specimen (see urine free cortisol). A container with a preservative is required for the urine.

Because a fatal episode of severe hypertension may be precipitated by a dye reaction in patients with pheochromocytoma, propranolol (Inderal) and phenoxybenzamine (Debenzyline) are usually given for several days before the test.

Adrenal venography

Adrenal venography aids in differential diagnosis of the causes of Cushing's syndrome and pheochromocytoma. A catheter is inserted through the femoral vein into the adrenal vein. Samples of venous blood can be taken from each adrenal and analyzed for aldosterone, androgens, and other substances. In Cushing's syndrome the blood is analyzed for plasma cortisol. If the plasma cortisol levels are higher in one adrenal than in the other, this indicates that a unilateral tumor is responsible for the syndrome. If plasma cortisol levels are bilaterally elevated, bilateral adrenal hyperplasia is responsible for Cushing's syndrome. Adrenal blood is analyzed for catecholamines. If the catecholamine levels are elevated on one side but not on the other, an unilateral pheochromocytoma is present on the side of the elevation. If adrenal specimens show no elevation in catecholamine levels, the pheochromocytoma is outside the adrenal gland.

Patient preparation

The patient is informed that the test aids in determining if symptoms are caused by abnormalities in the adrenal gland. The nurse assesses the patient for allergies to iodine, and if allergies exist, the patient may be given prednisone (5 mg four times per day) and diphenhydramine (25 mg four times per day) for 3 days before and after the test. The patient is told that a transient burning sensation may be experienced as the dye is injected. The nurse explains that the patient will be placed in a supine position and that the insertion site will be locally anesthetized. A signed consent is obtained. The nurse administers alpha-adrenergic blocking agents if ordered. These agents (propranolol and phenoxybenzamine) prevent the occurrence of a malignant hypertensive episode in patients who are suspected of having phenochromocytoma.

Aftercare

The nurse assesses the patient's vital signs and femoral venipuncture site frequently (see Chapter 29 for a discussion of care following an arteriogram). The physician is notified immediately if the patient shows signs and symptoms of malignant hypertension.

Scintigraphy

Scintigraphy using MIBG (^{131}I metaiodobenzylguanidine) is useful in detecting and diagnosing pheochromocytomas, especially when CT studies are negative or when metastasis or familial disease is considered likely. When pheochromocytomas are present, MIBG will concentrate sufficiently to produce an image using a scintillation camera.

Patient preparation

The nurse explains that a radioisotope is injected and that after injection of the radioisotope, a scanning camera will be passed over the patient repeatedly. The patient is reassured that the radiation exposure is minimal. The nurse assesses the patient for sensitivity to iodine, contrast dyes, and shellfish and obtains an informed consent.

Pituitary Function Tests

Serum studies

A number of serum studies are useful in evaluating the function of the pituitary (Table 59-4).

Roentgenogram of hand and wrist

Roentgenograms of the hand and wrist are useful in evaluating bone age and in comparing chronologic age with linear growth. Retarded bone age is found in hypopituitarism with GH deficiency, hypothyroidism, gonadal dysgenesis, and constitutional growth delay. Accelerated bone age is found with excess androgens or estrogens and with hyperthyroidism. The patient is instructed to remove all metal objects from the x-ray field.

Roentgenogram of sella turcica

An x-ray examination of the sella turcica permits diagnosis of ACTH-producing tumors of the pituitary gland. These tumors produce erosion and destruction of the sella turcica, which can be detected on x-ray film. The patient is told to remove all metal objects above the neck (such as hair ornaments and earrings) and dentures, because these interfere with visualization of the skull. If the patient has a glass eye, the nurse informs the radiology department, because this produces a confusing shadow.

Assessment of Hypoglycemia

Serum insulin

Serum insulin (plasma insulin assay) is useful in the diagnosis of insulinoma and abnormal lipid and carbohydrate metabolism. Normally, increasing glucose levels stimulate insulin production, and falling glucose levels inhibit the release of insulin. In patients with insulinoma, serum insulin levels remain normal or even elevated after fasting. The patient is instructed to fast 10 to 12 hours before the test and to withhold ACTH, oral contraceptives, epinephrine,

TABLE 59-4   Laboratory Studies for Pituitary Function

Test	Normal reference range (SI units)	Discussion of test
Growth hormone (GH), serum	Adult male: 0-2 ng/mL (0-2 μg/L) Female: 0-10 ng/mL (0-10 μg/L) Male > 60 years: 0-10 ng/mL (0.10 μg/L Female > 60 years: 0-14 ng/mL (0-14 μg/L	Measurement of growth hormone through radioimmunoassay is useful in differential diagnosis of growth disorders and in diagnosis of pituitary or hypothalamic disease GH levels. Elevated levels occur after ingestion of meats, during sleep, and with major surgery, stress, gigantism, acromegaly, diabetes mellitus, and anorexia nervosa. Decreased levels occur with pituitary insufficiency and dwarfism. Nurse instructs patient to fast overnight and to limit physical activity for 10 to 12 hours before test. Patient is told that fasting blood specimen is collected before arising in morning and that another sample will be drawn the following day for comparison. Patient should be relaxed and recumbent 30 to 60 minutes before sampling.
Insulin tolerance test (ITT)	Glucose falls < 40 mg/dL (< 2.2 mmol/L) Cortisol rises above baseline: < 7 μg/dL (> 0.19 μmol/L) GH rises above baseline: > 5 ng/mL (> 5 μg/L)	ITT measures serum levels of GH and ACTH after a loading dose of insulin and is useful in aiding with differential diagnosis of dwarfism and small stature and in obtaining information about reserve capacity of GH. ITT is contraindicated in patients with cerebrovascular disease, epilepsy, myocardial infarction, and low basal plasma cortisol levels. Patient is instructed to withhold food and fluids for 8 hours and to restrict physical activity for 10 to 12 hours before test. Specimens for glucose, cortisol, and GH are drawn before patient arises. Nurse gives insulin IV as ordered. Blood is drawn from venous catheter every 15 minutes for first hour and every 30 minutes for next 2 hours. At end of test, nurse ensures that patient receives a meal or IV dextrose in water. Levodopa and arginine may be used instead of insulin. If levodopa is used, nurse gives medication orally 60 to 90 minutes before blood samples are drawn. If arginine is used, medication is administered IV for 30 minutes after withdrawal of blood specimen. Three blood samples are then collected at intervals of 30 minutes.
Growth hormone suppression test (GH suppression test; glucose loading)	GH after glucose suppression to < 2 ng/mL (< 2 μg/L)	This test is useful in evaluating acromegaly or gigantism. Glucose suppresses GH secretion. In acromegaly, baseline values for GH are generally about 5 ng/mL and will not fall below this after glucose loading. Patient is told to limit activity and to fast for 10 to 12 hours before test. After blood sample for baseline GH level is withdrawn, nurse administers 100 g of glucose solution orally. A sample of blood is obtained every 30 minutes for 2 hours for GH assay. Drugs such as corticosteroids and phenothiazines will produce decreased levels of GH, whereas levels will be increased by amphetamines, estrogens, and arginine.

TABLE 59-4 Laboratory Studies for Pituitary Function—cont'd

Test	Normal reference range (SI units)	Discussion of test
Somatomedin-C assay	Male: 43-178 ng/mL (43-178 μg/L) Female: 24-153 ng/mL (24-153 μg/L)	Somatomedins are produced in liver and cause increased production of protein and increased sulfation of constituents of cartilage. Their secretion is controlled by GH. Somatomedin-C is measured by radioreceptor and immunoassay. This test is useful in screening for GH deficiency and pituitary insufficiency. Increased concentrations are found with acromegaly, and decreased concentrations occur with deficient GH in hypopituitarism, hypothyroidism, nutritional deficiency, and anorexia.
Serum prolactin (lactogen)	2-15 ng/mL Levels >300 ng/mL indicate pituitary tumors	Prolactin stimulates lactation in females and is stimulated by thyrotropin releasing hormone. Serum prolactin is particularly useful in screening for pituitary adenomas, since very high increases in prolactin levels are caused by this more than by anything else. Prolactin levels are also elevated with sleep, stress, pregnancy, and breastfeeding and by medications (chlorpromazine, haloperidol, reserpine, morphine, and estrogens). These medications should be withheld if possible before the test.
Testosterone, serum	Male: 52-280 pg/mL (180.4-971.6 pmol/L) Female: 1.6-6.3 pg/mL (5.6-21.9 pmol/L)	Testosterone is main androgen secreted by testes, and its production is under the control of luteinizing hormone from the anterior pituitary. Elevated levels are found with testicular tumors in men and with Stein-Leventhal syndrome, ovarian tumors, and adrenal tumors in women. Decreased levels are found with steroid therapy, primary and secondary hypogonadism in males, and estrogen therapy.

Estradiol, serum	Male: 12-34 pg/mL (44-124.8 pmol/L)
	Female (menstruating)
	  Early cycle: 24-68 pg/mL (88.1-249.6 pmol/L)
	  Mid cycle: 50-186 pg/mL (183.5-682.6 pmol/L)
	  Late cycle: 73-149 pg/mL (267.9-546.8 pmol/L)
	Female (postmenopausal): < 30 pg/mL (110 pmol/L)
		Estradiol, secreted by ovarian follicles during first half of menstrual cycle, by corpus luteum during second half of cycle, and during pregnancy, is most potent estrogen secreted during nonpregnant state. Increased levels are found with some types of ovarian, testicular, and adrenal tumors and with polycystic ovarian disease. Decreased levels occur with postmenopausal states, pituitary dysfunction, and primary ovarian malfunction. Levels vary with stage of menstrual cycle.

Progesterone, plasma	Male: 13-97 ng/dL (0.4-3.1 nmol/L)
	Female
	  Follicular phase: 15-70 ng/dL (0.5-2.2 nmol/L)
	  Luteal phase: 200-2500 ng/dL (6.4-79.5 nmol/L)
	  Menopausal: 10-22 ng/dL (0.32-0.7 nmol/L)
		Progesterone is a major female steroid hormone that is essential for preparation and maintenance of uterus during pregnancy and is synthesized by placenta during pregnancy. During nonpregnancy, it is synthesized by corpus luteum. In males, progesterone is a precursor for androgens and corticosteroids. Increased levels are found during and after ovulation and with adrenocortical hyperplasia. Decreased levels are found with nonovulatory menorrhea, toxemia, fetal death, and threatened abortion. Date of patient's last menstrual period or week of gestation should be indicated on laboratory slip.

Continued.

TABLE 59-4 Laboratory Studies for Pituitary Function—cont'd

Test	Normal reference range (SI units)	Discussion of test

Gonadotropins—follicle stimulating hormone; luteinizing hormone (FSH; LH)	FSH
	  Male: 1-7 mU/mL (1-7 U/L)
	  Female
	    Follicular phase: 1-9 mU/mL (1-9 U/L)
	    Ovulatory peak: 6-26 mU/mL) (6-26 U/L)
	    Luteal phase: 1-9 mU/mL (1-9 U/L)
	    Menopausal phase: 30-118 mU/mL (30-118 U/L)
	LH
	  Male: 6-23 mIU/mL
	  Female
	    Follicular phase: 5-30 mIU/mL
	    Midcycle phase: 75-150 mIU/mL
	    Luteal phase: 5-40 mIU/mL
	    Menopausal phase: 30-200 mIU/mL
		LH and FSH are gonadotropins that are secreted by the anterior pituitary. LH induces ovulation in women and stimulates testosterone secretion in men. FSH stimulates development of ovarian follicles, which produce estrogen, which in turn suppresses production of FSH. FSH induces spermatogenesis in males. FSH and LH levels are useful in diagnosing infertility and precocious puberty. Levels are decreased in pituitary insufficiency and increased with primary gonadal failure. Time of last menstrual period for females should be noted on laboratory slip.

Antidiuretic hormone serum (ADH, vasopressin)	1-5 pg/mL (1-5 ng/L)	ADH is produced by the posterior pituitary and is instrumental in water reabsorption in response to increased osmolality (water deficiency). With decreased osmolality (water excess), secretion of ADH is decreased, allowing increased excretion of water. Abnormally low levels of ADH occur with pituitary diabetes insipidus, and elevated levels occur with syndrome of inappropriate antidiuretic hormone secretion (SIADH). Normal ADH levels in presence of clinical evidence of diabetes insipidus may indicate a nephrogenic form of the disease. Blood sample is collected in a plastic syringe and tube, since glass causes degradation of ADH.

Osmolality, urine and serum	Serum: 275-295 mOsm/kg (same)
	  > 60 years: 280-301 mOsm/kg (same)
	Urine: random: 50-1200 mOsm/kg (same)
	  12-hour fluid restriction: > 850 mOsm/kg (same)
	  Osmolality ratio—urine and serum: 1-3 (same)
	  > 3 after 12-hour fluid restriction
		Osmolality is a test that measures concentration or number of particles in serum and urine. Particles include electrolyte ions, urea, glucose, protein, and creatinine. Serum creatinine reflects hydration levels. Increased serum values may be found with dehydration, primary aldosteronism, severe diabetes mellitus, diabetes insipidus, and hypernatremia. Serum values are decreased with Addison's disease, increased ADH secretion, water overload, hyponatremia, and liver failure. Urine osmolality values are determined either through random samples or a 24-hour collection. Urine specimens that cannot be analyzed immediately should be refrigerated. Elevated urine osmolality may be found with Addison's disease, dehydration, hyperglycemia, increased ADH secretion, and sodium overload. Decreased urine

TABLE 59-4	Laboratory Studies for Pituitary Function—cont'd	

Test	Normal reference range (SI units)	Discussion of test
		osmolality is found with primary aldosteronism, diabetes insipidus, renal failure, and water overload. Relationship between serum and urine values is important in interpreting findings. A ratio close to 1.0 (dilute urine) indicates advanced renal disease, and a ratio below 1.0 follows excessive water intake or excessive water loss as in diabetes insipidus. Fluid restriction may be necessary before collection of specimens for urine osmolality.
Water deprivation and vasopressin injection test (water deprivation test; water deprivation antidiuretic hormone stimulation test)	Decreased urine flow to < 0.5 mL/min Urine osmolality > 500 mOsm/L Serum osmolality < 300 mOsm/L Plasma ADH appropriate for serum osmolality	This test evaluates concentration of urine and serum after several hours (4 to 20 hours) of fasting and is diagnostic of diabetes insipidus. After fasting, urine specimen is collected for urine osmolality and blood is drawn for osmolality, sodium, and ADH level. Urine of patients with diabetes insipidus will not be concentrated, and serum osmolality will be high because of inability of kidneys to concentrate urine. If ADH (vasopressin) is then injected subcutaneously and samples of urine and blood are collected for osmolality 1 hour after injections, polyuria will be corrected and serum osmolality will decrease. The patient with severe diabetes insipidus should be hospitalized and monitored for signs of severe dehydration through observation of vital signs, urine output, serum osmolality, and body weight (before the test and every 3 hours). If weight loss is greater than or equal to 3% of total body weight, the loss is reported to physician.
Water loading test (water loading antidiuretic hormone suppression test)	Urine osmolality falls to < 100 mOsm/kg with > 90% of water load excreted in 4 hours Plasma ADH appropriate for serum osmolality	This test measures excretion of water load after ingestion of large amounts of water. Patients with SIADH will be unable to excrete urine in normal volumes (< 90% of water load is excreted), and serum osmolality will remain > 100 mOsm/kg. Test is started 2 hours after a light breakfast. Nurse obtains baseline samples for serum and urine osmolality. Patient is given water to drink (20 mL/kg) over 15 to 30 minutes. Soda crackers may be given with water as necessary. Nurse instructs patient to remain recumbent. Nurse collects samples every hour for 4 hours for serum and urine osmolality. Total urine output is measured.

and steroids. The nurse collects blood specimens for serum insulin and blood glucose (the insulin levels are compared with the glucose level). Usual reference range (in SI units) is less than 2 to 20 μU/mL (14 to 144 pmol/L).

C-peptide

C-peptide is measured by radioimmunoassay and is useful in evaluating hypoglycemia, insulinoma, and pancreatic beta-cell secretory function. C-peptide is an amino acid residue that is produced when proinsulin degrades. The other product of proinsulin degradation is insulin. When compared with serum insulin values, C-peptide values will vary directly with serum values. If one decreases, so will the other. The nurse instructs the patient to fast 8 to 12 hours before collection of the specimen of blood. Usual reference range is 1 to 2 ng/mL (fasting).

Prolonged fast

Prolonged (72-hour) fast is useful in determining if a patient has hypoglycemia during fasting or if hypoglycemia is caused by excessive insulin production. The test is performed if results of the serum insulin are inconclusive. The patient is hospitalized and is allowed only water for 3 days, or 72 hours. Blood is collected for glucose, insulin, and C-peptide levels every 6 hours and if the patient displays symptoms while fasting. The patient should be observed closely for signs of hypoglycemia. Normally, serum insulin levels fall steadily as glucose levels fall. In patients with insulinomas the serum insulin does not fall.

Diagnostic Tests for Diabetes Mellitus

Fasting blood glucose

Fasting blood sugar (FBS) helps detect diabetes mellitus and evaluate the status of patients with diabetes mellitus. A normal level, however, does not rule out diabetes mellitus. The utilization of glucose is related to circulating level of insulin and the ability of insulin to promote cellular metabolism of glucose. True glucose elevations indicate diabetes mellitus. However, hyperglycemia may also occur with acute stress, Cushing's disease, pancreatitis, myocardial infarction, and pregnancy. Many drugs cause blood sugar elevations in blood, such as furosemide, L-dopa, acetaminophen, ACTH, epinephrine, tetracycline, and phenytoin. Drugs such as ascorbic acid, chlorpropamide, and propranolol tend to decrease glucose values. The patient is instructed to fast for 8 to 12 hours before collection of the blood specimen. If the patient is on insulin, this should be administered after the blood sample has been drawn. Usual reference range (in SI units) for serum is 70 to 110 mg/dL (3.85 to 6.05 mmol/L), and for whole blood it is 60 to 100 mg/dL (3.30 to 5.50 mmol/L).

Two-hour postprandial glucose test

This test (2-hour PPG, 2-hour postprandial blood sugar, 2-hour PPBS, 2-hour p.c. blood sugar) screens for diabetes mellitus, and if results of this test are abnormal, a glucose tolerance test may be ordered. The test measures the level of glucose in a patient's body 2 hours after a meal. In a healthy patient the body responds to increased glucose levels with an increased secretion of insulin, so that blood glucose levels return to a premeal range 2 hours after a meal. In diabetic patients the blood glucose remains elevated at 2 hours. The nurse instructs the patient to eat a full meal and not to eat anything else until the sample is collected. The patient is told to avoid smoking, which increases blood glucose levels. Usual

reference range in SI units is less than 120 mg/dL (6.7 mmol/L).

Glycosylated hemoglobin test

Glycohemoglobin or **glycosylated hemoglobin** (HbA$_{1c}$) is a compound in which glucose is bound to hemoglobin A. Hemoglobin A accumulates within circulating erythrocytes and remains throughout their lifespan. The amount of glucose in the erythrocytes depends on the amount of glucose present in the plasma during the 120-day lifespan of the red blood cell. Glycohemoglobin gives a true indication of the degree of hyperglycemia present 2 or 3 months before the test. The greater the amount of glucose present, the greater the percentage of glycohemoglobin. The test is useful in evaluating the effectiveness of diabetic treatment and in determining the duration of hyperglycemia in newly diagnosed diabetics. However, the test is not responsive to short-term variations, such as exercise, stress, and food intake, and to recent changes in glucose levels and therefore is not useful in monitoring acute changes in the status of a diabetic patient. Falsely increased glycohemoglobin levels occur with the last trimester of pregnancy and with renal dialysis, and falsely decreased glycohemoglobin levels occur with hemolytic and pernicious anemias and with chronic renal failure. Usual reference range in SI units is 5.6% to 7.5% of total Hb (0.056% to 0.075% of total Hb).

Glucose tolerance test

The glucose tolerance test (GTT; oral glucose tolerance test, OGTT) is the most specific, sensitive, and complete test for diabetes mellitus. In this test the patient is given a standard oral glucose load, and serum and urine glucose specimens are obtained before the glucose load and then at 30 minutes, 1 hour, 2 hours, 3 hours, and sometimes 4 hours after administration of the glucose. Diabetic patients will not be able to tolerate this load, and glucose levels will remain elevated for longer than normal. Fasting blood glucose and glucose peak values also will be higher than normal. The test must be performed under rigidly controlled conditions if a true test response is to be obtained.

Patient preparation

The nurse instructs the patient to consume a high carbohydrate diet (at least 200 to 300 g) for at least 3 days before the test and to discontinue oral contraceptives, steroids, salicylates, and thiazide derivatives 3 days before the test. The patient is told to discontinue insulin or oral hypoglycemic agents on the day of the test. Fasting is required from midnight before the test and during the test period. Water is permitted, especially because several urine specimens are collected. Alcohol, coffee, and tea should be avoided 12 hours before testing. The nurse encourages the patient to bring materials for quiet activity during the test period, since even mild exercise will affect test results. The patient is cautioned not to smoke during the test period, since this will also affect test results.

The nurse ensures that the test begins between 7 and 9 AM (0700 and 0900 hr) and that the patient has been fasting for at least 8 and not more than 16 hours. Baseline urine and serum glucose specimens are collected. The nurse administers a 100 g carbohydrate load (usually in the form of a carbonated drink) and collects urine and blood specimens 30, 60, 120, and 180 minutes after the intake of the glucose. The specimens are labeled with the exact time of collection. The nurse monitors the patient for dizziness, faintness, sweating, tremors, excessive nausea, or vomiting and discontinues the procedure if necessary. Usual reference range in SI units—after ingestion of glucose is less than 115 mg/dL (6.3 mmol/L); at 30, 60, and 90 minutes it is less than 200 mg/dL (11 mmol/L); and at 120 minutes it is less than 140 mg/dL (7.7 mmol/L).

CRITICAL THINKING QUESTIONS

1 What are the categories of hormones secreted by the endocrine system? On what basis are they categorized?

2 Name three effects of cortisol.

3 Explain the process of negative feedback and give examples of it.

4 Design at least three questions to ask patients about risk factors in relation to the endocrine system.

5 Describe an effective approach to examining a painful thyroid gland.

6 Describe each of the tests that are used in the diagnosis of diabetes mellitus.

7 Outline what you would tell a patient who is undergoing adrenal venography, a thyroid scan, or a test for plasma renin activity.

BIBLIOGRAPHY

Current

1. Bates B: *A guide to physical examination and history-taking,* ed 4, Philadelphia, 1987, JB Lippincott Co.
2. Brunner LS, Suddarth DS: *Textbook of medical-surgical nursing,* Philadelphia, 1988, JB Lippincott Co.
3. Cella JH, Watson J.: *Nurse's manual of laboratory tests,* Philadelphia, 1989, FA Davis Co.

4. DeGowin RL: *DeGowin & DeGowin's bedside diagnostic examination,* ed 5, New York, 1987, Macmillan Publishing Co.
5. Hunt AH: Digital subtraction angiography: patient preparation and care, *J Neurosci Nurs* 19:4, 1987.
6. Lewis SM, Collier IC: *Medical-surgical nursing: assessment and management of clinical problems,* St Louis, 1987, Mosby–Year Book, Inc.
7. Malasanos L et al: *Health assessment,* ed 4, St. Louis, 1990, Mosby–Year Book, Inc.
8. McDonagh A: Getting your patient ready for a nuclear scan, *Nurs 91* 21:2, 1991.
9. *Nurse's ready reference: diagnostic tests,* Springhouse, Pa, 1991, Springhouse Corporation.
10. Sakiyama R: Common thyroid disorders, *Am Fam Physician* 38(1):227-238, 1988.
11. Seidel HM et al: *Mosby's guide to physical examination,* St Louis, 1991, Mosby–Year Book, Inc.
12. Sheps SG, Jiang NS, Klee GG: Diagnostic evaluation of pheochromocytoma, *Endocrinol Metab Clin North Am* 17:397, 1988.
13. Swartz MH: *Textbook of physical diagnosis,* Philadelphia, 1989, WB Saunders Co.
14. Taylor AL, Fishman LM: Corticotropin-releasing hormone, *N Engl J Med* 319:213, 1988.
15. Thompson JM et al: *Mosby's manual of clinical nursing,* ed 2, St Louis, 1989, Mosby–Year Book, Inc.
16. Tilkian SM, Conover MB, Tilkian AG: *Clinical implications of laboratory tests,* ed 4, St Louis, 1987, Mosby–Year Book, Inc.
17. Young WF, Klee GG: Primary aldosteronism: diagnostic evaluation, *Endocrinol Metab Clin North Am* 17:267, 1988.

Classic

18. Baberman S: *ABC's of interpretative laboratory data,* Greenville, 1984, Interpretative Laboratory Data, Inc.
19. Block G, Nolan J: *Health assessment for professional nursing: a developmental approach,* New York, 1986, Appleton-Century-Crofts.
20. Bowers A, Thompson J: *Clinical manual of health assessment,* St Louis, 1984, Mosby–Year Book, Inc.
21. Bryne CJ et al: *Laboratory tests: implications for nursing care,* Menlo Park, Calif, 1986, Addison-Wesley.
22. *Diagnostics,* Springhouse, Pa, 1981, Intermed Communications.
23. *Endocrine disorders,* Springhouse, Pa, 1984, Springhouse Corporation.
24. Fields W, McGinn-Campbell K: *Introduction to health assessment,* Reston, Va, 1983, Reston Publishing Co., Inc.
25. King RC: The fine art of giving a physical: exploring the neck and lymphatics, *RN,* pp 49, 99, June 1982.
26. Pagana KD, Pagana TJ: *Diagnostic testing and nursing implications: a case study approach,* St Louis, 1986, Mosby–Year Book, Inc.
27. Pagana KD, Pagana TJ: *Pocket nurse guide: laboratory and diagnostic tests,* St Louis, 1986, Mosby–Year Book, Inc.
28. Price S, Wilson L: *Pathophysiology,* New York, 1986, McGraw-Hill.
29. Tietz NW: *Textbook of clinical chemistry,* Philadelphia, 1986, WB Saunders Co.

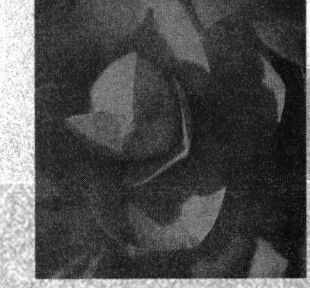

CHAPTER SIXTY

Nursing Management of Adults with Hypothalamus, Pituitary, or Adrenal Disorders

---

LEARNING OBJECTIVES

1 Describe the effects of excess glucocorticoids on adipose tissue distribution, protein and carbohydrate metabolism, the immune system, and the inflammatory response.

2 Explain the physiologic effects of deficiencies of cortisol, aldosterone, and gonadotropins.

3 Differentiate between the signs and symptoms of mineralocorticoid and glucocorticoid deficiencies.

4 Explain the general treatment principles of diseases caused by hormone deficiency or excess.

5 Differentiate between normal adrenal function and dysfunction.

6 Relate the pathophysiology of adrenal and pituitary diseases to the nursing management of patients with the diseases.

7 State the possible consequences of long-term steroid therapy.

8 Identify potential family pattern alterations and learning needs of patients experiencing Cushing's syndrome, acromegaly, hypopituitarism, and Addison's disease.

9 Develop a nursing care plan for the patient experiencing adrenal or pituitary dysfunction.

KEY TERMS

PATIENTS EXPERIENCING multiple changes in functional capacities may have endocrinologic diseases caused by dysfunction of the hypothalamus, pituitary, or adrenal glands. Careful nursing assessment of changes in the patient's behavior and functional capacities is paramount, because these diseases often have insidious courses and variable presentations. All of these diseases ultimately result in either excessive or deficient hormone production or secretion (Table 60-1).

HYPOTHALAMIC DYSFUNCTION
Definition/Etiology

The hypothalamus links the central nervous system with the endocrine system via the pituitary gland. Pituitary gland functioning is controlled by hypothalamic inhibiting and releasing hormones. Causes of hypothalamic dysfunction may be divided into three general categories: (1) internal responses to external stimuli, such as the neuroendocrine stress response; (2) drug effects on neurotransmitters, including those of tricyclic antidepressants and dopamine agonists; and (3) damage to the hypothalamus or surrounding tissue caused by tumor growth or internal hydrocephalus, trauma, surgery, infiltration, or infection.[2] Increased intracranial pressure effects are quite variable, depending on the extent of tissue or anatomic involvement and cerebral and collateral circulation.

Pathophysiology

Multiple homeostatic changes occur as a result of alterations in hypothalamic–pituitary gland neurosecretory connections, hypothalamic releasing and inhibitory factors (such as corticotropin-releasing hormone [CRH]), neuropeptides, and neurotransmitters. These homeostatic or endocrine disruptions may result in altered behavior, serum osmolality, temperature regulation, fluid volume, and thyroid, adrenal, and gonadal functioning.

Clinical Manifestations

Clinical signs and symptoms include disturbances in consciousness, behavior, and affect; alterations in body processes such as increased thirst, hyperphagia or increased appetite, and changes in temperature regulation; and pressure effects that result in headaches, visual field deficits, and third, fourth, and sixth cranial nerve palsies. These may be apparent as changes in accommodation and extraocular eye muscle movement. Classic signs and symptoms of increased intracranial pressure, such as headache, vomiting, and papilledema, are often absent when tumor growth is slow.

NURSING MANAGEMENT OF THE PATIENT WITH HYPOTHALAMIC DYSFUNCTION
Assessment

Nursing assessment of the patient with hypothalamic dysfunction includes evaluation of neurologic, physiologic, and psychosocial functioning; daily living and self-care resources; and coping abilities.[20] The data base begins with a nursing history focusing on the presenting symptom or chief complaint. A review of neurologic and endocrine systems includes functioning in relation to consciousness, thinking, speaking, moving, eating, elimination, sexual response, and coping with a chronic illness.[20] A full understanding of the patient's experience necessitates a discussion of preceding tests, procedures, therapies, medications, and self-treatment measures. Information regarding trauma, injuries, surgeries, chronic conditions, or family history of neurologic or endocrinologic disease is also obtained.

Most importantly, determine the impact of the symptom or disease on the patient and significant others by asking the patient to describe the symptom, its cause, and its meaning in relation to the current situation and the patient's family, significant others, and culture they share.[10,20]

Objective data are gathered by observing and examining nervous system, endocrine, and cardiovascular functioning. Alterations in consciousness, thinking skills, speech, movement, gait, cranial nerve functioning, sensation, and fluid volume status all require careful assessment.

Planning/Implementation

Nurses help patients and families cope with countless symptoms, procedures, medications, and body

TABLE 60-1 Pituitary and Adrenal Dysfunction

Disorders causing hypofunction	Disorders causing hyperfunction
PITUITARY DISORDERS	
Hypopituitarism	Hyperpituitarism
Diabetes insipidus	Syndrome of inappropriate ADH secretion (SIADH)
ADRENAL DISORDERS	
Adrenal insufficiency	Cushing's syndrome
	Hyperaldosteronism
	Pheochromocytoma

and daily living changes associated with endocrine disease. Diagnostic test results and the effects of medication are evaluated in terms of their impact on the patient's coping abilities and resources. Nursing care is altered as needed to help the patient understand and adapt to changes in role performance, self-concept, and identity.

Ongoing Care

Discharge planning is an essential part of nursing care. The patient and family are taught to cope with the demands of a chronic illness outside the hospital, often with limited support services. Nurses work collaboratively with the patient, family, and other health professionals to identify and utilize both internal and community resources.

Disorders of the Anterior Pituitary Gland

HYPOPITUITARISM
Definition

Diseases of the pituitary gland involve deficiencies of target organ hormones (such as cortisol) secondary to pituitary deficits of tropic hormones such as growth hormone and adrenocorticotropic hormone. **Hypopituitarism,** or underactivity of the anterior pituitary gland, is a relatively rare disorder. It is manifested by partial or complete deficiency of hormone secretion and usually involves multiple hormone deficiencies. The disorder may develop gradually or have an abrupt onset.

Etiology/Epidemiology

Neoplasms are the most common cause of hypopituitarism. Pituitary tumors are classified as functioning (hormonally active) or nonfunctioning, depending on whether a hormone is produced. Pituitary tumors are usually benign and commonly found in the anterior lobe. They are classified as microadenomas if they are less than 10 mm in diameter. One fourth of patients autopsied are found to have asymptomatic microadenomas. Other causes of hypopituitarism include the following[2]:

1. Suprasellar or parapituitary neoplasms
2. Congenital diseases or hereditary conditions including growth hormone deficiencies
3. Physical agents such as radiation, surgery, and trauma
4. Disrupted blood supply or postpartum hemorrhage causing pituitary necrosis (Sheehan's syndrome)
5. Inflammation or infections such as sarcoidosis, tuberculosis, abscess, and syphilis
6. Isolated idiopathic defects in hormone secretion

Pathophysiology

The diagnosis of hypopituitarism is often delayed, since three fourths of the gland has to be destroyed before signs and symptoms occur. Clinical findings may be quite variable, because they depend on both the etiologic process and the number and extent of hormone deficiencies.

A temporal sequence of hormone deficiencies occurs; growth hormone (GH) and luteinizing hormone (LH) fail first, followed by follicle-stimulating hormone (FSH) and thyroid-stimulating hormone (TSH), and last, by adrenocorticotropic hormone (ACTH). Prolactin deficiency is uncommon except in pituitary necrosis precipitated by hemorrhage or shock (Sheehan's syndrome). Antidiuretic hormone (ADH) deficiency is also uncommon, but it may occur after a head injury or an infection involving the posterior pituitary gland.

Advanced cases of hypopituitarism may be associated with hypoglycemia, hypothyroidism, hypothermia, and hypotension.

Clinical Manifestations

Most clinical findings result from hypogonadism (see box below), but hypothyroidism and hypoadrenalism (see box on p. 1658) can also produce widespread signs and symptoms. Adults show no obvious symptoms of GH deficiency, but deficiencies during childhood result in short stature with normal body proportions.

GONADOTROPIN DEFICIENCY

Female
Amenorrhea or menstrual irregularities
Infertility
Decreased libido
Breast and uterine atrophy
Loss of axillary and pubic hair
Vaginal dryness; dyspareunia or painful intercourse

Male
Decreased libido
Impotence
Small, soft testicles
Loss of axillary and pubic hair
Juvenile pattern of scalp hair

TSH AND ACTH DEFICIENCIES

TSH deficiency

Decreased energy
Constipation
Sensitivity to cold
Dry skin and hair
Fine wrinkling of the skin
Weight gain

ACTH deficiency

Inadequate response to stress
Weakness, tiredness
Postural hypotension
Pallor
Decreased skin and nipple pigmentation
Hypoglycemia

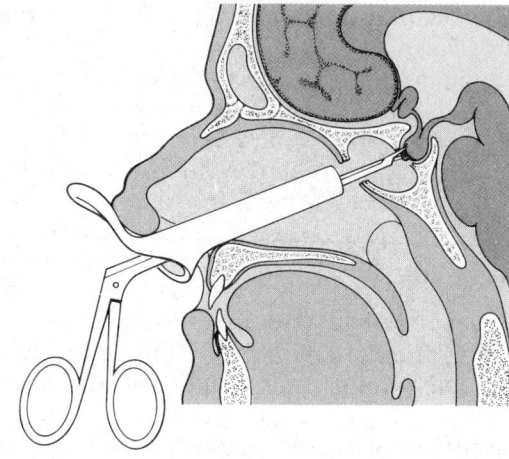

FIGURE 60-1   Transsphenoidal surgical approach.

Patients usually appear well nourished although severe, prolonged disease may be associated with weight loss and malnutrition. Pressure effects of tumors may vary from no symptoms to headaches, visual field deficits, cranial nerve palsies, and rhinorrhea. Chronic symptoms of fatigue, along with skin, body, and libido changes, often go undiagnosed and result in altered family and daily life functioning.

Diagnostic tests

Radiologic, neurologic, ophthalmologic, and endocrinologic diagnostic studies are used to evaluate pituitary and end organ functioning. Neuro-ophthalmologic evaluation includes testing of visual acuity, extraocular muscle functioning, funduscopy, and manual or computer-assisted plotting of visual fields.

Radiographic lateral and anteroposterior views of the pituitary fossa may show an increased size, appear normal, or show sellar erosion. Abnormalities may only be revealed by using computed tomography (CT) scanning or magnetic resonance imaging (MRI).

Anterior pituitary hormones, such as ACTH, are measured by radioimmunoassay before evaluating posterior pituitary function. This is done because decreased levels of ACTH and cortisol cause a decreased glomerular filtration rate, which masks the symptoms of diabetes insipidus. Radioimmunoassays of prolactin, TSH, thyroxine, cortisol, LH, FSH, estrogen (women), and testosterone (men) are also drawn. To determine the cause of hypopituitarism, pituitary hormones, specifically ACTH, TSH, LH, and

FSH, are drawn simultaneously with target organ hormones such as thyroxine and cortisol and the gonadal steroids estrogen and testosterone. Dynamic testing of reserve hormone levels such as the insulin hypoglycemia test may also be done.

Therapeutic Management

Treatments are individualized and depend on both the etiologic factor and the stage at which the disease or tumor is detected. Pituitary tumors require surgical removal or x-ray irradiation. A transsphenoidal surgical approach is used (Figure 60-1); craniotomy is rarely required. Recurrence after surgical treatment is common; therefore periodic CT scans are necessary. Target organ hormone replacement therapy is used before and during treatment and continued throughout the patient's life. Pituitary hormones and hypothalamic releasing factors are being evaluated for use in hypopituitarism.

Hormone replacement therapy

Hormone replacement therapy includes corticosteroids, thyroid hormone, and testosterone or estrogen. Corticosteroid replacement is undertaken with oral hydrocortisone, 20 mg in the morning and 10 mg in the early evening. Individual needs vary from 15 to 60 mg per day. Trauma, illness, surgery, or other stressors require increased, rapid-acting corticosteroid replacement. After corticosteroid replacement, levothyroxine (Synthroid) may be given if thyroid hormone replacement is needed. Thyroid hormone replacement is carried out gradually and carefully, especially in elderly persons, to prevent adrenal insufficiency, adrenal crisis, angina, or congestive heart failure. Thyroid hormone increases metabolic demands by increasing oxygen consumption and cardiac output, which compromises diminished adrenal cortisol reserves. Sexual functioning is maintained and osteoporosis prevented through the use of oral fluoxymesterone (Halotestin) or depot intramuscular testosterone (Depo-Testosterone) in men and ethinyl estradiol (Estinyl) or low-dose oral contraceptives in women. Attempts at restoring fertility include the use of gonadotropins and intermittent subcutaneous injections of gonadotropin-releasing hormone (GnRH).[21]

Emergency treatment

Patients may initially present with a severe headache, altered mental status, and rapid progressive visual loss or blindness as a result of tumor expansion and pressure on the optic chiasm. Tumor enlargement and hemorrhage may cause acute pituitary failure (pituitary apoplexy). These presenting symptoms require immediate plasma cortisol testing, assessment of fluid and electrolyte status, frequent monitoring of neurologic status and vital signs, and possible decompression. Temporary stabilization with high-dose intramuscular or intravenous corticosteroids is usually required. Acute infections or severe trauma requires early recognition and aggressive treatment of hypothyroidism or adrenal insufficiency.

NURSING MANAGEMENT OF THE PATIENT WITH HYPOPITUITARISM
Assessment

Patients with hypopituitarism may initially exhibit few or varied complaints, including headaches, visual changes, weakness, fatigue, cold intolerance, hair changes, menstrual changes, or alterations in sexual functioning. While establishing rapport with the patient, obtain a description of the onset (gradual or sudden) and course of the problem. Fully explore the problem by asking questions such as "Has your vision changed? Do you have frequent headaches? Do you have enough energy to carry out your work and daily activities? Have you noticed changes in your libido or sexual urges?" It is important to assess the patient's body image and self-esteem along with reactions of significant others to altered functioning and body changes. Hypopituitarism may be missed in elderly persons because of chronic, nonspecific symptoms that have gone unrecognized. The sensitive clinical cues in the younger individual that relate to loss of gonadal function are lost in postmenopausal women and older men experiencing a decreased libido because these symptoms are commonly attributed to "normal aging." Physical findings may include visual field deficits and changes in visual acuity, genital atrophy, hair loss, pallor, and skin dryness and wrinkling.

Nursing Diagnosis

Possible nursing diagnoses for a patient with hypopituitarism include the following:

Sensory/perceptual alterations (visual) related to tumor pressure effects

Pain related to tumor pressure effects

Body image disturbance related to changes in physical appearance and body functioning

Altered sexuality patterns related to gonadotropin deficiency

Altered role performance related to weakness and fatigue

Self-esteem disturbance related to changes in physical appearance and sexual functioning

Altered health maintenance related to lack of knowledge regarding the disease process, treatments, medications, and self-care

High risk for injury related to decreased vision

Planning

Patient-centered goals are initially directed at detecting signs and symptoms of possible pituitary insufficiency, referring patients for evaluation, and providing information and support during the diagnostic workup and treatment process. In the presence of tumor pressure effects, such as headache or visual or mental impairment, the goal is to maintain stable neurologic functioning and fluid volume. Major ongoing goals are to promote increased self-esteem and the use of cognitive and behavioral strategies, which help the patient cope with chronic endocrine dysfunction. The patient may need support, encouragement, and possible counseling to formulate or reprioritize personal, family, recreational, and vocational goals.

Nursing care for the patient with hypopituitarism is planned to meet the following outcomes:

Patient will demonstrate adaptive behaviors to visual changes

Patient will not experience injury

Pain will be controlled at an acceptable level

Patient will participate in desired role activities without fatigue

Patient will exhibit adaptive coping behaviors and verbalize reconciliation with mind-body alterations

Implementation

Early detection of visual and neurologic deficits, carrying out medical orders for intramuscular or intravenous corticosteroids, and preparing the patient for possible surgical decompression are all essential components of nursing care. Family dynamics, sexual concerns, and coping skills must be explored, since the disease may have profound effects on the patient and family. Physical or emotional stressors such as altered sleep, work, or dietary patterns, job loss, or the death of a close friend may all precipitate or exacerbate hypopituitarism. Support systems, relaxation strategies, and coping measures need to be developed and enhanced. Ongoing patient education promotes successful patient and family self-management of the disease. Optimal symptom control and disease management are attained through patient education regarding the nature of the disease; the dosage, timing, and side effects of medications (see box, p. 1676); signs and symptoms that require an increase in medication; and the need for lifelong hormone replacement and regular follow-up care.

Evaluation

The patient should experience relief of presenting symptoms. Observable patient responses indicating improved self-concept and understanding of the disease process may include positive self-statements, verbalization of daily accomplishments, and descriptions of coping strategies, as well as information regarding medication effects and side effects and symptoms requiring evaluation. Expected outcomes also include verbalization of feelings about the disease process and ongoing care, as well as satisfaction with family and vocational roles.

Documentation

The patient record should include documentation of assessments; all interventions; and the patient's feelings, coping strategies, and responses to the diagnosis and ongoing care. Follow-up care of the patient can be much more individualized and efficient if careful records of the patient's understanding of the disease process, medications, and activities are maintained.

Ongoing Care

Communication and coordination with community resources, counselors, and vocational rehabilitation agencies are essential to assist the patient in coping with a condition requiring lifelong medication and follow-up care.

ACROMEGALY
Definition

Acromegaly, a somewhat rare, chronic disease, results from excess pituitary growth hormone (GH) secretion occurring after puberty. Prepubertal GH excess results in gigantism, or an excess of longitudinal bone growth that occurs before epiphyseal closure.

Etiology/Epidemiology

Acromegaly is commonly caused by benign pituitary tumors; however, abnormal ectopic or hypothalamic stimulation may result in pituitary hyperplasia. Pituitary tumors fall into two major categories: macroadenomas, which often grow rapidly but contain less GH; and microadenomas, which grow more slowly but usually contain more GH. Ectopic, nonpituitary sources of growth hormone−releasing hormone (GH−RH) include adenomas of the pituitary and parathyroid glands and pancreas (multiple endocrine neoplasia type I, an autosomal dominant disease), carcinoid tumors of the pancreas or lungs, and hypothalmic tumors.

Pathophysiology

GH interacts with cell membrane receptors and increases collagen synthesis, resulting in enlargement of acral soft tissue and bones along with visceral organ growth. Bony enlargement is most prominent in the face, hands, and feet, because linear bone growth cannot occur after epiphyseal closure. Synovial overgrowth and cartilaginous thickening also contribute to joint enlargement (Figure 60-2).

Physiologic effects include elevated blood glucose and insulin resistance, hypercalcemia caused by increased calcium resorption from bones or parathyroid adenomas, increased urinary calcium excretion, and increased serum phosphate. Further, GH stimulation and pituitary stalk tumor pressure contribute to decreased TSH and ACTH reserves, resulting in fatigue, weakness, and myopathy.

Systemic pathophysiologic processes and diseases include the following[16]:

1. Kyphosis and premature arthritis of the weight-bearing joints as a result of vertebral collapse and cartilaginous degeneration
2. Peripheral neuropathy related to enlarged peripheral nerves and bony entrapment
3. Hyperhydrosis (excessive sweating) caused by elevated basal metabolic rate
4. Urinary calculi
5. Diabetes mellitus
6. Hypertension, either essential or related to pheochromocytoma or Conn's tumor (an adrenocortical adenoma)
7. Cardiomegaly related to hypertension, coronary artery disease, or cardiomyopathy
8. Impaired chest wall movement and lung function as a result of hypertrophy of small airways
9. Dyspnea, sleep apnea, and upper airway obstruction related to pharyngeal soft tissue hypertrophy

Oversecretion of other tropic hormones may also occur. Excess prolactin secretion, or hyperprolactinemia, may be caused by the tumor itself, a prolacti-

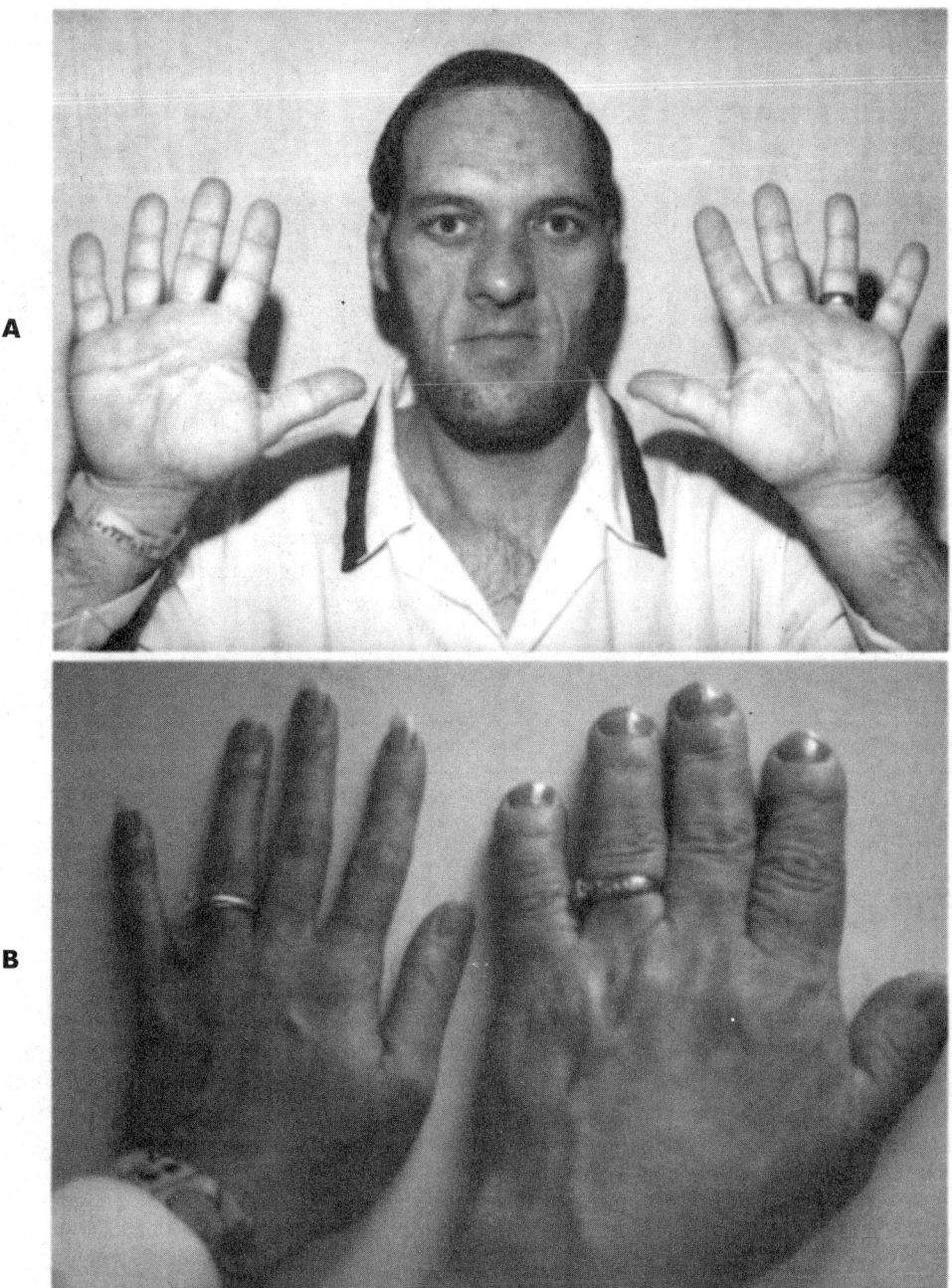

FIGURE 60-2   Patient with acromegaly. **A,** Typical appearance of adult patient with acromegaly. **B,** Healthy subject's hand *(left)* compared with hand *(right)* of patient with well-advanced acromegaly. (From Tindall GT, Barrow DL: *Disorders of the pituitary,* St Louis, 1986, Mosby–Year Book.)

noma, or interference with hypothalamic release of prolactin-inhibiting factor (PIF).

The presenting symptom in women may be amenorrhea, infertility, or galactorrhea (excessive or abnormal lactation). Men may experience impotence or lowered libido as a result of increased prolactin secretion and decreased gonadotropin production. Rarely, tumor impingement on the hypothalamus may cause diabetes insipidus.

Early diagnosis of acromegaly, although challenging, is important because of the high mortality associated with this disease.

Clinical Manifestations

Acromegaly is a slowly progressive disease; therefore clinical findings may become evident only with the passage of time. Signs and symptoms associated with acromegaly are given in the box on p. 1662.

CLINICAL MANIFESTATIONS OF ACROMEGALY

Growth hormone effects

Coarsened facial features
Soft tissue thickening of face and nose
Prognathism (forward projection of the lower jaw) with increased spacing of the lower teeth
Accentuated nasolabial folds
Macroglossia (enlargement of the tongue)
Prominence of the forehead and orbital ridges
Recurrent serous otitis media
Increased heel pad and skin thickness
Joint pain and enlargement
Arthritis, kyphosis, lumbar spondylosis (vertebral stiffening or fixation)
Lactation
Large, broad, "spadelike" hands
Broad feet
Hyperhydrosis
Hypertrichosis (excess growth of body hair)
Increased skin pigmentation
Seborrhea, acne, papillomas
Voice change

Paresthesias
Myopathy
Thyromegaly
Impaired glucose tolerance
Hypertension
Cardiac signs and symptoms such as dyspnea, paroxysmal nocturnal dyspnea, edema, and chest pain

Pituitary tumor effects

Radiographic sella turcica enlargement
Visual disturbances; photophobia; III, IV and VI cranial nerve palsies
Cerebrospinal fluid rhinorrhea

Growth hormone and hypopituitarism effects

Drowsiness, fatigue, lethargy
Amenorrhea
Decreased libido
Weakness

Diagnostic tests

Radiographic testing and biochemical testing, in addition to analysis of changes in physical appearance and body functioning, are used to diagnose acromegaly. Skull, hand, and foot x-ray studies, along with possible CT/MRI scans, are studied for pituitary fossa enlargement and characteristic bone changes of the skull and extremities. Visual field testing and funduscopy are performed to search for tumor pressure effects on the optic chiasm. Diagnosis is confirmed by hormonal testing.

Serum GH levels may be normal or elevated; however, levels of serum somatomedin-C (SM-C), a GH-dependent polypeptide, are elevated in almost all patients with acromegaly. Patients with acromegaly show a paradoxic rise in GH during a glucose tolerance test or after an intravenous injection of thyroid releasing hormone (TRH). Prolactin, blood sugar, and phosphate levels are also drawn.

Therapeutic Management

Treatment options are directed toward (1) returning GH levels to normal; (2) reversing the associated physiologic and metabolic abnormalities; (3) avoiding systemic complications, tumor enlargement, and hypopituitarism; and (4) preventing recurrence. These goals are not always achievable. Three therapeutic options—surgery, irradiation, and pharmacotherapy—are used singly or in combination to treat acromegaly. No therapy is ideal because of possible hypopituitarism and incomplete suppression of growth hormone levels.[9,11,12]

Surgery

Transsphenoidal microsurgery, often the treatment of choice for small tumors, is a relatively safe procedure with a mortality of 0% to 3%. Usually an incision is made in the mouth, between the upper gum and lip, and the sella turcica is entered through the floor of the nose and the sphenoid sinus (see Figure 60-1). A transfrontal craniotomy may be needed for large tumors. A combination of surgery and postoperative radiation may be required to normalize GH levels. Surgical side effects include intraoperative bleeding, CSF leakage, meningitis, optic nerve damage, and hypopituitarism.

Radiotherapy

Irradiation, often a successful treatment option, is carried out via linear accelerator, proton beam, or intrasellar implantation of yttrium 90 seeds. A major problem with the treatment is the slow onset of beneficial effects. It may take 10 years for GH to decrease to acceptable levels. Complications are rare but may include CSF rhinorrhea, meningitis, optic nerve damage, diabetes insipidus, and hypopituitarism.

Pharmacotherapy

Bromocriptine, a semisynthetic ergot alkaloid, is used as a secondary treatment in combination with surgery or radiation. It suppresses GH levels by binding with dopamine receptors and acting as a dopamine agonist. Dopamine agonists cause a paradoxic fall in GH levels in acromegalic patients. Normal GH levels are difficult to achieve, and the levels rise when the drug is discontinued. Side effects, including nausea, vomiting, and orthostatic hypotension, necessitate gradual dose increases. Other dopamine agonists are being developed and tested. Analogs of the hypothalamic hormone somatostatin also may be used to lower GH levels. Treatment of acromegaly often results in hypopituitarism; therefore target organ hormone replacement is essential.

NURSING MANAGEMENT OF THE PATIENT WITH ACROMEGALY
Assessment

The patient with acromegaly may note a change in appearance of the body, face, or hands along with headaches or visual changes, sweating, increased hair growth and oily skin, paresthesias, weight gain, weakness, and goiter. It is important to ask the patient if shoe, ring, or hat sizes have changed. Amenorrhea, decreased libido, galactorrhea, and infertility may also occur. Early diagnosis of acromegaly depends on careful analysis of both the clinical history and the patient's appearance. Detailed inspection of the skin, hair, face, joints, hands, and feet is essential. It is helpful to examine serial photographs of the patient. Cranial nerves are tested, the thyroid gland is palpated, and the cardiovascular and musculoskeletal systems are fully assessed. In particular, the patient's general appearance, body proportions, blood pressure, pulse, heart sounds, and muscle mass and strength are evaluated.

Nursing Diagnosis

Nursing diagnoses reflect physiologic manifestations of hormonal excess and the patient's emotional and psychologic responses to the changes in body functioning and appearance. Possible nursing diagnoses for a patient with acromegaly include the following:
- High risk for decreased cardiac output related to coronary artery disease, cardiomyopathy, hypertension, and cardiac dysrhythmias caused by sleep apnea
- High risk for ineffective breathing pattern related to dyspnea, sleep apnea, kyphosis, and small airway obstruction
- Sensory/perceptual alterations (visual, tactile) related to tumor pressure effects and nerve compression caused by growth of the cartilage and soft tissue
- High risk for injury related to diminished vision and sensation
- Activity intolerance related to weakness, myopathy, and joint pain
- Pain related to weakness, myopathy, paresthesias, joint pain, and headache
- Altered nutrition: less than body requirements caused by excess GH secretion
- Sleep pattern disturbance related to dyspnea and sleep apnea
- Body image disturbance related to musculoskeletal and integumentary changes and decreased gonadotropin production
- Altered sexuality patterns related to GH effects, decreased gonadotropin production, and possible increased prolactin secretion
- Altered health maintenance related to lack of understanding of the disease process and treatment measures

Planning

Specific goals are geared to the extent of the disease process and the individual situation of each patient. General goals for the patient with acromegaly include the following:
- Maximization of cardiac output through maintenance of normal blood pressure and reduction of fluid volume excess as measured by acceptable blood pressure, pulse rate, and rhythm; absence of an S_3 gallop; clear lungs; and weight loss (representing loss of water weight)
- Improved breathing pattern evidenced by a reduction in dyspneic episodes, comfortable respirations at a normal rate, and little or no use of the accessory muscles of respiration
- Prompt recognition of visual and neurologic deficits
- Prevention of accidental injuries caused by sensory/perceptual deficits
- Tolerance of daily activities without undue fatigue
- Increased comfort and reduced pain evident in the expression and appearance of the patient
- Maintenance of stable body weight and acceptable blood glucose levels
- Acceptable sleep pattern evident in the ability to sleep without dyspnea
- Adaptation to altered body image and increased self-acceptance demonstrated by positive self-statements, verbalized coping measures, and acceptance of physical appearance
- Expression and discussion of sexuality and feelings related to sexual functioning
- Adequate knowledge level and fully verbalized understanding of the disease process, treatment plan, and need for hormone replacement therapy

Implementation

Initial nursing interventions are threefold: (1) helping the patient understand and cope with the disease process, associated body changes, and treatment measures; (2) monitoring the patient for signs of compromised cardiopulmonary functioning or tumor pressure effects; and (3) maintaining a safe and restful environment. The patient should be encouraged to discuss the disease process and its impact on psychosocial functioning, daily activities, work, relationships, and sexual functioning.[5] Nurses must understand and work with the patient's reactions, feelings, and values and at the same time maintain the patient's sense of dignity while diagnostic studies are carried out.[5,20]

Respirations and breathing pattern are monitored during the day and throughout the night. Ask the patient if he or she has chest tightness, wheezing, dyspnea, or insomnia. Before auscultating lung fields make careful observations of respiratory rate and pattern, degree of effort, use of accessory muscles, and any abnormal movements of the chest wall. Breathing may be eased by placing the patient in semi-Fowler's position.

Cardiac functioning and fluid volume status are closely monitored via ongoing measurements of body weight and vital signs and through inspection, palpation, and auscultation of the neck, lungs, and heart. Abnormal lung sounds such as crackles, increased jugular venous pressure, an S_3, sustained or deviated apical impulse, and increasing edema are signs of fluid volume excess and congestive heart failure.

While assessing cardiopulmonary functioning, the nurse also carefully monitors the patient for changes in mental and neurologic status. Neurologic abnormalities or changing neurologic signs may indicate tissue and nerve compression caused by the tumor. Neurologic signs such as level of consciousness, pupillary equality and reactions, visual fields, and extraocular muscle functioning require frequent assessments. Changes in neurologic status or signs are promptly reported to the physician.

Peripheral numbness, tingling, paresthesias, and diminished sensations of the hands and feet are common and are due to peripheral nerve compression. These sensory alterations, along with possible visual field deficits, pain related to tumor pressure, myopathy, and bony overgrowth of the joints, put the patient at high risk for injuries or accidents. A safe environment must be maintained. Adequate lighting, clear walkways, use of nonskid shoes, and placement of objects within the patient's functional visual field are simple but important environmental alterations. Assess strength and fine and gross motor abilities along with the location, quality, radiation, and degree of any perceived discomfort.

Patient comfort and activity tolerance are promoted through maintenance of a calming environment, rest periods alternated with activity, timely use of pain medications, and measures such as imagery, music, and progressive relaxation. Dietary alterations can also counteract the fatigue associated with hyperglycemia secondary to the insulin antagonistic effects of GH. The prescribed diet is usually low in sodium, fat, and cholesterol. Helping the patient understand the increased energy benefit of blood sugar control will enhance adherence to the prescribed diet.

Patients receiving radiotherapy need information about the procedure and its safety. Pharmacotherapy patients require information regarding medication benefits and side effects. Patients undergoing transsphenoidal hypophysectomy need information about the procedure and postoperative care. Concerns about surgery, particularly anxiety and fear, must be discussed. Postoperative nursing care for transsphenoidal hypophysectomy patients is outlined in the box on p. 1665.

Evaluation

Effective treatment of the patient with acromegaly should result in improved cardiopulmonary and neurologic functioning and increased activity tolerance. Verbalizations related to body changes, altered sexual functioning, and treatment measures indicate the patient's level of psychologic adaptation to acromegaly.[5] The patient's understanding of the disease process, its treatment, and follow-up care should also be monitored.

Documentation

Accurate physical and psychologic baseline data are extremely important for documenting responses to interventions. Alterations in the therapeutic approach occur as the patient undergoes medical, surgical, or pharmacologic treatment. It is important to record the patient's understanding of verbal and written instructions about the disease, drugs, and long-term hormone replacement therapy.

Ongoing Care

Treatment of acromegaly is usually a lifelong process, requiring the promotion of patient autonomy through the development of self-care abilities in the home or community setting.[20] The nurse supports the patient and family throughout the diagnostic, treatment, and recovery periods and involves the family by teaching, providing community health nurse referrals, and arranging follow-up medical appointments as necessary. Ongoing medical supervision is essential to stabilize and monitor hormone levels.

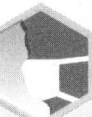

PREOPERATIVE AND POSTOPERATIVE NURSING INTERVENTIONS

Transsphenoidal Hypophysectomy

Intervention	Rationale
Compare postoperative neurologic status to preoperative neurologic examination	Neurologic assessments are most meaningful when compared with previous assessments; changes may indicate increased intracranial pressure (ICP)
Assess vital signs and neurologic status frequently—initially every 15 minutes	Hypovolemia and shock are complications of any surgical procedure
Carefully monitor facial expression and appearance, extraocular movements, visual acuity and fields, level of consciousness, speech, limb movements, sensation, and reflexes	Neurologic symptoms of increased ICP may develop rapidly or insidiously
Maintain head-of-bed elevation at 30 degrees	This decreases headaches by decreasing pressure on sella turcica and promoting venous return
Provide good oral hygiene and avoid tooth brushing	Nasal packing causes obligatory mouth breathing and drying of mucous membranes; surgical site must not be disturbed
Instruct patient to avoid blowing nose, sneezing, vigorous coughing, or straining at stool	These activities may cause a cerebrospinal fluid (CSF) leak
Observe for clear nasal drainage, constant swallowing, and severe, persistent, generalized or frontal headache	These signs and symptoms indicate CSF leak into sinuses
Test clear nasal drainage with glucose reagent strips (such as those used to test for glucose in urine)	A positive result indicates a CSF leak
Give antibiotics as ordered	Antibiotics may be ordered to prevent meningitis
Observe for weakness, weight loss, polydipsia, and polyuria	Loss of ADH and ACTH causes diabetes insipidus (often temporary) and adrenal insufficiency
Carry out fluid replacement orders	Diabetes insipidus requires aggressive fluid replacement
Administer cortisone and intramuscular vasopressin (Pitressin) as ordered	Hormone replacement therapy indicated
Educate patient regarding prescribed hormone replacement, use of Medic-Alert bracelet, and follow-up care	Follow-up care is important, since hormone replacement therapy may need adjustment and is required for life; ADH deficiency may resolve unless entire pituitary gland was removed
Instruct patient to avoid bending over, Valsalva's maneuver, or straining at stool for 2 months	These activities increase ICP and can disrupt surgical site and cause CSF leakage

Posterior Pituitary Dysfunction

DIABETES INSIPIDUS
Definition

Diabetes insipidus (DI) is a condition characterized by impaired renal conservation of water resulting from a deficiency of the antidiuretic hormone (ADH) arginine vasopressin. There are three basic forms of this disorder: (1) neurogenic or **central diabetes insipidus,** a defect of the pituitary gland or hypothalamus; (2) **nephrogenic diabetes insipidus,** a kidney tubular defect resulting in decreased water absorption; and (3) primary polydipsia, or excess water drinking, which can also result in impaired renal concentrating ability.[21]

Etiology/Epidemiology

Diabetes insipidus is an uncommon condition that often begins in childhood or early adult life and affects more males than females. Central DI may be a primary familial or idiopathic condition (50% of cases) or secondary to trauma, neurosurgery, tumors, granulomas, infections, and autoimmune or vascular conditions. Drugs such as alcohol and phenytoin (Dilantin) may also inhibit the release of ADH.

Nephrogenic DI may be inherited as an X-linked dominant trait, or it may be secondary to (1) chronic renal disease; (2) primary aldosteronism; (3) systemic diseases such as sickle cell anemia and multiple myeloma; (4) drugs, including some anesthetics, lithium, and mannitol; (5) hypercalcemia and hypokalemia; and (6) excessive water intake (primary polydipsia). A new form of vasopressin-resistant DI in pregnancy has also been documented.[17,21]

The syndromes of DI and nephrogenic diabetes insipidus are uncommon in elderly persons except that transient nephrogenic diabetes insipidus complicates mechanical relief of obstructive uropathy and hydronephrosis, the latter being more commonly seen in the older male.

Pathophysiology

Decreased or absent vasopressin secretion in central DI causes increased water loss in the urine and increased plasma osmolality and sodium levels. Increased thirst then stabilizes plasma osmolality and compensates for the increased urinary output.[2] Severe dehydration and hypernatremia can develop if thirst perception is diminished or if water is not available. Excessive, prolonged water intake along with systemic and renal diseases causes alterations in the renal osmotic gradient and countercurrent system. Familial nephrogenic DI, drugs, and hypercalcemia interfere with adenylate cyclase and cyclic adenosine monophosphate (cAMP), which inhibit membrane protein phosphorylation and prevent increased renal tubular reabsorption of solute-free water.[8,21] Pregnancy-induced DI is caused by placental degradation of vasopressin and possible mild deficiency of vasopressin.[21]

Clinical Manifestations

A triad of clinical symptoms—excessive thirst, polydipsia, and polyuria—occurs, often suddenly. Urine is dilute (specific gravity below 1.006), and serum osmolality is increased beyond 280 mOsm/L. Urine volume is increased in the range of 4 to 20 L/day, and frequent urination, often every 30 to 60 minutes, is common. Polydipsia (often a preference for cold drinks) usually normalizes hydration, but dehydration may occur as a result of fluid restriction, anesthesia, or trauma.

Diagnostic tests

After hypotonic polyuria (urine output greater than 200 mL/hr and specific gravity less than 1.006) has been documented, special diagnostic tests are used to differentiate the various forms of DI. Diagnostic studies include dehydration or water deprivation tests, osmotic stimulation, and administration of vasopressin or desmopressin (DDAVP). During these

tests serum osmolality and sodium and vasopressin levels are measured, along with urine osmolality. The studies require careful, frequent nursing assessments since severe dehydration can be induced by water deprivation, osmotic stimulation can cause congestive heart failure, and DDAVP can cause water intoxication and electrolyte imbalance. Hourly assessments of vital signs and body weight are made, and close observation is needed because of increased thirst and possible surreptitious drinking.

After differentiation of the type of DI, further studies are performed to determine the cause of the disease. Chest x-ray studies and CT/MRI brain scans may be ordered.

Therapeutic Management

Treatment of DI depends on the cause and is directed at improving urinary concentration and reducing urinary flow through the use of hormonal and nonhormonal agents. In addition to any necessary oral or intravenous fluid replacement, the drugs used to treat DI are summarized in Table 60-2. Nephrogenic diabetes insipidus is treated with thiazide diuretics in conjunction with salt restriction. These diuretics reduce the glomerular filtration rate and increase proximal tubular reabsorption of sodium. Thiazide diuretics may also be used in combination with chlorpropamide. Amiloride (Midamor) diuretics and prostaglandin synthesis inhibitors are also used to treat DI.[21]

NURSING MANAGEMENT OF THE PATIENT WITH DIABETES INSIPIDUS
Assessment

Patients with DI commonly complain of thirst, a desire for cold fluids, polydipsia, polyuria, and nocturia. These symptoms often occur abruptly. Insomnia as a result of nocturia may be a presenting complaint. Nocturia may also result in tiredness and malaise because of sleep pattern disturbance. The patient's fluid and electrolyte status is carefully monitored. In severe cases of ADH deficiency the nurse may observe a fluid intake and output of more than 12 L/day of hypotonic urine. Patients may also come to the hospital with severe dehydration or in altered states of consciousness as a result of fluid restriction or diminished thirst sensation. This condition can be quite serious in elderly patients who are unable to drink.[17]

Nursing Diagnosis

Individualized nursing diagnoses usually reflect alterations in fluid volume status and daily living patterns. Potential nursing diagnoses include the following:

TABLE 60-2   Pharmacology Summary: Drugs for Diabetes Insipidus

Drug	Dose	Indication	Limitations	Side effects
Desmopressin (DDAVP)	Intranasally (10 to 25 mg); subcutaneously (2 to 4 mg)	Central DI and vasopressin-resistant DI in pregnancy	High cost ($2000/yr)	Few (nasal congestion, headache, flushing of skin); severe hyponatremia may occur with overtreatment
Vasopressin (Pitressin)	5 to 10 U subcutaneously or intramuscularly	Acute central DI, short-term management	Very short duration of action (1 to 2 hours)	Sweating, tremor, "pounding" in head, abdominal cramps, nausea, angina, increased blood pressure, water intoxication
Lypressin (Diapid)	Intranasally qid	Central DI	Short duration of action (4 to 6 hours) does not prevent nocturia	Decreased absorption in presence of nasal congestion; irritation of nose, eyes, and lungs
Vasopressin tannate (Pitressin Tannate)	2.5 to 5 U intramuscularly (lasts 72 hours)	Chronic, severe central DI	Given by injection—synthetic hormones are usually preferred agents	Sweating, tremor, "pounding" in head, abdominal cramps, nausea, angina, increased blood pressure, water intoxication
Chlorpropamide (Diabinese)	250 to 500 mg/day	Mild, moderate, or severe central DI		Hypoglycemia and Antabuse-like reactions
Clofibrate (Atromide-S)	1 to 2 g/day	Mild, moderate, or severe central DI	Less potent than chlorpropamide	Cholelithiasis and cardiovascular complications
Carbamazepine (Tegretol)	200 to 400 mg/day	Mild or moderate central DI with detectable ADH levels	Serious side effects	Neurologic, hematopoietic, and cardiovascular side effects

Fluid volume deficit related to fluid restriction and polyuria

High risk for sleep pattern disturbance related to polydipsia, polyuria, and nocturia

High risk for altered role performance related to polyuria and nocturia

Altered health maintenance related to lack of knowledge regarding the disease process, diagnostic testing, treatment, and follow-up care

Planning

Goals related to maintenance of normal fluid volume status, life-style adjustments, and patient education include the following:

Patient understands and verbalizes the importance of fluid monitoring

Patient demonstrates accurate measurement and recording of fluid intake, fluid output, and urine specific gravity

Patient accurately records daily weight

Patient experiences acceptable sleep pattern evident in reduced episodes of nocturia

Patient carries out normal daily activities and roles with reduced complaints of polydipsia and polyuria

Patient possesses adequate knowledge level evident in ability to accurately discuss the disease process, medication usage, and signs of fluid volume alteration

Implementation

Provision of adequate fluid intake is important in preventing dehydration. Fluid volume status is assessed through the monitoring and accurate recording of mentation, vital signs, skin turgor, daily weights, intake, output, and urine specific gravity. Another primary responsibility of the nurse is patient education, which enables the patient to understand, cope with, and manage the disease by regularly using medications and by monitoring body weight and fluid intake and output. Before discharge the patient needs accurate information about drug administration, dosage, timing, and potential side effects. It is important to discuss the following aspects:

1. Self-injection techniques
2. The need to adequately warm and shake vials of vasopressin tannate suspended in oil
3. Avoidance of lung inhalation of nasal sprays because of pulmonary side effects
4. Increasing the dosage of nasal sprays when nasal congestion is present
5. The dangers of medication overdose

Evaluation

The effectiveness of the overall treatment plan will be demonstrated by stable body weight and the absence of polyuria. The patient should demonstrate an understanding of the disease process and its treatment, fluid balance principles, accurate measuring and recording of body weights and urine specific gravity, and correct administration of medications.

Documentation

Careful recording of assessment parameters reflecting fluid volume status ensures safe patient care and enables the physician to appropriately modify treatment. The patient should receive both verbal and written instructions about the disease, fluid balance measurements, and medications.

Ongoing Care

To manage the often lifelong illness of diabetes insipidus, patients need to know that medications will eradicate polyuria and nocturia and prevent excess water loss. It is important to teach the patient and family when to seek medical attention. Regular follow-up care and the use of a Medic-Alert bracelet and wallet card should be emphasized.

SYNDROME OF INAPPROPRIATE SECRETION OF ANTIDIURETIC HORMONE
Definition

The **syndrome of inappropriate secretion of antidiuretic hormone (SIADH),** in contrast to DI, is characterized by inappropriate, continued release of ADH. It results in water intoxication characterized by fluid volume expansion, hypotonicity of body fluids, and hyponatremia.

Etiology/Pathophysiology

Conditions and factors associated with SIADH include neoplastic tumors, respiratory disorders, central nervous system diseases, past neurologic surgery, and drugs. The exact pathogenesis of persistent and excessive ADH secretion is not fully understood. ADH-induced fixed antidiuresis and possible increased fluid intake cause fluid volume expansion, which inhibits adrenocortical secretion of aldosterone, causing salt loss in the urine and decreased proximal tubular reabsorption of sodium. Plasma osmolality is lowered; ADH continues to be secreted, causing water intoxication, hyponatremia, and initial cellular swelling.[17,21]

Clinical Manifestations

Signs and symptoms of SIADH depend on the degree of hyponatremia and rapidity of onset. Symptoms may include mental confusion, personality changes, lethargy, weakness, headache, weight gain, anorexia, abdominal cramping, nausea, and vomiting. Neurologic changes are more common at lower sodium levels and include stupor, seizures, or coma. Edema is absent because of salt loss and hyponatremia. Laboratory alterations indicative of SIADH include (1) a urinary sodium concentration greater than 20 mEq/L coupled with an elevated urine osmolality (above 100 mOsm/kg); (2) hyponatremia (less than 130 mEq/L) and hypo-osmolality (less than 280 mOsm/kg water); and (3) low or normal albumin levels and normal renal, thyroid, and adrenal function tests. Severe stress, pain, and hypovolemia interfere with the diagnosis of SIADH.[21]

Therapeutic Management

A simple treatment for SIADH is fluid restriction, to 500 mL or less per 24 hours. If fluid restriction and treatment of the underlying cause by surgical resection, irradiation, or chemotherapy are insufficient, pharmacotherapy may be used to inhibit the action of ADH. Demeclocycline (Declomycin), a tetracycline analog, and lithium (Lithium Carbonate) are effective because of their inhibition of cAMP synthesis in the renal tubule. Narcotic agonists, such as butorphanol (Stadol), are alternative drugs that change the osmoregulation of ADH.[17,21] Emergency situations may require the use of 3% or 5% intravenous saline solution and furosemide (Lasix) along with replacement of sodium, potassium, and magnesium. This treatment is undertaken gradually and carefully because rapid correction of hyponatremia may result in permanent brain damage from osmotic demyelination.

NURSING MANAGEMENT OF THE PATIENT WITH SIADH

Assessment

The nurse should carefully assess the mental and neurologic status, behavior, and personality of the patient at risk for developing SIADH. Physical assessment includes body weight, heart rate, and blood pressure. The patient is assessed for complaints of headache, abdominal pain, anorexia, nausea, vomiting, weakness, irritability, and muscle cramps. Water balance disorders in elderly patients may not be easily recognized because of coexistent medical illnesses.

Nursing Diagnosis

Nursing diagnoses for the patient with SIADH include the following:

Fluid volume excess related to inappropriate ADH secretion

High risk for injury related to hyponatremia and central nervous system alterations

Altered thought processes related to hyponatremia

Impaired verbal communication related to hyponatremia

Altered health maintenance related to lack of knowledge regarding the disease process and treatment regimen

Planning

Goals are individualized for each patient and usually include the following:

Patient maintains normal water balance as evidenced by normal weight and urine specific gravity

Mental alertness and stable emotional responses are restored as evidenced by a normal mental status examination and clear speech

Patient and family understand the disease process and treatment regimen

Implementation

Fluid restriction orders must be meticulously adhered to; intravenous saline, furosemide (Lasix), and electrolyte replacement administered; and daily weight records maintained. Alterations in mentation, behavior, and gastrointestinal and neuromuscular functioning are promptly communicated to the physician, and safety precautions are instituted if confusion, lethargy, or weakness is present.

Evaluation

Expected patient responses to treatment include fluid intake not to exceed urinary output and normal weight, urine specific gravity, and mental status.

Documentation

Vigilant documentation of baseline or admission assessment data and ongoing assessment parameters ensures that changes in vital signs, alertness, and behavior are promptly detected. Changes can be associated with worsening hyponatremia and the potential for grand mal seizures or respiratory arrest.

Ongoing Care

Chronic SIADH requires careful patient and family education regarding symptoms of fluid and electrolyte imbalance, dietary supplementation of sodium and potassium, fluid restriction, and pharmacotherapy. Periodic home visits may be required to monitor serum sodium levels and to identify potential toxic side effects of prescribed drugs.

Adrenal Gland Dysfunction

ADDISON'S DISEASE

Definition

Addison's disease, or insufficiency of the adrenal cortex, may be a primary disease of the adrenal cortex itself or adrenocortical failure caused by a deficiency of ACTH.

Etiology/Epidemiology

Primary adrenal disease, a relatively rare condition affecting both sexes equally, is commonly caused by autoimmune adrenalitis (70% of cases). Adrenalitis is often found in association with other autoimmune endocrine diseases such as diabetes mellitus, hypothyroidism, pernicious anemia, hypoparathyroidism, and ovarian or testicular failure. Addison's disease is uncommon in elderly persons; fewer than 5% of patients with this disease are over 60 years of age. Other causes of primary adrenal insufficiency include systemic infections or diseases such as tuberculosis and histoplasmosis, metastatic tumors, and surgical removal of the adrenal glands (bilateral adrenalectomy).[2,21] Secondary adrenocortical insufficiency is caused by either exogenous steroid withdrawal after long-term suppression of the hypothalamic-pituitary-adrenal axis or hypothalamic or pituitary infarction, tumors, or diseases.

Pathophysiology

Primary adrenal insufficiency is characterized by a lack of cortisol, mineralocorticoids (aldosterone), and androgens. Cortisol deficiency causes hypoglycemia because of decreased hepatic gluconeogene-

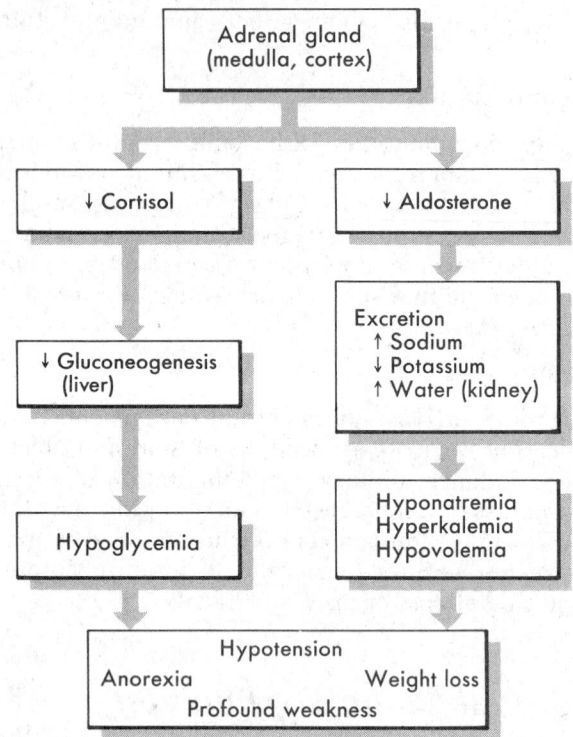

FIGURE 60-3 Pathologic alterations that accompany adrenocortical insufficiency.

sis and increased peripheral tissue sensitivity to insulin. Aldosterone deficiency causes increased sodium loss and potassium reabsorption in the kidneys. Sodium loss leads to water and volume depletion, hypotension (especially postural hypotension), and eventually shock. Hyperpigmentation is often present because of elevations of both ACTH and melanocyte-stimulating hormone (MSH).

Secondary adrenal insufficiency is not associated with hypoaldosteronism because of intact renin–angiotensin II production and potassium regulation of aldosterone. Both ACTH and cortisol levels are low, and hypogonadism and hypothyroidism are often present because of other tropic hormone deficiencies.

An acute adrenal crisis constitutes an emergency situation because of associated vascular collapse and electrolyte imbalances. It may be precipitated by stress such as infection, surgery, or trauma. Additional precipitating causes include failure to absorb steroids or withdrawal of exogenous steroids. The pathologic alterations accompanying adrenocortical insufficiency are diagramed in Figure 60-3.[7,14]

Clinical Manifestations

Clinical signs and symptoms of adrenocortical insufficiency are directly related to the hormone deficiencies and appear only after 90% of the glands have been destroyed[2,8] (see box above).

Diagnostic tests

Diagnostic tests and clinical signs such as skin pigmentation distinguish primary adrenal insufficiency from secondary adrenal insufficiency. Early morning cortisol and ACTH levels may be used for confirmation; however, more testing is required, since cortisol levels are often normal.

Baseline cortisol levels are drawn before and during a short ACTH stimulation test, during which a synthetic derivative of ACTH is given intramuscularly or intravenously and changes in cortisol and aldosterone are monitored. Both primary and secondary adrenocortical insufficiencies show no normal rise in plasma cortisol in response to ACTH.

Large depot injections or intravenous infusions of synthetic ACTH or cosyntropin (Cortrosyn) are used during prolonged stimulation tests to differentiate between primary and secondary insufficiency. Secondary insufficiency shows a gradual daily increase in cortisol, whereas primary insufficiency does not. Patients with primary disease require close monitoring and possible glucocorticoid administration during testing.

CLINICAL ALERT

Addisonian crisis occurs, sometimes quite suddenly, when adrenal hormone reserves are completely absent. Precipitants include infections, stress, trauma, adrenal hemorrhage, surgery, or abrupt withdrawal of exogenous glucocorticoid therapy. Signs and symptoms include weakness, abdominal pain, nausea, vomiting, diarrhea, and hypotension. Rapid replacement and stabilization of fluid volume, cortisol, and serum glucose levels are essential to prevent cardiac arrest, renal failure, or death. Careful and frequent nursing assessments of level of alertness, vital signs, fluid volume status, cardiovascular and respiratory functioning, and urinary output are required.

GERIATRIC CONSIDERATIONS

Adrenal Insufficiency

Elderly postsurgical or emergency room patients presenting with weakness and confusion need careful assessment regarding the possibility of adrenal insufficiency. Previous hospital records and medication lists of emergency room patients need to be requested, since a patient may have been taking corticosteroids for a chronic disease or may have recently been hospitalized for an acute stressful incident, such as a myocardial infarction or diabetic ketoacidosis, trauma, or surgery, that depleted adrenocortical reserves.

Therapeutic Management

All patients, whether they experience primary or secondary adrenal insufficiency, require replacement glucocorticoids. The drugs of choice are usually long-acting, synthetic glucocorticoids. The usual oral daily replacement dosages are 0.5 mg of dexamethasone or 5 mg of prednisone, daily at bedtime. Patients with primary adrenal insufficiency require both glucocorticoids and mineralocorticoids. Mineralocorticoid dosing is somewhat variable. Fludrocortisone (Florinef) is prescribed in a range from daily to three times per week along with adequate sodium intake.

Management of Addisonian Crisis

Acute adrenocortical insufficiency, or **addisonian crisis,** requires aggressive emergency management of vascular collapse and hypoglycemia. Intravenous saline and 5% dextrose solutions are rapidly infused along with intravenous dexamethasone sodium phosphate.[7,21] Electrolyte levels, blood sugar levels, and electrocardiograms (ECGs) are carefully monitored, and hemodynamic pressure monitoring may be instituted. Antibiotics are used to treat precipitating infections.

NURSING MANAGEMENT OF THE PATIENT WITH ADDISON'S DISEASE
Assessment

Changes that may be noted by the patient include decreased energy level and weight; altered gastrointestinal, cognitive, and emotional functioning; and increased skin pigmentation. Past health history may be positive for diabetes mellitus, thyroid disor-

ders, or other endocrinologic diseases. Behavioral alterations and coping measures should be carefully assessed. Postural hypotension and hyperpigmentation may be noted, but a patient may also exhibit pain, diarrhea, confusion, weakness, or actual coma and hypovolemic shock. Laboratory values may be normal in mild cases, but common abnormal findings include increased serum osmolality, hyponatremia, hyperkalemia, normocytic anemia, lymphocytosis, eosinophilia, and elevated renin levels.

Nursing Diagnosis

Possible diagnoses for a patient with adrenocortical insufficiency (Addison's disease) include the following:

High risk for fluid volume deficit related to aldosterone deficiency and gastrointestinal disturbances

High risk for injury related to electrolyte imbalance (hyperkalemia, hyponatremia) and hypoglycemia

Activity intolerance related to cortisol deficiency, hyperkalemia, and decreased cardiac output

High risk for ineffective individual coping related to decreased cortisol levels and associated emotional and physiologic instability

Altered health maintenance related to lack of knowledge regarding the disease, lifelong hormone replacement therapy, and ongoing care

Planning

Patient outcomes depend on success in maintaining normal fluid and electrolyte balance and in promoting increased physical strength and coping abilities. Goals for the patient include the following:

Normal fluid volume balance, evident in moist

 NURSING CARE PLAN *The Patient With Addison's Disease*

Nursing diagnosis/ Expected outcome	Interventions	Rationale
High risk for fluid volume deficit related to aldosterone deficiency and gastrointestinal disturbances • *Normal fluid volume balance, evident in moist mucous membranes, is established and maintained without orthostatic hypotension*	Monitor changes in mentation, respiration, vital signs, postural blood pressures, skin turgor, input and output, weight, sensation, and strength Promptly report signs and symptoms of hypovolemia During an acute episode of adrenal insufficiency, vital signs, mentation, and cardiac rhythm should be monitored at least every 30 minutes Administer intravenous dextrose, saline, glucocorticoids, mineralocorticoids, and antibiotics promptly and on schedule When foods are tolerated, provide regular meals and snacks and encourage intake of increased sodium, protein, and complex carbohydrates Encourage fluid intake of at least 3 L/day	Volume depletion may cause weakness, vascular collapse, and cardiac dysrhythmias Confusion, restlessness, hypotension, tachycardia, and fever may indicate impending adrenal crisis Physiologic changes occur quite rapidly, necessitating immediate corrective measures Prompt and careful management is required to prevent cardiac arrest, renal failure, or death Oral replacement of sodium losses is necessary, and maintenance of adequate blood glucose levels is required Fluid volume must be maintained until cortisol levels are stabilized
High risk for injury related to electrolyte imbalance (hyperkalemia, hyponatremia) and hypoglycemia • *Patient is free from injuries and maintains normal potassium and glucose levels*	Monitor serum potassium levels Promptly report signs and symptoms of hyperkalemia: weakness, paresthesias, nausea, abdominal pain and distention, and cardiac dysrhythmias or electrocardiogram (ECG) changes Monitor serum glucose levels Provide frequent between-meal and bedtime snacks; have patient avoid fasting	Decreased aldosterone secretion increases sodium and water excretion and decreases potassium excretion Muscle weakness, paresthesias, abdominal complaints, sharp peaked T waves, broad QRS complexes, prolonged Q-T intervals, and ventricular fibrillation or standstill are caused by high intracellular potassium levels Cortisol deficiency impairs hepatic gluconeogenesis and leads to hypoglycemia Patients do not tolerate fasting because of diminished liver storage of glycogen
Activity intolerance related to cortisol deficiency, hyperkalemia, and decreased cardiac output • *Patient is able to carry out daily activities without undue fatigue*	Assist with daily activities and utilize assistance and safety devices (walker, trapeze, siderails) Provide complete patient care during an acute episode of insufficiency Provide adequate rest periods and discontinue any activity if pain, weakness, fatigue, dyspnea, tachycardia, vertigo, dysrhythmias, or hypotension occurs	Cardiac output should be conserved to maintain cardiac functioning During episodes of acute adrenocortical insufficiency, the patient has no hormone reserves and cannot tolerate any physical or emotional stress Continued stress precipitates vascular collapse and addisonian crisis

NURSING CARE PLAN   *The Patient With Addison's Disease—cont'd*

Nursing diagnosis/ Expected Outcome	Interventions	Rationale
High risk for ineffective individual coping related to decreased cortisol levels and associated emotional and physiologic instability • *Patient verbalizes feelings and identifies coping strategies; behavioral responses show decreased tension and anxiety*	Maintain a calm and relaxing environment Explain all procedures and encourage patient participation in care planning. Avoid frequent changes of personnel and caregivers Encourage the patient to discuss feelings, fears, anxieties, and strengths Assist patient in investigating and utilizing stress management techniques such as imagery, medication, and progressive relaxation measures	Decreased cerebral perfusion, hypoglycemia, anxiety, and fear result in confusion and further vascular compromise A sense of control and familiarity with caregivers decreases the stress of hospitalization Open discussion of feelings and fears enhances the patient's coping abilities Stress management techniques reduce physiologic stress responses and may decrease adrenocortical hormone output
Altered health maintenance related to lack of knowledge regarding the disease, lifelong hormone replacement therapy, and ongoing care • *Patient verbalizes understanding of the disease process and the need for hormone replacement therapy and ongoing care*	Explain the basic disease process and associated emotional and physical changes Instruct the patient and family about steroid replacement therapy (see patient education guide, p. 1676) Ensure follow-up outpatient care appointments are scheduled	Information and the discussion of feelings and body changes enhance the patient's ability to cope with a lifelong illness Careful instruction regarding hormone replacement therapy reinforces patient self-responsibility for drug management Adrenocortical functioning will remain stable only if the patient adheres to the treatment regimen

mucous membranes, is established and maintained

Blood pressure is stable without orthostatic hypotension

Daily activities are tolerated without undue fatigue

Effective coping is demonstrated by use of adaptive coping methods and verbalization of increased self-esteem

Verbalizations demonstrate adequate knowledge and understanding of the disease process, hormone replacement therapy, and ongoing care

Implementation

Care of the patient with Addison's disease involves simultaneous monitoring and replacement of fluid volume, electrolytes, and glucose (Figure 60-4; also see "Nursing Care Plan: The Patient with Addison's Disease"). Once the patient has been stabilized, long-term nursing management focuses on helping the patient and family in coping with and managing a chronic disease requiring lifelong hormone replacement therapy. It is important to help the patient and family members understand that hormone replacement will alleviate physical signs and symptoms.

Patient education is essential and includes the need for lifelong daily medication; use of Medic-Alert cards or bracelets; increased glucocorticoid dosage during stressful minor illnesses; use of travel kits that include oral cortisone, along with intramuscular preparations for self-injection and intravenous vials for emergency injection by a physician; and the need for prompt evaluation and treatment of infections and illnesses.

Evaluation

The effectiveness of the overall treatment plan will be demonstrated by the maintenance of adequate fluid volume, the lack of orthostatic hypotension, and improved activity tolerance. The patient and family should demonstrate understanding of the disease process, hormone replacement therapy, and long-term follow-up.

Documentation

Careful documentation of clinical assessment parameters and responses to fluid and hormone replacement is essential in order to institute therapeutic alterations and to prevent life-threatening complications such as adrenal crisis.

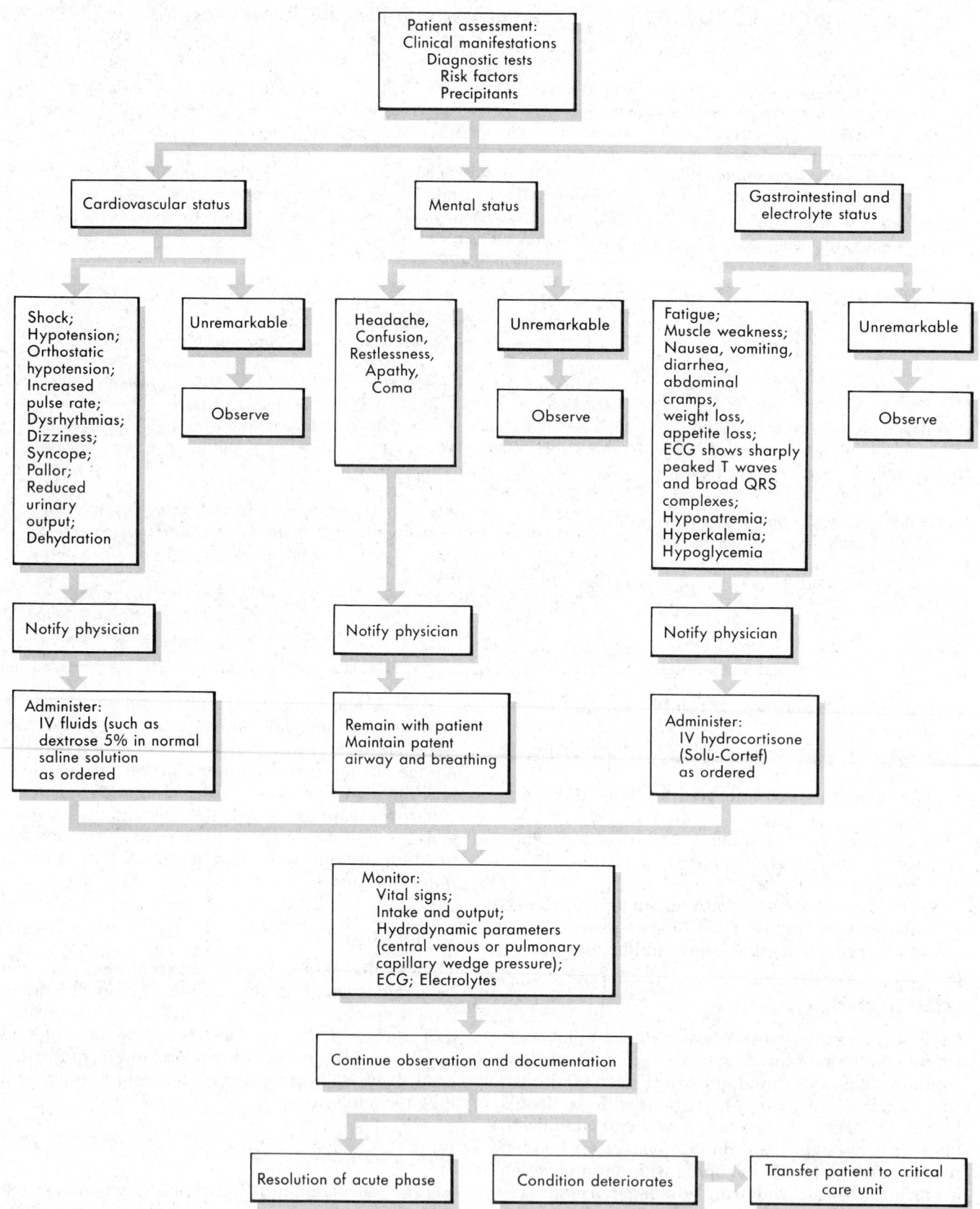

FIGURE 60-4   Critical Thinking Guide: the patient with adrenal crisis.

SIDE EFFECTS OF GLUCOCORTICOID THERAPY AND SIGNS OF POSSIBLE HORMONE EXCESS

Immunologic effects
Increased risk of infection
Masking of signs and symptoms of infection
Delayed healing

Fluid volume/cardiovascular effects
Increased blood volume, edema, hypotension, hypertension, congestive heart failure

Electrolyte alterations
Hypokalemia, hypocalcemia

Neurologic/emotional alterations
Mood alterations, depression, insomnia, anxiety, headache, psychosis

Musculoskeletal changes
Muscle wasting and weakness, osteoporosis, vertebral compression fractures

Gastrointestinal alterations
Nausea, abdominal pain, peptic ulcer

Ophthalmologic alterations
Glaucoma, cataracts, eye infections

Physical alterations
Moon face, thin extremities, truncal obesity

Endocrinologic alterations
Hyperglycemia, menstrual cycle changes, suppression of endogenous ACTH

Ongoing Care

Patient self-management of the disease, in conjunction with regular physician consultation, is essential, since medication dosages need to be altered during times of increased stress or illness. Nurses should be prepared to teach patients relaxation and stress management techniques or be able to refer patients to appropriate professionals for this training. Successful management of daily life stressors ensures a more homeostatic hormone balance and prevents undue stress on compromised adrenocortical reserves.

Since patients with Addison's disease are receiving replacement doses of glucocorticoids rather than the therapeutic doses used to treat diseases such as severe arthritis, asthma, or collagen vascular disorders, they are less likely to experience the more serious side effects of the drugs (see box above). Careful, individualized patient education regarding glucocorticoid replacement therapy, dosage adjustments in times of stress or illness, and signs and symptoms of excess or deficient hormone levels is essential (see patient education guide, p. 1676). Prioritized nursing diagnoses, goals, and interventions are outlined in the care plan on p. 1672.

CUSHING'S SYNDROME
Definition

Cushing's syndrome is a clinical condition caused by excessive amounts of the glucocorticoid cortisol.

Etiology/Epidemiology

The average age of onset is between 20 and 40 years. It occurs four times more commonly in women than men. Six distinct etiologic categories of Cushing's syndrome are known[2,21]:

1. Cushing's disease secondary to ACTH-producing pituitary microadenomas or hypothalamic lesions
2. Ectopic ACTH production by extrapituitary malignancies such as oat cell carcinoma of the lung
3. Slow-growing adrenal adenomas (more common in children and may indicate multiple endocrine neoplasia, an inherited disease of multiple endocrine organs)
4. Large, aggressive, adrenal carcinomas

CLINICAL ALERT

Prompt recognition of a hypertensive crisis or emergency is essential. These conditions are life threatening because of end organ damage and possible myocardial infarction, renal failure, and cerebrovascular accident or hemorrhage. Signs of severe blood pressure elevations include headache, nausea, vomiting, visual changes, chest pain, confusion or altered consciousness, and retinal hemorrhages, exudates, or papilledema.

PATIENT EDUCATION GUIDE *Corticosteroid Replacement Therapy*

1. Long-term management of your illness requires life-long steroid replacement therapy.
2. Continue your normal daily activities but take your medication every day without fail.
3. Do not alter your drug dosage or suddenly stop taking the medication—this could precipitate an acute adrenal crisis.
4. Take your medication with a meal or snack to avoid stomach irritation.
5. Take your daily medication at bedtime.
6. If you are taking two doses of medication, take the higher dose in the morning and the smaller dose in late afternoon or early evening (4 to 6 PM).
7. Keep an adequate supply of medication and carry extra medication when traveling.
8. Maintain your high-protein, high-carbohydrate, and adequate-sodium diet as ordered.
9. Promptly notify your physician if you experience severe stress; become ill or pregnant; or have an infection, an injury, a fever, a sore throat, a burning with urination, or a productive cough. These conditions may precipitate an adrenal crisis—your physician will recommend dosage adjustments or may order intramuscular injections.
10. Tell all health care providers (nurses, dentists, podiatrists) about your medication.
11. Avoid persons with infections (such as the flu or colds), and wash your hands regularly.
12. Report any of the following symptoms to your physician, since they may indicate hormone excess or deficiency: weakness, fatigue, depression, unusual weight change, dizziness, edema, back pain, decreased appetite, abdominal pain, black or bloody stools, and increased thirst or urination.
13. Exercise regularly, and practice daily relaxation or stress management techniques.
14. Always wear your Medic-Alert bracelet.
15. See your physician or health care provider regularly.

---

5. Exogenous, iatrogenic Cushing's syndrome, caused by chronic administration of corticosteroids
6. Alcohol-induced pseudo-Cushing's syndrome

Pathophysiology/Clinical Manifestations

Glucocorticoid administration or excess cortisol and possible androgen production may cause multiple metabolic consequences in every body system (Table 60-3). ACTH levels may be normal or elevated, as in pituitary-dependent or ectopic Cushing's syndrome. Common symptoms include weight gain, central obesity, and weakness.

Diagnostic tests

Diagnostic testing is used to confirm the diagnosis of Cushing's syndrome, to help differentiate the causes of it, and to search for the pituitary, adrenal, or ectopic sources of the hypercortisolism. Several tests may be performed because of false-positive and false-negative results, individual metabolic variations, and the effects of multiple external variables on cortisol secretion.

Plasma or urinary free cortisol levels, urinary 17-hydroxycorticoids, and 17-ketogenic steroids (17-KGS) may be normal or elevated. Obesity, alcoholism, stress, depression, and hyperthyroidism may cause elevated hormone levels. An insulin-induced hypoglycemia test does not cause the normal rise in cortisol. Plasma ACTH is elevated in pituitary disease or ectopic syndrome but not in adrenal Cushing's syndrome.

If clinical findings or laboratory tests suggest Cushing's syndrome, further tests are ordered. If a 2-day, low-dose dexamethasone suppression test does not show suppression of cortisol, a high-dose dexamethasone suppression test is ordered. Skull films, chest x-ray studies, CT/MRI scanning, ultrasonography, and venography are used to localize tumors.

Therapeutic Management

Without diagnosis and treatment, patients with endogenous Cushing's syndrome have a shortened life expectancy, often less than 5 years, with death commonly the result of cardiovascular disease.[2] Treatment modalities include surgery, irradiation, pharmacologic therapy, or a combination of these three approaches. Although there are no ideal treatments, attempts are made to normalize cortisol secretion, prevent insufficiencies, and minimize risks and continued need for medication.

A common, often preferred treatment of pituitary tumors is transsphenoidal surgical removal of the microadenoma (see Figure 60-1).[18,21] The surgery

TABLE 60-3   Cushing's Syndrome: Pathophysiologic Changes and Clinical Manifestations

Pathophysiologic changes	Clinical manifestations
Increased cortisol levels	Depression, apathy, mood changes, psychosis, cataracts
Sodium and water retention, potassium excretion	High blood pressure, hypokalemia, increased urinary potassium, metabolic alkalosis, edema
Increased androgen production	Acne, hirsutism, virilization, hyperpigmentation, amenorrhea, menstrual changes
Immunosuppression	Poor wound healing, leukocytosis, decreased lymphocyte and eosinophil production, increased erythropoiesis
Body fat redistribution	Moon facies, truncal obesity, "buffalo hump"
Increased protein catabolism and collagen loss	Skin and hair thinning, abdominal striae, muscle weakness, atrophy
Capillary fragility	Easy bruising
Gastric hyperacidity	Peptic ulcer formation
Increased calcium loss	Increased urinary calcium, osteoporosis, backache, pathologic fractures
Increased gluconeogenesis	Hyperglycemia

has a remission rate of 60% to 85%, but recurrences are possible. Other therapeutic options cause complete or partial pituitary gland destruction. These options include irradiation, implantation of yttrium 90 rods, cryotherapy, or hypophysectomy.[18,21]

Unilateral adrenalectomy is the treatment of choice for unilateral adrenal adenomas. Bilateral adrenalectomy is indicated for adrenal carcinoma or bilateral nodular hyperplasia of the adrenal glands. Pituitary irradiation or cryosurgery is usually combined with a bilateral adrenalectomy to prevent a condition known as Nelson's syndrome, which is characterized by pigmentation and an enlarging pituitary tumor after adrenalectomy. Ectopic ACTH-secreting tumors are removed surgically if possible.

Pharmacologic therapies are used, often in combination with irradiation, when surgery is contraindicated. Central agents used to treat pituitary Cushing's disease include cyproheptadine (Periactin), a serotonin antagonist that inhibits ACTH secretion, and bromocriptine (Parlodel).[21] Few patients respond to these drugs, and relapses are common after drug withdrawal. Adrenal enzyme inhibitors may be used in conjunction with irradiation or in preparation for surgery. These drugs block certain enzymatic reactions required for cortisol synthesis. The drugs most commonly used are aminoglutethimide (Elipten), metyrapone (Metopirone), mitotane (Lysodren), and ketoconazole (Nizoral).[18,21] Gastrointestinal and neurologic disturbances, skin rashes, and permanent adrenal cortical insufficiency are common drug side effects.

NURSING MANAGEMENT OF THE PATIENT WITH CUSHING'S SYNDROME
Assessment

Symptoms of Cushing's syndrome may be acute or chronic in onset and may include the following: weight gain, weakness, skin changes, emotional swings, change in libido, easy bruising, polydipsia, polyuria, nocturia, and edema. Vital signs are assessed, along with body habitus, muscle tone, and skin, while looking for clinical signs of Cushing's syndrome, especially fluid retention and hypertension (see Table 60-3). Clinical signs of Cushing's syndrome in elderly persons may be mistaken for normal signs of aging.[8] Nursing care is outlined in the nursing care plan on p. 1679. Vigilant postoperative nursing care is necessary for patients undergoing transsphenoidal hypophysectomy or adrenalectomy (see box).

Nursing Diagnosis

Potential nursing diagnoses for a patient with Cushing's syndrome include the following:

High risk for fluid volume excess related to excess glucocorticoids and fluid and sodium retention

High risk for infection related to immune system suppression from increased glucocorticoid output

Activity intolerance related to myopathy, weakness, and fatigue

High risk for injury related to cortisol excess, weakness, and fatigue

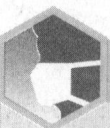

PREOPERATIVE AND POSTOPERATIVE NURSING INTERVENTIONS

Adrenalectomy

Intervention	Rationale
Perform frequent neurologic, cardiovascular, and renal assessments	Rapid and severe fluctuations in blood pressure and heart rate occur because of hormone release during surgery and sudden catecholamine depletion postoperatively
Continuously monitor cardiac rhythm and hemodynamic pressures	
Monitor vital signs and input and output frequently (at least every 4 hours)	Hemorrhage and hypovolemic shock may occur postoperatively because of manipulation of highly vascular tissues
Monitor serum electrolytes	Bilateral adrenalectomy causes sudden drop in adrenocortical hormones and catecholamines
Be alert for signs and symptoms of adrenal insufficiency: weakness, hypotension, fever, mental status changes	
Administer IV corticosteroids as ordered until oral intake is possible	High doses of IV cortisol are administered the day of surgery and afterward to enable the body to withstand stress of surgery
Be alert for signs of glucocorticoid excess or deficiency	Drug adjustment may be required to stabilize glucocorticoid levels
Use sterile dressing change techniques	Fluctuating cortisol and catecholamine levels put patient at risk for infection and thrombosis
Observe patient for signs and symptoms of infection and delayed wound healing	
Help patient in coughing, deep breathing, and leg exercises	

High risk for body image disturbance related to changes in appearance

Altered health maintenance related to lack of knowledge regarding the disease process, testing and treatment procedures, and ongoing care

Planning

Expected patient outcomes of nursing interventions include the following:

Patient exhibits a reduction in excess fluid volume as evidenced by loss of water weight and acceptable pulse and blood pressure

Patient remains free of infection, or infection is detected early

Patient tolerates daily activities without undue fatigue

Patient practices preventive injury safeguards

Patient adapts to altered body image by verbalizing feelings about body changes and strategies to deal with the changes

Patient verbalizes understanding of the disease process, treatment plans, and ongoing care

Implementation

Nursing care is outlined in the nursing care plan on p. 1679. The nurse monitors the patient for fluid volume excess, because sodium and water retention causes hypertension and possible congestive heart failure. Particular attention is paid to potassium levels, because hypokalemia can cause ventricular dysrhythmias. Vigilant postoperative nursing care is necessary for patients undergoing transsphenoidal hypophysectomy or adrenalectomy (see boxes).

Evaluation

Evaluation of the patient with Cushing's syndrome focuses on cardiopulmonary function, signs or symptoms of wound infection, the ability to perform activities of daily living, as well as the patient's adaptation to changes in body appearance.

Documentation

Proper documentation will alert other health team members to subtle changes in the patient's fluid balance and coping abilities. Written patient education

 NURSING CARE PLAN   *The Patient With Cushing's Syndrome*

Nursing diagnosis/ Expected outcome	Interventions	Rationale
High risk for fluid volume excess related to excess glucocorticoids and fluid and sodium retention • *Excess fluid volume is reduced as evidenced by loss of water and acceptable pulse and blood pressure*	Monitor and carefully record intake and output Record daily weight Assess jugular venous pressure, heart and breath sounds, and extremities for edema every 8 to 12 hours Monitor blood pressure and pulse every 8 hours and report elevations to the physician Maintain a high-potassium, low-sodium diet Administer diuretics and potassium supplements as ordered while monitoring potassium levels, weights, and vital signs	Excess cortisol production increases renal tubular reabsorption of sodium and water, causing fluid volume expansion Weight gain and decreased urinary output may serve as reliable indicators of fluid retention Signs of fluid expansion include increased jugular venous pressure, pulmonary crackles, S_3, and edema Hyperadrenocorticism may also be associated with increased mineralocorticoid activity, resulting in hypertension and altered cardiac output Decreased sodium intake decreases renal retention of sodium and water Non—potassium—sparing diuretics such as hydrochlorothiazide and furosemide (Lasix) cause increased urinary excretion of sodium, water, and potassium
High risk for infection related to immune system suppression from increased glucocorticoid output • *Risks of infection are minimized and infections that do occur are detected early*	Protect the patient from exposure to infected individuals Use proper handwashing and aseptic techniques Carefully monitor vital signs, fatigue-inducing activities, secretions, lung sounds, skin lesions, and white blood cell counts	Infections are more common because of immune system suppression Patients are at risk for infections via skin contamination, invasive procedures, and inhalation of pathogens Increased cortisol levels mask common signs of infection; fatigue or a feeling of general discomfort may indicate infection
Activity intolerance related to myopathy, weakness, and fatigue • *Patient demonstrates increased stamina and is able to carry out activities of daily living without undue stress*	Ensure adequate dietary intake of protein (0.8 to 1 g protein/kg/day) and vitamin C Encourage walking and other aerobic exercise as tolerated	Excess glucocorticoid output causes protein catabolism; adequate protein and vitamin C are needed for rebuilding collagen and muscle tissue Physical activity increases calcium metabolism and muscle tone and strength
High risk for injury related to cortisol excess • *Injuries are prevented*	Provide necessary safety devices and assistance, including adequate lighting, unobstructed walkways, an easily accessible call light, siderails, trapeze, and nonskid shoes Monitor patient for complaints of joint or low back pain and promptly report these symptoms to the physician	Spontaneous fractures and vertebral compression fractures may occur as a result of bone dissolution and osteoporosis Back and joint injuries can be minimized and prevented through daily muscle stretching and strengthening exercises Glucocorticoids inhibit the action of vitamin D and increase calcium excretion

Continued.

NURSING CARE PLAN *The Patient With Cushing's Syndrome—cont'd*

Nursing diagnosis/ Expected outcome	Interventions	Rationale
	Discuss a physical therapy consultation with the physician to promote back, joint, and muscle-strengthening exercises	Skin breakdown and bruising may occur secondary to decreased connective tissue and capillary fragility
	Ensure adequate intake of calcium and vitamin D	
	Pad bony prominences, provide good skin care, and use sheepskin or egg crate mattresses when necessary	
High risk for body image disturbance related to changes in appearance	Encourage expression of feelings regarding emotional and physical changes	Physical and emotional changes may precipitate anxiety and fear regarding responses of significant others
•*Patience verbalizes understanding of the disease process and accompanying physical and emotional changes and expresses personal feelings related to these changes*	Assess the patient's and family's understanding of the disease process	
	Encourage family members to share their perceptions and feelings about the patient's condition	
Altered health maintenance related to lack of knowledge regarding the disease process, testing and treatment procedures, and ongoing care	Assess the patient's and family's understanding of the disease process, medications, treatments, and ongoing care; provide needed information	Increased understanding of the disease, treatment measures, and follow-up care promotes self-care and adherence to the treatment regimen
•*Patient and family ask questions and demonstrate understanding of the disease process, treatment procedures, medications, and ongoing care*	Explain prescribed medications, use, side effects, and the signs and symptoms of hypoadrenalism and hyperadrenalism	Steroid replacement therapy after medical or surgical adrenalectomy requires careful monitoring to prevent hyperadrenalism
	Emphasize the importance of continuing medications, consulting with the physician regarding any over-the-counter medications, and maintaining regular outpatient follow-up care	Acute adrenal insufficiency may occur if steroids are discontinued

guides help the patient and family understand hormone replacement therapy.

Ongoing Care

Ongoing care is required and often includes continued treatment measures or medication adjustments. Treatment may cause pituitary or adrenal insufficiency necessitating lifelong hormone replacement therapy. Steroid replacement requires careful titration and altered dosages during times of stress, illness, or surgery (see Patient Education Guide, p. 1676). Nurses will often be performing telephone triage of these patients in the home and answering many questions related to medications, signs and symptoms, and illnesses.

HYPERALDOSTERONISM
Definition/Etiology/Epidemiology

Two categories of hyperaldosteronism exist, primary and secondary. In **primary hyperaldosteronism** (Conn's syndrome) the adrenal gland itself is the stimulus for excess aldosterone production. The incidence of primary hyperaldosteronism peaks at 50 years of age. There are four forms of primary hyperaldosteronism: (1) unilateral adrenal adenoma (60% to 70% of cases); (2) bilateral adrenal hyperplasia (30% to 40% of cases); (3) a rare familial reversible syndrome of bilateral adrenal hyperplasia; and (4) a rare adrenal carcinoma.[15,21] Primary hyperaldosteronism is twice as common in women as in men and in nonwhites as opposed to whites. Of all hypertensive patients, 1% to 2% may have primary hyperaldosteronism.

Adrenal tumors or adrenal hyperplasia may cause excess production of both corticoid precursors and androgens. Congenital or acquired virilizing adrenal hyperplasia is known as the adrenogenital syndrome.[2]

Secondary hyperaldosteronism occurs in response to nonadrenal activation of the renin-angiotensin system. Enhanced renin production and release occur in response to (1) sodium loss caused by restriction, diuretics, diarrhea, or volume depletion; (2) decreased afferent arteriolar pressure caused by an underlying edema disorder such as congestive heart failure, cirrhosis of the liver, or nephrotic syndrome; (3) renal arteriolar narrowing related to atherosclerosis, fibromuscular hyperplasia, arteriolar nephrosclerosis, or accelerated hypertension; and (4) a renin-producing tumor. A defect in chloride resorption in the ascending loop of Henle (Bartter's syndrome) also causes excessive aldosterone secretion.

Pathophysiology

Aldosterone is the major mineralocorticoid secreted by the zona glomerulosa of the adrenal cortex. Factors controlling aldosterone secretion include the renin-angiotensin system, ACTH, and plasma levels of potassium and sodium. Renin release is triggered by catecholamines, decreased perfusion pressure, and extracellular fluid volume deficit caused by sodium depletion. Renin release activates a cascade system in which angiotensin II is formed, which causes secretion of aldosterone from the adrenal glands to restore blood volume.[15]

Potassium plays a major role in aldosterone secretion. Small increases in plasma potassium, or hyperkalemia, stimulate aldosterone release, which results in increased tubular secretion of potassium (Figure 60-5). Acute administration of ACTH causes a transient increase in aldosterone secretion, whereas chronic ACTH release or administration results in low or normal aldosterone levels.[15]

Increased aldosterone secretion and aldosterone-producing adenomas and carcinomas increase renal tubular reabsorption of sodium in exchange for potassium and hydrogen. This causes sodium and water retention, urinary potassium loss, expansion of extracellular fluid volume, increased total peripheral vascular resistance, hypertension, hypokalemia, and mild metabolic alkalosis (Figure 60-6).

Clinical Manifestations

Patients with primary hyperaldosteronism are usually asymptomatic and have nonspecific physical signs. Clinical findings include hypertension, some-

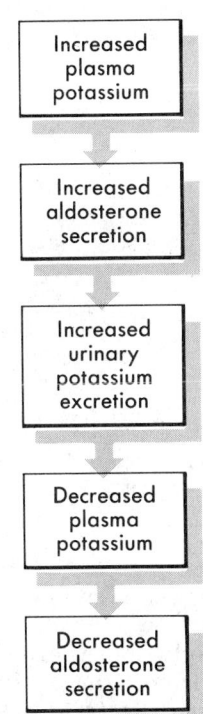

FIGURE 60-5   Interrelationships of plasma potassium levels and aldosterone secretion.

times severe, with associated headaches. Significant hypokalemia and metabolic alkalosis cause fatigue, muscle weakness, paresthesias, and cramping. Signs of tetany (Trousseau's and Chvostek's signs)[8,14] may be present because hydrogen ion shifts cause metabolic alkalosis and decrease plasma calcium levels. Polydipsia and polyuria may occur because of impaired renal concentrating ability. Edema is usually absent in primary hyperaldosteronism because of decreased absorption of sodium by the proximal nephron. The diagnosis of hyperaldosteronism depends on laboratory findings associated with changes in sodium and potassium rather than on clinical features.

Diagnostic tests

Tests used to diagnose and differentiate adenomas, hyperplasia, and the familial hyperplasia syndrome include the following: (1) measurement of 8 AM aldosterone, plasma renin activity (PRA), and cortisol in the supine position, followed by repeat blood sampling at noon after the patient has been standing for 4 hours; (2) plasma aldosterone and 24-hour urinary aldosterone measurements before and after volume expansion via high-salt intake or saline infusion (contraindicated in heart failure or hypokalemia); (3) measurement of plasma 18-hydroxycorticosterone (18-OHB), an aldosterone

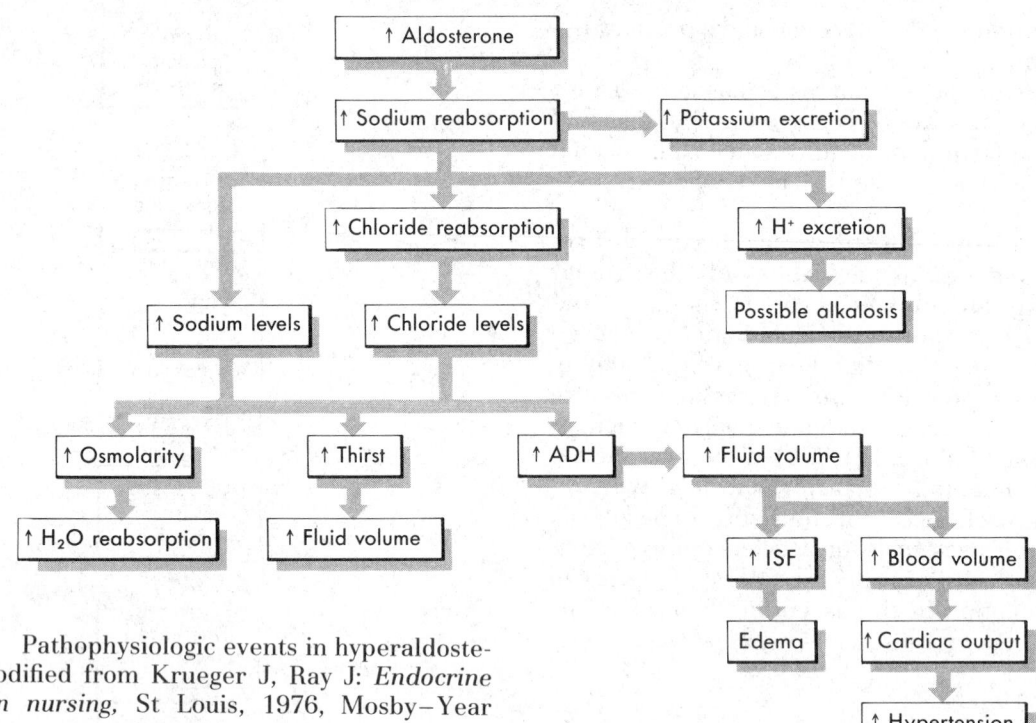

FIGURE 60-6   Pathophysiologic events in hyperaldosteronism. (Modified from Krueger J, Ray J: *Endocrine problems in nursing,* St Louis, 1976, Mosby–Year Book, Inc.)

precursor; (4) adrenal CT scanning; (5) adrenal vein catheterization studies; and (6) trials of dexamethasone suppression.[15]

Confounding the diagnostic evaluation in older subjects is the increasing frequency over the life span of nonfunctional adrenocortical adenomas. CT scan may reveal an initial impression of hyperaldosteronism; however, in elderly persons, induced hypokalemia from diuretic therapy for hypertension may be the cause.

Therapeutic Management

Treatment options include surgical removal of adrenal tumors, transluminal angioplasty, and various medications to control blood pressure and normalize potassium levels. Dexamethasone (Decadron) is used to treat the familial reversible syndrome of bilateral adrenal hyperplasia.[21]

Unilateral adrenal adenomas may be removed surgically after preoperative normalization of potassium and blood pressure. Spironolactone (Aldactone), an aldosterone antagonist, is commonly used preoperatively for blood pressure control. Transluminal angioplasty may be used to control blood pressure in various types of secondary hyperaldosteronism, including renal artery stenosis, fibromuscular hyperplasia, and atherosclerotic stenosis.

Many effective medications are available for medical treatment of renin-angiotensin-aldosterone-

induced hypertension. Primary hyperaldosteronism may be treated with a potassium-sparing diuretic such as amiloride (Midamor), which acts on the renal tubules.[15] Spironolactone is not useful in long-term therapy, because its effects wear off after several months and it is associated with gynecomastia and impotence in males. Angiotensin-converting enzyme (ACE) inhibitors, such as enalapril (Vasotec), are quite useful and effective because they block the conversion of angiotensin I to angiotensin II.[15,18]

NURSING MANAGEMENT OF THE PATIENT WITH HYPERALDOSTERONISM
Assessment

Presenting symptoms in patients with hyperaldosteronism include a history of headaches, paresthesias, muscle weakness, or fatigue. Few findings are noted on physical examination with the exception of diastolic hypertension without edema. Patients with hyperaldosteronism related to renal artery stenosis may have renal artery bruits, which are best heard over the lower back or in the upper quadrants of the abdomen. Long-standing hypertension may also cause cardiac and renal failure. Laboratory test results depend somewhat on the duration and severity of the potassium loss, but common findings include hypokalemia, hypernatremia, and a mild metabolic alkalosis. Potassium, PRA, and aldosterone levels are all affected by low-sodium diets and antihypertensive medications; therefore attempts are made to normalize diets and hold antihypertensive drugs 2 weeks before testing. When hyperaldosteronism is suspected, multiple screening and diagnostic tests may be ordered.

Nursing Diagnosis

Nursing diagnoses for the patient with hyperaldosteronism include the following:

Fluid volume excess related to sodium and water retention

Altered tissue perfusion related to hypertension and hypokalemia

Pain related to headache and paresthesias

Activity intolerance and potential for injury related to weakness and fatigue

Altered health maintenance related to lack of knowledge regarding the disease process, treatments, and ongoing care

Planning

Goals for the patient include the following:

Patient remains free of cardiovascular complications

Patient maintains normal blood pressure and serum potassium levels

Patient verbalizes knowledge of disease process and treatment

Patient protects self from injury

Implementation

Vital signs, intake and output, daily weights, and cardiac and lung sounds are regularly assessed and recorded. Signs and symptoms of hypokalemia, such as weakness, paresthesias, tetany, or dysrhythmias, are noted and promptly reported to the physician. A high-potassium, low-sodium diet is maintained, and potassium supplements and antihypertensive medications are administered as ordered. Patients require instruction regarding testing procedures, prescribed diet, medications and their side effects, and self-monitoring of blood pressure. The nursing care of a patient undergoing an adrenalectomy is outlined in the box on p. 1678.

Evaluation

Expected outcomes include normalization of blood pressure and serum potassium levels, patient verbalization of understanding of the disease process and medications, adherence to the prescribed diet and medications, and demonstrated patient ability to monitor blood pressure.

ADRENAL MEDULLARY DISEASE: PHEOCHROMOCYTOMA

Definition

Pheochromocytomas are highly vascular tumors that arise from adrenal medullary or sympathetic ganglion tissue and that produce, store, and secrete catecholamines.

Etiology/Epidemiology

Pheochromocytomas are usually curable but, if left untreated, are often fatal. They are rare, usually benign tumors occurring in 0.1% of hypertensive patients. Pheochromocytoma occurs most commonly in the middle adult years and is rare in elderly persons.[8,22]

Pathophysiology

Catecholamines produced by pheochromocytomas have both direct and indirect effects on the major organ systems, resulting in sympathetic nervous system stimulation characterized by peripheral vasoconstriction, increased heart rate and myocardial contractility and irritability, decreased intestinal motility, glycogenolysis, and pupillary dilation.

Clinical Manifestations

Increased circulatory levels of catecholamines cause a severe stress response or hypermetabolic panic. Recurrent, sustained, paroxysmal hypertensive attacks or crises occur with increasing frequency. Clinical features of the attacks include labile-resistant hypertension associated with headache, orthostatic hypotension, tachycardia, pallor or flushing, sweating, palpitations, anxiety, apprehension, chest or abdominal pain, and nausea and vomiting. Bladder wall pheochromocytomas cause bladder spasms and micturitional crises.

Stimuli that precipitate attacks include tumor palpation, emotional stress, exercise, intercourse, position change, Valsalva's maneuver, anesthesia, surgical procedures, and the intake of cheese, beer, or wine. Medications that stimulate tumor catecholamine release include beta blockers, histamine, glucagon, ACTH, opiates, nicotine, phenothiazines, tricyclic antidepressants, guanethidine, and succinylcholine.[2,8]

Complications of sustained catecholamine release include weight loss, impaired glucose tolerance, cholelithiasis, hypertensive encephalopathy, preeclampsia, angina, dysrhythmias, acute myocardial infarction, cerebral vascular accident, cardiomyopathy, and congestive heart failure.[2]

Diagnostic tests

Diagnostic tests include 24-hour (or less) urinary metanephrines, urinary and plasma catecholamines (norepinephrine, epinephrine, and dopamine), and urinary vanillylmandelic acid (VMA). These hormones and metabolites are elevated in 75% to 90% of patients with pheochromocytoma. Urinary tests may yield false results because of intake of certain antibiotics or hypertensive agents (see Chapter 59); foods such as cheese, chocolate, citrus fruit, or bananas; vitamins B and C; and beer, wine, and caffeine. A clonidine suppression test may be ordered, since patients with pheochromocytoma do not have suppression of plasma norepinephrine after administration of clonidine.

Methods used to localize tumors include CT/MRI scanning or scanning using meta-iodobenzylguanidine (MIBG), a material that concentrates in adrenergic vesicles. If the tumor cannot be located, blood samples for catecholamines are collected via venous catheterization.

Therapeutic Management

Surgery is the treatment of choice unless the patient is not a surgical candidate because of multiple tumor metastases or nonlocalization of the tumor. Acute treatment and preoperative preparation are required to control blood pressure and catecholamine release. Bed rest is indicated along with intravenous alpha-adrenergic and beta-adrenergic blocking drugs such as phentolamine (Regitine), nitroprusside (Nipride), and propranolol (Inderal). Oral agents that are given after stabilization and for ongoing medical treatment include propranolol (Inderal); calcium channel blocking drugs; phenoxybenzamine (Dibenzyline), an alpha-adrenergic blocker; and metyrosine (Demser), a hydroxylase inhibitor that blocks the conversion of tyrosine to norepinephrine. Surgery is scheduled only after the patient has been normotensive for at least 1 week. Ap-

CLINICAL ALERT

Prompt recognition of a hypertensive crisis or emergency is essential. These conditions are life threatening because of end organ damage and possible myocardial infarction, renal failure, cerebrovascular accident or hemorrhage, and death. Signs of severe blood pressure elevations include headache, nausea, vomiting, visual changes, chest pain, confusion or altered consciousness, and retinal hemorrhages, exudates, or papilledema.

proximately 25% of patients continue to have hypertension after surgery.[18,21]

Adrenalectomy, removal of one or both adrenal glands, involves significant intraoperative and postoperative surgical risks. Sudden, severe fluctuations in adrenal glucocorticoids, mineralocorticoids, and catecholamines cause changes in blood pressure, fluid volume, and electrolyte status. Bilateral adrenalectomy causes acute adrenal insufficiency. Complications include dysrhythmias, sudden alterations in fluid and electrolyte status, blood pressure swings, hypotension, hypoglycemia, myocardial infarction, congestive heart failure, infection, and bleeding.[7,22]

NURSING MANAGEMENT OF THE PATIENT WITH PHEOCHROMOCYTOMA
Assessment

Patients with pheochromocytoma often give a history of sustained or labile hypertension with recurrent episodes of headache, diaphoresis, and palpitations. The history may also be positive for other associated symptoms, including anxiety; various neurologic, respiratory, and cardiovascular complaints; and abdominal pain, nausea, vomiting, and weight loss. The health history may be positive for other endocrinologic diseases and glucose intolerance. Since the disorder can be inherited, the family history may be positive for pheochromocytoma, other endocrine tumors or diseases, or neurofibromatosis. Physical examination may reveal a thin, hypertensive patient with a forceful apical pulse, tachycardia, diaphoresis, and cool extremities. Palpation of the abdomen or masses may induce an attack.

Nursing Diagnosis

Possible nursing diagnoses for a patient with pheochromocytoma include the following:

Altered tissue perfusion related to catecholamine excess and severe hypertension

Decreased cardiac output related to hypertension and widespread severe vasoconstriction

Anxiety related to excess catecholamines

Pain related to headaches, apprehension, and decreased intestinal motility

Altered health maintenance related to lack of knowledge regarding the disease process and treatments

Planning

Goals for the patient include the following:

Tissue perfusion and cardiac output are within normal ranges

Patient evidences no neurologic or renal complications

Patient practices lifelong health promotion behaviors

Implementation

Prioritized nursing interventions, including frequent blood pressure and neurologic checks and cardiac auscultation, should be carried out in a calm and emotionally supportive manner.

Preoperative instructions include information about the surgical procedure, intravenous fluids and medications, and hemodynamic monitoring systems; and discussion and demonstration of coughing, deep breathing, leg exercises, and turning. Adrenergic blocking drugs and other antihypertensives used before surgery require close monitoring of cardiac rate and rhythm. Dietary requirements include increased protein and calories.

Evaluation/Documentation

Frequent nursing assessments and interventions should result in stabilization of blood pressure and fluid volume; prevention of neurologic, renal, or cardiac complications; and the patient's expression of comfort. During the acute phase of treatment, bedside neurologic and cardiovascular flow charts are used to promptly and accurately record patient assessments. Discharge planning includes in-depth discussion and teaching regarding stressful situations, signs of adrenal crisis, lifelong steroid replacement therapy, and ongoing health care.

Ongoing Care

The patient is assisted in identifying methods of reestablishing normal activities and roles while coping with the possibility of having to take lifelong medications. Nursing consultation with the endocrinologist and primary care physician is important to ensure correct and safe patient self-management instructions. Some patients may experience continued hypertension, so it is important that they and their families understand medications, blood pressure monitoring, and the need for ongoing care.

CRITICAL THINKING QUESTIONS

1 Describe the pathophysiologic changes associated with hypopituitarism, diabetes insipidus, SIADH, Cushing's syndrome, and Addison's disease.

2 Why are the signs and symptoms of mineralocorticoid deficiency different from those of glucocorticoid deficiency?

3 Explain the hormonal and physiologic differences between diseases of the adrenal cortex and those of the adrenal medulla.

4 What are the possible side effects and consequences of long-term steroid therapy?

5 Why is it important to assess coping skills and family functioning of patients with adrenal or pituitary diseases?

6 Outline the postoperative goals and nursing priorities for patients undergoing pituitary or adrenal surgery.

7 Mr. J, a 62-year-old black man, has had longstanding adrenal insufficiency and was recently admitted for treatment of pneumococcal pneumonia. His physician has written orders for intravenous fluids, intravenous cortisol, and stat electrolytes. What is the rationale for these orders? Identify three patient-centered goals, and prioritize your nursing interventions.

8 Ms. J, a 40-year-old woman, was recently admitted with a diagnosis of possible pheochromocytoma. After eating breakfast she complains of her heart "pounding" in her chest, sweating, and nausea. Identify and prioritize your nursing assessments and interventions.

9 Outline nursing care plans for patients with hypopituitarism, diabetes insipidus, Cushing's syndrome, and Addison's disease.

BIBLIOGRAPHY

1. Becker K: *Principles and practice of endocrinology and metabolism*, Philadelphia, 1990, JB Lippincott Co.
2. Besser G, Cudworth A: *Clinical endocrinology: an illustrated text*, Philadelphia, 1987, JB Lippincott Co.
3. Blackwell R: Hyperprolactinemia: evaluation and management, *Endocrinol Metabol Clin North Am* 21(1):105, 1992.
4. Chang-DeMoranville B, Jackson I: Diagnosis and endocrine testing in acromegaly, *Endocrinol Metabol Clin North Am* 21(3):649, 1992.
5. Ezzat S: Living with acromegaly, *Endocrinol Metabol Clin North Am* 21(3):753, 1992.
6. Hall P, Evared D: *Color atlas of endocrinology*, ed 2, Chicago, 1990, Year Book Medical Publishers.
7. Halloran T: Nursing responsibilities in endocrine emergencies, *Crit Care Nurs Q* 13(3):74, 1990.
8. Hershman J: *Endocrine pathophysiology: a patient oriented approach*, ed 3, Philadelphia, 1988, Lea & Febiger.
9. Jaffe C, Barkan A: Treatment of acromegaly with dopamine agonists, *Endocrinol Metabol Clin North Am* 21(3):713, 1992.
10. Kenney J: The consumer's views of health, *J Adv Nurs* 17:829, 1992.
11. Knappe G et al: Long-term results of acromegaly therapy and transsphenoidal adenomectomy, *Acta Endocrinol* 126(suppl 4):48, 1992.
12. Lamberts S, Reubi JC, Krenning E: Somastatin analogs in the treatment of acromegaly, *Endocrinol Metabol Clin North Am* 21(3):737, 1992.
13. Lehmert H et al: Family screening in pheochromocytoma:

is it worth the effort? *Acta Endocrinol* 126 (suppl. 4):159, 1992.

14. Loeb S, Cahill M: *Nurse review: endocrine problems,* Springhouse, Pa, 1990, Springhouse Corporation.

15. Melby J: Diagnosis of hyperaldosteronism, *Endocrinol Metabol Clin North Am* 20(2):247, 1992.

16. Molitch M: Clinical manifestations of acromegaly, *Endocrinol Metabol Clin North Am* 21(3):597, 1992.

17. Patterson L, Norian E: Diabetes insipidus versus syndrome of inappropriate antidiuretic hormone, *Dimen Crit Care Nurs* 8(4):226, 1989.

18. Rakel R: *Conn's current therapy,* Philadelphia, 1992, WB Saunders Co.

19. Reasner C: Anterior pituitary disease, *Crit Care Nurs Q* 13(3):62, 1990.

20. Register C: *Living with chronic illness,* New York, 1987, Bantam Books.

21. Wilson J, Foster D: *Williams textbook of endocrinology,* ed 8, Philadelphia, 1992, WB Saunders Co.

22. Winer N: Pheochromocytoma, *Crit Care Nurs Q* 13(3):14, 1990.

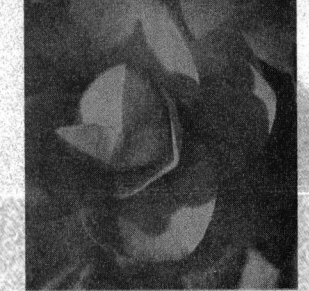

CHAPTER SIXTY-ONE

Nursing Management of Adults with Thyroid or Parathyroid Disorders

LEARNING OBJECTIVES

1 Correlate the pathophysiology of common thyroid and parathyroid disorders with their typical clinical manifestations.

2 Perform an appropriate nursing assessment for patients with thyroid or parathyroid disorders.

3 Identify nursing goals associated with the commonly encountered nursing diagnoses.

4 Develop strategies for nursing interventions aimed at meeting the defined goals, and discuss the rationale for the use of each strategy.

5 Discuss the nursing implications associated with common medications used to treat thyroid and parathyroid disorders.

6 Develop patient education guides for patients with common disorders of the thyroid or parathyroid glands.

7 Discuss the psychosocial implications of the symptoms associated with thyroid and parathyroid disorders.

8 Identify potential complications of thyroid and parathyroid disorders, and describe appropriate nursing assessment and intervention strategies.

KEY TERMS

DISORDERS of the thyroid and parathyroid glands are commonly encountered in clinical practice. The development and refinement of sophisticated diagnostic aids have enabled physicians to identify many asymptomatic and subclinical problems that previously went unrecognized. Thyroid and parathyroid hormones have wide-ranging and diverse effects in the body. Although multiple discrete disorders exist involving each gland, patients primarily experience symptoms related to either hormone excess or deficit and the complications produced by these imbalances. These disorders are generally managed on an outpatient basis.

Hyperthyroidism

Hyperthyroidism, or **thyrotoxicosis,** is a clinical syndrome that results from the metabolic effects of excess thyroid hormone at the cellular level. The syndrome usually results from hyperactivity of the thyroid gland as a primary disease state but can also occur as a secondary response to a problem in the stimulation and feedback loop of the pituitary hypothalamic axis (see Chapter 59).

GRAVES' DISEASE
Definition

Graves' disease (diffuse toxic goiter) is by far the most common form of hyperthyroidism and accounts for 60% to 70% of all clinical cases. It is a well-recognized disorder that has been described since the eighteenth century. Classic Graves' disease involves four separate components: (1) thyrotoxicosis, (2) thyroid enlargement, or goiter, (3) ophthalmopathy, and (4) dermopathy. Not every patient exhibits every component.

Etiology/Epidemiology

The exact cause of Graves' disease remains unknown. It is described as an autoimmune process of impaired immunoregulation that results from an as yet unidentified viral trigger. The incidence of Graves' disease is significantly associated with the presence of other autoimmune disorders, particularly pernicious anemia, insulin-dependent diabetes mellitus, myasthenia gravis, and rheumatoid arthritis. The disease follows a characteristic autoimmune pattern of exacerbations and remissions unless the gland is destroyed by radiation or surgery. The onset of Graves' disease is commonly associated with an episode of physical illness or significant physical or emotional stress.

The number of documented cases of Graves' disease has increased with improved diagnostic tools.

The disease affects women five times as often as men, and although it can occur at any age, the peak incidence is between the ages of 20 and 40 years. There is a strong familial predisposition to Graves' disease. It is estimated that 15% of patients with Graves' disease have a close relative with the disease, and 50% of the biologic relatives of these patients have thyroid antibodies in their blood.[10]

Pathophysiology

In Graves' disease the thyroid gland is stimulated into a state of sustained hypersecretion and autonomous function by the actions of a group of circulating immunoglobulins that are essentially nonsuppressible by the normal regulatory pathways.

It is theorized that the T-lymphocytes become sensitized to antigens within the thyroid gland and stimulate the B-lymphocytes to synthesize antibodies, which are called thyroid-stimulating immunoglobins (TSI). These antibodies attach themselves to the thyroid-stimulating hormone (TSH) receptor sites on the thyroid cell membrane and stimulate the cells to increase in size and activity. TSH is therefore displaced from its normal regulator role.

Thyroid hormone production in general may be increased tenfold, but the synthesis of triiodothyronine (T_3) is increased proportionately more than thyroxine (T_4). Since T_3 is metabolically up to four times more potent than T_4, the clinical effects of this imbalance in T_3 content of the thyroglobulin can be dramatic. Graves' disease represents one of the few known situations in which autoimmune antibodies stimulate organ function rather than acting in a purely destructive fashion.

Plasma cells and lymphocytes are also present in varying amounts throughout the thyroid gland, contributing to the classic clinical sign of thyroid enlargement, or **goiter.** This process is not confined to the thyroid gland itself. The infiltration of lymphocytes and plasma cells plus the accumulation of **mucopolysaccharides**, which form the intercellular matrix of connective tissue, contribute to the thickening of the skin and subcutaneous tissue, particularly over the lower tibia, that characterizes Graves' dermopathy. This infiltrative process also plays a part in the development of the classic Graves' ophthalmopathy, which is still poorly understood. The actual eye symptoms vary widely in severity but typically include inflammation and edema of the lids and conjunctiva, an increase in fatty tissue and muscle in the orbit that causes protrusion of the eye, and fibrous tissue infiltration, which may enlarge the extraocular muscles 10 to 20 times normal.

Muscle weakness and loss of muscle mass can be severe systemic effects of Graves' disease. They are believed to represent an acute myositis that results from a generalized cell-mediated immune reaction in the muscles. The pelvic and pectoral muscle girdles are particularly affected.

Thyroid hormone has marked chronotropic and inotropic effects on the heart, and many of the clinical symptoms of Graves' disease suggest a synergism between the actions of thyroxine and epinephrine. Although the circulating levels of catecholamines have been found to be normal in patients with Graves' disease, these individuals appear to be more sensitive to their action.

The metabolism of carbohydrates, fats, and proteins is also altered by hormone excess. The rates of glycogenolysis and glucogenesis are increased and can induce diabetes. Increased bone turnover depletes bone calcium stores and causes mild hypercalcemia.

Complications

Uncontrolled Graves' disease can produce serious and even life-threatening effects in vital organ systems. The rate of oxygen use by the tissues may be increased to the point where enormous stress is placed on the heart, resulting in systolic hypertension, angina, infarction, or heart failure. Patients with preexisting cardiovascular disease are at particular risk. The myositis can result in profound weakness and incapacity. Infiltrative eye disease can cause diplopia, corneal ulceration, and loss of vision. Metabolic hyperactivity can create acute anxiety and insomnia and even induce psychosis in some individuals.

Thyrotoxic crisis, or thyroid storm, is a rare but potentially fatal complication of Graves' disease that represents a breakdown in the body's tolerance to chronic hormone excess. This state of pronounced hypermetabolism and excessive adrenergic response can rapidly lead to heart failure and shock and is a true medical emergency. It is discussed later in this chapter.

Clinical Manifestations

Over 95% of patients with Graves' disease have palpable thyroid enlargement, or goiter.[18] It is generally diffuse and symmetric but may be asymmetric or, in rare cases, nodular. Symptoms of thyrotoxicosis are directly related to the basic abnormality of increased cell metabolism and are present in virtually all patients, although the range and severity may vary dramatically. A list of potential symptoms is provided in the box above. Young adults with moderate to severe disease typically experience weight loss despite hyperphagia, heat intolerance, diaphoresis, easy fatigability, nervousness and insomnia, and tachycardia and palpitations. In older patients the cardiovascular, muscular, or gastrointestinal symptoms typically predominate. In elderly

POSSIBLE SYMPTOMS OF THYROTOXICOSIS

Gastrointestinal
  Weight loss despite hyperphagia
  Abdominal pain or cramping
  Increased number of stools or diarrhea
Skin and hair
  Heat intolerance
  Diaphoresis
  Thin, brittle hair
  Plummer's nails
  Increased patchy pigmentation
  Graves' dermopathy
Neuromuscular
  Easy fatigability
  Muscle weakness, particularly pelvic and shoulder
    girdle
  Fine tremors
Cardiovascular
  Tachycardia
  Palpitations
  Systolic hypertension
  Dyspnea on exertion
Psychologic
  Anxiety and nervousness
  Insomnia and early awakening
  Difficulty concentrating
  Reduced tolerance to stress
Reproductive
  Oligomennorhea or amenorhea
  Decreased libido
Ocular
  Proptosis
  Upper lid retraction
  Periorbital edema
  Diplopia
  Redness of conjunctiva
  Visual loss

persons the classic signs are frequently absent. Apathy is very common and is often attributed to other causes with the thyroid disease overlooked.

The ophthalmopathy of Graves' disease may precede the symptoms of thyrotoxicosis, occur with them, or, in rare cases, occur in otherwise euthyroid (having a normally functioning thyroid gland) patients. Overt eye symptoms occur in approximately 30% to 40% of patients.[5] Patients may complain of dryness of the eyes, difficulty in focusing, or visual loss. Muscle weakness is a serious complication that can significantly interfere with the patient's vision. The combination of **proptosis** (bulging or forward displacement of the eye), periorbital swelling, and

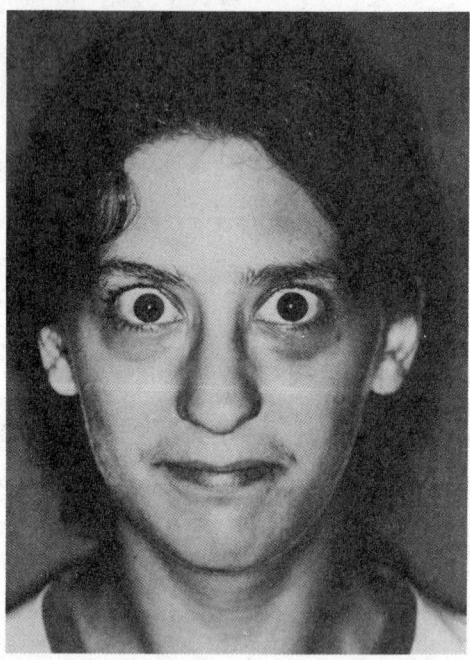

FIGURE 61-1   Classic Graves' ophthalmopathy. (From Rose LF, Kaye D: *Internal medicine for dentistry,* ed 2, St Louis, 1990, Mosby–Year Book, Inc.)

muscle involvement that characterizes Graves' ophthalmopathy is commonly termed **exophthalmos.** Figure 61-1 illustrates classic extensive ophthalmopathy.

Classic Graves' dermopathy occurs rarely, usually after many years, and in conjunction with ophthalmopathy. The infiltrative disease process causes the skin to be markedly thickened. It can occur anywhere, although the usual site is the lower tibial region.

The diagnosis of Graves' disease has been improved by recent advances in diagnostic technology that have increased the accuracy of thyroid screening. The sensitive TSH test uses monoclonal antibodies to significantly increase the diagnostic sensitivity to exclude 99% of euthyroid individuals and is the test of choice. It has eliminated the need for more expensive and time-consuming stimulation tests. Further workup may include serum measurements of T_3 and T_4, antithyroid antibodies, and thyroid imaging tests (see Chapter 59). In classic cases the clinical symptoms alone lead to a presumptive diagnosis. The box above summarizes common laboratory findings characteristic of Graves' disease.

Therapeutic Management

The management of Graves' disease is aimed at reducing the excess secretion of hormones, establishing a euthyroid state, and preventing or treating

DIAGNOSTIC TEST RESULTS CHARACTERISTIC OF GRAVES' DISEASE

Decreased sensitive TSH levels
Elevated serum T_4
Elevated serum T_3, T_3 resin uptake
Elevated thyroid radioactive iodine uptake
Presence of thyroid autoantibodies

complications. The treatment options are relatively simple and include drug therapy, surgery, and radioactive iodine treatment.

Drug therapy

Although drug therapy may be used as a primary mode of treatment for some patients with Graves' disease, it is increasingly playing a more supportive role in preparing patients for definitive treatment, controlling symptoms, and preventing complications. The major drugs in use are summarized in Table 61-1.

Iodide preparations are the oldest type of drug therapy for Graves' disease. They cause the thyroid to undergo temporary involution and decrease in size and vascularity. They promote storage of colloid material and quickly and effectively inhibit the release of thyroid hormones from glandular stores. The effects are transitory, however, and the thyroid will "escape" from the inhibitory effects within a few weeks.

The antithyroid drugs competitively inhibit the incorporation of iodide into metabolically active hormone and may be used as primary therapy for Graves' disease or to restore a euthyroid state before other definitive treatment. The major advantage of antithyroid drugs is that they cause no permanent damage to the gland itself. However, they are generally unable to sustain patients in a euthyroid state for prolonged periods, and the relapse rate is commonly greater than 50%.

Propylthiouracil (PTU) and methimazole (Tapazole) are the two drugs approved for use in the United States. They are taken up by the thyroid where they impair the synthesis of thyroxine by preventing the organic binding of iodine. PTU also partially inhibits the conversion of T_4 to T_3, and it is usually the drug of choice. Methimazole has a longer duration of action, however, which may make it preferable in situations where a single daily dose is desirable. Side effects are largely dose related. Agranulocytosis is an extremely serious side effect

TABLE 61-1   Pharmacology Summary: Graves' Disease

Drug	Action	Dosage	Side effects
Iodides	Inhibit release of thyroid hormones		
Lugol's solution		5 to 10 gtt by mouth (PO) 2 to 3 times daily	Strongly salty taste, possible gastrointestinal irritation
SSKI		1 to 2 gtt PO 2 to 3 times daily	
Propylthiouracil (PTU)	Inhibits synthesis of thyroxine by preventing organic binding of iodine	50 to 150 mg PO daily in divided doses (maintenance)	Mild gastrointestinal irritation Skin rash and pruritus Agranulocytosis (rare)
Methimazole (Tapazole)	Inhibits synthesis of thyroxine by preventing organic binding of iodine	5 to 15 mg PO daily (maintenance)	Mild gastrointestinal irritation Skin rash and pruritus Agranulocytosis (rare)
Propranolol (Inderal)	Blocks peripheral actions of thyroid hormones	10 to 80 mg PO 3 to 4 times daily	Depression or sleep disturbance Hypotension, bradycardia, heart block Gastrointestinal irritation Bronchospasm

that may occur in a few patients (less than 0.5%) during the first 3 months of therapy. If the condition is promptly recognized and the drug discontinued, it is usually self-limiting and completely reversible within 1 to 2 weeks.

It commonly requires 4 to 6 weeks to establish a euthyroid state, because T_4 has a serum half-life of 6 to 7 days and the thyroid gland has a large store of hormone that is unaffected by the drugs. Drug therapy is continued for at least 1 year after remission is achieved. Drug dosages are then gradually tapered, and the patient is closely monitored for relapses, which usually occur within 3 months.

Many of the clinical symptoms of Graves' disease resemble those of sympathetic overactivity, and the beta-adrenergic blockers play an essential role in symptom management. They rapidly and effectively relieve the tachycardia, palpitations, hypertension, and rhythm disturbances. They do not, however, directly affect the underlying hyperthyroid state. Propranolol (Inderal) remains the drug of choice, although the use of more selective agents such as nadolol (Corgard), atenolol (Tenormin), and metoprolol (Lopressor) continues to be researched.

Medical management

The use of sodium ^{131}I has gradually become the treatment of choice for most patients with Graves'

disease. Sodium ^{131}I treatment is contraindicated during pregnancy, but it has been found to be safe and effective in most other situations although caution is indicated in persons under 25 years of age. No statistically significant increase in cancer risk or teratogenesis has been demonstrated.[24]

Before treatment with sodium ^{131}I, antithyroid drug therapy is used to reduce glandular hormone stores and the amount of radionuclide required. Drugs are discontinued 5 to 7 days before treatment to facilitate thyroid uptake of the radionuclide. The actual dose of sodium ^{131}I varies and is based on an estimate of thyroid weight. The radionuclide is rapidly picked up by the thyroid gland and concentrated there. It emits strong beta particles that slowly destroy the hyperfunctioning thyroid tissue but have minimal effects on other body tissue since they are only capable of penetrating about 2 mm. The sodium ^{131}I not trapped by the thyroid is rapidly excreted in the urine and feces. The gland typically shrinks and becomes euthyroid within 6 to 12 weeks.

Hypothyroidism is the major side effect and is recognized as an acceptable treatment outcome. Approximately 5% to 25% become hypothyroid in the first year with an additional 1% to 3% in each subsequent year. Although the incidence of hypothyroidism is somewhat dose related, lowering the treatment dose does not reduce the risk of hypothyroidism, but it does significantly increase the risk of treatment failure. Careful follow-up of serum T_4 and TSH levels is important.

Patients may experience a brief episode of radiation thyroiditis 5 to 14 days after treatment, although acute side effects are uncommon. Tenderness in the neck is a common complaint. General comfort measures are usually adequate, but a brief course of glucocorticoids may be necessary if symptoms are severe. Hyperthyroid symptoms may also temporarily worsen from the release of stored hormones in the inflamed gland.

Treatment of ophthalmopathy

Graves' ophthalmopathy is a self-limiting condition that regresses with time to some degree. It is treated with supportive care using sodium restriction, diuretics, short-course corticosteroid therapy, eye lubricants, eye patches, and ocular muscle exercises. Super-voltage radiation or surgical decompression may be necessary in severe cases. Successful treatment of the underlying thyroid disease may or may not influence the course of the ophthalmopathy.

Surgical intervention

Thyroidectomy is the treatment of choice for patients with large goiters, pregnant women, or those reluctant to undergo sodium ^{131}I therapy. The procedure entails a negligible risk when performed by an experienced surgeon. Antithyroid drug therapy is used before surgery to induce a euthyroid state and reduce the size and vascularity of the gland. A few grams of tissue will be left intact on each side of the gland in the attempt to preserve adequate thyroid and parathyroid function. Total thyroidectomy is rarely indicated. The primary postoperative concerns are related to the effects of anesthesia, edema, bleeding, infection, and damage to the laryngeal nerves. Transient hypocalcemia occurs in up to 75% of all patients.

NURSING MANAGEMENT OF THE PATIENT WITH GRAVES' DISEASE
Assessment

Nursing assessment incorporates a wide range of factors. A thorough history is essential. It should include specific patient symptoms, how they have changed or progressed, and what treatment, if any, has been undertaken. A family history of goiter, hypothyroidism, hyperthyroidism, or any autoimmune disease process should also be explored. Enlargement of the gland itself may be visible on inspection or identifiable with gentle palpation.

Most patients with Graves' disease exhibit only a few of the clinical manifestations identified in the box on p. 1689, but they can all be important indicators. The patient's general physical appearance is assessed, as are recent changes in body weight, appetite, or bowel function. Abdominal complaints are particularly important in older patients.

Increased dermal blood flow and perspiration give the skin a soft, warm, moist, velvety feel. Facial flushing and palmar erythema are common. The skin over the lower tibia should be assessed for signs of Graves' dermopathy. Melanocyte-stimulating hormone (MSH) release may cause a generalized increase in skin pigmentation, or patchy vitiligo. The fingernails are often soft and friable and may separate from the nail bed at the distal margin (Plummer's nails). The patient may note that hair has become thin and fine and falls out in small patches.

The nurse should assess for signs of Graves' ophthalmopathy, including the adequacy of the patient's eyelid closure, the presence of diplopia or ptosis, and patient complaints of eye muscle weakness or dry, itchy eyes.

Tachycardia and systolic hypertension are common findings. Floppy mitral valve prolapse is also a common occurrence in Graves' disease, and the nurse may hear evidence of a systolic murmur or midsystolic click on auscultation.

The nurse should also assess for signs of thyrotoxic myopathy. Generalized fatigue, weakness, and dyspnea on exertion are common, and it may be possible to elicit specific problems with activities such as stair climbing, straight leg raises, or holding the arms above the head.

The patient's psychologic status should also be carefully assessed. It is common for patients to be nervous, anxious, and fidgety and have trouble concentrating. Patients often feel driven to be constantly active and yet are chronically fatigued, experiencing both insomnia and early morning awakening. The symptoms may be frightening and confusing and represent a real threat to psychologic equilibrium. Extreme mood lability is common. Hand tremors can make activities requiring fine motor control impossible.

It is essential to consider thyroid disease in elderly patients who rarely exhibit the classic signs of thyrotoxicosis. Vague complaints, exacerbations of chronic illnesses, and psychosocial changes may be nonspecific cues to thyroid disorders.

Nursing Diagnosis

Common diagnoses might include the following:
    Altered nutrition: less than body requirements, related to an intake less than metabolic needs secondary to an excessive metabolic rate
    Diarrhea related to increased peristalsis
    Activity intolerance related to muscle fatigue

Sleep pattern disturbance related to difficulty falling asleep or early morning awakening

Altered health maintenance related to lack of knowledge of Graves' disease and its treatment

High risk for injury: corneal damage related to inability to properly close eyelids secondary to proptosis

Anxiety related to perceived threat to self-concept and loss of control

Planning

Specific patient goals and their relative priority will reflect the patient's age and the severity of the symptoms. Outcome criteria might include the following:

Patient ingests sufficient balanced nutrients to achieve or maintain a desired body weight

Patient reestablishes and maintains a normal pattern of bowel elimination

Patient is able to participate in normal activities of daily living without experiencing excessive muscle fatigue or dyspnea

Patient obtains sufficient rest and sleep to meet perceived needs

Patient is knowledgeable about the disease process and treatment regimen and can state the potential risks and side effects of medications and treatment

Patient employs measures to protect the eyes and does not exhibit corneal damage

Patient can verbalize an understanding of behavior and does not exhibit signs of harmful anxiety

Implementation

There are no instant cures for Graves' disease, and its successful treatment may necessitate regimen adjustment over time. Patients are rarely hospitalized for the treatment of thyroid disorders and must be assisted to manage their disease successfully in the home. Nurses collaborate with patients and families in providing or planning care. General interventions revolve around increasing the patient's level of comfort in everyday living. A quiet, restful, and cool environment is ideal. For hospitalized patients a private or semiprivate room situated away from the activity of the central nursing station may be preferable. The nurse should discuss the need for increased rest with the patient and help the patient plan and space activities appropriately.

Hospitalized patients should be provided with the opportunity for frequent bathing and linen changes and should be offered help as needed to remain cool and comfortable. Providing help with self-care activities, ambulation, and laundry will also help conserve the patient's energy. These general comfort measures can also help the patient achieve restful

sleep, although sedatives or hypnotics may be necessary to augment the patient's rest.

The patient should eat a diet that is high in calories, protein, and carbohydrates and should drink extra fluid. Vitamin and mineral supplements should be added, particularly the water-soluble vitamins whose normal absorption is impaired. If diarrhea, abdominal cramping, or hypermotility is present, small frequent meals and snacks may be helpful, and the patient can be counseled to avoid high-fiber and gas-producing foods. Body weight is monitored regularly. Patients with insulin-dependent diabetes should be taught to increase the frequency of their blood testing.

Appropriate diversional activities are essential to help the patient deal with both anxiety and the boredom of enforced inactivity. Pursuing activities such as reading, watching TV, listening to music, and playing games successfully avoids muscle fatigue. Letter writing, needlework, and other close work may be very difficult or frustrating if the patient is experiencing tremors. The patient and family should be reassured that the psychologic symptoms are related to the disease process and will respond to treatment. Overstimulation and arguing should be avoided, and both the number of visitors and length of visits should be restricted. Empathetic understanding of the patient's mood swings can help the patient maintain control.

Eye care

Restricting the sodium content of the diet and having the patient sleep with the head of the bed elevated may help relieve periorbital edema. Comfort strategies include the use of physiological eye drops to counteract dryness, ophthalmic ointments for night use, tinted glasses to counter photophobia, and wraparound glasses to prevent injury from wind and airborne particles. Exercises for the extraocular muscles may prevent diplopia. The adequacy of eyelid closure should be assessed, and the patient should be advised to use hypoallergenic tape or eye patches during sleep as needed. The eyes should be inspected regularly for signs of corneal irritation or abrasion.

Drug therapy

The nurse is responsible for teaching the patient about medications and monitoring for side effects. Since hospitalization will involve minimal treatment time, if any, the emphasis must be on knowledgeable self-care. Patients should receive both written and oral instructions about all medications and associated side effects. The patient education guide on p. 1694 outlines the major points of patient education associated with the antithyroid drugs. Most

PATIENT EDUCATION GUIDE *Antithyroid Drugs*

Propylthiouracil and methimazole

Take the drug at the same time or times each day

Over-the-counter antihistamines may be used for mild skin rashes and itching

Report the abrupt occurrence of sore throat or fever immediately

Monitor body weight and other symptoms regularly

Do not increase or decrease drug dosage

SSKI or Lugol's solution

Take the drug after meals with a full glass of water, juice, or milk

Propranolol

Take the drug before meals

Take pulse daily and report if pulse is slower than baseline or irregular

Never abruptly stop taking the drug

Check body weight regularly and report the incidence of edema

If diabetic, monitor carefully for the occurrence of hypoglycemia

medications are broken down more rapidly in a hyperthyroid state, and the patient may need dosage adjustments for other prescribed drugs. Anticoagulant action is potentiated, and patients need careful assessment and follow-up.

Sodium ^{131}I therapy

The major nursing responsibilities associated with sodium ^{131}I therapy involve teaching and reassuring the patient about the safety of the treatment. The basic principles are summarized in the patient education guide below.

Preoperative care

General nursing care in the preoperative period continues all of the general comfort measures discussed under implementation. Surgery will not be attempted unless the patient is in a controlled, euthyroid state. Maintaining a quiet, restful environment in the hospital may be a major challenge. The nurse should pay particular attention to ensuring that the patient is in an optimal nutritional and fluid state to tolerate the stresses of surgery.

Immediate preoperative care involves patient education concerning the surgical procedure and the expected postoperative care. This includes general

PATIENT EDUCATION GUIDE *Outpatient Sodium ^{131}I Therapy*

The total body radiation exposure of sodium ^{131}I treatment is approximately equivalent to that of an intravenous pyelogram (IVP) or barium enema

The patient should fast the night before the isotope is administered to facilitate absorption of the isotope

Antithyroid drugs are discontinued at least 5 days before treatment

The isotope is administered orally in a colorless tasteless liquid as a one-time dose

The patient will remain in the outpatient department for about 2 hours to be monitored for vomiting; only very high-dose therapy necessitates hospitalization for isolation

Patients should avoid close body contact with infants, young children, or pregnant women during the first 24 hours after treatment; the radiation risk is minimal, however

Patients should increase their fluid intake to at least 2000 to 3000 ml/day for 2 to 3 days after treatment; flushing the toilet several times after use during this period reduces the risk of family exposure to the isotope

Tenderness in the neck is an expected side effect; acute symptoms should be promptly reported to the physician

measures such as turning and deep breathing routines, pain management, and the frequency of vital sign measurement. Specific instructions should address the expected appearance of the incision and dressings postoperatively and the importance of maintaining good alignment to avoid stress on the incision line. The patient should practice using hands and arms to stabilize and support the head and neck during movement.

Postoperative care

Immediate postoperative nursing care focuses on monitoring for complications associated with bleeding or edema. Although the expected blood loss from surgery is extremely small, the neck and thyroid gland are highly vascular areas, and serious bleeding can occur. Soft tissue swelling and compression are also possible, and tracheal, laryngeal, or glottal edema can result in respiratory distress or even obstruction.

The patient is placed in a semi-Fowler's position to facilitate breathing, and the nurse assesses vital signs and respiratory status frequently. The surgical dressing is inspected for tightness, compression, or signs of bleeding. The assessment should include the back of the patient's neck and pillow. Tightness may necessitate loosening the bulky dressings. Oxygen, suction apparatus, and a tracheostomy set should be readily available at the bedside. Frequent deep breathing is encouraged, although actual coughing should be done only as necessary to clear the airway of secretions. Other routine care includes en-

suring adequate pain relief and helping the patient with early ambulation. The nurse should remind the patient to maintain proper alignment of the head and neck and avoid both severe flexion and hyperextension, which could disrupt the patency of the incision.

Laryngeal nerve damage is possible during surgery, and the patient may experience immediate vocal impairment. Hoarseness that develops or worsens in the postoperative period is usually the result of laryngeal pressure or edema and will resolve within a few days. The patient's voice should be assessed at regular intervals for developing or worsening symptoms, but the patient should be reassured that the effects are transitory. Voice use should be limited in the immediate postoperative period. Food and fluid intake should also be introduced with caution because temporary dysphagia is common.

Transient hypocalcemia occurs commonly after thyroid surgery, and the nurse must assess for signs of incipient **tetany** frequently in the first 2 to 3 days after surgery. Early signs include tingling around the mouth and fingertips, muscle twitching or spasms, positive **Chvostek's** and **Trousseau's signs** (Figure 61-2), palpitations, or dysrhythmias. The physician should be informed of these symptoms immediately, and intravenous calcium should be available at the bedside.

The patient will advance to a soft, regular diet as soon as it can be tolerated, and the nurse encourages intake of adequate levels of protein and vitamin C to support wound healing. The incision is inspected daily, and the nurse encourages the patient

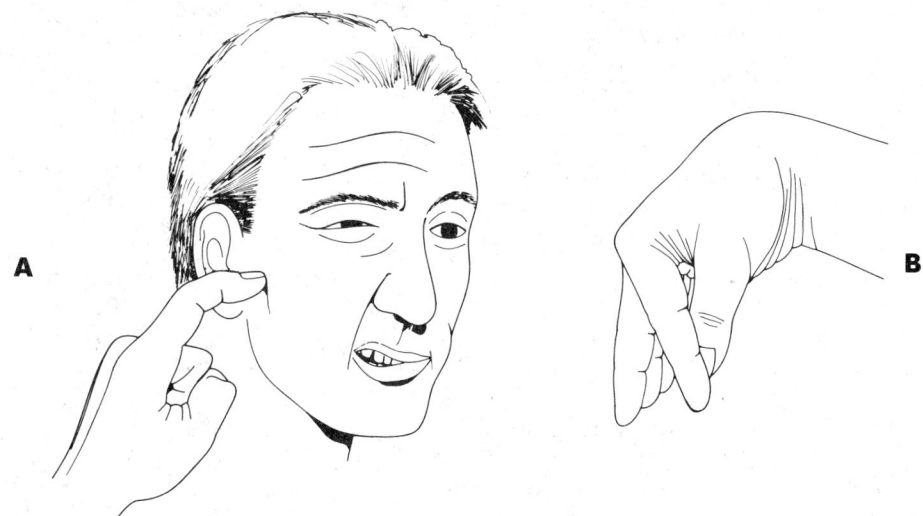

FIGURE 61-2 **A,** Chvostek's sign: a contraction of facial muscles elicited in response to a light tap over facial nerve in front of ear. **B,** Trousseau's sign: a carpopedal spasm induced by inflating a blood pressure cuff above systolic pressure.

NURSING CARE PLAN *Postoperative Thyroidectomy Patient*

Nursing diagnosis/ Expected outcome	Interventions	Rationale
High risk for ineffective breathing pattern related to tracheal compression and edema •*Breath sounds will be clear in all lung segments* •*Normal unlabored ventilation will be maintained*	Assess respiratory rate and depth every hour Auscultate lungs every 2-4 hours Encourage patient to deep breathe every hour Place patient in semi- to high-Fowler's position Help patient cough effectively to clear airway if needed Assess operative site for signs of swelling or compression; loosen dressings if necessary; monitor neck circumference every 4 hours Ensure that oxygen, suction, and a tracheostomy set are available on the unit or at the bedside	Postoperative edema and bleeding can contribute to the development of respiratory distress; deep breathing will support oxygenation and prevent atelectasis; coughing is minimized to prevent tissue damage and stress to the incision; an upright position facilitates air exchange; emergency equipment should be available in case of airway obstruction
High risk for injury: bleeding related to lack of incisional hemostasis •*Vital signs will remain at preoperative level* •*Postoperative bleeding will be promptly detected*	Monitor vital signs, skin color and level of consciousness every hour during first 24 hours Check dressing and area behind neck for bleeding	The first 24 hours is the period of greatest risk for surgical bleeding; bleeding may not be visible on the dressing, but drain down by gravity to the back of the neck
Acute pain related to incision and damaged neck muscles •*Postoperative pain will be adequately controlled*	Assess patient for pain regularly and offer prescribed analgesics as appropriate Maintain patient in semi-Fowler's position Maintain head and neck in good alignment; avoid hyperextension or extreme flexion Teach patient to support head and neck with hands when moving or changing position Teach patient to avoid abrupt or jarring movements	Adequate pain relief is essential to enable the patient to be out of bed and avoid complications of immobility; an upright position and support will reduce stress to the incision and minimize pain
High risk for impaired verbal communication related to laryngeal edema or nerve damage •*Patient will continue to speak in his normal voice*	Ask patient to speak his name each hour; assess for changes in pitch and tone or hoarseness Encourage voice rest and provide for alternate means of communication as needed Reassure patient that hoarseness that develops in the first day is transitory and will resolve	Tracheal intubation, postoperative edema, and surgical damage to the laryngeal nerves can all cause vocal changes; hoarseness that develops and worsens in the postoperative period is almost always reversible and not related to nerve damage
High risk for injury: physiologic related to the development of hypocalcemia secondary to surgical damage to parathyroid glands •*Serum calcium levels will remain within the normal range*	Assess for presence of Chvostek's and Trousseau's signs Observe for signs of muscle twitching or spasm Assess patient for numbness or tingling in lips or fingertips Have calcium available at the bedside for immediate IV administration	Parathyroid gland function may be disrupted by thyroid surgery; transient hypocalcemia occurs in most patients; the signs identified are those of early tetany

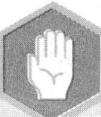

CLINICAL ALERT

Serious, even life-threatening complications such as laryngeal edema, tracheal obstruction, hypocalcemic tetany, and thyroid crisis are rare but potential complications of thyroid surgery. The nurse must monitor the patient's airway and vital signs frequently and be alert to signs of calcium imbalance. Emergency equipment must be readily available on the unit or at the bedside.

to gradually increase the extent of daily, gentle range-of-motion exercise for the neck. Abrupt jerking movements should be avoided. The nurse can discuss clothing modifications that will avoid irritation of the healing incision yet draw minimal attention to the scar. There is no hard evidence that creams or lotions in any way reduce the amount of scar tissue formed or improve its appearance.

The care plan on p. 1696 illustrates a general plan for a patient undergoing thyroidectomy.

Evaluation

Ongoing patient assessment helps the nurse evaluate the effectiveness of interventions. A successful treatment plan helps the patient maintain a stable body weight, maintain a normal elimination pattern, have sufficient energy to participate in normal daily activities, and achieve restful sleep at night. The patient will not experience diaphoresis, tachycardia, hypertension, or palpitations. The patient will use eye drops and positioning or patching as necessary to prevent eye injury. Most importantly, the patient will demonstrate knowledge of the disease process, treatment options, medications and how to manage their side effects, and the signs that indicate the need for medical assistance. Finally, the nurse will look for evidence that the patient feels in control of the situation and is able to problem solve appropriately.

Documentation

Documentation of care for the patient with Graves' disease primarily involves accurate recording of assessment data and interventions and validation of patient education. The recording of frequent, thorough physical assessments is essential while the treatment plan is being established and the patient's response is being evaluated. The patient's record

should contain accurate and detailed documentation of preoperative and postoperative care delivered. Since self-care is the foundation of treatment and the disease process requires long-term follow-up, the patient should receive both verbal and written instructions about the disease process and treatment plan.

Ongoing Care

Regardless of the treatment used, it is impossible to guarantee whether a patient will become or remain euthyroid. Careful ongoing follow-up is essential. It is important that the patient assume responsibility for self-care and know the symptoms that indicate disease recurrence or hypothyroidism. Uncomplicated Graves' disease rarely necessitates the involvement of community support agencies. The nurse assumes primary responsibility for patient and family education, which is summarized in the patient education guide on p. 1698.

THYROTOXIC CRISIS

Thyrotoxic crisis, or thyroid storm, is an acute, potentially life-threatening state of extreme thyroid overactivity that represents a breakdown in the body's tolerance to a chronic excess of thyroid hormones. The condition is rare, but most patients who experience crisis have had moderate to severe thyroid disease that has been untreated or inadequately treated. The syndrome is poorly understood, and patients cannot be identified by age, race, sex, or other demographic variables. Thyrotoxic crisis typically occurs during periods of severe physiologic or psychologic stress such as trauma, sepsis, delivery, or major surgery, but it also must be recognized as a potential complication following thyroidectomy. The syndrome should be acknowledged as a risk factor in critical care settings. It is currently theorized that an altered peripheral response to thyroid hormone and a heightened sensitivity of effector organs to adrenergic stimuli trigger the syndrome from as yet unknown mechanisms. T_3 and T_4 levels are not significantly elevated.

The diagnosis of thyrotoxic crisis is a clinical one, since no particular hormone levels confirm or deny it. Since the syndrome is rapidly fatal, the diagnosis must be made promptly. The clinical features include fever greater than 100° F, marked tachycardia, flushing and sweating, other exaggerated symptoms of thyrotoxicosis, and marked agitation and restlessness, which can lead to delirium and coma within 24 hours. Death typically occurs from dysrhythmias, shock, and heart failure, which responds poorly to digitalis therapy.

The goal is to treat the underlying disease process and effectively block the peripheral actions of the

PATIENT EDUCATION GUIDE   *Graves' Disease*

Objective: To modify behavior to promote patient comfort and knowledgeable self-care and prevent complications

General comfort measures

Establish quiet, cool, restful environments; use light clothing
Space activities throughout day
Plan frequent rest periods but avoid bed rest
Increase frequency of bathing and linen changes
Accept help with care activities to conserve energy
Ensure quiet atmosphere and cool temperatures to promote sleep

Diet and elimination

Eat a balanced high-calorie, high-protein, high-carbohydrate diet
Add extra fluids
Try eating small frequent meals and snacks
Take vitamin and mineral supplement daily
Weigh yourself twice each week
Avoid high-fiber and gas-producing foods
Take over-the-counter antidiarrheals as needed

Eye care

Restrict sodium in diet
Sleep with head of bed elevated
Use eye drops to keep eyes moist
Wear sunglasses when outdoors
Tape or patch eyes for sleep as needed

Diversion

Avoid stress and conflict where possible
Plan activities that do not cause muscle fatigue
Avoid activities requiring fine motor skills

Ongoing care

Monitor health status regularly; be alert to signs of recurring hyperthyroidism or hypothyroidism
See physician at regular intervals for ongoing evaluation of condition
Do not alter dosage or schedule for prescribed medications without consulting health care provider

---

thyroid hormones. Propranolol is administered by slow intravenous infusion. Iodides and intravenous propylthiouracil are given to block hormone synthesis and release. Steroids may also be administered to support the body's stress response and interfere with the peripheral conversion of T_4 to T_3. Gradual clearing of the mental symptoms is a good indication of clinical improvement.

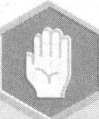

CLINICAL ALERT

Thyrotoxic crisis (thyroid storm) can occur in patients with preexisting thyroid disease who experience severe physiologic or psychologic stress. Symptoms include fever, tachycardia, agitation leading to delerium and coma, heart failure, and shock. The nurse monitors vital signs and level of consciousness frequently. Nursing interventions include decreasing environmental stimuli, reorienting and reassuring the patient, supporting cardiac and respiratory function, and reducing fever. Aspirin is avoided, because it reduces serum binding of T_4.

THYROIDITIS

Subacute thyroiditis is an acute inflammatory disorder of the thyroid gland usually caused by a viral infection. Once thought to be quite rare, subacute thyroiditis is being diagnosed more commonly. An antecedent sore throat or other upper respiratory tract infection is typical.

Symptoms of subacute thyroiditis include fever, malaise, soreness in the neck, and difficulty in swallowing. The gland is tender, exhibiting diffuse enlargement. Signs of local redness or heat may also be present. Symptoms of hyperthyroidism may be present because of the release of preformed thyroid hormones from the inflamed gland. Serum T_3 and T_4 values are typically elevated.

The disease is usually self-limiting, and complete recovery occurs over weeks or months. The hyperthyroid period may be followed by a hypothyroid phase once the pool of stored hormones has been exhausted, since new hormones are not yet being adequately synthesized. Hormone supplement may be necessary at this time to prevent recurrence of the disease. Treatment is basically symptomatic and supportive. Acetaminophen and propranolol can usually adequately control the symptoms, but a short course of steroids may be indicated in severe cases. The patient needs reassurance that the condition will resolve but should be closely followed until recovery is complete.

TOXIC ADENOMA (PLUMMER'S DISEASE)

In toxic adenoma a nodule begins to function autonomously, gradually increasing in size and suppressing normal gland function. Nodules are readily identifiable on palpation and appear as "hot" areas on thyroid scan. Thyrotoxicosis develops, and patients typically have rather severe adrenergic symptoms. The treatment options are the same as those for Graves' disease. Surgical lobectomy is often performed for large nodules.

Hypothyroidism

Hypothyroidism is a relatively common disorder, particularly in elderly persons, that can create a diffuse clinical syndrome resulting from the ongoing deficiency of thyroid hormones. The syndrome can occur from primary intrinsic thyroid disease or as a secondary problem related to hypothalamic imbalance or cellular resistance to thyroxine. Hypothyroidism primarily affects women between the ages of 30 and 60 years, and its effects may be overt or extremely subtle. It is estimated that subclinical forms of hypothyroidism may exist in as much as 2% to 9% of the general population and up to 15% of persons over 60 years. These patients have normal hormone levels, increased levels of TSH, and subtle nonspecific symptoms that are frequently dismissed as simple aging.

Hypothyroidism is of particular concern in patients over 50 years of age. Thus the classic signs and symptoms of hypothyroidism are well defined for this segment of the population. Important considerations are as follows:

- Because many of the signs and symptoms of hypothyroidism are consistent with normal aging (constipation, cold intolerance, psychomotor retardation, decreased exercise tolerance), they may be overlooked.
- Hypothyroidism is a cause of secondary hypertension, which may respond to thyroid hormone replacement.
- Mental status and emotional responses such as lethargy and depression are common presenting symptoms.

Thyroid hormone is essential to normal growth and development, and its absence or deficiency in infancy results in cretinism with profound and irreversible mental and physical consequences. Cretinism is rare in the United States where adequate prenatal and infant health care is available, but it is still a significant problem in third world areas. In adults thyroid hormone deficiency causes generalized slowing of the metabolic processes, which, if untreated, can result in the syndrome called **myxedema.** Symptoms depend less on the specific cause than on the age of the patient and the severity and duration of the deficiency and are largely reversible with adequate hormone replacement.

A deficiency of dietary iodine will cause a decrease in the production of thyroid hormones. This remains a significant cause of hypothyroidism in certain areas of the world, but it is a negligible cause of hypothyroidism in the United States. Surgery, sodium ^{131}I treatment, and the unmonitored use of antithyroid drugs, however, are all common causes of uncomplicated hypothyroidism in the United States.

HASHIMOTO'S THYROIDITIS
Etiology/Epidemiology

Hashimoto's thyroiditis is the most common cause of primary hypothyroidism in the United States. It is a relatively benign autoimmune disease that is characterized by slow but progressive degeneration of the thyroid gland. It has been identified in all age groups and both sexes but primarily affects middle-aged women. It exhibits a clear familial link and frequently occurs in association with other autoimmune disorders.

Pathophysiology

In Hashimoto's thyroiditis autoantibodies are developed against one or more components of the thyroid gland. At least one of the antibodies has a cytotoxic action in the gland. Massive lymphocyte infiltration can cause total destruction of the normal architecture of the thyroid gland in severe cases.

The gradual fall in T_3 and T_4 levels triggers a rise in TSH that stimulates compensatory growth or enlargement of the thyroid gland in the attempt to produce sufficient amounts of hormone. The lack of thyroid hormone decreases the metabolic rate and can produce widespread derangements in organ functioning. It causes disorders in virtually every form of lipid metabolism, including elevations in cholesterol and triglycerides. There is therefore an increased incidence and severity of hypertension and coronary artery disease, particularly in older patients. Myxedema coma is a rare but life-threatening end stage of progressively lowered body metabolism.

Clinical Manifestations

Because thyroid hormone influences most body metabolic processes, the clinical manifestations of hormone deficiency can be many and varied, as summarized in the box on p. 1700. They depend largely on the duration and severity of the deficiency. In its early stages Hashimoto's thyroiditis may produce a wide variety of vague symptoms that are not accom-

CLINICAL MANIFESTATIONS OF HYPOTHYROIDISM

Gastrointestinal

Flatulence, distention, and constipation*
Weight gain and fluid retention

Skin and hair

Intolerance to cold*
Skin changes*
   Coarsened, dry, and scaly
   Yellowish tone
Nonpitting edema of the face, hands, and lower legs
   Periorbital edema*
Thick, brittle nails
Hair fragility
   Loss of outer third of eyebrow

Neuromuscular

Generalized weakness and easy fatigability*
Cramps, paresthesias, and decreased deep tendon
   reflexes

Cardiovascular

Sinus bradycardia and increased diastolic pressure

Psychologic

Placid behavior, difficulty concentrating, and depression

Reproductive

Oligomenorrhea or menorrhagia

Other

Mild thyroid enlargement, painless or tender goiter*
Hoarse, husky voice
Enlarged tongue and slow, slurred speech
Shallow, slow respirations
Vertigo and conductive hearing loss

Laboratory

Increased TSH*
High titer thyroid antoantibodies*
Decreased serum T_3 and T_4
Anemia, elevated cholesterol and triglycerides, and
   hypoglycemia

*Common early signs.

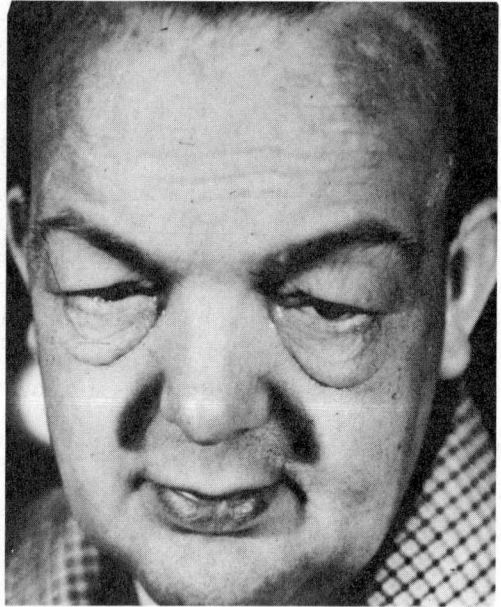

FIGURE 61-3   Typical facial appearance of myxedematous patients. (From Prior JA, Silberstein JS, Stang JM: *Physical diagnosis: the history and examination of the patient,* ed 6, St Louis, Mosby—Year Book, Inc.)

panied by objective physical findings. In middle-aged women these nonspecific complaints may be initially attributed to menopausal problems or adjustment problems associated with aging. A decreased metabolic rate causes typical complaints that include weakness, fatigue, cold intolerance, constipation, and weight gain. Mild to moderate painless goiter is also common, although in some cases the gland is quite tender.

As the hypothyroid state worsens, **glycosaminoglycans** are gradually deposited in the intracellular spaces of the skin and striated muscle. These substances accumulate, absorb fluid, and produce a nonpitting edema that becomes pronounced in the face, hands, and lower legs (Figure 61-3). Edema is often first noted around the eyes. Myxedema fluid collection causes widespread organ problems. Cardiomegaly and pericardial effusions are common, and glomerular filtration is decreased. Vertigo and conductive hearing loss result from middle and inner ear congestion. The respiratory center reacts sluggishly to altering blood gases, and there is decreased bellows action in the lung. Vocal cord congestion, tongue enlargement, and excess saliva cause a hoarse voice and a slurred speech pattern. Sinus bradycardia and decreased cardiac output occur, but actual heart failure is rare because overall oxygen demand is decreased.

Severe muscle weakness, cramping, paresthesias, neuropathies, and carpal tunnel syndrome are also common. Failure to ovulate and a lack of progesterone synthesis can lead to **oligomenorrhea.** Impotence and infertility in men are common. Reduced conversion of carotene to vitamin A gives the skin a yellowish tone. Nails are thickened and brittle, and the root shaft of the hair becomes fragile.

Although mental functioning initially remains intact, patients experience severe fatigue and lethargy. Placid behavior, slowed responses, difficulty concentrating, depression, and memory loss may all occur. In elderly patients these symptoms may be overlooked or attributed to developing senility.

The laboratory diagnosis of fully developed hypothyroidism is not difficult. An elevated TSH level is an important early indicator. Low serum T_3 and T_4 eventually occur, but these values remain normal during the compensatory stage. A high titer for thyroid autoantibodies is a classic sign.

Therapeutic Management

The goal of treatment is to increase the amount of thyroid hormones in the circulation, restoring a euthyroid state. If promptly identified, most of the tissue effects of hypothyroidism are reversible.

Drug therapy

The first successful use of sheep thyroid extract in 1891 established hormone replacement as the foundation for treatment of hypothyroidism.[22] A variety of hormone preparations are available, as summarized in Table 61-2. Levothyroxine sodium (Synthroid, Levothyroid) is the drug of choice for routine use. Young patients and individuals with mild dis-

ease can usually be safely treated with a full replacement dose. It requires about 2 months to restore hormone equilibrium. Full hormone replacement is often difficult or impossible to achieve in elderly patients or those with documented cardiac disease. Raising the metabolic rate dramatically increases demands on the heart and may trigger angina, dysrhythmia, or infarction in previously asymptomatic patients. Dosage adjustments are made gradually over several months. The results of hormone replacement are usually good, but lifelong monitoring is important.

NURSING MANAGEMENT OF THE PATIENT WITH HYPOTHYROIDISM
Assessment

A careful history is essential and should include data about the patient's current symptoms and the onset, course, and severity of the disease. Many of the symptoms are both subtle and subjective, and the patient may need help evaluating changes in feelings and behaviors. A positive family history of thyroid or autoimmune disease is significant as is a history of exposure to mild ionizing radiation such as that used to treat skin disorders.

The nurse assesses for changes in weight, appetite, bowel habits, energy level, muscle strength and

TABLE 61-2   Pharmacology Summary: Hypothyroidism

Generic name	Trade name	Composition	Usual daily dosage	Nursing implications
				ALL DRUGS
Levothyroxine	Synthroid, Levothyroid, Levoid	Synthetic isomer of T_4 Pure, stable, and inexpensive Half-life of 8 days; drug of choice for treatment	100 to 200 µg PO once daily, may be given IV	Establish regular schedule for taking drug Administer on empty stomach if feasible
Thyroid USP (dessicated)	Thyrar, Thyro-Teric	Animal derivative; T_3:T_4 ratio approximately 1:9; potency varies	60 to 180 mg PO once daily	Monitor for tachycardia, chest pain, or dyspnea during initial treatment period
Thyroglobulin	Proloid	Animal derivative; T_3:T_4 ratio approximately 1:2.5; potency varies, deteriorates rapidly	60 to 200 mg PO once daily	Monitor for improvement in energy, activity tolerance, level of alertness Teach patients signs of hormone excess
Liothyronine	Cytomel, Cytomine	Synthetic T_3 preparation; brief half-life, difficult to maintain sustained effect	25 to 75 µg PO in split doses	Reinforce importance of adherence with regimen and regular physician follow-up
Liotrix	Euthroid	Synthetic T_3 and T_4 product	60 to 180 µg of T_4	

tone, menstrual cycle, mood, or concentration. Physical assessment includes vital signs, weight, respiratory evaluation, and palpation of the thyroid, which is typically symmetrically enlarged with a soft, rubbery consistency. Classic changes in physical appearance include dry, coarse, yellowish skin and a puffy appearance to the face and hands. A small glistening bag of fluid may accumulate beneath the eye. Nails are thickened and brittle, whereas the hair is thin and fragile. The tongue is typically enlarged, and the voice is hoarse and husky with a slurred deliberate speech pattern.

Behavioral symptoms are often vague at the onset of the disease, and the patient may doubt his or her own perceptions. The nurse needs to be alert to the possibility of hypothyroidism in newly depressed patients and elderly patients who are exhibiting withdrawn or apathetic behavior.

Nursing Diagnosis

Appropriate nursing diagnoses will be determined by the severity of the hypothyroid state and the patient's response, but common diagnoses include the following:

Altered nutrition: more than body requirements, related to an intake greater than metabolic needs secondary to a reduced metabolic rate

Constipation related to a decreased metabolic rate and decreased activity

Activity intolerance related to muscle weakness and fatigue secondary to decreased metabolic rate

Altered health maintenance related to lack of knowledge of hypothyroidism and its treatment

Impaired verbal communication related to altered speech patterns and an enlarged tongue

Self-esteem disturbance related to altered physical appearance, altered thought processes, and communication problems

Planning

Specific goals will be developed to address the patient's individual situation and the severity of the symptoms. Outcome criteria will include the following:

Patient successfully adjusts diet to maintain a stable body weight and adequate balanced nutrient intake

Patient reestablishes a regular pattern of bowel elimination

Patient has sufficient energy to participate in the normal activities of daily living

Patient is knowledgeable about the disease process and treatment regimen and can state the side effects of medications

Patient compensates for the changes in voice and

tongue and communicates successfully with others

Patient accepts the disease-related changes in appearance and behavior and maintains a positive sense of self

Implementation

Restoration of proper hormone balance may require several months of therapy and, in some cases, is not completely feasible. Hypothyroidism is a lifelong process that needs to be successfully managed in the home environment, and it is essential that the patient assume responsibility for knowledgeable self-care.

General care

Environmental management is an important general intervention. Drafts are eliminated if possible, and extra blankets, sweaters, lap robes, bed socks, and warm drinks are employed to increase the patient's comfort.

The nurse helps the patient with self-care activities, carefully spacing activities and providing for periods of uninterrupted rest. Family and friends are encouraged to restrict visiting and avoid overtiring the patient. Local heat or massage may be useful in dealing with muscle cramps. Creams and moisturizers may improve the dryness of the skin. The patient should avoid harsh soaps and hot water and handle edematous skin with care.

The patient should receive education about a diet that is low in calories, cholesterol, and saturated fat yet meets the body's needs for balanced nutrients. The diet should include increased fiber, bulk, and fluids to counteract the tendency toward constipation. Stool softeners, bulk formers, or other laxatives may be needed. Accurate records of intake and output and bowel elimination should be maintained and the patient monitored for signs of fecal impaction. Daily weight should be recorded.

Vital signs are taken regularly, and the patient is assessed for dyspnea, angina, hypertension, or signs of heart failure. Frequent deep breathing is encouraged. The patient should be protected from infection, since the usual early physical symptoms of infection may be minimal or absent.

Appropriate sensory stimulation and diversion are incorporated into the patient's daily activities. The nurse assesses the patient's hearing and increases the level of stimulation if needed. Patients experiencing dizziness are assisted and monitored appropriately to prevent injury when out of bed.

Patient education about the disease process and treatment should take place in brief sessions and be repeated as necessary to facilitate the understanding and retention of information. Written materials are provided concerning the disease and hormone replacement. The patient should be knowledgeable about the signs of both hyperthyroidism and hypothyroidism, since replacement therapy will be lifelong and needs frequently fluctuate over time.

Drug therapy

The nurse teaches the patient about the drug being prescribed and monitors the patient's response. A regular schedule should be established for taking the drug. The hormones absorb faster and more completely on an empty stomach. The nurse teaches the patient to check and record pulse regularly. A resting pulse in excess of 100 beats/min probably indicates hormone excess. The patient should experience improved energy and activity tolerance, but nervousness, insomnia, or palpitations would indicate drug excess. The patient is monitored carefully for signs of chest pain or heart failure.

The concurrent use of other drugs can be dangerous, and the patient should be taught to inform all health care providers about his or her hypothyroid state. Many cases of myxedema coma can be attributed to the hypometabolism of drugs, and most drug doses need to be significantly reduced in the pres-

ence of hypothyroidism. The actions of digoxin and insulin, in particular, are potentiated by the hypothyroid state. Patient education for the patient with hypothyroidism is summarized in the box below.

Evaluation

The effectiveness of the overall treatment plan will be demonstrated by a reduction in the patient's edematous state and an improvement in energy, activity tolerance, and general well-being. The treatment response is gradual and occurs over a number of weeks. The patient's body weight should stabilize or decrease, and problems with constipation should be alleviated. The patient should demonstrate an understanding of the disease process and its treatment, be knowledgeable about all medications, and express an understanding of the need for long-term follow-up. Regimen adherence can become a problem as symptoms abate; thus reinforcement of the need for lifelong therapy is essential.

Documentation

Documentation of care involves the recording of accurate assessment data and the validation of appro-

---

 **PATIENT EDUCATION GUIDE**   *Hypothyroidism*

Objective: To modify the environment and patient routines to control symptoms and increase patient comfort; to prepare the patient for knowledgeable self-care

Environment

Increase room temperatures and eliminate drafts if possible

Use sweaters, lap robes, bed socks, and warm drinks to increase comfort

Activity

Space activities throughout the day; plan for rest periods

Ask for help as needed to conserve energy

Skin

Apply moisturizers and creams to counteract dryness

Avoid hot water and harsh soaps

Handle edematous skin with care

Diet

Follow a low-calorie, low-cholesterol, and low-saturated fat diet

Increase daily fluid intake

Monitor weight twice weekly

Bowels

Add fiber and bulk to the diet to prevent constipation

Increase activity to tolerance as condition improves

Use stool softeners and bulk formers as needed

Monitor bowel pattern, and use laxatives or suppositories if needed to maintain regularity

Medications

Take daily at same time

Take on an empty stomach

Take pulse twice weekly and call physician if greater than 100 beats/min

Check with physician before using any over-the-counter or prescription medication

Inform all health care providers of hypothyroid state and hormone replacement

Report the incidence of chest pain or shortness of breath to physician immediately

Report the return of symptoms or the development of nervousness, insomnia, or palpitations

Plan for regular long-term medical follow-up

Continue taking hormones as prescribed

priate patient education. Careful physical assessment is essential during the initial stages of hormone replacement and the patient should be monitored for signs of cardiac decompensation. The patient should receive both verbal and written instructions about the disease, drugs, and signs of hyperthyroidism and hypothyroidism for ongoing home management. It is important to revalidate the patient's understanding and retention of information since memory and concentration problems may impair learning.

Ongoing Care

Treatment of hypothyroidism is a lifelong process, and patients must be responsible for their own care at home. The disease may stabilize or worsen, and ongoing medical supervision is essential. The nurse assumes primary responsibility for patient education. The involvement of community agencies is rarely necessary, but the family should be involved in all teaching if possible to provide support and help the patient identify subtle variations in response.

MYXEDEMA COMA

Myxedema coma is the most severe manifestation of hypothyroidism, but the terms are not synonymous. Unrecognized or undertreated hypothyroidism can progress to myxedema in rare situations, particularly in the face of profound physiologic or psychological stress. When myxedema coma occurs it is an endocrine emergency that is often fatal. It usually occurs in elderly women who have received inadequate health care. It may be precipitated by heart failure, by pulmonary infections, or iatrogenically in response to the stress of diagnostic tests and procedures associated with hospitalization.

Like thyroid crisis, the underlying pathologic cause of myxedema coma is poorly understood. The

prolonged deficiency of thyroxine eventually causes inadequate production of thermal energy in the body and results in a significant fall in core body temperature. Cold weather may precipitate the crisis. Oxygen delivery to the tissues is impaired, and pronounced hypoxemia and hypercapnia occur. A dilutional hyponatremia develops that can be severe enough to induce seizures or coma.

Accurate diagnosis of the condition is the first step in treatment. Although speed is essential, the diagnosis must be made cautiously because aggressive thyroid hormone therapy in a euthyroid patient could be fatal. The diagnosis is usually made by assessing the history, physical symptoms, and laboratory findings and ruling out other possible causes of coma. Serum T_3 and T_4 values are low and TSH is elevated, but the actual values may not be dramatic. Dilutional hyponatremia, hypoglycemia, hypoxemia, and hypercapnia are all present.

Myxedema coma is typically preceded by the gradual onset of lethargy, which gradually worsens to stupor and outright coma. Core body temperature can fall as low as 75° F. The patient has bradycardia, hypoventilates, and has hypoactive bowel

CLINICAL ALERT

Myxedema coma is a rare but life-threatening complication of long-standing hypothyroidism that may occur in response to profound physiologic stress. Core body temperature falls to as low as 75° F, and the patient experiences bradycardia, hypoventilation, stupor, and coma. Treatment involves aggressive intravenous hormone replacement with careful monitoring of cardiac and respiratory response. Supportive care is provided, but active rewarming is contraindicated. Mortality can be as high as 50%.

TREATMENT OF MYXEDEMA COMA

Hormone replacement
Loading doses of intravenous levothyroxine because absorption is poor; adequate serum levels can be obtained in 24 hours

Respiratory care
Frequent assessment of respiratory status and adequacy
Intubation and mechanical ventilation are commonly necessary and should be aggressively used

Cardiac care
Continuous cardiac monitoring and frequent vital signs measurement
Serial blood gases
Monitoring for signs of cardiogenic shock

Fluids
Administered cautiously, free water restricted
Glucose solutions to combat hypoglycemia
Hydrocortisone to support the stress response
Accurate intake and output measurements

Rewarming
Active rewarming contraindicated
Monitor body temperature
General supportive care and comfort measures

sounds or frank ileus. Cerebellar symptoms such as clumsiness or ataxia may be present, or the patient may develop depression, paranoia, hallucinations, or other psychiatric symptoms.

Therapy revolves around hormone replacement, treatment of metabolic complications, and general supportive care. Patients are often acutely sensitive to the metabolic effects of hormone replacement, and the risks of cardiac damage or failure are quite real. Many patients have suffered irreversible brain damage before treatment is initiated, and full recovery is then unlikely. The prognosis is related to the length and depth of the coma. Despite aggressive treatment, mortality can be as high as 50%. Improvement in the patient's level of consciousness and a rise in core body temperature, which should occur naturally in response to hormone replacement, are good measures of the patient's response to treatment, outlined in the box on p. 1704.

NONTOXIC GOITER

Simple nontoxic goiter is a condition of idiopathic thyroid enlargement that usually represents compensated hypothyroidism. In regions of iodide defi-

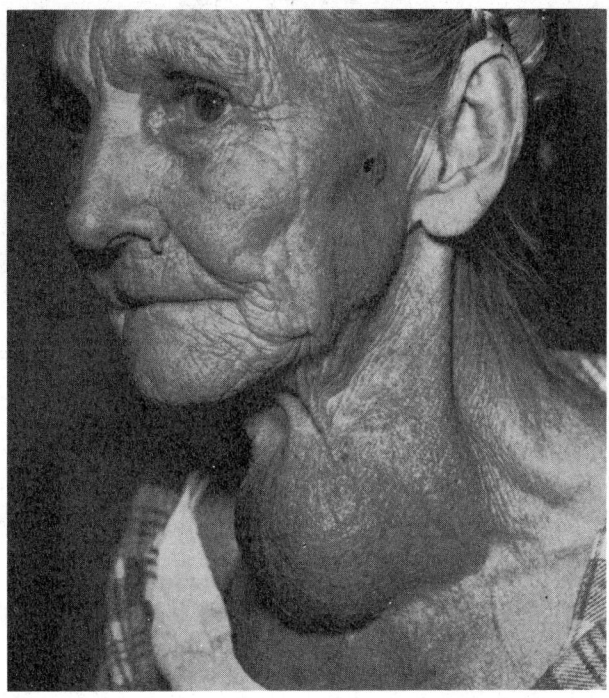

FIGURE 61-4   Massive thyroid enlargement caused by goiter. (From Prior JA, Silberstein JS, Stang JM: *Physical diagnosis: the history and examination of the patient,* ed 6, St Louis, Mosby–Year Book, Inc.)

ciency, simple goiter is a common condition that may affect up to 10% of the population. In developed countries, however, the cause is usually unknown. Inadequate hormone synthesis causes increased TSH stimulation and thyroid enlargement that is usually diffuse but may be nodular. Most patients are euthyroid and completely asymptomatic.

The size of the gland, degree of pressure exerted, and extent of cosmetic concern will dictate the treatment approach. The goiter may be mild or quite dramatic (Figure 61-4). If basically asymptomatic, the patient may be treated with levothyroxine. Exogenous hormone eliminates TSH stimulation and stops the growth of the goiter, even shrinking it at times. Large goiters may be treated with surgery and then suppressive therapy to prevent regrowth.

THYROID NODULES AND CANCER

Thyroid nodules occur quite commonly, especially in women. Since virtually all thyroid cancers initially appear as nodules, the primary concern is to differentiate between benign and malignant disease. This differentiation is not always easy in the early stages, but fortunately the incidence of thyroid cancer is extremely low. Nodules typically occur within the substance of the thyroid tissue. Approximately 80% are nonfunctioning, or "cold," nodules and are usually asymptomatic. Functional, or "hot," nodules tend to evolve into toxic adenomas and cause symptoms of hyperthyroidism. The treatment of benign nodules depends on their etiology, size, and the degree of pressure symptoms, if any. Cystic nodules usually require no treatment unless they reach significant size. Stable adenomas also require no treatment, although suppressive therapy may be used to inhibit their growth. Hot nodules are treated with drug therapy, radioactive iodine, or surgery as described under hyperthyroidism.

Thyroid cancers usually appear as solitary cold nodules. Most are papillary tumors that are slow-growing and confined to the gland, although they may grow more rapidly in older patients. The incidence of papillary tumors is associated with exposure to ionizing radiation, particularly in childhood; survival rates are good. Follicular, medullary, and undifferentiated tumors are virulent and resistant to treatment, but fortunately they are rare.

A lobectomy may be performed for small tumors or thyroidectomy for larger tumors. Gland destruction with high-dose sodium ^{131}I may also be used with large tumors. Chemotherapy has not been shown to be effective with thyroid cancer. Careful follow-up and assessment for metastasis are important.

HYPERPARATHYROIDISM

Definition

Hyperparathyroidism is a disorder of calcium, phosphate, and bone metabolism that is characterized by the hypersecretion of parathyroid hormone (PTH). The most common form is primary, reflecting a problem in the gland itself, but it can also occur in rare situations as a secondary response to disorders elsewhere in the body.

Etiology/Epidemiology

Hyperparathyroidism was once believed to be an extremely rare disorder but is now considered to be one of the most common endocrine disorders with incidence statistics estimated at as much as 1 to 3 per 1000 persons in the general population.[2] The incidence rate is two to four times greater in women and increases dramatically in both sexes after 50 years of age. Elderly women are at particular risk. Routine serum calcium screening has dramatically increased the identification of asymptomatic cases. Primary hyperparathyroidism is caused by a single-gland benign adenoma in 80% of the cases. The adenoma, which can vary in size from a slight increase to 100 times normal, secretes excess amounts of PTH. Multiple adenomas or a diffuse hyperplasia of all four glands occurs less commonly. A specific etiology for the glandular changes can rarely be determined. Cancer of the parathyroids is extremely rare.

Pathophysiology

Parathyroid hormone has three basic effects in the body: (1) to increase bone resorption, (2) to increase renal retention of calcium, and (3) to increase gastrointestinal absorption of calcium.

Hypercalcemia is the biochemical hallmark of hyperparathyroidism. Since greater than 90% of the body's calcium is found in the bones, the increased mobilization of this calcium is the most common cause of hypercalcemia. When excess PTH is present, it exaggerates normal bone turnover by disrupting the ratio of osteoblastic to osteoclastic activity.

The chronic excess of calcium produces the pathophysiologic characteristics of the disease. Fine crystallization of calcium deposits occurs in the interstitium of the kidney (**nephrocalcinosis**) and pro-

---

CLINICAL MANIFESTATIONS OF HYPERPARATHYROIDISM

Gastrointestinal
Anorexia*
Constipation*
Nausea and vomiting
Hyperacidity
Peptic ulcer disease
Pancreatitis

Renal
Polyuria, low urine specific gravity*
Increased urine acidity
Kidney calculi
Decreased glomerular filtration
Renal insufficiency

Cardiovascular
Shortened QT interval, increased contractility
Increased conduction, dysrhythmia
Heightened sensitivity to digitalis
Hypertension

Neuromuscular
Weakness or fatigue*
Muscle fiber atrophy
Depressed tendon reflexes

Skeletal
Diffuse osteopenia on x-ray examination
Diffuse bone pain
Easy fracture
Osteitis fibrosa cystica (rare)
Punched-out bony lesions (rare)

Behavioral
Depression
Memory change
Irritability
Confusion
Drowsiness and lethargy*
Stupor
Paranoid hallucination
Acute psychosis

Laboratory
Serum calcium above 10.8 mg/dL on at least three occasions*
Elevated immunoreactive PTH*

*Common early findings.

duces tubular damage, often decreasing the glomerular filtration rate. Nephrolithiasis can also occur with the production of calcium oxalate or phosphate stones. Both processes could eventually lead to kidney failure. Interference with the renal excretion of uric acid can also lead to gout.

Uninterrupted resorption in the bone causes the bone to be replaced by fibrous tissue and cysts. Severe osteoporosis may result. Chronic hypercalcemia appears to act as a physiologic stimulus for the release of gastrin, which can produce peptic ulcer disease. An acute hypercalcemic crisis can occur if serum calcium reaches life-threatening levels, usually greater than 15 mg/dL. An acute imbalance can lead to coma or fatal cardiac dysrhythmias.

Clinical Manifestations

Hyperparathyroidism is usually detected by routine blood chemistry screening, and the vast majority of patients are completely asymptomatic. When symptoms do occur, they are related to the presence of excess calcium. Slowly developing hypercalcemia is usually well tolerated until the imbalance becomes quite dramatic. The symptoms of calcium excess are diverse and nonspecific. Gastrointestinal symptoms are among the most common. Hypertension, from calcium's vasoconstrictive effects, occurs in as many as 50% of patients and does not completely resolve when the calcium level is reduced. The box on p. 1706 summarizes the symptoms that may accompany hyperparathyroidism.

When classic symptoms are present, the disease is quite easy to diagnose. Elevated fasting serum calcium is the most significant finding. Persistent elevation of the calcium above 10.8 mg/dL on at least three separate occasions is diagnostic of hypercalcemia.

Once the presence of hypercalcemia has been established the serum PTH level is measured to establish whether the parathyroid gland is the cause. Malignancy is the other common cause of hypercalcemia and should always be screened for, particularly in older patients. Malignancy can cause bone destruction and can occasionally cause the secretion of parathyrotropic substances that mimic the action of PTH on the bone. Measured PTH levels will be normal or decreased, however.

Therapeutic Management

The major therapeutic decision is whether to treat asymptomatic mild cases of hyperparathyroidism. The decision is a clinical one made in collaboration with the patient and will consider the patient's age, menopausal status, and osteoporosis risk profile. Patients may be monitored over time for evidence of progressive hypercalcemia or kidney or bone involvement. The presence of these factors supports the need for prompt surgical intervention. The prognosis is excellent with effective treatment.

Surgical management

Surgery is the only definitive therapy for primary hyperparathyroidism, and it is curative. The surgery is complicated by the nonspecific placement of the parathyroids within the thyroid gland. The skill of the surgeon is an important consideration. If a single adenoma is found, at least one other gland will be biopsied. If hyperplasia or multiple adenomas are found, three and one half glands or all four will be removed. Normal residual tissue may be allografted into the vascular muscle of the forearm.

A transient hypocalcemia, which should be self-limiting, is expected after surgery. If the serum calcium does not fall below 10 mg in the first 48 hours, it usually indicates that insufficient parathyroid tissue has been removed. In situations where the bone is seriously demineralized, the calcium level may fall dramatically after surgery. Recurrences are rare with single adenomas but common with multiple ones, and follow-up is required for at least 10 years.

Medical management

Conservative medical management may be used as a temporary measure for asymptomatic patients with mild hypercalcemia, but it is rarely an effective long-term approach. The aims of treatment are to increase the renal excretion of calcium and decrease gastrointestinal absorption and bone resorption. In the hospital setting high volumes of isotonic saline may be administered intravenously to increase the glomerular filtration of calcium supplemented by furosemide (Lasix) to block its reabsorption. Oral furosemide and a high daily fluid intake can adapt the treatment to more long-term management in the home environment. Dietary restriction of calcium will be used to augment treatment.

Conjugated estrogens or progestogens may be administered to limit postmenopausal bone loss by decreasing bone sensitivity to PTH. Research is ongoing into the use of diphosphonates for long-term inhibition of bone resorption in hypercalcemia, but the results are not yet consistent. Calcitonin or plicamycin may be given in situations of acute hypercalcemia, but they have transient effects and must be administered intravenously so they are not practical for long-term management.

NURSING MANAGEMENT OF THE PATIENT WITH HYPERPARATHYROIDISM
Assessment

Most patients with hyperparathyroidism are asymptomatic at the time of diagnosis. The nurse, however,

PATIENT EDUCATION GUIDE   *Hyperparathyroidism*

Objective: To help the patient manage disease symptoms and prepare for knowledgeable self-care

Activity

Space activities throughout the day; plan for periods of uninterrupted rest

Plan for at least 30 minutes of walking each day to support calcium movement into bones

Avoid bed rest

Use energy level as a guide to activity

Avoid high-impact activities or contact sports

Diet

Follow a low-calcium diet, limit milk products

Ensure at least 2 to 3 L of fluid each day

Eat small frequent meals and snacks if nauseated

Ensure adequate potassium and vitamin C in diet, especially if taking diuretics

Report the incidence of indigestion, epigastric pain, or blood in the stool

Elimination

Add bulk and fiber to the diet to prevent constipation

Use stool softeners and laxatives as needed to manage constipation

Medications

Take regularly as prescribed by physician

Report any change in symptoms to physician

Plan for regular medical follow-up

---

assesses for a positive family history of endocrine problems or a history of kidney disease or osteoporosis. The patient's dietary pattern is assessed for excess calcium content or use of multivitamin products containing vitamin D. The ongoing use of thiazide diuretics can also be a contributing factor, since they act to decrease tubular excretion of calcium. Common symptoms (see the box on p. 1706) such as changes in appetite, energy level, and bowel elimination pattern should also be considered. Physical assessment may be noncontributory, but the patient may exhibit mild hypertension, polyuria, and a decreased urine specific gravity. It is not possible to palpate even grossly enlarged parathyroid glands.

Nursing Diagnosis

Appropriate nursing diagnoses need to be individualized to each patient, since the range and severity of symptoms vary so much. Potential diagnoses include the following:

Constipation related to decreased peristalsis

Activity intolerance related to muscle weakness and fatigue

High risk for altered nutrition: less than body requirements, related to protracted anorexia or nausea

High risk for injury related to increased fracture risk secondary to bone demineralization

Altered health maintenance related to lack of knowledge of hyperparathyroidism and its treatment

Planning

Goals need to be developed for each patient, but outcome criteria related to commonly occurring problems might include the following:

Patient reestablishes a regular bowel elimination pattern and passes soft, formed stool

Patient experiences increased energy and is able to participate in usual activities without tiring

Patient maintains a stable body weight and ingests a balanced nutrient diet

Patient modifies environment and activities appropriately and does not experience accidental injury

Patient can accurately discuss the disease process, proposed treatment, and the safe use of all prescribed medications

Implementation

Patients with hyperparathyroidism are hospitalized only for surgery or the management of acute episodes of hypercalcemia. The nurse's primary responsibility is patient education that will enable the patient to modify daily routines and integrate knowledgeable disease management into the home environment (see box above). Patients and families should also be reassured that if behavioral symptoms are present they are related to the organic calcium excess and will resolve with effective treatment.

Preoperative and postoperative care

The nurse most commonly encounters the patient with primary hyperparathyroidism in the context of surgical care. Routine preoperative care and teaching are offered that are similar to those outlined for the patient undergoing thyroidectomy. The postoperative care also closely parallels that provided for the thyroidectomy patient. The patient is carefully monitored for signs of bleeding or edema in the neck, respiratory distress, vocal cord damage, or difficulty in swallowing. A fall in serum calcium is an expected outcome of surgery, and symptomatic hypocalcemia occurs in as many as 70% of patients.[4] The patient is assessed frequently for signs such as numbness and tingling or the development of a positive Chvostek's or Trousseau's sign, which would indicate latent tetany. Calcium gluconate must be readily available to replace needed calcium. The patient should be on a cardiac monitor during the first 48 hours. Mobility is encouraged to promote recalcification of the bones. The patient may need ongoing calcium replacement if the hypocalcemia persists.

Evaluation

The evaluation of care for patients treated by parathyroidectomy involves the assessment of appropriate wound healing and the reestablishment of a normal calcium balance. The patient's symptoms should be completely relieved, although ongoing routine follow-up will be necessary.

The evaluation for patients treated medically for overt hypercalcemia involves the resolution of symptoms such as weakness, anorexia, or constipation. The patient should be able to discuss the disease and its treatment, be knowledgeable about the symptoms of both hypercalcemia and hypocalcemia, and acknowledge the importance of ongoing care.

Documentation

Care documentation involves the recording of appropriate assessment and monitoring data and of all interventions. Patient education concerning diet, activity, disease process, and medications should be validated. The patient should receive written instructions about all medications and the symptoms of both hypercalcemia and hypocalcemia that would indicate a need for further medical attention. The patient's record should also include documentation of all preoperative and postoperative care delivered.

Ongoing Care

Hyperparathyroidism, except in cases of acute hypercalcemia, is managed by the patient in the home environment without the ongoing support of community agencies or services. The nurse is responsible for seeing that the patient is adequately prepared for knowledgeable self-care.

HYPOPARATHYROIDISM

Definition

Hypoparathyroidism is a rare disorder characterized by hypocalcemia and hyperphosphatemia that result from a lack of PTH or its effect. The primary disease state is theorized to result from an autoimmune process, although the etiologic factors are basically unknown and the small number of documented cases makes it difficult to draw any conclusions about populations at risk. The body has excellent adaptive mechanisms that ensure calcium conservation, which makes secondary hypocalcemia also very rare. The most common etiology of hypoparathyroidism is iatrogenic, caused by the inadvertent damage or removal of glands during thyroid surgery. In the absence of adequate PTH there is a decrease in bone resorption, a decrease in renal reabsorption of calcium, and a decrease in intestinal absorption of calcium. When renal excretion of calcium increases, there is a corresponding decrease in the excretion of phosphate. Hypocalcemia, hyperphosphatemia, and alkalosis result, producing widespread effects of neuromuscular excitability. If not reversed the condition can progress to full lifethreatening tetany.

Clinical Manifestations

The symptoms of hypoparathyroidism are highly variable and primarily related to the severity of calcium deficiency and the speed with which it develops. When the hypocalcemia develops gradually it is usually well tolerated and the patient remains asymptomatic. Increased neuromuscular excitability particularly affects the smooth muscle of the bronchi, intestine, gallbladder, and larynx, producing wheezing, abdominal cramping, and hoarseness. The assessment of Chvostek's and Trousseau's signs can be useful in detecting latent tetany (see Figure 61-2). Patients may also report numbness and tingling in the lips and fingertips, paresthesias, or heaviness and weakness in the muscles. Hypocalcemia lowers the seizure threshold, and the patient may experience focal, petit mal, or grand mal seizures. Laryngeal spasms represent the most serious danger, although dysrhythmia and heart block or failure are also possible. A serum calcium level below 6.5 mg/dL and a low or unmeasurable PTH level are usually present in symptomatic patients.

Therapeutic Management

Medical therapy involves replacing deficient calcium to restore serum levels to the normal range. Appropriate calcium replacement improves or reverses most signs of the disease. The patient is usually prescribed about 1.5 g of elemental calcium per day in divided doses in the form of calcium lactate, gluconate, or carbonate. Vitamin D preparations may be prescribed to augment intestinal absorption of the calcium. These preparations are quite potent and usually raise serum calcium levels quickly.

NURSING MANAGEMENT OF THE PATIENT WITH HYPOPARATHYROIDISM

Assessment

Most patients with hypoparathyroidism are asymptomatic, but the nurse needs to be alert to its occurrence in any patient who has undergone thyroid surgery or surgical exploration of the neck. Physical assessment will be the nurse's primary tool. The patient should be assessed regularly for signs of latent tetany, particularly numbness or tingling of the lips or fingertips or leg cramping. Chvostek's and Trousseau's signs are also important indicators.

Nursing Diagnosis

Two primary diagnoses apply to patients who develop hypocalcemia after surgery:

High risk for injury related to the risk of seizures, respiratory distress, and tetany secondary to hypocalcemia

Altered health maintenance related to lack of knowledge of hypocalcemia and its diet and drug treatment

Planning

Goals appropriate for the patient experiencing hypocalcemia include the following:

Patient does not experience physical injury related to incipient tetany

Patient can describe the disease process, proposed treatment, and the safe use of all medications

Implementation

Nursing strategies will be primarily focused on the prompt identification and treatment of tetany. An airway, suction and oxygen equipment, calcium gluconate, and a tracheostomy set should be readily available at the bedside of any patient with postoperative thyroid or parathyroid disease. If signs of latent tetany appear, the patient is continuously monitored for respiratory distress while therapy is initiated. Calcium gluconate will be given intravenously. The drug must be administered slowly because it is extremely irritating to the veins, and the patient ideally should be on a cardiac monitor during replacement. Patients receiving digoxin are at additional risk.

Seizure precautions are implemented, and anticonvulsant drugs may be needed. The experience of tetany can be extremely frightening for the patient, who should therefore receive calm reassurance

---

PATIENT EDUCATION GUIDE   *Hypoparathyroidism*

Objective: To help the patient successfully manage disease symptoms and prepare for self-care

Diet

Follow a calcium-rich diet; include adequate milk products

Restrict the amount of phosphorus in the diet, limiting meat, poultry, fish, eggs, cheese, and cereals

Take a phosphate binder (Amphojel) with or before meals

Elimination

Adjust quantities of dietary bulk, fiber, and fluids to manage hypermotility or constipation

Avoid increasing the quantities of whole grains and bran in the diet, which block calcium absorption

Use stool softeners or laxatives as needed to control constipation

Medications

Take regularly as prescribed by physician

Report the incidence of signs of hypercalcemia or hypocalcemia promptly

Schedule regular follow-up appointments with physician for monitoring calcium levels

about the nature of treatment. Anxiety can induce hyperventilation, which results in respiratory alkalosis from carbon dioxide loss. The alkalotic state decreases the solubility and ionization of calcium and worsens the tetany. Hyperventilation should be prevented, if necessary, by the use of a paper bag or rebreathing device. The general environment should be quiet and nonstimulating, but the patient should not be left unmonitored during the acute period.

Nursing intervention for chronic management primarily involves appropriate education about medications and the importance of regular medical follow-up. The box on p. 1710 summarizes the education appropriate for patients with hypoparathyroidism.

Evaluation

The treatment plan is considered effective if the patient does not experience tetany and learns how to successfully manage self-care. The patient should know the cause of the condition, the symptoms of both hypercalcemia and hypocalcemia, how to use prescribed medications safely, and the importance of ongoing medical follow-up.

Documentation

Care documentation primarily involves the recording of accurate physical assessment data and the interventions taken to avert or treat tetany. In addition the patient's record should reflect patient education concerning diet, medications, and the symptoms of hypercalcemia and hypocalcemia that would necessitate immediate medical intervention. Since the management of hypoparathyroidism is usually long-term, patient education should include both oral and written materials.

Ongoing Care

The patient will manage hypoparathyroidism in the home environment, and knowledgeable self-care is essential. The involvement of community agencies is rarely needed. It is important that the patient understand the importance and need for long-term therapy, be committed to regimen compliance, and understand the importance of physician follow-up because calcium levels may need to be monitored several times each year.

CRITICAL THINKING QUESTIONS

1 How does Graves' disease cause hypersecretion of thyroid hormone?
2 What diagnostic tests would be useful in diagnosing Graves' disease?
3 What are the classic symptoms of thyrotoxicosis?
4 What components should be included in a nursing history and assessment of Graves' disease?
5 What patient education is appropriate for patients receiving propylthiouracil?
6 What should be included in the care before and after surgery for a patient undergoing thyroidectomy?
7 What causes a goiter to develop?
8 What are some early symptoms of hypothyroidism?
9 What nursing strategies could be used to increase comfort for a patient with hypothyroidism?
10 Why do patients who develop myxedema coma have such low core body temperatures?
11 What is the goal of hormone replacement therapy in hypothyroidism?
12 How would you evaluate the effectiveness of the care for patients with hypothyroidism?
13 How does hyperparathyroidism produce symptoms of hypercalcemia?
14 What are the common symptoms of hypercalcemia?
15 How is acute hypercalcemia treated?
16 What patients are at risk for developing hypocalcemia?
17 What are the classic features of tetany?
18 What education should be given to the patient about the ongoing management of hypoparathyroidism?

BIBLIOGRAPHY

Current

1. Adlerberth A, Stenstrom G, Hasselgren PO: The selective B_1-blocking agent metoprolol compared with antithyroid drug and thyroxine as preoperative treatment of hyperthyroidism, *Ann Surg* 205(2):182, 1987.
2. Arnaud CD, Kolb FO: The calcitropic hormones and metabolic bone disease. In Greenspan FS, Forsham PH: *Basic and clinical endocrinology*, ed 3, East Norwalk, Conn, 1991, Appleton & Lange.
3. Calissendorff BM, Soderstrom M, Alveryd A: Ophthalmopathy and hyperthyroidism, *Acta Ophthalmol* 64:698, 1986.
4. Chapman I et al: Primary hyperparathyroidism: pathogenesis, diagnosis and management, *Comp Ther* 14(9):65, 1988.
5. Char DH: Advances in the management of thyroid related eye disease, *Int Ophthalmol Clin* 29(4):226, 1989.
6. Cooper DS, Ridgway EC: Clinical management of patients with hyperthyroidism, *Med Clin North Am* 69(5):953, 1985.
7. Federman DD: Hyperthyroidism in the geriatric population, *Hosp Pract* 26(2):61, 1991.
8. Felicetta JV: The aging thyroid: how it affects diagnosis and treatment in the elderly, *Consultant* 30(9):59, 1990.

9. Graves L: Disorders of calcium, phosphorus and magnesium, *Crit Care Nurs Q* 13(3):3, 1990.

10. Greenspan FS, Rapoport B: Thyroid gland. In Greenspan FS, Forsham PH: *Basic and clinical endocrinology,* ed 3, East Norwalk, Conn, 1991, Appleton & Lange.

11. Halloran TH: Nursing responsibilities in endocrine emergencies, *Crit Care Nurs Q* 13(3):74, 1990.

12. Helfand M, Crapo LM: Screening for thyroid disease, *Ann Intern Med* 112(11):840, 1990.

13. Isley WL: Thyroid disorders, *Crit Care Nurs Q* 13(3):39, 1990.

14. Jackson I, Cobb WE: Disorders of the thyroid. In Kohler PO: *Clinical endocrinology,* New York, 1986, John Wiley & Sons Inc.

15. Kabadi VM: Variability of L-thyroxine replacement dose in elderly patients with primary hypothyroidism, *J Fam Pract* 24(5):473, 1987.

16. Kannan CR: *Essential endocrinology: a primer for nonspecialists,* New York, 1986, Plenum Publishing Corp.

17. Lando MJ, Hoover LA, Zuckerbraun L: Surgical strategy in thyroid disease, *Arch Otolaryngol Head Neck Surg* 116(12):1378, 1990.

18. Larsen PR, Ingbar SH: The thyroid gland. In Wilson JD, Foster DW: *Williams' textbook of endocrinology,* ed 8, Philadelphia, 1992, WB Saunders Co.

19. McKenzie JM, Zakarija M: Hyperthyroidism. In DeGroot LJ: *Endocrinology,* Philadelphia, 1989, WB Saunders Co.

20. McMillan JY: Preventing myxedema coma in the hypothyroid patient, *Dimen Crit Nurs* 7(3):136, 1988.

21. Meek JC: Tests of thyroid function: update in the diagnosis and management of thyroid disease, *Comp Ther* 16(7):20, 1990.

22. Nordyke RA, Gilbert FI: Management of primary hypothyroidism, *Comp Ther* 16(7):28, 1990.

23. Pearsall HR, Altesman RI: The relationship of thyroid function to depression, *Hosp Med* 23(3):140, 1987.

24. Peele ME, Wartofsky L: A rational approach to the treatment of hyperthyroidism, *Comp Ther* 14(9):34, 1988.

25. Porat A, Sherwood LM: Disorders of mineral homeostasis and bone. In Kohler PO: *Clinical endocrinology,* New York, 1986, John Wiley & Sons Inc.

26. Sarsany SL: Thyroid storm, *RN* 51(7):46, 1988.

27. Stoffer SS, Szpunar WE: Thyroid disease in the elderly, *Postgrad Med* 84(6):133, 1988.

28. Utinger RD: Hypothyroidism. In DeGroot LJ: *Endocrinology,* Philadelphia, 1989, WB Saunders Co.

29. Yeatts RP, Clontz DM: Grave's ophthalmopathy, *J Ophthalmic Nurs Technol* 9(1):16, 1990.

30. Yeh SDJ: Symptoms, diagnosis and treatment of thyroid disease, *Comp Ther* 17(7):12, 1991.

31. Yeomans AC: Assessment and management of hypothyroidism, *Nurse Practitioner* 15(11):8, 1990.

Classic

32. Evangelisti JT, Thorpe CJ: Thyroid storm: a nursing crisis, *Heart Lung* 12(2):184, 1983.

33. Hellman R: The evaluation and management of hyperthyroid crisis, *Crit Care Q* 3:77, 1980.

34. Hoffman JTT, Newby TB: Hypercalcemia in primary hyperparathyroidism, *Nurs Clin North Am* 15(3):469, 1980.

35. Jenkins EH: Living with thyrotoxicosis, *Am J Nurs* 80(5):956, 1980.

36. Johnson D: Pathophysiology of thyroid storm: nursing implications, *Crit Care Nurse* 3(6):80, 1983.

37. Mathewson MK: Thyroid disorder, *Crit Care Nurse* 7(1), 1984.

38. Meek JC: Myxedema coma, *Crit Care Q* 3:131, 1980.

39. Muthe NC: *Endocrinology: a nursing approach,* Boston, 1981, Little, Brown & Co Inc.

40. Urbanic RC, Mazzaferri EL: Thyrotoxic crisis and myxedema coma, *Heart Lung* 7(3):435, 1978.

41. Wake MS, Brensinger JF: The nurses' role in hypothyroidism, *Nurs Clin North Am* 15(3):435, 1980.

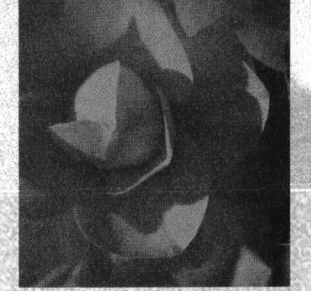

CHAPTER SIXTY-TWO

Nursing Management of Adults with Disorders of the Endocrine Pancreas

---

LEARNING OBJECTIVES

1 Explain the pathophysiology of diabetes mellitus.
2 Compare the classifications of diabetes in terms of pathophysiology, presenting symptoms, and therapeutic management.
3 Differentiate among the laboratory tests associated with the diagnosis or monitoring of diabetes mellitus.
4 Discuss the concept of metabolic control in relation to acute and chronic complications of diabetes mellitus.
5 Contrast the effects of diet and exercise on blood glucose control in insulin-dependent diabetes mellitus and noninsulin-dependent diabetes mellitus.
6 Compare the differences in action of common insulins and sulfonylureas.
7 Describe laboratory procedures currently used to follow diabetic patients.
8 Explain basic components of the teaching plan for insulin-dependent diabetes mellitus and noninsulin-dependent diabetes mellitus patients.
9 Relate the importance of the concept of self-management in diabetes care.
10 List available diabetes organizations for patient and family referrals.

THE GOAL OF THIS CHAPTER IS to provide the nurse with an understanding of diabetes from a physical, psychologic, and sociocultural perspective. Such an understanding requires the nurse to evaluate the effectiveness of disease management, not only in terms of patient compliance or physiologic parameters, but with regard for the patient's optimal health and well-being.

DIABETES MELLITUS
Definition

Diabetes mellitus is a metabolic disorder affecting a variety of physiologic systems, the most critical of which involves glucose metabolism. The term represents a generalization about a group of anatomic and chemical problems that result from a deficiency of insulin. The most striking abnormality of the disease is the development of fasting **hyperglycemia** (elevated blood sugar level), hyperlipidemia (elevated blood lipid level), and hyperaminoacidemia (elevated amino acid level).[15,30,48] Diabetes mellitus can be caused by an insufficient quantity of secreted insulin or resistance to insulin action.

There are three subclasses of diabetes mellitus. These are: (1) insulin-dependent diabetes mellitus (IDDM), or type I (previously called juvenile diabetes); (2) noninsulin-dependent diabetes mellitus (NIDDM), or type II (previously called maturity onset); and (3) other types, such as diabetes secondary to pancreatic disease or drugs or chemical agents. These classifications include diabetes associated with other physical conditions, impaired glucose tolerance, gestational diabetes mellitus, and increased risk of developing diabetes because of previous abnormality of glucose tolerance or potential abnormality of glucose tolerance.[42,44,58]

The majority of diabetic patients fall within the IDDM or NIDDM classification. The following outline shows how they differ in clinical manifestations and etiology:

I. Clinical types
  A. Diabetes mellitus
    1. Insulin-dependent (type I)
    2. Noninsulin-dependent (type II)
      a. Nonobese
      b. Obese
    3. Other types, including diabetes mellitus associated with certain conditions and syndromes:
      a. Pancreatic disease (i.e., pancreatectomy, cystic fibrosis)
      b. Endocrinopathies (i.e., acromegaly, Cushing's syndrome)
      c. Drug- or chemical-induced conditions (i.e., thiazide diuretics, glucocorticoids, psychoactive agents)
      d. Insulin receptor abnormalities
      e. Certain genetic syndromes (i.e., hyperlipidemia)
      f. Miscellaneous (i.e., malnutrition)
  B. Impaired glucose tolerance
    1. Nonobese
    2. Obese
    3. Impaired glucose tolerance associated with certain conditions and syndromes
    4. Age
  C. Gestational diabetes
II. Normal glucose tolerance but substantially increased risk of developing diabetes
    1. Previous abnormality of glucose tolerance (formerly "latent" diabetes)
    2. Potential abnormality of glucose tolerance (formerly "prediabetes")

Etiology/Epidemiology

From 1980 to 1987, the number of persons known to have diabetes increased by 1 million, for a total of nearly 7 million cases in the United States.[9] African Americans have a higher prevalence than Caucasians, and there is an increasing incidence among women older than 64.

Insulin-dependent diabetes mellitus

Patients with **insulin-dependent diabetes mellitus (IDDM)** generally have severely diminished insulin production. Endogenous insulin secretion is reduced from disease onset and throughout the clinical course. Peripheral insulin resistance, which is excessive amounts of circulating insulin antibodies that render insulin less effective, may also be present.

IDDM typically occurs before the age of 15 years and after the age of 6 months. Data regarding the incidence of IDDM after 30 years of age are minimal. There are about 1.6 cases of IDDM per 1,000 people under age 16 in the United States. Commonly, IDDM patients appear lean and often report a recent episode of weight loss with symptoms that mimic influenza.

IDDM may be slightly more prevalent in men than in women.[48,58] IDDM also tends to run in families. Siblings of children with IDDM have a 3% chance, or 10-fold increased risk, of developing the disease. The loss of insulin secretion in IDDM may be caused by many mechanisms. The role of several are described below.

Autoimmune mechanisms

It is becoming increasingly evident that IDDM is an autoimmune disease. IDDM has long been associated with autoimmune disorders, such as pernicious anemia and Addison's disease. Although the process is unclear, it appears that the immune system attacks and destroys the body's insulin-producing beta

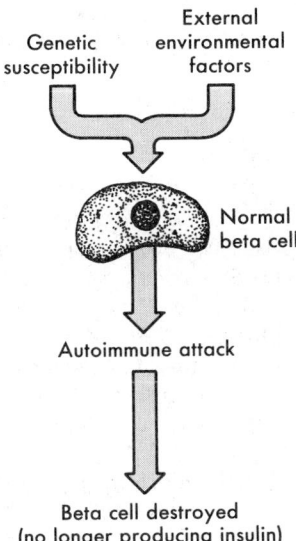

FIGURE 62-1   Current view of the pathogenesis of type I diabetes mellitus.

cells. Clinical evidence of autoimmune reactions in IDDM includes the presence of **insulitis,** or inflammation of pancreatic islets. The beta cells are selectively destroyed in IDDM, which becomes clinically apparent after 90% of the beta cells are lost.[49]

The triggering mechanism probably results from a combination of genetic and environmental factors (Figure 62-1). Genetic factors associated with histocompatibility antigens DR3 and DR4 are associated with a predisposition to immune activity against pancreatic islet tissues. A relationship between beta cell destruction and viral infections, most specifically the coxsackie B4 virus and the mumps virus, have been targeted as possible precipitants of the disease. There appears to be a seasonal incidence to IDDM, with midwinter and spring peaks, which occur during maximal incidences of viral and bacterial human infections.

Insulin autoantibodies
Insulin antibodies may result from beta cell destruction. In part, this belief is supported by the finding of insulin autoantibodies in 85% of children within 1 to 2 weeks of diagnosis, whereas only 1% to 2% of nondiabetic patients have such antibodies.

Noninsulin-dependent diabetes mellitus

By far the most common form of diabetes mellitus is **noninsulin-dependent diabetes mellitus (NIDDM),** with 80% of all diagnosed cases falling within this classification. NIDDM can occur at any age, but it usually occurs after the age of 40. Between 60% and 90% of patients are obese or have a history of obesity at the time of diagnosis. The degree of insulin deficiency in NIDDM results from a progressive loss of beta cell responsiveness to glucose.

The prevalence of diagnosed NIDDM is over 5 million persons or about 2.5% of the population. Prevalence is higher among American Indians, African Americans, and Hispanics, and increases with age and obesity. Because of the insidious nature of the disease, there are believed to be a large number of undiagnosed cases.[9] The increase in incidence and prevalence of NIDDM that has taken place over the past 20 years may be attributable to a broadening of diagnostic criteria.[48]

In comparison with IDDM patients with minimal or no beta cell functioning, NIDDM patients retain up to 50% of the normal beta cell mass. Hyperglycemia in NIDDM probably results from a combination of insulin resistance and impaired insulin secretion. Insulin resistance may be related to diminished plasma membrane receptors on target cells or some type of postreceptor block to glucose metabolism (see Table 62-1 for a comparison of IDDM and NIDDM).

Characteristic symptoms in older adults
The older adult with NIDDM may have symptoms of fatigue, weight loss, lethargy, weakness, or an instability of balance or shuffling gait. Skin pruritus, nocturia, or a vulvovaginitis may also occur. It is also possible for the first manifestation in the older patient to be peripheral neuropathy, renal dysfunction, or eye disorders.

Genetic mechanisms
The likelihood that NIDDM is hereditary is validated by the nearly 100% concordance rate in monozygotic twins.

Other types of diabetes

Other types of diabetes include those patients with hyperglycemia associated with another disease or drug therapy. Impaired glucose tolerance (IGT) occurs when a patient's glucose level is between normal and diabetic values (>140 mg/mL and <200 mg/mL). In the past, such patients were frequently called "borderline diabetics." Gestational diabetes (GD) is carbohydrate intolerance of variable severity with onset or first recognition during pregnancy that usually disappears after childbirth. Statistical risk class is a designation for individuals who have previously exhibited an elevated glucose level but are now normal. A final group includes those at potential risk for abnormality of glucose tolerance, including a monozygotic twin of a NIDDM patient, obese persons, and women whose children weighed more than 9 lb at birth.

TABLE 62-1   Comparison of Insulin-Dependent Diabetes Mellitus (IDDM) and Noninsulin-Dependent Diabetes Mellitus (NIDDM)

	IDDM	NIDDM
Clinical features		
Age at onset	Usually <30, but can occur at any age	Usually >35, but can occur at any age
Onset	Often rapid	Insidious
Weight	Nonobese, thin	Often obese, may be normal
Ketosis	Common	Rare
Symptoms	Polydipsia, polyphagia, polyuria	Frequently not recognized or less acute in presentation
Complications	Frequent	Frequent
Epidemiology		
Prevalence	0.5% of American population	2% of American population
Sex	Slight male prevalence	Female prevalence
Seasonal variation	Present	Unknown
Genetics		
Concordance in identical twins	<50%	>90%
HLA association	Present	Absent
Environmental factors	Virus, toxins, autoimmune stimulus	Obesity, nutrition
Pathology		
Control of diabetes	Often difficult with wide fluctuations of glucose	Variable; helped by dietary measures
Functioning islet cell	Severely reduced	Moderately reduced
Dietary management	Essential	Essential, may suffice for glucose control
Medication		
Insulin	Required for all	Required for 20% to 30%
Sulfonylurea	Not efficacious	Efficacious

Pathophysiology

Diabetes mellitus is associated with both insulin deficiency and an excess of counterinsulin hormones. The lack of insulin causes (1) lowered utilization of blood glucose by body cells resulting in increased blood glucose levels; (2) mobilization of fatty acids from fat stores resulting in abnormal fat metabolism; and (3) decreased protein disposition in body tissues due to the lack of protein anabolism, which insulin promotes under normal circumstances. These abnormalities lead to alterations in carbohydrates, fats (lipids), ketone bodies, and proteins (amino acids). Five hormones are involved in controlling blood glucose levels: insulin, glucagon, growth hormone, epinephrine, and cortisol. Of these hormones, insulin lowers the blood glucose level. The other four hormones, termed **counterregulatory hormones,** raise the blood glucose level. In poorly controlled diabetes mellitus and during other stresses, circulating glucagon, epinephrine, growth hormone, and cortisol are increased and the antiinsulin actions of each reinforce the actions of the others. A summary of the normal effects of pancreatic hormones can be found in Chapter 59. The pathophysiologic alterations of these hormones in diabetes follows.[30,48,58]

Insulin

The normal human pancreas contains approximately 200 units of insulin. Figure 62-1 demonstrates the pattern of insulin secretion in nondiabetic persons. In patients with IDDM, virtually no insulin is produced because of the immunologic destruction of cells. Patients with NIDDM exhibit variable reductions.[65]

Several factors affect tissue responses to insulin. Insulin receptors, located on the plasma membrane, bind insulin once it reaches target tissues. The number of receptors varies from tissue to tissue, with subtle differences in the characteristics and function of receptors among tissues. Decreased binding is associated with conditions such as obesity, and in NIDDM and IDDM patients.

Insulin resistance is another common finding in diabetes mellitus. Insulin resistance exists when a normal serum insulin concentration produces a subnormal response. There are multiple causes of insulin resistance which can occur singly or in combination. These include type II diabetes, obesity, diabetes due to antibodies to the insulin receptor, abnormal insulin secreted by the pancreas, hypersecretion of counterregulatory hormones, or antibodies to insulin.[15]

Insulin resistance is accompanied by an impaired ability of insulin to suppress glucose production and stimulate glucose use. This hyperglycemia renders the cells unable to use glucose, and results in intracellular starvation. The muscle tissue then uses free fatty acids (FFA) or ketone bodies to meet metabolic needs, because insulin is unavailable to decrease ketone body production by inhibiting lipolysis, stimulating fatty acid synthesis, and increasing use of ketone bodies.[15,47,48,61]

Counterregulatory hormones

Glucagon

Research suggests that a relative or absolute excess of glucagon is an essential factor in the development of diabetes mellitus. Glucagon, a hormone secreted by the islets of Langerhans, increases blood glucose concentration by (1) breakdown of glycogen (glycogenolysis), (2) increasing storage of glucose (**gluconeogenesis**), (3) increasing the conversion of amino acids to glucose (**glyconeogenesis**). Glucagon regulates liver-mediated mobilization of stored glucose to be used by organ tissues. High concentrations of blood glucagon result in the liver-mediated release of blood glucose, producing a persistent hyperglycemia. Glucagon also regulates the oxidation of fatty acids in the liver and the increased production of ketone bodies, and is the primary counterregulatory hormone responsible for restoration of **euglycemia** (normal blood glucose levels) once **hypoglycemia** (low blood sugar) has occurred.[61]

Epinephrine

The metabolism of carbohydrates, amino acids, lipids, and ketone bodies is influenced by catecholamines. In diabetic patients, catecholamine concentrations may be inappropriately increased (during hyperglycemia) or decreased (during hypoglycemia). Epinephrine is similar to glucagon, in that it can cause rapid increases in hepatic glucose production. Epinephrine can also impair glucose uptake by muscle and other insulin-sensitive tissues and stimulate lipolysis (release of free fatty acids from stored triglycerides). Studies have found epinephrine to have a modulating effect on insulin secretion, which may play a role in the severity of diabetes.[58,61,65]

Growth hormone

Diabetic patients tend to have increased growth hormone levels, which is significant for several reasons. Growth hormone appears to regulate tissue sensitivity to insulin. It is theorized that growth hormone may increase insulin requirements by decreasing the hepatic/extrahepatic response to insulin, and may also be involved in microvascular complications of diabetes mellitus. Growth hormone increases adipose tissue breakdown of triglycerides, releases fatty acids into the blood, and inhibits uptake and oxidation of glucose by body tissues.[15,58,61]

Cortisol

Cortisol is required for normal liver gluconeogenesis, and it helps the conversion of amino acids in liver glucose. Cortisol is a potent inhibitor of glucose uptake by tissues, resulting in elevation of blood glucose. Excessive cortisol activity is associated with insulin resistance. Cortisol excess impairs insulin's ability to suppress glucose production and stimulate use.[15,61]

Clinical Manifestations

Screening tests

The clinical manifestations of diabetes are summarized in Table 62-1. Screening tests are of value in many cases but should be limited to persons with a high risk for diabetes. Candidates for screening include those with a strong family history of diabetes mellitus; the markedly obese; those with obstetric history of babies weighing over 9 pounds at birth; and those with an obstetric history of miscarriage or fetal death. Pregnant women between 24 and 28 weeks gestation should be screened because of the incidence of gestational diabetes (between 60,000 and 90,000 women per year).[30,44]

Diagnostic tests

In 1978, the National Diabetes Data Group of the National Institutes of Health convened a work group designed to establish criteria for diagnosis of diabetes (see the box). Although the diagnostic criteria may vary slightly, depending on the organization or nation, these criteria are generally accepted as appropriate. Given these criteria, the prevalence of a false-positive diagnosis of diabetes is 4.2%.[30,44]

Other diagnostic procedures

Several general laboratory procedures are available to assist with the diagnosis or monitoring of diabetes mellitus.[1,30]

DIAGNOSTIC CRITERIA FOR DIABETES MELLITUS AND IMPAIRED GLUCOSE TOLERANCE

Nonpregnant adults
Criteria for diabetes mellitus

Diagnosis of diabetes mellitus in nonpregnant adults should be restricted to those who have *one* of the following signs:

- A random plasma glucose level of 200 mg/dL or greater plus classic signs and symptoms of diabetes mellitus, including polydipsia, polyuria, polyphagia, and weight loss
- A fasting plasma glucose level of 140 mg/dL or greater on at least two occasions
- A fasting plasma glucose level of less than 140 mg/dL plus sustained elevated plasma glucose level during at least two oral glucose tolerance tests; the 2-hour sample and at least one other between 0 and 2 hours after the 75 g glucose dose should be 200 mg/dL or greater; oral glucose tolerance testing is not necessary if the patient has a fasting plasma glucose level of 140 mg/dL or greater

Criteria for impaired glucose tolerance

Diagnosis of impaired glucose tolerance in nonpregnant adults should be restricted to those who have all of the following signs:

- A fasting plasma glucose level of less than 140 mg/dL
- A 2-hour oral glucose tolerance test plasma glucose level between 140 and 200 mg/dL
- An intervening oral glucose tolerance test plasma glucose value of 200 mg/dL or greater

Elderly adults
Criteria for diabetes mellitus

Approximately 50% of people over the age of 60 have abnormal glucose tolerance test results when measured by standards taken from a young population. When diagnosing the older patient use the following:

- Age-adjusted norms
- Out-patient testing, if necessary, to avoid the stress of hospitalization, diet alterations, physical inactivity, and multiple medications that may interfere with the results
- A fasting plasma glucose level about 140 mg/dL (or blood glucose level above 160 mg/dL) on more than one occasion

WHO SHOULD USE SMBG?

A policy statement of the American Diabetes Association indicates that SMBG should be mandatory for the following:
1. Pregnant women with diabetes
2. Any patient using an insulin-infusion pump
3. Any patient striving for excellent metabolic control

Other groups for which SMBG is most desirable include the following:
1. Patients who frequently experience episodes of hypoglycemia
2. Patients who are unable to recognize the usual hypoglycemic symptoms, perhaps because of autonomic neuropathy
3. Patients who have labile or brittle diabetes; SMBG can provide valuable information as to the degree or cause of the fluctuating state
4. Patients who are experiencing episodes of poor control, such as nocturnal hypoglycemia, and are interested in problem-solving regarding this
5. Patients who are interested in mastering their diabetes by documenting the glycemic pattern in ordinary life

Fasting plasma glucose

The recommended screening test for adults and children is the fasting plasma glucose test. Diagnostic testing is recommended in adults with a fasting plasma glucose level of 115 mg/dL or greater. Pregnant women with a fasting plasma glucose level above 105 mg/dL and a plasma glucose level of 150 mg/dL after an oral glucose tolerance test should receive further diagnostic testing.

Self-monitoring of blood glucose

Home self-monitoring of blood glucose (SMBG) provides an accurate means for the patient to self-monitor blood glucose levels. It provides a reading of the current blood glucose level, and is not dependent on often inaccurate urine testing. Since it can be done quickly using capillary blood, specific treatment plans can be individualized to current blood levels (see box on SMBG).

SMBG procedures require a drop of capillary blood, obtained by fingerstick, and placed on a reagent strip. The strip is impregnated with glucose oxidase, peroxidase, and a chromagen system. The glucose oxidase, as the glucose-specific enzyme, promotes the reaction, which ultimately gives a characteristic color proportional to the amount of glucose in the blood. Although the procedure varies slightly, depending on the manufacturer, most require the blood to remain on the strip for a prescribed time period (60 to 120 seconds) and then read. Lancets and automated devices for penetrating the finger are very effective means of obtaining an appropriate drop of blood. A variety of reagent strips are also available. Some strips can be used only for visual readings, whereas others can also be used with reflectance meters to provide more specific readings. Reagent strips vary slightly in colors produced by the glucose, or timing for visualizing the strips, and do not provide accurate readings if not done correctly.

Although SMBG is helpful for all diabetic patients, care should be taken to ensure that the patient has the appropriate visual skills to discriminate colors and to read the strip/meter accurately. A number of reflectance meters are available for interpretation of reagent strips. When accurately used, the magnitude of differences between meter and laboratory readings is small.

Glycosylated hemoglobin

Glycosylated hemoglobin (GH) has assumed an important role in the monitoring of long-term glucose control in diabetes. Glycosylated hemoglobin concentration reflects glycemic control during the life span of the molecule. Glycosylation of hemoglobin occurs throughout the life of the erythrocyte. Five minor components of hemoglobins are identifiable: A1a1, A1a2, A1B1, A1c, and HbF. About 5% of HgA1c is in red cells of a nondiabetic person, whereas diabetic persons are two to four times higher. Ranges for normal vary depending upon the type of assay used. General guidelines for ranges appear in Table 62-2.

The life span of erythrocytes is 120 days, so GH measurements are time-averaged values for blood glucose over the preceding 2 to 4 months. GH results provide the clinician with an overview of the metabolic control of the patient. This is particularly helpful, since patients may inaccurately record their own SMBG results and a few may falsify results or limit

food intake and increase insulin before an office visit.[15,30,48,58]

Serum fructosamine

Serum fructosamine is a colorimetric assay designed to measure serum glycosylated protein concentration. This assay correlates well with glycosylated hemoglobin and fasting plasma glucose concentration. It is useful for monitoring short-term glycemic control (3 to 6 weeks). The assay is relatively inexpensive and may prove especially useful for monitoring elderly patients.[5]

C-peptide

The C-peptide radioimmunoassay is useful when information is needed regarding endogenous insulin secretion. The connecting C-peptide of the insulin molecule is cleaned from insulin and packaged with secretory granules so that it is released during the insulin-secretion process. Partial suppression of insulin secretion by administration of exogenous insulin can be shown by C-peptide radioimmunoassay.[65]

Tests for ketone bodies

At the present time, tests for urinary ketones may be made quickly via Ketostix. For IDDM patients interested only in testing for ketones during periods of illness or prolonged hyperglycemia, such ketone-specific strips are cost effective and useful.

Urinary glucose measurements

Urine glucose measurement has many limitations and is too insensitive a tool for closely monitoring metabolic control.[1,58] These limitations can be summarized related to (1) renal threshold problems and (2) poor correlation between blood glucose and urine levels. Renal threshold refers to the level at which a patient will spill glucose into the urine. Some diabetic patients spill glucose at fairly low levels (<135 mg/dL), whereas others spill glucose at higher levels (>250 mg/dL).[58]

TABLE 62-2   Biochemical Indices of Metabolic Control: Top Limits*

Biochemical index	Normal	Acceptable	Fair	Poor
Fasting plasma glucose	115 mg/dL	150 mg/dL	200 mg/dL	>200 mg/dL
Postprandial plasma glucose	140 mg/dL	175 mg/dL	235 mg/dL	>235 mg/dL
Glycosylated hemoglobin	6%	8%	10%	10%
Fasting plasma cholesterol	200 mg/dL	225 mg/dL	250 mg/dL	>250 mg/dL
Fasting plasma triglyceride	150 mg/dL	175 mg/dL	200 mg/dL	>200 mg/dL

From The physician's guide to type II diabetes mellitus, diagnosis, and treatment. Reproduced with permission of the American Diabetes Association, Inc, Alexandria, Va.
*Adjust for normal laboratory values. Limits for elderly patients vary.

The most limiting aspect of urine testing is the poor correlation of urine glucose with blood glucose. The urine results reflect changes over a period of several hours, whereas blood glucose gives immediate readings. A more important limitation is that, even with a normal renal threshold, a negative urine glucose value cannot distinguish between euglycemia, moderate hyperglycemia, or hypoglycemia.

Therapeutic Management

The therapeutic management of patients with diabetes mellitus includes measures designed to promote euglycemia and prevent or reverse the complications resulting from chronic hyperglycemia (Figure 62-2).

This goal of complete normalization of glycemia is achievable. Current treatment emphasizes alleviation of symptoms, avoidance of acute complications of ketoacidosis, protection from untoward effects of the regimen, and prevention of chronic complications.[28] As a result, treatment regimens for all diabetic patients include balancing caloric intake and energy expenditure, and maintaining circulating concentrations of insulin to maintain normal plasma glucose levels with the goal of possibly preventing or delaying the development of chronic complications of macroangiopathy (e.g., coronary artery disease, cerebrovascular disease) and microangiopathy (e.g., retinopathy, nephropathy, neuropathy).

The therapeutic regimen should be *individualized,* and patients should be given the opportunity to set their own management goals. General criteria that guide regimen adjustments, include (1) maintaining circulating insulin levels to keep the blood glucose between 60 and 150 mg/dL most of the time; (2) keeping episodes of hypoglycemia infrequent and mild; and (3) keeping urine negative for ketones. Tests for glycemic control should be closely monitored and the regimen adjusted as needed to

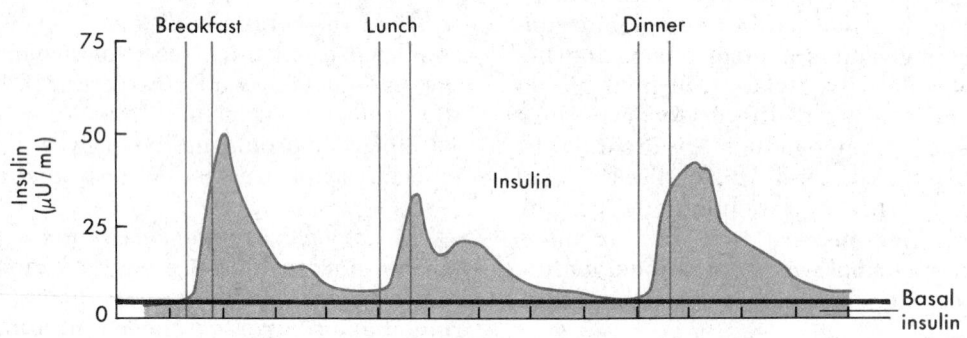

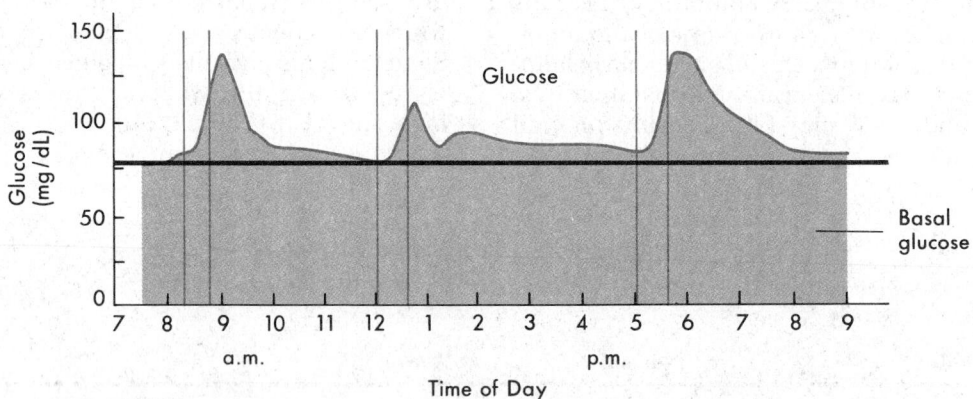

FIGURE 62-2   Pattern of insulin secretion in nondiabetic persons. Mean peripheral plasma insulin and glucose profiles in five nondiabetic subjects ingesting 630-kcal meals composed of 40% carbohydrate, 40% fat, and 20% protein. The meals took 15 minutes to ingest. All subjects were ambulatory but did not exercise. The plasma glucose concentration increased only 50% during the meals, whereas the plasma insulin concentration increased approximately 600%. The pattern of the rise in plasma insulin concentration closely matches that of the rise in plasma glucose concentration.

maintain appropriate levels. Some patients, despite strict adherence to their regimen, may have difficulty achieving these goals because of other problems beyond their control. Patients may also choose different goals from those prescribed by the therapeutic regimen.[52,53,65] In these cases, the guidelines are adjusted to avoid the feeling of failure in meeting prescribed therapeutic goals.

Diet

Although the dietary therapy is individualized to accomplish patient goals, there are nutritional criteria that guide management. Patients need to understand the relationship between food, insulin, and blood glucose levels and how to plan meals to reach and maintain weight goals. This generally involves extensive time with the dietitian. The nurse and other health care team members also need to ensure thorough assessment and positive outcomes related to nutrition education.[44,51,66]

All diabetic patients need to be taught to maintain appropriate blood glucose and blood cholesterol levels. They can also learn to maintain a reasonable weight by eating optimal calories for normal growth and development.

Nutrition assessment
A. Medical factors
　1. Type of diabetes (i.e., IDDM, NIDDM)
　2. Weight, height history
　3. Growth curve
　4. Medications (insulin, oral agents, other)
　5. Abnormal laboratory findings
　6. Significant physical findings
　7. Family history
B. Nutritional status
　1. Average pattern and intake of carbohydrate, protein, fat, and calories
　2. Saturated fat intake
　3. Alcohol intake
　4. Food preferences/allergies
　5. Special needs (i.e., growth, stress)
　6. Drug/diet interactions
C. Education status
　1. Reading level
　2. Learning preferences
D. Available support systems
　1. Facilities for food preparation
　2. Food budget
　3. Ethnic, cultural, social, religious background
　4. Life-style
　5. Support available from family and others

Nutrition planning
A meal plan that is medically and nutritionally sound and acceptable to the patient is important for main-

taining metabolic control. The basic daily meal plan provides adequate energy for daily activities, and is relatively consistent with regard to calories (total energy intake) and the distribution of carbohydrates, fats, and proteins. Variable meal plans might also be developed for regular changes in energy expenditure, such as weekly, monthly (with menses), and seasonal (spring versus winter) variation, and occasional changes (vacation).[66] Natural foods containing high fiber and unrefined carbohydrates should be encouraged.

The nurse has an important role in assuring a patient has adequate access to nutrition education. Once the nutrition plan is formulated, generally by the dietitian, the nurse monitors and follows-up on patient progress and response to the plan. In order to effectively fulfill this role, the nurse must understand the steps involved in formulating a nutritional plan.

The exchange system
To improve the dietary standards for care, the American Diabetes Association, in conjunction with the American Dietetic Association and the Public Health Service, developed the ADA exchange system. The exchange system divides food into six groups, according to the type and the amount of carbohydrate, protein, fat, and calories supplied by foods within that group.

TABLE 62-3   Summary of Exchange Lists (1986)

Exchange list	Carbohydrate (g)	Protein (g)	Fat (g)	Calories
Starch/bread	15	3	1*	80
Meats				
Lean		7	3	55
Medium fat		7	5	75
High fat		7	8	100
Vegetables	5	2		25
Fruits	15			60
Milk				
Skim	12	8	1*	90
Low fat	12	8	5	120
Whole	12	8	8	150
Fats			5	45

*In *Exchange Lists*, trace is listed. For calculation purposes, 1 g can be used. If patient always uses skim milk that is 0 fat and 80 cal, calculate it as such. If starches with >1 g fat are usually selected, then the nutrition counselor has the option of calculating with a different fat value if desired. See Table 4-3 and Appendix for the amount of fat in the various choices.

MEAL PLAN CALCULATION

A. Determine ideal body weight
> **Men**
> Medium frame   5 ft = 106 lb
> (plus 6 lb for each additional inch)
> Small frame (subtract 10%)
> Large frame (add 10%)
> **Women**
> Medium frame   5 ft = 100 lb
> (plus 5 lb for each additional inch)
> Small frame (subtract 10%)
> Large frame (add 10%)

B. Determine caloric needs
1. To estimate caloric needs
   a. Basal calories = 10 × desirable body weight
   b. Add activity calories
      (1) Sedentary—3 × desirable body weight
      (2) Moderate—5 × desirable body weight
      (3) Strenuous—10 × desirable body weight
2. Add calories for weight gain in pregnancy (+300 cal/day) or lactation (+500 cal/day)
3. Subtract calories for weight reduction (−500 cal/day; 3500 cal = 1 pound)

C. Determine percentage of carbohydrate, protein, and fat (1986 Nutritional recommendations for individuals with diabetes mellitus)
1. Carbohydrate—55% to 60% of total calories
2. Fat—<20% of total calories
3. Cholesterol—<300 mg/dL
4. Protein—8 g/kg body weight
5. Fiber—35 to 40 g/day

D. Determine calories of carbohydrates, protein, and fat
1. Carbohydrate calories = Total calories × 0.55 − 0.60
2. Protein calories = Total calories × 0.12 − 0.20
3. Fat calories = Total calories × 0.30

E. Conversion of calories into grams
1. Carbohydrate grams = Carbohydrate calories ÷ 4 cal/g
2. Protein grams = Protein calories ÷ 4 cal/g
3. Fat grams = Fat calories ÷ 9 cal/g

F. Determine number of servings from each food group
1. Determine carbohydrates from fruit and vegetable servings
   a. Query patients as to number of servings per day
   b. Add or subtract carbohydrates from these servings for total
   c. Repeat process for milk servings
2. Determine number of bread/starch servings
3. Determine number of meat/protein servings
   a. Add grams of protein from vegetable, bread, milk
   b. Subtract the protein value from total grams of protein
   c. Meat/protein servings = remaining protein ÷ 7 g protein serving
4. Determine number of fat servings
   a. Add grams of fat from milk, meat servings
   b. Subtract fat value from total grams to yield remaining fat
   c. Fat servings = remaining fat ÷ 5 g fat per serving

G. Distribute carbohydrate servings between meals and snacks

With the exchange group system, any food may be substituted in the proper amounts for any other listed food item within the same group. The exchange lists emphasize foods low in cholesterol and polyunsaturated fat. The system helps patients to understand the complexity of foods, their equivalents, and their categories and allows for flexibility in meal plans. Within each group, foods are listed in specific amounts called servings. Substitutions can be made for foods in the same food group but not from another food group. The exchange system provides patients with a reference point from which they can guide their dietary habits (Table 62-3). Although it is not appropriate for all patients, this is an important aid for teaching some patients how to manage their diabetes.[31,51]

The development of an individualized meal plan involves several steps (see boxes on meal plan calculation and sample meal plan). Although the meal plan is generally completed by a dietitian, the nurse can use this information to help the patient understand the rationale for certain dietary recommendations as well as communication with the dietitian.

Nutrition education

The nutritional aspect is the most difficult part of the diabetic regimen. Nutrition education conducted in a controlled atmosphere may not address the daily

SAMPLE MEAL PLAN WITH FOOD EXCHANGES FOR 1800-CALORIE DIET
Conversion of Exchanges into Meals and Snack

Meals	Exchanges	Food choices	Portions
Breakfast			
Fruit	1	Orange juice	cup
Starch/bread	2	Whole-wheat toast	2 slices
Milk	½	Milk, skim	½ cup
Fat	1	Margarine	1 tsp
Free	—	Coffee or tea, sugar substitute	1 tsp
Lunch			
Meat (medium fat)	3	Hamburger	3 oz
Starch/bread	3	Hamburger bun	1 medium
		Sherbet	¼ cup
Vegetable	1	Tomato	1 large
		with lettuce	as desired
Fat	1	Salad dressing, mayonnaise-type	2 tsp
Fruit	1	Pear	1 small
Free	—	Diet beverage, sugar-free	
Dinner			
Meat (medium fat)	3	Chicken breast (no skin)	4½ oz with bone
Starch/bread	4	Potato, baked	6 oz
		Whole-wheat bread	2 slices
Vegetable	1	Carrots	½ cup
Free	—	Lettuce	wedge
Free	—	Salad dressing, low calorie	2 tbs
Fat	1	Margarine	1 tsp
Fruit	1	Grapes	15 each
Milk	1	Milk, skim	1 cup
Free	—	Coffee or tea, sugar substitute	
Evening snack			
Milk	½	Milk, skim	½ cup
Starch/bread	1	Graham crackers	3 2½-inch squares

From Galloway JA et al: *Diabetes mellitus*, ed 9, Indianapolis, 1988, Eli Lilly Co.

stresses confronting an individual, such as social events, occupational or economic factors, ethnic concerns, changing caloric needs as part of normal growth, and boredom with the dietary regimen. Education needs to address these concerns so that patients are prepared to make informed choices and maintain metabolic goals. Some of the more common topics the nurse needs to discuss with the diabetic patient include the following[34]:

1. Special foods and sugar substitutes—The use of special and/or costly foods is not required, since the diabetic diet emphasizes healthful eating habits. As such, "dietetic" foods need not be purchased; in fact, these foods are often high in sodium as opposed to sucrose.

2. Alcohol—Alcohol tends to promote hypoglycemia, hypertriglyceridemia, and, with oral agents, may cause symptoms of palpitation, flushing, or facial tingling. If patients want alcohol, they should plan for small amounts and calculate this into the diet.

3. Eating out—Patients are instructed to make adjustments in total daily intake to plan for meals at restaurants or parties. Some useful strategies include ordering half portions, salads with dressing on the side, fresh fruit for dessert, and baked or steamed entrees. Cafeterias or buffets may also offer greater flexibility in keeping with the nutrition plan.

4. Food labels—Once the patient and dietitian

jointly develop a diet plan, the patient needs to learn about other tools to enhance food selection. One strategy is to teach the reading of food labels, looking at ingredients for carbohydrate and calorie contents. Such information is necessary for the patient to make independent and informed choices regarding food selection.

Pharmacologic interventions

The indications for treatment with insulin in IDDM are quite obvious, but in NIDDM the need for insulin is a more controversial decision. The indications for insulin treatment are as follows:

1. Patients with IDDM
2. Patients with NIDDM for whom metabolic control is not achieved with diet and exercise therapy alone
3. Patients of any age who have a history of diabetic ketoacidosis or nonketotic coma
4. Pregnant diabetic women unable to control hyperglycemia with diet therapy
5. Patients of any age with hyperglycemia, who may not usually require insulin, but who:
   a. Have a febrile illness
   b. Are receiving glucocorticoids
   c. Are undergoing major surgery
   d. Are under a period of extreme stress[50]

Insulins

There are a variety of insulins available, classified by purity, species, concentration, and action (Table 62-4). Although insulin is extracted from the pancreatic material of a variety of animals, cattle and pigs remain the two most common sources. The amino acid sequences of beef and pork insulins differ slightly from that of humulin insulin. This variation means that beef insulin, which differs by three amino acids, is more immunogenic in humans than pork insulin, which differs by one amino acid.

Extensive clinical trials have shown that humulin insulin is absorbed slightly more rapidly than beef or pork insulin. Humulin insulin has been useful in the treatment of patients with pork or beef allergies, although it has not been deemed superior to the animal insulins at this time. For the present, the following guidelines are recommended for initiating therapy with humulin insulins:

1. Newly diagnosed patients who have not previously been exposed to animal insulins
2. Persons who need temporary insulin therapy (e.g. gestational diabetes)
3. Those who are allergic to beef or pork
4. IDDM patients who require large daily doses because of insulin antibodies
5. Those with a personal preference
6. Persons whose religious beliefs prohibit consumption of animal products[15,65]

Routes of insulin delivery

There are several routes for insulin delivery, but the subcutaneous route is the one most frequently used. Subcutaneous insulin disappears from the injection site in about 60 minutes. It is therefore recommended that a meal be eaten 15 to 30 minutes after injection, so that the plasma glucose level and the plasma insulin level rise are coordinated. Problems associated with the subcutaneous administration include the varying rate of absorption, depending on injection site.

The intravenous route of insulin delivery is generally preferred during diabetic ketoacidosis since the subcutaneous route may yield erratic or diminished absorption with longer time of onset. The intramuscular site may also be used during diabetic ketoacidosis, but the pain associated with this

TABLE 62-4 Insulins by Relative Comparative Action Curves

Insulin	Onset (h)	Peak (h)	Usual effective duration (h)	Usual maximum duration (h)
Animal				
Regular	0.5-2.0	3-4	4-6	6-8
NPH	4-6	8-14	16-20	20-24
Lente	4-6	8-14	16-20	20-24
Ultralente	8-14	Minimal	24-36	24-36
Human				
Regular	0.5-1.0	2-3	3-6	4-6
NPH	2-4	4-10	10-16	14-18
Lente	3-4	4-12	12-18	16-20
Ultralente	6-10	?	18-20	20-30

method makes it inappropriate for daily use. The intraperitoneal route is being used for implantable insulin devices; however, this is still in the experimental phase. The oral, rectal, and nasal routes of insulin delivery are attractive possibilities for administration because of the potential ease of administration; but problems with absorption have limited these sites as potential routes for insulin delivery.[65]

Initiating insulin treatment

Treatment with insulin usually is initiated on an outpatient basis, especially if the patient did not have DKA at the time of diagnosis. In general, the starting dosage for a nonketotic person with IDDM is 0.6 unit per kilogram of body weight per day. This dosage may vary, depending on age, weight, and growth activity (i.e. adolescent growth spurts). The starting dosage should be much less than the expected optimal dose. Ordinarily the patient will be prescribed an initial starting dose and taught to SMBG, frequently increasing the insulin dosage by two units until the target blood glucose level is attained. The nurse closely follows the patient, usually with weekly clinic visits or daily telephone contact. The patterns of response to insulin vary slightly from patient to patient. Such variations need to be monitored so "fine tuning" can take place. The interval between dosage change should be at least 2 to 3 days, with adjustments made on the basis of blood glucose level patterns.[54] There are various reasons for increased insulin requirements, so careful assessment of such problems should be completed before the dosage is changed. Some of these include the following:

1. True resistance (greater than 200 U/day)
2. Inadequate activity
3. Overeating
4. Overdependence on specific insulin injection sites
5. Overdependence on one versus multiple injections

Insulin regimens

There are several basic patterns of insulin administration that provide successful management for the majority of patients. The initial choice of regimen depends on the type of diabetes and the degree of control desired. IDDM patients should strive to maintain plasma glucose concentrations in a normal range, or euglycemia, as a goal of insulin therapy. To accomplish this, multiple daily insulin injections are required. Many of these insulin regimens use split and mixed doses. The term *split dosage* refers to the administration of a total dose of insulin given in several injections over a certain time period. The term *mixed dosage* implies the use of various types of insulins in a given regimen (i.e., rapid- and

intermediate-acting insulins). Insulin regimens use this split and mixed method of insulin administration with combinations of rapid-, and intermediate-, and long-acting insulins that are designed to be administered in a multiple daily insulin injection format.

In more **conventional insulin therapy,** patients require a split-dosage regimen with two injections of an intermediate (i.e. NPH) insulin with or without regular insulin. Such regimens usually provide two thirds of the intermediate-acting insulin dose in the morning. To attain "tight" metabolic control, more intensive insulin regimens have been designed to mimic, as closely as possible, the normal physiologic pattern of the pancreas (see Chapter 59). In doing so, blood glucose levels are kept within a normal range as much as possible. The diabetic patient involved in this **intensive conventional therapy (ICT)** must be agreeable to two or more injections per day coupled with SMBG at least four or more times per day. Careful balancing of diet and activity and adherence to the regimen are critical. Patients are taught to adjust insulin dosages using algorithms, or guidelines, to meet target glucose levels. ICT is for patients who have had suboptimal control with conventional therapy and are knowledgeable, willing to do SMBG, want to have tight control, and have appropriately adapted to diabetes mellitus. There are numerous insulin protocols of varying sophistication. Some of the methods (Figure 62-3) most commonly used include:[8,20,50,52,53]

Two injections per day. The two injections per day method uses doses of rapid and intermediate-acting insulin before breakfast and supper. The rapid-acting insulin (i.e. regular) provides coverage of glycemic elevations after breakfast and supper, while the intermediate-acting insulin (i.e. NPH), with an evening dose of one half to one third of the morning dose, provides coverage after lunch and throughout the evening hours. This regimen is often chosen because it allows for increased glycemic control while requiring only two injections per day.

Disadvantages of this regimen are a direct result of the prolonged action of the intermediate-acting insulin. For example, an increase in the morning dose of intermediate-acting insulin, designed to combat after-lunch hyperglycemia, results in an overall increase in circulating insulin concentrations into the late afternoon and evening hours. The risk of hypoglycemia is then increased in the evening hours, following the administration of the second intermediate-acting insulin injection. Another concern with the prolonged action of the intermediate-acting insulin is that the patient must eat lunch and supper on time or risk a hypoglycemic reaction.

Three injections per day. The three injections per day method uses rapid- and intermediate-acting insulin for the prebreakfast dose, regular as a presup-

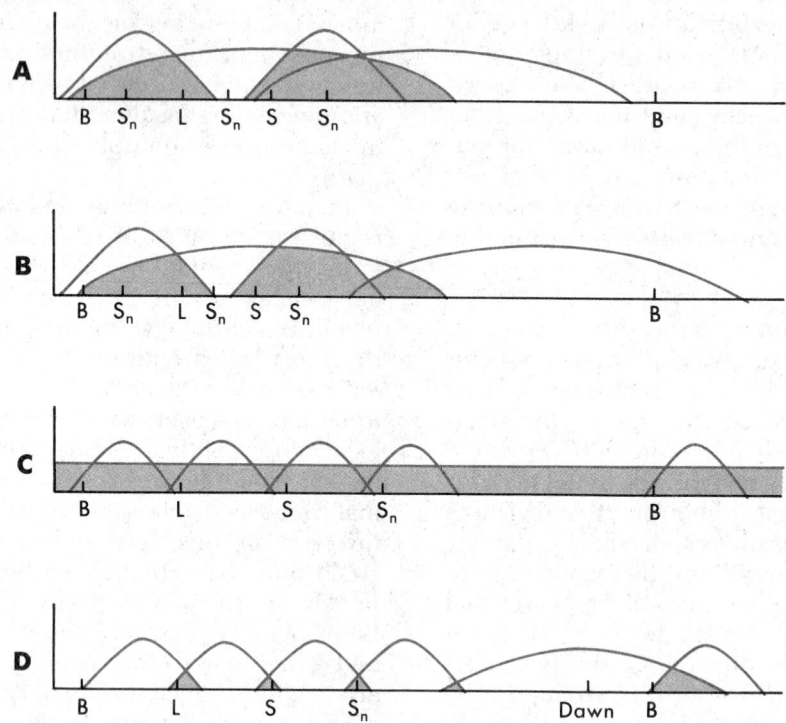

FIGURE 62-3   Insulin delivery protocols. **A,** Standard twice-daily insulin regimen (e.g., intermediate and short acting). **B,** Three-times-daily insulin regimen, suggested for patients with early-morning hypoglycemia followed by rebound hyperglycemia or for patients with early-morning hyperglycemia (dawn phenomenon). **C,** Multidose insulin regimen; 4 injections/day (short-acting insulin before meals and long-acting at bedtime). **D,** Alternative multidose regimen consisting of 5 injections (short-acting insulin premeal and intermediate-acting insulin at bedtime). *Shaded areas* illustrate overlap between insulin peaks.

per dose, and a small dose of NPH at bedtime. Because there is minimal overlap of the two intermediate-acting insulin doses, the inconsistency in timing of peak action and elevated concentrations of insulin are effectively managed. This method has also been found to be an effective means of maintaining acceptable blood glucose levels prebreakfast, since the bedtime intermediate dose is administered to accommodate elevations in blood glucose associated with hormonal activities.

Disadvantages of this regimen result from the elevated concentrations of insulin while the patient is sleeping, thus increasing the potential for nocturnal hypoglycemia. It is also necessary to monitor the *timing* of meals so that they coincide closely with the peak action of the intermediate-acting insulin to avoid hypoglycemia.

Multidose insulin. This therapy features 3 or 4 injections of short-acting insulin preceding meals coupled with longer-acting preparations designed to mimic basal insulin secretion. The regimen may consist of three preprandial doses of rapid-acting insulin coupled with a dose of bedtime lente or NPH. An-

other option involves injecting long-acting insulin (i.e. ultralente insulin) once a day or divided into two equal doses given before breakfast and supper. Doses of a rapid-acting insulin are administered preprandially (or prior to eating), which may or may not be a time that the long-acting insulin is given. This regimen usually requires three to five injections per day.

The long-acting insulin provides a basal insulin supply that is virtually peakless if administered in small doses. This gives the diabetic person a steady supply of insulin to accommodate metabolic needs at all times, and preprandial boluses of rapid-acting insulin may be preset for each meal or may be guided by a sliding scale, known as an algorithm, based on preprandial blood glucose levels. This regimen most mimics that of the insulin pumps, which provide basal insulin rates by continuous subcutaneous administration of short-acting insulin and supplement with preprandial boluses. The individual is free to alter timing and frequency of meals with the knowledge that a basal supply of circulating insulin will be available to maintain metabolic activities.

Insulin pumps. Insulin pumps are designed to provide a basal rate of regular insulin and bolus doses before mealtimes. Generally, the patient places the needle in subcutaneous abdominal tissue, changing the pump needle at least every 48 hours. The dangers associated with insulin pumps include insulin overdosage, insulin interruption, and continued insulin delivery during hypoglycemia. The pump is not for every patient; patients must be highly motivated, able to monitor frequently, and willing to adjust their regimen in conjunction with various insulin algorithms. Many patients can achieve the same results using ICT. The greatest advantage appears to be a perception of increased flexibility of lifestyle.[15,65]

Administration of insulin

The need for consistent and appropriate technique in insulin administration is critical to optimal metabolic control. Patients should demonstrate several steps in insulin administration, when reviewed by the nurse. These steps include preparing for injection using either single or mixed insulins, and insulin injection technique including appropriate site selection.

At present, all insulin types are generally designated in two different strengths: U-40 and U-100. There is a U-500 insulin, but its use is minimal. U-40 and U-100 syringes are available. The U indicates the number of units per milliliter. Insulin syringes will hold 1/20 or 1 mL, which would be 50 or 100 units of U-100 insulin.

The various sites available for insulin injection are depicted in Figure 62-4. Patients should rotate sites to avoid problems with hypertrophy, or lipodyatrophy.[30] Hypertrophy of subcutaneous tissue probably results from long-standing repeated injections at the same site. The fibrotic areas which result can become hard and disfiguring.

Lipoatrophy is a loss of fat at the site of repeated injections causing a disfiguring depression in the subcutaneous tissue. Lipoatrophy is rarely seen in patients treated with purified pork or human insulins. Patients can rotate injection sites in one area for 1 week until all sites have been used.

Specific steps must be carefully followed in insulin injection. Consistent methods and procedures are critical to accurate insulin injection as noted in the patient education guide on pp. 1732 and 1733.

When mixing insulins, there has been concern that altered absorption and action profiles occur between the mixed insulins. For example, it has been noted in some studies that premixing results in a potentiated effect of NPH/lente.[32,54,57] Although premixing remains a necessary component to insulin therapy, there are some guidelines which the nurse should give the patient, including the following:

1. Advise patient to be consistent; injecting im-

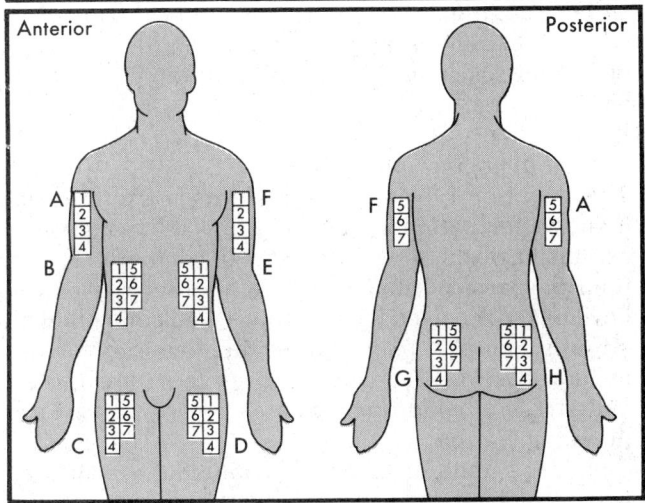

Injection record								
SITE		1	2	3	4	5	6	7
Right arm	A							
Right abdomen	B							
Right thigh	C							
Left thigh	D							
Left abdomen	E							
Left arm	F							
Left buttock	G							
Right buttock	H							

FIGURE 62-4   Injection record.

mediately after mixing one time and 60 minutes after another can make metabolic control difficult.

2. Use fast- and intermediate-acting insulins of the same brand; use the same brand consistently.

3. A mixture of regular plus NPH should be used within 5 minutes of mixing or wait 15 minutes after mixing (regular action may be slower 15 minutes after mixing).

4. Insulin can be stored at room temperature. Insulin can be stored mixed in a syringe (NPH/regular, lente/regular) for 14 days if refrigerated.

Insulin therapy in NIDDM

Recommendations for insulin therapy are based on several clinical studies, including the University Group Diabetes Program (UGDP) study.[22,53] Several recommendations regarding insulin therapy have been made by the ADA, including the following:

1. Insulin treatment does achieve euglycemia in NIDDM.

2. Newly diagnosed patients can be controlled on modest dosages once or several times per day.
3. Insulin requirements may increase over time.
4. There is an increase in insulin resistance in the NIDDM patient of several years' duration.
5. Although increased appetite and weight gain are seen, careful dietary management can lessen this potential problem.

The usual therapeutic regimen includes mixing a 2:1 ratio of rapid- and intermediate-acting insulin before breakfast and the same types of insulin in a 1:1 ratio before supper. For insulin dosages <30 U/day, a single injection may suffice. However, NIDDM patients may require >100 U/day because of insulin resistance. Therefore, multiple injections are common.[29,31]

Oral hypoglycemic agents

The use of oral hypoglycemic agents is often recommended for patients who meet the following criteria: onset of diabetes after age 40; diabetes of less than 5 years; normal weight or obese; those who have never received insulin or are well controlled on 40 units per day or less. Contraindications for use include IDDM, pregnancy, allergy to sulfonylureas, and stressful conditions such as myocardial infarction or infection.

A large number of NIDDM patients are treated with oral hypoglycemic agents. These agents augment beta cell secretion of insulin (Figure 62-5).

Oral hypoglycemic agents are divided into first and second generation agents. These agents differ in terms of potency, pharmacokinetics, and metabolism. The choice of agent depends on patient condition and nutritional status. Often, short-acting as opposed to longer-acting agents (such as chlorpropamide) are chosen to avoid episodes of hypoglycemia (Table 62-5).

The lowest effective oral agent dosage is initially prescribed for therapy. The dosage should be increased every week or two until control is achieved. If the patient does not respond initially, this is termed a primary failure. A secondary failure occurs if the selection of a second oral agent does not improve blood glucose levels. This occurs in 5% to 10% of patients, who must then begin insulin therapy.[29,30,44]

Combination therapy

At present, combination therapy of insulin and oral hypoglycemic agents is suggested only when glycemic control has not been achieved with diet and sulfonylureas and when reasonable control has not been apparent with insulin therapy.[11,50]

Exercise

Regular, aerobic exercise that involves using large muscle groups and that elevates the pulse rate to a level of 60% to 80% of maximum has the potential to lower serum triglycerides, lower blood glucose, increase insulin sensitivity, decrease blood pressure,

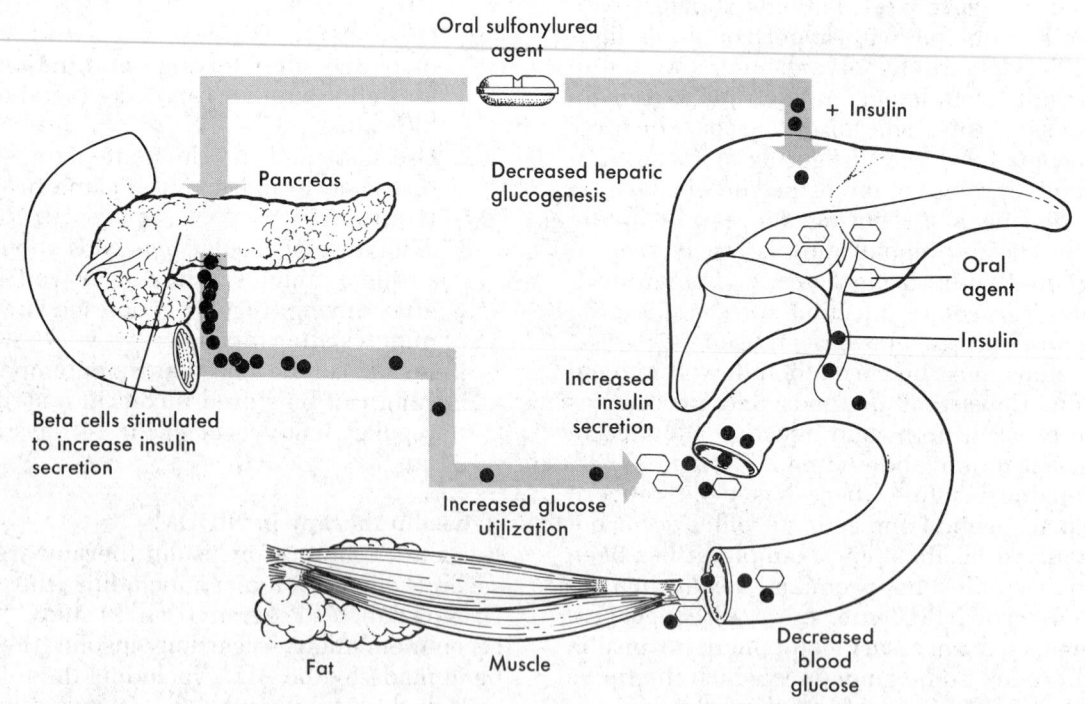

FIGURE 62-5 Mechanism of action of oral sulfonylurea agents.

TABLE 62-5   Pharmacology Summary: Sulfonylureas

Drug	Duration of action
FIRST GENERATION SULFONYLUREAS	
Tolbutamide (Orinase)	Short
Acetohexamide (Dymelor)	Medium
Tolazamide (Tolinase)	Medium
Chlorpropamide (Diabinese)	Long
SECOND GENERATION SULFONYLUREAS	
Glyburide (Micronase, DiaBeta)	Long
Glipizide (Glucotrol)	Medium

CLINICAL ADVANTAGES OF SECOND GENERATION ORAL HYPOGLYCEMIC AGENTS

More potent, so smaller doses effective

One dose a day is feasible because of 24-hour action

Less chance of hypoglycemia

Can be safely given to patients with moderate kidney function without risk of hypoglycemia

Effective in 25% of first generation primary failure patients

SIDE EFFECTS OF ORAL HYPOLGYCEMIC AGENTS

Skin rash

Gastrointestinal upset (e.g., nausea, vomiting, diarrhea)

Hematopoetic-leukopenia, thrombocytopenia, anemia

Hepatic toxicity

Alcohol sensitivity—particularly with chlorpropamide

Chlorpropamide-induced water retention and hyponatremia

---

increase the capacity to do physical work, and increase emotional well-being.

It is essential that adequate insulin is available for increased uptake of glucose from the blood. Exercise studies with IDDM subjects showed that inadequate circulating insulin (reflected by blood sugars above 250 mg/dL and elevated serum ketones) was associated with a worsening of serum ketone levels and a net increase, rather than a decrease in the blood glucose level. The blood glucose level can actually rise because, although muscle is responsible for using glucose in significant amounts during exer-

CLINICAL ALERT

Exercise in *poorly controlled* IDDM persons can lead to increased blood glucose levels and ketoacidosis. Patients need to be taught not to exercise with blood glucose level greater than 250 mg/dL and/or when positive for ketones.

cise, the liver is responsible for continuous repletion of the glucose pool. During the early phases of exercise, the liver increases its rate of glycogen breakdown to keep pace with muscle use. With prolonged exercise, gluconeogenesis accounts for an increasing amount of the glucose produced. These mechanisms permit a balance between glucose use and production that maintains blood glucose at a relatively constant level. A relative deficiency of insulin during exercise would then lead to an imbalance between muscle use (decreased) and liver production (increased), causing the paradoxical increase in the blood glucose level observed in the poorly controlled diabetic patient.[17,27]

Although the metabolic consequences of acute exercise in IDDM have been studied, the effect of exercise on NIDDM subjects has received less attention. However, most NIDDM patients are considered good candidates for an exercise program. Some of the benefits of exercise to NIDDM subjects include exercise-induced enhanced sensitivity to insulin and improvements in glucose tolerance. Additionally, obesity-associated peripheral resistance to insulin can be reversed or improved with physical activity.

Exercise planning

Exercise activity is often overlooked as a specific ingredient of the diabetic regimen. Although planned exercise is important, it is rarely discussed in terms of a prescribed program. However, there are also clear risks associated with more intensive exercise programs in patients with complications of diabetes. For this reason, every exercise plan needs to be carefully negotiated with the individual patient, and personal goals and preferences should be taken into account. Involvement of the physical therapist in this process is valuable to the patient.

Exercise intensity can be monitored by assessing the maximum heart rate during activity. To compute maximum heart rate, a carotid pulse, for a 10-second count, must be taken within 5 seconds of the activity having ended. Multiplying by 6 then yields heart rate. Maximum heart rate (100%) is approximately 220 minus age. To achieve benefits, an intensity of 60% to 80% of age-adjusted maximum heart rate should be achieved.[12,58]

Patients need to receive specific exercise information that addresses the type of exercise, how long, how frequent, and how intense. Walking is often selected as a program, because it involves little cost or equipment and is basically safe. Patients who have not been involved in an exercise program can begin at lower fitness levels and progress accordingly. A plan includes (1) establishing target goals that are specific, measurable, and realistic; (2) establishing weekly objectives designed to help patients reach their target goal in a realistic period of time; (3) establishing a schedule for activity that allows for specific and realistic time frames within which to carry out the activity (record keeping in an exercise log is helpful); and (4) measuring progress and making changes to adapt the system to individual goals and progress.[45]

Exercise precautions—IDDM

Exercise may potentiate the effects of insulin and therefore may cause blood glucose levels to decrease. To avoid hypoglycemia, patients should be taught that regular, sustained exercise requires glucose for energy. Because the decrease in blood glucose can last approximately 24 hours, hypoglycemia can be a problem for several hours. This requires careful monitoring and timing of meals and snacks. Patients must also be taught that on some occasions, the blood glucose level rises immediately after exercise and later drops. SMBG before and following exercise is therefore imperative. It should also be completed midway through intense exercise periods. The importance of providing the patient and family with this information cannot be overemphasized.

The best means to determine the correct amount of insulin with regard to exercise includes keeping an accurate record of the time of day of exercise, exercise duration, before and after blood glucose levels, time of injections in relation to food and exercise, food intake, number and times of reaction, and anecdotal information.

Calorie needs during exercise depend on the timing of exercise related to the insulin peak, the last meal, the patient's metabolism, and the propensity toward hypoglycemia. Patient exercise guidelines should include the following:

1. Do not exercise at times when a hypoglycemic reaction is likely
2. If you are exercising during a peak insulin time, eat an hour before the exercise and drink a carbohydrate liquid
3. Always carry a quick-acting carbohydrate with you
4. In case of a hypoglycemic reaction, always wear a Medic Alert identification tag

Exercise precautions—NIDDM

Aerobic activities are probably of greatest benefit to patients with NIDDM. Because the NIDDM patient still has some level of pancreatic response, the side effects of exercise are minimal. However, in some patients, oral hypoglycemic agent adjustments may need to be undertaken, because exercise does decrease insulin resistance and glucose intolerance.

NURSING MANAGEMENT OF THE PATIENT WITH DIABETES MELLITUS
Assessment

A thorough nursing assessment of the diabetic patient includes the collection of physical, psychosocial, and self-management data so that a nursing diagnosis can be adequately developed. Assessment should seek subjective patient statements, followed by objective findings. A systematic procedure needs to be consistently followed.[1,18,21]

The needs assessment might include:

- health and medical history
- medication and diet history
- mental status
- life-style practices such as occupation, social and cultural
- physical and psychologic factors (e.g., age, visual accuracy, hearing, ability to concentrate)
- barriers to education (e.g., literacy and motivation)
- family and social support
- previous diabetes education

The patient is encouraged to state perceptions of ability to cope with chronic illness. Such a technique respects the patient's knowledge and role as primary manager of diabetes. The nurse can then use the information to identify the appropriate and individual nursing diagnoses for the patient.

Nursing Diagnosis

The following nursing diagnoses may be appropriate for the patient with diabetes mellitus:

Knowledge deficit related to newly diagnosed diabetes mellitus

Ineffective individual coping related to stress of self-management

 **CLINICAL ALERT**

The role of the nurse in diabetes education is critical to quality care for the patient. The nurse must assess needs, teach, coordinate information, facilitate multidisciplinary team functioning, evaluate patient progress, and help the patient adhere to treatment.

Ineffective family coping related to changes imposed by treatment plan

Planning

Goals must be individualized to meet the needs and priorities of the patient. Outcome criteria include the following:

- Patient discusses key components of self-management of diabetes via diet, exercise, and medication management
- Patient demonstrates knowledge and skills related to diabetes self-management
- Patient verbalizes problems associated with diabetes care
- Patient and family discuss methods for problem-solving associated with diabetes care

Implementation

Nursing interventions need to focus on assisting the patient to achieve optimal self-management of diabetes. Educating the family must be emphasized, since the family is also impacted greatly by chronic disease.

The patient's readiness to learn must first be assessed prior to teaching. The patient must not be inundated with information or have inadequate information regarding his or her condition. To better organize the educational presentation, it is helpful to assess the content in terms of survival skills versus useful or additional information. After the patient is comfortable with "survival" information, he or she may have questions concerning insulin algorithms, eating away from home, or training for marathons. Education can then focus on integrating the regimen into the patient's life-style.

Survival education includes the basic nature of the disease and the importance of patient participation. The scope of education generally consists of the following:

  Relationship between nutrition, exercise, and medication in diabetes management
  Meal planning
  Self-monitoring for glycemic control
  Medication management (see the patient education guide on pp. 1732 and 1733)
  When to access professional assistance
  Close follow-up needs to be maintained so the patient has a person to call with questions.

Four to six weeks after diagnosis, the patient is usually ready for more in-depth education. More detail for patients on how to control their disease in usual and unusual circumstances, and how to follow a positive life-style. Suggested topics are listed in the box above.

Nurses need to work closely with the patient and family, to establish a rapport that encourages questions and the exchange of knowledge. Continuing diabetes education ensures maintenance of knowledge while facilitating information, recognizing technologic and other advances in diabetes care.

The need to carefully follow the prescribed regimen and avoid deviations (e.g. skipping medication) should also be emphasized. However, the nurse also discusses issues of patient nonadherence as a way of modifying the regimen to better suit patient needs. Evidence of nonadherence frequently means the regimen is based on inappropriate assessment information. It is often a symptom of the nurse and health care team's inadequate assessment, and therefore demands action and modification. Evidence of deviations from the regimen are carefully assessed and discussed with the patient.

Effective individual and family coping in diabetes must be promoted by first establishing a solid rapport with the patient and family. The need for counseling, based on the patient's perception of ability to manage diabetes in the home, work, or school environment should be assessed. The socioeconomic requirements are considered as a source of emotional and financial stress. Individualizing the regimen requirements to accommodate the psychosocial response of the patient and family is critical. Involving a social worker or psychologist as regular member of the health care team should also be encouraged by the nurse.

TOPICS FOR IN-DEPTH EDUCATION

Preventive health behaviors (e.g. eye care guidelines on p. 1746)
Updating nutritional concepts
Rationale and skills for monitoring blood glucose levels
Medications for control of blood glucose levels
Applying the exchange system of meal planning
Foot care
Recognition, treatment, and prevention of acute complications
Diabetes and exercise
Management of diabetes during short-term illness
Eating away from home
Using food labels for food selection
Modifying fat intake
Outlook for long-term complications
Planning for special occasions
Use of health care systems
Community resources
New technologies

PATIENT EDUCATION GUIDE   *How to Inject Insulin*

The nurse should provide the patient with the following instructions.

How to fill the syringe

1. In preparation for drawing and injecting insulin, gather all the supplies you will need: alcohol swab (or alcohol and cotton), syringe, and insulin bottle(s). Wash your hands thoroughly.
2. Mix the insulin by slowly rolling the bottle between your hands. *Never* shake the bottle; shaking causes air bubbles to form.
3. Clean the rubber stopper on the insulin bottle with an alcohol swab. Follow steps for *one* or *two* insulins.

If you are using only one *kind of insulin*

1. Draw *air* into the syringe by pulling out the plunger to the dose of insulin used.
2. Insert the needle into the rubber stopper and push in the plunger.

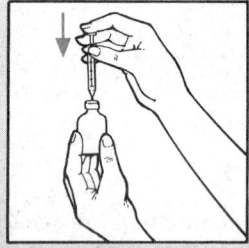

3. Turn over the bottle, with the syringe, and slowly pull the plunger down about 10 units past your dose (the extra units make adjusting the dose easier).

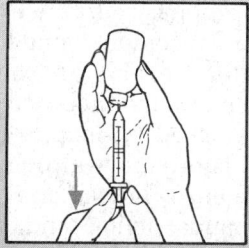

4. To remove air bubbles, flick or tap the syringe at the bubbles. When the bubbles go to the top of the syringe, push the plunger tip up to your exact dose. If bubbles remain, push the plunger until they disappear into the bottle. Then slowly pull back the plunger to your correct dose.

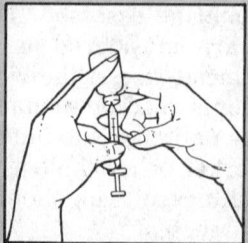

5. When the bubbles are gone and your dose is correct, remove the syringe from the upside-down bottle. Replace the cap to protect the needle. Place the syringe on a flat surface until ready to use.

If you are mixing two *kinds of insulin*

Remember to draw the *shorter-acting insulin* first. This is to avoid contaminating the vial and, thus, slowing the action time of future doses. You rely on the speedy action of short-acting insulin to combat high blood glucose levels quickly. Contaminating one insulin with another can alter the action of the contaminated insulin.

1. Draw air into the syringe by pulling the plunger out to the dose of your *longer-acting (cloudy)* insulin. Insert the needle into the *upright* bottle of *cloudy* insulin. Inject the air by pushing the plunger. Pull the needle out of the bottle without drawing up the insulin. (Keep the plunger down.)
2. Draw up air to equal the dose of the *short-acting (clear)* insulin. Insert the needle into the bottle of *short-acting* insulin and push down on the plunger to inject the air into the bottle.

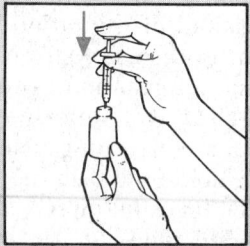

3. Turn over the bottle and syringe and slowly pull the plunger back to draw up the *short-acting* insulin plus 10 extra units. Remove air bubbles as directed in Step 4 under previous heading.

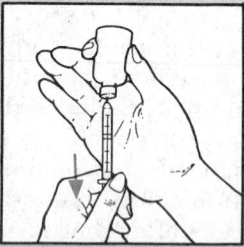

4. Adjust to the desired amount of short-acting insulin. Withdraw the needle.

PATIENT EDUCATION GUIDE   *How to Inject Insulin—cont'd*

5. Insert the needle into the upside-down bottle of *longer-acting* insulin and *slowly* draw out *only* the required dose. Do *not* pull out any extra units or you may contaminate the bottle when adjusting the dose. *The total amount of insulin in the syringe should equal the short-acting plus the longer-acting dose.* If you see air bubbles now, start over with a new syringe.

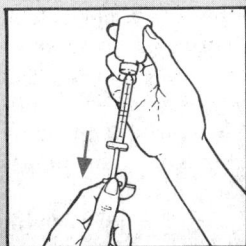

Remove the syringe from the bottle, cap the needle, and place the syringe on a flat surface until ready to use.

Six Steps of Injection

1. Prepare the injection site by cleansing with alcohol, Betadine or soap and water.
2. Carefully pick up the syringe and, with your free hand, pinch a 1- to 2-inch fold of skin between your thumb and forefinger. (When using your upper arm, a one-handed operation, pinch the skin by rolling your arm against the back of a chair or the edge of a table.)

3. Hold the syringe like a pencil and, using a dart-throwing kind of motion, insert the needle quickly into the skin.
4. The angle of the injection depends on how much fatty tissue you have. If you can pinch more than an inch, you can safely inject straight in at a 90-degree angle. Inject at a 45-degree angle if you have less than an inch of skin when you pinch.

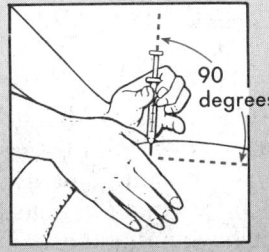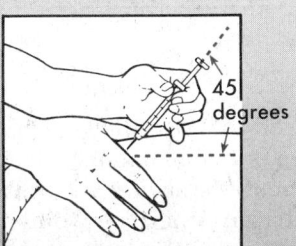

5. Inject the insulin. After completing the injection, pull the needle out quickly and immediately cover the site with cotton. Apply slight pressure for 5 to 8 seconds. *Do not rub.* Rubbing can cause too rapid absorption and may irritate the skin.

Replace the protective needle cover and follow the manufacturer's instructions for sterilizing glass syringes or destroying disposables to prevent their misuse.

The young adult

The diabetic adult is generally responsible for self-management. Often, the decisions he or she faces, including employment and personal relationships, are influenced by diabetes. Most jobs are open to diabetic individuals, although discrimination has been reported. Those who enter adulthood already diagnosed with diabetes mellitus should seek employment that does not require the operation of heavy equipment, driving long distances, or construction. Newly diagnosed individuals may have to change employment, which further contributes to the stress of the disease.

Patients who have adapted to their disease often continue to meet the challenges posed by normal growth and development. This includes establishing intimate relationships and perhaps starting a family. Those not adapting well may not have the confidence to establish such relationships.[11,41,56,66]

The elderly

Noninsulin-dependent diabetes mellitus is common in the elderly population. It is almost ten times as common among those over age 65 as those in the 20 to 44 age group. Based on the National Health Interview Survey (NHIS) data, it was estimated that from 1986 to 1988, 9.6% of all people in the United States over age 65 were diagnosed with diabetes. Alternately, roughly 43% of all people in the United States who were diagnosed with diabetes between 1986 and 1988 are over age 65. The NHIS data from

ETHICAL ISSUES

- Do individuals have a moral duty to take care of themselves in the best possible way?
- Should patients be given the authority to define the "best possible way?" Or should that be a professional definition?
- Should diabetic patients be encouraged to set their own parameters within which they will attempt to maintain control? Or should the disease management parameters be established by professionals, with patients considered noncompliant if they remain outside of them?

GERIATRIC CONSIDERATIONS

Diabetes

1. When compared with persons of the same age without diabetes, those with diabetes are 25 times more likely to be blind, 17 times more likely to develop kidney disease, 20 times more likely to develop gangrene, 15 times more likely to require an amputation and twice as likely to have a cerebrovascular accident or myocardial infarction. Older adults have a 70% higher rate of hospitalization.
2. Symptoms in older adults are often masked by other illnesses and present atypically. Urinary incontinence may mask polyuria, hunger is blunted by medication, and fatigue and weight loss often gradually occur. Adrenergic symptoms of hypoglycemia may be blunted or absent.
3. Assess for cognitive impairments which may cause inconsistent medication administration or erratic eating patterns.
4. Eating patterns can be variable in the elderly. When insulin is required, plan the dose to fit the patient's usual eating habits.
5. Accommodate visual or other sensory defects when modifying for functional limitations.
6. Diabetes is an expensive disease. Insurance coverage and cost of supplies must be considered.

1980 to 1987 showed that the prevalence of diabetes is higher among blacks than whites, with black females showing a rate twice that of white females. African American women over age 75 had the highest rate with almost one in four having diabetes.

Hospitalization rates and the rates for nursing home admissions are noted to be significantly higher for people with diabetes when compared with those without diabetes. Diabetes is the fifth ranking cause of death and reduces the life expectancy of men by 9 years and women by 7 years. Diabetes is especially serious in young persons. When one compares persons of the same age without diabetes, those with diabetes are 25 times more likely to become blind, 17 times more likely to develop kidney disease, 20 times more likely to develop gangrene, 15 times more likely to require an amputation, and twice as likely to have a cerebrovascular accident or myocardial infarction.

Diabetes often presents atypically in older adults. The classic symptoms of hyperglycemia in younger adults are polyuria, polydipsia, and polyphagia. These symptoms may be masked by other illnesses or entirely absent in older adults. For example, detection of polyuria may be confounded by urinary incontinence. Hunger and thirst may be blunted by the side effects of medication. Weight loss is sometimes profound but may be so gradual that it goes unnoticed for several years. Complications of diabetes, such as hyperglycemic hyperosmolar nonketotic coma, are relatively rare. However, efficient diagnosis and treatment to reduce mortality are often confounded by atypical presentations and the existence of other medical problems (see Table 62-6).[14]

Many elderly patients can be managed with dietary or oral hypoglycemic agent interventions. Regular opportunities for discussion of therapeutic management are as important for the elderly as they are for the young patient. Emphasis on lifetime manage-

ment is needed. The aging person must deal with a number of body changes that may contribute to loss in functional ability. The elderly person diagnosed with diabetes may view the disease as another assault on self-esteem or perceive it as making him or her useless. Such a diagnosis may enhance a sense of loneliness, especially in early widowhood, and result in accumulated or unresolved grief. Economic factors may contribute to the stress associated with disease diagnosis. It is critical to diabetes care to avoid stereotyping all elderly people as impaired. Careful assessment, education, and support are particularly needed in diagnosis of the elderly. The ability to comply with needed management is critical, so significant others might also be included to assist with regimen activities as needed.

Documentation

The documentation includes:
1. The patient's knowledge of pathophysiology; this must include patient understanding of the interaction of exercise, diet, and medication. Emphasis on lifetime management is needed.

TABLE 62-6	Hyperglycemic Hyperosmolar Nonketotic Coma	

History/symptoms	Signs	Treatment
Complains of fatigue, weakness	Orthostatic hypotension	Rehydration
Caretakers note confusion, lethargy or un-responsiveness	Tachycardia	Insulin
	Dry skin, tenting	Correct electrolytes and serum pH
Recent infection or other illness/injury		
	Poor skin turgor	
33% deny history of diabetes mellitus		Treat underlying problem
	Cold extremities	
	Glucose >600 mg/dL	
	Serum osmolarity >320 mOsm/L	

From Haire-Joshu D: *Management of diabetes mellitus: perspectives of care across the lifespan*, St Louis, 1992, Mosby–Year Book.

2. The patient's understanding of medication with name, dosage, care of insulin, expiration date, time of insulin action, and side effects; an evaluation of the patient's ability to self-administer the drug is noted.
3. The patient's knowledge and verbalization of how to manage acute diabetic complications; the causes, symptoms, treatment, and materials received by the patient concerning this is documented.
4. The patient's performance of monitoring techniques; including method and type of testing equipment, frequency, the recording, and patient interpretation of results.
5. Note the discharge activities, including dietary plan; the equipment and materials with which the patient was sent home; any written directions or pamphlets given to the patient and family; follow-up appointments or referrals; any special insulin devices (i.e. magnifiers for poor vision); and any other special services recommended to the patient.

Ongoing Care

The management of diabetes mellitus does not end when the patient is discharged from the hospital. In fact, the vast majority of diabetes care, including initiation of insulin therapy, occurs in an outpatient setting. This means that the nurse needs to encourage communication among a variety of health care agencies to ensure optimal patient care.

The use of community agencies should include the involvement of public health nurses on an as needed basis. The community health nurse is in a position to assess the patient in the home environment. This enables more accurate information that can be used to better tailor the regimen to meet individual needs. In addition, social workers can be very helpful in terms of counseling or assisting with identifying available financial aids to deal with the expense of diabetes mellitus. The cost of medication and materials is prohibitive to many patients. The availability of financial assistance is of critical concern to the patient and will have a major impact on adherence to the regimen. Psychologic or counseling services should also be identified so referrals can be made accordingly.

The patient always needs to have a 24-hour contact with a health care professional regarding the illness. This can be with a physician's office or a local hospital information service. Such contact increases the possibility of dealing with diabetic problems before they become severe, such as DKA, discussed below.

Other resources that need to be developed, and to which the patient should be referred, include local support groups sponsored by organizations concerned with diabetes care. Some of these organizations include the American Diabetes Association and the Joslin Diabetes Center. Many local hospitals and health care agencies offer diabetes support groups for patients and their families. Such resources should not be overlooked and should in fact be identified and cultivated.

Acute Complications of Diabetes

DIABETIC KETOACIDOSIS
Etiology/Epidemiology

Diabetic ketoacidosis (DKA) develops as a result of severe insulin deficiency and excess levels of the counterregulatory hormones. The cardinal symptoms of this disorder are hyperglycemia (elevated blood glucose > 350 mg/dL), elevated ketone levels, and acidosis (plasma bicarbonate < 9.0 mEq/L). The incidence of DKA generally results from undiagnosed diabetes and inadequacy of prescribed medication and dietary therapies. Physical stress, such as trauma, surgery, or illness, can also result in DKA. As of 1987 in the United States 110,000 people were hospitalized with DKA. The relative risk of developing DKA in those with diagnosed diabetes is higher in African Americans and has shown steady increase since 1980. However, mortality rates have declined during this same period.[9,12] The initial diagnosis of IDDM occurs as DKA in 25% of cases.[15,58]

Pathophysiology

DKA is the occurrence of ketoacidosis secondary to diabetes mellitus. Ketoacidosis is the result of insufficient cellular glucose utilization, intense lipolysis, and accelerated hepatic ketogenesis. As a result of insulin deficiency, plasma glucose, fatty acids, ketone, and hydrogen ion levels increase. This is because of increased gluconeogenesis from amino acids and glycogenolysis in the liver. At the same time, glucose uptake by insulin-sensitive tissues (i.e., muscle and adipose tissues) is diminished, resulting in hyperglycemia. This elevated glucose level results in water moving from the intracellular to the extracellular compartment. A dilutional hyponatremia results when the body then tries to compensate for this state by increasing water intake (polydipsia) and by excreting glucose by osmotic diuresis (polyuria). The diuresis results in increased loss of electrolytes (sodium, chloride, potassium). Insulin deficiency allows unrestrained lipolysis to occur, resulting in increased fatty acid production, and eventually in increased production of triglycerides. This large amount of fatty acids causes ketone bodies to accumulate in the absence of carbohydrate metabolism. The ketone bodies, in turn, mark an accumulation of hydrogen ions resulting in acidemia. The body also tries to adapt to elevated hydrogen ion levels via hyperventilation to lower P_{CO_2}. The body buffers excess hydrogen ions with bicarbonate and other buffering mechanisms and ultimately by excreting ketones via the kidney. A urine test showing heavy ketonuria is the result. A diagnosis of DKA is generally made if the patient's blood glucose level is > 350 mg/dL, bicarbonate level is less than 9 mg/L, and the pH is 7.2 or less, and plasma ketone levels are greater than 5 mmol/L.[12,30,66]

Complications and mortality

The most serious complications of DKA are the development of shock and coma. Each may lead to death. Delay in diagnosis or treatment may precipitate the likelihood of such an outcome. Currently,

TABLE 62-7 Common Presenting Symptoms and Signs in Diabetic Ketoacidosis

Symptoms	Signs
Nausea and vomiting	Tachycardia
Thirst and polyuria	Hypotension
Weakness and/or anorexia	Dehydration
Abdominal pain	Warm dry skin
Visual disturbances	Hyperventilation
Somnolence	Impaired consciousness/coma

the mortality rate for DKA is less than 5%. This decrease in mortality is attributable to the provision of optimal insulin, and successful fluid and electrolyte therapy during the early stages of DKA.[15,30]

Therapeutic Management

DKA syndrome consists of four abnormalities that must be corrected in a treatment program. These abnormalities are fluid depletion (resulting in dehydration), insulin deficiency (resulting in hyperglycemia), electrolyte depletion, and metabolic acidosis (resulting from an accumulation of hydrogen ions which are products of fat catabolism). Presenting signs and symptoms appear in Table 62-7. Treatment guidelines are given in the box on p. 1737.

NURSING MANAGEMENT OF THE PATIENT WITH DIABETIC KETOACIDOSIS
Assessment

Common symptoms of DKA should be documented; they appear in Table 62-7. Factors associated with diabetes, or related to the onset of diabetes (e.g., family history, recent flu-like symptoms, or infection), should be assessed.

Nursing Diagnosis

High risk for fluid volume deficit.
Altered patterns of urinary excretion due to DKA or hyperglycemia.
Anxiety.

Planning

- Correction of life-threatening abnormalities: dehydration, insulin and potassium deficiency.

CLINICAL PRESENTATION OF DIABETIC KETOACIDOSIS

Causes

Lack of adequate insulin

Incidental or minor factors may contribute, such as infections, cold, urinary tract infection

Major stresses associated with surgery, CVA, accident may precipitate

Signs and symptoms

Polydipsia, polyuria, weakness, malaise, nausea, abdominal pain

Symptoms may occur concurrently with other conditions (i.e. infections) and be difficult to distinguish

Without treatment, more classic symptoms appear, such as acetone odor on breath, Kussmaul's breathing, altered consciousness

Laboratory findings

Plasma glucose levels—350 to 1500 mg/dL

Ketonuria—large ketone bodies present

Venous blood pH—6.8 to 7.2

Serum bicarbonate—below 9 mEq/dL

Serum potassium (K)—results inversely proportional to pH

Treatment

Correct volume depletion—0.9% saline solution is generally used, because it is ideal for correcting extracellular fluid depletion

Follow-up fluids usually 0.45% saline and water

Administer intravenously via continuous, low-dose infusions

Generally 50 units regular in 500 mL normal saline or 1 unit/10 mL

Bolus IM or SC injections as needed hourly

Potassium replacement—loss of K^+ not reflected immediately in serum concentration and tends to change, depending on patient pH balance; frequent K^+ determinations are required

Administer for pH less than 7.0 mEq/L; initiate bicarbonate therapy very slowly and only in presence of severe acidosis

Follow-up care

Modify therapeutic regimen as needed to enhance adherence

Patient education regarding signs, symptoms, and treatment of preacidotic state (e.g., increase insulin, increase fluids, monitor)

Patient should be aware of available contact person for questions regarding diabetic illness

- Patient demonstrates adequate fluid volume and electrolyte balance.
- Patient demonstrates reduced anxiety level.
- Patient demonstrates effective coping skills.

Implementation

Carefully monitor the patient's fluid status. Fluid replacement, if late, leads to shock; if excessive, precipitates cardiac failure. Careful and frequent monitoring of blood glucose levels must be completed. Glucose may normalize quickly following IV insulin administration.

In addition, the nurse needs to be alert that:

- Glucose will be normalized more quickly than acidosis. Premature discontinuation of insulin may result in persistence and worsening of ketoacidosis.
- Too aggressive fluid replacement (particularly with isotonic saline) may induce congestive heart failure. Therefore, frequent auscultation of the lungs is mandatory.
- Nausea and vomiting from feeding the patient before gastric peristalsis has returned can result in aspiration pneumonia and further fluid and electrolyte imbalance. Therefore, solid foods are introduced cautiously.
- Hypoglycemia can occur if the insulin infusion is not supplemented with glucose when the blood glucose concentration is less than 300 mg/dL.
- Monitoring of potassium and bicarbonate replacement is critical. Assessment of mental status in light of possible cerebral edema, should be frequent and systematic.
- Monitoring of hourly output (should be at least 30 to 60 per hour) is crucial. Minimal output is reported to physician immediately.

Evaluation

Prompt and proper treatment of DKA should result in rapid resolution of the problem. Pursuit of the cause of DKA and intensive education to prevent further difficulties should be initiated.

Documentation

Careful documentation of the patient's mental status, as well as fluid and electrolyte status, must be maintained.

HYPERGLYCEMIC HYPEROSMOLAR NONKETOTIC COMA

Hyperglycemic hyperosmolar nonketotic coma (HHNK) is an often deadly complication of diabetes, distinguished by severe hyperglycemia, plasma hyperosmolality, dehydration, changed mental status, and lack of ketoacidosis. Serum sodium may be normal or low. Most patients are elderly, over age 60, and have a history of NIDDM. A sizeable minority are undiagnosed and/or untreated. Persons who are chronically ill, debilitated, have mild renal insufficiency, or lack either normal thirst mechanisms or access to water are at risk for developing HHNK. Acute conditions, such as surgery, cardiovascular diseases, etc., may precipitate HHNK. HHNK develops more insidiously than DKA. It is frequently associated with frank coma and other CNS symptoms. Treatment stresses fluid replacement and careful potassium and insulin therapy along the same protocols as DKA therapy. Mortality is around 40% to 50%, with death usually the result of shock or pulmonary embolus.[30]

NURSING MANAGEMENT OF THE PATIENT WITH HYPERGLYCEMIC HYPEROSMOLAR NONKETOTIC COMA
Assessment

A thorough history and physical assessment, with careful review of laboratory tests, is needed. This information is used not only for purposes of differentiation of diagnosis, but also serves as a baseline assessment. This is imperative given the rapid changes in clinical course which can result from either diagnosis.

Nursing Diagnosis

High risk for fluid volume deficit.
Knowledge deficit regarding diabetes care.
Altered health maintenance.

Planning

- The patient will maintain normal bicarbonate, potassium, and pH levels.
- The patient will maintain normal blood glucose levels.
- The patient will verbalize diabetes education survival skills.
- The patient will verbalize appropriate steps to take to avoid further problems related to diabetes.

Implementation

Provide an overview of diabetes and discuss the importance of routine diabetes care and careful monitoring of status (e.g. SMBG). Review medication and dietary plans with the patient, providing written materials and follow-up teaching as needed. Carefully review symptoms of acute complications including HHNK. Provide guidelines for the patient regarding contact with the diabetes health care team.

Evaluation

The patient verbally describes the diabetes management plan and discusses steps to take for acute illnesses.

HYPOGLYCEMIA (DIABETIC)
Definition

Episodes of low blood glucose levels or hypoglycemia caused by insulin constitute a major problem in the treatment of diabetes mellitus. This differs from hypoglycemia caused by organic, mechanical, or factitious reasons discussed later in the chapter. If euglycemia or metabolic control is to be attained, occasional mild hypoglycemic reactions are to be expected. However, episodes of severe hypoglycemia (e.g., coma, seizure, loss of consciousness) are *never* acceptable and must be avoided. Such attacks pose a serious health threat as well as psychosocial difficulties associated with employment problems or embarrassment.

COMMON CAUSES OF HYPOGLYCEMIA

Insulin errors (inadvertent or deliberate)
- reversal of morning and evening dosage
- reversal of short- and intermediate-acting insulin
- improper timing of insulin in relation to food
- excessive insulin dosage

Erratic or altered absorption of insulin
- more rapid absorption from exercising limbs
- unpredictable absorption from hypertrophied injection sites

Use of more purified insulin preparations or change from mixed species to single species or humulin insulin

Doses of oral hypoglycemic agents that are too high for need

Diet
- omitted or inadequate amounts of food
- timing errors: late snacks or meals

Exercise
- unplanned activity
- prolonged duration or increased intensity of activity

Alcohol and drugs
- impaired hepatic gluconeogenesis associated with alcohol intake
- impaired mentation associated with alcohol, marijuana, and cocaine

Etiology

Causes for hypoglycemic reactions are summarized in the box on p. 1738 and include delayed meals or lack of necessary amounts of food. Other causes include administration of excessive insulin or oral hypoglycemic agents and vomiting associated with illness or strenuous exercise, which may potentiate the effect of insulin. In particular, injection of insulin into an area that is to be exercised, facilitating absorption, may encourage a rapid fall in the blood glucose level. In some cases, the reaction may occur when the blood glucose level is still within normal limits. This usually occurs when the blood glucose level has decreased rapidly from a higher level, thus initiating the hypoglycemic symptoms despite a normal blood glucose level.

Clinical Manifestations

Signs and symptoms of insulin reactions vary among individuals, but are generally consistent for each person. Signs and symptoms usually progress through two stages: the adrenal and the cerebral stages. The adrenal stage occurs with the release of epinephrine; without adequate treatment, the patient progresses to the cerebral stage of hypoglycemia. In general, signs and symptoms are associated with the two groups: those the patient recognizes and those that appear without any perceived symptoms (hypoglycemia unawareness).

Blood glucose levels may fall below 40 mg/dL, precipitating seizures, without the patient perceiving any symptomatology. This lack of ability to perceive hypoglycemia is usually seen in patients who have had IDDM for more than 10 years. It is suspected that this lack of ability to perceive symptoms is associated with neuropathic changes, lack of counterregulatory hormone response (defective glucagon and epinephrine secretion), and diminished cerebral function caused by neuroglucopenia.[47,59]

Therapeutic Management

Hypoglycemic reactions have potentially long-term physiologic and psychosocial effects. Therefore, measures designed to prevent such reactions should

be stressed as a major component of diabetes management (see box). Treatment of mild hypoglycemic reactions is generally simple, involving 5 to 15 g of carbohydrate. This can often take the form of sugar, candy (i.e., six to eight Lifesavers), or orange juice; in patients who cannot swallow, glucagon may be administered subcutaneously or intramuscularly (0.5 to 1.0 mg). Packaged tubes of decorative icing can also be squeezed into the cheek of the patient if semi-conscious. Intravenous glucose is also a possibility for hospitalized patients. A critical thinking guide is presented in Figure 62-6.

Somogyi effect

In cases where episodes of hypoglycemia occur, especially during the night, there is an increased possibility of "hyperglycemic rebound" or Somogyi effect. The Somogyi effect results from excessive insulin administration, which results in blood glucose fluctuations. The hypoglycemia provokes secretion of the insulin antagonists (i.e., catecholamines, glucagon) which, coupled with the intake of carbohydrate to combat symptoms of low blood sugar, results in hyperglycemia. Many of the hypoglycemic episodes occur during sleep. However, an early morning hyperglycemia then results. The patient then "chases" elevated morning blood glucose levels with increased insulin doses, which can lead to increased hypoglycemic episodes. Symptoms of the nocturnal reaction include mild morning ketonuria, glycosuria, and possible headache or lethargy. Careful monitoring of the blood glucose level at night or over a period of time may document such a phenomenon, so that the cause and appropriate adjustments in insulin or an evening snack can take place.

CLINICAL ALERT

Family members, coworkers, and significant others must be taught to treat hypoglycemia, since the patient may be incapable of instituting appropriate measures.

PREVENTING HYPOGLYCEMIA

Daily consistency in diet, exercise, and medication

Dietary management including between-meal and bedtime snacks

Extra food before exercise, as determined by pre-exercise blood glucose levels

Regular and frequent blood glucose monitoring and urine testing

Adjustment of insulin program to ensure appropriate type, dosage, and timing of insulin

Routine carrying of rapid absorbing carbohydrate

Availability of glucagon in the home and work settings

Instructing coworkers and teachers, as well as family members, how to treat an insulin reaction

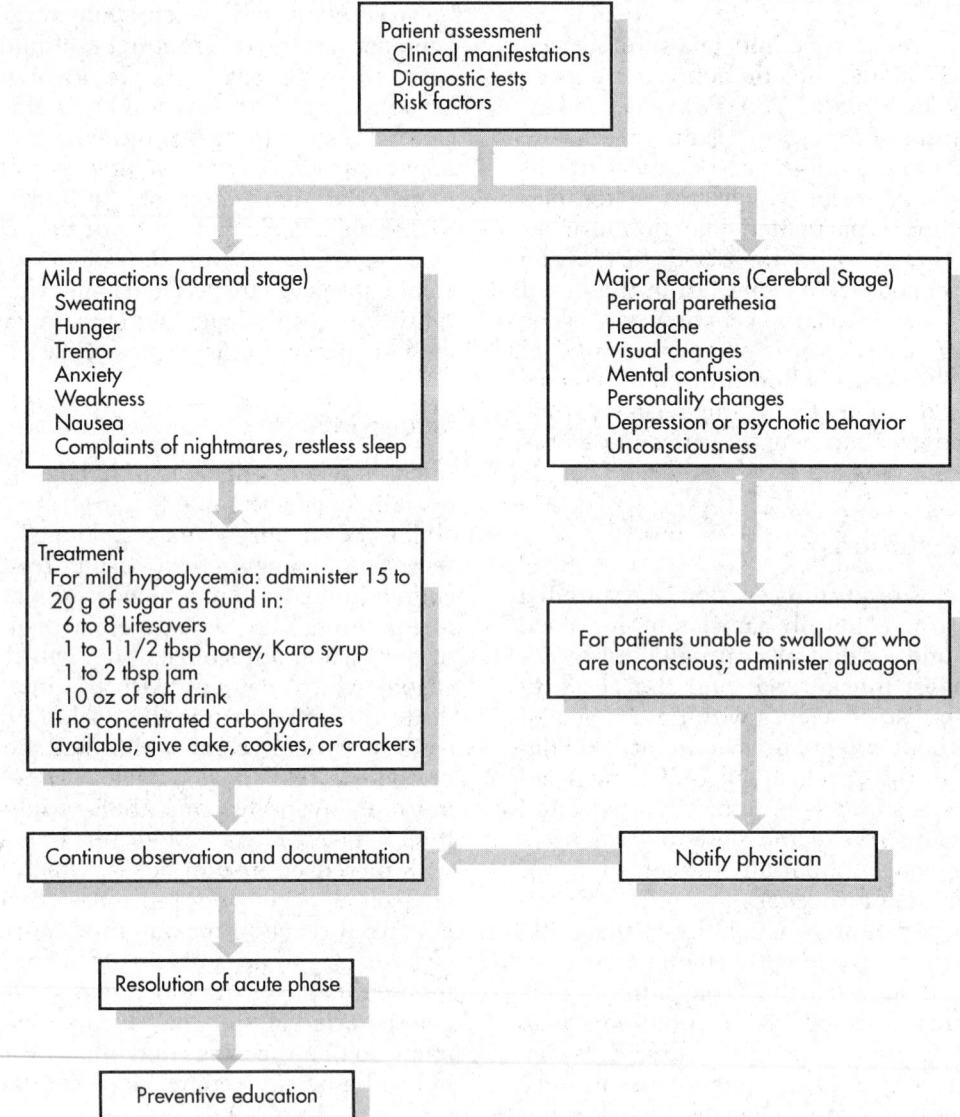

Patient assessment
Clinical manifestations
Diagnostic tests
Risk factors

Mild reactions (adrenal stage)
Sweating
Hunger
Tremor
Anxiety
Weakness
Nausea
Complaints of nightmares, restless sleep

Major Reactions (Cerebral Stage)
Perioral parethesia
Headache
Visual changes
Mental confusion
Personality changes
Depression or psychotic behavior
Unconsciousness

Treatment
For mild hypoglycemia: administer 15 to
20 g of sugar as found in:
6 to 8 Lifesavers
1 to 1 1/2 tbsp honey, Karo syrup
1 to 2 tbsp jam
10 oz of soft drink
If no concentrated carbohydrates
available, give cake, cookies, or crackers

For patients unable to swallow or who
are unconscious; administer glucagon

Continue observation and documentation

Notify physician

Resolution of acute phase

Preventive education

FIGURE 62-6   Critical Thinking Guide: the patient with hypoglycemia.

Dawn phenomenon

An elevation in blood glucose between 5:00 and 9:00 AM with no recorded episodes of nocturnal hypoglycemia is referred to as "dawn phenomenon." Although the cause of such activity is still being studied, the most popular belief is that such elevations result from a surge of cortisol or growth hormone.[54,57,61]

Brittle diabetes

Brittle diabetes can be characterized as rapid oscillations between hyperglycemia and hypoglycemia in the diabetic patient. In general, this patient is insulin dependent; however, patients with NIDDM might also present with "brittle" diabetes. Some of the more common causes and solutions associated with brittle diabetes are seen in the box on p. 1741.

Sick day

The key to good metabolic control is to balance nutrition, exercise, and medication for optimal maintenance of health. This goal can be achieved only when patients are prepared to manage their diabetes within the context of daily life. Factors such as illness can disrupt metabolic control. Even though food intake is diminished, insulin or oral agent dos-

BRITTLE DIABETES: CAUSES AND APPROACH

Causes	Approach
Overreliance on insulin preparations with broad activity peaks (i.e. 1 shot NPH)	Split and mixed insulin regimens allowing for a match between insulin requirements and availability
Variable time of insulin injection	Maintenance by the patient of a close log of timing of insulin injection in relation to meals, activity, and so on
Variations in insulin absorption	Patient demonstration of technique, emphasizing consistency in injection process
Variations in timing and amount of food eaten	Detailed diet history, suggesting causes of glycemic irregularities; emphasize consistency in amount and timing; avoid overtreatment of hypoglycemia
Disturbed glucose counterregulation	Set higher target glucose levels, encourage frequent SMBG
Altered insulin availability; insulin antibodies	Use highly purified or human insulins

ages must be taken or increased. It is important that patients be taught to take antidiabetic medications, because illness often elevates blood glucose.

NURSING MANAGEMENT OF THE PATIENT WITH DIABETIC HYPOGLYCEMIA

Assessment

The potential for the development of either acute or chronic complications in diabetes must be carefully scrutinized. Discuss the causes of acute complications (i.e., hyperglycemia, hypoglycemia) and ensure the patient and family's ability to manage. A discussion of terminologies, symptomatology, and treatment of hypoglycemia and hyperglycemia is needed. The importance of preventive measures associated with these occurrences is stressed.

The importance of early reporting of symptoms of any long-term complications (i.e. visual changes) should be emphasized. Preventive education in relation to macrovascular and microvascular disease should be a priority of care. Provide optimal health education that stresses appropriate dietary and exercise behaviors.

Nursing Diagnosis

Knowledge deficit related to diabetes self-management.
  High risk for injury.

Planning

• Patient demonstrates knowledge of relationship between nutrition, exercise, and medication.

• Patient demonstrates understanding of hyper- and hypoglycemia.
• Patient verbalizes appropriate steps to treatment of hypoglycemia.
• Patient demonstrates appropriate technique for self-monitoring of blood glucose (SMBG) and administration of insulin.
• Patient demonstrates appropriate steps for sick day management.

Implementation

Patient education is critical to the maintenance of normal blood glucose levels and the prevention of severe hypoglycemic episodes. Carefully assess and teach the patient about diabetes self-management including the causes of hypoglycemia as they relate to the individual. In addition, assist the patient in planning for the prevention of hypoglycemic episodes (e.g., if sleeping late, adjust p.m. insulin, appropriate planning and SMBG during exercise). Educate the patient and significant others regarding the use of glucagon. The nurse should see that every patient with diabetes mellitus has sick-day guidelines to follow. These guidelines need to address medication, diet, monitoring activities, and emergency measures as given in the patient education guide on p. 1742.

Evaluation

The patient discusses the components of therapeutic management in relation to diabetic control.

The patient records number of mild hypoglycemic episodes. Increases in such episodes should result in modification of the regimen.

PATIENT EDUCATION GUIDE *"Sick-Day" Management of Diabetes Mellitus*

"Sick" means having fever, vomiting, nausea, diarrhea, or congestion.

The nurse should provide the patient with the following instructions.

Insulin

If you take insulin shots, always take your insulin when you are sick, *even if you cannot eat your regular meals*. You may need extra insulin, for example:

1. If BG is 240-400 mg/dL add 2 to 4 units of regular insulin to the usual dose before meals and take the usual dose at bedtime.
2. If BG is 240-400 mg/dL and the urine is moderate to large for ketones, add 4 to 6 units of regular insulin to the usual dosage for *every* insulin dose until ketones are no longer moderate.

Medication

If you take a pill for diabetes, be sure to take it when you are sick. If vomiting, contact your physician or diabetes nurse educator.

Diet

If you are unable to eat your usual meals, try to drink fluids containing 10 g of carbohydrates every hour while awake. The following servings contain 10 g of carbohydrates:

½ cup ginger ale (not diet)
½ cup Coca-Cola (not diet)
½ cup chicken soup with noodles
¾ cup chilled Gatorade

If you *are able to eat* usual meals, then drink ½ cup of calorie-free fluid every hour while awake. The following are calorie-free:

Broth or bouillion
Decaffeinated tea
Sugar-free/caffeine-free soda, such as 7-Up or Sprite
Water

Urine/blood testing

Check your urine for ketones/acetone and check your blood glucose level every 4 hours

Seek professional advice if you have any of the following:

Diarrhea or vomiting for more than 6 hours
Moderate or large levels of ketones (++ or +++) in your urine even after two injections of regular insulin as instructed
Your blood tests for glucose are over 400 or urine tests for glucose are 2% to 5% even after two injections of regular insulin as instructed

---

The patient notifies the health care provider of any episodes of severe hypoglycemia requiring the use of glucagon.

The patient notifies the health care provider of acute illnesses which impact diabetes control.

Documentation

Careful documentation is needed of patterns of dietary intake, SMBG technique, blood glucose levels, activity, injection technique, and hypoglycemic episodes.

SURGERY IN DIABETES

Surgery in diabetic patients has all of the problems associated with surgery in general, plus the additional care needed to ensure the optimal physical condition of the patient. Preoperative management focuses on satisfactory control of the metabolic state, nutritional support, treatment of anemia, diagnosis and treatment of complicating diseases, and adequate hydration and electrolyte balance. Insulin-dependent patients (with IDDM or NIDDM) should be well-controlled for at least 7 days before their major surgery. The procedure of choice is to get a fasting blood glucose level the morning of surgery and, based on readings, begin the patient on an intravenous insulin drip. The blood glucose level should be monitored closely during and after the procedure. Because alterations in potassium levels are common, the fluid and electrolyte balance is strictly monitored.

Postoperative management encourages adequate wound healing, avoidance of cardiorespiratory problems, maintenance of adequate metabolic control, maintenance of adequate elimination, decreased risk of infection, and avoidance of neuropathic disorders that may compromise cardiopulmonary function during and after surgery. In patients with good metabolic control, wounds heal at the same rate as in nondiabetic patients. Optimal cardiorespiratory status can be promoted by good nursing care, such as patient mobilization, coughing, deep breathing exercises, spirometry, and chest physical therapy.[30,58]

In terms of diabetes management, care should be taken to avoid hypoglycemic episodes. Monitoring food intake is one means to avoid hypoglycemia. Intravenous dextrose can be used to supplement inadequate intake. Finally, since urinary bladder stasis occurs commonly in patients with long-term diabetes, careful monitoring of output is imperative. If the patient demonstrates frequency in voiding with small amounts, neuropathic bladder should be suspected.

NURSING MANAGEMENT OF THE PATIENT UNDERGOING SURGERY FOR DIABETES

Nursing Diagnosis

Altered fluid and electrolyte status.
    Infection related to surgery planning.

Planning

• Patient describes preoperative and postoperative procedures related to diabetes.

Implementation

Surgical procedures in diabetes demand that the nurse carefully maintain optimal aseptic technique. Before any procedure, the patient and family should receive extensive preoperative and postoperative teaching so that their cooperation is ensured. Awareness by the patient of symptoms that should be reported encourages quick response. Following surgery, strict measurement of intake and output and careful review of laboratory studies with emphasis on the blood glucose level is needed. A thorough nursing assessment is required, because symptoms of DKA or other acute aspects of poor control may have a short onset.

    Maintenance of appropriate fluids, with glucose-insulin-electrolyte solutions and potassium replace-ments, requires close bedside and laboratory monitoring. Strict aseptic techniques to promote healing and avoid infection are also observed. During recovery, resumption of oral feedings requires close scrutiny of blood glucose levels with further adjustment of insulin as needed.

Chronic Complications: Microvascular Disease

Long-term complications of diabetes mellitus are associated with the development of microvascular and macrovascular disease. Generally, eye and renal diseases predominate in patients diagnosed early in life (i.e. IDDM), whereas atherosclerotic diseases are more common in those later diagnosed (i.e. NIDDM).[15,44,52,66]

    One explanation for the development of diabetic complications may be the failure to normalize blood glucose. The degree of hyperglycemia over the years is related to increased risk and severity of diabetic complications. The Diabetes Control and Complications Trial (DCCT), a landmark multicenter trial completed in 1993, established the benefit of euglycemia, achieved through intensive therapy, in delaying the onset and progression of diabetic complications.

    An additional factor being studied as a possible contributor to complication development is genetic susceptibility. Although it is still controversial, susceptibility does help explain the conflict associated with metabolic control and complication development (Figure 62-7).[35]

    The **diabetic triopathy** includes the most frequently occurring complications of diabetes mellitus. These include retinopathy, nephropathy, and neuropathy. The main degenerative changes in dia-

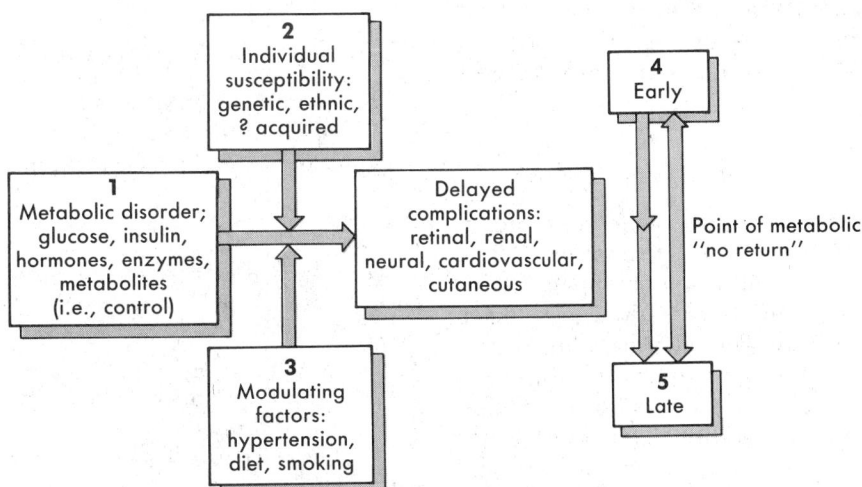

FIGURE 62-7 Etiology of diabetic complications.

betes occur because of a thickening of the capillary basement membrane. This thickened membrane, a characteristic lesion of microvascular disease, becomes weakened, more permeable, and structurally deficient. Another factor may be the effects of sorbitol in target tissues. During periods of chronic hyperglycemia, excess glucagon is converted to sorbitol, causing increased osmotic tonicity, cellular swelling, and diminished function. This sorbitol pathway is seen as a component in the development of complications. Changes in platelet adhesiveness have been found in persistent hyperglycemia, affecting coagulation and the cellular membrane. Because each of these changes are associated with chronic hyperglycemia, the degree of diabetic control may be related to the incidence and the severity of complications, although this has yet to be conclusively determined.[15,58]

RETINOPATHY

Diabetic **retinopathy** is a microvascular disease that results from microvascular occlusion, and is the leading cause of new blindness among Americans between the ages of 20 and 64. Diabetic retinopathy alone accounts for 12% of new cases of blindness annually.[9] Over the past 30 to 35 years, the prevalence of blindness from diabetic retinopathy has increased because of the lengthening life span of the diabetic patients. About 50% of patients with IDDM will develop retinopathy 7 to 10 years after diagnosis, with 95% having some form of retinopathy after 15 years. In NIDDM patients, the onset of retinopathy is less readily defined, and many manifest retinopathy at the time of diagnosis. However, it is also noted that in many of these cases, the patient is believed to have been glucose intolerant for years before being diagnosed.[44,64,66]

The presence of macular edema has been thought of as a manifestation of retinopathy in NIDDM. The presence of macular edema in IDDM suggests progressing disease not as responsive to treatment. Macular and generalized retinal edema also suggest renal disease.

Pathophysiology

There are five clinical pathologic processes recognized in diabetic retinopathy: (1) formation of microaneurysms (capillary wall outpouchings); (2) increased vascular permeability of retinal capillaries and arterioles; (3) closure of retinal capillaries and arterioles; (4) proliferation of new vessels; and (5) contraction of vitreous and fibrous glial proliferation with retinal detachment resulting. These processes are described clinically as nonproliferative, preproliferative (PPDR), and proliferative (PDR) retinopathy.[58,66]

Nonproliferative retinopathy

The hallmark of diabetic retinopathy is the capillary microaneurysm. The microaneurysm is an outpouching of the capillary wall that is seen through an ophthalmascope as a small, discrete dot, and is regarded as the first clinical sign of retinal involvement. Intraretinal hemorrhages and exudates also make up background diabetic retinopathy. These lesions result from either leakage of red blood cells or other blood components from microaneurysms or a weakened vasculature. Hard or waxy exudates appear yellow-white and resemble discrete deposits on the retina around the macula. Such exudates are the sign of a leaky capillary bed and, when found around the macula, are often called "diabetic maculopathy."

Preproliferative retinopathy

Preproliferative retinopathy is a special category of nonproliferative disease in which certain clinical findings (venous dilation, and intraretinal microvascular abnormalities) suggest the condition will advance to the next stage within 24 months. Clinical manifestations of this stage include presence of venous beading, large retinal blot hemorrhages, nerve fiber infarcts (also termed cotton wool spots), and intraretinal microvascular abnormalities.

Proliferative retinopathy

As the circulation in the retinal vessels becomes more stagnant, blood is shunted away from localized retinal areas. This results in further hypoxia, ischemia, and infarction. This new vascularization encourages abnormal vessel growth, which is dangerous because such new vessels are prone to bleeding, especially if the vitreous contracts. Patients may experience a major retinal hemorrhage, resulting in sudden and painful visual loss.[41,66]

Therapeutic Management

Photocoagulation, also called laser therapy, is an effective treatment of diabetic retinopathy. Photocoagulation often involves panretinal treatment that

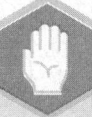

CLINICAL ALERT

Retinopathy is best treated before symptoms develop. The nurse arranges for patient consultation with an ophthalmologist for all diabetic patients and encourages patient follow-through on an annual basis.

places burns in a grid pattern across the eye while avoiding the macula and vital structures. Focal treatment is completed on the new vessel growth, sealing the vessels from leakage. Photocoagulation can reduce the risk of severe visual loss by about 60%, and is used to stop neovascularization before recurrent hemorrhages into the vitreous cause irreparable damage. Because of the risks associated with photocoagulation, only one eye at a time is treated, unless high-risk characteristics develop. Patients with high-risk proliferative diabetic retinopathy should receive immediate laser photocoagulation.

A second major advance in diabetic retinopathy has been the development of vitreous surgery. Removal of the blood-filled vitreous by suction through a small incision maintains the integrity of the eye, results in the removal of opacities, and releases the traction on the retina caused by proliferative vessel growth that causes retinal detachment. Those with severe visual impairment may be restored to sight with this method. Vitrectomy is an effective but risk-laden procedure with visual loss resulting from associated surgical complications.[41,64]

OTHER EYE DISORDERS

Persons with diabetes mellitus are subject to visual difficulties, including transitory refractive changes and cataracts.

Diabetic patients with transitory refractive changes have rapid changes in visual acuity on a hourly or daily basis. Although the cause of the disturbance is unclear, it is thought to be related to a variation in lens water content. Myopia is associated with marked hyperglycemia, whereas hyperopia is noted as blood sugar levels normalize. These changes are not serious and will subside, but are frustrating to the patient.

Cataracts are more common in persons with diabetes than in those without diabetes. There are two types of cataracts found in diabetes: metabolic cataracts and senile cataracts. Metabolic cataracts may develop at any age. They typically occur in newly diagnosed patients, commonly in very young children and disappear spontaneously when blood glucose control is attained. Senile cataracts occur with higher incidence and at an earlier age in diabetics than in persons without diabetes. Treatment is the same as for the nondiabetic patient (see Chapter 53).

NURSING MANAGEMENT OF THE PATIENT WITH DIABETIC EYE DISEASE
Assessment

Numerous epidemiologic studies have suggested that diabetic retinopathy and macular edema are associated with poor glycemic control and hyperten-

sion. The nurse works systematically with persons with diabetes to achieve optimal blood pressure and blood glucose control. While diabetic eye disease cannot be prevented, steps can be taken to assure early detection and treatment, as well as consistent follow-up. Nurses need to educate patients regarding these eye care principles and assist the patient as an advocate in the health care system.

Nursing Diagnosis

Knowledge deficit related to prevention of visual complications.
   Health seeking behaviors: routine eye care.

Planning

• The patient needs to be aware of principles of eye care and assure follow-up care.

Implementation

Teaching in accordance with the guidelines noted in the box on p. 1746 is recommended.

Evaluation

Monitor patient status regarding eye care at each visit.

DIABETIC NEPHROPATHY

Kidney involvement **(nephropathy)** is another microvascular complication of diabetes mellitus. Renal failure occurs in 46% of patients who develop diabetes before age 20, and in 6% with onset after age 40. Renal failure accounts for about 50% of deaths in patients who have had diabetes for 10 to 20 years. In adults who develop NIDDM, the incidence of nephropathy is approximately 3%.[15,48,58]

During the first few years after overt diabetic symptoms develop, the basement membrane of glomerular capillaries begins to thicken with a distinctive lesion that was first described in 1956 by Kimmelstiel and Wilson.[9] The earliest clinical change is an increased glomerular filtration rate that is reversible with adequate blood glucose control. Intermittent proteinuria, often evoked by physical activity, occurs and becomes persistent over time. After 15 years of diagnosed diabetes, almost one third of all IDDM patients will have persistent proteinuria. NIDDM patients tend to manifest proteinuria sooner than 15 years; however, this may be caused by years of undiagnosed diabetes.[25]

Nephropathy and retinopathy develop simultaneously in 25% to 30% of patients. This association is so well documented that, in the absence of retinopathy, it is doubtful as to whether there is a dia-

PATIENT EDUCATION GUIDE
Eye Care

Inform patients with diabetes that:

- sight-threatening eye disease is a common complication of diabetes mellitus and is often present even with good vision
- early detection and appropriate treatment of diabetic eye disease greatly reduces the risk of visual loss

People between 12 and 30 yr of age with diagnosis of diabetes mellitus of at least 5 yr duration should have a baseline ophthalmic examination including:

- history of visual symptoms
- measurement of visual acuity and intraocular pressure
- ophthalmoscopic examination through dilated pupils

People >30 yr of age should have baseline ophthalmic examinations, as specified in above, at the time of diagnosis of diabetes.

After the initial eye examination, people with diabetes mellitus should receive annual exams unless more frequent exams are indicated.

Women with insulin-dependent diabetes mellitus who are planning pregnancy within 12 mo should be examined by an ophthalmologist.

Those who become pregnant should have an examination for retinopathy by an ophthalmologist in the first trimester and thereafter at the discretion of the ophthalmologist.

Patients should be referred to the care of an ophthalmologist for:

- unexplained visual symptoms
- deterioration in visual acuity
- increased intraocular pressure
- any retinal abnormality
- any other ocular pathology that threatens vision

Patients should be referred to the care of a retinal specialist or other ophthalmologist for the following:

- preproliferative retinopathy
- proliferative retinopathy
- macular edema

Patients with functionally decreased visual acuity should undergo low-vision evaluation and rehabilitation

Laser photocoagulation therapy reduces the risk of visual loss and is generally effective in preventing blindness. Vitrectomy can restore vision in certain patients with diabetic eye disease.

CLINICAL ALERT

Radiologic procedures using dye contrast agents are associated with increased incidence of renal failure in diabetic patients.

betic precipitor to the patient's kidney disease.[48,58,62,63]

Pathophysiology

Diabetic nephropathy progresses through several phases. In the early (asymptomatic) stage, it is possible to identify renal abnormalities that may have begun very early in the diabetic process. Three changes that occur soon after diagnosis are hyperfiltration, nephromegaly, and microalbuminuria. Hyperfiltration, an elevated glomerular filtration rate (GFR), occurs in up to 40% of patients several months to years after diagnosis. Improved control of diabetes mellitus can sometimes improve GFR. Nephromegaly, an increase in renal volume, is not affected by metabolic control. Microalbuminuria, a subclinical rise in urinary albumin excretion rate, may be reduced by improved control. During this stage, which may last for 15 to 20 years, patients should be informed about the possibility of developing renal disease and about possible preventive measures, such as achieving optimal metabolic control and low-protein diets. Predisposing factors, such as hypertension and infection, should be vigorously treated.[37,62,63]

The transition from early, subclinical signs of renal disease is marked by the onset of clinical proteinuria and a falling GFR. During this clinical stage, proteinuria becomes constant and heavy. Plasma creatinine levels also begin to rise. The GFR declines linearly over time, with the rate of decline varying extensively. For example, patients may enter end-stage disease within 2 to 20 years after proteinuria is diagnosed. Anemia develops when renal function drops to 25% of normal. Anemia occurs when the erythropoietic effect on the bone marrow is inhibited because of retained nitrogenous wastes. Deficient blood clotting may also result. As renal failure develops, close monitoring of developing hypertension is imperative.[37,48,58]

Indications for Dialysis and Transplantation

End-stage renal disease is the natural course of declining function. End-stage renal disease is imminent when the serum creatinine level reaches 0.3 mg/mL. The results of such findings leave two options available: dialysis or transplantation (see Chapter 42).

NURSING MANAGEMENT OF THE PATIENT WITH DIABETIC NEPHROPATHY

Assessment

A careful review of the patient's clinical status, especially in regard to renal history, needs to be conducted. This includes review of routine urinalysis for presence of bacteria or white blood cells, annual review of urinary albumia and serum creatinine. Abnormal results, especially in conjunction with hypertension, suggest the need for referral to specialists.

Nursing Diagnosis

High risk for fluid volume alternations.

High risk for altered tissue perfusion related to renal disease.

Knowledge deficit related to preventive diabetes care and education.

Planning

- The patient will verbalize an understanding of pertinent cardiovascular risk factors.
- The patient will verbalize the need for glycemic control and routine renal care.

Implementation

Educate patients regarding principles of care of kidney disease. These include the following:

- inform patients about the potential renal complications of diabetes
- inform patients about the association between hypertension and accelerated renal disease
- discuss the need for regular blood pressure measurements and encourage patients to measure their own blood pressure at home
- stress the importance of treating hypertension
- explain the potential role that excessive protein in the diet may play in the pathogenesis and progression of diabetic nephropathy
- explain the possible relationship between poor glycemic control and the development of diabetic renal disease
- emphasize the strategies for achieving and maintaining ideal body weight as strategies for preventing hypertension and improving glycemic control
- review with patients the symptoms of urinary tract infection. Instruct patients to contact their health care provider if such symptoms occur
- review with patients which drugs are potentially nephrotoxic. Explain the danger of radiographic dye studies

Evaluation

The patient verbalizes principles of preventive renal care.

The patient receives routine preventive renal care.

DIABETIC NEUROPATHY

Diabetic **neuropathy** is a frequently recognized complication of diabetes that is yet to be adequately explained. Diabetic neuropathy is a heterogenous and overlapping group of neuropathic syndromes affecting the sensorimotor and autonomic nervous systems. The incidence of diabetic neuropathy reported in the literature ranges from 5% to 60%.[6,48] The discrepancies in reporting can be attributed to variations in criteria for diagnosis and to sensitivity of detection methods. Recent studies indicate that clinical signs of neuropathy can be detected in 8% of diabetic patients at the time of diagnosis, despite the lack of reported symptoms.[15,26]

In general it is believed that two broad groups of pathophysiologic disturbances are important in the pathogenesis of diabetic neuropathies: vascular lesions and metabolic derangements. Vascular lesions may result from small vessel occlusions caused by thickening of the vessel walls, and luminal plugging with aggregates of fibrin and platelets. Several biochemical abnormalities have been described with the Schwann cell, which inverts the axon with the myelin sheath. Damage to the Schwann cell may lead to demyelinization, followed by remyelinization. Over time, severe and irreversible nerve damage may result from this process. Genetic factors may increase susceptibility to neuropathy, whereas poor metabolic control also aggravates symptoms.

Two broad classifications of diabetic neuropathy are sensorimotor and autonomic. Despite the classification it is important to recall that generalizations *cannot* be made as to the clinical manifestations of neuropathies since they vary.

Sensorimotor Neuropathies

Diabetic polyneuropathy

Diabetic polyneuropathy is the most frequent form of diabetic neuropathy. It is distal, bilateral, and comparatively symmetrical. Clinical characteristics are quite variable. Patients exhibit distal **paresthesias** (uncomfortable sensations), or contact paresthesias. The sensory loss and motor weakness tend to affect the distal portion of the longest nerves first and do not conform to distribution of a nerve root or peripheral nerve. In most patients, absence of sensation is reported, as opposed to the pain that accompanies some of the other neuropathies. However, as symptomatology becomes more prolonged, the patient's complaints of painful paresthesias, such as episodic or burning pain, become more frequent. Progression of polyneuropathy follows a general course, beginning with involvement of the feet, progression to knees, involvement of hands and arms, abdominal involvement, and distal ends of intercostal nerves over midthorax.

Diabetic radiculopathy

Diabetic radiculopathy represents an infrequent form of peripheral neurologic involvement. The disorder is characterized by occasional to continual deep rooted pain, paresthesia, or sensory changes along a dermatomal distribution. Prognosis is excellent with recovery in several months.

Diabetic mononeuropathy

Diabetic mononeuropathy is common, often occurring as a result of a lesion or trauma to a specified nerve. Examples of some of the more common mononeuropathies include femoral mononeuropathy (with acute pain, deficit, and loss of reflexes), and sciatic mononeuropathy. Carpal tunnel syndrome, caused by median nerve involvement, is also common.

Cranial neuropathies

Cranial neuropathies belong to a category of mononeuropathies. The majority involve the third and sixth cranial nerves. Patients often complain of headache and diplopia associated with eye pain. However, the pupil is not affected, differentiating this neuropathy from carotid aneurysms. Recovery usually takes place within several weeks or months. Facial paralysis of the seventh nerve is another frequent finding with less favorable recovery than is found in nondiabetic patients.

Plexopathy

Plexopathy is characterized by pain extending from the hip to the anterior lateral surface of the thigh. It occurs periodically and more frequently at night. Treatment is supportive until recovery, which is generally complete.

Autonomic Neuropathies

The prevalence and incidence of autonomic dysfunction in diabetes are as difficult to determine as in the peripheral neuropathies. The prevalence ranges from 3% to 70% of all patients with peripheral neuropathy. Because the symptomatology is vague and tests for autonomic manifestations must be very specific, it is difficult to assess the correct percentage. However, it is believed that autonomic neuropathy is present for long periods in an asymptomatic state, and once the symptoms appear, they are irreversible. Symptoms can give major information regarding patient prognosis. Autonomic neuropathies usually present in three areas: gastrointestinal tract, genitourinary tract, and cardiovascular system.[6,15,48,58]

Gastrointestinal tract

Manifestations of autonomic gastrointestinal dysfunction often present as delayed gastric emptying, chronic diarrhea or constipation, and rectal incontinence. This symptomatology results from abnormalities involving extrinsic innervation from the vagus nerve. Although many of the subjective complaints are difficult to distinguish, complaints of early satiety, postprandial fullness, postprandial hypoglycemia, and erratic blood glucose levels are common. Diabetic diarrhea is also of serious concern to the patient. Although it is unpredictable in duration, it generally has a transient nocturnal component. Diagnosis is based on gastric emptying studies. Treatment focuses on instructing patients to eat smaller, more frequent meals of soft or liquid foods.

Genitourinary tract

Symptoms of genitourinary tract involvement often manifest as neurogenic bladder and sexual dysfunction. Neurogenic bladder is caused by a blunting of the sensation to void. Patients with hypotonic bladder complain of increasing intervals between voiding and of infections with progressive micturitional difficulty. Overflow incontinence may also be present. Treatment includes regular scheduling of voiding, cholinergic-stimulating drugs, and aggressive treatment of urinary tract infections.

Sexual dysfunction evidenced as impotence is estimated to occur in almost 50% of diabetic men. Vascular insufficiency is often reported as an etiologic factor in erectile failure. Other causes include psychogenic factors, alcohol, kidney failure, or medications associated with control of hypertension (i.e. methyldopa [Aldomet]). Treatment includes medications (e.g. papaverine) and erection aids and prosthetic devices surgically implanted in the corpus cavernosum (see Chapter 71). However, surgical implants (i.e., small carrion rod prosthesis or inflatable penile prosthesis) or sexual therapy should be considered only after extensive evaluation and education.[4,66,67]

Although sexual dysfunction in women has not been studied extensively, there is evidence of clitoral degenerative changes. Others report diminished libido and increased frequency of vaginitis. Further discussion of sexual dysfunction can be found in Chapter 69.

Cardiovascular system

The cardiovascular symptoms associated with autonomic neuropathy include resting tachycardia and postural hypotension. Although complaints of lightheadedness and visual disturbance upon rising may be noted, many patients are asymptomatic despite larger blood pressure decreases. The earliest manifestations of impaired autonomic innervation of the heart are caused by vagal denervation manifested by postural hypotension of 30 mm Hg or greater. The impact of autonomic neuropathy on cardiac reflexes is being examined as a potential cause of sudden death in diabetic patients.

Sudomotor dysfunction

Other autonomic neuropathies are associated with sweating disturbances associated with polyneuropathy of mixed nerves. Patients may complain of excessive perspiration within seconds of chewing food (gustatory sweating). Decreased sweating in the lower extremities, coupled with increased sweating in the upper trunk and extremities, is also bothersome to patients. Treatment with anticholinergic agents may be of benefit, but usually cause other side effects. Therapy generally aims toward symptom treatment and has limited success.

NURSING MANAGEMENT OF THE PATIENT WITH DIABETIC NEUROPATHY

Assessment

Careful history and physical to document clinical manifestations of neuropathy is needed. Precipitating factors and course of symptomatology should be assessed.

In addition, the nurse must carefully assess the patients' status regarding neuropathy at each visit. Interviews should determine the presence of pain, paresthesias, numbness, orthostatic changes, and gastrointestinal symptoms (e.g., vomiting or diarrhea). Physical assessment includes careful foot and neurologic examination.

Nursing Diagnosis

High risk for chronic pain.
  High risk for injury.
  High risk for activity intolerance.
  High risk for impaired mobility.
  High risk for sexual dysfunction.

Altered cerebral tissue perfusion, related to vascular complications.
  Sexual dysfunction related to diabetes mellitus.

Planning

- Patients will verbalize the possible relationship between poor glycemic control and the subsequent development of diabetic neuropathy.
- Patients will verbalize possible risk factors such as consumption of alcohol and smoking that may hasten the development or progression of diabetic neuropathy.
- Patients will verbalize that because sensory or motor neuropathy may be asymptomatic, routine evaluation is necessary even for those who have no symptoms of neuropathy.
- Patient will verbalize that diabetic neuropathy can contribute to the development of other complications, including loss of limb.
- Patient will discuss signs and symptoms of autonomic neuropathy.
- Patient relates the symptoms and treatment associated with acute/chronic complications of diabetes.
- Patient discusses all aspects of sexuality as impacted by diabetes.

Implementation

Studies have not firmly established that glucose control is effective in preventing or treating diabetic neuropathy. However, encouragement of good glycemic control seems prudent.

Treatment is dependent upon symptoms associated with the neuropathy, duration, and extent of interference with life-style. Educate the patient regarding specific therapies as needed. General patient education principles are stressed at each visit.

Evaluation

Follow-up of the patient regarding neuropathy should reveal appropriate preventive maintenance strategies. Treatment of symptomatology is assessed.

Chronic Complications: Macrovascular Disease

ATHEROSCLEROSIS

Macrovascular complications associated with atherosclerosis account for the majority of fatalities in the diabetic population. Endothelial injury is related to many factors, including hypertension, hy-

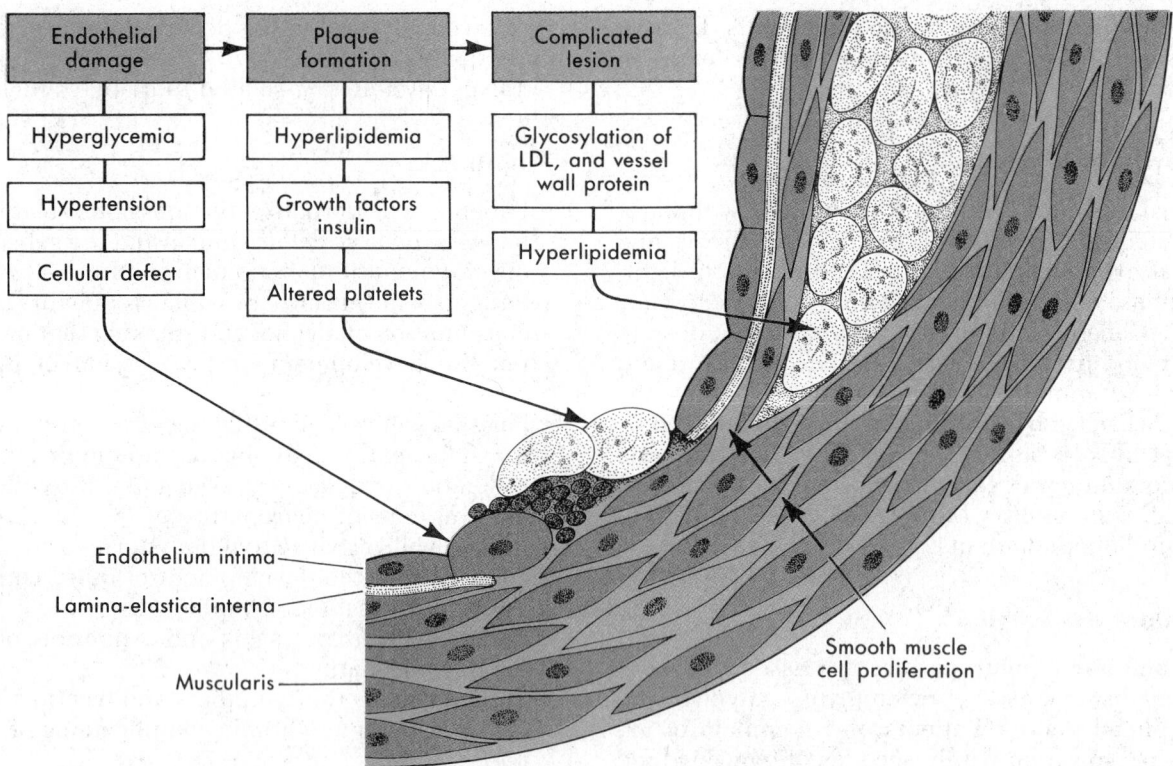

FIGURE 62-8 Possible pathogenic mechanisms of atherosclerosis in diabetes. Endothelial injury is brought about in several ways. The formation of the atherosclerotic plaque is promoted by hyperlipidemia (foam-cell formation, stimulation of smooth-muscle-cell growth), growth factors such as insulin, and adhesion and aggregation of platelets. Glycosylation of·lipoproteins and vessel wall proteins may be instrumental in stimulating lesion progression. Hyperlipidemia also enhances the accumulation of atherosclerotic debris and cholesterol crystals.

percholesterolemia, immunologic and viral assault, and local trauma. This is followed by platelet adhesion to the injury site, platelet aggregation, and release of intracellular materials. This release in turn causes further aggregation, vasoconstriction, and smooth muscle proliferation, with an accumulation of cholesterol and high-density lipoprotein (HDL). It has long been recognized that diabetic patients are prone to defects in lipid and lipoprotein levels. These are usually manifested as elevated plasma cholesterol and triglyceride levels. Another finding that is associated with the atherosclerotic process includes arterial wall stiffness, which contributes further to the atherosclerotic process[15,16] (Figure 62-8).

The pathophysiology of atherosclerosis remains under investigation. However, its relationship to various complications associated with diabetes is thoroughly documented. A summary of these complications follows.[5]

Coronary Artery Disease

The incidence of coronary artery disease (CAD) in the diabetic population is about twice as prevalent in comparison with the nondiabetic population. Prevalence rates increase with age and are higher in men. There is a striking increase in numbers associated with women. The incidence of congestive heart failure is approximately six times greater in diabetic patients than in the general population.[37,44,48]

The atherosclerotic process leading to coronary complications is the same as in the nondiabetic person. However, the left coronary artery is more frequently occluded in the diabetic person. Risk factors associated with increased likelihood of CAD include hypertension, hyperlipidemia, obesity, and smoking. These risk factors are particularly evident in the NIDDM group, which tends to be overweight and often presents with hypertension and hyperlipidemia. Treatment for diabetic persons with CAD is essentially the same as for the nondiabetic population. Extensive and early patient education focused on prevention is the best strategy with regard to this complication.[36]

The occurrence of CAD in the diabetic versus nondiabetic patient may be contrasted as follows:

1. Overall frequency is increased
2. Increase is striking among women
3. Disease is encountered more frequently in diabetes
4. Younger diabetic patients often are affected
5. Risk factors associated with increased likelihood of CAD include hypertension, hyperlipidemia, obesity, and smoking

Hypertension

Hypertension, defined as systolic pressure greater than 150 mm Hg and/or diastolic pressure greater than 94 mm Hg, is twice as common in the diabetic population as compared with nondiabetics. It is an early feature of nephropathy, and data suggest that hypertension promotes the microangiopathic changes seen in retinopathy and nephropathy. Causes of hypertension may be related to abnormalities of the sympathetic and parasympathetic systems, often seen in diabetes. Life-style, genetic background, and socioeconomic status contribute to the disease's progression.[24]

Hyperlipidemia

Hyperlipidemia is a metabolic abnormality with a reported prevalence in diabetes between 20% and 70%.[15,16] The extent of hyperlipidemia depends to a great extent on glycemic control, type and severity of diabetes, age, and nutritional habits. Hyperlip-

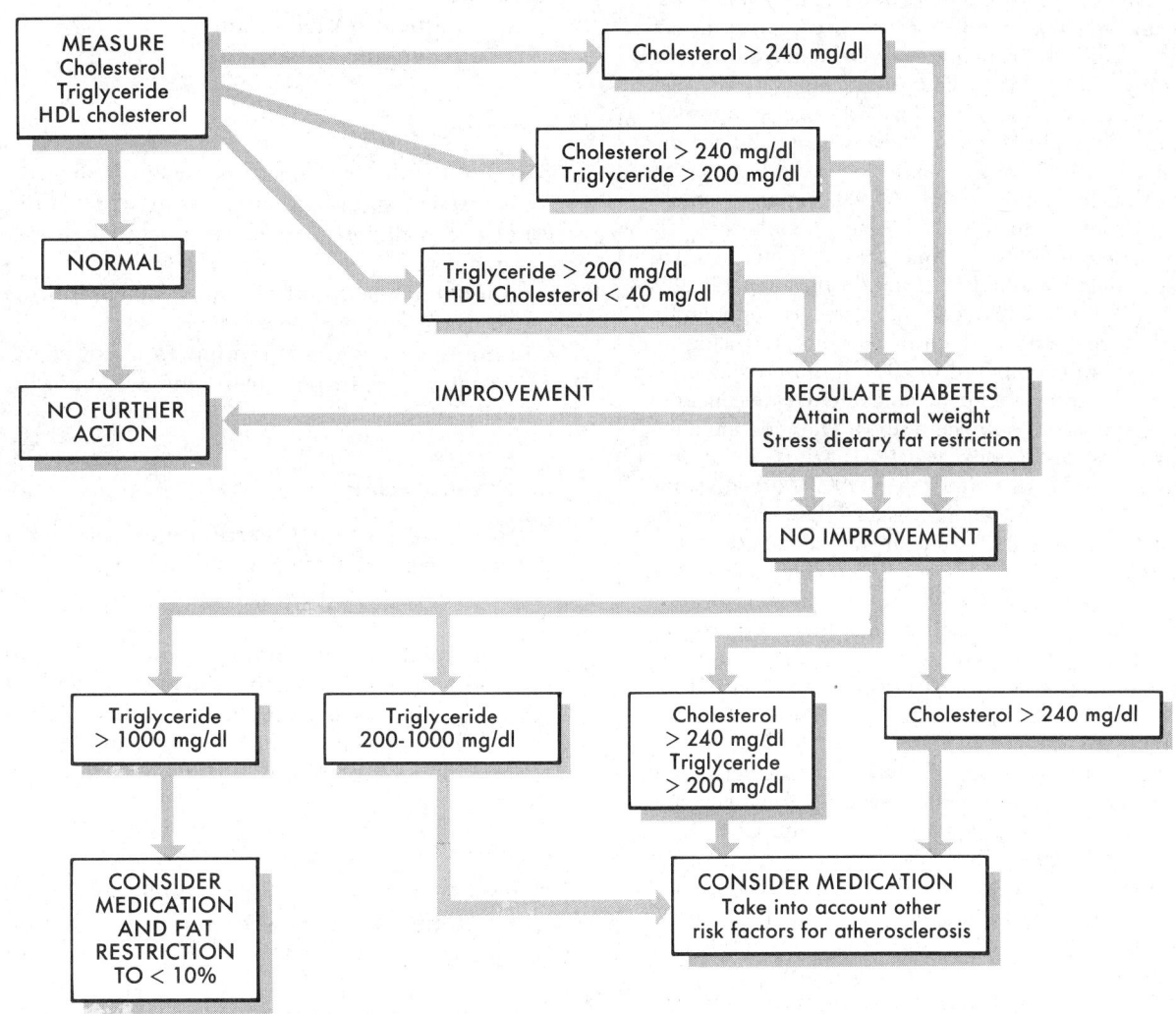

FIGURE 62-9   Approach to the patient with diabetes mellitus and hyperlipidemia. (From Galloway JA et al: *Diabetes mellitus,* ed 9, Indianapolis, 1988, Eli Lilly Co.)

RESEARCH BRIEF

The Prevalence and Impact of Smoking in Diabetic Subjects

Haire-Joshu, D: Smoking, cessation, and the diabetes health care team, *The Diabetes Educator* 17(1):54, 1991.

Smoking is a major cardiovascular risk factor for persons already at heightened risk due to a diagnosis of diabetes. This study determined the prevalence of smoking in a diabetic population and its relationship to physical complications of diabetes. Over a 12 month period, we reviewed the self-reported smoking status and diagnostic studies of all diabetic patients receiving an extensive physical examination through the clinical registry of our Diabetes Center. Data were obtained from 214 diabetic patients (X age = 44 years, M = 82, F = 135) with a X glycated hemoglobin of 12.5 mg/% (normal = 4.4-6.3 mg/%). The majority were prescribed insulin (87%) while the remainder were managed by oral therapy (13%). Mean body mass index (BMI) was 29, indicating a moderate level of obesity (approximately 25% above ideal body weight). Blacks accounted for 44% of the subjects.

Within this diabetic sample 32% reported smoking, in contrast to the 1989 Surgeon General's Report estimate of 29% in the general population. Diabetic males smoked at higher rates than females (M = 38%, F = 27%), exceeding general population prevalence. Forty percent of patients not using insulin smoked compared to 30% of those using insulin. Smoking occurred at equivalent rates in both black and white subjects (32%). Diabetic smokers above desirable body weight (BMI < 22.5) had higher systolic (t = 3.34, p = .003) and diastolic (t = 1.87, p = .05) blood pressure than ideal weight smokers (BMI < 22.5); for nonsmokers, weight was not related to blood pressure. Smokers were diagnosed more frequently with coronary artery disease (X^2 = 3.59, p = .05), with trends toward increased incidence of neuropathy (X^2 = 3.47, p = .06) and atherosclerosis (X^2 = 2.8, p = .08). Smokers did not show greater occurrences of hyperlipidemia or retinopathy.

Racial and other demographic characteristics of this sample may account for smoking prevalence exceeding that of the general population. Given that smoking increases the already substantial risk for cardiovascular complications, it is alarming that prevalence among diabetics approximates that of the general population. Moreover, smoking may be underestimated through underreporting. There is a need to identify issues that may encourage smoking in a diabetic population and to target cessation strategies.

idemia is a major factor in atheromatous events, and diabetic patients have higher low-density lipoprotein (LDL) levels but lower high-density lipoprotein (HDL) levels. Because many investigators believe HDL levels are inversely related to coronary risk, the diabetic patient is at considerable risk (Figure 62-9).[43]

NURSING MANAGEMENT OF THE PATIENT WITH DIABETIC ATHEROSCLEROSIS

Assessment

Careful assessment of modifiable risk factors related to the development of atherosclerotic disease should be conducted.

Nursing Diagnosis

Knowledge deficit related to understanding of risk factors.
Altered health maintenance.
Health-seeking behaviors.

Planning

- Patients will verbalize their risk of cardiovascular disease is higher than in persons without diabetes.
- Patients will verbalize the importance of not smoking.
- Patients will relate the importance of following appropriate dietary regimens.
- Patients will relate the importance of regular and consistent treatment from hypertension and hyperlipidemia.

Implementation

Educate the patient regarding general risk factors for cardiovascular disease. Additional information regarding specific patient factors should then be addressed.

Principles of prevention, including smoking prevention and cessation are stressed. Careful monitoring of blood pressure, plasma lipids, and glucose should be conducted. Follow-up with other health care team members should be coordinated.[19,23]

Evaluation

Annual evaluation of patient status is recommended with additional visits scheduled as warranted by condition.

PERIPHERAL VASCULAR DISEASE

The impact of peripheral vascular disease (PVD) in diabetes is enormous. It is estimated that PVD strikes diabetic persons with 30 times the frequency of nondiabetic persons. About 50% of amputations in this country are a result of PVD associated with diabetes. Risk factors of PVD are essentially the same as for the related vascular diseases, and treatment is focused toward prevention. This is especially critical since there is considerable evidence that, once vascular disease is reported, amputation of limbs is a likely outcome. Data also show a mortality rate of up to 57% of diabetic individuals within 3 years of amputation of a limb. This number rises to approximately 75% within 5 years.[26,38]

THE DIABETIC FOOT
Etiology

Persons with diabetes are prone to foot problems for a variety of reasons. Major precipitators of such problems include microvascular and macrovascular disease, which result in ischemia and delayed healing. Problems associated with neuropathy, including absence of sensation resulting in lack of pain awareness, contribute to the development of foot lesions. Of the diabetic persons admitted to the hospital in any given year, 20% require treatment for foot problems. Additionally, extended hospital stays are required for diabetic patients with foot problems.[26,38]

Pathophysiology

The risk associated with vascular disease mimics that which influences the development of vascular disease. Sensory changes usually appear as bilaterally symmetrical distal deficits. The classic Charcot joint (a loss of foot support caused by bone dissolution) results from repetitive trauma to insensitive bones and joints of the foot. Motor nerve disturbances lead to peripheral weakness, foot muscle atrophy and drop, and diminished reflexes (Table 62-8).

Clinical Manifestations

Most diabetic foot lesions result from a break in the skin leading to infections. These breaks often are caused by a loss of sensation that allows for prolonged painless trauma, encouraging foot lesion development. Some of the more common sources of breaks include (1) fissures, caused by dry skin; (2) blisters, caused by shoe friction and an ominous precursor to gangrenous lesions; (3) toenails which, because of inward curling or ingrown toenails, may become sources of infection; (4) corns and calluses, arising over bony prominences, are common sites of abscesses associated with osteomyelitis; and (5)

TABLE 62-8   Diabetic Feet: Warning Signs and Symptoms

	Signs	Symptoms
Vascular	Absent pedal, popliteal, or femoral pulses	Cold feet
	Femoral bruits	Intermittent claudication, calf or foot
	Dependent rubor, plantar pallor on elevation	Pain at rest (especially nocturnal), relieved by dependency
Neurologic	Sensory—deficits (vibratory and proprioceptive, then pain and temperature perception), hyperesthesia	Sensory—burning, tingling, or crawling sensations; pain; hypersensitivity
	Motor—diminished to absent deep tendon reflexes (Achilles then patellar), weakness	Motor—weakness (drop foot)
	Autonomic—diminished to absent sweating	Autonomic—diminished sweating
Musculoskeletal	Cavus feet with claw toes	Gradual change in foot shape
	Drop foot	Sudden, painless change in foot shape, with swelling, without history of trauma
	"Rocker-bottom" foot (Charcot joint)	
Dermatologic	Skin—abnormal dryness; chronic infections; keratonic lesions with or without hemorrhage (plantar or digital); trophic ulcer	Painless or exquisitely painful wounds
		Slow-healing or nonhealing wounds, or necrosis
	Hair—diminished to absent	Skin color changes (cyanosis, redness)
	Nails—trophic changes; onychomycosis; subungual ulceration or abscess; ingrown nails with paronychia	Recurrent infections (e.g., paronychia, athlete's foot)

From Diabetic foot problems: assessment and prevention, *Clinical Diabetes* 1:7, 1983. Reproduced with permission of the American Diabetes Association, Inc.

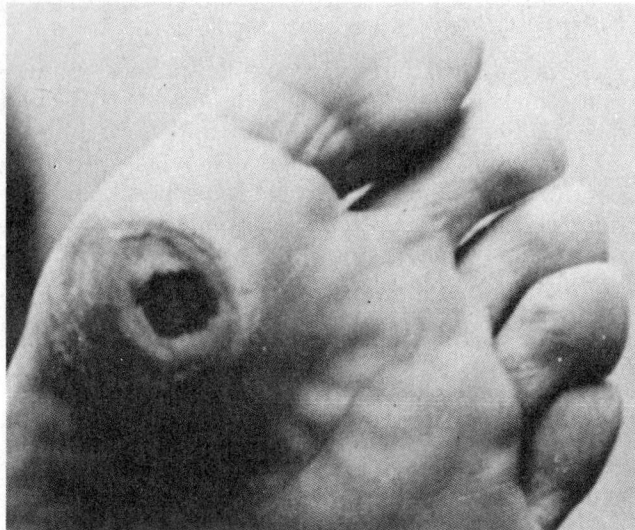

FIGURE 62-10 Classic neuropathic diabetic foot ulcer. Note ulceration in callus is well circumscribed. Lesion is painless. (From the Michigan Diabetes Research and Training Center, Ann Arbor, Mich, 1983, The University of Michigan.)

trauma, resulting from incompatibility of shoes or feet or foreign objects, such as stones (Figure 62-10).

Therapeutic Management

A major focus of the care of any diabetic patient should include extensive information on foot care and the opportunity to practice needed foot care skills. Because the majority of foot ulcers occur in patients over the age of 50, education needs to be stressed in particular with this group.

Follow-up visits should include comprehensive foot inspections to ensure that the skin on the foot is healthy. Regular podiatrist visits may also be recommended for foot care.

If ulceration occurs, medical care should begin immediately. Conservative treatment is rarely successful; intensive treatment is needed to avoid further complications associated with ulcerations. In general, therapeutic management involves (1) debridement of necrotic tissue; (2) culture of wound; (3) application of antibacterial solutions; (4) coverage of ulcer with gauze; and (5) placing patient on crutches to ensure a *no* weight-bearing situation. Daily changing of the dressing with regular debridement prevents pooling of exudate and encourages new tissue growth. Superficial ulcers that appear noninfected usually respond to local debridement.

After local swelling subsides, a walking plaster cast may be applied.

NURSING MANAGEMENT OF THE PATIENT WITH DIABETIC FOOT

Assessment

Physical assessment criteria are noted in Table 62-8.

Nursing Diagnosis

Knowledge deficit related to foot care.
Impaired physical mobility.
High risk for impaired skin integrity.
High risk for activity intolerance.
Altered health maintenance.
High risk for infection.

Planning

- The patient will discuss the importance of foot care.
- The patient will demonstrate appropriate foot care.
- The patient will discuss the relationship between neuropathy, peripheral vascular disease, and foot ulcers.
- The patient will avoid risk factors associated with neuropathy.
- The patient will be aware of special shoes for preventing/treating foot problems.

Implementation

The patient teaching plan describes steps for implementation.

Evaluation

The patient demonstrates good foot care without evidence of ulceration.

OTHER PERIPHERAL VASCULAR COMPLICATIONS
Skin Disorders

The condition of the skin provides clues to the presence of diabetes mellitus, such as frequency of infection, joint contractures, pruritus, and dryness. Compared with the nondiabetic person, the skin of the diabetic person is said to have structural differences, including increased numbers of mast cells in the dermis, increased capillary fragility, decreased temperature changes, and perhaps diminished circulation in the blood vessels of the skin. For these reasons, diabetic patients are more prone to skin in-

PATIENT EDUCATION GUIDE   *Foot Care*

The nurse should provide the patient with the following instructions.

Inspection

Look at your feet each day in a place with good light; use a mirror if you can't bend over to see the bottom of your feet.

Look for dry places and cracks in the skin, especially between the toes and around the heel; check for ingrown toenails, corns, calluses, discoloration, swelling, or sores.

If looking carefully at your feet is difficult for you, have a friend or family member help.

If corns, calluses, or other problems persist, see a foot doctor.

Bathing

Wash your feet daily in warm (not hot) water; always test the water temperature with your wrist or a bath thermometer to prevent burning yourself.

Do not soak your feet, because it will dry your skin.

Use a mild soap and rinse well; dry feet with a soft towel, making sure to dry between the toes.

To soften dry feet and keep the skin from cracking, use a cream or lotion such as Nivea, Eucerin, or Alpha Keri; do not put lotion between your toes.

If your feet sweat a lot, lightly dust with foot powder; wear cotton socks and change them several times a day.

Toenails

Trim your toenails only after bathing, when they are soft and easy to cut.

Always cut or file nails to follow the natural curve of your toe.

Avoid cutting nails shorter than the ends of your toes.

File sharp corners and rough edges of nails with an emery board so they do not cut the toes next to them.

Do not use sharp objects to poke or dig under the toenail or around the cuticle.

See a podiatrist for treatment of ingrown toenails and nails that are thick or tend to split when cut.

Corns and calluses

Control corn and callus build-up; after washing your feet, gently rub with a pumice stone.

Pad corns to reduce pressure.

Avoid using do-it-yourself corn or callus removers; they are caustic and may hurt healthy skin.

Never cut your corns and calluses with a razor blade; *no bathroom surgery.*

Socks

Wear clean, soft cotton or wool socks.

Socks should fit well and be free of seams and darns.

Never wear round garters or hose with elastic tops that might reduce the blood supply to your feet.

Shoes

Always wear shoes or slippers to cover and protect your feet.

Wear shoes that fit well. Shoes that do not fit well can cause sores, blisters, and calluses, but shoes that feel good have room for all the toes to be in their natural place; avoid pointed shoes that pinch the toes. The top part of the shoe should be soft and pliable; the lining should not have ridges, wrinkles, or seams; the toe box should be round and high to allow space for toe deformities; you may need to see an orthotic specialist for special shoes or to have your shoes adapted to your feet.

When you buy shoes, make an outline of each foot from stiff paper to insert in shoes.

Before you put on your shoes, carefully check for stones or rough spots that might hurt your feet.

Improve your circulation

Try to quit smoking if you smoke.

Exercise every day; take a brisk daily walk for ½ to 1 hour; if you are not able to walk or move about easily, ask your nurse or doctor what types of exercises are best for you.

Avoid being in the cold for long periods; wear wool socks.

Treatment of injuries

Look at your feet if you stumble or bump a hard object.

If your foot is hurt, do not keep walking on it, since that can cause more damage.

Cuts and scratches should be treated right away; wash with soap and water and apply a mild antiseptic such as Bactine or Johnson & Johnson First Aid Cream; never use strong chemicals such as boric acid.

Notify physician or podiatrist of any blisters or sores on your feet.

TABLE 62-9 Common Skin Disorders in Diabetes Mellitus

Skin disorder	Symptoms	Skin disorder	Symptoms
PRIMARY SKIN DISORDERS IN DIABETES MELLITUS		**INSULIN RESISTANCE**	
Diabetic dermopathy	Atrophic, red-brown, sharply circumscribed lesion; occurs on anterior skins in 50% of patients	Acanthosis nigricans	Hyperpigmented, evenly thickened and folded skin of flexural body regions
Joint contractures	Thick, waxy skin overlying joints; noted in almost 30% of IDDM patients	**ABNORMAL LIPID LEVELS**	
		Eruptive xanthomas	Multiple yellow-red and yellow-orange papules; located over joints, buttocks, and trunk; clears with good control
	Increased dermal collagen yields waxy texture; increased risk for microvascular disease (85% to 25% without finding)	Xanthelesma	Irregular plaques over eyelids
			Most common type of xanthoma
Necrobiosis lipoidica	Asymptomatic plaque on unilateral or bilateral skins; affects women more frequently than men		Begins as pinpoint-sized yellow-orange spots that coalesce and become thicker
Lipodystrophy	Mass of scar and fatty tissue caused by hypertrophy of subcutaneous fatty tissue leading to muscle hyperdevelopment	Xanthochromia	Yellowish skin discoloration accompanied by increase in carotene and blood cholesterol

fections than nondiabetics. This is particularly true during times of poor metabolic control (Table 62-9).

Infections

Although it is difficult to document an overall increase in infection frequency in diabetes, there are certain organisms to which diabetic persons appear more susceptible (e.g. influenza). In part, this may be caused by (1) an alteration in host defenses; (2) vascular insufficiency that limits infection-fighting factors; and (3) neurologic abnormalities such as neuropathy, which result in sensory nerve defects that limit the patient's awareness of trauma or inflammation. Some of the more common types of infection found in diabetes include urinary tract infections, vaginitis or vulvitis, and upper respiratory tract infections. There is also an increased susceptibility to foot infections.

The incidence of bacteriuria is approximately two to three times greater in diabetic women than in nondiabetics. This increase is associated with age and diabetic complications associated with longstanding diabetes. Common causes of the urinary tract infections include *Escherichia coli* and *Candida albicans.*

As with all such infections, preventive education, early detection, and follow-up are imperative. Patient instruction should be thorough, thus avoiding more acute health problems.[48]

Oral Complications

The principal oral complication associated with IDDM is periodontitis. Periodontitis is manifested by bone loss and tooth mobility, migration, and eventual loss. The disease is aggressive and severe in the diabetic patient. The microangiopathies associated with periodontal tissues of diabetic patients are well documented. The decrease in lumen size, followed by reduced vascular perfusion, may reduce oxygen consumption. This provides optimal conditions for anaerobic microorganism growth. Thus, dental education, care, and follow-up are critical to the overall health of the diabetic patient.[3,40]

NURSING MANAGEMENT OF THE PATIENT WITH OTHER PERIPHERAL VASCULAR COMPLICATIONS

Nursing Diagnosis

High risk for injury.
  High risk for infection.

Planning

- The patient will relate the importance of preventive strategies to avoid infection.
- The patient will discuss signs and symptoms associated with skin derangements, infections, and oral disorders.
- The patient will discuss the importance of good skin care.
- The patient will discuss specific preventive care strategies related to oral care.
- The patient will discuss strategies for early treatment of infections.

Implementation

The nurse reviews with the patient preventive education related to skin and oral care. Provision of specific guidelines for care, and early treatment of symptoms associated with acute derangements, should be provided. The importance of routine follow-up for diabetes care should also be stressed.

Evaluation

The patient receives regular, routine diabetes care.

HYPOGLYCEMIA (NONDIABETIC)

Definition

Hypoglycemia (not related to diabetes mellitus) is present when glucose concentrations decline progressively to concentrations of less than 50 mg/dL. When this decrease is rapid, symptoms of tachycardia, weakness, sweating, and hunger are noted. Gradual falls result in headache, blurred vision, and lethargy. After a period of time, patients may try to treat hypoglycemia by overeating, resulting in weight gain.

Etiology/Epidemiology

There are three classifications of hypoglycemia: organic, iatrogenic, and reactive. Organic hypoglycemia is a term that describes several types of hypoglycemia, including the following:

Insulinoma—Benign or malignant insulin producing tumors arising from the pancreatic beta cells, most often found in persons 40 to 60 years of age.

Islet cell differentiation—Also called nesidioblastosis; this form usually occurs during the first 6 months of life and results in neoformation of islet cells from pancreatic ducts.

Massive extrapancreatic tumors—Often located intraperitoneally or retroperitoneally; these tumors encourage hypoglycemia via excessive use of glucose.

Glycogen storage disorders—Very rare and may be found in infancy.

Counterregulation deficiency—For a variety of reasons, insulin secretion is not inhibited by counterregulatory hormones, such as cortisol and glucagon.

Dumping syndrome—Hypoglycemia following gastric surgery where normal stomach sphincter control is absent.

Leucine sensitivity—Found in infants following milk ingestion, which results in excessive insulin secretion.

Immune mediated hypoglycemia—An entity caused by antiinsulin receptor antibodies which occur spontaneously.

Iatrogenic hypoglycemia is associated with alcohol consumption, which interferes with the breakdown of liver glycogen, and drug reactions, often reflected by excessive salicylate ingestion, which results in severe hypoglycemia. Other drugs associated with this include beta blockers, sulfonylureas, and ethanol. Facetious insulin administration by patients with access to insulin may also be initiated for secondary gain.

Reactive hypoglycemia, which occurs within 5 minutes of meal ingestion, accounts for 75% of all cases of spontaneous hypoglycemia. Symptoms are transient and adrenergic.[58,59]

Pathophysiology

The extent of hypoglycemia in the general population is directly related to the pathophysiologic cause of the hypoglycemia. In general, if it is organic in nature (e.g. insulinoma), the amount of hypoglycemia is rare. Diagnosis is often based on the clinical history (i.e. gastric surgery) and plasma glucose or oral glucose tolerance test levels significantly lower than normal.

Therapeutic Management

Treatment is individualized to the patient, based on causative findings of hypoglycemia (e.g. surgical extraction of an insulinoma). If a medication is the causative factor, removal of the iatrogenic agent may be appropriate. In other cases, nutrition education regarding type and timing of meals (small, frequent feedings) is appropriate.

NURSING MANAGEMENT OF THE PATIENT WITH NONDIABETIC HYPOGLYCEMIA

Assessment

A thorough assessment, including a review of systems, can provide important information as to the type or cause of hypoglycemia. Laboratory tests generally include 5-hour glucose tolerance test, 72-hour fasting plasma glucose levels, insulin antibody levels, proinsulin and C-peptide and serum cortisol levels, and CAT scan. It is reasonable to monitor a patient with mild symptoms to validate results of modified dietary behaviors (i.e. alcohol ingestion) before embarking on expensive diagnostic studies.

Nursing Diagnosis

High risk for altered nutrition

Implementation

To combat hypoglycemia, the patient should be educated as to recommended dietary habits or other recommended therapeutic measures. In this manner, hypoglycemic episodes might be diminished.

Encourage the patient's understanding of the causes of hypoglycemia. Teach the patient the relationship between diet, meal timing and frequency, and hypoglycemia. Arrange for dietary consultations as needed and provide written materials regarding the designated regimen. The patient should discuss which symptoms are to be reported to the nurse, physician, or other designated professional.

Documentation

Document the patient's understanding of the disease pathophysiology, any dietary interventions or consultations, teaching of treatment measures, and materials provided. Patient response to diagnosis and follow-up interventions should also be noted.

CRITICAL THINKING QUESTIONS

1 Describe the process whereby diabetes mellitus results in hyperglycemia, hyperlipidemia, and hyperaminoacidemia.
2 Differentiate the therapeutic management of IDDM and NIDDM, explaining the rationale for each.
3 Discuss the major laboratory tests used to diagnose and monitor diabetes mellitus.
4 Explain the progression of microangiopathy and macroangiopathy in diabetes mellitus in relation to its impact on target organs.
5 What are the implications of achieving metabolic control in diabetes mellitus?
6 Compare dietary goals in IDDM versus NIDDM. What is the rationale for these goals?
7 Describe the exercise guidelines to be provided a patient with IDDM. How do these guidelines differ from those with NIDDM?
8 How does insulin action differ from that of the oral hypoglycemia agent?
9 What is the rationale for using insulin in patients with NIDDM?
10 Can oral hypoglycemic agents be used in IDDM? Why or why not?
11 What guidelines should be used in recommending SMBG in diabetes management?
12 Evaluate the extent to which SMBG impacts the therapeutic regimen in diabetes mellitus.
13 Describe the component of the following diabetic teaching plans: survival, indepth, continuing education.
14 Discuss the psychosocial implications of a diagnosis of diabetes mellitus on the patient and the psychosocial implications for the family.
15 What is the role of the nurse in diabetes education? The role of the patient?
16 Identify organizations available to assist the diabetic patient; the professional.

RESOURCES

1 AMERICAN DIABETES ASSOCIATION
1660 Duke St.
Alexandria, VA 22314
2 AMERICAN ASSOCIATION OF DIABETES EDUCATORS
500 N. Michigan, Suite 1400
Chicago, IL 60611
3 AMERICAN DIETETIC ASSOCIATION
216 West Jackson Blvd., Suite 800
Chicago, IL 60606
4 THE JOSLIN DIABETES CENTER
One Joslin Place
Boston, MA 02215
5 NATIONAL DIABETES INFORMATION CLEARINGHOUSE
Box NDIC
Bethesda, MD 20205

BIBLIOGRAPHY

Current
1. American Diabetes Association, Franz M et al: *Goals for diabetes education,* 1987, The Association.
2. Anderson JW, Gustafson NJ: Nutrition management of

hyperlipidemia in diabetes, *Practical Diabetology* 6(6):16, 1987.

3. Bartholomew GA, Roder N, Bell DS: Oral candidiasis in patients with diabetes mellitus: a thorough analysis, *Diabetes Care* 10(5):607, 1987.

4. Baum N, Neiman M, Lewis R: Evaluation and treatment of organic impotence in the male with diabetes mellitus, *Diabetes Educ* 14(2):123, 1988.

5. Biller J, Love BB: Diabetes and stroke, *Clinical Diabetes* 9(5):65, 1991.

6. Broadstone VL et al: Diabetic peripheral neuropathy. I. Sensorimotor neuropathy, *Diabetes Educ* 13(1):30, 1987.

7. Cefalie WT, Parker TB, Johnson CR: Validity of serum fructosamine as an index of short-term glycemic control in diabetic outpatients, *Diabetes Care* 11(8):662, 1988.

8. Davidson, MB: How to get the most out of insulin therapy, *Clinical Diabetes* 8(5):66, 1990.

9. Department of Health and Human Services, Public Health Service, Centers for Disease Control, Center for Chronic Disease Prevention and Health Promotion: *The prevention and treatment of complications of diabetes mellitus: A guide for primary care practitioners.*

10. Etzweiler D: Inpatient and outpatient hospital-based diabetes education programs, *Practical Diabetology* 6(6):1, 1987.

11. Flavin K, Still H, Haire-Joshu D: Role of the pharmacist in diabetes education, *J Consult Pharm*, 1987.

12. Fleckman, AM: Diabetic ketoacidosis, *Practical Diabetology* 10:1, 1991.

13. Franz MJ: Exercise and diabetes. In Haire-Joshu D, editor: *Management of diabetes mellitus: perspectives of care across the life span*, St. Louis, 1992, Mosby–Year Book.

14. Funnell MM, Merritt JH: Diabetes mellitus and the older adult, In Haire-Joshu D, editor: *Management of diabetes mellitus: perspectives of care across the life span.* St. Louis, 1992, Mosby–Year Book.

15. Galloway JA, editor: *Diabetes mellitus*, Indianapolis, 1988, Eli Lilly Co.

16. Goldberg AC: Cholesterol and diabetes: modifying risks of heart disease, *Clinical Diabetes* 6:84, 1988.

17. Greenlee G: Exercise options for patients with retinopathy and peripheral vascular disease, *Practical Diabetology* 6(4):9, 1987.

18. Haire-Joshu D: The process of evaluation in diabetes education. In Haire-Joshu D, editor: *Management of diabetes mellitus: perspectives of care across the life span*, St. Louis, 1992, Mosby–Year Book.

19. Haire-Joshu D: Smoking, cessation, and the diabetes health care team, *Diabetes Educ* 17(1):54, 1991.

20. Haire-Joshu D: Current issues in type II diabetes mellitus: continuing education series, *J Consult Pharm* 2(6):483, 1987.

21. Haire-Joshu D, Houston C: Promoting behavior change: teaching/learning strategies. In Haire-Joshu D, editor: *Management of diabetes mellitus: perspectives of care across the life span*, St. Louis, 1992, Mosby–Year Book.

22. Haire-Joshu D, Flavin K, Green S: Overview of type II diabetes, *J Consult Pharm* 2(5):413, 1987.

23. Haire-Joshu D, Morgan G, Fisher EB: Determinants of cigarette smoking, *Clin Chest Med* 12(4):711, 1991.

24. Howard WJ, Viberti GC: When to treat? A workshop to address the threshold of treatment of hypertension in diabetes, *Diabetes Care* 14(suppl 4):1, 1991.

25. Jerums G et al: Spectrum of proteinuria in type I and type II diabetes, *Diabetes Care* 10(4):419, 1987.

26. Levin ME, O'Neal LW: *The diabetic foot*, ed 4, St Louis, 1988, Mosby–Year Book.

27. MacDonald MJ: Postexercise late-onset hypoglycemia in insulin dependent diabetes mellitus, *Diabetes Care* 10(5):584, 1987.

28. Mitz R, Bennon JW: *Management and education of the diabetic patient*, Philadelphia, 1988, WB Saunders.

29. O'Connor PJ et al: Metabolic control in NIDDM: factors associated with patient outcomes, *Diabetes Care* 10(6):697, 1987.

30. Olson CO: *Diagnosis and management of diabetes mellitus*, New York, 1987, Raven Press.

31. Pederson O, Beck-Nielsen H: Insulin resistance and insulin dependent diabetes mellitus, *Diabetes Care* 10(4):516, 1987.

32. Peters AL, Davidson MB: Effect of storage on action of NPH and regular insulin mixtures, *Diabetes Care* 10(6):799, 1987.

33. Piuggi C: Nutrition education: teaching independent and responsible meal planning, *Practical Diabetology* 6(1):10, 1987.

34. Powers MA: Facilitating nutritional changes in "difficult" patients, *Diabetes Spectrum* 4(4):186, 1991.

35. Raskin P, Rosenstock J: Hyperglycemia, genetic susceptibility, and diabetic complication, *Clinical Diabetes* 5(6):135, 1987.

36. Rosenstock J et al: Reduction in cardiovascular risk factors with intensive diabetes treatment in IDDM, *Diabetes Care* 10(6):729, 1987.

37. Runyon JW: Coexisting hypertension and diabetes, *Practical Diabetology* 7(3):1, 1988.

38. Singer A: Peripheral vascular disease and the diabetic foot: clinical evaluation, *Practical Diabetology* 6(4):12, 1987.

39. Stone MB: Questions that diabetes patients ask, *Diabetes Educ* 13(3):298, 1987.

40. Wilson TG: Periodontal diseases and diabetes, *Diabetes Educ* 15(4):342, 1989.

41. Wilson LK, Jacobsen AM, Rand LJ: Psychosocial aspects of diabetic retinopathy, *Diabetes Care* 10(3):367, 1987.

42. Winter WE: Atypical diabetes in blacks, *Clinical Diabetes* 9(4):49, 1991.

43. Zeigler JA, Smith BM, Anderson JW: Glycemic control and serum lipids, *Practical Diabetology* 10:10, 1991.

Classic

44. American Diabetes Association: *The physician's guide to type II diabetes (NIDDM): diagnosis and treatment*, 1984, Upjohn Co.

45. Armstrong M, Wakat D: *The energetic diabetic: a personal fitness guide*, 1985, Brady Communication Co.

46. Berlin N et al: National standards for diabetes education programs, *Diabetes Educ* 12(3):292, 1986.

47. Cryer PE: Glucose counterregulation, hypoglycemia, and the intensive therapy of IDDM, *Clinical Diabetes* 2(5):108, 1984.

48. Davidson JK: *Clinical diabetes mellitus: a problem oriented approach*, New York, 1986, Thieme Medical Publishers.

49. Driscoll HK, Mordes JP, Rossini AA: IDDM and the immune system, *Clinical Diabetes* 4(3):51, 1986.

50. Flavin K, Haire-Joshu D: The pharmacologic repertoire, *Am J Nurs* 86:1244, 1986.

51. Goodman JI: A clinician's approach to the diabetic diet, *Practical Diabetology* 5(4):17, 1986.

52. Haire-Joshu D, Flavin K, Clutter W: Controlling the insu-

lin balance: contrasting type I and type II diabetes, *Am J Nurs,* 86:1239, 1986.

53. Haire-Joshu D, Flavin K, Santiago JV: Components of intensive conventional insulin therapy, *Am J Nurs,* 86:1244, 1986.

54. Haycock P: Insulin absorption: understanding the variables, *Clinical Diabetes* 4(5):97, 1986.

55. Leichter SB: Diabetes patient education in hospital settings, *Diabetes Educ* 12(3):277, 1986.

56. Lockwood D, et al: The biggest problem in diabetes, *Diabetes Educ* 12(1):30, 1986.

57. Lorber D: Increased insulin requirements: causes and correction, *Practical Diabetology* 4(6):1985.

58. Marble A et al: *Diabetes mellitus,* ed 12, Philadelphia, 1985, Lea & Febiger.

59. Musky S: Hypoglycemia, *Practical Diabetology* 4(2):16, 1985.

60. Raskin P: Self-monitoring: a practical guide to getting started, *Clinical Diabetes* 3(1):3, 1985.

61. Rizza RA, Zimmerman BR, Service JF: Brittle diabetes: tracking down its sources, *Clinical Diabetes* 3(3):58, 1985.

62. Rodman J: Preserving renal function in the patient with diabetes, *Practical Diabetology* 5(4):1, 1986.

63. Rosenstock J, Raskin P: Early diabetic nephropathy: assessment and potential therapeutic interventions, *Diabetes Care* 9(5):529, 1986.

64. Rosenthal JL, Rosenthal ML: Diabetic retinopathy in 1986, *Practical Diabetology* 5(2):1, 1986.

65. Schade DS et al: Intensive insulin therapy, *Excerpta Media,* 1983.

66. VanSon AR: *Diabetes and patient education: a daily nursing challenge,* New York, 1982, Appleton-Century-Crofts.

67. Zorgniotti AW: Vascular impotence and diabetes: an update, *Practical Diabetology* 4(2):1, 1985.

UNIT XV

The Gastrointestinal System

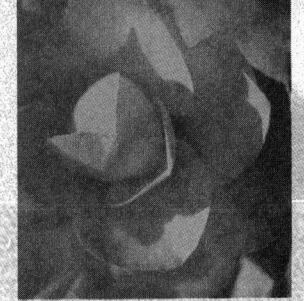

CHAPTER SIXTY-THREE

Nursing Assessment of the Gastrointestinal System

LEARNING OBJECTIVES

1 Understand the basic structures and functions of the gastrointestinal system.

2 Describe the process by which the body's nutrients are digested and absorbed.

3 Obtain relevant subjective information from the patient who has a gastrointestinal alteration.

4 Using correct technique, examine the patient to obtain appropriate objective information about the gastrointestinal system.

5 Differentiate abnormal from normal subjective and objective findings related to the gastrointestinal system.

6 Describe tests involved in the diagnosis of disorders of the gastrointestinal system.

7 Discuss the patient care that is required for each of the tests involved in the diagnosis of disorders of the gastrointestinal system.

THE MAIN FUNCTION of the gastrointestinal (GI) system is to provide the physical and chemical environment that is required to break up large complex food particles into less complex substances that can cross the mucous membrane of the GI tract and enter the circulatory system. Other functions of the GI tract include excretion of insoluble and unabsorbed food materials and the excretion of lipid-soluble waste products secreted by the liver. The GI tract flora also serves as a source of some food nutrients.

The assessment of the GI system is done in conjunction with an examination of the renal/urinary and reproductive systems (Chapters 41 and 68). This enables the nurse to better identify the organic source of pain when patients come to the hospital with vague complaints of abdominal discomfort.

GI alterations can occur at any age and have various causes. Older adults often report constipation as a result of decreased mobility and changing nutritional needs. Stress, inadequate rest, disturbed thought processes, and toileting delay may also lead to bowel dysfunction. GI alterations are commonly associated with paralysis of the lower extremities. The nurse must be alert to etiologic clues relative to the characteristics, sequence, duration, and persistence of GI discomfort.

ANATOMY AND PHYSIOLOGY
Structural Description

Mouth

The mouth begins the digestive process by masticating and lubricating the food and by adding an en-zyme to it. The mouth **(buccal cavity)** is made up of the lips, cheeks, hard and soft palates, tongue, salivary glands, and teeth.

Mastication of food is achieved by the cutting and grinding action of the teeth on the food as it is moved between them by the tongue and cheeks.

The adult has 32 teeth. They are anchored in the mandible and maxillary bones by their roots (Figure 63-1 *A* and *B*). The crown of a tooth is the visible portion that is protected from chemical and physical damage by hard dental enamel. The periodontal membrane covers and protects the root by forming the alveolar cavity surrounding each tooth. The health of the teeth depends on good hygiene, because food particles that become trapped under the periodontal membrane or between the teeth cause tooth decay and periodontal disease. Healthy teeth are important for good nutrition because they grind the food into small particles that are easily swallowed and have a larger surface area to facilitate digestion. Many of the nutritional problems of old age are exacerbated because the poor condition of the natural teeth or the discomfort produced by poorly fitting false teeth cause the individual to avoid hard foods such as raw fruits and vegetables, and some meats. Lubrication and moistening of the food are achieved by mixing it with the watery and mucus secretions of the salivary glands, as well as with the mucus secreted by the small glands that line the entire mouth.

The salivary glands are accessory digestive glands that lie outside the digestive tract and are connected to it by ducts. The parotid glands are the largest sal-

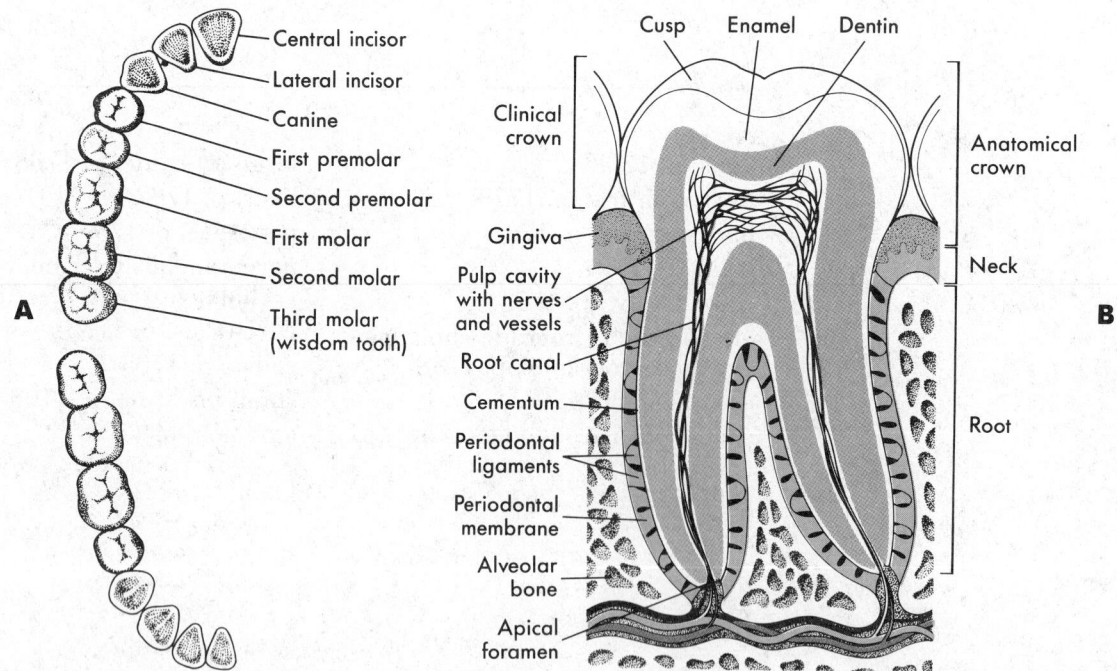

FIGURE 63-1   **A,** Adult teeth, and **B,** anatomic cross-section of molar.

ivary glands. They lie anterior to the ear lobe and secrete the enzyme ptyalin and a serous fluid. The parotid ducts open opposite the second upper molar teeth.

The submandibular glands lie adjacent to the mandible. They secrete serous fluid and mucus through ducts that empty close to the base of the tongue.

The sublingual glands are located beneath the floor of the mouth, and their secretions, which are primarily mucus, enter the buccal cavity through numerous small ducts.

Saliva neutralizes acid so that the ptyalin can function at its optimal pH. It also dissolves food ingredients so that they may be tasted. Taste buds for the four primary taste sensations are found on the surface of the tongue: sweetness is detected on the anterior surface and the tip of the tongue, sourness is detected on the two lateral sides, bitterness is detected on the superior dorsal surface, and saltiness is detected over the entire tongue. The palatability of food substances depends on the composite taste that results from the combination of the four primary sensations, on other factors such as the smell and fiber and fat content of the food, and on the appetite. (Food always tastes better when the individual is hungry.)

In addition to its purely digestive function, small amounts of saliva are produced constantly to keep the mouth moist and supple for speaking and to keep it clean. (The production of saliva is often deficient during sickness, and frequent mouth care is *essential* for the comfort and well-being of seriously ill patients.) Saliva contains IgA antibodies against the normal microorganisms in the environment. Despite the presence of antibodies, the normal mouth contains many resident microorganisms, and during disease, saliva can be a source of infection for illnesses such as measles, mumps, mononucleosis, and rabies.

Esophagus

The **esophagus** is a 25 cm long tube that passes through the thorax and diaphragm to the stomach. Like the rest of the GI tract, its walls are made up of four layers: (1) a mucous lining that, in the esophagus, is made up of nonkeratinized stratified squamous epithelium to protect it from abrasion; (2) a submucosal layer of connective tissue containing blood vessels and lymphatics; (3) a strong muscle layer that, in the upper quarter of the esophagus, is made up of voluntary skeletal muscle, and in the lower portion is mainly longitudinally directed smooth muscle, surrounding a smaller amount of circular smooth muscle; and (4) an outer layer of connective tissue, or adventitia, that binds the esophagus to surrounding structures of the mediastinum.

The chief function of the esophagus is to receive the bolus of food from the pharynx and propel it by peristalsis into the stomach. **Peristalsis** is a ring of relaxation followed by a ring of contraction that moves and propels material through the digestive tract.

Stomach

The **stomach** is J-shaped and lies just below the liver in the upper abdominal cavity (Figure 63-2). It is made up of the cardia, fundus, body, and pyloric regions. The cardia is the narrow region immediately below the esophageal opening, the fundus is the dome-shaped region to the left above the esophageal opening, the body is the central region, and the pylorus is the region close to the opening into the duodenum. The concave curvature of the J shape is referred to as the lesser curvature and the convex curvature is referred to as the greater curvature.

The stomach is supported by the lesser omentum, which passes from the lesser curvature to the inferior surface of the liver, and by the greater omentum, which passes from the greater curvature to the colon. These two membranes are extensions of the parietal peritoneum and they also store fat and reduce the spread of any infections that enter the peritoneal cavity.

The stomach continues the digestive process started in the mouth, stores the partly digested food, and controls the rate at which it enters the small intestine. Digestion and absorption are impaired when food passes too quickly into the intestines.

The smooth muscle of the stomach wall is made up of three layers: an inner oblique layer, a middle circular layer, and an outer longitudinal layer. As the stomach fills, the smooth muscle relaxes and the stomach is able to distend to contain a large meal without a significant increase in pressure. These muscles also contract and relax to churn the food and mix it with acid and enzymes secreted by the gastric glands.

The mucosa of the stomach is made up of columnar epithelium shaped into numerous rugae and folds that stretch easily with distention of the stomach. The parietal cells of the gastric glands secrete hydrochloric acid and the intrinsic factor necessary for the absorption of vitamin B_{12}, and the chief cells secrete enzymes (Table 63-1). These glands are most plentiful in the fundus and body of the stomach. Mucous glands are found throughout.

The secretion of hydrochloric acid is important because it reduces the pH of the stomach contents to pH_1, which kills most ingested microorganisms; its hydrogen ions break the chemical bonds holding the large molecules together; and it provides the optimum pH required by the gastric proteolytic enzymes.

The intrinsic factor is a polypeptide that is required for the absorption of vitamin B_{12} across the intestinal mucosa. Pernicious anemia develops in in-

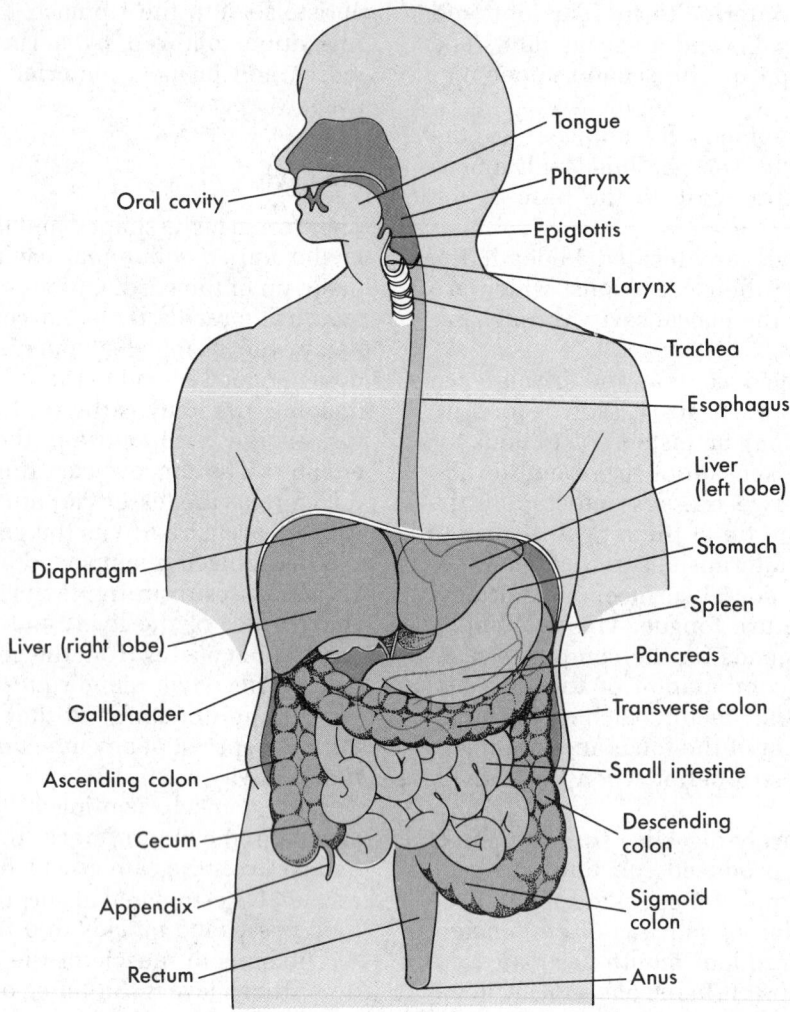

Oral cavity

Tongue

Pharynx

Epiglottis

Larynx

Trachea

Esophagus

Liver (left lobe)

Stomach

Spleen

Pancreas

Transverse colon

Small intestine

Descending colon

Sigmoid colon

Anus

Diaphragm

Liver (right lobe)

Gallbladder

Ascending colon

Cecum

Appendix

Rectum

FIGURE 63-2   Anatomy of the gastrointestinal system.

dividuals lacking intrinsic factor, and it is essential that affected individuals receive regular injections of vitamin B_{12}. Unfortunately, the production of intrinsic factor decreases and the incidence of pernicious anemia increases with age.

Mucus secretion is extremely important because it provides an alkaline protein covering that protects the mucosal cells from autodigestion of the stomach wall by gastric acid and proteolytic enzymes. Factors such as damage to the mucosa by overly abrasive or hot food, or chronic, stress-related reductions in gastric blood flow diminish the secretion of mucus and put the individual at risk of developing ulcers.

The gastric glands also contain endocrine cells that secrete gastrin, to control gastric secretion and motility, and other hormones (such as somatostatin and serotonin) whose significance is less well understood.

Pancreas and liver

The pancreas and liver are considered accessory organs of digestion (Figure 63-3). Their secretions enter the duodenum at the duodenal papilla, which contains sphincter muscles to prevent reflux of the intestinal contents into the common bile duct.

The **pancreas** is both an exocrine gland secreting sodium bicarbonate and enzymes and an endocrine gland secreting insulin, glucagon, and other hormones (Unit XIV). The pancreas lies horizontally along the posterior abdominal wall, and most of it lies outside the peritoneal cavity. (It is the somatic pain fibers that innervate the pancreas from the abdominal wall that are responsible for the intense and sharp nature of pancreatic pain.) Pancreatic secretions empty into the duodenum through the common bile duct and through the smaller accessory pancreatic duct.

TABLE 63-1   Chemical Digestion

Digestive juices and enzymes	Food enzyme digests (or hydrolyzes)	Resulting product*
Saliva		
Amylase (ptyalin)	Starch (polysaccharide or complex sugar)	Dextrins (short polysaccharides) and maltose (a disaccharide or double sugar)
Gastric juice		
Protease (pepsin: pepsinogen + hydrochloric acid)	Proteins, including casein	Proteoses and peptones (partially digested proteins)
Lipase (of little importance)	Emulsified fats (butter, cream, etc.)	*Fatty acids and glycerol*
Bile (contains no enzymes)	Large fat droplets (unemulsified fats)	Small fat droplets or emulsified fats
Pancreatic juice		
Protease (trypsin and chymotrypsin)†	Proteins (either intact or partially digested)	Proteoses, peptides, and *amino acids*
Lipase	Bile-emulsified fats	*Fatty acids and glycerol*
Amylase	Starch	Maltose
Intestinal juice: in brush border of cells of villi		
Peptidases‡	Peptides	*Amino acids*
Sucrase	Sucrose (cane sugar)	*Glucose and fructose* (simple sugars or monosaccharides)
Lactase	Lactose (milk sugar)	*Glucose and galactose* (simple sugars)
Maltase	Maltose (malt sugar)	*Glucose* (dextrose)

From Thibodeau GA: *Anthony's textbook of anatomy and physiology,* ed 13, St Louis, 1990, Mosby–Year Book.
*Substances in italic type are end products of digestion or, in other words, completely digested foods ready for absorption.
†Trypsin secreted in inactive form (trypsinogen) and converted to active form by trypsin itself and intestinal enzyme, enterokinase. Chymotrypsin secreted in inactive form (chymotrypsinogen) and converted to active form by action of trypsin and chymotrypsinogen.
‡Secreted in inactive form (pepsinogen); converted to active form (pepsin) by action of pepsin itself (autocatalysis) in acid environment provided by hydrochloric acid.

The **liver** is the largest gland in the body. It lies just under the diaphragm and occupies most of the right hypochondriac and the epigastric regions. It is made up of two lobes divided into smaller lobes. The functional units of the liver are microscopic hexagonal lobules separated from each other by numerous blood vessels and fibrous strands. Each lobule encloses a central venule and is surrounded by branches of the hepatic artery, hepatic portal vein, and bile duct. Arterial blood provides oxygen for the liver to produce bile and process the hepatic portal blood. For example, the liver maintains blood glucose and amino acid concentration by removing excess glucose and amino acids from the portal blood and secreting glucose when blood glucose levels fall; it synthesizes blood glucose, proteins, amino acids, and fats; it produces and secretes bile, which contains lipid-soluble bile pigments, metabolites, and cholesterol for excretion; and it secretes the detergent-like bile salts that aid in the digestion of fats.

The bile pigments are bilirubin and biliverdin.

(Biliverdin is the reduced form of bilirubin that gives bile its characteristic green color.) Bilirubin is formed from heme during the destruction of erythrocytes and hemoglobin. Blockage of the bile duct and hepatitis interfere with the secretion of bile and thus the excretion of bilirubin. During these conditions and when erythrocyte destruction is excessive, blood bilirubin concentration increases and is responsible for the characteristic yellow coloration of jaundice.

A portion of the lipid-soluble ingredients of bile, such as the bile salts and cholesterol, are reabsorbed from the intestines and returned to the liver. This recycling of bile ingredients is referred to as the enterohepatic circulation.

Bile enters the small bile ducts that join to form the hepatic duct and is delivered to the gallbladder via the cystic duct. The hepatic duct and the cystic duct merge to form the common bile duct, which opens into the duodenum at the ampulla of Vater (Figure 64-2).

The **gallbladder** is pear shaped and green like the

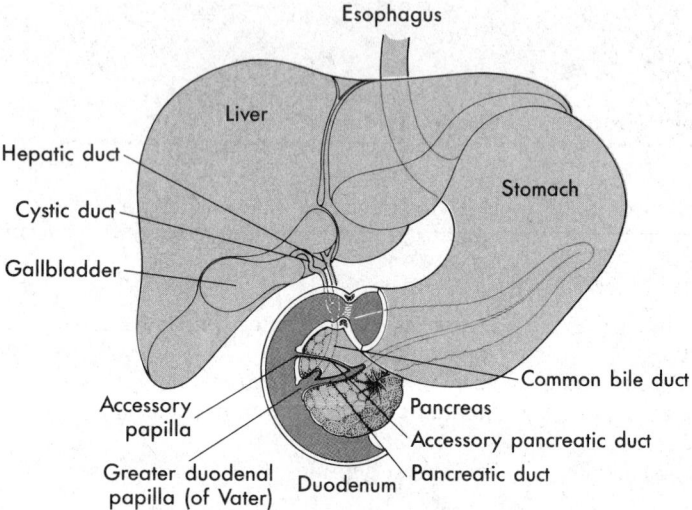

FIGURE 63-3   Liver, gallbladder, and pancreas.

bile it contains. It stores and concentrates bile and contracts to force bile into the duodenum during the digestion of fatty meals. During a lifetime, the reabsorption of water from the bile in the gallbladder may result in the formation of insoluble gallstones, especially if the bile contains higher-than-normal amounts of cholesterol.

Small intestine

The **small intestine** is made up of three regions: the duodenum, the jejunum, and the ileum. The duodenum is approximately 0.25 m long, the jejunum is approximately 2.5 m long, and the ileum is approximately 3.5 m long.

The surface area of the mucosa of the small intestine available for absorption is increased considerably by the provision of millions of villi, which are fingerlike projections of mucosa containing blood and lymph capillaries, and by the fine brush border of microvilli that forms the outer surface of the epithelial cells of the villi. New epithelial cells to replace those lost from the villi by wear and tear migrate from the crypts between the villi where they are produced. Enzymes and mucus are secreted by glands that empty into the crypts between the villi.

The acidity of the stomach contents is rapidly neutralized in the duodenum by the alkaline secretions of the liver and pancreas. The enzymes of the pancreas and intestinal glands continue the digestion of the ingested food nutrients, most of which are absorbed in the small intestine.

The contents of the intestines are mixed by rhythmic segmentation contractions of the circular muscle of the intestinal wall and by pendular movements created by the irregular contractions of the longitu-

dinal muscle. These movements continually expose the mucosa to unabsorbed nutrients and speed up their absorption as they are moved along the small intestines by peristalsis.

The peritoneum forms the mesentery that supports the intestines and their blood supply and lines the abdominal cavity. The visceral mesentery is fan-shaped, short where it is joined to the posterior wall of the abdominal cavity, and long where it is attached to the jejunum and ileum. The secretions of the peritoneum provide lubrication and allow the intestines to move freely against each other.

Large intestine

The **large intestine** has a larger diameter but shorter length than the small intestine, and its walls are puckered into pouches called haustra. It is made up of five parts: the ascending colon, the transverse colon, the descending colon, the sigmoid colon, and the rectum.

The ascending colon on the right side of the abdomen receives the intestinal contents through the ileocecal valve and directs them up to the transverse colon. The ileocecal valve prevents the contents of the large intestine and its potentially dangerous microorganisms from entering the ileum. (The appendix is a vestigial tube that opens off of the cecum, a sac at the inferior end of the ascending colon.)

The transverse colon lies horizontally between two 90-degree flexures and crosses the abdomen just below the liver and stomach. It passes its contents into the descending colon, which carries them vertically down the left side of the abdomen and delivers them into the sigmoid colon. The sigmoid colon is, as its name implies, S-shaped.

The rectum forms the final 20 cm of the intestinal tube. It ends in the anal canal, which is guarded by two sphincters, an internal, involuntary, smooth muscle sphincter and an outer, voluntary, striated muscle sphincter. The mucous membrane of the **anus** is made up of vertical folds to allow it to expand during defecation. Each fold possesses an artery and a vein. If the veins become enlarged they form varicosities called hemorrhoids, which may protrude through the anus and may strangulate and bleed. The smooth muscle of the colon is made up of an inner circular layer and an outer longitudinal layer.

Blood Supply

The stomach and pancreas receive their blood from a branch of the celiac artery, and the small intestine and most of the large intestine receive their blood from the superior or inferior mesenteric arteries. Blood from all these areas is collected into the hepatic portal vein and carried directly to the liver, where absorbed nutrients are processed before they enter the hepatic vein and the vena cava.

Chemical Digestion and Absorption of Nutrients

The enzymes contained in the various digestive juices, the food substances they break down, and the products that result are summarized in Table 63-1.

Carbohydrates

The digestion of starches is begun in the bolus of food produced in the mouth by the salivary enzyme ptyalin. However, this may not be important, because the action of ptyalin is stopped by the low pH of the stomach as soon as the bolus disintegrates. Most of the digestion of carbohydrate occurs in the intestines and is caused by the enzymes of the pancreatic and intestinal secretions: amylase, sucrase, maltase, and lactase.

The final products of carbohydrate digestion are monosaccharides. Glucose and galactose are absorbed from the intestines by an energy-requiring, active-transport mechanism. Fructose and other monosaccharides are absorbed by facilitated diffusion. Virtually no carbohydrates are able to be absorbed unless they first combine with specific carrier proteins.

Proteins

The digestion of protein begins in the stomach and continues in the intestine. The potent proteolytic enzymes of the GI tract are produced in an inactive form to prevent autodigestion of the glands, and they are only activated in the lumen of the tract, which is protected by mucus. The inactive gastric pepsinogen is converted to the active pepsin in the stomach lumen by hydrochloric acid; the inactive pancreatic trypsinogen is converted in the intestinal lumen to the active trypsin by the intestinal enzyme enterokinase, and similarly, the pancreatic precursors: chymotrypsinogen, procarboxypeptidase, and proelastase are activated in the intestinal lumen by trypsin. Autodigestion does occur when the mouth of the ducts relaxes and mucus secretion is deficient. This allows a reflux of the activated enzymes into the glands.

The final products of protein digestion are amino acids. They are absorbed from the intestines by extremely efficient active transport mechanisms located in the brush border of the epithelial cells.

Fats and fat-soluble vitamins

Although a small amount of fat is split into fatty acid and glycerol in the stomach, this reaction occurs mostly in the small intestine after the large fat droplets have been emulsified (i.e., broken down into small micelles) and thoroughly mixed with pancreatic lipase.

The fatty acids and glycerol are rapidly absorbed across the brush border of the epithelial cells because they are lipid soluble. They are reconstituted into neutral fat and secreted into the interior of the villi where they enter the blind-ended lymph capillaries (lacteals). This fat bypasses the liver and enters the general circulation via the thoracic duct.

Lipid-soluble vitamins and other substances are absorbed with the fatty acids and glycerol, and some fat should always be included in the diet to ensure that sufficient lipid-soluble vitamins are absorbed.

The lipid solubility of a number of carcinogens may provide a route for their absorption into the lymph capillaries and their distribution directly to the tissues. This may account for the relationship found between the amount of fat consumed and the incidence of certain cancers: more carcinogens may be absorbed by individuals eating high-lipid diets. Short-chain fatty acids may help protect the tissues from carcinogens because they enter the blood capillaries of the villi and are carried directly to the liver via the portal vein. Many of the carcinogens dissolved in this fat will be metabolized and excreted in bile before they can reach the tissues.

Ions

Specific carrier enzymes are responsible for the absorption of essential cations (e.g., sodium, potassium, calcium, magnesium, iron). Chloride and other small anions are electrostatically attracted to follow these ions, and chloride is also actively reabsorbed in the ileum and colon. Bicarbonate is converted into carbon dioxide and water by hydrogen ions secreted during the active reabsorption of sodium. The carbon dioxide then diffuses readily across the mucosa and can reform into (sodium) bicarbonate and provide additional hydrogen ions to be secreted in exchange for sodium.

Water and water-soluble vitamins

As dissolved substances are absorbed from the lumen of the intestine, the water follows them, attracted across the mucosa by the osmotic gradient that their absorption creates. Water-soluble vitamins are carried across the mucosa dissolved in the water or are carried across bound to special transport proteins.

A large volume of water is secreted during digestion. This water must be reabsorbed in addition to that contained in food and drink.

Control of Gastrointestinal Motility and Enzyme Secretion

The intrinsic activities of the GI tract are refined, coordinated, and controlled by neural and endocrine mechanisms.

Mouth

Mastication is a voluntary activity. However, the secretion of saliva is stimulated by the sight, smell, taste, and acidity of food, as well as by just thinking of eating. For any particular stimulus, more saliva is secreted when the individual is hungry.

Swallowing is initiated voluntarily by pushing the bolus of masticated food to the back of the mouth. However, once the food touches the pharyngeal walls, it initiates a reflex that propels the food into the esophagus. The swallowing reflex center lies in the medulla oblongata. In response to impulses from the walls of the pharynx and back of the mouth, the reflex center causes the larynx to rise and be closed by the epiglottis. This is especially important because it prevents the aspiration of food into the trachea. The reflex center also causes the nasal pharyngeal opening to be closed by elevation of the soft palate, the buccal cavity to be closed by the elevation of the tongue, and the contraction of the walls of the pharynx when all the openings except that to the esophagus have been closed. This contraction forces the food bolus into the esophagus, the only area open to it.

Esophagus

Like the entire GI tract, the esophageal smooth muscle contains an intrinsic plexus nervosus that coordinates its smooth muscle contraction. (Other areas of the GI tract also have a submucosal plexus that controls the activity of their glands.) Distention of the esophagus by a bolus of food stimulates peristalsis, which forces the bolus into the stomach.

Stomach

Contraction of the smooth muscle of the stomach results in a churning action, which mixes the stomach contents to increase the chemical breakdown of the food, and in peristalsis, which moves the stomach contents (chyme) through the stomach and into the duodenum. This innate activity is increased by the vagus nerve after stimulation caused by the sight, smell, taste, or chewing of food (cephalic phase); and it is also increased by the hormone gastrin, which is secreted by the gastric mucosa when the products of protein digestion are present in the stomach lumen (gastric phase). Secretion is inhibited when the pH of the gastric contents falls toward a pH of 1.0.

Gastric motility and enzyme secretion are decreased by the GI hormones, enterogastrone and gastric inhibitory peptide. Lipids contained in the chyme entering the duodenum provide the stimulus for the release of enterogastrone, and thus prolong the time that fatty foods spend in the stomach. The intrinsic movements of the stomach and the secretions of its glands are increased by the parasympathetic nervous system and inhibited by the sympathetic nervous system.

The two stomach openings are kept closed by muscular contraction. Contraction of the cardiac opening prevents the gastric contents from refluxing into the esophagus, and the pyloric sphincter controls the rate at which the stomach empties into the duodenum. Esophogeal and duodenal ulcers may result from relaxation of these stomach openings. The stomach normally empties into the duodenum in spurts when the pyloric sphincter relaxes as a result of strong waves of peristalsis passing over it. However, when the contents of the stomach irritate the mucosa or when the gastric control center in the medulla oblongata is irritated by emetics, the vomiting reflex is induced. The motor responses of this reflex empty the stomach through the esophagus. The larynx rises and is closed by the epiglottis. This is especially important because it prevents the aspiration of vomitus into the trachea. The nasal pharyngeal opening is closed by elevation of the soft palate. The gastric fundus and esophagus relax. After these stages are complete, a sudden and violent contraction of the abdominal muscles raises the pressure in the stomach and forces its contents up the esophagus and out of the mouth.

Pancreas and gallbladder

The secretion of pancreatic juice and bile is stimulated by neural reflexes and duodenal hormones. The hormone secretin is released in response to a fall in the pH of the duodenal contents when chyme enters from the stomach. This causes the pancreas to secrete copious amounts of sodium bicarbonate and the liver to secrete bile. The sodium bicarbonate neutralizes the acid and exerts a negative feedback effect on the secretion of secretin. The hormone cholecystokinin stimulates the secretion of pancreatic enzymes and the contraction of the gallbladder to secrete bile.

Intestines

Stretch of the intestinal wall elicits localized concentric contractions that produce segmentation of the lumen and its contents. The contracted areas relax and the relaxed areas contract alternately to mix the contents of the small intestine with its glandular secretions. Peristalsis is increased as chyme distends the duodenum (gastroenteric reflex), and its waves, which travel along the length of the intestine, are initiated and organized by the myenteric plexus. The movements of the small intestine and the secretions of its glands are increased by parasympathetic stimulation and decreased by sympathetic stimulation of the intrinsic plexus nervosus.

Colon

The movements of the **colon** are similar to those of the small intestine. However, the contents of the colon become progressively more solid as water is absorbed, and segmentation provides most of the propulsive force. Several times a day (particularly after breakfast) strong peristaltic waves cause a mass movement of fecal matter from the transverse colon into the sigmoid colon.

When fecal matter is moved into the rectum, the distention initiates the intrinsic rectal myenteric defecation reflex, which is weak. Stretch receptors in the rectum also initiate a parasympathetic reflex, which is sensed consciously; however, unless the external sphincter is relaxed voluntarily, defecation is prevented by the external sphincter. If the external sphincter prevents defecation, then the sensory receptors adapt and defecation is delayed until additional feces enter the rectum. Constipation often results when the urge to eliminate feces is consistently ignored, because the walls of the rectum (which is normally kept empty) become acclimatized to the presence of feces and thus the reflex mechanisms become less sensitive; and the contents of the colon become drier and harder to move when they stay longer in the colon, because more water is reabsorbed.

Diarrhea can result from irritation of the intestinal mucosa, which causes strong peristaltic waves to sweep the intestinal contents into and through the colon extremely rapidly. Infections and cathartics may also irritate the colon and promote water secretion instead of absorption, and the voluminous liquid contents of the colon are then swept out rapidly in the form of diarrhea.

ASSESSMENT
Subjective

Patients with a gastrointestinal disorder may experience symptoms such as abdominal pain, anorexia, nausea and vomiting, early satiety, or diarrhea.

For example, a patient's presenting symptoms may include vomiting. Vomiting may be secondary to urologic obstruction, increased intracranial pressure, drug toxicity, hepatobiliary disorder, gastroenteritis, pregnancy, or myocardial infarction. Abdominal pain can signal a multitude of problems related to the gastrointestinal, genitourinary, or cardiovascular systems (Figure 63-4).

As for any patient, an adequate system-specific history includes delineation of any positive findings (symptoms the patient complains of) through exploring various dimensions and a review of related systems. The box on p. 1772 provides a list of potential symptoms to review with the patient. In addition to specific symptoms, ask the patient about any history of weight loss, liver or gallbladder problems, irritable bowel syndrome, hepatitis, peptic ulcer disease, polyps, ulcerative colitis, Crohn's disease, hemorrhoids, fecal incontinence, trauma, exposure to infectious diseases, previous abdominal or urinary tract surgery, ostomy, renal disease, cardiac disease, arthritis, or cancer. If the patient is a woman, it may be necessary to determine the date

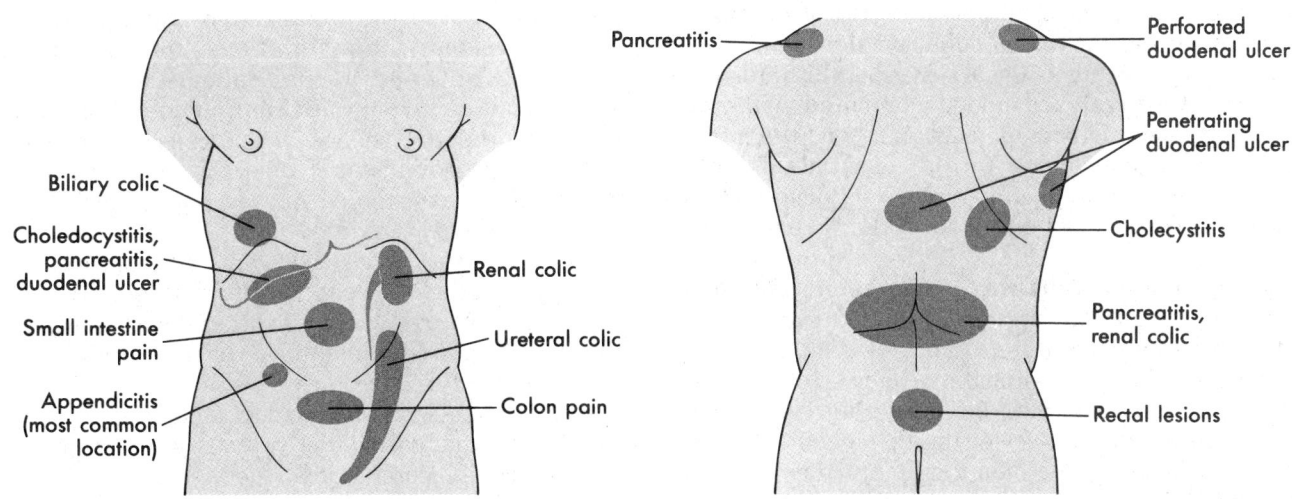

FIGURE 63-4   Common areas of referred abdominal pain.

GERIATRIC CONSIDERATIONS

Physiologic Changes in the Gastrointestinal System

The epithelial cells lining the digestive tract are subjected to constant friction and strong digestive enzymes. Therefore they need to reproduce at a rapid rate. This rate declines with age until it may be 25% slower in elderly individuals. Other aspects of digestive function also decline with age: the number of neurons in the intrinsic neural plexi; the secretion of digestive enzymes, acids, and bases; the gastric section of the intrinsic factor required for vitamin B_{12} absorption; and gut motility. The magnitude of these changes varies considerably from individual to individual. Some may not notice a reduction in digestive function; however, the loss of teeth makes it difficult for others to eat a balanced diet, and some experience a decline in their sense of taste. The frequency of swallowing difficulties and constipation and the incidence of pernicious anemia (inability to absorb sufficient vitamin B_{12}) increase with age. Because the epithelial cells of the gastrointestinal system are constantly being replaced by mitosis, they have a higher risk of developing mutations than less active tissues. Consequently, the risk of cancer increases with age.

POTENTIAL SYMPTOMS ASSOCIATED WITH GI DISORDERS

Abdominal distention
Abdominal pain
Anorectal pain
Anorexia
Belching or burping (eructation)
Black, tarry stools (melena)
Bloody emesis (hematemesis)
Changes in bowel patterns
Constipation
Diarrhea
Difficulty swallowing (dysphagia)
Epigastric discomfort after meals (dyspepsia)
Fecal incontinence
Flatulence (expelling intestinal gas)
Heartburn (pyrosis)
Hematochezia (bright-red blood in the stool or bright-red blood per rectum—BRBPR)
Hemorrhoids
Indigestion
Nausea
Vomiting

---

of the last normal menstrual period (LNMP) and the possibility of pregnancy. In addition, it is essential to determine usual dietary habits. One method is a 24-hour diet recall.

Include questions related to the oral cavity in the gastrointestinal system review (see box on p. 1773). In addition to these symptoms, ask about dental care, dental hygiene routines, and use of dentures or other appliances. Depending on the institution, clinician, and specific clinical situation, this information may be organized and documented with the head and neck history. In general, record the information in one category or the other, but not in both. Oral symptoms may manifest a variety of disorders that may or may not be related to the gastrointestinal system.

Determination of the appropriate related systems to review is guided by the nurse's knowledge of pathophysiology, treatment, and associated symptoms determined in delineating the gastrointestinal symptoms. For example, the patient may complain of abdominal pain. In reviewing the specific dimensions listed above, the pain may be further defined as sudden in onset, severe, sharp, located in the right lower quadrant, and associated with nausea

and vomiting. These symptoms could suggest an ectopic pregnancy, renal calculi, or appendicitis. Further assessment such as whether the pain has changed location since it began, the presence of urinary symptoms (frequency, urgency, dysuria), and the timing of the LNMP, sexual activity, and the use of contraception would assist in narrowing the scope.

Other appropriate history to explore includes major adult illnesses, hospitalizations, surgeries, injuries or accidents, immunizations, current medications, allergies, and habits. Patients with arthritis may be taking nonsteroidal antiinflammatory drugs (NSAIDs) that are well-known to cause gastritis and possibly gastrointestinal bleeding. Patients using digoxin may experience nausea and vomiting secondary to digoxin toxicity.

Family history that is relevant to the gastrointestinal system includes gallbladder disease, renal disease, colon cancer, malabsorption disorders, peptic ulcer disease, irritable bowel syndrome, and inflammatory bowel disease.

Personal/social history may include position in the family, marital status, support systems (formal and informal), coping strategies, educational level, home conditions, occupation, and religious preference. Economic background may also be explored.

POTENTIAL SYMPTOMS RELATED TO THE ORAL CAVITY

Bleeding or swelling of gums
Changes in or impairment of taste (dysgeusia)
Dry mouth (xerostomia)
Hoarseness
Mouth lesions
Pain with chewing
Sore throat (pharyngitis)
Tooth pain (secondary to caries, abscess, or sinusitis)

Objective

Physical assessment may involve several systems. Assessment needs may vary from patient to patient. In general, good lighting, a relaxed patient, and a calm approach will yield the best results. Have the patient in a supine position with the bladder empty. Stand at the patient's right side. Ask the patient to point to any areas of pain, and examine these potentially tender areas last. Monitor the examination by watching the patient's face for grimacing.

General assessment

General assessment includes vital signs, height, and weight. Note facial expression, apparent age as relative to chronologic age, nutritional status, general appearance, and stature. Any obvious abnormalities or assistive devices are also noted. In addition, record whether the patient appears to be comfortable or in distress.

Integumentary

Assessment of the skin is important with most any complaint because it obviously covers the entire body and can reflect systemic illness. Inspect and palpate the skin, noting temperature, color, moisture, turgor, integrity, and lesions. Evaluation of the hydration status of a patient presenting with vomiting and diarrhea should include assessment of skin turgor. The presence or absence of jaundice, a yellowing of the skin or sclera in association with an increased serum bilirubin, is important to note in patients with abdominal complaints.

Oral cavity and pharynx

Inspect the lips, noting symmetry, color, edema, and the presence of any lesions. If the patient is wearing lipstick, it should be removed. Lips should be symmetric, moist, pink, and without lesions. Inspect the teeth, noting number, condition, dental appliances, and occlusion. To observe occlusion, instruct the patient to clench his or her teeth. Normally, with the back molars together, there is a slight overriding of top teeth over bottom teeth. Inspect the oral/buccal mucosa. Instruct the patient to open his or her mouth. Using a light source such as a penlight, carefully observe the mucosa, noting moisture, lesions, color, and patency of the parotid duct orifices (Stenson's ducts). Inspect the gingivae, noting color and presence of hypertrophy or bleeding.

Inspect the tongue, noting moisture, symmetry, fasciculations, and lesions. Instruct the patient to stick out the tongue and move it side to side and up and down. Note if the tongue deviates to one side (CN XII). The tongue should normally protrude midline. Instruct the patient to touch the roof of the mouth with the tongue. Observe the floor of the mouth for vascularity and patency of the submaxillary duct orifices (Wharton's ducts). Note strength of the tongue by instructing the patient to push the tongue into each cheek against resistance.

Observe the hard palate for integrity. Observe the soft palate, noting gag reflex, movement of uvula with phonation (CN IX and X), and placement of the uvula. The uvula should be midline, and the uvula and soft palate should rise symmetrically with phonation.

To inspect the pharynx, instruct the patient to open the mouth widely, breathing through the nose. Adequate visualization may sometimes necessitate the use of a tongue depressor. Occasionally, asking the patient to "pant like a puppy-dog" may allow for adequate visualization. Note color, lesions, and the presence/absence of tonsils. Inspect the tonsils and record size, color, and presence/absence of exudate.

Cardiovascular

Observe the precordium for any pulsations, heaves, or lifts. Palpate the precordium for thrills and the apical impulse. Note the size and location of the apical impulse. Auscultate the precordium with both the bell and diaphragm, noting the rate, rhythm, the first heart sound (S1) and the second heart sound (S2) as well as any extra sounds. A patient with congestive heart failure may have an enlarged liver (hepatomegaly). (See Chapter 33 for a detailed description of the cardiac examination.)

Respiratory

Inspect the thorax, noting symmetry, configuration, and pattern of respirations, including depth, regularity, and ease of respirations. Palpate the thorax for tenderness and masses. Percuss the thorax generally for quality and symmetry. Auscultate the thorax,

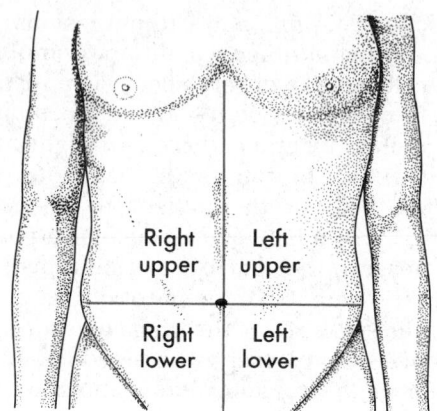
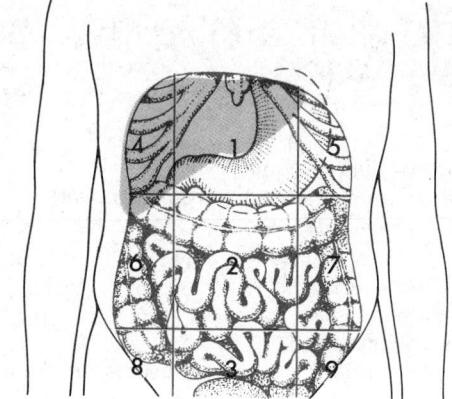

FIGURE 63-5   **A,** Four quadrants of the abdomen. **B,** Nine regions of the abdomen. *1,* Epigastric; *2,* umbilical; *3,* hypogastric (pubic); *4* and *5,* right and left hypochondriac; *6* and *7,* right and left lumbar; *8* and *9,* right and left inguinal.

noting breath sounds and any adventitious sounds such as crackles (rales), wheezes (rhonchi), or pleural friction rubs. A patient with right or left upper quadrant tenderness or guarding may have a lower lobe pneumonia. (See Chapter 25 for a complete discussion of respiratory assessment.)

Abdomen

Throughout inspection of the abdomen, the underlying organs (regions and/or quadrants) should be mentally visualized and used to describe findings (Figure 63-5). Inspect the abdomen, noting pigmentation, lesions, scars, striae, symmetry, umbilicus placement and contour, and any visible peristalsis or pulsations. Because the abdomen may sometimes be protected from the sun by clothing, it may serve as a baseline for comparison with the pigmentation of more tanned areas. Jaundice may be more readily observed in this area. Asymmetric distention of the abdominal wall may be a result of hernia, tumor, or bowel obstruction. Observe for diastasis recti (separation of the rectus abdominis muscles) while the patient raises his or her head.

Auscultate the abdomen before percussion or palpation or prevent disruption of auscultatory sounds. Note presence and timing of bowel sounds and presence of bruits or venous hums. Use the diaphragm to auscultate bowel sounds since they are high pitched. A rumbling noise or audible bowel sounds caused by gas in the intestine are called borborygmi. These may be heard normally as an occasional sound. High-pitched, splashing sounds may be heard in an early bowel obstruction. Always listen at least 2 minutes or longer before concluding that no bowel sounds are present. Use the bell to auscultate bruits or venous hums because those sounds are lower pitched. Auscultate in all four quadrants. Bruits may

arise from the renal, iliac, or femoral arteries or the abdominal aorta.

Percussion is first done generally throughout all quadrants to note tone (Figure 63-6). Normal abdominal percussion tone is tympanic with areas of dullness noted over organs or masses. Tympany reflects the presence of air in the stomach and intestines. This is followed with more specific percussion to determine liver span in the right midclavicular line (RMCL), splenic enlargement in the left midaxillary line (LMAL) or just anterior to the left midaxillary line, gastric air bubble, full bladder or enlarged uterus in the suprapubic area, and costovertebral angle tenderness (CVAT).

To percuss the liver span, begin at approximately the nipple line and percuss down the RMCL, stopping at the point in which the percussion notes change from the resonance of the lungs to the dullness associated with the liver. This is the upper border. Mark this top border. Be careful to percuss only in the intercostal spaces since percussion over a rib will elicit a dull or flat sound, thus creating an error in measurement of the liver span. Next, move down to the lower abdomen and begin percussion up the RMCL stopping at the point in which the percussion note changes from tympany of the abdomen to dullness. This is the lower border. Measure the distance between the two borders. This is the liver span in the RMCL. An expected liver span in the RMCL is within the range of 6 to 12 cm. If the lower border of the liver is greater than 2 to 3 cm below the costal margin, this may indicate enlargement or displacement. Liver span will vary, but it tends to be larger in tall men and smaller in short women (Figure 63-7).

To percuss for splenic dullness, reach across the patient just posterior to the LMAL. Percussion of one to two intercostal spaces of splenic dullness is an expected finding at about the level of the tenth rib.

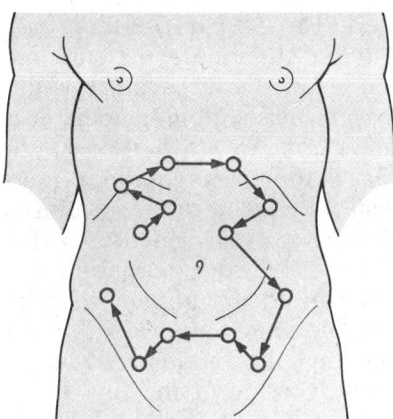

FIGURE 63-6   Systemic route for abdominal percussion.

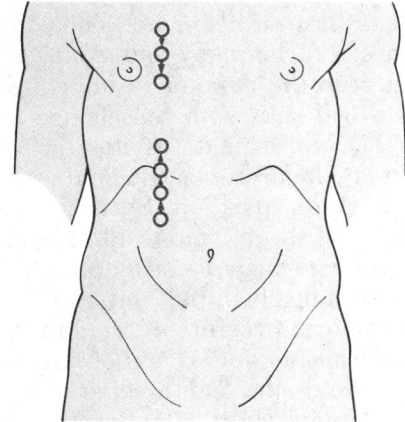

FIGURE 63-7   Liver percussion route.

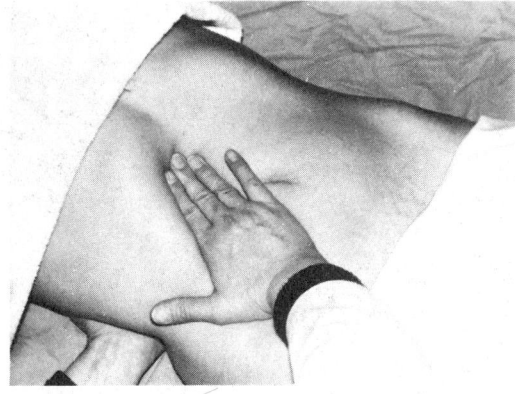

FIGURE 63-8   Palpation of the liver with left hand under eleventh and twelfth ribs and right hand parallel to right costal margin. (From Bowers AC, Thompson JM: *Clinical manual of health assessment*, ed 4, St Louis, 1992, Mosby–Year Book, Inc.)

More than this could indicate splenic enlargement. Evaluation of splenic dullness can be impaired by stomach or colon contents. Therefore it may be helpful to use another method of evaluating splenic enlargement. When the spleen enlarges, it does so in a downward anterior pattern. Percuss the last intercostal space in the anterior axillary line continuously as the patient takes deep breaths. The respiratory movement brings the spleen forward and downward during inspiration. Thus the percussion note would change to dullness on inspiration if the spleen were enlarged.

Following percussion, begin lightly palpating the abdomen to note muscle tone, areas of tenderness, hyperesthesia, or superficial masses (Figure 63-8). When examining the abdomen, having the patient flex the knees will facilitate relaxation of the abdominal musculature. Be gentle, and observe for grimacing or guarding.

Follow light palpation with deep palpation. It is sometimes helpful to use both hands with one hand placed over the other. Again, palpate all four quadrants of the abdomen, noting areas of tenderness or tension. Specifically identify liver and spleen borders, kidneys, and aorta if possible. Deep palpation may also be used to identify any masses.

To palpate the lower liver border, place your left hand, palmar surface up, under the patient's right flank. Place your right hand on the patient's abdomen, parallel to and just inferior to the right costal margin. Instruct the patient to take a deep breath. Using the palmar surface of the right hand, depress deeply at the costal margin or the area where the lower liver border was percussed. At the same time support and bring forward the liver with the left hand. The normal liver edge will slip under your fingers and feel firm and smooth. The hook or Middleton's technique can also be used in palpation of the liver (Figure 63-9) but is more uncomfortable for the patient.

The normal spleen is not palpable. To attempt to palpate the spleen, reach across the patient and place your left hand under the patient's left flank. Place your right hand on the patient's abdomen at the left costal margin. Instruct the patient to take a deep breath. With the right hand, palpate deeply and toward the anterior axillary line. At the same time, use the left hand to bring the spleen anteriorly. If the spleen was percussed as enlarged, palpate gently to avoid rupture.

Palpation of the kidneys is discussed in Chapter 41. In general, the kidneys are not usually palpable in the adult population.

If the patient gives a history of abdominal pain, determine the presence of rebound tenderness. Palpate deeply in an area of the abdomen away from the reported area of pain. Quickly release the pressure of deep palpation and, at the same time, ask

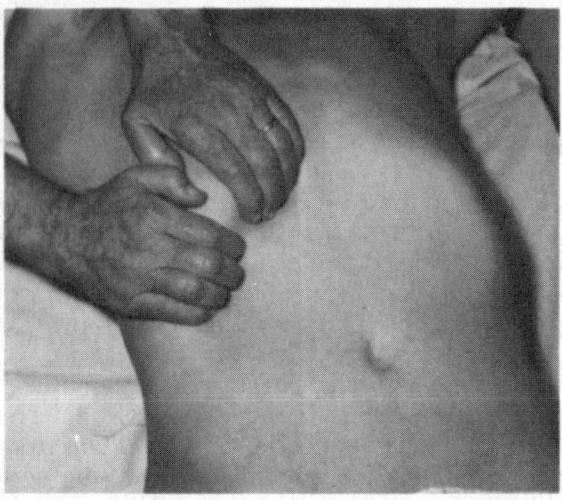

FIGURE 63-9   Liver palpation using Middleton or hook technique. (From Seidel HM et al: *Mosby's guide to physical examination,* ed 2, St Louis, 1991, Mosby–Year Book, Inc.)

the patient which hurts more, the pressure of deep palpation or the release of the pressure. Increased pain with quick release of pressure constitutes rebound tenderness. Rebound tenderness is generally associated with peritonitis. Because of the possibility of increasing the patient's level of pain, assessing for rebound tenderness should be performed at the end of the abdominal examination (Figure 63-10).

Two other tests may be used in assessing the patient with abdominal pain: the iliopsoas test and the obturator test. To perform the iliopsoas test, have the patient lie on the unaffected side and raise the contralateral leg at the hip against your resistance. A positive response is abdominal pain or an increase in abdominal pain. An alternative method to perform this test is to have the patient in a supine position and raise the leg at the hip against resistance. The obturator test is performed with the patient in a supine position. Instruct the patient to flex at the hip and knees. Hold the patient's leg immediately proximally to the knee and grasp the ankle. Rotate the lower leg medially and laterally while internally and externally rotating at the hip. Pain in the involved lower quadrant constitutes a positive obturator sign.

Evaluation of ascites may be done through percussion or palpation. Percussion is used to determine any areas of shifting dullness. With the patient in a supine position, map out the areas of tympany and dullness. Mark the areas of change. Then instruct the patient to turn on his or her side. Again determine the areas of tympany and dullness. Because fluid will shift to the dependent areas, the lines of demarcation will shift with the change in position (Figure 63-11). To evaluate ascites through palpation, determine the presence of a fluid wave with the patient in a supine position. Because this test requires the use of three hands, either another clinician or the patient may assist by placing the ulnar aspect of a hand firmly in the center of the patient's abdomen. The firm pressure exerted in the midline will prevent transmission of motion through subcutaneous adipose tissue. Tap the lateral aspect of the patient's abdomen while palpating the other side. Palpation of a fluid wave indicates ascites.

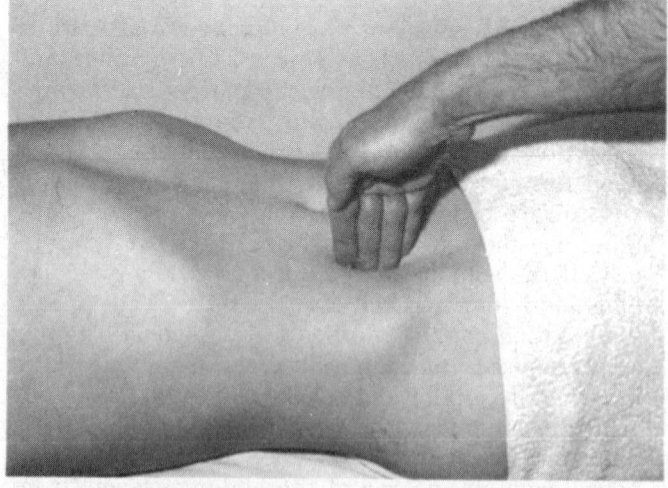
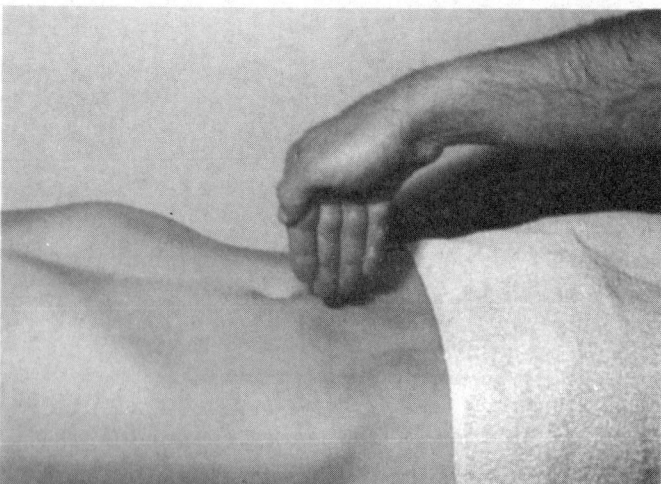

FIGURE 63-10   Testing for rebound tenderness. (From Seidel HM et al: *Mosby's guide to physical examination,* ed 2, St Louis, 1991, Mosby–Year Book, Inc.)

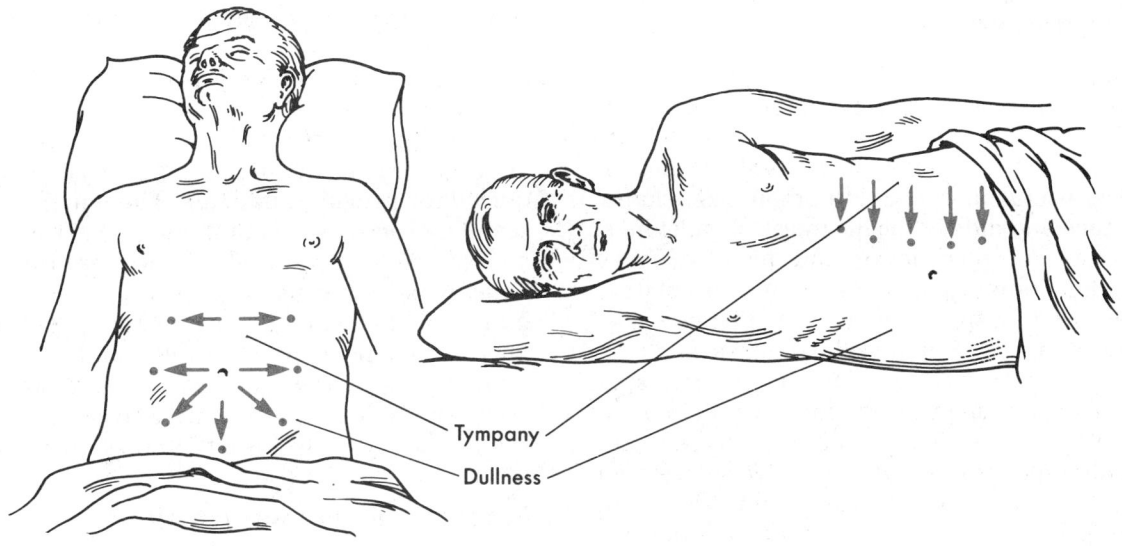

FIGURE 63-11   Test for shifting dullness.

Rectum

A rectal examination may be necessary, especially in the patient with abdominal pain or rectal bleeding. This examination is discussed in Chapter 68.

Genitalia

Examination of the male and female genitalia is discussed in Chapter 68. A patient with pelvic inflammatory disease, ovarian cyst or torsion, or an ectopic pregnancy may experience abdominal pain.

DIAGNOSTIC AND LABORATORY TESTS
Computed Tomography of the Abdomen

Computed tomography or computerized axial tomography (CT) provides detailed information of tissue densities and is used in the diagnosis of acute and chronic pancreatitis, pancreatic cysts, abnormalities of the common bile duct, cirrhosis of the liver, ascites, aneurysms, and pancreatic cancer. Computed tomography is preferred over ultrasonography when the patient is obese, since excessive fat hinders the transmission of ultrasound. Barium studies should precede computed tomography by at least 4 days, since barium may impede adequate visualization. The patient is placed inside a body scanner that passes radiation pulses through the patient's body, which are picked up by detectors, processed by a computer, reconstructed, and projected onto a screen. Water-soluble contrast dyes may be used to better delineate pancreatic margins. The patient must avoid oral intake for 4 hours before the study; otherwise no special preparation is required. The test takes 25 to 40 minutes.

GERIATRIC CONSIDERATIONS

Gastrointestinal Assessment
General approach

- Allow more time than for a younger adult
- Articulate clearly; the geriatric patient may be hearing impaired
- Impaired sight, comprehension, or mobility may result in less than optimum cooperation
- Provide clear, concise instructions

History collection

- Be alert for answers that do not seem appropriate; the patient may not have understood the question correctly because of impaired hearing or impaired comprehension
- Some questions may need to be repeated in a different manner
- The elderly patient may not complain of pain as a result of decreased pain sensations

Physical assessment

- The physical examination itself is not different, but the approach needs to be altered such that the appropriate information is assessed without undue discomfort or embarrassment for the patient
- Maintain an environment with minimal noise, distractions, and interruption
- The abdomen generally has less subcutaneous and adipose tissue as well as decreased muscle tone as a result of a decrease in muscle mass and connective tissue.
- Liver size may decrease after age 50
- Salivary gland secretions decrease in the elderly

Ultrasonography

Ultrasound involves transmission of high-frequency sound waves into the body area under examination. The echoes from the sound waves are converted into electrical energy and appear on an oscilloscope. Ultrasound is useful in evaluating organ size, shape, and structure and aids in the diagnosis of gallstones, differentiation of obstructive and nonobstructive jaundice, detection of pancreatic cysts and enlargement, detection of splenic cysts and splenomegaly, and in screening for hepatocellular disease. Ultrasonography is painless, safe, and has largely supplanted the cholecystogram and intravenous cholangiogram in the diagnosis of gallbladder disease. Endoscopic ultrasonography, which involves placement of a transducer into the posterior wall of the stomach shows promise in the early detection of pancreatic cancer.

The procedure is explained to the patient. The nurse instructs the patient to fast for 8 to 12 hours before the procedure to reduce bowel gas, which can hinder transmission of sound waves. If ultrasound of the gallbladder is desired, the patient is told to have a fat-free meal the evening before the procedure, so that bile will accumulate and enhance ultrasonic visualization. During the test, gallbladder contractility may be evaluated by giving the patient a fatty meal or an intravenous injection of sincalide. Sincalide may produce nausea, sweating, and flushing.

Scintigraphy

Scintigraphy, or nuclear imaging, involves intravenous injection of a small amount of radioactive isotope. A scintigraphic camera provides a two-dimensional representation of the gamma rays emitted by the nucleotide and measures the concentration of the radioisotope in a body site. The camera itself does not emit radiation; instead it detects the small and harmless amount of radiation emitted from the radioisotope as it localizes in the body. Radionucleotide scanning is used in the diagnosis of hepatocellular disease, hepatic metastases, biliary disease, lower gastrointestinal bleeding, gastric reflux, and Meckel's diverticulum. Nuclear imaging scans should be scheduled before tests involving barium since barium opacifies sites and blocks the exit of protons from the radionucleotides.

Patient preparation

The nurse informs the patient that the test allows visualization of the area of concern and that the patient will be required to lie still throughout the procedure. The patient is reassured that analgesics will be given, as ordered, to alleviate pain and facilitate the positioning. If the patient is especially anxious, someone can remain in the room throughout the procedure. Fasting is required for 3 to 4 hours for scans of the gallbladder, Meckel's diverticulum, and gastric emptying. Clear fluids are allowed before scans for gastrointestinal bleeding. Signed consents are required for investigational scans and may be required for pregnant patients. The length of time for scanning varies; scans of the liver, gastric emptying, and Meckel's diverticulum take approximately 1 hour, whereas scans of the gallbladder and gastrointestinal bleeding take several hours, and late views may be taken up to 24 hours following the initial scan. Following the scan, excreted amounts of radiation are minimal, and only universal precautions are necessary in disposing of body wastes.

Magnetic Resonance Imaging

Magnetic resonance imaging (MRI) is used primarily to create cross-sectional images of the liver and has more limited usefulness in imaging the biliary tree and the pancreas. The soft tissue detail and contrast of MRI is particularly useful in detecting focal lesions of the liver. During MRI an energy field is generated with a magnet and radio waves, and the subsequent absorption and release of energy is detected and changed to a visual image.

Patient preparation

The nurse explains that the test permits visualization of the abdominal organ under study and informs the patient that he or she will be placed on a narrow, padded, nonmetallic stretcher that is pushed inside a scanner tunnel. To minimize feelings of claustrophobia, fans inside the cylinder circulate air and mirrors provide a view of the room. The patient will hear metallic thumping noises that can be minimized through the use of earplugs. The patient is instructed to remove all jewelry, hair clips, and clothing with metal clips because these will produce artifacts. The MRI machine may deactivate pacemakers and implanted insulin pumps and move orthopedic or surgical clips, so the presence of these items must be reported. The machine may also interfere with the functioning of some IV drip regulators; therefore the nurse needs to check with MRI personnel about the infusion. No food or fluid restrictions are necessary. The test takes about 1 hour.

Diagnostic Tests for Disorders of the Upper Gastrointestinal System

Esophageal function studies

Several tests are useful in evaluating the functioning of the esophagus and aid in diagnosing the esophageal reflex. Before the tests, the patient swal-

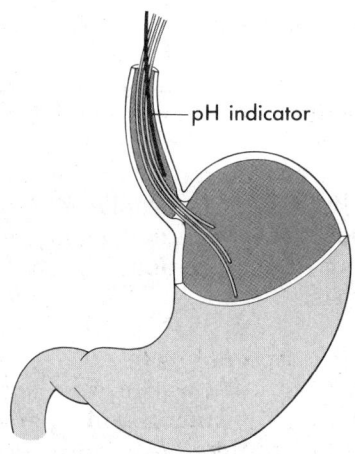

FIGURE 63-12   Esophageal function studies: placement of manometry tubes and pH probe within the esophagus.

lows three very thin tubes, the ends of which are 2 in (5 cm) apart (Figure 63-12). The distal ends of these tubes are initially passed into the stomach, and the proximal ends are attached to transducers. The tubes are used for five different studies of esophageal function.

Lower esophageal sphincter pressure—After insertion of the tubes into the stomach, they are slowly pulled backward. A rapid increase in pressure readings is indicative of the high-pressure zone of the lower esophageal sphincter (LES) (the value between the esophagus and the stomach). When the sphincter is unable to maintain a pressure greater than the tension of the stomach, acid flows back into the esophagus, producing the gastroesophageal reflex. Normal LES pressure is 10 to 20 mm Hg.

Swallowing pattern—With the three tubes in the esophagus, the patient is instructed to swallow, which normally registers a rapid rise and fall in pressure. Few, if any, swallowing waves are recorded on the graph if the patient has achalasia, whereas strong, propulsive, asynchronous waves are detectable with diffuse esophageal spasm.

Acid reflux—With the tubes in the stomach, a fourth tube that is a pH indicator is passed into the esophagus, and the stomach is filled with 100 mL of 0.1N hydrochloric acid. In patients with esophageal reflux, the esophageal pH will drop as acid refluxes from the stomach.

Acid clearing—The tubes are pulled back into the esophagus, and hydrochloric acid is instilled through them. The number of swallows that are required to completely clear the acid from the esophagus are counted. Patients with decreased esophageal motility will require more

than 10 swallows to clear the acid. (Normal values are less than 10 swallows.)

Bernstein test—In the **Bernstein test,** normal saline and 0.1N hydrochloric acid are alternately instilled through the tubes into the esophagus. The patient is unaware of which solution is being instilled. Discomfort that occurs with the instillation of hydrochloric acid is indicative of esophagitis or an ulcerated esophageal lesion. If pain continues after the acid has been discontinued an antacid is given for relief.

Patient preparation

The nurse explains that the purpose of the test is to evaluate the function of the esophagus. The patient is reassured that, although initial gagging may occur while the tubes are passed, no other real discomfort usually occurs. The nurse instructs the patient to fast past midnight. Sedation is not given because it will cause a drop in LES pressure, and the patient's participation is necessary.

Barium swallow

The barium swallow (esophagography) is a visualization of the esophagus, stomach, and small bowel using a contrast medium and fluoroscopy. Normally, the mucosa of the pharynx, esophagus, and duodenal bulb and the outline of the stomach appear smooth and regular, and the duodenal loop and jejunum are visualized in increasing numbers of folds. The deep folds of the jejunum produce a speckled pattern because of the barium lodged in them. This test is useful in detecting hiatal hernias, diverticula, varices, strictures, ulcers, tumors, and motility disorders, although more definitive diagnoses may require endoscopy or esophageal function studies. A barium swallow is not performed if a GI perforation is suspected, since a leak of the barium would produce an acute inflammatory reaction. It is also contraindicated when intestinal obstruction is suspected.

Patient preparation

The patient is informed that this test is an x-ray examination of the esophagus, stomach, and small bowel. The nurse tells the patient to drink a flavored barium mixture, 16 to 20 oz (480 to 600 mL) of which must be consumed if visualization is to be complete. The nurse describes the chalky taste and milkshake consistency of the mixture and explains that the patient will be secured to an x-ray table that will be tilted in various positions. The patient is instructed to fast for 8 to 12 hours before the test and to withhold most oral medications. The nurse ensures that the patient removes all metal objects and jewelry from the x-ray field. The test takes approximately 30 minutes. Since the barium may cause constipation and obstruction, the patient is instructed to monitor bowel movements and to notify the doctor if bowel movements have not occurred within 2 or 3 days. Stools will appear chalky and light colored.

Esophagogastroduodenoscopy

Esophagogastroduodenoscopy involves direct visualization of the lining of the esophagus, stomach, and duodenum with a flexible fiberoptic endoscope. The test is indicated for patients with epigastric pain, melena, or hematemesis and for obtaining biopsy samples of gastric ulcers, determining infection of esophageal varices, and removing foreign bodies and polypoid lesions.

Patient preparation

The patient is told that this test permits visualization of the esophagus, stomach, and upper duodenum and is reassured that the insertion of the scope through the mouth will not obstruct or interfere with breathing. The nurse explains that a local anesthetic may be sprayed onto the throat to prevent gagging and that the breath should be held while the spray is used. This anesthetic will taste unpleasant and make the tongue feel swollen. The patient is told not to swallow saliva once the throat has been anesthetized but to allow it to drain from the side of the mouth. The nurse explains that air may be insufflated into the stomach to flatten the walls for better visualization and that this may cause a feeling of fullness.

The patient is instructed to fast 6 to 12 hours before the test. The nurse obtains a signed consent, administers preoperative sedation as ordered, and ensures that dentures and all metal objects and jewelry are removed before the procedure.

Postprocedure care

The patient is assessed for a returning gag reflex by gently tickling the back of the throat. All food and fluids are withheld until the reflex does return. The nurse provides warm saline gargles for throat discomfort and monitors vital signs, including temperature, every 15 minutes for 4 hours. A sudden temperature spike may signal perforation. Perforation in the cervical portion of the esophagus produces pain on swallowing; thoracic perforation causes substernal or epigastric pain upon breathing or movement; diaphragmatic perforation causes shoulder pain; and gastric perforation causes back or abdominal pain.

Gastric analysis

Gastric analysis involves the examination of aspirated gastric juices. A gastric analysis may be per-

formed to evaluate the completeness of a vagotomy, confirm hypersecretion or achlorhydria, estimate acid secretory capacity, or assay for intrinsic factor. As a result of difficulties in maintaining accuracy, the value of gastric analysis has been questioned; however, it is still considered a worthwhile adjunct to other tests. Endoscopy has replaced gastric analysis in differentiating between malignant and benign lesions. Various determinations can be made from gastric analysis.

Basal gastric secretion rate

The determination of basal gastric secretion rate aids in measuring how much acid a patient secretes without intentional stimuli. After insertion of the nasogastric tube, gastric contents are aspirated while the patient assumes various positions, and this specimen is labeled "residual contents." The nasogastric tube is then connected to continuous low suction for 2 hours. A specimen is collected after 30 minutes, which may be discarded, and then specimens are collected in separate containers at 15-minute intervals for 1 hour. Gastric contents are measured at the end of each interval, and the color, odor, and presence of food, mucus, or bile is noted. A secretion rate of more than 6 mEq/hr is indicative of hypersecretion. A rate of 15 mEq/hr may be indicative of a hormonal abnormality affecting the parietal cells.

Gastric acid stimulation test

The gastric acid stimulation test measures the secretion of gastric acid after an injection of a drug such as histamine, Histalog, or Pentagastrin that stimulates gastric acid output. If parietal cells are damaged or destroyed, acid secretion will be decreased or absent. If the cells are hyperactive, acid secretion will increase in response to stimulation. Responses to stimulation aid in the diagnosis of duodenal ulcer, pernicious anemia, or Zollinger-Ellison syndrome. This test usually follows basal gastric secretion. The patient, with the nasogastric tube in place, receives a subcutaneous injection of the medication and after 15 minutes, a specimen of gastric contents is collected. Additional specimens are collected every 15 minutes for an hour. The specimens are labeled "stimulated contents" and are labeled in sequence. The color, odor, and quality of the gastric contents are observed and recorded. Normally, secretion rates vary from 11 to 21 mEq/hr for women and 18 to 28 mEq/hr for men.

Patient preparation

The patient is told that the test evaluates if the stomach is producing acid properly. The nurse describes the insertion of the nasogastric tube and reassures the patient that it will not prevent breathing. The patient is instructed to restrict foods, fluids, and smoking from midnight before the test. If histamine, Histalog, or Pentagastrin is to be injected, the patient is informed that flushing, dizziness, headache, faintness, and numbness of the extremities, and abdomen may result and is asked to report these changes immediately. Drugs such as cholinergics, anticholinergics, sedatives, and tranquilizers should be withheld for 24 to 48 hours before the test as ordered. If drugs are not discontinued, the nurse should note this on the laboratory slip. Following the procedure, soothing lozenges may be given to relieve throat discomfort. The test takes about 1 hour.

Small bowel biopsy

Small bowel biopsy involves removal of a tissue specimen from the small intestine for examination, and it aids in the diagnosis of diseases of the small intestine such as celiac sprue or lymphoma. A small biopsy tube is passed through the patient's mouth and is followed fluoroscopically until it reaches the desired location in the jejunum.

Patient preparation
The patient is told that the test helps identify and evaluate disorders of the small bowel. The nurse instructs the patient to go on a clear liquid diet 24 to 48 hours before the biopsy and to withhold all food and fluids after the evening meal before the biopsy. Ensure that coagulation test results are documented on the chart and that aspirin and anticoagulants are withheld, as ordered. A signed consent is obtained.

Procedure
The small bowel biopsy capsule and connecting tube are lubricated with water-soluble lubricant, the patient's throat is sprayed with local anesthetic, and then the capsule and tube are passed down the throat. Under fluoroscopy, the tube is advanced to the second and third bowel and past the ligament of Treitz. Suction is applied with a syringe attached to the exposed end of the tube, mucosal tissue is pulled into the capsule, and a specimen is obtained.

Postprocedure care
The patient's vital signs are monitored every 15 minutes for 1 hour, every 30 minutes for 1 hour, and every hour for 2 hours. The nurse reports any signs of abdominal bleeding (increased pulse, decreased blood pressure, dizziness, hematemesis, or coldness) immediately to the physician. Normal diet may resume with the return of the gag reflex.

Blood tests

A few blood tests have specific value in helping diagnose disorders of the upper GI area (Table 63-2).

Diagnostic Tests for Diseases of the Large Bowel

Barium enema

A barium enema involves fluoroscopic examination of the colon after rectal administration (enema) of a contrast medium. Air may also be insufflated after evacuation of the barium. The use of air and barium (double-contrast) technique is more precise especially in the detection of colonic neoplasms. If bowel perforation is suspected, a water-soluble agent such as diatrizoate meglumine (Gastrografin) is used instead of barium. A barium enema is useful in evaluating the colon for malignancies (Figure 63-13), polyps, diverticulitis, and inflammatory bowel disease. Complete preparation of the bowel is necessary before a barium enema, since the presence of stool in the bowel will interfere with visualization of the bowel. Bowel preparation will vary with the radiologist performing the study.

Patient preparation
The patient is informed that the test permits x-ray visualization of the large intestine after administra-

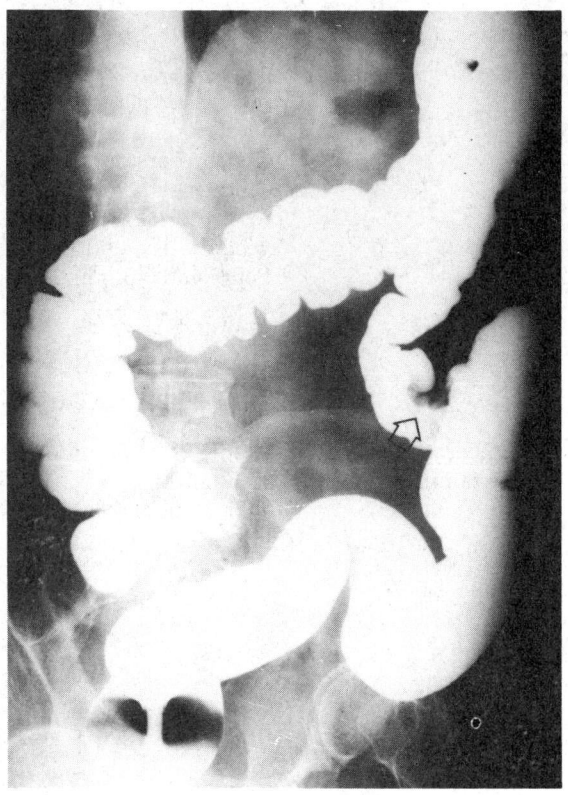

FIGURE 63-13   Barium enema. Cancer indicated by arrow in the descending colon. (From Pagana KD, Pagana TJ: *Pocket nurse guide to laboratory and diagnostic tests,* St Louis, 1986, Mosby–Year Book, Inc.)

TABLE 63-2 Blood Tests to Evaluate Upper Gastrointestinal System

Determination	Usual reference range (SI units)	Description of test
Serum gastrin	16-60 years M: <100 pg/mL (<100 ng/L) F: <75 pg/mL (<75 ng/L) >60 years <100 pg/mL (<100 ng/L)	Gastrin, secreted by the gastric antrum, stimulates the secretion of acid by the parietal cells of the stomach. Markedly elevated levels of serum gastrin are found with Zollinger-Ellison syndrome and pernicious anemia. The patient is instructed to avoid alcohol for at least 24 hours and to fast (except for water) for 12 hours before the test. The patient should be recumbent and relaxed for 30 minutes before the test since stress affects results.
Lactose tolerance test	Within 15 to 60 minutes after ingestion of lactose, plasma glucose levels rise >20 mg/dL (>1.1 mmol/L)	Lactose, a disaccharide found in dairy products, is broken down by the intestinal enzyme lactase into glucose and galactose. When lactase is absent, the lactose is not broken down and is not absorbed, which causes abdominal cramps and diarrhea. Decreased plasma glucose levels suggest a lactase deficiency. The patient is instructed to fast and to avoid strenuous activity for 8 hours before the test. The nurse administers 100 g of lactose orally, and ensures that blood samples for plasma glucose are drawn 30, 60, and 120 minutes after administration of the lactose.

D-Xylose absorption test	Blood levels: 25 to 40 mg/dL (1.7 to 2.7 mmol/L) in 2 hours
	Urine levels: >4 g excreted in 5 hours
	Adults 65 years or older
	  Blood levels: 25 to 40 mg/dL (1.7 to 2.7 mmol/L) in 2 hours
	  Urine levels: >3.5 g excreted in 5 hours and >5 g in 24 hours.
		D-Xylose, a monosaccharide, is given orally in water, and then its levels in the urine and blood are checked. Measurement of blood and urine levels helps evaluate the absorption qualities of the small intestine and aid in the diagnosis of malabsorption. The patient is instructed to fast for 10 to 12 hours before the test and to remain in bed during the test, since activity affects test results. Before administration of D-Xylose, the nurse collects a blood sample and a first-voided morning specimen. The D-Xylose is then administered, and all urine is collected for 5 to 24 hours. Venous blood is withdrawn 2 hours after administration of the D-Xylose.

Serum carotene and vitamin A	Carotene: 10 to 85 μg/dL (0.19 to 1.58 μmol/L) Vitamin A: 9.15-9.60 μg/mL (0.5-2.1 μmol/L)	Carotene is a fat-soluble precursor of vitamin A. When fat is poorly absorbed, absorption of carotene and vitamin A is impaired. Decreased carotene and vitamin A levels are found with malabsorption syndrome, febrile illness, and liver disease. Increased carotene levels are found with myxedema, diabetes mellitus, chronic nephritis, and excessive dietary intake of carrots.

tion of barium. The nurse stresses the importance of strict adherence to dietary restrictions, which usually consist of a low-fiber diet 1 to 3 days before the test. Clear liquids or water may be allowed 12 to 24 hours before the test. The patient's understanding of the dietary restrictions is verified. The nurse administers cathartics, such as bisacodyl, as ordered; a history of ulcerative colitis and active bleeding may be a contraindication to the administration of laxatives and enemas. If enemas are ordered the morning of the test, they should be repeated no more than three times, until the solution runs clear. The nurse explains the importance of keeping the anal sphincter tight around the rectal tube during instillation of the barium to prevent leakage of barium. The patient is instructed to take deep breaths to decrease the discomfort of cramps during instillation of the barium. The nurse stresses the need to take liquids freely after the procedure to facilitate passage of the barium and administers mild cathartics or enemas, if ordered. The patient needs to be reassured that a light-colored stool for 24 to 72 hours is expected.

Colonoscopy

Colonoscopy involves visualization of the entire colon from anus to cecum with the aid of a flexible fiberoptic tube. The tube is inserted through the anus into the large bowel. The bowel must be completely free of fecal material for successful visualization. Colonoscopy allows definitive evaluation of the mucosa of the colon, biopsy of mucosa and lesions in the colon, removal of polypoid lesions, and electrocautery of bleeding lesions. The procedure is contraindicated in patients who have profuse rectal bleeding.

Patient preparation
The nurse explains that the test permits visualization of the entire colon, and that it is a relatively safe procedure. The patient is told that he or she will be draped and placed in a left Sims position with legs drawn up. The nurse informs the patient that some "gas pains" may be experienced because air is insufflated for better visualization. The patient is instructed regarding dietary restrictions (usually a clear liquid diet is permitted 1 to 3 days before the procedure, and then oral intake is avoided for 8 hours immediately before the procedure). The nurse administers cathartics, enemas, and premedication as ordered.

An oral lavage of a saline osmotic laxative such as polyethylene glycol (GOLYTELY) may be better tolerated than the traditional dietary and enema routines. The patient drinks 240 mL of the laxative every 10 minutes over a 2-hour period or until stools

are clear liquid. No other special preparation is required.

Postprocedure care
The nurse monitors vital signs for 2 hours or until stable. Oral intake is withheld for 2 hours because of the possibility of perforation (signaled by tenderness, abdominal pain, and bloody stools). If a polyp has been removed, tell the patient that the stool may be tinged with blood.

Proctosigmoidoscopy

Proctosigmoidoscopy (sigmoidoscopy) involves direct visualization of the rectum and sigmoid colon with a rigid metal endoscope (flexible fiberscopes are replacing sigmoidscopes). The rigid metal scope is approximately 10 in (25 cm) long, whereas the flexible scope is approximately 24 in (60 cm) long.

Patient preparation
The procedure is described to the patient. The nurse prepares the patient to assume a knee-chest position or left lateral position and warns that the urge to defecate may occur as the scope is passed. Colicky pain or muscle spasm may be experienced as the instruments are passed. The patient is encouraged to take deep breaths and to allow the abdomen to go limp as the endoscope is passed. The nurse instructs the patient in dietary restrictions, if ordered, and administers an enema, if ordered, the morning of the procedure.

Examinations of the stool

Stool specimens are collected to aid in the detection of (1) occult blood; (2) ova, parasites, and blood (OPB); (3) microorganisms (culture and sensitivity); (4) fat; and (5) urobilinogen. Specimens are collected in a sterile container for culture and sensitivity and in a clean container for other examinations. A specimen of approximately 1 in (2.54 cm) in diameter is generally adequate unless the stool is being examined for tapeworm; in this examination, the entire stool is sent immediately to the laboratory.

Occult blood test

Testing the feces for occult blood is recommended on an annual basis for all persons 50 years or age or older by the American Cancer Society and aids in early diagnosis of colorectal cancer. It is also useful in detecting bleeding of the lower GI tract but has more limited usefulness in detecting bleeding from the upper GI tract because of alterations in hemoglobin as it passes through the tract.

Several different compounds have been used to

detect occult blood, the most common agent being guaiac. Guaiac is a naturally occurring substance that can be oxidized by hydrogen peroxide with an accompanying color change. Hemoccult II, the most widely used commercial guaiac test, requires that stool is placed on a guaiac-impregnated filter paper slide. Developer fluid is dropped on the slide, and the color is checked in 1 minute. A dark-blue reaction is indicative of occult blood. HemoQuant is a more expensive commercial test that is based on the conversion of heme to fluorescent porphyrins. HemoQuant has fewer requirements for dietary restrictions and can differentiate between heme that has been converted during transit through the gut and heme that has not.

Patient preparation

The nurse explains to the patient that the test helps detect bleeding in the GI tract and specifies whether three specimens or a random specimen is required. The nurse directs the patient to avoid red meat, poultry, fish, turnips, horseradish, and high peroxidase foods such as uncooked fruits and vegetables for 3 days before and during testing. If ordered, iron preparations, salicylates, nonsteroidal antiinflammatory drugs, vitamin C, rauwolfia derivatives, and steroids are withheld because they may alter test results. The patient is instructed not to mix toilet paper or urine with the specimen because this will also alter test results.

Stool culture

The stool can be examined for the presence of bacteria *(Salmonella, Shigella,* and *Staphylococcus aureus),* ova, and parasites. Stool samples for ova and parasites are obtained before barium examinations, because of excess crystalline material that is deposited in the stool. Insoluble diarrhea preparations, mineral oil, tetracyclines, and bismuth may also interfere with detection of ova and parasites. The patient is instructed not to mix urine with the specimen. The nurse uses gloves to obtain specimens and collects specimens in a clean, wide-mouthed specimen jar with a tight-fitting lid. A walnut-sized piece of feces is transferred into the collection jar, and mucus and blood streaks are included if present. A stool specimen for culture and sensitivity may also be collected using a sterile swab and transport medium. Stools for culture should be taken to the laboratory within 30 minutes of collection.

Fecal fat

Fecal fat occurs as a result of sloughed intestinal cells or unabsorbed dietary fat. The presence of large amounts of fecal fat is suggestive of inadequate bile and pancreatic secretions. In a qualitative test, a random stool specimen is collected for examination, whereas with a quantitative test, all stool for a 72-hour period is collected and refrigerated. Wax containers should not be used for collection. Stools for fecal fat should be collected before barium studies. Preparation for the test includes a high-fat diet for 3 days, and avoidance of alcohol, castor oil, and other laxatives. The usual reference range is <7 g/24 hr (<24 mmol/d).

Fecal urobilinogen

Fecal urobilinogen is responsible for the brown color of stools. Decreased amounts of fecal urobilinogen, which usually occur with biliary obstruction, result in a light, clay-colored stool. Specimens for urobilinogen should be collected in light-resistant containers and taken immediately to the laboratory, since urobilinogen readily breaks down. The usual reference range is 50 to 300 mg/24 hr.

Diagnostic Tests for Diseases of the Liver and Biliary System

Liver biopsy

A liver biopsy involves needle aspiration of a core of tissue for analysis and is useful in the diagnosis of primary liver disease. It is used less frequently for diagnosis of malignancy or metabolic disease. Because of its invasiveness and possible complications, other procedures have largely replaced the biopsy. Biopsy can identify liver disorders when other methods fail. The procedure should not be performed if the patient has a platelet count below 100,000 (SI units: 0.10×10^{12}/L). A biopsy may be performed with the patient under a local or general anesthetic. However, the procedure requires complete patient cooperation if performed without sedation

Patient preparation

The patient is informed that this test helps diagnose disorders of the liver. The nurse tells the patient who will perform the procedure and where, and that the needle remains in the liver approximately 1 second. If the patient is receiving local anesthetic, a supine position will be assumed with the right hand under the head. The patient is asked to remain as still as possible during the test. The nurse explains that even with the local anesthetic, a sensation similar to a punch in the right shoulder will be felt as the biopsy needle is inserted between the eighth and ninth intercostal space. The patient is instructed to refrain from breathing while the needle is inserted.

The nurse tells the patient to restrict food and fluids for 4 to 8 hours before the test. The patient's history is assessed for hypersensitivity to local anesthetics, and the nurse ensures that platelet count and prothrombin time tests have been performed. A signed consent is obtained. The patient should void immediately before the test, and baseline vital signs are recorded. The nurse administers sedation if ordered by the physician.

Postprocedure care

The patient is positioned on the right side with support under the costal margin to provide pressure. Vital signs are monitored every 15 minutes for 1 hour, then every 30 minutes for 4 hours, and every 4 hours for 24 hours. The nurse watches for symptoms of bleeding (tenderness around the biopsy site) and pneumothorax (increased respiratory rate, shoulder pain, pleuritic chest pain, and decreased breath sounds) and gives analgesics for pain.

Laboratory Tests for Liver Function

A number of tests are useful in evaluating liver function (Table 63-3).

Oral cholecystography

Oral cholecystography involves x-ray visualization of the gallbladder. After oral ingestion of a radiopaque, iodinated dye, the gallbladder will show up as a white-filled vesicle, whereas stones will appear dark. Whereas cholecystography is a reasonably accurate test for the diagnosis of pathologic gallbladder conditions, small gallstones may be missed, and the procedure is seldom effective if the serum bilirubin is greater than normal limits. Adequate visualization of the gallbladder depends on sufficient concentration of the dye, which depends on ingestion of the correct number of dye tablets; adequate absorption of dye from the GI tract (vomiting and diarrhea will prevent adsorption of the dye); abstinence from a fatty meal the morning of the test (a fatty meal will stimulate emptying of the gallbladder and subsequently of the dye before x-ray films are taken); a patent cystic duct (the dye enters the gallbladder through the cystic duct); and concentration of the dye within the gallbladder (a chronically inflamed gallbladder will not absorb the dye). Cholecystography is contraindicated in patients who are allergic to iodine dye or who are in early pregnancy. Ultrasonography is commonly performed in preference to cholecystography, because it is noninvasive, safe, and does not depend on adequacy of dye concentration.

Patient preparation

The patient is told that the procedure permits visualization of the gallbladder. The nurse instructs the patient to eat a fat-free meal the evening before the procedure and then to avoid oral intake except for water. The patient is assessed for hypersensitivity to contrast dyes, seafood, or iodine. The nurse administers 6 iopanoic acid tablets orally, 1 at a time at 5-minute intervals, with 1 or 2 mouthfuls of water, after the evening meal. The patient is observed for side effects of the dye administrations, such as abdominal cramps, vomiting, and diarrhea. The nurse reports such symptoms to the physician immediately. If the patient vomits after administration of the tablets of dye, the nurse examines the emesis for undigested tablets and notifies the physician so that the test can either be cancelled or the dye prescribed again. The patient is informed that he or she will be placed in various positions on the x-ray table and may then be given a high-fat meal or drink to stimulate emptying of the gallbladder. No other foods or fluids will be allowed until the test is complete.

Percutaneous transhepatic cholangiogram

Percutaneous transhepatic cholangiogram (PTC) involves insertion of a needle through the skin and directly into the liver under fluoroscopic guidance (Figure 63-14). Contrast medium is injected directly into a biliary nodule as the needle is slowly withdrawn. The outline of the biliary tree is then visible through fluoroscopy. This test is useful in evaluating the intrahepatic and extrahepatic ducts and until the advent of ERCP was the method of choice in evaluating obstructive jaundice. It is contraindicated in patients with iodine allergies, or who are uncooperative or poor surgical risks.

Patient preparation

The patient is informed that this test permits x-ray visualization of the biliary ducts. The nurse tells the

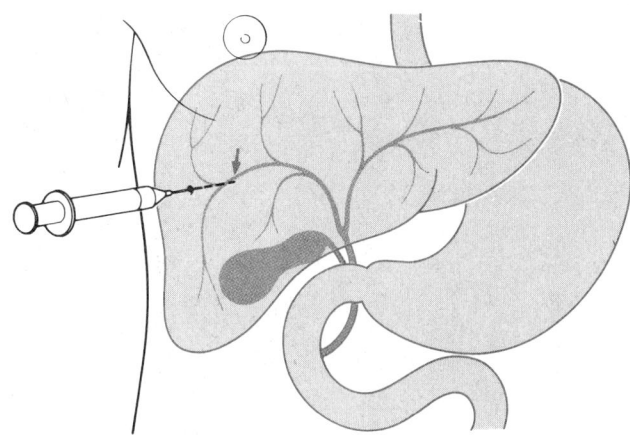

FIGURE 63-14 Insertion of a needle in a percutaneous transhepatic cholangiogram. (From Pagana KD, Pagana TJ: *Mosby's diagnostic and laboratory test reference*, St Louis, 1992, Mosby–Year Book, Inc.)

TABLE 63-3	Laboratory Assessment of Liver Functioning	

Test	Usual reference range (SI units)	Description of test
Plasma ammonia	M: 18-54 μmol/L F: 12-50 μmol/L	The liver synthesizes urea from ammonia, most of which comes from the GI tract. Most of the normal amount of ammonia in blood is in transit to the liver for synthesis. Elevations in plasma ammonia occur with liver damage or alteration to the blood flow to the liver. The venous blood specimen is collected in a heparinized tube, placed on ice, and taken immediately to the laboratory.
5'-Nucleotidase	1-11 U/L (17-183 nmol/sec/L)	5'-Nucleotidase is an enzyme that originates primarily in the hepatobiliary tract. If elevations occur, other liver function tests are necessary to establish the presence and cause of liver disease. The venous blood specimen should be handled gently to prevent hemolysis.
Serum bilirubin	Total: 0.1-1.2 mg/dL (1.7-20.5 μmol/L) *Conjugated (direct):* up to 0.3 mg/dL (up to 5.1 μmol/L) *Unconjugated (indirect):* 0.1-1 mg/dL (1.7-17.1 μmol/L)	Bilirubin, the main pigment in bile, is derived from biliverdin, which is formed in the breakdown of hemoglobin. After bilirubin is formed, it is bound to albumin and transported to the liver, where it is conjugated with glucuronide to form bilirubin diglucuronide, and excreted in bile. The total bilirubin is elevated in all forms of jaundice, but differential diagnosis is dependent on the type of bilirubin elevation (posthepatic, conjugated, direct, or prehepatic, unconjugated, indirect). In hemolytic jaundice, the hemolysis releases more unconjugated bilirubin than the liver can handle, so unconjugated bilirubin levels rise. In obstructive jaundice, levels of conjugated bilirubin rise, since the flow of bile is obstructed. With hepatic jaundice, liver cell jaundice causes all bilirubin values to rise. Yellow foods (yams and carrots), radiopaque contrast dyes, and numerous drugs (allopurinol, barbiturates, flurazepam, indomethacin, isoniazid, meperidine, morphine, oral contraceptives, sulfonamides, steroids, penicillin, and caffeine) influence bilirubin levels. The patient is instructed to fast for 4 hours before the test. The sample is protected from strong light, since light causes breakdown of bilirubin.
Urine bilirubin	Negative	Urine bilirubin produces yellow, smoky, or light brown coloration of the urine. The tests for urine bilirubin distinguish the appearance of urine from that caused by hemoglobin or myoglobin. If bilirubin is present in the urine, it is of the conjugated type, and therefore is useful in establishing the cause of jaundice.

TABLE 63-3   Laboratory Assessment of Liver Functioning—cont'd

Test	Usual reference range (SI units)	Description of test
		The patient is instructed in the collection of a random specimen of urine. Urine may be tested at the bedside (dipstick method or Ictotest tablet method) while it is fresh. Bilirubin breaks down on exposure to light or room temperature after 30 minutes.
Alanine aminotransferase (ALT); formerly serum glutamic-pyruvic transaminase (SGPT)	Adult: 8-20 U/L >60 y, M: 7-24 U/L F: 7-16 U/L	ALT is an enzyme that is found in highest concentrations in the liver. Serum ALT values are elevated 30 to 50 times normal in toxic hepatitis, and 20 times normal in infectious mononucleosis. Little or no elevation occurs with myocardial infarction. Drugs such as erythromycin, gentamicin, meperidine, morphine, codeine, digitalis, indomethacin, and salicylates cause decreased levels of ALT. Drugs that are being taken by the patient should be noted on the laboratory requisition.
Aspartate aminotransferase (AST); formerly serum glutamic-oxaloacetic transaminase (SGOT)	Adult: 8-20 U/L >60 y: 10-25 U/L	AST is an enzyme that is found in the pancreas, liver, heart muscle, skeletal muscle, and kidneys. AST levels are elevated within 8 to 12 hours of damage to the parenchymal cells of these organs. Serum levels peak in 24 to 36 hours after injury and fall to normal in 4 to 6 days. Because AST is found in so many different body organs, the specificity of the test is limited. Extreme elevations of AST occur with acute pancreatitis, severe fulminating hepatitis, severe liver necrosis, and acute myocardial infarction. Intramuscular injections and many drugs (salicylates, ampicillin, meperidine, erythromycin, oxacillin, digitalis, and flurazepam) interfere with test results. Drugs that are being taken by the patient should be noted on the laboratory slip.
Alkaline phosphatase (ALP)	Normal range varies with laboratory method used. SMA 1260 method 20-44 y, M: 102-122 U/L F: 98-112 U/L 45-64 y, M: 139-159 U/L F: 121-132 U/L 65+ y, M: 161-227 U/L F: 172-199 U/L	ALP is an isoenzyme that is relatively specific to bone, liver, intestine, and placenta. ALP is thought to be involved in the calcification of bone; the transport of metabolites across cell membranes and of lipids. Elevations of ALP occur with metastatic carcinoma to the liver, liver abscess, extrahepatic biliary tract obstruction, cirrhosis of the liver, active liver cell damage, rickets, and osteomalacia.
Platelet count	150,000-400,000/μL (0.15-0.4 × 10^{12}/L)	Platelets are tiny disc-shaped cells that largely control hemostasis. Many patients with liver disorders experience clotting disorders, and testing for hemostasis should precede any potentially traumatic or invasive procedure. For further discussion of the platelet count, see Chapter 37.

TABLE 63-3   Laboratory Assessment of Liver Functioning—cont'd

Test	Usual reference range (SI units)	Description of test
Partial thromboplastin time (PTT) or activated partial thromboplastin time (APTT)	25-38 seconds	APTT and PTT assess the intrinsic and common pathways of the coagulation process by measuring factors I, II, V, VIII, IX, X, XI, and XII. Since factors II, IX, and X are synthesized in the liver and are vitamin-K dependent, hepatic disorders or biliary obstruction may produce bleeding tendencies. See Chapter 37 for further details related to PTT and APTT.
Prothrombin time (PT; Protime)	11-12.5 seconds	PT assesses the extrinsic and common pathways of coagulation through measurement of the vitamin-K dependent factors II, V, VII, and X. Prolonged PT may indicate deficiencies in factors V, VII, or X; vitamin K deficiency; hepatic disease; oral anticoagulant therapy; or a number of medications (anabolic steroids, indomethacin, phenylbutazone, and thyroid hormones). A prolonged PT is associated with abnormal bleeding. For further details see Chapter 37.
Coagulation factor assays	Factor I: 0.15-0.35 q/dL (4.0-10.0 μmol/L) Factor II: 60%-150% (60-150 μmol/L) Factor V: 60%-150% (60-150 μmol/L) Factor VII: 65%-135% (65-135 μmol/L) Factor IX: 60%-140% (0.60-1.40 μmol/L) Factor X: 60%-130% (60-130 μmol/L)	Assays of the specific factors in the coagulation system are a useful follow-up to abnormal PT and APTT values. Hepatic disorders and vitamin K deficiencies will produce deficiencies of many of the factors such as I, II, III, V, VII, IX, and X, all of which are synthesized in the liver. For further details related to coagulation factor assays, see Chapter 37.

patient that the abdomen will be localized and that some pressure may occur as the needle is placed into the liver. The patient's history is assessed for hypersensitivity to contrast dyes or iodine. The nurse instructs the patient to fast for 8 hours before the test. If ordered, laboratory results are reviewed to ensure that bleeding, clotting, and prothrombin times, as well as platelet count, are normal. The nurse administers a laxative the evening before the test and a cleansing enema the morning of the test, if ordered.

A signed consent is obtained, and premedication administered, if ordered.

Postprocedure care

The nurse monitors the patient's vital signs closely for indications of hemorrhage and observes the needle insertion site for hemorrhage and bile leakage. A sandbag is placed over the insertion site, if ordered. The patient is maintained on bed rest and avoids oral intake, as ordered, in case surgery is necessary to control hemorrhage or bile extravasation. If a catheter is left in the biliary tract, the nurse establishes and maintains a sterile drainage system.

Diagnostic Tests for Diseases of the Pancreas

Endoscopic retrograde cholangiopancreatography

Endoscopic retrograde cholangiopancreatography (ERCP) involves endoscopic cannulation of the ampulla of Vater and retrograde injection of radiographic dye into the bile ducts. During the test, a fiberoptic duodenoscope is inserted through the oral pharynx, through the esophagus and stomach, and into the duodenum. The patient is given secretin intravenously to paralyze the duodenum and permit easier identification of the ampulla of Vater. A small catheter is passed down an accessory lumen of the scope and through the ampulla into the desired duct. Dye is injected and x-ray films are taken. The test aids in detection of strictures, intraductal stones, and malignant tumors, and is the method of choice in diagnosing pancreatic disorders. ERCP is contraindicated if the patient's bilirubin is greater than 3.5 mg/dL (61 μmol/L) or if the patient is uncooperative.

Patient preparation

The nurse explains that the test permits visualization of the common bile or pancreatic duct and takes approximately 1 hour. The necessity of remaining motionless during the test is stressed. The patient is reassured that no discomfort will be felt other than gagging as the duodenoscope is passed or an unpleasant taste if a local anesthetic is used to keep the patient from gagging. The patient is told that sedation will be administered intravenously to maintain comfort. The nurse instructs the patient to fast after midnight. A signed consent is obtained and baseline vital signs are recorded. The nurse administers premedication, as ordered.

Serum amylase and lipase

Amylase is a digestive enzyme for carbohydrates and is excreted by the pancreas, bowel, gynecologic system, and parotid glands. Levels of lipase secreted by the pancreas parallel elevations in amylase. Serum amylase is not elevated with chronic pancreatitis, but amylase and lipase levels are elevated with acute pancreatitis. Serum amylase is also elevated with mumps, pelvic inflammatory disease, and ischemic bowel disease. Usual reference range is amylase: Adult 25-125 U/L; >70 y 21-160 U/L; lipase: Adult 10-140 U/L; >60 y 18-180 U/L.

Urine amylase

Amylase is excreted into the GI tract and then into the blood. After glomerular filtration, amylase appears in the urine. Urine amylase values will usually rise in tandem with serum amylase values, but they will take 7 to 10 days to fall to normal after the onset of acute pancreatitis, whereas serum values will take 2 to 3 days to fall. The urine is collected for 2-, 6-, 8-, or 24-hour periods (see Chapter 41 for description of collection of 24-hour specimens) and is kept refrigerated. If the patient is catheterized, the catheter bag should be kept on ice. The usual reference range is 1 to 17 U/h.

CRITICAL THINKING QUESTIONS

1 What is peristalsis and how does it aid in the digestion and absorption of nutrients?
2 Describe the digestive process for each group of essential nutrients. In what GI tract organ does it begin and what are the final products of digestion?
3 Design at least three questions to discreetly ask patients about bowel patterns and characteristics of the stools.
4 Discuss psychologic and sociocultural factors to consider throughout the physical examination of the patient's abdomen.
5 Describe tests that are commonly used in the diagnosis of disorders of the gallbladder.
6 Of what complications must patients who undergo barium studies be warned?

BIBLIOGRAPHY

Current

1. Adam A: Imaging of the liver and biliary tract, *Medicine* 17:2127, Feb 1991.
2. Beck I: Investigating in pancreatic function, *Medicine* 17:2172, Feb 1991.
3. Beck I: Imaging and clinical approach to pancreatic disease, *Medicine* 17:2179, Feb 1991.
4. Bowers A, Thompson J: Clinical manual of health assessment, ed 3, St Louis, 1988, Mosby−Year Book, Inc.
5. Burrell LO: *Adult nursing in hospital and community settings,* Norwalk, 1992, Appleton & Lange.
6. *Diagnostic tests,* Springhouse PA, 1991, Springhouse Corporation.
7. Fleisher D et al: Detection and surveillance of colorectal cancer, *JAMA* 261(4):580, 1989.
8. Gallo JJ et al: *Handbook of geriatric assessment,* Rockville, Maryland, 1988, Aspen Publishers.
9. Gordon M: *Manual of nursing diagnosis,* New York, 1987, McGraw-Hill.
10. Kane RL et al: *Essentials of clinical geriatrics,* ed 2, New York, 1989, McGraw-Hill.
11. Knight K et al: Occult blood screening for colorectal cancer, *JAMA* 261(4):587, 1989.
12. Malasanos L et al: *Health assessment,* ed 4, St Louis, 1990, Mosby−Year Book, Inc.
13. Norman V: Bowel elimination alterations. In Snyder M, editor: *Guide to neurological nursing,* New York, 1989, John Wiley & Sons.
14. Pagana KD, Pagana TJ: *Diagnostic testing and implications,* St Louis, 1990, Mosby−Year Book, Inc.
15. Seidel HM et al: *Mosby's guide to physical examination,* ed 2, St Louis, 1991, Mosby−Year Book.
16. Semlacher EA, Shaffer EA: Jaundice: an approach to investigation and management, *Medicine* 17:2010, Feb 1991.
17. Silen W: *Cope's early diagnosis of the acute abdomen,* New York, Oxford University Press.
18. Swartz MH: *Textbook of physical diagnosis,* Philadelphia, 1989, WB Saunders.

Classic

19. Block G, Nolan J: *Health assessment for professional nursing: a developmental approach,* New York, 1986, Appleton-Century-Crofts.
20. Brunner LS, Suddartn DS: *Textbook of medical-surgical nursing,* Philadelphia, 1984, JB Lippincott.
21. Buschiazzo L, Naab G: Careful assessment of abdominal pain, *J Emerg Nurs* 12(2):72, 1986.
22. Carotenuto R, Bullock J: *Physical assessment of the gerontologic client,* Philadelphia, 1981, FA Davis Co.
23. Fields W, McGinn-Campbell K: *Introduction to health assessment,* Reston, Va, 1983, Reston Publishing Co.

24. Given BA, Simmons SJ: *Gastroenterology in clinical nursing,* St Louis, 1984, Mosby–Year Book, Inc.
25. McShane R, McLane A: Constipation: consensual and empirical validation, *Nurs Clin North Am* 20(4):801, 1985.
26. Murray R, Zentner S: Nursing assessment and health promotion through the life span, Englewood Cliffs, NJ, 1989, Prentice-Hall.
27. Prior JA, Silberstein JS, Stang J: Physical diagnosis: the history and examination of the patient, St Louis, 1981, Mosby–Year Book, Inc.

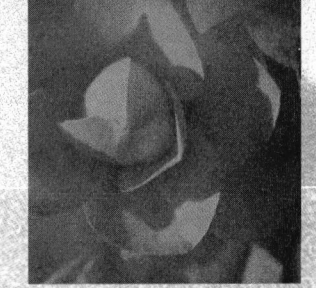

CHAPTER SIXTY-FOUR

Nursing Management of Adults with Disorders of the Mouth or Esophagus

---

LEARNING OBJECTIVES

1 Explain the cause, treatment, and prevention of dental problems.
2 Discuss the oral changes and nursing management of the aging patient.
3 Describe the common infections of the oral cavity and treatment.
4 Identify common products for oral hygiene.
5 Explain the etiology of oral cavity carcinoma.
6 Describe nursing interventions for the patient with esophageal disorders.
7 Differentiate between malignant and benign conditions of the esophagus.

KEY TERMS

achalasia, p. 1813
aphthous ulcers, p. 1796
bougienage, p. 1804
candidiasis, p. 1795
dysphagia, p. 1803
erythroplakia, p. 1798
gastroesophageal reflux (GERD), p. 1801
glossectomy, p. 1799

hiatal hernia, p. 1807
leukoplakia, p. 1798
lower esophageal sphincter (LES), p. 1801
odynophagia, p. 1803
periodontal disease, p. 1792
plaque, p. 1792
pyrosis, p. 1803
regurgitation, p. 1803

THE PROCESS of taking food and fluids into the body through the gastrointestinal tract begins in the mouth with mastication of food by the teeth. Food is swallowed and transported down the esophagus and into the stomach. This chapter discusses disorders of multifactorial origin that involve the mouth and esophagus. Oral disorders such as poor dental hygiene, infections, inflammations, and cancer interfere with dietary intake. Esophageal disorders such as dysphagia may also interfere with adequate nutrition.

Dental Problems

DENTAL CARIES
Definition

Dental caries (tooth decay) comprises an erosive process that develops when three conditions are present: (1) a susceptible tooth, (2) bacteria, and (3) a substrate.

Etiology/Epidemiology

Studies have shown that fluorides in community water supplies, individual use of dentifrices, mouth rinses, and well-balanced diets have decreased the prevalence of dental caries.[19] However, dental caries remains the greatest cause of tooth loss before 35 years of age and probably the most widespread human disease in the United States.

Pathophysiology

Caries develops when certain oral bacteria colonize on the surface of teeth in the form of a sticky gelatinous film that also contains mucus, desquamated cells, and food debris. This is called dental **plaque.** *Streptococcus mutans* organisms, the bacteria primarily responsible for dental decay, are seen in mouths with natural or artificial teeth, and their numbers are significantly lower before teeth erupt or after teeth are lost. It is also believed that *Lactobacillus acidophilus* bacteria play a minor role in acid production of plaque.

Dextran is produced by the fermenting of dietary sucrose by *S. mutans* and causes plaque to be sticky. Plaque bacteria, especially *S. mutans,* act on dietary fructose to produce lactic acid. At a pH of 5.5 or below, lactic acid decalcifies enamel. If carbohydrate intake is excessive, plaque bacteria can store intracellular polysaccharides. During periods of carbohydrate deficiency, the plaque bacteria can use this store to continue to produce lactic acid. Thus the development of caries depends on the plaque and dietary carbohydrates. The rate of caries development also depends on the susceptibility of enamel.

Clinical Manifestations

During the early stages, localized pain may result from exposure to hot or cold drinks. In later stages, abscesses form, leading to more severe pain and occasionally facial edema. The clinical appearance of caries begins with a chalky white area on enamel and progresses to a deep lesion. Early decay can be detected by clinical and x-ray examination.

PERIODONTAL DISEASE
Definition

Periodontal disease is not just a single disease but a group of disorders that for the most part are caused by bacteria. These diseases are initiated and sustained by plaque.

Etiology/Epidemiology

The most common cause of periodontal disease is poor dental hygiene. However, in some individuals causative factors are still unknown. Immunologic mechanisms have been implicated, and bacterial toxins and inflammation are the common denominators. Genetic factors do *not* play an important role. Tobacco use has been shown to increase the risk for gingivitis, periodontal disease, and early loss of teeth. Diabetes contributes to periodontal disease by suppression of local cell systems that control bacterial proliferation and inflammation. In addition, inflammation and hyperplasia of the gingiva, which may be related to periodontal disease, are caused by certain drugs. Drugs known to cause such changes are phenytoin (Dilantin) and oral contraceptives.

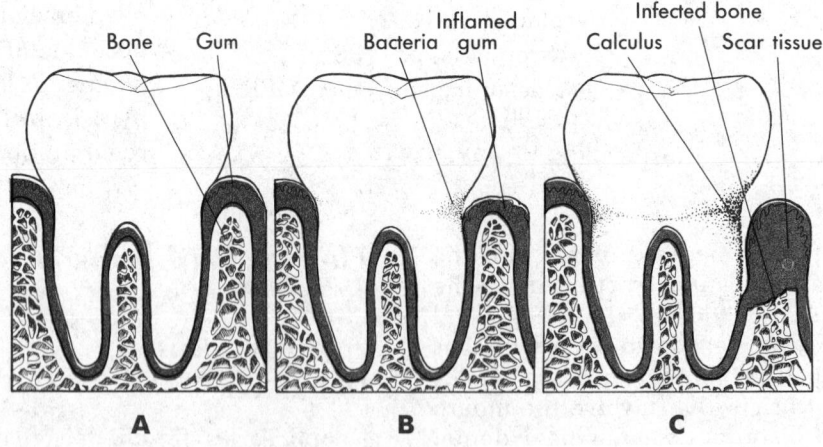

FIGURE 64-1   Progression of periodontal disease. **A,** Normal tooth, gum, and bone. **B,** Gingivitis with inflamed gum and bacterial plaque formation. **C,** Periodontitis with calculus (tartar) formation, loss of alveolar bone, and receding gum with scar tissue formation.

In the United States periodontal disease is responsible for more than 40% of all tooth extractions and is the major cause of tooth loss in people over 45 years of age. The insidious and progressive nature of the disease contributes to the problem, often being diagnosed only after extensive periodontal destruction has occurred.

Periodontal disease has not been extensively researched in the elderly population. The subjects in most studies have been people younger than 65 years old. Some people believe periodontal disease is not as serious a problem with elderly persons as it is with middle-aged persons. It is possible that periodontal problems in elderly persons tend to be quiescent, the principal tissue damage having occurred in previous years.[13]

Pathophysiology

In periodontal disease, plaque collects between the tooth and gum margins. With the collection of bacteria, saliva, and food debris in these spaces, the gum becomes inflamed; this is termed gingivitis (Figure 64-1). Calculus (a cementlike compound) accumulates in the gingival crevices, which worsens the inflammatory process and accelerates bone loss and loosening of the teeth. This stage is usually accompanied by bleeding, swelling, and pain. Frank pus sometimes exudes from under the gingival margin, accounting for the now outmoded term *pyorrhea*.

Clinical Manifestations

The symptoms of periodontal disease (chronic gingivitis or periodontitis) are usually so mild that they may go unnoticed. Patients may complain of discomfort from their teeth, bleeding of gums, difficulty when eating, looseness of teeth, and occasionally abscess formation. A lack of more severe symptoms permits the disease to progress to an irreversible stage before help is sought. In the past the loss of teeth was often considered a process of aging.

NURSING MANAGEMENT OF THE PATIENT WITH DENTAL PROBLEMS

Assessment

The nurse elicits a dental history regarding frequency of dental visits, dental problems, and the usual routine for toothbrushing and flossing. Since smoking is known to contribute to periodontal disease, it should be determined whether the patient smokes, the type of material, as well as frequency. Further questions focus on diet. A diet high in refined carbohydrates influences the formation of dental caries. During inspection of the mouth and teeth,

the nurse assesses and notes the following:
1. General appearance of the teeth
2. Plaque buildup on the teeth
3. Missing teeth
4. Gingival erythema and swelling
5. Purulent exudate
6. Dental caries
7. Halitosis

Dental caries can be detected by visual and x-ray examination. Periodontal disease is confirmed by examination for dental pockets and more accurately assessed by bone loss noted in x-ray films.

Nursing Diagnosis

Nursing diagnoses for the patient with dental problems include the following:

Knowledge deficit related to inability to prevent dental caries/periodontal disease

Noncompliance related to poor oral hygiene/dietary restrictions

Inadequate resources to provide dental maintenance care

Planning

The patient must understand the importance of proper dental hygiene. Patients' attitudes and feelings about whether they will perform the necessary actions to achieve the desired goal need to be determined. Cost of regular dental examination can be a problem. Perhaps the patient eats foods high in carbohydrates because of time constraints or poor eating habits. If the patient is ill and cannot perform the necessary aspects of oral hygiene, is there someone else who will assume responsibility? If the patient is hospitalized or in a nursing home, it is the caregiver's responsibility to perform the necessary action.

Outcomes for the patient with dental problems include:

Performs regular preventive dental hygiene

Follows dietary modifications such as reduced refined carbohydrates

Gets regular dental examinations

Identifies caregivers who can assist with oral hygiene

Implementation

Dental caries must be removed and replaced by suitable dental material. Dental office prophylaxis for periodontal disease includes removal of dental plaque and calculus by scaling the teeth. Once plaque is removed, it begins to form within 2 hours and is well established in 24 hours. It is essential to emphasize frequent removal for clinical success. A recommended program is brushing and the use of dental floss at least twice daily.

For advanced periodontal disease, surgical alterations of gingivae and alveolar bone, as well as splinting the teeth together, may help slow or prevent further deterioration. Prevention, however, is much more effective.

Oral hygiene

Proper hygiene to reduce dental plaque includes brushing the teeth after each meal, vigorous mouth rinsing, and flossing at least once each day. Plaque-disclosing solutions are extremely helpful because they allow patients to determine their own success with brushing by observing the amount of plaque left on the teeth.

Nutrition

Reducing refined carbohydrates, preferably sucrose-source foods, minimizes a major component of plaque formation. Limit between-meal snacks to decrease the contact time for debris left on and be-

---

GERIATRIC CONSIDERATIONS

Mouth Care in Elderly Persons

Oral changes

The oral structure and function change with aging. Severe wear of the teeth is common and increases in the presence of bruxism (grinding of teeth), exposure to abrasive dusts, and habits such as chewing tobacco. With increasing age, the motivation and physical dexterity needed for dental maintenance tend to decline.

Older patients continue to have an increased incidence of root caries. Decreased manual dexterity makes flossing impossible. Power and coordination are also decreased. Some of the muscle is replaced by connective tissue, and soreness and stiffness are common. Uncontrolled movements of the lips, tongue, and jaws make maintenance of oral hygiene more difficult. Atrophy of the mucosa causes it to become red and shiny. The epithelium becomes thinner but is more keratinized, resulting in thin lips and gingivae. Connective tissue is more loosely arranged, with a decrease in blood supply.

Extensive bone changes are found in older patients. Bone loss makes maintenance of denture function more costly and time consuming. Continued deterioration of the bone and atrophy of the gums necessitate correcting the denture fit every few years. Osteoporosis also contributes to degenerative bone changes that increase with age.

The amount and viscosity of salivary flow decrease with aging. Decreased lubrication makes the use of dentures more difficult. As salivary flow decreases, the incidence of caries increases and taste perception becomes altered. Aging also contributes to changes in microbiologic mouth flora. The prevalence of *Candida albicans* presents a common and difficult problem.

Nursing management

Neurologic assessment is necessary to determine the functional level; status of reflexes, tactile discrimination, recent memory, and muscle strength need to be assessed to see if the patient can perform the required care.

A health history is important to discover if chronic or debilitating diseases are contributing to oral symptoms. Use of multiple medications is common and may cause side effects. Tranquilizers often decrease salivary flow and cause tremors of the mouth and tongue.

Analysis of the patient's nutritional knowledge and subsequent counseling should be a routine part of the intervention program. Analysis of the basic food groups in terms of individual servings is an effective and efficient way to gather information about food intake. The patient can be taught how to choose proper foods and suggestions can be made for improvement. Promoting programs outside the home that provide a daily meal is an effective way to encourage patients to eat. People who live alone find it extremely difficult to prepare a meal that is eaten in isolation.

Microorganisms and poorly fitting dentures contribute to lesions in the oral cavity. The edentulous patient needs to be instructed to gently massage mouth tissues with a soft toothbrush. An inexpensive and effective cleaning agent for dentures is 2 teaspoons of water conditioner (Calgon) and 1 teaspoon of hypochlorite bleach (Purex) in an 8-ounce cup of water. Soaking for 30 minutes is required, and overnight soaking is recommended. Partial dentures with metal attachments should not be placed in this solution because it corrodes some metals.[19]

If teeth are present, proper toothbrushing with a soft toothbrush for teeth or dentures should be done daily. Daily flossing is recommended. Brushing with neutral 1.16% sodium fluoride gel daily greatly reduces root caries in the remaining teeth. If the patient cannot perform oral hygiene and has natural teeth, arrangements should be made to seek dental home care or routine trips to the dentist's office.[19]

tween the teeth and gums. Although a nutritious diet is important, this alone will not prevent periodontal disease.

Fluoride

Fluoride supplements produce a more acid-resistant tooth structure, enhance tooth remineralization, and interfere with bacterial growth. The success of fluoride depends on the amount present in the community water supply and the amount of water consumed daily. Most municipalities have enacted legislation to incorporate fluoridation of drinking water. Daily fluoride mouth rinses and topical applications by the dentist are effective supplements for children and adults who continue to have dental caries.[24] This is especially true for adults with reduced saliva production.

When the patient is ill, the nurse may need to assume complete responsibility for oral hygiene. Individuals with diminished salivary gland function because of certain illnesses, drugs, and irradiation are subject to serious alterations of the oral mucosa. In addition, the natural cleaning process of the teeth and mouth is less effective. In a normal healthy mouth, saliva lubricates and protects the oral mucosa, cleans the mouth, maintains the integrity of the teeth, and fights bacteria. When the normal ecology of the mouth is changed by a decrease in salivary composition, a previously healthy mouth can become vulnerable to decay. Dry and cracking oral soft tissues can be painful, and periodontal health can deteriorate. Recent research has indicated that no commercially available substitutes can compare with the natural lubricating features and viscosity of human saliva.[6]

Evaluation

The patient should be able to state causes of dental caries and periodontal disease, as well as measures to prevent their occurrence. It is important for the nurse to determine if the patient can comply with interventions and whether any changes have taken place as a result of following oral hygiene practices.

Disorders of the Oral Cavity

VINCENT'S INFECTION
Definition

Necrotizing ulcerative gingivitis is often referred to as Vincent's infection or *trench mouth*.

Etiology/Epidemiology

Vincent's infection seems to be associated with fusiform and spirochete organisms. Poor oral hygiene and nutrition are commonly found in these patients. Vincent's infection does not follow any epidemiologic patterns, nor does it seem to be contagious.

Clinical Manifestations

The patient usually has pain, fetid mouth odor, gingival erosion, and ulceration. A tendency toward bleeding may also be noted. Most of the time the patient has malaise but no fever or lymphadenopathy.

Therapeutic Management

The condition improves with hydrogen peroxide–saline mouth rinses (3% H_2O_2 diluted with equal parts of warm saline) and dental prophylaxis. Nystatin mouthwashes are not effective, since contact time with the oral mucosa is very short. Ketoconazole (Nizoral) taken systemically appears to offer an alternative to oral dissolution-type tablets, which some patients find objectionable. The patient is encouraged to eat a soft nutritious diet and to avoid smoking and alcoholic beverages.

CANDIDIASIS
Definition

Candida albicans is a fungus, normally part of the oral flora, that under certain circumstances produces an oral infection called **candidiasis,** also known as *moniliasis* and thrush.

Etiology/Epidemiology

Candidiasis tends to occur in the very young as well as the very old. Other susceptible individuals include those who are immunologically compromised and debilitated from diseases, such as leukemia, diabetes mellitus, and alcoholism. Other individuals at risk are those who are receiving long-term or large doses of antibiotics or steroids that disrupt the balance of mucosal flora, allowing *Candida* to flourish.

Clinical Manifestations

Symptoms of oral candidiasis vary, depending on the acute or chronic state of the infection. The classic clinical appearance includes the formation of white fungal plaques that have been compared with the appearance of milk curds (Figure 64-2). The patient may have either a solitary lesion or multiple lesions covering small or extensive areas of the mucosa. Removal of the plaque leaves an erythematous, painful, bleeding surface.

Therapeutic Management

Hydrogen peroxide–saline mouth rinses (3% H_2O_2 diluted with equal parts of warm saline) may pro-

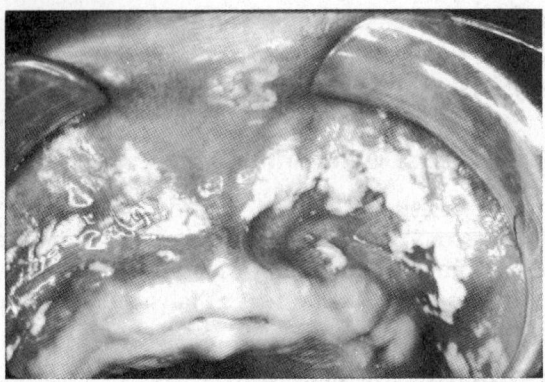

FIGURE 64-2 Acute pseudomembranous candidiasis. This is typical appearance of thrush: white flecks of candidal organisms can be removed relatively easily, leaving erythematous mucosal base. (From DeWeese DD et al: *Otolaryngology: head and neck surgery,* ed 7, St. Louis, 1988, Mosby–Year Book, Inc.)

vide some relief. Nystatin vaginal troches (100,000 units dissolved) or clotrimazole tablets (10 mg dissolved and taken five times daily) ingested orally have proven to be effective. Ketoconazole taken systemically appears to be equally effective. In addition, some patients object to oral dissolution and prefer taking tablets.

APHTHOUS ULCERS
Etiology/Epidemiology

Aphthous ulcers, such as *canker sores* and recurrent ulcerative stomatitis, have been associated with numerous causes: streptococci, trauma, emotional or physical stress, autoimmunity, allergy, and hormonal variations. Aphthous ulcers may affect patients of any age, although the most common age range is from 20 to 50 years, with females being affected twice as often as males. Approximately 30% of the population has been infected.

Clinical Manifestations

A prodromal period of several days usually precedes the outbreak of lesions. During this period the patient experiences a burning or itching sensation in the oral mucosal area. An erythematous macular or papular lesion then develops, which eventually erodes and ulcerates. The well-defined ulcers are approximately 2 to 10 mm in diameter and are surrounded by an intense erythematous halo. The base of the ulcer is covered by a grayish necrotic slough. Aphthous ulcers may occur in small groups or singularly in any area of the oral cavity. The ulcerations usually resolve in a 2-week period but may persist

if they are extremely large. The ulcerations heal without any notable scarring and may recur anytime from several days to years. Some studies have shown that aphthous stomatitis occurs less frequently among smokers than nonsmokers. It has been hypothesized that the constant irritation produced by smoking decreases sensitivity of the oral mucosa.

Therapeutic Management

Tetracycline aqueous oral suspension mouth rinses have been found to be quite helpful in reducing healing time and in controlling infection. Systemic therapy with tetracyclines does not seem to have a significant effect. Long-term users of tetracyclines should be carefully monitored for adverse reactions, especially if the rinses are swallowed.

The traditional approach for controlling signs and symptoms of this inflammation is the application of topical steroids four times per day after meals and at bedtime. Although mouth rinses and other topical preparations have been used, the best results have been achieved with the tetracycline mouthwashes and topical steroids in an emollient dental paste, used either separately or conjointly. Table 64-1 summarizes pharmacologic agents.

HERPES SIMPLEX VIRUS (HSV)
Definition

Herpes simplex virus (HSV) is manifested as a lesion called the *cold sore.*

Etiology/Epidemiology

The etiologic agent in oral herpetic lesions is *herpesvirus hominis, type I,* which may infect both mucosal and dermal tissues of the oral cavity. Herpetic infection may be primary (acute herpetic gingivostomatitis) or secondary (recurrent herpes simplex). Primary herpes simplex infection affects 90% of the population before puberty. Of the primary infections, 99% are asymptomatic, are mild, or appear as low-grade colds.

Clinical Manifestations

Signs and symptoms of HSV are fever, malaise, hypersalivation, acute regional lymphadenopathy, dysphagia, general soreness of the mouth, and painful, inflamed, erythematous gingivae. Several days after these symptoms develop, discrete oral lesions appear and the acute febrile episode subsides. Vesicular eruptions may occur on the tongue, buccal mucosa, and palate. Although the gingiva is not affected by vesicular eruption, it becomes intensely inflamed and painful. The vesicles rupture and clear fluid escapes, forming shallow erosions that eventu-

TABLE 64-1	Pharmacology Summary: Oral Infections and Inflammation	

Product	Description/dispensing form	Nursing implications
Amosam	Suspension	Mix with water (1:2 solution)
Carbamide peroxide (Gly-oxide)	Suspension	For canker sores and other painful lesions; apply directly to affected lesion for several minutes; expectorate; alternate with saline mouthwash every 2 hours
Clotrimazole (Lotrimin)	Lozenges	For *Candida* infections; must dissolve in mouth over 15 to 30 minutes
Diphenhydramine (Benadryl)	Anithistamine elixir	For painful oral mucosa; can be combined with antacid and antidiarrheal; may cause drowsiness
Dyclonine (Dyclone)	Local anesthetic, topical solution	For painful oral lesions; patient may be hypersensitive
Kaolin and pectin (Kaopectate)	Antidiarrheal liquid	To coat painful lesions; may be used as mouthwash
KY Jelly	Water-soluble lubricant	To coat lips or oral mucosa
Magnesium hydroxide (Milk of Magnesia)	Aqueous suspension	To coat oral mucosa; decreases oral acidity; may dry oral mucosa
Mineral oil	Liquid	To coat lips or oral mucosa; can cause lipid pneumonia if aspirated
Nystatin (Mycostatin)	Antifungal, antibiotic; oral suspension	For *Candida* (monilial) infections; may cause hypersensitivity
Hydrocortisone (Orabase HCA)	Oral paste	For temporary relief of minor lesions; systemic absorption has produced reversible symptoms
Lidocaine (Xylocaine 2% viscous solution)	Topical anesthetic liquid	For painful oral lesions; decreased sensitivity to hot foods and liquids; allergic reactions
Petroleum (Vaseline)	Lubricant	For dry lips: can cause lipid pneumonia if aspirated; use cautiously because topical bacterial growth may occur
Sucralfate suspension	Sucralfate, 12 g in 60 mL H_2O; Benylin syrup, 60 mL; Maalox suspension, 60 mL	For painful oral lesions; swish with 15 mL for 2 minutes, then swallow

ally ulcerate. The ulcerations are aggravated, and severe pain may occur with normal speech and mastication. Fetid mouth odor is present. Acute herpetic gingivostomatitis is usually resolved in about 2 weeks, although the regional lymphadenopathy may persist for several weeks. The virus is labile and highly contagious and is believed to be caused by contact and droplet infection; therefore contact restriction should be considered. The majority of primary infections are mild and may go unnoticed.

Secondary herpetic infections may occur regularly or sporadically. Burning or itching during the prodromal period may precede vesicular eruption by several hours or days. The most common site for recurrent infections (cold sores, fever blisters, herpes labialis) is the vermilion border (the junction of the pinkish red area of the lips and the surrounding skin). The same contact restrictions exist for secondary herpetic infections, since they are also contagious.

NURSING MANAGEMENT OF THE PATIENT WITH ORAL INFECTIONS
Assessment

Assessment includes whether the patient has had febrile episodes, bleeding from any part of the oral cavity, hypersalivation, malaise, and weakness. In addition, the patient is asked whether tenderness, burning, or pain occurs when talking or eating. Inspection of the mouth and lips is done to identify inflammation of the mucosa and whether vesicular eruptions or erythematous gingivae exist. Further inspection of the regional lymph nodes is necessary to determine generalized infection.

Implementation

General pain can be controlled with aspirin or acetaminophen. Antibiotics are usually not prescribed unless secondary infections occur. Prophylactic antibiotics may be needed if the patient has had repeated outbreaks. Nutrition is maintained by preparing balanced food combinations in a blender and having the patient drink some meals. Care should be taken to avoid foods and beverages containing refined carbohydrates, since these retard healing. Topical 2% viscous lidocaine mouth swishes and expectoration of the solution before meals alleviate pain. Lidocaine is not recommended for the very young or old patient because of general numbing of the oral cavity and potential swallowing difficulties. Immunosuppressed persons (e.g., those with cancer, kidney transplants, or AIDS) have an increased risk for developing primary herpetic gingivostomatitis. Acyclovir, a systemic antiviral agent, has been used with some success in controlling the symptoms. HSV is self-limiting, and signs and symptoms become progressively more severe for 1 week and disappear by the end of the second week.

CARCINOMA OF ORAL CAVITY
Etiology/Epidemiology

Carcinoma of the oral cavity has been linked to excessive alcohol consumption and all forms of tobacco use, including chewing tobacco and cigar, cigarette, and pipe smoking. Food carcinogens and HSV also have been implicated, but studies have not confirmed an associated risk factor.

Cancer of the oral cavity accounts for about 4% of all cancer deaths in the United States. Malignancies are most common in the sixth and seventh decades. As many as 80% of patients 45 years and older show some grossly visible pathologic process in tissues of the oral cavity. Atrophic lesions and benign tumors are common, as are ulcerative and hyperplastic lesions. There is a 2:1 male-to-female prevalence.

Clinical Manifestations

Leukoplakia is a white patch on the mouth or tongue mucosa that cannot be classified as another disease (Figure 64-3). The tissue cannot be rubbed off by simple mechanical force and is characterized by hy-

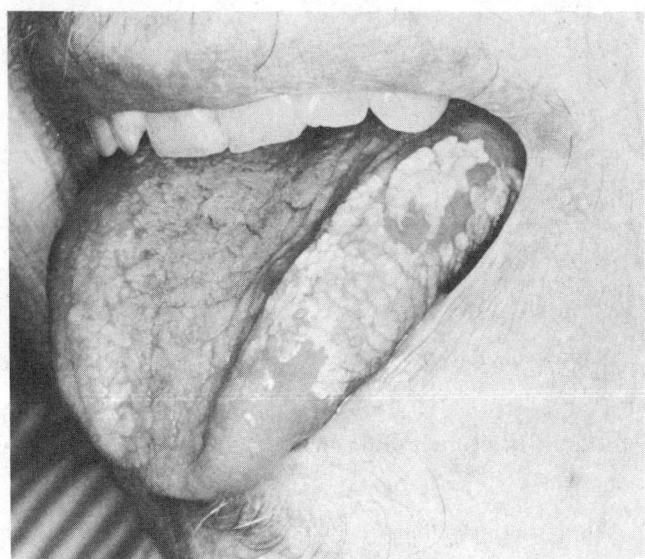

FIGURE 64-3 Leukoplakia of tongue. (From DeWeese DD et al: *Otolaryngology: head and neck surgery,* ed 7, St Louis, 1988, Mosby–Year Book, Inc.)

perkeratosis related to increased friction or irritation.

The lesions vary from localized single plaques to diffusely outlined patches with extensive involvement of the oral mucosa. Color, size, and elevation of the lesions may increase over time. Although many oral cancers are white patches, some are red. **Erythroplakia** is a red-appearing squamous cell carcinoma not well delineated with diffuse borders. A red lesion that is cancerous bleeds easily even when gently manipulated.

Many malignant lesions occur on the lower lip and present a more favorable prognosis, since they are easily visible in the early stages. Changes in the exposed mucosa and skin are called *actinic cheilitis* and are conducive to the development of a cancer. Patients with actinic cheilitis caused by long exposure to the ultraviolet spectrum of sunlight should be carefully examined at regular intervals to detect any change toward malignancy at an early stage.

In the early stages most oral cancers are painless. Another symptom of oral cancer is the feeling of firmness or hardness when the lesion is palpated. The length of time a lesion has been present may suggest a malignancy. A continuously growing lesion that has been present for several weeks or months is usually a sign of cancer. Paresthesia, particularly in the jaw, suggests an infiltrating malignant lesion. Hoarseness, a change in voice quality or tone, and dysphagia can all be symptoms of oral cancer.

Therapeutic Management

Specific diagnostic measures

An important component of the soft tissue examination is indirect laryngoscopy. This procedure is especially important for men 40 years of age or older who have dysphagia and persistent hoarseness. The patient experiences little discomfort and tolerates the procedure fairly well. Radiographic evaluation of the mandibular structures is also an essential part of the head and neck examination to rule out the presence of cancer. Excisional biopsy is the most accurate method of arriving at a definitive diagnosis. Oral exfoliative cytology, which involves scraping the lesion and placing the specimen on a slide, was initially believed to determine the difference between malignant and benign lesions. However, a negative smear can be obtained from a cancerous lesion. The chance of this false-negative finding is about 26%.

Toluidine blue in vivo staining is another method used to clinically distinguish between benign and malignant lesions of the oral cavity. In this test toluidine blue stain is painted on the lesion, which is then decolorized with a weak acetic acid. Toluidine blue supposedly stains the cancerous lesion but not the benign tissue; however, this technique has been judged unreliable.

Medical management

The 5-year survival rate for patients with oral cancers averages less than 50%. In addition, more than half the patients with oral cancers have cervical lymph node involvement at the time of diagnosis. Management of oral cancers includes radiation therapy, surgery, and, with more advanced cases, chemotherapy.

Surgical management

Several surgical procedures are used for removing oral cancers. Most are radical and involve removal of associated lymph nodes. Radical oral surgery with extensive tissue removal interferes with chewing, talking, and swallowing and produces some cosmetic deformity. Depending on the lesion site, the procedures used include a **glossectomy,** removal of the tongue; *hemiglossectomy,* removal of part of the tongue; *mandibulectomy,* removal of the mandible; and *total* or *supraglottic laryngectomy,* removal of the entire larynx or the portion above the true vocal cords. In many centers these surgeries are done in conjunction with lasers to decrease postoperative edema and exudate and the incidence of scarring.

Because oral cancers commonly metastasize to the cervical lymph nodes in the neck, a *radical neck dissection* is done either singularly or in conjunction with any of the above surgical procedures. This type of surgery is disfiguring and includes wide excision of the contents of the neck and removal of the regional and deep cervical lymph nodes and channels. In addition, other structures involved are the sternocleidomastoid muscle and closely related muscles, the external and internal jugular vein, the mandible, the submaxillary gland, and the spinal accessory nerve (cranial nerve XI). Frequently drains are placed in the incision and attached to suction to facilitate healing and prevent extensive hematoma formation. If the patient has had multiple surgical procedures, a tracheotomy also will be performed to maintain the airway. (See Chapter 27 for a complete discussion of radical neck dissection.)

To limit metastasis, a surgical procedure may require extensive revision that produces serious disfigurement of the head and neck. Plastic surgeons or otolaryngologists try to repair the damage by creating flaps from the surrounding tissue and using grafts from another part of the body for reconstruction.

Complications

Although the discomfort experienced by the patient is less than would be expected after extensive tissue removal, many complications can occur. Potential complications are airway obstruction, hemorrhage, tracheal aspiration, facial edema, fistula formation, and necrosis of the skin flaps. Because nerves are severed and manipulated during surgery, neurologic complications can also occur. The patient experiences shoulder droop if the spinal accessory nerve is removed and weakness of the upper lip if the mandibular portion of the facial nerve (cranial nerve VII) is damaged.

Radiation therapy is sometimes used before surgery to decrease the tumor size. Skin flap necrosis may occur postoperatively because the skin heals very slowly after radiation exposure and may place the patient at risk for carotid rupture. Radiation and chemotherapy may be used together postoperatively when the lesions are more advanced. When these treatments fail, palliative chemotherapy may be prescribed for the patient's comfort and relief of symptoms. If dysphagia becomes a problem because of edema or fistula formation, a gastrostomy may be performed so that nutritional intake is not compromised. Nursing measures for a gastrostomy tube are discussed in Chapter 16.

NURSING MANAGEMENT OF THE PATIENT WITH ORAL CANCER

Assessment

Mouth cancer has no reliable early signs or symptoms. As a result, the nurse assesses patients for contributing factors, such as tobacco use, alcohol consumption, and overexposure to sun and wind. The nurse also assesses patients for dental prophylaxis and oral hygiene habits.

The most common finding is that of a painful ulceration associated with induration. The patient should also be assessed for the following danger signals:

1. Appearance of white or red surface patches
2. Unusual bleeding in the mouth
3. Lumps or swelling in the neck
4. Irritations in the mouth that do not heal in 1 to 2 weeks
5. Hoarseness
6. Dysphagia

Nursing Diagnosis

Nursing diagnoses for the patient with oral cancer include the following:

Altered nutrition: less than body requirements related to oral pain or postoperative tissue loss

Body image disturbance related to visible postoperative disfigurement

Impaired verbal communication related to loss of structures for phonation

High risk for aspiration related to impaired swallowing

Planning/Implementation

The nurse plays a key role in the treatment process by formulating a care plan that starts preoperatively, continues through the postoperative stage, and ends when the patient is discharged. After assessing the patient's physical and psychologic status, the nurse must determine other sources available for gathering information and providing support. Family members, close friends, social workers, and pastoral care staff can contribute valuable information and assist in providing optimum care and support after the surgery. The care plan should be formulated at this time. It is important to assess the patient's knowledge of the disease, emotional response, and past coping mechanisms. This allows the nurse to determine what preoperative teaching needs to be done. Some patients want a great deal of information and want to learn about what will happen to them during and after the operation. Other patients, who may be having difficulties coping with the situation, may be limited in their ability to learn and integrate the information provided. Patients experiencing this devasting and potentially fatal disease need a great deal of emotional support and time to process information.

Antibiotic mouthwash may be used preoperatively to lessen the incidence of postoperative wound infection.[7]

Outcome criteria include the following:

Patient's intake and output will be in balance

The postoperative site will heal without fistula formation or infection

The patient demonstrates appropriate oral hygiene measures to prevent infection or irritation of oral tissues

The patient's weight will be maintained within 10% of preoperative status

Evaluation

In addition to the previously mentioned outcome criteria, other factors are considered in the patient's progress and rehabilitation. If the patient experiences shoulder drop or discomfort in the shoulder area, exercises need to be performed and evaluated to determine if they alleviate muscle function loss. Emotional adjustment needs continuous evaluation, depending on the extent of the cancer. During follow-up evaluations, the patient should be given information about cosmetic procedures that reduce disfigurement and allow for maximum function. Communication problems need to be continually assessed and alternate methods of speech encouraged. If the patient has had radiation therapy or chemotherapy, the effects of these treatments may produce serious complications that need ongoing interventions and evaluation.

Documentation

Routine examination of the oral cavity should be noted. Risk factors such as poor oral hygiene, smoking, and alcohol use should be recorded so that interventions may be instituted to achieve compliance. If the patient has surgical intervention, preoperative and postoperative care must be clearly stated. Full explanations regarding speech loss, as well as alternate methods of communication, are given to the patient and significant others and documented so the health team can evaluate the effectiveness of these interventions. It is essential to record explanations regarding any tubes that may go home with the patient, as well as tracheostomy care. If the patient lives alone, it is important to identify the caregiver who will be responsible for the patient. The chart should also contain the patient's psychologic reactions to treatment.

Ongoing Care

Altered appearance, swallowing, and speech pose great physical and emotional strains. A team of physicians, nurses, speech therapists, physical therapists, social workers, and prosthodontists is necessary to accomplish consistent and satisfactory rehabilitation.

Threats to the self-concept and diminished self-esteem can result from any damage or surgery to the face or head because of the high visibility of the area and the cultural value placed on physical attractiveness. Besides the visible disfigurement, the person with cancer of the oral cavity may have to contend with other changes in function and their resultant psychosocial adaptations. Some of these alterations are as follows:

1. Decreased or altered ability to communicate
2. Alternative methods for food intake
3. Self-imposed isolation or limits on social interactions
4. Anxiety over psychosexual role or function
5. Concerns over ability to resume previous employment or function within the family

The impact of the change on the individual's self-concept depends on several factors:

1. The prognosis or perceived chance of recovery from the surgery
2. The degree of disfigurement from the surgery
3. Individual strengths and coping mechanisms
4. Responses of family/significant others and caregivers
5. The personal meaning and significance of the physical change or changes

If the patient receives radiation therapy, mucositis usually develops in the oropharyngeal area. The quality and quantity of mucus produced generally change; long-term results involve dryness and thickening of mucus. As described earlier in the chapter, topical care of the affected area prevents mucositis from becoming a serious problem. Taste sensation may also be altered but usually resolves over time. Some patients may be left with permanent loss of taste, however.

Dysphagia may occur from the resultant mucositis or develop after radiation therapy. Weight loss needs to be carefully monitored to determine if the potential for negative nitrogen balance exists that may adversely affect healing of the surgical incision. Fibrosis may also cause neck stiffness and limit mobility. Physical therapy measures need to be instituted to prevent limited function. Nasopharyngeal regurgitation may occur if there is extensive scarring and fibrosis of the palate. Patients who have lost a substantial portion of the tongue and the supraglottis have a high risk for aspiration. The patient may have to undergo further surgery to prevent chronic pulmonary complications.

After radiation therapy, extremely painful ulcerations of the palate, tonsil, and base of the tongue may occur. Local topical therapy and meticulous oral hygiene are necessary to prevent infection and necrosis. (See Chapter 15 for discussion of treatment and related care.)

If further resection is necessary, planning and intervention with the patient and family are done to offer them a realistic expectation of results, function, and possible complications. The decision to undergo further surgery, radiation, or chemotherapy needs to be evaluated by the patient, the significant others, and the multidisciplinary health care team to maintain a balance between medical-surgical goals and empathetic support systems.

Esophageal Disorders

The esophagus provides a passageway for food from the oropharynx to the stomach. It is a muscular, pliable tube that is easily affected by intrathoracic or intra-abdominal pressures and volumes. Mucus-secreting glands lie along the length of the esophagus to lubricate the food bolus as it enters the stomach.

The esophagus is approximately 23 to 25 cm (8 to 10 inches) long and 1 to 2 cm (to 1 inch) wide. Approximately 5 cm above the esophageal entry to the stomach is a narrowed area called the gastroesophageal junction, or the **lower esophageal sphincter (LES)** (Figure 64-4). The LES is situated between the negative intrathoracic and positive intra-abdominal pressures. The LES normally remains constricted but relaxes when a peristaltic wave is conducted through it, allowing food to pass to the stomach. The LES is a high-pressure zone that acts to prevent acid reflux into the esophagus. Contraction of the LES seems to be mediated by the vagus nerve.

GASTROESOPHAGEAL REFLUX
Definition/Etiology/Epidemiology

Gastroesophageal reflux (GERD) refers to the reflux of stomach and duodenal contents into the esophagus. The frequency of GERD is unknown because the symptoms are variable and often nonspecific, but the condition is characterized by failure of the LES to remain normally closed between swallows. This functional disturbance permits excessive regurgitation through the LES. Chalasia (relaxation of the sphincter) is observed in normal infants, in patients with scleroderma, and in an idiopathic form in adults. Diabetes mellitus has also been found to be a predisposing condition for GERD. Lifting a heavy weight, a crushing chest injury, or an automobile accident may be followed by regurgitation, heartburn, and the diagnosis of pathologic reflux. GERD has also been known to follow surgical procedures involving the abdomen (e.g., vagotomy, gastrectomy). An increase in reflux has also been observed in patients with a tendency toward this problem when the LES pressure is decreased by anticholinergic drugs, cigarette smoking, caffeine, alcohol

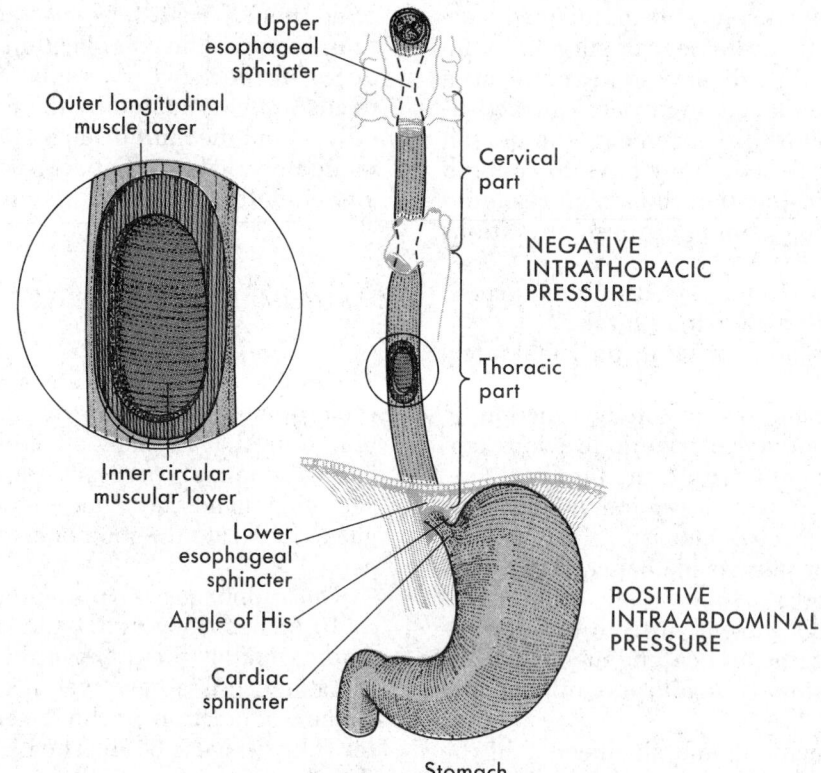

FIGURE 64-4   Normal anatomy of esophagus with cutaway to show muscle layers.

abuse, a high-fat diet, chocolate, and meperidine (Demerol). The box on p. 1803 lists agents that affect LES pressure.

Reflux during pregnancy, once believed to be caused by the increased abdominal pressure from the fetus, may be caused by reduced LES pressure as a result of extra production of estrogen and progesterone. Obese individuals appear to have extreme difficulties with reflux, which can be reversed by weight loss and physical conditioning. In addition, an incompetent LES may be aggravated by sudden increases in intra-abdominal pressure such as occur after ingesting a large meal, bending over, lifting, and wearing tight girdles or belts. Reflux esophagitis may also be the result of prolonged or repeated vomiting from various conditions or prolonged nasogastric intubation. Some patients with a hiatal hernia, which will be discussed further in this chapter, also have esophageal reflux.

Pathophysiology

The barrier to regurgitation of gastric contents into the esophagus is remarkably efficient. Normal, or physiologic, reflux may occur after meals when the stomach is distended. Although there is no discrete anatomic distal esophageal sphincter, a functional sphincter mechanism clearly exists at the gastroesophageal junction. The gastroesophageal junction is the point at which the muscular wall of the digestive tract changes from an esophageal to a gastric pattern. How this effective mechanism operates is still not fully established. Disorders of this mechanism lead to pathologic degrees of gastroesophageal reflux and related complications.[2]

The LES is composed of circular muscle at the distal end of the esophagus that is different from the rest of the esophagus both physically and pharmacologically. Normally when a person swallows, the LES relaxes, allowing food to enter the stomach. At other times the LES is contracted to prevent reflux of gastric contents back into the esophagus. LES pressure tends to be lower in persons with GERD.

GERD results because of alterations in the usual protective mechanisms:

1. Esophageal peristalsis and alkaline saliva fail to clear the lower esophagus of refluxed gastric contents.
2. The cardiac sphincter has inappropriate relaxation and a very low LES, allowing backup of gastric contents.
3. There is a decreased esophageal mucosal re-

AGENTS AFFECTING LES PRESSURE

Increase in pressure

Metoclopramide (Reglan)
Bethanechol (Urecholine)
Gastrin
Nonfat milk

Decrease in pressure

Alcohol
Anticholinergic drugs
Beta-adrenergic blocking drugs
Calcium channel blockers
Chocolate
Coffee
Meperidine (Demerol)
Estrogen
Fatty foods
Lidocaine
Morphine
Nicotine
Peppermint
Progesterone
Simethicone
Spearmint
Theophylline
Diazepam (Valium)

sistance to acid reflux usually seen with decreased secretion of bicarbonate and decreased mucosal blood flow.

4. There may be delayed gastric emptying or increased volume/production of gastric secretions.

The alterations listed in the second entry above are considered the hallmarks of the disease. Esophagitis has been found on endoscopy in approximately 50% of individuals with symptomatic GERD.[11] The esophageal squamous epithelium reacts to reflux by a thickening of the basal layer of the epithelium and changes in the vasculature. In more advanced GERD, inflammation and fibrosis result in an esophageal stricture.

Clinical Manifestations

The most common symptoms of gastroesophageal reflux are pyrosis and regurgitation. **Pyrosis** (heartburn) is a sensation of warmth or burning behind the sternum in the midline between the xiphoid and the manubrium seen in an estimated 75% of patients with GERD. It can spread to the interscapular region of the back, neck, jaws, and even down both arms.

The sensation may become a painful ache when intense. The patient usually experiences retrosternal burning shortly after eating, when bending over, or while lying down.

The duration is variable and usually has a wave-like moving quality. Relief is usually obtained within 3 to 5 minutes after taking a liquid antacid. Erosive esophagitis is believed to be present when interscapular pain is aggravated by ingestion of hot or cold liquids, coffee, citrus juices, or alcohol.[14]

Reflux is more likely to occur when the patient is lying on the right side. Position changes that compress the abdomen, such as an occupation requiring considerable bending or stooping, gardening, picking up objects off the floor, tying shoes, or lying flat after a full meal, may precipitate reflux symptoms. Heartburn is a symptom of esophageal dysfunction and is experienced as a result of abnormal motor activity of the esophagus, gastroesophageal regurgitation with acid, or direct mucosal irritation.

Regurgitation is the ejection of sour gastric contents from the mouth. It is distinguished from vomiting by the lack of preceding nausea and the small quantity of emesis ejected. Bending over or lying down facilitates the flow of gastric contents into the esophagus in the presence of an incompetent LES. The patient may awaken coughing or choking on a mouthful of fluid (called water brash, if it is salty saliva). Mucus, gastric contents, or bile may stain the pillow. Moving to an upright position provides relief. The patient may complain of "sour regurgitation" and an "acid" or bitter taste in the throat or mouth.[11]

Dysphagia, or difficulty in swallowing, may also occur when reflux causes an esophageal spasm, giving rise to difficulty in swallowing even when esophagitis is not present. This type of dysphagia can be experienced anywhere along the esophagus, whereas the feeling of obstruction because of edema and later fibrotic stenosis is usually localized to the lower esophagus. The patient may feel a fullness in the throat, have difficulty initiating swallowing, and experience excessive mucus secretion. The patient may make frequent attempts at swallowing to bring about relief. The swallowing difficulty in uncomplicated reflux esophagitis is for solid foods. Continued attempts to swallow usually result in passage of the bolus.

Odynophagia, or painful swallowing, may occur during exacerbations of reflux esophagitis. However, as the inflammation subsides, symptoms disappear for a short period. The ability to swallow deteriorates with each occurrence of esophagitis. Saliva may be swallowed with some difficulty, and the patient experiences difficulty in passing food through the esophagus.

With increasing discomfort associated with the intake of food, there will be significant weight loss. Bleeding is also a sign that esophagitis is present and may lead to more serious problems of stricture or stenosis at the gastroesophageal junction.

Another misleading symptom that can be caused solely by reflux is an angina-type chest pain. The patient may describe substernal pain radiating to the neck, mandible, shoulders, and upper arms. When reflux induced, this pain occurs more during rest, especially in the supine position, and is lessened by exercises. The picture may be further confused by the patient's response to nitrates. Nitrate drugs may alleviate pain from esophageal spasm, as well as pain from coronary spasm. It is important for the patient to have a complete cardiac evaluation to rule out the possibility of coronary artery disease. Prolonged ambulatory monitoring of esophageal pH is currently being proposed as the most reliable method for differentiating noncardiac chest pain from angina.[2]

Diagnostic Procedures

A barium swallow radiographic examination is generally the first study done when the patient has esophageal symptoms. This test allows visualization of the esophagus, stomach, and small intestine.

Continuous ambulatory 24-hour esophageal pH monitoring is used to confirm the diagnosis of GERD. This diagnostic measure will show the amount of acid reflux into the esophagus, under which specific circumstances this occurs, and the correlation with symptomatology. The monitor is portable, resembling the 24-hour cardiac monitor worn by patients; the esophageal probe is small and does not cause the patient major discomfort. The range of pH in the esophagus varies from 1 to 8, the normal being 6.5 to 7.0. Acid reflux is defined as a decreased pH of 4.0 in the esophagus.[2]

Manometry provides an assessment of pressures in the esophagus. Catheters are inserted into the esophagus to measure a variety of pressures during swallowing. Esophagoscopy is the most common method of examination to establish the diagnosis of reflux esophagitis and to determine its severity. This form of examination will establish the presence of visible esophagitis and provide information about the presence of a hiatal hernia, strictures, and neoplasms. Reflux of gastric contents into the esophagus may also be observed.

Therapeutic Management

Medical management

Not all persons with GERD have esophagitis. For the majority of these people, conservative measures to prevent reflux should be instituted and maintained indefinitely. The goal of pharmacologic therapy is twofold: (1) to administer antacids, which neutral-

ize esophageal contents, release endogenous gastrin, and increase LES pressure; and (2) to restore the ability of the esophagus to resist the irritating effects of refluxed gastric acid. Liquid antacids (Amphojel, Gelusil, Maalox, Mylanta, or combinations of these) selected on the basis of their effect on bowel regulation are given in doses of 15 to 30 mL between hourly feedings when the patient is awake. Antacids are discussed further in Chapter 65. The frequency of antacid administration may be reduced to 1 hour before and after meals and at bedtime when the patient has progressed to a six-meal regimen. If the symptoms are severe and persistent, an intra-esophageal milk-antacid drip is employed, which avoids overdistention of the stomach and neutralizes gastric acids effectively. If antacids alone do not control symptoms, histamine H_2 blockers may be added to the regimen. Intravenous cimetidine also provides relief and termination of bleeding.

Anticholinergic drugs are contraindicated in patients with reflux esophagitis. They delay stomach emptying, decrease LES pressure, and decrease the frequency of peristalsis that cleans the esophagus of acid contents. (See box on p. 1803.) Cholinergic drugs have shown some ability to increase LES pressure, acid clearance, and stomach emptying. Bethanechol (Urecholine), 25 mg four times daily (before meals and bedtime), has been used with some success to promote healing in reflux esophagitis. Metoclopramide (Reglan) also increases LES pressure, promotes increased gastric emptying and acid clearance, and has been observed to relieve symptoms of reflux problems. The effect of metoclopramide on LES pressure, however, is not as pronounced as bethanechol.

Complications

When deep ulcerations of the esophageal mucosa have occurred, a few patients develop esophageal strictures. These strictures may migrate over the years to the midesophageal area or above. The patient may have an esophageal obstruction from a narrowed esophageal lumen. Dysphagia is the common symptom of esophageal stricture formation. If the patient continues to have difficulty with swallowing and has no relief from the medicinal or dietary measures, **bougienage** should be employed. Bougienage is the use of various mercury-filled rubber tubes called *bougies* to dilate the esophagus (Figure 64-5). The dilators come in sets, with diameters increasing from 4.6 to 20 mm. The patient sits in a chair, and the smallest-caliber bougie is lubricated with a water-soluble material and passed through the nasopharynx into the esophagus until the point of resistance. Sedation is usually not required. Progressively larger bougies are passed until the resis-

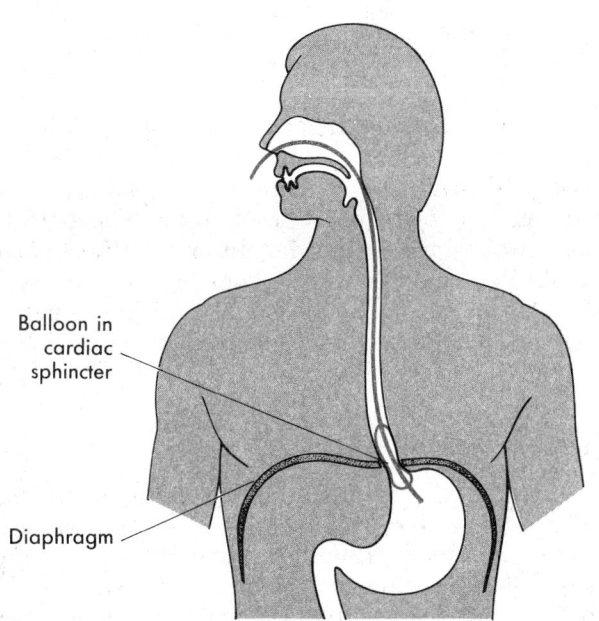

FIGURE 64-5   Bougienage relieves dysphagia by dilating lower esophageal sphincter.

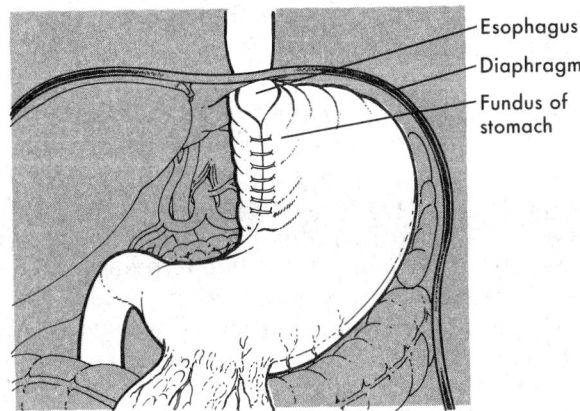

FIGURE 64-6   Nissen fundoplication for hiatal hernia showing fundus of stomach wrapped around distal esophagus and sutured to itself.

tance is overcome. The process takes several days, and only two or three bougies are passed each day. The process is repeated every 3 to 4 months. Bougienage is effective in relieving the dysphagia but may result in increased reflux with associated inflammation and fibrosis.

Perforation of the esophagus is a potential complication whenever dilation is attempted, and any bleeding should be reported immediately. In addition, infection may be a problem for patients with cardiac problems or immune deficiencies, and antibiotic prophylaxis may be required.

Any type of swallowing problem exposes the patient to risk of aspiration of ingested food or gastric secretions into the lungs. Respiratory symptoms are common in patients with esophageal reflux and have been found to account for 50% of surgical referrals. Respiratory symptoms may also occur without associated esophageal symptoms, such as dysphagia or regurgitation, which may create a delay in the actual diagnosis. Laryngitis or a chronic unexplained cough that awakens the patient at night is a common complaint. More serious changes include lung abscess, recurrent pneumonia, chronic bronchitis, and slowly progressive pulmonary fibrosis.

Surgical management

When medical management fails to control symptoms over a 6- to 12-month period, surgical correction of reflux should be considered. Candidates for antireflux surgery are those who (1) do not respond to medical therapy; (2) have recurrent esophageal ulceration, (3) have esophageal strictures, or (4) have a history of aspiration. Approximately 10% of patients with GERD will require an antireflux procedure.[3]

The goals for antireflux surgery are to restore sphincter competence by surrounding the lower end of the esophagus with a cuff of gastric fundal muscle (fundoplication). This involves wrapping the fundus of the stomach around the lower part of the esophagus. The techniques developed by Nissen[25] of Switzerland and Hill[23] of the United States are among the best known successful antireflux operations and are the most widely used (Figure 64-6). The Angelchik antireflux prosthesis was developed by Angelchik and Cohen in 1973 and presents an alternative to fundoplication. The procedure is easier to perform, consisting of a Silastic collarlike device placed around the distal part of the esophagus at the gastroesophageal junction. Each of the surgical procedures has had favorable results with 84% to 89% of patients experiencing good to excellent relief of symptoms.[1]

NURSING MANAGEMENT OF THE PATIENT WITH GASTROESOPHAGEAL REFLUX
Assessment

The first step is to identify symptoms the patient is experiencing that may be caused by gastroesophageal reflux. Is dysphagia, odynophagia, heartburn, or regurgitation present? Are tobacco and alcohol use contributing factors? Does a drug history reveal antagonizing agents such as anticholinergics, antibiotics, or aspirin? Does the patient have hematemesis, anemia (manifested by fatigue or pallor), or pulmonary symptoms such as a nocturnal cough or hoarseness on awakening? Is there a relationship of discomfort to the patient's position or activity; for example, does bending or stooping increase reflux? If the patient experiences chest pain when lying down, it may be caused by reflux. Do certain foods elicit or aggravate the symptoms? Peppermint and chocolate decrease LES pressure and may cause reflux. Does specific behavior alleviate symptoms? Activities such as chewing gum or sucking antacid tablets sometimes reduce reflux symptoms by stimulating alkaline saliva that lubricates the lower esophagus. Is the patient obese, or has there been a recent weight loss? All of these items are important in developing a nursing assessment specific to gastroesophageal reflux.

Nursing Diagnosis

Nursing diagnoses for the patient with GERD include the following:

Knowledge deficit related to dietary modification, postural therapy, antacid therapy, drug therapy, potential surgery

Pain related to regurgitation, odynophagia (painful swallowing), pyrosis (heartburn), or mucosal inflammation

Altered nutrition: less than body requirements related to dysphagia or odynophagia

Diarrhea or constipation related to administration of antacids

Noncompliance related to behavior modification regarding smoking, alcohol use, and weight reduction

Planning

It is important to determine if the patient is ready to learn preventive measures as part of a self-care regimen. If the patient has additional health problems, educational intervention may be more complicated when trying to implement a care plan in the presence of another disease process. Does the patient have a caregiver who is supportive of the regimen? For example, if the patient's partner has difficulty sleeping upright, the patient might abandon this position because the partner objects.

Outcome criteria for the patient include the following:

Patient will refrain or limit the use of alcohol and smoking

Patient will follow recommended dietary measures, postural therapy, and drug regimen

Weight will be maintained within 10% of ideal body weight

Patient will be free from epigastric discomfort

Implementation

Dietary management

The standard reflux diet restricts spicy, acidic, and fatty foods, as well as coffee, tea, and colas. Peppermint, spearmint, and chocolate should also be avoided.[10] Food should be thoroughly masticated and eaten slowly. Overdistention of the stomach should be avoided and the stomach not overloaded at any one meal.[10] Small low-fat meals are recommended to decrease gastric volume and control weight.

Postural therapy

The patient should not lie down immediately after eating. No food should be eaten for approximately 2 hours before bedtime. Sleeping with the chest elevated 6 to 8 inches and placing a pillow under the chest or the head on two pillows help prevent nocturnal reflux; however, using pillows or elevating the head of the bed may compress the stomach, thereby encouraging reflux. Six-inch wooden blocks placed under the legs at the head of the bed alleviate this problem. Bending forward, heavy lifting, straining at stool, or slumping in a chair, especially after eating, should be avoided. Tight girdles or belts should not be worn. Any clothing that increases intra-abdominal pressure should be avoided.

Behavior modification

Because smoking decreases LES pressure and increases gastric acid, attempts to quit smoking should be employed. In addition, coughing also causes reflux and a smoker's cough exacerbates the condition. Alcohol consumption also contributes to reflux, and hyperacidity and abstinence should be enforced. Exercise and diet are encouraged to decrease obesity and maintain weight within a normal range; most patients with GERD are encouraged to lose a minimum of 15 pounds.[11]

Drug therapy education

Antacids such as aluminum hydroxide and magnesium carbonate (Gaviscon), aluminum hydroxide and magnesium hydroxide (Maalox), aluminum hydroxide, magnesium hydroxide, or combinations of these drugs are selected on the basis of their effect on bowel regulation. Antacids are given 1 hour after meals and at bedtime for heartburn, regurgitation, and other symptoms of recurrent reflux. The nurse needs to determine how the patient tolerates these agents and any side effects of either diarrhea or constipation.

Gaviscon is used for relief of heartburn. This drug forms a cohesive foam that floats on the surface of stomach contents and neutralizes the acid. This neutralizing foam precedes stomach contents into the esophagus when reflux occurs, thus protecting the esophageal mucosa. To be effective, Gaviscon must be given when food is present in the stomach.

If reflux symptoms are severe and persist despite antacid therapy and life-style modifications, histamine H_2 blockers are added to the regimen. Cimetidine (Tagamet) or ranitidine (Zantac) is usually given after meals or at bedtime for approximately 4 to 6 weeks for patients with predominantly nocturnal symptoms.[10] The patient needs to be instructed about drug interactions and side effects from these agents, especially if prescribed for home use.

Motility drugs such as bethanechol (Urecholine) or metoclopramide (Reglan) may be prescribed for patients with poor LES pressure. Patients with hypertension need to be monitored for decreased blood pressure readings with bethanechol. Metoclopramide may accelerate absorption of drugs from the small bowel and diminish absorption of drugs from the stomach.

Anticholinergic drugs, such as chlordiazepoxide–clidinium bromide (Librax) and dicyclomine (Bentyl) are contraindicated in patients with gastroesophageal reflux. Simethicone (Mylicon) has also been found to decrease LES pressure that may contribute to exacerbation of symptoms. In addition, calcium channel blockers and aspirin may contribute to reflux. The patient should be questioned as to whether these medications exacerbate symptoms. Omeprazole (Prilosec), a gastric acid pump inhibitor, may be prescribed for severe symptoms. This drug is used to decrease the amount of gastric acid available for reflux into the esophagus.

Postoperative care

If medical management is refractory, the patient may be referred for fundoplication. A thoracic or abdominal approach may be used for any of the variations of fundoplication. The thoracic approach causes more postoperative discomfort than abdominal surgery and for a longer period. A chest tube is usually inserted. Assessment of closed chest drainage is essential to maintenance. (See Chapter 26.) The abdominal approach may predispose the patient to a greater risk of wound infection, and the nurse needs to assess the incision site for signs and symptoms of infection.

The patient will have a nasogastric tube, and tube patency must be maintained to avoid stomach distention. The nurse must continue to assess the drainage and provide oral and nasal care while the tube is in place. The nasogastric tube is on low suction for as long as 5 days to prevent overdistention while healing takes place. Drainage from the nasogastric tube is bloody for 8 to 12 hours after surgery and

gradually returns to the normal greenish yellow color. The use of straws, when the patient is allowed fluids, is contraindicated because of potential aerophagia (swallowing air). When peristalsis returns and the patient is allowed solid foods, small frequent feedings should be given to prevent overloading the stomach at any one time.

Postoperative breathing is painful, and the patient must be encouraged to cough, turn, and deep breathe to avoid respiratory complications. Whenever the incision site is close to the diaphragm, there is a potential for ventilatory problems. The use of narcotic medications that depress respirations such as morphine or meperidine is necessary to relieve the pain, but the nurse needs to monitor for this side effect.

After fundoplication, the patient may experience what is known as a *gas-bloat syndrome*. The wrap of the fundus may be too tight, causing discomfort from bloating and inability to eructate. Conversely, if the wraparound is too loose, the patient has the same symptoms as before surgical intervention. Also, if the wraparound slips down and encircles the body of the stomach, a partial gastric obstruction may occur.

Evaluation

Most patients who have GERD improve after 1 month of therapy with antacids and life-style modifications. If the symptoms continue, several questions need to be asked. Has the patient eliminated foods that exacerbate GERD? Even when the patient adheres to the appropriate dietary restrictions, is the quantity of food eaten in one sitting limited and eating or drinking avoided for at least 3 to 4 hours before lying down or sleeping? What progress did the patient make toward modifying behavior? Has the patient experienced additional symptoms that may not be associated with reflux, such as anemia and chest pain?

HIATAL HERNIA
Definition

A **hiatal hernia** is the herniation of the stomach and other abdominal viscera through an enlarged esophageal hiatus in the diaphragm. For years a variety of symptoms were attributed to gastric herniation through the hiatus when this condition was identified during a barium swallow examination. In the past hiatal hernias were frequently repaired surgically. However, recently it was found that the presence of a hiatal hernia is much less of a factor in GERD than previously believed. A person could have a pouch at the lower end of the esophagus without specific symptoms; conversely, a person could have severe symptoms of reflux without having a pouch at the end of the esophagus. A hiatal hernia is the most common problem of the diaphragm that affects the alimentary tract. Thus a hiatal hernia is not an illness but an anatomic condition. Today the common sliding, or type I, hiatal hernia is generally regarded as insignificant unless accompanied by symptoms of abnormal, unremitting GERD.

Etiology/Epidemiology

Hiatal hernias are categorized into two types (Figure 64-7). Type I, or sliding, hiatal hernia is a condition whereby a portion of the stomach herniates slightly upward into the enlarged diaphragmatic hiatus. It is believed that approximately 10% of adults in North America have a type I hiatal hernia. Most of the population are asymptomatic, and approximately 5% of persons diagnosed with a type I hiatal hernia also have symptoms of gastroesophageal reflux.[14]

In type II, or rolling, hiatal hernia, a portion of the stomach herniates alongside the esophagus and the herniated stomach extends above the gastroesophageal junction. Gastroesophageal reflux is usually not a clinical problem with this type of hernia, since the gastroesophageal junction is below the diaphragm. A type II hiatal hernia is larger and less common than the type I hernia.

Although the cause of most hiatal hernias is not known, it is believed that congenital or traumatic mechanisms play a role. Type I hernias have been seen in children early in life, whereas a type II hiatal hernia in infancy is extremely rare. When an individual has symptoms of GERD after trauma and a hiatal hernia is subsequently diagnosed, it is difficult to ascertain whether the accident caused the hernia or whether it predated the accident.

Clinical Manifestations

Most patients with a hiatal hernia are asymptomatic. Occasionally, the patient may have heartburn after overeating. Fullness and discomfort after eating are the usual presenting symptoms of a type II hernia; strangulation, infarction, and ulceration of the herniated stomach are the feared complications. So devastating are these complications that some physicians recommend surgical intervention for all type II hiatal hernias when discovered. If abnormal gastroesophageal reflux occurs in association with a hiatal hernia, the symptoms and complications are those of reflux that were discussed earlier in the chapter.

Therapeutic Management

Symptomatic hiatal hernias are easily diagnosed by a barium swallow examination. If the patient is asymptomatic, no treatment is required. When the patient has symptoms of GERD, the medical treatment and nursing management discussed earlier in the chapter should be instituted. If the hernia is large or there is constant risk of infarction, volvulus, or bleeding, repair of the hernia is recommended by one of the standard fundoplication techniques. The goal of surgery is to restore the hernia below the diaphragm, narrow the esophageal hiatus, and enhance LES function. Nursing care of the patient undergoing fundoplication is discussed earlier in the chapter.

CARCINOMA OF THE ESOPHAGUS
Definition

Carcinoma of the esophagus is categorized as either a squamous cell carcinoma or an adenocarcinoma of the esophageal epithelium.

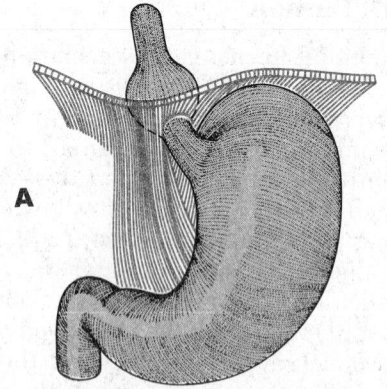
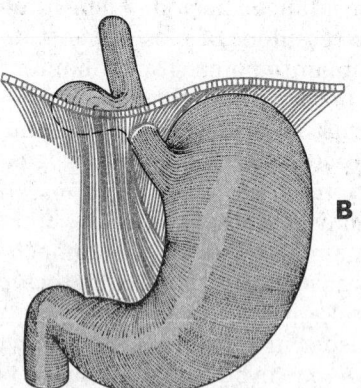

FIGURE 64-7 Hiatal hernia. **A,** Sliding hernia. **B,** Rolling hernia.

Etiology/Epidemiology

Esophageal cancer is usually discovered at a late stage, when surgery is no longer effective. Palliation rather than cure is the more realistic goal for most patients despite advances in surgery, radiation treatment, and chemotherapy. Ninety percent of esophageal cancers are squamous cell carcinomas, which are associated with both alcohol intake and tobacco use and possibly long-standing achalasia. Adenocarcinoma of the esophagus is associated with reflux esophagitis. Environmental carcinogens, nutritional deficiencies, chronic irritation, and mucosal damage have all been implicated as precursors to esophageal cancer. There have been 10,604 new cases of esophageal cancer diagnosed in the United States in 1990.[17] The incidence of cancer of the esophagus in the United States is 4 in 100,000; in the white male population, 3.5 in 100,000; and in black males, 13 in 100,000. It is prevalent in the age group 55 to 70 years.[20]

Pathophysiology

In the United States cancer of the esophagus is classified by its location: the upper third, the middle third, and the lower third. Twenty-four percent of esophageal cancers have been estimated to occur in the upper third, 47% in the middle third, and 29% in the lower third. The level at which the lesion is discovered does not influence the survival rate. Ninety percent of esophageal tumors are squamous cell carcinomas, with adenocarcinomas accounting for approximately 6%.[20] The extensive lymphatic network of the esophagus facilitates the rapid spread of tumor to varying local and distant sites. Carcinoma of the esophagus has an overall 5-year survival rate of 5%; this figure has remained relatively unchanged over the last 10 years.[22]

Clinical Manifestations

The most common clinical symptom is progressive dysphagia over a 6-month period with the sensation of food sticking in the throat. Initially the patient may experience difficulty in swallowing solid foods and within a few short months may be unable to swallow semisolid or soft foods, with a significant weight loss. Ultimately liquids and even the patient's own saliva produce a choking sensation or regurgitation. By the time the esophagus becomes obstructed, the cancer is far advanced.

Odynophagia (painful swallowing) is apparent in the majority of esophageal cancers. A steady, substernal, boring pain radiating to the back is associated with this lesion and indicates a poor prognosis. Other signs of advanced disease are regurgitation, vomiting, hoarseness, chronic cough, and iron-deficiency anemia. Weight loss may be directly related to the tumor, side effects of treatment, or the inability to swallow.

A barium swallow examination with fluoroscopy and endoscopy is used to detect esophageal cancer. A biopsy and cytologic examination provide a high degree of accuracy in the definitive diagnosis.

Once the cancer has been diagnosed, the question of tumor staging must be addressed. Staging is important to determine tumor size and patient management. For most patients with advanced disease, surgery is offered for palliative purposes to relieve dysphagia and restore continuity of the alimentary tract. Even patients who seem free of metastasis at the time of surgery only have a mean survival rate of 13 months.[8]

Therapeutic Management

Radiation therapy may be used for squamous cell carcinoma as both a curative and palliative treatment. The 5-year survival rate for patients without metastatic disease varies from less than 1% to 9%. Patients with obvious metastatic disease, fistulas, or large tumors receive radiation for palliation only. Fistulas create special problems for patients receiving radiation therapy. If a fistula develops, aspiration can be prevented with an esophageal prosthesis. An esophageal prosthesis is a silicone or latex rubber tube that can be placed in the esophagus to occlude the end of the fistula. If the patient experiences edema from radiation therapy, some improvement in swallowing and odynophagia usually takes place several weeks after the treatment has been discontinued. Following radiation, periodic dilation of the esophagus is usually required to maintain patency of the lumen.

Chemotherapy is also considered a palliative type of treatment for advanced cancer of the esophagus. Single-drug or combination-drug therapy may be used. Combination chemotherapy is most effective and produces longer periods of remission than single agents; however, combinations may be extremely toxic. Side effects include pulmonary toxicity, nephrotoxicity, nausea and vomiting, leukopenia, and sepsis.

Recently laser therapy has been used as palliation for esophageal obstruction from malignancies. Advantages include the following: (1) it can be performed with the patient under local anesthesia without the need for an operating room; (2) it may be used with other treatment methods without increasing the risk of side effects; (3) results are seen in days, and morbidity and mortality are lower than with other methods; and (4) it can be repeated indefinitely when other methods cannot be used. During endoscopy, initial debulking of the tumor by forceps may be necessary to allow for passage through

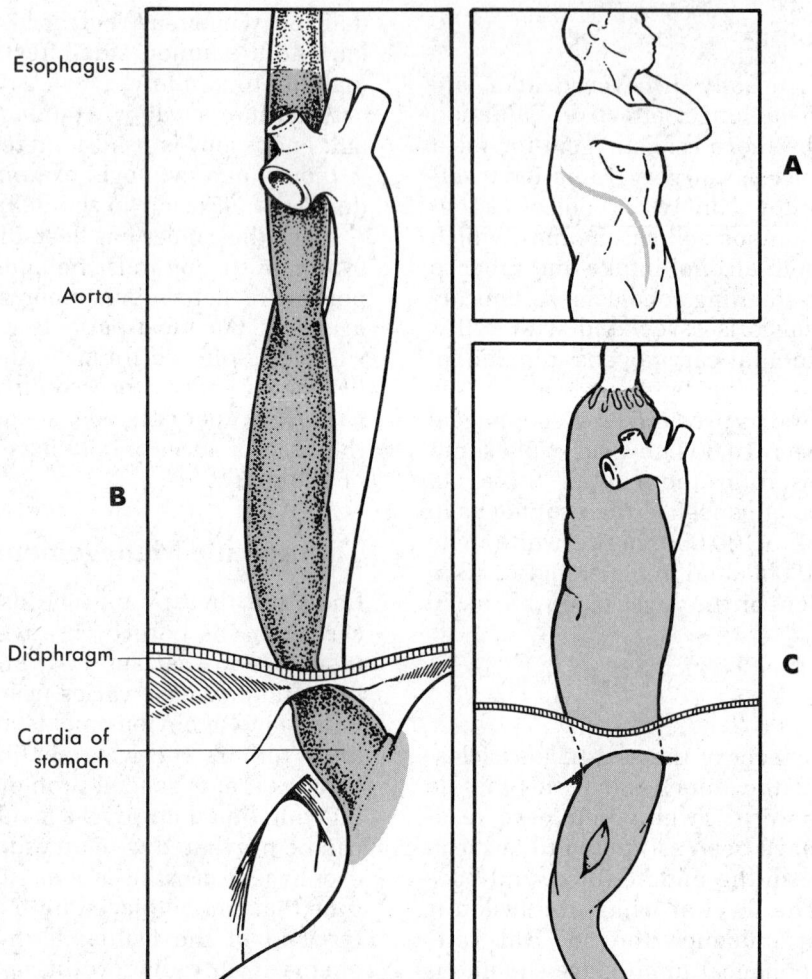

FIGURE 64-8 Esophagogastrectomy for lesions of lower and middle third of thoracic esophagus. **A,** Incision. **B,** Shaded portion to be resected. **C,** Completed reconstruction.

the narrowed lumen. Then the laser is used to vaporize the remains of the obstructing tumor, and suction is applied to evacuate gas and fluids. Complications are infrequent but include aspiration, hemorrhage, or perforation of the esophagus.[15]

Four types of surgical procedures can be performed (Figures 64-8 and 64-9):

1. *Esophagectomy* is removal of all or part of the esophagus using a Dacron graft to replace the parts resected.

2. *Esophagogastrostomy* involves resection of the lower portion of the esophagus and anastomosis of the remaining portion of the stomach.

3. *Esophagoenterostomy* is the resection of the esophagus and anastomosis to a portion of the colon.

4. With a *gastrostomy,* a catheter is inserted into the stomach and sutured to the abdominal wall. This procedure is performed when it is assumed the patient will not be able to take food orally.

NURSING MANAGEMENT OF THE PATIENT WITH ESOPHAGEAL CANCER
Assessment

The patient's skin is inspected frequently for leakage around the gastrostomy tube or from fistula formation. The assessment includes looking for signs of dehydration because of restrictions on oral intake and excessive drainage from the nasogastric tube. Because leakage may develop within the first week, the patient is assessed for any signs of infection: a low-grade temperature, fluid accumulation in the

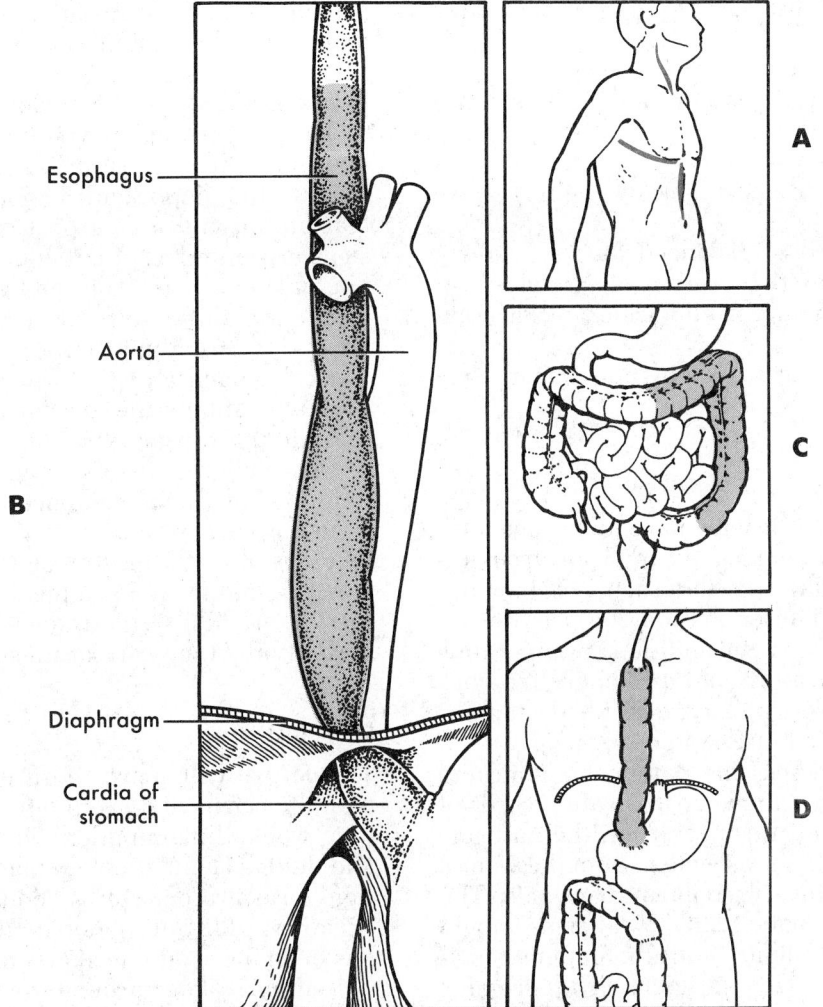

Esophagus

Aorta

B

Diaphragm

Cardia of
stomach

A

C

D

FIGURE 64-9 Esophagoenterostomy. **A,** Incision. **B,** Shaded area to be resected.
C, Portion of colon to be used. **D,** Completed reconstruction.

pleural space, and increased pulse respiratory rates.
Since the incision is near the diaphragm, the patient
will have difficulty coughing and breathing deeply,
making respiratory assessment essential. Nutritional status must be monitored continuously to determine the success of tube feedings. Support systems and previous patterns of coping also need to
be examined.

Nursing Diagnosis

Nursing diagnoses for the patient with esophageal
cancer include the following:
  High risk for impaired skin integrity related to the
    gastrostomy tube or fistula output
  High risk for fluid volume deficit related to the na-
    sogastric tube, wound drainage, or fistula out-
    put

High risk for infection and hemorrhage related to
  poor nutritional status, weakness, and impaired
  healing process
Ineffective breathing pattern related to incision
  pain and proximity to the diaphragm
Altered nutrition: less than body requirements related to dysphagia, decreased stomach capacity,
  gastrostomy tube

Planning

All aspects of care are discussed with the patient
and family before surgery. Feedback and time for
questions are planned. The nurse also determines
whether the diagnosis is known to the patient and
the patient's reactions to it. If the patient is to have
a permanent gastrostomy tube inserted, information
and reassurance are provided before surgery and a

plan is in place for follow-up care and support after surgery.

Outcome criteria include the following:

Skin integrity at gastrostomy tube insertion site will remain intact

The patient will show no signs of infection

The patient will state postoperative pain is under control

The patient will have balanced fluid/electrolyte status as indicated by serum electrolytes, 24-hour intake and output, and urine specific gravity

The patient will express feelings about changes in body image

Implementation

Candidates for surgery usually have numerous difficulties. Often they are emaciated and weak from impaired nutritional intake. Parenteral hyperalimentation (discussed in Chapter 18) may be used to improve nutritional status. In addition, preoperative teaching and preparation and postoperative care must be provided. Nursing measures for postoperative care are discussed in Chapter 26.

The nurse must assess the patient for fluid and electrolyte imbalances and keep accurate records of the intake and output. Drainage from the nasogastric or gastrostomy tubes, as well as from the wound or fistula, should be measured during each shift. The patient should be weighed daily. Vital signs should be monitored every 2 hours until the patient is stable and thereafter every 4 hours. The dressing should be checked frequently for signs of bleeding and during the postoperative period to determine if there is excessive drainage, odor, or separation of the suture line (see box below).

The patient will have reduced ability to cough and deep breathe because of incisional pain and proximity to the diaphragm. The nurse must pay particular attention to this aspect of care and report any signs or symptoms of pulmonary infection, pneumonia, or atelectasis. Pain medication is administered frequently and respiratory assessment made about effects on breathing pattern. If the patient is too weak to cough and perform breathing treatments, the nurse splints the incision while helping the patient do these exercises.

Obstruction of the esophageal lumen may lead to multiple nutritional complications. If the patient has a feeding gastrostomy, once peristalsis has returned, feedings of water or glucose in water are offered in small amounts. If no difficulties are encountered, food is gradually reintroduced. Tube feedings and gastrostomy tube care are discussed in Chapter 16.

Evaluation

The patient with a prosthesis or anastomosis is evaluated for signs and symptoms of leakage within the first week. Inflammation, low-grade temperature, and fluid accumulation are signs of leakage. The patient's respiratory status should be normal and no breathing difficulties noted. If a gastrostomy tube has been inserted, the skin must be continuously assessed for leakage around the tube and excoriation.

SKIN CARE: WOUND OR FISTULA DRAINAGE

1. Use aseptic or clean technique as appropriate.
2. Draw a pattern of the fistula opening. The pattern opening should be almost flush with the wound edge to prevent skin excoriation from contact with drainage.
3. Select a pectin-based skin barrier (e.g., Stomahesive, Karaya).
4. Trace the pattern opening on the skin barrier, making sure that the paper side of the skin barrier, which will be removed, is toward the patient's skin.
5. Cut an opening in the pectin-based skin barrier.
6. Select an ostomy pouch that has a spout or opening for liquid drainage.
7. Trace the pattern opening onto the adhesive backing of the ostomy pouch.
8. Cut an opening in the pouch ⅛ inch larger than the pattern.
9. Remove the adhesive backing on the pouch and attach the pouch to the shiny side of the pectin-based skin barrier.
10. Cleanse the patient's skin, making sure it is dry before securing the skin barrier.
11. Remove the adhesive backing on the skin barrier; press and seal the pectin-based barrier to the skin.
12. If skin is exposed, apply a paste (e.g., Karaya, Stomahesive) to the area.
13. Check to see if the liquid drainage is collecting in the ostomy bag.
14. Assess the skin frequently for signs of excoriation.
15. Empty the ostomy bag frequently, according to the amount of drainage, to prevent the bag from pulling against the skin barrier and breaking the seal.

Gastric erosion or pyloric obstruction by the balloon of the catheter must also be evaluated. The nurse should inquire as to whether the patient has had a fever or chills or experienced abdominal distention or constipation. Psychologic adjustment of the patient who is not able to ingest food orally is an ongoing aspect of evaluation. The patient may find the social implications of not being able to eat orally extremely distressing and need both physical and emotional support.

ACHALASIA

Definition

A motor disorder of the upper and lower esophageal sphincter, as well as the body of the esophagus, is known as **achalasia**.

Etiology/Epidemiology

Achalasia is a condition of decreased motility (dyssynergia) of the lower portion of the esophagus with absence of peristalsis and inability of the LES to relax completely during swallowing for entry of the bolus. This results in dilation of the lower, thoracic portion of the esophagus. The exact cause of achalasia is unknown, but the disorder reflects disturbances in neuromuscular activity of the esophagus. The disease affects both sexes and all ages but is more common in the 40- to 50-year-old age group. Studies have shown an association with autoimmune, familial, environmental, and infectious factors.

Pathophysiology

The esophagus is a muscular tube controlled by the upper and lower esophageal sphincters and by the muscles of the oropharynx. When any of these three components fails to work, a dysfunctional esophagus results. In achalasia the LES does not relax to allow foods to enter the stomach. The esophagus becomes dilated and the walls hypertrophy (Figure 64-10). When esophageal peristalsis is absent, no food can enter the stomach unless enough has accumulated to force its passage.

Manometry findings include (1) incomplete relaxation of the LES, (2) increased LES pressure, (3) absence of esophageal peristalsis, and (4) increased intraesophageal pressure.

Clinical Manifestations

The patient is unable to propel solids or liquids from the pharynx to the esophagus. Solids cause more difficulty than do liquids. Food may be regurgitated, including some from the previous meal. The symptoms are more prominent when the patient assumes a

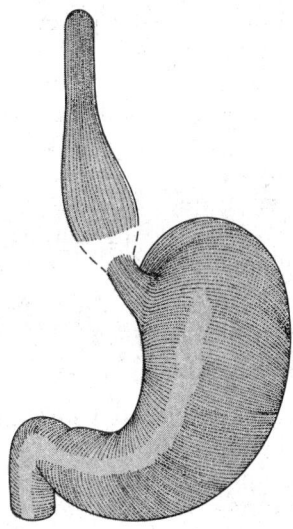

FIGURE 64-10   Achalasia showing dilation of esophagus above structure at cardia.

horizontal position and are relieved by moving around. Heartburn occurs in some individuals and is not usually relieved by antacids. Substernal chest pains may be felt at mealtime, and this pain is believed to be caused by esophagospasm. Weight loss occurs because of the discomfort and regurgitation associated with eating.

Esophagoscopy with biopsy is useful to rule out a malignancy. Radiography, manometry, and barium swallow are all measures to diagnose esophageal motor disorders.

Therapeutic Management

All forms of therapy are aimed at relieving the obstruction at the lower end of the esophagus. Complications include stasis esophagitis, carcinoma, and aspiration pneumonia. Temporary conservative treatment consists of nitrates (isosorbide dinitrate), calcium channel blockers (nifedipine), and terbutaline, which help relax the LES.[21] Much more effective treatment consists of forceful dilation with a pneumatic bag guided by radiographic control. Perforation from the attempt occurs in approximately 5% to 15% of patients. This procedure takes place after the esophagus has been cleared of contents. A dilator with a deflated balloon is passed down the esophagus. Under x-ray guidance, the balloon is inflated for 1 minute. The inflation may be repeated several times in order to stretch or tear enough LES tissue to allow the passage of food.

Surgical intervention may be necessary for patients in whom bag dilation fails or for those who are concerned about the risk of perforation. An esophagomyotomy, or Heller procedure, which consists of a transthoracic incision of the narrowed portion of the esophagus and part of the stomach, enlarges the esophageal mucosa, enabling food to pass more easily. A complication with this type of surgery is reflux esophagitis because of delayed gastric emptying and interruption of the gastroesophageal sphincter. The same nursing implications apply as with reflux esophagitis.

NURSING MANAGEMENT OF THE PATIENT WITH ACHALASIA

The patient is encouraged to drink fluids with meals to help push the bolus beyond the LES. Other symptomatic treatment includes sedatives, a semisoft bland diet, eating slowly and chewing food thoroughly, and anticholinergic drugs, which decrease LES pressure. Patients should also be instructed to sleep with the head of the bed elevated to prevent regurgitation or aspiration of food.

ESOPHAGEAL DIVERTICULUM

Esophageal diverticula are saclike outpouchings of one or more layers of the esophagus (Figure 64-11). As food is ingested, dysphagia occurs because food passes into the diverticulum and compresses the trachea. When a sufficient amount of food accumulates in the pocket, it overflows into the diaphragm and is regurgitated. Commonly the patient complains of a sour taste and a foul odor caused by stagnant food in the diverticulum. There is no specific treatment for diverticula. The diet may have to be liquids or semisoft foods to facilitate passage. When symptoms

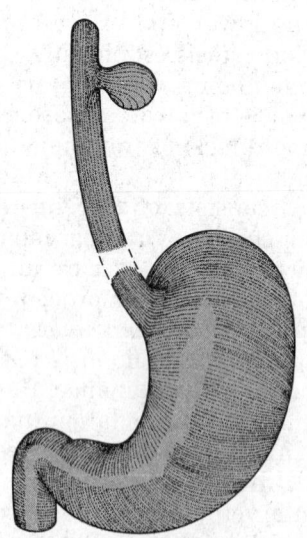

FIGURE 64-11   Esophageal diverticulum.

become severe, surgical removal of the herniated sac may be performed.

ESOPHAGEAL STRICTURES

Esophageal strictures are the result of inflammation and scarring from the ingestion of strong acids or alkali, reflux esophagitis, scleroderma, rheumatoid arthritis, and other connective tissue disorders. When the esophageal lumen has narrowed to the degree that dysphagia is a problem, dilation with a mechanical dilator will be necessary. When conservative treatment fails, surgery may be performed to resect the obstructed area.

CRITICAL THINKING QUESTIONS

1 Discuss the cause, treatment, and prevention of dental problems.
2 What oral changes occur with aging?
3 Name the common infections of the oral cavity and medications used to treat them.
4 Discuss appropriate nursing interventions for the patient with esophageal disorders.
5 What are the differences between malignant and benign conditions of the esophagus?
6 Discuss the long-term management and patient education for the person with GERD.

BIBLIOGRAPHY

Current

1. Cohen DJ, Starling JR: Surgery for reflux esophagitis: experience with the antireflux prosthesis, *AORN J* 43:858, 1986.
2. Dalton CB, Sinclair JW, Castell DO: Prolonged ambulatory esophageal pH monitoring, *Gastroenterol Nurs* 11(4):221-226, 1989.
3. DeMeester TR, Stein HJ: Surgical treatment of gastroesophageal reflux disease. In Castell DO: *The esophagus*, Boston, 1992, Little Brown & Co.
4. Frank-Stromborg M: The epidemiology and primary prevention of gastric and esophageal cancer, *Ca Nurs* 12(2):53-64, 1989.
5. Given BA, Simmons SJ: *Gastroenterology in clinical nursing*, ed 4, St Louis, 1984, Mosby–Year Book, Inc.
6. Hatton MN et al: Lubrication and viscosity features of human saliva and commercially available saliva substitutes, *J Oral Maxillofac Surg* 45:496, 1987.
7. Jones TR et al: Efficacy of an antibiotic mouthwash in contaminated head and neck surgery, *Am J Surg* 158:324-327, 1989.
8. Livstone EM, Skinner D: Tumors of the esophagus. In Berk JE, editor: *Bockus gastroenterology*, ed 4, Philadelphia, 1985, WB Saunders Co.
9. Maher KA et al: Intraesophageal balloon distention in the manometric evaluation of chest pain, *Gastroenterol Nurs* 13(1):4-8, 1990.
10. Managing acid reflux: a stepped up approach, *Patient Care*, p 72, April 15, 1986.
11. Marks R, Richter J: Gastroesophageal reflux disease. In

Zakim D, Dannenberg A, editors: *Peptic ulcer disease and other acid-related disorders,* New York, 1991, Academic Research Associates.

12. Medvec BR: Esophageal cancer, treatment and nursing interventions, *Semin Oncol Nurs* 4(4):246-256, 1988.
13. Page RC: Periodontal diseases in the elderly: a critical evaluation of current information, *Gerontology* 3:5, 1984.
14. Pope CE: The esophagus. In Sleisenger MH, Fordtran JS, editors: *Gastrointestinal disease,* ed 3, Philadelphia, 1983, WB Saunders Co.
15. Ragan JA: Lasers in gastroenterology, *Nurs Clin North Am* 25(3):685-696, 1990.
16. Schwartz SI et al: *Principles of surgery,* ed 5, New York, 1989, McGraw-Hill Book Co.
17. Silverberg E, Boring CC, Squires TS: Cancer statistics 1990, *CA* 40:9, 1990.
18. Silverman S, Gorsky M, Greenspan D: Current trends in occurrence of oral cancer: early detection of oral carcinoma, *J Dermatol Allergy* 6:26, 1983.
19. Swoope C, Smith DF, Kukens EM: Geriatric dentistry. In

Clark JW: *Clinical dentistry,* Philadelphia, 1986, Harper & Row, Publishers, Inc.
20. Taylor CR: Carcinoma of the esophagus: current imaging options, *Am J Gastroenterol* 81:1013, 1986.
21. Wong RKH et al: The effects of terbutaline sulfate, nitroglycerin and aminophylline on LES pressure and esophageal emptying in patients with achalasia, *J Clin Gastroenterol* 9:386, 1987.
22. Yakshe PN, Fleisher DS: Neoplasms of the esophagus. In Castell DO: *The esophagus,* Boston, 1992, Little, Brown & Co.

Classic
23. Hill LL: An effective operation for hiatal hernia: an eight-year appraisal, *Ann Surg* 166:681, 1967.
24. Leveret DH: Fluorides and the changing prevalence of dental caries, *Science* 217:26, 1982.
25. Nissen R: Gastropexy and fundoplication in surgical treatment of hiatal hernia, *Dig Dis Sci* 6:954, 1961.

CHAPTER SIXTY-FIVE

Nursing Management of Adults with Disorders of the Stomach or Duodenum

LEARNING OBJECTIVES

1 Describe the cause of acute and chronic gastritis.

2 Differentiate between chronic gastric and duodenal ulcer disease and acute stress ulcers.

3 Identify subjective data in the assessment of patients with peptic ulcer disease.

4 Compare actions and side effects of the agents used to treat peptic ulcer disease.

5 Describe areas of noncompliance for the patient with peptic ulcer disease.

6 Apply the nursing process to a patient who has peptic ulcer disease.

7 Identify preoperative nursing interventions for the patient undergoing gastric surgery.

8 Identify potential postoperative complications of gastric surgery.

9 Describe nursing interventions for a patient with gastrointestinal tract bleeding.

10 Develop a care plan for a patient experiencing the dumping syndrome.

11 Describe the care of the patient following gastric surgery.

KEY TERMS

DYSFUNCTION OF THE stomach or duodenum can adversely affect life-style and nutritional status. Digestion of nutrients, which begins in the mouth, continues in the stomach and duodenum. Protein breakdown and secretion of digestive juices begins in the stomach and duodenum. Many disorders of the stomach and duodenum are chronic and require the patient to make dietary and behavioral modifications. The nurse can identify risk factors and teach the patient about potential problems associated with these disorders.

ACUTE GASTRITIS
Definition

The term acute **gastritis** refers to transient inflammation of the gastric mucosa, mucosal hemorrhages, and erosion into the mucosal lining. Gastritis may occur when gastric acid secretion is excessive or absent.

Etiology/Epidemiology

Acute gastritis is commonly associated with alcoholism, aspirin ingestion, smoking, and stressful physical problems such as burns, central nervous system damage, chemotherapy, or radiation therapy. Additional causes of acute gastritis include ingestion of corrosive substances, viral infections, and food contaminated with *Staphylococcus* organisms. An epidemic form of acute gastritis of unknown cause has been found in persons with decreased acid secretion. The infectious organism has not been identified.

Pathophysiology

Vascular congestion, edema, acute inflammatory cell infiltration, and degenerative changes in the gastric epithelium occur in the presence of acute gastritis. Once mucosal injury has occurred and the gastric mucosal barrier has been disrupted, back diffusion of acid and pepsin occurs, contributing to the development of gastritis (see Figure 65-3). Acute gastritis is often limited to a single insult to the mucosa that resolves when the offending agent is removed.

Clinical Manifestations

Major manifestations of acute gastritis secondary to stress or ingestion of aspirin or nonsteroidal antiinflammatory agents are hematemesis, melena, pain, nausea, and vomiting. Persons experiencing severe nausea and vomiting and gastric bleeding may develop hypotension and dehydration. Some patients with gastritis are asymptomatic and require no treatment, whereas others with a mild form of the disease have discomfort relieved by eructation and defecation. Symptoms vary depending on the cause of the gastritis, but bleeding is more common with aspirin or NSAID-induced gastritis.[24]

Therapeutic Management

Most patients do not require treatment because the condition resolves when the cause is eliminated. For severe cases, however, antiemetics such as prochlorperazine (Compazine) or trimethobenzamide (Tigan) may be prescribed and intravenous fluids given to correct fluid and electrolyte imbalances. If the gastritis is caused by a bacterial agent, antibiotics may also be used. Patients who experience gastrointestinal bleeding from hemorrhagic gastritis require fluid and blood replacement and nasogastric lavage. A combination of antacids and cimetidine (Tagamet) or ranitidine (Zantac) may also be prescribed.

NURSING MANAGEMENT OF THE PATIENT WITH ACUTE GASTRITIS
Assessment

The nurse obtains information from the patient regarding the onset, frequency, and severity of gastrointestinal symptoms. The patient is assessed for dehydration and electrolyte imbalances. The nurse also determines the type and location of pain and relieving factors.

Nursing Diagnosis

Nursing diagnoses of the patient with acute gastritis include:

Fluid volume deficit related to vomiting, diarrhea, and blood loss

Pain related to epigastric discomfort, abdominal tenderness, and cramping

Planning

Many patients with gastritis are treated on an outpatient basis. Thus it is important to determine the patient's ability to identify factors causing the symptoms and to adhere to treatment methods for relieving them. Nursing care is planned to meet the following outcomes:

Relief of epigastric discomfort and related symptoms

Maintenance of adequate hydration and nutrition

Patient will use medications prescribed to relieve symptoms

Implementation

Usually food and fluids are withheld and oral intake restricted until the symptoms subside. The patient is observed for metabolic alkalosis and electrolyte imbalances, especially potassium, hydrogen, and chloride. Intake and output are recorded, especially if excessive vomiting occurs and nasogastric lavage is needed. Nasogastric lavage is discussed more completely later in the chapter. If antacids are administered hourly, the nurse needs to measure and maintain the pH of the gastric contents as ordered by the physician. When inflammation has subsided, clear liquids can be given at frequent intervals. The nurse needs to monitor the patient's tolerance of oral feedings. Once the patient can tolerate clear liquids and experiences no nausea or vomiting the diet is gradually advanced to solid foods.

CHRONIC GASTRITIS
Etiology/Epidemiology

Chronic gastritis is classified according to mucosal changes and the portion of the stomach involved. It is a slowly progressive disease that increases with advancing age. A specific cause of chronic gastritis is not likely. It occurs more frequently in women than in men and is seen more often in smokers. Reflux of duodenal contents into the stomach, immunologic injury, and genetic influences have an association with chronic gastritis. Other etiologic factors that have been implicated include long-term use of aspirin, NSAIDs, and alcohol. Increased episodes of acute gastritis do not cause chronic gastritis. Associations between chronic gastritis and gastric polyps and benign gastric ulcer and gastric cancer have been reported. Because gastric ulcers occur in the areas of chronic gastritis, it has been postulated that gastritis leads to gastric ulcer formation, but a direct cause-and-effect relationship has not been firmly established. Gastric cancer, however, is more likely to occur in persons with chronic gastritis.

Pathophysiology

Early pathologic changes include thickened mucous membranes with prominent rugae of the stomach. Degeneration occurs in varying degrees in the chief and parietal cells. As the disease advances, thinning and atrophy of the mucosa take place, further limiting the mucosal defense barrier, and the amount and concentration of secretions decrease. As gastric atrophy occurs, there is continued reduction in the mucosa, parietal, and chief cells, which decreases secretory activity even more.

Clinical Manifestations

Many patients with chronic gastritis are asymptomatic. Others have nausea, vomiting, and epigastric pain. Decreased gastric acid (hypochlorhydria) and pepsin secretions are also abnormal findings. Symptoms of vitamin B_{12} deficiency may develop. (Hematologic disorders are discussed in Chapter 38.)

Diagnosis is made by biopsy, endoscopy, and gastric analysis to evaluate secretions. Biopsy diagnosis is done to rule out the presence of gastric carcinoma.

Therapeutic Management

If pernicious anemia develops, the patient should receive vitamin B_{12} injections monthly and periodic evaluation of serum B_{12} levels. Glucocorticoids may induce parietal cell regeneration and reverse gastric mucosal changes in patients with pernicious anemia, but long-term corticosteroid therapy is neither practical nor safe.

NURSING MANAGEMENT OF THE PATIENT WITH CHRONIC GASTRITIS
Assessment

The nurse must obtain a medication history that includes over-the-counter medicines to determine whether these are contributing to irritation or ulceration of the gastric mucosa.

The nurse observes for signs and symptoms of anemia, such as fatigue, weakness, or pallor. It is also important to assess alcohol ingestion and smoking habits.

Nursing Diagnosis

Nursing diagnoses for the patient with chronic gastritis include:
    Pain related to epigastric distress and abdominal discomfort
    High risk for fatigue related to decreased vitamin B_{12} absorption
    Knowledge deficit related to lack of information about diet, medication regimen, and behavioral modification

Planning

The patient with chronic gastritis is treated symptomatically, and the nurse should plan to relieve symptoms and prevent acute exacerbations.

Implementation

The patient is taught to avoid drugs, such as salicylates and nonsteroidal antiinflammatory medications, or foods that seem to cause gastric irritation. If the patient believes certain foods cause irritation, those foods should be avoided. If pernicious anemia has been diagnosed, the nurse can be expected to administer vitamin B_{12} injections and to explain the need for this treatment method. The patient or significant person will be taught to administer the injection when at all possible. If heavy smoking and alcohol consumption contribute to chronic gastritis, behavioral modification is recommended. The diet regimen of small, frequent, bland feedings along with antacids after meals relieves symptoms of gastric irritation.

Evaluation

A reduction of the patient's symptoms is expected with adherence to the prescribed medication and dietary regimen. The patient will also demonstrate an increased activity level, as well as relief of epigastric and abdominal pain.

Documentation

The treatment and elimination of causative factors are noted. All medication and dietary regimens recommended for follow-up care will be documented, as well as the patient's response to interventions. In addition, if smoking and alcohol were noted as possible causative factors, the patient's compliance to eliminate these substances is recorded.

Peptic Ulcer Disease

Definition

Peptic ulcers are ulcerations that penetrate the mucosa or deeper structures of the gastrointestinal tract. Peptic ulcers can develop in the esophagus and jejunum, but more commonly occur in the stomach and duodenum. The term peptic ulcer has been used to describe both gastric and duodenal ulcers because it was believed that both were the result of acid and pepsin imbalances. It has been found that the incidence, physiology, and causes of gastric and duodenal ulcers are different and need to be discussed separately. However, the following generalities can be made:

1. All peptic ulcers require the presence of gastric acid.
2. The development of an ulcer reflects an imbalance of acid and pepsin and the natural ability of the gastrointestinal mucosa to protect itself from acid and pepsin.
3. Usually duodenal ulcers are caused by an increase in the aggressive factors (hypersecretion of acid), and gastric ulcers are a breakdown in the mucosal defense mechanisms.

Epidemiology

Although the incidence of peptic ulcer disease in the United States has decreased in recent years, it remains a major problem.[34] It is estimated that 25% of men and 17% of women have peptic ulcer disease, but only 5% to 10% of all individuals develop symptoms in their lifetime.[24] Peptic ulcer disease is com-

mon, although it rarely causes death. The incidence of symptomatic ulcer disease in the United States is approximately 18/1000 in adults, but the mortality is 2.5/100,000.[25] In the elderly, however, the risk of ulcer perforation has risen, possibly because of the increasing use of nonsteroidal antiinflammatory drugs. It has been estimated that one out of five patients on long-term NSAID therapy will experience peptic ulcer disease.[23] Approximately 30% to 50% of ulcers in the elderly are gastric.[33] The incidence of ulcers varies by age, sex, and site. In men and women the symptomatic duodenal ulcer is more common than the symptomatic gastric ulcer. Men are more likely to develop a duodenal ulcer but are equally as likely to develop a gastric ulcer. Recent studies have found that two thirds of patients with gastric and duodenal ulcers have an infection with *Helicobacter pylori.* This bacteria is found only on the gastric mucosa and is also associated with chronic gastritis. It is postulated that this bacteria is capable of digesting the protective mucosal lining, allowing ulceration to occur with epithelial exposure to the acid.[4] Studies are currently in progress using a combination drug therapy of two antibiotics, tetracycline and metronidazole, and bismuth, which appears to suppress the bacteria.

The peak occurrence of a duodenal ulcer is at age 40, with symptoms appearing between the ages of 25 to 55. The peak occurrence of a gastric ulcer is at age 50, with symptoms appearing most commonly between ages 40 and 70. Although most ulcers heal with drug therapy in 6 to 8 weeks, there is a high rate of recurrence (70% to 80% by the end of the first year and 95% at the end of 2 years).[6]

GASTRIC ULCERS
Etiology

In the past, multiple factors have been considered in the development of gastric ulcers, including dietary indiscretions and genetic predisposition. Currently, evidence strongly suggests a relationship between persons who ingest excessive amounts of NSAIDs, salicylates, or alcohol and the increased incidence of gastric ulcers. Cigarette smoking has been found to decrease prostaglandin synthesis, which alters the mucosal defense mechanism and predisposes the patient to ulcer formation as well as a slower rate of ulcer healing and a higher rate of ulcer-related complications.[22]

Pathophysiology

The most common site of a **gastric ulcer** is the distal half of the stomach (Figure 65-1). Although acid is essential for development of a gastric ulcer, the total amount does not appear to be important. Most persons with a gastric ulcer have a lower acid se-

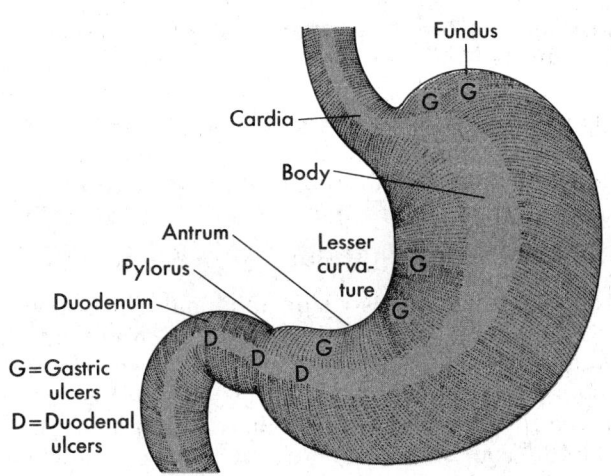

FIGURE 65-1   Common sites of peptic ulcer disease. Sixty percent of gastric ulcers occur on lesser curvature; twenty-five percent occur in prepyloric area.

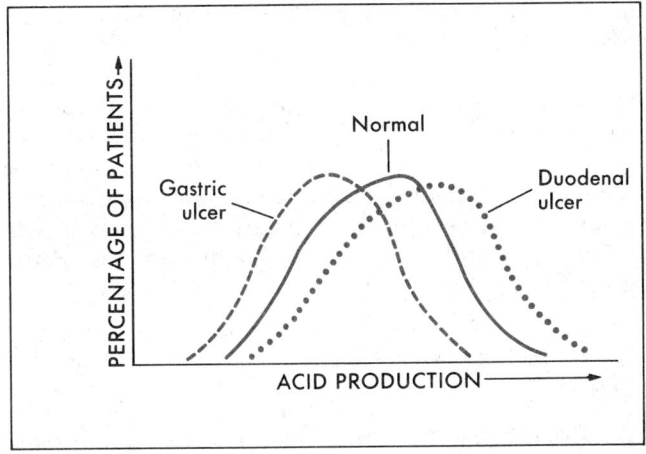

FIGURE 65-2   Comparison of acid production in gastric and duodenal ulcers. Acid production is lower than normal with gastric ulcers and higher than normal with duodenal ulcers.

cretion rate than persons with a duodenal ulcer and even lower than normal individuals (Figure 65-2). However, the usual problem is a failure in one or more of the mechanisms that protect the gastric mucosa from the highly concentrated gastric acid (pH 0.8 to 3). Several predisposing factors are believed to be responsible for the diminished gastric mucosal resistance.

The gastric mucosal barrier is a physiologic barrier formed by a layer of mucus. The secretion of mucus and bicarbonate act to maintain a near neutral pH on the gastric epithelium, protecting the lining from the corrosive effects of acid. If this mucus layer is interrupted for any reason, the highly concentrated hydrogen ions diffuse into the cells (back diffusion), and the cells release histamine (Figure 65-3). Histamine further stimulates acid secretion and capillary leakage of serum and blood. The back diffusion of hydrogen ions is associated with decreased acid and increased sodium levels. Once mucosal cells lose their blood and oxygen supply, the cells die and erosions and ulcers develop.

A cytoprotective effect is another mechanism at work in the gastric mucosal cells, assumed to be mediated in part by prostaglandins. Cytoprotection is the ability to confer mucosal protection without decreasing acid secretion. When the gastric mucosa has been exposed to any of several weak toxic stimuli, for example, dilute acid, base, or alcohol, the mucosal barrier develops an increased resistance to these offending agents. Antiprostaglandin drugs may compromise this cytoprotective effect, which partially explains why aspirin and nonsteroidal antiinflammatory drugs, inhibitors of prostaglandin synthesis, are major causes of gastric ulceration. It has been shown that gastric mucosal damage occurs as

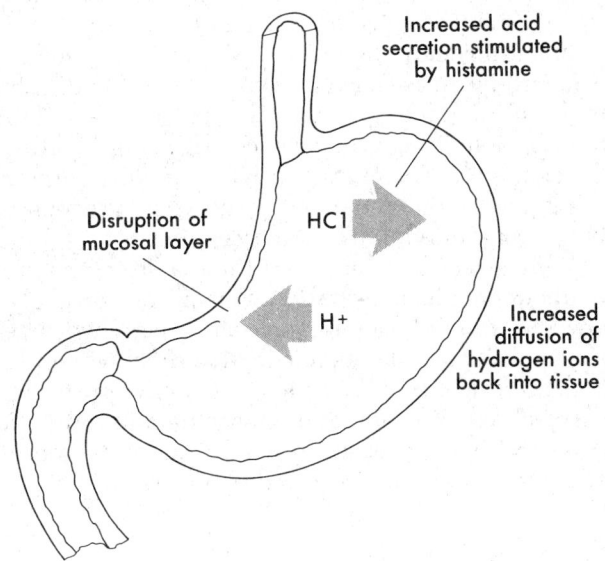

FIGURE 65-3   Back diffusion of hydrogen ions in gastric ulcers or acute gastritis.

rapidly as 1 hour after ingestion of acetylsalicylic acid. Erosions have been noted within 24 hours, and maximal injury has been reported within 3 to 7 days.[13]

Reflux of duodenal contents into the stomach may contribute to the chronic inflammatory process. Experimental studies have shown that reflux of bile acids from the duodenum under certain conditions can produce severe gastric mucosal damage.[22] It is believed that alkaline duodenal contents damage the protecting layer in the gastric mucus so that both acid and pepsin disrupt the epithelium and produce a gastric ulcer.

A gastric ulcer also may be superimposed on gastric cancer, particularly in the presence of gastric lymphomas. These ulcers presumably occur because of impairment of the blood supply to the tumor. A biopsy of all gastric ulcers should be done before treatment to exclude malignancy and treatment monitored endoscopically until healing is complete.[33]

DUODENAL ULCERS
Etiology

Duodenal ulcer is a blanket term for a heterogeneous group of disorders. Approximately 40% of duodenal ulcers are associated with actual hypersecretion of acid. Of this group, hypersecretion may be caused by the following:

1. Excessive parietal cell mass
2. Increased gastrin release after a meal
3. Increased sensitivity to gastrin
4. An uncontrolled source of gastrin release (Zollinger-Ellison syndrome)

For the remaining 60%, however, the amount of acid produced is normal. The reasons for development of duodenal ulcers in this category are multiple but definite characteristics are being identified; for example, accelerated gastric emptying with acid entering the duodenum at a rate that exceeds the buffering ability of alkaline secretions.

Pepsin seems to be one of the major contributors in duodenal ulcer formation. Pepsins are proteolytic enzymes found in gastric juice along with hydrochloric acid. Pepsin has its maximal activity when pH is at a level of 2 to 3.5 and loses its activity when the pH is above 5. In duodenal ulcer patients, the duodenal pH is lower than in normal patients, thereby allowing pepsin to damage the mucosa.

Pathophysiology

Patients who have duodenal ulcers because of increased parietal cell activity have been the subject of a great deal of research. The increased parietal cell mass causes hypersecretion of acid. The parietal cells have three types of receptors for acid-stimulating secretagogues. Acetylcholine, histamine, and gastrin are all secretagogues that stimulate the parietal cells to produce and release acid. Patients in this category also have a high level of circulating gastrin. Gastrin stimulates acid secretion by causing several events that precipitate histamine release, the most powerful stimulation for acid production. The defensive resistance of the mucosa depends on the mucosal integrity and regeneration. Ulceration occurs when the aggressive factors (those responsible for acid secretion) exceed the defensive factors.

Patients with increased amount of acid secretion have more rapid emptying of stomach contents than do normal persons. For these patients rapid emptying causes the acid load entering the duodenum to exceed the buffering ability of the alkaline secretions, further contributing to ulcer formation.

Clinical Manifestations

The symptoms of gastric or duodenal ulcers may be very similar (Table 65-1). Generally, however, the pain experienced by patients with a gastric ulcer usually follows the ingestion of food and is not relieved by food intake. The pain does not awaken the patient from sleep, nor does it produce the rhythmic discomfort associated with duodenal ulcers. On the other hand, the gnawing quality of pain radiating to the back has been described by patients with both types of ulcers. Nausea and vomiting may occur with gastric ulcers and results from gastric motility disturbances. Belching and bloating are common complaints classified as "dyspepsias" and described by patients with gastric or duodenal ulcers.

TABLE 65-1   Symptoms of Gastric Ulcers and Duodenal Ulcers

Symptom	Gastric ulcers (%)	Duodenal ulcers (%)
Anorexia	46-57	25-36
Belching*	48	59
Bloating*	55	49
Fatty food intolerance	—	14-72
Heartburn	19	27-59
Nausea	54-70	49-59
Pain		
Epigastric*	67	61-86
Radiation to back*	34	20-31
Frequently severe	68	53
Gnawing*	13	16
Episodic	16	56
At night	32-43	50-88
Increased by food	24	10-40
Food relief	2-48	20-63
Not related to food*	22-53	21-49
Relief with antacids*	36-87	39-86
Vomiting	38-73	25-57
Weight loss	24-61	19-45

Modified from Soll AH, Isenberg JI: Duodenal ulcer disease. In Sleisenger MH, Fordtran JS, editors: *Gastrointestinal diseases*, ed 3, Philadelphia, 1983, WB Saunders.
*Symptoms are similar for both types of ulcers.

The term dyspepsia is nonspecific and can include a variety of symptoms, such as nausea, vomiting, anorexia, fullness, bloating, pain, or discomfort. Hemorrhage is a common complication of gastric ulcers, and more gastric ulcers bleed than do duodenal ulcers. Bleeding from peptic ulcers stops spontaneously in 70% to 80% of patients.[19] The bleeding of duodenal ulcers is more likely to be chronic and duodenal ulcers are more likely to perforate than gastric ulcers.

Several approaches are used to diagnose peptic ulcers. Fiberoptic endoscopy can detect both gastric and duodenal ulcers. The endoscopist can identify erosion, strictures, and malignant neoplasms. The lesion can be photographed, a biopsy performed, and cell washings obtained for cytologic examination with this procedure.

Radiologic examination of the upper gastrointestinal tract using both standard and double air contrast studies is another common method for detecting peptic ulcers. Data suggest that small ulcerations may be missed using this procedure. It is also difficult to differentiate a malignant lesion from a benign lesion by radiology alone.

Stomach acid output, as well as serum gastrin levels, have been used in the past to gain additional information but have not been employed as much in recent years.

Complications

Gastrointestinal tract bleeding

Upper gastrointestinal (GI) tract bleeding occurs in 15% to 20% of patients with duodenal ulcers and 10% to 15% of patients with gastric ulcers. A common symptom of patients with active upper GI tract bleeding is vomiting blood (hematemesis). The emesis looks like coffee grounds because of the action of gastric acid on the hemoglobin molecule. Profuse upper GI tract hemorrhage may result in the passage of bright-red blood rectally **(hematochezia),** whereas tarry stools (melena) occur with slower rates of bleeding (but still above 50 mL/day).[9] If the patient has had peptic ulcers in the past and has recently ingested aspirin or alcohol, the possibility arises that erosive gastritis may be the cause of bleeding.

Hemorrhage

In the United States each year probably 100,000 patients with peptic ulcer bleed. The mortality has remained relatively unchanged over the past 15 years, averaging between 7% to 10%. Patients with significant bleeding from gastric ulcers are in the older age groups. Mucosal capillaries are superficial and tend to erode and break down readily. Bleeding from gastric ulcer is less likely to subside compared with bleeding from a duodenal ulcer.

Fiberoptic endoscopy with laser therapy can be performed to visualize and temporarily interrupt bleeding from large blood vessels until further corrective surgery can be done. Endoscopic laser photocoagulation has been used to seal off the bleeding vessels. Injection therapies with hypertonic saline, epinephrine, or alcohol have also been tried with positive results. Krejs reports that the most effective techniques are electrocoagulation or the heater probe used in conjunction with endoscopy to achieve immediate hemostasis.[19]

When patients have near-fatal hemorrhage, they should be prepared immediately for an emergency operation. In this situation, endoscopy may not locate the bleeding site because of the large amount of blood filling the gastric lumen. Patients with a bleeding gastric ulcer have signs and symptoms of shock but are usually alert and fully responsive. Surgery is indicated if the patient fails to stabilize after receiving blood over several hours. If the patient does stabilize several days later and rebleeding occurs, surgery is advised. If the patient has experienced one or more previous bleeding episodes, serious consideration is given to surgical intervention.

Perforation

When the ulcer crater penetrates the entire thickness of the wall of the stomach or duodenum, gastric acid, pancreatic enzymes, or bile is released into the peritoneal cavity, causing a chemical burn and peritonitis. Perforation is more likely to occur with long-standing peptic ulcer disease. A review of the past three decades shows that patients with perforated gastric ulcers had the following characteristics:[15]

1. Abdominal pain (92%)
2. Emesis (75%)
3. Fever (46%)
4. Hypotension (31%)
5. Hematemesis (24%)
6. No previous ulcer symptoms (43%)
7. Cigarette smoking (48%)
8. Ingestion of salicylates (27%)
9. Ingestion of diuretics (20%)
10. Ingestion of alcohol (19%)

Mortality from perforation is 5% to 15% for duodenal ulcers and somewhat higher for gastric ulcers. If the patient has a perforated gastric ulcer, the possibility of gastric cancer must be ruled out. Treatment consists of gastric resection, including ulcer removal with or without vagotomy, depending on the ulcer type. If the patient is extremely debilitated, only a biopsy and simple ulcer excision may be performed.

Penetration

Penetration occurs when the ulcer erodes through the wall of the gastric (pyloric) or duodenal area into adjacent organs. The most common site of penetration is the pancreas, with the main symptom being severe pain. Confirmation of the diagnosis is made by determination of the serum amylase, which will be elevated. Surgery is necessary to correct this situation. Penetration into surrounding viscera may also result in fistula of the colon, biliary tract, or liver, which also must be surgically repaired.

Obstruction

Gastric outlet obstruction is more common in patients who have an ulcer in the pyloric area, but it can occur in patients with a gastric ulcer as well. The occurrence in patients with peptic ulcer disease is about 5%. Repeated cycles of ulceration and healing can result in a buildup of scar tissue, especially at the pylorus. The resulting obstruction of the gastric outlet leads to gastric dilation and vomiting. Other clinical symptoms are nausea, epigastric fullness or bloating, anorexia, early satiety, and epigastric pain. Balloon dilation of the pylorus by endoscopy has been used in some centers to relieve this obstruction. Kozarek found that 70% of their 23 patients who had this procedure were asymptomatic 2½ years later.[18] All patients with gastric outlet obstruction should undergo preoperative gastric decompression for several days along with restoration of fluid and electrolyte balance. Operative results in patients with gastric outlet obstruction are usually highly satisfactory.

Therapeutic Management

Therapy is aimed at reducing symptoms, reducing or neutralizing acid secretions, and diminishing the risk of complications. The pharmacologic alteration of normal gastric acidity has become routine in patients with peptic ulcer disease, and the efficacy of this therapy has prompted widespread use.

Pharmacologic therapy

Drugs commonly used in the treatment of peptic ulcer disease include antacids (Table 65-2), histamine receptor antagonists, mucosal healing agents, prostaglandins, proton pump inhibitors, and occasionally anticholinergics (Table 65-3). Anticholinergics are used much less frequently since the induction of H_2 receptor antagonists in the treatment of the disease. They may still be used as adjunctive therapy, but will delay gastric emptying and allow the acid to be in prolonged contact with the damaged mucosa, thereby increasing the extent of ulceration.

Antacids

Antacids work by neutralizing or reducing the acidity of stomach contents. They have been shown to

RESEARCH BRIEF

Donowitz LG et al: Alteration of normal gastric flora in critical care patients receiving antacid and cimetidine therapy, *Infect Control* 7:23, 1986.

Normal gastric flora is altered in critical care patients receiving antacid and cimetidine therapy. One study included 153 critical care patients with documented cimetidine and antacid use. Those patients with altered gastric flora had an organism in their gastric flora 21% of the time preceding an episode of bacteremia and 27% of the time preceding an episode of pneumonia. A direct cause-and-effect relationship between administration of antacids, cimetidine therapy, and nosocomial bacteremias or pneumonias has not been firmly established, but the possibility remains that if this artificially maintained reservoir of organisms were not present, infections in critical care patients could be reduced.

heal both gastric and duodenal ulcers, although they are less successful with gastric ulcers. Antacids are easily obtained and do not require a prescription. They are relatively inexpensive even when taken in substantial doses.

The dosage and timing of antacid therapy are important. The quantity of antacid capable of neutralizing 80 to 90 mEq of acid (approximately 30 mL) is taken 1 to 3 hours before and after meals and at bedtime (seven doses per day).[12] The potency, content, and cost of different antacids vary greatly. Acid-neutralizing capacity is an important reason for selection of an antacid. Acid-neutralizing capacity is expressed as the milliequivalents of antacid required to keep the antacid suspension at a pH of greater than 3 for 2 hours in a laboratory test. Antacid therapy has several drawbacks, including diarrhea, constipation, drug interactions, and differences in absorption rates. Poor compliance is another problem because of the regimen of seven doses daily.

To reduce complications of drug interactions and altered absorption rates, patients taking antacids should wait 1 to 2 hours before ingesting other oral drugs. Because antacids lower gastric pH, enteric-coated drugs will be released while still in the stomach; these medicines should be given 1 hour apart. The nurse should be familiar with potency, side effects, and several brands of antacids to assist patients. Combination products (those containing aluminum and magnesium compounds) can minimize the side effects of constipation or diarrhea. The sodium content of antacids must also be considered. Patients with hypertension, congestive heart failure,

TABLE 65-2   Pharmacology Summary: Antacids

Trade name	Ingredients	Acid-neutralizing capacity per capsule, tablet, or 5 mL (meg)	Sodium content (mg)	Nursing implications
AlternaGel gel	Aluminum hydroxide	12	2	May decrease absorption of tetracyclines, phenytoin, corticosteroids, warfarin, isoniazid; inhibits gastric emptying; constipating
Aludrox	Aluminum hydroxide/ magnesium hydroxide	14	1.15	Same as above; may cause hypermagnesemia in persons with renal failure
Amphojel	Aluminum hydroxide	13-14	2.4	Can be used with low-phosphate diet to prevent urinary stones; inhibits gastric emptying; constipating; may decrease absorption of tetracyclines
Basal	Aluminum carbonate gel	13-14	2.8\E 2.1 2.4	Same as above
Gaviscon tablets	Aluminum hydroxide/ magnesium trisilicate, and sodium bicarbonate		19	May decrease absorption of tetracyclines; can cause rebound hyperacidity; inhibits gastric emptying
Gaviscon liquid	Aluminum hydroxide and magnesium carbonate		12.9	Decreased absorption of tetracyclines; may cause hypermagnesemia in persons with renal failure
Maalox	Aluminum/ magnesium hydroxide	13.5 (suspension) 8.5 (tablets)	1.35\E 1	May cause hypermagnesemia in persons with renal failure; may decrease absorption of tetracyclines, phenothiazines, iron salts, and isoniazid
Maalox Therapeutic concentrate	Aluminum hydroxide/ magnesium hydroxide	28.3	0.8	Same as above
Mylanta tablets	Aluminum hydroxide/ magnesium hydroxide/ simethicone	11.5	0.77	Same as above
Riopan	Magaldrate	13.5	0.3	Same as above
Rolaids	Dihydroxyaluminum	7.5-8	53	Hypercalcemia, constipation, rebound hyperacidity

Continued.

TABLE 65-2   Pharmacology Summary: Antacids—cont'd

Trade name	Ingredients	Acid-neutralizing capacity per capsule, tablet, or 5 mL (meq)	Sodium content (mg)	Nursing implications
Various brands	Sodium bicarbonate		27%	Not recommended as much because may lead to metabolic alkalosis with long-term use; may inhibit excretion of amphetamines or quinidine; rebound hyperacidity; sodium and water retention
Tums	Calcium carbonate	10	2.7	Not recommended for long-term therapy because of rebound hyperacidity, hypercalcemia; renal impairment decreased

or those on restricted or low-sodium diets should use only low-sodium antacids.

Histamine H₂ receptor blockers

Histamine H$_2$ receptor blockers, such as cimetidine (Tagamet) and ranitidine (Zantac), block the histamine H$_2$ receptors and decrease acid secretions. Acid production is not altogether stopped, but the concentration is reduced significantly to relieve symptoms and promote healing. Cimetidine has been used in more than 50 million patients, and its safety has been well established. The side effects reported are low even in high-risk hospitalized patients. There are less adverse reactions reported with ranitidine than with cimetidine.[8]

Drug interactions have been reported in patients receiving parenteral cimetidine or ranitidine therapy along with either theophylline, phenytoin, or warfarin. Since patients who are taking these drugs intravenously may have impaired renal or hepatic function, the levels of phenytoin and theophylline, as well as prothrombin time, should be monitored frequently.

Mucosal healing agents

Mucosal healing agents are those that heal ulcers in the absence of antisecretory properties. The exact mode of operation of mucosal healing agents is unknown. It is believed, however, that they achieve their effect by adhering to the proteins in the ulcer base.

Misoprostol is the first prostaglandin drug used to prevent ulcer formation in patients using long-term NSAID therapy. Prostaglandins inhibit the secretion of gastric acid and stimulate mucus and bicarbonate secretion on the mucosa of the stomach and small intestine, thereby helping to maintain the integrity of the mucosal lining.

The chemical structure of sucralfate (Carafate) stimulates the release of prostaglandins within the gastric mucosa, with prostaglandin E$_2$ reducing the acid attack, which allows healing to occur. Sucralfate does not have a significant acid-neutralization ability. The recommended dosage is 1 g, four times a day, 1 hour before meals and at bedtime. It has been shown that after 4 weeks of therapy, approximately 80% of ulcers have healed. The most common side effect is constipation.

Tripotassium dicitratobismuthate (De-nol), a bismuth compound, is not new but is not currently available in the United States. Proponents claim this drug is as effective as cimetidine for healing gastric and duodenal ulcers.[34] It is inexpensive, not absorbed in significant amounts, and has no serious side effects. Patients treated with De-nol have fewer relapses than those treated with cimetidine. It may discolor the teeth, tongue, and stools.[34]

Diet therapy

Traditionally, diet therapy was used in the belief that it would minimize acid secretion and promote

TABLE 65-3   Pharmacology Summary: Agents to Treat Peptic Ulcer Disease

Drug	Oral dosage	Uses	Side effects/nursing implications
Histamine H_2 receptor antagonist			
Cimetidine (Tagamet)	300 mg qid with or immediately after meals and hs or 400 mg bid or 800 mg hs	Gastric and duodenal ulcers, Zollinger-Ellison syndrome	Multiple drug interactions; antacids interfere with absorption; cigarette smoking reverses cimetidine-induced inhibition of nocturnal gastric secretion; may cause confusion in the elderly
Famotidine (Pepcid)	40 mg hs or 20 mg every 12 hr	Same as above	Same as above
Nizatidine (Axid)	300 mg hs 150 mg bid	Same as above	Same as above
Ranitidine (Zantac)	150 mg bid or 300 mg hs; drug absorption not affected by food	Same as above	Procainamide, glipizide, and warfarin drug interactions; antacids do not interfere with absorption; may cause headaches
Muscosal healing agents			
Sucralfate (Carafate)	1 g qid on empty stomach and hs	Duodenal ulcers	Given ½ hour before meals; tetracycline, phenytoin, digoxin, and cimetidine drug interactions; constipation; antacids should not be taken ½ hour before or after medication
Gastric acid pump inhibitor	20-40 mg/day	GERD	Give ½ hour before breakfast; may cause rash, itching and/or diarrhea
Omeprazole (Losec, Prilosec)	60 mg/day 20-40 mg/day	Hyperacidity Duodenal and gastric ulcers	
Prostaglandins			
Misoprostol (Cytotec)	100-200 mcg qid	NSAID-induced erosions	Can cause diarrhea and abdominal cramps that limit its use; may cause dysmenorrhea or other gynecologic dysfunction
Anticholinergics			
Pirenzephine (Gastrozepin)	50 mg bid	Duodenal ulcers	Dry mouth, multiple drug interactions; antacids may interfere with absorption
Propanthelin bromide (Probanthine)	15 mg tid and 30 mg hs	Peptic ulcers	Same as above
Glycopyrrolate (Robinul)	1 mg tid or 2 mg bid	Peptic ulcers	Same as above
Dicyclomine (Bentyl)	20-40 mg tid 30 mg hs	Peptic ulcers	Same as above

healing of ulcers. Studies have found limited benefit in diet modification and it may actually be harmful since milk is a potent gastric acid stimulant. Higher ulcer recurrence rates have been associated with low-fiber diets, and so there may be some value in increased fiber in the diet.

Modifications in diet are seldom recommended today with the exception of foods that have been found to cause discomfort in individual patients. Alcohol is limited, and a recent study found that black pepper and green pepper can produce gastric mucosal lesions.[21]

The milk-and-cream diet has had a long tradition in the treatment of peptic ulcers, and patients still ask about it. Nutrients play a complex role in ulcer physiology. Milk products do buffer gastric acid, but the protein and fat composition of milk actually stimulates further acid production through gastrin. Since all foods neutralize acid and stimulate gastric secretions, small feedings several times a day have the advantage of not increasing the degree of gastric motor activity caused by a larger meal. Patients should also avoid specific foods that worsen the symptoms, including caffeinated and decaffeinated coffee. Other agents known to aggravate the condition are cigarette smoking,[17] alcohol, and aspirin. Bland diets are not encouraged because of their uncertain compositions, questionable patient compliance, and lack of documentation in ulcer healing.

Surgical treatment

When medical management of peptic ulcer disease no longer relieves symptoms, surgery is usually recommended. It is estimated that 10% to 15% of all ulcer patients require surgery. Surgery is indicated in uncontrolled or life-threatening bleeding, perforation, penetration, or obstruction. The main goal of surgical intervention is the same as for medical treatment: to reduce acid secretion and allow healing.

Gastric resection

An **antrectomy** is the removal of the entire antrum, the gastrin-producing portion of the lower stomach. This eliminates one of the main stimuli to acid production. If only an antrectomy is performed, a truncal vagotomy is usually added, resulting in 90% reduction of both basal and maximal acid output and a very low ulcer recurrence rate. When the fundus of the stomach is directly anastomosed to the duodenum, the procedure is known as the **Billroth I,** or gastroduodenostomy. In this procedure, ulcers or cancer localized in the antrum of the stomach are removed (Figure 65-4). In the **Billroth II procedure,** or gastrojejunostomy, the duodenum is closed, and the fundus of the stomach is anastomosed into the jejunum. The Billroth II procedure removes ulcers

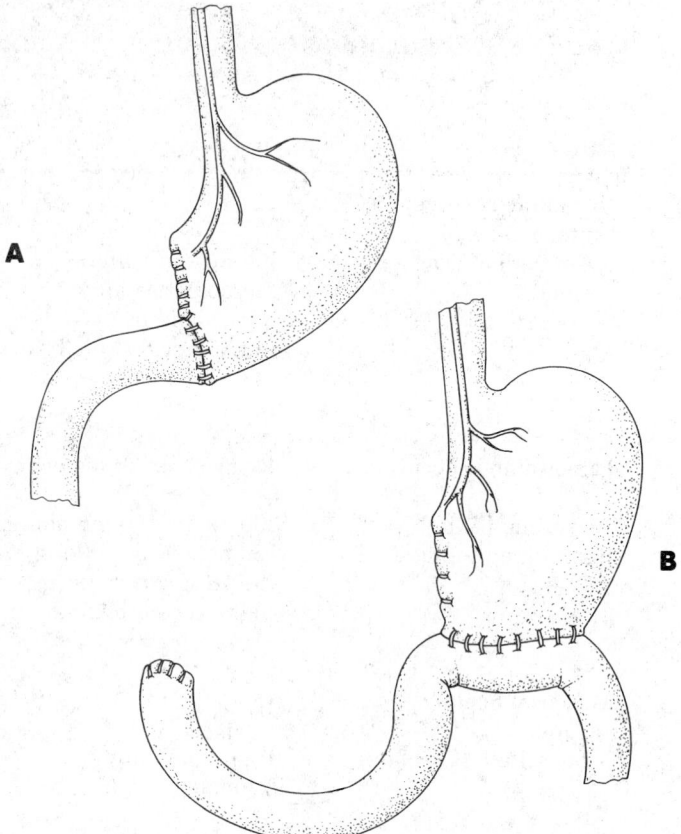

FIGURE 65-4 Surgical procedures in peptic ulcer disease. **A,** Billroth I procedure (gastroduodenostomy). **B,** Billroth II procedure (gastrojejunostomy). A vagotomy (severing of the vagus nerve) may be done to decrease acid production.

or cancer located in the body of the fundus. The Billroth surgeries are not used as much for peptic ulcer disease because of the associated operative morbidity and mortality. A total gastrectomy is rarely performed, except in patients with gastric cancer or the Zollinger-Ellison syndrome (an unusual condition that involves hypersecretion of acid with or without peptic ulcer disease).

Vagotomy

A **vagotomy** involves removal of the vagal innervation to the fundus, which interrupts the cephalic (vagal) pathway from producing acid in the parietal cells of the stomach. The most common procedure is the truncal vagotomy in which the entire trunk of both vagus nerves is severed below the diaphragm, resulting in denervation from the gastroesophagus to the midtransverse colon (Figure 65-5). The procedure is relatively easy to perform but may produce diarrhea and an increased incidence of gallstones. In addition, since the vagal supply to the antrum and

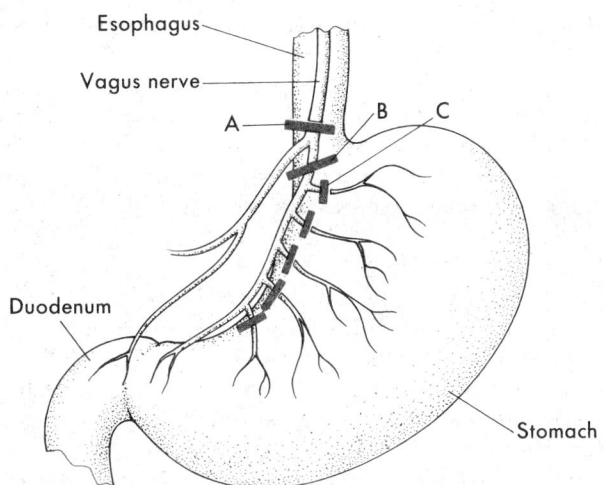

FIGURE 65-5   Vagotomy procedures. *A*, Truncal. *B*, Selective. *C*, Parietal cell vagotomy.

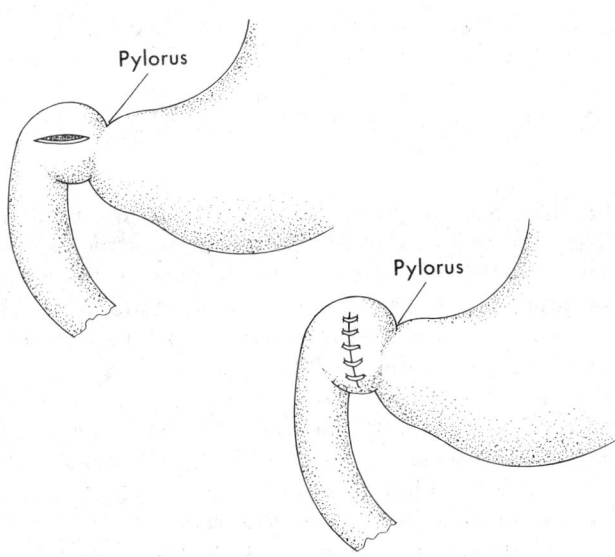

FIGURE 65-6   Pyloroplasty (Heinke-Mikulicz procedure). The pyloric outlet is widened and a vagotomy done to allow emptying of gastric contents.

pylorus is also interrupted, the stomach has delayed emptying. Therefore, it is usually necessary to perform either a pyloroplasty or gastrojejunostomy for increased drainage of the stomach contents. In a selective proximal vagotomy, only the fibers that supply the acid-secreting fundus are cut. This procedure produces few untoward effects, but is technically more difficult and reduces basal acid by only 80% and maximal acid by 50%. Ulcer recurrence is more likely following this procedure.

Pyloroplasty

Pyloroplasty, or surgical enlargement of the pylorus, is performed to provide drainage of the gastric contents. It is commonly combined with a vagotomy to increase gastric emptying (Figure 65-6).

Many controversies surround the decision to perform one procedure over another. Different criteria are used in selecting the type of surgery to be performed. Controlled studies continue to be undertaken to determine the most effective procedures to prevent recurrence. In addition, the improved medical management of peptic ulcers has greatly reduced the need for surgery.

Postoperative complications

Bleeding from the anastomosed suture line may occur up to 7 days after gastric surgery. Leakage may also occur from the anastomosis sites, as well as the blind end of the duodenal stump of the Billroth II procedure. The patient experiences abdominal rigidity, abdominal pain, an elevated temperature, and leukocytosis. Drainage from the incision may be bile stained. The patient must undergo surgical intervention for this complication.

Dumping syndrome

The **dumping syndrome** can occur after a pyloroplasty, gastroduodenostomy (Billroth I procedure), gastrojejunostomy (Billroth II procedure), truncal vagotomy, or antrectomy. The cause of the dumping syndrome is believed to be rapid gastric emptying whereby duodenal or jejunal distention is produced by a hypertonic bolus of food. Fluid accumulates in the gut from the hyperosmolar solution, and the blood volume subsequently decreases. As the duodenum or jejunum becomes more distended, increased intestinal motility and peristalsis occur. Further complications of the dumping syndrome occur several hours after the meal. Blood glucose levels rise rapidly after ingestion of a meal high in simple sugars. An exaggerated amount of insulin is released, followed by reactive hypoglycemia.

Clinical symptoms associated with the dumping syndrome are nausea, vomiting, epigastric pain, explosive diarrhea, borborygmi (noises made from gas passing through the liquid of the small intestine), and dyspepsia. Systemic symptoms include flushing, dizziness, tachycardia, diaphoresis, and orthostatic hypotension. Hypoglycemia occurs several hours after the meal.

Treatment of the dumping syndrome is mostly through dietary education. The patient should eat six small meals a day that are high in protein and fat and low in carbohydrates. Refined or concentrated carbohydrates should be avoided because they leave the stomach more quickly, pull fluid into the intestine, and increase insulin release. The patient should eat slowly and avoid drinking fluids during meals.

Anticholinergics may be prescribed to decrease stomach motility. The patient should also assume a recumbent position after meals for ½ to 1 hour to enhance digestion and relieve symptoms.

Diarrhea

Diarrhea may be a complication with any type of gastric surgery because of the changes in emptying time. However, it is most commonly found in patients who have had a truncal vagotomy with pyloroplasty, gastroenterostomy, or antrectomy. Diarrhea occurs more often in the early postoperative months and decreases within 1 year. A small minority of patients continue to have diarrhea that does not respond to medical treatment. Lactose and fluids should be eliminated during meals. If the condition persists, antidiarrheal agents such as diphenoxylate/atropine (Lomotil), loperamide (Imodium), paregoric, or codeine are often used. Cholestyramine, a bile acid-binding resin, has been shown to be helpful.

Reflux esophagitis

Any surgery involving the stomach may precipitate esophagitis. The symptoms occur most commonly among individuals who have had a vagotomy and pyloroplasty, a vagotomy and gastrectomy, or Billroth I and II procedures. Most patients are managed by medical means, but those whose condition is more severe may require fundoplication.

Nutritional deficits

The most commonly encountered complications of patients who have had gastric surgery are the vast nutritional deficits. Weight loss, malabsorption, anemia, and vitamin deficiency all represent serious threats to health.

Weight loss

Substantial weight loss occurs in nearly half of the patients who undergo surgery. More women than men have postoperative weight loss and in greater magnitude. The most significant reason for weight loss is decreased calorie intake because of a loss in the receptive relaxation of the stomach after a vagotomy, decreased reservoir size after gastric resection, alteration in gastric emptying (either too rapid or delayed), gastric reflux of bile, and early satiety.

Malabsorption

A large percentage of patients have some degree of malabsorption after gastric surgery. Steatorrhea occurs more commonly in persons who have had extensive operations, such as gastrojejunal anastomoses, and truncal vagotomy. Steatorrhea occurs in these patients because of inadequate mixing of food with bile and pancreatic juice producing lipolysis. Protein malabsorption may also accompany steator-

rhea, but this complication can be managed by increasing the protein and caloric intake. The patient is taught to avoid gluten and lactose. Dietary supplementation of vitamins and minerals is desirable in more severe cases of nutritional deficiency. If pancreatic insufficiency occurs, replacement of deficient pancreatic enzymes may be advisable.

Lactose deficiency

If a patient has a latent lactose deficiency, intolerance to milk and milk-derived dairy products may become more apparent after gastric surgery. Clinical manifestations are abdominal colic, diarrhea, and flatulence. The symptoms occur when lactose from the stomach is delivered to the small bowel too rapidly to be adequately digested by intestinal disaccharides. Treatment consists of a lactose-free diet. Many commercial, nutritionally complete, lactose-free liquid diets are available for food supplements or tube feedings. These formulas can easily be substituted for milk-based liquids and are palatable.

Vitamin and mineral deficiencies

The **intrinsic factor** in humans is produced exclusively by the stomach. Hepatic stores of vitamin B_{12} are usually adequate for 2 years. Pernicious anemia is a serious potential complication in any patient who has had a total gastrectomy or extensive resections. Without replacement therapy, serum B_{12} levels begin to fall 1 to 2 years after surgery, and pernicious anemia with subacute combined degeneration of the spinal cord is a potential risk.[31] It is recommended that all patients with a partial gastrectomy have vitamin B_{12} levels measured every 1 to 2 years so that replacement therapy can be instituted before the anemia appears.

Folic acid deficiency is more rare than vitamin B_{12} deficiency; decreased daily intake is the most common cause. Megaloblastic anemia results from folic acid deficiency and is also associated with pernicious anemia. Megaloblastic anemia indicates severe vitamin B_{12} or folic acid depletion. If 10% or more of the fundal mucosa remains after a gastrectomy, the intrinsic factor needed to prevent megaloblastic anemia will be produced. If atrophy of the remaining parietal cell mass progresses over the years, anemia may occur. Folic acid deficiency is corrected by exogenous replacement when vitamin B_{12} deficiency has been ruled out. (Hematologic disorders are discussed in Chapter 38.)

The most common cause of anemia after gastric surgery is iron deficiency because of impaired absorption. Iron absorption takes place only in the duodenum and proximal jejunum, and rapid gastric emptying may prevent adequate iron uptake. Replacement therapy consists of oral iron in the ferrous form. If patients are not responsive to oral replacement, parenteral administration of iron dextran is available. Iron deficiency anemia occurs in a large majority of premenopausal women and half of all men.

NURSING MANAGEMENT OF THE PATIENT WITH PEPTIC ULCER DISEASE
Assessment

Some patients may be asymptomatic, others experience weight loss, weakness, anorexia, and nausea. Typical symptoms are heartburn, dyspepsia, and pain in the midepigastric area or radiating to the back and arms. Usually pain occurs soon after ingestion of food and is relieved by antacids. Delayed gastric emptying may prompt complaints of fullness and distention.

The nurse must assess whether the patient smokes or drinks alcohol. In older patients it is important to investigate the medications they are taking to determine if the drugs are contributing to ulcer formation and to avoid drug interactions. A recent study of noninstitutionalized elderly patients indicates that each had at least five chronic illnesses and took an average of 11 medications. These medications would have been missed by the casual interviewer because 42% were nonprescription items.[26] Commonly used medications that are most likely to interact with antiulcer drugs are vitamins and minerals, analgesics, laxatives, and antacids.

Duodenal ulceration is clinically manifested by a rhythmic, deep midepigastric pain or burning that is relieved by ingestion of food, milk, or antacids and returns 1 to 3 hours later. Nocturnal pain is common in these patients and an important assessment parameter. Because of self-medication with antacids, these patients may also have a history of constipation or diarrhea, depending on the antacid therapy. It is also important to assess the character and color of stools. Guaiac-positive stools are tarry and soft and may be maroon tinged, if bleeding is moderate.

The nurse will determine the patient's attitude toward compliance with the therapeutic regimen. For example, administration of antacids, smoking cessation, and eating small, frequent meals are necessary modifications, and attitudes toward each need to be assessed to plan interventions that promote compliance.

Although anxiety is not a direct cause of peptic ulcer disease, it may aggravate symptoms. Thus physical, life-style, and situational assessments are necessary for holistic interventions.

Nursing Diagnosis

Nursing diagnoses of patients with peptic ulcer disease include:

Knowledge deficit (medications, diet, signs and symptoms of bleeding or perforation)

Pain related to potential ulceration of gastric or duodenal mucosa

Altered nutrition: less than body requirements related to pain, dyspepsia

Noncompliance with treatment and behavior modification

Anxiety related to the disease process

Constipation or diarrhea related to antacid therapy

Planning

Not all patients with peptic ulcer disease have the same needs. The nurse determines the severity of the symptoms, as well as past adherence to treatment, and identifies significant others who may contribute to and implement the plan of care. Potential compliance can be gauged with the following questions. Can the patient understand the treatment, and are there obstacles that would prevent action? For example, if sucralfate and an antacid regimen are prescribed, will the patient be able to afford the medications? Does the patient's life-style allow for the frequent dosages these agents require? In addition, the patient's level of anxiety is determined.

The four main outcomes to determine the effectiveness of nursing implementations are:

Ulcer healing as revealed by endoscopic examination

Relief of pain and other symptoms

Prevention of complications by adherence to the care plan

Prevention of recurrence

Implementation
Medications

Written information about antacid therapy is provided. To be maximally effective, these agents are taken in large doses (30 mL), seven times daily (1 and 3 hours after a meal and at bedtime). Potential problems with these agents include magnesium overload in the patient with renal failure, constipation or diarrhea, and noncompliance because of frequent dosing and disagreeable taste.

The nurse explains that sucralfate must be taken 1 hour before each meal and at bedtime. If taken immediately before eating, it is less effective because the food in the stomach interferes with binding of the molecule to the ulcer surface. The patient is advised that if the medication is not taken an hour before eating, it is best to delay the meal. Antacids should not be taken for 30 minutes before or after sucralfate because they inactivate the medication. The patient is also to be advised that certain medications, such as digoxin, warfarin, cimetidine, or ranitidine, may have decreased absorption when given simultaneously with sucralfate.[5]

The nurse instructs the patient about ranitidine and cimetidine. Both of these drugs are safe, and fewer than 5% of patients have side effects. The most common side effects are dizziness, somnolence, and mild lower GI upsets. Central nervous system disturbances such as headache and confusion occur in elderly or acutely ill patients with hepatic or renal dysfunction.

Numerous studies conducted to study the effectiveness of various antiulcer drugs have found that cigarette smoking retards ulcer healing even during the course of medication therapy. The patient is advised that smoking must be limited or eliminated in order for medications to be effective and for the ulcer to heal.

Diet

The patient is advised that most persons with gastric ulcers have basal and peak acid levels below those of normal subjects. Persons with duodenal ulcers generally exhibit normal or elevated basal and peak acid output. Since all foods both stimulate and buffer gastric acid, the current consensus is that small frequent meals during the day and no foods at bedtime are tolerated best for all patients with peptic ulcer. The patient should avoid specific foods that seem to worsen symptoms.

Bleeding/perforation

The nurse discusses medications associated with GI bleeding such as aspirin, nonsteroidal antiinflammatory agents, corticosteroids in high dosage, reserpine, and anticoagulants. The patient is asked to observe stools for melena (tarry stools), hematochezia (bright-red blood passed rectally), and emesis that has the appearance of coffee grounds or bright-red blood. The patient is also instructed to report such symptoms as fatigue and pallor.

Any patient with a history of peptic ulcer disease is instructed to report severe abdominal pain immediately. The symptoms of a perforated peptic ulcer are midepigastric or upper right quadrant pain of sudden and severe onset that may radiate to the right shoulder or scapula. The pain becomes generalized with a characteristic rigid, board-like abdomen as diffuse peritonitis develops. The patient may also have tachycardia, shallow respirations, abdominal guarding, and an elevated temperature.

Anxiety

Although emotional stress has not been documented to cause peptic ulcers, the patient may be anxious about potential recurrence and life-style changes. Sedatives are used to decrease anxiety, restlessness, and insomnia. In addition, careful explanations and reassurances need to be offered and feedback provided to determine the effectiveness of such interventions. If the patient continues to express anxiety, other treatment methods such as psychotherapy may be employed.

Evaluation

Although severe diet modification is not necessary except in the presence of dumping syndrome, the patient should know that a nutritious, well-balanced diet is important, not only for overall general health, but for wound and ulcer healing as well. The patient should know the medication routine and when to follow up with visits to the physician.

The nurse must not equate ulcer healing with cure. Most patients need ongoing evaluation, since management of peptic ulcer disease is a long-term process.

Documentation

Documentation of the care of the patient with peptic ulcer disease involves ongoing assessment and recording of drug interactions and side effects. This is especially important with elderly patients, who take many over-the-counter and prescription medications. It is also important to assess and chart compliance with the many forms of behavioral modification therapy, that is, diet, physical activity, and medication regimen. Any complications from the medical treatment or the development of symptoms are noted. If surgical treatment is necessary, a detailed report of preoperative and postoperative care is essential. The record should also reflect that patient teaching took place and the patient's response to information provided.

Ongoing Care

Because duodenal ulcers commonly recur, they are considered a chronic condition. Many patients require treatment repeatedly over a number of years. In some cases, after 10 or more years, the condition may "burn itself out." The two medical approaches include full-dose treatment with any of the successful antiulcer agents with each recurrence for 4 to 6 weeks or maintenance treatment with low-dose histamine H_2 blockers at bedtime. Maintenance treatment carries the long-term risk of side effects and drug interactions. In addition, once the drug is discontinued, the risk of recurrence increases. If recurrence is frequent, the patient may need surgical intervention.

As in duodenal ulcers, the recurrence rate of gastric ulcers is also high, and management depends on how many episodes occur. Maintenance therapy for gastric ulcers is less effective than for duodenal ulcers because the protective effects tend to wear off after about a year, even while the drug is being used.[3] Thus maintenance therapy is reserved for those patients who cannot tolerate surgery.

NURSING MANAGEMENT OF THE PATIENT WITH GASTROINTESTINAL BLEEDING

Assessment

Patients with active GI bleeding usually consult a physician when they vomit blood (hematemesis) (Figure 65-7). Sometimes the blood looks like coffee grounds because of the action of gastric acid on hemoglobin. Massive GI tract hemorrhage may result in the passage of bright-red blood through the rectum (hematochezia). Slower rates of bleeding cause the stool to turn black (melena). The nurse should be aware of hospitalized patients at risk for development of stress ulcers and possible hemorrhage. A careful physical examination and monitoring of vital signs may provide important data in the evaluation and management of active GI tract bleeding. "Postural" signs, caused by hemodynamic changes that occur after acute blood loss, are elicited by having the patient sit up from a supine position and evaluating changes in blood pressure and pulse.

Blood loss and peripheral vasoconstriction result in cool extremities and pallor of the conjunctivae, mucous membranes, nail beds, and palmar creases. During passage of stools on rectal examination, the character and color of the stool can be confirmed.

ASSESSMENT PARAMETERS ASSOCIATED WITH SIGNIFICANT BLOOD LOSS

- Systolic blood pressure <100 mm Hg
- Pulse rate >100 beats/min
- A 10 mm Hg orthostatic blood pressure drop
- Pale conjunctivae (hemoglobin level <10 g/dL)
- Pale palmar creases (hemoglobin level <6 g/dL)
- Red-maroon stool on digital rectal examination
- Bloody aspirate from NG tube

The box above lists assessment parameters that correlate with significant blood loss.

Nursing Diagnosis

Nursing diagnoses for patients with GI bleeding include:

High risk for injury: hypovolemia related to hemorrhage and dehydration from excessive fluid loss and inadequate fluid replacement

Altered electrolyte balance: hypernatremia, hypokalemia related to the body's attempt to compensate for lost fluid and massive gastric emptying or hematochezia

Altered tissue perfusion related to vasoconstriction associated with blood loss

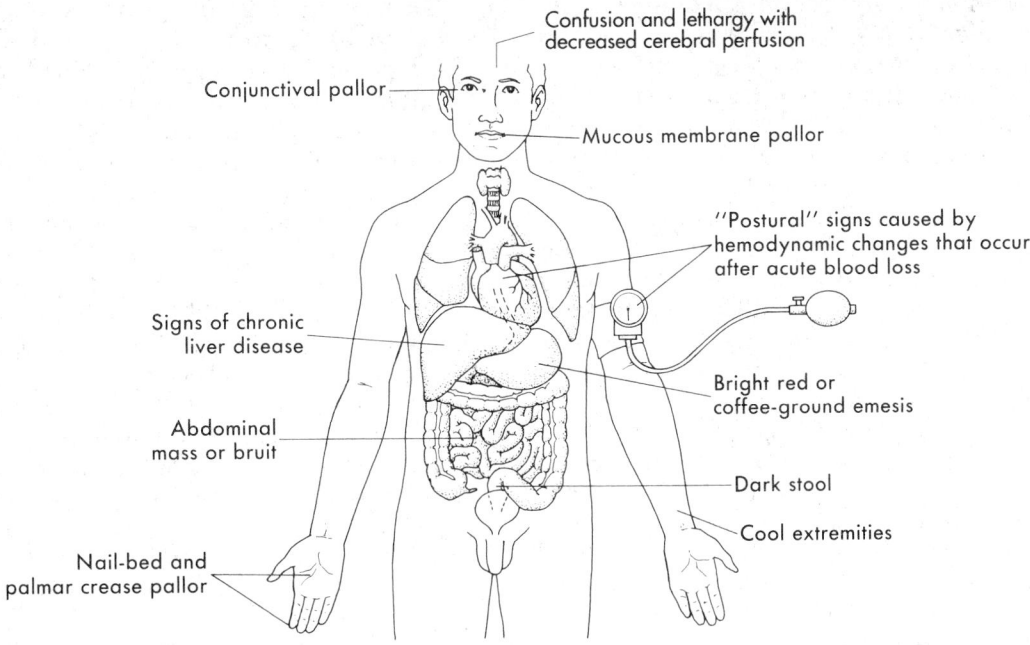

FIGURE 65-7   Clinical manifestations of upper GI tract bleeding.

Fluid volume deficit related to gastric lavage and hemorrhage

High risk for injury: altered clotting factors related to the body's attempt to restore hemostasis through clotting

Altered thought processes: confusion related to cerebral hypoxia associated with anemia, decreased oxygen capacity of citrated blood, and elevated ammonia levels

Anxiety related to hematemesis, abdominal pain, and uncertain outcome

Planning

The plan for the patient with GI bleeding is early detection and treatment of bleeding from the ulcer site, prevention of further bleeding and subsequent loss of circulating blood volume, and restoration of fluid volume. In addition, early recognition of electrolyte imbalances, as well as impaired cognitive function, prevent further injury.

The following outcomes provide a focus for nursing interventions:

1. Patient will be well-hydrated with serum electrolytes within normal range
2. There will be no further evidence of gastrointestinal bleeding
3. Hemoglobin and hematocrit will be within normal limits
4. The patient will demonstrate adequate cognitive function
5. Vital signs will be within baseline range

Implementation

Vital signs are monitored every 5 to 15 minutes. Systolic pressure must be kept above 90 mm Hg or no less than 20 to 30 mm Hg below baseline if the patient is hypertensive. If hypotension does occur, intravenous dopamine or another vasoconstrictor may be required to maintain tissue perfusion. The nurse obtains stool for guaiac testing and checks the color for prognostic value (red-maroon suggests more rapid bleeding than black or brown). At least one large-bore intravenous (IV) catheter (18 gauge) should be inserted for fluid and blood replacement. If the IV line is to be placed in an arm vein, the best choice is the right side because gastric lavage and possible endoscopy will be performed with the patient in the left lateral decubitus position. Blood can be drawn for the laboratory tests at the time of catheter insertion. Place the patient in the left lateral decubitus position with the head of the bed elevated 15 degrees. This helps support the patient's blood pressure and prevents aspiration of vomited gastric contents. The initial intravenous fluid will be a saline solution to restore blood pressure as soon as possible and preserve urine output until blood products are available. Oxygen is administered by mask or nasal cannula if cardiac output or perfusion is compromised.

Fluid intake and output should be carefully monitored throughout the acute phase of bleeding. A Foley catheter will probably be inserted and attached to gravity drainage with hourly urine output and specific gravity monitored. A drop in urine output to less than 30 mL/hr may represent acute renal failure. A specific gravity above 1.030 indicates dehydration. Peripheral edema, distended neck veins, moist rales, and elevated central venous pressure indicate fluid volume overload and impending pulmonary edema. Blood drawn during IV insertion is sent for type and crossmatch for whole blood. A flowsheet is set up to chart laboratory data, vital signs, nasogastric aspirate, blood transfused, and urine output.

A large-bore nasogastric (NG) tube (16 or 18 gauge) should be passed. The tube should be marked at 40, 50, and 60 cm from the tip to indicate when it has passed the lower esophageal sphincter (39 to 43 cm) and is correctly placed in the stomach. Low constant suction will be applied to clear the stomach of blood and to assess the rate of bleeding. If no fluid returns, the tube is left in place until bile-stained fluid is obtained, which is the only way to determine if the patient is not actively bleeding from the upper GI tract.

If the patient is bleeding and lavage is ordered, the NG tube will replaced with either a large-bore sump drain, an Ewald tube, or an Edlich 11 mm gastric-lavage tube. Again, the tube is measured and proper placement in the stomach confirmed.

The purpose of gastric lavage is to clear the stomach of blood and to assess the rate of bleeding. Once blood, clots, and intragastric materials are removed, the stomach walls can constrict, which may contribute to hemostasis. A great deal of controversy exists over the type and temperature of the solution to be used. Iced water decreases mucosal blood flow and temporarily stops bleeding long enough to permit visualization by endoscopy. On the other hand, iced solutions may cause the patient's core temperature to drop, may have an adverse effect on platelet function, and may prolong bleeding. At this time, tap water is recommended. It is less expensive and breaks up clots better than saline. Lavage should be done for no longer than 30 minutes because persistent blood return indicates continued bleeding. In addition, fluid overload is possible when lavage is continued for long periods. The water should not be suctioned out of the stomach but should drain by gravity. Forceful suction may cause mucosal damage and further bleeding.

The patient is monitored for mental changes, lethargy, confusion, drowsiness, and irritability as these signs are characteristic of decreased cerebral perfusion. If any of these signs are present, sedatives and tranquilizers should be avoided or used with caution.

The patient needs much emotional support and reassurance during this acute period. Most people are anxious at the sight of significant blood loss, and the apprehension can aggravate the severity of the pain that usually accompanies this bleeding ulcer.

Antacids may be added to the therapeutic regimen to neutralize gastric acid and control bleeding. Antacids are instilled through the NG tube in an attempt to titrate the intragastric pH above 3.5 (to inactivate pepsin) or preferably close to 7. The head of the bed should be elevated 45 degrees to prevent aspiration of antacids. The antacid regimen is as follows:

1. A dosage of 60 to 180 mL is administered through the NG tube.
2. Clamp the NG tube for 15 minutes.
3. Suction the aspirate and measure the pH.
4. Repeat this procedure every 15 minutes until the pH is 7.
5. When the pH reaches 7, reduce to an hourly interval and titrate the dosage to maintain the pH.

Histamine blockers are usually given parenterally, and elderly patients should be carefully monitored for renal insufficiency. If the patient cannot be stabilized or the bleeding is too rapid for visualization by endoscopy, emergency surgery is recommended.

Evaluation/Documentation

The nurse pays particular attention to recording vital signs in both the sitting and supine position and notes any changes. The color, amount, and frequency of emesis and stools are also important to record. Frequent assessment of the patient's color and body temperature are stated. Because large amounts of fluids are received with various interventions, an accurate recording of intake and output, as well as specific gravity, is critical to determine fluid volume excess. The patient's cognitive status must be documented during both the acute and recovery stages, including the patient's ability to participate in activities of daily living.

NURSING MANAGEMENT OF THE PATIENT WHO HAS UNDERGONE GASTRIC SURGERY

Indications for gastric surgery are uncontrolled or life-threatening bleeding, perforation, obstruction, and intractability.

Assessment

Bleeding is the most hazardous complication of peptic ulcer disease; assessment parameters have been discussed in the preceding paragraphs. Perforation of a peptic ulcer, either gastric or duodenal, is characterized by tachycardia in a normotensive or hypotensive patient. Sudden and severe abdominal pain is initially localized in the midepigastric area of the upper right quadrant. Respirations are shallow because of splinting and abdominal pain. The temperature is normal at first but rises several hours after perforation. Vomiting may be present but not in all cases. On palpation the abdomen is boardlike and rebound tenderness is noted. Bowel sounds are generally diminished or absent. Stool may be negative in the guaiac test because of rapid bleeding.

Nursing Diagnosis

Nursing diagnoses for the patient after gastric surgery include:

High risk for infection related to potential anastomotic leak, potential intestinal obstruction, impaired healing

Constipation related to decreased neuromuscular activity associated with gut manipulation and potential electrolyte imbalance

Fluid volume deficit related to NG decompression, NG irrigation, surgical drains, fistula formation

Pain related to surgical incision, abdominal distention, NG intubation, sore throat, mouth breathing, immobility

Altered nutrition: less than body requirements related to dumping syndrome

Anxiety related to increased nursing procedures

Planning

The patient's primary needs after gastric surgery involve prevention of infection, management of discomfort, gastric decompression, nutrition, and alleviating anxiety. The routine preoperative teaching plan is evaluated and measures taken to either reinforce or repeat information necessary for successful recovery (e.g., pulmonary toilet, use of the NG tube, and gradual return of peristalsis and early ambulation).

Outcome criteria for the patient who has had gastric surgery are as follows:

No evidence of infection or impaired healing process

The abdomen is soft and peristaltic movement can be auscultated

Electrolyte values are within the normal range

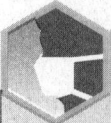

PREOPERATIVE AND POSTOPERATIVE NURSING INTERVENTIONS

Gastric Surgery

Preoperative

Interventions

1. Explain routine tests, procedures, and medications during immediate preoperative period (see Chapter 22).

2. Explain, demonstrate, and have patient practice splinting the wound with coughing and deep-breathing exercises.

3. Explain the presence of postoperative drainage tubes.

4. Complete the preoperative assessment.

Rationale

1. Decrease patient's fear of unknown. Give the patient a sense of control by informing him or her of routines and reasons for procedures, allowing choices and personal preference with some.

2. To gain cooperation with these maneuvers, preoperative practice is easier than postoperative, when the patient is in pain. High abdominal incision limits lung expansion because of postoperative pain.

3. Prepare the patient and family for a nasogastric tube, which reduces pressure on the anastomosis and decreases the incidence of nausea and vomiting. Postoperative incision drains may be present to decrease strain on abdominal suture line from accumulating drainage. Foreknowledge reduces the shock and anxiety of seeing a loved one with numerous tubes postoperatively.

4. Gives a baseline for monitoring psychologic and physical changes postoperatively.

Postoperative

Interventions

1. Encourage coughing and deep breathing with splinting of incision every 2 hours. Instruct patient in use of incentive spirometer as ordered. Auscultate lungs to determine effectiveness.

2. Give pain medication frequently (every 3 to 4 hours as patient requests) or before patient has to cough and deep breathe.

3. Encourage early ambulation (with physician's orders) after first 24 hours.

4. Careful monitoring of serum electrolytes and intake/output from N/G tube, incisional drains, catheter, and IV infusion. Report significant results to physician.

5. Maintain correct infusion rate for IV fluids.

6. Use swabs for mouth care (every 2 hours) with saline/H_2O_2 mixture. Brush teeth at least twice a day. Use water-soluble lubricant, Blistex, or Chapstick on lips. Inspect mucous membranes daily.

7. Assess for peristalsis and auscultate in all four quadrants of abdomen with NG suction off.

Rationale

1. Prevent atelectasis and pneumonia from retained secretions.

2. Narcotic analgesics are often required postoperatively because of the intensity of the pain.

3. Helps eliminate gas and fluid accumulation related to decreased peristalsis from manipulation of the small intestine during surgery.

4. Loss of fluid and electrolytes, particularly K+, from gastrointestinal drainage.

5. With NPO status, this is the only source for fluid and electrolyte replacement.

6. NG tube causes nasal stuffiness and patient will breathe through mouth. Saliva is decreased with no stimulus from food or fluid, resulting in cracking and/or herpes-type lesions in oral cavity and dry scaling of lips.

7. The return of bowel sounds indicates peristalsis is functional and the patient may be allowed to progress to fluids after NG tube is removed (NG tube usually in place for 3 to 4 days postoperatively). NG tube connected to suction "echoes" in upper quadrants and may mimic bowel sounds.

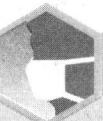

PREOPERATIVE AND POSTOPERATIVE NURSING INTERVENTIONS—cont'd

Interventions	*Rationale*
8. Flush NG tube gently every 4 hours with 30 to 50 mL normal saline. Assess quantity and character of NG aspirate; report bright-red bleeding to physician. Do not reposition NG tube.	8. Normal saline used so electrolytes are not "flushed out" in a hypotonic solution. Irrigation (i.e., withdrawal of flushing solution) may be contraindicated because of proximity of gastric suture line. Must maintain patency of nasogastric tube to prevent gas and fluid accumulation, which will disrupt anastamosis; drainage should be dark-red or coffee-ground in appearance.
9. When po intake is resumed, progress diet *slowly* from liquids to solids and assess patient's tolerance by: • auscultating bowel sounds • checking for abdominal distention • checking for nausea or vomiting	9. Small amounts of fluid are better tolerated initially. Stomach capacity is reduced as a result of surgery, so small meals 4 to 5 times/day are more easily tolerated. Paralytic ileus may be present; be aware of signs of increasing distention, nausea, and diminished bowel sounds.
10. Administer oxygen as ordered and assess patient's tolerance to the therapy: • increased activity tolerance • skin/mucous membranes appear well oxygenated • vital signs within preoperative baseline limits	10. Oxygen is frequently ordered by the physician to counteract effects of blood loss and resulting tissue hypoxia, which retards wound healing.
11. Keep head of bed elevated at least 30 degrees	11. Promotes aeration of lungs and decreases muscle strain on suture line.

No excess or deficit in fluid volume

Patient states that measures to relieve pain and discomfort have been successful

Nutritional status is stable as evidenced by no further weight loss

Decreased anxiety as evidenced by sleeping well and relating to significant persons

Implementation

If peritonitis develops and the patient exhibits abdominal distention, absent bowel sounds, rapid shallow breathing, and generalized abdominal pain, vital signs should be monitored for shock and hyperthermia. Antibiotics will be administered parenterally or through the NG tube. If an anastomotic leak is discovered, the patient will be taken back for further surgery and will need reassurance and emotional support. Strict aseptic technique should be used during dressing changes. The wound should be observed for redness, swelling, heat, localized tenderness, and pain.

The small intestine loses its peristaltic action for a few hours after surgery, and the large intestine takes several days to regain its function. The nurse needs to monitor the return of normal bowel function. Bowel sounds should be heard in all four quadrants, and the patient should be passing flatus. Measuring abdominal girth determines the extent of peristaltic activity. Until peristalsis returns, the patient's abdomen will be abnormally large, which is the result of intestinal distention caused by gas and fluid buildup. The measurements should be taken once per shift and the patient's abdomen marked where the measurements are taken to assure consistency. As normal bowel motility resumes, abdominal girth diminishes. After 3 to 4 days, the patient's intestines should resume normal function.

If abdominal distention persists and is accompanied by decreased or absent bowel sounds, nausea, vomiting, or elevated temperature, the patient may be experiencing a mechanical obstruction, abscess, hemorrhage, or metabolic disturbance such as potassium deficiency. Fluid and electrolyte imbalances are always a potential complication after gastric surgery. Patients lose fluids from NG decompression, surgical drains, or fistula formation. If an ileus persists, plasma may seep into the intestinal lumen and peritoneal cavity, causing fluid and electrolyte imbalances. Restriction of oral intake for several days causes fluid depletion, and the stress of surgery can lead to sodium and water retention, potassium loss, and a negative nitrogen balance. Monitoring urine intake and output is discussed in nursing implemen-

 NURSING CARE PLAN   *Patient Undergoing Gastric Surgery: Postoperative Care*

Nursing diagnosis/ *Expected outcome*	Interventions	Rationale
• *Patient will experience decreased pain as evidenced by statements of pain relief, relaxed facial expression, and increased participation in self-care*	signs of pain Administer pain medication as ordered Monitor for therapeutic and non-therapeutic effects of pain medication Instruct patient to splint the area and provide support during movement	have had major abdominal surgery is because of stretching of tissue and muscles during procedure and manipulation of abdominal viscera; local incisional pain is usually experienced when stress is placed on area; pain medications should be given as often as needed to provide comfort and effects monitored; splinting the area or providing support may also alleviate pain

Altered fluid and electrolyte balance related to nastogastric (NG) tube, gastric suction, drains, parenteral infusions, and restriction of oral intake
 	
• *Patient will have normal fluid balance as evidenced by:*
Stable weight
Blood pressure and pulse rate within normal limits and stable with position changes
No edema or distended neck veins
Normal serum osmolality
Balanced intake and output within 48 hr
Specific gravity within normal limits
Normal respirations
	Monitor the following:
	  Signs and symptoms of fluid excess or deficit
	  Weight gain or loss
	  Intake and output from NG tube, drains, catheter, intravenous infusion
	  Serum osmolality
	  Electrolyte levels
	  Rales or crackles
	  Record accurate intake and output
		Fluid balance is unstable because of gastric suction, intravenous fluids, and wound drainage; various parameters must be assessed to maintain fluid balance; water balance is also reflected by osmolality in correct range; loss of electrolytes is associated with NG tube and wound drainage

High risk for injury: infection, paralytic ileus • *Patient will be free from infection as evidenced by:* *No elevated temperature* *No redness or drainage at incision site* *Wound healing* • *Patient will have normal bowel sounds within 48 degrees* • *Patient will have no abdominal distention*	Monitor vital signs, especially temperature Frequently inspect incision Use sterile technique when changing dressings Keep skin clean and dry Record signs and symptoms of infection Measure abdominal girth from left to right anterior iliac crest Auscultate abdomen for presence of bowel sounds	Cross-infection between patients and patients and staff and autoinfection are primary sources of infection; aseptic technique and frequent handwashing reduce numbers of microorganisms; prevention is more effective than treatment with antimicrobial agents; paralytic ileus can occur after abdominal surgery; early detection may prevent further complications such as vomiting or strain on abdominal incision
Altered oral mucous membranes: dryness related to NG tube, mouth breathing, potential fluid volume deficit • *Patient will experience no sore throat, mouth lesions, or dysphagia* • *Patient will demonstrate no symptoms of bleeding, cracked lips, or foul breath*	Brush patient's teeth and rinse mouth with normal saline and hydrogen peroxide; if patient does not have gag reflex, use swabs to cleanse oral cavity Use water-soluble lubricant to moisten lips Inspect nares and apply water-soluble lubricant if dry or lesions noted	NG tube produces nasal irritation and potential for mucosal breakdown; because most patients with NG tube mouth breathe and have decreased stimulation of saliva, lips become cracked and oral mucosa dry; increased fluid losses because of NG suction and restriction of oral intake can result in dehydration, further contributing to oral mucosa problems

NURSING CARE PLAN *Patient Undergoing Gastric Surgery: Postoperative Care—cont'd*

Nursing diagnosis/ Expected outcome	Interventions	Rationale
Noncompliance related to difficulty modifying smoking and dietary regimen • *Patient demonstrates probability of future compliance as evidenced by statements of intentions to perform desired behavior*	Provide knowledge about eating small frequent meals and contribution of smoking to recurrence of peptic ulcers Assess patient's beliefs about smoking cessation and dietary modifications Plan interventions that strengthen positive beliefs and counter negative beliefs	All foods both neutralize and cause acid production; small frequent meals have been found to produce less acid Knowledge is necessary component for behavioral change, but knowledge alone does not produce compliance; patient's beliefs about each behavior must be assessed and interventions designed to either support or counter beliefs

tations for GI bleeding. Other interventions include meticulous recording of drainage from the NG tube, drains, and fistulas, as well as the amount of fluids used to irrigate tubes. Notify the physician of any abnormalities in electrolyte balance, administer supplemental electrolytes as ordered, and monitor the patient's response to replacement therapy.

The NG tube must be patent and the suction working properly. Without a physician's order, the NG tube should not be irrigated or repositioned by the nurse. To maintain patency, the NG tube is irrigated with 30 mL of sterile normal saline every 2 hours. Drainage from the tube is usually bloody after surgery and clots are most likely to block the suction mechanism, preventing decompression of gas and removal of fluid. If the NG tube becomes blocked, gas and fluid will accumulate, causing the abdomen to become distended. This will create tension on the surgical incision and dehiscence may occur. Should this happen, cover the incision with a sterile dressing moistened with normal saline until the physician arrives or the patient is taken to surgery. If after the immediate postoperative period (about 12 hours), the drainage becomes bright red, a hemorrhage should be suspected. Notify the physician immediately.

Measures for reducing anxiety may include thorough explanations and preparations for the patient and family. An explanation and description of the sensations experienced during and after the procedures or interventions lead to more accurate expectations. The sensory information includes explaining what the patient might feel, see, hear, smell, or taste. In addition, the nurse should allow the patient and family time for questions and realize that frequent repetitions may be necessary because increased anxiety interferes with information processing.

The dumping syndrome is a late postoperative complication which can develop 1 to 3 weeks after surgery and the patient and family should be given written instructions about dietary modification to control this problem. The dumping syndrome is discussed on p. 1829.

Documentation

It is important to record color, consistency, and amount of drainage from the NG tube, as well as other surgical drains. The incision is inspected frequently and signs and symptoms of infection recorded immediately. Documentation also reflects notification of the physician should any complication occur. It is also necessary to record the patient's response to pain medications. Any patient education is reflected in the chart, as well as patient or family concerns about treatment methods.

STRESS ULCERS
Definition/Etiology/Epidemiology

Stress ulcers are superficial gastroduodenal erosions resulting from physiologic stress–related mucosal damage in critically ill patients. Acute stress ulcers of the stomach are a different entity from chronic peptic ulcer disease. The stress lesions are more likely to occur in the mucosa of the fundus as opposed to the usual peptic ulcers in the duodenum and the gastric antrum. Clinical studies indicate that with severe stress, such as head injury or burns, the incidence of stress ulceration may approach 100%. The term "stress ulcers" is nonspecific and has included Curling's acute duodenal ulcer in the setting of burn injury and Cushing's gastroduodenal ulcers with head injury and a few superficial erosions confined to the mucosa.

Pathophysiology

The development of stress ulcers is believed to be the result of several factors including the hyposecretion of acid and a disruption of the gastric mucosal defense barrier. With severe physiologic stress, blood flow may be diverted away from the gut with resultant mucosal ischemia, which leads to the breakdown of the mucosal defense barrier and the cytoprotective effect. These factors are often associated with central nervous system injury. Other factors implicated are back diffusion of hydrogen ions and reflux of bile into the stomach.

Clinical Manifestations/Therapeutic Management

In the hospital setting the earliest sign of stress ulcers may be blood from the NG tube. Stress ulcers usually appear within 2 weeks of the precipitating stress. Hematemesis and melena are common manifestations and up to 10% of patients with stress ulcers have massive hemorrhage. Perforation may occur in as many as 15% of the patients.

Pain is not a predominant symptom of stress ulcers and when it does occur it more often signals perforation than bleeding. Medical treatment involves prophylactic therapy with cimetidine or ranitidine and antacids for prevention. When medical treatment is unsuccessful, the patient most likely will have to undergo surgical intervention.

NURSING MANAGEMENT OF THE PATIENT WITH STRESS ULCERS

The nurse should be aware of the potential for stress ulcers in patients who are at high risk, for example, those who have sustained central nervous system injury, burns, renal failure, major operative procedures, and trauma. Ongoing assessment of pallor, vital signs, aspirate, and stools is made. Gastric pH levels are also determined. Nursing management for patients with stress ulcers is similar to care of peptic ulcer disease and GI bleeding discussed earlier in this chapter.

GASTRIC CANCER
Etiology

The cause of gastric cancer remains unknown; however, numerous factors appear to be associated with the disease. It is also believed that exogenous factors in the environment, such as carcinogenic chemicals and oncogenic viruses may play an important part in gastric carcinoma.

Since the stomach has prolonged contact with food, dietary substances have been implicated. There appears to be a relationship with increased salt consumption. Ingestion of nitrates and nitrites in high-protein diets have given rise to the theory that carcinogenic compounds such as nitrosoamines and nitrosomides (nitroso compounds) can be formed by digestive action.

The marked reduction of gastric cancer in the United States over the past decades is believed to be the result of improved refrigeration that made available a wide assortment of fresh foods, including milk, vegetables, fruits, juices, beef, and fish, with a decrease in the consumption of preserved, salted, smoked, and spicy foods. Thus it is believed that both refrigeration and vitamin C (in fresh fruits and vegetables) can inhibit nitrosocarcinogens.

Genetic factors may play a role in the development of gastric cancer. Greater frequency exists in individuals of blood type A. Family history increases an individual's risk but only minimally. Only 4% of persons with gastric carcinoma have a family history of the disease.

Epidemiology

Approximately 23,800 new cases of gastric cancer are diagnosed annually in North America. [2] In 1991 the number of deaths in the United States from gastric cancer was estimated to be 13,400, less than half the number 35 years ago. [32] The highest incidence of gastric cancer (70/100,000 males) occurs in Japan, where the disease accounts for about 50% of all visceral cancers. Other countries with high morbidity and mortality (greater than 30/100,000 males) are Austria, Chile, Costa Rica, Ecuador, Federal Republic of Germany, Finland, Hungary, Iceland, Indonesia, and Italy. The cause of the high frequency in Japan and other countries is unknown.

Pathophysiology

Several factors are believed to be possible cancer precursors: polyps, pernicious anemia, postgastrectomy, chronic atrophic gastritis, and gastric ulcer. It is believed that gastric ulcer does not predispose individuals to gastric cancer but that gastric cancer may exist simultaneously with a gastric ulcer and not be discovered on the first diagnostic studies. [7]

Gastric cancer is an adenocarcinoma most often appearing as an irregular mass with deep central ulceration protruding into the lumen and invading the wall of the stomach. The tumor may infiltrate and cause a narrowing of the lumen, most often in the antrum. The infiltration can also extend throughout the entire stomach, resulting in a fixed nondistensible pouch with absence of normal folds and a narrowed lumen, but this is not very common. Polypoid lesions may also occur and be difficult to distinguish from benign polyps on x-ray examination. Cancer of the stomach may occur as a superficially spreading tumor involving only the mucosal surface and producing a granular appearance, although this is more rare. Approximately 75% of carcinomas are found in the distal third of the stomach. In addition to lymph node invasion, gastric carcinoma invades local structures, such as the lower end of the esophagus, pancreas, transverse colon, and peritoneum. Metastases occur in the lungs, pleura, liver, brain, and bone.

Clinical Manifestations

Unfortunately gastric cancer has no early symptoms, and physical examination will detect no findings. When the cancer is advanced, the patient has anorexia, abdominal pain, and weight loss. Clinical symptoms also differ, depending on the location of the lesion. If the tumor causes obstruction, the patient's symptoms resemble those of achalasia. When the tumor has ulcerated, some patients complain of pain similar to that of peptic ulcer, although the pain usually occurs after eating and is not relieved by food or antacids. Patients may also complain of symptoms arising from secondary metastases, ascites (liver), shortness of breath (lung), foul-smelling emesis (gastrocolic fistula), and back pain (pancreatic involvement).

With early gastric cancer, laboratory studies may be normal. More advanced disease may be accompanied by iron deficiency or anemia. Approximately 50% of patients show occult blood in the stool. Most have reduced amounts of gastric acid. Other diagnostic tests may reveal metastatic disease from the original tumor.

When the patient has signs and symptoms of gastric cancer, a thorough and systematic evaluation of the stomach by an endoscopist trained to detect subtle changes of texture and color is indicated. Multiple biopsies and cytologic studies are done if x-ray and endoscopic examinations reveal a suggestive lesion. Some of the other tests done in conjunction with endoscopy, biopsy, and cytology are gastric secretory studies to determine the presence of fasting achlorhydria, carcinoembryonic antigen (CEA) (serum CEA levels are frequently elevated in gastric cancer), and fetal sulfoglycoprotein antigen (FSA). FSA has been detected in the gastric juice of patients with gastric cancer.[37]

Therapeutic Management

Surgery is effective for patients with early gastric cancer. Surgery for advanced gastric cancer carries high morbidity and mortality. Approximately 80% of patients with gastric cancer undergo surgery for exploratory purposes, that is, to make certain the lesion is not resectable. Many surgeons believe that even in the presence of metastasis, patients are more comfortable and live longer with radical resections. However, no randomized control studies have been done to determine the effectiveness of such procedures. Thus there are many conflicting treatments for cancer of the stomach. If there is no evidence of distant metastasis, surgical resection for cure will be suggested. The choice of procedure depends on the tumor location and size. A complete gastrectomy, with anastomosis of the esophagus to the jejunum (esophagojejunostomy), is the choice for an extensive lesion (Figure 65-8). If there is evidence of local extension but no distant metastasis an exploratory laparotomy will be performed to evaluate the extent of the disease and attempt resection.

Gastric cancer is responsive to chemotherapy. There has been greater response rate and prolongation of survival time with combination chemotherapy than with individual agents alone. Radiation alone has been found to be ineffective because of the radioresistance of the tumor and the risk of proximal organ exposure. Radiation plus chemotherapy has been found to be more effective.

Patients with gastric cancer who receive no treatment have a mean survival time of approximately 11 months after the diagnosis.[37] In those who have undergone diagnostic exploratory laparotomy alone, the mean survival time is reported to be 4 to 5 months. Although this is less than the untreated group, it must be understood that these patients have added to the morbidity of surgery with extensive disease and confirmed unresectability.[36,37,39] Patients who had a palliative surgical procedure such as a simple bypass to relieve symptoms also have a mean survival time of 4 to 5 months.

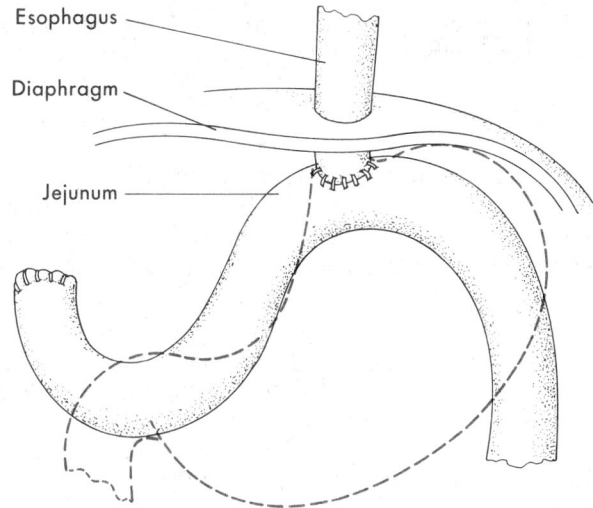

FIGURE 65-8   Total gastrectomy with esophagojejunostomy (anastomosis of the esophagus to the jejunum). Dotted lines indicate portions of the stomach and duodenum removed.

NURSING MANAGEMENT OF THE PATIENT AFTER SURGERY FOR GASTRIC CANCER

Assessment

Conditions that would indicate possible complications include a systolic blood pressure less than 90, elevated temperature (37.2° C or 99° F), hemorrhage through the incision, blood from chest tube drainage, pallor, dyspnea, cyanosis, tachycardia, increased respiratory rate, and chest pain. The nurse continuously assesses the patient to determine if any of these signs and symptoms have developed. In addition, it is important to frequently assess the patient's respiratory status and whether measures to alleviate pain are successful.

Nursing Diagnosis

Nursing diagnoses of the patient after surgery for gastric cancer include:

Ineffective breathing pattern related to pain, exploration of the chest cavity, abdominal distention

High risk for injury:

Pulmonary aspiration related to complete removal of the stomach

Infection, hemorrhage, anastomotic leak related to complete removal of stomach and anastomoses

Anemia, vitamin deficiency related to removal of stomach and loss of intrinsic factor

Altered nutrition: less than body requirements related to complete loss of stomach and jejunostomy feedings

Knowledge deficit (surgery, chemotherapy, and radiation therapy)

Ineffective individual coping related to depression, pain, extensive surgery, poor prognosis

Planning

The patient's nutritional status must be improved before surgery if at all possible using hyperalimentation or supplemental diet feedings. The major postoperative goals are to maintain nutrition, help the lungs expand, and prevent infection and pulmonary aspiration. The patient and family should be given an explanation of the disease and the surgical intervention. The nurse will also reinforce and clarify the physician's information. Opportunity should be provided for the patient and family to discuss their feelings and concerns about the diagnosis, various treatments, and the outcome.

Implementation

Nursing care for the patient with a total gastrectomy and esophagojejunostomy is different from other gastric surgeries because the chest cavity must be entered to anastomose the esophagus to the jejunum. The patient should be placed in a semi-Fowler position (30 to 45 degrees), which increases lung expansion and ventilation with minimal effort. It also facilitates chest tube drainage. The patient should be handled gently when turning and positioning because of the extensive surgery and the use of rib spreading retractors when the chest wall was entered.

Because the stomach has been completely removed, the patient will need replacement vitamin B_{12} for life. Other vitamin deficiencies and anemias may occur, thus it may be necessary to administer ascorbic acid, thiamine, riboflavin, nicotinic acid, vitamin K, and exogenous iron. The nurse observes the patient for signs and symptoms of anemia such as circumoral pallor and pallor of the nailbeds or conjunctivae.

If the patient does not have a feeding jejunostomy, a strict dietary regimen will have to be followed. The patient will experience the dumping syndrome. If the patient is to have an adjunct jejunostomy for feeding purposes, there are several types of jejunostomies used for feeding (see Chapter 16). Postoperative feedings may be initiated once the jejunostomy catheter has been verified by x-ray examination.

If feedings have not been instituted, the catheter is irrigated with 10 mL of sterile water or normal saline every 8 hours to avoid clogging.[14] Because the contents of the jejunum contain digestive enzymes, meticulous skin care of the stoma site is critical. Any drainage is identified and reported immediately. The use of karaya and stoma adhesive may protect the skin.

The patient and family are instructed regarding the rationale for combination therapies—surgery, chemotherapy, and radiation therapy in the treatment of gastric cancer. Written instructions in the simple form of "what to do" and "what not to do" during chemotherapy and radiation therapy, as well as potential side effects, are necessary. Patients and their families seldom remember all of the details presented to them and need frequent repetition as well as time for questions and feedback. The nurse provides a list of support groups (American Cancer Society, Make Today Count) and allows the patient to ventilate fears and anxieties when the opportunities present (see Chapter 20).

Evaluation

The patient should be relieved of pain and be comfortable. A thorough assessment is necessary to determine the location, nature, and duration of pain and if the patient is experiencing any side-effects from the pain medication. The respiratory status of the patient should be within preoperative baseline limits. The surgical incision should be healing with no signs or symptoms of infection. If the patient's stomach was removed completely, the nutritional status needs ongoing evaluation. The patient and significant person should demonstrate knowledge of potential problems with the dumping syndrome and care of a permanent feeding tube. If the prognosis is poor, it is important to determine if the family has adequate support mechanisms in place to minimize depression and anxiety. The patient and family should discuss openly the treatment, prognosis, and ongoing problems. The nurse is responsible for listening and reviewing the patient's progress and making referrals to rehabilitation services or community agencies as necessary. The patient will need supportive care when discharged from the hospital.

Documentation

The patient's record should clearly reflect the preoperative and postoperative status. Reports of pain, measures to relieve pain, and evaluation of the patient's response to nursing interventions are also an essential part of documentation. The surgical incision should be described and any signs or symptoms of infection noted. All tubes must be identified and patency and drainage recorded daily. The nutritional status and type of feeding the patient received must be identified. There is a strong possibility that the patient will be discharged with tubes in place; therefore the family and significant persons must be included in the discharge teaching plan. It is essential to describe their responses and note whether they understand instructions. It is also important to record psychologic reaction and adaptation to treatment and ongoing rehabilitation.

Ongoing Care

If radiation and chemotherapy are instituted, the patient must be frequently assessed to determine weight loss. One simple way to measure weight loss is to compare weight for height to ideal weight for height and calculate the percent deficit. Calories can be increased to counter the deficit. If the patient has a feeding jejunostomy, skin care will need to be evaluated to determine if further nursing measures are necessary to prevent skin excoriation. Radiation therapy may cause hypermotility of the GI tract and subsequent diarrhea. Management begins with an accurate record of the number of stools. If diarrhea persists, antidiarrheal agents or drugs that slow the GI tract may be prescribed. Abdominal distention or bloating may be a problem because of the resultant dumping syndrome, and further measures may need to be instituted to provide relief of symptoms.

As the patient becomes more debilitated and requires more care, other arrangements may be necessary. The nurse needs to involve other members of the health care team to determine alternative methods of care for the patient and family.

CRITICAL THINKING QUESTIONS

1 What are the causes of acute and chronic gastritis?
2 Differentiate between gastric and duodenal ulcer disease and stress ulcers.
3 List appropriate subjective data in the assessment of patients with peptic ulcer disease.
4 Discuss predisposing factors for gastric ulcer occurrence.
5 What are the actions and side effects of major antiulcer agents?
6 Discuss the administration and scheduling of major antiulcer agents.
7 What are complications that can occur from peptic ulcer disease?
8 Identify nursing interventions for the preoperative patient having gastric surgery.
9 What are the potential postoperative complications of gastric surgery?
10 What are the appropriate nursing interventions for a patient with GI bleeding?
11 Discuss postoperative care of the patient who has had surgery for gastric cancer.

BIBLIOGRAPHY

Current
1. Ahern HL, Rice KT: How do you measure gastric pH, *Am J Nurs* 5:70, May 1991.
2. Ayiomamitis A: The epidemiology of malignant neoplasms of the stomach in Canada during the period 1934-1984, *Gastroenterology* 83:26, 1987.
3. Barr GD et al: A two-year prospective controlled study of maintenance cimetidine and gastric ulcer, *Gastroenterology* 85:100, 1983.
4. Blaser MJ: Campylobacter-like organisms, gastritis and peptic ulcer disease, *Gastroenterology* 93:371, 1987.
5. Brockstein AJ: Peptic ulcer disease: new concepts, new and current therapies, *Consultant*, p 157, April 1986.
6. Bynum TE: Clinical presentation of ulcer disease. In Swabb EA, Szabo S, editors: *Ulcer disease, investigation and basis for therapy*, New York, 1991, Marcel Dekker.
7. Davis GR: Neoplasms of the stomach. In Berk JE, editor: *Bockus gastroenterology*, ed 4, Philadelphia, 1985, WB Saunders.
8. Donowitz LG et al: Alteration of normal gastric flora in critical care patients receiving antacid and cimetidine therapy, *Infect Control* 7:23, 1986.
9. Eastwood GL: Upper GI bleeding: differential diagnosis and management, *Hosp Med* 23:57, 1987.
10. Freston JW: Safety perspectives on parenteral H_2 receptor antagonists, *JAMA* 83:58, 1987.
11. Freston JW: Overview of medical therapy of peptic ulcer disease, *Gastroenter Clin North Am* 19(1):121, 1990.
12. Gebhard RL: New developments in the medical therapy of ulcers, *Soc Gastrointestinal Assistant J*, p. 4, Winter 1985.
13. Graham DY, Smith JL, Dobbs SM: Gastric adaptation oc-

curs with aspirin administration in man, *Dig Dis Sci* 28:1, 1983.

14. Grant J, Kennedy-Caldwell C: *Nutritional support in nursing,* Philadelphia, 1988, WB Saunders.

15. Herrington JR, Sawyers JL: Gastric ulcer, *Curr Probl Surg* 24:759, 1987.

16. Konapad E, Noseworthy T: Stress ulceration, a serious complication in the critically ill patient, *Heart Lung* 17(4):339, 1988.

17. Korman MG et al: Influence of cigarette smoking on healing and relapse in duodenal ulcer disease, *Gastroenterology,* 85:871, 1983.

18. Kozarek RA et al: Longterm follow-up in patients who have undergone balloon dilatation for gastric outlet obstruction, *Gastrointest Endosc* 36:558, 1990.

19. Krejs GJ: Endoscopic therapy in peptic ulcer disease. In Swabb EA, Szabo S, editors: *Ulcer disease, investigation and basis for therapy,* New York, 1991, Marcel Dekker.

20. McCarthy DM: Non-steroidal anti-inflammatory drug-induced ulcers, management by traditional therapies, *Gastroenterology* 96:662, 1989.

21. Myers BM, Smith JL, Graham DY: The effect of red and black pepper on the stomach, *Am J Gastroenterol* 82:211, 1987.

22. Quimby CF: Active smoking depresses prostaglandin synthesis in human gastric mucosa, *Ann Intern Med* 104:616, 1986.

23. Ritclie WP: Pathogenesis of acute gastric mucosal injury, *Viewpoint Dig Dis* 15:17, 1985.

24. Roth SH: Nonsteroidal anti-inflammatory drugs: gastropathy, death and medical practice, *Ann Intern Med* 109(5):353, 1988.

25. Schiller LW: Epidemiology, clinical manifestations and diagnosis. In Wyngaarden JB, Smith LH: *Cecil's textbook of medicine,* ed 17, Philadelphia, 1985, WB Saunders.

26. Shimp LA et al: Potential medication-related problems in noninstitutionalized elderly, *Drug Int Clin Pharmacol* 19:766, 1985.

27. Soll AH: Pathogenesis of peptic ulcer and implications for therapy, *N Engl J Med* 322(13):909, 1990.

28. Swartz ML: Cytotec, *Gastroenterol Nurs* 13(1):37, 1990.

29. Thomas JM, Misewicz G: Histamine H_2 receptor antagonists in the short- and long-term treatment of duodenal ulcer, *Clin Gastroenterol* 13:501, 1984.

30. Thompson JC: Choice of surgery for peptic ulcer, *Hosp Physician,* p. 103, June 1984.

31. Thomson AB, Mahachai V: *Medical management of uncomplicated peptic ulcer disease.* In Berk JE, editor: Bockus's gastroenterology, ed 4, Philadelphia, 1984, WB Saunders.

32. Vital Statistics of the United States, vol 2, *Mortality, part A* (1980), Hyattsville, Md, 1985, United States Department of Health and Human Services.

33. Walt R et al: Rising frequency of ulcer perforation in elderly people in the United Kingdom, *Lancet* 1:489, 1986.

34. Ward M: The management of the patient with peptic ulceration—an update, *Am Fam Physician* 16:383, 1987.

35. Wolosin JD et al: Gastric ulcer recurrence, follow up of a double blind placebo-controlled trail, *Clin Gastroenterol* 11:12, 1989.

Classic

36. Clark GC, Boulos PB, Ward NW: Cost-effectiveness in the treatment of gastric cancer, *Clin Oncol* 6:303, 1980.

37. Everson TC: Carcinoma of the stomach. In Everson TC, Warren J, editors: *Cancer of the digestive tract: clinical management,* New York, 1969, Appleton-Century-Crofts.

38. Langman MJ: What is happening to peptic ulcer, *Br Med J* 284:1063, 1982.

39. Yamanda E et al: The surgical treatment of cancer of the stomach, *Int Surg* 65:387, 1980.

CHAPTER SIXTY-SIX

Nursing Management of Adults with Intestinal Disorders

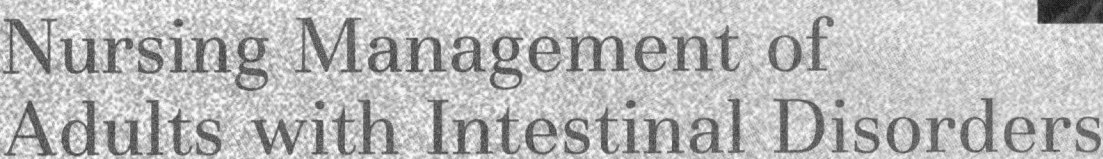

LEARNING OBJECTIVES

1 Identify nursing interventions to support the nutritional needs of patients with malabsorption syndromes.
2 Discuss the nursing care related to the prevention and management of intestinal infections.
3 Compare the disease processes of ulcerative colitis and Crohn's disease.
4 Discuss the long-term care requirements of the patient with inflammatory bowel disease.
5 Describe the preoperative care for the patient having bowel surgery.
6 Compare the different types of ostomies in terms of their function and care requirements.
7 Identify nursing interventions for irrigation and pouch application for a patient with an ostomy.
8 Discuss peristomal skin problems in terms of causes, prevention, and management.
9 Develop patient education guides for patients with ostomies.
10 Discuss the nursing management for a patient with diverticular disease.
11 Explain the pathophysiology of intestinal obstruction.
12 Identify the nurse's role in screening tests for colorectal cancer.

KEY TERMS

DISEASES THAT AFFECT the intestines span all age groups. Patients with disorders of the intestines can experience problems of nutrient absorption, fluid balance, and elimination. These diseases affect not only the function of the intestines but also the function of other body systems. Lifesaving treatment for some of these conditions can have a far-reaching impact on the individual's physiologic and psychologic recovery and return to a normal life. The patient and family are often required to make life-style adjustments. The patient having bowel diversion surgery must adapt to changes in elimination and in body image.

It is imperative that the nurse understand these diseases, treatments, and implications to act as caregiver, care coordinator, and patient advocate. Within these roles the nurse can effectively guide the patient through diagnosis, treatment, and rehabilitation with the least amount of distress and trauma.

Malabsorption is the failure of the gastrointestinal system to digest and then absorb one or more nutrients. The effect depends on the cause of the malabsorption and the nutrients not absorbed.

LACTOSE INTOLERANCE
Definition

Lactose intolerance is an inability to digest and absorb lactose, the disaccharide found in milk and milk products. The disorder occurs because of a deficiency of lactase, the enzyme needed for lactose breakdown.

Etiology/Epidemiology

The occurrence of lactose intolerance seems to be related to the ethnic background of the individual. The disorder is more frequent in people from Africa and the Orient and in Native Americans and Mexican Americans. It occurs less often in people of northern European descent. Lactose intolerance can become apparent at any age. A congenital or primary lactase deficiency may induce symptoms in the infant. However, it is not uncommon for the individual to remain symptom free until adulthood. Acquired lactase deficiency can develop after an injury to the intestinal mucosa. An acquired lactose intolerance may be temporary or permanent depending on the ability of the intestine to heal. Secondary lactose intolerance is seen in patients with inflammatory bowel disorders, infectious bowel diseases, and surgical resection of the small intestine.

Pathophysiology

The primary defect in lactose intolerance is a decrease in the amount of the digestive enzyme lactase.

This digestive enzyme is normally produced by the mucosal cells lining the intestine. When the enzyme is lacking, digestion of lactose is impaired. Diarrhea occurs because the presence of lactose increases the intestinal osmotic pressure. The increased osmotic pressure results in an increased fluid accumulation within the lumen. Fermentation of the lactose by intestinal bacteria leads to an increase in intestinal gas production.

Clinical Manifestations

Abdominal pain and diarrhea after the ingestion of milk or milk products are the primary symptoms of lactose intolerance. The patient may experience abdominal bloating and increased flatulence. Some patients have abdominal cramping with the diarrhea. Osteoporosis and dental caries may result from the decreased calcium intake.

Therapeutic Management

Dietary elimination of milk and milk products is the primary treatment. The level of the patient's lactose tolerance can be determined by gradually adding foods to the diet until symptoms reappear. Some patients benefit from the use of commercial lactase preparations (i.e., Lact-Aid). Calcium supplementation may be necessary if sufficient amounts cannot be obtained from the foods eaten.

ADULT CELIAC DISEASE
Definition/Etiology

Celiac disease, also called celiac sprue and nontropical sprue, is a permanent intolerance for gluten. Gluten is the protein substance found in grains such as barley, wheat, oats, and rye. Celiac disease leads to atrophy of the intestinal villi. This atrophy causes a decrease in the amount and activity of enzymes on the lining of the intestine. The end result is intestinal malabsorption. The true incidence of this disorder is unknown. Most patients with celiac disease have ancestors from northwestern Europe.

Pathophysiology

The cause of malabsorption in celiac disease is the diminished surface area of the intestinal villi. Changes in epithelial cell function, increased mucous production by the epithelial cells, and hypomotility also contribute to the malabsorption. These structural changes in the small intestine are the result of an inflammatory process stimulated by the presence of gluten. Fat and fat-soluble nutrients are primarily affected by the changes in celiac disease. When the proximal small intestine is involved, the patient will have problems related to the malabsorption of iron and calcium.

Clinical Manifestations

The patient with celiac disease has diarrhea of two or three mushy, light-colored, foul-smelling stools per day. The diarrhea is accompanied by explosive flatus. Laboratory examination of the stool will reveal increased fat content **(steatorrhea).** Because of problems of decreased nutrient absorption, these patients also experience severe weight loss, fatigue, and anorexia. The patient may have signs and symptoms of anemia because of decreased absorption of iron and fat-soluble vitamins. The patient's skin may show signs of increased bruising because of decreased absorption of vitamin K.

Therapeutic Management

Most patients with celiac disease will be symptom free if they eat a diet free of all wheat, rye, oats, and barley. Supplementation with vitamins and minerals may be necessary to make up for the severity of the dietary restrictions.

• • •

Tropical sprue occurs only in tropical climates. Bacterial infection is thought to be the underlying cause of this malabsorption. Clinically the patient shows manifestations similar to adult celiac disease.

Whipple's disease occurs primarily in men. It is thought to be caused by Gram-positive bacteria and the resulting accumulation of macrophages in the intestinal villi.[42] Patients experience diarrhea, steatorrhea, and weight loss. Arthritic-like symptoms and central nervous system symptoms may also occur in this disorder.

Surgically induced malabsorption syndrome is also called **short bowel syndrome.** After small bowel resections, varying degrees of malabsorption can occur, depending on the portion of bowel removed. An individual can tolerate removal of up to 40% of the small bowel if the duodenum, proximal jejunum, distal half of the ileum, and ileocecal valve are intact. However, significant malabsorption can occur when portions of the distal ileum are resected. The characteristics of the diarrhea and type of nutrient malabsorption depend on the section of bowel removed. For example, resection of 1 to 2 m of the distal ileum can result in malabsorption of vitamin B_{12}. Postoperatively the patient may have six to eight watery stools per day. Many patients are able to tolerate oral feedings over time as the remaining bowel adapts and resumes the absorptive function. Until nutritional needs can be met with oral feedings, some form of parenteral nutrition is necessary.

Many drugs produce diarrhea as a side effect and interfere with the absorption of specific nutrients. Prolonged use of antibiotics can disrupt the normal intestinal flora and contribute to the malabsorption of nutrients. The patient experiences diarrhea as the primary symptom. Overuse of aluminum hydroxide antacids can cause the malabsorption of nutrients such as iron, phosphorus, and fluoride. The aluminum in the antacid binds with the nutrient in the intestine, preventing its absorption.

NURSING MANAGEMENT OF THE PATIENT WITH MALABSORPTION SYNDROMES
Assessment

The nurse questions the patient about the pattern of bowel elimination. Identify the patient's normal pattern of defecation. A diet history helps to relate food intake to the occurrence of diarrhea. The nurse

TABLE 66-1 Laboratory Assessment for Malabsorption Syndromes

Test	Results

Complete blood count
  Hemoglobin
  Hematocrit
  Mean cell volume
	Anemia common in malabsorption of iron, folate, vitamin B_{12}

Coagulation profile Prothrombin time	Prolonged times related to vitamin K deficiency

Blood chemistries
  Albumin
  Cholesterol
  Calcium
  Iron
  Potassium
  Magnesium
  Phosphorus
	Decreased serum levels in malabsorption

Serum carotene	Decreased levels in fat malabsorption
Fecal fat determination (72-hour collection)	Requires measured intake of 100 g of fat per day; excretion of more than 6 to 7 g/day of fat in malabsorption
Xylose tolerance test	Urinary excretion of test dose decreased in malabsorption
Barium contrast x-ray studies	Dilation of small bowel; irregular mucosal folds; fragmentation of barium
Small bowel biopsy	Allows for accurate diagnosis based on mucosal changes
Hydrogen breath test	Elevated levels specific in lactose intolerance

inquires about changes in body weight and activity tolerance.

The clinical assessment of the patient includes observation of the characteristics of the patient's bowel movements. The nurse assesses the frequency, volume, consistency, color, and odor of the feces. Special attention is given to assessment of the patient's fluid balance. The nurse monitors daily weight, urine output, orthostatic blood pressures, skin turgor, and mucous membrane hydration. Dietary adequacy is also assessed (see Chapter 16).

Laboratory assessment of the patient with a malabsorption syndrome includes specific tests to determine the cause of the disorder. Table 66-1 summarizes the diagnostic procedures that may be included in the patient workup.

Nursing Diagnosis

The following nursing diagnoses may be appropriate for the patient with malabsorption disorders:

Diarrhea related to increased stool volume or dietary fat

Altered nutrition: less than body requirements related to malabsorption

Activity intolerance related to decreased absorption of foods for metabolism

Fluid volume deficit related to fluid loss into the intestine

Sensory/perceptual alterations related to neuromuscular irritability from decreased calcium

High risk for injury related to decreased bone density

Discomfort related to abdominal bloating and cramping

Impaired anal integrity related to irritation from diarrhea

Planning

Nursing care for the patient with malabsorption disorders is planned to meet the following outcomes:

The patient will have stools that are soft, formed, and of normal color and frequency

The patient will return to and maintain a desired weight

The patient will accomplish desired activities of daily living without fatigue or injury

The patient will prepare meals that are free of gluten or lactose and that provide sufficient nutrients

The patient will have fluids and electrolytes in balance

The patient will be free of abdominal bloating and cramping

GLUTEN-FREE DIET

Foods allowed

Milk, cheese, eggs
Meat, fish, poultry prepared without breading, creamed sauces, or wheat flour–thickened gravies
All fruits
Vegetables prepared without creamed sauces
Breads and cereals made from rice, corn, or gluten-free wheat flour
Gelatin desserts
Homemade ice cream, custard, rice pudding, and cornstarch pudding
Popcorn
Potato chips

Foods not allowed

Any homemade or commercial food that is breaded, creamed, or thickened with wheat flour or gluten stabilizers
Breads, crackers, muffins, rolls, cereals, pasta, macaroni, or spaghetti made from wheat, barley, oats, or rye grains and flours
Ale and beer
Mustard, soups
Instant coffee containing wheat
Cakes, cookies, and pastries made with gluten flours

Supplements needed

Iron, folate, or vitamin D

LACTOSE-FREE DIET

Foods allowed

Plain meat, fish, poultry, eggs
All vegetables and fruits prepared without lactose products
Vegetable oils and margarine, mayonnaise
Homemade recipes made with milk substitutes
Rice, noodles, macaroni, pasta, spaghetti
Lactose-free breads and cereals
Flavored gelatin
Lactose-free honey, sugar, jams, and jellies

Foods not allowed

Milk, cream, yogurt, cottage cheese, hard cheeses
Any creamed meat, vegetable, soup, or sauce
Organ meats (liver, sweetbreads, kidney, brains)
Ice cream, custard, pudding, ice milk
Butter, sour cream
Commercially prepared foods made with milk, milk by-products, butter, or lactose
Milk chocolate, toffee, caramels, butterscotch

The patient will maintain intact anal skin integrity

Implementation

The patient and family need instruction about a diet that is gluten free (see box, p. 1848) or lactose free (see box, p. 1848). Because the dietary changes required in many malabsorption syndromes are major alterations in eating habits the patient and family may need ongoing support to cope with these changes. The patient needs to understand that as long as the dietary causes are eliminated from the diet symptoms will not occur. Not adhering to the diet will result in the return of symptoms. Because gluten and lactose may be part of many processed and commercial foods, patients must learn to carefully read food product labels. The nurse may consider making a referral to a dietitian to help the patient and family in meal planning and food selection. The patient and family need to be educated about the use of nutritional supplements to ensure adequate intake of vitamins and minerals that may not be provided on a restricted diet.

Evaluation

As the patient responds to the dietary changes the frequency of bowel movements decreases. For patients with celiac disease the amount of fecal fat will decrease. The stool is formed. The patient begins to gain weight. As sufficient nutrients are absorbed the patient is able to increase activity levels without fatigue. Signs of fluid balance will be present as the frequency of diarrhea decreases.

Documentation

The nurse documents an accurate record of the frequency and characteristics of the patient's diarrhea. Changes in the patient's hydration status can be recorded on a flow chart that includes oral intake, urine and fecal output, mucous membrane condition, orthostatic blood pressure, and skin turgor. Record the patient's body weight as an indicator of nutritional status. The ability of the patient and family to plan meals within the dietary guidelines needs to be recorded as evidence of understanding and compliance.

Ongoing Care

As the bowel heals or adapts, the patient may begin to gradually increase consumption of gluten or lactose. In some cases, patients may be able to eat limited amounts of these foods and remain symptom free. Patients may need to continue using nutrient supplements such as vitamins and minerals as long as dietary intake is restricted. Periodic evaluation determines the adequacy of the patient's intake to support normal physiologic function.

INTESTINAL INFECTIONS
Etiology/Epidemiology

Infections of the gastrointestinal tract are among the most common infections in the general population. The development of an intestinal infection depends on the interaction of characteristics of the agent and the host. Agent factors that contribute to the development of an infection include the mode of entry into the body and the number of microbes that enter the body. The majority of infecting organisms that produce intestinal infections are acquired by the oral route. The source of the microorganism is contaminated food or water. Some intestinal infections occur as a result of person-to-person contact. The fecal-oral mode of transmission is commonly implicated in outbreaks of infectious diarrhea in institutions such as child-care centers and nursing homes. Among sexually active homosexual males protozoal infections are commonly implicated in the development of "gay bowel syndrome."

The number of microbes (inoculum) is also a factor in the development of infectious diarrhea. A large inoculum is required to produce symptoms with bacteria. This process requires prior multiplication of the bacteria in food or water before entry into the host. Protozoal infections require a smaller inoculum to produce diarrhea.

A variety of host factors attempt to protect the gastrointestinal tract from damage by microorganisms. The acid pH of the stomach kills most enteric pathogens. When the secretion of gastric acid is decreased or the pH is raised, the size of the inoculum necessary to produce infection is less. Food with a high acid-buffering capacity or high-fat content, such as mayonnaise, will protect a microbe from gastric acid. Liquids that pass through the stomach more

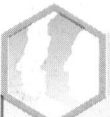

GERIATRIC CONSIDERATIONS

Diarrhea

Causative factors include foods, malabsorption, fecal impaction, low serum albumin, diverticulosis, infection, drugs (antibiotics, antidysrhythmics, aminophylline, digitalis, potassium supplements).
Can result in severe fluid and electrolyte imbalance, loss of nutrients, and fatigue. Hyponatremia and hypokalemia can occur.

quickly reduce the exposure of the microbe to gastric acid.

Small bowel motility affects the amount of time a pathogen is in contact with the intestinal wall. States of hypomotility increase the contact time and contribute to the development and duration of symptoms. The increased duration of symptoms with intestinal infections is commonly associated with the use of antidiarrheals and antispasmodic drugs that tend to decrease motility.

The normal intestinal bacterial flora offers protection against colonization by potentially pathogenic organisms. When the normal flora is disrupted, as occurs with prolonged antibiotic therapy, the person is more susceptible to infections of the intestines. The host immune system also contributes to resistance to intestinal infections. Immunocompromised patients who develop intestinal infections tend to have persistent infectious diarrhea instead of a self-limiting infection. The impaired immune response delays the body's ability to destroy invading pathogens.

Pathophysiology

The most common occurrence in infectious diarrhea is secretion of fluid into the intestinal lumen. Some bacteria produce enterotoxins in the small bowel that bind to mucosal receptors. The mucosal cells respond by increasing active secretion of water and electrolytes into the intestinal lumen. Changes in the ion pump cause active secretion of chloride and bicarbonate ions into the small intestine with inhibited reabsorption of sodium. To maintain isotonicity within the intestine, protein-rich fluid is secreted into the bowel. The amount of fluid secreted exceeds the ability of the large intestine to reabsorb the fluid into the vascular system.[41]

Another mechanism that produces diarrhea is related to inflammatory destruction of the intestinal lining by the infecting organism. Direct invasion by the microbe actually kills the mucosal cells.

Clinical Manifestations

The primary manifestation of an intestinal infection is diarrhea. The fecal output has increased water content. If the infecting organism acts by direct invasion of the intestinal mucosa, the feces may also contain blood and mucus. Patients may complain of rectal urgency and ineffective and painful straining with defecation (tenesmus). Other symptoms include fever greater than 102° F, nausea, vomiting, and abdominal cramping. Table 66-2 summarizes characteristics of intestinal infections associated with various infecting organisms.

TABLE 66-2   Intestinal Infections: Comparison of Clinical Manifestations Produced by Different Microorganisms

Agent	Onset	Incubation	Feces characteristics	Fever	Nausea/vomiting	Duration
Protozoa						
Giardia lamblia	Abrupt	2 wk	Watery	Uncommon	Common	Variable
Isospora belli	Abrupt	Unknown	Watery, blood, mucus	Rare	Rare	4-6 wk
Cryptosporidum	Abrupt	Unknown	Watery, blood, mucus	Rare	Rare	Variable
Entamoeba histolytica	Gradual	24 hr	Blood, mucus	Uncommon	Rare	3-14 days
Viruses						
Rotavirus	Abrupt	16-36 hr	Watery, blood, mucus	Uncommon	Common	1-2 days
Norwalk-like agent	Abrupt	16-36 hr	Watery, blood, mucus	Rare	Common	1-2 days
Bacteria						
Escherichia coli	Abrupt	4-96 hr	Watery, blood, mucus	Common	Rare	2-7 days
Vibrio cholerae	Abrupt	6-48 hr	Rice-water	Common	Uncommon	Variable
Staphylococcus aureus	Abrupt	1-6 yr	Watery, blood, mucus	Rare	Common	1 day
Clostridium perfringens	Abrupt	6-24 hr	Watery, blood, mucus	Rare	Rare	1 day
Shigella	Abrupt	24-72 hr	Blood, mucus	Common	Rare	2-20 days
Campylobacter jejuni	Abrupt	48-96 hr	Blood, mucus	Common	Uncommon	1-4 days
Salmonella	Abrupt	8-72 hr	Watery, blood, mucus	Common	Common	5-7 days
Yersinia enterocolitica	Variable	16-48 hr	Watery, blood, mucus	Common	Common	7-21 days
Vibrio parahaemolyticus	Abrupt	2-24 hr	Watery, blood, mucus	Uncommon	Common	1-3 days
Aeromonas hydrophila	Abrupt	Unknown	Watery	Rare	Common	1-7 days

Therapeutic Management

Many intestinal infections are self-limiting diseases. The administration of antibiotics is usually indicated for prolonged or severe diarrhea with a stool positive for leukocytes.

Fluid and electrolyte replacement is an essential part of the treatment program to offset the losses from the diarrhea. The oral route for fluid replacement is usually sufficient. If the patient is experiencing nausea and vomiting or is unable to consume sufficient fluids orally, the intravenous route is indicated. Once symptoms begin to subside the patient may begin to consume a soft, nonirritating diet as tolerated.

The use of antidiarrheals and antispasmodic agents in the treatment of infectious diarrhea is controversial. Use of these medications may actually increase the severity of the infection by increasing the contact time of the microbe with the intestinal wall. Intestinal absorbents containing kaolin and pectin (Kaopectate) may be used to increase stool consistency. Bismuth subsalicylate (Pepto-Bismol) can effectively decrease intestinal secretions and decrease the diarrhea volume. However, to be effective these agents may require large doses, as much as 30 to 60 mL every 30 to 60 minutes.

NURSING MANAGEMENT OF THE PATIENT WITH INTESTINAL INFECTIONS

Assessment

The interview of the patient with possible infectious diarrhea allows the nurse to collect information about the patient's symptom pattern. Inquire about the onset of the diarrhea. Questions about fecal characteristics include frequency of bowel movements, color, consistency, and amount. The nurse assesses the patient for associated symptoms such as fever, abdominal cramping, nausea, and vomiting. The patient may complain of anal burning or sensitivity as a result of tissue irritation from the diarrhea.

To assist in making an accurate diagnosis, the nurse inquires about recent drug use, especially antibiotics. Prolonged use of ampicillin, clindamycin, and the cephalosporins is associated with intestinal infections by *Clostridium difficile*. Ask the patient about recent travel and food intake. Diarrhea after foreign travel or after the ingestion of particular foods may suggest certain infecting organisms. For example, infections caused by *Salmonella* are associated with ingestion of contaminated eggs or poultry. Consumption of meat that has been cooked, cooled, and reheated can lead to infections by *Clostridium perfringens*.[41]

Thorough investigation of symptoms is necessary to differentiate infectious diarrhea from noninfectious causes of diarrhea. The causes of noninfectious diarrhea include heavy metal poisoning, monosodium glutamate, shellfish allergy, ingestion of toxic mushrooms, and fish toxins. Diarrhea from noninfectious causes is usually characterized by a short incubation period of minutes to hours after exposure. Patients with noninfectious diarrhea may also experience neurologic changes such as flushing and paresthesias. In food allergies, the patient may have itching and a skin rash.

Although the initial focus of the assessment is on the patient, the nurse includes questions about family members and co-workers who may have similar symptoms. The majority of gastrointestinal infections are communicable and represent a community health problem. The appropriate municipal and state officials may need to be notified about infections that originate in contaminated food and water or when the patient is a resident of a long-term care institution.

The nurse assesses the patient for indications of fluid volume imbalance. This aspect of the assessment is especially important for the elderly patient. The clinical assessment includes measurement of postural changes in blood pressure, skin turgor, mucous membrane hydration, and urine output.

The key laboratory assessment for patients with intestinal infections is a stool culture. Blood chemistries may be ordered to monitor changes in fluid and electrolyte status.

Nursing Diagnosis

Nursing diagnoses for the patient with an intestinal infection include the following:

Fluid volume deficit related to excessive losses from diarrhea and vomiting

Diarrhea related to intestinal inflammation

Abdominal pain related to intestinal inflammation

Altered nutrition: less than body requirements related to decreased intake and decreased absorption

Impaired anal skin integrity related to irritation from diarrhea

Planning

Nursing care for the patient with an intestinal infection is planned to achieve the following outcomes:

The patient will have decreased frequency and volume of bowel movements

The patient will maintain fluid and electrolyte balance

The patient will have adequate nutritional intake

The patient will verbalize relief of abdominal pain

The patient will have intact perianal skin

Implementation

Whenever possible the patient with infectious diarrhea should not share bathroom facilities with others until the diarrhea subsides. Careful hand washing after bowel movements is important to decrease the possible spread of the infection to others. The patient should not handle food that will be eaten by others.

Fluid intake is important to replace losses from diarrhea. When the patient can tolerate oral intake, clear liquids are usually given first because they will not stimulate further diarrhea. Apple juice, clear carbonated beverages, clear broth, electrolyte-containing beverages, and plain gelatin (i.e., Jell-O) can be included, as well as plain water. If vomiting is severe or the patient is unable to consume sufficient oral fluids, intravenous fluids with added electrolytes may be indicated. When diarrhea subsides the diet may progress to full fluids and then to a regular diet. Caution the patient to avoid milk, caffeine, and high-fiber foods, because they tend to increase intestinal irritation.

Measures to decrease the frequency of bowel movements are directed at reducing intestinal stimulation. When oral intake stimulates an increase in the diarrhea the patient receives nothing orally. Bed rest can contribute to the patient's level of comfort by decreasing peristalsis. If bismuth salts are used to decrease intestinal secretions, inform the patient that stools may turn black. Prolonged use of bismuth subsalicylate preparations can predispose the patient to salicylate toxicity.

The use of soothing ointments helps relieve the anal irritation from the diarrhea. Sitz baths, perineal washes, and the cautious use of a cool hair dryer rather than paper products after bowel movements can promote hygiene and prevent additional irritation.

Evaluation

The nurse monitors the patient for decreasing occurrence of symptoms as the illness resolves. Evaluation of the patient's response to fluid replacement includes stable blood pressure, moist mucous membranes, good skin turgor, and adequate urine output. Decreased abdominal cramping and frequency of bowel movements are noted.

Documentation

Documentation for a patient with an intestinal infection includes the frequency of bowel movements and the characteristics of the feces. Note changes in response to treatment. Record the patient's tolerance of oral intake.

Ongoing Care

Patient and family teaching becomes a major aspect of the ongoing care for intestinal infections. Hand washing after bowel movements is imperative to decrease the fecal-oral route of transmission. This aspect of hygiene is especially important for people who are responsible for food handling and preparation. Family members responsible for food preparation need to be made aware of the importance of proper methods of food preparation and storage to reduce the growth of infecting organisms.

INFLAMMATORY BOWEL DISEASE: ULCERATIVE COLITIS AND CROHN'S DISEASE

Definition

Inflammatory bowel disease is a chronic inflammatory disease of the small and/or large bowel. It is a perplexing problem in medicine, afflicting an estimated 2 million Americans with 10,000 new cases diagnosed each year.[28] Often those afflicted are young people in the beginning of their adult lives with education, careers, and the raising of families ahead of them. The term *inflammatory bowel disease* is used by many to include two intestinal disorders, **ulcerative colitis** and **Crohn's disease.** Crohn's disease is also called regional enteritis for disease in the ileum and Crohn's colitis for disease of the colon. These disorders have similarities, but 80% to 90% of cases can be differentiated by clinical, radiologic, and pathologic findings. Although similarities are evident and medical treatment may run the same course, surgical interventions may differ. This is a disease characterized by exacerbations and remissions.

Etiology

The etiology of inflammatory bowel disease is unknown. Genetic, environmental, microbial, and immunologic factors appear to be involved. The familial incidence of ulcerative colitis is 10% to 20%; for Crohn's disease there is a 20% to 40% incidence.[21] An environmental component is suggested by the geographic distribution. Inflammatory bowel disease is found more often in northern and urban areas. Reports indicating the occurrence of inflammatory bowel disease, especially ulcerative colitis, following an infectious process have been documented. Genetic, infectious, and autoimmune relationships to the disease are not clear.

Psychosomatic factors have been implicated in the etiology but not proven. Emotional factors play a role in the course of the disease unrelated to the cause. The chronic illness, social isolation, and frustration cause difficulties in effective coping. Emotional stress seems to increase bowel activity in these patients and plays a critical role in exacerbation of the disease.

Epidemiology

The peak incidence of inflammatory bowel disease occurs in the second and third decades. There are no consistent differences between the sexes. Ulcerative colitis and Crohn's disease have a definite increased incidence in the Jewish population and in higher socioeconomic groups. A lower incidence is found in the nonwhite population. There may be an intermingling of ulcerative colitis and Crohn's disease seen within the same family. The incidence of ulcerative colitis appears to be stable, whereas that of Crohn's disease is increasing in the United States. The incidence of inflammatory bowel disease is 5 to 10 cases per 100,000 individuals.[21]

Pathophysiology

According to Kirsner, "current evidence supports ulcerative colitis and Crohn's disease as independent but possibly distantly related diseases."[21] Distinction between the two diseases depends on pathologic features. In ulcerative colitis the disease is confined to the mucosa and submucosa of the colon. In Crohn's disease the inflammatory process involves all layers of the bowel and can occur throughout the gastrointestinal tract. Occasionally a patient may present features of both diseases, and it is difficult to make a definite diagnosis.

Ulcerative colitis is limited to the colon, generally starts on the left side of the colon at the rectosigmoid area, and progresses to the right side. In diffuse disease the entire colon is affected. In the early stages of ulcerative colitis tiny abscesses are formed in the tubular glands to produce the so-called crypt abscesses.[45] These abscesses coalesce, producing larger abscesses with purulent drainage, sloughing of the mucosa, and subsequent ulceration. Capillaries become friable and bleed, causing the characteristic diarrhea containing pus and blood. In longstanding disease the mucosa becomes diffusely and superficially ulcerated with pseudopolyps commonly present. Shortening of the colon occurs as a result of fibrosis.

In Crohn's disease all layers of the bowel are involved (transmural inflammation), and the disease process can occur in any area of the gastrointestinal tract. The entire colon may be involved, or only segments may be involved. The segmental involvement creates the characteristic "skip" pattern. Typically the disease starts in the ileum and right side of the colon and moves left.

In early Crohn's disease granulomas are found in lymphoid follicles of the mucosa. As the disease advances small ulcerations in the mucosa occur over the granulomas. As the granulomas increase, destruction of lymphatics occurs, producing edema and inflammation. These advance to deeper layers of the bowel wall with fibrosis and serositis. Penetrating narrow fistulous tracts lined by granulation tissue extend obliquely into the intestinal wall. Fibrosis results in thickening of the wall and narrowing of the lumen. Ulcers may coalesce to form deep longitudinal ulcers. Transverse fissures occur between these ulcers, creating the "cobblestone" pattern on the mucosa.[39] Fissures may extend through the entire bowel wall, creating a fistula into other segments of the bowel or the mesentery.

Clinical Manifestations

Clinical manifestations of inflammatory bowel disease depend on the pathologic findings of each disease. In ulcerative colitis the patient may exhibit initial symptoms of rectal bleeding to bloody diarrhea. Lower abdominal cramping is often followed by urgency and loose, bloody stools. Remission of the disease may occur, at which time the diarrhea improves. Other clinical features include weight loss, lethargy, and a sense of frustration and loss of control as a result of tenesmus and unpredictable bowel movements. In fulminant disease toxic megacolon may occur with destruction of circular and longitudinal muscles, marked dilation of the colon, and lack of peristalsis. Patients with toxic megacolon develop severe abdominal pain, abdominal distention, fever, tachycardia, and leukocytosis.

The onset of Crohn's disease is often insidious, with vague abdominal pain, unexplained anemia, lethargy, and fever. Rectal bleeding may be present. Diarrhea is more constant in Crohn's disease and is usually progressive with fewer periods of remission. As a result of intestinal fistulas or poor absorption of bile salts by the ileum, stools become very watery. Fever, weight loss, abdominal pain, and loss of appetite are common. Problems in the anal area, such as fissure or fistula in ano, are common manifestations. Crohn's disease, like ulcerative colitis, can progress to toxic megacolon.

Toxic megacolon, or toxic dilation of the large bowel, is a life-threatening complication of inflammatory bowel disease that occurs in less than 5% of patients. The bowel wall becomes so distended and thin that perforation is an immediate possibility. In the acutely ill patient this condition can occur quickly with the patient experiencing less diarrhea but increasing and diffuse pain. Abdominal distention develops, the patient's temperature rises to 104° F or more, and tachycardia is evident. Immediate

SIMILARITIES AND DIFFERENCES IN ULCERATIVE COLITIS AND CROHN'S DISEASE

Similarities

1. Afflicts young adults; higher social class; more in northern than southern areas; more urban than rural
2. Genetic considerations are similar—increased incidence in Jewish population, decreased incidence in blacks, some familial predisposition
3. Diarrhea, abdominal pain, fever, weight loss; bleeding may be common in ulcerative colitis
4. Remission and exacerbation of disease
5. Extracolonic complications (i.e., arthralgia, ocular uveitis, skin disorders)
6. Can advance in fulminant disease to toxic megacolon

Differences

1. Ulcerative colitis confined to mucosa and submucosa and extends in a continuous pattern left to right; Crohn's disease involves all structures of colon and progresses from terminal ileum to left side of bowel in skip pattern.
2. In ulcerative colitis, mucosa appears granular with pseudopolyps; in Crohn's disease, transverse fissures crossing each other produce a cobblestone appearance
3. In ulcerative colitis, bowel lumen narrows and colon usually shortens; in Crohn's disease, bowel wall is thickened as a result of lymphatic dilation; granuloma and fistulas may be seen

surgical intervention usually offers the best outcome. Toxic megacolon occurs less frequently with Crohn's disease than with ulcerative colitis. See the box on the similarities and differences in ulcerative colitis and Crohn's disease.

Long-term effects of the diseases

The development of carcinoma of the colon in longstanding cases of ulcerative colitis is a major concern. Patients who have had ulcerative colitis for 10 to 15 years are at high risk for development of colorectal cancer. About 40% to 50% of patients with total colonic involvement may ultimately develop colon cancer.[39] Recent studies suggest that patients with Crohn's disease are also at risk but to a lesser degree than those with ulcerative colitis. In either case, total **proctocolectomy** and bowel diversion may be necessary.

According to Harper and Fazio,[15] the relentless progression of Crohn's disease forces 40% to 50% of long-term patients to have some form of bowel diversion, such as an **ileostomy.** The incidence of obstruction, intestinal fistula, perianal disease, short bowel syndrome, and extracolonic complications makes the patient's future unpredictable.

Therapeutic Management

The medical management of these two diseases is symptomatic and supportive. The primary goal is to interrupt the inflammatory process. Management includes medication, diet intervention, and stress reduction. Drugs used in treatment are categorized into four groups: anti-inflammatory drugs, antibacterial drugs, drugs that affect the immune system, and antidiarrheal preparations. Treatment of the disease is based on the phase of the disease. For example, treatment of acute colitis differs from that of chronic and quiescent colitis. No known therapy will maintain a patient with Crohn's disease in remission.

Drug treatment

Sulfasalazine affects the inflammatory response and has some antibacterial activity. The acetylsalicylic acid activity of this drug is believed to depress prostaglandin synthesis at the colonic mucosa, thus decreasing inflammation. This is the drug of choice for mild chronic ulcerative colitis and is believed to reduce incidences of recurrence. Side effects include nausea, vomiting, epigastric distress, headaches, diarrhea, and generalized rash. Dosage is 3 to 4 g daily in divided doses during the acute phase. A maintenance dose is 1.5 to 2 g daily. Olsalazine sodium (Dipentum), a nonsulfa drug, is being used with good results and may prove to be the drug of choice for persons with a sensitivity to sulfa. Mesalamine (Rowasa), another nonsulfa drug, is being used in the form of a retention enema with good results.

Corticosteroids, another group of anti-inflammatory drugs, are not necessarily an ingredient in the treatment of mild colitis but are important drugs in the treatment of moderate and severe colitis. Steroids do not prevent recurrence of disease, but they do relieve symptoms in many cases. They can be given systemically or topically in the form of a retention enema. The retention enema is best suited for patients with disease of the descending colon and rectum. The drug given in this form is absorbed by the colonic mucosa and may produce side effects. The administration of prednisone in a sliding-scale dose according to disease activity seems to be an accepted regimen.

Metronidazole (Flagyl) is believed to be beneficial in Crohn's perianal disease. This drug is used in the treatment of bacterial infections caused by anaerobic microorganisms. It can be given orally or infused intravenously.

Antidiarrheal agents may help relieve some of the symptoms of inflammatory bowel disease. Antidiarrheals with anticholinergic agents (i.e., diphenoxylate [Lomotil]) are not recommended, because they can mask obstruction or contribute to toxic megacolon. Loperamide (Imodium) may be used to treat cramping and diarrhea in chronic ulcerative colitis and Crohn's disease.

Immunosuppressive drugs such as azathioprine (Imuran), 6-mercaptopurine, and cyclosporine have been used to decrease antibody-producing cells and may be used effectively to treat quiescent and chronic ulcerative colitis. They have proven most effective, however, in the treatment of Crohn's disease.[39] Studies are in progress to identify other drugs that stimulate the immune system (Table 66-3). Peppercorn predicts that cromolyn, chloroquine, methotrexate, and antitubercular agents may be found useful in the future.[27]

Some medical treatment includes exclusion of certain foods such as milk products and highly spiced foods. Approximately 20% of this patient population improves with dietary changes. Persons with moderate to severe disease may be nutritionally deficient, and a high-protein, high-calorie diet is recommended.

Stress is known to be a factor in the exacerbation of symptoms. Examination of stress factors in the patient's life and a realistic plan to reduce these factors and teach stress reduction coping mechanisms may help.

In some severe cases hospitalization for bowel rest is necessary. Total parenteral nutrition may be started for nutrition, fluid, and electrolyte replacement. Patients on bowel rest are given nothing by mouth. Nasogastric suction may be used if distention or severe diarrhea is present. Corticosteroids are given parenterally. Broad-spectrum antibiotics are used for toxic megacolon.

Surgical Management

Inflammatory bowel disease may require surgical treatment for two reasons. The first is an acute episode that does not respond to treatment or complications such as perforation, toxic colonic dilation, extracolonic complications, fissures, and abscesses. The second reason is the risk of cancer, which increases with the duration of ulcerative colitis and, to a lesser degree, with Crohn's disease.

Crohn's disease tends to have an unrelenting course and may necessitate surgical intervention. The surgical procedure depends on the area of involvement. Most surgeons prefer a conservative approach with limited resection and reanastomosis of the bowel. Unfortunately Crohn's disease tends to reappear proximal to the resected area or areas. If a major part of the colon is involved, including the rectum and perianal area, total proctocolectomy and permanent ileostomy is the treatment of choice (Figure 66-1). If the rectum is spared, an abdominal co-

TABLE 66-3   Pharmacology Summary: Inflammatory Bowel Disease

Drug	Action	Dosage/route	Side effects
Sulfasalazine (Azulfidine)	Anti-inflammatory, antibacterial	0.5 to 2 g four times daily orally	Nausea, vomiting, diarrhea, headache, rash, epigastric distress
Prednisone	Anti-inflammatory	Sliding scale according to disease (oral, intravenous, or rectal)	Euphoria, insomnia, gastrointestinal upset, acne, delayed wound healing, water retention, cataracts, ulcers, moon-faced appearance
Metronidazole (Flagyl)	Antibacterial	250 to 500 mg three times daily orally or intravenously	Nausea, vomiting, epigastric distress (do not take with alcohol)
Loperamide (Imodium)	Antidiarrheal	4 mg for one time, then 2 mg for each stool orally	Nausea, vomiting, constipation, drowsiness, fatigue, rash
Azathioprine (Imuran)	Immunosuppressant	1 mg/kg body weight daily orally	Leukopenia, bone marrow depression, nausea, vomiting, rash, stomatitis

lectomy and ileorectal anastomosis may be done.

When an operation is indicated for ulcerative colitis the surgical procedure may be dictated by the patient's physical condition, the type of complication, and the patient's personal preference. The operations of choice are a single-stage total proctocolectomy with construction of internal reservoir and valve **(Kock's pouch)** (Figure 66-2) or total proctocolectomy with **ileoanal anastomosis** with or without construction of an internal reservoir and temporary ileostomy (Figure 66-3). In the case of a poor-risk patient a subtotal colectomy with ileostomy may be performed. After the patient's recovery, in approximately 2 to 4 months, removal of the rectum or construction of an internal reservoir can be performed.

For years the surgical procedure of choice for acute ulcerative colitis was total proctocolectomy and permanent ileostomy. According to McLeod and

Fazio,[46] many patients view a permanent ileostomy as more forbidding than the disease itself. Despite reassurance, they prefer to live with the disease and long-term risk of cancer than undergo the procedure. On the other hand, some patients find that an ileostomy is a welcome relief to the frequent diarrhea. Patients will be most satisfied if they are fully informed and assist in the determination of the most appropriate surgical procedure.

Today ulcerative colitis patients have the choice and opportunity for a continence-saving procedure. Total abdominal colectomy and ileorectal anastomosis is a questionable procedure. It involves suturing the end of the small bowel to the top of the rectal stump.[43] Diseased tissue may remain in the rectum, and control of loose stools is unreliable. An alternative to this procedure is the total proctocolectomy and pull-through ileoanal anastomosis with pelvic reservoir. This involves removing all of the colon, the

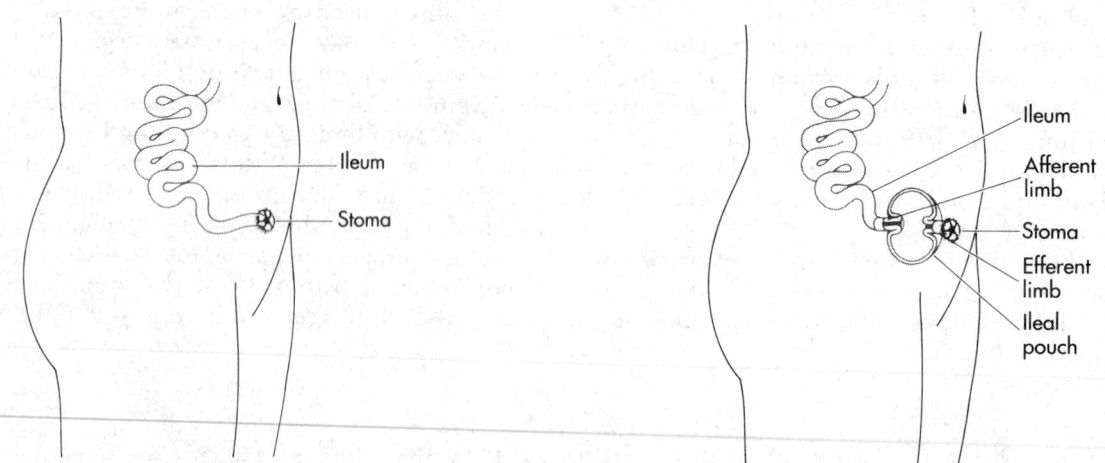

FIGURE 66-1   Total proctocolectomy with ileostomy.

FIGURE 66-2   Kock's continent ileostomy.

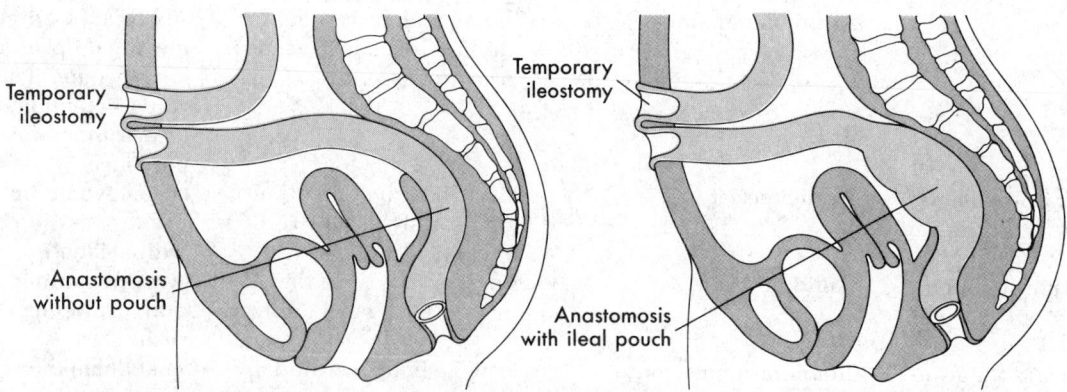

FIGURE 66-3   Ileoanal pull-through anastomosis with and without ileal pouch. Temporary ileostomy is formed until anastomosis heals.

upper part of the rectum, and the anal canal. The terminal portion of the ileum is anastomosed to the remaining portion of the anal canal. To prevent severe, debilitating diarrhea, an internal reservoir with a **J** shape, an **S** shape, or **W** shape is constructed from the ileum above the anus. To prevent pelvic infection and promote healing of the lines of anastomosis, a temporary abdominal loop ileostomy above the reservoir is constructed for bowel diversion. The ileostomy is closed 2 to 3 months after the initial surgery.

Crohn's disease accompanied by anal incontinence is a contraindication for the creation of an ileoanal reservoir. Crohn's disease can reappear in the reservoir with destructive results. The patient must be motivated by the possibility of not having a permanent ileostomy and be able to understand the disease process and available alternatives. Patients should understand the sometimes difficult and frustrating process of dealing with frequency and new bowel signals before they can attain continence. Complications include mucus discharge, frequency, night incontinence, bowel obstruction, pouchitis, bladder dysfunction, and other postoperative complications seen in abdominal surgery.

A secondary procedure, construction of Kock's pouch, involves the formation of a reservoir by suturing loops of adjacent ileum together to form a pouchlike structure. The bowel segment is then intussuscepted into the pouch and stapled in position. The result is the formation of a valve that holds the fecal contents in the pouch. The reservoir can store up to 500 mL of fluid, and the valve prevents involuntary evacuation until a tube is inserted to drain the pouch. A complication of Kock's pouch is breakdown of the valve, and an estimated 20% require additional surgery to correct this.[50] Other estimates put this complication rate at 40%.[43] Since this is a technically precise operation, complication rates may be related to the expertise of the surgical team. As a result of the above difficulties, the popularity of this procedure has decreased.

NURSING MANAGEMENT OF THE PATIENT WITH INFLAMMATORY BOWEL DISEASE
Assessment

The patient with inflammatory bowel disease is assessed for bowel elimination, knowledge of the disease process, support systems, coping abilities, nutritional status, pain, and ability to understand the disease process and treatment required.

Question the patient about previous bowel habits, including frequency and continence of stool. An understanding of the patient's past difficulties helps the nurse plan preoperative bowel preparation.

For the patient under medical management a complete understanding of the medical regimen is important. When the nurse is assessing the patient's knowledge, good questions to ask are "Tell me about your disease and your medicine" or "What has the doctor told you about your condition and treatment?" A knowledge deficit can often be identified with this type of questioning.

If surgery is planned, the nurse asks about the patient's understanding of the proposed surgery. At this time the nurse can assess the patient's expectations of the surgical outcome.

Before beginning to teach the patient assess the patient's ability to understand and comprehend a treatment program or surgical procedure. Sources of assessment data include the patient, family members, and other health care providers.

Pain management is essential during an acute phase of inflammatory bowel disease. The nurse might ask the patient about pain characteristics ("Is the pain constant, intermittent, relieved?"). Patients with Crohn's disease have abdominal pain when inflammation is present. Patients with ulcerative colitis have abdominal cramping and pain often relieved by defecation.

Family members and significant others can give helpful information about the patient concerning the home situation, habits, health, history, and ability to comply with treatment. This information will be necessary for long-term care planning. A lack of patient support systems may alter the patient's coping ability and compliance with a treatment program. Assess the patient's feelings about surgery. The patient may express feelings of anxiety, loss, powerlessness, and changes in body image.

When assessing nutritional status the nurse explores the patient's diet history. Give special attention to reports of anorexia, weight loss, and food intolerance (i.e., milk) that may aggravate the condition. Establish a baseline weight. Observe the patient's appearance for evidence of clinical signs of nutrient deficiencies. Assess serum electrolyte and albumin levels. Nutritional deficits can contribute to impaired healing and increased risk of infection.

During exacerbation of the disease observe for signs of dehydration and electrolyte imbalance. The patient may require hospitalization for fluid and electrolyte replacement and improvement of nutritional status.

Nursing Diagnosis

The following nursing diagnoses may be appropriate for the patient with inflammatory bowel disease during the preoperative phase of care:

Knowledge deficit of disease and treatment

Altered nutrition: less than body requirements related to bowel hypermotility and decreased absorption

Diarrhea related to bowel irritability

Fluid volume deficit related to diarrhea

Anxiety related to unknown disease outcomes

Powerlessness related to loss of control of body function

Impaired anal skin integrity related to frequency of diarrhea

Planning

Nursing care for the patient with inflammatory bowel disease is planned to achieve the following outcomes:

The patient will express understanding of the medical regimen

The patient will maintain a well-balanced diet

The patient will maintain fluid and electrolyte balance

The patient will have soft, formed stools

The patient will identify stressors and measures to reduce them

The patient will have control of intestinal function

The patient will have intact anal skin integrity

Implementation

Teach the patient the names of the medications, doses, routes, and when they are taken. Discuss side effects and who to call if a problem occurs. A complete understanding of the disease process and its implications increases treatment compliance and helps the patient in making appropriate decisions. If the patient is unable to understand, plan to instruct an appropriate caregiver. Patients with ulcerative colitis and Crohn's disease, in the acute phase, are often very ill and need a great deal of supportive nursing care and understanding. If there is little family support, identify community resources such as a community dietitian or home nursing service.

Interventions include examination of stressors in the patient's life and realistic ways to reduce them. Stress reduction exercises, such as progressive relaxation or cognitive therapy, may be therapeutic (see Chapter 3).

The patient in the acute phase may be weak enough to require assistance with activities of daily living. The nurse may need to help with basic hygiene and grooming needs. The patient's weakness may cause difficulty with mobility and require nursing assistance with ambulation. Have a bedpan or commode at the bedside available at all times. If odor is a problem as a result of frequent bowel movements, a room deodorizer may be used at the bedside. Supportive personnel and empathetic nursing care will ease the patient's adjustment through the diagnostic and treatment phases. Assist the patient with care of the anal area. Carefully cleanse and dry the area after each defecation. Breakdown

of anal tissue may require prescribed medications for treatment.

The patient with inflammatory bowel disease requires a high-protein, high-calorie, well-balanced diet. If the patient has diarrhea a low-fiber diet may be necessary to decrease peristalsis. Small frequent meals may be needed when poor appetite and intolerance to large amounts of food are noted. Monitor the patient's fluid balance and hydration. If lactose intolerance is suspected, eliminate milk products from the diet. The patient who is unable to tolerate oral foods may require total parenteral nutrition to sustain life.

It is best to use regularly scheduled analgesics during an acute exacerbation of the disease. Giving the pain medication on an as-needed basis may increase the anxiety level and decrease the pain threshold in an already anxious patient. Antianxiety drugs may help potentiate the effect of analgesics.

Preoperative care

When the decision for surgery has been made, specific goals for the patient might be as follows:

1. The patient will understand the proposed surgical alternatives and expected outcomes
2. The patient will demonstrate adaptive behaviors to cope with the surgical crisis
3. The patient will understand the reasons for preoperative bowel preparation

In preoperative teaching reinforce the physician's explanation of the surgical procedure and expected outcomes. The patient may need to discuss feelings and be reassured by the nurse that postoperative instruction on self-care will be done. If ostomy surgery is proposed, demonstrate the use and care of an ostomy pouch. Before surgery the patient's abdomen is marked for the appropriate stoma site. Stoma site selection can be done by the physician or by an enterostomal therapy nurse (see box on p. 1860). Reading material about ostomy care can be left for the patient and family.

The patient needs to know and understand that the physician may order a number of radiologic and laboratory tests to provide a baseline of the patient's physiologic function. Routinely a chest x-ray, urinalysis, complete blood count, and electrolyte studies are ordered before a major surgical procedure.[44] When cancer is suspected a more extensive workup including liver enzymes; liver, brain, or bone scans; computed tomography (CT scan); and carcinoembryonic antigen (CEA) titer may be ordered.

The decision to undergo surgery may be an extremely difficult one for the patient. The patient and the patient's support group may have lived through a series of disappointing remissions and exacerbations. Even with the knowledge that the surgery may cure, as in the case of ulcerative colitis, it is usually

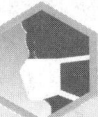

Ostomy Surgery

Nursing Interventions	Rationale
Assess knowledge of disease process and ostomy	Provides basis for teaching
Assess patient and family's internal resources and support	Need to know who can care for stoma; helpful to have assistance for patient if needed
Patient teaching: turn, cough, deep breathing, leg exercises; terms: ostomy, stoma, pouch	Prevention of postoperative complications
Determine stoma location	In rectus muscle, away from skin folds, umbilicus, bony prominences, scars; within field of vision
Assess sexuality patterns	Ostomy does not preclude previous patterns: cover stoma during sexual activity; empty pouch before encounters
Bowel preparation	Decreases postoperative wound infection and fistula development
Administer antibiotics	Decreases bacteria in intestinal lumen
Administer immunosuppressives, steroids	Decreases inflammatory response

Postoperative

Provide acceptance of patient and ostomy	Avoids or prevents feelings of rejection by nursing staff, family, friends
Assess vital signs	Hypotension possible from hypovolemia, blood loss
Assess electrolyte balance	Loss of H+ and K+ ions occurs with nasogastric suction
Monitor intake and output (urine, ostomy, tubes, drains)	Prevents fluid volume excess or deficit
Turn, cough, deep breathe, leg exercises	Prevents vascular and pulmonary complications
Pain management (medications, position, skin and wound care)	Permits patient to resume activities more quickly
Keep nasogastric tube patent	Prevents vomiting by keeping stomach decompressed
Provide oral hygiene	Prevents drying of mucous membranes
Assess for bowel sounds	Indicates return of bowel activity
Assess incisions for wound healing; aseptic dressing changes	Note color, healing, skin breakdown, redness, itching, burning
Skin care	Maintains skin integrity; may use skin barriers
Odor control	Rinse pouch daily with warm water and small amount of mouthwash; use room deodorizer; avoid asparagus, garlic, onions, fish, and eggs to decrease odor
Assist with ambulation	Promotes return of gastrointestinal function and improves circulation
Assess patient behaviors	Indicates coping abilities
Encourage verbalization of feelings	Establishes therapeutic relationship
Utilize dressing change and pouch change times for teaching stoma color and feel of stoma, skin appearance and cleansing, skin barrier, pouch application	Bright red to pink color is normal No nerve endings, no sensation
Encourage patient to participate in care	Promotes patient acceptance and independence
Teach ostomy care	Need for independence and control; independence promotes self-esteem
Advance diet as indicated	Intestinal tract must readjust postoperatively: avoid foods that produce gas and odor (yogurt and buttermilk decrease odor; well-balanced diet and protein needed for healing)
Diet: chew food thoroughly	Promotes more complete digestion
Administer medications in liquid form	Enteric-coated or timed-release medications may not be absorbed; liquid preparations readily absorbed from small intestine
Identify community resources; visit from an ostomate, United Ostomy Association	Provides information on life-style changes, adjustment

CRITERIA FOR STOMA SITE MARKING

Within the rectus abdominis muscle
Away from skin creases, folds, scars, or bony prominences
Where the patient can see the stoma
Either above or below the belt line

RESEARCH BRIEF

Hedrick JK: Effects of ET nursing intervention on adjustment following ostomy surgery, *J Enterostom Ther* 14:229, 1987.

The purpose of the study was to determine the enterostomal therapy (ET) nurse's impact on the ostomy patient's social readjustment and rehabilitation. The hypotheses were based on the theoretic model of crisis intervention. The treatment of the ostomy patient follows crisis theory and management. Within this framework it was hypothesized that short-term counseling by the ET nurse would improve the patient's level of adjustment 2 to 3 months postoperatively. The Maklebust Ostomy Adjustment Scale was used to measure the social readjustment of 40 postoperative ostomy patients. Half the subjects received counseling by the ET nurse, and half the subjects did not. The findings of the study supported the hypothesis that counseling and education by the ET nurse during the patient's hospitalization promoted feelings of well-being months after the crisis resolution. According to subject responses, the ET nurse plays a primary role in helping the patient toward successful postoperative social readjustment.

received as a shock. The patient may express feelings of anxiety, loss, and a sense of powerlessness. The most important need of the patient at this time is to be able to express feelings and misconceptions.[29] When an ostomy is required, a visitor from the United Ostomy Association can provide hope by representing someone who has traveled the same path and survived. The visitor is helpful in explaining information on life-style adjustments.

Based on findings that patients with a clean bowel have a lower incidence of postoperative sepsis, bowel preparation may be started 2 or 3 days preoperatively. This includes a low-residue to clear liquid diet and a bowel preparation of laxatives, an oral colonic lavage/electrolyte solution (i.e., GoLYTELY),[12] and enemas as ordered. The patient is given an antibiotic (neomycin or kanamycin) that is not absorbed systemically to decrease bacteria in the bowel. Before bowel preparation or any needed laboratory tests are done, explain how long they should take, what they are for, and what to expect.

Postoperative care

The immediate postoperative care of the patient who has undergone abdominal surgery initially involves primarily physical and metabolic assessment. Areas of assessment include bowel and urinary elimination, fluid balance, electrolyte balance, tissue perfusion, comfort/pain, nutrition, gas exchange, infection, and in the case of ostomy construction, assessment of the ileostomy and peristomal skin integrity.

Bowel elimination

After abdominal surgery bowel sounds and peristalsis may not resume for 3 to 5 days. Until this time the patient will require nasogastric suction to avoid nausea and vomiting of gastric secretions with potential aspiration and stress to the abdominal suture line. Nursing maintenance of the nasogastric tube with irrigation to provide patency may be required. When bowel function has resumed, accurately measure and record output. After an ileostomy, bowel

activity will begin within 24 to 48 hours postoperatively. Initiate appropriate ostomy care and teaching at this time.

Bowel diversion/ileostomy

Postoperative care of the patient with an ileostomy includes careful nursing observation of the stoma for color, size, type of stoma (loop or end), location on the abdomen, condition of the skin, and selection of an appliance.

The first pouch is placed over the stoma in the operating room. This pouch is clear for observation of the stoma and fecal contents.[29] Observe the stoma daily for change in color and size.

The healthy stoma will be red and slightly edematous. Report to the physician any color change from the normal red to dark blue or black or any rapid increase in stoma size. Because of high enzymatic content of the **effluent** (fecal discharge) select a pouch with a skin-protective barrier, adhesive backing, and pouch opening no more than ⅛ inch larger than the stoma.

When stool begins to pass into the pouch empty it when it is approximately one-third full. Allowing the pouch to fill to capacity can cause a break in the seal and pouch leakage. Because of the irritating effect of the effluent do not allow fecal matter to remain on the skin. Change a leaking pouch immediately.

The ileostomy effluent is liquid. The first drainage after surgery may be dark green and progress to yellowish brown as the patient is allowed to eat.

Nursing assessment with ostomy patients includes knowledge deficit, coping ability, grieving process, and sexual function. Helping the patient learn ostomy self-care, deal with the feelings of loss, and resume a normal life-style as a desirable person encompasses all of these areas.

The first step to ostomy self-care is having the patient look at the stoma. After this is accomplished gradually encourage the patient to assist with the care of emptying, cleaning, and changing the pouch until self-care is achieved. Teaching the pouch-change procedure in a systematic manner and with competence and compassion are vital nursing attributes. The patient often struggles with feelings of loss and faces learning something totally new. The nurse's acceptance of the patient and gentle guidance give the patient control of the situation and a sense of acceptability.

Promoting independence and self-care is vital but may not be possible if the patient is in a state of denial. Little learning can be done in this stage of the grief process. If the patient cannot progress to the point of willingness to learn, a caregiver needs to be taught the pouch-change procedure and care until the patient is ready to learn.

After discharge the patient changes the pouch every 5 to 7 days. This can be done before eating when the stoma is least active. At the time of the pouch change observe the skin for irritation or skin erosion. Use of an antacid, skin protective powder, or liquid skin barrier is appropriate if skin irritation is present.

Before discharge have the patient demonstrate cleaning and changing of the pouch and verbalize where to obtain ostomy supplies and for what to ask. Ensure that the patient has the name of a resource person in case of problems and the telephone number of the local ostomy support group.

The patient may shower or bathe with or without the pouch in place. After discharge the patient can resume normal activities except for lifting objects of more than 10 pounds. The stoma needs to be measured each time supplies are ordered to ensure that the pouch opening is the appropriate size. Stomas tend to shrink over time.

A special diet is not necessary, but the patient is encouraged to drink 8 to 10 glasses of fluid per day and to chew food well. Caution the patient to eat small amounts of such foods as peanuts, whole corn, celery, mushrooms, Chinese vegetables, and fresh fruit peels and pulp. These foods have been known to cause stomal blockage (see box). Encourage the

patient to eat potassium-rich foods. Removal of the colon disrupts water and electrolyte absorption. This places the patient at higher risk for dehydration and electrolyte imbalance.

The incidence of impotence as a result of nerve damage following total proctocolectomy for ulcerative colitis or Crohn's disease in the male is low if the surgery is done by a knowledgeable surgeon. Sexual relationships can be resumed when the physician deems it not harmful to the surgical area. The patient is cautioned to empty the pouch before intercourse and, if desired, wear a pouch cover or brief garment to detract notice from the appliance. Because an ostomy affects a person's self-concept and image, there may be a psychologic impact on sexual function. Fear of acceptability can decrease sexual ability and libido.[32] Counseling may be appropriate for these patients.

Kock's pouch

Postoperative care of the patient with Kock's pouch is similar to that for any patient undergoing major abdominal surgery. A drainage catheter is left in place in the pouch for 2 to 4 weeks. Nursing care includes irrigation of the catheter with 20 mL of saline every 3 to 4 hours. After the tube is removed teach the patient intermittent intubation using a 28 Fr catheter. Have the patient return the demonstration to ensure that all questions and concerns have been answered.

Ileoanal reservoir

The patient with an ileoanal reservoir will have a temporary ileostomy for 6 to 12 weeks and needs to be taught ostomy self-care. During this period there may be mucous discharge from the rectum. Teach the patient to gently cleanse, dry, and apply a protective ointment to the perirectal area. Irrigation of the reservoir with a catheter and syringe can be taught, as well as Kegel perineal and sphincter exercises to maintain muscle tone used for continence.

When the temporary ileostomy is closed, the patient will have frequent stools and will need aggressive prophylactic perianal skin care. Gentle cleansing, the cautious use of a hair dryer to dry the perianal area, and application of protective ointment or skin barrier is recommended. Sitz baths and Domeboro's solution soaks can help if skin irritation occurs.

Diet instruction after closure of the ileostomy includes elimination of foods known to increase bowel activity and the addition of foods that slow activity. Patients are encouraged to increase amounts of bananas, cheese, boiled rice, tapioca, and creamy peanut butter in their diets and to avoid highly spiced foods, raw foods, red wine, and fruit juices (see box on p. 1862). Some surgeons advocate increased fiber in the diet and decreased sugar intake. Diet lists are

DIETARY CONSIDERATIONS FOR THE OSTOMY PATIENT

Constipation may be a problem. If it occurs:
  Increase fluid intake
  Eat cooked fruits and vegetables, bran, raisins, or prunes
  Exercise
Foods that may cause diarrhea
  Green beans, broccoli, spinach, prunes, beans, cabbage
  Highly spiced foods
  Raw foods
  Red wines
If diarrhea occurs, avoid the diarrhea-causing foods listed above; eat:
  Bananas, applesauce
  Tapioca
  Boiled rice
  Creamy peanut butter
  Baked potatoes, white bread
  Hard cheese
  Tea
High-fiber foods that can cause blockage in the ileostomy patient
  Popcorn, corn on cob, whole corn
  Celery
  Fresh vegetables

  Wild rice, whole grains
  Chinese vegetables
  Coconut, dried fruit, fruit peels
  Potato skins
  Meat with casings
  Nuts and kernels
Foods that cause stoma odor
  Broccoli
  Baked beans
  Onions, asparagus, cabbage
  Eggs, fish
  Blue and cheddar cheese
  Alcohol/beer
  Turnips
Foods that cause gas
  Beans
  Mushrooms
  Cucumbers
  Onions
  Radishes
  Cabbage
  Milk and milk products
  Beer, carbonated beverages
  Cauliflower

helpful teaching aids. Leave these with the patient. Medications include bulk-forming agents such as psyllium hydrophilic mucilloid (Metamucil) and antidiarrheals. The patient is asked not to respond to every urge to defecate. With increased pouch capacity the number of bowel movements decreases. Night incontinence may occur, and a pad may need to be worn. The single greatest factor that seems to decrease the number of stools per day is time. As weeks pass, stools per day decrease.

The ileoanal reservoir is an alternative procedure to a permanent ileostomy, but it takes many months to accomplish continence and requires patience and a great desire not to wear a pouch.

Peristomal skin integrity

Nursing assessment of the peristomal skin is important. If the stoma site is not marked or placed in the best area for pouch adherence, the patient is at greater risk for damage to the epidermis in the per-isotomal peristomal area.

Loss of peristomal skin integrity may be associated with four primary factors: allergies, mechanical trauma, chemical reactions, and infection. Although less common, peristomal skin breakdown may be associated with the primary disease of the patient, such as fistulas from Crohn's disease.

Allergic response

Sensitivities to pouches, adhesives, skin barriers, powders, or belts may occur. When the nurse first observes the site, the skin will appear red, eroded, weeping, and bleeding. Generally the skin irritation will be limited to the area of contact. Look for a pattern effect, such as where taping is done or where the plastic of the pouch touches the skin. Avoidance of the irritant by changing the type of pouch, tape, or adhesive may resolve the problem.

Mechanical trauma

Mechanical trauma is attributed to pressure, friction, or stripping of adhesives and skin barriers from the skin. The most common causes are frequent pouch changes with stripping of the epidermis, overuse of adhesive tapes, and use of a belt worn too tightly. Change a secure pouching system once or twice per week. Use adhesive tape to picture frame the pouch judiciously. Wear a belt only when there are problems with the pouch seal leaking. Remove the pouch slowly and carefully while supporting the skin with the fingertips.

Chemical irritants

The most common chemical irritant is the stool from the stoma. Small bowel effluent contains proteolytic digestive enzymes. Exposure of the skin to the effluent can cause skin irritation in less than 1 hour. Nursing treatment is the application of an appropriate pouch that stays adhered 4 to 7 days. The use of a skin barrier (i.e., Stomahesive) cut to stoma size may be helpful. To treat weeping areas apply Stomahesive powder and liquid skin barrier (i.e., Skin Prep) before securing the pouch. The use of a "caulking paste" (i.e., Stomahesive Paste) may be needed to fill creases where leaking can occur.

Infection

A common infection of the peristomal skin is caused by *Candida albicans.*[7] The skin will, on initial nursing assessment, appear bright red with papular and vesicular lesions. Small satellite vesicles are common, giving the appearance of a rash on the outer perimeter of the infected area. The patient often complains of itching. Persons who have been taking antibiotics for 5 or more days are prone to this problem. When *Candida* is identified, assess other body areas, particularly skin folds and the perineal area, for infection. The physician will order nystatin powder or cream. When this medication is used, a liquid skin barrier is applied over the area before pouch application to ensure adherence of the adhesive.

Evaluate the treatment implemented in 2 or 3 days at the time of pouch removal. Daily contact with the patient in the hospital or by the home care nurse may be needed if there are still difficulties with the pouch seal.

Teach the patient or caregiver the appropriate care (i.e., pouch change, cleansing, irrigation, skin care) and observe a return demonstration. Provide the patient with a list of resource people, telephone numbers, where to obtain supplies, and what to ask for.

Evaluation

Evaluation of knowledge and understanding can be done by having the patient verbalize understanding of the disease and medical regimen. Support systems and coping abilities may be evaluated by discussion concerning treatment compliance with the patient or caregiver and asking about the general home situation. Evaluation of the nutritional status may continue with regular weights and reassessment of electrolyte and albumin levels.

When surgery is imminent and preoperative teaching has been implemented, evaluation may be done by having the patient verbalize understanding of the proposed surgery and expectations. Coping abilities may be evaluated by the patient's readiness to discuss surgery and willingness to participate in self-care.

Documentation

The nurse documents evidence of stability of vital signs, hydration status, bowel sounds, and the appearance of the stoma in the early postoperative period. Record the amount, color, and consistency of the stomal drainage. Record the patient's response to analgesics, tolerance of foods, and ability to select a well-balanced diet. Document the patient's participation in care of the stoma and peristomal skin, performance of acts of daily living, and the daily weight. Describe the patient's ability to cope with the stoma. Document questions the patient asks and the answers given. Describe the patient's and family's response to the teaching provided.

Ongoing Care

Many patients with inflammatory bowel disease or massive gastrointestinal resection experience months, years, or even a lifetime of inadequate nutrient absorption. For these people, programs are available to provide parenteral infusion in the home setting. Although cost is high, it is less expensive than hospitalization (see Chapter 16). The home care nurse is a resource for the care provided by the patient and family. Infusions, by pump, can be administered at night in an 8- to 12-hour period. This leaves the daytime for a normal life-style. The ostomy patient may need continued teaching after discharge until ready to assume self-care. The home care nurse is able to provide this on a short-term basis. Emphasis is placed on teaching ostomy self-care and promoting independence.[5]

ACUTE APPENDICITIS
Definition

Appendicitis, an inflammatory disease of the colon, refers to the inflammation of the appendix vermiformis.

It is rare before the age of 2 years and reaches a peak incidence in the second and third decades. The majority of patients are between the ages of 5 and 30 years. The disease is important, because it is common and curable. The difficulty lies in making a differential diagnosis.

Etiology

The initiating event in acute appendicitis appears to be obstruction, followed by increased intraluminal pressure, reduced venous drainage, thrombosis, hemorrhage, edema, and bacterial invasion of the wall of the appendix. As the process proceeds, the appendiceal artery becomes occluded as a result of the inflammation and venous stasis and perforation result.

Calculi are thought to be the most common cause of the initial obstruction. Obstruction by parasites, lymphoid hyperplasia, and twisting of the appendix by adhesions have also been incriminated.

Pathophysiology

In the early stages the appendix may appear only slightly swollen, but as the disease advances, it becomes hyperemic, warm, and covered with exudate. In the late stages it becomes gangrenous and may perforate. Microscopically, the picture ranges from acute inflammatory changes with superficial mucosal ulcerations to one or more perforations. Increased intraluminal pressure, transmural swelling, and inflammation eventually compromise the appendiceal end artery and cause perforation.

Clinical Manifestations

The history of a patient with appendicitis is of short duration—between 12 and 48 hours from onset to hospitalization. Most patients first report pain at onset, classically referred to the epigastric or periumbilical areas and later localized in the right lower quadrant at McBurney's point (midway between the umbilicus and the right anterior iliac crest). This sequence of pain location is found in about half of the patients. A significant number may have diffuse or lower abdominal pain or referred pain that makes the diagnosis more difficult. With perforation, pain may subside to generalized abdominal discomfort. Anorexia and nausea (with or without vomiting) are the second and third most common symptoms. Temperature may range from 100° to 101° F and increase if perforation occurs. The abdomen may be tender to touch. Blood studies show leukocytosis. A calcified fecalith in the right lower quadrant on flat film of the abdomen is helpful for diagnosis.

When diagnosis is difficult, appendicitis may be confused with other conditions causing acute abdominal pain such as diverticular abscess and rupture, ectopic pregnancy, or intestinal obstruction. In some cases, ultrasound and laparoscopy are used to diagnose appendicitis.

Therapeutic Management

Unless strongly contraindicated, the only therapy for acute appendicitis is prophylactic use of antibiotics and surgical removal of the appendix. Since mortality correlates with perforation and perforation correlates with duration of symptoms, early diagnosis and appendectomy are essential for the lowest acceptable morbidity and mortality. When surgery is performed early in the disease in an otherwise healthy individual, mortality is only slightly above that for general anesthesia.

If perforation is very likely, nasogastric suction is started and antibiotics are given. The decision to institute drainage of an abscess is made during surgery. Complications include wound infection, intraabdominal abscess, and mechanical small bowel obstruction.

NURSING MANAGEMENT OF THE PATIENT WITH ACUTE APPENDICITIS
Assessment

On admission the patient is placed on bed rest and is given nothing by mouth. Since the medical goal is to identify the problem or make a differential diagnosis several tests are ordered and a history and physical examination are performed.

Assessment of the patient's knowledge can be accomplished by questioning the patient and family about their understanding of the situation. The nurse can decrease the patient's and family's anxiety level by carefully explaining each test, what to expect, and the reason for the test. The nurse may fill in information or answer questions concerning possible outcomes of the testing.

A history of the patient's last oral intake and frequency of emesis is obtained. Serum electrolytes are assessed. The patient will be given nothing by mouth until the decision to do surgery is made. Intravenous fluids may be started. If vomiting is a problem a nasogastric tube is inserted, suction initiated, and the tube kept patent. If electrolyte studies show imbalances, intravenous medication corrections are ordered.

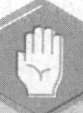 **CLINICAL ALERT**

Nurses are cautioned to avoid applying heating pads or administering cathartics, laxatives, or enemas to patients with acute appendicitis. The resulting stimulation of the bowel may precipitate rupture of the inflamed appendix, increase morbidity and mortality, and prolong hospitalization.

Pain is assessed as part of the differential diagnosis as previously discussed. Although the patient has pain, the physician may choose not to give pain medication because the analgesic may mask symptoms while a diagnosis is being made. Sudden cessation of pain may indicate that the appendix has ruptured.

The temperature, blood pressure, pulse, and respirations are monitored every hour. Symptoms of nausea, vomiting, pain, abdominal distention, leukocytosis, elevated temperature, tachycardia, diaphoresis, and hypotension may indicate peritonitis. Report any of the above symptoms to the physician, and document this information. Preoperative antibiotics will be ordered and given intravenously.

Nursing Diagnosis

The following nursing diagnoses may be appropriate for the patient with acute appendicitis:

Knowledge deficit related to disease process and surgery

Fluid volume deficit related to vomiting

Pain related to inflammation

High risk for infection related to rupture of appendix

Planning

Nursing care for the patient with appendicitis is planned to meet the following outcomes:

The patient will maintain fluid balance

The patient will express understanding of the disease process and the possibility of a surgical procedure

The patient will express understanding of the reason pain medication is withheld

The patient will be free of infection

Implementation

When peritonitis or abscess is not a problem, postoperative recovery is relatively uncomplicated. Areas addressed are fluid volume and nutritional deficit, pain, and the risk for infection.

The physician may order oral fluids and diet as tolerated 24 to 48 hours after surgery. If these are tolerated well, intravenous fluids are discontinued and medications are given orally. Urine output is measured to determine adequacy of intake and renal perfusion.

Pain medications are given intramuscularly or intravenously as ordered until the patient can take them orally. Instruct the patient to inform the nurse when pain occurs, and if pain medication is given, inquire if relief was obtained. Intravenous patient-controlled analgesia may be used until the patient can be given oral medications. This method of anal-

gesic administration is becoming more common, and studies have shown that pain is more controlled and the total narcotic amount used by patients is often less than with other methods of administration (see Chapter 14).

Nursing assessment includes body temperature, leukocyte count, and occurrence of pain, tenderness, or swelling at the incision site. Antibiotics may be ordered intravenously and then by mouth when tolerated. The patient needs to be instructed at discharge concerning medication, schedule, and dosage.

The patient is ambulated the first postoperative day and may be discharged on the third to fifth day if no problems arise. If abscess or peritonitis has occurred, the hospital stay will be longer. This patient may have drains and a nasogastric tube and require intravenous antibiotics for approximately 5 days. Monitor fluid volume and electrolyte balance as well as signs and symptoms of infection. The wound may be left open with orders to change the packing several times daily. During the packing change, assess for wound healing and evidence of infection. If the patient is discharged before complete closure of the wound, teach the patient or family how to change the packing and assess the wound. (See postoperative nursing management under ulcerative colitis.)

Documentation

For the patient with appendicitis or appendectomy document the location, intensity, frequency, and factors that relieve the pain. Record the patient's ability to ambulate and tolerate foods. Record the appearance of the wound (color, temperature, intactness, drainage). Describe the discharge and follow-up instructions given to the patient.

DIVERTICULAR DISEASE
Definition

Diverticular disease has two clinical forms, diverticulosis and diverticulitis. In **diverticulosis,** bulging pouches (diverticula) in the gastrointestinal wall push the mucosal lining through the surrounding muscle. The common sites for diverticula are in the descending and sigmoid colon, but they may develop anywhere from the proximal end of the pharynx to the anus. In **diverticulitis,** diverticula are inflamed and may cause obstruction, infection, and hemorrhage (Figure 66-4).

Diverticulosis is found in approximately 30 million people in the United States and is often asymptomatic. About 30% of the population over 60 years and 60% of the population over 80 years are found to have diverticular disease. The incidence is increasing.[14] Treatment is primarily medical. Technically, diverticulitis is a form of inflammatory bowel disease, although the literature for the most part does not use this terminology. It sometimes requires surgical intervention.

Etiology

Diverticular disease is most common over the age of 40 years and rarely occurs in younger persons. The incidence increases with age. Sex differentiation is unclear. The diverticula probably result from high intraluminal pressure on weak areas in the gastrointestinal wall where blood vessels enter. The left colon has more solid feces and decreased ability to move stool through the lumen.

Diet seems to play a large role in the development and prevention of diverticulosis. A diet high in fiber produces a large, bulky fecal mass that requires shorter transit time in the bowel and keeps intracolonic pressures within normal range. Fiber helps maintain a larger lumen and increases motility. The fact that diverticulosis is most prevalent in Western industrialized nations, where processing removes much of the roughage from foods, supports the theory that diverticula are encouraged by low-residue diets. In countries where food contains more natural bulk and fiber, diverticulosis is rare.

In diverticulitis undigested food mixes with bacteria and accumulates in the diverticular sac, forming a hard mass (fecalith). This mass cuts off the blood supply to the thin walls of the sac, making them more susceptible to attack by bacteria. Inflammation follows and may lead to perforation, abscess, peritonitis, obstruction, and hemorrhage. Occasionally, the inflamed colon may produce a fistula by adhering to the bladder or other organ.

Clinical Manifestations

Diverticulosis usually produces no symptoms but on occasion causes recurrent pain in the left lower quadrant without clinical evidence of acute diverticulitis. Such pain, often accompanied by constipation alternating with diarrhea, is often relieved by defecation or passing of flatus.

Common symptoms of diverticulitis include cramplike pain in the left lower quadrant of the abdomen or midabdominal pain radiating to the back; increased flatus; rectal bleeding; and signs of partial obstruction such as chronic constipation alternating with diarrhea, abdominal distention, anorexia, and low-grade fever. Nausea and vomiting may occur as the severity of the obstruction increases. A walled-off abscess will cause localized abdominal pain and tenderness. Rupture occurs in an estimated 20% of patients with diverticulitis.[14] These patients generally initially exhibit abdominal rigidity and pain in the left lower quadrant of the abdomen. Peritonitis occurs after fecal matter seeps from the rupture site

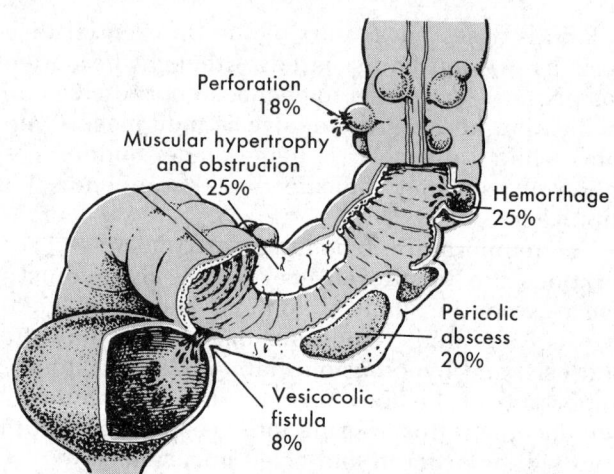

FIGURE 66-4   Complications of diverticulitis.

and causes sepsis with high fever, chills, hypotension, and elevated white blood cell count and erythrocyte sedimentation rate.

Peritonitis

Peritonitis is an inflammation of the abdominal peritoneum. Despite advances in antimicrobial therapy and supportive care, peritonitis remains a major contributor to the mortality of the patient with a disorder of the small or large bowel.

The development of peritonitis may be traced to one of two causes—bacterial invasion or chemical irritation. Bacterial invasion may be caused by a perforated or strangulated bowel. Examples include diverticular abscess and rupture, acute appendicitis with rupture, and strangulated hernia. Rupture of the intestine permits bowel contents and bacterial contaminants to enter the peritoneal cavity. This contamination quickly overwhelms the patient's defenses. Chemical irritation may be caused by materials such as blood, bile, necrotic tissue, pancreatic enzymes, talcum powder, or other foreign bodies. These materials cause a "sterile" inflammation and in the case of bacterial contamination can potentiate the problem.

Peritonitis occasionally heals spontaneously but usually requires aggressive therapy, including correction of the contamination, removal of the chemical irritant by surgery, and parenteral antibiotics. The formation of walled-off abscesses and development of extensive adhesions may be caused by peritonitis.

Therapeutic Management

Diagnosis of diverticulosis is made by barium enema. This procedure allows visualization of the outpouchings as well as distortions and narrowing of the lumen.[40] Barium enema needs to be done cautiously when diverticulitis is suspected. If bowel perforation is suspected a water-soluble contrast medium (i.e., Gastrografin or Hypaque) is used. These agents are absorbed from the peritoneal cavity. However, they have high osmolality and may dehydrate the patient and irritate the gastrointestinal mucosa. Colonoscopy may be of benefit in diagnosing certain cases, particularly in ruling out carcinoma. CT scan or ultrasound may be used to detect abscess formation.

The frequency of acute attacks can be reduced if the person is able to maintain soft stools at regular intervals. Hydrophilic colloids or bulk-forming laxatives (e.g., Metamucil) are good for this purpose. Diet management includes addition of fruits, vegetables, coarse cereal, bran, and plenty of fluids to increase bowel motility and decrease intraluminal pressures.[39] In the case of a mild attack with pain the patient may respond to a liquid or bland diet and stool softeners to minimize irritation. After pain subsides patients benefit from a high-fiber diet and bulk-forming medication.

During acute attacks conservative medical management such as antibiotics and bed rest is prescribed. Nothing by mouth is ordered to rest the bowel. Analgesics may be necessary. Morphine increases intracolonic pressure and is contraindicated in acute diverticular disease. Meperidine (Demerol) is preferred because it decreases intracolonic pressure.[14] The patient with diverticulitis exacerbation who does not respond to antibiotics and bed rest may require hospitalization with nasogastric drainage, parenteral fluids, and intravenous antibiotics.

Surgical treatment

Surgery is advised if long-term problems do not respond to medical management and is mandatory if complications such as hemorrhage, obstruction, abscesses, or perforation occur. A **colostomy** is surgically created by diverting the bowel to a stoma on the abdominal wall. When perforation, abscess, peritonitis, or fistula occurs, resection of the bowel with a temporary colostomy is required. Diversion of the stool allows for resolution of infection before closure of the colostomy.

Emergency surgery may not allow time for ideal bowel preparation or stoma site marking if a colostomy is necessary. In elective surgery a thorough bowel preparation is most important. The patient may be on a low-residue or clear liquid diet before surgery. Antibiotics are given orally and parenterally. Laxatives, enemas, or osmotic purgatives (GoLYTELY, Colyte, and Kleen-prep), as previously discussed, are given to cleanse the bowel.

Some controversy exists regarding the one-stage, two-stage, and three-stage surgical procedures. In the one-stage procedure resection of the affected bowel with anastomosis and without a diverting colostomy is performed. In the two-stage procedure resection of the diseased bowel is combined with a diverting colostomy. Colostomy closure is the second and final stage 6 weeks to several months later. The outmoded and little-used three-stage procedure includes a diverting colostomy, subsequent resection when inflammation has subsided, and closure when the anastomosis is healed. According to Finlay and Carter,[13] a multiple-stage procedure is generally much safer than a single-stage procedure, because

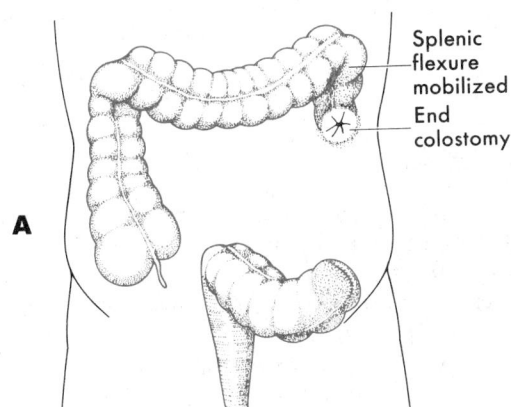
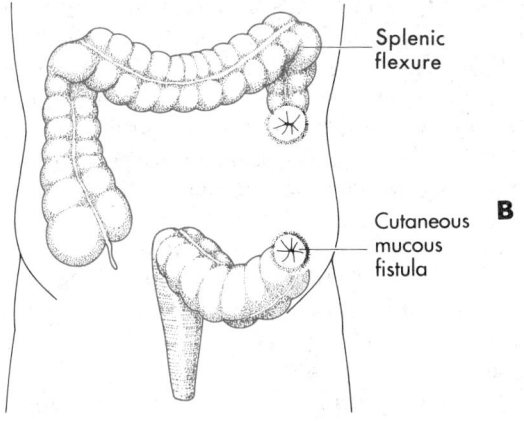

FIGURE 66-5 **A,** Hartmann's procedure. Descending colon is resected, and proximal end is brought to abdominal wall surface. **B,** Colon resection with proximal end colostomy and distal mucous fistula.

of the severe degree of inflammation usually present with diverticulitis and the difficulties this often causes in healing of an anastomosis. The two-stage procedure seems to be the most popular, since it requires only two surgeries while providing a safe, conservative approach to the situation.

Two types of bowel diversion can be used for resection with diverticulitis. The first is the descending colostomy with formation of either a **Hartmann's pouch** or a mucous fistula. In this instance the bowel is separated and the proximal end is brought up through the abdominal wall as an end colostomy. The distal portion (rectal stump) is either closed and stabilized in the pelvic cavity forming a blind Hartmann's pouch or is brought up to the abdominal surface and sutured to the skin forming a second (nonfunctioning) stoma called a mucous fistula (Figure 66-5).

The second, less-used procedure, is the loop colostomy (see Figure 66-9, *D*), which can be done anywhere proximal to the resected area but is usually placed in the transverse colon. When the loop colostomy is constructed the bowel is brought up through the abdominal surface, and a supporting rod or bridge is placed under the segment. At that time the bowel can be opened and sutured in surgery, or the bowel may be opened postoperatively by way of cautery. Removal of the affected bowel segment and reanastomosis of the bowel are done during the initial procedure.

NURSING MANAGEMENT OF THE PATIENT WITH DIVERTICULAR DISEASE
Assessment

The nurse assesses the patient for knowledge of the disease process, nutritional status, support systems, and pain. The patient's knowledge level about the disease is assessed. If surgery is planned ask about the patient's and family's understanding of the procedure and the patient's expected surgical outcome.

When assessing nutritional status the nurse explores the diet history and notes the patient's appearance, weight, hemoglobin, hematocrit, and albumin levels. Discuss and reinforce diet teaching concerning foods that aggravate diverticulitis (see boxes).

Identification of the patient's support system helps the nurse better understand the situation and include significant others in the care plan. A lack of support systems may decrease the patient's coping abilities and treatment compliance.

Abdominal pain is often the primary symptom of diverticulitis. The nurse may explore information about factors that appear to initiate pain. These factors may include certain types of food, whether the pain is constant or intermittent, and where the pain is located.

FOODS TO AVOID WITH DIVERTICULITIS

Popcorn, corn on cob, and whole corn
Celery
Fresh vegetables
Wild rice, whole grains
Chinese vegetables
Coconut, dried fruit, and fruit peels
Potato skins
Meat with casings
Nuts and kernels

Foods that cause stoma odor
Broccoli
Baked beans
Onions, asparagus, cabbage
Eggs, fish
Blue and cheddar cheese
Alcohol and beer
Turnips

HIGH-FIBER FOODS FOR DIVERTICULOSIS

Whole-grain cereals and breads
Beans
Peas
Fresh vegetables
Fresh fruit
Broccoli/brussels sprouts
Potatoes/potato skins, wild rice

Nursing Diagnosis

The following nursing diagnoses may be appropriate for the patient with diverticular disease in the preoperative phase of care:

Knowledge deficit related to disease process and treatment

Altered nutrition: less than body requirements related to decreased oral intake

Alteration in bowel elimination: constipation or diarrhea related to the inflammatory process

Abdominal pain related to obstruction of the bowel

Anxiety related to concerns about surgery

Planning

Nursing care for the patient with diverticulitis is planned to meet the following outcomes:

The patient will describe the diverticular disease process and treatment regimen

The patient will list foods to be included and avoided in a diet plan

The patient will have adequate nutritional intake

The patient will have absence of constipation or diarrhea

The patient will express relief of pain

The patient will describe the reason for surgery and its expected outcome

Implementation

Identification and inclusion of family or significant others in the teaching process are done by the nursing staff. Compliance with treatment often is affected by the person who prepares the meals and affects the patient's thoughts, feelings, and activity.

When instructing the patient and family the nurse includes an explanation of diverticula and how they form. The nurse ensures that the patient knows what signs and symptoms to watch for in an acute diverticulitis attack. Include a discussion of stool softeners and bulk-forming medications, how they are taken, and how often. The nursing staff or dietitian discusses the need for a well-balanced diet. Instruction in dietary roughage and encouragement of intake of food high in fiber is the basis of prevention in the medical phase. The patient avoids foods with seeds, because they may become trapped in the diverticula and initiate the inflammatory process. If the patient has inflammation, instruction about a bland, low-residue diet is provided.

The nurse can help the patient better understand the need for multiple procedures, a possible colostomy, and what that means. Include an explanation of all diagnostic tests (i.e., hematocrit, hemoglobin, electrolytes, x-ray studies), what they are for, what to expect, and how long the tests will take. General preoperative teaching includes deep breathing and leg exercises as well as pain control procedures.

Although the situation often is a surgical emergency in diverticular abscess or rupture, bowel preparation and stoma site marking are appropriate if time allows.

During the medical treatment phase of diverticular disease, a follow-up visit for evaluation of the treatment plan may be needed. At this time, careful review of the patient's and family's understanding of the treatment regimen can be done by having them verbalize their understanding of the treatment and how they have been following recommendations.

When surgery is planned have the patient verbalize reasons for surgery and the possibility of a temporary colostomy.

Postoperative care

The immediate postoperative nursing care for the patient with diverticular disease is as previously discussed in the section on inflammatory bowel disease. This section discusses the postoperative care in abdominal surgery that primarily involves physical and metabolic assessment as the patient recovers and the skin care of the peristomal area when an ostomy is performed. For nursing management of the patient with a temporary colostomy, see p. 1885. With the high incidence of fecal contamination, infection is a major concern for the patient undergoing surgery for diverticular abscess or rupture.

Infection

Observe for abscesses, purulent drainage, and fecal material around all wound and drain sites. Body temperature and white blood cell count are monitored, and any swelling, reddened, or painful area is reported. Often the abdominal wound is left open when peritonitis is present at the time of surgery, and meticulous wound care is mandatory. Because this wound may take weeks to close, wound care needs to be taught to the patient, family members, or caregivers for follow-up care after hospital discharge. Evaluation of wound care instruction is best done by having the caregiver/family return the demonstration as the nurse observes.

Evaluation

Evaluation of the patient includes determination of the return to normal body temperature and absence of abscess formation or drainage of purulent or fecal material from drain or wound sites. When a colostomy is performed the patient or caregiver needs to verbalize and demonstrate understanding of the ostomy care to the nurse. Have the patient and family demonstrate appropriate peristomal skin care and verbalize where to obtain ostomy supplies and support when needed.

Documentation

Document vital signs, hydration status, and daily weights. Describe the wound appearance and drainage with each dressing change. Record the patient's tolerance of ambulation, pain management strategies, and nutritional progress. Document patient teaching, return demonstrations, and the need for follow-up care or teaching.

Ongoing Care

Closure of the temporary colostomy is the desired goal in the case of diverticular disease. Usually this is done from 6 to 12 weeks after the initial surgical

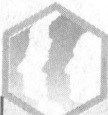

GERIATRIC CONSIDERATIONS

Colostomy Care

For the older person do not rush the teaching of colostomy care.[39] If discharge from the hospital is medically indicated before the patient has mastered colostomy care, there are several options. A family member may be taught to help the patient until self-care can be assumed, keeping in mind that the ultimate goal is patient independence. The expectation of independence may be more disruptive to the dependent family unit than simply resuming usual family routine. When no family member is available, the nurse may need to initiate a home care referral so the teaching process can go on after discharge. For the elderly patient, learning is often easier in a familiar environment. In some cases, referral to an extended care facility may be necessary to allow more time for recovery and learning.

procedure. Bowel preparation for closure includes a liquid diet several days before hospitalization for closure, laxatives, or intestinal lavage as previously mentioned, and the use of colostomy irrigation of the proximal and distal ends of the stoma for cleansing. A small amount of fluid used as a rectal enema may be appropriate. Fluid used for irrigation of the distal loop (mucous fistula) will usually return from both the distal opening and the rectum so placement of the patient on the toilet or bedpan is important during the procedure.

The patient will remain hospitalized for 5 to 8 days after closure depending on return of bowel activity. Remind the patient that intravenous fluids and a nasogastric tube will be used for the first few days postoperatively. Before discharge, a discussion and review of the high-fiber diet are appropriate.

ABDOMINAL WALL HERNIA
Definition

A **hernia** is a protrusion of the abdominal cavity contents through a congenital, acquired, or postoperative defect in the muscle wall of the abdomen. The most common sites for herniation are the inguinal, umbilical, femoral, and ventral or surgical incision areas (Figure 66-6).

Etiology/Clinical Manifestations

Most hernias result from congenital or acquired weakness of the abdominal wall, increased intraabdominal pressure from coughing or straining, or an enlarging lesion within the abdomen. Once the hernia has been formed, enlargement is usually progressive.

The term *reducible* refers to the ability to return the bulging hernia sac to the abdominal cavity when the patient is in a supine position. If the sac becomes larger than the opening in the muscle wall the hernia is nonreducible (incarcerated) and is at risk for circulatory restriction of the tissue (strangulation) with increased swelling, abdominal pain, necrosis, and bowel obstruction.

Inguinal hernias occur three times more frequently in men than women. The most common type is the indirect inguinal hernia. This type is caused by a weakness in the abdominal wall opening through which the spermatic cord emerges in men and the round ligament emerges in women. The hernia will extend down through the inguinal canal and onto the scrotum or labia. A direct inguinal hernia often occurs in older men and results from sac contents passing through the posterior inguinal wall. In either case abdominal contents, usually omentum or intestine, descend into the groin, scrotum, or labia, creating a mass. Pain and urinary frequency may occur.

An umbilical hernia is caused by a defect in the umbilicus at birth or a weakness in the rectus abdominis muscle. Small protrusions less than 1.5 cm may close spontaneously, but larger defects require surgical closure. Adult umbilical hernias are more common in women, are more commonly seen during pregnancy, and often are associated with obesity.

Femoral herniation is felt as a mass or bulge below the inguinal ligament and is more common in older women who have had children. The hernia is small with a narrow neck and prone to incarcerate and strangulate.

Ventral hernias occur in surgical incisions. Factors such as age, wound infection, malnutrition, obesity, increased intra-abdominal pressure, or abdominal distention influence the formation of ventral hernias. The location of the incision is also important. Transverse incisions are associated with fewer hernias than longitudinal incisions, and upper abdomen incisions are associated with fewer hernias than lower abdomen incisions. Incisional hernias associated with a colostomy or ileostomy may cause difficulty with bowel movement, colostomy irrigation, and ostomy pouch application.

Therapeutic Management

Hernias that cause no discomfort can often be left unrepaired, but the patient is warned about the importance of seeking medical advice promptly in the event of complications. Increasing size of herniation may lead to unsightly abdominal protrusion and activity restrictions. After reduction of the hernia the

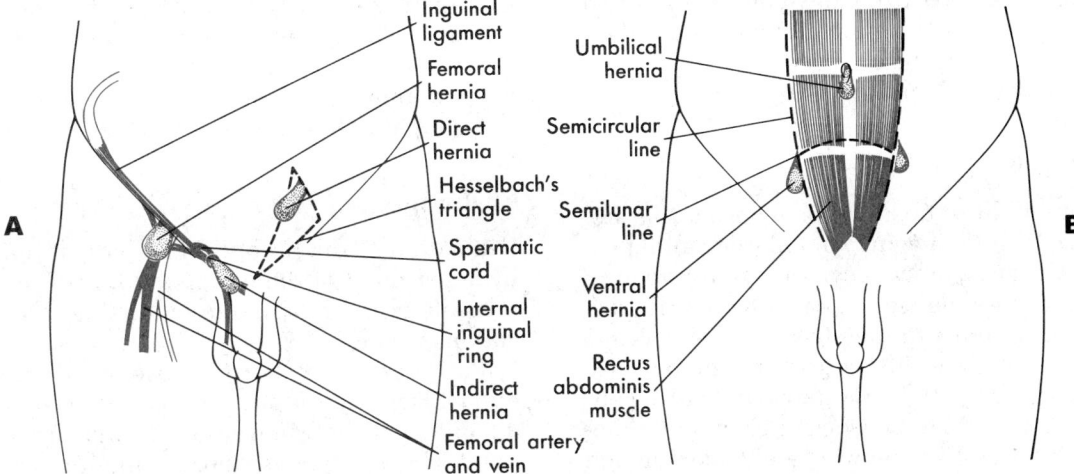

FIGURE 66-6   **A,** Inguinal hernia. **B,** Ventral hernia.

patient may elect to wear a truss or firm pad placed over the hernia site and held in place with a belt. This prevents the hernia from protruding and holds abdominal contents in place. The truss should be fitted by a qualified person or medical supplier to ensure proper fit.

Elective surgery for hernia repair (herniorrhaphy) may be done because of the inconvenience to the patient or constant risk of strangulation. The hernia defect is closed by approximating adjacent muscles or using a synthetic mesh. Uncomplicated hernia repair can be done safely, and the patient can be discharged the first or second day postoperatively. Some patients may use outpatient surgery for simple repairs. If incarceration or strangulation of the hernia results in bowel obstruction, hospitalization will be extended. Indications of incarceration and strangulation include abdominal pain, distention, changed bowel habits, temperature elevation, nausea, and vomiting. The patient may require an extensive abdominal procedure necessitating nasogastric drainage, intravenous fluids, and antibiotics. Complications of hernia repair include scrotal swelling, wound infection, urinary retention, and paralytic ileus.

NURSING MANAGEMENT OF THE PATIENT WITH ABDOMINAL WALL HERNIA
Assessment

When assessing the patient with a hernia, question the patient concerning knowledge of the disorder and treatment as well as experienced pain characteristics. Observe the hernia's location, size, limitations to clothing and activity, and the tissue perfusion of the area. An interview with the patient and significant others can elicit information about their understanding of herniation and the possible complications as well as past treatment (i.e., truss) and any complications experienced. From the information gathered the nurse will have a starting point from which to plan the nursing care.

Question the patient about pain or discomfort experienced. There is little correlation between the size of the hernia and the discomfort it produces. Small hernias tend to be more painful than larger ones but must be differentiated from strangulation. Note the size and location of the hernia. Initial assessment provides a baseline from which to judge enlargement. Assessment will indicate the limitation and inconvenience placed on the patient by the hernia.

If the hernia is nonreducible and accompanied by increased size and pain notify the physician immediately.

Nursing Diagnosis

Possible nursing diagnoses for the patient with hernia include the following:
   Knowledge deficit related to disease process
   Abdominal pain related to tissue swelling and obstruction
   Altered intestinal tissue perfusion related to strangulation of hernia
   Anxiety related to potential surgery and unknown outcomes

Planning

Nursing care for the patient with a hernia is planned to meet the following outcomes:
   The patient will demonstrate understanding of hernia formation and treatment choices
   The patient will experience abdominal pain relief

The patient will verbalize knowledge of signs and symptoms of incarceration and strangulation

The patient will verbalize reasons for surgery, expected outcomes, and follow-up care

Implementation

Instruct the patient to observe for a hernia that becomes nonreducible, begins to enlarge, and produces pain. Other significant symptoms are abdominal distention and change in bowel habits. Report any of these symptoms to the physician. Discourage prolonged standing and lifting or straining because they tend to aggravate the discomfort and hernia enlargement. If a truss is to be worn encourage the patient to have it fitted by a knowledgeable person and to give special attention to the skin under the truss and belt. Instruct the patient to keep these areas clean and dry and use talcum powder to prevent irritation. If surgery is to be performed instruct the patient and family about the procedure and expected outcomes.

Postoperative management

Address the following areas for the patient with an uncomplicated hernia repair.

Urinary retention is common postoperatively. If it persists longer than 8 hours intermittent catheterization or a Foley catheter may be ordered until the patient is able to void spontaneously.

In simple herniorrhaphy pain medication may be administered postoperatively by mouth every 3 to 4 hours as requested by the patient. To prevent pain at the incision site when coughing or sneezing teach the patient to splint the area with a pillow or pad or with interlaced fingers.

Wound infection rarely occurs. Assess the wound for erythema, tenderness, and discharge. If infection does develop it may require drainage and antibiotic therapy.

Scrotal swelling may occur after surgery and can be very painful. Elevating the scrotum on a rolled pad or towel and applying an ice pack are helpful. A jockstrap or jockey shorts may be worn for support.

The patient should be instructed to decrease activities for 5 or 6 days and discouraged from lifting heavy objects or straining with bowel movements. Application of an ice pack and scrotal support and the use of pain medication should be reviewed by the nurse with the patient before discharge. The patient is advised to report any redness or swelling of the surgical area or increased pain or drainage to the physician immediately.

With a strangulated hernia the repair may be extensive and the peritoneal cavity may be opened. In this instance the patient is prepared for surgery and managed after surgery as other abdominal surgery patients. These patients may require a longer hospitalization, nasogastric drainage, intravenous antibiotics, fluid and electrolyte replacement, and parenteral pain medication until peristalsis returns.

Evaluation

Evaluation of the preoperative patient may be done by assessment of the understanding of the disorder, possible risk factors, and actions needed if complications occur.

Postoperatively there is absence of infection, adequate urinary output, decreased scrotal swelling, adequate bowel movements, and freedom from pain. The patient verbalizes understanding of the avoidance of lifting and straining.

Documentation

Record the patient's vital signs and wound appearance. Describe the patient's comfort or discomfort and means to achieve comfort. Record patient teaching and follow-up instructions.

INTESTINAL OBSTRUCTION
Definition

Intestinal obstruction refers to the partial or complete impairment of the forward flow of intestinal contents. Intestinal obstructions usually involve actual blockage of the lumen. However, some conditions that decrease peristalsis, such as paralytic ileus, are not true obstructions.

Etiology/Epidemiology

Most obstructions occur in the ileum, which is the narrowest segment of the small intestine. The causes of obstruction are varied. Table 66-4 lists some of the situations that contribute to the development of an obstruction. Intestinal obstructions occur in people of all ages, and 90% of all obstructions result from adhesions or incarcerated hernias. Residues from foods high in fiber, such as raw coconut or fruit pulp, can obstruct the small bowel.

Pathophysiology

Normally, 7 to 8 L of electrolyte-rich fluids is secreted and then reabsorbed by the intestine each day. When the small intestine becomes obstructed, large amounts of fluid, bacteria, and swallowed air build up in the bowel proximal to the obstruction (Figure 66-7). Significant intestinal distention occurs as fluid and air accumulate. Besides secreted and ingested fluids, water and salts shift from the circulatory system into the intestinal lumen. Gases accumu-

TABLE 66-4 Causes of Intestinal Obstruction

Cause	Mechanism of obstruction
MECHANICAL	
Adhesions	Most common cause; fibrous bands of scar tissue constrict lumen
Hernias	Strangulated hernias become obstructed as a result of being irreducible and have a compromised blood supply
Volvulus	Twisting of bowel
Intussusception	Telescoping of bowel in proximal to distal direction; usually occurs in area of tumor or polyp in adult
Tumors	Frequent cause of obstruction in large intestine; develop slowly; fecal mass lodges at area of constriction
NEUROGENIC	
Paralytic ileus	Adynamic obstruction; occurs in postoperative patient and with pneumonia
VASCULAR	
Mesenteric artery occlusion	Leads to bowel infarction

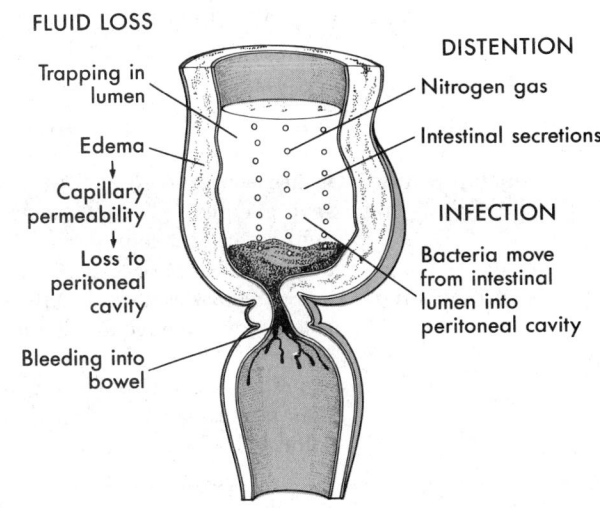

FIGURE 66-7 Pathophysiologic events in intestinal obstruction.

late from the nitrogen in swallowed air, which is poorly absorbed. Fermentation of intestinal contents by bacteria contributes to the gaseous distention.

Excessive fluid volume deficit characterizes intestinal obstruction. Fluid shifts occur by several mechanisms. Because of an increase in the intraluminal pressure, there is a decrease in the reabsorption of fluid from the intestine. Progressive edema of the bowel wall leads to severe intestinal distention. The distention causes venous compression and decreased venous return. As a result of the decreased venous return, venous pressure and capillary permeability are increased. Plasma movement into the bowel lumen and the peritoneal cavity increases as the capillaries become more permeable. Bacterial movement across the bowel wall into the peritoneal cavity may occur.

Clinical Manifestations

The early manifestations of intestinal obstruction occur as a result of the body's attempt to break up the obstruction. Spasms of cramping abdominal pain oc-

cur as peristaltic activity increases proximal to the obstruction. Obstructions high in the small intestine usually produce more severe pain than lower obstructions. The increased peristaltic activity produces an increase in auscultated bowel sounds. As the obstruction progresses, the intestine becomes hypoactive as a result of fatigue. The patient may experience periods of decreased bowel sounds and pain alternating with periods of increased pain.

As the intestinal lumen becomes distended proximal to the obstruction vomiting is likely. Characteristics of the emesis depend on the location of the obstruction. Table 66-5 compares the symptoms of obstruction based on location. The patient may exhibit symptoms of hypovolemia as a result of the shift in fluids out of the vascular system. Symptoms of peritonitis may develop as a result of bacterial movement.

The patient with a bowel obstruction may continue to have bowel movements. The colon distal to the obstruction continues to empty.

Therapeutic Management

Surgery is indicated to relieve mechanical obstructions caused by adhesions and hernias. If the patient is not stable enough for surgery, supportive therapy is instituted. In the past, long nasointestinal tubes were used in an attempt to provide intestinal decompression and avoid surgery. That process consumed valuable time and the majority of patients required surgery. According to Welch,[37] a significant number of patients whose bowel obstruction from adhesions resolved with intubation have recurrence of obstruction and many require surgery. Today the use of a nasogastric tube to decrease vomiting and surgery

TABLE 66-5   Comparison of Symptoms in Intestinal Obstruction

Obstruction	Vomiting	Distention	Oliguria	Pain
High small intestine	Occurs early and is severe; emesis is light green and copious; nonfecal odor	Appears late; limited to epigastric area	Present as a result of loss of fluid	Severe; upper quadrants
Low small intestine	Delayed; dark green color; may have fecal odor	Diffuse across abdomen	Less likely to occur	Severe; periumbilical
Colon	Occurs late in obstruction; usually has fecal color and odor	Diffuse	Not common	Less severe

before the patient decompensates from fluid and electrolyte loss and nutritional deficit is more usual. Fluid and electrolyte replacement is an essential part of treatment.

NURSING MANAGEMENT OF THE PATIENT WITH INTESTINAL OBSTRUCTION

Assessment

Subjective data collection includes information about the pattern of the patient's pain. Inquire about the onset, frequency, and characteristics of the pain. Many patients with obstruction will be able to recall the exact onset of the pain. Determining the location of the pain will be useful in determining the portion of bowel that is obstructed. Note any history of previous bowel disorders or abdominal surgeries. Ask the patient about any changes in bowel elimination.

Objective data collection begins with the assessment of the patient's abdomen. Inspect the abdominal surface for evidence of distention, hernias, scars indicating previous surgeries, or visible peristaltic waves. Auscultation of the abdomen may reveal characteristic changes in bowel sounds. An increase in frequency will be noted during episodes of pain. Bowel sounds may decrease between pain episodes. Late in the obstructive process, bowel sounds are hypoactive as the intestine becomes fatigued. The bowel sounds may resemble splashing similar to that made by the emptying of a narrow-necked bottle of water. The sound has a fine, metallic tinkling quality. The change is caused by gas bubbles breaking through the surface of the retained fluids. Eventually bowel sounds cease, and the abdomen becomes silent. The abdomen may be tender to light palpation, and muscle guarding may be present. As the abdominal distention increases, respiratory excur-

sion is jeopardized. Short, rapid respirations may be noted.

Laboratory assessment of the patient includes blood chemistries. Because of the fluid and electrolyte losses, the patient will have an elevated blood urea nitrogen (BUN), an indication of dehydration. Values for serum sodium, potassium, and magnesium will be decreased. The patient's hemoglobin and hematocrit may be increased because of hemoconcentration associated with the fluid volume deficit. If the patient has a high intestinal obstruction, metabolic alkalosis is likely to occur because of the loss of highly acidic gastric fluid with vomiting. If the obstruction occurs lower in the intestine, metabolic acidosis is more common as a result of vomiting of more alkaline fluid from the small bowel. (See Figure 66-8 for a critical thinking guide on intestinal obstruction.)

X-ray studies may be performed to determine the location of the obstruction. A flat plate of the abdomen may reveal unusual gas patterns in the bowel. When contrast studies are done, a barium enema is usually attempted first. If a barium swallow is done, the patient with a true obstruction would be unable to eliminate the barium. When an obstruction is suspected, water-soluble contrast medium is used for the upper gastrointestinal x-ray studies.

Nursing Diagnosis

Nursing diagnoses for the patient with an intestinal obstruction include the following:

Acute abdominal pain related to increased peristalsis

Fluid volume deficit related to increased losses from vomiting and third spacing

Decreased intestinal tissue perfusion related to hypovolemia

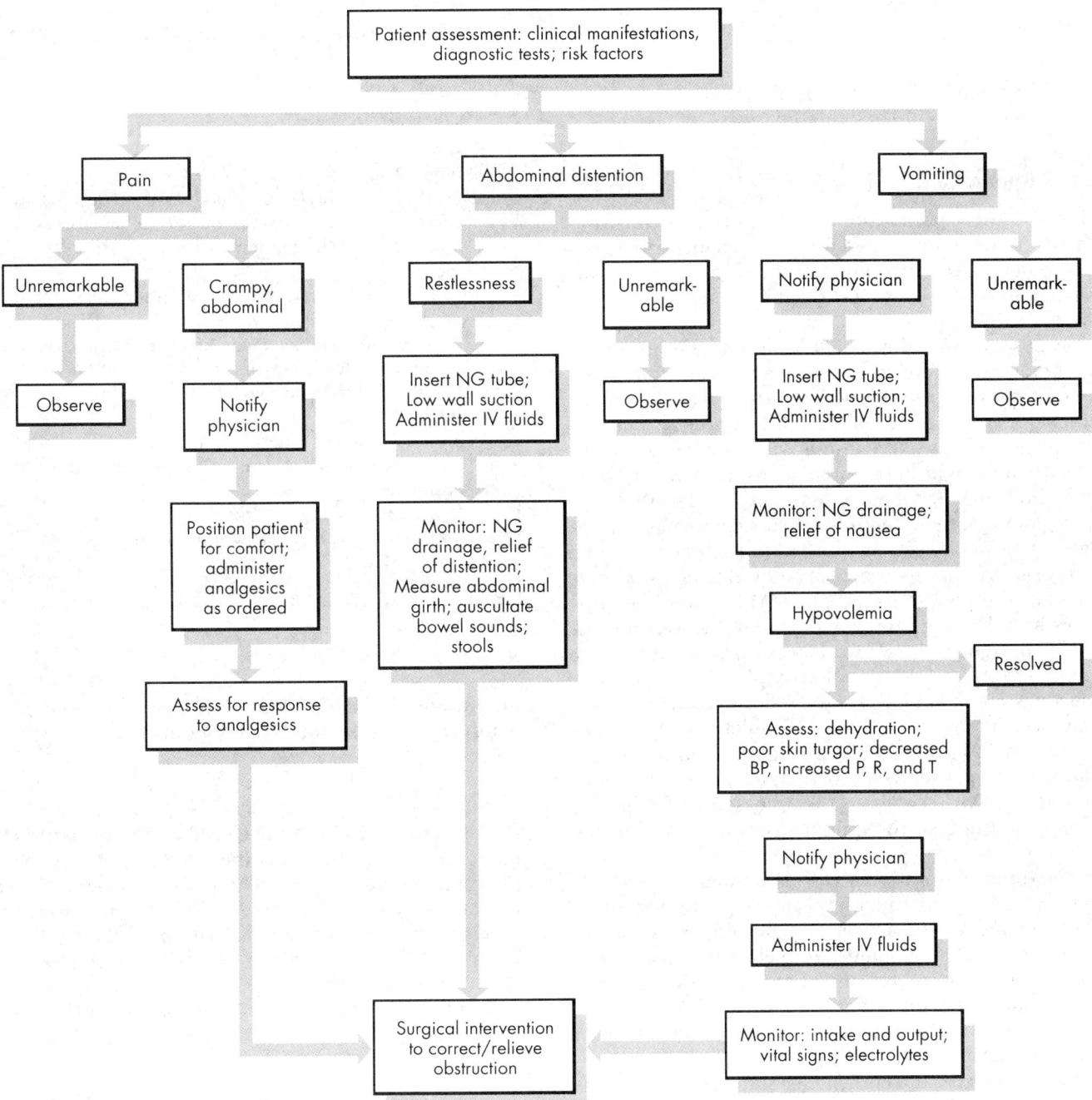

FIGURE 66-8   Critical Thinking Guide: intestinal obstruction.

Impaired gas exchange related to abdominal distention

Altered nutrition: less than body needs related to vomiting and obstruction

High risk for infection related to movement of intestinal flora into the peritoneal cavity

High risk for aspiration related to vomiting

Planning

Nursing interventions for the patient with an intestinal obstruction are planned to achieve the following outcomes:

  The patient will have return of normal bowel function

  The patient will maintain fluid and electrolyte balance

The patient will be free of pain

The patient will regain and maintain adequate nutrition

The patient will be free of infection

The patient will have adequate gas exchange

Implementation

Because the patient is to receive nothing orally, the intravenous route is used for fluid and electrolyte replacement. An indwelling urinary catheter is inserted to assist in accurate monitoring of the patient's urine output.

A nasogastric tube is usually attached to intermittent suction to relieve vomiting and distention. Normal saline is the solution of choice if periodic irrigations are required to maintain tube patency. The use of sterile water for irrigations will contribute to electrolyte and acid-base imbalances by washing out chloride ions. Frequent mouth care is essential.

If conservative treatment is not successful in relieving the obstruction, the patient is prepared for surgery. Preoperative preparation includes explanations of the procedure at a level the patient can understand. Detailed teaching may not be appropriate if the patient is in acute distress. However, family members may find detailed explanations helpful. Nasogastric drainage, an indwelling urinary catheter, and intravenous fluid and electrolyte replacement are maintained before surgery. Emotional support for the patient is important, because the patient is not only experiencing the stressors of pain and vomiting, but also the added stressor of emergency surgery.

Postoperative nursing care is similar for any patient who has had abdominal surgery. Nursing interventions include measures to maintain fluid balance, bowel rest, comfort, and gas exchange. Nasogastric drainage is continued until bowel activity returns. Some patients require temporary bowel diversion to manage the obstruction. Total parenteral nutrition may be necessary for patients at risk for further nutritional deficit, especially those patients who are already compromised.

Evaluation

Successful relief of the obstruction will be evidenced by a relief of abdominal distention and return of normal bowel activity. Periodic monitoring of bowel sounds is important. The patient's hydration status will return to normal. For the patient with surgical intervention, the incision will heal without complications.

Documentation

Record the return of bowel sounds, relief of abdominal distention, and bowel elimination patterns. Doc-

GERIATRIC CONSIDERATIONS

Constipation

1. Bowel programs stress dietary fiber, adequate fluids, and regular exercise.
2. Change fiber or fluid intake slowly. Diminished cardiac reserves make the elderly person less able to adapt to sudden increases in blood volume.
3. Bran is an effective source of fiber, but add it gradually to decrease nausea and distention.
4. Risk factors predisposing elderly persons to constipation include depression, decreased mobility, low-fiber diet, hypothyroidism, and poor fluid intake.
5. Select a regular time for bowel elimination, and adhere to schedule, since bowel elimination is patterned.
6. Impaction should be suspected if a feeling of pressure without passing stool in the rectum or watery diarrhea occurs.

ument data indicating fluid and electrolyte balance, comfort, nutrition status, and wound healing.

Ongoing Care

Patient teaching about measures to decrease the recurrence of obstruction is included in the discharge planning for the patient. The patient needs to learn measures to prevent constipation (see box on constipation in elderly persons). In cases where there is a possibility of recurring obstructions the patient and family need to be aware of what symptoms to report to a health care provider. For the patient with a temporary ostomy, follow-up care is necessary as plans are made for closure of the stoma.

POLYPS
Definition

Polyps are growths on the mucosal lining of the colon. These projections into the bowel lumen can easily be removed during colonoscopy, and biopsy samples can be obtained. Although the larger percentage of polyps are benign and require no treatment, patients who are predisposed to this condition are advised to have them removed and are observed for possible malignant changes. In certain hereditary diseases of the colon, polyp formation is rapid and has a high incidence of malignant change.

The distinction between Gardner's syndrome and familial polyposis coli is arbitrary. Whether the two conditions are distinct entities or differing manifestations of a single disorder remains unanswered. A common feature of both is diffuse colonic polyps with a high propensity for neoplastic transformation.

Etiology

Familial polyposis, an autosomal dominant trait, is transmitted by an affected parent. A 50% chance of receiving this dominant gene exists for each child. Both sexes have the potential to be affected equally, since the trait shows no sexual predisposition. Approximately 1 in 8000 people will develop the disease.[44] Gardner's syndrome accounts for 10% of patients with familial polyposis.

Pathophysiology

The lesions of familial polyposis are precancerous adenomatous polyps that begin as small swellings on the mucosa of the large intestine. These polyps gradually increase in size and number until the entire colon is studded with hundreds of polyps. Unlike the polyps in familial polyposis, which blanket the colon, the polyps in Gardner's syndrome are scattered along the colon. They may be found anywhere in the gastrointestinal tract, although they are rarely found in the small intestine. The polyps in the large intestine, like those found in familial polyposis, tend to become cancerous 10 to 15 years after the first manifestation of the disease.

Clinical Manifestations

Some of the clinical manifestations for the diseases are the same. The patient may report mild to moderate diarrhea, bleeding, increased mucus in the stools, and crampy abdominal pain. Gardner's syndrome is also associated with a myriad of other manifestations including cancer of the thyroid; cancer of the ampulla of Vater; cancer of the small intestine; osteomas; connective tissue tumors; and cutaneous, sebaceous, or dermoid cysts.

The average age of onset of polyp development is 25 years. First symptoms may appear at 33 years with a diagnosis of cancer at 39 years.[47] The patient's chance of developing cancer, if left untreated, is estimated to be 80% to 100%. The diagnosis is made by rectal examination, colonoscopy, air-contrast barium enema, and biopsy, as well as an accurate family history. No preventive measures are known, but regular checkups for people with a family history of these diseases are essential.

Therapeutic Management

Surgical intervention for familial polyposis and Gardner's syndrome is essential to the survival of the patient. Since restorative proctocolectomy or subtotal colectomy with ileoanal anastomosis is the treatment of choice, the patient, while asymptomatic, must make the decision about having the colon removed. Asymptomatic individuals who feel well have a difficult time making a choice that has emotional as well as physical implications. The treatment of Gardner's syndrome is the same as for familial polyposis. A total colectomy with ileostomy or internal reservoir may be indicated if extensive polyps are found. At times a subtotal colectomy with ileorectal anastomosis may be adequate, although if the entire colon mucosa is not removed the patient may still be at risk. Appropriate alternative choices for the familial polyposis and Gardner's syndrome patient include the following:

1. Total proctocolectomy and pull-through ileoanal anastomosis with a pelvic reservoir
2. Subtotal colectomy with ileorectal anastomosis
3. Continent ileostomy (Kock's pouch)
4. Total proctocolectomy with permanent ileostomy

NURSING MANAGEMENT OF THE PATIENT WITH FAMILIAL POLYPOSIS AND GARDNER'S SYNDROME

Assessment

Preoperative nursing care for the patient with familial polyposis and Gardner's syndrome is the same as for the ulcerative colitis patient. In addition, the patient and family require education and counseling about the disease. Assess their knowledge concerning the disease, and then a plan can be formulated to meet their needs.

Nursing Diagnosis

Nursing diagnoses for the patient with familial polyposis and Gardner's syndrome include the following:

Knowledge deficit related to disease process
Anxiety related to concerns about surgery and ongoing care

Planning

Nursing care for the patient with hereditary colon polyps is planned to achieve the following outcome:

The patient will participate in treatment choices and preventive measures

Implementation

Once a trusting relationship with the patient and family is developed the nurse can provide information about the disease process and where the polyps are located. Discuss the genetic component of this disease and suggest genetic counseling before starting a family. Assessment of all family members and follow-up evaluations are necessary to detect the disease as early as possible.

ISCHEMIC DISORDERS OF THE COLON
Definition

Visceral vascular occlusion as a result of trauma; emboli; hypovolemia; spasm; iatrogenesis; or thrombi that affect the celiac axis, superior mesenteric plexus, and inferior mesenteric vessels may result in ischemia progressing to necrosis and perforation of the abdominal viscera.[39]

Etiology

Vascular changes in the bowel as a result of arteriosclerosis are common in the older age group and diabetes mellitus population. Occlusion of the mesenteric vessels may occur with resultant infarction of the affected bowel. During resection of an abdominal aortic aneurysm, the inferior mesenteric artery may need to be ligated with resultant iatrogenic left-colon ischemia. Other occurrences of ischemia may be seen in drug-overdose patients after treatment for hypovolemic shock and spasm of the vascular system.

Clinical Manifestations

Initial signs and symptoms are vague and appear as generalized abdominal discomfort. This may be ignored or minimized by the health care team in view of other patient needs. Signs and symptoms initially include leukocytosis and advance to sudden onset of severe, left lower quadrant abdominal pain often out of proportion to diagnostic findings. The patient may then develop abdominal distention, nausea, vomiting, and shock. The patient may have marked abdominal guarding; rapid, shallow respirations; fever; and fluid and electrolyte imbalance.

The patient with mesenteric angina (spasms of the mesenteric vessels) will report progressively worsening symptoms. The initial symptom is abdominal pain after eating. This is followed by profound progressive weight loss and all the accompanying symptoms of nutritional deficit.

Therapeutic Management

Prompt surgical intervention is essential when mesenteric occlusion and bowel infarction have occurred. Treatments vary. One method of management is the "second look" procedure. In this procedure, when vascular compromise is diagnosed, a laparotomy is performed and the necrotic portion of the bowel is removed. Because it is difficult to determine the viability of the mucosal layer of the remaining bowel, a second laparotomy in 6 to 12 hours may be indicated. Correction of the underlying cause is essential. One of the main complications of the surgery is failure of the bowel anastomosis, and often a temporary ostomy is indicated.[50]

For the patient with chronic bowel ischemia, arteriography may be indicated and a conservative approach considered. Bowel rest, total parenteral nutrition, anticoagulants, and papaverine infusions to decrease visceral spasm may be used.

NURSING MANAGEMENT OF THE PATIENT WITH ISCHEMIC DISORDERS OF THE COLON

The nursing implications for preoperative and postoperative nursing care are generally the same as those for the patient with diverticular abscess and rupture. Another consideration is that patients with mesenteric angina may have been through many diagnostic tests without diagnosis. These patients may become frustrated and frightened. As a result of the vague and insidious onset of the disease they may have been referred for a psychiatric evaluation because no other diagnosis could be substantiated. Postoperatively, these patients may require total parenteral nutrition and bowel rest until adequate bowel function returns.

Assessment

The elderly patient, most often affected with ischemic bowel disease, may have undergone changes in mental status as a result of arteriosclerotic disease and may be incapable of learning independent care. Careful assessment of the patient's coping abilities, limitations, and support systems is necessary.

Nursing Diagnosis

Nursing diagnoses for the patient with ischemic disorders of the colon include the following:
  Altered nutrition: less than body requirements related to abdominal pain
  Anxiety related to unconfirmed diagnosis
  Abdominal pain related to ischemia
  Fluid volume deficit related to third spacing
  Impaired intestinal tissue perfusion related to the ischemic process

Planning

Nursing care for the patient with ischemic bowel disease is planned to achieve the following outcomes:

The patient will express understanding of the disease process and the treatment regimen

The patient will regain and maintain adequate nutritional status

The patient will express relief of pain

The patient will regain and maintain adequate hydration

The patient will regain adequate intestinal tissue perfusion

Implementation

If the patient is unable to learn self-care the nurse teaches the caregiver and makes appropriate referrals until the colostomy is closed. Skilled nursing facilities and home health care agencies may be appropriate referrals.[39]

BLUNT AND PENETRATING TRAUMA
Definition

Each year in the United States some 50 million people incur accidental injuries with over 100,000 people losing their lives.[39] Trauma is the leading cause of death between the ages of 1 and 37 years and ranks third as the cause of death in all ages. The liver is the most commonly injured abdominal organ in blunt and penetrating trauma.[9] Solid organs bleed profusely when injured. Hypovolemia occurs early with this type of injury, and peritonitis may occur later. With hollow organ penetration, peritonitis occurs early, and hypovolemia, as a result of fluid volume shifts, occurs later.

Etiology

The gunshot wound is the most common penetrating abdominal injury seen in most urban trauma centers. Every abdominal organ is at risk for damage, but the four organs most commonly violated are the liver, small bowel, stomach, and colon. Mortality is directly related to the number of organs injured and the resulting vascular damage. Immediate threats include hemorrhage and hypovolemic shock. Later, subsequent bacterial peritonitis may lead to systemic sepsis. Any penetrating wound between the nipples and pubic hair area must be assumed to have intraperitoneal injury and requires exploratory laparotomy. The stab wound is the second most common penetrating injury. They usually produce minimal tissue damage and carry a lower mortality than gunshot wounds,[39] which carry an 8 to 10 times greater mortality than stab wounds.[9]

Automobile or pedestrian accidents cause 50% to 70% of blunt abdominal injuries.[39] Damage is done by crushing, shearing, or bursting forces as a result of visceral compression or rapid deceleration. Burst injuries are caused by a transient closed loop obstruction with sudden increase in the intraluminal pressure. The organ injured most frequently in blunt trauma is the spleen.[31]

Clinical Manifestations

Morbidity with colon wounds is primarily related to fecal contamination of the peritoneal cavity and subsequent intraperitoneal sepsis. Management of colon trauma includes control of hemorrhage, minimization of fecal contamination, and prevention of continuous fecal peritoneal soilage if the suture line dehisces.

Immediately after the injury, a diagnostic peritoneal lavage may be used to diagnose intraperitoneal bleeding. Before the diagnostic peritoneal lavage a nasogastric tube and a Foley catheter are inserted to decompress the stomach and the urinary bladder. The diagnostic peritoneal lavage involves the instillation of a crystalloid solution into the peritoneal cavity with a gravity siphon to return the fluid. The siphoned fluid is examined for white blood cells, red blood cells, amylase, bile, bacteria, and foreign matter in the peritoneal cavity.

In general, indications for exploratory laparotomy include evidence of significant internal bleeding, suspicion of major vascular injury, spreading peritonitis, or any penetrating abdominal wound that has entered the peritoneal cavity.

Therapeutic Management

The surgeon has several options when managing colon injuries. These are primary resection with anastomosis, closure of the colon wound with proximal loop colostomy, primary closure with exteriorization of the wound as a colostomy stoma, or resection of the injured colon with an end colostomy and Hartmann's pouch.

Factors that influence the type of closure are the extent of injury and amount of contamination, interval from injury to repair, and physical stability of the patient. Wounds of the cecum may require diversion of the stool by cecostomy tube or a proximal loop ileostomy until satisfactory healing and resolution of infection have occurred.

Wounds of the left side of the colon that require resection are best treated with a proximal loop colostomy or end colostomy with mucous fistula or Hartmann's pouch (Figure 66-9). Closure of these temporary ostomies can usually be performed within 6 to 12 weeks after the initial surgery.

Antibiotic treatment may be instituted before or after the surgery, according to the physician's preference. Some of the intravenous medications used in a 5-day regimen with emergency colon surgery

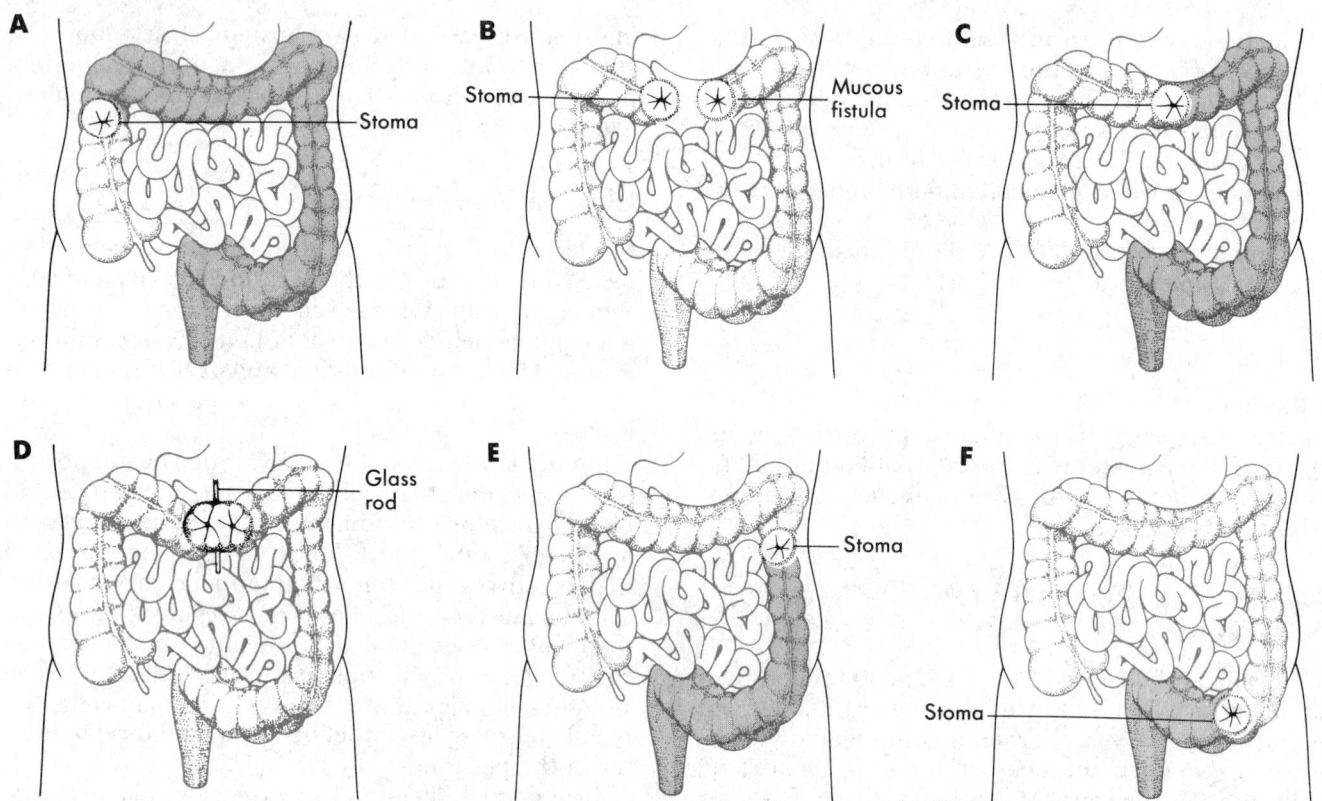

FIGURE 66-9   **A,** Ascending colostomy. **B,** Double-barrel colostomy. **C,** Traverse colostomy. **D,** Loop colostomy. **E,** Descending colostomy. **F,** Sigmoid colostomy.

are clindamycin (Cleocin), gentamicin, ampicillin, and metronidazole (Flagyl).

NURSING MANAGEMENT OF THE PATIENT WITH BLUNT AND PENETRATING TRAUMA

Assessment

Surgery for traumatic injury is usually performed on an emergency basis. The patient has little time to prepare for the idea of an ostomy. Often the need for an ostomy is not absolutely determined until surgical exploration reveals the full extent of the injury. Even though the patient may have signed a consent form listing the possibility of ostomy surgery, the crisis situation generally hampers full awareness of the implications should this become necessary. The sudden necessity of the crisis situation can produce extreme anxiety. The best nursing intervention may be smoothing the path to surgery by physical support of body functions, obtaining appropriate preoperative tests and consent forms, answering questions of patient and family when possible, and giving reassurance concerning treatment and postoperative care.

Emergency assessment by the physician and nurse includes the areas of gas exchange, tissue perfusion, fluid volume and electrolyte balance, excretory function, risk for infection/contamination, fear/anxiety, and neurologic deficit.

Any penetrating wound is considered contaminated, and penetration of the peritoneal cavity is an indication for exploratory laparotomy. Peritoneal lavage or endoscopy can be used to ascertain contamination of the peritoneal cavity by feces or bacteria in the case of blunt trauma.

Nursing Diagnosis

The following nursing diagnoses may be appropriate for the patient with blunt or penetrating abdominal trauma:

Altered tissue perfusion related to blood loss
Fluid volume deficit related to blood loss and third spacing
Abdominal pain related to tissue injury
Anxiety and fear related to unknown surgical outcomes
High risk for infection related to fecal contamination of abdominal cavity

Planning

Nursing care for patients with abdominal trauma is planned to achieve the following outcomes:

The patient will maintain adequate gas exchange and have normal blood gas values

The patient will regain and maintain normal fluid volume and electrolyte levels

The patient will have adequate blood flow with vital signs within normal range

The patient will express a decreased or reduced level of pain

The patient will maintain adequate urinary output

The patient will have wound healing without infection

The patient will show a reduction of fear and anxiety

Implementation

A nasotracheal or endotracheal tube may be needed for controlled mechanical ventilation. Assess for sucking thoracic wounds, and if present, apply an occlusive petroleum gauze pressure dressing. A chest tube may be inserted to evacuate blood and air from the pleural space. Arterial blood gases are drawn to evaluate gas exchange.

A large-gauge catheter is inserted in a peripheral vein to obtain blood samples for appropriate laboratory tests and type and crossmatch for blood. Intravenous fluid replacement, as needed, is then started. A peripheral intravenous line is maintained to replace fluid volume and electrolyte loss. A nasogastric tube is inserted to evacuate the stomach. If the patient is unable to void, an indwelling catheter is placed in the bladder. The physician will order an intravenous antibiotic to be given preoperatively. Appropriate x-ray studies are done.

Explanation to the patient and family of what is about to happen and what to expect can be done as treatment progresses. The patient and family may not have questions but will need reassurance that whatever is needed will be done. Family members may need time to talk about their fears and feelings while the patient is prepared for surgery.

Evaluation

Evaluation of gas exchange, tissue perfusion, fluid and electrolyte balance, urinary function, and neurologic status can be done by reassessment of the above areas. Infection may not be as easily evaluated until 2 or 3 days into the postoperative period. The nurse can evaluate the patient's and family's fear and anxiety by active listening and observing their adaptive behaviors.

Documentation

The nurse records breath sounds and the patient's ability to maintain adequate gas exchange, hydration, and urinary and gastrointestinal output. Document wound healing and drainage. Vital signs, intake and output, ambulation, and neurologic status are appropriate data to record on a flow sheet. Describe the patient's and family's concerns regarding the extent of injury, need for life-style changes, coping abilities, and the teaching provided.

Ongoing Care

Areas of assessment are as previously discussed in the chapter under inflammatory bowel disease and involve physical and metabolic assessment as the patient recovers. In addition, assess bowel elimination/ stomal assessment, knowledge deficit, and coping abilities. (See the discussion of stomal assessment and colostomy care under colon cancer.)

Assessment of the patient's understanding and knowledge can be done by discussion. The patient is informed about the surgery and why it was done, as well as the care and changing of the ostomy pouch. If the abdominal wound is left open teach the patient and family the dressing procedure and signs and symptoms of infection. Ensure that the patient has the physician's name and telephone number, knows when to see the physician again, knows where to obtain supplies, and has the names of other resource people, such as an enterostomal therapist, home care agencies, and medical suppliers.

Often with trauma the patient has feelings of fear, helplessness, anger, and guilt. Assess the patient's ability to cope with these feelings as well as the general situation while providing care. The nurse's empathetic attitude will often encourage the sharing of these feelings and attitudes toward the situation. Inclusion of the family in these sessions may be appropriate and is needed in the teaching sessions. In some cases, the patient and family may need psychologic services, and a nursing referral to a psychiatric clinical nurse specialist or other disciplines will be appropriate.

CANCER OF THE COLON
Definition

The incidence of colon cancer in the United States ranks third after prostate and lung cancer in men and second after breast cancer in women. It has an estimated 50% cure rate, and the annual incidence is in excess of 155,000 cases.[8]

In the colon, two thirds of all growths are seen in the rectosigmoid and rectum. Cancer of the colon is seen in almost all age groups, but the highest incidence occurs in ages 60 years and above.[39]

RISK FACTORS FOR DEVELOPMENT OF COLON CANCER

Over 40 years of age
Family history of colorectal cancer
Previous history of colorectal cancer
Adenomatous polyps
Family history of familial polyposis
Ulcerative colitis
Crohn's disease
Previous pelvic irradiation

From Broadwell D, Jackson B: *Principles of ostomy care*, St Louis, 1982, Mosby–Year Book, Inc.

FIVE-YEAR SURVIVAL RATE BY DUKES' STAGING[3]

Dukes' Stage	Patients Alive after 5 Years (%)
A	90
B	60-80
C	20-50
D	<5

Overall 5-year survival for all patients with colorectal cancer is 50%

Etiology

The cause of colorectal cancer remains unknown. Certain predisposing and risk factors have been identified. Neoplastic polyps or adenomas may undergo malignant change and become frank carcinomas. Gardner's syndrome and familial polyposis (discussed earlier in this chapter) are genetic diseases that are related to the incidence of colon or rectal cancer when the polyps of these diseases are allowed to remain a long time. Risk factors include familial colon cancer and ulcerative colitis (see box above). Other factors implicated in colorectal cancer include lack of bulk in the diet, high-fat intake, and high bacterial counts. These factors have encouraged diet changes to decrease animal fat, increase complex carbohydrates, and increase dietary fiber as primary preventive measures.

Pathophysiology

Microscopically, colorectal cancers are graded according to cellular differentiation. These gradings are (1) well differentiated, (2) moderately well differentiated, (3) poorly differentiated, and (4) anaplastic. Prognosis can be related to the grade. Grade 1 is more favorable in terms of patient survival.

Tumor spread can occur in a number of ways, including (1) spread within the layers of the bowel wall; (2) spread to the lymphatic system and lymph nodes; (3) bloodstream spread; (4) transperitoneal spread; and (5) spread to suture lines, abdominal incisions, or drain sites.[39] Tumor growth can produce secondary effects, including obstruction of the bowel lumen and ulceration of the bowel wall leading to hemorrhage. Tumor penetration may result in abscess or fistula formation and secondary tumor deposit in the other tissues.

One of the most widely used classifications of postoperative staging is Dukes' method. In this method, stage A refers to cancer confined to the bowel wall; in stage B the cancer has penetrated the bowel into the extrarectal tissue without lymph node involvement; in stage C lymph nodes are involved and may include growth through the bowel wall; and stage D generally refers to nonresectable growths (see box).

Clinical Manifestations

Rectal bleeding is the most frequent presenting symptom of colon cancer, and the color may vary from dark to bright red, depending on the location of the neoplasm. Chronic occult bleeding can lead to anemia, lethargy, and shortness of breath. A history of a change in bowel habits may be reported alternating between constipation and diarrhea. Constipation more frequently results from descending colon cancer, whereas ascending colon cancer may occur without change in bowel habits (Figure 66-10). Rectal cancer can produce a sense of incomplete evacuation. Some patients report spasmlike rectal pain of the sphincter muscles. Other symptoms seen in the later stages of colon cancer are abdominal pain, nausea, vomiting, weight loss, cachexia, and abdominal distention or ascites.

Therapeutic Management

Diagnostic testing

The most important factors influencing survival and recurrence are the biologic potential of the tumor (whether it is slow growing and invades locally or is aggressive with a tendency to metastasize) and early diagnosis before onset of symptoms and the metastatic process.

Digital examination can identify 15% of colorectal cancers. Proctosigmoidoscopy increases that number to 66%. The advent of flexible fiberoptic sigmoidoscopy has made examination of the sigmoid

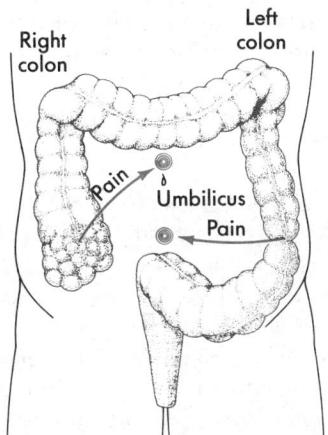

FIGURE 66-10   Pattern of referred pain related to location of tumor in colon cancer.

and descending colon more comfortable and acceptable to the patient. Fecal occult blood examination followed by proctosigmoidoscopy remains the most reliable tool for screening.

Colonoscopy allows for examination of the entire colon and remains the most accurate tool for detecting cancer throughout the colon. Screening for rectal cancer is recommended for everyone beginning at 40 years of age. The American Cancer Society recommends the following screening for asymptomatic individuals: annual digital rectal examination beginning at 40 years; annual examination of stool for occult blood beginning at 50 years; and proctosigmoidoscopy every 3 to 5 years beginning at 50 years.[2]

A barium enema can be used to examine for cancer or polyps, but in the case of an imperfectly prepared bowel, results may not be accurate. An air-contrast barium enema can provide more thorough delineation of the intestinal lining.

Active malignancy within the body can be assayed by a blood test when cancer and metastasis are suspected. The carcinoembryonic antigen (CEA) is a specific glycoprotein antigen in adenocarcinomas of the gastrointestinal tract. Antibodies to this antigen are measured. If a rising CEA is found, the patient may have scans of suspected areas of metastasis. If liver involvement is suspected, the serum alkaline phosphatase or bilirubin levels are assessed for elevation.

Radiation therapy

Radiation therapy as an adjunct to surgery and as primary treatment is being increasingly employed for rectal cancer. Radiation may be used as an adjunct for patients with bulky or fixed tumors and for patients at high risk for local recurrence. Intracavitary radiation may be used as the primary treatment.[16] In addition, intraoperative radiation therapy has been employed for patients with locally advanced disease.

Radiation therapy is used preoperatively to decrease the chance of cancer cell implantation at the time of resection. Radiation, by destroying cancer cells, reduces the size of the tumor and decreases the rate of lymphatic involvement. A moderate radiation dose is given over 5 to 6 weeks before surgery. This dose (4500 to 5000 cGy) results in few side effects and is associated with fewer complications after surgery.

Postoperatively, those patients at high risk for recurrence or persons who have Dukes' stages B and C may receive the same dose (4500 to 5000 cGy) administered over 4 to 6 weeks. Postoperative radiation may be delayed to allow healing. These patients experience side effects such as diarrhea, tenesmus, fatigue, and radiation enteritis.

Radiation used as a primary treatment is only for patients with limited disease (stage A). The radiation may be applied by way of proctoscope directly into the tumor. High doses of radiation can be delivered directly into the tumor during surgery when the abdomen is open. This is for tumors at high risk for recurrence and reduces the risk of normal tissue destruction.

The many side effects of radiation therapy include skin inflammation, diarrhea/colitis, anemia, leukopenia, thrombocytopenia, fibrosis or scarring of tissue, and fistulization to other structures. Other effects include tissue friability, poor healing and circulation in the treated area, spasticity of the bladder with urinary incontinence, and alteration in sexual and reproductive abilities.

Chemotherapy

Chemotherapy is given to the patient with systemic disease that is incurable by surgery or radiation alone. Postoperatively it is used as an adjunct for those who are suspected of having micrometastases that are not clinically detectable.[40] In addition, it may be used as palliative therapy to reduce tumor size or relieve symptoms of the disease, such as obstruction or pain.

Although many drugs have been tested in the treatment of colon cancer, primarily two are used, namely, 5-fluorouracil (5-FU) and mitomycin. Folinic acid is sometimes added to potentiate the action of 5-FU. The effectiveness of the chemotherapy drugs on colon cancer is questionable, and patient response varies. Physician opinion on the treatment of colon cancer by chemotherapy also varies.

Side effects of 5-FU include nausea, vomiting, diarrhea, alopecia, myelosuppression, stomatitis, dermatitis, leukopenia, thrombocytopenia, and anemia.

Mitomycin side effects include stomatitis, myelosuppression, liver dysfunction, renal failure, thrombocytopenia, leukopenia, and hypertension. These drugs are given intravenously in a 3- to 5-day cycle.

Surgical management

Many factors are involved in choosing the appropriate operative procedure. These include location of the tumor, obstruction or perforation of the bowel, possible metastasis, fitness of the patient, and the surgeon's preferences.

For carcinoma of the colon without obstruction the procedure will vary according to location of the tumor. A portion of the bowel on either side of the tumor is removed, and an end-to-end anastomosis connects the divided ends. The amount and extent of bowel removed depend on the location of the tumor and the blood supply to that segment. Special care is taken to approximate ends without tension and to remove surrounding lymph nodes with ligation of the lymphovascular pedicles.[48]

Several different procedures are used for carcinoma of the rectum. The location of the tumor in the rectum is the most important factor. If the tumor is near the anorectal sphincter it may be impossible for the surgeon to perform a resection with adequate margins to prevent recurrence. Any tumor located less than 2 to 2.5 cm from the anal verge may not be resectable while still preserving sphincter function. In this case a wide resection of the rectum, levator ani muscle, and area of lymphatic drainage is done with formation of a permanent colostomy.

If the tumor can be resected with removal of only the sigmoid colon and upper or middle rectum with adequate margins the surgeon may select a sphincter-preserving technique. Two of the more commonly used techniques are stapled end-to-end anastomosis and the pull-through procedure. In the end-to-end anastomosis the anastomosis is done with an end-to-end anastomotic stapler. This stapler is time saving, provides a secure suture line, and is readily used for a difficult low anastomosis. The second procedure, the pull-through operation, allows for the attachment of the proximal colon to the rectal cuff with the least amount of damage to the sphincter.

If the surgeon is unable to do an anastomosis, an abdominoperineal resection may be done. This refers to removal of the colon through the abdomen and the rectum by way of the perineum. A wide resection is done to decrease the possibility of metastasis by direct lymphatic routes, and a permanent colostomy is performed. It also results in a perineal wound that may be closed with a drain in place or packed and left open to heal by secondary intention. Major complications of this procedure are sexual dysfunction and failure of the wound to heal.

If the patient is a surgical risk or develops cardiovascular problems during surgery the surgeon may choose the Hartmann's pouch procedure. This procedure oversews the rectal stump and leaves it in situ. A permanent colostomy is then created.

NURSING MANAGEMENT OF THE PATIENT WITH CANCER OF THE COLON

Assessment

The areas to be assessed by the nurse for the patient with colon cancer are knowledge deficit, coping abilities, grief process, and nutritional status.

Assessment of the patient's and family's knowledge can often be done by discussing questions focused on the patient's knowledge, thoughts, feelings, and misconceptions concerning the disease. Coping abilities are affected by several factors, including the patient's ability to adaptively deal with loss, as well as a history of loss adaptation. Additional factors include decreased visual acuity, hearing disability, and decreased mobility with arthritic changes. The absence of support systems may affect ability to cope with the situation.

Many losses accompany colon cancer surgery. Paramount may be the real or perceived loss of life as well as loss of a function. Other perceived losses may be employment, social status, and love. Just opening the topic in an empathetic manner may bring forth a flood of feelings from the patient. Nursing assessment of the stage of the grief process is often difficult. Patients may jump from stage to stage. If the patient is in the stage of denial it is difficult to intervene in the knowledge deficit area.

As previously discussed, nutritional status is an important variable in the susceptibility to infection and the postoperative healing process. The patient with a tumor may report weight loss in past months and loss of appetite. If the bowel is partially obstructed, a pattern of alternating constipation and diarrhea, nausea, and vomiting may have been present.

Nursing Diagnosis

The following nursing diagnoses may be appropriate for the patient with colon cancer:

Knowledge deficit related to disease process and treatment

Fatigue related to tumor growth and anorexia

Altered nutrition: less than body requirements related to anorexia

Sexual dysfunction related to postoperative complications and body image disturbance

Anticipatory grieving related to loss of body function and disease process

Hopelessness related to diagnosis of cancer

Powerlessness related to loss of control of bowel elimination

Body image disturbance related to presence of colostomy

Planning

Nursing care for the patient with cancer of the colon is planned to achieve the following outcomes:

The patient will express understanding of the disease process and planned treatment

The patient will participate in the care plan and make adaptive decisions concerning care

The patient will discuss feelings about the disease, potential loss, body image, and sexual dysfunction

The patient will maintain adequate nutritional status

Implementation

Patient teaching

The patient and family should understand that certain operative findings may demand a variation in the planned procedure. If an ostomy is a possibility, the nurse can give as much information as desired by the patient either verbally or in written format for later reading. If radiation or chemotherapy is planned, discussion of the treatment with information concerning what to expect is appropriate.

The usual preoperative teaching concerns what the patient can expect regarding the nasogastric tube, intravenous line, Foley catheter, dressings, pain medications, deep breathing, and leg exercises. Preoperative bowel preparation is done at this time. If ostomy surgery is a possibility, the stoma site is marked, preferably by the enterostomal therapist.

Fear of change from independence to dependence and curtailment of activity may be anxieties that the nurse can help allay by active listening, discussion, and reassurance. Inclusion of family or significant others in the care plan may reduce the patient's anxiety and sense of isolation.

Four major areas of life are affected when a person is diagnosed as having cancer. These are self-esteem, sexuality, family, and work. These areas pertain to ostomy surgery as well. Cancer and anticancer therapies affect the physical self, the psychologic self, and the social self in the immediate future and over time.[32] The empathetic nurse can give the patient an opportunity to discuss feelings of loss and the sense of sadness loss incurs.

If a nutritional deficit is determined, include discussion of a high-protein diet and ways of making foods more palatable. Nutritional liquid supplements (e.g., Ensure) may be encouraged. A nutritional consultation can be helpful.

Postoperative care

The immediate postoperative care involves physical and metabolic assessment as the patient recovers. Areas of assessment are bowel and urinary elimination, fluid and electrolyte balance, tissue perfusion, nutrition, comfort/pain, gas exchange, infection, and peristomal skin integrity. These areas were discussed previously in the chapter. The assessment, care, and appliance selection for the temporary or permanent colostomy are important and are applicable to ostomies performed for varied reasons.

Long-term complications indigenous to the abdominal resection with permanent colostomy are urinary retention or incontinence, pelvic abscess, failure of perineal wound healing or infection, and sexual dysfunction.

Stoma assessment

If surgery is performed under emergency conditions stoma placement and construction may not be optimal. The nurse will want to observe the stoma and peristomal area frequently after surgery for type of stoma (loop or end), as well as color, size, and location of the stoma and the condition of the peristomal skin. Common stomal and peristomal complications in the immediate postoperative period are necrosis, retraction, and abscess.

Compromised blood flow to the stoma may cause color change and necrosis. The stoma will appear pale and dusty to black. If the level of ischemia is not below the fascia, conservative management can be employed. Ischemia below the fascia requires surgical revision of the stoma to prevent fecal spillage into the peritoneal cavity. If the nurse notes a change in stoma color, notification of the surgeon and documentation in the medical record are mandatory.

Tension at the stoma site, where it is sutured to the skin, can create poor healing or necrosis of the stomal-skin edge. This can result in retraction of the stoma into the abdomen. This occurs most often when the abdomen is obese. If retraction occurs below the level of the fascia the surgeon must revise the stoma; if not the stoma can be treated conservatively with the nurse fitting a flexible pouch and skin barrier. If retraction occurs, physician notification and documentation are necessary.

Stoma placement too close to the wound, retention sutures, and drains in the area create challenging pouching situations. The nurse may want to use a flexible pouch, skin barrier, and Stomahesive paste and powder to bridge indentations. If the nurse determines the need for these products, the pouching procedure should be included in the care plan and each pouch change documented.

Temporary colostomy

The nurse can determine the location of the opening in the bowel from the surgical record and by observation of the location of the stoma on the abdomen. Effluent consistency is directly related to location of the diversion (Figure 66-9). The effluent from a stoma in the ascending colon will be liquid, in the transverse colon it will be loose to semiformed, and in the descending/sigmoid areas the consistency will be close to normal. The care plan and type of pouch selected by the nurse depend on the stoma location and consistency of the effluent.

Effluent consistency of the transverse loop colostomy is usually loose and output is unpredictable, requiring a drainable ostomy pouch. The inclusion of a skin barrier on the back of the pouch is desirable. Special attention should be given to keeping the opening of the pouch not more than ⅛ inch larger than the stoma. Teach the patient to empty the pouch when it is no more than one-third full and to cleanse the pouch from the bottom with a squeeze bottle filled with soapy water. The pouch can be changed every 4 to 7 days depending on the stability of the adhesive seal.

The patient with a temporary descending or sigmoid colostomy can wear a pouch and empty it as needed or can be taught to do colostomy irrigations for 24-hour control of output. Colostomy irrigation should be taught only if the patient desires to learn this form of control.

Permanent colostomy

In an abdominoperineal resection, the colostomy is created in the descending colon and usually placed in the left lower abdominal quadrant. The patient with a permanent descending colostomy can be taught two forms of colostomy management. The first is wearing a drainable pouch at all times and allowing the bowels to move spontaneously. The pouch may be emptied and cleansed from the bottom opening and changed once or twice per week (see patient education guide above). The second form of management is the colostomy irrigation. Colostomy irrigation has two purposes: to establish regularity and to relieve constipation. This procedure is reserved for patients who have sigmoid or descending colostomies. The nurse can give the patient a choice of management, with both forms being discussed and taught. The patient can then make the decision about care. This encourages a sense of independence.

Daily irrigation is for regulation of the bowel and for the convenience of having bowel elimination at a predictable time and place. Water serves as a stimulus for peristalsis. Irrigation is not an exact procedure and should serve the patient's needs. It is for the patient's convenience, and when it is judged inconvenient, nonproductive, or undesirable, it should not be forced into the patient's routine. Bowel elimination occurs with or without irrigation.

PATIENT EDUCATION GUIDE
Pouch Change Procedure

Gather Materials

Drainable pouch—opening not more than ⅛ inch larger in diameter than the stoma (use pouch with skin barrier backing if available)

Liquid skin barrier (skin preparation)

Washcloth and towel

Soap and water

Tissue

Disposable gloves

Trash bag

Procedure

Apply gloves

Gently remove old pouch by supporting skin with one hand as you slowly remove the pouch adhesive with the other

Wash and dry the peristomal area (note any skin irritation or changes in size or color of the stoma and document)

Apply liquid skin barrier to peristomal skin and allow to dry

Remove paper from back of ostomy pouch to expose adhesive surface; center opening over stoma and press into place

Tape may be used in a picture-frame fashion but usually is not necessary

Discard old pouch, tissue, and gloves in trash bag; seal and discard

---

Most patients are able to control elimination with dietary regulation.

When assessing the patient as a candidate for irrigation, these factors are considered[49]:

1. Past bowel habits: frequency of stools (the person with a history of frequent stools or irritable bowel is not an appropriate candidate)
2. Location of a colostomy: transverse colostomy may not regulate as a result of loose effluent
3. Age of patient: independence is important; the patient can do the irrigation without assistance
4. General health of the patient: is the patient ill or becoming more ill (e.g., metastatic cancer)? does the procedure leave the patient exhausted?
5. Patient's personal preference: would the patient prefer to empty and clean a drainable pouch? (See patient education guide above.)

If for some reason irrigation of the colostomy is not convenient or desirable at a particular time (e.g., family emergency, diarrhea), then it can be skipped

PATIENT EDUCATION GUIDE   *Colostomy Irrigation*

Procedure

Place 1 quart of warm tap water into the vinyl water bag. Let water run through the tube, then clamp off. This removes air from the tube.

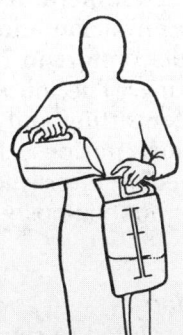

Hang the water bag so that the bottom of the bag is at shoulder level when sitting on the toilet.

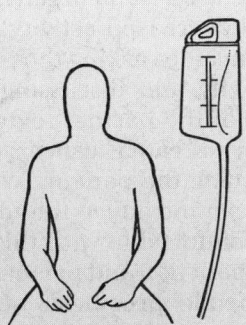

Put belt, with face plate assembly, around body and attach. Place sleeve (cut to proper length) between the legs and into the toilet.

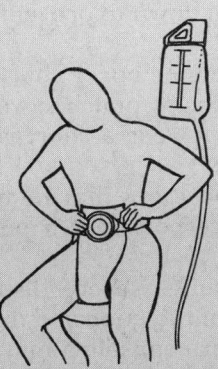

Lubricate the Uni-Tip Cone and insert through the top of the open sleeve into the stoma. Hold in place.

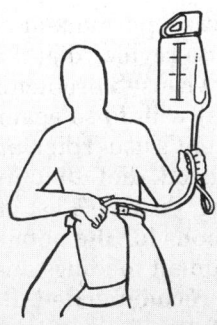

Open clamp and allow water to flow. The water bag should empty in 7 to 10 minutes. Remove catheter or Uni-Tip and close top of the open sleeve by folding down and attaching clips.

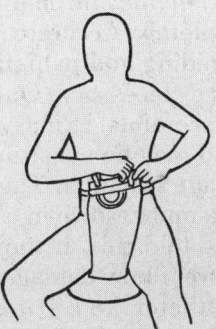

Elimination generally occurs within 20 to 25 minutes. After irrigation is completed, all parts should be washed in cold water and hung to dry. NOTE: You do not eat the same food daily, therefore the time required and amount of elimination may vary, but usually only 1 quart of warm tap water is necessary for an irrigation.

Used with permission of Smith and Nephew United, Inc., Largo, Fla.

and a drainable pouch worn until the patient is able to resume the usual routine.

The appliance choice for the permanent colostomy depends on the form of management. The patient who chooses not to irrigate wears a drainable pouch. The patient who irrigates and has good control from one irrigation to the next can wear a small closed security pouch, stoma cap, or piece of gauze over the stoma.

The patient with a permanent colostomy may be encouraged to eat a regular diet if able to do so previously. Foods that caused problems in the past (e.g., gas-forming foods) will do so again.

Assess the patient's usual diet, and, if needed, discuss a well-balanced diet that includes adequate protein for healing. Provide a list of gas-forming and odor-producing foods for the patient. If the appetite is poor, small frequent feedings and nutritional supplements may be recommended. Referral to a dietitian may be helpful.

Urinary elimination

As a result of the large amount of tissue removed in the abdominoperineal resection, nerves that control the bladder may be damaged and bladder support altered. Postoperatively, after the Foley catheter is removed, the patient may be unable to void or empty the bladder completely. Accurate recording and documentation of voiding and palpation of the bladder for distention are necessary. Question the patient about bladder discomfort. Urinary incontinence may be a problem and may be upsetting to the patient in an already difficult situation. The problem may be caused by edema and resolve in a few days. The patient needs to be told this. If there has been parasympathetic nerve fiber damage the patient may need a Foley catheter and a urology consultation may be required.

Infection

With any type of colon surgery there is always a chance of contamination of the abdominal cavity during the surgery. Certainly, when a large amount of tissue is removed, as in an abdominoperineal resection, and a cavity is left as sanctuary for bacteria there is increased risk of infection. Assessment of the perineal wound includes monitoring of the drain site for increased pain, redness, and purulent drainage, as well as monitoring body temperature for elevation.

The perineal wound may be closed in one of three ways. The first is the closed wound with a drain to suction. This form has a high risk for abscess formation. The second is the semiclosed wound, which is partially closed with either a Jackson-Pratt, Davol, or Penrose drain in place. The last is the open wound that is packed with gauze.

In the closed wound the drain to suction is left in place for 3 to 5 days. After drain removal sitz baths may be ordered two or three times daily for comfort and to promote healing. In the semiclosed wound the drains are left in longer, but the surgeon may choose to shorten the drains over time. In the open wound, after the packing is removed, physician-ordered irrigations and sitz baths are implemented by the nurse. This wound may be slow to heal. Observation for change in drainage color and odor and temperature elevation should be reported to the physician and documented. The patient will have discomfort in the area and much difficulty with sitting. The nurse may provide a pillow or cushion for sitting and expect the patient to sit for only short periods. If perineal wound irrigations are needed after discharge teach the family or caregiver meticulously clean wound irrigation technique.

Sexual dysfunction

Sexual dysfunction related to removal of the rectum can best be defined in men as an inability to obtain full erection, orgasm, emission, and ejaculation. In women sexual dysfunction is defined as a decrease or absence of the orgasmic sensations during intercourse that they had before surgery.[39] Contributing factors are partial to complete disruption of the nerve's supply to the genital organs, psychologic factors, or age and decreased activity.

Assessment includes asking the patient about normal sexual activity and discussing misconceptions about reactions of the partner, extent of sexual impairment, ability to "catch" cancer, and fears of sexual activity harming the patient. With an open attitude the nurse can introduce the topic of sex. If the patient seems comfortable with this topic the nurse can discuss the patient's and partner's fears, give information on penile prosthesis surgery, and give simple suggestions to both partners that may decrease anxiety concerning intercourse,[49] including the following:

1. Odor is not a problem unless the pouch is leaking.
2. Empty the pouch before a sexual encounter.
3. Tape pouch down to prevent distracting pouch movement.
4. Pouch covers or boxer shorts for men may be worn to keep pouch away from partner; women may wear a short gown or crotchless underwear.
5. Different positions may be tried.
6. Rehearse responses if a pouch seal leak occurs.

Some patients suffer severe disturbances of body image with fear of rejection and depression. In these cases, referral for counseling may be needed.

Body image

Cancer and the anticancer therapies, including surgery, have a great effect on the patient's body image. The person's value of beauty may be assaulted, as well as the value of body function control. Weight loss, hair loss, skin reactions to treatment, scars, and stomas may leave a patient feeling unattractive, undesirable, and unloved. Fatigue, illness, and loss of control of a body function when an ostomy is constructed may generate feelings of powerlessness, hopelessness, and despair.

The nurse can give the patient an opportunity to talk about these feelings. Above all, the nurse's silent communication of touch and eye contact can give the patient a message of acceptance and value.

Evaluation

Evaluation of the patient's care plan includes that the patient is able to make informed, adaptive decisions about care and is able to consume sufficient nutritional intake to maintain body weight. The patient demonstrates deep breathing and leg exercises and verbalizes pain control methods and expected surgical outcomes. Postoperatively the patient or caregiver verbalizes and demonstrates understanding of the ostomy care to the nurse. The patient and family verbalize where to obtain supplies and support when needed.

Documentation

Record vital signs, intake and output, response to comfort measures, ambulation, and wound healing. Describe the patient's response to the stoma and participation in the care of the stoma. Record the patient's tolerance of oral foods, diet progression, and ability to plan and prepare a well-balanced diet to meet the needs of an ostomy patient. Document patient/family concerns, responses to teaching, expressions of ability to cope with life-style changes, and the support systems available for ostomy patients.

Assess family needs and concerns along with those of the patient. The patient may adapt better and feel less isolated when family members are included in the teaching. Because family needs and support have been determined to be vital to healthy psychosocial adaptation of not only the patient but also all family members it becomes incumbent on nurses to include family needs and goals in the care

ETHICAL ISSUES

- If disability and disfigurement can be destructive of self as well as body, what is the nurse's role in preventing damage to the patient's self? Is a damaged self an inevitable consequence of illness or injury?

plan.[13] Support groups are available to the cancer patient. Groups such as the United Ostomy Association can be meaningful. Provide the patient with telephone numbers and addresses of appropriate groups before hospital discharge.

THERAPEUTIC COMMUNICATION GUIDE

Colostomy

Assessment

Determine patient's feelings regarding care.

Example	*Nurse:*	"You will be going home soon, Mr. Kinney. How comfortable do you feel in managing your colostomy?"
	Patient:	"Well, I'm not sure I can do it. I've been able to take care of it in the hospital, but at home I won't have any help."

Intervention

Provide reassurance and clarify need for further instruction.

Example	*Nurse:*	"It's normal to feel a little unsure of yourself. You've done so well in the hospital. Is there anything I can help you with before you leave?"
	Patient:	"No, I understand what I need to do."

Recognize patient's feelings. Offer additional resources and support.

Example	*Nurse:*	"You still seem a little anxious. Would it help if I find a nurse to visit you for a while at your home?"
	Patient:	"I'd like that. I'd feel better knowing I wasn't all alone."

Offer familiar source of support and help.

Example	*Nurse:*	"I will give you our telephone number at the hospital. Whenever you like, you can call us and we can help."

Ongoing Care

After hospital discharge, the patient may be faced with a plethora of problems: dealing with an unhealed perineal or abdominal wound, chemotherapy or radiation and its side effects, lack of support systems, poor appetite, and minimal knowledge about self-care. A home care referral is appropriate for the patient of any age, but it may be particularly needed with the geriatric patient. Older patients may be poorly motivated or confused while hospitalized, but once they are home the activities of rehabilitation become more meaningful. Teach the elderly person in a consistent manner; it is best if each session is conducted by the same nurse. The activity or procedure can be taught in a step-by-step, routine manner. It is helpful to provide written instructions to the patient.

A major factor in survival time for the metastatic cancer patient seems to be a sense of hope and a will to live. Removal of this sense of hope leaves the patient nothing but the wait for death. Nurturing the understanding that each individual day has meaning and is an opportunity to do important things or spend time with family can give quality to the patient's days.

HEMORRHOIDS

Definition

Hemorrhoids are one of the most common health problems seen in humans. All humans are born with an internal and external set of hemorrhoids. Hemorrhoids are cushions of vascular tissue in the anal canal.[3] The lay term is "piles." The hemorrhoids progressively enlarge and may become symptomatic with aging. Incidence is greatest during active adulthood from age 20 to 50 years.

Etiology/Pathophysiology

Etiologic factors include straining at stool with resultant increased intra-abdominal and hemorrhoidal venous pressures. Formed stool in the rectal ampulla is believed to result in obstruction of retrograde venous flow. Repeated and lengthy exposure of the hemorrhoids to increased pressure and obstructed venous flow leads to a permanent dilation. Factors implicated are heredity, constipation, diarrhea, obesity, pregnancy, congestive heart failure, portal hypertension, and prolonged sitting and standing.

Clinical Manifestations

The most common symptoms associated with enlarged, abnormal hemorrhoids are prolapse and bleeding. Bright red bleeding and prolapse usually

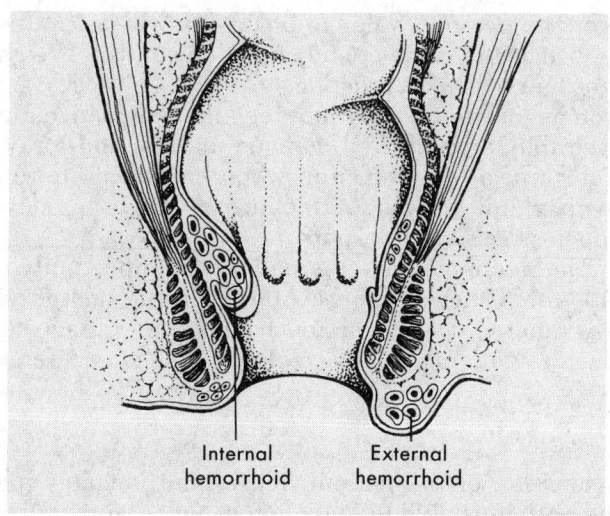

FIGURE 66-11   Internal and external hemorrhoids.

occur at the time of defecation. The internal hemorrhoids appear above the internal sphincter and are not apparent unless prolapsed (Figure 66-11). The external hemorrhoids are those that appear outside the anal sphincter and are less likely to bleed and cause pain unless thrombosis occurs. Thrombosis, or clotting of blood within the hemorrhoid, can occur at any time and is manifested by intense pain, edema, and inflammation. These thrombosed hemorrhoids may become ischemic and ulcerated.

Classification of internal hemorrhoids is done by a staging system to help determine how invasive a procedure is necessary to correct the disorder:

Stage 1: enlarged but not prolapsing; some bleeding present

Stage 2: prolapse during defecation but spontaneously reduce; bleeding present

Stage 3: prolapse and require manual reduction; bleeding, discomfort, soiling present

Stage 4: enlarged, prolapsed, swollen, and cannot be reduced; bleeding, pain, ischemia, and thrombosis may occur

Therapeutic Management

Medical therapy is based on modification of the stools to decrease the need to strain at defecation. To counteract the hard stool, use of bulk stool softeners such as Metamucil, bran, and natural food fiber is advocated. Consumption of at least 8 to 10 glasses of water daily will help to prevent constipation. Often this is all that is required for first- or small second-stage hemorrhoids. Topical creams with hydrocortisone are valuable only if itching is present.

Therapeutic interventions include sclerotherapy, rubber-band ligation, cryotherapy, infrared photocoagulation, laser excision, and operative hemorrhoidectomy. In sclerotherapy a needle is inserted at the apex of the hemorrhoidal column and a sclerosing solution is injected. The inflammation created by the solution causes fixation to underlying muscles, thereby preventing prolapse. This procedure may cause pain, necrosis, and ulceration at the injection site. The rubber-band ligation is a popular and easy method of treatment. A rubber band is placed at the base of the hemorrhoid tissue. This causes strangulation, sloughing, and scarring. Infection is of concern in this procedure.

Cryotherapy, another method of tissue destruction, is achieved by freezing. Freezing may result in deep ulcers and cause superficial sloughing. Pain and slow healing may accompany the procedure. Infrared photocoagulation is the destruction of tissue by creation of a small burn. Subsequent inflammation and scarring create fixation. Pain and bleeding may be complications of this procedure. The Nd-YAG laser has been used for fixation and excision of hemorrhoids. Postoperative complications include hemorrhage, abscess, and pain.

The hemorrhoidectomy has been the standard against which all other treatments have been compared. After removal of the hemorrhoid, wounds can be left open or closed, although closed wounds are reported to heal faster. Complications of hemorrhoidectomy include hemorrhage, local infection, pain, urinary retention, and abscess.

NURSING MANAGEMENT OF THE PATIENT WITH HEMORRHOIDS

Often these patients are seen on an outpatient basis in the clinic or office setting, where time is limited. These patients require that their needs be addressed, and it is important that the nurse take the time to do this.

Assessment

Areas of assessment are knowledge, pain/comfort, tissue perfusion, and nutrition/diet. Postoperative assessment includes infection, bowel elimination, and urinary elimination.

The nurse assesses the knowledge level by asking the patient about the condition, what information has been provided about treatment, and what treatments have been done before surgery and why. Rectal conditions can be embarrassing to the patient. The nurse's direct but concerned attitude can decrease embarrassment. Questions about pain, as well as swelling and prolapse, can elicit information about the patient's comfort level. Ask the patient to report any postoperative pain or discomfort. The patient may have great anxiety concerning the first defecation and may want to discuss this.

Assess the prolapsed hemorrhoid for swelling, thrombosis, and ischemia. If thrombosis is present, the patient will have a great deal of pain. Ischemic tissue will be dark red to necrotic. Assess hematocrit and hemoglobin levels, because long-term rectal bleeding can result in anemia. Postoperatively the nurse should assess for hemorrhage.

Assessment of the patient's diet habits may be an indicator of cause. A low-bulk diet contributes to chronic constipation. Observe for swelling, increased pain at the surgical site, abscess formation, purulent drainage, and temperature elevation. The patient is assessed for the first bowel movement after surgery. Urinary retention is predominantly a postoperative problem for male patients. Assess for ability to void and to empty the bladder.

Nursing Diagnosis

The following nursing diagnoses may be appropriate for the patient with hemorrhoids:

Rectal pain related to swelling, inflammation, and/or prolapse

Knowledge deficit related to the disease process, treatment, diet, and prevention

Altered nutrition/anemia related to chronic rectal bleeding

Planning

Nursing care for the patient with hemorrhoids is planned to meet the following outcomes:

The patient will report a decrease in rectal pain

The patient will have an understanding of how hemorrhoids develop and the treatment regimen

The patient will identify when swelling, prolapse, and thrombosis occur and take corrective action

The patient will verbalize ways to increase bulk in the diet

The patient will verbalize care of the surgical area and discharge instructions

The patient will verbalize diet and medication regimen to maintain soft stools

The patient will describe ways to prevent recurrence of hemorrhoids

Implementation

Teach the patient about hemorrhoids and their etiologic factors. Reinforce dietary adherence to the high-residue diet. Stress the importance of keeping the stool soft but formed to help prevent formation of stricture, as well as keeping the rectal area clean. Encourage the patient to wash the anal area after defecation and to pat dry with a soft cloth rather than irritate the tissues with toilet paper. Local moist heat applied to the anal area and sitz baths are soothing. Local anesthetics (i.e., Nupercainal ointment or Tucks pads) may give temporary relief. Manual reduction of prolapsed hemorrhoids may be demonstrated. The patient needs to know the symptoms of thrombosis. When hemorrhoids thrombose an ice pack may be applied to prevent further swelling and pain. Incision of the hemorrhoid may be needed to release encased blood clots.

Diet instruction including bulk-forming foods such as fresh fruit, vegetables, and bran cereals as well as encouraging 8 to 10 glasses of fluid per day, unless contraindicated, is necessary. If the patient is anemic, discussion of foods high in iron such as red meats, liver, and dark green leafy vegetables can be included. The patient may be placed on an iron supplement. After surgery the patient is advised to eat a diet high in roughage, to exercise moderately, to drink plenty of fluids, and to establish a routine time for a daily bowel movement. Remind the patient to cleanse the area gently after each bowel movement.

To prevent pressure on the anal area postoperatively, a cushion may be used for sitting or the patient may prefer to lie on the back or side. Warm compresses may be used postoperatively for the first 48 hours. Sitz baths can be given twice or more daily. Pain medication is given as ordered.

Hemorrhage may occur within 24 hours after surgery. It can also occur between the seventh and tenth postoperative days when the sutures slough and separate from the pedicle. The physician may order pressure applied to the area by way of an inflated Foley catheter if hemorrhage occurs. Rectal tubes and the taking of rectal temperatures are avoided.

The incidence of wound infection is slight after rectal surgery but is most likely to occur if bowel action is delayed and healing tissue becomes adhered. If the patient is fearful of having a bowel movement, stool softeners, laxatives, and an analgesic may be needed before the first movement. Emotional support and a warm sitz bath immediately after the first bowel movement are helpful.

The patient can eat a full diet immediately after surgery. This stimulates elimination. If a spontaneous bowel movement does not occur in 2 to 3 days postoperatively, laxatives may be increased and an oil retention enema followed by a cleansing enema may be given carefully through a small rectal tube.

Urinary retention is a frequent complication in men. Postoperatively, to promote urination, the patient is told to feel free to strain as he normally would to urinate. If he cannot void, he should sit in a warm tub bath up to the waist and void in this position. If retention occurs, intermittent catheterization can be used, and if the problem continues, a catheter may be inserted for 48 hours and then removed. Patients usually void spontaneously after this.

Evaluation

Have the patient demonstrate understanding of the diet recommendation, care of the affected area, and indications to watch for by return demonstration and verbalization of understanding.

Evaluation of interventions can be done postoperatively by having the patient demonstrate knowledge of the care of the surgical area and verbalize understanding of increased bulk in the diet. Evaluation of pain is done by patient feedback. Tissue perfusion, infection, and bowel and urinary elimination can be evaluated by observation and patient feedback.

Documentation

Record rectal drainage, pain control, ambulation, vital signs, and hydration status. Pay particular attention to urinary and bowel elimination. Record urinary output and any problems the patient has with urination. Document the first and subsequent bowel movements and the results of enemas if administered. Document the frequency and effectiveness of sitz baths. Record patient teaching and follow-up plans.

ANAL FISSURE AND FISTULA

An anal fissure is a slitlike ulcer resembling a crack in the lining of the anal canal or below the anorectal line. Usually it is the result of trauma caused by hard-formed stool that overstretches the anal lining. Another form of trauma is anal sexual intercourse. The ulcer does not heal readily. Defecation initiates spasm of the anal sphincter and pain. Slight bleeding may occur. If the lesion does not heal spontaneously, the tract is excised surgically. An anal fistula is an inflammatory sinus or tract with a primary opening in the anal crypt and a secondary opening on the anal or perineal skin or in the rectal mucous membrane. It results from rupture or drainage of an anal abscess. The anal fistula is usually a chronic condition. Treatment of this condition is a fistulectomy or fistulotomy with either removal or opening of the fistula tract. The postoperative care required for a patient who has had repair of an anal fissure or fistula is similar to the patient who has had a hemorrhoidectomy.

CRITICAL THINKING QUESTIONS

1 Describe the relationship between the intake of lactose and gluten and the development of malabsorption syndromes.

2 Outline a teaching plan for the patient with a malabsorption syndrome.

3 Describe how agent-host factors play a role in the development of an intestinal infection.

4 Identify the nursing interventions for the management of a patient with an intestinal infection.

5 Compare and contrast the disease processes of ulcerative colitis and Crohn's disease.

6 Describe the preoperative preparation for the patient having bowel surgery.

7 Identify the primary differences between an ileostomy and a colostomy in terms of function and care requirements.

8 Describe how the nurse can prevent and manage peristomal skin problems.

9 Develop a teaching plan for the patient with a permanent ostomy.

10 Describe some of the psychologic effects of bowel diversion surgery.

11 Explain the problems experienced by the patient with diverticular disease.

12 Relate the assessment findings in intestinal obstruction to the pathophysiologic process.

13 Identify the primary screening examinations for colorectal cancer.

14 Describe the nursing care for a patient with hemorrhoids.

RESOURCES

1 AMERICAN CANCER SOCIETY TOWER PLACE 3340 Peachtree Rd., N.E. Atlanta, GA 30026 (404) 320-3333 Local offices are listed in telephone books.

2 CROHN'S AND COLITIS FOUNDATION OF AMERICA, INC. 444 Park Ave., South New York, NY 10016-7374 (212) 285-3440

3 INTERNATIONAL ASSOCIATION FOR ENTEROSTOMAL THERAPY 500 Birch St. P.O. Box 2690, Suite 175 Newport Beach, CA 92660 (714) 476-0268

4 UNITED OSTOMY ASSOCIATION 36 Executive Park, Suite 120 Irvine, CA 92714 (714) 660-8624

BIBLIOGRAPHY

Current

1. Alterescu K: Colostomy, *Nurs Clin North Am* 22(2):281, 1987.
2. Baird SB, editor: *A cancer source book for nurses,* Atlanta, 1991, American Cancer Society.
3. Beck DE, Welling DR, editors: *Patient care in colorectal surgery,* Boston, 1991, Little, Brown & Co.
4. Benham KJ: Gardner's syndrome: an overview and case history, *J Enterostom Ther* 14(6):287-288, 1987.
5. Black M: Crohn's disease, pathophysiology, diagnosis, and management, *Gastroenterol Nurs* 11:259-262, 1989.
6. Broadwell DC: Gastrointestinal system. In Thompson JM et al, editors: *Mosby's manual of clinical nursing,* ed 2, St Louis, 1989, Mosby–Year Book, Inc.
7. Broadwell DC: Peristomal skin integrity, *Nurs Clin North Am* 22(2):321, 1987.
8. *Cancer facts & figures, 1992,* Atlanta, 1992, American Cancer Society.
9. Cardona VD et al: *Trauma nursing: from resuscitation through rehabilitation,* Philadelphia, 1988, WB Saunders.
10. Cooke DM: Inflammatory bowel disease: primary health care management of ulcerative colitis and Crohn's disease, *Nurse Pract* 16(8):27, 1991.
11. Cooper BT et al: *Manual of gastroenterology,* New York, 1987, Churchill Livingstone, Inc.
12. Dueholm S, Rubinstein E: Preparation for elective colorectal surgery, *Dis Colon Rectum,* p 360, May 1987.
13. Finlay I, Carter D: A comparison of emergency resection and staged management in perforated diverticular disease, *Dis Colon Rectum,* p 929, Dec 1987.
14. Gordon PH, Nivatvongs S: *Principles and practice of surgery for the colon, rectum, and anus,* St Louis, 1992, Quality Medical Publishers.
15. Harper P, Fazio M: The long-term outcome in Crohn's disease, *Dis Colon Rectum,* p 174, March 1987.
16. Hassey K: Radiation therapy for rectal cancer and the implications for nursing, *Cancer Nurs* 10(6):311, 1987.
17. Hassey K: Skin care for patients receiving radiation therapy for rectal cancer, *J Enterostom Ther* 14(5):197, 1987.
18. Heimann T, Geleont I: Familial polyposis coli: results of mucosal proctectomy with ileoanal anastomosis, *Dis Colon Rectum,* p 424, June 1987.
19. Hennessy K: Nutritional support and gastrointestinal disease, *Nurs Clin North Am* 24(2):373-382, 1989.
20. Herberth L, Gosnell D: Nursing diagnosis for oncology nursing practice, *Cancer Nurs* 19(1):41, 1987.
21. Kirsner JB: Inflammatory bowel disease. I. Nature and pathogenesis, *Dis Mon* 37(10):605-666, 1991.
22. Meize-Grochowski AR: When the diagnosis is Crohn's disease . . . diagnosis, *RN* 54(2):52-56, 1991.
23. McConnell E: Meeting the challenge of intestinal obstruction, *Nurs 87* 17(7):34-41, 1987.
24. Motta GJ: Life span changes: implication for ostomy care, *Nurs Clin North Am* 22(2):333, 1987.
25. Nurses GI handbook, *Nurs 80* 20(11):65-80, 1990.
26. O'Toole MT: Advanced assessment of the abdomen and gastrointestinal problems, *Nurs Clin North Am* 25(4):771-776, 1990.
27. Peppercorn MA: Advances in drug therapy for inflammatory bowel disease, *Ann Intern Med* 112(1):50-60, 1990.
28. Peppercorn MA: *Therapy of inflammatory bowel disease: new medical and surgical approaches,* New York, 1990, Marcel Dekker, Inc.
29. Rideout BW: The patient with an ileostomy, *Nurs Clin North Am* 22(2):253, 1987.
30. Rolstad B: Innovative surgical procedure and stoma care in the future, *Nurs Clin North Am* 22(2):341, 1987.
31. Sheehy SB et al: *Manual of clinical trauma care: the first hour,* St Louis, 1989, Mosby–Year Book, Inc.
32. Shipes E: Psychosocial issues: the person with an ostomy, *Nurs Clin North Am* 22(2):291, 1987.
33. Shipes E: Sexual function following ostomy surgery, *Nurs Clin North Am* 22(2):303, 1987.
34. Sitzman JV: Favorable response to parenteral nutrition and medical therapy in Crohn's disease, *Gastroenterology* 99(6):1647-1652, 1990.
35. Skidmore-Roth L: *Mosby's 1992 nursing drug reference,* St Louis, 1992, Mosby–Year Book, Inc.
36. Swartz ML: Beyond the scope: a nursing view of extraintestinal manifestations of inflammatory bowel disease, *Gastroenterol Nurs* 12:3-9, 1989.
37. Welch JP: *Bowel obstruction: differential diagnosis and clinical management,* Philadelphia, 1990, WB Saunders.

38. Williams SR: *Nutrition and diet therapy,* ed 6, St Louis, 1989, Mosby–Year Book, Inc.

Classic

39. Broadwell D, Jackson B, editors: *Principles of ostomy care,* St Louis, 1982, Mosby–Year Book, Inc.
40. Click C: Chemotherapy and the ostomy patient, *J Enterostom Ther* 7(5):10, 1980.
41. DeHovitz JA et al: Gastrointestinal infections. In Roberts RB, editor: *Infectious diseases: pathogenesis, diagnosis, and therapy,* Chicago, 1986, Year Book Medical Publishers, Inc.
42. Eastwood GL: Malabsorption syndrome. In Eastwood GL, editor: *Core textbook of gastroenterology,* Philadelphia, 1984, JB Lippincott Co.
43. Goligher J: Alternatives to conventional ileostomy in the surgical treatment of ulcerative colitis, *J Enterostom Ther* 10(3):79, 1983.
44. Kellock G: The disease of familial polyposis: its impact on families, *J Enterostom Ther* 8(5):12, 1981.
45. Kodner I, Fry R: Inflammatory bowel disease, *Clin Symp* 34:1982.
46. McLeod R, Fazio V: The continent ileostomy: an acceptable alternative, *J Enterostom Ther* 11(4):140, 1984.
47. Postier R, O'Malley V: Continence-preserving operations for ulcerative colitis and familial polyposis, *J Enterostom Ther* 11(6):237, 1984.
48. Rodriquez D: Radiotherapy and the ostomy patient: special considerations, *J Enterostom Ther* 8(4):21, 1981.
49. Smith D: Colostomy irrigations—so simple, *J Enterostom Ther* 10(6):22, 1983.
50. Spencer M, Parnett W: The continent ileal reservoir (Kock pouch): a new approach, *J Enterostom Ther* 9(5):8, 1982.

CHAPTER SIXTY-SEVEN

Nursing Management of Adults with Disorders of the Liver, Biliary Tract, or Exocrine Pancreas

---

LEARNING OBJECTIVES

1 Relate the pathophysiology and clinical manifestations to the therapeutic management of cirrhosis and its complications.

2 Describe the nursing management for a patient with cirrhosis and its complications.

3 Compare the causative factors, routes of infection, incubation period, severity, clinical manifestations, and therapeutic management of the various types of hepatitis.

4 Describe the nursing management for a patient with hepatitis.

5 Describe the nursing management for a patient with cancer of the liver.

6 Describe the indications for liver transplantation and care of the patient postoperatively.

7 Differentiate among cholecystitis, cholelithiasis, cholecystectomy, choledocholithiasis, and lithotripsy.

8 Describe the etiology, epidemiology, pathophysiology, clinical manifestations, and therapeutic management of patients with cholecystitis and cholelithiasis.

9 Specify the nursing management for patients with disorders of the gallbladder.

10 Describe the etiology, epidemiology, pathophysiology, clinical manifestations, and therapeutic management of the patient with pancreatitis.

11 Plan the nursing management for the patient with pancreatitis.

12 Describe the nursing management for the patient with cancer of the pancreas.

THIS CHAPTER DISCUSSES disorders of the accessory organs of digestion, namely, the liver, gallbladder, and exocrine pancreas. These organs assist in digestion in various ways. When an alteration occurs in the normal function of any one of these organs, not only is digestion affected, but also other problems can occur, possibly even death. Nursing care can be as simple as teaching a patient about a special diet or as complex as intensive care monitoring. In most cases, quality nursing care can make the difference between the patient surviving or dying.

CIRRHOSIS
Definition

Cirrhosis is a chronic degenerative disease of the liver causing liver enlargement and subsequent contraction that result in loss of normal liver architecture and function.

Etiology/Epidemiology

Most people associate cirrhosis with alcoholism. However, several forms of cirrhosis are caused by factors other than alcoholism, such as hepatitis or chemicals.

Laennec's cirrhosis (portal, nutritional, fatty, or alcoholic cirrhosis) is the most common form of cirrhosis in the Western world. It is the fourth leading cause of death in the United States. It affects twice as many males as females. A major cause of Laennec's cirrhosis is nutritional deprivation, especially a decrease in protein intake. This is a common finding in alcoholics. In fact, approximately 80% of patients with Laennec's cirrhosis have a history of chronic ingestion of alcohol.

Postnecrotic cirrhosis (posthepatic, toxic, or nodular cirrhosis) is the most common form of cirrhosis worldwide. It is caused by viral hepatitis, exposure to hepatotoxins (i.e., industrial chemicals), or infection. Primary biliary cirrhosis develops when the small bile ducts are destroyed. The incidence of this form of cirrhosis is much higher in females than males. The other forms of cirrhosis are very rare. Secondary biliary cirrhosis is caused by chronic biliary tree obstruction, such as gallstones, a tumor, or biliary atresia, or severe, recurrent, right-sided congested heart failure. Pigment cirrhosis is caused by diseases such as hemochromatosis, a rare iron storage disease. Finally, idiopathic cirrhosis has no known specific cause.

Pathophysiology

The type of cirrhosis a person has determines the beginning morphologic changes in the liver, but the liver will mainly progress through the following stages: destruction, inflammation, fibrotic regeneration, and hepatic insufficiency. Because of the damage to the liver's parenchymal cells, the liver becomes inflamed and enlarged, called **hepatomegaly** (Figure 67-1). The body attempts to regenerate the damaged hepatocytes, but fibrosis occurs. As the disease progresses the liver becomes small, hard, and nodular. Eventually, the normal architecture of the liver is lost, as is the structure of the vasculature and lymphatics. These changes ultimately cause hepatic insufficiency.

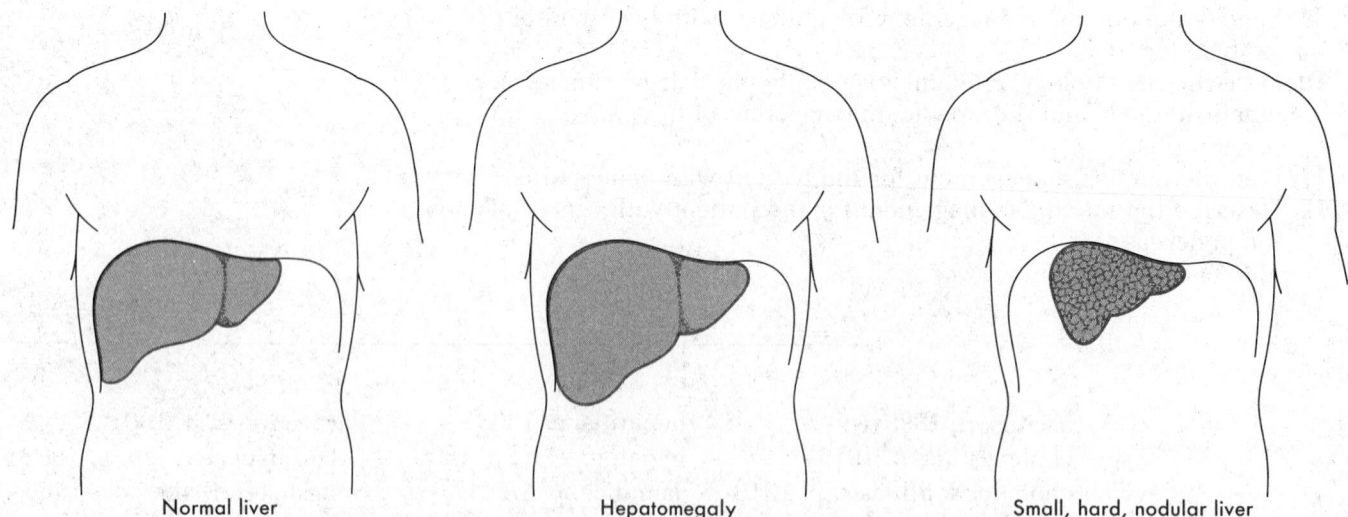

Normal liver   Hepatomegaly   Small, hard, nodular liver

FIGURE 67-1   Changes in structure of liver with cirrhosis.

Clinical Manifestations

Early symptoms

The signs and symptoms of cirrhosis are similar for all types, regardless of the cause. Early clinical manifestations are vague and parallel flulike symptoms or other gastrointestinal disorders. These symptoms include general weakness, fatigue, anorexia, indigestion, abnormal bowel function (either constipation or diarrhea), flatulence, nausea, vomiting, and abdominal discomfort, especially in the epigastric region or in the right upper quadrant. These symptoms are caused by the alteration in the metabolic functioning of the liver or by changes in the venous flow to the gastrointestinal mucosa from the congestion of blood. The pain is caused by the inflammation of the liver, swelling of the liver capsule, or vascular or biliary spasm. Because of the vagueness of these symptoms, patients usually do not seek medical attention in the early stages.

Hepatic insufficiency

Hepatic insufficiency and its complications cause many clinical manifestations that affect the entire body (Figure 67-2). Collateral circulation develops in an attempt to maintain normal blood flow. The newly expanded vessels are found at the cardia of the stomach up to the esophagus, in the paraumbilical vein, and at the anus in the hemorrhoidal veins. The new veins are not able to handle the blood volume passing through them and therefore become varicosed, causing the patient to have esophageal varices, varicose paraumbilical veins, and hemorrhoids. The liver continues to fail, causing ascites and portal hypertension to develop. The portal hypertension may cause splenomegaly and variceal hemorrhage. The patient usually loses weight and has muscle atrophy, but this sign is not as noticeable because of the accumulation of abdominal fluid.

As the ascites increases, pressure is placed on the diaphragm and limits the ability of the chest to expand. The patient suffers from dyspnea. There may be interference with CO_2 and O_2 exchange, which will lead to hypoxia.

Skin

The skin of the patient with cirrhosis yellows, which is termed **jaundice,** because of the liver's inability to metabolize bilirubin after the destruction of red blood cells. The jaundice may range from a slight yellow tint of the sclera to a deep bronze yellow overall. The amount of jaundice depends on the severity of the cirrhosis: the more severe the cirrhosis, the more severe the jaundice. The patient will suffer from pruritus (itching) caused by the accumulation of bile salts. The skin will be dry, and skin le-

sions may be present. Spider angiomas (spider nevi, telangiectasis, or vascular spiders) and palmar erythema are also present in patients with cirrhosis. Spider angiomas are small, red, dilated, pulsating arterioles that have a bright red central point with vessels branching out from the central point. They disappear when pressure is applied. Palmar erythema is redness of the palms that blanches with pressure. Both lesions are believed to be caused by an increase in estrogen levels.

Vitamin synthesis

A patient with cirrhosis will be deficient in vitamins A, D, K, and B complex. Fat-soluble vitamins (A, D, and K) require bile salts to be absorbed from the gastrointestinal tract. A damaged liver does not form bile salts, so fat-soluble vitamins cannot be absorbed. The normal liver also stores many vitamins, including B-complex vitamins. When a liver becomes injured, its ability to store vitamins is lost. Vitamin K is essential for the synthesis of prothrombin and clotting factors VII, IX, and X. The healthy liver also produces several clotting factors (fibrinogen, prothrombin, and factors VII, IX, and X). The cirrhotic liver is unable to absorb vitamin K or produce the clotting factors. This causes the patient with cirrhosis to have bleeding tendencies. The patient may bleed from the gums from a simple task such as brushing teeth. Epistaxis may occur from nose blowing. Bruising occurs very easily, and hematuria is often present. Continued hepatic damage may lead to disseminated intravascular coagulation (DIC). (Refer to Chapter 38 for further information on DIC.)

Hematopoietic changes

Anemia is also a problem for the patient with cirrhosis. Alcohol is toxic to the bone marrow, so the normal production of red blood cells is altered. The spleen becomes enlarged secondary to portal hypertension. It will not function appropriately and does not produce an adequate number of platelets. The patient with esophageal varices may lose copious amounts of blood from varices that rupture. The above alterations are manifested by paleness, purpura, leukopenia, and thrombocytopenia. The liver loses its phagocytic function. This along with the leukopenia makes the patient less resistant to infection.

Endocrine/metabolic changes

Several endocrine problems arise when the liver is damaged. The metabolism and activation of the hormones from the adrenal cortex, ovaries, and testes (aldosterone, antidiuretic hormone [ADH], estrogen, testosterone) are altered. Women have men-

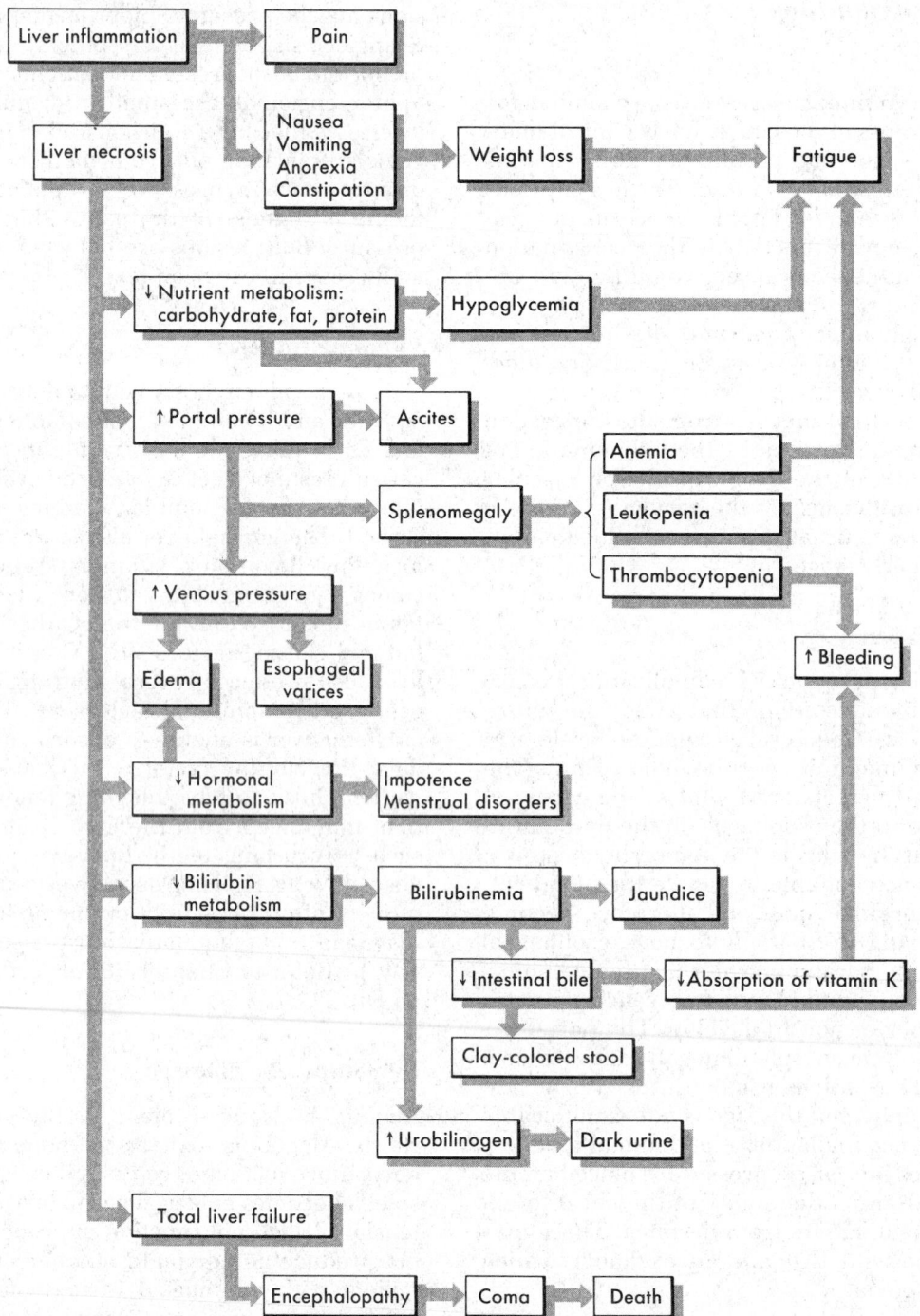

FIGURE 67-2 Pathophysiologic events related to liver failure.

strual irregularities. Men experience gynecomastia (excessive development or enlargement of one or both breasts in men); loss of hair from the chest, axilla, and pubic area; and impotence.

Cirrhosis can cause hepatorenal syndrome (functional renal failure). The cause of the renal failure is unknown. Hepatorenal syndrome is marked by ol-

iguria, decreased urine sodium, increased urine/plasma creatinine, and a urine/plasma osmolality ratio higher than 1.0.[35] The patient with cirrhosis becomes increasingly weak with muscle atrophy. Pain occurs in the upper right abdominal quadrant that increases when sitting or bending forward. The patient may have a sweet, musty breath odor known

TABLE 67-1   Alterations in Laboratory Values with Cirrhosis

Test	Normal value	Alteration
SGOT	10 to 40 mU/mL	Increased
SGPT	7 to 35 mU/mL	Increased
Alkaline phosphatase	20 to 90 mU/mL	Increased
Serum albumin	3.5 to 5.0 g/dL	Decreased
Bilirubin		Increased
Total	0.3 to 1.0 mg/dL	
Direct	0.1 to 0.4 mg/dL	
Prothrombin time (PT)	Less than 2 seconds' deviation from control	Prolonged
Partial thromboplastin time (PTT)	25 to 37 seconds	Prolonged
Serum ammonia	80 to 110 µg/dL	Increased
Total protein	6.0 to 8.4 g/dL	Decreased
Sodium	135 to 145 mEq/L	Decreased
Potassium	3.5 to 5.0 mEq/L	Decreased
Chloride	100 to 106 mEq/L	Decreased
Magnesium	1.5 to 2.0 mEq/L	Decreased
Cholinesterase	0.5 pH U/hr or greater	Decreased
Hemoglobin	Men: 13 to 18 g/dL Women: 12 to 16 g/dL	Decreased
Hematocrit	Men: 45% to 52% Women: 37% to 48%	Decreased
Urine urobilinogen	Up to 1.0 Ehrlich U/2 hr	Increased
Fecal urobilinogen	40 to 280 mg/24 hr	Decreased

as fetor hepaticus caused by the injured liver's inability to metabolize methionine.

The liver's inability to metabolize bilirubin causes changes in the urine and stool. The kidneys excrete excessive amounts of bilirubin (urobilinogen), causing the urine to become a dark amber color. The damaged liver is unable to convert bilirubin into bile. The lack of bile in the gastrointestinal tract causes the stool to be clay colored. Many alterations occur in the laboratory studies of patients with cirrhosis (Table 67-1).

Therapeutic Management

Treatment is designed to eliminate or relieve causative factors (i.e., alcohol or right-sided congestive heart failure), treat any problems that have occurred as a result of liver damage, prevent further liver damage, and provide supportive care.

Abstinence from alcohol and any other hepatotoxins (i.e., acetaminophen) is essential to prevent further liver damage. Diet therapy is aimed at correcting the patient's negative nitrogen balance and malnutrition, promoting the regeneration of functional liver tissue, and compensating for the liver's inability to store vitamins while at the same time avoiding fluid retention and hepatic encephalopathy. A well-balanced, high-calorie (2500 to 3000 calories/day), moderately high-protein (75 g of high-quality protein per day), low-fat, low-sodium (200 to 1000 mg/day) diet with additional vitamins and folic acid usually meets the needs of the patient with cirrhosis and improves deficiencies that exist. The increased number of calories provides the patient with the energy that is needed to help heal the damaged liver. The protein helps facilitate cellular regeneration, but the patient needs to be closely monitored for changes in mental status that could indicate impending hepatic encephalopathy. Fat is usually not tolerated well by the patient with liver damage, because the liver is not producing the bile that is necessary for digestion of fats. The decreased amount of sodium assists with preventing fluid retention. The vitamins and folic acid are necessary for healing and to replace those products that are not being produced by the liver.

If a patient is having difficulty with nausea or vomiting, antiemetics may be prescribed. Caution is used when administering antiemetics to patients with liver damage, because many of the medications rely on the liver for detoxification. Diphenhydramine (Benadryl) or dimenhydrinate (Dramamine) may be given, whereas prochlorperaxine maleate (Compazine), hydroxyzine pamoate (Vistaril), and hydroxyzine hydrochloride (Atarax) are medications that should be avoided.

Complications

Ascites and edema

Ascites is the presence of excessive fluid in the peritoneal cavity. A variety of factors cause ascites. Cirrhosis causes parenchymal cell failure. The damaged liver is unable to form as much albumin as it normally forms, causing the amount of albumin in the blood to decrease. Normally, serum albumin helps maintain the oncotic pressure within the plasma. When serum albumin decreases, plasma oncotic pressure decreases. When oncotic pressure is low, fluid is able to leave the plasma. In the case of the patient with cirrhosis, the fluid leaves the plasma and enters the peritoneal cavity, causing ascites. Fluid also accumulates in dependent areas such as the ankles and presacral area.

Cirrhosis also causes changes in the hepatic vasculature. The vessels within the portal system become obstructed, increasing the pressure within the system. When portal venous pressure is elevated, the capillary hydrostatic pressure increases as does the pressure within the liver. Fluid is then allowed to ooze into the peritoneal cavity. The circulating plasma volume decreases (hypovolemia). The hypovolemia is sensed by the kidneys, causing secretion of the enzyme renin. The vasopressor angiotensin is then formed within the body in attempts to increase the resistance of the flow of blood. The adrenal cortex secretes aldosterone and the hypothalamus secretes ADH to conserve the fluid within the vasculature. These factors lead to the retention of sodium and water, increasing the amount of ascitic fluid and edema. Figure 67-3 summarizes this process.

The severity of fluid retention determines the treatment. The patient with excessive amounts of fluid retention is placed on bed rest with accurate monitoring of intake and output. Patients are restricted to 500 to 1000 mL of fluid per day and to 200 to 1000 mg of sodium per day. These restrictions are continued until an adequate response occurs.

If the regimen of fluid and sodium restriction does not decrease the amount of ascites and fluid retention within 4 to 5 days, diuretic therapy is begun. Spironolactone (Aldactone) is often the initial drug of choice. The patient may be started on approximately 300 mg/day, and dosages may be increased up to a maximum of 1000 mg/day. If spironolactone therapy does not produce adequate diuresis, furosemide (Lasix) or hydrochlorothiazide (HydroDiuril) is added to the treatment regimen.[10]

Salt-poor albumin may be administered in attempts to restore plasma volume if the intravascular volume has significantly decreased. It is also used

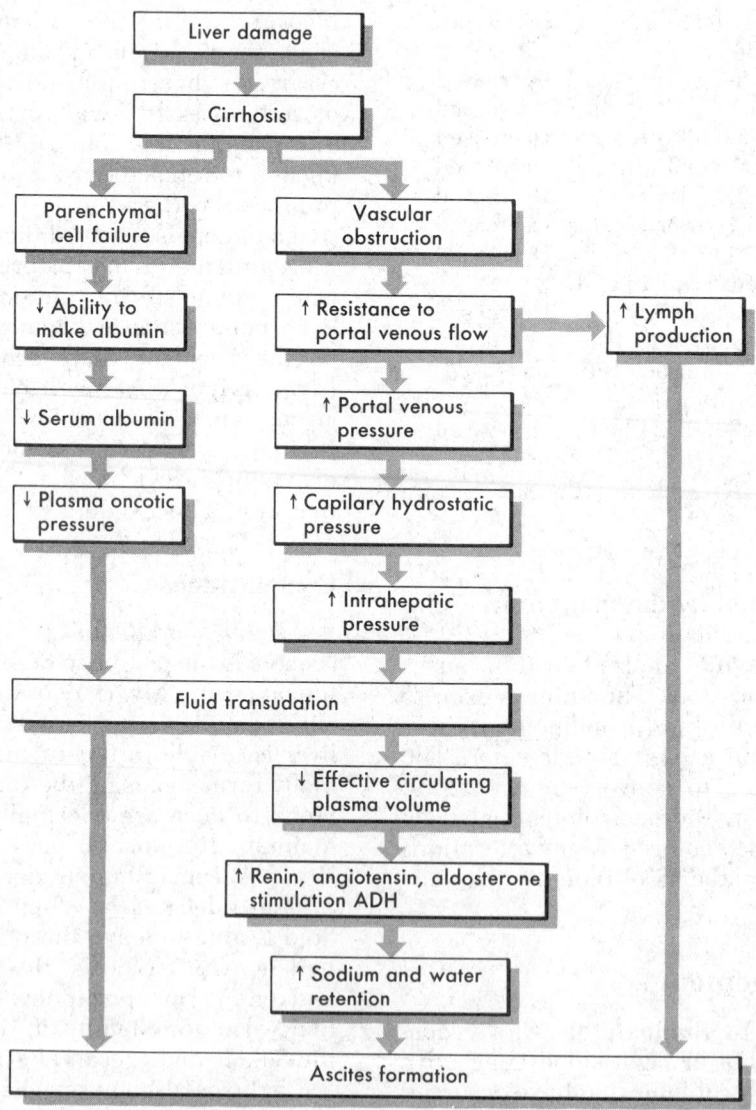

FIGURE 67-3   Pathogenesis of ascites.

to retain the plasma volume and to enhance diuresis by draining fluid from the interstitial area into the intravascular area.

LeVeen shunt

A **LeVeen shunt** (peritoneovenous shunt) (Figure 67-4), first introduced in 1962, may need to be inserted for intractable ascites. This procedure allows for the continuous shunting of ascitic fluid from the abdominal cavity through a one-way, pressure-sensitive valve, into a silicone tube that empties into the superior vena cava. It should not be performed on patients who have varices, infections, or coagulation disorders or patients who are in congestive heart failure or a coma. While the patient is under anesthesia, the valve is implanted into the abdominal wall. A long tubing with many openings is inserted into the abdominal cavity, and the silicone tube is threaded under the subcutaneous tissue up to the jugular vein and then to the superior vena cava. The one-way, pressure-sensitive valve opens when the pressure within the abdominal cavity increases by 3 cm of water pressure. Such a change occurs during inhalation as the diaphragm pushes down. Pressure in the abdominal cavity increases, whereas pressure in the superior vena cava decreases. The ascitic fluid then enters the venous system via the superior vena cava. When the patient exhales, the pressure within the abdomen decreases

and the pressure in the superior vena cava increases, thus closing off the valve and ceasing the flow of ascitic fluid. The valve will not open if the pressure in the superior vena cava is greater than the pressure within the abdominal cavity. This condition occurs if the patient develops congestive heart failure after the LeVeen shunt is inserted. In this case the shunt's built-in safety feature prevents fluid overload into the vascular system. Patients remain on diuretic therapy even with the shunt in place.

Several complications may occur from the LeVeen shunt, including congestive heart failure and hemodilution from the ascitic fluid, leakage of the ascitic fluid, infection at the insertion sites, peritonitis, septicemia, subcutaneous bleeding, disseminated intravascular coagulation (DIC), gastrointestinal bleeding, and shunt thrombosis. Because of these complications the patient with a LeVeen shunt needs to be monitored very closely.

Paracentesis

Paracentesis (Figure 67-5) is only done for patients with ascites when the large volume of ascitic fluid compromises the patient's respirations, causes abdominal discomfort, or poses a threat of rupturing an umbilical hernia or for diagnostic purposes. It is only a temporary method of removing fluid, and the ascitic fluid tends to reaccumulate.

The patient urinates before insertion of the tro-

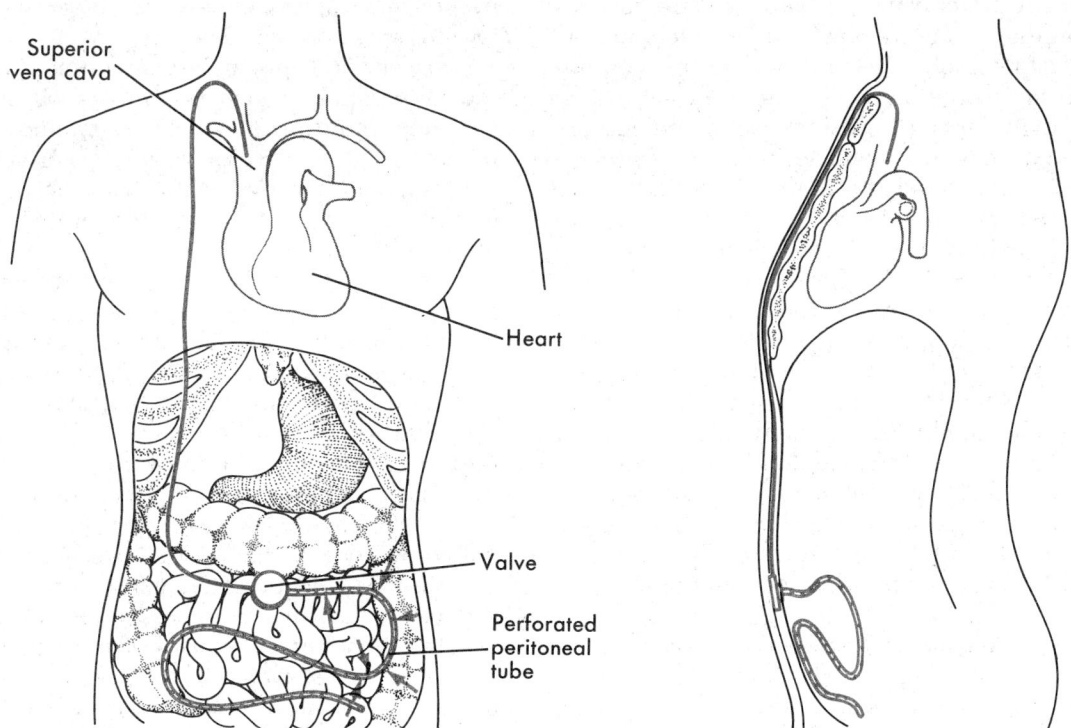

FIGURE 67-4   LeVeen continuous peritoneal jugular shunt.

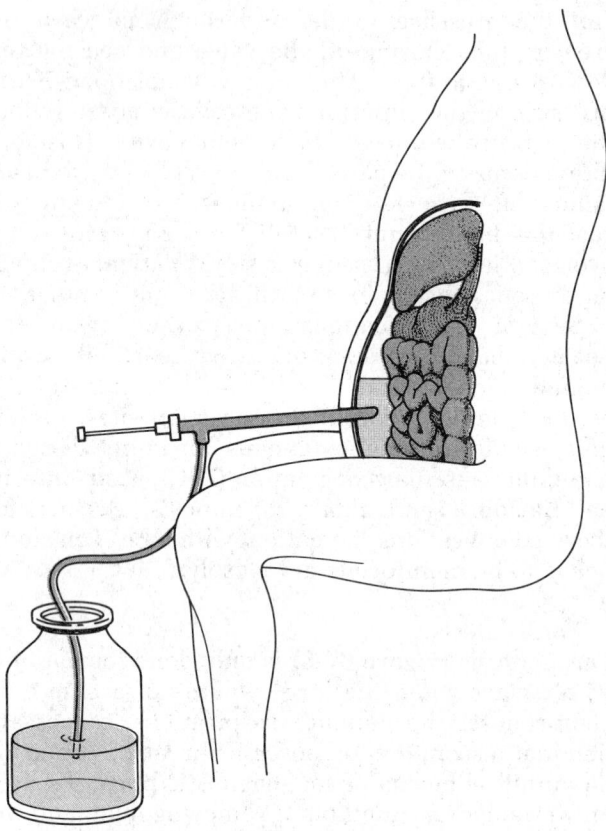

FIGURE 67-5   Paracentesis.

car to prevent puncturing the bladder. The patient then sits on the side of the bed with both feet firmly on the floor, footstool, or chair. If the patient cannot tolerate sitting at the side of the bed, he or she is placed in high Fowler's position. The abdominal area is prepared with povidone-iodine (Betadine), an incision is made below the umbilicus, and the trocar is inserted. The metal guide is removed, and the remaining plastic cannula from the trocar is connected to a drainage tube. The ascitic fluid is then withdrawn either by gravity or vacuum. The removal of too much fluid can cause hypovolemia. The fluid should be removed over 30 to 90 minutes to prevent sudden changes in blood pressure, which could lead to syncope. This fluid is high in protein and electrolytes, and the body can become depleted of these vital components. The patient will be monitored for signs of hypovolemia and electrolyte imbalances. A dressing will be applied over the insertion site and should be observed for bleeding and leakage.

Portal hypertension and esophageal varices

Changes in the structure of the portal venous system that occur with cirrhosis cause an increase in pressure within the portal vein and portal vein branches, resulting in **portal hypertension.** When

CLINICAL ALERT

Nursing Priorities for the Patient with Bleeding Esophageal Varices

- Contact physician
- Maintain airway
- Start 2 intravenous lines with 18-gauge catheters
- Draw blood for type and crossmatch
- Prepare for administration of vasopressin
- Prepare for insertion of Sengstaken-Blakemore tube

measured directly during a surgical procedure, the pressure is normally 7 to 14 mm Hg. Portal hypertension exists when this pressure exceeds 20 to 22 mm Hg. Portal pressure can also be measured percutaneously via a transhepatic route. When measured by this method, portal hypertension exists if the portal pressure is more than 8 mm Hg higher than the pressure of the inferior vena cava.

In most instances, portal hypertension caused by cirrhosis is irreversible. Many times portal hypertension is not recognized until the patient has an esophageal varix hemorrhage. This major complication of cirrhosis requires immediate medical attention because the varix hemorrhage is life threatening. Approximately 60% of the patients who have esophageal varices experience bleeding or hemorrhaging from the varices.

Varices can rupture from anything that increases the abdominal venous pressure such as coughing, sneezing, vomiting, or Valsalva's maneuver. Rupture may occur slowly over several days or suddenly and without pain. An endoscopy may be performed to identify the varices or to rule out bleeding from other sources.

A ruptured esophageal varix poses a medical emergency. The patient's airway must be maintained while attempts are made to control the bleeding varices. Intubation should take place if there is a threat of aspiration or if a Sengstaken-Blakemore tube (SB tube) is to be inserted. The patient is admitted to the intensive care unit. Two intravenous lines are started using large-bore catheters. Blood is drawn and sent to the laboratory for type and crossmatching. The hormone vasopressin will probably be administered intravenously or directly into the superior vena cava to decrease or stop the hemorrhaging. Vasopressin causes vasoconstriction of the splenic arteries, which in turn causes a decrease in portal venous flow and pressure. However, many complications occur with the use of vasopressin, including decreased coronary blood flow, decreased heart rate, and increased blood pressure. Therefore some institutions currently use vasopressin along with nitroglycerin during sclerotherapy. The nitroglycerin seems to reverse the unwanted effects of the vasopressin.

Vasopressin will temporarily control the esophageal bleeding in approximately 60% of the patients. About half of the patients whose hemorrhaging is controlled with vasopressin will have a recurrence of the bleeding. Therefore balloon tamponade may be used. Balloon tamponade controls bleeding by applying pressure against the esophageal veins. A Sengstaken-Blakemore tube may be used. It is effective in temporarily controlling the esophageal bleeding in approximately 40% to 90% of the patients.

Sengstaken-Blakemore tube

The **Sengstaken-Blakemore tube (SB tube)** (Figure 67-6) has an esophageal balloon, a gastric balloon, and three lumens: one for gastric lavage, one for inflating the gastric balloon, and one for inflating the esophageal balloon. Patency of all balloons is checked before insertion of the tube. The well-lubricated tube is inserted through the nose into the stomach. The gastric balloon is inflated with 200 to 300 cc of air and gently pulled back to ensure that it is against the cardiac orifice of the stomach. If the bleeding continues after the gastric balloon is inflated, the bleeding is assumed to be esophageal. The esophageal balloon is then inflated to attain a pressure between 20 and 40 mm Hg. Traction is applied to the Sengstaken-Blakemore tube to prevent the gastric balloon from slipping away from the cardiac orifice of the stomach. The patient's nose is protected by a foam rubber block called a nasal cuff. This block also serves to secure the tube. If the tube is inflated too much or for a prolonged period of time, the patient can get an ulcer secondary to necrosis at the site. Necrosis is prevented by periodically deflating the esophageal balloon every 12 hours and the gastric balloon every 24 to 36 hours. Flow sheets are maintained to document periodic release of the balloon.

The head of the bed is elevated 30 to 45 degrees to prevent aspiration of gastric contents and to help the patient breathe. Continuous monitoring of the balloon pressures and traction is mandatory. The esophageal balloon can slip, occluding the patient's airway. If this happens, the tube is cut immediately below the nose block. A pair of scissors must be kept at the patient's bedside specifically for this purpose.

Gastric lavage is performed to remove any swallowed blood from the stomach. Removal of this blood helps to prevent the degradation of the blood into ammonia. Some institutions prefer the use of iced, isotonic saline solutions for the lavage, whereas other institutions use room temperature solutions. The cold temperature of the iced solutions aids in vasoconstriction. However, if a piece of ice enters the tubing it can occlude or tear the tube.

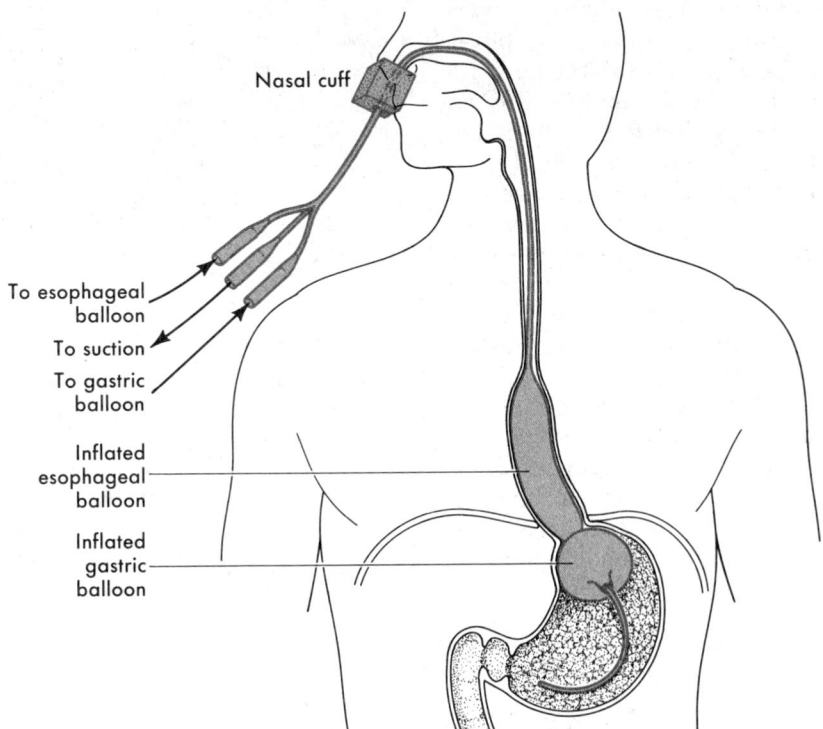

FIGURE 67-6   Sengstaken-Blakemore tube.

Balloon tamponade has many complications, including aspiration, reflux, airway obstruction, esophageal necrosis, and esophageal rupture. Of the complications that occur, 5% to 20% result in death. Once the bleeding is controlled, the pressure in the balloons is gradually decreased. The Sengstaken-Blakemore tube is removed by the physician. Because 40% to 60% of the patients will have another bleeding episode, they must be closely monitored for any signs of bleeding.

Endoscopic injection sclerotherapy is another method to control bleeding esophageal varices. After getting nothing by mouth for 6 hours, the patient receives a sedative along with a local anesthetic. An endoscope is placed into the esophagus where the varices are located. Sclerosing solutions such as ethanolamine oleate or sodium morrhuate are injected into the varices or into the submucosa next to the varices. The process is repeated as the endoscope is withdrawn and other varices are located. The sclerosing agents usually cause thrombosis and sclerosis within 5 minutes. This procedure may be repeated if the first attempt is unsuccessful.

Transhepatic cannulation and thrombosis constitute another method to control bleeding. A catheter is threaded into the left gastric vein and the gastroesophageal variceal plexus. The vessels are injected with solutes that cause thrombosis, such as thrombin. Once thrombosis occurs, the bleeding ceases.

Once an esophageal varix has hemorrhaged, other measures must be taken to prevent hypovolemic shock and complications from the bleeding. Oxygen may be administered to increase oxygen in the blood. Hemoglobin, hematocrit, sodium, and potassium samples should be drawn to determine the need for blood or electrolyte replacements. Caution must be exercised when replenishing blood and electrolytes. Excessive replacement and fluid overload must be avoided. If blood transfusions are necessary, fresh whole blood or fresh frozen plasma is used. Fresh blood products are used because the damaged liver has difficulty removing the citrate that is added as a preservative to stored blood. Fresh blood products also contain more clotting factors than blood that has been stored.

Cathartics and enemas are administered to remove any blood that has entered the intestinal tract before ammonia is formed. Neomycin will be administered. This antibiotic destroys colonic bacteria and prevents the formation of ammonia. These treatments assist in preventing hepatic encephalopathy.

Portacaval shunt

Surgical shunting of the blood from the portal system to the venous system (Figure 67-7) may be used as a method to reduce the portal pressure in patients with portal hypertension and esophageal varices. The portacaval shunt diverts blood from the portal

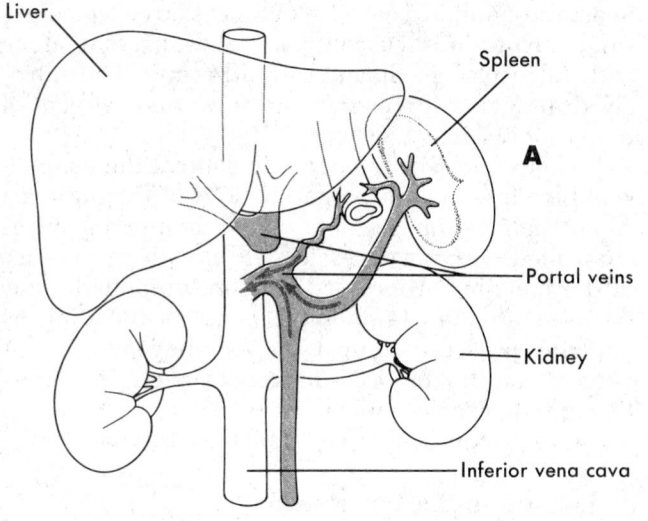

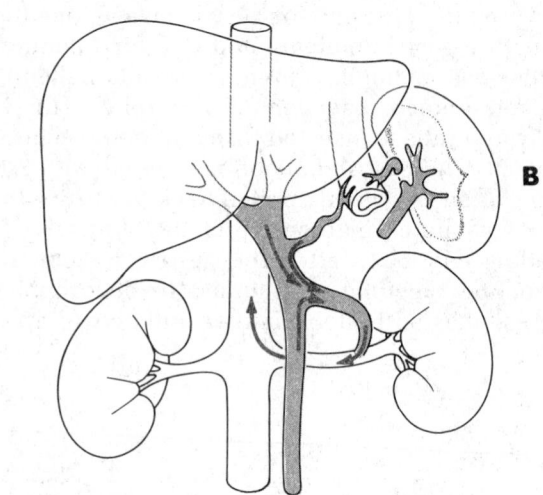

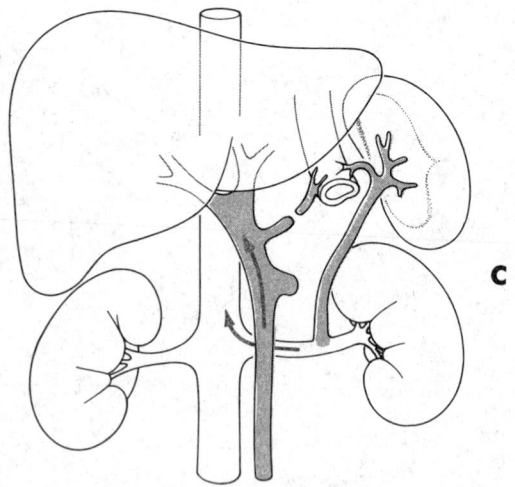

FIGURE 67-7 Shunting procedures for portal hypertension. **A,** End-to-side portacaval shunt. **B,** Splenorenal shunt. **C,** Distal splenorenal shunt.

vein to the inferior vena cava. The splenorenal shunt involves a splenectomy with anastomosis of the splenic vein to the left renal vein. The mesocaval shunt involves anastomosis of the superior mesenteric vein to the inferior vena cava. These procedures have a high mortality and may be performed in an emergency situation hemorrhage or in a therapeutic situation when a patient has already hemorrhaged. The incidence of hepatic encephalopathy, gastrointestinal bleeding, ascites, and liver failure is high in patients who have surgical shunting procedures. These procedures should not be used prophylactically because of the many complications and the fact that patients' chances for survival rarely improve.

Hepatic encephalopathy

Ammonia is produced by the bacterial degradation of protein and other nitrogenous compounds in the intestinal tract. When the liver is damaged, it is unable to metabolize substances that can be toxic to the brain, such as ammonia, mercaptans, and amino acid. The exact pathogenesis is unclear, but it is believed that the build-up of these toxic substances in the brain causes a disorder known as hepatic encephalopathy or portal-systemic encephalopathy. The patient presents with various central nervous system alterations. These alterations tend to follow four stages (Table 67-2).

Careful observation of the patient with cirrhosis is imperative to assess any changes in mental status. Patients in stages I (prodromal) and II (impending) will have their dietary protein restricted. If their condition deteriorates, protein is eliminated from the diet. Protein is added to the diet, 10 to 20 g/day every 3 to 5 days up to a maximum of 60 mg/day, as the patient's condition improves. Usually the vegetable proteins, such as soybeans or legumes, are better tolerated. Lactulose or neomycin may be given. Lactulose decreases the bowel's pH, decreases the production of ammonia by bacteria within the bowel, and functions as a cathartic. Neomycin inhibits protein synthesis in bacteria, thereby decreasing the production of ammonia. These effects cleanse the bowel and decrease the serum ammonia.

NURSING MANAGEMENT OF THE PATIENT WITH CIRRHOSIS

Assessment

A thorough nursing history gives insight into possible causes of cirrhosis and the length of time the patient has been having problems. Recall that the early manifestations of cirrhosis are subtle, resembling flulike symptoms. The chief complaint is determined. Obtain more information about any current health problems. Ask the patient if any symptoms, either past or present, have occurred that might in-

TABLE 67-2 Stages of Hepatic Encephalopathy	
Stage	**Clinical manifestations**
Stage I (prodromal)	Disorientation, decreased attention span, decreased response time, forgetfulness, slurred speech, restlessness, irritability, change in sleep patterns, normal electroencephalogram (EEG)
Stage II (impending)	Asterixis, confusion, lethargy, drowsiness, apraxia
Stage III (stuporous)	Asterixis, stupor, incoherence but patient becomes noisy and abusive when aroused, hyperventilation
Stage IV (coma)	Positive Babinski's reflex, decerebrate/decorticate posturing, fetor hepaticus, coma

dicate cirrhosis, such as changes in bowel habits or menstrual irregularities. A family health history is also important in determining if there is a family history of liver disorders or alcohol abuse. Information is obtained concerning the patient's past and present work and home environment. This provides information on possible exposure to hepatotoxins, such as carbon tetrachloride.

A thorough physical examination provides information on the stage of disease and helps the nurse plan the overall nursing care. The patient's mental status is important to observe. Note response time to questions and how appropriate the responses are. The general appearance of the patient is also noted. Weigh the patient, and assess the appropriateness of the patient's weight. Are there signs of muscle atrophy? Is the patient's abdomen protruding? Assess the patient's skin, scleras, and mucous membranes, observing for signs of jaundice, bruising, spider angiomas, and palmar erythema. The degree and location of any discoloration are documented. Note if the skin is dry and if it appears to be scratched.

Observe the patient's trunk. Gynecomastia should be noted. Observe the abdomen for distention, an everted umbilicus, and caput medusae. Measure the abdominal girth. Auscultate the abdomen, assessing for hypoactive, hyperactive, or normal bowel sounds. Gently palpate the abdomen, noting any tenderness or discomfort. Palpate for hepatomegaly by gently rolling the fingers under the right costal margin. The liver is normally soft and can be felt under the costal margin (see Chapter 63). The cirrhotic liver is firm and enlarged. If ascites is present the nurse will note a shifting dullness when the abdomen is percussed.

While assessing the patient's upper extremities, test for asterixis (liver flap or flapping tremor). The patient's arm should be stretched out. The patient is then instructed to hyperextend the wrist with the fingers separated, relaxed, and extended. The patient in stages II (impending) and III (stuporous) of hepatic encephalopathy has a rapid, irregular flexion and extension (flapping) of the wrist. This reaction can also be elicited in the feet and is believed to be a peripheral response to the alterations of the central nervous system caused by the liver's impaired metabolic function.

Nursing Diagnosis

The nursing diagnoses for a patient with cirrhosis and its complications include the following:

Activity intolerance related to fatigue and anemia

Constipation related to the liver's inability to metabolize food products and to lack of activity

Ineffective individual coping related to prognosis

Diarrhea related to the failing liver's inability to metabolize food products

Fluid volume deficit related to nausea, vomiting, and diarrhea

Fluid volume excess related to fluid retention associated with increased ADH and aldosterone secretion, increased hydrostatic pressure, and decreased colloidal osmotic pressure from ascites

Ineffective breathing patterns related to pressure on diaphragm from enlarging liver and ascites

High risk for infection related to thrombocytopenia and malnutrition

High risk for injury related to decreased clotting factors, inability to metabolize vitamin K, and weakness

Knowledge deficit related to cirrhosis, treatments, and complications

Altered nutrition: less than body requirements related to anorexia, nausea, vomiting, and diarrhea

Pain related to enlarging liver and spasm of the biliary ducts

Personal identity disturbance related to physical appearance (gynecomastia, ascites, jaundice)

Self-care deficit related to fatigue

Sexual dysfunction related to alterations in the metabolism of and inactivation of hormones from the adrenal cortex, ovaries, and testes

Impaired skin integrity related to pruritus, ascites, and generalized fluid retention

Altered thought processes related to build-up of ammonia

High risk for violence directed at others related to the build-up of ammonia and the subsequent manifestations of hepatic encephalopathy

Planning

The nurse plans interventions that will prevent any further damage to the liver and improve the patient's overall physical and mental condition. Nursing care for the patient with cirrhosis is planned to achieve the following outcomes:

Patient performs activities of daily living without becoming fatigued

Patient has normal respiratory function and is free from dyspnea

Patient is free from discomfort, both itching and pain

Patient has a decrease or absence of fluid retention and ascites

Patient is free from injuries and bleeding

Patient abstains from alcohol

Patient reports an increase in appetite

Patient reports a decrease in nausea and vomiting

Patient is oriented to person, place, and time

Patient's skin remains intact

Patient and family demonstrate appropriate family interaction

Patient and family work with support groups

Implementation

Nursing interventions for the patient with cirrhosis are numerous. Individualized, supportive therapy is essential, with emphasis being placed on preventing the complications that commonly occur with cirrhosis. Nurses must include family members or significant others in all teachings, stressing the importance of strict maintenance to the patient's treatment regimen. The patient is encouraged to rest. The patient usually lacks energy reserves and must learn to conserve strength to decrease the demands that basic activities of daily living and exercise place on the liver. Activities are based on tolerance and the presence of complications. The nurse assesses the patient's tolerance of activities and identifies activities that cause fatigue. Bed rest is recommended until the patient regains strength. Activity level is increased gradually as the patient's condition improves.

Precautions are taken to avoid infection and circulatory problems that often occur in patients on bed rest. Encourage the patient to take deep breaths and cough at regular intervals to prevent pneumonia. Turn the patient at least every 2 hours, and have the patient move in bed, flexing and extending extremities to prevent thrombophlebitis.

The patient with cirrhosis has bleeding tendencies because of the lack of vitamin K and certain clotting factors. Therefore the nurse assesses for bleeding and takes measures to avoid such occurrences. Assess the patient's gums for any bleeding. Encourage the use of a soft-bristle toothbrush. If bleeding at the gums becomes severe, discontinue use of a toothbrush and use cotton-tipped applicators or sponges for oral hygiene. An electric razor is used when shaving. Stools and emesis are assessed for frank blood and checked for occult blood. Aspirin is avoided because of its anticoagulant effects. The patient should abstain from vigorous nose blowing, coughing, and straining while having a bowel movement. Such activities can lead to severe bleeding. Normal saline nose drops may be necessary if nasal congestion is a problem. Stool softeners are administered if the patient is constipated.

Special precautions are taken if the patient must receive an intramuscular injection. The smallest-gauge needle possible is used. Gentle pressure is applied after the injection to prevent any bleeding. Too much pressure can cause trauma to the underlying tissue and subcutaneous bleeding.

All potential injuries must be recognized and then avoided. If the patient is restless, the siderails must be up and padded. Assist the patient with ambulation, and prevent any trauma that could result in a bruise or bleed. As always, have the patient's call bell within reach.

If the patient has bleeding esophageal varices, the nurse assists the physician in measures to control the hemorrhaging, including monitoring the Sengstaken-Blakemore tube. The nurse must know the correct amount of pressure in each balloon and the correct amount of traction to be applied to prevent ulceration or airway obstruction. The nurse performs gastric lavage, noting the amount and color of the return. Maintaining patient comfort is another nursing intervention. The patient may have abdominal pain. Noninvasive techniques such as positive imagery or distraction should be attempted. If these methods fail, analgesics may be administered. As stated previously, caution must be taken when administering analgesics to patients with cirrhosis because of the damaged liver's inability to metabolize and detoxify many medications. The medications may alter the patient's mental and neurologic status and cause false assessment and evaluation of hepatic encephalopathy.

Pruritus is another problem for the patient with cirrhosis. The nurse must assess for signs of scratching, because vigorous scratching can cause a subcutaneous bleed. Soap and rubbing alcohol should be avoided because they will cause further drying of the skin. The skin should be patted and not rubbed while washing and drying. Washcloths, towels, gowns, and bed linens should be soft to avoid irritating the skin. Moisturizing lotions may be beneficial in keeping the skin soft. Antihistamines, such as diphenhydramine (Benadryl), may be administered if itching is severe.

The patient's fluid and electrolyte status must be assessed frequently. Accurate monitoring of intake and output is essential. The patient is weighed on the same scale and in the same type of clothing twice each day. The nurse assesses for fluid retention and ascites, noting any presacral, ankle, or peripheral edema. The abdomen is palpated, noting any fluid wave. Measuring of abdominal girth is done at least once per shift, recording the girth and the point at which the girth was measured (i.e., at the umbilicus). The nurse is responsible for administering any diuretics, noting the patient's response to the medication, and observing for any side effects. The nurse observes for any clinical manifestations of electrolyte imbalances such as hypokalemia or hyponatremia.

The importance of frequent, thorough evaluation of the neurologic and mental status of patients with cirrhosis cannot be overemphasized. Accurate assessment is the key to recognizing a patient going into hepatic coma. The nurse's observations should be charted every 2 hours, using flow sheets for consistent measurement. Changes in mental status are often very subtle and may be recognized only if the nurse has cared for the patient daily. Family members may comment on changes in the patient's personality. Nursing personnel must note these comments and be alert to any further deterioration in the patient's condition.

The nurse monitors the patient's intake of dietary protein. If the patient's mental or neurologic condition deteriorates, the amount of dietary protein is decreased or even totally eliminated. The nurse explains the dietary restrictions to the patient and the patient's family and enforces adherence to such restrictions.

Throughout all interactions with the patient and family, the nurse is nonjudgmental and provides emotional and psychologic support. The diagnosis of cirrhosis and its complications causes fear and anxiety. The patient and family require education and guidance concerning treatments, potential problems, and interventions that may occur. The nurse must continually reinforce the abstinence of alcohol. The patient must know that any ingestion of alcohol could be physically and psychologically detrimental. The nurse may set up consultations with a psychologist or a social worker. Referring the patient and family to support groups such as Alcoholics Anonymous and Al-Anon may be beneficial.

Evaluation

The evaluation of nursing interventions requires periodic assessment of the patient for symptom relief. The nurse observes for improvement in skin color and activity tolerance. Changes in body weight should occur as nutritional intake increases and retained fluid is eliminated. The nurse monitors the response of the patient and family to resources for alcohol abuse treatment.

Documentation

Thorough, accurate documentation is vital to the care of both the patient with cirrhosis and the patient's family. Proper documentation will key others into any changes that may occur, no matter how subtle the changes. The nurse documents the assessment of the patient, interventions that are performed, and the patient's response to these interventions. The nursing care plan is reviewed and updated frequently to provide the patient with the best and most consistent care possible.

Ongoing Care

Prognosis for the patient with cirrhosis is poor. Over 50% of patients without complications die within 5 years. Between 70% and 90% of patients die within 5 years after the onset of ascites, and 75% to 95% of patients with bleeding esophageal varices die within 5 years. Survival can be improved with permanent adherence to treatment regimens and abstinence from hepatotoxins, especially alcohol.

Discharge instructions given to the patient and family emphasize the importance of adherence to treatment regimens. The patient and family should be given information on the signs and symptoms of impending complications. They should be encouraged to seek medical attention should any complications occur. Frequent medical follow-up is also recommended. Visits from a community or home health nurse are helpful in monitoring the patient's progress and answering any questions that the patient or family members have. The nurse can assess and evaluate the patient's progress and provide physical and emotional support to the patient and family. Detoxification programs may assist the patient and family dealing with the problems that arise from abusing alcohol. The patient and family should be encouraged to continue in treatment even after the patient has withdrawn from alcohol.

HEPATITIS
Definition

Hepatitis is an inflammation of the liver resulting from viral agents, bacterial agents, or exposure to hepatotoxins or drugs such as carbon tetrachloride or acetaminophen.

Etiology/Epidemiology

Five major agents cause viral hepatitis: hepatitis viruses A, B, C, D, and E. The first four types are the most prevalent in the United States; type E has been seen in Asia, Africa, and Mexico.

Hepatitis A, also referred to as infectious hepatitis, is caused by an RNA virus that is transmitted through feces, contaminated water, or contaminated food. Its incubation period is 2 to 6 weeks. Hepatitis B is caused by a DNA virus that is transmitted parenterally (blood transfusions or contaminated needles) or by direct contact (sexual partners or health care professionals). Its incubation period is between 4 weeks and 6 months. Hepatitis C, formerly called hepatitis non-A, non-B, is caused by an RNA virus. It is the major cause of posttransfusion hepatitis. Its incubation period is between 5 and 10 weeks. Hepatitis D (delta agent) is caused by an incomplete RNA virus. It occurs as a complication of hepatitis B. Hepatitis E is caused by an RNA virus with an incubation period of 2 to 9 weeks. Health officials are required by law to report all cases of viral hepatitis to the Centers for Disease Control in Atlanta, Georgia. Approximately 60,000 to 70,000 cases are reported annually. The incidence of hepatitis is believed to be much higher, however, because a number of asymptomatic cases are never diagnosed. Hepatitis A is the most common form of viral hepatitis. However, with the increasing number of intravenous drug abusers, the incidence of hepatitis B is rising.

Pathophysiology

The basic pathologic findings in all forms of viral hepatitis are very similar. The virus invades the portal tracts, periportal space, and lobules of the liver, causing inflammation of the liver and destruction of the liver parenchymal cells. This results in necrosis, degeneration, and autolysis of individual hepatocytes. Infiltration of the liver by leukocytes and histiocytes also occurs. Liver enzymes are released, and liver function decreases. The damaged hepatocytes are removed by phagocytosis, and regeneration of the cells occurs. Residual damage depends on the severity of the course of the illness. Usually recovery can be expected with only mild liver damage. However, viral hepatitis can cause cirrhosis, chronic hepatitis, or even death.

Clinical Manifestations

The clinical manifestations of viral hepatitis vary greatly, from no symptoms to hepatic failure or hepatic encephalopathy. Symptomatology is generally divided into three stages: the preicteric (prodromal) stage, the icteric stage, and the posticteric (convalescent) stage.

Before the onset of jaundice (preicteric stage), the patient experiences flulike symptoms. These include general malaise, lassitude and weakness, headaches, mild fever (38° to 39° C), chills, cough, coryza, rhinitis, anorexia, intermittent nausea and vomiting, and diarrhea or constipation. The patient may also experience a decreased sense of smell, moderate to severe dyspepsia, an intolerance of fats, dull pain and tenderness in the right upper quadrant, hepatomegaly, lymphadenopathy, myalgia, photophobia, urticaria, and weight loss (5 kg). The person who drinks coffee or smokes may have an aversion to the smells and tastes of coffee, tobacco, or other strong odors. This preicteric stage lasts approximately 1 week and then subsides as the jaundice appears.

The icteric stage usually lasts 2 to 6 weeks, peaking at 2 weeks. Jaundice appears because of the damaged liver's inability to metabolize bilirubin. The patient has yellow skin, scleras, and mucous membranes; dark amber urine; and clay-colored stools. The increased levels of bilirubin cause pruritus, which may be severe enough to cause excoriation of the skin from the patient scratching. During the icteric stage the abdominal pain, dyspepsia, fatigue, and lassitude usually continue. The liver remains enlarged and becomes increasingly tender.

The posticteric stage begins as the jaundice subsides, lasting 2 to 6 weeks. The patient remains fatigued. The liver decreases in size but remains tender. The patient's appetite usually returns during this stage. A relapse may occur during the posticteric stage. The previously described symptoms reappear but in a milder form. Complete recovery is expected within 6 months. Leukopenia is common in patients with hepatitis. Patients have an elevated direct bilirubin, serum glutamic oxaloacetic transaminase (SGOT), serum glutamic pyruvic transaminase (SGPT), and alkaline phosphatase and a decreased serum albumin. Hypoglycemia is present in approximately 50% of patients with hepatitis. Patients with severe cases of hepatitis also have a prolonged prothrombin time.

Therapeutic Management

No specific treatment exists for patients with viral hepatitis other than supportive therapy for existing symptoms and preventing the transmission of the disease. A majority of patients are managed at home. The patients who do require hospitalization are usually dehydrated from protracted nausea and vomiting, have very prolonged prothrombin time, or have developed life-threatening complications.

Bed rest is usually prescribed for 1 to 2 weeks if the patient is fatigued. The patient's activity may be increased as tolerated. Patients with hepatitis must abstain from ingesting alcohol and continue such abstinence for a minimum of 1 year after all clinical and laboratory manifestations return to normal. Most patients will tolerate a low-fat, high-carbohydrate diet best with the largest meal in the morning. The patient may find that anorexia prevents an adequate fluid and caloric intake. In such cases, small frequent meals with increased amounts of clear liquids are advisable. If the nausea becomes severe, dimenhydrinate (Dramamine) or trimethobenzamide (Tigan) may be given one-half hour before meals. If dehydration becomes a problem, intravenous fluids are started. Vitamin C is administered to aid healing. Vitamin B complex is administered to compensate for the damaged liver's inability to absorb this fat-soluble vitamin. Vitamin K is administered if prothrombin time is prolonged.

Controversy exists as to the benefit of corticosteroids in the treatment of hepatitis. If they are used, it should be sparingly.

Prevention of the spread of hepatitis is a primary concern of health care professionals. The patient, family, and health care providers must be knowledgeable about routes of transmission of the virus and take steps to avoid such transmission. Proper personal hygiene and good sanitation will help prevent the spread of hepatitis A. Patients with hepatitis A are most contagious in the early stages of the disease, often before a diagnosis is made. Therefore personnel must always handle excretions from patients with care. Patients hospitalized with hepatitis A should be placed in a private room and their stool and urine isolated and disposed of properly. Disposable dishes should be used.

Regular immune serum globulin (immune serum globulin or gamma globulin) is given as soon as possible to persons who have been in direct contact with a person with hepatitis A during the infectious period (2 weeks before and 1 week after the onset of symptoms). The dosage of 0.02 mL/kg of body weight given intramuscularly is effective in 80% to 90% of the cases.

Hepatitis B immune globulin (HBIg) is given to prevent hepatitis B. It should be administered to individuals who were exposed to hepatitis B virus via a needle puncture, contact with feces or oral secretions, or sexual contact. A dose of 0.06 mL/kg of body weight is administered intramuscularly as quickly after exposure as possible. This dose is repeated 1 month later.

A vaccine against hepatitis B is also available. It is recommended that persons at high risk for developing hepatitis B be vaccinated. Such persons include high-risk health care personnel (emergency room, operating room, intensive care unit, and dialysis employees; phlebotomists; and laboratory technicians), persons with high-risk life-styles (drug addicts, homosexuals, and prostitutes), and infants born to mothers who are hepatitis B surface antigen (HB_sAg) positive. Before administration of the vaccine, the person is screened to see if he or she is already immune to hepatitis B. If immunity exists, the vaccine is not administered. Three vaccinations will be given to those who show no immunity: an initial vaccination, a vaccination 1 month later, and a third vaccination 6 months after the first injection. The hepatitis B vaccine has been shown to provide protection for 3 to 5 years in approximately 90% of the persons treated.

Hepatitis C is mainly spread through blood transfusions. Therefore prevention of this form of hepatitis is best achieved by only using blood products when truly necessary. The blood should be received from volunteer donors rather than persons who are paid for a blood donation. The transfusion should also be screened for elevated SGPT and hepatitis B core (anti-HB_c).

NURSING MANAGEMENT OF THE PATIENT WITH HEPATITIS

Assessment

The nurse obtains a thorough health history including information on exposure to causative agents of hepatitis such as contaminated needles, blood transfusions, industrial chemicals, or infected individuals. While obtaining the health history, the nurse should gain insight into any recent changes in the patient's tolerance of activities of daily living and should note the patient's tolerance to the interview. Recall that people with hepatitis become easily fatigued.

The nursing assessment focuses on the presence of the previously discussed clinical manifestations including fever and gastrointestinal disturbances. Any changes in the patient's sense of smell or taste are noted. Assess the color of the patient's skin, scleras, mucous membranes, urine, and stool. Observe for any bleeding that might indicate a prolonged prothrombin time. The abdomen should be palpated, noting any hepatomegaly, tenderness, or pain.

Nursing Diagnosis

Nursing diagnoses for a patient with hepatitis include the following:

Ineffective individual coping related to diagnosis and potential long-term problems
Diarrhea related to liver's inability to metabolize food products
Altered family processes related to isolation procedures
Fatigue related to increased energy demands
Fluid volume deficit related to vomiting and diarrhea
Impaired skin integrity related to pruritus resulting from bile salt deposits beneath the skin
High risk for infection related to the disease process and transmission of hepatitis
High risk for injury related to altered clotting mechanisms
Altered health maintenance related to knowledge deficit of hepatitis, its treatment regimens, and prevention of spread
Altered nutrition: less than body requirements related to nausea and vomiting and the difficulty of digesting fats because of diminished bile flow
Pain related to pruritus and liver inflammation
Personal identity disturbance related to physical appearance from jaundice
Self-care deficit related to fatigue
Impaired skin integrity related to scratching secondary to pruritus
Social isolation related to isolation protocols

Planning

Outcome criteria for the patient include the following:

No spread of hepatitis in the hospital or to persons in contact with the patient who has hepatitis
Patient reports an increase in appetite
Patient's weight is maintained
Patient is free from gastrointestinal problems associated with hepatitis
Patient is free from pain and discomfort
Patient resumes normal activity
Patient understands hepatitis and the ways that it is spread
Patient has normal liver function
Patient is free from complications associated with hepatitis

Implementation

Nurses must take actions to prevent the spread of hepatitis. Universal precautions are used for all patients. Isolation precautions such as blood/body fluid precautions and enteric precautions are used. As with all patients, needles used on the patient with hepatitis should never be recapped. The needle is disposed of in a labeled impermeable needle disposal container located within the patient's room. Gowns and gloves are worn by anyone having contact with contaminated items such as bedpans. Hand washing is imperative while caring for the patient with hepatitis.

The person with hepatitis is usually tired. Therefore the nurse must assist the patient in getting an adequate amount of rest. Nursing interventions are planned to allow the patient longer periods of uninterrupted rest. The patient who is extremely fatigued will need to turn, cough and deep breathe, and do passive range of motion exercises to prevent complications that occur from bed rest, such as pneumonia or thrombophlebitis. A patient may feel uncomfortable asking visitors to leave, even if the patient is very tired. The nurse may need to intervene and explain to visitors the importance of the patient getting adequate rest. The patient's activity level may be increased as strength increases. The nurse monitors this activity, noting the patient's tolerance to an increase in mobility.

Nursing personnel must protect the patient from injury caused by the patient's prolonged bleeding times. Siderails may need to be padded. The nurse provides assistance for the patient when the patient is up to prevent injury. Electric razors and soft toothbrushes are used.

The patient with hepatitis is generally anorexic and suffers from nausea and vomiting. Usually a high-carbohydrate, low-fat diet is best tolerated. Avoid giving the patient large amounts of food at a time. This will only decrease appetite. Small frequent meals seem to be tolerated best. Antiemetics may be administered 30 minutes before meals if nausea and vomiting become a severe problem. The patient's reaction to the medication is documented. The patient should take in at least 2500 to 3000 mL of fluid per day. Provide the patient with a variety of beverages, fruit juices, and carbonated soft drinks. If the patient is unable to drink the necessary amount of fluid, an intravenous line is started to avoid dehydration. The patient will be on strict intake and output. Weights are measured daily using the same scale with the patient wearing approximately the same weight clothing. The nurse observes and records the amount and color of urine and the amount, color, and consistency of the stool.

If the patient's bilirubin level is elevated, pruritus may occur. Soap and rubbing alcohol are avoided, because they will further dry the skin. The skin is patted and not rubbed while washing and drying it. All clothes, towels, and bed linens should be soft to avoid further irritation to the skin. Moisturizing lotions may be helpful in keeping the skin soft. If the itching is severe, antihistamines such as diphenhydramine (Benadryl) may be administered. The nurse documents the patient's response to the medication.

The majority of patients with hepatitis are managed at home. The nurse educates the patient and family about the prevention of hepatitis. Personal care items and drinking glasses should not be shared. Intimate contact should be avoided during the infectious period. The patient's clothes should be laundered separately. If an automatic dishwasher is available, it should be used with the water temperature increased. If possible, the person with hepatitis should use separate bathroom facilities. If this is not a possibility, the shared bathroom should be cleansed daily with a chlorine solution. The patient and family are taught symptoms of relapse. They are encouraged to seek medical assistance immediately if such symptoms occur. The patient should have frequent check-ups for at least 1 year. Abstinence from alcohol is mandatory to avoid further damage to the recovering liver.

Evaluation

To evaluate interventions for the patient with hepatitis, the nurse needs to monitor the patient's food intake and body weight. Increasing activity tolerance can be evaluated by subjective reports of increased energy. Objectively, the patient's cardiovascular response to activity will be within normal limits. The patient and family should be able to identify measures to prevent the spread of hepatitis.

Documentation

Thorough, accurate documentation is vital in the care of patients with hepatitis. Nurses must document their assessments as accurately as possible. Documenting the color of the patient's skin, scleras, mucous membranes, urine, and stool helps to identify the stages the patient is going through. Nurses' notes will guide the patient's treatments. For example, the nurse may assess the patient's intolerance to being out of bed. The patient will then be encouraged to remain on bed rest. The written observations of a nurse may be the key to recognizing a patient who is developing complications from hepatitis such as hepatic encephalopathy.

Ongoing Care

The prognosis for patients with hepatitis is very good, but relapses do occur. Therefore the patient must have frequent medical follow-up examinations, including laboratory tests such as bilirubin, globulin, and liver enzyme studies. The patient is encouraged to seek medical attention if he or she notes a relapse or the presence of any manifestations that would indicate hepatitis. Throughout the year after diagnosis, the patient should carry identification stating when the onset of hepatitis occurred. Patients requiring medical or dental care during the first year after diagnosis should inform health care professionals of the date that the patient had hepatitis. The patient with hepatitis may not donate blood during the first year after diagnosis.

The importance of abstinence from alcohol ingestion for at least 1 year cannot be overemphasized. The patient must be aware of the severe complications that can arise from the ingestion of alcohol and be encouraged to adhere to this restriction. Depending on the cause of hepatitis, the patient may require counseling and psychologic help. Drug addicts and alcoholics can benefit from rehabilitation programs. Visits from the community or home health nurse are also beneficial. The nurse may be able to educate the patient and family about unsanitary conditions that exist in the home environment. The nurse will also be able to observe the patient's recovery period and assess for clinical manifestations indicating relapse of the disease.

CANCER OF THE LIVER
Definition

The hepatic system, like all other areas of the human body, can be invaded with malignant cells. It is rare to have a hepatic malignancy that originates within the biliary system. Such primary tumors may originate within the liver itself (hepatocellular) or within the bile ducts (cholangiomas). Most hepatic malignancies, however, originate elsewhere and metastasize to the liver. Cancers of the lungs, breast, stomach, colon, pancreas, kidneys, bladder, and skin are the most common forms to metastasize to the liver.

Etiology/Epidemiology

As with most cancers, the exact cause of primary carcinoma of the liver is unknown. However, many predisposing factors are seen in these patients, including cirrhosis, hepatitis B, hepatitis C, hemochromatosis, androgenic steroids, and type II glycogen storage disease. Metastasis to the liver occurs because of the vast capillary circulation within the liver. Malignant cells will get into the bloodstream and migrate and lodge within the liver.

The American Cancer Society estimates that there will be 15,800 new cases of cancer of the liver and biliary passages in the United States in 1993.[3] Primary hepatic carcinomas account for less than 2% of all malignancies. These primary malignancies occur more often in men than in women and rarely occur before the fifth decade of life.

Pathophysiology

Malignancies within the liver occur and progress like malignancies in other areas of the body. Cancer cells proliferate and rob healthy cells of nutrients and oxygen. The malignant tumor grows and compresses normal liver cells, causing the liver to enlarge. These cells also extend into the vascular bed of the liver, further compromising the liver of oxygen and nutrients and leading to hemorrhaging. Eventually malignant cells outnumber normal cells, and the liver is unable to function. The malignant cells often invade surrounding areas of the liver including the gallbladder, peritoneum, and diaphragm, causing alterations in their normal processes.

Clinical Manifestations

Primary carcinomas of the liver are difficult to diagnose in the early stage. Patients may be asymptomatic, or they may be extremely ill. Common presenting manifestations include the presence of a right upper quadrant mass, abdominal pain, and weight loss. Liver function tests may be altered, but in some patients they are normal. Alpha-fetoprotein levels may be elevated as the disease progresses. Patients with metastatic liver disease show signs of deterioration including weight loss, anorexia, and weakness. Continued progression of the disease causes symptoms that are associated with liver failure, including hepatomegaly, jaundice, ascites with subsequent weight gain, hepatic bruits, and possible esophageal varices. Ultrasound, computed tomography (CT) scanning, and magnetic resonance imaging (MRI) are often useful in detecting hepatic tumors. Liver biopsy is necessary for definitive diagnosis of cancer of the liver.

Therapeutic Management

Patients with liver cancer have a very poor prognosis; most die within 6 months of diagnosis. Surgical removal of the tumor is the only cure for liver cancer. This procedure, however, is rarely successful, because most cancers of the liver are well advanced before diagnosis. Liver transplantation has also been attempted with patients with liver cancer, but the survival rate remains poor. Because of the poor prognosis, treatment focuses on support. The management is very similar to the patient with cirrhosis, since both diseases cause liver failure. The patient will be on a well-balanced, low-sodium, high-carbohydrate diet. Protein is necessary for cellular regeneration but can be fatal in patients with severe liver damage. The patient with liver failure has difficulty metabolizing the ammonia that is produced by the deamination of amino acids. The buildup of ammonia in the brain leads to hepatic encephalopathy. Therefore the amount of protein that these patients receive depends on their mental status. Antiemetics may be prescribed if the person is nauseated or vomiting.

Pain management is very important and difficult. All attempts must be made to make the patient comfortable. This is often difficult because the damaged liver is unable to metabolize and detoxify many medications. Chemotherapy has been used to slow down the growth of tumors of the liver. Some chemotherapy is delivered systemically, whereas other types are administered directly into the hepatic artery. Although tumor growth decreases, patient survival rates have not increased. Other treatments, such as radiation therapy, hormonal therapy, and hepatic artery ligation, have been attempted. None of these therapies have increased survival time.

NURSING MANAGEMENT OF THE PATIENT WITH LIVER CANCER

Assessment

The nurse obtains an accurate and thorough history from the patient suspected of having liver cancer. The patient's past medical history can be particularly important, especially if the patient previously had cirrhosis, hepatitis B, hepatitis C, or another form of cancer. Changes in weights and appetite should also be noted. A head-to-toe assessment is performed paying specific attention to the abdominal area. Abdominal masses or pain can indicate liver cancer. Blood for alpha fetoprotein and liver function tests is drawn. The nurse must be able to interpret the results.

Nursing Diagnosis

Nursing diagnoses for a patient with cancer of the liver include the following:

Activity intolerance related to fatigue and weakness caused by increased metabolic demands and treatments

Anxiety related to poor health status secondary to diagnosis of cancer

Body image disturbances related to physical appearance from weight loss and ascites

Ineffective individual coping related to situational crisis secondary to diagnosis of terminal disease

Fatigue related to nausea, vomiting, and increased metabolic demands

Fluid volume excess related to altered metabolism of antidiuretic hormone and aldosterone secondary to ascites caused by liver failure

Anticipatory grieving related to potential loss of health and life secondary to diagnosis of terminal disease

Impaired home maintenance management related to fatigue and weakness secondary to cancer

Altered health maintenance related to knowledge deficit concerning diagnosis, treatments, procedures, and management of cancer

High risk for infection related to decreased immune system secondary to cancer of the liver

Altered nutrition: less than body requirements related to anorexia, nausea, vomiting, and increased metabolic demands

Pain related to enlarging liver secondary to spread of cancer

Altered protection related to decreased immune system and the damaged liver's inability to form clotting factors secondary to metastasis

Planning

The nurse plans interventions to meet the following goals:

The patient will be free from pain

The patient and family will verbalize their feelings and concerns about the diagnosis and prognosis of this disease

The patient and family will have decreased anxiety and fear, making them able to cope with the diagnosis and prognosis of this disease

The patient will have an adequate intake of fluids and nutrients to provide for nutritional needs and thus maintain weight

The patient will be free of infection

The patient will be able to do activities of daily living without becoming fatigued

The patient will have adequate rest

Implementation

Caring for the patient with liver cancer is difficult. The loss of a loved one is inevitable, and the nurse can assist and guide the patient and family in ventilating their feelings about this loss. Meeting the physical needs of the patient with liver cancer is very similar to meeting the needs of the patient with cirrhosis, since both of the diseases lead to liver failure. Refer to the section on managing the patient with cirrhosis for this information.

Evaluation

Evaluation of the patient with cancer may be done by assessing the patient and family's understanding of the disease process and its prognosis. The evaluation of nursing interventions requires continual assessment of the patient's pain relief and patient feedback about various methods used for pain relief. The evaluation should conclude that the patient has an adequate nutritional intake, weight is being maintained, and an adequate amount of rest and sleep is obtained.

Documentation

The nurse accurately documents the patient's physical and psychosocial condition. Nursing interventions are noted, as is the patient's response to such interventions. Patient and family interactions may also be documented so that interventions can be implemented as needed.

Ongoing Care

Prognosis for the patient with liver cancer is very poor. The patient and family must continually be supported. Education continues as the disease progresses. The patient and family may be referred to an area hospice organization for support.

LIVER TRANSPLANTATION
Definition

Two forms of liver transplantation are orthotopic liver transplantation and heterotopic liver transplantation. Orthotopic liver transplantation is replacement of the patient's failed or diseased liver with the donated liver. Heterotopic liver transplantation is grafting of the donated liver to an ectopic site with the failed or diseased liver remaining in place. Orthotopic liver transplantation is the preferred method. The surgical procedure of transplantation takes between 8 and 10 hours.

Etiology/Epidemiology

The first liver transplant was performed in 1963 by Dr. Thomas Starzl at the University of Colorado in Denver. Since that day the art and science of liver transplantation have undergone many changes that have saved thousands of lives.

The United Network for Organ Sharing (UNOS) reports that 3056 liver transplants were performed in the United States in 1992. As of June 1993, 2676 patients were registered with UNOS awaiting liver transplantation.

As with all organ/tissue transplantation, selection of a recipient is an extremely difficult task. The box below lists the indications for adult liver transplantation. Patients selected as potential recipients must undergo physical and psychosocial screenings. Physically, the severity of the liver disease must be confirmed. Contraindications for transplantation need to be identified. A battery of tests is performed including ABO typing, hepatitis B and HIV screening, liver function tests, alpha-fetoprotein levels, VDRL, cytomegalovirus (CMV) serology, and HTLV-1. Routine laboratory work is also done, including a complete blood count (CBC), serum electrolytes, blood urea nitrogen (BUN), creatinine, ammonia, cholesterol, triglycerides, and a urinalysis. A chest x-ray, electrocardiogram (ECG), pulmonary function tests, abdominal ultrasound, and abdominal computed tomography (CT) scanning are also done.

Psychosocial evaluations are performed. The patient must be psychologically stable. Patients must realize that they will be on daily medications for the remainder of their lives and must prove willing to comply with such a regimen. Family members are also screened, since their support is an important aspect of successful transplantation.

Some patients will have to relocate to a nearby transplant center. This can be another stressful situation for the patient and family, but it is necessary to make the transplant process go as quickly as possible. A patient proven to be a good candidate for transplantation is placed on UNOS's waiting list with information about blood type and size. The patient and family then await the call informing them that a liver has become available. This can be an exasperating time. Many patients die while they are waiting.

Almost all liver donations are obtained from patients who are brain dead, thus making donation of such organs an ethical issue. Transplant teams will not use organs from anyone unless the family agrees to such procedures. Even if a person has signed an organ donor's permit or provision on the back of the driver's license, organs will not be retrieved without total family permission. Therefore it is very important for individuals to make their wishes known when they are alive and healthy. This will help alleviate such difficult decisions during a very stressful time. The matching of a recipient and donor is initially based on ABO compatibility and liver size. The ABO barrier can be crossed with liver transplantation but is not a desirable action. Liver size is an important consideration when matching donors and recipients. If the liver is too small, difficulties may arise when attempting to anastomose the vessels of the patient with the donated liver. When the patient's abdomen is too small to accommodate a larger liver, pressure may be placed on the grafted liver, resulting in necrosis. The large liver may also place pressure on the patient's diaphragm, resulting

---

INDICATIONS FOR ADULT LIVER TRANSPLANTATION

Primary biliary cirrhosis
Laennec's cirrhosis (alcohol-induced cirrhosis)
Chronic active hepatitis
Sclerosing cholangitis
Drug-induced liver failure
Primary hepatic carcinomas that are confined to the liver
Hemochromatosis
Wilson's disease
Budd-Chiari syndrome
Alpha$_1$-antitrypsin deficiency

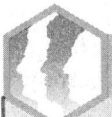

GERIATRIC CONSIDERATIONS

Organ Donation

Traditionally, anyone over 55 years of age was not considered a potential organ donor. The limited number of organs available for transplantation has resulted in physicians being more willing to use organs from individuals 60 to 80 years old. The National Organ Procurement and Transplantation Network reports a fourfold increase in the number of organ donors over 65 years of age since 1988. Aging does not necessarily mean that organs have suffered too much wear and tear for transplantation. The important factor in determining if an organ can be donated is the overall health of the donor at the time of death, not the donor's age.

in respiratory failure. Attempts have been made to transplant partially resected livers, but this is only done in a very few institutions.

Once a recipient and donor are matched, activation of the transplant begins. The recipient needs to get to the hospital as soon as possible so that the transplant can take place before any damage occurs to the donated liver.

Therapeutic Management

Postoperatively, the patient will be in an intensive care unit (ICU). The patient may arrive on the unit hypothermic from being exposed in a cold environment (the operating room) for an extended period of time or from medications that the person receives. The patient is warmed gradually to avoid vasodilation, which can lead to cardiovascular instability.

The stress on the body after a transplant can affect many systems. The cardiovascular system can be affected from the fluid shifts that occur during surgery. The patient may lose blood during transplantation, creating hypovolemia that affects the cardiovascular system.

The patient arrives on the ICU intubated and needs mechanical ventilation. The weaning process should occur based on the patient's blood gases and respiratory effort. During the postoperative period the patient may develop atelectasis or pneumonia. Suctioning and chest physiotherapy help prevent these pulmonary complications (refer to Chapter 26).

Renal insufficiency may result from the fluid shifts and the cardiovascular instability. It may also occur

from cyclosporin toxicity. Urine output and laboratory studies (BUN, serum creatinine, and creatinine clearance) assist in identifying problems of the renal system. The patient's electrolytes may be altered as a result of the stress of surgery and the fluids and drugs given to the patient during surgery. Careful monitoring for alterations in electrolytes helps to prevent these problems. As with all major abdominal surgeries, the patient will have a functional ileus. Abdominal assessment is imperative. Bowel sounds and the passage of flatus must be documented.

Many transplant patients develop infections because of the immunosuppressive therapy that they are required to take to prevent organ rejection. Careful monitoring of the patient's temperature and observing for signs of infection can help control this complication.

One of the most feared complications after liver transplantation is that of organ rejection. Four types of rejection are possible. Hyperacute rejection occurs during surgery when circulation is established to the donated organ. Accelerated rejection occurs from 1 to 5 days after transplantation. These two forms of rejection rarely occur in patients who undergo liver transplantation. If they do occur, the only way to treat them is to remove the transplanted liver and immediately retransplant with a new liver. Acute rejection occurs 1 to 2 weeks after transplant. This form of rejection is treated by increasing the doses of immunosuppressive agents. Chronic rejection occurs months to years after a transplantation. This type of rejection may also require retransplantation.

The major goal after a transplant is to prevent all forms of rejection. This is done by massive doses of immunosuppressive agents. Usually a triple immunosuppressive regimen is instituted. The patient receives calculated amounts of cyclosporine, prednisone, and azathioprine (Imuran). The amounts of these agents are altered according to the patient's needs.

Patients who undergo transplantation often suffer major psychologic trauma from the stress of the transplantation, the medications that are administered, the changes in body image, or a host of other reasons. Special attention and intervention must be taken to prevent psychologic complications. Referrals to psychiatry, psychology, social services, and/or pastoral care can be valuable in the prevention or treatment of psychologic problems.

GALLSTONES
Definition

Cholecystitis is an acute or chronic inflammation of the gallbladder. **Cholelithiasis** is the formation or presence of stones or calculi in the gallbladder. **Cho-**

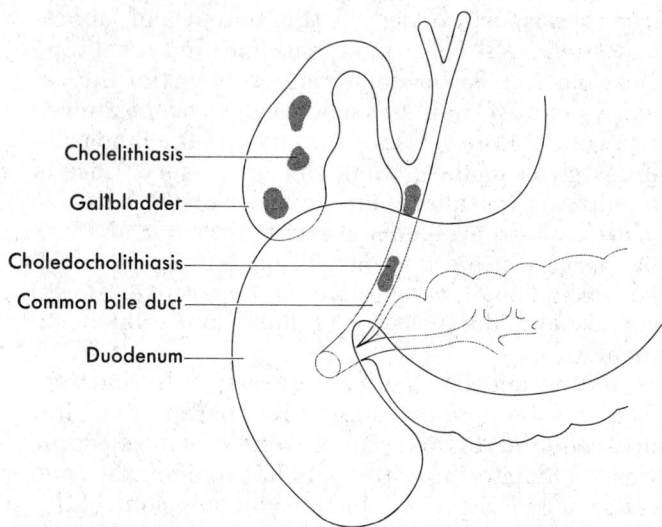

FIGURE 67-8   Common locations of gallstones.

ledocholithiasis is the presence of stones or calculi in the common bile duct (Figure 67-8).

Etiology/Epidemiology

Twenty to twenty-five million Americans have gallstones, with approximately 1 million new cases being diagnosed each year. Over 500,000 patients have biliary tract operations each year, making cholecystectomy the third most common general surgical procedure in the United States. Cholelithiasis is three to four times more common in women until menopause, after which the differences in occurrence decrease. The incidence is also higher in Native Americans and whites than in Asians and blacks. A noted difference also exists between blacks in the Western world and blacks in Africa with the incidence being lower in blacks in Africa.

Cholelithiasis occurs more frequently in obese people, pregnant women, people with diabetes, multiparous women, and women who use birth control pills. The exact etiology of gallstones and the common bile duct is not known. They are believed to be caused by an alteration in lipid metabolism.

The role of female sex hormones in the formation of gallstones is unknown. However, statistics show that the incidence of stones is higher in women than men, particularly in women with multiple pregnancies, those who are pregnant, and those who use birth control pills. These statistics suggest that the female sex hormones may contribute to the formation of gallstones.

Over 90% of the cases of cholecystitis are caused by gallstones. Other etiologic factors include bacteria (Staphylococcus, Escherichia coli, Streptococcus, or Salmonella), chemical irritants, kinking of the neck of the gallbladder, mucous obstruction, fasting, and trauma. Acute cholecystitis is more common during middle adulthood, whereas chronic cholecystitis is more prevalent among elderly persons.

Pathophysiology

The two types of gallstones are cholesterol stones and pigment stones. Cholesterol stones are much more prevalent in the United States than are pigment stones. Cholesterol stones are composed entirely of cholesterol, or cholesterol is the major component of the stone. The stones are light in color (usually a pale yellow) and are radiolucent. Pigment stones are composed of polymerized bilirubin or calcium bilirubin. They are black or brown and are radiopaque. Cholesterol stones form when the bile within the gallbladder or common bile duct becomes supersaturated with cholesterol. After this, nucleation and precipitation of cholesterol monohydrate crystals occur. The crystals begin to congregate, increase in size, and form macroscopic stones.

Much less is known about the pathogenesis of pigment stones. Patients with pigment stones tend to have higher concentrations of unconjugated bilirubin. Calcium bilirubin stones are associated with infections. However, the exact mechanism of pigment stone formation is unknown.

The majority of the cases of cholecystitis begin with stone formation. The lodged stone blocks the drainage of bile from the gallbladder. The gallbladder becomes inflamed, edematous, and distended. The enlarged gallbladder causes venous congestion and alters the normal circulatory pattern to the gallbladder.

The bile that is trapped within the gallbladder acts as an irritant, causing cellular infiltration of the gallbladder wall after 3 to 4 days. The vascular occlusion along with the bile stasis causes the mucosal lining of the gallbladder to become necrotic. Initially the bile in the gallbladder is sterile. The bacterial growth is secondary to the ischemia and occurs usually within a few days.

Clinical Manifestations

Many patients with gallstones are asymptomatic. The gallstones may be discovered during an examination for another problem such as an abdominal CT scan or during abdominal surgery unrelated to the gallbladder. Such "silent" gallstones may never cause problems.

A patient with symptomatic cholelithiasis or acute cholecystitis generally displays the same basic symptoms. Usually there is a history of indigestion after eating foods high in fat. When an attack occurs, the patient will have pain and tenderness in the right subcostal region or in the epigastric region. The pain begins gradually and over a period of approximately 30 minutes builds to an intense pain. This pain often radiates to the back at the scapular level or to the shoulder. The pain, which can last several hours, is often accompanied by anorexia, nausea, vomiting, and flatulence. The patient will have an increased heart rate and respiratory rate. Diaphoresis will be present. The patient may think that a heart attack is occurring. The gallbladder is generally palpable. However, with palpation, the pain will increase, causing the patient to have a transient inspiratory arrest (temporarily holding one's breath). This is known as positive Murphy's sign. The patient may have a low-grade (38° C) fever. The leukocyte count may be slightly elevated (10,000 to 15,000 cells/mm^3). If the count is much higher than 20,000 cells/mm^3, the patient may have empyema (a pus-filled gallbladder) or the gallbladder may have perforated.

The patient with a stone lodged in the common bile duct will have mild jaundice. The stool may contain fat (steatorrhea) and be clay colored because of the lack of bile in the intestinal tract. The kidneys try to remove the excess bilirubin from the bloodstream, resulting in urobilinogen and dark amber-colored urine.

Patients with chronic cholecystitis are usually less severely ill than patients with acute cholecystitis. Therefore the patient may not seek medical attention until symptoms of biliary tract obstruction develop, such as jaundice. The patient realizes an intolerance to spicy foods or foods with a high fat content and avoids such foods. The pain that is experienced is more of a dull ache in the epigastric region or the right upper quadrant of the abdomen. The pain generally lasts a few minutes and subsides. Residual soreness remains in the area where the pain was located. Nausea, vomiting, and flatulence do not occur as often with chronic cholecystitis as they do with acute cholecystitis or cholelithiasis.

Therapeutic Management

Patient with "silent" gallstones will usually be made aware of the gallstones' presence. They are taught to recognize the symptoms of an attack or obstruction and are instructed to seek medical attention should any symptoms appear. Occasionally such patients undergo an elective cholecystectomy, or removal of the gallbladder.

Symptomatic patients with cholelithiasis and acute cholecystitis are placed on bed rest. A nasogastric tube is inserted and connected to low suction; the patient is given nothing by mouth to allow the gastrointestinal tract and thus the gallbladder to rest. An intravenous line is started, and fluid resuscitation is begun to rehydrate the patient and to replace drainage from the nasogastric tube. If nausea remains a problem, antiemetics are administered.

Analgesics and antispasmodics are administered to decrease the patient's pain. Meperidine hydrochloride (Demerol) is the drug of choice, because the incidence of spasms of the sphincter of Oddi is decreased as compared with the opiates. Ampicillin, cephalosporin, or tetracycline is given prophylactically to prevent infection of the biliary tree or as treatment for an already present infection. If empyema or perforation occurs, gentamicin, tobramycin, and clindamycin are administered.

Further therapeutic management depends on the patient's condition and the physician. If the patient's condition greatly improves by giving the gastrointestinal tract a rest, treatment is conservative, with dietary restrictions such as avoidance of spicy and high-fat foods.

Removal of the gallstones is usually recommended. This may be done early in the course of the illness or postponed to a future date. There are many approved methods of removing gallstones, and other methods are currently under investigation.

Nonsurgical stone removal

Nonsurgical methods include dissolution therapy, endoscopic retrograde cholangiopancreatography (ERCP), and extracorporeal shock-wave lithotripsy. Dissolution therapy is a nonsurgical method of removing gallstones. It is accomplished by administering bile salts such as ursodiol (ursodeoxycholic acid) orally to a patient in an attempt to dissolve the gallstones. Certain criteria must be met before a patient is considered eligible to receive dissolution therapy. The gallstones must be cholesterol stones measuring less than 15 mm. Pigment gallstones or large gallstones will not dissolve with this therapy. The gallbladder must have adequate circulation of bile before ursodiol treatment can begin. The patient takes ursodiol from 6 to 24 months and must be committed to continue with the therapy for that length of time. Gallstones may re-form even after extended treatment with ursodiol, since the gallbladder is still intact and continues to concentrate and store bile. The use of ursodiol is contraindicated during pregnancy and while breast feeding.

Endoscopic retrograde cholangiopancreatography (ERCP) is another nonsurgical method of diagnosing and treating gallstones in the common bile duct. The patient receives lidocaine to prevent gagging and is instructed to swallow the end of an endoscope. The physician guides the endoscope cannula into the common bile duct. Dye is injected, and x-rays are taken to locate the stone. If the stone is in the common bile duct, an endoscopic papillotomy (EPT) can be performed. The cannula of the endoscope is replaced with an electric surgical cutter. The sphincter of Oddi can be enlarged by cutting it open (sphincterotomy). A basket is passed through

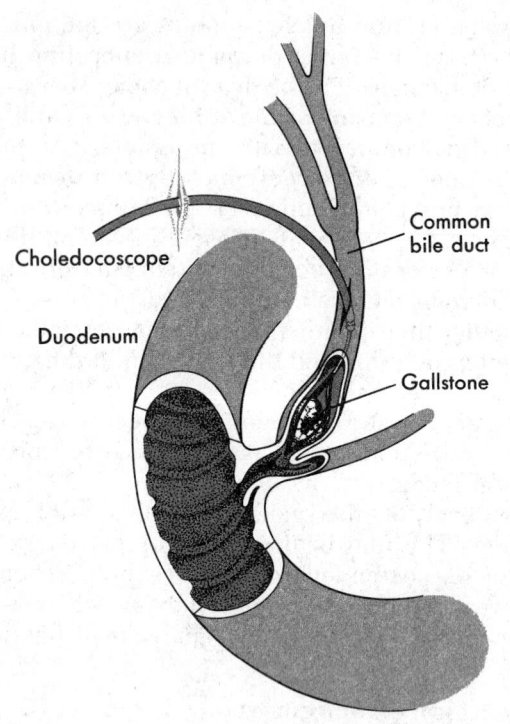

FIGURE 67-9   Endoscopic retrograde cholangiopancreatography (ERCP) for gallstone removal.

the endoscope to retrieve the stone (Figure 67-9). The stone can then be placed into the duodenum and passed naturally in the stool or removed in the basket. The opening of the bile duct will retain its new width, allowing the same size stones or smaller stones to pass through it should they recur.

Extracorporeal shock-wave lithotripsy has been performed in the United States since 1988. This noninvasive, outpatient procedure involves the use of shock waves to break up gallstones into sandlike particles, making them small enough to pass through the common bile duct and into the gastrointestinal tract. The shock waves are produced by a machine called a lithotriptor (Figure 67-10). A water bag is placed on the patient's right upper quadrant. The water within the bag amplifies the shock waves. Analgesics and sedatives may be administered to relax the patient and to decrease the discomfort of the shock waves. A conductive gel is applied to the patient's abdomen, and the patient lies prone on the water bag. Multiple shock waves are given until the stones are small enough to pass through the gastrointestinal tract. The patient may eat, drink, and resume normal activity immediately after the procedure. This form of treatment does not eliminate the cause of cholelithiasis; thus stone formation may recur.

Surgical management

Laparoscopic laser cholecystectomy is a method of removing the gallbladder without performing major

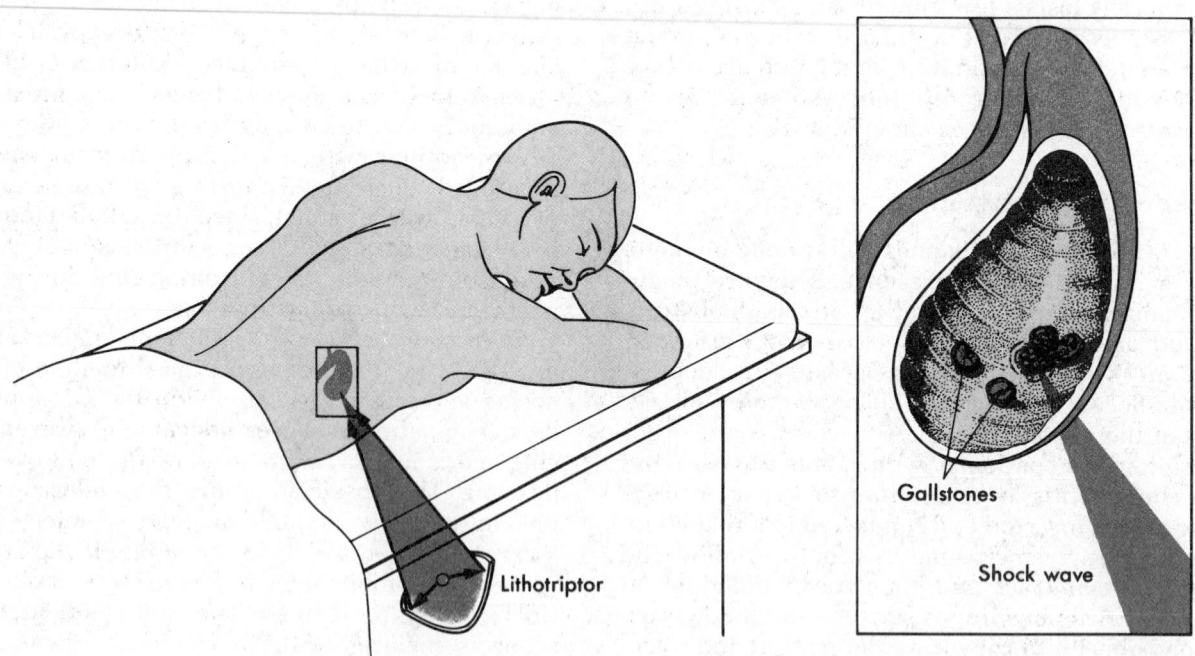

FIGURE 67-10   Extracorporeal shock-wave lithotripsy.

abdominal surgery. This method eliminates the large scar, postoperative complications, and extended recovery that occur with open cholecystectomy. The patient is given nothing orally after midnight the day of surgery. After the patient receives general anesthesia, an intravenous line is started, and a nasogastric tube and Foley catheter are inserted. The abdomen is prepared and draped. The surgeon makes a 10 mm puncture above the umbilicus. The abdominal cavity is inflated with carbon dioxide. A laparoscope, which has a microscopic video camera attached to it, is inserted into this site. Two additional 5 mm punctures are made, one at the right anterior axillary line and one at the midclavicular line. Forceps are then inserted through these punctures to grasp the gallbladder. A final 10 mm puncture is made to the right of the midline. The dissection laser is placed in this site. While monitoring the procedure with the video camera, the surgeon dissects the gallbladder with the laser and removes it through the midline puncture with the forceps. The carbon dioxide is evacuated, the puncture sites are closed, and a dressing is applied. The nasogastric tube and Foley catheter are removed. The patient will then go to the postanesthesia area. The patient wakes up quickly and will receive clear liquids. If these are tolerated, the intravenous line is removed and the patient is offered a regular diet. Ambulation is encouraged as soon as possible.

The patient must have stable vital signs, tolerate food, and ambulate well before discharge. Discharge instructions include resuming moderate activity in 2 to 3 days and contacting the physician if discomfort increases or if signs of infection develop (fever, redness, drainage). A cholecystectomy (removal of the gallbladder) is usually the treatment of choice. This may be done either by doing a laparoscopic cholecystectomy or in the more traditional manner of an abdominal cholecystectomy.

When an abdominal cholecystectomy is performed, the gallbladder is removed and the cystic duct, vein, and artery are ligated. A nasogastric tube is in place as a prophylactic means of decreasing abdominal distention and preventing vomiting. It is usually removed 36 to 48 hours postoperatively when bowel sounds return and the patient is not nauseated or vomiting.

A Jackson-Pratt drain or a Penrose drain may be inserted. The Jackson-Pratt drain or Penrose drain should produce less than 50 mL of blood-tinged drainage per shift. This drain is removed when the drainage is minimal.

If stones are in the common bile duct and edema is present, a biliary drainage tube or T tube is inserted to keep the duct open and to allow for drainage of the bile until the swelling resolves. The short end of the tube is placed in the common bile duct, and the longer end of the tube is brought out to the

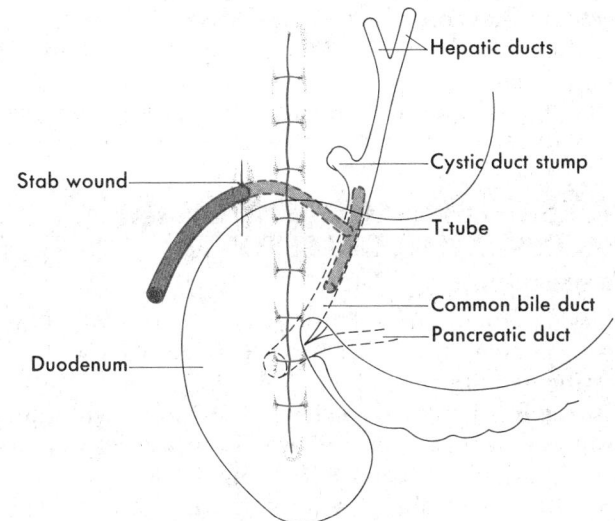

FIGURE 67-11 T tube.

surface through a stab wound (Figure 67-11). The long end is attached to a closed drainage system (bile bag) placed below the level of the common bile duct. Initially the drainage is blood tinged. The wound normally drains up to 500 mL during the first 24 hours and decreases in amount as the edema of the common bile duct resolves. This amount should be accurately recorded. If drainage is excessive, the patient may need to receive bile. If this is the case, the bile bag must be kept on ice. It should be disguised and preferably given via a nasogastric tube. If the patient does not receive his or her own bile, bile salts, such as florantyrone or dehydrocholic acid, are given orally. The T tube is clamped for 1 to 2 hours before meals and unclamped 1 to 2 hours after the patient eats. This allows the bile to drain from the liver into the duodenum. The bile then facilitates digestion. The patient may show signs of distress during this clamping procedure, including abdominal pain, nausea, vomiting, amber-colored urine, and clay-colored stools. If distress occurs, the T tube is unclamped immediately. The time that the T tube remains clamped is increased as the patient tolerates the procedure. Approximately 7 days after the operation, the physician injects dye into the common bile duct (cholangiogram) and assesses its patency. The T tube is removed 24 hours after the cholangiogram if the edema is resolved and the bile ducts appear normal. This 24-hour waiting period allows for the dye to drain out of the ducts. If the duct remains edematous and bile is not draining properly, the patient is discharged with the T tube in place. In such cases the patient is given instructions for the care of the T tube. The T tube is removed at a follow-up visit with the surgeon.

Patients at high risk for not surviving a cholecystectomy may need a cholecystostomy (forming an opening into the gallbladder through the abdominal wall). This can be done using local anesthetic. The opening provides a means of removing pus and possibly the stone. It also allows drainage of bile.

NURSING MANAGEMENT OF THE PATIENT WITH GALLSTONES

Assessment

Nursing assessment of the patient with cholelithiasis or cholecystitis must be performed accurately to distinguish the clinical manifestations of gallbladder disease from other disorders with similar symptomatology, such as liver disease. The first step is obtaining a patient history. The nurse must obtain information regarding the onset of symptoms. Inquire about precipitating factors such as ingestion of high-fat foods. Any relationship among food intolerance, pain and subsequent anorexia, nausea, vomiting, or flatulence should be noted. An accurate description of the quality and quantity of pain is helpful in accurately assessing the patient with gallbladder disease.

A physical examination is performed. The patient's vital signs are measured, noting any alterations from normal such as hyperthermia, tachycardia, or tachypnea. The nurse notes any signs of jaundice. The skin, sclera, mucous membrane, urine, and stool are observed for alterations in the presence of bilirubin. The abdomen is inspected, auscultated, and palpated. Any tenderness, swelling, or pain is documented, as is the presence of positive Murphy's sign and bowel sounds.

Nursing Diagnosis

Nursing diagnoses for patients with cholelithiasis or cholecystitis include the following:

Fluid volume deficit related to anorexia, nausea, vomiting, and nasogastric tube drainage

Impaired skin integrity related to surgical incision and secretions from drainage tubes

Ineffective breathing patterns related to difficulty breathing postoperatively because of abdominal incision and distention

Altered health maintenance related to a knowledge deficit concerning cholelithiasis or cholecystitis, treatments, and complications

Noncompliance with prescribed therapy related to lack of desire to change eating habits

Alteration in nutrition: less than body requirements related to nausea and vomiting secondary to cholecystitis and to NPO status while the gallbladder is resting

Alteration in nutrition: more than body requirements related to lack of knowledge about appropriate nutrition

Pain related to inflammation of the gallbladder, obstruction of the biliary drainage, and spasms of the ducts

Sleep pattern disturbance related to pruritus and pain

Planning

Outcome criteria for patients with cholelithiasis and cholecystitis include the following:

Patient is free from pain and discomfort

Patient's fluid and electrolyte levels are balanced

Patient is free from clinical manifestations of jaundice

Patient verbalizes correct dietary measures to avoid further attacks of cholelithiasis or cholecystitis

Surgical patient is free from postoperative complications

Obese patient will reduce weight

Implementation

Analgesics are administered to provide relief from pain. As always, the nurse must observe the patient for side effects and adverse reactions from the medication. The response to the medication (pain relief) is noted. The nurse enforces the patient's NPO status. A nasogastric tube is inserted and anchored properly to avoid nasal irritation or necrosis. The nasogastric tube is connected to low suction and monitored for amount, color, and consistency of any output. If nausea is a problem even after the insertion of the nasogastric tube, antiemetics may be administered.

An intravenous line is started for replacement of fluids and electrolytes lost from vomiting and from the draining nasogastric tube. The intravenous line is also used for the administration of antibiotics. The patient's intake and output are closely monitored, noting the color of the urine and the stool.

Further nursing care is based on the patient's response to treatments. If the patient is managed conservatively, the nurse teaches the patient causative factors of cholelithiasis and cholecystitis attacks and ways to avoid such attacks, mainly through dietary restriction of fatty, high-cholesterol, and spicy foods. Obese patients are advised about weight reduction. The nurse arranges for a dietician to counsel the patient regarding proper nutrition.

Preoperative care

Patients undergoing surgery require preoperative teaching. They need to be taught ways of preventing postoperative complications. The nurse teaches the patient how to use an incentive spirometer. The patient is also instructed to turn, cough, and take deep breaths at least every 2 hours after surgery. Giving the patient instructions on how to splint the abdomen when coughing and teaching repositioning and ambulation techniques that avoid straining abdominal muscles help to ease postoperative discomfort. The nurse informs the patient that pain medications are available if needed. Many patients are now being placed on patient-controlled anesthesia (PCA). These patients need to be given instructions on how to operate the machines. The patient needs to know about the drainage tubes that will be in place. Information is also given to the patient concerning postoperative procedures, such as dressing changes and nasogastric tube irrigations. Vitamin K may be given preoperatively to prevent hemorrhaging during surgery.

Postoperative care

Patients recovering from gallbladder surgery require routine postoperative care including frequent assessment of their respiratory, cardiovascular, and central nervous systems and assessment of the operative site. The physician is notified immediately should there be any significant change in the patient's vital signs or neurologic status or if the amount of drainage from the operative site is excessive.

The patient returns from surgery with a nasogastric tube in place as a prophylactic means of decreasing abdominal distention and preventing vomiting. The nurse is responsible for verifying placement of the nasogastric tube, maintaining its patency, monitoring its output, and preventing any complications from the tube. A Jackson-Pratt or Penrose drain will be in place. The patient is placed in low Fowler's position. This promotes bile drainage, preventing pressure and fluid accumulation under the diaphragm. The nurse monitors the amount and color of the drainage from the tubes. Initially, there should be less than 50 mL of blood-tinged drainage per shift. The surgeon is notified if the drainage is excessive, contains bile, or is bright red.

If a T tube is in place, its drainage bag is at the level of the common bile duct to prevent the reflux of bile. Special care must be taken not to kink or pull the T tube. A gauze roll is placed under the tube, anchoring it to the patient's abdomen. The nurse is responsible for monitoring the amount and character of the drainage from the T tube, reporting any alterations to the surgeon immediately. The drainage may be slightly blood tinged during the first few hours; then it will be green. The T tube will drain up to 500 mL during the first 24 hours. The amount should decrease as the edema resolves and bile begins flowing through the common bile duct. If there is an excessive amount of bile drainage, the nurse may need to replace the bile either orally or via a

nasogastric tube. This helps to improve the patient's digestion. The bile should be disguised in juice, such as tomato or grape juice. If the patient does not receive bile, bile salts, such as florantyrone or dehydrocholic acid, are given orally.

Even with a T tube there may be drainage from the operative site. Nurses must monitor any drainage from the operative site, because the leakage of bile can be very irritating to the skin. The dressings need to be changed whenever drainage is noted. Montgomery straps make this frequent task easier to perform. Each time the dressing is changed, the skin should be thoroughly cleansed. An antimicrobic agent, such as povidone-iodine (Betadine) ointment, is applied around the insertion site to prevent infection. Skin barriers, such as karaya, may be placed on the skin to protect it from digestion by the bile. The nasogastric tube is removed once bowel

---

DRESSING CHANGE FOR A PATIENT WITH A T TUBE

Prevent kinking of the tube; tape a gauze roll to the patient's abdomen at the side of the insertion site of the T tube; place the T tube over the gauze roll, and secure it in place with adhesive tape

Keep the bile drainage bag below the insertion site to prevent the backflow of bile

Carefully empty the collection container; do not contaminate the openings

Record the amount and color of the drainage

Wash your hands thoroughly

Remove the old dressing, pulling the skin away from the tape

Inspect the old dressing for signs of infection; estimate the amount of drainage on this dressing

Inspect the insertion site for swelling, inflammation, erythema, warmth, drainage, dehiscence, or evisceration

Put on sterile gloves

Cleanse the area around the insertion site with sterile 4 × 4s moistened with normal saline; start at the insertion site, and cleanse the area in concentric circles

Apply an antimicrobial agent, such as Betadine ointment, around the insertion site

Apply a protective agent, such as karaya, on the skin to protect it from irritation from the bile

Make a slit in a 4 × 4 gauze sponge, and place the gauze sponge around the T tube

Apply additional 4 × 4s over the T tube, being careful not to occlude the T tube

Secure the dressing with hypoallergenic tape or Montgomery straps

Document the findings in the nurse's notes

sounds resume and the patient is not nauseated. This is usually between 36 and 48 hours postoperatively. The patient begins drinking low-fat liquids followed by a bland diet. The nurse notes the color of the patient's stool. Clay-colored stool and steatorrhea should alert the nurse to the lack of bile in the intestinal tract. This may be caused by an obstruction. The surgeon is notified of the existence of such manifestations.

The nurse is responsible for the care of the T tube (see box). Dressing changes continue until the T tube is removed. The nurse will clamp the T tube 1 to 2 hours before meals and unclamp the tube 1 to 2 hours after meals. The nurse monitors the patient for complications caused by clamping the T tube. The physician is notified immediately if any complications arise.

The Jackson-Pratt or Penrose drain is removed when the drainage is minimal. The T tube is removed when the edema has subsided and the flow of bile has resumed. Patients discharged with a T tube are taught how to care for the tube. Emphasis is placed on not dislodging the tube. The area around the tube is cleansed when needed. The nurse may arrange for a follow-up visit from the community or home health nurse, who will be able to monitor the drainage from the tube and answer any questions that may arise once the patient is home. The patient returns to the surgeon's office to have the T tube removed.

Patients who have had cholecystectomies are usually discharged in 5 to 7 days. The nurse gives the patient discharge instructions that include care of the suture line and any drainage tubes still in place. The activity of the patient depends on how the patient feels. The patient can resume normal activities but should not lift heavy objects for at least 6 weeks.

There are no dietary restrictions once the patient is discharged, but most patients will stay on a low-fat diet for approximately 6 months. The patient needs to be aware that bile is still being produced but is no longer stored since the gallbladder has been removed. Since bile is being produced, the patient may later develop symptoms of biliary tract disease. The patient is instructed to seek medical attention if symptoms reappear.

Evaluation

As the patient recovers from an acute pain episode, the nurse evaluates the patient's response to food intake. The patient should be pain free after meals. The nurse monitors the patient's food selections for compliance with a prescribed diet. For the patient managed surgically, the nurse evaluates the incision for healing, the signs of respiratory complications, and the ability to return to preoperative level of activity.

Documentation

Accurate documentation of the patient's history of the illness and current symptoms is imperative to avoid confusing cholecystitis and cholelithiasis with other gastrointestinal disorders. The nurse also documents the patient's intake and output and responses to therapy. These documentations provide information for the proper care of each patient.

Ongoing Care

Patients who are managed conservatively require continual dietary restrictions of their consumption of fatty foods. They should avoid such foods as fried foods, cream, whole milk, butter, margarine, peanut butter, nuts, chocolate, pastries, and gravies. Patients who are managed surgically will occasionally have a recurrence of stones elsewhere in the biliary system, such as in the common bile duct. Patients must be made aware of this possibility and encouraged to seek medical attention if any symptoms reappear.

PANCREATITIS
Definition

Pancreatitis is acute or chronic inflammation of the pancreas.

Etiology/Epidemiology

The exact etiology of pancreatitis is unknown. However, many predisposing factors are thought to produce it (see box on p. 1923). Alcoholism and biliary tract disease are the two most commonly associated factors with pancreatitis. Patients who have biliary tract disorders as a precipitating factor are usually women, whereas those with alcoholism as a precipitating factor are generally male.

Pathophysiology

The pathophysiologic process of pancreatitis is the same regardless of the predisposing factor. Stimulation of the pancreas occurs, causing secretion of digestive enzymes. The enzymes are unable to follow their normal course because of the blockage of the ducts by edema or stones. The pancreatic enzymes build up and cause an increase in pressure within the duct. The duct ruptures, releasing the enzymes. The enzymes begin digesting the pancreas. The mechanism that provokes this autodigestion process is unknown. In chronic pancreatitis, protein precipitates within the pancreatic duct cause the duct to become plugged. The duct becomes dilated, leading to atrophy of the acinar tissue, which is replaced by fibrotic tissue. Necrosis of the pancreas occurs. A

PREDISPOSING FACTORS FOR PANCREATITIS

Alcoholism*
Biliary tract disease*
Trauma
  Postsurgical
  Abdominal trauma
Pancreatic carcinoma
Drugs
  Immunosuppressive agents: corticosteroids
  Diuretics: thiazides, furosemide
  Opiates
  Oral contraceptives
Infections
  Mumps
  Coxsackievirus B
  Mycoplasma
Metabolic conditions
  Pregnancy
  Hyperlipidemia
  Hyperparathyroidism (hypercalcemia)
Duodenal ulcers
Vascular disease
  Lupus erythematosus
Heredity
Idiopathic causes

*Most common factors.

pseudocyst may develop as a complication of pancreatitis (Figure 67-12). After autodigestion occurs, the pancreas and occasionally surrounding organs form walls around cystic fluid and necrotic debris. The cyst also contains pancreatic enzymes. These pseudocysts may then develop into an abscess.

Clinical Manifestations

Clinical manifestations vary greatly and depend on the severity of the attack. Some patients are virtually asymptomatic, whereas others are in extreme distress. Ranson's prognostic indicators are often used to recognize severe pancreatitis. These indicators and their relationship to morbidity and mortality are listed in the box on p. 1924. Abdominal pain is the hallmark of acute pancreatitis. A problem arises when trying to distinguish the abdominal pain of pancreatitis from the abdominal pain experienced in other gastrointestinal disorders. Pancreatitis causes a steady pain localized to the epigastrium or left upper quadrant. This pain is caused by the enlargement of the pancreatic capsule, an obstruction, or the chemical irritation from the enzymes. As the pain progresses, it becomes diffuse and radiates to the back and flanks. The back pain is caused by retroperitoneal irritation. The pain may last several days. The back pain decreases when the trunk is flexed, so patients tend to get into a fetal position. Eating exacerbates the pain.

Of the patients with pancreatitis, 70% to 90% will vomit. Vomiting relieves the pain initially but causes an increase in pain as the vomiting continues. The abdomen is tender to touch, but there is little if any abdominal rigidity or guarding. A large amount of blood and plasma may pool into the retroperitoneal

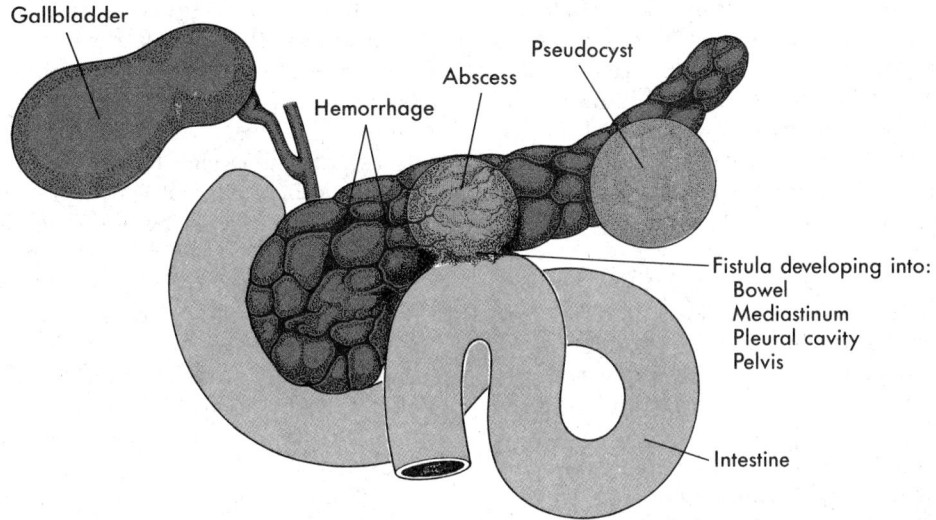

FIGURE 67-12   Complications of pancreatitis.

PROGNOSTIC INDICATORS FOR PANCREATITIS

Signs present on admission

Age > 55 years
White blood cell count > 16,000/mm³
Serum glucose level > 200 mg/dL
Serum lactate dehydrogenase (LDH) level > 350 IU/L
SGOT > 250 IU/L

Signs that develop within 48 hours

Fall in hematocrit > 10%
BUN rise > 5 mg/dL
Serum calcium level < 8 mg/dL
Base deficit > 4 mEq/L
Arterial Po_2 < 60 mm Hg
Estimated fluid sequestration > 6 L

Relationship of indicators to morbidity/mortality

0.9% die when zero to two signs are present
15% die when three or four signs are present
40% die when five or six signs are present
100% die when seven or more signs are present

and peritoneal spaces (third spacing), which can cause hypovolemia and shock.

Other symptoms that may be present but are nonspecific to pancreatitis include low-grade fever, tachycardia, malaise, and restlessness. Laboratory tests reveal an increased serum and urine amylase. Serum amylase rises within a few hours and begins falling after 2 days. Amylase is excreted in the urine by the kidneys. Patients who do not seek medical attention for 2 or 3 days may have a normal serum amylase but an elevated urine amylase. An increased serum lipase, leukocytosis, and hematocrit, as well as a decreased serum calcium and albumin, are also present. If the pancreatitis spreads into the islets of Langerhans, the patient may develop hyperglycemia. Abdominal CT and ultrasound show an enlarged pancreas.

The patient with chronic pancreatitis demonstrates the symptoms previously described as well as steatorrhea caused by decreased production of lipase by the damaged pancreas. Fats are not absorbed properly by the intestinal tract and remain in the stool.

Patients with small pseudocysts may be asymptomatic. Patients with larger cysts experience hyperthermia, abdominal discomfort, and abdominal tenderness. The mass is palpable in approximately half of the cases. It is diagnosed by use of a CT scan or ultrasonography.

Therapeutic Management

Treatment for patients with pancreatitis centers on alleviating the precipitating cause of the disease (if possible), supporting the patient, and preventing or treating complications. A cholecystectomy may be indicated if the precipitating factor is biliary tract disease; otherwise, treatment is medical in nature. The patient needs relief from pain. This is usually accomplished with the administration of 50 to 100 mg of meperidine (Demerol) every 4 to 6 hours. Morphine may cause spasms of the sphincter of Oddi and should be avoided.

Shock is the leading cause of death in patients with pancreatitis, so measures must be taken to avoid this complication. Patients whose condition is unstable may require the insertion of a central venous pressure line for accurate assessment of hemodynamic status. All patients will have a peripheral intravenous line. Colloids or fresh whole blood is administered to replace the fluids lost into the peritoneal or retroperitoneal cavities. Sodium bicarbonate is administered if the patient is in metabolic acidosis. Patients with hyperglycemia from islet cell damage receive insulin. A Foley catheter may be inserted to provide a more accurate assessment of output and to provide information on the need for fluid replacement.

Interventions are employed to decrease the activity of the pancreas, thereby suppressing its secretions. The patient is given nothing orally. A nasogastric tube may be inserted to treat or prevent nausea and vomiting and to decrease abdominal distention. Parenteral anticholinergic medications, such as atropine or propantheline, will assist in decreasing pancreatic activity. Patients who remain NPO for an extended period require hyperalimentation.

Patients with pancreatitis may develop stress ulcers when the gastric pH decreases. Antacids or H_2 histamine receptor antagonists, such as cimetidine, may be given as a preventive measure. Cimetidine controls intragastric pH more effectively if given as a continuous intravenous infusion rather than orally.

Controversy exists as to the value of antibiotics as a prophylactic measure in treating pancreatitis, but they are administered if the patient develops a secondary infection. The patient remains on a strict treatment regimen until the pain subsides, pancreatic enzymes return to normal, and laboratory values return to normal. This may take over 1 week. Therefore the nurse must assess for complications of prolonged bed rest, such as pneumonia and thrombophlebitis.

Once the acute attack is over, treatments are aimed at preventing further attacks. The patient will

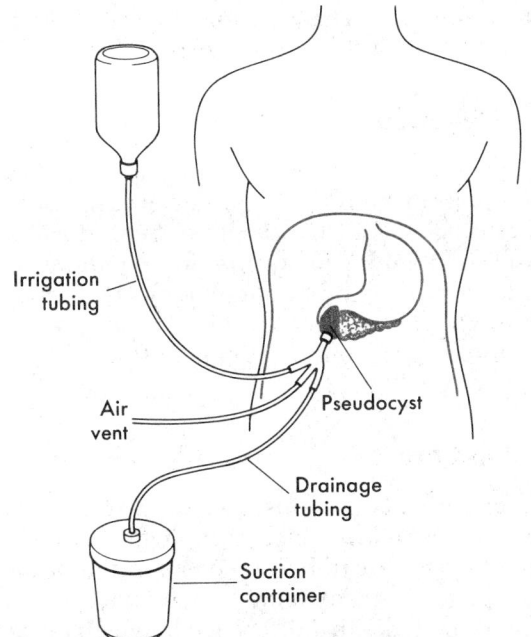

FIGURE 67-13   Pancreatic sump tubes.

be on a bland, low-fat, high-protein, high-carbohydrate diet. Abstinence from alcohol and gastric stimulants such as coffee is mandatory. Patients with chronic pancreatitis may require bile salts to aid in digestion and promote absorption of fat-soluble vitamins. They may also need oral hypoglycemic agents or insulin if there is destruction of the islets of Langerhans.

Large pseudocysts that rupture, get infected, or hemorrhage require surgery to drain the area and evacuate the cyst cavity. A soft sump tube with multiple openings is inserted through a stab wound of the skin (Figure 67-13). The sump tube resembles a Foley catheter with three lumens. One is an air vent, one is for infusion of irrigation solution, and one is for the drainage of debris. Multiple sump tubes will be used depending on the number of cysts. The sump is attached to suction for drainage of the cysts. After 12 hours the area will begin to be irrigated via the sump with normal saline or lactated Ringer's. The amount of fluid that drains from the sump should equal or exceed the amount of fluid instilled from sump irrigation. The irrigation process continues until the CT scan reveals pancreatic healing.

NURSING MANAGEMENT OF THE PATIENT WITH PANCREATITIS
Assessment

Pancreatic disorders are often mistaken for other gastrointestinal disorders. A thorough history and physical assessment are vital in correctly diagnosing

pancreatitis. If this is the first attack, the nurse obtains information concerning the history of predisposing factors, such as alcohol abuse or biliary tract disease. An accurate description of the pain and its relationship to meals, location, quality, and measures that relieve it is noted. The patient is asked if vomiting has occurred and, if so, whether the vomiting relieved the pain.

The nurse monitors the patient's vital signs, noting any alterations from normal. Close attention is paid to signs that may indicate shock, such as hypotension; weak, thready pulse; pale-colored skin; cool, clammy skin; tachypnea; decreased urine output; and altered mental status. The nurse observes the patient closely for signs of metabolic alterations, such as hyperglycemia or hypocalcemia. Laboratory results are assessed.

Nursing Diagnosis

The nursing diagnoses for patients with pancreatitis include the following:

Fluid volume deficit related to vomiting and nasogastric tube drainage

Impaired health maintenance related to knowledge deficit concerning the disease and treatment regimen

Altered nutrition: less than body requirements, related to anorexia, vomiting, and impaired digestion secondary to the loss of enzymes necessary for the digestive process

Pain related to stimulation of nerve endings associated with obstruction of the pancreatic tract

Planning

Outcome criteria for the patient with pancreatitis include the following:

Patient reports freedom from discomfort and pain

Patient's fluid and electrolyte status is balanced

Patient's vital signs are stable

Patient verbalizes understanding of the dietary regimen

Patient and family verbalize factors that may cause recurrence of the disease

Patient reports abstinence from alcohol

Patient and family work with a support group as needed

Implementation

Vital signs are measured at least every hour during acute attacks. The nurse carefully monitors all aspects of vital signs and notifies the physician of changes that may indicate the development of complications, such as shock. Many patients with pancreatitis who also have a history of alcoholism are assessed as being manipulative when they ask for pain medications. Pancreatitis is extremely painful, and the nurse should administer analgesics to provide relief from this pain. As always, when administering medications, the nurse observes for side effects and adverse reactions from the medication. The nurse needs to document the patient's response to the medication, such as relief from pain. Other methods to relieve pain, such as repositioning or positive imagery, should be used.

An intravenous line is started for the administration of fluid and electrolyte replacements or volume expanders. The nurse is responsible for the correct infusion of the fluid and noting the patient's response to the replacement. The intravenous line must be observed frequently for edema, erythema, or other signs of infiltration. The patient may be receiving sodium bicarbonate, and it is very damaging to tissue when infiltration occurs.

The patient is given nothing orally, and a nasogastric tube is inserted to provide rest for the patient's digestive system. The nurse must assess the amount and color of the drainage and prevent complications from the nasogastric tube such as necrosis of the ala nasi from improper taping techniques. Antacids may be administered via the nasogastric tube. The nasogastric tube is clamped for 20 to 30 minutes after the instillation of the medication.

The patient needs continuous nutritional support. This will be provided with hyperalimentation (TPN) if the patient requires such intervention. The nurse is responsible for monitoring the effects of the hyperalimentation. Once oral nutrition is permitted the nurse assesses the patient's tolerance to food, observing for the recurrence of nausea, vomiting, or abdominal distention. The patient needs to be educated about diets that are bland, low in fat, and high in protein and carbohydrates. A dietary consultation is often beneficial.

If the complication of an abscess from a pseudocyst arises, the nurse is responsible for the care of the pancreatic sump tubes, including irrigation of the tube, monitoring its input and output, dressing the stab wounds, and observing for signs of infection. Patients who are addicted to alcohol may go through withdrawal. The nurse must be aware of this in order to protect the patient from injury and provide supportive care to the patient and family. Referral to an alcohol treatment center may be beneficial.

Evaluation

The evaluation of nursing care for the patient with pancreatitis focuses on the patient's response to measures to relieve symptoms and prevent complications. The patient's pain should be relieved. As the patient recovers from an acute episode, vital signs should be within normal limits. Laboratory tests will indicate fluid and electrolyte balance. The patient should be able to tolerate oral intake without discomfort. Serum amylase, urine amylase, and serum glucose levels will be within normal ranges.

Documentation

Accurate documentation of the nursing assessment can be a great help to the physician in making the correct diagnosis of pancreatitis. Such documentation aids in planning the proper interventions to take with each individual patient. Noting changes in output and vital signs can alert health care professionals to impending complications and possibly alleviate severe problems.

Ongoing Care

Patients with pancreatitis will remain on a bland, low-fat, high-calorie, high-carbohydrate diet after discharge. There can be no consumption of alcohol or beverages with caffeine. Compliance to such a regimen can make the difference between full recovery or recurrence of the disease. The patient may require rehabilitative treatment if alcohol is abused. Support groups for both the patient and family are the best form of treatment.

CANCER OF THE PANCREAS
Definition

Cancer of the pancreas occurs when malignant cells proliferate within the pancreas.

Etiology/Epidemiology

As with most forms of cancer, the cause of pancreatic cancer remains unknown. It is far more common in persons over the age of 60 years, especially males. Patients with hereditary pancreatitis or diabetes have an increased incidence of developing pancreatic cancer. Other risk factors include cigarette smoking, high-fat consumption, and exposure to chemicals such as coke and benzidine. Pancreatic cancer is the fifth leading cause of death from cancer. The incidence of pancreatic cancer has greatly increased over the past decade. This disease kills approximately 25,000 people each year in the United States. It is estimated that there were more than 27,000 new cases of pancreatic cancer diagnosed in 1993. Five-year survival rates are very poor, with only 3% of patients with pancreatic cancer surviving.[3] Total survival rates are just as ominous, with the average life expectancy after diagnosis being an additional 4 to 8 months.

Pathophysiology

As with all cancers, pancreatic cancer begins with an alteration at the cellular level. A malignant cell divides into two malignant cells. This process continues as the malignant cells invade the pancreas, taking over its normal functions. Most pancreatic tumors are fast growing and invade the fat, lymph, blood vessels, and perineural areas.

Clinical Manifestations

Clinical manifestations vary according to the location of the invading tumor. The majority of patients suffer from nonspecific, vague pain caused by the tumor invading the perineural area. Patients describe the pain in various ways from intermittent to persistent and a dull ache to radiating back pain. Often the pain occurs at night, awakening the patient. It is occasionally relieved by lying on the side or in a fetal position. Obstruction of the bile ducts occurs when the malignancy invades the head of the pancreas. This obstruction causes the patient to become jaundiced, the stools to become clay colored, and the urine to be dark amber (urobilinogen). It also leads to malabsorption of nutrients, nausea, vomiting, and subsequent weight loss and weakness. Patients with pancreatic cancer may experience glucose intolerance when the beta cells of the pancreas are affected. Diagnosis of pancreatic cancer is usually not accomplished until the malignancy has advanced. It is difficult to distinguish pancreatic cancer from pancreatitis. Both cause elevated serum lipase, amylase, and glucose. A tumor can be seen with ultrasound, computed tomography (CT), or endoscopic retrograde cholangiopancreatography (ERCP). Pancreatic biopsy is necessary for a definitive diagnosis of pancreatic cancer.

Therapeutic Management

Surgical removal of a malignancy offers the only hope for curing pancreatic cancer. This is only possible in a minimal number of patients where the tumor is localized to the head of the pancreas. When the tumor has spread to the body and tail of the pancreas, metastasis to other areas is likely, making surgical resection useless. Even with surgical resection, 5-year survival rates remain poor.

Pancreaticoduodenectomy, or **Whipple's procedure** (Figure 67-14), is the radical surgery of choice. This procedure involves resecting the proximal head of the pancreas, the adjoining duodenum, the distal portion of the stomach, and the distal segment of the common bile duct. An anastomosis of the jejunum to the pancreatic duct (pancreatojejunostomy), common bile duct (choledochojejunostomy), and stomach (gastrojejunostomy) is done.

A cholecytojejunostomy may be done as a palliative measure to relieve biliary obstruction and the clinical manifestations that this obstruction causes. This procedure does not increase the survival rate. Patients undergoing pancreatic surgery must be stabilized. Parenteral feedings are administered to im-

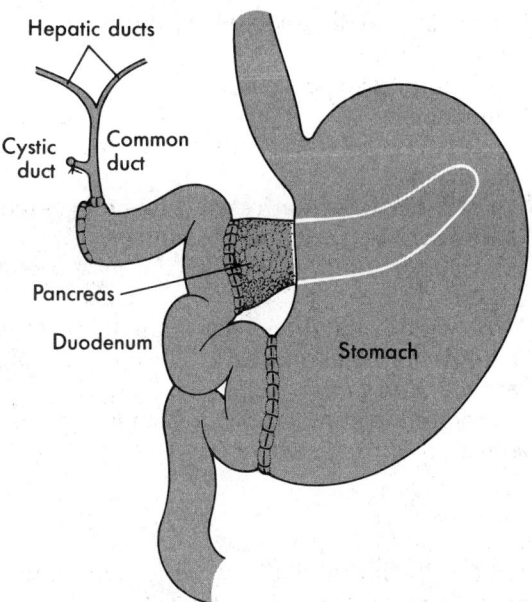

FIGURE 67-14 Whipple's procedure, or radical pancreas resection, entails resection of proximal pancreas, adjoining duodenum, distal portion of stomach, and distal segment of common bile duct. Anastomosis of pancreatic duct, common bile duct, and stomach to jejunum is done.

prove the patient's nitrogen balance. Electrolyte imbalances are corrected, as well as any anemias.

NURSING MANAGEMENT OF THE PATIENT WITH PANCREATIC CANCER

Assessment

A detailed history is elicited from the patient with suspected pancreatic cancer. Important information should include, but not be limited exclusively to, a familial history of pancreatitis and a patient history of diabetes mellitus. The nurse should also inquire about the patient's exposure to suspected pancreatic carcinogens (e.g., cigarette smoke) and increased amounts of fats or chemicals. Assessment includes an accurate description of the pain pattern as well as a physical assessment of signs and symptoms of pancreatic obstruction. These signs and symptoms vary according to the location of the tumor. Some of them include nausea, vomiting, weight loss, weakness, jaundice, clay-colored stool, urobilinogen, and glucose intolerance.

Nursing Diagnosis

The nursing diagnoses for patients with pancreatic cancer include the following:

  Ineffective coping related to pain, depression, and poor prognosis secondary to diagnosis of cancer of the pancreas

Fluid volume deficit related to anorexia, nausea, and vomiting

Anticipatory grieving related to poor prognosis of the disease

Hopelessness related to the diagnosis of a terminal disease

High risk for infection related to suppressed immune system secondary to cancer

High risk for injury related to decreased platelet count

Alteration in nutrition: less than body requirements related to anorexia, nausea, vomiting, diarrhea, and pain

Pain related to stimulation of the nerve ending associated with obstruction

Planning

Outcome criteria for patients with pancreatic cancer might include the following:

The patient and family will verbalize an understanding of pancreatic cancer and its treatments and prognosis

The patient has a minimal amount of pain and discomfort

The patient will maintain an adequate intake of fluid and food

The patient will be free from infection

The patient will be free from bleeding

The patient and family will verbalize concerns and feelings

The patient and family will successfully grieve

Implementation

Nursing interventions for the patient with pancreatic cancer are individualized. Because of the very poor prognosis, most of the interventions are physically and psychosocially supportive. Many nursing interventions for the patient with pancreatic cancer are similar to the interventions carried out for the patient with pancreatitis. The nurse caring for the patient with pancreatic cancer participates in educating the patient and family about cancer of the pancreas and its prognosis. Referrals are made to appropriate sources, such as pastoral care departments and hospices. Another focus of nursing care includes pain management. Initially, pain control may not be necessary, but as the disease progresses, it becomes a major part of the patient's care.

The patient's weight is monitored. The nurse incorporates the patient's nutritional needs into the care plan. Efforts are made to stimulate the patient's appetite. Small frequent feedings that are low in fat and not spicy may be tolerated best. Consultation with a dietitian is beneficial.

If surgery is the treatment of choice, preoperative patient education includes standard information about postoperative pain management, abdominal splinting, turning, coughing, and deep breathing. Patients who undergo surgery for pancreatic cancer also need education about their surgery. Allow them time to discuss the surgery and ask questions. All questions should be addressed in an honest, straightforward manner.

Postoperatively, the patient is in the intensive care unit. During this time the patient should receive the treatments that one would carry out on all patients with major abdominal surgery, including closely monitoring vital signs, observing the incision site for drainage and infection, administering antibiotics and pain medications, and monitoring the nasogastric tube for patency and drainage. The patient's blood sugar also must be monitored. Blood glucose levels are sent to the laboratory and/or fingersticks are done at the bedside. Should the patient show signs of hyperglycemia, a fast-acting insulin is administered. The nurse is also responsible for postoperative wound care, performing sterile dressing changes and observing for signs and symptoms of infection. Any fever, abdominal pain, drainage, swelling, or redness at the suture site is documented and reported to the physician immediately.

Evaluation

The evaluation of the nursing care for patients with pancreatic cancer can best be done by allowing the patient and family to verbalize their understanding of the disease and its management and prognosis. The patient will verbalize effective methods of controlling pain. Continuous evaluation of the patient's nutritional status will take place by routinely weighing the patient and monitoring intake and output. The nurse also evaluates how the patient and family are coping. They must receive continuous support and assistance while going through the grieving process. Spiritual needs may be identified during this evaluation process.

Documentation

The patient history and physical are accurately documented. Response to treatments, especially analgesia, is recorded. Weights and intake and output are also documented.

Ongoing Care

Patients with pancreatic cancer do not survive very long, having a life expectancy of less than 6 months. Therefore they must be made as comfortable as possible for the remainder of their lives. Encourage the patient and family to express themselves and their concerns and fears. The American Cancer Society organizes and supports many programs. Supplying the family with names and telephone numbers of support groups may be of assistance. Local hospice organizations are also beneficial. Such organizations can supply the patient and family with additional educational materials and support.

CRITICAL THINKING QUESTIONS

1 What is the nursing management of the patient with cirrhosis?

2 Compare and contrast the causative factors, routes of infection, incubation period, severity, clinical manifestations, and therapeutic management of type A, type B, and type non-A, non-B hepatitis.

3 What is the nursing management of the patient with hepatitis?

4 Describe the postoperative care for the patient having a liver transplant.

5 Discuss the differences among cholecystitis, cholelithiasis, cholecystectomy, steatorrhea, and choledocholithiasis.

6 Discuss the nursing management of the patient with pancreatitis.

7 Compare the nursing management of the patient with pancreatitis to that of the patient with pancreatic cancer.

BIBLIOGRAPHY

Current

1. Adinaro D: Liver failure and pancreatitis: fluid and electrolyte concerns, *Nurs Clin North Am* 22(4):843, 1987.
2. Akdamar K: Control of gastrointestinal bleeding by endoscopy: an overview, *Curr Concepts Gastroenterol* 8(6):6, 1986.
3. American Cancer Society: Cancer statistics—1993, *Cancer* 43(1):18, 1993.
4. Anderson FD: The cirrhotic process in the alcoholic, *Crit Care Q* 8(4):74, 1986.
5. Anderson FD: Portal-systemic encephalopathy in the chronic alcoholic, *Crit Care Q* 8(4):74, 1986.
6. Birdsall C, Fiore-Lopez N: How do you manage pancreatic sump tubes? *Am J Nurs* 87(6):770, 1987.
7. Black M: Primary biliary cirrhosis, *Hosp Med* 22(5):184, 1986.
8. Brown A: Acute pancreatitis: pathophysiology, nursing diagnosis, and collaborative problems, *Focus Crit Care* 18(2):121, 1991.
9. Burns SM, Martin MJ: VP/NTG therapy in the patient with variceal bleeding, *Crit Care Nurse* 10(9):42, 1990.
10. Chopra S: *Disorders of the liver*, Philadelphia, 1988, Lea & Febiger.
11. Dobberstein K: The liver: to know it is to love it, *Am J Nurs* 87(1):74, 1987.
12. Dudley SL, Starin RB: Cholelithiasis: diagnosis and current therapeutic options, *Nurse Pract* 16(3), 1991.
13. Gallo UE, Fontanarosa PB: Acute cholecystitis, *Emerg Care Q* 5(3):84, 1989.
14. Gauwitz DF: Endoscopic cholecsytectomy: the patient-friendly alternative, *Nurs 90* 20(12):58, 1990.

15. Griefzu S, Dest V: When the diagnosis is pancreatic cancer, *RN* 54(8):38, 1991.
16. Groer MW, Shekleton ME: *Basic pathophysiology: a holistic approach*, ed 3, St Louis, 1989, Mosby–Year Book, Inc.
17. Hauser SC: Answers to questions on gallbladder disease, *Hosp Med* 23(6):44, 1987.
18. Hornbaker AE: Hematologic disorders in the critically ill alcoholic, *Crit Care Q* 8(4):29, 1986.
19. Jaffe MS: *Medical-surgical nursing care plans: nursing diagnosis and intervention*, ed 2, Norwalk, Conn, 1992, Appleton & Lange.
20. Jeffres C: Complications of acute pancreatitis, *Crit Care Nurse* 9(4):38, 1989.
21. Jensen DM: Portal-systemic encephalopathy and hepatic coma, *Med Clin North Am* 70(5):1081, 1986.
22. Jermier BJ, Treloar DM: Bringing your patient through gallbladder surgery, *RN* 49(11):18, 1986.
23. Johnson D: Fluid and electrolyte dysfunction in alcoholism, *Crit Care Q* 8(4):53, 1986.
24. Jurf JB et al: Cholecystectomy made easier, *Am J Nurs* 90(12):38, 1990.
25. Maloney JP: Surgical intervention in the alcoholic patient with portal hypertension, *Crit Care Q* 8(4):63, 1986.
26. Munn NC: When the bile duct is blocked, *RN* 52(1):50, 1989.
27. Pierce JD et al: Acute esophageal bleeding and endoscopic injection sclerotherapy, *Crit Care Nurse* 10(9):67, 1990.
28. Sabesin S: Countering the dangers of acute pancreatitis, *Emerg Med* 19(17):71, 1987.
29. Sheets L: Liver transplantation, *Nurs Clin North Am* 24(4):881, 1989.
30. Smith A: When the pancreas self-destructs, *Am J Nurs* 91(9):38, 1991.
31. Smith SL, Ciferni ML: Liver transplantation, *Crit Care Nurs Clin North Am* 4(1):131, 1992.
32. Throwe AN: Families and alcohol, *Crit Care Q* 8(4):79, 1986.
33. United Network for Organ Sharing, *UNOS Update* 8(2), 1992.
34. Williams SR: *Nutrition and diet therapy*, ed 7, St Louis, 1993, Mosby–Year Book, Inc.
35. Wyngaarden JB, Smith LH, editors: *Cecil textbook of medicine*, ed 19, Philadelphia, 1992, WB Saunders Co.

Classic

36. Dodd RP: Ascites: when the liver can't cope, *RN* 47(10):26, 1984.
37. Fredette SL: When the liver fails, *Am J Nurs* 84(1):64, 1984.
38. Gitlin N, Heyman MB: Nutritional support in liver disease, *Nutritional Support Services* 4(6):14, 1984.
39. Given BA, Simmons SJ: *Gastroenterology in clinical nursing*, ed 4, St Louis, 1984, Mosby–Year Book, Inc.
40. Greenberger NJ: Etiology and pathogenesis of chronic pancreatitis, *Hosp Pract* 20(9):83, 1985.
41. Kirkman-Liff B, Dandoy S: Hepatitis B: what price exposure? *Am J Nurs* 84(8):988, 1984.
42. LaSala C: Caring for the patient with a transhepatic biliary decompression catheter, *Nurs 85* 15(2):52, 1985.
43. Miller B, Gavant ML: Biliary catheter care, *Am J Nurs* 85(10):1115, 1985.
44. Peternel E: A high-tech approach to a GI problem, *RN* 48(6):44, 1985.
45. Quinless F: Portal hypertension: physiology, signs and symptoms, *Nurs 84* 14(1):52, 1984.

UNIT XVI

Reproductive System

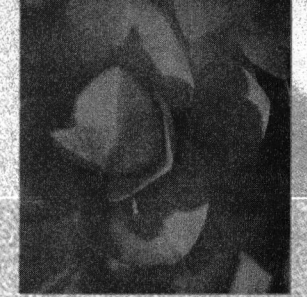

CHAPTER SIXTY-EIGHT

Nursing Assessment of the Reproductive System

LEARNING OBJECTIVES

1 Know the basic anatomical structure and functions of the male and female reproductive systems.
2 Obtain relevant subjective information from the patient who has a reproductive alteration.
3 Using correct technique, examine the patient to obtain appropriate objective information about the reproductive system.
4 Differentiate abnormal from normal subjective and objective findings related to the reproductive system.
5 Describe the tests and procedures that are involved in the diagnosis of disorders of the male and female reproductive systems.
6 Describe the care for patients undergoing each of the tests and procedures that diagnose reproductive alteration.

KEY TERMS

THE FUNCTION of the male and female reproductive systems is to reproduce new members of the species and ensure that the species survives. Both men and women produce gametes by a random selection of the chromosomes of their parents, and their reproductive systems provide for the mating of the gametes, the successful development of the offspring within the woman, the birth, and early nutrition. The reproductive hormones are responsible for the maintenance of the reproductive organs and for the development of secondary sexual characteristics.

ANATOMY AND PHYSIOLOGY
Female Reproductive System

The female reproductive system (Figure 68-1) is designed to produce ova at regular intervals and to provide the reproductive organs necessary for fertilization, implantation, and growth and maturation of the embryo; to expel the fetus; and to provide milk for the newborn infant's nutrition. The primary sex organs of the female are the ovaries.

Ovaries

The **ovaries** are two irregular ovoid structures that lie in the abdominal cavity close to the infundibulum of the fallopian tube. They are made up of a stroma of connective tissue in which many follicles are embedded. The stroma is surrounded by a layer of cuboidal epithelium from which the ovarian follicles were originally formed in the early months of gestation.

The maturation of the reproductive tract at puberty, the maintenance of the reproductive organs of the mature adult, the development of the secondary sexual characteristics, and the ability to reproduce are functions of the ovarian hormones. These hormones are controlled by follicle stimulating hormone (FSH) and luteinizing hormone (LH) secreted by the anterior lobe of the pituitary gland, which is in turn controlled by the hypothalamus.

Secondary sex organs

The female reproductive tract is made up of the uterus and fallopian tubes, the vagina, the external genitalia, and the glands.

The **uterus** provides the support and blood supply for the growing fetus. It is a hollow, pear-shaped organ, which in the nongravid state (7 × 5 cm long) lies in the pelvic region. It has a dome-shaped fundus, a body, and a constricted neck called the cervix. The uterus lies between two broad ligaments or sheets attached to the lateral abdominal wall, and by a thickened portion (cardinal ligaments) to the pelvic floor. The broad ligaments lie in the frontal plane and cover and support the uterus, the fallopian tubes, and the ovaries. The cardinal ligaments contain smooth muscle, uterine nerves, and blood vessels. Other supporting ligaments include the two round ligaments, which extend from the upper outer angles of the uterus to the labia majora, a posterior ligament and an anterior ligament, which connect the uterus with the posterior and anterior walls of the abdominal cavity, and the uterosacral ligaments, which extend from the sacrum to the cervix and enclose the rectum. Assisted by the muscles of the pelvic floor, these ligaments support the uterus and prevent it from prolapsing into the vagina.

The uterine wall is made up of three layers of smooth muscle (myometrium) with fibers arranged in longitudinal, circular, and spiral directions. The myometrium, which is much thicker in the fundus than in the neck (cervix) of the uterus, is capable of considerable hypertrophy during pregnancy. The cervix normally has a very small lumen: the uterine inner opening is called the internal os, the outer opening to the vagina is called the external os.

The inner lining of the uterus (endometrium) is made up of two layers: a superficial layer of columnar epithelium and glands, supported by a basal layer of connective tissue, and the deeper regions of the glands.

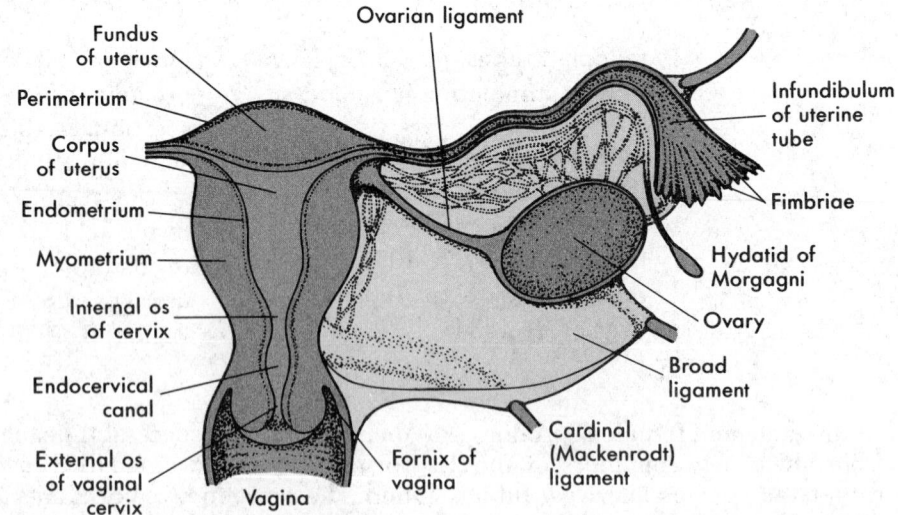

FIGURE 68-1   Female reproductive system. Cross section of uterus, adnexa, and upper vagina.

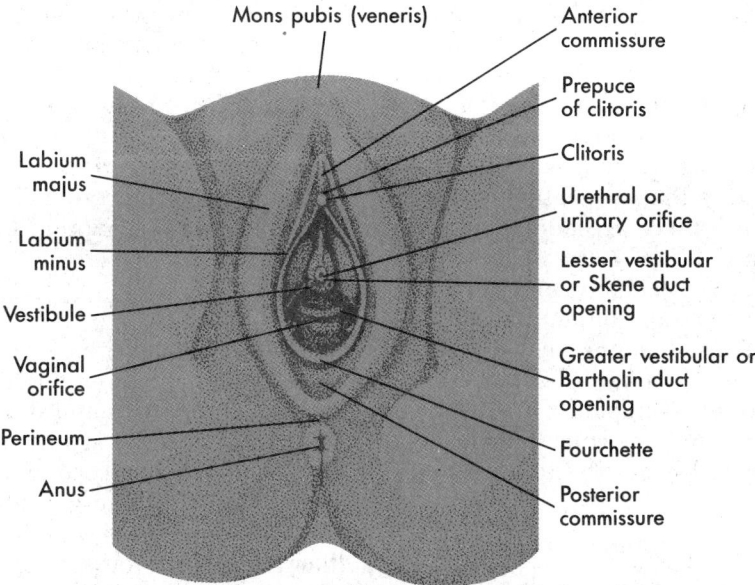

Mons pubis (veneris)

Anterior commissure

Prepuce of clitoris

Clitoris

Urethral or urinary orifice

Lesser vestibular or Skene duct opening

Greater vestibular or Bartholin duct opening

Fourchette

Posterior commissure

Labium majus

Labium minus

Vestibule

Vaginal orifice

Perineum

Anus

FIGURE 68-2   External female genitalia.

The two **fallopian tubes,** or uterine tubes, are continuations of the uterus. Each is about 10 cm long and stretches from the uterus to a funnel-shaped structure (infundibulum), close to but not enclosing, an ovary. They have a muscular wall and are lined with ciliated columnar epithelium. The cilia move the contents of the tubes toward the uterus.

The **vagina** serves to receive the penis during sexual intercourse and as a birth canal during parturition. It is made up of an outer fibrous layer, an inner smooth muscle layer containing bands of connective tissue, and an inner mucosal layer of stratified squamous epithelium arranged in folds, or rugae.

The external genitalia (Figure 68-2) surround the external vaginal opening. They are called the vulva, and they include the mons pubis, labia majora, labia minora, clitoris, vestibule, and vestibular glands. The mons pubis is the area covering the symphysis pubis, which becomes covered with hair at puberty. The labia majora are two thickened folds of skin, connective tissue, and smooth muscle that surround the smaller labia minora, the clitoris, and the vaginal orifice. The clitoris is a small cylindrical, erectile structure (approximately 3 cm anterior to the vagina) that originates from the same tissues that develop into the penis of the male fetus. It consists of a glans, a body, and two crura, and it is partly covered by the anterior ends of the labia minora. It and the surrounding tissues enlarge by becoming engorged with blood in response to tactile and sexual stimulation. The clitoris is the center of the erotic sensations that lead to orgasm in the female. The area between the labia minora contains the vaginal orifice and the urethral opening and is called the vestibule. The perineum refers to the area around the vaginal opening between the anus and the mons pubis.

The vestibular glands (Bartholin's glands) lie close to the vaginal orifice. They lubricate the vestibule by secreting mucus during sexual excitement.

Menstrual cycle and gonadal hormones

Throughout the reproductive period, the ovaries and reproductive tract undergo cyclical changes that last about 28 days and are under the control of the hypothalamic and hypophyseal hormones.

Ovarian cycle

At the beginning of each **menstrual cycle** approximately six primordial follicles begin to grow under the influence of **follicle stimulating hormone** (FSH). Most of them regress and die after a few days leaving the largest one to mature into a fluid-filled graafian follicle, which secretes estrogen. About midcycle (day 14), the follicle ruptures and releases its ovum into the peritoneal cavity. The secretion of FSH and ovulation are controlled by the concentration of the hypothalamic luteinizing hormone releasing−hormone (LHRH) and by the negative feedback effects of estrogen.

Some of the follicle cells remain in the ovary following ovulation. They reproduce and form the corpus luteum, a yellow structure that secretes estrogen and progesterone during the remaining 14 days of the cycle. If the ovum is not fertilized, the corpus luteum degenerates and the secretion of estrogen and progesterone declines, bringing the cycle to an end.

Ovarian cycles begin at puberty when the secretion of LHRH increases under the influence of a "biological clock." They become irregular and cease at menopause, because there are no longer primordial follicles that can respond to the stimulation of FSH. After menopause, because there are no developing follicles, there is also a deficiency of estrogen and progesterone. This deficiency leads to some involution of the reproductive tract and diminution of the protective mucus secretions of glands, such as those lining the walls of the vagina and uterus. An increase in the secretion of FSH at menopause results because of the reduction in pituitary gonadotropin inhibition normally provided by the ovarian steroids.

Uterine cycle
Menstruation phase
Menstruation is bleeding (usually lasting 4 to 5 days) that results from the shedding of the superficial layer of endometrium. The endometrium degenerates because the amount of estrogen and progesterone secreted by the corpus luteum declines. The first day on which menstrual bleeding occurs is clearly identifiable and is called day 1 of the menstrual cycle.

Proliferative phase
Estrogen, secreted by the developing graafian follicle in the ovary, stimulates the regrowth of the superficial layer of the endometrium by stimulating the proliferation of the columnar cells lining the glands of the basal layer, and the cells of the connective tissue surrounding the glands. Estrogen also renders the myometrium more sensitive to stimulation and therefore more likely to contract when stimulated. This part of the menstrual cycle is referred to as the proliferative phase, or the estrogen phase, and its duration is the most variable of the three phases. The cervical mucus secretions thicken during ovulation, which marks the end of this phase.

Secretory phase
The duration of the secretory phase shows less variation. It normally lasts 14 days regardless of the length of the proliferative phase. After ovulation, the follicle cells that remain in the ovary reproduce and form the corpus luteum, which secretes estrogen and progesterone. The corpus luteum is controlled by luteinizing hormone secreted by the adenohypophysis. Progesterone stimulates the endometrial glands to become secretory, and like estrogen it increases the water content and thickness of the endometrium. Unlike estrogen, progesterone decreases the sensitivity of the myometrium to nervous or hormonal stimulation, and thus it is less likely to contract in the presence of progesterone.

When the corpus luteum degenerates, the endo-metrium deteriorates, and menstruation marks the end of one menstrual cycle and the beginning of the next. The feedback effects of estrogen and progesterone are not fully understood and may vary with concentration. Estrogen may have a positive feedback on the secretion of LHRH before ovulation. Certainly progesterone has a negative feedback effect upon the secretion of LH and FSH.

Secondary sexual characteristics
Secondary sexual characteristics begin to develop at puberty under the influence of the gonadal hormones. The growth and development of the breasts (mammary glands) are the most obvious of these in the female. Other secondary sexual characteristics include lighter bone growth, thinner skin, broader smoother hip bones, and the growth of pubic and axillary hair. (In women the pubic hair grows in an area shaped like a shield and does not extend above the mons pubis.) Some of these characteristics are attributable to the lower levels of androgens found in women, and others to the effects of estrogen and progesterone.

The breasts, which secrete colostrum and milk to nourish the infant, lie over the muscles above the second to sixth ribs. Each breast is made up of 15 to 20 lobes, supported by connective tissue and adipose tissue. The adipose tissue is largely responsible for the difference in size of the breasts in comparisons made between individuals (Figure 68-3). The devel-

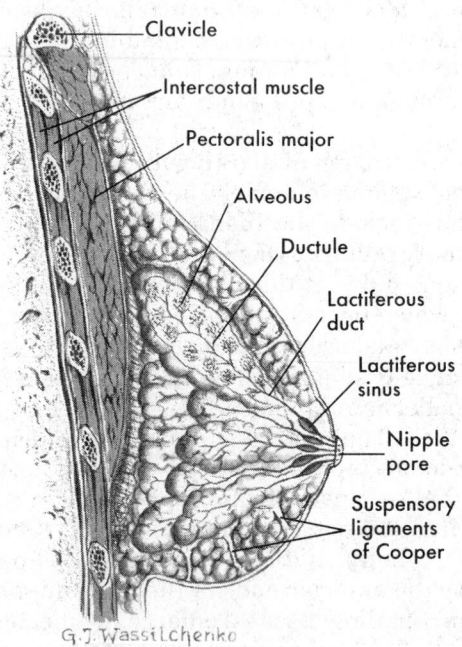

Clavicle

Intercostal muscle

Pectoralis major

Alveolus

Ductule

Lactiferous duct

Lactiferous sinus

Nipple pore

Suspensory ligaments of Cooper

G. J. Wassilchenko

FIGURE 68-3 Structure of the breast. (From Thompson JM et al: *Mosby's manual of clinical nursing*, ed 2, St Louis, 1989, Mosby–Year Book, Inc.)

opment of the mammary glands is stimulated by estrogen and progesterone which are secreted by the corpus luteum after puberty until menopause and by the placenta during pregnancy. The production of milk is stimulated by prolactin, secreted by the anterior lobe of the pituitary gland. Milk is normally produced only after the birth of a baby in response to suckling. Lactation at other times is abnormal (galactorrhea) and is usually due to excess prolactin secretion. Prolactin secretion is controlled by a hypothalamic prolactin-inhibiting hormone. Forcing milk out of the mammary gland alveoli to the nipple area is a function of oxytocin. Oxytocin is secreted by the posterior lobe of the pituitary gland when the baby suckles, during labor, and during orgasm. It also causes the uterine muscles to contract unless their contraction is inhibited by progesterone.

Male Reproductive System

The male reproductive system is designed to produce and constantly maintain an adequate supply of gametes (sperm) and place them in the vagina of the female. Starting at puberty, sperm are produced in the testes and stored in the epididymis. They are delivered to the penis by the vas deferens along with the secretions of the reproductive glands. The reproductive tract and the secondary sexual characteristics develop, and are maintained, under the influence of the gonadal hormones, especially testosterone. The primary sex organs of the male are the testes.

Testes

The **testes** are ovoid structures that lie outside the body in the scrotum (Figure 68-4). They are made up of seminiferous tubules and the interstitial cells

that pack the spaces between them. The cells forming the seminiferous tubules are of two kinds: the spermatogonia, which constantly divide and produce haploid sperm (i.e., with half the usual number of chromosomes) by meiosis; and the Sertoli, or nurse, cells, which form the outer layer of the tubule and secrete nutrients for the immature sperm embedded in pouches around them. The Sertoli cells form a blood-testes barrier and control the substances reaching the spermatogonia and sperm. Once the sperm reach the center of the lumen of the seminiferous tubules, they are moved and stored in the epididymis.

The **sperm** consists of a body largely made up of chromosomes and a flagellum, or tail. Despite the presence of a tail, they do not become motile until mixed with the secretions of the accessory glands, especially those of the prostate gland. They must also undergo capacitation in the female reproductive tract before they are capable of fertilizing the ovum.

The **scrotum** is a pouch suspended behind the **penis** in the perineal region. It is supported by smooth muscle (dartos) in the subcutaneous tissue. The blood and lymph vessels, the vas deferens, the nerves, and a continuation of the internal oblique abdominal muscle (cremaster) pass into the abdomen through the inguinal canals. The relaxation of the dartos and cremaster muscles lower the scrotum away from the body during high environmental temperatures. The temperature of the testes is maintained about 2° C below body temperature for optimum sperm viability.

Secondary sex organs

The epididymis is a single, tightly coiled tube lying close to the testes and enclosed in a fibrous capsule. It is responsible for the nutrition and maturation of

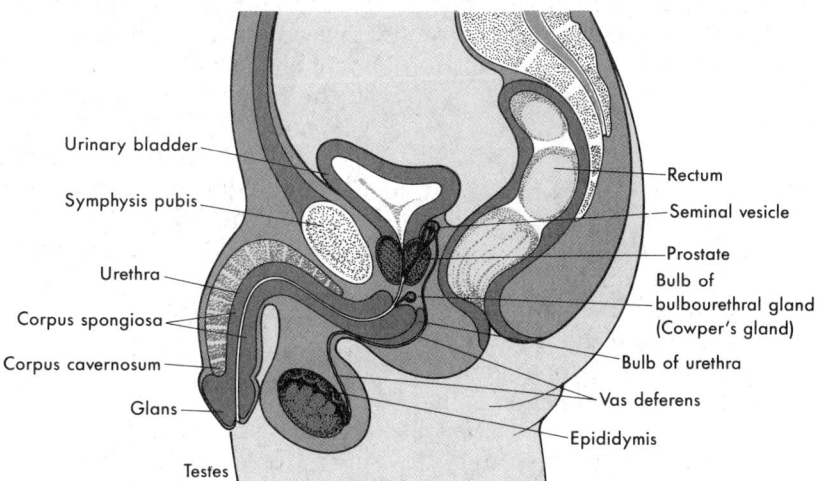

FIGURE 68-4   Male reproductive system. (From Anthony CP, Thibodeau GA: *Textbook of anatomy and physiology,* ed 12, St Louis, 1987, Mosby–Year Book, Inc.)

the sperm, which it stores for 3 to 6 weeks. The epididymis reabsorbs components of the fluid that originates in the seminiferous tubules and secretes other substances into the fluid that surrounds and supports the sperm.

The vas deferens is a tube that has thick smooth-muscle walls and can propel the sperm from the epididymis to the ejaculatory duct. After entering the abdominal cavity, it passes up and over the ureter where it enters the bladder. This circuitous route develops when the testes, formed near the origin of the kidneys, descend to enter the scrotum when the fetus is about 28 weeks of age.

The seminal vesicles are two convoluted glands that lie close to the bladder. They produce a viscous liquid, rich in fructose to provide energy for the sperm, that is forced into the ejaculatory duct when peristalsis conducts the sperm along the vas deferens.

The prostate gland lies below the bladder and surrounds the urethra. It produces a thin alkaline fluid that is secreted into the urethra through many small ducts during ejaculation. Because it neutralizes the acidity of the urethra and vagina, this fluid serves to protect the sperm from death and also to promote the sperm's motility.

The bulbourethral glands are two pea-shaped glands that lie at the base of the penis and drain into the urethra. They are stimulated during sexual excitement, and before ejaculation they secrete a mucoid fluid that coats the urethra and protects the sperm from acid urine residues.

Semen is made up of the sperm and the secretions of the testes and epididymis, the seminal vesicles (approximately 60% of semen by volume), the prostate glands (approximately 35%), and the bulbourethral glands. Normally 1.5 to 5 mL of semen is ejaculated, containing 60 to 150 million sperm per milliliter. Lower sperm counts are associated with infertility because sperm mortality is high, and because many sperm are needed to reduce the outer covering of the ovum sufficiently for one sperm to penetrate and fertilize it.

Male hormones

Testosterone is produced in the interstitial cells of the testes and in the adrenal cortex. In the testes it is produced in response to adenohypophyseal **luteinizing hormone** (LH, or interstitial cell secreting hormone). LH is in turn secreted due to stimulation of the adenohypophysis by hypothalamic gonadotropin-releasing hormone. This gonadotropin also appears to control the secretion of follicle stimulating hormone (FSH), which stimulates spermatogenesis in the male.

Large amounts of testosterone are secreted by the testes in the male fetus because of the high concen-

GERIATRIC CONSIDERATIONS

Aging and Reproductive Function

The health of the reproductive system is dependent upon the concentration of gonadal hormones in the blood. This concentration declines gradually after middle age in males but sperm production and reproductive function continue and elderly men may sire children. However, for women the ability to give birth ceases after menopause when there are no longer sufficient ova to mature and secrete estrogen and progesterone in response to FSH and LH. This reduction in estrogen and progesterone concentration leads to a decline in the thickness of the reproductive tract walls and its secretory capacity; however, a women's desire and ability to be a partner in coitus continues. Hormone replacement reverses the effects of menopause and slows its associated bone loss and decline in the secondary sexual characteristics.

trations of maternal chorionic gonadotropin. This is essential for the normal growth and development of the male reproductive tract. In the absence of testosterone the baby will have a female phenotype (appearance). After birth, testosterone is produced in very small quantities. At *puberty* the amount of gonadotropin secreted by the hypothalamus increases markedly and stimulates the secretion of testosterone by the testes.

Testosterone stimulates the growth and maturation of the testes and reproductive tract and the development and maintenance of the secondary sex characteristics. In the male these are increased rate of bone growth, and earlier maturation of the epiphyseal plates and cessation of growth in length; increased muscle and skin growth (the muscles of the male are usually stronger and the skin thicker than in the female); increased growth in size of the larynx, and hence a deepening of the voice; hair growth on the face, chest, and axillary and pubic regions (the pubic hair is diamond-shaped, reaching up toward the navel); and the development of baldness by men who have inherited baldness genes.

ASSESSMENT
Subjective

Patients may present with symptoms such as vaginal, breast, or penile discharge, genital pruritus, or breast or genital lesions. Patients may also present with dysuria, dysmenorrhea, postmenopausal bleeding, infertility, stress incontinence, or abdominal pain.

POTENTIAL SYMPTOMS ASSOCIATED WITH REPRODUCTIVE DISORDERS

Reproductive symptoms: female

Amenorrhea
Dysmenorrhea
Dysuria
Incontinence
Oligomenorrhea
Polymenorrhea
Dyspareunia
Metrorrhagia
Menorrhagia
Genital lesions
Genital pruritus
Mood swings
Premenstrual syndrome (PMS)
Night sweats

Reproductive symptoms: breast

Discharge
Discomfort
Lumps or masses
Dimpling

Reproductive symptoms: male

Dysuria
Genital lesions
Hematuria
Infertility
Impotency
Incontinence
Groin mass or swelling
Lump or swelling in scrotum
Penile discharge
Testicular pain or mass

The box above provides a list of potential symptoms to review with the patient. In addition to specific symptoms, ask the patient about any history of reproductive cancer, hepatitis B, blood transfusions, sexually transmitted diseases (gonorrhea, chlamydia, syphilis, HPV or genital warts, herpes, trichomonas, HIV or AIDS), sexual activity, numbers of partners, age of first intercourse, and method(s) of birth control. Also inquire regarding any history of diabetes mellitus.

Ask women about previous pregnancies, abortions (spontaneous, therapeutic, and elective), menstrual history, frequency of PAP smears, last PAP and pelvic examination (date and results), gynecological procedures or surgery, onset of menopause (if appropriate) and breast self-examination (knowledge and practice). Inquire regarding mammograms, dates, and results.

Ask men about any history of prostate problems or symptoms such as difficulty starting or stopping stream or change in force or size of stream. Ask if testicular self-examination is done. Inquire regarding any previous surgeries such as vasectomy, transurethral prostatectomy, or hernia repair.

Medications such as antihypertensives, antidepressants, narcotics, or antipsychotics may cause impotence or decreased libido. Inquiry into habits is very important to facilitate determination of risk-taking behaviors associated with sexually transmitted diseases such as human immunodeficiency virus or hepatitis B.

Family history that is relevant to the reproductive system includes cancer of reproductive organs, fibrocystic disease of the breasts, diabetes mellitus, hernias, and infertility. For women, inquire regarding maternal exposure to DES.

Objective

Physical examination of the patient with a reproductive complaint may involve more than the breast and genital area based on the patient's history and the nurse's knowledge of pathophysiology. In general, a relaxed patient and a calm approach will yield the best results.

Breast

Inspect the breasts with the patient in the following positions: sitting with arms relaxed at sides, sitting with hands on hips and the pectoralis muscles contracted, sitting with arms over head, and supine with arm behind head and pillow under the shoulder being examined. Observe the breasts for symmetry, size, contour, integrity (presence of lesions), edema (peau d'orange), erythema, and obvious venous patterns. Observe the nipples for symmetry, eversion, or inversion. Observe for supernumerary nipples. Discharge may be noted on observation, but is generally more commonly noted on palpation. Note the appropriateness of breast development related to the woman's age.

Palpate the breasts using the pads of the fingers with the patient supine (see Figure 68-5). Some clinicians advocate palpation both in the sitting and supine positions. Palpate in an organized manner so that no portion of the breast is missed. Some clinicians prefer to examine the breasts in concentric circles while others prefer to examine the breasts in a "spokes of the wheel" pattern. The exact pattern of choice is not an issue, but palpating the breast in a complete and methodical manner is imperative. Note any masses including location, size, shape, consistency, tenderness, mobility, borders, and retrac-

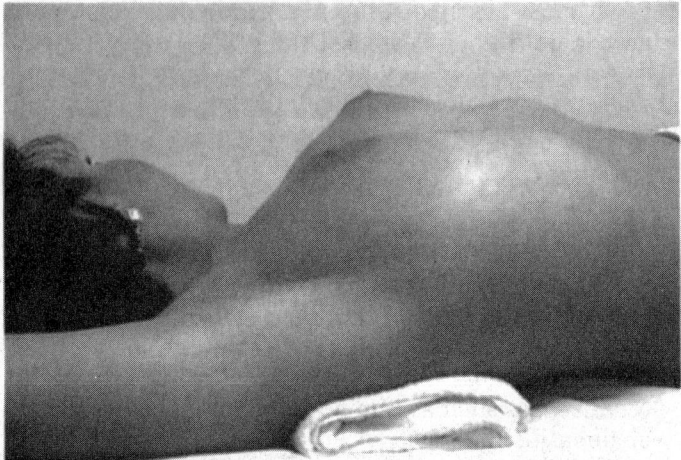

FIGURE 68-5 Supine position for breast palpation. (From Seidel HM et al: *Mosby's guide to physical examination,* ed 2, St Louis, 1991, Mosby–Year Book, Inc.)

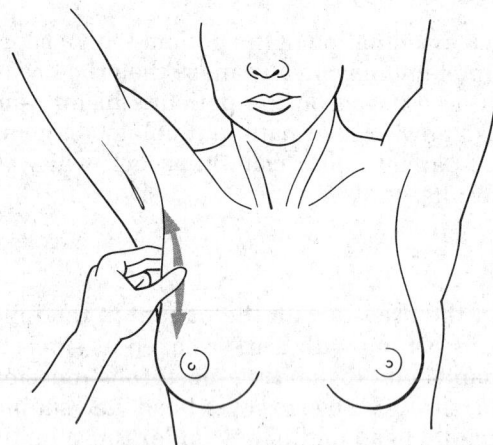

FIGURE 68-6 Palpating the tail of Spence.

tion of the overlying skin. Squeeze the nipples and note any discharge. The examiner may ask the patient if she prefers to do this part of the exam as she may be more proficient at expressing discharge if it is present. If discharge is present, record color, if unilateral or bilateral, and if one or more ducts appear to be involved. Include the tail of Spence and axillary lymph nodes in palpation (see Figure 68-6). See the box above for a summary of the breast examination.

During the examination of the breasts, it is important to teach the patient breast self-examination (BSE) if the patient has not been previously instructed in the technique (see Chapter 69). Also, breast exam should be performed on both males and females in a similar manner.

SUMMARY OF BREAST EXAMINATION

Inspection

- in multiple positions
  - —sitting with arms hanging loosely at sides
  - —arms extended over the head
  - —hands pressed on hips or hands pushed together in front of chest
  - —seated and leaning over
  - —supine
- size, symmetry, contour, retractions or dimpling, skin color, texture, or any changes, venous patterns, supernumerary nipples
- nipples and areolae for shape, symmetry, color, texture, size, nipple inversion, eversion, or retraction

Palpation

- in the sitting and supine positions
- systematically in all four quadrants, over the areolae, in the axillae, and in the supraclavicular and infraclavicular areas for lymph nodes, masses, or tenderness
- palpate the nipples and compress to observe for discharge

Abdominal examination

If the patient's complaint includes abdominal pain, an assessment of the abdomen precedes the assessment of the genitalia. Inspect the abdomen for skin characteristics, abnormal vascular patterns, contour, symmetry, surface motion, obvious masses. Auscultate for bowel sounds, friction rubs, and bruits. Percuss the abdomen in all quadrants for general tone (tympanic), liver span, and splenic enlargement. Lightly palpate in all quadrants for guarding, tenderness, and masses saving the area of discomfort for last. Deeply palpate in all quadrants for masses, tenderness, and organomegaly (liver, spleen, kidneys, aorta, gravid or abnormally enlarged uterus). Finally, assess for costovertebral angle tenderness on the back. See Chapter 63 for a detailed discussion of the abdominal examination.

Female genitalia

Examination of the female genitalia is not usually done by the bedside nurse. This is a skill which requires much practice and therefore develops over time. Nurses who do perform this examination are usually in an expanded role such as a nurse practitioner or nurse clinician with advanced training and education.

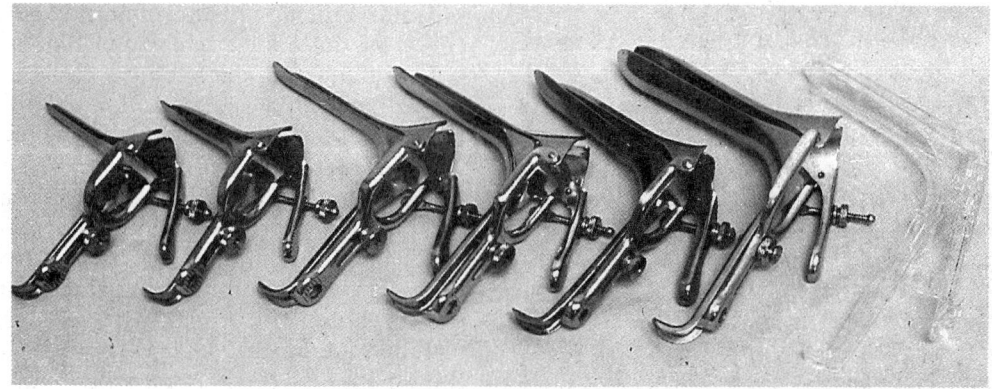

FIGURE 68-7   Vaginal specula. (From Malasanos LM et al: *Health assessment*, ed 4, St Louis, 1990, Mosby–Year Book, Inc.)

The examiner should place all needed equipment in an easily accessible location prior to having the patient assume the lithotomy position. Equipment includes exam gloves; light source (mobile and bright); specula (have choices of size and style available—see Figure 68-7); PAP smear collection accessories (brush, spatula, slide, fixative); culture media for gonorrhea, chlamydia, and herpes; potassium hydroxide (KOH) and saline (NaCl) solutions, slides, and cover slips for examination of abnormal discharge; scopettes, and water-soluble lubricant. Prior to beginning the examination, the examiner puts on two pair of clean exam gloves so that both hands remain gloved throughout the examination.

External genitalia

The patient is examined in a lithotomy position after emptying her bladder. If this is the patient's first pelvic examination, explain the procedure to her prior to placing her in the lithotomy position. If she has had previous exams, reassure her that you will tell her what you are doing as you proceed. Tell the patient that you are going to touch her. Use the back of your hand to touch the medial aspect of the thigh. Inspect and palpate the external genitalia noting hair distribution related to the woman's age, lesions, swelling, erythema, and presence of nits, lice, or excoriation. Palpate in the inguinal area along the inguinal ligament for lymphadenopathy. Small (less than 0.5 cm), mobile, nontender nodes are commonly present.

Tell the patient you are going to spread the labia and do so using your dominant thumb and index finger. Examine the vulva and vaginal introitus for inflammation, lesions (e.g., warts), discharge, trauma, swelling, atrophic changes, or masses. Inspect the clitoris for inappropriate size (normally 3 to 4 mm) and lesions. Inspect the urethral meatus and the skenes or paraurethral glands. Observe for inflammation or discharge in the paraurethral area. Insert the index finger in the vagina and exert pressure anteriorly on the urethra observing for discharge from the urethra or Skenes glands or tenderness.

Inform the patient that you are now going to palpate for enlargement or tenderness of the Bartholin glands. Using the dominant thumb and index finger, place the index finger in the vagina and the thumb outside at approximately 7 to 8 o'clock on each side of the vaginal introitus and palpate for tenderness, swelling, or purulent discharge. Bartholin glands are normally not seen or felt.

The examination of the external genitalia is completed with inspection of the perineum and anus for masses (hemorrhoids), scars, fissures, fistulas, or inflammation. Prior to beginning the speculum examination, the examiner should also assess for pelvic relaxation. With the labia spread, instruct the patient to "bear down as if having a bowel movement or cough." If vaginal relaxation is present, ballooning of the anterior vaginal wall (cystocele) or of the posterior vaginal wall (rectocele) may be observed. The presence of vaginal relaxation will be confirmed via speculum and bimanual examinations. If uterine prolapse is present, the cervix may protrude with straining.

Speculum examination

Prior to beginning this part of the examination, choose the appropriate speculum (e.g., Pederson for nulliparous or not postmenopausal female and Graves for the multiparous female). Tell the patient she will feel your fingers pressing down on the muscle inside her vagina (place index and middle fingers of nondominant hand in the introitus and press on the perineal muscle) and she should try to relax the muscle. With the closed speculum in the dominant hand, slowly insert it obliquely over the two fingers in the introitus with posterior pressure on the speculum as it is inserted. Introduce the speculum into the vagina as far as it will go, rotate it into a transverse

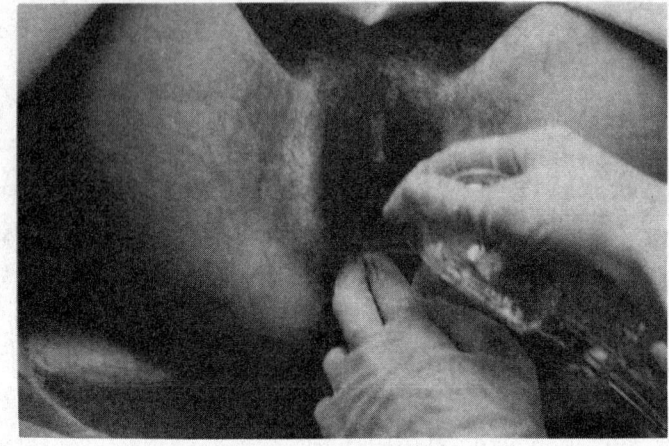

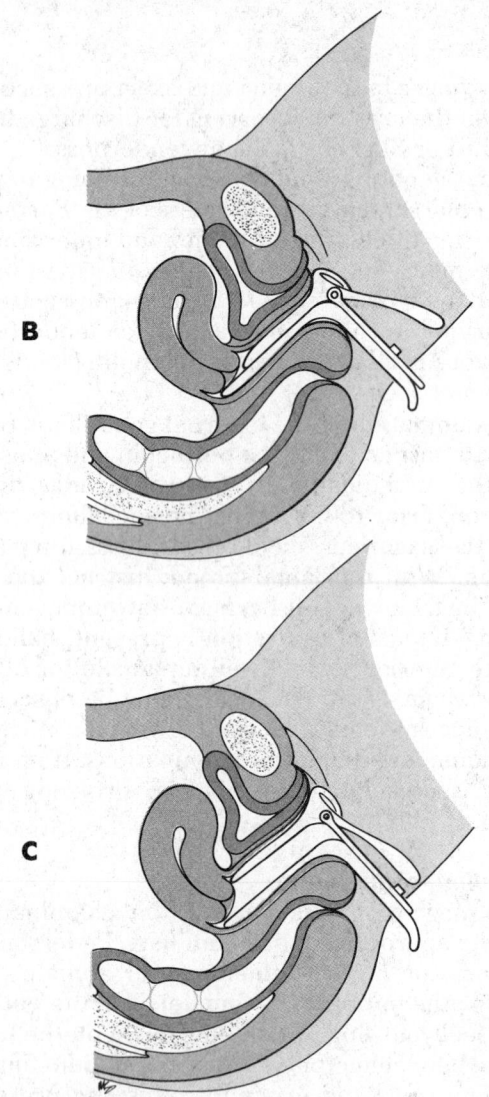

FIGURE 68-8 Speculum examination. **A,** Apply downward pressure in posterior vaginal opening with two fingers; **B,** direct speculum downward at 45-degree angle; and **C,** speculum in place, locked, and stabilized. (From Seidel HM et al: *Mosby's guide to physical examination,* ed 2, St Louis, 1991, Mosby–Year Book, Inc.)

position, and slowly open the blades to visualize the cervix at the end between the blades and the vaginal walls on the sides. Once the cervix and vagina are adequately visualized, tighten the screw on the handle to keep the speculum open and in place while you complete the examination. If the cervix is not visualized when the blades are opened, *gently* turn the blades in various directions in an attempt to visualize the cervix, being careful not to pinch the patient. The most common reasons for not visualizing the cervix are not inserting the speculum far enough or being too far anterior or posterior (depending on the position of the uterus) (see Figure 68-8).

Inspect the cervix for erythema, lesions, masses, color changes (blueness secondary to the congestion of pregnancy or large tumor), discharge, ulceration, eversion versus erosion, and contour of the cervical os. A linear os is characteristic of a woman who has had a vaginal delivery while the nulliparous woman's cervical os is circular. Eversion is a normal finding in multiparous females and is present when the squamocolumnar cells of the endocervix and the squamocolumnar junction (transformation or T-zone) are clearly visible on the ectocervix. To the unexperienced examiner, the appearance of the ectropion cervix can be confused with erosion or inflammation secondary to cervicitis.

After inspection of the cervix, gonorrhea, chlamydia, and herpes cultures as well as a PAP smear are obtained if desired. Cultures are done prior to the PAP smear, and the PAP smear is obtained using a spatula to obtain ectocervical cells and the brush to obtain endocervical cells. The cultures and PAP are placed in/on the appropriate collection media and sent to the lab. The preparation/fixation techniques vary from one institution to another. If abnormal vaginal discharge is noted (green, gray, amine or stale odor, white adherent to erythematous vaginal walls) a saline (NaCl) and potassium hydroxide (KOH) slide of the discharge can be prepared and examined under the microscope for the presence of hyphae (candidal vaginitis), clue cells (bacterial vaginosis), or trichomonads (*Trichomonas vaginalis*).

The patient is informed that the speculum will now be removed. The screw is loosened and the speculum is withdrawn slowly, maintaining posterior pressure at all times and allowing the blades to close slowly as the speculum is removed. Be careful not to pinch the vaginal walls or vulva between the blades. Observe the vaginal walls as the speculum is withdrawn for erythema, lesions, lacerations, masses, and relaxation of anterior or posterior walls.

Bimanual examination

The purpose of the bimanual examination is to evaluate the cervix, uterus, and adnexae (ovaries, fallopian tubes). The outside glove is removed from the nondominant hand, which will be placed on the patient's abdomen, and lubricant is applied to the dominant gloved hand (this hand still has two gloves on at this time) of which the index and middle fingers will be placed into the vagina. Stand between the patient's wide-spread legs and tell her that you will be placing two lubricated fingers in her vagina and one hand on top of her abdomen to examine her uterus and ovaries.

As the fingers are introduced into the vagina, palpate the vaginal walls on all sides (being sure to include the fornices) for masses, relaxation, and tenderness. To evaluate the tone of the vaginal muscles, instruct the patient to squeeze your fingers by contracting her muscles as if to hold or stop her urine flow. Rotate the hand with the palm facing upward and begin the exam of the cervix for masses, consistency, tenderness at rest or with motion (CMT or cervical motion tenderness accompanies pelvic inflammatory disease), and integrity of the os. The abdominal hand is placed on the abdomen one-third the way to the umbilicus. The pelvic hand is used to displace the uterus and ovaries toward the abdomen so the abdominal hand can then palpate the uterus and ovaries. While palpating the uterus, the examiner notes size, shape, symmetry, consistency, mobility, tenderness, and position (see Figure 68-9). If

the uterus is in a retroverted or retroflexed position, palpation on vaginal exam will be minimal, but it should be felt well on rectovaginal exam. The right and left adnexae are palpated assessing for the presence of ovaries and masses (see Figure 68-10). If ovaries are felt, the size, contour, presence of masses, tenderness, mobility, and consistency should be ascertained. If a mass is found, its size, shape, mobility, tenderness, consistency, and location should be described. In many individuals, adnexal structures are not palpable and especially by the novice examiner. In thin women the adnexal structures are more easily palpated than in full-figured or obese women. Ovaries *should not* be palpable in postmenopausal women, and if they are, an ovarian malignancy should be suspected.

After completion of the examination of the ovaries and adnexae, the hand is slowly and gently withdrawn. The glove on the dominant hand is removed, being careful not to contaminate the clean glove on the nondominant hand. One clean glove remains on each hand at this time.

Rectovaginal examination
The rectovaginal exam is a necessary step in every pelvic exam though often omitted by the examiner. This exam allows you to assess the rectum, rectovaginal septum, adnexae, uterus (especially if it is ret-

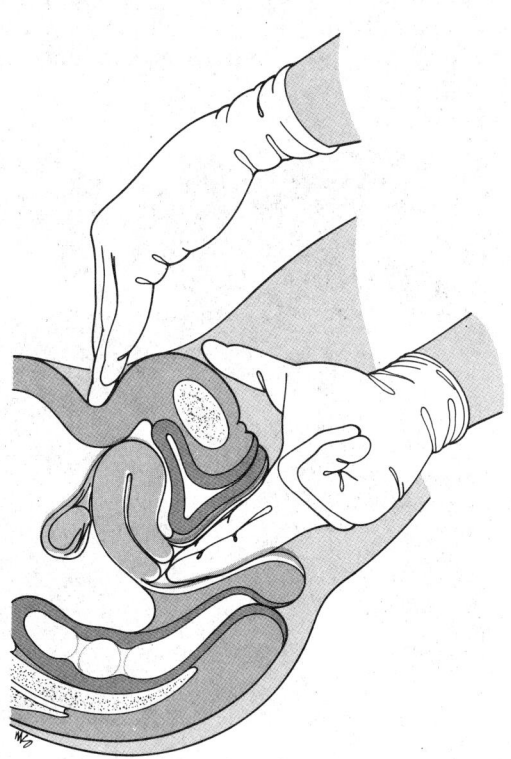

FIGURE 68-9   Bimanual palpation of the uterus.

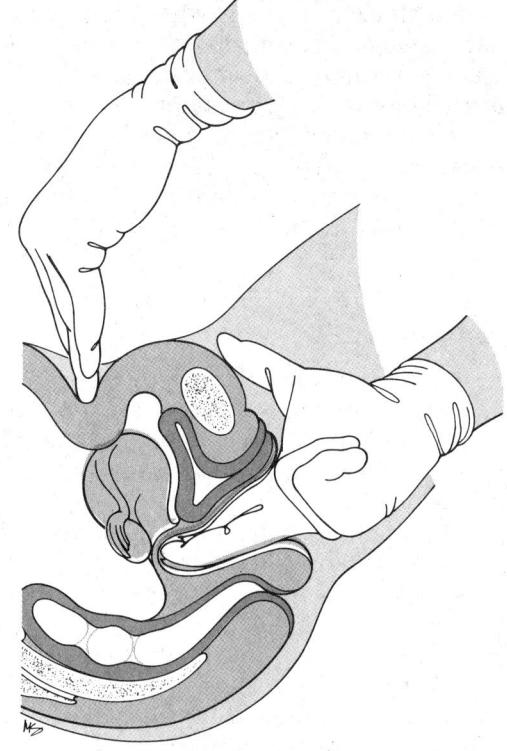

FIGURE 68-10   Bimanual palpation of the adnexae.

roverted or retroflexed), and the cul-de-sac. Explain to the patient that you will be placing one finger in her rectum and one in her vagina and repeating the exam just as you did in her vagina. Tell her it may be somewhat uncomfortable, but should not be painful and may make her have the urge to defecate but she will not.

Apply lubricant to the index and middle fingers of the dominant hand, visually locate the vaginal and rectal orifices, and tell the patient you are now placing one finger at the opening of the vagina (the index) and the rectum (the middle). As you insert the fingers simultaneously into the vagina and rectum, have the patient "bear down as if having a bowel movement" which relaxes the rectal sphincter and allows your finger to enter more easily and less uncomfortably. Be sure to insert the fingers slowly and follow the path of the vagina and rectum.

Systematically note rectal sphincter tone, masses in the rectum, the rectovaginal septum for thickness, nodularity, tenderness, or confirmation of rectocele if previously felt on vaginal exam, uterus for position, shape, size, symmetry, mobility, consistency, and tenderness, adnexae for masses or enlargement or abnormalities of ovaries, and finally for stool (presence and hard versus soft). Withdraw your fingers simultaneously and tell the patient the examination is completed. If stool is present on the glove, examine it for color and presence of blood or pus. Tan or gray stool may indicate obstructive jaundice and black tarry stool indicates upper gastrointestinal bleeding. If indicated and if available you may place some stool from the glove of the rectal finger on a stool guaiac card to assess for occult blood. Stool guaiac would be indicated in patients over age 40 and patients with a complaint or history of gastrointestinal bleeding. At this time be sure to offer the patient a washcloth or tissues and allow her to get dressed. The pelvic examination should always be performed as the last part of a physical examination.

Male genitalia

As previously stated in relation to the examination of the female genitalia, the examination of the male genitalia is not usually performed by the bedside nurse, but rather a nurse in an expanded role such as a nurse practitioner or advanced clinician. The only equipment necessary for examination of the male genitalia is latex gloves, lubricant, and culture media for gonorrhea, chlamydia, and herpes if indicated. Many novice examiners fear that the patient will have an erection during the examination. However, this rarely occurs since the patient is just as nervous as the examiner or more nervous in most cases. As long as the examination is performed in a professional manner, it should not be a source of stimulation to the patient.

The examination of the male genitalia can be performed with the patient in the lying or standing position or both. If only one position is to be included and the patient is not debilitated, the standing position is the position of choice because hernias or scrotal masses may not be apparent in the supine position. The examination includes inspection, palpation, hernia examination, and rectal examination including examination of the prostate. Always put on clean examination gloves prior to beginning the examination.

Inspection

Inspect the groin skin for the presence of a superficial fungal infection (jock itch), excoriation (scabies), or other rashes or lesions (condyloma, syphilitic chancre, or herpes). Observe for male distribution of hair related to the man's age, and for the presence of pubic lice or nits (eggs) attached to the hairs.

Assess the penis noting the presence or absence of circumcision. If the patient is uncircumcised, retract the foreskin or have the patient retract the foreskin to examine the glans. The cheesy white material found under the foreskin near the corona is called smegma and is normal. Normally the foreskin should slide easily over the glans. Phimosis exists when the foreskin (prepuce) cannot be retracted over the glans and paraphimosis exists when the foreskin is retracted and cannot be returned over the glans. The glans is inspected for inflammation, lesions, and the position of the urethra. The urethra should be located centrally on the glans (Figure 68-11). Occasionally the urethra will be located on the ventral surface of the penis (hypospadias) or less

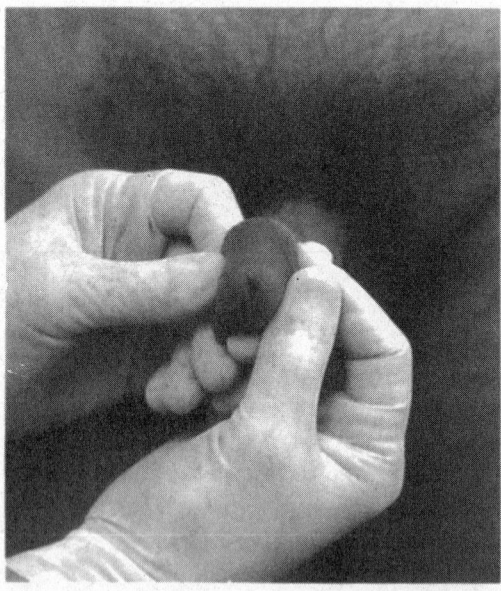

FIGURE 68-11   Palpation of the urethra. (From Seidel HM et al: *Mosby's guide to physical examination*, ed 2, St Louis, 1991, Mosby–Year Book, Inc.)

commonly on the dorsal surface of the penis (epispadias). The meatus should also be assessed for inflammation, discharge, or lesions. Observe the overall size of the penis and scrotum compared to the man's age.

Inspect the scrotum for lesions, rashes, swelling, and symmetry. Normally the left testicle is lower than the right but the sizes are very similar. Pinpoint, dark red, slightly raised telangiectatic lesions on the scrotum called angiokeratomas are commonly found in patients over the age of 50 and are benign lesions.

Palpation

Palpate in the inguinal area along the inguinal ligament for the presence of inguinal lymphadenopathy. Small (less the 0.5 cm), mobile, nontender nodes are commonly present in this area.

Palpate the penis from the glans to the base, noting tenderness or masses. Palpate the urethra from the external meatus through the corpus spongiosum to its base. If discharge is present, cultures for gonorrhea and chlamydia should be obtained and the discharge can also be examined microscopically if desired. The urethra can be "milked" or "stripped" either by the patient or the examiner to facilitate the collection of the discharge. Gonorrhea and chlamydia cultures may also be obtained in asymptomatic men whose partners have been diagnosed with either gonorrhea or chlamydia.

Palpation of the scrotum includes palpation of the testes, epididymis, and vas deferens (see Figure 68-

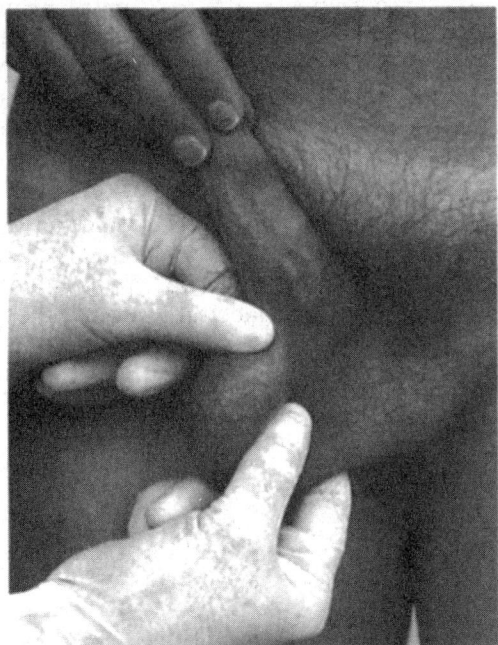

FIGURE 68-12   Palpation of the scrotum. (From Seidel HM et al: *Mosby's guide to physical examination,* ed 2, St Louis, 1991, Mosby–Year Book, Inc.)

12). Note size, shape, consistency, presence of masses or nodularity, and tenderness of each testis. Normal testes have a firm, rubbery consistency without nodularity. If a mass is present, try to determine if it is arising from within the scrotum (e.g., from the testis) or from above the scrotum in the abdominal cavity (e.g., inguinal hernias). If you can get your fingers above the mass it is probably within the scrotum, but if you cannot palpate the superior border of the mass it is most likely originating from the abdominal cavity.

Locate the epididymis on the posterior aspect of the testis and palpate for tenderness, nodularity, or masses. The spermatic cords (the most prominent structure being the vas deferens) are palpated for tenderness, symmetry, and nodularity from the epididymis superiorly to the external abdominal ring. The vas deferens are firm cords about 2 to 4 mm in diameter and feel like partially cooked spaghetti. An absent vas deferens on a side may be associated with the absence of the kidney on the corresponding side.

A common enlargement of the spermatic cord is a varicosity called a varicocele. These are usually located on the left side and feel like a "bag of worms" when palpated. Varicoceles are seen and palpated best in the standing position.

If a scrotal mass is identified, it should be transilluminated in a dark room with a flashlight or penlight. Vascular structures, tumors, blood, hernias, and normal testes do not transilluminate. Transillumination of the light as a red glow indicates the presence of serous fluid such as a hydrocele (abnormal collection of clear fluid in the tunica vaginalis) or a spermatocele (pea-sized, nontender, mass containing spermatozoa usually attached to the upper pole of the epididymus).

Hernia examination

The inguinal and femoral areas are assessed via inspection and palpation for the presence of hernias. Ninety percent of all hernias are located in the inguinal area. Commonly, hernias are better seen than felt. Ask the patient to turn his head to the side and cough or strain down as if having a bowel movement (valsalva maneuver). As the patient coughs or strains, observe the inguinal and femoral areas for any sudden swelling or bulging, which may indicate a hernia. If the patient complains of pain while coughing, evaluate the area of discomfort.

Palpation for inguinal hernias is performed by having the examiner place the dominant index finger (with the nail facing the examiner) in the scrotum above the testis and invaginating the scrotal skin. The examiner's finger should follow the spermatic cord laterally into the inguinal canal parallel to the inguinal ligament and superiorly toward the external inguinal ring. With the finger in the inguinal canal or against the external inguinal ring, instruct the patient to cough or strain (see Figure 68-13). If a her-

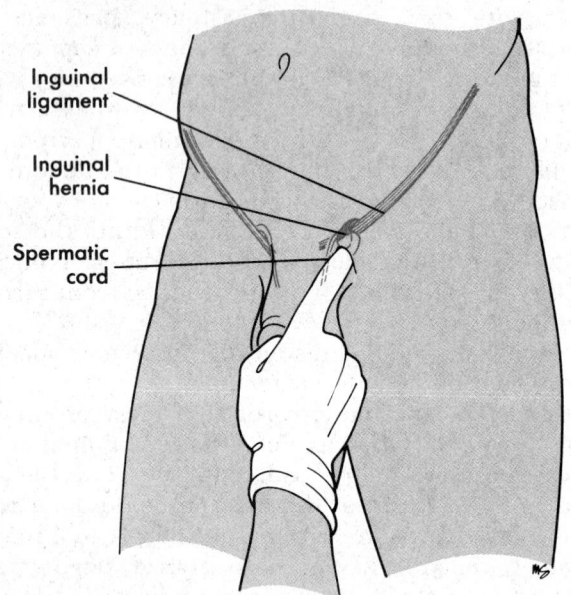

FIGURE 68-13   Examination of the male client for indirect inguinal hernias.

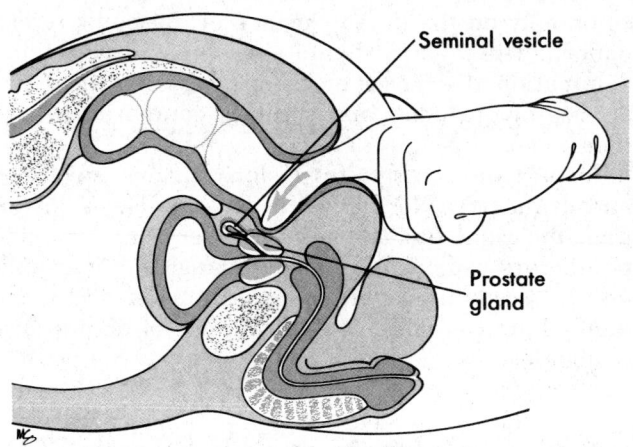

FIGURE 68-14   Palpation of the prostate gland.

nia is present, a sudden bulging against the finger will be felt with the straining maneuver. Both sides of the scrotum should be assessed. An indirect inguinal hernia may present as a large scrotal mass that does not transilluminate over which bowel sounds can be auscultated with a stethoscope.

While doing the male genitalia examination, you should teach the patient self-genital examination if he has not been previously instructed. See Chapter 69 for a complete discussion of genital self-examination of the male.

Rectal examination

Even though the rectal examination is uncomfortable and often embarrassing, it provides valuable information about the rectum, the peritoneal cavity at the end of the rectum, and the prostate gland. Be sure to explain to the patient what you plan to do before and during the examination and use a slow and gentle approach. The rectal examination can be performed with the patient in any of the following positions: the knee-chest, left lateral with knees and hips flexed, or standing with the hips flexed and the upper body supported by the examination table or bed. The standing position is probably the position of choice. A good light source should be available to aid in inspection of the external area.

Once the patient is positioned, carefully inspect the perianal area for masses, rashes, inflammation, excoriation, or scars. Spread the buttocks apart and observe the anus for lesions (warts), skin tags, external hemorrhoids, fissures, and fistulas. Tell the

patient that you are now going to insert a lubricated finger into his rectum and that he may feel the urge to defecate but he will not.

With the palmar surface of the index finger toward the anterior rectal wall, palpate the posterior surface of the prostate (see Figure 68-14). Tell the patient he may feel the urge to urinate, but he will not. Note the size, contour, consistency, mobility, and tenderness of the prostate. The gland should feel smooth, firm, nontender, and slightly mobile. A normal prostate has a diameter of about 4 cm and protrudes less than 1 cm into the rectum. Greater protrusion denotes prostate enlargement. Prostate enlargement is classified by the amount of projection into the rectum with grade I being 1 to 2 cm of protrusion; grade II being 2 to 3 cm of protrusion; grade III being 3 to 4 cm of protrusion; and grade IV being more than 4 cm of protrusion. An enlarged prostate that is rubbery or boggy in nature indicates benign prostatic hypertrophy, whereas a stone-hard, nodular prostate may indicate carcinoma, prostatic calculi, or chronic fibrosis.

Withdraw your finger and examine it for fecal material which should be brown and soft and without blood or pus. Tan or gray stool could indicate obstructive jaundice and black tarry stool indicates upper gastrointestinal bleeding. If the patient is 40 years or older or has a complaint of gastrointestinal or rectal bleeding, you should check the stool for occult blood with the guaiac test.

DIAGNOSTIC AND LABORATORY TESTS
Diagnostic Tests for Conditions of the Female Reproductive System

Papanicolaou test

The Papanicolaou test (Pap test, Pap smear) involves microscopic examination of exfoliated cells that

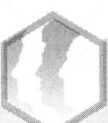

GERIATRIC CONSIDERATIONS

Reproductive Assessment

General approach
* allow more time than for a younger adult
* articulate clearly; the geriatric patient may be hearing impaired
* impaired sight, comprehension, or mobility may result in less than optimum cooperation
* provide clear, concise instructions

History collection
* be alert for answers which do not appear appropriate; the patient may not have understood the question correctly due to impaired hearing or impaired comprehension
* some questions may need to be repeated in a different manner
* elderly women may complain of dyspareunia secondary to vaginal dryness as a result of decreased estrogen

Physical assessment
* the physical examination itself is not different, but the approach needs to be altered so that the appropriate information is assessed without undue discomfort or embarrassment for the patient
* maintain an environment with minimal noise, distractions, and interruption
* because of decreased connective and adipose tissue in the breasts, masses may be more easily appreciated
* gynecomastia in the elderly male may be a result of a possible cancer or thyroid disease
* the prostate gland in the elderly male is frequently enlarged but should still feel firm, not hard, and be without nodularity
* elderly women may have dryness of the vagina and experience vaginal or urinary tract infections secondary to decreased estrogen
* palpable ovaries are *never* normal in an elderly postmenopausal female

of the physician. Women who have a family history of cervical cancer or venereal disease or whose mothers took diethylstilbestrol (DES) during their pregnancies may require more frequent testing. Studies suggest that women at greatest risk for cervical cancer are least likely to seek screening or follow-up to abnormal Pap tests. If findings from examination are abnormal, a culposcopy or biopsy is done to confirm the diagnosis.

Patient preparation
The patient is told that the test involves collecting cells from the cervix and that, although slight discomfort may be felt during insertion of the speculum, there will be no actual pain. The nurse determines if the patient has douched, had sexual intercourse, is menstruating, has used a lubricant, or has taken a tub bath in the 24 hours before the test, because these may affect accuracy of test results.

The patient is asked to void and then remove her clothes from the waist down. The nurse asks the patient to drape herself and to lie on the examining table with buttocks at the edge of the table and heels in the stirrups.

Procedure
Ideally, the sample should include cells from the vaginal portion of the cervix, the squamocolumnar junction of the external os, and the endocervical epithelium. If the patient is perimenopausal or postmenopausal, the vaginal pool should be sampled, as cells from the endometrium, tubes, and ovaries slough onto the vaginal floor. Samples are collected using a cotton applicator stick, spatula or endometrial brush. The sample material is wiped immediately and thinly across a glass slide and either sprayed with a commercial fixative or hairspray or immersed in a fixative solution. The nurse labels the slide and sends it to the laboratory.

Postprocedure care
The patient is informed as to how and when test results may be obtained. The nurse is particularly alert to questions and concerns that the patient may have.

Vaginal smear

The vaginal smear is useful in the detection of vaginitis. Cells collected with a cotton-tipped swab or wooden spatula are smeared on opposite ends of a glass slide. Cells at one end are treated with normal saline, and those at the other end with potassium hydroxide. Epithelial and white cells, *Trichomonas* organisms, and bacteria will appear at the saline-treated end and *Candida* at the end treated with potassium. If *Haemophilus vaginalis* is suspected, the discharge is placed on a dry slide and examined for clue cells and the organism. When *herpes genitalis*

have been obtained from the cervix and vagina. This test is particularly useful in the early detection of cellular changes associated with premalignant or malignant conditions, although it is also used to identify fungal and viral infections and to monitor the effects of hormonal therapy. The American Cancer Society recommends that women who are or who have been sexually active or who are 18 years of age have a Pap smear annually. If the woman has three or more negative examinations, the Pap smear may be performed less frequently at the discretion

is suspected, a smear is taken from lesions or ulcerations. Specimens must be examined microscopically immediately after collection.

Biopsy

Biopsy involves removal of a small amount of tissue for the microscopic examination of the structure of tissues and cells. When an abnormal tissue mass is small and easily removed, as may occur in breast tissue, an excisional biopsy is performed with the aid of a scalpel, cutting or aspiration needle, or a punch.

Biopsy may occur on an outpatient basis or in hospital. A signed consent is required before biopsy.

Endometrial biopsy
Endometrial biopsy involves removal of tissue from the walls of the uterus and is primarily useful in detecting if endometrial buildup has occurred following progesterone secretion after ovulation. Endometrial biopsy may also be used to aid in the diagnosis of endometrial cancer, tuberculosis, polyps, and inflammatory conditions and as a predictor of ovulation in infertility workups. Endometrial biopsy is contraindicated in patients with cervical abnormalities or who have had cervical surgeries, patients with cervical or vaginal infections and in uncooperative patients. Samples are obtained through curettage (scraping the endometrium) or by aspiration or suction. Aspiration is the most accurate method at this time in the outpatient diagnosis of endometrial cancer.

Patient preparation
The patient is told that the test involves removal of a small amount of tissue from the inner wall of the uterus, and that some menstrual-like cramps may be felt during the procedure. The nurse reassures the patient that the discomfort is temporary.

Procedure
Following a pelvic examination, a tenaculum is placed on the cervix, and a small metal probe (sound) is inserted to determine the size of the uterus. A thin, hollow curet or aspirator is then inserted, and the specimen obtained.

Postprocedure care
The patient is instructed to wear a pad because some vaginal bleeding is normal. The nurse cautions the patient to avoid heavy lifting for 24 hours and to avoid douching and intercourse for 72 hours. The patient is told to report any heavy vaginal bleeding or temperature elevations that occur within 48 hours after biopsy.

Cervical biopsy
Cervical biopsies (cervical punch biopsies) are useful in evaluating cervical lesions as a follow-up procedure to an abnormal Pap smear and in the histologic diagnosis of cervical cancer. The biopsy usually involves multiple specimens from the cervix and is performed when the cervix is least vascular (shortly after menses). The Schiller iodine test may be performed during the biopsy as a means of identifying abnormal tissue. Iodine stains normal squamous epithelium a dark mahogany, but it fails to stain abnormal tissue, which does not contain glycogen. Iodine is applied to the cervix with a long cotton applicator stick that has been dipped in Schiller iodine solution.

Procedure
The patient is placed in a lithotomy position and a speculum is inserted, after which a colposcope, a magnifying instrument, may be inserted for direct visualization. Specimens are obtained, and bleeding is controlled with application of silver nitrate solution, cautery, or sutures, and insertion of a tampon or packing. Usually, only mild discomfort is felt, although some individuals report considerable discomfort during the procedure. The procedure takes approximately 15 minutes.

Postprocedure care
The nurse instructs the patient to rest, to avoid heavy lifting for 24 hours, and to report heavy bleeding. Packing or tampons are left in for the recommended time (usually 8 to 24 hours). The patient is told to report bleeding that is heavier than menstrual bleeding to her physician. Continued use of tampons is to be avoided as it may provide irritation and provoke bleeding; a foul-smelling grayish discharge may occur following the biopsy and is normal for up to 3 weeks. Intercourse and douching are to be avoided until the physician indicates that they are permissible.

Cervical conization
Cervical conization is usually performed when a Pap smear is abnormal and no lesion is visible. A cone-shaped sample of squamocolumnar tissue is removed from the cervix for examination. This procedure requires anesthesia and surgical facilities. The patient is instructed to rest and to avoid heavy lifting for at least 3 days following the cone biopsy.

Breast biopsy
A breast biopsy is particularly useful in confirming or ruling out cancer of the breast and is indicated if a patient has palpable masses, suspicious masses on mammography, bloody discharge from the nipples, or persistently inflamed breast lesions. A combination of mammography and fine biopsy provides a relatively simple and sensitive method for early diagnosis of breast cancer. Biopsy may be performed through open or needle methods. Needle biopsy has

limited value because the sample is small, may be unrepresentative, and may fail to provide precise information about cell type. Since accuracy of results may be further limited by inaccurate placement of the fine, flexible needle, ultrasound may be used to guide placement of the needle. Both needle and open biopsies can be performed on an outpatient basis if the patient is cooperative, because only local anesthesia is required. Fasting is required if general anesthetic is used.

Patient preparation

The nurse tells the patient who will perform the procedure and where. The patient is informed that the test allows microscopic examination of breast tissue. Unless the biopsy is performed under general anesthesia, no fasting is necessary. A signed consent is obtained prior to the procedure. The patient is informed that a small bandage may be placed over the biopsy site, and that some pain may be noted following the procedure. Verbalization and discussion of fears are encouraged. The patient is given specific information as to how and when results may be obtained.

Visual examinations

Colposcopy

Colposcopy involves direct visualization of the vagina and cervix using an instrument with a magnifying lens and a light (colposcope), and is usually performed on an outpatient basis. Colposcopy is useful in the evaluation of vaginal and cervical lesions and cellular dysplasia and is used as a follow-up procedure in patients who have abnormal Pap smears or whose mothers took DES (diethylstilbestrol) during pregnancy. A biopsy may be taken during colposcopy. The procedure takes approximately 10 to 15 minutes.

Patient preparation

The nurse informs the patient that this test enables magnified visualization of the cervix and vagina and answers questions with concrete, objective information. The procedure is described as similar to any pelvic examination, and the patient is told that it produces no real discomfort. If a biopsy is to be performed, the patient should be prepared for the probability of vaginal flow following the procedure.

Culdoscopy/culdotomy

Culdoscopy involves direct visualization of the peritoneal cavity, and especially of the uterus, fallopian tubes, and ovaries under spinal or local anesthesia. A small incision is made into the posterior fornix of the cul-de-sac, and a culdoscope is inserted. This test is particularly useful as part of an infertility workup. The procedure takes about 1 hour.

Patient preparation

The nurse explains that the procedure involves visualization of reproductive structures through a small incision made into the vagina. The patient is informed that foods and fluids are to be withheld before the surgery and that preoperative sedation will be given. A signed consent is obtained.

Postprocedure care

The nurse observes the patient's vital signs and monitors the patient for vaginal bleeding and discomfort. The patient is instructed to avoid douching and sexual intercourse for 1 or 2 weeks or until healing has occurred.

Laparoscopy

Laparoscopy (peritoneoscopy) involves direct visualization of the uterus, ovaries, and tubes using a fiberoptic light. The laparoscope is inserted through a small abdominal incision. Laparoscopy takes about 15 to 30 minutes.

Patient preparation

The nurse explains that the procedure involves examination of internal reproductive organs through a small slit near the umbilicus. The patient is instructed to withhold foods and fluids from the midnight prior to the surgery. The patient is told that rest is important for 2 to 7 days following the procedure, and that shoulder pain may be experienced during this period if air or gas is injected into the abdomen to enhance visualization during surgery. This pain should disappear within 24 to 36 hours following the procedure and can be relieved with analgesic. The nurse obtains a signed consent, prepares the abdomen for surgery, and administers preoperative sedation as ordered.

Hysteroscopy

Hysteroscopy involves direct visualization of the cervical canal and intrauterine cavity with a lighted telescopic instrument (hysteroscope) and is used in the evaluation of abnormal bleeding, primary or secondary infertility, habitual abortions, and detection of foreign bodies, such as IUDs. Contraindications to hysteroscopy include pregnancy, profuse bleeding, and acute pelvic inflammatory disease. The presence of infection is ruled out before the procedure. The procedure is best performed after menstrual flow has ceased for at least 2 to 3 days so that menstrual products are not carried into the oviduct.

The procedure may be performed using a pericervical anesthetic block or general anesthesia. Following cleansing of the vulva, vagina, and cervix, the hysteroscope is introduced, and the uterus is dilated with 32% dextran, 5% dextrose in water, normal saline, or carbon dioxide. Visualization of the uterine cavity takes approximately 3 to 5 minutes. Hysteroscopy has been combined with diagnostic cannulation of the fallopian tubes, allowing assessment of tubal factor infertility.

Patient preparation

The nurse explains to the patient that the procedure allows direct visualization of the interior of the uterus. If local anesthesia is to be used, the patient is reassured that little or no discomfort will occur. If general anesthesia is to be used, the patient is told to withhold foods and fluids past midnight. The nurse reassures the patient that she will be draped during the procedure. A signed consent is obtained. The patient is instructed to void before the procedure.

Radiography

Hysterosalpingography (uterutubogram)

Hysterosalpingography involves radiographic visualization of the uterine cavity and fallopian tubes following injection of a contrast medium through the cervix. While largely replaced by ultrasonography it is still primarily useful in the evaluation of tubal patency and it is also used to evaluate uterine abnormalities. Dye is inserted into the cervix through a cannula placed into the cervical os. It is more accurate than the Rubin test. Hysterosalpingography is usually performed 4 to 5 days following the cessation of menses so that there is less possibility of debris occluding the tubes and to avoid inducing abortion in an unknown pregnancy.

Patient preparation

The nurse explains to the patient that the test allows visualization of the uterus and fallopian tubes through x-ray visualization. The patient is told that she may experience some mild cramping during the procedure, which takes about 15 minutes. The nurse instructs the patient to take a laxative the evening before the test and an enema or suppository the morning of the study so that gas and feces will not distort the x-ray image.

The patient is assessed for allergy to iodine preparations. The nurse administers mild sedatives or antispasmodics, if ordered. The patient is encouraged to void and is assisted into a lithotomy position on the x-ray table.

Postprocedure care

The nurse assesses the patient for nausea, faintness, and discomfort and administers analgesics as ordered. The patient is instructed to apply a perineal pad for several hours because the radiopaque dye may stain clothing and to be alert to signs of infection such as fever, malaise, or muscle ache. Severe pain and bleeding that exceeds two or three pads may indicate perforation of the uterus and must be reported immediately.

Mammography

Mammography is a low-energy radiographic examination of breast tissue that is a useful screening device for breast malignancy, evaluation of palpable and nonpalpable masses, and differentiation between malignant and benign breast disease. This procedure has a high false positive result rate and a 10% to 20% false negative rate. However, in combination with physical examination, the diagnostic accuracy of mammography is 90% or higher and is recommended by the American Cancer Society on an annual or biannual basis for women aged 40 to 49 and annually for women over 50 years. Studies suggest that cost, failure of health care professionals to recommend mammography, and a belief that mammography was unimportant to them act as significant deterrants to women in seeking mammography.

During the mammography the patient rests one of her breasts on an examination table and a compressor is placed on the breast. While the patient holds her breath, a radiograph is taken of the superior to inferior view and then of the lateral view. The procedure is repeated with the second breast. Well-delineated clear spots suggest cysts, whereas diffusely outlined areas are suggestive of cancer. Xeromammography involves recording of the radiographic images on a selenium-coated plate and transferring the images to a special paper. This process enables enhancement of edges and sharpening of images.

Contrast mammography involves injection of a radiopaque dye into the breast duct and is useful in detecting nonpalpable intraductal papillomas.

Patient preparation

The procedure is explained to the patient and the patient is advised that the test has a high rate of false-positive results. The patient is told that the test takes 15 to 30 minutes and that compression of the breast may produce a transient, vicelike discomfort. If contrast medium is being used, an assessment for allergies to the dye is conducted. Before the test, the patient is directed to remove all jewelry and clothing above the waist and dress in a gown that is open in the front. Skin creams and powders should be removed prior to the test.

Ultrasonography

Ultrasonography (ultrasound) involves passing high-frequency sound waves through tissue, which are then reflected to a transducer and converted to electrical energy. Images are then formed on an oscilloscope screen. Ultrasound is useful in detecting foreign bodies (such as IUDs), distinguishing between cystic and solid tumor bodies of the breast of pelvis, evaluating fetal growth and viability, detecting fetal abnormalities, and detecting ectopic pregnancies. Ultrasound generally is noninvasive, safe, and painless. Transducers may be placed directly into the vaginal canal if abdominal examination or visualization is inconclusive, such as during diagnosis of ectopic pregnancies or miscarriage. This form of ultrasound is invasive.

During ultrasound of the breast, the patient lies face down on the examining table while each breast is immersed in warm, chlorinated water. During emersion, a transducer emits ultrasonic waves, which are transmitted through the water and reflected off the breast. The examination takes about 15 minutes.

Patient preparation

The test is described to the patient. The nurse explains that the pelvic area will be coated with water-soluble jelly to increase sound conduction and that a transducer crystal will be passed over this area unless the transducer is placed directly into the vaginal canal. If an ultrasound examination of the pelvic area has been ordered, the patient is instructed to drink and not to void for 1½ to 2 hours before the procedure. The nurse stresses that a full bladder is essential to the accuracy of the test.

For breast sonography, instruct the patient to strip to the waist and to remove lotions or powders. The patient's history is checked for evidence of back problems, since this makes maintenance of the position during examination uncomfortable.

Pregnancy test

All pregnancy tests, regardless of method, are based on detection of human chorionic gonadotropin (HCG), which is secreted after the fertilization of the ovum. Newer methods such as radioreceptor assay (RRA) for serum HCG are relatively quick and can detect pregnancy 6 to 8 days after conception. Regardless of method, it is important to know that the tests do not indicate whether or not a pregnancy is normal. HCG is also present with hydatidiform moles and chorioepithelioma (male and female). False positive results may occur in premenopausal or perimenopausal patients with gonadal hormone deficiencies and in the presence of certain tranquilizers. If urine samples are required, the patient should be instructed to collect a first-voided morning specimen, since this specimen contains the highest concentration of HCG.

Diagnostic Tests for Diseases of the Male Reproductive System

Infusion cavernosography

Infusion cavernosography is an invasive procedure used to detect insufficiencies in the venous supply to the corpus cavernosum in patients with a history of impotence. Generally, infusion cavernosography is indicated in patients who have had abnormal nocturnal penile tumescence testing and who are unable to maintain erections. Infusion is accomplished by inserting a small-gauge needle into the cavernosum and infusing normal saline or radiopaque dye, or both.

Patient preparation

The procedure is described to the patient. The nurse assesses for sensitivities to contrast media and informs the patient that no fasting is required.

Nocturnal penile tumescence test

The nocturnal penile tumescence (NPT) test evaluates the frequency, duration, and rigidity of nocturnal penile erection over a 2- to 3-night period. The test may be performed in the hospital or at home. Changes in penile circumference are measured by two strain gauges that are placed on the penis, one near the tip and the other at the base. The gauges are attached to a chart recorder. Findings from polygraphic and penile-circumference monitoring are compared with reports given by the patient. Since NPT assessments are not totally reliable, results are particularly valuable if they mimic the findings of the patient. Normally, men experience three to five erections, each lasting 25 to 35 minutes during nighttime sleep. In patients who report impotence yet have normal NPT tracings, an underlying psychogenic problem might be suspected.

Semen analysis

Semen analysis involves collection of semen for measurement of seminal volume, sperm counts, and microscopic examination. The procedure is inexpensive and technically simple and enables evaluation of male fertility and the effectiveness of male sterilization. The procedure may also be used to detect semen on the body or clothing of rape victims.

Patient preparation

The patient is instructed to provide a sample either through masturbation (which provides the most desirable specimen), coitus interruptus, or use of a condom. If the patient is using a condom, the condom should be washed thoroughly in soap and water, rinsed, and dried completely, since the condom may contain spermicidal lubricants or powders. The patient is told to tie the condom after collection and place it in a glass or jar for transport to the laboratory. The nurse instructs patients who are collecting semen through the processes of masturbation or coitus interruptus to deposit the specimen into a clean plastic specimen container, and to transport it to the laboratory within 2 hours of collection. Any loss or spillage of semen should be reported by the patient because this is important to volume and counts. The patient is informed that the specimen must not be exposed to direct sunlight or to extremes of temperature. The nurse instructs the patient to avoid sexual intercourse for the period recommended by the doctor, because the sperm count may be affected by continence.

If the patient is a rape victim, the nurse directs her to place damp clothing in a paper bag (plastic will promote molding) and prepares her for collection of a vaginal specimen. To obtain a dried smear from skin, the nurse washes the skin with gauze moistened with normal saline and applies the smear to a glass slide that is immediately placed in loplin jars containing 95% ethanol. Gloves are recommended for the handling of specimens. The nurse provides emotional support during examination and refers the victim to an appropriate agency or professional for counselling.

Prostatic specific antigen

Prostatic specific antigen (PSA) is a glycoprotein that is found only in the cytoplasm of the epithelial cells of the prostate. Levels above 4 ng/mL may indicate benign hypertrophy, and significantly elevated levels may indicate cancer of the prostate. The test involves collection of a blood sample and should be collected either before digital prostate examination or at least 48 hours following to avoid falsely elevated levels.

Alkaline phosphatase

Alkaline phosphatase (ALP) is an isoenzyme thought to be influential in bone calcification and metabolite and lipid transport. Total serum ALP levels reflect the alkaline phosphatase isoenzymes in bone, liver, intestine, kidneys, and placenta. Elevated levels also occur with cirrhosis, extrahepatic biliary tract obstruction, hyperparathyroidism, rickets, Paget's disease, osteomalacia, the third trimester of pregnancy, and certain drugs, such as intravenous albumin, oxacillin, penicillin, phenothiazines, tolbutamide, and allopurinal. Reference ranges vary with laboratory method used; general reference levels for adults are 20 to 90 U/L.

Patient preparation

The patient is informed that the test involves collection of a blood specimen to evaluate bone and liver function. The nurse instructs the patient to fast 8 to 12 hours before withdrawal of the specimen since food may elevate ALP levels by 25%. A medication history is obtained from the patient, because the physician may wish medications such as vitamin preparations or drugs that influence liver function withheld for 24 hours.

Acid phosphatase

Acid phosphatase (ACP, prostatic acid phosphatase {PAP}) is a group of phosphatase enzymes found in most body tissues, but is 1000 times more concentrated in prostatic tissue. The test is particularly useful in detecting prostatic carcinoma and in monitoring responses to the treatment of carcinoma. Elevated levels may also occur with benign prostatic hypertrophy, nonprostatic metastases to the bone, Paget's disease, primary hyperthyroidism, and thrombocytosis. Radioimmunoassay is used to determine the prostatic fraction in serum or the major isoenzyme that is secreted by the prostate. Patients need not restrict food or fluids before the collection of the serum sample. Levels may be decreased by alcohol, fluorides, and oxalates and increased with clofibrate. The test should not be performed if extensive palpation of the prostate or a transurethral resection has been performed within 24 hours of collection of the specimen. The specimen must be handled gently and refrigerated immediately to avoid hemolysis. The normal reference range for men is 0.15 to 0.65 BLB (Bersey, Lowry, and Brock) units/mL. and for women is 0.02 to 0.55 BLB units/mL.

Alpha-fetoprotein

Alpha-fetoprotein (AFP, alpha-FP) is produced primarily by embryonic and fetal liver cells. AFP levels are elevated with testicular cancer, primary liver cancer, pregnancy, abortion, cirrhosis, hepatitis, Hodgkin's disease, lymphoma, or renal tumor. Both serum AFP and serum human chorionic gonadotrophin (HCG) levels are useful in monitoring responses to therapy for carcinoma. The normal reference range is <25 ng/mL or <25 µg/L (SI units).

Ultrasonography

Ultrasonography of the scrotum is the preferred method for differential diagnosis of questionable scrotal masses or chronic scrotal swelling and is useful in diagnosing hydrocele, spermatocele, and scrotal abscess. The test is relatively noninvasive and is performed while the patient is on his back with his penis taped to the abdominal wall.

Ultrasonography of the prostate is particularly useful in diagnosing prostatic cancer when combined with rectal examination and prostatic-specific antigen. In benign prostatic hypertrophy, ultrasound will reveal a sharply defined capsule, whereas in prostatic cancer, ultrasound will show an asymmetric prostate capsule. Ultrasound of the prostate may be performed by passing a transducer slowly over the abdomen or bladder, or by inserting a probe with an ultrasound transducer into the patient's rec-

TABLE 68-1	Diagnostic Tests for Sexually Transmitted Diseases	
Test	**Type**	**Description**
Venereal Disease Research Laboratory Test (VDRL)	Serum	The VDRL is a widely used screening test for syphilis. An antigen complex of cardiolipin, lecithin, and cholesterol is added to serum, and the sample is rotated, then examined microscopically. If flocculation is present, the sample is diluted until no further reaction occurs. This provides a measure of the amount of reagin present in the patient's serum. Reagin is a nontreponemal antibody to the lipoidal antigen that results from infection by *Treponema pallidum,* the spirochete that causes syphilis. Because false positive results may be caused by viral or bacterial infections, immunization, drug addiction, pregnancy, lupus erythematosus, or rheumatoid arthritis, the fluorescent treponemal antibody absorption test is used for verification of VDRL results. A negative reaction may not rule out syphilis because immunologic changes cannot be detected for 14 to 21 days after infection. Patients should abstain from alcohol for 24 hours before collection of the serum sample.
CSF-VDRL	Cerebrospinal fluid	An examination of the CSF for reactivity in the VDRL is recommended for anyone who has had syphilis for an unknown period to rule out asymptomatic neurosyphilis. The CSF-VDRL is very specific and rarely yields false positive results. The CSF specimen is collected during a lumbar puncture (see Chapter 44).
Rapid plasma reagin (RPR), flocculation RPR	Serum	RPR, like the VDRL, is a nontreponemal test but is a newer test and more sensitive than VDRL in early primary syphilis. In the RPR test, the patient's serum is mixed with a cardiolipin on a plastic card, rotated, and examined for flocculation. If flocculation occurs, the sample is diluted until no visible reaction is detected. This provides a titer of the reagin antibody. Because the RPR has a high false positive rate, RPR-reactive serum needs to be examined using a confirmatory treponemal test such as FTA-ABS.
Fluorescent treponemal antibody absorption (FTA-ABS), FTA	Serum	The FTA-ABS is the most commonly used treponemal test, and is used for verification of nontreponemal reactive test results. The FTA-ABS will nearly always be positive in individuals with past or present syphilis. In FTA-ABS, *Treponema pallidum* is added to the patient's serum. If antibodies to *Treponema pallidum* are present in the serum, they will coat the *Treponema* organisms. The slide containing the patient's serum and *Treponema* organisms is then stained with a fluorescein-labeled antiglobulin. This antiglobulin attaches to the coated *Treponema,* making them fluorescent under a microscope with ultraviolet light. False positive reactions in FTA are uncommon but may occur in patients with abnormal globulins.
Fluorescein monoclonal antibodies	Lesion exudate	Exudate is taken from a lesion and placed on a slide. Highly specific monoclonal antibodies will react only with pathogenic treponemes. Fluorescein antiserum binds to the antigen specific antibodies, making the pathogenic treponeme visible under a fluorescent microscope. This test is highly specific compared with

Continued.

TABLE 68-1 Diagnostic Tests for Sexually Transmitted Diseases—cont'd

Test	Type	Description
		darkfield microscopy and other serologic tests for syphilis and can be used for all lesions including those from the oral mucosa, but is not widely used clinically.
Darkfield microscopy (microscopic darkfield examination)	Exudate from a moist lesion (particularly of genitals, trunks, and extremities)	Exudate from a moist lesion is placed on a slide and sent immediately to the laboratory because the test depends on motile organisms. A test is considered positive if at least one motile organism is detected. Before a lesion can be considered darkfield negative, slides taken over a period of days must reveal no motile *Treponema pallidum.* Examination of oral lesions by darkfield microscopy is not useful because it is difficult to distinguish *T. pallidum* from oral treponemes.
Immunofluorescence	Serum	Immunofluorescence is useful in the diagnosis of AIDS, cytomegalovirus, *Chlamydia, Mycoplasma pneumoniae,* and herpes simplex types I and II. The antigen is detected by fluorochrome-labeled, specific antibodies (direct method) or by using a virus-specific antibody to bind with the antigen in the specimen.
Cell culture for gonorrhea, chlamydia	Swab from cervix (women), urethra (men), anus (if anal intercourse has occurred), or throat (if oral intercourse has occurred)	Cultures of discharge from lesions are necessary in the definitive diagnosis of gonorrhea and chlamydia and the detection of yeast. The detection of gonorrhea is more reliable than the detection of chlamydia, in which culture yields a high rate of false negative results. Urethral specimens are obtained by inserting a sterile cotton swab or platinum loop into the anterior urethra before patient voids, and immediately inoculating a modified Thayer-Martin or Transgrow medium. Cervical swabs are obtained after first wiping excess mucus from the external os. Patient should avoid douching before collection of the swab. Anal swabs are obtained by inserting a sterile swab 1 inch (2.54 cm) into the anal canal. If stool is present on the swab, the swab must be repeated. All swabs must be placed immediately into appropriate transport media.
Gram stain	Swab from purulent discharge	Gram-stained smears of purulent discharge from male urethras, in particular, are useful in the rapid detection of gonorrhea. Smears are not usually sufficient in chronic infections to demonstrate the presence of gonococci.
Tzanck smear	Swab from vesicular skin lesions	The Tzanck smear is particularly useful in the diagnosis of genital herpes. Tzanck smears of vesicular skin lesions show the intranuclear inclusions and/or multinucleated giant cells of herpes simplex and varicella zoster.
Chlamydiazine	Serum	Chlamydiazine is a specific enzyme immunoassay test (see ELISA) used in the detection of chlamydia. It is more rapid but less reliable than cell culture.
Microtrak	Serum	Microtrak is a direct fluorescent antibody test (see immunofluorescence) used in the detection of chlamydia. It is more rapid but less reliable than cell culture.
Whiff test (Smith test)	Swab from vagina	The Whiff test is useful in the detection of bacterial vaginosis. The discharge from the vaginal area is swabbed, the discharge is placed immediately on a glass slide, and 10% KON is added to the slide. The presence of a fishy odor is indicative of bacterial vaginosis. Patients should not douche before examination.

tum. A condom, filled with water, covers the probe and creates a transmission medium between the probe and prostate. The transducer emits sound waves through the prostate, which are reflected back to the transducer and converted to electrical impulses that are displayed on a screen. Ultrasonography of the prostate and scrotum takes approximately 30 to 60 minutes.

Patient preparation for ultrasound (transrectal) of the prostate

The nurse explains that the test allows visualization of the prostate and that during the test the patient will be asked to be on the left side with knees bent. The nurse explains that some mild pressure may be felt as the probe is inserted rectally. Approximately an hour prior to the procedure a self-administered enema is given to eliminate fecal matter from the rectum.

Testicular scintigraphy

Testicular scintigraphy is a nuclear medicine scan that is useful in differentiating acute testicular torsion from acute epididymo-orchitis. With torsion, there is decreased uptake of the nucleotide whereas with acute epididymo-orchitis there is increased flow and uptake of the nucleotide.

During the test $^{99m}TcO_4$ is administered intravenously while the patient lies under a scintillation camera. The patient's penis is taped to the abdomen and the testis are spread apart. After injection of the radionucleotide, rapid sequential images are taken over a period of 6 minutes.

Biopsy of the prostate gland

Biopsy of the prostate gland is useful in confirming prostatic cancer; in diagnosing benign prostatic hypertrophy, prostatitis, and tuberculosis; and in evaluating suspicious nodules discovered during prostatic examination. Needle biopsy is performed if a perineal or a transrectal approach is used whereas an endoscope and a cutting loop are employed in a transurethral route. Specimens are placed into 10% formalin.

Patient preparation

The nurse explains that the test enables microscopic examination of prostatic tissue and facilitates exploration of questions and concepts. The nurse explains that the patient will assume a left lateral position during the procedure. If a perineal approach is used, local anesthetic will be given during the procedure so that it is necessary to check the patient's history for hypersensitivity to anesthetic agents. If a transrectal approach is used, the nurse administers enemas until clear the morning of the examination. The

nurse checks vital signs and administers a sedative, if ordered, prior to the procedure. A signed consent is necessary.

Postprocedure care

The nurse checks vital signs immediately after the procedure, every 15 minutes for an hour, and then every hour until stable. If needle biopsy has been performed, the puncture site is checked for hematoma formation and the patient is instructed to wash the area with soap and water after bowel movements to reduce the chance of infection. The nurse instructs the patient to report fever as this may indicate infection and to check the voiding pattern for 2 to 3 days for frequency, amount, and bleeding. The nurse reassures that some bleeding is normal. The patient is given specific information as to how and when results may be obtained.

Diagnostic Tests for Sexually Transmitted Diseases

A number of tests are performed for the evaluation and diagnosis of sexually transmitted diseases (Table 68-1), many of which are specific to a particular disease. Gloves are recommended during collection of specimens. Follow-up diagnosis of sexual partners is necessary with positive findings.

CRITICAL THINKING QUESTIONS

1 What are the primary and secondary reproductive organs, and how do the reproductive hormones function to develop and maintain them?
2 Design at least three questions to discreetly ask patients about reproductive symptoms.
3 Discuss psychologic and sociocultural factors to consider throughout the physical examination of the patient's reproductive system.
4 Describe tests that are used in the detection of chlamydia.

BIBLIOGRAPHY

Current

1. Barsevick AM, Lauver D: Women's information needs about colposcopy, *Image* 22(1):22, 1990.
2. Bowers A, Thompson J: *Clinical manual of health assessment*, ed 2, St Louis, 1988, Mosby–Year Book, Inc.
3. Burrell LO: *Adult nursing in hospital and community settings*, Norwalk, Conn, 1992, Appleton & Lange.
4. Diagnostic tests, Springhouse, 1991, Springhouse Corporation.
5. Drukker BH, deMendonca WC: In Sciarra JJ, editor: *Gynecology and obstetrics*, vol 1, Philadelphia, 1988, JB Lippincott.
6. Fischbach F: *A manual of laboratory and diagnostic tests*, Philadelphia, 1992, JB Lippincott.

7. Gallo JJ et al: *Handbook of geriatric assessment,* Rockville, Md, 1988, Aspen Publishers.

8. Gordon M: *Manual of nursing diagnosis,* New York, 1987, McGraw-Hill.

9. Kane RL et al: *Essentials of clinical geriatrics,* ed 2, New York, 1989, McGraw Hill.

10. Lotocki RJ: Cold-knife cervical cone biopsy (conization), *Journal SOGC* 13(1):51, 1992.

11. Loucks A: *Chlamydia: an unheralded epidemic, AMJ Nursing* 87:923, 1987.

12. McComb P: Hysteroscopy, *Journal SOGC* 14(3):17, 1992.

13. Malasanos L et al: *Health assessment,* ed 4, St Louis, 1990, Mosby–Year Book.

14. Mason DR: Erectile dysfunctions: assessment and care, *Nurse Practitioner* 14(12):23-34, 1989.

15. Morra M, Blumberg B: Women's perceptions of early detection in breast cancer. How are we doing? *Semin Oncol Nurs* 7(3):151, 1991.

16. Murray R, Zentner S: *Nursing assessment and health promotion through the life span,* Englewood Cliffs, NJ, 1989, Prentice-Hall Inc.

17. Nettina S, Kauffman FH: Diagnosis and management of sexually transmitted lesions, *Nurse Pract* 15(1):20, 1990.

18. O'Leary TJ: Utilization of screening mammography by primary care physicians, *Appl Radiology* 18(12):28, 1989.

19. Pagana KD, Pagana TJ: *Diagnostic testing and nursing implications,* ed 3 St. Louis, 1991, Mosby–Year Book, Inc.

20. Roitt I: *Essential immunology,* London, 1988, Blackwell Scientific Publications.

21. Screening for breast cancer in elderly women, *American Geriatrics Society* 37(9):883, 1989.

22. Seidel HM et al: *Mosby's guide to physical examination,* ed 2, St. Louis, 1991, Mosby–Year Book, Inc.

23. Strax P: In Sciarra JJ, editor: *Gynecology and obstetrics,* vol 1, Philadelphia, 1988, JB Lippincott.

24. Sturgeon D: New marker will help track prostatic cancer, *Can Clin Lab* Aug/Sept, 1987.

25. Swartz MH: *Textbook of physical diagnosis,* Philadelphia, 1989, WB Saunders.

26. Tilkoan SM, Conover MB, Tilkan AG: *Clinical implications of laboratory tests,* St. Louis, 1987, Mosby–Year Book, Inc.

27. Trahan Regier P: Monoclonal antibodies, *Am J Nurs* 87(4):469, 1987.

28. Young H, McMillan M, editors: *Immunological diagnosis of sexually transmitted diseases,* New York, 1988, Dekker.

29. Zabriskie V, Lukehart SA: In Sciarra JJ, editor: *Obstetrics and gynecology,* vol 1, Philadelphia, 1988, JB Lippincott.

Classic

30. Baberman S: *ABCs of interpretative laboratory data,* Greenville, S.C., 1984, Interpretative Laboratory Data Inc.

31. Block G, Nolan J: *Health assessment for professional nursing: a developmental approach,* New York, 1986, Appleton-Century-Crofts.

32. Buschiazzo L, Naab G: Careful assessment of abdominal pain, *JEN* 12(2), 72, 1986.

33. Carotenuto R, Bullock J: *Physical assessment of the gerontologic client,* Philadelphia, 1981, FA Davis.

34. Dougherty CM, Pastorek JG: In Sciarra JJ, editor: *Gynecology and obstetrics,* vol 1, Philadelphia, 1984, JB Lippincott.

35. Fields W, McGinn-Campbell K: *Introduction to health assessment,* Reston, Va, 1983, Reston Publishing Co.

36. Hadii M et al: Prostatic specific antigen: an immunohistologic marker for prostatic neoplasm, *Cancer* 48(5):1229, 1981.

37. Jevtich MJ, Maxwell DD: In Krane RJ, Sirokyim MB, Goldstein I, editors: *Male sexual dysfunction,* Boston, 1983, Little, Brown & Co.

38. Krane RJ: In Walsh, PC et al, editors: *Campbell's urology,* Philadelphia, 1986, WB Saunders.

39. Peeling WB, Griffiths CJ: Imaging of the prostate by ultrasound, *J Urol* 132:217, 1984.

40. Sedlis A, Chen P: In Sciarra JJ, editor: *Gynecology and obstetrics,* vol 1, Philadelphia, 1986, JB Lippincott.

41. Valle RF, Sciarra JJ: In Sciarra JJ, editor: *Obstetrics and gynecology,* vol 1, Philadelphia, 1986, JB Lippincott.

42. Wagner AL: In Sciarra JJ, editor: *Obstetrics and gynecology,* vol 1, Philadelphia, 1986, JB Lippincott.

43. Wingerson L: Two new tests for chlamydia get quick results without culture, *JAMA* 250:2257, 1983.

CHAPTER SIXTY-NINE

Sexuality and Reproductive Health

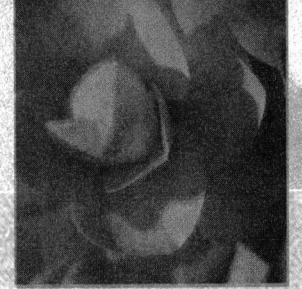

LEARNING OBJECTIVES

1 Define sexual health.
2 Discuss sexual development throughout the life span.
3 Describe the human sexual response cycle in women and men.
4 Discuss older adult sexual health issues.
5 Discuss gay and lesbian sexual health issues.
6 Describe the components of a sexual health assessment.
7 Discuss health promotion practices.
8 Contrast the value and side effects of various common forms of contraception.
9 Differentiate between the major alterations in sexual function based on the phase of sexual response that is affected.

---

anorgasmia, p. 1974
contraception, p. 1966
dyspareunia, p. 1972
erectile dysfunction, p. 1969
homosexuality, p. 1960
hypogonadism, p. 1968
orgasm, p. 1959

Papanicolaou (Pap) smear, p. 1965
premature ejaculation, p. 1976
sexual arousal disorders, p. 1970
sexual desire disorders, p. 1967
sexual health, p. 1958
sexuality, p. 1957
vaginismus, p. 1972

TODAY nurses are placing a greater emphasis on the importance of the sexual nature of individuals in the delivery of holistic care. Assessments of sexual health, sexual counseling, and patient education related to promoting or restoring sexual health are now looked at as essential components of comprehensive nursing care.[14] However, nurses cannot effectively deal with the sexual problems of their patients until they have a basic understanding of sexuality and their own sexual nature.

SEXUALITY AND SEXUAL HEALTH

Human **sexuality** has been defined as a complex phenomenon that encompasses the totality of human beings, influencing their ego, their self-image, and their feelings about themselves and others.[30] In addition, sexuality forms the biologic basis for sexual pleasure and influences our relationships with each other. Sexuality involves the interaction of the biologic, psychologic, sociologic, spiritual, and cultural aspects of our lives. According to Maslow,[47]

1957

sexuality is part of a broader category known as *stimulation needs*. Maslow's belief that sexual needs are of basic importance to the individual is represented by the fact that the stimulation category is second only to the survival category in Maslow's hierarchy of motivated needs.

In 1975 the World Health Organization (WHO) proposed that the standard definition of **sexual health** include "the integration of the somatic, emotional, intellectual, and social aspects of the sexual being in ways that are positively enriching and that enhance personality, communication, and love."[49] This definition, by identifying the importance of the interaction of the various components, illustrates the complexity of human sexuality.

SEXUAL DEVELOPMENT

The evolution of human sexuality begins in the womb and continues throughout life. Physiologic and psychologic sexual development normally proceeds through each growth and developmental stage. However, sexual development may be affected by the impact of cultural and social norms. According to Brink,[11] cultural teaching about sex and sexuality, called social enculturation, has a profound effect on sexuality by mandating values or rules regarding the relationship of sex and love and the acceptability of specific sexual behaviors. Injuries, illnesses, birth anomalies, or surgical modifications may further affect the sexual development of an individual. Consequently, the development of human sexuality is a very individualized process.

The adult years, from 21 to 45 years old, are typically filled with career development activities, the search for a partner, and the development of a fulfilling and stable sexual relationship. As a result, a new feeling of responsibility for sexual behavior usually begins to develop. The fulfillment of sexual needs during this period is often based on the individual's definition of adult sexuality and an internally defined gender role behavior formed during adolescence. Males are likely to reach the peak of their sexuality early in this developmental period. Females are more likely to reach their sexual peak in their late 30s or early 40s.[30] Values related to acceptable adult sexual behavior have become more liberal over the last few years. The availability of contraceptives, as well as effective treatments for most sexually transmitted diseases, has further influenced the sexual practices of today's young adults. However, the current acquired immune deficiency syndrome (AIDS) epidemic is likely to dramatically affect the sexual behavior practiced by individuals in this age group.

The middle adult years, from 46 to 65 years old, represent the time when decreased hormone production may result in changes in sexual desire and sexual response. Both men and women may find that increased stimulation is required for orgasm, and sexual excitement may be less intense.[30] External physical changes may result in fears related to an individual's sexual attractiveness, especially in U.S. society, which seems to place a special value on a youthful appearance. Resolving the resulting self-esteem vs. despair issue is a major goal of individuals of this age group and a major factor in their obtaining sexual fulfillment. Many women who have reached midlife have completed their child rearing responsibilities and do not plan on additional pregnancies. Contraceptive choices for these women are more limited and pregnancies are more risky.[26] The fear of unwanted pregnancy may bring additional anxiety and stress to the sexual encounter.

SEXUAL RESPONSE CYCLE

According to Masters and Johnson, male and female sexual response cycles are basically the same. The cycle can be divided into four general phases preceded by a preexcitement, or desire, phase.[30] Figure 69-1 depicts the male and female sexual response cycles. Accurate sexual assessment and comprehensive nursing care require that the nurse have a general understanding of sexual stimulation and the major physiologic factors that accompany each phase of the sexual response cycle. Masters and Johnson suggest that there is basically only one pattern for men: a rapid excitement phase followed by a short plateau, then orgasm and resolution (Figure 69-1, *B*). Women, by contrast, appear to experience a variety of sexual response patterns. Figure 69-1, *A*, depicts three of the most prevalent patterns for women. Pattern A illustrates a response characterized by multiple orgasmic peaks. Pattern B shows fluctuating levels of excitement throughout the plateau phase but no distinct orgasm. Pattern C is characterized by interruptions of the excitement phase followed by an intense orgasm and rapid resolution.

Preexcitement Phase

The preexcitement phase is a precursor to the first phase of the sexual response cycle. During this phase the individual may fantasize about or wish to actually engage in sexual activities. The intensity of the resultant desire for sexual activity appears to be mediated by the level of circulating androgens and their effect on cells in the central and peripheral nervous systems.

Excitement or Arousal Phase

The excitement phase in men and women has both physiologic and psychologic origins. Vasocongestion in the genital area is the major physiologic change that occurs in this phase. In men, penile erection occurs secondary to the rapid influx and retention of

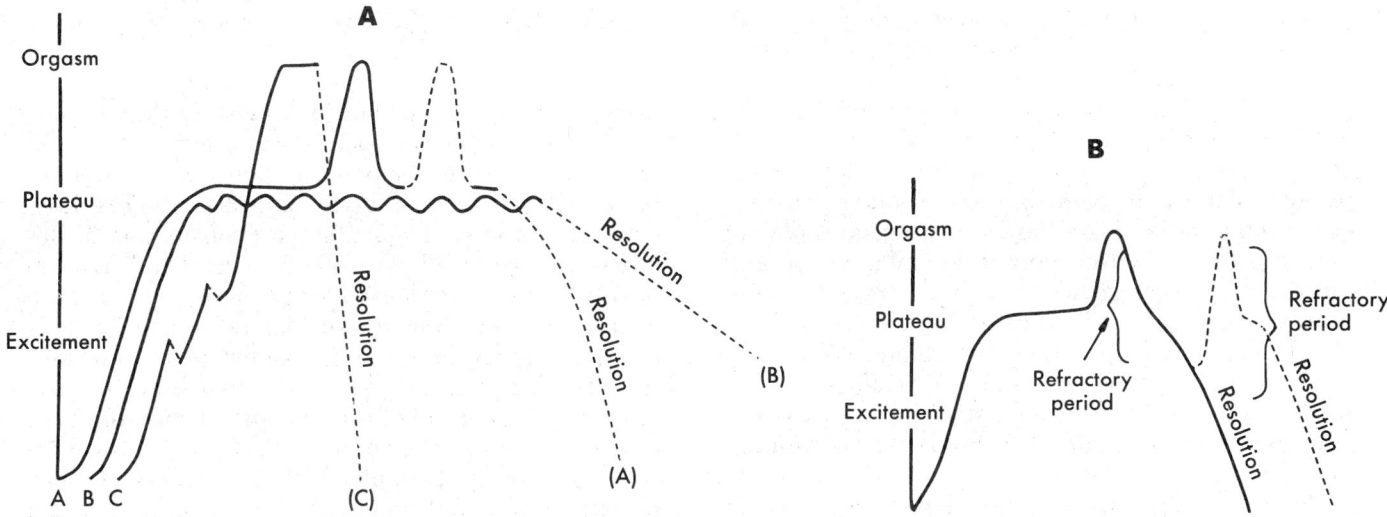

FIGURE 69-1   **A,** Female sexual response cycle. **B,** Male sexual response cycle. (**A** from Masters W, Johnson V: *Human sexual response,* Boston, 1966, Little, Brown & Co Inc; **B** from Woods NF: Human sexuality: an overview. In Woods NF, editor: *Human sexuality in health and illness,* ed 3, St Louis, 1984, Mosby–Year Book, Inc.)

blood in the spongy tissues of the penis. Erection can be induced by two separate stimuli: (1) psychic stimuli initiating a neurologic response via the cortical pathway and mediated by sympathetic and parasympathetic nerves and (2) tactile stimulation initiating a neurologic response via a reflex through the sacral spinal cord. A thickening and tensing of the scrotal skin occur, elevating the scrotal sac; the spermatic cords also shorten. The testes increase in size and elevate.

In some women, vaginal lubrication can occur within seconds during this phase, whereas other women take much longer to achieve lubrication. Lubrication results from vasoconstriction in and around the vagina that causes fluid to pass through the tissues comprising the vaginal walls. The external genitalia swell and the clitoris increases in size, becomes erect, and is increasingly more sensitive. The vaginal vault balloons and lengthens.[30]

In both men and women the heart rate, blood pressure, and respirations increase. Myotonia, or muscular tension, develops throughout the body, especially in the thighs, abdomen, and pelvic area. Breasts enlarge and nipples may become erect because of involuntary muscle fiber contraction in the areola. A flush or rash may appear on the trunk and spread to the face.[30]

Plateau Phase

The plateau phase is a natural extension of the excitement phase. In men the penis increases in diameter and may take on a deeper hue at the glans. Testes continue to elevate and thicken because of vasoconstriction. An emission of a few drops of seminal

fluid containing sperm may occur at this time from the corpus glands. In women the labia minora take on a deeper hue and the tissues around the nipples may swell. The clitoris retracts under the clitoral hood. The opening to the vagina decreases in size related to the engorgement of surrounding tissues.

Orgasm

It is important to note that not every sexual encounter will terminate in an actual orgasm for both partners. During this phase sexual pleasure peaks. In men, **orgasm** is usually accompanied by ejaculation or ejection of seminal fluid in response to the contraction of the vas deferens, prostate, and seminal vesicles. Contractions of the pelvic floor occur in conjunction with the closure of the internal sphincters of the bladder, which prevents retrograde ejaculation or discharge of the seminal fluid into the bladder rather than outside through the urethra.

In women, rhythmic contractions of the vagina and uterus occur during this phase. An all-over warmth and a throbbing sensation in the pelvis are experienced. Some women ejaculate a fluid that is similar to the male's prostatic fluid from the urethra at the time of orgasm.[2,40] Muscles in the pelvic floor and rectal sphincter contract, forcing pooled blood out of engorged blood vessels and relieving pelvic tension.

Resolution Phase

The final phase of the human sexual response cycle is resolution. The resolution phase is accompanied by a sense of well-being and relaxation. Vital signs slowly return to normal in both men and women. In men, loss of erection begins immediately following ejaculation. Testes and scrotal tissue return to their relaxed state. If nipples were erect during the sexual excitement phase, they slowly lose their erect state. A refractory period occurs at resolution during which the man is unable to respond to further sexual stimulation. The length of time the man remains in the refractory period depends on age and individual characteristics.[30]

In women the external genitalia, uterus, and vagina return to their prestimulation state. Women do not experience the same type of physiologic refractory period as men. Consequently, they may experience multiple orgasms with appropriate stimulation.[30]

Sexual satisfaction does not necessarily depend on completion of the entire sexual response cycle. Of greater importance is the person's sense of fulfillment with the total experience.[30,45]

OLDER ADULT SEXUAL HEALTH ISSUES

Some normal changes occur with aging that require accommodation; however, sexual expression is appropriate and should be encouraged in older adults.[42] The sexual response cycle is intact, and there is no known intrinsic biologic limitation to sexual capacity related to aging. Nurses can play an important role as the facilitators who support individual sexual expression in the older person.

Physiologic Changes in Elderly Persons

Physiologic changes of aging women include a reduction or absence of breast engorgement during arousal, although nipple sensitivity remains normal; the sex flush just before orgasm may lessen or disappear; engorgement of the labia minora is reduced, although the clitoris retains its sensitivity.[30] The mucosa of the vagina thins, providing less protection for the bladder and urethra during intercourse. The increased trauma inflicted on the cells of the bladder and urethra during intercourse results in a higher incidence of cystitis in sexually active older women.[13]

Vaginal lubrication is reduced in amount, and the time it takes to be produced is prolonged. Decreased vaginal lubrication can make penetration uncomfortable or even painful (dyspareunia).[44] The lining of the bladder and urethra becomes thinner in the aged woman, and this may result in irritability and feelings of needing to urinate during or after sexual activity. The phases of the sexual response cycle may take longer to occur. The orgasmic phase may be shortened and the force and number of orgasmic contractions reduced. However, women who maintain an active sex life complain of little difficulty, indicating that lack of sexual activity may result in

changes that can affect sexual enjoyment in later life.[30]

Older men may find that achieving an erection takes an increased period of time and that tumescence (the hardness of penile engorgement) as well as the sensitivity of the penis is reduced. The amount of semen produced and the sperm count are lessened. The force of ejaculatory contractions is decreased by reduced prostatic contractility.[44] On the positive side the increased length of time it takes the aging man to become prepared may in fact afford his partner greater time for enjoyment of the encounter. Men are often able in old age to achieve a much more satisfying level of erectile and ejaculatory control than they had as young men. Better control increases their ability to please their partners. Retired partners often have more time for loving stimulation before sexual activity, and thus both can achieve their desired level of sexual expression in a more relaxed atmosphere.

GAY AND LESBIAN SEXUAL HEALTH ISSUES

Homosexuality may be defined as a lifelong physical and psychologic attraction to members of one's own sex, whether that attraction is acted on or not. According to Kus,[29] homosexuality is determined by sexual orientation rather than sexual behavior. Consequently, homosexual activity may be sporadic, transitory, nonexistent, or continual throughout the individual's lifetime.[17] The term *homosexual* is rarely used today by members of gay and lesbian communities. It is viewed as having negative connotations and is used primarily by heterosexual individuals lacking in awareness, understanding, and sensitivity.[29]

Because of their life-styles, gay and lesbian Americans face some special health care issues. These same issues may exist for bisexual individuals. Societal misperceptions frequently place all members of gay and lesbian communities in one category, thus suggesting that they all have the same needs.[17] Nurses should be aware of the dangers resulting from such generalizations. Since sexual preference and affiliative choice are highly individual, health care providers must avoid labeling and categorizing individuals on the basis of sexuality.

Young gay and lesbian individuals may experience severe guilt, feelings of isolation, fear of rejection, and low self-esteem as they attempt to come to grips with their sexuality. This psychologic distress frequently occurs as a result of the need for these men and women to hide their sexual orientation from a society that stigmatizes, rejects, and discriminates against any departure from the majority norm.[24,29] These negative feelings may manifest themselves in isolation, depression, drug and alco-

GERIATRIC CONSIDERATIONS

Sexuality and the Older Adult

Nurses can support elderly persons in the fulfillment of their sexual needs by maintaining a nonjudgmental attitude toward sexuality. Viewing elderly persons in terms of their strengths rather than weaknesses and assisting them to maximize their strengths are imperative in maintaining their overall health. Myths and taboos about sexuality and aging should be discussed and refuted. Most of those myths can be grouped together into the following general category: elderly people are not desirable, desirous of sex, or capable of sex.[28]

Educating elderly persons to understand that physiologic changes are a normal part of aging and not necessarily a negative process is an important function for nurses. Helping elders explore the new meanings of sexuality is a holistic way of viewing healthy aging. Nurses can encourage elderly persons to appreciate their bodies and their sexual urges.[41] An emphasis should be placed on healthy bodies and a healthy lifestyle to enhance and promote sexual health. Nurses can help elderly persons feel comfortable in discussing sexual issues and finding solutions for problems as they arise.[28]

Older women may need information about the use of water-soluble lubricant gels and estrogen replacement to ensure continued enjoyment of the sex act. These lubricants can be inserted before sexual activity, or the insertion may be included in the couple's foreplay.[44] Participating in intercourse on a regular basis can also increase the woman's natural secretions.[28]

Both men and women may experience a decreased sexual drive because of medications they are taking. The nurse should help them understand that medications may be available that afford similar therapeutic effect without the loss of sexual desire. They need to be encouraged to tell their health care provider if loss of sexual urge or erectile problems are inhibiting their normal sexual responses. Medications can often be adjusted to decrease negative side effects. If erection problems in the male or vaginal atrophy in the female results from treatments or medications that cannot be changed, the nurse should help the elderly couple explore alternate methods of sexual expression that will enable them to continue a healthy relationship.

Touching, whether sexual or not, is known to be important for health. Older individuals in caring relationships should be encouraged to touch each other. Patting the hand, touching the shoulder, and rubbing the back are all legitimate ways to express feelings. This form of touching does not have explicit sexual connotations, but it assists a person in maintaining the self-esteem so important to people of all ages.

A lack of privacy may also be a problem for older couples. Many older couples live with their children and have little private space to themselves. Other older couples live in institutional settings where they may be assigned to separate rooms. Families and institutional caregivers frequently have little sensitivity for the sexual needs of older adults. Nurses who understand the normal sexual needs of aged persons should be advocates for those elders who no longer live in the privacy of their own homes so that their needs for sexual expression are not neglected.

As long as elderly persons are comfortable and happy with their modes of sexual expression, sexuality need not cease for them; quite the contrary—sexual fulfillment in the aged is known to be a factor in their continued good health.

---

hol addiction, or suicidal ideation. Nurses who identify one or more of these problems in a patient should make referrals to appropriate counselors or community support groups. The fear of discovery and subsequent stigmatization may lead gay and lesbian patients to delay seeking professional help for health-related problems. Further, if nurses initially communicate negative attitudes regarding homosexuality, gay and lesbian patients are less likely to trust that they will be accepted and receive sensitive and unbiased care.[24]

Lack of acceptance may then result in gay and lesbian patients withholding information essential to correct diagnosis of sex-related problems. This is especially true in the case of sexually transmitted diseases. Because of a high incidence of anal intercourse, gay men may also have more frequent gastrointestinal infections and rectal tears. In addition, gay and bisexual men currently represent the population group with the highest incidence of AIDS. Further, alcoholism and drug abuse are chronic problems that affect gays and lesbians in percentages similar to those seen in the overall population of the United States.

Finally, sensitive and unbiased care of gay and lesbian patients requires that nurses confront and work through their own ideas and feelings regarding sexuality. Projection of personal values onto a patient can seriously interfere with the nurse-patient interaction and may result in inconsistent patient adherence to treatment plans.

SEXUAL HEALTH ASSESSMENT

The interpretation of a patient's sexual health is an important part of any comprehensive nursing assessment. Sexual evaluation requires collection of both historic and physical data. The sensitive nature of the information obtained during this type of assessment requires strictest confidentiality.

Sexual History

The extent of the sexual history should be related to the patient's diagnosis or sex-related questions and comments. Since sexual topics are often difficult to discuss, the nurse will frequently have to be alert to subtle clues provided by the patient and ask questions related to those clues. Nonthreatening questions should be asked first as a way to put the patient at ease (see boxes). Care should be taken to ensure that the interview is conducted in a private, relaxed atmosphere. Sufficient time without interruptions should be provided to allow all questions

to be answered and any misconceptions to be discussed fully. The nurse should ensure that all verbal and nonverbal communications are designed to provide the patient with assurance of complete confidentiality. An objective, empathetic, nonjudgmental attitude is maintained throughout the assessment. Vocabulary should be on the patient's level of understanding, and patient input should be solicited and used in developing the patient care plan.

Physical Examination

In some instances, nurses may be responsible for performing the physical examination, or they may

---

GUIDELINES FOR A COMPREHENSIVE SEXUAL HISTORY

A comprehensive sexual history includes documentation of the following topics of general information:

1. Information about significant others (sources of support or lack of support and types of support)
2. History of acute and chronic health problems
3. History of the use of prescription drugs
4. Childhood sexual activity—introduction to sexuality, family attitude toward sex, childhood and adolescent sexual experiences
5. Adult sexual activity—sexual experience, previous sexual dysfunctions, conditions that resulted secondary to sexual practices (i.e., venereal disease, pregnancy, abortion)
6. Current sexual activity—current sexual experience, sexual self-concept, and the use of safer sexual practices
7. Current sexual problems—when problems started, what treatments have been tried, and the results that were achieved from those treatments
8. History of nonprescriptive drugs and alcohol use and how these substances have affected or affect the patient's sexual functioning
9. What the patient's goals are related to the treatment of the problem or problems and what the patient thinks would help meet those goals

---

SEXUAL HISTORY GUIDELINES

1. The patient may be uncomfortable with this topic of conversation. Provide privacy, ensure confidentiality, and try to put the patient at ease. Only ask questions related to the diagnosis or sexually related comments or suggestions that the patient has made.
2. Be aware that you may be uncomfortable with the topic. Your discomfort is not a reason to ignore this area of concern. Practice and patience, along with additional information about the topic of sexuality, will increase your comfort with this topic.
3. Begin with the less sensitive questions (i.e., "Who do you have for support?" and "How is your relationship with your spouse or partner?").
4. After the patient is less anxious, you may move to more explicit questions. These questions should be presented in a nonthreatening format (i.e., "Sometimes individuals who have had a heart attack are worried about how their heart condition will affect their sexual relationship with their partner. Do you have this concern?" or "Older men are sometimes troubled by an inability to obtain or maintain an erection. Is this a problem that you are experiencing?").
5. Be open and nonjudgmental. Negative body language such as a lack of eye contact, fidgeting, or physically moving away from the patient when he or she asks questions about sexual problems will be interpreted to mean that this is an inappropriate topic for discussion. Be informed and frank about your responses. Answer questions in terms that the patient will understand.
6. Provide sufficient time for questions to be answered and solutions explored fully. Because of the sensitive nature of these questions, the question and answer period may take some additional time. However, this part of the sexual history should never be rushed.

assist another health care provider. No matter what the specific role, the first concern of the nurse is the comfort of the patient. This includes psychologic reassurance, attention to physical comfort measures, and careful draping to protect the patient's sense of modesty. The physical examination includes a careful examination of the external genitalia of both male and female patients to rule out the presence of disease or anatomic abnormality. It also includes a pelvic examination for the female patient and a prostate and rectal examination for the male. Laboratory work will be specific for suspected diagnoses.

HEALTH PROMOTION PRACTICES

Routine practices designed to ensure the early detection of disease and to promote sexual and reproductive health should be discussed with all patients. Interactions during health assessments provide nurses with an ideal opportunity to explain and demonstrate preventive procedures to patients. At the same time, the patient's level of knowledge can be determined and written materials given to reinforce learning. The following sections contain a discussion of common preventive practices that frequently appear in nursing care plans.

Breast Self-Examination

Breast cancer is one of the most common malignancies affecting women today (see Chapter 70). We generally think of women when we think of breast cancer, but men may develop this malignancy as well. Breast cancer can occur at any age. In women, however, it tends to occur more frequently in the perimenopausal years.

The most effective way of dealing with this type of cancer is early detection. Breast self-examination (BSE) is one of the most effective and inexpensive methods available for the early detection of malignancy. Nurses can play a key role in health promotion by teaching all patients how to perform this simple procedure and by reminding patients that a monthly BSE is important in protecting their health. The self-examination technique is easy to learn and takes a minimum amount of time to perform each month. However, despite its simplicity and the availability of information describing the procedure, many adults still do not routinely perform BSE.

Initially, some patients may experience discomfort at touching their own breasts. They should, however, be encouraged to perform the examination routinely so that they become familiar with the appearance and texture of their own breast tissue. The individual will then be better prepared to identify any changes that may occur.

The technique of BSE is best taught through demonstration and patient participation. The box on

RESEARCH BRIEF

Lashley ME: Predictors of breast self-examination practice among elderly women, *Adv Nurs Sci* 9(4):25, 1987.

The author uses the health belief model as the theoretic framework for this study. Subjects were 65 years of age or over and participants in a senior citizens' center. The findings revealed that 61% of this sample of 101 reported doing a monthly BSE; 15% reported doing the procedure bimonthly. The best predictor of BSE was the perceived barriers concept. The author notes that this finding is in conflict with the health belief model prediction.

p. 1964 serves as a guideline for this procedure. If patients are already performing self-examinations, they should be asked to demonstrate their technique. Women need to be told that female breasts may have a tendency to become swollen, painful, and lumpy before the start of the menstrual period and that the best time to perform the examination is 7 to 10 days after menses. Further, the examination should be done on the same day each month to ensure regular performance. Men, postmenopausal women, and women who have had hysterectomies should simply pick a specific day of the month and regularly perform their BSE on that day. When women become familiar with how their breasts normally feel at a given time in their cycle, they will quickly note any changes that occur.[6]

Pamphlets describing the actual examination, educational films, and breast models are available from several sources such as the American Cancer Society to help the patient learn to perform the procedure.[6] Some type of written instructions should be sent home with the patient for later reference, and plenty of time should be allowed for the patient to ask questions.

Mammography

Mammography is a highly sensitive radiographic test used to detect tumors in the breast. However, mammography is not meant to take the place of breast self-examination and professional examination in the early detection of breast cancer. Optimal early detection depends on a combination of all three measures.[3] Mammography's unique contribution to the screening process is its ability to detect preclinical lesions at a stage of high curability.[21] Patient preparation for this test is described in Chapter 68. The American Cancer Society has developed routine

PATIENT EDUCATION GUIDE   *Breast Self-examination*

Many good reasons exist for doing a breast self-examination each month. One reason is that breast cancer is most easily treated and cured when it is found early. Another is that the more you do it, the better you will get at it. When you get to know how your breasts normally feel, you will quickly be able to feel any change. Another reason is that it is easy to do.

The best time to do a breast self-examination is after your period, when breasts are not tender or swollen. If you do not have regular periods or sometimes skip a month, do it on the same day every month.

How to do a breast self-examination (see A)

1. Lie down with a pillow under your right shoulder. Place your right arm behind your head.
2. Use the finger pads of your middle three fingers on your left hand to feel for lumps or thickening. Your finger pads are the top third of each finger.

3. Press firmly enough to know how your breast feels. If you are not sure how hard to press, ask your health care provider, or try to copy the way your health care provider uses finger pads during a breast examination. Learn how your breasts feel most of the time. A firm ridge in the lower curve of each breast is normal.
4. Move around the breast in a set way. You can choose either the circle (see **B**), the up and down line (see **C**), or the wedge (see **D**). Do it the same way every time. It will help you to make sure that you've gone over the entire breast area and to remember how your breast feels each month.
5. Now examine your left breast using right-hand finger pads.
6. If you find any changes, see your health care provider right away.

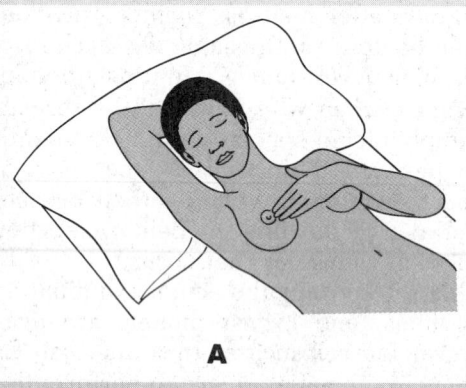

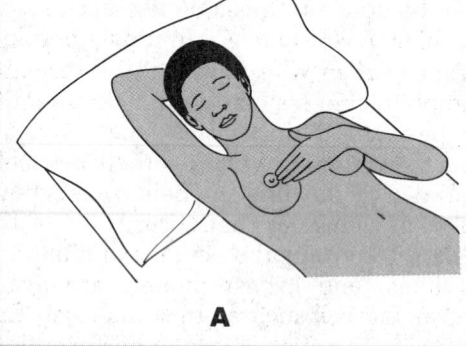

A

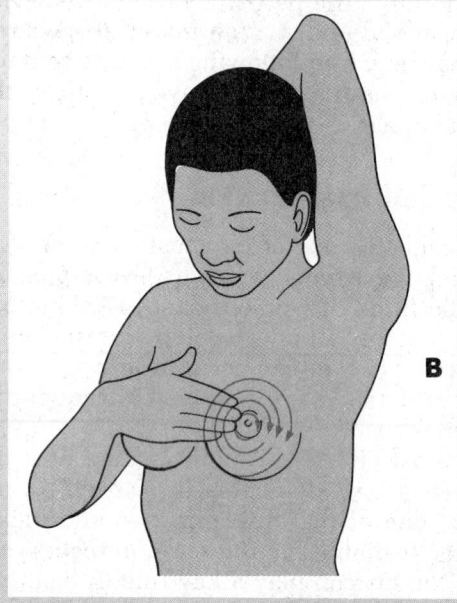

B

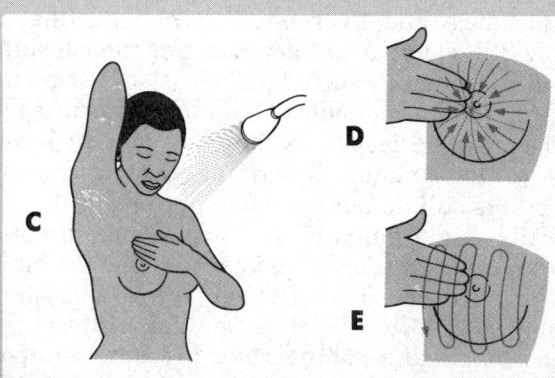

C

D

E

For added safety (see E)

1. You might want to check your breasts while standing in front of a mirror right after you do your breast self-examination each month. See if there are any changes in the way your breasts look, for example, dimpling of the skin, changes in the nipple, or redness and swelling.
2. You might also want to do an extra breast self-examination while you are in the shower. Your soapy hands will glide over the wet skin making it easy to check how your breasts feel (see **D**).

Courtesy American Cancer Society, 1990.

mammography guidelines for women who are asymptomatic. These guidelines are based on the age of the woman. It is recommended that patients have a baseline mammogram between the ages of 35 and 40 years. Women between 40 and 49 years old should have a mammogram every 1 to 2 years and those 50 years or older should have a mammogram every year.

Papanicolaou (Pap) Smear

Invasive epidermoid carcinoma is one of the most common cancers of the reproductive organs (see Chapter 70). Early detection of cancer has been shown to significantly reduce mortality. Cervical cancer is almost 100% curable, and endometrial cancer is nearly 90% curable when detected and treated early.[4] The **Papanicolaou (Pap) smear** is currently the best available test for the early detection of cervical cancer.[4]

The Pap smear is not as accurate in the detection of endometrial cancer as it is in the diagnosis of cervical cancer. Additional protection can be provided, however, by taking a sample of endometrial tissue and examining the cells under a microscope at the same time the Pap smear is obtained. The American Cancer Society guidelines for the recommended frequency of Pap smears is shown in the box below. Patients should be made aware of the importance of this test in the early detection of cervical cancer (see Chapter 68).

GUIDELINES FOR PAPANICOLAOU SMEAR

According to the American Cancer Society, the following guidelines are to be used by practitioners for obtaining Papanicolaou smears (Pap tests):

1. All women who have reached the age of 18 years should have a pelvic examination and a Pap smear.
2. Pap smears should be obtained on an annual basis until the woman has had three or more consecutive satisfactory, normal tests.
3. After three or more normal tests, the test may be performed less frequently, at the discretion of the physician.
4. Annual Pap smears are necessary for women who are sexually active.
5. If a woman has a warning signal such as irregular or excessive bleeding, bleeding after regular periods have stopped, or an unusual vaginal discharge, she should see her health care provider right away.

Courtesy American Cancer Society, 1989.

Testicular Self-examination

Regular testicular self-examination (TSE) is currently recommended by many experts as an effective method for detecting the early stages of scrotal cancer. Scrotal cancer is the most common neo-

PATIENT EDUCATION GUIDE
Testicular Self-examination

According to the American Cancer Society, the following examination will take approximately 3 minutes each month to perform and is the individual's best hope for early detection of testicular cancer.

1. Pick a day of the month and perform the examination on the same day of each month.
2. Perform the examination after a warm bath or shower when the scrotal skin is most relaxed.
3. Hold the scrotum in one hand.
4. Examine each testicle separately by gently rolling it between the thumb and fingers of the other hand.
5. Check for hard lumps or knots.
6. The examination should not be painful.
7. Promptly report any abnormal finding to your health care provider such as a slight enlargement of one of the testes, a change in its consistency, a dull ache in the lower abdomen and groin, together with a sensation of dragging and heaviness.

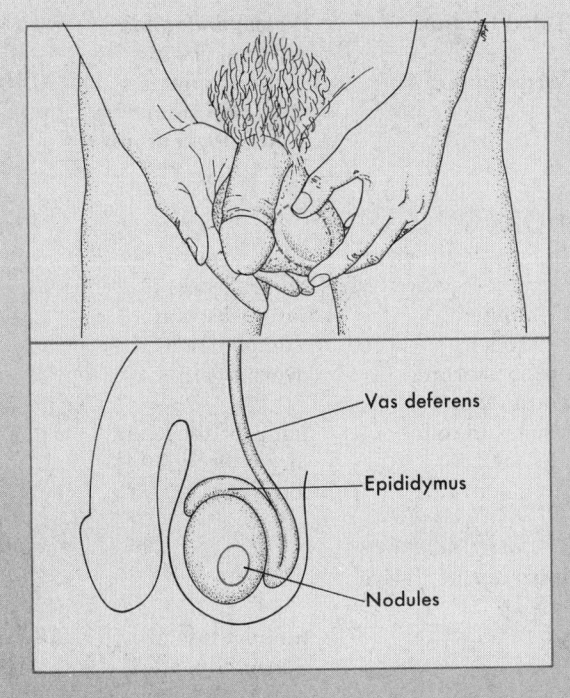

Courtesy American Cancer Society, 1990.

plasm in males between the ages of 15 and 34 years (see Chapter 71). Prognosis is good if the cancer is detected early. The survival rate for the most common type of testicular cancer, seminoma, is nearly 100% in cases detected and treated early.[5]

Through patient education, nurses can play a significant role in the early detection of this type of cancer. All males beyond the age of adolescence should be provided with instructions on this simple examination. Routine physicals are usually good times to introduce the patient to TSE. Males should be asked whether they perform TSEs on a regular basis. If not, information and a demonstration can be provided by a nurse who is comfortable with the topic, skilled in the examination, and sensitive to the possibility of embarrassment for the patient (see the box on p. 1965).

If regular TSEs are already being performed, the nurse may ask the patient to demonstrate the method he is currently using. The nurse should provide sufficient time to answer any questions the patient may have about the examination, concerns about his genitalia, or any unusual findings noted in previous examinations. Written material can be provided for later reference. Finally, nurses are responsible for maintaining strict privacy during the examination and protecting the patient's confidentiality.

CONTRACEPTION

Contraception is defined as the purposeful avoidance of unplanned or unwanted pregnancy using devices or medications.[22] Contraception can be distinguished from birth control, which encompasses all methods including abortion and abstinence, by its focus on prevention of pregnancy. All contraceptive methods have some risks and are subject to limitations or failures (Table 69-1).

A variety of contraceptive devices are currently in use. Further information describing contraceptive devices or medications may be obtained from any of the sources referred to in this chapter and most obstetric/gynecologic nursing textbooks. The nurse's responsibility as it relates to contraception may include one or more of the following: patient education, counseling, physical assessment, and long-term follow-up care to promote continued success with the chosen contraceptive method.

One form of contraception that has recently become available in the United States is a reversible

TABLE 69-1   Contraceptive Risk and Failure Rates

Type of contraception	Inherent risks/problems	Failure rate (%)	Type of contraception	Inherent risks/problems	Failure rate (%)
SURGICAL			**MECHANICAL/PHARMACOLOGIC**		
Tubal ligation	Typical abdominal surgical risks	0.04	Cervical cap	Local irritation	8
Vasectomy	Bruising, edema, pain, infection, psychologic problems	0.15	Diaphragm with spermicide	Toxic shock syndrome; advance planning required, local irritation	18
HORMONAL			Sponge with spermicide	Same as above	18 to 28
Injectable progestin	Allergy/sensitivity to drug	0.3	**PHARMACOLOGIC**		
Combined estrogen/ progesterone oral tablet	Cardiovascular complications, weight gain	2.0	Foams, creams, jellies, vaginal suppositories	Local irritation; advance planning required	21
Progestin-only tablet	Same as above and breakthrough bleeding	2.5	**OTHER**		
			Douche	Infection, local irritation	40
MECHANICAL			Rhythm method	Advance planning required; daily self-testing	20
Intrauterine device (IUD)	Infection	6			
Condom	Minimal loss of sensitivity; advance planning required	12			

Modified from Hatcher RA et al: *Contraceptive technology: 1988-1989,* ed 14, New York, 1988, Irvington Publisher Inc.

implant contraceptive system known as the Norplant System. The Norplant System involves six flexible Silastic capsules containing long-term, low-dose progestin designed to prevent ovulation. The capsules are inserted subdermally in the woman's upper arm using a local anesthetic. The device can be removed at any time and provides an extremely low failure rate (1%) for the individual during the time it is in place. However, the Norplant devices are expensive, and the woman is likely to experience irregular menstrual bleeding during the first 6 months after insertion.

Alterations in Sexual Function

The alterations in sexual functioning for which patients seek assistance are known as sexual disorders.[7] There are four major groups of sexual disorders: (1) physiologic disorders, (2) psychosexual disorders, (3) gender identification variations, and (4) paraphilias. The physiologic and psychosexual disorders are alterations in sexual desire, alterations in sexual arousal, pain related to sexual activity, and alterations in orgasm.

The gender identity disorders category includes several conditions such as childhood gender identity disorder, adolescent gender identity disorder, and adult gender identity disorder (nontranssexual) and transsexualism. The paraphilia disorder category includes sexual disorders related to nonnormative variations in the choice of sexual objects.[30] This chapter does not discuss gender identity disorders or paraphilia disorders. Complete discussions of these disorders can be found in texts on psychiatric nursing. The information contained in this chapter is designed only to introduce the reader to these conditions.

ALTERATIONS IN SEXUAL DESIRE
Definition

Disorders of the first phase of the sexual cycle are labeled **sexual desire disorders** according to the Diagnostic and Statistical Manual of Mental Disorders (DSM III-R). Diagnoses within this category include several separate problems labeled hypoactive sexual desire disorder and sexual aversion.

According to Kaplan,[45] a large percentage of marital problems are concerned with sexual desire disorders. Although there are no established normal levels of sexual desire, there is agreement that a (1) lack of fantasizing about sex, (2) lack of impulse to masturbate, (3) failure of erection, and (4) lack of nocturnal emissions in the young man are hallmarks of sexual desire disorders. In women a (1) lack of sexual fantasies, (2) lack of masturbation, and (3)

failure to respond to sexual stimulation are frequently present in individuals presenting with this problem. Patients may seek help at the request of their partner or based on a change in their interest in sexual activities that they have noticed and are concerned about.[35]

Hypoactive sexual desire disorders (HSDD) are defined as "persistently or recurrently deficient or absent sexual fantasies and desire for sexual activity."[7] Disorders of the desire phase of the sexual response cycle affect both men and women. Hypoactive sexual desire is the diagnostic category used when the etiology of the problem is unknown.[45] Sexual aversion disorder is the diagnostic category used when persistent avoidance of all or nearly all genital contact with a sexual partner exists.[7]

Etiology

The etiology of sexual desire disorders includes both physiologic and psychologic problems (see the box below). Psychic problems such as subclinical and clinical manifestations of depression may contribute to sexual desire disorders as well as stress, anxiety, and a lack of energy.

ETIOLOGY OF ALTERATIONS IN SEXUAL DESIRE (HSDD)

Congenital hypogonadism
Primary (hypergonadotropic hypogonadism)
  Klinefelter's syndrome
  Reifenstein's syndrome
  Sertoli cell–only syndrome
  Anorchism (absence of testicles)
  Male Turner's syndrome
Secondary (hypogonadotropic hypogonadism)
  Kallman's syndrome
  Female Turner's syndrome
  Isolated luteinizing hormone (LH) deficiency
  Isolated follicle-stimulating hormone (FSH) deficiency
  Prader-Willi syndrome

Acquired hypogonadism
Alcohol or drug abuse
Effects of irradiation
Orchitis
Trauma
Tumors (gonadal or pituitary)

Other causes of HSDD
Depression (clinical and subclinical levels)
Marital strife
Anxiety/frustration

Pathophysiology

The group of physiologic problems most frequently related to alterations in sexual desire result from a condition known as hypogonadism.[20] **Hypogonadism** is defined as a defective internal secretion of the gonads and is usually not diagnosed until 16 or 17 years of age when a delay of puberty or changes in secondary sex characteristics can be ascertained. The condition occurs in either of two forms—congenital or acquired—and is characterized by diminished testicular or ovarian function.

Some causes of alteration in sexual desire disorders are psychologic in origin. In the case of either subclinical or clinical depression, energy for sexual activity is decreased, impeding the desire to be sexually active. With relief of the depression, energy for all activities, including sexual responses, can be expected to return.[35] Marital strife, anxiety, lack of sleep, and frustrations can also sap the strength and energy available for sexual activity and lead to a reduced sexual desire. Resolution of these problems and the concerns attending them can be expected to restore interest in sex.

Clinical Manifestations

Clinical manifestations depend on the etiology of the problem. Clinical signs and symptoms of hypogonadism may include immature sexual development or gradual atrophy and loss of the secondary sex characteristics of the individual. These findings, coupled with a loss of sexual desire, suggest the need for further investigation and basic hormone tests. Patients experiencing anxiety and stress may appear nervous, be unable to sit still, have short attention spans, or express strong emotions with little or no stimulus. Patients who are depressed may look sad and complain of a loss of appetite, insomnia, lack of energy, and weight loss.

Therapeutic Management

Medical treatment is based on the etiology of the problem. Treatment of endocrine system–based sexual dysfunction may include hormone replacement or surgical intervention in the case of tumors.[42] Counseling and patient education will also be required.

Where chronic alcohol abuse has altered sexual desire, therapy is directed at treatment of the alcoholism through counseling as well as individual and group therapy, including couples therapy.[32] Psychologic problems may require counseling, and psychotherapy may be needed when psychiatric problems are the basis for the sexual dysfunction. In many cases sexual therapy will help resolve sexual desire disorders.[30]

NURSING MANAGEMENT OF THE PATIENT WITH SEXUAL DESIRE DISORDER

Assessment

The nursing assessment of a patient with sexual desire disorders includes a thorough patient history and physical examination. The history includes documentation of the individual's attitude toward sex, sexual preference, sexual desire, sexual performance, and previous sexual response patterns. The patient is asked about support systems, self-esteem, body image, and medication history.

Nursing Diagnosis

The nursing diagnoses for patients with sexual desire disorders may include one or more of the following:

Sexual dysfunction: decreased sexual desire disorder related to illness

Sexual dysfunction: decreased sexual desire disorder related to hormone imbalance

Sexual dysfunction: decreased sexual desire disorder related to depression

Sexual dysfunction: decreased sexual desire disorder related to ineffective coping

Sexual dysfunction: decreased sexual desire disorder related to substance abuse

High risk for anxiety: altered body function

Planning

The overall goals for the patient with sexual desire disorder are the presence of an increased sexual desire and the resumption of acceptable levels of sexual activity. Short-term goals include outcome criteria such as the following:

Patient will have an understanding of the factors that have had an impact on his or her sexual behavior and the treatments available for that type of problem

Patient will seek professional help for substance abuse

Patient will seek professional help for depression

Patient will reduce stressors and develop a constructive coping pattern

Patient will alter his or her life-style to allow time for more rest and relaxation

Patient will be able to discuss his or her sexual problem with significant others

Implementation

Nursing interventions for patients with sexual desire disorders are based on the identified goals. When medical treatment involves hormone replacement, careful counseling and nursing follow-up assessment should occur. Hormones are powerful chemicals and may produce profound side effects. Patients receiving hormone replacement may experience pronounced behavioral changes from their usual relatively passive behavior patterns to greater assertiveness or aggressiveness. Nursing care includes helping these patients understand the changes occurring in their feelings and how to control aggressive tendencies that could lead to antisocial acts or social humiliation. Special care should be taken to respond to the developmental needs of young adults, especially those with endocrine-related diagnoses who may have concerns regarding delayed physical development complicating their overall sexual problem.[25]

Sexual desire disorders associated with chronic alcoholism and drug abuse require nursing care directed toward assisting newly recovering patients in developing supportive relationships. Ongoing nursing care assists patients in focusing on the relationship aspect of their life before resuming sexual activity.[33]

Generally, however, nursing interventions involve gentle probing and open-ended questions about the person's life. This commonly results in the person disclosing problems of a psychic or emotional nature, allowing the nurse to intervene or make referral for sex therapy. Nonjudgmental, active listening is often the best assessment and therapeutic technique since problems that have advanced to a stage in which sexual function is impaired are often paramount in the patient's thinking. The nurse informs the patient about the therapeutic possibilities available and assists the patient in decisions regarding forms of therapy that might be helpful.

Evaluation

The nurse monitors the patient's responses to the treatment plan to ensure that it continues to meet individual needs. The nurse evaluates the success of the interventions based on whether the patient resumes sexual activity at a level that he or she perceives as acceptable.

Documentation

Accurate documentation of the history of the illness and current symptoms is essential in the determination of the etiology of the problem. The nurse documents the patient's goals for future sexual functioning in order to individualize the patient care plan. Documentation also contains information about the supportive and educational interventions provided and the patient's perception of changes that occurred in sexual patterns during the course of the treatment. Each expected outcome is also evaluated.

ERECTILE DYSFUNCTION
Definition

Erectile dysfunction may be defined as persistent or recurrent and partial or complete failure to maintain an erection until completion of sexual activity. Persistent or recurrent inability to experience excitement and pleasure during sexual activity is also characteristic of the disorder.

Etiology

Erectile dysfunction may occur in males of any age and may result from either physiologic or psychologic problems. Erectile dysfunction may eventually result in up to 25% to 60% of all males with diabetes mellitus.[12] Occlusive vascular disease, which causes diminished blood flow to the internal pudendal arteries, may also result in a partial or complete failure to attain or maintain an erection. Neurologic disease, endocrine disorders, and problems related to substance abuse may also affect the ability of the male to attain and maintain an erection.[23] External events and internal psychologic events may also result in erection problems. When males are stressed, are angry, or become preoccupied and anxious about their performance they are less likely to be able to successfully perform.[9,32,36]

Pathophysiology

It is suspected that many of the main physiologic causes for erectile dysfunction have a vascular basis. Inhibited sexual excitement has been associated with large, medium, and small vessel disease.[23] Trauma and the chemical influences of alcohol and drugs are also known to be causative or contributing factors to temporary and permanent erectile dysfunction by decreasing the neural transmissions between the brain and the sexual organs. Emotions can also inhibit neural transmissions and result in an erectile disorder.

Clinical Manifestations

Clinical manifestations may include signs and symptoms of vascular disease, cirrhosis, or chronic renal failure. The presence of an endocrine disease such as diabetes mellitus may also be identified during the physical examination. Evidence of substance abuse or trauma may be suspected after close observation of the patient. Findings from arterial blood flow and nerve conduction tests may reveal complications in those systems.

Therapeutic Management

Treatment of the disorder may be medically oriented, be psychotherapeutic, or involve surgical implantation of a penile prosthesis depending on the etiology of the problem (see Chapter 71 for further discussion of erectile dysfunction and related treatment).

NURSING MANAGEMENT OF THE PATIENT WITH ERECTILE DYSFUNCTION
Assessment

The nursing assessment contains information related to the patient's perception of previous sexual behavior, desire for a change in sexual performance, and current self-image. Additional information includes a detailed sexual history including sexual preference, history of erection problems, premature ejaculation, spontaneous morning emissions, past partners, and types of erotic stimulation used in the past. The physical examination includes information about the patient's circulatory system, nervous system, endocrine system, cardiovascular system, and anatomic anomalies of the genitalia.

Nursing Diagnosis

The nursing diagnoses for persons with erectile dysfunction may include one or more of the following:
 Sexual dysfunction: erectile dysfunction related to illness
 Sexual dysfunction: erectile dysfunction related to performance anxiety
 Sexual dysfunction: erectile dysfunction related to substance abuse
 Sexual dysfunction: erectile dysfunction related to ineffective coping
 Sexual dysfunction: erectile dysfunction related to substance abuse
 High risk for anxiety: altered body function

Planning

The overall goal for the patient with erectile dysfunction will be the resumption of normal sexual performance or the development of alternate strategies for achieving sexual satisfaction if the erection problems are irreversible. Short-term goals may include one or more of the following:
 Patient will be comfortable discussing his problem
 Patient will maintain a positive attitude toward his sexuality
 Patient will be able to understand the etiology of his erection problems and the treatments available for that type of problem
 Patient will develop strategies for dealing with his temporary erectile dysfunction
 Patient will develop alternative means for achieving sexual satisfaction if erections are no longer possible
 Patient will participate in counseling or sex therapy

Implementation

The nurse must establish a therapeutic relationship with the patient that allows for discussion of feelings, perceptions, and emotional distress. The nurse must also educate patients about alternative ways to express love and affection. The patient should be encouraged to seek appropriate professional evaluation and therapy. When medical treatment involves medications or surgery, nursing care involves helping patients understand their medication regimen and supporting patients through the perioperative period.

Evaluation

The nurse evaluates the patient's progress on the basis of expected outcomes. The patient will discuss his problem in a positive way, and he will show that he has the knowledge and skills to function sexually in a way that will bring pleasure to himself and his partner.

Documentation

Accurate documentation of the history of the illness is essential in the determination of the etiology of the problem. The nurse must also document the patient's goals for future sexual functioning in order to individualize the patient care plan. Documentation should also contain information about the supportive and educational interventions that were provided and the patient's perception of changes that occurred in his ability to attain and maintain an erection during the course of treatment. Patient comments related to interactions with significant others should also be included in the charting if they are pertinent to the treatment regimen.

FEMALE SEXUAL AROUSAL DISORDER
Definition

Female **sexual arousal disorder** is characterized by persistent or recurrent inability to become physiologically ready for sexual activity or inability to experience a subjective sense of sexual excitement or pleasure. Female sexual arousal consists of two phases: physiologic arousal and subjective arousal. Females may fail to display the physiologic signs of arousal (engorgement and lubrication) but still experience a subjective sense of readiness for sexual activity.[38] This may lead to the practitioner overlooking the real problem.

Etiology

Alterations in female arousal may be neglected because more women complain of anorgasmia.[38] However, arousal disorders may be the primary problem leading to anorgasmia. The body-mind interaction is probably where alterations in sexual arousal originate; therefore they may be either transient or prolonged. Transient alterations in sexual arousal can be traced to factors such as fatigue, anxiety, stress, and substance abuse.[38] Physiologic changes related to the long-term use of oral contraceptives and other prescription medications, chronic illness, and substance abuse may also result in a decreased sexual desire disorder for the female. Prolonged problems may have a deeper psychologic basis.

Pathophysiology

The main factor related to alterations in female sexual arousal appears to be psychogenic. The presence of strong emotional factors prevents neural impulses from getting from the brain to the vagina. Physiologic conditions may also interfere with neural transmissions or result in low energy levels. Low energy levels mean that the individual has no energy for sexual activities or anything else.

Clinical Manifestations

Clinical manifestations of female sexual arousal dysfunction frequently include vague complaints of an inability to achieve orgasm. Most patients are not aware of or do not mention the real problem, which is a lack of sexual arousal. Physical findings are frequently normal.

Therapeutic Management

Treatment of female sexual arousal disorder may include counseling and psychotherapy to discover the underlying causes. Changes in the individual's medications may be initiated, and chronic illness should be evaluated and treated. Extended sexual therapy may be necessary if the problem is long-standing.

NURSING MANAGEMENT OF THE PATIENT WITH FEMALE SEXUAL AROUSAL DISORDER

Assessment

A complete sexual history may contain clues to the presence of alterations in sexual arousal. The woman may give indications that she has been unable to become ready for sexual activity, but that fact may be lost in the health professional's focus on her lack of orgasm. Complaints of discomfort with sexual activity may also mask the fact that the woman

is unable to achieve sexual arousal. Careful listening and attention to the clues to this elusive problem are necessary to its diagnosis.

Nursing Diagnosis

The nursing diagnoses for patients with female sexual arousal disorder depend on the etiology of the problem. However, these diagnoses are common:
    Sexual dysfunction: anxiety
    Sexual dysfunction: mental trauma (i.e., spouse abuse, child sexual abuse, rape)
    Sexual dysfunction: lack of sufficient rest
    Sexual dysfunction: substance abuse
    High risk for anxiety: altered body function

Planning

The overall goal for the patient with female sexual arousal disorder will be the resumption of an acceptable level of sexual arousal so that sexual activity can be enjoyed. Short-term goals will include one or more of the following outcomes depending on the etiology of the problem:
    Patient will be able to discuss the etiology of her sexual problem
    Patient will understand the treatments available for this problem
    Patient will seek counseling or sex therapy
    Patient will alter her life-style to provide more time for rest and relaxation
    Patient will decrease the stress in her life

Implementation

The nursing care of the individual with female sexual arousal disorder is based on the ability of the nurse to form a therapeutic relationship with the patient. Patients are likely to be vague in their description of the problem and very sensitive to the responses of the nurse. The nurse must be able to sift through the general information and select relevant clues. Treatment of female sexual arousal disorder may include counseling the patient regarding the need to obtain additional rest and relaxation, stress reduction, and relief of situational anxiety. It may also include counseling related to substance abuse.[10] Prolonged forms of the problem may require psychotherapy to discover the underlying causes. Extended sexual therapy may be necessary if the problem is long-standing. Child abuse, spouse abuse, and other complicated psychologic problems that can affect sexual arousal may require long-term therapy.

Evaluation

The nurse evaluates the patient based on whether she is able to return to an acceptable level of sexual activity. The nurse also evaluates the patient on her responses to treatment and each of the outcome criteria.

Documentation

Accurate documentation of the history of the illness and the presenting symptoms is essential in the determination of the etiology of the problem. The nurse must also individualize the patient care plan based on the etiology of the problem. Documentation contains information about the supportive and educational interventions that were provided and the patient's perception of the changes that occurred in her ability to become sexually aroused during the course of the treatment. Patient comments related to interactions with significant others are also documented when pertinent.

DYSPAREUNIA AND VAGINISMUS
Definition

Dyspareunia is defined as difficulty or discomfort associated with sexual activity.[34] It may affect either sex; however, more commonly women experience the problem. **Vaginismus** is involuntary and intense muscular spasms of genital musculature that interfere with coitus.[16] Women of any age may be afflicted. The severity of the problem varies from a mild form in which discomfort is experienced but intercourse can be tolerated to highly intense pain as a result of which the vaginal orifice is so tightly clamped shut that not even a finger may be inserted.[30] In men, dyspareunia results in painful ejaculation.[31]

Etiology

The etiology of dyspareunia or vaginismus may be psychologic or physiologic. Physiologic problems may include pathologic conditions of the uterus, cervix, ovaries, or fallopian tubes in the female. In males, pathologic problems of the reproductive organs or the urinary tract may also result in dyspareunia.

Psychologic problems, such as phobias, may be at the root of either dyspareunia or vaginismus.[34] Painful or traumatic experiences such as rape or sexual molestation may also be predisposing factors. Other sources of these problems may be deep and often inaccessible, such as guilt about intercourse or erotic thoughts. Women may fear penile penetration, whereas men may fear entering the vagina. Individuals may also have health concerns that include fear of (1) pregnancy, (2) venereal disease, (3) cancer, or (4) AIDS. Finally, marital problems or anger at the partner may be present.

Pathophysiology

Psychologic problems may result in the individual being unable to relax during coitus. Fear and anxiety can inhibit arousal, which can in turn result in a lack of vaginal lubrication for the woman. Once established, the cycle of anxiety and pain can increase with each attempt at penetration. Physiologic causes include growths at the opening of the vagina (either benign or malignant), endometriosis, and other pelvic pathologic conditions, any of which may cause pain. Insufficient vaginal lubrication may lead to discomfort or pain during sexual activity. In addition, vaginal and urinary infections may result in dyspareunia.

Men may experience pain related to carcinoma of the prostate; stenosis of the ejaculatory ducts; urethritis; prostatitis; seminal vesiculitis[31]; inflammations, infections, or tumors of the testes; epididymis; and urinary or pelvic organs.[30] Allergic reactions, skin irritations, and mucous membrane sensitivity to some spermicidal jellies or creams may cause genital pain, irritation, and edema for both sexes.

Clinical Manifestations

Pelvic pathologic conditions may be found during a physical examination. Signs and symptoms of infections may also be present. The patient may appear anxious and fearful.

Therapeutic Management

Treatment depends on the etiology. Physiologic problems such as infections, allergic reactions, pelvic conditions, and growths on the genitalia are treated with appropriate medications. Often removing these causes will relieve dyspareunia. If necessary, in the case of vaginismus, vaginal dilation with relaxation exercises may be prescribed. In this treatment a set of graded dilators is introduced by the patient into the vagina according to a prescribed schedule until insertion of the largest dilator is possible.[30] Pain on ejaculation for men will be treated by treating the basic cause either medically (infection or inflammation) or surgically (prostatic carcinoma) according to the physician's decision.[31]

Women seeking assistance for alterations in sexual arousal may experience discomfort during vaginal penetration because of a lack of natural vaginal lubrication. All physiologic causes of pain must be ruled out before psychologic interventions are considered.[34] Psychologic problems should be referred to a qualified therapist or counselor for treatment. Long-term follow-up may be required to coordinate the care for this patient and prevent a recurrence of the problem.

NURSING MANAGEMENT OF THE PATIENT EXPERIENCING DISCOMFORT RELATED TO SEXUAL ACTIVITY

Assessment

A complete and careful physical examination including a pelvic examination for women and a gentle testicular, rectal, and prostate examination for men is done to determine any physical cause for pain. Laboratory examinations of blood, urine, and vaginal or penile discharges are important; if prostatic carcinoma is suspected, an acid phosphatase determination is done to check for metastasis.[19] A detailed sexual history is obtained. Attention is focused on evidence of rape or traumatic sexual incidents in the person's life. The nurse attempts to determine whether these patients have ever been able to tolerate sexual activity or if the problem has developed in relation to some specific event in their history.

Nursing Diagnosis

The nursing diagnoses for the patient experiencing discomfort related to sexual activity may include one or more of the following:

Sexual dysfunction: pain related to previous traumatic experiences

Sexual dysfunction: pain related to fear of pregnancy

Sexual dysfunction: pain related to fear of infections

Sexual dysfunction: pain related to infection

Sexual dysfunction: pain related to insufficient vaginal lubrication

Sexual dysfunction: pain related to allergic reactions

Planning

Planning is directed at assisting the patient to have sexual intercourse without pain. The outcome criteria may include one or more the following:

Patient will seek counseling or sex therapy

Patient will understand how to prevent unwanted pregnancies and infections

Patient will understand the etiology of the problem and will know what treatments are available

Patient will understand what vaginal lubrications are available and how to use them

Patient will be provided with information about vaginal products that do not cause allergic reactions

Implementation

Nursing interventions include patient teaching related to the phases of the sexual response cycle, with specific attention on methods of individual preparation for enjoying sexual expression. Teaching for female patients includes an explanation of the relationship between the use of feminine hygiene products and a decrease in natural flora and secretions in the vagina. Patient teaching also includes instructions about good hygiene practices related to the foreskin of uncircumcised males and the irritation that can sometimes develop when the male external genitalia come into contact with vaginal hygiene products and contraceptive medications. Emotional support during therapy is very important. The patient should be given uninterrupted, private time with the nurse in an unhurried atmosphere so that he or she can discuss feelings. When dilation of the vaginal orifice is part of medical therapy, careful teaching is important to prevent needless pain. The teaching plan includes information about the need for a water-soluble lubricating gel during dilation and sexual activity. New long-lasting vaginal moisturizers appear to be the best solution for decreased vaginal lubrication problems.

Evaluation

The nurse will evaluate the responses of the patient to treatment and each of the outcome criteria. The nurse will also evaluate whether sexual behavior has resumed without further pain.

Documentation

Accurate documentation of the history of the illness and the presenting symptoms is essential in the determination of the etiology of the problem. The nurse must also individualize the patient care plan based on the etiology of the problem. Documentation contains information about the supportive and educational interventions that were provided and the patient's perception of the changes in discomfort that occurred related to sexual intercourse during the course of the study.

INHIBITED FEMALE ORGASM
Definition

Alterations in orgasm in the female may be defined as "persistent or recurrent delay in, or absence of, orgasm following a normal sexual excitement phase during sexual activity of sufficient intensity, focus, and duration."[7]

Orgasm is related to sexual relief that usually accompanies, but does not always accompany, sexual activity. Although a great deal of concern surrounds the lack of orgasm, what is more important is satisfaction with the sexual experience. Both men and women can suffer from inhibited orgasm. When a total lack of orgasm is a problem in satisfying sexual expression, it is called **anorgasmia.**

Orgasmic disorders can be divided into five subgroups. Primary orgasmic disorder is present when an individual has never experienced an orgasm; secondary orgasmic failure occurs when an individual who has previously experienced orgasm experiences inhibition or loss of previously normal responses. Situational anorgasmia is diagnosed when orgasm occurs only under certain conditions. Coital anorgasmia is present when orgasm is not achieved through coitus. Finally, in random anorgasmia, there are few orgasms, which occur only in unpredictable situations.[30]

Etiology

A number of problems can lead to inhibited orgasm for the woman. Physiologic and psychologic sources are both implicated in these problems, but no particular cause is etiologic of any anorgasmic subgroup.

Pathophysiology

Physiologic causes of inhibited female orgasm include chronic endocrine diseases such as diabetes complicated by neuropathy that may render the genital organs insensitive to orgasm. Neurologic diseases such as multiple sclerosis may produce unpredictable periods of insensitivity because the disease progresses erratically.

Fatigue, anxiety, and stress are also influential in anorgasmia. Short-term disinterest in sex because of simple tiredness is frequent when an individual is heavily involved in work, family, or school activities. However, chronic fatigue and stress can disrupt the enjoyment of sex entirely and form a pattern of orgasmic dysfunction.

Discord in the couple relationship may be a factor in coital anorgasmia. Such problems as failure to communicate, hostility, fear of abandonment by the partner, ambivalence toward the relationship, and power struggles may be related problems.[45] Insensitivity, lack of skill, and unattractiveness of the partner may also result in lack of orgasms.[30,45] Substance abuse may result in orgasmic dysfunction.

Clinical Manifestations

Women with this type of disorder are usually able to describe their problem. However, in the absence of chronic disease, the physical examination generally yields few clues. The patient may appear tired, stressed, or anxious. Patients experiencing marital discord may be very emotional or express no emotions at all depending on how they are coping with the situation.

Therapeutic Management

Masters and Johnson[30] developed a method of therapy for primary orgasmic disorders that focuses on exploring sensual pleasure and assisting the person or couple to learn what stimuli are pleasurable to each other before any genital contact occurs. Engaging the whole body in nongenital pleasuring frees the couple from the need to perform until each is comfortable with the sensual aspect of their sexuality.

The treatment of primary orgasmic disorders may include exercises in self-stimulation, fantasies, relaxation, and muscle and breath control. Secondary and other forms of anorgasmia are usually treated using anxiety and stress reduction exercises and sensate-focusing exercises. Counseling and psychotherapy may be necessary when deep-seated fears and problems are involved. Therapists may treat the patient alone or may involve the partner either from the beginning or later when the patient is deemed ready.

NURSING MANAGEMENT OF THE PATIENT EXPERIENCING INHIBITED FEMALE ORGASM
Assessment

A health history includes a complete psychosexual history, which includes information about sex education, the patient's previous patterns of sexual response, and her feelings about sexual relationships and sex in general. Any instances of incest or rape, as well as homosexual and heterosexual experiences, should be elicited. The patient's ability to pleasure herself to orgasm through masturbation should be elicited. Contraceptive practices and goals for reproduction are important information. Assessments of self-esteem and body image are important elements of the health history. Finally, any history of psychiatric or psychologic disturbance or participation in therapeutic treatment programs is noted.

Nursing Diagnosis

Nursing diagnoses for the patient experiencing female orgasmic dysfunction include the following:
  Sexual dysfunction: inhibited female orgasm related to illness
  Sexual dysfunction: inhibited female orgasm related to anxiety
  Sexual dysfunction: inhibited female orgasm related to fatigue

Sexual dysfunction: inhibited female orgasm related to substance abuse

High risk for anxiety: altered body function

Planning

Planning will be related to the individualized nursing diagnoses. However, the long-term goal for the patient experiencing orgasmic dysfunction is that the patient experience orgasm. Short-term goals will depend on the etiology of the problem but may include one or more of the following:

- Patient will have an understanding of her problem and will be able to discuss it with her significant other
- Patient will maintain a positive attitude toward her sexuality
- Patient will understand the treatment for her problem
- Patient will participate in counseling or sex therapy

Implementation

The nursing care of the patient with orgasmic dysfunction is based on the ability of the nurse to form a therapeutic relationship with the patient. Patients may be shy and are likely to be uncomfortable discussing their problems, and the interview must be conducted in an area that ensures their privacy. Treatment may include counseling the patient regarding the need to obtain additional rest and relaxation, stress reduction, and the relief of situational anxiety. Information related to the mechanics of arousal and orgasm is provided. The need to communicate what feels good to the partner should be discussed. Treatment may also include counseling related to substance abuse if that is the cause of the problem. Prolonged forms of the problem may require psychotherapy to discover the underlying causes. Extended sexual therapy may be necessary if the problem is long-standing.

Evaluation

The nurse evaluates the responses of the patient to treatment and each of the outcome criteria. The nurse also evaluates whether the patient perceives that she is now able to achieve orgasm with sexual activity.

Documentation

Accurate documentation of the history of the illness is essential. Documentation should contain information about the supportive and educational interventions that were provided and the patient's percepation of the changes that have occurred in her ability to achieve orgasm since beginning treatment.

INHIBITED MALE ORGASM
Definition

Several disorders are included in the category of inhibited male orgasm. Delayed ejaculation is found when the man has a history of never having been able to ejaculate into the vagina. A secondary form of the problem occurs when ejaculatory ability has been lost.

Etiology

Most frequently, ejaculatory problems relate to fatigue, stress, the effects of alcohol and drugs, or performance anxiety. Performance anxiety has been defined as the inability to relax and "let go."

Pathophysiology

Fatigue and stress decrease the individual's energy levels. Alcohol and drugs decrease the neural transmissions between the brain and the sexual organs. Performance anxiety interferes with the individual's ability to relax.

Clinical Manifestations

The patient may present with signs of anxiety, stress, or fatigue. The use of alcohol and drugs may also be evident on examination.

Therapeutic Management

Medical treatment is based on the etiology of the problem. Where chronic substance abuse has altered sexual function, therapy is directed at treatment of the alcohol or drug abuse through counseling as well as individual and group therapy, including couples therapy. The frequency of delayed ejaculation further dictates the treatment. Rest, stress reduction, relaxation, and sensitivity exercises as defined by Masters and Johnson may help. Sexual counseling may be prescribed to treat the primary form of the disease.[30]

NURSING MANAGEMENT OF THE PATIENT WITH INHIBITED MALE ORGASM
Assessment

The nursing assessment of a patient with inhibited male orgasm includes a thorough patient history and physical examination. The history includes documentation of the individual's attitude toward sex, sexual preference, sexual desire, sexual performance, and previous sexual response patterns. The patient is asked about his support systems, self-esteem, body image, and medication history. A thorough physical assessment is done, and preexisting causes are ruled out. The nursing history includes information such as (1) whether the problem is continual or intermittent, (2) whether there has been a change in ejaculatory pattern, (3) the presence of life-style factors such as drug or alcohol abuse, or (4) the presence of stress, anxiety, or depression.

Nursing Diagnosis

Common nursing diagnoses include the following:
Sexual dysfunction: inhibited male orgasm related to substance abuse
Sexual dysfunction: inhibited male orgasm related to fatigue
Sexual dysfunction: inhibited male orgasm related to anxiety
High risk for anxiety: altered body function

Planning

Goals will depend on the etiology of the problem but may include one or more of the following:
Patient will have an understanding of his problem and will be able to discuss it with his significant other
Patient will maintain a positive attitude toward his sexual ability
Patient will understand the treatment for his problem
Patient will participate in counseling or sex therapy
Patient will experience normal ejaculatory ability

Implementation

Treatment may include counseling the patient regarding the need to obtain additional rest and relaxation, stress reduction, and the relief of situational anxiety. It may also include counseling related to substance abuse. Prolonged forms of the problem may require psychotherapy to discover the underlying causes. Extended sexual therapy may be necessary if the problem is long-standing.

Evaluation

The nurse evaluates the responses of the patient to treatment and each of the outcome criteria. The nurse will also evaluate whether the patient perceives that he is now able to achieve orgasm with sexual activity.

PREMATURE EJACULATION
Definition

Premature ejaculation is an alteration in sexual function occurring during the orgasmic phase. It can be defined as a persistent or recurrent ejaculation with minimal sexual stimulation. It may also be defined as ejaculation before, on, or shortly after penetration and before the person wishes it.[7] It is probably the most common sexual dysfunction in the male population and is related to a man's inability to properly sense the late stage of excitement.[30] Kaplan[45] has found that those who are afflicted with premature ejaculation experience an atypically steep curve of excitation resulting in uncontrollable orgasmic response.

Etiology

When premature ejaculation is present, several psychologic factors can intensify the problem or prevent its relief. Performance anxiety can block the individual's ability to prolong sexual performance. Physiologic changes such as those associated with degenerative neurologic diseases may make neuromuscular control impossible and may be the basis of the problem. For example, males with multiple sclerosis may have no sensation of approaching orgasm.[30] Inflammatory processes such as posterior urethritis and prostatitis may make the urethra so sensitive that ejaculatory control is difficult. In both of these conditions, the pain related to the inflammation may irritate the bladder and urethral mucosa, triggering ejaculation and preventing normal control.

Clinical Manifestations

Initially, a complete and thorough physical assessment is essential. In cases of infection or inflammation, generally, pain and urinary bleeding will prompt the male to seek medical assistance before premature ejaculation becomes a long-standing problem. A thorough neurologic examination is necessary when there is a pattern of erratic loss of ejaculatory control and erectile failure. Multiple sclerosis or other neurologic impairments may be detected in this examination.

Therapeutic Management

Medical treatment will be directed at the root cause of the problem. Counseling and sexual therapy are usually necessary when physiologic causes for premature ejaculation have been ruled out. Techniques to delay ejaculation were developed by Masters and Johnson.[30] In addition, newer techniques have been developed to deal with erection problems. In some settings the nurse may do the teaching. Sexual activity should be freed of all performance anxiety to ensure the greatest therapeutic effect. Drugs are not recommended to reduce premature ejaculation nor are anesthetic creams and gels.[30]

NURSING MANAGEMENT OF THE PATIENT WITH PREMATURE EJACULATION

Assessment

The nursing assessment of a patient with premature ejaculation includes a thorough patient history and physical examination. The history includes documentation of the individual's attitude toward sex, sexual preference, sexual desire, sexual performance, and previous sexual response patterns. The patient is asked about his support systems, self-esteem, body image, and medication history. A thorough physical assessment is done, and preexisting causes are ruled out. The nursing history includes information such as (1) whether the problem is continual or intermittent, (2) whether there has been a change in ejaculatory patterns, (3) the presence of life-style factors such as drug or alcohol abuse, or (4) the presence of stress, anxiety, or depression.

Nursing Diagnosis

Common nursing diagnoses include the following:
   Sexual dysfunction: premature ejaculation related to substance abuse
   Sexual dysfunction: premature ejaculation related to fatigue
   Sexual dysfunction: premature ejaculation related to anxiety
   Potential for anxiety: altered body function

Planning

Planning will be related to the individualized nursing diagnoses. However, the long-term goal for the patient experiencing premature ejaculation is that the patient experience the ability to voluntarily control ejaculation. Short-term goals will depend on the etiology of the problem but may include one or more of the following:
   Patient will have an understanding of his problem and will be able to discuss it with his significant other
   Patient will maintain a positive attitude toward his sexuality
   Patient will understand the treatment for his problem
   Patient will participate in counseling or sex therapy

Implementation

The nursing care of the patient with premature ejaculatory problems will include education about the relationship between thoughts and feelings and the sexual response cycle. If appropriate, the nurse should counsel the patient regarding the need to obtain additional rest and relaxation, initiate stress reduction, or seek relief from situational anxiety. Counseling may also be related to the contribution of substance abuse to sexual dysfunction. Prolonged forms of the problem may require psychotherapy to discover the underlying causes. Extended sexual therapy may be necessary if the problem is long-standing and related to serious conflicts in the patient's relationship with his significant other.

Evaluation

The nurse evaluates the responses of the patient to treatment and each of the outcome criteria. The nurse also evaluates whether the patient perceives that he is now able to ejaculate when he wishes.

CRITICAL THINKING QUESTIONS

1 Discuss the topic of sexual health as it relates to the individual.
2 Trace sexual health through each of the developmental phases from young adulthood through older adulthood.
3 Identify and discuss each phase of the human response cycle.
4 Identify psychologic and social biases that impede older adults in enacting their sexuality.
5 Discuss reasons that nurses should be sensitive and supportive when assisting gay and lesbian patients with sexual health issues.
6 List the basic information necessary to formulate the sexual assessment. Discuss information important to nursing assessment of specific sexual needs.
7 List and describe preventive health practices related to sexuality and reproductive health.
8 In counseling patients about contraceptives, list major factors that should be considered. Pay attention to side effects that could be physically dangerous or life-threatening. List chronic health conditions in which specific contraceptives should not be prescribed.
9 List specific sexual disorders according to when they occur in the sexual cycle. List the major medical interventions for each sexual disorder.
10 Describe nursing interventions that might make the experience more comfortable and

supportive for patients requiring treatment for sexual disorders.

BIBLIOGRAPHY

Current

1. Allen ME: A holistic view of sexuality and the aged, *Holistic Nurs Pract* 1(4):76, 1987.
2. Alzate H, Hoch Z: The "G spot" and "female ejaculation": a current appraisal, *J Sex Marital Ther* 12(3):211, 1986.
3. American Cancer Society: *Mammography found my breast cancer early,* New York, 1988, The Society.
4. American Cancer Society: *Stay healthy: learn about uterine cancer,* New York, 1989, The Society.
5. American Cancer Society: *For men only,* New York, 1990, The Society.
6. American Cancer Society: *How to do breast self-examination,* New York, 1990, The Society.
7. American Psychiatric Association: *Diagnostic and statistical manual of mental disorders,* ed 3, Washington, DC, 1987, The Association.
8. Barker LR, Burton JR, Zieve PD: *Principles of ambulatory medicine,* ed 3, Baltimore, 1990, Williams & Wilkins Co.
9. Barlow DH: Causes of sexual dysfunction: the role of anxiety and cognitive interference, *Consult Clinical Psychologists* 54:140-148, 1986.
10. Boston Women's Health Collective: *The new our bodies, ourselves,* New York, 1990, Simon & Schuster Inc.
11. Brink PJ: Cultural aspects of sexuality, *Holistic Nurs Pract* 1(4):12, 1987.
12. Bullock BL, Rosendahl PP: *Pathophysiology,* ed 2, Glenview, Ill, 1988, Scott, Foresman & Co.
13. Burnside IM: *Psychosocial nursing care of the elderly,* ed 3, New York, 1988, McGraw-Hill Inc.
14. Cox HC et al: *Nursing diagnosis,* Philadelphia, 1989, FA Davis Co.
15. Danielson R: Counseling for young men: what does it do? *Reprod Health* 22(3):115-121, 1990.
16. DeSantis L, Thomas JT: Parental attitudes toward adolescent sexuality: transcultural perspectives, *Nurse Pract* 12(8):43, 46, 48, 1987.
17. Dubay W: *Gay identity: the self under ban,* Jefferson, NC, 1987, McFarland & Co Inc. Publishers.
18. Ellis G: *Infertility: medical and social choices,* Washington, DC, 1988, Office of Technology Assessment.
19. Fishback F: *A manual of laboratory diagnostic tests,* ed 3, Philadelphia, 1988, JB Lippincott Co.
20. Gooren LJG et al: Estrogen-induced prolactinoma in a man, *J Clin Endocrinol Metabol* 66(2):444, 1988.
21. Hamwi DA: Screening mammography: increasing the effort toward breast cancer detection, *Nurse Pract* 15(12):27, 30-32, 1990.
22. Hatcher RA et al: *Contraceptive technology: 1988-1989,* ed 14, New York, 1988, Irvington Publishers Inc.
23. Heller JE, Gleich P: Erectile impotence: evaluation and management, *J Family Pract* 26:321, 1988.
24. Hitchcock JM, Wilson HS: Personal risking: lesbian self-disclosure of sexual orientation to professional health care providers, *Nurs Res* 41(3):178-183, 1992.
25. Howe CL: Developmental theory and adolescent sexual behavior, *Nurse Pract* 11(2):65, 68, 71, 1986.
26. Jarrett ME, Lethbridge DJ: The contraceptive needs of midlife women, *Nurse Pract* 15(12):34-39, 1990.
27. Jensen MD, Bobak IM: *Maternity and gynecologic care,* St Louis, 1989, Mosby–Year Book, Inc.
28. Johnson B: *Sexuality and aging.* (Unpublished manuscript.)
29. Kus RJ: From grounded theory to clinical practice: cases from gay research. In Chenitz WC, Swanson JM, editors: *From practice to grounded theory,* Menlo Park, Calif, 1986, Addison-Wesley Publishing Co Inc.
30. Masters WH, Johnson VE, Kolodny RC: *On sex and human loving,* Boston, 1988, Little, Brown & Co Inc.
31. Montague DK, Corriere NJ, Jr: Painful orgasm, *Consultant* 27:21, 1987.
32. National Institute on Alcohol Abuse and Alcoholism (NIAAA): *Alcohol and health,* Rockville, Md, 1987, The Institute.
33. Reed RC, Blaine DA: Sexual addictions, *Holistic Nurs Pract* 2(4):75, 1988.
34. Sarazin SK, Seymour SF: Causes and treatment options for women with dyspareunia, *Nurse Pract* 16(10), 1991.
35. Stuart GW, Sundeen SJ: *Principles and practice of psychiatric nursing,* ed 3, St Louis, 1987, Mosby–Year Book, Inc.
36. United States Federal Bureau of Investigation: *Uniform crime reports,* Washington, DC, 1990, US Government Printing Office.
37. Walz TH, Blum NS: *Sexual health in later life,* Lexington, Mass, 1987, DC Heath & Co.
38. Woods NF: Toward a holistic perspective of human sexuality: alterations in sexual health and nursing diagnoses, *Holistic Nurs Pract* 1(4):1, 1987.
39. Zilbergeld B: *The new male sexuality: the truth about men, sex, and pleasure,* New York, 1992, Bantam Press.

Classic

40. Addiego F: Female ejaculation: a case study, *J Sex Res* 17(1):13, 1981.
41. Butler RN, Lewis MI: *Sex after sixty,* St Louis, 1976, Mosby–Year Book, Inc.
42. Capuzzi D: Sexuality and aging: an overview for counselors, *Personnel Guidance J* 61(1):31, 1982.
43. Jacobsen L: Illness and human sexuality, *Nurs Outlook* 32(1):50, 1978.
44. Kain CD, Reilly N, Schultz ED: The older adult: a comparative assessment, *Nurs Clin North Am* 25(4):833-848, 1990.
45. Kaplan HS: *The new sex therapy: disorders of sexual desire,* vol 2, New York, 1979, Brunner/Mazel Inc.
46. Kelly S: Some social and psychological aspects of organic sexual dysfunction in men, *Sexuality Disability* 4:123-128, 1981.
47. Maslow AH: *Motivation and personality,* New York, 1954, Harper & Row, Publishers Inc.
48. Weisberg M: Developments in sexual research: a doubting ob-gyn is convinced, *Sex Med Today* 14, 1982.
49. World Health Organization: *Definition of sexual health,* New York, 1975, The Organization.

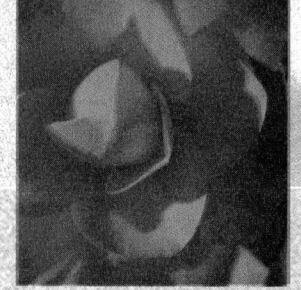

CHAPTER SEVENTY

Nursing Management of Women with Reproductive System Disorders

---

LEARNING OBJECTIVES

1 List common disorders of the female reproductive tract.
2 Identify risk factors for gynecologic disorders.
3 List common nursing diagnoses for patients with gynecologic disorders.
4 Develop a care plan for a patient undergoing gynecologic surgery.
5 Identify a treatment plan and follow-up care for patients with a specific benign gynecologic disorder.
6 Identify the two most common benign breast disorders.
7 List the risk factors for breast cancer.
8 Identify the current therapies for breast cancer.
9 List the nursing interventions for patients with metastatic breast cancer.

KEY TERMS

DISORDERS OF THE female reproductive system encompass primary and secondary sex organs. The impact of these disorders for the woman is far reaching; beyond the physical alterations, the patient experiences a threat to her self-concept, body image, and sexuality. The woman's image of herself as a sexual being is affected by the diseases and their treatment. The treatment outcomes also affect the patient's family. The nurse plays a major role in teaching women about measures for prevention, risk factors, early detection, and treatment of the disorders.

Disorders of the Female Genital Tract

VULVOVAGINITIS

Definition

Vulvovaginitis is an inflammation of the vulva and vagina. Normally, the vagina is protected from infection by its pH of 3.5 to 4.5, the presence of Doderlein's bacillus, which is a normal part of the vaginal flora, and the hormone estrogen.

Etiology

If the vaginal pH is altered, if the invading organisms are numerous, or if the woman's resistance is decreased by aging, malnutrition, stress, disease, or the use of broad-spectrum antibiotics, her risk of infection is increased (see box for other risk factors). Those risk factors explain why some women harboring infectious organisms, including *Candida albicans, Trichomonas vaginalis, Neisseria gonorrhoeae, Chlamydia* species, and the herpes simplex virus (see Chapter 11 for a discussion of specific organisms), develop an infection whereas other women are resistant.

RISK FACTORS FOR VULVOVAGINAL INFECTIONS

Dermatologic allergies
Use of broad-spectrum antibiotics
Diabetes mellitus
Frequent douching
Intercourse with an infected partner
Low estrogen levels
Poor perineal hygiene
Tight, nonabsorbent, and heat-retaining clothing

Epidemiology

Organisms causing infection of the vulva and vagina are usually introduced from outside sources, such as clothing, hands, or douche nozzles, or during sexual intercourse. In sexually active women, reinfection may occur after treatment unless their sexual partners are also treated. Women of menopausal and postmenopausal age are often predisposed to atrophic or senile vaginitis. Decreased estrogen production causes thinning of the vaginal mucosa and makes vaginal secretions more alkaline, changing the vaginal pH and allowing the invasion of organisms. Pyogenic bacterial invasion of the thin vaginal mucosa produces symptoms of burning, pruritus, and leukorrhea.

Clinical Manifestations

The common signs of infection of the vulva and vagina are inflammation of the tissues; abnormal discharge from the vagina, urethra, or Bartholin's glands; and itching. The discharge may be purulent, white, curdlike, greenish yellow, or grayish white. Each of the organisms that cause vaginitis is usually associated with a specific type of vaginal discharge, and each might produce slightly different symptoms. Itching is common to most organisms but is usually especially intense in the vulva with *Trichomonas vaginalis* infection. Severe itching may also be present because of menopausal changes in the epithelium, high urinary sugar content as a result of diabetes mellitus, allergies, irritation from a chronic discharge, or cancer of the vulva. With severe pruritus, there are usually excoriations of the skin caused by scratching, and secondary infection may result. Diagnostic studies for vulvovaginitis include direct visual examination of the vulva and vagina, culture of the organism, and bimanual examination to assess for inflammation of the vagina and its surrounding tissues. Dysuria may occur as a consequence of local irritation of the urinary meatus.

Therapeutic Management

Vulvar and vaginal infections can be treated by a variety of methods. The major goals are to cure the infection, prevent reinfection, prevent complications, and prevent infection of the sexual partner or partners. Vaginitis is usually treated with warm douches, such as 1 tablespoon of vinegar mixed with 1 quart of water. An estrogen preparation, given orally or applied intravaginally, may help to restore the vaginal epithelium to a normal state. However, because of the link between estrogen use in menopausal women and endometrial cancer, this therapy should be used with caution. Abscesses require incision and drainage, which are usually done at the time the woman first seeks medical attention. Some lesions may require biopsy, and antibiotics may be given if systemic effects of another infection are present. Relief from pain occurs almost immediately after incision and drainage. However, the woman may experience soreness for a day or two.

NURSING MANAGEMENT OF THE PATIENT WITH VULVOVAGINITIS

Assessment

Ask the patient to give a history of her symptoms, including duration and attempts at relief, as well as information about sexual practices and signs of infection in the sexual partner. Predisposing factors, patterns of repeated infections, and additional underlying medical problems must be identified. The vulva and vagina are inspected and palpated. A smear or culture may also be taken.

Nursing Diagnosis

Possible nursing diagnoses may include the following:

  Knowledge deficit related to vulvovaginitis
  High risk for impaired skin integrity related to vulvar infection and vaginal drainage on the perineal skin
  Discomfort related to pruritus, burning, and leukorrhea

Planning

The woman is able to do the following:

  Patient implements habits that improve or promote health
  Patient explains how infections occur and are spread
  Patient explains ways to prevent reinfection
  Patient identifies choices for therapy and their expected results
  Patient expresses feeling of comfort
  Patient remains free from infection or seeks appropriate treatment when symptoms occur

Implementation

Douching is frequently prescribed for treatment of vaginal infections, but local applications of vaginal suppositories, ointments, or creams are also common. The nurse advises the woman of the importance of washing her hands before and after each application. Because the substances used to treat vaginitis melt with body heat, the patient should lie down after insertion to help distribute the medication in the vaginal canal and to prevent loss of medication from the vagina. These medications are best administered at bedtime. The patient should wear a sanitary pad, not a tampon, as long as she is being treated for the infection. Heat increases circulation, promotes healing, and provides comfort. Applications of heat may be prescribed in the form of douches, perineal irrigations, or sitz baths, and the patient may require instruction in these procedures (see patient education guide).

Most women who have vaginal infections are asked to abstain from sexual intercourse during the period of treatment. The male partner's use of a condom until symptoms of infection disappear may be suggested. The patient is also advised that her sexual partner should be treated if infection recurs.

Ongoing Care

The patient assumes responsibility for self-care. With patients who have recurrent vulvovaginal infections, risk factors as well as proper hygienic care should be discussed fully and as often as necessary.

PELVIC INFLAMMATORY DISEASE

Definition

Pelvic inflammatory disease (PID) is an infection of the fallopian tubes, ovaries, pelvic peritoneum, pelvic veins, or connective tissue. The infection may be confined to one structure, or it may involve all of the pelvic structures. Inflammation of the fallopian tube is known as salpingitis, and inflammation of the ovary is known as oophoritis.

Etiology/Epidemiology

The infection is usually bacterial, but it may also be caused by a virus, fungus, or parasite. It may

PATIENT EDUCATION GUIDE

Perineal Care

Instruct the patient to do the following:
1. Wash hands.
2. Fill perineal bottle with solution of half hydrogen peroxide and half warm water.
3. Sit on commode.
4. Squeeze perineal bottle containing solution over perineal area starting from front to back.
5. Pat area dry, using 4- × 4-inch gauze or toilet tissue and wiping in one direction from front to back. A hair dryer on cool setting may be used to dry area if it is too sore to touch.
6. Perform perineal irrigations in the morning and at bedtime or more often as desired.
7. Wash hands.

be acute, subacute, recurrent, or chronic and may be localized or widespread. *Gonococcus, Chlamydia, Haemophilus, Streptococcus, Mycoplasma,* and anaerobes can cause severe or recurrent salpingitis (see Chapter 11 for a discussion of specific organisms). These organisms invade the pelvic organs during sexual intercourse, childbirth, the postpartum period, or abortion. The rupture of structures adjacent to the uterus may spill organisms into the pelvic cavity, thus causing an infection. PID is reported to occur five times more often among women using intrauterine devices than among those using other methods of birth control.

Risk factors are important considerations in the clinical management and prevention of upper genital tract infections. The menstruating teenager who has multiple sexual partners, does not use contraception, and lives in an area with a high prevalence of sexually transmitted disease has the highest risk. Seventy-five percent of PID cases occur in women less than 25 years of age. Hospitalized women, who usually have a decreased resistance to infection, are also at risk for PID. Surgery on the reproductive tract, childbearing, and abortion all lower resistance and provide portals of entry for pathogens. To prevent PID and its serious consequences, it is important to prevent infections of the vulva, vagina, and cervix and to treat promptly any infections that occur. Cleanliness and asepsis are essential.

Pathophysiology

Pathogenic organisms are usually introduced from the vagina, ascending through the cervical canal into the uterus. They pass into the pelvis by the fallopian tubes through thrombosed uterine veins or through the lymphatics of the uterus. Many of the organisms causing PID lodge in the fallopian tubes. The terms salpingitis and PID are often considered synonymous. Adhesions form, and strictures or sterility may result. Infertility is one of the most serious consequences of PID. Obstruction of the fallopian tubes resulting from inflammation may be complete or partial. Complete obstruction of the tubes makes conception impossible. Partial tubal obstruction predisposes the woman to ectopic pregnancy, because although the sperm have been able to pass through the stricture, the fertilized ovum cannot reach the uterus. Although generalized peritonitis can occur, the infection usually remains confined to the lower abdomen and the pelvis. An abscess in the cul-de-sac of Douglas is common. Other complications include bacteremia with septic shock and thrombophlebitis with possible embolization.

Clinical Manifestations

Signs and symptoms of PID include severe abdominal pain or pressure, lower abdominal cramping, intermenstrual spotting, metrorrhagia, dyspareunia (painful intercourse), fever and chills, malaise, nausea, and vomiting. Sometimes a foul-smelling, purulent vaginal discharge may also be present. The symptoms last for a variable period of time and may temporarily subside. Some cases of PID are never reported to a nurse or physician. Diagnostic studies for PID include a culture and Gram stain of purulent secretions and laparoscopic or ultrasonographic visualization of the pelvic inflammation. Leukocyte count and erythrocyte sedimentation rate are also assessed to confirm an infectious process.

Therapeutic Management

During a physical examination, most sexually active women should have a routine cervical smear or culture taken to screen for gonorrhea. Women need to be educated about preventing infection, recognizing infection in their sexual partners, and what to do when they suspect that infection has occurred (see Chapter 11). The goal of therapy is to control and eradicate the infection by preventing the infection from spreading to other body systems in the patient or to other persons. Even before the specific infective organism is determined, the patient is placed on broad-spectrum antibiotic therapy. Women with mild to moderate infections are usually treated as outpatients; however, patients who are acutely ill may be hospitalized.

NURSING MANAGEMENT OF THE PATIENT WITH PELVIC INFLAMMATORY DISEASE
Assessment

The nurse assesses the patient for abdominal and pelvic pain, low back pain, dyspareunia, metrorrhagia, constipation, dysuria, malaise, nausea and vomiting, vaginal drainage, and pruritic vulva. Other signs of PID include identification of the organism through culture or Gram stain of purulent secretions, elevated leukocyte count, increased erythrocyte sedimentation rate, visualization of inflammation through laparoscopic examination, visualization of abscess or inflammation through ultrasonography, rebound tenderness in abdomen, normal bowel sounds progressing to ileus in untreated persons, excoriation of vulva from vaginal discharge, and elevated temperature.

Nursing Diagnosis

Possible nursing diagnoses may include the following:

Knowledge deficit related to PID

High risk for fluid volume deficit related to nausea and vomiting

High risk for impaired skin integrity related to excoriation of the vulva from vaginal drainage and pruritus

High risk for pain related to generalized peritonitis

Altered sexuality patterns related to the possibility of spreading infection during intercourse

Planning

The woman with PID is able to do the following:

Patient verbalizes knowledge about PID

Patient identifies appropriate treatment regimens for PID

Patient complies with treatment regimen

Patient verbalizes relief of pain

Patient explains the rationale for increased fluid intake during the infectious process

Patient explains the cause of vaginal drainage and pruritus if present

Patient shares concerns regarding her sexual partner as a possible source of infection

Implementation

In the hospital, patients are usually placed on bed rest in semi-Fowler's position to provide dependent drainage so that abscesses will not form high in the abdomen where they might rupture and cause generalized peritonitis. Intravenous fluids may be indicated. It is recommended that sexual partners of women with PID be treated as possible sources of infection. Analgesics may be necessary to alleviate pain. The amount, color, and odor of vaginal discharge and changes in pain level are assessed and the temperature monitored every 4 hours until fever subsides. Catheterization and use of tampons are avoided to prevent the spread of infection (see patient education guide).

Evaluation

The patient reports no lower abdominal pain and no vaginal drainage, pruritus, inflammation, or excoriation of the vulva. The patient remains afebrile and takes medications at the time and dosage prescribed. She describes the symptoms of PID and shows her intent to notify a health care provider if symptoms recur.

Documentation

Assessment data, nursing interventions, and validation of patient teaching are put in the patient's record.

Ongoing Care

The patient verbalizes preventive measures for recurrence of PID. Follow-up care and teaching for the patient with PID emphasize the patient's ability to verbalize her intent to prevent venereal disease if PID is caused by gonorrhea or *Chlamydia* organisms; to avoid douching, intercourse, or use of tampons for at least 1 week after completion of therapy; to ask the sexual partner to be examined; to describe the symptoms of PID; and to notify the health care provider if symptoms recur.

PATIENT EDUCATION GUIDE   *Pelvic Inflammatory Disease*

The patient and significant other should be informed about the following:

1. The effects of PID on general health and on the functioning of the reproductive organs
2. The method by which organisms gain entry into the body (e.g., during sexual intercourse or after pelvic surgery, abortion, or childbirth) and how the infection spreads
3. The greater susceptibility to PID caused by use of intrauterine devices
4. The treatment regimen for PID, including the medications prescribed
5. Proper perineal care, especially wiping from front to back
6. The importance of follow-up observation as needed and of yearly gynecologic examinations

Patients should also be taught the following:

1. To avoid frequent douching, which reduces natural flora that combat infectious organisms
2. To avoid strong soaps, bubble baths, sprays, powders, and deodorants, which may be irritating to the perineal skin
3. To wear clean, loose-fitting cotton undergarments
4. To wear pads or tampons no longer than 6 hours, preferably changing them every 4 hours
5. To remove diaphragms within 6 hours after insertion
6. To insist that a sexual partner wear a condom if there is any possibility of infection
7. To report to the physician signs, such as the return of symptoms and any unusual vaginal discharge or odor

TOXIC SHOCK SYNDROME
Definition

Toxic shock syndrome (TSS), first identified in the late 1970s, is an acute bacterial infection caused by the bacterium *Staphylococcus aureus.*

Etiology/Epidemiology

TSS usually occurs in women who are menstruating, using tampons (particularly superabsorbent tampons), and changing tampons less frequently than every 6 hours. Women at increased risk for TSS include those who insert tampons with their fingers rather than with the inserters provided with many brands of tampons; those who have had a chronic vaginal infection; and those with genital herpes. TSS has also occurred in nonmenstruating women and in men and has been associated with cellulitis, surgical wound infections, and subcutaneous abscesses.

Pathophysiology

With TSS, *Staphylococcus* bacteria from the vagina or cervix enter the uterus and then the bloodstream. Tampons, especially when they are absorbent and not changed often, provide an environment for the bacteria to multiply and produce poisonous toxins. It is unclear whether TSS is caused by a direct effect of secreted toxin on host cells, endogenous mediators released by a toxin, or other factors. The role of blood, magnesium, and other heavy metals and tampon components in producing the toxin is even less clear.[4]

Clinical Manifestations

Most women experience a prodromal flulike illness for the first 24 hours. Between days 2 and 4 of the menstrual period, the patient may experience symptoms such as a sudden high fever (up to 102° F [38.9° C]), vomiting, diarrhea, myalgia, hypotension, and signs suggestive of the onset of septic shock. Sore throat, headache, and a red macular palmar or diffuse rash followed by desquamation of the skin of the hands and feet often develop. Urinary output is decreased, and the urea nitrogen level becomes elevated. Disorientation may occur from dehydration and the release of toxins; pulmonary edema and inflammation of the mucous membranes may also occur. Blood tests indicate leukocytosis, thrombocytopenia, and elevated levels of bilirubin, urea nitrogen, creatinine, serum glutamic oxaloacetic transaminase (SGOT), serum glutamic pyruvic transaminase (SGPT), and creatine phosphokinase (CPK). Blood and urine cultures should be taken along with throat cultures when appropriate, and vaginal and cervical specimens should be evaluated.[61]

Therapeutic Management

Treatment of TSS varies because of the range in type and severity of symptoms. However, because all isolates of *S. aureus* from persons with TSS have been penicillin resistant, beta lactamase–resistant penicillins or cephalosporins are usually administered. A basic aspect of medical care is to carefully look for and document symptoms as they develop. It is important to observe the conjunctiva for reddening and the skin for redness and rash, to maintain a record of fluid status including measurement of vomitus and diarrhea for replacement therapy and of urine for signs of renal failure, and to look for swelling and impaired mobility in the joints and for peripheral edema. Evaluate laboratory data for electrolyte imbalance secondary to vomiting and diarrhea, elevated BUN suggesting renal impairment, elevated enzymes reflecting hepatic dysfunction, and decreased platelet count indicating possible disseminated intravascular coagulation (DIC).

NURSING MANAGEMENT OF THE PATIENT WITH TOXIC SHOCK SYNDROME
Assessment

When taking the patient's history the nurse determines if the patient has recently used tampons. The nurse notes what kind she used, how long she used a single tampon before changing it, and whether she noted any problems when inserting the tampon. Assess the patient also for symptoms of TSS, including the presence of a high fever, myalgia, vomiting, diarrhea, sore throat, headache, and fatigue. Assess the extremities for edema. Check the palms and soles for the presence of an erythematous rash. Desquamation and sloughing usually occur 1 to 2 weeks after the rash. Note the patient's level of consciousness, as well as the presence of disorientation or any intermittent confusion. Hypotension, nonpurulent inflammation of the conjunctiva, and hyperemia of the oropharynx and vagina are also signs of TSS.

Nursing Diagnosis

Nursing diagnoses may include the following:
    Anxiety related to TSS
    High risk for fluid volume deficit related to vomiting and diarrhea
    Pain related to myalgia
    High risk for injury related to possible disseminated intravascular coagulation
    Altered renal/gastrointestinal tissue perfusion related to the disease process

Planning

The woman with TSS is able to do the following:

Patient verbalizes reduction of anxiety and emotional stress

Patient experiences less vomiting and diarrhea

Patient verbalizes relief of discomfort

Patient experiences fewer complications

Patient verbalizes awareness of self-care measures

Implementation

The patient is placed on bed rest and given antibiotics. Close monitoring of vital signs and fluid status is important. If there is respiratory distress, oxygen therapy is instituted. Since disseminated intravascular coagulation (DIC) has been observed in patients with TSS, the nurse assesses the patient for hematomas, petechiae, cyanosis, oozing from puncture sites, and coolness of the fingers and toes.

Evaluation

Vaginal cultures are negative for the organism. The patient no longer has any symptoms of TSS and demonstrates knowledge of TSS and the intent to practice behaviors that will prevent reinfection.

Documentation

Documentation of care of the TSS patient involves recording of the assessment data, the nursing interventions, and the patient teaching of signs and symptoms to report to a health care provider as well as knowledge of preventive measures.

Ongoing Care

Women who are menstruating and develop a sudden high fever accompanied by vomiting or diarrhea are counseled by the nurse to seek immediate medical treatment. If the woman is wearing a tampon, she should remove it immediately. Since the use of tampons during menstruation has been linked to TSS, it is recommended that superabsorbent tampons not be used. If tampons are used, women should alternate their use with pads, change them frequently (every 4 hours), and insert them carefully to avoid abrasions. Applicators with rough edges should not be used. Patients who have TSS are instructed not to use tampons. Teach the patient the following:

To avoid using tampons until clearance from a physician

To wash hands thoroughly before inserting a tampon

To avoid the use of high-absorbency tampons

To change tampons frequently during the day and to wear sanitary napkins at night

To report signs of recurrence to a health care provider immediately

ABNORMAL UTERINE BLEEDING

Definition

Abnormal uterine bleeding is often termed infrequent uterine bleeding, excessive bleeding, prolonged menses, or intermenstrual bleeding. Infrequent uterine bleeding is defined as oligomenorrhea if the intervals between bleeding episodes vary from 35 days to 6 months and defined as amenorrhea if there are no menses for at least 6 months. **Hypermenorrhea** is excessive bleeding at the time of the regular menstrual flow. **Metrorrhagia** is the appearance of uterine bleeding between the regular menstrual periods or after menopause.

Etiology

In younger women, hypermenorrhea may be attributable to endocrine disturbances, but in older women it is usually attributable to inflammatory disturbances or tumors of the uterus. Emotional or psychologic disturbances may also affect bleeding. A woman with hypermenorrhea should inform her gynecologist. The severity of hypermenorrhea is usually estimated in terms of numbers of pads or tampons used in excess of those used for the regular menstrual flow. Metrorrhagia merits early diagnosis and treatment, since it may be symptomatic of cancer or benign tumors of the uterus.

Pathophysiology

Abnormal uterine bleeding is usually divided into two major categories: organic and dysfunctional (en-

---

DIAGNOSTIC STUDIES FOR UTERINE BLEEDING

Complete blood count: to determine degree of anemia

Thyroid function tests: to assess thyroid function

Dilation and curettage: to assess endometrium for carcinoma, polyps, etc.

Hysterogram: to identify endometrial polyps, leiomyomas, endometrial carcinoma, adnexal masses

Hysteroscopy: to identify intrauterine abnormalities

Endocrine profile: to assess functioning of the adrenal glands, ovaries, and pituitary glands

Tests confirming ovulation

   Endometrial biopsy

   Basal body temperatures

   Examination of cervical mucus

   Cytologic examination of consecutive vaginal smears

   Serum or urine progesterone levels

docrinologic). The organic causes can be subdivided into systemic disease and reproductive tract disease. Systemic disorders include leukemia, severe sepsis, idiopathic thrombocytopenic purpura, and von Willebrand's disease. Reproductive tract disorders include complications of pregnancy such as an incomplete abortion or ectopic pregnancy, trophoblastic disease, and malignancies of any part of the genital tract. After organic and systemic causes of the abnormal bleeding are ruled out, the diagnosis of **dysfunctional uterine bleeding (DUB)** can be made (see box for diagnostic studies). In most patients with DUB, ovulation fails to occur. There is continuous estradiol production without corpus luteum formation. The estrogen stimulation leads to a continuously proliferating endometrium. The most common causes of amenorrhea are diminished body fat seen in female athletes and women with anorexia nervosa.

Clinical Manifestations

The clinical manifestations of abnormal uterine bleeding are listed in the box below.

Therapeutic Management

After routine speculum examination and pelvic examination, the primary methods used to diagnose these gynecologic causes of hypermenorrhea and metrorrhagia are endometrial biopsy and dilation and curettage (D & C). In the absence of an organic cause of abnormal uterine bleeding, it is preferable to use medical instead of surgical treatment if the patient wants to retain her uterus for future child-

bearing. Several methods are accepted for treatment of DUB, including estrogens, progestins, nonsteroidal anti-inflammatory agents, antifibrinolytic agents, and danazol. Progestin therapy is usually the treatment of choice for patients with DUB because it reestablishes ovulation. Medroxyprogesterone acetate in a dosage of 10 mg daily for 10 days each month is a therapeutic regimen that produces regular bleeding on withdrawal in patients with adequate amounts of endogenous estrogen to cause endometrial growth.

NURSING MANAGEMENT OF THE PATIENT WITH ABNORMAL UTERINE BLEEDING

Assessment

Early diagnosis and prompt management are necessary if reproductive and genital problems are to be prevented. Areas to be assessed include the following:

1. Bleeding: amount of menstrual flow, presence of bleeding between periods, regularity of menstrual cycle
2. Pain: presence and severity of menstrual cramps or pain with menses, midcycle cramping or pain suggestive of ovulation
3. Vaginal secretions: color and consistency, especially at midcycle
4. Presence of anemia
5. Psychosocial concerns

Nursing Diagnosis

Nursing diagnoses include the following:
  Body image disturbance related to DUB
  Pain related to menstrual cramping
  Sexual dysfunction related to DUB

Planning

The woman with DUB is able to do the following:
  Patient demonstrates adaptive responses to self-concept
  Patient verbalizes pain controlled with analgesics
  Patient communicates to her partner concerns related to sexual dysfunction

Implementation

The nurse interprets the meaning of the uterine bleeding for the patient and encourages the woman to express her feelings. The nurse explains the importance of recording dates, type of flow, and number of sanitary pads or tampons used. Further, she teaches the patient pain-relieving techniques and explains the importance of sharing concerns with her partner.

COMMON TYPES OF ABNORMAL UTERINE BLEEDING AND CAUSES

Midcycle spotting: midcycle estradiol fluctuation associated with ovulation

Delayed menstruation with excessive bleeding: anovulation or threatened abortion

Frequent bleeding: pelvic inflammatory disease, endometriosis, anovulation, DUB

Profuse menstrual bleeding: cervical and endometrial polyps, DUB, intrauterine device, leiomyomas

Intermenstrual or irregular bleeding: endometrial polyps, uterine or cervical cancer, DUB, oral contraceptive use

Postmenopausal bleeding: endometrial hyperplasia, estrogen therapy, or endometrial cancer

Evaluation

The patient demonstrates adaptive responses to self-concept; states that she has discussed sexual concerns with her partner; keeps a record of bleeding dates and amount of flow; and uses analgesics as prescribed, achieving comfort.

Documentation

Record the amount of menstrual flow (number of pads or tampons used), date of last menstrual period, presence of metrorrhagia, regularity of cycle, and presence and severity of menstrual cramps. Patient teaching and evidence of learning are also documented.

Ongoing Care

The causes of abnormal bleeding differ in women during the childbearing years compared with postmenopausal women. In the latter group, carcinoma is one of the most common reasons for uterine bleeding. Women of all ages need to be educated about the importance of follow-up care when dysfunctional uterine bleeding is first detected.

PREMENSTRUAL SYNDROME
Definition

Premenstrual syndrome (PMS) is the presence of somatic and psychologic symptoms during premenstruum or early menstruation with the absence of postmenstrual symptoms. Identical symptoms must occur in three consecutive cycles to confirm a diagnosis of PMS.

Etiology

The exact cause of PMS is unknown. However, PMS may be related to decreasing estrogen and progesterone concentrations. Other theories suggest vitamin deficiencies, excessive prostaglandins, abnormal magnesium metabolism, endorphin malfunction, and multiple psychologic disturbances.[12] Symptoms vary widely from one woman to another and from one cycle to the next in the same person. A generally stressful life appears to intensify physical symptoms. PMS has been reported in more than 25% of all reproductive age groups, but women more than 30 years of age are most likely to seek treatment. This could indicate that symptoms increase with age, aging enhances one's sensitivity to the symptoms of PMS, or women over 30 years old have better access to health care.[21]

Pathophysiology

The pathophysiologic cause of PMS is unknown.[30]

RESEARCH BRIEF

Winter E, Ashton D, Moore D: Dispelling myths: a study of PMS and relationship satisfaction, *Nurse Pract* 16(5):34-45, 1991.

Twenty-six PMS patients and twenty-six non-PMS patients completed three questionnaires about satisfaction with personal relationships. Statistically, PMS patients reported significantly more dissatisfaction with marital and sexual relationships. No differences linked to age were found. These findings may assist nurses in assessing and treating patients with PMS more effectively.

Clinical Manifestations

Symptoms may include behavioral changes (tension, irritability, mood swings, anxiety, crying, depression, insomnia), fatigue, signs of water and sodium retention (edema, weight gain, breast enlargement and tenderness, and abdominal bloating), palpitations, increased appetite, headache, and backache.

Therapeutic Management

PMS has no single treatment and no specific medication. Some physicians prescribe pain relievers, diuretics, and progesterone. The patient's diet is reviewed, and a high-protein, well-balanced diet is suggested.

NURSING MANAGEMENT OF THE PATIENT WITH PREMENSTRUAL SYNDROME
Assessment

Assess the patient for tension, irritability, mood swings, anxiety, crying spells, depression, insomnia, fatigue, and food cravings. Other symptoms may include weight gain, breast tenderness, oliguria, diarrhea or constipation, styes, headache, vertigo, and backache.

Nursing Diagnosis

Nursing diagnoses may include the following:
Anxiety related to PMS
Knowledge deficit related to PMS and its management

Planning

The woman is able to do the following:
Patient verbalizes that her symptoms are temporary and not related to a disease

Patient identifies therapies to minimize symptoms of PMS

Implementation

The nurse assists women with PMS by acknowledging the existence of the syndrome and its symptoms, which may be severe for some women. Because some women have been made to feel that the symptoms are nonexistent or exaggerated, the nurse encourages patients to keep a menstrual symptom calendar to document the cycle and nature of the symptoms. Encourage women to plan activities during the symptom-free part of their cycles.

The patient also assumes responsibility for following a dietary plan that may minimize the symptoms of PMS. This plan includes eating small meals and eliminating or restricting sugar, alcohol, caffeine, and nicotine. Supplements of vitamin B_6, calcium, and magnesium may be prescribed. Daily exercise and relaxation are encouraged. Self-help groups and literature help some women gain some control over their bodies. Group support also tends to reduce stress.

Evaluation

The patient verbalizes her symptoms of PMS, acknowledges that the symptoms are temporary, and lists therapies to minimize the symptoms of PMS.

DYSMENORRHEA

Definition

Dysmenorrhea is uterine pain with menstruation, commonly called "menstrual cramps."

Etiology

Primary dysmenorrhea unassociated with any pelvic pathologic condition usually develops when ovulatory function is established (less than 20 years of age), and there is no underlying organic disease. Often it will disappear or decline after pregnancy or by the woman's late 20s. Secondary dysmenorrhea is painful menstruation caused by organic disease such as pelvic inflammatory disease or endometriosis and most often occurs in women older than 20 years of age (see box above).

More than 50% of menstruating women have some degree of dysmenorrhea, with 5% to 20% of women being incapacitated.[48] Studies in industries and schools have shown it to be the greatest single cause of absenteeism among women. It affects 10% of high school girls each month, and an estimated 140 million work hours are lost annually.[34] It is one of the most common health problems for which women seek treatment. Dysmenorrhea has been re-

CAUSES OF SECONDARY DYSMENORRHEA
Endometriosis Pelvic infection Endometrial or endocervical polyps Leiomyomas Cervical stenosis Congenital abnormalities Use of an intrauterine device (IUD)

ported to be significantly increased among mothers and sisters of women with dysmenorrhea.

Pathophysiology

Primary dysmenorrhea is produced by a high concentration of uterine prostaglandin that stimulates the frequency and strength of uterine contractions, which cause the pain.

Clinical Manifestations

Besides the primary pain of the uterine contractions, many women also have systemic symptoms of breast tenderness, abdominal distention, nausea and vomiting, headache, dizziness, palpitations, perspiration, and hot flashes. The systemic effects are thought to result from prostaglandin absorption into the bloodstream. Secondary dysmenorrhea is suspected if dysmenorrhea begins after the age of 20 years. Secondary dysmenorrhea is described as a steady or cramping pain and may be specific to the site of pelvic disorder. Diagnostic studies to rule out organic causes for dysmenorrhea include pelvic examination, laparoscopy, dilation and curettage, and hysterosalpingography. Conditions that cause general debilitation such as inadequate diet, minimal exercise, anemia, and fatigue are often related to dysmenorrhea.

Therapeutic Management

Treatment of secondary dysmenorrhea is aimed at the organic cause. Surgical and pharmacologic interventions may be appropriate, depending on the severity and type of pathologic condition. If no organic cause of dysmenorrhea can be found, the woman is instructed to exercise and eat nutritious foods, especially those high in fiber, to avoid constipation. Local application of heat and mild analgesics are prescribed. Aspirin is a prostaglandin inhibitor that causes vasodilation of blood vessels, thereby increasing the blood flow and relieving ischemia, increasing the rate of menstrual flow, and decreasing hypertonus of the muscles. Prostaglandin inhibitors like ibuprofen and naproxen are effective when begun at the onset of menses. Oral contraceptives are also used to suppress ovulation by inhibiting prostaglandin levels.

NURSING MANAGEMENT OF THE PATIENT WITH DYSMENORRHEA

The nurse assesses the woman for colicky and cyclic pain or dull pain in the lower pelvis radiating toward the perineum and back. Pain may be experienced 24 to 48 hours before menses or at the start of menses, and dysmenorrhea may also be associated with symptoms of premenstrual syndrome.

The nurse teaches the woman to use pain-relieving techniques such as relaxation, local application of heat, and abdominal massage. The woman is instructed about the effective dosage and administration of prostaglandin antagonists or other medications.

Good posture, exercise, and good nutrition can decrease the incidence of dysmenorrhea. Positive attitudes can be encouraged; a woman who regards menstruation as normal is less likely to experience it as an illness. Women who are unable to engage in activities because of dysmenorrhea are urged to seek health care.

MENOPAUSE AND CLIMACTERIC
Definition

The **climacteric,** which lasts for 12 to 18 months, is a normal and self-limiting transitional phase between reproductive and nonreproductive ability. Climacteric is characterized by menses becoming scanty, irregular, and spaced further apart until they cease. Menopause is said to have occurred when there has been no menstrual flow for 1 year (although some women have periods even after 1 year of amenorrhea). Natural menopause may occur between 35 and 60 years of age, with the average age at 52 years. If a woman stops menstruating before 40 years of age, the condition is called premature ovarian failure.

Etiology

Factors associated with early menopause are excessive exposure to radiation, poor general health, breast feeding, inadequate spacing between pregnancies, frequent spontaneous or therapeutic abortions, and hypothyroidism with severe obesity. Cessation of menstruation may be artificially induced by irradiation of the ovaries, surgical removal of both ovaries, or hysterectomy. In addition, surgical removal of both ovaries results in the more pronounced physiologic changes characteristic of menopause. When the uterus is removed and the ovaries are left in place, menstruation ceases, but the ovaries continue to produce estrogen and progesterone, provided climacteric has not been reached.

Pathophysiology

During the climacteric there is a gradual decline in ovarian function, since the ovaries gradually cease to produce ova and estrogen. The lack of ovarian function produces amenorrhea and sterility. Women can enjoy sexual activity during climacteric and menopause, since sexual function does not depend on the release of ova or hormones.

Clinical Manifestations

Approximately 10% of women have pronounced symptoms during menopause as a result of hormonal changes. Vasomotor reactions such as hot flashes or flushes are associated with a lack of estrogen, increased levels of luteinizing hormone, increased prostaglandins, and high levels of follicle-stimulating hormone.

Hot flashes are felt as waves of warmth accompanied by perspiration and flushing of the skin, especially in the face, neck, and arms. Situations that increase heat production such as exercising, experiencing excitement, eating, drinking alcoholic beverages, or wearing warm clothing may induce hot flashes. Hot flashes are the most common symptom for which menopausal women seek treatment (about 75% of all women experience them). Lasting from seconds to minutes, they are usually most disturbing during sleep and may be associated with feelings of dizziness, chills, chest pains, and inability to concentrate. Obese individuals are less likely to develop hot flashes, since they do not have as great a decrease in estrogen levels.

Decreased hormones cause thinning of the vaginal mucosa. Consequently, many women may have dyspareunia, vaginal dryness, burning, itching, and occasional bleeding after menopause. The lack of estrogen causes vaginal secretions to become more alkaline, leading to an increase in vaginal infections.

Estrogen helps retain calcium in the bone. With menopause and the gradual decrease in estrogen, there is a depletion of bone mass. Osteoporosis is defined as a reduction in the quantity of structural bony material, characterized by reductions in the bone mineral content and bone calcium. Women begin to lose bone at a rate of 0.75% to 1.0% per year between the ages of 30 and 35 years. The rate of loss increases with age; by the time women reach menopause they may be losing from 2% to 3% yearly. About 1 out of every 4 women more than 65 years of age will develop osteoporosis. This number is expected to increase as the population ages.[27]

Therapeutic Management

There is much debate about the advantages and disadvantages of postmenopausal estrogen replacement therapy. The increased risk of endometrial cancer with estrogen therapy has been documented, but adding progestin minimizes this increased risk.[19] Only a few studies have demonstrated a relationship between estrogen use and breast cancer. However, current research indicates that oral estrogen use will not increase this risk; yet it is recommended that a mammogram be obtained to rule out subclinical breast cancer before estrogen therapy is initiated. Estrogen therapy has been effective in treating hot flashes, vaginal atrophy, and osteoporosis, and in protecting against heart disease.

Typically, oral estrogen therapy is administered cyclically; that is, 0.625 mg of conjugated equine estrogen is taken from days 1 to 25, and 10 mg of medroxyprogesterone acetate is taken from days 15 to 25. Thereafter, this cycle is repeated. It is usually best to use the lowest dose possible that relieves symptoms, with the goal of gradual and complete withdrawal of medication. Absolute contraindications to estrogen replacement therapy are cerebrovascular, gallbladder, liver, and pancreatic disease; sickle cell anemia; and a history of myocardial infarction, deep vein thrombosis, pulmonary embolism, or estrogen-dependent tumors of the uterus or breast. Transdermal estradiol (Estraderm) is also being evaluated as a long-term modality for osteoporosis.

Calcium absorption declines with age as well as with estrogen deficiency, prompting some physicians to recommend prophylactic use of 1000 to 1500 mg/day of calcium, especially in patients with osteoporosis. However, this is still an area of controversy. Calcium supplementation does not cause hypercalcemia or renal stones in healthy people, but it can exacerbate constipation. Calcium supplements are available in many forms, but the generic calcium carbonate products are the most cost effective.

NURSING MANAGEMENT OF THE PATIENT DURING CLIMACTERIC
Assessment

Assess the patient for symptoms of menopause including hot flashes (flushes), night sweats, and diaphoresis; insomnia, vertigo, and fatigue; lack of appetite or weight gain, and abdominal fat deposition; nausea or vomiting, headache, palpitations, and tachycardia; irritability, nervousness, depression, crying spells, forgetfulness, and difficulty in concentrating; and dyspareunia, decreasing labial fat, de-

PATIENT EDUCATION GUIDE

Kegel Exercises

Kegel exercises are performed to help strengthen and tighten muscles that support the pelvic organs. These muscles (pelvic floor) are used to stop the flow of urine. To perform Kegel exercises while standing or sitting, tighten the pelvic floor muscles as hard as you can. Hold for 5 seconds, then release. Repeat at least 10 times. This exercise can be done many times throughout the day. Next lie with your back on the floor and place a pillow under your knees. With your ankles crossed squeeze your buttocks together, drawing in the anus, as if to prevent a bowel movement. Keep your knees pressed firmly together. Hold for 5 seconds, then relax. Repeat at least 10 times.

creased size of vagina, reduction in breast size, and loss of pubic and axillary hair.

Nursing Diagnosis

Nursing diagnoses for the menopausal woman may include the following:

Knowledge deficit related to menopause

Self-esteem disturbance related to the aging process and menopause

Alteration in comfort related to hot flashes, diaphoresis

Altered patterns in sexuality related to decreased libido and atrophic vagina

Planning

The woman undergoing menopause is able to do the following:

Patient explains the physiologic process of climacteric and menopause

Patient expresses to the nurse any concerns about femininity, sexuality, and aging

Patient verbalizes feelings of comfort

Patient verbalizes satisfying sexual relationships

Implementation

Education regarding menopause should precede its onset. Most women have heard of the "change of life." However, the negative image of menopause is reinforced by the media, health professionals, and the general public. Many women appreciate opportunities made by nurses to discuss menopause. Women approaching menopause need to know what

 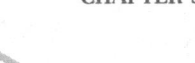

PATIENT EDUCATION GUIDE *Menopause*

Emphasize the following factors:

1. The climacteric period is normal and self-limiting.
2. A nutritious diet and weight control will improve the physical condition. Reduce calories as needed; increase intake of calcium, phosphorus, and vitamin D; avoid red meats, coffee, tea, chocolate, and excess alcohol.
3. An exercise program (such as 45 minutes of exercise three times per week) promotes vitality.
4. Interest and participation in activities will help decrease anxiety and tension.
5. Menopause does not end the patient's sex life.
6. Side effects of estrogen replacement therapy include weight gain, nausea, vomiting, unusual vaginal bleeding, and breast lumps. Report to a health professional any bleeding that occurs 6 months or more after the last menstrual period.

7. Skin creams and lotions can be used to prevent drying, itching, and cracking skin.
8. Breast self-examination should be performed monthly.
9. Calcium intake must be monitored, since calcium requirements increase as the woman ages. Milk and calcium supplements may be necessary to offset osteoporosis.
10. To prevent pregnancy, contraceptives should be used for 1 year after the last menstrual period. Since menstrual cycles are irregular, the rhythm method is an unreliable method of birth control.
11. For itching or burning vulvar areas, a prescription can be obtained for a cortisone cream.
12. Perineal muscle tone and bladder control can be improved by practicing Kegel exercises daily (see box).
13. A water-soluble lubricant should be used to prevent dyspareunia during coitus.
14. An annual physical examination is important for maintaining good health.

it is, why it occurs, what effect it has on reproductive and sexual ability, what can be done to make it more comfortable, and what symptoms require medical attention.

The nurse and the patient plan an exercise program in which movement and weight-bearing are emphasized. Walking is an excellent weight-bearing exercise that prevents the accelerated bone loss of immobility. Other beneficial exercises are bicycling, stationary cycling, and aerobic dancing. The patient avoids activities such as jogging that add pressure to weight-bearing joints.

Because falls are often an immediate cause of osteoporosis-related fractures, fall prevention is important. The proper use of assistive devices and the need to assess the home for such hazards as throw rugs and poorly lighted stairs can protect the patient from fall-related fractures (see patient education guide).

Evaluation

The patient verbalizes the process of climacteric and menopause; the importance of exercise, eating a well-balanced diet, avoiding fatigue, and continuing contraception; and an understanding of prescribed medications. The patient is able to discuss alterations in body image and self-concept resulting from menopause, and she identifies adaptive responses to

these changes and verbalizes a movement toward acceptance of the physiologic and psychologic changes associated with menopause.

Documentation

Record the menopausal symptoms and physiologic changes the woman is experiencing, and note the patient teaching and the woman's understanding of menopause and of the desired health behaviors.

Ongoing Care

Many communities today have women's centers with special programs directed toward menopausal women. Self-help networks are being formed. Many colleges have an increased enrollment of older women students and are trying to respond to their special needs. In the past the few books available about menopause were written by physicians. Today scores of popular books are available. All of these activities represent ways in which women are coping in a positive way with problems that occur during menopause. Education serves to teach a woman what to expect during menopause and how to deal with problems that may occur. Self-help and discussion groups help some women redefine themselves and find better ways to relate to family members. Proper diet and exercise are also important in stressful situations. Women who establish good health practices will be better able to manage problems that arise.

ENDOMETRIOSIS
Definition

Endometriosis is a condition in which endometrial cells, which normally line the uterus, are seeded throughout the pelvis and extend to the umbilicus (Figure 70-1).

Etiology/Epidemiology

Endometriosis appears to be increasing, although this may be a result of better diagnosis. It is not known how endometriosis develops.

There is some evidence that women have about a sevenfold greater chance of developing endometriosis if a sister or mother has it. The highest incidence of endometriosis is among white women, 25 to 35 years of age, who are in higher socioeconomic classes and postpone childbearing until the later reproductive years.

Endometriosis is a disease not only of great individual variability, but also of contrasting pathophysiologic processes. It is a benign disease yet has the characteristics of a malignancy: it is locally infiltrative, invasive, and widely disseminating. There may also be an inverse relationship between the extent of pelvic endometriosis and the severity of pelvic pain. Women with extensive endometriosis may be asymptomatic, whereas women with minimal endometriosis may have incapacitating pain.

Clinical Manifestations

Endometriosis usually progresses gradually and first becomes symptomatic in the woman between 30 and 40 years of age. The characteristic symptom of endometriosis is pelvic pain and discomfort that occur 1 to 2 days before menstruation and last 2 to 3 days. They may be unilateral or bilateral and may radiate to the lower back, legs, and groin. Other symptoms of endometriosis are a feeling of fullness in the lower abdomen, dyspareunia, hypermenorrhagia, irregular menstrual cycles, exhaustion, and poor general health. Advanced disease may cause no symptoms at all. Approximately 40% to 50% of women with endometriosis are infertile, and the disease is sometimes first detected when a woman seeks medical attention because of an inability to conceive. Laparoscopy with a biopsy of the lesions may confirm the diagnosis.

Therapeutic Management

The response of endometriosis to treatment is still variable and poorly understood. Antiovulatory drugs that induce a state physiologically similar to pregnancy and hence suppress menstruation are frequently prescribed. Oral contraceptives with potent progestins and minimal estrogen are used to produce endometrial atrophy and to decrease the endometrial flow into the peritoneal cavity. However, irregular bleeding, as well as the symptoms of early pregnancy such as nausea, vomiting, depression, and fatigue, may still occur.

Synthetic androgens that suppress ovarian activity such as danazol may be prescribed. Danazol is used to arrest proliferation of the endometrium, to prevent ovulation, and thus to produce atrophy of the ectopic endometrium. Side effects from this expensive therapy may include hot flashes, mild acne, oily skin, a dry vagina, depression, and weight gain.

Some women find that endometriosis disappears spontaneously, and some women who become pregnant remain asymptomatic after their pregnancy. For minimal symptoms, treatment with mild analgesics may be sufficient. Regular pelvic examinations are recommended to monitor the progression of endometriosis.

When the involvement is severe, surgery may be necessary. A laparoscopy may be performed to remove endometrial implants and to lyse adhesions. Lasers may be used to vaporize the small implants of endometrial tissue, thereby destroying them. A total hysterectomy, oophorectomy, and salpingectomy may also be done. Removal of the ovaries prevents further bleeding of endometrial implants that cannot be removed. If the woman is premenopausal and the ovaries are removed, very small amounts of estrogen may be given. The disease is incurable, but menopause stops its progression.

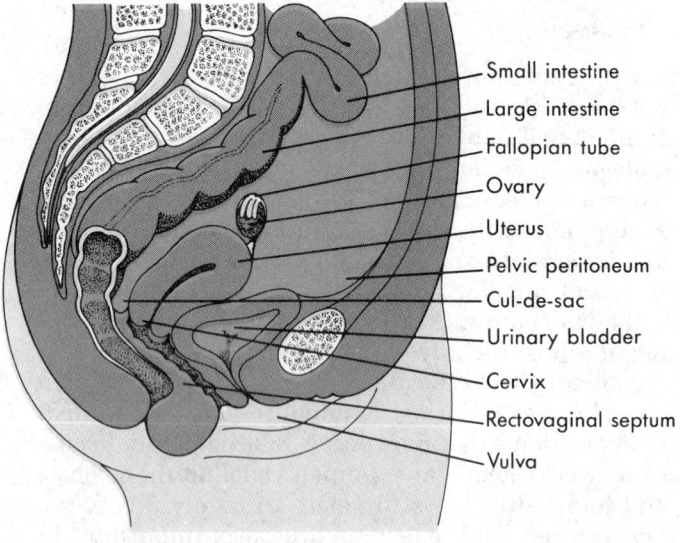

- Small intestine
- Large intestine
- Fallopian tube
- Ovary
- Uterus
- Pelvic peritoneum
- Cul-de-sac
- Urinary bladder
- Cervix
- Rectovaginal septum
- Vulva

FIGURE 70-1　Common sites of endometriosis.

NURSING MANAGEMENT OF THE PATIENT WITH ENDOMETRIOSIS

Assessment

Ask the patient to give a history of her symptoms, including pelvic pain with menstruation, aching, cramping, bearing-down sensation in the pelvis or lower back, dyspareunia, and hypermenorrhea.

Nursing Diagnosis

Possible nursing diagnoses are as follows:
> Knowledge deficit related to endometriosis
> Pain related to endometriosis
> Situational low self-esteem related to endometriosis

Planning

The woman with endometriosis is able to do the following:
> Patient explains the causes and treatment of endometriosis
> Patient verbalizes pain control with analgesics
> Patient demonstrates adaptive responses to self-concept and self-esteem

Implementation

The nurse reinforces the physician's explanation of the expected results of treatment, teaches the patient pain-relieving techniques, instructs the patient about the dosage and possible side effects of prescribed medications, emphasizes the importance of receiving regular checkups and reporting any abnormal vaginal bleeding, and encourages the patient to express her feelings. Encouraging the woman not to delay childbearing may necessitate a different family planning schedule. The nurse provides support and listens as the patient discusses these concerns.

The characteristic symptom of endometriosis is pain and discomfort accompanying menstruation that become progressively worse. The fact that such pain was not present at the onset of menses alerts the nurse to encourage the patient to see a gynecologist at once. Many women with severe pain related to menstruation have been labeled as neurotic, when in fact they have been suffering from endometriosis. The nurse is in a key position to reassure these patients and help them with adaptive responses to self-concept.

LEIOMYOMA
Definition

Leiomyomas, or fibroid tumors of the uterus, are benign tumors arising from the muscle tissue of the uterus. They include myomas, fibromas, and fibromyomas.

Etiology/Epidemiology

It has been estimated that 20% to 25% of women more than 30 years of age develop uterine fibroid tumors (myomas). They are more common in black women and in women who have never been pregnant. Because their growth is stimulated by ovarian hormones, uterine fibroids tend to disappear spontaneously with menopause. They rarely become malignant.

Pathophysiology

The cause of uterine myomas is unknown. Because they regress after menopause, it has been suggested that they are stimulated by estrogen. The size and number of myomas vary. Most are found in the body of the uterus, but some occur in the cervix or may involve the broad ligament. When the growths are larger, they may produce actual uterine enlargement. Submucosal tumors may impinge on blood vessels of the endometrium and cause bleeding. As they grow larger, they may impinge on the opposite uterine wall and distort the cavity of the uterus as well.

Clinical Manifestations

The symptoms related to myomas are primarily pressure from an enlarging pelvic mass: pain (including dysmenorrhea), abnormal uterine bleeding, infertility, and pregnancy complications (including abortion, premature labor, and dystocia). The severity of symptoms is often directly related to the number, location, and size of the myomas. However, most women are asymptomatic. Diagnostic tests for leiomyomas may include a pregnancy test, dilation and curettage, laparoscopy, and ultrasonography. The pregnancy test rules out pregnancy as a cause of symptoms. Dilation and curettage detect submucosal leiomyomas, whereas laparoscopy visualizes subserous leiomyomas. The ultrasonography differentiates between inflammatory masses or endometriosis from lower pedunculated or subserous leiomyomas.

Therapeutic Management

The treatment of fibroid tumors depends on the symptoms and the age of the patient, whether more children are desired, and how near the woman is to menopause. If the symptoms are not severe, the woman may simply need close health supervision. If the tumor is near the outer wall of the uterus, a myomectomy (surgical removal of the tumor) may be performed. This operation leaves the muscle walls of the uterus relatively intact. If bleeding or obstruction is severe, a hysterectomy may be necessary. Occasionally, if surgery is contraindicated or the

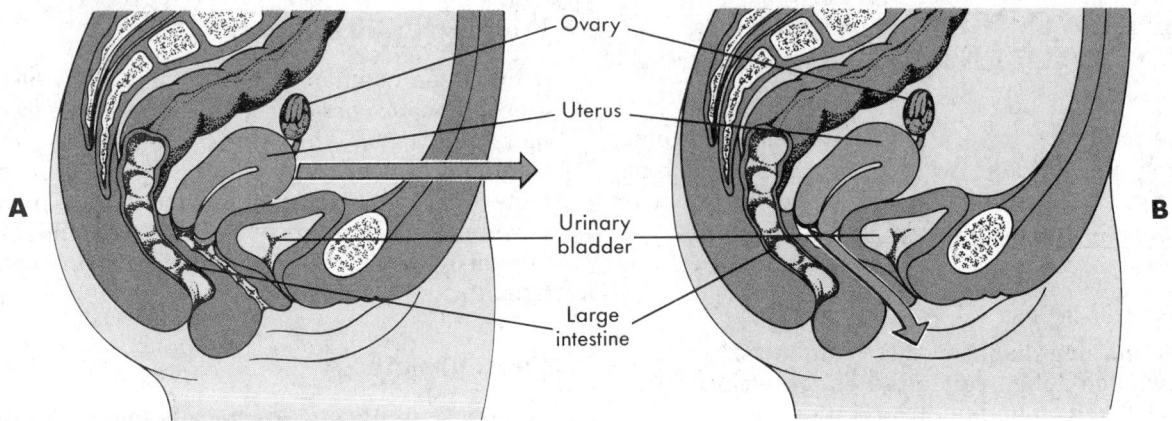

Ovary

Uterus

Urinary
bladder

Large
intestine

FIGURE 70-2   In an abdominal hysterectomy, **A,** uterus is removed through an abdominal incision. In a vaginal hysterectomy, **B,** uterus is removed through vagina. There is no abdominal incision.

woman is approaching menopause, radiation may be used to reduce the size of the tumor and to stop vaginal bleeding.

Small, symptomless leiomyomas do not require treatment. However, regular pelvic examinations are important to see if the leiomyoma is growing too large. After menopause, when estrogen levels decline, leiomyomas tend to get smaller.

Hysterectomy

A hysterectomy, an operation to remove the uterus and the cervix, is performed for many conditions, such as dysfunctional uterine bleeding, endometriosis, malignant and nonmalignant growths of the uterus and cervix, and problems of pelvic relaxation and prolapse. With total hysterectomy the entire uterus is removed. Estrogens are still released, and menopause will occur naturally. A total abdominal hysterectomy with bilateral salpingo-oophorectomy (TAH-BSO) includes the removal of the uterus, fallopian tubes, and ovaries. Beyond TAH-BSO, a radical hysterectomy also removes the pelvic lymph nodes. Because the ovaries are removed with these last two operations, menopause is surgically induced. In all cases the vagina remains intact, and intercourse is possible even though childbearing is not.

A hysterectomy can be performed from two surgical approaches. The abdominal approach is used if the fallopian tubes and ovaries are to be removed or if it is necessary to explore the pelvic cavity (Figure 70-2). A vaginal hysterectomy approach is used when the uterus is prolapsed or when the patient is unable to tolerate abdominal surgery. In this case there is no abdominal incision; the uterus is removed through the vagina.

NURSING MANAGEMENT OF THE PATIENT WITH LEIOMYOMA
Assessment

Ask the patient to give a history of her symptoms, which may include dull, aching, colicky pain; acute pain if torsion of a pedunculated leiomyoma has occurred; cramps; dysmenorrhea; pelvic fullness or heaviness; constipation; urinary frequency or urgency; and hypermenorrhea.

Nursing Diagnosis

Possible nursing diagnoses are as follows:
   Pain related to leiomyomas
   Self-esteem disturbance related to the presence of leiomyomas

Planning

The woman with leiomyoma is able to do the following:
   Patient verbalizes pain controlled with analgesics
   Patient demonstrates adaptive responses to self-concept and self-esteem if a hysterectomy is performed

Implementation

The nurse working with a patient who has leiomyoma should do the following:
   1. Reinforce the physician's explanation of treatment plan
      a. Myomectomy to preserve uterus for childbearing in young women
      b. Total hysterectomy
      c. Pelvic examinations at regular intervals to monitor status of leiomyoma

NURSING CARE PLAN   *Hysterectomy Patients*

Nursing diagnosis/ Expected outcome	Interventions	Rationale
Knowledge deficit related to perioperative period • *Patient will verbalize preoperative teaching and perioperative routines*	Obtain feedback of patient's knowledge of surgery and preoperative routines Clarify any misconceptions related to outcome of the surgical procedure (i.e., sexual myths, "sex life is over," "dry up like a prune," "constant mood swings") Provide information related to surgically induced menopause Allow time for questions from both patient and her partner Provide emotional support and reassurance to patient and her partner	A patient's concerns, fears, and unanswered questions will affect her physical and mental recovery
Fluid volume deficit related to internal hemorrhage • *Patient will be free from continuous bright red bleeding from incisional site or sites*	Assess vital signs every 4 hours for 48 hours and then every shift Assess incision and vagina for bleeding and drainage every 4 hours Record number of pads used per shift Monitor laboratory values (hemoglobin, hematocrit) for anemia	Internal hemorrhage is a major complication that causes circulating blood volume loss and fluid volume depletion
Altered peripheral tissue perfusion related to bed rest, thrombophlebitis • *Patient will be free of signs of thrombophlebitis*	Assess legs for redness, increased temperature, tenderness along vein, severe cramping, and Homan's sign every shift Assess proper placement of antiembolic stockings every 4 hours if ordered Remove antiembolic stockings for 30 minutes twice daily Do not elevate bed at knee gatch Assist in passive and active leg exercises every shift	Manipulation and trauma of pelvic blood vessels during surgery predispose patient to thrombophlebitis Postoperative pain also inhibits patient from normal activities and increases risk of thrombophlebitis Interventions are aimed at enhancing circulation and increasing venous blood return
Pain related to abdominal incision or gas pains • *Patient will verbalize effective pain control*	Assess patient's pain history (include prior pain medication, dosage, frequency, and response) Assess postoperative pain and medication 1 or 2 hours following administration Administer analgesia before ambulation	Adequate pain relief is important to enable patient to be out of bed and avoid complications of immobility

Knowledge deficit concerning self-care after discharge
 	
• *Patient verbalizes full understanding of restrictions, diet, wound care, pain control, and limitations in sexual activity*
	Patient/family education:
	  Avoid tampons or douches until approved by physician
	  Avoid sexual intercourse until approved by physician; it will be permitted once healing of abdominal wound and vaginal vault has occurred (approximately 4 to 6 weeks)
		To provide a complete recovery and prevent complications, woman who has undergone hysterectomy needs to know what changes she should expect in herself and what care she needs when she goes home

Continued.

NURSING CARE PLAN   *Hysterectomy Patients—cont'd*

Nursing diagnosis/ Expected outcome	Interventions	Rationale
	Limit stair climbing for 1 to 2 weeks and gradually increase to normal Limit heavy housework and lifting of heavy objects for 4 weeks (objects that cannot be lifted with one hand are considered heavy objects) Maintain fluid intake of at least 2000 mL/day Maintain high-protein diet to promote healing Notify physician if temperature is above 101° F or if redness, pain, or swelling occurs at suture line Take mild oral analgesics to maintain pain control	
Body image disturbance after surgery as evidenced by decrease in self-esteem, perception of self as asexual *Patient verbalizes adaptation to altered body image as evidenced by absence of weeping, irritability, verbalization of discomfort with present body, and attempt at difficult physical or mental tasks despite limitations*	Encourage expression of feelings regarding loss of uterus, "I'm wondering how you feel about having had your uterus removed." Identify normal reactions to total abdominal hysterectomy, "Many women become concerned about their femininity or womanhood after they have had this surgery." Encourage short-term, realistic goals: "How about planning a manicure for tomorrow morning?" Encourage constructive use of support systems 　Exchanging feelings with partner: "Have you shared your feelings with your husband?" 　Clarifying partner's perception of surgical experience: "How do you think the surgical experience will affect your wife?"	Hysterectomy is often accompanied by some degree of emotional upset; women may worry about sterility, mutilation, losing sexual attractiveness, and cancer; grief-like responses to loss of a body part may occur

2. Teach the patient pain-relieving techniques
3. Instruct the patient about the dosage of prescribed medications and possible side effects
4. Instruct the patient with hypermenorrhea to include extra iron in her diet to prevent iron-deficiency anemia that may occur because of blood loss
5. Emphasize the importance of regular checkups to monitor the status of leiomyoma
6. Encourage the patient to express her feelings and assist her with appropriate coping measures

Care of the patient undergoing a hysterectomy is given in the nursing care plan. The average hospital stay for a hysterectomy varies according to the type of hysterectomy performed; however, it is usually 3 to 10 days. Depending on the medical condition of the patient and on the type of hysterectomy performed, the patient may enter the hospital the day before or the day of surgery.

Evaluation

Pain-relieving techniques and analgesics are effective. The patient expresses her feelings about the diagnosis and treatment plan and identifies possible coping strategies.

Documentation

Assessment data and nursing interventions are recorded with validation of the patient's knowledge of leiomyomas and comprehension of the subject matter taught.

Ongoing Care

Before discharge, tell the patient that her body will need several weeks to fully recover, and she will probably tire easily. Low-impact exercise such as walking, frequent breaks, and rest periods will be helpful. If an abdominal incision was used, strenuous physical activities such as heavy housework (vacuuming) and heavy lifting (anything over 10 lb) are to be avoided until approved by the physician. The patient's physician informs her when she can start having sexual relations and begin douching. Sexual relations can be resumed about 4 to 6 weeks after a total abdominal hysterectomy and 2 to 3 weeks after a vaginal hysterectomy. Discuss sexuality information with the patient.

Serosanguineous vaginal drainage is normal for about 2 to 4 weeks after an abdominal hysterectomy. Initially the drainage is bloody and continuous, and it then diminishes to serous and spotty before completely stopping. Teach perineal care to patients with vaginal drainage. The patient will have no dietary restrictions other than those she might have had for other medical reasons before surgery. A well-balanced diet will promote healing. Encourage the patient to avoid wearing tight clothing such as a girdle or knee-high hose, which might constrict circulation to the surgical site and cause venous stasis. Signs of infection to report to the physician if they occur are as follows:

1. Redness, swelling, drainage, or increased soreness along the surgical incision site
2. Increased or odorous vaginal discharge or bleeding
3. A temperature of 101° F (38.3° C) or more
4. Any urinary problems such as burning or difficulty urinating, frequent urination, or passing small amounts of urine

CERVICAL POLYPS
Definition/Etiology

Endocervical and cervical polyps are the most common benign growths of the cervix. Cervical polyps are grapelike growths that form when an area of the cervical mucosa proliferates and are seen most often in multiparous women in their 40s or 50s.

Pathophysiology

Cervical polyps generally arise from the endocervical tissue but occasionally are found on the outer cervix, or ectocervix. These growths are usually visible at the cervical os as bright red, vascular, fragile areas. They are most often pedunculated and appear to protrude from the cervical canal. Polyps may occur singly or in clusters and can be from a few millimeters up to 4 cm in diameter.

Clinical Manifestations

Bleeding is a common symptom because of the vascularity of the polyp. The characteristics of the bleeding associated with polyps closely resemble the signs of early cervical cancer. The amount of bleeding is small and occurs between menstrual periods. Also, contact bleeding produced by coitus, douching, or vaginal examination may occur.

Therapeutic Management

The pedicle by which the polyp is attached is quite small so that the polyp can easily be removed by twisting the pedicle at its base or using biopsy forceps or a sharp curette. Tissue examination of the removed polyp is important, since epidermoid cancer arises from cervical polyps in a small percentage of cases.

NURSING MANAGEMENT OF THE PATIENT WITH CERVICAL POLYPS

Assess the amount of bleeding before polyp removal, and counsel the patient after the results of the tissue examination.

ENDOMETRIAL POLYPS
Definition/Etiology

Endometrial polyps are localized overgrowths of endometrial glands and stroma that project beyond the surface of the endometrium. Polyps occurring in the endometrium are associated with endometrial hyperplasia. This is most often a result of excess estrogen. Endometrial polyps occur most frequently in premenopausal women when anovulatory cycles become more frequent. They may also result from the use of exogenous estrogen therapy for menopausal symptoms. Women with anovulatory cycles throughout their menstrual life are also susceptible.

Pathophysiology

Endometrial polyps are soft and pliable and may be single or multiple. Most polyps arise from the fundus of the uterus. They vary from a few millimeters to several centimeters in diameter (Figure 70-3).

Clinical Manifestation/Therapeutic Management

Endometrial polyps are frequently asymptomatic. If present, symptoms include intermenstrual or postmenopausal spotting or bleeding. A woman with persistent, irregular bleeding should have a dilation and curettage (D & C). If polyps are found, they can usually be removed by the use of polyp forceps.

Dilation and curettage

The most common method of obtaining endometrial cells for study is dilation and curettage (D & C). This procedure is done to obtain endometrial or endocervical tissue for histologic examination of a suspected malignancy, to study the influence of ovarian hormones on the endometrial cells in evaluating causes of infertility, to treat excessive uterine bleeding, to induce abortion, or to prevent hemorrhage after a spontaneous incomplete abortion by removing early products of conception. Preoperative care includes informing the woman what will be done and why and preparing her for anesthesia. The D & C can be performed with the patient under local or general anesthesia, depending on the patient's age, health

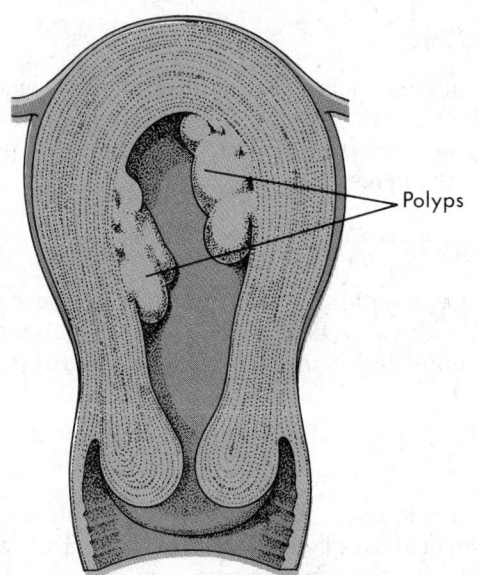

FIGURE 70-3   Endometrial polyps.

status, and ability to cooperate and on the indication for the procedure.

For a D & C, metal dilators of graduated sizes are inserted into the cervical canal. Once the cervix is dilated, curettes having a sharp surface are used to remove endometrial tissues (Figure 70-4). The operation takes between 30 and 60 minutes. The major complications of a D & C are hemorrhage and perforation of the uterus. Postoperative uterine bleeding and pelvic and back pain are normal.

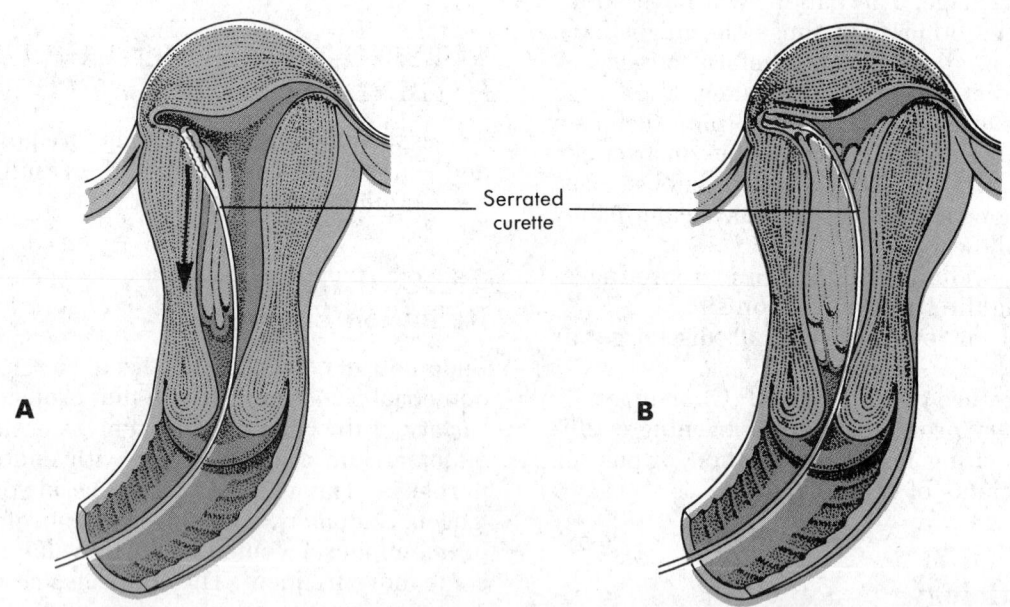

FIGURE 70-4   Dilation and curettage of uterine cavity. **A,** Anterior, posterior, and lateral walls are curetted with curette followed by, **B,** top of cavity.

NURSING MANAGEMENT OF THE PATIENT UNDERGOING DILATION AND CURETTAGE

Postoperatively, assess for excessive bleeding and give analgesics for the pelvic discomfort. Most women are discharged on the day of surgery or the following day. Normal daily activities can be resumed, although vigorous exercise is discouraged. Patients are instructed not to have sexual intercourse, not to douche, and not to wear tampons for 1 week. If the woman is taking birth control pills, she is to continue to take them as prescribed. Her menstrual cycle will continue as before, and the possibility of pregnancy will remain. All vaginal bleeding should disappear in 7 to 10 days. Women are instructed to report recurrence of vaginal bleeding or the development of a vaginal discharge with odor.

UTERINE DISPLACEMENTS
Definition/Etiology

The uterus and the cervix normally lie at a right angle to the long axis of the vagina, with the body of the uterus tilted slightly forward. However, the uterus is freely movable because of the requirements of pregnancy. Uterine displacements (Figure 70-5) are simple uterine anatomic variations with no clinical significance. The most common variation is retroversion, which may be acquired after childbirth or may be congenital.

Pathophysiology/Clinical Manifestations

Uterine displacements may be caused by the weakening of pelvic muscles. The displacements may be retrograde, with retroversion or retroflexion, or forward, with anteflexion or anteversion. Uterine displacements may be uncomfortable. The woman with a retrograde displacement may complain of fatigue, backache, muscle strain, and leukorrhea. Uterine displacements may cause dysmenorrhea and infertility. The displacements are diagnosed by pelvic examination and x-ray films.

Therapeutic Management

The displacements may be corrected by muscle strengthening exercises, support of the uterus by a pessary, or surgical shortening of uterine ligaments. Pessaries (Figure 70-6) are instruments of hard rubber or plastic that maintain the uterus in a forward position by exerting pressure on ligaments that are attached to the posterior wall of the cervix. Surgery

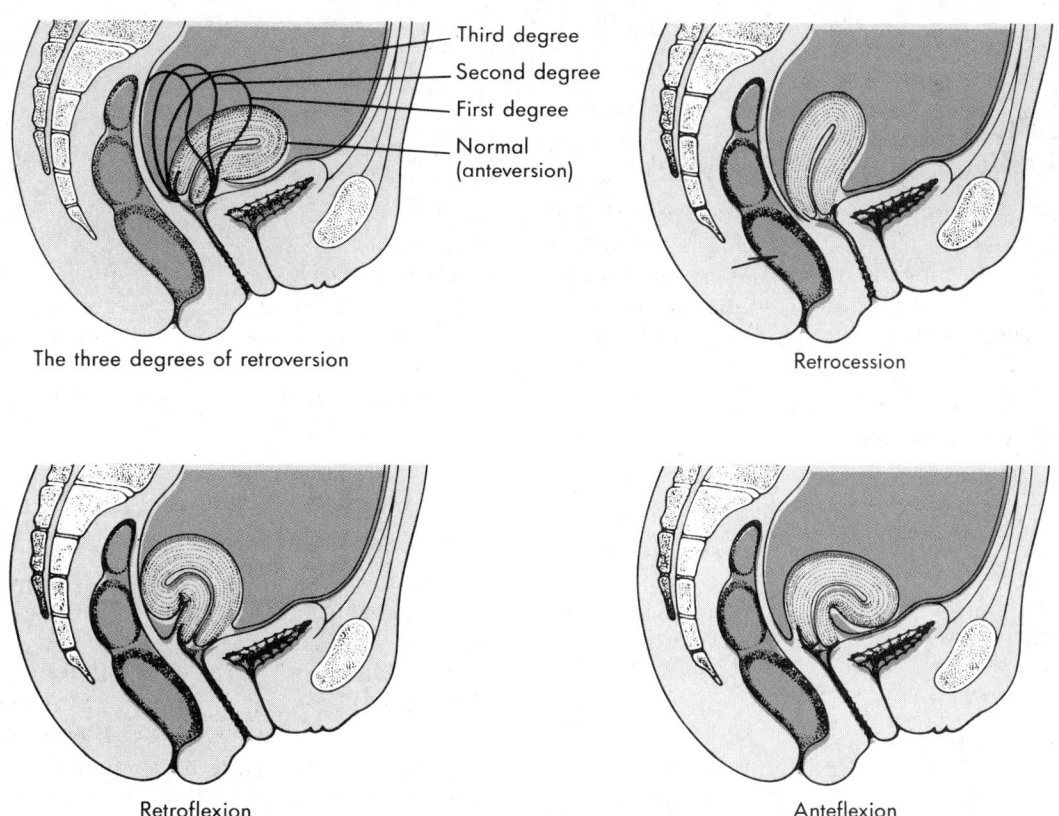

Third degree
Second degree
First degree
Normal (anteversion)

The three degrees of retroversion

Retrocession

Retroflexion

Anteflexion

FIGURE 70-5   Uterine displacements.

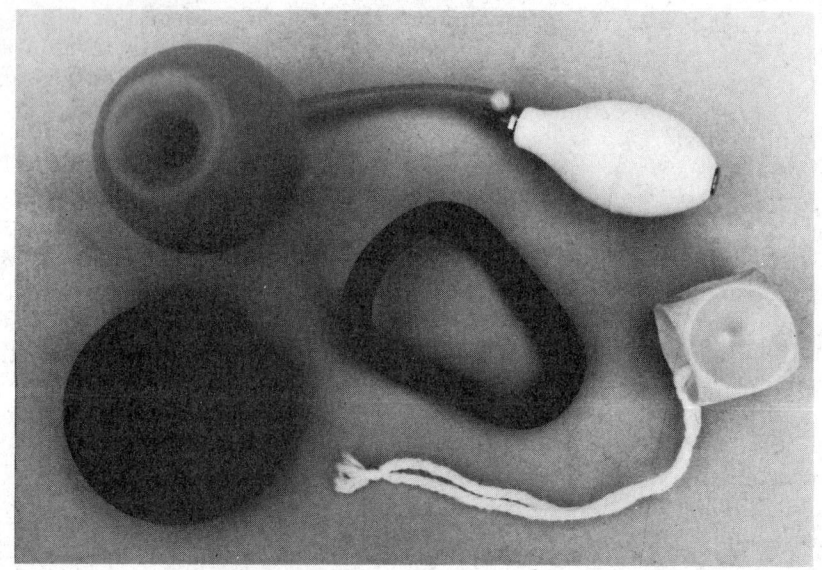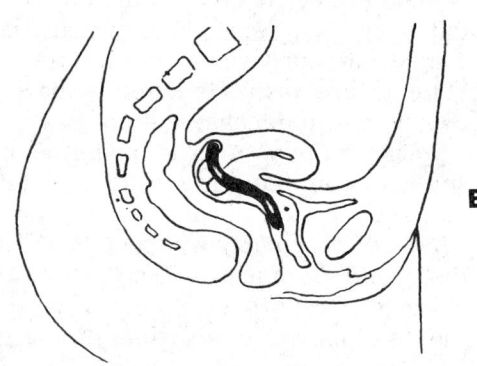

FIGURE 70-6   **A,** Examples of pessaries (Smith-Hodge, donut, inflatable types). **B,** Pessary in place to hold posterior vaginal fornix and, with it, attached cervix wall backward and upward in pelvis. (**A** from Droegemuller W et al: *Comprehensive gynecology,* St Louis, 1987, Mosby–Year Book, Inc. **B** from Beacham DW, Beacham WD: *Synopsis of gynecology,* ed 10, St Louis, 1982, Mosby–Year Book, Inc.)

for backward displacements is done only if the condition is incapacitating.

UTERINE PROLAPSE
Etiology/Pathophysiology

The internal reproductive organs of the woman are supported by pelvic muscles. When these muscles atrophy with age or become weakened by childbearing, they are no longer able to provide support. The uterus may collapse into the vagina (prolapse) (Figure 70-7, *A*) and impinge on other structures.

Clinical Manifestations

The woman with a uterine prolapse may complain of urinary incontinence, retention, constipation, backache, and vaginal discharge from the increased pressure exerted by the prolapsed uterus. The symptoms may increase with coughing or prolonged standing. The diagnosis is confirmed with a pelvic examination.

Therapeutic Management

If the woman is unable to withstand surgery, a pessary may be used to support the uterus. However, a hysterectomy is the preferred treatment.

CYSTOCELE

A cytocele is the protrusion of the bladder through the vaginal wall because of weak pelvic musculature (Figure 70-7, *B*). The woman complains of voiding problems such as frequency, urgency, and stress incontinence. The cystocele can be diagnosed by visual inspection during the pelvic examination. The cystocele is corrected by tightening the pelvic muscles to provide more support to the bladder. Correction is achieved by surgically shortening the muscles that support the bladder. The surgery, known as anterior colporrhaphy or anterior repair, is performed using a vaginal approach.

RECTOCELE

A rectocele is the protrusion of the rectum through the vaginal wall (Figure 70-7, *C*). The woman complains of symptoms of rectal pressure such as constipation, heaviness, and hemorrhoids. The rectocele is diagnosed by pelvic examination and x-ray films of the lower gastrointestinal tract. Surgery is indicated to strengthen the weakened muscles. The operation is called a posterior colporrhaphy. If it is done at the same time that a cystocele is repaired, it is called an anteroposterior colporrhaphy (anteroposterior repair).

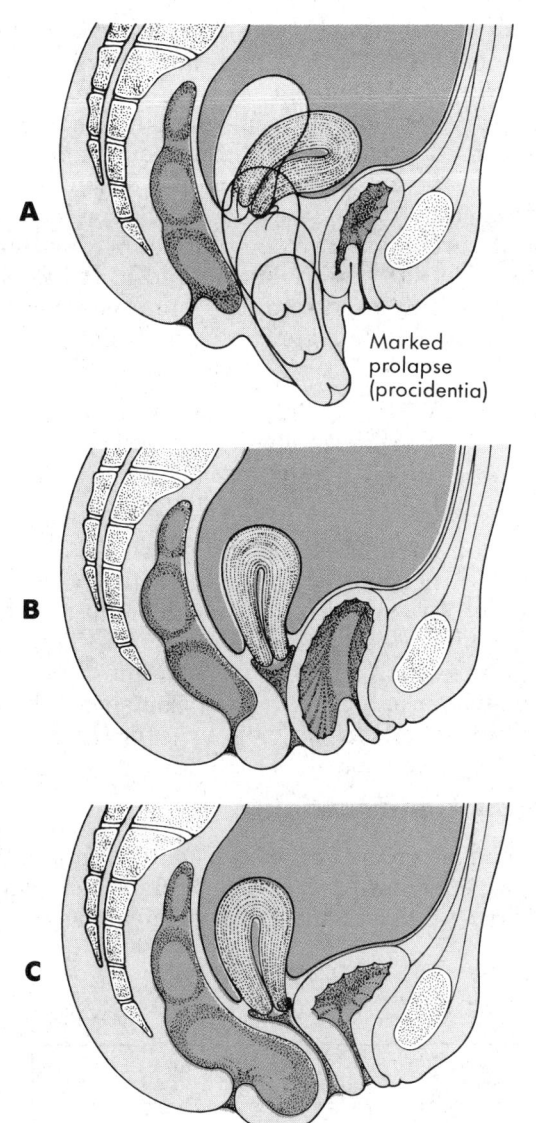

FIGURE 70-7   **A,** Uterine prolapse. **B,** Cystocele. **C,** Rectocele.

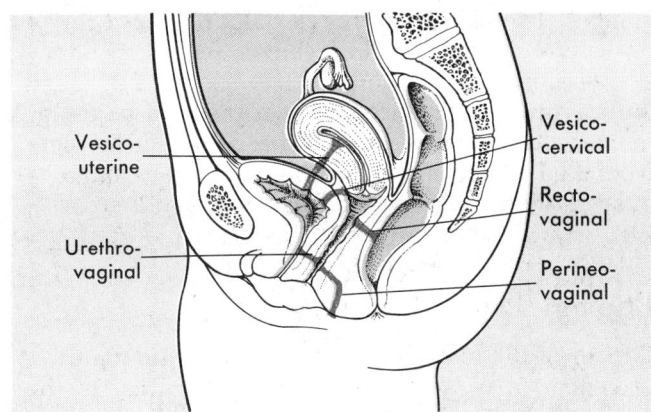

FIGURE 70-8   Sites of vaginal fistula formation.

NURSING MANAGEMENT OF THE PATIENT WITH UTERINE DISPLACEMENT

Many of the problems related to relaxation of the pelvic muscles (uterine displacements, uterine prolapse, cystocele, rectocele) are preventable. Perineal exercises are taught so that the woman develops the ability to tighten and relax gluteal and perineal floor muscles. Learning to start and stop the urinary stream also increases perineal muscle tone. If the patient is to have a pessary, teach her how to insert it, when to remove it, how to clean it, and how to reinsert it. Usually the patient can be taught to remove the pessary at bedtime and to reinsert it in the morning. If it remains in place, the patient should have it removed, cleaned, and reinserted by the physician or nurse practitioner periodically.

VAGINAL FISTULAS
Definition/Pathophysiology

A fistula is an abnormal connection through openings in two organs. Fistulas of the female reproductive tract occur between the vagina and rectum (rectovaginal fistula), vagina and bladder (vesicovaginal fistula), and vagina and ureter (ureterovaginal fistula) (Figure 70-8). Fistulas may be caused by radiation therapy, surgery, weakness caused by pregnancies, or disease such as cancer.

Clinical Manifestations

Fistulas are recognized by vaginal drainage containing urine or stool. Odor and irritation of the vagina and vulva are common. Fistulas are diagnosed by pelvic examination and radiography (fistulogram).

Therapeutic Management

If the fistula is small, it may heal spontaneously. However, if it does not heal, surgery is necessary to close the openings. The surgical approach may be similar to an anterior or posterior colporrhaphy. Fistulas that are difficult to repair or very large may require urinary or fecal diversion.

NURSING MANAGEMENT OF THE PATIENT WITH A VAGINAL FISTULA

Effective nursing measures to assist the woman whose fistula cannot be repaired must be aimed at relieving discomfort, preventing infection, and improving the patient's self-perception and self-care abilities. Frequent sitz baths, douches, and frequent changing of perineal pads and undergarments are needed. The skin in this area must be cared for to prevent excoriation; mild creams or cornstarch may be soothing. The patient with a fistula may need long-term physical care and assistance in adjusting to her altered body image. She may feel helpless from the lack of control over body functions and may express these feelings and frustrations to the nurse.

CANCER OF CERVIX
Etiology/Pathophysiology

Cancer of the cervix is the sixth most common form of cancer in women, ranking behind cancer of the breast, colon and rectum, lung, endometrium, and ovary.[5] The incidence is greater among blacks and Hispanics than in whites. Women who become sexually active in their teens are at a higher risk for cancer of the cervix, as are those who have had multiple sexual partners, those who have given birth more than once, and those of low socioeconomic status. The incidence of cervical cancer is also higher in women whose sexual partners have these risk factors.

Over the past 20 years, the incidence of invasive genital neoplasia has decreased, while that of pre-invasive neoplasia has increased. The increase in genital human papillomavirus (HPV) and increased screening such as Pap smears may be factors in this increase.[24,33] It has been shown that the presence of human papillomavirus—the same agent responsible for the venereal wart—can result in neoplastic changes in the cervix. Intercourse without condom protection in young teenage girls exposes an immature cervix to potentially carcinogenic factors.

Of cervical carcinomas, 95% are of squamous cell origin, 4% are of adenocarcinoma origin, and 1% are from rare cell types. The precursor lesions of cervical carcinoma have been identified as dysplasia. **Cervical intraepithelial neoplasia (CIN)** is the term commonly used to define the precursor state. CIN has been subdivided into the following three stages:

CIN I   Mild dysplasia
CIN II   Moderate dysplasia
CIN III   Severe dysplasia to
          carcinoma in situ

The continuum that begins with mild dysplasia and that, if not interrupted, ends with invasive carcinoma has a variable time schedule with each patient (see Figure 70-9 for stages of CIN). The tumor usually spreads by direct extension into the vagina, parametrium, or pelvis. It may also spread by way of the lymphatics to the lung, liver, or bone.

Clinical Manifestations

Early cancer of the cervix is usually asymptomatic. The two chief symptoms are **leukorrhea** (vaginal discharge) and irregular vaginal bleeding or spot-

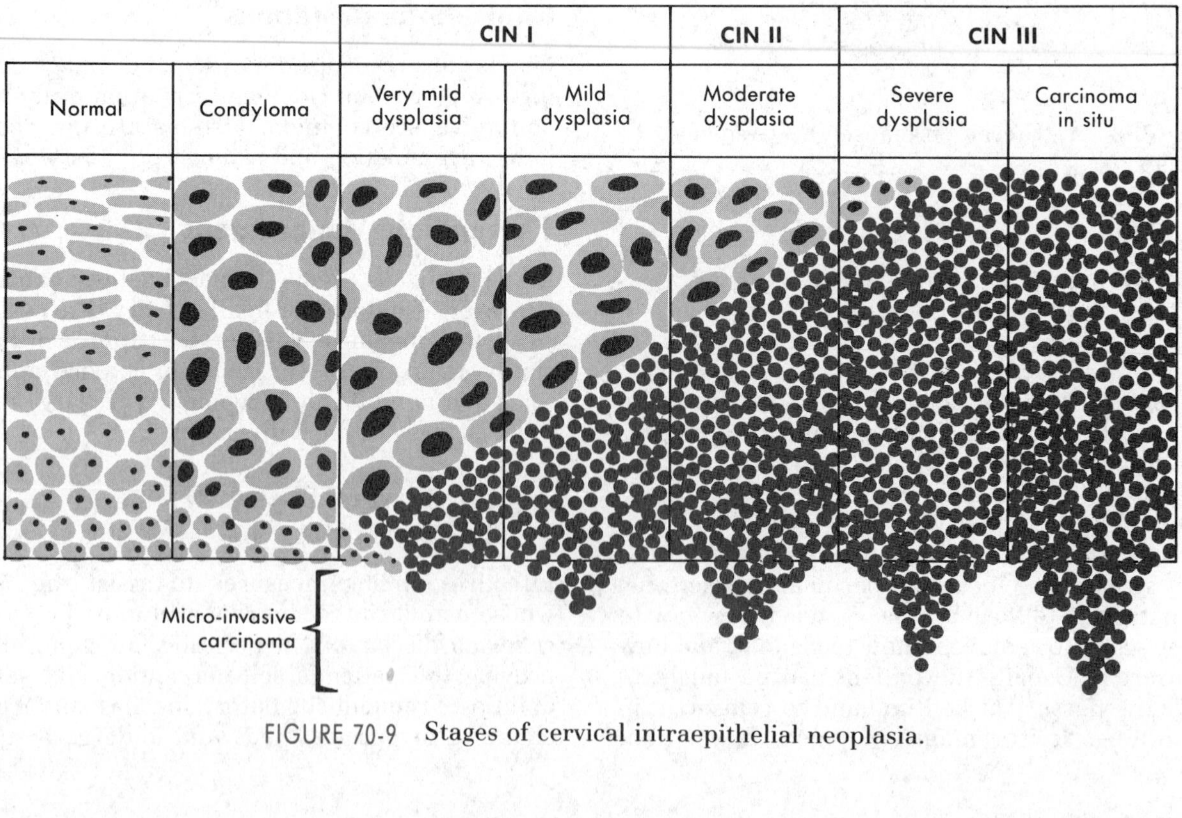

FIGURE 70-9   Stages of cervical intraepithelial neoplasia.

FIGO STAGING SYSTEM FOR CANCER OF THE CERVIX UTERI

Stage I

Carcinoma is strictly confined to cervix (extension to corpus should be disregarded)

Stage I-A Preclinical carcinomas of cervix, that is, those diagnosed only by microscope

Stage I-A1 Minimal microscopically evident stroma invasion

Stage I-A2 Lesions detected microscopically that can be measured; upper limit of the measurement should not show a depth of invasion more than 5 mm from base of epithelium (origin) to a second dimension (horizontal spread) and should not exceed 7 mm; larger lesions should be staged as I-B

Stage I-B Lesions larger than with stage I-A2 whether seen clinically or not; preformed space involvement should not alter staging but should be specifically recorded for future decisions

Stage II

Carcinoma has extended beyond cervix but has not extended to pelvic wall; carcinoma involves upper two thirds of vagina but does not extend into lower third

Stage II-A No obvious parametrial involvement

Stage II-B Obvious parametrial involvement

Stage III

Carcinoma has extended to pelvic wall and lower third of vagina, hydronephrosis has occurred, or patient has nonfunctioning kidney

Stage III-A No extension to pelvic wall

Stage III-B Extension to pelvic wall, hydronephrosis, or nonfunctioning kidney

Stage IV

Carcinoma has extended beyond true pelvis or has clinically involved mucosa of bladder or rectum

---

ting. The vaginal discharge increases gradually in amount and becomes watery and, finally, dark and foul smelling because of necrosis and infection of the tumor mass. The bleeding occurs at irregular intervals, between periods (metrorrhagia), or after menopause. It is usually noted after intercourse, douching, or defecation. As the disease progresses, the bleeding may become constant and increase in amount.

Therapeutic Management

The gynecologist and radiation oncologist jointly perform the evaluation and staging of the patient with carcinoma of the cervix. Application of the staging system developed by the International Federation of Gynecology and Obstetrics (see box above) is based on several diagnostic studies: clinical evaluation, cytologic and colposcopic studies, endocervical curettage and biopsies, and radiographic studies (see box for diagnostic studies).

Carcinoma in situ is treated by removal of the affected area. This removal can be accomplished by cryosurgery, electrocautery, laser, conization, or hysterectomy. Cryosurgery, electrocautery, and laser treatments require special skills and close follow-up study to be sure that the entire lesion has been destroyed. Cryotherapy and laser therapy have proven successful in treating cervical dysplasias.[46] Conization, the conical removal of a large portion of the exocervix and endocervix, is considered conservative management for women who want to have more children.[50] Hysterectomy is the treatment of choice for patients who do not desire fertility. The decision to remove the ovaries depends on the age of the patient and the condition of the ovaries.

Early carcinoma of the cervix can be treated with a hysterectomy or intracavitary radiation (Figure 70-10). However, whether to do a simple or radical hysterectomy with pelvic lymphadenectomy is a controversial question. When the depth of tumor invasion is 3 mm or less, a lymph node dissection or pelvic irradiation is not required, since the incidence of lymph node metastasis is 1% or less.[55] Wertheim's radical hysterectomy with pelvic lymphadenectomy may be required with more extensive lesions. A radical hysterectomy involves removal of the uterus,

DIAGNOSTIC STUDIES FOR CERVICAL CANCER

Pap smear
Physical examination
Multiple cervical biopsy specimens
Colposcopy if indicated to obtain biopsies
Endocervical curettage
Conization if indicated to obtain tissue sample
Cystoscopy
Sigmoidoscopy
Intravenous pyelogram
Chest x-ray examination

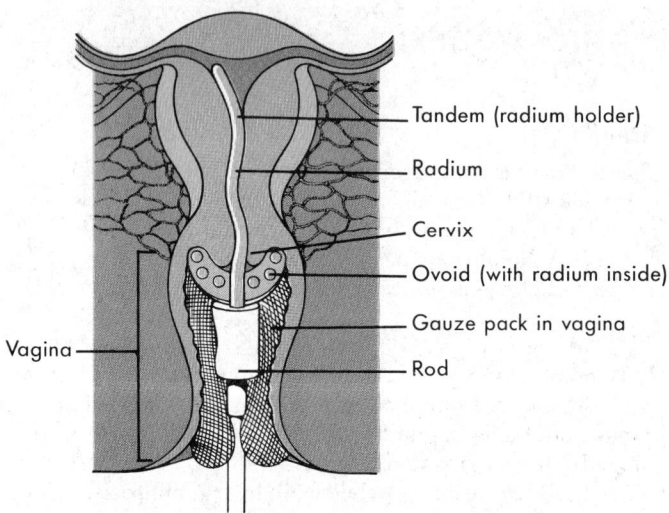

FIGURE 70-10 Intracavitary irradiation of cervix for treatment of cervical cancer.

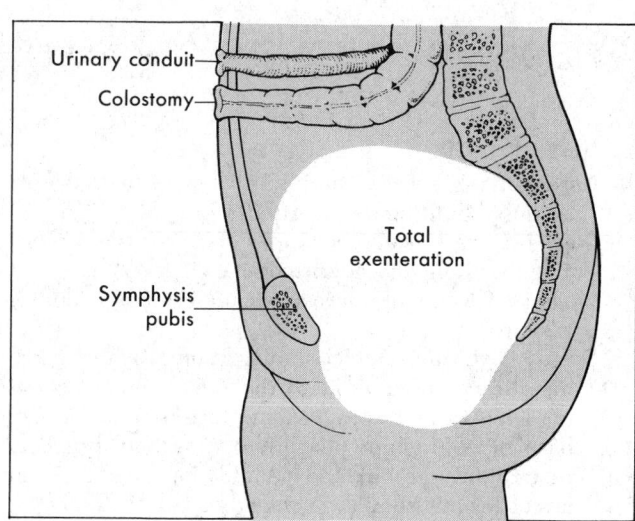

FIGURE 70-11 Total pelvic exenteration, showing placement of urinary stoma and colostomy.

proximal vagina, and pelvic lymph nodes. Bilateral pelvic lymphadenectomy involves removal of the common iliac, hypogastric, and obturator lymphatics and nodes.

Patients with stage II-B, III, or IV-A cervical cancer are treated with irradiation alone. External irradiation and intracavitary therapy are used in various combinations. The treatment plan is tailored to each patient based on the extent of disease.

Chemotherapy

The cure of recurrent cervical cancer has not significantly improved with the progress of modern chemotherapy. One reason is that approximately 95% of cervical cancers are squamous cell, which are less responsive to most chemotherapeutic agents. In addition, recurrent cancers often appear within a previously irradiated area that is fibrotic and avascular. The perfusion of this area is marginal, and therefore it is difficult to obtain a high tissue concentration of the drug in the neoplasm. Finally, many drugs are nephrotoxic and have limited usefulness because of the ureteral obstruction associated with advanced cervical cancers.[52] No evidence exists that cervical cancers are sensitive to hormonal manipulation.[53]

Recurrent disease

Once treatment by radiation therapy has failed, further radiation is not useful. Selected patients may be candidates for pelvic exenteration (Figure 70-11). In women this involves removal of the perineum, pelvic floor, levator muscles, and all reproductive or-

gans. Additionally, the lymph nodes, rectum, distal sigmoid colon, urinary bladder, and distal ureters are excised. A colostomy and urinary conduit are created, and vaginal reconstruction may be done during this initial procedure.[20]

NURSING MANAGEMENT OF THE PATIENT WITH CANCER OF THE CERVIX
Assessment

The nurse assesses the patient for unusual vaginal bleeding, discharge, malodorous discharge, the presence of lymphedema, back and leg pain, and a feeling of rectal pressure.

Nursing Diagnosis

Possible nursing diagnoses include the following:
 Anxiety related to diagnosis
 Pain related to cervical tumor
 High risk for impaired skin integrity related to vulvar excoriation from vaginal discharge
 Altered sexuality patterns related to treatment

Planning

The woman with cervical cancer is able to do the following:
 Patient verbalizes fears or concerns related to diagnosis of cancer
 Patient verbalizes pain control with analgesics
 Patient identifies methods to maintain skin hygiene

Implementation

Nursing care for the patient with cervical cancer includes the following:

1. Introducing her to persons who have successfully undergone the same experience
2. Involving the family as much as possible
3. Positioning the patient comfortably and changing her position slowly
4. Maintaining the patient's body alignment
5. Applying heating pads to the lower abdomen
6. Providing the pain relief measure of the patient's choice
7. Changing the patient's dressings and sanitary pads frequently
8. Assessing the skin for irritation
9. Assessing the color, odor, and amount of vaginal drainage

An essential aspect of the nursing care of the cervical cancer patient is teaching. Refer to sections in the text regarding nursing management of the hysterectomy and implant patients. Explanations regarding female anatomy, alteration in body function, and impact on sexual function should be included in the teaching sessions. Many teaching plans are also available in the literature for patients undergoing pelvic exenteration.[51,62] The psychologic aspects are immense. Adaptation includes changes in body image, life-style, and sexual relations. Nurses are in key positions to assist these patients to redevelop and adjust their lives to what they consider worthwhile and acceptable levels of functioning.

Evaluation

Anxiety is reduced, and pain is controlled. The patient is able to express her fears and concerns. Skin hygiene is maintained.

Documentation

Documentation involves recording the assessment data and nursing interventions, including validation of the patient's knowledge of cervical cancer and her comprehension of the treatment plan.

Ongoing Care

Dramatic decreases in cancer deaths are associated with early detection and treatment. To save more lives through diagnosis and treatment, it is important to determine the population at risk and then to provide them with information on frequent, inexpensive screening. Nurses take an active role in the prevention and detection of cervical cancer. Nurses can both educate and encourage their patients to assume responsibility for their health by routinely participating in screening programs.

NURSING MANAGEMENT OF THE PATIENT UNDERGOING INTERNAL IRRADIATION

Assessment

Assess the patient for side effects of radiation therapy such as nausea, vomiting, anorexia, diarrhea, dry skin reactions, moist desquamation, blistering, and sloughing of skin surfaces.

Nursing Diagnosis

Possible nursing diagnoses include the following:

Knowledge deficit related to internal irradiation

Social isolation related to radiation exposure

Potential for injury related to irradiation

Sexual dysfunction related to effects of irradiation on female reproductive organs

Impaired physical mobility related to being on bed rest during implantation

Planning

The patient is able to do the following:

Patient defines the purpose and side effects of internal irradiation

Patient defines radiation precautions

Patient complies with restrictions on mobility during implantation

Patient identifies changes in the vagina produced by the radiation

Patient lists home care instructions before hospital discharge

Implementation

While the patient is undergoing a radium or cesium implant, diligent nursing care is provided. Since these implants are sealed sources, no precautions with excreta are necessary. Although the nursing staff must try to reduce the radiation exposure to themselves as much as possible, the patient is carefully observed and attended. (Refer to Chapter 15 for additional information on time, distance, and shielding during patient radiation.) Contacts with the nurse provide a good opportunity for the patient to talk about her fear and anxiety. To minimize her own radiation exposure, the nurse stands at the head of the bed or at the entrance to the room. Visitors are limited to 30 minutes per day in the radiation area. No children or pregnant women are allowed to visit the patient. Diversional activities are encouraged during this time of limited visitations.

A recent development in major medical centers in the United States is the use of remote afterloading brachytherapy equipment rather than manual afterloading brachytherapy. Remote afterloading precludes exposure of nursing personnel to radiation, because the radioactive sources are withdrawn pneumatically into a shielded container whenever someone enters the room. As a result, time spent with the patient can be focused on the patient's needs rather than on the risk of personal radiation exposure.[37]

During the application the patient is on absolute bed rest. She may log roll from side to side, and the head of the bed may be raised to 45 degrees. The patient is encouraged to practice deep breathing and coughing exercises and to flex and extend the feet to promote venous return.

Usually the patient is on a low-fiber diet to prevent frequent bowel movements, a side effect of irradiation. A urinary catheter is placed to prevent bladder distention. Observe the patient for evidence of temperature elevation, nausea, and vomiting. These symptoms are reported, since they may indicate infection or perforation of the uterus. Although perineal care is omitted, any profuse vaginal drainage is reported immediately.

Irradiation causes scarring and fibrosis of the vagina with a decrease in normal vaginal secretions. Sexual activity after internal irradiation can be resumed in about 1 week. However, teach the patient to use a water-soluble lubricant during sexual intercourse since the normal vaginal lubrication is decreased. If the patient is not sexually active, vaginal closure may occur because of fibrosis and scarring. Teach the patient to use a vaginal dilator once she is discharged from the hospital (Figure 70-12). The dilator may be warmed under running water and lubricated with a water-soluble lubricant to ease insertion. The dilator is inserted once or twice each day for 5 minutes. Progressive ambulation is recommended after the implants are removed. A Fleet's enema and douche may be prescribed for cleaning, and the urinary catheter is removed. The patient is usually discharged from the hospital that same day.

Evaluation

Radiation precautions are maintained. The patient verbalizes an understanding of and rationale for ra-

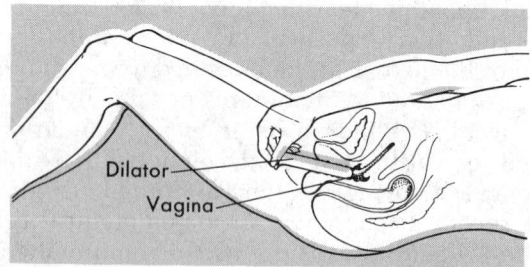

FIGURE 70-12   Use of a vaginal dilator after intracavitary implant for cervical cancer.

diation precautions. Restricted mobility is maintained during implant, with the patient remaining on bed rest with the head of the bed elevated 45 degrees. Postimplant care is instituted. The patient understands instructions about vaginal douching, resuming sexual intercourse, and use of the dilator.

Documentation

Record the assessment data and nursing interventions, noting validation of the patient's knowledge and comprehension of the treatment plan.

Ongoing Care

The nurse plays a key role in radiotherapy. Essentially she prepares the patient for therapy, promotes radiation safety by observing radiation precautions, and psychologically supports the patient and family before and throughout the administration of radiotherapy. The nurse in the community assists by assessing the patient for side effects of therapy and ensuring compliance with the prescribed treatment regimen. Printed home care instructions are helpful in providing the link between hospital and home and are reviewed with the patient before discharge.

CANCER OF ENDOMETRIUM
Etiology

Endometrial cancer primarily occurs in women more than 50 years of age, but the incidence among younger women is increasing. It is the most common malignancy of the female genital tract.[5,53] Several prevalent factors have been identified in high-risk groups: obesity, nulliparity, diabetes, hypertension, uninterrupted estrogen stimulation, menses continuing past 50 years of age, history of dysfunctional uterine bleeding, and history of anovulation.[44]

Pathophysiology

Endometrial tumors are of adenocarcinoma, adenoacanthoma, and adenosquamous carcinoma origin. Most adenocarcinomas are well differentiated and less invasive than the other types. Adenoacanthoma refers to an adenocarcinoma with squamous metaplasia. In adenosquamous carcinoma the squamous component is malignant and poorly differentiated. Local extension of endometrial tumors may involve the myometrium, paravaginal tissues, and paracervical tissues. Usually the disease is advanced before the lymph nodes are involved. The cancer may penetrate the uterine wall and spread to the abdominal cavity or to the liver, lungs, brain, or bone. It may also spread by lymphatic or hematogenous routes.

HOME CARE GUIDE   *After Intracavitary Implant*

1. You may resume your usual diet unless instructed otherwise by your physician. If you have problems with diarrhea, you will need to follow a low-fiber diet.
2. It is common to feel tired for a couple of weeks. Take frequent breaks and rest periods. Daily exercise such as walking is good for you.
3. If you have a vaginal discharge, you may douche daily with 2 tablespoons of povidone-iodine (Betadine) or vinegar in a quart of water. Report any excessive vaginal discharge or bleeding to your physician.
4. The following need to be reported to your physician should they occur:
   a. Extreme nausea or vomiting, or both.
   b. Any unusual problems with urinating, including urinating small amounts, urinating more frequently than usual, burning with urinating, or blood in the urine.
   c. Any unusual problems with bowel habits such as diarrhea, constipation, or rectal bleeding.
   d. Any unusual or prolonged abdominal or back pain.
5. Begin using the vaginal dilator when insertion is comfortable, usually 1 to 3 days after surgery (Figure 71-6). Use the dilator once or twice a day for 5 minutes to prevent closure of your vagina. The dilator may be warmed under running water and lubricated before insertion with water-soluble lubricant such as K-Y jelly. Do *not* use the dilator if you had a hysterectomy after your radium implant. When you return to the clinic, ask your physician how long you need to use the dilator.
6. Sexual activity may be resumed as soon as it is comfortable (about 7 to 10 days) or as indicated by your physician. Again you may need to use a water-soluble lubricant such as K-Y jelly.
7. Bathing may be resumed as soon as the applicator is removed, although a shower is preferable to a tub bath.
8. Take your medications as prescribed, and if you have any concerns or problems, do not hesitate to call your physician. Many physicians collaborate with nurse practitioners or clinical nurse specialists who can also provide information. Return for your follow-up clinic appointment at the scheduled date and time.

Clinical Manifestations

About 50% of patients with postmenopausal bleeding have cancer of the uterus. Its progress is slow, metastasis occurs late, and the symptom of irregular vaginal bleeding often appears early enough to allow for cure of the disease. In the premenopausal or climacteric woman, abnormal bleeding or spotting may be interpreted as normal menopausal symptoms. However, during this time the menstrual periods should become lighter and farther apart. Any other bleeding pattern is referred to the physician.

Therapeutic Management

Staging is done jointly by the gynecologist and radiation oncologist. The history and physical, bimanual pelvic and rectal examinations, and a fractional D & C are the primary procedures for diagnosing and evaluating endometrial cancer. The staging system most commonly used is the FIGO staging system. Most patients will have stage I disease, and over 90% of the tumors will be adenocarcinomas.

Surgery is the primary treatment for endometrial cancer. The treatment for stage I adenocarcinomas is a total abdominal hysterectomy and bilateral salpingo-oophorectomy. Patients with stage I-A and I-B and grade I and II carcinomas may also receive intracavitary radiation followed by a hysterectomy and bilateral salpingo-oophorectomy. Patients with stage II disease may receive an additional boost of 4000 centiGrey (cGy) of whole pelvis irradiation to cause tumor shrinkage and help prevent spread. Afterward the patient will undergo a hysterectomy. Stage III and IV diseases are uncommon, and the treatment plan is tailored to each patient based on age, medical condition, and the volume and extent of disease.

Hormonal therapy

Response to hormonal therapy depends on the grade of the tumor and the presence or absence of estrogen and progesterone receptors. Progestins usually cause no serious side effects and are generally recommended instead of chemotherapy for patients with recurrent disease.

Chemotherapy

Doxorubicin was the first drug to be systematically used in treating endometrial cancer. Drugs used in combination may be more effective. One such combination includes cyclophosphamide, doxorubicin, and cisplatin. Generally, cytotoxic chemotherapy is reserved for patients in whom hormonal therapy has been unsuccessful.[54]

CANCER OF THE OVARY
Etiology

Ovarian cancer is the fifth most frequent cause of cancer death in women and is the leading cause of gynecologic death in the United States.[5,43] Malignant neoplasms of the ovaries occur at all ages, including infancy and childhood. The major histologic types occur in distinctive age ranges. Malignant germ cell tumors are most common in women in their 20s and 30s, whereas epithelial cancers of the ovary are primarily seen in perimenopausal women. The greatest number of cases of ovarian cancer are found in women 50 to 59 years old. The highest rates of ovarian cancer are in highly industrialized areas such as the United States and Europe but not Japan. It is most common in the white population but rare in Asian women. Incidence among blacks is less than among whites, but it has been increasing. The rate is higher among Jewish women than among non-Jewish women and among nulliparous women than among parous women.

Although epidemiologic studies suggest that environmental factors may influence the development of ovarian cancer, no strong association with any one factor has been documented. Postulated risk factors are talc and asbestos, but definite correlations have not been established.

Pathophysiology

Hormonal factors seem to influence the incidence of ovarian cancer. Risk factors are ovarian dysfunction, irregular menses, and infertility. Risk decreases with the use of oral contraceptives and with each pregnancy.[36] Other risk factors include genetic ones (a familial association of carcinoma of the ovary and the breast), high-dose irradiation to the pelvis, endometriosis, and multiple primary cancers.

Classification of malignant ovarian tumors is complex because of the difficulty in identifying specific embryologic cell types. Frequently, ovarian tumors are composed of a combination of cell types. Histologic classification by the World Health Organization includes epithelial tumors (which account for ap-

proximately 90% of the ovarian malignancies), germ cell tumors, and stromal tumors.

Clinical Manifestations

The early diagnosis of an ovarian neoplasm is usually made by chance because of frequent screening. There is no known method for detecting ovarian cancer at an early stage; however, specific tumor markers such as CA-125 are being evaluated. The signs and symptoms of advanced disease include ascites, abdominal pain and pressure, nausea and vomiting, constipation, and urinary frequency. An ovarian enlargement should be suspected of being an ovarian malignancy. Palpable ovaries in premenarchal or postmenopausal women are an abnormal physical finding. To assess the extent of disease, the surgeon looks at the abdomen and pelvis and explores the area by palpation. Cytologic and biopsy specimens are also used to determine the stage of disease.

Therapeutic Management

A patient suspected of having ovarian cancer undergoes surgery as soon as the diagnostic workup is complete. Ovarian cancer commonly spreads by peritoneal seeding and implantation. Common sites of metastasis are the peritoneum, omentum, and bowel surfaces, although spread to other pelvic organs does occur (Figure 70-13).

A total abdominal hysterectomy and bilateral salpingo-oophorectomy with tumor debulking is generally the treatment of choice. The smaller the volume of tumor remaining, the better the response to adjuvant therapy. Generally, patients with a residual tumor less than 2 cm in diameter have a better prognosis than those with residual disease greater than 2 cm.[57]

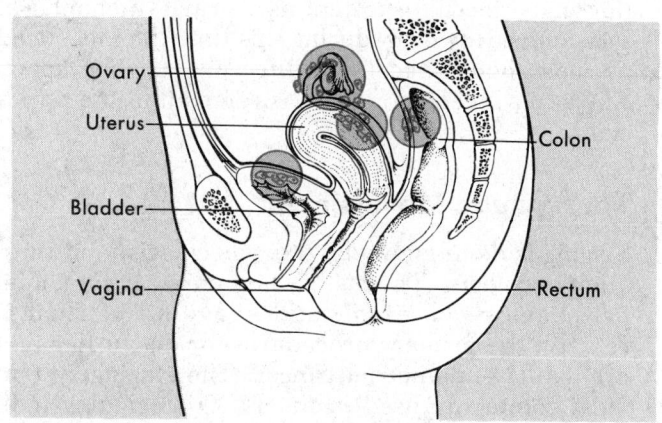

FIGURE 70-13 Sites of metastasis with ovarian cancer.

Chemotherapy

Approximately two thirds of women with ovarian cancer have stage III and IV disease that is not surgically curable.[15] Thus, following tumor-reductive surgery, patients with epithelial ovarian tumors usually receive chemotherapy. The overall response rate to combination chemotherapy is between 60% and 90% with a complete response rate of 40% to 60%.[15] (Refer to Chapter 15 for a discussion of chemotherapy response rate.) A commonly used drug combination is cisplatin and cyclophosphamide. Patients usually receive 6 to 12 courses of this drug regimen. The clinical value of intraperitoneal chemotherapy is under investigation.

Second-look surgery

Second-look surgery is a technique used to determine the response of the disease to chemotherapy and whether therapy is continued. If there is no evidence of disease either macroscopically or microscopically, the chemotherapy is stopped and the patient is monitored for recurrent disease. If the tumor volume has decreased, chemotherapy with the same agents may be continued once the patient recovers from the surgery. If there is evidence of progressive disease, the chemotherapeutic agents are changed.[45]

Radiation therapy

External radiation therapy is effective as an adjuvant therapy following a tumor-debulking procedure that leaves residual tumor nodules no larger than 1.5 to 2 cm. The radiation dose varies from institution to institution but is usually 2000 to 3000 cGy to the abdomen and 4500 to 5000 cGy to the pelvis over 6 to 8 weeks. Potential complications associated with radiation therapy include radiation enteritis, myelosuppression, and nausea.

NURSING MANAGEMENT OF THE PATIENT WITH OVARIAN CANCER
Assessment

To increase the chance of detecting ovarian cancer while it is in early, more treatable stages, the nurse pays close attention to women who are 40 years of age or older and who complain of vague gastrointestinal discomfort, increased abdominal girth, abnormal bowel or bladder functions, or abnormal vaginal bleeding.

Nursing Diagnosis

Primary nursing diagnoses are related to the extent of the tumor and the pressure of ascites and include

the following:
  Pain
  Ineffective breathing pattern
  Fluid volume excess
  Anticipatory grieving related to the poor prognosis of the disease
Other nursing diagnoses may be important, depending on the patient's presenting symptoms.

Planning

The goals for the woman with ovarian cancer include the following:
  Patient's pain is relieved
  Patient's breathing patterns are comfortable
  Patient maintains fluid balance
  Patient accepts the terminal nature of the disease

Implementation

Teaching the patient about the diagnosis, surgery, and adjuvant therapy for ovarian cancer is an important aspect of patient care. Teaching begins in the clinical setting and continues through the course of adjuvant treatment.[28] Ovarian cancer patients are managed similar to patients undergoing abdominal hysterectomy and patients receiving chemotherapy and external radiation therapy. Since ovarian cancer is generally at an advanced stage at the time of diagnosis despite the woman's sense of well-being, the nurse supports and encourages the woman to comply with the treatment regimen. As the disease progresses, the nurse becomes involved in activities that increase the patient's comfort.

Evaluation

Pain is controlled with analgesics, and the patient breathes easily for her level of activity. A paracentesis is performed periodically to decrease the amount of ascitic fluid so as to help maintain fluid balance and facilitate movement of the diaphragm during respiration. The patient discusses her disease with her family and with health care providers and uses appropriate coping mechanisms to resolve fears.

Documentation

Documentation involves recording the assessment data and nursing interventions, with validation of the patient's knowledge of ovarian cancer and of the treatment plan.

Ongoing Care

Nursing care focuses on the psychologic impact of ovarian cancer. The artificial menopause that may occur when the ovaries are removed and the poor prognosis associated with the disease involve feelings about self-worth, femininity, sexuality, mutilation, and even death. The nurse in the inpatient and outpatient setting as well as in the community needs to be aware of such concerns and to provide emotional support and education about physical and psychologic expectations after therapy.

CANCER OF THE VULVA
Etiology

Cancer of the vulva is not a common cancer, accounting for only 3% to 4% of all gynecologic cancers. It occurs rarely in women under 50 years of age, with two thirds of the cases found in women more than 60 years of age. In the United States it appears at a younger age in black women than in white women and is more common in women of a poorer socioeconomic class. However, in general, incidence is not influenced by parity, race, or culture. The incidence is gradually rising, possibly because of the increasing numbers of elderly women. As with cervical cancer, there is strong evidence that vulvar cancer and its precursors are a result of an infection with the sexually transmitted human papilloma virus.

Pathophysiology

Most of the lesions arise in the labia, although one fourth may occur in the vestibule and periurethral area. Approximately 86% of vulvar cancers are of the squamous cell type. The vulva is covered with a thin layer of skin; therefore any malignancy that appears elsewhere on the skin can occur here. For example, malignant melanoma of the vulva may occur.

The lesion tends to spread submucosally, with the larger masses becoming ulcerated and secondarily infected. Metastasis may occur to the inguinal lymph nodes, liver, lung, brain, or gastric mucosa.

Clinical Manifestations

The disease is usually localized and well-demarcated. The most common complaints are vulvar itching (pruritus) and burning. On inspection, an ulcer may be noted; abnormal pigmentation or lack of pigmentation (leukoplakia) and asymmetry may also be detected.

Therapeutic Management

The diagnosis of vulvar cancer can only be made by biopsy and histologic examination of the tissue. Surgery is the primary treatment for cancer of the vulva, and the extent of the procedure depends on the disease stage (Figure 70-14).

Stage 0

In recent years the incidence of carcinoma in situ of the vulva has been increasing. Nearly half the patients are 20 to 40 years of age. Approximately one third of the affected patients have associated papilloma virus infection of the cervix, vagina, and vulva.[10] However, studies indicate that the risk of progression of carcinoma in situ to invasive disease may be low in these younger women.[58,60] Treatment is individualized to preserve vulvar anatomy. Usually a local excision or partial vulvectomy with excision of the upper 3 to 5 mm of tissue is necessary. Laser vaporization has also been used.

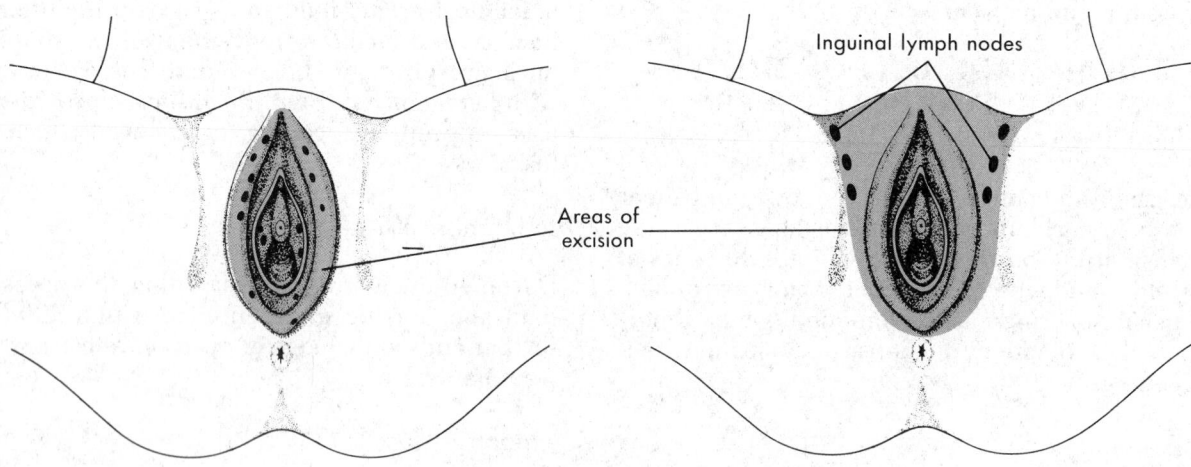

FIGURE 70-14 Types of vulvectomy.

Stage I

The standard treatment for stage I cancer of the vulva is radical vulvectomy. However, treatment that minimizes the extent of radical surgery is being evaluated. In many institutions wide local excisions are already being used as a replacement for radical surgery.

Stages II and III

The radical vulvectomy, which consists of bilateral inguinal lymphadenectomy and an en bloc removal of the entire vulva from the perineal body to the upper margins of the mons pubis, is the standard treatment for invasive carcinoma of the vulva. In addition, a vaginal resection may be required, and if there is urethral involvement, the distal third of the urethra may be excised. The urethral meatus is usually left intact.[54]

Stage IV

Tumors that involve the bladder or rectal mucosa are treated with a radical vulvectomy and pelvic exenteration. However, patients with metastasis or unresectable disease are treated palliatively for symptomatic control.

Radiation therapy

Radiation therapy has played a minor role in the treatment of vulvar cancers, because the cure rates from surgery alone are high and problems with vulvar skin tolerance to radiation have been noted. However, with present methods of radiation therapy producing minimal adverse effects, radiation may offer an acceptable alternative to surgery and may also have a palliative role in advanced disease. Results from chemotherapy have been disappointing; no treatment regimen has yielded a good response rate.

NURSING MANAGEMENT OF THE PATIENT WITH CANCER OF VULVA

Assessment

Assess the patient for white, thickened skin in the vulvar area, long-standing pruritus, chronic inflammation, irritation of the vulva, unusual discharge, bleeding, or lesions in the vulvar area.

Nursing Diagnosis

Possible nursing diagnoses include the following:
  High risk for infection related to surgical incision
  Constipation related to fear of dehiscence and pain

Altered patterns of urinary elimination related to surgical incision
Sexual dysfunction related to vulvectomy
Body-image disturbance from loss of sexual organ
Knowledge deficit related to convalescent care

Planning

Goals for the patient include the following:
  Patient maintains adequate elimination
  Patient remains free from preventable infection
  Patient adapts positively to altered body image
  Patient states methods of home convalescent care

Implementation

The woman requiring a vulvectomy has some special nursing needs in addition to routine preoperative and postoperative care. Measures are taken to prevent contamination of the vulvar wound and to prevent the need for straining to defecate. Enemas are given preoperatively, and the patient is placed on a low-fiber diet after surgery. A urinary catheter is used for drainage. When the catheter is removed, the patient may be unable to void because of difficulty in relaxing the perineum; sitz baths may help. A hair dryer on a cool, continuous setting is used to keep the vulvar wound dry. Large amounts of tissues are removed from the vulva and groin during the operation, and the sutures are usually taut, causing discomfort. The patient will generally need frequent analgesic medication to relieve the discomfort.

Wound breakdown is often a complication. The vulvar wound is frequently left exposed. The wound is cleaned two or three times per day with normal saline or other solutions. After this, a hair dryer on a cool setting is used to dry the area. Home care instructions after vulvectomy and lymphadenectomy are important to ensure proper wound healing and prevent infection. Because the vulvar wounds may heal slowly, the woman may become discouraged. Privacy is ensured, and the woman is encouraged to express her feelings concerning this disfiguring surgery. Some women may feel that their femininity has been irreparably damaged or that the disfigurement may end their sexual life. Sexual intercourse can usually be resumed after complete wound healing or in about 4 to 6 weeks.

Evaluation

The patient exhibits normal inflammation and ecchymosis at the surgical site; passes soft, formed stool; can urinate without difficulty; expresses feelings related to the surgery and its impact on her body image; and identifies proper home care requirements.

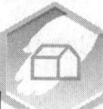

HOME CARE GUIDE   *Radical Vulvectomy Patients*

1. Avoid sexual activity for 4 to 6 weeks or as indicated by your physician.
2. Avoid activities such as driving a car and heavy housework such as vacuuming or heavy lifting until approved by your physician. Walking is good for you. You may still tire easily, and frequent rest periods may be necessary.
3. Avoid periods of prolonged sitting, standing, or crossing your legs. Also avoid wearing tight clothing such as girdles or knee-high hose.
4. Report to your physician any redness, swelling, drainage, odor, or increased soreness along suture lines.
5. Report any temperature over 101° F to your physician.
6. Any unusual problems with elimination should be reported. This includes difficulty urinating (such as burning with small amounts, increased frequency, or blood in urine), bowel problems, constipation, and diarrhea.
7. Keep perineal area as clean and dry as possible. Wash perineum with a solution such as peroxide and water after each urination or defecation. Pat area dry.
8. You may resume your usual diet unless specified by your physician or dietitian. Try to eat a well-balanced diet so as to promote healing.
9. Take your medications as prescribed, and if you have any concerns or problems, don't hesitate to call your physician or the nurse practitioner. Return for your clinic appointment at the scheduled date and time.

Documentation

Documentation involves the recording of the assessment data and nursing interventions, with validation of the patient's knowledge of vulvar cancer and comprehension of the treatment plan.

Ongoing Care

As the patient recovers from the surgical procedure, she begins to accept her altered body image. Often a community nurse will be visiting the patient to assist her in her recovery at home. The patient is encouraged to share her concerns as she convalesces and assumes increasing self-care. Gradual resumption of physical and social activities is emphasized.

Breast Disorders

BENIGN BREAST DISORDERS
Etiology/Epidemiology

The breast evolves continuously from puberty through menopause in response to the hormonal cycles regulating menses. Similarly, many benign breast disorders vary according to developmental stages of the woman's life (Table 70-1). Benign breast disease is no longer an acceptable term; more acceptable terms are disorders or changes. The rate of occurrence of benign breast changes is unknown, because in many women the abnormality may be so slight as to go unnoticed, or the physician may note benign breast changes but decide that a biopsy or treatment is unnecessary.

Pathophysiology

The cause of a benign breast disorder is not fully known. Some evidence points to differences in hormonal patterns that may cause nodularity and mastalgia (pain in the mammary gland), but the specific mechanism has not been identified conclusively.[31] The hormone estrogen is responsible for development of the ductal epithelium, whereas progesterone is responsible for lobular-alveolar proliferation in the breast. An imbalance of these hormones during the luteal phase of ovulation may cause nodularity and mastalgia. Benign breast changes occur more commonly during menarche and menopause when hormones are most unstable and produce anovulatory cycles. Other hormones may be involved in breast changes, and studies to determine the causes continue.[31]

Clinical Manifestations

Many women routinely experience swelling and tenderness during the cyclic hormonal changes of their reproductive years. Nodularity and mastalgia may result if the swelling and tenderness persist and intensify. Nodularity may be described as granular or discrete lumpiness, often associated with tender-

TABLE 70-1   Benign Disorders of the Breast

Classification	Disorder	Life stage
Developmental conditions	Subareolar lumps	Neonatal
	Neonatal breast abscess	
	Solitary lump under areola	Peripubertal
	Congenital abscess and retraction of nipple	
	Polymastia	
Benign tumors	Fibroadenoma	Early reproductive
	Intraductal papilloma	phase
Disorders of lactation	Fissure of nipple	Reproductive phase
	Peripheral breast abscess	
	Galactocele	
Cystic changes	Fibrocystic disorders	Late premenopausal
	Gross cysts	
	Duct ectasia	Perimenopausal and menopausal
	Periductal mastitis	

Adapted from Preece PE: Nomenclature of benign breast disease with particular reference to national differences in approach. In L'Etang HJ, editor: *Benign breast disease,* London, 1983, The Royal Society of Medicine.

ness. Nodularity may be bilateral, but usually one breast is more nodular than the other. Mastalgia is felt as a continuous burning or aching—a diffuse and persistent sensation that may grow more intense with ovulation and premenstruation. Mastalgia becomes more intense during a woman's third decade. It may be relieved by hormonal manipulation or eventually by menopause.[31]

Distinct lumps are diagnosed as benign or cancerous. Benign distinct lumps are usually persistent and unchanging and may be gross cysts, fibrocystic, galactoceles, or fibroadenomas. Diagnosis is based on physical, mammographic, and ultrasonographic examination; needle aspiration of tissue with cytologic assay; or biopsy examination of a tissue.

Nipple discharge, also an unusual finding, often occurs in women over 50 years old. Medications such as insulin and hormones may promote breast secretions. Galactorrhea is an excessive spontaneous secretion of a milky discharge and is associated with pituitary and thyroid disorders. A bloody or clear, sticky discharge should be examined cytologically for malignant cells, although carcinoma is an infrequent cause of abnormal nipple discharge.[14,31] Inflammation of the breast may also cause a thick white, green, greenish brown, or blood-streaked nipple discharge. Infections of the breast are rare, but they occur most frequently during postpartum changes in the breast when obstruction of the ducts with continued milk secretion may create a locus for bacterial infection.

The three most common benign breast disorders are **fibrocystic disorder,** fibroadenoma, and mammary duct ectasia. Fibrocystic changes in the breast are more common, although they cause the greatest discomfort; specific therapeutic measures can alleviate symptoms. Fibroadenoma and mammary duct ectasia are not usually treated. The nursing management is the same for all benign breast conditions.

FIBROCYSTIC DISORDER
Definition

The most common benign disorder of the breast is fibrocystic changes in the fibrous tissue of the breast, often with fluid-filled cysts.

Clinical Manifestations

The breast changes include lumpy breasts, mastalgia, and sometimes nipple discharge. The lumpiness and tenderness are more apparent before menses. When palpated the cysts (lumps) are soft, well differentiated, and movable; when the cysts are deep, they may feel hard. The cysts may be singular or multiple and may have a "mirror image" in the opposite breast. Fibrocystic changes occur most often in women from 30 years of age to menopause or when administration of hormones is discontinued.[14]

Therapeutic Management

Diagnosis is based on the patient's history and physical examination. Mammography and ultrasonography are used to differentiate a cyst from a solid tumor. As a therapeutic measure the cyst is aspirated by needle and syringe to empty it and the fluid is sent for cytologic examination. The fluid volume may vary from 0.5 to 50 mL. When cysts recur in the same area and repeated aspirations are ineffective, the cyst may be surgically excised. In rare instances, after all other methods to control the symptoms are unsuccessful, a simple mastectomy may be indicated.[31]

Dietary measures

Fibrocystic breasts are usually treated conservatively. The usefulness of eliminating methylxanthines (caffeine and theophylline) is still controversial, but it is the least expensive therapy. Many women have reported a lessening of symptoms, even though clinical findings by palpation and mammography were not significantly changed.[14] Vitamin E (400 to 600 units daily) has helped diminish symptoms and nodularity in some patients.[2]

Hormones

Although hormones have been effective in reducing symptoms, they may produce side effects that are more traumatic than the symptoms. Danazol, an anterior pituitary suppressant, may cause weight gain, hot flashes, menstrual irregularities, hirsutism, and deepening of the voice. Tamoxifen, an antiestrogen drug, may cause side effects of vaginitis, decreased libido, nausea, or anorexia. Both danazol and tamoxifen significantly reduce symptoms of fibrocystic disorders, however, and are indicated when the patient has severe symptoms.[14] Oral contraceptives may also be tried for 3 to 4 months, with progesterone added for the last 5 days if needed.[2]

Other methods

Diuretic drugs taken immediately before menstruation when the woman experiences breast pain and increased breast fullness have provided relief. Analgesics may be indicated to relieve painful symptoms, and anti-inflammatory agents such as ibuprofen have been useful in relieving swelling and tenderness.

FIBROADENOMA
Definition

The second most common benign breast disorder is **fibroadenoma,** which is a lump of fibrous and glandular tissue.

Clinical Manifestations

Fibroadenoma is the most common breast lump in women less than 25 years old and may be related to the hormonal changes of menarche. Fibroadenomas are well circumscribed, movable, firm, rounded masses, but they may become calcified and feel hard. They are influenced by the menstrual cycle and may increase in size during premenses and pregnancy. Diagnosis is made by physical examination and history. Mammography may be used to observe the characteristics of a particular patient's mass. When a mass is questionable, it is examined by biopsy to rule out malignancy. Fibroadenomas do not seem to respond to medications or dietary regimens and may be excised if their symptoms are severe.[14]

MAMMARY DUCT ECTASIA
Definition

Mammary duct ectasia occurs when the ducts are dilated and fluid is retained in them.

Clinical Manifestations

Mammary duct ectasia is characterized by inflammation of the duct behind the nipple and by ductal enlargement caused by debris and fluid. Although the condition begins with inflammation of the ducts, this resolves and is followed by ductal fibrosis and enlargement.

Major symptoms vary according to the patient's menopausal state. Premenopausal women experience breast pain and a palpable mass; perimenopausal women usually have a thick, sticky nipple discharge; and postmenopausal women usually experience nipple retraction as a result of fibrotic changes. Other symptoms may include itching of the nipple and subareolar pain that may increase before menses. The nipple discharge, usually intermittent without a cyclic pattern, may be serous or thick and is white, green, greenish brown, or blood streaked.[14] This condition usually requires no treatment, but if the ducts become infected, antibiotics may be needed. Any abscess that develops must be drained.

NURSING MANAGEMENT OF THE PATIENT WITH BENIGN BREAST DISORDERS
Assessment

Nursing assessment begins with careful history taking as the woman describes her symptoms. Nipple discharge, pain, changes in the breast, and the date of the woman's last menstrual period are noted. The best time to do an examination is on days 7 to 10 of the menstrual cycle for those women still menstruating. Thorough inspection and palpation of the breast, axilla, and supraclavicular nodes are performed to detect any masses or changes in the breast tissue. The breast is "milked" to detect discharge; in the case of discharge, the specimen is sent for cytologic examination. Assess the woman's self-examination techniques. (See Chapter 68 for a complete discussion of the breast self-examination [BSE].) Assess the woman's fears, anxiety, and coping mechanisms. Note any verbal and nonverbal behaviors that suggest anxiety.

Nursing Diagnosis

Benign breast changes are often considered normal. Depending on the woman's symptoms, the following diagnoses may apply:

Knowledge deficit related to specific benign breast changes and their treatment

Anxiety related to fear of having breast cancer

Pain related to increased swelling accompanying menses

Planning

Goals related to the diagnoses and nursing care are identified:

Patient is able to relate information about benign breast changes, diet plan, specific medications, and side effects of medications

Patient's anxiety is decreased

Patient is able to maintain a normal life-style without excessive pain

Implementation

The nurse provides explicit information about benign breast changes, including signs and symptoms, so the woman will know what is normal for her; about the technique of and need for BSE; and about the therapeutic effects of diet change, diuretics, or hormones, along with their side effects. Provide written instructions to supplement verbal instructions.

If the woman is undergoing diagnostic procedures, the nurse teaches her what to expect before and after these procedures. Instruct her to refrain from using deodorant on the day of a mammogram because the aluminum in many products may give a false-positive reading in the axillary area. In the case of biopsy examination and needle aspirations, which are often done with the patient under local anesthesia and requires no preparation, assure the woman that the procedure provides identification of her disease and is a step toward eliminating her symptoms.

Provide emotional support to all who are experiencing breast changes that may be interpreted as breast cancer. Assure women that approximately 80% of the lumps found are benign. Adequate knowledge about benign disorders will help to alleviate fear and anxiety.

Evaluation

Benign breast disorders do not require routine follow-up observation. If symptoms are not alleviated or the condition changes, the woman seeks further medical therapy. The woman is less anxious after being taught about the benign condition and her medical management. She performs BSE monthly using an appropriate technique and has a professional breast examination appropriate for her age.

Documentation

Document the findings of breast assessment and interventions, noting the woman's ability to understand the material. When she returns for a follow-up examination, her response to teaching, her performance of BSE, and her alleviation of symptoms are recorded.

Ongoing Care

The woman with a benign breast condition maintains follow-up care with a health professional and seeks further therapy if her condition changes.

CANCER OF THE BREAST
Etiology/Epidemiology

Breast cancer remains the leading cancer in women in the United States, at 32% of all cancers in women. In 1993 approximately 182,000 women and 1000 men are projected to get breast cancer, and 46,000 women and 300 men will die of this disease.[6] The estimate is that breast cancer occurs by age 85 in 1 of every 9 women in the United States.[1] Although men get breast cancer, the material in this chapter is directed to women. The findings for breast cancer and treatment measures are similar for men and women, although men are often diagnosed at a later stage of the disease.

Women at a higher risk for developing breast cancer are over 50 years, have a family history of breast cancer, had a prior breast disease, began menarche before 12 years, began menopause after 50 years, are nulliparous, experienced their first live birth after 30 years, drink alcohol daily, or are Jewish.[1,47] Studies show that drinking alcohol increases the risk for breast cancer. Some studies implicate and some studies deny any increased risk with dietary fat, obesity, body shape, diet additives, total calorie intake, birth control pills, and hormone replacement medications.[25] A woman's ultimate risk of breast cancer is growing older, especially if the woman had early menarche with menopause after 55 years.[40] However, it is estimated that 80% of all breast cancers have no correlation with risk factors.[32,38] Therefore BSE should be a monthly health practice for all women.

Pathophysiology

Breast cancer is usually an adenocarcinoma that originates in epithelial tissue of the breast and occurs in the ducts (ductal carcinoma) or lobes (lobular carcinoma). Cancers developing in other areas of the breast are labeled miscellaneous or in situ. The invasiveness of breast cancers is determined by pathologic studies seeking to show whether the mass is penetrating the duct wall or breast tissue outside the tumor mass; the cancer is considered noninvasive or noninfiltrating when no infiltration of cells is found outside the tumor mass. The most frequently diagnosed tumor cell is invasive intraductal carcinoma.[23,38] The box below shows the major and some rare classifications of carcinomas of the breast.[41]

Carcinoma in situ, including Paget's disease, denotes noninvasive tumors 4 cm or smaller.[22] These tumors are curable. However, tumors labeled noninvasive have been known to recur as invasive lesions.[26]

Multiple studies are done on the tumor to give information beyond cell type. Histologic grading (1 through 4) includes determining the cell's appearance (differentiated vs. poorly differentiated) and mitotic rate. Nuclear grade (3 to 1) evaluates how differentiated the cell's nucleus appears. Lymphatic and blood vessels adjacent to the tumor are also evaluated for tumor involvement. Estrogen and progesterone receptor studies are done to determine the presence or absence of estrogen receptor and progesterone receptor proteins in the breast cancer cells. These studies combined with tumor classification, stage, and number of positive lymph nodes (discussed in this chapter) provide more information about the potential for recurrence of breast cancer and the type of adjuvant therapy (chemotherapy or radiation therapy) to be used. Newer studies being done on the tumor cells include DNA flow cytometry and oncogene determination.[23]

Clinical Manifestations

Tumors obvious under a microscope may be difficult to palpate. A dominant mass or thickening in the breast or axilla may be found on physical examination. The tumor may be felt as a hard, round, fixed mass or as soft and spongy. It may have discrete or irregular borders and may be fixed to the skin causing retraction (dimpling) of the skin or nipple. Some tumors produce a bloody or clear discharge from the nipple. Paget's disease is marked by persistent eczema or encrustation over the areola or nipple. Inflammatory breast cancer is characterized by swelling, inflammation, and skin edema causing peau d'orange, a dimpled condition of the skin.[7] About half of all breast cancers occur in the upper outer quadrant of the breast. The second most common site (18%) is around and under the nipple (Figure 70-15).[49] Tumors occur more frequently in the left than in the right breast.

CARCINOMAS OF THE BREAST

Carcinoma in situ
Lobular
Ductal
Paget's disease

Noninvasive carcinoma
Intraductal
Intracystic
Solid duct
Lobular

Invasive carcinoma
Infiltrating ductal (not otherwise specified)
    Comedo
    Medullary
    Mucinous
    Papillary
    Scirrhous
Infiltrating lobular
Infiltrating tubular

Rare carcinomas
Tubular
Inflammatory
Apocrine
Lipid rich

Adapted from Teng PK: Pathology of breast cancer. In Ariel IM, Cleary JB, editors: *Breast cancer: diagnosis and treatment,* New York, 1987, McGraw-Hill Book Co.

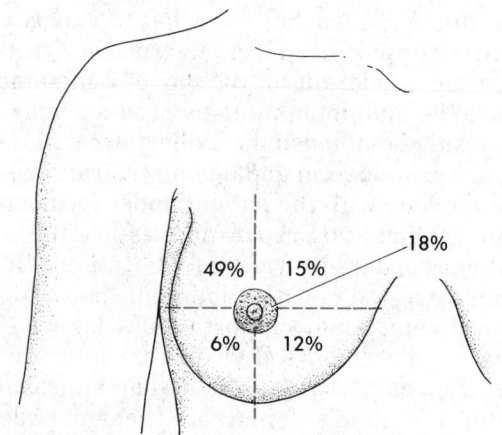

FIGURE 70-15   Incidence of tumors in breast.

Diagnostic studies

Breast tumors of about 1 cm in diameter can be detected by palpation, but other studies must be done to detect smaller ones, and definitive diagnosis can be made only by biopsy. Women should practice monthly BSE to note any subtle changes in the breast tissue, supraclavicular nodes, or axilla. Postmenopausal and pregnant women should set a specific day for BSE each month. If a woman notes changes, she should be examined by a professional health care provider. It is recommended that every woman between 20 and 40 years old receive a professional physical breast examination every 3 years, and women more than 40 years old receive the examination annually.[1] The physician or nurse who examines the woman can validate the woman's findings, determine whether the breast is normal or not, and decide whether further studies are needed.

Mammography is the most commonly used diagnostic tool for detecting breast cancer. If the screening mammogram indicates a problem or the woman has a breast mass, a xeromammogram is done. The xeromammogram provides a uniform image of the breast with a wide exposure, which compensates for the breast's dense tissue. There is a 5% to 10% margin of error even with a xeromammogram.

The American Cancer Society's guidelines for mammography are as follows:

1. Baseline mammogram for women between 35 and 39 years of age
2. Annual or biennial mammogram for women 40 to 49 years of age
3. Annual mammogram for women 50 years and older[1]

The possibility of a cancerous mass in the breast requires a definitive diagnostic biopsy. The three types of biopsies are needle, incision, and excision.

Further surgery after an excisional biopsy with a 2 cm margin may not be done if the patient and physician choose to treat the tumor with primary radiation therapy. If the tumor is 4 cm or larger, an incisional biopsy of the mass is done to determine malignancy. In a one-stage procedure, surgery is begun to retrieve the biopsy specimen and progresses if a frozen-section examination confirms malignancy. In a two-stage procedure, tissue is obtained by a needle biopsy, an excisional biopsy, or an incisional biopsy and the patient and physician discuss treatment options if the final pathology report confirms malignancy. Then the operation specific for the size of the tumor is done.[8]

Therapeutic Management

Surgery

Tumor size and nodal involvement help determine cancer stage (as defined in this section) and appropriate therapeutic measures. Therefore lumpectomy, segmental resection (partial mastectomy), or simple mastectomy is usually accompanied by axillary dissection of the lymph nodes. Axillary dissection involves taking a sample of 10 to 15 lymph nodes from the anatomic distribution of nodes at locations lateral and inferior to the pectoralis minor muscle, levels I and II (Figure 70-16). Positive nodes and nodes fixed to the muscle increase the person's stage of disease.[9,23]

If the tumor can be completely removed by excisional biopsy or lumpectomy (Figure 70-17), the patient and physician may decide to use local irradiation of the breast to destroy any potentially microscopic cancer cells in the area. If the tumor is determined to be too large for lumpectomy, more extensive surgery may be done.

Segmental mastectomy is removal of the tumor and adjacent tissue while the nipple, areola, and most of the breast remain intact (Figure 70-18). Another term used to describe this procedure is quadrantectomy, which is removal of a quadrant of the breast along with the overlying skin. In a total or simple mastectomy, all breast tissue is removed, and both pectoralis major and pectoralis minor muscles are left intact (Figure 70-19). A subcutaneous mastectomy is done to remove all breast tissue but to preserve the nipple and areola; this procedure often precedes immediate reconstruction.[9,26]

A modified radical mastectomy (Figure 70-20) is performed if the tumor is 4 cm or larger, if it is invasive, or if the patient and physician decide this procedure is in the patient's best interest. There are various definitions of modified radical mastectomy, including one by Danforth and Lippman[9] described as the Patey method. In this operation all breast tis-

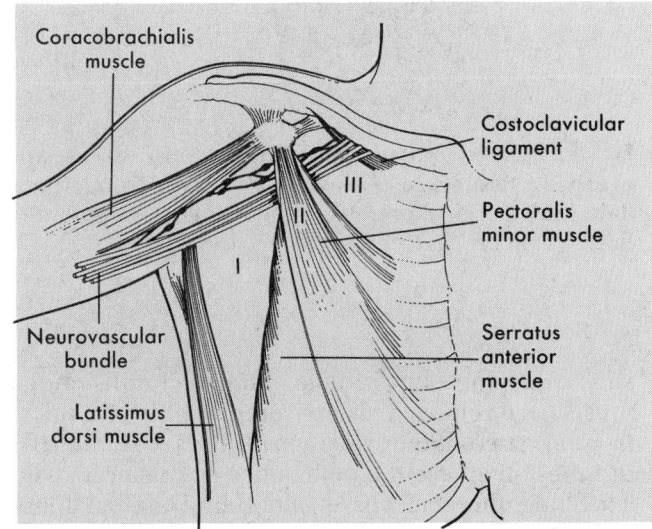

FIGURE 70-16   Anatomic levels of axilla.

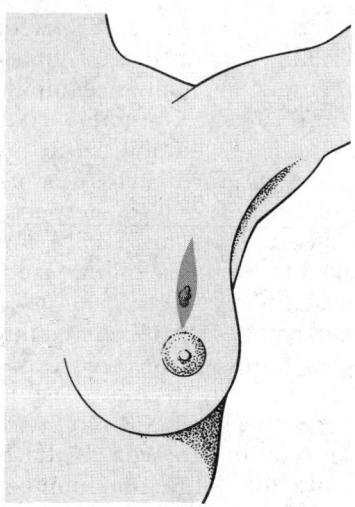

FIGURE 70-17   Excisional biopsy, or lumpectomy. Tumor is removed to diagnose cancer (biopsy) or as conservative surgery for cancer treatment (lumpectomy). (Redrawn from Romsdahl MM: Surgical options in the primary treatment of breast cancer, *Cancer Bull* 35:66, 1983.)

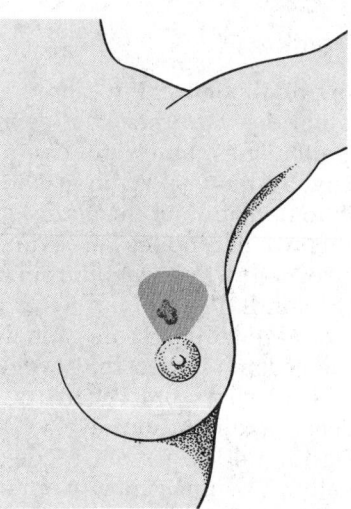

FIGURE 70-18   Segmental mastectomy. Tumor is removed along with segment of normal tissue surrounding it. (Redrawn from Romsdahl MM: Surgical options in the primary treatment of breast cancer, *Cancer Bull* 35:66, 1983.)

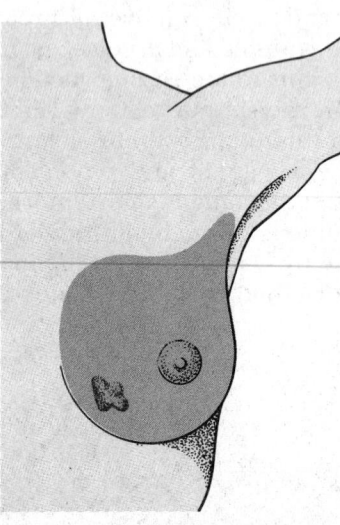

FIGURE 70-19   Total or simple mastectomy. Breast and overlying tissue are removed. (Redrawn from Romsdahl MM: Surgical options in the primary treatment of breast cancer, *Cancer Bull* 35:67, 1983.)

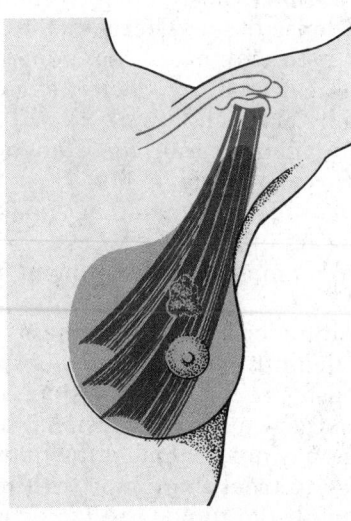

FIGURE 70-20   Modified radical mastectomy. Breast is removed along with portion of axillary lymph nodes, skin overlying breast, and often pectoralis minor muscle. (Redrawn from Romsdahl MM: Surgical options in the primary treatment of breast cancer, *Cancer Bull* 35:67, 1983.)

sue, overlying skin, nipple, and pectoralis minor muscle are removed, as are samples of lymph nodes from all surrounding positions (levels I, II, and III); at times all adjacent lymph nodes are also removed. The long thoracic nerve and thoracodorsal blood vessels are preserved to maintain full use of adjacent muscles. Currently the Halsted or radical mastectomy is not done in the United States because re-

fined techniques of pathologic evaluation, radiation therapy, and chemotherapy have made it unnecessary in most cases.

Staging

After breast surgery and axillary dissection, the staging process is completed. The universal staging and classification system for breast cancer agreed on in 1987, the TNM (tumor, node, metastasis) system, is based on clinical and pathologic evaluations (see box below). Staging depends on size of tumor, size and presence or absence of nodal malignancy, or absence of distant metastasis. Tumor in situ that has no nodal or metastatic involvement and is noninvasive is stage 0. A stage I tumor is 2 cm or smaller with no nodal or metastatic involvement. Stage II has five subgroupings, describing a tumor 2 to 5 cm with or without nodal involvement and with no metastasis. Stage III has six subgroupings, describing a tumor 5 to 10 cm and usually with lymph node involvement and no metastasis. Stage IV denotes a tu-

UICC/TNM AND AJCC STAGING OF BREAST CANCER

T: tumor

T_x: primary tumor cannot be assessed
T_0: no evidence of primary tumor
T_{is}: carcinoma in situ
T_1: tumor 2.0 cm or less
  T_{1a}: 0.5 cm or less
  T_{1b}: > 0.5 cm but not more than 1 cm
  T_{1c}: > 1.0 cm but not more than 2 cm
T_2: tumor > 2.0 cm but not more than 5.0 cm
T_3: tumor > 5.0 cm
T_4: tumor any size with direct extension to chest wall or skin
  T_{4a}: extension to chest wall
  T_{4b}: edema or ulceration of skin of breast or satellite skin; nodular, confined to the same breast
  T_{4c}: both T_{4a} and T_{4b}
  T_{4d}: inflammatory carcinoma

N: node

N_x: regional lymph nodes cannot be assessed
N_0: no regional lymph node metastasis
N_1: metastasis to movable ipsilateral axillary lymph nodes
N_2: metastasis to ipsilateral axillary lymph nodes fixed to one another or to other structures
N_3: metastasis to ipsilateral internal mammary lymph nodes

M: distant metastasis

M_x: presence of distant metastasis cannot be assessed
M_0: no distant metastasis
M_1: distant metastasis (includes metastasis to ipsilateral supraclavicular lymph nodes)

Stage groupings   Classification

Stage	T	N	M
0	T_{is}	N_0	M_0
1	T_1	N_0	M_0
IIA	T_0	N_1	M_0
	T_1	N_1	M_0
	T_2	N_0	M_0
IIB	T_2	N_1	M_0
	T_3	N_0	M_0
IIIA	T_0	N_2	M_0
	T_1	N_2	M_0
	T_2	N_2	M_0
	T_3	N_1, N_2	M_0
IIIB	T_4	Any N	M_0
	Any T	N_3	M_0
IV	Any T	Any N	M_1

From American Joint Committee on Cancer (AJCC): *Manual for staging of cancer*, ed 4, Philadelphia, 1992, JB Lippincott.

mor of any size, with or without nodal involvement but with distant metastasis.[3]

NURSING MANAGEMENT OF THE PATIENT UNDERGOING BREAST CANCER SURGERY

Nursing care for patients who undergo surgery includes the usual preoperative preparation and coping issues (see nursing care plan). The patient's assessment begins preoperatively before biopsy and continues through recovery from surgery. Before biopsy the nurse records the location, size, discreteness, and hardness of the changed tissue; the presence and characteristics of nipple discharge; the appearance of the breast and nipple; any signs of dimpling or retraction of the breast or nipple; inflammation or swelling of breast tissue; enlargement of axillary nodes; and breast pain and tenderness.

The patient's emotional state is recorded. Anxiety is usually present before diagnosis and may be intensified after diagnosis. If possible, the nurse and patient discuss the patient's usual coping mechanisms as well as her available support systems. This assessment is accomplished by attentive listening to the patient's spoken and unspoken needs, fears, questions, and understanding of the procedures and treatment goals. The nurse may need to answer questions as the patient tries to understand all information the surgeon has given her. Booklets specifically concerning breast operations, radiation therapy, chemotherapy, and breast reconstruction address questions related to other treatment plans (see Resources). The nurse reviews the literature with the patient and answers questions as they arise to help the patient understand her treatment options.

Postoperative care includes maintaining good lung ventilation, preventing infection of the surgical site, and achieving early ambulation. Patients who have had some type of breast surgery will usually have a wound catheter for incisional drainage attached to suction. Provide the patient emotional support for body image changes, and give instructions about arm care to prevent lymphedema and frozen shoulder.

Postoperatively the patient may have pain and tenderness at the surgical site, the shoulder, and the affected arm. Shoulder and arm pain may result from her position on the surgical table, manipulation of the nerves during the procedure, and sometimes placement of the wound catheter against nerves. Restriction of arm and muscular movements on the affected side depends on the surgical procedure. The patient may need to be referred to a physical therapist if the operation has been extensive or if the patient protects her arm movement too much.

During her first postoperative evaluation, teach the patient postoperative BSE including the surgical incision, all chest wall tissue, and her normal breast. Teach her to notify the physician of any changes in the surgical area that indicate recurrence, such as redness, rash, lumps, swelling, or a break in the skin integrity. Refer the patient or family if they need assistance with their grieving process.

Radiation therapy

Patients who have had an excision biopsy or lumpectomy may determine with their physician that external radiation therapy is their primary therapy choice. This provides local therapy while preserving the breast tissue. Radiation therapy is given over 5 to 6 weeks for a total of 5000 to 5300 cGy.[35] A radiation boost may be given to the tumor area by electron beam or by a needle implant of iridium 192 (^{192}Ir). The latter is inserted surgically and left in place for 48 hours.[16] Visitors and health care team members should observe radiation precautions when ^{192}Ir is in place (see Figure 15-7). The electron beam method is used more commonly, because it is noninvasive and the results are similar to those of ^{192}Ir.[18]

Radiation therapy may also be used postoperatively to provide more protection for the patient by destroying microscopic cancer cells in adjacent breast tissue, especially if the tumor was an invasive carcinoma. If the tumor was located medially, radiation therapy may be recommended for the area overlying the internal mammary lymph nodes, because these nodes usually drain the medial area of breast tissue and cannot be surgically removed.

Postoperative radiation therapy is usually delivered to the patient over 5 to 5½ weeks for a total dose of 5000 cGy, with a further boost to the tumor bed. Evaluation of the size and location of the tumor and of the presence of positive axillary lymph nodes is made before therapy to determine the sites and depth of irradiation.[29,42] (See Chapter 15 for further discussion of radiation therapy.)

NURSING MANAGEMENT OF THE PATIENT UNDERGOING RADIOTHERAPY

Nursing intervention during radiation therapy may be limited, since this therapy is maintained by a physician radiotherapist and a radiation technician. Patients who receive radiation therapy have specific areas of need related to treatment and psychosocial needs in which nurses may provide care, such as skin changes, anemia, fatigue, and swelling of the breasts[59] (see Chapter 15). The patient should maintain good skin care and notify her radiotherapist if skin changes occur.

NURSING CARE PLAN   *The Patient With Breast Cancer*

Nursing diagnosis/ Expected outcome	Interventions	Rationale
PREOPERATIVE		
Coping related to unknown events surrounding breast • *Patient will explain surgical procedure and perioperative routine*	Assess patient's prior surgical experiences Obtain feedback of patient's knowledge of this surgery and perioperative routine Provide specific information to resolve misconceptions Allow time for questions and concerns, especially about loss of her breast Provide emotional support to patient and partner	Patients who have knowledge and who are able to cope with their fears or concerns will recover more rapidly
POSTOPERATIVE		
High risk for infection in wound because of removal of lymph channels and presence of wound drainage system • *Patient will have decreased wound drainage and removal of drains about 7 to 10 days after surgery with no signs of infection*	Assess drainage system for patency; color, amount, and type of secretions; and proper suctioning Instruct patient on care of wound drainage system: cleaning site and catheter insertion site; emptying infection collection device; recording amount, color, and type of drainage; maintaining suction collection device Have patient give return demonstration on home care of wound drainage system Have patient report signs of infection: fever, redness at surgical site, or purulent drainage	Patients who are able to care for themselves recover more rapidly; maintaining suction reduces risk of a seroma; cleaning wound and catheter insertion sites reduces risk of infection
Grieving over body alteration • *Patient and partner will adjust normally to altered breast appearance*	Assess patient's ability to inspect her breast after surgery Assist patient in looking at surgical site if needed Listen attentively to patient's and partner's concern to provide emotional support Request Reach to Recovery visit for in the hospital or after discharge	Emotional healing to loss of a breast takes time for most women
Altered tissue perfusion related to removal of some lymph nodes in surgical site • *Patient will verbalize care for her arm on surgical side to prevent or control lymphedema*	Instruct patient to avoid heavy lifting; getting a blood pressure, intravenous fluids, laboratory studies on affected arm; infections from burns, sewing, or gardening injuries in hospital or after discharge	Some patients are prone to develop lymphedema; prevention is less difficult and costly than treating lymphedema
Immobility related to loss of motion while surgical drains are in place • *Patient will retain full motion of arm and shoulder on surgical site*	Instruct patient to begin gentle exercises when drains are still in place, such as brushing her hair, hand to shoulder Instruct to increase exercises after drains are removed to include raising arm above head (using a pulley or climbing the wall) and full rotation of arm Request Reach to Recovery volunteer to teach exercises appropriate for postmastectomy patients	Patients may continue to keep arm immobile after surgical drains are removed; frozen shoulder is very difficult and painful to treat

Chemotherapy

Chemotherapy provides systemic therapy to all regions of the body to which malignant cells may travel. It has been determined that tumor cell control occurs best when the tumor is small.

Adjuvant chemotherapy is often given to patients with stage I, II, or III breast cancer. Studies have demonstrated that patients with stage I benefit from adjuvant chemotherapy; the National Cancer Institute has strongly recommended that this treatment be given to all patients.[11] Many combinations of agents are used for first-line adjuvant chemotherapy, the two main combinations being 5-fluorouracil/doxorubicin/cyclophosphamide and 5-fluorouracil/methotrexate/cyclophosphamide. To intensify therapy, other agents such as vincristine, prednisone, or tamoxifen may be added. Adjuvant chemotherapy may be given every 3 weeks over a 6-month period. The drugs usually given to outpatients may be administered by push or bolus intravenous infusion or by continuous infusion therapy over 48 to 96 hours. Various regimens are used throughout the world based on the experience of physicians and nurses who manage the regimens. With the advent of central venous catheter placement, chemotherapy is easier to deliver and provides less risk of extravasation of vesicant agents. Nausea, vomiting, changes in bowel and bladder function, and myleosuppression are common side effects.

Patients with stage III cancer with skin or chest wall involvement may receive chemotherapy preoperatively (neoadjuvant chemotherapy). This program of care provides the same combination drugs as adjuvant chemotherapy, but three or more courses are given before surgery to reduce the size of the tumor. Chemotherapy is completed after the operation, and radiation therapy may then be prescribed.

Patients with primary stage IV breast cancer (metastatic disease at the time of diagnosis) receive chemotherapy as primary medical management. These patients have had a biopsy to confirm the diagnosis but usually do not have the breast removed. They will be treated with a specific chemotherapy regimen until they no longer respond to that particular therapy; then another combination is usually administered. Various experimental trials of new drugs are being conducted throughout the world to find better treatments for breast cancer patients (see Chapter 15).

Drug trials show that combination chemotherapy or tamoxifen alone compared with no adjuvant chemotherapy improves survival rates of all women.[13] Long-term tamoxifen use (2 to 5 years) is more effective than short-term use. Survival rates and protection of the contralateral breast were highly significant during the years the patients received tamoxifen and up to 10 years (the longest time studied). Tamoxifen, an antiestrogen, is especially effective in patients who are estrogen receptor positive.[13]

Some patients receiving chemotherapy or hormonal therapy experience side effects that may affect their self-image. These include hair loss from chemotherapy, weight gain, and temporary menopausal symptoms from either chemotherapy or hormonal therapy. Sexuality may be a concern for many breast cancer patients. Libido usually decreases during myelosuppression and may be further decreased by cytotoxic or hormonal suppression of the ovaries. Advise patients of potential changes in their sexual functioning so that they may feel free to ask questions regarding areas such as birth control measures and ways of expressing love if sexual intercourse becomes too painful during chemotherapy or hormonal therapy. Often the vaginal wall becomes thin and dry; water-soluble lubricants can be used to decrease dyspareunia. Use of estrogen cream is not advised because of its hormonal content. Nonhormonal drugs are available to help reduce hot flashes caused by the therapy.

Reconstruction

The patient whose disease is limited to the breast may benefit from reconstructive surgery, which can be done any time after the original operation. Some patients have reconstruction done at the time of the original procedure; others must wait until they have completed adjuvant chemotherapy or radiation therapy to ensure that the area is free of disease. (See Chapter 76 for a complete discussion of reconstruction.)

Recurrent breast cancer metastasis

Although patients with stage 0 and stage I breast cancers have very good prognoses, about 50% of all patients with breast cancer will have metastasis within 10 years. In a few cases the disease may metastasize even 30 years after diagnosis, although most patients who relapse do so within 2 years of their diagnosis.

Metastasis may occur in any part of the body, the most common sites of recurrence being bone, lung, pleura, breast surgery site, central nervous system, and liver, in that order.[22,29] Metastasis in the bone and surgical site causes many treatment problems but is not life threatening, whereas metastasis in the other sites listed, being vital organs, is life threatening.[39] With bone metastasis the patient may have intractable bone pain, become hypercalcemic, or have a pathologic fracture of a weight-bearing bone or a compression fracture of the vertebrae. Regardless of site, metastasis changes the patient's quality of life. Currently, metastatic breast cancer is considered incurable.[39]

Medical management is directed to the site of metastasis and the symptoms related to it. Chemotherapy is the usual means of controlling the spread of cancer cells throughout the body, with radiation therapy used at specific sites (brain, spinal cord, or bone) for tumor cell destruction or pain control. Each patient is treated according to site of disease, previous chemotherapy exposure, and the drugs useful in her case. Although metastatic breast cancer is incurable, many patients live comfortable lives for several years while their cancer is under control. Routine follow-up studies are necessary so that early detection of a recurrence will lead to early treatment.

NURSING MANAGEMENT OF THE PATIENT WITH METASTATIC BREAST CANCER

Assess patients with recurrent or metastatic breast cancer to determine signs of disease that may be present but are not recognized. The nurse provides psychologic support during this time. Teach the patient management of the disease process. Teach the patient her risks for fractures in the bones affected by metastasis. Weight bearing may continue, even when degenerating bone lesions are present in the long bones, as long as pain does not limit the patient's mobility. Although pathologic fractures may occur regardless of the care given to the patient, nurses should be aware of the sites of bone metastasis and protect the patient during transfer procedures. The patient's bony extremities should not be used when moving her up in bed or onto a stretcher; instead, a lift sheet or a transfer board should be used. An overhead trapeze may be ordered if there is no risk of humerus or vertebral fracture. Pain medication should be adequate to control the pain, which may be intense. Documenting the patient's pain level, amount of drug, the duration of pain relief, and amount of pain relief will help the nurse determine if a sufficient level of relief is maintained for the patient. The patient should be mobile as long as possible.

Chest wall or breast lesions may cause the patient great physical and emotional distress. Dry, itching nodules may be treated with an emollient cream or lotion. If the lesions become open or are draining, they may be cleansed with normal saline solution followed by a wet-to-wet dressing of normal saline solution. If the lesions are malodorous and draining, sodium hypochlorite solution at one-fourth strength or other debriding agents may be used. At times, charcoal-impregnated gauze outside the dressing may help reduce odor. The patient may need to use

a power spray to clean the lesion if it has multiple crevices. The basic problem of cancer to the chest wall will not be resolved with this care, but local care may reduce infection and provide comfort for the patient.[17]

A patient with lung or pleural metastasis may have great difficulty breathing. She should be placed in a comfortable position and instructed to space her activities to allow adequate rest. Assess her breathing capacity and changes in breathing patterns, and document her abilities as well as limitations. Oxygen may be needed at home to help her maintain a near-normal living pattern.

Patients with central nervous system (CNS) metastasis may have many cranial, cerebral, or spinal abnormalities that require nursing and medical care. The nurse must be aware of what is normal for a specific patient so that she may identify any changes and treat them as early as possible. Steroids should be given around the clock rather than four times daily to control inflammation of the tumor at the site of CNS metastasis. The patient may repeatedly require reorientation to her surroundings. Instruct the patient's family regarding safety measures when the patient is disoriented.

Liver metastasis may cause major body image problems with jaundice; dry, flaking skin; ascites; and muscle wasting. Good skin care with body lotion and bath oils provides comfort. Ascites is managed medically; however, the nurse assists the patient in reaching a comfortable breathing position and encourages small frequent feedings.

A patient whose disease process is advancing may become less able to carry on her normal life-style. The patient and her family may find accompanying role changes difficult to accept. New coping patterns may emerge and should be encouraged. The nurse who has been a supportive person may now help the patient and family find a referral service for home care or for outpatient or inpatient hospice care. When the disease continues to progress and death is imminent, support for the family as well as the patient is important. Many families are able to organize their own support and do not need a hospice referral, but many patients and families benefit from this vital service.

CRITICAL THINKING QUESTIONS

1 How is the vagina normally protected from infection?

2 What are four risk factors for developing vulvovaginal infections?

3 What is the most serious consequence of pelvic inflammatory disease?

4 What laboratory values are elevated in toxic shock syndrome?

5 What patient teaching is appropriate for the patient with toxic shock syndrome?

6 What is dysfunctional uterine bleeding?

7 What are some theories about the cause of premenstrual syndrome?

8 What dietary modifications can be used to decrease the symptoms of premenstrual syndrome?

9 What is the greatest single cause of absenteeism among women?

10 List several physiologic changes that occur in women as a result of menopause.

11 What patient teaching is appropriate for the woman going through the "change of life"?

12 List a common nursing diagnosis for the woman with endometriosis.

13 What dietary modifications are important in the patient with leiomyomas?

14 What should be included in the postoperative care for a patient undergoing hysterectomy?

15 What is the most common method for obtaining endometrial cells for study?

16 How is cervical cancer treated?

17 What patients are at risk for developing endometrial cancer?

18 What patient teaching is appropriate for a patient receiving internal irradiation?

19 What nursing strategies could be used to increase comfort in a patient with a vulvectomy?

20 What are the two most common benign breast disorders?

21 What diagnostic tools are used to differentiate between breast cancer and benign breast disorders?

22 What are five risk factors for breast cancer?

23 What are the three therapeutic modalities for breast cancer?

24 What nursing measures are used for a patient who is newly diagnosed with breast cancer?

25 What are the nursing interventions for post-mastectomy patients?

26 What are the most common sites of breast cancer metastasis? What are two nursing measures to be taken for each site?

RESOURCES

1 AGENCY FOR HEALTH CARE POLICY AND RESEARCH PUBLICATIONS CLEARINGHOUSE P.O. Box 8547 Silver Spring, MD 20907 1-800-358-9295 "Urinary Incontinence in Adults" guidelines are available free; future guidelines will be sent as they are developed if you request

2 AMERICAN ASSOCIATION OF SEX EDUCATORS, COUNSELORS, AND THERAPISTS Eleven Dupont Circle, N.W. Washington, DC 20036-1207 1-202-462-1171 Agency to certify practitioners in the field of human sexuality

3 AMERICAN CANCER SOCIETY (contact your local agency) Provides "Reach to Recovery," "I Can Cope," sometimes ostomy supplies, ostomy visitors, other services, and information for patients with cancer or cancer information for health professionals

4 CANCER INFORMATION SERVICE 1-800-4-CANCER A nationwide toll-free program sponsored by National Cancer Institute

5 ICI PHARMA P.O. Box 30000 Philadelphia, PA 19103-9620 Provides videotapes on lumpectomy and mastectomy, nursing literature

6 NATIONAL CENTER FOR PMS AND MENSTRUAL DISTRESS 15 Smith Road Bedford, NH 03102

7 NATIONAL HEALTH INFORMATION CLEARINGHOUSE P.O. Box 1133 Washington, DC 1-800-336-4797

8 NATIONAL ORGANIZATION FOR WOMEN (NOW) Check phone book for local chapter

9 NATIONAL PMS SOCIETY Box 11467 Durham, NC 27703

10 NATIONAL SEXUALLY TRANSMITTED DISEASE HOTLINE 1-800-227-8922

11 OFFICE OF CANCER COMMUNICATIONS National Cancer Institute Building 31, Room 10A24 Bethesda, MD 20892 Provides booklets and other information about cancer for health professionals and clients

12 PATIENT INFORMATION LIBRARY PAS Publishing 345-G Serramonte Plaza Daly City, CA 99015 1-415-994-1150 Many pamphlets related to women's health that may be purchased for a small fee.

13 SEX INFORMATION AND EDUCATION COUNCIL OF THE U.S. 130 West 42nd Street, Suite 2500 New York, NY 10036 1-212-819-9770

14 SUSAN G. KOMEN FOUNDATION I'm Aware Line answers questions about breast cancer 1-800-462-9273

15 UNITED OSTOMY ASSOCIATION, INC. 36 Executive Park, Suite 120 Irvine, CA 92714 1-800-826-0826 Provides educational information, magazines, and referrals for support groups

16 Y-ME 1-800-221-2141 Former breast cancer patients provide support and answer questions about breast cancer

17 YWCA local association may have the ENCORE program, an exercise and discussion group for women who have been treated for breast cancer

BIBLIOGRAPHY

Current

1. American Cancer Society: *Cancer facts and figures—1993*, Atlanta, 1993, The Society.
2. Ariel IM, Teng PK, Prudente R: Fibrocystic breasts: diagnosis, treatment, and association with cancer. In Ariel IM, Cleary JB, editors: *Breast cancer: diagnosis and treatment*, New York, 1987, McGraw-Hill Book Co.
3. Beahrs OH et al: *Manual for staging of cancer*, ed 3, New York, 1988, JB Lippincott Co.
4. Bergdoll M, Chesney P: *Toxic shock syndrome*, Boca Raton, Fla, 1991, CRC Press.
5. Boring CC, Squires TS, Tong T: Cancer statistics, 1991, *CA* 41:19, 1991.
6. Boring CC, Squires TS, Tong T: Cancer statistics, 1993, *CA* 43:7, 1993.
7. Cleary JB: Breast biopsy. In Ariel IM, Cleary JB, editors: *Breast cancer: diagnosis and treatment*, New York, 1987, McGraw-Hill Book Co.
8. Danforth DN, Lichter AS, Lippman ME: The diagnosis of breast cancer. In Lippman ME, Lichter AS, Danforth DN, editors: *Diagnosis and management of breast cancer*, Philadelphia, 1988, WB Saunders Co.
9. Danforth DN, Lippman ME: Surgical treatments of breast cancer. In Lippman ME, Litchter AS, Danforth DN, editors: *Diagnosis and management of breast cancer*, Philadelphia, 1988, WB Saunders Co.
10. Deppe G, Lawrence W: Vulvar dystrophy and neoplasia. In Gusberg S, Shingleton H, Deppe G, editors: *Female genital cancer*, New York, 1988, Churchill Livingstone.
11. Dorr FA, Friedman MA: The role of chemotherapy in the management of primary breast cancer, *CA* 41:231, 1991.
12. Droegemueller W et al: *Comprehensive gynecology*, St Louis, 1987, Mosby–Year Book, Inc.
13. Early Breast Cancer Trialist Collaborative Group: Systematic treatment of early breast cancer by hormonal, cytotoxic, or immune therapy, *Lancet* 339:1, 1992.
14. Ellerhorst-Ryan JM, Turba EP, Stahl DL: Evaluating benign breast disease, *Nurse Pract* 13(9):13, 1988.
15. Eriksson J, Walczak J: Ovarian cancer, *Semin Oncol Nurs* 6:214, 1990.
16. Findlay PA: Radiation therapy as definitive treatment of breast cancer. In Lippman ME, Lichter AS, Danforth DN, editors: *Diagnosis and management of breast cancer*, Philadelphia, 1988, WB Saunders Co.
17. Gilmore MA: Symptomatic treatment of an ulcerating breast mass in a patient with advanced carcinoma of the breast, *Cancer Bull* 43:461, 1991.
18. Goodman RL: *Perspectives in diagnosing and treating early breast cancer*. Teleconference, 1988, Hospital Satellite Network, CME-T5219.
19. Greendale G, Carlson K, Schiff I: Estrogen and progestin therapy to prevent osteoporosis: attitudes and practices of general internists and gynecologists, *J Gen Intern Med* 5:464, 1990.
20. Gurganus S, Morris J: Pelvic exenteration: the challenge of rehabilitation in a patient with multiple psychosocial problems, *J Enter Ther* 18(2):52, 1991.
21. Hsia L, Long M: Premenstrual syndrome: current concepts in diagnosis and management, *J Nurse Midwifery* 35:351, 1990.
22. Hutter RVP: At last—worldwide agreement on the staging of breast cancer, *Arch Surg* 122:1235, 1987.
23. Hutter RVP: The role of the pathologist in the management of breast cancer, *CA* 41:283, 1991.
24. Jobson V: Cryotherapy and laser treatment for intraepithelial neoplasia of the cervix, vagina, and vulva, *Oncology* 5(8):69, 1991.
25. Kelsey JL, Gummon MD: The epidemiology of breast cancer, *CA* 41:146, 1991.
26. Kinne DW: The surgical management of primary breast cancer, *CA* 41:71, 1991.
27. Kirkpatrick M, Edwards M, Finch N: Assessment and prevention of osteoporosis through use of a client self-reporting tool, *Nurse Pract* 16(7):16, 1991.
28. Lamb M: Psychosexual issues: the woman with gynecologic cancer, *Semin Oncol Nurs* 6:237, 1990.
29. Lichter AS: Technical aspects of the treatment of breast cancer with radiation therapy. In Lippman ME, Lichter AS, Danforth DN, editors: *Diagnosis and management of breast cancer*, Philadelphia, 1988, WB Saunders Co.
30. Lindow K: Premenstrual syndrome: family impact and nursing implications, *J Obstet Gynecol Nurs* 20:135-138, 1991.
31. Love SM et al: Benign breast disorders. In Harris JR et al, editors: *Breast diseases*, Philadelphia, 1987, JB Lippincott Co.
32. Mettlin C: Breast cancer risk factors. In Ariel IM, Cleary JB, editors: *Breast cancer: diagnosis and treatment*, New York, 1987, McGraw-Hill Book Co.
33. Nolte S, Hanjani P: Intraepithelial neoplasia of the lower genital tract, *Semin Oncol Nurs* 6:181, 1990.
34. *Nursing '87 books. Diseases: causes and diagnosis, current therapy*, ed 2, Springhouse, Pa, 1987, Nursing Management Nurses Reference Library.
35. Pierce SM, Harris JR: The role of radiation therapy in the management of primary breast cancer, *CA* 41:85, 1991.
36. Piver S et al: Epidemiology and etiology of ovarian cancer, *Semin Oncol* 18:177, 1991.
37. Ratliff C: Brachytherapy revolution: the selection ^{137}CS unit, *Nurs News Today* 2(5):9, 1990.
38. Scanlon EF: Breast cancer. In Holleb AI, Fink DJ, Murphy GP, editors: *American Cancer Society textbook of clinical oncology*, Atlanta, 1991, American Cancer Society.
39. Smith IE: Recurrent disease. In Harris JR et al, editors: *Breast diseases*, Philadelphia, 1987, JB Lippincott Co.
40. Stewart JA, Foster RS: Breast cancer and aging, *Semin Oncol* 16:41, 1989.
41. Teng PK: Pathology of breast cancer. In Ariel IM, Cleary JB, editors: *Breast cancer: diagnosis and treatment*, New York, 1987, McGraw-Hill Book Co.
42. Yarold JR, Bloom HJG: Radiation after limited and radical surgery. In Hoogstraten B, Burn I, Bloom HJG, editors: *Breast cancer*, New York, 1989, Springer-Verlag.
43. Zimny M: Ovarian cancer: a nursing overview, *Oncology* 5:147, 1991.

Classic

44. Barber H: *Manual of gynecologic oncology*, Philadelphia, 1980, JB Lippincott Co.
45. Barber H: Ovarian cancer: diagnosis and surgical management. In Forastiere A, editor: *Gynecologic cancer*, New York, 1984, Churchill Livingstone.
46. Beecham J et al: Tumors of the female reproductive organs. In Rubin P, editor: *Clinical oncology for medical students and physicians*, New York, 1983, American Cancer Society.
47. Berkowitz CS: Risk factors. In Merchant DJ, editor: *Breast disease*, vol 1. *Contemporary issues in obstetrics and gynecology*, New York, 1986, Churchill Livingstone.

48. Bouchard R, Owens N: *Nursing care of the cancer patient,* ed 4, St Louis, 1980, Mosby–Year Book, Inc.

49. Case C, editor: *The breast cancer digest,* ed 2, Bethesda, Md, 1984, National Cancer Institute.

50. Coppleson M: *Gynecologic oncology,* Edinburgh, 1981, Churchill Livingstone.

51. Crosson K: A patient teaching aid for the pelvic exenteration patient, *Oncol Nurs Forum* 8:53, 1981.

52. DiSaia P, Rich W: Advanced and recurrent carcinoma of the cervix. In Coppleson M, editor: *Gynecologic oncology,* Edinburgh, 1981, Churchill Livingstone.

53. Griffith M et al: *Oncology nursing: pathophysiology, assessment and intervention,* New York, 1984, MacMillan Publishing Co.

54. Morrow P, Townsend D: *Synopsis of gynecologic oncology,* New York, 1981, John Wiley & Sons.

55. Perez C et al: Gynecologic tumors. In DiVita V, Hellmann S, Rosenberg S, editors: *Cancer principles and practice of oncology,* Philadelphia, 1985, JB Lippincott Co.

56. Preece PE: Nomenclature of benign breast disease, with particular reference to national difference in approach. In L'Etang HJ, editor: *Benign breast disease,* London, 1983, The Royal Society of Medicine.

57. Robertson C, Moreland B: Overview of ovarian cancer, *Dimen Oncol Nurs* 1:11, 1985.

58. Rutledge F: Prognostic factors in epidermoid cancer of the vulva, *Obstet Gynecol* 37:892, 1971.

59. Weichselbaum RR et al: Radiotherapy in the treatment of breast cancer. In Pfeiffer CH, Mulliken JB, editors: *Caring for the patient with breast cancer: an interdisciplinary/multidisciplinary approach,* Reston, Va, 1984, Reston Publishing Co.

60. Wharton J et al: Microinvasive cancer of the vulva, *Am J Obstet Gynecol* 118:159, 1974.

61. Wroblewski S: Toxic shock syndrome, *Am J Nurs* 81:82, 1981.

62. Yarbrough B: Teaching plan for patient undergoing pelvic exenteration, *Oncol Nurs Forum* 2:36, 1981.

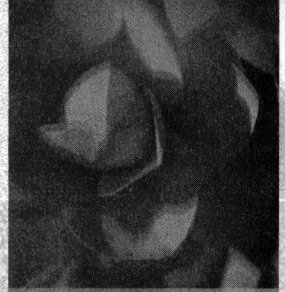

CHAPTER SEVENTY-ONE

Nursing Management of Men with Reproductive System Disorders

LEARNING OBJECTIVES

1 Identify the principal pathophysiologic process associated with benign prostatic hypertrophy.
2 List four common clinical manifestations of benign prostatic hypertrophy.
3 Describe the purpose of the voiding diary in patients with benign prostatic hypertrophy.
4 Identify three complications of hormonal therapy for prostatic cancer.
5 List three nursing strategies for preventing disruption of the urethrovesical anastomosis after radical prostatectomy.
6 Describe an exercise regimen for the patient with stress urinary incontinence after radical prostatectomy.
7 Explain the elements of testicular self-examination.
8 Identify three nursing strategies for reducing nausea and vomiting in the patient undergoing chemotherapy for testicular cancer.
9 State the most common presenting symptom of testicular cancer.
10 Outline the elements of a teaching plan for the patient learning to inject a vasodilator for erectile dysfunction.

DISORDERS OF THE male reproductive system affect the penis, urethra, prostate, and seminal vesicles, as well as the scrotum and its contents. Because of their proximity, the rectum and the upper and lower urinary tracts also may be affected. The nursing management of patients with reproductive system diseases centers on the signs and symptoms of a specific disorder and the disorder's impact on the patient's general health and well-being.

BENIGN PROSTATIC HYPERTROPHY
Definition

Benign prostatic hypertrophy (BPH), also called benign prostatic hyperplasia, is the enlargement of the glandular and stromal portions of the prostate. Symptoms of prostatism occur in the aging man when enlargement of the gland and hypertrophy of the smooth muscle of the prostatic capsule obstruct the outflow of urine from the bladder.

Etiology/Epidemiology

The etiology of BPH remains unclear. Prostatic hyperplasia requires two conditions: aging and functioning testes. BPH is relatively rare among men under 40 years of age, but its incidence rises steadily as males pass their fifth decade of life. Although microscopic hyperplasia may be noted in males as young as 35 years of age, clinically significant bladder outlet obstruction occurs in as many as 51% of men between 60 and 69 years of age.[27] The incidence rises to 75% among males entering the eighth decade of life.[11] Men have a 1 in 4 chance of requiring surgical or medical intervention for BPH as they pass the fifth decade of life.[62]

Pathophysiology

To understand the pathogenesis of BPH, the nurse considers factors that predispose the gland to enlargement and subject the bladder to the effects of outlet obstruction.

Endocrine control and prostatic hyperplasia

Circulating androgens, produced or influenced by the testes, are necessary for the production, progression, and maintenance of BPH. In the aging man dihydrotestosterone levels decline, whereas levels of endogenous estradiol remain relatively unaffected. This hormonal imbalance may increase the likelihood of developing BPH.

Bladder outlet obstruction

Enlargement of the prostate gland is not always clinically significant; it is the symptoms and complications of bladder outlet obstruction that produce **obstructive uropathy** and that warrant intervention.

Obstruction occurs when anatomic or physiologic factors such as prostate enlargement partially block the bladder outlet. This blockage forces the bladder to exert more energy to empty itself and decreases urinary flow. This condition interferes with efficient bladder emptying and ultimately causes obstructive uropathy.

Obstruction from BPH adversely affects the three bladder mechanisms necessary for efficient voiding: urethral diameter, urethral funneling, and detrusor muscle contraction strength. Enlargement of the prostatic lobes directly compromises the urethral outflow tract by decreasing the diameter of the prostatic urethra.

Prostatic enlargement also compromises the urethral sphincter's ability to funnel and allow free passage of urine. During bladder filling the proximal urethral wall must remain rigid to maintain a watertight seal and to ensure continence. In contrast, the urethral wall must expand and distend during micturition to allow the free passage of urine needed for complete bladder emptying. When BPH encroaches on the bladder neck and the proximal urethral wall, the urethra's ability to expand in response to micturition is compromised and urinary flow is reduced.

Prolonged obstruction of the bladder further compromises lower urinary tract function by lessening the efficiency of detrusor muscle contraction. The normal detrusor muscle is composed of smooth muscle bundles interspersed with connective tissue. Obstruction may increase the ratio of connective tissue to smooth muscle (trabeculation), which decreases the efficiency of detrusor muscle contraction, or it may lead to overdistention of the bladder wall and loss of muscle tone.[72]

The obstructive uropathy produced by BPH affects all levels of the urinary system. Inefficient bladder emptying results in urinary stasis, which renders the bladder more susceptible to infection. Over a prolonged period recurrent infections and changes in bladder muscle function affect the efficiency of ureteral peristalsis, which ultimately compromises renal function. Early signs of obstructive uropathy are **trabeculation** of the bladder (thickening of the bladder muscle with a loss of contractility) and lower urinary tract infection. Late complications include hydroureteronephrosis (abnormal enlargement of the upper urinary tracts) and upper urinary tract infection. If the condition goes untreated, renal function may fail, resulting in death.

Clinical Manifestations

An altered urinary elimination pattern is the cardinal symptom. Changes include decreased force of urinary stream, hesitancy, urinary frequency (voids at least every 2 hours), **nocturia** (awakened by urgency to void two or more times), and postvoid dribble. Urgency, frequency, and nocturia may be exacerbated by detrusor instability (uncontrolled contractions of the detrusor muscle that cause a precipitous desire to urinate or urge incontinence).[8] The risk of detrusor instability increases with the magnitude of obstruction and is thought to arise from changes in the bladder wall produced by obstruction.[5] Other clinical manifestations include complications of urinary obstruction such as urinary tract infection, urinary stones, hematuria, and signs of renal insufficiency including nausea, vomiting, weight loss, and oliguria or polyuria.

Abnormal laboratory values include an elevated serum creatinine (greater than 2.0 mg/dL) and an elevated blood urea nitrogen (BUN) (greater than 20 mg/dL).

Therapeutic Management

The timing of interventions for BPH remains controversial. When symptoms of bladder outlet obstruction are mild or moderate, a period of "watchful waiting" may occur during which the prostate is routinely assessed and the progression of symptoms is monitored without intervention. Clinicians may use a symptoms score or other tool to monitor the progression of bladder outlet obstruction caused by BPH. When symptoms of obstruction are severe or when complications such as urinary tract infection, compromised renal function, or acute urinary retention occur, prompt intervention is warranted.[11,27]

Medical interventions

Traditionally, open or transurethral surgery has been the mainstay of the medical management of BPH. More recently, however, pharmacologic agents have enjoyed more widespread use.

Recently, the agent finestaride (Proscar) has been tested and approved for use by the U.S. Food and Drug Administration. Finestaride inhibits the enzyme 5-alpha reductase that blocks the uptake and utilization of androgens by the prostate gland, causing reduction of glandular hyperplasia and prostatic size.[23]

Other medications alleviate symptoms of bladder outlet obstruction by reducing urethral resistance to urinary flow. The bladder neck and prostatic urethra are richly supplied by alpha-adrenergic receptors that are excited by norepinephrine. Medications that block or antagonize these receptors relax the bladder outlet and reduce symptoms of obstruction caused by hypertonicity of the proximal urethra. Three agents may be used: prazosin, terazosin, and doxazosin. Terazosin (Hytrin) has enjoyed particu-

larly widespread use for BPH, because it effectively relieves bladder outlet obstruction while producing minimal effects on systemic blood pressure.[8]

Surgical interventions

Surgical interventions for BPH should relieve bladder outlet obstruction while preserving continence and normal erectile function. Transurethral resection of the prostate gland and open prostatectomy have been traditionally used to relieve prostatic obstruction. Other interventions, including transurethral prostate incision, transurethral laser interstitial prostatectomy, microwave therapy, balloon dilation, and intraurethral stents (Table 71-1), have been used as alternatives to transurethral or open prostatectomy.

Transurethral resection of the prostate typically is preferred to open resection, since an abdominal incision and prolonged period of general anesthesia are avoided[11] (Figure 71-1). The goal of surgery is to relieve obstruction of the bladder outlet by disrupting the prostatic capsule. Prostatic incision allows more efficient funneling of the proximal urethra during voiding. The potential advantages of this approach are preservation of antegrade ejaculation and avoidance of complications associated with transurethral resection of the prostate.

Open resection for BPH typically is reserved for cases in which hypertrophy is advanced and encroaches on the bladder base or when BPH is complicated by bladder pathologic conditions such as a significant bladder wall diverticulum or calculus. Suprapubic, retropubic, or perineal prostatectomy then is performed by removing the prostate through the bladder vesicle or via a lower abdominal incision. The principal advantage of open prostatectomy is the ability to resect particularly enlarged prostate glands. Open surgery typically is avoided in less severe cases, because the transurethral approach avoids the risks of open surgery with prolonged general anesthesia.[11]

NURSING MANAGEMENT OF THE PATIENT WITH BENIGN PROSTATIC HYPERTROPHY
Assessment

Symptoms of benign prostatic hypertrophy (BPH) caused by bladder irritation and obstruction are assessed using a symptom scoring tool (see box on p. 2032). The nurse assesses BPH via rectal examination. The prostate is noted under the anterior rectal wall; a healthy prostate is walnut-shaped, about 4 cm in diameter, with two palpable posterior lobes. It should cause a protrusion of 1 cm or less into the rectum. The hypertrophied prostate is symmetrically enlarged with a uniform, boggy presentation.

TABLE 71-1   Alternative Treatments for Benign Prostatic Hypertrophy

Treatment	Description	Complications	Potential advantages
Transurethral prostate incision	Limited transurethral incisions of prostatic capsule from bladder neck to lateral or upper border of verumontanum; typically limited to patients with mild enlargement	Significant bleeding is rare complication	Less extensive resection reduces morbidity associated with classic transurethral resection technique; bleeding typically is minimal
Microwave therapy	Transurethral application of heat using microwave technology in single or multiple applications	Transient but severe local inflammation with intensification of irritative voiding symptoms; acute urinary retention requiring catheter drainage	Beneficial for patients who are poor candidates for surgical resection
Transurethral laser incision prostate	Transurethral incision of the prostatic tissue and capsule using a laser	Transient local inflammation, urinary retention	Superior control of bleeding during resection, diminished morbidity, and rapid recovery following laser resection
Intraurethral stent	Transurethral placement of titanium wire mesh (stent) that remains securely fixed in prostatic urethra; in time, urethra epithelializes device	Migration, dislodgment of device, infection or calculus formation, local inflammation with irritative voiding symptoms	Surgical resection and associated complications of hemorrhage and acute retention are avoided; device may be removed if local inflammation or infection occurs*

From Grayhack and Kozlowski[11]; Lepor.[16]
*Not approved for this use by the U.S. Food and Drug Administration.

There should be no discrete, hard nodules or asymmetric differences in lobe size.

A bladder chart is used to obtain objective, reliable documentation of bladder elimination patterns. The chart documents urinary frequency, voided volumes, presence and frequency of nocturia, and patterns of incontinence (Figure 71-2). A record of simultaneous fluid intake is included. Urinary residual volumes are recorded for men on an intermittent catheterization program. These volumes often are compared with voided volume to assess the bladder's efficiency in emptying.

Assessment of urinary elimination patterns is complemented by observation of the voided urinary stream. Simultaneous electronic recording of a urinary flow rate is helpful but not always necessary. The key to success when observing the urinary stream is minimization of anxiety and careful avoidance of any environmental distractions. The stream is assessed for force, caliber, constancy, and trimness. The normal stream should be relatively constant, have a caliber approximately equal to a pencil lead, and have enough force to clear the patient's feet and reach a toilet within several inches of the penis. The stream should be relatively uninterrupted and should not spray to the side of the penis. Several drops are expelled from the penis at the termination of micturition; excessive postvoid dribbling occurs when the patient continues to dribble urine from the penis for several minutes after micturition is terminated. The nurse should ask the patient to compare this with his usual voiding pattern at home.

Psychosocial assessment of BPH focuses on the patient's perception of himself with regard to pros-

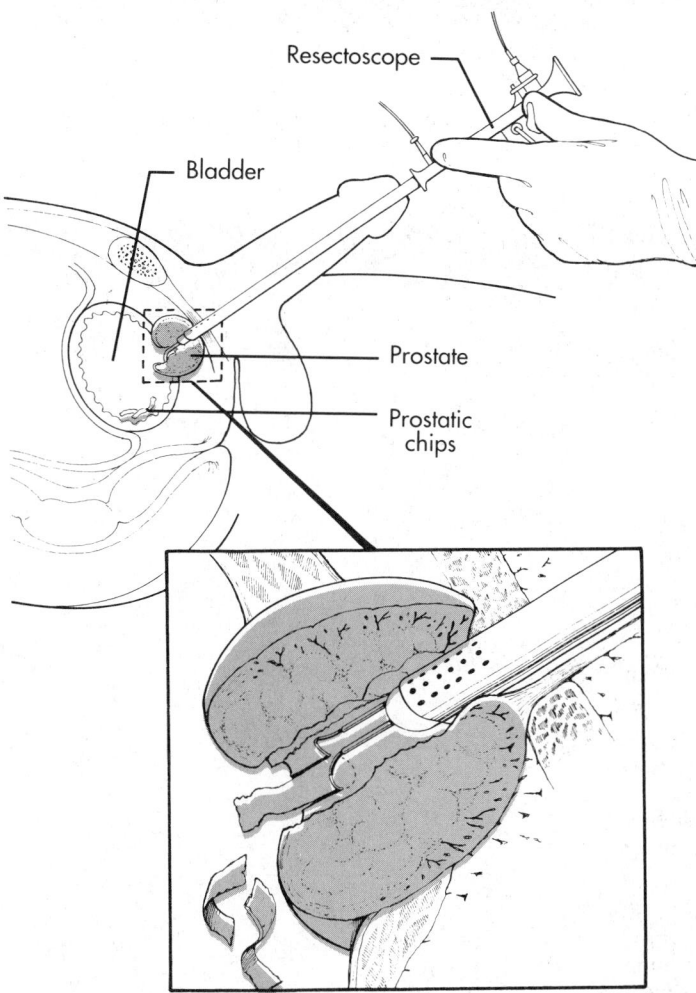

FIGURE 71-1   Transurethral resection of prostate (TURP). (From Gray M: *Genito-urinary disorders,* St Louis, 1992, Mosby–Year Book, Inc.)

tatism and on exploration of his fears about potential side effects of surgical or medical treatment. The nurse explores the patient's perceptions of the causes of BPH. Myths about a relationship between BPH and sexual activity, diet, and alcohol consumption may evoke feelings of guilt and should be dispelled. Expectations concerning surgery or medications are discussed with the patient and his family or partner.

Nursing Diagnosis

Several nursing diagnoses are appropriate for the patient with BPH, depending on the severity of symptoms and the medical management. Common diagnoses are as follows:

Altered patterns of urinary elimination related to bladder outlet obstruction

Urge incontinence related to detrusor instability caused by bladder outlet obstruction

Urinary retention related to bladder outlet obstruction or acute urinary retention with inability to void

High risk for urinary tract infection related to urinary stasis

Altered peripheral tissue perfusion related to surgical resection of prostatic vascular bed

Fluid volume excess, electrolyte imbalance related to absorption of irrigation fluid into vascular bed during transurethral prostatectomy

Sexual dysfunction related to erectile dysfunction and/or ejaculatory dysfunction

Planning

Specific patient goals vary according to the severity of BPH and the patient's treatment regimen. Postoperative goals might include the following:

Patient maintains a regular schedule of complete bladder emptying: every 2 to 4 hours during waking hours and two or fewer episodes of nocturia per night

INTERNATIONAL PROSTATE SYMPTOM SCORE

Patient name:

	Not at all	Less than one time in five	Less than half the time	About half the time	More than half the time	Almost always	
1. Incomplete emptying Over the past month, how often have you had a sensation of not emptying your bladder after you finish urinating?	0	1	2	3	4	5	
2. Frequency: Over the past month, how often have you had to urinate again less than 2 hours after you finished urinating?	0	1	2	3	4	5	
3. Intermittency: Over the past month, how often you you found it difficult to postpone urination?	0	1	2	3	4	5	
4. Urgency: Over the past month, how often have you found it difficult to postpone urination?	0	1	2	3	4	5	
5. Weak stream: Over the past month, how often have you had a weak urinary stream?	0	1	2	3	4	5	
6. Straining Over the past month, how often have you had to push or strain to begin urination?	0	1	2	3	4	5	

	None	One time	Two times	Three times	Four times	Five times	
7. Nocturia: Over the past month, how many times did you most typically get up to urinate from the time you went to bed at night until the time you got up in the morning?	0	1	2	3	4	5	

TOTAL I-PPS score:
(Scores range from 0 to 35, with 0 being symptomatic and 35 indicating severe symptoms)

	Delighted	Pleased	Mostly satisfied	Mixed—Equally satisfied and dissatisfied	Mostly dissatisfied	Unhappy	Terrible
Quality of life as a result of urinary symptoms If you were to spend your life with your urinary symptoms the way they are now, how would you feel?	0	1	2	3	4	5	6

SOURCE: The I-PSS was developed by the Measurement Committee of the American Urological Association. The International Concensus, under the patronage of the World Health Organization, recommends its use for the evaluation of all patients experiencing prostatism.

VOIDING DIARY

Name: _John Q Patient_____

Date: ____/____/_____

Time	Amount voided	Leakage	Amount consumed
8:00 AM	140 cc	✔	
9:00 AM	120 cc		480 cc (breakfast)
9:20 AM	90 cc		
10:00 AM	60 cc		
11:40 AM	150 cc		360 cc (lunch)
12:25 PM	120 cc		
1:50 PM	120 cc		
3:30 PM	150 cc		
6:00 PM	175 cc	✔	600 cc (dinner)
6:20 PM	60 cc		
6:35 PM	60 cc		120 cc (coffee)
7:00 PM	60 cc		
8:30 PM	140 cc		120 cc (coffee c̄ snack)
9:30 PM	120 cc		
11:00 PM	160 cc in bed	✔	
2:00 AM	120 cc in bed		
4:00 AM	120 cc in bed		
6:15 AM	100 cc in bed		

FIGURE 71-2   Excerpt from a voiding diary of a patient with BPH. Patient is given a graduated urine container, and he records time and amount he voids, volume of fluids consumed, and any comments. Urinary leakage is noted by placing a check mark in appropriate column. This chart demonstrates small functional bladder capacity (60 to 150 mL), since urinary frequency is associated closely with fluid intake. Nocturia and urge incontinence also are noted.

Patient prevents acute urinary retention or describes a strategy for managing it should it occur

Patient identifies risk factors for urinary tract infection and uses measures to prevent occurrence

Patient identifies expected effects and potential side effects of treatment regimen and describes measures to cope with these effects

Implementation

Nursing care focuses on alleviating the symptoms of altered patterns of urinary elimination and on preventing and managing complications. A man typically seeks help for BPH when urinary symptoms be-

come severe enough to interfere with his daily activities. Medical or surgical intervention may be indicated immediately, or it may be delayed because of the potential for spontaneous resolution of symptoms.

The nurse helps the patient formulate strategies to alleviate and cope with symptoms of altered urinary elimination patterns. Regularly scheduled voiding (every 2 hours) and **double voiding** (instruct the patient to void, wait several minutes, then void again to maximize bladder emptying) may be used to alleviate diurnal frequency. Fluid intake also is altered; the patient should be instructed to avoid consuming large amounts of fluid with meals while ensuring a daily intake of approximately 1500 to 2000 mL unless other medical conditions warrant fluid restriction. Fluids are limited to 240 to 360 mL at mealtimes, and sipping beverages between meals throughout the day is recommended. Nocturia often is alleviated (but rarely eliminated) if the patient avoids fluid intake for 2 to 3 hours before going to bed.

The nurse teaches the patient to recognize, prevent, and manage complications of BPH. Perhaps the most distressing complication is acute urinary retention. The patient is advised of the association between retention and alcohol intake, chilling, and urinary tract infection. The nurse reviews the patient's medications and, if necessary, advises him to consult a physician concerning use of prescription drugs such as anticholinergic, spasmolytic, antidepressant, or antianxiety agents. The patient is taught to avoid nonprescription medications containing decongestants that may interfere with bladder neck funneling and cause acute retention. The nurse teaches the patient not to postpone micturition and to avoid a large fluid intake when a toilet is not readily accessible.

The patient is instructed that urinary retention requires urgent medical attention. Inability to pass urine despite an intense desire to void initially is managed by having the patient try to relax in a quiet, private bathroom with both feet firmly on the floor. The patient should drink warm tea to assist in his attempts to void. If these measures are unsuccessful, the patient tries to void in a tub filled with warm water or while taking a warm shower; this often promotes further relaxation of the pelvic floor muscles, with subsequent micturition. If micturition does not occur after 6 hours, the patient should go to an immediate care clinic or hospital emergency department for relief via catheterization.

Urinary retention with marked urinary frequency and nocturia also may be relieved temporarily through intermittent catheterization, which is undertaken in consultation with a physician. The goal is to provide regular, complete bladder emptying, which reduces voiding symptoms and prevents complications related to urinary retention. The patient is instructed in the use of a clean technique to catheterize; scheduling is determined in consultation with the physician.

The patient and his family must be taught to recognize other complications of bladder outlet obstruction and the strategies for managing them if they arise. Urinary tract infection is a common complication requiring prompt treatment. The cardinal signs of this infection are urinary urgency, frequency, nocturia, and dysuria. A urinary tract infection associated with a fever may be a sign of pyelonephritis and may require hospitalization.

Urge incontinence also may be associated with bladder outlet obstruction caused by BPH. Patients with this condition complain of urinary frequency and nocturia associated with marked urgency to urinate and leakage before reaching the toilet. The nurse assesses the patient's mobility, environment, clothing, and access to a toilet. Diurnal frequency and incontinence are managed by using a timed voiding schedule with a fluid control regimen and by providing an environment and clothing that promote optimal movement onto the toilet. Nocturia exacerbated by urge incontinence is managed by having the patient avoid fluids for 2 to 3 hours before sleep. A bedside or hand-held urinal further reduces the risk of nighttime incontinence or falls caused by rushing to the toilet.

An insidious onset of nausea, vomiting, and loss of appetite may indicate renal insufficiency; the patient is instructed to report these symptoms to his physician promptly.

Postoperative care

Nursing care of the patient undergoing transurethral or open surgery for BPH centers on managing and preventing complications. Before surgery the patient is instructed that altered ejaculatory function (retrograde ejaculation) is expected after prostatectomy and that this will decrease his fertility potential. He also is reassured that he should continue to experience the sensations associated with ejaculation and that the surgery is not expected to impair his ability to generate and maintain an erection.

Immediately after prostatic resection the patient's bladder is drained by a three-way Foley catheter. The patient is assessed every 1 to 2 hours to ensure the catheter's patency and to assess blood loss. Gentle traction, created by taping the catheter against the thigh, provides hemostasis of affected prostatic vessels (Figure 71-3). Nonetheless, even a small amount of blood will color all catheter output light red or pink, so the patient is reassured that even a large volume of red-tinged urine does not necessarily indicate excessive blood loss. The patient's vital signs are monitored regularly, and the physician is promptly informed if the patient shows systemic signs of excessive blood loss (rapid pulse with declining blood pressure). Intake and output are carefully documented, and the irrigation system is assessed every hour for signs of obstruction to prevent bladder overdistention or rupture. Gentle irrigation, using saline and a catheter-tipped syringe or continuous irrigation, is used if clots impede adequate catheter drainage (Figure 71-4).

Continuous or intermittent irrigation, if used, typically is discontinued after 24 hours, and often the catheter is removed 36 to 72 hours after surgery. After the catheter is removed, the patient's urinary output must be assessed regularly for volume of output and residual bleeding. The patient should be informed that he can expect mild to moderate dysuria

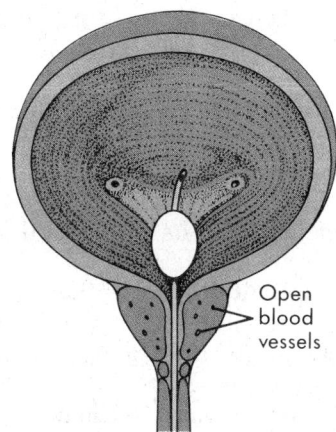
Open blood vessels

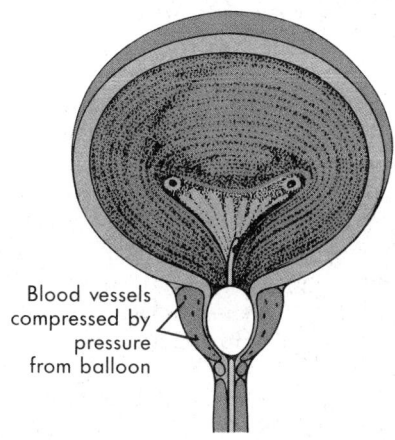
Blood vessels compressed by pressure from balloon

FIGURE 71-3   Gentle traction is maintained against prostatic vascular bed to prevent excessive bleeding following transurethral resection.

after catheter removal and that this discomfort progressively resolves by repeated micturition over 1 to 2 days. The patient should be given several bottles to collect his urine; each voiding should appear progressively clearer until the urine regains its normal yellow color. The patient should be encouraged to drink fluids to help relieve initial dysuria and to resolve hematuria.

Pain after prostate surgery commonly is associated with bladder distention, irritation from the catheter or irrigation solution, or bladder spasm. Maintaining catheter patency greatly reduces both the discomfort associated with bladder distention and the risk of painful bladder spasm. The physician should be consulted about the use of smooth muscle relaxants if bladder spasms persist despite adequate drainage. Pain caused by irritation from the catheter is alleviated by minimizing catheter manipulation and by promoting adequate rest.

Because of the significant risk of deep vein thrombosis after transurethral prostate surgery, the patient should be given antiembolic stockings before the procedure. This risk is further reduced by ensuring adequate hydration via oral or intravenous fluids in the immediate postoperative period. Also during this period the foot of the bed should be raised 20 to 30 degrees, and the patient should be encouraged to perform passive leg exercises. The radius of the calf is documented every 4 hours if thrombosis is suspected.

Medical therapy

The nurse teaches the patient receiving pharmacologic therapy for BPH to take medications regularly and to identify and manage potential side effects. The principal side effects of antiandrogenic medica-

tions are decreased sperm production and loss of libido; the potential side effects of estrogens include those for antiandrogenic drugs as well as nausea, "feminization" of the male body habitus, and thromboembolic complications such as pulmonary embolus, thrombophlebitis, stroke, and myocardial infarction.

Any patient receiving a medication that alters hormonal aspects of BPH is given written and verbal instructions on drug use and potential adverse effects. The patient is taught to take estrogens or antiandrogenic medications with meals to avoid nausea and to recognize the signs of potential thromboembolic complications, including tenderness, swelling, and redness of an extremity; severe chest pain; shortness of breath; indigestion that cannot be relieved by usual measures; sudden headache; slurring of speech; or visual changes. The patient should seek immediate care if these symptoms occur.

Patients receiving prazosin or terazosin also are taught to monitor their medications and to recognize and manage adverse side effects. The principal untoward effects are postural hypotension and potential erectile dysfunction. The patient is taught to rise slowly from the supine position to avoid dizziness. Dangling the legs and exercising the ankles before arising also may alleviate postural hypotension. The medication may have to be discontinued to reverse the erectile dysfunction.

Evaluation

The patient with BPH requires continual evaluation to assess the effectiveness of nursing interventions. A successful care plan helps the patient establish an acceptable pattern of urinary elimination that allows him to continue his daily activities and to enjoy rel-

CLINICAL ALERT

During the first 24 hours after prostate surgery the nurse assesses the patient to prevent transurethral resection (TUR) syndrome, which occurs when excessive absorption of irrigating solution causes fluid volume excess and associated electrolyte imbalance. The patient's vital signs and mental alertness are assessed regularly, and symptoms of bradycardia, hypertension, tachypnea, confusion, agitation, vomiting, headache, and tremor are reported promptly to the physician. Extra care must be taken with the geriatric patient, because these symptoms may be misinterpreted as acute confusion related to surgical intervention rather than signs of significant fluid and electrolyte imbalance. Successful reversal of the syndrome requires rapid intervention to prevent convulsion and possibly death from the electrolyte imbalance.

atively uninterrupted sleep at night. The patient should be able to identify and describe ways to manage complications of bladder outlet obstruction, including urinary tract infection, acute urinary retention, and urge incontinence. Patients undergoing surgery for BPH should identify the goals of surgery and have realistic expectations about fertility potential and erectile function. Patients undergoing medical therapy for BPH must demonstrate knowledge of medication regimens and potential side effects.

Documentation

In documenting the care of the patient with BPH before medical or surgical therapy, the nurse records both the assessment of altered urinary elimination patterns and patient teaching about managing symptoms of bladder outlet obstruction and potential complications. The records also document instructions related to medical or surgical management of BPH.

Ongoing Care

Long-term management of the patient who has undergone surgery for BPH involves continual assessment of sexual and urinary function. The man is allowed to express his concerns about sexual function openly, and the nurse assesses for perceptions of altered self-esteem and sexuality. The patient who receives medications for BPH is reassured that the side effects of erectile dysfunction, loss of libido, or altered body habitus resolve when the medications are discontinued. The patient who undergoes sur-

gery for BPH is advised that he may resume sexual activity 6 to 8 weeks after surgery and that retrograde ejaculation will not limit his ability to engage in sexual intercourse. Resolution of issues related to self-concept and sexuality may require 6 to 12 months, and optimal erectile function also may require 12 months. Detailed assessment of altered sexual function may be required if dysfunction persists beyond this time.

The patient's urinary function also may be altered by prostate surgery. Men who undergo surgery for BPH generally note a significant improvement in their ability to empty the bladder with diminution of daytime urinary frequency and nocturia. However, some patients experience stress urinary incontinence after surgery. These patients are taught to use an appropriate urinary containment device. Pads that adhere to the undergarments or a urinary dribble pouch is used when leakage is mild to moderate; a condom catheter is used when leakage is severe. The patient is reassured that leakage may be temporary and may disappear within the first year following surgery. Any patient who experiences urinary leakage following surgery is taught to perform pelvic muscle exercises. The patient is taught to isolate and contract the pelvic muscles and to refrain from contracting distant muscle groups such as the thigh or abdominal muscles. Pelvic muscle exercises consist of muscle contractions designed to increase endurance and maximal strength. The patient is taught to contract the pelvic muscles maximally for a 10-second period followed by a 10-second rest period, or he is taught to contract the muscles maximally for an 8-second period for improving maximal strength and 30 seconds using steady contraction to improve endurance. The patient is given a graded exercise program beginning with 10 repetitions every other day with steady progression to 35 to 50 repetitions.[8]

When symptoms of incontinence persist for longer than 12 months the patient is advised to consult a urologist for correction of this incontinence. Several alternative treatment modalities may be used. Alpha sympathomimetics increase smooth muscle tone at the bladder neck and proximal urethra, minimizing stress urinary incontinence. Several agents, including pseudoephedrine and phenylpropanolamine, are available in over-the-counter or prescription preparations. Sudafed S.A. capsules are a long-acting form of pseudoephedrine; one capsule is administered in the morning. Dexatrim without caffeine capsules contain phenylpropanolamine; they are also administered in the morning. Ornade spansules or Entex L.A. capsules are administered by prescription only. Imipramine (Tofranil) is a tricyclic antidepressant that exerts a mild anticholinergic and alpha-sympathomimetic effect. This agent is administered three or four times per day. The

Nursing diagnosis/ *Expected outcome*	Interventions	Rationale
Altered peripheral, prostatic bed tissue perfusion • *Patient experiences minimal blood loss; vital signs, hematocrit and hemoglobin levels remain at preoperative levels* • *Hematuria resolves within 7 to 10 days of prostate resection*	Before catheter removal: Monitor urinary drainage bag for bright red blood clots Compare postoperative hematocrit and hemoglobin levels for evidence of significant blood loss Monitor vital signs (pulse, blood pressure, respirations) for signs of significant blood loss Monitor catheter drainage system to ensure maintenance of gentle traction against prostatic urethra After catheter removal: Provide patient with several bottles to monitor hematuria; after catheter removal, voided urines should progress from visibly blood tinged to clear yellow Advise patient that small flecks of burgundy-colored "scabs" or clots may be shed for 7 to 10 days after catheter removal and that these should clear within 24 to 48 hours	Excessive blood loss may occur after prostatectomy; gentle traction on drainage catheter balloon allows hemostasis; indwelling catheter is left in place until prostatic capsule heals; mild hematuria persists for 7 to 10 days after resection
Potential urinary retention • *Urinary output remains at preoperative levels (1500 to 2000 mL/day)*	Monitor catheter drainage for patency; monitor continuous drainage system every hour for patency; straighten any kinked tubes Gently irrigate clots or debris from catheter, using catheter-tipped syringe with saline, after consulting with physician Ensure adequate fluid intake (1500 to 2000 mL/day)	Urinary retention may occur if catheter becomes occluded with blood clots or other sediment from surgical resection; retention must be rapidly recognized and alleviated to prevent acute bladder overdistention and potential infection caused by retention of urine and other debris from prostatectomy
Pain related to bladder spasm • *Patient remains free of bladder spasm*	Maintain patent urinary drainage system while catheter is in place Alleviate urethral irritation; minimize catheter manipulation and promote adequate rest during immediate postoperative period before catheter removal Administer anticholinergic medications in consultation with physician if nonpharmacologic measures fail to prevent or relieve bladder spasms	Bladder spasms are caused by unstable bladder contractions, causing pain at bladder, bladder outlet, and urethra; maintaining a relatively empty bladder and minimizing urethral irritation from an indwelling catheter often will prevent spasms; anticholinergic medications will help relieve painful bladder spasms if nonpharmacologic management fails to prevent unstable contractions
Altered peripheral, lower extremity tissue perfusion related to deep vein thrombosis • *Patient remains free of symptoms of deep vein thrombosis (pain, pallor of affected extremity)* • *Peripheral perfusion assessed by physical examination and Doppler assessment remains within normal limits*	Provide patient with antiembolic stockings before prostate surgery Ensure adequate hydration during immediate postoperative period (1500 to 2000 mL/day) by means of oral or intravenous fluids	Venous stasis and subsequent thrombus formulation may occur after prostate resection, because legs are placed in stirrups for a prolonged period during surgery; antiembolic stockings minimize risk of thrombosis by promoting venous return in legs; adequate fluid hydration reduces risk of thrombus formation by preventing hemoconcentration

Continued.

NURSING CARE PLAN   *Postprostatectomy Patient—cont'd*

Nursing diagnosis/ Expected outcome	Interventions	Rationale
Potential fluid volume excess related to TUR syndrome • *Patient remains free of symptoms of TUR syndrome (bradycardia, tachypnea, confusion, vomiting, agitation, headache, and tremor)* • *Serum electrolyte laboratory values remain at preoperative levels*	Monitor patient for symptoms of TUR syndrome; promptly report any changes to physician Maintain adequate fluid intake (1500 to 2000 mL/day) by means of intravenous or oral fluids	TUR syndrome occurs when excessive irrigating solution is absorbed through prostatic vascular bed; signs of altered mental status, changed vital signs, and tremor progress rapidly to convulsion and possible death unless measures are taken to reverse electrolyte and fluid imbalances

nurse teaches the patient to selectively administer alpha-sympathomimetic medications during the day since protection from stress urinary incontinence is not required during sleep and since these agents often interfere with sleep. The nurse assesses the blood pressure before and during therapy because these agents may increase blood pressure, particularly among older individuals with preexisting hypertension.[8]

An artificial urinary sphincter is a prosthetic device that is implanted surgically. The device consists of a cuff that substitutes for the man's sphincter mechanism, an abdominal reservoir, and a pump that is placed under the loose skin of the scrotum. Following activation, the cuff remains in a closed position opposing urethral leakage. When the man wishes to urinate, he compresses the pump mechanism, opening the sphincter and allowing micturition. Periurethral bulking agents are injected under the mucosa of the urethra to mechanically improve the urethral sphincter mechanism's ability to close and prevent urinary leakage. GAX collagen, Polytef paste, or autologous fat may be injected into the urethra for bulking. Collagen and Polytef paste are undergoing clinical trials for use in males with postprostatectomy incontinence.[8]

Symptoms of bladder obstruction occasionally recur, possibly indicating regrowth of the prostate gland. The patient should be advised to undergo rectal assessment of his prostate gland annually and to report the recurrence of symptoms to his physician.

CANCER OF THE PROSTATE
Definition

Cancer of the prostate is the uncontrolled spread of poorly differentiated, abnormally proliferative malignant cells. Prostatic cancer occurs as a primary tumor from the organ or as a metastasis from a distant site. Adenocarcinoma of the prostate accounts for approximately 95% of all malignancies of the gland, whereas transitional or squamous cell carcinomas, sarcomas, and metastatic lesions constitute only 5% of prostatic tumors.

Etiology/Epidemiology

The cause of prostatic carcinoma remains unclear. However, there is a strong association between prostatic cancer and aging; the disorder is rare among males under 50 years of age, but the incidence climbs steadily after the fifth decade. Four factors may contribute to the development of prostatic cancer: genetic factors, including familial or racial predisposition[40,68,76]; endogenous hormonal influences; exposure to environmental elements[45,71,75]; and coexisting sexually transmitted pathogens.[43,56]

Adenocarcinoma of the prostate is the third leading cause of cancer-related deaths among men in the United States, after lung and colorectal malignancies.[70] The prevalence of prostatic carcinoma increases with age; as many as 30% of males between the ages of 70 and 79 years are found to have evidence of carcinoma at autopsy, and as many as 67% of males who live to the age of 80 to 89 years may be affected.[64] Based on these observations, prostatic cancer may be the most prevalent form of malignancy among older men.[4]

Pathophysiology

The pathophysiologic changes of prostatic carcinoma are the result of local tumor growth, extension of cancer cells into adjacent pelvic structures, and metastatic spread to distant organ systems. Carcinoma of the prostate arises from the acinar portion of the gland or from components of the ductal system that drain these acini. Most malignancies are multifocal and arise as one or more palpable, hardened nodules typically noted in the posterior lobe of the gland. In some cases the prostate becomes indurated rather than developing detectable nodules.[4]

Tumor growth disrupts the normal architecture of the prostatic glandular system, causing the organ to enlarge and progressively obstruct the bladder outlet. As a result, urinary elimination patterns are altered and pathologic changes occur in the upper and lower urinary tracts.

Prostatic tumors may invade adjacent anatomic structures. Tumor cells sometimes penetrate the prostatic capsule and involve the bladder base, causing ureteral obstruction. Occasionally the tumor spreads to the pelvic floor musculature; invasion of the rectum is rare.

Metastases from prostatic cancers spread via the body's vascular and lymphatic channels. The obturator lymph nodes are most commonly affected.[59] Hematogenous metastases affect the skeletal system first; bony metastases are noted in 85% of patients who die of prostatic carcinoma. These lesions cause the severe, chronic pain often associated with advanced cases of prostatic carcinoma.[12] Other distant sites affected by metastasis from prostatic cancer are the central nervous system, liver, lungs, and adrenal glands.[4] The box below outlines the clinical stages used to guide diagnosis and treatment of prostatic cancer.

Clinical Manifestations

Prostatic carcinoma often has no early symptoms and may be discovered by microscopic examination of tissue chips produced during transurethral resection of the prostate for benign prostatic hyperplasia.

WHITMORE-JEWETT STAGES OF PROSTATIC CANCER

A1—Tumor unsuspected: 3 or fewer chips; 1 lobe involved

A2—Tumor unsuspected: 3 or more chips; more than 1 lobe

B1—Palpable node in prostate: palpable node 1 cm or less in diameter; low grade; 1 lobe

B2—Palpable node in prostate: 1 cm or more in diameter; high grade; more than 1 lobe

C —Tumor palpable beyond prostatic capsule: local extension of tumor

D1—Tumor palpable: pelvic nodes involved

D2—Tumor palpable: distant metastasis

From Catalona WJ, Scott WM: Carcinoma of the prostate. In Walsh PC et al: *Campbell's urology*, Philadelphia, 1986, WB Saunders Co.

Among younger males (ages 40 to 50 years) an abrupt change in urinary elimination patterns (urgency, urinary frequency, nocturia) that is unrelated to urinary tract infection may indicate prostatic cancer. The symptoms of advanced disease include altered urinary elimination patterns (urinary frequency, decreased force of stream, postvoid dribble, feelings of incomplete bladder emptying, and nocturia), hematuria (nonacinar tumors), and bone pain (metastasis present).

Laboratory findings include elevated acid phosphatase, elevated alkaline phosphatase, and elevated prostatic-specific antigen (PSA). If there is a residual tumor after radical prostatectomy, the PSA remains elevated.

Therapeutic Management

Radiotherapy

Medical management of prostatic cancer varies according to the type of tumor and its stage. The goal of radiotherapy is to eradicate the rapidly proliferating tumor cells while leaving nonmalignant, more stable cells unaffected.[7]

Radiotherapy for prostatic cancer consists of either placing irradiated seeds directly into the gland or exposing the prostate and pelvic lymph nodes to relatively high doses of external beam radiation (6600 to 7000 rad). ^{125}I seed therapy is used alone or in combination with external beam radiotherapy. The seeds are implanted transperineally under transrectal ultrasound guidance or during open surgery.[21]

External beam radiotherapy consists of a series of measured doses given over 6 to 8 weeks. The patient lies in a prone position during the procedure so that the small bowel is pushed away from the irradiated area. The side effects of radiotherapy include diarrhea and radiation-induced cystitis (characterized by urinary frequency, urgency, nocturia, and occasional urge incontinence). A prolonged change in bowel habits and irritative bladder symptoms are the most common long-term adverse effects of treatment.[7]

Surgical interventions

Open or laparoscopic lymphadenectomy of the pelvic nodes may be used to stage prostatic adenocarcinoma before radical surgery. An open lymphadenectomy is accomplished through a midline or Pfannenstiel incision, and the pelvic lymph nodes are examined and dissected. In a laparoscopic dissection the peritoneum is entered with a laparoscope, and a pneumoperitoneum is created using carbon dioxide after initial inspection of the peritoneum for adhesions or unexpected pathologic conditions. The pelvic nodes are examined and dissected under laparoscopic control, avoiding an open incision.[28]

Radical prostatectomy is the complete removal of the prostate, seminal vesicles, and prostatic capsule followed by surgical reanastomosis of the bladder and remaining urethra. Different surgical approaches—suprapubic (retropubic), perineal, and transcoccygeal—are used. Radical prostatectomy typically is limited to cases in which the tumor is confined to the prostatic capsule, as is noted with stage A2, B1, and B2 lesions.[3,4]

The complications of radical prostatectomy include those related to anesthesia as well as postoperative stress urinary incontinence, stricture at the site of surgical anastomosis, and rectal trauma.[52] Lymphocele, lymphadenopathy, and wound infections occur less often.[4]

Hormonal therapy

Exogenous hormones may be used to slow or reverse tumor growth by suppressing the release of luteinizing hormone (LH) from the pituitary, by inhibiting androgen synthesis in the testes and adrenals, or by blocking androgenic responses in the prostate and other target tissues. Estrogens are commonly used and are given in one of three forms: diethylstilbestrol, estradiol, or the synthetic estrogen chlorotrianisene (Tace). Complications of estrogen use in men include cardiovascular toxicity and nausea.

Surgery also may be used to slow tumor growth by means of hormonal manipulation. Removing the testes, adrenals, or pituitary gland prevents production of androgens needed for tumor growth. Orchiectomy, the removal of one or both testes, is commonly employed.

Other therapeutic strategies have been used on a more limited basis. Systemic chemotherapy, for example, has played only a minor role in the treatment of prostatic cancer. A variety of agents have been used, since no one regimen offers a clear advantage. Immunotherapy, cryotherapy, and cryosurgery have limited value in prostatic cancer because of a lack of clearly identified tumor-specific antigens capable of inducing an immune response to fight tumor cells.[4]

Relief of obstruction by means of transurethral resection of the prostate often is used as a palliative measure in advanced disease. See discussion of benign prostatic hypertrophy, p. 2029.

NURSING MANAGEMENT OF THE PATIENT WITH CANCER OF THE PROSTATE
Assessment

The nurse assesses for prostatic cancer by digital rectal examination of the prostate, which reveals a discrete, hard nodule or indurated area. Pain assessment is crucial for the man with advanced prostatic cancer and bony metastasis. The impact of pain on the patient's life is assessed through use of a diary, which is kept for 5 to 7 days. During this time the patient records the time and date of pain episodes and estimates the magnitude of the pain and its effect on activities of daily living, quality of sleep, energy level, social interactions, perceptions of self-worth, and sexual activity.[33] Objective physiologic parameters also are continually assessed, including blood pressure, pulse, respirations, muscle tone, skin temperature, and impairment of movement, as well as x-ray films and other evidence of the presence and severity of specific metastatic lesions.

A man with prostatic cancer faces issues of self-concept related to altered genitourinary function and anxiety and fear about possible loss of libido and erectile function as a result of surgical or hormonal treatments. Men with advanced cancer may face psychosocial issues associated with chronic pain and dying. The nurse can best assess these issues by listening carefully and by judiciously using open-ended, structured questions rather than brief, highly structured interviews.

Nursing Diagnosis

Several nursing diagnoses are appropriate for the patient with prostatic cancer, depending on the tumor stage, presence of complications, and medical management strategy. Common diagnoses include the following:

Altered patterns of urinary elimination related to bladder outlet obstruction

Diarrhea related to external beam radiotherapy

High risk for fluid volume deficit related to diarrhea

Altered peripheral tissue perfusion related to potential for disruption of surgically created urethrovesical anastomosis

Sexual dysfunction related to transurethral resection of prostate, radical prostatectomy, or hormonal therapy

Stress incontinence related to radical prostatectomy

Chronic pain related to bony metastasis

Anxiety related to prognosis associated with advanced prostatic cancer

Planning

Specific patient goals are determined by the patient's age, the medical management plan, and the severity of symptoms. General goals include the following:

Patient maintains an acceptable routine of complete bladder elimination every 2 to 4 hours during waking hours and has two or fewer episodes of nocturia per night

Patient demonstrates knowledge of strategies for coping with bouts of diarrhea related to radiotherapy

Patient consumes 2000 to 2500 mL of fluid per day during episodes of diarrhea

Patient maintains the integrity of the urethrovesical anastomosis after radical prostatectomy

Patient demonstrates knowledge of potential sexual dysfunctions related to prostatectomy or medical or surgical hormonal therapy

Patient demonstrates knowledge of strategies for eliminating or containing stress incontinence, including pelvic floor exercises

Patient demonstrates knowledge of methods to control chronic pain, including proper analgesic use and nonpharmacologic pain reduction strategies

Patient demonstrates knowledge of prognosis related to prostatic cancer and demonstrates behavior that helps him cope with issues related to chronic pain and dying

Implementation

Nursing care of the patient with prostatic cancer varies according to the stage of the tumor, the severity of associated symptoms, the medical management plan, and the presence of adverse effects of medical interventions.

Radiotherapy

Nursing care of the patient undergoing external beam or interstitial radiation therapy focuses on detecting and preventing potential complications. Diarrhea and irritative voiding symptoms are common. The patient is reassured that diarrhea is transient, and the nurse helps the patient maintain an adequate fluid intake (2000 to 2500 mL/day) during episodes of diarrhea. The patient is encouraged to drink fluids such as Gatorade or clear fruit juices, which supply the electrolytes lost during diarrhea. Beverages containing caffeine are avoided because of their propensity to increase bowel motility and the urge to urinate. The patient with severe diarrhea is advised to eat several small meals of bland foods and to avoid fatty or fried foods.

Irritative voiding symptoms also may be transient. The patient is encouraged to maintain an adequate fluid intake to avoid dehydration and to flush the urinary system. The physician is consulted about the use of urinary analgesics such as phenazopyridine (Pyridium) or spasmolytic medications such as propantheline (Pro-Banthine) or oxybutynin (Ditropan).

Radical prostatectomy

Nursing care of the patient undergoing radical prostatectomy centers on preventing potential complications related to open surgery and helping the patient reestablish acceptable patterns of urinary elimination and sexual function. Preoperative preparation includes shaving the perineum, external genitalia, and upper thighs the night before surgery. The patient should be placed on a low-residue diet 24 to 48 hours before surgery to reduce the amount of fecal material in the bowel. Cleansing enemas are given until the lower bowel is purged of fecal material. The patient should be informed that he will return from the operating room with a urethral catheter that probably will remain in place for 10 to 14 days and that he will have a perineal dressing that must be changed frequently during the first 48 hours.[9,57] The nurse also should reinforce teaching concerning potentially altered sexual function. Loss of fertility is expected; erectile function may or may not be adversely affected.[36]

The urethral catheter is monitored every 1 to 2 hours during the first postoperative day for bleeding and patency. The patient is reassured that urinary drainage will be red tinged and that this does not indicate excessive bleeding. The wound dressing is assessed every 2 to 4 hours during the first 24 to 48 hours for urine, blood, or serosanguineous drainage. Vital signs are monitored regularly for evidence of excessive bleeding, and catheters are monitored for kinks or clots causing loss of patency. The catheter is gently irrigated or maintained on continuous irrigation only after consultation with the physician (Figure 71-4).

The delicate urethrovesical anastomosis is meticulously maintained during the first 10 to 14 days while initial healing occurs. The catheter is carefully maintained in position to avoid disrupting the surgical site. It is secured against the thigh, but no traction is put against it. The physician is consulted about the use of anticholinergic or spasmolytic medications to prevent bladder spasms that cause discomfort and put stress on the urethrovesical anastomosis.

The patient is maintained on a low-residue diet, and adequate fluid intake (1500 to 2000 mL/day) is encouraged to avoid stressing the anastomosis by straining for a bowel movement. The physician is consulted about the use of codeine or a diphenoxylate-atropine preparation (Lomotil) to prevent bowel movements during the first 5 days. No foreign objects, including enema syringes, suppositories, or rectal temperature probes, are inserted into the rectum until the urethrovesical anastomosis heals.

Normal bowel patterns usually resume within 5 to 7 days. The patient then is advanced to a regular diet, and medications to prevent bowel movements are discontinued. The patient is encouraged to ingest 2000 to 2500 mL of fluid per day; prune juice or apple juice may be offered to assist in softening the stool. The physician is consulted about the use

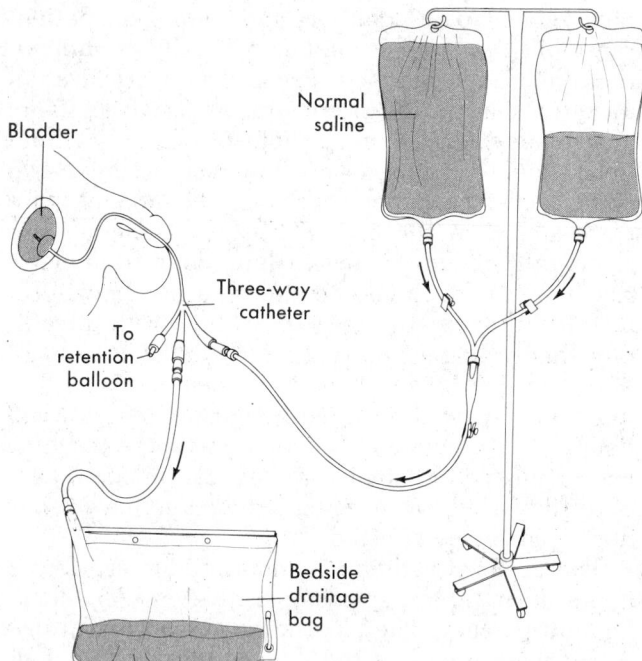

Bladder

Normal saline

Three-way catheter

To retention balloon

Bedside drainage bag

FIGURE 71-4   Continuous irrigation of bladder requires a three-way Foley catheter that allows simultaneous infusion and drainage of an irrigating solution (normal saline) through bladder. Solution is infused rapidly into bladder, and bedside drainage bag is assessed for evidence of excessive bleeding and then drained every 1 to 2 hours.

of stool cathartics or softeners if dietary measures do not produce a normally formed, soft bowel movement.

The catheter typically is removed within 10 to 14 days. The patient is informed that dysuria is transitory and is relieved by ingesting fluids and repeated voiding. Urinary output is assessed for adequate volume and hematuria. The patient also is informed that burgundy-colored material related to shedding of "scabs" at the surgical site may be passed and that some hematuria may persist for 4 to 8 weeks.[9] Dysuria may persist beyond the first 24 hours after removal of the catheter because of urethritis or urinary tract infection. The nurse should obtain a medical order for urine culture and consult the physician about the use of a urinary analgesic if needed.

The principal long-term adverse effects of radical prostatectomy are stress urinary incontinence[36] and sexual dysfunction.[46] The patient who experiences stress urinary incontinence should be reassured that leakage typically is temporary. The patient is taught to perform exercises for the pelvic floor muscles to hasten the recovery of continence.

The patient also is informed that he may safely resume sexual activity 6 to 8 weeks after discharge from the hospital. The patient is encouraged to express his concerns and fears about altered sexual function and to explore strategies for coping with any erectile dysfunction. He is advised that reversible erectile dysfunction is common during the first 6 to 12 months.

Hormonal therapy

The nurse assumes primary responsibility for teaching the patient undergoing hormonal therapy to take oral medications and to monitor himself for any adverse effects. The nurse also teaches the patient who undergoes surgery how to recognize and cope with potential adverse effects related to reduced endogenous androgens.

The nurse explains to the patient that hormonal therapy should arrest the spread of prostate cancer by affecting the tumor's reliance on androgens. The patient also is informed that hormonal therapy may affect his libido and erectile function. The patient is encouraged to express his feelings and concerns about sexual dysfunction and potential changes in body image.

The nurse and patient discuss strategies for coping with infertility and erectile dysfunction. The possibility of banking sperm before therapy is begun is explored if fertility is a concern. The patient is reassured that the changes in libido and erectile function may be reversible when medications are discontinued. The nurse discusses surgical, medical, or mechanical options to correct persistent erectile dysfunction.

The nurse should not be dissuaded if the patient shows no interest in issues related to sexual function; patients often refuse to admit to such concerns because of denial, anxiety, or depression. Patient education by the nurse provides the patient with knowledge and the opportunity to address and cope with sexual dysfunctions when he deems appropriate.[12]

The patient is taught to identify and manage other potential adverse effects of pharmacologic agents used to treat prostatic cancer. Estrogens or antiandrogenic agents may cause nausea and should be taken with food. Potentially serious thromboembolic side effects may occur. Symptoms such as headache, slurred speech, shortness of breath, chest pain with indigestion and edema, and warmth and pain in an extremity may indicate stroke, myocardial infarction, pulmonary embolus, or thrombophlebitis and warrant emergent medical care.

Evaluation

The patient's responses to nursing care must be evaluated continuously to assess the effectiveness of interventions. A successful care plan for the man undergoing radiotherapy helps the patient cope with transient irritative voiding symptoms and diarrhea and prevents excessive fluid loss. Successful nursing care of the patient undergoing radical prostatectomy helps the patient avoid both disrupting the urethrovesical anastomosis and complications from excessive bleeding, urinary retention, or infection. Successful nursing care of the patient undergoing hormonal therapy helps the patient take medications on the appropriate schedule and avoid or manage side effects, including sexual dysfunction.

Documentation

Documenting altered urinary and bowel elimination patterns is important in the nursing care of patients with prostatic cancer. With patients suffering chronic pain from bony metastasis, a pain management program should be documented in detail.

Ongoing Care

Long-term care of the patient with prostatic cancer typically focuses on four aspects: altered sexual function, altered urinary elimination patterns, chronic pain, and, in patients with advanced tumors, issues relating to dying.

When symptoms of incontinence persist for longer than 12 months the patient is advised to consult a urologist. Several alternative treatment modalities may be used. Alpha sympathomimetics increase smooth muscle tone at the bladder neck and proximal urethra, minimizing stress urinary incontinence. Several agents, including pseudoephedrine and phenylpropanolamine, are available in over-the-counter or prescription preparations. Sudafed S.A. capsules are a long-acting form of pseudoephedrine; one capsule is administered in the morning. Dexatrim without caffeine capsules contain phenylpropanolamine; they are also administered in the morning. Ornade spansules or Entex L.A. capsules are administered by prescription only. Imipramine (Tofranil) is a tricyclic antidepressant that exerts a mild anticholinergic and alpha-sympathomimetic effect. This agent is administered three or four times per day. The nurse teaches the patient to selectively administer alpha-sympathomimetic medications during the day, since protection from stress urinary incontinence is not required during sleep and since these agents often interfere with sleep. The nurse assesses the blood pressure before and during therapy, because these agents may increase blood pressure, particularly among older individuals with pre-existing hypertension.[8]

An artificial urinary sphincter is a prosthetic device that is implanted surgically. The device consists of a cuff that substitutes for the man's sphincter mechanism, an abdominal reservoir, and a pump that is placed under the loose skin of the scrotum.

Following activation, the cuff remains in a closed position, opposing urethral leakage. When the man wishes to urinate, he compresses the pump mechanism, opening the sphincter and allowing micturition. Periurethral bulking agents are injected under the mucosa of the urethra to mechanically improve the urethral sphincter mechanism's ability to close and prevent urinary leakage. GAX collagen, Polytef paste, or autologous fat may be injected into the urethra for bulking. Collagen and Polytef paste are undergoing clinical trials for use in males with post-prostatectomy incontinence.[8]

Nursing care of the patient with erectile dysfunction resulting from prostatic cancer involves both the patient and his partner. Providing emotional support and empathy and encouraging communication with his partner profoundly affect the patient's perceptions about sexual function. The nurse facilitates communication between partners while providing opportunities for each to express concerns about sexuality and intimacy. Both partners should be informed that erectile dysfunction may resolve within 6 to 12 months after surgery. The nurse also should reinforce the importance of sexual expressions other than intercourse. Physical intimacy, hugging, kissing, and massage will help the man express sexual feelings and will promote his partner's sexual satisfaction during the convalescent period after surgery or during hormonal therapy. The patient should be advised to consult his urologist for assessment and treatment if sexual dysfunction persists beyond an acceptable period.

The patient with reduced bone integrity and chronic pain caused by bony metastasis presents a particularly difficult nursing challenge. He is instructed that he is at greater risk of injury from falls or spontaneous pathologic bone fracture, and the nurse should help him obtain appropriate aids for walking, such as a walker or cane. The home environment is assessed and the patient assisted in reducing environmental factors that may contribute to a fall, such as loose rugs on the floor, poorly lit hallways, or inadequate house slippers. The nurse helps the patient identify activities that lessen or exacerbate pain and helps him devise strategies for reducing it. Family members are enlisted to help the patient reorder his daily activities in a way that allows him optimal time and energy to cope with his pain. The nurse helps the patient and his family identify realistic goals for pain management and helps the patient realize these goals. The nurse should praise the patient when goals are attained and should encourage family members to assist in this strategy to alleviate the feelings of low self-worth that often accompany chronic pain.[33]

This treatment is supplemented with appropriate nonpharmacologic strategies for reducing pain (see Chapter 14). The physician is consulted about the use of pharmacologic or neurosurgical treatments for managing pain.

A detailed discussion of the nursing care of the dying patient is provided in Chapter 20. The patient who is terminally ill with prostatic cancer often faces issues related to dying while struggling with chronic pain caused by bony metastasis. The patient's family and social network are assessed continually for signs that the patient is becoming isolated from significant others. The nurse should be aware that depression, chronic pain, and anxiety may lead some patients to consider or attempt suicide. The patient is encouraged to talk to his family and health care providers about feelings of depression and suicidal fantasies. The nurse should help such patients and their families devise strategies for coping with depression and suicidal ideations. If appropriate, the patient is referred for mental health care.

TESTICULAR CANCER

Definition

Testicular cancer arises from the testis and its appendages or is the product of metastasis from distant sites.

Etiology/Epidemiology

The cause of testicular tumors is unknown; common associated factors are testicular atrophy,[60] failure of one or both testes to descend (cryptorchidism), and scrotal trauma.[32] Testicular atrophy may occur as a result of a viral or pyogenic orchitis or as the result of uncorrected cryptorchidism. Both the cryptorchid and contralateral testes have a greater potential for developing a malignant tumor. A history of scrotal trauma also has been noted in up to 25% of all patients with testicular tumors.[55] Viruses and exposure to certain chemicals may contribute to development of testicular tumors, but conclusive evidence of these suspicions has not yet been established.[32]

Testicular tumors are the second most common malignancy among men 20 to 35 years of age, and they account for 1% to 2% of all tumors in men.[41] Metastatic tumors of the testis are relatively rare; renal cell and prostatic carcinomas are most likely to metastasize to the testis.[49]

Pathophysiology

Testicular tumors arise from two distinct histologic components of the testis. Germ cell tumors arise from the portion of the testis that controls spermiogenesis; these tumors account for more than 90% of all testicular cancers.[63] Non–germ cell tumors arise from other testicular structures; they constitute 5% to 10% of all testicular cancers.[32]

RESEARCH BRIEF

Scott DW, Oberst MT, Bookbinder MI: Stress-coping response to genitourinary cancer in men, *Nurs Res* 33(6):325, 1984.

A descriptive study of the stress-coping responses of 30 men with noninvasive bladder cancer was undertaken during a routine hospitalization for invasive assessment (cystoscopy). A stress-coping conceptual model was used, which postulated that a person will cope with any life-threatening event by examining the magnitude of the threat, adjusting emotional responses, and engaging in coping behaviors to neutralize the threat. Anxiety, problem-solving ability, and concurrent stress were assessed by appropriate tools. The predominant coping strategy used was identified and correlated with these variables. Analysis of the data revealed that most subjects did not consider a diagnostic hospitalization for a genitourinary tumor to be a major crisis and did not state concerns over the long-range implications of their cancer. Men with greater problem-solving ability and higher education seemed to cope best with the diagnosis, whereas men with less education and problem-solving ability were most likely to experience dysphoric stress.

Germ cell tumors

Several tumors arise from the germ cell structures of the testis. Seminomas account for 30% to 40% of all testicular tumors. Three types of seminomas have been noted: anaplastic; typical, or classic; and spermatocytic. These tumors arise from the germ cells that line the seminiferous tubules of the testis and that differentiate into spermatids and eventually mature sperm cells.[9] Typical, anaplastic, and spermatocytic seminomas are distinguished by differences in the cytologic characteristics of the cells that compose the tumors and by differences in response to therapy.

Embryonal cell carcinoma also arises from the germ cells. It is highly aggressive and malignant and accounts for approximately 20% of all testicular tumors. These tumor cells may differentiate into several malignant forms. They commonly differentiate into incomplete forms of embryonic cells or extraembryonic (yolk sac trophoblastic) cells. They are thought to have the potential for malignant differentiation into a tumor called teratoma.

A teratoma is composed of tissue from all three germ cell layers that line the seminiferous tubule. Mature teratomas account for approximately 5% to 10% of testicular tumors. Two types of teratomas occur. The neonatal tumor is slow growing and rarely metastasizes. In contrast, teratomas that develop during adulthood show significant malignancy and require aggressive treatment. A teratocarcinoma has elements of both embryonal cell carcinoma and teratoma.

Choriocarcinoma is an extraembryonal malignancy that rarely occurs as a pure tumor.[63] The yolk sac testicular tumor typically occurs in boys under 3 years of age.[60] Polyembryoma and simple epidermoid cysts are rare forms of germ cell tumors.[32]

Germ cell tumors invade adjacent structures and metastasize via hematogenous or lymphatic routes. Local invasion is particularly significant, because it exposes many lymphatic channels to tumor invasion. The most common sites of lymphatic metastasis are the mediastinal and supraclavicular nodes.[60] Bloodborne metastases are likely to affect the lungs, bones, or liver.[63]

Non–germ cell tumors

Non–germ cell tumors of the testis account for only 5% to 10% of testicular malignancies. Leydig (interstitial) cell tumors, Sertoli cell tumors, or gonadal blastoma tumors (also called gonadoblastomas) may occur. Clear parameters of neoplasia (malignant tendencies) have not yet been established.[26] The box below lists the clinical stages of testicular tumors used to guide diagnosis and treatment.

Clinical Manifestations

The symptoms of early disease include an enlarged scrotum (a cardinal sign), a sensation of scrotal fullness (may be perceived as pain), and gynecomastia (painful enlargement of the breasts).

With seminoma, a symmetric mass, either hard or soft, may be felt in the scrotum; with embryonal cell carcinoma, the mass is asymmetric and smaller.

The symptoms of advanced disease are cough, dyspnea, and hemoptysis (lung metastasis); enlarged supraclavicular lymph nodes (lymphatic metastasis); abdominal mass; and back pain or numbness.

Abnormal laboratory values include elevated serum alpha-fetoprotein and elevated serum beta human chorionic gonadotropin.

Therapeutic Management

Surgical management

Surgical management of testicular cancer is determined by the type and stage of the tumor. Inguinal orchiectomy is combined with or followed by radical retroperitoneal lymphadenectomy to stage the tumor and guide subsequent care.[44] Dissection typically includes ipsilateral or bilateral inguinopelvic and para-aortic lymph nodes. Because extensive surgery causes loss of ejaculatory function, only limited dissection is done if nodes are not obviously enlarged.[31]

Radiotherapy and chemotherapy

Radiotherapy or chemotherapy is used if a retroperitoneal tumor is found. Radiotherapy is the usual treatment for cases of nonadvanced seminoma (stages A, B1, and B2). External beam radiotherapy consists of 2500 to 3500 rad delivered to the inguinopelvic and para-aortic nodes over a 3-week period.[26] Chemotherapy is used for tumors with mixed histology (more than one form of tumor) or for non–germ cell tumors. Chemotherapy is used for high-stage seminomas, tumors with mixed histology (more than one form of tumor), and non–germ cell tumors. Cisplatin, bleomycin, vinblastin, cyclophosphamide, vincristine, and dactinomycin are used in various combinations.[30] Two courses of adjuvant chemotherapy are given 3 weeks apart. Although the patient is exposed to potentially harmful side effects with these drugs, the rate of recurrence is low with this regimen.[31]

Advanced disease

Traditionally, advanced testicular tumors complicated by metastases have been treated with wide surgical excision of the tumor and metastatic lesions; this treatment has a survival rate of approximately 43%.[61] Combining surgical resection with adjuvant chemotherapy has significantly increased the survival rate for these patients.[47] If these treatments fail, the patient undergoes additional courses of chemotherapeutic drugs, called salvage regimens, and attempts are made to debulk the tumor surgically.[31]

CLINICAL STAGES OF TESTICULAR TUMORS

A—Tumor limited to testis

B1—Tumor in testis and retroperitoneal lymph nodes

B2—Tumor in retroperitoneal lymph nodes 2 to 6 cm in diameter as assessed by computed tomography (CT) scan

B3—Tumor in retroperitoneal lymph nodes larger than 6 cm as assessed by CT scan

C—Tumor above the diaphragm or involving solid abdominal organs

NURSING MANAGEMENT OF THE PATIENT WITH TESTICULAR CANCER

Assessment

The nurse examines the testes and scrotum to detect a testicular tumor (see Chapter 68). Such a tumor will cause enlargement and tenderness of the affected testis and hemiscrotum. In cases of seminoma the enlarged testes may be fairly symmetric and soft, or they may be symmetric and hardened if the tumor has a significant fibrous component. Asymmetric testicular enlargement may indicate embryonal cell carcinoma. The supraclavicular, inguinal, and pelvic lymph nodes are palpated to detect lymphatic spread. Abdominal palpation may reveal a mass in cases of advanced disease with extensive para-aortic node enlargement and tumor extension.

Psychosocial assessment of the patient with testicular cancer centers on issues stemming from fear of cancer, altered sexual function, and changes in body image caused by the disease and its treatment. The nurse explores the patient's understanding of testicular cancer and dispels any myths he might hold about a relationship between sexual activity and malignancy. The nurse also assesses the patient's goals and feelings about his altered reproductive potential, including his partner in these discussions whenever possible.

Nursing Diagnosis

Common diagnoses may include the following:

Pain related to testicular tumor

Anxiety related to presence of testicular tumor and treatment strategies

Sexual dysfunction related to altered ejaculatory function (reduced fertility potential) and potential altered erectile function

Diarrhea related to side effects of radiotherapy, chemotherapy

Altered nutrition: less than body requirements related to side effects of chemotherapy

Body image disturbance related to side effects of chemotherapy, removal of tumor

Altered pulmonary tissue perfusion related to lung metastases

Planning

Specific patient goals are determined with the help of the patient and his family or significant others. These goals are influenced by the patient's age and plans and goals for family planning, as well as by the severity of disease, the presence of local invasion or distant metastasis, and the medical management plan. General goals include the following:

Patient experiences minimal discomfort from the presence or physical manipulation of the testicular tumor

Patient expresses anxieties and fears about testicular cancer and states realistic goals concerning treatment

Patient and partner state strategies for coping with altered fertility potential

Patient and partner state strategies for coping with altered erectile function, if necessary, including ways to express sexual intimacy other than intercourse

Patient reestablishes normal bowel elimination routine after radiotherapy or chemotherapy

Patient consumes sufficient nutrients to maintain a desired body weight during and after chemotherapy

Patient demonstrates knowledge of potential loss of muscle mass and hair in response to chemotherapy and identifies strategies for coping with these changes

Patient's respirations and blood pressure remain within normal limits, and pulmonary embolus is avoided

Implementation

The first priority for nursing in the care of patients who have or are at risk for tumor of the testis is early detection of cancer by testicular self-examination (see Chapter 69). Young men should be taught to perform self-examination monthly beginning at 15 years of age.[15] Nurses should strive to teach all males over age 15 to examine their testes. Special emphasis is given to men with identified risk factors for testicular tumor, including cryptorchidism or a history of cryptorchidism or viral or bacterial orchitis.

When a testicular tumor is suspected, the man is advised to seek immediate care. Because the disease commonly affects otherwise healthy young men, anxiety is common. Patient education about testicular cancer and potential treatments is begun immediately after a tumor is confirmed. The nurse helps the patient who has received such a diagnosis to identify support persons and to contact them if necessary. The nurse also explains all tests in concrete terms and emphasizes what the patient will experience, as well as how the results of procedures will contribute to care.

Pain from testicular enlargement is exacerbated by physical manipulation and by anxiety stemming from discovery of a tumor. Physical examination or manipulation of the scrotum for diagnostic or therapeutic procedures is performed slowly and gently. Discomfort may be relieved by applying heat to the scrotum with a heating pad set at the lowest temperature setting or by means of a warm bath or compress. The patient is advised to use a scrotal support when active to relieve discomfort. Analgesics are provided in consultation with the physician. The nurse continues to assess the patient for chest, abdominal, or back pain that may become apparent after scrotal discomfort is relieved. Findings are reported to the physician, since discomfort in these areas may indicate metastatic disease.

Surgery

Orchiectomy, which often is performed near the time of retroperitoneal lymph node dissection, is the principal procedure for removing a testicular tumor. Preoperative teaching includes (1) reviewing findings from diagnostic tests (intravenous pyelogram, blood tests for alpha-fetoprotein and beta human chorionic gonadotropin, chest x-rays, and CT scans) and (2) explaining the dual therapeutic and diagnostic value of surgery. The patient is instructed that orchiectomy involves removing the primary tumor, whereas retroperitoneal lymph node dissection is performed to remove affected nodes and to assist in determining the stage of the tumor. The nurse explains that staging a testicular neoplasm helps determine medical and nursing treatment.

The nurse helps the patient cope with anxieties about altered body image and sexual function and emphasizes that unilateral orchiectomy will not cause significant redistribution of the patient's body fat or hair and will not destroy his potential for reproduction. Nonetheless, the nurse should explain to the patient that his potential for fertility may be affected by the extent of the disease and by other treatment, including retroperitoneal lymph node dissection, radiotherapy, and chemotherapy. The patient is advised that using a prosthetic device will disguise the scrotal deformity created by removing a testis.

The patient will return from surgery with a dressing over the scrotal wound; a catheter may be in place. The nurse regularly assesses the dressing for drainage or other signs of wound infection, including a temperature higher than 101° F. No surgical drains are used with routine orchiectomy, and discharge from the dressing should be minimal.

The patient is provided with adequate scrotal support to relieve discomfort caused by movement and postoperative edema. The nurse helps him maintain a position that avoids discomfort at the surgical site. Analgesic medications are provided after consulting the physician. Discomfort at the wound site usually persists only 24 to 48 hours. The physician is notified if significant scrotal pain persists for longer than 48 hours.[57]

Retroperitoneal lymphadenectomy may be performed with orchiectomy and may alter the patient's fertility potential by impeding ejaculatory function. The nurse assesses the patient's goals and desires concerning family planning and includes the patient's partner in these discussions whenever possible. The patient and his partner are introduced to alternate strategies for having children. Options include adoption, insemination with donor sperm, sperm banking, and electroejaculation stimulation, which is a procedure to gather semen when retrograde ejaculation causes infertility.[8]

The patient who undergoes lymph node dissection will return from the operating room with a midline thoracoabdominal wound and a nasogastric tube connected to suction. Oral intake is avoided for approximately 1 to 2 days, and fluids are administered intravenously to avoid fluid volume or short-term nutritional deficits. After signs of peristalsis return (regular bowel sounds assessed by auscultation and passage of flatus), the nasogastric tube is removed and the patient is allowed to have a clear liquid diet. The diet is slowly advanced to solid foods according to the patient's tolerance.

A midline abdominal or thoracoabdominal dressing is left in place after surgery. Discharge from the wound is not uncommon and may require frequent dressing changes for the first several days. The wound is assessed regularly for signs of infection, including fever. Pain from the incision typically is more severe than that experienced after orchiectomy alone. The nurse teaches the patient to splint his chest and abdomen when coughing or turning and administers analgesics after consulting the physician.

Radiotherapy and chemotherapy

Nursing care of patients receiving external beam radiotherapy to lymphatic nodes in the abdomen, pelvis, or thorax or of those receiving intravenous chemotherapy focuses on preventing and managing side effects. Fluid volume or nutritional deficits may arise because of diarrhea or because nutritional intake is inadequate as a result of suppressed appetite or stomatitis. The patient is encouraged to sip small amounts of electrolyte-rich fluids (i.e., Gatorade, clear fruit juices), to eat several small meals each day, and to avoid fatty or fried foods. This regimen minimizes nausea while ensuring adequate fluid and nutritional intake.

Antiemetics or antidiarrheal drugs are used if nonpharmacologic measures fail to control nausea and vomiting (see Chapter 15).

Immunosuppression is a common side effect of both radiotherapy and chemotherapy. The patient is taught that he is at greater risk for infection because of this condition and that he should avoid large crowds or excessive contact with individuals suffering from upper respiratory infections or the flu.

Evaluation

Continual evaluation helps the nurse monitor the effectiveness of patient teaching and interventions. A successful treatment program will help the patient demonstrate knowledge of testicular self-examination and ensure that he knows he must seek health care if a suspicious area is found. Pain after surgery will be minimized, and the incision will remain infection free. The patient will identify the principal untoward effects of radiotherapy or chemotherapy and will maintain an adequate body weight and state of hydration. Evaluation also includes evidence that the patient has reasonable expectations about his fertility potential and that he can identify strategies for coping with infertility if necessary.

Documentation

Documenting the patient's response to treatment regimens and maintaining an adequate fluid volume and nutritional status are essential to the nursing care of a patient with testicular cancer.

Ongoing Care

The long-term care of men with testicular cancer focuses on preventing tumor recurrence and reestablishing adequate sexual function and self-concept. All men with testicular cancer should be taught testicular self-examination and to recognize the symptoms of tumor recurrence. The nurse emphasizes the importance of follow-up evaluations.

Fertility and ejaculatory function have become increasingly important issues as the survival rate for men with testicular cancer grows. The patient is informed that sperm production may remain suboptimal for approximately 2 years after chemotherapy or radiotherapy. Detailed assessment is indicated if symptoms persist beyond this period. The patient who has ejaculatory dysfunction or persistent subfertility is informed about treatments for infertility. Alternatives to fertilization through intercourse include artificial insemination through donor sperm, electroejaculation stimulation with intrauterine insemination, and hyperstimulation of the ovaries in combination with in vitro fertilization or related procedures. The couple may need to be referred to a nurse specialist or physician specialist to obtain detailed information about these family planning programs.

ERECTILE DYSFUNCTION
Definition

Erectile dysfunction or impotence is the failure to achieve penile tumescence of adequate rigidity or duration for successful intercourse.

Etiology/Epidemiology

Erectile dysfunction typically has many causes. Common contributing factors are hormonal disorders, neurologic and other medical disorders, and surgical and traumatic disorders.[2] Drug-induced,[51] vascular,[73] and psychogenic[17] causes also are common. The incidence of dysfunction increases in the presence of these factors and with increasing age. The absolute incidence of erectile dysfunction is unknown, because reporting is incomplete due to cultural and societal values concerning sexual behavior.[9]

Pathophysiology

Erectile dysfunction may arise from a single cause, although a multifactorial etiology is most common. The endocrine system modulates libido and tumescence over a prolonged period. Functioning testicular tissue and an adequate supply of androgens are necessary for the development and maintenance of erectile and fertility functions of the reproductive system and secondary male characteristics. Nonetheless, an individual erection is a neurovascular rather than a hormonally modulated event. The psychogenic factors that determine sexuality also affect erectile function, profoundly influencing both individual erectile events and the individual's lifelong responses to sexual intimacy.

Hormonal disorders

Hormonal disorders that disturb the hypothalamic-pituitary-gonadal axis typically cause erectile dysfunction ranging from mild loss of libido to hypogonadism and organic impotence.[9] Hypogonadism that occurs before puberty delays or arrests the onset of pubescent changes, whereas hypogonadism occurring after puberty produces a loss of testicular and penile size, impaired libido, gynecomastia (feminization of the male breast), and changes in the body soma (habitus or shape) reflecting a more feminine distribution of hair and fatty tissue.[2]

Vascular disorders

Vascular disorders affect erectile dysfunction by interfering with the arterial or venous events needed to attain or sustain tumescence. Arterial abnormalities may affect the inflow of blood into the penis needed to attain an erection. Arteriosclerosis and atherosclerosis affect erectile activity when they compromise arterial flow in the penile, internal pudendal, or internal iliac arteries. Cigarette smoking affects erectile activity when it produces small vessel changes that compromise arterial inflow needed for an erection.[54]

Venous defects affect erectile function when the venules and larger veins that drain the erectile bodies allow excessive runoff of blood, making the individual unable to sustain an erection. Pelvic trauma, cigarette smoking, and other unknown factors contribute to venous incompetence and erectile dysfunction.[54]

Neurologic disorders

Any neurologic disorder that affects the brain, spinal cord, or peripheral nervous system has the potential to contribute to erectile dysfunction. Individuals who experience neuropathic disorders find themselves unable to initiate an erection.

Disorders of the brain, including traumatic injuries, multiple sclerosis, or tumors, may affect erectile dysfunction, particularly when they cause profound personality changes or altered mentation. Spinal cord disorders, including traumatic injuries, myelodysplastic defects, tabes dorsalis, spinal cord tumors, amyotrophic lateral sclerosis, and multiple sclerosis, may affect the ability to attain an erection when desired even though "reflex" (involuntary or uncontrolled) erections may be noted. Peripheral polyneuropathies such as those associated with diabetes mellitus, renal insufficiency, amyloidosis, or related metabolic disorders may contribute to erectile dysfunction, particularly when peripheral neuropathies coexist with vascular disease.[8]

Other medical disorders

Nonneurologic medical disorders associated with erectile dysfunction include heart disease and chronic obstructive pulmonary disease.[9]

Surgical and traumatic disorders

Surgical procedures affect erectile function by unavoidably compromising the peripheral neural or vascular erectile apparatus. Extensive surgical procedures of the abdomen and pelvis such as ileostomy, colostomy, and abdominoperineal resection are associated with erectile dysfunction. Radical prostatectomy may cause impotence, particularly if the perineal approach is used.[74]

Trauma to the lower urinary tract and pelvis also can cause erectile dysfunction. Up to half of men with a pelvic fracture and injury to the bladder or proximal urethra experience erectile dysfunction caused by vascular or peripheral neurologic disturbance.

Drugs

Many drugs are associated with erectile dysfunction (see box below). Antihypertensives that affect the autonomic and central nervous system often result in erectile dysfunction. The thiazides and spironolactone may cause erectile dysfunction by depress-

---

DRUGS ASSOCIATED WITH ERECTILE DYSFUNCTION

Antihypertensive agents
Sympatholytics (alpha-methyldopa, clonidine)
Alpha-adrenergic blocking agents (prazosin, phenoxybenzamine)
Beta-adrenergic blocking agents (propranolol, atenolol)
Vasodilators (hydralazine)
Diuretics (spironolactone, other thiazides)

Psychotropic agents
Major tranquilizers/antipsychotics (chlorpromazine, thioridazine)
Antidepressants (imipramine, amitriptyline)
Antianxiety agents (diazepam, chlordiazepoxide)

Illicit or abused substances
Alcohol
Cocaine
Narcotics
Heroin
Nicotine

Hormonal agents
Androgens
Antiandrogens
Estrogens

Anticholinergic agents
Propantheline
Methantheline bromide

Antacids
Cimetidine

Cardiac agents
Digoxin

From Wein AJ, van Arsdalen KN: Drug-induced male sexual dysfunction, *Urol Clin North Am* 15(1):23, 1988.

ing libido and altering endocrine balance. Methyl-dopa (Aldomet) causes erectile dysfunction by stimulating prolactin production via a sedative, depressant effect that suppresses libido.[65]

Antidepressant and antipsychotic drugs cause erectile dysfunction via effects on the central and peripheral nervous systems.[2] Alcohol and recreational drugs also exert an effect on erectile function. Alcohol causes the suppression of serum testosterone levels and, at particularly high levels, will depress libido and impair performance. Other recreational drugs that commonly compromise erectile function include marijuana, cocaine, nicotine, amphetamines, barbiturates, and opiates.

Psychogenic dysfunction

Sexual function is a combination of physiologic processes and psychologic and sociocultural factors. Successful sexual arousal, initiation of an erection, and maintenance of an erection correlate with affectual events that provide positive feedback, promoting the cascade of behaviors that result in a satisfying sexual encounter. Adverse pyschosocial events may interfere with this cascade of events and render a man unable to sustain or maintain an erection with or without the presence of organic dysfunction.[35]

Three factors needed to obtain an erection from the psychosocial perspective are (1) adequate physiologic responses, (2) adequate stimulation, and (3) repeated positive reinforcement toward sexual expression. Psychosocial factors may adversely affect these factors. Stress results in increased fatigue, muscle tension, and anxiety. Anxiety may decrease sexual performance by preoccupying the man as he seeks to identify and cope with stressors in his environment. Anxiety and depression are commonly noted in men with erectile dysfunction. These factors may lead to impotence, or they may coexist with organic dysfunction.[35]

Four psychosocial factors can be identified that distinguish affected men from men with normal sexual function. They are (1) differences in affect during sexual stimulation, (2) a tendency to lack appreciation of arousal during stimulation, (3) a tendency to be distracted during sexual experiences, and (4) adverse reactions to anxiety experienced during a sexual encounter. Men with psychogenic impotence fail to develop or lose sight of the positive feedback loop that enhances the normal sexual response. Instead, they interpret physiologic and psychosocial aspects of sexual behavior in a negative way that inhibits their performance rather than allowing enjoyment of this human response.[35]

Clinical Manifestations

The clinical manifestations of erectile dysfunction include loss of ability to generate erections, loss of ability to maintain erections, insufficient rigidity for vaginal penetration, impaired libido, loss of testicular size with feminization of the male body habitus, and failure of external genitalia and secondary sex characteristics to develop.

Therapeutic Management

Hormonal therapy

Therapeutic management is based on careful assessment of the causative factors. Hormonal abnormalities may be managed by administering exogenous androgens. Parenteral testosterone is used and occasionally is combined with beta human chorionic growth hormone if infertility and impotence coexist.

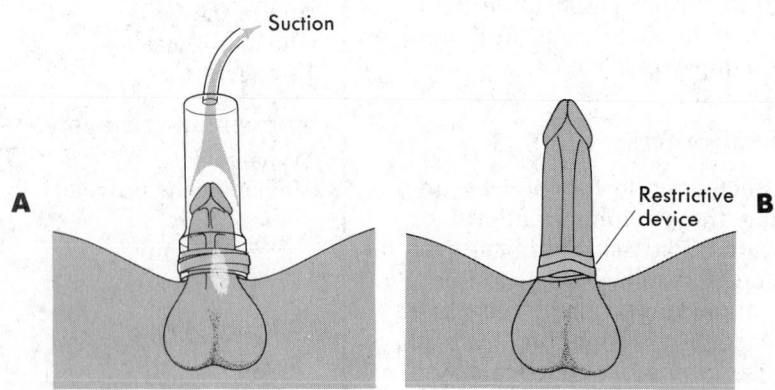

FIGURE 71-5   **A,** Mechanical devices create a vacuum to shunt blood into penis. **B,** A tourniquet or restrictive device for maintaining penile engorgement must be used for successful intercourse.

The side effects include liver toxicity, polycythemia, paradoxic feminization, and suppression of spermiogenesis.[22]

Therapy for vascular disorders

In some patients vascular surgery of the major vessels that supply the penis and other organs in the pelvis and trunk may correct erectile dysfunction, prevent catastrophic vascular emergencies, and improve circulation to affected areas.[18,73] Other patients are taught to inject a vasodilator (papaverine, prostaglandin E, phentolamine) into the corporeal bodies of the penis to correct vascular impotence.[34] The preparation is injected directly into a cavernous body near the base of the penis. Minoxidil cream also has been used as a vasoactive agent; the agent is massaged into the penis over the cavernous body. Side effects of injectable vasodilators include priapism (painful, sustained erection) and development of fibrous plaques at injection sites. Minoxidil cream is undergoing clinical trials to determine its efficacy for erectile dysfunction.

Mechanical devices

A vacuum-pump device also can be used to treat erectile dysfunction. The device uses suction to mechanically draw blood into the cavernous bodies. A restriction device is placed at the base of the penis to trap blood and thus prevent loss of erection (Figure 71-5). These devices provide a noninvasive, reversible method for obtaining erection. Potential complications include ischemia to the penis and painful ejaculation when semen is trapped in the proximal urethra.[38]

Prosthetic therapy

Prosthetic devices are surgically implanted in the corporeal bodies on either side of the penis (Figure 71-6). Semirigid or flexible devices were developed first and are relatively easy to implant. They are easy for the patient to use but difficult to conceal in clothing. The principal complications with these devices are infection and erosion of the device through the skin.[64]

An inflatable **penile prosthesis** is more difficult to implant and to use than a semirigid device, but it has several advantages. It is easier to conceal in clothing and more esthetically pleasing for most patients because it has a flaccid state and an erect state (Figure 71-7).[48] Complications from these devices include infection, erosion of the implant through the skin, and mechanical failure.

Psychologic therapy

Psychologic therapy is indicated when psychogenic impotence is diagnosed, or it may be used as an adjunct in cases of organic dysfunction. Behavioral therapy and counseling help the patient alter behavior that impedes sexual encounters and develop a more positive attitude toward behavior that constitutes a satisfying and successful male sexual response.

NURSING MANAGEMENT OF THE PATIENT WITH ERECTILE DYSFUNCTION
Assessment

The nurse assesses the patient's body habitus and external genitalia for evidence of hormonal abnor-

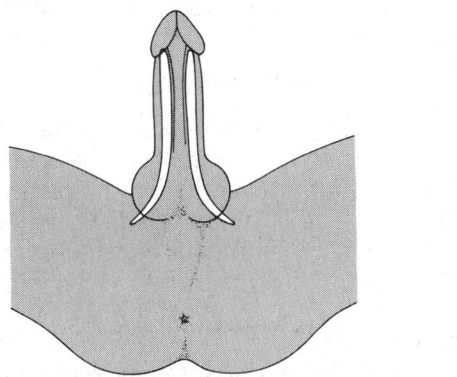
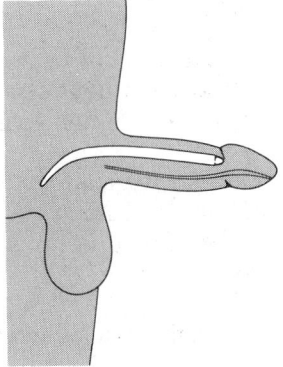

FIGURE 71-6   A semirigid prosthesis is implanted in corpora cavernosa and remains in an erect position that may be difficult to hide in clothing.

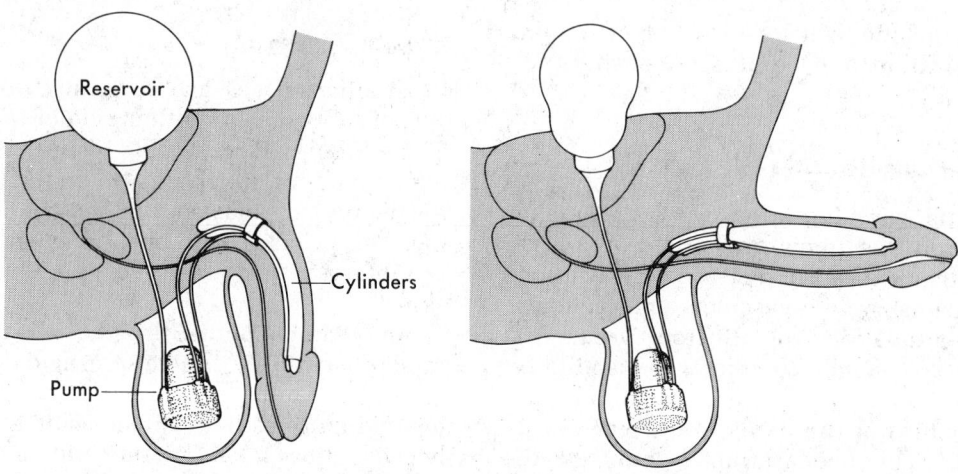

FIGURE 71-7   The Scott Inflatable Prosthesis has both erect and flaccid positions designed to mimic normal erectile function.

malities that might contribute to erectile dysfunction. The distribution of body hair, fat, and general body morphology are examined. The genitalia are examined, including measuring testicular and penile size. The erect penis also is examined if assessment is undertaken within the context of a sleep laboratory for male sexual dysfunction. This examination is performed only in the presence of another health care professional.

Nursing Diagnosis

Several nursing diagnoses are used, including diagnoses related to the disorders that cause impotence. Common nursing diagnoses directly related to erectile dysfunction are as follows:

Sexual dysfunction related to erectile dysfunction

Altered sexuality patterns related to erectile dysfunction

Body image disturbance related to endocrine abnormality with altered body habitus

Planning

Specific patient goals vary according to the severity of the dysfunction, the medical treatment strategy, and related disorders or diseases. Common goals include the following:

Patient describes alternate strategies for coping with erectile dysfunction, including various medical and surgical treatment options and forms of sexual expression other than intercourse

Patient and his partner describe a sexually satisfying relationship

Patient shows evidence of satisfaction with or acceptance of body habitus

Implementation

Nursing management focuses both on the affected male and his partner whenever possible.

Hormonal therapy

The nurse is responsible for teaching the patient to administer hormonal medications (testosterone) and to watch for side effects.

The patient is instructed to check his weight daily during the initial weeks after androgens are given and when dosages are changed. Rapid weight gain may indicate significant sodium and water retention and may require consultation with the physician about lowering the dosage or using a diuretic. The nurse explains to the patient that response to therapy will be slow. The diabetic patient is advised that testosterone will enhance the action of insulin and that he should be sensitive to signs of hypoglycemia (diaphoresis, tremor, anxiety, and pallor). Such episodes are treated immediately by consuming carbohydrates, and testosterone dosages may have to be changed to prevent recurrence.

Vascular therapy

A specialist nurse typically assumes primary responsibility for instructing men to inject vasodilators for impotence. The principal side effect of injectable vasodilators is priapism, and the patient is advised to seek immediate treatment if it occurs.[6]

Mechanical devices

The nurse often assumes principal responsibility for assisting in the selection of a mechanical device for impotence. The choice is based on the couple's ability to manipulate the device. For example, some devices require suction provided by the patient and are best avoided if the patient and his partner are easily fatigued when blowing up a balloon. Other systems involve manipulating a tourniquet-type device and require a certain level of manual dexterity and strength. Selection of a device also requires careful assessment of the preferences of the patient and his partner. Both partners are taught to use the device with written and verbal coaching and, whenever possible, by example and return demonstration. The patient is advised to remove the tourniquet device after intercourse is completed to prevent ischemia.

Penile prosthesis care

The care of patients undergoing placement of a penile prosthesis focuses on preoperative instruction concerning use of the device and ensuring adequate follow-up care. Preoperative teaching centers on the care and use of the device to be implanted. The nurse helps the patient with a semirigid device to develop strategies for concealing his prosthesis in clothing. The patient should wear elastic briefs that contain the implant. The penis ideally is placed at a 45-degree angle from the base rather than facing directly upward or outward from the abdominal wall. The patient is instructed to avoid tight slacks or boxer shorts that emphasize the presence of the implant. Before surgery the nurse obtains a model of an inflatable device and allows the patient and his partner to practice activating and deactivating it. If the couple lack the manual dexterity to use the device properly, the surgeon is consulted about the need for further instruction before implantation or about use of an alternative device.

Surgical implantation of a penile prosthesis may be a "day stay" procedure or may require hospitalization for 5 to 10 days, depending on the patient and the type of device used. The patient returns from surgery with a penile or scrotal incision. Drainage from the wound should be minimal, and the nurse assesses for signs of infection and amount and characteristics of drainage with each dressing change. She also assesses regularly for signs of systemic infection. The physician is consulted if the patient's temperature rises above 101° F.

The patient is advised that penile and scrotal swelling will be noted for 3 to 5 days and that the hematoma will persist for approximately 2 weeks. The patient should avoid strenuous activity for 3 weeks and operate the inflatable device under direct supervision until he masters its proper use.

The patient is instructed to avoid sexual contact for approximately 21 days to allow sufficient healing. Inflatable devices may be partially inflated and deflated following implantation to promote formation of a fibrous sheath. The patient is instructed

about the signs of implant erosion (thinning and stretching of the skin beneath the glans or hematuria and dysuria), and he is advised to seek medical care if this occurs. The patient also is advised of the signs and symptoms of infection of the implant, including tenderness of the penis, fever, dysuria, and signs of urinary tract infection. The nurse educates the patient to seek care promptly if infection occurs.[9]

Evaluation

Continual evaluation of a strategy to correct erectile dysfunction helps the patient and his partner identify and implement ways to resume a mutually satisfying sexual relationship. The patient should demonstrate knowledge of proper self-injection techniques, of routines for taking oral medication, or of the use of a mechanical or surgically implanted device. Ideally, the patient's partner demonstrates equal knowledge of a care program, including strategies for coping with potential complications.

Documentation

Documenting patient and partner education concerning use of injectable or other medications, an implantable prosthesis, or a mechanical device forms the most important record of care for the impotent male.

Ongoing Care

Care of a patient with erectile dysfunction requires continual assessment of altered behavioral patterns and assistive devices used to alleviate the condition. The couple also is encouraged to explore expressions of sexual intimacy other than intercourse.

Ongoing care of men who use oral or parenteral medications requires routine monitoring of the success of therapy and prevention of complications. The nurse reassures the man who is taking oral testosterone that response to therapy is slow. She also should point out objective signs of response to therapy throughout ongoing care and should restate realistic goals of therapy as needed.

Ongoing assessment of men who inject their penises with vasodilators is essential for this form of treatment to succeed. The nurse systematically assesses the patient by means of telephone conversations and clinic appointments to assure that the patient has no complications and is satisfied with self-injection. She should discuss alternative strategies with patients who become dissatisfied with self-injection therapy.

Ongoing care of the patient with a surgically implanted penile prosthesis centers on education in the use of the device and prevention of delayed complications. The nurse reinforces for the couple the teaching of implant use and strategies for smoothly integrating activation of the device during intercourse. The patient is advised to consult his physician about using prophylactic antibiotics before urologic instrumentation (catheterization, cystourethroscopy) is performed after implantation. The patient also is advised to seek prompt medical care if symptoms of prosthetic infection develop such as fever with urinary tract infection and hematuria.

CRITICAL THINKING QUESTIONS

1 How does BPH alter urinary elimination patterns? What complications are associated with urinary obstruction?

2 What is the goal of transurethral resection? What is the nursing care of a three-way Foley catheter after surgery?

3 What can the nurse do to help the patient alleviate and cope with symptoms of altered urinary elimination?

4 How can the nurse assess for bleeding after surgery? How can she assess for TUR syndrome?

5 What kinds of instruction should the nurse give the patient before discharge regarding stress urinary incontinence? recurrence of bladder obstruction?

6 Describe a nursing strategy for assessing pain in the patient with prostatic cancer and bony metastasis.

7 What symptoms are common after radiotherapy, and how may the nurse minimize them?

8 What are the two major long-term effects of radical prostatectomy, and what are the related nursing interventions?

9 What are the four major aspects of nursing care during long-term rehabilitation of a patient with prostatic cancer? Describe the major interventions for each.

10 What are the symptoms of testicular tumors? How can the nurse teach patients to detect possible warning signs of cancer?

11 Outline the nursing care of the patient after radiotherapy and chemotherapy and after surgery.

12 What factors are involved in erectile dysfunction? How can the nurse assess the effect of dysfunction on the patient and his partner? Describe the nursing care of the patient with a penile prosthesis. What must the nurse teach the patient to assure continual care?

BIBLIOGRAPHY

Current

1. Belcher AE: Neoplasia. In Thompson JM et al: *Mosby's clinical nursing,* St Louis, 1989, Mosby–Year Book, Inc.
2. Benson GA, Boileau agileau MA: The penis: sexual function and dysfunction. In Gillenwater JY et al: *Adult and pediatric urology,* Chicago, 1987, Year Book Medical Publishers, Inc.
3. Brendler CB: Perioperative care. In Walsh PC et al: *Campbell's urology,* Philadelphia, 1986, WB Saunders Co.
4. Catalona WJ, Scott WM: Carcinoma of the prostate. In Walsh PC et al: *Campbell's urology,* Philadelphia, 1986, WB Saunders Co.
5. Cucci A: Detrusor instability in prostatic outlet obstruction in relation to urethral opening pressure, *Neurourol Urodynamics* 9:17-24, 1990.
6. Duffy LM, Sidi AA, Lange PH: Vasoactive intracavernous pharmacotherapy: the nursing role in teaching self-injection therapy, *Urology* 138:1198, 1986.
7. Findlay PA, Glatstein E: Principles of radiation therapy. In Graham SD: *Urologic oncology,* New York, 1986, Raven Press.
8. Gray ML: *Genitourinary disorders,* St Louis, 1992, Mosby–Year Book, Inc.
9. Gray ML, Dobkin KA: Genitourinary system. In Thompson JM et al: *Mosby's clinical nursing,* St Louis, 1989, Mosby–Year Book, Inc.
10. Gray ML, Dougherty MC: Urinary incontinence—pathophysiology and treatment, *J Enterostom Ther* 14(4):152, 1987.
11. Grayhack JT, Kozlowski JM: Benign prostatic hyperplasia. In Gillenwater JY et al, editors: *Adult and pediatric urology,* St Louis, 1991, Mosby–Year Book, Inc.
12. Henrich-Rynning T: Prostatic cancer treatments and their effects of sexual functioning, *Oncol Nurs Forum* 14(6):37, 1987.
13. Klein FA: Prostatic carcinoma: interstitial radiation therapy. In Graham SD: *Urologic oncology,* New York, 1986, Raven Press.
14. Krane RJ: Penile prostheses, *Urol Clin North Am* 15(1):77, 1988.
15. La Follette S: Perioperative care of the testis tumor patient, *AUAA J* 8(3):12, 1988.
16. Lepor H: What will replace TURP? *Contemp Urol* 4(2):30-41, 1992.
17. Levine SB: The psychological evaluation and therapy of psychogenic impotence. In Seagraves RT, Schoenberg HW: *Diagnosis and treatment of erectile disturbances: a guide for clinicians,* New York, 1985, Plenum Publishing Corp.
18. Lewis RW: Venous surgery for impotence, *Urol Clin North Am* 15(1):115, 1988.
19. Linehan WM, Andriole GL: Endocrine aspects of urologic oncology. In Graham SD: *Urologic oncology,* New York, 1986, Raven Press.
20. MacElveen-Hoehn P, McCorkle R: Understanding sexuality in progressive cancer, *Semin Oncol Nurs* 1(1):56, 1985.
21. Marinelli D et al: Follow-up prostate biopsy in patients with carcinoma of the prostate treated by [192]iridium template irradiation plus supplemental external beam radiation, *J Urol* 147:922, 1992.
22. McClure RD: Endocrine evaluation and therapy of erectile dysfunction, *Urol Clin North Am* 15(1):53, 1988.

23. McConnell JD et al: An inhibitor of 5 alpha reductase (MK-906) suppresses prostatic dihydrotestosterone in men with benign prostatic hyperplasia, *J Urol* 141(part 2), 1989.

24. Meuller SC, Lue TF: Evaluation of vasculogenic impotence, *Urol Clin North Am* 15(1):65, 1988.

25. Morales A et al: Oral and transcutaneous pharmacologic agents in the treatment of impotence, *Urol Clin North Am* 15(1):87, 1988.

26. Morse MJ, Whitmore WF: Neoplasms of the testis. In Walsh PC et al: *Campbell's urology*, Philadelphia, 1986, WB Saunders Co.

27. Narayan P: Neoplasms of the prostate gland. In Tanagho EA, McAninch JW, editors: *Smith's general urology*, Norwalk, Conn, 1992, Lange Medical Books.

28. Parra R, Andruss C, Boullier J: Staging laparoscopic pelvic lymph node dissection: comparison of results with open pelvic lymphadenectomy, *J Urol* 147:875-878, 1992.

29. Paulson DF: Principles of oncology. In Walsh PC et al: *Campbell's urology*, Philadelphia, 1986, WB Saunders Co.

30. Presti JC, Herr HW: Genital tumors. In Tanagho EA, McAninch JW, editors: *Smith's general urology*, Norwalk, Conn, 1992, Lange Medical Books.

31. Rowland RG: Management of carcinoma of the testicle. In Graham SD: *Urologic oncology*, New York, 1986, Raven Press.

32. Rowland RG, Donohue JP: Scrotum and testis. In Gillenwater JY et al: *Adult and pediatric urology*, Chicago, 1987, Year Book Medical Publishers, Inc.

33. Schroeder PM, Gunta KE: Comfort. In Thompson JM et al: *Clinical nursing*, St Louis, 1986, Mosby–Year Book, Inc.

34. Sidi AA: Vasointracavernous pharmacotherapy, *Urol Clin North Am* 15(1):95, 1988.

35. Smith AD: Psychologic factors in multidisciplinary evaluation and treatment of erectile dysfunction, *Urol Clin North Am* 15(1):41, 1988.

36. Walsh PC: Benign prostatic hyperplasia. In Walsh PC et al: *Campbell's urology*, Philadelphia, 1986, WB Saunders Co.

37. Wein AJ, van Arsdalen KN: Drug-induced male sexual dysfunction, *Urol Clin North Am* 15(1):23, 1988.

38. Witherington R: Suction device therapy in the management of erectile impotence, *Urol Clin North Am* 15(1):123, 1988.

Classic

39. Birkhoff JD: The natural history of benign prostatic hypertrophy. In Hinman F: *Benign prostatic hypertrophy*, New York, 1983, Springer-Verlag New York, Inc.

40. Blair A, Fraumeni JF: Geographic patterns of prostate cancer in the United States, *National Cancer Institute* 61:1379, 1978.

41. Blandy JP, Hope-Stone HF, Dayan AD: *Tumors of the testicle*, New York, 1970, Grune & Stratton, Inc.

42. Boller F, Frank E: Clinical syndromes. In Boller F, Frank E: *Sexual dysfunction in neurological disorders*, New York, 1982, Raven Press.

43. Centifano YM et al: Herpesvirus particles in prostatic carcinoma cells, *J Virol* 12:1608, 1973.

44. Donohue JP: Retroperitoneal lymphadenectomy, *Urol Clin North Am* 4:509, 1977.

45. Dunn JE: Cancer epidemiology in populations in the United States with emphasis on Hawaii, California and Japan, *Cancer Res* 35:3240, 1975.

46. Eggleston JC, Walsh PC: *Nerve sparing radical retropubic prostatectomy: pathologic findings in the first 100 cases.* Paper presented at the annual meeting of the American Urological Association, Abstract No. 511, 1981.

47. Einhorn LH, Donohue JP: Improved chemotherapy in disseminated testicular cancer, *J Urol* 117:65, 1977.

48. Furlow WL: Use of inflatable penile prosthesis in the management of erectile dysfunction, *Urol Clin North Am* 8(1):181, 1981.

49. Hannash KA: Metastatic tumors to the testicle, *Prog Clin Biol Res* 203:61, 1984.

50. Jacobs SC: Spread of prostatic cancer to bone, *Urology* 21:337, 1983.

51. Jarowencko MV, Bennett AH: Pharmacology of impotence—sexual dysfunction. In Libertino AJ: *International perspectives in urology*, vol 5, Baltimore, 1982, Williams & Wilkins.

52. Jewett HJ et al: The palpable nodule of prostatic cancer: results 15 years after radical excision, *JAMA* 203:115, 1968.

53. Kakkar VV et al: Natural history of preoperative deep vein thrombosis, *Lancet* 2:230, 1969.

54. Kedia KR: Vascular disorders and male erectile dysfunction, *Urol Clin North Am* 8:153, 1981.

55. Kimbrough JC, Denslow JC: Malignant disease of the testis, *J Urol* 65:611, 1951.

56. Lang DJ, Kummer JF, Hartley DP: Cytomegalovirus in semen: persistence and demonstration in extracellular fluid, *N Engl J Med* 291:121, 1974.

57. Lerner J, Khan Z: Manual of urological nursing, St Louis, 1982, Mosby–Year Book, Inc.

58. Martin D: Malignancy in the cryptorchid testis, *Urol Clin North Am* 9(3):371, 1982.

59. McLaughlin AP et al: Prostatic carcinoma: incidence and location of unsuspected lymphatic metastases, *J Urol* 115:89, 1976.

60. Merrin C: Seminoma, *Urol Clin North Am* 4(3):379, 1977.

61. Merrin C et al: Combination radical surgery and sequential chemotherapy for treatment of advanced carcinoma of the testis (stage III), *Cancer* 37:2029, 1976.

62. Moore RA: Benign hypertrophy and carcinoma of the prostate, *Surgery* 16:152, 1944.

63. Mostofi FK: Testicular tumors: epidemiologic, etiologic and pathologic features, *Cancer* 32:1186, 1973.

64. Narayan P, Lange PH: Semirigid penile prosthesis in the management of erectile impotence, *Urol Clin North Am* 8(1):169, 1981.

65. Papadoupalous C: Cardiovascular drugs and sexuality, *Arch Intern Med* 140:1341, 1980.

66. Paulson DF, Kane RD: A prospective study in the pharmaceutical management of benign prostatic hyperplasia, *J Urol* 113:811, 1975.

67. Rango RE, MeLeod PJ, Reudy J: Treatment of benign prostatic hypertrophy with medrogestone, *Clin Pharmacol Ther* 12:658, 1971.

68. Schuman LM et al: Epidemiologic study of prostatic cancer, *Cancer Treat Rep* 61:181, 1977.

69. Scott DW, Oberst MT, Bookbinder MI: Stress-coping response to genitourinary cancer in men, *Nurs Res* 33(6):325, 1984.

70. Silverberg E, Lubera JA: A review of American Cancer Society estimates of cancer cases and deaths, *Cancer* 33:2, 1983.

71. Staszewski J, Hanszel J: Cancer mortality among the Polish born in the United States, *National Cancer Institute* 35:291, 1965.

72. Turner-Warwick RT: Bladder outflow obstruction in the male. In Mundy AR, Stephenson TP, Wein AJ: *Urodynamics: principles, practice, and application,* London, 1984, Churchill Livingstone.

73. Virag R: Arterial and venous hemodynamics in male impotence. In Bennett A: *Management of male impotence,* Baltimore, 1982, Williams & Wilkins.

74. Wagner G, Green R: General medical disorders and erection failure. In Wagner G, Green R: *Impotence,* New York, 1981, Plenum Publishing Corp.

75. Winkelstein W, Ernster VL: Epidemiology and etiology. In Murphy GP: *Prostatic cancer,* Littleton, Mass, 1979, PSG Publishing Co, Inc.

76. Woolf CM: An investigation of the familial aspects of carcinoma of the prostate, *Cancer* 13:739, 1960.

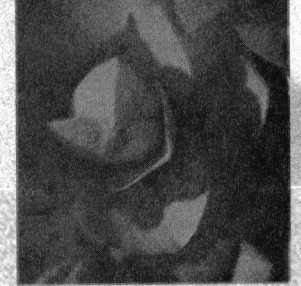

CHAPTER SEVENTY-TWO

Nursing Management of Adults with Sexually Transmitted Diseases

---

DESPITE MEDICAL ADVANCES in the diagnosis and treatment of communicable diseases, the incidence of infections transmitted through intimate or sexual activities continues to increase worldwide. This chapter discusses the medical and nursing management of sexually transmitted diseases. Note that acquired immune deficiency syndrome (AIDS) is covered in Chapter 40.

SEXUALLY TRANSMITTED DISEASES
Definition

Sexually transmitted diseases (STDs) are infections that are primarily transmitted during sexual intercourse. These diseases may have other routes of transmission (e.g., perinatally from mother to fetus). STDs can occur with or without symptoms and may have long periods of asymptomatic infection. STDs were previously referred to as venereal diseases (VD).[6]

Epidemiology

Any sexually active person may be at risk for an STD. The major risk factors for STDs appear to be multiple sexual partners, high rate of new sexual partners within a short period, high rate of partner change, casual sexual partners, combination of drug use and sexual activity, and unprotected sexual contact. However, the essential risk factor for STDs is exposure to a person with an STD. In the United States, STDs characteristically occur in urban, poor, and minority populations, particularly among adolescents and males.[2] Because some STDs persist and have long incubation periods, even persons in mutually monogamous sexual relationships are at some risk. Health care behaviors that can reduce the risk of acquiring STDs or prevent complications include "safer sex" practices, early diagnosis and treatment, compliance with therapy, and partner referral. The advent of acquired immune deficiency syndrome (AIDS) and an increase in STDs produced a new, urgent reason to educate sexually active individuals on risk reduction.

STDs reportable to the Centers for Disease Control (CDC) are AIDS, chancroid, gonorrhea, granuloma inguinale, lymphogranuloma venereum, syphilis, and hepatitis B virus. The number of reportable STDs continues to increase in the United States. Gonorrhea is estimated to infect 250 million people worldwide and nearly 3 million in the United States each year. There were 602,577 reported cases of gonorrhea in 1991.[7] Annual syphilis incidence is about 50 million cases worldwide and 250,000 cases in the United States. The CDC had 41,006 reported cases of syphilis in 1991.[7] Although reporting of STDs is performed, there are unreported cases and delays in reporting the statistics to the CDC. There are limited statistics on the "new generation" of STDs such as chlamydia, *Trichomonas, Candida,* herpes, genital warts, and molluscum contagiosum. In addition, bowel pathogens such as *Salmonella, Giardia, Amoeba, Shigella, Campylobacter,* hepatitis A and B, the herpes viruses, cytomegalovirus (CMV), and Epstein-Barr virus (EBV) may be sexually transmitted. Recently cervical cancer, which shares the epidemiologic characteristics of an STD, has been strongly associated with herpes virus, human papillomavirus, and HIV infection.

STDs continue to be among the world's most common communicable diseases. Four main factors are responsible:

1. Unprotected sexual contact with multiple partners. The sexual revolution of the 1960s in the mobile societies of North America and Western Europe increased available heterosexual and homosexual partners.
2. Widespread use of oral contraceptive pills decreased the use of barrier contraceptives (condoms and diaphragms) and altered the perceived susceptibility of women to some pathogens.
3. Antibiotic resistance. The indiscriminate use of antibiotics has increased the prevalence of bacterial strains less sensitive to these medications. Antibiotic resistance continues to increase, complicating treatment of gonorrhea and chancroid. In 1989, 3.2% of gonorrhea

cases in the United States were penicillin resistant and 4.9% of the cases were tetracycline resistant, which increases morbidity and requires retreatment.[11]

4. Treatment delay. In societies with a wide variety of conflicting viewpoints regarding sexuality, both health care workers and patients continue to have difficulty dealing with STDs. Patients may be reluctant to seek treatment; health care workers may find it difficult to be objective and supportive. Also, the signs and symptoms of STDs may not seem significant to laypersons and uninformed medical professionals and may appear to resolve spontaneously. Some individuals may be asymptomatic carriers and unaware that they need treatment.

Clinical Manifestations

Clinical manifestations depend on the specific STD and are listed later in the chapter.

Therapeutic Management

Therapeutic management related to STDs includes both pharmacologic treatment of individuals diagnosed with STDs and education geared toward future prevention. Effective management of STDs begins with accessible, low-cost, confidential diagnostic and treatment facilities with well-equipped clinical laboratories able to perform complete blood counts (CBCs), wet mounts, urinalyses, Gram stains, bacterial cultures, and serologies. Return appointments after initial treatment are important for three reasons. First, documenting cure with repeat culture demonstrates that the patient is no longer infectious. Second, early identification and treatment of resistant strains, multiple infections, or reinfection decrease the duration of symptoms and infectivity. Third, detecting relapses or complications by systematic monitoring of chronic conditions promotes early medical intervention.

NURSING MANAGEMENT OF THE PATIENT WITH A SEXUALLY TRANSMITTED DISEASE
Assessment

Because coinfection with multiple STDs is common, a complete sexual and STD history is essential (refer to box). The duration and character of presenting symptoms should be noted in relationship to the individual's last sexual contact, especially if the exposure was to new or anonymous partners or to known infected partners during the previous 6 months. Knowing sexual orientation (heterosexual,

SEXUAL HISTORY ASSESSMENT QUESTIONNAIRE

General patient population

1. Are you currently sexually active?
2. Are you currently sexually active with more than one partner?
3. In the past, what were your sexual practices (sexual behaviors)?
4. What are your current sexual practices (sexual behaviors)?
5. Would you like to share your sexual orientation/ preference?
6. How has your present illness affected your sexual relationships?
7. Do you have any concerns about changes in your sexual activity?
8. Have you ever had a sexually transmitted disease?

Patients with sexually transmitted diseases

1. How old were you when you first became sexually active?
2. Are you currently sexually active?
3. When you engage in sexual activity, is it with men, women, or both?
4. Are you currently sexually active with more than one partner?
5. What type of sexual practices do you engage in?
6. What type of protection or prevention methods do you practice?
7. Have you ever had a sexually transmitted disease?

THERAPEUTIC COMMUNICATION GUIDE

Sexually Transmitted Disease

Assessment

Assess the patient's feelings of guilt or shame.

Example   *Patient:*   "I'm so ashamed. I've disgraced my whole family. I was so bad that God gave me this illness to punish me."

Intervention

Gently introduce reality.

Example   *Nurse:*   "Tom, gonorrhea is a common infectious disease that can be treated. I'm sorry you feel ashamed, but it is not a punishment for your behavior."

---

homosexual, or bisexual) and practices (penile-vaginal, penile-anal, penile-oral, vulvar-oral, or anal-oral) can help the examiner direct collection of laboratory specimens. Patient use of barrier protection (condoms) decreases the transmission risk of some routes. Prior history of STDs, including specific disease, extent of illness, treatment, and complications, may help determine current risk. It is important to check for allergies to antibiotics, especially penicillin. Systemic symptoms such as fever, chills, diaphoresis, myalgia, arthralgia, and headache may indicate primary infection as in herpes simplex virus or disseminating disease.

Patients' physical symptoms are commonly complicated by their emotional responses. Complaints of depression, anger, fear, and guilt are common and need to be addressed if education and treatment are to be effective. Outcome is also influenced by educational and income level, primary language, cul-

tural orientation, health insurance coverage, and support network.

In women, menstrual irregularities may occur, and therefore it is important to record the date of the last menstrual period and Papanicolaou (Pap) examination. The duration and character of accompanying symptoms such as sore throat, vaginal discharge, vulvar itching or discomfort, urinary urgency or frequency, dysuria, genital lesions, rectal discharge, itching, pain, and bleeding help in differentiating multiple infections and involved sites from each other. Ascending disease may cause abdominal or pelvic pain, especially with intercourse (dyspareunia). Skin rashes, itching, and lesions may be the only manifestation of systemic disease. Noting the location, size, and tenderness of enlarged lymph nodes helps to determine the extent of the invasion and stage of some progressive diseases.

Men should be interviewed about urethral discharge, dysuria, genital lesions, itching, scrotal pain, and pelvic discomfort. Description of lymphadenopathy is useful in men and women. In addition, homosexual and bisexual men may have sore throat from gonorrheal pharyngitis and rectal symptoms or diarrhea from proctitis.

Physical examination begins with vital signs; temperature and heart rate may be elevated with systemic disease. In women the pharynx is observed for lesions of herpes simplex virus or syphilis and the erythema and exudates of gonorrhea. The abdomen is auscultated for bowel sounds and palpated for masses and tenderness associated with pelvic inflammatory disease. Skin rashes, especially distribution on the palms and soles, are commonly the presenting symptom of secondary syphilis. Details of genital, cervical, and rectal lesions including size, shape, and location are often diagnostic and deserve careful observation. The amount, color, consistency, and odor of vaginal, cervical, and rectal discharge vary with etiology and may be diagnostic. Cervical mobility is commonly decreased because of pain in pelvic inflammatory disease and may be accompanied by masses in the fallopian tubes or near the ovaries. Inguinal and femoral lymphadenopathy accompanies many acute and chronic STDs, including herpex simplex, pelvic inflammatory disease, lymphogranuloma venereum, and donovanosis.

Men are examined for perioral lesions of herpes simplex and syphilis and the same skin rashes as women. Genital lesions in men are commonly more easy to diagnose than in women and should be accurately described. Urethral discharge may be spontaneous as in gonorrhea or require manual expression from the penis, as is often true with *Chlamydia*. Lymphadenopathy in the inguinal and femoral chains is common and may be tender or nontender, acute or chronic. Examine homosexual men for pharyngeal lesions, erythema, and exudates; abdominal tenderness; and rectal discharge, itching, bleeding, and lesions.

Nursing Diagnosis

Nursing diagnoses for patient with STDs include the following:

Pain related to oral, genital, or rectal lesions

Altered skin integrity: genital or rectal lesions related to STD

Altered bowel elimination: constipation or diarrhea related to rectal lesions, inflammation, or pain

Altered urinary elimination related to local inflammation or sacral nerve involvement

High risk for infection related to genital or rectal lesions

Knowledge deficit related to routes of transmission, STD prevention, and follow-up

Self-esteem disturbance related to guilt and anger at route of transmission or sexual orientation

Anxiety related to partner notification/contact tracing or disclosing sexual orientation

Fear related to diagnosis of STD and implications for life-style

Planning

Nursing goals for the patient with an STD are as follows:

Patient will practice safe sex and avoid risky behaviors that may lead to infection of self or others

---

 PATIENT EDUCATION GUIDE *STD Prevention*

1. Reduce the number of people the patient has sex with (preferably to one person), and avoid sexual contact with individuals who have multiple partners or partners from high-risk groups
2. Find out as much as possible about a potential partner's present and past sexual activities and avoid contact with individuals known to be infected or who are at high risk of infection
3. Examine the genital area for sores, pus, or rashes before having sex, and avoid sexual contact if any of these signs are present (however, a person can have an STD without any symptoms)
4. Wash hands and genital/rectal area before and immediately after sex to reduce the presence of germs and secretions (germs that cause syphilis and gonorrhea are sensitive to soap and water)
5. Wash the foreskin that covers the head of the penis daily since germs may become trapped there

6. Use a mouthwash or gargle with hydrogen peroxide (one part to three parts of water) or Listerine Antiseptic (26.9% alcohol) to possibly slightly reduce the risk of oropharyngeal STD infection
7. Use latex condoms with all sexual partners
8. Use a water-based lubricant such as KY Jelly
9. Use vaginal spermicidal contraceptives that have germicidal and viricidal properties
10. Urinate after intercourse to reduce the risk of contracting some forms of STDs
11. Avoid excessive douching to maintain a normal bacterial balance in the vagina
12. Seek medical help if the patient has any suspicion that he or she might have contracted an STD, and give the practitioner information about past STDs, present symptoms, current medications, and sexual activities involving the throat or rectum
13. Seek an STD examination twice per year or more often if needed

From American Foundation for the Prevention of Veneral Disease Inc: *Venereal disease prevention for everyone,* New York, 1985, Foundation Press.

Patient will avoid contact of painful areas with aggravating items

Patient will display healing of skin lesions

Patient will exhibit normal bowel function

Patient will exhibit normal urinary elimination

Patient will maintain intact skin and mucous membranes

Patient will verbalize feelings about STD diagnosis

Patient will verbalize rationale for early identification and treatment of self and partners

Patient will comply with medical/treatment regimen

Implementation

The primary goals of STD treatment are to alleviate symptoms and decrease transmission. Since misinformation about STDs is common, simple, clearly written information on routes of transmission, risk reduction, proper latex condom use, signs and symptoms of infection, treatment course, and treatment options needs to be reinforced often (see box on STD prevention). Safer sex guidelines should be incorporated in the STD prevention education (see box on safer sex practices).

Genital lesions are commonly infectious and uncomfortable. They should be kept clean and dry to avoid secondary infection. Wash hands thoroughly after touching a lesion. Loose, absorbent cotton underclothing is usually more comfortable than close-fitting clothing. Sitz baths decrease lesional discomfort and enhance urinary and bowel elimination. Sexual intercourse during active lesions increases the risk of transmission and may also be painful. Future sexual partners and health care providers should be advised of recurring or latent infections that may be transmitted during sexual contact or have the potential to affect a fetus or an infant.

Reducing the number of sexual partners and partners from high-risk groups and latex condom use are the next best steps to sexual abstinence. The risk of STDs is directly related to the number of sexual partners, the number of partners that those partners have experienced, and the sexual behaviors practiced. Therefore knowing any sexual partner well, including past and present sexual practices, is very important.

The patient or the patient's partner or partners may have a strong emotional response to the diagnosis. Many times one of the partners is unaware that the other partner is engaging in intimate contact with another. The issue is further compounded if the partner is having contact with a member of the same sex. This is especially true for women who become HIV infected from a bisexual partner and unknowingly become pregnant.

Patients with STDs are sometimes immobilized by strong negative feelings such as anger, fear, and guilt. Patients with herpes simplex will have a lifelong problem with infection as repeated attacks occur. This may affect their desirability as a sexual partner.

Patients commonly stop taking their medication

PATIENT EDUCATION GUIDE   *Safer Sex Practices*

Golden Rules

1. Know your partner
2. Reduce the number of sexual partners
3. Practice only safe or moderately safe practices
4. Avoid the exchange of blood or body fluids
5. Do not mix sex and drugs
6. Have regular physical examinations

Safe

1. Abstinence
2. Fantasy, voyeurism
3. Hugging
4. Body massage
5. Social (dry) kissing
6. Frottage (body to body rubbing)
7. Solo masturbation, masturbation without contact of body fluids

Moderately Safe

1. French (wet) kissing
2. Anal intercourse with latex condom
3. Vaginal intercourse with latex condom
4. Fellatio interruptus (oral-genital sex without ejaculation)
5. Cunnilingus (oral-vaginal sex)
6. Water sports (urine contact)

Unsafe

1. Anal intercourse without latex condoms
2. Vaginal intercourse without latex condoms
3. Fisting (manual-anal intercourse)
4. Fellatio with semen ingestion
5. Rimming (oral-anal contact)
6. Blood contact
7. Urine ingestion

From Bennett J, Gee G: *AIDS: concepts and nursing practice,* Baltimore, 1988, Williams, & Wilkins.

as soon as their symptoms are gone. Since the symptoms of STDs commonly disappear quite rapidly after antibiotics have been started, patients should be warned that symptoms will reappear unless the medication is taken as directed until it is finished. Patients should also be told to avoid alcohol during the treatment. A combination of some medications, such as metronidazole, and alcohol has been known to result in severe gastric distress. Alcohol has been shown to irritate the genitourinary system and actually retard healing. Alcohol also reduces a person's inhibitions, which can result in unsafe sex.

In addition, to ensure the effective treatment of STDs, it is essential that all sexual partners be treated at the same time as the patient. Sexual or intimate contact should be avoided until the follow-up examination confirms the effectiveness of the treatment. Since many of the treatments require multiple-dose therapy, the nurse must emphasize the importance of returning for repeat cultures or tests to determine if treatment is effective.

Infectious lesions need to be kept clean and dry. Symptomatic relief for some lesions may include general comfort measures such as heat lamps or lotions. The nurse should emphasize the importance of hygiene measures such as frequent hand washing. Douching, unless ordered by the physician, should be avoided, since it may spread the infection. The nurse teaches the patient to wear clean, loose, cotton underwear. Microwaving washed underwear will kill the bacteria; however, only cotton undergarments can be heated in the microwave. As part of the emphasis on hygiene the nurse encourages frequent bathing and changing of undergarments.

Evaluation

The nurse evaluates whether the patient has avoided transmission to others, uses barrier protection correctly, and returns for tests or follow-up and whether sexual partners received treatment. To assess understanding of disease transmission and prevention methods, the nurse asks questions about STD prevention and safer sex practices. The nurse asks whether treatment has minimized lesion pain and/or drainage and evaluates the lesion's appearance. The nurse also evaluates whether the patient has maintained formed, easily eliminated stools and comfortable urinary elimination. Psychosocial aspects such as self-esteem, anger, and guilt should be evaluated.

Documentation

The nurse documents both developing problems and the response to intervention. Current symptoms, sexual practices, and emotional state may all affect outcome and plan. Labeling specimens and recording test results, treatment regimen, and patient compliance are also important, especially if the expected cure is not obtained. Noting reasons for noncompliance may help the practitioner readjust the treatment plan. Any side effects of therapy or development of allergy should be carefully entered in the medical record. The nurse also documents reporting of communicable diseases.

Ongoing Care

The nurse provides written and verbal instructions in long-term physical and emotional effects of STDs. Referrals to private and community resources are provided to patients needing emotional support or infertility evaluation.

HERPES GENITALIS
Definition

Herpes genitalis is an infection of the genital tract with herpes simplex virus (HSV). HSV can also infect mucous membranes of the mouth and rectum. Herpes genitalis is a treatable, but not curable, viral disease characterized by recurrent episodes of acute, painful, red-based, vesicular eruptions (blisters).[8]

Etiology/Epidemiology

The two closely related forms of HSV, types I and II, are specialized in their ability to infect the oral (HSV-I) or the genital (HSV-II) region. Most persons with HSV are infected in infancy with type I during feeding or kissing by adults and have infrequent recurrences around the lips. Because prior infection with HSV I confers relative immunity to HSV II, many persons completely resist or have less dramatic HSV II infections based on their prior immunity from HSV I. Persons with no prior HSV I who are infected with HSV II as their first HSV infection may have more severe primary symptoms and more frequent recurrences. HSV II is usually acquired sexually after puberty in the genital or anal region but also causes 10% to 20% of the lesions above the waist from oral-oral or oral-genital contact. Likewise, about 10% to 20% of the genital or anal lesions are caused by HSV I.[8]

Pathophysiology

HSV I or II produces vesicular lesions that contain infectious virus and giant cells formed by the fusion of many infected cells 2 to 12 days after entering the mucous membranes of the vagina, urethra, mouth, or anus or after penetrating damaged skin.[3] Virus is also transported up the sensory nerves to the sensory ganglia of the sacral spinal cord or trigeminal nerves where it establishes latency. Inactive infection may persist for a lifetime or be interrupted by recurrent episodes of reactivation at or near the original site of entry. The immune response controls primary infection in 1 to 4 weeks and reactivation of previous infection in 3 to 10 days but cannot eliminate latency.[8]

A patient is considered infectious as long as there is virus shedding.[3] Secretions of HSV in the saliva have been reported for as long as 7 days. Primary genital lesions are infective for 7 to 12 days after lesion development. Asymptomatic oral and genital lesions with virus shedding are common.

Immunosuppressed patients or newborns suffer more serious disease because they lack protective immunity. In immunosuppressed adults (e.g., HIV-infected persons) local reactivation may progress to form deep painful ulcers. Neonates suffer widespread and often fatal systemic disease, because their immature immune system cannot control the virus.

Individuals can be contagious without significant symptoms, and unnoticed lesions may occur in the cervix, vagina, or urethra. Recurrences usually become less frequent or stop after a few years. HSV may spread from active lesions to other parts of the body. The eye is particularly vulnerable; there the virus produces a characteristic, dendritic corneal lesion. If the virus is improperly treated, loss of vision can result from corneal scarring.

Approximately two thirds of infected individuals will have one to five recurrences annually, with the first recurrence 1 to 3 months after the primary infection. Reactivation of HSV may be precipitated by stress, trauma, immunosuppression, sexual activity, or the menstrual cycle and is usually more localized, smaller, and shorter than the primary infection. HSV is also associated with an increased incidence of cervical cancer. It is recommended that infected women have a Pap test every 6 months.

Clinical Manifestations

After an incubation period of 2 to 12 days, primary herpes genitalis may begin with both local and systemic symptoms (fever, malaise, and anorexia). Locally, itching and erythema evolve into clusters of 2 to 8 mm blisters that break, producing painful ulcers. Complications include urinary retention resulting from effects on the ulcer, constipation, painful enlargement of regional lymph nodes, or rarely, symptoms of meningitis (headache, stiff neck, or photophobia). Healing may require several weeks.[8]

Recurrent attacks may be preceded by a prodrome of tingling, itching, or burning pain lasting a few hours to 1 week before skin lesions begin. Vaginal, urethral, or rectal discharge may be the only symptom when lesions lie deeper. Lesions last for 3

to 10 days and may heal without scarring. Virus may be transferred to the cornea, producing keratitis, or infect the nail bed or fingers, causing herpetic whitlow.

Diagnosis can be made by medical history alone in recurrent disease or by appearance and location of lesions. Herpes can be grown in tissue culture within 24 to 48 hours from vesicular fluids or cells scraped from the base of the ulcer. A more rapid presumptive diagnosis is based on finding multinucleated giant cells in these fluids (Tzanck test). HSV antibodies specific for each type can be measured and should appear and increase in titer during primary attack. Antibody tests are not helpful in diagnosing recurrent disease beyond documenting past exposure to the virus.

Therapeutic Management

Latent infection of the sensory ganglia remains incurable. The oral antiviral drug acyclovir reduces viral shedding and the length and severity of symptoms dramatically in primary infection but only marginally in recurrent disease in healthy patients (Table 72-1). Most immunocompromised patients with chronic, progressive reactivation disease respond well to similar short 5- to 10-day courses of therapy but have frequent recurrences.

Primary genital lesions are treated with oral acyclovir. Topical acyclovir is effective for mild or moderate infection. Severe infection is treated with in-

TABLE 72-1 Pharmacology Summary: Herpes Genitalis

Drug	Dosage and frequency
Acyclovir (Zovirax)	5% ointment q4h 5 times daily for 5 days
Acyclovir sodium	200 mg PO q4h 5 times daily for 10 days for initial outbreak and 5 days for recurrent episodes
Acyclovir (severe disease)	5 mg/kg of body weight IV q6h for 5-7 days
Acyclovir (suppression)	200 mg PO 2-5 times per day
Burrow's solution (soaks)	q4-5h prn for pain
Aspirin	600 mg PO q6h prn for pain
Codeine	30 mg PO q6h prn for pain
Phenazopyridine (Pyridium)	200 mg PO q6-8h prn for pain

From Centers for Disease Control: Sexually transmitted diseases: treatment guidelines, *MMWR* 38 (S-8):1, 1989.

travenous acyclovir. Recurrent genital lesions are best treated with intravenous acyclovir; topical acyclovir is usually not effective.

Continuous prophylaxis of both healthy and immunocompromised patients at reduced doses (200 mg three times per day orally) has decreased the rate of recurrences. Prophylactic oral acyclovir, 400 to 800 mg/day, is efficacious for adults with six or more episodes of herpes genitalis per year.[4] Strains of HSV resistant to acyclovir have appeared but remain uncommon.

NURSING MANAGEMENT OF THE PATIENT WITH HERPES GENITALIS
Assessment

In addition to the routine nursing assessment for patients with STDs, the patient should be assessed for itching, vesicles, or painful ulcers.

Implementation

In addition to the routine nursing implications for patients with STDs, the following special needs exist for patients diagnosed with herpes genitalis:

  Examine the external genitalia and vagina for characteristic lesions; if lesions are noted, location and appearance should be documented

  Gonococcal culture and Venereal Disease Research Laboratory (VDRL) tests should be obtained because of the frequency of concurrent STDs

  HIV antibody testing should be obtained because of the strong association between HIV infection and genital ulcer disease

  If the patient is hospitalized, lesions should be kept clean and dry using wound and skin precautions; Burrow's solution soaks can be administered every 4 hours to reduce pain

  If the patient is seen in an outpatient setting, instruct on the care of vesicles and good hand washing techniques

  Discuss the role of stress, poor nutrition, and insufficient rest as they relate to recurrences of the symptoms related to herpes infections

  If the patient is a woman, instruct her on the need for yearly Pap tests because of the possible increased risk of cervical cancer associated with herpes genitalis

  Counsel female patients regarding the threat an outbreak poses for newborns and the need to inform practitioners in the event of future pregnancies so that the course of the disease can be monitored closely

  Provide pregnant women with information about the possibility of spontaneous abortions and the signs and symptoms requiring immediate medical attention

  If the virus is present in the amniotic fluid, provide the pregnant patient with nonjudgmental support during the time she attempts to decide about abortion

  Instruct on safer sex practices and STD prevention methods

  Provide the patient with a contact number for the local herpes support group if one is available in the community

Evaluation

In addition to the evaluation for STDs, the nurse assesses the vesicle or ulcer for a decrease in size and improvement in skin integrity.

SYPHILIS
Definition/Etiology

Syphilis is a chronic, multisystemic disease primarily affecting the skin, nervous system, heart, or aorta but capable of appearing in any organ. Syphilis is known by laypersons as bad blood, lues, pox, and syph.[3,20] The disease progresses through four stages (primary, secondary, latent, and tertiary) and may persist for years without symptoms. The bacterial agent of syphilis is the spiral spirochete Treponema pallidum, which is transmitted almost exclusively during the primary or secondary stages of disease by direct contact. The secondary stage is the most infectious stage. Transmission to the fetus in utero causes congenital deformities, and transmission to neonates during birth may also occur. After dramatically decreasing with the introduction of penicillin in the 1940s, the incidence of syphilis quadrupled in the United States in the past 30 years. As a result of sexual behavior changes associated with AIDS, syphilis has declined among homosexual men, once the highest risk group. Syphilis has increased among heterosexuals, especially in cities, among poor persons, and in poor minorities.

Pathophysiology

The spirochete penetrates skin or mucous membranes and then disseminates in the lymphatics and blood. In the primary stage, local production causes a painless ulcer (chancre) in about 3 weeks, which heels spontaneously (Figure 72-1). The secondary stage (dissemination), characterized by systemic symptoms and rash, is again controlled after a few weeks to months but may relapse (Figure 72-2). A prolonged latent phase provides an asymptomatic period. During the tertiary stage, severe and irreversible disease of the nervous system or heart and aorta develops. Not all patients progress to the next stage, and previously inapparent infection may present at any stage.

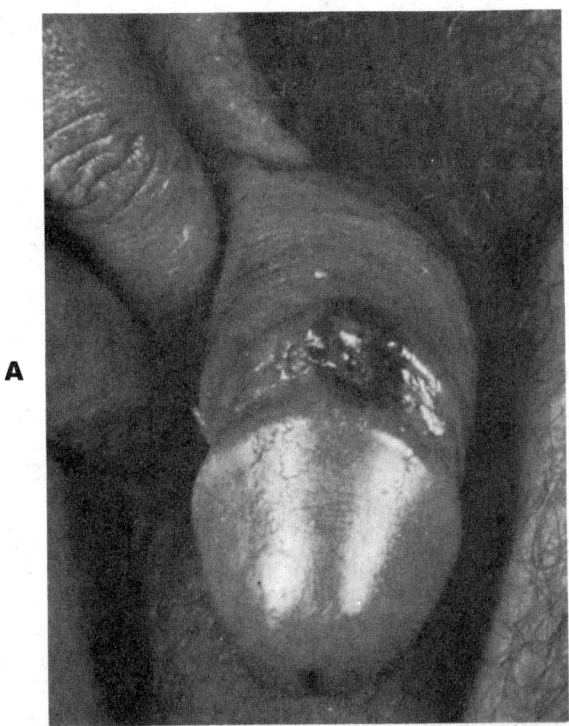

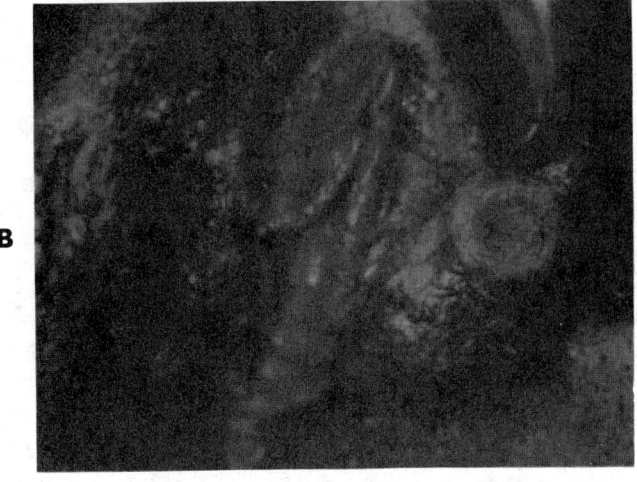

FIGURE 72-1   Primary syphilis. **A,** Chancre of penis. **B,** Chancre of vulva. (From Wehrle PF, Top FH: *Communicable and infectious diseases,* ed 9, St Louis, 1981, Mosby–Year Book, Inc.)

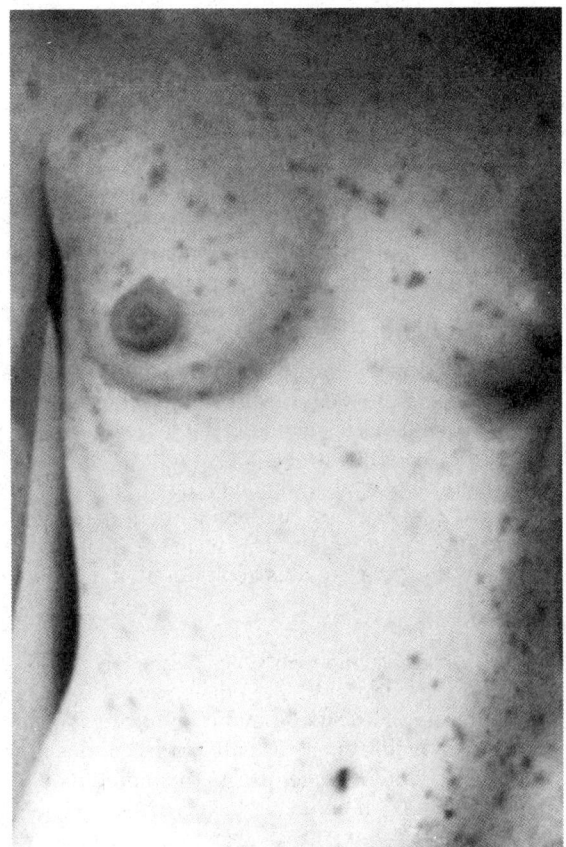

FIGURE 72-2   Rash of secondary syphilis. (From Ellner PD, Neu HC: *Understanding infectious disease,* St Louis, 1992, Mosby–Year Book, Inc.)

Clinical Manifestations

The primary chancre usually appears as a painless, indurated ulcer with serous exudate on the skin or mucous membrane and is least likely to be noted in the vagina or rectum. Secondary syphilis presents as a maculopapular rash, often involving the palms and soles. Other secondary symptoms are moist, raised, gray to pink lesions of the genital and perirectal skin, enlarged lymph nodes, fever, fatigue, or infections of the eyes, bones, liver, or meninges. A wide variety of nervous system syndromes including dementia, pain in the legs, loss of sensation in the legs, and destruction of the aorta occur in the late (10 to 25 years later) stages of syphilis. Destructive inflammatory masses (gummas) can appear in any organ (see box).

A nonspecific but useful test for antibodies to lipids (VDRL and rapid plasma reagin [RPR]) is positive within a few weeks, remains positive for years, and becomes negative with successful treatment. Because other diseases may cause reactive VDRL and RPR tests, tests for specific antitreponemal antibodies (fluorescent treponemal antibody, absorbed [FTA-ABS]) are used to confirm the diagnosis. These tests have the disadvantages of not being useful in testing cerebrospinal fluid and remaining positive despite successful treatment. Dark-field or antibody staining of exudates from lesions or aspirates can be used to confirm syphilis in primary or secondary stages.

STAGES OF SYPHILIS

Primary stage

Occurs 10 to 90 days after contact and involves one or more painless, firm, buttonlike chancres at the site of initial contact; chancres disappear in 2 to 6 weeks without treatment; regional, nontender lymphadenopathy is usually present

Secondary stage

Occurs 4 to 6 weeks after the chancre and involves a symmetric mucocutaneous nonpruritic rash on the body, including palms of hands and soles of feet; may also include alopecia, flulike symptoms, and generalized lymphadenopathy that disappears in 2 to 12 weeks with or without treatment; condylomata lata may also be present on moist parts of the body such as genital and anal areas

Latent stage

May last up to 20 or more years, when *Treponema pallidum* remains hidden; in the early latent stage, patients may be asymptomatic or have relapsing lesions; individuals are usually not infectious during the late latent stage; pregnant women may infect their unborn children during this stage

Tertiary stage

Occurs in 1 to 10 years in 30% of untreated patients; benign, gummatous lesions are present; exists in three general forms: late benign, cardiovascular, and neurosyphilitic; individuals are usually not infectious during this stage; late complications include insanity, blindness, deafness, heart disease, ulcerous tumors, seizures, coma, and death

---

TABLE 72-2   Pharmacology Summary: Syphilis

Drug	Dosage and frequency
PRIMARY, SECONDARY, OR LATENT SYPHILIS OR WITHIN 1 YR OF CONTACT WITH INFECTED PARTNER	
Penicillin G benzathine	2.4 mU IM in single injection
Doxycycline	500 mg PO bid for 2 wk
Tetracycline or erythromycin	500 mg PO qid for 15 days
IF MORE THAN 1 YR DURATION	
Penicillin G benzathine	2.4 mU IM for 3 successive wk
Doxycycline	100 mg PO bid for 4 wk
Tetracycline or erythromycin	500 mg PO q6h for 30 days
SYPHILIS INVOLVING NERVOUS SYSTEM	
Aqueous penicillin	2 mU q4h IV for 10-14 days
followed by penicillin G benzathine	2.4 mU weekly IM for 3 wk
Penicillin G procaine	2.4 mU weekly IM for 10-14 days
plus probenecid	500 mg q6h PO
followed by penicillin G benzathine	2.4 mU weekly IM for 3 wk

From Centers for Disease Control: Sexually transmitted diseases: treatment guidelines, *MMWR* 38 (S-8):1, 1989.

Therapeutic Management

Penicillin is the drug of choice for syphilis, but the treatment regimen varies according to the stage of the disease (Table 72-2). Erythromycin or tetracycline is used when the patient is allergic to penicillin. Because of the long-term consequences of inadequate treatment, penicillin is usually given intramuscularly or intravenously, especially in syphilis of the nervous system or secondary syphilis. Adverse reactions to treatment include the usual allergic reactions to penicillin and two other reactions easily misunderstood as allergies. The procaine reaction occurs within minutes of accidental intravenous injection of procaine penicillin and is an unusual consequence of intramuscular injection. Acute hyperventilation, fever, tachycardia, vomiting, or convulsions may occur. A second type of nonallergic reaction begins within 4 hours of treatment as fever, headache, malaise, increased rash, or convulsions and is called the Jarisch-Herxheimer reaction. It is presumably a reaction to toxins released by killed organisms. Both reactions are self-limited. They may be difficult to diagnose when drugs are given for other reasons for patients with undiagnosed syphilis.

NURSING MANAGEMENT OF THE PATIENT WITH SYPHILIS
Assessment

In addition to routine nursing assessment for patients with STDs, assess for painless ulcers, maculopapular rashes, and nervous system changes.

Implementation

In addition to the previously discussed nursing implications for patients with STDs, a number of special needs exist for individuals diagnosed with syphilis:

1. In cases of late syphilis, assess patient according to organs involved:
   a. Cardiovascular: decreased cardiac output, pulmonary congestion
   b. Neurosyphilitic: level of consciousness, mood, coherence, behavior, presence of ataxia
2. Instruct patient of need to get repeat VDRL checks every 3 months for 1 year; should see fourfold decrease in titer; less than fourfold decrease or increase in titer suggests relapse (following treatment for latent syphilis, patient needs repeat checks every 6 months for 2 years)
3. Instruct patient to avoid sexual intercourse until lesions are resolved
4. Check for allergy to penicillin; if unknown, administer penicillin and have patient wait 30 minutes before leaving office or clinic

Evaluation

In addition to evaluation of patients with STDs, the ulcers should decrease in size, rash should fade, and mental changes should improve or stabilize.

GONORRHEA
Definition

Gonorrhea is a sexually transmitted disease caused by an intracellular, Gram-negative diplococcal bacterium know as gonococcus or *Neisseria gonorrhoeae.* Gonorrhea is know by laypersons as white, the drips, the strain, clap, or the dose.[3,20] It is primarily an infection of the genital or rectal mucosa, commonly resulting in cervicitis, urethritis, or proctitis, but it may also invade the deeper genital tract or the bloodstream to cause pelvic inflammatory disease or disseminated disease.[11]

Etiology/Epidemiology

Gonorrhea is one of the most commonly reported sexually transmitted diseases. However, like most STDs, it is largely a disease of poor, young, nonwhite men and their sexual partners. Reported cases are 10 times higher in nonwhites than whites. The majority of cases occur in persons 20 to 24 years of age. The incidence of gonorrhea is seasonal, with the highest rates in late summer and lowest rates in late winter and early spring. Women are commonly asymptomatic carriers.

In addition, pelvic inflammatory disease, a serious complication of gonorrhea and other STDs, develops in approximately 20% to 40% of infected women.[11] Gonococcal PID is a major cause of involuntary infertility and ectopic pregnancy despite effective treatments.

Over the past 40 years the gonococcus bacterium has become increasingly resistant to penicillin, requiring higher doses of penicillin for cure. Penicillinase-producing *Neisseria gonorrhoeae* (PPNG) organisms have acquired total resistance by making penicillinase, an enzyme that renders penicillin inactive. PPNG is spreading worldwide but remains responsive to other antibiotics. However, gonococci are also becoming relatively resistant to tetracyclines, penicillins, and other drugs.

Pathophysiology

The gonococcus is usually transmitted through intimate sexual contact with an infected partner. The incubation period is 2 to 7 days. *N. gonorrhoeae* adheres to the mucosal cells. Progressive mucosal cell damage and invasion of the site with leukocytes, submucosal microabcess formation, and exudation of purulent fluid occur in the lumen of the infected organ. After reproducing at the urethral, cervical, anal, or pharyngeal mucosa to cause local symptoms, the microorganism may ascend the reproductive tract of women to cause salpingitis and pelvic peritonitis, or in men it may cause epididymitis. Some strains can invade the blood to cause arthritis, dermatitis, or other deep infections. Infected women may transmit the gonococcus to the eyes of their newborns (gonococcal ophthalmia neonatorum) during birth, and gonococcal conjunctivitis can occur through autoinoculation in adults.

Clinical Manifestations

Most men experience a spontaneous purulent discharge, severe dysuria, penile itching, and redness at the urethral opening. If untreated, the infection can spread to the epididymis, causing pain and swelling. Complications of gonococcal urethritis include epididymitis, acute or chronic prostatitis, seminal vesiculitis, and infection of Cowper's and Tyson's glands. Women are more likely to be asymptomatic. Copious, greenish yellow, mucopurulent discharge from the cervix, dysuria, and itching and burning of the vulva may cause women to seek treatment. Untreated, the infection may spread via the uterus to the fallopian tubes and pelvic peritoneum causing fever and pelvic pain acutely and can be complicated by tubal obstruction and ectopic pregnancy. It may cause involuntary infertility in the future.

Men and women may also have tonsillitis, pharyngitis, conjunctivitis, and rectal inflammation with bloody mucopurulent discharge. Although pharyngeal gonorrhea is most commonly asymptomatic, erythematous and edematous pharynx and tonsillar vesicles may be present.

With extragenital dissemination the patient develops fever, pustular skin lesions, and migratory polyarthralgia and polyarthritis. Purulent arthritis of one or a few joints may follow and, if untreated, lead to progressive joint destruction.

A Gram stain of urethral, cervical, or rectal pus may confirm the presence of Gram-negative diplococci but may not detect the gonococcus, especially in women. Gram stain is usually sufficient to confirm the diagnosis in men and begin treatment. Culture from the infected site on selective antibiotic-containing media provides a conclusive diagnosis, because it increases the likelihood of growing gonococci by suppressing the growth of normal flora. Use of cotton swabs (which contain inhibitors) to obtain the specimen, recent urination, vaginal douching, and some vaginal speculum lubricants may inhibit the growth of the gonococcus. Confirmation of gonococcal arthritis requires seeing or growing the Gram-negative diplococci in joint fluid or blood.

Therapeutic Management

Successful treatment of gonorrhea has been accomplished through the concurrent use of probenecid and penicillin (Table 72-3). A variety of other choices are available to treat PPNG, including spectinomycin and ceftriaxone and in areas where penicillin and tetracycline resistance is common may be the primary treatment of choice.

NURSING MANAGEMENT OF THE PATIENT WITH GONORRHEA

Assessment

In addition to assessment for patients with STDs, assess for vaginal, cervical, and urethral discharge associated with genital itching or burning.

Implementation

In addition to routine nursing implications for patients with STDs, use of loose, absorbent underclothes, changed frequently after perineal/penile irrigation, enhances cleanliness and comfort. Sitz baths decrease lower abdominal discomfort and dysuria. Intercourse encourages migration of some bacteria from the lower to upper reproductive tract and infection of partners and should be avoided. Patients must be aware that fertility may be altered. Other special needs for gonorrhea are as follows:

Obtain specimens for chlamydia and urine culture to rule out concurrent infections

TABLE 72-3 Pharmacology Summary: Gonorrhea	
Drug	**Dosage and frequency**
Ampicillin*	3.5 g PO in single dose
Amoxicillin*	3 g PO in single dose
Penicillin G procaine*	4.8 mU IM in single dose
ACCOMPANIED BY PROBENECID*	
Tetracycline	500 mg PO qid for 7 days
Doxycycline	100 mg PO bid for 7 days
FOR PROVEN OR SUSPECTED PPNG (PENICILLIN-RESISTANT STRAINS)	
Ceftriaxone	250 mg IM once
Doxycycline	100 mg PO bid for 7 days
Spectinomycin	2.0 mg IM once

From Centers for Disease Control: Sexually transmitted diseases: treatment guidelines, *MMWR* 38 (S-8):1, 1989.
*Single-dose regimens should be followed by 7 days of tetracycline for coexisting chlamydial infections.

Remove intrauterine device (IUD) if indicated and discuss alternative birth control methods

Discuss the need to notify present and past sexual partners of the diagnosis and the need for them to promptly seek medical care

Evaluation

In addition to evaluation for patients with STDs, the urethral discharge should not be present.

CHANCROID
Definition/Etiology

Chancroid is an acute, localized infectious disease that results in a painful genital ulcer with uneven borders, also known as a "soft chancre," and purulent lymphadenitis. *Haemophilus ducreyi*, a small, slow-growing bacterium, causes this relatively uncommon STD. Outbreaks of chancroid in North America and its development of penicillin resistance have recently attracted more interest. About 1000 cases are reported annually in the United States, but it remains an important problem in much of the tropical world where it is often transmitted by prostitutes. Uncircumcised men appear to be at increased risk. No perinatal transmission is documented.[8]

Pathophysiology

The organism is found in both the local ulcer and regional lymph nodes and is seen within phagocytic cells and free in exudate. The lymph nodes are filled with vast numbers of neutrophils, but they are apparently unable to eliminate the organism. *H. ducreyi* probably enters through the skin and then enters the circulation and lymphatic system. Systemic sequelae are not evident.

Clinical Manifestations

The primary lesion at the site of inoculation consists of one or more small, painful papules occurring 3 to 7 days after exposure. Papules progress to pustules and then flat, soft ulcers that are malodorous, bleed easily, and may become so painful that contact with clothing is intolerable. In contrast, the chancre of syphilis is clean and painless and has a hard base. Unilateral lymphadenitis with overlying erythema may develop into an abscess.[17] Laboratory diagnosis is often difficult, and treatment is usually based on a clinical diagnosis.

Therapeutic Management

The treatment of choice is erythromycin, but multiple other antibiotics are also effective (Table 72-4). Fluctuant buboes may require needle aspiration and drainage.

NURSING MANAGEMENT OF THE PATIENT WITH CHANCROID
Assessment

In addition to routine nursing assessment for patients with STDs, assess for a painful ulcer with uneven borders and purulent lymphadenitis.

Implementation

In addition to routine nursing implications for patients with STDs, instruct patients diagnosed with chancroid to wash the genital area more frequently with soap and water, especially after sexual contact, to reduce the risk of contracting STDs in the future. Counsel patients that they can become reinfected with chancroid, because a previous episode does not provide future immunity.

Evaluation

In addition to the evaluation for patients with STDs, the ulcer should decrease in size and then disappear.

TABLE 72-4 Pharmacology Summary: Chancroid

Drug	Dosage and frequency
Erythromycin or	0.5 g PO qid for 7 days
Ceftriaxone	250 mg IM once in single dose
Trimethoprim/ sulfamethoxazole	1 double-strength tablet PO for 10-14 days
Amoxicillin and	500 mg daily for 7 days
clavulanic acid	125 mg daily for 7 days
Ciprofloxacin	500 mg PO bid for 3 days

From Centers for Disease Control: Sexually transmitted diseases: treatment guidelines, *MMWR* 35 (S-8):1, 1989.

CHLAMYDIA
Definition/Etiology

Chlamydia trachomatis, a Gram-negative, intracellular bacterium, causes several common sexually transmitted diseases. Cervicitis and urethritis are the most common, but chlamydia also causes epididymitis, proctitis, salpingitis, endometritis, and Reiter's syndrome. Chlamydia may be the most common STD agent in the United States. Although both men and women may have asymptomatic infection, women are more likely to be asymptomatic carriers despite deep pelvic infection. Untreated chlamydia results in extension of infection to the fallopian tubes and pelvic inflammatory disease, potentially causing infertility.

Pathophysiology

Non–lymphogranuloma venereum chlamydial infections in men usually appear as either nongonococcal urethritis (NGU) or postgonococcal urethritis (PGU). As the name of the latter condition (PGU) suggests, coinfection with chlamydia is commonly recognized only after penicillin treatment for gonorrhea fails to resolve the patient's symptoms. Untreated, infection can spread from the urethra, causing epididymitis, which presents as a tender scrotal swelling.[19] In women, *Chlamydia trachomatis* is one of the main causes of cervicitis and urethral symptoms. As in the male urethra, chlamydia and gonococcus often infect the cervix.

Clinical Manifestations

Symptoms of chlamydial urethritis in men include a scanty, white or clear discharge, burning or itching around the meatus, urinary frequency, and mild dysuria. The urethral discharge may be observable only after penile milking or at the urethral meatus after a long period without urination. Symptoms of cervicitis in women may include one or more of the following: vaginal itching or burning, dull pelvic pain, low-grade fever, vaginal discharge, and irregular bleeding. Asymptomatic infected women may have hypertrophic erosion of the cervix.

Chlamydia is easy to treat. Although chlamydia cultures are sensitive, they are also expensive, not easily available, and slow (2 to 6 days). Gram stain of urethral or cervical discharge demonstrating polymorphonuclear leukocytes but no diplococci is helpful but nonspecific. The fluorescein-labeled monoclonal antibody test is available for screening high-risk populations. Results can be obtained rapidly, and the cost is approximately half that of culture. The specimen is placed directly on a slide, stained, and examined under a fluorescein microscope, giving a test result within 20 to 30 minutes. Treatment can be initiated promptly based on confirmed diagnosis.[19]

Therapeutic Management

The drug of choice for chlamydia treatment is tetracycline. Doxycycline, a more expensive form of tetracycline requiring less frequent dosing, is interchangeable and may increase compliance. Pregnant patients or patients allergic to tetracycline can be treated with erythromycin. Penicillin, the drug of choice for gonorrhea, may suppress the multiplication of chlamydia temporarily but usually does not provide a cure.[19]

NURSING MANAGEMENT OF THE PATIENT WITH CHLAMYDIA
Assessment

In addition to assessment for patients with STDs, assess for white or clear discharge and signs of urethritis.

Evaluation

In addition to evaluation for patients with STDs, the discharge should decrease and then stop, and symptoms of urethritis should also be alleviated.

GENITAL WARTS
Definition/Etiology

Venereal or **genital warts** (condylomata acuminata) are raised, rough, cauliflower-like growths on the vulva, perianal area, vaginal or rectal walls, penis, or cervix caused by sexual transmission of human papillomavirus. Genital warts are common among sexually active adults. Lesions develop 6 to 8 weeks after infection with the papillomavirus in moist areas of the genitalia of 60% to 70% of individuals exposed. Pregnancy, heavy perspiration, poor personal hygiene, and immunosuppression increase the rate of growth of warts. Condylomata acuminata often accompany other STDs, and papillomavirus can be transmitted to infants during birth. Human papillomaviruses are typed and have been found to infect specific parts of the body. External genital lesions are often caused by types 6 and 11, whereas types 16 and 18 have been associated with flat growths in the cervical canal and cervical cancers. Types 1 and 2 are associated with warts on the skin.

Pathophysiology

Genital warts usually start as a single, tiny, pink papule that enlarges, spreads to adjoining areas, and may coalesce, producing a cauliflower appearance. Some strains of papillomavirus may cause cervical cancer, but these are not the same strains that cause most genital warts.

Clinical Manifestations

Most patients present with soft, pink, fleshy, irregularly surfaced growths in the anal or genital area. Growths may itch and become excoriated from scratching. Vaginal discharge, dysuria, and bleeding during or after intercourse may also occur. Venereal warts can mimic other lesions and must be differentiated from carcinoma and syphilis. Diagnosis is usually made on clinical symptoms. However, biopsy is helpful in atypical cases. Culposcopy is necessary to diagnose the flat cervical warts associated with dysplasia and cervical cancer.

Therapeutic Management

Treatment is optional, because they usually disappear spontaneously. If treatment is indicated, topical chemotherapy, freezing, or surgical removal may be used (Table 72-5). All partners should be treated concurrently to reduce the risk of reinfection. Pap smears every 6 months are essential in monitoring women with flat cervical warts.

NURSING MANAGEMENT OF THE PATIENT WITH GENITAL WARTS
Assessment

In addition to assessment of patients with STDs, assess for raised, rough, cauliflower-like growths in or on the genitalia.

TABLE 72-5 Therapeutic Management: Condylomata Acuminata (Genital Warts)	
Treatment	Comments
SMALL VULVAR OR PENILE WARTS	
Podophyllin	Wash off after 2 to 6 hours; do not use during pregnancy or on bleeding lesion
	Protect surrounding skin with petroleum jelly
LARGE (> 2 CM) VAGINAL AND RECTAL WARTS	
CO$_2$ laser	
Electrocautery	Requires local or general anesthesia
Surgical excision	
Cryosurgery	
MULTIPLE (> 10) OR RESISTANT WARTS	
Topical 5-fluorouracil	One-half applicator of 5% fluorouracil every night for 5 nights; tampon to prevent leakage onto external genitalia
	Zinc oxide ointment to protect introitus and vulva

Implementation

In addition to nursing implications for patients with an STD, the following are special needs for patients with genital warts:

Obtain specimen for pregnancy test if indicated (prodophyllin is contraindicated in pregnancy)

Advise the patient that treatment may require several visits

If podophyllin is used, advise the patient to wash the area with soap and water when treatment is complete (usually 2 to 6 hours)

Advise the patient to keep area clean and dry except for prescribed medication

Counsel patient to wash genital area frequently with soap and water, especially following intercourse

Discuss the need to contact present and past sexual partners and encourage them to seek medical care

Evaluation

In addition to evaluation for patients with STDs, the warts should disappear spontaneously or with treatment.

LYMPHOGRANULOMA VENEREUM
Definition/Etiology

Lymphogranuloma venereum (LGV) is a chronic, progressively destructive, and usually curable infection of the lymphatics with three stages: a transient, primary genital lesion; secondary lymphadenitis with bubo formation; and chronic lymphedema of the genitalia and rectum caused by destruction of lymphatics. LGV is caused by a few of the more invasive strains of *Chlamydia trachomatis,* an intracellular bacterium. Although LGV is endemic throughout the world, only 500 to 1000 cases are reported in the United States annually. Most cases are in homosexual men, travelers from endemic areas, or low socioeconomic persons in the southeastern United States. Men are diagnosed three times more frequently than women.[13]

Pathophysiology

After an incubation period of 3 to 12 days, a small, painless, herpetic ulcer forms at the site of inoculation.[3] Painful, inflamed regional lymphadenopathy develops 2 to 6 weeks after infection, which may become abscessed and form draining fistulas to the skin, vagina, or rectum. Progressive, destructive, local ulceration or obstruction of lymphatics may cause permanent deformity or lymphedema.[13]

Clinical Manifestations

The primary lesion appears at the site of initial infection, 1 to 3 weeks after intercourse, but is noticed in only 10% to 40% of cases, because it is asymptomatic and disappears by itself in 2 to 3 days. The second stage begins 10 to 30 days later when lymph nodes draining the site of infection become tender, swollen, and matted. Systemic symptoms (fever, malaise, myalgias, and arthralgias) may occur at the same time. Rupture of the abscessed lymph nodes (buboes) relieves pain and fever. In LGV, proctitis, perianal pruritus, mucopurulent rectal discharge, and perirectal lymph node enlargement may be the presenting symptoms of second-stage disease. The proctitis becomes chronic and invasive in the third stage of LGV. Perirectal abscess, perineal fistulas, rectal strictures, stenosis, and adhesions are painful complications that may interfere with normal bowel movements.

A serologic (complement fixation) test greater than 1:16 is considered diagnostic. Lower titers may be suggestive but not diagnostic because the test cross reacts with other strains of chlamydia. Isolation of the organism in aspirated pus is diagnostic.[13] A clinical diagnosis can be made based on the presence of buboes.

Therapeutic Management

Tetracycline, 500 mg by mouth every 6 hours for 2 to 4 weeks, is rapidly effective in both primary and secondary manifestations of LGV. Drainage of buboes may be necessary.

NURSING MANAGEMENT OF THE PATIENT WITH LYMPHOGRANULOMA VENEREUM

Assessment

In addition to routine assessment of patients with STDs, assess for a painful lymphadenopathy in the genital area.

Implementation

In addition to routine nursing implications for patients with STDs, individuals diagnosed with LGV have some special needs:

- If the patient is hospitalized, maintain clean, dry lesions using skin and wound precautions
- If the patient is seen in an outpatient setting, instruct the patient on the importance of skin care and good hand washing
- Instruct patient to use sitz baths or cool compresses every 6 hours to decrease discomfort and for cleansing
- Instruct patient to cover ruptured fistulas with nonadherent dressings
- Instruct patient in the need for biannual pelvic examinations to detect possible malignant changes
- Sexual contacts of known or suspected cases should be referred for prophylactic treatment

Evaluation

In addition to routine evaluation for patients with STDs, the lymph nodes should decrease in size and any drainage should stop.

DONOVANOSIS
Definition/Etiology

Donovanosis is a chronic, progressive bacterial infection of the genital area. Donovanosis is also known as granuloma inguinale, granuloma contagiosa, granuloma Donovani, and sclerosing granuloma. The causative organism is *Calymmatobacterium granulomatis*. This is a rare infection in the United States.[3,10]

Pathophysiology

The incubation period is 8 to 80 days. The infection is mildly contagious, usually requiring multiple exposures. New lesions can occur by autoinoculation.

The primary lesion appears as an indurated nodule, which erodes to a beefy, exuberant, granulomatous ulcer. Lesions are usually in warm, moist areas. The granulomatous ulcer progresses slowly, and there is swelling around the ulcer, producing a pseudolymphadenopathy.[3,10]

Clinical Manifestations

Lesions bleed readily on contact. Phimosis or lymphedema is common and may mimic buboes (pseudobuboes). In females, lesions occur commonly on the labia, cervix, and vaginal wall. In males, lesions commonly occur on the prepuce or glans.[10] Diagnosis is suggested by clinical signs. Definitive diagnosis is made by the presence of Donovan bodies (clusters of blue- or black-staining organisms with a safety pin appearance) with Wright's or Giemsa's stain.

Therapeutic Management

Tetracycline, 0.5 g orally every 6 hours, is the most common treatment. Alternative drugs are chloramphenicol, 0.5 g orally every 8 hours, and ampicillin, 0.5 g orally four times per day. Erythromycin, 0.5 g orally every 6 hours, is used during pregnancy. Clinical response is evidenced by a shrinking lesion in about 7 days.

NURSING MANAGEMENT OF THE PATIENT WITH DONOVANOSIS

Nursing management for donovanosis is the same as for lymphogranuloma venereum.

TRICHOMONIASIS
Definition/Etiology

Trichomoniasis is a genitourinary tract infection caused by a parasitic protozoan affecting both men and women but usually presenting as vaginal discharge in women. *Trichomonas vaginalis* is an oval, flagellated, motile protozoan that readily attaches to mucous membranes and other surfaces. It is transmitted sexually and rarely on moist clothing or towels. Both men and women may be asymptomatic. The highest incidence occurs in females aged 16 to 35 years.[3]

Pathophysiology

The incubation period of trichomoniasis varies from 4 to 20 days, averaging 7 days. Inflammation of vaginal epithelium by invading organisms may extend to include the endocervix, urethra, and Skene's glands. Host susceptibility, organism virulence, and coinfection are some factors contributing to the clinical severity of disease.

Clinical Manifestations

The characteristic malodorous, thin, frothy, greenish gray or yellow vaginal discharge may be accompanied by intense vulvar irritation and itching. Urinary frequency, dysuria, and dyspareunia are also common. Petechiae may be present on the cervix or vagina. Men are more commonly asymptomatic than women but may have urethral discharge and mild urethral irritation after urination or intercourse. Diagnosis is made by large numbers of white blood cells and distinctive, flagellated organisms easily identified in microscopic examination of a saline wet mount of vaginal or urethral discharge.

Therapeutic Management

Metronidazole, 250 mg orally three times daily for 7 days, is the treatment of choice for *Trichomonas* infection. Metronidazole has an Antabuse-like effect, producing mild to severe nausea and vomiting in individuals taking the drug and ingesting alcohol. Abstaining from alcohol 24 hours before and 48 hours after metronidazole treatment usually avoids this reaction. A few individuals have this Antabuse-like effect when exposed to topical alcohols in perfumes and colognes.

NURSING MANAGEMENT OF THE PATIENT WITH TRICHOMONIASIS
Assessment

In addition to routine assessment of patients with STDs, assess for malodorous, thin, frothy, greenish gray discharge with itching.

Implementation

In addition to routine nursing implications for patients with STDs, the following are special needs:
- Counsel the patient to avoid alcohol during treatment (especially if metronidazole is the treatment medication)
- Inform patients taking metronidazole that their urine may turn dark orange or brown
- Counsel patient to avoid douches, sprays, and powders that might affect the pH of the vagina
- Instruct the patient how to disinfect douche nozzles, applicators, diaphragms, and the toilet area
- Instruct the patient to wear loose-fitting clothing and cotton underwear
- Discuss the importance of routine Pap smears (especially if the patient is sexually active with more than one partner)
- Based on the diagnosis, discuss the need to contact sex partners so they can be treated concurrently

Evaluation

In addition to routine evaluation for patients with STDs, assess whether the discharge and itching stop.

BACTERIAL VAGINOSIS
Definition/Etiology

Bacterial vaginosis is a noninvasive, sexually transmitted bacterial infection. *Gardnerella vaginalis,* perhaps in synergistic combination with certain anaerobic bacteria, appears epidemiologically to be the causative organism of bacterial vaginosis. However, this infection is believed to be caused by various organisms, both aerobic and anaerobic. Symptoms often arise 5 to 10 days after sexual contact, although simultaneous treatment of asymptomatic partners is not usually necessary to cure women.[18]

Pathophysiology

The relationship between *Gardnerella* and vaginitis is not completely clear. Although it is isolated in 98% of women with nontrichomonal, noncandidal vaginal symptoms, *Gardnerella* can also be cultured from 30% to 70% of asymptomatic women. Vaginal epithelial cells may become studded with the *Gardnerella* coccibacillus (clue cells) and are seen in about 90% of patients. The distinctive odor described by most patients has recently been associated with aromatic amines produced by anaerobic bacteria but not *Gardnerella.*

Clinical Manifestations

Bacterial vaginosis is characterized by scant to moderate, malodorous, nonirritating, thin, grayish vaginal discharge, occasionally accompanied by mild, nonfocal abdominal discomfort; it may closely resemble other vaginal infections. Severe pruritus rarely occurs. Clue cells are seen on wet mount, and a whiff test (KOH added to vaginal discharge produces a distinctive amine fishlike odor) is positive in about 70% of patients. Of the cases of bacterial vaginosis, 90% are cured with one course of metronidazole, 500 mg by mouth two times daily for 7 days. Alternative therapies are ampicillin, 500 mg orally four times per day for 7 days, or amoxicillin, 500 mg orally three times per day for 7 days. Ampicillin and amoxicillin are less effective than metronidazole.[18]

NURSING MANAGEMENT OF THE PATIENT WITH BACTERIAL VAGINOSIS
Assessment

In addition to routine assessment for patients with STDs, assess for malodorous, nonirritating, thin, grayish discharge with mild abdominal discomfort.

Implementation

In addition to routine nursing implications for patients with STDs the following are special needs:

Counsel the patient to avoid alcohol during treatment with metronidazole

Inform patient to avoid douching and tampon use during infection

Discuss the need to contact sexual partners so they can be treated concurrently

Evaluation

In addition to evaluation for patients with STDs, the discharge should disappear and abdominal discomfort diminish.

CANDIDIASIS
Definition/Etiology

Candidiasis is a common vaginal infection sometimes transmitted sexually and caused by overgrowth of a yeastlike fungus, usually caused by an altered vaginal environment. Infection with *Candida albicans* commonly occurs in women without sexual contact. Asymptomatic colonization of the penis, however, is common in men with infected female partners, resulting in potential cross infection. Newborns with oral candidiasis (thrush) are probably infected at birth.

Pathophysiology

Candida albicans is a normal inhabitant of the vagina, mouth, and digestive tract of most adult women. Altered vaginal pH by prolonged use of antibiotics, steroids, oral contraceptives, excessive douching, diabetes, or pregnancy produces conditions favorable to rapid yeast reproduction. Pseudohyphae form networks that invade vaginal epithelium, causing extensive inflammation of the internal and external genitalia with itching, burning, and pain. Immunosuppressed individuals have frequent recurrences of oral and perigenital candidiasis. Extension of oral candidiasis to the esophagus in AIDS is not uncommon, although esophagitis may develop without oral symptoms. Vaginal candidiasis is a common finding in HIV-infected women.

Clinical Manifestations

Intense vulvovaginal pruritus, soreness, and irritation may extend to the inner thighs. Vaginal mucosa is diffusely erythematous, and usually a thick, white "cottage cheese" discharge is present with removable white patchy exudates. Although men are usually asymptomatic, they may experience inflammation or rash of the external genitalia. Uncircumcised men may harbor *Candida* under the foreskin. Yeast spores or pseudohyphae are easily identified on a potassium hydroxide (KOH) preparation of vaginal discharge.

Therapeutic Management

Effective antifungal agents are available in topical and systemic preparations. Topical creams and tablets are usually tried first, reserving systemic therapy for persistent or frequent recurrent infections. Agents used to treat candidiasis include miconazole nitrate, clotrimazole, nystatin (Mycostatin), ketoconazole, amphotericin B, and fluconazole.

NURSING MANAGEMENT OF THE PATIENT WITH CANDIDIASIS
Assessment

In addition to routine assessment of patients with STDs, assess for pruritus, erythema, and thick, white discharge.

Implementation

In addition to routine nursing implications for patients with STD, the following are special needs:

Encourage strict perineal hygiene

Teach to assess perineal area for white growth

Evaluation

In addition to routine evaluation of patients with STDs, the discharge, itching, and erythema should be alleviated.

MOLLUSCUM CONTAGIOSUM
Definition/Etiology

Molluscum contagiosum is a mildly contagious, benign skin disease transmitted by both sexual and nonsexual contact. Molluscum is caused by a poxvirus that is commonly transmitted in some (especially tropical) areas by nonsexual contact in children. When the growth occurs on or near the genitalia of sexually active adults, it is usually transmitted through sexual contact. Autoinoculation can also occur.[3]

Pathophysiology

The small epithelial tumors can develop anywhere on the skin after contact with an infected individual. Tumors grow slowly or may regress spontaneously but may spread rapidly and extensively in immunosuppressed patients (e.g., AIDS patients).

Clinical Manifestations

Lesions are small, discrete, waxy pink, dome-shaped growths with depressed centers. These growths are normally painless and contain a soft, cheesy material within the central depression. Any one lesion has a life span of 2 to 3 months.

Diagnosis is usually made on clinical appearance alone. However, fluid from the tumor center can be expressed onto a slide and viewed under the microscope. A positive diagnosis is made from the appearance of large "molluscum bodies" or "Henderson-Patterson bodies" (masses of virus). Diagnosis may be confirmed by biopsy.

Therapeutic Management

Treatment includes curetting (scraping out) the contents of the central depression with or without adjunctive use of chemicals, freezing, or electrocautery. Treatment of sexual partners at the same time prevents reinfection. The prognosis is good whichever treatment is selected, because most lesions disappear in 6 to 24 months.[3]

NURSING MANAGEMENT OF THE PATIENT WITH MOLLUSCUM CONTAGIOSUM

Assessment

In addition to routine assessment of patients with STDs, assess for dome-shaped lesions with depressed centers.

Implementation

In addition to routine nursing implications for patients with STDs, the following are special needs:

Teach patient to avoid touching small tumors
Encourage good hand washing
Inform the patient not to share personal items, that is, towels and washcloths

Evaluation

In addition to routine evaluation for patients with STDs, the lesions should disappear without spreading.

CRITICAL THINKING QUESTIONS

1 Compare the signs and symptoms of vaginitis with the signs and symptoms of pelvic inflammatory disease.
2 Explain what tests you would expect to see used to diagnose syphilis, herpes, and gonorrhea.
3 Describe the important patient care needs that should be addressed in a care plan for a patient diagnosed with herpes.
4 What should be included in a teaching plan for a patient with a sexually transmitted disease?
5 Outline the major nursing interventions for a patient with a sexually transmitted disease.
6 Describe the psychologic reaction to an STD diagnosis and the nursing interventions required.

RESOURCES LIST

1 American Red Cross National Headquarters 1709 New York Ave. Washington, DC 20006
2 Centers for Disease Control Sexually Transmitted Diseases 1600 Clifton Road, NE Atlanta, GA 30333
3 Gay Men's Health Crisis, Inc. 129 West 20th St. New York, NY 10011
4 Herpes Hotline:(415) 328-7710
5 Sex Information and Education Council of the United States 32 Washington Pl. New York, NY 10003
6 Sexually Transmitted Diseases Control Program Call Box STD, Caparra Heights Sta. San Juan, Puerto Rico 00922
7 STD Hotline: 1-800-227-8922
8 The National Foundation for Infectious Diseases 4733 Bethesda Ave., Suite 750 Bethesda, MD 20814

BIBLIOGRAPHY

Current

1. American College Health Association: *What are sexually transmitted diseases?* Rockville, Md, 1989, The Association.
2. Aral SO, Holmes KK: Epidemiology of sexual behavior and sexually transmitted diseases. In Holmes KK et al, editors: *Sexually transmitted diseases*, New York, 1990, McGraw-Hill Book Co.
3. Benenson AS: *Control of communicable diseases in man*, Washington, DC, 1990, American Public Health Association.
4. Bennett J, Gee G: *AIDS: concepts and nursing practice*, Baltimore, Md, 1988, Williams & Wilkins Co.
5. Centers for Disease Control: Condoms for prevention of sexually transmitted disease, *Morbid Mortal Weekly Rep* 37(9):133, 1988.
6. Centers for Disease Control: Sexually transmitted diseases treatment guidelines, *Morbid Mortal Weekly Rep* 38(S-8):1, 1989.
7. Centers for Disease Control: Notifiable diseases, *Morbid Mortal Weekly Rep* 40(51, 52):899-901, 1991.
8. Corey L: Genital herpes. In Holmes KK et al, editors: *Sexually transmitted diseases*, New York, 1990, McGraw-Hill Book Co.
9. Hart G: Donovanosis. In Holmes KK et al, editors: *Sexu-*

ally transmitted diseases, New York, 1990, McGraw-Hill Book Co.

10. Hook EW, Handsfield HH: Gonococcal infections in the adult. In Holmes KK et al, editors: *Sexually transmitted diseases,* New York, 1990, McGraw-Hill Book Co.

11. Kaminester LH: *Sexually transmitted diseases: an illustrated guide to differential diagnosis,* Triangle Park, NC, 1991, Burroughs Wellcome Co.

12. Perine PL, Osoba AO: Lymphogranuloma venereum. In Holmes KK et al, editors: *Sexually transmitted diseases,* New York, 1990, McGraw-Hill Book Co.

13. Public Health Service: *Sexually transmitted diseases statistics.* Pub No 00-5306, Atlanta, 1987, US Government Printing Office.

14. Quinn TC: *Clinical management of sexually transmitted diseases,* Triangle Park, NC, 1989, Burroughs Wellcome Co.

15. Redfield RR, Burke DS: HIV infection: The clinical picture, *Sci Am* 259:90-98, 1988.

16. Ronald AR, Albritton W: Chancroid and *Haemophilus ducreyi.* In Holmes KK et al, editors: *Sexually transmitted diseases,* New York, 1990, McGraw-Hill Book Co.

17. Secor RM: Bacterial vaginosis: a comprehensive review, *Nurs Clin North Am* 23(4):865-876, 1988.

18. Stamm WE, Holmes KK: *Chlamydia trachomatis* infections of the adult. In Holmes KK et al, editors: *Sexually transmitted diseases,* New York, 1990, McGraw-Hill Book Co.

19. Thorn GW et al: *Harrison's principles of internal medicine,* New York, 1989, McGraw-Hill Book Co.

20. Weber J, Weiss RA: HIV infection: the cellular picture, *Sci Am* 259:101, 1988.

Classic

21. American Foundation for the Prevention of Venereal Disease: *Venereal disease prevention for everyone,* New York, 1985, Foundation Press.

22. Braude Al, Davis CE, Fierer J: *Infectious diseases and medical microbiology,* ed 2, Philadelphia, 1986, WB Saunders Co.

23. Centers for Disease Control: STD treatment guidelines, *Morbid Mortal Weekly Rep* 34(4S):755, 1985.

24. Emmons J, Courter P: Towards control of chlamydial infections, *Nurse Pract* 10(11):15, 1985.

25. Mandel GL, Doublas, RG, Bennett JE: *Principles and practices of infectious diseases,* ed 2, New York, 1985, John Wiley & Sons Inc.

26. Public Health Service: *Guidelines for STD education.* Pub No 00-4672, Atlanta, 1985, US Government Printing Office.

UNIT XVII

Integumentary System

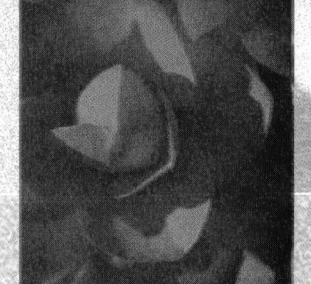

CHAPTER SEVENTY-THREE

Nursing Assessment of the Integumentary System

LEARNING OBJECTIVES

1 Know the structure of the skin and its main functions.
2 Obtain relevant subjective information from the patient who has an integumentary alteration.
3 Using correct technique, examine the patient to obtain appropriate objective information about the integumentary system.
4 Differentiate abnormal from normal subjective and objective findings related to the integumentary system.
5 Describe diagnostic procedures that are involved in the diagnosis and detection of skin disorders.
6 Discuss patient preparation and care related to the procedures for diagnosing skin disorders.

KEY TERMS

biopsy, p. 2087
ceruminous glands, p. 2081
core temperature, p. 2082
dermis, p. 2081
epidermis, p. 2080
immunofluorescence, p. 2088
intradermal skin test, p. 2088

melanin, p. 2080
patch test, p. 2088
primary lesions, p. 2084
sebaceous glands, p. 2081
secondary lesions, p. 2084
sudoriferous glands, p. 2081
Wood's light, p. 2087

THE SKIN IS THE largest organ of the body, accounting for approximately 7% of the body weight. It protects the body against excessive water loss and agents in the environment such as bacteria, viruses, chemicals, and ultraviolet radiation. The integument resists mechanical forces such as friction, vibration, and pressure, and it detects physical changes in the external environment, thereby enabling the individual to avoid noxious stimuli. The skin has the extremely important function of regulating the amount of heat lost by the body, and it also synthesizes vita-

min D, excretes some waste materials and toxins, and reacts immunologically to microorganisms and chemicals.

The assessment of the integumentary system, which is always integrated into the assessment of all body systems, includes an examination of the skin, mucous membranes, body hair, and nails. Its focus is a determination of whether the skin and appendages are intact and functional. A thorough integumentary assessment includes questions about nutrition and elimination, health care practices, history

2079

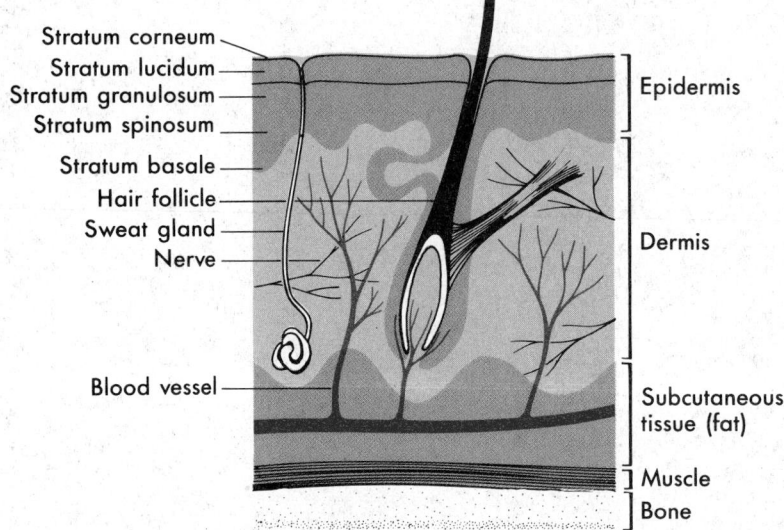

Stratum corneum
Stratum lucidum
Stratum granulosum
Stratum spinosum
Stratum basale
Hair follicle
Sweat gland
Nerve
Blood vessel

Epidermis
Dermis
Subcutaneous tissue (fat)
Muscle
Bone

FIGURE 73-1   Structures of the skin.

of illness and treatment, and life-style. An adept examination requires the nurse to be aware of ethnic differences.

ANATOMY AND PHYSIOLOGY
Structural Description

The human skin is made up of two layers, the epidermis and the dermis, bonded together and lying over the hypodermis or subcutaneous layer. The skin contains a number of accessory structures derived from epidermal cells, including the nails, hair, and a variety of glands.

Epidermis

The **epidermis** (Figure 73-1) is made up of stratified squamous epithelium, which can be subdivided into four or five layers depending on its location in the body. New cells are constantly being formed by the germinal layer next to the dermis, and the older cells are pushed upward by the younger cells. As the cells are pushed further away from the dermis with its rich blood supply, their metabolism changes and they synthesize and become filled with a protein called keratin. They also become dehydrated and flattened until the outermost layer, the stratum corneum, is made up of many layers of dead, flattened, scalelike cells that are constantly being rubbed off by friction with the environment. The stratum corneum becomes thick in areas of the body that are subjected to a lot of friction, such as the hands and feet. Calluses are an extreme example of the epidermis in a high friction area.

The epidermis lacks its own blood supply and only possesses a few simple receptor nerve endings in the lowest layers close to the dermis. Apart from the upper portions of the hair follicles and the duct of glands that pass through the epidermis from the dermis, the epidermis is almost entirely made up of densely packed cells tightly bonded together.

The normal color of the skin is a result of the presence or absence of a number of factors, such as melanin, carotene, and the amounts of oxyhemoglobin and deoxyhemoglobin in the superficial layers of the dermis. Melanocytes, found in the epidermal layers near the dermis, produce **melanin** granules. The larger the number of granules and the more the melanin is dispersed through the epidermis, the darker the appearance of the skin. Carotene is a yellowish pigment, found in foods such as carrots and apricots, that is stored in the fatty tissues of the body. When it is present to excess, it gives the skin a yellowish tinge, which, unlike true jaundice, does not involve the whites of the eyes. The white-red component of the skin's color is proportional to the amount of blood in the dermal blood vessels. The skin will appear red or pink when the hemoglobin is saturated with oxygen, and it will appear blue (cyanotic) when the partial pressure of oxygen is low and the absolute amount of deoxygenated hemoglobin exceeds 5 g/100 mL.

The skin shows many ridges and creases. The smallest of these are seen as fingerprints or heel prints, and they can be used for identification purposes, because they are unique for each individual. Their small ridges, which originate in the papillary layer of the dermis, anchor the epidermis to the dermis. Larger ridges can be seen on the palms and knuckles. Ridges and folds that develop prenatally are supported and maintained by the elastic fibers in the dermis. However, as the individual ages, additional creases develop as these elastic fibers lose some of their elasticity. This process is accelerated in individuals who smoke heavily, because (1) nicotine causes vasoconstriction, which reduces the amount of blood flowing in the skin and deprives it of its nutrition, and (2) chemicals and free radicals in the smoke accelerate the loss of elasticity that is normally associated with aging.

Dermis

The **dermis** (see Figure 73-1) is made up of dense fibrous connective tissue well supplied with blood vessels that also provide the nutrition for the lower layers of the epidermis. The arteries enter the skin and form a deep subcutaneous plexus from which arterioles rise to supply capillary loops in the papillary layer and in the accessory skin structures. The amount of blood flowing through the superficial layers of the dermis is controlled by dilating or constricting special arteriovenous anastomoses. The skin is well supplied with lymph vessels, which originate in lymph capillaries in the papillary layer.

The strength of the skin is provided by collagen fibers that are attached to the epidermis and oriented to produce the characteristic ridges of the papillae. Many different types of cells are found in the dermis: the fibrocytes that produce the collagen and elastin fibers; macrophages, lymphocytes, and mast cells that are important in protecting the individual from injury and disease; and a number of other specialized cells.

The dermis is well supplied with motor nerves to control the caliber of the blood vessels and the tension in the smooth muscle of the skin. It is also supplied with a wide variety of sensory receptors (see Unit XI) and nerves to monitor the skin and the external environment.

Hair, nails, and glands

The skin possesses a number of accessory structures (hair, nails, and glands), which are produced in the dermis from invaginated epithelial cells and pass through the epidermis to the exterior.

Hair (see Figure 73-1) has a limited protective function. On the scalp it protects against heat and cold, whereas the eyelashes and hair in the nose protect the eyes and nose from airborne particles. Hair also serves an ornamental function and adds to sexual attractiveness. Each hair is formed from a papilla of epithelial cells that surround a capillary tuft at the base of a follicle lined with epithelium. As the epithelial cells divide, they are pushed upward and form the hair shaft as they become keratinized and die. The life span of a hair varies with its location.

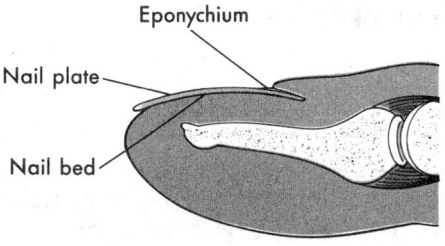
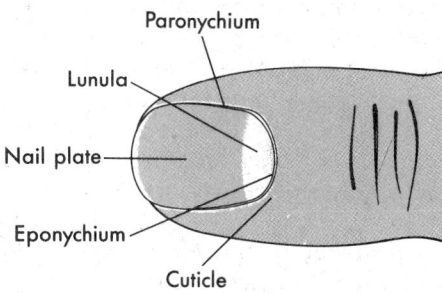

FIGURE 73-2   Structures of the nail.

(Scalp hair may last 3 to 4 years before it is pushed out and replaced.) Hair follicles are lubricated by the secretions of the associated sebaceous glands. Smooth muscle attached to the follicles can alter the angle at which the hair leaves the skin surface. When the tension in the smooth muscle increases, the hair is pulled more erect and causes small bumps on the skin surface around the hairs. These bumps are associated with feeling cold (goose bumps).

Nails (Figure 73-2) are found on the distal dorsal surface of the fingers and toes where they serve as a protection and aid in grasping and picking up small objects. They are made up of transparent epithelial cells that grow and are pushed up from the root growth areas of the matrix and the lunula of the nail bed.

The glands of the skin are sebaceous glands, ceruminous glands, and sudoriferous glands. **Sebaceous glands** secrete an oily substance (sebum) into the hair follicles, which lubricates the follicle and keeps the skin supple. **Ceruminous glands** are only found in the external auditory meatus. They secrete a waxy substance (cerumen) that protects the eardrum from drying out. **Sudoriferous glands** (sweat glands) secrete a watery fluid to aid in keeping the body cool, and in doing so they also excrete some waste products. A specialized type of apocrine sweat gland develops at puberty that produces a particularly odoriferous secretion. These glands are most prevalent in the axillary and pubic regions, and their secretion is usually related to sexual activity. (The mammary glands, or breasts, are also specialized modifications of sweat glands.)

Functions of Skin

Protection from dehydration and mechanical injury

The keratin of the epidermis and the sebum secreted by the sebaceous glands are hydrophobic and render the skin impervious to water. This prevents undue water loss. The insensible (invisible) water lost through the skin amounts to approximately 350 mL/day. Additional water may be lost through the sweat glands. However, this water loss is deliberate and forms an essential part of the homeostasis of body temperature. Water loss through the skin can cause dehydration where large areas of the epidermis are denuded by burns or other injuries or where environmental temperatures are excessive. In addition to protecting the body against dehydration, the epidermis protects the body from dehydration when it is in an aqueous environment.

Unlike water, lipid-soluble substances can enter the body through the skin easily by simple diffusion. Normally this is not a problem. However, many pesticides and herbicides are lipid soluble, and poisoning can occur when adequate precautions are not taken. Some lipid-soluble medications are now administered through the skin by applying them in the form of skin patches.

The epidermis also protects the underlying structures from mechanical abrasion. Its thickness in any particular location depends on the normal stresses that the area is subjected to. For example, the skin on the palmar surfaces of the hands and feet is thicker than it is on the face, because it is subjected to more friction. However, unusual friction can cause blistering and abrasion of the skin and can tear the epidermis and underlying tissues.

Epidermal cells increase their rate of reproduction when they are not surrounded by other epidermal cells. Thus whenever skin is damaged or torn, new skin is formed from the epidermal cells at the cut edge of the wound and from glandular cells that remain in the dermis. The new epithelial cells continue to reproduce at a fast rate until they cover underlying connective tissue and completely close the gap. However, they can only do this if sufficient connective tissue remains to support them and if the blood and oxygen supply is adequate. If the dermis is destroyed, the epidermis will not regrow until the dermis has been replaced for new epithelial cells to grow on.

The extremely important inflammation and immune reactions that allow the skin to form the first line of defense against microorganisms are reviewed in Chapter 11.

Temperature control

The skin plays an extremely important role in the homeostasis of body temperature, which must be kept constant because it affects the metabolic rate. All the chemical reactions speed up as body temperature increases, and this leads to the loss of excessive amounts of energy, body water, and salts. Conversely, if body temperature falls too low, metabolism and the activity of the brain and heart slow down. Ultimately this leads to drowsiness, which may progress through coma to death.

Two reflex centers in the hypothalamus are responsible for temperature control. One senses an increase in the core temperature, and one senses a decrease.

Core temperature is the temperature of the blood in the chest, abdomen, and head. It rises when heat production exceeds heat loss and falls when heat production is less than heat loss. To remain constant, heat loss must equal heat production.

Heat is lost through the skin by conduction, convection, radiation, and evaporation. The amount of heat lost depends on the difference in temperature between the skin and its surroundings. In addition, the amount of heat lost by evaporation depends on the wetness of the skin and the relative humidity of the air. Skin temperature is controlled by involuntary mechanisms. It can be changed by passing more or less blood through the superficial blood vessels of the dermis. When core temperature falls, the amount of blood in the skin is reduced by vasodilation of cutaneous arteriovenous shunts. This diverts blood away from the superficial layers of the dermis back to the venous system and reduces the warmth transferred to the skin by blood. Consequently, the skin cools down and less heat is lost by conduction, convection, radiation, and evaporation. Receptors in the skin make the cerebral cortex aware of this cooling, and this encourages the individual to put on more clothes or find a warmer place.

Heat production is proportional to the metabolic rate. It can be increased by increased muscle tone, by shivering, and as a result of increased secretion of hormones such as epinephrine and thyroxine.

When core temperature falls, body temperature is returned to normal by (1) increasing heat production by increasing muscle tone or by promoting shivering and (2) reducing heat loss by reducing the temperature of the skin until heat loss is equal to heat production.

When core temperature rises it is difficult to reduce heat production significantly, and most of the control is exerted by increasing the amount of heat lost through the skin. When core temperature rises, the amount of blood in the skin is increased by closing the arteriovenous shunts. This warms the skin and increases heat lost to the surroundings when they are cooler than the skin. The sympathetic nervous system also stimulates the sweat glands to secrete sweat, and the energy required to evaporate the water in sweat is taken from the skin. Thus the skin temperature falls.

When the environment is warmer than the skin, the only method available for eliminating surplus heat is the evaporation of sweat. However, evaporation is not effective when the relative humidity is high (i.e., the air cannot hold any additional water). Under very hot and humid conditions, the individual runs the risk of heat exhaustion even at low levels of activity.

A fever is an unusual increase in core temperature. Body temperature (approximately 37° C [98.6° F] by mouth) is well controlled, and although it exhibits normal diurnal fluctuations for any individual, it remains fairly constant. However, the temperature control centers in the hypothalamus are sensitive to the metabolic by-products of infection or large-scale tissue damage. These substances alter the sensitivity of the control centers so that the set point for temperature control is raised. Once this happens, all the processes that raise body temperature will be initiated, the skin will be cool and pale, and shivering may occur. Once the new core temperature is reached, it will be maintained, and the resulting fever can be detected with a thermometer. When the infection is over, the control centers return to their normal setting and the fever ends. When this happens all the processes that lower body temperature will be initiated. The skin will be flushed and warm, and sweating will occur. Sometimes during the course of the fever the effect on the reflex centers is intermittent. In this case (e.g., malaria), bouts of shivering and sweating alternate.

Prostaglandins are involved in resetting the reflex control centers to higher temperatures, and antiprostaglandin medications, such as aspirin, return body temperature to normal by inhibiting the prostaglandin-mediated effects of the metabolic by-products. High body temperatures may protect the body against some infections, and over-the-counter medications should not be used routinely to control minor fevers.

Other functions

The skin has a number of other functions. The melanin in the epidermis absorbs high-energy ultraviolet light and reduces its damaging effect on the subepidermal layers. However, the germinal layer of the epidermis is susceptible to damage by ultraviolet radiation, particularly in individuals with a fair complexion. These individuals have less melanin and have a greater risk of skin cancer than dark-skinned individuals. This risk is proportional to the intensity and duration of the individual's exposure to the sun's ultraviolet radiation.

The skin synthesizes vitamin D from dehydrocholesterol, which supplements the vitamin D taken in with food. Vitamin D is especially important when the rate of growth is high, as it is in children and adolescents. Bone growth is poor when children who

GERIATRIC CONSIDERATIONS

Physiologic Changes in the Integumentary System

The elasticity of the integumentary system declines with age. This can be seen in the increased number of wrinkles that form in the skin and are particularly noticeable on the faces of heavy smokers and individuals subjected to excessive amounts of ultraviolet light. The skin of elderly persons is thinner than that of younger individuals. There is a decline in the number of glands and the quantity of sebum and sweat secreted. This often results in drier skin and an increased sensitivity to heat. The number of melanocytes declines with age; this can be seen in a reduced ability to tan and in graying of the hair. As with all systems the rate at which the skin ages varies considerably from individual to individual. It is affected by exposure to varying amounts of damaging ultraviolet waves and to chemical and physical stressors in the environment and by each individual's genetic inheritance.

have a vitamin D–deficient diet are not sufficiently exposed to the sun, perhaps as a result of poor weather or premature entry into the work force.

The skin is also used for communication. Blushing communicates embarrassment, and facial expressions caused by the contraction of muscles attached to the skin communicate a wide range of emotions, such as surprise, anger, happiness, and sadness. The odor of the secretions of the apocrine sweat glands plays a role in sexual communication.

Although excretion is not a primary function of the skin, its secretions do contain a variety of waste products, and odor can give the health care professional additional clues as to health status and cleanliness.

ASSESSMENT
Subjective

Patients may present with symptoms such as pruritus, rash, or changes in pigmentation. Integumentary changes or lesions may be a result of a disorder primarily of the skin, or they may be a result of disorders of other systems. Patients with liver disease may be jaundiced, and patients with renal failure may have pale, ashen, dry, pruritic skin with uremic frost. Patients may exhibit hair changes or loss (alopecia) secondary to endocrine problems, psychologic problems, or chemotherapy for cancer.

The box on p. 2084 lists potential symptoms to review with the patient. In addition to specific symp-

POTENTIAL SYMPTOMS RELATED TO INTEGUMENTARY SYSTEM

Systemic
Arthralgias (pain in joints)
Fever
Malaise

Skin
Dryness
Ecchymoses (bruising)
Edema or swelling
Erythema (redness)
Hives
Lesions
Masses
Pain
Petechiae (pinpoint-sized, nonraised, purplish red spots)
Pruritus (itching)

Hair
Hair loss (alopecia)
Changes in texture

Nails
Changes in texture
Changes in shape
Changes in color
Changes in adherence to nail bed
Inflammation
Pain or tenderness

toms, ask the patient about hay fever, asthma, any recent travel, and exposure to chemicals, plants, insects, pets, or other people with rashes.

Other appropriate history to explore includes major adult illnesses, hospitalizations, surgeries, injuries or accidents, immunizations, current medications, allergies, and habits. Specific adult illnesses to review include diabetes mellitus, peripheral vascular disease, connective tissue disorders, or sexually transmitted diseases such as syphilis, gonorrhea, or human immune virus (HIV), since these diseases may involve integumentary changes.

Family history that is relevant to the integumentary system includes skin cancer; infestations; bacterial, fungal, or viral infections; psoriasis; eczema; asthma; and hay fever. Some family members may have hay fever, whereas others have asthma, and still others have eczema, asthma, and hay fever. This is known as atopy, a familial predisposition to develop an allergic response. The specific clinical form (e.g., hay fever or asthma) is not inherited.

Objective

Physical assessment of the patient with an integumentary complaint may involve examination of the skin, nails, and hair. In addition, if the history suggests a viral infection, examination of the head and neck (including eyes, ears, nose, and throat) as well as heart and lungs may also be indicated.

General assessment

General assessment is included for any patient and refers to the examiner's overall impression of the patient's health. General assessment includes vital signs, height, and weight. Note facial expression, apparent age relative to chronologic age, nutritional status, general appearance, and stature. Any obvious abnormalities or assistive devices should also be noted. In addition, record whether the patient appears to be comfortable or in distress.

Skin

Inspect the skin in good lighting. Side lighting may be helpful in detecting an elevation or depression as well as surface characteristics (smooth, uneven, rough). Note color, integrity, variation in pigmentation, lesions, vascularity, and hygiene. If lesions are present, note site, color, distribution, configuration or arrangement, size of individual lesions, number, tenderness, and discharge.

Lesions may be subdivided into two groups: primary and secondary. **Primary lesions** are de novo without any antecedent lesions and are caused directly by a disease process. **Secondary lesions** are primary lesions modified as a result of trauma, healing, or other external factors. Figure 73-3 illustrates primary and secondary lesions.

Palpate for thickness, temperature, tenderness, turgor, edema, mobility, and moisture. Turgor refers to the elasticity of the skin. To evaluate turgor, pick up the skin and let it go, observing how quickly it returns or rebounds to its previous position (Figure 73-4). A dehydrated individual exhibits loss of turgor, and "tenting" may occur.

Skin moisture varies from area to area of the body as well as in various systemic states. For example, increased moisture may be noted with increased activity, fever, warm environment, obesity, or anxiety and may be concentrated on the palms, scalp, forehead, and axillae. Closely evaluate intertriginous areas in obese patients such as folds of pendulous breasts, axillae, thighs, or groin areas for evidence of increased moisture with tenderness and erythema.

Hair

Inspect and palpate the hair, noting distribution, quantity, and texture (coarse or fine). Note appro-

Mascule—flat; nonpalpable; circumscibed; less than 1 cm in diameter; brown, red, purple, white, or tan in color
Examples: Freckles; flat moles; rubella; rubeola; drug eruptions

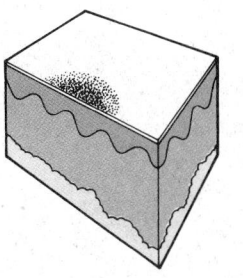

Vesicle—elevated; circumscribed; superficial; filled with serous fluid; less than 1 cm in diameter
Examples: Blister varicella

Papule—elevated; palpable; firm; circumscribed; less than 1 cm in diameter; brown, red, pink, tan, or bluish red in color
Examples: Warts; drug-related eruptions; pigmented nevi; eczema

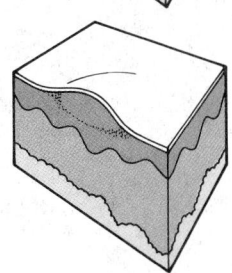
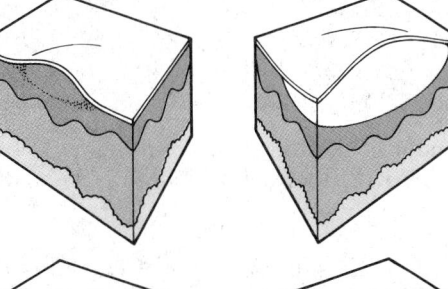
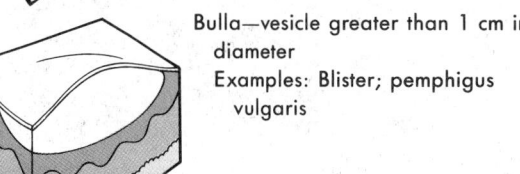

Bulla—vesicle greater than 1 cm in diameter
Examples: Blister; pemphigus vulgaris

Plaque—elevated; flat topped; firm; rough; superficial papule greater than 1 cm in diameter, may be coalesced papules
Example: Psoriasis; seborrheic and actinic keratoses; eczema

Pustule—elevated superficial; similar to vesicle but filled with purulent fluid
Examples: Impetigo; acne; variola; herpes zoster

Wheal—elevated, irregular-shaped area of cutaneous edema; solid, transient, changing variable diameter; pale pink in color
Examples: Urticaria; insect bites

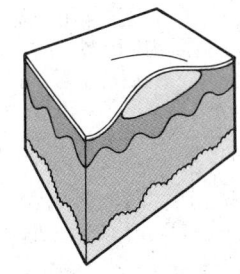

Cyst—elevated; circumscribed; palpable; encapsulated; filled with liquid or semi-solid material
Example: Sebaceous cyst

Noble—elevated; firm; circumscribed; palpable; deeper in dermis than papule; 1 to 2 cm in diameter
Examples: Erythema nodosum; lipomas

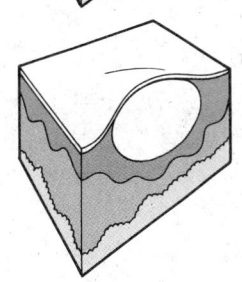

Scale—heaped-up keratinized cells; flaky exfoliation; irregular; thick or thin; dry or oily; varied size; silver, white, or tan in color
Examples: Psoriasis; exfoliative dermatitis

Tumor—elevated; solid; may or may not be clearly demarcated; greater than 2 cm in diameter; may or may not vary from skin color
Example: Neoplasms

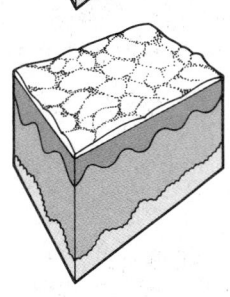
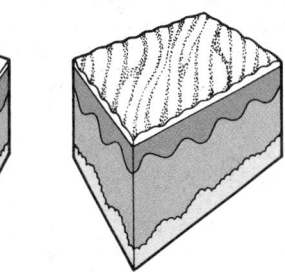

Lichenification—rough, thickened epidermis; accentuated skin markings due to rubbing or irritation; often involves flexor aspect of extremity
Example: Chronic dermatitis

FIGURE 73-3   Skin lesions.

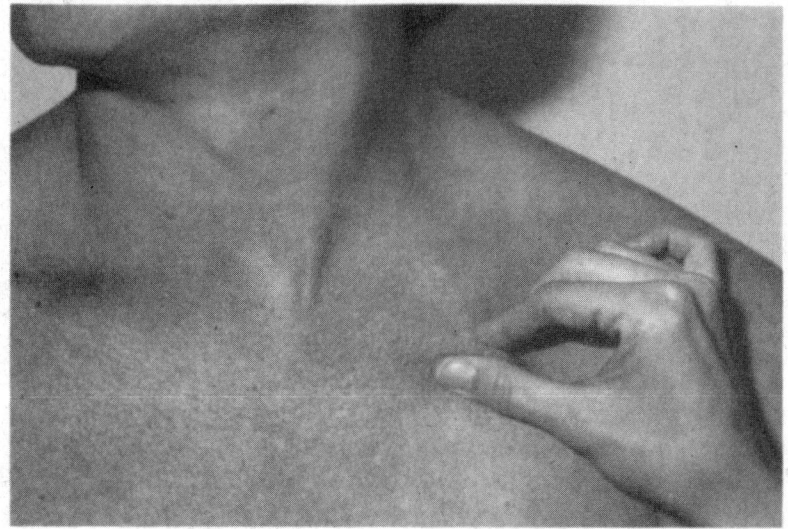

FIGURE 73-4   Assessment of skin turgor. (From Seidel HM et al: *Mosby's guide to physical examination,* ed 2, St Louis, 1991, Mosby–Year Book, Inc.)

priate male/female pattern and quantity. Hirsutism is an increased hair growth in a male distribution pattern in a female, which may be associated with heredity, hormone imbalances, or some medications. Hypertrichosis is an excessive hair growth over all the body.

Also observe for parasites. Pediculosis is not related to the state of personal hygiene. Head lice may be determined by observing for nits (pearly white,

oval capsules firmly attached to the hairs, close to the scalp surface, especially in the cervical area). In the setting of body lice, inspect the seams of clothing for the nits.

Nails

Inspect and palpate the nails, noting presence or absence, growth, curvature, adhesion, color, and thick-

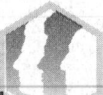

GERIATRIC CONSIDERATIONS

Integumentary Assessment

General approach

Allow more time than for a younger adult

Articulate clearly; the geriatric patient may be hearing impaired

Impaired sight, comprehension, or mobility may result in less than optimum cooperation

Provide clear, concise directions

History collection

Be alert for answers that do not appear appropriate; the patient may not have understood the question correctly because of impaired hearing or comprehension

Some questions may need to be repeated in a different manner

Physical assessment

The physical examination itself is not different, but the approach needs to be altered such that the appropriate information is assessed without undue discomfort or embarrassment for the patient

Maintain an environment with minimal noise, distractions, and interruption

Decreased elasticity (turgor) is found even in patients with adequate hydration and causes wrinkles

Dry skin is common secondary to decreased sweat and sebaceous gland production

Hyperpigmented macules may frequently be observed and are sometimes referred to as "age" or "liver" spots

Progressive thinning of all body hair occurs

Thinning of the epidermis and dermis leads to capillary fragility and therefore easy bruising

Onychomycosis, a fungal condition of the nails, is a common finding

ness. Clubbing is an overcurvature of the nail caused by loss of the angle between the posterior nail fold and the nail plate. Clubbing occurs in chronic pulmonary disease, carcinoma of the bronchus, or congenital heart disease. Nails may be spoon shaped (koilonychia) from iron deficiency or possibly from local irritants. Note any pitting, transverse ridges, or longitudinal ridges of the nails. Pitting of the nails may be associated with psoriasis or eczema. Transverse ridges may be associated with cessation of growth related to a severe illness, whereas longitudinal ridges may be associated with a fungal infection or a variation of normal.

ASSESSMENT OF SKIN IN DARK-SKINNED INDIVIDUALS

1. Inspection and palpation are equally important in assessing the dark-skinned patient. Skin color changes are best observed in the sclera, conjunctiva, oral mucosa, tongue, lips, nail beds, palms, and soles. Normal variations in pigmentation should be considered when assessing for skin color changes. The oral mucosa may have areas of darker pigmentation in the gums, the cheeks, and borders of the tongue. The lips may have a normal dark blue color. The presence of edema may cause dark skin to appear lighter in color. Changes in skin texture assessed by palpation may be the only indication of the presence of skin rashes.

2. In dark-skinned patients, pallor results in the loss of normal red tones in the skin. The brown-skinned person may have yellow-tinged skin when pallor is present. In the black-skinned patient, pallor produces an "ashen gray" color.

3. Jaundice is best observed in the sclera closest to the center of the eye. The dark-skinned patient may have normal yellow pigmentation present in the sclera. Inspection of the hard palate for a yellow color can confirm the presence of jaundice.

4. Cyanosis may be difficult to detect in the dark-skinned patient. Inspection in areas of lightest pigmentation will often indicate the presence of cyanosis, such as the nail beds, conjunctivae, palms, and soles.

5. Petechiae are best observed in the conjunctiva and oral mucosa. They may also be seen in areas of lighter pigmentation over the abdomen, gluteal folds, or inner aspect of the forearm.

6. Erythema is determined by palpating for increased skin temperature that is usually associated with conditions that produce this skin color change.

DIAGNOSTIC AND LABORATORY TESTS
Biopsy

Biopsy of skin lesions involves removal of a small sample of skin, using a punch or a scalpel. A punch biopsy involves the use of a small instrument with a terminal end of 3 to 8 mm ($\frac{1}{8}$ to $\frac{5}{16}$ inches) that is applied firmly and rotated to yield a round skin specimen. Raised or elevated skin lesions may be shaved with a scalpel and the scrapings sent for biopsy. Skin areas may also be excised or incised to yield tissue for biopsy. Excision biopsy is preferred if a lesion is rapidly growing or if comparison of the lesion and surrounding normal skin is desired. If the patient has a fungal or viral infection, cells may be obtained by pressing a clean glass slide firmly to the lesion (touch preparation). A fixative is applied to the slide immediately afterward.

Patient preparation

The patient is informed that a small specimen of tissue will be removed for examination, and a consent is obtained as required. The nurse cleanses the area with an antibacterial solution before biopsy. Direct pressure is applied to the area to stop bleeding after the procedure. The nurse instructs the patient in wound care and suggests contacting the physician for results of the biopsy.

Scrapings

Skin areas are scraped to the dermis with a sharp scalpel, and the scrapings are examined for the presence of fungal infection and ectoparasites after the addition of 10% to 40% KOH (potassium hydroxide). Specimens of hair and from nails may also be used. Brittle, broken hair strands should be used. Nails, including nail beds, should be vigorously scraped. Skin and nail areas are cleansed with alcohol and air dried before scraping.

Culture

Swab samples are collected from the affected area and placed immediately in appropriate culture media. Note recurrent or current antibiotic therapy on the laboratory slip.

Wood's Light

Wood's light is a high-pressure mercury light that transmits long-wave ultraviolet wavelengths ("black light"). Wood's light is used to directly visualize skin in a darkened room. The various and characteristic fluorescent colors that are produced are useful in detecting bacterial and fungal infections, porphyria, and pigmentary alterations. The nurse instructs the patient to avoid shampooing, bathing, and application of makeup to the area under examination for 24 hours before the test.

Cytology

Cells that are collected are stained with Giemsa or Wright's stain and viewed microscopically after staining.

Immunofluorescence

In **immunofluorescence,** fluorescent dyes are attached to antibody molecules. The antibody appears as a colored fluorescence when complexed with an antigen and viewed under the microscope. In direct immunofluorescence, the fluorescein-tagged antibody reacts with the antigen specific to it. In indirect immunofluorescence a fluorescein-tagged antiglobulin reacts with an unlabeled antibody-antigen complex. The antiglobulin then binds with the unlabeled antibody. Both tests are useful in detecting bacterial and viral antigens involved in infections of the skin.

Skin Tests for Allergies

Skin tests are a useful, convenient, sensitive, and economic means of determining if a patient has specific sensitivities to environmental allergens. Tests include patch, scratch, and intradermal methods. The patient is informed that the test will help determine the substance to which the allergic reaction has occurred.

Patch test

In the **patch test** a suspected allergen is applied to the skin under a nonabsorbent adhesive patch. The patient is instructed not to remove the patch and to keep the area dry for 48 hours. A positive reaction consists of erythema, vesicles, and some induration. The patient is directed to return immediately if itching and burning develop before the end of the 48-hour period. The nurse removes the patch and reinspects in 72 hours.

Intradermal skin test

For the **intradermal skin test,** the nurse prepares a site that is several fingerwidths from the antecubital space with an alcohol swab. Hairy or blemished areas should be avoided, as should rubbing to the extent that the skin becomes reddened. The nurse uses the nondominant hand to stretch the patient's skin and inserts the needle, bevel up, at an angle almost parallel to the skin. The allergen is slowly injected until a small wheal forms. If a wheal does not form, the needle may be more than 3 mm (⅛ inch) below the surface.

CRITICAL THINKING QUESTIONS

1 How do the epidermis and dermis differ in structure?
2 How does the skin help regulate body temperature?
3 Design at least three questions to discreetly ask patients about skin breakdown in the perineal area.
4 Discuss psychologic and ethnic factors to consider throughout the physical examination of the patient's integument.
5 Discuss special considerations in regard to skin integrity in older adults.
6 Describe the care and preparation of a patient who is undergoing skin biopsy.
7 Describe the procedure for an intradermal skin test.

BIBLIOGRAPHY

Current

1. Ashton R et al: *Differential diagnosis in dermatology,* Philadelphia, 1990, JB Lippincott Co.
2. Bates B: *A guide to physical examination and history-taking,* ed 4, Philadelphia, 1987, JB Lippincott Co.
3. Bowers A, Thompson J: *Clinical manual of health assessment,* ed 3, St Louis, 1988, Mosby–Year Book, Inc.
4. Epstein E: *Common skin disorders,* ed 3, Oradell, NJ, 1988, Medical Economics Books.
5. Gallo JJ et al: *Handbook of geriatric assessment,* Rockville, Md, 1988, Aspen Publishers.
6. Kane RL et al: *Essentials of clinical geriatrics,* ed 2, New York, 1989, McGraw-Hill Book Co.
7. LeFever Kee J: *Handbook of laboratory and diagnostic tests with nursing implications,* Philadelphia, 1990, JB Lippincott Co.
8. Malasanos L et al: *Health assessment,* ed 4, St Louis, 1990, Mosby–Year Book, Inc.
9. Pagana KD, Pagana TJ: *Diagnostic testing and nursing implications: a case study approach,* St Louis, 1990, Mosby–Year Book, Inc.
10. Seidel HM et al: *Mosby's guide to physical examination,* ed 2, St Louis, 1991, Mosby–Year Book, Inc.
11. Swartz MH: *Textbook of physical diagnosis,* Philadelphia, 1989, WB Saunders Co.
12. Thompson JM et al: *Mosby's manual of clinical nursing,* ed 2, St Louis, 1989, Mosby–Year Book, Inc.

Classic

13. Bloch B, Hunter M: Teaching physiological assessment of black persons, *Nurse Educ* 6(1):24, 1981.
14. Block G, Nolan J: *Health assessment for professional nursing: a developmental approach,* New York, 1986, Appleton-Century-Crofts.
15. Bryne CJ et al: *Laboratory tests: implications for nursing care,* Menlo Park, NJ, 1986, Addison-Wesley Publishing Co, Inc.
16. Carotenuto R, Bullock J: *Physical assessment of the gerontologic client,* Philadelphia, 1981, FA Davis Co.
17. Prior JA et al: *Physical diagnosis: the history and examination of the patient,* St Louis, 1981, Mosby–Year Book, Inc.

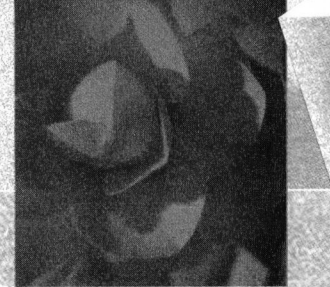

CHAPTER SEVENTY-FOUR

Nursing Management of Adults with Skin Disorders

LEARNING OBJECTIVES

1 Describe the general treatment modalities for skin disorders.

2 Help the patient and family cope with the psychologic trauma of dermatologic disorders.

3 Discuss nursing care for the patient with pruritus.

4 Use the nursing process to provide care for patients with inflammatory, infectious, autoimmune, or neoplastic skin disorders.

5 Discuss patient education needs in secretory disorders.

6 Discuss the pathophysiology and treatment of psoriasis.

7 Contrast extrinsic and intrinsic risk factors related to the development of pressure ulcers.

8 Develop a plan of care for the patient with a risk of developing pressure ulcers.

9 Compare the types of neoplastic skin disorders.

10 Identify special considerations for the elderly patient, the black patient, and the patient with HIV.

KEY TERMS

THE SKIN IS OFTEN THE first body organ to show signs of medical problems. Hospitalized patients commonly have preexisting skin problems that flare up or need continuing care during the hospital stay. Other skin problems occur during the course of a disease or as a result of a reaction to therapy.

Common Interventions for Skin Disorders

TOPICAL MEDICATIONS

Topical medications are used to lubricate or dry the skin, to reduce inflammation, or as a vehicle to provide medication. They are chosen both for direct delivery of medication to the skin and for the vehicle in which the medication is suspended. Vehicles with a drying effect such as powders, aerosols, and suspensions are used on open, weeping lesions such as eczema. Extremely dry, scaling lesions benefit from an occlusive ointment-based medication which will hydrate the skin, while a less scaly condition will benefit from either an oil-in-water or water-in-oil preparation. The vehicle and the medication must be chosen carefully; for example, if an ointment were applied to an open, weeping lesion, the skin could macerate from excess moisture. The rule of thumb when choosing a vehicle is that when the lesion is wet, use something drying, when the lesion is dry, use something that will wet.

Topical medication is absorbed more readily by inflamed skin, so the dosage may need to be reduced for safety. When increased absorption is desired, topical medication may be applied to hydrated skin or covered with wet or occlusive dressings. These dressings promote absorption by increasing hydration of the stratum corneum. In cases where there is generalized involvement of the skin, hydration of the stratum corneum is easily attained by using therapeutic baths.

During application of topical medications the nurse can convey many messages to a patient. Before the introduction of universal precautions, it was advocated that all topicals with nonsystemic effects be applied with an ungloved hand. This conveyed a strong message of acceptance to the patient. Now with universal precautions it is necessary to wear gloves when applying topical medications. The patient can still have a feeling of acceptance if the nurse is careful to explain that wearing gloves is a way to protect the patient and is not being done out of fear or lack of understanding. Since medications such as mercury, anthralin, juniper tar, or nitrogen mustard can be absorbed into the nurse's skin, their application poses a risk. Gloves are, therefore, worn at all times. Application of topicals must be done to avoid irritation of hair follicles. The medication is applied with the palms of the hands, using long, smooth strokes that follow the direction of hair growth. The medication should never be applied in circular motions, against the direction of hair growth, or patted into the skin.

CORTICOSTEROIDS

Corticosteroids are one of the most commonly used medications. Their antiinflammatory action alleviates pruritus (itching) and inflammation, while their antimitotic action inhibits rapid cell growth. Corticosteroids are beneficial in both acute and chronic conditions. In chronic conditions, steroid use, particularly the more potent fluorinated steroids, have the potential for producing side effects. Complications include skin atrophy, striae, telangiectasia, dermatitis, exacerbation of acne, or infections, and systemic effects with long-term use. Steroids applied under occlusive dressings or on the face, neck, or intertriginous areas (skin surfaces that are in contact, such as skin folds) require special precautions, since these situations increase medication absorption and thereby increase the potential for side effects.

Nursing precautions and patient education for steroid use are essential. Topical steroids should be applied evenly and in a thin coat. Patients who will be self-medicating must be instructed on proper application. The nurse observes for and educates the patient to observe for side effects. Any side effects must be reported. The nurse cautions the patient that steroids should only be applied as instructed and only to the areas of the body noted. Fluorinated steroids should not be applied to the face, groin, or axillae due to the increased absorption of medications in this area and the potential for serious side effects.

THERAPEUTIC BATHS

When the entire skin surface is involved with disease, a bath is a means to provide topical treatment to all the skin quickly and efficiently. Patients with pruritic skin may benefit from a tepid bath that lubricates and hydrates the skin. Products such as oilated oatmeal provide a soothing, antipruritic action while lubricating dry skin. Patients with weeping lesions may benefit from a bath with drying and cooling effects such as potassium permanganate. In general, the water temperature should be 96° F. Towels can be placed over the chest and shoulders during the bath to keep the skin moist. Patients with dry, mildly scaling conditions should gently use their bare hands, rather than a washcloth, to cleanse their skin. Use of a washcloth, can increase inflammation and itching. Soap should only be used when necessary and should only be used on the soles of the feet, in the axillae, and in the groin. The soap should be pH balanced so as not to alter the acid mantle of the skin, and should be fragrance free. Removal of thick scales or plaques, as in psoriasis, may be done by scrubbing the area with a washcloth being mindful of the possibility of eliciting pruritus. Rubbing of the skin may be beneficial, but caution must be taken not to elicit the "itch-scratch-itch" cycle by stimulating the skin. This is particularly true in atopic patients. Even though baths can be therapeutic, they may also be detrimental. For example, an atopic who is not in flare will do better to avoid frequent bathing as this will dry the skin, lead to pruritus, which will lead to the "itch-scratch-itch" cycle, and eventuate into a full blown exacerbation of the disease. Specific agents for therapeutic baths are discussed in Table 74-1.

DRESSINGS
Open Dressings

Certain disorders require treatment with open, wet dressings to cool the skin, increase evaporative water loss, control itching, allow infected lesions to drain, and facilitate penetration of topical medicaments. The usual dressing material is gauze, terry cloth towels, or flannel bath blankets: for dressings at home, old, clean bed linens may be used. Dressings should be two to four layers thick to hold the

solution on the skin. Cotton-filled dressings should not be used on open wounds, since the cotton lint stays on the wound. Dressings generally are applied after the therapeutic bath and followed with the prescribed topical medication. The dressing should be soaked in the prescribed, warmed solution, wrung out until just damp, applied to the body, and secured in place. To secure dressings for a "mummy wrap" (total body), a bath blanket, or other soft blanket works very well. The patient should be kept warm while extensive dressings are being applied to prevent hypothermia. Heat lamps and blankets help reduce heat loss. Wet dressing should never be covered with occlusive material such as plastic, or incontinence pads. Occlusive material prevents air from reaching the skin, and skin **maceration** (abnormal softening) may result.

Occlusive Dressings

Occlusive dressings are used to hydrate the skin and to apply topical medication, usually steroids. The dressings are applied to the skin after the medication has been applied and then covered with an airtight wrap such as plastic film. Between dressing changes the nurse must assess the skin for atrophy, maceration, inflamed hair follicles (folliculitis), and dilated blood vessels. The dressings may be applied

---

TABLE 74-1   Therapeutic Baths

Type of agent	Rationale	Nursing interventions
Saline or tap water	Used in generalized skin problems Cooling	Determine that bathwater is at proper temperature (96° F); do not allow water to cool excessively
Colloidal		
Oatmeal (Aveeno)	Antipruritic	Disperse medication properly for maximum effect
Cornstarch	Antipruritic lubricating	May be slippery; use bath mats or pads and railings
Soda bicarbonate	Cooling	Avoid contact with eyes
Tar	Antipruritic	Use old linens and towels, since medication stains
Balnetar	Keratolytic	May be slippery
Zetar	Lubricates	Will cause sensitivity to sunlight
Emollient	Softens skin	May be slippery; use bath mats or pads and railings
Alpha-Keri	Hydrates skin	
Lubath	Antipruritic	Observe for itching, indicating an allergy to the agent's perfume
Potassium permanganate	Disinfectant Deodorizing Astringent	Dissolve all crystals before using bath; undissolved crystals may cause a chemical burn. Use old linens and towels, since medication stains permanently

for up to 12 out of 24 hours; however, if side effects develop, the frequency may have to be decreased. Extreme caution should be taken in occluding an open wound, or a wound that may be infected.

Common Skin Disorders

PRURITUS

Pruritus (itching) is one of the most common skin problems. The sensation of itching is a form of pain, as the nonmyelinated C fibers carry both pain and itch perception. Itching and scratching are protective responses to irritating substances such as woolen clothing, soap, or chemicals. Itching also can be a symptom of systemic disease such as severe liver or renal disease. It may follow drug hypersensitivity or blood reactions, and it may occur in the elderly as a result of dry skin. Heat and low humidity also induce pruritus. During the winter months use of a moisturizer and increasing room humidity with a cool mist vaporizer are advantageous. Itching also may be caused by emotional factors or may occur without any apparent skin lesion. Scratching may cause skin damage such as wheals, excoriation (abrasion of the epidermis), redness, skin infections, and open, draining areas. These skin disorders in turn cause tissue anoxia, vasodilation, and inflammation, causing more itching. This process is called the "itch-scratch-itch" cycle. Left untreated, severe pruritus can be disabling.

NURSING MANAGEMENT OF THE PATIENT WITH PRURITUS
Assessment

The nurse asks the patient about any factors that cause itching. The nurse also asks the patient to describe the itching (i.e., does it demonstrate a pattern or occur on skin that is touching the bed linens?). Itching often worsens at night, and the patient may be unable to sleep, since no distractions are available to take his or her mind off the sensation. Therefore the patient's ability to sleep should also be assessed. The assessment focuses on the pattern of skin eruption or excoriation caused by the scratching. The nurse should also investigate whether the eruption was present at the time pruritus began. A patient who complains that the itching begins before the rash is noticeable may be an atopic or may have a systemic cause for the pruritus with the clinical rash only a reaction to the physical scratching of the skin. The skin should be closely examined for any clinical signs of infection, either as a cause of pruritus or as a result of scratching. Infestation must be ruled out in complaints of pruritus.

Nursing Diagnosis

A nursing diagnosis for patients with pruritus is alteration in comfort caused by itching related to inflammation, irritation, or an unknown cause. A second diagnosis may be impaired skin integrity related to open areas secondary to scratching.

Planning

Patient goals are (1) to have the patient express relief from itching and (2) to restore comfort within 1 hour if the itching is acute or within 24 hours if the itching is chronic. Unfortunately some patients cannot be successfully treated for their pruritus. In these cases the goal is to alleviate the itching as much as possible to make it tolerable. The goal for the patient with open areas is to promote healing of those areas, as evidenced by formation of granulation tissue, decreasing drainage, reduction in wound size, and decreasing erythema.

Implementation

Interventions for control of itching include cooling the skin with wet compresses or medicated baths. Antipruritic colloids such as oatmeal, starches, or bath oils may relieve itching for patients with dry, flaky skin or other generalized pruritic skin disorders. The patient will also benefit from keeping the skin lubricated and cool. He or she is taught to use tepid water, not hot water, for bathing and to pat the skin to a moist dry instead of rubbing completely dry. A lubricant is applied immediately after the bath while the skin is still damp to help increase hydration of the stratum corneum. Applying pressure, or an ice pack to "trigger" areas may reduce pruritus. Acute histamine-mediated itching such as from a drug allergy may be treated with antihistamines such as diphenhydramine (Benadryl) or topical steroids, or a combination. Restraints or mittens may be required if the urge to scratch cannot be controlled. Patients who habitually scratch (as in chronic pruritus) may require behavior modification to break the cycle. Fingernails should be trimmed and kept clean. Open wounds may require dressings, topical or systemic antibiotics to treat infection.

Evaluation

Goal attainment is measured by assessing for data that indicate the pruritus has subsided. These include the patient's assurance that he or she does not itch anymore, makes less use of antipruritics, scratches less, or has improved sleep. Goal attainment for patients with open skin lesions is measured by formation of granulation tissue, decreasing drainage, reduction in wound size, and decreasing erythema, as these signs indicate healing.

Inflammatory Skin Disorders

DERMATITIS

The terms *eczema* and *dermatitis* are used interchangeably, although they do have slightly different meanings. Eczema is not a disease; it is a reaction pattern in the skin similar to the reaction patterns of blistering and swelling. **Dermatitis** is inflammation of the skin caused by an allergic response, a stress response, or an unknown factor.

Some common dermatoses such as contact dermatitis can develop into eczema. Contact dermatitis has two sources: a normal allergic reaction to something the skin has touched (a primary irritant) or an allergic reaction and hypersensitivity in patients who are sensitive to a particular substance (an allergic sensitizer). Typical primary irritants include perfumes, soaps, cosmetics, plants, solvents, clothing, shoes, metals (especially nickel), dyes, and preservatives. An allergic sensitizer reaction involves the cell-mediated reaction and a delayed hypersensitivity response. The T cell lymphocyte becomes sensitized when the individual comes in contact with allergens, such as poison ivy or poison oak. The initial response may occur in 5 to 21 days, but exposure a second time evokes a faster reaction, in as little as 12 hours (see Figure 74-1).

Seborrheic dermatitis is an erythema and scaling of the intertriginous areas, such as beneath the breasts and between the fingers. The skin may develop eczema as a result of increased oiliness and perspiration.

NURSING MANAGEMENT OF THE PATIENT WITH DERMATITIS
Assessment

Nursing assessment commonly reveals pruritus, pain, and burning. In mild reactions the skin appears

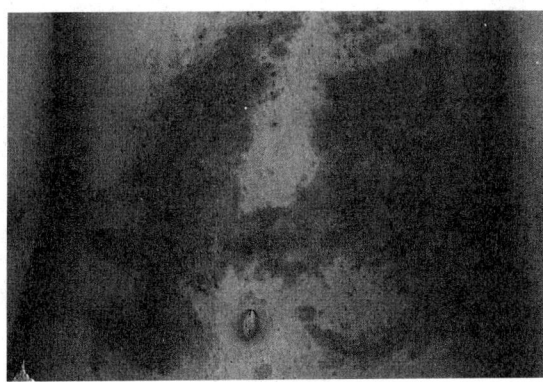

FIGURE 74-1 Contact dermatitis caused by contact with poison ivy. (From Habif TP: *Clinical dermatology: a color guide to diagnosis and treatment*, St Louis, 1985, Mosby–Year Book, Inc.)

red and may have vesicles and oozing. In more severe reactions the skin may develop bullae, erosions, or ulcerations. The patient also may develop systemic reactions such as generalized edema, fever, and malaise. Chronic exposure to allergens may produce red, dry skin with scales, fissures, lichenification, and hypopigmentation. The nurse also assesses for stressful events in the patient's life.

Nursing Diagnosis

Nursing diagnoses include:
  Pain related to itching and inflammation of the skin
  Body image disturbance related to skin lesions
  Impaired skin integrity related to scratching
  Knowledge deficit related to lack of information about causative factors

Planning

The main goals for the patient are to increase comfort and reduce itching, as evidenced by the patient's statements. Other goals are:
  Patient uses less medication for itching
  Patient returns to normal sleep patterns
  Patient has a positive self-concept, as evidenced by positive self-report or activities involving others without covering the exposed areas
  Skin integrity is improved, as evidenced by decreasing size of lesions

Implementation

Interventions for dermatitis are based on the severity of reactions. If the skin is open and weeping, Burrow's solution (aluminum acetate) dressings may be prescribed to dry and heal the skin. Systemic corticosteroids may be prescribed to reduce inflammation or to suppress the allergic response. Once vesicles have dried, steroids can be applied topically. Aveeno baths can soothe generalized dermatitis. Patients with open lesions may require antibiotics to prevent infection. The condition is not contagious, and isolation is not required unless there is documented infection or the patient has HBV or HIV. As with any procedure in which the nurse comes in contact with body fluids, universal precautions must be used. Stress management techniques (see Chapter 3) may be used to reduce or to help the patient cope with stress.

EXFOLIATIVE DERMATITIS

Exfoliative dermatitis (also known as exfoliative erythroderma) is a serious condition involving progressive inflammation of the skin with erythema and scaling. The skin loses its outermost layer (the stratum corneum, or horny layer) causing loss of fluids and protein through capillary walls, resulting in a negative nitrogen balance. Patients with exfoliative dermatitis in the absence of a history of underlying skin disease should have a complete workup to rule out systemic disease such as malignancy.

The condition starts acutely as patchy or generalized red eruptions on the skin. The skin first appears pink and then changes to a dark red. This is due to vasodilation. Within a week the skin *exfoliates* (sheds) thin white or yellow scales, leaving new, smooth red skin. The patient often has a fever, malaise, and flu-like symptoms. Patients may lose hair, have breast enlargement, and have elevated serum uric acid levels. The generalized vasodilation can lead to high cardiac output failure secondary to the shunting of blood to the skin. Exudation secondary to leakage of fluid can lead to fluid and electrolyte imbalance. Anemia is also common, caused by low serum albumin and protein loss. The patient often requires fluids and volume expanders to maintain circulation, as fluids are escaping through the skin. Antibiotics may be prescribed to treat infection, and/or steroids to reduce inflammation. Topically, medicated baths and topical steroids under wet wraps (mummy wraps) are used to help reduce erythema through vasoconstriction. The baths, topical steroids, and wraps also help to make the patient more comfortable.

NURSING MANAGEMENT OF THE PATIENT WITH EXFOLIATIVE DERMATITIS
Assessment

The patient's temperature is assessed frequently for signs of instability. Hypothermia can occur as a result of increased blood flow to the skin and increased loss of heat through convection and evaporation. Patients with exfoliative dermatitis will have chills in the absence of fever due to the loss of the thermoregulatory function of their skin.

The nurse assesses for signs of infection in the skin and reports them if noted. Changes in skin hue, increased drainage, and changes in the color of non-involved skin may be signs of infection. Serum white blood cell counts may rise, and a left shift in the differential may be noticed. Fever is not a reliable sign of infection, as the patient's temperature is unstable.

High output congestive heart failure may be a significant problem related to hyperemia and increased blood flow to the skin. The nurse frequently assesses for symptoms of heart failure. Lung sounds may indicate crackles and rhonchi; cough or orthopnea may be present. The patient may have sacral or leg edema and weight gain. Also, the patient may report itching, dyspnea, leg cramps from hypokalemia, and fatigue. The patient's nutritional status is assessed, since both protein and iron are lost with exfoliation.

Nursing Diagnosis

Common nursing diagnoses include:
  High risk for infection related to loss of skin barrier
  Pain related to itching and skin inflammation
  Hypothermia related to loss of skin
  Impaired skin integrity related to loss of skin surface
  Fluid volume deficit related to evaporation and excretion from open skin

Planning

Goals include stabilizing the patient's fluid volume, as evidenced by stable vital signs, normal serum potassium (3.5 to 5 mEq/L), urine output of 30 mL/hr, normal skin turgor at 3 seconds, and stabilization of body weight within 48 hours of beginning therapy. Also the patient should be more comfortable, as evidenced by less use of analgesia and by verbal statements. The patient should have no clinical signs of skin infection, as evidenced by a normal white blood cell count and absence of fever. A purple or dark hue to the skin may persist secondary to erythroderma in the absence of clinical infection.

Implementation

If exfoliative dermatitis is caused by a medication, the skin symptoms may begin to clear rapidly after discontinuance of the drug, but may persist for up to 2 weeks. Other benign cutaneous causes, such as psoriasis, atopic dermatitis, or malignant causes such as T-cell lymphoma, cannot be cleared as rapidly. Skin care may include frequent tub baths and lubricants to control itching, promote comfort, and enhance absorption of topical medications. Topical steroids in varying strengths are used along with wraps as indicated. Antihistamines, as well as mild sedatives, are commonly used to control pruritus. Bedside cool mist humidifiers, which increase room humidity and help to keep the skin from becoming too dry, may also offer some relief for pruritus.

Volume expanders may be necessary to maintain the patient's blood pressure and urine output. The patient should be kept in a warm room (90 degrees F) to maintain body temperature, and should wear full pajamas (preferably cotton or cotton flannel). The patient should also be reminded to try not to scratch or rub the skin, and that nails should be kept trimmed and clean. Diversional activities may be required to reduce the desire to scratch.

ECZEMA

Eczema is classified as an acute or chronic inflammatory condition. Primary skin changes in acute eczema include tiny red vesicles; secondary changes include scaling and weeping of serous or purulent material, crusting, excoriation, and secondary infection. With chronic eczema, scaling and lichenification also occur at 3 weeks or later.

Atopic eczema is the most severe and the most common form of eczema. Patients with atopic eczema develop macular or papular lesions in response to scratching. These individuals have an itch that rashes, rather than a rash that itches. Their skin is extremely sensitive and there may be identifiable "trigger factors" that start the "itch-scratch-rash" cycle. With continued scratching the macules and papules will develop into vesicles and further into open lesions. In chronic eczema the skin develops scales, crusts, fissures, and lichenification. The cause of atopic eczema is unknown, but it occurs primarily in patients with personal or family history of atopic diseases such as hay fever, asthma, urticaria, or migraine headaches. Of patients who have a history of genetic predisposition to allergy, 30% have atopic eczema.

NURSING MANAGEMENT OF THE PATIENT WITH ECZEMA

Assessment

The subjective symptom of atopic eczema is severe paraoxysmal itching. In adults the objective finding is lichenified brown or gray lesions. Sometimes the lesions are oozing, crusting vesicles. The lesions are very dry unless scratched, rubbed, or torn open. Patients with atopic eczema have very dry skin, since they do not have normal skin lipids or a normal ability to sweat. Also, these patients have a lower resistance to cutaneous viral and bacterial infections; herpes simplex and vaccinia are most dangerous. Drug allergies and sensitivities are common. Serum IgE is elevated, and eczematic patients may have an intolerance of heat and cold. The incidence of cataracts in atopic patients is approximately 10%. The reason for cataract development is not clearly understood. Development may be due to the increased amounts of steroids, both systemic and prolonged topical use, or to keratoconus.[16] When the cataract requires surgical removal, the operation is performed when the eczema is quiescent.

Nursing Diagnosis

The common nursing diagnoses are:
  Impaired skin integrity: high risk for infection
  Pain: itching related to inflammatory process and open wounds
  Knowledge deficit related to lack of information about aggravating factors
  Body image disturbance related to presence of visible lesions

Planning

The immediate goal is to alleviate the patient's itching. Other goals are restoring skin integrity without infection and educating the patient about aggravating factors, as evidenced by the patient's being able to plan how to avoid these factors in everyday life.

Implementation

Interventions begin with eliminating aggravating factors such as extremes of heat, cold, rapid temperature changes, woolen fabrics, friction, emotional stress, fatigue, viruses, and identifiable foods and inhalants to which the individual may be allergic. Vaccinations should be given with caution. The patient should have a dust-free environment and wear clean, loosely fitting pajamas. The skin should be lubricated regularly, especially after hydration in a bath. Bathing restrictions may be instituted during remission to avoid overdrying with water. Only superfatted or neutral soaps should be used for cleansing. Use of soap should be limited to odor producing areas of the body, axillae, groin, and feet. Topical steroids prescribed during exacerbation, emollients, and a good skin care regimen during remission should be stressed. Systemic steroids may be needed during severe exacerbations. Occlusive dressings are employed when patients are in an acute flare (exacerbation). This helps to "cool down" the skin, allow for vasoconstriction, and increase absorption of topical steroids. If food allergies have been identified, a diet program to avoid these allergens should be implemented.

An important activity in a person's normal day, exercise should be done carefully to avoid excessive sweating. The patient is educated on how to care for skin when participating in exercise. Emollients and antihistamines are used to help maintain these activities, if necessary.

Evaluation/Documentation

Goal attainment is evaluated by assessing for relief of itching and restoration of skin integrity. The patient should be able to describe ways to reduce stress that provokes the symptoms. The condition of the skin and the patient's psychologic status are recorded daily. The pain management program should be described, and the effect on the patient's comfort of eliminating aggravating factors should be identified. The teaching plan for long-term self-care should be recorded, as well as the patient's understanding of potential compliance with the program.

Ongoing Care

Before dismissal the patient should be able to discuss plans for eliminating the factors that aggravate the disease. These patients often are asked to alter several aspects of their lives simultaneously. The nurse is sensitive to the stress induced by the need for rapid changes in life-style and assesses the patient's risk for noncompliance.

PSORIASIS
Definition

Psoriasis is a common, chronic disease of rapid epidermal cell production (6 to 9 times the normal cell turnover rate) without cellular maturation of the skin. The normal progression of a cell from the basal cell layer at the bottom of the epidermis to the stratum corneum occurs in 26 to 28 days; in the patient with psoriasis this process occurs in 3 to 4 days. Because of the rapid cell passage to the upper layer of skin, the normal cellular maturation cannot occur.

Etiology

Psoriasis is a genetically determined disease of epidermal proliferation. Although the disease is inherited, it may skip generations making identification of other affected family members difficult. Psoriasis can appear at any age and affects men and women equally.[7] There are several types of psoriasis. Psoriasis vulgaris, or plaque psoriasis, is the most common form; guttate, pustular, and exfoliative psoriasis are other types. Guttate psoriasis usually follows a streptococcal or viral infection (see Figure 74-2).

The pustular and exfoliative forms of the disease are the worst forms.

Clinical Manifestations

Psoriatic lesions appear as red, raised papules that may coalesce into large plaques covered by silvery scale. The plaques are well circumscribed, with the lesions being symmetrical (e.g., both elbows or knees). The scales can be lifted off easily leading to punctate bleeding, or Auspitz sign. Involvement of nails exhibits as pitting, yellow color and may be distorted and separated from the nail bed. Psoriasis may involve the scalp which may lead to alopecia. A form of arthritis has been associated with psoriasis, psoriatic arthritis. The arthritis flares in conjunction with exacerbation of the skin disease and is usually nonsymptomatic during periods of remission. Psoriatic arthritis most commonly affects the hands and the sacroiliac joints, but may affect any joint.

Psoriasis vulgaris exhibits with well circumscribed erythematous lesions with silver scale (Figure 74-3). The lesions are seen most often on the elbows, knees, gluteal folds, sacrum, and scalp. Guttate psoriasis exhibits with a droplike pattern. The lesions are small and coinlike, erythematous and scaly.

In pustular psoriasis, pustules may form on any area of the body, and when they coalesce, form "lakes" of pus. The pustules are sterile, but individuals with this form of the disease are very sick. They are febrile, have problems with thermoregulation, and may develop high cardiac output failure. These individuals require hospitalization and intensive nursing care, including medicated tub baths followed by topical steroids and wet wraps. Exfoliative psoriasis (also categorized as exfoliative erythro-

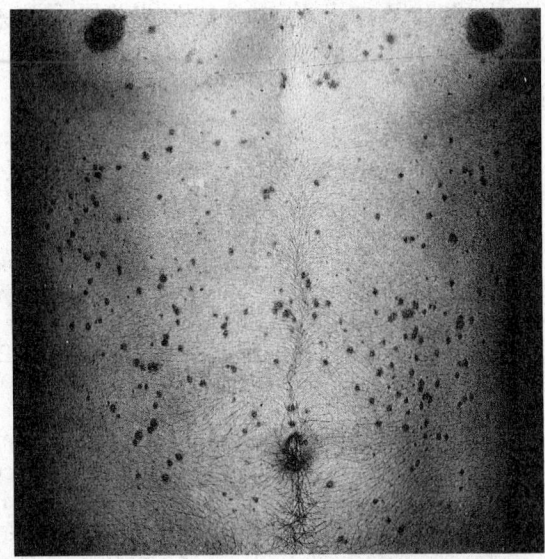

FIGURE 74-2 Guttate psoriasis. Numerous uniformly small lesions may abruptly occur following streptococcal infection. (From Habif TP: *Clinical dermatology: a color guide to diagnosis and treatment,* ed 2, St Louis, 1990, Mosby–Year Book, Inc.)

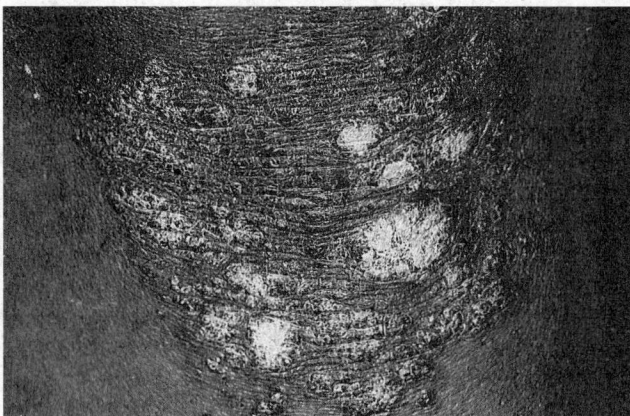

FIGURE 74-3 Psoriasis vulgaris. Typical oval plaque with well-defined borders and silver scale. (From Habif TP: *Clinical dermatology: a color guide to diagnosis and treatment,* ed 2, St Louis, 1990, Mosby–Year Book, Inc.)

derma) is the other serious form of the disease. These individuals, like the pustular patients, require intensive nursing care, with baths, topical steroids, and wet wraps. Since both exfoliative and pustular psoriasis are unstable forms of the disease patients must be monitored closely. In both forms the patient can lose fluid and electrolytes, iron, and up to 9 g of protein a day. Patients can exhibit prostration, fever, and severe tenderness of the skin. In addition high cardiac output failure, pulmonary emboli, exhaustion, pneumonia, and sepsis are possible serious complications. Any form of psoriasis affects the patient psychologically and physically.

Therapeutic Management

The treatment of psoriasis varies; both systemic and topical therapies are used. Because there is no cure for the disease, the goal is limited to controlling the lesions by slowing epidermal cell turnover. Since psoriasis is a chronic problem, the treatment plan must be one the patient understands and can comply with for a lifetime.

One of the oldest treatments is Goeckerman therapy. Coal tar preparations are applied to the skin (avoiding face, groin, and axillae) after the patient has soaked in a medicated tar bath. Tar acts as an antimitotic. After the tar is applied to the skin the patient is exposed to ultraviolet B light, which enhances the action of the tar. After the light treatment, a occlusive lubricant (such as Eucerin or Aquaphor) is applied liberally to the skin surface to enhance the absorption of the tar and to lubricate. In cases where the plaques are extremely thick, a keratolytic may be used to help decrease the thickness of the plaque, which allows for better penetration of topical medicine. Topical steroids and lubricants are used liberally in patients who are in an acute flare (exacerbation). Systemic steroids are very rarely used to treat psoriasis. Even though systemic steroids will quickly stop a flare, upon withdrawal of the steroids a rebound effect occurs. This steroid rebound will cause an immediate flare, or worse, convert the plaque or exfoliative type psoriasis to pustular. Other topical treatments include anthralin, salicylic acid, and photochemotherapy. Anthralin is very irritating and must be applied carefully, avoiding noninvolved skin. It works to help decrease the thickness of the plaques, but the therapy may take an extended period of time. It is generally used when the disease is not progressing with other modalities. Salicylic acid is another irritating modality that is used like anthralin. Photochemotherapy (PUVA) is the use of *P*soralen and *U*ltraviolet *A*. The patient is given psoralen 2 hours before exposure to the ultraviolet light. This treatment is generally successful, but takes a long time before results are seen.

It works best as a maintenance modality after a patient has gone into remission.

In cases that are not responsive to conservative topical treatment, methotrexate or Etretinate (vitamin A derivative) may be used. Methotrexate is used because it inhibits DNA synthesis and acts on the rapidly dividing epidermal cells in the psoriatic lesion. Patients receiving methotrexate must be monitored for renal, hematologic, or hepatic changes. Etretinate is effective in the treatment of palmar-plantar-pustular, erythrodermic and pustular psoriasis, as well as the symptoms of arthritis. Etretinate has some serious side effects and should be used with caution, and only in severe, recalictrant cases. Research on the use of cyclosporine for treatment of severe psoriasis has demonstrated effectiveness; however, there are serious side effects.

NURSING MANAGEMENT OF THE PATIENT WITH PSORIASIS

Assessment findings include psoriatic plaques, guttate lesions, pustules or erythroderma, nail pitting and/or disfigurement, and possible arthritis. The scalp should be examined carefully for involvement. The patient may or may not report itching or associated pain. Exacerbating factors should be explored, such as a recent period of psychologic or physical stress (illness, surgery). The patient's mental status should be assessed, since psoriasis may cause depression and despair.

The treatment of psoriasis varies and the nurse educates the patient about the treatment plan. The patient's knowledge of the disease, its trajectories, and the patient's life-style are assessed before a treatment plan is developed.

The chronicity of the disease is emphasized. A regular skin care program is developed, taking into consideration the patient's life-style. Skin lesions generally can be controlled, and this should be emphasized to the patient. Lesions commonly worsen whenever the skin has been injured or irritated (cuts, scrapes, sunburn). This is known as the Koebner reaction. Physical illness, particularly streptococcal infections, may induce a flare. Emotional stress has also been identified as a factor that may induce a flare. Certain drugs such as beta blockers, lithium, and indocin also can cause exacerbations. It is important that the patient understand the importance of not picking at or scratching the lesions. The patient should also know that, in general, the disease is better managed if his or her life is balanced, with time for work, sleep, exercise, and relaxation. The patient should be taught daily skin care. He or she should be taught to avoid washing too often or overuse of soap and to maintain skin hydration with lubricants.

Infectious Skin Disorders

FOLLICULITIS, FURUNCLES, AND CARBUNCLES

Folliculitis is a staphylococcal infection of hair follicles. It can also be caused by irritation of the hair follicle from use of occlusive topical medications. Small pustules commonly are seen on the shaved body areas such as the face and legs. The hair shaft cannot pierce the skin and turns back into the epidermis, causing infection and inflammation. **Furuncles** (boils) are a dermal form of folliculitis. Furuncles commonly occur on the neck, axillae, and buttocks. A furuncle begins as a small pimple-like area that progresses and deepens. Redness, tenderness, and swelling develop in the area, and within a few days the boil comes to a point of yellow or black color. **Carbuncles** are more invasive furuncles that go deep into the subcutaneous tissue. Patients with carbuncles can become ill with fever, pain, and leukocytosis, because the infection does not limit itself to a confined area. Draining boils should be covered with a dressing. Universal precautions should always be employed when dealing with suppurative lesions.

NURSING MANAGEMENT OF THE PATIENT WITH FOLLICULITIS, FURUNCLES, AND CARBUNCLES

The involved area should not be "popped" since the infection may quickly spread into surrounding tissues. The wall holding the pus apart from normal body tissues can easily break with pressure. The areas can be treated with hot compresses, which help localize the boil or "bring it to a head." At this point the boil can be opened with a sterile scalpel. The incision allows the boil to drain without risk of the wall rupturing. Patients should be taught to use dressings to control drainage on linens and clothing. They also may benefit from daily showers with antibiotic soap to reduce skin bacteria. If a man has folliculitis on the face, he should stop shaving until the condition resolves. The nurse should instruct the patient on prescribed medication, emphasizing the need to complete the entire course of the medication even if he or she feels well.

Healing begins after the lesion has drained, and the skin should have the same appearance as the surrounding skin. A dark red and purple area of scar over the lesion is not uncommon and may require a year to subside.

The condition of the patient's skin and the teaching plan are recorded. The patient's stated understanding or demonstration of the self-care plan provides further documentation of care given.

CELLULITIS

Cellulitis is a diffuse, acute streptococcal or staphylococcal infection of the skin and subcutaneous tissue. Cellulitis occurs most commonly in the lower extremities, usually beginning in an open wound. However, many cases of cellulitis have no obvious source of bacterial entry to the skin. The infection may spread through the lymphatic system from infection sites. Locally, the infection spreads as a result of the release of enzymes produced by the bacteria. The enzymes prevent the normal body responses that would reduce local spread of infection, such as walling off the site. The skin is red, hot to the touch, tender, and swollen. Pitting edema or an orange peel appearance (peau d'orange) may be present. Lymphangitic streaks may extend proximally from the site of infection.

Treatment of cellulitis begins with identifying the infecting organism through tissue or blood cultures. Systemic antibiotics, commonly penicillin or erythromycin, are given and continued for 1 week after signs appear that the infection is clearing. The affected extremity is immobilized and elevated to improve venous return and reduce edema.

NURSING MANAGEMENT OF THE PATIENT WITH CELLULITIS

The nurse inspects the skin for redness, and the skin should be palpated for changes in temperature. Open draining areas may indicate infection. The nurse should assess for edema by measuring the circumference of the extremities and for pain. The affected extremity should be elevated to reduce edema and improve venous return. Aseptic technique and universal precautions must be used for wound care, and isolation may be required. The patient should be assessed for signs of spreading systemic infection (see Chapter 13 for a discussion of septic shock). Pain may be controlled with cool compresses for open lesions or warm compresses for intact and swollen skin. Intravenous antibiotics are administered as ordered, and analgesics are given as needed.

HERPES ZOSTER
Definition/Etiology

Herpes zoster or shingles is a viral infection that causes painful skin vesicles along the nerve distribution (Figure 74-4). It is caused by the varicella virus, the same virus that causes chickenpox. It is assumed that herpes zoster is a reactivation of a latent form of the virus occurring in patients with lowered immunity. Individuals who have not had chickenpox may acquire the disease by exposure to an individual with herpes zoster.

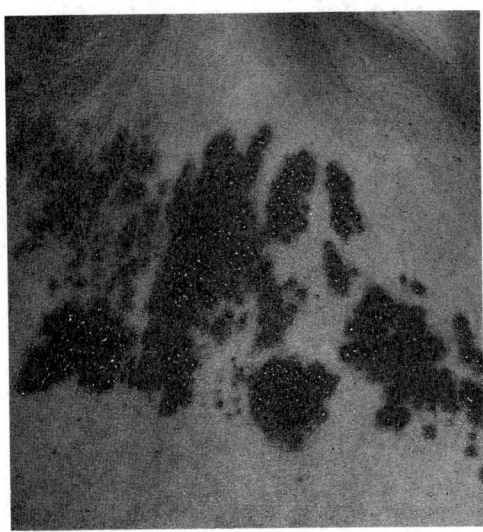

FIGURE 74-4   Herpes zoster. Diffuse involvement of a dermatome. (From Habif TP: *Clinical dermatology: a color guide to diagnosis and treatment*, St Louis, 1985, Mosby–Year Book, Inc.)

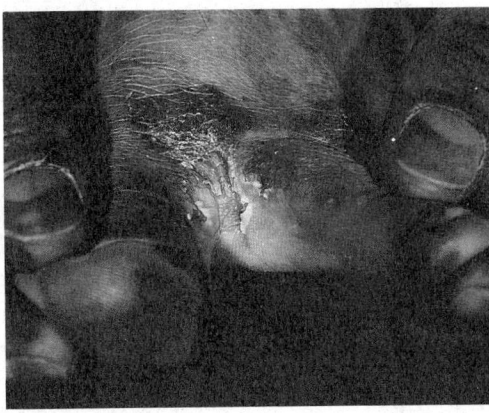

FIGURE 74-5   Tinea pedis. (From Habif TP: *Clinical dermatology: a color guide to diagnosis and treatment*, ed 2, St Louis, 1990, Mosby–Year Book, Inc.)

Clinical Manifestations

The disease begins with pain in nerve dermatome distribution areas or with gastrointestinal distress. The pain may be burning, stabbing, cutting, or aching. The slightest touch or even a breeze may provoke pain. Vesicles appear on the skin in bandlike strips around the body along dermatomal distribution lines. Herpes zoster rarely crosses the midline. If lesions do cross the midline, or become generalized, the patient should be worked up for possible malignancy. Evolution of the lesions is exhibited by rupture of the vesicles and the formation of crusts.

Therapeutic Management

The goal of treatment is to relieve pain, prevent infection and scarring, and reduce the possibility of postherpetic neuralgia. Oral analgesics are prescribed and have been shown to reduce the incidence of persistent pain. The lesions also may be injected with steroids. Acyclovir, if started early, may reduce the severity of herpes zoster. Wet dressings or shake lotions may be used to help dry the lesions and control pain. Silver sulfadiazine may also be used to prevent secondary infection.

NURSING MANAGEMENT OF THE PATIENT WITH HERPES ZOSTER

Patients should be taught how to apply topical medications, correctly take systemic medications, and apply wet dressings. Universal precautions help control the spread of the infectious fluid found in the lesions. Linens should be washed separately, and separate bath linen should be used. Children and individuals who have not had chickenpox should be kept away from the patient during outbreaks.

FUNGAL INFECTIONS

Most fungal skin infections are easily treated; in contrast, systemic fungal infections can be lethal. The common name for fungal infections is "ringworm"; other names are "athlete's foot" and "jock itch." Tinea infections, often called ringworm, are summarized in Table 74-2. (Also see Figure 74-5 for an illustration of tinea pedis.)

PARASITIC SKIN DISORDERS

Parasitic skin disorders are more common in patients from low socioeconomic backgrounds and in the elderly. These groups of patients may have poor hygienic practices because they are unable to obtain materials for hygiene. The infestation may occur in families with children who become infected at school or in day care. Lice can transmit rickettsial diseases such as typhus.

Pediculosis

Pediculosis is infestation of the body, skin, or hair by lice. Lice appear as small, silvery, shiny, oval eggs along the back of the head, behind the ears, or in the hair. When the eggs hatch, the lice bite for food, which leads to intense itching. The scratching may lead to secondary infection, crusts, or matted hair. Hair lice are contagious and spread through shared combs, brushes, hats, and bed linens. Head lice infestation is treated with lindane (Kwell) shampoo.

TABLE 74-2   Summary of Tinea

Type	Distribution	Occurrence	Clinical features
Tinea corporis	Nonhairy parts of body; face; neck; extremities	More common in hot and humid climates; more common in rural than in urban settings; occurs in both adults and children	Pruritus; papulosquamous annular lesions with raised borders; lesions expand peripherally with central clearing
Tinea cruris	Groin; inner thigh; scrotum or labia not involved	More common in adult men; tends to recur; flare-ups common in summer; aggravated by tight clothes, perspiration, and physical activity	Pruritus; hypopigmented; well-demarcated lesions; dryness and scaling; pustules present at margins; central clearing sometimes present; secondary bacterial or candidal infection and maceration common
Tinea capitis	Scalp	More common in children; contagious	Lesions vary; small, gray scaly patches with short broken hairs; mild erythematous papules; raised, boggy, inflamed nodules dotted with perifollicular abscesses; thick, yellow, suppurative lesions; lesions may be small coalesced, or cover entire scalp; hairless patches
Tinea pedis	Feet; begins in third and fourth interdigital spaces and spreads to involve plantar surface; may involve nails	Rare in children; not transmitted by simple exposure	Lesions vary; maceration, scaling, fissuring of interdigital space; vesicular scaling, erythema of plantar surface; chronic, noninflamed, diffuse scaling; nails brittle, discolored; pruritus
Tinea unguium	Toenails and (less commonly) fingernails	—	Nails thickened, lusterless, and discolored; subungual debris; nail plate crumbling or absent

From Thompson JM et al: *Mosby's manual of clinical nursing*, ed 2, St. Louis, 1989, Mosby–Year Book, Inc.

After shampooing, any eggs (nits) should be picked from the hair. Pediculosis corporis is infestation with body lice, usually along the trunk and neck. Lice live and may been seen on clothing. Pediculosis pubis is genital lice infestation and is spread by sexual contact. The lice often leave red brown excretions on the patient's underwear. Lice may be seen on the hair. Body or pubic lice infestation may be treated with lindane, permethrin, or crotamiton.

Scabies

Scabies is infestation of the skin by the itch mite. The patient reports severe itching, especially at night. When the skin is examined, small, raised burrows may be seen. The female mite burrows into the skin and lays eggs. A burrow may look like a thread on the skin, most commonly seen in the finger webs and on the wrists, but any body part may be involved. Lindane is used to treat the infestation.

NURSING MANAGEMENT OF THE PATIENT WITH PARASITIC SKIN DISORDERS

The patient and family are taught measures to prevent the infestation from spreading. For head lice, comb and hair brushes should be cleaned with hot water and lindane. Linens should be washed in hot water (130° F). Furniture, rugs, and floor should be thoroughly cleaned. Clothing must be machine washed or dry cleaned. The patient and family may need the opportunity to ventilate their concerns about being labeled as dirty or unclean.

Autoimmune Disorders

PEMPHIGUS VULGARIS

Pemphigus vulgaris is an autoimmune disease that causes blistering in the epidermis. Patients have large, flaccid, blisters (bullae). Because the blisters are in the epidermis, they have a very thin covering of skin and break easily, leaving large denuded areas of skin. On initial exam, patients may have crusting areas instead of intact blisters. The lesions are painful, open, bleed easily, and heal slowly. The fluid that drains from the bullae is serum and very foul smelling. Bacterial infection of the open areas is common. Patients often have blisters in the mouth, anus, vagina, pharynx, and larynx. Pemphigus usually appears in patients in their 40s and 50s. It can be fatal.

Pemphigus is treated with steroids, immunosuppressive drugs (Cytoxan, Imuran, gold), and plasmapheresis. Adrenocortocotropic hormone (ACTH) also may be prescribed in acute stages of the disease. Once the acute phase has passed, immunosuppressive drugs may be used for control. These drugs require 3 to 4 weeks to take effect and therefore are not prescribed for early treatment of the disease. Plasmapheresis is the removal and reinfusion of treated plasma cells. The process reduces the circulating levels of antibodies, thereby reducing the immune reaction. Plasmapheresis is used as maintenance therapy.

NURSING MANAGEMENT OF THE PATIENT WITH PEMPHIGUS VULGARIS

Assessment

The patient's skin is assessed daily for new blisters or signs of local or systemic infection. The skin adjacent to the blistered areas is examined first. Nikolsky's sign, the ability to blister and slough the epidermis with lateral finger pressure, frequently is present. The mouth and mucous membranes are evaluated for color, pain, and consistency of saliva (thin or thick). The mouth is checked for white patches of *Candida* infection, as such infections are common in patients taking steroids. The foul odor and the patient's pain make this dermatologic problem difficult to treat. The nurse is sensitive to the patient's feelings of anger and embarrassment. It is important for the nurse to control feelings about the smell of the drainage while with the patient.

Nursing Diagnosis

Common nursing diagnoses include:

Impaired skin integrity related to loss of skin barrier from broken blisters

Pain related to open wounds

Fluid volume deficit related to fluid loss through open skin

Altered nutrition; less than body requirements related to impaired mucous membranes

Altered mucous membranes related to open draining lesions

Body image disturbance related to the reaction of others to wounds

Planning

Goals for the patient include restoring skin integrity within 7 to 10 days, as evidenced by no new blister formation, healing, dry skin, and no clinical signs of infection: improving the patient's comfort, as evidenced by his statements and decreasing use of analgesics; assuring adequate nutrition and fluids, as evidenced by stable body weight and fluid balance: and improving the patient's self-esteem.

Implementation

Mouth care every 2 hours with half strength mouthwashes and water begins on admission. Commercial mouthwashes are not used since they are concentrated and can cause burning. Viscous xylocaine may help reduce pain before eating and drinking. If the patient's mouth does not receive proper care, nutritional intake will decrease, resulting in delayed healing. The lips should be kept moist with petrolatum or lip balm.

Infection is the leading cause of death in patients with pemphigus, and nurses must be careful to assess for infection and institute measures that reduce the risk for infection. Patients with pemphigus are most often on steroids which can mask the symptoms of infection. Therefore the nurse must pay particular attention to more subtle signs of infection such as changes in vital signs. Serum exudate and body secretions should be examined for changes in color, and the results of culture and sensitivity tests must be reported so that appropriate antibiotics can be prescribed. Universal precautions must be observed at all times.

Evaluation/Documentation

The degree of goal attainment is evaluated by assessing for (1) improved skin and mucous membrane integrity; (2) improved patient comfort, as demonstrated by his statements and a decrease in the amount of analgesia required, (3) adequate caloric intake for body size; and (4) a stable fluid balance, with urinary output of 30 mL/hr. The patient also should be making positive statements about himself or herself and should be able to look at the skin lesions without negative facial or verbal expressions. The condition of the skin, presence of infection, and response to the treatment plan is recorded. Subtle signs of infection may be the only cues, and the nurse should be astute in assessing the patient.

Ongoing Care

Upon dismissal the patient and family should know about any follow-up needed for medications. Steroids require a specific taper schedule to prevent adrenal crisis. Because immunosuppressive drugs can alter liver function and blood cell production, follow-up liver studies and blood cell counts are necessary. Long-term use of immunosuppressive drugs also has been shown to increase the risk of carcinoma. The patient usually finds that heat and sweating worsen the condition, so he or she is instructed to stay cool and avoid wearing clothes on the involved open areas.

TOXIC EPIDERMAL NECROLYSIS

Toxic epidermal necrolysis (TEN) is a severe skin reaction to drug ingestion or viral infection. Drugs most commonly associated with TEN are barbiturates, antibiotics, sulfonamides, hydantoins, and allopurinol. The cause of TEN is unknown, but it may be linked to the immune system. Initial symptoms of the disease are burning sensations in the eyes, skin tenderness, fever, malaise, and joint pain. Within a few hours to 2 days, the skin develops a rash that evolves into generalized skin erythema and sloughing. Patients with TEN are critically ill, and the disease has a high mortality, ranging from 25% to 50%.[7] The major cause of death is sepsis from infection of the skin and mucousal surfaces. If the loss of skin is through the dermis, scarring is possible. Skin loss may be as high as 100%. Treatment is similar to that for exfoliative dermatitis and burns. All nonessential drugs are discontinued immediately.

NURSING MANAGEMENT OF THE PATIENT WITH TOXIC EPIDERMAL NECROLYSIS

Nursing care of the patient with TEN is similar to that for exfoliative dermatitis, pemphigus, and burns. The patient's skin is very fragile and will tear off with harsh handling. Intake and output must be monitored carefully along with electrolyte balance. Due to the incapacitating aspect of the disease, the patients must be monitored carefully for atelectasis;

their barrier function must be maintained until their skin regenerates. Air-fluidized beds reduce the risk of skin tears by reducing the amount of direct handling of the patient. Oral mucosa require care every 2 hours with prescribed mouthwashes and water. Maintaining adequate nutrition is a challenge and viscous xylocaine may be used before eating to help with discomfort. If the patient is unable to ingest food normally, parenteral nutrition should be instituted.

SCLERODERMA

Scleroderma is an autoimmune disorder with alteration and fibrosis of connective tissue in skin and internal organs. The disease has both systemic and local forms. It is more common in women and usually begins in the 30s. Systemic sclerosis has two major subsets, diffuse scleroderma and CREST (*C*alcinosis cutis, *R*aynaud's phenomenon, *E*sophageal involvement, *S*clerodactyly, *T*elangiectasia).

Diffuse sclerosis may be rapidly progressive and fatal due to extensive fibrosis and degenerative changes in internal organs. Organs most often affected include lungs, kidneys, esophagus, intestinal tract and heart. CREST syndrome is slowly progressive, with the skin being the major organ involved. Involvement of internal organs usually is delayed. In systemic sclerosis, the skin initially has hard, smooth, round, ivory-colored plaques that are immobile and bound tightly to the underlying structures. As the disease progresses, the areas atrophy and the skin becomes smooth, yellowish, and firm. The earliest symptoms occur in the hands and face. In advanced disease the face becomes masklike, the fingers clawlike and useless (Figure 74-6). Autoamputation of digits is possible as the disease progresses. Patients have symptoms of Raynaud's disease, the gastrointestinal tract may be become involved, and the patient has difficulty with digestion, diarrhea, and constipation. The fibrosis will extend to the heart, lungs, and kidneys.

Localized scleroderma is restricted to skin involvement. Raynaud's phenomenon, acrosclerosis, and involvement of internal organs are not seen with localized scleroderma. Three forms of localized scleroderma have been identified. They are morphea, linear scleroderma, and en coup de sabre. Morphea can occur at any age, but is most often seen after the age of 30. It begins spontaneously with thickening of the skin. The skin becomes bound down and the skin color changes to a purple, which eventually evolves into an ivory-colored area of involvement. Theses areas will enlarge over time and show no signs of improvement. Linear scleroderma consists of bands of sclerosis that cross joint lines. Eventually they may lead to mild, or occasionally severe, joint contractures. Linear morphea, unlike

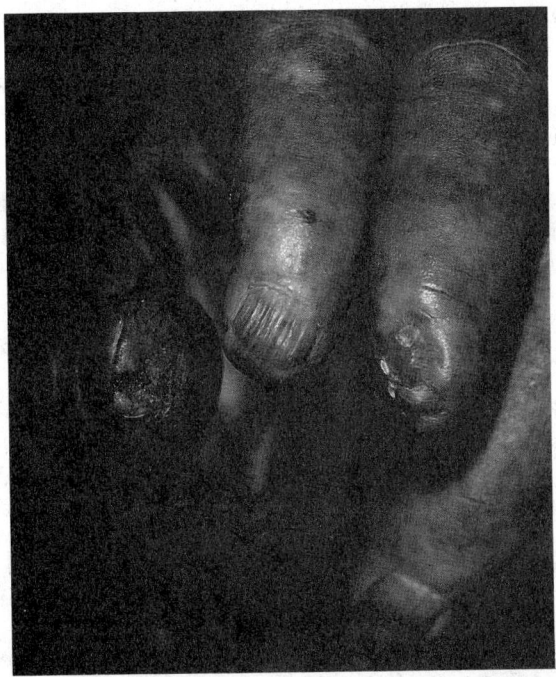

FIGURE 74-6 Scleroderma. Fingertips are narrowed and the fingers are shortened as a result of distal bone resorption. (From Habif TP: *Clinical dermatology: a color guide to diagnosis and treatment*, ed 2, St Louis, 1990, Mosby–Year Book, Inc.)

morphea, may involve the subcutaneous tissue and muscle. The last form of localized scleroderma is en coup de sabre. The clinical appearance is that of a sharp, deep, vertical line of sclerosis on the face such as would be caused by the blade of a sabre. Atrophy of one side of the face may evolve over time.

NURSING MANAGEMENT OF THE PATIENT WITH SCLERODERMA

Management of scleroderma is not well defined, and there is no known cure. Several medications have been tried, but none seem to arrest or slow the disease process. Management is aimed at reducing the symptoms and making the patient as comfortable as possible. Physical therapy is the most beneficial treatment for patients with scleroderma. Penicillamine has been proven effective in reducing skin thickness and slowing progression of visceral disease. Topical steroids with occlusion, or infusion of injectable steroids directly into the plaques, may be beneficial in morphea. Multiple lesions that are in an active inflammatory stage may be treated with hydroxychloroquine sulfate. Linear scleroderma is treated with early and aggressive physical therapy.

Patients with symptoms of Raynaud's phenomenon may be helped with vasodilators. Patients with digestive problems may be treated with tetracycline, as the symptoms are worsened by bacterial growth in the intestine. Mastication is difficult. Patients should be placed in reverse Trendelenburg position to facilitate swallowing and digestion.

DERMATOMYOSITIS

Dermatomyositis is a rare autoimmune disease causing skin and muscle inflammation. Onset may be acute or insidious, but most often it is acute. The patient usually reports weakness of the proximal and girdle muscles. He or she may report inability to climb stairs, rise from a low chair, raise arms over the head, or turn over in bed. The cause of the disease is unknown, it may occur at any age, and it is equally as prevalent in women as men. Dermatomyositis in adults can be associated with malignancy and collagen vascular disease. In adults, the course may be acute, chronic, recurrent, or cyclic. The skin signs of dermatomyositis include the diagnostic heliotrope (violaceous discoloration around the eyes), Gottron's papules (smooth, violaceous-to-red, flat-topped papules over the knuckle), a photosensitive violaceous eruption (usually over bony prominences), periungual telangiectasia, and poikiloderma (finely mottled white and brown pigmented areas, telangiectasia, and atrophy in sun-exposed areas).[16]

Treatment includes high doses of steroids to reduce inflammation. If the patient does not respond to the systemic steroids, then immunosuppressive drugs, such as methotrexate or azathioprine, are substituted or used in conjunction with the steroids. Antimalarials (hydroxychloroquine sulfate or chloroquine phosphate) can be effective in treating the cutaneous lesions but have no effect on the muscle disease.[16] Plasmapheresis also has been used to remove serum components responsible for the symptoms. Rest is critical to reduce muscle damage. Physical therapy, except for ROM exercises to prevent contractures, should be started after muscle inflammation has subsided.

NURSING MANAGEMENT OF THE PATIENT WITH DERMATOMYOSITIS

During acute stages of the disease, the patient needs total care. A patient with dermatomyositis does not appear as ill as other patients needing total care (e.g., stroke patients), but he or she is very weak and should not be left alone to transfer to the chair or to perform any care unless the nurse is sure the patient has the strength and endurance. A chair and toilet with a high seat should be used to facilitate rising up from it. The patient is not encouraged to perform self-care because muscle damage can occur in acute stages of the disease. The patient often requires assistance with eating and cannot eat quickly because of dysphagia.

Pressure-Related Conditions

PRESSURE ULCERS
Definition

Pressure ulcer is the term used to describe localized tissue destruction that is directly related to prolonged pressure. Pressure causes interference of the blood supply leading to vascular insufficiency and ultimately tissue anoxia and death. Pressure ulcers may range in size from small (dime-sized) and shallow (partial thickness) to large (grapefruit-sized) and deep (full thickness) (see Table 74-3). Pressure ulcers are also called decubitus ulcers (from the Latin word *decumbere,* to lie down) because they are commonly seen in bedridden individuals. It is now known that a patient does not have to be bedridden to develop a pressure ulcer.

Etiology

Pressure ulcers may develop in any position that is constantly maintained. The most common sites for ulcer development are sacrum, coccyx, ischial tuberosities, greater trochanters, elbows, heels, scapulae, occipital bone, sternum, ribs, iliac crests, patellae, lateral malleoli, and medial malleoli. Pressure alone is not the only causative factor in ulcer formation. Pressure acts along with any of the following: fric-

tion, shear, moisture, poor nutrition, presence of an underlying disease state, elevated temperature, infection, or incompetent circulation. Muscle tissue is more sensitive to ischemia than skin tissue, consequently deep muscle tissue may be necrotic by the time overlying skin is affected.

All risk factors mentioned above must be considered in the etiology of pressure ulcers. Friction is the action of two surfaces moving across one another. In hospitalized or bedridden patients, friction can result from being pulled across the bed sheet during repositioning. This action can "rub" away (abrade) the stratum corneum, which results in loss of barrier function. Shear is the tearing or stretching of tissue. This may occur when a patient "slides" down in bed while in a sitting position. This sliding results in the outer tissues staying in place by sticking to the bed linen while deeper tissues slide downward. The tissues are being pulled in opposite directions, resulting in stretching, obstruction, or tearing of tissue.

Moisture due to incontinence, wound drainage, or diaphoresis can macerate the skin. Macerated skin erodes easily and allows for softening of connective tissue. Patients who are immobile have the greatest risk of ulcer formation. These patients need to have their position changed frequently, and appropriate pressure-relieving devices should be employed. Malnutrition states put a patient at risk for pressure ulcer formation due to decreased tissue tolerance. Nutritional intake is not only directly related to the quality of body tissue but also to ability to heal. Patients' nutritional intake and serum albumin levels are monitored closely.

TABLE 74-3   Stages of Pressure Ulcers

Stage	Description	Goal of intervention
I	A reddened area that returns to normal skin color after 15 to 20 minutes of pressure relief (e.g., turning to other side). The skin is intact, but the area may appear pale when pressure first is removed.	To cover and protect.
II	Area in which the top layer of skin is missing. The ulcer usually is shallow with a pinkish red base, and white or yellow eschar may be present.	To cover, protect, hydrate, insulate, and absorb.
III	Deep ulcers that extend into the dermis and subcutaneous tissues. White, gray, or yellow eschar usually is present at the bottom of the ulcer and the ulcer crater may have a lip or edge. Purulent drainage is common.	To cover, protect, hydrate, insulate, absorb, cleanse, prevent infection, and promote granulation.
IV	Deep ulcers that extend into muscle and bone. These ulcers have a foul smell and the eschar is brown or black. Purulent drainage is common.	To cover, protect, hydrate, insulate, absorb, cleanse, prevent infection, obliterate dead space, and promote granulation.

Increased temperature either due to febrile states, or from exogenous sources such as sun lamps, can be contributing factors for pressure ulcer formation and delayed healing. Elevations in temperature increase metabolic rate and the need for oxygen and nutrients. This increased demand in an already compromised pressure site is detrimental. Infection increases metabolic rate, as does temperature elevation, thus having similar effects on tissue.

Compromised circulation, as in peripheral vascular disease, increases a patient's risk for pressure ulcer development because of decreased tissue oxygenation. Other underlying disease states, such as diabetes mellitus, can put a patient at risk. In diabetes patients may have poor circulation or neuropathies, which will increase risk for ulcer formation. Diabetics generally have impaired wound healing, which also increases their risk factors. Elderly individuals are at higher risk for development of pressure ulcers due to any of the factors mentioned. In addition, aging skin has less subcutaneous tissue, elastin, and collagen fibers, and decreased moisture. All of these factors contribute to skin friability and decrease the ability of the skin to withstand pressure, friction, and shear.

NURSING MANAGEMENT OF THE PATIENT WITH PRESSURE ULCERS
Assessment

To assess the patient's risk of forming pressure ulcers, the nurse must know the causes of pressure sores. Several assessment guides are currently available for use (e.g., Gosnell or Braden). The factors common to most are mobility, activity, mental status, medications that cause changes in blood flow or cognitive ability, continence, nutritional status, age, and chronic illnesses (Table 74-4). Patients are assessed and given a score, which can range from 5 to 20. The higher the score, the greater the risk of developing pressure ulcers. Other descriptive data such as vital signs also are requested in the assessment.

Common areas of skin breakdown (pressure points) are assessed a minimum of every 2 hours in patients at risk. Tissue temperature may be elevated over areas of released pressure with reactive hyperemia. The skin may feel cold over areas of actual necrosis.[9]

Assessment of risk for pressure ulcers is complex and extensive. Data gathered on admission do not accurately predict the risk of pressure ulcers.[19] Patients should be reassessed as their condition changes. In assessing a pressure sore, the nurse collects data on the location and size of the sore, the presence of eschar or exudate, and whether the wound has sinus tracts. Sinus tracts are open tunnels through the surrounding skin caused by bacteria and drainage; they indicate that the ulcer is severe and requires additional care. If the ulcer is covered with necrotic tissue (eschar), the necrotic tissue must be removed before the ulcer may be staged or assessed for appropriate treatment. Eschar also may slow or inhibit healing all together. New tissue, or granulation tissue, migration is slowed by the presence of necrotic tissue. The most important aspects in the treatment of ulcers is to keep the wound moist, free of exudate and necrotic tissue, and protect with artificial barriers (dressings) to allow for healing.

Nursing Diagnosis

A nursing diagnosis for patients at risk of forming pressure ulcers is high risk for impaired skin integrity related to a specific factor such as prolonged immobility. A nursing diagnosis for a patient with a pressure ulcer is impaired skin integrity. The nurse indicates the stage of the ulcer as part of the problem statement. The cause will reflect the risk factors that contributed to development of the sore.

Planning

Nursing care is planned to achieve the following outcomes:
   Skin remains intact
   Ulcers are free of necrotic tissue/infection
   Granulation tissue forms in ulcers
   Wound becomes smaller
   Ulcers heal

Implementation

Prevention

Preventive measures to provide relief from prolonged pressure cannot be overemphasized. Pressure points are inspected, even if the patient must be lifted off the bed to see the buttocks. Patients are turned or lifted a minimum of every 2 hours. If a patient is developing reddened areas that do not disappear within 10 minutes after a change in position, the schedule is increased. Even small shifts in body weight at unscheduled intervals reduce the incidence of ulcer formation.[17] Massage should be used cautiously. If tissue is reddened (hyperemic) massage may cause maceration and damage to ischemic tissue. Deep massage may angulate and tear vasculature, resulting in a decrease in the delivery of oxygen and nutrients.[12]

Turn patients so that they are not lying directly on the acromial process or greater trochanter. They should rest on pillows supporting the body at a 30- to 45-degree angle to the bed. The smaller angle reduces the direct pressure on the hips and shoulders.

TABLE 74-4 Pressure Sore Risk Assessment Ratings and Classifications

Variable	Rating				
	1	2	3	4	5
Mental status: An assessment of one's level of response to environment	Alert: Oriented to time, place, and person. Responsive to all stimuli, and understands explanations.	Apathetic: Lethargic, forgetful, drowsy, passive, and dull. Sluggish, depressed. Able to obey simple commands. Possibly disoriented to time.	Confused: Partial and/or intermittent disorientation to time, place, and person. Purposeless response to stimuli. Restless, aggressive, irritable, anxious, and may require tranquilizers or sedatives.	Stuporous: Total disorientation. Does not respond to name, simple commands, or verbal stimuli.	Unconscious: Nonresponsive to painful stimuli.
Continence: The amount of bodily control of urination and defecation.	Fully controlled: Total control of urine and feces.	Usually controlled: Incontinent of urine and/or of feces not more often than once every 48 hours or has Foley catheter and is incontinent of feces.	Minimally controlled: Incontinent of urine or feces at least once every 24 hours.	Absence of control: Consistently incontinent of both urine and feces.	
Mobility: The amount and control of movement of one's body.	Full: Able to control and move all extremities at will. May require the use of a device but turns, lifts, pulls, balances, and attains sitting position at will.	Slightly limited: Able to control and move all extremities but a degree of limitation is present. Requires assistance of another person to turn, pull, balance, and/or attain a	Very limited: *Can assist another person* who must initiate movement via turning, lifting, pulling, balancing, and/or attaining a sitting position (contractures, paralysis may be	Immobile: Does not assist self in any way to change position. Is unable to change position without assistance. Is completely dependent on others for movement.	

	sitting position at will but self-initiates movement or request for help to move.		present).
Activity: The ability of an individual to ambulate.	**Ambulatory:** Is able to walk unassisted. Rises from bed unassisted. With the use of a device such as cane or walker is able to ambulate without the assistance of another person.	**Walks with help:** Able to ambulate with assistance of another person, braces, or crutches. May have limitation of stairs.	**Chairfast:** Ambulates only to a chair, requires assistance to do so or is confined to a wheelchair.	**Bedfast:** Is confined to bed during entire 24 hours of the day.
Nutrition: The process of food intake.	Eats some food from each basic food category every day and the majority of each meal served or is on tube feeding.	Occasionally refuses a meal or frequently leaves at least half of a meal.	Seldom eats a complete meal and only a few bites of food at a meal.	

Vital signs: The temperature, pulse, respiration, and blood pressure to be taken and recorded at the time of every assessment rating.

Skin appearance: A description of observed skin characteristics: color, moisture, temperature, texture.

Diet: Record the specific diet order.

24-hour fluid balance: The amount of fluid intake and output during the previous 24-hour period should be recorded.

Medications: List name, dosage, frequency and route for all prescribed medications. In a PRN order, list the pattern for the period since last assessment.

Interventions: List all devices, measures, and/or nursing care activity being used for the purpose of pressure sore prevention.

Comments: Use this space to add explanation or further detail regarding any of the previously recorded data, patient condition, etc. or to describe anything which you believe to be of importance but not accounted for previously.

From Gosnell D: Assessment and evaluation of pressure sores, *Nurs Clin North Am* 22(2):399, 1987.

Pillows also can be placed to relieve pressure from any point. The general position of the patient in bed or in the chair should be assessed, and pillows should be used to support anatomic alignment. Patients should not be pulled up to the head of the bed by their arms, since this greatly increases the risk of shearing injury to the sacrum. Patients also should not remain in a semi-Fowler position for extended periods, since the sacral skin shears easily from the prolonged pressure. With each position change the skin is assessed and skin care given. Lotions lubricate the skin during back rubs. Rubbing alcohol does not toughen the skin, as once thought; rather, it dries the skin and should not be used in skin care.

There are many devices for relieving pressure. They are not substitutes for nursing care, but they may lengthen the interval between skin care and repositioning. The effectiveness of any device is based on studies done measuring surface-tissue interface pressures. These pressures must be low enough to allow capillary blood flow.[10,12] Pressure-relieving devices work by redistributing pressure, particularly at bony prominences. Devices range from mattress overlays such as foams, gel, and water- or air-filled cushions to specialized beds such as air-fluidized or low air loss.[12]

Wound management

Wound cleansing

All wounds must be clean to heal. Any necrotic tissue must be removed, because necrotic tissue is a perfect host for bacteria and increases the risk of systemic bacterial infection. The goal of wound cleansing is removal of bacteria and surface contaminates (foreign bodies, purulent exudate, slough), and protection of the wound.[4] Some wound cleansing agents, particularly topical antiseptics, may be deleterious to wound healing. Such things as hexachlorophene, chlorhexidene, and povidone-iodine scrubs have proven to be damaging to healing wounds, therefore indiscriminate use is avoided.[12] Normal saline may be used as a safe method of wound cleansing in most cases. Gentle flushing, in order to not disturb new epithelial cells, is always preferable over forced irrigation. The goal of cleansing a necrotic or infected wound is to remove debris and bacteria while minimizing tissue damage. Surfactant cleansers, saline, or selective topical antiseptics can be used. Topical antiseptics may be cytotoxic and should only be used in a heavily contaminated wound.[4]

Debridement

Debridement is the removal of devitalized tissue and is extremely important in the management of a contaminated wound. Debridement can be accomplished by one of three methods: mechanical, chemical, or autolytic. Mechanical, or sharp surgical debridement, is very effective and preserves more tissue. Wet-to-dry dressings may be used for mechanical debridement, but this method indiscriminately removes healthy tissue along with the necrotic tissue. Chemical debridement is accomplished with topical enzymes. These enzymes act on collagen and liquefy necrotic debris. Autolytic debridement is accomplished with the use of occlusive and semiocclusive dressings. By occluding the wound, the body's own enzymes are allowed to act on necrotic tissue.

Wound dressings

Choosing the appropriate dressing is a critical step in wound healing (Table 74-5), and the nurse must decide which of the many products available best fits the patient's needs. The nurse considers the location of the ulcer, the stage of the wound, the amount of drainage, the presence of infection or necrotic tissue, the frequency of dressing changes, the cost, the ease of use, and the patient's comfort.

Nonabsorptive thin films are excellent for treating stage I and stage II ulcers and skin tears. Because these films usually are coated with adhesive on one side and are permeable to fluids, they create a desirable moist environment that speeds healing. Absorptive gel wafers also work well on stage I and stage II ulcers. Deep ulcers, stages III and IV, require packing that reduces infection and debrides the

---

TABLE 74-5 Appropriate Wound Coverings

	Stage of wound*		Eschar slough		
	I	II		III	IV
Ointments	E	S	O	O	O
Plasticized coatings	E	E	O w	O w/d	O w	w
Gauze: wet, wet/dry	O	S	S	S	S
Thin films (nonabsorptive)	E	E	S	S	S
Thick wafers (absorptive)	E	E	S	S	S
Absorptive gels	O	E	S	E	E
Enzymatic debriding agents	O	O	E	O	O
Lubricating sprays	E	E	O	E	E

From Fowler E: Equipment and products used in treatment of pressure ulcers, *Nurs Clin North Am* 22(2):449, 1987.
*O, not appropriate or not used; E, excellent; S, satisfactory; w, wet; w/d, wet/dry.

wound upon removal. Dead space must be filled in any wound before an outer dressing is applied. This may be accomplished with the use of fillers such as granules, dextromer beads, or packing.

Surgery

Surgery is an alternative to the long process of cleaning an ulcer and supporting it while it heals. Surgical repair is performed on stage III and stage IV ulcers, on ulcers larger than 2 cm in diameter, and in patients who can tolerate surgery.[2] In stage III ulcers, normal tissue near the wound is rotated to cover it. Deep stage IV ulcers often require myocutaneous flaps to replace missing tissue.

Evaluation

The degree of goal attainment should be evaluated for patients with impaired skin integrity or high risk for impairment. Patients with high risk for impaired skin integrity are assessed for intact skin with no signs of prolonged redness over pressure areas.

Goal attainment for patients with pressure ulcers depends on the ulcer; stage I ulcers should have intact skin and reduced risk of breakdown; stage II, stage III, and stage IV ulcers should have a clean wound with granulation tissue appearing, a reduction in wound size, and reduced wound drainage.

Documentation

Accurate documentation of thorough assessment, planning, and intervention is critical. All areas of risk, including changes in or reduction of risk factors, are charted every 4 hours in the high-risk patient. The lower-risk patient should have documentation at least twice daily.

Ongoing Care

The changeable risk factors should be monitored to determine the continued risk. The patient or family should be aware of the risk factors and should understand how to reduce the risk of skin breakdown. For example, a patient who is malnourished requires continual nutritional support. A patient with reduced sensation should be fitted with an individual chair or wheelchair cushion. However, the cushion does not eliminate the need for continued movement, and the patient is taught how and when to move about in the chair. A paraplegic patient is taught to examine his or her skin upon arising and before going to bed. If reddened areas are noted, the patient, should not rest on that area for 30 minutes and should shift the body more often. Quadriplegic and hemiplegic patients require the same care, but it usually is performed by a family member.

Skin Cancer

Skin cancer is the most common form of cancer in the United States, affecting one in six individuals. Individuals who are fair-haired and light-skinned have a 1 in 3 risk of developing skin cancer. Fortunately, the tumors are easily seen and therefore may be treated early and successfully. Ninety percent of all skin cancers are caused by exposure to the sun. Individuals who live in areas with high sun exposure (e.g., Arizona and Florida) have higher incidences of skin cancer than do residents of northern states or Canada. Other, less common causes of skin cancer include overexposure to x-rays and exposure to certain chemicals such as arsenic, tar, and coal. Burn scars can develop skin cancer many years after the burn injury, as can any site of tissue trauma.

BASAL CELL CARCINOMA

Basal cell carcinoma (also known as basal cell epithelioma) is the most common form of skin cancer. It derives its name from the layer of the skin in which it originates, the basal cell layer. Basal cells can be classified as nodular or noduloulcerative, pigmented, fibrosing, fibroepithelioma, and superficial. It may also may appear as a spot or patch that continues to itch, hurt, crust, scab, or bleed. An open sore or wound that does not heal, or persists for more than 4 weeks, or closes and then reopens should also be suspect.[14] The most common form is nodular or noduloulcerative. The lesion appears as a small, waxy-looking nodule with a rolled, pearly, or translucent border. As the lesion progresses, the center develops ulcers or crusts. Pigmented basal cells appear more in people with dark hair and eyes. The lesions are similar to the nodular form and may be mistaken for a malignant melanoma. Fibrosing basal cells may resemble lesions of scleroderma and are uncommon. A rare type of basal cell is the fibroepithelioma. It presents a slightly elevated, reddish lesion and may resemble a skin tag. The last and least common form is the superficial basal cell. It may resemble psoriasis, eczema, or a fungal infection. If these conditions are diagnosed, treated, and do not respond to conventional treatment, then biopsy should be performed to rule out cancer.

The most common sites of basal cell carcinomas are the exposed area of the face and neck. The cancer is slow growing and seldom metastasizes, but it can grow so large that the entire nose, lip, or ear must be removed and reconstructed. (See Figure 74-7.)

SQUAMOUS CELL CARCINOMA

Squamous cell carcinoma occurs less frequently than basal cell carcinoma and is more aggressive.

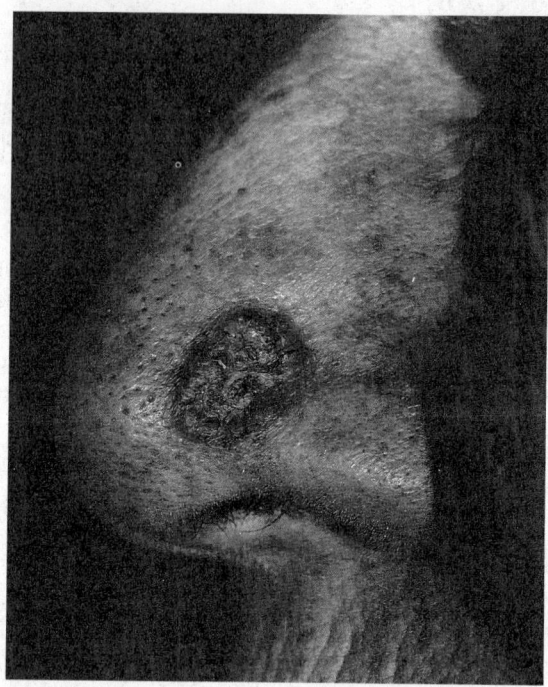

FIGURE 74-7   Basal cell carcinoma. Center has ulcerated and is covered with a crust. (From Habif TP: *Clinical dermatology: a color guide to diagnosis and treatment,* ed 2, St Louis, 1990, Mosby–Year Book, Inc.)

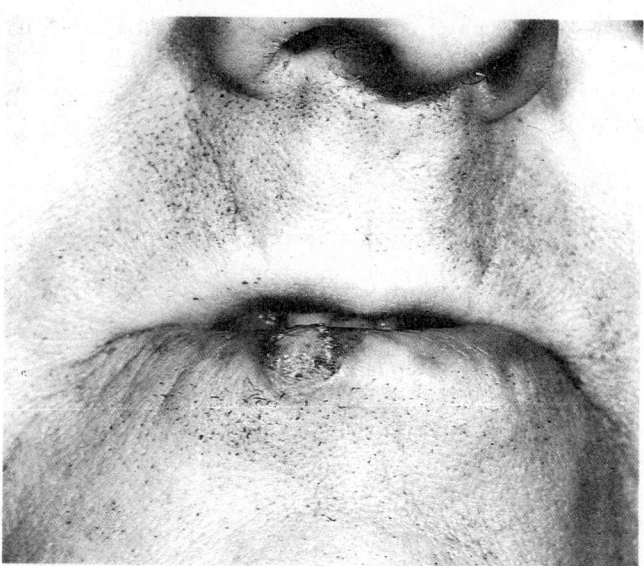

FIGURE 74-8   Squamous cell carcinoma. The sun-exposed lower lip is a common site for squamous cell carcinoma. (From Habif TP: *Clinical dermatology: a color guide to diagnosis and treatment,* ed 2, St Louis, 1990, Mosby–Year Book, Inc.)

The lesions appear on sun-exposed areas or on mucous membranes but can occur on nonexposed skin. They may also appear in areas damaged by some other condition and rarely arise on normal appearing skin. Squamous cell carcinoma grows faster than basal cell carcinoma and is more likely to metastasize to other body areas. Squamous cell carcinoma can be fatal, making early detection and treatment extremely important. They may develop from actinic keratoses or leukoplakia. (See Figure 74-8.)

Squamous cells that arise on skin exhibiting wrinkling, pigmentation, loss of elasticity, or actinic keratoses are secondary to sun exposure. Squamous cell lesions may also appear on burn and scar sites, areas of chronic inflammation (particularly in dark-skinned individuals), or on radiation-damaged skin.[16] Clinically, squamous cells exhibit as thick, rough, horny, shallow lesions initially. They may ulcerate, and have a raised border and a crusted surface covering a pebbly, granular base. A squamous cell carcinoma should be suspected when a bump or open sore develops in an area of chronic inflammation. Blacks do not have a high incidence of skin cancer, but squamous cell carcinoma represents greater than two-thirds of all skin cancers seen in blacks. These lesions are particularly aggressive in blacks, therefore any suspect lesion warrants immediate attention.[27]

MALIGNANT MELANOMA
Definition/Etiology

Malignant melanoma, commonly called melanoma, is cancer of the melanocyte cells in the skin (see Figure 74-9). Melanoma comprises 5% of all skin cancers. It is estimated that by the year 2000 one in ninety individuals will develop a melanoma. Melanoma is seen at an earlier age than other skin cancers and affects both sexes equally.[14] It is an aggressive cancer that requires aggressive therapy to control its rapid spread.

The cause of melanoma is unknown. Sun exposure is strongly suspected, as is a genetic predisposition, the presence of many moles, previous malignancy, exposure to chemical carcinogens, giant congenital nevi, dysplastic nevi, history of painful sunburns, exposure to environmental pollutants, or oncogenic viruses. There are many theories about etiology with some thought being that it is a combination of factors. In general, patients with fair complexions, blue eyes, and blonde or red hair are the most susceptible. The incidence of melanoma is highest in the sun-exposed climates.

Clinical Manifestations

Melanoma has many types: superficial spreading melanoma, which appears as a circular lesion with irregular borders, usually on the trunk or lower extremities; nodular melanoma, berrylike nodules

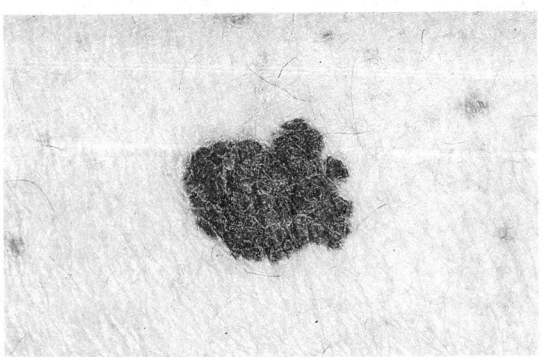

FIGURE 74-9 Lentigo malignant melanoma. (From Habif TP: *Clinical dermatology: a color guide to diagnosis and treatment,* ed 2, St Louis, 1990, Mosby–Year Book, Inc.)

ABCDs AND WARNING SIGNS OF MALIGNANT MELANOMA

A—Asymmetry
B—Border irregularity
C—Color variegation (brown, black, blue, red, white)
D—Diameter (>5 mm)
Moles that change in: size
                            color
                            shape
                            elevation
                            surrounding skin
                            surface
                            sensation
                            consistency

with blue-black color, which frequently invades the dermis and subcutaneous tissue; lentigo maligna, which appears on sun-exposed surfaces and appears as a flat lesion that slowly turns black; and acral lentigious melanoma, which occurs on skin not exposed to the sun and appears as irregular pigmented macules that develop nodules. The Skin Cancer Foundation has published the ABCDs of malignant melanoma and warning signs (see the box above). If an individual notices any of the characteristics listed in this table he or she should seek medical attention immediately.

Therapeutic Management

Medical management involves surgery to excise the tumor completely, including a border of normal skin. Regional lymph node dissection may be required to identify the extent of spread and to reduce spread through the lymphatic network. Metastatic disease can be treated, but in general the results are marginal. The use of immunotherapy is still experimental in the treatment of metastatic melanoma. The best treatment is prevention and/or early detection. Individuals should examine their skin on a regular basis. The total skin surface including scalp, intertriginous areas, and toe and finger webs should be examined. Sunscreens with a minimum SPF (Sun Protection Factor) of 15 should always be used. Sun exposure should be limited and suspect lesions should be biopsied for diagnosis.

NURSING MANAGEMENT OF THE PATIENT WITH MALIGNANT MELANOMA

Assessment

Patients with melanoma are assessed for the presence of other suspicious skin lesions. Lesions that are very dark with an irregular border should be reported. The groin and axillae should be palpated for masses. Laboratory tests usually include alkaline phosphatase and lactate dehydrogenase.

Nursing Diagnosis

Common nursing diagnoses include:
    Defensive coping related to fear of malignancy, disfigurement, or death
    Anxiety related to unknown outcome
    Knowledge deficit (planned treatments) related to new diagnosis

Planning

The goal for the patient is a positive coping style, as evidenced by focusing on the disease and its management, a reduction of anxiety, and evidence of knowledge about the plan for care.

Implementation

Nursing interventions center on reducing anxiety before surgery. Anxiety is best treated by providing the patient with information and by reviewing information or spending time with the patient expressing awareness of his or her fears. Postoperative care depends on the extent of the resection. Large wounds often must be closed with skin grafting. (See care of the skin graft in Chapter 76.) Patients are taught about photoprotection. Table 74-6 lists sun protection needs for types of skin.

Evaluation/Documentation

The degree of goal attainment is evaluated by assessing for positive self-statements, realistic fears, re-

TABLE 74-6   Photoprotection Needs For Skin Types

Skin type	Physical appearance	Tanning history	Photoprotection needed
I	Very fair skin, freckles Gray/green or blue eyes Red, blond, or brown hair	Sunburns easily and usually with severe peeling	15 or more
II	Fair skin Blue, brown, gray, or green eyes Brown, red, or blond hair	Minimal sun tanning Sunburns easily and painfully	15 or more
III	Moderately fair skin Usually brown hair and eyes	Gradual sun tanning, does burn	8-10
IV	Light brown unexposed skin Dark hair and eyes	Tans with initial sun exposure	6-8
V	Brown unexposed skin	Easy skin tanning, rarely sunburns	4
VI	Black unexposed skin	Never sunburns	0

duced anxiety, and knowledge of planned treatment. The excision site should be healing without evident infection or delayed healing. The appearance of the lesion and surgical site is documented on each shift. The patient's reaction to the diagnosis and prognosis and understanding of follow-up care are recorded.

Ongoing Care

Long-term follow-up care involves monthly self-assessment of the skin, having suspicious lesions examined by a professional, having family members with suspicious lesions see a physician, limiting sun exposure, and using sun screens when outdoors.

Special Patient Populations

Elderly patients, black patients, and patients with HIV have special needs for skin care and diagnosis.

THE GERIATRIC PATIENT
Changes Associated with Aging

The skin of the geriatric patient is different from skin in other age groups. As the skin ages it loses dermal collagen, blood vessels, fat, and elastin fibers. The body hair thins, sweat ducts and sebaceous glands decrease in density leading to decrease in lubrication and decrease in sweat production, and the epidermis thins. Wrinkling, the most obvious sign of skin aging, occurs because the collagenous fibers in the dermis become more stable and less flexible, the elastic fibers fray from continued stress causing the skin to lose its elasticity and resiliency.

The fluid content of the skin decreases causing dryness. Dryness causes itching that can be aggravated during winter months by hot, dry, air produced by heaters. Lubricating the skin with a moisturizer, and utilizing a cool mist vaporizer to raise room humidity will help alleviate the problem. Loss and redistribution of subcutaneous fat increases the risk of pressure sores.

Skin Growths in the Elderly

Many years of exposure to the environment and the normal process of aging produce a number of skin growths that are common to elderly patients. Most of these growths are benign. *Seborrheic keratoses* are small, discrete, raised, darkly pigmented lesions that have a greasy, "stuck on" appearance. They appear on the chest and back and often on the neck and face. They may pose a cosmetic problem but can be removed easily. *Senile lentigines* are the so-called liver spots of older age. They are areas of pigmentation that range from pinpoint size to slightly larger. They typically appear on areas of the skin that have been exposed to the sun. *Acrochordon,* or skin tags, are flesh-colored, raised fibromas commonly seen around the neck, chest, upper back, axillae, and groin. These can be unsightly and can be removed for cosmetic reasons. *Cherry angiomas* are pinpoint red lesions typically seen on the chest and back. They actually are small collections of capillaries.

THE BLACK PATIENT

The diagnosis of skin disease is heavily dependent on the clinician's eye. Knowing this, it is imperative that there be some discussion about how skin disease manifests in the black patient. Equally as im-

GERIATRIC CONSIDERATIONS

Skin Conditions

- The aging skin is prone to developing skin cancers. Basal cell carcinoma accounts for 80%.
- Changes in the skin occur slowly and gradually.
- Carcinomas appear frequently on the nose, eyelid, or cheek from sun exposures.
- Seborrheic keratoses are benign epidermal growths frequently seen on face, scalp, trunk, and upper extremities.
- Xerosis (dry skin) is the most common skin problem. Emollients such as mineral oil, lanolin, or white petroleum jelly help seal in moisture.

portant as recognizing disease is the recognition of normal variants in black skin. There are also those conditions that are seen more commonly in black patients, or may be unique to blacks.

Common Conditions

There are several conditions that may manifest in black individuals that may cause concern but are only normal variants. A condition known as Futcher's or Voight's lines exhibits clinically as a demarcation between darkly pigmented skin and lightly pigmented skin. This condition is generally on the upper arms, with the darker segment anterolaterally and the lighter segment anteromedially. This skin manifestation is common in all ages and both sexes.[27] There are nail manifestations that may also be disconcerting to patients, but are again only normal variants. Longitudinal linear, dark bands may be seen in the nail plate. They vary in size from one to several millimeters and may be single or multiple. These pigmented bands are generally due to melanin deposition. Even though this pigmentation is generally a normal variant, all other possible causes must be ruled out. Other possible causes include trauma, postirradiation melanonychia, subungual melanoma (or nevus), topical application of silver- or mercury-containing compounds, ingestion of antimalarials, paronychia, Addison's disease, and pigmentation due to Peutz-Jeghers syndrome. In addition, hyperpigmentation of either lateral or posterior nail folds, or both, may be secondary to inflammation (paranychia) or a cutaneous marker for systemic disease, such as dermatomyositis.[27]

In addition to normal variants, some common skin disorders have distinct clinical manifestations in black skin. Atopic dermatitis exhibits with follicular lesions. These lesions may precede the classic li-

chenified lesions seen in other skin colors. Pityriasis rosea, which is seen in all racial groups, exhibits clinically in a specific way in black skin. The characteristic lesions are generally salmon-pink in color, but due to the darker pigmentation in black skin, salmon-pink is not a possibility. The clinical lesion is more of a dull reddish brown to deep, dark brown. The lesions will have abundant fine scaling which is very obvious in black skin, while almost unapparent in whites. Pityriasis rosea generally clears without residual skin manifestations, but in blacks may leave significant postinflammatory pigmentary changes.

Psoriasis, though uncommon, is also seen in individuals with black skin. The distribution is the same, but as in pityriasis rosea, the typical bright red color seen in plaques will exhibit differently. Plaques will exhibit with a violaceous to bluish black hue. Postinflammatory pigmentary changes may be seen with this condition.

In addition to common skin diseases with different manifestations, there are some skin conditions that are more commonly seen in black individuals. Fox-Fordyce disease, a chronic, pruritic dermatosis is seen more commonly in black individuals. The lesions are seen in the apocrine-bearing regions of the body. Apocrine sweat ducts become plugged with keratinous material leading to rupture of the intraepidermal duct. The lesions are follicular papules seen in the axillae, areolae, and the pubic areas of the body. The course is chronic and persistent, and hormone therapy may provide some relief.

Hair disorders seen more commonly in black individuals include hot comb alopecia, and traction alopecia. Well-defined patches of incomplete scalp alopecia is the characteristic sign of hot comb alopecia. Hair loss is irreversible and seen most in young black females who utilize a heated comb in conjunction with petrolatum to straighten the hair. It is important to differentiate hot comb alopecia from other causes of alopecia such as lupus erythematosus, scleroderma, pseudopelade of Brocq, and lichen planopilaris.

Traction alopecia exhibits as patchy hair loss which has been gradual. It results from the cumulative effects of prolonged traction on scalp hair during styling (e.g., corn rows). If caught early the alopecia is reversible. Parents should be discouraged from braiding the hair of children and leaving the hair in this style for prolonged periods of time.

Pomade acne is another dermatologic condition that is more commonly seen in black individuals. As the name implies, the acne develops secondary to the application of greasy creams and oils to the hair and scalp. These preparations are comedogenic. The best treatment is to discontinue the use of these preparations, but it is difficult to break established cultural customs.

Acne keloidalis nuchae, dermatosis papulosis

nigra, pseudofolliculitis, and sickle-cell leg ulcers are just some of the skin conditions that are nearly unique to blacks. Acne keloidalis nuchae is a deep follicular inflammatory process seen on the nape of the neck. The etiology is unknown. The process begins with firm, discrete, globoid follicular and perifollicular papules. Because of the location on the nape of the neck, these lesions are irritated by shirt collars. The papules become confluent, and ingrown hairs become evident. Permanent alopecia, along with hypertrophic or keloidal scarring follows. Sinus tracts, abscesses, and chronic drainage may be a later development. This condition must always be differentiated from an infectious process (particularly fungal), and because of the scarring aspect of the disease, the lesion should be monitored for the development of squamous cell carcinoma.

Dermatosis papulosa nigra is unique to black individuals. The etiology is unknown, but some theories are hereditary, a nevoid condition, or a variant of seborrheic keratosis. It appears earlier in life than seborrheic keratosis, generally appearing near puberty. Clinically the lesions exhibit as pigmented, pedunculate, and verrucous papules. They are found on the malar areas of the face, but may be found on the chest, neck and back. These lesions do not have a malignant tendency, but because they may be numerous, a malignant tumor may be overlooked.

The hair of black individuals has a coiled nature which may cause the free end to reenter the skin. When this happens an inflammatory process begins. This is particularly true in the beard area. Shaving of the beard only worsens the condition by sharpening the end of the free hair which allows for easier reentry into the skin. When the condition occurs in males it is given the name pseudofolliculitis barbae. The clinical lesion is an irritated papular and pustular eruption on the mandible, chin, and neck. Discontinuance of shaving is the best treatment, but there have been some advances made in shaving equipment. A straight razor has been developed especially for black men in order to help prevent this condition.

Lastly, leg ulcers in black individuals may be caused by sickle cell anemia. These ulcers may be single or multiple, unilateral or bilateral, and are characteristically on the lower third of the leg at or near the malleoli. Clinically the ulcers are chronic, well defined, may have a slightly raised border, and appear to be "punched out." Leg ulcers with no other apparent etiology should make the diagnostician suspicious of sickle cell.

THE PATIENT WITH HIV

Kaposi's sarcoma is the most commonly known skin manifestation in patients with HIV, but there are other dermatologic manifestations that clinicians should know. The severity of the dermatosis can generally be correlated with the degree of immune dysfunction. These dermatoses generally present as papulosquamous lesions.

In general the skin of HIV patients is drier and the dryness worsens with the advance of the disease. As the T-cell counts drop the skin conditions worsen. Xerosis and asteatotic eczema will worsen causing pruritus and the development of erythematous patches. Treatment is with emollients containing alpha hydroxyl acids or urea, and topical corticosteroids. Seborrheic dermatitis is another common papulosquamous condition seen in HIV patients. Again the severity of the skin condition correlates with the severity of immunosuppression. Seborrheic dermatitis may be the initial presentation of HIV infection. The clinical manifestation of seborrheic dermatitis in these patients is atypical in that the lesions are frequently annular patches and plaques with fine yellow, greasy scale, pigmentary changes, or hyperkeratotic plaques which may be crusted and resemble psoriasis. The scalp, body folds (axilla and groin), trunk, and extremities may be involved. Treatment is with low- or medium-potency corticosteroids. Ketoconazole topically, systemically or in shampoos may be helpful.[18]

With an impaired immune system, a psoriasiform dermatitis may be seen. The presentation of the dermatitis is very much like psoriasis, but the lesions generally are flatter, redder, and more irregular in shape. Scale is present, but is finer than in typical psoriasis. The classic areas of presentation for this psoriasiform dermatitis are axilla, groin, genitals, face, scalp, palms, soles, and nails. The spectrum of the cutaneous manifestations are similar to regular psoriasis; it may be pustular, erythrodermic, guttate, or plaque type. Treatment is a challenge in that the common treatments for psoriasis are immunosuppressive, corticosteroids, tars, and ultraviolet phototherapy.

An HIV-associated papular eruption and eosinophilic pustular folliculitis (EPF) has been reported in patients with HIV. The lesions are papular and may erode, or become lichenified. The distribution is follicular and pruritus varies from mild to extreme. Treatment is with ultraviolet phototherapy B. Norwegian scabies exhibit with hyperkeratotic lesions that are intensely pruritic. Characteristically the lesions are found on the hands, in the body folds, and on the genitalia. Conventional treatment is employed. Patients with HIV have a higher rate of cutaneous drug eruptions. The characteristic lesions are macular and maculopapular. There is a variable degree of pruritus. Drug reactions are treated as any other drug reaction would be treated; withdraw the suspected drug, treat symptomatically.

It must be emphasized that anytime a "common" skin condition manifests in an unusual manner, or does not respond to conventional treatment, a thorough history must be obtained from the patient. At all times universal precautions should be employed. Most importantly all patients should be treated with compassion and caring. For further information on care of the HIV patient, see Chapter 40.

CRITICAL THINKING QUESTIONS

1 Describe the nurse's responsibility for the general aspects of dermatologic care (i.e., dressings, phototherapy, photoprotection).

2 Discuss your feelings about caring for patients with open, draining skin lesions. How could you help the patient improve his or her self-concept?

3 Pruritus is a common aspect of skin disorders. Develop a plan of care for the patient with acute pruritus; chronic pruritis.

4 Describe how infection can be contained in patients with pemphigus; scabies.

5 Your patient has been diagnosed with psoriasis. Plan a teaching strategy for the patient, who will be discharged in 3 days.

6 List and describe the intrinsic and extrinsic factors related to pressure ulcers. How could the risk factors be modified?

7 Your patient is a 30-year-old quadriplegic who has undergone surgical repair of a pressure ulcer. Develop a teaching plan for him to prevent recurrence and allow the flap to heal.

8 Describe the skin cancers and their appearance.

9 Your patient is a 35-year-old mother of two who is to have a wide excision of a melanoma on her leg. Plan her care, using nursing and interpersonal processes.

BIBLIOGRAPHY

Current

1. Barnes S: Patient/family education for the patient with pressure necrosis, *Nurs Clin North Am* 22(2):463, 1987.
2. Black J, Black S: Surgical management of pressure ulcers, *Nurs Clin North Am* 22(2):429, 1987.
3. Bobel L: Nutritional implications in the patient with pressure sores, *Nurs Clin North Am* 22(2):379, 1987.
4. Bryant R: *Acute and chronic wounds: nursing management,* St Louis, 1992, Mosby–Year Book.
5. Coleman D et al: A worst-case guide for any case of psoriasis, *RN* March: 39, 1988.
6. Eisenbaum S, Black J: Melanoma, *Plast Surg Nurs* 8:42, 1988.
7. Fitzpatrick T et al: *Dermatology in general medicine,* ed 3, New York, 1987, McGraw-Hill.
8. Fowler E: Equipment and products used in management and treatment of pressure ulcers, *Nurs Clin North Am* 22(2):449, 1987.
9. Gosnell D: Assessment and evaluation of pressure sores, *Nurs Clin North Am* 22(2):399, 1987.
10. Habif T: *Clinical dermatology: a color guide to diagnosis and treatment,* St Louis, 1990, Mosby–Year Book.
11. Maklebust J: Pressure ulcers: etiology and prevention, *Nurs Clin North Am* 22(2):359, 1987.
12. Maklebust J, Sieggreen M: *Pressure ulcers: guidelines for prevention and nursing management,* West Dundee, Illinois, 1991, S-N Publications.
13. Paletta C, Jurkiewicz M: Hidradenitis suppurativa, *Clin Plast Surg* 14:383, 1987.
14. *Pressure ulcers in adults: prediction and prevention,* Pub No 92-0047, Rockville, MD, 1992, US Department of Health and Human Services, Agency for Health Care Policy and Research.
15. Prigel C: How to spot melanoma, *Nurs '87* 17(6):60, 1987.
16. Robins P: *Sun sense: a complete guide to: prevention, early detection and treatment of skin cancer,* New York, 1990, Skin Cancer Foundation.
17. Rosen T, Lanning M, Hill M: *Nurse's atlas of dermatology,* Boston, 1983, Little, Brown, Inc.
18. Sanchez M, de los Santos L, Arond J: HIV-associated papulosquamous diseases, *Dermatol Nurs* 4(4):253, 1992.
19. Stotts N, Paul S: Pressure ulcer development in surgical patients, *Decubitus* 1(3):24, 1988.

Classic

20. Baron M: The skin and wound healing, *Top Clin Nurs* 5(2):11, 1983.
21. Bennett L, Lee BY: Pressure versus shear in pressure sore causation. In Lee BY: *Chronic ulcers of the skin,* New York, 1985, McGraw-Hill.
22. Blom D: Dramatic decrease in decubitus ulcers, *Geriatr Nurs* March:84, 1985.
23. Brown M et al: Nursing innovation for prevention of decubitus ulcers in long term care facilities, *J Plast Reconstr Surg Nurs* 2:51, 1981.
24. Curtin L: Wound management: care and cost—an overview, *Nurs Manage* 15(2):22, 1984.
25. DeLisa J, Mikulic M: Pressure ulcers—what to do if prevention fails, *Postgrad Med* 77(60):209, 1985.
26. Melski J, Arndt K: Topical therapy for acne, *N Engl J Med* 302:503, 1980.
27. Rosen T, Martin S: *Atlas of black dermatology,* Boston, 1981, Little, Brown Inc.

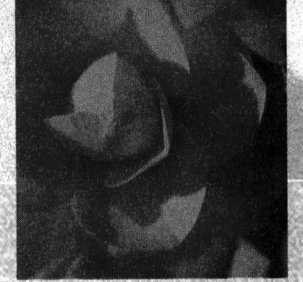

CHAPTER SEVENTY-FIVE

Nursing Management of Adults with Burns

LEARNING OBJECTIVES

1 Differentiate superficial partial-thickness, deep partial-thickness, and full-thickness injury in relation to the level and severity of injury.

2 Define eschar and describe its effects on the healing of burn wounds.

3 Describe the physiologic alterations in selected body systems caused by thermal, electrical, or chemical burns.

4 Using the nursing process, outline the care of the patient with a minor burn injury who is undergoing outpatient treatment.

5 Discuss the care of the patient in the emergent, acute, and rehabilitation phases of a moderate to severe burn.

6 Discuss the needs and contributions of the family or significant others in the care and successful recovery of the burn patient.

7 Discuss the nurse's role in fluid resuscitation of the burn patient.

8 Outline the nursing care requirements related to the psychosocial needs of the burn patient.

9 Describe the nursing responsibilities related to surgical and nonsurgical wound care, including debridement, excision, and graft care.

KEY TERMS

A MAJOR BURN is one of the most traumatic events that an individual and family can endure. Unlike serious injuries or debilitating diseases that run their course, a severe burn may have psychologic, physiologic, and social consequences that permanently alter the quality of a person's life.

BURN INJURY
Etiology

Fire is one of the most common causes of accidental death in the United States. Approximately 2 million people suffer burn injuries each year, and in about 6000 cases these injuries prove fatal.[15] Men suffer the most burn injuries, although statistically children and the elderly also seem to be at great risk. Topical chemical exposure and radiation as well as fire can cause severe burns. An electrical current can cause devastating burn injuries to internal structures while appearing to cause only minor surface injuries. Many severe burn injuries and fatalities occur in individuals who do not have an obvious burn wound. In these patients inhalation of smoke, smoke products, and chemicals during a fire results in potentially fatal damage to the respiratory system.

Pathophysiology

All severe burn injuries, regardless of origin, can alter the function of several body systems (see Figure 75-1).

Integumentary system

A burn destroys the epidermis, allowing tissue fluids to escape and potential pathogens to enter. If the lowest layer of the epidermis is destroyed, the wound will not heal without scarring. Because all epidermal appendages (such as the hair follicles and sebaceous and sweat glands) arise in the dermis, an injury that extends through the dermis destroys these appendages' ability to regenerate. Since skin thickness and exposure to the source of the burn may vary, it is not uncommon to see a patient with several burn wounds of different depths (see Figure 75-2). Historically, the depth of burn was classified as first-degree, second-degree, third-degree, or fourth-degree. However, burns are more precisely described as superficial partial-thickness, deep partial-thickness, and full-thickness.

A superficial **partial-thickness burn** (first-degree) is best exemplified by a sunburn. This type of burn affects the superficial epidermis. The injury leaves the skin pink or red, dry, and painful. There is no blistering, but a slight edema may develop. The affected epidermis sheds in approximately 1 week without leaving a residual scar. Unless this type of burn is extensive, it does not require hospitalization.

Deep partial-thickness burns (second-degree) involve both the epidermis and the dermis. They are caused by prolonged exposure (longer than 10 seconds) to intense heat flashes or by prolonged contact with hot liquids or objects. Deep partial-thickness burns produce a wound that is blistered or wet if the blister has been broken. The wound is red; it blanches and refills when pressure is applied. These wounds are quite painful. Local superficial edema develops, and such edema also may be present in unburned areas if the burn covers a large area. This type of wound heals in 2 to 3 weeks without surgical intervention and usually does not scar unless infected or traumatized. If the wound extends into the deep layers of the dermis, skin grafting of the affected area may be necessary to achieve the best result.

A **full-thickness burn** (third-degree) destroys the epidermis and dermis; thus the skin cannot regenerate (see Figure 75-3). All dermal structures are destroyed and cannot be replaced or regenerated. An extensive full thickness burn can involve subcutaneous structures and may include fat, fascia, tendon, and bone (fourth-degree). This burn varies in color from white to black or charred and may have dark networks of thrombosed capillaries. The wound appears dry and leathery as a covering of denatured protein called **eschar** develops. If reddened, third-degree wounds do not blanch with pressure. The wound itself may not be painful, since the superficial nerve endings within it have been destroyed. However, wound margins are extremely painful and reflect the presence of intact nerves. This type of wound requires skin grafting for closure, because the skin layers have no base from which to regenerate (see Figure 75-4).

Cardiovascular system

A burn injury causes a massive outpouring of catecholamines, which in turn cause the peripheral blood vessels to constrict. However, because of the injury these vessels have become more permeable, allowing fluids and colloids to leak into the surrounding tissues. The more severe the injury, the greater the impact on the vascular system.

The leaking fluid becomes trapped in the interstitial space, causing the edema characteristic of burn. If the burn is relatively minor, the edema is primarily local; however, when the burn is extensive (15% to 20% of total body surface area [TBSA]), this change in vascular permeability is a systemic response, causing edema throughout the body. Soon after the burn occurs, colloids cross into the interstitial space, causing more fluid to follow as a result of changes in oncotic pressures. The greater the blood flow to a given area, the more colloid and fluid can cross the vessel walls into the interstitial space.

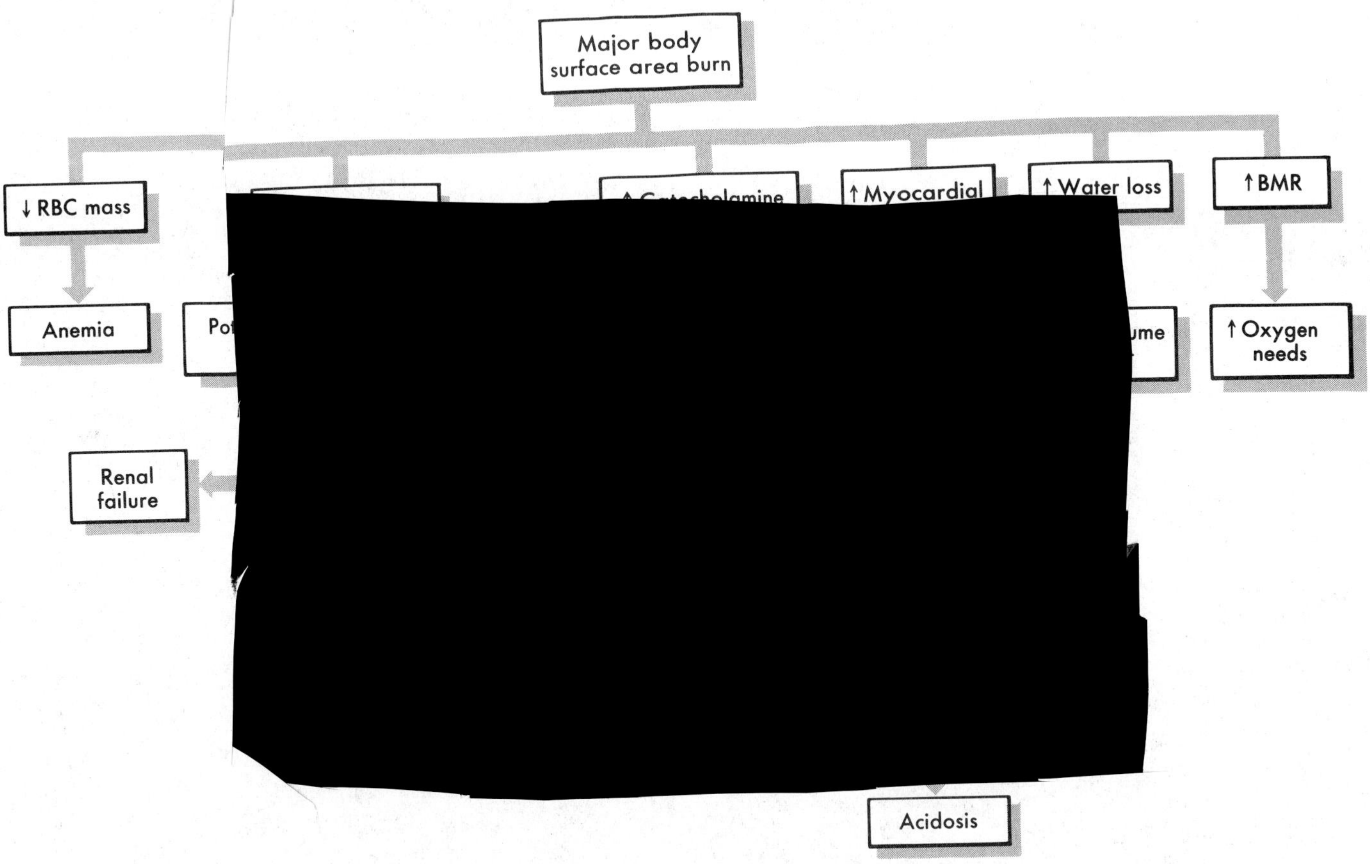

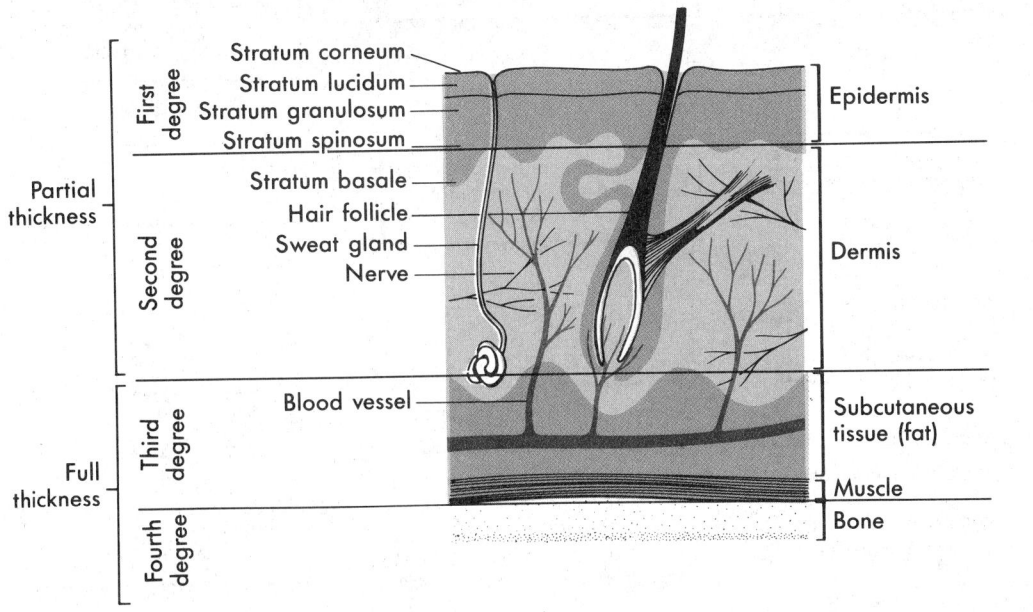

Major body
surface area burn

↓ RBC mass

↑Myocardial

↑Water loss

↑BMR

Anemia

Pot

ume

↑Oxygen
needs

Renal
failure

Acidosis

FIGURE 75-1   Pathophysiologic events contributing to organ system failure in the burn patient.

Stratum corneum
Stratum lucidum
Stratum granulosum
Stratum spinosum
First degree

Epidermis

Stratum basale
Hair follicle
Sweat gland
Nerve
Second degree

Partial
thickness

Dermis

Blood vessel
Third degree

Subcutaneous
tissue (fat)

Full
thickness

Muscle

Fourth degree

Bone

FIGURE 75-2   Layers of the skin involved in burn injury.

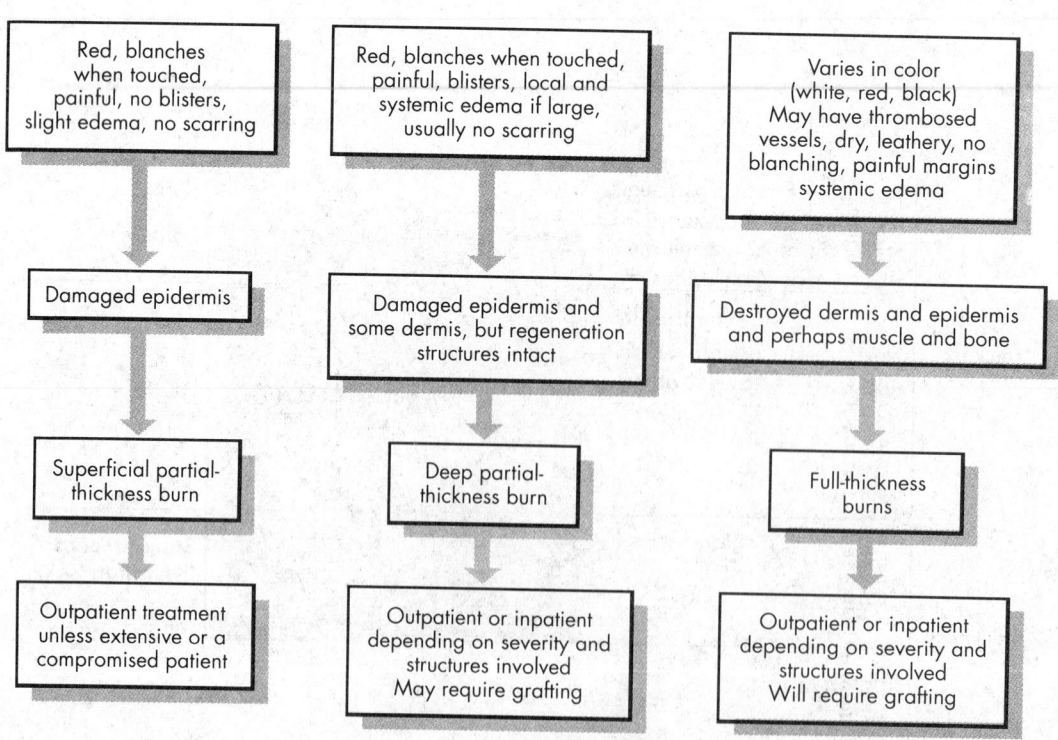

Red, blanches when touched, painful, no blisters, slight edema, no scarring	Red, blanches when touched, painful, blisters, local and systemic edema if large, usually no scarring	Varies in color (white, red, black) May have thrombosed vessels, dry, leathery, no blanching, painful margins systemic edema
Damaged epidermis	Damaged epidermis and some dermis, but regeneration structures intact	Destroyed dermis and epidermis and perhaps muscle and bone
Superficial partial-thickness burn	Deep partial-thickness burn	Full-thickness burns
Outpatient treatment unless extensive or a compromised patient	Outpatient or inpatient depending on severity and structures involved May require grafting	Outpatient or inpatient depending on severity and structures involved Will require grafting

FIGURE 75-4   Critical Thinking Guide: classifying burn injury.

Consequently, a relative hypovolemia may ensue within several hours. If fluid resuscitation succeeds, cardiac output begins to return to normal at the end of the first 24 hours postburn, becoming hypermetabolic during the second 24 hours. Capillary integrity is restored completely sometime between the third and fifth postburn day and diuresis begins.

The initial vasoconstriction may trap red blood cells, making them unavailable to the body. The fluid losses to the environment and into the interstitial space cause a relative hemoconcentration, as blood cells are too large to cross the permeable capillary membrane. This hemoconcentration causes the hematocrit to rise and the viscosity of the blood to increase, causing the blood flow to slow. This alteration in blood flow can affect the body in several ways, including altering peripheral tissue oxygenation and nutrition and venous stasis, possibly leading to further tissue destruction. Destruction of red blood cells may begin in the wound at the time of the burn, and may continue as hemolyzed cells die and decompose.

The reduction in circulating blood volume decreases cardiac output and may lead to inadequate tissue perfusion. Cellular hypoxia shifts cellular metabolism from aerobic to anaerobic, with a net result of acidosis from the buildup of lactic acid. This accumulation of acid can cause further structural damage and irreversible shock.

Acid-base homeostasis normally is maintained by three mechanisms, blood-borne buffers, the lungs, and the renal tubules, but fluid shifts disrupt these controls. Plasma, which carries the blood-borne buffering agents, escapes into the interstitial space, thus removing the buffers from the vascular space. The normal respiratory function of expelling carbon dioxide can be altered by irritation from smoke inhalation or by thoracic constriction from circumferential eschar, which can cause hypoventilation. Renal tubular function can be impaired by the decrease in cardiac output, causing excessive elimination of bicarbonate.

Normally, sodium is the main cation in extracellular fluid, including intravascular fluid. Potassium is the main cation in the intracellular space. When cells are destroyed in a burn wound and intracellular fluid is released, serum potassium levels can rise considerably, resulting in potentially life-threatening cardiac dysrhythmias. Once capillary integrity has been restored, however, the kidneys eliminate vast amounts of potassium, and the patient may lose 80 to 200 mEq of potassium per day.

Pulmonary system

Facial or neck edema caused by burns or smoke inhalation may threaten the airway and if severe may necessitate intubation. Pulmonary edema may develop as a result of fluid shifts aggravated by fluid replacement therapy and hypoproteinemia. These problems subside when diuresis begins and resolve within a few weeks if no damage has occurred from smoke inhalation.

Because of the body's protective mechanisms (e.g., closure of the glottis), burns of the pulmonary parenchyma are rare and usually occur only if steam is inhaled. The upper airway can be damaged if an individual breathes very hot air; this also may cause burns of the oral mucosa, palate, and pharynx. Inhalation injury is the most common cause of lung damage. One autopsy study indicated that 70% of burn patients expiring within 12 hours of injury also had suffered an inhalation injury.[14]

Inhaling smoke, soot, and/or chemicals released when substances such as plastic or insulation materials burn causes mucosal sloughing, changes in pulmonary capillary permeability, inflammation, and eventually pulmonary edema. Initially, asphyxia is secondary to the fire's consumption of all available oxygen and the patient's subsequent inhalation of carbon monoxide. By-products of incomplete combustion induce coughing, bronchospasm, and eventually tracheobronchitis, which further decreases oxygenation capacity.[14] Inhalation of smoke causes diminished surfactant and atelectasis, decreasing the surface area for gas exchange. Edema formation, increased by fluid resuscitation, decreases the tracheal width and therefore the volume of air exchange. Fluid resuscitation, in the face of changes in capillary permeability and an increased pulmonary blood flow, also can increase the amount of fluid accumulating in the lungs.[12] The increase in fluid in the lung fields combined with the presence of foreign substances puts the patient with an inhalation injury at great risk of developing bronchopneumonia. This may develop at any time as a result of the initial injury or as atelectasis or aspiration or inhalation of airborne microorganisms occurs.[14]

Renal system

The hypovolemia that develops immediately after the burn occurs causes the renal arteries to constrict. It is first seen as oliguria caused by a decrease in the glomerular filtration rate. This situation is further compromised by secretion of antidiuretic hormone from the posterior pituitary as the body tries to conserve blood volume. Initially, hematuria may be observed as a result of red blood cell destruction at the time of injury. If hematuria persists longer than 24 hours, during which fluid resuscitation takes place, acute glomerular or tubular damage may be the cause. Further, if the burn extends into muscle, myoglobin, released from the muscle cells, may be present. Myoglobin in the urine can lead to acute tubular necrosis.[12] Adequate fluid resuscitation allows the kidneys to flush the glomeruli and eliminate these waste products. Glycosuria also may develop initially and may clear spontaneously with resuscitation. Burn patients with preexisting renal disorders have a high risk of developing renal insufficiency during the postburn period. This may first be manifested by decreased urine output accompanied by elevated serum creatinine and blood urea nitrogen levels. Total renal failure caused either by decreased renal blood flow or by preexisting renal disease carries a poor prognosis for recovery.[12]

Gastrointestinal system

The hypovolemia induced by the initial burn injury causes gastric dilation and paralytic ileus during the immediate postburn period. This may resolve within 24 to 36 hours, only to recur secondary to sepsis. The burn patient also is at risk for developing a gastroduodenal stress ulcer, known as Curling's ulcer. Intestinal blood may be overtly or covertly present in the stool; black stools are not uncommon. Early in the burn course gastric bleeding is more common, whereas later the source of bleeding usually is duodenal. Both conditions are thought to be caused by local capillary engorgement accompanied by mucosal sloughing secondary to ischemia and irritation.

Additional system derangements

Within the hemopoietic system, the rapid destruction of red blood cells in the wound and the gradual hemolysis of damaged cells cause the bone marrow to release new erythrocytes. The white blood cell count rises in the first few days after the burn occurs because of the release of catecholamines. (In the presence of a transient reaction to the topical ointment Silvadene there may be a transient decrease in the white cell count.) The cells adhere and may become trapped in the intravascular fluid, altering their phagocytic function. In the early postburn period, platelets are rapidly destroyed, but they increase in number after the first 5 days, posing the additional risk of vascular thrombosis.[29] Neurologically, the patient may exhibit a variety of mental states produced by the hypoxia of hypovolemia or inhalation injury and the psychogenic shock of the burn trauma. Mental changes constitute one of the primary indicators of the adequacy of circulating blood volume or the incidence of carbon monoxide poisoning. The stress of the burn stimulates the anterior lobe of the pituitary to produce adrenocorticotrophic hormone (ACTH). This in turn stimulates the adrenal cortex, leading to a rise in glucose levels. ACTH also stimulates the adrenal medulla, producing epinephrine and norepinephrine. This causes the symptoms of the "fight or flight" response.

Hypermetabolism, increased glucose flow, and severe protein and fat wasting are characteristic of the response to major trauma and infection. This response is most severe in burn injury. Patients with other serious disorders or trauma demonstrate metabolic rates of 20% to 75% above normal. Patients with burns covering more than 40% of TBSA have demonstrated metabolic rates of up to 200% of normal. Such severely burned patients can lose protein at a rate of up to 2 to 3 g per percentage of TBSA per day in addition to having a marked negative nitrogen balance from the hypermetabolic state.[3]

Glucose production and use in the burn patient are abnormal. Because of the increase in catecholamines, patients demonstrate a type of "insulin resistance" similar to diabetic individuals. The burn wound consumes large amounts of glucose through anaerobic metabolism, with new glucose being derived from muscle protein in the wound.[3]

The energy requirements for maintaining weight, nitrogen balance, and energy equilibrium have been estimated from analysis of weight change versus predicted dietary intake in a group of adults with large burns. This study produced the Curreri formula for caloric requirements (see the Nursing Care Plan). In some cases caloric need can surpass 5000 kcal/24 hr to offset the massive protein breakdown.[3] If the high caloric and protein load is not achieved, wound healing is delayed or is abnormal, with defects in fibroblast and white cell function.

Electrical Burns

An **electrical burn** produces a cutaneous injury that represents only a fraction of the damage sustained (see Figure 75-5). Low-voltage electricity flows along the path of least resistance. High-voltage electricity tends to take a direct path. Different tissues offer different resistance, ranging from least to greatest as follows: nerve, blood, muscle, skin, tendon, fat, and bone. The more resistant the tissue, the greater the heat produced as the electricity passes through.[2]

With true electrical injury, a current is passed through the skin after contact with a conductor (usually a body part). This injury produces the characteristic entry and exit wounds, with significant deep-tissue destruction. The entry wound usually is charred and has adherent eschar. The exit wound usually is larger than the entry wound and may appear as if the electricity exploded out the site. The exit wound marks the place where the patient was "grounded." The areas the current passed through initially may appear viable. Electrical injury differs from other burn injuries in that the tissue damage is progressive along the path of the electrical current. The level of tissue injury may not be finally determined for a number of days.[2]

Electrical burns affect many body systems simi-

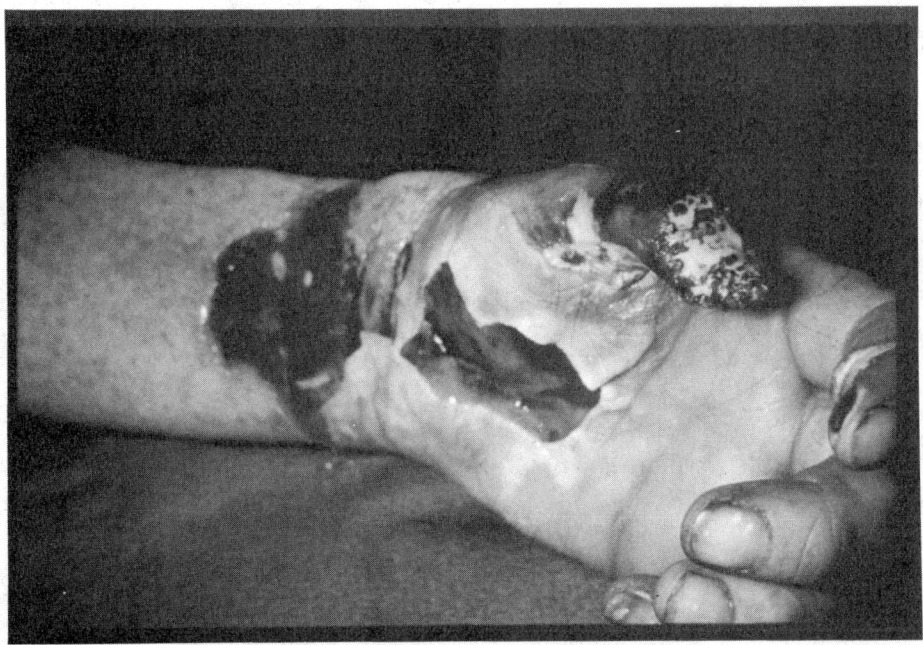

FIGURE 75-5   Electrical burn.

larly to true thermal injury caused by sparks that alight on clothing, but they also have characteristic sequelae. The cardiac abnormalities associated with an electrical injury usually occur at the time of contact with the electrical source. Minor dysrhythmias or complete arrest may occur, depending on the strength of the current and the duration of contact. Respiratory abnormalities can occur, such as anoxia from muscle tetany. Blood vessels and the contained vascular fluids provide the easiest pathway for the current. Heat degrades vessel walls, and extensive vascular damage can occur. Delayed hemorrhage from large vessels can occur in an area of extensive necrosis. As great numbers of red blood cells are destroyed, the debris from cellular membranes and intracellular contents are circulated through the kidneys. Hematuria may occur and may last for several days. Because of the massive muscle injury associated with electrical injury, large amounts of myoglobin are released from the damaged or destroyed muscle cells. The presence of myoglobin is an indicator of underlying nonobservable muscle damage. Circulating myoglobin must be eliminated by the kidneys and may cause direct damage to the glomeruli and tubule system. The bowel adjacent to a high-voltage contact point may be damaged, and perforation may be spontaneous or delayed. The classic "stress" ulcer also may occur. The pancreas, gallbladder, and liver also may be involved as a result of the heat generated during muscle destruction.

Changes in the electroencephalogram (EEG) and occasional unconsciousness have been noted after an electrical insult. Less frequently, true spinal cord injury has occurred. Motor deficits are more common than sensory deficits and may not be noted until the patient is ambulated and neuromuscular imbalances are identified. Fractures also may occur, either from a fall at the time of injury or from severe muscle contraction.[12] Cataract formation is a complication of electrical injury and has been known to occur as long as 3 years following electrical injury, therefore consistent ophthalmologic examinations are necessary.[4]

Chemical Burns

A **chemical burn** and burns from materials that adhere to the skin, such as tar, differ from thermal injury in the duration of tissue destruction. The chemical agent reacts with the tissue to form thermal energy that denatures the protein in the cells. The injury may range from minor blisters to cell damage and sloughing. The amount of tissue damage depends on the concentration of the agent, quantity of agent, length of exposure, mechanism of action, and depth of penetration.[18] Some chemicals such as tannic acid cause organ toxicity in addition to surface damage. This internal damage may be restricted to one organ or may cause systemic damage. Inhaled chemicals may damage the respiratory system and also may be more difficult to neutralize and treat.[18] Because of their affinity for tissue, alkaline agents are more difficult to remove and may cause more damage than acids.[4]

NURSING CARE PLAN   *Nutritional Deficit in the Burn Patient*

Nursing diagnosis/ Expected outcome	Interventions	Rationale
Altered nutrition, less than body requirement related to increased caloric demand of burn injury	Consult with dietitian regarding caloric allotment	Dietitian is the expert in this area and a valuable member of the burn team.
•*Patient maintains caloric intake sufficient to promote healing and maintain ideal body weight based on the Curreri formula (25 kcal × wt. (kg) + 40 kcal × %burn = daily caloric requirements) as evidenced by maintenance of weight and progressive healing*	Assess level of pain before eating and medicate accordingly	Pain commonly diminishes appetite.
	Schedule potentially painful procedures to avoid mealtimes	Anxiety from impending procedures as well as pain from procedures already performed will diminish the appetite.
	Eliminate noxious environmental stimuli (odors, noises, wound care materials)	Unpleasant stimuli decrease the desire to eat.
	Allow ample time for completion of the meal	The physical act of eating may be difficult; a relaxed atmosphere enhances the appetite.
	Provide assistive devices to promote self-feeding (feeding blocks, plate rails)	Self-feeding fosters independence and enhances self-concept, which promotes participation at meals.
	Allow selection of preferred foods within prescribed nutritional framework (15% to 25% protein, 45% to 55% carbohydrates, 20% to 40% fat)	Self-selection of preferred foods diminishes feelings of powerlessness and provides palatable, pleasurable calories and nutrients.
	Provide high-calorie snacks between meals (milk shakes, protein drinks, juice)	High-calorie snacks increase total caloric intake, and may be easier to tolerate in combination with average sized meals. Anorexia can occur if a large quantity of food is presented at each meal.
	Weigh daily at the same time on the same scale	Daily weights give a gross indication of nutritional status.

Infection

Infection is a leading cause of death in individuals who have survived the burn injury itself. The injury destroys the body's protective cover, its frontline defense against foreign invasion. In addition, inhalation injuries frequently result in pulmonary infections.[6] In the wounds themselves, the eschar, a leathery covering of denatured protein on a full-thickness burn, is an excellent medium for the growth of microorganisms. It is difficult to treat with systemic antimicrobial agents. There is some belief that the source of the infection may be the patient's own microbial flora, since the wounds commonly become infected 3 to 5 days after admission.[11] Trauma, including minor thermal injury, induces an inflammatory response. Severe burns initiate further changes, such as venous stasis, microthrombi formation, and immunosuppression.[8] In burn injury the viscosity and flow of the blood changes and a barrier develops between the bacteria and the body's own phagocytes. This barrier alters the delivery of oxygen, antibodies, and phagocytic cells to the injured area. The burned patient's serum reflects impairment of neutrophils and macrophages. The neutrophils are altered so that bacteria may be phagocytized but not killed. Bacteria can reside and divide within the neutrophil and are protected from antimicrobials by the cell membrane. The end result is an excellent environment for harboring and propagating infectious organisms, regardless of the source.

Healing

The ultimate solution for the multiple-system problems of the burn patient is an intact covering of skin. Partial-thickness injuries heal through the migration of epithelial cells from the wound margins and from the small pieces of epithelium remaining in hair follicles and sweat glands. As healing progresses, epithelial islands appear. The newly formed epithelium is very delicate and easily damaged and must be carefully protected.

Deeper wounds heal through a cascade of events. Mast cells, located in the dermis, secrete histamine, causing an accumulation of exudate over the wound surface. White blood cells are chemotactically attracted to the area, phagocytizing wound debris and bacteria. Marginal epithelial cells migrate from the periphery of the wound. Fibroblasts secrete collagen, and injured venules bud, forming capillary networks. These processes create granulation tissue, which, when healthy, is beefy red and highly vascular.

If the wound is not disrupted, its edges pull together and wound contracture ensues. Fibroblasts continue to infiltrate, but the layers of collagen are not uniformly laid down, so scarring will occur. The surrounding epithelium continues to encroach from the margins inward. Ultimately, a closed wound with an elevated scar results.

Therapeutic Management

A multidisciplinary team can most effectively devise the comprehensive treatment plan that burn patients require. The team comprises physicians, nurses, occupational therapists, dietitians, social workers, and psychologists. The team works with the patient to accomplish five primary objectives: (1) to preserve body function, (2) to prevent infection, (3) to restore skin integrity, (4) to provide support and comfort, and (5) to restore a normal living pattern to the patient. The American Burn Association (ABA) has developed a general classification system, the Injury Severity Grading System, that categorizes all burn injuries as major, moderate, or minor (Table 75-1).

The physical environment in which care is given is an important factor in the patient's survival. A severe burn causes the individual to lose heat through evaporation and convection. To decrease the caloric demand for maintaining the patient's body temperature, the room temperature is kept between 82° F and 92° F with an ambient humidity of greater than 80%. Infection control is a serious problem in the care of burn patients. The use of scrub suits and individual dressing care items, as well as readily available facilities for handwashing and waste disposal, helps minimize the risk of infection; isolation helps alleviate the danger of nosocomial infection. Equipment is individualized, and the caregiver must not be caring for another infectious or compromised patient.

The three phases of burn care are the emergent,

TABLE 75-1 Burn Classification (American Burn Association)

Severity of burn	Criteria	Recommended treatment facility
Minor	Partial thickness of <15% TBSA; no full thickness; no involvement of eyes or ears	Emergency rooms; outpatients
Moderate	Partial thickness of 15% to 25% TBSA; full thickness <10% TBSA not involving the hands, face, eyes, ears, feet, or genitalia	General hospital; may be outpatients
Major	Partial thickness of >25% TBSA; full thickness >10% TBSA; true electrical injuries; injury to hands, face, eyes, ears, feet, or genitalia; complications of inhalation injury, fracture, or other concomitant trauma; poor-risk patients	Burn unit of hospital; burn center

or resuscitative phase, the acute phase, and the rehabilitation phase. The emergent phase generally encompasses the period from the time the burn was incurred to the point at which the patient is considered physiologically stable, usually within 48 hours after injury. The acute phase lasts until all full-thickness burns are covered with skin. The rehabilitation period for adults lasts approximately 5 years and includes reintegration into society.

Medical personnel obtain a brief history at the scene if possible; the complete medical and nursing history is completed later in the acute care facility. The initial information includes a description of the circumstances of the injury, any other injury sustained, the chemical agents or type of materials involved in the fire, and whether the fire occurred in a confined space (indicating the possibility of an inhalation injury). Known allergies and preexisting medical conditions also are valuable pieces of information that are best obtained as early as possible.

THE ABCs OF LIFE SUPPORT

A: Establish **A**irway.
B: Ensure **B**reathing.
C: Provide **C**irculation.

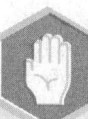

CLINICAL ALERT

Although the patient may have been brought to the emergency room by experienced personnel, it is not uncommon for patients to have some areas of clothing or skin that are still smoldering, meaning that the last vestiges of the burning process remain. The nurse must carefully check a recent burn victim to ensure that all burning has been stopped and cooled.

Prehospital care

At the scene of the burn injury, emergency personnel are primarily concerned with separating the patient from the source of the injury and providing the ABCs (see box) of trauma care as needed until the patient arrives at the emergency room. In addition, measures to keep the patient warm and minimize further contamination of the wound are instituted.

Emergency department care

On arrival in the emergency facility, the care begun at the scene continues at a rapid pace. Arterial blood gases usually are the first laboratory evaluation performed after admission to establish levels of pulmonary function. Carboxyhemoglobin levels are assessed for the possibility of carbon monoxide poisoning.

Additional blood evaluations may include serum electrolytes, creatinine, blood urea nitrogen, colloid oncotic pressure, total protein, albumin, and trace elements such as calcium and magnesium. These levels characteristically reveal the changes in fluid composition in the various compartments. Admission cultures of the blood, urine, and sputum usually are ordered as documentation of baseline status. Wound surface swab (qualitative) cultures from various sites also may be obtained. Large burn injuries require massive amounts of fluid as quickly as possible to prevent hypovolemic shock. At least two intravenous lines using entry ports larger than 18 gauge are established immediately. The longer the patient goes without fluid support, the greater the peripheral vasoconstriction, making placement of peripheral lines more difficult. If intravenous catheters were inserted under nonsterile conditions, they must be replaced. Intravenous access is best obtained through intact skin, but burned sites are used if necessary. A Foley catheter is inserted and the patient's weight obtained to assess the adequacy of fluid resuscitation. A nasogastric tube is inserted to decompress the stomach in anticipation of possible ileus and to evaluate the pH of gastric contents. Urinalysis and culture and sensitivity are performed after the catheter is inserted. Peripheral pulses are evaluated for presence and character, particularly in circumferential injuries. If the pulses are absent (as assessed by ultrasonic monitoring devices) or if the patient is having respiratory difficulty because of a tight band of circumferential eschar around the thorax, an incision may be made through the eschar **(escharotomy)** to ease the constriction. Since the incision is made only through the eschar, very little blood is noted. Deeper burn wounds may require an incision to the fascia **(fasciotomy),** causing greater blood loss because the wound extends into living tissue.[27] Once initial assessments have been made and life-threatening dysfunctions have been addressed, pain medication can be administered if necessary. Narcotics administered intravenously are the initial drugs of choice, because absorption from the musculature is erratic and an ileus may be present.[12] Antianxiety agents may be used. Drugs (e.g., Narcan) to reverse these medications must be available if respiratory depression develops. Tetanus toxoid also is administered at this time because of the high probability of anaerobic burn wound contamination.[7]

Inhalation injury

Inhalation injuries are most common when the fire occurs in a closed space. The findings of facial burns, singed nasal hairs, and sputum tinged with carbon, as well as auscultation of wheezing and rales, suggest an inhalation injury. Any patient with a suspected inhalation injury receives 100% humidified oxygen in case an inhalation injury becomes apparent within the first few days. An endotracheal tube is inserted at the first signs of respiratory distress caused by smoke inhalation or an edematous airway.[14] In the case of an edematous airway, the patient may remain intubated only a few days until the edema subsides. A tracheostomy is not performed unless a severe respiratory emergency develops, because any invasive procedure increases the risk of infection.[12] The serum carboxyhemoglobin is a valuable indicator of the carbon monoxide content of the blood. Because hemoglobin has a greater affinity for

AREA	AGE – YEARS					% 2°	% 3°	% TOTAL
	0 – 1	1 – 4	5 – 9	10 – 15	ADULT			
Head	19	17	13	10	7			
Neck	2	2	2	2	2			
Ant. Trunk	13	13	13	13	13			
Post. Trunk	13	13	13	13	13			
R. Buttock	2 1/2	2 1/2	2 1/2	2 1/2	2 1/2			
L. Buttock	2 1/2	2 1/2	2 1/2	2 1/2	2 1/2			
Genitalia	1	1	1	1	1			
R.U. Arm	4	4	4	4	4			
L.U. Arm	4	4	4	4	4			
R.L. Arm	3	3	3	3	3			
L.L. Arm	3	3	3	3	3			
R. Hand	2 1/2	2 1/2	2 1/2	2 1/2	2 1/2			
L. Hand	2 1/2	2 1/2	2 1/2	2 1/2	2 1/2			
R. Thigh	5 1/2	6 1/2	8 1/2	8 1/2	9 1/2			
L. Thigh	5 1/2	6 1/2	8 1/2	8 1/2	9 1/2			
R. Leg	5	5	5 1/2	6	7			
L. Leg	5	5	5 1/2	6	7			
R. Foot	3 1/2	3 1/2	3 1/2	3 1/2	3 1/2			
L. Foot	3 1/2	3 1/2	3 1/2	3 1/2	3 1/2			
					TOTAL			

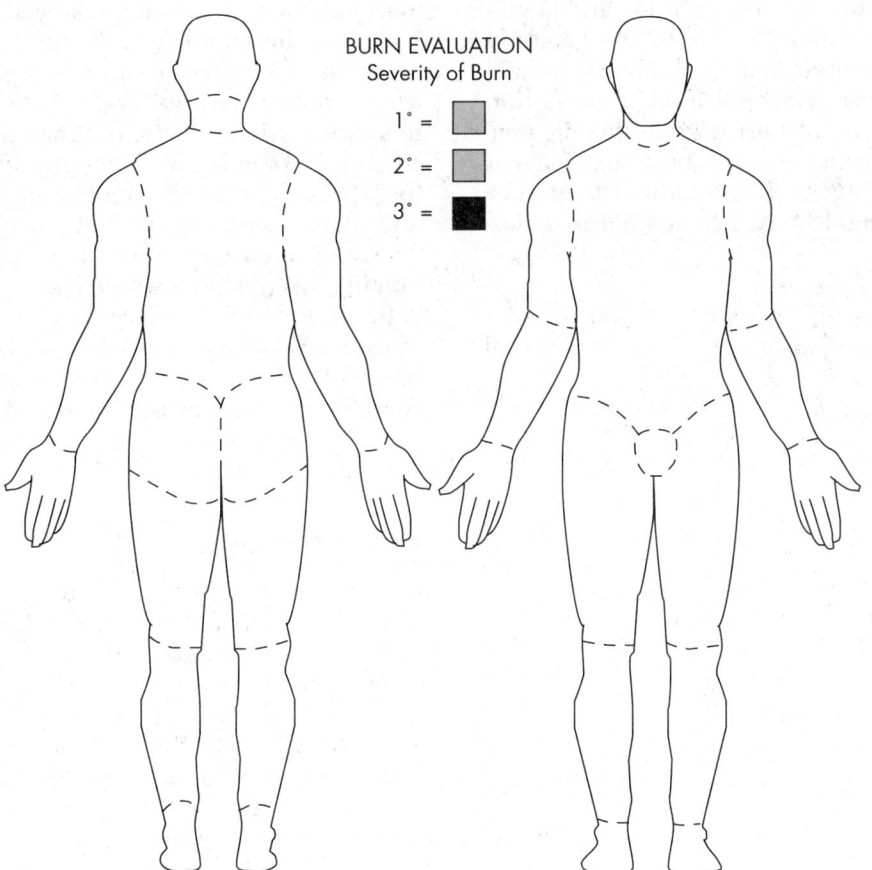

BURN EVALUATION
Severity of Burn

1° =
2° =
3° =

FIGURE 75-6 Lund and Browder burn assessment chart. (From Lund CC, Browder NC: The estimate of areas of burns, *Surg Gynecol Obstet* 79:352, 1944. By permission of *Surg Gynecol Obstet*.)

carbon monoxide than for oxygen, an elevated carboxyhemoglobin level indicates that less oxygen is being delivered to all vital tissues. The patient may exhibit depressed mental status and may even be stuporous as a result of the anoxia caused by elevated carboxyhemoglobin levels. The physician uses the fiberoptic bronchoscope to visualize the upper airway structures and to confirm the presence of airway edema and inflammation, mucosal sloughing, and carbonaceous material in the airway. In many institutions the patient also undergoes a xenon ventilation-perfusion scan to help define the areas of injury.

Burn assessment

The sites of injury can most easily be documented by using a line drawing of the body, shading areas of partial and full thickness injury. The extent of the burn can be calculated by using a nomogram denoting the relative percentages of the various body parts. The most widely used tool is the Lund and Browder chart (see Figure 75-6).[30] Burn size can be roughly estimated by using the "rule of nines," which assigns 9% of the total body surface area to the head and each arm, 18% to each leg, anterior and posterior trunk, and the remaining 1% to the genitalia (Figure 75-7).[10] It is important to obtain a good assessment of burn area, since all fluid resuscitation formulas are functions of burn size, either in percentage of body surface area or in actual burned body surface area (BBSA). If the patient is neither over nor under normal body size, standard nomograms are useful for calculating total body surface. These nomograms use the patient's height and weight to calculate body surface area in square meters.

Fluid resuscitation

Over the years various formulas have been developed to guide the fluid resuscitation of burn patients. The Parkland formula (lactated Ringer's 4 mL/kg × BBSA, 0 colloid, 0 water) is probably the most commonly used for the resuscitation of the adult burn patient. The primary solution used after initial resuscitation is 5% dextrose, and the goal is to maintain a serum sodium concentration at 140 Eq/L. Hypertonic saline has been used to treat shock states, including burns, but it is not widely used. Table 75-2 summarizes other formulas used for fluid resuscitation. Administration of colloid during the initial postburn period is controversial. Immediately after injury, the serum albumin and total protein levels are elevated because of the rapid loss of plasma fluids. As fluid resuscitation is implemented, both the albumin and total protein levels decrease, reflecting the dilution of existing intravascular proteins. Capillary integrity is partly restored within 12 to 24 hours of injury, and colloid-containing solutions may be added to the resuscitation regimen at this time to normalize serum levels. Fresh plasma, whole blood, or salt-poor albumin may be used to replace colloid, depending on the physician's preference. Initial resuscitation is considered complete 24 hours after treatment begins, but evaporative fluid loss from the open burn wounds is still massive. Additionally, evaporative water losses can be as high as 250 mL/day for every degree of body temperature above normal. Fluid maintenance requirements decrease as the patient's wounds heal or become biologically closed. However, factors that further compromise the patient, such as sepsis or renal failure, may increase fluid requirements.

Wound treatment

As soon as the initial assessments have been made and analgesia has taken effect, the burn wounds are cleaned and debrided, either by immersion or in a shower. Blisters are removed, the area is cleansed, and nonadherent tissue is removed. Once the wounds have been cleaned and debrided, the extent and depth of the injury are reassessed. Frequently, additional areas of injury are discovered. Care is taken to examine the scalp and all skin folds. All remaining hair is clipped short or shaved from surrounding skin to decrease surface contamination. After the second assessment, a topical antimicrobial agent is applied. The introduction of topical antimicrobial agents has been associated with a dramatic

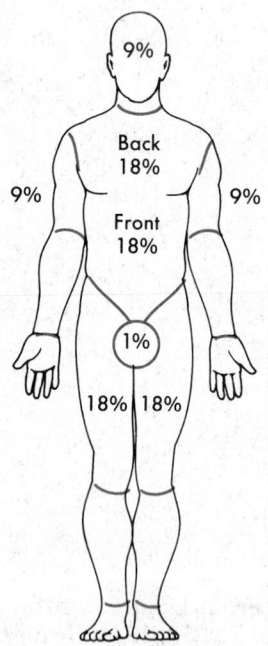

FIGURE 75-7 Rule of nines.

TABLE 75-2   Calculating Fluid Needs in Burn Patients

Name	First 24 hours	Solutions, amounts, and rates, second 24 hours
Brooke (modified) 1970	2 mL lactated Ringer's solution/% BBSA/kg	Colloid 0.5 mL/% BBSA/kg
		+
	½ given over first 8 hr	D_5W maintenance
	½ given over next 16 hr	
Burnett Burn Center	3 ml isotonic or hypertonic alkaline sodium solution/% BBSA/kg	Colloid 0.5 mL/% BBSA/kg
		+
		Additional colloid as needed
	½ as *guide* for first 8 hr	+
	½ as *guide* for next 16 hr	D_5 ¼ normal saline maintenance
	Calculated volumes are used as "starting points" for IV rate, but actual rates are titrated to individual patient response.	+
		D_5 (% BBSA)(TBSA M^2)

Adapted from Rubin M et al: Fluid resuscitation of the thermally injured patient, *Clin Plast Surg* 13(1):13, 1986.

decline in the mortality of burn injuries. The two most widely used antimicrobial agents are silver sulfadiazine (Silvadene, Flint SSD) and mafenide acetate (Sulfamylon), which have different properties and indications. Systemic antibiotics usually are reserved for systemic infections to avoid the development of resistant pathogens.[11] See Figure 75-8 for an illustration of the application of silver sulfadiazine and wrap.

Gastrointestinal system

The gut reacts to trauma and subsequent catecholamine release by decreasing enteric circulation and slowing or stopping peristalsis. Intestinal gases accumulate and may cause nausea and vomiting, with the risk of aspiration. For this reason a nasogastric tube must be used to accomplish gastric decompression. Gastric hyperacidity accompanies the gas accumulation, and an antacid regimen is initiated as soon as possible, usually in an amount that depends on gastric pH. Systemic alkalinizers usually are prescribed before surgery for debridement or grafting if the patient's intake of all other oral or nasogastric fluids is limited. Gastric alkalinization therapy is continued until the wound is almost healed, especially if the patient's oral intake remains limited. The histamine H_2-receptor antagonists (used to treat peptic ulcer disease) may be used prophylactically for burn-related stress ulcer. Cimetidine and ranitidine are the most commonly prescribed drugs. They exert their action on the parietal cells by competitively inhibiting the action of histamine and reducing the amount of gastric acid secreted.

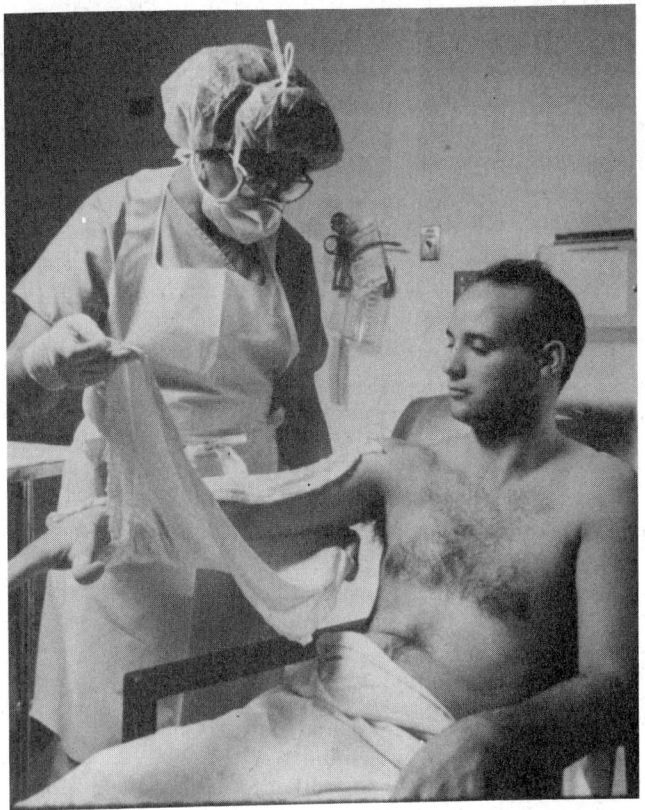

FIGURE 75-8   Applying silver sulfadiazine and wrap.

Musculoskeletal system

Rehabilitative care begins on the day of the injury. The goals of rehabilitation are to limit or prevent loss of motion, prevent or minimize anatomical deformities, prevent loss of body weight (especially muscle mass), and return the patient to work and normal activity as soon as possible. Active range of motion is the most important factor in preventing loss of motion and muscle mass and anatomical deformity in burned patients, but adjunctive measures also may be necessary. Proper positioning is critical for maintaining joint motion. The benefit gained from frequent exercise can be lost after sleeping briefly in a "comfortable" position (see Table 75-3).

Management of concomitant fractures in a burn injury presents special problems. Simple fractures usually can be kept immobile in splints, but more complicated fractures require further stabilization. Because routine casts of plaster or fiberglass interfere with proper wound care, fractures may require external fixation devices. The pins represent additional sources of contamination, but topical antimicrobial agents can be applied to pin sites. External fixation also allows direct visualization of the surface wounds, and even skin grafting can be accomplished around the pin sites.

Hands and wrists must be splinted early in the postburn course. Flexion is considered the position of comfort for the wrist. The problems associated with this position are the tendency for the metacarpal-phalangeal joints to hyperextend with flexion of the interphalangeal joints and loss of thumb abduction or rotation. These usually are overcome if the wrist is placed in extension (20 to 40 degrees).[32]

Pain control

The pain of a burn wound depends on its extent and depth and the stage of healing. Partial-thickness wounds have exposed nerve endings that can cause excruciating pain, even when touched by air currents. In contrast, in full thickness injuries the nerve endings in the wound have been destroyed but the margins are hypersensitive to pain. The severely burned patient also may feel deep muscle pain caused by inflammation and ischemia. The most common intervention for pain control is pharmacologic. Almost all burn units use narcotic analgesics, some combining them with psychotropic drugs. The initial drug of choice is morphine, but other drugs such as methadone, codeine, and hydromorphone may be used. Narcotics are given intravenously until fluid resuscitation is completed and gastric motility restored. Patient-controlled analgesia (PCA) pumps have been used with some success in the burn patient by alleviating pain while allowing the patient a measure of environmental control. Dosages of analgesia vary according to the individual patient, and are most effective when administered with some flexibility that is based on the patient's unique situation.[2]

A mixture of nitrous oxide and oxygen (Nitronox) can be delivered through mask or mouthpiece to alleviate the most painful procedural situations. Its use is currently somewhat limited due to the lack of information regarding long-term usage.[7]

It is important to remember that any manipulation of the patient causes pain. Activities of daily living, which cause the patient to move, pull at the wound and produce cracks, rubs, and bleeding. Splints are cumbersome, uncomfortable, and heavy. Hydrotherapy, wound debridement, and dressing changes all cause significant pain. Respiratory depression caused by use of narcotics can be a problem, although it is infrequent. The availability of medications that reverse the action of narcotics (e.g., Narcan) and equipment that provides respiratory support if needed lessens the risk of narcotics use.

TABLE 75-3	Positioning the Burn Patient
Area burned	**Position**
Upper extremities	No pillow under neck
	Towel roll under cervical spine
	Neck splint
	90-degree abduction, neutral rotation
	Elbow splint to maintain position
	Abduction with 10- to 15-degree forward flexion and external rotation
	Support abducted arm with suspension from IV pole or bedside table
	Extension of elbow
	Hand splint
Lower extremities	Hip extension with neutral rotation
	Supine with leg extended
	Prone-lying (if medically appropriate)
	Trochanter roll
	Foam wedge along lateral aspect of thigh
	Knee or long leg splint
	Knee extension
	Patient out of bed with legs extended and elevated
	Ankle splint
	Padded footboard with heels free of pressure

CLINICAL ALERT

A pillow for the head is contraindicated in burn injuries of the lower face or anterior neck. Pillows encourage the development of flexion contractures of the neck, often accompanied by a deformity of the lower face. The neck is placed in extension during rest and sleep periods. The position of comfort is the position of contracture.

Nonsurgical treatment

A wound left to heal without surgical intervention must be kept clean and free of devitalized tissue, as epithelial migration is impeded by these physical obstructions. This is accomplished through hydrotherapy, mechanical wound debridement, and removal of serous crusts and nonadherent tissue from the wound's surface. Applying topical agents provides the wound with some protection and aids in the removal of eschar through bacterial action and the release of collagenase from migrating epithelial cells. A number of topical agents can be used, depending on the physician's preference, the desired result, and the risk of potential side effects. Enzymatic agents (Travase) that are proteolytic and act to shorten the time of eschar separation may be used to achieve more rapid wound closure and decrease the risk of infection.[19] The patient must be observed for side effects specific to each topical agent such as hemodynamic alterations, electrolyte imbalances, and pain. Burn wounds contract and heal from migration of epithelium. The healing process is very slow, scars develop, and contractures may be permanent.

Surgical management

Surgical therapy follows two principal techniques. One is staged removal of dead tissue (usually at 7- to 10-day intervals). The other is excision of all dead tissue as soon as the patient is hemodynamically stable (usually within 4 days.) The highest excisional priority is early joint mobilization, particularly in the hands. These areas frequently are excised and grafted early in the burn course. Maximal preservation of facial contour usually calls for serial debridement with delayed excision and grafting.

Types of excision

There are two basic methods of excision, tangential and fascial. Frequently, both methods are used on the same patient for excision of different body parts. **Tangential excision** involves gradual planing of the

burn to the level of viability, which is demonstrated by diffuse, punctate capillary bleeding. Tangential excision attempts to preserve as much viable tissue as possible; however, if it is used early in the burn course (within 4 to 5 days of injury), zones of the wound that might have recovered in time are lost. If the injury is severe enough, tangential excision to fat may occur. Because tangential excision can cause massive blood loss, only a small area of skin can be planed during one procedure.

Because fat has limited vascularity, split-thickness skin grafts do not adhere well. In these cases the surgeon may perform a **fascial excision** in which all denatured tissue is removed with the underlying fat layer. This method is used chiefly with large, full-thickness injuries. By removing the fat bed an extremely vascular tissue (fascia) is revealed, and thus graft take is almost assured. However, removing the fat layer is extremely disfiguring, as fat gives the body shape and contour. Blood loss with fascial excision is less than that of tangential excision.[25]

Grafts

Surgical excision of a burn wound requires wound closure. This can be achieved with a variety of synthetic and biologic dressings. Permanent closure can be accomplished only with **autografts.** These are grafts harvested from uninjured areas of the patient's body. Occasionally donor skin can be harvested from an identical twin. The sites of choice for donor harvesting are areas usually hidden from plain view such as the buttocks, thighs, upper arms, lower abdomen, and scalp. However, if necessary any area with intact skin can and will be harvested. There are two types of grafts: split-thickness skin grafts (STSG) and full-thickness skin grafts (FTSG). Split-thickness skin grafts are taken only through some layers of the epidermis. Donor areas are actually surgically created partial-thickness injuries that heal spontaneously in 7 to 14 days. Split-thickness grafts are applied to wounds in two forms, as sheet grafts or meshed grafts. **Sheet grafts** are applied just as they are harvested. They produce the best cosmetic result and generally are applied to highly visible areas such as the face and back of the hands. Sheet grafts are also used in areas that undergo the most stress, such as joint areas. Sheet grafts are laid on the wound and secured with staples or sutures. They may then be left open to the air so that they can be easily monitored. With **meshed grafts,** a mesh pattern, or lattice, of small slits is created with a mechanical device after the skin is harvested. The meshing allows the donor skin to be expanded to cover a larger surface area than the original donor site. Meshed grafts are placed on the wound bed and secured with sutures, staples, or dressings. The grafts can be expanded to cover large wounds or left unexpanded to allow for maximal drainage of a small area. Because the graft is fragile, a layer of fine mesh gauze is placed over the graft after it has been positioned. The gauze may be impregnated with various solutions to prevent the dressing from drying out or adhering to the wound and to prevent or control infection. A bulky dressing is then applied to absorb drainage. Orthotic splints may be applied to prevent movement of the grafted area. Surgical dressings usually are left intact for 3 to 4 days if no bleeding or signs of infection are noted. Full-thickness skin grafts are used primarily for reconstructive procedures, although they are becoming more common with primary grafting. Skin is taken through all epidermal layers so that the donor site does not epithelialize. The donor site can then be primarily closed or can be closed with a split-thickness skin graft. Full-thickness skin grafts are used in areas such as the face where the best cosmetic effect is desired. The newest type of autograft is cultured epithelium. Single cells taken from unburned skin are placed on a growth medium and will grow to between 50 and 70 times the size of the initial sample. Within 3 to 4 weeks, enough skin can be grown to cover an adult. The skin is adhered to a backing of vaseline gauze and applied to the recipient bed in the operating room.[8]

Biologic and synthetic skin substitutes

Biologic dressings are temporary organic coverings for burn wounds. They are valuable because they have many of the properties of skin and provide many of the same functions. Biologic dressings minimize fluid loss, decrease pain, and keep the wound's surface moist for future graft application. In a partial-thickness wound they allow for healing underneath. Biologic dressings for clinical use are described as **homograft** (allograft), which comes from another human being; **xenograft** (heterograft), which comes from other animal species; and synthetic wound barriers. Homograft comes from living people other than the recipient, such as parents or siblings, but most frequently it comes through anatomical donations. Homograft may harbor any number of communicable diseases, including HIV and hepatitis B, but potential donations are carefully screened before they are accepted.[6] Homograft is considered a biologic dressing, but unlike other such dressings it may be left in place for as long as 8 days. Homograft is covered with a dressing of fine mesh gauze impregnated with antimicrobials. The gauze may be changed as often as every 8 hours to evaluate the homograft and site. Human amnionic membranes (amnion) have been used for years as temporary wound coverings. After placement amnion may be left on the wound until it is sloughed. Because amnion has bacteriostatic properties, a topical antimicrobial is not needed. The main disadvantages of amnion are its limited shelf life and the preparation required before it can be applied to a burned patient. Heterografts (skin from other animal species) have been used for many years. Porcine xenograft is readily available from several commercial sources, is easy to store, sterile, and adheres well to wound beds. The biggest disadvantage of porcine xenograft is that it is easily digested by wound collagenase, leaving the wound open to bacterial invasion. One of the most recently developed synthetic skin substitutes is the collagen dressing (e.g., Epigard and Biobrane). Collagen offers many of the advantages sought in a skin substitute. Synthetic skin provides results at least as acceptable as those of homograft in covering split-thickness defects. These dressings close the wound and protect it from bacterial penetration, so topical antimicrobials are not necessary. Synthetic skin can decrease pain and encourage healing in partial-thickness injuries, but it is not as effective as homograft in preparing a granulation bed for later autografting.

Electrical burns

After adequate fluid resuscitation has been assured, attention is directed to the wounds themselves. If edematous muscles, vessels, and nerves are compressed, a fasciotomy (incision through skin into fascia around muscle) may be required. In these cases the patient frequently is taken into the operating room after admission so that muscle exploration can be performed. All obviously dead muscle is excised, and the wound is left open, although it is covered with an antimicrobial to keep it moist and to minimize infection. In an electrical injury, the thrombosed vasculature deprives tissues of their blood supply, and tissue death may follow. The wound is inspected every 6 hours to identify any additional areas of necrosis. As many as three or four debridements carried out over a week or more may be necessary before all necrotic tissue has been excised. Amputation of the involved extremity may be required. Open wounds are treated with a topical antimicrobial drug such as silver sulfadiazine or bacitracin. Nonexcised areas such as entry and exit wounds may be treated with mafenide acetate, since it can penetrate devitalized tissue. After all necrotic tissue has been removed, the wounds are closed, primarily or with a graft. Full-thickness skin grafts or tissue flaps frequently are used to cover electrical injuries and may be used in conjunction with amputations to produce the best possible base for a prosthetic device.

Chemical burns

The key to treating almost any chemical burn is copious lavage with plain water or an isotonic solution. Dilution with water decreases the concentration, removes the chemical from bodily contact, and decreases the chemical's rate of reaction with tissue.[18] After the chemical has been diluted and removed, standard burn therapies of fluid resuscitation, wound debridement, and local wound care are implemented. Laboratory analysis of serum contents may be ordered to check for any systemic toxicity, such as hepatic damage from topical tannin. Because chemical injuries of the eyes have a high incidence of permanent damage, prompt attention is essential. Copious lavage with physiologic saline may be required for up to 48 hours after injury. Corneal perforation may occur as a late complication. Close daily observation, preferably by an ophthalmologist, is desirable. Prophylactic instillation of a bland ophthalmic ointment usually is prescribed until edema resolves sufficiently for a full corneal evaluation to be performed.

Tar burns

The burn injury caused by contact with tar will vary in severity depending on the temperature of the tar. The removal of the tar is not a treatment priority. Cooling the tar with water should be done immediately in order to stop the process of tissue destruction. Ointment with a petroleum base is then applied and the area is dressed. This promotes emulsification of the tar and its eventual removal. The dressing is changed on a schedule to best promote the removal of the tar. Once the tar is totally eliminated, the burn is assessed and care begun accordingly.[4,16]

NURSING MANAGEMENT OF THE PATIENT WITH BURNS
Assessment

In the emergent phase, assessment is constant during the immediate postburn and early stabilization activities. The nurse may perform the initial physical assessment in conjunction with the physician, and several assessments may be going on at once. Initial evaluations include the airway, breathing, and circulation (ABCs). The nurse must assess the vital signs, including respiratory rate, temperature, peripheral blood pressure, and apical and peripheral pulses. These values point to alterations in hemodynamic status and to circulatory compromise caused by edema or eschar. After the immediate stability of the patient's condition has been assured, additional assessments are performed system by system (see box above).

When all other assessments have been completed, the physician and nurse evaluate the size and depth of the burn wound. During the initial period after injury, the wound itself does not endanger the patient's life. The most imminent threat is cardiovascular compromise or pulmonary deficit mani-

---

NURSING INTERVENTION SUMMARY

Assessments for a Moderate or Severe Burn

1. Control the airway, breathing, and circulation.
2. Obtain baseline vital signs and weight.
3. Physical assessment

Respiratory—Observe for singed nasal hairs, circumoral burns, conjunctivitis, sooty/bloody sputum, and hoarseness; observe for symmetry and use of accessory muscles of respiration; auscultate for rales, rhonchi, wheezing, and inspiratory stridor; palpate ribs for tenderness

Cardiac—Ausculate for rate, rhythm, and quality; compare apical and radial pulses; observe ECG for ectopy; palpate limbs for circulation, edema, and capillary refill

Genitourinary—Observe urine for color, quantity, quality, and specific gravity

Gastrointestinal—Observe abdomen for distention; auscultate for bowel sounds; palpate for tenderness

Musculoskeletal—Observe for unusual limb position; palpate for fractures (including head, neck, and limbs)

Neurologic—Assess orientation and level of consciousness; assess pain status

Integumentary—Assess depth, size, and location of all burn wounds; assess entry and exit wounds in electrical burns

---

fested as shock or respiratory distress. Constant nursing assessment continues when the patient moves into the acute phase. Each system is routinely assessed to determine any changes in the patient's status. Additional areas of assessment reflect the concerns of the acute phase: nutritional status, splinting, positioning, and wound care. Wound care is most critical during this phase. Most patients undergo some grafting procedures. As these procedures are completed and areas are grafted and debrided, the wounds are assessed with each dressing change for healing, drainage, wound margins, and the presence or absence of signs of infection. In many of these areas assessment is similar to assessment of other surgical wounds. Areas of granulation with an obvious blood supply indicate wound healing, whereas necrotic tissue or foul-smelling, purulent drainage indicates an infection. A particularly important area of assessment is the patient's level of pain and the adequacy of the pain control measures used (see Chapter 14).

NURSING CARE PLAN   *The Patient with a Major Burn*

Nursing diagnosis/ Expected outcome	Interventions	Rationale
Fluid volume deficit related to increased capillary permeability and increased fluid loss through burn wound (emergent phase) •*Patient will maintain an adequate urine output (30 mL/hr minimum), vital signs within expected limits, electrolytes within normal limits and clear mental status.*	Vital signs q1h Intake and output q1h and observe for trends Weigh daily Monitor electrolytes as drawn (usually q12h) Assess level of consciousness hourly	Monitoring objective physical data frequently will alert caregivers to subtle condition changes that may be crucial to the patient's recovery, or indicate a needed change in the therapeutic regimen.
Infection, high risk for, related to impaired skin integrity and presence of burn wound, impaired immune response, presence of intravenous lines and multiple invasive treatments (emergent, acute phases)	Observe IV site qd for signs of infection Change dressing according to unit protocol	IV insertion site prime location for infection because of frequent manipulation. Consistent monitoring and care will decrease chances of significant infection developing.
•*Patient will remain free of infection as evidenced by temperature 99°-101°F (R), absence of swelling, pain, phlebitis at IV site, absence of infectious organisms in burn wound, urine, blood, and sputum*	Instruct patient to report pain or discomfort Maintain aseptic technique when cleansing burn wounds and changing dressings Monitor wounds for evidence of infection; culture wounds as indicated unit policy Monitor temperature q4h. Rectal probe may be used if consistent monitoring is desired Limit patient contact with individuals who are harboring infectious organisms Maintain universal precautions	Patient may be first to note developing abnormality. Aseptic technique will limit the number of potentially harmful organisms in the burn wound. Close assessment of the wounds and systematic culturing will aid in prompt identification of an infection beginning. Alterations in temperature may be the first sign of an impending infection. Exposure to individuals harboring infections may cause the compromised burn patient to contract an infection. Universal precautions, particularly scrupulous hand washing and gloving when dealing with bodily fluids, is the best way to limit the spread of infectious organisms.
Pain, acute related to exposed nerve endings and frequent dressing changes and debridement (emergent, acute, rehab phases) • *Patient will report pain at a consistently manageable level, 3 or less on a scale of 1 to 10*	Assess need for pain relief every 1 to 2 hours through evaluation of verbal responses, body language, and vital signs. Administer prescribed analgesic promptly when needed; administer before known painful experiences such as dressing changes and debridement	Frequent assessment of pain status provides information related to the unique pain experience for each patient, and allows interventions to be planned accordingly. Prompt administration aids in the alleviation of pain before it becomes severe and less responsive to analgesia. Medication administered before a procedure is more effective in alleviating pain. Anticipating and acting on a patient's needs create a caring atmosphere which aids in alleviating discomfort.

NURSING CARE PLAN   *The Patient with a Major Burn—cont'd*

Nursing diagnosis/ Expected outcome	Interventions	Rationale
	Discuss with patient the effectiveness of the analgesics received; if ineffective in terms of desired outcome, discuss alternate analgesics with physician	Every patient's response to pain and medication is somewhat unique. Evaluation for effectiveness of the medication and altering it as needed improves the chances for a positive outcome.
	If possible, supply patient with a system for patient-controlled analgesia (PCA)	Patient-controlled analgesia has been proven to be very effective in the management of severe pain.
	If possible, teach the patient alternative methods of pain control to augment pharmacologic agents (relaxation, deep breathing, self-hypnosis, guided imagery) and assist with implementation of these methods	Adjunct methods of pain control are very effective in potentiating or replacing pharmaceutical analgesics in many people.
	Discuss procedures to be performed with patient, and allow as much patient participation in each procedure as possible	Environmental control is very effective in decreasing anxiety, which aids in pain relief.
Family processes, altered, high risk for, related to burn injury and resultant physical, economic, and role changes (emergent, acute, rehab phases)	Assist the family in assessing causative factors of family stressors	Identifying specific areas of concern will aid in identifying individual interventions.
•The patient and family will talk about their feelings related to the experience with health care professionals and each other; the family will participate in the care of the patient; the family will access external sources of assistance; the patient will begin to move from the sick role.	Create a supportive environment for family, including private space, awareness of hospital routine, and identification of caregivers	Identification of a specific area will make the environment more familiar and decrease stress. Familiarity with routine helps to normalize an abnormal situation.
	Involve family members in the care of the patient as much as possible	Involving the family members in providing physical care helps to promote closeness between members.
	Support family in decisions to spend time outside the hospital	Decreasing stress within the family by promoting rest will be beneficial for the patient and assist the return to routine behavior.
	Facilitate the family in accessing organizations and individuals who can act as supports	Many organizations exist that provide support and assistance to families in crisis. Other former burn patients may be available to offer assistance.
	Assist the family in communicating with the patient as needed	Experience with many burn patients may offer the nurse unique insights to the burn experience which can facilitate communication.

Nursing Diagnosis

As with all patients, the burn patient requires individualized assessment to determine all areas that would respond to nursing care. The nursing diagnosis for each patient must be reevaluated as the patient's condition changes. Nursing diagnoses related to burn injuries will change in priority to reflect the patient's progress through the phases of burn care. Because burn injury is the classic example of multiple trauma, the individual experience of the patient is crucial to the construction of a useful nursing care plan (see care plan).

Planning

The outcomes for the patient are specific to the nursing diagnoses assigned and tailored to the patient's needs. Short-term goals, as well as long-term goals, are identified to provide benchmarks for patient achievement. Sharing goals with the patient and family when possible may help diminish the powerlessness that burn patients commonly feel.

Implementation

Care of the burn patient, implemented through the nursing care plan, involves diverse activities that are closely related to the patient's needs and condition.

Emergent phase

During the emergent phase, immediately after injury, nursing care focuses on the stabilization of the patient's condition and aiding the patient and family as they begin to cope with a highly stressful situation. When the patient enters the emergency department or clinic, the nurse's first tasks are related to the primary concerns of maintaining an airway, checking for and controlling bleeding, and evaluating and reestablishing circulation. The next priority in the initial care of the patient is initiating one or more venous access sites. These serve as routes for fluid resuscitation and for administration of narcotics for pain management, and the initial dose may be given at this time. Blood and other specimens are then obtained to aid in delineating the patient's status. A Foley catheter is inserted to measure urine output and obtain specimens, and a nasogastric tube is inserted to aid in gastric decompression and analysis. Once the patient's systemic status is relatively stable, nursing care centers on the wound. The patient's baseline weight is obtained, and the wounds are bathed and debrided by the nurse and burn team members, either in a shower or tank depending on institutional policy. Once the wounds are cleansed, the nurse applies the ordered topical agent and the patient is put to bed and allowed to rest. Tetanus prophylaxis, if it has not already been administered, and additional pain medication may be given at this time.

Acute phase

When the patient moves into the acute phase, nursing care is based even more on individual needs, while still reflecting established standards. Some nursing interventions are unique to burn patients and serve as the basis for creative, individualized nursing care.

Infection control

The nurse initiates measures to compensate for the patient's compromised ability to fight infection upon entering the burn unit. This can be upgraded to strict isolation if the burn wound becomes infected. Nursing staff and other members of the health care team routinely wear scrubs as the duty uniform to minimize contamination, since scrubs can be changed when soiled. Additional precautions are taken when the chance for contamination is greatest, such as during hydrotherapy, wound debridement, and linen changes. In these situations the nurse can use a cover gown or plastic apron. Shoe covers may also be worn to decrease contamination of footwear. Anyone coming into direct contact with the burn wounds must observe aseptic technique and don sterile gloves to perform dressing changes and wound debridement. Hair must be restrained and may be additionally protected with a cap. Clean gloves are worn to protect the caregiver from body excretions when performing routine tasks such as taking vital signs, aspirating nasogastric tubes, or collecting urine.

Comfort and pain management

The most common nursing intervention in pain relief is administering prescribed narcotics and instituting comfort measures. Distraction and other cognitive measures such as relaxation techniques, guided imagery, and hypnosis can augment the analgesic effect. In addition to pain, severe pruritus is

ETHICAL ISSUES

- How should the nurse respond to a person with massive burns who refuses further treatment?
- How can a nurse continue to treat a person with burns when the treatment always causes great pain for the patient?

RESEARCH BRIEF

Bell L et al: Pruritus in burns, *J Burn Care Rehabil* 9(3):305, 1988.

This descriptive study by the staff at the Oregon Burn Center was conducted to determine if itching was viewed as a significant problem among all nurses practicing burn care, and to identify patterns among treatment modalities. An 18-item questionnaire was sent to all nurses working in 158 burn centers throughout the United States and Canada. The study found that nurses considered itching to be a significant problem for the patients, particularly at night, and particularly with patients having partial-thickness burns. The most common treatments were the use of Benadryl and antipruritic lotions. All suggested treatments provided some relief to the patients, but none was completely effective. Further research to compare specific treatment methods was suggested.

a significant problem for the burn patient as healing begins. If not controlled, the frequent, severe scratching can destroy fragile grafts and open new areas that may require coverage. Applying lotion and administering antipruritics may be of some help, but the patient needs a great deal of reinforcement to stop scratching.

Splinting and positioning

On admission, consideration is given to preventing loss of motion and anatomical deformity, and a plan for splinting and positioning is developed. Proper positioning is essential for preventing contracture. The position of comfort is frequently the position of contracture. In the past it was not uncommon for patients to develop contractures of both burned and unburned joints. The incidence of contracture in healing patients has been reduced through use of active range of motion (AROM) or appropriate passive range of motion (PROM) and proper resting positions. Burn patients and their families must be taught the importance of early active exercise and proper positioning during rest and sleep. Standing and ambulating must be instituted as soon as possible. Such exercise can reduce the loss of muscle mass, help stimulate appetite, and increase the patient's sense of normalcy. The joints of all extremities are exercised throughout the 24-hour day unless there is a strong contraindication (e.g., fracture or open joints). The burn patient begins active exercise early each day with a schedule of planned activities.

During the first few days exercise periods can last only 3 to 5 minutes per hour. AROM can be encouraged by allowing the patient to accomplish all possible activities of daily living. However, even with the most cooperative patients, AROM programs may not prevent deformities and contractures. In these situations passive motion, serial splinting, and proper positioning are necessary. The principles and considerations in using splints are the same as those for proper positioning. Splints are indicated for preventing further damage to certain structures (e.g., exposed tendons, open joints) and with nerve damage, comatose patients, edematous anatomical areas (e.g., hands), and minor fractures. Splints are worn only when the patient is resting, and AROM is encouraged at other times. Splints frequently are applied to freshly grafted extremities to maintain position for optimal graft adherence. In these cases, splints are applied in the operating room after a dressing has been put on the fresh graft. Range of motion of the affected extremity is curtailed for 4 to 5 days. After this period PROM is instituted, with great care taken so as not to shear the new graft. The patient usually can perform AROM in 7 to 10 days.

Fluid resuscitation

One of the prime objectives of care of the burn patient is restoring fluid balance through fluid resuscitation. The nurse participates in this effort by initiating and maintaining the appropriate fluid therapy as ordered by the physician. Half of the calculated requirements is administered during the first 8 hours after injury. The adequacy of the resuscitation effort is determined by evaluating vital signs (every 15 to 30 minutes) and, more importantly, urine output. The nurse evaluates urine output every 15 minutes for the first hour so that the fluid can be titrated to produce a minimum output of 0.5 mL/kg/hr. Fluid formulas are adjusted to the patient's needs. After the first 8 hours, as the patient's condition stabilizes, the nurse can decrease the frequency of monitoring to hourly and evaluate the urine specific gravity, which is a valuable indicator of glomerular filtration. Fluid resuscitation is considered complete after 24 hours; however, fluid requirements remain high as long as the wounds are open. Nursing responsibilities concerned with maintaining the intravenous line continue as long as the line is present.

Nutrition

A burn patient's metabolic processes create a greater need for calories, protein, carbohydrates, and fat. Wound healing and maintaining homeostasis require a massive caloric intake. The physician usually prescribes some nutritional supplementation. Even with the usual supplements, it is essential for the patient's well-being that regular meals be eaten when possible. The nurse is responsible for devising a treatment plan that encourages consumption of meals. (See Nursing Care Plan for Nutritional Deficit in the burn patient.) In some cases supplements may be given through tube feedings at intervals. Total parenteral nutrition has been used on occasion, but it presents another opportunity for infection.

Gastrointestinal management

Burn patients commonly have diarrhea, usually secondary to the hyperosmolar solutions needed to provide an adequate amount of calories. However, the type of antacid administered to combat stress ulcers can contribute to the development of diarrhea. Magnesium-based antacids can cause diarrhea, and aluminum-based antacids can cause constipation. Balanced antacids generally are available, and ideally these would be the types prescribed for prolonged administration. However, if these are unavailable, alternating the two types of antacid can accomplish the same goal. In addition, the use of continuous tube feedings at a low infusion rate decreases the need for large doses of antacid, thereby avoiding some of the negative results. Opioids as well as antacids can cause constipation. In burn patients, morphine and its derivatives usually are the drugs of choice for pain management. However, using a nonopiate-based drug decreases the potential for constipation. Bulk-forming agents (e.g., bran) or stool softeners are also prescribed to assist in normalizing bowel function.

Wound care

The wound may be cleaned by hydrotherapy or shower in which the topical agents are removed and the eschar is softened. The wound is debrided by mechanical removal of eschar by the nurse or through the use of wet-to-dry dressings, which are changed two or three times a day. Both techniques are very painful to the patient and generate great anxiety. Medications for pain are mandatory before all dressing changes or wound manipulation. Once the wound is clean, either an open or closed method of wound dressing may be used. With the open method the nurse applies the topical agents in a thin layer and the wound is left open to the air. This method allows greater visualization of the wound but leads to some heat loss. The closed method uses bulky dressings soaked with antimicrobial solution. This method generally is reserved for patients with documented allergies to topical agents, some of which are sulfa based. In such cases dressings are changed at least daily to evaluate the wound's con-

dition. Once the wounds are free of eschar, surgery is scheduled if the burns are deep enough to require grafting. Preoperative care of the burn patient involves teaching about the procedure and reviewing respiratory care and the expected routine after surgery. Burn patients commonly undergo several procedures and require interventions to ease their anxiety, which may be aggravated by anticipating increased pain and by periods of extreme immobility. Postoperative care of the burn patient involves evaluation of vital signs, respiratory and fluid status, and overall system recovery, much like any other surgical recovery period. The difference lies in the care that is specific to the type of grafting done and the donor site used.

Sheet grafts

Because sheet grafts are not perforated, any wound drainage accumulates beneath the sheet graft. The accumulated drainage interferes with graft adherence and thus must be evacuated. One technique is called "rolling out" in which a cotton-tipped applicator is used to very gently push the accumulated fluid to a small opening in the graft made by a needle puncture or a small incision. Fluid that has accumulated in the center of the graft must not be rolled out to the edges, as this would disrupt any capillary infiltration of the graft that is proximal to the edges. Center accumulations may also be evacuated by gentle aspiration with a tuberculin syringe and a fine needle (smaller than 20 gauge). The sheet graft must be rolled every 15 minutes immediately after surgery and until drainage becomes minimal, usually no longer than 2 to 3 hours. The graft then can be rolled as needed, but its fluid accumulation must be assessed at least hourly during the first 24 hours after surgery. The graft edges must be kept moist to prevent tissue death, and a thin layer of a topical antimicrobial such as bacitracin or Polysporin may be applied with a sterile cotton-tipped applicator around all the edges of the graft until the graft has fully adhered, usually 5 to 7 days after surgery.

Mesh grafts

Split-thickness skin grafts can be perforated with small slits to allow for expansion of the graft to fully cover the open wound. The created "holes" allow the wound to drain, preventing the graft from floating or not adhering to the recipient bed. These grafts usually are left with the surgical dressings intact for 3 to 5 days after surgery to allow for optimal adherence. If the grafts are left open (i.e., without surgical dressings), care must be taken to keep them moist by using a topical antimicrobial agent impregnated into fine mesh gauze or moist saline compresses. Topical antimicrobial agents are left in place for at least 12 hours. Saline compresses are replaced before they are completely dry to avoid adherence to the new graft or recipient site. Care must be taken to minimize manipulation of the graft. Gentle range of motion of the grafted part can safely be restarted 5 to 7 days after surgery but care must be taken to avoid shearing forces on this area. Even after fully adherent, the graft site is delicate and easily broken down until the wound has fully matured.

Donor site

Donor sites are surgically created partial-thickness injuries. There are a number of dressing techniques employed to facilitate healing of these areas. Xeroform gauze may be placed on the donor site in the operating room and the area covered with a bulky dressing, which is left in place for 24 hours. The area is then redressed with fine mesh gauze impregnated with an antimicrobial and another bulky dressing, which is then changed every 12 hours.[8] Biobrane, a synthetic skin substitute, may also be used. This consists of collagen fibers that adhere to the wound and is removed in about 7 days. Fine mesh gauze impregnated with scarlet red (a mixture of lanolin, olive oil, and petroleum), or with antimicrobial solution is a more traditional method.[7] The donor site with the gauze in place is exposed to the air and kept as dry as possible, using heat lamps if necessary. The desired appearance is a firm, scablike dressing. Patients usually complain of moderate to severe pain in this area that subsides in a few days. In general, donor sites heal spontaneously in 7 to 14 days and may leave a residual skin color change which fades over time.

Outpatient care of minor burn wounds

If a total assessment of the burn patient has revealed a minor wound and few or no concomitant injuries, care of the burned areas can be completed on an outpatient basis. The injured areas are bathed with warm water and mild soap. Blisters may be left intact if they are in areas where they would not interfere with activities of daily living. If the blister is in an area of high mobility where it would be ruptured, it is gently debrided and a dressing is applied. Wounds are treated with a topical antimicrobial, usually silver sulfadiazine (Silvadene). Occasionally, a triple antibiotic (Polysporin) is used. Fine mesh gauze is applied to hold the ointments or creams in contact with the wound, and a bulky dressing is used to protect the area from trauma or environmental contamination. Elastic wraps may be applied to further stabilize and protect the dressing. If environmental contamination of the wound is possible, the physician may prescribe an antibiotic regimen, usually oral penicillin or erythromycin. The patient is given tetanus toxoid and tetanus immune globulin if the last tetanus injection was more than 10 years ago. These patients may also need prescriptions for antipruritics and a mild analgesic. Despite the rapid pace of an emergency department, the nurse must set aside time for patient teaching (see the patient education box below). The patient may return to work as soon as desired and the injury will not interfere with job performance. The nurse must advise the patient of any side effects of prescribed drugs, particularly with regard to mind-altering

---

PATIENT EDUCATION GUIDE   *Outpatient Burn Care*

Objective: Prior to discharge from the emergency department, the patient or caregiver is able to describe procedures that promote healing and prevent complication in a minor burn wound.

Hygiene

Bathe daily to reduce surface bacteria

Wound care

Clean wound three or four times a day with mild soap and water to reduce surface bacteria and debris

Examine wound daily for color changes, odor, drainage, and alterations in wound borders to detect possible early signs of infection

Redress wounds as prescribed (ointment or dry dressing)

Keep affected limbs elevated to promote comfort by decreasing dependent edema

Return to clinic or see physician as instructed

Medication

Follow medication orders as instructed (appropriate times, dosages, indications, and duration)

Activity

Resume normal activity, using comfort and the physician's instructions as a guide

Exercise affected limb four times a day or as directed by the physician to promote circulation, increase muscle tone, and decrease complications of immobility

Allow periods of rest during the day (healing burn wounds require high metabolic demand, increasing the need for rest)

Nutrition

Eat a properly balanced diet that includes protein and vitamin C

pharmaceuticals, which may create a safety hazard in the workplace or during the patient's daily activities.

Evaluation

The evaluation phase of the nursing process involves consideration of the patient's present situation in light of the goals that were originally established with each nursing diagnosis. At the times specified, the patient's progress is compared to the outcome criteria and the plan is evaluated accordingly. It is one of the responsibilities of the nurse caring for the patient who has been burned to evaluate the patient's status on a regular basis. The actual time for evaluation and reflection on the patient's progress will differ according to the patient and the nursing diagnosis involved. Evaluation of the identified problems and interventions will result in the care plan being continued, revised, or resolved. If the plan has no major flaws and patient seems to be progressing toward the established goal, the plan is continued. If the goal was inappropriate, or the nursing diagnosis incorrect, or perhaps the interventions were insufficient, the plan is revised. Resolution of the plan occurs when the patient has achieved the established goal, and the area of concern is no longer problematic. In the care of the burn patient, many of the established nursing diagnoses will be current long after the patient is discharged. Use of the plan by the home care nurse as well as the nurse in the burn unit can facilitate continuity of care.

Documentation

The initial assessment data must be recorded as a baseline for care. A human outline may be used to delineate the type and size of the initial burn wound. Other information, including a history of the injury, medications, and fluids administered, can be recorded in a flow chart or narrative notes, depending on institutional policy. Characteristics of the wounds may be charted as frequently as twice a day. This also is institutional policy reflecting the patient population. The nursing diagnoses may be recorded as a standardized care plan, with interventions for the particular patient added as needed. These nursing care plans are documented so that progress in the areas identified can be noted at regular intervals. Home-going care and instruction also are documented. This gives the entire burn team information about the patient's

---

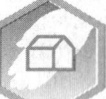

HOME CARE GUIDE *Burn Care*

Before discharge, the patient and family or other caregiver must be taught proper care of the patient and his or her wounds to ensure proper healing and to help the patient begin readjustment into society.

General care

Patient or family should notify the physician if any of the following occur:
1. Change in wound status (open, draining, enlarging, blisters, edema, redness)
2. Signs of infection (temperature above 99° F, foul-smelling or copious wound drainage)
3. Difficulty with dressings or pressure garments

Skin care

Daily care of the skin includes:
1. Daily gentle bathing with mild soap
2. Application of moisturizer to healed burn areas as ordered by the physician
3. Dressing changes on open areas
   a. Wash hands
   b. Wear gloves
   c. Dispose of old dressing
   d. Cleanse areas with mild soap and water and clean washcloth
   e. Apply dressing as specified (may be open or closed method)
   f. Disinfect basin or tub

Daily living

Activities are resumed in conjunction with the patient's ability and the physician's orders, but in general the patient is reminded to:
1. Take protective measures in sunlight, since skin is much more sensitive
   a. Use a sunscreen with a sun protection factor (SPF) higher than 15
   b. Wear long-sleeved shirts, pants, and a hat
   c. Avoid direct, intense sunlight
2. Avoid shearing of the skin
   a. Wear soft clothing, and wash new clothing before wearing
   b. Be aware of instances when the skin may be damaged and use caution (cleaning, cooking, ironing)
3. Eat a well-balanced diet
4. Avoid excess weight gain or loss, since pressure garments will be affected
5. Take in ample fluids (64 ounces or more per day)
6. Exercise injured limbs and joints at least four times a day
7. Increase endurance with aerobic activity
8. Take medications as prescribed (side effects, indications, and dosages are reviewed before discharge)
9. Clean pressure garments daily in mild soap
10. Return to clinic or physician when scheduled

readiness to assume care and areas that need to be covered before discharge.

Ongoing Care

The teaching plan initiated early in the hospital course to allow the patient and family to participate in care continues with a slightly different focus. Areas to review and reinforce include skin care, care of any remaining wounds, diet, exercise, medications, and the need for follow-up care in the future (see home care guide).

Psychologic adaptation

The family or significant others are included in the treatment regimen from the time of admission. Immediate family and friends are encouraged to visit the patient. These meetings are best held in a waiting or visiting area, which allows separation from the patient care area and renews the patient's sense of familial belonging. Visiting the patient in the hospital allows the family to observe wound healing and changes in the patient's appearance. The family can begin to adjust to changes in the patient's physical functioning, and they can come to understand the patient's day-to-day struggles. They also can gain insight into the problems and goals of rehabilitation, emotional as well as physical. The patient is aided in making a healthy emotional adjustment to the reality of the injuries and in preparing realistically for life outside the hospital. Patients need guidance in making realistic appraisals of their conditions, with emphasis on their abilities rather than disabilities. Honest discussion of the patient's feelings about home care offers the nurse an opportunity to anticipate and circumvent possible problems before they occur. The patient must be encouraged to discuss fears related to disfigurement, and the nurse and other members of the burn team can assist in the grieving process. The patient's self-esteem is fostered through performing self-care, assisting with other patients, and taking part in constructing the plan of care.

Rehabilitation

Pressure dressings can decrease the occurrence of hypertrophic scarring, which usually develops when collagen is inappropriately deposited in the wound during healing. Hypertrophic scarring is known to occur more often in individuals with darker complexions, but the actual cause is unknown. The scar becomes elevated and has a "Swiss cheese" appearance. Elastic wraps, stockinettes with elastic reinforcements, or custom-made pressure garments are applied to all burned areas to decrease hypertrophic scar formation. Elastic garments are worn constantly and may be removed only for bathing. Two garments are obtained for each patient so that a clean one is available after the daily bath. This practice continues until the scar has fully matured, which takes 1 to 2 years. Scar maturation is signaled by the loss of scar erythema and by softening of the scarred area. Until the scar matures, further hypertrophic scarring and subsequent joint contracture are possible. The decline in emotional problems 1 year after injury coincides with physical improvement and concomitant social improvements. Skin and scar maturation, which usually is complete within 12 to 24 months after healing, means an increase in physical functioning, improved appearance of the skin, and near-normal skin sensation.

Reintegration

The burn victim's reemergence into society depends on several factors. Psychological adjustment, the degree of disfigurement, sexual adjustment, education, vocational rehabilitation, and outpatient care all affect reintegration. Frustration with the long rehabilitative period is not unusual, as the emotional adjustments may take longer than the physical treatment. Psychologic reactions vary with the patient's stage of development. However, all patients are concerned about their perception by others. An accepting environment, with adequate familial support, usually allows the patient to finally accept the body changes that followed the injury. In some cases the caregivers may perceive something as a problem, whereas the patient does not. For example, a patient who was seen in an outpatient clinic with a severe hypertrophic scar on his face was asked to submit his choice for a primary reconstruction project. The caregiver thought the patient would want the facial scar removed, but the patient only wanted a slight contracture of the ankle corrected so he could play football more easily. The patient can best define the way to make an adjustment, and is a vital component of any long-term treatment plan.

CRITICAL THINKING QUESTIONS

1   What layers of the skin are altered in a full-thickness burn? A partial-thickness burn? Describe each of these burns, including color, blister formation, and severity.

2   What does eschar look like? Why is it important to remove it from the burn wound?

3   What are the basic nursing activities in outpatient burn care? What areas are to be covered in the outpatient teaching plan?

4   Name three areas that require assessment by the nurse when treating the severely burned patient, and explain what information can be gathered from the assessment.

5   Write two sample nursing interventions re-

lated to the nursing diagnosis "Pain related to the burn injury."

6 Write one long-term goal and one short-term goal appropriate to the nursing diagnosis in question 5.

7 Using the Brooke formula, calculate the fluid requirements of a patient with 75% third-degree burns who weighed 230 pounds on admission.

8 What nursing interventions could be implemented for the family of a burn patient? What kind of information would be valuable for the nurse gather about the family?

9 What is the difference between a split-thickness and mesh skin graft? Describe the nursing care requirements of each.

10 What are some important factors in the successful rehabilitation of the burn patient? What factors are most detrimental to the burn patient?

11 Describe the environmental considerations necessary for the burn patient, and discuss the rationale for each.

RESOURCES

1 AMERICAN BURN ASSOCIATION SE 1130 East McDowell, B-2 Phoenix, AZ 85006

2 BURN FOUNDATION 1311 Chancellor Street Philadelphia, PA 19107

3 JOBST INSTITUTE (Pressure garments) Box 653 Toledo, OH 43694

4 NATIONAL INSTITUTE FOR BURN MEDICINE 909 East Ann St Ann Arbor, MI 48104

5 PHOENIX SOCIETY (Burn rehabilitation) 11 Rust Hill Road Levittown, PA 19056

BIBLIOGRAPHY

Current

1. American Burn Association: Hospital and prehospital resources for optimal care of patients with burn injury: guidelines for operation and development of burn centers, *J Burn Care Rehabil* 11:97, 1990.
2. Bingham H: Electrical burns, *Clin Plast Surg* 13(1):75, 1986.
3. Burdge J, Conkright M, Ruberg R: Nutritional and metabolic consequences of thermal injury, *Clin Plast Surg* 13(1):49, 1986.
4. Burgess M: Initial management of a patient with extensive burn injury, *Critical Care Nurs Clin North Am* 3(2):165, 1991.
5. Carlson D, Jordan B: Implementing nutritional therapy in the thermally injured patient, *Critical Care Nurs Clin North Am* 3(2):221, 1991.
6. Cioffi W, Rue L: Diagnosis and treatment of inhalation injuries, *Critical Care Nurs Clin North Am* 3(2):191, 1991.
7. Dalen K, Elster S: Nursing role in management: burn client. In Lewis S, Collier I, editors: *Medical surgical nursing assessment and management of clinical problems*, St Louis, 1992, Mosby-Year Book, Inc.

8. Duncan D, and Driscoll D: Burn wound management, *Critical Care Nurs Clin North Am* 3(2):199, 1991.
9. Dyer C, Roberts D: Thermal trauma, *Nurs Clin North Am* 25(1):85, 1990.
10. Halloway N: *Nursing the critically ill adult*, Menlo Park, 1988, Addison-Wesley Publishing Co.
11. Heggers JP, Robson MC: Infection control in burn patients, *Clin Plast Surg* 13(1):39, 1986.
12. Helvig B: Trauma to the integument: burns. In Howell E, Widia L, Hill M, editors: *Comprehensive trauma nursing theory and practice*, Glenview, Ill, 1988, Scott, Foresman.
13. Herndon DN, Parks DH: Comparison of serial debridement and early massive excision with cadaver skin overlay in the treatment of large burns in children, *Trauma* 26(2):149, 1986.
14. Herndon DN et al: Incidence, mortality, pathogenesis and treatment of pulmonary injury, *J Burn Care Rehabil* 7(2):184, 1986.
15. Nebraska Burn Institute: Advanced burn life support course manual, Lincoln, 1990, The Institute.
16. Pruitt B, Goodwin CW: Thermal & environmental injury. In Moore EE, editor: *Early care of the injured patient*, ed 4, Philadelphia, 1990, BC Decker.
17. Rue L, Cioffi W: Resuscitation of thermally injured patients, *Critical Care Nurs Clin North Am* 3(2):181, 1991.
18. Saydjari R et al: Chemical burns, *J Burn Care Rehabil* 7(5):404, 1986.
19. Silverstein P, Maxwell P, Duckett L: Enzymatic debridement. In Boswick JA Jr, editor: *The art and science of burn care*, Rockville, Md, 1987, Aspen Publishers.
20. Van der Does W: Pain and anxiety ratings during burn care, *Nursing Times* 86(53), 1990.
21. Warden GD: Outpatient care of thermal injuries, *Surg Clin North Am* 67(1):147, 1987.

Classic

22. Artz CP, Moncrief JA, Pruitt BA Jr, editors: *Burns: a team approach*, Philadelphia, 1979, WB Saunders.
23. Curreri PW et al: Dietary requirements of patients with major burns, *J Am Diet Assoc* 65:415, 1974.
24. Demling RH: Fluid and electrolyte management, *Crit Care Clin* 1(1):27, 1985.
25. Desai MH: Epidemiology, assessment and treatment of burn injuries, *Emerg Care Q* 1(3):51, 1985.
26. Foley FD: The burn autopsy: fatal complications of burns, *Am J Clin Pathol* 52(1):1, 1969.
27. Jacoby F: Care of the massive burn wound, *CCQ* 7(3):44, 1984.
28. Jonason A: Complications of burn injury, *Occup Health Nurs* (7):24, 1983.
29. Kenner CV: Burn injury. In Kenner CV, Guzzetta CE, Dossey M, editors: *Critical care nursing body-mind-spirit*, Boston, 1985, Little, Brown & Co.
30. Lund CC and Browder NC: The estimate of areas of burns, *Surg Gynecol Obstet* 79:352, 1944.
31. Marshall WG Jr, Dimick AR: The natural history of major burns with multiple subsystem failure, *Trauma* 23(2):102, 1983.
32. Nadel E, Kozerefski PM: Rehabilitation of the critically ill burn patient, *CCQ* 7(3):19, 1984.
33. Robinson K, Cross P, Terry J: The crucial first days, *Am J Nurs* 85(1):30, 1985.
34. Wachtel TL: Epidemiology, classification and administrative considerations for critically burned patients. In Wachtel TL, editor: *Critical care clinics: burns*, Philadelphia, 1985, WB Saunders.

CHAPTER SEVENTY-SIX

Nursing Management of Adults Undergoing Cosmetic or Reconstructive Surgery

---

LEARNING OBJECTIVES

1 Explain the intended outcomes of cosmetic and reconstructive surgery.
2 Discuss the effects of plastic surgery on body image.
3 Describe the preoperative teaching and evaluation measures for the cosmetic or reconstructive surgery patient.
4 Identify postoperative nursing care for the cosmetic and reconstructive surgical patient.
5 Describe the changes in physical appearance that occur with the various types of cosmetic and reconstructive surgery.
6 Discuss the nursing interventions to detect and prevent common postoperative complications of cosmetic and reconstructive surgery.
7 State the goals and interventions for major nursing diagnoses after cosmetic and reconstructive surgery.
8 Describe home care instructions for the cosmetic and reconstructive surgical patient.

KEY TERMS

abdominoplasty, p. 2155
augmentation mammoplasty, p. 2159
breast reconstruction, p. 2166
blepharoplasty, p. 2145
blow-out fracture, p. 2170
flaps, p. 2161

malocclusion, p. 2170
mentoplasty, p. 2149
rhinoplasty, p. 2147
rhytidectomy, p. 2149
skin graft, p. 2161
suction assisted lipectomy (SAL), p. 2157

THERE ARE TWO major areas of plastic surgery—cosmetic (aesthetic) and reconstructive. Cosmetic or aesthetic surgery refers to surgical techniques performed to improve the appearance of a body part. Reconstructive surgery focuses on the healing and restoration of patients with injury, disfigurement, or scarring that resulted from trauma, disease, or congenital defects.

Plastic surgery, especially cosmetic surgery, has been called the surgery of the psyche because of its effect on the patient's psychosocial functioning. A plastic surgical procedure cannot be determined successful based solely on a good technical result. Patients must positively incorporate the physical changes into their body image. Their perception of the outcome is what actually determines a successful surgical result. The primary challenge facing the nurse who cares for the plastic surgical patient involves promoting a positive adaptation to the altered body image.

Whatever reason the patient gives for considering cosmetic surgery, it is valid to that individual. Nurses must be objective and nonjudgmental, both verbally and nonverbally, and must support the patient physiologically, psychologically, and socially.

GENERAL NURSING MANAGEMENT

Plastic surgery is performed in the inpatient setting, as well as in a variety of outpatient settings. Factors that determine the surgical setting include the patient and surgeon's preference, the specific procedure, the type of anesthesia selected, the patient's health and emotional status, the availability of adequate postoperative care, and the patient's financial situation. A majority of plastic surgical procedures are performed today in the outpatient setting.

Preoperative Nursing Management

The nurse plays a major role in helping the patient and significant other achieve realistic expectations of what the surgery offers. Preoperative teaching and evaluation of the teaching are done by the nurse.

During the initial appointments, the patient is informed of the realities of the surgical experience. Much of this information is provided by the surgeon when the patient is first seen, but it is the nurse's responsibility to reinforce and clarify this information, answer questions, and address the patient's concerns. The nurse plays a major role in helping the patient and significant other achieve realistic expectations of what the surgery offers. The patient may be shown before and after pictures of former patients who have had the same surgery. Computer imaging may also be used to project the person's appearance after surgery.

The patient needs to be in good general health and any preexisting conditions must be stable and controlled. For example, diabetes and hypertension are not contraindications to cosmetic surgery as long as the conditions are well-managed and stable.

It is important that the patient understands the time needed for healing. Healing and hence the results depend on the age, state of health, nutritional status, whether a smoker or nonsmoker, and skin type of the patient. Other factors affecting wound healing are the patient's stress level, preexisting conditions, and overall physical and psychologic health. Some surgeries take a full year before the re-

sults of the surgery can be assessed. Many patients will become discouraged during this prolonged time. In some procedures, time off from work and away from public scrutiny is necessary during early healing, especially when swelling and bruising are prominent. The nurse can assist the patient in scheduling the best time for surgery, based on job and social considerations.

Preoperative nursing care of all patients having cosmetic or reconstructive surgery is similar in some ways.

Postoperative Nursing Management

Nursing care in the postoperative period focuses on the physical and emotional comfort of the patient, physiologic homeostasis, and health teaching to the patient and significant other. Many of the cosmetic surgeries are not especially painful. Analgesics are ordered and usually control pain.

Infection is usually not a problem after cosmetic surgery. However, the nurse still asseses for signs and symptoms of infection after every operation. In teaching for home care, the patient and significant other need to know the basic principles in preventing infection and who to notify if signs and symptoms of infection should occur.

After discharge, several office visits are necessary for follow-up. This is a prime time for the nurse to evaluate the effectiveness of health teaching, answer any questions the patient has, and offer continued emotional support.

Some major potential nursing diagnoses for the patient in the postoperative period may include (1) body image disturbance related to edema and ecchymosis of the operative site or related to delayed desired results; (2) pain related to edema and severed nerve endings; and (3) high risk for infection related to invasion of foreign pathogens. Goals include helping the patient in achieving a positive self-image, minimizing pain, and preventing infection.

Cosmetic Surgery

The purpose of cosmetic surgery is to improve appearance, not attain perfection. Patients must have realistic expectations about what cosmetic surgery can and cannot accomplish. They must be willing to accept the creation of a scar in exchange for the change in appearance they are seeking. They also must be willing to endure discomfort and varying degrees of pain in order to achieve the desired outcome. Patients who are satisfied with the result of cosmetic surgery feel the risks are minimal compared to the enhanced body image and self-concept they experience once healing is complete. Patients elect to have cosmetic surgery to improve appearance, restore a previously satisfactory appearance, attain the physical endowments they perceive others to have, escape being regarded as different, and avoid the social stigma attached to the effects of aging.

BLEPHAROPLASTY
Definition

Blepharoplasty involves the removal of loose skin and protruding periorbital fat of the upper and lower eyelids. Blepharoplasty is often performed with a rhytidectomy (face-lift).

Etiology

With the aging process, a sagging or relaxation of the eyelid skin and orbital septum occurs (Figure 76-1). As the orbital septum becomes weaker, periorbital fat begins to bulge. Lid redundancy and fat protrusion may also be a result of heredity.

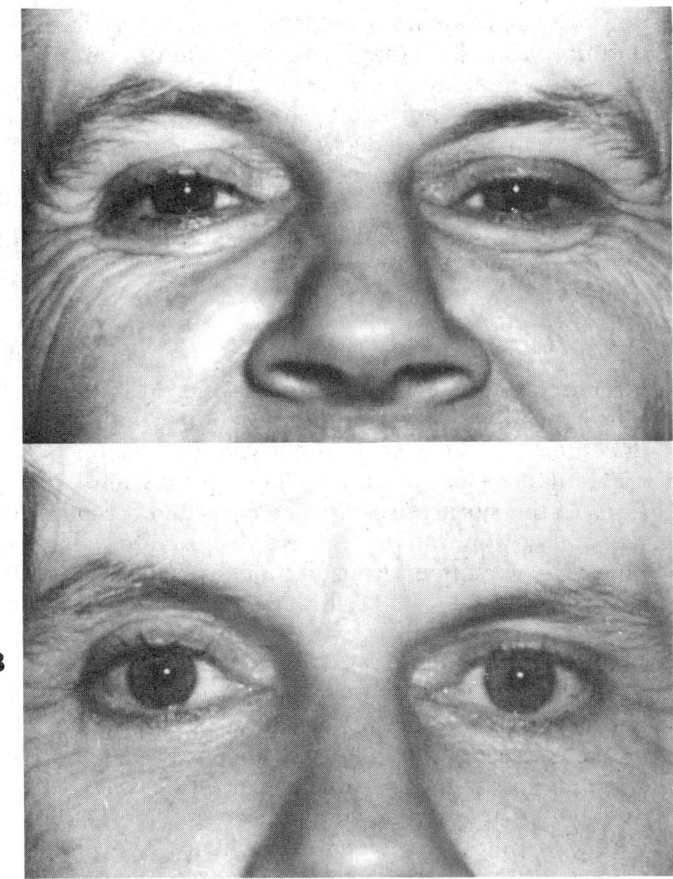

FIGURE 76-1 **A,** Preoperative and **B,** postoperative views of a blepharoplasty patient.

Clinical Manifestations

The patient has a chronically tired appearance. The relaxation of the skin can be so severe that it may hamper the patient's field of vision. Even patients in their late 20s may request blepharoplasty because of early signs of ptosis and the inability to wear eye makeup to their satisfaction.

Therapeutic Management

The patient is given a local anesthetic for blepharoplasty unless other operations are going to be conducted concurrently. The procedure removes loose skin and excess fat from the upper and/or lower eyelids. The suture line of the upper lid is made in the crease of the eyelid, while the lower lid suture line is immediately below the lash margin (Figure 76-2). Both incisions heal with a nearly imperceptible scar. Suture removal is usually done 4 to 5 days after surgery to reduce additional scarring that may occur around the suture sites.

Complications are rare but may include visual loss from bleeding, dry eyes, corneal abrasion, scarring that pulls the eyelid into an abnormal shape, hematoma, extraocular muscle paresis, ectropion, which is an eversion of the edge or margin of the eyelid, lash alopecia, and an undesirable aesthetic result.

NURSING MANAGEMENT OF THE PATIENT UNDERGOING BLEPHAROPLASTY
Assessment

Preoperatively the nurse conducts a history and physical to rule out thyroid disease, chronic allergy, and kidney disease, because these health alterations can cause puffiness around the eye. History of preexisting eye disease, eyelid abnormalities, and scars from previous eye surgery must be assessed. Vision is also evaluated, since one of the possible complications of this surgery is vision loss. Vision is assessed with glasses or contacts if the patient wears them. A Schirmer's (tear) test is done to rule out dry eye syndrome. Visual problems should be referred to an ophthalmologist or optometrist. Preoperative teaching and evaluation are done.

Postoperatively the patient is assessed for marked swelling, bruising, bleeding, and eye pain. The function of the extraocular muscles is also assessed. Gross vision should be assessed by asking the patient to count fingers on the nurse's hand or identify easily recognizable objects.

Nursing Diagnosis

Postoperative nursing diagnoses include:
   High risk for injury related to altered vision from
      eyelid surgery

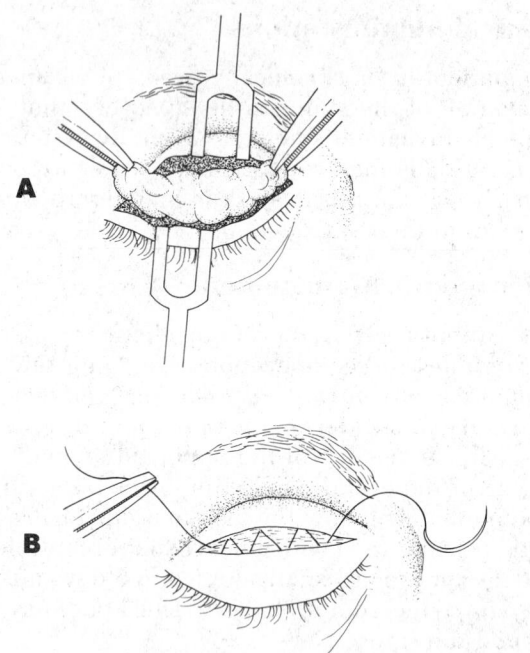

FIGURE 76-2   Blepharoplasty procedure. **A,** Removal of excess fat from upper eye lid. **B,** Wound closure.

Sensory/perceptual alteration (visual) related to retrobulbar hemorrhage, edema, or corneal injury

Impaired tissue integrity related to surgical manipulation of eyelid tissue

Alteration in comfort related to invasive procedure, edema, ecchymosis, incisions, and sensory deprivation

Alteration in body image related to actual and perceived change in appearance

Impaired home maintenance management related to inadequate knowledge of care and expectations

Planning

Patient goals include the following:

Patient will be free of injury from falling or walking into objects

Patient will have reestablished preoperative visual acuity and no evidence of bleeding

Patient will maintain intact eye tissue integrity with optimal wound healing

Patient will have minimal or controlled discomfort/pain

Patient will progress toward a positive integration of physical changes into body image

Patient will understand and follow home care instructions

Implementation

Nursing care includes elevating the head of the bed to reduce edema. Iced eye compresses are applied using clean technique. Gauze pads are used, since cotton may stick and pull the skin when removed. The compresses should be changed every 30 minutes for the first 4 hours. Observe eye edema, ecchymosis, and suture site. Mild pain is expected after surgery. The patient may state that his or her eyes feel dry and itch. Cold compresses will help alleviate this. An ophthalmic ointment may be ordered also. Hemorrhaging, which can result in severe eye pain or loss of vision, must be reported immediately to the surgeon. The patient also must be instructed to avoid the Valsalva maneuver, which increases intrathoracic pressure and increases blood pressure in the head and eye, thereby increasing the risk of hemorrhage. Patients are usually discharged when they are fully awake and have stable vital signs. Sutures are removed 4 to 5 days after surgery.

Evaluation

Nursing interventions are evaluated by monitoring patient outcomes. The patient should be free from injury as a result of temporary altered vision postoperatively. Evaluate eye tissue integrity for signs of optimal wound healing. Pain, discomfort, and response to analgesics are assessed. Since blepharoplasty is usually performed on an outpatient basis, the patient's knowledge of postoperative care is evaluated and reinforced with written instructions. The patient and family reactions to the alterations in eye appearance and body image are evaluated with each postoperative visit.

Documentation

Documentation includes an assessment of the eyelids. Verbal and written home care instructions are documented along with the patient's response to teaching. The patient/family perceptions and reactions to the surgical results are recorded. Preoperative and postoperative photographs provide valuable objective documentation of the physical results of surgery.

Ongoing Care

Self-care instruction includes the continuation of iced compresses for 24 hours. Because lying on one side increases the possibility of swelling in the dependent eye area, the patient should sleep supine with two pillows to elevate the head. The patient should understand the importance of not bending over at the waist for the first 48 hours after discharge because this increases pressure to the operative area.

The patient should refrain from vigorous activities, such as sports, for 1 month. Light activities, such as short walks and shopping, can be resumed after 1 week. The nurse encourages the patient to wear sunglasses to prevent eye squinting when in bright sunlight. Sunglasses may also be desired by the patient to conceal swelling and bruising. Eye makeup may be used after suture removal and if there are no open areas. Insertion of contact lenses should be delayed for 2 weeks. Earlier manipulation of lids to insert contacts could cause wound separation.

RHINOPLASTY

Definition

Rhinoplasty corrects nasal structure deformities that can be congenital, hereditary, or traumatic. Depending on the nature of the deformity, rhinoplasty surgery can be cosmetic or reconstructive.

Etiology

This procedure is performed for cosmetic reasons when the patient is dissatisfied with the appearance of the nose. Reconstructive rhinoplasty and/or septoplasty is performed when there is a perforated septum caused by traumatic irritation, repeated cauterization for epistaxis, or penetrating septal injury.

This procedure is also performed to correct a deviated septum from nasal trauma resulting from a fall, blow to the nose, or previous surgery.

Clinical Manifestations

The nose has a significant role in body image with ties to culture and heredity. Postoperatively, the patient's body image and self-esteem may be enhanced, because results of this procedure are often satisfactory and pleasing to the patient (Figure 76-3).

Therapeutic Management

For rhinoplasty, the patient usually receives a local anesthetic in combination with intravenous sedation or a general anesthetic. Incisions are made inside the nose, so scars are not visible. Occasionally, small external excisions at the lateral wall of each nostril and near the nasal bridge are made to narrow the nose. The nasal bone is fractured, excess tissue is removed, and cartilage and bone are remolded into the desired shape. The mucous membranes are held in place with internal packings of petrolatum gauze and the bones with an external splint. The packings are removed the next morning, and the splint remains in place for 1 week. Complications may include slight bleeding to frank hemorrhage, infection, tear duct injury, displacement of nasal bones, and an undesirable aesthetic result.

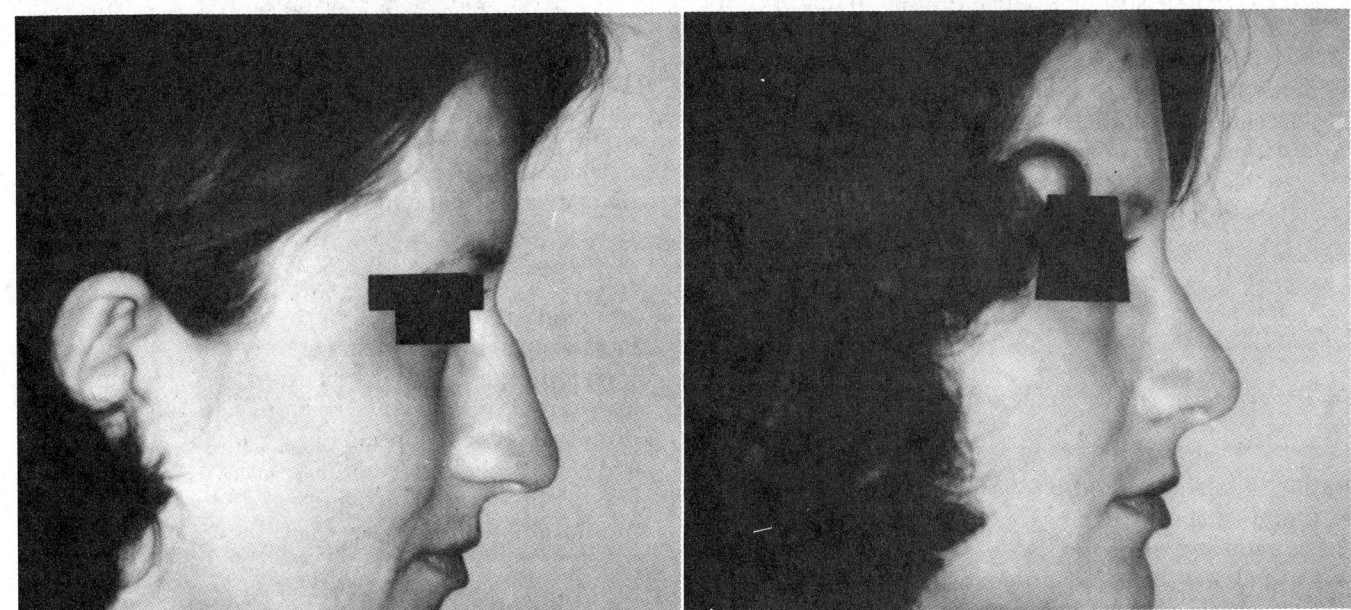

FIGURE 76-3   **A,** Preoperative and **B,** postoperative views of rhinoplasty.

NURSING MANAGEMENT OF THE PATIENT UNDERGOING RHINOPLASTY

Assessment

Preoperative assessment includes obtaining information about the patient's family support. Sometimes significant others cannot understand why "Aunt Jane is unhappy with her nose." This lack of support may make postoperative recovery difficult.

Physical examination of the nose includes making observations of its relationship to other features of the face. The status of the internal nares and anterior airway is important, since deviations of the turbinates or septum may also require repair to achieve a patent airway and the desired physical change in the nose. Inspecting the nasal mucosa with a bright light and nasal speculum is necessary. In recent years, nasal surgery has been sought to reconstruct the nose after the use of recreational inhalation drugs. The internal structures of the nose can be destroyed by drugs, and little can be accomplished through surgical repair.

Preoperative instructions include avoiding aspirin, alcohol, and sunburn for at least 2 weeks before surgery. The night before surgery, the patient may be instructed to wash the face with a cleansing solution. Cosmetics or toiletries are not worn the morning of surgery.

Postoperative assessment focuses on hemorrhage, edema, pain, discoloration, and unstable vital signs.

Nursing Diagnosis

Postoperative nursing diagnoses include:

Ineffective breathing pattern related to disruption of the normal breathing pathway

Impaired tissue integrity related to surgical manipulation of nasal tissue

Alteration in comfort related to invasive procedure, nasal packing, and eye edema and ecchymosis

Alteration in body image related to facial edema, ecchymosis, nasal splint, and actual and perceived change in appearance

Impaired home maintenance management related to inadequate knowledge of care and expectations

Planning

Patient goals include the following:

Patient will have no respiratory distress and will mouth breathe

Patient will maintain intact tissue integrity with optimal wound healing

Patient will have minimal or controlled discomfort

Patient will progress toward a positive integration of the physical change in appearance of the nose into body image

Patient will understand and follow home care instructions

Implementation

Nursing care is directed at controlling pain, reducing edema, and preventing hemorrhage and infection. The surgical procedure and the packings can be uncomfortable, and analgesics will be ordered. The area around the patient's eyes is edematous and ecchymotic, and iced eye compresses are applied. The patient is positioned with the head elevated at a 30-degree angle to minimize edema and to promote drainage. The nurse should provide an emesis basin and instruct the patient to expectorate any blood. Bleeding may not always be visible, because the blood may run down the back of the throat. Patients should be assessed for frequent swallowing, since it may be the only sign of bleeding. Some blood on the external nasal dressing (dripstrip) is expected. The dripstrip, a small dressing placed under the nose and taped to the cheeks, can be changed by the nurse without a physician's order. The amount and characteristics of the drainage are noted and documented in the chart.

Evaluation

Nursing interventions are evaluated by monitoring patient outcomes. The patient will maintain optimal respiratory patterns by adjusting to mouth breathing. Nasal drainage will be minimal. Eyelid and nasal edema and ecchymosis will begin to decrease within 7 to 10 days postoperatively. Pain, discomfort, and response to analgesics are assessed. The patient's knowledge of postoperative care is evaluated and reinforced with written instructions. The patient and family reactions to the alterations in appearance and body image are evaluated with each postoperative visit.

Documentation

Documentation includes an assessment of the eyelids, nasal splint, and nasal bleeding. Verbal and written home care instructions are documented along with the patient's response to teaching. The patient/family perceptions and reactions to the surgical results are recorded. Preoperative and postoperative photographs provide valuable objective documentation of the physical results of surgery.

Ongoing Care

The patient is taught to sleep on two pillows to elevate the head and reduce edema. The patient should avoid bending over, because this increases intracranial pressure, which may result in nasal bleeding. A cold air humidifier decreases the dry throat associated with mouth breathing. The dripstrip may be changed as needed. The nasal splint should not be removed, even though the patient may feel uncomfortable and have itching. Because the nasal bone and cartilage are moldable for weeks, use of the nasal splint can help prevent an undesirable aesthetic result. The patient should be instructed to sneeze through the mouth and not blow through the nose. Cool compresses applied to the eyes are continued for approximately 48 hours. A soft diet should be eaten for about 1 week. After the nasal packing and splint are removed, the nose will remain swollen for as long as 3 to 4 weeks. The patient is instructed to gently cleanse the nares and upper lip. Patients need to be instructed that ecchymosis will last approximately 2 weeks and the nose and upper lip may be numb for approximately 6 months. It may be several months before final results can be judged.

MENTOPLASTY

Mentoplasty or genioplasty is the surgical reshaping of the chin. It is frequently formed in combination with rhinoplasty in order to achieve a balanced profile. Mentoplasty may be accomplished by inserting a prosthesis or splitting the mandible and moving it forward. The latter is often done in combination with surgery to correct dental malocclusion.

This section will discuss mentoplasty with a prosthesis. The most commonly used prostheses are made of biologically inert silicone or alloplast. The incision may be made inside the mouth or externally underneath the chin. A pressure dressing is applied postoperatively to prevent edema and fluid collection.

Mentoplasty is usually performed on an outpatient basis. Patients are instructed to keep the dressing dry and intact. With an oral incision, meticulous oral hygiene is essential. Gentle brushing and/or a Water Pik are encouraged. Patients will progress from a liquid to a soft diet. Chewing is discouraged for the first few days to decrease chin movement. Oral sutures will dissolve in 7 to 10 days. Complications of mentoplasty include infection, nerve damage, and asymmetry of the chin.

RHYTIDECTOMY
Definition

Rhytidectomy is the redistribution and/or removal of facial skin and fat from the face, jaw line, and neck (Figure 76-4). This procedure restores a more youthful and rested appearance. The results of this procedure are not permanent, and many patients will return for subsequent face-lifts. The correction

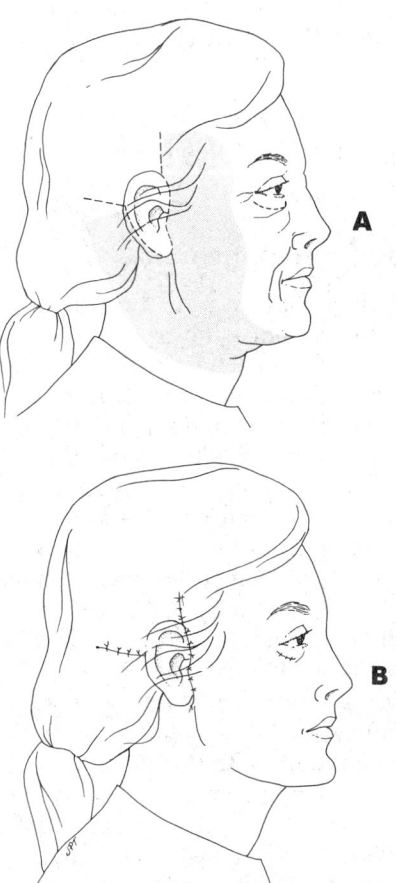

FIGURE 76-4 Rhytidectomy and blepharoplasty. **A,** Shaded area shows where tissue is undermined and pulled toward the incision lines. Excess skin is excised. Note the incision lines around the ear and scalp. **B,** Postoperative result, with tightened facial and neck tissue.

can last as long as 10 years, although results vary with each individual. This procedure does not remove fine wrinkles around the mouth, forehead, or corners of the eyes. For this reason, a chemical peel or dermabrasion may be performed in conjunction with rhytidectomy.

Etiology

A loose, wrinkled facial and neck appearance results from age, sun and wind exposure, poor nutrition, smoking, excessive alcohol use, weight loss, heredity, obesity, and generalized loss of elasticity in aging skin. Patients will also seek rhytidectomy for (1) redundant soft tissue from dermatitis, such as smallpox or acne scarring, (2) asymmetric redundancy as in facial palsy, (3) redundant soft tissue resulting from trauma, and (4) preauricular lesions.

Clinical Manifestations

The loose skin associated with the aging process is especially noticeable in the jowl areas and just beneath the chin. Patients frequently complain of looking tired and worried.

Therapeutic Management

This procedure can be outpatient or inpatient surgery, and the patient is given a local or general anesthetic. The patient shampoos, and the male patient shaves the hair on his face. Incisions are made in the temporal area (hidden in the hairline), extending in front of the ear, around the ear lobe, upward in the crease behind the ear, then angling in the hair toward the back of the head (Figure 76-4). Patients must be reassured that only small amounts of hair, if any, are shaved around the incision lines. There will be no bald spots postoperatively. After surgery, the face is wrapped in large bulky dressings to hold the skin tight and reduce the risk of hematoma. Subcutaneous drains may be used to facilitate drainage and prevent infection. The patient experiences minimal pain with this procedure. On the fifth to tenth postoperative day, the sutures are removed.

Complications can include hematoma (especially in the first 24 to 48 hours), transient visual impairment caused by eyelid edema, hair loss, nerve injury, infection, and an undesirable aesthetic result. Infection is not a common complication, but some surgeons may prescribe antibiotics prophylactically. Hair loss is usually temporary and occurs from decreased blood supply to the hair follicles. Nerve injury causing paralysis of the lip is a rare but serious complication. Most often paralysis is caused by nerve swelling, and function returns in a few weeks when the edema has subsided.

NURSING MANAGEMENT OF THE PATIENT UNDERGOING RHYTIDECTOMY

Assessment

Preoperative nursing assessment focuses on the expectations of the surgical outcome and physical ability to undergo the operation. Hypertensive and diabetic patients can undergo this surgery if the disorder is well-controlled.

Postoperatively the nurse assesses the patient for hematoma, which is manifested as facial asymmetry with pain or tightness on one side of the face. The nurse also assesses the patient for sensory deficits, especially if blepharoplasty was concurrently performed. The large bulky dressing and edema may impair hearing, sight, and sensation. Nerve damage is also assessed by asking the patient to wrinkle the forehead and nose, purse the lips, smile, and squint the eyes.

Nursing Diagnosis

Postoperative nursing diagnoses include:
  Impaired tissue integrity related to tissue transfer and severed blood vessels of the face and neck
  Alteration in comfort related to invasive procedure, head dressing, edema, ecchymosis, and incisions
  Alteration in body image related to edema, ecchymosis, and perceived change in appearance
  Sensory/perceptual alteration (visual, auditory, tactile) related to edema and facial dressing
  Impaired home maintenance management related to inadequate knowledge of care and expectations

Planning

Patient goals include the following:
  Patient will maintain intact tissue integrity with optimal wound healing and no hematoma
  Patient will have minimal or controlled discomfort/pain
  Patient will progress toward a positive integration of physical changes into body image
  Patient will return to preoperative state of sensory/perceptual input
  Patient will understand and follow home care instructions

Implementation

The head of the bed should be elevated to prevent excessive edema and prevent stress on the suture line. The patient may be discharged the day of surgery or spend the first postoperative night in the hospital. The nurse assesses for hematoma by observing for facial pain or swelling. The patient will feel facial tightness under the dressing. This requires frequent assessment for any indication of hematoma or excessive edema. Blood pressure is monitored and controlled as needed to maintain systolic pressure below 160 mm Hg. This helps prevent impaired peripheral perfusion. Hypertensive patients should resume their prescribed antihypertensive medications after surgery.

With the bulky head dressing, patients will have decreased hearing. The edema will also cause pressure on the nerve endings and numbness will result. If the patient has had a blepharoplasty, there will be an alteration in vision. It is difficult to wear glasses with the bulky head dressing. These temporary distortions should be explained to the patient and significant other(s). All needed objects should be placed within the patient's reach. Head and neck movement should be limited. Patients are instructed to move the head, neck, and shoulders as a unit from the waist. They also should be instructed to move slowly and not to nod "yes" or "no."

Dressings and drains are removed 1 to 3 days after surgery. Hair may be washed at this time. Ears are cleansed of blood and drainage. Suture removal begins approximately 4 days after surgery. Crusting along the incision lines is normal during the first 2 weeks. These crusts should not be manually removed, since scarring can result. An antibiotic ointment may be ordered to soften the crusts and aid in their separation. The nurse can assist the patient in increasing self-esteem and body image perception by emphasizing the temporary nature of the swelling and bruising.

Evaluation

Nursing interventions are evaluated by monitoring patient outcomes. Evaluate facial and neck tissue for edema, ecchymosis, and signs of optimal wound healing. Pain, discomfort, and response to analgesics are assessed. The patient's knowledge of postoperative care is evaluated and reinforced with written instructions. The patient and family reactions to the alterations in appearance and body image are evaluated with each postoperative visit.

Documentation

Documentation includes an assessment of the face and neck. Verbal and written home care instructions are documented along with the patient's response to teaching. The patient/family perceptions and reactions to the surgical results are recorded. Preoperative and postoperative photographs provide valuable objective documentation of the physical results of surgery.

Ongoing Care

Education is provided to the patient and significant other who will be assisting in home care. The patient and caregiver are instructed in the necessity of assessing the dressings and surrounding skin area. Signs and symptoms of infection are taught. The caregiver must also know the importance of postoperative nutrition and pain management of the patient.

The patient should sit up at home to reduce facial edema and should continue to sleep on two pillows for 1 week to elevate the head. Patients should consume full liquids and soft foods with the highest nutritional content possible until the dressings are

removed. Sexual activity increases blood flow to the face and should be avoided for at least 1 week postoperatively to avoid prolonged swelling or precipitate a hematoma. Once the sutures are removed, women can wear makeup, which helps minimize the appearance of the suture lines. Men can apply shaving lotions and creams. No permanent waves or hair dye/bleaching is permitted for 4 to 6 weeks postoperatively.

BROW/FOREHEAD LIFT

With aging, the forehead and brow lose their elasticity and begin to sag, causing a tired and worried appearance. Brow and forehead lifts can be performed for a rejuvenating effect without any visible scars. A brow lift or browpexy involves the excision of a strip of skin above the eyebrows. The incisions are made parallel to the hair follicles. A brow lift alleviates some eyelid redundancy and ptosis. A forehead lift alleviates eyelid redundancy, brow and temple ptosis, and forehead furrows. Incisions are usually made in the hairline, or at the top of the forehead along the hairline.

Headaches may be experienced postoperatively because of the dilation of blood vessels in the head as a result of surgical trauma. They can be relieved with ice packs and analgesics. Complications include hematoma, alopecia, and asymmetry of expression. Nursing management is similar to that for a patient with rhytidectomy.

CHEMICAL FACE PEEL
Definition

A chemical face peel uses topical caustic agents to produce a controlled burn, which removes fine facial wrinkles and skin blemishes. There are several different chemicals or chemical mixtures that are commonly used for face peeling. Chemical peel is not a substitute for rhytidectomy, because the peel does not remove folds of skin. Chemical face peeling can be used in combination with rhytidectomy to remove wrinkles around the mouth, on the forehead, and near the corners of the mouth and eyes. The desired final result is removal of the small wrinkles of the face, generation of a new superficial layer of skin, and a tightening of the deeper skin layers. The facial skin appears smooth, fine, and more youthful.

Etiology

Indications for chemical face peeling include fine wrinkles from the aging process, alterations in pigmentation such as chloasma from a previous pregnancy, radiation skin damage, freckles, and superficial acne scarring.

Clinical Manifestations

The ideal patient for this surgical procedure is one who is middle-aged and fair-skinned. The peeling solution lightens the skin. If used in dark-skinned patients, it could leave permanent skin color changes.

Therapeutic Management

Phenol peel

A solution of buffered phenol or trichloroacetic acid, sterile water, croton oil, and septisol is applied with a sterile applicator to the wrinkled areas. Waterproof adhesive tape may be applied to all of the treated areas except the mouth, eyes, and nose, creating a masklike dressing. This mask stays in place for 24 to 48 hours. Then the dressing is carefully removed from the face while the patient is sedated. The facial skin is open and weeping and resembles skin that has sustained a second-degree burn. Excess exudate is removed with gauze, and a thymol iodine powder is applied with applicators to promote drying. A superficial eschar develops and is removed with antibiotic ointment over 3 to 4 days. Redness is present for about 6 to 8 weeks, and a pink hue to the skin will be noticeable for several months. Once healing is complete, makeup and shaving products can be used. Makeup with a purple hue will help conceal the erythema. Because phenol is absorbed into the bloodstream and can cause systemic toxicity, this procedure is performed in the operating room with an electrocardiogram machine attached to the patient to monitor dysrhythmias.

TCA peel (trichloroacetic acid)

This procedure begins with washing the face with soap, rinsing with water, then scrubbing with acetone or ether. The trichloroacetic acid is rubbed into the skin, wrinkles, and skin folds. The acid produces a white blanching or frosting of the skin, producing a chemical burn. Immediately after the peel, the skin may be covered with antibiotic ointment, alternating with a mild steroid lotion to relieve itching. Following this period of "weeping" of the skin where sloughing of the superficial epidermis occurs, a period of flakiness and skin peeling will occur. Moisturizers, sunscreens, and sometimes pigment inhibitors are recommended at this time.

Complications after face peeling may include pain, prolonged erythema, scarring, milia (white papules), and an undesirable aesthetic result. Erythema usually lasts 6 to 10 weeks but can last as long as 3 to 4 months. Because the skin color after the peel is lighter, a difference in skin color between the treated and untreated areas can occur.

NURSING MANAGEMENT OF THE PATIENT UNDERGOING A CHEMICAL FACE PEEL

Assessment

Preoperatively the nurse assesses the patient's knowledge of chemical peel and the postoperative responsibilities that should continue after discharge.

Postoperatively the patient requires assessment of blood pressure and heart rhythm because of the complications of the absorbed phenol. Hypertension and dysrhythmias must be reported. Because the face and eyes swell, the patient's physical safety must be considered.

Nursing Diagnosis

Postoperative nursing diagnoses include:

Impaired skin integrity related to chemical peel procedure

Alteration in comfort related to the procedure, itching, and burning sensations

Alteration in body image related to the actual and perceived change in appearance

High risk for decreased cardiac output related to ineffective pumping of the heart caused by systemic phenol absorption

Impaired home maintenance management related to inadequate knowledge of care and expectations

Planning

Patient goals include the following:

Patient will maintain intact skin integrity of the face with optimal healing

Patient will have minimal or controlled discomfort, itching, and pain

Patient will progress toward a positive integration of physical changes into the body image

Patient will experience blood pressure and heart rhythm within acceptable limits

Patient will understand and follow home care instructions

Implementation

Elevating the head of the bed will help prevent edema. Edema is most likely to occur in the eyelid areas, resulting in limited vision. The patient should avoid excessive movement of the mouth and should be discouraged from talking and chewing to avoid excessive pressure and tension on the skin. Paper and pen can be used for communication. A full liquid diet, incorporating as many vitamins, minerals, and protein as possible, should be given through a straw.

Evaluation

Nursing interventions are evaluated by monitoring patient outcomes. Evaluate facial tissue for redness, edema, ecchymosis, and signs of optimal wound healing. Pain, itching, discomfort, and response to analgesics are assessed. Blood pressure and heart rhythm are evaluated. The patient's knowledge of postoperative care is evaluated and reinforced with written instructions. The patient and family reactions to the alterations in appearance and body image are evaluated with each postoperative visit.

Documentation

Documentation includes an assessment of the facial tissue. Blood pressure and heart rhythm are recorded. Verbal and written home care instructions are documented along with the patient's response to teaching. The patient/family perceptions and reactions to the surgical results are recorded. Preoperative and postoperative photographs provide valuable objective documentation of the physical results of surgery.

Ongoing Care

Milia may appear during the first 6 to 8 postoperative weeks and can be removed by washing the face with a washcloth. Patients must stay out of the sun for 6 months, because the melanin in the skin is reduced. If sun exposure is encountered during this time, unsightly hyperpigmentation can occur. The final results do not appear for many weeks, and the patient may become discouraged. Psychologic support from significant others and the health care team is important during this time.

DERMABRASION
Definition

Dermabrasion is the removal of facial epidermis and a portion of the superficial dermis to smooth scars and reduce surface irregularities. This is considered the preferred treatment for acne and other depressed scars.

Etiology

Surface irregularities can occur from acne scars, chickenpox scars, or other depressed scars. Dermabrasion can smooth fine wrinkle lines. Tattoos caused by foreign bodies, such as gunpowder, may also be removed by dermabrasion.

Clinical Manifestations

The patient has high points or elevations of the face. The goal of dermabrasion is to smooth the high areas so the low areas appear less deep.

Therapeutic Management

The patient receives a local or general anesthetic while dermabrasion is performed, usually on an outpatient basis. Most dermabrasion is performed with a motor-driven wheel and diamond-impregnated burrs. Due to the large amount of aerosolized blood products created, the use of masks and goggles is especially important. The abraded surfaces are irrigated with saline during the operation, and the patient's face is dressed with an antibiotic ointment and gauze. The timing of the removal of the gauze varies with the surgeon. The abraded skin heals by first forming a coagulum from serum. The eschar (crusting) forms in 2 to 3 days and starts to separate in 7 to 10 days. The epithelium that lines the hair and sweat gland follicles comes to the skin surface and creates a new epithelial layer. A thin epidermis begins to form, and collagen is laid down by the third to fourth postoperative day. The skin develops pigmentation 3 to 4 weeks after the abrasion. Possible complications of dermabrasion include milia, infection, and pigmentation changes.

NURSING MANAGEMENT OF THE PATIENT UNDERGOING DERMABRASION
Assessment

Preoperative assessment focuses on the patient's motivation for the procedure and the ability to continue the necessary care at home. The nurse assesses the patient postoperatively for excessive edema and the presence of pruritus.

Nursing Diagnosis

Postoperative nursing diagnoses include:
- Impaired skin integrity related to surgical procedure
- Alteration in comfort: pain related to surgical procedure, itching, and burning sensations
- Alteration in body image related to actual and perceived change in appearance
- Impaired home maintenance management related to inadequate knowledge of care and expectations

Planning

Patient goals include the following:
- Patient will maintain intact skin integrity with optimal healing

Patient will have minimal or controlled discomfort and pain

Patient will progress toward a positive integration of changed appearance into body image

Patient will understand and follow home care instructions

Implementation

An essential nursing intervention after the procedure is to keep the abraded areas dry during the first postoperative week. Gentle heat from a hair dryer may be used.

Evaluation

Nursing interventions are evaluated by monitoring patient outcomes. Evaluate facial tissue for redness, edema, ecchymosis, and signs of optimal wound healing. Pain, itching, discomfort, and response to analgesics are assessed. The patient's knowledge of postoperative care is evaluated and reinforced with written instructions. The patient and family reactions to the alterations in appearance and body image are evaluated with each postoperative visit.

Documentation

Documentation includes an assessment of the facial tissue. Verbal and written home care instructions are documented along with the patient's response to teaching. The patient/family perceptions and reactions to the surgical results are recorded. Preoperative and postoperative photographs provide valuable objective documentation of the physical results of surgery.

Ongoing Care

The patient should be told to expect some swelling of the face. To prevent further edema, the patient is taught to keep the head elevated, especially when sleeping. Talking, smiling, and chewing are to be kept to a minimum to avoid tension to the treated areas. Clear liquids using a straw are prescribed for the first 2 days. The superficial eschar is assisted to dry, and gentle heat from a 60-watt bulb or hairdryer may be used. An antibiotic ointment may be prescribed twice daily and should be applied to the eschar. Once the eschar falls off, the patient may experience pruritus. Topical ice, antihistamines, and steroids may be required. Some physicians may prescribe medications to hasten maturation of the epidermis. Exposure to the sun must be avoided for 2 to 4 months to prevent hyperpigmentation. Sunscreens and a head covering such as a wide-brimmed hat are used when the patient is outdoors.

COLLAGEN INJECTION
Definition

Collagen suspension can be injected in soft tissue to elevate a depressed area such as that created by acne scars. Collagen can also be injected into small wrinkles of the forehead, upper lip, and near the eyes. Small amounts of collagen are injected into the dermis and act as a framework into which new cells can grow. The first treatment causes a slight inflammatory reaction that leads to some scar formation. This is the desired effect since the scar tissue raises the skin, minimizing the defect or the wrinkles. It is not a substitute for rhytidectomy or a permanent correction for wrinkles or defects. Injections need to be repeated every 6 to 12 months as collagen is reabsorbed.

Etiology

Patients seeking collagen injections have experienced disease; trauma, such as acne scars; or skin wrinkles from aging.

Clinical Manifestations

The patient has minor depressions or wrinkles in the soft tissue of the skin.

Therapeutic Management

Collagen is injected intradermally with a 30-gauge needle. Collagen injection is performed in the physician's office, and the patient goes home the same day. Complications include prolonged swelling, hard, round areas known as induration, redness at the injection site, infection, herpes eruption, allergic reaction, and partial loss of vision if injected in the blood vessels around the eye.

NURSING MANAGEMENT OF THE PATIENT UNDERGOING COLLAGEN INJECTIONS
Assessment

The nurse assesses the patient's motivation for the procedure and expectations of the results. In taking the history of the patient, the nurse asks if there is

 **CLINICAL ALERT**

Every patient undergoing collagen injections should receive an intradermal test dose of collagen to identify potential sensitivity reactions.

a history of autoimmune disorders. Patients with autoimmune disorders are not treated with collagen, since the foreign protein may exacerbate the disorder. A test dose of a small amount of collagen is given to determine if the patient will have an adverse response to the exogenous collagen. The nurse administers 0.1 mL collagen intradermally into the forearm. The patient is observed for a positive reaction, such as erythema, induration, pruritus, tenderness, or swelling at the test site appearing days or even weeks later. The test site is reevaluated in 4 weeks. Careful follow-up is important, because some patients will conceal a positive skin reaction to be considered a candidate for the procedure.

Nursing Diagnosis

Posttreatment nursing diagnoses include:
- Alteration in body image related to actual and perceived change in appearance
- Impaired home maintenance management related to inadequate knowledge of care and expectations

Planning

Patient goals include the following:
- Patient will progress toward a positive integration of physical changes into the body image
- Patient will understand and follow home care instructions

Implementation

The nurse provides measures that make the immediate postoperative period physiologically and psychologically comfortable for the patient.

Evaluation

Nursing interventions are evaluated by monitoring patient outcomes. Evaluate facial tissue for edema, ecchymosis, allergic response, and signs of optimal healing. Pain or discomfort are assessed. The patient's knowledge of postoperative care is evaluated and reinforced with written instructions. The patient and family reactions to the alterations in appearance and body image are evaluated with each postoperative visit. They are reminded that the results of collagen therapy are temporary and will need to be repeated.

Documentation

Documentation includes an assessment of the face and neck. Verbal and written home care instructions are documented along with the patient's response to teaching. The patient/family perceptions and reactions to the surgical results are recorded. Preoperative and postoperative photographs provide valuable objective documentation of the physical results of collagen injection. Also included in documentation is the product name, dosage, lot number, and expiration date.

Ongoing Care

The patient is taught not to wash the face or apply makeup, facial creams, or lotions for 3 to 4 hours after the procedure. After this period, normal skin care can resume. Exposure to strong sunlight, alcohol, and excessive exercise can cause mild swelling and should be avoided for 1 week after the injection. Patients need to be reminded that the effects of collagen treatments are temporary. As the collagen begins to be reabsorbed, some patients feel their wrinkles or scars look worse than before treatment. Photographs before and after the procedure are very helpful in providing reassurance and reinforcing reality.

ABDOMINOPLASTY
Definition

Abdominoplasty corrects lax abdominal tissue and skin and repairs the abdominal wall to improve the contour and appearance of the abdominal area. To some extent it also improves the physiologic function of the abdomen.

Etiology

The loose and stretched skin of the abdomen has elastic fibers that were destroyed, and weight loss will not restore its integrity. Multiple pregnancies may cause abdominal muscles to separate and the abdominal fascia to become permanently loosened. Patients with a large weight loss may also have large folds of skin remaining on their abdomen, arms, thighs, and buttocks. Weight loss reduces the amount of adipose tissue, but it does not reduce distended and stretched skin.

Clinical Manifestations

Individuals who seek abdominoplasty may have deformities of the abdomen ranging from skin excess to large fatty aprons of skin hanging from the abdomen to as far as the knees. This tissue may be so excessive that it interferes with walking.

Therapeutic Management

The operation is performed with the patient supine and the hips flexed. Hip flexion allows the maximum excision of abdominal tissue. Incisions are made along the pubic hairline, curving to the inguinal skin creases. The tissues are lifted off the abdominal wall to the xiphoid process, and the excess tissue is pulled down and removed. The umbilicus is repositioned by making a small incision in the midline of the abdomen, pulling the umbilicus through the incision, and suturing it in place.

Complications include hematoma, seroma (collection of serosanguineous fluid), fat necrosis, skin necrosis, wound dehiscence, infection, pulmonary embolism, undesirable scarring, and hernia.

NURSING MANAGEMENT OF THE PATIENT UNDERGOING ABDOMINOPLASTY
Assessment

The ideal candidate for abdominoplasty is one who is at a preferred body weight with an abdominal deformity between the xiphoid process and symphysis pubis. Individuals must be willing to accept the inevitable scar that this surgery will produce. Women who have had multiple pregnancies as the cause of this condition must be reasonably certain they no longer wish to bear children. This surgery is not for weight loss. In most cases, it would not be performed on an obese patient who is unwilling to lose weight through diet and exercise. Poor candidates for this surgery include patients with poor posture, those who are thin with a protruding abdomen, and those with multiple abdominal scars from previous surgeries. During the preoperative assessment, abdominal surgery scars are noted, such as from a cholecystectomy or cesarean section. Old scars may alter blood flow to the flap after surgery.

Postoperative assessment includes auscultation of the lungs for clear bilateral breath sounds. Atelectasis may occur as a postoperative complication because of a decreased respiratory effort after anesthesia. The nurse also auscultates the abdomen for return of bowel sounds.

The incision is assessed for blanch response, pallor, or cyanosis. Signs of hematoma include increasing discomfort, edema, ecchymosis, and skin flap pallor. Wound drains must be assessed for patency and drainage color and amount. Urinary voiding patterns are to be assessed until normal voiding patterns resume. If the patient does not void within 6 to 8 hours after surgery, a straight catheter may be ordered by the physician to empty the bladder and decrease tension on the suture line.

Nursing Diagnosis

Postoperative nursing diagnoses include:
  Impaired tissue integrity related to surgical manipulation of tissue and incisions

  Alteration in tissue perfusion related to decreased mobility, pain, and position
  Alteration in comfort: pain related to invasive procedure, incision, dressing, and position
  Alteration in elimination patterns related to positioning and decreased mobility
  Alteration in body image related to actual and perceived change in appearance
  Impaired home maintenance management related to inadequate knowledge of care and expectations

Planning

Patient goals include the following:
  Patient will have intact tissue integrity with optimal wound healing
  Patient will maintain normal respiratory function
  Patient will maintain peripheral perfusion without complications from venous stasis
  Patient will have minimal or controlled discomfort and pain
  Patient will maintain adequate urinary and bowel elimination
  Patient will progress toward a positive integration of physical changes into the body image
  Patient will understand and follow home care instructions

Implementation

Postoperative nursing interventions are similar to those for other general surgery patients. Most patients have a urinary catheter inserted in the operating room. If not, the patient must be assessed closely for urinary retention. The patient must remain with the head of the bed elevated, and the knees and hips flexed (similar to sitting in a reclining chair). This position decreases tension on the abdominal area. Decreased tension helps maintain blood supply to the tissues. An abdominal binder may be applied during surgery to keep the abdominal wall flap positioned against the fascia (a fibrous membrane that covers, supports, and separates muscles and unites the skin with underlying tissue). A suction wound drain is usually placed in surgery.

To prevent skin breakdown due to immobility, an eggcrate, foam, or air mattress should be used. Patients are permitted to ambulate the day after surgery, because this will prevent respiratory complications, improve peristalsis, and improve circulatory status. Walking in a slouched position minimizes tension on the suture line. The reclining chair position may contribute to incisional edema, which may lead to venous stasis and thrombophlebitis. The patient is encouraged to perform leg exercises while in bed, at least every 2 hours. Antiembolism hose are usually worn.

Evaluation

Nursing interventions are evaluated by monitoring patient outcomes. Evaluate abdominal tissue for intact skin integrity and signs of optimal wound healing. Pain, discomfort, and response to analgesics are assessed. Peripheral perfusion is assessed to detect venous stasis. Urinary and bowel elimination is evaluated. The patient's knowledge of postoperative care is evaluated and reinforced with written instructions. The patient and family reactions to the alterations in appearance and body image are evaluated with each postoperative visit.

Documentation

Documentation includes an assessment of the abdominal tissue. Verbal and written home care instructions are documented along with the patient's response to teaching. The patient/family perceptions and reactions to the surgical results are recorded. Preoperative and postoperative photographs provide valuable objective documentation of the physical results of surgery.

Ongoing Care

Patients are discharged from the hospital in 3 to 4 days. Patients should continue to walk in a slouched position for 5 days after discharge. Patients may wear an elasticized leotard from the waist to the ankles or elasticized pantyhose for support and compression. Showers are usually permitted 3 or 4 days after the procedure. Sutures are removed approximately 2 weeks after surgery. Normal activity can be resumed slowly, and resumption of the patient's activity level can begin in 6 to 8 weeks. Patients may remain on antibiotics and must be taught to avoid aspirin and aspirin-containing compounds because of their anticoagulant effect. Cigarette smoking must also be avoided because of its vasoconstrictive effect.

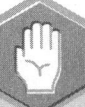

CLINICAL ALERT

The ideal patient is a young, relatively thin individual who has localized fatty deposits. The average patient is 30 to 45 years old, 5 to 10 pounds overweight, with modest skin relaxation from prior pregnancy or weight fluctuations.

SUCTION ASSISTED LIPECTOMY
Definition

Suction assisted lipectomy (SAL) or liposuction is the removal of subcutaneous fat deposits using a long, blunt suction cannula (Figure 76-5). The goal of this procedure is to improve the contour of the abdomen, hips, thighs, knees, ankles, chin, upper arms, or buttocks. It is used alone to remove fat deposits that are resistant to diet and exercise, to debulk flaps, and to remove lipomas. SAL is also used in combination with other procedures such as abdominoplasty, rhytidectomy, and reduction mammoplasty to enhance anatomic contours and produce a more desirable aesthetic result.

Etiology

Most patients who seek this procedure have localized fatty deposits on their hips, thighs, buttocks, or other areas that are not reduced through diet or exercise.

Therapeutic Management

The patient receives a local or general anesthetic and the procedure is usually done on an outpatient

RESEARCH BRIEF

Courtiss E, Donelan M: Skin sensation after suction lipectomy: a prospective study of 50 consecutive patients, *Plast Reconstr Surg* 81(4):550, 1988.

The major purpose of this study was to evaluate skin sensation after suction lipectomy. Critics of this cosmetic surgical procedure suggest that damage to blood vessels and nerves occurs because lipectomy is performed blindly. Pain was measured before and after surgery, using a device that emits a controlled electric current. All patients had pain in the areas to be treated by suction lipectomy, but often the degree of pain was variable and patchy. After surgery, initial pain was decreased in all treated areas. Sensation began to return to preoperative levels at 1 month. Depending on the size of the area treated, some patients did not have the return of full preoperative sensation for 1 year or longer. Basically, the larger the treated area, the larger area and greater degree of decreased sensation and the slower the return of pain. Despite the negative pressure of the suction pumps and the trauma caused by the suction cannulas, the authors of this study conclude that suction lipectomy does not permanently damage sensory nerves, which mediate pain.

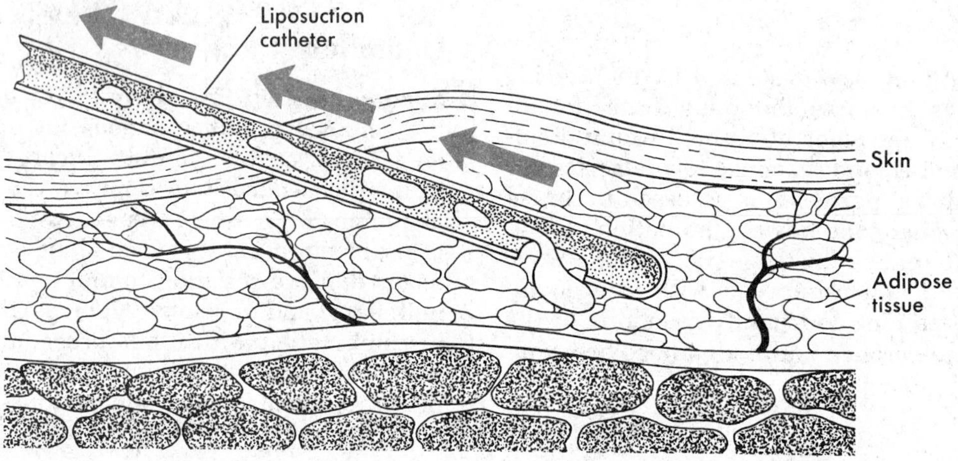

FIGURE 76-5 Suction assisted lipectomy. The blunt cannula removes adipose tissue.

basis. The major advantage of the procedure is that fatty tissue is removed through many small (½ inch) incisions. A blunt-tipped cannula is inserted through these incisions, and the adipose tissue is removed. To reduce the possibility of postoperative bleeding and serum accumulation, a supportive garment or dressing is used.

After suction lipectomy, there can be large fluid shifts into the operative and nonoperative tissue. This potential fluid shift is treated by intravenous fluids during surgery. Patients who have over 1000 mL of fat removed are generally considered for inpatient treatment. Other complications include loss of sensation in certain areas of the treated skin, fat embolism, hematoma, infection, and an undesirable aesthetic result related to contour deformities, ripples, bumps, and asymmetry of the treated areas.

NURSING MANAGEMENT OF THE PATIENT UNDERGOING SUCTION ASSISTED LIPECTOMY

Assessment

Peripheral pulses are assessed for rate and quality before the procedure. The nurse should assess the patient's use of anticoagulant medications, history of inflammatory fat disease, uncontrolled hypertension, diabetes mellitus, and poor cardiovascular status, because these factors are possible contraindications to suction lipectomy. Postoperative nursing assessment for this patient includes monitoring vital signs, assessing the surgical areas for edema and hemorrhaging, and assessing for pain. Signs of these complications include increasingly tight dressings, pallor of the extremity, and loss of peripheral pulses. The nurse must also be aware of any signs of hypovolemic shock, caused by the large fluid shifts from

the vascular compartment, and fat embolism, caused by release of fat globules into the bloodstream.

Nursing Diagnosis

Postoperative nursing diagnoses include:
  Impaired tissue integrity related to surgical manipulation of tissue
  Alteration in fluid volume: deficit related to loss of fluid from wounds and fluid shift
  Alteration in comfort: pain related to invasive procedure, incision, dressing, and position
  Alteration in body image related to actual and perceived change in appearance
  Impaired home maintenance management related to inadequate knowledge of care and expectations

Planning

Patient goals include the following:
  Patient will maintain intact tissue integrity without infection or other complications
  Patient will maintain adequate fluid volume with hemodynamic stability
  Patient will have minimal or controlled discomfort and pain
  Patient will progress toward a positive integration of physical changes into the body image
  Patient will understand and follow home care instructions

Implementation

Nursing interventions include elevating the patient's legs to improve venous return and reduce dependent edema if suction lipectomy was performed on the lower extremities. Intravenous fluids will be administered based on the amount of tissue removed. Removal of a large amount of adipose tissue, such as 3000 mL, may require a blood transfusion to restore adequate fluid volume. The patient will have dressings and a compression garment over the treated areas to minimize edema, prevent hemorrhaging, and press the loose skin onto the underlying tissue to ensure a smooth surface. It is important that dressings remain smooth and uniform to prevent uneven pressure on the tissue which could cause uneven skin contour. Before discharge, the patient must void to ensure adequate renal perfusion.

Evaluation

Nursing interventions are evaluated by monitoring patient outcomes. Evaluate the surgical area for intact skin integrity and signs of optimal wound healing. Pain, discomfort, and response to analgesics are assessed. Adequate fluid volume is evaluated with vital signs, sensorium, and intake and output. The patient's knowledge of postoperative care is evaluated and reinforced with written instructions. The patient and family reactions to the alterations in appearance and body image are evaluated with each postop visit.

Documentation

Documentation includes an assessment of the surgical area. Verbal and written home care instructions are documented along with the patient's response to teaching. The patient/family perceptions and reactions to the surgical results are recorded. Preoperative and postoperative photographs provide valuable objective documentation of the physical results of surgery.

Ongoing Care

The patient must be instructed to keep the dressings dry. Generally the pressure dressing remains in place for 1 week and then a support garment is worn. The patient is encouraged to eat foods high in iron. An iron supplement may be prescribed for anemia caused by blood loss. The patient is taught the signs and symptoms of infection and electrolyte imbalance. The patient needs to understand that the final appearance may not occur for several months to 1 year. Because of this delayed result, the patient may feel depressed and disappointed in the results. Encouragement from the nurse and significant others often helps the patient during this time.

AUGMENTATION MAMMOPLASTY
Definition

Augmentation mammoplasty is the surgical enlargement of the breasts and is one of the most common cosmetic surgical procedures performed. A silicone-filled or saline-filled breast prosthesis is used to enlarge the breast (Figure 76-6).

Etiology

Breast augmentation is performed for aesthetic reasons and also as reconstructive surgery for female patients without breast development (amastia) and for those with unilateral breast maldevelopment from Poland syndrome.

Clinical Manifestations

Breasts that the patient perceives as small are usually associated with an altered self-concept, altered self-esteem, self-consciousness, and embarrassment.

Therapeutic Management

The surgical procedure involves enlarging the breast by inserting a prosthesis beneath the breast tissue or beneath the pectoralis chest muscles if no or minimal tissue is present. Most implants today are Silastic envelopes filled with fluid such as saline. There has been much controversy about silicone-filled prostheses and their long-term effects. At present, their usage is limited to controlled research studies.

This surgery is most frequently an outpatient procedure. A local anesthetic with sedation is adequate, although a general anesthetic can be used if the pa-

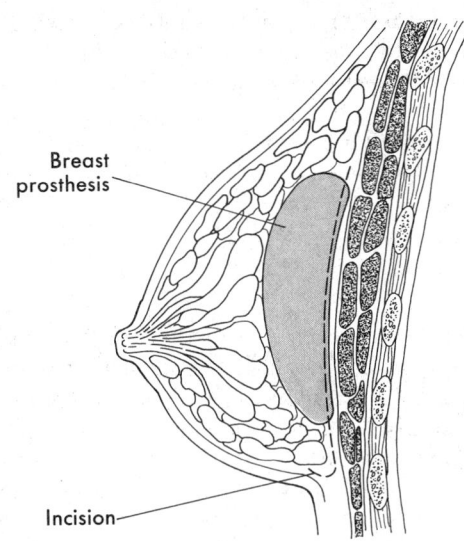

FIGURE 76-6   Augmentation mammoplasty. A prosthesis is used to enlarge the breast.

tient prefers. The incision is made under the breast, around the areola, or in the axilla. The implant is inserted through the incision. To prevent local tissue irritation, the implants are kept wrapped until needed and rinsed with saline before insertion. Implants must be handled with caution to prevent damage or contamination in the operating room. The incision is sutured closed, and a light gauze dressing is applied. The surgeon may order a bra or an elastic bandage for support.

Complications of breast augmentation include hematoma, infection, leakage of the implant, implant rupture, and an undesirable aesthetic result. Large hematomas are drained. Antibiotics usually control infection. Sometimes the implant is removed until the infection is under control. Ruptured implants need to be removed. A thorough irrigation of the breast pocket must be done before replacement with a new implant.

Capsular contracture is the development of a firm, fibrous scar formed around the breast implant. The breast has a hard, spherical appearance. The natural movement of the breast is restricted and can progress to a fixed position on the chest wall. Capsules can be reduced by placing manual pressure on the breast. If manual pressure does not release the capsule, it must be excised. The cause of capsules is unknown but seems to be related to tissue reaction to a foreign body, hematoma formation, contamination of the implant, too small a pocket formed in the breast during surgery, subclinical infection, or leakage of silicone from a damaged implant. The incidence of capsular contracture can be reduced with daily massage that disrupts fibrous tissue as it develops. Prevention of capsules with cortisone and vitamin E is being studied.

NURSING MANAGEMENT OF THE PATIENT UNDERGOING AUGMENTATION MAMMOPLASTY

Assessment

Preoperatively the nurse must assess the patient's motivation for the surgery. Women who are having breast augmentation for a significant other instead of for their own self-image are poor candidates. The desired size for breast enlargement can be estimated preoperatively by trying on a bra filled with breast implants. The preoperative history and examination focus on preexistent breast diseases, past breast surgery, and family history of breast cancer. Breast implants may interfere with accurate readings of future mammograms.

Assessment of the patient after surgery includes assessment of the breasts for pallor, swelling, and pain. These signs may indicate a hematoma. Generally, patients have moderate pain after this surgery. Patients who have had subpectoral implants will

have greater discomfort and muscle spasms. Symptoms of infection include swelling, erythema, increasing pain (usually unilaterally), and temperature above 100° F.

Nursing Diagnosis

Postoperative nursing diagnoses include:

Impaired skin integrity related to stretched breast skin and severed blood vessels

Alteration in body image related to actual and perceived change in breast appearance

Impaired home maintenance management related to inadequate knowledge of care and expectations

Planning

Patient goals include the following:

Patient will maintain intact skin integrity with optimal wound healing and no evidence of capsular contracture

Patient will progress toward a positive integration of the breast changes into the body image

Patient will understand and follow home care instructions

Implementation

Nursing interventions include elevating the head of the bed to reduce swelling. Some surgeons may have the patient wear a bra postoperatively to increase comfort and decrease suture tension. Other surgeons prefer the patient not to wear a bra, because this allows the breast skin to stretch and develop a normal position and sag. Not wearing a bra may also help reduce the risk for capsular contracture. The patient's temperature is also monitored. Dressings are changed under a physician's order using sterile technique. The patient is assured that the appearance of the breast will improve when the sutures are removed and healing is complete. Shoulder and arm movements may be curtailed for several weeks. Activities of daily living can be resumed gradually during this time.

Evaluation

Nursing interventions are evaluated by monitoring patient outcomes. Evaluate the breast area for intact skin integrity and signs of optimal wound healing. Pain, discomfort, and response to analgesics are assessed. The patient's knowledge of postoperative care is evaluated and reinforced with written instructions. Return demonstration of breast massage is observed, if applicable. The patient and family reactions to the alterations in appearance and body image are evaluated with each postoperative visit.

Documentation

Documentation includes an assessment of the breasts. Verbal and written home care instructions are documented along with the patient's response to teaching. The patient/family perceptions and reactions to the surgical results are recorded. Preoperative and postoperative photographs provide valuable objective documentation of the physical results of surgery. Documentation also includes (in both intraoperative and office records) the manufacturer, style, size, and lot numbers of the implants.

Ongoing Care

The patient should be encouraged to continue monthly breast self-examinations and routine mammography after the age of 35. Mammography technicians should be informed of the presence of breast implants by the patient before the study is performed. Thus additional appropriate views will be included.

Reconstructive Surgery

The purpose of reconstructive surgery is to improve form or function of a body part/area. The ultimate goal is to increase patients' ability to interact successfully with their environment, both physically and psychosocially. Reconstructive surgery may be performed as a life-saving measure such as a person with an amputated arm. It may restore function to the person with a lacerated tendon of the hand. Reconstructive surgery may correct congenital deformities and ablate cancerous lesions of the head and neck. It frequently involves the use of healthy tissue such as a flap or graft to reconstruct the defect. Reconstructive surgery aims to correct a defect while at the same time provide the best aesthetic result possible. While reconstruction for head and neck cancer, craniofacial anomalies, hand injuries, and burns are considered components of the plastic surgery specialty, they are discussed in other chapters of this book.

SKIN GRAFTS

A **skin graft** is used in reconstructive surgery to cover an open wound and provide protection to the underlying structures. One example of this is the surgical repair of decubitus ulcers when healing by primary or secondary intention is not feasible. The area where the skin graft is taken from is called the donor site. The area where the skin graft is placed is called the recipient site. Donor tissue nearest the defect will provide the best match for skin color, texture, and thickness. Skin grafting is used in reconstructive surgery to provide protection to underlying areas.

A skin graft is created when a portion of the epidermis and dermis is surgically removed from its blood supply before being transplanted to another area. A split-thickness skin graft, otherwise known as a partial-thickness skin graft, is composed of the epidermis and only a portion of the dermis. A full-thickness skin graft contains the epidermis and all of the dermis. Both of these grafts are used to cover large surface defects. Skin grafts are transferred without an established blood supply and initially survive by getting oxygen from serum. The survival of the skin graft depends on the growth of blood vessels in the area where the graft is transplanted. Providing an optimal "bed" on which the transplanted graft will lie is critical. Nurses play a major role in preventing the accumulation of any substance between the graft and the bed that would prevent adherence of the new graft. This includes preventing a hematoma or wound exudate. Often a special dressing that exerts even pressure and facilitates contact between the graft and the bed is placed over this site.

FLAPS

Flaps involve the transfer of tissue from one area of the body to an adjacent area while maintaining a continuous blood supply through its base. Flaps are used to replace tissue loss, and cover an exposed wound, bone, tendon, or nerve. Flaps may be used to cover areas with poor vascularity. This is seen when extra padding is needed, as in reconstructive surgery for pressure ulcers or when cartilage and bone must be covered.

There are several types of flaps. A pedicle flap consists of skin and subcutaneous tissue with its own blood supply. Muscle flaps consist of muscle and their own blood supply. Musculocutaneous (or myocutaneous) flaps transfer muscle, skin, and subcutaneous tissue with their own blood supply. These flaps are used to repair pressure ulcers, leg defects, and breast reconstruction. Omental flaps consist of the omentum (the fatty tissue over the abdomen) and are rotated to cover a wound. They are used to cover chest wall defects, axillary defects, and carotid arteries that are exposed. A skin graft is required over an omental flap to provide external coverage of the omentum.

A free flap involves the transfer of tissue with its blood supply from the donor site to the recipient site. The blood vessels and nerves of the donor tissue are anastomosed to the recipient site through a microsurgical technique. A free flap is used when the tissue adjacent to the defect is inappropriate as a result of poor vascularity or inappropriate tissue

NURSING CARE PLAN   *Patient with Postoperative Flaps and Grafts*

Nursing diagnosis/ Expected outcome	Interventions	Rationale
Impaired tissue integrity related to surgical manipulation of tissue, disrupted circulation, and incisions • *Patient will maintain intact tissue integrity with reestablishment of adequate circulation and optimal wound healing*	Assess flap/graft for circulation—color, temperature, sensation, capillary refill, Doppler Assure there is no pressure on the site or kinking of the flap Assess wound for drainage—color, amount, odor, infection, hematoma, edema, and degree of healing Keep wound/dressing dry	Constant assessment of the flap/graft site is necessary to promote postoperative healing. Decreased tissue perfusion may occur because of edema or poor positioning. Wound drainage may indicate the presence of infection or complications such as graft death. Pallor, cyanosis, coolness, or edema may indicate inadequate tissue perfusion. Pressure, kinking, and stretching may decrease blood supply to the graft.
	Observe drainage and maintain intact/patent wound drains	Assessment of the drainage device is necessary to prevent hematoma formation or to assure that fluid is not collecting in the tissue.
	Observe approximation of incision lines	The incision line should remain intact with progressive healing. The survival of the skin graft depends on the growth of a new blood supply on the area or "bed" on which the graft lies. Any accumulation between the graft and "bed" prevents adherence. Dependent positioning promotes edema and swelling
	Monitor vital signs, including temperature Keep bed covers off surgical site, use bed cradle	

	No coffee, tea, chocolate, or caffeine-containing carbonated beverages
	No smoking in room
	Keep room temperature warm
	If face or trunk:
	  Elevate head of bed
	  Keep off the operative site
	If upper extremity:
	  Elevate extremity above heart level
	  Use a sling when up or elevate extremity using an IV pole
	  Monitor color, warmth, movement, and sensation of fingers every 2 hours for first 24 hours, then every 4-8 hours
	If lower extremity:
	  Elevate extremity at all times
	  Monitor color, warmth, movement, and sensation of toes every 2 hours for first 24 hours, then every 4-8 hours
		Caffeine and nicotine cause venous constriction and may decrease blood flow to the surgical site

Modified from Goodman, T. ed.: *Core curriculum for plastic and reconstructive surgical nursing*, Pitman, NJ, 1989, Anthony J. Jannetti, p 91.

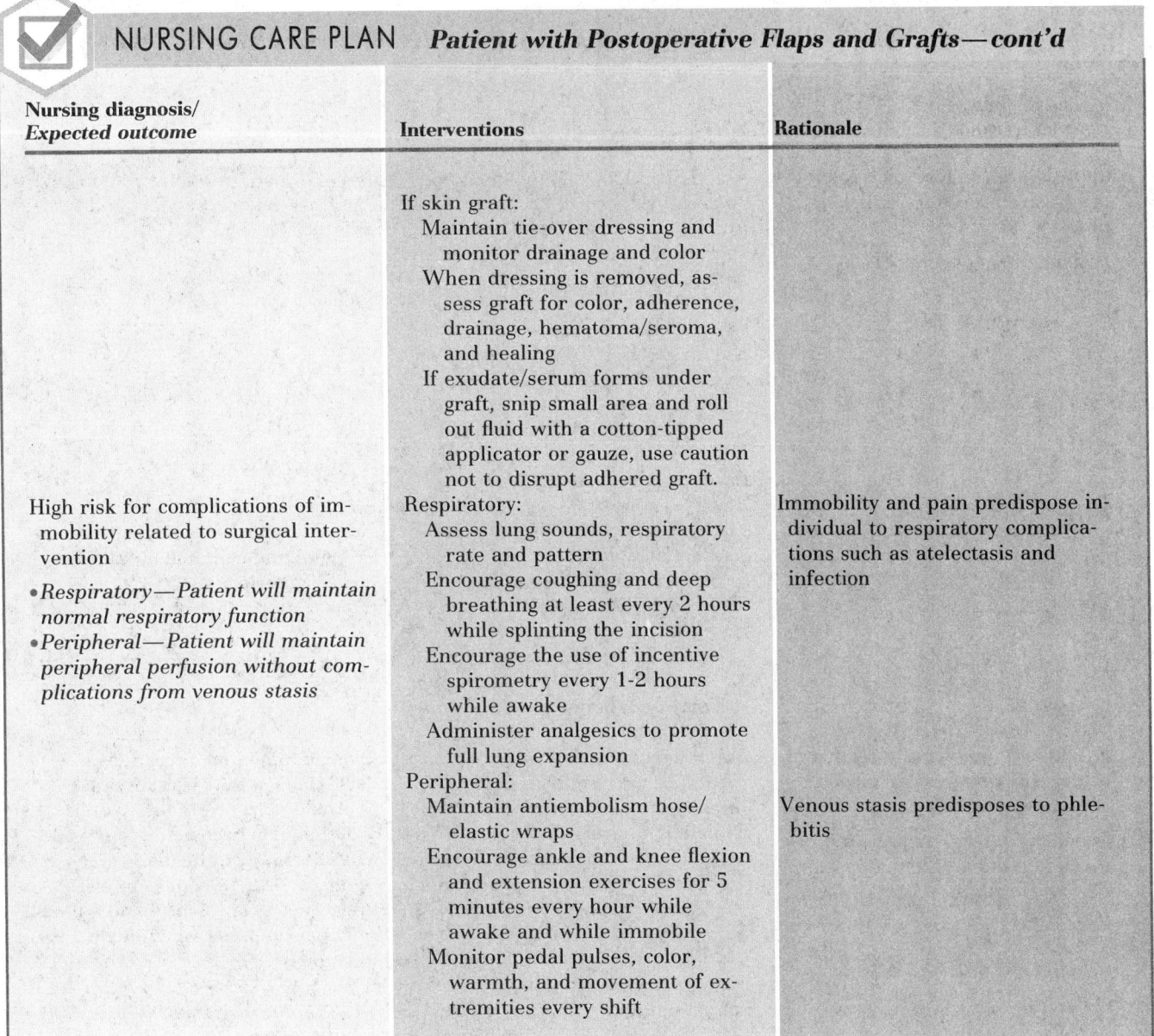

NURSING CARE PLAN   *Patient with Postoperative Flaps and Grafts—cont'd*

Nursing diagnosis/ Expected outcome	Interventions	Rationale

High risk for complications of immobility related to surgical intervention
 	
• *Respiratory—Patient will maintain normal respiratory function*
• *Peripheral—Patient will maintain peripheral perfusion without complications from venous stasis*
	If skin graft:
	  Maintain tie-over dressing and monitor drainage and color
	  When dressing is removed, assess graft for color, adherence, drainage, hematoma/seroma, and healing
	  If exudate/serum forms under graft, snip small area and roll out fluid with a cotton-tipped applicator or gauze, use caution not to disrupt adhered graft.
	Respiratory:
	  Assess lung sounds, respiratory rate and pattern
	  Encourage coughing and deep breathing at least every 2 hours while splinting the incision
	  Encourage the use of incentive spirometry every 1-2 hours while awake
	  Administer analgesics to promote full lung expansion
	Peripheral:
	  Maintain antiembolism hose/ elastic wraps
	  Encourage ankle and knee flexion and extension exercises for 5 minutes every hour while awake and while immobile
	  Monitor pedal pulses, color, warmth, and movement of extremities every shift
		Immobility and pain predispose individual to respiratory complications such as atelectasis and infection
		
		Venous stasis predisposes to phlebitis

Continued.

integrity. An example of a free flap is the transfer of the gluteus muscle for breast reconstruction.

NURSING MANAGEMENT OF THE PATIENT WITH FLAPS AND GRAFTS

Various types of flaps and grafts are used extensively in reconstructive surgery. Therefore a nursing care plan is presented for a patient with these procedures.

TISSUE EXPANSION

Tissue expansion may be an alternative to flap and graft procedures in selected cases. The procedure involves the insertion of an inflatable device under the tissue to create a redundancy of tissue. This technique stretches the tissue in the same manner as pregnancy stretches the abdomen to accommodate the growing fetus. Expansion is useful in any area of the body where there is a shortage of tissue.

Advantages of tissue expansion over other reconstructive procedures such as flaps and grafts include a better match of skin in color, texture, and hair-bearing characteristics; easier procedure with less operating time and anesthesia; better circulation and better quality tissue; and no need for the creation of a donor site with an additional scar.

Indications for tissue expansion include breast reconstruction prior to implant insertion, reconstruction of burn scars and defects subsequent to tumor removal, tattoos, wound scars, and large birthmarks.

NURSING CARE PLAN   *Patient with Postoperative Flaps and Grafts—cont'd*

Nursing diagnosis/ Expected outcome	Interventions	Rationale

Alteration in comfort: pain related to invasive procedure, incision, dressing, and position
 	
•*Patient will report pain relief*
	Assess pain for type, location, and severity
	Administer analgesics as needed/ ordered and observe effectiveness
	Instruct on relaxation techniques and imagery
	Offer back care at least every 4 hours
	Assist in changing position at least every 2 hours
	Use egg crate on bed or air fluidized bed
	Encourage early ambulation
	Bowel:
	   Assess bowel sounds and abdominal distention
	   Monitor bowel elimination
	   Provide a low residue diet for 4 days in order to reduce the need for bowel movements. Also, constipating medications may be administered, depending on location of flap
		Relief of pain promotes physiologic and psychologic comfort and healing
		
		A low residue diet may help to prevent wound contamination from fecal material

Alteration in body image related to actual and perceived change in appearance •*Patient will progress toward a positive integration of temporary and permanent physical changes into body image*	Assess reactions to changed appearance and willingness to look at area and perform wound care Explain temporary distortions in appearance and sensation (edema, erythema, ecchymosis, numbness) to patient and significant other[s]) Encourage verbalization of feelings of patient and significant other(s) Encourage support of significant other(s) Provide realistic reassurance and encourage patience Assess and explore sexual issues	Clues to potential alterations in self-concept may be expressed verbally or nonverbally Patients may become discouraged. Results may not be determined for up to a year for some surgeries. Appearances may change and will continue to improve when healing is complete
Impaired home maintenance management related to inadequate knowledge of care and expectations •*Patient and significant other(s) will understand and follow home care instructions*	Provide instructions for home care Instruct to observe for signs and symptoms of infection Assist patient with use of special support garments as ordered Reinforce previous teaching regarding postoperative course, medications, possible complications, desired results, and activity limitations	Education provides information to the patient and significant other who will be assisting in home care to promote completion of healing process

NURSING CARE PLAN   *Patient with Postoperative Flaps and Grafts—cont'd*

Nursing diagnosis/ Expected outcome	Interventions	Rationale
	Offer encouragement and support if complications occur	
	Stress importance of follow-up office visits	
	Provide written home care instructions	
	Assist patient with return to lifestyle activities (e.g., return to work)	
	Instruct on skin care to prevent breakdown in other areas (e.g., decubitus ulcers with immobile patients)	
	If donor site:	
	Keep bed covers off site	
	Monitor dressing or skin substitute for color, drainage, and degree of healing	
	If Xeroform/Scarlet Red, etc., keep area dry and exposed to air	
	Heat lamp to site for 30 minutes every 4 hours, may use blow dryer to dry	
	Remove dressing/skin substitute in 7-10 days when donor site is healed, then apply lubricating cream of choice	

Tissue expansion requires one surgical procedure to implant the expander as close to the defect as possible without expanding the defect. The expander contains an injection reservoir. At various intervals, the reservoir is injected with saline to further stretch the tissue. These serial injections are continued until adequate tissue expansion is achieved. This usually requires 3 to 6 months. A second surgical procedure is then required to remove the expander and reconstruct the defect.

Tissue expansion may be performed on an outpatient or inpatient basis. Serial injections are done in the physician's office. Nursing interventions center on assisting the patient to cope with body image alterations that occur with the temporary distorted appearance caused by the expansion. The patient needs support and reinforcement that the change in appearance is temporary. A bluish or pink discoloration of the expanded area is expected and also temporary. Modifications in clothing, the use of wigs, or the use of other camouflage techniques may be suggested. Support and understanding of the significant other(s) is especially important at this time.

Pain or discomfort can be relieved with analgesics. Discomfort immediately following each serial expansion usually subsides within 2 to 12 hours. Patients must be instructed in wound care and to observe the expanded area for changes in appearance, signs of infection, or extrusion of the implant. Complications include infection, hematoma/seroma, exposure and kinking of the expander, necrosis of expanded tissue, and device failure (unexpected expander deflation).

REPLANTATION

Replantation is the reattachment of an amputated limb or digit. The part is reattached through the use

TABLE 76-1	Assessment of Vascular Occlusion	
	ARTERIAL	**VENOUS**
Skin color	Pale, mottled blue	Cyanotic, blue
Capillary refill	Sluggish (>3 seconds)	Brisk (<3 seconds)
Tissue turgor	Prunelike, then hollow	Tense, swollen, distended
Temperature	Cool	Cool
Dermal bleeding	Scant amount of dark blood	Rapid bleeding, dark blood

of a microscope. Vessels, bone, tendons, and nerves can be anastomosed to reattach the amputated part. The primary goals of replantation are to restore function and to enhance the quality of life. A replantation purely for cosmetic purposes is rarely attempted.

Indications for replantation include multiple digit injuries, thumb amputation, and major extremity injuries. The degree of success of a replantation depends on the type of injury. A sharp separation injury that has a nearly clean surgical edge with minimal damage to vessels, nerves, and tendons is best suited for a successful replantation. More severe injuries such as crush and avulsion injuries are least suited.

Management of the amputated part begins at the site of injury by rinsing the part with saline, wrapping it in a damp, saline sponge, sealing it in a plastic bag or container, and placing the container in an ice chest. Caution must be used not to place the amputated part directly on ice since this will cause irreversible cellular damage. The part is then transported with the patient as quickly as possible. Stump bleeding must be controlled and measures instituted to minimize infection. Speed is essential in dealing with these patients in order to reduce ischemia time (the length of time the amputated part is starved of a blood supply). The shorter the ischemia time, the greater the chance of a successful replantation.

Postoperatively, several parameters of replant viability must be monitored. These include color, capillary refill, temperature, tissue turgor, and Doppler pulses. Of these parameters, temperature is the most indicative of early circulatory problems. Temperature monitors/probes are used to detect subtle changes. A temperature of 34° to 36° C is considered optimal. A decrease of 2 or more degrees in an hour or a decline to 32° C demands immediate attention. Vascular compromise may be assessed by using the chart in Table 76-1. Postoperative medications may include aspirin as an anticoagulant, antibiotics, and dextran to improve capillary blood flow and reduce viscosity.

Other nursing management considerations are similar to the care of the patient undergoing flaps and grafts. Rehabilitation involves months of physical and occupational therapy. Patients need continual reinforcement of their progress. They must be taught to reduce or avoid any chance of vasoconstriction. Also, since sensation to the replanted part has been disrupted, care must be taken to avoid potential problems such as burns, pressure areas, and cuts.

BREAST RECONSTRUCTION

Definition

Breast reconstruction surgery is performed for abnormalities of the breast tissue that are congenital or acquired. Congenital abnormalities include athelia (absence of the nipple), amastia (lack of breast development), polymastia (more than two breasts), polythelia (more than two nipples), macromastia (disproportionately large breasts), or ectopic breast tissue usually found in the axilla. Acquired abnormalities include burns and trauma to the breast, surgical procedures, radiation, or removal of the breast because of cancer. Men may develop breasts, known as gynecomastia, and a simple mastectomy is performed once liver and endocrine alterations are ruled out.

Mastectomy for breast cancer causes disfigurement and psychologic depression. (See Chapter 70 for a complete discussion of management of women with breast cancer.) Knowledge of breast reconstruction has a positive psychologic effect and will often give a patient the strength to tolerate chemotherapy or radiation therapy.

Contraindications to breast reconstruction include large invasive tumors, extensive chest wall or axillary metastasis, and body system metastasis. Patients receiving chemotherapy are usually advised to complete the regimen and wait at least 1 month before having surgery. Patients having radiation therapy are usually advised to wait 1 week for every radiation therapy treatment they have had.

Etiology

Breast cancer is a major factor in the mortality of women in the United States. Mastectomies are still performed despite a trend toward less radical surgery for treatment of breast cancer. A good candidate for breast reconstruction is a woman who has a good chance of having the cancer arrested, but this is not an absolute criterion.

Clinical Manifestations

Patients who have pliable chest tissue remaining and have a horizontal incision can be considered optimal candidates for reconstruction. Patients with little chest tissue or muscle and with vertical scars can also be reconstructed.

Therapeutic Management

Breast reconstruction can be performed at the same time as the mastectomy. However, there is greater risk of hematoma and decreased tissue perfusion with immediate reconstruction because of the extensive surgery in one body area. For this reason, some surgeons prefer to wait at least 6 weeks after mastectomy, until the scar is healed and the patient has had radiation or chemotherapy treatment.

There are several surgical procedures for breast reconstruction, from a simple approach to complex. One approach is to insert a breast implant under the muscle. For individuals without adequate tissue, a tissue expander can be used to stretch the skin and muscle for eventual implant insertion. The use of implants in breast reconstruction is contraindicated when there are large cancerous lesions, when radiation may be used, and with inflammatory cancer.

For patients in whom the pectoralis muscle of the chest wall has been excised during mastectomy, the latissimus dorsi muscle and a section of skin from the back can be brought through the axilla to cover the chest defect (Figure 76-7). This procedure provides for the missing muscle and the skin. An implant is placed under the muscle. The transverse rectus abdominis myocutaneous (TRAM) flap consists of the rectus abdominis muscle and skin flap from the lower abdomen (Figure 76-8). This procedure creates breast tissue from the adipose tissue of the lower abdomen, and usually there is no need for an implant. An added benefit with this procedure is an abdominoplasty.

If the back and lower abdominal muscles are not usable, a free flap can be used for breast reconstruction. The gluteus muscle has been used for this procedure.

A nipple and areola can be created for the reconstructed breast by taking tissue from the nipple on the opposite breast or using dark skin from the labia or inner thigh. Tattooing an areola on the breast

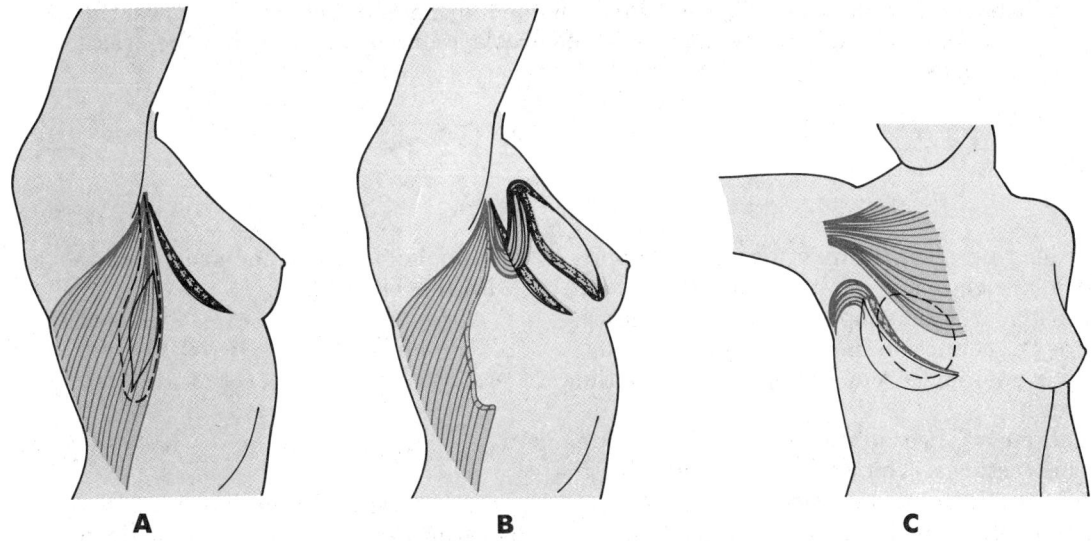

A   **B**   **C**

FIGURE 76-7   Latissimus dorsi flap. **A,** Latissimus dorsi flap is designed using pattern of breast pocket. **B,** Skin and strip of latissimus muscle with nerve and blood supply is tunneled through the axilla to the chest. **C,** Flap is rotated into place on the chest. A breast implant is then inserted under the muscle.

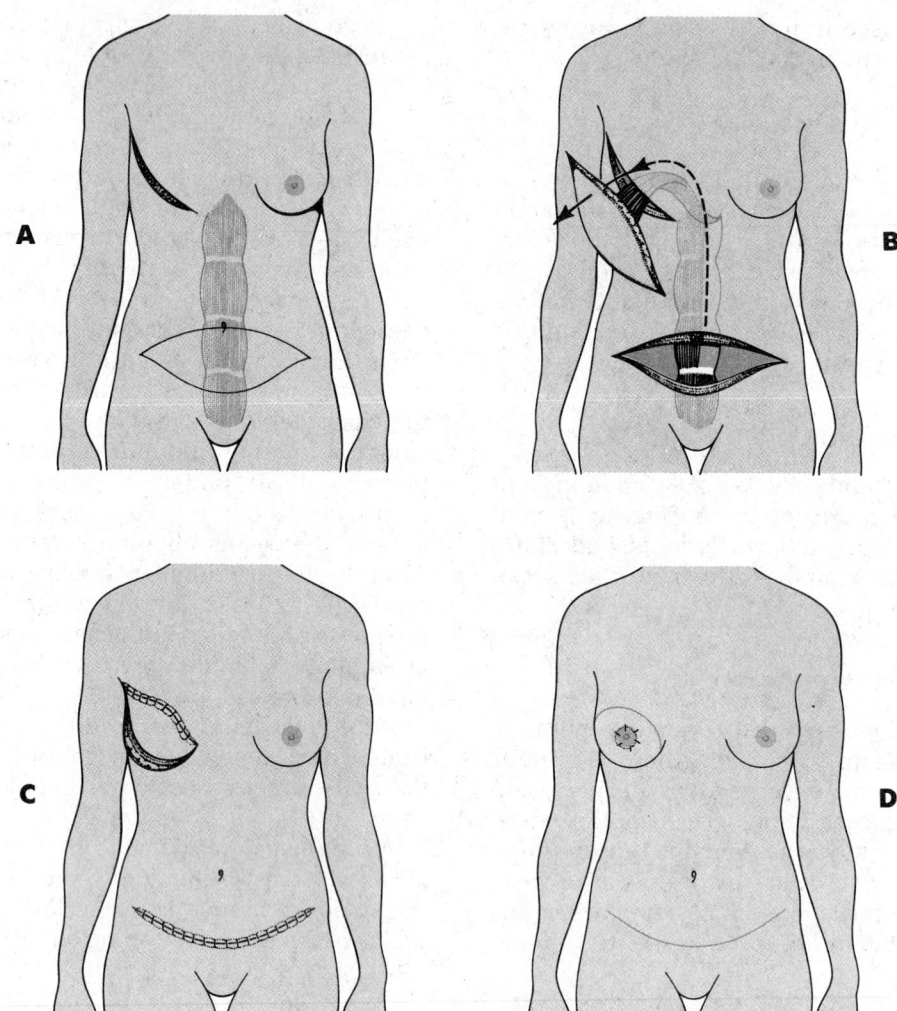

FIGURE 76-8 TRAM flap. **A,** TRAM flap is planned. **B,** The abdominal tissue, while attached to the rectus muscle, nerve, and blood supply, is tunneled through the abdomen to the chest. **C,** The flap is trimmed to shape the breast. The lower abdominal incision is closed. **D,** Nipple and areola are reconstructed after the breast is healed.

mound can also be used. In most cases, the opposite breast also needs surgery to match the newly created breast's size and shape. To achieve symmetry, mastopexy, reduction mammoplasty, or augmentation mammoplasty may be performed for the opposite breast.

Complications of breast reconstruction include capsular contractures. The response to a foreign body is the formation of a fibrous capsule around the implant. If an infection, hematoma, or trauma occurs, excessive capsular formation will develop, resulting in a deformed breast. Other complications include skin ulceration, hypertrophic scar formation, intercostal neuralgia, infection, hematoma, flap necrosis, and an undesirable aesthetic result. Ab-

dominal hernia has been reported as a complication with the TRAM flap.

NURSING MANAGEMENT OF THE PATIENT UNDERGOING BREAST RECONSTRUCTION
Assessment

Before surgery the patient is assessed for the usual surgical risks, expectations of the surgery, status of cancer treatment, and her feelings about her diagnosis of known or suspected breast cancer (where a biopsy will be done). As with the aesthetic surgical patient, the expectations the patient has about the outcome of the surgery must be explored. It is important that the patient understand that the reconstructed breast will not feel or look completely normal. Current techniques do not offer lactation, nipple sensation, or nipple erectility in the reconstructed breast. The newly recreated breast will never be a premastectomy breast, but from the patient's perspective, it does offer an improvement over the mastectomy scar. Reconstruction assists the patient in feeling "complete" or "whole" once again. Breast reconstruction also permits the patient to wear clothing without a prosthesis. Significant others may not be completely supportive and may express feelings that the patient "is alive and that should be good enough, why go through more surgery?" The nurse needs to explore these feelings with the patient and significant others and make referrals for continued counseling when necessary.

Assessment of the patient after the surgery centers on having an adequate blood supply to the transferred tissues. The nurse must be aware of the graft and protect it from pressure, kinking, and stretching. The breast should be observed for color, capillary refill, temperature, and drainage. Pallor, cyanosis, coolness, or delayed capillary filling should be reported to the surgeon, because it may indicate an inadequate blood supply.

The patient is assessed for body image adjustment. Nurses should assess verbal comments and willingness to look at and touch the breast. It may be necessary to assure the patient that the appearance of the breast will continue to improve when the sutures are removed and healing is complete.

Nursing Diagnosis

Postoperative nursing diagnoses include:
   Impaired tissue integrity related to surgical manipulation of tissue and incisions
   Alteration in tissue perfusion related to decreased mobility, pain, and chest incisions
   Alteration in comfort: pain related to invasive procedure, incisions, and dressings
   Alteration in elimination related to decreased mobility, analgesics, and abdominal surgery (for TRAM flap only)
   Alteration in body image related to actual and perceived change in breast appearance and effects on sexuality
   Impaired home maintenance management related to inadequate knowledge of care and expectations

Planning

Patient goals include the following:
   Patient will maintain intact tissue integrity with optimal wound healing
   Patient will maintain normal respiratory function
   Patient will maintain peripheral perfusion without complications from venous stasis

   Patient will have minimal or controlled discomfort and pain
   Patient will maintain adequate urinary and bowel elimination
   Patient will progress toward a positive integration of physical changes and sexuality concerns into the body image
   Patient will understand and follow home care instructions

Implementation

The patient is placed in Fowler's position and is usually permitted to turn to the nonoperative side, which elevates the newly reconstructed breast and improves drainage. Patients who had breast reconstruction using the latissimus dorsi muscle are discouraged initially from moving the affected arm, although pain usually prevents extreme motion. Drains are usually in place to help prevent hematoma formation, and the nurse must assess patency of the drainage device to assure that fluid is not collecting in the tissues. The drainage is also assessed for color and odor, which could indicate postoperative infection. The patient's temperature is also monitored at least once every 8 hours in the immediate postoperative period.

The flap is assessed for color, temperature, and capillary refill. Assessment of the nipple areola is made, and dressings are designed so this area can be observed. Areolae that are deep-red, purple, dusky, or black around the edge are reported to the surgeon immediately. Dressings are changed as needed using sterile technique. Once the dressings are removed, patients wear a front closing brassiere without stays or underwiring. This in itself has a psychologic lift, making the patient feel "normal," which facilitates a return to wellness and enhanced body image.

Evaluation

Nursing interventions are evaluated by monitoring patient outcomes. Evaluate the breast area for intact skin integrity and signs of optimal wound healing. Pain, discomfort, and response to analgesics are assessed. Respiratory function and peripheral perfusion are monitored and evaluated. The patient's knowledge of postoperative care is evaluated and reinforced with written instructions. The patient and family reactions to the alterations in appearance and body image are evaluated with each postoperative visit.

Documentation

Documentation includes an assessment of the breasts, and respiratory and peripheral vascular status. Verbal and written home care instructions are documented along with the patient's response to teaching. The patient/family perceptions and reactions to the surgical results are recorded. Preoperative and postoperative photographs provide valuable objective documentation of the physical results of surgery.

Ongoing Care

The patient can resume light activity, such as short walks and cooking, 2 weeks after surgery. At 3 weeks, driving a car and carrying light parcels are permitted. At 6 weeks, the patient may return to full activity including regular exercise. Sexual activity can resume as soon as the breast feels comfortable and the patient is without pain. The nurse can refer the patient to community support groups. These groups can be of assistance in helping the patient cope with problems and concerns, such as clothing, bras, emotions, and sexuality.

REDUCTION MAMMOPLASTY

Reduction mammoplasty removes excess breast tissue and overlying skin from large, pendulous breasts. There is reconstruction of breast contour, size, shape, and symmetry. Large breasts result in part from heredity, pregnancy, breast-feeding, and an exaggerated hormone response in puberty.

Most women seek breast reduction for relief of back and neck pain, bra strap grooves in the shoulders, inability to wear backless or strapless clothes, or for relief of intertriginous dermatitis, which manifests as a rash under the breasts from perspiration and skin chafing. Patients with large breasts also encounter ridicule from others because of the appearance and sexual connotations associated with large breasts.

Breast reduction is usually performed through keyhole incisions around the nipple and areola, and incisions under the breast. The lower portion of the breast is removed and the sides brought down to form the new breast. The nipple is carried to the reconstructed breast on a pedicle of tissue from the underside. The lactation ducts may be severed, and the woman may not be able to breast-feed.

Nursing management is similar to that for a patient undergoing breast reconstruction. Length of recovery is shorter, however, because of the fact that the chest muscles are undisturbed.

MAXILLOFACIAL TRAUMA
Facial Fractures

Facial bone fractures often occur with facial injury. Any of the facial bones may fracture, either individually or in combination.

Nasal Fractures

Fractures of the nasal bones can occur with or without dislocation of the nasal cartilages. Reduction (restoring to a normal position) of a nasal fracture is usually performed by closed reduction with the patient receiving topical and local anesthetics. Usually this closed reduction is accomplished by digital and instrumental manipulation. At times it is necessary to perform an open reduction using wire fixation.

Mandibular Fractures

The mandible is the most commonly fractured bone. Many mandibular fractures occur in two places. A fracture will occur at the site of impact and on the opposite side. The opposite side of impact is often fractured as well because of the arched shape of the bone. When there is a fracture of the mandible or lower jaw, the biting surfaces of the teeth may not meet properly. This is known as **malocclusion.** Some mandibular fractures can be corrected using closed reduction and fixation between the jawbones, which is commonly known as "wiring the jaw" (intermaxillary fixation). Most of these fractures require open reduction with internal wires and/or plating and supplementary intermaxillary fixation.

Maxillary Fractures

Like a mandibular fracture, a maxillary fracture also results in malocclusion. If a maxillary fracture is severe, it can also result in a deformity of the middle face. In this situation, the middle face has a flattened or "smashed in" appearance. The goal of surgery is to restore occlusion and correct any facial deformity.

Zygomatic Fractures

Zygomatic (cheekbone) bone fractures are common because of the prominence of the cheek on the face. Fractures of the zygoma may interfere with the patient's ability to open and close the mouth properly. These fractures also result in a flattening of the cheek on the involved side. The goal of surgery is to elevate the depressed fracture and maintain the reduction. Depending on the severity of the fracture, closed or open reduction with internal fixation is performed.

Orbital Floor Fractures

The eye and periorbital tissue rests on the orbital floor. The bones of the orbital floor are eggshell thin. Orbital floor fractures often occur with maxillary and zygomatic fractures. If an orbital floor fracture occurs without a maxillary or zygomatic fracture, this is known as a **blow-out fracture.** The goal of surgery is to restore the orbital floor and correct the placement of the eyeball. If the floor cannot be surgically corrected by elevating the bony fragments, an implant will be used. This implant may be cartilage, bone, or synthetic material.

NURSING MANAGEMENT OF THE PATIENT WITH FACIAL FRACTURES

Assessment

Preoperatively the nurse assesses for skin integrity, hydration, oxygenation, edema, oral hygiene, nutrition, communication, and vision. Postoperatively the nurse assesses for facial swelling, asymmetry of the facial structures, and abnormal facial bone movement. In addition, the nurse also assesses the patient for vision, noting unequal eye movement and diplopia. When rhinorrhea (thin, watery discharge from the nose) or otorrhea (ear inflammation with purulent discharge) is noted, there is the possibility of cerebrospinal fluid (CSF) leakage through the fractures. The fluid is assessed for sugar using Testape or Ketostix. Cerebrospinal fluid contains sugar, whereas rhinorrhea does not. Cerebrospinal fluid dries on bed linens in concentric, halo-like rings and does not crust.

Nursing Diagnosis

Postoperative nursing diagnoses include:
  Ineffective airway clearance related to wired jaws, increased secretions, and swelling
  Impaired tissue integrity related to surgical manipulation of tissue and bone, and incisions
  Alteration in comfort: pain related to invasive procedure, wired jaws, and swelling
  Alteration in nutrition related to surgical procedure, altered eating patterns, and pain
  Alteration in body image related to actual and perceived change in appearance and function
  Impaired home maintenance management related to inadequate knowledge of care and expectations

Planning

Patient goals include the following:
  Patient will maintain a patent airway
  Patient will maintain intact tissue integrity with optimal healing
  Patient will have minimal or controlled discomfort and pain
  Patient will maintain adequate nutrition to promote wound healing and maintain body functioning
  Patient will progress toward a positive integration of physical changes into the body image

Patient will understand and follow home care instructions

Implementation

Patients with intermaxillary fixation after surgery require some special assessment and care. Once the jaw is wired, patients are reminded they cannot open the mouth and should not try to do so. If patients become very distressed and panic, the nurse helps them relax and reminds them to breathe through their nose. Suction equipment and a wire cutter are kept at the bedside at all times. In the event of vomiting, the patient is turned to the side or helped to a full sitting position with the head tipped forward. Suction is used to remove the vomitus that is not expelled through the nose or mouth. Wires holding the jaw together should be cut only if the patient cannot expel the vomitus. If ineffective airway clearance develops, the nurse should not hesitate to cut the wires connecting the upper and lower teeth.

Nursing interventions also include oral care with a soft toothbrush or toothswabs. More aggressive mouth care, such as using a Water Pik, may be ordered.

Evaluation

Nursing interventions are evaluated by monitoring patient outcomes. Evaluate for a patent airway and observe the operative area for signs of optimal wound healing. Pain, discomfort, and response to analgesics are assessed. The nutritional status is evaluated in order to promote wound healing. The patient's knowledge of postoperative care is evaluated and reinforced with written instructions. The patient and family reactions to the alterations in appearance and body image are evaluated with each postoperative visit.

Documentation

Documentation includes an assessment of the operative area. Verbal and written home care instructions are documented along with the patient's re-

CLINICAL ALERT

Wire cutters and suction equipment are kept at the bedside of a patient with intermaxillary fixation. If ineffective airway clearance occurs, the nurse should cut the wires immediately and establish a patent airway.

sponse to teaching. The patient/family perceptions and reactions to the surgical results are recorded. Preoperative and postoperative photographs provide valuable objective documentation of the physical results of surgery.

Ongoing Care

On discharge the patient should be able to perform the needed suture line care. The patient must notify the nurse or physician if the wound becomes infected. If discharged with intermaxillary fixation, the patient should carry a wire cutter at all times. The patient and significant other need to know which wires to cut if an emergency occurs, such as vomiting, choking, or cardiac arrest. The patient needs to know how to prepare a high-calorie, high-protein liquid diet. Liquid multivitamins may be helpful. The patient should avoid carbonated beverages and alcohol. Carbonated beverages fizz in the back of the throat and interfere with the airway. Alcohol can cause nausea and vomiting when combined with analgesia. A 10-pound weight loss is not uncommon while the jaws are wired.

Patients should use a Water Pik and soft toothbrush at home. The gums will be tender at first and may bleed. The ends of the wires may irritate the mucosa and can be lined with paraffin wax. Water-related activities, such as swimming, should be avoided. The airway cannot be cleared of water rapidly when the jaws are wired, and there is an increased risk of drowning. Sutures are usually removed after 5 days. Follow-up revisions may be necessary to align scars with normal skin folds and lines.

CRITICAL THINKING QUESTIONS

1 What are the intended outcomes of cosmetic and reconstructive surgery?

2 What determines a successful surgical result?

3 What effect does plastic surgery have on body image?

4 List factors that determine the surgical setting for a plastic surgical procedure.

5 Why do patients elect to have cosmetic surgery?

6 What are the preoperative teaching interventions for the cosmetic and reconstructive surgical patient?

7 Identify the necessary factors to evaluate the psychosocial status of the plastic surgery patient.

8 List five major nursing diagnoses that are most appropriate for patients who will undergo cosmetic and reconstructive surgery.

Discuss the goals and nursing interventions for each diagnosis.

9 List five major nursing diagnoses that are most appropriate for patients in the immediate postoperative period of cosmetic and reconstructive surgery. Discuss the goals and nursing interventions for each diagnosis.

10 What are the expected changes in physical appearance that occur with the various types of cosmetic and reconstructive surgery?

11 List nursing interventions to detect and prevent common complications of cosmetic and reconstructive surgery.

12 Describe home care instructions for the various cosmetic and reconstructive surgical procedures.

BIBLIOGRAPHY

Current

1. Baptist G: Abdominoplasty: surgical technique and nursing care, *Plast Surg Nurs* 7:41, 1987.
2. Bergstrom N, Demuth P, Braden B: A clinical trial of the Braden scale for predicting pressure sore risk, *Nurs Clin North Am* 22:417, 1987.
3. Binger J: Liposuction/suction lipectomy, *Perioper Nurs Q* 2:82.
4. Black J: Planning reconstruction, *Plast Surg Nurs* 7:20, 1987.
5. Black J, Black S: Surgical management of pressure ulcers, *Nurs Clin North Am* 22:429, 1987.
6. Cohen L: Free-flap surgery: nurses make it work, *RN* 51:26, 1988.
7. Conflitti M: Bilateral breast reduction: from the nurse as a patient perspective, *Plast Surg Nurs* 7:18, 1987.
8. Fowler E: Equipment and products used in management and treatment of pressure ulcers, *Nurs Clin North Am* 22:449, 1987.
9. Georgiade N et al: *Essentials of plastic, maxillofacial and reconstructive surgery,* Baltimore, 1987, Williams & Wilkins.
10. Goodman, T, ed: *Core curriculum for plastic and reconstructive surgical nursing,* Pitman, NJ, 1989, Anthony J Jannetti.
11. Hutcheson H: Breast reconstruction using abdominal tissue: a nursing diagnoses approach, *Plast Surg Nurs* 7:11, 1987.
12. Lisman R, Hyde K, Smith B: Complications of blepharoplasty, *Clin Plast Surg* 15(2):309, 1988.
13. Maklebust J: Pressure ulcers: etiology and prevention, *Nurs Clin North Am* 22:359, 1987.
14. Salisbury C, Kaye B: Complications following rhytidectomy, *Plast Surg Nurs* 7:76, 1987.
15. Sohn S: *Fundamentals of aesthetic plastic surgery,* Baltimore, 1987, Williams & Wilkins.
16. Williams K: The expanding role of tissue expansion, *Plast Surg Nurs* 7:87, 1987.

Classic

17. Baj P: Collagen for implantation: patient selection and education, *AORN J* 41(2):362, 1985.
18. Barrett, B, ed: *Manual of patient care in plastic surgery,* Boston, 1982, Little, Brown & Co.

19. Bernstein N: *Emotional care of the facially burned and disfigured,* Boston, 1976, Little, Brown & Co.
20. Black J, Arnold P: Facial fractures, *AJN* 82:1086, 1982.
21. Coley ME: Collagen injection: technique and patient selection, *Plast Surg Nurs* 5:46, 1985.
22. Dinner M, Coleman C: Breast reconstruction: use of autogenous tissue, *AORN J* 42:490, 1985.
23. Georgiade G: Immediate reconstruction of the breast following modified radical mastectomy for carcinoma of the breast, *Clin Plast Surg* 11:383, 1984.
24. Goin J, Goin M: *Changing the body: psychological effects of plastic surgery,* Baltimore, 1981, Williams & Wilkins.
25. Grossman J: Abdominoplasty: indications and technique, *AORN J* 44:582, 1986.
26. Hutcheson H, Hartrampf C: Breast reconstruction using abdominal tissue, *Plast Surg Nurs* 6:97, 1986.
27. Knapp T, Vistnes L: The augmentation of soft tissue with injectable collagen, *Clin Plast Surg* 12:2, 1985.
28. Kole T, Mladick R: Intraoperative care of the lipoplasty patient, *Plast Surg Nurs* 6:105, 1986.
29. Lawson E: Success with lipoplasty as an outpatient procedure, *Plast Surg Nurs* 5:94, 1985.
30. Lawson E: Psychological aspects of the lipoplasty patient, *Plast Surg Nurs* 6:108, 1986.

31. Mangan M: Patient education with tissue expanders . . . to educate the professionals, *Plast Surg Nurs* 6:76, 1986.
32. Mathes S, Nahai F: *Clinical applications for muscle and musculocutaneous flaps,* St. Louis, 1982, Mosby–Year Book, Inc.
33. McCraw J, Arnold P: *McCraw and Arnold's atlas of muscle and musculocutaneous flaps,* Norfolk, Virginia, 1986, Hampton Press.
34. Navara T: Why turn our backs on plastic surgery patients? *RN* 49:67, 1986.
35. Neuberger G, Reckling J: A new look at wound care, *Nurs '85* 15:34, 1985.
36. Roy D: Caring for the self-esteem of the cosmetic patient, *Plast Surg Nurs* 6:138, 1986.
37. Salisbury C: Demonstration of a "capsule" and subsequent external decompression, *Plast Surg Nurs* 6:141, 1986.
38. Vinnik M: Self-imposed isolation as a factor in depression following cosmetic surgery, *Plast Surg Nurs* 6:144, 1986.
39. Watts V et al: When your patient has jaw surgery, *RN* 48(10):44, 1985.

Special Concerns of the Critically Ill Adult

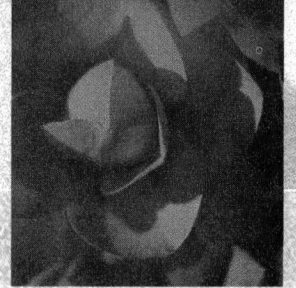

CHAPTER SEVENTY-SEVEN

The Critically Ill Adult with Multisystem Organ Failure

LEARNING OBJECTIVES

1 Identify psychologic and physiologic consequences of admission to a critical care unit.

2 Define multisystem organ failure (MSOF) and the clinical conditions (etiology) associated with its development.

3 Outline the pathophysiology of MSOF, including mediator release, maldistribution of circulating volume, imbalance of oxygen supply and demand, and alterations in metabolism.

4 Describe the role of translocation of bacteria in the development and progression of MSOF.

5 Explain the assessment findings of the hyperdynamic state.

6 State the goals of management for the MSOF patient based on the pathophysiologic changes.

7 Develop a nursing care plan for the MSOF patient, including nursing diagnoses, expected patient outcomes, and nursing interventions.

8 List potential discharge planning needs for the critically ill patient.

WITH THE AVERAGE age of patients increasing and the length of hospital stays decreasing, the number of patients with catastrophic illnesses and injuries requiring intensive care both in the intensive care unit (ICU) and on the general medical-surgical units is steadily increasing. The use of more sophisticated monitoring and therapy requires a thorough preparation by nurses in the areas of assessment, anatomy and physiology, pathophysiology, pharmacology, nutrition, and the use of advanced technologic equipment. Because of the highly technologic environment, it is easy for the patient to get lost in the "machines" and the nurse to focus on equipment and numbers. Therefore the nurse must make every effort to focus on the patient as a human being. Nurses must be supportive and caring as patients and families cope with catastrophic illness and the use of high technology.

CRITICAL CARE PRACTICE

The American Association of Critical Care Nurses (AACN) defines **critical care nursing** as "that specialty within nursing which deals specifically with human responses to life-threatening problems."[51] AACN's Conceptual Model for Critical Care Nursing contains five major components: (1) scope of practice, (2) principles of practice, (3) standards for nursing care of the critically ill, (4) the nursing process, and (5) the provision of quality care for the critically ill patient.[2]

According to AACN, the scope of critical care nursing encompasses the dynamic interaction of the critical care nurse, the critically ill patient, and the critical care environment. The American Association of Critical Care Nurses has developed standards of care specific to critical care nursing (see box below). The nursing process provides a systematic method of patient care, especially care of the critically ill.[1] Continual assessment and monitoring are major components of the ICU nurse's role. Early identification of complications or deterioration requires the knowledge of anatomy and physiology, current assessment techniques, and normal values for particular laboratory tests and hemodynamic variables. Assessment findings of the critically ill patient must not just be compared to a set of "normal" values but judged according to the patient's baseline. What is normal for a particular patient may not be normal for another patient, even though the medical diagnoses are the same. Emphasis is placed on repeated measures and changes rather than on absolute values.

Through collaboration with other members of the health care team, the nurse develops a plan of care based on significant assessment findings and the patient's response to therapy. Nursing diagnoses and collaborative problems are documented together with expected patient outcomes and appropriate interventions. Once again, outcomes should be specific and individualized for each patient based on his or her baseline status and response to therapy.

CRITICAL CARE ENVIRONMENT

The critically ill patient is characterized by "the presence of real or potential life-threatening health problems and by the requirement for continuous observation and intervention to prevent complications and restore health."[19] The critical care environment is any designated area equipped for the care of critically ill patients.

The critical care area is fast paced, highly specialized, and requires highly technical equipment. Electrocardiographic monitors are at each bedside. These display continuous electrocardiographic tracings that are also displayed on a central console at the nurses' station. Various pressure channels, such as pulmonary artery pressures, arterial blood pressure, and intracranial pressure, also may be displayed on the bedside monitor. Patients who need respiratory support have mechanical ventilators. Other specialized equipment may include the intraaortic balloon pump, hemodialysis or peritoneal dialysis equipment, and pulse oximeters. Necessary supplies, such as oxygen, suction apparatus, intravenous fluids and pumps, medications, and emergency equipment, must be easily accessible. Special carts for emergency equipment are present in the critical care area and contain defibrillators, emergency medications, intubation equipment, oxygen, and other necessary supplies. The nurse/patient ratio is often one-to-two or one-to-one, depending on the severity of the patient's condition.

The critical care nurse is an integral member of the critical care team and is involved in intense collaboration with other members of the team, including the physician, respiratory therapist, pharmacist, social worker, dietitian, and other health care professionals who provide care and support for the patient. Interdependent nursing interventions planned through multidisciplinary collaboration are imperative. The critical care nurse is the one constant in the critical care environment and thus serves as the coordinator of the critical care team, planning and individualizing care to best meet the needs of the patient and family.

Ethical Considerations

Although the ability to sustain life by artificial means has dramatically increased, mortality rates remain high for many critically ill patients with syndromes such as septic shock and multisystem organ failure.

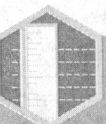

STANDARDS OF CRITICAL CARE NURSING

- Data shall be collected continuously on all patients.
- Identification of patient problems and needs and their priority shall be based on collected data.
- An appropriate plan of nursing care shall be formulated.
- The plan of nursing care shall be implemented according to the priority of identified problems and needs.
- The results of nursing care shall be continuously evaluated.

From the American Association of Critical Care Nursing (AACN).

RESEARCH BRIEF

Baggs JG et al: The association between interdisciplinary collaboration and patient outcomes in a medical intensive care unit, *Heart and Lung* 21:18, 1992.

A study examining interdisciplinary collaboration between ICU nurses and physicians found that nurses' reports of collaboration were significantly associated with positive patient outcome. The study examined decision-making concerning patient transfers from the ICU to a general medical-surgical unit. In situations where the nurse reported collaboration with resident staff, negative outcomes (readmission to the ICU or death on the medical-surgical unit) decreased from 16% to 5% (p<0.02 based on logistic multiple regression analysis). No significant relationship was found between residents' reports of collaboration and patient outcomes. Also, the amount of collaboration reported by residents was poorly correlated with the amount of collaboration reported by nurses about the same decisions.

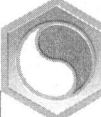

ETHICAL ISSUES

Should patients be considered incapable of competent decision-making during a period of physiologic crisis?

Should a patient who is lucid and rational and has suffered a trauma from which survival is unprecedented be allowed to refuse treatment? If the patient has suffered a trauma from which recovery is assured?

Patient and family wishes concerning "heroic" measures often present numerous ethical and legal dilemmas in the ICU. As controls over availability of resources tighten and critical care costs skyrocket, care decisions regarding limiting or withdrawing treatment are presently being made earlier in the patient's course than in the past. Costs approaching $200,000 have been quoted for a 21-day stay in the ICU. To address these problems, some institutions are developing specialty services designed to meet the needs of families and patients who are terminally ill. While in the past these services have focused on chronic illness, the preterminal state associated with acute critical illness such as multisystem organ failure is now also being addressed.[22] Patient and family preferences regarding heroic measures, physical comfort, psychosocial comfort, and family support are incorporated into decision-making. A major goal of the team is to transfer the patient from the ICU to the general medical-surgical unit. Moving patients out of the ICU increases patient/family interaction and enhances patient dignity and privacy.[31]

Psychosocial Effects

Admission to the critical care unit can be an extremely stressful event to both the patient and family. Preconceived ideas and past experiences with friends or family in an ICU may increase the pa-

tient's and family's anxiety beyond a functional level. The ICU environment along with the disease process itself affects many psychosocial elements. Environmental factors such as sensory overload, sensory deprivation, sleep deprivation, and stress may decrease the patient's ability to use his or her own functional coping mechanisms effectively.

Sources of sensory overload include excessive noise, glaring lights, numerous faces, invasive and painful procedures, and lack of routine schedule. Patients may exhibit anxiety, confusion, disorientation, hallucinations, or restlessness as evidence that they are sensory overloaded. Sensory overload is often compounded by sleep deprivation. Because of the intense and frequent monitoring done in many critical care units, patients rarely get long periods of rest, even through the night. It is not uncommon in many critical care units to do baths and daily weights on the night shift, further interrupting a patient's ability to get extended periods of sleep.

Sensory deprivation can actually be present, even if the patient is also suffering from sensory overload in other areas. Lack of familiar faces, immobility, and physical isolation all contribute to sensory deprivation. Conditions altering sensory input, such as spinal cord injuries or visual and hearing losses can compound the sensory deprivation. Initially, patients may not have their glasses, hearing aids, or false teeth with them that they normally wear at home, often making them unable to interact with those around them (both staff and family).

Along with physical environmental factors, emotional and behavioral changes related to illness and hospitalization are also common.[56] Because the visiting hours in many units are very limited, the patient's feelings of loneliness are magnified. Lack of familiar sights, sounds, and faces further increases loneliness and sensory deprivation. Because of the severity of the patient's condition and intensity of the ICU environment, feelings of helplessness and powerlessness are common. If the patient's prognosis is poor or involves loss of limb or other body alterations, feelings of anger, denial, and depression emerge. Changes in self-concept are common because of the lack of privacy, the numerous invasive devices, and any alterations caused by the disease process itself, such as severe edema or extensive scarring.

Strategies to decrease sensory overload include private, glassed-in rooms, reducing the volume on bedside alarms and other equipment in the unit such as phones and paging equipment, and planning the patient's schedule to allow longer periods of rest, especially at night. Along with decreasing sensory overload, efforts should also be made to decrease sensory deprivation. Increased visiting hours and ambulation or carriage outside the unit may alleviate some of the sensory deprivation. See Chapter 17 for further discussion on sensory overload, sensory deprivation, and sleep deprivation.

Teaching and provision of information help decrease the stressors faced by both the patient and family. Information concerning ICU admission and stay, such as rules of the unit (visiting hours, phone calls), explanation of equipment, and planned therapies has been shown to alleviate anxiety levels.[56] In areas of the country where multiple languages are commonly spoken, translators and printed information (if the patient can read) in the patient's native language are helpful.

Feelings of powerlessness and helplessness are common in any hospitalized patient, and the critical care environment may increase these feelings even more in the critically ill patient. The multitude of daily activities and interventions and the increased separation from family further exacerbate helplessness and anxiety. The critical care nurse must not only provide experienced technologic care, but must also demonstrate interpersonal caring as well. Developing a relationship with the patient and family based on mutual respect and trust fosters a more positive experience for both patient and family. Also, primary nursing and consistency in care givers also fosters trust and helps alleviate anxiety.

Lack of verbal communication is often a major obstacle to interacting with the patient in the ICU. Methods of nonverbal communication include frequent touching and remaining at the patient's bedside or in line of vision as much as possible. Picture board and hand signals can also be used to allow the intubated patient an avenue to express wants and needs. Chapter 18, Caring and the Emotional Response to Illness, provides further assessment and interventional strategies to minimize psychosocial stressors for the hospitalized patient. Above all, the nurse must constantly focus on the patient as an individual and not just an entity connected to numerous lines and monitoring devices.

The psychosocial impact of the unit on the patient and family should not be underestimated. A patient who is restless, anxious, or in pain requires more oxygen delivery. The critically ill patient may be unable to meet this increased demand; therefore physiologic progress may be slowed or halted. Every effort should be made to minimize psychosocial stressors both for patient and family comfort, as well as improvement of the patient's condition.

Physiologic Effects

The critically ill or injured patient has suffered a major physiologic insult. Whether that insult be traumatic, ischemic, or infectious, significant changes occur in the body as it tries to protect and heal itself and maintain its normal function. Not only do the insult and the patient's previous state of health determine the extent of damage and prognosis, but the critical care unit itself places the patient at added risk for serious complications.[32] Both the physical

---

ENVIRONMENTAL FACTORS AFFECTING PHYSIOLOGIC RESPONSES

Physical environment

Stressors
  Noise level
  Painful procedures
  Lack of family contact
  Severity of disease process
Increased exposure to pathogens
Immobility

Immunosuppressant factors

Stress
Pain
Trauma
General anesthesia
Pharmacologic agents
  Immunosuppressive drugs
  Sedation
  Sensorium-altering medications
Hemorrhage
Blood transfusions

Therapeutic interventions

Invasive lines, catheters, and devices
Invasive diagnostic procedures
Inadequate nutritional support
Antibiotic therapy
Pharmacologic agents

environment (such as the noise level and glaring lights) and therapeutic interventions (such as multiple invasive lines and nephrotoxic antibiotics) contribute to the development of secondary complications (see the box on p. 2180).

Because infectious and inflammatory complications are some of the most common and most deadly complications in the unit, risk factors must be identified that predispose a patient to infectious complications or overwhelming inflammation. Risk factors for infection include both immunosuppression as well as increased exposure to microorganisms and their products, such as endotoxin from gram-negative bacteria. Other complications that trigger an inflammatory response are noted in the box below.

Host-related factors including age (over 65 years), chronic disease states, and immunosuppression may increase the risk of infection. Iatrogenic factors such as invasive lines and catheters, immunosuppressant therapy, surgical procedures, and antibiotic therapy may predispose the patient to the development of sepsis and thus MSOF.[10] The skin and mucosal surfaces provide the first line of defense against microbial invasion. If they are breached by invasive devices and procedures or decubiti, bacterial colonization can occur. Invasive devices such as intravenous lines, endotracheal tubes, and urinary catheters may serve as reservoirs for the colonization and spread of organisms. Assessment and prevention focus on the environment, the natural host defenses, laboratory values, and the therapeutic regimen.[27] Therapeutic benefits must be weighed against any increased risk to the patient, such as infection. For example, antibiotic therapy not only kills pathogenic organisms but the normal flora of the body as well. When the balance of the normal flora is altered, more pathogenic organisms can multiply unchecked. Vaginal yeast infections and oral candidiasis are examples. Antibiotics and other pharmacologic agents can be toxic to the inner ear, the kidney, and the bone marrow. Coagulopathies and changes in mental status may be related to certain drug regimens rather than the disease process itself.

Another iatrogenic complication involves lack of enteral feeding (either oral or via feeding tubes). When a patient is not fed enterally, the gut mucosal lining atrophies. When this occurs, the gut is thought to lose its ability to prevent bacterial migration from the gut and into the blood. Normally, the normal flora of the bowel is contained by numerous gut defense mechanisms, but lack of feeding harms the integrity of the mucosal barrier. Contamination of the lungs and blood can then result.

Obviously, the more severe the insult, the more likely the patient will develop complications. Also, in patients with altered defense mechanisms or increased severity of insult, normal regulatory and clearance mechanisms are more likely to be overwhelmed. One of the most deadly complications associated with critical illness is the development of multisystem organ failure. It is becoming increasingly more frequent in the ICU due to increased survival rates following initial insults, frequent antibiotic use, and the increased use of invasive devices and procedures.

COMPLICATIONS OF CRITICAL ILLNESS THAT TRIGGER INFLAMMATION

Mechanical tissue damage
  Burns
  Crush injuries
  Surgical procedures
Abscesses
  Intraabdominal
  Intracranial
  Other
Ischemic/necrotic tissue
  Myocardial infarction
  Pancreatitis
  DIC
Microbial invasion
  Immunosuppressed states

Surgery/trauma
Community exposure
Nosocomial exposure
Endotoxin release
  Gram-negative sepsis
  Translocation of bacteria from gut
Global perfusion deficits
  Shock states
  Cardiopulmonary arrest
Regional perfusion deficits
  Vascular injury
  Vascular repair procedures
  Thromboembolic events

MULTISYSTEM ORGAN FAILURE
Definition

Multisystem organ failure (MSOF) is a nonspecific expression of critical illness involving progressive, sequential dysfunction (and/or failure) of two or more organ systems. MSOF is not a series of isolated failures but a systemic process that has the potential to damage every organ. It is not individual problems in individual organs, but a total body problem in which each of the organs becomes a victim. The sequential organ failure of MSOF is not only related to the insult itself but also to associated therapeutic interventions and secondary complications.* Multisystem organ failure (MSOF) is also called multiple organ failure, sequential organ failure, and, more recently, multiple organ dysfunction syndrome. MSOF often follows successful resuscitation of patients with severe trauma, major surgery, intraabdominal sepsis, and other forms of critical illness.[33,55] Overall mortality rates of 60% to 90% have been reported, and MSOF is the major cause of death following septic, burn, and traumatic insults. Research reports a high correlation between the number of organs involved and percent mortality. Mortality approaches 100% when three or more organs have failed.[23,37]

Two major categories of MSOF have been described (Figure 77-1).[34,38] In Type I, the insult itself, along with resuscitative measures, contributes directly to the development of rapid respira-

*References 15, 24, 26, 30, 53.

tory failure, followed by renal and cardiovascular failure. Infection may or may not be present, and death ensues within 2 to 4 days of admission. Direct pulmonary trauma (hemothorax/pneumothorax, pulmonary contusion, or aspiration), severe head injury, and delayed or inadequate resuscitative measures greatly contribute to the early, rapid MSOF picture.[34,38]

In Type II, secondary complications, such as persistent inflammation and ischemia, contribute to loss of gut barrier function,[17] hypermetabolism,[34] and overwhelming inflammation.[25] Pulmonary failure usually occurs first, followed by liver/GI dysfunction, renal failure, and cardiovascular instability. The central nervous system and hematologic system may also be involved. MSOF is the final outcome, often accompanied by late mortality (defined as 14 to 21 days after insult). DeCamp and Demling[15] have staged the MSOF continuum (Table 77-1).

Etiology

The three major causes of MSOF are infection, poor perfusion (ischemia), and persistent inflammation (see the box below). Septic shock remains the most common single etiologic factor causing MSOF, although, positive blood cultures and clinical infection are not required to initiate the MSOF process. Forty percent to fifty percent of MSOF patients do not

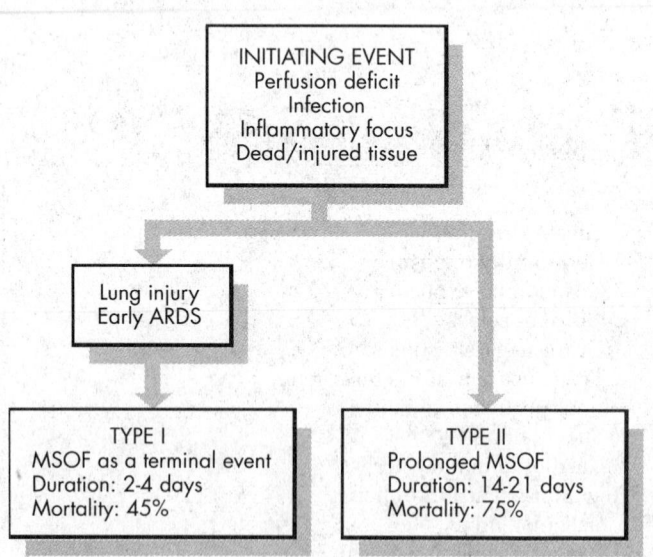

FIGURE 77-1 Classification of multisystem organ failure. (From Lekander BJ, Cerra FB: The syndrome of multiple organ failure, *Crit Care Nurs Clin North Am* 2:332, 1990.)

ETIOLOGY OF MSOF

Ischemia
Cardiac arrest
Disseminated intravascular coagulation
Shock
Thromboembolic events
Vascular injury

Inflammation
Abscesses
Ischemia
Pancreatitis
Surgical procedures
Thermal injury
Tissue trauma

Infection
Gram-negative
Gram-positive
Viral
Fungal
Rickettsial

TABLE 77-1   Multisystem Organ Failure Progression

Stage	Onset after injury	Clinical observations
Sepsis	2-7 days	Fever and leukocytosis
		Decreased systemic vascular resistance
		Increased cardiac output and oxygen consumption
Early MSOF	7-14 days	Acute respiratory failure
		Impaired oxygen extraction
		Hypermetabolism with or without jaundice
		Ileus and thrombocytopenia
		Leukocytosis or leukopenia
		Possible mental status changes
Established MSOF	2 weeks to months	Progressive adult respiratory distress syndrome
		Hemodynamic instability
		Hypermetabolism and lactic acidosis
		Jaundice and azotemia with or without oliguria
		Possible stress gastrointestinal tract bleeding
		Disseminated intravascular coagulation
Preterminal MSOF	Weeks to months	Hypodynamic cardiovascular state refractory to inotropic or alpha adrenergic support
		Minimal oxygen extraction
		Worsening lactic acidosis

Reprinted with permission from DeCamp MM, Demling RH: Posttraumatic multisystem organ failure. *JAMA* 260:532, 1988. Copyright 1988, American Medical Association.

have positive blood cultures or a documented source of infection.[15,17] Even classically "noninfectious" states such as hypovolemic shock or cardiac arrest trigger the inflammatory response because inflammation is the body's initial response to insult. Aseptic abscesses, ischemic tissue, and necrotic tissue continually trigger the inflammatory response.

Although designed to be a protective response, the inflammatory response has the potential to cause tissue destruction. Just as coagulation is a physiologic response when it occurs at the site of injury, inflammation protects the body as long as the inflammatory response is controlled and localized. If clotting is uncontrolled, damage occurs in the body. Likewise, if inflammation is uncontrolled, tissue and organ damage occur.

Because the involved organs in the patient with MSOF display similar patterns of tissue damage and are often remote from the initial injury site or septic source,[40] theories concerning the pathophysiologic mechanism involved in MSOF focus on common pathways and interactions between the organ systems, rather than on isolated processes.[4,20,42] Inflammation and inflammatory mediators are a focal point of clinical research and therapy.

A **mediator** is any substance in the circulation or tissue that causes biologic activity, i.e., carries out the functions of a response. Inflammatory mediators cause the inflammatory response to occur. Sympathetic mediators, including epinephrine and norepinephrine, carry out the actions of the sympathetic response. Examples of inflammatory mediators include complement, bradykinin, and tumor necrosis factor. MSOF is now recognized as a systemic syndrome mediated by numerous plasma enzyme cascades, cellular elements, and other mediators commonly released and activated in inflammation and/or infection.[4,20,25]

Pathophysiology

Following bodily insult, specific early events occur that trigger the release of mediators into the circulation from various sources as the body suffers insult, seeks to protect itself, and recovers from the insult. If the body loses control of these systems and mediators, which are designed to protect and defend the patient, organ damage can occur. The major danger of the MSOF syndrome appears to be its ability to keep itself going. Once the inflammatory response becomes overly activated, it may keep itself "turned on" despite the removal of initial stimuli such as abscesses, microbes, or necrotic tissue[15,42]; therefore prevention of and early identification of complications or patient deterioration are crucial in this patient population. Special attention must be given to recognition of early markers of infection, inflammation, and ischemia. Exaggerated and overwhelming

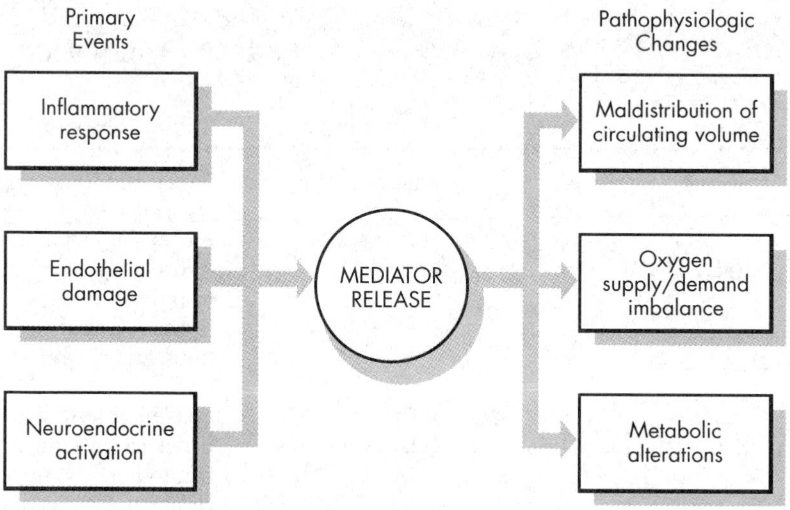

Primary
Events

Inflammatory
response

Endothelial
damage

Neuroendocrine
activation

MEDIATOR
RELEASE

Pathophysiologic
Changes

Maldistribution of
circulating volume

Oxygen
supply/demand
imbalance

Metabolic
alterations

FIGURE 77-2 Interaction of primary events, mediator release, and pathophysiologic changes. (From Secor VH: Mediators of coagulation and inflammation: Relationship and clinical significance, *Crit Care Nurs Clin North Am* 5:422, 1993.)

inflammation leads to maldistribution of circulating volume, imbalance of oxygen supply and demand, and alterations in metabolism (Figure 77-2).

Neuroendocrine activation

One of the earliest responses to injury is the triggering of the stress response (see Chapter 3). This response involves the nervous system and endocrine system and is referred to as neuroendocrine activation. Following an insult, activation of the neuroendocrine system stimulates the release of numerous substances into the circulation, including ACTH from the anterior pituitary, glucocorticoids from the adrenal cortex, epinephrine from the adrenal medulla, and norepinephrine from sympathetic nerves.[52] Pituitary and CNS endorphin, growth hormone, and prolactin levels are also increased following exposure to stressful stimuli. The secretion of "stress hormones" prepares the body for fight or flight from the insult. The hormones also allow the body to compensate for complications occurring secondary to the insult, such as fluid losses, hypotension, and microbial invasion. Other changes, including increased blood flow, increased capillary permeability, and increased blood glucose, provide an environment necessary for adequate tissue repair and healing. If hemorrhage or massive leakage of fluid to the tissues occurs, other mediators responsible for maintaining circulating volume and perfusion pressures will also be released, such as aldosterone and renin.

Inflammatory response

Activation of the inflammatory response represents a major physiologic event in the body. Following an insult, multiple inflammatory mechanisms are activated to protect the patient from invading microor-

ganisms, limit the extent of injury, and promote rapid healing of involved tissues. Microorganisms do not have to be present to stimulate an inflammatory response. Tissue damage, alone, triggers the inflammatory cascade. A series of complex interactions occur through plasma cascades, cells, and various mediators (Table 77-2).[46,47] While the process is initiated to protect the patient, lack of appropriate regulation can lead to uncontrolled inflammation that ultimately harms the patient.[4,42] This overwhelming activation of inflammation at the systemic level has been recently entitled the **systemic inflammatory response syndrome (SIRS).**[3]

Many inflammatory mediators, normally produced by activated white blood cells and endothelial cells, carry out the protective functions of the inflammatory and immune responses, but these same mediators can damage tissues and vessels and are associated with many signs and symptoms seen in MSOF.[8,18,57] Tumor necrosis factor (TNF), interleukin-1 (IL-1), oxygen-derived free radicals (ODFR), arachidonic acid metabolites (AA), and proteases are examples of mediators produced by active white blood cells.

Because inflammation or severe infection often leads to activation of coagulation or alterations in hemostasis, DIC and other coagulopathies are common in the septic patient or the patient experiencing a major inflammatory insult, such as soft tissue damage, burn injury, or pancreatitis.[6] The microvascular thrombi of DIC further obstruct blood flow to the organ beds and thus contribute to ischemic organ damage and MSOF.[39]

Loss of endothelial integrity

The endothelium is a single layer of specialized cells that lines the entire vascular system from the aorta, arteries, and capillary beds, through the venules and

TABLE 77-2 Inflammatory Mediators and Activities

Mediator	Activity
Complement	Induction of inflammation
	Vasodilation
	Increased capillary permeability
	Enhanced neutrophil aggregation at injury site
	Opsonization (coating of bacteria)
Kinin	Vasodilation
	Increased capillary permeability
	Enhanced neutrophil aggregation
	Smooth muscle contraction
Tumor necrosis factor (TNF) and Interleukin-1 (IL-1)	Produced primarily by activated macrophages
	Enhanced immune cellular function
	Fever
	Endothelial damage
	Increased capillary permeability
	Decreases body's response to catecholamines
Arachidonic acid metabolites (prostaglandins, thromboxanes, leukotrienes)	Produced primarily by WBCs and endothelial cells
	Variable activity (dependent on specific prostaglandin acting)
	Vasoconstriction or vasodilation
	Increased or decreased platelet aggregation
	Increased capillary permeability
Oxygen-derived free radicals (ODFR)	Endothelial damage
	Denaturation of proteins
	Cell membrane damage
	Tissue damage
	Increased capillary permeability
Other mediators	Clotting factors, colony stimulating factors, Hageman factor, heparin, histamine, interferon, plasminogen, plasminogen activators, platelet activating factor, proteases, and tissue factor

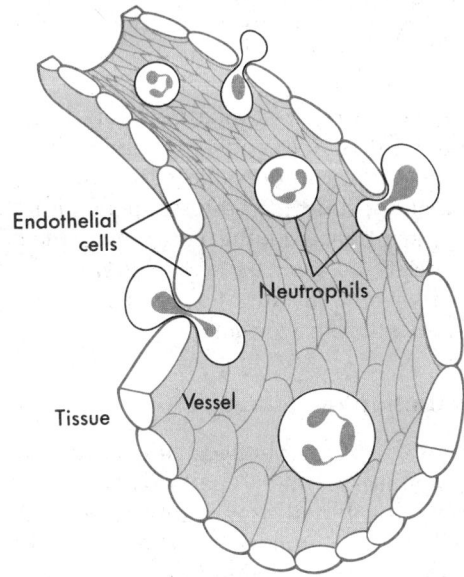

FIGURE 77-3 Migration of WBCs (neutrophils) from the circulation to the tissue.

veins, and back through the vena cava to the heart. The endothelium is not just an inert barrier between the blood and the tissue; it is actually the synthesis site for numerous mediators related to hemostasis and other metabolic functions of the body.

If the endothelium suffers damage or has an increase in permeability, changes occur in coagulation and blood flow. In response to mediators such as complement, histamine, and kinin, endothelial cells retract and their junctions widen, leading to the increased capillary permeability (capillary leak) and edema commonly seen in inflammation. These widened junctions or gaps also allow for the movement of plasma proteins and white blood cells from the blood to the tissue site of injury (Figure 77-3). Once again, the initial response is protective; it allows necessary substances to move to the injured area. But if the body loses control of the response, the changes occur not only locally but systemically as well. Therefore instead of having local edema and clotting, the patient experiences disseminated clotting (and possibly DIC) and widespread edema, both in the periphery and in the major organ beds.

The endothelium is very susceptible to damage by a variety of factors, especially white blood cells and their mediators. The white blood cells make toxic mediators (such as proteases and other enzymes) to kill bacteria, but these same mediators can also damage the patient's own living tissue as well.[54] Although the endothelium has the potential to repair itself and maintain normal function, extensive damage or mediator activity overwhelms the endothelium's repair mechanisms, resulting in widespread permeability and coagulation abnormalities.[39] The increased capillary permeability, necessary in the initial stages of localized inflammation, begins to occur throughout many capillary beds in the systemic circulation and promotes fluid loss to the tissues. This leakage of fluid into the tissues yields the generalized peripheral edema commonly observed in these patients as well as organ edema. As tissues continue to swell, vascular flow is further obstructed and tissue ischemia worsens.

Maldistribution of volume

Because of the many changes caused by the numerous inflammatory and sympathetic mediators in the circulation, the blood flow is often redistributed or maldistributed. Changes in the circulation that maldistribute the circulating volume include increased capillary permeability, vasodilation, selective vasoconstriction, and vascular obstruction.

Maldistribution of volume occurs at the systemic, organ, and local level. Even though the cardiac output is often increased in severe inflammation or infection, perfusion may be inadequate in some tissue beds. Patchy areas of low blood flow may exist in an organ (due to localized vasoconstriction or thrombi in various areas of the organ itself) even when the organ's overall flow is normal or increased.[41,42] The vascular changes and thrombi are related to the activity and damage caused by many of the circulating inflammatory mediators.

Without adequate blood flow, oxygen delivery is inadequate to meet the tissue oxygen demands; therefore the balance of oxygen supply and demand is disrupted. The tissues become hypoxic and organ dysfunction and damage occur. This is not just a low blood pressure problem. The sustained inflammatory response actually affects blood flow and vascular patency in the organ beds.

Imbalance of oxygen supply/demand

The imbalance in oxygen supply and demand occurs because of a decreased oxygen supply and an increased demand for oxygen by the body. A decreased use of oxygen by the cells and failure of the compensatory mechanisms designed to protect the body also contribute to the imbalance between oxygen supply and demand. Oxygen delivery is determined primarily by arterial oxygen saturation (Sao_2), cardiac output, and hemoglobin level. Because of problems with ventilation and/or perfusion in the lungs secondary to ARDS, Sao_2 is usually low (<90%). Myocardial dysfunction and poor volume resuscitation may contribute to an inadequate cardiac output. Hemorrhage or laboratory phlebotomy may lead to the development of a low hematocrit.

Drawing a large number of blood samples is often an unaccounted source of blood loss.

Sources of increased oxygen demand include increased work of breathing, fever, shivering, pain, anxiety, hypermetabolism, and tachycardia. If oxygen demand is high and supply is low, an imbalance occurs, particularly if the compensatory mechanisms of increasing flow and extraction are not working adequately. Tissue oxygen demands are not met, anaerobic metabolism occurs, tissue ischemia develops, and lactic acidosis often ensues. Changes in the distribution of blood flow and obstruction of flow by vasoconstriction and thrombi at the microcirculatory level compound the supply and demand imbalance (Figure 77-4).

Alterations in metabolism

Another factor in both the pathophysiology and survival rates of MSOF is the nutritional status of the patient, both before and after admission to the hospital. The hypermetabolic state that often occurs in

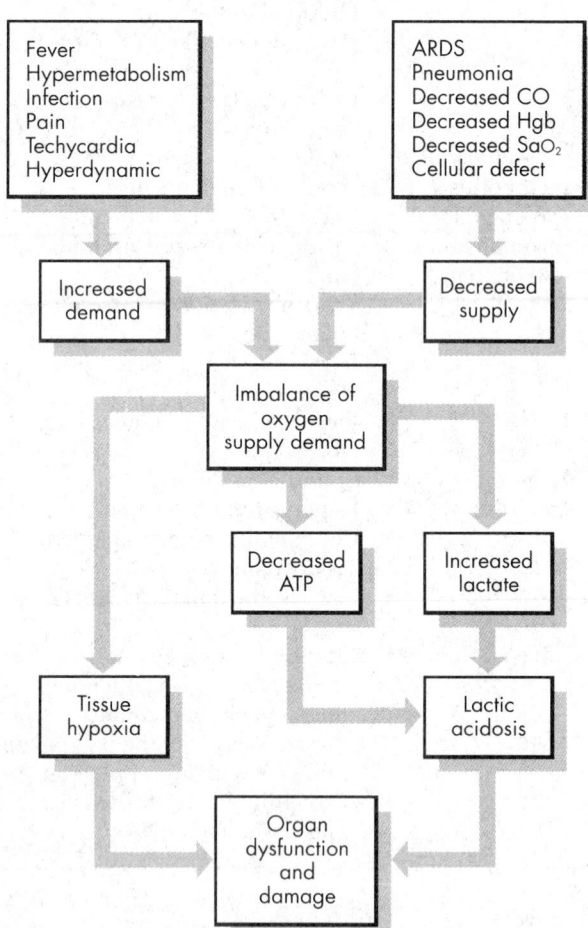

FIGURE 77-4   Causes and effects of the imbalance between oxygen supply and demand.

critically ill patients is a primary pathophysiologic mechanism in MSOF.[13] In hypermetabolism, the body does not metabolize carbohydrates, proteins, and lipids in the normal manner. Gluconeogenesis (formation of glucose from noncarbohydrate sources, such as lipids or proteins) increases. The muscle mass and visceral protein stores are severely depleted as the body uses the protein and amino acids from these stores to feed the gluconeogenesis pathway in the liver. Massive protein catabolism (breakdown) affects immunologic function, diaphragmatic muscle strength, mobility, and organ system integrity. Because the liver is involved in metabolic and immunologic function, liver dysfunction compounds the immune dysfunction and metabolic abnormalities.

Clinical Manifestations

The MSOF syndrome is complex and involves all systemic processes and major body systems. The MSOF patient progresses through various stages of clinical presentation during the development and progression of the syndrome. Although actual failure of the individual organ systems often represents the preterminal phase of this syndrome, the initial presentation and early findings are quite different from the final, preterminal state. The patient initially presents and progresses in the **hyperdynamic state.**

The patient may remain in the hyperdynamic phase for days to weeks, depending on the magnitude (severity) of the septic challenge, the patient's physiologic reserve, resuscitative measures (particularly fluid resuscitation), and the ability to eradicate the initiating source. Table 77-3 summarizes the assessment findings in the patient in the hyperdynamic state of MSOF.

Cardiovascular system

The earliest definitive signs of the hyperdynamic state are elevated cardiac output (CO) and decreased systemic vascular resistance (SVR). With sympathetic stimulation, venous return and preload increase. Along with tachycardia, the increased preload increases CO. Due to the expanded capacity of the vascular system secondary to the vasodilation accompanied by a fluid resuscitation, the CO rises secondary to the larger circulating volume now present. The SVR is decreased secondary to the vasodilatory action of many of the mediators, such as complement and bradykinin. The low SVR and relative volume deficit contribute to the hypotension. Decreased central pressures such as pulmonary artery pressures, pulmonary capillary wedge pressure (PCWP), and central venous pressure (CVP) reflect the volume deficit. Skin is often flushed and warm in the hyperdynamic state and thus may provide a false sense of security that tissue perfusion is adequate. Although vasodilation is occurring in the periphery, there are actually areas of vasoconstriction and low blood flow in some of the organ vascular beds. To compensate for the hypotension, heart rate increases. Sympathetic stimulation, fever, and pain also contribute to the tachycardia. In the latter stages of MSOF, increased ectopy accompanies the tachycardia, and the patient is likely to decompensate and become bradycardic during endotracheal suctioning or disconnection from the ventilator.

Pulmonary system

Because of the presence of ARDS and pneumonia, ventilation and perfusion are not adequately matched, and poor arterial oxygen saturation occurs. Crackles and wheezes are common especially in the presence of increased secretions, such as pneumonia or cardiogenic pulmonary edema. Sputum is often malodorous, tenacious, and creamy yellow or green if infection is present. With inadequate oxygen delivery, anaerobic metabolism occurs, and pH drops. In the early stages of MSOF, the patient will attempt to compensate by increasing respiratory rate; therefore too much CO_2 may be blown off, and respiratory alkalosis occurs. As the lungs become more stiff (decreased ability to distend), compliance decreases and peak inspiratory pressure increases. Gas exchange worsens and blood gas values continue to deteriorate. Respiratory acidosis then develops as the lungs cannot adequately remove the circulating CO_2.

The mixed venous oxygen saturation (Svo_2) may actually be elevated in septic shock and severe inflammation. Due to changes in the microcirculation and tissue oxygen extraction, the tissues may not be able to extract the oxygen they need and the blood returns to the right side of the heart still carrying most of its oxygen and thus displaying a high Svo_2. The Svo_2 becomes difficult to interpret in this situation, because the elevated value may actually reflect poor tissue oxygenation rather than the adequate oxygenation a high value usually reflects. In other words, high concentrations of oxygen are being returned to the right heart because the tissues cannot "get it out." They need it. Their oxygenation is not adequate, but they are unable to get the oxygen they need. The Svo_2 must be interpreted in light of other variables of tissue oxygenation such as oxygen delivery and oxygen consumption. At the terminal stage, Svo_2 is usually low, as CO, Sao_2, and Hgb decrease.

Gastrointestinal system

The GI tract and liver suffer many significant changes along with the other organs. Hepatic dys-

TABLE 77-3 Clinical Assessment of the Hyperdynamic State

System	Assessment findings	
Cardiovascular	Increased cardiac output*	Warm, flushed skin*
	Decreased SVR	Peripheral edema
	Tachycardia	Petechiae
	Hypotension	Increased Svo_2
	Decreased PCWP, CVP	Fever*
Respiratory	Tachypnea/bradypnea	Respiratory alkalosis (early) changing to respiratory acidosis if ARDS severe
	Dyspnea, diaphoresis	
	Use of accessory muscles	Decreased Pao_2 and Sao_2
	Wheezes, crackles	
	Infiltrates on CXR	
	Ventilatory dependence	
	V/Q mismatch or true shunt	
Central nervous system	Decreased level of consciousness	Irregularities in temperature, cardiovascular and respiratory responses
	Decreased Glasgow coma score	
	Irritability, confusion, restlessness, agitation	
Renal	Adequate to decreased urine output	Fluid overload state as renal failure worsens
	Metabolic acidosis	Increased BUN and Cr
	Decreased bicarbonate	Increased potassium
Gastrointestinal	Decreased bowel sounds	Abdominal distention
	Diarrhea	Stress ulceration
	Upper and lower GI bleeding	Mucosal atrophy
		Stools positive for blood
Hepatic	Increased liver function tests	Decreased drug clearance leading to toxicity
	Increased total bilirubin	Increased PT/PTT
	Decreased plasma proteins, such as albumin	Coagulopathies
Laboratory findings	Leukocytosis*	Decreased fibrinogen
	Hyperglycemia	Increased FDPs
	Increased lactate	Decreased platelets
	Metabolic acidosis	

*Many patients who succumb to the disease either die in the hyperdynamic state or remain in the hyperdynamic state until the very preterminal state, when cardiac output, temperature, and white blood count fall and the other signs and symptoms listed above become even more severe. The hyperdynamic state, however, is the focal clinical presentation of MSOF.

function can lead to coagulopathies, hepatic encephalopathy, decreased synthesis of vital proteins, such as albumin, and poor drug clearance. Findings include increased PT/PTT, disorientation, decreased albumin levels, and increased toxic levels of drugs normally metabolized by the liver. Because the liver is responsible for filtering the blood draining from the GI circulation, liver dysfunction can increase the incidence of septicemia, because the liver cannot clear bacteria and their toxins that may be leaking from the injured gut.

In the critically ill patient, the gut has a tendency to atrophy, especially if the patient is not being fed enterally. When this occurs, the bacteria that normally reside in the gut may move across the gut wall and gain access to the systemic circulation either directly or indirectly through the lymphatics. Gut ischemia and necrosis can initiate GI bleeding or actual perforation. Clinical findings include diarrhea, gross or occult blood in the stool, abdominal pain, and distention. Gross or occult blood may also be found in the NG aspirate as well. In critically ill patients, upper GI bleeding is commonly related to stress ulceration of the gastric mucosa. An ileus is very common in the critically ill patient, and is accompanied by decreased to absent bowel sounds and increased NG drainage.

Central nervous system

The patient in shock and MSOF demonstrates restlessness, agitation, and decreases in level of consciousness. Decreased oxygen delivery, damage by mediators, and alterations in fluid and electrolytes have all been implicated in CNS damage. Fever occurs in response to changes in the hypothalamus induced by the inflammatory mediators. An increase in temperature may also be related to the increased metabolic rate and excess heat production. At the terminal stage, temperature may actually be below normal secondary to hypothalamic damage and metabolic failure.

Renal system

Acute tubular necrosis is common in the patient with MSOF. Clinically, a decrease in urine output accompanied by increases in BUN and creatinine are the classic signs of renal failure, although urine output may remain adequate or elevated in the early stages. Renal failure also contributes to the metabolic acidosis and electrolyte abnormalities common in these patients. Excessive tissue damage, rhabdomyolysis, and cell death damage the renal tubules and predispose the patient to renal failure. A falling urine output is also indicative of a volume deficit, especially if BUN and creatinine are not elevated above the patient's baseline. Because of the systemic vasodilatation, more volume is actually needed to maintain adequate circulation and organ perfusion.

Hematologic system

White blood counts are initially elevated secondary to normal stress responses and immune mechanisms. In the terminal stages, the counts may decrease, even in the presence of gross infection, due to mass consumption and bone marrow exhaustion. WBCs that are circulating are often immature (shift to the left) as the bone marrow attempts to supply the body's demands. Platelet counts may also be decreased secondary to accelerated coagulation and consumption.

Laboratory values

Hyperglycemia that is often resistant to insulin therapy often heralds the onset of infection and inflammation. Glucose levels increase in response to sympathetic nervous system activation and increased gluconeogenesis. During infection and inflammation, an insulin resistance is thought to occur that also contributes to elevated glucose levels. Hypoglycemia may be seen in the terminal stages secondary to liver dysfunction and metabolic failure. Following accelerated coagulation, excessive fibrinolysis is initiated. Increased fibrin degradation products (FDPs) are seen, usually accompanied by an elevated PT/PTT.

Therapeutic Management

The management of the patient with MSOF remains difficult and controversial. It requires a multidisciplinary approach including nursing, medicine, respi-

ratory therapy, nutritional support, physical therapy, occupational therapy, social services, pastoral care, and rehabilitation. Collaborative management concentrates on five major goals:[5,16]

1. Prevention and early identification of infectious/inflammatory stimuli
2. Restoration of oxygen supply/demand balance
3. Provision of nutritional support and metabolic requirements
4. Individual organ support
5. Psychologic support of the patient and family

Once triggered, the inflammatory response can continue uncontrolled, if regulation is lost. Even aggressive treatment of the initial insult may not halt the vicious cycle of inflammation and mediator release once the system becomes overwhelmed. Therefore, the ultimate and most effective weapon against MSOF is prevention. Early interventions must focus on infection control, prevention and early identification of complications, and prompt, aggressive resuscitation and ongoing therapy.[27,28] Upon the patient's admission, all treatable injuries are managed. For example, removal of all necrotic tissue, early debridement of burn eschar, and prompt stabilization of fractures minimize further soft tissue damage, inflammation, and infection.[5,16] Antibiotic therapy is based on initial Gram stain results and the patient's clinical status and changed according to patient response and culture reports. Global interventions to prevent infection or stimulation of inflammation such as handwashing, aseptic technique, and nutrition are certainly helpful. However, they may not be enough to protect the critically ill patient exposed to resistant environmental pathogens, breakdown of natural defense barriers, or overwhelming inflammation. More aggressive support of tissue oxygenation and nutrition may have to be instituted.

Oxygen supply/demand balance

Increasing oxygen supply and decreasing oxygen demand aid in restoring the balance between oxygen supply and demand. Although arterial blood gases (ABGs) provide crucial patient information, they assess only the amount of oxygen brought into the body, not that actually delivered to the tissues. Oxygen transport formulas, such as oxygen delivery (DO_2) and oxygen consumption (VO_2), provide the clinician with much more valid information concerning oxygen delivery and tissue oxygenation because they include not only the oxygen content of the blood but also cardiac output. A high arterial saturation (Sao_2) does not benefit the patient if cardiac output is so low that oxygen cannot be delivered to the tissues. Likewise, assessing oxygen delivery without considering the amount of oxygen that tissues actually consume (VO_2) leads to misinterpretation of assessment findings and clinical condition. Cardiac output, hemoglobin, and arterial saturation are principal variables in both DO_2 and VO_2 formulas; therefore, aggressive efforts are aimed at optimizing cardiac output, hemoglobin, and arterial saturation in MSOF, and often increasing them to supranormal (above normal) values to maximize oxygen delivery and consumption.[44]

Cardiac output

Pulmonary artery catheterization is often necessary to accurately monitor fluid status and cardiac function. Due to the low SVR, large volumes of fluid are usually necessary to maintain adequate preload. Adequate preload also increases the accuracy of pulmonary artery measurements taken during mechanical ventilation.[35] The optimal type of fluid for volume resuscitation remains controversial. Crystalloids tend to cause fewer complications, but they do third-space more easily than the colloids. A larger volume of crystalloids is usually required for adequate resuscitation, and edema formation is often significant. The colloids have also been implicated in complications such as renal failure, hypotension, coagulopathies, and glucose abnormalities. Because each patient has different underlying pathologies and complications, choice of fluid is guided by individual patient response to fluid challenge. Along with volume infusion, inotropic agents are used to counteract myocardial depression and increase cardiac output. Dobutamine is often used to increase cardiac output and thus increase DO_2.

If fluid and inotropic therapy do not maintain adequate cardiac output and perfusion pressures, vasopressor therapy is begun. Vasopressors must be judiciously titrated to avoid excessive vasoconstriction. Extreme vasoconstriction hinders flow to select organs, especially in the splanchnic and renal circulation. Increasing the afterload also increases myocardial oxygen demands and contributes to myocardial fatigue and ischemia. Dopamine is often used as a vasopressor agent, but other vasopressor agents such as Neo-Synephrine and Levophed are now being used to induce vasoconstriction and increase SVR, so the dopamine can be infused at lower doses to enhance renal, gut, and inotropic support. For the patient who does develop an elevated SVR, nitroprusside may be used to reduce afterload and myocardial oxygen demands.[11]

Hemoglobin

Since oxygen is bound to Hgb, adequate levels of Hgb are necessary for sufficient oxygen delivery to the tissues. Conversely, if Hgb levels are too high, increased transit time and sludging (which promotes the development of microthrombi) could occur in the microcirculation. A hemoglobin of 10 to 12 g/dL is frequently recommended.

Arterial saturation

Along with cardiac output and hemoglobin, the third major variable in the oxygen transport formulas is SaO_2. Along with pulmonary damage and poor gas exchange, the critically ill patient often exhibits respiratory depression and a decrease in level of consciousness. Measures to improve oxygen saturation include ventilatory support, prevention of nosocomial pneumonia, and frequent position changes. Intubation and mechanical ventilation are often necessary to maintain a patent airway, achieve adequate minute ventilation, and maintain $SaO_2 > 90\%$. Positive end-expiratory pressure (PEEP) may be added to improve gas exchange, particularly if an intrapulmonary shunt is present. Although mechanical ventilation may be a requirement for adequate oxygen delivery, intubation does represent another insult to the patient as it bypasses upper respiratory tract defense mechanisms and increases the patient's levels of stress and anxiety. High levels of FIO_2 can lead to oxygen toxicity and the production of substances that can cause further lung damage.

Decrease oxygen demand

Because oxygen demand is greater than supply, any patient condition that increases demand such as fever, pain, shivering, and tachycardia places a severe strain on an already compromised balance. While fever enhances immune system function, excessive body temperatures ($>102°$ F or $39°$ C) increase oxygen demand and need to be reduced and controlled. Pain medication and antianxiety medication not only increase patient comfort, but also decrease restlessness, tachycardia, and work of breathing, thus "freeing up" additional oxygen for use by the major organ beds. Analgesics also enhance toleration of invasive procedures and interventions such as turning, suctioning, dressing changes, and line insertions.

Nutritional support

Because the patient with MSOF is so hypermetabolic, early nutritional support is vital to prevent complications, such as gut atrophy and severe muscle catabolism (breakdown). Primary goals of nutritional support focus on support of organ structure and function and maintenance of nitrogen equilibrium. Enteral feedings are encouraged because they are associated with fewer complications than parenteral nutrition, and they maintain gut integrity.[7] Advantages of early enteral feedings include: (1) enhancement of enteral barrier function, (2) prevention of GI atrophy and maintenance of mucosal integrity, thus aiding in prevention of bacterial translocation, (3) decrease in bile sludging, which minimizes the risk of cholestasis and cholecystitis, (4) decrease in stress ulceration, and (5) support of hepatic function. The use of jejunostomy tubes has promoted the use of early enteral feedings and minimized the risk of aspiration.

Because standard stress bleeding prophylaxis of H_2-blockers and antacids has been associated with an overgrowth of bacteria in the stomach and increased incidence of nosocomial pneumonia secondary to migration of these bacteria and gastric reflux, clinicians are examining other therapies for mucosal protection. In several studies, sucralfate and/or continuous infusions of H_2-blockers provided gastric mucosal protection and decreased the incidence of nosocomial pneumonia in the intubated patient in comparison with standard therapy (antacids and H_2-blockers).[21,49] Sucralfate provides mucosal protection without greatly altering the gastric pH.

Individual organ support

The fourth major goal of therapy is support of individual organs; however, supportive care treats manifestations and does not remove the underlying problem. The treatment of the patient must focus on the entire patient, including the disease process and underlying problems, such as infection, ischemia, and inflammation.

Investigational therapies

Investigational therapies for the patient with MSOF are extremely broad in scope. With the changed emphasis in looking at MSOF as an inflammatory process as well as a hypoperfusion problem, much of the drug research of the last several years is aimed at altering the inflammatory response. Pharmacologic agents that are being aggressively studied include nonsteroidal anti-inflammatory agents such as indomethacin and ibuprofen; antibodies to specific mediators such as anti-endotoxin antibodies and anti-TNF antibodies; and combinations of vasoactive agents that aid in the redistribution of volume. Knowledge of the inflammatory response is not only vital for understanding the pathophysiology of clinical conditions but also for ensuring safe, effective delivery of pharmacologic agents and accurate assessment of the patient's response to therapy.[12,48] The high mortality rates associated with MSOF reflect the inadequacy of even the highly technologic monitoring and interventions available to the critical care team at the present. Until newer therapies that can control the inflammatory process without increasing the risk of infection are fully developed, efforts must be focused on prevention and early identification of inflammation and infection.

NURSING MANAGEMENT OF THE CRITICALLY ILL PATIENT
Assessment

Nursing assessment of the critically ill patient begins with a thorough assessment of all the major body systems. Although the critically ill patient is often connected to numerous lines and monitoring devices, physical assessment findings continue to provide valuable and often early information regarding patient progress or the development of complications. The critical care nurse then integrates the assessment findings with data obtained from the numerous monitoring devices. Numbers and assessment findings are only part of the picture; the patient is viewed as a whole, not as a collection of bits and pieces of information.

Central nervous system

Level of consciousness (LOC) and orientation are frequently assessed in the ICU to grossly monitor CNS function and cerebral perfusion. The nurse may have to rely on a family member's assessment of patients whose baseline LOC is unknown, such as the elderly. Assessing LOC is more difficult in the intubated patient, since verbal responses are not possible. The use of picture boards and the ability to follow commands give evidence of the patient's LOC. Restlessness and agitation are also noted, since they often signify decreased cerebral perfusion, pain, or neurologic impairment.

Cardiovascular system

Heart rate and blood pressure are often measured hourly in many critical care units. A central line may be present to measure CVP, or the patient may have a pulmonary artery catheter. These catheters allow the measurement of cardiac output, pulmonary artery pressures, and pulmonary capillary wedge pressures. The thermistor on the catheter also allows for the measure of core body temperature. Once the CO is obtained, the SVR can then be calculated, along with oxygen delivery and oxygen consumption. Because the patient often has leaky capillaries, edema is usually present and should also be assessed.

Respiratory system

The chest is auscultated bilaterally to assess for bilateral breath sounds and proper artificial airway placement. Any crackles or wheezes are also noted. The ventilator setting should be double-checked against the ordered settings. The rate, depth, and rhythm of respirations are noted, along with the use of accessory muscles or diaphoresis. Arterial blood gases are frequently drawn to assess arterial oxygenation and saturation and acid base balance. The color, consistency, and odor of the sputum is described. The position and security of the artificial airway (ETT, NTT, trach) is assessed often. The condition of the skin and mucous membranes around the tube is examined.

Renal system

Urine output is measured hourly using a urimeter to get accurate readings. The volume, color, and clarity of the urine are examined. Specific gravity may also be measured. The urine is often tested for glucose, ketones, and protein with dipsticks designed specifically for that purpose.

Gastrointestinal system

The abdomen is auscultated for bowel sounds every 4 to 8 hours. If abdominal distention is noted, abdominal girth measurements are often taken each shift or each day. The patency and placement of the NGT is checked, and the amount, color, and consistency of the NG aspirate is noted. The gastric aspirate is often checked for the presence of blood and the pH is also recorded. The amount, color, and consistency of any stools are also recorded. The stool may also be checked for occult blood. Because the patient is receiving IV antibiotics, the normal flora of the gut becomes altered, and the patient may have an overgrowth of more pathogenic species. The stool may also be checked for bacterial load.[13]

Laboratory

Following completion of the physical assessment and hemodynamic monitoring, laboratory specimens are usually sent, including electrolyte levels, complete blood counts, glucose, BUN, creatinine, and ABGs. If the patient has coagulopathies, a PT/PTT and fibrin degradation products may also be sent. All other invasive devices including intravenous lines, arterial lines, chest tubes, drains, and external fixation devices must be checked for their effect on the patient's skin integrity and functional ability. The critical care nurse is not only responsible for the assessment of the patient, but also the monitoring equipment associated with that patient. Knowledge of proper procedure, calibration, and usage is imperative. It becomes easy to rely on the equipment rather than astute assessment skills, but remember equipment can be faulty. Proper troubleshooting is imperative to get an accurate assessment of the patient's condition.

Psychosocial

As mentioned previously in this chapter, the patient in the ICU environment suffers from many psychosocial stressors as well as physiologic stressors. Psychosocial assessment findings include feelings of powerlessness, helplessness, fear, anxiety, alteration in self-concept and depersonalization. For the patient unable to speak or answer questions, pertinent information can also be gathered from family and significant others. Changes in vital signs such as increased heart rate, blood pressure, and respiratory rate can also signal emotional changes such as increased fear or anxiety.

Nursing Diagnosis

The patient with MSOF has numerous problems and complications. Many nursing diagnoses apply to the MSOF patient during the clinical course. Frequently cited nursing diagnoses and associated etiologies are as follow:

Altered tissue perfusion related to maldistribution of circulating volume secondary to capillary permeability, tissue edema, microvascular thrombi, hemorrhage, vascular plugging with platelets and white blood cells, loss of autoregulation, vasodilation, vasoconstriction, myocardial depression, and low perfusion pressures.

Fluid volume deficit related to vasodilation, increased capillary permeability, hemorrhage, decreased intake, inadequate fluid resuscitation, increased insensible losses (NGT, ETT, diaphoresis), excessive wound drainage, fistulas, and diarrhea.

Fluid volume excess related to renal failure, congestive heart failure, liver failure (ascites), endocrine disorders (SIADH), and iatrogenic volume overload.

Impaired gas exchange related to vasoconstriction, increased capillary permeability, alterations in pulmonary endothelium, atelectasis, decreased functional residual capacity, secretion accumulation, intrapulmonary shunting secondary to ARDS, and pulmonary edema secondary to biventricular failure and pneumonia.

High risk for infection related to invasive techniques, immunocompromise, antibiotic administration, and immunosuppressant therapy.

Altered nutrition related to hypermetabolism secondary to mediator activity and inadequate nutritional support.

Altered skin integrity related to malnutrition, invasive devices, volume status, dehydration, edema, obesity, excessive diaphoresis, poor perfusion, frequent dressing changes, neuropathies, preexisting chronic diseases such as peripheral vascular disease or diabetes, and immobility secondary to ICU environment, restraints, extent of injury, muscle atrophy, and neuromuscular blockade.

Decreased cardiac output related to hypovolemia, ischemic dysfunction, and myocardial depression secondary to mediators, acidosis, and exhaustion.

Anxiety related to prognosis, ICU environment, procedures, neuromuscular blockade, and pain.

Alteration in comfort related to injuries, invasive devices, immobility, invasive procedures, hyperthermia, and hypothermia.

Hyperthermia/hypothermia related to mediator activity in the hypothalamus and metabolic abnormalities.

Impaired communication related to artificial airway and decreased level of consciousness secondary to head injury, poor cerebral perfusion, liver failure, and sedation.

Ineffective family coping related to prognosis, severity of insult, ICU environment, infrequent visiting hours, previous coping strategies, financial burdens, role change, and fear.

Planning

The critical care nurse collaborates with all members of the critical care team to develop a plan of care that is patient-specific and goal-oriented. Assessment and treatment of the patient with this complex syndrome focuses primarily on minimizing infectious/inflammatory stimuli, maintaining adequate preload and circulating volume, enhancing oxygen delivery and consumption, minimizing oxygen demand, and meeting metabolic requirements.[36,43] Understanding the patient and the disease process enhances clinical decision-making as one integrates assessment findings, trends in patient response to therapy, and knowledge of underlying pathophysiologic derangements into developing an individualized plan of care. The plan of care should focus on prompt recognition and treatment of secondary complications. The priority of interventions focuses on those complications that pose the greatest threat to the patient's life. These priorities are constantly reevaluated and reorganized as the patient's condition changes. In the ICU, priorities may change hourly, depending on the condition of the patient.

Implementation

Meticulous line, site, and catheter care and observation, along with aggressive wound and skin care decrease iatrogenic complications related to invasive devices. Hand washing remains a key factor in prevention of nosocomial colonization and infection. All catheters, line sites, and wounds should be assessed every 24 to 48 hours for edema, erythema, warmth, pain, and drainage. Mucous membranes (oral and vaginal) are common sites for secondary infections such as *Candida,* and should be assessed when providing oral and perineal care. The skin is a vital barrier against the invasion of pathogens. By maintaining its integrity, the nurse can minimize microbial access into the body. Proper nutritional support, skin care, positioning, and dressing placement are all necessary to keep the skin intact.

A secure airway and frequent oral care are crucial in reducing aspiration and nosocomial pneumonia. Strict aseptic technique must be followed to minimize pulmonary contamination. If secretions are thick or the patient does not have the strength to mobilize them, suctioning is indicated. Both secretions and suctioning predispose the patient to atelectasis and pneumonia, so care must be taken to ensure absolute sterile technique in the suctioning procedure. Recent research supports the use of ventilator breaths over the use of manual resuscitation bags in maintaining Sao_2 for hyperoxygenation and hyperventilation during routine suctioning.[45] A closed ventilator circuit also minimizes contamination. Unnecessary suctioning at frequent intervals is associated with increased risk for hypoxemia, airway collapse, and infection. The nurse's decision to suction the patient is based on careful auscultation of the lungs.

Removing intubated patients from the ventilator during pulmonary artery measurements often compromises ventilatory status, gas exchange, and arterial saturation; therefore, the patient should remain on the ventilator during measurements. Turning and repositioning also aid in redistribution of flow through the lungs, enhancing V/Q matching and preventing venous stasis.

Astute assessment and prompt intervention in the case of cardiovascular instability, poor perfusion, and inflammatory or infectious complications are crucial in the prevention of MSOF. Hypotension, tachycardia, and weak pulses all indicate cardiovascular instability. Poor urine output, changes in level of consciousness, poor capillary refill, and GI bleeding are often indications of poor organ perfusion and should be monitored frequently. Along with the psychosocial interventions carried out by the nurse at the bedside, consults are also obtained with social services and pastoral care according to patient and family wishes. Social services can provide information concerning financial consideration, long-term patient care facilities, and temporary housing for the family. Each of these areas may be major sources of stress and anxiety for the patient and family. Patients not only need someone to treat them in the

NURSING CARE PLAN   *The Patient with Multisystem Organ Failure*

Nursing diagnosis/ Expected outcome	Interventions	Rationale

Impaired gas exchange related to atelectasis, secretions, pulmonary edema, pulmonary microthrombi, and vasoconstriction
 	
•*ABGs at baseline*
•*Respiratory rate: 16-20/min*
•*Regular, unlabored respirations*
•*Clear bilateral breath sounds*
•*Clear, thin secretions*
•*Clear CXR*
	Auscultate breath sounds q2h and PRN
	Assess respiratory rate, depth, rhythm q2h and PRN
	Enhance secretion removal by:
	  Turn and deep breathe q2h. By placing injured or congested lung up, you promote ventilation/perfusion matching.
	  Suction PRN. Note amount, color, character, and odor of the aspirate.
	  Ensure adequate hydration to aid in secretion removal.
	Maintain patent airway. Keep HOB at 30-45 degrees.
	Administer supplemental oxygen as ordered.
	If patient requires mechanical ventilation:
	  Monitor ventilator settings—FIO$_2$, mode, tidal volume, rate, humidity, and temperature.
	  Monitor respiratory parameters—peak inspiratory pressure, static effective compliance, exhaled tidal volume.
	Administer antibiotics as ordered.
	Administer pain medication to increase comfort and ease of respirations. Observe for adverse effects on cardiopulmonary status after administration: respiratory distress, shallow respirations, decreased BP.
		Change in breath sounds or respiratory rate, depth, and rhythm could signal respiratory distress related to pneumonia, pulmonary edema, or endotracheal dislodgement.
		Increased secretions increase the risk of pneumonia and poor gas exchange.
		
		Appropriate ventilator settings help promote alveolar ventilation and prevent atelectasis. An artificial airway such as an endotracheal tube or nasotracheal tube bypasses the usual warming and humidification that takes place in the nasopharynx. Humidification is necessary to prevent viscous secretions.
		Increased peak inspiratory pressure indicates stiffening lungs or airway obstruction related to secretions, bronchoconstriction, or a kink in the endotracheal tube.
		Pain medication increases patient comfort and cooperation in deep breathing and coughing maneuvers.

Cardiac output: decreased related to decreased circulating volume, myocardial depression, and ventricular dysfunction
 	
•*CO > 8.0 L/min*
•*CI > 4.0 L/min/m²*
•*MAP > 70 mm Hg*
•*Heart rate 60-100/min*
•*Strong pulses bilaterally*
•*Warm, dry skin*
•*Capillary refill < 3 seconds*
•*PCWP > 12 mm Hg or higher depending on the patient*
•*Urine output 0.5 mL/kg/hr*
•*Intact sensorium*
	Obtain PAP, PCWP, CO, SVR, PVR q 2-4 hr.
	Vital signs q 1 hr with continuous monitoring of cardiac rhythm.
	Administer intravenous fluids as ordered. Observe for signs and symptoms of fluid overload: PCWP>18, crackles, edema, weight gain, dyspnea, pink frothy sputum.
	Administer vasoactive agents as ordered.
	  Monitor infusion rates and titrate to set parameters.
	  Closely check solution, concentration, rate.
	  Monitor changes in SVR, PVR, CO, CI.
	Administer inotropic agents as ordered. Evaluate patient's response to therapy by monitoring hemodynamics.
		Hemodynamic variables such as CO and SVR greatly affect oxygen delivery (DO$_2$) and oxygen consumption (VO$_2$). The CO and SVR are manipulated to enhance perfusion and oxygen delivery to the tissues. Supranormal (above normal) values are frequently the goal of therapy in an attempt to further increase DO$_2$.
		Intravenous fluids increase circulating volume and ventricular preload, thus increasing CO. If the patient has poor myocardial or renal function, fluid overload can occur and lead to pulmonary edema.
		Vasoactive agents affect SVR and tissue perfusion. A patient with a very low SVR may have a poor BP and/or poor perfusion to the tissues. Vasopressor agents are used

Nursing diagnosis/ Expected outcome	Interventions	Rationale
	Document accurate intake and output. Administer sodium bicarbonate per order to treat acidosis. Enhance tissue perfusion	to increase SVR and BP. A very high SVR indicates vasoconstriction, which can actually hinder flow to the organ beds. In this case, vasodilators are used. Inotropic agents increase cardiac contractility, which is a major determinant of CO. Severe acidosis can affect cardiovascular performance and the patient's responsiveness to certain drugs, particularly sympathetic agents, such as dopamine and epinephrine.

Altered tissue perfusion related to decreased circulating volume, microthrombi, decreased cardiac output, maldistribution of circulating volume, and altered cellular function
 	
• *Intact sensorium*
• *Heart rate 60-100/min*
• *Strong pulses bilaterally*
• *SBP ± 20 mm Hg baseline*
• *Warm, dry skin*
• *Baseline ABGs & pH*
• *Urine output > 0.5 mL/kg/hr*
• *Baseline BUN and creatinine*
• *Bowel sounds*
• *Absence of GI bleeding*
• *CO > 8.0 L/min*
• *PCWP 8-12 mm Hg*
• *SaO$_2$ > 90%*
• *SvO$_2$ 60%-80%*
• *Electrolytes within normal limits*
	Assess organ perfusion by:
	  Assess LOC q 1h.
	  Monitor cardiac rhythm and BP continuously.
	  Obtain PA, PCWP, CO q 4h and PRN.
	  Obtain labs as ordered.
	  Measure urine output hourly.
	  Assess bowel sounds and NGT aspirate q 4h. Guaiac all stools.
	  Assess pulses for regularity, amplitude, rate.
	  Assess skin for temperature, color, dryness, and turgor.
	Enhance gas exchange.
	Enhance cardiac output.
	Administer antiarrhythmic agents. Monitor for side-effects.
	Provide individual organ support as necessary: mechanical ventilation, hemodialysis, vasoactive agents.
	Administer sucralfate, antacids, H$_2$ blockers per order to decrease incidence of stress ulceration.
	Monitor DO$_2$ and VO$_2$ to assess adequacy of oxygen delivery for tissue oxygen demands.
		Decreased perfusion in an organ bed leads to ischemia, tissue damage and further activation of the inflammatory response. If perfusion is not adequate, organ dysfunction and failure can result
		
		Stress ulcers often lead to upper GI bleeding and increased morbidity and mortality.
		Antacids and H$_2$-blockers may promote bacterial overgrowth in the stomach, which may then reflux into the oropharynx and be aspirated into the lungs, causing pneumonia; therefore they should be used with caution and the patient monitored closely for evidence of pneumonia.
		DO$_2$ and VO$_2$ are more accurate measures of tissue oxygenation than an ABG because they look at not only SaO$_2$, but also CO and Hgb, both important determinants of oxygen delivery and consumption.

Continued.

NURSING CARE PLAN *The Patient with Multisystem Organ Failure—cont'd*

Nursing diagnosis/ Expected outcome	Interventions	Rationale

High risk for infection related to invasive lines and procedures, altered host defenses, and prolonged antibiotic therapy
 	
• *WBC 5000-10,000/mm³*
• *Normal differential*
• *Temperature 98.6° F ± 1*
• *Heart rate 60-100/min*
• *Clear urine*
• *Thin, clear sputum*
• *Glucose 70-110 mg/dL*
• *Absence of purulence, erythema, edema, excessive warmth, or pain at line sites or wounds*
• *Pink, moist mucous membranes*
	WASH YOUR HANDS.
	Prompt recognition of inflammation or infection:
	  Assess all catheters, lines sites, and wounds daily for edema, erythema, warmth, pain, drainage.
	  Monitor oral mucous membranes daily for *Candida* and other supra-infections.
	  Follow daily WBC, CXR, glucose.
	  Observe urine, sputum, and wound for changes in color and character.
	
	  Monitor temperature q 1-2 hours or continuously via a rectal probe or PA catheter.
	Change lines and dressings per unit protocol.
	Use strict aseptic technique with line and catheter placement and care.
	Remove traces of blood from stopcork ports and keep ports covered with sterile end caps.
	Remove potential contaminants from the environment (cut flowers, soil, standing water).
	Secure airway to prevent aspiration and enhance oxygen delivery.
	Provide frequent oral care to reduce the risk of aspiration of contaminated oropharyngeal secretions.
		Inflammation at the catheter site is associated with the development of infection and/or thrombophlebitis.
		Prolonged antibiotic therapy or altered host defenses may allow for the overgrowth of opportunistic organisms such as *Candida*.
		
		Increased temperature often indicates the presence of infection or inflammation.
		Risk of infection increases with increased duration of line placement.
		
		Old blood promotes bacterial growth.
		Bacteria can enter open ports and contaminate the system.
		Soil and water can be contaminated with pseudomonas and other bacteria and fungi that can then be transmitted to the patient.
		The cuff on the ETT does not prevent all secretions from reaching the lungs. Because the patient does not have intact pulmonary defense mechanisms, even small amounts of contaminated aspirate can lead to pneumonia.

Altered nutrition related to lack of nutritional support, hypermetabolic state, diarrhea, and altered GI function
 	
• *Baseline weight ± 3 lb*
• *Total serum protein 6.0-8.0 g/dL*
• *Electrolytes within normal limits*
• *Maintain muscle mass and strength*
• *Positive nitrogen balance*
• *Serum glucose 70-110 mg/dL*
• *Positive bowel sounds*
• *Calorie and protein intake at levels recommended by nutritional support consult*
• *Skin pink and intact*
	Nutritional support consult within 24 hours of admission.
	Assess bowel sounds and abdomen q 4h.
	Record daily weights at the same time each day, using same scale, same clothing, etc.
	Observe for effects of malnutrition:
	  Poor wound healing.
	  Clotting abnormalities.
	  Muscle wasting and weakness.
	  Electrolyte imbalances.
	  Skin breakdown.
	  Gut atrophy (GI bleeding, diarrhea, increased WBC and temperature).
		Nutritional support teams are specialized in dealing with nutritional needs of patients, especially critically ill patients with complex problems.
		The patient with systemic inflammation and multiple organ dysfunction has increased metabolic demands which must be met early or the patient may develop complications of malnutrition very quickly.

NURSING CARE PLAN   *The Patient with Multisystem Organ Failure—cont'd*

Nursing diagnosis/ Expected outcome	Interventions	Rationale
	Administer nutrition enterally if possible. If TPN is necessary, check rate, solution, additives for accuracy.	TPN does not adequately nourish the mucosa of the gut lumen and gut atrophy occurs, which can lead to the translocation of bacteria from the gut into the bloodstream. Enteral feedings maintain a more effective GI barrier and healthier GI function.
	Meticulous tube, line, and site care. Both enteral and parenteral feeding are associated with infectious complications.	
	Monitor electrolytes, glucose, nutritional support labs q 4-8 hr or as ordered.	
	Send 24-hour urine for UUN and assessment of nitrogen balance 1-2 times/week.	
	Monitor for complications of TPN: catheter sepsis, hyperglycemia, infiltration, fluid and electrolyte imbalances, mucosal atrophy.	The high glucose content of TPN provides a rich medium for bacterial growth, so infection is a major complication of TPN administration.
	Monitor for complications of enteral nutrition: aspiration, distention, tube dislodgement, diarrhea, fluid and electrolyte imbalances.	
Anxiety related to ICU environment, severity of disease, separation from family and significant others, pain, and respiratory insufficiency	Minimize overstimulation.	Removal of stimuli allows the patient to relax and regain control.
	Allow periods of rest.	Sleep deprivation decreases the patient's ability to deal with stressful events.
	Explain all procedures and equipment *before* beginning.	
• *Verbalization of decreased anxiety*	Explain ICU environment to patient and family: alarms, equipment, visiting hours.	Fear of the unknown and feelings of "loss of control of one's own body" increase anxiety.
• *Communicates specific fears to RN/MD/social worker*	Provide pain and/or anti-anxiety agents PRN.	
• *Heart rate < 100/min*	Assess signs and symptoms of anxiety. Answer questions and concerns.	Discovering source of anxiety provides a basis for intervention.
• *BP at baseline*	Avoid discussing patient condition "over" the patient.	Discussing "over" the patient increases the patient's feelings of helplessness and lack of control. Often hearing is intact even when a patient is not very responsive. Patient may hear and not understand. This can increase patient anxiety as he makes up information to fill in the gaps that he doesn't understand.
• *Respiratory rate < 20*	Identify baseline anxiety level and coping mechanisms from patient and family.	
	Promote stable respiratory status.	
	Consider social work consult in the presence of financial, family, or discharge concerns.	
	Minimize noise.	Hypoxemia/hypoxia increases restlessness and agitation.

ICU, but also to care for them. Nurses at the bedside 24 hours a day play the key role in creating a nurturing environment. See also the nursing interventions summary box on MSOF.

Evaluation

Evaluation is an ongoing process in the ICU. The nurse continually evaluates the patient's response to the plan of care and communicates those responses to the critical care team, both in written and verbal formats. Evaluation focuses on the expected patient outcomes developed in the planning stage. If the expected patient outcomes are not being met as the patient progresses, changes may have to be made not only in the interventions but also in the stated outcomes. Are the outcomes realistic? achievable? Evaluation of stated outcomes occurs simultaneously with evaluation of patient responses to the plan of care. Constant, ongoing assessment and evaluation

---

NURSING INTERVENTIONS SUMMARY   *The Patient With MSOF*

Prevention and early identification of inflammatory stimuli

WASH YOUR HANDS before and after patient contact

Thorough history and physical to prevent overlooking injuries or other significant information

Rapid resuscitation to decrease shock and ischemic time

Surgical debridement/drainage of necrotic tissue or abscesses

Early stabilization of fractures to prevent further tissue damage and promote early ambulation

Replace within 12 to 24 hours lines inserted in the field

Secure airway to prevent aspiration and enhance oxygen delivery

Frequent oral care to minimize oropharyngeal contamination and risk of silent aspiration

Meticulous handwashing, line, site, catheter care, observation, and documentation

Maintain closed systems: capped ports, fewer stopcocks, inline suctioning, manual ventilator breaths for hyperoxygenation/hyperventilation

Meticulous wound care

Prompt recognition: cultures, WBC, fever, radiographic changes

Intravenous antibiotic administration based on Gram stain, patient condition, culture reports and patient response

Remove potential contaminants: cut flowers, standing water

Ensure proper terminal cleaning of bedside and other reusable equipment

Early, aggressive supportive therapy: nutrition, intravenous fluids, mobilization, pulmonary toilet

Restoration of oxygen supply/demand

Optimize cardiac output
  Pulmonary artery catheterization
  Fluid resuscitation
  Inotropic therapy
  Vasoactive therapy
  Control severe acidosis

Optimize hemoglobin
  Maintain level at 10-12 gm/dL
  Monitor CBC
Optimize SaO_2
  Ventilatory support
  Prevent nosocomial pneumonia
    Sterile technique with suctioning
    Frequent oral care
    Consider sucralfate for stress bleeding prophylaxis
    Monitor for aspiration of gastric contents, tube feedings, oral secretions
  Frequent position changes and early mobility

Nutritional support

Early tube feedings if possible

Total parenteral nutrition as necessary to meet metabolic needs

Individual organ support as indicated

Mechanical ventilation

Hemodialysis/continuous arteriovenous hemofiltration

Inotropic and vasoactive agents

Therapeutic beds

Psychosocial support of patient and family

Explain unit environment, equipment, and regulations

Explain all procedures and answer all questions if possible

Institute primary nursing

Social services and pastoral care consult

Involve patient in as much decision-making as possible

Establish form of communication, either verbal or nonverbal as necessary

Minimize sensory overload and deprivation

Abbreviations: WBC, white blood count; gm/dL, grams per deciliter; CBC, complete blood count.

are crucial in restoring the patient to optimal health and minimizing life-threatening complications.

Documentation

To deliver effective care, the nurse constantly interacts with all levels of the health care delivery team to coordinate the therapy required by the patient to reach the therapeutic goals necessary for recovery. This interaction is carried out both verbally and in written form through thorough and adequate documentation which focuses on expected patient outcomes, patient responses to therapy, changes in patient status, and around-the-clock recording of hemodynamic variables, pulmonary parameters, and laboratory values. In the critical care unit, many signs are recorded hourly, such as heart rate, blood pressure, respiratory rate, and urine output. Intake and output are also recorded hourly in many units. Due to the instability of many patients, changes can occur very rapidly and trends are noted very carefully.

Ongoing Care

Transfer out of the ICU to either a step-down unit or general medical-surgical floor can provoke extreme anxiety in both the patient and family. The patient has usually been in the ICU for an extended time and has come to rely heavily on the nurses in the unit. The patient may miss being monitored closely once on the general unit and may actually fear an arrest situation, especially if one has previously occurred.

Patients moving to the floor from the ICU will usually have central lines in place and are often on supplemental oxygen. In some institutions, mechanical ventilators may be allowed on the general floors. Due to the absence of much of the "high-tech" monitoring equipment available in the unit, caring for a critically ill patient on the floor requires a high degree of competence in clinical assessment. The priorities are still the same: airway, breathing, and circulation. Depending on the physical layout of the unit, patients are often not visible from the nursing station as they are in the ICU; therefore, great care must be taken to ensure all alarms needed are turned on and set with appropriate limits and that the call light is within reach of the patient. Involvement of the family in the care of the patient and notification of bedside nurse in case of patient deterioration provides further protection for the patient on the general unit.

The key signs and symptoms warning of impending organ dysfunction and damage primarily relate to adequacy of tissue perfusion and cardiovascular stability. Although these patients are stable, they are not out of danger. Many patients developing MSOF

TABLE 77-4   Evidence of Impending Organ Dysfunction

System	Assessment findings
Cerebral	Changes in level of consciousness
	Irregular respirations
	Pupillary changes
Cardiovascular	Hypotension
	Tachycardia
	Weak pulses
	Increased or decreased CVP
Pulmonary	Hyperventilation or hypoventilation
	Bradypnea or tachypnea
	Dyspnea
	Diaphoresis
	Use of accessory muscles
	Wheezes
	Crackles
	Thick and malodorous sputum
Renal	Decreased urine output
	Elevated CVP
	Increased daily weight
Liver	Jaundice
	Ascites
	Coagulopathies

have experienced a successful resuscitation and may even appear stable for several days following the insult. Evidence of impending damage is outlined in Table 77-4. Cardiovascular instability and poor tissue perfusion both lead to ischemia, tissue damage, organ dysfunction, and ultimately organ failure. Prompt recognition of these signs and symptoms allows earlier intervention and possibly prevention of further damage.

Discharge planning

Efforts to decrease length of stay, improve appropriate bed utilization, and maximize cost containment have lead to earlier discharge of complex patients from the ICU and medical-surgical units.[9] Early, effective discharge planning provides continuity of care and decreases readmissions. Traditionally, discharge and discharge planning occurred from the medical-surgical units, but with the increasing availability of highly technologic home care, more patients are discharged directly from the ICU. Therefore, discharge planning is the responsibility of the ICU nurse and critical care team (see box on p. 2200). Upon discharge, the patient may still require highly technologic home care. The presence of central lines, major dressing changes, and possibly even

DISCHARGE PLANNING CONSIDERATIONS

Conditions requiring intervention and planning

Wound care
Oxygen therapy
Home ventilator
Nutritional support
Pain control
Intravenous line care
Infection control
Medications

Types of information needed

Technical information (skills, use of equipment)
Potential complications and emergency measures
Parameters to notify health care personnel
Source of supplies
Contact person

Discharge planning

Assess home health care needs of patient
Assess knowledge base of patient and family
Organization of multidisciplinary conferences (nursing, medicine, pharmacy, social service, respiratory care, physical/occupational therapy, home health agency, dietary, pastoral care, family or other home caregivers)
Implement teaching plan days to weeks before discharge
Reevaluate patient status and knowledge base and skill level of patient and family prior to discharge

a ventilator requires intense patient and family education and collaboration with home health care agencies and the department of social services. Communication must be accurate and thorough to ensure that the agencies involved are clearly aware of the patient's acuity and specific needs. Not all home health care agencies provide the pharmaceutical and technologic services required by some patients on discharge. Once again, anxiety can be a major factor in hindering a smooth discharge. A thorough assessment of patient and family knowledge must be completed so an appropriate teaching plan can be developed.

CRITICAL THINKING QUESTIONS

1 Define multisystem organ failure (MSOF) in relation to the inflammatory response.

2 A patient is moved from the general medical-surgical unit to the ICU. How does this transfer increase the risk of infection and other complications?

3 List the primary events that contribute to the release of mediators into the circulation.

4 Describe the factors that contribute to the development of each major pathophysiologic change listed below.
   a. Maldistribution of circulating volume
   b. Imbalance of oxygen supply/demand
   c. Alterations in metabolism

5 Explain the etiology and pathophysiology of the following assessment findings of the hyperdyamic state.
   a. Increased cardiac output
   b. Decreased SVR
   c. Tachycardia
   d. Hypotension

6 What is the major goal of therapy for the critically ill patient?

7 Mr. Lee is septic and has a cardiac output of 10 L/min. Because myocardial depression occurs early in septic shock and MSOF, an increase in contractility cannot be the cause of the increased cardiac output. What other factors contribute to Mr. Lee's elevated cardiac output?

8 Mr. Smith has generalized peripheral edema, yet his PCWP and urine output are low. Therefore, he is not volume overloaded: what is the source of his edema?

9 You receive this report on the patient you are to care for this shift:
   a. She is febrile (103° F) and shivering
   b. She is fighting the ventilator and breathing rapidly over the set rate
   c. Her cardiac output is 10 L/min, heart rate is 140 bpm, and BP is 95/50
   d. She is agitated and in pain
      Which of the above findings increase oxygen demand? What can you do to decrease that demand?

10 A patient develops nosocomial pneumonia 6 days after admission to the ICU. The critical care team decided the stress ulcer prophylaxis of antacids and H_2-blockers may have predisposed the patient to the development of the pneumonia and the patient is switched to sucralfate. What is the connection between the prophylaxis and the pneumonia? Why is sucralfate preferred?

11 The culture report on a 25-year-old patient shows gram-negative organisms growing in the blood and sputum, but the patient's temperature is 96° F and his WBC count is less

than 1000/mm^3. Why would his temperature and WBC be decreased if he is still infected?

12 Discuss appropriate nursing interventions for three of the nursing diagnoses common to the MSOF patient.

13 Why is individual organ support (e.g., hemodialysis and mechanical ventilation) alone not effective in the treatment of MSOF?

BIBLIOGRAPHY

Current

1. Alfaro R: Applying the nursing process to the critically ill patient. In Shoemaker WC et al: *Textbook of critical care*, ed 2, Philadelphia, 1989, WB Saunders.
2. Alspach JG: *AACN's Core curriculum for critical care nursing*, ed 4, Philadelphia, 1991, WB Saunders.
3. American College of Chest Physicians/Society of Critical Care Medicine Consensus Conference: Definitions for sepsis and organ failure and guidelines for the use of innovative therapies in sepsis, *Crit Care Med* 20:864, 1992.
4. Anderson BO, Harken AH: Multiple organ failure: inflammatory priming and activation sequences promote autologous tissue injury, *J Trauma* 30:S44, 1990.
5. Baue AE: *Multiple organ failure: Patient care and prevention*, St. Louis, 1990, Mosby–Year Book, Inc.
6. Bell TN: Disseminated intravascular coagulation and shock: multisystem crisis in the critically ill, *Crit Care Nurs Clin North Am* 2:255, 1990.
7. Bessey PQ: Nutritional support in critical illness. In Deitch EA, editor: *Multiple organ failure: pathophysiology and basic concepts of therapy*, New York, 1990, Thieme Medical Publishers.
8. Beutler B: Cachectin in tissue injury, shock, and related states, *Crit Care Clin* 5:353, 1989.
9. Bigler BR: Critical care nursing: Expanding roles and responsibilities within the community, *Crit Care Nurs Clin North Am* 2:493, 1990.
10. Browder W, Williams D: Immunosuppression in the surgical patient, *J Nat Med Assoc* 80:531, 1988.
11. Burns KM: Vasoactive drug therapy in shock, *Crit Care Nurs Clin North Am* 2:167, 1990a.
12. Byram DA: Future expectations for critical care nurses: Competence in immunotherapy, *Crit Care Nurs Clin North Am* 1:797, 1989.
13. Cerra FB: Metabolic manifestation of multiple systems organ failure, *Crit Care Clin* 5:119, 1989.
14. Collins AS: Gastrointestinal complications in shock, *Crit Care Nurs Clin North Am* 2:269, 1990.
15. DeCamp MM, Demling RH: Posttraumatic multisystem organ failure, *JAMA* 260:530, 1988.
16. Deitch EA: Multiple organ failure: Summary and overview. In Deitch EA, editor: *Multiple organ failure: pathophysiology and basic concepts of therapy*, New York, 1990, Thieme Medical Publishers.
17. Deitch EA: The role of intestinal barrier failure and bacterial translocation in the development of systemic infection and multiple organ failure, *Arch Surg* 125:403, 1990.
18. Dinarello CA: Biology of interleukin 1, *FASEB J* 2:108, 1988.
19. Disch J: Scope of practice defined, *Focus on AACN* 7:18, 1980.
20. Dorinsky PM, Gadek JE: Multiple organ failure, *Clin Chest Med* 11:581, 1990.
21. Driks MR: Nosocomial pneumonia in intubated patients given sucralfate as compared with antacids or histamine type 2 blockers, *N Engl J Med* 317:1376, 1987.
22. Field BE, Devich LE, Carlson RW: Impact of a comprehensive supportive care team on management of hopelessly ill patients with multiple organ failure, *Chest* 96:353, 1989.
23. Fry DE: Multiple system organ failure, *Surg Clin North Am* 68:107, 1988.
24. Goodwin CW: Multiple organ failure: clinical overview of the syndrome, *J Trauma* 30:S163, 1990.
25. Goris RJ: Multiple organ failure: whole body inflammation?, *Schweizerische Medizinische Wochenschrift* 119:347, 1989.
26. Hotter AN: The pathophysiology of multi-system organ failure in the trauma patient, *Clin Issues Crit Care Nurs* 1:465, 1990.
27. Hoyt NJ: Host defense mechanisms and compromises in the trauma patient, *Crit Care Nurs Clin North Am* 1:7535-766, 1989.
28. Hoyt NJ: Preventing septic shock: Infection control in the intensive care unit, *Crit Care Nurs Clin North Am* 2:287, 1990.
29. Huddleston VB: Multisystem organ failure: What you need to know, *Nurs* 91:34, 1991.
30. Huddleston VB, editor: *Multisystem organ failure: pathophysiology and clinical implications*, St. Louis, 1992, Mosby–Year Book, Inc.
31. Jillings CR: Shock: Psychosocial needs of the patient and family, *Crit Care Nurs Clin North Am* 2:325, 1990.
32. Khansari DN, Murgo AJ, Faith RE: Effects of stress on the immune system, *Immunol Today* 11:170, 1990.
33. Knaus WA, Wagner DP: *Multiple systems organ failure: epidemiology and prognosis*, *Crit Care Clin* 5:221, 1989.
34. Lekander BJ, Cerra FB: The syndrome of multiple organ failure, *Crit Care Nurs Clin North Am* 2:331, 1990.
35. Lookinland S: Comparison of pulmonary vascular pressures based on blood volume and ventilator status, *Nurs Res* 38:68, 1989.
36. Macho JR, Luce JM: Rational approach to the management of multiple systems organ failure, *Crit Care Clin* 5:379, 1989.
37. Marshall JC, Meakins JL: Multiorgan failure. In Wilmore DW, editor: *American College of Surgeons: Care of the surgical patient*. vol 1. *Critical care*, New York, 1989, Scientific American.
38. Meakins JL: Etiology of multiple organ failure, *J Trauma* 30:S165, 1990.
39. Müller-Berghaus G: Pathophysiologic and biochemical events in disseminated intravascular coagulation: Dysregulation of procoagulant and anticoagulant pathways, *Semin Thromb Hemost* 15:58, 1989.
40. Nuytinck HKS et al: Whole-body inflammation in trauma patients, *Arch Surg* 123:1519, 1988.
41. Parillo JE et al: Septic shock in humans: Advances in the understanding of pathogenesis, cardiovascular dysfunction, and therapy, *Ann Intern Med* 113:227, 1990.
42. Pinsky MR, Matuschak GM: Multiple systems organ failure: Failure of host defense homeostasis, *Crit Care Clin* 5:199, 1989.
43. Sheagren JN: Mechanism-oriented therapy for multiple systems organ failure, *Crit Care Clin* 5:393, 1989.
44. Shoemaker WC et al: Prospective trial of supranormal values of survivors as therapeutic goals in high risk surgical patients, *Chest* 94:1176, 1988.
45. Stone KS: Ventilator versus manual resuscitation bag as the method for delivering hyperoxygenation before endo-

tracheal suctioning, *Clin Issues Crit Care Nurs* 1:289, 1990.

46. Stroud M, Swindell B, Bernard GR: Cellular and humoral mediators of sepsis syndrome, *Crit Care Nurs Clin North Am* 2:151, 1990.

47. Tracey KJ, Lowry SF: The role of cytokine mediators in septic shock, *Adv Surg* 23:21, 1990.

48. Tribett D: Immune system function: Implications for critical care nursing practice, *Crit Care Nurs Clin North Am* 1:725, 1989.

49. Tryba M: Side effects of stress bleeding prophylaxis, *Amer J Med* 86:85, 1989.

50. Wilmore DW: The gut: A central organ after surgical stress, *Surgery* 104:917, 1988.

Classic

51. AACN: Definition of Critical Care Nursing, Newport Beach, Calif, 1984, AACN.

52. Axelrod J, Reisine TD: Stress hormones: Their interaction and regulation, Science 224:452, 1984.

53. Baue AE: Multiple, progressive, or sequential systems failure: A syndrome of the 1970s, *Arch Surg* 110:779, 1975.

54. Brigham KL: Role of free radicals in lung injury, *Chest* 89:859, 1986.

55. Carrico CJ et al: Multiple-organ-failure syndrome [Panel discussion-Surgical Infection Society], *Arch Surg* 121:196, 1986.

56. Roberts SL, editor: *Behavioral concepts and the critically ill patient,* ed 2, Norwalk, Conn, 1986, Appleton-Century-Crofts.

57. Tracey KJ et al: Shock and tissue injury induced by recombinant human cachectin, *Science* 234:470, 1986.

Index

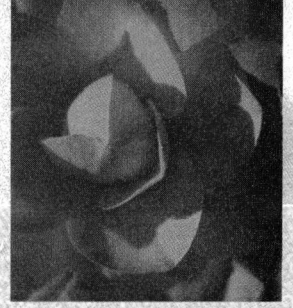

SMAST; *see* Short Michigan Alcoholism
  Screening Test
SMBG; *see* Self-monitoring of blood glucose
Smear
  Papanicolaou, 1946-1947
    in cancer detection, 287
    in genital warts, 2070
    in health promotion practices, 1965
  Tzanck, 1954
  vaginal, 1947-1948
Smith test, 1954
Smoke inhalation, 2121
Smokeless tobacco, 727
Smoking, 58
  in aneurysm, 712
  in arterial insufficiency, 706, 707
  in atherosclerosis, 694, 695, 698
  cancer and, 282-283
    lung, 58, 660
    prevention of, 286
  cessation of, 664
  in chronic obstructive pulmonary disease, 619
  in deep-vein thrombosis, 751
  diabetes and, 1752
  dysplasia and, 279
  hypertension and, 724, 726-727
  metaplasia and, 279
  preoperative assessment in, 467
  in Raynaud's disease, 716
Smooth muscle
  peripheral vascular, 217
  of stomach, 1765
  tumors of, 284
Snellen chart, 1418, 1419
SNF; *see* Skilled nursing facilities
So you have high blood cholesterol, 913
Social enculturation, 1958
Social Services for Medicaid, 1243
Society of Military Widows, 435
Sodium
  in burns, 2128
  in cardiomyopathy, 894, 896
  in cirrhosis, 1899
  in Graves' disease, 1691, 1694
  in headache, 1239
  homeostasis of, 1059-1060
  in hypertension, 725, 726, 733-734
  imbalances of, 183-187
  in nutrition support, 362
  in pericarditis, 889
  in polycythemia vera, 969
  in renal function, 1072
  in renal tuberculosis, 1086
  in shock, 223
  in valvular disease, 928-929
Sodium bicarbonate
  in cardiopulmonary resuscitation, 853
  in duodenal ulcers, 1825, 1826
  in hyperkalemia, 189
  in metabolic acidosis, 205
  in oral care, 318
  in pancreatitis, 1924
  in shock, 233
  in tumor lysis syndrome, 976
  in ventricular fibrillation, 816
Sodium chloride
  in hypermagnesemia, 197
  in hypernatremia, 184
  in hypertension, 734
  in loop of Henle, 1058
Sodium citrate, 471
Sodium hypochlorite, 2023
Sodium nitroprusside, 839
Sodium-potassium pump, 168, 169
Sodium tetradecyl sulfate, 747
Soft chancre, 2068
Solu-Medrol; *see* Methylprednisolone
Solute, 167
Solvents, 1097
Somatomedin, 1631, 1649
Somatosensory evoked potential, 1316
Somnolence, 384-385
Somnothane; *see* Halothane
Somogyi effect, 1739
Sore throat, 593
Sotradecal, 747
Sound transmission, 1469-1470
Spacer device, 631
Spasticity, 1317
Spatial disorders, 1291

Spectinomycin, 2068
Speculum examination, 1941-1942
Speech pathology, 100
Speech reception threshold, 1477
Sperm, 1937
Spermatogonia, 295
Spherocyte, 953
Sphincter
  artificial urinary, 1131, 1132
    in benign prostatic hypertrophy, 2038
    in prostatic cancer, 2043
  lower esophageal, 1779, 1801-1802
Spinal accessory nerve, 1171, 1182, 1185
Spinal administration of analgesics, 267
Spinal anesthesia, 481, 499
Spinal cord
  compression of, 325
  disorders of, 1361-1390
    degenerative, 1262
    injury in, 1362-1383; *see also* Spinal cord,
      injury to
    intervertebral disk disease in, 1386-1389
    tumors in, 1383-1386
  functions of, 1172-1173
  injury to, 1362-1383
    clinical manifestations of, 1364-1366
    definition of, 1362
    etiology and epidemiology of, 1362-1364
    functional goals in, 1382
    management in, 1369-1374
    neurogenic shock and, 234
    pathophysiology of, 1364, 1365
    rehabilitation in, 1374-1383
    therapy in, 1366-1369
  ischemia of, 713
  in pain transmission, 252, 253
  pathways in, 1173
  radiation therapy and, 295
  structure of, 1169-1172
Spinal muscular atrophy, 1262-1267
Spinal nerves, 1163, 1165-1169, 1171, 1172
Spinal shock, 1366
Spindles, muscle, 1514
Spine
  abscess of, 1309
  assessment of, 1520
  curvature of, 1517
  roentgenography of, 1192-1193
Spinothalamic tract, 252, 253
Spiral fracture, 1537, 1538
Spiritual care needs, 330-331
Spiritual counselor, 101
Spirometry
  in mechanical ventilation weaning, 578-579
  in respiratory assessment, 534
  in respiratory disorders, 540-542
Spironolactone
  in dilated cardiomyopathy, 894
  drug interactions with, 733
  in erectile dysfunction and, 2049
  fluid and electrolyte balance and, 177
Spleen, 686, 1010
Splenectomy, 1024
Splinting
  in burns, 2137
  in fracture, 1540
  hand, 1288, 1289
  nasal, 603
  in soft tissue trauma, 1531
Split-thickness skin graft, 2131, 2161
Spondaic word threshold, 1477
Spondee threshold test, 1477
Spongiform encephalitis, 1311
Spongioblastoma, 1346
Spongy bone, 1510
Spontaneous pneumothorax, 620
Sports injuries, 1535-1537
Sprain, 1530, 1558
Sputum examination, 535
Squamous cell carcinoma
  of larynx, 605
  of lung, 660
  of skin, 2109-2110
ST segment, 799, 800
STA-MCA; *see* Superficial middle temporal
      artery to middle cerebral artery bypass
Stable angina pectoris, 860
Stadol; *see* Butorphanol
Staging
  of laryngeal cancer, 605

Staging—cont'd
  of tumors, 289
Stain, Gram
  in gonorrhea, 2068
  for sexually transmitted diseases, 1954
Stallones' definition of epidemiology, 53
Stapes, 1468, 1494
Staphylococcus, 152
  in infective endocarditis, 916
  in meningitis, 1301
Staphylococcus aureus, 648
  in bacterial pneumonia, 649
  in intestinal infection, 1850
  methicillin-resistant, 156
  in otitis media, 1492
  in toxic shock syndrome, 1984
Starr-Edwards prosthetic valve, 931
State anxiety, 396
State nursing practice act, 129-130
Static equilibrium, 1470-1471
Statistical bias, 60
Statistical power analysis, 60
Statistical risk classes, 1715
Status asthmaticus, 629
Status epilepticus, 1231, 1232
STD Hotline, 2075
STDs; *see* Sexually transmitted diseases
Steatorrhea, 339
Stellate ganglion nerve block, 271
Stem cells, 1009
Stenosis
  aortic, 924-925
  mitral, 921-922
  tricuspid, 927
Stents
  in coronary artery disease, 866
  intraurethral, 2030
Stepped care approach in hypertension, 59,
      729-730
Sternbach's study on anxiety, 250
Sternocleidomastoid muscle, 184
Sterognosis, 1187
Steroids
  in acoustic neuroma, 1500
  in dermatitis, 2093
  in dermatomyositis, 2103
  in exfoliative dermatitis, 2094
  in facial nerve paralysis, 1407
  in glaucoma, 1431
  in glomerulonephritis, 1083
  in head injury, 1338-1339
  in headache, 1238
  in hypertension, 723
  in intervertebral disk disease, 1387
  in myocardial infarction, 876
  in pemphigus, 2101
  in psoriasis, 2097
  in radiation therapy, 295
  in renal disorders, 1089
  in restrictive lung disease, 634
  side effects of, 2090
  in sinusitis, 591
  in skin disorders, 2090
  in thyroiditis, 1698
  in uremic pericarditis, 1102
  in uveitis, 1461
Sterotaxic surgery, 1349
Stimulants
  abuse of, 442-446
  in pain management, 268
Stimulation
  sensory; *see* Sensory stimulation
  transcutaneous electrical nerve; *see*
      Transcutaneous electrical nerve
      stimulation
Stimulus
  pacemaker, 825-827
  stress as, 38
Stocking, compression, 752-754, 755
Stoma
  in cancer
    bladder, 1155, 1156
    colon, 1885
  care of, 611
  marking sites of, 1860
Stomach; *see also* Gastrointestinal system
  chemical digestion in, 1766, 1767
  disorders of, 1817-1844
    gastric cancer in, 1840-1843
    gastric surgery in, 1835-1839

PATTERN EDUCATION GUIDES

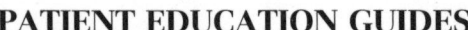